Stockley's Drug Interactions

A source book of interactions, their mechanisms, clinical importance and management

Seventh edition

Edited by

Karen Baxter

BSc, MSc, MRPharmS

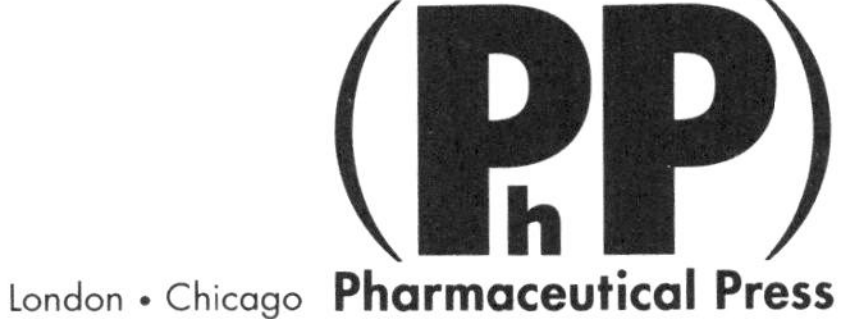

London • Chicago Pharmaceutical Press

Published by the Pharmaceutical Press
Publications division of the Royal Pharmaceutical Society of Great Britain

1 Lambeth High Street, London SE1 7JN, UK
100 South Atkinson Road, Suite 206, Grayslake, IL 60030-7820, USA

First edition 1981
Sixth edition 2002
Seventh edition 2006

Printed and bound in Great Britain by William Clowes Ltd, Beccles, Suffolk

ISBN 0 85369 624 1

A catalogue record for this book is available from the British Library

Stockley's Drug Interactions

Contents

Preface

The aim of Stockley's Drug Interactions is to inform busy doctors, pharmacists, surgeons, nurses and other healthcare professionals, of the facts about interactions, without their having to do the time-consuming literature searches and full assessment of the papers for themselves. These therefore are the practical questions which this book attempts to answer:

- Are the drugs in question known to interact or is the interaction only theoretical and speculative?
- If they do interact, how serious is it?
- Has it been described many times or only once?
- Are all patients affected or only a few?
- Is it best to avoid these two drugs altogether or can the interaction be accommodated in some way?
- And what alternative and safer drugs can be used instead?

To précis the mass of literature into a concise and easy-to-read form, the text has been organised into a series of individual monographs, all with a common format. If you need some insight into the general philosophy underlying the way all this information is handled in this book, you should have a look at the section, 'Before using this book. . .'.

All of the existing monographs have been reviewed, updated and revalidated, and many new ones have been added since the last edition making a total in excess of 2800. One of the major changes of this edition is the restructuring of the information resulting in the creation of 11 new chapters. This is to allow better representation of the cardiovascular and anti-infective drugs, by separating out the main therapeutic groups, and to allow the inclusion of new chapters covering growing therapeutic areas, such as lipid-regulating drugs. Greater attention has also been given to information provided by drug regulatory bodies in other countries, and this is reflected in the citation of much more US prescribing information. The brief outline of the most common mechanisms of interaction in Chapter 1 remains but it has been updated and now, among other things, includes a discussion of the drug transporter proteins, which look to become increasingly important in explaining the mechanisms of drug interactions.

Aside from the editorial staff many other people have contributed to this publication and the Editor gratefully acknowledges the assistance and guidance they have provided. Working within Martindale Publications the Stockley staff have had access both to the databases and the considerable expertise of the Martindale staff, which has of course been invaluable. Thanks are due to John Wilson and Tamsin Cousins who have handled various aspects of the production of this book, and Suzanne Armour for helping us sift through the literature. Thanks are also due to Charles Fry, for his support.

The full text of Stockley is available on MedicinesComplete and abridged versions are available in various other digital products and so thanks goes to Julie McGlashan and all those who have been involved in the development of these products. The staff of the Pharmacy Department at Walsgrave Hospital also deserve mention for allowing me to keep in touch with clinical pharmacy, answering my questions, and providing feedback on content.

Finally, this publication would not be complete without acknowledging the support of Ivan Stockley, who has guided us through this edition and continues to be a good source of advice and feedback on all of the various Stockley products. We are truly grateful.

Anyone who wishes to contact the Stockley team can do so at the following address: *stockley@rpsgb.org*

London, September 2005

Abbreviations

ACE—angiotensin-converting enzyme
ADP—adenosine diphosphate
AIDS—acquired immunodeficiency syndrome
ALL—acute lymphoblastic leukaemia
ALT—alanine aminotransferase
am—*ante meridiem* (before noon)
AML—acute myeloid leukaemia
aPPT—activated partial thromboplastin time
AST—aspartate aminotransferase
AUC—area under the time–concentration curve
$AUC_{0-12\ h}$—area under the time–concentration curve measured over 0 to 12 hours
AV—atrioventricular
BNF—British National Formulary
BP—blood pressure
BP—British Pharmacopoeia
BPC—British Pharmaceutical Codex
BPH—benign prostatic hyperplasia
bpm—beats per minute
BUN—blood urea nitrogen
CAPD—continuous ambulatory peritoneal dialysis
CDC—Centers for Disease Control (USA)
Cmax—maximum serum concentration
CNS—central nervous system
COPD—chronic obstructive pulmonary disease
CPR—cardiopulmonary resuscitation
CSF—cerebrospinal fluid
CSM—Committee on Safety of Medicines (UK)
ECG—electrocardiogram
ECT—electroconvulsive therapy
ED_{50}—the dose at which 50% of subjects respond
EEG—electroencephalogram
e.g.—*exempli gratia* (for example)
EMEA—The European Agency for the Evaluation of Medicinal Products
FDA—Food and Drug Administration (USA)
FEF_{25-75}—maximum expiratory flow over the middle 50% of the vital capacity
FEV_1—forced expiratory volume in one second
ft—foot (feet)
FVC—forced vital capacity
GGT—gamma glutamyl transpeptidase
g—gram(s)
h—hour(s)
HAART—highly active antiretroviral therapy
HCV—hepatitis C virus
HIV+—human immunodeficiency virus positive
HRT—hormone replacement therapy
i.e.—*id est* (that is)
im—intramuscular
INR—international normalised ratio
ITU—intensive therapy unit
IU—International Units
iv—intravenous
IUD—intra-uterine device
kg—kilogram(s)
l—litre
lbs—pound(s) avoirdupois
LDL—low-density lipoproteins
µg—microgram(s)
m—metre(s)
MAC—minimum alveolar concentration
MAOI—monoamine oxidase inhibitor
MAOI-A—monoamine oxidase inhibitor, type A
MAOI-B—monoamine oxidase inhibitor, type B
MCA—Medicines Control Agency
MHRA—Medicines and Healthcare products Regulatory Agency
MIC—minimum inhibitory concentration
mEq—milliequivalent(s)
meq—milliequivalent(s)
mg—milligram(s)
min—minute(s)
ml—millilitre(s)
mmHg—millimetre(s) of mercury
µmol—micromole
mmol—millimole
mol—mole
MRSA—methicillin-resistant *Staphylococcus aureus*
ms—millisecond(s)
msec—millisecond(s)
ng—nanogram(s)
nM—nanomole
nmol—nanomole
NNRTI—non-nucleoside reverse transcriptase inhibitor
NRTI—nucleoside reverse transcriptase inhibitor
NSAID—non-steroidal anti-inflammatory drug
OTC—over-the-counter (i.e. obtainable without a prescription)
PABA—para-amino benzoic acid
PCP—*Pneumocystis carinii* pneumonia
pH—the negative logarithm of the hydrogen ion concentration
pm—*post meridiem* (after noon)
pO_2—plasma partial pressure (concentration) of oxygen
PPI—proton pump inhibitor
ppm—parts per million
PTT—partial thromboplastin time
PUD—peptic ulcer disease
s—second(s)
sbp—systolic blood pressure
SSRI—selective serotonin reuptake inhibitor
STD—sexually transmitted disease
SVT—supraventricular tachycardia
TSH—thyroid-stimulating hormone
UK—United Kingdom
US and USA—United States of America
USP—The United States Pharmacopeia
UTI—urinary tract infection
Vd—volume of distribution
Vmax—maximum velocity

Before using this book . . .

. . . you should read this short explanatory section so that you know how the drug interaction data have been set out here, and why – as well as the basic philosophy that has been followed in presenting it.

The monographs

This publication has over 2800 monographs with a common format, which are subdivided into sections like these:

- An abstract or summary for quick reading.
- **Clinical evidence**, detailing one, two or more illustrative examples of the interaction, followed by most or all of other supportive clinical evidence currently available.
- **Mechanism**, in brief.
- **Importance and management**, a short discussion designed to aid rapid clinical decision making. For example:
  – Is the interaction established or not?
  – What is its incidence?
  – How important is it?
  – How can it be managed?
  – And what, if any, are the non-interacting alternatives?
- **References**, a list of all of the relevant references. The length of the references list gives a very fair indication of the extent of the documentation. A long list indicates a well documented interaction, whereas a short list indicates poor documentation.

Some of the monographs have been compressed into fewer subsections instead of the more usual five, simply to save space where information is limited or where there is little need to be more expansive.

The monographs do not carry the drug interaction Hazard/Severity ratings as used in the electronic *Stockley Interactions Alerts* because of the difficulties of applying them to monographs that cover multiple pairs of drug–drug interactions, but what is written in each monograph should speak for itself.

Quality of information on interactions

The data on interactions are of widely varying quality and reliability. The best come from clinical studies carried out on large numbers of patients under scrupulously controlled conditions. The worst are anecdotal, uncontrolled, or based solely on *animal* studies. Sometimes they are no more than speculative and theoretical scaremongering guesswork, hallowed by repeated quotation until they become virtually set in stone.

The aim has been to filter out as much useless noise as possible, so wherever possible 'secondary' references are avoided, and 'primary' references which are available in good medical and scientific libraries are used instead – although sometimes unpublished, good quality, in-house reports on drug company files have been used where the drug company has kindly allowed access to the information. Product literature (the Summary of Product Characteristics in the UK and the Prescribing Information in the US) rather than the research reports that lie behind them are also cited because they are the only source of published information about new drugs.

The quality of drug company literature is very variable. Some of it is excellent, helpful and very reliable, but regrettably a growing proportion contains a welter of speculative and self-protective statements, probably driven more by the company's medico-legal policy than anything else, and the nervousness of drug regulatory authorities. It is almost unbelievable (but true all the same) that drug companies that are scrupulous in the way they do their research, come out with statements about possible interactions that are little more than guesswork.

When drawing your own conclusions

The human population is a total mixture, unlike selected batches of laboratory animals (same age, weight, sex, and strain etc.). For this reason human beings do not respond uniformly to one or more drugs. Our genetic make up, ethnic background, sex, renal and hepatic functions, diseases and nutritional states, ages and other factors (the route of administration, for example) all contribute towards the heterogeneity of our responses. This means that the outcome of giving one or more drugs to any individual for the first time is never totally predictable because it is a new and unique 'experiment'. Even so, some idea of the probable outcome of using a drug or a pair of drugs can be based on what has been seen in other patients: the more extensive the data, the firmer the predictions.

The most difficult decisions concern isolated cases of interaction, many of which only achieved prominence because they were serious. Do you ignore them as 'idiosyncratic' or do you, from that moment onwards, contraindicate the use of the two drugs totally?

There is no simple 'yes' or 'no' answer to these questions, but one simple rule-of-thumb is that isolated cases of interaction with old and very well-tried pairs of drugs are unlikely to be of general importance, whereas those with new drugs may possibly be the tip of an emerging iceberg and should therefore initially be taken much more seriously until more is known. The delicate balance between these two has then to be set against the actual severity of the reaction reported and weighed up against how essential it is to use the drug combination in question.

When deciding the possible first-time use of any two drugs in any particular patient, you need to put what is currently known about these drugs against the particular profile of your patient. Read the monograph. Consider the facts and conclusions, and then set the whole against the backdrop of your patients unique condition (age, disease, general condition, and so forth) so that what you eventually decide to do is well thought out and soundly based. We do not usually have the luxury of knowing absolutely all the facts, so that an initial conservative approach is often the safest.

1

General considerations and an outline survey of some basic interaction mechanisms

A. What is a drug interaction?

An interaction is said to occur when the effects of one drug are changed by the presence of another drug, herbal medicine, food, drink or by some environmental chemical agent. Much more colourful and informal definitions by patients are that it is "... when medicines fight each other...", or "... when medicines fizz together in the stomach ...", or "...what happens when one medicine falls out with another..."

The outcome can be harmful if the interaction causes an increase in the toxicity of the drug. For example, there is a considerable increase in risk of severe muscle damage if patients on statins start taking azole antifungals (see 'Statins + Azoles', p.831). Patients taking monoamine oxidase inhibitor antidepressants (MAOIs) may experience an acute and potentially life-threatening hypertensive crisis if they eat tyramine-rich foods such as 'cheese', (p.876).

A reduction in efficacy due to an interaction can sometimes be just as harmful as an increase: patients on warfarin given rifampicin need more warfarin to maintain adequate and protective anticoagulation (see 'Anticoagulants + Rifamycins', p.311), while patients taking 'tetracyclines', (p.244) or 'quinolones', (p.232) need to avoid antacids and milky foods (or separate their ingestion) because the effects of these antibacterials can be reduced or even abolished if admixture occurs in the gut.

These unwanted and unsought-for interactions are adverse and undesirable but there are other interactions that can be beneficial and valuable, such as the deliberate co-prescription of antihypertensive drugs and diuretics in order to achieve antihypertensive effects possibly not obtainable with either drug alone. The mechanisms of both types of interaction, whether adverse or beneficial, are often very similar, but the adverse interactions are the focus of this publication.

Definitions of a drug interaction are not rigidly adhered to in this publication because the subject inevitably overlaps into other areas of adverse reactions with drugs. So you will find in these pages some 'interactions' where one drug does not actually affect another at all, but the adverse outcome is the simple additive effects of two drugs with similar effects (for example the combined effects of two or more CNS depressants, or two drugs which affect the QT interval). Sometimes the term 'drug interaction' is used for the physico-chemical reactions that go on if drugs are mixed in intravenous fluids, causing precipitation or inactivation. The long-established and less ambiguous term is 'pharmaceutical incompatibilities'. Incompatibilities are not covered by this publication.

B. What is the incidence of drug interactions?

The more drugs a patient takes the greater the likelihood that an adverse reaction will occur. One hospital study found that the rate was 7% in those taking 6 to 10 drugs but 40% in those taking 16 to 20 drugs, which represents a disproportionate increase.[1] A possible explanation is that the drugs were interacting.

Some of the early studies on the frequency of interactions uncritically compared the drugs that had been prescribed with lists of possible drug interactions, without appreciating that many interactions may be clinically trivial or simply theoretical. As a result, an unrealistically high incidence was suggested. Most of the later studies have avoided this error by looking at only potentially clinically important interactions, and incidences of up to 8.8% have been reported.[2-4] Even so, not all of these studies took into account the distinction that must be made between the incidence of potential interactions and the incidence of those where clinical problems actually arise. The simple fact is that some patients experience quite serious reactions while taking interacting drugs, while others appear not to be affected at all.

A screening of 2422 patients over a total of 25,005 days revealed that 113 (4.7%) were taking combinations of drugs that could interact, but evidence of interactions was observed in only seven patients, representing only 0.3%.[2] In another hospital study of 44 patients over a 5-day period taking 10 to 17 drugs, 77 potential drug interactions were identified, but only one probable and four possible adverse reactions (6.4%) were detected.[5] A further study among patients taking anticonvulsant drugs found that 6% of the cases of toxicity were due to drug interactions.[6] These figures are low compared with those of a hospital survey that monitored 927 patients who had received 1004 potentially interacting drug combinations. Changes in drug dosage were made in 44% of these cases.[7] A review of these and other studies found that the reported incidence rates ranged from 2.2 to 70.3%, and the percentage of patients actually experiencing problems was less than 11.1%. Another review found a 37% incidence of interactions among 639 elderly patients.[8] Yet another review of 236 geriatric patients found an 88% incidence of clinically significant interactions, and a 22% incidence of potentially serious and life-threatening interactions.[9] A 4.1% incidence of drug interactions on prescriptions presented to community pharmacists in the USA was found in a further survey,[10] whereas the incidence was only 2.9% in another American study,[11] and just 1.9% in a Swedish study.[12] An Australian study found that about 10% of hospital admissions were drug-related, of which 4.4% were due to drug interactions.[13] A very high incidence (47 to 50%) of potential drug interactions was found in a study carried out in an Emergency Department in the US.[14] One French study found that 16% of the prescriptions for a group of patients taking antihypertensive drugs were contraindicated or unsuitable,[15] whereas another study on a group of geriatrics found only a 1% incidence.[16] The incidence of problems would be expected to be higher in the elderly because ageing affects the functioning of the kidneys and liver.[17,18]

These discordant figures need to be put into the context of the under-reporting of adverse reactions of any kind by medical professionals, for reasons that may include pressure of work or the fear of litigation. Both doctors and patients may not recognise adverse reactions and interactions, and some patients simply stop taking their drugs without saying why. None of these studies give a clear answer to the question of how frequently drug interactions occur, but even if the incidence is as low as some of the studies suggest, it still represents a very considerable number of patients who appear to be at risk when one thinks of the large numbers of drugs prescribed and taken every day.

1. Smith JW, Seidl LG, Cluff LE. Studies on the epidemiology of adverse drug reactions. V. Clinical factors influencing susceptibility. *Ann Intern Med* (1969) 65, 629.
2. Puckett WH, Visconti JA. An epidemiological study of the clinical significance of drug-drug interaction in a private community hospital. *Am J Hosp Pharm* (1971) 28, 247.
3. Shinn AF, Shrewsbury RP, Anderson KW. Development of a computerized drug interaction database (Medicom) for use in a patient specific environment. *Drug Inf J* (1983) 17, 205.
4. Ishikura C, Ishizuka H. Evaluation of a computerized drug interaction checking system. *Int J Biomed Comput* (1983) 14, 311.
5. Schuster BG, Fleckenstein L, Wilson JP, Peck CC. Low incidence of adverse reactions due to drug-drug interaction in a potentially high risk population of medical inpatients. *Clin Res* (1982) 30, 258A.
6. Manon-Espaillat R, Burnstine TH, Remler B, Reed RC, Osorio I. Antiepileptic drug intoxication: factors and their significance. *Epilepsia* (1991) 32, 96–100.
7. Haumschild MJ, Ward ES, Bishop JM, Haumschild MS. Pharmacy-based computer system for monitoring and reporting drug interactions. *Am J Hosp Pharm* (1987) 44, 345.
8. Manchon ND, Bercoff E, Lamarchand P, Chassagne P, Senant J, Bourreille J. Fréquence et gravité des interaction médicamenteuses dans une population âgée: étude prospective concernant 639 malades. *Rev Med Interne* (1989) 10, 521–5.
9. Lipton JL, Bero LA, Bird JA, McPhee SJ. The impact of clinical pharmacist' consultations on physicians' geriatric drug prescribing. *Med Care* (1992) 30, 646–58.

10. Rupp MT, De Young M, Schondelmeyer SW. Prescribing problems and pharmacist interventions in community practice. *Med Care* (1992) 30, 926–40.
11. Rotman BL, Sullivan AN, McDonald T, DeSmedt P, Goodnature D, Higgins M, Suermond HJ, Young CY, Owens DK. A randomized evaluation of a computer-based physician's workstation; design considerations and baseline results. *Proc Annu Symp Comput Appl Med Care* (1995) 693–7.
12. Linnarsson R. Drug interactions in primary health care. A retrospective database study and its implications for the design of a computerized decision support system. *Scand J Prim Health Care* (1993) 11, 181–6.
13. Stanton LA, Peterson GM, Rumble RH, Cooper GM, Polack AE. Drug-related admissions to an Australian hospital. *J Clin Pharm Ther* (1994) 19, 341–7.
14. Goldberg RM, Mabee J, Chan L, Wong S. Drug-drug and drug-disease interactions in the ED; analysis of a high-risk population. *Am J Emerg Med* (1996) 14, 447–50.
15. Paille R, Pissochet P. L'ordonnance et les interactions medicamenteuses: etude prospective chez 896 patients traites pour hypertension arterielle en medicine generale. *Therapie* (1995) 50, 253–8.
16. Di Castri A, Jacquot JM, Hemmi P, Moati L, Rouy JM, Compan B, Nachar H, Bossy-Vassal A. Interactions medicamenteuses: etude de 409 ordannances etablies a l'issue d'une hospitalisation geriatrique. *Therapie* (1995) 50, 259–64.
17. Cadieux RJ. Drug interactions in the elderly. *Postgrad Med* (1989) 86, 179–86.
18. Tinawi M, Alguire P. The prevalence of drug interactions in hospitalized patients. *Clin Res* (1992) 40, 773A.

C. How seriously should interactions be regarded and handled?

It would be very easy to conclude after browsing through this publication that it is extremely risky to treat patients with more than one drug at a time, but this would be an over-reaction. The figures quoted in the previous section illustrate that many drugs known to interact in some patients, simply fail to do so in others. This partially explains why some quite important drug interactions remained virtually unnoticed for many years, a good example of this being the increase in serum digoxin levels seen with quinidine (see 'Digitalis glycosides + Quinidine', p.709).

Examples of this kind suggest that patients apparently tolerate adverse interactions remarkably well, and that many experienced physicians accommodate the effects (such as rises or falls in serum drug levels) without consciously recognising that what they are seeing is the result of an interaction.

One of the reasons it is often difficult to detect an interaction is that, as already mentioned, patient variability is considerable. We now know many of the predisposing and protective factors that determine whether or not an interaction occurs but in practice it is still very difficult to predict what will happen when an individual patient is given two potentially interacting drugs. An easy solution to this practical problem is to choose a non-interacting alternative, but if none is available, it is frequently possible to give interacting drugs together if appropriate precautions are taken. If the effects of the interaction are well-monitored they can often be allowed for, often simply by adjusting the dosages. Many interactions are dose-related so that if the dosage of the causative drug is reduced, the effects on the other drug will be reduced accordingly. Thus a non-prescription dosage of cimetidine may fail to inhibit the metabolism of phenytoin, whereas a larger dose may clearly increase phenytoin levels (see 'Phenytoin + H_2-blockers', p.368).

The dosage of the affected drug may also be critical. For example, isoniazid causes the levels of phenytoin to rise, particularly in those individuals who are slow acetylators of isoniazid, and levels may become toxic. If the serum phenytoin levels are monitored and its dosage reduced appropriately, the concentrations can be kept within the therapeutic range (see 'Phenytoin + Antituberculars', p.363). Some interactions can be accommodated by using another member of the same group of drugs. For example, the serum levels of doxycycline can become subtherapeutic if phenytoin, barbiturates or carbamazepine are given, but other 'tetracyclines' (p.243) do not seem to be affected. Erythromycin causes serum lovastatin levels to rise because it inhibits its metabolism, but does not affect pravastatin levels because these two statins are metabolised in different ways (see 'Statins', (p.827)). It is therefore clearly important not to uncritically extrapolate the interactions seen with one drug to all members of the same group.

It is interesting to note in this context that a study in two hospitals in Maryland, USA, found that when interacting drugs were given with warfarin (but not theophylline) the length of hospital stay increased by a little over 3 days, with a rise in general costs because of the need to do more tests to get the balance right.[1] So it may be easier, quicker and cheaper to use a non-interacting alternative drug (always provided that its price is not markedly greater).

The variability in patient response has lead to some extreme responses among prescribers. Some clinicians have become over-anxious about interactions so that their patients are denied useful drugs that they might reasonably be given if appropriate precautions are taken. This attitude is exacerbated by some of the more alarmist lists and charts of interactions, which fail to make a distinction between interactions that are very well documented and well established, and those that have only been encountered in a single patient, and which in the final analysis are probably totally idiosyncratic. 'One swallow does not make a summer', nor does a serious reaction in a single patient mean that the drugs in question should never again be given to anyone else.

Table 1.1 Some drug absorption interactions

Drug affected	*Interacting drugs*	*Effect of interaction*
Digoxin	Metoclopramide	Reduced digoxin absorption
	Propantheline	Increased digoxin absorption (due to changes in gut motility)
Digoxin Levothyroxine Warfarin	Colestyramine	Reduced absorption due to binding/complexation with colestyramine
Ketoconazole	Antacids H_2-blockers Proton pump inhibitors	Reduced ketoconazole absorption due to reduced dissolution
Penicillamine	Antacids (containing Al^{3+} and/or Mg^{2+}), iron preparations, food	Formation of less soluble penicillamine chelates resulting in reduced absorption of penicillamine
Methotrexate	Neomycin	Neomycin-induced malabsorption state
Quinolone antibiotics	Antacids (containing Al^{3+} and/or Mg^{2+}), milk, Zn^{2+}(?), Fe^{2+}	Formation of poorly absorbed complexes
Tetracyclines	Antacids (containing Al^{3+}, Ca^{2+}, Mg^{2+}, and/or Bi^{2+}), milk, Zn^{2+}, Fe^{2+}	Formation of poorly soluble chelates resulting in reduced antibiotic absorption (see Fig. 1.1, p.3)

At the other extreme, there are some health professionals who, possibly because they have personally encountered few interactions, fail to consider drug interactions, so that some of their patients are potentially put at risk. An example of this is the fact that cisapride continued to be prescribed with known interacting drugs, even after the rare risk of fatal torsade de pointes arrhythmias, which can cause sudden death, was well established[2] (see 'Cisapride + Miscellaneous', p.732). The responsible position lies between these two extremes, because a very substantial number of interacting drugs can be given together safely, if the appropriate precautions are taken. There are relatively few pairs of drugs that should always be avoided.

1. Jankel CA, McMillan JA, Martin BC. Effect of drug interactions on outcomes of patient receiving warfarin or theophylline. *Am J Hosp Pharm* (1994) 51, 661–6.
2. Smalley W, Shatin D, Wysowski DK, Gurwitz J, Andrade SE, Goodman M, Chan KA, Platt R, Schech SD, Ray WA. Contraindicated use of cisapride: impact of food and drug administration regulatory action. *JAMA* (2000) 284, 3036–9.

D. Mechanisms of drug interaction

Some drugs interact together in totally unique ways, but as the many examples in this publication amply illustrate, there are certain mechanisms of interaction that are encountered time and time again. Some of these common mechanisms are discussed here in greater detail than space will allow in the individual monographs, so that only the briefest reference need be made there.

Mechanisms that are unusual or peculiar to particular pairs of drugs are detailed within the monographs. Very many drugs that interact do so, not by a single mechanism, but often by two or more mechanisms acting in concert, although for clarity most of the mechanisms are dealt with here as though they occur in isolation. For convenience, the mechanisms of interactions can be subdivided into those that involve the pharmacokinetics of a drug, and those that are pharmacodynamic.

1. Pharmacokinetic interactions

Pharmacokinetic interactions are those that can affect the processes by which drugs are absorbed, distributed, metabolised and excreted (the so-called ADME interactions).

1.1. Drug absorption interactions

Most drugs are given orally for absorption through the mucous membranes of the gastrointestinal tract, and the majority of interactions that go on within the gut result in reduced rather than increased absorption. A clear distinction must be made between those that decrease the *rate* of absorption and those that alter the *total amount* absorbed. For drugs that are given chronically on a multiple dose regimen (e.g. the oral anticoagulants) the rate of absorption is usually unimportant, provided the total amount of drug absorbed is not markedly altered. On the other hand for drugs that are given as single doses, intended to be absorbed rapidly (e.g. hypnotics or analgesics), where a rapidly achieved high concentration is needed, a reduction in the rate of absorption may result in failure to achieve an adequate effect. 'Table 1.1', (p.2) lists some of the drug interactions that result from changes in absorption.

(a) Effects of changes in gastrointestinal pH

The passage of drugs through mucous membranes by simple passive diffusion depends upon the extent to which they exist in the non-ionised lipid-soluble form. Absorption is therefore governed by the pKa of the drug, its lipid-solubility, the pH of the contents of the gut and various other parameters relating to the pharmaceutical formulation of the drug. Thus the absorption of salicylic acid by the stomach is much greater at low pH than at high. On theoretical grounds it might be expected that alterations in gastric pH caused by drugs such as the H_2-blockers would have a marked effect on absorption, but in practice the outcome is often uncertain because a number of other mechanisms may also come into play, such as chelation, adsorption and changes in gut motility, which can considerably affect what actually happens. However, in some cases the effect can be significant. Rises in pH due to 'proton pump inhibitors', (p.138), 'H_2-blockers and antacids', (p.135) can markedly reduce the absorption of ketoconazole.

(b) Adsorption, chelation and other complexing mechanisms

Activated charcoal is intended to act as an adsorbing agent within the gut for the treatment of drug overdose or to remove other toxic materials, but inevitably it can affect the absorption of drugs given in therapeutic doses. Antacids can also adsorb a large number of drugs, but often other mechanisms of interaction are also involved. For example, the tetracycline antibacterials can chelate with a number of divalent and trivalent metallic ions, such as calcium, aluminium, bismuth and iron, to form complexes that are both poorly absorbed and have reduced antibacterial effects (see 'Figure 1.1', (below)).

These metallic ions are found in dairy products and antacids. Separating the dosages by 2 to 3 hours goes some way towards reducing the effects of this type of interaction. The marked reduction in the bioavailability of penicillamine caused by some antacids seems also to be due to chelation, although adsorption may have some part to play. Colestyramine, an anionic exchange resin intended to bind bile acids and cholesterol metabolites in the gut, binds to a considerable number of drugs (e.g. digoxin, warfarin, levothyroxine), thereby reducing their absorption. 'Table 1.1', (p.2) lists some drugs that chelate, complex or adsorb other drugs.

(c) Changes in gastrointestinal motility

Since most drugs are largely absorbed in the upper part of the small intestine, drugs that alter the rate at which the stomach empties can affect absorption. Propantheline, for example, delays gastric emptying and reduces 'paracetamol (acetaminophen)' absorption, (p.123), whereas 'metoclopramide', (p.127), has the opposite effect. However, the total amount of drug absorbed remains unaltered. Propantheline also increases the absorption of 'hydrochlorothiazide', (p.729). Drugs with anticholinergic effects decrease the motility of the gut, thus the tricyclic antidepressants can increase the absorption of 'dicoumarol', (p.316), probably because they increase the time available for dissolution and absorption but in the case of 'levodopa', (p.513), they may reduce the absorption, possibly because the exposure time to intestinal mucosal metabolism is increased. The same reduced levodopa absorption has also been seen with 'homatropine', (p.505). These examples illustrate that what actually happens is sometimes very unpredictable because the final outcome may be the result of several different mechanisms.

(d) Induction or inhibition of drug transport proteins

The oral bioavailability of some drugs is limited by the action of drug transporter proteins, which eject drugs that have diffused across the gut lining back into the gut. At present, the most well characterised drug transporter is 'P-glycoprotein', (p.8). Digoxin is a substrate of P-glycoprotein, and drugs that induce this such as rifampicin, may reduce the bioavailability of 'digoxin', (p.711).

(e) Malabsorption caused by drugs

Neomycin causes a malabsorption syndrome, similar to that seen with non-tropical sprue. The effect is to impair the absorption of a number of drugs including 'digoxin', (p.683) and 'methotrexate', (p.475).

1.2. Drug distribution interactions

(a) Protein-binding interactions

Following absorption, drugs are rapidly distributed around the body by the circulation. Some drugs are totally dissolved in the plasma water, but many others are transported with some proportion of their molecules in solution and the rest bound to plasma proteins, particularly the albumins. The extent of this binding varies enormously but some drugs are extremely highly bound. For example, dicoumarol has only four out of every 1000 molecules remaining unbound at serum concentrations of 0.5 mg%. Drugs can also become bound to albumin in the interstitial fluid, and some, such as digoxin, can bind to the heart muscle tissue.

The binding of drugs to the plasma proteins is reversible, an equilibrium being established between those molecules that are bound and those that are not. Only the unbound molecules remain free and pharmacologically active, while those that are bound form a circulating but pharmacologically inactive reservoir which, in the case of drugs with a low-extraction ratio, is temporarily protected from metabolism and excretion. As the free molecules become metabolised, some of the bound molecules become unbound and pass into solution to exert their normal pharmacological actions, before they, in their turn are metabolised and excreted.

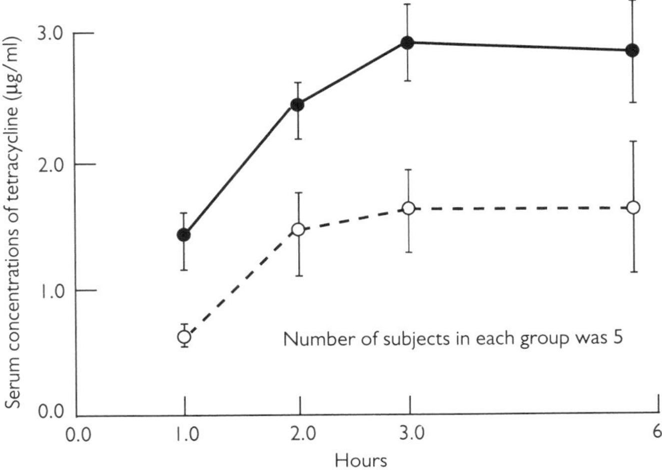

Fig. 1.1 A drug chelation interaction. Tetracycline forms a less-soluble chelate with iron if the two drugs are allowed to mix within the gut. This reduces the absorption and depresses the serum levels and the antibacterial effects (after Neuvonen PJ, *BMJ* (1970) 4, 532, with permission). The same interaction can occur with other ions such as Al^{3+}, Ca^{2+}, Mg^{2+}, Bi^{2+} and Zn^{2+}.

Depending on the concentrations and their relative affinities for the binding sites, one drug may successfully compete with another and displace it from the sites it is already occupying. The displaced (and now active) drug molecules pass into the plasma water where their concentration rises. So for example, a drug that reduces the binding from 99 to 95% would increase the unbound concentration of free and active drug from 1 to 5% (a fivefold increase). This displacement is only likely to raise the number of free and active molecules significantly if the majority of the drug is within the plasma rather than the tissues, so that only drugs with a low apparent volume of distribution (V_d) will be affected. Examples include the sulphonylureas, such as tolbutamide (96% bound, V_d 10 litres), oral anticoagulants, such as warfarin (99% bound, V_d 9 litres), and phenytoin (90% bound, V_d 35 litres). However, another important factor is clearance. Clinically important protein-binding interactions are unlikely if only a small proportion of the drug is eliminated during a single-passage through the eliminating organ (low-extraction ratio drugs), since any increase in free fraction will be effectively cleared. Most drugs that are extensively bound to plasma proteins and subject to displacement reactions (e.g. warfarin, sulphonylureas, phenytoin, methotrexate, and valproic acid) have low-extraction ratios, and drug exposure is therefore independent of protein-binding.

An example of displacement of this kind happens when patients stabilised on warfarin are given cloral hydrate because its major metabolite, trichloroacetic acid, is a highly bound compound that successfully displaces warfarin. This effect is only very short-lived because the now free and active warfarin molecules become exposed to metabolism as the blood flows through the liver, and the amount of drug rapidly falls. This transient increase in free warfarin levels is unlikely to change the anticoagulant effect of warfarin because the clotting factor complexes that are produced when warfarin is taken have a very long half-life, and thus take a long time to reach a new steady state. Normally no change in the warfarin dosage is needed (see 'Anticoagulants + Cloral and derivatives', p.276).

In vitro many commonly used drugs are capable of being displaced by others but in the body the effects seem almost always to be buffered so effectively that the outcome is not normally clinically important. It would therefore seem that the importance of this interaction mechanism has been grossly over-emphasised,[1-3] It is difficult to find an example of a clinically important interaction due to this mechanism alone. It has been suggested that this interaction mechanism is likely to be important only for drugs given intravenously that have a high-extraction ratio, a short pharmacokinetic-pharmacodynamic half-life and a narrow therapeutic index. Lidocaine has been given as an example of a drug fitting these criteria.[3] Some drug interactions that were originally assumed to be due to changes in protein binding have subsequently been shown to have other interaction mechanisms involved. For example, inhibition of metabolism has subsequently been shown to be important in the 'warfarin/phenylbutazone interaction', (p.301), and the 'tolbutamide/sulphonamide interaction', (p.422).

However, knowledge of altered protein binding is important in therapeutic drug monitoring. Suppose for example a patient taking phenytoin was given a drug that displaced phenytoin from its binding sites. The amount of free phenytoin would rise but this would be quickly eliminated by metabolism and excretion thereby keeping the amount of free active phenytoin the same. However, the total amount of phenytoin would now be reduced. Therefore if phenytoin was monitored using an assay looking at total phenytoin levels it may appear that the phenytoin is subtherapeutic and that the dose may therefore need increasing. However, as the amount of free active phenytoin is unchanged this would not be necessary and may even be dangerous.

Basic drugs as well as acidic drugs can be highly protein bound, but clinically important displacement interactions do not seem to have been described. The reasons seem to be that the binding sites within the plasma are different from those occupied by acidic drugs (alpha-1-acid glycoprotein rather than albumin) and, in addition, basic drugs have a large V_d with only a small proportion of the total amount of drug being within the plasma.

(b) Induction or inhibition of drug transport proteins

It is increasingly being recognised that distribution of drugs into the brain, and some other organs such as the testes, is limited by the action of drug transporter proteins such as P-glycoprotein. These proteins actively transport drugs out of cells when they have passively diffused in. Drugs that are inhibitors of these transporters could therefore increase the uptake of drug substrates into the brain, which could either increase adverse CNS effects, or be beneficial. For more information see 'Drug transporter proteins', (p.8).

1. MacKichan JJ. Protein binding drug displacement interactions. Fact or fiction? *Clin Pharmacokinet* (1989) 16, 65–73.
2. Sansom LN, Evans AM. What is the true clinical significance of plasma protein binding displacement interactions? *Drug Safety* (1995) 12, 227–33.
3. Benet LZ, Hoener B-A. Changes in plasma protein binding have little clinical relevance. *Clin Pharmacol Ther* (2002) 71, 115–121.

Table 1.2 Drugs affecting or metabolised by the cytochrome P450 isoenzyme CYP1A2

Inhibitors	Cimetidine	Fluvoxamine
	Fluoroquinolones	Ipriflavone
	Ciprofloxacin	Mexiletine
	Enoxacin	Tacrine
	Grepafloxacin	Zileuton
Inducers	Barbiturates	Phenytoin
	Lansoprazole	Tobacco smoke
Substrates	Caffeine	*Tricyclic antidepressants*
	Clozapine	Amitriptyline
	Duloxetine	Clomipramine
	Flecainide	Imipramine
	Olanzapine	*Triptans*
	Tacrine	Frovatriptan
	Theophylline*	Zolmitriptan
		R-Warfarin

* Considered the preferred *in vivo* substrate, see Bjornsson TD, Callaghan JT, Einolf HJ, *et al*. The conduct of *in vitro* and *in vivo* drug–drug interaction studies: a PhRMA perspective. *J Clin Pharmacol* (2003) 43, 443–69.

1.3. Drug metabolism (biotransformation) interactions

Although a few drugs are lost from the body simply by being excreted unchanged in the urine, most are chemically altered within the body to less lipid-soluble compounds, which are more easily excreted by the kidneys. If this were not so, many drugs would persist in the body and continue to exert their effects for a long time. This chemical change is called 'metabolism', 'biotransformation', 'biochemical degradation' or sometimes 'detoxification'. Some drug metabolism goes on in the serum, the kidneys, the skin and the intestines, but the greatest proportion is carried out by enzymes that are found in the membranes of the endoplasmic reticulum of the liver cells. If liver is homogenised and then centrifuged, the reticulum breaks up into small sacs called microsomes which carry the enzymes, and it is for this reason that the metabolising enzymes of the liver are frequently referred to as the 'liver microsomal enzymes'.

We metabolise drugs by two major types of reaction. The first, so-called Phase I reactions (involving oxidation, reduction or hydrolysis), turn drugs into more polar compounds, while Phase II reactions involve coupling drugs with some other substance (e.g. glucuronic acid) to make usually inactive compounds.

The majority of phase I oxidation reactions are carried out by the haem-containing enzyme cytochrome P450. Cytochrome P450 is not a single entity, but is in fact a very large family of related isoenzymes, about 30 of which have been found in human liver tissue. However, in practice, only a few specific subfamilies seem to be responsible for most (about 90%) of the metabolism of the commonly used drugs. The most important isoenzymes are: CYP1A2, CYP2C9, CYP2C19, CYP2D6, CYP2E1 and CYP3A4. Other enzymes involved in phase I metabolism include monoamine oxidases and epoxide hydrolases.

Less is known about the enzymes responsible for phase II conguation reactions. However, UDP-glucuronyltransferases (UGT), methyltransferases, and N-acetyltrasferases (NAT) are examples.

Although metabolism is very important in the body removing drugs, it is increasingly recognised that drugs can be adsorbed, distributed, or eliminated by transporters, the most well understood at present being 'P-glycoprotein', (p.8).

(a) Changes in first-pass metabolism

(i) Changes in blood flow through the liver

After absorption in the intestine, the portal circulation takes drugs directly to the liver before they are distributed by the blood flow around the rest of the body. A number of highly lipid-soluble drugs undergo substantial biotransformation during this first-pass through the gut wall and liver and there is some evidence that some drugs can have a marked effect on the extent of first pass metabolism by altering the blood flow through the liver. However, there are few clinically relevant examples of this, and many can be explained by other mechanisms, usually altered hepatic metabolism (see (ii) below). One possible example is the increase in rate of absorption of dofetilide with 'verapamil', (p.169), which has resulted in an increased incidence of torsade de pointes.

Another is the increase in bioavailability of high-extraction beta-blockers with 'hydralazine', (p.637), possibly caused by altered hepatic blood flow, or altered metabolism.

(ii) Inhibition or induction of first-pass metabolism

The gut wall contains metabolising enzymes, principally the cytochrome P450 isoenzymes. In addition to the altered metabolism caused by changes in hepatic blood flow (see (i) above) there is evidence that some drugs can have a marked effect on the extent of first-pass metabolism by inhibiting or inducing the cytochrome P450 isoenzymes in the gut wall or in the liver. An example is the effect of grapefruit juice, which seems to induce the cytochrome P450 isoenzyme CYP3A4, mainly in the gut, and therefore increases the metabolism of oral 'calcium channel blockers', (p.11). Although altering the amount of drug 'absorbed', these interactions are usually considered drug metabolism interactions.

(b) Enzyme induction

When barbiturates were widely used as hypnotics it was found necessary to keep on increasing the dosage as time went by to achieve the same hypnotic effect, the reason being that the barbiturates increase the activity of the microsomal enzymes so that extent of metabolism and excretion increases. This phenomenon of enzyme stimulation or 'induction' not only accounts for the need for an increased dose but if another drug that is metabolised by the same range of enzymes is also present, its enzymatic metabolism is similarly increased and larger doses are needed to maintain the same therapeutic effect. However, note that not all enzyme-inducing drugs induce their own metabolism (a process known as auto-induction). The metabolic pathway that is most commonly induced is phase I oxidation mediated by the cytochrome P450 isoenzymes. The main drugs responsible for induction of the most clinically important cytochrome P450 isoenzymes are listed in 'Table 1.2', (p.4), 'Table 1.3', (p.6), 'Table 1.4', (p.6). 'Figure 1.2', (below) shows the reduction in trough ciclosporin levels when given with the enzyme inducing agent, St John's wort. 'St John's wort', (p.799), induces the metabolism of ciclosporin by induction of CYP3A4 and possibly also P-glycoprotein. 'Figure 1.3', (above) shows the effects of another enzyme inducing agent, rifampicin (rifampin) on the serum levels of 'ciclosporin', (p.777), presumably via its effects on CYP3A4. Phase II glucuronidation can also be induced. An example is when rifampicin induces the glucuronidation of 'zidovudine', (p.592).

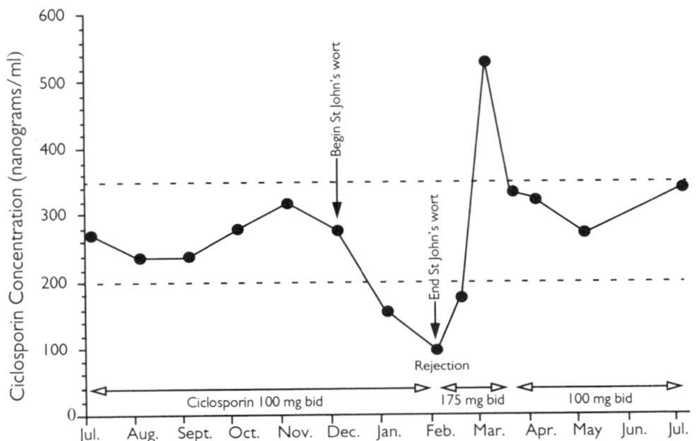

Fig. 1.2 Chronology of ciclosporin trough concentrations (—●—) in a patient self-medicating with St John's wort. ---------- = desired ciclosporin therapeutic range (after Barone GW, Gurley BJ, Ketel BL, Lightfoot ML, Abul-Ezz SR. Drug interaction between St. John's Wort and Cyclosporine. *Ann Pharmacother* (2000) 34: 1013–16, with permission).

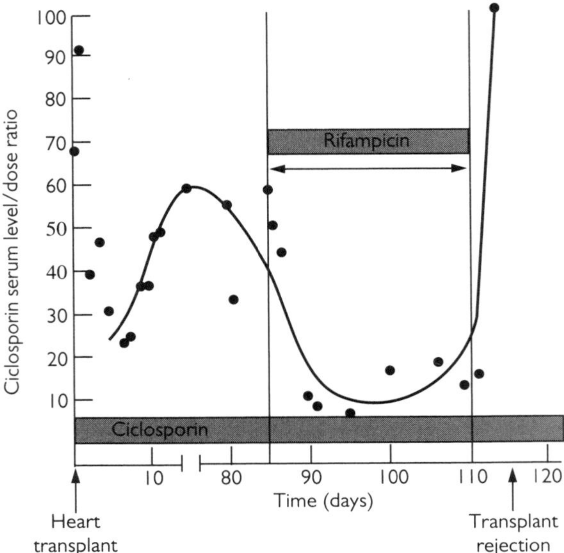

Fig. 1.3 An enzyme induction interaction. Rifampicin (600 mg daily plus isoniazid) increased the metabolism of ciclosporin (cyclosporin) in this patient, thereby reducing the trough serum levels. He subsequently died because his heart transplant was rejected (after *Transplant Proc*, 16, Van Buren D, Wideman CA, Ried M, Gibbons S, Van Buren CT, Jarowenko M, Flechner SM, Frazier OH, Cooley DA, Kahan BD. The antagonistic effect of rifampicin upon cyclosporine bioavailability. 1642–5, Copyright (1984), with permission from Elsevier).

The extent of the enzyme induction depends on the drug and its dosage, but it may take days or even 2 to 3 weeks to develop fully, and may persist for a similar length of time when the inducing agent is stopped. This means that enzyme induction interactions are delayed in onset and slow to quiesce. Enzyme induction is a common mechanism of interaction and is not confined to drugs; it is also caused by the chlorinated hydrocarbon insecticides such as dicophane and lindane, and smoking tobacco.

If one drug reduces the effects of another by enzyme induction, it may be possible to accommodate the interaction simply by raising the dosage of the drug affected, but this requires good monitoring, and there are obvious hazards if the inducing drug is eventually stopped without remembering to reduce the dosage again. The raised drug dosage may be an overdose when the drug metabolism has returned to normal.

(c) Enzyme inhibition

More common than enzyme induction is the inhibition of enzymes. This results in the reduced metabolism of an affected drug, so that it may begin to accumulate within the body, the effect usually being essentially the same as when the dosage is increased. Unlike enzyme induction, which may take several days or even weeks to develop fully, enzyme inhibition can occur within 2 to 3 days, resulting in the rapid development of toxicity. The metabolic pathway that is most commonly inhibited is phase I oxidation by the cytochrome P450 isoenzymes. The main drugs responsible for inhibition of the most clinically important cytochrome P450 isoenzymes are listed in 'Table 1.2', (p.4), 'Table 1.3', (p.6), 'Table 1.4', (p.6). For example a marked increase occurred in the plasma levels of a single dose of sildenafil after 7 day's of ritonavir, probably because ritonavir inhibits the metabolism of sildenafil via CYP3A4 (see 'Sildenafil + Protease inhibitors', p.1030).

An example of inhibition of phase I hydrolytic metabolism, is the inhibition of epoxide hydrolase by valpromide, which increases the levels of 'carbamazepine', (p.350). Phase II conjugative metabolism can also be inhibited. Examples are the inhibition of carbamazepine glucuronidation by 'sodium valproate', (p.348), and the inhibition of methyltransferase by

Table 1.3 Drugs affecting or metabolised by the CYP2 family of cytochrome P450 isoenzymes

Isoenzyme	*Inhibitors*	*Inducers*	*Substrates*
CYP2B6	Thiotepa	Phenobarbital	Cyclophosphamide
		Phenytoin	Ifosfamide
CYP2C8	Gemfibrozil		Repaglinide
CYP2C9	Amiodarone	Rifampicin	Irbesartan
	Azoles		Losartan
	Fluconazole		*NSAIDs*
	Miconazole		Celecoxib
	Voriconazole		Diclofenac
	SSRIs		Etoricoxib
	Fluvoxamine		Rofecoxib
	Fluoxetine		Phenytoin
	Ticlopidine		*Statins*
	Zafirlukast		Fluvastatin
			Rosuvastatin
			Tolbutamide*
			S-Warfarin*
CYP2C19	Fluvoxamine		Cilostazol
	Isoniazid		Diazepam
	Proton pump inhibitors		Escitalopram
	Esomeprazole		Phenytoin
	Omeprazole		Proguanil
	Ticlopidine		*Proton pump inhibitors*
	Valdecoxib		Omeprazole
CYP2D6	Amiodarone	Rifampicin	*Anticholinesterases, centrally-acting*
	Bupropion		Donepezil
	Cimetidine		Galantamine
	Dextropropoxyphene		*Antipsychotics*
	Diphenhydramine		Clozapine
	Duloxetine		Risperidone
	Propafenone		Thioridazine
	Quinidine		*Beta-blockers*
	Ritonavir		Carvedilol
	SSRIs		Labetolol
	Fluoxetine		Metoprolol
	Paroxetine		Propranolol
	Sertraline		Timolol
	Valdecoxib		Cyclobenzaprine
			Flecainide
			Mexiletine
			Opioids
			Codeine
			Dihydrocodeine
			Hydrocodone
			Oxycodone
			Dextromethorphan*
			Propafenone
			Tamoxifen
			Tolterodine
			Tricyclics
			Desipramine
			Imipramine
			Nortriptyline
			Trimipramine
			Venlafaxine
CYP2E1	Disulfiram	Alcohol	Chlorzoxazone*
		Isoniazid	Paracetamol

* Considered the preferred *in vivo* substrates, see Bjornsson TD, Callaghan JT, Einolf HJ, *et al*. The conduct of *in vitro* and *in vivo* drug–drug interaction studies: a PhRMA perspective. *J Clin Pharmacol* (2003) 43, 443–69.

Table 1.4 Drugs affecting or metabolised by the cytochrome P450 isoenzyme CYP3A4

Inhibitors	Aprepitant	Imatinib
	Azoles	*Macrolides*
	Itraconazole	Clarithromycin
	Ketoconazole	Erythromycin
	Delavirdine	Troleandomycin
	Diltiazem	Nefazodone
	Grapefruit juice	*SSRIs*
	HIV-protease inhibitors	Fluoxetine
	Amprenavir	Verapamil
	Indinavir	
	Nelfinavir	
	Ritonavir	
	Saquinavir	
Inducers	Bosentan	Phenytoin
	Carbamazepine	Rifabutin
	Dexamethasone	Rifampicin
	Efavirenz	St John's wort (*Hypericum perforatum*)
	Nevirapine	
Substrates	Amiodarone	Ergot derivatives
	Anticholinesterases, centrally-acting	*Estrogens*
	Donepezil	Combined oral contraceptives
	Galantamine	*HIV-protease inhibitors*
	Antihistamines	Amprenavir
	Astemizole	Indinavir
	Terfenadine	Nelfinavir
	Antineoplastics	Ritonavir
	Docetaxel	Saquinavir
	Ifosfamide	Imatinib
	Irinotecan	Lidocaine, oral
	Teniposide	*Opioids*
	Vincristine	Alfentanil
	Vinblastine	Fentanyl
	Aprepitant	Buprenorphine
	Azoles	Methadone
	Itraconazole	Pimozide
	Benzodiazepines	*Progestogens*
	Alprazolam	Oral contraceptives
	Triazolam	Propafenone
	Midazolam*	Quetiapine
	Bosentan	Quinidine
	Buspirone*	Reboxetine
	Calcium channel blockers	Rifabutin
	Diltiazem	Sibutramine
	Felodipine*	Sildenafil
	Lercanidipine	Sirolimus
	Carbamazepine	Solifenacin
	Ciclosporin	*Statins*
	Cilostazol	Atorvastatin
	Cisapride	Lovastatin
	Corticosteroids	Simvastatin*
	Budesonide	Tacrolimus
	Dexamethasone	Tadalafil
	Fluticasone	Tamoxifen
	Hydrocortisone	Tolterodine
	Methylprednisolone	*Tricyclics*
	Dapsone	Amitriptyline
	Delavirdine	Imipramine
	Disopyramide	Toremifene
	Dutasteride	Vardenafil
	Eletriptan	Voriconazole
	Eplerenone	Zolpidem
		Zopiclone

* Considered the preferred *in vivo* substrates, see Bjornsson TD, Callaghan JT, Einolf HJ, *et al*. The conduct of *in vitro* and *in vivo* drug–drug interaction studies: a PhRMA perspective. *J Clin Pharmacol* (2003) 43, 443–69.

aminosalicylates causing raised levels of 'azathioprine', (p.492).

The clinical significance of many enzyme inhibition interactions depends on the extent to which the serum levels of the drug rise. If the serum levels remain within the therapeutic range the interaction may not be clinically important.

(d) Genetic factors in drug metabolism

An increased understanding of genetics has shown that some of the cytochrome P450 isoenzymes are subject to 'genetic polymorphism', which simply means that some of the population have a variant of the isoenzyme with different (usually poor) activity. The best known example is CYP2D6, for which a small proportion of the population have the variant with low activity and are described as being poor metabolisers (about 5 to 10% in white caucasians, 0 to 2% in Asians and black people). Which group any particular individual falls into is genetically determined. The latter, smaller group, cannot metabolise drugs that normally use this isoenzyme and are therefore called 'slow metabolisers' while the majority who possess the isoenzyme are called 'fast or extensive metabolisers'. You can find out which group any particular individual falls into by looking at the way a single dose of a test or 'probe' drug is metabolised. This varying ability to metabolise certain drugs may explain why some patients develop toxicity when given an interacting drug while others remain symptom free. CYP2D6, CYP2C9 and CYP2C19 also show polymorphism, whereas CYP3A4 does not, although there is still some broad variation in the population without there being distinct groups. At present, genotyping is primarily a research tool and is not used clinically. In the future, it may become standard clinical practice and may be used to individualise drug therapy.[1]

(e) Cytochrome P450 isoenzymes and predicting drug interactions

It is interesting to know which particular isoenzyme is responsible for the metabolism of drugs because by doing *in vitro* tests with human liver enzymes it is often possible to explain why and how some drugs interact. For example, ciclosporin is metabolised by CYP3A4, and we know that rifampicin (rifampin) is a potent inducer of this cytochrome, whereas ketoconazole inhibits its activity, so that it comes as no surprise that the former reduces the effects of ciclosporin and the latter increases it.

What is very much more important than retrospectively finding out why two drugs interact, is the knowledge such *in vitro* tests can provide about forecasting which other drugs may possibly also interact. This may reduce the numbers of expensive clinical trials in subjects and patients and avoids waiting until significant drug interactions are observed in clinical use. A lot of effort is being put into this area of drug development.[2-6] However, at present such prediction is, like weather forecasting, still a somewhat hit-and-miss business because we do not know all of the factors that may modify or interfere with metabolism. It is far too simplistic to think that we have all the answers just because we know which liver isoenzymes are concerned with the metabolism of a particular drug, but it is a very good start.

'Table 1.2', (p.4), 'Table 1.3', (p.6), 'Table 1.4', (p.6) are lists of drugs that are inhibitors, inducers, or substrates of the clinically important cytochrome P450 isoenzymes, and each drug has a cross reference to a monograph describing a drug interaction thought to occur via that mechanism. If a new drug is shown to be an inducer, or an inhibitor, and/or a substrate of a given isoenzyme, these tables could be used to predict likely drug interactions. However, what may happen *in vitro* may not necessarily work in clinical practice because all of the many variables which can come into play are not known (such as how much of the enzyme is available, the concentration of the drug at the site of metabolism, and the affinity of the drug for the enzyme). Remember too that some drugs can be metabolised by more than one cytochrome P450 isoenzyme; some drugs (and their metabolites) can both induce a particular isoenzyme and be metabolised by it; and some drugs (or their metabolites) can inhibit a particular isoenzyme but not be metabolised by it. With so many factors possibly impinging on the outcome of giving two or more drugs together, it is very easy to lose sight of one of the factors (or not even know about it) so that the sum of 2 plus 2 may not turn out to be the 4 that you have predicted.

For example, ritonavir and other protease inhibitors are well know potent inhibitors of CYP3A4, and in clinical use increase the levels of many drugs that are substrates of this isoenzyme. Methadone is a substrate of CYP3A4, and some *in vitro* data show that ritonavir (predictably) increased methadone levels. However, unexpectedly, in clinical use the HIV protease inhibitors seem to decrease methadone levels, by a yet unknown mechanism (see, 'Opioids; Methadone + Protease inhibitors', p.116).

Another factor complicating the understanding of metabolic drug interactions is the finding that there is a large overlap between the inhibitors/inducers and substrates of P-glycoprotein (a 'drug transporter protein', (p.8)) and those of CYP3A4. Therefore, both mechanisms may be involved in many of the drug interactions previously thought to be due to effects on CYP3A4.

1. Phillips KA, Veenstra DL, Oren E, Lee JK, Sadee W. Potential role of pharmacogenomics in reducing adverse drug reactions: a systematic review. *JAMA* (2001) 286, 2270–79.
2. Bjornsson TD, Callaghan JT, Einolf HJ, Fischer V, Gan L, Grimm S, Kao J, King SP, Miwa G, Ni L, Kumar G, McLeod J, Obach RS, Roberts S, Roe A, Shah A, Snikeris F, Sullivan JT, Tweedie D, Vega JM, Walsh J, Wrighton SA. The conduct of in vitro and in vivo drug-drug interaction studies: a PhRMA perspective. *J Clin Pharmacol* (2003) 43, 443–69.
3. Bachmann KA, Ghosh R. The use of *in vitro* methods to predict *in vivo* pharmacokinetics and drug interactions. *Curr Drug Metab* (2001) 2, 299–314.
4. Yao C, Levy RH. Inhibition-based metabolic drug–drug interactions: predictions from *in vitro* data. *J Pharm Sci* (2002) 91, 1923–35.
5. Worboys PD, Carlile DJ. Implications and consequences of enzyme induction on preclinical and clinical drug development. *Xenobiotica* (2001) 31, 539–56.
6. Venkatakrishnan K, von Moltke LL, Obach RS, Greenblatt DJ. Drug metabolism and drug interactions: application and clinical value of *in vitro* models. *Curr Drug Metab* (2003) 4, 423–59.

1.4. Drug excretion interactions

With the exception of the inhalation anaesthetics, most drugs are excreted either in the bile or in the urine. Blood entering the kidneys along the renal arteries is, first of all, delivered to the glomeruli of the tubules where molecules small enough to pass through the pores of the glomerular membrane (e.g. water, salts, some drugs) are filtered through into the lumen of the tubules. Larger molecules, such as plasma proteins, and blood cells are retained within the blood. The blood flow then passes to the remaining parts of the kidney tubules where active energy-using transport systems are able to remove drugs and their metabolites from the blood and secrete them into the tubular filtrate. The renal tubular cells additionally possess active and passive transport systems for the reabsorption of drugs. Interference by drugs with renal tubular fluid pH, with active transport systems and with blood flow to the kidney can alter the excretion of other drugs.

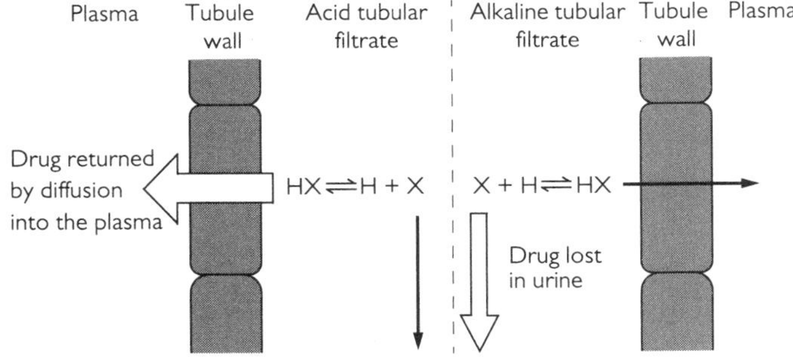

Fig. 1.4 An excretion interaction. If the tubular filtrate is acidified, most of the molecules of weakly acid drugs (HX) exist in an un-ionised lipid-soluble form and are able to return through the lipid membranes of the tubule cells by simple diffusion. Thus they are retained. In alkaline urine most of the drug molecules exist in an ionised non-lipid soluble form (X). In this form the molecules are unable to diffuse freely through these membranes and are therefore lost in the urine.

(a) Changes in urinary pH

As with drug absorption in the gut, passive reabsorption of drugs depends upon the extent to which the drug exists in the non-ionised lipid-soluble form, which in its turn depends on its pKa and the pH of the urine. Only the non-ionised form is lipid-soluble and able to diffuse back through the lipid membranes of the tubule cells. Thus at high pH values (alkaline), weakly acid drugs (pKa 3 to 7.5) largely exist as ionised lipid-insoluble molecules, which are unable to diffuse into the tubule cells and will therefore be lost in the urine. The converse will be true for weak bases with pKa values of 7.5 to 10.5. Thus pH changes that increase the amount in the ionised form (alkaline urine for acidic drugs, acid urine for basic drugs) increase the loss of the drug, whereas moving the pH in the opposite direction will increase their retention. 'Figure 1.4', (p.7) illustrates the situation with a weakly acidic drug. The clinical significance of this interaction mechanism is small, because although a very large number of drugs are either weak acids or bases, almost all are largely metabolised by the liver to inactive compounds and few are excreted in the urine unchanged. In practice therefore only a handful of drugs seem to be affected by changes in urinary pH (possible exceptions include changes in the excretion of 'quinidine', (p.187) or 'high-dose aspirin', (p.79), due to alterations in urinary pH caused by antacids, and the increase in the clearance of 'methotrexate', (p.484), with urinary alkalinisers. In cases of overdose, deliberate manipulation of urinary pH has been used to increase the loss of drugs such as methotrexate and salicylates.

Table 1.5 Examples of interactions probably due to changes in renal transport

Drug affected	*Interacting drug*	*Result of interaction*
Cefalosporins Dapsone Methotrexate Penicillins Quinolones	Probenecid	Serum levels of drug affected raised; possibility of toxicity with some drugs
Methotrexate	Salicylates and some other NSAIDs	Methotrexate serum levels raised; serious methotrexate toxicity possible

(b) Changes in active renal tubular excretion

Drugs that use the same active transport systems in the renal tubules can compete with one another for excretion. For example, probenecid reduces the excretion of penicillin and other drugs. With the increasing understanding of drug transporter proteins in the kidneys, it is now known that probenecid inhibits the renal secretion of many other anionic drugs via organic anion transporters (OATs).[1] Probenecid possibly also inhibits some of the ABC transporters in the kidneys. The ABC transporter, P-glycoprotein, is also present in the kidneys, and drugs that alter this may alter renal drug elimination, although there are no clear examples of this yet. See, 'Drug transporter proteins', (below) for further discussion. Some examples of drugs that possibly interact via altered renal transport are given in 'Table 1.5', (above).

(c) Changes in renal blood flow

The flow of blood through the kidney is partially controlled by the production of renal vasodilatory prostaglandins. If the synthesis of these prostaglandins is inhibited the renal excretion of some drugs may be reduced. An interaction where this is the suggested mechanism is the rise in serum lithium seen with some NSAIDs, see 'Lithium + NSAIDs', p.854.

(d) Biliary excretion and the entero-hepatic shunt

(i) Enterohepatic recirculation

A number of drugs are excreted in the bile, either unchanged or conjugated (e.g. as the glucuronide) to make them more water soluble. Some of the conjugates are metabolised to the parent compound by the gut flora and are then reabsorbed. This recycling process prolongs the stay of the drug within the body, but if the gut flora are diminished by the presence of an antibacterial, the drug is not recycled and is lost more quickly. This may possibly explain the rare failure of the oral contraceptives that can be brought about by the concurrent use of penicillins or tetracyclines, but see Mechanism in 'Oral contraceptives + Antibacterials; Penicillins', p.746. Antimicrobial-induced reductions in gut bacteria may reduce the activation of 'sulfasalazine', (p.739). Reduction of bacterial flora has also been suggested as the reason why in some patients quinolone antibacterials increase the levels of 'digoxin', (p.710).

(ii) Drug transporters

Increasing research shows that numerous drug transporter proteins (both from the ABC family and SLC family, see 'Drug transporter proteins', (below)) are involved in the hepatic extraction and secretion of drugs into the bile.[2] The relevance of many of these to drug interactions is still unclear, but the bile salt export pump (ACBB11) is known to be inhibited by a variety of drugs including ciclosporin, glibenclamide, and bosentan. Inhibition of this pump may increase the risk of cholestasis, and the maker of bosentan says they should be avoided in patients on bosentan (see 'glibenclamide', (p.424) and 'ciclosporin', (p.784)).

1. Lee W, Kim RB. Transporters and renal drug elimination. *Annu Rev Pharmacol Toxicol* (2004) 44, 137–66.
2. Faber KN, Müller M, Jansen PLM. Drug transport proteins in the liver. *Adv Drug Deliv Rev* (2003) 55, 107–24.

1.5. Drug transporter proteins

Drugs and endogenous substances are now known to cross biological membranes not just by passive diffusion but by carrier-mediated processes, often known as transporters. Significant advances in the identification of various transporters have been made, although the contribution of many of these to drug interactions in particular, is still unclear.[1,2] The most well known is P-glycoprotein, which is a product of the MDR1 gene (ABCB1 gene) and a member of the ATP-binding cassette (ABC) family of efflux transporters.[1] Its involvement in drug interactions is discussed in (a) below.

Another ABC transporter is sister P-glycoprotein, otherwise called the bile salt export pump (BSEP or ABCB11).[1] It has been suggested that inhibition of this pump may increase the risk of cholestasis, see Drug transporters under 'Drug excretion interactions', (p.7).

Other transporters that are involved in some drug interactions are the organic anion transporters (OATs), organic anion-transporting polypeptides (OATPs) and organic cation transporters (OCTs), which are members of the solute carrier superfamily (SLC) of transporters.[1] The best known example of an OAT inhibitor is probenecid, which affects the renal excretion of a number of drugs, see Changes in active kidney tubule excretion under 'Drug excretion interactions', (p.7).

Table 1.6 Some possible inhibitors and inducers of P-glycoprotein shown to alter the levels of P-glycoprotein substrates in clinical studies[1]

Inhibitors		*Inducers*
Atorvastatin	Ketoconazole	Rifampicin
Clarithromycin	Propafenone	St John's wort (*Hypericum perforatum*)
Dipyridamole	Quinidine	
Erythromycin	Valspodar	
Itraconazole	Verapamil	

1. Mizuno N, Niwa T, Yotsumoto Y, Sugiyama. Impact of drug transporter studies on drug discovery and development. *Pharmacol Rev* (2003) 55, 425–61.

(a) P-glycoprotein interactions

More and more evidence is accumulating to show that some drug interactions occur because they interfere with the activity of P-glycoprotein. This is an efflux pump found in the membranes of certain cells, which can push metabolites and drugs out of the cells and have an impact on the extent of drug absorption (via the intestine), distribution (to the brain, testis, or placenta) and elimination (in the urine and bile). So, for example, the P-glycoprotein in the cells of the gut lining can eject some already-absorbed drug molecules back into the intestine resulting in a reduction in the total amount of drug absorbed. In this way P-glycoprotein acts as a barrier to absorption. The activity of P-glycoprotein in the endothelial cells of the blood-brain barrier can also eject certain drugs from the brain, limiting CNS penetration and effects.

The pumping actions of P-glycoprotein can be induced or inhibited by some drugs. So for example, the induction (or stimulation) of the activity of P-glycoprotein by rifampicin (rifampin) within the lining cells of the gut causes digoxin to be ejected into the gut more vigorously. This results in a fall in the plasma levels of digoxin (see 'Digitalis glycosides + Rifamycins', p.711). In contrast, verapamil appears to inhibit the activity of P-glycoprotein, and is well known to increase digoxin levels (see 'Digitalis glycosides + Calcium channel blockers; Verapamil', p.692). Ketoconazole also has P-glycoprotein inhibitory effects, and has been shown to increase CSF levels of ritonavir, possibly by preventing the efflux of ritonavir from the CNS (see 'Protease inhibitors + Azoles', p.609). Thus the induction or inhibition of P-glycoprotein can have an impact on the pharmacokinetics of some drugs. Note that there is evidence that P-glycoprotein inhibition may have a greater impact on drug distribution (e.g. into the brain) than on drug absorption (e.g. plasma levels).[2]

There is an overlap between CYP3A4 and P-glycoprotein inhibitors, inducers and substrates. Therefore, both mechanisms may be involved in many of the drug interactions traditionally thought to be due to changes in CYP3A4. 'Table 1.6', (p.8) lists some possible P-glycoprotein inhibitors and inducers. Many drugs that are substrates for CYP3A4 (see 'Table 1.4', (p.6)) are also substrates for P-glycoprotein. Digoxin and talinolol are examples of the few drugs that are substrates for P-glycoprotein but not CYP3A4.

P-glycoprotein is also expressed in some cancer cells (where it was first identified). This has led to the development of specific P-glycoprotein inhibitors, such as valspodar, with the aim of improving the penetration of cytotoxic drugs into cancer cells.

1. Mizuno N, Niwa T, Yotsumoto Y, Sugiyama Y. Impact of drug transporter studies on drug discovery and development. *Pharmacol Rev* (2003) 55, 425–61.
2. Lin JH, Yamazaki M. Clinical relevance of P-glycoprotein in drug therapy. *Drug Metab Rev* (2003) 35, 417–54.

2. Pharmacodynamic interactions

Pharmacodynamic interactions are those where the effects of one drug are changed by the presence of another drug at its site of action. Sometimes the drugs directly compete for particular receptors (e.g. beta-2 agonists such as salbutamol and beta-blockers such as propranolol) but often the reaction is more indirect and involves interference with physiological mechanisms. These interactions are much less easy to classify neatly than those of a pharmacokinetic type.

2.1. Additive or synergistic interactions

If two drugs that have the same pharmacological effect are given together the effects can be additive. For example, alcohol depresses the CNS and, if taken in moderate amounts with normal therapeutic doses of any of a large number of drugs (e.g. sedatives, tranquillisers, etc.), may cause excessive drowsiness. Strictly speaking (as pointed out earlier) these are not interactions within the definition given in 'What is a drug interaction?', (p.1). Nevertheless, it is convenient to consider them within the broad context of the clinical outcome of giving two drugs together.

Additive effects can occur with both the main effects of the drugs as well as their adverse effects, thus an additive 'interaction' can occur with anticholinergic antiparkinson drugs (main effect) or butyrophenones (adverse effect) that can result in serious anticholinergic toxicity (see 'Antipsychotics + Anticholinergics', p.529).

Sometimes the additive effects are solely toxic (e.g. additive ototoxicity, nephrotoxicity, bone marrow depression, QT interval prolongation). Examples of these reactions are listed in 'Table 1.7', (below). It is common to use the terms 'additive', 'summation', 'synergy' or 'potentiation' to describe what happens if two or more drugs behave like this. These words have precise pharmacological definitions but they are often used rather loosely as synonyms because in practice it is often very difficult to know the extent of the increased activity, that is to say whether the effects are greater or smaller than the sum of the individual effects.

(a) The serotonin syndrome

In the 1950s a serious and life-threatening toxic reaction was reported in patients on iproniazid (an MAOI) when they were treated with 'pethidine (meperidine)', (p.869). The reasons were then not understood and even now we do not have the full picture. What happened is thought to have been due to over-stimulation of the 5-HT_{1A} and 5-HT_{2A} receptors and possibly other serotonin receptors in the central nervous system (in the brain stem and spinal cord in particular) due to the combined effects of these two drugs. It can occur exceptionally after taking only one drug, which causes over-stimulation of these 5-HT receptors, but much more usually it develops when two or more drugs (so-called serotonergic or serotomimetic drugs) act in concert. The characteristic symptoms (now known as the 'serotonin syndrome') fall into three main areas, namely altered mental status (agitation, confusion, mania), autonomic dysfunction (diaphoresis, diarrhoea, fever, shivering) and neuromuscular abnormalities (hyperreflexia, incoordination, myoclonus, tremor). These are the 'Sternbach diagnostic criteria' named after Dr Harvey Sternbach who drew up this list of clinical features and who suggested that at least three of them need to be seen before classifying this toxic reaction as the 'serotonin syndrome' rather than the 'neuroleptic malignant syndrome'.[1]

The syndrome can develop shortly after one serotonergic drug is added to another, or even if one is replaced by another without allowing a long enough washout period in between, and the problem usually resolves within about 24 hours if both drugs are withdrawn and supportive measures given. Non-specific serotonin antagonists (cyproheptadine, chlorpromazine, methysergide) have also been used for treatment. Most patients recover uneventfully, but there have been a few fatalities.

Table 1.7 Additive, synergistic or summation interactions

Drugs	*Result of interaction*
Antipsychotics + Anticholinergics	Increased anticholinergic effects; heat stroke in hot and humid conditions, adynamic ileus, toxic psychoses
Antihypertensives + Drugs causing hypotension (Phenothiazines, Sildenafil)	Increased antihypertensive effects; orthostasis
Beta-agonist bronchodilators + Potassium-depleting drugs	Hypokalaemia
CNS depressants + CNS depressants Alcohol + Antihistamines Benzodiazepines + Anaesthetics, general Opioids + Benzodiazepines	Impaired psychomotor skills, reduced alertness, drowsiness, stupor, respiratory depression, coma, death
Drugs that prolong the QT interval + Other drugs that prolong the QT interval Amiodarone + Disopyramide	Additive prolongation of QT interval, increased risk of torsade de pointes
Methotrexate + Antibacterials; Co-trimoxazole	Bone marrow megaloblastosis due to folic acid antagonism
Nephrotoxic drugs + Nephrotoxic drugs (e.g. Aminoglycosides, Cisplatin, Ciclosporin, Vancomycin	Increased nephrotoxicity
Neuromuscular blockers + Drugs with neuromuscular blocking effects (e.g. Aminoglycosides)	Increased neuromuscular blockade; delayed recovery, prolonged apnoea
Potassium supplements + Potassium-sparing drugs (e.g. ACE inhibitors, Angiotensin II receptor antagonists, Potassium-sparing diuretics)	Hyperkalaemia

Following the first report of this syndrome, many other cases have been described involving 'tryptophan and MAOIs', (p.874), the 'tricyclic antidepressants and MAOIs', (p.873), and, more recently, the 'SSRIs', (p.984) but other serotonergic drugs have also been involved and the list grows every year (see 'SSRIs + St John's wort (*Hypericum perforatum*)', p.987).

It is still not at all clear why many patients can take two, or sometimes several serotonergic drugs together without problems, while a very small number develop this serious toxic reaction, but it certainly suggests that there are as yet other factors involved that have yet to be identified. The full story is likely to be much more complex than just the simple additive effects of two drugs.

1. Sternbach H. The serotonin syndrome. *Am J Psychiatry* (1991) 148, 705–13.

2.2. Antagonistic or opposing interactions

In contrast to additive interactions, there are some pairs of drugs with activities that are opposed to one another. For example the oral anticoagulants can prolong the blood clotting time by competitively inhibiting the effects of dietary vitamin K. If the intake of vitamin K is increased, the effects of the oral anticoagulant are opposed and the prothrombin time can return to normal, thereby cancelling out the therapeutic benefits of anticoagulant treatment (see 'Anticoagulants + Vitamin K', p.321). Other examples of this type of interaction are listed in 'Table 1.8', (below)).

Table 1.8 Opposing or antagonistic interactions

Drug affected	*Interacting drugs*	*Results of interaction*
ACE inhibitors or Loop diuretics	NSAIDs	Antihypotensive effects opposed
Anticoagulants	Vitamin K	Anticoagulant effects opposed
Antidiabetics	Glucocorticoids	Hypoglycaemic effects opposed
Antineoplastics	Megestrol	Cytotoxic effects possibly opposed
Levodopa	Antipsychotics (those with dopamine antagonist effects)	Antiparkinsonian effects opposed
Levodopa	Tacrine	Antiparkinsonian effects opposed

2.3. Drug or neurotransmitter uptake interactions

A number of drugs whose actions occur at adrenergic neurones can be prevented from reaching those sites of action by the presence of other drugs. The tricyclic antidepressants prevent the re-uptake of noradrenaline (norepinephrine) into peripheral adrenergic neurones. Thus patients on tricyclics given parenteral noradrenaline have a markedly increased response (hypertension, tachycardia) (see 'Tricyclic antidepressants + Sympathomimetics; Directly-acting', p.1001). Similarly, the uptake of guanethidine and related drugs (guanoclor, betanidine, debrisoquine, etc.) is blocked by 'chlorpromazine, haloperidol, tiotixene', (p.670), a number of 'indirectly-acting sympathomimetic amines', (p.669) and the 'tricyclic antidepressants', (p.671) so that the antihypertensive effect is prevented. The antihypertensive effects of clonidine are also prevented by the tricyclic antidepressants, one possible reason being that the uptake of clonidine within the CNS is blocked (see 'Clonidine + Tricyclic and related antidepressants', p.667). Some of these interactions at adrenergic neurones are illustrated in 'Figure 1.5', (below).

E. Drug-herb interactions

The market for herbal medicines and supplements in the Western world has markedly increased in recent years, and, not surprisingly, reports of interactions with 'conventional' drugs have arisen. The most well known and documented example is the interaction of St John's wort (*Hypericum perforatum*) with a variety of drugs, see (a) below. There have also been isolated reports of other herbal drug interactions, attributable to various mechanisms, including additive pharmacological effects.

Based on these reports, there are a growing number of reviews of herbal medicine interactions, which seek to predict likely interactions based on the, often hypothesised, actions of various herbs. Many of these predictions seem tenuous at best.

Rather than add to the volume of predicted interactions, at present, *Stockley's Drug Interactions* includes only those interactions for which there are published reports.

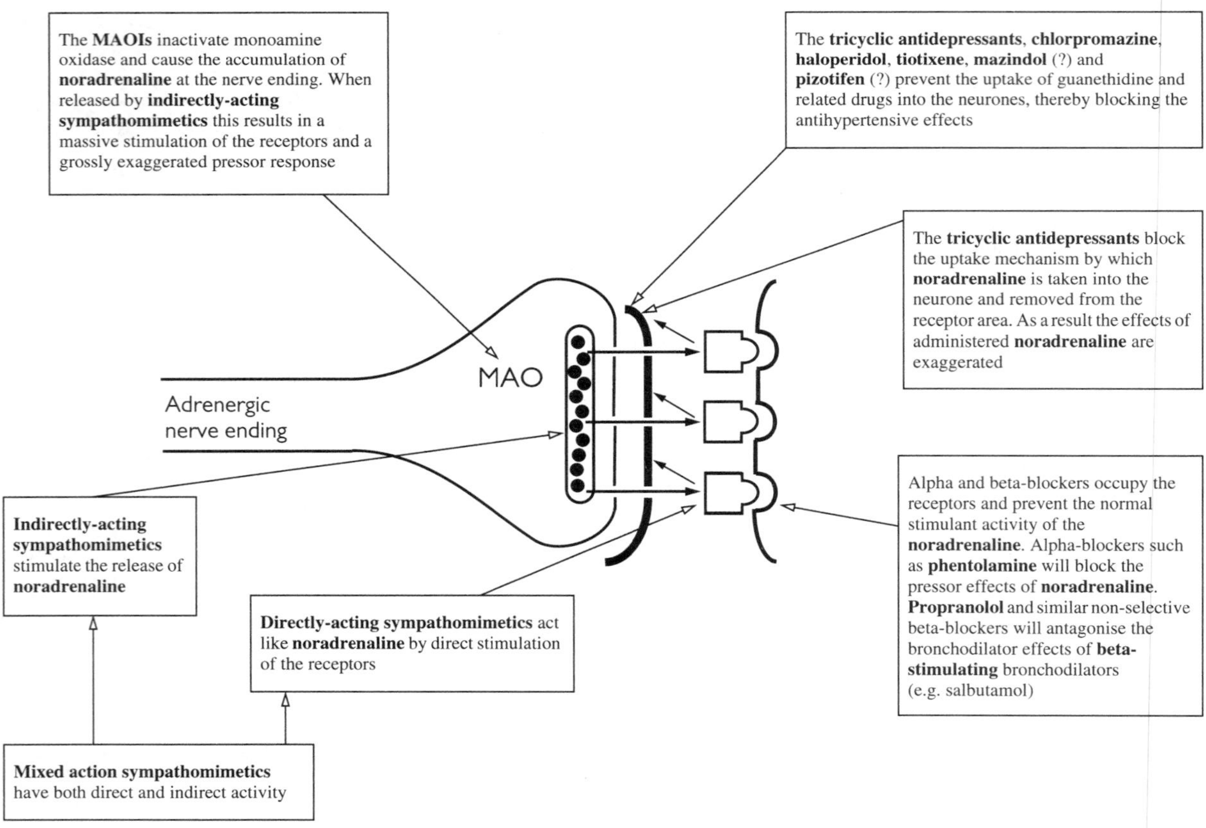

Fig. 1.5 Interactions at adrenergic neurones. A highly simplified composite diagram of an adrenergic neurone (molecules of noradrenaline (norepinephrine) indicated as (●) contained in a single vesicle at the nerve-ending) to illustrate in outline some of the different sites where drugs can interact. More details of these interactions are to be found in individual monographs.

To aid collection of data in this area, health professionals should routinely ask patients about their use of herbal medicines and supplements, and report any unexpected responses to treatment.

An additional problem in interpreting these interactions, is that the interacting constituent of the herb is usually not known and is therefore not standardised for. It could vary widely between different products, and batches of the same product.

(a) St John's wort

An increasing number of reports have implicated St John's wort (*Hypericum perforatum*) in drug interactions. Evidence has shown that the herb can induce the cytochrome P450 isoenzyme CYP3A4, and can also induce 'P-glycoprotein', (p.8). Hence St John's wort decreases the levels of 'ciclosporin', (p.799) and 'digoxin', (p.712), respectively. Other less certain evidence suggests that CYP2E1 and CYP1A2 may also be induced. St John's wort has serotonergic properties, and this has resulted in a pharmacodynamic interaction with the 'SSRIs', (p.987), namely the development of the serotonin syndrome. St John's wort contains many possible constituents that could be responsible for its pharmacological effects. The major active constituents are currently considered to be hyperforin (a phloroglucinol) and hypericin (a naphthodianthrone). Hypericin is the only constituent that is standardised for, and then only in some St John's wort preparations.

General references

1. Miller LG. Herbal medicinals. Selected clinical considerations focusing on known or potential drug-herb interactions. *Arch Intern Med* (1998) 158, 2200–11.
2. Fugh-Berman A. Herb-drug interactions. *Lancet* (2000) 355, 134–8. Erratum *ibid.* 1020.
3. Wang Z, Gorski JC, Hamman MA, Huang S-M, Lesko LJ, Hall SD. The effects of St John's wort (*Hypericum perforatum*) on human cytochrome P450 activity. *Clin Pharmacol Ther* (2001) 70, 317–26.
4. Williamson EM. Drug interactions between herbal and prescription medicines. *Drug Safety* (2003) 26, 1075–92.
5. Henderson L, Yue QY, Bergquist C, Gerden B, Arlett P. St John's wort (*Hypericum perforatum*): drug interactions and clinical outcomes. *Br J Clin Pharmacol* (2002) 54, 349–56.
6. Gurley BJ, Gardner SF, Hubbard MA, Williams DK, Gentry WB, Cui Y, Ang CYW. Cytochrome P450 phenotypic ratios for predicting herb-drug interactions in humans. *Clin Pharmacol Ther* (2002) 72, 276–87.
7. Dresser GK, Schwarz UI, Wilkinson GR, Kim RB. Coordinate induction of both cytochrome P4503A and MDR1 by St John's wort in healthy subjects. *Clin Pharmacol Ther* (2003) 73, 41–50.

F. Drug-food interactions

It is well established that food can cause clinically important changes in drug absorption through effects on gastrointestinal motility or by drug binding, see 'Drug absorption interactions', (p.3). In addition, it is well known that tyramine (present in some foodstuffs) may reach toxic concentrations in patients on 'MAOIs', (p.876). With the growth in understanding of drug metabolism mechanisms, it has been increasingly recognised that some foods can alter drug metabolism. Currently, grapefruit juice causes the most clinically relevant of these interactions, see (b) below.

(a) Cruciferous vegetables and charcoal-broiled meats

Cruciferous vegetables, such as brussels sprouts, cabbage, and broccoli, contain substances that are inducers of the cytochrome P450 isoenzyme CYP1A2. Chemicals formed by 'burning' meats additionally have these properties. These foods do not appear to cause any clinically important drug interactions in their own right, but their consumption may add another variable to drug interaction studies, so complicating interpretation. In drug interaction studies where alteration of CYP1A2 is a predicted mechanism, it may be better for patients to avoid these foods during the study.

(b) Grapefruit juice

By chance, grapefruit juice was chosen to mask the taste of ethanol in a study of the effect of ethanol on felodipine, which led to the discovery that grapefruit juice itself markedly increased felodipine levels, see 'Calcium channel blockers + Grapefruit juice', p.655. In general, grapefruit juice inhibits intestinal CYP3A4, and only slightly affects hepatic CYP3A4. This is demonstrated by the fact that intravenous preparations of drugs that are metabolised by CYP3A4 are not much affected, whereas oral preparations of the same drugs are. These interactions result in increased drug levels.

Some drugs that are not metabolised by CYP3A4 show decreased levels with grapefruit juice, such as 'fexofenadine', (p.428). The probable reason for this is that grapefruit juice is an inhibitor of some drug transporters (see 'Drug transporter proteins', (p.8)), and possibly affects organic anion-transporting polypeptides (OATPs), although inhibition of P-glycoprotein has also been suggested.

The active constituent of grapefruit juice is uncertain. Grapefruit contains naringin, which degrades during processing to naringenin, a substance known to inhibit CYP3A4. Because of this, it has been assumed that whole grapefruit will not interact, but that processed grapefruit juice will. However, subsequently some reports have implicated the whole fruit. Other possible active constituents in the whole fruit include bergamottin and dihydroxybergamottin.

General references

1. Ameer B, Wientraub RA. Drug interactions with grapefruit juice. *Clin Pharmacokinet* (1997) 33, 103–21.

G. Conclusions

It is now quite impossible to remember all the known clinically important interactions and how they occur, which is why this reference publication has been produced, but there are some broad general principles that need little memorising:

- Be on the alert with any drugs that have a narrow therapeutic window or where it is necessary to keep serum levels at or above a suitable level (e.g. anticoagulants, anticonvulsants, antihypertensives, anti-infectives, antineoplastic cytotoxics, digitalis glycosides, hypoglycaemic agents, immunosuppressants, etc.).
- Remember some of those drugs that are key enzyme inducing agents (e.g. phenytoin, barbiturates, rifampicin, etc) or enzyme inhibiting agents (e.g. azole antifungals, HIV-protease inhibitors, erythromycin, SSRIs).
- Think about the basic pharmacology of the drugs under consideration so that obvious problems (additive CNS depression for example) are not overlooked, and try to think what might happen if drugs that affect the same receptors are used together. And don't forget that many drugs affect more than one type of receptor.
- Keep in mind that the elderly are at risk because of reduced liver and renal function on which drug clearance depends.

2

ACE inhibitors and angiotensin II receptor antagonists

ACE inhibitors (angiotensin-converting enzyme inhibitors) prevent the production of angiotensin II from angiotensin I, whereas the angiotensin II receptor antagonists are more selective, and target the angiotensin II type I (AT_1) receptor, which is responsible for the pressor actions of angiotensin II.

Angiotensin II is involved in the renin-angiotensin-aldosterone system, which regulates blood pressure, sodium and water homoeostasis by the kidneys, and cardiovascular function. Angiotensin II stimulates the synthesis and secretion of aldosterone and raises blood pressure via a direct vasoconstrictor effect.

Angiotensin converting enzyme (ACE) is identical to bradykinase, so ACE inhibitors may additionally reduce the degradation of bradykinin and affect enzymes involved in the production of prostaglandins.

Many of the interactions of the ACE inhibitors or angiotensin II receptor antagonists involve drugs that affect blood pressure. Consequently in most cases the result is either an increase in the hypotensive effect (e.g. alcohol) or a decrease in the hypotensive effect (e.g. indometacin).

In addition, due to their effects on aldosterone, the ACE inhibitors and angiotensin II antagonists may increase potassium concentrations and can therefore have additive hyperkalaemic effects with other drugs that cause elevated potassium levels. Furthermore, drugs that affect renal function may potentiate the adverse effects of ACE inhibitors and angiotensin II antagonists on the kidneys.

Most ACE inhibitor and angiotensin II receptor antagonist interactions are pharmacodynamic, that is, interactions result in an alteration in drug effects rather than drug disposition, so in most cases interactions of individual drugs will be applicable to the group.

'Table 2.1', (p.13) lists the ACE inhibitors and the angiotensin II receptor antagonists and some of their proprietary names. Although most of the interactions of the ACE inhibitors or angiotensin II receptor antagonists are covered in this section, if the ACE inhibitor or angiotensin II receptor antagonist is the affecting drug, the interaction is dealt with elsewhere.

Table 2.1 ACE inhibitors and angiotensin II receptor antagonists

Generic names	*Proprietary names*
ACE inhibitors	
Benazepril	Benace, Boncordin, Briem, Cibace, Cibacen, Cibacene, Labopal, Lotensin, Tensanil, Zinadril
Captopril	ACE-Hemmer, Acenorm, Aceomel, Acepress, Acepril, Aceprilex, Aceril, Aceten, Adocor, Alkadil, Alopresin, Antasten, Apo-Capto, Apuzin, Atrisol, Biodezil, Bugazon, Calpix, Capace, Capin, Capostad, Capoten, Capotena, Capotril, Capril, Capti, Captil, Capto, capto-basan, Captobeta, Captodan, Captodoc, Capto-dura M, Captoflux, Captogamma, Captohexal, Captolane, Captol, Captomax, Captomed, Captomerck, Captomin, Capton, Captopiril, Captopress, Captor, Captoser, Captosina, Captosol, Captotec, Captotyrol, Captral, Captrizin, Cardiace, Cardiagen, Cardipril, Carencil, Catona, Catonet, Catoplin, Catoprol, Cesplon, Convertal, cor tensobon, Coronorm, Cryopril, Dardex, Debax, Dexacap, Dilabar, Ductopril, Ecapresan, Ecaten, Ecopace, Epicordin, Epsitron, Ftonavil, Garanil, Gemzil, Geroten, Hipertex, Hipertil, Hipoten, Hipotensil, Huma-Captoril, Hypotensor, Inhibace, Jucapt, Kaplon, Katopil, Kenolan, Keyerpril, Kimafan, Lenpryl, Lopirin, Lopril, Maxipril, Mereprine, Midrat, Mundil, Neo-Ipertas, Normapril, Normolose, Novapres, Novo-Captoril, Nu-Capto, Odupril, Pertacilon, Pressomax, Prilovase, Properil, Reductel, Rilcapton, Romir, Ropril, Sancap, Sigacap Cor, Tenpril, Tensiomin, Tensiomin-Cor, Tensobon, Tensoprel, Tensopril, Tensostad, Topace, Toprilem, Venopril, Vidapril, Zapto
Cilazapril	Dynorm, Inhibace, Inibace, Initiss, Inocar, Justor, Vascace, Vascase
Delapril	Adecut, Cupressin, Delaket, Delakete
Enalapril	Acepril, Acetec, Acetensil, Agioten, Alacor, Alapren, Alapril, Alphapril, Amprace, Analept, Anapril, Angiopril, Antiprex, Atens, Auspril, Bajaten, Balpril, Baripril, Benalapril, Berlipril, Bionafil, Bitensil, Blocatril, BQL, Cetampril, Ciplatec, Clipto, Controlvas, Converten, Convertin, Corodil, Corprilor, Corvo, Crinoren, Dabonal, Danssan, Defluin, Denapril, Dilvas, Ditensor, Ecaprilat, E-Cor, Ednyt, Elpradil, Ena, ena-basan, Enabeta, Enac, EnAce, Enacodan, enadura, Enahexal, Enalabal, Enalabell, Enaladex, Enaladil, Enalafel, Enalagamma, Enalamed, Enaldun, EnaLich, Enalind, Enaloc, Enalprin, Enalten, Enam, Enap, Enapirex, Enapren, Enapril, Enaprotec, Ena-Puren, Enaran, Enarenal, Enaril, Enasifar, Enatec, Enatral, Enatrial, Enatyrol, Enoval, Envas, Epril, Erxetilan, Esalfon, Eupressin, Feliberal, Gadopril, Glioten, Gnostocardin, Grifopril, Herten, Hiperson, Hipertin, Hipoartel, Hipten, Iecatec, Iecatec , Imotoran, Innovace, Insup, Invoril, Istopril, Jutaxan, Kaparlon-S, Kenopril, Kinfil, Kontic, Korandil, Lapril, Leovinezal, Linatil, Lipraken, Lotrial, Lowpress, Malen, Megapress, Mepril, Nacor, Nalapril, Nalaprix, Nalopril, Naprilene, Narapril, Naritec, Neolapril, Neotensin, Norpril, Nuril, Octorax, Ofnifenil, Palane, Pharmapress, Pres, Presi Regul, Pressitan, Pressotec, Prilan, Priltenk, Protal, Pulsol, Quimalan, Rablas, Reca, Renalapril, Renipress, Renipril, Renistad, Renitec, Reniten, Sanvapress, Stadelant, Sulocten, Supotron, Tensazol, Ulticadex, Vapresan, Vasocor, Vasolat, Vasopren, Vasopril, Vasotec, Virfen, Vitobel, Xanef
Fosinopril	Dynacil, Eliten, Fosinil, Fosinorm, Fosipres, Fositen, Fositens, Fovas, Fozitec, Hiperlex, Monopril, NewAce, Sinopril, Staril, Tenso Stop, Tensocardil, Tensogard, Vasopril
Imidapril	Cardipril, Hipertene, Tanatril
Lisinopril	Acemin, Acepril, Acerbon, Acerdil, Acetan, Adicanil, Alapril, Alfaken, Axelvin, Biopril, Carace, Cipril, Conpres, Coric, Dapril, Diroton, Doneka, Doxapril, Ecapril, Farpresse, Fibsol, Gnostoval, Icoran, Iricil, Irumed, Lanatin, Landolaxin, Leruze, Likenil, Linoril, Linvas, Liprace, Lipreren, Lipril, Lisdene, Lisdene, Lisi, Lisi Lich, Lisibeta, Lisigamma, Lisihexal, Lisinal, Lisinobell, Lisinogen, Lisinospes, Lisinostad, Lisinotyrol, Lisipril, Lisi-Puren, Lisitril, Lisodur, Lisodura, Lisopress, Lisopril, Lisoril, Lispril, Listril, Nafordyl, Normopril, Novatec, Perenal, Presokin, Press-12, Pressuril, Prilosin, Prinil, Prinivil, Ranopril, Renotens, Secubar, Sedotensil, Sinopren, Sinopril, Tensikey, Tensopril, Tensopril, Terolinal, Tersif, Thriusedon, Tivirlon, Tonotensil, Vasojet, Vercol, Veroxil, Vivatec, Z-Bec, Zesger, Zestan, Zestril, Zetomax, Zinopril
Moexipril	Femipres, Fempress, Moex, Perdix, Tensotec, Univasc
Pentopril	
Perindopril	Aceon, Acertil, Coverene, Coverex, Coversum, Coversyl, Noliprel, Perigard, Prestarium, Prexum, Procaptan
Quinapril	Accupril, Accuprin, Accupro, Accupron, Acequin, Acuitel, Acuprel, Acupril, Acuretic, Asig, Conan, Ectren, Korec, Lidaltrin, Quinazil, Quinil, Vasocor
Ramipril	Acovil, Altace, Carasel, Cardace, Corpril, Delix, Hopecard, Hypren, Lostapres, Naprix, Pramace, Preface, Quark, Ramace, Ramcor, Ramipres, Remik, R-Pril, Stiebenyl, Triatec, Tritace, Unipril, Vesdil
Spirapril	Cardiopril, Quadropril, Renormax, Renpress, Setrilan
Temocapril	Acecol
Trandolapril	Afenil, Gopten, Mavik, Odric, Odrik, Preran, Udrik
Angiotensin II receptor antagonists	
Candesartan	Amias, Atacand, Bilaten, Blopress, Blox, Candesar, Dacten, Kenzen, Parapres, Ratacand, Tiadyl
Eprosartan	Epratenz, Futuran, Navixen, Regulaten, Teveten, Tevetens, Tevetenz
Irbesartan	Aprovel, Avapro, Irban, Irovel, Karvea
Losartan	Alsartan, Aradois, Aratan, Cartan, Corodin, Corus, Cosaar, Covance, Cozaar, Cozaarex, Enromic, Klosartan, Loctenk, Loortan, Lorista, Lorsacor, Lortaan, Lorzaar, Losacar, Losacor, Losanorm, Losapres, Losaprex, Losartec, Losatal, Lozap, Lozitan, Neo-Lotan, Niten, Nu-Lotan, Ocsaar, Paxon, Prelertan, Redupress, Sanipresin, Simperten, Tacardia, Tenopres, Zart
Olmesartan	Alteis, Benetor, Benicar, Olmes, Olmetec, Omesar, Votum
Tasosartan	
Telmisartan	Gliosartan, Kinzal, Kinzalmono, Micardis, Pritor, Pritoral, Samertan, Telma
Valsartan	Angiosan, Dalzad, Diovan, Diovane, Kalpress, Miten, Nisis, Provas, Redutensil, Sarton, Starval, Tareg, Valpression, Vals, Varexan, Vartalan

ACE inhibitors + Albumin-containing plasma protein solution

Acute hypotension has been seen in patients taking enalapril when rapidly infused with albumin-containing stable plasma protein solution (SPPS). Captopril appears to interact similarly.

Clinical evidence

A woman on **enalapril** 10 mg in the morning, underwent surgery for groin lymph node resection under spinal and general anaesthesia. When rapidly infused with 500 ml of the albumin solution, **stable plasma protein solution (SPPS,** *Commonwealth Serum Laboratories, Melbourne, Australia*), her pulse rose to 90 to 100 bpm and systolic blood pressure fell from 100 to 60 mmHg and a red flush was noted on all exposed skin. The blood pressure was controlled at 90 to 95 mmHg with metaraminol 4.5 mg, given over 10 minutes. When the **SPPS** was finished, the blood pressure and pulse rate spontaneously restabilised.[1]

Two very similar cases have been recorded in patients on **enalapril** when given **SPPS**.[2,3] The maker of **SPPS** notes that **captopril** has also been involved in this hypotensive interaction.[4]

Mechanism

Not fully established, but it is believed that SPPS contains low levels of pre-kallikrein activator, which stimulates the production of bradykinin, which can cause vasodilatation and hypotension. Normally the bradykinin is destroyed by kininase II (ACE), but this is delayed by the ACE inhibitor so that the hypotensive effects are exaggerated and prolonged.[3,5]

Importance and management

An established interaction of clinical importance. Other ACE inhibitors would be expected to interact similarly. The author of one report suggested that if rapid expansion of intravascular volume is needed in patients taking ACE inhibitors, an artificial colloid might be a safer choice than SPPS.[1] The maker of SPPS also recommended using an alternative plasma volume expander, including other albumin solutions.[4] It should be noted that following these reports SPPS was withdrawn from the Australasian market.[6]

1. McKenzie AJ. Possible interaction between SPPS and enalapril. *Anaesth Intensive Care* (1990) 18, 124–6.
2. Young K. Enalapril and SPPS. *Anaesth Intensive Care* (1990) 18, 583.
3. Young K. Hypotension from the interaction of ACE inhibitors with stable plasma protein solution. *Anaesthesia* (1993) 48, 356.
4. Schiff P. SPPS, hypotension and ACE inhibitors. *Med J Aust* (1992) 156, 363.
5. Bönner G, Preis S, Schunk U, Toussaint C, Kaufmann W. Hemodynamic effects of bradykinin on systemic and pulmonary circulation in healthy and hypertensive humans. *J Cardiovasc Pharmacol* (1990) 15 (Suppl 6), S46–S56.
6. McKenzie AJ. ACE inhibitors, colloid infusions and anaesthesia. *Anaesth Intensive Care* (1998) 26, 330.

ACE inhibitors + Allopurinol

Three cases of Stevens-Johnson syndrome (one fatal) and two cases of hypersensitivity have been attributed to the use of captopril with allopurinol. Anaphylaxis and myocardial infarction occurred in one man on enalapril when given allopurinol. The combination of ACE inhibitors and allopurinol may increase the risk of leucopenia and serious infection.

Clinical evidence

An elderly man with hypertension, chronic renal failure, congestive heart failure and mild polyarthritis on multiple drug treatment, which included **captopril** 25 mg twice daily and diuretics, developed fatal Stevens-Johnson syndrome about 5 weeks after starting to take allopurinol 100 mg twice daily.[1] The authors of the report noted that the maker of **captopril** was aware of 2 other patients who developed the syndrome 3 to 5 weeks after allopurinol was started.[1] Another report describes fever, arthralgia and myalgia in a diabetic man with chronic renal failure who was similarly treated. He improved when the **captopril** was withdrawn.[2] Exfoliatory facial dermatitis occurred in another patient with renal failure who was taking **captopril** and allopurinol.[3] A man on **enalapril** had an acute anaphylactic reaction with severe coronary spasm, culminating in myocardial infarction, within 20 minutes of taking allopurinol 100 mg. He recovered and continued to take **enalapril** without allopurinol.[4]

The maker of **captopril** also warns that neutropenia/agranulocytosis, resulting in serious infection, has occurred in patients on **captopril** and other ACE inhibitors, and that concurrent treatment with allopurinol may be a complicating factor, especially in those with renal impairment.[5]

No significant pharmacokinetic changes were seen in 12 healthy subjects given allopurinol and **captopril** alone and in combination.[6]

Mechanism

Not understood. It is uncertain whether these are interactions because allopurinol alone can cause severe hypersensitivity reactions, particularly in the presence of renal failure and in conjunction with diuretic use. Captopril can also induce a hypersensitivity reaction.

Importance and management

These interactions are not clearly established, and the reaction appears to be rare and unpredictable. All that can be constructively said is that patients on both drugs should be very closely monitored for any signs of hypersensitivity (e.g. skin reactions) or low white cell count (sore throat, fever), especially if they have renal impairment. The maker of captopril recommends that differential white blood cell counts should be performed before combined therapy with allopurinol, then every 2 weeks during the first 3 months of therapy, and periodically thereafter.[5] The makers of several other ACE inhibitors also state in their prescribing information that concomitant administration of ACE inhibitors and allopurinol may lead to an increased risk of leucopenia. For other interactions with ACE inhibitors that result in leucopenia see also 'ACE inhibitors + Azathioprine', p.18 and 'ACE inhibitors + Procainamide', p.30.

1. Pennell DJ, Nunan TO, O'Doherty MJ, Croft DN. Fatal Stevens-Johnson syndrome in a patient on captopril and allopurinol. *Lancet* (1984) i, 463.
2. Samanta A, Burden AC. Fever, myalgia, and arthralgia in a patient on captopril and allopurinol. *Lancet* (1984) i, 679.
3. Beeley L, Daly M, Stewart P. *Bulletin of the West Midlands Centre for Adverse Drug Reaction Reporting* (1987) 24, 9.
4. Ahmad S. Allopurinol and enalapril. Drug induced anaphylactic coronary spasm and acute myocardial infarction. *Chest* (1995) 108, 586.
5. Capoten (Captopril). E. R. Squibb & Sons Ltd. UK Summary of product characteristics, February 2003.
6. Duchin KL, McKinstry DN, Cohen AI, Migdalof BH. Pharmacokinetics of captopril in healthy subjects and in patients with cardiovascular diseases. *Clin Pharmacokinet* (1988) 14, 241–59.

ACE inhibitors + Antacids

Antacids are said to reduce the bioavailability of a number of ACE inhibitors but this seems unlikely to be clinically important. The bioavailability of fosinopril is reduced by about one third by *Mylanta*.

Clinical evidence, mechanism, importance and management

An antacid containing **aluminium/magnesium hydroxide** and **magnesium carbonate** reduced the AUC of a single 50-mg dose of **captopril** in 10 healthy subjects by about 40% compared with the fasting state. However, this did not alter the extent of the reduction in blood pressure.[1] Another study found that ***Mylanta*** [probably containing **aluminium/magnesium hydroxide**] similarly reduced the bioavailability of **fosinopril** 20 mg by about one-third.[2] The mechanism of this interaction is uncertain, but is unlikely to be due to elevated gastric pH since cimetidine did not have a similar effect.[2] Note that greater decreases in **captopril** bioavailability (caused by food) were found not to be clinically relevant (see 'ACE inhibitors + Food', p.24), therefore, it is unlikely these changes will be clinically important. However, the makers of **fosinopril** suggest[3,4] separating administration of **fosinopril** and antacids by at least 2 hours. Several other makers of ACE inhibitors also warn that antacids may reduce the bioavailability of ACE inhibitors, quite possibly based on the way these named ACE inhibitors interact, but there seems to be no evidence of a clinically significant interaction in practice. It is briefly noted in a review that **antacid** administration did not affect the pharmacokinetics of ramiprilat, the active metabolite of **ramipril**.[5]

1. Mäntylä R, Männistö PT, Vuorela A, Sundberg S, Ottoila P. Impairment of captopril bioavailability by concomitant food and antacid intake. *Int J Clin Pharmacol Ther Toxicol* (1984) 22, 626–9.
2. Moore L, Kramer A, Swites B, Kramer P, Tu J. Effect of cimetidine and antacid on the kinetics of the active diacid of fosinopril in healthy subjects. *J Clin Pharmacol* (1988) 28, 946.

3. Staril (Fosinopril), E. R. Squibb & Sons Ltd. UK Summary of product characteristics, June 2005.
4. Monopril (Fosinopril). Bristol-Myers Squibb Company. US Prescribing information, July 2003.
5. Todd PA, Benfield P. Ramipril. A review of its pharmacological properties and therapeutic efficacy in cardiovascular disorders. *Drugs* (1990) 39, 110–35.

ACE inhibitors + Antipsychotics

Marked postural hypotension occurred in a patient given chlorpromazine and captopril. The hypotensive adverse effects of antipsychotics such as the phenothiazines may be additive with the effects of ACE inhibitors.

Clinical evidence, mechanism, importance and management

A patient fainted and developed marked postural hypotension (standing blood pressure 66/48 mmHg) when given **captopril** 6.25 mg twice daily and **chlorpromazine** 200 mg three times daily. He had previously taken **chlorpromazine** with nadolol, prazosin and hydrochlorothiazide without any problems, although his blood pressure was poorly controlled on this therapy. Since the patient's blood pressure was quite elevated when on **chlorpromazine** or **captopril** alone, there appeared to be a synergistic hypotensive effect between the two drugs.[1]

The makers of several ACE inhibitors warn that ACE inhibitors may enhance the hypotensive effects of certain antipsychotics, and that postural hypotension may occur. Some of these warnings are based, not unreasonably, on the adverse reactions seen with other ACE inhibitors or antihypertensives, but not necessarily on direct observations.[2] Warn patients to lay down and elevate their legs if they feel faint or dizzy, and to get up slowly. Dosage adjustments may be necessary to accommodate this interaction.

1. White WB. Hypotension with postural syncope secondary to the combination of chlorpromazine and captopril. *Arch Intern Med* (1986) 146, 1833–4.
2. Knoll Ltd. Personal communication,1993.

ACE inhibitors + Aprotinin

Aprotinin suppressed the hypotensive action of captopril and enalapril in *rats*.

Clinical evidence, mechanism, importance and management

A study in spontaneously hypertensive *rats* found aprotinin suppressed the hypotensive responses of **captopril** and **enalapril**.[1] Aprotinin is a proteolytic enzyme inhibitor that has many actions including antagonism of the kallikrein-kinin system, which in turn affects bradykinins and renin. It would therefore be expected to have complex interactions with the ACE inhibitors,[2] which also affect these proteins.

1. Sharma JN, Amrah SS, Noor AR. Suppression of hypotensive responses of captopril and enalapril by the kallikrein inhibitor aprotinin in spontaneously hypertensive rats. *Pharmacology* (1995) 50, 363–9.
2. Waxler B, Rabito SF. Aprotinin: a serine protease inhibitor with therapeutic actions: its interaction with ACE inhibitors. *Curr Pharm Des* (2003) 9, 777–87.

ACE inhibitors + Aspirin

The antihypertensive efficacy of captopril and enalapril may be reduced by high-dose aspirin in about 50% of patients. Low-dose aspirin (less than or equal to 100 mg daily) appears to have little effect. It is unclear whether aspirin attenuates the benefits of ACE inhibitors in coronary artery disease and heart failure. The likelihood of an interaction may depend on disease state. Renal failure has been reported in a patient taking captopril and aspirin.

Clinical evidence

(A) Effects on blood pressure

(a) Captopril

Aspirin 600 mg six-hourly for 5 doses did not significantly alter the blood pressure response to a single 25 to 100-mg dose of captopril in 8 patients with essential hypertension. However, the prostaglandin response to captopril was only blocked in 4 of the 8, and in these patients the blood pressure response to captopril was blunted.[1] In another study, aspirin 75 mg daily did not alter the antihypertensive effects of captopril 25 mg twice daily in 15 patients with hypertension.[2]

(b) Enalapril

Two groups of 26 patients, one with mild to moderate hypertension on enalapril 20 mg twice daily and the other with severe primary hypertension on enalapril 20 mg twice daily (plus nifedipine 30 mg and atenolol 50 mg daily), were additionally given test doses of aspirin 100 and 300 mg daily for 5 days. The 100-mg dose of aspirin did not alter the efficacy of the antihypertensive drugs, but the 300-mg dose reduced the antihypertensive efficacy in about half the patients in both groups. In these patients, the antihypertensive effects were diminished by 63% in those with mild to moderate hypertension and by 91% in those with severe hypertension.[3] In contrast, another study in 7 patients with hypertension taking enalapril (mean daily dose 12.9 mg) found that aspirin 81 mg or 325 mg daily for 2 weeks did not have any significant effect on blood pressure.[4] A further study also found that aspirin 100 mg daily for 2 weeks did not alter the antihypertensive effect of enalapril 20 or 40 mg daily in 18 patients.[5]

(B) Effects in coronary artery disease and heart failure

Various studies have looked at the short-term effects of the combination of ACE inhibitors and aspirin on haemodynamic parameters. In one study in 40 patients with decompensated heart failure, aspirin 300 mg given on the first day and 100 mg daily thereafter antagonised the short-term haemodynamic effects of **captopril** 50 mg given every 8 hours for 4 days. It was found that aspirin antagonised the short-term haemodynamic effects of **captopril** (the **captopril**-induced increase in cardiac index and the reduction in peripheral vascular resistance and pulmonary wedge pressure were all abolished).[6] Another study, in 15 patients with chronic heart failure receiving treatment with ACE inhibitors (mainly **enalapril** 10 mg twice daily), demonstrated that aspirin in doses as low as 75 mg impaired vasodilatation induced by arachidonic acid.[7] In yet another study, aspirin 325 mg daily worsened pulmonary diffusion capacity and made the ventilatory response to exercise less effective in patients taking **enalapril** 10 mg twice daily, but did not exert this effect in the absence of ACE inhibitors.[8] However, results from studies are inconsistent. In a review,[9] five of 7 studies reported aspirin did not alter the haemodynamic effects of ACE inhibitors whereas the remaining two did. In one of these studies showing an adverse interaction between aspirin and **enalapril**, **ticlopidine** did not interact with **enalapril**.[10]

A retrospective study involving 576 patients with heart failure requiring hospitalisation, showed a trend towards an increased incidence of early re-admissions (within 30 days after discharge) for heart failure among subjects treated with ACE inhibitors and aspirin compared with those treated with ACE inhibitors without aspirin (16% vs 10%). In patients without coronary artery disease the increase in readmissions was statistically significant (23% vs 10%).[11] However, long-term survival in heart failure was not affected by the use of aspirin with ACE inhibitors. Furthermore, among patients with coronary artery disease there was a trend towards improvement in mortality in patients treated with the combination compared with ACE inhibitor without aspirin (40% vs 56%).[12] Similarly, a lack of adverse interaction was found in a retrospective study involving 14 129 elderly patients who survived a hospitalisation for acute myocardial infarction. However, the added benefit of the combination over patients who received either aspirin or ACE inhibitors alone was not statistically significant.[13]

A number of large trials have used ACE inhibitors with aspirin. There have been sub-group analyses or retrospective reviews of these trials to examine the potential interaction. The results are summarised in 'Table 2.2', (p.16). However, the trials vary in the initiation and duration of aspirin/ACE inhibitor treatment and the length of follow-up, the degree of heart failure/ischaemia and the prognosis of the patients, and the final end point (whether compared with placebo or with the benefits of aspirin or ACE inhibitors). The conclusions are, therefore, conflicting and an editorial[14] disputes the findings of one of these studies.[15]

(C) Effects on renal function

Acute renal failure developed in a woman on **captopril** when she started to take aspirin for arthritis. Renal function improved when both were stopped.[16]

(D) Pharmacokinetic studies

A single-dose study in 12 healthy subjects found that the pharmacokinetics of **benazepril** 20 mg and aspirin 325 mg were not affected by concurrent use.[17]

Table 2.2 Sub-group analyses of clinical trials assessing the interaction between aspirin and ACE inhibitors

Trial and patients	*Aspirin dose*	*ACE inhibitor*	*Follow-up*	*Finding*	*Refs*
Evidence of an interaction					
SOLVD 6512 patients treated for heart failure or prevention of heart failure	Not reported	Enalapril	37 to 41 months	Combined treatment associated with reduced benefits compared with enalapril alone.	1
CONSENSUS II 6090 patients with acute MI	Not reported	Enalapril	6 months	Effect of enalapril less favourable in those taking aspirin at baseline.	2
GUSTO-I 31 622 post-MI patients without heart failure	Not reported	Not reported	11 months (starting 30 days post MI)	Combined use associated with higher mortality than aspirin alone (mortality rates 3.3 vs 1.6%).	3
EPILOG 2619 patients undergoing coronary angioplasty	325 mg daily	Not reported	12 months	Combined use associated with higher mortality than aspirin alone (mortality rates 3.7 vs 1.2%).	3
AIRE 1986 patients after acute MI, with heart failure	Not reported	Ramipril 2.5 to 5 mg twice daily started 3 to 10 days after MI	15 months (average)	Trend towards greater benefit of ramipril in those not receiving aspirin.	4
No evidence of an interaction					
BIP Secondary prevention of MI in 1197 patients with coronary artery disease	250 mg daily	Captopril or Enalapril	5 years (average)	Lower death rate in those on combined therapy than those on ACE inhibitor alone (19 vs 27%).	5
SAVE 2231 patients with left ventricular dysfunction after MI	Not reported	Captopril 75 to 150 mg daily	42 months (average)	Trend towards greater benefits of captopril when taken with aspirin.	6
HOPE Prevention of cardiovascular events in 9297 patients without left ventricular dysfunction or heart failure	Not reported	Ramipril 10 mg daily	About 4.5 years	Benefits of ramipril not affected by aspirin.	7
CATS Early treatment of acute MI in 298 patients	80 to 100 mg daily	Captopril	1 year	Benefits of captopril not affected by aspirin. Better prognosis in those on aspirin.	8
ISIS-4 Early treatment of acute MI in 58 050 patients	Not reported	Captopril 100 mg daily	At 5 weeks and 1 year	Benefits of captopril not affected by aspirin.	9
Meta analysis of AIRE, SAVE, SOLVD and TRACE 12 763 patients with left ventricular dysfunction or heart failure with or without MI	Not reported	Captopril, enalapril, ramipril, trandolapril	35 months (average)	Benefits of ACE inhibitors observed even if aspirin given.	10
Meta analysis of CCS-1, CONSENSUS II, GISSI-3, and ISIS-4 Early treatment of MI in 96 712 patients	160 to 325 mg daily	Captopril, enalapril, lisinopril	30 days	ACE inhibitor reduced 30-day mortality from 15.1 to 13.8%. Ace inhibitor plus aspirin reduced 30-day mortality from 6.7 to 6.3%.	11
TRACE 1749 patients with left ventricular dysfunction after acute MI	Not reported	Trandolapril 1 to 4 mg daily	24 to 50 months	Trend towards greater benefit of trandolapril in those receiving aspirin (mortality of 45% with ACE inhibitor, and 34% with ACE inhibitor plus aspirin.	12
SMILE 1556 patients with acute MI	Not reported	Zofenopril 7.5 mg increasing to 30 mg twice daily for 6 weeks	At 6 weeks and 1 year	Benefits of zofenopril not significantly affected by aspirin.	13
HOPE 22 060 patients with left ventricular dysfunction or heart failure without MI or coronary artery disease without left ventricular dysfunction acute MI	Not reported	Captopril, enalapril, ramipril, trandolapril	More than 3 years	Benefits of ACE inhibitors observed even if aspirin given.	14

1. Al-Khadra AS, Salem DN, Rand WM, Udelson JE, Smith JJ, Konstam MA. Antiplatelet agents and survival: a cohort analysis from the Studies of Left Ventricular Dysfunction (SOLVD) trial. *J Am Coll Cardiol* (1998) 31, 419–25.
2. Nguyen KN, Aursnes I, Kjekshus J. Interaction between enalapril and aspirin on mortality after acute myocardial infarction: subgroup analysis of the Cooperative New Scandanavian Enalapril Survival Study II (CONSENSUS II). *Am J Cardiol* (1997) 79, 115–19.
3. Peterson JG, Topol EJ, Sapp SK, Young JB, Lincoff AM, Lauer MS. Evaluation of the effects of aspirin combined with angiotensin-converting enzyme inhibitors in patients with coronary artery disease. *Am J Med* (2000) 109, 371–7.
4. The Acute Infarction Ramipril Efficacy (AIRE) Study Investigators. Effect of ramipril on mortality and morbidity of survivors of acute myocardial infarction with clinical evidence of heart failure. *Lancet* (1993) 342, 821–8.

Table 2.2 Sub-group analyses of clinical trials assessing the interaction between aspirin and ACE inhibitors *(continued)*

5. Leor J, Reicher-Reiss H, Goldbourt U, Boyko V, Gottlieb S, Battler A, Behar S. Aspirin and mortality in patients treated with angiotensin-converting enzyme inhibitors. A cohort study of 11,575 patients with coronary artery disease. *J Am Coll Cardiol* (1999) 33, 1920–5.
6. Pfeffer MA, Braunwald E, Moyé LA, Basta L, Brown EJ, Cuddy TE, Davis BR, Geltman EM, Goldman S, Flaker GC, Klein M, Lamas GA, Packer M, Rouleau J, Rouleau JL, Rutherford J, Wertheimer JH, Hawkins CM, on behalf of the SAVE Investigators. Effect of captopril on mortality and morbidity in patients with left ventricular dysfunction after myocardial infarction. Results of the survival and ventricular enlargement trial. *N Engl J Med* (1992) 327, 669–77.
7. The Heart Outcomes Prevention Evaluation Study Investigators. Effect of an angiotensin-converting-enzyme inhibitor, ramipril, on cardiovascular events in high-risk patients. *N Engl J Med* (2000) 342, 145–53.
8. Oosterga M, Anthonio RL, de Kam PJ, Kingma JH, Crijns HJ, van Gilst WH. Effects of aspirin on angiotensin-converting enzyme inhibition and left ventricular dilation one year after myocardial infarction. *Am J Cardiol* (1998) 81, 1178–81.
9. ISIS-4 (Fourth International Study of Infarct Survival) Collaborative Group. ISIS-4: a randomised factorial trial assessing early oral captopril, oral mononitrate, and intravenous magnesium sulphate in 58,050 patients with suspected acute myocardial infarction. *Lancet* (1995) 345; 669–85.
10. Flather MD, Yusuf S, Køber L, Pfeffer M, Hall A, Murray G, Trop-Pedersen C, Ball S, Pogue J, Moyé L, Braunwald, for the ACE-inhibitor Myocardial Infarction Collaborative. Long-term ACE-inhibitor therapy in patients with heart failure or left-ventricular dysfunction: a systematic overview of data from individual patients. *Lancet* (2000) 335, 1575–81.
11. Latini R, Tognoni G, Maggioni AP, Baigent C, Braunwald E, Chen Z-M, Collins R, Flather M, Franzosi MG, Kjekshus J, Køber L, Liu L-S, Peto R, Pfeffer M, Pizzetti F, Santoro E, Sleight P, Swedberg K, Tavazzi L, Wang W, Yusuf S. Clinical effects of early angiotensin-converting enzyme inhibitor treatment for myocardial infarction are similar in the presence and absence of aspirin. *J Am Coll Cardiol* (2000) 35 1801–7.
12. Køber L, Torp-Pedersen C, Carlsen JE, Bagger H, Eliasen P, Lyngborg K, Videbæk J, Cole DS, Auclert L, Pauly NC, Aliot E, Persson S, Camm AJ, for the Trandolapril Cardiac Evaluation (TRACE) Study Group. A clinical trial of the angiotensin-converting-enzyme inhibitor trandolapril in patients with left ventricular dysfunction after myocardial infarction. *N Engl J Med* (1995) 333, 1670–6.
13. Ambrosioni E, Borghi C, Magnani B, for the Survival of Myocardial Infarction Long-Term Evaluation (SMILE) Study Investigators. The effect of the angiotensin-converting-enzyme inhibitor zofenopril on mortality and morbidity after anterior myocardial infarction. *New Engl J Med* (1995) 332, 80–5.
14. Teo KK, Yusuf S, Pfeffer M, Kober L, Hall A, Pogue J, Latini R, Collins R, for the ACE Inhibitors Collaborative Group. Effects of long-term treatment with angiotensin-converting-enzyme inhibitors in the presence or absence of aspirin: a systematic review. *Lancet* (2002) 360, 1037–43.

Mechanism

(A). Some, but not all the evidence suggests that prostaglandins may be involved in the hypotensive action of ACE inhibitors, and that aspirin, by inhibiting prostaglandin synthesis, may partially antagonise the effect of ACE inhibitors. This effect appears to depend on the dose of aspirin and may also be dependent on sodium status and plasma renin, therefore it does not occur in all patients.

(B). Uncertain. The beneficial effects of ACE inhibitors in heart failure and ischaemic heart disease are thought to be due, in part, to the inhibition of the breakdown of kinins, which are important regulators of prostaglandin and nitric oxide synthesis. Such inhibition promotes vasodilatation and afterload reduction. Aspirin may block these beneficial effects by inhibiting cyclo-oxygenase (COX) and thus prostaglandin synthesis, causing vasoconstriction, decreased cardiac output and worsening heart failure.[9,18]

Importance and management

(A). Low-dose aspirin (less than or equal to 100 mg daily) does not alter the antihypertensive efficacy of captopril and enalapril. No special precautions would therefore seem to be required with ACE inhibitors and these low doses of aspirin. A high dose of aspirin (2.4 g daily) has been reported to interact in 50% of patients in a single study. Aspirin 300 mg daily has been reported to interact in about 50% of patients in another study, whereas 325 mg daily did not interact in further study. Thus, at present, it appears that if an ACE inhibitor is used with aspirin in doses higher than 300 mg daily, blood pressure should be monitored more closely, and the ACE inhibitor dosage raised if necessary. Intermittent use of aspirin should be considered as a possible cause of erratic control of blood pressure in patients on ACE inhibitors.

(B). Both ACE inhibitors and aspirin are used in coronary artery disease and heart failure, and the information about a possible interaction is conflicting. This may be due to much of the clinical data being obtained from retrospective non-randomised analyses.[18] It may also be a factor of different disease states. For example, an interaction may be less likely to be experienced in patients with heart failure of ischaemic aetiology than those with non-ischaemic causes, because of the added benefits of aspirin in ischaemic heart disease.[19] The available data, and its implications, have been extensively reviewed.[9,14,18-23] Some commentators have advised that, if possible, aspirin should be avoided in patients requiring long-term treatment for heart failure, particularly if heart failure is severe.[14,21] Others suggest avoiding aspirin in heart failure unless there are clear indications such as atherosclerosis.[9,18,22,23] The use of lower doses of aspirin (80 to 100 mg daily rather than greater than or equal to 325 mg daily) in those with heart failure on ACE inhibitors has also been suggested.[19,20,22] Conversely, an advisory council in the USA[24] has stated that, "Many physicians believe that the data supporting the existence of an adverse interaction between aspirin and ACE inhibitors are not sufficiently compelling to justify altering the current practice of prescribing the two agents together." Others are in general agreement with this.[19,25] Data from ongoing randomised trials may provide further insight. Until these are available, combined low-dose aspirin and ACE inhibitors may continue to be used where there is a clear indication for both.

(C). An increased risk of deterioration in renal function or acute renal failure appears to occur rarely with the combination of aspirin and ACE inhibitors. The routine monitoring of renal function, which is advised with ACE inhibitors, should be sufficient to detect any interaction.

1. Moore TJ, Crantz FR, Hollenberg NK, Koletsky RJ, Leboff MS, Swartz SL, Levine L, Podolsky S, Dluhy RG, Williams GH. Contribution of prostaglandins to the antihypertensive action of captopril in essential hypertension. *Hypertension* (1981) 3, 168–73.
2. Smith SR, Coffman TM, Svetkey LP. Effect of low-dose aspirin on thromboxane production and the antihypertensive effect of captopril. *J Am Soc Nephrol* (1993) 4, 1133–9.
3. Guazzi MD, Campodonico J, Celeste F, Guazzi M, Santambrogio G, Rossi M, Trabattoni D, Alimento M. Antihypertensive efficacy of angiotensin converting enzyme inhibition and aspirin counteraction. *Clin Pharmacol Ther* (1998) 63, 79–86.
4. Nawarskas JJ, Townsend RR, Cirigliano MD, Spinler SA. Effect of aspirin on blood pressure in hypertensive patients taking enalapril or losartan. *Am J Hypertens* (1999) 12, 784–9.
5. Polónia J, Boaventura I, Gama G, Camões I, Bernardo F, Andrade P, Nunes JP, Brandão F, Cerqueira-Gomes M. Influence of non-steroidal anti-inflammatory drugs on renal function and 24 h ambulatory blood pressure-reducing effects of enalapril and nifedipine gastrointestinal therapeutic system in hypertensive patients. *J Hypertens* (1995) 13, 925–31.
6. Viecili PR, Pamplona D, Park M, Silva SR, Ramires JAF, da Luz PL. Antagonism of the acute hemodynamic effects of captopril in decompensated congestive heart failure by aspirin administration. *Braz J Med Biol Res* (2003) 36, 771–80.
7. Davie AP, Love MP, McMurray JJV. Even low-dose aspirin inhibits arachidonic acid-induced vasodilation in heart failure. *Clin Pharmacol Ther* (2000) 67, 530–7.
8. Guazzi M, Pontone G, Agostoni P. Aspirin worsens exercise performance and pulmonary gas exchange in patients with heart failure who are taking angiotensin-converting enzyme inhibitors. *Am Heart J* (1999) 138, 254–60.
9. Mahé I, Meune C, Diemer M, Caulin C, Bergmann J-F. Interaction between aspirin and ACE inhibitors in patients with heart failure. *Drug Safety* (2001) 24, 167–82.
10. Spaulding C, Charbonnier B, Cohen-Solal A, Juillière Y, Kromer EP, Benhamda K, Cador R, Weber S. Acute hemodynamic interaction of aspirin and ticlopidine with enalapril. Results of a double-blind, randomized comparative trial. *Circulation* (1998) 98, 757–65.
11. Harjai KJ, Nunez E, Turgut T, Newman J. Effect of combined aspirin and angiotensin-converting enzyme inhibitor therapy versus angiotensin-converting enzyme inhibitor therapy alone on readmission rates in heart failure. *Am J Cardiol* (2001) 87, 483–7.
12. Harjai KJ, Solis S, Prasad A, Loupe J. Use of aspirin in conjunction with angiotensin-converting enzyme inhibitors does not worsen long-term survival in heart failure. *Int J Cardiol* (2003) 88, 207–14.
13. Krumholz HM, Chen Y-T, Wang Y, Radford MJ. Aspirin and angiotensin-converting enzyme inhibitors among elderly survivors of hospitalization for an acute myocardial infarction. *Arch Intern Med* (2001) 161, 538–44.
14. Hall D. The aspirin—angiotensin-converting enzyme inhibitor tradeoff: to halve and halve not. *J Am Coll Cardiol* (2000) 35, 1808–12.
15. Latini R, Tognoni G, Maggioni AP, Baigent C, Braunwald E, Chen Z-M, Collins R, Flather M, Franzosi MG, Kjekshus J, Køber L, Liu L-S, Peto R, Pfeffer M, Pizzetti F, Santoro E, Sleight P, Swedberg K, Tavazzi L, Wang W, Yusuf S, on behalf of the Angiotensin-converting Enzyme Inhibitor Myocardial Infarction Collaborative Group. Clinical effects of early angiotensin-converting enzyme inhibitor treatment for acute myocardial infarction are similar in the presence and absence of aspirin. Systematic overview of individual data from 96,712 randomized patients. *J Am Coll Cardiol* (2000) 35 1801–7.

16. Seelig CB, Maloley PA, Campbell JR. Nephrotoxicity associated with concomitant ACE inhibitor and NSAID therapy. *South Med J* (1990) 83, 1144–8.
17. Sioufi A, Pommier F, Gauducheau N, Godbillon J, Choi L, John V. The absence of a pharmacokinetic interaction between aspirin and the angiotensin-converting enzyme inhibitor benazepril in healthy volunteers. *Biopharm Drug Dispos* (1994) 15, 451–61.
18. Massie BM, Teerlink JR. Interaction between aspirin and angiotensin-converting enzyme inhibitors: real or imagined. *Am J Med* (2000) 109, 431–3.
19. Nawarskas JJ, Spinler SA. Update on the interaction between aspirin and angiotensin-converting enzyme inhibitors. *Pharmacotherapy* (2000) 20, 698–710.
20. Stys T, Lawson WE, Smaldone GC, Stys A. Does aspirin attenuate the beneficial effects of angiotensin-converting enzyme inhibition in heart failure? *Arch Intern Med* (2000) 160, 1409–13.
21. Cleland JGF, John J, Houghton T. Does aspirin attenuate the effect of angiotensin-converting enzyme inhibitors in hypertension or heart failure? *Curr Opin Nephrol Hypertens* (2001) 10, 625–31.
22. Peterson JG, Lauer MS. Using aspirin and ACE inhibitors in combination: why the hullabaloo? *Cleve Clin J Med* (2001) 68, 569–74.
23. Olson KL. Combined aspirin/ACE inhibitor treatment for CHF. *Ann Pharmacother* (2001) 35, 1653–8.
24. Consensus recommendations for the management of chronic heart failure. On behalf of the membership of the Advisory Council To Improve Outcomes Nationwide in Heart Failure [ACTION HF]. *Am J Cardiol* (1999) 83 (2A), 1A–38A.
25. Peterson JG, Topol EJ, Sapp SK, Young JB, Lincoff AM, Lauer MS. Evaluation of the effects of aspirin combined with angiotensin-converting enzyme inhibitors in patients with coronary artery disease. *Am J Med* (2000) 109, 371–7.

ACE inhibitors + Azathioprine

Anaemia has been seen in patients given azathioprine and enalapril or captopril. Leucopenia occasionally occurs with captopril and azathioprine.

Clinical evidence

(a) Anaemia

Nine out of 11 kidney transplant patients taking ACE inhibitors (**enalapril** or **captopril**) showed a haematocrit fall from 34 to 27%, and a haemoglobin fall from 11.6 to 9.5 g/dl when ciclosporin was replaced by azathioprine. Two patients were switched back to ciclosporin, and had a prompt rise in their haematocrit. Another 10 patients on both drugs similarly showed some anaemia when compared with 10 others not taking an ACE inhibitor (haematocrit of 33% compared with 41%, and haemoglobin 11.5 g/dl compared with 13.9 g/dl).[1] A later study by the same group of workers (again in patients on **enalapril** and **captopril**) confirmed these findings: no pharmacokinetic interaction was found between **enalapril** and azathioprine.[2]

(b) Leucopenia

A patient whose white cell count fell sharply when treated with both **captopril** 50 mg daily and azathioprine 150 mg daily, did not develop leucopenia when given each drug separately.[3] Another patient who was given **captopril** (increased to 475 mg daily [sic] then reduced to 100 mg daily) immediately after discontinuing azathioprine, developed leucopenia. She was later successfully treated with **captopril** 4 to 6 mg daily [sic].[4] Other patients have similarly shown leucopenia when given both drugs;[5,6] in one case this did not recur when rechallenged with captopril alone (at a lower dose).[6]

Mechanism

The anaemia appears to be due to suppression of erythropoietin by the ACE inhibitors, and azathioprine may cause patients to be more susceptible to this effect.[2] The cause of the leucopenia is unknown. It may just be due to the additive effects of both drugs.

Importance and management

Anaemia caused by captopril and enalapril has been seen in kidney transplant patients and in dialysis patients (see 'ACE inhibitors or Angiotensin II receptor antagonists + Epoetin', p.23). The evidence that this effect can be potentiated by azathioprine is limited, but it would be prudent to monitor well if these drugs are used together. The evidence that the concurrent use of ACE inhibitors and azathioprine increases the risk of leucopenia is also limited. However, the maker of captopril recommends that captopril should be used with extreme caution in patients on immunosuppressant therapy, especially if there is renal impairment. They advise that differential white blood cell counts should be performed prior to therapy, then every 2 weeks in the first 3 months of captopril therapy, and periodically thereafter.[7] The makers of a number of other ACE inhibitors also state in their prescribing information that concurrent administration of ACE inhibitors and **cytostatic** or **immunosuppressive agents** may lead to an increased risk of leucopenia. For other interactions with ACE inhibitors that lead to leucopenia see also 'ACE inhibitors + Allopurinol', p.14 and 'ACE inhibitors + Procainamide', p.30.

1. Gossmann J, Kachel H-G, Schoeppe W, Scheuermann E-H. Anemia in renal transplant recipients caused by concomitant therapy with azathioprine and angiotensin-converting enzyme inhibitors. *Transplantation* (1993) 56, 585–9.
2. Gossmann J, Thürmann P, Bachmann T, Weller S, Kachel H-G, Schoeppe W, Scheuermann E-H. Mechanism of angiotensin converting enzyme inhibitor-related anemia in renal transplant recipients. *Kidney Int* (1996) 50, 973–8.
3. Kirchertz EJ, Gröne HJ, Rieger J, Hölscher M, Scheler F. Successful low dose captopril rechallenge following drug-induced leucopenia. *Lancet* (1981) i, 1363.
4. Case DB, Whitman HH, Laragh JH, Spiera H. Successful low dose captopril rechallenge following drug-induced leucopenia. *Lancet* (1981) i, 1362–3.
5. Elijovisch F, Krakoff LR. Captopril associated granulocytopenia in hypertension after renal transplantation. *Lancet* (1980), i, 927–8.
6. Edwards CRW, Drury P, Penketh A, Damluji SA. Successful reintroduction of captopril following neutropenia. *Lancet* (1981) i, 723.
7. Capoten (Captopril). E. R. Squibb & Sons Ltd. UK Summary of product characteristics, February 2003.

ACE inhibitors + Beta-blockers

No clinically important pharmacokinetic interactions have been seen between bisoprolol and imidapril, or between propranolol and cilazapril, fosinopril, quinapril, or ramipril. No clinically significant interaction has been found between captopril or trandolapril and unnamed beta-blockers.

Clinical evidence, mechanism, importance and management

Propranolol 80 mg three times daily did not affect the pharmacokinetics of a single 20-mg dose of **quinapril** in 10 healthy subjects.[1] The pharmacokinetics of **ramipril** 5 mg daily were unaffected by **propranolol** 40 mg twice daily.[2] Similarly, the maker of **fosinopril** reports that the bioavailability of fosinoprilat, the active metabolite, was not altered by **propranolol**.[3,4] Another study found no significant pharmacokinetic interaction between **cilazapril** 2.5 mg daily and **propranolol** 120 mg daily, but the reductions in blood pressure were more pronounced and long-lasting.[5,6] In a single-dose, placebo-controlled, crossover study in 16 healthy men, **bisoprolol** 5 mg given with **imidapril** 10 mg did not significantly influence the pharmacokinetics of its active metabolite **imidaprilat**, and the pharmacodynamic effects, including blood pressure and heart rate reductions, were mainly additive.[7] The maker of **captopril** states that it has been safely given with other commonly used antihypertensive agents e.g. beta-blockers.[8] Similarly, the makers of **trandolapril** note that in patients with left ventricular dysfunction after myocardial infarction, no clinical interaction has been found between **trandolapril** and beta-blockers (not named).[9]

No important adverse interaction seems to occur, and the combination of these ACE inhibitors and **propranolol** or other beta-blockers are clinically useful.

1. Horvath AM, Pilon D, Caillé G, Colburn WA, Ferry JJ, Frank GJ, Lacasse Y, Olson SC. Multiple-dose propranolol administration does not influence the single dose pharmacokinetics of quinapril and its active metabolite (quinaprilat). *Biopharm Drug Dispos* (1990) 11, 191–6.
2. van Griensven JMT, Seibert-Grafe M, Schoemaker HC, Frölich M, Cohen AF. The pharmacokinetic and pharmacodynamic interactions of ramipril with propranolol. *Eur J Clin Pharmacol* (1993) 45, 255–60.
3. Staril (Fosinopril). E. R. Squibb & Sons Ltd. UK Summary of product characteristics, June 2005.
4. Monopril (Fosinopril). Bristol-Myers Squibb Company. US Prescribing information, July 2003.
5. Belz GG, Essig J, Kleinbloesem CH, Hoogkamer JFW, Wiegand UW, Wellstein A. Interactions between cilazapril and propranolol in man; plasma drug concentrations, hormone and enzyme responses, haemodynamics, agonist dose-effect curves and baroreceptor reflex. *Br J Clin Pharmacol* (1988) 26, 547–56.
6. Belz GG, Essig J, Erb K, Breithaupt K, Hoogkamer JFW, Kneer J, Kleinbloesem CH. Pharmacokinetic and pharmacodynamic interactions between the ACE inhibitor cilazapril and β-adrenoceptor antagonist propranolol in healthy subjects and in hypertensive patients. *Br J Clin Pharmacol* (1989) 27, 317S–322S.
7. Breithaupt-Grögler K, Ungethüm W, Meurer-Witt B, Belz GG. Pharmacokinetic and dynamic interactions of the angiotensin-converting enzyme inhibitor imidapril with hydrochlorothiazide, bisoprolol and nilvadipine. *Eur J Clin Pharmacol* (2001) 57, 275–84.
8. Capoten (Captopril). E. R. Squibb & Sons Ltd. UK Summary of product characteristics, February 2003.
9. Gopten (Trandolapril). Abbott Laboratories Ltd. UK Summary of product characteristics, September 2004.

ACE inhibitors + Calcium channel blockers

No clinically important adverse interactions have been seen between amlodipine and benazepril or captopril; between felodipine and ramipril; between manidipine and delapril; between

nicardipine and spirapril; between nilvadipine and imidapril; or between nifedipine and fosinopril, lisinopril, moexipril, or trandolapril.

Clinical evidence, mechanism, importance and management

No evidence of either a pharmacokinetic or adverse pharmacodynamic interaction was seen in 12 healthy subjects given single doses of **nifedipine** retard 20 mg and **lisinopril** 20 mg; the effects on blood pressure were additive.[1] The maker of **fosinopril** notes that the bioavailability of fosinoprilat, the active metabolite, was not altered by **nifedipine**.[2,3] Similarly, the maker of **moexipril** notes that no clinically important pharmacokinetic interaction occurred with **nifedipine** in healthy subjects but in patients, the antihypertensive effect was enhanced. If **moexipril** is added to **nifedipine**, they recommend a reduced starting dose of **moexipril**.[4] The maker of **trandolapril** has data on file showing that there is no significant interaction between single doses of **trandolapril** and sustained-release **nifedipine** in healthy subjects.[5] They also note that in patients with left ventricular dysfunction after myocardial infarction, no clinical interaction has been found between **trandolapril** and calcium channel blockers (not named).[6]

A study in 12 healthy subjects indicated that there was no pharmacokinetic interaction between single doses of **amlodipine** 5 mg and **benazepril** 10 mg.[7] No clinically important adverse interactions were seen in 29 hypertensive patients on **captopril** 25 mg twice daily when given **amlodipine** 10 mg daily; blood pressure control was significantly improved.[8] The maker of **captopril** says that it has been safely given with other commonly used antihypertensive agents e.g. long-acting calcium channel blockers,[9] and the maker of **amlodipine** says that it has been safely given with ACE inhibitors, and no **amlodipine** dosage changes are needed.[10]

No pharmacokinetic interaction occurred between single doses of **felodipine** 10 mg and **ramipril** 5 mg in healthy subjects. The blood pressure lowering effect of the combination was greater, and **ramipril** attenuated the reflex tachycardia caused by **felodipine**.[11] The maker of **spirapril** briefly noted in a review that **nicardipine** increased **spirapril** plasma concentrations by about 25% and those of its active metabolite spiraprilat by about 45%, and reduced **nicardipine** bioavailability by 30%. It was assumed that the interaction took place at the absorption site. However, the changes were not considered clinically relevant.[12] In a single-dose, placebo-controlled, crossover study in 16 healthy subjects, no pharmacokinetic interaction occurred between **nilvadipine** 8 mg and **imidapril** 10 mg, and the pharmacodynamic effects, including blood pressure reduction and decrease in total peripheral resistance, were mostly additive.[13]

In another single-dose crossover study in 18 healthy subjects, concurrent use of **manidipine** 10 mg and **delapril** 30 mg did not significantly alter the pharmacokinetics of either drug or their main metabolites.[14] A number of products combining an ACE inhibitor with a calcium channel blocker are available. It is generally advised that ACE inhibitor/calcium channel blocker combination products are only used in patients who have already been stabilised on the individual components in the same proportions.

1. Lees KR, Reid JL. Lisinopril and nifedipine: no acute interaction in normotensives. *Br J Clin Pharmacol* (1988) 25, 307–13.
2. Staril (Fosinopril). E. R. Squibb & Sons Ltd. UK Summary of product characteristics, June 2005.
3. Monopril (Fosinopril). Bristol-Myers Squibb Company. US Prescribing information, July 2003.
4. Perdix (Moexipril). Schwarz Pharma Ltd. UK Summary of product characteristics, May 2005.
5. New horizons in antihypertensive therapy. Gopten® Trandolapril. Knoll AG, 1992.
6. Gopten (Trandolapril). Abbott Laboratories Ltd. UK Summary of product characteristics, September 2004.
7. Sun JX, Cipriano A, Kern JC, Chan K, John VA. Drug interaction study of benazepril and amlodipine in healthy subjects. *Pharm Res* (1992) 9 (10 Suppl), S313.
8. Maclean D, Mitchell ET, Wilcox RG, Walker P, Tyler HM. A double-blind crossover comparison of amlodipine and placebo added to captopril in moderate to severe hypertension. *J Cardiovasc Pharmacol* (1988) 12 (Suppl 7), S85–S88.
9. Capoten (Captopril). E. R. Squibb & Sons Ltd. UK Summary of product characteristics, February 2003.
10. Istin (Amlodipine besilate). Pfizer Ltd. UK Summary of product characteristics, April 2005.
11. Bainbridge AD, MacFadyen RJ, Lees KR, Reid JL. A study of the acute pharmacodynamic interaction of ramipril and felodipine in normotensive subjects. *Br J Clin Pharmacol* (1991) 31, 148–53.
12. Grass P, Gerbeau C, Kutz K. Spirapril: pharmacokinetic properties and drug interactions. *Blood Pressure* (1994) 3 (Suppl 2), 7–13.
13. Breithaupt-Grögler K, Ungethüm W, Meurer-Witt B, Belz GG. Pharmacokinetic and dynamic interactions of the angiotensin-converting enzyme inhibitor imidapril with hydrochlorothiazide, bisoprolol and nilvadipine. *Eur J Clin Pharmacol* (2001) 57, 275–84.
14. Stockis A, Gengler C, Goethals F, Jeanbaptiste B, Lens S, Poli G, Acerbi D. Single oral dose pharmacokinetic interaction study of manidipine and delapril in healthy volunteers. *Arzneimittelforschung* (2003) 53, 627–34.

ACE inhibitors + Capsaicin

An isolated report describes a cough in a woman taking an ACE inhibitor each time she used a topical cream containing capsaicin.

Clinical evidence, mechanism, importance and management

A 53-year-old woman who had been taking an unnamed ACE inhibitor for several years, complained of cough each time she applied *Axsain*, a cream containing capsaicin 0.075%, to her lower extremities. Whether this reaction would have occurred without the ACE inhibitor was not determined,[1] but cough is a recognised adverse effect of ACE inhibitors and pre-treatment with an ACE inhibitor has been shown to enhance the cough caused by inhaled capsaicin.[1] This potential interaction is probably of little general clinical importance.

1. Hakas JF. Topical capsaicin induces cough in patient receiving ACE inhibitor. *Ann Allergy* (1990) 65, 322.

ACE inhibitors + Clonidine

Potentiation of the antihypertensive effect of clonidine by ACE inhibitors can be clinically useful.[1] However, limited evidence suggests that the effects of captopril may be delayed when patients are switched from clonidine.[2] Note that sudden withdrawal of clonidine may cause rebound hypertension.

1. Catapres (Clonidine hydrochloride). Boehringer Ingelheim Ltd. UK Summary of product characteristics, November 2003.
2. Gröne H-J, Kirchertz EJ, Rieger J. Mögliche Komplikationen und Probleme der Captopriltherapie bei Hypertonikern mit ausgeprägten Gefäßschäden. *Therapiewoche* (1981) 31, 5280–7.

ACE inhibitors + Co-trimoxazole or Trimethoprim

Two reports describe serious hyperkalaemia, apparently caused by the concurrent use of trimethoprim and enalapril or quinapril in association with renal impairment.

Clinical evidence

A 40-year-old woman with transplanted lungs (taking ciclosporin, azathioprine, prednisolone, **enalapril**, gentamicin inhalation, salbutamol and acetylcysteine) developed life-threatening hyperkalaemia of 6.8 mmol/l when she was treated with high-dose co-trimoxazole 120 mg/kg daily for suspected *Pneumocystis carinii* pneumonia. The co-trimoxazole and **enalapril** were stopped and she was treated with sodium chloride 0.9%, mannitol and furosemide. After 12 hours her serum potassium had decreased to 4.6 mmol/l and she began to recover over a period of a week, but she then developed fatal septic shock with multi-organ failure.[1] In another case, an elderly man treated with **quinapril** 20 mg daily for essential hypertension was found to have hyperkalaemia (serum potassium 7 to 7.4 mmol/l) and azotaemia after 20 days treatment with co-trimoxazole for mild acute pyelonephritis. Co-trimoxazole and **quinapril** were stopped, and nifedipine was given to control blood pressure. After treatment with dextrose, insulin, sodium polystyrene sulfonate and calcium gluconate, the azotaemia and hyperkalaemia resolved over 36 hours.[2]

Mechanism

Hyperkalaemia has been reported in patients receiving co-trimoxazole alone. This is attributed to the trimethoprim component, which can have a potassium-sparing effect on the distal part of the kidney tubules. ACE inhibitors reduce aldosterone synthesis, which results in reduced renal loss of potassium. The interaction is probably due to the additive effects of these two mechanisms, compounded by impaired renal function.[1,2]

Importance and management

Clinical examples of this interaction seem to be few, but the possibility of hyperkalaemia with either trimethoprim or ACE inhibitors alone, particularly with other factors such as renal impairment, is well documented.

Thus it may be prudent to monitor potassium levels if this combination is used. It has been suggested that trimethoprim should probably be avoided in elderly patients with chronic renal impairment taking ACE inhibitors, and that patients with AIDS taking an ACE inhibitor for associated nephropathy should probably discontinue this treatment during high-dose co-trimoxazole therapy.[2]

1. Bugge JF. Severe hyperkalaemia induced by trimethoprim in combination with an angiotensin-converting enzyme inhibitor in a patient with transplanted lungs. *J Intern Med* (1996) 240, 249–52.
2. Thomas RJ. Severe hyperkalemia with trimethoprim-quinapril. *Ann Pharmacother* (1996) 30, 413–14.

ACE inhibitors + Dialysis or Transfusion membranes

An anaphylactoid reaction can occur in patients on ACE inhibitors within a few minutes of starting haemodialysis using high-flux polyacrylonitrile membranes ('AN 69'). Anaphylactoid reactions have also been reported in patients on ACE inhibitors undergoing low-density lipoprotein apheresis. In addition, hypotensive reactions associated with blood transfusions through leucoreduction filters have occurred in patients on ACE inhibitors.

Clinical evidence, mechanism, importance and management

(a) High-flux dialysis

In a retrospective study, 9 of 236 haemodialysis patients treated with **high-flux polyacrylonitrile membranes ('AN 69')** were found to have had anaphylactoid reactions (severe hypotension, flushing, swelling of face and/or tongue, and dyspnoea) within 5 minutes of commencing haemodialysis. Treatment with an ACE inhibitor had been recently started in all 9 patients (7 **enalapril**, 1 **captopril**, 1 **lisinopril**). The anaphylactoid reactions disappeared in all 6 patients who discontinued the ACE inhibitor. Two other patients were given a filter rinsing procedure (the 'Bioprime' rinse method) and a new dialysis membrane, and in the final patient further anaphylactoid reactions were prevented by cellulose-triacetate haemofiltration while ACE inhibitor therapy was continued.[1] Similar reactions have been reported elsewhere and are thought to be bradykinin mediated.[2,3] The UK Committee on Safety of Medicines has advised that the combination of ACE inhibitors and such membranes should be avoided, either by substituting an alternative membrane or an alternative antihypertensive drug.[4]

(b) Lipoprotein apheresis

Anaphylactoid reactions occurred in 2 patients on ACE inhibitors during removal of low-density lipoproteins (LDL apheresis) with dextran sulfate adsorption.[5] Further reactions were reported in 6 patients treated with either **captopril** or **enalapril** and dextran sulfate apheresis. When the interval between the last dose of ACE inhibitor and the apheresis was prolonged to 12 to 30 hours no further adverse reactions occurred.[6] However, other workers found lengthening the interval to be ineffective in one patient.[7] The makers of **enalapril** suggests temporarily withholding the ACE inhibitor therapy prior to each apheresis,[8] but other makers of ACE inhibitors recommend using a different class of antihypertensive drug[9-11] or changing the method of lipoprotein reduction.[9,12]

(c) Transfusion reactions

A report describes 8 patients receiving ACE inhibitors and blood transfusions through bedside **leucoreduction filters** who experienced severe hypotensive reactions. The reactions were attributed to bradykinin generation during blood filtration and prevention of bradykinin breakdown due to the ACE inhibitors. Six of the patients tolerated subsequent transfusions, but 3 had discontinued their medication the day before the planned transfusion and one received washed (plasma-depleted) components. One patient experienced a second reaction, but then received washed red cells and had no reaction.[13]

1. Verresen L, Waer M, Vanrenterghem Y, Michielsen P. Angiotensin-converting-enzyme inhibitors and anaphylactoid reactions to high-flux membrane dialysis. *Lancet* (1990) 336, 1360–2.
2. Tielemans C, Madhoun P, Lenaers M, Schandene L, Goldman M, Vanherweghem JL. Anaphylactoid reactions during hemodialysis on AN69 membranes in patients receiving ACE inhibitors. *Kidney Int* (1990) 38, 982–4.
3. Tielemans C, Vanherweghem JL, Blumberg A, Cuvelier R, de Fremont JF, Dehout F, Dupont P, Richard C, Stolear JC, Wens R. ACE inhibitors and anaphylactoid reactions to high-flux membrane dialysis. *Lancet* (1991) 337, 370–1.
4. Committee on Safety of Medicines. Anaphylactoid reactions to high-flux polyacrylonitrile membranes in combination with ACE inhibitors. *Current Problems* (1992) 33, 2.
5. Olbricht CJ, Schaumann D, Fischer D. Anaphylactoid reactions, LDL apheresis with dextran sulphate, and ACE inhibitors. *Lancet* (1992) 340, 908–9.
6. Keller C, Grützmacher P, Bahr F, Schwarzbeck A, Kroon AA, Kiral A. LDL-apheresis with dextran sulphate and anaphylactoid reactions to ACE inhibitors. *Lancet* (1993) 341, 60–1.
7. Davidson DC, Peart I, Turner S, Sangster M. Prevention with icatibant of anaphylactoid reactions to ACE inhibitor during LDL apheresis. *Lancet* (1994) 343, 1575.
8. Innovace (Enalapril). Merck Sharp & Dohme Ltd. UK Summary of product characteristics, July 2004.
9. Capoten (Captopril). E. R. Squibb & Sons Ltd. UK Summary of product characteristics, February 2003.
10. Tanatril (Imidapril). Trinity Pharmaceuticals Ltd. UK Summary of product characteristics, May 2003.
11. Perdix (Moexipril). Schwarz Pharma Ltd. UK Summary of product characteristics, May 2005.
12. Accupro (Quinapril). Pfizer Ltd. UK Summary of product characteristics, June 2004.
13. Quillen K. Hypotensive transfusion reactions in patients taking angiotensin-converting-enzyme inhibitors. *N Engl J Med* (2000) 343, 1422–3.

ACE inhibitors + Diuretics; Loop, thiazide or related

The combination of captopril or other ACE inhibitors with loop or thiazide or related diuretics is normally safe and effective, but 'first dose hypotension' (dizziness, lightheadedness, fainting) can occur, particularly if the dose of diuretic is high, and often in association with various predisposing conditions. A few cases of renal insufficiency, and even acute renal failure, have been reported in patients taking ACE inhibitors and diuretics, possibly associated with sodium depletion. A case of severe hyponatraemia has been reported. Diuretic-induced hypokalaemia may still occur when ACE inhibitors are used with potassium-depleting diuretics.

Clinical evidence

(a) First dose hypotensive reaction

The concurrent use of **captopril** or other ACE inhibitors and loop or thiazide or related diuretics is normally safe and effective, but some patients experience 'first dose hypotension' (i.e. dizziness, lightheadedness, fainting) after taking the first one or two doses of an ACE inhibitor. This appears to be associated with, and exaggerated by, certain conditions (heart failure, renovascular hypertension, haemodialysis, high levels of renin and angiotensin, low-sodium diet, dehydration, diarrhoea or vomiting, etc.) and/or hypovolaemia and sodium depletion caused by diuretics, particularly in high doses. A study describes one woman whose blood pressure of 290/150 mmHg failed to respond to **furosemide** 10 mg intravenously. After 30 minutes she was given **captopril** 50 mg orally and within 45 minutes her blood pressure fell to 135/60 mmHg, and she required an infusion of saline to maintain her blood pressure.[1] In another study, a man developed severe postural hypotension shortly after **furosemide** was added to **captopril** treatment.[2]

Starting with a low dose of ACE inhibitor reduces the risk of first-dose hypotension. In a study in 8 patients with hypertension, treated with a diuretic (mainly **furosemide** or **hydrochlorothiazide**) for at least 4 weeks, **captopril** was started in small increasing doses from 6.25 mg. Symptomatic postural hypotension was seen in 2 of the 8 patients, but was only mild and transient.[3]

Hypotension is more common in patients with heart failure who are receiving large doses of diuretics. In a study in 124 patients with severe heart failure, all receiving **furosemide** (mean dose 170 mg daily; range 80 to 500 mg/day) and 90 also receiving the potassium-sparing diuretic spironolactone, the addition of **captopril** caused transient symptomatic hypotension in 44% of subjects. The **captopril** dose had to be reduced, and in 8 patients it was later discontinued. In addition, four patients developed symptomatic hypotension after 1 to 2 months of treatment, and **captopril** was also discontinued in these patients.[4]

There is some evidence that in patients with heart failure the incidence of marked orthostatic hypotension requiring treatment discontinuation in the first 36 hours was lower with **perindopril** 2 mg once daily than **captopril** 6.25 mg three times daily (6 of 357 cases versus 16 of 368 cases, respectively).[5]

(b) Hypokalaemia

Although ACE inhibitors can maintain potassium levels, the concurrent use of loop or thiazide or related diuretics can result in hypokalaemia. In one analysis, 7 of 21 patients on diuretics given ACE inhibitors for heart failure developed hypokalaemia. This was corrected by potassium supplementation in 2 cases, an increase in the ACE inhibitor dose in 3 cases, and use of a potassium-sparing diuretic in the remaining 2 cases.[6]

(c) Hyponatraemia

An isolated report describes a patient who developed severe hyponatraemia 3 days after **bendroflumethiazide** 10 mg daily was added to antihypertensive treatment with **enalapril** 20 mg daily and atenolol 100 mg daily. However, on 2 other occasions she only developed mild hyponatraemia when treated with **bendroflumethiazide** alone.[7] An earlier study reported changes in sodium balance due to **captopril** in all 6 patients with renovascular hypertension and in 11 of 12 patients with essential hypertension; loss of sodium occurred in 12 of the 18 patients.[1]

(d) Impairment of renal function

The risk of ACE inhibitor-induced renal impairment in patients with or without renovascular disease can be potentiated by diuretics.[8-11] In an analysis of 74 patients who had been treated with **captopril** or **lisinopril**, reversible acute renal failure was more common in those who were also treated with a diuretic (**furosemide** and/or **hydrochlorothiazide**) than those who were not (11 of 33 patients compared with 1 of 41 patients).[10] Similarly, in a prescription-event monitoring study, **enalapril** was associated with raised creatinine or urea concentrations in 75 patients and it was thought to have contributed to deterioration in renal function and subsequent deaths in 10 of these patients. However, 9 of these 10 were also receiving loop or thiazide diuretics, sometimes in high doses.[12] Retrospective analysis of a controlled study in patients with hypertensive nephrosclerosis identified 8 of 34 patients who developed reversible renal insufficiency when treated with **enalapril** and various other antihypertensives including a diuretic (**furosemide** or **hydrochlorothiazide**). In contrast, 23 patients treated with placebo and various other antihypertensives did not develop renal insufficiency. Subsequently, **enalapril** was tolerated by 7 of the 8 patients without deterioration in renal function and 6 of these patients later received diuretics.[13] One patient was again treated with **enalapril** with recurrence of renal dysfunction, but discontinuation of the diuretics (**furosemide**, **hydrochlorothiazide**, and **triamterene**) led to an improvement in renal function despite the continuation of **enalapril**.[14]

Renal impairment in patients on ACE inhibitors and diuretics has also been described in patients with heart failure. A patient with congestive heart failure and moderate renal insufficiency developed acute non-oliguric renal failure while on **enalapril** 20 mg daily and **furosemide** 60 to 80 mg daily, which resolved when the sodium balance was restored.[15] In a study involving 90 patients with severe congestive heart failure who were receiving **furosemide** and spironolactone, a decline in renal function occurred in 18 patients during the first month after initiation of **captopril** treatment; mean serum creatinine levels rose from 220 to 300 micromol/l. All the patients were receiving high daily doses of **furosemide** and all had renal dysfunction before receiving the first dose of **captopril**.[4]

Acute, fatal, renal failure developed in 2 patients with cardiac failure within 4 weeks of being treated with **enalapril** and **furosemide**, and in 2 similar patients renal impairment developed over a longer period.[16] Reversible renal failure has also been described in a patient with congestive heart failure when treated with **captopril** and **metolazone**.[17]

(e) Pharmacokinetic and diuresis studies

A study in healthy subjects given single doses of **enalapril** and **furosemide** found no evidence of any pharmacokinetic interaction between these drugs.[18] Another study in hypertensive patients found that **captopril** did not affect the urinary excretion of **furosemide**, nor its subsequent diuretic effects.[19] However, a further study in healthy subjects showed that, although **captopril** did not alter urinary excretion of **furosemide**, it did reduce diuresis.[20] Yet another study in healthy subjects found that **captopril** reduced the urinary excretion of **furosemide**, and reduced the diuretic response during the first 20 minutes to approximately 50%, and the natriuretic response to almost 30%, whereas **enalapril** and **ramipril** did not significantly alter the diuretic effects of **furosemide**.[21] **Lisinopril** did not alter plasma levels or urinary excretion of **furosemide**, nor did it alter urinary electrolyte excretion.[22] Similarly, **furosemide** did not affect the pharmacokinetics of **lisinopril** either in single-dose or multiple-dose regimens.[23]

In a single-dose, randomised, crossover study in 19 elderly patients the pharmacokinetics of **enalapril** 10 mg were unaffected by **hydrochlorothiazide** 25 mg. However, there was a significant reduction in renal clearance and a significant increase in the AUC of its metabolite, enalaprilat, resulting in higher serum levels of the active drug. This acute interaction was not thought to be clinically significant for long-term use.[24] No significant pharmacokinetic interaction occurred between **imidapril** and **hydrochlorothiazide** in healthy subjects[25] and neither **captopril** nor **ramipril** altered the diuresis induced by **hydrochlorothiazide**.[21] The maker of **spirapril** briefly noted in a review that there was no clinically relevant pharmacokinetic interaction between **spirapril** and **hydrochlorothiazide**.[26] Furthermore no pharmacokinetic interaction was found when **spirapril** and **hydrochlorothiazide** were administered together as a bi-layer tablet.[27] The maker of **moexipril** also notes that there was no clinically important pharmacokinetic interaction when **moexipril** was given with **hydrochlorothiazide** in healthy subjects.[28,29]

Mechanisms

The first dose hypotension interaction is not fully understood. One suggestion is that if considerable amounts of salt and water have already been lost as a result of using a diuretic, the resultant depletion in the fluid volume (hypovolaemia) transiently exaggerates the hypotensive effects of the ACE inhibitor.

The cases of hypokalaemia are simply a result of the potassium-depleting effects of the diuretics.

Thiazides can cause hyponatraemia, but this enhanced effect may have been due to an alteration in renal haemodynamics caused by the ACE inhibitor; sustained angiotensin-converting enzyme blockade can produce natriuresis.[1]

Marked decreases in blood pressure may affect renal function, and in addition, the renin-angiotensin system plays an important role in the maintenance of the glomerular filtration rate when renal artery pressure is diminished.[9] However, diuretic-induced sodium depletion may also be an important factor in the renal impairment sometimes observed with ACE inhibitors.

Importance and management

The 'first dose hypotension' interaction between ACE inhibitors and diuretics is well established. The risk is higher when the dose of diuretic is greater than furosemide 80 mg daily or equivalent, and in those with various conditions[30] (see section (a) in 'Clinical Evidence'). In patients on these doses of diuretic, consideration should be given to temporarily stopping the diuretic or reducing its dosage a few days before the ACE inhibitor is added. If this is not considered clinically appropriate, the first dose of the ACE inhibitor should be given under close supervision. In all patients on diuretics, therapy with ACE inhibitors should be started with a very low dose, even in patients at low risk (e.g. those with uncomplicated essential hypertension on low-dose thiazides). To be on the safe side, all patients should be given a simple warning about what can happen and what to do when they first start concurrent use. The immediate problem (dizziness, lightheadedness, faintness), if it occurs, can usually be solved by the patient lying down. Taking the first dose of the ACE inhibitor just before bedtime is also preferable.[31] Any marked hypotension is normally transient, but if problems persist it may be necessary temporarily to reduce the diuretic dosage. There is usually no need to avoid the combination just because an initially large hypotensive response has occurred.

A number of products combining an ACE inhibitor with a thiazide diuretic are available for the treatment of hypertension. These products should be used only in those patients who have been stabilised on the individual components in the same proportions.

The use of ACE inhibitors in patients on potassium-depleting diuretics does not always prevent hypokalaemia developing. Serum potassium should be monitored.

This is only an isolated report, but be aware that ACE inhibitors may affect the natriuresis caused by diuretics.

The cases cited emphasise the need to monitor renal function in patients on ACE inhibitors and diuretics. If increases in blood urea and creatinine occur, a dosage reduction and/or discontinuation of the diuretic and/or ACE inhibitor may be required. In a statement, the American Heart Association comments that acute renal failure complicating ACE inhibitor therapy is almost always reversible and repletion of extracellular fluid volume and discontinuation of diuretic therapy is the most effective approach. In addition, withdrawal of interacting drugs, supportive management of fluid and electrolytes, and temporary dialysis where indicated are the mainstays of therapy.[11]

The possibility of undiagnosed renal artery stenosis should also be considered.

None of the pharmacokinetic changes observed appear to be clinically significant.

1. Case DB, Atlas SA, Laragh JH, Sealey JE, Sullivan PA, McKinstry DN. Clinical experience with blockade of the renin-angiotensin-aldosterone system by an oral converting-enzyme inhibitor (SQ 14,225, captopril) in hypertensive patients. *Prog Cardiovasc Dis* (1978) 21, 195–206.
2. Ferguson RK, Vlasses PH, Koplin JR, Shirinian A, Burke JF, Alexander JC. Captopril in severe treatment-resistant hypertension. *Am Heart J* (1980) 99, 579–85.
3. Koffer H, Vlasses PH, Ferguson RK, Weis M, Adler AG. Captopril in diuretic-treated hypertensive patients. *JAMA* (1980) 244, 2532–5.
4. Dahlström U, Karlsson E. Captopril and spironolactone therapy for refractory congestive heart failure. *Am J Cardiol* (1993) 71, 29A–33A.
5. Haïat R, Piot O, Gallois H, Hanania G. Blood pressure response to the first 36 hours of heart failure therapy with perindopril versus captopril. French General Hospitals National College of Cardiologists. *J Cardiovasc Pharmacol* (1999) 33, 953–9.
6. D'Costa DF, Basu SK, Gunasekera NPR. ACE inhibitors and diuretics causing hypokalaemia. *Br J Clin Pract* (1990) 44, 26–7.
7. Collier JG, Webb DJ. Severe thiazide-induced hyponatraemia during treatment with enalapril. *Postgrad Med J* (1987) 63, 1105–6.
8. Watson ML, Bell GM, Muir AL, Buist TAS, Kellett RJ, Padfield PL. Captopril/diuretic combinations in severe renovascular disease: a cautionary note. *Lancet* (1983) ii, 404–5.
9. Hoefnagels WHL, Strijk SP, Thien T. Reversible renal failure following treatment with captopril and diuretics in patients with renovascular hypertension. *Neth J Med* (1984) 27, 269–74.
10. Mandal AK, Markert RJ, Saklayen MG, Mankus RA, Yokokawa K. Diuretics potentiate angiotensin converting enzyme inhibitor-induced acute renal failure. *Clin Nephrol* (1994) 42, 170–4.
11. Schoolwerth AC, Sica DA, Ballermann BJ, Wilcox CS. Renal considerations in angiotensin converting enzyme inhibitor therapy. A statement for healthcare professionals from the Council on the Kidney in Cardiovascular Disease and the Council for High Blood Pressure Research of the American Heart Association. *Circulation* (2001) 104, 1985–91.
12. Speirs CJ, Dollery CT, Inman WHW, Rawson NSB, Wilton LV. Postmarketing surveillance of enalapril. II: Investigation of the potential role of enalapril in deaths with renal failure. *BMJ* (1988) 297, 830–2.
13. Toto RD, Mitchell HC, Lee H-C, Milam C, Pettinger WA. Reversible renal insufficiency due to angiotensin converting enzyme inhibitors in hypertensive nephrosclerosis. *Ann Intern Med* (1991) 115, 513–19.
14. Lee H-C, Pettinger WA. Diuretics potentiate the angiotensin converting-enzyme inhibitor-associated acute renal dysfunction. *Clin Nephrol* (1992) 38, 236–7.
15. Funck-Brentano C, Chatellier G, Alexandre J-M. Reversible renal failure after combined treatment with enalapril and frusemide in a patient with congestive heart failure. *Br Heart J* (1986) 55, 596–8.
16. Stewart JT, Lovett D, Joy M. Reversible renal failure after combined treatment with enalapril and frusemide in a patient with congestive heart failure. *Br Heart J* (1986) 56, 489–90.
17. Hogg KJ, Hillis WS. Captopril/metolazone induced renal failure. *Lancet* (1986) 1, 501–2.
18. Van Hecken AM, Verbesselt R, Buntinx A, Cirillo VJ, De Schepper PJ. Absence of a pharmacokinetic interaction between enalapril and frusemide. *Br J Clin Pharmacol* (1987) 23, 84–7.
19. Fujimura A, Shimokawa Y, Ebihara A. Influence of captopril on urinary excretion of furosemide in hypertensive subjects. *J Clin Pharmacol* (1990) 30, 538–42.
20. Sommers De K, Meyer EC, Moncrieff J. Acute interaction of furosemide and captopril in healthy salt-replete man. *S Afr Tydskr Wet* (1991) 87, 375–7.
21. Toussaint C, Masselink A, Gentges A, Wambach G, Bönner G. Interference of different ACE-inhibitors with the diuretic action of furosemide and hydrochlorothiazide. *Klin Wochenschr* (1989) 67, 1138–46.
22. Sudoh T, Fujimura A, Shiga T, Tateishi T, Sunaga K, Ohashi K, Ebihara A. Influence of lisinopril on urinary electrolytes excretion after furosemide in healthy subjects. *J Clin Pharmacol* (1993) 33, 640–3.
23. Beermann B. Pharmacokinetics of lisinopril. *Am J Med* (1988) 85 (Suppl 3B) 25–30.
24. Weisser K, Schloos J, Jakob S, Mühlberg W, Platt D, Mutschler E. The influence of hydrochlorothiazide on the pharmacokinetics of enalapril in elderly patients. *Eur J Clin Pharmacol* (1992) 43, 173–7.
25. Breithaupt-Grögler K, Ungethüm W, Meurer-Witt B, Belz GG. Pharmacokinetic and dynamic interactions of the angiotensin-converting enzyme inhibitor imidapril with hydrochlorothiazide, bisoprolol and nilvadipine. *Eur J Clin Pharmacol* (2001) 57, 275–84.
26. Grass P, Gerbeau C, Kutz K. Spirapril: pharmacokinetic properties and drug interactions. *Blood Pressure* (1994) 3 (Suppl 2), 7–13.
27. Schürer M, Erb K, Junge K, Schäfer HF, Schulz H-U, Amschler S, Krupp S, Hermann R. Drug interaction of spirapril hydrochloride monohydrate and hydrochlorothiazide. *Arzneimittelforschung* (2003) 53, 414–19.
28. Perdix (Moexipril). Schwarz Pharma Ltd. UK Summary of product characteristics, May 2005.
29. Univasc (Moexipril). Schwarz Pharma. US Prescribing information, May 2003.
30. British National Formulary. 49th ed. London: The British Medical Association and The Pharmaceutical Press; 2005. p. 98–9.
31. Capoten (Captopril). E. R. Squibb & Sons Ltd. UK Summary of product characteristics, February 2003.

ACE inhibitors + Diuretics; Potassium-sparing

Combining ACE inhibitors with potassium-sparing diuretics (amiloride, spironolactone, triamterene) can result in clinically relevant or severe hyperkalaemia, particularly if other important risk factors are present.

Clinical evidence

(a) Hyperkalaemia

(i) Spironolactone. Twenty-five of 262 patients treated with ACE-inhibitors and spironolactone, and admitted to hospital for medical emergencies, were found to have serious hyperkalaemia (serum potassium levels greater than 6 mmol/l, and at least 8 mmol/l in 11 patients). These 25 patients were elderly (mean age 74 years) and being treated for hypertension, heart failure, diabetic nephropathy, proteinuria, or nephrotic syndrome; 22 had associated renal impairment and 12 had signs of volume depletion. Combined treatment had been started an average of 25 weeks before the admission. The ACE inhibitors involved were **enalapril**, **captopril**, **lisinopril** or **perindopril,** and the average dose of spironolactone was 57 mg daily; 10 were also receiving a loop or thiazide diuretic. Nineteen patients had ECG changes associated with hyperkalaemia; 2 of them died, 2 required temporary pacing for third-degree heart block, and 2 survived after sustained ventricular tachycardia and fibrillation. Of the 19 patients, 17 required at least one haemodialysis session and 12 were admitted to intensive care.[1]
Similar findings were found in an analysis of 44 patients with congestive heart failure who were taking spironolactone and ACE inhibitors or angiotensin II receptor antagonists, and were admitted for treatment of life-threatening hyperkalaemia. Their mean age was 76 years, the mean dose of spironolactone was 88 mg daily (range 25 to 200 mg daily) and 40 patients also received loop diuretics. In addition, 35 had type II diabetes. Haemodialysis was given to 37 patients, but in 6 patients renal function did not recover and 2 patients developed fatal complications.[2] A number of other cases of serious hyperkalaemia have been described in patients on ACE inhibitors (**captopril, enalapril, lisinopril**), spironolactone, and loop (furosemide or bumetanide) or thiazide (hydroflumethiazide) diuretics.[3-8] Many of the patients were elderly and were receiving 50 to 100 mg of spironolactone daily,[3,4,7] but one diabetic patient with moderate renal impairment was receiving just 25 mg daily.[6] In one report, the 4 cases had associated **enalapril**-induced deterioration in renal function and died.[3] Another patient died from complete heart block.[4]
One of the factors that affect the incidence of hyperkalaemia appears to be the dose of spironolactone. In a preliminary investigation for the Randomised Aldactone Evaluation Study (RALES), 214 patients with congestive heart failure taking an ACE inhibitor and a loop diuretic with or without digitalis, were randomised to receive placebo or various doses of spironolactone for 12 weeks. The incidence of hyperkalaemia (serum potassium level of 5.5 mmol/l or greater) was 5% for the placebo group, whereas it was 5%, 13%, 20% and 24% when spironolactone was given in single daily doses of 12.5, 25, 50, or 75 mg, respectively.[9] The main RALES study involving 1663 patients showed a 30% reduction in the risk of mortality in patients with severe heart failure when given spironolactone in addition to treatment including an ACE inhibitor, a loop diuretic and in most cases digoxin. During the first year of follow-up, the median creatinine concentration in the spironolactone group increased by about 4 to 9 micromol/l and the median potassium concentration increased by 0.03 mmol/l, but there was a low incidence of serious hyperkalaemia (2% in the spironolactone group compared with 1% in the placebo group). However, the dose of spironolactone was fairly low (mean dose 26 mg daily; range 25 mg every other day to 50 mg daily depending on serum potassium levels and response). In addition, patients with a serum creatinine concentration of more than 221 micromol/l or a serum potassium concentration of more than 5 mmol/l were excluded.[10] A higher incidence of hyperkalaemia (serum potassium levels greater than 5 mmol/l) has been reported in 15 of 42 patients hospitalised for heart failure and prescribed spironolactone. It was suggested that spironolactone may be a precipitating cause of dehydration and renal dysfunction and that the high incidence of hyperkalaemia may be due to the excessively large doses of spironolactone prescribed.[11]

(ii) Other potassium-sparing diuretics. The serum potassium levels of two patients taking furosemide and unnamed potassium-sparing diuretics and potassium supplements showed rises of 18% and 24% when given **captopril** 37.5 to 75 mg daily. The rises occurred within one or two days. No clinical signs or symptoms of hyperkalaemia were seen, but one of the patients had an increase in serum potassium to above the upper limits of normal for the laboratory.[12] In a postmarketing survey, 2 patients who had **enalapril**-associated renal impairment and died were also receiving **amiloride** and furosemide; one was also taking potassium supplements.[3] Four diabetic patients, with some renal impairment, developed life-threatening hyperkalaemia with severe cardiac arrhythmias and deterioration of renal function, within 8 to 18 days of having an **amiloride**/hydrochlorothiazide diuretic added to their **enalapril** treatment. Two suffered cardiac arrest and both died. Potassium levels were between 9.4 and 11 mmol/l. A fifth diabetic patient with normal renal function developed hyperkalaemia soon after receiving **amiloride**/hydrochlorothiazide and **captopril** in combination.[13] A further case of hyperkalaemia and cardiac arrest was associated

with **enalapril** and furosemide/**amiloride**.[14] In a brief report, the makers of **enalapril** noted that, of 47 serious cases of hyperkalaemia, 25 patients were on one or more (unnamed) potassium-sparing agents.[15]

(b) Serum potassium levels unchanged

A retrospective comparison of 35 patients treated for congestive heart failure found no differences in the serum potassium levels of 16 patients on furosemide, **amiloride** and **enalapril** when compared with another group of 19 patients on furosemide and **amiloride** alone. Patients were excluded from the comparison if they had significant renal impairment or were taking other drugs likely to affect serum potassium.[16] Another retrospective analysis found that **captopril**, given to 6 patients on ***Dyazide*** (hydrochlorothiazide/**triamterene**), had not increased the potassium levels.[17]

(c) Potentiation of effect

The manufacturer of **spironolactone** warns that since ACE inhibitors decrease aldosterone production they should not routinely be used with spironolactone, particularly in patients with marked renal impairment.[18] However, a beneficial effect has been found in severe heart failure, see the RALES study in *(a)* above. **Spironolactone** can cause potentiation of the effect of antihypertensive drugs and their dosage may need to be reduced.[18] For reports of hypotension associated with diuretics and ACE inhibitors see, 'ACE inhibitors + Diuretics; Loop, thiazide or related', p.20.

Mechanism

ACE inhibitors reduce the levels of aldosterone, which results in the retention of potassium. This would be expected to be additive with the potassium-retaining effects of amiloride, spironolactone and triamterene, leading to hyperkalaemia, but usually only if other risk factors are present (see 'Importance and management' below).

Importance and management

Hyperkalaemia with ACE inhibitors and potassium-sparing diuretics is fairly well documented and well established. Its incidence is uncertain, but if it occurs it can be serious and potentially life threatening. Important hyperkalaemia usually only appears to develop if one or more other risk factors are also present, particularly renal impairment. Other risk factors include advanced age[7] and diabetes[2] (hyperkalaemia has been found to be relatively common in both non-insulin-dependent and insulin-dependent diabetics).[19] In addition, doses of spironolactone greater than 25 mg daily increase the risk of hyperkalaemia.

Because ACE inhibitors have potassium-sparing effects, potassium-sparing diuretics such as amiloride and triamterene should normally not be given concurrently. If, however, the use of both drugs is thought to be appropriate the serum potassium levels should be closely monitored so that any problems can be quickly identified. Note that the concurrent use of a potassium-depleting diuretic (a loop diuretic or a thiazide) with the potassium-sparing diuretic may not necessarily prevent the development of hyperkalaemia. The combination of an ACE inhibitor and spironolactone in heart failure is beneficial, but close monitoring of serum potassium is needed, especially with any changes in treatment or in the patient's clinical condition.

1. Schepkens H, Vanholder R, Billiouw J-M, Lameire N. Life-threatening hyperkalemia during combined therapy with angiotensin-converting enzyme inhibitors and spironolactone: an analysis of 25 cases. *Am J Med* (2001) 110, 438–41.
2. Wrenger E, Müller R, Moesenthin M, Welte T, Frölich JC, Neumann KH. Interaction of spironolactone with ACE inhibitors or angiotensin receptor blockers: analysis of 44 cases. *BMJ* (2003) 327, 147–9.
3. Speirs CJ, Dollery CT, Inman WHW, Rawson NSB, Wilton LV. Postmarketing surveillance of enalapril. II: Investigation of the potential role of enalapril in deaths with renal failure. *BMJ* (1988) 297, 830–2.
4. Lakhani M. Complete heart block induced by hyperkalaemia associated with treatment with a combination of captopril and spironolactone. *BMJ* (1986) 293, 271.
5. Lo TCN, Cryer RJ. Complete heart block induced by hyperkalaemia associated with treatment with a combination of captopril and spironolactone. *BMJ* (1986) 292, 1672.
6. Odawara M, Asano M, Yamashita K. Life-threatening hyperkalaemia caused by angiotensin-converting enzyme inhibitor and diuretics. *Diabet Med* (1997) 14, 169–70.
7. Vanpee D, Swine C. Elderly heart failure patients with drug-induced serious hyperkalemia. *Aging Clin Exp Res* (2000) 12, 315–19.
8. Dahlström U, Karlsson E. Captopril and spironolactone therapy for refractory congestive heart failure. *Am J Cardiol* (1993) 71, 29A–33A.
9. The RALES Investigators. Effectiveness of spironolactone added to an angiotensin-converting enzyme inhibitor and a loop diuretic for severe chronic congestive heart failure (The Randomized Aldactone Evaluation Study [RALES]). *Am J Cardiol* (1996) 78, 902–7.
10. Pitt B, Zannad F, Remme WJ, Cody R, Castaigne A, Perez A, Palensky J, Wittes J, for the Randomized Aldactone Evaluation Study Investigators. The effect of spironolactone on morbidity and mortality in patients with severe heart failure. *N Engl J Med* (1999) 341, 709–17.
11. Berry C, McMurray J. Life-threatening hyperkalemia during combined therapy with angiotensin-converting enzyme inhibitors and spironolactone. *Am J Med* (2001) 111, 587.
12. Burnakis TG, Mioduch HJ. Combined therapy with captopril and potassium supplementation. A potential for hyperkalemia. *Arch Intern Med* (1984) 144, 2371–2.
13. Chiu T-F, Bullard MJ, Chen J-C, Liaw S-J, Ng C-J. Rapid life-threatening hyperkalemia after addition of amiloride HCl/hydrochlorothiazide to angiotensin-converting enzyme inhibitor therapy. *Ann Emerg Med* (1997) 30, 612–15.
14. Johnston RT, de Bono DP, Nyman CR. Preventable sudden death in patients receiving angiotensin converting enzyme inhibitors and loop/potassium sparing diuretic combinations. *Int J Cardiol* (1992) 34, 213–15.
15. Brown C, Rush J. Risk factors for the development of hyperkalemia in patients treated with enalapril for heart failure. *Clin Pharmacol Ther* (1989) 45, 167.
16. Radley AS, Fitzpatrick RW. An evaluation of the potential interaction between enalapril and amiloride. *J Clin Pharm Ther* (1987) 12, 319–23.
17. Schuna AA, Schmidt GR, Pitterle ME. Serum potassium concentrations after initiation of captopril therapy. *Clin Pharm* (1986) 5, 920–3.
18. Aldactone (Spironolactone). Pharmacia Ltd. UK Summary of product characteristics, March 2004.
19. Jarman PR, Keheley AM, Mather HM. Life-threatening hyperkalaemia caused by ACE inhibitor and diuretics. *Diabet Med* (1997) 14, 808.

ACE inhibitors or Angiotensin II receptor antagonists + Epoetin

Epoetin may cause hypertension and thereby reduce the effects of antihypertensive drugs. An additive hyperkalaemic effect is theoretically possible with ACE inhibitors or angiotensin II receptor antagonists and epoetin. It is not entirely clear whether captopril, enalapril, fosinopril or other ACE inhibitors affect the efficacy of epoetin or not, but any interaction may take many months to develop.

Clinical evidence

(A) Antihypertensive effects opposed

The most frequent adverse effect of epoetin is an increase in blood pressure, so it is important to control any existing hypertension before epoetin is started (the makers contraindicate epoetin in uncontrolled hypertension). Blood pressure should be monitored before and during epoetin treatment, and if necessary antihypertensive drug treatment should be started or increased if the pressure rises.[1]

(B) Epoetin efficacy

(a) Decreased epoetin effects

In a retrospective analysis of 43 haemodialysis patients given epoetin regularly for about 10 months, the dose of epoetin was not significantly different between patients on **captopril** (20 patients) and a control group (23 patients) who did not receive any ACE inhibitors (116.7 versus 98.3 units/kg per week, respectively). However, the haemoglobin and haematocrit values were significantly less at 6.2 mmol/l and 29.3% in the **captopril** group than the values of 7.1 mmol/l and 33.3% in the control group.[2] Another retrospective study of 40 dialysis patients found that the 20 patients taking an ACE inhibitor (**captopril** 12.5 to 75 mg daily, **enalapril** 2.5 to 5 mg daily or **fosinopril** 10 to 20 mg daily) showed some evidence of increased epoetin requirements after 1 year when compared with the control group. However, this was not significant until 15 months when the cumulative epoetin dosage requirements were about doubled (12092 versus 6449 units/kg).[3] Similarly, a prospective study with a 12-month follow-up period found that 20 patients receiving **enalapril** 5 to 20 mg daily required significantly higher doses of epoetin compared with 20 patients receiving nifedipine or 20 patients receiving no antihypertensive therapy.[4] Higher epoetin requirements with ACE inhibitors were also reported in a small study in peritoneal dialysis patients.[5] Furthermore, another prospective study found that 15 patients in whom ACE inhibitors (**enalapril**, **captopril**, or **perindopril**) were withdrawn and replaced with amlodipine, felodipine or doxazosin, showed an increase in mean haematocrit level and a decrease in mean epoetin dose requirement.[6]

(b) No interaction

A retrospective review of 14 haemodialysis patients receiving epoetin, compared the haematocrit and dosage of epoetin for 16 weeks before and 16 weeks after starting ACE inhibitors (8 on **captopril,** mean dose 35 mg daily and 6 on **enalapril,** mean dose 7.85 mg daily). This study failed to find any evidence of a clinically significant interaction when ACE inhibitors were added.[7] Another study involving 17 patients on chronic haemodialysis found that ACE inhibitors (5 **captopril**, 12 **enalapril**) for 3 and 12 months did not increase the epoetin dose requirements or reduce the haematocrits.[8] However, given the results of the study[3] reported in *(a)* above, it is possible that these studies were not continued for long enough to detect an effect. Another study in 14 haemodialysis patients found no difference in epoetin requirements between patients receiving **losartan**

25 mg daily or placebo,[9] but again the **losartan** was only given for 3 months. A further study [length not specified] involving 604 dialysis patients also found that the use of ACE inhibitors or angiotensin II receptor blockers was not associated with epoetin resistance.[10]

(c) ACE inhibitors compared with Angiotensin II receptor antagonists

In a prospective study in 25 patients who had been undergoing haemodialysis for more than one year, 12 patients were given **temocapril** 2 mg daily and 13 patients received **losartan** 25 to 50 mg daily for 12 months. **Temocapril** significantly decreased blood haemoglobin levels from 9.8 to 9.1 g/dl at 3 months and reached a minimum of 9 g/dl at 6 months; haemoglobin levels recovered to 9.7 g/dl at the end of the study by increasing the dosage of epoetin. In contrast, no change was found in haemoglobin values in the patients receiving **losartan.** The dosage of epoetin was gradually increased from 76 to 121 units/kg per week in the **temocapril** group, but in the **losartan** group the epoetin dose was not significantly increased (94 versus 101 units/kg per week).[11] Similar results were found with **captopril** and **losartan**.[12]

(C) Hyperkalaemia

The maker of epoetin beta comments that potassium elevation has been reported in a few uraemic patients receiving epoetin and that serum potassium levels should be monitored regularly.[1] An additive hyperkalaemic effect is, therefore, theoretically possible with patients also receiving ACE inhibitors or angiotensin II receptor antagonists.

Mechanism

(A). Epoetin can cause hypertension, possibly associated with haemodynamic changes produced by the increase in haematocrit.[13]

(B). It has been argued that ACE inhibitors might possibly reduce the efficacy of epoetin in haemodialysis patients for several reasons. Firstly, because patients with chronic renal failure show haematocrit falls when given ACE inhibitors, secondly because ACE inhibitors reduce polycythaemia following renal transplantation, and thirdly because ACE inhibitors reduce the plasma levels of endogenous erythropoietin.[2,7,14] Many other factors have also been proposed.[15]

(C). Drugs that block angiotensin II cause reduced levels of aldosterone, which results in the retention of potassium. This would be expected to be additive with other drugs that cause hyperkalaemia.

Importance and management

Blood pressure should be routinely monitored on patients on epoetin, and this monitoring would seem sufficient to detect any adverse interaction with ACE inhibitors. The dose of ACE inhibitor may need to be increased, but if blood pressure rises cannot be controlled, a transient interruption of epoetin therapy is recommended. Potassium levels should also be monitored if epoetin is given with ACE inhibitors. If potassium levels rise, consider ceasing epoetin until the level is corrected.[1]

The overall picture of the effect of ACE inhibitors on epoetin resistance is unclear, and it would seem that an interaction, if it happens, takes a long time to develop. As epoetin dosage is governed by response, no immediate intervention is necessary. The major implication of this interaction is probably cost, as ultimately higher doses of epoetin appear to be needed in patients on ACE inhibitors. More long-term study is needed. Preliminary evidence suggests that **losartan** may not interact,[11,15] but the evidence is too slim to draw any definite conclusions.

1. NeoRecormon (Epoetin beta). Roche Products Ltd. UK Summary of product characteristics, February 2004.
2. Walter J. Does captopril decrease the effect of human recombinant erythropoietin in haemodialysis patients? *Nephrol Dial Transplant* (1993) 8, 1428.
3. Heß E, Sperschneider H, Stein G. Do ACE inhibitors influence the dose of human recombinant erythropoietin in dialysis patients? *Nephrol Dial Transplant* (1996) 11, 749–51.
4. Albitar S, Genin R, Fen-Chong M, Serveaux M-O, Bourgeon B. High dose enalapril impairs the response to erythropoietin treatment in haemodialysis patients. *Nephrol Dial Transplant* (1998) 13, 1206–10.
5. Mora C, Navarro JF. Negative effect of angiotensin-converting enzyme inhibitors on erythropoietin response in CAPD patients. *Am J Nephrol* (2000) 20 248.
6. Ertürk Ş, Nergizoğlu G, AteŞ K, Duman N, Erbay B, Karatan O, Ertuğ AE. The impact of withdrawing ACE inhibitors on erythropoietin responsiveness and left ventricular hypertrophy in haemodialysis patients. *Nephrol Dial Transplant* (1999) 14, 1912–16.
7. Conlon PJ, Albers F, Butterly D, Schwab SJ. ACE inhibitors do not affect erythropoietin efficacy in haemodialysis patients. *Nephrol Dial Transplant* (1994) 9, 1358.
8. Schwenk MH, Jumani AQ, Rosenberg CR, Kulogowski JE, Charytan C, Spinowitz BS. Potential angiotensin-converting enzyme inhibitor–epoetin alfa interaction in patients receiving chronic hemodialysis. *Pharmacotherapy* (1998) 18, 627–30.
9. Chew CG, Weise MD, Disney APS. The effect of angiotensin II receptor antagonist on the exogenous erythropoietin requirement of haemodialysis patients. *Nephrol Dial Transplant* (1999) 14, 2047–9.
10. Saudan P, Halabi G, Perneger T, Wasserfallen J-B, Wauters J-P, Martin P-Y. Use of ace inhibitors or angiotensin II receptors blockers is not associated with erythropoietin resistance in dialysis patients. *J Am Soc Nephrol* (2002) 13, 443A.
11. Kato A, Takita T, Furuhashi M, Takahashi T, Maruyama Y, Hishida A. No effect of losartan on response to erythropoietin therapy in patients undergoing hemodialysis. *Nephron* (2000) 86, 538–9.
12. Schiffl H, Lang SM. Angiotensin-converting enzyme inhibitors but not angiotensin II AT 1 receptor antagonists affect erythropoiesis in patients with anemia of end-stage renal disease. *Nephron* (1999) 81, 106–8.
13. Sweetman SC, editor. Martindale: The complete drug reference. 34th ed. London: Pharmaceutical Press; 2005. p. 747.
14. Pratt MC, Lewis-Barned NJ, Walker RJ, Bailey RR, Shand BI, Livesey J. Effect of angiotensin converting enzyme inhibitors on erythropoietin concentrations in healthy volunteers. *Br J Clin Pharmacol* (1992) 34, 363–5.
15. Macdougall IC. ACE inhibitors and erythropoietin responsiveness. *Am J Kidney Dis* (2001) 38, 649–51.

ACE inhibitors + Food

Food has little or no effect on the absorption of the ACE inhibitors cilazapril, enalapril, fosinopril, lisinopril, quinapril, ramipril, spirapril, and trandolapril. Although food may reduce the absorption of captopril and moexipril, this does not appear to be clinically important. Food reduced the absorption of imidapril, and reduced the conversion of perindopril to perindoprilat, and the makers recommend these drugs be administered before food.

Clinical evidence, mechanism, importance and management

(a) No interaction

Although food reduced the AUC of **captopril** 25 to 100 mg by up to 56%[1-4] this had no effect on the maximum decrease in blood pressure.[1,3,4] One study in 10 healthy subjects reported a one-hour delay in the maximum hypotensive effect.[1] Another study, in 10 hypertensive patients, found that the extent and duration of antihypertensive efficacy of **captopril** 50 mg twice daily for one month was not affected by whether the drug was taken before or after food.[5] However, decreasing the dose of an ACE inhibitor might reduce the duration of the hypotensive effect and it has been suggested that these results should be confirmed with lower doses of **captopril**.[5]

Other single-dose studies have shown that food had no statistically significant effect on the pharmacokinetics of **enalapril**, and its active metabolite, enalaprilat,[6] or on **lisinopril**.[7] Similarly, food had minimal effects on the pharmacokinetics of **cilazapril** (AUC decreased by only 14%).[8] Food caused small, but statistically significant increases in the time to reach maximum plasma concentrations for **quinapril** and its active metabolite However, as the increase was less than 30 minutes this is not expected to alter the therapeutic effect.[9] Likewise, the makers of **spirapril** briefly mention in a review that food delayed the absorption of **spirapril** by 1 hour, but did not affect the bioavailability of **spirapril** or spiraprilat, its active metabolite.[10] Other makers state that food had no effect on the absorption of **fosinopril**,[11,12] or **ramipril**.[13,14]

(b) Possible interaction

In one study food reduced the AUC of **moexipril** by 40 to 50%.[15] Food did not reduce **moexipril**-induced ACE-inhibition and therefore the reduced bioavailability was not expected to be clinically relevant.[16] However, the US makers suggest taking moexipril 1 hour before food.[17] Although food did not significantly affect the pharmacokinetics of a single 4-mg oral dose of **perindopril,** the AUC of its active metabolite perindoprilat was reduced by 44%.[18] The blood-pressure lowering effects were not assessed, but it seems possible that they would not be affected (see captopril, above). Nevertheless, the maker recommends that **perindopril** should be taken before a meal.[19] The maker of **imidapril** states that a fat-rich meal significantly reduces the absorption of **imidapril**, and recommends that the drug be taken at the same time each day, about 15 minutes before a meal.[20]

1. Mäntylä R, Männistö PT, Vuorela A, Sundberg S, Ottoila P. Impairment of captopril bioavailability by concomitant food and antacid intake. *Int J Clin Pharmacol Ther Toxicol* (1984) 22, 626–9.
2. Singhvi SM, McKinstry DN, Shaw JM, Willard DA, Migdalof BH. Effect of food on the bioavailability of captopril in healthy subjects. *J Clin Pharmacol* (1982) 22, 135–40.
3. Öhman KP, Kågedal B, Larsson R, Karlberg BE. Pharmacokinetics of captopril and its effects on blood pressure during acute and chronic administration and in relation to food intake. *J Cardiovasc Pharmacol* (1985) 7 (Suppl 1), S20–S24.
4. Müller H-M, Overlack A, Heck I, Kolloch R, Stumpe KO. The influence of food intake on pharmacodynamics and plasma concentration of captopril. *J Hypertens* (1985) 3 (Suppl 2), S135–S136.

5. Salvetti A, Pedrinelli R, Magagna A, Abdel-Haq B, Graziadei L, Taddei S, Stornello M. Influence of food on acute and chronic effects of captopril in essential hypertensive patients. *J Cardiovasc Pharmacol* (1985) 7 (Suppl 1), S25–S29.
6. Swanson BN, Vlasses PH, Ferguson RK, Bergquist PA, Till AE, Irvin JD, Harris K. Influence of food on the bioavailability of enalapril. *J Pharm Sci* (1984) 73, 1655–7.
7. Mojaverian P, Rocci ML, Vlasses PH, Hoholick C, Clementi RA, Ferguson RK. Effect of food on the bioavailability of lisinopril, a nonsulfhydryl angiotensin-converting enzyme inhibitor. *J Pharm Sci* (1986) 75, 395–7.
8. Massarella JW, DeFeo TM, Brown AN, Lin A, Wills RJ. The influence of food on the pharmacokinetics and ACE inhibition of cilazapril. *Br J Clin Pharmacol* (1989) 27, 205S–209S.
9. Ferry JJ, Horvath AM, Sedman AJ, Latts JR, Colburn WA. Influence of food on the pharmacokinetics of quinapril and its active diacid metabolite, CI-928. *J Clin Pharmacol* (1987) 27, 397–9.
10. Grass P, Gerbeau C, Kutz K. Spirapril: pharmacokinetic properties and drug interactions. *Blood Pressure* (1994) 3 (Suppl 2), 7–13.
11. Staril (Fosinopril). E. R. Squibb & Sons Ltd. UK Summary of product characteristics, June 2005.
12. Monopril (Fosinopril). Bristol-Myers Squibb Company. US Prescribing information, July 2003.
13. Tritace (Ramipril). Aventis Pharma Ltd. UK Summary of product characteristics, July 2003.
14. Altace (Ramipril). Monarch Pharmaceuticals Inc. US Prescribing information, September 2004.
15. Perdix (Moexipril). Schwarz Pharma. Product Monograph, October 1995.
16. Stimpel M, Cawello W. Pharmacokinetics and ACE-inhibition of the new ACE-inhibitor moexipril: is coadministration with food of clinical relevance? *Hypertension* (1995) 25, 1384.
17. Univasc (Moexipril). Schwarz Pharma. US Prescribing information, May 2003.
18. Lecocq B, Funck-Brentano C, Lecocq V, Ferry A, Gardin M-E, Devissaguet M, Jaillon P. Influence of food on the pharmacokinetics of perindopril and the time course of angiotensin-converting enzyme inhibition in serum. *Clin Pharmacol Ther* (1990) 47, 397–402.
19. Coversyl (Perindopril). Servier Laboratories Ltd. UK Summary of product characteristics, February 2003.
20. Tanatril (Imidapril). Trinity Pharmaceuticals Ltd. UK Summary of product characteristics, May 2003.

ACE inhibitors + Garlic

A patient on lisinopril developed marked hypotension and became faint after taking garlic capsules.

Clinical evidence, mechanism, importance and management

A man whose blood pressure was 135/90 mmHg while on **lisinopril** 15 mg daily began to take garlic 4 mg daily (*Boots odourless garlic oil capsules*). After 3 days he became faint on standing and was found to have a blood pressure of 90/60 mmHg. Stopping the garlic restored his blood pressure to 135/90 mmHg within a week. The garlic on its own did not lower his blood pressure. The reasons for this interaction are not known, although garlic has been reported to cause vasodilatation and blood pressure reduction.[1] This seems to be the first and only report of this reaction, so its general importance is small. There seems to be nothing documented about garlic and any of the other ACE inhibitors.

1. McCoubrie M. Doctors as patients: lisinopril and garlic. *Br J Gen Pract* (1996) 46, 107.

ACE inhibitors + Gold

Peripheral vasodilatation has occurred in some patients on gold therapy when given ACE inhibitors.

Clinical evidence, mechanism, importance and management

A report describes 4 patients on long-term gold therapy for rheumatoid arthritis who developed nitritoid reactions (adverse effects associated with **sodium aurothiomalate** treatment consisting of facial flushing, nausea, dizziness, and occasionally, hypotension, as a result of peripheral vasodilatation). These reactions occurred soon after starting treatment with an ACE inhibitor (**captopril**, **enalapril**, or **lisinopril**). All the patients had been receiving a monthly injection of **sodium aurothiomalate** 50 mg for at least 2 years and none had ever had such a reaction before. The reactions were controlled by changing treatment to aurothioglucose (1 patient), discontinuing the ACE inhibitor (2), or reducing the dose of **sodium aurothiomalate** to 25 mg (1).[1] There appear to be few reports of this interaction, possibly because the nitritoid reaction is an established adverse effect of gold therapy. However, a possible interaction should be borne in mind if a patient experiences these reactions and is also taking an ACE inhibitor.

1. Healey LA, Backes MB, Mason V. Nitritoid reactions and angiotensin-converting-enzyme inhibitors. *N Engl J Med* (1989) 321, 763.

ACE inhibitors + H_2-blockers

No clinically important adverse interactions have been seen between cimetidine and captopril, enalapril, fosinopril, moexipril, quinapril or spirapril, or between H_2-blockers and cilazapril. Cimetidine modestly reduced the bioavailability of temocapril.

Clinical evidence, mechanism, importance and management

Cimetidine did not appear to alter the pharmacokinetics or pharmacological effects of **captopril**[1] or **enalapril**,[2] or the pharmacokinetics of **fosinopril**[3] or **quinapril**[4] in healthy subjects. The makers of **cilazapril** found no clinically significant interaction following the use of H_2-blockers[5] and the makers of **moexipril** say that no important pharmacokinetic interaction occurred with **cimetidine**.[6,7] The makers of **spirapril** briefly note in a review that **cimetidine** did not alter the plasma concentrations of **spirapril** or its active metabolite spiraprilat.[8] None of these pairs of drugs appears to interact to a clinically relevant extent, and no special precautions appear to be necessary.

Preliminary findings suggest **cimetidine** 400 mg twice daily had no effect on the metabolism of **temocapril** 20 mg daily in 18 healthy subjects, but the AUC was reduced by 26% on the fifth day of concurrent treatment.[9] The clinical relevance of this is uncertain, bear this interaction in mind if the effects of **temocapril** seem inadequate.

1. Richer C, Bah M, Cadilhac M, Thuillez C, Giudicelli JF. Cimetidine does not alter free unchanged captopril pharmacokinetics and biological effects in healthy volunteer. *J Pharmacol* (1986) 17, 338–42.
2. Ishizaki T, Baba T, Murabayashi S, Kubota K, Hara K, Kurimoto F. Effect of cimetidine on the pharmacokinetics and pharmacodynamics of enalapril in normal volunteers. *J Cardiovasc Pharmacol* (1988) 12, 512–9.
3. Moore L, Kramer A, Swites B, Kramer P, Tu J. Effect of cimetidine and antacid on the kinetics of the active diacid of fosinopril in healthy subjects. *J Clin Pharmacol* (1988) 28, 946.
4. Ferry JJ, Cetnarowski AB, Sedman AJ, Thomas RW, Horvath AM. Multiple-dose cimetidine administration does not influence the single-dose pharmacokinetics of quinapril and its active metabolite (CI-928). *J Clin Pharmacol* (1988) 28, 48–51.
5. Vascace (Cilazapril). Roche Products Ltd. UK Summary of product characteristics, November 2002.
6. Perdix (Moexipril). Schwarz Pharma Ltd. UK Summary of product characteristics, May 2005.
7. Univasc (Moexipril). Schwarz Pharma. US Prescribing information, May 2003.
8. Grass P, Gerbeau C, Kutz K. Spirapril: pharmacokinetic properties and drug interactions. *Blood Pressure* (1994) 3 (Suppl 2), 7–13.
9. Trenk D, Schaefer A, Eberle E, Jähnchen E. Effect of cimetidine on the pharmacokinetics of the ACE-inhibitor temocapril. *Eur J Clin Pharmacol* (1996) 50, 556.

ACE inhibitors or Angiotensin II receptor antagonists + Heparins

Heparin may increase the risk of hyperkalaemia with ACE inhibitors or angiotensin II receptor antagonists.

Clinical evidence, mechanism, importance and management

An extensive review of the literature found that heparin (both **unfractionated** and **low molecular weight heparins**) and **heparinoids** inhibit the secretion of aldosterone, which can cause hyperkalaemia.[1] The UK Committee on Safety of Medicines suggests that plasma-potassium concentrations should be measured in all patients with risk factors (including those taking potassium sparing drugs) before starting heparin, and monitored regularly thereafter, particularly if heparin is to be continued for more than 7 days.[2] Some workers[1] have suggested that the monitoring interval should probably be no greater than 4 days in patients at relatively high risk for hyperkalaemia. Other risk factors include renal insufficiency, diabetes mellitus, pre-existing acidosis or raised plasma potassium.[2] Most makers of ACE inhibitors and angiotensin II receptor antagonists also recommend monitoring potassium levels, but some UK makers recommend avoiding concurrent use,[3,4] although this seems to be somewhat of an over-reaction.

If hyperkalaemia occurs, the offending drugs should be stopped (although this may not be practical in the case of heparin). When the hyperkalaemia has been corrected (by whatever medical intervention is deemed appropriate) the drugs can cautiously be reintroduced.

1. Oster JR, Singer I, Fishman LM. Heparin-induced aldosterone suppression and hyperkalemia. *Am J Med* (1995) 98, 575–86.
2. Committee on Safety of Medicines/Medicines Control Agency. Suppression of aldosterone secretion by heparin. *Current Problems* (1999) 25, 6.

3. Aprovel (Irbesartan). Sanofi Synthelabo. UK Summary of product characteristics, August 2004.

4. Olmetec (Olmesartan). Sankyo Pharma UK Ltd. UK Summary of product characteristics, August 2004.

ACE inhibitors + Insect allergen extracts

There is an increased risk of anaphylactoid reactions in patients receiving ACE inhibitors during desensitisation with bee or wasp venom.

Clinical evidence, mechanism, importance and management

A report describes 2 cases of **enalapril**-induced anaphylactoid reactions during **wasp venom immunotherapy**. In one patient generalised pruritus and severe hypotension occurred within a few minutes of the first administration of the **venom**. Desensitisation was achieved after the **enalapril** was stopped, and then the immunotherapy was maintained by discontinuing the **enalapril** 24 hours before the monthly **venom** injection. However, on one occasion, when the **enalapril** had not been stopped, the patient experienced a severe anaphylactoid reaction 30 minutes after the **venom** injection. In the other patient an anaphylactoid reaction occurred after the second dose of **venom**. The ACE inhibitor was replaced with nifedipine so that **venom immunotherapy** could be achieved. It was thought that a decrease in the breakdown of bradykinin due to the ACE inhibitor combined with increased histamine release during immunotherapy could have caused the anaphylactoid reactions.[1]

Several makers of ACE inhibitors warn that life-threatening anaphylactoid reactions have been rarely reported in patients undergoing desensitising treatment with **Hymenoptera** (bee or wasp) **venom** whilst also receiving an ACE inhibitor and therefore caution should be used in such patients. It has also been suggested that similar reactions may occur after an insect bite.[2] Some makers advise temporarily withholding the ACE inhibitor prior to each desensitisation, while others suggest substitution of a different antihypertensive agent e.g. a calcium channel blocker. Beta-blockers are not recommended because they may reduce the efficacy of adrenaline (epinephrine) in the treatment of hypersensitivity reactions.[3]

1. Tunon-de-Lara JM, Villanueva P, Marcos M, Taytard A. ACE inhibitors and anaphylactoid reactions during venom immunotherapy. *Lancet* (1992) 340, 908.

2. Tanatril (Imidapril). Trinity Pharmaceuticals Ltd. UK Summary of product characteristics, May 2003.

3. Sweetman SC, editor. Martindale: The complete drug reference. 34th ed. London: Pharmaceutical Press; 2005. p. 853.

ACE inhibitors + Interleukin-3

Marked hypotension can occur when patients on ACE inhibitors are given interleukin-3.

Clinical evidence, mechanism, importance and management

Twenty-six patients with ovarian or small-cell undifferentiated cancers were treated with chemotherapy followed by recombinant human interleukin-3. Three of the 26 were taking ACE inhibitors (not named) and all three developed marked hypotension (WHO toxicity grade 2 or 3) within 1 to 4 hours of the first interleukin-3 injection. Their blood pressures returned to normal while continuing the interleukin-3 when the ACE inhibitors were stopped. When the interleukin-3 was stopped, they once again needed the ACE inhibitors to control their blood pressure. None of the other 23 patients showed hypotension except one who did so during a period of neutropenic fever.[1] The authors of the report suggest (and present some supporting evidence) that the drugs act synergistically to generate large amounts of nitric oxide in the blood vessel walls. This relaxes the smooth muscle in the blood vessel walls causing vasodilatation and consequent hypotension.[1] Information seems to be limited to this single report, but it would be prudent to monitor blood pressure even more closely in patients receiving interleukin-3 while taking ACE inhibitors.

1. Dercksen MW, Hoekman K, Visser JJ, ten Bokkel Huinink WW, Pinedo HM, Wagstaff J. Hypotension induced by interleukin-3 in patients on angiotensin-converting enzyme inhibitors. *Lancet* (1995) 345, 448.

ACE inhibitors + Iron compounds

Serious systemic reactions occurred in three patients given infusions of ferric sodium gluconate while taking enalapril. Oral ferrous sulfate may decrease absorption of captopril, but this is probably of little clinical importance.

Clinical evidence

(a) Intravenous iron

A man with iron-deficiency anaemia on furosemide and digoxin was given 125 mg of **ferric sodium gluconate** (*Ferlixit*) intravenously in 100 ml of saline daily. Four days later, **enalapril** 5 mg daily was started. After the infusion of only a few drops of his next dose of **ferric sodium gluconate**, he developed diffuse erythema, abdominal cramps, hypotension, nausea and vomiting. He recovered after being given hydrocortisone 200 mg. Three days later, in the absence of the **enalapril**, he recommenced the iron infusions for a further 10 days without problems, and was later treated uneventfully with the **enalapril**.[1] Two other patients taking **enalapril** reacted similarly when given intravenous infusions of **ferric sodium gluconate**. Neither was given any more intravenous iron and later had no problems while taking **enalapril** alone. During the same 13-month period in which these three cases occurred, 15 other patients, who were not taking ACE inhibitors, also received intravenous iron therapy with no adverse reactions.[2] In contrast, a randomised, crossover study involving 1117 dialysis patients given a placebo or a single intravenous dose of 125 mg of **ferric sodium gluconate complex** (*Ferrlecit*) in sucrose, found no evidence of any significant interaction in the 308 patients taking ACE inhibitors.[3]

(b) Oral iron

A double-blind study in 7 healthy subjects, given single 300-mg doses of **ferrous sulfate** or placebo with **captopril** 25 mg, found that the AUC of unconjugated plasma **captopril** (the active form) was reduced by 37% although the maximum plasma levels were not substantially changed. The AUC of total plasma **captopril** was increased by 43%, although this was not statistically significant. There were no significant differences in blood pressure between treatment and placebo groups.[4]

Mechanism

(a). Uncertain. Intravenous iron may cause a variety of systemic reactions including fever, myalgia, arthralgia, hypotension, nausea and vomiting, which are believed to be due to the release of various inflammatory mediators such as bradykinin, caused by iron-catalysed toxic free radicals. The authors of the report suggest that ACE inhibitors like enalapril decrease the breakdown of kinins so that the toxic effects of the iron become exaggerated.[2]

(b). Reduced levels of unconjugated captopril in the plasma are probably due to reduced absorption resulting from a chemical interaction between ferric ions and captopril in the gastrointestinal tract.[4]

Importance and management

(a). The interaction with intravenous iron is not firmly established because about 25% of all patients given iron by this route develop a variety of systemic reactions, ranging from mild to serious anaphylactoid reactions. In addition, other workers have not found any interaction. However, be aware that there may be an increased risk of anaphylactoid reactions if intravenous iron is given to patients taking any ACE inhibitor.[2]

(b). There is limited evidence that orally administered iron may reduce the absorption of captopril. The clinical relevance of this is unknown, but probably small. Information about the effect of oral iron on other ACE inhibitors is lacking.

1. Rolla G. Personal communication, 1994.

2. Rolla G, Bucca C, Brussino L. Systemic reactions to intravenous iron therapy in patients receiving angiotensin converting enzyme inhibitor. *J Allergy Clin Immunol* (1994) 93, 1074–5.

3. Warnock DG, Adkinson F, Coyne DW, Strobos J, Ferrlecit® Safety Study Group. ACE inhibitors and intravenous sodium ferric gluconate complex in sucrose (SFGC): lack of any significant interaction. *J Am Soc Nephrol* (2000) 11, 170A.

4. Schaefer JP, Tam Y, Hasinoff BB, Tawfik S, Peng Y, Reimche L, Campbell NRC. Ferrous sulphate interacts with captopril. *Br J Clin Pharmacol* (1998) 46, 377–81.

ACE inhibitors + Moracizine

Moracizine causes some moderate alterations in the pharmacokinetics of free captopril, but these are unlikely to be clinically important.

Clinical evidence, mechanism, importance and management

In a pharmacokinetic study, 19 healthy subjects were given moracizine 250 mg or **captopril** 50 mg, both 8-hourly, either alone or together, for 3 treatment periods of 22 doses. When taken together the pharmacokinetics of the moracizine and total **captopril** remained unchanged, but the maximum blood levels of the free **captopril** and its AUC decreased by 32 and 14%, respectively. The half-life of the free **captopril** was shortened by 44%.[1] These modest changes are unlikely to be clinically relevant. There seem to be no reports of adverse reactions when both drugs have been used together.

1. Pieniaszek HJ, Shum L, Widner P, Garner DM, Benedek IH. Pharmacokinetic interaction of moricizine and captopril in healthy volunteers. *J Clin Pharmacol* (1993) 33, 1005.

ACE inhibitors + NSAIDs

Although some variation between drugs occurs, on the whole, the NSAIDs appear to slightly affect the blood pressure lowering effects of the ACE inhibitors. Indometacin appears to have the most significant effect. The combination of NSAID and ACE inhibitor may increase the risk of renal impairment. Rarely, hyperkalaemia has been associated with the combination.

Clinical evidence

(A) Effects on blood pressure

(a) Celecoxib

In a double-blind study in hypertensive patients treated with **lisinopril** 10 to 40 mg daily, celecoxib did not have a clinically or statistically significant effect on blood pressure. The 24-hour blood pressure increased by 2.6/1.5 mmHg in 91 patients treated with celecoxib 200 mg twice daily for 4 weeks compared with 1/0.3 mmHg in 87 patients receiving placebo.[1] In another study involving 810 elderly patients with osteoarthritis and controlled hypertension given either celecoxib 200 mg or rofecoxib 25 mg daily for 6 weeks, approximately 40% of the patients randomised to the celecoxib group were receiving ACE inhibitors. Systolic blood pressure increased by a clinically significant amount (greater than 20 mmHg) in 11% of patients receiving celecoxib,[2] while in another study, only 4 of 87 (4.6%) of hypertensive patients stabilised on ACE inhibitors had clinically significant increases in blood pressure after taking celecoxib 200 mg twice daily for 4 weeks.[3] A further study in 25 hypertensive patients with osteoarthritis stabilised on trandolapril (with or without hydrochlorothiazide) found that the 24-hour blood pressure was not significantly increased by celecoxib 200 mg daily but at its peak activity celecoxib increased diastolic and systolic blood pressure by about 5/4 mmHg respectively.[4]

(b) Ibuprofen

Ibuprofen 400 mg every 8 hours has been found to interfere with the efficacy of **antihypertensive drugs** in some patients with mild-moderate hypertension, when compared with paracetamol or placebo.[5] The addition of ibuprofen therapy for 4 weeks in 90 patients stabilised on ACE inhibitors resulted in clinically significant increases in blood pressure in 15 of the patients. For the group as a whole, diastolic blood pressure was increased by 3.5 mmHg.[3] In one single-dose study, ibuprofen 800 mg or indometacin 50 mg abolished the hypotensive effect of **captopril** 50 mg in 8 healthy subjects when they were on a high sodium diet, but not when they were on a low sodium diet.[6] A case report describes attenuation of the antihypertensive effects of **captopril** by ibuprofen in an elderly woman.[7] However, a study in 17 black women found that ibuprofen 800 mg three times daily for one month did not alter the antihypertensive effect of **fosinopril** 10 to 40 mg daily when given with hydrochlorothiazide 25 mg daily. It was thought that the diuretic might have enhanced salt depletion and renin stimulation making the antihypertensive action of the combination less prostaglandin dependent.[8]

(c) Indometacin

(i) Captopril. In a randomised, double-blind study, 105 patients with hypertension received captopril 25 to 50 mg twice daily for 6 weeks, which reduced their blood pressure by a mean of 8.6/5.6 mmHg. Indometacin 75 mg once daily was then added for one week, which caused a rise in blood pressure in the group as a whole of 4.6/2.7 mmHg (an attenuation of the effect of captopril of about 50%). Clear attenuation was seen in 67% of the patients, and occurred regardless of baseline blood pressure.[9] This same interaction has been described in numerous earlier studies in patients with hypertension and in healthy subjects given indometacin.[6,10-17] A case is described of a man whose blood pressure was well controlled on captopril 75 mg daily. His blood pressure rose from 145/80 mmHg to 220/120 mmHg when he self-medicated with indometacin suppositories 200 mg daily.[18] In contrast, a randomised, placebo-controlled, crossover study in 11 patients found that indometacin 50 mg twice daily did not alter the antihypertensive efficacy of captopril 50 mg twice daily.[19]

(ii) Enalapril. Indometacin 50 mg twice daily for 1 week significantly reduced the antihypertensive effect of enalapril 20 to 40 mg once daily by about 18 to 22% in 9 patients with hypertension.[20] In another study in 18 patients, indometacin 25 mg three times daily attenuated the antihypertensive effect of enalapril 20 to 40 mg daily. The reduction in hypotensive effect was about 42% when assessed by 24-hour ambulatory blood-pressure monitoring (9.4/4.1 mmHg increase in BP with indometacin), and 12 to 23% when assessed by clinic blood pressure monitoring.[21] Similar results were found in other studies.[22-25] A further study in 10 normotensive subjects maintained on fixed sodium intake and given enalapril 20 mg daily with or without indometacin 50 mg twice daily for one week, demonstrated that indometacin reduced the natriuretic response to the ACE inhibitor.[26] A single case report describes a patient on enalapril 10 mg daily whose hypertension failed to be controlled when indometacin 100 mg daily in divided doses was added.[27] However, other studies found indometacin did not significantly alter the blood pressure response to enalapril.[16,19,28]

(iii) Lisinopril. In a placebo-controlled, crossover study, indometacin 50 mg twice daily for 2 weeks produced mean blood pressure increases of 5.5/3.2 mmHg in 56 patients on lisinopril 10 to 20 mg daily.[29] Similarly, results of an earlier study found indometacin increased the blood pressure of 9 patients on lisinopril.[23] In contrast, indometacin 50 mg twice daily for 4 weeks was found to have little effect on the antihypertensive efficacy of lisinopril 40 mg daily in 16 patients when compared with 20 patients who received lisinopril and placebo.[30]

(iv) Other ACE inhibitors. A placebo-controlled, randomised, crossover study in 16 hypertensive patients found that indometacin 50 mg twice daily reduced the blood pressure lowering effects of **cilazapril** 2.5 mg daily. The reduction was greater when **cilazapril** was added to **indometacin** therapy than when indometacin was added to **cilazapril** therapy (approximately 60% vs 30% reduction in hypotensive effect measured 3 hours after the morning dose).[31] The antihypertensive effects of **perindopril** 4 to 8 mg daily were also found to be reduced by about 30% by indometacin 50 mg twice daily in 10 hypertensive patients.[32] A brief mention is made in a review that the pharmacodynamics of **ramipril** were unaffected by 3 days of indometacin (dosage not stated) in healthy subjects.[33] Indometacin 25 mg three times daily did not alter the hypotensive effects of **trandolapril** 2 mg daily in 17 hypertensive patients.[34]

(d) Rofecoxib

The maker of rofecoxib notes that in patients with mild-to-moderate hypertension, administration of rofecoxib 25 mg daily with **benazepril** 10 to 40 mg daily, for four weeks, was associated with a small attenuation of the antihypertensive effect (average increase in mean arterial pressure of 2.8 mmHg) compared with the ACE inhibitor alone.[35] Similarly, a case report describes a patient on **lisinopril** 10 mg daily whose blood pressure rose from 127/78 to 143/89 mmHg when given rofecoxib 25 mg daily. His blood pressure was controlled by increasing the dose of **lisinopril** to 20 mg daily.[36]

In another study involving 810 elderly patients with osteoarthritis and controlled hypertension given either celecoxib 200 mg or rofecoxib 25 mg daily for 6 weeks, approximately 29% of the patients randomised to the rofecoxib group were receiving ACE inhibitors. Systolic blood pressure increased by a clinically significant amount (greater than 20 mmHg) in 17% of the patients receiving rofecoxib.[2]

(e) Sulindac

In one study, sulindac 200 mg twice daily given to patients taking **captopril** 100 to 200 mg twice daily caused only a small rise in blood pressure (from 132/92 to 137/95 mmHg).[12] Sulindac 150 mg twice daily did not attenuate the blood pressure response to **captopril** when substituted for ibuprofen in an elderly woman.[7] Similarly, sulindac 200 mg twice daily did not blunt the antihypertensive effect of **enalapril** in 9 patients with hypertension.[28] A study in 17 black women also found that sulindac 200 mg twice daily for one month did not alter the antihypertensive effect of **fosinopril** 10 to 40 mg daily when given with hydrochlorothiazide 25 mg daily.[8]

(f) Other NSAIDs

A single dose of **lornoxicam** 8 mg was found to have no effect on the systolic blood pressure of 6 hypertensive patients on **enalapril**, but a small rise in diastolic pressure (from 88.2 to 93.3 mmHg) occurred after 2 hours.[22] **Oxaprozin** 1.2 g daily for 3 weeks did not affect the pharmacodynamics of **enalapril** 10 to 40 mg daily in 29 patients with hypertension.[37] Twenty-five hypertensive patients with osteoarthritis and stabilised on trandolapril 2 to 4 mg daily (with or without hydrochlorothiazide) had increases in diastolic and systolic blood pressure of about 3/4 mmHg respectively,during concurrent treatment with **diclofenac** 75 mg twice daily.[4] A study found that only 5 of 91 (5.5%) hypertensive patients stabilised on ACE inhibitors had clinically significant increases in blood pressure during concurrent treatment with **nabumetone** 1 g twice daily for 4 weeks.[3] A study in 17 black women found that **nabumetone** 1 g twice daily for one month did not alter the antihypertensive effect of **fosinopril** 10 to 40 mg daily when given with hydrochlorothiazide.[8]

(B) Effects on renal function

In a retrospective analysis, 3 of 162 patients who had been treated with ACE inhibitors and NSAIDs developed reversible renal failure compared with none of 166 treated with just ACE inhibitors and none of 2116 treated with just NSAIDs. One patient was treated with **naproxen** or **salsalate** and had a progressive decline in renal function over 19 months after **captopril** was started. Another man treated with unnamed **NSAIDs** developed reversible renal failure 4 days after starting to take **captopril**.[38] In another similar analysis, in patients aged over 75 years, 2 out of 12 patients given an **ACE inhibitor** and an **NSAID** developed acute renal failure (1 died) and a further 4 showed deterioration in renal function. All of these 6 patients were also taking **diuretics** but of the 6 with unaffected renal function, only two were taking diuretics.[39] A randomised, crossover study in 17 black patients receiving **fosinopril** with hydrochlorothiazide and **NSAIDs** for a month, found acute renal failure (a decrease in GFR of greater than or equal to 25%) occurred in 4 of the 17 patients when receiving **ibuprofen**, 1 of 17 receiving **sulindac** and 0 of 17 receiving **nabumetone**.[8] In contrast, another retrospective analysis found no evidence that the adverse effects of **ACE inhibitors** on renal function were greater in those taking **NSAIDs**.[40] A further study in 17 hypertensive patients with normal baseline renal function, found that **indometacin** 25 mg three times daily did not adversely affect renal function when used with **trandolapril** 2 mg daily for 3 weeks.[41]

(C) Hyperkalaemia

Hyperkalaemia, resulting in marked bradycardia, was attributed to the use of **loxoprofen** in an elderly woman on **imidapril**.[42] A 77-year-old woman with mild hypertension and normal renal function on **enalapril** 2.5 mg daily arrested and died 5 days after starting treatment with **rofecoxib** for leg pain. Her potassium was found to be 8.8 mmol/L. Although an infection and dehydration could have contributed to the hyperkalaemia in this patient the possibility of a potentially serious interaction, especially in the elderly, should be borne in mind.[43]

(D) Pharmacokinetic studies

The maker of **spirapril** briefly noted in a review that there was no relevant pharmacokinetic interaction between **spirapril** and **diclofenac**.[44] **Oxaprozin** 1.2 g daily for 3 weeks did not affect the pharmacokinetics of **enalapril** 10 to 40 mg daily in 29 patients with hypertension.[37] A brief mention is made in a review that the pharmacokinetics of **ramipril** were unaffected by 3 days of **indometacin** administration (dosage not stated) in healthy subjects.[33]

Mechanism

Some, but not all the evidence suggests that prostaglandins may be involved in the hypotensive action of ACE inhibitors, and that NSAIDs, by inhibiting prostaglandin synthesis, may partially antagonise the effect of ACE inhibitors. Another suggestion is that NSAIDs promote sodium retention and so blunt the blood pressure lowering effects of several classes of antihypertensive drugs including ACE inhibitors. This interaction may be dependent on sodium status and on plasma renin, and so drugs that affect sodium status e.g. diuretics may possibly influence the effect. Therefore, the interaction does not occur in all patients. It may also depend on the NSAID, with indometacin being frequently implicated, and sulindac less so, as well as on the dosing frequency.[4]

Both NSAIDs and ACE inhibitors alone can cause renal impairment. In patients whose kidneys are underperfused, they may cause further deterioration in renal function when used together.[45]

Importance and management

The interaction between indometacin and ACE inhibitors is well established, with several studies showing that indometacin can reduce the antihypertensive effect of a number of ACE inhibitors. The interaction may not occur in all patients. If indometacin is required in a patient on any ACE inhibitor, it would be prudent to monitor blood pressure. In comparative studies, indometacin has been shown to have less effect on the calcium channel blockers amlodipine, felodipine, and nifedipine, than on enalapril.[21,24,25] See also, 'Calcium channel blockers + NSAIDs', p.659. Therefore, a calcium channel blocker may sometimes be an alternative to an ACE inhibitor in a patient requiring indometacin.

Limited information suggests that sulindac has little or no effect on ACE inhibitors and may, therefore, be less likely to cause a problem.

Although information about other NSAIDs is limited the mechanism suggests that all of them are likely to interact similarly. Until more is known, it may be prudent to increase blood pressure monitoring when any NSAID is added or discontinued in a patient on any ACE inhibitor. Intermittent use of NSAIDs should be considered as a possible cause of erratic control of blood pressure in patients on ACE inhibitors. In addition, sodium status and, therefore, diuretic use may affect any interaction.

There is an increased risk of deterioration in renal function or acute renal failure with the combination of NSAIDs and ACE inhibitors, especially if poor renal perfusion is present. Renal function should be monitored periodically in patients on ACE inhibitors and NSAIDs, particularly in volume depleted patients. In a statement, the American Heart Association comments that acute renal failure complicating ACE inhibitor therapy is almost always reversible and repletion of extracellular fluid volume and discontinuation of diuretic therapy is the best approach. In addition, withdrawal of interacting drugs, supportive management of fluid and electrolytes, and temporary dialysis where indicated are the mainstays of therapy.[46]

Combined use of NSAIDs and ACE inhibitors may increase the risk of hyperkalaemia, but this appears to be rare.

1. White WB, Kent J, Taylor A, Verburg K, Lefkowith JB, Whelton A. Effects of celecoxib on ambulatory blood pressure in hypertensive patients on ACE inhibitors. *Hypertension* (2002) 39, 929–34.
2. Whelton A, Fort JG, Puma JA, Normandin D, Bello AE, Verburg KM, for the SUCCESS VI Study Group. Cyclooxygenase-2-specific inhibitors and cardiorenal function: a randomized, controlled trial of celecoxib and rofecoxib in older hypertensive osteoarthritis patients. *Am J Ther* (2001) 8, 85–95.
3. Palmer R, Weiss R, Zusman RM, Haig A, Flavin S, MacDonald B. Effects of nabumetone, celecoxib, and ibuprofen on blood pressure control in hypertensive patients on angiotensin converting enzyme inhibitors. *Am J Hypertens* (2003) 16, 135–9.
4. Izhar M, Alausa T, Folker A, Hung E, Bakris GL. Effects of COX inhibition on blood pressure and kidney function in ACE inhibitor-treated blacks and hispanics. *Hypertension* (2004) 43, 573–7.
5. Radack KL, Deck CC, Bloomfield SS. Ibuprofen interferes with the efficacy of antihypertensive drugs. A randomized, double-blind, placebo-controlled trial of ibuprofen compared with acetaminophen. *Ann Intern Med* (1987) 107, 628–35.
6. Goldstone R, Martin K, Zipser R, Horton R. Evidence for a dual action of converting enzyme inhibitor on blood pressure in normal man. *Prostaglandins* (1981) 22, 587–98.
7. Espino DV, Lancaster MC. Neutralization of the effects of captopril by the use of ibuprofen in an elderly woman. *J Am Board Fam Pract* (1992) 5, 319–21.
8. Thakur V, Cook ME, Wallin JD. Antihypertensive effect of the combination of fosinopril and HCTZ is resistant to interference by nonsteroidal antiinflammatory drugs. *Am J Hypertens* (1999) 12, 925–8.
9. Conlin PR, Moore TJ, Swartz SL, Barr E, Gazdick L, Fletcher C, DeLucca P, Demopoulos L. Effect of indomethacin on blood pressure lowering by captopril and losartan in hypertensive patients. *Hypertension* (2000) 36, 461–5.
10. Moore TJ, Crantz FR, Hollenberg NK, Koletsky RJ, Leboff MS, Swartz SL, Levine L, Podolsky S, Dluhy RG, Williams GH. Contribution of prostaglandins to the antihypertensive action of captopril in essential hypertension. *Hypertension* (1981) 3, 168–73.
11. Swartz SL, Williams GH. Angiotensin-converting enzyme inhibition and prostaglandins. *Am J Cardiol* (1982) 49, 1405–9.
12. Salvetti A, Pedrinelli R, Magagna A, Ugenti P. Differential effects of selective and non-selective prostaglandin-synthesis inhibition on the pharmacological responses to captopril in patients with essential hypertension. *Clin Sci* (1982) 63, 261S–263S.
13. Silberbauer K, Stanek B, Templ H. Acute hypotensive effect of captopril in man modified by prostaglandin synthesis inhibition. *Br J Clin Pharmacol* (1982) 14, 87S–93S.
14. Witzgall H, Hirsch F, Scherer B, Weber PC. Acute haemodynamic and hormonal effects of captopril are diminished by indomethacin. *Clin Sci* (1982) 62, 611–15.

15. Ogihara T, Maruyama A, Hata T, Mikami H, Nakamaru M, Naka T, Ohde H, Kumahara Y. Hormonal responses to long-term converting enzyme inhibition in hypertensive patients. *Clin Pharmacol Ther* (1981) 30, 328–35.
16. Koopmans PP, Van Megen T, Thien T, Gribnau FWJ. The interaction between indomethacin and captopril or enalapril in healthy volunteers. *J Intern Med* (1989) 226, 139–42.
17. Fujita T, Yamashita N, Yamashita K. Effect of indomethacin on antihypertensive action of captopril in hypertensive patients. *Clin Exp Hypertens* (1981) 3, 939–52.
18. Robles Iniesta A, Navarro de León MC, Morales Serna JC. Bloqueo de la acción antihipertensiva del captoprilo por indometacina. *Med Clin (Barc)* (1991) 96, 438.
19. Gerber JG, Franca G, Byyny RL, LoVerde M, Nies AS. The hypotensive action of captopril and enalapril is not prostacyclin dependent. *Clin Pharmacol Ther* (1993) 54, 523–32.
20. Salvetti A, Abdel-Haq B, Magagna A, Pedrinelli R. Indomethacin reduces the antihypertensive action of enalapril. *Clin Exp Hypertens A* (1987) 9, 559–67.
21. Polónia J, Boaventura I, Gama G, Camões I, Bernardo F, Andrade P, Nunes JP, Brandão F, Cerqueira-Gomes M. Influence of non-steroidal anti-inflammatory drugs on renal function and 24 h ambulatory blood pressure-reducing effects of enalapril and nifedipine gastrointestinal therapeutic system in hypertensive patients. *J Hypertens* (1995) 13, 925–31.
22. Walden RJ, Owens CWI, Graham BR, Snape A, Nutt J, Prichard BNC. NSAIDs and the control of hypertension: a pilot study. *Br J Clin Pharmacol* (1992) 33, 241P.
23. Duffin D, Leahey W, Brennan G, Johnston GD. The effects of indomethacin on the antihypertensive responses to enalapril and lisinopril. *Br J Clin Pharmacol* (1992) 34, 456P.
24. Morgan T, Anderson A. Interaction of indomethacin with felodipine and enalapril. *J Hypertens* (1993) 11 (Suppl 5), S338–S339.
25. Morgan TO, Anderson A, Bertram D. Effect of indomethacin on blood pressure in elderly people with essential hypertension well controlled on amlodipine or enalapril. *Am J Hypertens* (2000), 13, 1161–7.
26. Fricker AF, Nussberger J, Meilenbrock S, Brunner HR, Burnier M. Effect of indomethacin on the renal response to angiotensin II receptor blockade in healthy subjects. *Kidney Int* (1998) 54, 2089–97.
27. Ahmad S. Indomethacin-enalapril interaction: an alert. *South Med J* (1991) 84, 411–2.
28. Oparil S, Horton R, Wilkins LH, Irvin J, Hammett DK. Antihypertensive effect of enalapril in essential hypertension: role of prostacyclin. *Am J Med Sci* (1987) 294, 395–402.
29. Fogari R, Zoppi A, Carretta R, Veglio F, Salvetti A: Italian Collaborative Study Group. Effect of indomethacin on the antihypertensive efficacy of valsartan and lisinopril: a multicentre study. *J Hypertens* (2002) 20: 1007–14.
30. Shaw W, Shapiro D, Antonello J, Cressman M, Vlasses P, Oparil S. Indomethacin does not blunt the antihypertensive effect of lisinopril. *Clin Pharmacol Ther* (1987) 41, 219.
31. Kirch W, Stroemer K, Hoogkamer JFW, Kleinbloesem CH. The influence of prostaglandin inhibition by indomethacin on blood pressure and renal function in hypertensive patients treated with cilazapril. *Br J Clin Pharmacol* (1989) 27, 297S–301S.
32. Abdel-Haq B, Magagna A, Favilla S, Salvetti A. Hemodynamic and humoral interactions between perindopril and indomethacin in essential hypertensive subjects. *J Cardiovasc Pharmacol* (1991) 18 (Suppl 7), S33–S36.
33. Quoted as data on file (Hoechst) by Todd PA, Benfield P. Ramipril. A review of its pharmacological properties and therapeutic efficacy in cardiovascular disorders. *Drugs* (1990) 39, 110–35.
34. Pritchard G, Lyons D, Webster J, Petrie JC, MacDonald TM. Indomethacin does not attenuate the hypotensive effect of trandolapril. *J Hum Hypertens* (1996) 10, 763–7.
35. Vioxx (Rofecoxib). Merck Sharp & Dohme Ltd. UK Summary of product characteristics, August 2003.
36. Brown CH. Effect of rofecoxib on the antihypertensive activity of lisinopril. *Ann Pharmacother* (2000) 34, 1486.
37. Noveck RJ, McMahon FG, Bocanegra T, Karem A, Sugimoto D, Smith M. Effects of oxaprozin on enalapril and enalaprilat pharmacokinetics, pharmacodynamics: blood pressure, heart rate, plasma renin activity, aldosterone and creatinine clearances, in hypertensive patients. *Clin Pharmacol Ther* (1997), 61, 208.
38. Seelig CB, Maloley PA, Campbell JR. Nephrotoxicity associated with concomitant ACE inhibitor and NSAID therapy. *South Med J* (1990) 83, 1144–8.
39. Adhiyaman V, Asghar M, Oke A, White AD, Shah IU. Nephrotoxicity in the elderly due to co-prescription of angiotensin converting enzyme inhibitors and nonsteroidal anti-inflammatory drugs. *J R Soc Med* (2001) 94, 512–14.
40. Stürmer T, Erb A, Keller F, Günther K-P, Brenner H. Determinants of impaired renal function with use of nonsteroidal anti-inflammatory drugs: the importance of half-life and other medications. *Am J Med* (2001) 111, 521–7.
41. Pritchard G, Lyons D, Webster J, Petrie JC, MacDonald TM. Do trandolapril and indomethacin influence renal function and renal functional reserve in hypertensive patients? *Br J Clin Pharmacol* (1997) 44, 145–9.
42. Kurata C, Uehara A, Sugi T, Yamazaki K. Syncope caused by nonsteroidal anti-inflammatory drugs and angiotensin-converting enzyme inhibitors. *Jpn Circ J* (1999) 63, 1002–3.
43. Hay E, Derazon H, Bukish N, Katz L, Kruglyakov I, Armoni M. Fatal hyperkalaemia related to combined therapy with a COX-2 inhibitor, ACE inhibitor and potassium rich diet. *J Emerg Med* (2002) 22, 349–52.
44. Grass P, Gerbeau C, Kutz K. Spirapril: pharmacokinetic properties and drug interactions. *Blood Pressure* (1994) 3 (Suppl 2), 7–13.
45. Sturrock NDC, Struthers AD. Non-steroidal anti-inflammatory drugs and angiotensin converting enzyme inhibitors: a commonly prescribed combination with variable effects on renal function. *Br J Clin Pharmacol* (1993) 35, 343–8.
46. Schoolwerth AC, Sica DA, Ballermann BJ, Wilcox CS. Renal considerations in angiotensin converting enzyme inhibitor therapy. A statement for healthcare professionals from the Council on the Kidney in Cardiovascular Disease and the Council for High Blood Pressure Research of the American Heart Association. *Circulation* (2001) 104, 1985–91.

ACE inhibitors and other antihypertensives + Orlistat

Orlistat has been found in a handful of cases to oppose the effects of enalapril and losartan and other antihypertensive drugs (amlodipine, atenolol, hydrochlorothiazide) resulting in marked increases in blood pressure, hypertensive crises and, in one case, intracranial haemorrhage.

Clinical evidence, mechanism, importance and management

The Argentinian System of Pharmacovigilance identified the following 3 cases. An obese man whose hypertension was controlled at 120/80 mmHg with daily doses of **losartan** 100 mg, **atenolol** 100 mg and **hydrochlorothiazide** 12.5 mg developed a hypertensive crisis (BP 260/140 mmHg) 7 days after starting to take orlistat 120 mg three times daily. The orlistat was stopped and the crisis was controlled. When later rechallenged with orlistat, his diastolic blood pressure rose to 100 to 110 mmHg after 5 days, but the systolic increased only slightly. His blood pressure returned to baseline values 3 days after stopping the orlistat.[1]

Two other patients reacted similarly. One whose blood pressure was controlled at 130/85 mmHg on daily doses of **enalapril** 20 mg and **losartan** 50 mg developed an intracranial haemorrhage and hypertension (160/100 mmHg) with occasional systolic peaks of around 200 mmHg one week after starting orlistat 120 mg three times daily. The other patient who was stable on daily doses of **enalapril** 20 mg and **amlodipine** 5 mg began to develop hypertensive peaks (180/120 mmHg) 60 days after starting orlistat 120 mg twice daily. The hypertension responded to a change to **losartan/hydrochlorothiazide**, but 20 days later new hypertensive peaks developed (180/110 to 120 mmHg). When the orlistat was withdrawn, the hypertension was controlled within 48 hours.[1]

The Uppsala Adverse Drug Reaction database has two reports of aggravated hypertension in women on antihypertensives and orlistat.[1] Transitory hypertension has also been reported in previously normotensive healthy individuals on orlistat.[2,3] However, the maker has found no evidence of an association between orlistat and hypertension.[4] They also reported no interaction between orlistat and **losartan**[5] and no clinically significant pharmacokinetic interactions between orlistat and **captopril**, **atenolol**, **furosemide** or **nifedipine** in healthy subjects.[6]

Mechanism

Not understood. Suggestions include a decrease in the absorption of the drugs due to accelerated gastrointestinal transit, increased defaecation, diarrhoea, or an increase in the amount of fat in the chyme.[1] An explanation for the difference between the clinical and pharmacokinetic studies may be that the latter tended to be single-dose studies and in healthy subjects only.

Importance and management

The antihypertensive/orlistat interactions seem to be confined to the reports cited here, and their general significance is unclear. Given that the makers report that specific drug interaction studies have not found any evidence of an interaction[4-6] it seems likely to be small.

1. Valsecia ME, Malgor LA, Farías EF, Figueras A, Laporte J-R. Interaction between orlistat and antihypertensive drugs. *Ann Pharmacother* (2001) 35, 1495–6.
2. Persson M, Vitols S, Yue Q-Y. Orlistat associated with hypertension. *BMJ* (2000) 321, 87.
3. Persson M, Vitols S, Yue Q-Y. Orlistat associated with hypertension. Author's reply. *BMJ* (2001) 322, 111.
4. Huber MH. Orlistat associated with hypertension. Roche concludes that there is no evidence of a causal association. *BMJ* (2001) 322, 110.
5. Xenical (Orlistat). Roche Products Ltd. UK Summary of product characteristics, June 2005.
6. Weber C, Tam YK, Schmidtke-Schrezenmeier G, Jonkmann JHG, van Brummelen P. Effect of the lipase inhibitor orlistat on the pharmacokinetics of four different antihypertensive drugs in healthy volunteers. *Eur J Clin Pharmacol* (1996) 51, 87–90.

ACE inhibitors + Pergolide

An isolated report describes severe hypotension when a patient on lisinopril was given pergolide.

Clinical evidence, mechanism, importance and management

A man successfully treated for hypertension with **lisinopril** 10 mg daily, experienced a severe hypotensive reaction within four hours of taking a single 50-microgram dose of pergolide for periodic leg movements during sleep. He needed hospitalisation and treatment with intravenous fluids. It is not clear whether this patient was extremely sensitive to the pergolide or whether what occurred was due to an interaction. The authors of this report suggest that in patients on antihypertensives the initial dose of pergolide should be 25 micrograms.[1] It would seem prudent to monitor the initial use of pergolide and ACE inhibitors.

1. Kando JC, Keck PE, Wood PA. Pergolide-induced hypotension. *Ann Pharmacother* (1990) 24, 543.

ACE inhibitors + Potassium compounds

ACE inhibitors maintain serum potassium levels. Hyperkalaemia is therefore a possibility if potassium supplements or potassium-containing salt substitutes are given, particularly in those patients where other risk factors are present, such as decreased renal function.

Clinical evidence

(a) Potassium levels increased by concurrent use

(i) Potassium supplements. The serum potassium levels of a patient on a potassium supplement rose by 66% when **captopril** was added, with signs of a deterioration in renal function. Four others taking potassium supplements and furosemide (2 also taking unnamed potassium-sparing diuretics) showed rises in potassium levels of only 8 to 24% when given **captopril**. The rises occurred within 1 or 2 days. No clinical signs or symptoms of hyperkalaemia were seen, but 3 of the 5 patients had rises to above the upper limits of normal for the laboratory.[1] A postmarketing survey identified 10 patients in whom **enalapril** appeared to have been associated with renal function impairment and death. Eight of them were also taking potassium supplements and/or potassium-sparing diuretics, and hyperkalaemia appeared to have been the immediate cause of death in two of them.[2] In a review of 47 patients treated with **enalapril** for heart failure and who experienced serious hyperkalaemia, 8 had received concurrent potassium supplements.[3]
In another survey of 53 patients on ACE inhibitors who had hyperkalaemia in the absence of significant renal impairment, less than 5% were taking a potassium supplement, but 30% were using a potassium-containing **salt substitute** (see *(ii)* below).[4]

(ii) Dietary potassium. Two patients with renal impairment, one on **lisinopril** and the other on **enalapril**, developed marked hyperkalaemia shortly after starting to take ***'Lo salt'*** (a **salt substitute** containing 34.6 g potassium in every 100 g). One developed a life-threatening arrhythmia.[5] A similar report describes a man on **captopril** who developed hyperkalaemia and collapsed 2 weeks after starting to use a **salt substitute** containing potassium.[6] A further report of severe hyperkalaemia in a patient taking **lisinopril** 10 mg daily and on a very-low-calorie diet with a protein supplement. The protein supplement contained 48 mmol of potassium and salad topped with lemon juice and potassium chloride salt added at least another 72 mmol daily.[7] In 53 patients on ACE inhibitors who had hyperkalaemia in the absence of significant renal impairment, 30% were using a **salt substitute**, and 72% were eating a moderate-to-high potassium diet, consisting of 2 or more servings of a potassium-rich food daily.[4] Hyperkalaemia and acute renal failure has also been reported in a diabetic patient taking **lisinopril** 20 mg twice daily following the use of a potassium-based water softener.[8]

(b) Potassium levels unaltered by concurrent use

A retrospective analysis of 14 patients without renal impairment taking potassium supplements and either furosemide or hydrochlorothiazide, found that the levels of serum potassium, during a 4-year period, had not significantly increased after the addition of **captopril**.[9] Another study in 6 healthy subjects found that intravenous potassium chloride caused virtually the same rise in serum potassium levels in those given **enalapril** as in those given a placebo.[10]

Mechanism

The potassium-retaining effects of ACE inhibitors (due to reduced aldosterone levels) are additive with increased intake of potassium, particularly when there are other contributory factors such as poor renal function or diabetes.

Importance and management

The documentation of this interaction appears to be limited, but it is well established. In practice, a clinically relevant rise in potassium levels usually occurs only if other factors are also present, the most important of which is impaired renal function. In practice, because ACE inhibitors have potassium-sparing effects, potassium supplements should not routinely be given concurrently. If a supplement is needed serum potassium should be closely monitored. This is especially important where other possible contributory risk factors are known to be present.

Other sources of dietary potassium should also be borne in mind. Patients with heart disease and hypertension are often told to reduce their salt (sodium) intake. One way of doing this is to use potassium-containing salt substitutes. However, it appears that there is some risk associated with excess use, especially in patients taking ACE inhibitors.

1. Burnakis TG, Mioduch HJ. Combined therapy with captopril and potassium supplementation. A potential for hyperkalemia. *Arch Intern Med* (1984) 144, 2371–2.
2. Speirs CJ, Dollery CT, Inman WHW, Rawson NSB, Wilton LV. Postmarketing surveillance of enalapril. II: Investigation of the potential role of enalapril in deaths with renal failure. *BMJ* (1988) 297, 830–2.
3. Brown C, Rush J. Risk factors for the development of hyperkalemia in patients treated with enalapril for heart failure. *Clin Pharmacol Ther* (1989) 45, 167.
4. Good CB, McDermott L, McCloskey B. Diet and serum potassium in patients on ACE inhibitors. *JAMA* (1995) 274, 538.
5. Ray KK, Dorman S, Watson RDS. Severe hyperkalaemia due to the concomitant use of salt substitutes and ACE inhibitors in hypertension: a potentially life threatening interaction. *J Hum Hypertens* (1999) 13, 717–20.
6. Packer M, Lee WH. Provocation of hyper- and hypokalemic sudden death during treatment with and withdrawal of converting-enzyme inhibition in severe chronic congestive heart failure. *Am J Cardiol* (1986) 57, 347–8.
7. Stoltz ML, Andrews CE. Severe hyperkalemia during very-low-calorie diets and angiotensin converting enzyme use. *JAMA* (1990) 264, 2737–8.
8. Graves JW. Hyperkalemia due to a potassium-based water softener. *N Engl J Med* (1998) 339,1790–1.
9. Schuna AA, Schmidt GR, Pitterle ME. Serum potassium concentrations after initiation of captopril therapy. *Clin Pharm* (1986) 5, 920–3.
10. Scandling JD, Izzo JL, Pabico RC, McKenna BA, Radke KJ, Ornt DB. Potassium homeostasis during angiotensin-converting enzyme inhibition with enalapril. *J Clin Pharmacol* (1989) 29, 916–21.

ACE inhibitors + Probenecid

Probenecid decreases the renal clearance of captopril, but this is probably not clinically important. Probenecid raises enalapril serum levels.

Clinical evidence, mechanism, importance and management

Steady-state levels of unchanged and total **captopril**, given by intravenous infusion, were slightly increased (14% and 36%, respectively) by the use of probenecid in 4 healthy subjects. Renal clearance of unchanged **captopril** decreased by 44%, but total clearance was reduced by only 19%.[1] These moderate changes are unlikely to be clinically important. Probenecid 1 g twice daily for 5 days increased the AUC of **enalapril** and enalaprilat by about 50% after a single 20-mg oral dose in 12 healthy subjects. Renal clearance of **enalapril** decreased by 73%.[2] A moderate increase in the hypotensive effects might be expected, but there do not appear to be any reports of adverse effects.

1. Singhvi SM, Duchin KL, Willard DA, McKinstry DN, Migdalof BH. Renal handling of captopril: effect of probenecid. *Clin Pharmacol Ther* (1982) 32, 182–9.
2. Noormohamed FH, McNabb WR, Lant AF. Pharmacokinetic and pharmacodynamic actions of enalapril in humans: effect of probenecid pretreatment. *J Pharmacol Exp Ther* (1990) 253, 362–8.

ACE inhibitors + Procainamide

The combination of captopril or other ACE inhibitors and procainamide possibly increases the risk of leucopenia. No pharmacokinetic interaction occurs between captopril and procainamide.

Clinical evidence, mechanism, importance and management

The pharmacokinetics of **captopril** 50 mg twice daily and procainamide 250 mg three-hourly were unaffected by concurrent use in 12 healthy subjects.[1] However, the maker of **captopril** notes that neutropenia/agranulocytosis and serious infection have occurred in patients on **captopril**, and concurrent treatment with procainamide may be a complicating factor. They recommend the combination be used with caution, especially in patients with impaired renal function. They suggest that differential white blood cell counts should be performed before therapy, then every 2 weeks in the first 3 months of **captopril** therapy and periodically thereafter.[2] The makers of a number of other ACE inhibitors suggest that concurrent use of ACE inhibitors and procainamide may lead to an increased risk of leucopenia. For reports of other interactions with ACE inhibitors that result in leucopenia see also 'ACE inhibitors + Allopurinol', p.14 and 'ACE inhibitors + Azathioprine', p.18.

1. Levinson B, Sugerman AA, McKown J. Lack of kinetic interaction of captopril (CP) and procainamide (PA) in healthy subjects. *J Clin Pharmacol* (1985) 25, 460.
2. Capoten (Captopril). E. R. Squibb & Sons Ltd. UK Summary of product characteristics, February 2003.

ACE inhibitors + Rifampicin (Rifampin)

An isolated report describes a rise in blood pressure in one hypertensive patient, which was attributed to an interaction between enalapril and rifampicin. Rifampicin may reduce the plasma levels of the active metabolites of imidapril and spirapril.

Clinical evidence, mechanism, importance and management

A man on **enalapril** and a variety of other drugs (warfarin, acebutolol, bendroflumethiazide, dipyridamole, metoclopramide and *Gaviscon*) developed a fever. He was given streptomycin, oxytetracycline and rifampicin (rifampin), because of a probable *Brucella abortus* infection, whereupon his blood pressure rose from 164/104 to 180/115 mmHg over the next 5 to 6 days. It was suspected that an interaction with the rifampicin was possibly responsible. Subsequent studies in the same patient showed that after stopping and then restarting the rifampicin, the 7-hour AUC of enalaprilat, the active metabolite of **enalapril**, was reduced by 31%, although the AUC of **enalapril** was unchanged.[1] There is also the hint of this interaction in another report, where **enalapril** failed to control blood pressure in a patient on rifampicin.[2] The maker of **spirapril** briefly noted in a review that the use of rifampicin with **spirapril** modestly decreased plasma **spirapril** concentrations and those of its active metabolite spiraprilat.[3] The maker of **imidapril** notes that rifampicin reduced plasma levels of imidaprilat, the active metabolite of **imidapril**.[4]

The mechanism of this interaction is not clear because rifampicin is a potent liver enzyme inducing agent which might have been expected to cause the production of more, rather than less, of the active metabolites of these ACE inhibitors. However, the authors of one of the reports postulated that the rifampicin might have increased the loss of the enalaprilat in the urine,[1] and others suggested that rifampicin stimulates the elimination of spiraprilat non-specifically.[3]

The general importance of these interactions is uncertain. The isolated reports with **enalapril** suggest minor clinical relevance. The makers of **spirapril** did not consider the modest pharmacokinetic changes to be clinically relevant.[3] However, the makers of **imidapril** state that rifampicin might reduce the antihypertensive efficacy of **imidapril**,[4] but this awaits clinical assessment.

1. Kandiah D, Penny WJ, Fraser AG, Lewis MJ. A possible drug interaction between rifampicin and enalapril. *Eur J Clin Pharmacol* (1988) 35, 431–2.
2. Tada Y, Tsuda Y, Otsuka T, Nagasawa K, Kimura H, Kusaba T, Sakata T. Case report: nifedipine-rifampicin interaction attenuates the effect on blood pressure in a patient with essential hypertension. *Am J Med Sci* (1992) 303, 25–7.
3. Grass P, Gerbeau C, Kutz K. Spirapril: pharmacokinetic properties and drug interactions. *Blood Pressure* (1994) 3 (Suppl 2), 7–13.
4. Tanatril (Imidapril). Trinity Pharmaceuticals Ltd. UK Summary of product characteristics, May 2003.

ACE inhibitors + Sibutramine

Sibutramine had only a minimal effect on blood pressure control with ACE inhibitors.

Clinical evidence, mechanism, importance and management

In a randomised, double-blind study over 52 weeks involving 220 obese, hypertensive patients, whose hypertension was well controlled with an ACE inhibitor (**benazepril**, **enalapril** or **lisinopril**) with or without concurrent thiazide diuretic therapy, two-thirds of the patients were additionally given sibutramine and one third were given placebo. Sibutramine 20 mg daily caused small increases in mean blood pressure compared with placebo (133.1/85.5 compared with 130.4/82.8, at 52 weeks, respectively), but overall hypertension remained well controlled.[1]

1. McMahon FG, Weinstein SP, Rowe E, Ernst KR, Johnson F, Fujioka K, and the Sibutramine in Hypertensives Clinical Study Group. Sibutramine is safe and effective for weight loss in obese patients whose hypertension is well controlled with angiotensin-converting enzyme inhibitors. *J Hum Hypertens* (2002) 16, 5–11.

ACE inhibitors + Sympathomimetics

The antihypertensive effects of ACE inhibitors may be reduced by sympathomimetics.

Clinical evidence, mechanism, importance and management

A randomised, double-blind, crossover study in 13 patients with hypertension controlled with various antihypertensive agents including ACE inhibitors in 6 patients, found that a single dose of ***Dimetapp Extentabs*** (**phenylpropanolamine** 75 mg with brompheniramine 12 mg) caused only a minor systolic/diastolic blood pressure rise (1.7/0.9 mmHg) over 4 hours. This was not considered to be clinically important, although (as the authors point out) these results do not necessarily apply to different doses and immediate-release preparations.[1] Several makers of ACE inhibitors warn that the antihypertensive effects of ACE inhibitors may be reduced by sympathomimetics.

1. Petrulis AS, Imperiale TF, Speroff T. The acute effect of phenylpropanolamine and brompheniramine on blood pressure in controlled hypertension. *J Gen Intern Med* (1991) 6, 503–6.

Angiotensin II receptor antagonists + Antacids

Irbesartan and olmesartan do not appear to interact with antacids.

Clinical evidence, mechanism, importance and management

A single-dose, crossover study in 18 healthy subjects demonstrated that there was no clinically meaningful pharmacokinetic interaction between **irbesartan** 300 mg and an antacid containing **aluminium/magnesium hydroxides** (***Unimaalox***) given with, or 2 hours before, the **irbesartan**.[1]

The bioavailability of **olmesartan** 20 mg daily was slightly lower when it was given 15 minutes after an **aluminium/magnesium hydroxide** antacid, compared with **olmesartan** alone, but this was not considered to be clinically significant.[2]

1. Marino MR, Vachharajani NN. Drug interactions with irbesartan. *Clin Pharmacokinet* (2001) 40, 605–14.
2. Laeis P, Püchler K, Kirch W. The pharmacokinetic and metabolic profile of olmesartan medoxomil limits the risk of clinically relevant drug interaction. *J Hypertens* (2001) 19 (Suppl 1), S21–S32.

Angiotensin II receptor antagonists + Azoles

Fluconazole reduces the conversion of losartan to its active metabolite and decreases the metabolism of irbesartan, but does not appear to influence the pharmacokinetics of eprosartan; candesartan and valsartan also seem unlikely to interact. Itraconazole does not significantly affect the pharmacokinetics or antihypertensive effects of losartan. Ketoconazole does not affect the pharmacokinetics of eprosartan or losartan.

Clinical evidence, mechanism, importance and management

(a) Fluconazole

In a study of 32 healthy subjects, half were given **losartan** 100 mg daily and half were given **eprosartan** 300 mg twice daily for 20 days. Fluconazole 200 mg daily was additionally given to both groups on days 11 to 20. Fluconazole increased the AUC and maximum plasma levels of **losartan** by 69 and 31%, respectively, and reduced those of E-3174, **losartan's** active metabolite, by 41 and 54%, respectively. However, fluconazole had no significant effect on the pharmacokinetics of **eprosartan**.[1] In a randomised, crossover study, 11 healthy subjects were given a single 50-mg dose of **losartan** after 4 days of fluconazole (400 mg on day 1 and 200 mg daily on days 2 to 4) or placebo. The AUC of **losartan** was increased by 27% while its maximum plasma level was reduced by 23% by fluconazole. The AUC and the maximum plasma levels of E-3174 were reduced by 47% and 77%, respectively. However, no significant changes in the hypotensive effect of **losartan** were noted.[2]

It is thought that fluconazole inhibits the conversion of **losartan** to its active metabolite mainly by inhibiting the cytochrome P450 isoenzyme CYP2C9,[1-4] although other isoenzymes may play a minor role. The lack of pharmacodynamic changes suggests that this pharmacokinetic interaction may not be clinically important, but this requires confirmation in the clinical setting because E-3174 has greater pharmacological activity than **losartan**,[5,6] and so the possibility of a decreased therapeutic effect should be kept in mind.[2]

Irbesartan is primarily metabolised by CYP2C9.[4] A study in 15 healthy subjects given **irbesartan** 150 mg daily for 20 days found that the steady-state AUC and maximum blood levels were increased by about 55 % and 18% respectively by fluconazole 200 mg daily on days 11 to 20, probably as a result of CYP2C9 inhibition.[7] These modest increases were considered unlikely to be clinically relevant and a dosage reduction would not generally be required.[8]

Following *in vitro* experiments, the role of CYP enzymes in the metabolism and interactions of sartans (**candesartan**, **eprosartan**, **irbesartan**, **losartan** and **valsartan**) was considered to be small, although **losartan**, **irbesartan** and, to a minor extent, **candesartan** are metabolised by CYP2C9. Only **losartan** and **irbesartan** were considered to have a theoretical potential for pharmacokinetic drug interactions involving the CYP2C9 enzyme.[4]

(b) Itraconazole

The pharmacokinetics and hypotensive effects of a single 50-mg dose of **losartan** and its active metabolite E-3174 were not significantly affected by itraconazole 200 mg daily for 4 days in 11 healthy subjects.[2] Inhibition of the cytochrome P450 isoenzyme CYP3A4 alone (caused by itraconazole) does not appear to prevent the conversion of **losartan** to E-3174. No special precautions would appear to be needed if these drugs are used concurrently.

(c) Ketoconazole

A placebo-controlled, crossover study in 11 healthy subjects given a single 30-mg intravenous dose of **losartan**, found that ketoconazole 400 mg daily for 4 days did not affect the conversion of **losartan** to its active metabolite, E-3174, nor the plasma clearance of **losartan**.[9] Inhibition of the cytochrome P450 isoenzyme CYP3A4 alone (caused by ketoconazole) does not appear to prevent the conversion of **losartan** to E-3174.

The plasma clearance of a 20-mg intravenous dose of E-3174 was also unaffected by pretreatment with ketoconazole.[9] Similar results were found in a study involving 27 healthy subjects. Ketoconazole 200 mg daily for 5 days was found to have no effect on the pharmacokinetics of **eprosartan** or **losartan** and its active metabolite.[6] No special precautions would appear to be needed if these drugs are used concurrently.

1. Kazierad DJ, Martin DE, Tenero D, Boike SC, Ilson B, Freed MI, Etheredge R, Jorkasky DK. Fluconazole significantly alters the pharmacokinetics of losartan but not eprosartan. *Clin Pharmacol Ther* (1997) 61, 203.
2. Kaukonen K-M, Olkkola KT, Neuvonen PJ. Fluconazole but not itraconazole decreases the metabolism of losartan to E-3174. *Eur J Clin Pharmacol* (1998) 53, 445–9.
3. Parnell K, Rodgers J, Graff D, Allen T, Hinderliter A, Patterson J, Pieper J. Inhibitory effect of fluconazole and erythromycin plus fluvastatin on losartan disposition in normal volunteers. *Clin Pharmacol Ther* (2000) 67, 121.
4. Taavitsainen P, Kiukaanniemi K, Pelkonen O. In vitro inhibition screening of human hepatic P_{450} enzymes by five angiotensin-II receptor antagonists. *Eur J Clin Pharmacol* (2000) 56, 135–40.
5. Sweetman SC, editor. Martindale: The complete drug reference. 34th ed. London: Pharmaceutical Press; 2005. p. 948
6. Blum RA, Kazierad DJ, Tenero DM. A review of eprosartan pharmacokinetic and pharmacodynamic drug interaction studies. *Pharmacotherapy* (1999) 19, 79S–85S.
7. Kovacs SJ, Wilton JH, Blum RA. Steady state pharmacokinetics of irbesartan alone and in combination with fluconazole. *Clin Pharmacol Ther* (1999) 65, 132.
8. Marino MR, Vachharajani NN. Drug interactions with irbesartan. *Clin Pharmacokinet* (2001) 40, 605–14.
9. McCrea JB, Lo MW, Furtek CI, Ritter MA, Carides A, Waldman SA, Bjornsson TD, Goldberg MR. Ketoconazole does not effect the systemic conversion of losartan to E-3174. *Clin Pharmacol Ther* (1996) 59, 169.

Angiotensin II receptor antagonists + Beta-blockers

There appears to be no clinically significant pharmacokinetic interaction between atenolol and tasosartan or valsartan, and concurrent use enhances the hypotensive effects. Irbesartan has been given safely with beta-blockers.

Clinical evidence, mechanism, importance and management

A study in 17 patients with essential hypertension found that **atenolol** 50 mg daily reduced the peak plasma levels and the AUC of **tasosartan** 50 mg daily by 24% and 16% respectively over 14 days, but the pharmacokinetics of its active metabolite enoltasosartan were not affected. The peak plasma levels and AUC of **atenolol** were decreased by 22% and 18%, respectively. The reduction in diastolic pressure was greater with **tasosartan** plus **atenolol** than after either treatment alone. The pharmacokinetic interaction was not considered of primary clinical importance, and the drug combination was not associated with any particular adverse events.[1] In a single-dose, crossover study in 12 healthy subjects, the pharmacokinetics of **valsartan** 160 mg and **atenolol** 100 mg were not significantly altered by concurrent use. The combination showed some additive effects on resting blood pressure.[2] The makers say that **irbesartan** has been safely given with antihypertensives such as beta-blockers.[3]

Although information is limited, and apparently limited to the drugs discussed here, no significant adverse interaction would be expected between angiotensin II receptor antagonists and beta-blockers.

1. Andrawis NS, Battle MM, Klamerus KJ, Burghart PH, Neefe L, Weinryb I, Mayer P, Abernethy DR. A pharmacokinetic and pharmacodynamic study of the potential drug interaction between tasosartan and atenolol in patients with stage 1 and 2 essential hypertension. *J Clin Pharmacol* (2000) 40, 231–41.
2. Czendlik CH, Sioufi A, Preiswerk G, Howald H. Pharmacokinetic and pharmacodynamic interaction of single doses of valsartan and atenolol. *Eur J Clin Pharmacol* (1997) 52, 451–9.
3. Aprovel (Irbesartan). Sanofi Synthelabo. UK Summary of product characteristics, August 2004.

Angiotensin II receptor antagonists + Calcium channel blockers

No significant pharmacokinetic interactions occur between nifedipine and candesartan or irbesartan, or between amlodipine and telmisartan or valsartan. Calcium channel blockers have been given safely with eprosartan or irbesartan.

Clinical evidence, mechanism, importance and management

Nifedipine 30 mg daily did not significantly affect the pharmacokinetics of **candesartan** 16 mg daily in 12 healthy subjects; the AUC for **nifedipine** was decreased by 10 to 15%, but this was not statistically significant.[1]

In vitro studies indicated that **nifedipine** (an inhibitor of the cytochrome P450 isoenzyme CYP2C9) inhibited the oxidation of **irbesartan**.[2] However, a randomised, crossover study in 11 healthy subjects given **irbesartan** 300 mg daily alone or with the addition of **nifedipine** 30 mg daily for 4 days, found that **nifedipine** did not alter the pharmacokinetics of **irbesartan**.[2] The maker says that **irbesartan** has been safely given with antihypertensives such as long-acting calcium channel blockers.[3] Similarly the maker of **eprosartan** notes that it has been safely given with calcium channel blockers (e.g. sustained-release **nifedipine**).[4]

In a study in 12 healthy subjects, **telmisartan** 120 mg daily had no clinically relevant effect on the pharmacokinetics of **amlodipine** 10 mg daily for 9 days, and there was no evidence of any marked effect of **amlodipine** on the pharmacokinetics of **telmisartan**. Although there were no serious adverse effects, mild to moderate adverse events (most commonly headache) occurred slightly more frequently with the combination compared with **amlodipine** alone (19 compared with 12 events).[5] The pharmacokinetics of single oral doses of **valsartan** 160 mg or **amlodipine** 5 mg, in 12 healthy subjects, were not significantly changed when the drugs were given together, although the pharmacokinetics of **valsartan** showed wide variations between subjects.[6]

No special precautions would therefore appear to be necessary if any of these drugs are given together, although an increase in adverse effects may occur.

1. Jonkman JHG, van Lier JJ, van Heiningen PNM, Lins R, Sennewald R, Högemann A. Pharmacokinetic drug interaction studies with candesartan cilexetil. *J Hum Hypertens* (1997) 11 (Suppl 2), S31–S35.
2. Marino MR, Hammett JL, Ferreira I, Ford NF, Uderman HD. Effect of nifedipine on the steady-state pharmacokinetics and pharmacodynamics of irbesartan in healthy subjects. *J Cardiovasc Pharmacol Ther* (1998) 3, 111–17.
3. Aprovel (Irbesartan). Sanofi Synthelabo. UK Summary of product characteristics, August 2004.
4. Teveten (Eprosartan). Solvay Healthcare Ltd. UK Summary of product characteristics, December 2003.
5. Stangier J, Su C-APF. Pharmacokinetics of repeated oral doses of amlodipine and amlodipine plus telmisartan in healthy volunteers. *J Clin Pharmacol* (2000) 40, 1347–54.
6. Novartis Pharmaceuticals Ltd. Data on file, Protocol 37.

Angiotensin II receptor antagonists + Diuretics; Loop, thiazide or related

Symptomatic hypotension may occur when an angiotensin II receptor antagonist is started in patients on high-dose diuretics. No clinically relevant pharmacokinetic interactions appear to occur between candesartan, eprosartan, irbesartan, losartan, telmisartan or valsartan and hydrochlorothiazide, although the bioavailability of hydrochlorothiazide may be modestly reduced.

Similarly, there is no clinically significant pharmacokinetic interaction between valsartan and furosemide.

Clinical evidence, mechanism, importance and management

(a) Hypotension

Angiotensin II receptor antagonists and thiazide or related diuretics have useful additive effects in the control of hypertension and are generally well tolerated. A double-blind, placebo-controlled study involving 604 patients found that **losartan** 50 mg given with **hydrochlorothiazide** 12.5 mg once daily produced an additive reduction in trough sitting systolic and diastolic blood pressure and no statistically significant differences in adverse experiences compared with placebo were observed.[1] Similarly, the makers of **eprosartan** and **irbesartan** note that they have been safely given with thiazide diuretics.[2,3] However, a study in 13 healthy subjects given **telmisartan** and **hydrochlorothiazide** found that the most frequently reported adverse event was postural hypotension with associated lightheadedness.[4] Symptomatic hypotension, especially after the first dose, may occur when angiotensin II receptor antagonists are started in patients with sodium and/or volume depletion such as those on **high-dose diuretics**. It is recommended that any volume and/or sodium depletion should be corrected before the angiotensin II receptor antagonist is given. Some makers suggest that the dose of diuretic should be reduced and some makers recommend using a lower starting dose of the angiotensin II receptor antagonist.

Consider also 'ACE inhibitors + Diuretics; Loop, thiazide or related', p.20.

(b) Pharmacokinetic studies

The concurrent use of **hydrochlorothiazide** 25 mg daily and **candesartan** 12 mg daily for 7 days in 18 healthy subjects increased the AUC and maximum serum levels of **candesartan** by 18 and 23% respectively, and reduced the AUC of **hydrochlorothiazide** by 14%, but these changes were not considered to be clinically relevant.[5] **Eprosartan** 800 mg also decreased the AUC of **hydrochlorothiazide** 25 mg by about 20% in 18 healthy subjects, but again this was not considered to be clinically important. In addition, **hydrochlorothiazide** had no effect on **eprosartan** pharmacokinetics.[6] Similarly, in a study of 12 patients with mild or moderate hypertension given **losartan** 50 mg alone or with **hydrochlorothiazide** 12.5 mg daily for 7 days, the AUC of **hydrochlorothiazide** decreased by 17% during concurrent use (not clinically significant) while the pharmacokinetics of **losartan** were unchanged.[7] A single-dose study in 12 healthy subjects found that **valsartan** 160 mg reduced the systemic availability of **hydrochlorothiazide** 25 mg (AUC decreased by 31%), but the mean amount of **hydrochlorothiazide** excreted in the urine did not seem to change significantly. The pharmacokinetics of **valsartan** were not significantly affected by **hydrochlorothiazide**.[8]

In a randomised, crossover study in 13 healthy subjects, **telmisartan** 160 mg daily was given with **hydrochlorothiazide** 25 mg daily for 7 days. There was no difference in AUC and maximum plasma concentrations of either drug compared with when they were given alone.[4] Similarly, no pharmacokinetic interactions were found between **irbesartan** and **hydrochlorothiazide**.[9]

The relative bioavailability of **furosemide** 40 mg was reduced by about 26% when it was given with **valsartan** 160 mg in 12 healthy subjects. However, this pharmacokinetic interaction had no influence on the diuretic effect of **furosemide**. Simultaneous use of **valsartan** and **furosemide** did not modify the pharmacokinetics of **valsartan**.[10]

The changes in **furosemide** and **hydrochlorothiazide** pharmacokinetics appear to be of no practical importance, and the combination with an angiotensin II receptor antagonist can produce a significant and useful additional reduction in blood pressure.

1. MacKay JH, Arcuri KE, Goldberg AI, Snapinn SM, Sweet CS. Losartan and low-dose hydrochlorothiazide in patients with essential hypertension. A double-blind, placebo-controlled trial of concomitant administration compared with individual components. *Arch Intern Med* (1996) 156, 278–85.
2. Teveten (Eprosartan). Solvay Healthcare Ltd. UK Summary of product characteristics, December 2003.
3. Aprovel (Irbesartan). Sanofi Synthelabo. UK Summary of product characteristics, August 2004.
4. Yong C-L, Dias VC, Stangier J. Multiple-dose pharmacokinetics of telmisartan and of hydrochlorothiazide following concurrent administration in healthy subjects. *J Clin Pharmacol* (2000) 40, 1323–30.
5. Jonkman JHG, van Lier JJ, van Heiningen PNM, Lins R, Sennewald R, Högemann A. Pharmacokinetic drug interaction studies with candesartan cilexetil. *J Hum Hypertens* (1997) 11 (Suppl 2), S31–S35.
6. Blum RA, Kazierad DJ, Tenero DM. A review of eprosartan pharmacokinetic and pharmacodynamic drug interaction studies. *Pharmacotherapy* (1999) 19, 79S–85S.
7. McCrea JB, Lo M-W, Tomasko L, Lin CC, Hsieh JY-K, Capra NL, Goldberg MR. Absence of a pharmacokinetic interaction between losartan and hydrochlorothiazide. *J Clin Pharmacol* (1995) 35, 1200–6.
8. Novartis Pharmaceuticals Ltd. Data on file, Protocol 07.
9. Marino MR, Vachharajani NN. Drug interactions with irbesartan. *Clin Pharmacokinet* (2001) 40, 605–14.
10. Bindschedler M, Degen P, Flesch G, de Gasparo M, Preiswerk G. Pharmacokinetic and pharmacodynamic interaction of single oral doses of valsartan and furosemide. *Eur J Clin Pharmacol* (1997) 52, 371–8.

Angiotensin II receptor antagonists + Diuretics; Potassium-sparing

There may be a risk of hyperkalaemia if angiotensin II receptor antagonists are given with potassium-sparing diuretics (amiloride, spironolactone, triamterene), particularly if other risk factors are also present.

Clinical evidence, mechanism, importance and management

Life-threatening hyperkalaemia occurred in 6 patients with congestive heart failure who were taking **spironolactone** and an angiotensin II receptor antagonist (**candesartan**, **losartan** or **telmisartan**). Analysis of these patients together with another 38 similar patients, who had received ACE inhibitors, identified certain conditions that may lead to the development of severe hyperkalaemia in such patients: advanced age, dose of **spironolactone** greater than 25 mg, reduced renal function and type II diabetes.[1] Based on evidence from other drugs that affect the renin-angiotensin system (e.g. ACE inhibitors), the makers of angiotensin II receptor antagonists warn that concurrent use of potassium-sparing diuretics (e.g. **amiloride**, **spironolactone**, **triamterene**), or other drugs that increase potassium levels, may increase serum potassium. There is a greater risk of hyperkalaemia if renal impairment is present and/or heart failure or diabetes. Some makers recommend that the combinations be used cautiously and that serum potassium should be monitored regularly. However, other makers advise against the concurrent use.

Consider also 'ACE inhibitors + Diuretics; Potassium-sparing', p.22.

1. Wrenger E, Müller R, Moesenthin M, Welte T, Frölich JC, Neumann KH. Interaction of spironolactone with ACE inhibitors or angiotensin receptor blockers: analysis of 44 cases. *BMJ* (2003) 327, 147–9.

Angiotensin II receptor antagonists + Erythromycin

The pharmacokinetics and blood-pressure lowering effect of losartan do not seem to be affected by erythromycin.

Clinical evidence, mechanism, importance and management

When 10 healthy subjects were given **losartan** 50 mg daily for a week and then, after a 6-day washout period, **losartan** 50 mg daily plus erythromycin 500 mg four times daily for a week, it was found that erythromycin had no significant effect on the pharmacokinetics of **losartan** or its active metabolite, E-3174. In addition, erythromycin did not alter the blood pressure lowering effect of **losartan**.[1] Inhibition of the cytochrome P450 isoenzyme CYP3A4 alone does not appear to prevent the conversion of losartan to E-3174. There would therefore appear to be no reason to take any special precautions if both drugs used concurrently.

1. Williamson KM, Patterson JH, McQueen RH, Adams KF, Pieper JA. Effects of erythromycin or rifampin on losartan pharmacokinetics in healthy volunteers. *Clin Pharmacol Ther* (1998) 63, 316–23.

Angiotensin II receptor antagonists + Food or Drinks

Food modestly increases the bioavailability of eprosartan and slightly reduces the bioavailability of telmisartan. Food appears to have little or no effect on candesartan, irbesartan, losartan, olmesartan and valsartan. Grapefruit juice has a minor effect on the pharmacokinetics of losartan and its active metabolite E-3174.

Clinical evidence, mechanism, importance and management

(a) Food

Food delays **eprosartan** absorption, and modestly increases the AUC and maximum serum concentrations by up to 25%. The UK maker recommends that **eprosartan** is given with food,[1] but the US maker suggests that this is not clinically significant.[2] Food reduces the AUC of **telmisartan** by about 6 to 20% depending on dose,[3] but this is not expected to cause a reduction in therapeutic efficacy.[4]

A study in 16 healthy men found that a **high-fat breakfast** had no clinically relevant effects on the bioavailability of a single 300-mg dose of **irbesartan**.[5] The makers of **candesartan**,[6,7] **losartan**,[8] **olmesartan**[9] and **valsartan**[10] state that these drugs may be given with or without food.

(b) Grapefruit juice

A study in 9 healthy subjects found that grapefruit juice approximately doubled the time for a single 50-mg dose of **losartan** to be detected in the serum (from 0.6 to 1.3 hours) and reduced the AUC of the active metabolite of **losartan**, E-3174, by 21%. **Losartan** is partly metabolised by the cytochrome P450 isoenzyme CYP3A4 and transported by P-glycoprotein, both of which can be affected by grapefruit juice. This may explain the changes seen.[11] However, this interaction is unlikely to be clinically relevant.

1. Teveten (Eprosartan). Solvay Healthcare Ltd. UK Summary of product characteristics, December 2003.
2. Teveten (Eprosartan). Biovail Pharmaceuticals Inc. US Prescribing information, January 2004.
3. Micardis (Telmisartan). Boehringer Ingelheim Pharmaceuticals Inc. US Prescribing information, May 2004.
4. Micardis (Telmisartan). Boehringer Ingelheim Ltd. UK Summary of product characteristics, December 2004.
5. Vachharajani NN, Shyu WC, Mantha S, Park J-S, Greene DS, Barbhaiya RH. Lack of effect of food on the oral bioavailability of irbesartan in healthy male volunteers. *J Clin Pharmacol* (1998) 38, 433–6.
6. Amias (Candesartan). Takeda UK Ltd. UK Summary of product characteristics, December 2004.
7. Atacand (Candesartan). AstraZeneca. US Prescribing information, February 2005.
8. Cozaar (Losartan). Merck Sharp & Dohme Ltd. UK Summary of product characteristics, July 2003.
9. Benicar (Olmesartan). Sankyo. US Prescribing information, March 2003.
10. Diovan (Valsartan). Novartis Pharmaceuticals UK Ltd. UK Summary of product characteristics, September 2004.
11. Zaidenstein R, Soback S, Gips M, Avni B, Dishi V, Weissgarten Y, Golik A, Scapa E. Effect of grapefruit juice on the pharmacokinetics of losartan and its active metabolite E3174 in healthy volunteers. *Ther Drug Monit* (2001) 23, 369–73.

Angiotensin II receptor antagonists + H_2-blockers

Cimetidine may cause a small rise in plasma concentrations of valsartan, but this is unlikely to be clinically significant. Cimetidine did not significantly affect the pharmacokinetics and blood-pressure lowering effect of losartan. Ranitidine did not significantly alter the pharmacokinetics of eprosartan.

Clinical evidence, mechanism, importance and management

(a) Cimetidine

A 2-period, randomised, crossover study in 8 healthy subjects given **losartan** 100 mg alone and after taking cimetidine 400 mg four times daily for 6 days, found that the pharmacokinetics and pharmacodynamics of the **losartan** and its active metabolite, E-3174, were not changed to a clinically relevant extent by the cimetidine, although there was a modest increase of 18% in the AUC of **losartan**.[1] No special precautions are needed if these drugs are used concurrently.

In a single-dose, crossover study cimetidine 800 mg, given one hour before **valsartan** 160 mg, increased the initial rate of absorption of valsartan (attributed to a raised gastric pH) resulting in a roughly 50% increase in maximum plasma concentration. However, the AUC was only slightly increased and there were large inter-subject variations in the pharmacokinetics of **valsartan**.[2] The changes in **valsartan** pharmacokinetics seen with cimetidine appear to have little or no clinical relevance, but the UK makers[3] cautiously suggest that the systemic exposure to **valsartan** may be marginally increased. However, the US makers suggest that no clinically significant interaction is likely to occur.[4]

(b) Ranitidine

Seventeen healthy subjects were given a single 400-mg dose of **eprosartan** alone and after taking ranitidine 150 mg twice daily for 3 days. The ranitidine caused some slight, but statistically insignificant changes in the pharmacokinetics of the **eprosartan** (maximum plasma concentration and AUC reduced by approximately 7% and 11%, respectively).[5]

1. Goldberg MR, Lo M-W, Bradstreet TE, Ritter MA, Höglund P. Effects of cimetidine on pharmacokinetics and pharmacodynamics of losartan, an AT_1-selective non-peptide angiotensin II receptor antagonist. *Eur J Clin Pharmacol* (1995) 49, 115–19.
2. Schmidt EK, Antonin K-H, Flesch G, Racine-Poon A. An interaction study with cimetidine and the new angiotensin II antagonist valsartan. *Eur J Clin Pharmacol* (1998) 53, 451–8.
3. Diovan (Valsartan). Novartis Pharmaceuticals UK Ltd. UK Summary of product characteristics, September 2004.
4. Diovan (Valsartan). Novartis Pharmaceuticals Corporation. US Prescribing information, November 2003.
5. Tenero DM, Martin DE, Ilson BE, Boyle DA, Boike SC, Carr AM, Lundberg DE, Jorkasky DK. Effect of ranitidine on the pharmacokinetics of orally administered eprosartan, an angiotensin II antagonist, in healthy male volunteers. *Ann Pharmacother* (1998) 32, 304–8.

Angiotensin II receptor antagonists + Mannitol

A report describes mannitol-induced acute renal failure in a diabetic patient on losartan.

Clinical evidence, mechanism, importance and management

A man with diabetic nephropathy receiving **losartan** 25 mg twice daily for hypertension developed acute renal failure after being given a total of 420 g of mannitol intravenously over 4 days for haemorrhagic glaucoma. The patient recovered after the mannitol and **losartan** were discontinued and haemodialysis was performed.[1] The mechanism is not fully understood, but the combination may result in a marked decrease in glomerular filtration rate. Caution is recommended.[1] For comment on the potentiation of ACE inhibitor-induced renal damage by diuretics, see 'ACE inhibitors + Diuretics; Loop, thiazide or related', p.20.

1. Matsumura M. Mannitol-induced toxicity in a diabetic patient receiving losartan. *Am J Med* (2001) 110, 331.

Angiotensin II receptor antagonists + NSAIDs and other analgesics

Indometacin may attenuate the antihypertensive effect of losartan, valsartan, or other angiotensin II receptor antagonists. However, low-dose aspirin does not appear to alter the antihypertensive effect of losartan. No clinically relevant pharmacokinetic interactions occur between telmisartan and ibuprofen or paracetamol (acetaminophen), or between valsartan and indometacin.

Clinical evidence

(a) Aspirin

A double-blind placebo-controlled study in 10 patients with hypertension taking **losartan** (mean daily dose 47.5 mg) found that neither aspirin 81 mg nor 325 mg daily for 2 weeks had any significant effect on blood pressure.[1] The maker of **olmesartan** warns that aspirin at doses greater than 3 g daily may act synergistically with angiotensin II receptor antagonists in decreasing glomerular filtration and therefore increase the risk of acute renal failure.[2]

(b) Ibuprofen

In a cross-over study in 12 healthy subjects, **telmisartan** 120 mg daily had no effect on the pharmacokinetics of ibuprofen 400 mg three times a day for 7 days. Similarly, the pharmacokinetics of **telmisartan** were unaffected by the concurrent use of ibuprofen compared with previous studies of **telmisartan** alone.[3] For mention of ibuprofen interfering with the antihypertensive effect of an ACE inhibitor and other antihypertensive agents, see 'ACE inhibitors + NSAIDs', p.27.

(c) Indometacin

In a study in 111 patients with hypertension, **losartan** 50 mg once daily for 6 weeks reduced their blood pressure by a mean of 7.9/5.3 mmHg. Indometacin 75 mg once daily was then added for one week and this caused a rise in blood pressure in the group as a whole of 3.8/2.2 mmHg (approximately 45% reduction in the effect of **losartan**). A rise in ambulatory diastolic blood pressure was seen in 69% of the **losartan**-treated patients during indometacin use.[4] In contrast, a much smaller study in 10 patients with essential hypertension treated with **losartan** found that indometacin 50 mg twice daily for one week caused sodium and fluid retention, but did not significantly attenuate the antihypertensive effects of losartan.[5]

In a placebo-controlled, crossover study in 56 hypertensive patients whose blood pressure was adequately controlled by **valsartan** 80 to 160 mg daily, the addition of indometacin 50 mg twice daily for 2 weeks produced an increase in mean blood pressure of 2.1/1.9 mmHg.[6] A study in normotensive subjects maintained on fixed sodium intake and given **valsartan** 80 mg daily with or without indometacin 50 mg twice daily for one week, demonstrated that indometacin reduced the natriuretic response to the angiotensin receptor blockade.[7] In 12 healthy subjects the pharmacokinetics of single oral doses of **valsartan** 160 mg or indometacin 100 mg were not significantly changed when the drugs were given together, although the pharmacokinetics of **valsartan** showed wide variations between subjects.[8]

(d) Paracetamol (Acetaminophen)

Telmisartan 120 mg had no effect on the pharmacokinetics of paracetamol 1 g in a single-dose study in 12 healthy subjects. The pharmacokinetics of **telmisartan** were also unaffected by paracetamol compared with previous studies of **telmisartan** alone.[3]

Mechanism

Some evidence suggests that prostaglandins may be partially involved in the hypotensive action of angiotensin II receptor antagonists, and that NSAIDs, by inhibiting prostaglandin synthesis, may antagonise their effects. However, a non-specific mechanism such as sodium retention may also be involved as indometacin has been shown to reduce the hypotensive effect of other classes of antihypertensive drugs.[6,7]

Importance and management

Several makers of angiotensin II receptor antagonists caution that, as with other antihypertensive agents, the antihypertensive effect may be attenuated by NSAIDs such as indometacin. Patients on losartan or valsartan or other angiotensin II receptor antagonists, who require indometacin and probably related NSAIDs, should be monitored for alterations in blood pressure control. Poor renal perfusion may increase the risk of renal failure if angiotensin II receptor antagonists are given with NSAIDs and so regular hydration of the patient and monitoring of renal function is recommended.[2]

For details of similar interactions involving ACE inhibitors, see 'ACE inhibitors + Aspirin', p.15 and 'ACE inhibitors + NSAIDs', p.27.

1. Nawarskas JJ, Townsend RR, Cirigliano MD, Spinler SA. Effect of aspirin on blood pressure in hypertensive patients taking enalapril or losartan. *Am J Hypertens* (1999) 12, 784–9.
2. Olmetec (Olmesartan). Sankyo Pharma UK Ltd. UK Summary of product characteristics, August 2004.
3. Stangier J, Su C-APF, Fraunhofer A, Tetzloff W. Pharmacokinetics of acetaminophen and ibuprofen when coadministered with telmisartan in healthy volunteers. *J Clin Pharmacol* (2000) 40, 1338–46.
4. Conlin PR, Moore TJ, Swartz SL, Barr E, Gazdick L, Fletcher C, DeLucca P, Demopoulos L. Effect of indomethacin on blood pressure lowering by captopril and losartan in hypertensive patients. *Hypertension* (2000) 36, 461–5.
5. Olsen ME, Thomsen T, Hassager C, Ibsen H, Dige-Petersen H. Hemodynamic and renal effects of indomethacin in losartan-treated hypertensive individuals. *Am J Hypertens* (1999) 12, 209–16.
6. Fogari R, Zoppi A, Carretta R, Veglio F, Salvetti A: Italian Collaborative Study Group. Effect of indomethacin on the antihypertensive efficacy of valsartan and lisinopril: a multicentre study. *J Hypertens* (2002) 20: 1007–14.
7. Fricker AF, Nussberger J, Meilenbrock S, Brunner HR, Burnier M. Effect of indomethacin on the renal response to angiotensin II receptor blockade in healthy subjects. *Kidney Int* (1998) 54, 2089–97.
8. Ciba. Data on file, Protocol 43.

Angiotensin II receptor antagonists + Phenobarbital

Phenobarbital minimally alters plasma concentrations of losartan and its active metabolite.

Clinical evidence, mechanism, importance and management

In a placebo-controlled study involving 15 healthy subjects, phenobarbital 100 mg daily for 16 days significantly reduced the AUC of **losartan** and its active metabolite, E-3174, after a single 100-mg dose of **losartan**. For both **losartan** and its metabolite, the AUC during phenobarbital use was about 20% less than the AUC before phenobarbital, but this was not considered to be clinically significant.[1]

1. Goldberg MR, Lo MW, Deutsch PJ, Wilson SE, McWilliams EJ, McCrea JB. Phenobarbital minimally alters plasma concentrations of losartan and its active metabolite E-3174. *Clin Pharmacol Ther* (1996) 59, 268–74.

Angiotensin II receptor antagonists + Potassium compounds

There may be a risk of hyperkalaemia if angiotensin II receptor antagonists are given with potassium supplements or potassium-containing salt substitutes, particularly in those patients where other risk factors are present such as decreased renal function.

Clinical evidence, mechanism, importance and management

In placebo-controlled clinical studies, significantly elevated serum potassium concentrations were noted in 0.9% of patients treated with **eprosartan** compared with 0.3% of patients who received placebo.[1,2] **Losartan** has also been shown to cause hyperkalaemia; an incidence of 1.5% was found in hypertension clinical trials, but in a study in type II diabetic patients with nephropathy, the incidence was 9.9%.[3]

Based on evidence from other drugs that affect the renin-angiotensin system (e.g. ACE inhibitors), the makers of angiotensin II receptor antagonists warn that concurrent use of potassium supplements, **salt substitutes** or other drugs that increase potassium levels may increase serum potassium. Some makers advise against co-medication. However, if concurrent use is considered necessary, potassium levels should be closely monitored, particularly in those with renal impairment; other risk factors include diabetes mellitus or heart failure. For reports of hyperkalaemia associated with ACE inhibitors and dietary potassium, see 'ACE inhibitors + Potassium compounds', p.30.

1. Teveten (Eprosartan). Solvay Healthcare Ltd. UK Summary of product characteristics, December 2003.
2. Teveten (Eprosartan). Biovail Pharmaceuticals Inc. US Prescribing information, January 2004.
3. Cozaar (Losartan). Merck Sharp & Dohme Ltd. UK Summary of product characteristics, July 2003.

Angiotensin II receptor antagonists + Rifampicin (Rifampin)

Rifampicin increases the metabolism of losartan and its active metabolite, E-3174, which may result in reduced antihypertensive effects.

Clinical evidence, mechanism, importance and management

Ten healthy subjects were given **losartan** 50 mg daily for a week and then, after a 6-day washout period, **losartan** 50 mg daily plus rifampicin 300 mg twice daily for a week. It was found that the rifampicin reduced the **losartan** AUC by 36%, reduced its half-life from 2 to 0.9 hours, and increased its clearance by 60%. The AUC of the active metabolite, E3174, was reduced by 41% and its half-life was reduced from 5.1 to 2.5 hours. Diastolic blood pressure was significantly reduced by **losartan** alone, but not by the combination.[1] The presumed reason for this interaction is that rifampicin (a recognised enzyme inducer) increases the metabolism of the **losartan** by the cytochrome P450 isoenzyme CYP2C9.

The clinical importance of this interaction still awaits assessment, but it would seem likely that the antihypertensive effects of the **losartan** would be reduced by rifampicin. If both drugs are used, be alert for the need to increase the **losartan** dosage. More study is needed.

1. Williamson KM, Patterson JH, McQueen RH, Adams KF, Pieper JA. Effects of erythromycin or rifampin on losartan pharmacokinetics in healthy volunteers. *Clin Pharmacol Ther* (1998) 63, 316–23.

3

Alcohol

For social and historical reasons alcohol is usually bought from a store or in a bar or restaurant, rather than from a pharmacy, because it is considered to be a drink and not a drug. However, pharmacologically speaking it has much in common with medicinal drugs that depress the central nervous system. Objective tests show that as blood-alcohol levels rise, the ability to perform a number of skills gradually deteriorates as the brain becomes progressively disorganised. The myth that alcohol is a stimulant has arisen because at parties and social occasions it helps people to lose some of their inhibitions and it allows them to relax and unwind. Professor JH Gaddum put it amusingly and succinctly when, describing the early effects of moderate amounts of alcohol, he wrote that "logical thought is difficult but after dinner speeches easy." The expansiveness and loquaciousness that are socially acceptable, can lead on, with increasing amounts of alcohol, to unrestrained behaviour in normally well-controlled individuals, through to drunkenness, unconsciousness, and finally death from respiratory failure. These effects are all a reflection of the progressive and deepening depression of the CNS.

'Table 3.1', (p.37) gives an indication in very broad terms of the reactions of men and women to different amounts and concentrations of alcohol.

On the whole women have a higher proportion of fat in which alcohol is not very soluble, their body fluids represent a smaller proportion of their total body mass, and their first-pass metabolism of alcohol is less than men because they have less alcohol dehydrogenase in their stomach walls. Consequently if a man and woman of the same weight matched each other, drink for drink, the woman would finish up with a blood alcohol level about 50% higher than the man. The values shown assume that the drinkers regularly drink, have had a meal and weigh between 9 and 11 stones (55 to 70 kg). Higher blood alcohol levels would occur if drunk on an empty stomach and lower values in much heavier individuals. The liver metabolises about one unit per hour so the values will fall with time.

Since alcohol impairs the skills needed to drive safely, almost all national and state authorities have imposed maximum legal blood alcohol limits (see 'Table 3.2', p.37). In the UK and a number of other countries this has been set at 80 mg/100 ml (35 micrograms per 100 ml in the breath) but impairment is clearly detectable at lower concentrations, for which reason some countries have imposed much lower legal limits.

Probably the most common drug interaction of all occurs if alcohol is drunk by those taking other drugs that have CNS depressant activity, the result being even further CNS depression. Blood alcohol levels well within the legal driving limit may, in the presence of other CNS depressants, be equivalent to blood alcohol levels at or above the legal limit in terms of worsened driving and other skills. This can occur with some antihistamines, analgesics, antidepressants, cough, cold and influenza remedies, hypno-sedatives and others (see 'Alcohol + CNS depressants', p.48). This section contains a number of monographs that describe the results of formal studies of alcohol combined with a number of recognised CNS depressants, but there are still many other drugs that await study of this kind, and which undoubtedly represent a real hazard.

A less common interaction that can occur between alcohol and some drugs, chemical agents, and fungi is the flushing (*Antabuse*) reaction. This is exploited in the case of disulfiram (*Antabuse*) as a drink deterrent, but it can occur unexpectedly with some other drugs and can be both unpleasant and possibly frightening, but it is not usually dangerous.

Table 3.1 Reactions to different concentrations of alcohol in the blood

Amounts of alcohol drunk				
Man 11 stones (70 kg)	*Woman 9 stones (55 kg)*	*Blood-alcohol levels mg% (mg per 100 ml)*	*Reactions to different % of alcohol in the blood*	
2 units	1 unit	25–30	Sense of well-being enhanced. Reaction times reduced	
4 units	2 units	50–60	Mild loss of inhibition, judgement impaired, increased risk of accidents at home, at work and on the road; no overt signs of drunkenness	
5 units	3 units	75–80	Physical co-ordination reduced, more marked loss of inhibition; noticeably under the influence; at the legal limit for driving in the UK	
7 units	4 units	100+	Clumsiness, loss of physical control, tendency to extreme responses; definite intoxication	
10 units	6 units	150	Slurred speech, possible loss of memory the following day, probably drunk and disorderly	
24 units	14 units	360	Dead drunk, sleepiness, possible loss of consciousness	
33 units	20 units	500	Coma and possibly death	
1 unit	= half pint (300 ml medium strength beer)	= glass wine (100 ml)	= single sherry or martini (a third of a gill (50 ml))	= single spirit one-sixth gill (25 ml)
	3–4% alcohol	11% alcohol	17–20% alcohol	37–40% alcohol

After *Which?* October 1984, page 447 and others.

Table 3.2 Maximum legally allowable blood alcohol limits when driving in various countries

80 mg%	Canada,* Cape Verde, Central African Republic, Ghana, Guatemala, Ireland, Kenya, Luxembourg, Malaysia, Malta, Mauritius, Mexico, New Zealand,* Nicaragua, Niger, Paraguay, Seychelles, Singapore, Suriname, Switzerland, Uganda, United Kingdom, United States of America,* Uruguay, Zambia
70 mg%	Bolivia, Ecuador, Honduras
60 mg%	Brazil, Sri Lanka
52 mg%	Republic of Korea
50 mg%	Argentina, Australia,* Austria, Belarus, Benin, Bosnia & Herzegovina, Bulgaria, Cambodia, Croatia, Denmark, El Salvador, Finland, France, French Polynesia, Germany, Greece, Guinea-Bissau, Iceland, Israel, Italy, Kyrgyzstan, Micronesia (Federated States of), Namibia, Netherlands, Peru, Philippines, Portugal, Slovenia, South Africa, Spain, Thailand, The former Yugoslav Republic of Macedonia, Turkey, United Republic of Tanzania, Venezuela
49 mg%	Chile, Costa Rica, Latvia
40 mg%	Lithuania
35 mg%	Jamaica
33 mg%	Turkmenistan
30 mg%	Georgia, India, Japan, Republic of Moldova
20 mg%	Estonia, Mongolia, Norway, Poland, Sweden
10 mg%	Algeria, Guyana, Palau
0 mg%	Armenia, Azerbaijan, Colombia, Czech Republic, Equatorial Guinea, Eritrea, Gambia, Guinea, Hungary, Islamic Republic of Iran, Jordan, Kazakhstan, Malawi, Nepal, Nigeria, Panama, Romania, Russian Federation, Slovakia
No legislation	China, Comoros, Congo (Brazzaville), Dominican Republic, Ethiopia, Lao People's Democratic Republic, Togo, Ukraine

Note: For easy comparison the legally allowable blood alcohol limits have all been expressed as mg%. Thus: blood alcohol levels of 80 mg% = 80 mg of alcohol in 100 ml blood = 0.8 g/l.

*Variations occur within these countries e.g. in Australia there are the following limits – 0.0% for drivers of heavy, dangerous goods, public transport vehicles; learners and drivers under 25 years of age for first three years of driving.

WHO Global Alcohol database, Geneva, 2003.

Alcohol + Abacavir

Alcohol reduces the metabolism of abacavir.

Clinical evidence, mechanism, importance and management

A study in 24 HIV+ patients found that alcohol 0.7 g/kg increased the AUC of a single 600-mg dose of abacavir by 41%. The half life of abacavir was increased by 26% from 1.42 to 1.79 hours. The pharmacokinetics of alcohol were not affected by concurrent abacavir.[1] Alcohol may inhibit the formation of abacavir carboxylate resulting in a trend towards increased abacavir glucuronide formation and reduced abacavir metabolism. The increase in exposure to abacavir was not considered to be clinically significant, since it is within levels seen in other studies using higher doses, which demonstrated no additional safety concerns at doses of up to three times the recommended daily dose of abacavir.[1] No special precautions therefore appear to be necessary.

1. McDowell JA, Chittick GE, Stevens CP, Edwards KD, Stein DS. Pharmacokinetic interaction of abacavir (1592U89) and ethanol in human immunodeficiency virus-infected adults. *Antimicrob Agents Chemother* (2000) 44, 1686–90.

Alcohol + Amfetamines

Dexamfetamine can reduce the deleterious effects of alcohol to some extent, but some impairment still occurs making it unsafe to drive. Another report suggests the combination of metamfetamine and alcohol produces an increase in perceived total intoxication, and may also increase cardiac adverse effects.

Clinical evidence

Alcohol 0.85 g/kg (2 ml/kg of 100 proof vodka in orange juice) worsened the performance of a SEDI task (Simulator Evaluation of Drug Impairment) in 12 healthy subjects.[1] This task is believed to parallel the skills needed to drive safely, and involves tests of attention, memory, recognition, decision making and reaction times. When the subjects were additionally given 0.09 or 0.18 mg/kg **dexamfetamine**, the performance of the SEDI task was improved (dose related), but the subjective assessment of intoxication was unchanged. Blood alcohol levels reached a maximum of about 100 mg% at an hour. The bioavailability of the alcohol was slightly increased.[1]

Earlier reports using different testing methods found that in some tests **dexamfetamine** modified the effects of alcohol,[2,3] but the total picture was complex, and other reports found no antagonism.[4,5] Another study found that in stress situations, where relief of fatigue or boredom alone will not produce improved performance, **dexamfetamine** failed to improve attentive motor performance made worse by alcohol.[6] A later study found that, while the combination of alcohol and **metamfetamine** diminished the subjective feelings of alcohol intoxication, there was actually an increase in feelings of total intoxication.[7]

Mechanism

Not understood. Although alcohol is a CNS depressant and the amfetamines are CNS stimulants, there is no simple antagonism between the two.[3] The combination of alcohol and metamfetamine may increase cardiac work load and toxicity.[7]

Importance and management

Clearcut conclusions cannot be drawn from the evidence presented in the reported studies. There is some evidence that the effects of alcohol are modified or reduced, but driving skills appear to remain impaired to some extent. There is also evidence of an increased risk of adverse cardiac effects. The increase in perceived total intoxication noted in one report has been suggested as a possible reason for the popularity of the illicit use of the combination.[7] See also 'Alcohol + Ecstasy (MDMA, 3,4-methylenedioxymethamfetamine)', p.50.

1. Perez-Reyes M, White WR, McDonald SA, Hicks RE. Interaction between ethanol and dextroamphetamine: effects on psychomotor performance. *Alcohol Clin Exp Res* (1992) 16, 75–81.
2. Harger RN, ed. Dextro-amphetamine, alcohol, and dextro-amphetamine-alcohol combination and mental performance; in Alcohol and traffic safety. Bloomington, Indiana: Indiana Univ Press; 1966 P. 211–14.
3. Wilson L, Taylor JD, Nash CW, Cameron DF. The combined effects of ethanol and amphetamine sulfate on performance of human subjects. *Can Med Assoc J* (1966) 94, 478–84.
4. Hughes FW, Forney RB. Dextro-amphetamine, ethanol and dextro-amphetamine-ethanol combinations on performance of human subjects stressed with delayed auditory feedback (DAF). *Psychopharmacologia* (1964) 6, 234–8.
5. Newman HW, Newman EJ. Failure of dexedrine and caffeine as practical antagonists of the depressant effect of ethyl alcohol in man. *Q J Stud Alcohol* (1956) 17, 406–10.
6. Harger RN, ed. Effect of d-amphetamine and alcohol on attentive motor performance in human subjects; in Alcohol and traffic safety. Bloomington, Indiana: Indiana Univ Press; 1966 P. 215–19.
7. Mendelson J, Jones RT, Upton R, Jacob P. Methamphetamine and ethanol interactions in humans. *Clin Pharmacol Ther* (1995) 57, 559–68.

Alcohol + Aminosalicylic acid

Alcohol can abolish the lipid-lowering effects of aminosalicylic acid.

Clinical evidence, mechanism, importance and management

The effectiveness of PAS-C (purified aminosalicylic acid recrystallised in vitamin C) and diet on the treatment of hyperlipidaemia types IIa and IIb was studied in a group of 63 subjects. It was noted that when 3 of the subjects drank unstated amounts of alcohol (beer or cocktails), the effects of the PAS-C on lowering serum cholesterol, triglyceride and LDL-cholesterol levels were completely abolished.[1] The reasons are not understood.

Patients given aminosalicylic acid to reduce lipid levels should avoid alcohol. There seems to be no evidence that alcohol affects the treatment of tuberculosis with aminosalicylic acid.

1. Kuo PT, Fan WC, Kostis JB, Hayase K. Combined para-aminosalicylic acid and dietary therapy in long-term control of hypercholesterolemia and hypertriglyceridemia (types II_a and II_b hyperlipoproteinemia). *Circulation* (1976) 53, 338–41.

Alcohol + Anticholinergics

Propantheline appears not to affect blood alcohol levels, whereas atropine may cause a modest reduction. Marked impairment of attention can occur if alcohol is taken in the presence of atropine or glycopyrronium (glycopyrrolate), probably making driving more hazardous. No adverse interaction appears to occur with transdermal hyoscine and alcohol.

Clinical evidence, mechanism, importance and management

Oral **propantheline** (15 mg four times daily or 30 mg three times daily for 5 days and 30 mg or 60 mg 2 hours before alcohol) did not affect blood alcohol levels in 3 subjects, whereas a single 3-mg oral dose of **atropine** 2 hours before alcohol reduced the AUC of alcohol by a modest 20% in 3 subjects.[1] Another study in healthy subjects of the effects of oral **atropine** 500 micrograms or **glycopyrronium** 1 mg in combination with alcohol 0.5 g/kg showed that, while reaction times and co-ordination were unaffected or even improved, there was a marked impairment of attention, which was large enough to make driving more hazardous.[2] Patients should be warned.

A double-blind crossover study in 12 healthy subjects showed that a transdermal **hyoscine** preparation (*Scopoderm-TTS*) did not alter the effects of alcohol on the performance of several psychometric tests (Critical Flicker Fusion Frequency, Choice Reaction Tasks), nor was the clearance of alcohol or **hyoscine** changed. Blood alcohol levels of up to 80 and 130 mg% were studied.[3] No special precautions seem necessary.

1. Gibbons DO, Lant AF. Effects of intravenous and oral propantheline and metoclopramide on ethanol absorption. *Clin Pharmacol Ther* (1975) 17, 578–84.
2. Linnoila M. Drug effects on psychomotor skills related to driving: interaction of atropine, glycopyrrhonium and alcohol. *Eur J Clin Pharmacol* (1973) 6, 107–12.
3. Gleiter CH, Antonin K-H, Schoenleber W, Bieck PR. Interaction of alcohol and transdermally administered scopolamine. *J Clin Pharmacol* (1988) 28, 1123–7.

Alcohol + Anticonvulsants

Moderate social drinking does not appear to affect the serum levels of carbamazepine, ethosuximide or phenytoin. Some small changes are seen in serum phenobarbital and sodium valproate

levels, but no changes in the control of epilepsy seem to occur. No pharmacokinetic interaction was detected between tiagabine and alcohol, and tiagabine did not alter the cognitive effect of alcohol.

Clinical evidence, mechanism, importance and management

A study in 29 non-drinking epileptics found that when they drank 1 to 3 glasses of an alcoholic beverage (1 to 3 units) over a 2-hour period, twice a week, for 16 weeks, the serum levels of **carbamazepine**, **ethosuximide** and phenytoin were unchanged when compared with those from a control group of 23 epileptics given drinks without alcohol. There was a marginal change in **phenobarbital** levels, and some increase in serum **valproate** levels. However, this effect is hard to interpret as **valproate** levels are known fluctuate and are hard to reproduce. Other anticonvulsants used were **clonazepam**, **primidone** and **sultiame**, but too few patients used these for a valid statistical analysis to be carried out. Maximum blood alcohol levels ranged from 5 to 33 mg%. More important than any changes that occurred in serum anticonvulsant levels, was the finding that this social drinking had no effect on the frequency of tonic-clonic convulsions, partial complex seizures, or on the epileptic activity as measured by EEGs.[1] Another study in healthy subjects excluded any pharmacodynamic or pharmacokinetic interaction between **tiagabine** and alcohol. In this study, **tiagabine** 4 mg three times daily did not alter the effect of a single dose of ethanol as assessed in a range of cognitive tests.[2]

There would therefore seem to be no reason for epileptics on the above drugs to avoid alcohol in moderate social amounts. Some anticonvulsants have sedative effects, which may be additive with those of alcohol, see 'Alcohol + Barbiturates', p.42. Consider also 'Alcohol + Anticonvulsants; Phenytoin', p.39.

1. Höppener RJ, Kuyer A, van der Lugt PJM. Epilepsy and alcohol: the influence of social alcohol on seizures and treatment in epilepsy. *Epilepsia* (1983) 24, 459–71.
2. Kastberg H, Jansen JA, Cole G, Wesnes K. Tiagabine: absence of kinetic or dynamic interactions with ethanol. *Drug Metabol Drug Interact* (1998) 14, 259–73.

Alcohol + Anticonvulsants; Phenytoin

Chronic heavy drinking reduces serum phenytoin concentrations so that above-average doses of phenytoin may be needed to maintain adequate levels.

Clinical evidence

(a) Acute alcohol ingestion

In a study designed to test the effects of acute alcohol intoxication in epileptics, 25 patients were given a 12 oz (about 340 ml drink) of 25% alcohol. Blood alcohol levels ranged from 39 to 284 mg%. All patients had signs of alcohol intoxication without any effect on seizure frequency.[1] The metabolism of a single dose of phenytoin was not affected in one study in healthy subjects by the acute ingestion of alcohol.[2]

(b) Heavy drinking

Blood phenytoin levels measured 24 hours after the last dose of phenytoin in a group of 15 drinkers (consuming a minimum of 200 g ethanol daily for at least 3 months) were approximately half those of 76 non-drinkers. The phenytoin half-life was reduced by 30%.[3]

Another study confirmed that alcoholics without liver disease have lower than usual plasma levels of phenytoin after taking standard doses while drinking.[4] A report describes a chronic alcoholic who was resistant to large doses of phenytoin,[5] and another describes a reduction in serum phenytoin levels accompanied by seizures in a man when his consumption of alcohol increased.[6]

(c) Moderate social drinking

A study in non-drinking epileptics (17 in the experimental group, 14 in the control group) found that the serum levels of phenytoin were unchanged by moderate drinking, and there was no influence on tonic-clonic convulsions or partial complex seizures. The experimental group drank 1 to 3 glasses of an alcoholic beverage (equivalent to a glass of beer containing 9.85 g ethanol) over a 2-hour period, twice a week, for 16 weeks, and their maximum blood alcohol levels ranged from 5 to 33 mg%.[7]

Mechanism

Supported by *animal* data,[8] the evidence suggests that repeated exposure to large amounts of alcohol induces liver microsomal enzymes so that the rate of metabolism and clearance of phenytoin from the body is increased.

Importance and management

An established and clinically important interaction although the documentation is limited. Heavy drinkers may need above-average doses of phenytoin to maintain adequate serum levels. However, be aware that patients with liver impairment usually need lower doses of phenytoin, so the picture may be more complicated. Moderate drinking appears to be safe in those on phenytoin.[1,7] Consider also 'Alcohol + Anticonvulsants', p.38.

1. Rodin EA, Frohman CE, Gottlieb JS. Effect of acute alcohol intoxication on epileptic patients. *Arch Neurol* (1961) 4, 115–18.
2. Schmidt D. Effect of ethanol intake on phenytoin metabolism in volunteers. *Experientia* (1975) 31, 1313–14.
3. Kater RMH, Roggin G, Tobon F, Zieve P, Iber FL. Increased rate of clearance of drugs from the circulation of alcoholics. *Am J Med Sci* (1969) 258, 35–9.
4. Sandor P, Sellers EM, Dumbrell M, Khouw V. Effect of short- and long-term alcohol use on phenytoin kinetics in chronic alcoholics. *Clin Pharmacol Ther* (1981) 30, 390–7.
5. Birkett DJ, Graham GG, Chinwah PM, Wade DN, Hickie JB. Multiple drug interactions with phenytoin. *Med J Aust* (1977) 2, 467–8.
6. Bellibas SE, Tuglular I. A case of phenytoin-alcohol interaction. *Therapie* (1995) 50, 487–8.
7. Höppener RJ, Kuyer A, van der Lugt PJM. Epilepsy and alcohol: the influence of social alcohol intake on seizures and treatment in epilepsy. *Epilepsia* (1983) 24, 459–71.
8. Rubin E, Lieber CS. Hepatic microsomal enzymes in man and rat: induction and inhibition by ethanol. *Science* (1968) 162, 690–1.

Alcohol + Antihistamines

Some antihistamines cause drowsiness, which can be increased by alcohol. The detrimental effects of alcohol on driving skills are considerably increased by the use of the older more sedative antihistamines and appear to be minimal or absent with the newer non-sedating antihistamines. Some of the more sedative antihistamines are common ingredients of cough, cold and influenza remedies. See 'Table 13.1', (p.425), which lists antihistamines by their sedative potential.

Clinical evidence

(a) Non-sedating antihistamines

Acrivastine 4 and 8 mg, given with and without alcohol, was found in a study to behave like **terfenadine** (which interacts minimally or not at all).[1] A double blind study found that **terfenadine** 60 to 240 mg alone did not affect psychomotor skills, nor did it affect the adverse effects of alcohol.[2] Another study had similar findings.[3] However, a later study found that **terfenadine** 240 mg slowed brake reaction times in the laboratory when given either alone or with alcohol.[4] Other studies have shown that **astemizole** 10 to 30 mg daily,[5-7] **desloratadine**,[8] **ebastine** 20 mg,[9] **fexofenadine** 120 to 240 mg,[10] **levocabastine** 2 nasal puffs of 0.5 mg/ml,[11] **loratadine** 10 to 20 mg[3,12] and **mizolastine** 10 mg[13] do not interact with alcohol. **Cetirizine** 10 mg also appeared not interact with alcohol in two studies[13,14] but some slight additive effects were detected in another.[12]

(b) Sedative antihistamines

Significant impairment of psychomotor performance was seen in healthy subjects given 12 mg of **chlorphenamine** with alcohol 0.5 g/kg.[5] Alcohol 0.75 g/kg and **dexchlorpheniramine** 4 mg/70 kg given to 13 healthy subjects significantly impaired their performance of a number of tests (standing steadiness, reaction time, manual dexterity, perception, etc.).[15] Other studies in *animals* also describe this interaction.[16] **Diphenhydramine** in doses of 25 or 50 mg was shown to increase the detrimental effects of alcohol on the performance of choice reaction and co-ordination tests in subjects who had taken 0.5 g/kg alcohol;[17] the interaction between **diphenhydramine** in doses of 50, 75 or 100 mg and alcohol in doses of 0.5 to 0.75 g/kg has been confirmed in other reports.[2,18-21] A marked interaction can also occur with **promethazine**.[22] A very marked deterioration in driving skills was clearly demonstrated in a test of car drivers given 20 ml of *Beechams Night Nurse* (**promethazine** with **dextromethorphan**), 10 ml of *Benylin* (**diphenhydramine** with **dextromethorphan**), or 30 ml of *Lemsip Night time flu medicine* (**chlorphenamine** with **dextromethorphan**). Very poor scores were seen when they were additionally given a double **Scotch whiskey** about 1.5 hours later.[23] In 19 healthy subjects **emedastine** in oral doses of 2 or 4 mg twice daily was found to be sedating and impair driving ability. The addition of alcohol increased this impairment.[24]

The effects of alcohol (blood levels about 50 mg%) and antihistamines, alone or together, on the performance of tests designed to assess mental and motor performance were examined in 16 subjects. **Clemizole** 40 mg or **tripelennamine** 50 mg alone did not significantly affect the performance under the stress of delayed auditory feedback, neither did they potentiate the effect of alcohol.[18] **Clemastine** in 3-mg doses also affected co-ordination, whereas 1.5 mg and 1 mg did not.[17,25] A study in 5 subjects showed that the detrimental effects of 100 ml of **whiskey** on the performance of driving tests on a racing car simulator (blood alcohol estimated as less than 80 mg% were not increased by 50 mg **cyclizine**.[26] However 3 of the subjects experienced drowsiness after **cyclizine**, and other studies have shown that **cyclizine** alone causes drowsiness in the majority.[27] A study in 17 subjects of the effects of alcohol and **mebhydrolin** 0.71 mg/kg found that the performance of a number of tests on perceptual, cognitive and motor functions was impaired to some extent.[28] No interaction was detected in one study of the combined effects of **pheniramine aminosalicylate** 50 mg or **cyproheptadine hydrochloride** 4 mg and alcohol 0.95 ml/kg.[29] **Triprolidine** 10 mg alone can significantly affect driving performance,[3] and marked deterioration in driving skills has been demonstrated with 10 ml of *Actifed Syrup* (**triprolidine** with **pseudoephedrine**) alone and with a double **whiskey**.[23]

Mechanism

When an interaction occurs it appears to be due to the combined or additive central nervous depressant effects of both the alcohol and the antihistamine. The authors of one study found that the sedating effects of cetirizine and emedastine were more marked in women than in men, and they noted that they had also previously seen this with mizolastine, acrivastine and clemastine.[24] The reason for this is not established although it has been suggested that a smaller volume of distribution in women may result in higher plasma antihistamine levels.

Importance and management

An adverse interaction between alcohol and the **most sedative antihistamines** (diphenhydramine, promethazine) is well established and clinically important. Marked drowsiness can occur with these antihistamines taken alone, which makes driving or handling other potentially dangerous machinery much more hazardous. This can be further worsened by alcohol. Remember that some of these antihistamines appear 'in disguise' as antiemetics, sedatives and as components of cough/cold and influenza remedies (e.g. *Benylin*, *Lemsip*, *Night Nurse*), which can be bought over the counter. Patients should be strongly warned. Emedastine may also cause marked sedation when used orally, but it is usually given as eye drops.

The situation with some of the **less sedative antihistamines** (clemastine, clemizole, cyclizine, cyproheptadine, mebhydrolin, pheniramine, tripelennamine and triprolidine) is less clear cut, and tests with some of them failed to detect an interaction with normal doses and moderate amounts of alcohol, however it has been clearly seen with *Actifed Syrup* (containing triprolidine). It would therefore be prudent to issue some cautionary warning, particularly if the patient is likely to drive.

The **non-sedating antihistamines** (acrivastine, astemizole, cetirizine, ebastine, fexofenadine, levocabastine, loratadine, mizolastine, terfenadine) seem to cause little or no drowsiness in most patients and the risks if taken alone or with alcohol appear to be minimal or absent. Nevertheless, patients should be advised to be alert to the possibility of drowsiness if they have not taken the drug before. Any drowsiness would be apparent after the first few doses.

The possible interactions of alcohol with other antihistamines not cited here do not seem to have been formally studied, but increased drowsiness and increased driving risks would be expected with any that cause some sedation. Patients should be warned. The risks with non-sedating antihistamines (e.g. **azelastine**, **epinastine**, **setastine**) are probably minimal, but this needs confirmation.

1. Cohen AF, Hamilton MJ, Peck AW. The effects of acrivastine (BW825C), diphenhydramine and terfenadine in combination with alcohol on human CNS performance. *Eur J Clin Pharmacol* (1987) 32, 279–88.
2. Moser L, Hüther KJ, Koch-Weser J, Lundt PV. Effects of terfenadine and diphenhydramine alone or in combination with diazepam or alcohol on psychomotor performance and subjective feelings. *Eur J Clin Pharmacol* (1978) 14, 417–23.
3. O'Hanlon JF. Antihistamines and driving performance: The Netherlands. *J Respir Dis* (1988) (Suppl), S12–S17.
4. Bhatti JZ, Hindmarch I. The effects of terfenadine with and without alcohol on an aspect of car driving performance. *Clin Exp Allergy* (1989) 19, 609–11.
5. Hindmarch I, Bhatti JZ. Psychomotor effects of astemizole and chlorpheniramine, alone and in combination with alcohol. *Int Clin Psychopharmacol* (1987) 2, 117–19.
6. Bateman DN, Chapman PH, Rawlins MD. Lack of effect of astemizole on ethanol dynamics or kinetics. *Eur J Clin Pharmacol* (1983) 25, 567–8.
7. Moser L, Plum H, Bückmann M. Interaktionen eines neuen Antihistaminikums mit Diazepam und Alkohol. *Med Welt* (1984) 35, 296–9.
8. Rikken G, Scharf M, Danzig M, Staudinger H. Desloratadine and alcohol coadministration: no increase in impairment of performance over that induced by alcohol alone. Poster at EAACI (European Academy of Allergy and Clinical Immunology) Conference, Lisbon, Portugal. 2-4 July 2000.
9. Mattila MJ, Kuitunen T, Plétan Y. Lack of pharmacodynamic and pharmacokinetic interactions of the antihistamine ebastine with ethanol in healthy subjects. *Eur J Clin Pharmacol* (1992) 43, 179–84.
10. Vermeeren A, O'Hanlon JF. Fexofenadine's effects, alone and with alcohol, on actual driving and psychomotor performance. *J Allergy Clin Immunol* (1998) 101, 306–11.
11. Nicholls A, Janssens M, James R. The effects of levocabastine and ethanol on psychomotor performance in healthy volunteers. *Allergy* (1993) 48 (Suppl 16), 34.
12. Ramaekers JG, Uiterwijk MMC, O'Hanlon JF. Effects of loratadine and cetirizine on actual driving and psychometric test performance, and EEG during driving. *Eur J Clin Pharmacol* (1992) 42, 363–9.
13. Patat A, Stubbs D, Dunmore C, Ulliac N, Sexton B, Zieleniuk I, Irving A, Jones W. Lack of interaction between two antihistamines, mizolastine and cetirizine, and ethanol in psychomotor and driving performance in healthy subjects. *Eur J Clin Pharmacol* (1995) 48, 143–50.
14. Doms M, Vanhulle G, Baelde Y, Coulie P, Dupont P, Rihoux J-P. Lack of potentiation by cetirizine of alcohol-induced psychomotor disturbances. *Eur J Clin Pharmacol* (1988) 34, 619–23.
15. Franks HM, Hensley VR, Hensley WJ, Starmer GA, Teo RKC. The interaction between ethanol and antihistamines. 1: Dexchlorpheniramine. *Med J Aust* (1978) 1, 449–52.
16. Smith RB, Rossie GV, Orzechowski RF. Interactions of chlorpheniramine ethanol combinations: acute toxicity and antihistaminic activity. *Toxicol Appl Pharmacol* (1974) 28, 240–7.
17. Linnoila M. Effects of antihistamines, chlormezanone and alcohol on psychomotor skills related to driving. *Eur J Clin Pharmacol* (1973) 5, 247–54.
18. Hughes FW, Forney RB. Comparative effect of three antihistaminics and ethanol on mental and motor performance. *Clin Pharmacol Ther* (1964) 5, 414–21.
19. Baugh R, Calvert RT. The effects of diphenhydramine alone and in combination with ethanol on histamine skin response and mental performance. *Eur J Clin Pharmacol* (1977) 12, 201–4.
20. Burns M, Moskowitz H. Effects of diphenhydramine and alcohol on skills performance. *Eur J Clin Pharmacol* (1980) 17, 259–66.
21. Burns M. Alcohol and antihistamine in combination: effects on performance. *Alcohol Clin Exp Res* (1989) 13, 341.
22. Hedges A, Hills M, Maclay WP, Newman-Taylor AJ, Turner P. Some central and peripheral effects of meclastine, a new antihistaminic drug, in man. *J Clin Pharmacol* (1971) 11, 112–19.
23. Carter N. Cold cures drug alert. *Auto Express* (1992) November Issue 218, 15–16.
24. Vermeeren A, Ramaekers JG, O'Hanlon JF. Effects of emedastine and cetirizine, alone and with alcohol, on actual driving of males and females. *J Psychopharmacol* (2002) 16, 57–64.
25. Franks HM, Hensley VR, Hensley WJ, Starmer GA, Teo RKC. The interaction between ethanol and antihistamines. 2. Clemastine. *Med J Aust* (1979) 1, 185–6.
26. Hughes DTD, Cramer F, Knight GJ. Use of a racing car simulator for medical research. The effects of marzine and alcohol on driving performance. *Med Sci Law* (1967) 7, 200–4.
27. Brand JJ, Colquhoun WP, Gould AH, Perry WLM. (–)-Hyoscine and cyclizine as motion sickness remedies. *Br J Pharmacol Chemother* (1967) 30, 463–9.
28. Franks HM, Lawrie M, Schabinsky VV, Starmer GA, Teo RKC. The interaction between ethanol and antihistamines. 3. mebhydrolin. *Med J Aust* (1981) 2, 447–9.
29. Landauer AA, Milner G. Antihistamines, alone and together with alcohol, in relation to driving safety. *J Forensic Med* (1971) 18, 127–39.

Alcohol + Antihypertensives

Chronic moderate to heavy drinking raises the blood pressure and reduces, to some extent, the effectiveness of antihypertensive drugs. A few patients may experience postural hypotension, dizziness and fainting shortly after having a drink. Alpha blockers may enhance the hypotensive effect of alcohol in subjects susceptible to the alcohol flush syndrome.

Clinical evidence, mechanism, importance and management

(a) Hypertensive reaction

A study in 40 men with essential hypertension (treated with **diuretics**, **beta-blockers**, **verapamil**, **prazosin**, **captopril** or **methyldopa**) who were moderate to heavy drinkers, found that when they reduced their drinking over a 6-week period from an average of 450 ml ethanol weekly (about 6 drinks daily) to 64 ml ethanol weekly, their average blood pressure fell by 5/3 mmHg.[1] The reasons are uncertain. These findings are consistent with those of other studies in hypertensive[2] and normotensive[3] men. It seems likely that this effect will occur with any antihypertensive. Patients with hypertension who are moderate to heavy drinkers should be encouraged to reduce their intake of alcohol. It may then become possible to reduce the dosage of the antihypertensive. It should be noted that epidemiological studies show that regular light to moderate alcohol consumption is associated with a *lower* risk of cardiovascular disease.[4]

(b) Hypotensive reaction

A few patients taking some antihypertensives feel dizzy or begin to 'black out' or faint if they stand up quickly or after exercise. This orthostatic and exertional hypotension may be exaggerated in some patients shortly after drinking alcohol, possibly because it can lower the output of the heart (noted in patients with various types of heart disease[5,6]). Patients just beginning antihypertensive treatment should be warned.

A study in 10 Japanese hypertensive patients found that alcohol 1 ml/kg decreased blood pressure for several hours. Treatment with **prazosin** 1 mg three times daily caused a significant reduction in blood pressure and enhanced alcohol-induced hypotension.[7] These effects may be restricted to Orientals. The reason being that the alcohol flush syndrome, caused by accumulation of vasodilative acetaldehyde due to a genetic alteration in aldehyde dehydrogenase, is rare in whites and blacks.[7] The clinical significance is uncertain as the dose of **prazosin** in the study was relatively small. Also the dose of alcohol was relatively large and the findings may not apply to more moderate drinking.

(c) CNS effects

For mention of the possibility of increased sedation with indoramin and alcohol, see 'Alcohol + Indoramin', p.55. For mention of the disulfiram-like reaction when tolazoline is given with alcohol, see 'Alcohol + Tolazoline', p.65. For the possible CNS effects of other antihypertensives and alcohol, see 'Alcohol + Calcium channel blockers', p.45 and 'Alcohol + Beta-blockers', p.44.

1. Puddey IB, Beilin LJ, Vandongen R. Regular alcohol use raises blood pressure in treated hypertensive subjects. A randomised controlled trial. *Lancet* (1987) i, 647–51.
2. Potter JF, Beevers DG. Pressor effect of alcohol in hypertension. *Lancet* (1984) i, 119–22.
3. Puddey IB, Beilin LJ, Vandongen R, Rouse IL, Rogers P. Evidence for a direct effect of alcohol on blood pressure in normotensive men — a randomized controlled trial. *Hypertension* (1985) 7, 707–13.
4. Sesso HD. Alcohol and cardiovascular health: recent findings. *Am J Cardiovasc Drugs* (2001) 1, 167–72.
5. Gould L, Zahir M, DeMartino A, Gomprecht RF. Cardiac effects of a cocktail. *JAMA* (1971) 218, 1799–1802.
6. Conway N. Haemodynamic effects of ethyl alcohol in patients with coronary heart disease. *Br Heart J* (1968) 30, 638–44.
7. Kawano Y, Abe H, Kojima S, Takishita S, Omae T. Interaction of alcohol and an α_1-blocker on ambulatory blood pressure in patients with essential hypertension. *Am J Hypertens* (2000) 13, 307–12.

Alcohol + Antipsychotics

The detrimental effects of alcohol on the skills related to driving are made worse by chlorpromazine and to a lesser extent by flupentixol and thioridazine, and possibly by prochlorperazine. Any interaction with amisulpride, haloperidol, sulpiride or tiapride seems to be mild or relatively unimportant. There is evidence that drinking can precipitate the emergence of extrapyramidal side-effects in patients taking antipsychotics.

Clinical evidence

(a) Effect on driving and other skills

No significant pharmacokinetic interactions were seen in 18 healthy subjects given single 50- and 200-mg doses of **amisulpride** with 0.8 g/kg alcohol, nor were the detrimental effects of alcohol on performance increased by the **amisulpride**.[1]

Twenty-one subjects showed a marked deterioration in the performance of a number of skills related to driving when given **chlorpromazine** 200 mg daily and alcohol (blood levels 42 mg%). Many complained of feeling sleepy, lethargic, dull, groggy, and poorly coordinated; and most considered themselves more unsafe to drive than with alcohol alone.[2] A later study confirmed these findings with **chlorpromazine** 1 mg/kg and blood alcohol levels of 80 mg%.[3] Increased sedation was clearly seen in another study with alcohol and chlorpromazine,[4] and another showed clear impairment of psychomotor skills related to driving.[5]

Single 0.5-mg doses of **haloperidol** or **flupentixol** strongly impaired attention, but did not significantly interact with alcohol in one study.[6] However, a double-blind study in subjects given **flupenthixol** 0.5 mg three times a day for 2 weeks found that when combined with 0.5 g/kg alcohol their performance of a number of tests (choice reaction, coordination, attention) was impaired to such an extent that driving or handling other potentially dangerous machinery could be hazardous.[7]

A study in 12 healthy subjects found that **prochlorperazine** 5 mg three times daily (no alcohol) for 3 days caused carelessness and slowing of a weaving test while driving a car, with little subjective appreciation of the deterioration. No changes could be detected in the performance of kinetic visual acuity or simple reaction time tests.[8] Alcohol would be expected to increase this impairment, but nobody seems to have checked on this yet, nevertheless patients should be warned.

Sulpiride 50 mg three times daily for 2 weeks caused only a mild decrease in psychomotor skills with alcohol in healthy subjects.[5] **Thioridazine** 25 mg caused some additive effects with alcohol, with a moderately deleterious effect on attention.[6] Another study found that **thioridazine** and alcohol affected skills related to driving, but not as much as the effects seen with **chlorpromazine**.[3] A further study found no difference between the effects of **thioridazine** and a placebo with alcohol.[5,9]

A study in 9 alcoholics given 400 to 600 mg of **tiapride** daily showed that wakefulness was not impaired when combined with alcohol 0.5 g/kg and in fact appeared to be improved, but the effect on driving skills was not studied.[10]

(b) Precipitation of extrapyramidal side-effects

A report describes in detail 7 patients who developed acute extrapyramidal side-effects (akathisia, dystonia) while taking **trifluoperazine**, **fluphenazine**, **perphenazine**, or **chlorpromazine** when they drank alcohol.[11] The author stated that these were examples of numerous such alcohol-induced toxicity reactions observed by him over an 18-year period involving phenothiazines and butyrophenones. Elsewhere he describes the emergence of drug-induced parkinsonism in a woman taking **perphenazine** and amitriptyline when she began to drink.[12] Eighteen cases of **haloperidol**-induced extrapyramidal reactions among young drug abusers, in most instances associated with the ingestion of alcohol, have also been described.[13]

(c) Reduced fluphenazine levels

A study in 7 schizophrenics found that when given 40 g of alcohol to drink at about the same time as their regular injection of fluphenazine decanoate (25 to 125 mg every 2 weeks), their serum fluphenazine levels were depressed by 30% at 2 hours and by 16% at 12 hours.[14]

Mechanism

Uncertain.

(a) Additive CNS depressant effects are one explanation of this interaction.

(b) One suggestion to account for the emergence of the drug side-effects is that alcohol lowers the threshold of resistance to the neurotoxicity of these drugs. In addition it seems possible that alcohol impairs the activity of tyrosine hydroxylase so that the dopamine/acetylcholine balance within the corpus striatum is upset.[12]

Importance and management

The documentation is limited.

(a) Warn patients that if they drink while on chlorpromazine, and to a lesser extent thioridazine or flupentixol (probably other related drugs as well) they may become very drowsy, and should not drive or handle other potentially dangerous machinery. Some risk is possible with prochlorperazine as well, but the effects of alcohol with amisulpride, haloperidol, sulpiride and tiapride appear to be minimal.

(b) The author of the reports describing the emergence of serious adverse effects to antipsychotics in those who drink, considers that patients should routinely be advised to abstain from alcohol during antipsychotic treatment.

(c) The clinical importance of reduced fluphenazine levels is uncertain. This needs more study.

1. Mattila MJ, Patat A, Seppälä T, Kalska H, Jalava M-L, Vanakoski J, Lavanant C. Single oral doses of amisulpride do not enhance the effects of alcohol on the performance and memory of healthy subjects. *Eur J Clin Pharmacol* (1996) 51, 161–6.
2. Zirkle GA, King PD, McAtee OB, Van Dyke R. Effects of chlorpromazine and alcohol on coordination and judgement. *JAMA* (1959) 171, 1496–9.
3. Milner G, Landauer AA. Alcohol, thioridazine and chlorpromazine effects on skills related to driving behaviour. *Br J Psychiatry* (1971) 118, 351–2.
4. Sutherland VC, Burbridge TN, Adams JE, Simon A. Cerebral metabolism in problem drinkers under the influence of alcohol and chlorpromazine hydrochloride. *J Appl Physiol* (1960) 15, 189–96.
5. Seppälä T, Saario I, Mattila MJ. Two weeks' treatment with chlorpromazine, thioridazine, sulpiride, or bromazepam: actions and interactions with alcohol on psychomotor skills related to driving. *Mod Probl Pharmacopsychiatry* (1976) 11, 85–90.
6. Linnoila M. Effects of diazepam, chlordiazepoxide, thioridazine, haloperidole, flupenthixole and alcohol on psychomotor skills related to driving. *Ann Med Exp Biol Fenn* (1973) 51, 125–32.
7. Linnoila M, Saario I, Olkoniemi J, Liljequist R, Himberg JJ, Mäki M. Effect of two weeks' treatment with chlordiazepoxide or flupenthixole, alone or in combination with alcohol, on psychomotor skills related to driving. *Arzneimittelforschung* (1975) 25, 1088–92.
8. Betts T, Harris D, Gadd E. The effects of two anti-vertigo drugs (betahistine and prochlorperazine) on driving skills. *Br J Clin Pharmacol* (1991) 32, 455–8.
9. Saario I. Psychomotor skills during subacute treatment with thioridazine and bromazepam, and their combined effects with alcohol. *Ann Clin Res* (1976) 8, 117–23.
10. Vandel B, Bonin B, Vandel S, Blum D, Rey E, Volmat R. Étude de l'interaction entre le tiapride et l'alcool chez l'homme. *Sem Hop Paris* (1984) 60, 175–7.
11. Lutz EG. Neuroleptic-induced akathisia and dystonia triggered by alcohol. *JAMA* (1976) 236, 2422–3.

12. Lutz EG. Neuroleptic-induced parkinsonism facilitated by alcohol. *J Med Soc New Jers* (1978) 75, 473–4.
13. Kenyon-David D. Haloperidol intoxication. *N Z Med J* (1981) 93, 165.
14. Soni SD, Bamrah JS, Krska J. Effects of alcohol on serum fluphenazine levels in stable chronic schizophrenics. *Hum Psychopharmacol* (1991) 6, 301–6.

Alcohol + Aspirin or Salicylates

A small increase in the gastrointestinal blood loss caused by aspirin occurs in patients if they drink, but any increased damage to the lining of the stomach is small and appears usually to be of minimal importance in most normal individuals. Some limited information suggests that aspirin can raise or lower blood alcohol levels.

Clinical evidence

(a) Alcohol + aspirin: effect on blood loss

The mean daily blood loss from the gut of 13 healthy men was 0.4 ml while taking no medication, 3.2 ml while taking 2100 mg of soluble **unbuffered aspirin** (*Disprin*) and 5.3 ml while also taking 180 ml of **Australian whiskey** (31.8% alcohol). In this study, alcohol alone did not cause gastrointestinal bleeding.[1]

A similar study showed that the daily gastrointestinal blood loss increased from 2.15 to 5.32 ml when the subjects drank 120 ml of **vodka** (40% alcohol) followed by 200 ml of table **wine** in addition to **aspirin** 600 mg four times daily.[2] An epidemiological study of patients admitted to hospital with gastrointestinal haemorrhage showed a statistical association between bleeding and the ingestion of **aspirin** alone, and the combination with alcohol produced a significant synergistic effect.[3] A more recent case-control study, involving 1224 patients admitted to hospital with upper gastrointestinal bleeding and 2945 controls, found that alcohol alone may cause gastrointestinal bleeding, and the concurrent use of **aspirin** with alcohol was associated with an increased risk for all levels of alcohol consumption. The risk of bleeding with regular use of **aspirin** at doses greater than 325 mg was increased sevenfold among all drinkers.[4] Endoscopic examination revealed that **aspirin** and alcohol have additive damaging effects on the gastric mucosa (not on the duodenum), but the extent is small.[5] However, a further case-control study found that large amounts of red wine (roughly over 500 ml of wine daily) increased the risk of upper gastrointestinal bleeding associated with low-dose **aspirin**, and small amounts of red wine (roughly less than 200 ml of wine daily) reduced this risk.[6] Another study using gastric mucosal potential difference as a measure of mucosal damage found that aspirin with alcohol caused additive damage to the mucosa.[7] In a review of the evidence, it was considered that while more study was needed, data available are highly suggestive that the gastrointestinal toxicity of alcohol and aspirin are combined in individuals who are truly heavy daily drinkers and heavy aspirin users.[8] See also 'Alcohol + NSAIDs', p.59.

No increased gastrointestinal bleeding occurred in 22 healthy subjects given three double **gins** or **whiskies** (equivalent to 142 ml of 40% ethanol) and 728 mg of buffered **sodium acetylsalicylate** (*Alka-Seltzer*).[9]

(b) Alcohol + aspirin: effect on blood alcohol levels

Five healthy subjects were given a standard breakfast with and without **aspirin** 1 g followed by 0.3 g/kg alcohol an hour later. The **aspirin** increased the peak blood alcohol levels by 39% and the AUC by 26%.[10] Similarly, in another study 28 healthy subjects were given a midday meal (two sandwiches and a cup of tea or coffee), followed 90 minutes later by 600 mg of **aspirin** or a placebo, and then half-an-hour later by two standard drinks (35.5 ml of 37.5% **vodka** (21.6 g alcohol) plus 60 ml of orange juice), which were drunk within a 15-minute period. The blood alcohol levels of the men were raised by 31% after 1 hour (from 24.29 to 31.85 mg%) and by 18% (from 20.82 to 24.57 mg%) after 2 hours. The blood alcohol levels of the women subjects were raised by 32% (from 37.39 to 49.23 mg%) after 1 hour and by 21% (from 37.56 to 45.54 mg%) after 2 hours.[11]

However, a later study (effectively a repeat of a study[10] above) in 12 healthy subjects failed to find any effect on blood alcohol levels, but peak **aspirin** levels were reduced 25%.[12] A crossover trial in 10 healthy male subjects found that after taking 75 mg of **aspirin** daily for a week, their mean blood alcohol AUC following a 0.3 g/kg dose was reduced by 23%, but this was not statistically significant. Individual maximum blood levels varied; one subject showed a rise, two were unchanged, and five were lowered, but overall the reduction was 23% and this was statistically significant.[13]

Mechanism

(a). Aspirin and alcohol can damage the mucosal lining of the stomach, one measure of the injury being a fall in the gastric potential difference. Once the protective mucosal barrier is breached, desquamation of the cells occurs and damage to the capillaries follows. Aspirin causes a marked prolongation in bleeding times, and this can be increased by alcohol.[14] The total picture is complex.

(b). The increased blood alcohol levels in the presence of food and aspirin may possibly occur because the aspirin reduces the enzymic oxidation of the alcohol by alcohol dehydrogenase in the gastric mucosa, so that more remains available for absorption.[10] Any decreases with low dose aspirin may possibly be due to delayed gastric emptying.[13]

Importance and management

The combined effect of aspirin and alcohol on the stomach wall is established. Aspirin 3 g daily for a period of 3 to 5 days induces an average blood loss of about 5 ml or so. Some increased loss undoubtedly occurs with alcohol, but it seems to be quite small and unlikely to be of much importance in most normal individuals using moderate doses. In one study it was found that alcohol was a mild damaging agent or a mild potentiating agent for other damaging drugs.[5] On the other hand it should be remembered that chronic and/or gross overuse of salicylates and alcohol may result in gastric ulceration, and also that diflunisal may cause drowsiness, so additive CNS depression could result from taking it with alcohol. See also, 'Alcohol + NSAIDs', p.59.

Information about the increase in blood alcohol levels caused by aspirin after food is very limited and contradictory, and of uncertain practical importance. However no practically relevant interaction has been seen with other drugs such as the 'H_2-blockers', (p.53)), which have been extensively studied, and which appear to interact by the same mechanism. The pattern for these drugs is that the increases in blood alcohol levels are appreciable with small doses of alcohol, but usually they become proportionately too small to matter with larger doses of alcohol (i.e. those that give blood and breath levels at or around the legal driving limit in the UK).

1. Goulston K, Cooke AR. Alcohol, aspirin, and gastrointestinal bleeding. *BMJ* (1968) 4, 664–5.
2. DeSchepper PJ, Tjandramaga TB, De Roo M, Verhaest L, Daurio C, Steelman SL, Tempero KF. Gastrointestinal blood loss after diflunisal and after aspirin: effect of ethanol. *Clin Pharmacol Ther* (1978) 23, 669–76.
3. Needham CD, Kyle J, Jones PF, Johnston SJ, Kerridge DF. Aspirin and alcohol in gastrointestinal haemorrhage. *Gut* (1971) 12, 819–21.
4. Kaufman DW, Kelly JP, Wiholm B-E, Laszlo A, Sheehan JE, Koff RS, Shapiro S. The risk of acute major upper gastrointestinal bleeding among users of aspirin and ibuprofen at various levels of alcohol consumption. *Am J Gastroenterol* (1999) 94, 3189–96.
5. Lanza FL, Royer GL, Nelson RS, Rack MF, Seckman CC. Ethanol, aspirin, ibuprofen, and the gastroduodenal mucosa: an endoscopic assessment. *Am J Gastroenterol* (1985) 80, 767–9.
6. Lanas A, Serrano P, Bajador E, Fuentes J, Guardia J, Sainz R. Effect of red wine and low dose aspirin on the risk or upper gastrointestinal bleeding. A case-control study. *Gastroenterology* (2000) 118 (Suppl. 2) A251.
7. Murray HS, Strottman MP, Cooke AR. Effect of several drugs on gastric potential difference in man. *BMJ* (1974) 1, 19–21.
8. Pfau PR, Lichtenstein GR. NSAIDs and alcohol: never the twain shall mix? *Am J Gastroenterol* (1999) 94, 3098–3101.
9. Bouchier IAD, Williams HS. Determination of faecal blood-loss after combined alcohol and sodium acetylsalicylate intake. *Lancet* (1969) i, 178–80.
10. Roine R, Gentry T, Hernández-Munõz R, Baraona E, Lieber CS. Aspirin increases blood alcohol concentrations in humans after ingestion of ethanol. *JAMA* (1990) 264, 2406–8.
11. Sharma SC, Feeley J. The influence of aspirin and paracetamol on blood concentrations of alcohol in young adults. *Br J Clin Pharmacol* (1996) 41, 467P.
12. Melander O, Lidén A, Melander A. Pharmacokinetic interactions of alcohol and acetylsalicylic acid. *Eur J Clin Pharmacol* (1995) 48, 151–3.
13. Kechagias S, Jönsson K-Å, Norlander B, Carlsson B, Jones AW. Low-dose aspirin decreases blood alcohol concentrations by delaying gastric emptying. *Eur J Clin Pharmacol* (1997) 53, 241–6.
14. Rosove MH, Harwig SSL. Confirmation that ethanol potentiates aspirin-induced prolongation of the bleeding time. *Thromb Res* (1983) 31, 525–7.

Alcohol + Barbiturates

Alcohol and the barbiturates are CNS depressants, which together can have additive and possibly synergistic effects. Activities requiring alertness and good co-ordination, such as driving a car or handling other potentially dangerous machinery, will be made more difficult and more hazardous. Alcohol may also continue to interact the next day if the barbiturate has hangover effects.

Clinical evidence

A study in man of the effects of a single 0.5-g/kg dose of alcohol, taken in the morning after a dose of **amobarbital** 100 mg every night for 2 weeks showed that the performance of co-ordination skills was much more impaired than with either drug alone.[1]

This increased CNS depression due to combined use has been described in a number of other clinical studies,[2-4] and has featured very many times in coroners' reports of fatal accidents and suicides.[5] A study of the fatalities due to this interaction indicated that with some barbiturates the CNS depressant effects are more than additive.[6] There is also some evidence that blood alcohol levels may be reduced in the presence of a barbiturate.[3,7,8]

Mechanism

Both alcohol and the barbiturates are CNS depressants, and simple additive CNS depression provides part of the explanation. Thermodynamics have been used to account for the more than additive effects.[9] Acute alcohol ingestion may inhibit the liver enzymes concerned with the metabolism of the barbiturates.[10]

Importance and management

Few formal studies in normal clinical situations have been made of the alcohol/barbiturate interactions, but the effects (particularly those that result in fatalities) are very well established, serious and of clinical importance. The most obvious hazards are increased drowsiness, lack of alertness and impaired co-ordination, which make the handling of potentially dangerous machinery (e.g. car driving), and even the performance of everyday tasks (e.g. walking downstairs) more difficult and dangerous. Only amobarbital is specifically referenced here, but this interaction would be expected with all of the barbiturates. Some barbiturate hangover effects may be present the next morning and may therefore continue to interact significantly with alcohol. Patients should be warned.

1. Saario I, Linnoila M. Effect of subacute treatment with hypnotics, alone or in combination with alcohol, on psychomotor skills relating to driving. *Acta Pharmacol Toxicol (Copenh)* (1976) 38, 382–92.
2. Kielholz P, Goldberg L, Obersteg JI, Pöldinger W, Ramseyer A, Schmid P. Fahrversuche zur Frage der Beeinträchtigung der Verkehrstüchtigkeit durch Alkohol, Tranquilizer und Hypnotika. *Dtsch Med Wochenschr* (1969) 94, 301–6.
3. Morselli PL, Veneroni E, Zaccala M, Bizzi A. Further observations on the interaction between ethanol and psychotropic drugs. *Arzneimittelforschung* (1971) 21, 20–3.
4. Wegener H, Kötter L. Analgetica und Verkehrstüchtigkeit: wirkung einer Kombination von 5-Allyl-5-isobutylsäure, Dimethylaminophenazon und Coffein nach einmaliger und wiederholter applikation. *Arzneimittelforschung* (1971) 21, 47–51.
5. Gupta RC, Kofoed J. Toxicological statistics for barbiturates, other sedatives, and tranquillizers in Ontario. *Can Med Assoc J* (1966) 94, 863–5.
6. Stead AH, Moffat AC. Quantification of the interaction between barbiturates and alcohol and interpretation of fatal blood concentrations. *Hum Toxicol* (1983) 2, 5–14.
7. Mould GP, Curry SH, Binns TB. Interaction of glutethimide and phenobarbitone with ethanol in man. *J Pharm Pharmacol* (1972) 24, 894–9.
8. Mezey E, Robles EA. Effects of phenobarbital administration on rates of ethanol clearance and on ethanol-oxidizing enzymes in man. *Gastroenterology* (1974) 66, 248–53.
9. King LA. Thermodynamic interpretation of synergism in barbiturate/ethanol poisoning. *Hum Toxicol* (1985) 4, 633–5.
10. Rubin E, Gang H, Misra PS, Lieber CS. Inhibition of drug metabolism by acute ethanol intoxication. A hepatic microsomal mechanism. *Am J Med* (1970) 49, 801–6.

Alcohol + Benzodiazepines and related drugs

Benzodiazepine and related tranquillisers increase the CNS depressant effects of alcohol to some extent. The risks of car driving and handling other potentially dangerous machinery are increased. The risk is heightened because the patient may be unaware of being affected. Some benzodiazepines used at night for sedation are still present in appreciable amounts the next day and therefore may continue to interact if the patient carries on drinking.

Clinical evidence

It is very difficult to assess and compare the results of the very many studies of this interaction because of the differences between the tests, their duration, the dosages of the benzodiazepines and alcohol, whether given chronically or acutely, and a number of other variables. However, the overall picture seems to be that **diazepam**[1-13] has a more marked effect than **chlordiazepoxide**,[1,14-18] **medazepam**,[19] or **oxazepam**,[8] but possibly the same as **triazolam**.[20,21] The effects of **lormetazepam** may be greater than **diazepam**.[22] The potencies of **alprazolam**,[23,24] **bromazepam**,[25] **brotizolam**,[26] **clobazam**,[27] **lorazepam**,[12,28-30] **oxazolam**,[31] **metaclazepam**,[32] **potassium clorazepate**[33] and **zopiclone**[34,35] are unclear. Patients taking **lorazepam** and **triazolam** may be unaware of the extent of the impairment that occurs,[20,29] and the anxiolytic effects of **lorazepam** may be opposed by alcohol.[30] **Alprazolam** and alcohol together may possibly increase behavioural aggression.[36]

The benzodiazepines that are used primarily to aid sleep: **flurazepam**,[37-39] **nitrazepam**,[4,40] **temazepam**[38] and **flunitrazepam**,[34,41] when taken the night before alcohol or in the evening with alcohol, can still interact with alcohol the next morning, but **midazolam**,[42] **triazolam**,[35] and **zopiclone**[35] appear not to do so. One study has found that either **temazepam** or **triazolam** with alcohol produced greater performance impairment and sedation than that found with either drug or alcohol alone.[43] The sedative effects of **midazolam** alone have been shown to have dissipated within 4 hours, and to not be affected by alcohol after this time[44] (see also 'Alcohol + Fentanyl-midazolam', p.52). Alcohol may mitigate the effects of **loprazolam** and may possibly have less of a hangover effect.[45] Alcohol appears to have minimal effects on the pharmacokinetics of **zopiclone**[46] and zolpidem.[47]

Mechanism

The CNS depressant actions of the benzodiazepines and alcohol are additive. Alcohol also increases the absorption and raises the serum levels of some benzodiazepines.[27,48-50] It has been suggested that clearance of benzodiazepines via phase I metabolism tends to be more affected by alcohol intake than that of drugs such as lorazepam, oxazepam or lormetazepam that only undergo phase II conjugation.[50]

Importance and management

Extensively studied, well established and clinically important interactions. The overall picture is that these drugs worsen the detrimental effects of alcohol.[51] Up to a 20 to 30% increase in the impairment of psychomotor function has been suggested.[20] The deterioration in skills will depend on the particular drug in question (see 'Clinical evidence' above), its dosage and the amounts of alcohol taken. With modest amounts of alcohol the effects may be quite small in most patients (although a few may be more markedly affected[13]), but anyone taking any of these drugs should be warned that their usual response to alcohol may be greater than expected, and their ability to drive a car, or carry out any other tasks requiring alertness, may be impaired. They may be quite unaware of the deterioration. Benzodiazepines and alcohol are frequently found in the blood of car drivers involved in traffic accidents which suggests that the risks are real.[51-53]

1. Dundee JW, Isaac M. Interaction of alcohol with sedatives and tranquillisers (a study of blood levels at loss of consciousness following rapid infusion). *Med Sci Law* (1970) 10, 220–4.
2. Morselli PL, Veneroni E, Zaccala M, Bizzi A. Further observations on the interaction between ethanol and psychotropic drugs. *Arzneimittelforschung* (1971) 21, 20–3.
3. Linnoila M, Häkkinen S. Effects of diazepam and codeine, alone and in combination with alcohol, on simulated driving. *Clin Pharmacol Ther* (1974) 15, 368–73.
4. Linnoila M. Drug interaction on psychomotor skills related to driving: hypnotics and alcohol. *Ann Med Exp Biol Fenn* (1973) 51, 118–24.
5. Missen AW, Cleary W, Eng L, McMillan S. Diazepam, alcohol and drivers. *N Z Med J* (1978) 87, 275–7.
6. Laisi U, Linnoila M, Seppälä T, Himberg J-J, Mattila MJ. Pharmacokinetic and pharmacodynamic interactions of diazepam with different alcoholic beverages. *Eur J Clin Pharmacol* (1979) 16, 263–70.
7. Palva ES, Linnoila M, Saario I, Mattila MJ. Acute and subacute effects of diazepam on psychomotor skills: interaction with alcohol. *Acta Pharmacol Toxicol (Copenh)* (1979) 45, 257–64.
8. Molander L, Duvhök C. Acute effects of oxazepam, diazepam and methylperone, alone and in combination with alcohol on sedation, coordination and mood. *Acta Pharmacol Toxicol (Copenh)* (1976) 38, 145–60.
9. Curry SH, Smith CM. Diazepam-ethanol interaction in humans: addition or potentiation? *Commun Psychopharmacol* (1979) 3, 101–13.
10. Smiley A, Moskowitz H. Effects of long-term administration of buspirone and diazepam on driver steering control. *Am J Med* (1986) 80 (Suppl 3B), 22–9.
11. Erwin CW, Linnoila M, Hartwell J, Erwin A, Guthrie S. Effects of buspirone and diazepam, alone and in combination with alcohol, on skilled performance and evoked potentials. *J Clin Psychopharmacol* (1986) 6, 199–209.
12. Aranko K, Seppälä T, Pellinen J, Mattila MJ. Interaction of diazepam or lorazepam with alcohol. Psychomotor effects and bioassayed serum levels after single and repeated doses. *Eur J Clin Pharmacol* (1985) 28, 559–65.
13. van Steveninck AL, Gieschke R, Schoemaker HC, Pieters MSM, Kroon JM, Breimer DD, Cohen AF. Pharmacodynamic interactions of diazepam and intravenous alcohol at pseudo steady state. *Psychopharmacology (Berl)* (1993) 110, 471–8.
14. Hughes FW, Forney RB, Richards AB. Comparative effect in human subjects of chlordiazepoxide, diazepam, and placebo on mental and physical performance. *Clin Pharmacol Ther* (1965) 6, 139–45.
15. Linnoila M. Effects of diazepam, chlordiazepoxide, thioridazine, haloperidole, flupenthixole and alcohol on psychomotor skills related to driving. *Ann Med Exp Biol Fenn* (1973) 51, 125–32.
16. Linnoila M, Saario I, Olkoniemi J, Liljequist R, Himberg JJ, Mäki M. Effect of two weeks' treatment with chlordiazepoxide or flupenthixole, alone or in combination with alcohol, on psychomotor skills related to driving. *Arzneimittelforschung* (1975) 25, 1088–92.
17. Hoffer A. Lack of potentiation by chlordiazepoxide (Librium) of depression or excitation due to alcohol. *Can Med Assoc J* (1962) 87, 920–1.

18. Kielholz P, Goldberg L, Obersteg JI, Pöldinger W, Ramseyer A, Schmid P. Fahrversuche zur frage der beeinträchtigung der verkehrstüchtigkeit durch Alkohol, Tranquilizer und Hypnotika. *Dtsch Med Wochenschr* (1969) 94, 301–6.
19. Landauer AA, Pocock DA, Prott FW. The effect of medazepam and alcohol on cognitive and motor skills used in car driving. *Psychopharmacologia* (1974) 37, 159–68.
20. Dorian P, Sellers EM, Kaplan HL, Hamilton C, Greenblatt DJ, Abernethy D. Triazolam and ethanol interaction: kinetic and dynamic consequences. *Clin Pharmacol Ther* (1985) 37, 558–62.
21. Ochs HR, Greenblatt DJ, Arendt RM, Hubbel W, Shader RI. Pharmacokinetic noninteraction of triazolam and ethanol. *J Clin Psychopharmacol* (1984) 4,106–7.
22. Willumeit H-P, Ott H, Neubert W, Hemmerling K-G, Schratzer M, Fichte K. Alcohol interaction of lormetazepam, mepindolol sulphate and diazepam measured by performance on the driving simulator. *Pharmacopsychiatry* (1984) 17, 36–43.
23. Linnoila M, Stapleton JM, Lister R, Moss H, Lane E, Granger A, Eckardt MJ. Effects of single doses of alprazolam and diazepam, alone and in combination with ethanol, on psychomotor and cognitive performance and on autonomic nervous system reactivity in healthy volunteers. *Eur J Clin Pharmacol* (1990) 39, 21–8.
24. Rush CR, Griffiths RR. Acute participant-rated and behavioral effects of alprazolam and buspirone, alone and in combination with ethanol, in normal volunteers. *Exp Clin Psychopharmacol* (1997) 5, 28–38.
25. Seppälä T, Saario I, Mattila MJ. Two weeks' treatment with chlorpromazine, thioridazine, sulpiride, or bromazepam: actions and interactions with alcohol on psychomotor skills relating to driving. *Mod Probl Pharmacopsychiatry* (1976) 11, 85–90.
26. Scavone JM, Greenblatt DJ, Harmatz JS, Shader RI. Kinetic and dynamic interaction of brotizolam and ethanol. *Br J Clin Pharmacol* (1986) 21, 197–204.
27. Taeuber K, Badian M, Brettel HF, Royen T, Rupp K, Sittig W, Uihlein M. Kinetic and dynamic interaction of clobazam and alcohol. *Br J Clin Pharmacol* (1979) 7, 91S-97S.
28. Allen D, Baylav A, Lader M. A comparative study of the interaction of alcohol with alpidem, lorazepam and placebo in normal subjects. *Int Clin Psychopharmacol* (1988) 3, 327–41.
29. Seppälä T, Aranko K, Mattila MJ, Shrotriya RC. Effects of alcohol on buspirone and lorazepam actions. *Clin Pharmacol Ther* (1982) 32, 201–7.
30. Lister RG, File SE. Performance impairment and increased anxiety resulting from the combination of alcohol and lorazepam. *J Clin Psychopharmacol* (1983) 3, 66–71.
31. Hopes H, Debus G. Untersuchungen zu kombinationseffekten von Oxazolam und Alkohol auf leistung und befinden bei gesunden Probanden. *Arzneimittelforschung* (1984) 34, 921–6.
32. Schmidt V. Experimentelle untersuchunger zur wechselwirkung zwischen Alkohol und Metaclazepam. *Beitr Gerichtl Med* (1983) 41, 413–7.
33. Staak M, Raff G, Nusser W. Pharmacopsychological investigations concerning the combined effects of dipotassium clorazepate and ethanol. *Int J Clin Pharmacol Biopharm* (1979) 17, 205–12.
34. Seppälä T, Nuotto E, Dreyfus JF. Drug–alcohol interactions on psychomotor skills: zopiclone and flunitrazepam. *Pharmacology* (1983) 27 (Suppl 2), 127–35.
35. Kuitunen T, Mattila MJ, Seppala T. Actions and interactions of hypnotics on human performance: single doses of zopiclone, triazolam and alcohol. *Int Clin Psychopharmacol* (1990) 5 (Suppl 2), 115–30.
36. Bond AJ, Silveira JC. Behavioural aggression following the combination of alprazolam and alcohol. *J Psychopharmacol* (1990) 4, 315.
37. Saario I, Mattila M. Effect of subacute treatment with hypnotics alone or in combination with alcohol on psychomotor skills related to driving. *Acta Pharmacol Toxicol (Copenh)* (1976) 38, 382–92.
38. Betts TA, Birtle J. Effect of two hypnotic drugs on actual driving performance next morning. *BMJ* (1982) 285, 852.
39. Hindmarch I, Gudgeon AC. Loprazolam (HR158) and flurazepam with ethanol compared on tests of psychomotor ability. *Eur J Clin Pharmacol* (1982) 23, 509–12.
40. Saario I, Linnoila M, Mäki M. Interaction of drugs with alcohol on human psychomotor skills related to driving: effect of sleep deprivation or two weeks' treatment with hypnotics. *J Clin Pharmacol* (1975) 15, 52–9.
41. Linnoila M, Erwin CW, Brendle A, Logue P. Effects of alcohol and flunitrazepam on mood and performance in healthy young men. *J Clin Pharmacol* (1981) 21, 430–5.
42. Hindmarch I, Subhan Z. The effects of midazolam in conjunction with alcohol on sleep, psychomotor performance and car driving ability. *Int J Clin Pharmacol Res* (1983) 3, 323–9.
43. Simpson CA, Rush CR. Acute performance-impairing and subject-rated effects of triazolam and temazepam, alone and in combination with ethanol, in humans. *J Psychopharmacol* (2002) 16, 23–34.
44. Lichtor JL, Zacny J, Korttila K, Apfelbaum JL, Lane BS, Rupani G, Thisted RA, Dohrn C. Alcohol after midazolam sedation: does it really matter? *Anesth Analg* (1991) 72, 661–6.
45. McManus IC, Ankier SI, Norfolk J, Phillips M, Priest RG. Effects on psychological performance of the benzodiazepine, loprazolam, alone and with alcohol. *Br J Clin Pharmacol* (1983) 16, 291–300.
46. Larivière L, Caillé G, Elie R. The effects of low and moderate doses of alcohol on the pharmacokinetic parameters of zopiclone. *Biopharm Drug Dispos* (1986) 7, 207–10.
47. Wilkinson CJ. The acute effects of zolpidem, administered alone and with alcohol, on cognitive and psychomotor function. *J Clin Psychiatry* (1995) 56, 309–18.
48. MacLeod SM, Giles HG, Patzalek G, Thiessen JJ, Sellers EM. Diazepam actions and plasma concentrations following ethanol ingestion. *Eur J Clin Pharmacol* (1977) 11, 345–9.
49. Laisi U, Linnoila M, Seppälä T, Himberg J-J, Mattila MJ. Pharmacokinetic and pharmacodynamic interactions of diazepam with different alcoholic beverages. *Eur J Clin Pharmacol* (1979) 16, 263–70.
50. Tanaka E, Misawa S. Pharmacokinetic interactions between acute alcohol ingestion and single doses of benzodiazepines, and tricyclic and tetracyclic antidepressants–an update. *J Clin Pharm Ther* (1998) 23, 331–6.
51. Schuster R, Bodem M. Evaluation of ethanol-benzodiazepine-interactions using blood sampling protocol data. *Blutalkohol* (1997) 34, 54–65.
52. Chan AWK. Effects of combined alcohol and benzodiazepine: a review. *Drug Alcohol Depend* (1984) 13, 315–41.
53. Staub C, Lacalle H, Fryc O. Présence de psychotropes dans le sang de conducteurs responsables d'accidents de la route ayant consommé en même temps de l'alcool. *Soz Praventivmed* (1994) 39, 143–9.

Alcohol + Beta-blockers

The effects of atenolol and metoprolol do not appear to be changed by alcohol. Some preliminary evidence suggests that the effects of alcohol and atenolol/chlortalidone or propranolol are additive on the performance of some psychomotor tests, but the importance of this is uncertain. There is some evidence that alcohol modestly reduces the haemodynamic effects of propranolol. Some of the effects of sotalol may also be changed by alcohol.

Clinical evidence, mechanism, importance and management

No clinically significant changes in blood pressure, pulse rate or the pharmacokinetics of single 100-mg doses of **atenolol** or **metoprolol** occurred in 8 healthy subjects 6 hours after drinking the equivalent of 200 ml absolute alcohol.[1] The performance of a number of psychomotor tests was found to be impaired by alcohol 0.6 g/kg in 12 normal subjects and by one tablet of *Tenoretic* (**atenolol** 100 mg with chlortalidone 25 mg). When alcohol and *Tenoretic* were taken together there was some evidence of additive effects but the practical importance of this is not clear.[2]

Propranolol 40 mg every 6 hours had no effect on the alcohol-induced impairment of performance on a number of psychomotor tests in 12 healthy subjects given 50 ml/70 kg bodyweight of alcohol, except that **propranolol** antagonised the effect of alcohol in one test (pursuit meter).[3] However, in another study, **propranolol** enhanced the effects of alcohol on some tests (inebriation and divided attention).[4]

A study in 6 healthy subjects found that alcohol (sufficient to maintain blood levels of 800 mg/l) raised the mean AUC of a single 80-mg oral dose of **propranolol** by 17.4% in 5 of them and decreased it by 37% in the other subject, but this was considered unlikely to be clinically important. No changes in heart rate or blood pressure were seen.[5] In contrast, a double-blind study in 14 healthy subjects found that alcohol (equivalent to 32 to 72 ml absolute alcohol) increased the clearance of a single 80-mg dose of **propranolol** and diminished its ability to lower blood pressure. **Propranolol** was not able to abolish the alcohol-induced rise in heart rate.[6] Similarly, another study found that alcohol decreased the rate of absorption and increased the rate of elimination of **propranolol**, but the clinical significance of this small alteration was not assessed.[7]

A further study in 6 healthy subjects found that although the blood pressure lowering effects of **sotalol** 160 mg were increased by alcohol, **sotalol** did not cancel out the alcohol-induced rise in heart rate.[6]

It would seem prudent to be alert for changes in response to beta-blockers that may be due to alcohol. The authors of one of the studies advise patients on **propranolol** to take an extra dose (a quarter to a third of their usual daily dose) if they develop angina or tachycardia after consuming alcohol.[6] See also, 'Alcohol + Antihypertensives', p.40.

1. Kirch W, Spahn H, Hutt HJ, Ohnhaus EE, Mutschler E. Interaction between alcohol and metoprolol or atenolol in social drinking. *Drugs* (1983) 25 (Suppl 2), 152.
2. Gerrard L, Wheeldon NM, McDevitt DG. Psychomotor effects of combined atenolol/chlorthalidone administration: interaction with alcohol. *Br J Clin Pharmacol* (1994) 37, 517P–518P.
3. Lindenschmidt R, Brown D, Cerimele B, Walle T, Forney RB. Combined effects of propranolol and ethanol on human psychomotor performance. *Toxicol Appl Pharmacol* (1983) 67, 117–21.
4. Alkana RL, Parker ES, Cohen HB, Birch H, Noble EP. Reversal of ethanol intoxication in humans: an assessment of the efficacy of propranolol. *Psychopharmacology (Berl)* (1976) 51, 29–37.
5. Dorian P, Sellers EM, Carruthers G, Hamilton C, Fan T. Propranolol-ethanol pharmacokinetic interaction. *Clin Pharmacol Ther* (1982) 31, 219.
6. Sotaniemi EA, Anttila M, Rautio A, Stengård J, Saukko P, Järvensivu P. Propranolol and sotalol metabolism after a drinking party. *Clin Pharmacol Ther* (1981) 29, 705–10.
7. Grabowski BS, Cady WJ, Young WW, Emery JF. Effects of acute alcohol administration on propranolol absorption. *Int J Clin Pharmacol Ther Toxicol* (1980) 18, 317–19.

Alcohol + Bromocriptine

There is some very limited evidence that the adverse effects of bromocriptine may possibly be increased by alcohol.

Clinical evidence, mechanism, importance and management

Intolerance to alcohol, which improved on continued treatment, has been briefly mentioned in a report about patients taking bromocriptine for acromegaly.[1] In another report two patients with high prolactin levels were said to have developed the side-effects of bromocriptine, even in low doses, while continuing to drink. When they abstained, the frequency and the severity of the side-effects fell, even with higher doses of bromocriptine.[2] This, it is suggested, may be due to some alcohol-induced increase in the sensitivity of dopamine receptors.[2] There would seem to be little reason, on the basis of this extremely sparse evidence, to tell all patients on bromocriptine not to drink, but it would be reasonable to warn them to try avoiding alcohol if side-effects develop.

1. Wass JAH, Thorner MO, Morris DV, Rees LH, Mason AS, Jones AE, Besser GM. Long-term treatment of acromegaly with bromocriptine. *BMJ* (1977) 1, 875–8.
2. Ayres J, Maisey MN. Alcohol increases bromocriptine's side effects. *N Engl J Med* (1980) 302, 806.

Alcohol + Buspirone

Buspirone with alcohol may cause drowsiness and weakness, although it does not appear to cause much impairment of performance.

Clinical evidence, mechanism, importance and management

A study in 12 healthy subjects showed that, in contrast to lorazepam, buspirone 10 or 20 mg did not appear to interact with alcohol (i.e. worsen the performance of certain psychomotor tests), but it did make the subjects feel drowsy and weak.[1,2] Similarly, another study in 13 healthy subjects found that combining buspirone (15 and 30 mg/70 kg) and alcohol caused sedation, but very little impairment of performance. In this study, the sedative effects were broadly similar to those seen with alprazolam plus alcohol, but alprazolam plus alcohol clearly impaired performance.[3] Similar findings were reported in another earlier comparison with diazepam.[4] The UK maker notes that there is no information on higher therapeutic doses of buspirone combined with alcohol, and they suggest that it would be prudent to avoid alcohol while taking buspirone.[5] They also caution patients of the potential hazards of driving or handling other potentially dangerous machinery until they are certain that buspirone does not adversely affect them.[5]

1. Mattila MJ, Aranko K, Seppala T. Acute effects of buspirone and alcohol on psychomotor skills. *J Clin Psychiatry* (1982) 43, 56–60.
2. Seppälä T, Aranko K, Mattila MJ, Shrotriya RC. Effects of alcohol on buspirone and lorazepam actions. *Clin Pharmacol Ther* (1982) 32, 201–7.
3. Rush CR, Griffiths RR. Acute participant-rated and behavioral effects of alprazolam and buspirone, alone and in combination with ethanol, in normal volunteers. *Exp Clin Psychopharmacol* (1997) 5, 28–38.
4. Erwin CW, Linnoila M, Hartwell J, Erwin A, Guthrie S. Effects of buspirone and diazepam, alone and in combination with alcohol, on skilled performance and evoked potentials. *J Clin Psychopharmacol* (1986) 6, 199–209.
5. Buspar (Buspirone hydrochloride). Bristol-Myers Pharmaceuticals. UK Summary of product characteristics, July 2005.

Alcohol + Butyraldoxime

A disulfiram-like reaction can occur in those exposed to *N*-butyraldoxime if they drink alcohol.

Clinical evidence, mechanism, importance and management

Workers in a printing company complained of flushing of the face, neck, and upper trunk; shortness of breath, tachycardia, and drowsiness, very shortly after drinking quite small quantities of alcohol (1.5 oz (about 45 ml) of **whiskey**), and were found to have increased levels of acetaldehyde in their blood. The reason appeared to be that the printing ink they were using contained *N*-butyraldoxime, an antioxidant which, like disulfiram, can inhibit the metabolism of alcohol causing acetaldehyde to accumulate (see 'Alcohol + Disulfiram', p.50).[1] It is possible that it is a metabolite of *N*-butyraldoxime that causes this effect, rather than *N*-butyraldoxime itself.[2] This reaction would seem to be more unpleasant and socially disagreeable than serious. No treatment normally seems necessary.

1. Lewis W, Schwartz L. An occupational agent (N-butyraldoxime) causing reaction to alcohol. *Med Ann Dist Columbia* (1956) 25, 485–90.
2. DeMaster EG, Redfern B, Shirota FN, Crankshaw DL, Nagasawa HT. Metabolic activation of *n*-butyraldoxime by rat liver microsomal cytochrome P450. A requirement for the inhibition of aldehyde dehydrogenase. *Biochem Pharmacol* (1993) 46, 117–23.

Alcohol + Caffeine

Despite popular belief, objective tests show that caffeine does not counteract the effects of alcohol. It does not sober up those who have drunk too much, and may even make them more accident-prone.

Clinical evidence, mechanism, importance and management

A study in a large number of healthy subjects given caffeine 300 mg/70 kg, either alone or with alcohol 0.75 g/kg, found that caffeine did not antagonise the deleterious effect of alcohol on the performance of psychomotor skill tests. Only reaction times were reversed.[1] Two other studies also found that caffeine did not antagonise the effects of alcohol in a variety of tests.[2,3] Yet another test carried out in 8 subjects found that, contrary to expectations, caffeine increased the frequency of errors in the performance of a serial reaction time task.[4] A further study found no evidence that caffeine opposed the actions of alcohol, instead it appeared to increase its detrimental effects.[5] The reasons are not understood.

Despite the long standing and time-hallowed belief in the value of strong black coffee to sober up those who have drunk too much, it seems that it is not effective, except possibly that the time taken to drink the coffee gives the liver just a little more time to metabolise some of the alcohol. **Coffee** and other sources of caffeine do not make it safe to drive or handle dangerous machinery, and it may even make drivers more accident-prone.

1. Franks HM, Hagedorn H, Hensley VR, Hensley WJ, Starmer GA. The effect of caffeine on human performance, alone and in combination with alcohol. *Psychopharmacologia* (1975) 45, 177–81.
2. Nuotto E, Mattila MJ, Seppälä T, Konno K. Coffee and caffeine and alcohol effects on psychomotor function. *Clin Pharmacol Ther* (1982) 31, 68–76.
3. Newman HW, Newman EJ. Failure of dexedrine and caffeine as practical antagonists of the depressant effect of ethyl alcohol in man. *Q J Stud Alcohol* (1956) 17, 406–10.
4. Lee DJ, Lowe G. Interaction of alcohol and caffeine in a perceptual-motor task. *IRCS Med Sci* (1980) 8, 420.
5. Oborne DJ, Rogers Y. Interactions of alcohol and caffeine on human reaction time. *Aviat Space Environ Med* (1983) 54, 528–34.

Alcohol + Calcium carbimide

Alcohol causes a disulfiram-like reaction in patients taking calcium carbimide. Calcium carbimide has been used as an alcohol deterrent.

Clinical evidence, mechanism, importance and management

Calcium carbimide interacts with alcohol in a similar way to disulfiram and by a similar mechanism (see 'Alcohol + Disulfiram', p.50). Both of them bind to aldehyde dehydrogenase, but calcium carbimide is said to have fewer adverse effects because it does not bind to dopamine beta hydroxylase. Like disulfiram it is used to deter alcoholics from continuing to drink.[1,2]

1. Peachey JE, Brien JF, Roach CA, Loomis CW. A comparative review of the pharmacological and toxicological properties of disulfiram and calcium carbimide. *J Clin Psychopharmacol* (1981) 1, 21–6.
2. Monteiro MG. Pharmacological treatment of alcoholism. *Aust N Z J Med* (1992) 22, 220–3.

Alcohol + Calcium channel blockers

Blood alcohol levels can be raised and may remain elevated for a much longer period of time in patients taking verapamil. Alcohol may also increase the bioavailability of felodipine and nifedipine, but amlodipine appears not to interact.

Clinical evidence

(a) Alcohol serum levels and effects increased

Ten healthy subjects given **verapamil** 80 mg three times daily for 6 days were additionally given alcohol 0.8 g/kg on day 6. Peak blood alcohol levels were found to be raised by 16.7% (from 106.45 to 124.24 mg%) and the 12-hour AUC was raised by almost 30%. The time that blood alcohol levels exceeded 100 mg% was prolonged from 0.2 to 1.3 hours and the subjects said they felt more intoxicated.[1] In another study no evidence was found that **verapamil** 80 or 160 mg antagonised the effects of alcohol.[2]

(b) Alcohol pharmacokinetics unchanged

A study in 30 healthy subjects found that single and multiple doses of **amlodipine** 10 mg (with or without lisinopril and simvastatin) for 15 days had no effect on the pharmacokinetics of alcohol 0.8 g/kg nor on subjective psychological performance. Alcohol did not alter the pharmacokinetics of **amlodipine**.[3]

(c) Felodipine and nifedipine effects increased

A study in 8 healthy subjects given enough alcohol to maintain their blood levels at 0.8 to 1.2 mg% found that their blood **felodipine** levels (following a single 10-mg oral dose) were approximately doubled (AUC increased by 77%, maximum blood levels increased by 98%). Diuresis was approximately doubled and heart rates were increased.[4] Alcohol (75 ml of 94% alcohol with 75 ml of orange juice) given to ten healthy subjects increased the AUC of single 20-mg doses of **nifedipine** by 54%, but no significant changes in heart rate or blood pressure were seen.[5] In another study no evidence was found that **nifedipine** 10 or 20 mg antagonised the effects of alcohol.[2]

Mechanism

Not understood. It seems possible that verapamil inhibits the metabolism of alcohol by the liver, thereby reducing its loss from the body. Alcohol also appears to inhibit the metabolism of nifedipine, and to increase the bioavailability of felodipine.

Importance and management

Information seems to be limited to these reports and they need confirmation. An alcohol concentration rise of almost 17% as caused by verapamil is quite small, but it could be enough to raise legal blood levels to illegal levels if driving. Moreover the intoxicant effects of alcohol may persist for a much longer period of time (five times longer in this instance).[1] The clinical significance of the nifedipine/alcohol and felodipine/alcohol interaction is uncertain. Amlodipine appears not to interact. Note that long-term moderate to heavy drinking can impair the efficacy of antihypertensives, see 'Alcohol + Antihypertensives', p.40.

1. Bauer LA, Schumock G, Horn J, Opheim K. Verapamil inhibits ethanol elimination and prolongs the perception of intoxication. *Clin Pharmacol Ther* (1992) 52, 6–10.
2. Perez-Reyes M, White WR, Hicks RE. Interaction between ethanol and calcium channel blockers in humans. *Alcohol Clin Exp Res* (1992) 16, 769–75.
3. Vincent J, Colangelo P, Baris B, Willavize S. Single and multiple doses of amlodipine do not alter the pharmacokinetics of alcohol in man. *Therapie* (1995) (Suppl) 50, 509.
4. Pentikainen PJ, Virolainen T, Tenhunen R, Aberg J. Acute alcohol intake increases the bioavailability of felodipine. *Clin Pharmacol Ther* (1994) 55, 148.
5. Qureshi S, Laganière S, Caillé G, Gossard D, Lacasse Y, McGilveray I. Effect of an acute dose of alcohol on the pharmacokinetics of oral nifedipine in humans. *Pharm Res* (1992) 9, 683–6.

Alcohol + Cannabis

Smoking cannabis (marijuana) may alter the bioavailability of alcohol. The effects of drinking alcohol and smoking cannabis appear to be at least additive on driving performance. However, there is some evidence that regular cannabis use *per se* does not potentiate the effects of alcohol.

Clinical evidence, mechanism, importance and management

Fifteen healthy subjects given alcohol 0.7 g/kg developed peak plasma alcohol levels of 78.25 mg% at 50 minutes, but if they smoked a cannabis cigarette 30 minutes after the drink, their peak plasma alcohol levels were only 54.8 mg% and they occurred later, at 105 minutes. In addition, their subjective experience of the drugs decreased when used together.[1] One study in 14 regular cannabis users (long-term daily use) and 14 infrequent cannabis users found that regular use reduced the disruptive effects of alcohol on some psychomotor skills relevant to driving, whereas infrequent use did not have this effect. In this study, neither group had smoked any cannabis in the 12 hours before the alcohol test.[2] In contrast, simultaneous use of alcohol and oral **Δ^9-tetrahydrocannabinol** (the major active ingredient of cannabis) reduced the performance of psychomotor tests, suggesting that those who use both drugs together should expect the deleterious effects to be additive.[3] In a further study, subjects smoked cannabis containing 100 or 200 micrograms/kg of **Δ^9-tetrahydrocannabinol** and drank alcohol (to achieve an initial blood level of 70 mg% and booster doses to maintain levels at 40 mg%) or placebo 30 minutes before driving. They found that cannabis, even in low to moderate doses, negatively affected driving performance in real traffic situations. Further, the effect of combining moderate doses of both alcohol and cannabis resulted in dramatic performance impairment as great as that observed with blood levels of alcohol 140 mg% alone.[4,5] Concurrent use of cannabis and alcohol before driving should therefore be avoided.

1. Lukas SE, Benedikt R, Mendelson JH, Kouri E, Sholar M, Amass L. Marihuana attenuates the rise in plasma ethanol levels in human subjects. *Neuropsychopharmacology* (1992) 7, 77–81.
2. Wright KA, Terry P. Modulation of the effects of alcohol on driving-related psychomotor skills by chronic exposure to cannabis. *Psychopharmacology (Berl)* (2002) 160, 213–19.
3. Bird KD, Boleyn T, Chesher GB, Jackson DM, Starmer GA, Teo RKC. Intercannabinoid and cannabinoid-ethanol interactions and their effects on human performance. *Psychopharmacology (Berl)* (1980) 71, 181–8.
4. National Highway Traffic Safety Administration. Marijuana and alcohol combined severely impede driving performance. *Ann Emerg Med* (2000) 35, 398–9.
5. Jolly BT. Commentary: drugged driving—different spin on an old problem. *Ann Emerg Med* (2000) 35, 399–400.

Alcohol + Carmofur

A disulfiram-like reaction occurred in a patient on carmofur when he was given coeliac plexus blockade with alcohol.

Clinical evidence, mechanism, importance and management

A man with pancreatic carcinoma treated with carmofur 500 mg daily for 25 days experienced a disulfiram-like reaction (facial flushing, diaphoresis, hypotension with BP 60/30 mmHg, and tachycardia of 128 bpm) within 30 minutes of being given coeliac plexus alcohol blockade for pain relief. Blood acetaldehyde levels were found to have risen sharply, supporting the belief that the underlying mechanism is similar to the disulfiram-alcohol interaction (see 'Alcohol + Disulfiram', p.50). It is suggested that alcohol blockade should be avoided for 7 days after treatment with carmofur.[1]

1. Noda J, Umeda S, Mori K, Fukunaga T, Mizoi Y. Disulfiram-like reaction associated with carmofur after celiac plexus alcohol block. *Anesthesiology* (1987) 67, 809–10.

Alcohol + Cephalosporins

Disulfiram-like reactions can occur in those taking cefamandole, cefmenoxime, cefoperazone, cefotetan, latamoxef (moxalactam) and possibly cefonicid after drinking alcohol or following an injection of alcohol. This is not a general reaction of the cephalosporins, but is confined to those with particular chemical structures.

Clinical evidence

A young man with cystic fibrosis was given 2 g of **latamoxef** intravenously every 8 hours for pneumonia. After 3 days' treatment he drank, as was his custom, a can of **beer** with lunch. He rapidly became flushed with a florid macular eruption over his face and chest. This faded over the next 30 minutes but he complained of severe nausea and headache. A woman patient also on **latamoxef** became flushed, diaphoretic and nauseated after drinking a cocktail of **vodka** and tomato juice.[1] This reaction has also been described in two subjects who drank alcohol while receiving **latamoxef**,[2] two of 10 subjects given **latamoxef** and alcohol,[3] and a patient on **latamoxef** given theophylline elixir containing 20% alcohol.[4] It has also been seen in a patient on **latamoxef** following the injection of alcohol into the para-aortic space for coeliac plexus block.[5]

The symptoms experienced have included flushing of the face, arms and neck, shortness of breath, headache, tachycardia, dizziness, hyper- and hypotension, nausea and vomiting.

Similar reactions have been described in patients or subjects on **cefamandole**,[6,7] **cefoperazone**,[5,8-15] **cefmenoxime**,[16] **cefonicid**[17] and **cefotetan**,[18] after drinking **wine**, **beer**, or other alcoholic drinks, and after the ingestion of an 8.5% alcoholic elixir.[16]

Mechanism

These reactions appear to have the same pharmacological basis as the disulfiram/alcohol reaction (see 'Alcohol + Disulfiram', p.50). Three of these cephalosporins (latamoxef, cefamandole and cefoperazone) can raise blood acetaldehyde levels in *rats* when alcohol is given, but to a lesser extent than disulfiram.[2,11,19] It appears that it normally only occurs with cephalosporins that possess a methyltetrazolethiol group in the 3-position on the cephalosporin molecule,[11,20] but it has also been seen with cefonicid, which possesses a methylsulfonthiotetrazole group instead.[17]

Importance and management

Established but unpredictable interactions of varying incidence. Two out of 10 subjects given latamoxef and alcohol reacted in one study,[3] five out of 8 on cefotetan reacted,[18] and 8 out of 9 on cefoperazone reacted.[14,15] The reaction appears normally to be more embarrassing or unpleasant and frightening than serious, with the symptoms subsiding spontaneously after a few hours. There is evidence that the severity varies; in one study cefoperazone was said to be worse than latamoxef, which in turn was said to be worse than **cefmetazole**.[21] Treatment is not usually needed but there are two reports[4,6] of two elderly patients who needed treatment for hypotension, which was life-threatening in one case;[4] plasma expanders and dopamine have been used as treatment.[4,6]

Because the reaction is unpredictable, warn all patients taking these potentially interacting cephalosporins that it can occur during and up to three days after the course of treatment is over. Advise them to avoid alcohol. Those with kidney or liver disease in whom the drug clearance is prolonged should wait a week. It should not be forgotten that some foods and pharmaceuticals contain substantial amounts of alcohol, and a reaction with some topically applied products cannot be excluded (see 'Alcohol + Disulfiram', p.50).

This disulfiram-like reaction is not a general reaction of all the cephalosporins. One study found no interaction in those taking **cefpirome** and alcohol,[22] and in another **ceftizoxime** was reported not to interact with alcohol.[23] No interaction was seen with cefonicid and alcohol in one placebo-controlled study,[24] however a case report describes a disulfiram-reaction in one patient taking the combination.[17]

A number of other cephalosporins are possible candidates for this reaction because they possess the methyltetrazolethiol group in the 3-position. These include, **ceforanide**, **cefotiam**, and **cefpiramide**.[11,20]

1. Neu HC, Prince AS. Interaction between moxalactam and alcohol. *Lancet* (1980), i, 1422.
2. Buening MK, Wold JS, Israel KS, Kammer RB. Disulfiram-like reaction to β-lactams. *JAMA* (1981) 245, 2027–8.
3. Elenbaas RM, Ryan JL, Robinson WA, Singsank MJ, Harvey MJ, Klaasen CD. On the disulfiram-like activity of moxalactam. *Clin Pharmacol Ther* (1982) 32, 347–55.
4. Brown KR, Guglielmo BJ, Pons VG, Jacobs RA. Theophylline elixir, moxalactam, and a disulfiram-like reaction. *Ann Intern Med* (1982) 97, 621–2.
5. Umeda S, Arai T. Disulfiram-like reaction to moxalactam after celiac plexus alcohol block. *Anesth Analg* (1985) 64, 377.
6. Portier H, Chalopin JM, Freysz M, Tanter Y. Interaction between cephalosporins and alcohol. *Lancet* (1980), ii, 263.
7. Drummer S, Hauser WE, Remington JS. Antabuse-like effect of β-lactam antibiotics. *N Engl J Med* (1980) 303, 1417–18.
8. Foster TS, Raehl CL, Wilson HD. Disulfiram-like reaction associated with parenteral cephalosporin. *Am J Hosp Pharm* (1980) 37, 858–9.
9. Allaz A-F, Dayer P, Fabre J, Rudhardt M, Balant L. Pharmacocinétique d'une novelle céphalosporine, la céfopérazone. *Schweiz Med Wochenschr* (1979), 109, 1999–2005.
10. Kemmerich B, Lode H. Cefoperazone – another cephalosporin associated with a disulfiram type alcohol incompatibility. *Infection* (1981) 9, 110.
11. Uri JV, Parks DB. Disulfiram-like reaction to certain cephalosporins. *Ther Drug Monit* (1983) 5, 219–24.
12. Bailey RR, Peddie B, Blake E, Bishop V, Reddy J. Cefoperazone in the treatment of severe or complicated infections. *Drugs* (1981) 22 (Suppl 1), 76–86.
13. Ellis-Pegler RB, Lang SDR. Cefoperazone in Klebsiella meningitis: A case report. *Drugs* (1981) 22 (Suppl 1), 69–71.
14. Reeves DS, Davies AJ. Antabuse effect with cephalosporins. *Lancet* (1980) ii, 540.
15. McMahon FG. Disulfiram-like reaction to a cephalosporin. *JAMA* (1980), 243, 2397.
16. Kannangara DW, Gallagher K, Lefrock JL. Disulfiram-like reactions with newer cephalosporins: cefmenoxime. *Am J Med Sci* (1984) 287, 45–7.
17. Marcon G, Spolaor A, Scevola M, Zolli M, Carlassara GB. Effetto disulfiram-simile da cefonicid: prima segnalazione. *Recenti Prog Med* (1990) 81, 47–8.
18. Kline SS, Mauro VF, Forney RB, Freimer EH, Somani P. Cefotetan-induced disulfiram-type reactions and hypoprothrombinemia. *Antimicrob Agents Chemother* (1987) 31, 1328–31.
19. Yanagihara M, Okada K, Nozaki M, Tsurumi K, Fujimura H. Cephem antibiotics and alcohol metabolism. Disulfiram-like reaction resulting from intravenous administration of cephem antibiotics. *Folia Pharmacol Japon* (1982) 79, 551–60.
20. Norrby SR. Adverse reactions and interactions with newer cephalosporin and cephamycin antibiotics. *Med Toxicol* (1986) 1, 32–46.
21. Nakamura K, Nakagawa A, Tanaka M, Masuda H, Hayashi Y, Saionji K. Effects of cephem antibiotics on ethanol metabolism. *Folia Pharmacol Japon* (1984) 83, 183–91.
22. Lassman HB, Hubbard JW, Chen B-L, Puri SK. Lack of interaction between cefpirome and alcohol. *J Antimicrob Chemother* (1992) 29 (Suppl A), 47–50.
23. McMahon FG, Noveck RJ. Lack of disulfiram-like reactions with ceftizoxime. *J Antimicrob Chemother* (1982) 10 (Suppl C), 129–33.
24. McMahon FG, Ryan JR, Jain AK, LaCorte W, Ginzler F. Absence of disulfiram-type reactions to single and multiple doses of cefonicid: a placebo-controlled study. *J Antimicrob Chemother* (1987) 20, 913–8.

Alcohol + Ciprofloxacin

Ciprofloxacin does not significantly affect the pharmacokinetics of alcohol or the psychomotor performance observed with alcohol alone. There is an isolated report of a cutaneous reaction to ciprofloxacin, which may have been precipitated by alcohol ingestion.

Clinical evidence, mechanism, importance and management

A 3-day course of ciprofloxacin 500 mg twice daily had no significant effect on the pharmacokinetics of a single oral dose of **alcohol** (30 g/75 ml **vodka**) in 12 healthy subjects, nor was the performance of a number of psychomotor tests affected.[1]

There is an isolated report of red blotches developing on the face and body of a tetraplegic patient on ciprofloxacin 250 mg twice daily within 10 minutes of drinking 2 cans of beer containing 4.7% alcohol. He did not feel unwell or drowsy and the blotches faded over a period of 30 minutes. Previous courses of ciprofloxacin had not produced any side effects and the same brand of alcohol caused no problems in the absence of ciprofloxacin.[2] The general clinical importance of this report is unknown.

1. Kamali F. No influence of ciprofloxacin on ethanol disposition: a pharmacokinetic-pharmacodynamic interaction study. *Eur J Clin Pharmacol* (1994) 47, 71–4.
2. Vaidyanathan S, Singh G, Sett P, Watt JWH, Soni BM, Oo T. Cutaneous adverse reaction to ciprofloxacin precipitated by ingestion of alcohol in a tetraplegic patient. *Spinal Cord* (1999) 37, 663–4.

Alcohol + Clomethiazole

Long-term use of alcohol with clomethiazole can cause serious, even potentially fatal, CNS depression due to additive CNS depressant effects, which are associated with increased clomethiazole bioavailability.

Clinical evidence, mechanism, importance and management

The following is taken from an editorial in the British Medical Journal, which was entitled 'Chlormethiazole and alcohol: a lethal cocktail':[1]

Clomethiazole is commonly used to treat withdrawal from alcohol because of its hypnotic, anxiolytic and anticonvulsant effects. It is very effective if a rapidly reducing dosage regimen is followed over six days, but if it is used long term and drinking continues it carries several serious risks.

Alcoholics readily transfer dependency to clomethiazole and may visit several practitioners and hospitals to get their supplies. Tolerance develops so that very large amounts may be taken (up to 25 g daily). Often alcohol abuse continues and the combination of large amounts of alcohol and clomethiazole can result in coma and even fatal respiratory depression, due mainly to simple additive CNS depression. Other factors are that alcohol increases the bioavailability of clomethiazole (probably by impairing first pass metabolism),[2] and in the case of those with alcoholic cirrhosis, the systemic bioavailability may be increased tenfold because of venous shunting.[3]

It is suggested that clomethiazole should not be given long term. If prescribers choose to manage detoxification at home, it should be done under very close supervision, issuing prescriptions for only one day's supply to ensure daily contact and to minimise the risk of abuse. And if the patient shows evidence of tolerance or clomethiazole dependency or of continuing to drink, the only safe policy is rapid admission for inpatient care.[1]

Nobody appears to have checked on the combined effects of clomethiazole and alcohol on driving and related skills, but concurrent use would be expected to increase the risks.

1. McInnes GT. Chlormethiazole and alcohol: a lethal cocktail. *BMJ* (1987) 294, 592.
2. Neuvonen PJ, Pentikäinen PJ, Jostell KG, Syvälahti E. The pharmacokinetics of chlormethiazole in healthy subjects as affected by ethanol. *Clin Pharmacol Ther* (1981) 29, 268–9.
3. Pentikäinen PJ, Neuvonen PJ, Tarpila S, Syvälahti E. Effect of cirrhosis of the liver on the pharmacokinetics of chlormethiazole. *BMJ* (1978) 2, 861–3.

Alcohol + Cloral hydrate

Both alcohol and cloral hydrate are CNS depressants, and their effects may be additive, possibly even more than additive. Some patients may experience a disulfiram-like flushing reaction if they drink after taking cloral hydrate for several days.

Clinical evidence

Studies in 5 healthy subjects given cloral hydrate 15 mg/kg and alcohol 0.5 g/kg found that both drugs given alone impaired their ability to carry out complex motor tasks. When taken together, the effects were additive, and possibly even more than additive. After taking cloral for 7 days, one of the subjects experienced a disulfiram-like reaction (bright red-purple flushing of the face, tachycardia, hypotension, anxiety and persistent headache) after drinking alcohol.[1,2]

The disulfiram-like reaction has been described in other reports.[3] Note that the earliest report was published more than a century ago in 1872 and described two patients on cloral hydrate who experienced this reaction after drinking only half a bottle of **beer**.[2]

Mechanism

Alcohol, cloral and trichloroethanol (to which cloral hydrate is metabolised) are all CNS depressants. During concurrent use, the metabolic pathways used for their elimination are mutually inhibited: blood-alcohol levels rise because the trichloroethanol competitively depresses the oxidation of alcohol to acetaldehyde, while trichloroethanol levels also rise because its production from cloral hydrate is increased and its further conversion and clearance as the glucuronide is inhibited. As a result the rises in the blood levels of alcohol and trichloroethanol are exaggerated, and their effects are accordingly greater.[1,2,4] In one subject, blood levels of acetaldehyde during the use of cloral hydrate with alcohol were only 50% of those after alcohol alone, so that the flushing reaction, despite its resemblance to the disulfiram reaction, may possibly have a partially different basis.[2]

Importance and management

A well-documented and established interaction. Only a few references are given here. A comprehensive bibliography can be found in the references by Sellers.[1,2] Patients given cloral hydrate should be warned about the extensive CNS depression that can occur if they drink, and of the disulfiram-like reaction that may occur after taking cloral for a period of time. Its incidence is uncertain. The legendary Mickey Finn, which is concocted of cloral hydrate and alcohol, is reputed to be so potent that deep sleep can be induced in an unsuspecting victim within minutes of ingestion, but the evidence seems largely to be anecdotal. Very large doses of both would be likely to cause serious and potentially life-threatening CNS depression.

It seems likely that **cloral betaine**, **triclofos** and other compounds closely related to cloral hydrate will interact with alcohol in a similar manner, but this requires confirmation.

1. Sellers EM, Lang M, Koch-Weser J, LeBlanc E, Kalant H. Interaction of chloral hydrate and ethanol in man. I. Metabolism. *Clin Pharmacol Ther* (1972) 13, 37–49.
2. Sellers EM, Carr G, Bernstein JG, Sellers S, Koch-Weser J. Interaction of chloral hydrate and ethanol in man. II. Hemodynamics and performance. *Clin Pharmacol Ther* (1972) 13, 50–8.
3. Bardoděj Z. Intolerance alkohlu po chloralhydrátu. *Cesk Farm* (1965) 14, 478–81.
4. Wong LK, Biemann K. A study of drug interaction by gas chromatography–mass spectrometry—synergism of chloral hydrate and ethanol. *Biochem Pharmacol* (1978) 27, 1019–22.

Alcohol + CNS depressants

The concurrent use of small or moderate amounts of alcohol and therapeutic doses of drugs that are CNS depressants can increase drowsiness and reduce alertness. These drugs include analgesics, anticonvulsants, antidepressants, antihistamines, antipsychotics, antinauseants, appetite suppressants, hypno-sedatives, opioid analgesics, and others. This increases the risk of accident when driving or handling other potentially dangerous machinery, and may make the performance of everyday tasks more difficult and hazardous.

Clinical evidence, mechanism, importance and management

Alcohol is a CNS depressant (see 'alcohol', (p.36)). With only small or moderate amounts of alcohol and with blood-alcohol levels well within legal driving limits, it may be quite unsafe to drive if another CNS depressant is being taken concurrently. The details of most of the drugs that have been tested are set out in the monographs in this section, but there are others that nobody seems to have tested formally. The summary above contains a list of some of those that commonly cause drowsiness. Quite apart from driving, almost everyone meets potentially dangerous situations every day at home, in the garden, in the street and at work. Crossing a busy street or even walking downstairs can become much more risky under the influence of CNS depressant drugs and drink. A cause for concern is that patients may be partially or totally unaware of the extent of the deterioration in their skills. Patients should be warned.

Alcohol + Cocaine

Alcohol increases blood levels of cocaine as well as its physiological and subjective effects.

Clinical evidence, mechanism, importance and management

A study in 8 cocaine users found that intranasal cocaine 100 mg and alcohol 0.8 g/kg produced greater euphoria and increase in heart rate than cocaine alone, and reduced alcohol sedation without altering the feeling of drunkenness. In addition, the combination resulted in higher plasma levels of cocaine and the appearance of cocaethylene, a metabolite produced by the interaction of the two drugs.[1] A further similar study with intranasal cocaine 1 mg/kg every 30 minutes for 4 doses and oral alcohol 1 g/kg reported very similar findings.[2] It was concluded that the enhanced physiological effects may lead to use of larger amounts of the combination with an increased risk for toxic effects,[2] such as cardiotoxicity.[1]

1. Farré M, de la Torre R, González ML, Terán MT, Roset PN, Menoyo E, Camí J. Cocaine and alcohol interactions in humans: neuroendocrine effects and cocaethylene metabolism. *J Pharmacol Exp Ther* (1997) 283, 164–76.
2. McCance-Katz EF, Kosten TR, Jatlow P. Concurrent use of cocaine and alcohol is more potent and potentially more toxic than use of either alone--a multiple-dose study. *Biol Psychiatry* (1998) 44, 250–9.

Alcohol + Codeine

Codeine, in 50-mg doses, both alone and with alcohol, impairs the ability to drive safely. This is probably less of a problem with the relatively small amounts of codeine in most non-prescription compound analgesic preparations, but if these make the patient drowsy, alcohol should be avoided.

Clinical evidence, mechanism, importance and management

Double blind studies on a very large number of professional army drivers found that 50 mg of codeine and alcohol 0.5 g/kg, both alone and together, impaired their ability to drive safely on a static driving simulator. The number of 'collisions', neglected instructions and the times they 'drove off the road' were increased.[1,2] Codeine dosages of this order are given in the form of Codeine Phosphate Tablets BP (30 to 60 mg dose), higher doses of Codeine Linctus BP (30 mg dose) and a variety of other elixirs, linctuses and compound proprietary preparations. These preparations, particularly with alcohol, are likely to make drivers more accident-prone. However, in the UK only relatively small amounts of codeine (5 to 8 mg per dose of analgesic, up to 15 mg per dose of cough mixture) are found in preparations that can be sold to the public without prescription, and the effect of these doses with alcohol do not appear to have been studied. Nevertheless, even these products generally carry the warning that they may cause drowsiness and that if affected the patient should not drive or operate machinery, and that alcoholic drinks should be avoided. Alcohol appears not to affect the pharmacokinetics of codeine.[3]

1. Linnoila M, Häkkinen S. Effects of diazepam and codeine, alone and in combination with alcohol, on simulated driving. *Clin Pharmacol Ther* (1974) 15, 368–73.
2. Linnoila M, Mattila MJ. Interaction of alcohol and drugs on psychomotor skills as demonstrated by a driving simulator. *Br J Pharmacol* (1973) 47, 671P–672P.
3. Bodd E, Beylich KM, Christophersen AS, Mørland J. Oral administration of codeine in the presence of ethanol: a pharmacokinetic study in man. *Pharmacol Toxicol* (1987) 61, 297–300.

Alcohol + Co-dergocrine mesilate (Ergoloid mesylates)

Co-dergocrine mesilate (ergoloid mesylates) causes a very small reduction in blood alcohol levels.

Clinical evidence, mechanism, importance and management

Thirteen subjects were given 0.5 g/kg of 25% alcohol in orange juice after breakfast, before and after taking 4.5 mg of co-dergocrine mesilate (ergolide mesylates, *Hydergine*) every 8 hours for nine doses. The co-dergocrine caused a small reduction in blood alcohol levels (maximum serum levels reduced from 59 to 55.7 mg%, clearance reduced from 0.11 to 0.10 g/kg/h).[1] The reason is not understood. This interaction is almost certainly not of clinical importance.

1. Savage IT, James IM. The effect of Hydergine on ethanol pharmacokinetics in man. *J Pharm Pharmacol* (1993) 45 (Suppl 2), 1119.

Alcohol + Cycloserine

A brief report describes an enhancement of the effects of alcohol in 2 patients on cycloserine.[1] The clinical significance of this case report is unclear. However, the makers of cycloserine state that it

is 'incompatible' with alcohol because of an increased risk of epileptic episodes, and contraindicate its use in alcohol abuse.[2]

1. Glaß F, Mallach HJ, Simsch A. Beobachtungen und Untersuchungen über die gemeinsame Wirkung von Alkohol und D-Cycloserin. *Arzneimittelforschung* (1965) 15, 684–8.
2. Cycloserine. King Pharmaceuticals Ltd. UK Summary of product characteristics, March 2001.

Alcohol + Cyproterone acetate

Cyproterone acetate's usual efficacy appears to be lost in those drinking alcohol to excess, but there seems to be no evidence that normal social amounts of alcohol interact.

Clinical evidence, mechanism, importance and management

The makers of cyproterone acetate say that alcohol appears to reduce its effects, and so it is of no value in chronic alcoholics.[1] This appears to be based solely on a simple and unelaborated statement in an abstract of studies[2] on 84 men whose hyper- or abnormal sexuality was treated with cyproterone acetate, which stated that "antiandrogens do not inhibit male sexual behaviour during alcohol excess."

The suggested reasons for this reaction are unknown, but it may possibly be due several factors. These include enzyme induction by the alcohol, which could possibly increase the metabolism and loss of the cyproterone from the body; increased sexual drive caused by alcohol, which might oppose the effects of cyproterone; and reduced compliance by alcoholic patients who forget to take their tablets while drinking to excess.[3]

It seems therefore that cyproterone may not be effective in alcoholic patients, but there is nothing to suggest that the effects of cyproterone are opposed by normal moderate social amounts of alcohol.

1. Androcur (Cyproterone acetate). Schering Health Care Ltd. UK Summary of product characteristics, April 2004.
2. Laschet U, Laschet L. Three years clinical results with cyproterone-acetate in the inhibiting regulation of male sexuality. *Acta Endocrinol (Copenh)* (1969) 138 (Suppl), 103.
3. Schering Health Care Limited. Personal communication, January 1997.

Alcohol + Dextropropoxyphene (Propoxyphene)

The CNS depressant effects of alcohol are only modestly increased by normal therapeutic doses of dextropropoxyphene. In deliberate suicidal overdosage the CNS depressant effects appear to be additive, and can be fatal.

Clinical evidence

Alcohol alone (blood levels of 50 mg%) impaired the performance of various psychomotor tests (motor co-ordination, mental performance and stability of stance) in 8 healthy subjects given more than 65 mg of dextropropoxyphene alone. When given together there was some evidence that the effects were greater than with either alone, but in some instances the impairment was no greater than with just alcohol. The effect of alcohol clearly predominated.[1]

Another study found that the effects of alcohol (3 double measures of vodka) on the performance of two psychomotor tests were not altered in subjects who had also been given two tablets of *Distalgesic* (dextropropoxyphene 32.5 mg + paracetamol (acetaminophen) 325 mg in each tablet).[2] A further study found no change in the psychomotor effects of alcohol (0.5 g/kg) following the addition of dextropropoxyphene 130 mg but the bioavailability of the dextropropoxyphene was raised by 25%.[3] Yet another study[4] found a 31% increase in bioavailability of dextropropoxyphene with blood alcohol levels of about 80 to 100 mg%.

Mechanism

Not understood. Both drugs are CNS depressants, and there may be enhanced suppression of the medullary respiratory control centre.[5-7] In overdosage the fatal dose of dextropropoxyphene is reduced by the presence of alcohol.[5-7] This is possibly also due to increased bioavailability of dextropropoxyphene.[7]

Importance and management

Numerous reports describe the severe and sometimes fatal respiratory depression that can follow alcohol/dextropropoxyphene overdosage, but information about moderate social drinking and therapeutic doses of dextropropoxyphene is limited. The objective evidence is that the interaction with moderate doses of both is quite small. Even so it would seem prudent to warn patients that dextropropoxyphene can cause drowsiness and this may be exaggerated to some extent by alcohol. They should be warned that driving or handling potentially hazardous machinery may be more risky, but total abstinence from alcohol does not seem to be necessary.

1. Kiplinger GF, Sokol G, Rodda BE. Effects of combined alcohol and propoxyphene on human performance. *Arch Int Pharmacodyn Ther* (1974) 212, 175–80.
2. Edwards C, Gard PR, Handley SL, Hunter M, Whittington RM. Distalgesic and ethanol-impaired function. *Lancet* (1982) ii, 384.
3. Girre C, Hirschhorn M, Bertaux L, Palombo S, Dellatolas F, Ngo R, Moreno M, Fournier PE. Enhancement of propoxyphene bioavailability by ethanol: relation to psychomotor and cognitive function in healthy volunteers. *Eur J Clin Pharmacol* (1991) 41, 147–52.
4. Sellers EM, Hamilton CA, Kaplan HL, Degani NC, Foltz RL. Pharmacokinetic interaction of propoxyphene with ethanol. *Br J Clin Pharmacol* (1985) 19, 398–401.
5. Carson DJL, Carson ED. Fatal dextropropoxyphene poisoning in Northern Ireland: review of 30 cases. *Lancet* (1977) i, 894–7.
6. Whittington RM, Barclay AD. The epidemiology of dextropropoxyphene (Distalgesic) overdose fatalities in Birmingham and the West Midlands. *J Clin Hosp Pharm* (1981) 6, 251–7.
7. Williamson RV, Galloway JH, Yeo WW, Forrest ARW. Relationship between blood dextropropoxyphene and ethanol levels in fatal co-proxamol overdosage. *Br J Clin Pharmacol* (2000) 50, 388–9.

Alcohol + Dimethylformamide

A disulfiram-like reaction can occur in about 20% of those who drink alcohol after being exposed to dimethylformamide vapour.

Clinical evidence

A 3-year study in a chemical plant where dimethylformamide (DMF) was used found that about 20% (19 out of 102 men) exposed to DMF vapour experienced flushing of the face, and often of the neck, arms, hands, and chest, after drinking alcohol. Sometimes dizziness, nausea and tightness of the chest also occurred. A single glass of **beer** was enough to induce a flush lasting 2 hours. The majority of the men experienced the reaction within 24 hours of exposure to DMF, but it could occur even after 4 days.[1] Three further cases of this interaction are described in other reports.[2,3]

A further study in 126 factory workers exposed to DMF and 54 workers who had no contact with DMF indicated that DMF adversely affected liver function, and that concurrent alcohol had a synergistic effect, although individual differences in tolerance to the interaction were observed.[4]

Mechanism

Men exposed to DMF vapour develop substantial amounts of DMF and its metabolite (*N*-methylformamide) in their blood and urine.[1] This latter compound in particular has been shown in *rats* given alcohol to raise their blood acetaldehyde levels by a factor of five, so it would seem probable that the *N*-methylformamide is similarly responsible for this disulfiram-like reaction in man (see 'Alcohol + Disulfiram', p.50).[5] Both agents are hepatotoxic.[4]

Importance and management

An established interaction, with the incidence said to be about 20%.[1] Those who come into contact with DMF, even in very low concentrations, should be warned of this possible interaction with alcohol. It would appear to be more unpleasant than serious in most instances, and normally requires no treatment. Further studies are required on the hepatotoxic effects.

1. Lyle WH, Spence TWM, McKinneley WM, Duckers K. Dimethylformamide and alcohol intolerance. *Br J Ind Med* (1979) 36, 63–6.
2. Chivers CP. Disulfiram effect from inhalation of dimethylformamide. *Lancet* (1978) i, 331.
3. Reinl W, Urban HJ. Erkrankungen durch dimethylformamid. *Int Arch Gewerbepathol Gewerbehyg* (1965) 21, 333–46.
4. Wrbitzky R. Liver function in workers exposed to *N,N*-dimethylformamide during the production of synthetic textiles. *Int Arch Occup Environ Health* (1999) 72, 19–25.
5. Hanasono GK, Fuller RW, Broddle WD, Gibson WR. Studies on the effects of *N,N'*-dimethylformamide on ethanol disposition and monoamine oxidase activity in rats. *Toxicol Appl Pharmacol* (1977) 39, 461–72.

Alcohol + Disulfiram

The ingestion of alcohol while taking disulfiram will result in flushing and fullness of the face and neck, tachycardia, breathlessness, giddiness, and hypotension, nausea and vomiting. This is called the Disulfiram or Antabuse reaction. It is used to deter alcoholic patients from drinking. A mild flushing reaction of the skin may possibly occur in particularly sensitive individuals if alcohol is applied to the skin or if the vapour is inhaled.

Clinical evidence

One of the early descriptions of this toxic interaction was made in 1937 by Dr EE Williams[1] who noted it amongst workers in the rubber industry who were handling **tetramethylthiuram disulphide**:

"Even beer will cause a flushing of the face and hands, with rapid pulse, and some of the men describe palpitations and a terrible fullness of the face, eyes and head. After a glass of beer (six ounces) the blood pressure falls about 10 points, the pulse is slightly accelerated and the skin becomes flushed in the face and wrists. In 15 minutes the blood pressure falls another 10 points, the heart is more rapid, and the patient complains of fullness in the head."

The later observation[2] by Hald and his colleagues of the same reaction with the ethyl congener (disulfiram) led to its introduction as a drink deterrent. Patients experience throbbing in head and neck, giddiness, sweating, nausea, vomiting, thirst, chest pain, difficulty in breathing, and headache. The severity of the reaction can depend upon the amount of alcohol ingested, but some individuals are extremely sensitive. Respiratory depression, cardiovascular collapse, cardiac arrhythmias, unconsciousness, and convulsions may occur. There have been fatalities.[3] An unusual and isolated report describes painful, intermittent and transient myoclonic jerking of the arms and legs as the predominant manifestation of the disulfiram reaction in one patient.[4] Another unusual case has been reported in which a woman with a history of bipolar disorder, and alcoholism which was treated with disulfiram, was admitted to hospital with a 3- to 4-day history of changes in her mental state, including difficulties with orientation and concentration and visual hallucinations. The confusional state was attributed to alcohol consumption while taking disulfiram and the probability of this was supported by an earlier similar, though shorter, episode experienced by the patient.[5]

A mild disulfiram reaction is said to occur in some patients who apply alcohol to the skin, but it is probably largely due to inhalation of the vapour.[6] It has been reported after using **after-shave lotion** (50% alcohol),[6] **tar gel** (33% alcohol)[7] and a **beer-containing shampoo** (3% alcohol).[8] A **contact lens wetting solution** (containing **polyvinyl alcohol**) used to irrigate the eye has also been implicated in a reaction,[9,10] although the probability of an interaction with this secondary alcohol has been disputed.[11] It has also been described in a patient who inhaled vapour from paint in a poorly ventilated area and from the inhalation of '**mineral spirits**'.[12] A woman on disulfiram reported vaginal stinging and soreness during sexual intercourse, and similar discomfort to her husband's penis, which seemed to be related to the disulfiram dosage and how intoxicated her husband was.[13]

Mechanism

Partially understood. Alcohol is normally rapidly metabolised within the liver, firstly to acetaldehyde (by acetaldehyde dehydrogenase) and then by a series of biochemical steps to water and carbon dioxide. Disulfiram inhibits this first enzyme so that the acetaldehyde accumulates. Prostaglandin release may also be involved.[14] Not all of the symptoms of the reaction can be reproduced by injecting acetaldehyde so that some other biochemical mechanism(s) must also be involved. For example, it is thought that the inhibition of dopamine-beta-hydroxylase may have some part to play. It has been suggested that the mild skin flush that can occur if alcohol is applied to the skin is not a true disulfiram reaction.[15]

Importance and management

An extremely well-documented and important interaction exploited therapeutically to deter alcoholics from drinking. Initial treatment should be closely supervised because an extremely intense and potentially serious reaction occurs in a few individuals, even with quite small doses of alcohol. Apart from the usual warnings about drinking, patients should also be warned about the unwitting ingestion of alcohol in some pharmaceutical preparations.[16] The risk of a reaction is real. It has been seen following a single-dose of an alcohol-containing **cough mixture**,[17] whereas the ingestion of small amounts of **communion wine** and the absorption of alcohol from a **bronchial nebuliser spray** or **ear drops** did not to result in any reaction in 3 individuals.[18] (See also 'Alcohol-containing ritonavir oral solution (Norvir) + Disulfiram or Metronidazole', p.50). Patients should also be warned about the exposure to alcohol from certain foods, cosmetics, solvents etc.

Treatment

The disulfiram reaction can be treated, if necessary, with ascorbic acid. A dose of 1 g given orally is reported to be effective in mild cases (heart rate less than 100 bpm and general condition good). It works within 30 to 45 minutes. Moderately severe cases (heart rate 100 to 150 bpm, blood pressure 150/100 mmHg) can be treated with 1 g of intravenous ascorbic acid and this is effective within 2 to 5 minutes. Critically ill patients may need other standard supportive emergency measures.[19]

1. Williams EE. Effects of alcohol on workers with carbon disulfide. *JAMA* (1937) 109, 1472.
2. Hald J, Jacobsen E, Larsen V. The sensitizing effects of tetraethylthiuramdisulphide (Antabuse) to ethylalcohol. *Acta Pharmacol* (1948) 4, 285–96.
3. Kwentus J, Major LF. Disulfiram in the treatment of alcoholism: a review. *J Stud Alcohol* (1979) 40, 428–46.
4. Syed J, Moarefi G. An unusual presentation of a disulfiram-alcohol reaction. *Del Med J* (1995) 67, 183.
5. Park CW, Riggio S. Disulfiram-ethanol induced delirium. *Ann Pharmacother* (2001) 35, 32–5.
6. Mercurio F. Antabuse®-alcohol reaction following the use of after-shave lotion. *JAMA* (1952) 149, 82.
7. Ellis CN, Mitchell AJ, Beardsley GR. Tar gel interaction with disulfiram. *Arch Dermatol* (1979) 115, 1367–8.
8. Stoll D, King LE. Disulfiram-alcohol skin reaction to beer-containing shampoo. *JAMA* (1980) 244, 2045.
9. Newsom SR, Harper BS. Disulfiram-alcohol reaction caused by contact lens wetting solution. *Contact Intraocul Lens Med J* (1980) 6, 407–8.
10. Newsom SR. Letter to the editor. *Contact Intraocul Lens Med J* (1981) 7, 172.
11. Refojo MF. Letter to Editor. *Contact Intraocul Lens Med J* (1981) 7, 172.
12. Scott GE, Little FW. Disulfiram reaction to organic solvents other than ethanol. *N Engl J Med* (1985) 312, 790.
13. Chick JD. Disulfiram reaction during sexual intercourse. *Br J Psychiatry* (1988) 152, 438.
14. Truitt EB, Gaynor CR, Mehl DL. Aspirin attenuation of alcohol-induced flushing and intoxication in oriental and occidental subjects. *Alcohol Alcohol* (1987) 22 (Suppl 1), 595–9.
15. Haddock NF, Wilkin JK. Cutaneous reactions to lower aliphatic alcohols before and during disulfiram therapy. *Arch Dermatol* (1982) 118, 157–9.
16. Parker WA. Alcohol-containing pharmaceuticals. *Am J Drug Alcohol Abuse* (1982–3) 9, 195–209.
17. Koff RS, Papadimas I, Honig EG. Alcohol in cough medicines: hazards to the disulfiram user. *JAMA* (1971) 215, 1988–9.
18. Rothstein E. Use of disulfiram (Antabuse) in alcoholism. *N Engl J Med* (1970) 283, 936.
19. McNichol RW, Sowell JM, Logsdon SA, Delgado MH, McNichol J. Disulfiram: a guide to clinical use in alcoholism treatment. *Am Fam Physician* (1991) 44, 481–4.

Alcohol-containing ritonavir oral solution (Norvir) + Disulfiram or Metronidazole

The makers suggest the possibility of a disulfiram-reaction with disulfiram or metronidazole and an alcohol-containing preparation of Norvir (ritonavir).

Clinical evidence, mechanism, importance and management

The UK makers of the oral solution of ritonavir (*Norvir*) say that since it contains 43% alcohol the preparation should not be taken with disulfiram or other drugs such as metronidazole because a disulfiram reaction is possible,[1] (for details of this reaction see, 'Alcohol + Disulfiram', p.50). However in practice the risk is probably fairly small because the recommended dose of ritonavir in this form is only 7.5 ml. No interaction will occur with ritonavir capsules because they do not contain alcohol.

1. Norvir Oral Solution (Ritonavir). Abbott Laboratories Ltd. UK Summary of product characteristics, January 2005.

Alcohol + Ecstasy (MDMA, 3,4-methylenedioxymethamfetamine)

Alcohol may slightly increase the plasma levels of ecstasy while alcohol levels may be slightly reduced by concurrent administration. Ecstasy may reduce subjective sedation associated with alcohol without reversing the effects of alcohol on psychomotor skills. Alcohol may enhance the transient immune dysfunction associated with ecstasy.

Clinical evidence, mechanism, importance and management

A study in 9 healthy subjects found that alcohol 0.8 g/kg increased the maximum plasma levels of a single 100-mg dose of ecstasy by 13%, with no change in AUC. The AUC and maximum plasma levels of alcohol were reduced by 9% and 15% after ecstasy administration. The combination induced a longer lasting euphoria and sense of well-being than either ecstasy or alcohol alone. Ecstasy reversed the subjective feelings of sedation associated with alcohol, but did not reverse feelings of drunkenness, or the effects of alcohol on psychomotor performance. This may have implications for road safety, as subjects may consider they are driving better when actual performance is impaired by alcohol.[1] More study is needed. See also 'Alcohol + Amfetamines', p.38.

Another study in 6 healthy subjects found that a single dose of ecstasy produced a time-dependent immune dysfunction. Ecstasy impaired CD4 T-cell function, which is responsible for cellular immunity. Alcohol alone may produce a decrease in T-helper cells and in B lymphocytes, which are responsible for humoral immunity. Concurrent ecstasy and alcohol increased the suppressive effect of ecstasy on CD4 T-cells and increased natural killer cells. It was suggested that the transient defect in immunological homoeostasis could have clinical consequences such as increased susceptibility to infectious diseases.[2] More study is needed.

1. Hernández-López C, Farré M, Roset PN, Menoyo E, Pizarro N, Ortuño J, Torrens M, Camí J, de la Torre R. 3,4-Methylenedioxymethamphetamine (Ecstasy) and alcohol interactions in humans: psychomotor performance, subjective effects, and pharmacokinetics. *J Pharmacol Exp Ther* (2002) 300, 236–44.
2. Pacifici R, Zuccaro P, Hernández López C, Pichini S, Di Carlo S, Farré M, Roset PN, Ortuño J, Segura J, de la Torre R. Acute effects of 3,4-methylenedioxymethamphetamine alone and in combination with ethanol on the immune system in humans. *J Pharmacol Exp Ther* (2001) 296, 207–15.

Alcohol + Edible fungi

A disulfiram-like reaction can occur if alcohol is taken after eating the smooth ink(y) cap fungus (*Coprinus atramentarius*) or certain other edible fungi.

Clinical evidence

A man who drank 3 pints of **beer** 2 hours after eating a meal of freshly picked and fried **ink(y) caps** (***Coprinus atramentarius***) developed facial flushing and a blotchy red rash over the upper half of his body. His face and hands swelled and he became breathless, sweated profusely, and vomited during the 3 hours when the reaction was most severe. On admission to hospital he was tachycardic and 12 hours later he was in atrial fibrillation, which lasted for 60 hours. The man's wife who ate the same meal but without an alcoholic drink did not show the reaction.[1]

This reaction has been described on many occasions in medical and pharmacological reports[2-4] and in books devoted to descriptions of edible and poisonous fungi. Only a few are listed here. Mild hypotension and "...alarming orthostatic features..." are said to be common symptoms[5] but the arrhythmia seen in the case cited here[1] appears to be rare. Recovery is usually spontaneous and uncomplicated. A similar reaction has been described after eating ***Boletus luridus***,[6] and other fungi including ***Coprinus micaceus***, ***Clitocybe claviceps*** and certain **morels**.[6] An African relative of ***Coprinus atramentarius*** – ***Coprinus africanus*** – which also causes this reaction, is called the **Ajeimutin** fungus by the Nigerian Yoruba people. The literal translation of this name is the 'eat-without-drinking-alcohol' mushroom.[7]

Mechanism

An early and attractive idea was that the reaction with *Coprinus atramentarius* was due to the presence of disulfiram (one group of workers actually claimed to have isolated it from the fungus[8]), but this was not confirmed by later work,[9,10] and it now appears that the active ingredient is coprine (*N*-5-(1-hydroxycyclopropyl)-glutamine).[11,12] This is metabolised in the body to 1-aminocyclopropanol, which appears, like disulfiram, to inhibit aldehyde dehydrogenase (see 'Alcohol + Disulfiram', p.50). The active ingredients in the other fungi are unknown.

Importance and management

An established and well documented interaction. It is said to occur up to 24 hours after eating the fungus. The intensity depends upon the quantity of fungus and alcohol consumed, and the time interval between them.[1,4] Despite the widespread consumption of edible fungi and alcohol, reports of this reaction in the medical literature are few and far between, suggesting that even though it can be very unpleasant and frightening, the outcome is usually uncomplicated. Treatment appears normally not to be necessary.

The related fungus ***Coprinus comatus*** (the '**shaggy ink cap**' or '**Lawyers wig**') is said not to interact with alcohol,[5,13] nor is there anything to suggest that it ever occurs with the **common field mushroom** (***Agaricus campestris***) or the cultivated variety (***Agaricus bisporis***).[13]

1. Caley MJ, Clarke RA. Cardiac arrhythmia after mushroom ingestion. *BMJ* (1977) 2, 1633.
2. Reynolds WA, Lowe FH. Mushrooms and a toxic reaction to alcohol: report of four cases. *N Engl J Med* (1965) 272, 630–1.
3. Wildervanck LS. Alcohol en de kale inktzwam. *Ned Tijdschr Geneeskd* (1978) 122, 913–14.
4. Buck RW. Mushroom toxins—a brief review of literature. *N Engl J Med* (1961) 265, 681–6.
5. Broadhurst-Zingrich L. Ink caps and alcohol. *BMJ* (1978) 1, 511.
6. Budmiger H, Kocher F. Hexenröhrling (Boletus luridus) mit Alkohol: ein kasuistischer beitrag. *Schweiz Med Wochenschr* (1982) 112, 1179–81.
7. Oso BA. Mushrooms and the Yoruba people of Nigeria. *Mycologia* (1975) 67, 311–19.
8. Simandl J, Franc J. Isolace tetraethylthiuramdisulfidu z hníku inko ustového (*Coprinus atramentarius*). *Chem Listy* (1956) 50, 1862–3.
9. Vanhaelen M, Vanhaelen-Fastré R, Hoyois J, Mardens Y. Reinvestigation of disulfiram-like activity of *Coprinus atramentarius* (Bull. *ex* Fr.) Fr. extracts. *J Pharm Sci* (1976) 65, 1774–6.
10. Wier JK, Tyler VE. An investigation of *Coprinus atramentarius* for the presence of disulfiram. *J Am Pharm Assoc* (1960) 49, 426–9.
11. Hatfield GM, Schaumberg JP. Isolation and structural studies of coprine, the disulfiram-like constituent of *Coprinus atramentarius*. *Lloydia* (1975) 38, 489–96.
12. Lindberg P, Bergman R, Wickberg B. Isolation and structure of coprine, the *in vivo* aldehyde dehydrogenase inhibitor in *Coprinus atramentarius*; syntheses of coprine and related cyclopropanone derivatives. *J Chem Soc* (1977) (6) 684–91.
13. Radford AP. Ink caps and mushrooms. *BMJ* (1978) 1, 112.

Alcohol + Erythromycin

Alcohol can cause a moderate reduction in the absorption of erythromycin ethylsuccinate. There is some evidence that intravenous erythromycin can raise blood alcohol levels but the extent and the practical importance of this is unknown.

Clinical evidence, mechanism, importance and management

(a) Effects on alcohol

A study in 10 healthy subjects found that erythromycin base 500 mg three times daily did not alter the pharmacokinetics of oral alcohol 0.8 g/kg and the subjects' perception of intoxication was unaltered.[1] In contrast, another study in 8 healthy subjects, primarily investigating the effects of intravenous erythromycin lactobionate 3 mg/kg on gastric emptying, found that when they were given a liquid meal of orange juice, alcohol 0.5 g/kg and lactulose 10 g immediately after a solid meal, the mean peak blood alcohol levels were raised by about 40% and the AUC over the first hour was increased by 33%. After that the curve was virtually the same as that seen with a saline placebo. The authors suggest that the increased blood alcohol levels are a result of erythromycin causing more rapid gastric emptying, so that the alcohol is exposed to metabolism by the gastric mucosa for a shorter time.[2]

What this means in terms of an increase in the effects of alcohol (e.g. on driving) is not known, but more study of this interaction is needed using oral erythromycin.

(b) Effects on erythromycin

When single 500-mg doses of erythromycin ethylsuccinate were taken by 9 healthy subjects with two 150-ml of alcoholic drinks (one immediately and the other 150 minutes later) the erythromycin AUC was decreased by about 27% and the absorption was delayed. One subject showed a 185% *increase* in absorption. The alcoholic drink was pisco sour, which contains lemon juice, sugar and pisco (a traditional brandy-like liqueur distilled from grapes grown in Chile or Peru). Blood alcohol levels achieved were about 50 mg%.[3]

The reason for the reduced absorption of erythromycin is not understood but it is suggested that the slight delay occurs because alcohol delays gastric emptying, so erythromycin reaches its absorption site in the duodenum a little later.[3] The extent to which this reduced absorption might affect the control of an infection is uncertain.

1. Min DI, Noormohamed SE, Flanigan MJ. Effect of erythromycin on ethanol's pharmacokinetics and perception of intoxication. *Pharmacotherapy* (1995) 15, 164–9.
2. Edelbroek MAL, Horowitz M, Wishart JM, Akkermans LMA. Effects of erythromycin on gastric emptying, alcohol absorption and small intestinal transit in normal subjects. *J Nucl Med* (1993) 34, 582–8.
3. Morasso MI, Chávez J, Gai MN, Arancibia A. Influence of alcohol consumption on erythromycin ethylsuccinate kinetics. *Int J Clin Pharmacol Ther Toxicol* (1990) 28, 426–9.

Alcohol + Ethionamide

A psychotoxic reaction has been seen in a patient on ethionamide attributed to the heavy consumption of alcohol.[1] It is unclear whether this represents a clinically meaningful interaction but it appears to be the only case on record.

1. Lansdown FS, Beran M, Litwak T. Psychotoxic reaction during ethionamide therapy. *Am Rev Respir Dis* (1967) 95, 1053–5.

Alcohol + Fentanyl-midazolam

The residual effects of fentanyl-midazolam appear not to interact adversely with alcoholic drinks taken several hours later.

Clinical evidence, mechanism, importance and management

A study in 12 healthy subjects concluded that the residual effects of fentanyl 2 micrograms/kg with **midazolam** 0.1 mg/kg given intravenously for surgery were unlikely to interact significantly in outpatients if they drank when they arrived home about 4 hours later. The subjects were given alcohol 0.7 g/kg to achieve blood levels of about 60 mg%.[1] The effects of **midazolam** alone have also been shown to have dissipated within 4 hours, and are not affected by alcohol after this time, see 'Alcohol + Benzodiazepines and related drugs', p.43.

1. Lichtor JL, Zacny J, Apfelbaum JL, Lane BS, Rupani G, Thisted RA, Dohrn C, Korttila K. Alcohol after sedation with i.v. midazolam–fentanyl: effects on psychomotor functioning. *Br J Anaesth* (1991) 67, 579–84.

Alcohol + Fluvastatin

Alcohol does not significantly interact with fluvastatin.

Clinical evidence, mechanism, importance and management

Ten healthy subjects took a single 40-mg dose of fluvastatin and 70 g of alcohol diluted in lemonade. This acute ingestion of alcohol had no effect on the peak serum levels of fluvastatin or its AUC, but the half-life was reduced by almost one-third. The lipid profile was hardly changed.[1] In a second related study, 20 patients with hypercholesterolaemia were given 40 mg of fluvastatin and 20 g of alcohol daily for 6 weeks. The AUC of fluvastatin was slightly increased and the half-life was increased by almost a third, but the lipid profile with fluvastatin plus alcohol was little different from fluvastatin alone.[1,2] The conclusion was reached that although long-term moderate drinking has some small effect on the pharmacokinetics of fluvastatin, its safety and efficacy are unaltered.[1] There would seem to be no reason for patients on fluvastatin to avoid alcohol.

1. Smit JWA, Wijnne HJA, Schobben F, Sitsen A, de Bruin TWA, Erkelens DW. Effects of alcohol consumption on pharmacokinetics, efficacy, and safety of fluvastatin. *Am J Cardiol* (1995) 76, 89A–96A.
2. Smit JW, Wijnne HJ, Schobben F, Sitsen A, De Bruin TW, Erkelens DW. Effects of alcohol and fluvastatin on lipid metabolism and hepatic function. *Ann Intern Med* (1995) 122, 678–80.

Alcohol + Food

Food reduces the absorption of alcohol and therefore its intoxicant effects. Foods rich in serotonin (e.g. bananas) taken with alcohol may produce adverse effects such as diarrhoea and headache.

Clinical evidence, mechanism, importance and management

(a) Alcohol absorption

In a study 24 healthy subjects were given alcohol 0.3 g/kg either 1 hour before or after an **evening meal**. It was found that the maximum alcohol levels were increased by 87% from 21.3 to 39.9 mg%, and the AUC was increased by 63% when given in the fasting rather than the fed state. However there was large inter and intra-individual variability in alcohol bioavailability.[1] Other studies have shown similar effects,[2,3] and shown that this is not limited to specific components of food,[3] as well as demonstrating that food also reduces the feeling of intoxication.[2] Milk has also been shown to have this effect, see 'Alcohol + Milk', p.58. The rate of gastric emptying is slower after food, and this allows greater first-pass metabolism of alcohol. Thus, the effects of alcohol are greatest when taken on an empty stomach.

(b) Alcohol + Dietary serotonin

Serotonin (**5-HT**) is excreted in the urine as 5-hydroxyindole-3-acetic acid (5-HIAA) and **5-hydroxytryptophol** (**5-HTOL**) and the ratio of **5-HTOL** to 5-HIAA is normally very low (less than 0.01). A study in 10 healthy subjects found that 4 hours after alcohol 0.5 g/kg the ratio was increased about 70-fold. When the same amount of alcohol was given with 3 **bananas**, a food rich in 5-HT, the ratio was increased about 100-fold at 4 hours and was still significantly raised at 24 hours. Within 4 hours, seven of the 10 subjects experienced adverse effects including diarrhoea, headache and fatigue. The symptoms were attributed to high levels of **5-HTOL**, which is usually a minor metabolite of **serotonin**. Other foods rich in **serotonin** such as **pineapple**, **kiwi fruit** or **walnuts** may produce similar effects if taken with even moderate amounts of alcohol.[4]

1. Fraser AG, Rosalki SB, Gamble GD, Pounder RE. Inter-individual and intra-individual variability of ethanol concentration-time profiles: comparison of ethanol ingestion before or after an evening meal. *Br J Clin Pharmacol* (1995) 40, 387–92.
2. Jones AW, Jönsson KÅ. Food-induced lowering of blood-ethanol profiles and increased rate of elimination immediately after a meal. *J Forensic Sci* (1994) 39, 1084–93.
3. Jones AW, Jönsson KÅ, Kechagias S. Effect of high-fat, high-protein, and high-carbohydrate meals on the pharmacokinetics of a small dose of ethanol. *Br J Clin Pharmacol* (1997) 44, 521–6.
4. Helander A, Some M. Dietary serotonin and alcohol combined may provoke adverse physiological symptoms due to 5-hydroxytryptophol. *Life Sci* (2000) 67, 799–806.

Alcohol + Furazolidone

A disulfiram-like reaction may occur in patients taking furazolidone if they drink alcohol.

Clinical evidence

A patient taking furazolidone 200 mg four times daily complained of facial flushing, lachrymation, conjunctivitis, weakness, and light-headedness within 10 minutes of drinking **beer**. It occurred on several occasions and lasted 30 to 45 minutes.[1]

A man prescribed furazolidone 100 mg four times daily and who had taken only three doses, developed intense facial flushing, wheezing and dyspnoea (lasting an hour), within one hour of drinking 2 oz (about 60 ml) of **brandy**. The same thing happened again the next day after drinking a **Martini cocktail**. No treatment was given.[2] A report originating from the makers of furazolidone stated that by 1976, 43 cases of a disulfiram-like reaction had been reported, of which 14 were produced experimentally using above-normal doses of furazolidone.[3] A later study in 1986 described 9 out of 47 patients (19%) who complained of a disulfiram-like reaction after drinking alcohol while taking furazolidone 100 mg four times daily for 5 days.[4] The report does not say whether all of them drank.[4]

Mechanism

Uncertain. It seems possible that furazolidone acts like disulfiram by inhibiting the activity of acetaldehyde dehydrogenase (see 'Alcohol + Disulfiram', p.50).

Importance and management

An established and clinically important interaction of uncertain incidence. One report suggests that possibly about 1 in 5 may be affected.[4] Reactions of this kind appear to be more unpleasant and possibly frightening than serious, and normally need no treatment, however patients should be warned about what may happen if they drink.

1. Calesnick B. Antihypertensive action of the antimicrobial agent furazolidone. *Am J Med Sci* (1958) 236, 736–46.
2. Kolodny AL. Side-effects produced by alcohol in a patient receiving furazolidone. *Md State Med J* (1962) 11, 248.
3. Chamberlain RE. (Eaton Laboratories, Norwich Pharmacal Co.) Chemotherapeutic properties of prominent nitrofurans. *J Antimicrob Chemother* (1976) 2, 325–36.
4. DuPont HL, Ericsson CD, Reves RR, Galindo E. Antimicrobial therapy for travelers' diarrhea. *Rev Infect Dis* (1986) 8, (Suppl 2), S217–S222.

Alcohol + Ginseng

Ginseng increases the clearance of alcohol from the body and lowers blood alcohol levels.

Clinical importance, mechanism, importance and management

Fourteen healthy subjects, each acting as their own control, were given oral alcohol (72 g/65 kg as a 25% solution) with and without a ginseng extract (3 g/65 kg) mixed in with it. They drank the alcohol or the alcohol/ginseng mixture over a 45-minute period in 7 portions, the first four at 5-minute intervals and the next three at 10-minute intervals. Measurements taken 40 minutes later showed that the presence of the ginseng lowered blood alcohol levels by an average of 38.9%. The levels of 10 subjects were lowered by 32 to 51% by the ginseng, 3 showed reductions of 14 to 18% and one showed no changes at all.[1]

The reasons for this interaction are uncertain, but it is suggested that ginseng possibly increases the activity of the enzymes (alcohol and aldehyde dehydrogenase),[2] which are concerned with the metabolism of the alcohol, thereby increasing the clearance of the alcohol from the body. What this means in practical terms is not clear but the authors of the report suggest the possibility of using ginseng to treat alcoholic patients and those with acute alcohol intoxication.[1]

1. Lee FC, Ko JH, Park KJ, Lee JS. Effect of *Panax ginseng* on blood alcohol clearance in man. *Clin Exp Pharmacol Physiol* (1987) 14, 543–6.
2. Choi CW, Lee SI, Huh K. Effect of ginseng on the hepatic alcohol metabolizing enzyme system activity in chronic alcohol-treated mice. *Korean J Pharmacol* (1984) 20, 13–21.

Alcohol + Glutethimide

The combination of glutethimide and alcohol resulted in greater impairment in some psychomotor tests, but improvement in others. Alcohol does not interact with glutethimide taken the previous night.

Clinical evidence, mechanism, importance and management

In a series of studies, blood alcohol levels were raised a mean of 11% by glutethimide, while plasma and urinary glutethimide levels were reduced.[1] Neither glutethimide nor alcohol significantly impaired reaction times, but the combination did. However, in two other tests (tracking efficacy and finger tapping) impairment was greatest after glutethimide alone and reduced by the presence of alcohol.[1] In contrast, a later study found that glutethimide did not subjectively or objectively impair the performance of a number of psychomotor skill tests related to driving, and did not interact with alcohol given the morning after the glutethimide dose.[2] Both drugs are CNS depressants and their effects would be expected to be additive.

The information is limited and somewhat contradictory, nevertheless patients should be warned about the probable results of taking glutethimide and alcohol together. Driving, handling dangerous machinery or undertaking any task needing alertness and full co-ordination is likely to be made more difficult and hazardous. There is no evidence of a hangover effect, which could result in an interaction with alcohol the next day.[2]

1. Mould GP, Curry SH, Binns TB. Interactions of glutethimide and phenobarbitone with ethanol in man. *J Pharm Pharmacol* (1972) 24, 894–9.
2. Saario I, Linnoila M. Effect of subacute treatment with hypnotics, alone or in combination with alcohol, on psychomotor skills related to driving. *Acta Pharmacol Toxicol (Copenh)* (1976) 38, 382–92.

Alcohol + Glyceryl trinitrate (Nitroglycerin)

Patients who take glyceryl trinitrate while drinking may feel faint and dizzy.

Clinical evidence, mechanism, importance and management

The results of studies[1,2] on the combined haemodynamic effects of alcohol and glyceryl trinitrate give support to earlier claims that concurrent use increases the risk of exaggerated hypotension and fainting.[3,4] Their vasodilatory effects[5] would appear to be additive. The greatest effect was seen when the glyceryl trinitrate was taken 1 hour or more after starting to drink.[1] It is suggested that this increased susceptibility to postural hypotension should not be allowed to stop patients from using glyceryl trinitrate if they want to drink, but they should be warned and told what to do if they feel faint and dizzy (i.e. sit or lie down).[1]

1. Kupari M, Heikkilä J, Ylikahri R. Does alcohol intensify the hemodynamic effects of nitroglycerin? *Clin Cardiol* (1984) 7, 382–6.
2. Abrams J, Schroeder K, Raizada V, Gibbs D. Potentially adverse effects of sublingual nitroglycerin during consumption of alcohol. *J Am Coll Cardiol* (1990) 15, 226A.
3. Shafer N. Hypotension due to nitroglycerin combined with alcohol. *N Engl J Med* (1965) 273, 1169.
4. Opie. LH. Drugs and the heart. II. Nitrates. *Lancet* (1980) i, 750–3.
5. Allison RD, Kraner JC, Roth GM. Effects of alcohol and nitroglycerin on vascular responses in man. *Angiology* (1971) 22, 211–22.

Alcohol + Griseofulvin

An isolated case report describes a very severe disulfiram-like reaction after a man on griseofulvin drank a can of beer. Other isolated reports note flushing and tachycardia. A few others have shown increased alcohol effects.

Clinical evidence

(a) Disulfiram-like reaction

A man took griseofulvin 500 mg daily for about 2 weeks without problems. Subsequently he drank a can of **beer**, took his usual dose of griseofulvin about an hour later, and within 30 to 60 minutes developed a severe disulfiram-like reaction (flushing, severe nausea, vomiting, diarrhoea, hypotension and paraesthesias of all extremities). He was successfully treated with intravenous sodium chloride 0.9%, potassium and dopamine, and intramuscular promethazine.[1]

Other isolated cases of flushing and tachycardia attributed to concurrent use have also been described.[2]

(b) Increased alcohol effects

The descriptions of this response are very brief. One of them describes[3] a man who had "... decreased tolerance to alcohol and emotional instability manifested by crying and nervousness so severe that the drug was stopped." Another[4] states that "... a possible potentiation of the effects of alcohol has been noted in a very small number of patients."

Mechanism

Not understood. The reaction (a) described above possibly has the same pharmacological basis as the disulfiram/alcohol reaction (see 'Alcohol + Disulfiram', p.50).

Importance and management

The documentation is extremely sparse, which would seem to suggest that adverse interactions between alcohol and griseofulvin are uncommon. Concurrent use need not be avoided but it may be prudent to warn patients. The disulfiram-like reaction described was unusually severe.

1. Fett DL, Vukov LF. An unusual case of severe griseofulvin-alcohol interaction. *Ann Emerg Med* (1994) 24, 95–7.
2. Robinson MM. Griseofulvin therapy of superficial mycoses. *Antibiot Annu* (1959–60) 7, 680–6.
3. Drowns BV, Fuhrman DL, Dennie CC. Use, abuse and limitations of griseofulvin. *Mo Med* (1960) 57, 1473–6.
4. Simon HJ, Randz LA. Untoward reactions to antimicrobial agents. *Annu Rev Med* (1961) 12, 119–20.

Alcohol + H_2-blockers

Although some studies have found that blood alcohol levels can be raised to some extent in those taking some H_2-blockers and possibly remain elevated for longer than usual, others report that no significant interaction occurs. Drinking may worsen the gastrointestinal disease for which these H_2-blockers are being given. Hypoglycaemia associated with alcohol may be enhanced by H_2-blockers.

Clinical evidence

(a) Evidence of an interaction

A double-blind study in 6 healthy subjects showed that after taking **cimetidine** 300 mg four times daily for 7 days, the peak plasma alcohol levels following the ingestion of 0.8 g/kg alcohol were raised by about 12% (from 146 to 163 mg%). The AUC was increased by about 7%. The subjects assessed themselves as being more intoxicated while taking **cimetidine** and alcohol than with alcohol alone.[1]

An essentially similar study[2,3] found that the blood alcohol levels were raised by 17% (from 73 to 86 mg%) by **cimetidine** but not by **ranitidine**. A later study in 6 healthy subjects found that **cimetidine** 400 mg twice daily for a week approximately doubled the AUC following a single 0.15-g/kg oral dose of alcohol and raised peak levels by about 33%. No changes were seen when the alcohol was given intravenously.[4] Another study in healthy subjects given **cimetidine** or **ranitidine** for only two days showed that peak plasma alcohol levels were raised by 17 and 28% respectively, and the time that blood levels remained above the 80 mg% mark (the legal driving limit in the UK and some other countries) was prolonged by about one-third.[5] **Nizatidine** was said to inhibit the metabolism of alcohol in man, but little detail was given in the report.[6] A further study in subjects given 0.75 g/kg alcohol found that single doses of **cimetidine** 800 mg, **nizatidine** 300 mg, or **ranitidine** 300 mg raised blood alcohol levels at 45 minutes by 26% (from 75.5 to 95.2 mg%), 17.5% (from 75.5 to 88.7 mg%) and 3.3% (75.5 to 78 mg%) respectively, and the AUCs at 120 minutes were increased by 25%, 20% and 9.8% respectively. Each of the subjects said they felt more inebriated after taking **cimetidine** or **nizatidine**.[7] Another study found that **cimetidine** almost doubled peak alcohol blood levels, whereas **ranitidine** raised the levels by about 50%.[8] In subjects with substantial first-pass metabolism of alcohol, **cimetidine** increased the blood levels of repeated small drinks of alcohol to a greater degree than that which occurred after an equivalent single dose. The levels reached were associated with psychomotor impairment.[9]

In contrast, in one study, a combination of chlorphenamine (an H_1-blocker) and **cimetidine** reduced the rate of absorption and peak blood alcohol levels, and suppressed alcohol-induced flushing.[10]

(b) Evidence of no interaction

The makers of cimetidine have on file three unpublished studies that did not find any evidence to suggest that **cimetidine** or **ranitidine** significantly increased the blood levels of alcohol. One study was in 6 healthy subjects given single 400-mg doses of **cimetidine**, another in 6 healthy subjects given **cimetidine** 1 g daily for 14 days, and the last in 10 healthy subjects given either **cimetidine** 400 mg twice daily or **ranitidine** 150 mg twice daily.[11] A number of other studies also failed to demonstrate significant interactions involving either **cimetidine, ranitidine**, **famotidine**, or **nizatidine**, and a number of different alcoholic drinks (low to high dose), either on an empty stomach or after eating.[12-25] Two other studies showing an interaction between other H_2-blockers and alcohol found that **famotidine** had no significant effect on blood alcohol levels.[7,8]

(c) Hypoglycaemia

A study in 10 healthy subjects given alcohol 0.5 g/kg before and after 7 days administration of **cimetidine** 400 mg twice daily, **ranitidine** 150 mg twice daily, or **famotidine** 40 mg once daily found that hypoglycaemia following alcohol ingestion was enhance by all three H_2-blockers. The effect was especially marked with **famotidine**.[26]

Mechanism

(a) and (b) It would appear that the interacting H_2-blockers inhibit the activity of alcohol dehydrogenase (ADH) in the gastric mucosa so that more alcohol passes unmetabolised into the circulation, thereby raising the levels.[27-31] It has been suggested that most of the studies assessing the interaction of H_2-blockers with larger quantities of alcohol fail to show an interaction. The decrease in first pass metabolism with increasing amounts of alcohol could explain this, as it implies that a significant interaction with H_2-blockers would be more likely with smaller quantities of alcohol.[9,32] Other factors that affect the first pass metabolism of alcohol, such as fasting, chronic alcoholism and female gender may also affect the outcome. The increase in blood alcohol levels with cimetidine or ranitidine and low alcohol dose may also be explained by the effect of H_2-blockers or alcohol on gastric emptying times.[23,32] In one study the decrease in first-pass metabolism correlated with a ranitidine-induced increase in the rate of gastric emptying and an increase in blood alcohol levels.[33] However, with small quantities of alcohol the magnitude of the effect on peak levels may be too small to increase effects on psychomotor performance,[32,34] although one study suggested that an effect may occur.[9]

(c) The hypoglycaemic effect is not considered to be due to effects on alcohol absorption but may be an effect of H_2-blockers on glucose metabolism.[26]

Importance and management

The contrasting and apparently contradictory results cited here clearly show that this interaction is by no means established. Extensive reviews of the data concluded that the interaction is, in general, clinically insignificant.[31,32,35,36] Under conditions mimicking social drinking there is some evidence that H_2-blockers may[26] or may not[25] increase blood alcohol levels to those associated with impairment of psychomotor skills. However, as yet, there are insufficient grounds to justify any general warning regarding alcohol and H_2-blockers. But note that many of the conditions for which H_2-blockers are used may be made worse by alcohol, so restriction of drinking may be needed.

1. Feely J, Wood AJJ. Effects of cimetidine on the elimination and actions of alcohol. *JAMA* (1982) 247, 2819–21.
2. Seitz HK, Bösche J, Czygan P, Veith S, Simon B, Kommerell B. Increased blood ethanol levels following cimetidine but not ranitidine. *Lancet* (1983) i, 760.
3. Seitz HK, Veith S, Czygan P, Bösche J, Simon B, Gugler R, Kommerell B. *In vivo* interactions between H_2-receptor antagonists and ethanol metabolism in man and in rats. *Hepatology* (1984) 4, 1231–4.
4. Caballeria J, Baraona E, Rodamilans M, Lieber CS. Effects of cimetidine on gastric alcohol dehydrogenase activity and blood ethanol levels. *Gastroenterology* (1989) 96, 388–92.
5. Webster LK, Jones DB, Smallwood RA. Influence of cimetidine and ranitidine on ethanol pharmacokinetics. *Aust N Z J Med* (1985) 15, 359–60.
6. Palmer RH. Cimetidine and alcohol absorption. *Gastroenterology* (1989) 97, 1066–8.
7. Guram M, Howden CW, Holt S. Further evidence for an interaction between alcohol and certain H_2-receptor antagonists. *Alcohol Clin Exp Res* (1991) 15, 1084–5.
8. DiPadova C, Roine R, Frezza M, Gentry T, Baraona E, Lieber CS. Effects of ranitidine on blood alcohol levels after ethanol ingestion: comparison with other H_2-receptor antagonists. *JAMA* (1992) 267, 83–6.
9. Gupta AM, Baraona E, Lieber CS. Significant increase of blood alcohol by cimetidine after repetitive drinking of small alcohol doses. *Alcohol Clin Exp Res* (1995) 19, 1083–7.
10. Tan OT, Stafford TJ, Sarkany I, Gaylarde PM, Tilsey C, Payne JP. Suppression of alcohol-induced flushing by a combination of H_1 and H_2 histamine antagonists. *Br J Dermatol* (1982) 107, 647–52.
11. Smith Kline and French. Personal communication, February 1989.
12. Dobrilla G, de Pretis G, Piazzi L, Chilovi F, Comberlato M, Valentini M, Pastorino A, Vallaperta P. Is ethanol metabolism affected by oral administration of cimetidine and ranitidine at therapeutic doses? *Hepatogastroenterology* (1984) 31, 35–7.
13. Johnson KI, Fenzl E, Hein B. Einfluß von Cimetidin auf den abbau und die wirkung des Alkohols. *Arzneimittelforschung* (1984) 34, 734–6.
14. Tanaka E, Nakamura K. Effects of H_2-receptor antagonists on ethanol metabolism in Japanese volunteers. *Br J Clin Pharmacol* (1988) 26, 96–9.
15. Holtmann G, Singer MV. Histamine H_2 receptor antagonists and blood alcohol levels. *Dig Dis Sci* (1988) 33, 767–8.
16. Holtmann G, Singer MV, Knop D, Becker S, Goebell H. Effect of histamine-H_2-receptor antagonists on blood alcohol levels. *Gastroenterology* (1988) 94, A190. (abs).
17. Fraser AG, Prewett EJ, Hudson M, Sawyerr AM, Rosalki SB, Pounder RE. The effect of ranitidine, cimetidine or famotidine on low-dose post-prandial alcohol absorption. *Aliment Pharmacol Ther* (1991) 5, 263–72.
18. Jönsson K-Å, Jones AW, Boström H, Andersson T. Lack of effect of omeprazole, cimetidine, and ranitidine on the pharmacokinetics of ethanol in fasting male volunteers. *Eur J Clin Pharmacol* (1992) 42, 209–12.
19. Fraser AG, Hudson M, Sawyerr AM, Smith M, Rosalki SB, Pounder RE. Ranitidine, cimetidine, famotidine have no effect on post-prandial absorption of ethanol 0.8 g/kg taken after an evening meal. *Aliment Pharmacol Ther* (1992) 6, 693–700.
20. Fraser AG, Prewett EJ, Hudson M, Sawyerr AM, Rosalki SB, Pounder RE. Ranitidine has no effect on post-prandial absorption of alcohol (0.6 g/kg) after an evening meal. *Eur J Gastroenterol Hepatol* (1992) 4, 43–7.
21. Kendall MJ, Spannuth F, Walt RP, Gibson GJ, Hale KA, Braithwaite R, Langman MJS. Lack of effect of H2-receptor antagonists on the pharmacokinetics of alcohol consumed after food at lunchtime. *Br J Clin Pharmacol* (1994) 37, 371–4.
22. Pipkin GA, Mills JG, Wood JR. Does ranitidine affect blood alcohol concentrations? *Pharmacotherapy* (1994) 14, 273–81.
23. Bye A, Lacey LF, Gupta S, Powell JR. Effect of ranitidine hydrochloride (150 mg twice daily) on the pharmacokinetics of increasing doses of ethanol (0.15, 0.3, 0.6 g kg^{-1}). *Br J Clin Pharmacol* (1996) 41, 129–33.
24. Hindmarch I, Gilburt S. The lack of CNS effects of nizatidine, with and without alcohol, on psychomotor ability and cognitive function. *Hum Psychopharmacol* (1990) 5, 25–32.
25. Brown ASJM, James OFW. Omeprazole, ranitidine and cimetidine have no effect on peak blood ethanol concentrations, first pass metabolism or area under the time–ethanol curve under 'real-life' drinking conditions. *Aliment Pharmacol Ther* (1998) 12, 141–5.
26. Czyżyk A, Lao B, Szutowski M, Szczepanik Z, Muszyñski J. Enhancement of alcohol-induced hypoglycaemia by H_2-receptor antagonists. *Arzneimittelforschung* (1997) 47, 746–9.
27. Caballería J. Interactions between alcohol and gastric metabolizing enzymes: practical implications. *Clin Ther* (1991) 13, 511–20.
28. Fiatarone JR, Bennett MK, Kelly P, James OFW. Ranitidine but not gastritis or female sex reduces the first pass metabolism of ethanol. *Gut* (1991) 32, A594.
29. Caballería J, Baraona E, Deulofeu R, Hernández-Muñoz R, Rodés J, Lieber CS. Effects of H_2-receptor antagonists on gastric alcohol dehydrogenase activity. *Dig Dis Sci* (1991) 36, 1673–9.
30. Brown ASJM, Fiatarone JR, Day CP, Bennett MK, Kelly PJ, James OFW. Ranitidine increases the bioavailability of postprandial ethanol by the reduction of first pass metabolism. *Gut* (1995) 37, 413–17.
31. Gulger R. H_2-antagonists and alchol: Do they interact? *Drug Safety* (1994) 10, 271–80.
32. Fraser AG. Is there an interaction between H_2-antagonists and alcohol? *Drug Metabol Drug Interact* (1998) 14, 123–145.

33. Amir I, Anwar N, Baraona E, Lieber CS. Ranitidine increases the bioavailability of imbibed alcohol by accelerating gastric emptying. *Life Sci* (1996) 58, 511–18.
34. Baraona E, Gentry RT, Lieber CS. Bioavailability of alcohol: role of gastric metabolism and its interaction with other drugs. *Dig Dis* (1994) 12, 351–57.
35. Levitt MD. Review article: lack of clinical significance of the interaction between H_2-receptor antagonists and ethanol. *Aliment Pharmacol Ther* (1993) 7, 131–8.
36. Monroe ML, Doering PL. Effect of common over-the-counter medications on blood alcohol levels. *Ann Pharmacother* (2001) 35, 918–24.

Alcohol + HRT

Acute ingestion of alcohol markedly increases the levels of circulating estradiol in women using oral HRT. A smaller increase is seen with transdermal HRT. Estradiol does not affect blood alcohol levels.

Clinical evidence mechanism, importance and management

Twelve healthy postmenopausal women on HRT (**estradiol** 1 mg daily and **medroxyprogesterone acetate** 10 mg daily for 10 out of each 25 days) were given an alcoholic drink (0.7 g/kg bodyweight, a dose shown to achieve mean peak alcohol serum levels of 21 mmol/L after about 1 hour) during the oestrogen-only phase of the HRT cycle. It was found that their peak **estradiol** levels rose threefold and were significantly above the baseline for 5 hours. No significant increases in the levels of circulating estrone (an oestrogen secreted by the ovaries) were seen, and blood alcohol levels were not changed.[1] A similar smaller 1.2-fold increase in peak **estradiol** levels was seen in another study when women on **transdermal estradiol** were given alcohol.[2]

The reasons for these changes are not understood, and their clinical significance is unknown. However, alcohol can increase *endogenous* **estradiol** levels in postmenopausal women. Since both alcohol and HRT are linked with a small increase in breast cancer risk, it has been postulated that the combination of HRT and alcohol could be additive. Indeed, some have even suggested that women taking HRT should limit their alcohol intake.[3] More study is needed to confirm any interaction and its importance. Note that alcohol does not affect ethinylestradiol levels, see 'Alcohol + Oral contraceptives', p.60.

1. Ginsburg ES, Mello NK, Mendelson JH, Barbieri RL, Teoh SK, Rothman M, Gao X, Sholar JW. Effects of alcohol ingestion on estrogens in postmenopausal women. *JAMA* (1996) 276, 1747–51.
2. Ginsburg ES, Walsh BW, Gao X, Gleason RE, Feltmate C, Barbieri RL. The effect of acute ethanol ingestion on estrogen levels in postmenopausal women using transdermal estradiol. *J Soc Gynecol Investig* (1995) 2, 26–9.
3. Gorins A. Responsabilité croisée des estrogènes et de l'alcool dans le cancer du sein. *Presse Med* (2000) 29, 670–2.

Alcohol + Hydromorphone

A single case report describes a fatality due to the combined CNS depressant effects of hydromorphone and alcohol.

Clinical evidence, mechanism, importance and management

A young man died from the combined cardiovascular and respiratory depressant effects of hydromorphone and alcohol.[1] He fell asleep, the serious nature of which was not recognised by those around him. Post-mortem analysis revealed alcohol and hydromorphone concentrations of 90 mg% and 100 nanograms/ml, neither of which is particularly excessive. This case emphasises the importance of warning patients about the potentially hazardous consequences of drinking while taking potent CNS depressants of this kind.

1. Levine B, Saady J, Fierro M, Valentour J. A hydromorphone and ethanol fatality. *J Forensic Sci* (1984) 29, 655–9.

Alcohol + Indoramin

The serum levels of both indoramin and alcohol may be raised by concurrent use. The increased drowsiness may possibly increase the risks when driving.

Clinical evidence

When 10 healthy subjects were given a single 50-mg oral dose of indoramin together with alcohol 0.5 g/kg in 600 ml of alcohol-free lager, the AUC of indoramin was increased by 25% and the peak levels raised by 58%.[1,2] When the subjects were given a single 175-microgram/kg intravenous dose of indoramin together with the same oral dose of alcohol, a 26% rise in blood alcohol levels occurred during the first 1.25 hours after dosing, but no change in indoramin pharmacokinetics were seen. The combination of alcohol and indoramin caused more sedation than either drug alone.[2]

Mechanism

Uncertain. Increased absorption of the indoramin from the gut or reduced liver metabolism may be responsible for the raised indoramin serum levels. The increase in sedation would appear to be due to the additive sedative effects of the two drugs.

Importance and management

Information is limited but the interaction appears to be established. The clinical importance of the raised serum indoramin and alcohol levels is uncertain, however since indoramin sometimes causes drowsiness when it is first given, there is the possibility that alertness will be reduced, which could increase the risks of driving or handling other machinery. Patients should be warned. More study is needed. For mention of the effect of moderate to heavy drinking on the efficacy of antihypertensives in general, see 'Alcohol + Antihypertensives', p.40.

1. Abrams SML, Pierce DM, Franklin RA, Johnston A, Marrott PK, Cory EP, Turner P. Effect of ethanol on indoramin pharmacokinetics. *Br J Clin Pharmacol* (1984) 18, 294P–295P.
2. Abrams SML, Pierce DM, Johnston A, Hedges A, Franklin RA, Turner P. Pharmacokinetic interaction between indoramin and ethanol. *Hum Toxicol* (1989) 8, 237–41.

Alcohol + Isoniazid

Isoniazid increases the hazards of driving after drinking alcohol. Isoniazid-induced hepatitis may also possibly be increased by alcohol, and the effects of isoniazid are possibly reduced.

Clinical evidence, mechanism, importance and management

The effects of isoniazid 750 mg with 0.5 g/kg alcohol were examined in 100 volunteers given various psychomotor tests, and in a further 50 drivers using a driving simulator. No major interaction was seen in the psychomotor tests, but the number of drivers who 'drove off the road' on the simulator was increased.[1,2] There would therefore appear to be some extra risks for patients on isoniazid who drink and drive, but the effect does not appear to be large. Patients should nevertheless be warned. The incidence of severe progressive liver damage due to isoniazid is said to be higher in those who drink regularly,[3,4] and the clinical effects of isoniazid are also said to be reduced by heavy drinking in some patients.[3]

1. Linnoila M, Mattila MJ. Effects of isoniazid on psychomotor skills related to driving. *J Clin Pharmacol* (1973) 13, 343–50.
2. Linnoila M, Mattila MJ. Interaction of alcohol and drugs on psychomotor skills as demonstrated by a driving simulator. *Br J Pharmacol* (1973) 47, 671P–672P.
3. Anonymous. Interactions of drugs with alcohol. *Med Lett Drugs Ther* (1981) 23, 33–4.
4. Kopanoff DE, Snider DE, Caras GJ. Isoniazid-related hepatitis. *Am Rev Respir Dis* (1978) 117, 991–1001.

Alcohol + Ivermectin

Alcohol may increase the bioavailability of ivermectin.

Clinical evidence, mechanism, importance and management

Anecdotal reports from Nigeria suggest that ivermectin is more potent when taken with **palm wine**, a local alcoholic drink, and a few cases of ataxia and postural hypotension occurring with ivermectin were considered to be due to an interaction with alcohol.[1] Ivermectin formulated as an alcoholic solution has been found to have about twice the systemic availability of tablets and capsules.[2] In another study, 20 healthy subjects were given ivermectin 150 micrograms/kg with either 750 ml of **beer** (4.5% alcohol) or 750 ml of water. Plasma levels of ivermectin at 1 to 4 hours were increased by about 51% to 66% when it was given with **beer** rather than water. No side effects were reported in either group.[1] More study is needed.

1. Shu EN, Onwujekwe EO, Okonkwo PO. Do alcoholic beverages enhance availability of ivermectin? *Eur J Clin Pharmacol* (2000) 56, 437–8.
2. Edwards G, Dingsdale A, Helsby N, Orme MLE, Breckenridge AM. The relative systemic bioavailability of ivermectin after administration as capsule, tablet, and oral solution. *Eur J Clin Pharmacol* (1988) 35, 681–4.

Alcohol + Kava

There is some evidence that kava may worsen the CNS depressant effects of alcohol.

Clinical evidence, mechanism, importance and management

Forty healthy subjects underwent a number of cognitive tests and visuomotor tests after taking alcohol alone, kava (Kava-Kava; the pepper plant *Piper methysticum*) alone, or both together. The subjects took 0.75 g/kg alcohol (enough to give blood alcohol levels above 50 mg%) and the kava dose was 1 g/kg. The kava drink was made by mixing middle grade Fijian kava with water and straining it to produce about 350 ml of kava liquid. It was found that kava alone had no effect on the tests, but when given with alcohol it potentiated both the perceived and measured impairment that occurred with alcohol alone.[1]

No very strong conclusions can be drawn from the results of this study, but they do suggest that car driving and handling other machinery may possibly be more hazardous if kava and alcohol are taken together. The outcome of taking different doses of alcohol and kava seems not to have been studied.

1. Foo H, Lemon J. Acute effects of kava, alone or in combination with alcohol, on subjective measures of impairment and intoxication and on cognitive performance. *Drug Alcohol Rev* (1997) 16, 147–55.

Alcohol + Ketoconazole

A few cases of disulfiram-like reactions have been seen in patients who drank alcohol while taking ketoconazole.

Clinical evidence, mechanism, importance and management

One patient, out of group of 12, taking ketoconazole 200 mg daily experienced a disulfiram-like reaction (nausea, vomiting, facial flushing) after drinking.[1] No further details are given, and the report does not say whether any of the others drank alcohol. A woman on ketoconazole 200 mg daily developed a disulfiram-like reaction when she drank.[2] Another report describes a transient 'sunburn-like' rash or flush on the face, upper chest and back of a patient taking ketoconazole 200 mg daily when she drank modest quantities of **wine** or **beer**.[3] The reasons for the reactions are not known but it seems possible that ketoconazole may act like disulfiram and inhibit the activity of acetaldehyde dehydrogenase (see 'Alcohol + Disulfiram', p.50). The incidence of this reaction appears to be very low (these appear to be the only reports) and its importance is probably small. Reactions of this kind are usually more unpleasant than serious.

1. Fazio RA, Wickremesinghe PC, Arsura EL. Ketoconazole treatment of *Candida esophagitis*—a prospective study of 12 cases. *Am J Gastroenterol* (1983) 78, 261–4.
2. Meyboom RHB, Pater BW. Overgevoeligheid voor alcoholische dranken tijdens behandeling met ketoconazol. *Ned Tijdschr Geneeskd* (1989) 133, 1463–4.
3. Magnasco AJ, Magnasco LD. Interaction of ketoconazole and ethanol. *Clin Pharm* (1986) 5, 522–3.

Alcohol + Lithium

Some limited evidence suggests that lithium carbonate combined with alcohol may make car driving more hazardous.

Clinical evidence, mechanism, importance and management

Alcohol 0.5 g/kg raised the serum levels of lithium in 9 out of 10 healthy subjects by 16% after they took a single 600-mg dose of lithium carbonate. Four subjects had at least a 25% increase in lithium levels. However these rises were not considered to be clinically important.[1] In contrast a study in 20 healthy subjects given lithium carbonate (to achieve lithium serum levels of 0.75 mmol/l) and alcohol 0.5 g/kg, and who were subjected to various psychomotor tests (choice reaction, coordination, attention) to assess any impairment of skills related to driving, indicated that lithium carbonate both alone and with alcohol may increase the risk of accident. In this study, lithium did not affect blood alcohol levels.[2] Information is very limited but patients should be warned.

1. Anton RF, Paladino JA, Morton A, Thomas RW. Effect of acute alcohol consumption on lithium kinetics. *Clin Pharmacol Ther* (1985) 38, 52–5.
2. Linnoila M, Saario I, Maki M. Effect of treatment with diazepam or lithium and alcohol on psychomotor skills related to driving. *Eur J Clin Pharmacol* (1974) 7, 337–42.

Alcohol + Liv. 52

Liv. 52, an Ayurvedic herbal remedy, appears to reduce the hangover symptoms after drinking, reducing both urine and blood alcohol and acetaldehyde levels at 12 hours. However it also raises the blood alcohol levels of moderate drinkers for the first few hours after drinking.

Clinical evidence

Nine healthy subjects who normally drank socially (alcohol 40 to 100 g weekly) took six tablets of *Liv. 52* two hours before drinking alcohol (four 60 ml doses of **whiskey**, equivalent to 90 g of alcohol). Their blood alcohol levels at 1 hour were increased by 15% (from 75 to 86.2 mg%). After taking three tablets of *Liv. 52* daily for two weeks, their 1-hour blood alcohol levels were raised by 27% (from 75 to 95.3 mg%).[1] The blood alcohol levels of 9 other moderate drinkers were raised over the first 2 hours by about 28 to 44% after taking three tablets of *Liv. 52* twice daily for two weeks, and by 19% and 17% respectively over the following 2 hours.[2] Only a minor increase in the blood alcohol levels of 8 occasional drinkers occurred.[2] Acetaldehyde levels in the blood and urine were markedly lowered at 12 hours, and hangover seemed to be reduced.[1]

Mechanism

Not understood. *Liv. 52* contains the active principles from *Capparis spinosa*, *Cichorium intybus*, *Solanum nigrum*, *Cassia occidentalis*, *Terminalia arjuna*, *Achillea millefolium*, *Tamarix gallica* and *Phyllanthus amarus*.[1] These appear to increase the absorption of alcohol, or reduce its metabolism by the liver, thereby raising the blood-alcohol levels. It is suggested that the reduced hangover effects may possibly occur because it prevents the binding of acetaldehyde to cell proteins allowing a more rapid elimination.[1]

Importance and management

Direct experimental evidence seems to be limited to these two studies.[1,2] *Liv. 52* appears to reduce the hangover effects after drinking, but at the same time it can significantly increase the blood alcohol levels of moderate drinkers, for the first few hours after drinking. Increases of up to 30% may be enough to raise the blood alcohol from legal to illegal levels when driving. Moderate drinkers should be warned. Occasional drinkers appear to develop higher blood alcohol levels than moderate drinkers but *Liv. 52* seems not to increase them significantly.[1]

1. Chauhan BL, Kulkarni RD. Alcohol hangover and Liv.52. *Eur J Clin Pharmacol* (1991) 40, 187–8.
2. Chauhan BL, Kulkarni RD. Effect of Liv.52, a herbal preparation, on absorption and metabolism of ethanol in humans. *Eur J Clin Pharmacol* (1991) 40, 189–91.

Alcohol + Mefloquine

Mefloquine does not normally appear to interact with alcohol. An isolated report describes two incidents of severe psychosis and depression in a man on mefloquine who drank large quantities of alcohol.

Clinical evidence, mechanism, importance and management

Mefloquine 250 mg or placebo was given to two groups of 20 healthy subjects on days 1, 2, 3, 8, 15, 22 and 29. They were tested on days 4, 23 and 30 after taking enough alcohol to achieve blood levels of about 35 mg%. Mefloquine did not affect blood alcohol levels, nor did it increase the effects of alcohol on two real-highway driving tests or on psychomotor tests done in the laboratory. In fact, the mefloquine group actually drove better than the placebo group.[1]

A 40-year old man with no previous psychiatric history taking mefloquine 250 mg weekly for malarial prophylaxis had no problems with the first 2 doses. However, on two separate occasions when taking the third and fourth doses he concurrently drank about half a litre of whisky, whereupon he developed severe paranoid delusions, hallucinations and became suicidal. When he stopped drinking he had no further problems while taking subsequent doses of mefloquine. He was used to drinking large amounts of alcohol and had experienced no problems while previously taking proguanil/chloroquine.[2]

The broad picture is that mefloquine appears not to worsen the effects of moderate amounts of alcohol and it seems unlikely that it will have a marked effect with larger doses, but this needs confirmation. Just why an unusual toxic reaction developed in one individual is not known.

1. Vuurman EFPM, Muntjewerff ND, Uiterwijk MMC, van Veggel LMA, Crevoisier C, Haglund L, Kinzig M, O'Hanlon JF. Effects of mefloquine alone and with alcohol on psychomotor and driving performance. *Eur J Clin Pharmacol* (1996) 50, 475–82.
2. Wittes RC, Saginur R. Adverse reaction to mefloquine associated with ethanol ingestion. *Can Med Assoc J* (1995) 152, 515–17.

Alcohol + Meprobamate

The intoxicant effects of alcohol can be considerably increased by the presence of normal daily doses of meprobamate. Driving or handling other potentially dangerous machinery is made much more hazardous.

Clinical evidence

A study in 22 subjects, given meprobamate 400 mg four times daily for a week, showed that with blood alcohol levels of 50 mg% their performance of a number of coordination and judgement tests was much more impaired than with either drug alone.[1] Four of the subjects were quite obviously drunk while taking both and showed marked incoordination and social disinhibition. Two could not walk without assistance. The authors say this effect was much greater than anything seen with alcohol alone.

Other studies confirm this interaction, although the effects appeared to be less pronounced.[2-6]

Mechanism

Both meprobamate and alcohol are CNS depressants, which appear to have additive effects. There is also some evidence that alcohol may inhibit or increase meprobamate metabolism, depending on whether it is taken acutely or chronically, but the contribution of this to the enhanced CNS depression is uncertain.[7,8] Meprobamate does not appear to increase blood alcohol levels.[5]

Importance and management

A well-documented and potentially serious interaction. Normal daily dosages of meprobamate in association with relatively moderate blood-alcohol concentrations, well within the UK legal limit for driving, can result in obviously hazardous intoxication. Patients should be warned.

1. Zirkle GA, McAtee OB, King PD, Van Dyke R. Meprobamate and small amounts of alcohol: effects on human ability, coordination, and judgement. *JAMA* (1960) 173, 1823–5.
2. Reisby N, Theilgaard A. The interaction of alcohol and meprobamate in man. *Acta Psychiatr Scand* (1969) 208 (Suppl), 5–204.
3. Forney RB, Hughes FW. Meprobamate, ethanol or meprobamate-ethanol combinations on performance of human subjects under delayed audiofeedback (DAF). *J Psychol* (1964) 57, 431–6.
4. Ashford JR, Cobby JM. Drug interactions. The effects of alcohol and meprobamate applied singly and jointly in human subjects. III. The concentrations of alcohol and meprobamate in the blood and their effects on performance; application of mathematical models. *J Stud Alcohol* (1975) (Suppl 7), 140–61.
5. Cobby JM, Ashford JR. Drug interactions. The effects of alcohol and meprobamate applied singly and jointly in human subjects. IV. The concentrations of alcohol and meprobamate in the blood. *J Stud Alcohol* (1975) (Suppl 7), 162–76.
6. Ashford JR, Carpenter JA. Drug interactions. The effects of alcohol and meprobamate applied singly and jointly in human subjects. V. Summary and conclusions. *J Stud Alcohol* (1975) (Suppl 7), 177–87.
7. Misra PS, Lefèvre A, Ishi H, Rubin E, Lieber CS. Increase of ethanol, meprobamate and pentobarbital metabolism after chronic ethanol administration in man and in rats. *Am J Med* (1971) 51, 346–51.
8. Rubin E, Gang H, Misra PS, Lieber CS. Inhibition of drug metabolism by acute ethanol intoxication: a hepatic microsomal mechanism. *Am J Med* (1970) 49, 801–6.

Alcohol + Methaqualone ± Diphenhydramine

The CNS depressant effects of alcohol and its detrimental effects on the skills relating to driving or handling other potentially dangerous machinery are increased by the concurrent use of methaqualone with or without diphenhydramine.

Clinical evidence

(a) Methaqualone

A retrospective study of drivers arrested for driving under the influence of drugs and/or drink showed that, generally speaking, those with blood methaqualone levels of 1 mg/l or less showed no symptoms of sedation, whereas those with levels above 2 mg/l demonstrated staggering gait, drowsiness, incoherence and slurred speech. These effects were increased if the drivers had also been drinking alcohol. The authors state that the levels of methaqualone needed for driving skills to become impaired are considerably lowered by alcohol, but no precise measure of this is presented in the paper.[1]

(b) Methaqualone with diphenhydramine

A double-blind study in 12 healthy subjects given two *Mandrax* tablets (methaqualone 250 mg with diphenhydramine 25 mg) showed that the resulting sedation and reduction in cognitive skills were enhanced by alcohol 0.5 g/kg. Residual amounts of a single-dose of *Mandrax* continued to interact for as long as 72 hours. Methaqualone blood levels are also raised by regular moderate amounts of alcohol.[2] Enhanced effects were also seen in another study.[3]

Mechanism

Alcohol, methaqualone and diphenhydramine are all CNS depressants, the effects of which are additive. The diphenhydramine/alcohol interaction is discussed under 'Alcohol + Antihistamines', p.39. A hangover can occur because the elimination half-life of methaqualone is long (10 to 40 hours).

Importance and management

An established interaction of importance. Those taking either methaqualone or methaqualone/diphenhydramine should be warned that handling machinery, driving a car, or any other task requiring alertness and full coordination, will be made more difficult and hazardous if they drink. Levels of alcohol below the legal driving limit with normal amounts of methaqualone may cause considerable sedation. Patients should also be told that a significant interaction may possibly occur the following day, because methaqualone taken on the previous day is likely to still persist in the body.

1. McCurdy HH, Solomons ET, Holbrook JM. Incidence of methaqualone in driving-under-the-influence (DUI) cases in the State of Georgia. *J Anal Toxicol* (1981) 5, 270–4.
2. Roden S, Harvey P, Mitchard M. The effect of ethanol on residual plasma methaqualone concentrations and behaviour in volunteers who have taken Mandrax. *Br J Clin Pharmacol* (1977) 4, 245–7.
3. Saario I, Linnoila M. Effect of subacute treatment with hypnotics, alone or in combination with alcohol, on psychomotor skills related to driving. *Acta Pharmacol Toxicol (Copenh)* (1976) 38, 382–92.

Alcohol + Methotrexate

There is some inconclusive evidence that the consumption of alcohol may increase the risk of methotrexate-induced hepatic cirrhosis and fibrosis.

Clinical evidence, mechanism, importance and management

It has been claimed that alcohol can increase the hepatotoxic effects of methotrexate.[1] Two reports indicate that this may be so; in one, 3 out of 5 patients with methotrexate-induced cirrhosis were reported to have taken alcohol concurrently (2 patients greater than 85 g, one patient 25 to 85 g ethanol per week),[2] and in the other, the subject was known to drink excessively.[3] However, the evidence is by no means conclusive and no direct causal relationship has been established. The makers of methotrexate advise the avoidance of drugs, including alcohol, which have hepatotoxic potential.[4]

1. Almeyda J, Barnardo D, Baker H. Drug reactions XV. Methotrexate, psoriasis and the liver. *Br J Dermatol* (1971) 85, 302–5.

2. Tobias H, Auerbach R. Hepatotoxicity of long-term methotrexate therapy for psoriasis. *Arch Intern Med* (1973) 132, 391–400.
3. Pai SH, Werthamer S, Zak FG. Severe liver damage caused by treatment of psoriasis with methotrexate. *N Y State J Med* (1973) 73, 2585–7.
4. Methotrexate. Wyeth Laboratories. UK Summary of product characteristics, May 2000.

Alcohol + Metoclopramide

There is some evidence that metoclopramide can increase the rate of absorption of alcohol, raise maximum blood alcohol levels, and possibly increase alcohol-related sedation.

Clinical evidence, mechanism, importance and management

A study in 7 subjects found that 20 mg of intravenous metoclopramide increased the rate of alcohol absorption, and the peak blood levels were raised from 55 to 86 mg%. Similar results were seen in 2 healthy subjects given metoclopramide orally.[1] Another study in 7 healthy subjects found that 10 mg of intravenous metoclopramide accelerated the rate of absorption of alcohol 70 mg/kg given orally, and increased its peak levels but not to a statistically significant extent. Blood alcohol levels remained below 12 mg%. More importantly the sedative effects of the alcohol were increased.[2] The reasons are not fully understood, but it appears to be related to an increase in gastric emptying. These two studies were done to find out more about intestinal absorption mechanisms rather than to identify daily practicalities, so the importance of the findings is uncertain, but it seems possible that the effects of alcohol will be increased. Metoclopramide alone can cause drowsiness, and if affected, patients should not drive or operate machinery.

1. Gibbons DO, Lant AF. Effects of intravenous and oral propantheline and metoclopramide on ethanol absorption. *Clin Pharmacol Ther* (1975) 17, 578–84.
2. Bateman DN, Kahn C, Mashiter K, Davies DS. Pharmacokinetic and concentration-effect studies with intravenous metoclopramide. *Br J Clin Pharmacol* (1978) 6, 401–7.

Alcohol + Metronidazole

A disulfiram-like reaction has occurred in a few patients on oral metronidazole who drank alcohol. There is one report of its occurrence when metronidazole was applied as a vaginal insert, and another when metronidazole was given intravenously. Some clinical trials have not confirmed the interaction, and its existence is disputed in some reports. The interaction is alleged to occur with all other 5-nitroimidazoles (e.g. tinidazole).

Clinical evidence

A man who had been in a drunken stupor for three days was given two metronidazole tablets (a total of 500 mg) one hour apart by his wife in the belief that they might sober him up. Twenty minutes after the first tablet he was awake and complaining that he had been given disulfiram (which he had taken some months before). Immediately after the second tablet he took another drink and developed a classic disulfiram-like reaction with flushing of the face and neck, nausea and epigastric discomfort.[1] Other individual cases have been reported.[2]

All 10 alcoholic patients in a test of the value of metronidazole 250 mg twice daily as a possible drink-deterrent experienced some disulfiram-like reactions of varying intensity (facial flushing, headaches, sensation of heat, fall in blood pressure, vomiting).[3] The majority of 60 other patients, given 250 to 750 mg metronidazole daily, developed mild to moderate disulfiram-like reactions.[4] The incidence in other reports is said to be lower: 24%,[5] 10%[6] and 2%.[7] Other preparations are also implicated. The reaction has been seen in a patient treated with intravenous metronidazole and a trimethoprim-sulfamethoxazole (co-trimoxazole) preparation containing 10% alcohol as a diluent,[8] and has also been reported in association with metabolic acidosis in an intoxicated man 4 hours after being given intravenous metronidazole as prophylaxis following injury.[9] Another report describes a reaction with a metronidazole vaginal insert.[10] A fatality occurred in a frail 31-year old woman attributed to cardiac arrhythmia caused by acetaldehyde toxicity resulting from the alcohol/metronidazole interaction, linked to autonomic distress caused by a physical assault.[11] Alcohol is also said to taste unpleasant[1,3] or to be less pleasurable[7] while taking metronidazole. Some drug abusers apparently exploit the reaction for 'kicks'.[12] In contrast, there are other reports, including two well-controlled studies, showing that metronidazole has no disulfiram-like effects.[13-15]

Mechanism

Not fully understood. Metronidazole, like disulfiram, can inhibit the activity of acetaldehyde dehydrogenase, xanthine oxidase and aldehyde dehydrogenase.[16] The accumulation of acetaldehyde may be responsible for most of the symptoms (see 'Alcohol + Disulfiram', p.50). However, recent studies indicate a lack of a disulfiram-like reaction,[13,14] and it has been suggested that if such a reaction does occur it may be by a mechanism other than the inhibition of hepatic acetaldehyde dehydrogenase.[15]

Importance and management

A reasonably well studied interaction, but it remains a controversial issue. The incidence is variously reported as between 0 and 100%, with more recent reports disputing its existence.[15,17] Nevertheless because of the uncertainty, all patients given metronidazole by mouth should be warned about what may happen if they drink. The reaction, when it occurs, normally seems to be more unpleasant and possibly frightening than serious, and usually requires no treatment, although one report describes a serious reaction when intravenous metronidazole was given to an intoxicated man,[9] and one possible fatality has been reported.[11] The risk of a reaction with metronidazole used intravaginally seems to be small because the absorption is low (about 20% compared with about 100% orally), but evidently it can happen, even if only rarely.[10] Patients should be warned. It has been alleged that the disulfiram-like reaction with alcohol occurs with all of the related 5-nitroimidazoles,[18,19] but there do not appear to be any published reports of it occurring with **nimorazole**, **ornidazole**, **secnidazole** or **tinidazole**. The maker of **tinidazole** notes that abdominal cramps, flushing and vomiting have occurred when **tinidazole** has been taken together with alcohol, and recommends that the combination should be avoided.[20]

1. Taylor JAT. Metronidazole—a new agent for combined somatic and psychic therapy for alcoholism: a case study and preliminary report. *Bull Los Angel Neuro Soc* (1964) 29, 158–62.
2. Alexander I. 'Alcohol—Antabuse' syndrome in patients receiving metronidazole during gynaecological treatment. *Br J Clin Pract* (1985) 39, 292–3.
3. Ban TA, Lehmann HE, Roy P. Rapport préliminaire sur l'effect thérapeutique du Flagyl dans l'alcoolisme. *Union Med Can* (1966) 95, 147–9.
4. Sansoy OM. Evaluation of metronidazole in the treatment of alcoholism. A comprehensive three-year study comprising 60 cases. *Rocky Mtn Med J* (1970) 67, 43–7.
5. de Mattos H. Ralações entre o alcoolismo e aparelho digestivo. Experiência com metronidazol. *Hospital (Rio J)* (1968) 74, 1669–76.
6. Channabasavanna SM, Kaliaperumal VG, Mathew G, Itty A. Metronidazole in the treatment of alcoholism: a controlled trial. *Indian J Psychiatry* (1979) 21, 90–3.
7. Penick SB, Carrier RN, Sheldon JB. Metronidazole in the treatment of alcoholism. *Am J Psychiatry* (1969) 125, 1063–6.
8. Edwards DL, Fink PC, Van Dyke PO. Disulfiram-like reaction associated with intravenous trimethoprim–sulfamethoxazole and metronidazole. *Clin Pharm* (1986) 5, 999–1000.
9. Harries DP, Teale KFH, Sunderland G. Metronidazole and alcohol: potential problems. *Scott Med J* (1990) 35, 179–180.
10. Plosker GL. Possible interaction between ethanol and vaginally administered metronidazole. *Clin Pharm* (1987) 6, 189 and 192–3.
11. Cina SJ, Russell RA, Conradi SE. Sudden death due to metronidazole/ethanol interaction. *Am J Forensic Med Pathol* (1996) 17, 343–6.
12. Giannini AJ, DeFrance DT. Metronidazole and alcohol—potential for combinative abuse. *J Toxicol Clin Toxicol* (1983) 20, 509–15.
13. Goodwin DW. Metronidazole in the treatment of alcoholism: a negative report. *Am J Psychiatry* (1967) 123, 1276–8.
14. Gelder MG, Edwards G. Metronidazole in the treatment of alcohol addiction: a controlled trial. *Br J Psychiatry* (1968) 114, 473–5.
15. Visapää J-P, Tillonen JS, Kaihovaara PS, Salaspuro MP. Lack of disulfiram-like reaction with metronidazole and ethanol. *Ann Pharmacother* (2002) 36, 971–4.
16. Fried R, Fried LW. The effect of Flagyl on xanthine oxidase and alcohol dehydrogenase. *Biochem Pharmacol* (1966) 15, 1890–4.
17. Williams CS, Woodcock KR. Do ethanol and metronidazole interact to produce a disulfiram-like reaction? *Ann Pharmacother* (2000) 34, 255–7.
18. Koren G, Prober CG, Gold R, eds. Nitroimidazoles: in Antimicrobial therapy in infants and children. New York: Marcel Dekker; 1988 P. 729–745.
19. Andersson KE. Pharmacokinetics of nitromidazoles. Spectrum of adverse reactions. *Scand J Infect Dis* (1981) 26 (Suppl), 60–7.
20. Fasigyn (Tinidazole). Pfizer Ltd. UK Summary of product characteristics, November 1998.

Alcohol + Milk

Blood levels of alcohol and its intoxicant effects are reduced if milk has been drunk.

Clinical evidence, mechanism, importance and management

Ten subjects were given 25 ml of alcohol (equivalent to a double **whiskey**) after drinking a pint and a half of water or milk during the previous 90 minutes. Blood alcohol levels at 90 minutes were reduced by about

40% and at 120 minutes by about 25%, by the presence of the milk. The intoxicant effects of the alcohol were also clearly reduced.[1] The reasons are not understood, but a possible explanation is that the presence of milk in the stomach delays gastric emptying so increasing the first-pass metabolism of alcohol, see also, 'Alcohol + Food', p.52. These findings appear to confirm a long and widely held belief among drinkers, but whether this interaction can be regarded as advantageous or undesirable is a moot point.

1. Miller DS, Stirling JL, Yudkin J. Effect of ingestion of milk on concentrations of blood alcohol. *Nature* (1966) 212, 1051.

Alcohol + Niclosamide

Alcohol may possibly increase the adverse effects of niclosamide.

Clinical evidence, mechanism, importance and management

The makers of niclosamide advise avoiding alcohol while taking niclosamide. The reasoning behind this is that while niclosamide is virtually insoluble in water, it is slightly soluble in alcohol, which might possibly increase its absorption by the gut, resulting an increase in its adverse effects. There are no formal reports of this but the maker says that they have some anecdotal information that is consistent with this suggestion.[1]

1. Bayer. Personal communication, July 1992.

Alcohol + Nicotinic acid (Niacin)

An isolated report describes delirium and metabolic acidosis in a patient taking nicotinic acid for hypercholesterolaemia after ingesting about one litre of wine. Delirium had occurred on a previous similar occasion after he drank beer while on nicotinic acid. It is suggested that the nicotinic acid may have caused liver dysfunction, which was exacerbated by the large amount of alcohol. The patient did have some elevations in liver enzymes.[1] No general conclusions can be drawn from this single case.

1. Schwab RA, Bachhuber BH. Delirium and lactic acidosis caused by ethanol and niacin coingestion. *Am J Emerg Med* (1991) 9, 363–5.

Alcohol + Nitrofurantoin

There appears to be no good clinical evidence for an alleged interaction between alcohol and nitrofurantoin.

Clinical evidence, mechanism, importance and management

Despite claims in some books and reviews, an extensive literature survey failed to find any experimental or clinical evidence for an alleged disulfiram-like reaction between alcohol and nitrofurantoin.[1] A study in healthy subjects failed to demonstrate any such interaction[2] and a survey of the reports in the maker's database also failed to find good evidence for alcohol intolerance.[3] It is concluded that this 'interaction' is erroneous.[1]

1. Rowles B, Worthen DB. Clinical drug information: a case of misinformation. *N Engl J Med* (1982) 306, 113–4.
2. Miura K, Reckendorf HK. The nitrofurans. *Prog Med Chem* (1967) 5, 320–81.
3. D'Arcy PF. Nitrofurantoin. *Drug Intell Clin Pharm* (1985) 19, 540–7.

Alcohol + NSAIDs

NSAIDs may increase the risk of gastrointestinal haemorrhage associated with alcohol. The skills related to driving are impaired by indometacin and phenylbutazone. Additive sedation occurs if patients drink while taking phenylbutazone, but this does not appear to occur with indometacin. A few isolated reports attribute acute renal failure to concurrent NSAIDs and acute excessive alcohol consumption. Dipyrone appears not to interact with alcohol.

Clinical evidence, mechanism, importance and management

(a) Gastrointestinal complications

In healthy subjects the concurrent use of alcohol with **ibuprofen** 2400 mg over 24 hours increased the damaging effect of ibuprofen on the stomach wall, although this did not reach statistical significance.[1] A case-control study involving 1224 patients admitted to hospital with upper gastrointestinal bleeding and 2945 controls found that alcohol consumption was associated with a threefold increase in the incidence of acute upper gastrointestinal haemorrhage from light to heavy drinking. There was some evidence to suggest that the risk of upper gastrointestinal bleeding was increased by concurrent **ibuprofen**.[2] Another case-control study found that the use of prescription NSAIDs or over-the-counter **naproxen** or **ibuprofen** in those with a history of alcohol abuse produced a risk ratio of adverse gastrointestinal effects that was greater than the expected additive risk. Both NSAID use and excessive alcohol consumption carry the risk of gastrointestinal adverse effects. This information suggests that NSAIDs should be used with caution in heavy drinkers.[3] See also 'Alcohol + Aspirin or Salicylates', p.42.

(b) Psychomotor skills and alcohol levels

A study on a large number of healthy subjects showed that the performance of various psychomotor skills related to driving (choice reaction, coordination, divided attention tests) were impaired by single doses of **indometacin** 50 mg or **phenylbutazone** 200 mg. Alcohol 0.5 g/kg made things worse in those taking **phenylbutazone**, but the performance of those taking **indometacin** was improved to some extent.[4] The reasons are not understood. The study showed that the subjects were subjectively unaware of the adverse effects of **phenylbutazone**. Information is very limited, but patients should be warned if they intend to drive. In two studies, **ibuprofen** 800 mg had no significant effect on blood alcohol levels of healthy subjects.[5,6]

The pharmacokinetics of alcohol 1 g/kg and the results of performance tests were found to be similar in subjects given **dipyrone** 1 g or a placebo.[7] No special precautions seem to be necessary.

(c) Renal complications

After taking **ibuprofen** 400 mg the evening before, 400 mg the following morning, and then 375 ml of **rum** later in the day, followed by two further 400-mg tablets of **ibuprofen**, a normal healthy young woman with no history of renal disease developed acute renal failure.[8] Another similar case was reported in a 22-year-old woman who had taken **ibuprofen** 1200 mg the morning after binge drinking.[9] Both recovered.[8,9] A further case has been reported in a young woman after concurrent **ketoprofen** 600 mg and binge drinking.[10] It is suggested that volume depletion caused by the alcohol (and compounded by vomiting) predisposed these patients to NSAID-induced renal toxicity.[9,10] The general importance of these isolated cases remains to be determined.

1. Lanza FL, Royer GL, Nelson RS, Rack MF, Seckman CC. Ethanol, aspirin, ibuprofen, and the gastroduodenal mucosa: an endoscopic assessment. *Am J Gastroenterol* (1985) 80, 767–9.
2. Kaufman DW, Kelly JP, Wiholm B-E, Laszlo A, Sheehan JE, Koff RS, Shapiro S. The risk of acute major upper gastrointestinal bleeding among users of aspirin and ibuprofen at various levels of alcohol consumption. *Am J Gastroenterol* (1999) 94, 3189–96.
3. Neutel CI, Appel WC. The effect of alcohol abuse on the risk of NSAID-related gastrointestinal events. *Ann Epidemiol* (2000) 10, 246–50.
4. Linnoila M, Seppälä T, Mattila MJ. Acute effect of antipyretic analgesics, alone or in combination with alcohol, on human psychomotor skills related to driving. *Br J Clin Pharmacol* (1974) 1, 477–84.
5. Barron SE, Perry JR, Ferslew KE. The effect of ibuprofen on ethanol concentration and elimination rate. *J Forensic Sci* (1992) 37, 432–5.
6. Melander O, Lidén A, Melander A. Pharmacokinetic interactions of alcohol and acetylsalicylic acid. *Eur J Clin Pharmacol* (1995) 48, 151–3.
7. Badian LM, Rosenkrantz B. Quoted as personal communication by Levy M, Zylber-Katz E, Rosenkranz B. Clinical pharmacokinetics of dipyrone and its metabolites. *Clin Pharmacokinet* (1995) 28, 216–34.
8. Elsasser GN, Lopez L, Evans E, Barone EJ. Reversible acute renal failure associated with ibuprofen ingestion and binge drinking. *J Fam Pract* (1988) 27, 221–2.
9. Johnson GR, Wen S-F. Syndrome of flank pain and acute renal failure after binge drinking and nonsteroidal anti-inflammatory drug ingestion. *J Am Soc Nephrol* (1995) 5, 1647–52.
10. Galzin M, Brunet P, Burtey S, Dussol B, Berland Y. Nécrose tubulaire après prise d'anti-inflammatoire non stéroïdien et intoxication éthylique aiguë. *Nephrologie* (1997) 18, 113–15.

Alcohol + Olanzapine

Postural hypotension and possibly drowsiness may be increased when alcohol is given with olanzapine.

Clinical evidence, mechanism, importance and management

The makers say that patients on olanzapine have shown an increased heart rate and accentuated postural hypotension when given a single-dose of alcohol (amount not stated).[1] No pharmacokinetic interaction has been seen.[1,2] In practical terms this means that patients should be warned of the risk of faintness and dizziness if they stand up quickly. The makers also say that olanzapine can cause drowsiness, and they warn about driving or operating dangerous machinery.[3] and it would be expected that alcohol might worsen this effect. The patient information leaflet produced by the makers[4] says that patients should not drink alcohol with olanzapine because of the potential drowsiness that would result.

1. Zyprexa (Olanzapine). Eli Lilly. Clinical and Laboratory Experience A Comprehensive Monograph, August 1996.
2. Zyprexa (Olanzapine). Eli Lilly and Company. US Prescribing information, September 2004.
3. Zyprexa (Olanzapine). Eli Lilly and Company Ltd. UK Summary of product characteristics, February 2005.
4. Zyprexa (Olanzapine). Lilly. Patient information sheet, November 2004.

Alcohol + Oral contraceptives

The detrimental effects of alcohol may be reduced to some extent in women on oral contraceptives, but blood alcohol levels are possibly unaltered. Alcohol does not affect the pharmacokinetics of ethinylestradiol.

Clinical evidence mechanism, importance and management

(a) Effect of oral contraceptives on alcohol

A controlled study in 54 women showed that those taking a combined oral contraceptive (30, 35 or 50 micrograms **oestrogen**) unexpectedly tolerated the effects of alcohol better than those not taking oral contraceptives (as measured by a reaction-time test and a bead-threading test), but their blood-alcohol levels and its rate of clearance were unchanged.[1] The authors say that they do not recommend women on oral contraceptives to drink more than usual, since even if alcohol is tolerated better, blood levels are not reduced.[1] In contrast, two other studies suggest that peak blood alcohol levels and alcohol clearance may be reduced in those taking oral contraceptives.[2,3]

(b) Effect of alcohol on oral contraceptives

Alcohol ingestion did not have any significant effect on **ethinylestradiol** pharmacokinetics in 9 healthy women taking a combined oral contraceptive (ethinylestradiol/gestodene 30/75 micrograms). In this study, alcohol was given as a single dose of 0.4 g/kg (2 to 3 standard drinks) on day 14 then 0.4 g/kg twice daily for 7 days. The findings of this study contrast with those of the effect of alcohol on estradiol in postmenopausal women (see 'Alcohol + HRT', p.55). This may be because the ethinyl group in **ethinylestradiol** confers protection from the effects of alcohol.[4]

1. Hobbes J, Boutagy J, Shenfield GM. Interactions between ethanol and oral contraceptive steroids. *Clin Pharmacol Ther* (1985) 38, 371–80.
2. Jones MK, Jones BM. Ethanol metabolism in women taking oral contraceptives. *Alcohol Clin Exp Res* (1984) 8, 24–8.
3. Zeiner AR, Kegg PS. Menstrual cycle and oral contraceptive effects on alcohol pharmacokinetics in caucasian females. *Curr Alcohol* (1981) 8, 47–56.
4. Sarkola T, Ahola L, von der Pahlen B, Eriksson CJP. Lack of effect of alcohol on ethinylestradiol in premenopausal women. *Contraception* (2001) 63, 19–23.

Alcohol + Orlistat

A study in healthy subjects found that orlistat for 6 days had no significant effect on the pharmacokinetics of alcohol.[1] There is nothing to suggest that alcohol should be avoided while taking orlistat.

1. Melia AT, Zhi J, Zelasko R, Hartmann D, Güzelhan C, Guerciolini R, Odink J. The interaction of the lipase inhibitor orlistat with ethanol in healthy volunteers. *Eur J Clin Pharmacol* (1998) 54, 773–7.

Alcohol + Paracetamol (Acetaminophen)

Many case reports describe severe liver damage, fatal in some instances, in some alcoholics and persistent heavy drinkers who take only moderate doses of paracetamol. However, controlled studies have found no association between alcoholism and paracetamol-induced hepatotoxicity. There is controversy about the use of paracetamol in alcoholics. Some consider standard therapeutic doses can be used, whereas others recommend the dose of paracetamol should be reduced, or paracetamol avoided. Occasional and moderate drinkers do not seem to be at any extra risk.

Clinical evidence

(a) Increased hepatotoxicity

Three chronic alcoholic patients developed severe liver damage after taking paracetamol. They had AST levels of about 7000 to 10 000 units. Two of them had taken 10 g of paracetamol over 24 or 48 hours before admission (normal dosage is up to 4 g daily), and the third patient had taken about 50 g of paracetamol over 72 hours. One of them died in hepatic coma and post mortem revealed typical paracetamol toxicity. Two of them also developed renal failure.[1]

There are other numerous other case reports of liver toxicity in alcoholics attributed to the concurrent use of alcohol and paracetamol. In the reports cited here, which include a total of about 30 patients, about one-third had been taking daily doses of up to 4 g daily, and one-third had taken doses within the range 4 to 8 g daily.[2-18] Fasting possibly makes things worse.[19] A later survey reviewed a total of 94 cases from the literature, and described a further 67 patients, 64% of whom were alcoholics, who developed liver toxicity after taking paracetamol. In 60% of cases the paracetamol dose did not exceed 6 g daily and in 40% of cases the dose did not exceed 4 g daily. More than 90% of the patients developed AST levels ranging from 3000 to 48 000 units.[20]

(b) No effect on hepatotoxicity

In a retrospective review of 553 cases of paracetamol-induced severe hepatotoxicity treated at a liver failure unit over a 7-year period, there was no association between the level of alcohol consumption and the severity of the hepatotoxicity (mean INR and serum creatinine levels in the first 7 days after overdose). Alcohol consumption was categorised into 4 groups ranging from non-drinkers to heavy drinkers (greater than 60 g of alcohol daily in men and 40 g daily in women).[21]

In a randomised, placebo-controlled study, there was no difference in measures of hepatotoxicity (mean AST levels, mean INR) between 102 alcoholic patients who received paracetamol 1g four times daily for 2 days, and 99 who received placebo. In this study, patients had entered an alcohol detoxification centre, and were given paracetamol immediately after stopping alcohol use (the assumed time of greatest susceptibility, see Mechanism, below).[22] A systematic review by the same research group concluded that the use of therapeutic doses of paracetamol in alcoholic patients is not associated with hepatic injury.[23]

(c) Effect on alcohol levels

Paracetamol 1 g was found to have no effect on the single-dose pharmacokinetics of alcohol in 12 healthy subjects.[24] Another study found that blood alcohol levels were raised by 1 g of paracetamol but this was not statistically significant.[25]

Mechanism

Uncertain. Paracetamol is normally predominantly metabolised by the liver to non-toxic sulfate and glucuronide conjugates. Persistent heavy drinking stimulates a normally minor biochemical pathway involving the cytochrome P450 isoenzyme CYP2E1, which allows the production of unusually large amounts of highly hepatotoxic metabolites. Unless sufficient glutathione is present to detoxify these metabolites (alcoholics often have an inadequate intake of protein), they become covalently bound to liver macromolecules and damage results. In fact alcoholics may possibly be most susceptible to toxicity during alcohol withdrawal because, while drinking, alcohol may possibly compete with the paracetamol for metabolism and even inhibit it. Acute ingestion of alcohol by non-alcoholics appears to protect them against damage because the damaging biochemical pathway is inhibited rather than stimulated. However, induction of CYP2E1 in humans appears to be only modest and short-lived, and most studies have failed to show an increase in hepatotoxic metabolites in alcoholics.[26]

Importance and management

The incidence of unexpected paracetamol toxicity in chronic alcoholics is uncertain, but possibly fairly small, bearing in mind the very wide-spread use of paracetamol and alcohol. Note that all the evidence for an interaction comes from anecdotal case reports and case series, albeit in large numbers. However, the damage, when it occurs, can be serious and therefore some have advised that alcoholics and those who persistently drink heavily should avoid paracetamol or limit their intake considerably.[20] The normal daily recommended 'safe' maximum of 4 g is said to be too high in some alcoholics.[20] Because of this, the US Food and Drug Administration have required that all paracetamol-containing products bear the warning that those consuming 3 or more alcoholic drinks every day should ask their doctor whether they should take paracetamol.[27] However, others consider that the evidence does not prove that there is an increase in paracetamol hepatotoxicity in alcoholics,[23,26] and is insufficient to support any change in paracetamol use or dose in alcoholics.[23,28] They note that the alternatives, aspirin and NSAIDs, are associated with a greater risk of gastrointestinal adverse effects in alcoholics,[23] see 'Alcohol + NSAIDs', p.59'. Further study is needed. The risk for non-alcoholics, moderate drinkers and those who very occasionally drink a lot appears to be low.

It is still prudent to consider patients who are alcoholics as being at high risk of hepatotoxicity after a paracetamol overdose, and to treat them with acetylcysteine at lower plasma-paracetamol concentrations.[26] Possible malnutrition in these patients would further support the need for such treatment.

1. McClain CJ, Kromhout JP, Peterson FJ, Holtzman JL. Potentiation of acetaminophen hepatotoxicity by alcohol. *JAMA* (1980) 244, 251–3.
2. Emby DJ, Fraser BN. Hepatotoxicity of paracetamol enhanced by ingestion of alcohol. *S Afr Med J* (1977) 51, 208–9.
3. Goldfinger R, Ahmed KS, Pitchumoni CS, Weseley SA. Concomitant alcohol and drug abuse enhancing acetaminophen toxicity. *Am J Gastroenterol* (1978) 70, 385–8.
4. Barker JD, de Carle DJ, Anuras S. Chronic excessive acetaminophen use and liver damage. *Ann Intern Med* (1977) 87, 299–301.
5. O'Dell JR, Zetterman RK, Burnett DA. Centrilobular hepatic fibrosis following acetaminophen-induced hepatic necrosis in an alcoholic. *JAMA* (1986) 255, 2636–7.
6. McJunkin B, Barwick KW, Little WC, Winfield JB. Fatal massive hepatic necrosis following acetaminophen overdosage. *JAMA* (1976) 236, 1874–5.
7. LaBrecque DR, Mitros FA. Increased hepatotoxicity of acetaminophen in the alcoholic. *Gastroenterology* (1980) 78, 1310.
8. Johnson MW, Friedman PA, Mitch WE. Alcoholism, nonprescription drugs and hepatotoxicity. The risk from unknown acetaminophen ingestion. *Am J Gastroenterol* (1981) 76, 530–3.
9. Licht H, Seeff LB, Zimmerman HJ. Apparent potentiation of acetaminophen hepatotoxicity by alcohol. *Ann Intern Med* (1980) 92, 511.
10. Black M, Cornell JF, Rabin L, Shachter N. Late presentation of acetaminophen hepatotoxicity. *Dig Dis Sci* (1982) 27, 370–4.
11. Fleckenstein JL. *Nyquil* and acute hepatic necrosis. *N Engl J Med* (1985) 313, 48.
12. Gerber MA, Kaufmann H, Klion F, Alpert LI. Acetaminophen associated hepatic injury: report of two cases showing unusual portal tract reactions. *Hum Pathol* (1980) 11, 37–42.
13. Leist MH, Gluskin LE, Payne JA. Enhanced toxicity of acetaminophen in alcoholics: report of three cases. *J Clin Gastroenterol* (1985) 7, 55–9.
14. Himmelstein DU, Woolhandler SJ, Adler RD. Elevated SGOT/SGPT ratio in alcoholic patients with acetaminophen hepatotoxicity. *Am J Gastroenterol* (1984) 79, 718–20.
15. Levinson M. Ulcer, back pain and jaundice in an alcoholic. *Hosp Pract* (1983) 18, 48N, 48S.
16. Seeff LB, Cuccherini BA, Zimmerman HJ, Adler E, Benjamin SB. Acetaminophen hepatotoxicity in alcoholics. A therapeutic misadventure. *Ann Intern Med* (1986) 104, 399–404.
17. Florén C-H, Thesleff P, Nilsson Å. Severe liver damage caused by therapeutic doses of acetaminophen. *Acta Med Scand* (1987) 222, 285–8.
18. Edwards R, Oliphant J. Paracetamol toxicity in chronic alcohol abusers – a plea for greater consumer awareness. *N Z Med J* (1992) 105, 174–5.
19. Whitcomb DC, Block GD. Association of acetaminophen hepatotoxicity with fasting and ethanol use. *JAMA* (1994) 272, 1845–50.
20. Zimmerman HJ, Maddrey WC. Acetaminophen (paracetamol) hepatotoxicity with regular intake of alcohol: analysis of instances of therapeutic misadventure. *Hepatology* (1995) 22, 767–73.
21. Makin A, Williams R. Paracetamol hepatotoxicity and alcohol consumption in deliberate and accidental overdose. *Q J Med* (2000) 93, 341–9.
22. Kuffner EK, Dart RC, Bogdan GM, Hill RE, Casper E, Darton L. Effect of maximal daily doses of acetaminophen on the lever of alcoholic patients: a randomized, double-blind, placebo-controlled trial. *Arch Intern Med* (2001) 161, 2247–52.
23. Dart RC, Kuffner EK, Rumack BH. Treatment of pain or fever with paracetamol (acetaminophen) in the alcoholic patient: a systematic review. *Am J Ther* (2000) 7, 123–4.
24. Melander O, Lidén A, Melander A. Pharmacokinetic interactions of alcohol and acetylsalicylic acid. *Eur J Clin Pharmacol* (1995) 48, 151–3.
25. Sharma SC, Feely J. The influence of aspirin and paracetamol on blood concentrations of alcohol in young adults. *Br J Clin Pharmacol* (1996) 41, 467P.
26. Prescott LF. Paracetamol, alcohol and the liver. *Br J Clin Pharmacol* (2000) 49, 291–301.
27. Food and Drug Administration. FDA announces new alcohol warnings for pain relievers and fever reducers. HHS News. Available at: http://www.fda.gov/bbs/topics/NEWS/NEW00659.html (accessed 08/06/04).
28. Rumack BH. Acetaminophen hepatotoxicity: the first 35 years. *J Toxicol Clin Toxicol* (2002) 40, 3–20.

Alcohol + Paraldehyde

Both alcohol and paraldehyde have CNS depressant effects, which can be additive. Their concurrent use in the treatment of acute alcohol intoxication has had a fatal outcome.

Clinical evidence, mechanism, importance and management

A report describes 9 patients who died suddenly and unexpectedly after treatment for acute alcohol intoxication with 30 to 90 ml paraldehyde (the authors quote a normal dose range of 8 to 30 ml; fatal dose 120 ml or more, usually preceded by coma). None of the patients had hepatic impairment, although one did have some fatty changes.[1] Both are CNS depressants and may therefore be expected to have additive effects at any dosage, although an *animal* study suggested that it might be less than additive.[2]

1. Kaye S, Haag HB. Study of death due to combined action of alcohol and paraldehyde in man. *Toxicol Appl Pharmacol* (1964) 6, 316–20.
2. Gessner PK, Shakarjian MP. Interactions of paraldehyde with ethanol and chloral hydrate. *J Pharmacol Exp Ther* (1985) 235, 32–6.

Alcohol + Penicillins

No adverse interaction normally occurs between alcohol and phenoxymethylpenicillin or amoxicillin.

Clinical evidence, mechanism, importance and management

A long-standing and very common belief among members of the general public (presumably derived from advice given by doctors and pharmacists) is that alcohol should be strictly avoided while taking any antibiotic. It has been claimed that alcohol increases the degradation of penicillin in the gut and reduces the amount available for absorption.[1] However, one study showed that the pharmacokinetics of **phenoxymethylpenicillin (penicillin V)** were unaffected by alcoholic drinks,[2] and another study found that alcohol delayed the absorption of **amoxicillin** but did not affect the total amount absorbed.[3] There seems to be no evidence to support claims of an adverse interaction.

1. Kitto W. Antibiotics and ingestion of alcohol. *JAMA* (1965) 193, 411.
2. Lindberg RLP, Huupponen RK, Viljanen S and Pihlajamäki KK. Ethanol and the absorption of oral penicillin in man. *Int J Clin Pharmacol Ther Toxicol* (1987) 25, 536–8.
3. Morasso MI, Hip A, Márquez M, González C, Arancibia A. Amoxicillin kinetics and ethanol ingestion. *Int J Clin Pharmacol Ther Toxicol* (1988) 26, 428–31.

Alcohol + Procainamide

Alcohol may modestly increase the clearance of procainamide.

Clinical evidence, mechanism, importance and management

Alcohol 0.73 g/kg increased the clearance (by 34%) and decreased the elimination half-life (by 25%) of a single 10-mg/kg oral dose of procainamide in healthy subjects. This was due to increased acetylation of procainamide to its active metabolite *N*-acetylprocainamide.[1] The clinical relevance of these modest changes is probably small.

1. Olsen H, Mørland J. Ethanol-induced increase in procainamide acetylation in man. *Br J Clin Pharmacol* (1982) 13, 203–8.

Alcohol + Procarbazine

A flushing reaction has been seen in patients on procarbazine who drank alcohol.

Clinical evidence

One report describes 5 patients taking procarbazine whose faces became very red and hot for a short time after drinking **wine**.[1] Another says that flushing occurred in 3 patients on procarbazine after drinking **beer**.[2] Two out of 40 patients taking procarbazine in a third study complained of facial flushing after taking a small alcoholic drink, and one patient thought that the effects of alcohol were markedly increased.[3] Yet another describes a 'flush syndrome' in 3 out of 50 patients who drank alcohol while taking procarbazine.[4]

Mechanism

Unknown, but it seems possible that in man, as in *rats*,[5] the procarbazine inhibits acetaldehyde dehydrogenase in the liver causing a disulfiram-like reaction (see 'Alcohol + Disulfiram', p.50).

Importance and management

An established interaction but of uncertain incidence. It seems to be more embarrassing, possibly frightening, than serious and if it occurs it is unlikely to require treatment, however patients should be warned.

1. Mathé G, Berumen L, Schweisguth O, Brule G, Schneider M, Cattan A, Amiel JL, Schwarzenberg L. Methyl-hydrazine in the treatment of Hodgkin's disease and various forms of haematosarcoma and leukaemia. *Lancet* (1963) ii, 1077–80.
2. Dawson WB. Ibenzmethyzin in the management of late Hodgkin's disease. In 'Natulan, Ibenzmethyzin'. Report of the proceedings of a symposium, Downing College, Cambridge, June 1965. Jelliffe AM and Marks J (Eds). Bristol: John Wright; 1965. P. 31–4.
3. Todd IDH. Natulan in management of late Hodgkin's disease, other lymphoreticular neoplasms, and malignant melanoma. *BMJ* (1965) 1, 628–31.
4. Brulé G, Schlumberger JR, Griscelli C. *N*-isopropyl-α-(2-methylhydrazino)-*p*-toluamide, hydrochloride (NSC-77213) in treatment of solid tumors. *Cancer Chemother Rep* (1965) 44, 31–8.
5. Vasiliou V, Malamas M, Marselos M. The mechanism of alcohol intolerance produced by various therapeutic agents. *Acta Pharmacol Toxicol (Copenh)* (1986) 58, 305–10.

Alcohol + Proton pump inhibitors

Lansoprazole, omeprazole and pantoprazole do not interact with alcohol.

Clinical evidence

(a) Lansoprazole

A study in 30 healthy subjects given 0.6 g/kg alcohol before and after taking lansoprazole for 3 days found that the pharmacokinetics of alcohol were not significantly changed and blood alcohol levels were not raised by lansoprazole.[1]

(b) Omeprazole

A number of studies have shown that omeprazole does not affect blood alcohol levels.[2-5]

(c) Pantoprazole

Pantoprazole 40 mg or placebo were given daily to 16 healthy subjects for 7 days. On day 7 they were also given alcohol 0.5 g/kg in 200 ml of orange juice 2 hours after a standard breakfast. The maximum serum levels and the AUC of alcohol were not significantly changed by pantoprazole.[6]

Mechanism

The proton pump inhibitors do not affect alcohol dehydrogenase activity[3,7] (compare with the 'H_2-blockers', (p.53)), and would not be expected to alter the first-pass metabolism of alcohol.

Importance and management

The proton pump inhibitors do not appear to interact with alcohol, and no special precautions are necessary with concurrent use. But note that some of the conditions for which these drugs are used may be made worse by alcohol, so restriction of drinking may be needed.

1. Girre C, Coutelle C, David P, Fleury B, Thomas G, Palmobo S, Dally S, Couzigou P. Lack of effect of lansoprazole on the pharmacokinetics of ethanol in male volunteers. *Gastroenterology* (1994) 106, A504.
2. Guram M, Howden CW, Holt S. Further evidence for an interaction between alcohol and certain H_2-receptor antagonists. *Alcohol Clin Exp Res* (1991) 15, 1084–5.
3. Roine R, Hernández-Muñoz R, Baraona E, Greenstein R, Lieber CS. Effect of omeprazole on gastric first-pass metabolism of ethanol. *Dig Dis Sci* (1992) 37, 891–6.
4. Jönsson K-Å, Jones AW, Boström H, Andersson T. Lack of effect of omeprazole, cimetidine, and ranitidine on the pharmacokinetics of ethanol in fasting male volunteers. *Eur J Clin Pharmacol* (1992) 42, 209–212.
5. Minocha A, Rahal PS, Brier ME, Levinson SS. Omeprazole therapy does not affect pharmacokinetics of orally administered ethanol in healthy male subjects. *J Clin Gastroenterol* (1995) 21, 107–9.
6. Heinze H, Fischer R, Pfützer R, Teyssen S, Singer MV. Lack of interaction between pantoprazole and ethanol: a randomised, double-blind, placebo-controlled study in healthy volunteers. *Clin Drug Invest* (2001) 21, 345–51.
7. Battiston L, Tulissi P, Moretti M, Pozzato G. Lansoprazole and ethanol metabolism: comparison with omeprazole and cimetidine. *Pharmacol Toxicol* (1997) 81, 247–52.

Alcohol + Quetiapine

Quetiapine does not appear to affect the pharmacokinetics of alcohol, although their sedative effects are possibly additive.

Clinical evidence, mechanism, importance and management

A randomised crossover study in 8 men with psychotic disorders found that the mean breath concentration of alcohol after taking 0.8 g/kg alcohol in orange juice was unaffected by quetiapine 250 mg three times daily. Some statistically significant changes in the performance of psychomotor tests were seen, but these were considered to have little clinical relevance. Despite this the makers caution against the use of quetiapine in combination with other centrally acting drugs and alcohol.[1,2] This is probably because drowsiness is the most common adverse effect of quetiapine, occurring in 18% of patients.[2] This drowsiness might be expected to be worsened by alcohol.

1. Seroquel (Quetiapine fumarate). AstraZeneca UK Ltd. UK Summary of product characteristics, June 2005.
2. Seroquel (Quetiapine fumarate). AstraZeneca Pharmaceuticals LP. US Prescribing information, June 2005.

Alcohol + Retinoids

There is evidence that the consumption of alcohol may increase the serum levels of etretinate in patients taking acitretin. A single case report describes a marked reduction in the effects of isotretinoin following the acute intake of alcohol.

Clinical evidence, mechanism, importance and management

(a) Acitretin

A study in 10 patients with psoriasis taking acitretin found that concurrent intake of alcohol seemed to be associated with an increase in the formation of its metabolite etretinate, which has a much longer half-life than acitretin. The implications of this study are not known, but it is suggested that it may have some bearing on the length of the period after acitretin therapy during which women are advised not to conceive.[1]

(b) Isotretinoin

A former alcoholic, who normally no longer drank, was treated for acne conglobata with some success for 3 months with 60 mg of isotretinoin daily. When for 2 weeks he briefly started to drink again as part of his job (he was a **sherry** taster) his skin lesions reappeared and the isotretinoin adverse effects (mucocutaneous dryness) vanished. When he stopped drinking his skin lesions became controlled again and the drug side-effects re-emerged. The following year while on another course of isotretinoin the same thing happened when he started and stopped drinking. The reasons are not known, but one suggestion is that the alcohol briefly induced the liver microsomal enzymes responsible for the metabolism of isotretinoin, thereby reducing both its therapeutic and adverse effects.[2] The general importance of this apparent interaction is not known.

1. Larsen FG, Jakobsen P, Knudsen J, Weismann K, Kragballe K, Nielsen-Kudsk F. Conversion of acitretin to etretinate in psoriatic patients is influenced by ethanol. *J Invest Dermatol* (1993) 100, 623–7.
2. Soria C, Allegue F, Galiana J, Ledo A. Decreased isotretinoin efficacy during acute alcohol intake. *Dermatologica* (1991) 182, 203.

Alcohol + Sibutramine

There does not seem to be a clinically relevant interaction between sibutramine and alcohol.

Clinical evidence, mechanism, importance and management

In a randomised study, 20 healthy subjects were given 20 mg of sibutramine with 0.5 g/kg of alcohol diluted in ginger beer, or placebo. Sibutramine did not potentiate the cognitive or psychomotor effects of alcohol, and in one test, sibutramine slightly reduced the impairment caused by alcohol.[1] However, the maker notes that the consumption of alcohol is generally not compatible with recommended adjuvant dietary modification.[2]

1. Wesnes KA, Garratt C, Wickens M, Gudgeon A, Oliver S. Effects of sibutramine alone and with alcohol on cognitive function in healthy volunteers. *Br J Clin Pharmacol* (2000) 49, 110–17.
2. Reductil (Sibutramine). Abbott Laboratories Ltd. UK Summary of product characteristics, February 2004.

Alcohol + Sodium cromoglicate (Cromolyn sodium)

No adverse interaction occurs between sodium cromoglicate and alcohol.

Clinical evidence, mechanism, importance and management

A double-blind crossover trial in 17 healthy subjects found that the inhalation of 40 mg of sodium cromoglicate had little or no effect on the performance of a number of tests on human perceptual, cognitive and motor skills, whether taken alone or with alcohol 0.75 g/kg. Nor did it affect blood alcohol levels.[1] This is in line with the common experience of patients, and no special precautions seem to be necessary.

1. Crawford WA, Franks HM, Hensley VR, Hensley WJ, Starmer GA, Teo RKC. The effect of disodium cromoglycate on human performance, alone and in combination with ethanol. *Med J Aust* (1976) 1, 997–9.

Alcohol + SSRIs and related drugs

Citalopram, duloxetine, fluoxetine and sertraline in therapeutic doses do not appear to interact with alcohol, but some modest interaction possibly occurs with fluvoxamine.

Clinical evidence, mechanism, importance and management

(a) Citalopram

The makers of citalopram say that no pharmacodynamic interactions have been noted in clinical studies in which citalopram was given with alcohol.[1]

(b) Duloxetine, Fluoxetine

Concurrent duloxetine 60 mg and alcohol, in a dose sufficient to produce blood levels of about 100 mg%, did not worsen the psychomotor impairment observed with alcohol alone in a single-dose study in healthy subjects.[2]

Neither fluoxetine 30 to 60 mg nor alcohol (4 oz **whiskey**) affected the pharmacokinetics of the other in healthy subjects, and fluoxetine did not alter the effect of alcohol on psychomotor activity (stability of stance, motor performance, manual co-ordination).[3] Similarly, blood alcohol levels of 80 mg% impaired the performance of a number of psychomotor tests in 12 healthy subjects, but the addition of fluoxetine 40 mg daily taken for 6 days before the alcohol had little further effect.[4] Another study also found no change in the performance of a number of psychophysiological tests when fluoxetine was combined with alcohol.[5] No problems were found in a study of 76 patients on fluoxetine 60 mg daily when they drank alcohol.[6]

(c) Fluvoxamine

One study found that fluvoxamine 150 mg daily with alcohol impaired alertness and attention more than alcohol alone,[7] whereas another study in subjects given 40 g of alcohol (blood alcohol levels up to 70 mg% failed to find evidence that the addition of fluvoxamine 50 mg twice daily worsened the performance of the psychomotor tests used, and it even appeared to reverse some of the effects.[8] Another study similarly found no significant interaction.[9] The pharmacokinetics of alcohol were hardly affected by fluvoxamine, but the steady state maximum plasma levels of the fluvoxamine were increased by 20%, although the fluvoxamine AUC was unchanged.[8] The situation with fluvoxamine is therefore less clear than with the drugs listed in (a) above, but it would seem prudent to give patients some warning that the effects of alcohol may possibly be modestly increased.

(d) Paroxetine

Studies in human subjects[10,11] found that paroxetine alone caused little impairment of a series of psychomotor tests related to car driving, and with alcohol the effects were unchanged except for a significant decrease in attentiveness and reaction time.[10] Another study suggested that the alcohol-induced sedation was antagonised by paroxetine.[12] No special precautions seem to be necessary.

(e) Sertraline

Sertraline (in doses of up to 200 mg for nine days) was found not to impair cognitive or psychomotor performance, and it also appeared not to increase the effects of alcohol.[13] This suggests that no special precautions would seem necessary, even so the makers do not recommend concurrent use.[14]

1. Cipramil (Citalopram). Lundbeck Ltd. UK Summary of product characteristics, April 2003.
2. Skinner MH, Weerakkody G. Duloxetine does not exacerbate the effects of alcohol on psychometric tests. *Clin Pharmacol Ther* (2002) 71, 53.
3. Lemberger L, Rowe H, Bergstrom RF, Farid KZ, Enas GG. Effect of fluoxetine on psychomotor performance, physiologic response, and kinetics of ethanol. *Clin Pharmacol Ther* (1985) 37, 658–64.
4. Allen D, Lader M, Curran HV. A comparative study of the interactions of alcohol with amitriptyline, fluoxetine and placebo in normal subjects. *Prog Neuropsychopharmacol Biol Psychiatry* (1988) 12, 63–80.
5. Schaffler K. Study on performance and alcohol interaction with the antidepressant fluoxetine. *Int Clin Psychopharmacol* (1989) 4 (Suppl 1), 15–20.
6. Florkowski A, Gruszczyñski W. Alcohol problems and treating patients with fluoxetine. *Pol J Pharmacol* (1995) 47, 547.
7. Duphar Laboratories. Study of the effects of the antidepressant fluvoxamine on driving skills and its interaction with alcohol. Data on file, 1981.
8. van Harten J, Stevens LA, Raghoebar M, Holland RL, Wesnes K, Cournot A. Fluvoxamine does not interact with alcohol or potentiate alcohol-related impairment of cognitive function. *Clin Pharmacol Ther* (1992) 52, 427–35.
9. Linnoila M, Stapleton JM, George DT, Lane E, Eckardt MJ. Effects of fluvoxamine, alone and in combination with ethanol, on psychomotor and cognitive performance and on autonomic nervous system reactivity in healthy volunteers. *J Clin Psychopharmacol* (1993) 13, 175–80.
10. Cooper SM, Jackson D, Loudon JM, McClelland GR, Raptopoulos P. The psychomotor effects of paroxetine alone and in combination with haloperidol, amylobarbitone, oxazepam, or alcohol. *Acta Psychiatr Scand* (1989) 80 (Suppl 350), 53–55.
11. Hindmarch I, Harrison C. The effects of paroxetine and other antidepressants in combination with alcohol on psychomotor activity related to car driving. *Acta Psychiatr Scand* (1989) 80 (Suppl 350), 45.
12. Kerr JS, Fairweather DB, Mahendran R, Hindmarch I. The effects of paroxetine, alone and in combination with alcohol on psychomotor performance and cognitive function in the elderly. *Int Clin Psychopharmacol* (1992) 7, 101–8.
13. Warrington SJ. Clinical implications of the pharmacology of sertraline. *Int Clin Psychopharmacol* (1991) 6 (Suppl 2), 11–21.
14. Lustral (Sertraline). Pfizer Ltd. UK Summary of product characteristics, December 2003.

Alcohol + Sulfiram

Disulfiram-like reactions have been seen in at least three patients who drank alcohol after using a solution of sulfiram on the skin for the treatment of scabies.

Clinical evidence

A man who used undiluted *Tetmosol* (a solution of sulfiram) for 3 days on the skin all over his body developed a disulfiram-like reaction (flushing, sweating, skin swelling, severe tachycardia and nausea) on the third day after drinking three double **whiskies**. The same thing happened on two subsequent evenings after drinking.[1] Similar reactions have been described in two other patients after drinking while using *Tetmosol* or *Ascabiol* (also containing sulfiram).[2,3]

Mechanism

Sulfiram (tetraethylthiuram *monosulphide*) is closely related to disulfiram (tetraethylthiuram *disulphide*) and can apparently undergo photochemical conversion to disulfiram when exposed to light. The longer it is stored, the higher the concentration.[4,5] The reaction with alcohol (inhibition of aldehyde dehydrogenase) appears therefore to be largely due to the presence of disulfiram[6] (see 'Alcohol + Disulfiram', p.50).

Importance and management

An established interaction. The makers of sulfiram preparations and others advise abstention from alcohol before, and for at least 48 hours after application, but this may not always be necessary. The writer of a letter,[7] commenting on the first case cited,[1] wrote that he had never encountered this reaction when using a diluted solution of *Tetmosol* on patients at the Dreadnought Seamen's Hospital in London who ". . . are not necessarily abstemious." This would suggest that the reaction is normally uncommon and unlikely to occur if the solution is correctly diluted (usually with 2 to 3 parts of water), thereby reducing the amount absorbed through the skin. However, one unusually sensitive patient is said to have had a reaction (flushing, sweating, tachycardia) after using diluted *Tetmosol*, but without drinking alcohol. It was suggested that she reacted to the alcohol base of the formulation passing through her skin.[8] Patients should be warned.

1. Gold S. A skinful of alcohol. *Lancet* (1966) ii, 1417.
2. Dantas W. Monosulfiram como causa de síndrome do acetaldeído. *Arq Cat Med* (1980) 9, 29–30.
3. Blanc D, Deprez Ph. Unusual adverse reaction to an acaricide. *Lancet* (1990) 335, 1291–2.
4. Lipsky JJ, Mays DC, Naylor S. Monosulfiram, disulfiram, and light. *Lancet* (1994) 343, 304.

5. Mays DC, Nelson AN, Benson LM, Johnson KL, Naylor S, Lipsky JJ. Photolysis of monosulfiram: a mechanism for its disulfiram-like reaction. *Clin Pharmacol Ther* (1994) 55, 191.
6. Lipsky JJ, Nelson AN, Dockter EC. Inhibition of aldehyde dehydrogenase by sulfiram. *Clin Pharmacol Ther* (1992) 51, 184.
7. Erskine D. A skinful of alcohol. *Lancet* (1967) i, 54.
8. Burgess I. Adverse reactions to monosulfiram. *Lancet* (1990) 336, 873.

Alcohol + Sumatriptan

Alcohol does not alter the pharmacokinetics of sumatriptan.

Clinical evidence, mechanism, importance and management

Single 0.8-g/kg doses of alcohol were given to 16 healthy subjects, followed 30 minutes later by 200 mg of sumatriptan. No statistically significant changes were seen in the pharmacokinetics of sumatriptan.[1] There is nothing to suggest that alcohol should be avoided while taking sumatriptan.

1. Kempsford RD, Lacey LF, Thomas M, Fowler PA. The effect of alcohol on the pharmacokinetic profile of oral sumatriptan. *Fundam Clin Pharmacol* (1991) 5, 470.

Alcohol + Tetracyclic antidepressants

Mianserin and maprotiline can cause drowsiness and impair the ability to drive or handle other dangerous machinery, particularly during the first few days of treatment. This impairment is increased by alcohol. Pirlindole appears not to interact with alcohol.

Clinical evidence

(a) Maprotiline

A double blind crossover trial in 12 healthy subjects found that single 75-mg oral doses of maprotiline subjectively caused drowsiness, which was increased by 1 g/kg of alcohol. The performance of a number of psychomotor tests was also worsened after the addition of alcohol.[1] However, in a later study the same group did not find that maprotiline 50 mg twice daily increased the detrimental effects of alcohol.[2]

(b) Mianserin

A double-blind crossover study in 13 healthy subjects given 10 to 30 mg of mianserin twice daily for 8 days, with and without alcohol 1 g/kg, showed that their performance in a number of psychomotor tests (choice reaction, coordination, critical flicker frequency) were impaired by mianserin alone and by concurrent use with alcohol. The subjects were aware of feeling drowsy, muzzy, and less able to carry out the tests.[3]

These results confirm the findings of other studies.[4,5]

(c) Pirlindole

A study in healthy subjects given pirlindole 75 to 150 mg daily for 4 days indicated that it did not affect the performance of a number of psychomotor tests, with or without 0.4 g/kg of alcohol.[6]

Mechanism

The CNS depressant effects of mianserin, and possibly maprotiline, appear to be additive with those of alcohol.

Importance and management

Drowsiness is a frequently reported side-effect of mianserin, particularly during the first few days of treatment. Patients should be warned that driving or handling dangerous machinery will be made more hazardous if they drink. It would seem prudent (at the risk of being overcautious) to warn patients taking maprotiline of the possible increased risk if they drink and then drive or handle potentially dangerous machinery.[2] Pirlindole appears not to interact.

1. Strömberg C, Seppälä T, Mattila MJ. Acute effects of maprotiline, doxepin and zimeldine with alcohol in healthy volunteers. *Arch Int Pharmacodyn Ther* (1988) 291, 217–228.
2. Strömberg C, Suokas A, Seppälä T. Interaction of alcohol with maprotiline or nomifensine: echocardiographic and psychometric effects. *Eur J Clin Pharmacol* (1988) 35, 593–99.
3. Seppälä T, Strömberg C, Bergman I. Effect of zimeldine, mianserin and amitriptyline on psychomotor skills and their interaction with alcohol: a placebo controlled cross-over study. *Eur J Clin Pharmacol* (1984) 27, 181–9.
4. Seppälä T. Psychomotor skills during acute and two-week treatment with mianserin (Org GB 94) and amitriptyline, and their combined effects with alcohol. *Ann Clin Res* (1977) 9, 66–72.
5. Strömberg C, Mattila MJ. Acute comparison of clovoxamine and mianserin, alone and in combination with ethanol, on human psychomotor performance. *Pharmacol Toxicol* (1987) 60, 374–9.
6. Ehlers T, Ritter M. Effects of the tetracyclic antidepressant pirlindole on sensorimotor performance and subjective condition in comparison to imipramine and during interaction of ethanol. *Neuropsychobiology* (1984) 12, 48–54.

Alcohol + Tetracyclines

Doxycycline serum levels may fall below minimum therapeutic concentrations in alcoholic patients, but tetracycline is not affected. There is nothing to suggest that moderate amounts of alcohol have a clinically relevant effect on the serum levels of any tetracycline in non-alcoholic subjects.

Clinical evidence

(a) Alcoholic patients

A study into the effects of alcohol on **doxycycline** and **tetracycline** found that the half-life of **doxycycline** was 10.5 hours in 6 alcoholics (with normal liver function) compared with 14.7 hours in 6 healthy subjects. The serum **doxycycline** levels of 3 of the alcoholic patients fell below the minimum inhibitory concentration (said to be the generally accepted level) at 24 hours. The half-life of tetracycline was the same in both groups. All of the subjects were given **doxycycline** 100 mg daily after a 200 mg loading dose, and **tetracycline** 500 mg twice daily after an initial 750 mg loading dose.[1]

(b) Non-alcoholic patients

Single 500-mg doses of **tetracycline** were given to 9 healthy subjects with water or alcohol 2.7 g/kg. The alcohol caused a 33% rise in the maximum serum **tetracycline** levels from 9.3 to 12.4 micrograms/ml, and a 50% rise in the **tetracycline** AUC.[2] The clinical relevance of this rise is unknown.

Another study in healthy subjects found that cheap red wine, but not whisky (both 1 g/kg) postponed the absorption of **doxycycline**, probably because of the presence of acetic acid, which slows gastric emptying. However, the total absorption was not affected. The authors concluded[3] that acute intake of alcoholic beverages have no clinically relevant effects on the pharmacokinetics of **doxycycline**.

Mechanism

Heavy drinkers can metabolise some drugs much more quickly than non-drinkers due to the enzyme-inducing effects of alcohol.[4] The interaction with doxycycline would seem to be due to this effect, possibly allied with some reduction in absorption from the gut.

Importance and management

Information is limited, but the interaction between doxycycline and alcohol appears to be established and of clinical significance in alcoholics but not in non-alcoholic individuals. One possible solution to the problem of enzyme induction is to give alcoholic subjects double the dose.[5] Alternatively tetracycline could be used because it appears not to be affected. There is nothing to suggest that moderate or even occasional heavy drinking has a clinically relevant effect on any of the tetracyclines in non-alcoholic subjects.

1. Neuvonen PJ, Penttilä O, Roos M, Tirkkonen J. Effect of long-term alcohol consumption on the half-life of tetracycline and doxycycline in man. *Int J Clin Pharmacol Biopharm* (1976) 14, 303–7.
2. Seitz C, Garcia P, Arancibia A. Influence of ethanol ingestion on tetracycline kinetics. *Int J Clin Pharmacol Ther* (1995) 33, 462–4.
3. Mattila MJ, Laisi U, Linnoila M, Salonen R. Effect of alcoholic beverages on the pharmacokinetics of doxycycline in man. *Acta Pharmacol Toxicol (Copenh)* (1982) 50, 370–3.
4. Misra PS, Lefèvre A, Ishii H, Rubin E, Lieber CS. Increase of ethanol, meprobamate and pentobarbital metabolism after chronic ethanol administration in man and rats. *Am J Med* (1971) 51, 346–51.
5. Neuvonen PJ, Penttilä O, Lehtovaara R and Aho K. Effect of antiepileptic drugs on the elimination of various tetracycline derivatives. *Eur J Clin Pharmacol* (1975) 9, 147–54.

Alcohol + Tianeptine

Alcohol reduced the absorption of tianeptine and lowered plasma levels by about 30%.

Clinical evidence, mechanism, importance and management

The absorption and peak plasma levels of tianeptine after a single 12.5-mg dose were reduced by about 30% in 12 healthy subjects by alcohol. The subjects were given vodka diluted in orange juice to give blood alcohol levels between 77 and 64 mg%. The plasma levels of the major metabolite of tianeptine were unchanged.[1] No behavioural studies were done so that the clinical significance of these studies is as yet uncertain.

1. Salvadori C, Ward C, Defrance R, Hopkins R. The pharmacokinetics of the antidepressant tianeptine and its main metabolite in healthy humans — influence of alcohol co-administration. *Fundam Clin Pharmacol* (1990) 4, 115–25.

Alcohol + Tolazoline

A disulfiram-like reaction may occur in patients on tolazoline if they drink.

Clinical evidence, mechanism, importance and management

Seven healthy subjects were given tolazoline 25 mg daily for 4 days. Within 15 and 90 minutes of drinking 90 ml of **port wine** (18.2% alcohol), 2 hours after the last dose of tolazoline, 6 experienced tingling over the head, and 4 developed warmth and fullness of the head.[1] The reasons are not understood, but this reaction is not unlike a mild disulfiram reaction, and may possibly have a similar mechanism (see 'Alcohol + Disulfiram', p.50). Patients given tolazoline should be warned about this reaction if they drink, and advised to limit their consumption. Reactions of this kind with drugs other than disulfiram are usually more unpleasant or frightening than serious, and treatment is rarely needed.

1. Boyd EM. A search for drugs with disulfiram-like activity. *Q J Stud Alcohol* (1960) 21, 23–5.

Alcohol + Trazodone

Trazodone makes driving or handling other dangerous machinery more hazardous, and further impairment may occur with alcohol.

Clinical evidence

A study in 6 healthy subjects comparing the effects of single-doses of amitriptyline 50 mg and trazodone 100 mg found that both drugs impaired the performance of a number of psychomotor tests, causing drowsiness and reducing 'clearheadedness' to approximately the same extent. Only manual dexterity was further impaired when the subjects on trazodone were given sufficient alcohol to give blood levels of about 40 mg%.[1]

Another study similarly found that the impairment of psychomotor performance by trazodone was increased by alcohol.[2]

Mechanism

Uncertain. Simple additive depression of the CNS seems a likely explanation.

Importance and management

An established interaction, and of practical importance. Patients should be warned that their ability to drive, handle dangerous machinery or to do other tasks needing complex psychomotor skills may be impaired by trazodone, and further worsened by alcohol.

1. Warrington SJ, Ankier SI, Turner P. Evaluation of possible interactions between ethanol and trazodone or amitriptyline. *Neuropsychobiology* (1986) 15 (Suppl 1), 31–7.
2. Tiller JWG. Antidepressants, alcohol and psychomotor performance. *Acta Psychiatr Scand* (1990) (Suppl 360), 13–17.

Alcohol + Trichloroethylene

A flushing skin reaction similar to a mild disulfiram reaction can occur in those exposed to trichloroethylene when they drink alcohol.

Clinical evidence

An engineer from a factory where trichloroethylene was being used as a degreasing agent, developed facial flushing, a sensation of increased pressure in the head, lachrymation, tachypnoea and blurred vision within 12 minutes of drinking 85 ml of **bourbon whiskey**. The reaction did not develop when he was no longer exposed to the trichloroethylene. Other workers in the same plant reported the same experience.[1]

Vivid red blotches in a symmetrical pattern on the face, neck, shoulders and back were seen in other workers when they drank about 2 pints of **beer**[2] after having been exposed for a few hours each day for 3 weeks to increasing concentrations of trichloroethylene vapour (up to 200 ppm). Note that this was twice the permitted maximum permissible level for trichloroethylene in air at that time.[3] This reaction has been described as the 'degreasers flush'.[2] There is also some evidence that short-term exposure to the combination may possibly reduce mental capacity.[4]

Mechanism

Uncertain. One suggested mechanism is a disulfiram-like inhibition of acetaldehyde metabolism by trichloroethylene (see 'Alcohol + Disulfiram', p.50).

Importance and management

An established interaction. It would seem to be more unpleasant and socially disagreeable than serious, and normally requires no treatment.

1. Pardys S, Brotman M. Trichloroethylene and alcohol: a straight flush. *JAMA* (1974) 229, 521–2.
2. Stewart RD, Hake CL, Peterson JE. "Degreasers' Flush": dermal response to trichloroethylene and ethanol. *Arch Environ Health* (1974) 29, 1–5.
3. Smith GF. Trichloroethylene: a review. *Br J Ind Med* (1966) 23, 249–62.
4. Windemuller FJB, Ettema JH. Effects of combined exposure to trichloroethylene and alcohol on mental capacity. *Int Arch Occup Environ Health* (1978) 41, 77–85.

Alcohol + Tricyclic antidepressants

The ability to drive, to handle dangerous machinery or to do other tasks requiring complex psychomotor skills may be impaired by amitriptyline, and to a lesser extent by doxepin, particularly during the first few days of treatment. This impairment is increased by alcohol. Amoxapine, clomipramine, desipramine, imipramine, and nortriptyline appear to interact with alcohol only minimally. Information about other tricyclics appears to be lacking. There is also evidence that alcoholics may need larger doses of desipramine and imipramine to control depression.

Clinical evidence

(a) Amitriptyline

Amitriptyline 0.8 mg/kg impaired the performance of three motor skills tests related to driving in 21 healthy subjects. When additionally given alcohol to produce blood levels of about 80 mg% the performance was even further impaired.[1]

Similar results have been very clearly demonstrated in considerable numbers of subjects using a variety of psychomotor skill tests,[1-6] the interaction being most marked during the first few days of treatment, but tending to wane as treatment continues.[5] There is also some limited evidence from *animal* studies that amitriptyline may possibly enhance the fatty changes induced in the liver by alcohol,[7] but this still needs confirmation from human studies. Unexplained blackouts lasting a few hours have also been described in 3 women after drinking only modest amounts;[8] they had been taking amitriptyline or **imipramine** for only a month.

(b) Doxepin

A double-blind crossover trial in 20 healthy subjects given various combinations of alcohol and either doxepin or a placebo showed that with blood alcohol levels of 40 to 50 mg% their choice reaction test times were prolonged and the number of mistakes increased. Coordination was obviously impaired after 7 days treatment with doxepin, but not after 14 days.[3] In an earlier study doxepin appeared to cancel out the deleterious effects of alcohol on the performance of a simulated driving test.[9]

(c) Other tricyclics

Studies in subjects with blood alcohol levels of 40 to 60 mg% showed that **clomipramine** and **nortriptyline** had only slight or no effects on various choice reaction, coordination, memory and learning tests.[3,10-12] The interaction between **amoxapine** and alcohol is said to be slight,[13] but two patients have been described who experienced reversible extrapyramidal symptoms (parkinsonism, akathisia) while taking **amoxapine**, apparently caused by drinking.[14] Tests in subjects given 100 mg of **desipramine** indicated that no significant interaction occurred with alcohol,[15] but **imipramine** 150 mg daily tended to increase the sedative-hypnotic effects of alcohol.[16]

The half-lives of oral **imipramine** and **desipramine** were about 45% and 30% lower respectively, in recently detoxified alcoholics (without liver disease) compared with healthy subjects, and the intrinsic clearances were 200% and 60% greater, respectively.[17]

Mechanism

Part of the explanation for the increased CNS depression is that both alcohol and some of the tricyclics, particularly amitriptyline, cause drowsiness and other CNS depressant effects, which can be additive with the effects of alcohol.[6] The sedative effects are said in one review to be amitriptyline> doxepin> imipramine> nortriptyline> desipramine> **protriptyline**.[18] In addition alcohol causes marked increases (100 to 200%) in the plasma concentrations of amitriptyline, probably by inhibiting its first pass metabolism.[4] The lower serum levels of imipramine and desipramine seen in abstinent alcoholics is attributable to induction by alcohol of the cytochrome P450 isoenzymes.[17]

Importance and management

The increased CNS depression resulting from the amitriptyline/alcohol interaction is well documented and clinically important. Warn patients that driving or handling dangerous machinery may be made more hazardous if they drink, particularly during the first few days of treatment, but the effects of the interaction diminish during continued treatment. The alcohol/doxepin interaction is less well documented and the information is conflicting, but to be on the safe side a similar warning should be given. Amoxapine, clomipramine, desipramine, imipramine and nortriptyline appear to interact only minimally with alcohol. Direct information about other tricyclics seems to be lacking, but there appear to be no particular reasons for avoiding concurrent use. However, prescribers may feel it appropriate to offer some precautionary advice, because during the first 1 to 2 weeks of treatment many tricyclics (without alcohol) may temporarily impair the skills related to driving.[13]

Also be aware that alcoholic patients (without liver disease) may need higher doses of imipramine (possibly doubled) and desipramine to control depression, and if long-term abstinence is achieved the dosages may then eventually need to be reduced. Information about other tricyclics seems to be lacking.

1. Landauer AA, Milner G, Patman J. Alcohol and amitriptyline effects on skills related to driving behavior. *Science* (1969) 163, 1467–8.
2. Seppälä T. Psychomotor skills during acute and two-week treatment with mianserin (ORG GB 94) and amitriptyline, and their combined effects with alcohol. *Ann Clin Res* (1977) 9, 66–72.
3. Seppälä T, Linnoila M, Elonen E, Mattila MJ, Mäki M. Effect of tricyclic antidepressants and alcohol on psychomotor skills related to driving. *Clin Pharmacol Ther* (1975) 17, 515–22.
4. Dorian P, Sellers EM, Reed KL, Warsh JJ, Hamilton C, Kaplan HL, Fan T. Amitriptyline and ethanol: pharmacokinetic and pharmacodynamic interaction. *Eur J Clin Pharmacol* (1983) 25, 325–31.
5. Seppälä T, Strömberg C, Bergman I. Effects of zimeldine, mianserin and amitriptyline on psychomotor skills and their interaction with ethanol: a placebo controlled cross-over study. *Eur J Clin Pharmacol* (1984) 27, 181–9.
6. Scott DB, Fagan D, Tiplady B. Effects of amitriptyline and zimelidine in combination with alcohol. *Psychopharmacology (Berl)* (1982) 76, 209–11.
7. Milner G, Kakulas BA. The potentiation by amitriptyline of liver changes induced by ethanol in mice. *Pathology* (1969) 1, 113–18.
8. Hudson CJ. Tricyclic antidepressants and alcoholic blackouts. *J Nerv Ment Dis* (1981) 169, 381–2.
9. Milner G, Landauer AA. The effects of doxepin, alone and together with alcohol in relation to driving safety. *Med J Aust* (1973) 1, 837–41.
10. Hughes FW, Forney RB. Delayed audiofeedback (DAF) for induction of anxiety: effect of nortriptyline, ethanol, or nortriptyline-ethanol combinations on performance with DAF. *JAMA* (1963) 185, 556–8.
11. Liljequist R, Linnoila M, Mattila M. Effect of two weeks' treatment with chlorimipramine and nortriptyline, alone or in combination with alcohol, on learning and memory. *Psychopharmacology (Berl)* (1974) 39, 181–6.
12. Berlin I, Cournot A, Zimmer R, Pedarriosse A-M, Manfredi R, Molinier P, Puech AJ. Evaluation and comparison of the interaction between alcohol and moclobemide or clomipramine in healthy subjects. *Psychopharmacology (Berl)* (1990) 100, 40–5.
13. Wilson WH, Petrie WM, Ban TA, Barry DE. The effects of amoxapine and ethanol on psychomotor skills related to driving: a placebo and standard controlled study. *Prog Neuropsychopharmacol* (1981) 5, 263–70.
14. Shen WW. Alcohol, amoxapine, and akathisia. *Biol Psychiatry* (1984) 19, 929–30.
15. Linnoila M, Johnson J, Dubyoski K, Buchsbaum MS, Schneinin M, Kilts C. Effects of antidepressants on skilled performance. *Br J Clin Pharmacol* (1984) 18, 109S–120S.
16. Frewer LJ, Lader M. The effects of nefazodone, imipramine and placebo, alone and combined with alcohol, in normal subjects. *Int Clin Psychopharmacol* (1993) 8, 13–20.
17. Ciraulo DA, Barnhill JG, Jaffe JJ. Clinical pharmacokinetics of imipramine and desipramine in alcoholics and normal volunteers. *Clin Pharmacol Ther* (1988) 43, 509–18.
18. Marco LA, Randels RM. Drug interactions in alcoholic patients. *Hillside J Clin Psychiatry* (1981) 3, 27–44.

Alcohol + Trinitrotoluene

Men exposed to trinitrotoluene (TNT) in a munitions factory were found to have a greater risk of TNT-induced liver damage if they had a long history of heavy drinking than if they were non-drinkers.[1]

1. Li J, Jiang Q-G, Zhong W-D. Persistent ethanol drinking increases liver injury induced by trinitrotoluene exposure: an in-plant case-control study. *Hum Exp Toxicol* (1991) 10, 405–9.

Alcohol + Venlafaxine

No important interaction normally appears to occur between venlafaxine and alcohol.

Clinical evidence, mechanism, importance and management

Venlafaxine 50 mg every 8 hours was found to have some effect on psychomotor tests (digit symbol substitution, divided attention reaction times, POM scales) in 16 healthy subjects, but these changes were small and not considered to be clinically significant. No pharmacodynamic or pharmacokinetic interactions occurred when alcohol 0.5 g/kg was added.[1] There would seem to be no reason for avoiding concurrent use.

1. Troy SM, Turner MB, Unruh M, Parker VD, Chiang ST. Pharmacokinetic and pharmacodynamic evaluation of the potential drug interaction between venlafaxine and ethanol. *J Clin Pharmacol* (1997) 37, 1073–81.

Alcohol + Xylene

Some individuals exposed to xylene vapour, who subsequently drink alcohol, may experience dizziness and nausea. A flushing skin reaction has also been seen.

Clinical evidence, mechanism, importance and management

Studies in subjects exposed to *m*-xylene vapour at concentrations of 140 or 250 ppm for 4 hours who were then given 0.8 g/kg of alcohol showed that about 10% experienced dizziness and nausea.[1] One subject exposed to 300 ppm *m*-xylene vapour developed a conspicuous dermal flush on his face, neck, chest and back. He also showed some erythema with alcohol alone. The reasons for these reactions are not understood, but it is possible that xylene plasma levels are increased because alcohol impairs its metabolic clearance, and that acetaldehyde levels may also transiently increased.

1. Riihimäki V, Laine A, Savolainen K, Sippel H. Acute solvent-ethanol interactions with special reference to xylene. *Scand J Work Environ Health* (1982) 8, 77–9.

4

Alpha blockers

The selective and non-selective alpha blockers are categorised and listed in 'Table 4.1', (below). The principal interactions of the alpha blockers are those relating to enhanced hypotensive effects. Early after the introduction of the selective alpha blockers it was discovered that in some individuals they can cause a rapid reduction in blood pressure on starting treatment (also called the 'first-dose effect' or 'first-dose hypotension'). The risk of this may be higher in patients already on other antihypertensive drugs. The first-dose effect has been minimised by starting with a very low dose, and then escalating the dose slowly over a couple of weeks. In addition, some of the makers recommend giving the first dose on retiring to bed. If symptoms such as dizziness, fatigue or sweating develop, patients should be warned to lie down, and to remain lying flat until they abate completely.

It is unclear whether there are any real differences between the alpha blockers in their propensity to cause this first-dose effect. With the exception of indoramin, postural hypotension, syncope, and dizziness are listed as adverse effects of the alpha blockers available in the UK and for most it is recommended to start with a low dose and titrate as required. Tamsulosin is reported to have some selectivity for the alpha receptor 1A subtype, which are found mostly in the prostate, and therefore have less effect on blood pressure and initial titration of the dose is therefore not considered to be necessary. Nevertheless, it would be prudent to exercise caution with all the drugs in this class.

Alpha blockers are also used to increase urinary flow-rate and improve obstructive symptoms in benign prostatic hyperplasia. In this setting, their effects on blood pressure are more of an adverse effect, and their additive hypotensive effect with other antihypertensives may not be beneficial.

The index should be consulted for a full listing of the interactions of the alpha blockers, since those interactions where the alpha blocker is affecting another drug are generally covered elsewhere.

Table 4.1 Alpha blockers

Drug	*Principal indications*	*Proprietary names*
Selective alpha$_1$ blockers (Alpha blockers)		
Alfuzosin	BPH	Alfetim, Benestan, Dalfaz, Mittoval, Urion, UroXatral, Xatral
Bunazosin	Hypertension	Andante, Detantol
Doxazosin	BPH; Hypertension	Alfadil, Alfadoxin, Alfamedin, Angicon, Ascalan, Benur, Cadex, Cardoral, Cardosin, Cardoxan, Cardular, Cardura, Carduran, Dedralen, Diblocin, Dorbantil, Dosan, Doxacar, Doxacard, Doxacor, Doxadura, Doxagamma, Doxaloc, Doxamax, Doxano, Doxapress, Doxa-Puren, Doxasin, Doxasyn, Doxatan, Doxatensa, DoxaUro, Doxazoflo, Doxazomerck, Doxolbran, Hibadren, Jutalar, Kamiren, Maguran, Magurol, Normothen, Pencor, Prodil, Progandol, Prostadilat, Prostazosina, Supressin, Tonocardin, Unoprost, Uriduct, Vazosin, Zoflux, Zoxan
Indoramin	BPH; Hypertension; Migraine	Baratol, Doralese, Vidora, Wydora, Wypresin
Prazosin	BPH; Heart failure; Hypertension; Raynaud's syndrome	Adversuten, Alpress, Anapres, Apo-Prazo, Atodel, CP-Prazo, Decliten, Deprazolin, duramipress, Hexapress, Huma-Prazin, Hypotens, Hypovase, Hyprosin, Kentovase, Lopress, Minipres, Minipress, Minison, Mizosin, Novo-Prazin, Nu-Prazo, Parabowl, Peripress, Polypress, Pratsiol, Prazac, Prazocip, Pressin, Sinozzard
Tamsulosin	BPH	Aclosan, Alna, Expros, Flomax, Harnal, Josir, Mapelor, Omic, Omix, Omnic, Pradif, Prostall, Reduprost, Secotex, Urimax, Urolosin
Terazosin	BPH; Hypertension	Adecur, Alfaprost, Benaprost, Benph, Blavin, Deflox, Dysalfa, Eglidon, Ezosina, Flotrin, Flumarc, Fosfomik, Heitrin, Hyron, Hytrin, Hytrin BPH, Hytrine, Hytrinex, Ibiprovir, Isontyn, Itrin, Kornam, Magnurol, Olyster, Prostatil, Setegis, Sinalfa, Sutif, Tazusin, Tera, Terafluss, Teranar, Teraprost, Teraumon, Terazid, Terazoflo, Unoprost, Urodie, Uroflo, Vicard, Zayasel, Zytrin
Other drugs with alpha-blocking actions		
Phenoxybenzamine	Hypertensive episodes in phaeochromocytoma; Neurogenic bladder; Shock	Dibenyline, Dibenzyline, Dibenzyran, Fenoxene
Phentolamine	Erectile dysfunction; Hypertensive episodes in phaeochromocytoma	Herivyl, Regitin, Regitina, Regitine, Rogitine, Z-Max
Urapidil	Hypertension	Ebrantil, Elgadil, Eupressyl, Mediatensyl

BPH = Benign prostatic hyperplasia

Alpha blockers + ACE inhibitors

Severe first-dose hypotension, and synergistic hypotensive effects that occurred in a patient on enalapril when given bunazosin have been replicated in healthy subjects. The first-dose effect seen with other alpha blockers (particularly alfuzosin, prazosin and terazosin) is also likely to be potentiated by ACE inhibitors. In one small study tamsulosin did not have any clinically relevant effects on blood pressure that was already well controlled by enalapril.

Clinical evidence

After a patient on **enalapril** developed severe first-dose hypotension when given **bunazosin**, this interaction was further studied in 6 healthy subjects. When given **enalapril** 10 mg or **bunazosin** 2 mg, their systolic/diastolic blood pressures over 6 hours were reduced by 9.5/6.7 mmHg. When **bunazosin** was given one hour after **enalapril** the pressure fall was 27/28 mmHg, and still fell by 19/22 mmHg, even when the dose of **enalapril** was reduced to 2.5 mg.[1]

The makers of **alfuzosin**[2] and **prazosin**[3,4] warn that patients receiving antihypertensive drugs are at particular risk of developing postural hypotension after the first dose of alpha blocker.

Retrospective analysis of a large multinational study in patients given 5 or 10 mg of **terazosin** daily found that **terazosin** only affected the blood pressure of patients taking ACE inhibitors (**enalapril**, **lisinopril** or **perindopril**) if the blood pressure was uncontrolled. No change in blood pressure was seen in those with normal blood pressure (i.e. those without hypertension and those with hypertension controlled by ACE inhibitors). The most common adverse effect in the 10-week **terazosin** phase was dizziness, and the incidence of this appeared to be lower in those on antihypertensives (13% to 16%) than those not (21% to 25%).[5] However, the maker of **terazosin** notes that the incidence of dizziness in patients with BPH treated with **terazosin** was higher when they were also receiving an ACE inhibitor.[6]

In a small placebo-controlled study in 6 hypertensive men with blood pressure well controlled by **enalapril**, the addition of **tamsulosin** 400 micrograms daily for 7 days then 800 micrograms daily for a further 7 days had no clinically relevant effects on blood pressure (assessed after 6 and 14 days of **tamsulosin**). In addition, no first-dose hypotensive effect was seen on the day **tamsulosin** was started, or on the day the dose was increased.[7]

Mechanism

The first-dose effect of alpha blockers (see 'Alpha blockers', (p.67)) may be potentiated by ACE-inhibitors. Tamsulosin possibly has less effect on blood pressure since it has some selectivity for alpha receptors in the prostate.

Importance and management

Direct information is limited. Acute hypotension (dizziness, fainting) sometimes occurs unpredictably with the first dose of some $alpha_1$-blockers (particularly, alfuzosin, prazosin and terazosin; but see 'Alpha blockers', (p.67)), and this can be exaggerated if the patient takes or is already taking a beta-blocker or a calcium channel blocker (see 'Alpha blockers + Beta-blockers', below, and 'Alpha blockers + Calcium channel blockers', p.69). It would therefore seem prudent to apply the same precautions to ACE inhibitors, namely reducing the dose of the other antihypertensive to a maintenance level, then starting the alpha blocker at the lowest dose, with the first dose given at bedtime. Note that the acute hypotensive reaction appears to be short-lived. There is limited evidence that terazosin and tamsulosin may not cause an additional hypotensive effect in the longer term in patients with BPH who have hypertension already well-controlled with ACE inhibitors. Nevertheless, caution should be exercised in this situation, and a dose reduction of the ACE inhibitor may be required.

1. Baba T, Tomiyama T, Takebe K. Enhancement by an ACE inhibitor of first-dose hypotension caused by an $alpha_1$-blocker. *N Engl J Med* (1990) 322, 1237.
2. Xatral (Alfuzosin). Sanofi-Aventis. UK Summary of product characteristics, March 2003.
3. Hypovase (Prazosin). Pfizer Ltd. UK Summary of product characteristics, December 2004.
4. Minipress (Prazosin). Pfizer Inc. US Prescribing information, September 2000.
5. Kirby RS. Terazosin in benign prostatic hyperplasia: effects on blood pressure in normotensive and hypertensive men. *Br J Urol* (1998) 82, 373–9.
6. Hytrin (Terazosin). Abbott Laboratories Ltd. UK Summary of product characteristics, October 2000.
7. Lowe FC. Coadministration of tamsulosin and three antihypertensive agents in patients with benign prostatic hyperplasia: pharmacodynamic effect. *Clin Ther* (1997) 19, 730–42.

Alpha blockers + Beta-blockers

The risk of first-dose hypotension with prazosin is higher if the patient is already taking a beta-blocker. This is likely to be true of other alpha blockers, particularly alfuzosin, bunazosin and terazosin. In a small study tamsulosin did not have any clinically relevant effects on blood pressure that was already well controlled by atenolol. Alpha blockers and beta-blockers may be combined for additional lowering of blood pressure in patients with hypertension.

Clinical evidence

A marked hypotensive reaction (dizziness, pallor, sweating) occurred in 3 out of 6 hypertensive patients on **alprenolol** 400 mg twice daily when they were given the first 500-microgram dose of **prazosin**. All 6 patients had a greater reduction in blood pressure after the first **prazosin** dose than after 2 weeks of treatment with 500 microgram three times daily (mean reduction 22/11 mmHg compared with 4/4 mmHg). A further 3 patients already taking **prazosin** 500 microgram three times daily had no unusual fall in blood pressure when given the first dose of **alprenolol** 200 mg.[1] The severity and the duration of the first-dose effect of **prazosin** was also found to be increased in healthy subjects given a single dose of **propranolol** concurrently.[2] In a placebo-controlled study in 8 hypertensive men with blood pressure well controlled by **atenolol**, the addition of **tamsulosin** 400 micrograms daily for 7 days then 800 micrograms daily for a further 7 days had no clinically relevant effect on blood pressure (assessed after 6 and 14 days of **tamsulosin**). No hypotension was seen with the first dose of **tamsulosin** or when the dose of **tamsulosin** was increased.[3]

Retrospective analysis of a large multinational study in patients given 5 or 10 mg of **terazosin** daily found that **terazosin** only affected the blood pressure of patients taking beta blockers (**atenolol**, **labetalol**, **metoprolol**, **sotalol**, and **timolol**) if the blood pressure was uncontrolled. No change in blood pressure was seen in those with normal blood pressure (i.e. those without hypertension and those with hypertension controlled by beta blockers). The most common adverse effect in the 10-week **terazosin** phase was dizziness, and the incidence of this appeared to be lower in those on antihypertensives (13% to 16%) than those not (21% to 25%).[4]

No pharmacokinetic interaction occurred between **alfuzosin** 2.5 mg and **atenolol** 100 mg in a single-dose study in 8 healthy subjects.[5] The maker notes that postural hypotension may occur in patients receiving antihypertensives when they start **alfuzosin**.[6,7] Similarly, the maker of **indoramin** states that concurrent use with beta-blockers may enhance their hypotensive action, and that titration of the dose of the beta-blocker may be needed.[8]

The maker of **doxazosin** states that no adverse drug interaction has been observed between **doxazosin** and beta-blockers,[9,10] although they do note that the most common adverse reactions associated with **doxazosin** are of a postural hypotension type.[9]

Mechanism

The normal cardiovascular response (a compensatory increased heart output and rate) that should follow the first-dose hypotensive reaction to alpha blockers is apparently compromised by the presence of a beta-blocker. The problem is usually only short-lasting because some physiological compensation occurs within hours or days, and this allows the blood pressure to be lowered without falling precipitously. Tamsulosin possibly has less effect on blood pressure since it has some selectivity for alpha receptors in the prostate (see 'Alpha blockers', (p.67)). Two studies have shown that the pharmacokinetics of prazosin are not affected by either alprenolol[1] or propranolol.[11]

Importance and management

An established interaction. Some patients experience acute postural hypotension, tachycardia and palpitations when they begin to take prazosin or other alpha blockers (particularly alfuzosin, bunazosin and terazosin; but see also 'Alpha blockers', (p.67)). A few patients even collapse in a sudden faint within 30 to 90 minutes, and this can be exacerbated if they are already taking a beta-blocker. It is recommended that those already on beta-blockers should have their dose of beta-blocker reduced to a maintenance dose and begin with a low-dose of these alpha blockers, with the first dose taken just before going to bed. They should also be warned about the possibility of postural hypotension and how to manage it (i.e. lay down, raise the legs and get up slowly). Similarly, when adding a beta-blocker to an alpha blocker, it may be prudent to decrease the dose of the alpha blocker and re-titrate as necessary. There is limited evidence that terazosin and tamsulosin may not cause an additional hypotensive effect in the longer term in patients with BPH who have hypertension already well-controlled with beta-blockers. Nevertheless, caution should be exercised in this situation, and a dose reduction of the beta-blocker may be required.

1. Seideman P, Grahnén A, Haglund K, Lindström B, von Bahr C. Prazosin first dose phenomenon during combined treatment with a β-adrenoceptor in hypertensive patients. *Br J Clin Pharmacol* (1982) 13, 865–70.
2. Elliott HL, McLean K, Sumner DJ, Meredith PA, Reid JL. Immediate cardiovascular reponses to oral prazosin-effects of β-blockers. *Clin Pharmacol Ther* (1981) 29, 303–9.
3. Lowe FC. Coadministration of tamsulosin and three antihypertensive agents in patients with benign prostatic hyperplasia: pharmacodynamic effect. *Clin Ther* (1997) 19, 730–42.
4. Kirby RS. Terazosin in benign prostatic hyperplasia: effects on blood pressure in normotensive and hypertensive men. *Br J Urol* (1998) 82, 373–9.
5. Bianchetti G, Padovani P, Coupez JM, Guinebault P, Hermanns P, Coupez-Lopinot R, Guillet P, Thénot JP, Morselli PL. Pharmacokinetic interactions between hydrochlorothiazide, atenolol, and alfuzosin: a new antihypertensive drug. *Acta Pharmacol Toxicol (Copenh)* (1986) 59 (Suppl 5), 197.
6. Xatral (Alfuzosin). Sanofi-Aventis. UK Summary of product characteristics, March 2003.
7. Uroxatral (Alfuzosin). Sanofi-Synthelabo Inc. US Prescribing information, June 2003.
8. Doralese (Indoramin). GlaxoSmithKline UK. UK Summary of product characteristics, December 2003.
9. Cardura (Doxazosin). Pfizer Ltd. UK Summary of product characteristics, May 2003.
10. Cardura (Doxazosin). Pfizer Inc. US Prescribing information, April 2002.
11. Rubin P, Jackson G, Blaschke T. Studies on the clinical pharmacology of prazosin. II: The influence of indomethacin and of propranolol on the action and the disposition of prazosin. *Br J Clin Pharmacol* (1980) 10, 33–9.

Alpha blockers + Calcium channel blockers

Blood pressure may fall sharply when calcium channel blockers are first given to patients already taking alpha blockers (particularly prazosin and terazosin), and vice versa. In a small study, tamsulosin did not have any clinically relevant effects on blood pressure well controlled by nifedipine. Verapamil may increase the AUC of prazosin and terazosin. Alpha blockers and calcium channel blockers may be combined for additional blood pressure lowering in patients with hypertension.

Clinical evidence

(a) Dihydropyridine calcium channel blockers

Although there was a tendency for first-dose hypotension no serious adverse events or postural symptoms were seen in 6 normotensive subjects given **nifedipine** 20 mg twice daily for 20 days, with **doxazosin** 2 mg once daily for the last 10 days. The same results were noted in 6 other normotensive subjects given the drugs in the opposite order. No pharmacokinetic interactions were found.[1]

Two patients with severe hypertension given **prazosin** 4 or 5 mg experienced a sharp fall in blood pressure shortly after being given **nifedipine** *sublingually*. One of them complained of dizziness and had a fall in standing blood pressure from 232/124 to 88/48 mmHg about 20 minutes after taking **nifedipine** 10 mg. However, in a further 8 patients with hypertension taking prazosin the reduction in blood pressure 20 minutes after the addition of *sublingual* nifedipine was smaller (mean reduction of 25/12 mmHg when lying and 24/17 mmHg when standing).[2] However, it is not clear what contribution **prazosin** had to the effect seen with *sublingual* **nifedipine**, since the experiment was not repeated using a **prazosin** placebo but these patients' blood pressure had earlier remained unchanged 1 hour after taking prazosin alone. Note that *sublingual* **nifedipine** alone may cause dangerous falls in blood pressure.

Retrospective analysis of a large multinational study in patients given 5 or 10 mg of **terazosin** daily found that **terazosin** only affected the blood pressure of patients taking calcium channel blockers (**amlodipine**, **felodipine**, **flunarizine**, **isradipine** and **nifedipine**) if the blood pressure was uncontrolled. No change in blood pressure was seen in those with normal blood pressure (i.e. those without hypertension and those with hypertension controlled by calcium channel blockers). The most common adverse effect in the 10-week **terazosin** phase was dizziness, and the incidence of this appeared to be lower in those on antihypertensives (13% to 16%) than those not (21% to 25%).[3]

In a placebo-controlled study in 7 hypertensive men, with blood pressure well controlled by **nifedipine**, the addition of **tamsulosin** 400 micrograms daily for 7 days then 800 micrograms daily for a further 7 days had no clinically relevant effect on blood pressure (assessed after 6 and 14 days of **tamsulosin**). In addition, no first-dose hypotension was seen on the first day of **tamsulosin**, or on increasing the dose.[4]

(b) Verapamil

A study in 8 normotensive subjects given single 1-mg doses of **prazosin** showed that the peak serum **prazosin** levels were raised by 85% (from 5.2 to 9.6 nanograms/ml) and the **prazosin** AUC increased by 62% when it was given with a single 160-mg dose of verapamil. The standing blood pressure, which was unchanged after verapamil alone, fell from 114/82 to 99/81 mmHg when **prazosin** was given alone, and was further reduced to 89/68 mmHg when both drugs were given together.[5] A similar pharmacokinetic interaction was noted in another study in hypertensive patients.[6] In this study, the first 1-mg dose of **prazosin** alone caused a 23 mmHg fall in standing systolic blood pressure, and half the patients (3 of 6) experienced symptomatic postural hypotension. A similar fall in blood pressure occurred when the first 1-mg dose of **prazosin** was given to 6 patients who had been taking verapamil for 5 days, and 2 patients experienced symptomatic postural hypotension.[6]

When verapamil 120 mg twice daily was added to **terazosin** 5 mg daily in 12 hypertensive patients, the peak plasma levels and the AUC of the **terazosin** were increased by about 25%. In contrast, no changes in verapamil pharmacokinetics occurred when **terazosin** (1 mg increased to 5 mg daily) was added to verapamil 120 mg twice daily in another 12 patients.[7] Both groups of patients had significant falls in standing blood pressure when the combination therapy was first started. Symptomatic orthostatic hypotension (which lessened within about 3 weeks) occurred in 4 patients when verapamil was first added to **terazosin**, and in 2 patients when **terazosin** was first added to verapamil.[7]

Mechanism

Not fully understood. It would seem that the vasodilatory effects of the alpha blockers and the calcium channel blockers can be additive or synergistic, particularly after the first dose.[1,8] The fall in blood pressure seen with prazosin and verapamil may, in part, result from a pharmacokinetic interaction.[8] Tamsulosin possibly has less effect on blood pressure since it has some selectivity for alpha receptors in the prostate (see 'Alpha blockers', (p.67)).

Importance and management

The interaction between calcium channel blockers and alpha blockers would appear to be established and of clinical importance, although the documentation is limited. Marked additive hypotensive effects can occur when concurrent therapy is started, particularly with alfuzosin, bunazosin, prazosin and terazosin; but see also 'Alpha blockers', (p.67). It is recommended that patients already on calcium channel blockers should have their dose of calcium channel blocker reduced and begin with a low-dose of alpha blocker, with the first dose taken just before going to bed. Caution should also be exercised when calcium channel blockers are added to established alpha-blocker therapy. Patients should be warned about the possibilities of exaggerated hypotension, and told what to do if they feel faint and dizzy. There is limited evidence that terazosin and tamsulosin may not cause an additional hypotensive effect in the longer term in patients with BPH who have hypertension already well-controlled with calcium channel blockers. Nevertheless, caution should be exercised in this situation, and a dose reduction of the calcium channel blocker may be required.

1. Donnelly R, Elliott HL, Meredith PA, Howie CA, Reid JL. The pharmacodynamics and pharmacokinetics of the combination of nifedipine and doxazosin. *Eur J Clin Pharmacol* (1993) 44, 279–82.
2. Jee LD, Opie LH. Acute hypotensive response to nifedipine added to prazosin in treatment of hypertension. *BMJ* (1983) 287, 1514.
3. Kirby RS. Terazosin in benign prostatic hyperplasia: effects on blood pressure in normotensive and hypertensive men. *Br J Urol* (1998) 82, 373–9.
4. Lowe FC. Coadministration of tamsulosin and three antihypertensive agents in patients with benign prostatic hyperplasia: pharmacodynamic effect. *Clin Ther* (1997) 19, 730–42.
5. Pasanisi F, Elliott HL, Meredith PA, McSharry DR, Reid JL. Combined alpha adrenoceptor antagonism and calcium channel blockade in normal subjects. *Clin Pharmacol Ther* (1984) 36, 716–23.
6. Elliott HL, Meredith PA, Campbell L, Reid JL. The combination of prazosin and verapamil in the treatment of essential hypertension. *Clin Pharmacol Ther* (1988) 43, 554–60.

7. Lenz ML, Pool JL, Laddu AR, Varghese A, Johnston W, Taylor AA. Combined terazosin and verapamil therapy in essential hypertension. Hemodynamic and pharmacodynamic interactions. *Am J Hypertens* (1995) 8, 133–45.
8. Meredith PA, Elliott HL. An additive or synergistic drug interaction: application of concentration-effect modeling. *Clin Pharmacol Ther* (1992) 51, 708–14.

Alpha blockers + Cimetidine

No important interaction occurs with cimetidine and either alfuzosin or tamsulosin.

Clinical evidence, mechanism, importance and management

Cimetidine 1 g daily in divided doses for 20 days was found to have minimal effects on the pharmacokinetics of single 5-mg doses of **alfuzosin** in 10 healthy subjects. The maximum serum levels and the AUC were increased by up to 24%, (not statistically significant) and the half-life was shortened by 14%. Cimetidine did not appear to increase the incidence of postural hypotension seen with **alfuzosin**.[1] These changes are not clinically relevant, and there would seem to be no reason for avoiding concurrent use.

The UK maker of **tamsulosin** notes that concurrent use of cimetidine causes a rise in plasma levels of **tamsulosin**, but as levels remain within the normal range, they consider that no dosage adjustment is necessary.[2] However, note that the US makers say that caution should be used, particularly with doses greater then 400 micrograms.[3]

1. Desager JP, Harvengt C, Bianchetti G, Rosenzweig P. The effect of cimetidine on the pharmacokinetics of single oral doses of alfuzosin. *Int J Clin Pharmacol Ther Toxicol* (1993) 31, 568–71.
2. Flomax MR (Tamsulosin). Yamanouchi Pharma Ltd. UK Summary of product characteristics, July 2001.
3. Flomax (Tamsulosin). Boehringer Ingelheim Pharmaceuticals Inc. US Prescribing information, August 2002.

Alpha blockers + Diuretics

Patients with congestive heart failure, who have had large doses of diuretics, should start prazosin treatment with low doses. Alpha blockers and diuretics may be combined for additional blood pressure lowering in patients with hypertension. An increased incidence of dizziness has been noted with the combination of terazosin and a diuretic. In patients with BPH, terazosin, in the presence or absence of diuretics, had no additional antihypertensive effect in those with controlled blood pressure, but did reduce blood pressure in those with uncontrolled hypertension.

Clinical evidence, mechanism, importance and management

The acute first-dose hypotension that can occur with alpha blockers such as **prazosin** can be exacerbated by beta-blockers and calcium channel blockers (see 'Alpha blockers + Beta-blockers', p.68 and 'Alpha blockers + Calcium channel blockers', p.69), but there seems to be no direct evidence that diuretics normally do the same. However, the maker of **prazosin** suggests that it is particularly important that patients with congestive heart failure who have undergone vigorous diuretic treatment should be given the initial dose of **prazosin** at bedtime and the lowest dose (500 micrograms two to four times daily) to start with. The reason is that left ventricular filling pressure may decrease in these patients with a resultant fall in cardiac output and systemic blood pressure.[1,2] There seems to be no reason for avoiding concurrent use if these precautions are taken.

Retrospective analysis of a large multinational study in patients given 5 or 10 mg of **terazosin** daily found that **terazosin** only affected the blood pressure of patients taking diuretics (**amiloride**, **bendroflumethiazide**, **chlortalidone**, **hydrochlorothiazide** and **spironolactone**) if the blood pressure was uncontrolled. No change in blood pressure was seen in those with normal blood pressure (i.e. those without hypertension and those with hypertension controlled by diuretics). The most common adverse effect in the 10-week **terazosin** phase was dizziness, and the incidence of this appeared to be lower in those on antihypertensives (13% and 16%) than those not (21% and 25%).[3] However, the UK maker of **terazosin** notes that the incidence of dizziness in patients with benign prostatic hyperplasia treated with **terazosin** was higher when they were also receiving a diuretic.[4] Similarly, in clinical trials in patients with hypertension, a higher proportion experienced dizziness when treated with **terazosin** plus a diuretic compared with placebo plus a diuretic (20% vs 13%).[5] The maker states that when **terazosin** is added to a diuretic, dose reduction and retitration may be necessary.[4,6]

No pharmacokinetic interaction occurred between **alfuzosin** 5 mg and **hydrochlorothiazide** 25 mg in a single-dose study in 8 healthy subjects.[7] The maker notes that postural hypotension may occur in patients receiving antihypertensive medications when they start **alfuzosin**.[8] Similarly, the maker of **indoramin** states that concurrent use with diuretics may enhance their hypotensive action, and that titration of the dose of the diuretic may be needed.[9]

The maker of **tamsulosin** states that concomitant **furosemide** decreases plasma levels of **tamsulosin**, but that as levels remain within the normal range no change in dosage is necessary.[10,11]

The maker of **doxazosin** notes that no adverse drug interaction has been observed between **doxazosin** and **thiazides**[12,13] or **furosemide**.[12]

1. Invicta Pharmaceuticals. Personal communication, 1995.
2. Hypovase (Prazosin). Pfizer Ltd. UK Summary of product characteristics, December 2004.
3. Kirby RS. Terazosin in benign prostatic hyperplasia: effects on blood pressure in normotensive and hypertensive men. *Br J Urol* (1998) 82, 373–9.
4. Hytrin (Terazosin). Abbott Laboratories Ltd. UK Summary of product characteristics, October 2000.
5. Rudd P. Cumulative experience with terazosin administered in combination with diuretics. *Am J Med* (1986) 80 (Suppl 5B), 49–54.
6. Hytrin (Terazosin). Abbott Laboratories. US Prescribing information, February 2001.
7. Bianchetti G, Padovani P, Coupez JM, Guinebault P, Hermanns P, Coupez-Lopinot R, Guillet P, Thénot JP, Morselli PL. Pharmacokinetic interactions between hydrochlorothiazide, atenolol, and alfuzosin: a new antihypertensive drug. *Acta Pharmacol Toxicol (Copenh)* (1986) 59 (Suppl 5), 197.
8. Xatral (Alfuzosin). Sanofi-Aventis. UK Summary of product characteristics, March 2003.
9. Doralese (Indoramin). GlaxoSmithKline UK. UK Summary of product characteristics, December 2003.
10. Flomax MR (Tamsulosin). Yamanouchi Pharma Ltd. UK Summary of product characteristics, July 2001.
11. Flomax (Tamsulosin). Boehringer Ingelheim Pharmaceuticals Inc. US Prescribing information, August 2002.
12. Cardura (Doxazosin). Pfizer Ltd. UK Summary of product characteristics, May 2003.
13. Cardura (Doxazosin). Pfizer Inc. US Prescribing information, April 2002.

Alpha blockers + Miscellaneous

The makers of prazosin say that there is clinical experience of it being administered without any adverse interactions with the following drugs: antiarrhythmics (procainamide, quinidine), antigout agents (allopurinol, colchicine, probenecid), benzodiazepines (diazepam, chlordiazepoxide), dextropropoxyphene (propoxyphene), hypoglycaemic agents (insulin, chlorpropamide, phenformin, tolazamide, tolbutamide) and phenobarbital.[1,2] Similarly, the makers of doxazosin say that no adverse interactions have been observed with oral hypoglycaemic drugs[3,4] or uricosuric agents.[3]

1. Hypovase (Prazosin), Pfizer Ltd. UK Summary of product characteristics, December 2004.
2. Minipress (Prazosin). Pfizer Inc. US Prescribing information, September 2000.
3. Cardura (Doxazosin). Pfizer Ltd. UK Summary of product characteristics, May 2003.
4. Cardura (Doxazosin). Pfizer Inc. US Prescribing information, April 2002.

Alpha blockers + NSAIDs

Indometacin reduces the blood-pressure lowering effects of prazosin in some individuals. Other alpha blockers appear not to interact with NSAIDs.

Clinical evidence

A study in 9 healthy subjects found that **indometacin** 50 mg twice daily for 3 days had no statistically significant effect on the hypotensive effect of a single 5-mg dose of **prazosin**. However, in 4 of the subjects it was noted that the maximum fall in the mean standing blood pressure due to the **prazosin** was 20 mmHg less when they were taking **indometacin**. Three of these 4 felt faint when given **prazosin** alone, but not while taking the **indometacin** as well.[1]

Mechanism

Not established. It seems probable that indometacin inhibits the production of hypotensive prostaglandins by the kidney.

Importance and management

Direct information seems to be limited to this study but what occurred is consistent with the way indometacin reduces the effects of many other different antihypertensives (e.g. see 'ACE inhibitors + NSAIDs', p.27, and 'Beta-blockers + Aspirin or NSAIDs', p.626). It apparently does not affect every subject. If indometacin is added to established treatment with prazosin, be alert for a reduced antihypertensive response, although it is not known exactly what happens in patients taking both drugs long-term. However, the makers say that prazosin has been given with indometacin (and also **aspirin** and **phenylbutazone**) without any adverse interaction in clinical experience to date.[2,3] Other makers also note that no adverse interaction has been seen between **doxazosin** or **terazosin** and NSAIDs (unspecified),[4,5] or **aspirin**, **ibuprofen**, or indometacin.[6,7]

1. Rubin P, Jackson G, Blaschke T. Studies on the clinical pharmacology of prazosin. II: The influence of indomethacin and of propranolol on the action and disposition of prazosin. *Br J Clin Pharmacol* (1980) 10, 33–9.
2. Hypovase (Prazosin). Pfizer Ltd. UK Summary of product characteristics. December 2004.
3. Minipress (Prazosin). Pfizer Inc. US Prescribing information, September 2000.
4. Cardura (Doxazosin). Pfizer Ltd. UK Summary of product characteristics, May 2003.
5. Hytrin (Terazosin). Abbott Laboratories Ltd. UK Summary of product characteristics, October 2000.
6. Cardura (Doxazosin). Pfizer Inc. US Prescribing information, April 2002.
7. Hytrin (Terazosin). Abbott Laboratories. US Prescribing information, February 2001.

Bunazosin + Rifampicin (Rifampin)

Rifampicin markedly reduces bunazosin serum levels.

Clinical evidence, mechanism, importance and management

A 7-day course of rifampicin (rifampin) 600 mg daily reduced the mean maximum serum levels of bunazosin 6 mg daily in 15 healthy subjects by 82% (from 11.6 to 2.1 nanograms/ml). The bunazosin AUC was reduced more than sevenfold (from 151 to 20 micrograms/l). The duration of blood-pressure lowering effect was shortened, the heart rate increase was less pronounced, and some adverse effects of bunazosin treatment (fatigue, headache) disappeared.[1,2] The probable reason is that the rifampicin (a recognised, potent liver-enzyme inducing agent) increases the metabolism of the bunazosin by the liver so that it is lost from the body much more quickly.

The evidence seems to be limited to this study, but anticipate the need to raise the bunazosin dosage if rifampicin is added. Information about other alpha-blockers does not seem to be available.

1. Al-Hamdan Y, Otto U, Kirch W. Interaction of rifampicin with bunazosin, an alpha$_1$-adrenoceptor antagonist. *J Clin Pharmacol* (1993) 33, 998.
2. Nokhodian A, Halabi A, Ebert U, Al-Hamdan Y, Kirch W. Interaction of rifampicin with bunazosin, an α_1-adrenoceptor antagonist, in healthy volunteers. *Drug Invest* (1993) 6, 362–4.

Indoramin + Miscellaneous

The makers of indoramin warn about additive sedative effects with CNS depressants. Based on early theoretical considerations, they contraindicated its use with MAOIs.

Clinical evidence, mechanism, importance and management

Indoramin sometimes causes drowsiness, and this effect may possibly be additive with that of other **CNS depressants**, including **alcohol** (see also 'Alcohol + Indoramin', p.55).

Concurrent use of **MAOIs** is contraindicated by the makers of indoramin.[1] This was included in the datasheet at the time indoramin was first licensed, and was based on a theoretical suggestion that the effects of noradrenaline (norepinephrine) may be potentiated,[2] leading to vasoconstriction with a possible increase in blood pressure. However, the pharmacology of these drugs suggests just the opposite, namely that hypotension is the more likely outcome. (Note that the hypertensive effects of noradrenaline (norepinephrine) may be treated with a non-selective alpha blocker such as phentolamine.) The makers are not aware of any reported interactions between indoramin and **MAOIs**.[2] Note that the **MAOIs** are not contraindicated with any of the other alpha blockers.

1. Doralese (Indoramin). GlaxoSmithKline UK. UK Summary of product characteristics, December 2003.
2. GlaxoSmithKline. Personal communication, August 2003.

5

Analgesics and NSAIDs

The drugs dealt with in this section include aspirin and other salicylates, non-aspirin NSAIDs, opioid analgesics, and the miscellaneous analgesics nefopam and paracetamol. 'Table 5.1', (p.73) contains a listing, with further classification, and proprietary names.

Interactions

(a) Aspirin and NSAIDs

Aspirin and the NSAIDs generally undergo few pharmacokinetic interactions. The majority are highly protein bound, and have the potential to interact with other drugs via this mechanism. However, with a few exceptions, most of these interactions are not clinically important (see 'Protein binding interactions', (p.3)). Of the newer NSAIDs, celecoxib is metabolised by the cytochrome P450 isoenzyme CYP2C9, and inhibits CYP2D6.

Most of the important interactions with NSAIDs and aspirin are pharmacodynamic. Aspirin and all non-selective NSAIDs inhibit platelet aggregation, and so can increase the risk of bleeding and interact with other drugs that have this effect. NSAIDs that are highly selective for cyclo-oxygenase-2 (COX-2) do not inhibit platelet aggregation.

Aspirin and all NSAIDs (including COX-2 selective NSAIDs) affect the synthesis of renal prostaglandins, and so can cause salt and water retention. This can increase blood pressure and affect antihypertensive therapy.

Aspirin and non-selective NSAIDs prevent the mechanisms to protect the gastrointestinal mucosal and so cause gastrointestinal toxicity. COX-2 selective NSAIDs (coxibs) are less likely to have this effect.

(b) Opioids

Morphine is metabolised by glucuronidation by UDP-glucuronyltransferases, mainly to one active and one inactive metabolite. The glucuronidation of morphine can be induced or inhibited by various drugs. Morphine is not affected by the cytochrome P450 isoenzymes. The semi-synthetic morphine analogues, hydromorphone and oxymorphone, are also principally metabolised by glucuronidation and are not affected by cytochrome P450 isoenzymes.

Codeine, dihydrocodeine, and hydrocodone are probably pro-drugs, and require metabolic activation, possibly by CYP2D6 or UGT enzymes. Inhibitors of these enzymes may therefore reduce their efficacy. Oxycodone is also metabolised by CYP2D6 and CYP3A4. Buprenorphine is metabolised by CYP3A4.

Methadone is principally metabolised by CYP3A4 and CYP2D6, although CYP2C8 may also play a role.

Alfentanil is extensively metabolised by CYP3A4, and has been used as a probe drug for assessing CYP3A4 activity. Fentanyl and sufentanil are also metabolised, but because they are high-hepatic-extraction drugs (see 'Changes in first-pass metabolism', (p.4)) they show less effect with inhibitors or inducers of CYP3A4, although this may still be clinically important.

(c) Paracetamol

Paracetamol is not absorbed from the stomach, and the rate of absorption is well correlated with the gastric emptying rate. Paracetamol has therefore been used as a marker drug in studies of gastric emptying. Paracetamol is primarily metabolised by the liver to a variety of metabolites, principally the glucuronide and sulfate conjugates. Hepatotoxicity of paracetamol is thought to be due to a minor metabolite, N-acetyl-p-benzoquinone imine (NAPQI), which is inactivated with glutathione and excreted as mercapturate and cysteine conjugates. When the liver stores of glutathione are depleted, and the rate of production of NAPQI exceeds the rate of production of glutathione, excess NAPQI attaches to liver protein and causes liver damage. CYP2E1 may be involved in the formation of this hepatotoxic metabolite.

General references

1. Brouwers JRBJ, de Smet PAGM. Pharmacokinetic-pharmacodynamic drug interactions with nonsteroidal anti-inflammatory drugs. *Clin Pharmacokinet* (1994) 27, 462–5.
2. Rumack BH. Acetaminophen hepatotoxicity: the first 35 years. *J Toxicol Clin Toxicol* (2002) 40, 3–20.
3. Armstrong AC, Cozza KL. Pharmacokinetic drug interactions of morphine, codeine, and their derivatives: theory and clinical reality, Part I. *Psychosomatics* (2003) 44, 167–71.
4. Armstrong AC, Cozza KL. Pharmacokinetic drug interactions of morphine, codeine, and their derivatives: theory and clinical reality, Part II. *Psychosomatics* (2003) 44, 515–20.

Table 5.1 Analgesics and NSAIDs

Generic names	*Proprietary names*
Aspirin and oral salicylates	
Aloxiprin	Superpyrin
Aspirin	AAS, Acekapton, Acenterine, Acesal, Aceticil, Acetin, Acetosal, Acitab, Actorin, Acylpyrin, Adiro, Adprin-B, Aggrenox, Albyl minor, Albyl-E, Alcacyl instantanee, Alka-Seltzer, Analgesin, Angettes, Anopyrin, Antacsal, Antifebrin, Apo-Asa, Arthritis Pain Formula, ASA, Asaflow, Asaphen, ASA-ratio, Ascot, Ascriptin, ASL, Aspec, Aspegic, Aspent, Aspergum, Aspicalm, Aspicot, Aspidol, Aspiglicina, Aspilets, Aspiricor, Aspirin Cardio, Aspirin Protect, Aspirin with Stomach Guard, Aspirina, Aspirina 03, Aspirine, Aspirine Cardio, Aspirine pH8, Aspirine Protect, Aspirinetas, Aspirinetta, Aspirisucre, Aspisol, Asprimox, Aspro, ASS, Astrix, Bamyl, Bamyl S, Bayaspirina, Bayer Low Adult Strength, Bioplak, Buffered Pirin, Bufferin, Buffex, Caas, Cama Arthritis Pain Reliever, Caparin, Caprin, Cardegic, Cardioaspirin, Cardioaspirina, Cardioaspirine, Cardiosolupsan, Cardiprin, Cardirene, Cartia, Casprin, Catalgine, Cemirit, Cimaas, Claragine, Colfarit, Colsprin, Coraspir, Corplus, Decitriol, Delisprin, Desenfriolito, Disgren, Disperin, Dispril, Disprin, Disprin Direct, Disprina, Dolorosan, Dusil, Easprin, Ecasil, Ecoprin, Ecosprin, Ecotrin, Egicalm, Emotpin, Empirin, Enprin, Entrarin, Entrophen, Equate, Extra Strength Bayer Plus, Flectadol, Geniol AP, Geniol SC sin Cafeina, Geniolito, Genprin, Globoid, Glyprin, Godamed, Godasal, Halfprin, Hassapirin Puro, Herz ASS, HerzASS, Herzschutz ASS, Hipotermal, Hjerdyl, Hjertemagnyl, Idotyl, Inyesprin, Istopirin, Juridin, Jusprin, Kalmopyrin, Kardegic, Kardiren, Kilios, LAsprin, Lisaspin, Lowasa, Magnaprin, Magnecyl, Magnyl, Micropirin, Midolen, Migraspirina, Miniasal, Myoprin, Norwich Extra Strength, Novasen, Nuevapina, Nu-Seals, Okal, PostMI, Primaspan, Propirin, Pure Health, Regular Strength Bayer, Resprin, Rhonal, Rivasa, Salicil, Salimont, Salospir, Salycilina, Santasal N, Saspryl, Sedergine, Seferin, Solprin, Somalgin, Spren, St. Joseph Adult Chewable, Tevapirin, Therasa, Thrombace Neo, Thrombo AS, Thrombo ASS, Thrombostad, Tiatral 100 SR, Tiplac, Togal ASS, Togal Mono, Toldex, Tri-Buffered ASA, Tromalyt, Trombyl, Upsalgin-N, Upsarin, V-AS, Vincent's Powders, ZORprin
Benorilate	Benoral, Duvium, Salipran
Choline salicylate	Aldo Otico, Applicaine, Arthropan, Audax, Bonjela, Bucagel, Cholisal, Dercolina, Dermojela, Dinnefords Teejel, Earex Plus, Gelora, Givalex, Mundisal, Ora-Sed, Ora-Sed Jel, Paidoterin Descongestivo NF, Pansoral, Seda-Gel, Soragel, Teejel, Tenderol, Zytee
Diflunisal	Analeric, Artrodol, Diflusal, Dolobid, Dolocid, Donobid, Flunidor, Fluniget
Ethenzamide	
Lysine aspirin	Alcacyl instantanee, ASL, Aspegic, Aspegic Codeine, Aspicalm, Aspidol, Aspisol, Cardegic, Cardiosolupsan, Cardirene, Coraspir, Corplus, Decitriol, Dolorosan, Dolotol 12, Egicalm, Flectadol, Inyesprin, Kardegic, Kardiren, Lisaspin, Migpriv, Migrafin, Migraprim, Premig, Tiplac
Magnesium salicylate	Backache Maximum Strength Relief, Bayer Select Maximum Strength Backache, Cholagol, Doans, Extra Strength Doans PM, Magan, Mobidin, Mobigesic, Momentum Muscular Backache Formula, Novasal, Nuprin Backache, Painaid BRF Back Relief Formula, Rati Salil E, Tetra-Mag
Salsalate	Amigesic, Argesic-SA, Artha-G, Disalcid, Marthritic, Salflex, Salsitab
Sodium salicylate	A Saude da Mulher, Angino-Rub, Antiseptic Mouthwash, Brulex, Colphen, Cystex, Doans Backache Pills, Dodds, Gly Thymol, Glyco-Thymoline, Hairscience Shampoo, Ilvico, Jackson's Pain & Fever, Pilulas De Witt's, Plax, Saliject, Scot-Tussin Original 5-Action, TCP, Theinol, Tussirex
NSAIDs	
Fenamates	
Floctafenine	Idarac
Flufenamic acid	Algesalona, Assan, Mobilisin, Movilisin, Rheugesal, Dignodolin, Rheuma Lindofluid
Meclofenamic acid	Lenidolor, Movens
Mefenamic acid	Acinic, Aidol, Algifemin, Artriden, Beafemic, Conamic, Coslan, Dolcin, Dolfenal , Femen, Fenamic, Fenamin, Flipal, Gandin, Hamitan, Hostan, Lysalgo, Manic, Manomic , Masafen , Medicap, Mednil, Mefa, Mefac, Mefamic, mefe-basan, Mefen, Mefenacide, Mefenan, Mefenix, Mefic, Melur, Mephadolor, Namic, Namifen, Napan, Painnox, Panamic, Parkemed, Ponac, Ponalar, Ponalgic, Ponmel, Ponnesia, Ponstan, Ponstel, Ponstil, Ponstyl, Pontacid, Pontalon, Pontin, Prostan, Pynamic, Sefmic, Sicadol, Spiralgin, Tanston, Templadol, Vidan
Tolfenamic acid	Bifenac, Clotam, Fenamic, Flocur, Gantil, Migea, Polmonin, Purfalox, Rociclyn, Tolfamic, Turbaund
Indole- and indene-acetic acids	
Acemetacin	Acemetadoc, Acemix, Emflex, Espledol, Gamespir, Oldan, Rantudal, Rantudil, Rheutrop, Solart, Tilur
Indometacin (Indomethacin)	Acuflex, Adco-Indogel, Aflamin, Agilex, Agilisin, Aliviosin, Ammi-Indocin, Antalgin, Arthrexin, Artrinovo, Autritis, Begincalm, Betacin, Bonidon, Bucin, Catlep, Chrono-Indocid, Cidomel, Confortid, Docin , Dolcidium, Dolcispray, Dolovin, Dometin, Elmego, Elmetacin, Flamaret, Flamecid, Flexidin, Flexin Continus, Flexono, Flogoter, Fortathrin, Grindocin, Hastel, Idc, Idicin, IM 75, Inacid, Indo, Indo Top, Indobene, Indocaf, Indocap, Indocarsil, Indocid, Indocid Colirio, Indocid PDA, Indocin, Indocolir, Indocollirio, Indocollyre, Indocontin, Indohexal, Indolar SR, Indolgina, Indom, Indoman, Indomax, Indomed, Indomee, Indomelan, Indomen, Indomethol, Indometin, Indomet-ratiopharm, Indomod, Indonilo, Indono, Indopaed, Indophtal, Indoptol, Indotard, Indotex, Indotrin, Indovis, Indoxen, Inflamate, Inflam, Infree, Inthacine, Italon, Itapredin, Klonametacina, Liometacen, Luiflex, Malival, Mederreumol, Mediflex, Metacen, Metacidil, Methocaps, Metindo, Mobilat Akut Indo, Moviflex, Neo Decabutin, Nisaid, Novo-Methacin, Nu-Indo, Pardelprin, Ralicid, Restameth-SR, Reumacid, Reumadolor, Reusin, Rheubalmin Indo, Rheumacin, Rhodacine, Rimacid, Rothacin, Satogesic, Slo-Indo, Vonum Cutan
Sulindac	Aclin, Algocetil, Apo-Sulin, Arthrocine, Artribid, Bio-Dac, Cenlidac, Clinoril, Copal, Daclin, Kenalin, Novo-Sundac, Sulindal

Continued

Table 5.1 Analgesics and NSAIDs *(continued)*

Generic names	*Proprietary names*
Oxicams	
Lornoxicam	Acabel, Artok, Bosporon, Lorcam, Lornox, Noxon, Taigalor, Telos, Xefo, Xefocam
Meloxicam	Aflamid, Alivian, Anposel, Bioflac, Coxflam, Dormelox, Ecax, Exel, Flexidol, Hyflex, Inicox, Isox, Leutrol, Lonaflam, Loxam, Loxibest, Loxiflam, Loxiflan, Loxitan, Loxitenk, Masflex, Melflam, Mel-OD, Melodol, Melosteral, Melotec, Melox, Meloxigran, Meloxil, Melpor, Melstar, Merapiran, Mevamox, Miogesil, Mobec, Mobex, Mobic, Mobicox, Movacox, Movalis, Movatec, Movicox, Movoxicam, Parocin, Rafree, Skudal, Telaroid, Tenaron, Uticox, Ziloxican, Zix
Piroxicam	Algoxam, Ammidene, Anartrit, Androxicam, Anflene, Antiflog, Arthremin, Artinor, Artroxicam, Artyflam, Axis, Baxo, Benisan, Bioximil, Bleduran, Brexecam, Brexicam, Brexic-DT, Brexidol, Brexin, Brexine, Brexinil, Brexivel, Brexodin, Brionot, Bruxicam, Calmapir, Candyl-D, Cicladol, Ciclafast, Citoken T, Clevian, clinit, Conzila, CP-Pirox, Cycladol, Dexicam, Dixonal, Doblexan, Dolonex, Dolzycam, durapirox, Erazon, Euroxi, Exipan, Fabopxicam, Fabudol, Facicam, Felcam, Feldegel, Felden, Feldene, Feldox, Felrox, Felxicam, Finalgel, Flamexin, Flamic, Flamostat, Flexar, Flexase, Flodeneu, Flodol, Flogene, Flogocan, Flogosine, Flogoxen, Floxicam, Foldox, Geldene, Glandicin, Homocalmefyba, Hotemin, Huma-Pirocam, Ifemed, Improntal, Inflaced, Inflamene, Inflanan, Inflanox, Inflax, Ipsoflog, Jenapirox, Ketazon, Lampoflex, Lisedema, Manoxicam , Maswin, Micar, Mobicam DT, Mobilat Akut Piroxicam, Mobilis, Movon, Moxicam, Nac, Nalgesic, Neo Axedil, Neogel, Neotica, Notagol, Novo-Pirocam, Nu-Pirox, Osteocalmine, Osteral, Oxicam, Oxicanol, Painrelipt-D, PC-20, Pedifan, Pemar, Pericam, Piram, Piram-D, Pirax, Piro, Piro KD, Piroalgin, Pirobeta, Pirocal, Pirocam, Pirodax, Pirofix, Piroflam, Piroftal, Pirohexal-D, Pirom, Pirorheum, PirorheumA, Pirosol, Pirox, Piroxal, Piroxan, Piroxcin, Piroxen, Piroxene, Piroxica, Piroxifen, Piroxiflam, Piroxil, Piroxin, Piroxiplus, Piroxistad, Piroxsil, Pixicam, Polipirox, Polyxicam, Posedene, Pricam, Prodoxidil, Proponol, Pro-Roxikam, Proxalyoc, Pyrocaps, Pyroxy, Reucam, Reumador, Reumagil, Reumoxican, Reutricam, Rheugesic, Rheumaplus, Rheumitin, Riacen, Roccaxin, Rosiden, Roxazin, Roxene, Roxenil, Roxicam, Roxiden, Roxifen, Roxium, Roxycam, R-Tyflam, Rumadene, Rumaxicam , Ruvamed, Salvacam, Sasulen, Sefdene, Sinartrol, Sindrolen, Solicam, Solocalm, Sotilen, Spirox, Suganril, Synoxicam, Tirovel, Tonimed, Tricifa, Truxa, Truxa R, Uphaxicam, Valopon, Vefren, Velaned, Vidapirocam, Vitaxicam, Xicam, Xycam, Zerospam, Zitumex
Tenoxicam	Admiral, Alganex, Algin-Vek, Amcinafal, Ampirovix, Artriunic, Artroxicam, Artruic, Aspagin, Avancel, Biodruff, Bioflam, Bioreucam, Calibral, Docticam, Dolmen, Doxican, Dranat, Hobaticam, Indo-bros, Istotosal, Liaderyl, Mefenix, Memzotil, Mitrotil, Mobiflex, Nadamen, Neo-adlibamin, Neo-antiperstam, Neo-endusix, Octiveran, Oxytel, Ponsolit, Recaflex, Redac, Reutenox, Rexalgan, Seftil, Sinoral, Soral, Teconam, Teflan, Tenalgin, Tenax, Tenocam, Tenotec, Tenox, Tenoxen, Tenoxil, Tentepanil, Texicam, Tilatil, Tilcitin, Tilcotil, Tiloxican, Tobitil, Tonox, Toscacalm, Velasor, Voir, Zibelant
Phenylacetic acid derivatives	
Alclofenac	
Diclofenac	3-A, 3A Ofteno, Abitren, Acoflam, Agilomed, Agofenac, Ainedif, Aktiosan, Algefit, Algosenac, Allvoran, Almiral, Alsidexten, Amminac, Ammi-Votara, Ana-Flex, Analpan, Anthraxiton, Apo-Diclo, Arcanafenac, Arclonac, Arthotec, Arthrotec, Arthru-Derm, Artotec, Artren, Artrenac, Artrenac Pro, Artrotec, Athrofen, Atomo Desinflamante Geldic, Augelit, Autdol, Banoclus, Bel-Gel, Benevran, Betaren, Biofenac, Blokium, Cataflam, Catanac, Chinclonac, Clo-Far, Clofaren, Clofec, Clofenac, Clofenak, Clofen, Clofon, Clonac, Clonodifen, Cofenac, Curinflam, Damixa, Dealgic, Declofon, Dedolor, Defanac, Deflamat, Deflamm, Deflox, Delimon, Deltaflogin, Deltaren, Demac, Denaclof, Desinflam, Desinflex, Dexomon, DFN, Di Retard, Diastone, Dicfafena, Diclac, Diclax, Diclaxol, Diclo P, Diclo-B, diclo-basan, Diclobene, Diclocular, Diclodan, Diclo-Denk, Diclo, Diclo-Divido, Diclodoc, Diclofan, Diclofen, Diclofenbeta, Dicloflex, Dicloftal, Dicloftil, Diclo-Gel, Diclogenom, Diclogesic, Diclogrand, Diclohexal, Diclolan, Diclomar, Diclomax, Diclomel, Diclomelan, Diclometin, Diclomex, Diclomol, Diclomol, Diclon, Diclonac, Diclophlogont, Dicloplast, Diclo-Puren, Dicloral, Dicloran, Diclorengel, Dicloreum, Diclo-saar, Diclosian, Diclosifar, Diclostad, Diclosyl, Diclotears, Diclovit, Diclovol, Diclozip, Dicogel, Difelene, Difenac, Difenan, Difend, Difen, Difene, Difenet, Difeno, Difenol, Difnal, Difnan, Dignofenac, Dinac, Dinaclon, Dinefec, Dioxaflex, Dirret, Disipan, Dnaren, Dofen, Doflex, Dolaren, Dolaut, Dolflam, Dolgit-Diclo, Dolmina, Dolo Nervobion, Dolo Tomanil, Dolocide K, Dolocide Plus, Dolotren, Dolo-Voltaren, Dolpasse, Dorcalor, Dorflan, Dorgen, Doriflan, Doroxan, Dosanac, duravolten, Ecofenac, Econac, Effekton, Effigel, Elitiran, Esgipyrin DS, Evadol, Evinopon, Exflam, Eyeclof, Feloran, Fenac, Fenactol, Fenadium, Fenadol, Fenaflan, Fenagel, Fenaren, Fenburil, Fender, Fenil-V, Fenlodac, Fenoclof, Fensaide, Figrel, Fisioren, Flamatak, Flameril, Flamrase, Flanakin, Flanaren, Flankol, Flector, Flexagen, Flexamina, Flogan, Flogesic, Flogiren, Flogofenac, Flogoken, Flogonac , Flotac, Fluxpiren, Forgenac, Fortedol, Fortenac, Fortfen, Fustaren, Galedol, Gel Antiinflamatorio, Grofenac, Huma-Difenac, I-Gesic, Imanol, Imflac, Inac, Indofeno, Infla-Ban, Infladoren, Inflamac, Inflamax, Inflanac, Jenafenac, Jonac, Jutafenac, K-Fenac, Kindaren, Klonafenac, Lenitil, Lertus, Lesflam, Levedad, Leviogel, Lexobene, Lifenac, Liroken, Lisiflen, Lodyfen, Lofenac, Lofensaid, Luase, Luparen, Mafena, Magluphen, Masaren, Merpal, Merxil, Metaflex NF, Misofenac, Modifenac, Molfenac, Monoflam, Motifene, Myfenax , Myogit, Myonac, Nac, Nacgel, Naclof, Naklofen, Natura Fenac, Neocoflan, Neo-Pyrazon, Neotaflan, Neotaren, Normulen, Novapirina, Novo-Difenac, Noxiflex, Nu-Diclo, Oftic, Olfen, Optobet, Ortoflan, Ostaren, Otriflu, Oxa, Oxalgin, Oxaprost, Painex, Panamor, Pengon, Pennsaid, Pharmaflam, Pirexyl, Piroflam, Posnac, Practiser, Primofenac, Pro Lertus, Probenxil, Profenac, Rapten Rapid, Reactine, Relaxyl, Relipain, Remafen, Remethan, Rewodina, Rhemofenax, Rheumabene, Rheumatac, Rheumavek, Rhewlin, Rhumalgan, Rhumanol, Rodinac, Rumatab, Ruvominox, Selectofen, Sfinac, Sintofenac, Sipirac, Slofenac, Solaraze, Solunac, Still, Subsyde, Taks, Tomanil, Topfans, Trabona, Tratul, Tricin, Tromagesic, Tromax, Turbogesic, Ultrafen, Uniclophen, Uniren, Urigon, Vartelon, Veenac, Veltex, Vendrex, Veral, Vesalion, Vicmafen, Vifenac, Vilacril, Vilonit, Vimultisa, Voldal, Volfenac, Volnac, Vologen, Volraman, Volsaid, Volta, Voltaflan, Voltaflex, Voltanac, Voltaren, Voltaren Colirio, Voltaren Dolo, Voltaren Emulgel, Voltaren Ophta, Voltaren Ophtha, Voltaren T, Voltarene, Voltarol, Voltarol Ophtha, Voltfast, Voltrix, Volverac, Voren, Vostar, Votalen, Votamed, Voveran, Vurdon, Xedenol, Xenid, Xinia, Zeroflog, Zolterol, Zymamed

Continued

Table 5.1 Analgesics and NSAIDs *(continued)*

Generic names	*Proprietary names*
Propionic acid derivatives	
Dexketoprofen	Adolquir, Badyket, Desketo, Dexalgin 25, Dexoket, Enangel, Enantyum, Keral, Ketesse, Nosatel, Pyrsal, Quiralam, Quirgel, Stadium, Sympal
Fenoprofen	Expron, Fenopron, Nalfon, Trandor
Flurbiprofen	Acustop Cataplasma, Ansaid, Antadys, Bedice, Benactiv, Bonatol-R, Cebutid, Clinadol, Distex, Dobrofen, Edolfene, Fladolef-B, Flugalin, Flurbid, Flurofen, Fluroptic, Flurozin, Froben, Inflaflur, Luarprofeno, Neo Artrol, Novo-Flurprofen, Ocufen, Ocufen , Ocuflur, Reupax, Ropion, Strefen, Strepfen, Strepsils Intensive, Tantum Activ Gola, Targus, Tolerane, TransAct, Transact Lat, TransActLAT
Ibuprofen	ACT-3, Actiprofen, Adex, Adulfen Lysine, Advil, Aktren, Aktren, Algiasdin, Algidrin, Algiflex, Algifor, Algioprofen, Algofen, Algoflex, Algofren, Alindrin, Alogesia, Altior, Ambufen, Anadin Ibuprofen, Anadin Ultra, Anadvil, Anbifen, Antalgil, Antalisin, Antarene, Apain, Aprofen, Arfen, Arthrofen, Artofen, Artril, Avallone, Babefen Sus, Babypiril, Bediatil, Benflogin, Bestafen, Betagesic, Betaprofen, Bifen, Bistryl, Bladex, Borafen, Borakid, Brufen, Brunal, Bruprin, Brusil, Bufigen, Bumed, Bupogesic, Burana, Buscofen, Butafen, Butidiona, Calmine, Calprofen, Cefen, Cibalgina Due Fast, Cipgesic, Citalgan, Contraneural, Copiron, Cuprofen, Dalsy, Days, Deucodol, Dibufen, Diltix, Diprodol, Dismenol N, Dismenol Neu, Doctril, Dolgit, Dolibu, Dolo Sanol, Dolocyl, Dolo-Dismenol, Dolodoc, Dolofast, Dolofort, Dolo-Puren, Dolorac, Dolormin, Dolorsyn, Dolorub, Dolo-Spedifen, Dolprin, Dolprofen, Doltaque, Dolval, Dolver, Doraplax, Doretrim , Dorival, Druisel, Duafen, Duran, Ebufac, Ecoprofen, Edenil, Emflam, Epsilon, Ergix, Espidifen, Esprenit, Eudorlin Extra, Eudorlin Migrane, Expanfen, Extrapan, Faspic, Febratic, Femapirin, Feminalin, Fenbid, Fenopine, Fenpaed, Fenpic, Feverfen, Flexafen, Fortapal, Galprofen, Ganaprofene, Gelofeno, Gelufene, Genpril, G-Fen, Ginenorm, Greatofen, Grefen, Gyno-Neuralgin, Hedex Ibuprofen, Heidi, Hemagene Tailleur, Huma-Profen, Ibalgin, Iboflam, Ibosure, Ibrofen, Ibrufhalal, Ibu, Ibu Benuron, Ibu Evanol, Ibu-4, Ibu-6, ibu-Attritin, Ibubeta, Ibubex, Ibucler, Ibu-4, -6, -8, Ibudol, Ibudolor, Ibufabra, Ibufac, Ibufem, Ibufen, Ibufen-L, Ibufix, Ibuflam, Ibuflex, Ibufran, Ibugan, Ibugel, Ibugesic, Ibuhexal, Ibu-Lady, Ibulan, Ibuleve, Ibulgan, Ibulos, Ibumac, Ibumar, Ibumax, Ibumed, Ibumerck, Ibumetin, Ibumousse, Ibu-Novalgina, Ibupax, Ibupen, Ibupirac, Ibupiretas, Ibupril, Ibuprof, Ibuprofan, Ibuprox, Ibu-ratiopharm, Iburem, Iburen, Ibureumin, Ibusal, Ibusi, Ibusifar, Ibu-Slow, Ibuspray, Ibusumal, Ibu-Tab, Ibutad, Ibutenk, Ibutop, Ibutop Cuprofen, Ibutop Ralgex, Ibux, Ibuxin, Ibuzidine, Imbun, Intralgis, Inza, Ipren, Iproben, Iprogel, Ipson, Irfen, Isdibudol, Isdol, Jenaprofen, Junifen, Kesan, Kin, Kontagripp, Kratalgin, Librofem, Lombalgina, Malafene, Mandafen, Manorfen, Medifen, Melabon, Melfen, Menadol, Mensoton, Mentholatum Ibuprofen, Midol Cramp & Body Aches, Migrafen, Migranin Ibuprofen, Moment, Motrax, Motrin, Neobrufen, Neutropain, Niofen, Nodolfen, Norflam T, Norvectan, Novaprin, Novartril, Novo-Profen, Nuprilan, Nuprin, Nureflex, Nurofen, Nurofen Migraine, Nurofen Stopgrip, Oberdol, Obifen, Offeno, Optalidon, Optifen, Opturem, Orbifen, Ostofen, Oxibut, Ozonol, Pabiprofen, Pacifene, Pakurat, Panafen, Paraflex Crema, Parartrin, Parsal, Pediaprofen, Perofen, Perviam, Pfeil, P-Fen, Phor Pain, Phorpain, Pippen, Pirexin, Pironal, Ponstil Mujer, Ponstin, Proartinal, Probufen, Profen, Profeno, Profinal, Proflex, Pyriped, Quadrax, Radian-B Ibuprofen, Rafen, Ranfen, ratioDolor, Realdrax, Relcofen, Remidol, Rheumanox, Rimafen, Roco, Rozovin, Rumasian, Rumatifen, Rupan, Saetil, Saleto-200, Saridon N, Schmerz-Dolgit, Schufen, Sindol, Siprofen, Skelan IB, Solfen, Solpaflex, Solufen, Solvium, Spalt, Spedifen, Spidifen, Spidufen, Spifen, Sporfen, Subitene, Tabalon, Tabcin, Takigrip, Tifen, Tispol Ibu-DD, Tofen, Togal Ibuprofen, Trauma-Dolgit, Trifene, Tri-Profen, Trofen, Uniprofen, Upfen, Urem, Urgo, Zafen
Ketoprofen	Actron, Alket, Alrheumun, Apo-Keto, Arcental, Artrinid, Artrofene, Artrosil, Artrosilene, Bi-Profenid, Birofenid, Ceprofen, Deflogix, Dolgosin, Dolofar, Dolo-Ketazon, Efiken, Euketos, Extraplus, Farbovil, Fastum, Flexen, Flogofin, Gabrilen, Helenil, Ibifen, Kaprofen , Keduril, Kefentech, Kenhancer, Keprodol, Ketartrium, Ketobene, Ketocid, Keto, Ketodol, Ketodur, Ketofene, Ketoflam, Ketomex, Ketonal, Ketop, Ketoplus, Ketorin, Ketoselect, Ketosolan, Ketotop, Ketovail, Ketum, K-Profen, Larafen, Lasonil CM, Menaril, Meprofen, Mohrus, Myproflam, Novo-Keto, Oki, Orofen, Orudis, Orugesic, Oruvail, Oscorel, Phardol Schmerz, Powergel, Prodon, Profenid, Profinject, Prontoket, Provail, Relatene, Reuprofen, Rhodis, Rhovail, Rofenid, Rofepain, Salicrem K, Siduro, Spondylon, Talflex, Tiloket, Togal Mobil-Gel mit ketoprofen , Topfena, Toprec, Toprek, Totifen, Zon
Naproxen	Actiquim, Acusprain, Aleve, Algioprux, Algonapril, Alidase, Aliviomas, Alpoxen, Anaprox, Anapsyl, Annoxen, Antalgin, Aperdan, Apo-Napro-Na, Apranax, Artagen, Arthroxen, Artron, Bioxan, Bonyl, Bumaflex N, Causalon Pro, Congex, Crysanal, Dafloxen, Debril, Deflamox, Denaxpren, Deucoval, Diferbest, Dolormin mit Naproxen, Dolxen, Dysmenalgit, Easy Dayz, Eurogesic Gel, Fabralgina, Fadalivio, Femme Free, Fibroxyn, Flanax, Flexen, Flogen, Floginax, Flogocefal, Floxalin, Fuxen, Genalgen, Gerinap, Gibixen, Gynestrel, Inveoxel, Inza, Iqfasol, Laser, Ledox, Lorexen, Lundiran, Melgar, Miranax, Momen , Momendol, Monarit, Nafasol, Naflapen, Nalgesin, Napflam, Napmel, Napratec, Naprelan, Napren, Naprius, Naprobene, Naprocet, Naprocoat, Naprodil, Naprofidex, Naprogen, Naprogesic, Naprometin, Napromex, Naprontag, Naprorex, Naprosian, Naprosyn, Naprosyne, Naproval, Naprovite, Naprox, Naproxi, Naprux, Napsen, Napsyn, Napxen, Narocin, Narzen, Naxen, Naxopren, Naxyn, Neo Eblimon, Neonaxil, Neuralprona, Nitens, Nixal, Noflam-N, Novaxen, Novo-Naprox, Nu-Naprox, Nuprafen, Nycopren, Pactens, Point, Polyxen, Prevacid NapraPAC, Prexan, prodolor, Pronat, Pronaxen, Pronaxil, Pronoxen, Proxagol, Proxalin, Proxen, Reprost, Reuxen, Seladin, Sertrixen, Serviproxan, Sicadentol Plus, Soden, Sodixen, Sonap , Soproxen, Sunprox, Synalgo, Synflex, Tacron, Tandax, Tanizona, Ticoflex, Traumox, Triox NF, Tundra, U-Proxyn, Velsay, Veradol, Vinsen, Xenar, Xenobid, Xicane, Zynal
Oxaprozin	Alvo, Danoprox, Daypro, Dayrun, Deflam, Duraprox, Walix
Tiaprofenic acid	Fengam, Flanid, Surgam, Surgamyl, Thialgin, Tiaprofen
Pyrazolone derivatives	
Azapropazone	Debelex, Prolixan, Rheumox
Feprazone	Brotazona, Zepelin
Kebuzone	Ketazon

Continued

Table 5.1 Analgesics and NSAIDs *(continued)*

Generic names	*Proprietary names*
Metamizole sodium (Dipyrone)	Algiopiret, Algirona, Algopyrin, Alnex, Anador, Analgesil, Analgex, Analgin, Analgine, Anaprol, Apiron, Apixol, Avafontan, Avaldrian, Ayoral Simple, Baralgin M, Baralgina M, Berlosin, Centagin, Conmel, Dalsin, Deparon, Dioxadol, Dipigrand, Dipimax, Dipirex, Dipiron, Dipironax, Dipydol, Ditral, Dofisan, Dolgan, Dolofur, Domenal, Dorilan, Dornal, Dorona, Exalgin, Exodalina, Fandall, Fardolpin, Findor, Genergin, Inalgon Neu, Indigon, Integrobe, Invoigin, Kno-Paine, Macodin, Magnil, Magnol, Magsons, Maxiliv, Mecoten, Mermid, Metapirona, Mezabox, Midelin, Minalgin, Minoral, Mizoltec, Neo Melubrina, Neomelin, Neo-Melubrina, Nivagin, Nofebrin, Nopain, Novacler, Novalgin, Novalgina, Novalgine, Novaminsulfon, Novemina, Olan-Gin, Optalgin, Paleodina, Panalgorin, Phanalgin, Piramagno, Pirandall, Pirinovag, Pirogina, Piromebrina, Poloren, Prodolina, Pyranol, Spasmo Inalgon Neu, Suprim, Termonal, Termonil, Termoprin, Termopriona, Unibios Simple, Utidol, V-Talgin
Oxyphenbutazone	Edefen, Redolet
Phenylbutazone	Ambene, Basireuma, Bloken, Bresal, Butadion, Butalen, Butazolidin, Butazolidina, Butazolidine, Butazolon, Butazona, Butazonil, Delbulasa, exrheudon OPT, Fezona, Inflazone, Kadol, Lorfenil, Neo Butazol
Selective inhibitors of cyclo-oxygenase-2 (Coxibs)	
Celecoxib	Artilog, Celcox, Celebra, Celebrex, Celedol, Celemax, Celib, Cobix, Coxel, Coxtenk, Niflam, Orthocel, Solexa, Tisorek, Ultracele, Zycel
Etodolac	Acudor, Articulan, Dualgan, Eccoxolac, Ecridoxan, Etonox, Etopan, Hypen, Lodine, Lodot, Lonine, Metazin, Sodolac, Todolac
Etoricoxib	Algix, Arcoxia, Auxib, Ebov, Ecoxib, Etoxib, Etozox, Exxiv, Kretos, Tauxib
Meloxicam	See under Oxicams
Nimesulide	Aflogen, Ainex, Aldoron, Alencast, Algimesil, Algolider, Algosulid, Algover, Amocetin, Antalgo, Antiflogil, Aponil, Areuma, Aulin, Auromelid, Beta Nicip, Chemisulide, Cimelide, Cliovyl, Coxtral, Deflogen, Degorflan, Delfos, Deltaflan, Dimesul, Discorid, Doloc, Doloctaprin, Dolostop, Doloxtren, Domes, Donulide, Edemax, Edrigyl, Efridol, Elinap, Erlecit, Erreflog, Eskaflam, Eudolene, Fansidol, Fansulide, Fasulide, Fladalgin, Flamide, Flogilid, Flogostop, Flogovital NF, Flolid, Gerilide, G-Revm, Idealid, Inflalid, Isodol, Jabasulide, Kartal, Lalide, Ledolid, Ledoren, Lemesil, Lizepat, Londopon, Lusemin, Melicat, Melicate, Melimont, Mesulid, Mesupon, Metaflex, Migraless, Min-A-Pon, Mosuolit, Multiformil, Myxina, Neosulida, Nerelid, Nexen, Niberan, Nicip, Nide, Nidol, Nilide , Nimalgex, Nimed, Nimedex, Nimelide, Nimenol, Nimepast, Nimes , Nimesil, Nimesilam, Nimesul, Nimesulene, Nimesulix, Nimesulon, Nimesyl, Nimesyl Gel, Nimex, Nimfast, Nimica, Nimind, Nimm, Nimodol, Nims, Nimulid, Nimulid , Nimusyp, Nimutab, Nisalgen, Nise, Nisuflex, Nisulid, Nisural, Noalgos, Noxalide, Redaflam, Remov, Resulin, Ristolzit, Ritamine, Rolaket, Scaflam, Scalid, Severin, Sintalgin, Solving, Specilid, Sudinet, Sulidamor, Sulimed, Tranzicalm, Ventor, Virobron, Volonten, Willgo
Parecoxib	Bextra, Bioval-P, Dynastat, Dynastat , Rayzon, Valcox, Valdixx, Valus-P, Vorth-P
Rofecoxib	Algioxib, Antidol, Arofexx, Befol, Blokium Cox, Coxiro, Coxxil, Dolostop, Doxtran, Foldoxx, Miraxx, Peroxx, Rofeb, Rofetab, Rofixx, Rofiz, Silfox, Toloxane, Unicalm, Versatil, Viartril, Vioxx
Valdecoxib	Bioval, Valdiff, Valdixx, Valus, Vorth
Other	
Benzydamine hydrochloride	Afloben, Agilona, Andolex, Benflogin, Benzirin, Benzitrat, Bucco-Tantum, Ciflogex, Difflam, Difflam Anti-inflammatory Lozenges, Difflam Anti-inflammatory Throat Spray, Difflam Solution, Easy gel, Ernex, Flogin-Ped, Flogo Rosa, Flogoral, Fonergoral, Fulgium, Ginesal, Lonol, Momen, Multum, Neoflogin, Opalgyne, Rosalgin, Sandival Desleible, Saniflor Collutorio, Tantum, Tantum Rosa, Tantum Verde, Tantum Verde, Tantumar, Tantum, Vantal, Verax, Xentafid
Felbinac	Dolinac, Dolo Target, Seltouch, Spalt Schmerz-Gel, Target, Traxam
Ketorolac	Acular, Aculare, Acularen, Algikey, Alidol, Brodifac, Burten, Cadolac, Celfax, Cetrolac, Dilox, Dolac, Dolgenal, Dolotor, Dolten, Droal, Elipa, Estopein, Findedol, Findol, Glicima, Kelac, Kemanat, Kerarer, Ketanov, Ketlur, Keto, Ketodrops, Ketonic, Ketopharm, Klenac, Lixidol, Netaf, Nolarac, Onemer, Poenkerat, Sinalgico, Supradol, Syndol, Taradyl, Tenkdol, Toloran, Tonum, Topadol, Tora-Dol, Toral, Torolac, Tromedal
Nabumetone	Aflex, Akratol, Anfer, Anfer , Artaxan, Balmox, Bumetone , Elitar, Ethyfen, Listran, Mebutan, Mevedal, Nabone, Nabonet, Nabuco, Nabucox, Nabuflam, Nabuser, Nabuton, Naditone, Naflex, Nametone, No-Ton , Relafen, Relif, Relifen, Relifex, Religer, Relisan, Relitone, Rodanol S
Phenazone (Antipyrine)	Aurone, Erasol, Migrane-Kranit, Oto-Phen, Tropex
Tolmetin	Artrocaptin, Tolectin
Opioid and related analgesics	
Anaesthetic adjuncts	
Alfentanil	Alfast, Alfenta, Brevafen, Fanaxal, Fentalim, Limifen, Rapifen
Fentanyl	Actiq, Duragesic, Durogesic, Fenodid, Fentabbott, Fentanest, Fentax, Haldid, Leptanal, Nafluvent, Sintenyl, Sublimaze, Talgesil, Tanyl, Trofentyl
Remifentanil	Ultiva
Sufentanil	Fastfen, Fentatienil, Sufenta

Continued

Table 5.1 Analgesics and NSAIDs *(continued)*

Generic names	*Proprietary names*
Mild to moderate pain	
Codeine	Actacode, Antitussivum Burger, Bepro, Bisoltus, Bromophar, Bronchicum Extra Sterk, Bronchicum Mono Codein, Bronchosedal, Codant, Codedrill, Codeisan, Codenfan, codi OPT, Codical, Codicaps mono, Codicaps Neo, Codicompren, Codifos, Codinex, Codipertussin, Codipront Mono, Codipront N, Coditard, Eulyptan, Fludan Codeina, Galcodine, Gloceda, Glottyl, Histaverin, Makatussin Codein, Makatussin nouvelle formule, Neo-Codion, Neo-Codion, Omnopon, Optipect Kodein, Paderyl, Perduretas Codeina, Rekod, Toseina , Toularynx, Tricodein, Tryasol, Tussoret
Dextropropoxyphene (Propoxyphene)	Abalgin, Darvon, Darvon Simple, Darvon-N, Deprancol, Depronal, Dexofen, Doloxene, Liberen, Parvodex, Romidon, Zideron
Dihydrocodeine	Codicontin, Codidol, Condugesic, Contugesic, DF 118, DHC, DHC Continus, Dicodin, Didor, Hydrocodeinon, Hydrocodin, Paracodin, Paracodin N, Paracodina, Paracodine, Remedacen, Rikodeine, Tiamon Mono, Tosidrin
Moderate to severe pain	
Partial agonists and agonists/antagonists	
Buprenorphine	Anorfin, Bupren, Buprenex, Buprex, Buprine, Magnogen, Nopan, Norphin, Pentorel, Prefin, Subutex, Temgesic, Transtec
Butorphanol	Beforal, Butrum, Moradol, Stadol
Meptazinol	Meptid, Meptidol
Nalbuphine	Bufigen, Bufilem, Intapan, Nalcryn, Naltrox, Nubain, Nubaina, Nubak, Onfor
Pentazocine	Fortal, Fortalgesic, Fortral, Fortralin, Fortwin, Ospronim, Pangon, Pentawin, Sosegon, Sosenol, Talwin, Talwin NX
Pure agonists	
Dextromoramide	Palfium
Diamorphine (Heroin)	Diaphin
Dipipanone	Diconal, Wellconal
Hydrocodone	Biocodone, Dicodid, Hycodan
Hydromorphone	Dilaudid, Dolonovag, Hydal, Hydromorph, Opidol, Palladon, Palladone, Sophidone
Morphine	Actiskenan, Algedol, Amidiaz, Analfin, Analmorph, Anamorph, Astramorph PF, Avinza, Capros, Compensan, Contalgin, DepoDur, Depolan, Dimorf , Dolcontin, Doltard, Duralmor, Duramorph, Filnarine, GNO, Graten, Infumorph, Kadian, Kapabloc, Kapanol, LA Morph, M-beta, MCR, M-Dolor, M-Eslon, MIR, M-long, Morapid, Morcap, Morcontin, Moretal, Morph, Morphanton, Morphex, Morphgesic, MOS, Moscontin, MS Contin, MS Mono, MSI, MSIR, MS-Long, MSP, MSR, MST, MST Continus, MST Unicontinus, MST Uno, M-Stada, Mundidol, MXL, Neocalmans, Noceptin, Oglos, Omnopon, Oramorph, Ordine, RA Morph, RMS, Roxanol, Sevredol, Sevre-Long, Skenan, Slovalgin, SRM-Rhotard, Statex, Stellorphinad, Stellorphine, Substitol, Twice, Vendal, Zomorph
Oxycodone	Endocodone, Endone, Oxanest, Oxinovag, Oxy IR, Oxycod, Oxycontin, Oxyfast, Oxygesic, OxyIR, Oxynorm, Percolone, Proladone, Roxicodone, Supeudol
Oxymorphone	Numorphan
Papaveretum	Omnopon
Pethidine (Meperidine)	Alodan, Cluyer, Demerol, Dolantin, Dolantina, Dolantine, Dolargan, Dolestine, Dolosal, Dolsin, Meperol
Tramadol	Acugesic, Adamon, Adolonta, Amadol, Ammitram, Anadol, Analab, Biodalgic, Biodol, By-Madol, Calmador, Ceparidin, Contramal, Dolol, Dolzam, Dromadol, Ecodolor, Fortradol, Fraxidol, Jutadol, Lanalget, Larapam, Mabron, Madol, Madola, Mandolgin, Minidol, Monocrixo, Nobligan, Nycodol, Paindol, Paxilfar, Pengesic, Pharmadol, Prontalgin, Prontofort, Protradon, Rofy , Sefmal, Sensitram, Sylador, Takadol, Tamolan, Theradol, Tial, Timarol, Timasen, Tioner, Tiparol, T-long, Topalgic, Trabar, Trabilin, Tracine, Tradol, Tradolan, Tradolgesic, Tradonal, Tralgiol, Tralgit, Tralic, Trama, Tramabene, Tramabeta, Tramacip, Tramada, Tramadex, Tramadin, Tramadoc, Tramadol-Dolgit, Tramadolor, Tramadon, Tramadura, Tramagetic, Tramagit, Tramahexal, Tramake, Trama-Klosidol, Tramal, Tramalan, Tramalgic, Tramamed, Tramapine, Tramastad, Tramazac, Trambo, Tramelene, Tramex, Tramium, Tramo, Tramoda, Tramundal, Tramundin, Trasedal, Travex, TRD-Contin, Trexol, Trosic, Ultram, Urgendol, Veldrol, Volcidol-S, Xymel, Zamadol, Zamudol, Zodol, Zumalgic, Zydol, Zytram
Opioid dependence	
Levacetylmethadol	
Methadone	Aldolan, Amidona, Aptus Methadone, Biodone, Deperidol, Dolmed, Dolophine, Eptadone, Gobbidona, Hepatadon, Ketalgine, Martindale Methadone Mixture DTF, Metadol, Metadon, Metasedin, Methadose, Methatabs, Pallidone, Phymet DTF, Physeptone, Pinadone DTF, Symoron, Synastone

Continued

Table 5.1 Analgesics and NSAIDs *(continued)*

Generic names	*Proprietary names*
Miscellaneous	
Nefopam	Acupan, Oxadol, Silentan
Paracetamol (Acetaminophen)	Abdine Cold Relief, Abenol, Abrol, Abrolet, Acamol, Acamoli, Acephen, Acertol, Acet, Aceta, Acetafen, Acetalgine, Acetamol, Acetasil, Acetif, Acetofen, Acetolit, Actron, Adol, Aldolor, Algogen, Algostase Mono, Alpirex, Alsiphene, Alvedon, A-Mol , Amolgen, Anadin Paracetamol, Anadin-3, Anatyl, Andopan, Andox, Angenol, Antalgic, Antidol, Apacet, Apap, Apiretal, Apotel, Apra, Apracur Antifebril, Arfen, Arthritis Pain Formula Aspirin Free, Artritol, Asafen Nueva Formula, Aspirin Free Anacin, Aspirin Free Pain Relief, Atasol, Atralidon, Bandol, Becetamol, Ben-u-ron, Biogesic, Boots Pain Relief Suspension 6 Years Plus, Bromo Seltzer, Brunomol, Calinofen, Calpol, Captin, Causalon, Cefabrina, Cefecon D, Cemol, Cephanol, Cetafrin, Cetinject, Childrens Dynafed Jr, Childrens Feverhalt, Childrens Mapap, Childrens Panadol, Childrens Panadol Drops for Infants, Christamol, Claradol, Contac Erkaltungs-Trunk, Contradol, Contre-Douleurs P, Coriver, Cotibin Compuesto, Crocin, Cryogenine Plus, Cupanol, Curadon, Curpol, Custodial, Dafalgan, Daga, Daimeton, Dalminette, Daro, Datril, Depon, Depon Maximum, Dexamol, Dexamol Kid, Dhamol, Dirox, Dismifen, Disprin Paracetamol, Disprol, Dolal, Dolgesic, Doliprane, Dolitabs, Dolko, Dolol-Instant, Dolono, Dolorol, DoloStop nouvelle formule, Dolostop, Dolotec, Dolotemp, Dolprone, Doluvital, Dolviran, Dorfen, Dorico, Dorvan,Dristancito, Duaneo, Duorol, Dymadon, Dynafed EX, Efferalgan, Efferalganodis, Empaped, Enelfa, Expandox, Farpik, Febran, Febrectal, Febrectol, Febridol, Fenn, Fennings Childrens Cooling Powders, Fensum, Fevamol, Feverall, Fibrexin, Fibrimol, Fiebrolito, Finimal Junior, Frilen, Galpamol, Gelocatil, Geluprane, Genapap, Genebs, Geniol-P, Gewamol, Go-Pain P, Gripeonil, Gripotermon, Grippostad, Grippostad Heissgetrank, Guemusin, Halenol, Hedex, Icetazol, Icolid Plus , Ifutemp, Infadrops, Infalgina, Infantaire, Influbene N, Kafa, Kinder Finimal, Kitadol, Kit-Syrup, Kratofin simplex, Lagalgin, Lemsip Children's Cold Relief, Lemsip Cold & Flu Original, Cold & Flu Max, Lemsip, Levadol, Liquiprin, Lonarid Aplo, Lotemp, Magnidol-Plus, Malex, Malidens, Mandanol, Mapap, Maranox, Masferol, Meda, Medinol, Medipyrin, Medpramol, Mejoral, Mejoralito, Melabon Infantil, Mexalen, Miradol, Momentum, Mono Praecimed, Multifebrin, Multi-gesic, Mypara, Napa, Napamol, Naprex, Nasa, Neodol, Neodolito, Nina, Nodipir, Nodolex, Normaflu, Notem, Novo-Gesic, Nutamol, Obimol, Oraphen-PD, Ordov Febrigesic, Osa Suppositoires contre douleurs et fievre, Pacemol, Pacimol, Paedialgon, Pain Aid Free, Painamol, Paldesic, Pamol, Panado, Panadol, Panagesic, Panaleve, Panam, Panamax, Panasorbe, Panitone, Panodil, Para Z Mol, Paracap, Paracare, Paracet, Paracets, Paracin, Paracip, Paraclear, Paradco, Parafizz, Para-G , Parahexal, Parakapton, Paralen, Paralgen, Paralgin, Paralief, Paralink, Paralyoc, Paramed, Paramol TP, Paramolan, Paramol, Paranal-L, Parapaed, Paraspeed, Para-Suppo, Parat, Para-Tabs, Paratol, Paratral, Parmol, Parox Meltab, Parsel, Partamol, Paximol, PCM, Pediatrix, Peinfort, Pemol, Perdolan, Perfalgan, Perfusalgan, PH 4 Plus, Pharmacard Family Douleurs & Fievre, Pharmacen, Pinex, Piramin, Plovacal, Poro, Predualito, Progesic, Prolief, Puernol, Pyracon, Pyradol, Pyretal, Pyrexon, Pyrigesic, Pyrimel, Ramol, Rapidol, Redutemp, Reliv, Remedol, Resakal, Ridenol, Robigesic, Rokamol, Rubophen, Salzone, Sara, Sedalito, Seranex N, Serimol , Setamol, Silapap, Sinaspril-Paracetamol, Sinedol, Siniphen Nouvelle formule, Sinmol, Sinpro N, Sons Piral, Sudis, Supofen, Tachipirina, Tafirol, Tantaphen, Tapanol, Tapsin sin Cafeina, Temperal, Tempire, Tempofin, Tempra, Temzzard, Termalgin, Termofren, Termol, Termo-Ped, Termotrin, Tiffy, Tilekin, Togal, Treupel Dolo, Treuphadol, Tumdi, Tunelzin, Tylenol, Tylephen, Tylex, Tylidol, Tymol, Ultragin, UN-Aspirin, Uni-Ace, Uni-Febrin, Unigrip, Unimol, Uphamol, Varipan, Vick Vitapyrena, Vicks Paracetamol, Viclor, Vimoli, Winasorb, Winpain, Xebramol, Xumadol, Zaramol, Zolben

Aspirin or other Salicylates + Antacids or Urinary alkalinisers

The serum salicylate concentrations of patients taking large doses of aspirin or other salicylates as anti-inflammatory agents can be reduced to subtherapeutic levels by some antacids.

Clinical evidence

A child with rheumatic fever taking aspirin 600 mg five times daily had a serum salicylate concentration of between 8.2 and 11.8 mg/dl while taking 30 ml of *Maalox* (**aluminium/magnesium hydroxide** suspension). When the *Maalox* was withdrawn, the urinary pH fell from a range of 7 to 8 down to a range of 5 to 6.4, whereupon the serum salicylate level rose three- to fourfold to about 38 mg/dl, which required a dosage reduction.[1] An associated study in 13 healthy subjects taking aspirin 4 g daily for a week found that **sodium bicarbonate** 4 g daily reduced serum salicylate levels by 44%, from 27 to 15 mg/dl. This reflected a rise in the urinary pH from a range of 5.6 to 6.1 up to around 6.2 to 6.9.[1,2] Similar changes have been reported in other studies with: aspirin or **choline salicylate** and **aluminium/magnesium hydroxides**; aspirin and **magnesium trisilicate/aluminium hydroxide**; and aspirin or **sodium salicylate** and **sodium bicarbonate**.[3-7] There is some evidence that this effect does not occur at low serum salicylate levels,[4,5] or if the pH of the urine is unchanged.[5]

Mechanism

Aspirin and other salicylates are acidic compounds that are excreted by the kidney tubules and are ionised in solution. In alkaline solution, much of the drug exists in the ionised form, which is not readily reabsorbed, and therefore is lost in the urine. If the urine is made more acidic (e.g. with ammonium chloride), much more of the drug exists in the un-ionised form, which is readily reabsorbed, so that less is lost in the urine and the drug is retained in the body.[6,7]

In vitro data show that magnesium oxide and aluminium hydroxide strongly adsorb aspirin and sodium salicylate.[8] However, in two of the studies above aluminium hydroxide-containing antacids had no effect on the extent of absorption of salicylate.[3,5]

Importance and management

A well established and clinically important interaction for those on long-term treatment with large doses of salicylates because the serum salicylate level may become subtherapeutic. This interaction can occur with both 'systemic' antacids (e.g. sodium bicarbonate) as well as some 'non-systemic' antacids (e.g. magnesium/aluminium hydroxides), but only occurs if there is an increase in urinary pH. Care should be taken to monitor serum salicylate levels if any antacid is started or stopped in patients where the control of salicylate levels is critical.

No important adverse interaction would be expected in those taking occasional doses of aspirin for analgesia. Some aspirin formulations actually include antacids as buffering agents to increase absorption rates and raise peak serum levels,[9] which gives more rapid analgesia, and/or in an attempt to decrease gastric irritation. Note that antacids may also increase the rate of absorption of aspirin given as enteric-coated tablets.[10]

1. Blondheim SH, Alkan WJ, Brunner D, eds. Frontiers of Internal Medicine. 12th Int Congr Intern Med, Tel Aviv, 1974. Basel: Karger; 1975 p. 404–8.
2. Levy G, Leonards JR. Urine pH and salicylate therapy. *JAMA* (1971) 217, 81.
3. Levy G, Lampman T, Kamath BL, Garrettson LK. Decreased serum salicylate concentration in children with rheumatic fever treated with antacid. *N Engl J Med* (1975) 293, 323–5.
4. Hansten PD, Hayton WL. Effect of antacid and ascorbic acid on serum salicylate concentration. *J Clin Pharmacol* (1980) 20, 326–31.
5. Shastri RA. Effect of antacids on salicylate kinetics. *Int J Clin Pharmacol Ther Toxicol* (1985) 23, 480–4.
6. Macpherson CR, Milne MD, Evans BM. The excretion of salicylate. *Br J Pharmacol* (1955) 10, 484–9.
7. Hoffman WS, Nobe C. The influence of urinary pH on the renal excretion of salicyl derivatives during aspirin therapy. *J Lab Clin Med* (1950) 35, 237–48.
8. Naggar VF, Khalil SA, Daabis NA. The in-vitro adsorption of some antirheumatics on antacids. *Pharmazie* (1976) 31, 461–5.
9. Nayak RK, Smyth RD, Polk A, Herczeg T, Carter V, Visalli AJ, Reavey-Cantwell NH. Effect of antacids on aspirin dissolution and bioavailability. *J Pharmacokinet Biopharm* (1977) 5, 597–613.
10. Feldman S, Carlstedt BC. Effect of antacid on absorption of enteric-coated aspirin. *JAMA* (1974) 227, 660–1.

Aspirin + Caffeine

Caffeine modestly increases the bioavailability, rate of absorption and plasma levels of aspirin.

Clinical evidence, mechanism, importance and management

Caffeine citrate 120 mg given to healthy subjects with a single 650-mg dose of aspirin increased the aspirin AUC by 36%, increased the maximum plasma levels by 15%, and increased the rate of absorption by 30%.[1] This confirms the results of a previous study.[2] Both of these studies suggest that caffeine may modestly potentiate the efficacy of aspirin via a pharmacokinetic mechanism.

1. Thithapandha A. Effect of caffeine on the bioavailability and pharmacokinetics of aspirin. *J Med Assoc Thai* (1989) 72, 562–6.
2. Yoovathaworn KC, Sriwatanakul K, Thithapandha A. Influence of caffeine on aspirin pharmacokinetics. *Eur J Drug Metab Pharmacokinet* (1986) 11, 71–6.

Aspirin or other Salicylates + Carbonic anhydrase inhibitors

A severe and even life-threatening toxic reaction can occur in those on high dose salicylate treatment if they are given carbonic anhydrase inhibitors (acetazolamide, diclofenamide).

Clinical evidence

An 8-year-old boy with chronic juvenile arthritis, stable on prednisolone, indometacin and **aloxiprin**, was admitted to hospital with drowsiness, vomiting and hyperventilation (diagnosed as metabolic acidosis) within a month of increasing the **aloxiprin** dosage from 3 to 3.6 g daily and adding **diclofenamide** 25 mg three times daily for glaucoma.[1]

Other cases of toxicity (metabolic acidosis) have included a 22-year-old woman on **salsalate** given **acetazolamide** 250 mg four times daily,[1] and in 2 elderly women on large doses of aspirin given **acetazolamide** or **diclofenamide**.[2] Salicylate poisoning developed in a man on **diclofenamide** within 10 days of starting to take aspirin 3.9 g daily.[3] Coma developed in an 85-year-old woman taking aspirin 3.9 g daily when the dosage of **acetazolamide** was increased from 500 mg to 1 g daily,[4,5] and toxicity was seen in a very elderly man given both drugs.[5] Levels of unbound **acetazolamide** were found to be unusually high.[5] An elderly man became confused, lethargic, incontinent and anorexic when treated with **acetazolamide** and **salsalate**. He needed intravenous hydration.[6] A 50-year-old woman treated with **acetazolamide** for glaucoma was admitted to hospital with confusion and cerebellar ataxia, associated with hyperchloraemic acidosis, 14 days after starting to take aspirin for acute pericarditis.[7]

Mechanism

Not fully established. One idea is that these carbonic anhydrase inhibitors (acetazolamide, diclofenamide) affect the plasma pH, so that more of the salicylate exists in the un-ionised (lipid-soluble) form, which can enter the CNS and other tissues more easily, leading to salicylate toxicity.[2] However, carbonic anhydrase inhibitors also make the urine more alkaline, which increases the loss of salicylate[8] (see also 'Aspirin or other Salicylates + Antacids or Urinary alkalinisers', above). *Animal* studies confirm that carbonic anhydrase inhibitors increase the lethal toxicity of aspirin.[3] An alternative suggestion is that because salicylate inhibits the plasma protein binding of acetazolamide and its excretion by the kidney, acetazolamide toxicity, which mimics salicylate toxicity, may occur.[5]

Importance and management

Although there are few clinical reports on record, the interaction between carbonic anhydrase inhibitors and salicylates is established, well confirmed by *animal* studies, and potentially serious. One study recommended that carbonic anhydrase inhibitors should probably be avoided in those on high dose salicylate treatment.[5] If they are used, the patient should be well monitored for any evidence of toxicity (confusion, lethargy, hyperventilation, tinnitus) because the interaction may develop slowly and insidiously.[2] In this context other non-steroidal anti-inflammatory drugs may be safer. Naproxen proved to be a satisfactory substitute in one case.[1] The authors of one study suggest that **methazolamide** may possibly be a safer alternative to acetazolamide because it is minimally bound to plasma proteins. They also suggest paracetamol (acetaminophen) as an alternative to salicylate in patients taking acetazolamide.[5] The reports cited here concern carbonic anhydrase inhibitors given orally, not as eye drops. It is not known whether the latter interact similarly, but there appear to be no reports.

1. Cowan RA, Hartnell GG, Lowdell CP, McLean Baird I, Leak AM. Metabolic acidosis induced by carbonic anhydrase inhibitors and salicylates in patients with normal renal function. *BMJ* (1984) 289, 347–8.
2. Anderson CJ, Kaufman PL, Sturm RJ. Toxicity of combined therapy with carbonic anhydrase inhibitors and aspirin. *Am J Ophthalmol* (1978) 86, 516–19.
3. Hurwitz GA, Wingfield W, Cowart TD, Jollow DJ. Toxic interaction between salicylates and a carbonic anhydrase inhibitor: the role of cerebral edema. *Vet Hum Toxicol* (1980) 22 (Suppl), 42–4.
4. Chapron DJ, Brandt JL, Sweeny KR, Olesen-Zammett L. Interaction between acetazolamide and aspirin — a possible unrecognized cause of drug-induced coma. *J Am Geriatr Soc* (1984) 32, S18.
5. Sweeney KR, Chapron DJ, Brandt JL, Gomolin IH, Feig PU, Kramer PA. Toxic interaction between acetazolamide and salicylate: case reports and a pharmacokinetic explanation. *Clin Pharmacol Ther* (1986) 40, 518–24.
6. Rousseau P, Fuentevilla-Clifton A. Acetazolamide and salicylate interaction in the elderly: a case report. *J Am Geriatr Soc* (1993) 41, 868–9.
7. Hazouard E, Grimbert M, Jonville-Berra A-P, De Toffol M-C, Legras A. Salicylisme et glaucome: augmentation réciproque de la toxicité de l'acétazolamide et de l'acide acétyl salicylique. *J Fr Ophtalmol* (1999) 22, 73–5.
8. Macpherson CR, Milne MD, Evans BM. The excretion of salicylate. *Br J Pharmacol* (1955) 10, 484–9.

Aspirin + Colestipol or Colestyramine

Colestyramine and colestipol do not appear to have any clinically important effects on the absorption of aspirin.

Clinical evidence, mechanism, importance and management

(a) Colestipol

The extent of absorption of a single 650-mg dose of aspirin was unaffected by colestipol 10 g in 12 healthy subjects. However, the rate of aspirin absorption was increased by colestipol: at 60 minutes after the dose the plasma level was increased by about 40%.[1] No particular precautions seem to be necessary during concurrent use.

(b) Colestyramine

A study in 3 healthy subjects and 3 patients, and a later study in 7 healthy subjects, found that colestyramine 4 g delayed the absorption of a single 500-mg dose of aspirin (peak levels extended from 30 to 60 minutes) but the total amount absorbed was only reduced by 5 to 6%. Some of the subjects had slightly higher serum aspirin levels while taking colestyramine.[2] Similar results were reported in another study (a 31% lower plasma aspirin level at 60 minutes, but no difference in total absorption).[1] There would seem to be little reason for avoiding concurrent use unless rapid analgesia is needed.

1. Hunninghake DB, Pollack E. Effect of bile acid sequestering agents on the absorption of aspirin, tolbutamide, and warfarin. *Fedn Proc* (1977) 35, 996.
2. Hahn K-J, Eiden W, Schettle M, Hahn M, Walter E, Weber E. Effect of cholestyramine on the gastrointestinal absorption of phenprocoumon and acetylosalicylic acid in man. *Eur J Clin Pharmacol* (1972) 4, 142–5.

Aspirin or other Salicylates + Corticosteroids or Corticotropin

Serum salicylate levels are reduced by corticosteroids and therefore they may rise, possibly to toxic concentrations, if the corticosteroid is withdrawn without first reducing the salicylate dosage. Concurrent use increases the risk of gastrointestinal bleeding and ulceration. Consider also 'Corticosteroids + NSAIDs', p.807.

Clinical evidence

A 5-year-old boy on long-term **prednisone**, at least 20 mg daily, was given **choline salicylate** 3.6 g daily, and the **prednisone** was gradually tapered off to 3 mg daily over a 3-month period. Severe salicylate toxicity developed, and in a retrospective investigation of the cause, using frozen serum samples drawn for other purposes, it was found that the serum salicylate levels had risen from about 10 mg% to 90 mg% during the withdrawal of the **prednisone**.[1] Later studies in 3 other patients on **choline salicylate** or aspirin and either **prednisone** or another unnamed corticosteroid, found about a threefold rise during corticosteroid withdrawal.[1] **Hydrocortisone** was also found to increase the clearance of **sodium salicylate** in 4 other patients.[1]

A serum salicylate rise of similar proportions has been described in a patient on **aloxiprin** when **prednisolone** was withdrawn.[2] Other studies in both adults and children show that **prednisone, methylprednisolone, betamethasone** and **corticotropin** reduce serum salicylate levels.[3-5] Two studies also found that intra-articular **dexamethasone**, **methylprednisolone**, and **triamcinolone** transiently reduced serum salicylate levels in patients given enteric-coated aspirin.[6,7] However one study in patients found that **prednisone** 12 to 60 mg daily had no effect on the clearance of single doses of **sodium salicylate**.[8]

Mechanism

Uncertain. One idea is that the presence of the corticosteroid increases the glomerular filtration rate, which increases salicylate clearance. When the corticosteroid is withdrawn, the clearance returns to normal and the salicylate accumulates. Another suggestion is that the corticosteroids increase the metabolism of the salicylate.[3]

Importance and management

Well established interactions. Concurrent use is very common but patients should be monitored to ensure that salicylate levels remain adequate when corticosteroids are added[4] and do not become excessive if they are withdrawn. It should also be remembered that concurrent use may increase the incidence of gastrointestinal bleeding[9] and ulceration. See also 'Corticosteroids + NSAIDs', p.807.

1. Klinenberg JR, Miller F. Effect of corticosteroids on blood salicylate concentration. *JAMA* (1965) 194, 601–4.
2. Muirden KD, Barraclough DRE. Drug interactions in the management of rheumatoid arthritis. *Aust N Z J Med* (1976) 6 (Suppl 1), 14–17.
3. Graham GG, Champion GD, Day RO, Paull PD. Patterns of plasma concentrations and urinary excretion of salicylate in rheumatoid arthritis. *Clin Pharmacol Ther* (1977) 22, 410–20.
4. Bardare M, Cislaghi GU, Mandelli M, Sereni F. Value of monitoring plasma salicylate levels in treating juvenile rheumatoid arthritis. *Arch Dis Child* (1978) 53, 381–5.
5. Koren G, Roifman C, Gelfand E, Lavi S, Suria D, Stein L. Corticosteroids-salicylate interaction in a case of juvenile rheumatoid arthritis. *Ther Drug Monit* (1987) 9, 177–9.
6. Edelman J, Potter JM, Hackett LP. The effect of intra-articular steroids on plasma salicylate concentrations. *Br J Clin Pharmacol* (1986) 21, 301–7.
7. Baer PA, Shore A, Ikeman RL. Transient fall in serum salicylate levels following intraarticular injection of steroid in patients with rheumatoid arthritis. *Arthritis Rheum* (1987) 30, 345–7.
8. Day RO, Harris G, Brown M, Graham GG, Champion GD. Interaction of salicylate and corticosteroids in man. *Br J Clin Pharmacol* (1988) 26, 334–7.
9. Carson JL, Strom BL, Schinnar R, Sim E, Maislin G, Morse ML. Do corticosteroids really cause upper GI bleeding? *Clin Res* (1987) 35, 340A.

Aspirin + Dapsone

Dapsone does not significantly affect the pharmacokinetics of aspirin.

Clinical evidence, mechanism, importance and management

A comparison of the pharmacokinetics of aspirin in 8 healthy subjects and 8 patients with uncomplicated lepromatous leprosy found that the pharmacokinetics of a single 600-mg dose of aspirin was not affected by either leprosy, or treatment with dapsone 100 mg daily for 8 days.[1]

1. Garg SK, Kumar B, Shukla VK, Bakaya V, Lal R, Kaur S. Pharmacokinetics of aspirin and chloramphenicol in normal and leprotic patients before and after dapsone therapy. *Int J Clin Pharmacol* (1988) 26, 204–5.

Aspirin + Food

Avoid food if rapid analgesia is needed because it delays the absorption of aspirin.

Clinical evidence, mechanism, importance and management

A study in 25 subjects given aspirin 650 mg in five different aspirin preparations showed that food roughly halved their serum salicylate levels when measured 10 and 20 minutes later, compared with those seen when the same dose was taken while fasting.[1] Similar results were found in subjects given calcium aspirin 1.5 g.[2] Another study in 8 healthy subjects who were given effervescent aspirin 900 mg, serum salicylate levels were roughly halved by food at 15 minutes, but were more or less unchanged after an hour.[3] A possible reason for the reduced rate of absorption is that food delays gastric emptying. Thus if rapid analgesia is needed, aspirin should be taken without food, but if aspirin is needed long-term, giving it with food is thought to help to protect the gastric mucosa.

1. Wood JH. Effect of food on aspirin absorption. *Lancet* (1967) ii, 212.
2. Spiers ASD and Malone HF. Effect of food on aspirin absorption. *Lancet* (1967) i, 440.
3. Volans GN. Effects of food and exercise on the absorption of effervescent aspirin. *Br J Clin Pharmacol* (1974) 1, 137–41.

Aspirin + Griseofulvin

An isolated report describes a marked fall in serum salicylate levels in a child given aspirin and griseofulvin.

Clinical evidence, mechanism, importance and management

An 8-year-old boy with rheumatic fever on aspirin 110 mg/kg daily and furosemide, digoxin, captopril, potassium, aluminium/magnesium hydroxide and iron, had a very marked fall in serum salicylate levels (from a range of 18.3 to 30.6 mg/dl to less than 0.2 mg/dl) within 2 days of starting griseofulvin 10 mg/kg daily. Two days after the griseofulvin was stopped, the salicylate levels were back to their former levels. The reasons for this effect are not known, but some interference with the salicylate absorption is suggested.[1] This appears to be the first and only report of this interaction so that its general importance is uncertain, but it would be prudent to monitor the effects in any patient if substantial doses of salicylates are given with griseofulvin.

1. Phillips KR, Wideman SD, Cochran EB, Becker JA. Griseofulvin significantly decreases serum salicylate concentrations. *Pediatr Infect Dis J* (1993) 12, 350–2.

Aspirin + Kaolin-pectin

Kaolin-pectin causes a small reduction in the absorption of aspirin, which is not clinically relevant.

Clinical evidence, mechanism, importance and management

The absorption of aspirin 975 mg in 10 healthy subjects was reduced by 5 to 10% by 30 or 60 ml of kaolin-pectin.[1] A likely explanation is that the aspirin becomes adsorbed by the kaolin so that the amount available for absorption through the gut wall is reduced. This small reduction in absorption is unlikely to be of clinical importance.

1. Juhl RP. Comparison of kaolin-pectin and activated charcoal for inhibition of aspirin absorption. *Am J Hosp Pharm* (1979) 36, 1097–8.

Aspirin + Laxatives

Sodium sulphate and castor oil used as laxatives can cause a modest, but probably clinically unimportant, reduction in aspirin absorption.

Clinical evidence, mechanism, importance and management

In an experimental study of the possible effects of laxatives on drug absorption, healthy subjects were given 10 to 20 g of oral **sodium sulfate** and 20 g of **castor oil** (doses sufficient to provoke diarrhoea). Absorption, measured by the amount of drug excreted in the urine, was decreased at 4 hours. The reduction was 21% for **castor oil** and aspirin, and 27% for **sodium sulfate** and aspirin. However, serum levels of aspirin were relatively unchanged. The overall picture was that while these laxatives can alter the pattern of absorption, they do not seriously impair the total amount of drug absorbed.[1] More study is needed in a clinical situation.

1. Mattila MJ, Takki S, Jussila J. Effect of sodium sulphate and castor oil on drug absorption from the human intestine. *Ann Clin Res* (1974) 6, 19–24.

Aspirin + Levamisole

A rise in salicylate levels occurred in a patient on aspirin when levamisole was given, but this effect was not confirmed in a subsequent controlled study.

Clinical evidence, mechanism, importance and management

A preliminary report of a patient who showed an increase in salicylate levels when levamisole was given with aspirin[1] prompted a study of this possible interaction. Sustained-release aspirin 3.9 g daily in two divided doses was given to 9 healthy subjects over a period of 3 weeks, with levamisole 50 mg three times a day for a week, each subject acting as his own control. No significant changes in plasma salicylate levels were found.[2]

1. Laidlaw D'A. Rheumatoid arthritis improved by treatment with levamisole and L-histidine. *Med J Aust* (1976) 2, 382–5.
2. Rumble RH, Brooks PM, Roberts MS. Interaction between levamisole and aspirin in man. *Br J Clin Pharmacol* (1979) 7, 631–3.

Aspirin + Pentazocine

Renal papillary necrosis occurred in man regularly taking large doses of aspirin when he was given pentazocine.

Clinical evidence, mechanism, importance and management

An isolated report describes renal papillary necrosis in a man, regularly taking aspirin 1.8 to 2.4 g daily, within 6 months of additionally starting to take pentazocine 800 to 850 mg daily. He developed abdominal pain, nausea and vomiting, and passed tissue via his urethra. Before starting the pentazocine and after it was stopped, no necrosis was apparent. The postulated reason for this reaction is that the pentazocine-induced reduction in blood flow through the kidney potentiated the adverse effects of the chronic aspirin use.[1] The general importance of this case is uncertain, but it emphasises the risks of long-term use (possibly abuse) of aspirin with pentazocine.

1. Muhalwas KK, Shah GM, Winer RL. Renal papillary necrosis caused by long-term ingestion of pentazocine and aspirin. *JAMA* (1981) 246, 867–8.

Aspirin + Phenylbutazone

Phenylbutazone reduces the uricosuric effects of high-dose aspirin. Concurrent use is likely to be associated with an increased risk of gastrointestinal damage.

Clinical evidence

The observation that several patients given aspirin and phenylbutazone developed elevated serum urate levels, prompted a study in 4 patients without gout. This showed that aspirin 2 g daily had little effect on the excretion of uric acid in the urine, but marked uricosuria occurred with aspirin 5 g daily. When phenylbutazone 200, 400 and then 600 mg daily over 3 days was also given the uricosuria was abolished. Serum uric acid levels rose from an average of 4 to 6 mg%. The interaction was confirmed in a patient with tophaceous gout. The retention of uric acid also occurs if the phenylbutazone is given first.[1]

Mechanism

Not understood. It seems almost certain that some interference occurs within the kidney tubules. Phenylbutazone is structurally related to sulfinpyrazone, which interacts similarly, see 'Aspirin or other Salicylates + Sulfinpyrazone', p.82.

Importance and management

An established but sparsely documented interaction. If serum urate measurements are taken in patients on aspirin and phenylbutazone for diagnostic purposes, this interaction should be considered in their interpretation. The potential problems arising from this interaction should also be recognised in any patient given both drugs. Although there does not appear to be any specific evidence for phenylbutazone, concurrent use of aspirin and NSAIDs increases the risk of gastrointestinal damage and is not recommended, see also 'NSAIDs + Aspirin; Anti-inflammatory dose', p.83.

1. Oyer JH, Wagner SL, Schmid FR. Suppression of salicylate-induced uricosuria by phenylbutazone. *Am J Med Sci* (1966) 225, 40–5.

Aspirin or other Salicylates + Probenecid

The uricosuric effects of high doses of aspirin or other salicylates and probenecid are not additive as might be expected but are mutually antagonistic. Low dose, enteric-coated aspirin appears not to interact.

Clinical evidence

(a) High-dose aspirin or other salicylates

A study found that the average urinary uric acid excretion in 24 hours was 673 mg with a single 3-g daily dose of probenecid, 909 mg with a 6-g daily dose of **sodium salicylate**, but only 114 mg when both drugs were given.[1] Similar antagonism has been seen in other studies in patients given 2.6 to 5.2 g aspirin daily.[2-4] No antagonism is seen until serum salicylate levels of 5 to 10 mg/dl are reached.[4]

(b) Low-dose aspirin

A crossover study in 11 patients with gouty arthritis, stabilised on probenecid, found that enteric-coated aspirin 325 mg daily, taken either with probenecid or 6 hours after probenecid, had no effect on serum urate levels or on the 24-hour urate excretion.[5]

Mechanism

Not understood. The interference probably occurs at the site of renal tubular secretion, but it also seems that both drugs can occupy the same site on plasma albumins.

Importance and management

A well established and clinically important interaction. Regular dosing with substantial amounts of salicylates should be avoided if this antagonism is to be avoided, but small very occasional analgesic doses probably do not matter. Serum salicylate levels of 5 to 10 mg/dl are necessary before this interaction occurs. Low-dose aspirin (325 mg or less daily) does not seem to interact.

1. Seegmiller JE, Grayzel AI. Use of the newer uricosuric agents in the management of gout. *JAMA* (1960) 173, 1076–80.
2. Pascale LR, Dubin A, Hoffman WS. Therapeutic value of probenecid (Benemid®) in gout. *JAMA* (1952) 149, 1188–94.
3. Gutman AB, Yü TF. Benemid (*p*-di-*n*-propylsulfamyl-benzoic acid) as uricosuric agent in chronic gouty arthritis. *Trans Assoc Am Physicians* (1951) 64, 279–88.
4. Pascale LR, Dubin A, Bronsky D, Hoffman WS. Inhibition of the uricosuric action of Benemid by salicylate. *J Lab Clin Med* (1955) 45, 771–7.
5. Harris M, Bryant LR, Danaher P, Alloway J. Effect of low dose daily aspirin on serum urate levels and urinary excretion in patients receiving probenecid for gouty arthritis. *J Rheumatol* (2000) 27, 2873–6.

Aspirin or other Salicylates + Sulfinpyrazone

The uricosuric effects of the salicylates and sulfinpyrazone are not additive, as might be expected, but are mutually antagonistic.

Clinical evidence

When **sodium salicylate** 6 g was given with sulfinpyrazone 600 mg daily to one patient the average urinary uric acid excretion in 24 hours was 30 mg, whereas when each drug was used alone in the same doses the average 24-hour urinary excretion was 281 and 527 mg for **sodium salicylate** and sulfinpyrazone respectively.[1] A later study in 5 men with gout given a sulfinpyrazone infusion for about an hour (300 mg bolus followed by 10 mg/minute) found that the additional infusion of **sodium salicylate** (3 g bolus followed by 10 to 20 mg/minute) virtually abolished the uricosuria. When the drugs were given in the reverse order to 3 other patients the same result was seen.[2]

In another study, the uricosuria caused by sulfinpyrazone 400 mg daily was found to be completely abolished by aspirin 3.5 g.[3] The clearance of a single 400-mg dose of sulfinpyrazone was modestly increased by 12 to 27% in 5 healthy subjects given four doses of aspirin 325 mg over 24 hours.[4]

Mechanism

Not fully understood. Sulfinpyrazone competes successfully with salicylate for secretion by the kidney tubules so that salicylate excretion is reduced, but the salicylate blocks the inhibitory effect of sulfinpyrazone on the tubular reabsorption of uric acid causing the uric acid to accumulate within the body.[2]

Importance and management

An established and clinically important interaction. Concurrent use for uricosuria should be avoided. Doses of aspirin as low as 700 mg can cause an appreciable fall in uric acid excretion,[3] but the effects of an occasional small dose are probably of little practical importance.

1. Seegmiller JE, Grayzel AI. Use of the newer uricosuric agents in the management of gout. *JAMA* (1960) 173, 1076–80.
2. Yu TF, Dayton PG, Gutman AB. Mutual suppression of the uricosuric effects of sulfinpyrazone and salicylate: a study in interactions between drugs. *J Clin Invest* (1963) 42, 1330–9.
3. Kersley GD, Cook ER, Tovey DCJ. Value of uricosuric agents and in particular of G.28 315 in gout. *Ann Rheum Dis* (1958) 17, 326–33.
4. Buchanan MR, Endrenyi L, Giles AR, Rosenfeld J. The effect of aspirin on the pharmacokinetics of sulfinpyrazone in man. *Thromb Res* (1983) (Suppl 4), 145–52.

Aspirin + *Tamarindus indica*

***Tamarindus indica* fruit extract markedly increases the absorption and serum levels of aspirin.**

Clinical evidence, mechanism, importance and management

A study in 6 healthy subjects found that the bioavailability of a single 600-mg dose of aspirin was increased when taken with a meal containing *Tamarindus indica* fruit extract. The aspirin AUC rose sixfold, the maximum serum levels rose almost threefold (from 10.04 to 28.62 mg/ml) and the half-life increased moderately (from 1.04 to 1.5 hours).[1] The reasons are not known, nor has the clinical importance of these large increases been evaluated, but this interaction should be borne in mind if high doses of aspirin are taken with this fruit extract. There would seem to be the possible risk of aspirin toxicity.

1. Mustapha A, Yakasai IA, Aguye IA. Effect of *Tamarindus indica L.* on the bioavailability of aspirin in health human volunteers. *Eur J Drug Metab Pharmacokinet* (1996) 21, 223–6.

Nefopam + Miscellaneous

Nefopam should not be given to patients taking MAOIs. Be cautious with tricyclic antidepressants, anticholinergics and sympathomimetics. The intensity and incidence of adverse effects are somewhat increased when nefopam is given with codeine, pentazocine or dextropropoxyphene (propoxyphene).

Clinical evidence, mechanism, importance and management

Detailed information about adverse interactions between nefopam and other drugs does not seem to be available, but convulsions have been seen in a few patients and the makers say that nefopam is contraindicated in patients with a history of convulsive disorders.[1] Caution should be exercised with the **tricyclic antidepressants** because these lower the convulsive threshold. In addition, the anticholinergic adverse effects of nefopam may be additive with those of **tricyclics** and other drugs with anticholinergic effects.[1] For example, the UK Committee on Safety of Medicines has a number of reports of urinary retention caused by nefopam[2], which would be expected to be worsened by drugs with anticholinergic activity. Nefopam appears to have sympathomimetic activity and the makers say it should not be given with the **MAOIs**.[1]

A controlled trial was conducted in 45 healthy subjects divided into nine groups of five, each given nefopam 60 mg three times daily for 3 days with either **aspirin** 650 mg, **diazepam** 5 mg, **phenobarbital** 60 mg, **dextropropoxyphene** (**propoxyphene**) 65 mg, **codeine** 60 mg, **pentazocine** 50 mg, **indometacin** 25 mg or **hydroxyzine** 50 mg (all three times daily). The only changes were a possible additive increase in the intensity and incidence of adverse effects with nefopam and **codeine**, **pentazocine** or **dextropropoxyphene**. There was no evidence that the bioavailability of nefopam was change by the other drugs.[3] The incidence of sedation with nefopam is 20 to 30% which, depending on the circumstances, may present a problem if given with other **sedative drugs**.[4]

1. Acupan (Nefopam). 3M Health Care Ltd. UK Summary of product characteristics, November 2000.

2. Committee on Safety of Medicines (CSM). Nefopam hydrochloride (Acupan). Current Problems No 24, January 1989.
3. Lasseter KC, Cohen A, Back EL. Nefopam HCl interaction study with eight other drugs. *J Int Med Res* (1976) 4, 195–201.
4. Heel RC, Brogden RN, Pakes GE, Speight TM, Avery GS. Nefopam: a review of its pharmacological properties and therapeutic efficacy. *Drugs* (1980) 19, 249–57.

NSAIDs + Allopurinol

Allopurinol does not affect indometacin or phenylbutazone levels.

Clinical evidence, mechanism, importance and management

Allopurinol 300 mg each morning was given to 8 patients for 5 days with **indometacin** 50 mg every 8 hours. The allopurinol had no significant effect on the AUC of **indometacin** and the amounts of **indometacin** excreted in the urine were not significantly altered.[1]

Allopurinol 100 mg three times daily for a month had no effect on the elimination of a 200-mg daily dose of **phenylbutazone** in 6 healthy subjects, and no effect on the steady-state plasma levels of **phenylbutazone** in 3 patients taking 200 or 300 mg daily.[2] In another study in 8 patients with acute gouty arthritis it was found that allopurinol 100 mg every 8 hours produced small but clinically unimportant effects on the half-life of **phenylbutazone** 6 mg/kg.[3]

There seems to be no reason for avoiding concurrent use of these NSAIDs and allopurinol.

1. Pullar T, Myall O, Haigh JRM, Lowe JR, Dixon JS, Bird HA. The effect of allopurinol on the steady-state pharmacokinetics of indomethacin. *Br J Clin Pharmacol* (1988) 25, 755–7.
2. Rawlins MD, Smith SE. Influence of allopurinol on drug metabolism in man. *Br J Pharmacol* (1973) 48, 693–8.
3. Horwitz D, Thorgeirsson SS, Mitchell JR. The influence of allopurinol and size of dose on the metabolism of phenylbutazone in patients with gout. *Eur J Clin Pharmacol* (1977) 12, 133–6.

NSAIDs + Aspirin; Anti-inflammatory dose

The combined use of aspirin and NSAIDs increases the risk of gastrointestinal damage. There is no clinical rationale for the combined use of anti-inflammatory/analgesic doses of aspirin and NSAIDs and such use should be avoided. See also 'NSAIDs + Aspirin; Antiplatelet dose', p.84. There are numerous early pharmacokinetic studies of aspirin and NSAIDs, many of which showed that aspirin reduced the levels of NSAIDs.

Clinical evidence

A. Gastrointestinal damage

The risk of upper gastrointestinal bleeding or perforation was increased by slightly more than an additive effect in users of both aspirin and NSAIDs (8.2-fold) when compared with aspirin alone (2.4-fold) or NSAIDs alone (3.6-fold) in a case-control study of data from 1993 to 1998 in the UK General Practice Research Database. The specific NSAIDs were not mentioned.[1] Another study provided similar findings,[2] as have studies specifically looking at low-dose aspirin (325 mg or less daily), see 'NSAIDs + Aspirin; Antiplatelet dose', p.84. Analysis of Yellow Card reports to the UK Committee on Safety of Medicines of gastrointestinal perforation/obstruction, ulceration or bleeding with **diclofenac**, **naproxen** and **ibuprofen** revealed that 28% of the patients were receiving concurrent aspirin (dose not stated).[3]

The one pharmacodynamic study below, that also measured gastrointestinal blood loss, found increased bleeding for the combination of anti-inflammatory doses of aspirin and **sodium meclofenamate**.[4]

A case report described acute ulcerative colitis in a woman on **rofecoxib** 25 mg daily who took aspirin as self-medication.[5] Note that there is some evidence that low-dose aspirin attenuates any gastrointestinal benefits of **celecoxib**, see 'NSAIDs + Aspirin; Antiplatelet dose', p.84.

B. Pharmacokinetic and pharmacodynamic studies

Early studies evaluating non-aspirin NSAIDs in rheumatoid arthritis commonly permitted the concurrent use of aspirin, which was then in wide use for this condition. The unexpected finding that **indometacin** was no more effective than placebo in patients on aspirin in one study led to a number of pharmacokinetic studies with this combination (see (d) **Indometacin**, below), and subsequently other NSAID/aspirin combinations. These studies generally have little clinical relevance to current clinical practice where anti-inflammatory doses of aspirin are not used in combination with NSAIDs because of the increased risk of gastrointestinal bleeding (see above) and lack of proven additional benefit. However, they are briefly summarised below.

(a) Diclofenac

Aspirin 900 mg reduced the AUC of diclofenac 50 mg by about one-third in a single-dose study.[6] In a clinical study, there was no significant difference in efficacy between diclofenac 50 mg three times daily or diclofenac plus aspirin 900 mg three times daily.[7]

(b) Fenamates

A study in 20 healthy subjects given aspirin 600 mg and **sodium meclofenamate** 100 mg both three times daily for 14 days found no significant reductions in plasma salicylate levels, but plasma **meclofenamate** levels were reduced to some extent. However, gastrointestinal blood loss was approximately doubled compared with either drug alone.[4]

(c) Ibuprofen and related drugs

Aspirin 1.3 to 3.6 g daily more than halved the serum levels of ibuprofen 800 mg to 2.4 g daily,[8,9] without affecting salicylate levels.[9] There was little additional clinical benefit from the combination.[9] Similarly, aspirin reduced the AUC of **flurbiprofen** by about two-thirds,[10] but without any clear changes in clinical effectiveness.[11] The pharmacokinetics of the aspirin were unchanged by **flurbiprofen**.[10] Aspirin 3.9 g daily also virtually halved the AUC of **fenoprofen** 2.4 g daily,[12] and reduced the AUC of **ketoprofen** 200 mg daily[13] by about one-third. The AUC of **naproxen** was only minimally reduced, by 10 to 15%).[14,15] **Choline magnesium trisalicylate** increases the clearance of **naproxen** by 56% and decreases its serum levels by 26%.[16]

(d) Indometacin

The overall picture with aspirin and indometacin is confusing and contradictory. One early study found that indometacin was no more effective than placebo in patients already on aspirin.[17] Consequently, a number of studies were conducted to see if there was a drug interaction. Some studies reported that aspirin reduced serum indometacin levels[12,18-20] or its efficacy,[21] or that the combination was no more effective than either drug alone.[22] Others report that no change in indometacin levels occurred[23-25] Further studies using buffered aspirin claimed that it increased the rate of absorption of indometacin and is associated with an increase in adverse effects (tiredness, lack of coordination).[26,27]

(e) Oxicams

Aspirin 3 g daily increased the maximum plasma levels of **meloxicam** 30 mg daily by 25% and its AUC by 10%.[28] Plasma levels of **piroxicam** 40 mg then 20 mg daily were not significantly affected by aspirin 3.9 g daily, and salicylate levels were unaffected by **piroxicam**.[29] Aspirin 2.6 to 3.9 g daily more than halved the serum levels of **tenoxicam** 20 mg daily.[30]

(f) Miscellaneous NSAIDs

Aspirin 600 mg four times daily caused a 15% fall in the plasma levels of **diflunisal** 250 mg twice daily for 3 days.[31] Single-dose studies have shown that the absorption of **nabumetone** 1 g is not significantly altered by aspirin 1.5 g.[32] The plasma levels of **tolmetin** 1.2 g daily were slightly reduced by aspirin 3.9 g daily.[33]

Mechanism

The damaging effects of aspirin and NSAIDs on the gut appear to be additive. The mechanisms behind the pharmacokinetic changes have not been resolved. Changes in the rates of absorption and renal clearance and competition for plasma protein binding have been proposed.

Importance and management

The additive risk of gastrointestinal damage from combining aspirin and NSAIDs is established. Because of this, and the lack of clear benefit from the combination, the use of anti-inflammatory/analgesic doses of aspirin with NSAIDs should be avoided. For information on low-dose aspirin and NSAIDs see 'NSAIDs + Aspirin; Antiplatelet dose', p.84. Consider also 'NSAIDs + NSAIDs', p.90.

1. García Rodríguez LA, Hernández-Díaz S. The risk of upper gastrointestinal complications associated with nonsteroidal anti-inflammatory drugs, glucocorticoids, acetaminophen, and combinations of these agents. *Arthritis Res* (2001) 3, 98–101.

2. Mellemkjaer L, Blot WJ, Sørensen HT, Thomassen L, McLaughlin JK, Nielsen GL, Olsen JH. Upper gastrointestinal bleeding among users of NSAIDs: a population-based cohort study in Denmark. *Br J Clin Pharmacol* (2002) 53, 173–81.
3. Committee on Safety of Medicines/Medicines Control Agency. Non-steroidal anti-inflammatory drugs (NSAIDs) and gastrointestinal safety. *Current Problems* (2002) 28, 5.
4. Baragar FD, Smith TC. Drug interaction studies with sodium meclofenamate (Meclomen®). *Curr Ther Res* (1978) 23 (April Suppl), S51–S59.
5. Charachon A, Petit T, Lamarque D, Soulé J-C. Colite aiguë hémorragique chez une malade traitée par rofécoxib associé à une auto-médication par aspirine. *Gastroenterol Clin Biol* (2003) 27, 511–13.
6. Willis JV, Kendall MJ, Jack DB. A study of the effect of aspirin on the pharmacokinetics of oral and intravenous diclofenac sodium. *Eur J Clin Pharmacol* (1980) 18, 415–8.
7. Bird HA, Hill J, Leatham P, Wright V. A study to determine the clinical relevance of the pharmacokinetic interaction between aspirin and diclofenac. *Agents Actions* (1986) 18, 447–9.
8. Albert KS, Gernaat CM. Pharmacokinetics of ibuprofen. *Am J Med* (1984) 77(1A), 40–6.
9. Grennan DM, Ferry DG, Ashworth ME, Kenny RE, Mackinnon M. The aspirin-ibuprofen interaction in rheumatoid arthritis. *Br J Clin Pharmacol* (1979) 8, 497–503.
10. Kaiser DG, Brooks CD, Lomen PL. Pharmacokinetics of flurbiprofen. *Am J Med* (1986) 80 (Suppl 3A), 10–15.
11. Brooks PM, Khong TK. Flurbiprofen-aspirin interaction: a double-blind crossover study. *Curr Med Res Opin* (1977) 5, 53–7.
12. Rubin A, Rodda BE, Warrick P, Gruber CM, Ridolfo AS. Interactions of aspirin with nonsteroidal antiinflammatory drugs in man. *Arthritis Rheum* (1973) 16, 635–45.
13. Williams RL, Upton RA, Buskin JN, Jones RM. Ketoprofen-aspirin interactions. *Clin Pharmacol Ther* (1981) 30, 226–31.
14. Segre EJ, Chaplin M, Forchielli E, Runkel R, Sevelius H. Naproxen-aspirin interactions in man. *Clin Pharmacol Ther* (1974) 15, 374–9.
15. Segre E, Sevelius H, Chaplin M, Forchielli E, Runkel R, Rooks W. Interaction of naproxen and aspirin in the rat and in man. *Scand J Rheumatol* (1973) (Suppl 2), 37–42.
16. Furst DE, Sarkissian E, Blocka K, Cassell S, Dromgoole S, Harris ER, Hirschberg JM, Josephson N, Paulus HE. Serum concentrations of salicylate and naproxen during concurrent therapy in patients with rheumatoid arthritis. *Arthritis Rheum* (1987) 30, 1157–61.
17. The Cooperating Clinics Committee of the American Rheumatism Association. A three-month trial of indomethacin in rheumatoid arthritis, with special reference to analysis and inference. *Clin Pharmacol Ther* (1967) 8, 11–37.
18. Kaldestad E, Hansen T, Brath HK. Interaction of indomethacin and acetylsalicylic acid as shown by the serum concentrations of indomethacin and salicylate. *Eur J Clin Pharmacol* (1975) 9, 199–207.
19. Jeremy R, Towson J. Interaction between aspirin and indomethacin in the treatment of rheumatoid arthritis. *Med J Aust* (1970) 3, 127–9.
20. Kwan KC, Breault GO, Davis RL, Lei BW, Czerwinski AW, Besselaar GH, Duggan DE. Effects of concomitant aspirin administration on the pharmacokinetics of indomethacin in man. *J Pharmacokinet Biopharm* (1978) 6, 451–76.
21. Pawlotsky Y, Chales G, Grosbois B, Miane B, Bourel M. Comparative interaction of aspirin with indomethacin and sulindac in chronic rheumatic diseases. *Eur J Rheumatol Inflamm* (1978) 1, 18–20.
22. Brooks PM, Walker JJ, Bell MA, Buchanan WW, Rhymer AR. Indomethacin—aspirin interaction: a clinical appraisal. *BMJ* (1975) 3, 69–71.
23. Champion D, Mongan E, Paulus H, Sarkissian E, Okun R, Pearson C. Effect of concurrent aspirin (ASA) administration on serum concentrations of indomethacin (I). *Arthritis Rheum* (1971) 14, 375.
24. Lindquist B, Jensen KM, Johansson H, Hansen T. Effect of concurrent administration of aspirin and indomethacin on serum concentrations. *Clin Pharmacol Ther* (1974) 15, 247–52.
25. Barraclough DRE, Muirden KD, Laby B. Salicylate therapy and drug interaction in rheumatoid arthritis. *Aust N Z J Med* (1975) 5, 518–23.
26. Turner P,Garnham JC. Indomethacin-aspirin interaction. *BMJ* (1975) 2, 368.
27. Garnham JC, Raymond K, Shotton E, Turner P. The effect of buffered aspirin on plasma indomethacin. *Eur J Clin Pharmacol* (1975) 8, 107–13.
28. Busch U, Heinzel G, Narjes H, Nehmiz G. Interaction of meloxicam with cimetidine, Maalox or aspirin. *J Clin Pharmacol* (1996) 36, 79–84.
29. Hobbs DC, Twomey TM. Piroxicam pharmacokinetics in man: aspirin and antacid interaction studies. *J Clin Pharmacol* (1979) 19, 270–81.
30. Day RO, Paull PD, Lam S, Swanson BR, Williams KM, Wade DN. The effect of concurrent aspirin upon plasma concentrations of tenoxicam. *Br J Clin Pharmacol* (1988) 26, 455–62.
31. Schulz P, Perrier CV, Ferber-Perret F, VandenHeuvel WJA, Steelman SL. Diflunisal, a new-acting analgesic and prostaglandin inhibitor: effect of concomitant acetylsalicylic acid therapy on ototoxicity and on disposition of both drugs. *J Int Med Res* (1979) 7, 61–8.
32. von Schrader HW, Buscher G, Dierdorf D, Mügge H, Wolf D. Nabumetone — a novel anti-inflammatory drug: the influence of food, milk, antacids, and analgesics on bioavailability of single oral doses. *Int J Clin Pharmacol Ther Toxicol* (1983) 21, 311–21.
33. Cressman WA, Wortham GF, Plostnieks J. Absorption and excretion of tolmetin in man. *Clin Pharmacol Ther* (1976) 19, 224–33.

NSAIDs + Aspirin; Antiplatelet dose

There is some evidence that non-selective NSAIDs such as ibuprofen antagonise the antiplatelet effects of low-dose aspirin, but that COX-2-selective NSAIDs (coxibs) do not. Some, but not other, epidemiological studies have shown that non-selective NSAIDs reduce the cardioprotective effects of low-dose aspirin. Combined use of NSAIDs and low-dose aspirin increases the risk of gastrointestinal bleeds. This seems to apply equally to coxibs.

Clinical evidence

(a) Cardioprotective effects

A pharmacodynamic study in healthy subjects found that **ibuprofen** 400 mg daily given 2 hours before aspirin 81 mg daily for 6 days reduced the degree of thromboxane inhibition and blocked the inhibition of platelet aggregation. Conversely, when the aspirin was given 2 hours before the daily **ibuprofen** dose, there was no reduction in the antiplatelet effects of aspirin. However, **ibuprofen** 400 mg three times daily (with the first dose taken 2 hours after the daily aspirin dose) inhibited the antiplatelet effect of aspirin. Inhibition of the antiplatelet effects of aspirin was not seen with **diclofenac** 75 mg twice daily, nor with single 25-mg daily doses of **rofecoxib**, or **paracetamol** (acetaminophen) 1 g taken 2 hours before or after the aspirin.[1]

Similarly, in other studies **celecoxib** 200 mg twice daily[2] and **parecoxib** 40 mg twice daily[3] did not alter the antiplatelet effect of aspirin 325 mg, and the makers say that at steady-state **etoricoxib** 120 mg daily did not affect the antiplatelet activity of aspirin 81 mg daily.[4]

As a consequence of these pharmacodynamic studies, various cohort/case-control studies or sub-group analyses have been conducted to see if **ibuprofen** and/or other NSAIDs reduce the cardioprotective effect of low-dose aspirin in patients, see 'Table 5.2', (p.85). Because these studies are neither prospective nor randomised, their findings are suggestive only, nevertheless they provide some useful insight. One study appeared to confirm the pharmacodynamic data in that patients on **ibuprofen** and aspirin had a higher mortality than those on aspirin alone, aspirin plus **diclofenac**, or aspirin plus another NSAID.[5] Another study found that regular, but not intermittent, use of NSAIDs was a problem.[6] However, two other studies did not find that NSAIDs, or **ibuprofen** in particular, reduced the benefit of aspirin on mortality post-myocardial infarction.[7,8]

(b) Gastrointestinal effects

Low-dose aspirin alone (300 mg or less daily) was associated with an increased risk of hospitalisation for bleeding peptic ulcer in a case-control study. The odds ratios were 2.3 for aspirin 75 mg daily, 3.2 for 150 mg daily, and 3.9 for 300 mg daily. Use of NSAIDs combined with low-dose aspirin was associated with a greater risk of bleeding (odds ratio 7.7) than use of either NSAIDs alone (5.4) or low-dose aspirin alone (3.3).[9] Similar findings were reported in a cohort study (rate ratio for gastrointestinal bleed for low dose aspirin 2.6, and for combined use with NSAIDs, 5.6).[10]

Patients taking low-dose aspirin (325 mg or less daily) with **celecoxib** had a higher frequency of gastrointestinal complications than those taking **celecoxib** alone. Moreover, there was no difference in frequency of gastrointestinal complications between those taking low-dose aspirin with **celecoxib** and those taking low-dose aspirin with **ibuprofen** or **diclofenac**. This was despite **celecoxib** alone being associated with a lower frequency of gastrointestinal adverse effects than **ibuprofen** or **diclofenac** alone.[11] Similarly, the makers of **valdecoxib** note that use with low-dose aspirin increased the risk of gastrointestinal bleeds.[12]

Mechanism

Aspirin irreversibly blocks the production of thromboxane A2 by binding to cyclo-oxygenase (COX-1) in platelets, and so inhibits platelet aggregation. The beneficial cardiovascular effects are attributed to this effect. Other NSAIDs that are COX-1 inhibitors also have this effect, but it is more short-lived since they bind reversibly. These NSAIDs can therefore competitively inhibit the blinding of aspirin to platelets (a fact that was shown *in vitro* as early as the 1980's[13]). When these NSAIDs are present in sufficient quantities at the time a daily low-dose of aspirin is given, they therefore reduce its antiplatelet effect. *In vitro* study confirms that COX-2 selective NSAIDs have less effect.[14]

It is well known that aspirin and NSAIDs have additive gastrointestinal adverse effects (see 'NSAIDs + Aspirin; Anti-inflammatory dose', p.83). This occurs even at the low doses of aspirin used for antiplatelet effects (doses as low as 75 mg daily).[9]

Importance and management

The evidence currently available on the antagonism of antiplatelet effects is insufficient to recommend that ibuprofen is not used with low-dose aspirin. Nevertheless, some have concluded that when patients taking low-dose aspirin for cardioprotection require long-term NSAIDs for inflammatory conditions, the use of diclofenac would seem preferable to ibuprofen.[15] A coxib might also be an alternative.[15] However the increased risk of serious cardiovascular effects with the coxibs (as a class[16]) probably preclude this.

It is important to also consider the possible increased risk of gastrointestinal adverse effects from any combination. From a gastrointestinal perspective, the lowest dose of aspirin should be used (75 mg).[9] However, when combined with low-dose aspirin, the available evidence indicates that there is no gastrointestinal benefit to be obtained from using a coxib as opposed to diclofenac or ibuprofen.[11] Note that the UK Committee on Safety of Medicines has advised that the combination of a non-aspirin

Table 5.2 Summary of studies on the effect of NSAIDs on the cardioprotective effect of antiplatelet dose aspirin

Study type	*Criteria*	*Outcome*	*Drugs*	*Comments*	*Refs*
Studies showing a decrease in the cardioprotection of aspirin with NSAIDs					
Retrospective cohort	Discharge after CVD	Mortality	Aspirin alone (6285) Aspirin + Ibuprofen (187) Aspirin + Diclofenac (206) Aspirin + other NSAID (429)	Increased all-cause mortality and cardiovascular mortality in those on aspirin + ibuprofen compared with the other groups	1
Subgroup analysis of an RCT	Male physicians randomised to aspirin 325 mg on alternate days or placebo	First MI	Aspirin alone (5273) Aspirin + intermittent NSAID (5147) Aspirin + regular NSAID (598)	Use of NSAIDs for 60 days or more per year was associated with an increased risk of MI in those on aspirin	2
Case-control		First non-fatal MI	Aspirin alone (288) NSAIDs (170) Ibuprofen (104) Naproxen (24)	Both aspirin alone, and NSAIDs alone were associated with a reduced risk of MI, but combined use was not	3
Studies showing no effect of NSAIDs on the cardioprotection of aspirin					
Retrospective cohort	Discharge after MI	Death in first year	Aspirin alone (36 211) NSAID alone (736) Aspirin + NSAID (2096) Neither (9541)	Risk of death reduced to a similar extent by aspirin, NSAIDs, and the combination	4
Retrospective cohort	Discharge after MI and on aspirin	Death in first year	Aspirin alone (66 739) Aspirin + Ibuprofen (844) Aspirin + other NSAID (2733)	Risk of death comparable between the 3 groups	5

1. MacDonald TM, Wei L. Effect of ibuprofen on cardioprotective effect of aspirin. *Lancet* (2003) 361, 573–4.
2. Kurth T, Glynn RJ, Walker AM, Chan KA, Buring JE, Hennekens CH, Gaziano JM. Inhibition of clinical benefits of aspirin on first myocardial infarction by nonsteroidal antiinflammatory drugs. *Circulation* (2003) 108, 1191–5.
3. Kimmel SE, Berlin JA, Reilly M, Jaskowiak J, Kishel L, Chittams J, Strom BL. The effects of nonselective non-aspirin non-steroidal anti-inflammatory medications on the risk of nonfatal myocardial infarction and their interaction with aspirin. *J Am Coll Cardiol* (2004) 43, 985–90.
4. Ko D, Wang Y, Berger AK, Radford MJ, Krumholz HM. Nonsteroidal antiinflammatory drugs after acute myocardial infarction. *Am Heart J* (2002) 143, 475–81.
5. Curtis JP, Wang Y, Portnay EL, Masoudi FA, Havranek EP, Krumholz HM. Aspirin, ibuprofen, and mortality after myocardial infarction: retrospective cohort study. *Br Med J* (2003) 327, 1322–3.

NSAID and low-dose aspirin should be used only if absolutely necessary.[17,18] They state that patients on long-term aspirin should be reminded to avoid NSAIDs, including those bought without prescription.[18] If concurrent use is necessary, where appropriate, the use of a proton pump inhibitor may be considered for prophylaxis of NSAID-induced gastrointestinal damage.

1. Catella-Lawson F, Reilly MP, Kapoor SC, Cucchiara AJ, De Marco S, Tournier B, Vyas SN, FitzGerald GA. Cyclooxygenase inhibitors and the antiplatelet effects of aspirin. *N Engl J Med* (2001) 345, 1809–17.
2. Wilner KD, Rushing M, Walden C, Adler R, Eskra J, Noveck R, Vargas R. Celecoxib does not affect the antiplatelet activity of aspirin in healthy volunteers. *J Clin Pharmacol* (2002) 42, 1027–30.
3. Noveck RJ, Kuss ME, Qian J, North J, Hubbard RC. Parecoxib sodium, injectable COX-2 specific inhibitor, does not affect aspirin-mediated platelet function. *Reg Anesth Pain Med* (2001) 26 (Suppl), 19.
4. Arcoxia (Etoricoxib). Merck Sharp & Dohme Ltd. UK Summary of product characteristics, May 2005.
5. MacDonald TM, Wei L. Effect of ibuprofen on cardioprotective effect of aspirin. *Lancet* (2003) 361, 573–4.
6. Kurth T, Glynn RJ, Walker AM, Chan KA, Buring JE, Hennekens CH, Gaziano JM. Inhibition of clinical benefits of aspirin on first myocardial infarction by nonsteroidal antiinflammatory drugs. *Circulation* (2003) 108, 1191–5.
7. Ko D, Wang Y, Berger AK, Radford MJ, Krumholz HM. Nonsteroidal antiinflammatory drugs after acute myocardial infarction. *Am Heart J* (2002) 143, 475–81.
8. Curtis JP, Wang Y, Portnay EL, Masoudi FA, Havranek EP, Krumholz HM. Aspirin, ibuprofen, and mortality after myocardial infarction: retrospective cohort study. *BMJ* (2003) 327, 1322–3.
9. Weil J, Colin-Jones D, Langman M, Lawson D, Logan R, Murphy M, Rawlins M, Vessey M, Wainwright P. Prophylactic aspirin and risk of peptic ulcer bleeding. *BMJ* (1995) 310, 827–30.
10. Sorensen HT, Mellemkjaer L, Blot WJ, Nielsen GL, Steffensen FH, McLaughlin JK, Olsen JH. Risk of upper gastrointestinal bleeding associated with use of low-dose aspirin. *Am J Gastroenterol* (2000) 95, 2218–24.
11. Silverstein FE, Faich G, Goldstein JL, Simon LS, Pincus T, Whelton A, et al. Gastrointestinal toxicity with celecoxib versus nonsteroidal anti-inflammatory drugs for osteoarthritis and rheumatoid arthritis: the CLASS study: a randomized controlled trial. *JAMA* (2000) 284, 1247–55.
12. Bextra (Valdecoxib). Pharmacia Ltd. UK Summary of product characteristics, May 2004.
13. Parks WM, Hoak JC, Czervionke RL. Comparative effect of ibuprofen on endothelial and platelet prostaglandin synthesis. *J Pharmacol Exp Ther* (1981) 219: 415–19.
14. Ouellet M, Riendeau D, Percival MD. A high level of cyclooxygenase-2 inhibitor selectivity is associated with a reduced interference of platelet cyclooxygenase-1 inactivation by aspirin. *Proc Natl Acad Sci U S A* (2001) 98, 14583–8.
15. FitzGerald GA. Parsing an enigma: the pharmacodynamics of aspirin resistance. *Lancet* (2003) 361, 542–4.
16. FitzGerald GA. Coxibs and cardiovascular disease. *N Engl J Med* (2004) 351, 1709–11.
17. Committee on Safety of Medicines/Medicines Control Agency. Non-steroidal anti-inflammatory drugs (NSAIDs) and gastrointestinal safety. *Current Problems* (2002) 28, 5.
18. Committee on Safety of Medicines/Medicines and Healthcare products Regulatory Agency. Reminder: Gastrointestinal toxicity of NSAIDs. *Current Problems* (2003) 29, 8–9.

NSAIDs + Colestipol or Colestyramine

Simultaneous colestyramine markedly reduced the oral absorption of diclofenac and sulindac, modestly reduced the absorption of ibuprofen, but only delayed and did not reduce the extent of absorption of naproxen. Administration of colestyramine three or more hours after oral sulindac, piroxicam, or tenoxicam still markedly reduced their plasma levels. Markedly reduced oxicam levels have also been found when colestyramine is given after intravenous meloxicam or tenoxicam. Simultaneous colestipol modestly reduced the oral absorption of diclofenac, but had no effect on ibuprofen absorption.

Clinical evidence

(a) Diclofenac

A single-dose crossover study in 6 healthy fasting subjects found that the simultaneous use of **colestyramine** 8 g markedly reduced the AUC of a single 100-mg oral dose of enteric coated diclofenac by 62% and reduced its maximum plasma levels by 75%. **Colestipol** 10 g reduced the diclofenac AUC by 33% and its maximum plasma levels by 58%.[1]

(b) Ibuprofen and related drugs

A single-dose crossover study in 6 healthy fasting subjects found that the simultaneous use of **colestyramine** 8 g modestly reduced the AUC of a single 400-mg oral dose of ibuprofen by 26% and reduced its maximum serum levels by 34%. The rate of absorption was also reduced. Conversely, **colestipol** 10 g had no significant effect on the pharmacokinetics of ibuprofen.[2]

The absorption of a single 250-mg dose of **naproxen** was delayed but not reduced in 8 healthy fasting subjects by simultaneous **colestyramine** 4 g in 100 ml of orange juice. The amount absorbed after 2 hours was reduced from 96 to 51%, but was complete after 5 hours.[3]

(c) Oxicams

A study in 12 healthy subjects found that **colestyramine** 4 g taken 2 hours before a 30 mg *intravenous* dose of **meloxicam** increased its clearance by 49% and reduced its mean residence time in the body by 39%.[4]

Another study in 8 healthy subjects found that **colestyramine** increased the clearance of a single 20-mg oral dose of **piroxicam** and a single 20-mg *intravenous* dose of **tenoxicam** by 52% and 105% respectively, and reduced their half-lives by 40% and 52% respectively. In this study, **colestyramine** 4 g three times daily was started 2 hours before the intravenous **tenoxicam** and 3.5 hours after the oral **piroxicam**.[5] In another multiple-dose study, **colestyramine** 4 hours after oral **piroxicam** or oral **tenoxicam** gave similar results,[6] as did a study starting **colestyramine** 24 hours after the last dose of a 14-day course of **piroxicam** 20 mg daily.[7] The elimination half-life of both analgesics was roughly doubled by **colestyramine** 24 g daily.[6]

(d) Sulindac

Colestyramine 4 g twice daily with meals was found to reduce the AUC of a simultaneous single 400-mg dose of sulindac by 78% and of its sulphide metabolite by 84% in 6 healthy subjects. Even when the sulindac was given 3 hours before the **colestyramine**, its AUC was reduced by 44% and that of its sulphide metabolite by 55%.[8]

Mechanism

The studies of simultaneous oral use suggest that the anion exchange resin colestyramine, and to a lesser extent colestipol, bind anionic NSAIDs (e.g. diclofenac) in the gut, so reducing their absorption. The studies showing reduced plasma levels when colestyramine was given after intravenous oxicams or separated by at least 3 hours from some oral NSAIDs, suggest that colestyramine can reduce the enterohepatic recirculation of these drugs.

Importance and management

Established interactions. Colestyramine markedly reduces the initial absorption of some NSAIDs (shown for diclofenac), and if these NSAIDs also undergo enterohepatic recirculation, their clearance will also be increased (shown for meloxicam, piroxicam, sulindac, and tenoxicam). This latter interaction cannot be avoided by separating the doses, and it may be best not to use these drug combinations. Colestyramine can be used to speed the removal of piroxicam and tenoxicam following overdosage.[3] Diclofenac has been formulated with colestyramine in an attempt to reduce gastric mucosal damage by reducing direct mucosal contact: 140 mg of diclofenac-colestyramine is considered equivalent to 70 mg of diclofenac.[9]

The reduction in absorption of ibuprofen with colestyramine is probably not clinically important, and naproxen is not affected. Nevertheless, colestyramine delayed the absorption of both ibuprofen and naproxen, which may be relevant if they are being taken for the management of acute pain. Information on many other NSAIDs appears to be lacking. Animal studies suggest that **mefenamic acid**, **flufenamic acid** and **phenylbutazone** will also be affected by colestyramine.[10,11] Note that it is usually recommended that other drugs are given 1 hour before or 4 to 6 hours after colestyramine. The reduction in diclofenac absorption with colestipol may be clinically relevant—if the combination is required monitor well. Note that it is usually recommended that other drugs are given 1 hour before or 4 hours after colestipol.

1. Al-Balla SR, El-Sayed YM, Al-Meshal MA, Gouda MW. The effects of cholestyramine and colestipol on the absorption of diclofenac in man. *Int J Clin Pharmacol Ther* (1994) 32, 441–5.
2. Al-Meshal MA, El-Sayed YM, Al-Balla SR, Gouda MW. The effect of colestipol and cholestyramine on ibuprofen bioavailability in man. *Biopharm Drug Dispos* (1994) 15, 463–71.
3. Calvo MV, Dominguez-Gil A. Interaction of naproxen with cholestyramine. *Biopharm Drug Dispos* (1984) 5, 33–42.
4. Busch U, Heinzel G, Narjes H. The effect of cholestyramine on the pharmacokinetics of meloxicam, a new non-steroidal anti-inflammatory drug (NSAID), in man. *Eur J Clin Pharmacol* (1995) 48, 269–72.
5. Guentert TW, Defoin R, Mosberg H. The influence of cholestyramine on the elimination of tenoxicam and piroxicam. *Eur J Clin Pharmacol* (1988) 34, 283–9.
6. Benveniste C, Striberni R, Dayer P. Indirect assessment of the enterohepatic recirculation of piroxicam and tenoxicam. *Eur J Clin Pharmacol* (1990) 38, 547–9.
7. Ferry DG, Gazeley LR, Busby WJ, Beasley DMG, Edwards IR, Campbell AJ, Enhanced elimination of piroxicam by administration of activated charcoal or cholestyramine. *Eur J Clin Pharmacol* (1990) 39, 599–601.
8. Malloy MJ, Ravis WR, Pennell AT, Hagan DR, Betagari S, Doshi DH. Influence of cholestyramine resin administration on single dose sulindac pharmacokinetics. *Int J Clin Pharmacol Ther* (1994) 32, 286–9.
9. Suárez-Otero R, Robles-San Román M, Jaimes-Hernández J, Oropeza-de la Madrid E, Medina-Peñaloza RM, Rosas-Ramos R, Castañeda-Hernández G. Efficacy and safety of diclofenac-cholestyramine and celecoxib in osteoarthritis. *Proc West Pharmacol Soc* (2002) 45, 26–8.
10. Rosenberg HA, Bates TR. Inhibitory effect of cholestyramine on the absorption of flufenamic and mefenamic acids in rats. *Proc Soc Exp Biol Med* (1974) 145, 93–8.
11. Gallo D G, Bailey K R, Sheffner A L. The interaction between cholestyramine and drugs. *Proc Soc Exp Biol Med* (1965) 120, 60–5.

NSAIDs + Dextropropoxyphene (Propoxyphene)

No pharmacokinetic interaction occurs between dextropropoxyphene and meclofenamate, and dextropropoxyphene does not alter sulindac plasma levels.

Clinical evidence, mechanism, importance and management

In healthy subjects dextropropoxyphene 260 mg daily and **sodium meclofenamate** 400 mg daily for a week was found to have no effect on the plasma levels of either drug.[1]

The maker of **sulindac** notes that dextropropoxyphene had no effect on the plasma levels of **sulindac** or its sulfide metabolite.[2]

1. Baragar FD, Smith TC. Drug interaction studies with sodium meclofenamate (Meclomen®). *Curr Ther Res* (1978) 23 (April Suppl), S51–S59.
2. Clinoril (Sulindac). Merck Sharp & Dohme Ltd. UK Summary of product characteristics, November 2003.

NSAIDs + Food

Food reduces the rate of absorption, but has no important effect on the extent of absorption, of aceclofenac, celecoxib, dexketoprofen, diclofenac, etodolac, etoricoxib, flurbiprofen, ibuprofen, indometacin, piroxicam, sulindac and tenoxicam. Food delayed the rate and extent of absorption of ketoprofen. Food increased the initial amount of nabumetone absorbed, and the initial absorption of a sustained release preparation of ibuprofen. Food had no effect on the pharmacokinetics or efficacy of naproxen and is reported to have no effect on the pharmacokinetics of rofecoxib or valdecoxib.

Clinical evidence

(a) Coxibs

The maker of **celecoxib** notes that a **high-fat meal** delayed absorption by about one hour.[1] Similarly, a **high-fat meal** reduced the maximum level of **etoricoxib** by 36% and delayed it by 2 hours, without affecting the extent of absorption.[2] However, the makers note that concurrent food intake does not affect the pharmacokinetics of **rofecoxib**[3] or **valdecoxib**.[4]

(b) Diclofenac

Thirteen healthy subjects were given single 105-mg doses of diclofenac potassium suspension (*Flogan*l) while fasting and after food. The pharmacokinetics of diclofenac were not changed to a clinically relevant extent by food, except that absorption was delayed (time to maximum level increased by about 30 minutes).[5] Similar findings (an increase in time to maximum level of 1.5 to 3 hours) were reported for single doses of enteric-coated diclofenac tablets.[6] However, there was no difference in steady state levels of diclofenac 50 mg twice daily when given before or after food.[6]

(c) Ibuprofen and related drugs

The makers state that the rate, but not the extent, of **aceclofenac** absorption was reduced by food.[7]

Food slightly increased the maximum plasma level and AUC of sustained-release **flurbiprofen** (*Froben SR*) by 15 and 25%, respectively, but delayed the time to achieve the maximum level by about 5 hours.[8]

Food had no effect on the pharmacokinetics of the *(S)*- and *(R)*-enantiomers of ibuprofen in one study.[9] However, in another study, food significantly delayed the absorption of both enantiomers of ibuprofen, but slightly increased the ratio of the *(S)*- to *(R)*-enantiomer.[10] In a further study, food increased the maximum plasma level of sustained-release ibuprofen (*Brufen Retard*) by 42% without affecting the time to achieve the maximum level.[8]

Food significantly decreased the rate and extent of absorption of **ketoprofen** in both single and multiple dose studies in healthy subjects. The AUC was decreased by about 40% and the time to maximum levels decreased by about 5 hours.[11] In another study, the absorption of **ketoprofen** (200 mg daily, as a gastric-juice resistant, sustained-release formulation, given 4 hours before the first meal of the day) was about 15 to 24% greater when 16 healthy subjects were given a **low-calorie/low-fat diet** rather than a **high-calorie/high-fat diet**.[12] The absorption of a single 25-mg dose of dexketoprofen was delayed by food (maximum level reduced by 45% and time to maximum level delayed by about 1 hour), but the AUC was not affected.[13]

Food did not have any clinically relevant effect on the pharmacokinetics of sustained-release **naproxen** in two studies.[14,15] Taking a single 550-mg dose of **naproxen sodium** with **a meal** had no effect on its analgesic efficacy in postoperative pain when compared with the fasted state.[16]

(d) Indometacin and sulindac

Studies in patients and healthy subjects, given single or multiple oral doses of indometacin, found that food delayed and reduced peak serum indometacin levels, but fluctuations in levels were somewhat reduced.[17] The maker of sulindac notes that food delayed the time to achieve peak plasma levels of the active metabolite by 1 to 2 hours.[18]

(e) Oxicams

Food caused some delay in the time to reach maximum levels of **piroxicam** in a single-dose study, but had no effect on total absorption.[19] In another study, the steady-state plasma levels of **piroxicam** 20 mg daily were unaffected by food.[20] The bioavailability of **tenoxicam** 20 mg was unaffected by food in 12 healthy subjects, although the time taken to reach peak serum levels was delayed by about 4 hours.[21] The rate (time to peak serum levels) and extent (AUC) of absorption of **meloxicam** 30 mg was not altered by food intake.[22]

(f) Miscellaneous NSAIDs

The absorption of a single 1-g dose of **nabumetone** was increased by food and **milk**, as shown by an increase of about 50% in the maximum levels and a 40% increase in the 0 to 24-hour AUC. However, the 0 to 72-hour AUC was not significantly increased.[23]

When 18 healthy subjects were given **etodolac** 400 mg after a **high-fat meal**, peak serum levels were roughly halved, and delayed from 1.4 to 3.8 hours, but the total amount absorbed was not markedly changed when compared to the fasting state.[24]

Mechanism

Food delays gastric emptying, therefore frequently affects the rate, but not the extent, of absorption of the NSAIDs.

Importance and management

Food reduces the rate of absorption, but has no or little effect on the extent of absorption, of most of the NSAIDs studied. This will have no clinical relevance when these drugs are being used regularly to treat chronic pain and inflammation. However, if these drugs are being used for the treatment of acute pain, administration on an empty stomach would be preferable in terms of onset of effect, and is suggested by the maker of dexketoprofen[25] and etoricoxib.[2] However, administration with or after food is a usual recommendation for NSAIDs in an attempt to minimise their gastrointestinal adverse effects.

Food delayed the rate and extent of absorption of ketoprofen, nevertheless, administration with food is recommended, and the dose is best titrated to effect.[26]

Note that the effect of food can be altered by the formulation. Food delayed the rate of absorption of ibuprofen from one conventional formulation, but had no effect on the rate, and actually increased the maximum level from a sustained release preparation.

1. Celebrex (Celecoxib). Pharmacia Ltd. UK Summary of product characteristics, March 2003.
2. Arcoxia (Etoricoxib). Merck Sharp & Dohme Ltd. UK Summary of product characteristics, May 2005.
3. Vioxx (Rofecoxib). Merck Sharp & Dohme Ltd. UK Summary of product characteristics, August 2003.
4. Bextra (Valdecoxib). Pharmacia Ltd. UK Summary of product characteristics, May 2004.
5. Poli A, Moreno RA, Ribiero W, Dias HB, Moreno H, Muscara MN, De Nucci G. Influence of gastric acid secretion blockade and food intake on the bioavailability of a potassium diclofenac suspension in healthy male volunteers. *Int J Clin Pharmacol Ther* (1996) 34, 76–9.
6. Sioufi A, Stierlin H, Schweizer A, Botta L, Degen PH, Theobald W, Brechbühler S. Recent findings concerning clinically relevant pharmacokinetics of diclofenac sodium. In: Voltarol — New Findings, ed Kass E. Proc Int Symp Voltarol, Paris June 22nd, 1981. 15th Int Congress of Rheumatology. p 19–30.
7. Preservex (Aceclofenac). UCB Pharma Ltd. UK Summary of product characteristics, June 2003.
8. Pargal A, Kelkar MG, Nayak PJ. The effect of food on the bioavailability of ibuprofen and flurbiprofen from sustained release formulation. *Biopharm Drug Dispos* (1996) 17, 511–19.
9. Levine MA, Walker SE, Paton TW. The effect of food or sucralfate on the bioavailability of S(+) and R(-) enantiomers of ibuprofen. *J Clin Pharmacol* (1992) 32, 1110–14.
10. Siemon D, de Vries JX, Stötzer F, Walter-Sack I, Dietl R. Fasting and postprandial disposition of R(-)- and S(+)-ibuprofen following oral administration of racemic drug in healthy individuals. *Eur J Med Res* (1997) 2, 215–19.
11. Caillé G, du Souich P, Besner JG, Gervais P, Vèzina M. Effects of food and sucralfate on the pharmacokinetics of naproxen and ketoprofen in humans. Am J Med (1989) 86 (Suppl 6A) 38–44. Correction. *ibid. (1990) 89, 838.*. (1990) 89, 838..
12. Le Liboux A, Teule M, Frydman A, Oosterhuis B, Jonkman JHG. Effect of diet on the single- and multiple-dose pharmacokinetics of sustained-release ketoprofen. *Eur J Clin Pharmacol* (1994) 47, 361–6.
13. McEwen J, De Luca M, Casini A, Gich I, Barbanoj MJ, Tost D, Artigas R, Mauleón D. The effect of food and an antacid on the bioavailability of dexketoprofen trometamol. *J Clin Pharmacol* (1998) 38 (Suppl), 41S–45S.
14. Mroszczak E, Yee JP, Bynum L. Absorption of naproxen controlled-release tablets in fasting and postprandial volunteers. *J Clin Pharmacol* (1988) 28, 1128–31.
15. Palazzini E, Cristofori M, Babbini M. Bioavailability of a new controlled-release oral naproxen formulation given with and without food. *Int J Clin Pharmacol Res* (1992) 12, 179–84.
16. Forbes JA, Sandberg RÅ, Bood-Björklund L. The effect of food on bromfenac, naproxen sodium, and acetaminophen in postoperative pain after orthopedic surgery. *Pharmacotherapy* (1998) 18, 492–503.
17. Emori HW, Paulus H, Bluestone R, Champion GD, Pearson C. Indomethacin serum concentrations in man. Effects of dosage, food, and antacid. *Ann Rheum Dis* (1976) 35, 333–8.
18. Clinoril (Sulindac). Merck Sharp & Dohme Ltd. UK Summary of product characteristics, November 2003.
19. Ishizaki T, Nomura T, Abe T. Pharmacokinetics of piroxicam, a new nonsteroidal anti-inflammatory agent, under fasting and postprandial states in man. *J Pharmacokinet Biopharm* (1979) 7, 369–81.
20. Tilstone WJ, Lawson DH, Omara F, Cunningham F. The steady-state pharmacokinetics of piroxicam: effect of food and iron. *Eur J Rheumatol Inflamm* (1981) 4, 309–13.
21. Day RO, Lam S, Paull P, Wade D. Effect of food and various antacids on the absorption of tenoxicam. *Br J Clin Pharmacol* (1987) 24, 323–8.
22. Busch U, Heinzel G, Narjes H. Effect of food on pharmacokinetics of meloxicam, a new non steroidal anti-inflammatory drug (NSAID). *Agents Actions* (1991) 32, 52–3.
23. von Schrader HW, Buscher G, Dierdorf D, Mügge H, Wolf D. Nabumetone — a novel anti-inflammatory drug: the influence of food, milk, antacids, and analgesics on bioavailability of single oral doses. *Int J Clin Pharmacol Ther Toxicol* (1983) 21, 311–21.
24. Troy S, Sanda M, Dressler D, Chiang S, Latts J. The effect of food and antacid on etodolac bioavailability. *Clin Pharmacol Ther* (1990) 47, 192.
25. Keral (Dexketoprofen trometamol). A. Menarini Pharmaceuticals UK Ltd. UK Summary of product characteristics, March 2001.
26. Orudis (Ketoprofen). Hawgreen Ltd. UK Summary of product characteristics, January 2002.

NSAIDs or Aspirin + Ginkgo biloba

An isolated report describes spontaneous bleeding from the iris associated with the use of aspirin and a *Ginkgo biloba* extract. Another describes fatal intracerebral bleeding with *Ginkgo biloba* and ibuprofen, and another prolonged bleeding and subdural haematomas with *ginkgo biloba* and rofecoxib.

Clinical evidence

A 70-year-old man developed spontaneous bleeding from the iris into the anterior chamber of his eye within a week of starting to take a *Ginkoba* tablet twice daily. He experienced recurrent episodes of blurred vision in one eye lasting about 15 minutes, during which he could see a red discoloration through his cornea. Each *Ginkoba* tablet contained 40 mg of concentrated (50:1) extract of *Ginkgo biloba*. He was also taking aspirin 325 mg daily, which he had taken uneventfully for 3 years since having coronary bypass surgery. He stopped taking the *Ginkoba* but continued with the aspirin, and 3 months later had experienced no recurrence of the bleeding.[1] In an analysis of supplement use, 23% of 123 patients were currently taking supplements, and 4 patients were found to be taking ginkgo and aspirin. However, no problems from this use were found on review of the patients' notes.[2]

A case of fatal intracerebral bleeding has been reported in a 71-year-old patient taking a *Ginkgo biloba* supplement (*Gingium*) 4 weeks after he started to take **ibuprofen** 600 mg daily.[3] A 69-year-old man on a ginkgo biloba supplement and **rofecoxib** had a subdural haematoma after a head injury, then recurrent small spontaneous haematomas. He was subsequently found to have a prolonged bleeding time, which returned to normal one week after stopping the ginkgo biloba supplement and **rofecoxib**, and remained normal after restarting low-dose **rofecoxib**.[4]

Mechanism

The reason for the bleeding is not known, but *Ginkgo biloba* extract contains ginkgolide B, which is a potent inhibitor of platelet-activating factor, which is needed for arachidonate-independent platelet aggregation. On their own, *Gingko biloba* supplements have been associated with prolonged bleeding times,[5,6] left and bilateral subdural haematomas,[5,7] a right parietal haematoma,[8] post-laparoscopic cholecystectomy bleeding,[9] and subarachnoid haemorrhage.[6] The authors of the first report suggest that the use of aspirin, which is also an inhibitor of platelet aggregation, may have had an additional part to play in what happened. Ibuprofen is also an inhibitor of platelet aggregation, but selective inhibitors of COX-2 such as rofecoxib have no effect on platelets and would not be expected to potentiate any bleeding effect of *Ginkgo biloba*.

Importance and management

The evidence from these reports is too slim to forbid patients taking aspirin or NSAIDs and *Ginkgo biloba* concurrently, but some do recommend caution.[10] Medical professionals should be aware of the possibility of increased bleeding tendency with *Ginkgo biloba*, and report any suspected cases.[8] Consider also 'Antiplatelet drugs + Herbal medicines', p.520.

1. Rosenblatt M, Mindel J. Spontaneous hyphema associated with ingestion of *Ginkgo biloba* extract. *N Engl J Med* (1997) 336, 1108.
2. Ly J, Percy L, Dhanani S. Use of dietary supplements and their interactions with prescription drugs in the elderly. *Am J Health-Syst Pharm* (2002) 59, 1759–62.
3. Meisel C, Johne A, Roots I. Fatal intracerebral mass bleeding associated with *Ginkgo biloba* and ibuprofen. *Atherosclerosis* (2003) 167, 367.
4. Hoffman T. Ginko, Vioxx and excessive bleeding – possible drug-herb interactions: case report. *Hawaii Med J* (2001) 60, 290,
5. Rowin J, Lewis SL. Spontaneous bilateral subdural hematomas associated with chronic *Ginkgo biloba* ingestion. *Neurology* (1996) 46, 1775–6.
6. Vale S. Subarachnoid haemorrhage associated with *Ginkgo biloba*. *Lancet* (1998) 352, 36.
7. Gilbert GJ. *Ginkgo biloba*. *Neurology* (1997) 48, 1137.
8. Benjamin J, Muir T, Briggs K, Pentland B. A case of cerebral haemorrhage – can *Ginkgo biloba* be implicated? *Postgrad Med J* (2001) 77, 112–13.
9. Fessenden JM, Wittenborn W, Clarke L. Gingko biloba: a case report of herbal medicine and bleeding postoperatively from a laparoscopic cholecystectomy. *Am Surg* (2001) 67, 33–5.
10. Griffiths J, Jordan S, Pilon S. Natural health products and adverse reactions. *Can Adverse React News* (2004) 14, 2–3.

NSAIDs or Aspirin + Gold

Gold appears to increase the risk of aspirin-induced liver damage. The use of gold with fenoprofen seems to be safer with regard to liver toxicity. An isolated report suggested that naproxen may have contributed to gold-induced pneumonitis.

Clinical evidence, mechanism, importance and management

A study in rheumatoid patients given aspirin 3.9 g or **fenoprofen** 2.4 g daily suggested that gold induction therapy (**sodium aurothiomalate**, by intramuscular injection, to a total dose of 985 mg over 6 months) increased aspirin-induced hepatotoxicity. Levels of AST, LDH and alkaline phosphatase were higher during aspirin than during **fenoprofen** treatment. These indicators of liver dysfunction suggest that **fenoprofen** is safer than aspirin in this context. Combined treatment with gold and NSAIDs was more effective than the NSAIDs alone.[1]

A patient with rheumatoid arthritis on gold (**sodium aurothiomalate**) developed pneumonitis soon after **naproxen** 500 mg twice daily was added. An *in vitro* study suggested the pneumonitis was due to hypersensitivity to gold. However, the patient's condition continued to deteriorate despite stopping the gold, then showed marked improvement when the **naproxen** was discontinued as well. The authors suggest that the **naproxen** may have altered the patient's immune system in some way to make them more sensitive to the gold.[2] This appears to be the only report of such an effect, and is therefore unlikely to be of general relevance.

1. Davis JD, Turner RA, Collins RL, Ruchte IR, Kaufmann JS. Fenoprofen, aspirin, and gold induction in rheumatoid arthritis. *Clin Pharmacol Ther* (1977) 21, 52–61.
2. McFadden RG, Fraher LJ, Thompson JM. Gold-naproxen pneumonitis: a toxic drug interaction? *Chest* (1989) 96, 216–18.

NSAIDs or Aspirin + H_2-blockers

The H_2-blockers (cimetidine, famotidine, nizatidine, ranitidine) have no effect or cause only modest and normally clinically unimportant changes in the serum levels of aspirin, diclofenac, flurbiprofen, ibuprofen, indometacin, ketoprofen, lornoxicam, meloxicam, naproxen, piroxicam, rofecoxib and tenoxicam. More importantly they may protect the gastric mucosa from the irritant effects of the NSAIDs.

Clinical evidence

(a) Aspirin

Cimetidine 300 mg, given 1 hour before aspirin 1.2 g caused only a modest increase in the serum salicylate levels of 3 out of 6 healthy subjects.[1] When 13 patients with rheumatoid arthritis taking enteric-coated aspirin were given **cimetidine** 300 mg four times daily for 7 days the total amount of aspirin absorbed was unaltered, but serum levels were slightly raised, from 161 to 180 micrograms/ml.[2] The pharmacokinetics of a single 1-g dose of aspirin were largely unchanged in 6 healthy subjects given **ranitidine** 150 mg twice daily for a week.[3] **Famotidine** has been found to cause some small changes in the pharmacokinetics of aspirin, but this is of doubtful clinical importance.[4]

(b) Azapropazone

A randomised pharmacokinetic study in 12 healthy subjects found that after taking **cimetidine** 300 mg every 6 hours for 6 days the AUC of a single 600-mg dose of azapropazone was increased by 25%, and the AUC of **cimetidine** was increased by 16%. No significant changes in laboratory values (blood counts, enzyme levels) were seen, and adverse effects were minor (headaches in 3 subjects).[5]

(c) Diclofenac

Famotidine 40 mg raised the peak plasma levels of enteric-coated diclofenac 100 mg from 5.84 to 7.04 mg/l in 14 healthy subjects. Peak plasma diclofenac levels also occurred more rapidly (2 versus 2.75 hours). The extent of the absorption was unchanged.[6] Diclofenac did not affect the pharmacokinetics of **ranitidine** nor its ability to suppress gastric pH.[7] Another study also found that the pharmacokinetics of diclofenac were unaffected by **ranitidine**.[8]

(d) Flurbiprofen

Cimetidine 300 mg three times daily for 2 weeks increased the maximum serum level of flurbiprofen 150 to 300 mg daily in 30 patients with rheumatoid arthritis, but **ranitidine** 150 mg twice daily had no effect. The efficacy of the flurbiprofen (assessed by Ritchie score, 50 ft walking time, grip strength) was not altered.[9] Another study in healthy subjects found that **cimetidine** 300 mg four times daily slightly increased the serum levels of a single 200-mg dose of flurbiprofen, and raised the flurbiprofen AUC by 13%.[10] However, no significant interaction occurred with **ranitidine** 150 mg twice daily.[10]

(e) Ibuprofen

Cimetidine 400 mg three times daily raised the peak serum levels and AUC of a 600-mg dose of ibuprofen by 14% and 6% respectively. No changes were seen with **ranitidine** 300 mg daily.[11] Another study found larger increases (AUC for *R*-ibuprofen of 37% and for *S*-ibuprofen of 19%, but these were not statistically significant).[12] However, 5 other studies with ibuprofen found no interaction with **cimetidine** or **ranitidine**,[13-17] or **nizatidine**.[14] However, analysis of the results of one study showed that peak serum ibuprofen levels in black subjects (USA) were 54% higher and occurred sooner, whereas in white subjects (USA) they were 27% lower and delayed.[15,18]

(f) Indometacin

Cimetidine 1 g daily for 2 weeks was given to 10 patients with rheumatoid arthritis on indometacin 100 to 200 mg daily for over a year. The plasma indometacin levels fell by an average of 18%, but there was no significant change in the clinical effectiveness of the anti-inflammatory treatment (as measured by articular index, pain, grip strength and erythrocyte sedimentation rate).[19] Another study found no changes in the pharmacokinetics of indometacin in healthy subjects given **ranitidine**.[20] No marked changes in the bioavailability of either **cimetidine** or **ranitidine** was seen when given with indometacin in a single-dose study in healthy subjects.[21]

(g) Ketoprofen

Cimetidine 600 mg twice daily was found not to affect the pharmacokinetics of enteric-coated ketoprofen 100 mg twice daily in 12 healthy subjects.[22]

(h) Lornoxicam

Cimetidine 400 mg twice daily increased the maximum serum levels and AUC of lornoxicam 8 mg twice daily by 28% and 9% respectively in 12 healthy subjects. **Ranitidine** 150 mg twice daily had no significant effect on lornoxicam pharmacokinetics in these same subjects, except that one subject showed a very marked increase in serum lornoxicam levels while taking both drugs. He dropped out of the trial after 6 days because of severe gastric irritation. It is not clear what part, if any, the **ranitidine** had to play.[23]

(i) Meloxicam

In an open, randomised, crossover study a group of 9 healthy subjects was given meloxicam 30 mg alone, or with **cimetidine** 200 mg four times daily for 5 days. **Cimetidine** had no significant effect on the pharmacokinetics of the meloxicam.[24]

(j) Naproxen

One study found no adverse interaction between naproxen and **cimetidine** and no alteration in the beneficial effects of **cimetidine** on gastric acid secretion,[25] but another study found a moderate 39 to 60% decrease in the naproxen half-life.[26,27] In one of these studies the half-life of naproxen was reduced by about 40% by **ranitidine** and 50% by **famotidine**.[27] A further study found that **nizatidine** does not affect the pharmacokinetics of naproxen.[28]

(k) Piroxicam

Cimetidine 300 mg four times daily for 7 days slightly increased the half-life and the AUC of a single 20-mg dose of piroxicam by 8 and 16% respectively in 10 healthy subjects.[29] Another study found that **cimetidine** caused a 15% rise in the AUC of piroxicam.[30] In 12 healthy subjects the half-life and AUC of a single-dose of piroxicam were increased by 41% and 31% respectively by **cimetidine** 200 mg three times daily, and the plasma levels were raised accordingly.[31] For example, at 4 hours they were raised by almost 25%.[31] **Ranitidine** does not affect the pharmacokinetics of piroxicam.[32] No clinically significant changes occurred in the steady-state serum levels of piroxicam in a further study when either **cimetidine** or **nizatidine** were given.[33]

(l) Rofecoxib

The maker notes that **cimetidine** 800 mg twice daily increased the AUC of rofecoxib by 23% and increased the maximum level by 21%. These minor changes were not considered clinically relevant.[34]

(m) Tenoxicam

The pharmacokinetics of a single 20-mg oral dose of tenoxicam was unaltered in 6 healthy subjects after they took **cimetidine** 1 g daily for 7 days.[35]

Mechanism

Uncertain. Piroxicam and lornoxicam serum levels are possibly increased because their metabolism is reduced by the cimetidine.[23,31]

Importance and management

Most of these interactions between the NSAIDs and cimetidine, famotidine, nizatidine or ranitidine appear to be of no particular clinical importance. The general relevance of the case of increased lornoxicam levels and severe gastric irritation with ranitidine is uncertain, but probably small. The H_2-blockers as a group may protect the gastric mucosa from the irritant effects of the NSAIDs and concurrent use may therefore be advantageous.

1. Khoury W, Geraci K, Askari A, Johnson M. The effect of cimetidine on aspirin absorption. *Gastroenterology* (1979) 76, 1169.
2. Willoughby JS, Paton TW, Walker SE, Little AH. The effect of cimetidine on enteric-coated ASA disposition. *Clin Pharmacol Ther* (1983) 33, 268.
3. Corrocher R, Bambara LM, Caramaschi P, Testi R, Girelli M, Pellegatti M, Lomeo A. Effect of ranitidine on the absorption of aspirin. *Digestion* (1987) 37, 178–83.
4. Domecq C, Fuentes A, Hurtado C, Arancibia A. Effect of famotidine on the bioavailability of acetylsalicylic acid. *Med Sci Res* (1993) 21, 219–20.
5. Rainsford KD, ed. Azapropazone: 20 years of clinical use. Kluwer Academic Pub; 1990 p. 136–45.
6. Suryakumar J, Chakrapani T, Krishna DR. Famotidine affects the pharmacokinetics of diclofenac sodium. *Drug Invest* (1992) 4, 66–8.
7. Blum RA, Alioth C, Chan KKH, Furst DE, Ziehmer BA, Schentag JJ. Diclofenac does not affect the pharmacodynamics of ranitidine. *Clin Pharmacol Ther* (1992) 51, 192.
8. Dammann HG, Simon-Schultz J, Steinhoff I, Damaschke A, Schmoldt A, Sallowsky E. Differential effects of misoprostol and ranitidine on the pharmacokinetics of diclofenac and gastrointestinal symptoms. *Br J Clin Pharmacol* (1993) 36, 345–9.
9. Kreeft JH, Bellamy N, Freeman D. Do H_2-antagonists alter the kinetics and effects of chronically-administered flurbiprofen in rheumatoid arthritis? *Clin Invest Med* (1987) 10 (4 Suppl B), B58.
10. Sullivan KM, Small RE, Rock WL, Cox SR, Willis HE. Effects of cimetidine or ranitidine on the pharmacokinetics of flurbiprofen. *Clin Pharm* (1986) 5, 586–9.
11. Ochs HR, Greenblatt DJ, Matlis R, Weinbrenner J. Interaction of ibuprofen with the H-2 receptor antagonists ranitidine and cimetidine. *Clin Pharmacol Ther* (1985) 38, 648–51.
12. Li G, Treiber G, Klotz U. The ibuprofen-cimetidine interaction. Stereochemical considerations. *Drug Invest* (1989) 1, 11–17.
13. Conrad KA, Mayersohn M, Bliss M. Cimetidine does not alter ibuprofen kinetics after a single dose. *Br J Clin Pharmacol* (1984) 18, 624–6.
14. Forsyth DR, Jayasinghe KSA, Roberts CJC. Do nizatidine and cimetidine interact with ibuprofen? *Eur J Clin Pharmacol* (1988) 35, 85–8.
15. Stephenson DW, Small RE, Wood JH, Willis HE, Johnson SM, Karnes HT, Rajasekharaiah K. Effect of ranitidine and cimetidine on ibuprofen pharmacokinetics. *Clin Pharm* (1988) 7, 317–21.
16. Evans AM, Nation RL, Sansom LN. Lack of effect of cimetidine on the pharmacokinetics of R(-)- and S(+)-ibuprofen. *Br J Clin Pharmacol* (1989) 28, 143–9.
17. Small RE, Wilmot-Pater MG, McGee BA, Willis HE. Effects of misoprostol or ranitidine on ibuprofen pharmacokinetics. *Clin Pharm* (1991) 10, 870–2.
18. Small RE, Wood JH. Influence of racial differences on effects of ranitidine and cimetidine on ibuprofen pharmacokinetics. *Clin Pharm* (1989) 8, 471–2.
19. Howes CA, Pullar T, Sourindhrin I, Mistra PC, Capel H, Lawson DH, Tilstone WJ. Reduced steady-state plasma concentrations of chlorpromazine and indomethacin in patients receiving cimetidine. *Eur J Clin Pharmacol* (1983) 24, 99–102.
20. Kendall MJ, Gibson R, Walt RP. Co-administration of misoprostol or ranitidine with indomethacin: effects on pharmacokinetics, abdominal symptoms and bowel habit. *Aliment Pharmacol Ther* (1992) 6, 437–46.
21. Delhotal-Landes B, Flouvat B, Liote F, Abel L, Meyer P, Vinceneux P, Carbon C. Pharmacokinetic interactions between NSAIDs (indomethacin or sulindac) and H_2-receptor antagonists (cimetidine or ranitidine) in human volunteers. *Clin Pharmacol Ther* (1988) 44, 442–52.
22. Verbeeck RK, Corman CL, Wallace SM, Herman RJ, Ross SG, Le Morvan P. Single and multiple dose pharmacokinetics of enteric coated ketoprofen: effect of cimetidine. *Eur J Clin Pharmacol* (1988) 35, 521–7.
23. Ravic M, Salas-Herrera I, Johnston A, Turner P, Foley K, Rosenow DE. A pharmacokinetic interaction between cimetidine or ranitidine and lornoxicam. *Postgrad Med J* (1993) 69, 865–66.
24. Busch U, Heinzel G, Narjes H, Nehmiz G. Interaction of meloxicam with cimetidine, Maalox or aspirin. *J Clin Pharmacol* (1996) 36, 79–84.
25. Holford NHG, Altman D, Riegelman S, Buskin JN, Upton RA. Pharmacokinetic and pharmacodynamic study of cimetidine administered with naproxen. *Clin Pharmacol Ther* (1981) 29, 251–2.
26. Vree TB, van den Biggelaar-Martea M, Verwey-van Wissen CPWGM, Vree ML, Guelen PJM. The pharmacokinetics of naproxen, its metabolite *O*-desmethylnaproxen, and their acyl glucuronides in humans. Effect of cimetidine. *Br J Clin Pharmacol* (1993) 35, 467–72.
27. Vree TB, van den Biggelaar-Martea M, Verwey-van Wissen CPWGM, Vree ML, Guelen PJM. The effects of cimetidine, ranitidine and famotidine on the single-dose pharmacokinetics of naproxen and its metabolites in humans. *Int J Clin Pharmacol Ther Toxicol* (1993) 31, 597–601.
28. Satterwhite JH, Bowsher RR, Callaghan JT, Cerimele BJ, Levine LR. Nizatidine: lack of drug interaction with naproxen. *Clin Res* (1992) 40, 706A.
29. Mailhot C, Dahl SL, Ward JR. The effect of cimetidine on serum concentrations of piroxicam. *Pharmacotherapy* (1986) 6, 112–17.
30. Freeman DJ, Danter WR, Carruthers SG. Pharmacokinetic interaction between cimetidine and piroxicam in normal subjects. *Clin Invest Med* (1988) 11, C19.
31. Said SA, Foda AM. Influence of cimetidine on the pharmacokinetics of piroxicam in rat and man. *Arzneimittelforschung* (1989) 39, 790–2.
32. Dixon JS, Lacey LF, Pickup ME, Langley SJ, Page MC. A lack of pharmacokinetic interaction between ranitidine and piroxicam. *Eur J Clin Pharmacol* (1990) 39, 583–6.
33. Milligan PA, McGill PE, Howden CW, Kelman AW, Whiting B. The consequences of H_2 receptor antagonist-piroxicam coadministration in patients with joint disorders. *Eur J Clin Pharmacol* (1993) 45, 507–12.
34. Vioxx (Rofecoxib). Merck & Co, Inc. US Prescribing information, March 2004.
35. Day RO, Geisslinger G, Paull P, Williams KM. Neither cimetidine nor probenecid affect the pharmacokinetics of tenoxicam in normal volunteers. *Br J Clin Pharmacol* (1994) 37, 79–81.

NSAIDs or Aspirin + HRT or Oral contraceptives

The loss of diflunisal from the body in women is increased by oral contraceptives to the level normally seen in men. One study showed modestly reduced levels of ibuprofen with oral contraceptives, but another study did not. Oral contraceptives reduced the levels of aspirin, but not phenylbutazone. There are no clinically relevant changes in the pharmacokinetics of oxaprozin with conjugated oestrogens. See also 'Oral contraceptives + Etoricoxib or Rofecoxib', p.759.

Clinical evidence, mechanism, importance and management

(A) Effect on NSAIDs

(a) Aspirin

The AUC of single-doses of aspirin 300 mg and 600 mg was lower in 10 women after they started to take a combined oral contraceptive (**ethinylestradiol/norethisterone** 30 micrograms/1 mg). After the oral contraceptive had been discontinued, the pharmacokinetics of aspirin returned to baseline values.[1]

(b) Diflunisal

The clearance of a single 250-mg dose of diflunisal was 53% higher in 6 women on oral contraceptives than in 6 control women, but was similar to the clearance value in 6 men.[2] This difference is unlikely to be of clinical importance.

(c) Ibuprofen

In one study, the pharmacokinetics of (*R*)-ibuprofen did not differ between women on combined oral contraceptives, control women, and control men.[3] However, in another study, the median 0 to 12-hour AUC of (*S*)-ibuprofen lysinate was 29% lower in users of oral contraceptives, and pain-intensity was higher (possibly due to reduced pain tolerance).[4]

(d) Oxaprozin

There was no difference in the pharmacokinetics of a single 1.2-g dose of oxaprozin in 11 women on **conjugated oestrogens** (*Premarin*) than in 11 control women, except that the time to peak concentration was shorter (4 versus 8.9 hours).[5] This difference is unlikely to be of clinical importance.

(e) Phenylbutazone

The pharmacokinetics of a single 400-mg dose of **phenylbutazone** did not change in 10 women after they started to take a combined oral contraceptive containing **ethinylestradiol/norethisterone** 30 micrograms/1 mg.[1]

1. Gupta KC, Joshi JV, Hazari K, Pohujani SM, Satoskar RS. Effect of low estrogen combination oral contraceptive on metabolism of aspirin and phenylbutazone. *Int J Clin Pharmacol Ther Toxicol* (1982) 20, 511–13.
2. Macdonald JI, Herman RJ, Verbeeck RK. Sex-difference and the effects of smoking and oral contraceptive steroids on the kinetics of diflunisal. *Eur J Clin Pharmacol* (1990) 38, 175–9.
3. Knights KM, McLean CF, Tonkin AL, Miners JO. Lack of effect of gender and oral contraceptive steroids on the pharmacokinetics of (R)-ibuprofen in humans. *Br J Clin Pharmacol* (1995) 40, 153–6.
4. Warnecke J, Pentz R, Siegers C-P. Effects of smoking and contraceptives on the pharmacokinetics and pharmacodynamics of S(+)-ibuprofen lysinate in humans. *Naunyn Schmiedebergs Arch Pharmacol* (1996) 354 (Suppl 1), R33.
5. Scavone JM, Ochs HR, Greenblatt DJ, Matlis R. Pharmacokinetics of oxaprozin in women receiving conjugated estrogen. *Eur J Clin Pharmacol* (1988) 35, 105–8.

NSAIDs or Aspirin + Mazindol

Mazindol does not appear to interact adversely with indometacin or salicylates.

Clinical evidence, mechanism, importance and management

An 8-week, placebo-controlled, double-blind study, mazindol was given to 26 patients with obesity and arthritis, 15 of whom were on **salicylates**, 11 on **indometacin** and one on dextropropoxyphene (propoxyphene) with paracetamol (acetaminophen). Additional analgesic and anti-inflammatory drugs used were ibuprofen (4 patients), phenylbutazone (1), dextropropoxyphene (7) and paracetamol (3). No symptoms attributable to salicylism or **indometacin** toxicity (gastric intolerance, headache) were observed.[1]

1. Thorpe PC, Isaac PF, Rodgers J. A controlled trial of mazindol (Sanjorex, Teronac) in the management of obese rheumatic patients. *Curr Ther Res* (1975) 17, 149–55.

NSAIDs or Aspirin + Metoclopramide

Metoclopramide increases the rate of absorption of aspirin and tolfenamic acid. Conversely, metoclopramide reduces the bioavailability of ketoprofen.

Clinical evidence

(a) Aspirin

In one study, intramuscular metoclopramide given before oral effervescent aspirin increased the rate of aspirin absorption during a migraine attack to that seen when aspirin was given alone when headache free.[1] Similarly, in another study, intramuscular or oral metoclopramide 10 mg increased the rate of absorption of aspirin in patients with migraine.[2] However, in another study, there was no difference in the pharmacokinetics of aspirin when given with oral metoclopramide to healthy subjects.[3] In addition, in one clinical trial there was no difference in analgesic efficacy between aspirin with metoclopramide (*Migravess*) and aspirin alone (*Alka-Seltzer*) for migraine attacks.[4]

(b) Ketoprofen

In a single-dose study in 4 healthy subjects, there was a 28% reduction in the AUC of a 50-mg capsule of ketoprofen when taken with metoclopramide 10 mg. The maximum plasma levels were almost halved and the time to reach this maximum was prolonged by 30%.[5]

(c) Tolfenamic acid

Rectal metoclopramide 20 mg, given to 8 healthy subjects 30 minutes before oral tolfenamic acid 300 mg, caused a threefold increase in the serum tolfenamic acid levels at 45 minutes. There was no change in the maximum level or the AUC.[6] In another study, rectal metoclopramide similarly enhanced the rate of oral absorption of tolfenamic acid when given during a migraine attack.[7]

Mechanism

Metoclopramide speeds up gastric emptying. The relatively poorly soluble ketoprofen spends less time in the stomach where it dissolves, and as a result less is available for absorption in the small intestine. Conversely, the absorption rate of tolfenamic acid is increased, without a change in the extent of absorption.

Importance and management

The clinical importance of the reduction in ketoprofen levels is unknown, but the authors of the study recommend that ketoprofen (and possibly other NSAIDs that are poorly soluble) should be taken 1 to 2 hours before metoclopramide. Conversely, for aspirin, tolfenamic acid, and other NSAIDs, metoclopramide can be used to increase the rate of absorption, and therefore possibly speed up the onset of analgesic effect in conditions such as migraine.

1. Volans GN. The effect of metoclopramide on the absorption of effervescent aspirin in migraine. *Br J Clin Pharmacol* (1975) 2, 57–63.
2. Ross-Lee LM, Eadie MJ, Heazlewood V, Bochner F, Tyrer JH. Aspirin pharmacokinetics in migraine: the effect of metoclopramide. *Eur J Clin Pharmacol* (1983) 24, 777–85.
3. Manniche PM, Dinneen LC, Langemark M. The pharmacokinetics of the individual constituents of an aspirin-metoclopramide combination ('Migravess'). *Curr Med Res Opin* (1984) 9, 153–6.
4. Tfelt-Hansen P, Olesen J. Effervescent metoclopramide and aspirin (Migravess) versus effervescent aspirin or placebo for migraine attacks: a double-blind study. *Cephalalgia* (1984) 4, 107–11.
5. Etman MA, Ismail FA, Nada AH. Effect of metoclopramide on ketoprofen pharmacokinetics in man. *Int J Pharmaceutics* (1992) 88, 433–5.
6. Tokola RA, Anttila V-J, Neuvonen PJ. The effect of metoclopramide on the absorption of tolfenamic acid. *Int J Clin Pharmacol Ther Toxicol* (1982) 20, 465–8.
7. Tokola RA, Neuvonen PJ. Effects of migraine attack and metoclopramide on the absorption of tolfenamic acid. *Br J Clin Pharmacol* (1984) 17, 67–75.

NSAIDs + NSAIDs

The combined use of NSAIDs increases the risk of gastrointestinal damage, and because there is no clinical rationale for the combined use of different NSAIDs, such use should be avoided. Diflunisal raises serum indometacin levels about twofold. Indometacin and flurbiprofen appear not to affect each other's pharmacokinetics. Naproxen levels are not altered by diflunisal. Floctafenine does not alter diclofenac levels. Indometacin caused renal impairment in a patient recovering from phenylbutazone-induced acute renal failure.

Clinical evidence

(a) Gastrointestinal effects

The risk of serious upper gastrointestinal bleeding was increased by the use of more than one NSAID in a meta-analysis of data from three case-controlled studies (odds ratio 4.9 with one NSAID and 10.7 with two).[1] Another study provided similar findings: the odds ratio was 7.1 with one NSAID and 12.3 with two or more NSAIDs.[2] Similar findings have been reported with aspirin and NSAIDs, see 'NSAIDs + Aspirin; Anti-inflammatory dose', p.83. Analysis of yellow card reports to the UK Committee on Safety of Medicines of gastrointestinal perforation, obstruction, ulceration or bleeding with **diclofenac**, **naproxen** and **ibuprofen** revealed that 6% of the patients were receiving another non-aspirin NSAID.[3]

One pharmacodynamic study in healthy subjects found that gastric instillation of a solution of **diflunisal** before an **indometacin** solution prevented the fall in transmucosal potential difference seen with **indometacin** alone. This was interpreted as evidence that **diflunisal** protects the human gastric mucosa against the damaging effects of **indometacin**.[4] However, the relevance of this test to the adverse effects of NSAIDs used clinically is unknown. Note that fatal gastrointestinal haemorrhage has been reported in a patient treated with **diflunisal** and **indometacin**.[5]

(b) Pharmacokinetic studies

No clinically significant changes in the pharmacokinetics of either **indometacin** 75 mg daily or **flurbiprofen** 150 mg daily occurred when both drugs were given to patients.[6]

Diflunisal 250 mg twice daily had no effect on plasma levels or urinary excretion of **naproxen** 250 mg twice daily.[7]

A study in 16 healthy subjects showed that **diflunisal** 500 mg twice daily raised the steady-state plasma levels and the AUC of **indometacin** 50 mg twice daily about twofold. Combined use was associated with more gastrointestinal and CNS adverse effects, but there was no clear effect on blood loss in the faeces.[8] Another study produced similar findings.[9]

No change in free **diclofenac** levels was seen when 6 healthy subjects were given **floctafenine** 400 mg with **diclofenac** 75 mg daily for a week.[10]

(c) Renal effects

An isolated report describes deterioration in renal function in a patient during recovery from **phenylbutazone**-induced renal failure when **indometacin** 25 mg three times a day was given. The **indometacin** was discontinued with improvement of renal function.[11]

Mechanism

The damaging effects of the NSAIDs on the gut appear to be additive. Diflunisal may inhibit the glucuronidation of indometacin, or could compete for renal clearance of unmetabolised indometacin.[9] All NSAIDs have the propensity to cause renal impairment.

Importance and management

The gastrointestinal toxicity of the NSAIDs is well documented, and it appears that combined use increases this risk. The UK Committee on Safety of Medicines state that not more than one NSAID should be used concurrently.[3,12] The marked rise in plasma levels of indometacin with diflunisal gives an additional reason why this combination in particular should not be used. Some NSAIDs cause more gastrointestinal toxicity than others, a suggested broad 'rank order' of seven NSAIDs commonly used in the UK is as follows. Highest risk (**azapropazone**); intermediate risk (diclofenac, indometacin, **ketoprofen** and naproxen, with **piroxicam** more risky than the others); lowest risk (ibuprofen),[12] which has been borne out in a more recent analysis.[3] The ranking was based on epidemiological studies and the yellow card database. **Ketorolac** may also be particularly associated with gastrointestinal bleeding, and concurrent use with other NSAIDs has been identified as a risk factor,[13] therefore the makers consequently specifically contraindicate its use with other NSAIDs.[14]

1. Lewis SC, Langman MJS, Laporte J-R, Matthews JNS, Rawlins MD, Wiholm B-E. Dose-response relationships between individual nonaspirin nonsteroidal anti-inflammatory drugs (NANSAIDs) and serious upper gastrointestinal bleeding: a meta-analysis based on individual patient data. *Br J Clin Pharmacol* (2002) 54, 320–6.
2. Anon. Do not combine several NSAIDs. *Prescrire Int* (2003) 12, 20.
3. Committee on Safety of Medicines/Medicines Control Agency. Non-steroidal anti-inflammatory drugs (NSAIDs) and gastrointestinal safety. *Current Problems* (2002) 28, 5.
4. Cohen MM. Diflunisal protects human gastric mucosa against damage by indomethacin. *Dig Dis Sci* (1983) 28, 1070–77.
5. Edwards IR. Medicines Adverse Reactions Committee: eighteenth annual report, 1983. *N Z Med J* (1984) 97, 729–32.
6. Rudge SR, Lloyd-Jones JK, Hind ID. Interaction between flurbiprofen and indomethacin in rheumatoid arthritis. *Br J Clin Pharmacol* (1982) 13, 448–51.
7. Dresse A, Gerard MA, Quinaux N, Fischer P, Gerardy J. Effect of diflunisal on human plasma levels and on the urinary excretion of naproxen. *Arch Int Pharmacodyn Ther* (1978) 236, 276–84.
8. Van Hecken A, Verbesselt R, Tjandra-Maga TB, De Schepper PJ. Pharmacokinetic interaction between indomethacin and diflunisal. *Eur J Clin Pharmacol* (1989) 36, 507–12.
9. Eriksson L-O, Wåhlin-Boll E, Liedholm H, Seideman P, Melander A. Influence of chronic diflunisal treatment on the plasma levels, metabolism and excretion of indomethacin. *Eur J Clin Pharmacol* (1989) 37, 7–15.
10. Sioufi A, Stierlin H, Schweizer A, Botta L, Degen PH, Theobald W, Brechbühler S. Recent findings concerning clinically relevant pharmacokinetics of diclofenac sodium. In: Voltarol — New Findings, ed Kass E. Proc Int Symp Voltarol, Paris June 22nd, 1981. 15th Int Congress of Rheumatology. p 19–30.
11. Kimberly R, Brandstetter RD. Exacerbation of phenylbutazone-related renal failure by indomethacin. *Arch Intern Med* (1978) 138, 1711–12.
12. Committee on the Safety of Medicines/Medicines Control Agency. Relative safety of oral non-aspirin NSAIDs. *Current Problems* (1994) 20, 9–11.
13. Committee on Safety of Medicines/Medicines Control Agency. Ketorolac: new restrictions on dose and duration of treatment. *Current Problems* (1993) 19, 5–6.
14. Toradol (Ketorolac trometamol). Roche Products Ltd. UK Summary of product characteristics, October 2002.

NSAIDs or Aspirin + Paracetamol (Acetaminophen)

Paracetamol levels are increased by diflunisal. Diclofenac, nabumetone and sulindac pharmacokinetics are not affected by paracetamol. There is no pharmacokinetic interaction between ibuprofen and paracetamol. Propacetamol increases the antiplatelet effects of diclofenac, although the clinical relevance of this is uncertain.

One epidemiological study found that paracetamol alone, and particularly when combined with NSAIDs, was associated with an increased risk of gastrointestinal bleeding, but other studies have not found such an effect.

Two isolated case reports describe renal toxicity in 3 patients on ibuprofen or flurbiprofen in which paracetamol use was a theoretical contributing factor.

Clinical evidence, mechanism, importance and management

(a) Antiplatelet effects

Combining single doses of intravenous **propacetamol** 30 mg/kg and **diclofenac** 1.1 mg/kg augmented the platelet inhibitory effect of **diclofenac** by about a third at 90 minutes post dose in healthy subjects. At 5 minutes, the inhibitory effect of both **diclofenac** alone and the combination was 100%, and by 22 to 24 hours, neither **diclofenac** alone nor the combination had any inhibitory effect.[1] In a previous study, the authors had shown that **propacetamol** (which is hydrolysed to paracetamol) also inhibited platelet function, and they suggest that the effects of **diclofenac** and **propacetamol** are additive.[1] The clinical relevance of these findings is unclear, but the authors say it should be considered when assessing the risk of surgical bleeding.[1] Further study is needed.

(b) Gastrointestinal damage

The risk of upper gastrointestinal bleeding or perforation was slightly increased in users of both aspirin and paracetamol (relative risk 3.3) when compared with aspirin alone (2.4) or paracetamol alone (2.4) in a case-control study of the UK General Practice Research Database from 1993 to 1998. Moreover, the risk was markedly increased in those using NSAIDs and paracetamol (16.6) when compared with NSAIDs alone (3.6). The paracetamol doses used were at least 2 g daily. Paracetamol in doses of less than 2 g daily was not associated with an increased risk. Other drug doses and specific NSAIDs were not mentioned.[2] However, other epidemiological studies have not found any increased risk of upper gastrointestinal bleeding with paracetamol at any dose.[3] Paracetamol is usually considered not to increase the risk of upper gastrointestinal adverse effects, and the results of this case-control study are probably insufficient to change prescribing practice. Further studies are needed, controlled for dose of NSAID and indication for treatment.

(c) Pharmacokinetic studies

(i) Diclofenac. Diclofenac 25 mg given with paracetamol 500 mg, both three times daily for 14 days, had no effect on the pharmacokinetics of diclofenac in 6 healthy subjects.[4]

(ii) Diflunisal. Diflunisal significantly raised serum paracetamol levels by 50% but the total bioavailability was unchanged in healthy subjects. Diflunisal levels were not affected.[5,6] This interaction has not been shown to be clinically important. Nevertheless, the makers of diflunisal recommend

that the combination should be used with caution, because of the association of high levels of paracetamol with hepatotoxicity.[6]

(iii) Ibuprofen. Ibuprofen 400 mg given with paracetamol 650 mg, both every 6 hours for 2 days, had no effect on the pharmacokinetics of either drug in a crossover study in 20 healthy subjects.[7]

(iv) Nabumetone. In a single-dose study, the absorption of nabumetone 1 g was not significantly altered by paracetamol 1.5 g.[8]

(v) Sulindac. The makers of sulindac note that paracetamol had no effect on the plasma levels of sulindac or its sulfide metabolite.[9]

(d) Renal effects

Two children (aged 12 and 14 years) developed acute flank pain and reversible renal function impairment during the short-term use of **flurbiprofen** or **ibuprofen**. They had also taken paracetamol.[10] Similarly, a 14-month-old infant with febrile status epilepticus was treated with an alternating regimen of paracetamol and **ibuprofen**, and subsequently developed acute renal failure.[11] NSAIDs can cause renal toxicity, whereas paracetamol is less likely to cause renal toxicity, except perhaps in overdose.[12] The authors of the first case report proposed that tubular toxicity of NSAIDs and paracetamol are theoretically synergistic.[10] This is because NSAIDs inhibit the production of glutathione (needed to prevent the accumulation of toxic metabolites of paracetamol) and renal ischaemia (possibly induced by NSAIDs, or by dehydration) might lead to the accumulation of paracetamol in the renal medulla.[10]

A review concluded that the available evidence does not support an increased risk of renal toxicity with the use of combination products of aspirin and paracetamol when compared with either drug alone.[13] Paracetamol is often combined with NSAIDs in the management of chronic pain. In addition, paracetamol and **ibuprofen** are often used concurrently (as alternating doses) in the management of fever, particularly in children. This latter practice has become controversial. Opponents cite the lack of efficacy data to support combined use (rather than appropriate doses of single agents), and the theoretical increased risk of overdose and renal toxicity.[14,15] Others consider that, in the absence of true safety issues, professional judgement should be used for recommending combined treatment.[16] Further study is clearly needed.

1. Munsterhjelm E, Niemi TT, Syrjälä MT, Ylikorkala O, Rosenberg PH. Propacetamol augments inhibition of platelet function by diclofenac in volunteers. *Br J Anaesth* (2003) 91, 357–62.
2. García Rodríguez LA, Hernández-Díaz S. The risk of upper gastrointestinal complications associated with nonsteroidal anti-inflammatory drugs, glucocorticoids, acetaminophen, and combinations of these agents. *Arthritis Res* (2001) 3, 98–101.
3. Lewis SC, Langman MJS, Laporte J-R, Matthews JNS, Rawlins MD, Wiholm B-E. Dose-response relationships between individual nonaspirin nonsteroidal anti-inflammatory drugs (NANSAIDs) and serious upper gastrointestinal bleeding: a meta-analysis based on individual patient data. *Br J Clin Pharmacol* (2002) 54, 320–6.
4. Sioufi A, Stierlin H, Schweizer A, Botta L, Degen PH, Theobald W, Brechbühler S. Recent findings concerning clinically relevant pharmacokinetics of diclofenac sodium. In: Voltarol — New Findings, ed Kass E. Proc Int Symp Voltarol, Paris June 22nd, 1981. 15th Int Congress of Rheumatology. p 19–30.
5. Merck Sharp & Dohme Ltd. Personal communication, 1988.
6. Dolobid (Diflunisal). Merck Sharp & Dohme Ltd. UK Summary of product characteristics, March 2000.
7. Wright CE, Antal EJ, Gillespie WR, Albert KS. Ibuprofen and acetaminophen kinetics when taken concurrently. *Clin Pharmacol Ther* (1983) 34, 707–10.
8. von Schrader HW, Buscher G, Dierdorf D, Mügge H, Wolf D. Nabumetone — a novel anti-inflammatory drug: the influence of food, milk, antacids, and analgesics on bioavailability of single oral doses. *Int J Clin Pharmacol Ther Toxicol* (1983) 21, 311–21.
9. Clinoril (Sulindac). Merck Sharp & Dohme Ltd. UK Summary of product characteristics, November 2003.
10. McIntire SC, Rubenstein RC, Gartner JC, Gilboa N, Elllis D. Acute flank pain and reversible renal dysfunction associated with nonsteroidal anti-inflammatory drug use. *Pediatrics* (1993) 92, 459–60.
11. Del Vecchio MT, Sundel ER. Alternating antipyretics: is this an alternative? *Pediatrics* (2001) 108, 1236–7.
12. Whelton A. Renal effects of over-the-counter analgesics. *J Clin Pharmacol* (1995) 35, 454–63.
13. Bach PH, Berndt WO, Delzell E, Dubach U, Finn WF, Fox JM, Hess R, Michielsen P, Sandler DP, Trump B, Williams G. A safety assessment of fixed dose combinations of acetaminophen and acetylsalicylic acid, coformulated with caffeine. *Ren Fail* (1998) 20, 749–62.
14. Carson SM. Alternating acetaminophen and ibuprofen in the febrile child: examination of the evidence regarding efficacy and safety. *Pediatr Nurs* (2003) 29, 379–82.
15. Anon. No evidence for practice of alternating doses of paracetamol and ibuprofen in children with fever. *Pharm J* (2004) 272, 4.
16. Conroy S, Tomlin S, Soor S. Unsubstantiated alarmist declarations need to be examined. *Pharm J* (2004) 272, 152.

NSAIDs + Phenobarbital

Phenobarbital modestly increases the loss of fenoprofen and phenylbutazone from the body.

Clinical evidence, mechanism, importance and management

Pretreatment with phenobarbital 15 or 60 mg every 6 hours for 10 days reduced the AUC of a single 200-mg dose of **fenoprofen** in 6 healthy subjects by 23% and 37% respectively.[1]

The half-life of a single 6-mg/kg dose of **phenylbutazone** was reduced by 38% after pretreatment with phenobarbital 2 to 3 mg/kg daily for 3 weeks in 5 healthy subjects.[2] Other studies confirm that phenobarbital increases the loss of **phenylbutazone** from the body.[3,4]

The probable reason is that the phenobarbital increases the metabolism of these NSAIDs by the liver, thereby hastening their clearance.

The clinical importance of these interactions is uncertain (probably small) but be alert for any evidence of reduced NSAID effects if phenobarbital is added.

1. Helleberg L, Rubin A, Wolen RL, Rodda BE, Ridolfo AS, Gruber CM. A pharmacokinetic interaction in man between phenobarbitone and fenoprofen, a new anti-inflammatory agent. *Br J Clin Pharmacol* (1974) 1, 371–4.
2. Anderson KE, Peterson CM, Alvares AP, Kappas A. Oxidative drug metabolism and inducibility by phenobarbital in sickle cell anemia. *Clin Pharmacol Ther* (1977) 22, 580–7.
3. Levi AJ, Sherlock S, Walker D. Phenylbutazone and isoniazid metabolism in patients with liver disease in relation to previous drug therapy. *Lancet* (1968) i, 1275–9.
4. Whittaker JA, Price Evans DA. Genetic control of phenylbutazone metabolism in man. *BMJ* (1970) 4, 323–8.

NSAIDs + Probenecid

Probenecid reduces the loss of dexketoprofen, diflunisal, ketoprofen, ketorolac, indometacin, naproxen, sodium meclofenamate, tenoxicam and tiaprofenic acid from the body, and raises their serum levels. Increased clinical effects have been seen for indometacin, but indometacin toxicity has also occurred. Ketorolac and probenecid are specifically contraindicated. The uricosuric effects of probenecid are not affected by indometacin. The active metabolite of sulindac was not affected by probenecid, and sulindac slightly reduced the uricosuric effects of probenecid.

Clinical evidence

(a) Diflunisal

Probenecid 500 mg twice daily increased the steady-state plasma levels of diflunisal 250 mg twice daily by 65% in 8 healthy subjects, and reduced the clearances of the glucuronide metabolites.[1]

(b) Indometacin

A study in 28 patients with osteoarthritis, taking indometacin 50 to 150 mg daily orally or rectally, showed that probenecid 500 mg to 1 g daily roughly doubled their indometacin plasma levels and this paralleled the increased effectiveness (relief of morning stiffness, joint tenderness and raised grip strength indices). However, 4 patients developed indometacin toxicity.[2]

Other studies have also demonstrated the marked rise in plasma indometacin levels caused by probenecid.[3-5] Clear signs of indometacin toxicity (nausea, headache, tinnitus, confusion and a rise in blood urea) occurred in a woman with stable mild renal impairment when given probenecid.[6] The uricosuric effects of probenecid were not altered.[3]

(c) Ketoprofen and Dexketoprofen

Probenecid 500 mg every 6 hours reduced the clearance of ketoprofen 50 mg every 6 hours by 67% in 6 healthy subjects.[7] The maker of dexketoprofen notes that plasma levels may be increased by probenecid, and adjustment of the dose of dexketoprofen is required.[8]

(d) Ketorolac

Probenecid 500 mg four times daily for 4 days increased the total AUC of a single 10-mg dose of ketorolac in 8 subjects by more than threefold, increased its half-life from 6.6 to 15.1 hours, raised its maximum plasma levels by 24% and reduced its clearance by 67%.[9]

(e) Meclofenamate

Single-dose studies in 6 healthy subjects on the pharmacokinetics of sodium meclofenamate 100 mg found that pretreatment with probenecid [dosage unstated] increased its AUC and reduced its apparent plasma clearance by 60%, primarily due to a decrease in non-renal clearance.[10]

(f) Naproxen

Probenecid 500 mg twice daily increased the plasma levels of naproxen 250 mg twice daily by 50% in 12 healthy subjects.[11]

(g) Sulindac

The makers of sulindac note that probenecid increased plasma levels of sulindac and its sulfone metabolite, but had little effect on the active sulfide metabolite. Sulindac produced a modest reduction in the uricosuric action of probenecid,[12,13] which is said not to be clinically significant in most circumstances.[13]

(h) Tenoxicam

Probenecid 1 g twice daily for 4 days increased the maximum serum levels of a single 20-mg oral dose of tenoxicam by 25%. None of the other pharmacokinetic parameters was significantly altered.[14]

(i) Tiaprofenic acid

Probenecid appeared to reduce the urinary excretion of tiaprofenic acid in one healthy subject. The maximum urinary excretion rate was reduced by 66% and delayed by 2 hours.[15]

Mechanism

Probenecid is a known substrate for renal glucuronidation, and possibly competitively inhibits the renal glucuronidation of these NSAIDs.[8,16]

Importance and management

The interaction between indometacin and probenecid is established and adequately documented. Concurrent use should be well monitored because, while clinical improvement can undoubtedly occur, some patients may develop indometacin toxicity (headache, dizziness, light-headedness, nausea, etc.). This is particularly likely in those with some impaired renal function. Reduce the indometacin dosage as necessary. Information about other NSAIDs is limited, but these interactions also appear to be established. The clinical importance of most of them is uncertain, but probably small. Reports of adverse effects seem to be lacking, but it would still be prudent to be alert for any evidence of increased adverse effects. Reduce the NSAID dosage if necessary. The exception is ketorolac, which its makers[17] say should be avoided with probenecid because of the marked increases seen in its plasma levels.

1. Macdonald JI, Wallace SM, Herman RJ, Verbeeck RK. Effect of probenecid on the formation and elimination kinetics of the sulphate and glucuronide conjugates of diflunisal. *Eur J Clin Pharmacol* (1995) 47, 519–23.
2. Brooks PM, Bell MA, Sturrock RD, Famaey JP, Dick WC. The clinical significance of indomethacin-probenecid interaction. *Br J Clin Pharmacol* (1974) 1, 287–90.
3. Skeith MD, Simkin PA, Healey LA. The renal excretion of indomethacin and its inhibition by probenecid. *Clin Pharmacol Ther* (1968) 9, 89–93.
4. Emori W, Paulus HE, Bluestone R, Pearson CM. The pharmacokinetics of indomethacin in serum. *Clin Pharmacol Ther* (1973) 14, 134.
5. Baber N, Halliday L, Littler T, Orme ML'E, Sibeon R. Clinical studies of the interaction between indomethacin and probenecid. *Br J Clin Pharmacol* (1978) 5, 364P.
6. Sinclair H, Gibson T. Interaction between probenecid and indomethacin. *Br J Rheumatol* (1986) 25, 316–17.
7. Upton RA, Williams RL, Buskin JN, Jones RM. Effects of probenecid on ketoprofen kinetics. *Clin Pharmacol Ther* (1982) 31, 705–12.
8. Keral (Dexketoprofen trometamol). A. Menarini Pharmaceuticals UK Ltd. UK Summary of product characteristics, March 2001.
9. Mroszczak EJ, Combs DL, Goldblum R, Yee J, McHugh D, Tsina I, Fratis T. The effect of probenecid on ketorolac pharmacokinetics after oral dosing of ketorolac tromethamine. *Clin Pharmacol Ther* (1992) 51, 154.
10. Waller ES. The effect of probenecid on the disposition of meclofenamate sodium. *Drug Intell Clin Pharm* (1983) 17, 453–4.
11. Runkel R, Mroszczak E, Chaplin M, Sevelius H, Segre E. Naproxen-probenecid interaction. *Clin Pharmacol Ther* (1978) 24, 706–13.
12. Clinoril (Sulindac). Merck Sharp & Dohme Ltd. UK Summary of product characteristics, November 2003.
13. Clinoril (Sulindac). Merck & Co Inc. US Prescribing information, July 1998.
14. Day RO, Geisslinger G, Paull P, Williams KM. Neither cimetidine nor probenecid affect the pharmacokinetics of tenoxicam in normal volunteers. *Br J Clin Pharmacol* (1994) 37, 79–81.
15. Jamali F, Russell AS, Lehmann C, Berry BW. Pharmacokinetics of tiaprofenic acid in healthy and arthritic subjects. *J Pharm Sci* (1985) 74, 953–6.
16. Vree TB, van den Biggelaar-Martea M, Verwey-van Wissen CPWGM, van Ewijk-Beneken Kolmer EWJ. Probenecid inhibits the glucuronidation of indomethacin and *O*-desmethylindomethacin in humans: a pilot experiment. *Pharm World Sci* (1994) 16, 22–6.
17. Toradol (Ketorolac trometamol). Roche Products Ltd. UK Summary of product characteristics, October 2002.

NSAIDs or Aspirin + Prostaglandins

Misoprostol increases the incidence of abdominal pain and diarrhoea when used with diclofenac or indometacin. Isolated cases of neurological adverse effects have been seen with naproxen or phenylbutazone given with misoprostol. No important pharmacokinetic interactions seem to occur between aspirin, diclofenac, ibuprofen or indometacin and misoprostol. NSAIDs are reported not to affect the abortive effects of intravaginal misoprostol.

Clinical evidence, mechanism, importance and management

(A) Oral misoprostol

(a) Gastrointestinal adverse effects

A higher incidence of abdominal pain, diarrhoea, nausea and dyspepsia occurred when **diclofenac** was combined with misoprostol.[1,2] Concurrent use of **indometacin** and misoprostol also resulted in an increase in frequency and severity of abdominal symptoms, frequency of bowel movements and a decrease in faecal consistency.[3] The most frequent adverse effect of misoprostol alone is diarrhoea, and this may limit the dose tolerated. When using misoprostol with NSAIDs, warn patients about the possibility of increased stomach pain and diarrhoea. Preparations combining **diclofenac** or **naproxen** with misoprostol are available.

(b) Neurological adverse effects

A man with rheumatoid arthritis on long-term **naproxen** developed ataxic symptoms a few hours after starting misoprostol. He said he felt like a drunk person, staggering about and vomiting. He rapidly improved when he stopped the misoprostol but the adverse symptoms recurred on two further occasions when he restarted misoprostol.[4]

Adverse effects developed in 3 patients taking **phenylbutazone** 200 to 400 mg daily when they took misoprostol 400 to 800 micrograms daily.[5] One had headaches, dizziness and ambulatory instability that disappeared and then reappeared when the misoprostol was stopped and then restarted. No problems occurred when the **phenylbutazone** was replaced by **etodolac** 400 mg daily. The other 2 patients developed symptoms including headache, tingles, dizziness, hot flushes and transient diplopia.[5,6] No problems developed when one of them was given **naproxen** and misoprostol.[6] The reasons for this reaction are not understood but theoretically it could possibly be due to a potentiation of the adverse effects of **phenylbutazone**. The general relevance of these few reports is unclear, but bear them in mind should unexpected neurological effects occur.

(c) Pharmacokinetic studies

No clinically important pharmacokinetic interactions have been found to occur between aspirin 975 mg and misoprostol 200 micrograms,[7] or between **ibuprofen** and misoprostol.[8] One study found that misoprostol 800 micrograms daily decreased the AUC of a single 100-mg dose of **diclofenac** by a modest 20%.[2] However, other studies have found that misoprostol had no effect on steady-state **diclofenac** pharmacokinetics.[9] Similarly, the bioavailability of **diclofenac** and misoprostol from a combination tablet (*Arthrotec*) was similar to that seen when the two drugs were given separately.[10]One study found that misoprostol 200 micrograms raised the steady-state levels of **indometacin** 50 mg three times daily by about 30%,[11] whereas another found that **misoprostol** 400 micrograms twice daily reduced the AUC of **indometacin** 50 mg twice daily by 13% after one dose and reduced the maximum steady-state plasma concentration by 24%.[3] These modest changes in serum **indometacin** levels are unlikely to be clinically important.

(B) Vaginal prostaglandins

NSAIDs and aspirin are frequently avoided before the use of **prostaglandins** for induction of uterine contractions, because of the theoretical concern that they may inhibit efficacy.[12] For example, the UK makers of **dinoprostone** say that NSAIDs including aspirin should be stopped before giving intravaginal **dinoprostone** for induction of labour.[13] However, a study involving 416 women given intravaginal misoprostol to induce early abortion found that the concurrent use of oral NSAIDs did not interfere with the efficacy of misoprostol,[12] and the US makers of **dinoprostone** do not list NSAIDs or aspirin as possible interacting drugs.[14] Further study is needed. Consider also 'Mifepristone + Aspirin or NSAIDs', p.1024.

1. Gagnier P. Review of the safety of diclofenac/misoprostol. *Drugs* (1993) 45 (Suppl 1), 31–5.
2. Dammann HG, Simon-Schultz J, Steinhoff I, Damaschke A, Schmoldt A, Sallowsky E. Differential effects of misoprostol and ranitidine on the pharmacokinetics of diclofenac and gastrointestinal symptoms. *Br J Clin Pharmacol* (1993) 36, 345–9.
3. Kendall MJ, Gibson R, Walt RP. Co-administration of misoprostol or ranitidine with indomethacin: effects on pharmacokinetics, abdominal symptoms and bowel habit. *Aliment Pharmacol Ther* (1992) 6, 437–46.
4. Huq M. Neurological adverse effects of naproxen and misoprostol combination. *Br J Gen Pract* (1990) 40, 432.
5. Jacquemier JM, Lassoued S, Laroche M, Mazières B. Neurosensory adverse effects after phenylbutazone and misoprostol combined treatment. *Lancet* (1989) 2, 1283.
6. Chassagne Ph, Humez C, Gourmelen O, Moore N, Le Loet X, Deshayes P. Neurosensory adverse effects after combined phenylbutazone and misoprostol. *Br J Rheumatol* (1991) 30, 392.
7. Karim A, Rozek LF, Leese PT. Absorption of misoprostol (Cytotec), an antiulcer prostaglandin, or aspirin is not affected when given concomitantly to healthy human subjects. *Gastroenterology* (1987) 92, 1742.

8. Small RE, Wilmot-Pater MG, McGee BA, Willis HE. Effects of misoprostol or ranitidine on ibuprofen pharmacokinetics. *Clin Pharm* (1991) 10, 870–2.
9. Karim A. Pharmacokinetics of diclofenac and misoprostol when administered alone or as a combination product. *Drugs* (1993) 45 (Suppl 1), 7–14.
10. Karim A, Smith M. Biopharmaceutical profile of diclofenac misoprostol combination tablet Arthrotec. *Scand J Rheumatol* (1992) 96 (Suppl), 37–48.
11. Rainsford KD, James C, Hunt RH, Stetsko PI, Rischke JA, Karim A, Nicholson PA, Smith M, Hantsbarger G. Effects of misoprostol on the pharmacokinetics of indomethacin in human volunteers. *Clin Pharmacol Ther* (1992) 51, 415–21.
12. Creinin MD, Shulman T. Effect of nonsteroidal anti-inflammatory drugs on the action of misoprostol in a regimen for early abortion. *Contraception* (1997) 56, 165–8.
13. Propess (Dinoprostone). Ferring Pharmaceuticals Ltd. UK Summary of product characteristics, February 1998.
14. Prostin E2 (Dinoprostone). Pharmacia & Upjohn Company. US Prescribing information, March 2003.

NSAIDs or Aspirin + Proton pump inhibitors

The antiplatelet activity and the pharmacokinetics of aspirin do not appear to be affected by omeprazole. There was no pharmacokinetic interaction between omeprazole and diclofenac, naproxen or piroxicam, or between pantoprazole and diclofenac or naproxen, or between esomeprazole and naproxen or rofecoxib.

Clinical evidence

(a) Aspirin

In a preliminary study in 11 healthy subjects, **omeprazole** 20 mg daily for 2 days reduced the serum levels of salicylic acid at 30 and 90 minutes after a single 650-mg dose of aspirin by 40 to 52% respectively.[1] However, another study in 14 healthy subjects given **omeprazole** 20 mg daily for 4 days with a final dose one hour before a single 125-mg dose of aspirin found that **omeprazole** did not significantly affect the plasma levels of either aspirin or salicylic acid. **Omeprazole** also did not affect the antiplatelet effects of aspirin.[2] Similarly, **omeprazole** had no effect on the bioavailability of aspirin (uncoated or enteric-coated tablets) in another study, although it increased the rate of absorption of aspirin from enteric-coated tablets.[3]

(b) Diclofenac

A single 105-mg dose of diclofenac potassium suspension (*Flogan*) was given to 13 healthy subjects while fasting and after gastric acid secretion blockade with **omeprazole**. The pharmacokinetics of the diclofenac were not changed to a clinically relevant extent by **omeprazole**.[4] Similarly, **omeprazole** 20 mg daily given with diclofenac 50 mg twice daily for one week had no effect on the pharmacokinetics of either drug in 24 healthy subjects.[5]

In another study a single 40-mg oral dose of **pantoprazole** and diclofenac 100 mg as enteric-coated *Voltarol* were given to 24 healthy subjects together and separately. Neither drug affected the pharmacokinetics of the other.[6]

(c) Naproxen

Naproxen 250 mg twice daily given to healthy subjects with **omeprazole** 20 mg daily,[5] **pantoprazole** 40 mg daily,[7] or **esomeprazole** 40 mg daily[8] for one week had no effect on the pharmacokinetics of either naproxen or the proton pump inhibitor.

(d) Piroxicam

Omeprazole 20 mg daily given to 24 healthy subjects with piroxicam 10 mg daily for one week had no effect on the pharmacokinetics of either drug.[5]

(e) Rofecoxib

Esomeprazole 40 mg daily given to 32 healthy subjects with rofecoxib 12.5 mg daily for one week had no effect on the pharmacokinetics of either drug apart from a slight increase in the maximum level of rofecoxib.[9]

Mechanism

Data from *animal* studies suggest that the absorption and thus the effects of aspirin and NSAIDs can be reduced by omeprazole and H_2-blockers via a pH dependent mechanism.[10,11] However, note that clinical trials have not found H_2-blockers to have any important effect on the pharmacokinetics of aspirin or NSAIDs, see 'NSAIDs or Aspirin + H_2-blockers', p.88. It was suggested that reducing gastric acidity with omeprazole results in the earlier disruption of enteric-coated tablets, and an increased absorption rate.[3]

Importance and management

The interaction between aspirin and omeprazole is not established. The balance of evidence suggests that omeprazole is unlikely to have an important effect on the pharmacokinetics and efficacy of aspirin. However, because of the uncertainty generated by the *animal* and preliminary clinical data,[1,10,11] it would be of benefit to confirm this in further studies.[2,12]

No pharmacokinetic interactions have been identified between any of the other NSAIDs and PPIs cited here, and no special precautions are needed during concurrent use. For mention that valdecoxib raises plasma levels of omeprazole see 'NSAIDs; Parecoxib or Valdecoxib + Miscellaneous', p.101. Note that omeprazole and other proton pump inhibitors are widely used in the management of the gastrointestinal complications of aspirin and NSAIDs.

1. Anand BS, Sanduja SK, Lichtenberger LM. Effect of omeprazole on the bioavailability of aspirin: a randomized controlled study on healthy volunteers. *Gastroenterology* (1999) 116: A371.
2. Iñarrea P, Esteva F, Corudella, Lanas A. Omeprazole does not interfere with the antiplatelet effect of low-dose aspirin in man. *Scand J Gastroenterol* (2000) 35, 242–6.
3. Nefesoglu FZ, Ayanoglu-Dülger G, Ulusoy NB, Imeryüz N. Interaction of omeprazole with enteric-coated salicylate tablets. *Int J Clin Pharmacol Ther* (1998) 36, 549–53.
4. Poli A, Moreno RA, Ribiero W, Dias HB, Moreno H, Muscara MN, De Nucci G. Influence of gastric acid secretion blockade and food intake on the bioavailability of a potassium diclofenac suspension in healthy male volunteers. *Int J Clin Pharmacol Ther* (1996) 34, 76–9.
5. Andersson T, Bredberg E, Lagerström P-O, Naesdal J, Wilson I. Lack of drug-drug interaction between three different non-steroidal anti-inflammatory drugs and omeprazole. *Eur J Clin Pharmacol* (1998) 54, 399–404.
6. Bliesath H, Huber R, Steinijans VW, Koch HJ, Wurst W, Mascher H. Lack of pharmacokinetic interaction between pantoprazole and diclofenac. *Int J Clin Pharmacol Ther* (1996) 34, 152–6.
7. Schulz H-U, Hartmann M, Krupp S, Schuerer M, Huber R, Luehmann R, Bethke T, Wurst W. Pantoprazole lacks interaction with the NSAID naproxen. *Gastroenterology* (2000) 118 (Suppl 2), A1304.
8. Hassan-Alin M, Nilsson-Pieschl C, Naesdal J, Langstrom G, Lundgren M, Nyman L. Lack of drug-drug interaction between esomeprazole and naproxen in healthy subjects. Digestive Disease Week Abstracts and Itinerary Planner May 17-22, 2003 FL, Orlando, USA, Abstract T1651.
9. Hassan-Alin M, Nilsson-Pieschl C, Naesdal J, Langstrom G, Lundgren M, Nyman L. Lack of drug-drug interaction between esomeprazole and rofecoxib in healthy subjects. Digestive Disease Week Abstracts and Itinerary Planner May 17-22, 2003 FL, Orlando, USA, Abstract T1650.
10. Lichtenberger LM, Ulloa C, Romero JJ, Vanous AL, Illich PA, Dial EJ. Nonsteroidal anti-inflammatory drug and phospholipid prodrugs: combination therapy with antisecretory agents in rats. *Gastroenterology* (1996) 111, 990–5.
11. Giraud M-N, Sanduja SK, Felder TB, Illich PA, Dial EJ, Lichtenberger LM. Effect of omeprazole on the bioavailability of unmodified and phospholipid-complexed aspirin in rats. *Aliment Pharmacol Ther* (1997) 11, 899–906.
12. Fernández-Fernández FJ. Might proton pump inhibitors prevent the antiplatelet effects of low- or very low-dose aspirin. *Arch Intern Med* (2002) 162, 2248.

NSAIDs + Rifampicin (Rifampin)

The plasma levels of celecoxib, diclofenac, etoricoxib and rofecoxib are reduced by rifampicin. Some increase in dosage may be needed. Metamizole (dipyrone) increased the maximum level of rifampicin.

Clinical evidence

(a) Celecoxib

Pretreatment with rifampicin 600 mg daily for 5 days reduced the AUC of a single 200-mg dose of celecoxib by 64% and increased the clearance by 185% in 12 healthy subjects.[1]

(b) Diclofenac

A study in 6 healthy subjects found that after taking rifampicin 450 mg daily for 6 days, the maximum serum levels of diclofenac, measured 8 hours after a single 100-mg dose of enteric coated tablets, was reduced by 43% and the AUC was reduced by 67%.[2]

(c) Etoricoxib

The makers note that rifampicin has been found to reduce the serum levels of etoricoxib by 65%.[3]

(d) Metamizole sodium (Dipyrone)

A study in untreated patients with leprosy showed that the pharmacokinetics of a single 600-mg dose of rifampicin were not markedly changed by 1 g of metamizole sodium (dipyrone), but peak serum rifampicin levels occurred sooner (at 3 instead of 4 hours) and were about 50% higher.[4]

(e) Rofecoxib

The makers note that rifampicin produced about a 50% decrease in rofecoxib plasma levels.[5]

Mechanism

Rifampicin is a potent inducer of hepatic enzymes, and it is likely that it increased the metabolism of these NSAIDs.

Importance and management

Although information is limited, these pharmacokinetic interactions appear to be established. Their clinical relevance remains to be determined, but it seems likely that the efficacy of these NSAIDs will be reduced by rifampicin. Combined use should be well monitored, and the NSAID dosage increased if necessary. See also 'NSAIDs; Parecoxib or Valdecoxib + Miscellaneous', p.101. The clinical relevance of the increase in rifampicin maximum levels with metamizole is uncertain.

1. Jayasagar G, Krishna Kumar M, Chandrasekhar K, Madhusudan RY. Influence of rifampicin pretreatment on the pharmacokinetics of celecoxib in healthy male volunteers. *Drug Metabol Drug Interact* (2003) 19, 287–95.
2. Kumar JS, Mamidi NVSR, Chakrapani T, Krishna DR. Rifampicin pretreatment reduces bioavailability of diclofenac sodium. *Indian J Pharmacol* (1995) 27, 183–5.
3. Arcoxia (Etoricoxib). Merck Sharp & Dohme Ltd. UK Summary of product characteristics, May 2005.
4. Krishna DR, Appa Rao AVN, Ramanakar TV, Reddy KSC, Prabhakar MC. Pharmacokinetics of rifampin in the presence of dipyrone in leprosy patients. *Drug Dev Ind Pharm* (1984) 10, 101–110.
5. Vioxx (Rofecoxib). Merck Sharp & Dohme Ltd. UK Summary of product characteristics, August 2003.

NSAIDs or Aspirin + Sucralfate

Sucralfate appears not to have a clinically important effect on the pharmacokinetics of aspirin, choline-magnesium trisalicylate, diclofenac, ibuprofen, indometacin, ketoprofen, piroxicam or naproxen.

Clinical evidence, mechanism, importance and management

Sucralfate 2 g was given to 18 healthy subjects 30 minutes before single-doses of **ketoprofen** 50 mg, **indometacin** 50 mg, or **naproxen** 500 mg. Some significant changes were seen (modestly reduced maximum serum concentrations of **ketoprofen**, **naproxen** and **indometacin**, reduced rate of absorption of **naproxen** and **indometacin**, increased time to achieve maximal serum concentrations with **indometacin**) but no alterations in bioavailability occurred.[1] A delay, but no reduction in the total absorption of **naproxen** is described in two studies.[2,3] It is unlikely that its clinical efficacy will be reduced.[2] Sucralfate 1 g four times daily for 2 days was found not to decrease the rate of absorption of a single 400-mg dose of **ibuprofen**[4] or of a single 650-mg dose of **aspirin**.[5] Sucralfate 5 g in divided doses did not significantly alter the absorption of a single 600-mg dose of **ibuprofen**.[6] Similarly, another study also found that sucralfate had no important effect on the pharmacokinetics of **ibuprofen** enantiomers.[7] In one study, sucralfate 2 g was found not to affect significantly the pharmacokinetics of either **piroxicam** 20 mg or **diclofenac** 50 mg.[8] However, in another study, sucralfate 2 g twice daily modestly reduced the 0 to 8-hour AUC and maximum serum levels of a single 105-mg dose of **diclofenac potassium** by 20% and 38% respectively.[9] Sucralfate 1 g every 6 hours was found not to affect the pharmacokinetics of **choline-magnesium trisalicylate** 1.5 g every 12 hours.[10]

Single dose studies do not necessarily reliably predict what will happen when patients take drugs regularly, but most of the evidence available suggests that sucralfate is unlikely to have an adverse effect on treatment with these NSAIDs.

1. Caillé G, Du Souich P, Gervais P, Besner J-G. Single dose pharmacokinetics of ketoprofen, indomethacin, and naproxen taken alone or with sucralfate. *Biopharm Drug Dispos* (1987) 8, 173–83.
2. Caille G, du Souich P, Gervais P, Besner JG, Vezina M. Effects of concurrent sucralfate administration on pharmacokinetics of naproxen. *Am J Med* (1987) 83 (Suppl 3B), 67–73.
3. Lafontaine D, Mailhot C, Vermeulen M, Bissonnette B, Lambert C. Influence of chewable sucralfate or a standard meal on the bioavailability of naproxen. *Clin Pharm* (1990) 9, 773–7.
4. Anaya AL, Mayersohn M, Conrad KA, Dimmitt DC. The influence of sucralfate on ibuprofen absorption in healthy adult males. *Biopharm Drug Dispos* (1986) 7, 443–51.
5. Lau A, Chang C-W, Schlesinger PK. Evaluation of a potential drug interaction between sucralfate and aspirin. *Clin Pharmacol Ther* (1986) 39, 151–5.
6. Pugh MC, Small RE, Garnett WR, Townsend RJ, Willis HE. Effect of sucralfate on ibuprofen absorption in normal volunteers. *Clin Pharm* (1984) 3, 630–3.
7. Levine MAH, Walker SE, Paton TW. The effect of food or sucralfate on the bioavailability of S(+) and R(-) enantiomers of ibuprofen. *J Clin Pharmacol* (1992) 32, 1110–14.
8. Ungethüm W. Study on the interaction between sucralfate and diclofenac/piroxicam in healthy volunteers. *Arzneimittelforschung* (1991) 41, 797–800.
9. Pedrazzoli J, Pierossi M de A, Muscará MN, Dias HB, da Silva CMF, Mendes FD, de Nucci G. Short-term sucralfate administration alters potassium diclofenac absorption in healthy male volunteers. *Br J Clin Pharmacol* (1997) 43, 104–8.
10. Schneider DK, Gannon RH, Sweeney KR, DeFusco PA. Influence of sucralfate on trisilate bioavailability. *J Clin Pharmacol* (1991) 31, 377–9.

NSAIDs + Tobacco smoking

The clearance of diflunisal and phenylbutazone from the body is greater in smokers than in non-smokers.

Clinical evidence, mechanism, importance and management

(a) Diflunisal

The clearance of a single 250-mg dose of diflunisal was 35% higher in 6 women who smoked 10 to 20 cigarettes a day than in 6 non-smoking women.[1] This change does not appear to be large enough to be of clinical importance.

(b) Phenylbutazone

The half-life of a single 6-mg/kg dose of phenylbutazone was 37 hours in a group of smokers (10 or more cigarettes daily for 2 years) compared with 64 hours in a group of non-smokers. The metabolic clearance was roughly doubled.[2] The conclusion to be drawn is that those who smoke may possibly need larger or more frequent doses of phenylbutazone to achieve the same therapeutic response, but this needs confirmation.

1. Macdonald JI, Herman RJ, Verbeeck RK. Sex-difference and the effects of smoking and oral contraceptive steroids on the kinetics of diflunisal. *Eur J Clin Pharmacol* (1990) 38, 175–9.
2. Garg SK, Kiran TNR. Effect of smoking on phenylbutazone disposition. *Int J Clin Pharmacol Ther Toxicol* (1983) 20, 289–90.

NSAIDs; Acemetacin + Miscellaneous

Acemetacin is a glycolic acid ester of indometacin, and its major metabolite is indometacin. Therefore the interactions of indometacin would be expected.

NSAIDs; Azapropazone + Antacids or Laxatives

A study in 15 patients taking azapropazone 300 mg three times daily found that antacids (dihydroxyaluminium sodium carbonate, aluminium magnesium silicate), bisacodyl or anthraquinone laxatives only caused a minor (5 to 7%) reduction in azapropazone plasma levels.[1] No special precautions would seem to be needed if any of these drugs are given together with azapropazone. Consider also 'NSAIDs; Miscellaneous + Antacids', p.99.

1. Faust-Tinnefeldt G, Geissler HE, Mutschler E. Azapropazon-Plasmaspiegel unter Begleitmedikation mit einem Antacidum oder Laxans. *Arzneimittelforschung* (1977) 27, 2411–12.

NSAIDs; Azapropazone + Chloroquine

The plasma levels of azapropazone are not significantly changed by chloroquine.

Clinical evidence, mechanism, importance and management

A study in 12 subjects given azapropazone 300 mg three times daily found that the plasma levels of azapropazone, measured at 4 hours, were not affected by chloroquine 250 mg daily for 7 days.[1] No special precautions would seem to be needed if these drugs are given together.

1. Faust-Tinnefeldt G, Geissler HE. Azapropazon und rheumatologische Basistherapie mit Chloroquin unter dem Aspekt der Arzneimittelinteraktion. *Arzneimittelforschung* (1977) 27, 2170–4.

NSAIDs; Coxibs + Antacids

Antacids [unspecified] do not affect the pharmacokinetics of etoricoxib or rofecoxib to a clinically relevant extent according to the makers.[1,2] Aluminium/magnesium hydroxides had no clinically significant effect on the rate or absorption of celecoxib[3,4] or valdecoxib.[5,6]

1. Arcoxia (Etoricoxib). Merck Sharp & Dohme Ltd. UK Summary of product characteristics, May 2005.
2. Vioxx (Rofecoxib). Merck Sharp & Dohme Ltd. UK Summary of product characteristics, August 2003.
3. Celebrex (Celecoxib). Pharmacia Ltd. UK Summary of product characteristics, March 2003.
4. Celebrex (Celecoxib). Pfizer Inc. US Prescribing information, February 2005.
5. Bextra (Valdecoxib). Pharmacia Ltd. UK Summary of product characteristics, May 2004.
6. Bextra (Valdecoxib). Pfizer Inc. US Prescribing information, November 2004.

NSAIDs; Coxibs + Azoles

Fluconazole markedly raises celecoxib levels, and the dose should be reduced but ketoconazole has no effect on celecoxib levels. Fluconazole and ketoconazole moderately increase valdecoxib levels, and the lowest recommended doses should be used to start with. Ketoconazole moderately raises etoricoxib serum levels, but this is unlikely to be of clinical relevance.

Clinical evidence

(a) Celecoxib

The maker notes that **fluconazole** 200 mg daily increased the AUC of a single 200-mg dose of celecoxib by 130% and increased the maximum level by 60%. Conversely, **ketoconazole** had no effect on the pharmacokinetics of celecoxib.[1]

(b) Etoricoxib

The makers note that **ketoconazole** 400 mg daily for 11 days increased the AUC of a single 60-mg dose of etoricoxib by 43% in healthy subjects.[2]

(c) Rofecoxib

The makers note that **ketoconazole** had no effect the pharmacokinetics of rofecoxib.[3]

(d) Valdecoxib and parecoxib

The makers of parecoxib and valdecoxib report a study in which **fluconazole** increased the plasma levels of valdecoxib by 19% and raised its AUC by 62%.[4-6] **Ketoconazole** had a similar, but more moderate effect on the levels of valdecoxib (maximum plasma levels increased by 24%, AUC increased by 38%).[4-6]

Mechanism

Fluconazole is a potent inhibitor of the cytochrome P450 isoenzyme CYP2C9 and ketoconazole inhibits CYP3A4. Celecoxib is extensively metabolised by CYP2C9, and therefore shows marked rises in plasma levels when given with fluconazole. Etoricoxib is partially metabolised by CYP3A4, therefore shows moderate rises in plasma levels with ketoconazole. Valdecoxib is metabolised by both CYP2C9 and CYP3A4, therefore was modestly affected by both fluconazole and ketoconazole. Parecoxib is a valdecoxib prodrug, and interacts similarly. Rofecoxib does not generally undergo oxidation by cytochrome P450 isoenzymes, and was therefore not affected by ketoconazole.

Importance and management

These pharmacokinetic interactions are established, although their effect in clinical practice has not been assessed. The marked rise in celecoxib levels with fluconazole could be important, and the UK maker recommends that the dose of celecoxib should be halved in patients receiving fluconazole,[1] whereas the US maker suggests starting with the lowest recommended dose.[7] The rise in valdecoxib with fluconazole is less marked, nevertheless the maker recommends that for parecoxib the dosage should be reduced (but they do not suggest by how much),[5] and for valdecoxib to start with the lowest recommended dose.[4]

For ketoconazole, the makers say that no parecoxib dosage adjustments should be needed,[5] but valdecoxib should be started at the lowest recommended dose.[4] Conversely, the makers of etoricoxib do not consider the moderate rise in serum levels with ketoconazole to be clinically relevant.[2] Rofecoxib is not affected by ketoconazole, and would not be expected to be affected by fluconazole either.

1. Celebrex (Celecoxib). Pharmacia Ltd. UK Summary of product characteristics, March 2003.
2. Arcoxia (Etoricoxib). Merck Sharp & Dohme Ltd. UK Summary of product characteristics, May 2005.
3. Vioxx (Rofecoxib). Merck Sharp & Dohme Ltd. UK Summary of product characteristics, August 2003.
4. Bextra (Valdecoxib). Pharmacia Ltd. UK Summary of product characteristics, May 2004.
5. Dynastat injection (Parecoxib sodium). Pharmacia Ltd. UK Summary of product characteristics, April 2004.
6. Bextra (Valdecoxib). Pfizer Inc. US Prescribing information, November 2004.
7. Celebrex (Celecoxib). Pfizer Inc. US Prescribing information, February 2005.

NSAIDs; Diclofenac + Antacids

The absorption of diclofenac is not affected by aluminium hydroxide, magnesium hydroxide, or the combination.

Clinical evidence, mechanism, importance and management

Two teaspoonfuls of a 5.8% suspension of **aluminium hydroxide** had no effect on the bioavailability of a single 50-mg dose of diclofenac in 7 healthy subjects.[1] In another study, 10 ml of **magnesium hydroxide** suspension (850 mg) was found to have no significant effect on the rate or extent of absorption of a single 50-mg dose of diclofenac in 6 healthy fasted subjects.[2] However, there was a tendency to an increased rate of absorption. *Aluco Gel* (**aluminium/magnesium hydroxide**) had no effect on the extent of absorption of enteric-coated diclofenac, but may have reduced the rate of absorption.[3] No particular precautions would seem to be needed if these antacids are given with diclofenac.

1. Schumacher A, Faust-Tinnefeldt G, Geissler HE, Gilfrich HJ, Mutschler E. Untersuchungen potentieller Interaktionen von Diclofenac-Natrium (Voltaren) mit einem Antazidum und mit Digitoxin. *Therapiewoche* (1983) 33, 2619–25.
2. Neuvonen PJ. The effect of magnesium hydroxide on the oral absorption of ibuprofen, ketoprofen and diclofenac. *Br J Clin Pharmacol* (1991) 31, 263–6.
3. Sioufi A, Stierlin H, Schweizer A, Botta L, Degen PH, Theobald W, Brechbühler S. Recent findings concerning clinically relevant pharmacokinetics of diclofenac sodium. In: Voltarol — New Findings, ed Kass E. Proc Int Symp Voltarol, Paris June 22nd, 1981. 15th Int Congress of Rheumatology. p 19–30.

NSAIDs; Diclofenac + Cephalosporins or Doxycycline

Doxycycline and cefadroxil do not alter the pharmacokinetics of diclofenac. The biliary excretion of ceftriaxone is increased by diclofenac.

Clinical evidence, mechanism, importance and management

The pharmacokinetics of diclofenac 100 mg daily were unaffected by either **cefadroxil** 2 g daily (8 patients) or doxycycline 100 mg daily (7) for one week.[1] No special precautions are needed while taking either of these drugs and diclofenac.

A pharmacokinetic study in 8 patients who had undergone cholecystectomy and who had a T-drain in the common bile duct, found that diclofenac 50 mg every 12 hours increased the excretion of intravenous **ceftriaxone** 2 g in the bile by about fourfold and roughly halved the urinary excretion.[2] The clinical importance of this is uncertain, but probably small.

1. Schumacher A, Geissler HE, Mutschler E, Osterburg M. Untersuchungen potentieller Interaktionen von Diclofenac-Natrium (Voltaren) mit Antibiotika. *Z Rheumatol* (1983) 42, 25–7.
2. Merle-Melet M, Bresler L, Lokiec F, Dopff C, Boissel P, Dureux JB. Effects of diclofenac on ceftriaxone pharmacokinetics in humans. *Antimicrob Agents Chemother* (1992) 36, 2331–3.

NSAIDs; Diclofenac + Pentazocine

An isolated report describes grand mal seizures in a patient given diclofenac and pentazocine.

Clinical evidence, mechanism, importance and management

A man with Buerger's disease had a grand mal seizure while watching television 2 hours after being given a single 50-mg suppository of diclofenac. He was also taking pentazocine 50-mg three times daily. He may possibly have had a previous seizure some months before after taking a single 100-mg slow-release diclofenac tablet.[1] The reasons for this reaction are not known, but on rare occasions diclofenac alone has been associated with seizures (incidence said to be 1 in 100 000) and seizures have also been seen with pentazocine alone. It is not clear what part the disease itself, or watching television, had in the development of this adverse reaction.[1]

No interaction between diclofenac and pentazocine is established, but be aware of this case if concurrent use is being considered, particularly in patients who are known to be seizure-prone.

1. Heim M, Nadvorna H, Azaria M. With comments by Straughan J and Hoehler HW. Grand mal seizures following treatment with diclofenac and pentazocine. *S Afr Med J* (1990) 78, 700–1.

NSAIDs; Diclofenac topical + Miscellaneous

Topical diclofenac intended for use on the skin is very unlikely to interact adversely with any of the drugs known to interact with the diclofenac given orally.

Clinical evidence, mechanism, importance and management

The makers of *Pennsaid* (a 1.5% topical solution of diclofenac in 45% (w/w) dimethyl sulfoxide) say that when the maximum dosage of 1 ml is used on the skin, the maximum serum levels of diclofenac achieved are less than 10 nanograms/ml.[1] This is 50 times lower than the maximum serum levels achieved with the oral diclofenac 25 mg. Despite these very low concentrations, the makers list all the interactions that have been observed after systemic administration of diclofenac sodium (**aspirin**, **digoxin**, **lithium**, **oral hypoglycaemic agents**, **diuretics**, **NSAIDs** including other **diclofenac** preparations, **methotrexate**, **ciclosporin**, **quinolones** and **antihypertensives**).[1] They note that the risk of these interactions in association with topical use is not known, but is probably low.[1] None of the drugs listed have yet been reported to interact with topical diclofenac.

1. Pennsaid (Diclofenac). Dimethaid International. UK Summary of product characteristics, February 2004.

NSAIDs; Diflunisal + Antacids

Antacids containing aluminium with or without magnesium can reduce the absorption of diflunisal by up to 40%, but no important interaction occurs if food is taken at the same time. Magnesium hydroxide can increase the rate of diflunisal absorption.

Clinical evidence

A study in 4 healthy fasted subjects found that when given three 15-ml doses of *Aludrox* (**aluminium hydroxide**), 2 hours before, together with, and 2 hours after, a single 500-mg oral dose of diflunisal, the diflunisal AUC was reduced about 40%.[1] Another study showed that the AUC of a single 500-mg dose of diflunisal was reduced by 13% by a single 30-ml dose of *Maalox* (**aluminium/magnesium hydroxide**), by 21% when given 1 hour after the antacids, and by 32% when the antacid was given four times daily.[2] However, in another study, **aluminium/magnesium hydroxide** had no effect on the AUC diflunisal when the diflunisal was given 30 minutes after food.[3] This study found that the AUC of diflunisal was reduced by 26% by 15 ml of **aluminium hydroxide** gel in fasted subjects, but not when the diflunisal was given after food.[3] **Magnesium hydroxide** suspension markedly increased the rate of diflunisal absorption in fasted subjects. The plasma diflunisal level was increased by 130% at 30 minutes, and by 64% at one hour but the AUC was only increased by a modest 10%.[3]

Mechanism

Just how aluminium antacids reduce the absorption of diflunisal is not clear, but adsorption or formation of insoluble salts has been suggested. Food appears to reduce this effect.[3] By raising the pH, magnesium hydroxide may promote the dissolution of diflunisal, so increasing its absorption.[3] Consider also 'NSAIDs; Fenamates + Antacids', below.

Importance and management

Aluminium-containing antacids appear to reduce the absorption of diflunisal in the fasted state, but not if taken with food. Since NSAIDs should be taken with or after food, it appears that this interaction has little clinical relevance. See also 'NSAIDs; Miscellaneous + Antacids', p.99. Magnesium hydroxide increases the absorption of diflunisal in the fasted state, which may improve the onset of analgesia. However, note that magnesium hydroxide increased the endoscopically-detected gastric toxicity of ibuprofen in one study, see 'NSAIDs; Ibuprofen and related drugs + Antacids', p.98.

1. Verbeeck R, Tjandramaga TB, Mullie A, Verbesselt R, De Schepper PJ. Effect of aluminium hydroxide on diflunisal absorption. *Br J Clin Pharmacol* (1979) 7, 519–22.
2. Holmes GI, Irvin JD, Schrogie JJ, Davies RO, Breault GO, Rogers JL, Huber PB, Zinny MA. Effects of Maalox on the bioavailability of diflunisal. *Clin Pharmacol Ther* (1979) 25, 229.
3. Tobert JA, DeSchepper P, Tjandramaga TB, Mullie A, Buntinx AP, Meisinger MAP, Huber PB, Hall TLP, Yeh KC. Effect of antacids on the bioavailability of diflunisal in the fasting and postprandial states. *Clin Pharmacol Ther* (1981) 30, 385–9.

NSAIDs; Etoricoxib + Miscellaneous

The makers of etoricoxib recommend care when using etoricoxib with drugs that are metabolised by human sulfotransferases (they name oral salbutamol and minoxidil). This is because etoricoxib is an inhibitor of human sulfotransferase activity, and may increase the levels of these drugs. The increase in ethinylestradiol levels with etoricoxib is thought to be via this mechanism.[1] See 'Oral contraceptives + Etoricoxib or Rofecoxib', p.759.

1. Arcoxia (Etoricoxib). Merck Sharp & Dohme Ltd. UK Summary of product characteristics, May 2005.

NSAIDs; Fenamates + Antacids

The absorption of mefenamic acid and tolfenamic acid is markedly accelerated by magnesium hydroxide in the fasted state. The absorption of tolfenamic acid is retarded by aluminium hydroxide alone or combined with magnesium hydroxide/magnesium carbonate, but is not affected by sodium bicarbonate.

Clinical evidence

Studies in 6 healthy fasted subjects given a single 500-mg dose of **mefenamic acid** or 400 mg **tolfenamic acid** showed that **magnesium hydroxide** accelerated the absorption of both drugs (the **mefenamic acid** AUC after 1 hour was increased threefold and the **tolfenamic acid** AUC sevenfold) but the total bioavailability was only slightly increased. In contrast, **aluminium hydroxide,** alone and in combination with **magnesium hydroxide/magnesium carbonate** (*Medisan Forte*), markedly retarded the rate of absorption of **tolfenamic acid** without causing a marked change in the total amount absorbed. **Sodium bicarbonate** 1 g did not significantly alter the absorption of **tolfenamic acid.**[1]

Mechanism

Uncertain. It is suggested that magnesium hydroxide increases the solubility of acidic drugs such as the fenamates, possibly by forming a soluble salt and therefore enhancing their dissolution. In contrast, aluminium antacids may form insoluble salts of the drug. Note that food may reduce these effects, see 'NSAIDs; Diflunisal + Antacids', above.

Importance and management

Information is very limited but it would appear that if rapid analgesia is needed with either mefenamic acid or tolfenamic acid, magnesium hydroxide can be given concurrently but aluminium hydroxide should be avoided. However, note that this applies to the fasted state, whereas NSAIDs are usually taken with or after food. Also note that magnesium hydroxide increased the endoscopically-detected gastric toxicity of ibuprofen in one study, see 'NSAIDs; Ibuprofen and related drugs + Antacids', p.98. Aluminium hydroxide markedly retards the speed of absorption. Sodium bicarbonate does not interact. Consider also 'NSAIDs; Miscellaneous + Antacids', p.99.

1. Neuvonen PJ, Kivistö KT. Effect of magnesium hydroxide on the absorption of tolfenamic and mefenamic acids. *Eur J Clin Pharmacol* (1988) 35, 495–501.

NSAIDs; Ibuprofen and related drugs + Antacids

Magnesium hydroxide increased the initial absorption of ibuprofen and flurbiprofen, but had no effect on ketoprofen. Unexpectedly, a pharmacodynamic study showed increased gastric erosions when ibuprofen was formulated with magnesium hydroxide.

A small reduction in ketoprofen absorption occurred with aluminium-magnesium hydroxide, but dexketoprofen, ibuprofen and flurbiprofen were not affected, and naproxen showed a slight increase in rate and extent of absorption. Aluminium phosphate had no effect on ketoprofen absorption.

Sodium bicarbonate increased the rate of naproxen absorption, and aluminium hydroxide and magnesium oxide decreased it. Dimeticone did not affect ketoprofen.

Clinical evidence

(a) Dexketoprofen

An **aluminium/magnesium hydroxide** antacid (*Maalox*) had no effect on the rate or extent of absorption of a single 25-mg dose of dexketoprofen in 24 healthy subjects, although the maximum level was slightly (13%) lower.[1]

(b) Flurbiprofen

Maalox (**aluminium/magnesium hydroxide**) 30 ml, taken 30 minutes before a single 100-mg dose of flurbiprofen, was found to affect neither the rate nor extent of flurbiprofen absorption in a group of young and old fasting healthy subjects. Similarly, the antacid had no effect on steady-state flurbiprofen pharmacokinetics when both drugs were given 90 minutes before food.[2] Another study found that **magnesium hydroxide** increased the 0 to 2-hour AUC by 61%, but the 0 to 8-hour AUC was not changed in fasted subjects, which demonstrated an increased rate of flurbiprofen absorption.[3]

(c) Ibuprofen

An antacid containing **aluminium/magnesium hydroxide**, given before, with and after a single 400-mg dose of ibuprofen, did not alter the pharmacokinetics of ibuprofen in 8 healthy fasted subjects.[4] In another study, the absorption of ibuprofen formulated with **aluminium** was delayed and reduced compared to that of ibuprofen without **aluminium**.[5] Another study in 6 healthy fasted subjects found that 850 mg of **magnesium hydroxide** increased the 0 to 1-hour AUC and the peak concentration of a single 400-mg dose of ibuprofen by 65% and 31% respectively. The time to the peak was shortened by about 30 minutes and the total bioavailability was unchanged.[6] In a pharmacodynamic study in healthy subjects, a 400-mg ibuprofen tablet buffered with 200 mg of **magnesium hydroxide**, given at a dose of two tablets three times daily for 5 days resulted in about a threefold increase in number of endoscopically-detected gastric erosions when compared with the same dose of conventional ibuprofen tablets.[7]

(d) Ketoprofen

Five healthy fasted subjects had a 22% reduction in the absorption of a 50-mg dose of ketoprofen (as measured by the amount excreted in the urine) when they were given a 1-g dose of **aluminium hydroxide**.[8] Conversely, **aluminium phosphate** 11 g (as a single then a daily dose) had no effect on the pharmacokinetics of ketoprofen 100 mg in 10 patients.[9] Another study in 12 healthy fasted subjects showed that **dimeticone** did not significantly affect the bioavailability of a single 100-mg dose of ketoprofen.[10] In another study 10 ml of **magnesium hydroxide** suspension (equivalent to 850 mg) was found to have no significant effect on the rate or extent of absorption of ketoprofen 50 mg in fasted subjects, although the rate of ketoprofen absorption was already noted to be fast.[6]

(e) Naproxen

Sodium bicarbonate 700 or 1400 mg increased the rate of absorption of single 300-mg doses of naproxen in 14 healthy fasted subjects, whereas **magnesium oxide** or **aluminium hydroxide** 700 mg had the opposite effect, and reduced the rate of absorption. **Magnesium carbonate** had little effect.[11] On the other hand when 15 or 60 ml of **aluminium/magnesium hydroxide** (*Maalox*) was given, the rate and extent of absorption were slightly increased.[11]

Mechanism

Magnesium hydroxide appears to improve the rate of absorption of some acidic NSAIDs (which become more soluble as the pH rises) such ibuprofen and flurbiprofen. Why this increased the gastric toxicity of ibuprofen in the one pharmacodynamic study is unclear.[7] Sodium bicarbonate appears to have a similar effect on rate of absorption. Aluminium antacids do not produce soluble salts with these NSAIDs, and may therefore reduce the rate/extent of absorption. Food may reduce the effects of antacids on NSAIDs.

Importance and management

It would appear that the initial absorption of both ibuprofen and flurbiprofen is increased by magnesium hydroxide, but not if aluminium hydroxide is present as well. Thus if rapid analgesia is needed, an antacid containing magnesium hydroxide but without aluminium hydroxide could be used with these NSAIDs. However, the unexpected finding that magnesium hydroxide increased the endoscopically-detected gastric toxicity of ibuprofen[7] suggests that caution may be warranted, particularly on long-term use. Further study is needed.

Sodium bicarbonate and aluminium hydroxide appear to have a similar effect on naproxen, namely an increased and decreased effect on rate of absorption. However, note that these effects were seen in the fasted state, and may not apply when the NSAIDs are taken with or after food (as is usual). This is also the case with 'diflunisal', (p.97).

No particular precautions would seem to be needed if dimeticone, aluminium phosphate or magnesium hydroxide are given with ketoprofen, and it seems doubtful if the effects of ketoprofen will be reduced to any great extent by aluminium hydroxide.

1. McEwen J, De Luca M, Casini A, Gich I, Barbanoj MJ, Tost D, Artigas R, Mauleón D. The effect of food and an antacid on the bioavailability of dexketoprofen trometamol. *J Clin Pharmacol* (1998) 38 (Suppl), 41S–45S.
2. Caillé G, du Souich P, Vézina M, Pollock SR, Stalker DJ. Pharmacokinetic interaction between flurbiprofen and antacids in healthy volunteers. *Biopharm Drug Dispos* (1989) 10, 607–15.
3. Rao TRK, Ravisekhar K, Shobha JC, Sekhar EC, Naidu MUR, Krishna DR. Influence of magnesium hydroxide on the oral absorption of flurbiprofen. *Drug Invest* (1992) 4, 473–6.
4. Gontarz N, Small RE, Comstock TJ, Stalker DJ, Johnson SM, Willis HE. Effect of antacid suspension on the pharmacokinetics of ibuprofen. *Clin Pharm* (1987) 6, 413–16.
5. Laska EM, Sunshine A, Marrero I, Olson N, Siegel C, McCormick N. The correlation between blood levels of ibuprofen and clinical analgesic response. *Clin Pharmacol Ther* (1986) 40, 1–7.
6. Neuvonen PJ. The effect of magnesium hydroxide on the oral absorption of ibuprofen, ketoprofen and diclofenac. *Br J Clin Pharmacol* (1991) 31, 263–6.
7. Mäenpää J, Tarpila A, Jouhikainen T, Ikävalko H, Löyttyniemi E, Perttunen K, Neuvonen PJ, Tarpila S. Magnesium hydroxide in ibuprofen tablet reduces the gastric tolerability of ibuprofen. *J Clin Gastroenterol* (2004) 38, 41–5.
8. Ismail FA, Khalafallah N, Khalil SA. Adsorption of ketoprofen and bumadizone calcium on aluminium-containing antacids and its effect on ketoprofen bioavailability in man. *Int J Pharmaceutics* (1987) 34, 189–96.
9. Brazier JL, Tamisier JN, Ambert D, Bannier A. Bioavailability of ketoprofen in man with and without concomitant administration of aluminium phosphate. *Eur J Clin Pharmacol* (1981) 19, 305–7.
10. Presle N, Lapicque F, Gillet P, Herrmann M-A, Bannwarth B, Netter P. Effect of dimethicone (polysilane gel) on the stereoselective pharmacokinetics of ketoprofen. *Eur J Clin Pharmacol* (1998) 54, 351–4.
11. Segre EJ, Sevelius H, Varady J. Effects of antacids on naproxen absorption. *N Engl J Med* (1974) 291, 582–3.

NSAIDs; Indometacin or Sulindac + Antacids

Aluminium hydroxide with magnesium carbonate or magnesium hydroxide caused a small reduction in the extent of indometacin absorption. Aluminium hydroxide alone reduced the rate of indometacin absorption, and sodium bicarbonate tended to increase it. Aluminium/magnesium hydroxide had no effect. These changes are probably not clinically important. Aluminium/magnesium hydroxide had no effect on sulindac absorption.

Clinical evidence

The AUC of a single 50-mg dose of indometacin was reduced by 35% in 12 healthy fasted subjects when formulated with 80% *Mergel* (an antacid formulation of **aluminium/magnesium hydroxide**, and **magnesium carbonate**) and by 18% when taken with 90% *Mergel*.[1]

In another single-dose study in 6 healthy fasted subjects, **aluminium hy-**

droxide suspension 700 mg reduced the rate of indometacin absorption, and reduced the peak indometacin plasma levels. Conversely, **sodium bicarbonate** 1.4 g increased the rate of absorption (this did not reach significance because of wide inter-individual variation).[2] In a further study 30 ml of **aluminium/magnesium hydroxide** caused only slight changes in the absorption of a 50-mg dose of indometacin in fasted subjects.[3]

The makers of sulindac note that an antacid (**aluminium/magnesium hydroxide** suspension) had no effect on the absorption of sulindac.[4]

Mechanism

Not known. Aluminium compounds might form insoluble salts with indometacin.[2] Food might reduce this effect, see 'NSAIDs; Diflunisal + Antacids', p.97.

Importance and management

Adequately but not extensively documented. Some small reduction in plasma indometacin levels is possible with some aluminium containing antacids. Despite this the makers of indometacin recommend that it be taken with food, milk or an antacid to minimise gastrointestinal disturbances. Sulindac absorption is not affected.

1. Galeazzi RL. The effect of an antacid on the bioavailability of indomethacin. *Eur J Clin Pharmacol* (1977) 12, 65–8.
2. Garnham JC, Kaspi T, Kaye CM and Oh VMS. The different effects of sodium bicarbonate and aluminium hydroxide on the absorption of indomethacin in man. *Postgrad Med J* (1977) 53, 126–9.
3. Emori HW, Paulus H, Bluestone R, Champion GD, Pearson C. Indomethacin serum concentrations in man. Effects of dosage, food and antacid. *Ann Rheum Dis* (1976) 35, 333–8.
4. Clinoril (Sulindac). Merck Sharp & Dohme Ltd. UK Summary of product characteristics, November 2003.

NSAIDs; Indometacin + Cocaine

An isolated report describes marked oedema, anuria and haematemesis in a premature child attributed to an interaction between the cocaine and indometacin taken by the mother before the birth.

Clinical evidence, mechanism, importance and management

A woman who was a cocaine abuser and who was in premature labour was unsuccessfully treated with terbutaline and magnesium sulfate. Indometacin proved to be more effective, but after being given 400 mg over 2 days she gave birth to a boy estimated at 34 to 35 weeks. Before birth the child was noted to be anuric and at birth showed marked oedema, and later haematemesis. The suggested reasons are that the anuria and oedema were due to renal vascular constriction of the foetus caused by the cocaine combined with some interference by the indometacin with ADH-mediated water reabsorption. Both drugs can cause gastrointestinal bleeding, which would account for the haematemesis. The authors of this report point out that one of the adverse effects of cocaine is premature labour, and that the likelihood is high that indometacin may be used to control it. They advise screening likely addicts in premature labour for evidence of cocaine usage before indometacin is given.[1]

1. Carlan SJ, Stromquist C, Angel JL, Harris M, O'Brien WF. Cocaine and indomethacin: fetal anuria, neonatal edema and gastrointestinal bleeding. *Obstet Gynecol* (1991) 78, 501–3.

NSAIDs; Indometacin + Vaccines

Some very limited evidence suggests that the response to immunisation with live vaccines may be more severe than usual in the presence of indometacin.

Clinical evidence, mechanism, importance and management

A man with ankylosing spondylitis on indometacin 25 mg three times daily had a strong primary-type reaction 12 days after **smallpox vaccination**. He experienced 3 days of severe malaise, headache and nausea, as well as enlarged lymph nodes. The scab that formed was unusually large (3 cm in diameter) but he suffered no long term ill-effects.[1] The suggestion was that indometacin alters the response of the body to viral infections, whether originating from vaccines or not.[1] For example, a child taking indometacin developed haemorrhagic chickenpox during a ward outbreak of the disease.[2] These appear to be isolated reports, and of little general importance. Note that NSAIDs such as indometacin may mask the signs and symptoms of infection.

1. Maddocks AC. Indomethacin and vaccination. *Lancet* (1973) ii, 210–11.
2. Rodriguez RS, Barbabosa E. Hemorrhagic chickenpox after indomethacin. *N Engl J Med* (1971) 285, 690.

NSAIDs; Ketorolac + Pentoxifylline

Pentoxifylline may increase the risk of bleeding with ketorolac, and the combination should be avoided.

Clinical evidence, mechanism, importance and management

A review of bleeding events associated with the use of postoperative ketorolac revealed that a small number of patients were also taking pentoxifylline.[1] The makers therefore recommend that this drug combination should be avoided.[2]

1. Syntex Pharmaceuticals Limited. Personal communication, January 1995.
2. Toradol (Ketorolac trometamol). Roche Products Ltd. UK Summary of product characteristics, October 2002.

NSAIDs; Ketorolac + Vancomycin

An isolated report describes temporary acute renal failure and gastrointestinal bleeding following the use of ketorolac and vancomycin.

Clinical evidence, mechanism, importance and management

A previously healthy middle-aged man developed complete kidney shut down and subsequent gastrointestinal bleeding following uncomplicated surgery when treated with ketorolac trometamol and vancomycin. The reason for the temporary kidney failure is not known, but the authors of the report suggest that the ketorolac inhibited the normal production of the vasodilatory renal prostaglandins so that renal blood flow was reduced. This would seem to have been additive with nephrotoxic effects of the vancomycin.[1] Ketorolac alone can cause dose-related and transient renal dysfunction.[1] It has also been suggested that the trometamol component may be associated with hyperkalaemia.[2] The gastrointestinal bleeding appeared to be due to the direct irritant effects of the ketorolac, possibly made worse by the previous use of piroxicam[1] (see also 'NSAIDs + NSAIDs', p.90). The general importance of this interaction is uncertain, but it may be prudent to monitor renal function during concurrent use.

1. Murray RP, Watson RC. Acute renal failure and gastrointestinal bleed associated with postoperative Toradol and vancomycin. *Orthopedics* (1993) 16, 1361–3.
2. Waters JH. Ketorolac-induced hyperkalaemia. *Am J Kidney Dis* (1995) 26, 266.

NSAIDs; Miscellaneous + Antacids

The rate and extent of absorption of ketorolac, metamizole and tolmetin was not significantly affected by aluminium/magnesium hydroxide. Nabumetone absorption was not affected by aluminium hydroxide, and an unspecified antacid did not affect etodolac absorption.

Clinical evidence

(a) Etodolac

A study in 18 healthy fasted subjects found that when given a single 400-mg dose of etodolac with 30 ml of an unnamed antacid neither the rate nor the extent of etodolac absorption were altered.[1]

(b) Ketorolac

The AUC of oral ketorolac 10 mg was found to be reduced by 11% (not statistically significant) when taken with an unstated amount of **aluminium/magnesium hydroxide** suspension (*Maalox*) in 12 healthy fasted subjects. The rate of absorption was not affected.[2]

(c) Metamizole sodium (Dipyrone)

The concurrent use of 20 ml of *Maaloxan* (**aluminium/magnesium hydroxide** gel) was reported to have had no effect on the pharmacokinetics of the metabolites of metamizole sodium (dipyrone).[3]

(d) Nabumetone

The absorption of a single 1-g dose of nabumetone (as assessed by AUC and maximum plasma level) was not significantly altered by 160 ml of **aluminium hydroxide** suspension (*Aludrox*) in 15 healthy fasted subjects.[4]

(e) Tolmetin

A pharmacokinetic study in 24 healthy fasted subjects showed that **aluminium/magnesium hydroxide** suspension (*Maalox*), given as a single 20-ml dose four times daily for 3 days, had no significant effect on the absorption of a single 400-mg dose of **tolmetin**.[5]

Mechanism

None.

Importance and management

Although information is limited, no particular precautions would seem to be needed if aluminium or aluminium/magnesium antacids are given with any of these antacids. Note that antacids have been frequently given with NSAIDs to reduce their gastric irritant effects. Consider also 'coxibs', (p.96), 'diclofenac', (p.96), 'diflunisal', (p.97), 'ibuprofen and related drugs', (p.98), 'indometacin', (p.98), 'fenamates', (p.97), and 'oxicams', (below) for information about the interaction of other NSAIDs with antacids.

1. Troy S, Sanda M, Dressler D, Chiang S, Latts J. The effect of food and antacid on etodolac bioavailability. *Clin Pharmacol Ther* (1990) 47, 192.
2. Mroszczak EJ, Jung D, Yee J, Bynum L, Sevelius H, Massey I. Ketorolac tromethamine pharmacokinetics and metabolism after intravenous, intramuscular, and oral administration in humans and animals. *Pharmacotherapy* (1990) 10 (Suppl 6), 33S–39S.
3. Scholz W, Rosenkrantz B. Clinical pharmacokinetics of dipyrone and its metabolites. *Clin Pharmacokinet* (1995) 28, 216–34.
4. von Schrader HW, Buscher G, Dierdorf D, Mügge H, Wolf D. Nabumetone — a novel anti-inflammatory drug: the influence of food, milk, antacids, and analgesics on bioavailability of single oral doses. *Int J Clin Pharmacol Ther Toxicol* (1983) 21, 311–21.
5. Ayres JW, Weidler DJ, MacKichan J, Sakmar E, Hallmark MR, Lemanowicz EF, Wagner JG. Pharmacokinetics of tolmetin with and without concomitant administration of antacid in man. *Eur J Clin Pharmacol* (1977) 12, 421–8.

NSAIDs; Naproxen + Amoxicillin

An isolated report describes acute interstitial nephritis with nephrotic syndrome associated with the use of naproxen and amoxicillin.

Clinical evidence, mechanism, importance and management

A man without any previous renal problems developed acute interstitial nephritis with nephrotic syndrome after taking naproxen for 4 days (total 4 g) and amoxicillin for 10 days (total 24 g). He appeared to recover when the drugs were stopped, but 3 months later he developed renal failure and needed haemodialysis.[1] This is not only a rare syndrome (reported to be only 55 cases in the world literature in 1988)[1] but this is the first case involving both of these drugs. No special precautions would normally seem to be necessary.

1. Nortier J, Depierreux M, Bourgeois V, Dupont P. Acute interstitial nephritis with nephrotic syndrome after intake of naproxen and amoxycillin. *Nephrol Dial Transplant* (1990) 5, 1055.

NSAIDs; Naproxen + Sulglicotide

Sulglicotide does not affect the absorption of naproxen.

Clinical evidence, mechanism, importance and management

Sulglicotide 200 mg had no significant effects on the pharmacokinetics of single 500-mg doses of naproxen in 12 healthy subjects.[1] Sulglycotide may therefore be used to protect the gastric mucosa from possible injury by naproxen without altering its absorption.

1. Berté F, Feletti F, De Bernardi di Valserra M, Nazzari M, Cenedese A, Cornelli U. Lack of influence of sulglycotide on naproxen bioavailability in healthy volunteers. *Int J Clin Pharmacol Ther Toxicol* (1988) 26, 125–8.

NSAIDs; Oxicams + Antacids

The pharmacokinetics of the oxicams were not affected by aluminium/magnesium hydroxide antacids. Similarly, aluminium hydroxide alone had no effect on piroxicam or tenoxicam. Lornoxicam pharmacokinetics were not altered by tripotassium dicitratobismuthate or aluminium hydroxide with calcium carbonate.

Clinical evidence, mechanism, importance and management

(a) Lornoxicam

Neither 10 ml of *Maalox* (**aluminium/magnesium hydroxide**) nor 10 g of *Solugastril* (**aluminium hydroxide** with **calcium carbonate**) had any effect on the pharmacokinetics of a 4-mg lornoxicam film-coated tablet in 18 healthy fasted subjects.[1] A later study similarly found no changes in the absorption or pharmacokinetics of a lornoxicam film-coated tablet given with **bismuth chelate** (**tripotassium dicitratobismuthate**) 120 mg twice daily.[2] There would seem to be no reason for avoiding concurrent use.

(b) Meloxicam

In an open, randomised, crossover study 9 healthy fasted subjects were given meloxicam 30 mg alone or with *Maalox* suspension (**aluminium/magnesium hydroxide** 900/600 mg) four times daily for 4 days. *Maalox* had no significant effect on the pharmacokinetics of the meloxicam.[3] Therefore no adjustments of the dosage of meloxicam are needed if given with this type of antacid.

(c) Piroxicam

A multiple-dose study in 20 healthy subjects found that *Mylanta* (**aluminium/magnesium hydroxide**) and *Amphojel* (**aluminium hydroxide**) did not significantly affect the bioavailability of piroxicam 20 mg daily taken after food.[4] Concurrent use need not be avoided.

(d) Tenoxicam

The bioavailability of tenoxicam 20 mg was found to be unaffected in 12 healthy subjects by **aluminium hydroxide** (*Amphojel*) or **aluminium/magnesium hydroxide** (*Mylanta*) whether taken before, at the same time, or after the tenoxicam, and in the fasted state or with food.[5] No special precautions seem necessary.

1. Dittrich P, Radhofer-Welte S, Magometschnigg D, Kukovetz WR, Mayerhofer S, Ferber HP. The effect of concomitantly administered antacids on the bioavailability of lornoxicam, a novel highly potent NSAID. *Drugs Exp Clin Res* (1990) 16, 57–62.
2. Ravic M, Johnston A, Turner P, Foley K, Rosenow D. Does bismuth chelate influence lornoxicam absorption? *Hum Exp Toxicol* (1992) 11, 59–60.
3. Busch U, Heinzel G, Narjes H, Nehmiz G. Interaction of meloxicam with cimetidine, Maalox or aspirin. *J Clin Pharmacol* (1996) 36, 79–84.
4. Hobbs DC, Twomey TM. Piroxicam pharmacokinetics in man: aspirin and antacid interaction studies. *J Clin Pharmacol* (1979) 19, 270–81.
5. Day RO, Lam S, Paull P, Wade D. Effect of food and various antacids on the absorption of tenoxicam. *Br J Clin Pharmacol* (1987) 24, 323–8.

NSAIDs; Oxyphenbutazone or Phenylbutazone + Anabolic steroids

Serum oxyphenbutazone levels are raised about 40% by the use of methandienone (methandrostenolone). Phenylbutazone appears to be unaffected.

Clinical evidence

The serum levels of oxyphenbutazone 300 to 400 mg daily for 2 to 5 weeks were raised by 43% (range 5 to 100%) in 6 subjects given **methandienone**. Neither prednisone 5 mg nor dexamethasone 1.5 mg daily were found to affect oxyphenbutazone levels.[1]

Two other studies confirm this interaction with oxyphenbutazone.[2,3] One of them found no interaction with phenylbutazone.[2]

Mechanism

Uncertain. One idea is that the anabolic steroids alter the distribution of oxyphenbutazone between the tissues and plasma so that more remains in circulation. There may also possibly be some changes in metabolism.

Importance and management

The interaction is established but its importance is uncertain. There seem to be no reports of toxicity arising from concurrent use but the possibility should be borne in mind.

1. Weiner M, Siddiqui AA, Shahani RT, Dayton PG. Effect of steroids on disposition of oxyphenbutazone in man. *Proc Soc Exp Biol Med* (1967) 124, 1170–3.
2. Hvidberg E, Dayton PG, Read JM, Wilson CH. Studies of the interaction of phenylbutazone, oxyphenbutazone and methandrostenolone in man. *Proc Soc Exp Biol Med* (1968) 129, 438–43.
3. Weiner M, Siddiqui AA, Bostanci N, Dayton PG. Drug interactions.The effect of combined administration on the half-life of coumarin and pyrazolone drugs in man. *Fedn Proc* (1965) 24, 153.

NSAIDs; Parecoxib or Valdecoxib + Miscellaneous

Both parecoxib and valdecoxib are available as commercial preparations, but as parecoxib is rapidly metabolised to valdecoxib, the interactions of both drugs are discussed together, usually by considering the effects of valdecoxib. Phenytoin modestly decreased valdecoxib levels, but this is not thought to be clinically relevant. However, because of this interaction the makers do caution the concurrent use with carbamazepine, dexamethasone and, particularly, rifampicin. Valdecoxib increases the levels of dextromethorphan and omeprazole. Because of these interactions, caution is advised with drugs that are metabolised by the same isoenzymes, namely flecainide, metoprolol, propafenone, omeprazole, diazepam, imipramine and phenytoin. No interaction appears to occur between parecoxib or valdecoxib and alfentanil, fentanyl or midazolam.

Clinical evidence, mechanism, importance and management

Parecoxib is a parenteral drug that is rapidly metabolised in the liver to the active COX-2 inhibitor valdecoxib. Valdecoxib is available as an oral preparation, and is predominantly metabolised by the cytochrome P450 isoenzymes CYP3A4 and CYP2C9. The interactions of both drugs are discussed together, usually by considering the effects of valdecoxib.

(a) Cytochrome P450 isoenzyme CYP3A4 inducers

The makers say that after giving **phenytoin** 300 mg daily and valdecoxib 40 mg twice daily for 12 days the AUC of valdecoxib was decreased by 27%[1,2] but this was not considered to be clinically significant.[1] The possible effects of other enzyme inducers on parecoxib and valdecoxib have not been studied, but the makers suggest that the metabolism of valdecoxib may possibly be increased by drugs such as **carbamazepine** and **dexamethasone**, and they particularly advise caution with **rifampicin**, which is known to be a potent inducer of CYP3A4, and which may therefore have more effect than **phenytoin**.[1] This might potentially result in a reduction in the effects of parecoxib, but there is, as yet, no evidence to confirm that this is clinically important. For the theoretical possibility that valdecoxib may increase **phenytoin** levels, see below.

(b) Miscellaneous interactions via the cytochrome P450 isoenzyme system

The makers have done several interaction studies to find out whether parecoxib or valdecoxib can inhibit or induce the cytochrome P450 isoenzymes CYP2C9, CYP2D6, CYP2C19, and CYP3A4 and thereby determine their potential to interact with drugs metabolised by these isoenzymes.

(i) CYP2C19. The makers say that the AUC of a single 40-mg dose of **omeprazole** was increased by 46% by valdecoxib 40 mg twice daily for a week (see also 'NSAIDs or Aspirin + Proton pump inhibitors', p.94). This indicates that valdecoxib is an inhibitor of CYP2C19 and although the makers consider it to be a weak inhibitor[3] they suggest that caution should be observed with drugs that have a narrow therapeutic margin and are known to be metabolised by CYP2C19. They list **diazepam**, **imipramine** and **phenytoin**.[1,4] The implication is that the serum levels of these drugs and their effects may possibly be increased. However, studies listed by the US maker found that the plasma exposure of **diazepam** is increased by 28% and the pharmacokinetics of **phenytoin** were not significantly altered by valdecoxib.[2] For the minor effect of **phenytoin** on valdecoxib see (a) above.

(ii) CYP2D6. The makers say that treatment with 40 mg of valdecoxib twice daily for a week caused a threefold increase in the serum levels of **dextromethorphan**. This indicates that valdecoxib is an inhibitor of CYP2D6, and although the makers consider it to be a weak inhibitor[2,3] they suggest that caution should be observed with drugs that have a narrow therapeutic margin and are known to be predominantly metabolised by CYP2D6. They list **flecainide**, **metoprolol** and **propafenone**.[1,4] The implication is that the serum levels of these drugs and their effects may possibly be increased, but so far there appears to be no direct clinical reports of any problems with concurrent use.

(iii) CYP3A4. A study in 12 healthy adults found no significant changes in the pharmacokinetics of **midazolam** 70 micrograms/kg given an hour after receiving 40 mg of intravenous parecoxib. Valdecoxib also had no effect on the metabolism of oral **midazolam**.[1,5] This suggests that parecoxib and valdecoxib are unlikely to inhibit or induce the activity of CYP3A4. This means that parecoxib should not have metabolic interactions with other drugs that are metabolised by CYP3A4.[3]

1. Bextra (Valdecoxib). Pharmacia Ltd. UK Summary of product characteristics, May 2004.
2. Bextra (Valdecoxib). Pfizer Inc. US Prescribing information, November 2004.
3. Pharmacia Ltd. Personal communication, May 2002.
4. Dynastat injection (Parecoxib sodium). Pharmacia Ltd. UK Summary of product characteristics, April 2004.
5. Ibrahim AE, Karim A, Feldman J, Kharasch ED. Effects of parecoxib, a parenteral COX-2 specific inhibitor, on the disposition of midazolam. American Society of Anesthesiologists. 51st Annual Meeting San Francisco, California, 14–18 October 2000.

NSAIDs; Phenazone (Antipyrine) + Miscellaneous

Changes in the half-life of phenazone (reduced by liver enzyme-inducers, prolonged by liver enzyme-inhibitors) are used to detect the possible effects of drugs on liver enzyme activity.

Clinical evidence, mechanism, importance and management

Phenazone is metabolised by mixed function oxidase enzymes in the liver, for which reason it is extensively used as a model drug for studying whether other drugs induce or inhibit liver enzymes. For example, **barbiturates** reduce the half-life of phenazone. In one study **phenobarbital** caused about a 40% reduction thereby demonstrating that the liver enzymes were being stimulated to metabolise the phenazone more rapidly.[1] In contrast, other drugs that are enzyme inhibitors cause the half-life of phenazone to be prolonged, which shows that the activity of the metabolising enzymes is reduced (e.g. **ticlopidine**, see 'Ticlopidine + Miscellaneous', p.525). Thus phenazone often features in drug interaction studies because it provides predictive information about whether a particular drug is likely or not to stimulate or inhibit the metabolism of other drugs. Phenazone itself is now little used for its analgesic and antipyretic effects.

1. Vesell ES, Page JG. Genetic control of the phenobarbital-induced shortening of plasma antipyrine half-lives in man. *J Clin Invest* (1969) 48, 2202–9.

NSAIDs; Phenylbutazone + Methylphenidate

Methylphenidate significantly increased [amount not stated] the serum levels of phenylbutazone 200 to 400 mg daily in 5 out of 6 patients, due, it is suggested, to inhibition of liver metabolising enzymes.[1] The clinical importance of this is uncertain.

1. Sellers EM ed. Clinical Pharmacology of Psychoactive Drugs. Ontario: Addiction Research Foundation, 1973. p183–202.

NSAIDs; Phenylbutazone + Pesticides

Chronic exposure to lindane and other chlorinated pesticides can slightly increase the rate of metabolism of phenylbutazone.

Clinical evidence, mechanism, importance and management

The plasma half-life of phenylbutazone in a group of men who regularly used **chlorinated insecticide** sprays (mainly **lindane**) as part of their work, was found to be 20% shorter (51 hours) than in a control group (64 hours), due, it is believed, to the enzyme-inducing effects of the **pes-**

ticides.[1] This modest increase in rate of metabolism is of doubtful direct clinical importance, but it illustrates the changed metabolism that can occur in those exposed to environmental chemical agents.

1. Kolmodin-Hedman B. Decreased plasma half-life of phenylbutazone in workers exposed to chlorinated pesticides. *Eur J Clin Pharmacol* (1973) 5, 195–8.

NSAIDs; Phenylbutazone or Oxyphenbutazone + Tricyclic antidepressants

The tricyclic antidepressants can delay the absorption of phenylbutazone and oxyphenbutazone from the gut, but their antirheumatic effects are probably not affected.

Clinical evidence, mechanism, importance and management

The absorption of a single 400-mg dose of phenylbutazone in 4 depressed women was considerably delayed (time to maximum level, 4 to 10 hours compared with 2 hours), but the total amount absorbed (measured by the urinary excretion of oxyphenbutazone) remained unchanged when they were pretreated with **desipramine** 75 mg daily for 7 days.[1] In another 5 depressed women the half-life of oxyphenbutazone was found to be unaltered by 75 mg of **desipramine** or **nortriptyline** daily.[2] *Animal* studies have confirmed that the absorption of phenylbutazone and oxyphenbutazone are delayed by the tricyclic antidepressants, probably because their anticholinergic effects reduce the motility of the gut,[3,4] but there seems to be no direct clinical evidence that the antirheumatic effects of either drug are reduced by this interaction. No particular precautions appear to be needed.

1. Consolo S, Morselli PL, Zaccala M, Garattini S. Delayed absorption of phenylbutazone caused by desmethylimipramine in humans. *Eur J Pharmacol* (1970) 10, 239–42.
2. Hammer W, Mårtens S, Sjöqvist F. A comparative study of the metabolism of desmethylimipramine, nortriptyline, and oxyphenylbutazone in man. *Clin Pharmacol Ther* (1969) 10, 44–9.
3. Consolo S. An interaction between desipramine and phenylbutazone. *J Pharm Pharmacol* (1968) 20, 574–5.
4. Consolo S, Garattini S. Effect of desipramine on intestinal absorption of phenylbutazone and other drugs. *Eur J Pharmacol* (1969) 6, 322–6.

NSAIDs; Sulindac + Dimethyl sulfoxide (DMSO)

A single case report describes a patient on sulindac who developed a serious peripheral neuropathy when he applied DMSO to his skin.

Clinical evidence, mechanism, importance and management

A man with a long history of degenerative arthritis was treated uneventfully with sulindac 400 mg daily for 6 months until, without his doctor's knowledge, he began regularly to apply a topical preparation containing 90% DMSO to his upper and lower extremities. Soon afterwards he began to experience pain, weakness in all his extremities, and difficulty in standing or walking. He was found to have both segmental demyelination and axonal neuropathy. He made a partial recovery but was unable to walk without an artificial aid.[1] The reason for this reaction is not known, but studies in *rats* have shown that DMSO can inhibit a reductase enzyme by which sulindac is metabolised,[2] and it may be that the high concentrations of unmetabolised sulindac increased the neurotoxic activity of the DMSO. Although there is only this case on record, its seriousness suggests that patients should not use sulindac and DMSO-containing preparations concurrently.

1. Reinstein L, Mahon R, Russo GL. Peripheral neuropathy after concomitant dimethyl sulfoxide use and sulindac therapy. *Arch Phys Med Rehabil* (1982) 63, 581–4.
2. Swanson BN, Mojaverian P, Boppana VK, Dudash M. Dimethylsulfoxide (DMSO) interaction with sulindac (SO). *Pharmacologist* (1981) 23, 196.

Opioids + Benzodiazepines

Diazepam appears not to alter the respiratory depressant effects of pethidine (meperidine). However, a case report describes antagonism of the respiratory depressant effects of diamorphine and phenoperidine by lorazepam and diazepam. Midazolam enhances the sedative and analgesic effects of morphine. However, diazepam has been shown to antagonise the analgesic effect of morphine. Morphine and pethidine delay gastric emptying so that the rate of absorption of diazepam given orally may be reduced. Dextropropoxyphene (propoxyphene) reduced the loss of alprazolam from the body, but had no effect on the pharmacokinetics of diazepam and lorazepam. Use of benzodiazepines may be a risk factor in the sudden death of patients using/abusing opioids. Consider also 'methadone', (p.114) and 'fentanyl', (p.111).

Clinical evidence, mechanism, importance and management

(a) Analgesia

In one study, low-dose **midazolam** (given to achieve levels of 50 nanograms/ml) reduced the dose of **morphine** required for postoperative analgesia in the first 12 hours.[1] However, in another study postoperative pain scores were higher in patients premedicated with oral **diazepam** 10 mg than with placebo.[2] In yet another study, the benzodiazepine antagonist flumazenil enhanced **morphine** analgesia in patients who had been premedicated with **diazepam**.[3] It is suggested that benzodiazepines antagonise the analgesic effect of opioids via their effect on supraspinal GABA receptors. Why this has been shown in some studies, but not others, is unclear. Benzodiazepines and opioids are commonly used in surgical anaesthesia, and the relevance of these findings to clinical practice is uncertain.

(b) Overdose

Sudden deaths in patients who abuse opioids are frequently associated with ingestion of other CNS depressants, particularly **benzodiazepines**. Cases have been reported with **buprenorphine**,[4] **oxycodone**,[5] and **tramadol**[6] with various **benzodiazepines**. For **buprenorphine**, it is considered most likely that excessive CNS depression is solely due to combined pharmacological effects, and not to any pharmacokinetic interaction.[7,8]

(c) Pharmacokinetics

Intramuscular **pethidine** 100 mg and intramuscular **morphine** 10 mg delayed the absorption of oral **diazepam** 10 mg. **Diazepam** levels were found to be lower and peak levels were not reached in the 90-minute study period compared with the peak level at 60 minutes in the control group.[9] The underlying mechanism is that the opiate analgesics delay gastric emptying so that the rate of absorption of the **diazepam** is reduced. The maximal effect of **diazepam** would be expected to be delayed in patients on these opioids.

Another study in healthy subjects showed that **dextropropoxyphene** 65 mg every 6 hours prolonged the **alprazolam** half-life from 11.6 to 18.3 hours, and decreased the clearance from 1.3 to 0.8 ml/minute/kg. The pharmacokinetics of single-doses of **diazepam** and **lorazepam** were not significantly affected.[10] It would seem that **dextropropoxyphene** inhibits the metabolism (hydroxylation) of the **alprazolam** by the liver, thereby reducing its loss from the body, but has little or no effect on the *N*-demethylation or glucuronidation of the other two benzodiazepines. The clinical importance of this is uncertain, but the inference to be drawn is that the CNS depressant effects of **alprazolam** will be increased, over and above the simple additive CNS depressant effects likely when other benzodiazepines and **dextropropoxyphene** are taken together. More study is needed.

(d) Respiratory depression

A 14-year-old boy with staphylococcal pneumonia secondary to influenza developed adult respiratory distress syndrome. It was decided to suppress his voluntary breathing with opiates and use assisted ventilation and he was therefore given **phenoperidine** and **diazepam** for 11 days, and later **diamorphine** with **lorazepam**. Despite receiving **diamorphine** 19.2 mg in 24 hours his respiratory drive was not suppressed. On day 17, despite serum **morphine** and **lorazepam** levels of 320 and 5.3 micrograms/ml respectively, he remained conscious and his pupils were not constricted.[11] Later *animal* studies confirmed that **lorazepam** opposed the respiratory depressant effects of **morphine**.[11]

In contrast, intravenous **diazepam** 0.15 mg/kg did not alter the respiratory depressant effect of intravenous **pethidine** 1.5 mg/kg in a study in healthy subjects[12] or in patients with chronic obstructive pulmonary disease.[13] Moreover, in the setting of overdose (see (b) above), benzodiazepines might increase the respiratory depressant effects of opioids.

(e) Sedation

The sedative effects of **midazolam** and **morphine** were additive in a study in patients given these drugs intravenously prior to surgery.[14]

1. Gilliland HE, Prasad BK, Mirakhur RK, Fee JPH. An investigation of the potential morphine sparing effect of midazolam. *Anaesthesia* (1996) 51, 808–11.
2. Caumo W, Hidalgo MPL, Schmidt AP, Iwamoto CW, Adamatti LC, Bergmann J, Ferreira MBC. Effect of pre-operative anxiolysis on postoperative pain response in patients undergoing total abdominal hysterectomy. *Anaesthesia* (2002) 57, 740–6.
3. Gear RW, Miaskowski C, Heller PH, Paul SM, Gordon NC, Levine JD. Benzodiazepine mediated antagonism of opioid analgesia. *Pain* (1997) 71, 25–9.
4. Reynaud M, Petit G, Potard D, Courty P. Six deaths linked to concomitant use of buprenorphine and benzodiazepines. *Addiction* (1998) 93, 1385–92.
5. Burrows DL, Hagardorn AN, Harlan GC, Wallen EDB, Ferslew KE. A fatal drug interaction between oxycodone and clonazepam. *J Forensic Sci* (2003) 48, 683–6.
6. Clarot F, Goullé JP, Vaz E, Proust B. Fatal overdoses of tramadol: is benzodiazepine a risk factor of lethality? *Forensic Sci Int* (2003) 134, 57–61.
7. Ibrahim RB, Wilson JG, Thorsby ME, Edwards DJ. Effect of buprenorphine on CYP3A activity in rat and human liver microsomes. *Life Sci* (2000) 66, 1293–8.
8. Kilicarslan T, Sellers EM. Lack of interaction of buprenorphine with flunitrazepam metabolism. *Am J Psychiatry* (2000) 157, 1164–6.
9. Gamble JAS, Gaston JH, Nair SG, Dundee JW. Some pharmacological factors influencing the absorption of diazepam following oral administration. *Br J Anaesth* (1976) 48, 1181–5.
10. Abernethy DR, Greenblatt DJ, Morse DS, Shader RI. Interaction of propoxyphene with diazepam, alprazolam and lorazepam. *Br J Clin Pharmacol* (1985) 19, 51–7.
11. McDonald CF, Thomson SA, Scott NC, Scott W, Grant IWB, Crompton GK. Benzodiazepine-opiate antagonism — a problem in intensive-care therapy. *Intensive Care Med* (1986) 12, 39–42.
12. Zsigmond EK, Flynn K, Martinez OA. Diazepam and meperidine on arterial blood gases in healthy volunteers. *J Clin Pharmacol* (1974) 14, 377–81.
13. Zsigmond EK, Shively JG, Flynn K. Diazepam and meperidine on arterial blood gases in patients with chronic obstructive pulmonary disease. *J Clin Pharmacol* (1975) 15, 464–68.
14. Tverskoy M, Fleyshman G, Ezry J, Bradley EL, Kissin I. Midazolam-morphine sedative interaction in patients. *Anesth Analg* (1989) 68, 282–5.

Opioids + Dexamfetamine or Methylphenidate

Dexamfetamine and methylphenidate increase the analgesic effects of morphine and other opioids and reduce their sedative and respiratory depressant effects.

Clinical evidence, mechanism, importance and management

Dexamfetamine increased the analgesic effect of **morphine** and reduced its respiratory depressant effects to some extent in studies during postoperative analgesia[1] and in healthy subjects.[2] Methylphenidate 15 mg daily similarly increased the analgesic effects of various opioids (**morphine**, **hydromorphone**, **levorphanol**, **oxycodone**) and reduced the sedative effects in patients with chronic pain due to advanced cancer.[3] Therefore, the analgesic dose of an opioid may be lower than expected in patients on these drugs.

1. Forrest WH, Brown BW, Brown CR, Defalque R, Gold M, Gordon HE, James KE, Katz J, Mahler DL, Schroff P, Teutsch G. Dextroamphetamine with morphine for the treatment of postoperative pain. *N Engl J Med* (1977) 296, 712–15.
2. Bourke DL, Allen PD, Rosenberg M, Mendes RW, Karabelas AN. Dextroamphetamine with morphine: respiratory effects. *J Clin Pharmacol* (1983) 23, 65–70.
3. Bruera E, Chadwick S, Brenneis C, Hanson J, MacDonald RN. Methylphenidate associated with narcotics for the treatment of cancer pain. *Cancer Treat Rep* (1987) 71, 67–70.

Opioids + H_2-blockers

No clinically significant interaction appears to occur between cimetidine and intranasal butorphanol, morphine, pethidine or tramadol, and between ranitidine and morphine or pethidine. However, isolated reports describe adverse reactions in patients on methadone, morphine or mixed opium alkaloids and cimetidine, or morphine and ranitidine. Consider also 'Opioids; Fentanyl and related drugs + H_2-blockers', p.111.

Clinical evidence

(a) Butorphanol

The pharmacokinetics of intranasal butorphanol 1 mg every 6 hours and oral **cimetidine** 300 mg every 6 hours for 4 days were not significantly altered by concurrent use in 16 healthy subjects, except for a moderate increase in elimination half-life of **cimetidine**.[1]

(b) Methadone

A brief mention is made in the introduction to an *in vitro* study of an elderly patient on methadone 25 mg daily who developed apnoea 2 days after starting **cimetidine** 1200 mg daily.[2] Another elderly patient on methadone 5 mg every 8 hours and subcutaneous morphine 8 mg every 3 hours also developed apnoea (respiratory rate 2 breaths per minute) after receiving intravenous **cimetidine** 300 mg every 6 hours for 6 days. This was controlled with naloxone. The patient had previously shown no ill effects from the administration of morphine during combined **cimetidine** and methadone therapy.[3]

(c) Morphine

(i) Cimetidine. Cimetidine 300 mg four times daily for 4 days given to 7 healthy subjects had no effect on the pharmacokinetics of a single 10-mg dose of intravenous morphine. The extent and duration of the morphine-induced pupillary miosis was also unchanged.[4] In other healthy subjects, cimetidine 600 mg, given 1 hour before a 10-mg dose of intramuscular morphine prolonged the respiratory depression due to morphine, but the extent was small and considered clinically insignificant.[5]

In contrast, an acutely ill patient with grand mal epilepsy, gastrointestinal bleeding and an intertrochanteric fracture who was undergoing haemodialysis three times a week, was being treated with cimetidine 300 mg three times daily. After being given the sixth dose of intramuscular morphine (15 mg every 4 hours) he became apnoeic (three breaths per minute), which was controlled with naloxone. He remained confused and agitated for the next 80 hours with muscular twitching and further periods of apnoea controlled with naloxone. He had received nine 10-mg intramuscular doses of morphine on a previous occasion in the absence of cimetidine without problems. About a month later he experienced the same adverse reactions when given opium alkaloids while still taking cimetidine (see (d) below).[6]

(ii) Ranitidine. A man with terminal cancer on intravenous ranitidine 150 mg every 8 hours became confused, disorientated and agitated when given the ranitidine after an intravenous infusion of morphine 50 mg daily was started. When the ranitidine was stopped his mental state improved but worsened when he was given ranitidine again 8 hours and 16 hours later. He again improved when the ranitidine was stopped.[7]

Similarly, another report describes hallucinations in a patient on ranitidine and sustained-release morphine followed by rectal methadone, but the author discounted the possibility of an interaction.[8]

(d) Opium Alkaloids, Mixed

A patient on **cimetidine** 150 mg twice daily developed apnoea, confusion, and muscle twitching after receiving 7 doses of intramuscular *Pantopon* (hydrochlorides of mixed opium alkaloids) postoperatively. He required 4 doses of naloxone over the next 24 hours.[6]

(e) Pethidine (Meperidine)

Cimetidine 600 mg twice daily for one week reduced the total body clearance of single 70-mg intravenous doses of pethidine in 8 healthy subjects by a modest 22%.[9] In a similar study by the same research group, **ranitidine** 150 mg twice daily had no effect on pethidine pharmacokinetics.[10]

(f) Tramadol

In an unpublished study on file with the makers, **cimetidine** increased the AUC of tramadol by 15% to 27% and decreased the total body clearance by 14% to 22% in healthy subjects.[11] The makers say that these changes are clinically insignificant.[12]

Mechanism

Cimetidine inhibits the activity of the liver enzymes concerned with the *N*-demethylation of methadone[2] and pethidine[9,10] so they could accumulate in the body, thereby exaggerating their respiratory depressant effects. Liver impairment might possibly have contributed towards, or even been largely responsible for the cases with methadone, because both patients were elderly.

In vitro studies have shown that the conjugation of morphine is not affected by cimetidine or ranitidine.[13] The isolated cases of possible interactions remain unexplained.[6,7]

Importance and management

The virtual absence of a generally important interaction between morphine and cimetidine interaction is adequately documented. Concurrent use normally causes only a slight and normally unimportant prolongation of the respiratory depression due to morphine, but it might possibly have some importance in patients with pre-existing breathing disorders. *In vitro* evidence suggests that ranitidine is unlikely to interact with morphine.[6] Information about the interaction between pethidine and cimetidine is very limited, and its clinical importance is uncertain, but probably small given the minor changes in pharmacokinetics. Ranitidine has been shown not to interact.

It also seems doubtful if the interaction between methadone and cimetidine is of any general importance when the two isolated reports cited here are viewed against the background of the wide-spread use of both of these two drugs for a good number of years and the lack of other published adverse reports. There is no clinically important pharmacokinetic interaction between intranasal butorphanol and oral cimetidine, or between tramadol and cimetidine. Consider also 'Opioids; Fentanyl and related drugs + H_2-blockers', p.111.

1. Shyu WC, Barbhaiya RH. Lack of pharmacokinetic interaction between butorphanol nasal spray and cimetidine. *Br J Clin Pharmacol* (1996) 42, 513–17.
2. Dawson GW, Vestal RE. Cimetidine inhibits the *in vitro* N-demethylation of methadone. *Res Commun Chem Pathol Pharmacol* (1984) 46, 301–4.
3. Sorkin EM, Ogawa GS. Cimetidine potentiation of narcotic action. *Drug Intell Clin Pharm* (1983) 17, 60–1.
4. Mojaverian P, Fedder IL, Vlasses PH, Rotmensch HH, Rocci ML, Swanson BN, Ferguson RK. Cimetidine does not alter morphine disposition in man. *Br J Clin Pharmacol* (1982) 14, 809–13.
5. Lam AM, Clement JL. Effect of cimetidine premedication on morphine-induced ventilatory depression. *Can Anaesth Soc J* (1984) 31, 36–43.
6. Fine A, Churchill DN. Potentially lethal interaction of cimetidine and morphine. *Can Med Assoc J* (1981) 124, 1434–6.
7. Martinez-Abad M, Delgado Gomis F, Ferrer JM, Morales-Olivas FJ. Ranitidine-induced confusion with concomitant morphine. *Drug Intell Clin Pharm* (1988) 22, 914–5.
8. Jellema JG. Hallucination during sustained-release morphine and methadone administration. *Lancet* (1987) ii, 392.
9. Guay DRP, Meatherall RC, Chalmers JL, Grahame GR. Cimetidine alters pethidine disposition in man. *Br J Clin Pharmacol* (1984) 18, 907–14.
10. Guay DRP, Meatherall RC, Chalmers JL, Grahame GR, Hudson RJ. Ranitidine does not alter pethidine disposition in man. *Br J Clin Pharmacol* (1985) 20, 55–9.
11. Data on file. Cited in: Raffa RB, Nayak RK, Liao S, Minn FL. The mechanism(s) of action and pharmacokinetics of tramadol hydrochloride. *Rev Contemp Pharmacother* (1995) 6, 485–97.
12. Zydol (Tramadol). Pharmacia Ltd. UK Summary of product characteristics, December 2002.
13. Knodell RG, Holtzman JL, Crankshaw DL, Steele NM, Stanley LN. Drug metabolism by rat and human hepatic microsomes in response to interaction with H_2-receptor antagonists. *Gastroenterology* (1982) 82, 84–8.

Opioids + Ondansetron

Ondansetron reduces the analgesic efficacy of tramadol and at least double the dose was required in one clinical study. This resulted in more vomiting despite the ondansetron. In contrast, in a study in healthy subjects, ondansetron had no effect on the analgesic potency of morphine.

Clinical evidence

(a) Morphine

A double-blind, placebo-controlled study in 12 healthy subjects found that a single 16-mg intravenous dose of ondansetron given 30 minutes after a single 10-mg intravenous dose of morphine did not alter the pharmacokinetics of morphine or its metabolites, morphine-3- and morphine-6-glucuronides. The analgesic effect of morphine (as measured by a contact thermode system) was also unaffected by ondansetron.[1]

(b) Tramadol

Patients who received a single 4-mg dose of ondansetron given one minute before induction of anaesthesia required 26 to 35% more tramadol by patient controlled analgesia from 1 to 4 hours post-operatively than those who received placebo.[2] Similarly, a 1-mg/hour ondansetron infusion increased the dose of post-operative tramadol used during patient controlled analgesia by two- to threefold in 30 patients when compared with placebo in 29 patients. Moreover, in this study the group receiving ondansetron actually experienced more vomiting, probably because they used more tramadol, which caused an emetic effect not well controlled by the ondansetron.[3]

Mechanism

On theoretical grounds ondansetron (a 5-HT_3 receptor antagonist) might be expected to decrease the effects of anti-nociceptive drugs because serotonin (5-HT) is thought to cause anti-nociception via presynaptic 5-HT_3 receptors on primary afferent nociceptive neurones in the spinal dorsal horn. This has been demonstrated for tramadol, which is not a pure opioid and also acts by enhancing the effects of serotonin and noradrenaline (norepinephrine). However, ondansetron had no effect on morphine analgesia in healthy subjects.

Importance and management

The interaction between ondansetron and tramadol appears to be established and of clinical importance. Ondansetron may double the dose requirement of tramadol, and so result in increased emetic effects, consequently ondansetron does not appear to be the best antiemetic to use with tramadol.[1] Although not tested, other 5-HT_3 receptor antagonists would be expected to interact similarly. Ondansetron appears to have no effect on morphine, and can be used with this, and presumably other similar opioids. Consider also 'Opioids; Alfentanil + Ondansetron', p.107.

1. Crews KR, Murthy BP, Hussay EK, Passannante AN, Palmer JL, Maixner W, Brouwer KLR. Lack of effect of ondansetron on the pharmacokinetics and analgesic effects of morphine and metabolites after single-dose morphine administration in healthy volunteers. *Br J Clin Pharmacol* (2001) 51, 309–16.
2. De Witte JL, Schoenmaekers B, Sessler DI, Deloof T. The analgesic efficacy of tramadol is impaired by concurrent administration of ondansetron. *Anesth Analg* (2001) 92, 1319–21.
3. Arcioni R, della Rocca M, Romanò S, Romano R, Pietropaoli P, Gasparetto A. Ondansetron inhibits the analgesic effects of tramadol: a possible 5-HT_3 spinal receptor involvement in acute pain in humans. *Anesth Analg* (2002) 94, 1553–7.

Opioids + Opioids

Opioids with mixed agonist/antagonist properties (e.g. buprenorphine, butorphanol, nalbuphine, pentazocine) may precipitate opioid withdrawal symptoms in patients on pure opioid agonists such as fentanyl, methadone and morphine (see 'Table 5.1', (p.73), for other examples).

Opioids + Oral contraceptives

The clearance of morphine is roughly doubled by combined oral contraceptives. Combined oral contraceptives do not appear to alter the pharmacokinetics of pethidine.

Clinical evidence, mechanism, importance and management

(a) Morphine

The clearance of intravenous morphine 1 mg and oral morphine 10 mg was increased by 75% and 120% respectively in 6 young women taking a combined oral contraceptive.[1] The suggested reason is that the oestrogen component of the contraceptive increases the activity of the liver enzyme (glucuronyl transferase) concerned with the metabolism of morphine. This implies that the dosage of morphine would need to be increased to achieve the same degree of analgesia. Whether this is so in practice requires confirmation.

(b) Pethidine (Meperidine)

One early study suggested that 4 of 5 women taking a combined oral contraceptive (**mestranol** with **noretynodrel** or **norethisterone**) excreted more unchanged pethidine in the urine than a control group of 4 women not taking contraceptives who were found to excrete more of the demethylated metabolite.[2] However a later, well controlled, comparative study in 24 healthy subjects (8 women taking a combined oral contraceptive containing **ethinylestradiol/norgestrel** 50/500 micrograms, and 8 women and 8 men not taking contraceptives) found no differences between the plasma levels or excretion patterns of pethidine between the three groups.[3] No special precautions appear to be needed during concurrent use.

1. Watson KJR, Ghabrial H, Mashford ML, Harman PJ, Breen KJ, Desmond PV. The oral contraceptive pill increases morphine clearance but does not increase hepatic blood flow. *Gastroenterology* (1986) 90, 1779.
2. Crawford JS, Rudofsky S. Some alterations in the pattern of drug metabolism associated with pregnancy, oral contraceptives, and the newly-born. *Br J Anaesth* (1966) 38, 446–54.
3. Stambaugh JE, Wainer IW. Drug interactions I: meperidine and combination oral contraceptives. *J Clin Pharmacol* (1975) 15, 46–51.

Opioids + Promethazine

Promethazine reduces the anaesthetic and analgesic dose requirements of many opioid analgesics. It has potent sedative effects which would be expected to be additive with CNS depressant effects of the opioids.

Clinical evidence, mechanism, importance and management

The maintenance doses of a variety of opioid analgesics (**morphine**, **pethidine** (**meperidine**), **oxymorphone**, **hydromorphone**, **fentanyl**, **pentazocine**) required during surgical anaesthesia were reduced by 28% to 46% when 132 patients were pre-medicated with intramuscular promethazine, 50 mg/70 kg of body-weight when compared with control patients. Similarly, on-demand **pentazocine** requirements post-Caesarean section were reduced by 32% in women given promethazine as soon as the cord was clamped.[1] This possible advantageous interaction would be expected to be accompanied by increased sedation since promethazine is a potent CNS depressant, which would have additive effects with the CNS depressant effects of the opioids. Consider also 'Opioids; Pethidine (Meperidine) + Phenothiazines', p.121.

1. Keèri-Szàntò M. The mode of action of promethazine in potentiating narcotic drugs. *Br J Anaesth* (1974) 46, 918–24.

Opioids + Rifampicin (Rifampin)

Rifampicin markedly increases the metabolism of codeine and morphine, and reduces their pharmacological effects.

Clinical evidence, mechanism, importance and management

(a) Codeine

A study in 9 extensive metabolisers and 6 poor metabolisers of the cytochrome P450 isoenzyme CYP2D6 found that after taking rifampicin 600 mg daily for 3 weeks, the metabolism of a single 120-mg oral dose of codeine phosphate was markedly increased in both phenotypes. The AUC of codeine was decreased by 79.4% in extensive metabolisers and 83.5% in poor metabolisers and the *N*-demethylation and glucuronidation metabolic pathways were induced in both types of subject. However, the *O*-demethylation of codeine (mediated by the cytochrome P450 isoenzyme CYP2D6) was induced only in extensive metabolisers. In extensive metabolisers, there was a 56% reduction in the AUC of morphine, which is considered the main active metabolite of codeine, and a 173% increase in the AUC of another active metabolite normorphine. Note that morphine and its metabolites were not detected in poor metabolisers, either before or after rifampicin was given. Rifampicin reduced the respiratory and psychomotor effects of the codeine in extensive metabolisers, but not in poor metabolisers. In contrast, rifampicin did not alter the pupillary effect of codeine in extensive metabolisers, but decreased it in poor metabolisers. The clinically more relevant question of whether, and to what extent, the analgesic effects of the codeine were reduced by this interaction was not addressed by this study.[1] However, some reduction in effect might be expected. Therefore, if these drugs are used concurrently, be alert for the need to raise the codeine dosage. More study is needed.

(b) Morphine

In a randomised, double-blind crossover study, 10 healthy subjects were given either oral morphine sulfate 10 mg or a placebo on days 1, 4, 15 and 18, with rifampicin 600 mg daily on days 5 to 18. It was found that the rifampicin increased the clearance of the morphine by 49% and its analgesic effects (using a modified cold pressor test) were abolished.[2] The mechanism of this interaction is uncertain since morphine is principally metabolised by glucuronidation (see 'opioids', (p.72)), but the findings of this study could not be attributed to rifampicin induction of glucuronosyltransferases (UGTs).[2] You should be alert for the need to use an increased dosage of morphine in patients treated with rifampicin. More study is needed.

1. Caraco Y, Sheller J, Wood AJJ. Pharmacogenetic determinants of codeine induction by rifampin: the impact on codeine's respiratory, psychomotor and miotic effects. *J Pharmacol Exp Ther* (1997) 281, 330–6.
2. Fromm MF, Eckhardt K, Li S, Schänzle G, Hofmann U, Mikus G, Eichelbaum M. Loss of analgesic effect of morphine due to coadministration of rifampin. *Pain* (1997) 72, 261–7.

Opioids + Ritonavir

The makers of ritonavir predict that it will decrease the serum levels of morphine, but this has not been assessed. Ritonavir decreased pethidine and increased norpethidine levels, which may possibly increase toxicity on long-term use. Consider also 'Opioids; Methadone + Protease inhibitors', p.116, and 'Opioids; Fentanyl and related drugs + Ritonavir', p.113.

Clinical evidence, mechanism, importance and management

(a) Morphine

The makers of ritonavir say that, although pharmacokinetic data on the concurrent use of morphine and ritonavir are not available, they have unpublished data indicating that ritonavir will induce the hepatic enzymes responsible for the glucuronidation of morphine (its principal route of metabolism), and their prediction is that morphine serum levels will be decreased.[1] However there seems to be no confirmatory clinical evidence of this interaction and no published data to show whether this interaction is important or not.

(b) Pethidine (Meperidine)

Ritonavir 500 mg twice daily for 10 days decreased the AUC of a single 50-mg dose of oral pethidine by 67% and increased the AUC of norpethidine by 47% in 8 healthy subjects.[2]

It is suggested that ritonavir increased the metabolism of pethidine to its metabolite, although the mechanism is unclear. Norpethidine is pharmacologically active, and is possibly less effective an analgesic than the parent compound, and more likely to cause CNS effects such as seizures. It has a longer half-life than pethidine. The short-term use of oral pethidine with ritonavir is unlikely to be a problem, but the increased levels of norpethidine suggest an increased risk of toxicity on longer-term use.[1]

The pharmacokinetic findings with oral pethidine may not apply to parenteral pethidine, and this needs to be studied separately.

1. Abbott Laboratories Ltd (UK). Personal communication, March 1998.
2. Piscitelli SC, Kress DR, Bertz RJ, Pau A, Davey R. The effect of ritonavir on the pharmacokinetics of meperidine and normeperidine. *Pharmacotherapy* (2000) 20, 549–53.

Opioids + SSRIs

Short-term fluoxetine use decreased the analgesic effect of morphine, but a single-dose very slightly increased it. No pharmacokinetic interaction occurs between morphine and fluoxetine. An isolated report describes a marked reduction in the analgesic effects of oxycodone in a patient when starting fluoxetine. Short-term fluoxetine appears not to alter the analgesic effects of pentazocine.

A case of probable serotonin syndrome has been reported in a patient on sertraline after dramatically increasing the dose of oxycodone, and in a man on fluoxetine when given a single-dose of pentazocine.

Clinical evidence

(a) Morphine

A double-blind placebo-controlled study in 35 patients found that oral **fluoxetine** 10 mg daily for 7 days pre-operatively reduced the analgesic effect of intravenous morphine given for postoperative dental pain.[1] In contrast, a double-blind crossover study in 15 healthy subjects found that a single 60-mg dose of **fluoxetine** slightly improved (by 3 to 8%) the analgesic effect (as assessed by dental electrical stimulation) of morphine sulfate in doses tailored to produce and maintain steady-state plasma levels of 15, 30 and 60 nanograms/ml for 60 minutes. Plasma levels of morphine were not affected by **fluoxetine**, and morphine was found not to affect plasma levels of **fluoxetine** or norfluoxetine. The subjects experienced less nausea and drowsiness, but the psychomotor and respiratory depressant effects of morphine were not altered.[2]

(b) Oxycodone

A man with advanced multiple sclerosis found that when he began to take **fluoxetine** 20 mg daily for depression he needed to increase his analgesic dosage of oxycodone (for painful muscle spasms) about fourfold, from 65 to 75 mg daily to about 250 to 275 mg daily.[3]

A bone-marrow transplant recipient on, amongst other drugs, **sertraline** 50 mg daily, ciclosporin 75 mg daily, and oxycodone 10 mg as needed, developed severe tremors and visual hallucinations. This coincided with him taking oxycodone 200 mg over 48 hours for severe pain. An adverse reaction to ciclosporin was initially suspected (although serum levels were not high), and this was temporarily discontinued along with the oxycodone. The visual hallucinations decreased but the tremors continued, and did not lessen until **sertraline** was discontinued and cyproheptadine given. It was concluded that the patient was experiencing a form of the serotonin syndrome as a result of markedly increased opioid use while on an SSRI.[4]

(c) Pentazocine

A double-blind placebo-controlled study in 35 patients has shown that oral **fluoxetine** 10 mg daily for 7 days pre-operatively did not to reduce the analgesic effects of pentazocine 45 mg given intravenously for postoperative dental pain.[1]

A man who had been taking **fluoxetine** 20 mg daily for 10 days, later increased to 40 mg daily, was given a single 100-mg oral dose of pentazocine (*Talwin Nx* containing pentazocine 50 mg and naloxone 500 micrograms) for a severe headache. Within 30 minutes he complained of lightheadedness, anxiety, nausea and paraesthesias of the hands. He was diaphoretic, flushed, and ataxic, and had a mild tremor of his arms. His blood pressure was 178/114 mmHg, pulse 62 bpm and respiration 16 breaths per minute. He was given intramuscular diphenhydramine 50 mg and recovered over the following 4 hours.[5]

Mechanism

Fluoxetine inhibits the activity of the cytochrome P450 isoenzyme CYP2D6 within the liver so that the metabolism of oxycodone to an active metabolite oxymorphone is reduced (see also 'Opioids; Codeine and related drugs + Quinidine', p.108, but compare 'Opioids; Methadone + SSRIs', p.118). However, in the one of the reported cases the patient was a poor metaboliser of CYP2D6 (see 'Genetic factors', (p.4)), suggesting that other isoenzymes may be involved.[3] Morphine is not metabolised by CYP2D6, so would not be expected to be affected. It has been suggested that the reason for the reduced analgesia may have something to do with the initial effects of SSRIs on serotonergic neurotransmission.[2] The serotonin syndrome seems to develop unpredictably in a few patients given two or more serotonergic drugs, in this cases, opioids and SSRIs. See also 'the serotonin syndrome', (p.9).

Importance and management

Short-term fluoxetine appears not to have an important effect on the analgesic efficacy of pentazocine, and no special precautions seem to be needed. However, short-term fluoxetine appears to reduce the efficacy of morphine, whereas a single-dose of fluoxetine slightly increased it. The relevance of these findings to clinical practice remains to be determined, and further studies are required, particularly in patients on long-term fluoxetine. Nevertheless, bear the possibility of reduced morphine efficacy in mind in patients who have recently started fluoxetine. Similarly, the isolated report with oxycodone suggests that some patients may experience a marked reduction in analgesic efficacy when given fluoxetine. Bear this in mind in the event of an unexpected lack of efficacy. Further study is needed. Note that SSRIs may increase the effects of 'methadone', (p.118).

The incidence of serotonin syndrome-like reactions with opioids and SSRIs is rare, and the general importance of the cases with oxycodone and sertraline or pentazocine and fluoxetine is uncertain. However, the possibility of the serotonin syndrome should be considered in patients experiencing altered mental status, autonomic dysfunction and neuromuscular adverse effects while on these drugs. The serotonin syndrome had also been reported with 'tramadol and SSRIs', (p.123).

1. Gordon NC, Heller PH, Gear RW, Levine JD. Interactions between fluoxetine and opiate analgesia for postoperative dental pain. *Pain* (1994) 58, 85–8.
2. Erjavec MK, Coda BA, Nguyen Q, Donaldson G, Risler L, Shen DD. Morphine-fluoxetine interactions in healthy volunteers: analgesia and side effects. *J Clin Pharmacol* (2000) 40, 1286–95.
3. Otton SV, Wu D, Joffe RT, Cheung SW, Sellers EM. Inhibition by fluoxetine of cytochrome P450 2D6 activity. *Clin Pharmacol Ther* (1993) 53, 401–9.
4. Rosebraugh CJ, Flockhart DA, Yasuda SU, Woosley RL. Visual hallucination and tremor induced by sertraline and oxycodone in a bone marrow transplant patient. *J Clin Pharmacol* (2001) 41, 224–7.
5. Hansen TE, Dieter K, Keepers GA. Interaction of fluoxetine and pentazocine. *Am J Psychiatry* (1990) 147, 949–50.

Opioids + Tobacco smoking or Environmental pollution

Dextropropoxyphene and pentazocine are less effective as analgesics in smokers than in non-smokers. Atmospheric pollution has a similar effect on pentazocine. Codeine metabolism was not affected to a clinically relevant extent by smoking.

Clinical evidence

(a) Codeine

The metabolism of a single 25-mg dose of codeine did not differ between 9 heavy smokers (greater than 20 cigarettes daily) and 9 non-smoking control subjects, except that smokers had a slightly higher rate of glucuronidation.[1] This is unlikely to be clinically important. No differences in the efficacy of codeine are expected between smokers and non-smokers, although this requires confirmation.

(b) Dextropropoxyphene (Propoxyphene)

A study in 835 patients who were given dextropropoxyphene for mild or moderate pain or headache showed that its efficacy as an analgesic was decreased by smoking. The drug was rated as ineffective in 10.1% of 335 non-smokers, 15% of 347 patients who smoked up to 20 cigarettes daily, and 20.3% of 153 patients who smoked more than 20 cigarettes daily.[2]

(c) Pentazocine

A study in which pentazocine was used to supplement nitrous oxide relaxant anaesthesia found that patients who came from an urban environment needed about 50% more pentazocine than those who lived in the country (3.6 compared with 2.4 micrograms/kg per minute). Roughly the same difference was seen between those who smoked and those who did not (3.8 compared with 2.5 micrograms/kg per minute).[3] In another study it was found that pentazocine metabolism was 40% higher in smokers than in non-smokers.[4]

Mechanism

It is thought that tobacco smoke contains compounds that increase the activity of the liver enzymes concerned with the metabolism of dextropropoxyphene and pentazocine, which increases its loss from the body and diminishes its effectiveness as an analgesic.[2] However, the metabolism of codeine was minimally affected by smoking.

Importance and management

The interaction appears to be well established. Prescribers should be aware that dextropropoxyphene is twice as likely to be ineffective in those who smoke more than 20 cigarettes a day (1 in 5) as in those who do not smoke (1 in 10). Similarly, smokers and urban dwellers from polluted areas may need about 40 to 50% more pentazocine than country dwellers and non-smokers to achieve the equivalent amount of analgesia. In contrast, codeine metabolism does not appear to be affected to a clinically important extent by smoking.

1. Yue Q-Y, Tomson T, Säwe J. Carbamazepine and cigarette smoking induce differentially the metabolism of codeine in man. *Pharmacogenetics* (1994) 4, 193–8.
2. Boston Collaborative Drug Surveillance Program. Decreased clinical efficacy of propoxyphene in cigarette smokers. *Clin Pharmacol Ther* (1973) 14, 259–63.
3. Keeri-Szanto M, Pomeroy JR. Atmospheric pollution and pentazocine metabolism. *Lancet* (1971) i, 947–9.
4. Vaughan DP, Beckett AH, Robbie DS. The influence of smoking on the intersubject variation in pentazocine elimination. *Br J Clin Pharmacol* (1976) 3, 279–83.

Opioids + Tricyclic antidepressants; Amitriptyline

No marked increase in the psychomotor effects of buprenorphine, oxycodone or pentazocine occurred when amitriptyline was given. However, respiratory depression was somewhat increased when amitriptyline was given with buprenorphine and pentazocine. Consider also 'Opioids; Morphine + Tricyclic antidepressants', p.120, and 'Opioids; Tramadol + Tricyclic antidepressants', p.123.

Clinical evidence

(a) Buprenorphine

A study in 12 healthy subjects found that both buprenorphine 400 micrograms given sublingually and amitriptyline 50 mg given orally impaired the performance of a number of psychomotor tests (digit symbol substitution, flicker fusion, Maddox wing, hand-to-eye coordination, reactive skills), and the subjects felt drowsy, feeble, mentally slow and muzzy. When amitriptyline 30 mg, increased to 75 mg daily was given for 4 days before a single dose of buprenorphine, the psychomotor effects were not significantly increased, but the respiratory depressant effects of the buprenorphine were enhanced.[1]

(b) Oxycodone

Pretreatment with amitriptyline 10 mg increased to 50 mg daily for 4 days caused no major changes in the psychomotor effects of a single 0.28-mg/kg oral dose of oxycodone in 9 healthy subjects.[2] Respiratory effects were not assessed.

(c) Pentazocine

Both pentazocine and amitriptyline given alone caused 11 healthy subjects to feel drowsy, muzzy and clumsy, and reduced the performance of a number of psychomotor tests. However, when they were given intramuscular pentazocine 30 mg after taking amitriptyline 50 mg daily for a week, the combination of drugs appeared not to impair driving or occupational skills more than either drug given alone.[3] Respiratory depression was increased more by the combination than either drug alone. Amitriptyline modestly decreased pentazocine plasma levels by about 20% at 1.5 and 3.5 hours.[3]

Mechanism

The CNS depressant effects of opioids and drugs such as amitriptyline are expected to be additive.

Importance and management

Based on these available studies it appears that amitriptyline does not cause any important additional impairment in psychomotor performance when added to buprenorphine, oxycodone or pentazocine. Nevertheless, patients should be warned about the sedative effects of both these classes of drugs (see also 'Tricyclic antidepressants + Dextropropoxyphene (Propoxyphene)', p.995). Moreover, respiratory depressant effects were increased somewhat, and this may be clinically important in patients with a restricted respiratory capacity.[3] Combined use may be beneficial in the management of pain, see 'Opioids; Morphine + Tricyclic antidepressants', p.120.

1. Saarialho-Kere U, Mattila MJ, Paloheimo M, Seppälä T. Psychomotor, respiratory and neuroendocrinological effects of buprenorphine and amitriptyline in healthy volunteers. *Eur J Clin Pharmacol* (1987) 33, 139–46.
2. Pöyhiä R, Kalso E, Seppälä T. Pharmacodynamic interactions of oxycodone and amitriptyline in healthy volunteers. *Curr Ther Res* (1992) 51, 739–49.
3. Saarialho-Kere U, Mattila MJ, Seppälä T. Parenteral pentazocine: effects on psychomotor skills and respiration, and interactions with amitriptyline. *Eur J Clin Pharmacol* (1988) 35, 483–9.

Opioids; Alfentanil + Diltiazem

Diltiazem delayed tracheal extubation in patients undergoing surgery.

Clinical evidence, mechanism, importance and management

A 24% increase in the AUC of alfentanil and a 50% increase in half-life was seen in 15 patients anaesthetised with midazolam and alfentanil (induced with 50 micrograms/kg, then maintained with 1 microgram/kg per minute) when pretreated with diltiazem 60 mg orally 2 hours before induction, then an infusion for 23 hours starting at induction. Tracheal extubation was performed on average 2.5 hours later in the patients receiving diltiazem than in a placebo-group.[1] Diltiazem is an inhibitor of the cytochrome P450 isoenzyme CYP3A4, which is responsible for the metabolism of alfentanil. Diltiazem may delay recovery from anaesthesia after large doses of alfentanil.[1] Caution is required.

1. Ahonen J, Olkkola KT, Salmenperä M, Hynynen M, Neuvonen PJ. Effect of diltiazem on midazolam and alfentanil disposition in patients undergoing coronary artery bypass grafting. *Anesthesiology* (1996) 85, 1246–52.

Opioids; Alfentanil + Ondansetron

Ondansetron had no effect on the analgesic potency, sedative, or respiratory depressant effects of alfentanil.

Clinical evidence, mechanism, importance and management

Single-doses of intravenous ondansetron 8 or 16 mg in healthy subjects were found to have no effect on the sedation or ventilatory depression due to alfentanil (a continuous infusion of 0.25 to 0.75 micrograms/kg following a 5 microgram/kg bolus dose) and had no effect on the rate of recovery.[1] Similarly, in another study, intravenous ondansetron 8 mg had no effect on the reaction of 8 healthy subjects to pressure, cold or electrical stimulation, nor did it oppose the analgesic effect of intramuscular alfentanil 30 micrograms/kg.[2] No special precautions would seem to be necessary during concurrent use. Consider also 'Opioids + Ondansetron', p.104.

1. Dershwitz M, Di Biase PM, Rosow CE, Wilson RS, Sanderson PE, Joslyn AF. Ondansetron does not affect alfentanil-induced ventilatory depression or sedation. *Anesthesiology* (1992) 77, 447–52.
2. Petersen-Felix S, Arendt-Nielsen L, Bak P, Bjerring P, Breivik H, Svensson P, Zbinden AM. Ondansetron does not inhibit the analgesic effect of alfentanil. *Br J Anaesth* (1994) 73, 326–30.

Opioids; Alfentanil + Reserpine

An isolated report describes ventricular arrhythmias in a patient on reserpine when given alfentanil during anaesthesia.

Clinical evidence, mechanism, importance and management

A hypertensive woman on reserpine 250 micrograms daily was given intravenous alfentanil 800 micrograms over 5 minutes, before anaesthesia with thiopental and suxamethonium (succinylcholine). During surgery she was given nine 100-microgram doses of alfentanil and 70% N_2O/O_2. Bradycardia developed and frequent unifocal premature ventricular contractions occurred throughout the surgery, but they disappeared 3 to 4 hours afterwards. The reasons are not understood.[1]

1. Jahr JS, Weber S. Ventricular dysrhythmias following an alfentanil anesthetic in a patient on reserpine for hypertension. *Acta Anaesthesiol Scand* (1991) 35, 788–9.

Opioids; Alfentanil + Rifampicin (Rifampin)

Alfentanil clearance is markedly increased by rifampicin.

Clinical evidence, mechanism, importance and management

A study in 9 healthy subjects found that when they were given intravenous alfentanil 20 micrograms/kg after taking rifampicin 600 mg orally for 5 days, alfentanil clearance was increased almost threefold (13.2 compared with 4.9 ml/kg per minute for the controls).[1] The reason appears to be that rifampicin increases the activity of the cytochrome P450 isoenzyme CYP3A4 in the liver, which is concerned with the metabolism of alfentanil (see 'opioids', (p.72)). This study was primarily designed to investigate the role of CYP3A4 in the metabolism of alfentanil, but it also provides good evidence that alfentanil will be much less effective in patients treated with rifampicin. A much larger dose will almost certainly be needed. See also 'Opioids + Rifampicin (Rifampin)', p.105.

1. Kharasch ED, Russell M, Mautz D, Thummel KE, Kunze KL, Bowdle A, Cox K. The role of cytochrome P450 3A4 in alfentanil clearance: implications for interindividual variability in disposition and perioperative drug interactions. *Anesthesiology* (1997) 36–50.

Opioids; Buprenorphine + Antiretrovirals

Preliminary evidence suggests that buprenorphine does not affect antiretroviral efficacy, nor does it alter zidovudine pharmacokinetics.

Clinical evidence, mechanism, importance and management

There was no difference in antiviral efficacy, as measured by viral load, between 83 patients on highly-active antiretroviral therapy (HAART) and 20 other patients on HAART and buprenorphine in a preliminary study.[1] In another study, there was no difference in the pharmacokinetics of oral **zidovudine** between patients on buprenorphine and control subjects.[2] Buprenorphine is not expected to cause **zidovudine** toxicity.

The effect of antiretrovirals on buprenorphine does not appear to have been studied, nevertheless the makers predict that inhibitors of the cytochrome P450 isoenzyme CYP3A4, such as the protease inhibitors **ritona-**

vir, **indinavir**, and **saquinavir**, may increase the exposure to buprenorphine and norbuprenorphine. They suggest halving the starting dose of buprenorphine in patients on these drugs.[3] However, note that **ritonavir** unexpectedly decreased methadone levels, see 'Opioids; Methadone + Protease inhibitors', p.116.

1. Carrieri MP, Vlahov D, Dellamonica P, Gallais H, Lepeu G, Spire B. Obadia Y, the Manif-2000 study group. Use of buprenorphine in HIV-infected injection drug users: negligible impact on virologic response to HAART. *Drug Alcohol Depend* (2000) 60, 51–4.
2. McCance-Katz EF, Rainey PM, Friedland G, Kosten TR, Jatlow P. Effect of opioid dependence pharmacotherapies on zidovudine disposition. *Am J Addict* (2001) 10, 296–307.
3. Subutex (Buprenorphine hydrochloride). Schering-Plough Ltd. UK Summary of product characteristics, September 2003.

Opioids; Buprenorphine + Ketoconazole

Ketoconazole raises levels of buprenorphine, and the dose should be reduced.

Clinical evidence, mechanism, importance and management

The makers of buprenorphine note that an interaction study with ketoconazole found a 50% increase in the AUC of buprenorphine and a 70% increase in its maximum level, and smaller increases in the levels of the metabolite norbuprenorphine.[1] Ketoconazole is an inhibitor of the cytochrome P450 isoenzyme CYP3A4, which is involved in the metabolism of buprenorphine.[2] The maker recommends that the dose of buprenorphine should be halved when starting treatment with ketoconazole, and then further titrated as clinically indicated. They say that a similar dose-reduction should be considered with other inhibitors of CYP3A4. They specifically name **gestodene**, **troleandomycin**, **ritonavir**, **indinavir** and **saquinavir** (see 'Antiretrovirals', (p.107)).[1]

1. Subutex (Buprenorphine hydrochloride). Schering-Plough Ltd. UK Summary of product characteristics, September 2003.
2. Iribarne C, Picart D, Creano Y, Bail JP, Berthou F. Involvement of cytochrome P450 3A4 in N-dealkylation of buprenorphine in human liver microsomes. *Life Sci* (1997) 60, 1953–64.

Opioids; Buprenorphine + Ketorolac

A single case report describes marked respiratory depression in a man on buprenorphine when ketorolac was added.

Clinical evidence, mechanism, importance and management

A man underwent thoracotomy for carcinoma of the middle third of his oesophagus. An hour after transfer to the recovery ward he complained of severe pain at the operative site and was given epidural buprenorphine 150 micrograms (3 micrograms/kg), and 2 hours later intramuscular ketorolac 30 mg because of continued pain. During the next hour he became more drowsy, stopped obeying commands and his respiratory rate dropped to 6 breaths per minute. He recovered after 6 hours of mechanical ventilation. The authors of this report suggest that it may be necessary to use less buprenorphine in the presence of ketorolac to avoid the development of these respiratory depressant effects.[1] This appears to be the only report of this possible interaction.

1. Jain PN, Shah SC. Respiratory depression following combination of epidural buprenorphine and intramuscular ketorolac. *Anaesthesia* (1993) 48, 898–9.

Opioids; Butorphanol + Metoclopramide

No clinically important pharmacokinetic interaction occurs between intranasal butorphanol and oral metoclopramide. Nausea associated with butorphanol was reduced by metoclopramide.

Clinical evidence, mechanism, importance and management

The pharmacokinetics of a single 1-mg intranasal dose of butorphanol were unaffected by a single 10-mg oral dose of metoclopramide in 24 healthy women. The pharmacokinetics of metoclopramide were also not affected, except for a delay in the time to reach maximum plasma levels (increased from 1 to 2 hours), which was probably due to reduction of gastrointestinal motility by butorphanol.[1] The lack of a pharmacokinetic interaction was attributed to the involvement of different metabolic pathways for the two drugs. Metoclopramide reduced the nausea associated with butorphanol, probably by antagonism of central and peripheral dopamine receptors.[1] Information seems to be limited to this report but where the drugs are used together, such as in the treatment of migraine, no dosage adjustments would appear to be necessary.

1. Vachharajani NN, Shyu WC, Barbhaiya RH. Pharmacokinetic interaction between butorphanol nasal spray and oral metoclopramide in healthy women. *J Clin Pharmacol* (1997) 37, 979–85.

Opioids; Codeine + Carbamazepine

Carbamazepine appears to increase the production of a more potent metabolite of codeine, normorphine.

Clinical evidence, mechanism, importance and management

An experimental study in 7 epileptic patients to find out if carbamazepine induces the enzymes concerned with the metabolism of codeine found that it increased *N*-demethylation (to norcodeine and normorphine) by two- to threefold, but did not affect *O*-demethylation (to morphine). The patients were given a single 25-mg dose of codeine before and 3 weeks after starting treatment with carbamazepine 400 to 600 mg daily.[1] Normorphine is an active metabolite, so that the authors of this study suggest those taking both codeine and carbamazepine may possibly experience a stronger analgesic effect.[1] However, this needs further study. There would seem to be no reason for avoiding concurrent use.

1. Yue Q-Y, Tomson T, Säwe J. Carbamazepine and cigarette smoking induce differentially the metabolism of codeine in man. *Pharmacogenetics* (1994) 4, 193–8.

Opioids; Codeine + Diclofenac

Diclofenac did not affect the pharmacokinetics or analgesic effects of codeine in healthy subjects.

Clinical evidence, mechanism, importance and management

A single 50-mg dose of diclofenac sodium did not have an important effect on the pharmacokinetics of a single 100-mg dose of codeine phosphate in a placebo-controlled crossover study in 12 healthy subjects. There was no effect on the metabolic clearance of morphine, and only a slight (about 5% to 10%) increase in the levels of glucuronide metabolites. In addition, diclofenac did not alter the analgesic effects of codeine as assessed in a cold pressor test (a test in which opioids, but not NSAIDs, are effective).[1]

These findings are in contrast to an earlier *in vitro* study by the same research group, which found that diclofenac markedly inhibited the glucuronidation of codeine in human liver tissue.[2]

Although this interaction perhaps requires confirmation in a multiple-dose study in a clinical setting, the findings in healthy subjects suggest that no special precautions are required during the concurrent use of diclofenac and codeine.

1. Ammon S, Marx C, Behrens C, Hofmann U, Mürdter T, Griese E-U, Mikus G. Diclofenac does not interact with codeine metabolism in vivo: a study in healthy volunteers. *BMC Clin Pharmacol* (2002) 2, 2.
2. Ammon S, von Richter O, Hofmann U, Thon KP, Eichelbaum M, Mikus G. In vitro interaction of codeine and diclofenac. *Drug Metab Dispos* (2000) 28, 1149–52.

Opioids; Codeine and related drugs + Quinidine

The analgesic effects of codeine, and probably also dihydrocodeine and hydrocodone, are reduced or abolished by quinidine. Quinidine altered the metabolite profile of oxycodone, but not its pharmacodynamic effects. Consider also 'fentanyl', (p.112), 'morphine', (p.120), and 'tramadol', (p.122).

Clinical evidence

(a) Codeine

Codeine 100 mg was given to 16 extensive metabolisers of sparteine with and without single 200-mg doses of quinidine. The quinidine reduced the peak morphine levels by about 80% (from a mean of 18 nanomol/l to less than 4 nanomol/l). Codeine given alone increased the pain threshold (pin-prick pain test using an argon laser) but no significant analgesic effects were detectable when the quinidine was also present.[1] Another study found that the effects of codeine after using quinidine in extensive metabolisers of the cytochrome P450 isoenzyme CYP2D6 were virtually the same as codeine alone in poor metabolisers.[2]

These studies confirm the preliminary findings of a previous study using codeine 100 mg and quinidine 50 mg.[3] The quinidine reduced the peak morphine plasma levels by more than 90% (by 92% in 7 extensive metabolisers, and by 97% in one poor metaboliser) and similarly abolished the analgesic effects.[3]

(b) Dihydrocodeine

A study in which 4 extensive metabolisers of the cytochrome P450 isoenzyme CYP2D6 were given dihydrocodeine 40 or 60 mg found that when pretreated with quinidine 200 mg almost none of the morphinoid metabolites of dihydrocodeine normally present in the serum could be detected.[4] The same authors found essentially the same results in a later study in 10 extensive metabolisers of the cytochrome P450 isoenzyme CYP2D6 given dihydrocodeine 60 mg and quinidine 50 mg.[5]

(c) Hydrocodone

In a comparative study, 5 extensive metabolisers and 6 poor metabolisers of the cytochrome P450 isoenzyme CYP2D6 were given hydrocodone, and 4 extensive metabolisers were given hydrocodone after pre-treatment with quinidine. The metabolism of the hydrocodone to its active metabolite hydromorphone was found to be high in the extensive metabolisers who described 'good opiate effects' but poor in the poor metabolisers and the extensive metabolisers pre-treated with quinidine who described 'poor opiate effects'.[6]

(d) Oxycodone

Quinidine, given as 200 mg 3 hours before and 100 mg 6 hours after a single 20-mg dose of oxycodone almost completely inhibited the formation of the metabolite, oxymorphone in 10 healthy extensive metabolisers of the cytochrome P450 isoenzyme CYP2D6. Despite this, the psychomotor and subjective effects of oxycodone were not altered (note that analgesia was not assessed). The AUC of the metabolite noroxycodone was increased about 85%, and the oxycodone AUC was slightly increased by 13%.[7] Similar results were given in the preliminary report of another study.[8]

Mechanism

The evidence available shows that the conversion of codeine, dihydrocodeine and hydrocodone to their active analgesic metabolites in the body (morphine, morphinoid metabolites and hydromorphone respectively) probably depends upon the activity of the cytochrome P450 isoenzyme CYP2D6 in the liver. If this isoenzyme is inhibited by quinidine, these conversions largely fail to occur and the analgesic effects are reduced or lost. This interaction is only likely to occur in extensive metabolisers, and not in poor metabolisers, who have minimal CYP2D6 activity and who therefore probably receive minimal benefit from these analgesics in any case.[2] Quinidine also blocks conversion of oxycodone to oxymorphone, but it appears this is not important for the pharmacodynamic effects of this drug.

Importance and management

The interaction between codeine and quinidine is well established and clinically important. Codeine will be virtually ineffective as an analgesic in extensive metabolisers taking quinidine. An alternative analgesic (not dihydrocodeine or hydrocodone, see below) should be used. No interaction would be expected in poor metabolisers (about 7% of Caucasians), but codeine is probably unlikely to be effective in these patients in any case. Whether the antitussive effects of codeine are similarly affected is not established, but it seems likely. Note that this interaction has been used clinically in an attempt to treat codeine dependence.[9]

The interactions of dihydrocodeine and hydrocodone are less well established, but the evidence suggests that their analgesic effects will similarly be reduced or lost if quinidine is given. Further study is needed.

The available evidence suggests that the efficacy of oxycodone may not be affected by quinidine, but this needs confirmation. Consider also 'fentanyl', (p.112), 'quinidine', (p.120) and 'tramadol', (p.122).

1. Sindrup SH, Arendt-Nielsen L, Brøsen K, Bjerring P, Angelo HR, Eriksen B, Gram LF. The effect of quinidine on the analgesic effect of codeine. *Eur J Clin Pharmacol* (1992) 42, 587–92.
2. Caraco Y, Sheller J, Wood AJ. Pharmacogenetic determination of the effects of codeine and prediction of drug interactions. *J Pharmacol Exp Ther* (1996) 278, 1165–74.
3. Desmeules J, Dayer P, Gascon M-P, Magistris M. Impact of genetic and environmental factors on codeine analgesia. *Clin Pharmacol Ther* (1989) 45, 122.
4. Hufschmid E, Theurillat R, Martin U, Thormann W. Exploration of the metabolism of dihydrocodeine via determination of its metabolites in human urine using micellar electrokinetic capillary chromatography. *J Chromatogr B Biomed Appl* (1995) 668, 159–70.
5. Hufschmid E, Theurillat R, Wilder-Smith CH, Thormann W. Characterization of the genetic polymorphism of dihydrocodeine O-demethylation in man via analysis of urinary dihydrocodeine and dihydromorphine by micellar electrokinetic capillary chromatography. *J Chromatogr B Biomed Appl* (1996) 678, 45–51.
6. Otton SV, Schadel M, Cheung SW, Kaplan, Busto UE, Sellers EM. CYP2D6 phenotype determines the metabolic conversion of hydrocodone to hydromorphone. *Clin Pharmacol Ther* (1993) 54, 463–72.
7. Heiskanen T, Olkkola KT, Kalso E. Effects of blocking CYP2D6 on the pharmacokinetics and pharmacodynamics of oxycodone. *Clin Pharmacol Ther* (1998) 64, 603–11.
8. Colucci R, Kaiko R, Grandy R. Effects of quinidine on the pharmacokinetics and pharmacodynamics of oxycodone. *Clin Pharmacol Ther* (1998) 63, 141.
9. Fernandes LC, Kilicarslan T, Kaplan HL, Tyndale RF, Sellers EM, Romach MK. Treatment of codeine dependence with inhibitors of cytochrome P450 2D6. *J Clin Psychopharmacol* (2002) 22, 326–9.

Opioids; Dextromoramide + Troleandomycin

An isolated report describes a marked increase in the effects of dextromoramide and coma in a man treated with troleandomycin.

Clinical evidence, mechanism, importance and management

A man on dextromoramide developed signs of overdosage (a morphine-like coma, mydriasis and depressed respiration) 3 days after starting treatment with troleandomycin for a dental infection. He recovered when given naloxone. A possible explanation is that the troleandomycin reduced the metabolism of the dextromoramide, thereby reducing its loss from the body and increasing its serum levels and effects.[1] The general importance of this interaction is uncertain but concurrent use should be well monitored. It is not clear whether other macrolides can interact similarly. Compare also 'Opioids; Fentanyl and related drugs + Macrolides', p.112.

1. Carry PV, Ducluzeau R, Jourdan C, Bourrat Ch, Vigneau C, Descotes J. De nouvelles interactions avec les macrolides? *Lyon Med* (1982) 248, 189–90.

Opioids; Dextropropoxyphene (Propoxyphene) + Food

Food can delay the absorption of dextropropoxyphene, but the total amount absorbed may be slightly increased.

Clinical evidence, mechanism, importance and management

A study in healthy subjects given a single 130-mg dose of dextropropoxyphene (as capsules) showed that while fasting, peak plasma dextropropoxyphene levels were reached after about 2 hours. **High-fat** and **high-carbohydrate meals** delayed peak serum levels by about 1 hour, and **high protein** by about 2 hours. Both the **protein and carbohydrate meals** caused a small 25 to 30% increase in the total amount of dextropropoxyphene absorbed.[1] Likely reasons for the delay in absorption are that food delays gastric emptying. Avoid food if rapid analgesic effects are needed. See also 'Opioids; Morphine + Food', p.119.

1. Musa MN and Lyons LL. Effect of food and liquid on the pharmacokinetics of propoxyphene. *Curr Ther Res* (1976) 19, 669–74.

Opioids; Dextropropoxyphene (Propoxyphene) + Orphenadrine

An alleged adverse interaction between dextropropoxyphene and orphenadrine, which is said to cause mental confusion, anxiety, and tremors, seems to be very rare, if indeed it ever occurs.

Clinical evidence, mechanism, importance and management

The makers of orphenadrine used to state in their package insert that mental confusion, anxiety and tremors have been reported in patients receiving both orphenadrine and dextropropoxyphene. The makers of dextropropoxyphene issued a similar warning. However, in correspondence with both makers, two investigators[1] of this interaction were told that the basis of these statements consisted of 6 anecdotal reports from clinicians to one maker and 7 to the other (some could represent the same cases). Of the 7 cases to one maker, 4 occurred where patients had received twice the recommended dose of orphenadrine. In every case the adverse reactions seen were similar to those reported with either drug alone. A brief study in 5 patients given both drugs to investigate this alleged interaction failed to reveal an adverse interaction.[2] One case has been reported separately.[3]

The documentation is therefore sparse, and no case of interaction has been firmly established. The investigators calculated that the two drugs were probably being used together on 300 000 prescriptions a year, and that these few cases would be less than significant.[1] There seems therefore little reason for avoiding concurrent use, although prescribers should know that the advisability of using the two drugs together has been the subject of some debate.

1. Pearson RE, Salter FJ. Drug interaction? — Orphenadrine with propoxyphene. *N Engl J Med* (1970) 282, 1215.
2. Puckett WH, Visconti JA. Orphenadrine and propoxyphene (cont.). *N Engl J Med* (1970) 283, 544.
3. Renforth W. Orphenadrine and propoxyphene. *N Engl J Med* (1970) 283, 998.

Opioids; Diamorphine + Pyrithyldione

A single case report describes a fatality due to the combined CNS depressant effects of diamorphine and pyrithyldione.

Clinical evidence, mechanism, importance and management

A heroin (diamorphine) addict was found dead after taking pyrithyldione (a sedative and hypnotic) and diamorphine. His blood pyrithyldione and brain morphine levels were found to be 590 nanograms/ml and 0.06 nanograms/g respectively, suggesting that he had taken only a therapeutic dose of the pyrithyldione and a moderate dose of diamorphine. The presumed cause of death was the combined CNS depressant effects of both drugs. The authors of the report draw the conclusion that the pyrithyldione potentiated the effects of the diamorphine.[1]

1. Jorens PG, Coucke V, Selala MI, Schepens PJC. Fatal intoxication due to the combined use of heroin and pyrithyldione. *Hum Exp Toxicol* (1992) 11, 296–7.

Opioids; Fentanyl + Anticonvulsants

Patients on anticonvulsants appear to need more fentanyl than those not on anticonvulsants.

Clinical evidence, mechanism, importance and management

Twenty-eight patients, undergoing craniotomy for seizure focus excision and on long-term treatment with anticonvulsants in various combinations, needed 48 to 144% more fentanyl during anaesthesia than a control group of 22 patients who were not on anticonvulsants.[1] The fentanyl maintenance requirements in micrograms/kg per hour were:

- 2.7 in the control group,
- 4 in patients on **carbamazepine**,
- 4.7 in patients on **carbamazepine** and **phenytoin** or **sodium valproate**,
- 6.3 in patients on **carbamazepine**, **sodium valproate** and either **phenytoin** or **primidone**).

Similar results were reported by the same authors in a study involving 61 patients.[2]

The suggested reason is that these anticonvulsants are potent enzyme inducing agents (with the exception of **sodium valproate**), which increase the metabolism of fentanyl by the liver, so that it is cleared from the body more quickly.[1] Changes in the state of opiate receptors induced by chronic anticonvulsant exposure may also be involved.[2] A marked increase in the fentanyl requirements should therefore be anticipated in any patient on long-term treatment with these interacting anticonvulsants, but not **sodium valproate**.

1. Tempelhoff R, Modica P, Spitznagel E. Increased fentanyl requirement in patients receiving long-term anticonvulsant therapy. *Anesthesiology* (1988) 69, A594.
2. Tempelhoff R, Modica PA, Spitznagel EL. Anticonvulsant therapy increases fentanyl requirements during anaesthesia for craniotomy. *Can J Anaesth* (1990) 37, 327–32.

Opioids; Fentanyl and related drugs + Azoles

Some patients may experience prolonged and increased alfentanil effects if they are given fluconazole. Fentanyl does not usually interact with itraconazole, but one case of possible opioid toxicity has been reported.

Clinical evidence

(a) Alfentanil + Fluconazole

A double-dummy randomised crossover study in 9 healthy subjects given intravenous alfentanil 20 micrograms/kg after receiving fluconazole 400 mg, orally or by infusion, found that fluconazole reduced alfentanil clearance by about 60%. Both the alfentanil-induced ventilatory depression and its subjective effects were increased.[1]

(b) Fentanyl + Itraconazole

The pharmacokinetics and pharmacodynamics of a single 3-micrograms/kg intravenous dose of fentanyl were not altered by itraconazole 200 mg once daily for 4 days in a crossover study in 10 healthy subjects.[2] However, a case report describes a man with cancer and severe oropharyngeal candidiasis on transdermal fentanyl 50 micrograms/hour who developed signs of opioid toxicity (agitated delirium, bilateral myoclonus of muscles in the hand) the day after starting oral itraconazole 200 mg twice daily.[3]

Mechanism

Fluconazole and itraconazole inhibit the cytochrome P450 isoenzyme CYP3A4 in the liver, which is concerned with the metabolism of alfentanil and fentanyl. However, fentanyl has a high hepatic extraction, and therefore even large changes in the isoenzymes responsible for its metabolism are considered unlikely to cause much change in its pharmacokinetics. **Sufentanil** also has a high hepatic extraction, see 'Opioids; Fentanyl and related drugs + Macrolides', p.112.

Importance and management

The interaction of alfentanil with fluconazole appears to be established and clinically important. *In vitro* data indicate that **ketoconazole** and itraconazole may interact in a similar way.[4,5] Alfentanil should be given with care to those who have recently had these drugs, and it may be necessary to use a lower alfentanil dose.[5] Be alert for evidence of prolonged alfentanil effects and respiratory depression.

Fentanyl was not affected by itraconazole in healthy subjects, but the single case report introduces a note of caution, particularly in those with unstable advanced disease. Further study is needed.

1. Palkama VJ, Isohanni MH, Neuvonen PJ, Olkkola KT. The effect of intravenous and oral fluconazole on the pharmacokinetics and pharmacodynamics of intravenous alfentanil. *Anesth Analg* (1998) 87, 190–4.
2. Palkama VJ, Neuvonen PJ, Olkkola KT. The CYP3A4 inhibitor itraconazole has no effect on the pharmacokinetics of i.v. fentanyl. *Br J Anaesth* (1998) 81, 598–600.
3. Mercadante S, Villari P, Ferrera P. Itraconazole–fentanyl interaction in a cancer patient. *J Pain Symptom Manage* (2002) 24, 284–6.
4. Labroo RB, Thummel KE, Kunze KL, Podoll T, Trager WF, Kharasch ED. Catalytic role of cytochrome P4503A4 in multiple pathways of alfentanil metabolism. *Drug Metab Dispos* (1995) 23, 490–6.
5. Rapifen (Alfentanil hydrochloride). Janssen-Cilag Ltd. UK Summary of product characteristics, March 2000.

Opioids; Fentanyl + Baclofen

The effects of fentanyl are increased by baclofen.

Clinical evidence, mechanism, importance and management

A study in three groups of 10 patients showed that pretreatment with baclofen 0.6 mg/kg, either in four intramuscular doses for 5 days, or intravenously in 100 ml of glucose 5% 45 minutes before surgery, prolonged the duration of fentanyl anaesthesia from 18 to 30 minutes (fentanyl plus nitrous oxide in oxygen). The baclofen reduced the amounts of fentanyl needed by 30 to 40%.[1] The reasons are not known but a suggestion is that what happens is connected in some way with the action of baclofen on

GABA receptors.[1] This appears to be the only report of this effect, but bear in mind that baclofen may potentiate the effects of fentanyl.

1. Panerai AE, Massei R, De Silva E, Sacerdote P, Monza G, Mantegazza P. Baclofen prolongs the analgesic effect of fentanyl in man. *Br J Anaesth* (1985) 57, 954–5.

Opioids; Fentanyl and related drugs + Benzodiazepines

The combined use of midazolam with fentanyl or related drugs is synergistic in the induction of anaesthesia. Respiratory depression and hypotension have occurred in adults when fentanyl was used in conjunction with diazepam or midazolam, or when sufentanil was used with midazolam or lorazepam. This has also occurred in neonates when fentanyl was used with midazolam. Increased sedation has been seen when alfentanil was used with midazolam. Retrospective evidence suggests that midazolam can increase the dose requirement of sufentanil, but midazolam did not alter the analgesic efficacy of fentanyl in healthy subjects. Consider also 'Opioids + Benzodiazepines', p.102.

Clinical evidence

(a) Anaesthetic induction

Combining **midazolam** and **alfentanil** or fentanyl for the induction of anaesthesia reduces the dose required of both the benzodiazepine and the opioid, when compared with either drug alone.[1-3] The interaction is synergistic (more than additive).[2]

(b) Analgesic effects

An analysis of 43 patients who were mechanically ventilated following major trauma, and who were given infusions of **sufentanil** alone or **sufentanil** plus **midazolam**, found that **midazolam** appeared to reduce the efficacy of the **sufentanil**. The rate of **sufentanil** infusion in the group given both drugs (21 patients) was increased more than 50% above the group given **sufentanil** alone (22 patients). It was found possible to reduce the **sufentanil** infusion in 8 of patients given **sufentanil** alone, whereas this was possible in only one patient given both drugs.[4]

Conversely, in a study in healthy subjects, intravenous **midazolam** 500 micrograms to 2 mg per 70 kg did not affect the analgesia produced by intravenous fentanyl 100 micrograms per 70 kg in a cold pressor test.[5]

(c) Hypotension and respiratory depression

(i) Neonates. Hypotension occurred in 6 neonates with respiratory distress who were given **midazolam** (a bolus of 200 micrograms/kg and/or an infusion of 60 micrograms/kg per hour) for sedation during the first 12 to 36 hours of life. Five of them were also given fentanyl either as an infusion (1 to 2 micrograms/kg per hour) or a bolus (1.5 to 2.5 micrograms/kg), or both. Blood pressures fell from an average of 55/40 mmHg to 36/24 mmHg in 5 of them, and from 42/28 to less than 20 mmHg in one.[6] Another report describes respiratory arrest in a child of 14 months when given both drugs.[7]

(ii) Adults. **Midazolam** 50 micrograms/kg alone caused no episodes of apnoea or hypoxaemia in 12 healthy subjects, whereas fentanyl 2 micrograms/kg alone caused hypoxaemia in 6 subjects but no apnoea. When used together 6 subjects had apnoea and 11 subjects had hypoxaemia.[8] Similarly, fentanyl plus **diazepam** caused more respiratory depression in 12 healthy subjects than either drug alone.[9] Hypotension has also been seen in adult patients given fentanyl with **midazolam**[10] or **diazepam**.[11]

A case of acute hypotension has also been described in a man on clonidine, captopril and furosemide who was premedicated with intramuscular **midazolam** 5 mg and anaesthetised with **sufentanil** 150 micrograms.[12] This is consistent with another report of sudden hypotension during anaesthetic induction in 4 patients given high-dose **sufentanil** who had received **lorazepam** prior to induction.[13]

(d) Sedation

A study of patients having abdominal hysterectomies under **alfentanil** and **midazolam** anaesthesia found that although the pharmacokinetics of **midazolam** were unchanged but postoperative sedation was more pronounced, when compared with a group of patients that did not receive **alfentanil**.[14]

Mechanism

Uncertain. The additional use of other CNS depressants may produce additive respiratory depressant and sedative effects. Why midazolam might increase the analgesic dose requirement for sufentanil is unknown.

Importance and management

Increased sedative and respiratory depressant effects are to be expected when benzodiazepines are used with opioids such as fentanyl and related drugs. When used for the induction of anaesthesia, dose requirements of both agents are reduced. Case reports suggest that clinically important hypotension may unexpectedly occur, and it would now seem prudent to be alert for this. More study is needed.

Whether the use of midazolam has any effect on the dose requirement of sufentanil and other opioids in the intensive care setting requires further study. Midazolam did not alter fentanyl analgesia in healthy subjects.

1. Ben-Shlomo I, Abd-El-Khalim H, Ezry J, Zohar S, Tverskoy M. Midazolam acts synergistically with fentanyl for induction of anaesthesia. *Br J Anaesth* (1990) 64, 45–7.
2. Vinik HR, Bradley EL, Kissin I. Midazolam–alfentanil synergism for anesthetic induction in patients. *Anesth Analg* (1989) 69, 213–17.
3. Kissin I, Vinik HR, Castillo R, Bradley EL. Alfentanil potentiates midazolam-induced unconsciousness in subanalgesic doses. *Anesth Analg* (1990) 71, 65–9.
4. Luger TJ, Hill HF, Schlager A. Can midazolam diminish sufentanil analgesia in patients with major trauma? A retrospective study with 43 patients. *Drug Metabol Drug Interact* (1992) 10, 177–84.
5. Zacny JP, Coalson DW, Klafta JM, Klock PA, Alessi R, Rupani G, Young CJ, Patil PG, Apfelbaum JL. Midazolam does not influence intravenous fentanyl-induced analgesia in healthy volunteers. *Pharmacol Biochem Behav* (1996) 55, 275–80.
6. Burtin P, Daoud P, Jacqz-Aigrain E, Mussat E, Moriette G. Hypotension with midazolam and fentanyl in the newborn. *Lancet* (1991) 337, 1545–6.
7. Yaster M, Nichols DG, Deshpande JK, Wetzel RC. Midazolam-fentanyl intravenous sedation in children: case report of respiratory arrest. *Pediatrics* (1991) 86, 463–6.
8. Bailey PL, Moll JWB, Pace NL, East KA, Stanley TH. Respiratory effects of midazolam and fentanyl: potent interaction producing hypoxemia and apnea. *Anesthesiology* (1988) 69, 3A, A813.
9. Bailey PL, Andriano KP, Pace NL, Westenskow DR, Stanley TH. Small doses of fentanyl potentiate and prolong diazepam induced respiratory depression. *Anesth Analg* (1984) 63, 183.
10. Heikkïlä J, Jalonen J, Arola M, Kanto J, Laaksonen V. Midazolam as adjunct to high-dose fentanyl anaesthesia for coronary artery bypass grafting operation. *Acta Anaesthesiol Scand* (1984) 28, 683–89.
11. Tomicheck RC, Rosow CE, Philbin DM, Moss J, Teplick RS, Schneider RC. Diazepam-fentanyl interaction — hemodynamic and hormonal effects in coronary artery surgery. *Anesth Analg* (1983) 62, 881–4.
12. West JM, Estrada S, Heerdt M. Sudden hypotension associated with midazolam and sufentanil. *Anesth Analg* (1987) 66, 693–4.
13. Spiess BD, Sathoff RH, El-Ganzouri ARS, Ivankovich AD. High-dose sufentanil: four cases of sudden hypotension on induction. *Anesth Analg* (1986) 65, 703–5.
14. Persson MP, Nilsson A, Hartvig P. Relation of sedation and amnesia to plasma concentrations of midazolam in surgical patients. *Clin Pharmacol Ther* (1988) 43, 324–31.

Opioids; Fentanyl and related drugs + H_2-blockers

Cimetidine, but not ranitidine, increases the plasma levels of alfentanil. Some preliminary observations suggest that the effects of fentanyl may be increased by cimetidine.

Clinical evidence, mechanism, importance and management

(a) Alfentanil

A pharmacokinetic study in 19 intensive care patients[1] intravenous **cimetidine** 1.2 g daily for 2 days was given with a single 125-microgram/kg intravenous dose of alfentanil. The cimetidine increased the alfentanil half-life by 75 or 62%, and reduced the clearance by 64 or 54% when compared with an oral aluminium/magnesium hydroxide antacid and intravenous **ranitidine** 300 mg daily respectively. The alfentanil plasma levels were significantly raised by the **cimetidine**, probably because **cimetidine** inhibits the metabolism of the alfentanil, thereby reducing its loss. Whether the alfentanil effects are increased to a clinically important extent awaits assessment. However, be alert for increased alfentanil effects because pharmacokinetic changes of this size are known to be clinically important in some patients (see 'macrolides', (p.112) and 'azoles', (p.110). **Ranitidine** did not interact.

(b) Fentanyl

The terminal half-life of fentanyl 100 micrograms/kg was reported to be more than doubled, from 155 to 340 minutes by pretreatment with **cime-**

tidine (10 mg/kg the night before and 5 mg/kg 90 minutes before the fentanyl dose). The possible reason is that the **cimetidine** inhibits the metabolism of fentanyl by the liver, thereby delaying its clearance from the body.[2] The clinical importance of this interaction has not been assessed, but if both drugs are used concurrently, be alert for increased and prolonged fentanyl effects.

1. Kienlen J, Levron J-C, Aubas S, Roustan J-P, du Cailar J. Pharmacokinetics of alfentanil in patients treated with either cimetidine or ranitidine. *Drug Invest* (1993) 6, 257–62.
2. Unpublished data quoted by Maurer PM, Barkowski RR. Drug interactions of clinical significance with opioid analgesics. *Drug Safety* (1993) 8, 30–48.

Opioids; Fentanyl and related drugs + Macrolides

Some patients may experience prolonged and increased alfentanil effects if they are given erythromycin or particularly troleandomycin. Troleandomycin also interacts with fentanyl but to a lesser extent. Erythromycin appears not to interact with sufentanil. Consider also 'Opioids; Dextromoramide + Troleandomycin', p.109.

Clinical evidence

(a) Erythromycin

Erythromycin 500 mg twice daily for 7 days increased the mean half-life of **alfentanil** in 6 subjects from 84 to 131 minutes and decreased the clearance by 26%. The two most sensitive subjects had considerable changes with only one day of erythromycin treatment, and overall showed a marked change. The other 4 subjects had only small or moderate changes.[1]

A 32-year old man undergoing exploratory laparotomy was given erythromycin 1 g and neomycin 1 g, both three times daily, on the day before surgery. He was given pancuronium, **alfentanil** and thiopental for induction, followed by suxamethonium (succinylcholine) and N_2O/O_2. Anaesthesia was maintained with **alfentanil**. Altogether he received 20.9 mg of **alfentanil**. An hour after recovery he was found to be unrousable and with a respiratory rate of only 5 breaths per minute. He was successfully treated with naloxone.[2] Another patient given **alfentanil** and erythromycin is said to have developed respiratory arrest during recovery.[3]

In contrast, 7 days' treatment with erythromycin 500 mg twice daily in 6 healthy subjects was found not to affect the pharmacokinetics of intravenous **sufentanil** 3 micrograms/kg in the 9 hours following administration.[4] Two of the subjects were the same as those who had shown an alfentanil/erythromycin interaction cited above.

(b) Troleandomycin

A study in 9 healthy subjects given troleandomycin 500 mg orally found that the clearance of intravenous **alfentanil** 20 micrograms/kg was reduced by almost 70% when compared to subjects given placebo.[5] Another study found that troleandomycin (500 mg starting 105 minutes before alfentanil then 250 mg every 6 hours for 3 doses) reduced the clearance of **alfentanil** by 88%.[6] This study found that troleandomycin only reduced **fentanyl** clearance by 39%.

Mechanism

Troleandomycin, and to a lesser extent erythromycin, inhibit the cytochrome P450 isoenzyme CYP3A4 in the liver, which is involved in the metabolism of alfentanil, sufentanil and fentanyl. However, in contrast to alfentanil, sufentanil and fentanyl are high extraction drugs (see 'Changes in first-pass metabolism', (p.4)) and are therefore less likely to be affected by changes in liver metabolism.[6,7]

Importance and management

The interactions of alfentanil with erythromycin and troleandomycin appear to be established and clinically important. Alfentanil should be given in reduced amounts or avoided in those who have recently had either of these drugs.[1] Be alert for evidence of prolonged alfentanil effects and respiratory depression. The interaction appears not to affect all patients given erythromycin. Alternatively, sufentanil in doses of 3 micrograms/kg or less can be used instead, but much larger doses of sufentanil should be given with caution.[4] Fentanyl is another alternative for use with erythromycin, but should probably be used with caution with troleandomycin. Consider also 'Opioids; Dextromoramide + Troleandomycin', p.109.

1. Bartkowski RR, Goldberg ME, Larijani GE and Boerner T. Inhibition of alfentanil metabolism by erythromycin. *Clin Pharmacol Ther* (1989) 46, 99–102.
2. Bartkowski RR, McDonnell TE. Prolonged alfentanil effect following erythromycin administration. *Anesthesiology* (1990) 73, 566–8.
3. Yate PM, Thomas D, Short TSM, Sebel PS, Morton J. Comparison of infusions of alfentanil or pethidine for sedation of ventilated patients on ITU. *Br J Anaesth* (1986) 58, 1091–9.
4. Bartkowski RR, Goldberg ME, Huffnagle S, Epstein RH. Sufentanil disposition. Is it affected by erythromycin administration? *Anesthesiology* (1993) 78, 260–5.
5. Kharasch ED, Russell M, Mautz D, Thummel KE, Kunze KL, Bowdle A, Cox K. The role of cytochrome P450 3A4 in alfentanil clearance: implications for interindividual variability in disposition and perioperative drug interactions. *Anesthesiology* (1997) 87, 36–50.
6. Ibrahim AE, Feldman J, Karim A, Kharasch ED. Simultaneous assessment of drug interactions with low- and high-extraction opioids. Application to parecoxib effects on the pharmacokinetics and pharmacodynamics of fentanyl and alfentanil. *Anesthesiology* (2003) 98, 853–61.
7. Kharasch ED, Thummel KE. Human alfentanil metabolism by cytochrome P450 3A3/4. An explanation for the interindividual variability in alfentanil clearance? *Anesth Analg* (1993) 76, 1033–9.

Opioids; Fentanyl and related drugs + Parecoxib or Valdecoxib

Parecoxib had no effect on the pharmacokinetics of alfentanil or fentanyl.

Clinical evidence, mechanism, importance and management

Parecoxib 40 mg intravenously given one hour before and 12 hours after an infusion of **alfentanil** 15 micrograms/kg or fentanyl 5 micrograms/kg had no effect on the pharmacokinetics of these opioids in a crossover study in 12 healthy subjects.[1] Pupil diameter versus time curves were not affected by parecoxib. This interaction was investigated because both valdecoxib (for which parecoxib is a prodrug) and **alfentanil** are substrates of the cytochrome P450 isoenzyme CYP3A4. The study suggests there should be no interaction during concurrent use.

1. Ibrahim AE, Feldman J, Karim A, Kharasch ED. Simultaneous assessment of drug interactions with low- and high-extraction opioids. Application to parecoxib effects on the pharmacokinetics and pharmacodynamics of fentanyl and alfentanil. *Anesthesiology* (2003) 98, 853–61.

Opioids; Fentanyl + Quinidine

Quinidine appears to increase the oral absorption and therefore the effects of fentanyl, but does not significantly alter intravenous fentanyl-induced miosis. See also 'morphine', (p.120), and compare 'codeine', (p.108).

Clinical evidence, mechanism, importance and management

Quinidine sulfate 600 mg given one hour before an infusion of fentanyl 2.5 micrograms/kg did not alter the fentanyl-induced miosis in healthy subjects. However, the same dose of quinidine given before *oral* fentanyl 2.5 micrograms/kg (with ondansetron as an antiemetic) did increase fentanyl-induced miosis. This increase was considered proportionate to the increase in the AUC of fentanyl (160%). There was no change in the elimination half-life of fentanyl.[1]

It was suggested that quinidine inhibits the intestinal drug efflux pump P-glycoprotein and so allows an increase in oral fentanyl absorption, and a consequent increase in effect. The effects on miosis indicate that quinidine did not alter brain access of fentanyl.[1]

The clinical importance of this finding to the use of *buccal* fentanyl citrate (of which a significant proportion is swallowed) remains to be determined, but be aware that effects may be increased. See also 'Opioids; Morphine + Quinidine', p.120, and compare 'Opioids; Codeine and related drugs + Quinidine', p.108.

1. Kharasch ED, Hoffer C, Altuntas TG, Whittington D. Quinidine as a probe for the role of P-glycoprotein in the intestinal absorption and clinical effects of fentanyl. *J Clin Pharmacol* (2004) 44, 224–33.

methadone (an indicator of increased *N*-demethylation) when given disulfiram 500 mg daily for 7 days. However, there was no effect on the degree of opiate intoxication, nor were withdrawal symptoms experienced.[1] No special precautions would seem to be necessary.

1. Tong TG, Benowitz NL, Kreek MJ. Methadone-disulfiram interaction during methadone maintenance. *J Clin Pharmacol* (1980) 20, 506–13.

Opioids; Methadone + Fusidic acid

There is evidence that long-term fusidic acid may modestly reduce the effects of methadone.

Clinical evidence, mechanism, importance and management

A drug abuser with AIDS needed an increase in levomethadone (*R*-methadone) dosage from 60 to 80 mg daily within 6 months of starting to take fusidic acid 1.5 g daily.[1] The patient showed evidence of liver enzyme induction (using antipyrine as a marker of induction), from which it was concluded that fusidic acid increases the metabolism and loss of methadone from the body.[1] A subsequent study confirmed that fusidic acid 500 mg daily for 28 days increased antipyrine clearance in 10 patients on levomethadone, and some of them developed clinical signs of underdosage. In contrast, fusidic acid 500 mg daily for 14 days had no effect in another 10 patients on levomethadone.[2]

Information appears to be limited to these reports. Bear them in mind in the event of any unexpected reduction in efficacy of methadone in a patient treated with long-term fusidic acid.

1. Brockmeyer NH, Mertins L, Goos M. Pharmacokinetic interaction of antimicrobial agents with levomethadon in drug-addicted AIDS patients. *Klin Wochenschr* (1991) 69, 16–18.
2. Reimann G, Barthel B, Rockstroh JK, Spatz D, Brockmeyer NH. Effect of fusidic acid on the hepatic cytochrome P450 enzyme system. *Int J Clin Pharmacol* (1999) 37, 562–6.

Opioids; Methadone + NNRTIs

Methadone plasma levels can be markedly reduced by efavirenz or nevirapine and withdrawal symptoms have been seen. In one study methadone had no effect on delavirdine levels.

Clinical evidence

(a) Delavirdine

The pharmacokinetics of delavirdine 600 mg twice daily did not differ between 16 HIV-negative subjects on methadone maintenance therapy and 15 healthy control subjects.[1]

(b) Efavirenz

An HIV+ woman who had been on methadone for over a year began to complain of discomfort within 4 weeks of having nelfinavir replaced by efavirenz 600 mg daily, and by 8 weeks typical methadone withdrawal symptoms were occurring late in the afternoon. It was found that the levels of (*R*)-methadone (the active enantiomer) had fallen from 168 to 90 nanograms/ml, and those of the (*S*)-methadone from 100 to 28 nanograms/ml. The methadone dosage had to be increased from 100 mg to 180 mg daily before the symptoms disappeared.[2] A further case is reported in which a man on maintenance methadone stopped taking efavirenz 600 mg daily because of the occurrence of withdrawal symptoms in spite of increased methadone dosage.[3] Another report describes a man who required a 133% increase in methadone dose over 4 weeks after starting efavirenz, and mentions two other patients who complained of opioid abstinence shortly after starting efavirenz. They also required methadone dose increases.[4]

In a pharmacokinetic study, 11 patients on methadone 35 to 100 mg daily were given efavirenz plus dual nucleoside analogues. Nine of the patients developed methadone withdrawal symptoms and needed dose increases of 15 to 30 mg (mean 22%). A pharmacokinetic study of these patients showed that 3 weeks after starting efavirenz their mean methadone AUCs were reduced by 57% and their maximum plasma levels by 48%.[5] In another retrospective study, 6 out of 7 patients needed methadone dosage increases of 8% to 200% within 2 weeks to 8 months of starting an efavirenz-based regimen.[6]

(c) Nevirapine

A retrospective review revealed 7 cases of patients on methadone maintenance who developed withdrawal symptoms after starting regimens including nevirapine. The symptoms developed within 4 to 8 days, and methadone dose increases of 21% to 186% were required. Despite this, 3 patients did not respond, and elected to discontinue nevirapine, and in 2 of these somnolence developed within 2 weeks, and the methadone dosage was reduced back down. Methadone plasma levels were available in 2 patients, and these revealed a decrease of about 90% in methadone levels after starting nevirapine.[7] In a pilot study of a once daily nevirapine-containing regimen, 30% of patients required an increase in methadone dosage.[8] Others reported that 4 of 5 patients on methadone developed withdrawal symptoms on starting nevirapine-including regimens and two refused further nevirapine despite an increase in methadone dose. Another 2 patients were successfully treated with increases in their methadone doses of 33% and 100%.[9] Two other similar cases have been reported.[3,10]

In a pharmacokinetic study, 8 patients on methadone maintenance (dose range 30 to 120 mg daily) had methadone levels measured before and 14 days after starting antiretroviral therapy including nevirapine 200 mg daily. The methadone AUC decreased by 52%, and the maximum level by 36%. Six patients complained of symptoms of methadone withdrawal, and required a mean increase in methadone dose of 16%.[11]

Mechanism

Efavirenz and nevirapine induce the metabolism of methadone (possibly by the cytochrome P450 isoenzyme CYP3A4, or CYP2B6[12]), the effect of which would be to increase its loss from the body, thereby reducing its effects. In contrast, delavirdine is an inhibitor of various cytochrome P450 isoenzymes, and might therefore be expected to inhibit the metabolism of methadone, but this requires confirmation.

Importance and management

Established interactions of clinical importance. If efavirenz or nevirapine are added to established treatment with methadone, be alert for evidence of opiate withdrawal, and raise the methadone dose accordingly. Some patients may require an increase in methadone dose frequency to twice daily.[9] Some authors have found that the dosage increase required is much less than that predicted based on the reduction in methadone levels,[5,11] whereas others have questioned this.[4,13] It may be important not to confuse the adverse effects of the NNRTIs with withdrawal symptoms.[5] In patients who subsequently discontinue the NNRTI, the methadone dose should be gradually reduced.[5,7]

1. Booker B, Smith P, Forrest A, DiFrancesco R, Morse G, Cottone P, Murphy M, McCance-Katz E. Lack of effect of methadone on the pharmacokinetics of delavirdine & N-delavirdine. *Intersci Conf Antimicrob Agents Chemother* (2001) 41, 14.
2. Marzolini C, Troillet N, Telenti A, Baumann P, Decosterd LA, Eap CB. Efavirenz decreases methadone blood concentrations. *AIDS* (2000) 14, 1291–2.
3. Pinzani V, Faucherre V, Peyriere H, Blayac J-P. Methadone withdrawal symptoms with nevirapine and efavirenz. *Ann Pharmacother* (2000) 34, 405–7.
4. Boffito M, Rossati A, Reynolds HE, Hoggard PG, Back DJ, di Perri G. Undefined duration of opiate withdrawal induced by efavirenz in drug users with HIV infection and undergoing chronic methadone treatment. *AIDS Res Hum Retroviruses* (2002) 18, 341–2.
5. Clarke SM, Mulcahy FM, Tjia J, Reynolds HE, Gibbons SE, Barry MG, Back DJ. The pharmacokinetics of methadone in HIV-positive patients receiving the non-nucleoside reverse transcriptase inhibitor efavirenz. *Br J Clin Pharmacol* (2001) 51, 213–7.
6. Tashima K, Bose T, Gormley J, Sousa H, Flanigan TP. The potential impact of efavirenz on methadone maintenance. Poster presented at 9th European Conference on Clinical Microbiology and Infectious Diseases, Berlin, March 23rd 1999 (Poster PO552).
7. Altice FL, Friedland GH, Cooney EL. Nevirapine induced opiate withdrawal among injection drug users with HIV infection receiving methadone. *AIDS* (1999) 13, 957–62.
8. Staszewski S, Haberl A, Gute P, Nisius G, Miller V, Carlebach A. Nevirapine/didanosine/lamivudine once daily in HIV-1 infected intravenous drug users. *Antivir Ther* (1998) 3 (Suppl 4), 55–6.
9. Otero M-J, Fuertes A, Sánchez R, Luna G. Nevirapine-induced withdrawal symptoms in HIV patients on methadone maintenance programme: an alert. *AIDS* (1999) 13, 1004–5.
10. Heelon MW, Meade LB. Methadone withdrawal when starting an antiretroviral regimen including nevirapine. *Pharmacotherapy* (1999) 19, 471–2.
11. Clarke SM, Mulcahy FM, Tjia J, Reynolds HE, Gibbons SE, Barry MG, Back DJ. Pharmacokinetic interactions of nevirapine and methadone and guidelines for use of nevirapine to treat injection drug users. *Clin Infect Dis* (2001) 33, 1595–7.
12. Gerber JG, Rhodes RJ, Gal J. Stereoselective metabolism of methadone N-demethylation by cytochrome P4502B6 and 2C19. *Chirality* (2004) 16, 36–44.
13. Calvo R, Lukas JC, Rodriguez M, Carlos MA, Suarez E. Pharmacokinetics of methadone in HIV-positive patients receiving the non-nucleoside reverse transcriptase efavirenz. *Br J Clin Pharmacol* (2002) 53, 211–14.

Opioids; Methadone + NRTIs

Zidovudine had no effect on methadone levels in one study, but there is one report of a patient requiring a modest increase in

methadone dose after starting zidovudine. Methadone can increase zidovudine serum levels, and reduce levels of didanosine from the tablet formulation, but not the enteric-coated capsule preparation. Small decreases in stavudine levels may occur. Similarly, small changes in the pharmacokinetics of abacavir and methadone occur on concurrent use, and there is a report of two patients requiring increases in methadone dose. The clinical relevance of all these changes is uncertain. A single dose of zidovudine/lamivudine had no effect on methadone pharmacokinetics.

Clinical evidence

(a) Abacavir

Eleven patients given methadone with abacavir had a 23% increase in the rate of methadone clearance but no change in the half-life or renal clearance. In addition, there was a 34% decrease in the peak concentration of abacavir, which occurred later, but no change in abacavir clearance or half-life.[1] Of 3 patients on methadone maintenance who started treatment with abacavir, lamivudine and zidovudine, 2 required methadone dosage increases (31% and 46%). The abacavir was thought to be responsible.[2]

(b) Didanosine

A study in 17 subjects on methadone maintenance found that the AUC and maximum levels of didanosine tablets was 57% and 66% lower respectively when compared with 10 control subjects. Trough levels of methadone did not differ from historical controls, suggesting that didanosine had no effect on methadone pharmacokinetics.[3] A later study showed that there was no reduction in the AUC of didanosine given as enteric-coated capsules.[4]

(c) Stavudine

A study in 17 subjects on methadone maintenance found that the AUC and maximum levels of stavudine were 23% and 44% lower respectively when compared with 10 control subjects. Trough levels of methadone did not differ from historical controls suggesting that stavudine had no effect on methadone pharmacokinetics.[3]

(d) Zidovudine

(i) Methadone effects reduced or unaffected. A drug abuser with AIDS needed an increase in his levomethadone (*R*-methadone) dosage from 40 to 60 mg daily, within a month of beginning treatment with zidovudine 1 g daily.[5]
In contrast, a study found no evidence of any change in the pharmacokinetics of methadone in HIV+ patients on methadone maintenance 14 days after they started zidovudine 200 mg every 4 hours. No methadone withdrawal symptoms occurred.[6] Another study in 16 patients on methadone maintenance found that a single-dose of a fixed combination of zidovudine 300 mg with lamivudine 150 mg *(Combivir)* had no effect on the pharmacokinetics of methadone, and there was no evidence of withdrawal or toxicity.[7]

(ii) Zidovudine effects increased. In one study the AUC of zidovudine was increased on average by 43% by methadone, and in 4 of 9 patients it was doubled.[6] In another study, 8 HIV+ patients starting methadone maintenance found a 29% increase in the AUC of oral zidovudine and a 41% increase in the AUC of intravenous zidovudine.[8] Decreased zidovudine clearance in patients on methadone is described in another report.[9]

Mechanism

Uncertain. It appears that methadone reduces the bioavailability of didanosine, and to a lesser extent, stavudine, possibly because it delays gastric emptying. Thus, the enteric-coated didanosine preparation appears not to be affected.[3,4] Conversely, methadone apparently reduces the glucuronidation of the zidovudine by the liver, resulting in an increase in its serum levels.[10] Methadone may also reduce renal clearance of zidovudine.[8]

Importance and management

The increase in zidovudine levels with methadone is established, although the clinical relevance is uncertain. Be alert for any increase in zidovudine adverse effects. The balance of evidence suggests that zidovudine is unlikely to reduce methadone levels, and the one case reported remains unexplained. However, note that some of the adverse effects of zidovudine may be mistaken for opioid withdrawal effects.

The reduction in didanosine levels with methadone may be clinically relevant, and the authors suggest increasing the dose of the tablet formulation. Monitor virological response. The enteric-coated didanosine preparation is not affected.

The reduction in stavudine levels and the changes in abacavir peak levels with methadone are probably not clinically relevant, but again, further data are required. The reports with abacavir suggest that it would be prudent to monitor methadone dose requirements when this drug is started.

1. Sellers E, Lam R, McDowell J, Corrigan B, Hedayetullah N, Somer G, Kirby L, Kersey K, Yuen G. The pharmacokinetics of abacavir and methadone following coadministration: CNAA1012. *Intersci Conf Antimicrob Agents Chemother* (1999) 39, 663.
2. Pardo López MA, Pastor C, Pérez Hervás MP, Fernández Villalba E. Síndrome de abstinencia a opiáceos tras la administración de zidovudina + lamivudina + abacavir en pacientes infectados por el virus de la inmunodeficiencia humana en tratamiento con metadona. *Rev Clin Esp* (2003) 203, 407–8.
3. Rainey PM, Friedland G, McCance-Katz EF, Andrews L, Mitchell SM, Charles C, Jatlow P. Interactions of methadone with didanosine and stavudine. *J Acquir Immune Defic Syndr* (2000) 24, 241–8.
4. Friedland G, Rainey P, Jatlow P, Andrews L, Damle B, McCance-Katz E. Pharmacokinetics of didanosine from encapsulated enteric coated bead formulation vs chewable tablet formulation in patients on chronic methadone therapy. XIV International AIDS Conference, Barcelona, 2002. Abstract TuPeB4548.
5. Brockmeyer NH, Mertins L, Goos M. Pharmacokinetic interaction of antimicrobial agents with levomethadon in drug-addicted AIDS patients. *Klin Wochenschr* (1991) 69, 16–18.
6. Schwartz EL, Brechbühl A-B, Kahl P, Miller MA, Selwyn PA, Friedland GH. Pharmacokinetic interactions of zidovudine and methadone in intravenous drug-using patients with HIV infection. *J Acquir Immune Defic Syndr* (1992) 5, 619–26.
7. Rainey PM, Friedland GH, Snidow JW, McCance-Katz EF, Mitchell SM, Andrews L, Lane B, Jatlow P. The pharmacokinetics of methadone following co-administration with a lamivudine/zidovudine combination tablet in opiate-dependent subjects.*Am J Addict* (2002) 11, 66–74.
8. McCance-Katz EF, Rainey PM, Jatlow P, Friedland G. Methadone effects on zidovudine disposition (AIDS clinical trials group 262). *J Acquir Immune Defic Syndr Hum Retrovirol* (1998) 18, 435–43.
9. Burger DM, Meenhorst PL, ten Napel CHH, Mulder JW, Neef C, Koks CHW, Bult A, Beijnen JH. Pharmacokinetic variability of zidovudine in HIV-infected individuals: subgroup analysis and drug interactions. *AIDS* (1994) 8, 1683–9.
10. Cretton-Scott E, de Sousa G, Nicolas F, Rahmani R, Sommadossi J-P. Methadone and its metabolite N-demethyl methadone, inhibit AZT glucuronidation in vitro. *Clin Pharmacol Ther* (1996) 59, 168.

Opioids; Methadone + Protease inhibitors

Methadone serum levels can be reduced by amprenavir, nelfinavir, lopinavir/ritonavir, ritonavir/saquinavir, and possibly ritonavir. An increased methadone dosage may be needed in some patients to prevent opiate withdrawal. No interaction appears to occur with indinavir or possibly saquinavir alone.

Clinical evidence

(a) Amprenavir

Methadone levels were reduced by 35% (range 28% to 87%) in 5 patients within 17 days of starting to take amprenavir 1200 mg twice daily and abacavir 600 mg twice daily. Two patients reported nausea before their daily methadone dose, which can be a sign of opiate withdrawal.[1] Note that abacavir may modestly reduce methadone levels, and could therefore have contributed to this effect, see 'Opioids; Methadone + NRTIs', p.115.

(b) Indinavir

A multiple dose, randomised, two-period, crossover study in 12 patients on methadone maintenance found that the pharmacokinetics of methadone were unchanged by indinavir 800 mg every 8 hours for 8 days. A small decrease in indinavir peak levels and a small increase in trough levels was noted when compared with historical controls.[2] Another study in 6 HIV+ patients on methadone and two nucleoside analogues similarly found that methadone serum levels remained unchanged when indinavir was added.[3,4]

There are also clinical reports about 2 patients whose methadone levels appeared to be unaltered while taking indinavir, but who later had reduced levels when treated with nelfinavir or ritonavir (see (b) and (c) below).[5,6] This would seem to confirm that indinavir does not have a clinically relevant effect on maintenance treatment with methadone.

(c) Lopinavir/ritonavir

Lopinavir/ritonavir 400 mg/100 mg twice daily for 7 days decreased the AUC of methadone by 26% and increased its clearance by 42% in 15 healthy subjects on methadone maintenance therapy. Four of the subjects had clinically important increases in opiate-withdrawal scores, and were all found to have subtherapeutic trough methadone levels.[7] [Note that the same dose of ritonavir alone had no effect on methadone levels, see (e) below]. Similarly, in another study, lopinavir/ritonavir based antiretroviral therapy reduced the AUC of methadone by 36% after 14 days' treatment in 8 HIV+ patients on methadone maintenance. However, none of these patients experienced methadone withdrawal during the study or during 6 weeks of follow-up.[8] In another study (that did not measure methadone levels), none of 18 patients experienced methadone withdrawal during the 28 days after starting lopinavir/ritonavir.[9]

In another study, methadone appeared to have no effect on lopinavir pharmacokinetics, and no effect on ritonavir pharmacokinetics when given with lopinavir.[10]

(d) Nelfinavir

An HIV+ man who had been stable on methadone 100 mg daily for several years and taking indinavir 800 mg and zalcitabine 750 micrograms three times daily, developed opiate withdrawal symptoms within 6 weeks of starting stavudine and nelfinavir 750 mg three times daily. His methadone dosage was increased to 285 mg daily before therapeutic serum levels were achieved. When his antiretroviral treatment was withdrawn, his methadone dosage was successfully reduced to 125 mg daily.[6] Two other patients on nucleoside analogues had a 40 to 50% fall in serum methadone levels when nelfinavir was added.[3,4] Similarly, the makers of nelfinavir say that in a pharmacokinetic study nelfinavir reduced the concentrations of methadone and its metabolites by 29 to 47%. However, despite this reduction none of the subjects developed withdrawal symptoms.[11] Conversely, 4 of 6 patients in another study developed symptoms of methadone withdrawal within 5 to 7 days of starting nelfinavir-based therapy. They had mean reductions in methadone AUC of 56%.[12]

In another study looking at the levels of nelfinavir and its metabolite M8, methadone tended to increase the exposure to nelfinavir, and reduced the AUC of M8 by 47%.[13]

(e) Ritonavir

A patient on lamivudine and zidovudine had a marked decrease in methadone serum levels when ritonavir was added.[3,4]

Eleven healthy subjects were given a single 20-mg dose of methadone on day 1 of a study, followed by a 2-week washout period and then ritonavir on days 15 to 28. On day 25 a single 5-mg dose of methadone was given. It was found that the ritonavir reduced the maximum serum levels of the methadone by 37.8% and the AUC by 36.3%.[14] However, in another study, ritonavir 100 mg twice daily for 7 days had no significant effect on methadone pharmacokinetics in 15 healthy subjects on methadone maintenance.[7]

In a further study, methadone apparently increased ritonavir exposure by 60%, but had no effect on ritonavir pharmacokinetics when this was given with lopinavir.[10]

(f) Ritonavir/Saquinavir

A patient taking methadone 90 mg daily with indinavir, lamivudine and zidovudine, developed withdrawal symptoms and was hospitalised within a week of stopping these HIV drugs and starting ritonavir 400 mg, saquinavir 400 mg and stavudine 40 mg twice daily. The patient was eventually re-stabilised on methadone 130 mg daily.[5]

A later study in 12 HIV+ subjects on methadone maintenance found that ritonavir/saquinavir 400/400 mg twice daily decreased the (*S*)-methadone AUC by 40% and the (*R*)-methadone AUC by 32%. However, when these decreases were corrected for changes in protein binding, the free (*R*)-methadone AUC was decreased by only 19.6%, and the free (*S*)-methadone AUC by 24.6%. None of the subjects experienced methadone withdrawal or required a change in their methadone dosage.[15] Similarly, in another study ritonavir/saquinavir 100/1600 mg twice daily caused no clinically relevant changes in total or free levels of either enantiomer of methadone in 12 HIV-negative subjects on methadone maintenance therapy. No subjects experienced methadone withdrawal.[16]

(g) Saquinavir

A study in an HIV+ patient on methadone and two nucleoside analogues found that methadone serum levels remained unchanged when saquinavir was added.[3,4]

Mechanism

Not known. The findings are the opposite of those originally predicted based on *in vitro* data showing *inhibition* of methadone metabolism (mediated by the cytochrome P450 isoenzyme CYP3A).[17] It is possible that these protease inhibitors induce the activity of other isoenzymes or act via other mechanisms (e.g. glucuronyltransferases). The reduction in methadone levels has not always correlated with clinical effects, and it has been suggested that this may be because of enantiomer selective changes in pharmacokinetics and/or altered protein binding.

Importance and management

Information is limited but the interactions with amprenavir, nelfinavir, lopinavir/ritonavir, saquinavir/ritonavir, and probably ritonavir would appear to be established. However the picture seems to be that not all patients experience withdrawal symptoms if given these drugs. Monitor well so that those who do need a dosage increase can be identified. Indinavir appears not to interact, and very limited evidence suggests that saquinavir alone does not interact either. Consider also 'Opioids + Ritonavir', p.105.

1. Bart P-A, Rizzardi PG, Gallant S, Golay KP, Baumann P, Pantaleo G, Eap CB. Methadone blood concentrations are decreased by the administration of abacavir plus amprenavir. *Ther Drug Monit* (2001) 23, 553–5.
2. Cantilena L, McCrea J, Blazes D, Winchell G, Carides A, Royce C, Deutsch P. Lack of a pharmacokinetic interaction between indinavir and methadone. *Clin Pharmacol Ther* (1999) 65, 135.
3. Touzeau D, Beauverie P, Bouchez J, Poisson N, Edel Y, Dessalles M-C, Lherm J, Furlan V, Lagarde B. Méthadone et nouveau anti-rétroviraux. Résultats du suivi thérapeutique. *Ann Med Interne (Paris)* (1999) 150, 355–6.
4. Beauverie P, Taburet A-M, Dessalles M-C, Furlan V, Touzeau D. Therapeutic monitoring of methadone in HIV-infected patients receiving protease inhibitors. *AIDS* (1998) 12, 2510–11.
5. Geletko SM, Erickson AD. Decreased methadone effect after ritonavir initiation. *Pharmacotherapy* (2000) 20, 93–4.
6. McCance-Katz EF, Farber S, Selwyn PA, O'Connor A. Decrease in methadone levels with nelfinavir mesylate. *Am J Psychiatry* (2000) 157, 481.
7. McCance-Katz EF, Rainey PM, Friedland G, Jatlow P. The protease inhibitor lopinavir-ritonavir may produce opiate withdrawal in methadone-maintained patients. *Clin Infect Dis* (2003) 37, 476–82.
8. Clarke S, Mulcahy F, Bergin C, Reynolds H, Boyle N, Barry M, Back DJ. Absence of opioid withdrawal symptoms in patients receiving methadone and the protease inhibitor lopinavir-ritonavir. *Clin Infect Dis* (2002) 34, 1143–5.
9. Stevens RC, Rapaport S, Maroldo-Connelly L, Patterson JB, Bertz R. Lack of methadone dose alterations or withdrawal symptoms during therapy with lopinavir/ritonavir. *J Acquir Immune Defic Syndr* (2003) 33, 650–1.
10. Smith P, McCance-Katz E, Sarlo J, Di Francesco R, Morse GD. Methadone increases ritonavir exposure when administered alone but not lopinavir/RTV combination. *Intersci Conf Antimicrob Agents Chemother* (2003) 43, 339.
11. Viracept (Nelfinavir mesilate). Roche Products Ltd. UK Summary of product characteristics, June 2005.
12. Clarke S, Mulcahy F, Bergin C, Tjia J, Brown R, Barry M, Back DJ. The pharmacokinetic interaction between methadone and nelfinavir [abstract P276]. *AIDS* (2000) 14 (Suppl 4), S95.
13. Smith PF, Booker BM, Di Francesco R, Morse GD, Cottone PF, Murphy MK, McCance-Katz, E. Effect of methadone or LAAM on the pharmacokinetics of nelfinavir & M8. *Intersci Conf Antimicrob Agents Chemother* (2001) 41, 14.
14. Hsu A, Granneman GR, Carothers L, Dennis S, Chiu Y-L, Valdes J, Sun E. Ritonavir does not increase methadone exposure in healthy volunteers. 5th Conference on Retroviruses and Opportunistic Infection, Chicago, Feb 1–5, 1998, abstract 342.
15. Gerber JG, Rosenkranz S, Segal Y, Aberg J, D'Amico R, Mildvan D, Gulick R, Hughes V, Flexner C, Aweeka F, Hsu A, Gal J. Effect of ritonavir/saquinavir on stereoselective pharmacokinetics of methadone: Results of AIDS Clinical Trials Group (ACTG) 401. *J Acquir Immune Defic Syndr* (2001) 27, 153–60.
16. Shelton MJ, Cloen D, DiFrancesco R, Berenson CS, Esch A, de Caprariis PJ, Palic B, Schur JL, Buggé CJL, Ljungqvist A, Espinosa O, Hewitt RG. The effects of once-daily saquinavir/minidose ritonavir on the pharmacokinetics of methadone. *J Clin Pharmacol* (2004) 44, 293–304.
17. Iribarne C, Berthou F, Carlhant D, Dreano Y, Picart D, Lohezic F, Riche C. Inhibition of methadone and buprenorphine *N*-dealkylations by three HIV-1 protease inhibitors. *Drug Metab Dispos* (1998) 26, 257–60.

Opioids; Methadone + Rifamycins

Serum methadone levels can be markedly reduced by rifampicin, and withdrawal symptoms have occurred in some patients. Rifabutin appears to interact to a lesser extent, so fewer patients are likely to be affected. Consider also 'Opioids + Rifampicin (Rifampin)', p.105.

Clinical evidence

(a) Rifabutin

A study in 24 HIV+ patients on methadone maintenance found that after taking rifabutin 300 mg daily for 13 days the pharmacokinetics of the methadone were minimally changed. However 75% of the patients reported at least one mild symptom of methadone withdrawal, but this was not enough for any of them to withdraw from the study. Only 3 of them asked for and received an increase in methadone dosage. The authors offered the opinion that over-reporting of withdrawal symptoms was likely to be due to the warnings that the patients had received.[1]

(b) Rifampicin

The observation that former heroin addicts on methadone maintenance complained of withdrawal symptoms when given rifampicin, prompted a study in 30 patients on methadone. Withdrawal symptoms developed in

21 of the 30 within 1 to 33 days of starting rifampicin 600 to 900 mg daily and isoniazid daily. In 6 of the 7 most severely affected, the symptoms developed within a week, and their plasma methadone levels fell by 33 to 68%. None of 56 other patients on methadone and other anti-tubercular treatment (which included isoniazid but not rifampicin) developed withdrawal symptoms.[2-4]

Other cases of this interaction have been reported.[5-9] Some patients needed two to threefold increases in the methadone dosage while taking rifampicin to control the withdrawal symptoms.[6,7,9]

Mechanism

Rifampicin is a potent enzyme-inducing agent, which increases the activity of the liver enzymes concerned with the metabolism of methadone, resulting in a marked increase in its clearance from the body. In 4 patients in the study cited, the urinary excretion of the major metabolite of methadone rose by 150%.[2] Rifabutin has only a small enzyme inducing effect.

Importance and management

The interaction between methadone and rifampicin is established, adequately documented and of clinical importance. The incidence is high. Two-thirds of the narcotic-dependent patients in the study cited[2] developed this interaction, 14 of whom were able to continue treatment. Withdrawal symptoms may develop within 24 hours. The analgesic effects of methadone would also be expected to be reduced. Concurrent use need not be avoided, but the effects should be monitored and appropriate dosage increases (as much as two to threefold) made where necessary.

Rifabutin appears to interact to a very much lesser extent so that fewer patients may need a methadone dosage increase.

1. Brown LS, Sawyer RC, Li R, Cobb MN, Colborn DC, Narang PK. Lack of a pharmacologic interaction between rifabutin and methadone in HIV-infected former injecting drug users. *Drug Alcohol Depend* (1996) 43, 71–7.
2. Kreek MJ, Garfield JW, Gutjahr CL, Giusti LM. Rifampin-induced methadone withdrawal. *N Engl J Med* (1976) 294, 1104–6.
3. Garfield JW, Kreek MJ, Giusti L. Rifampin-methadone relationship. 1. The clinical effects of rifampin-methadone interaction. *Am Rev Respir Dis* (1975) 111, 926.
4. Kreek MJ, Garfield JW, Gutjahr CL, Bowen D, Field F, Rothschild M. Rifampin-methadone relationship. 2. Rifampin effects on plasma concentration, metabolism, and excretion of methadone. *Am Rev Respir Dis* (1975) 111, 926–7.
5. Bending MR, Skacel PO. Rifampicin and methadone withdrawal. *Lancet* (1977) i, 1211.
6. Van Leeuwen DJ. Rifampicine leidt tot onthoudingsverschijnselen bij methadongebruikers. *Ned Tijdschr Geneeskd* (1986) 130, 548–50.
7. Brockmeyer NH, Mertins L, Goos M. Pharmacokinetic interaction of antimicrobial agents with levomethadon in drug-addicted AIDS patients. *Klin Wochenschr* (1991) 69, 16–18.
8. Holmes VF. Rifampin-induced methadone withdrawal in AIDS. *J Clin Psychopharmacol* (1990) 10, 443–4.
9. Raistrick D, Hay A, Wolff K. Methadone maintenance and tuberculosis treatment. *BMJ* (1996) 313, 925–6.

Opioids; Methadone + SSRIs

Methadone serum levels may rise if fluvoxamine is added, sometimes resulting in increased adverse effects. Sertraline, paroxetine, and possibly fluoxetine, may also modestly increase methadone levels. Caution is warranted during combined use.

Clinical evidence

(a) Fluoxetine

Methadone 30 to 100 mg daily, and fluoxetine 20 mg daily were given to 9 patients (two of them were also taking fluvoxamine). Although there were possible compliance problems with some of the patients, the methadone plasma/dose ratio of the group as a whole was not altered by the addition of the fluoxetine.[1] This is consistent with the results of two other studies, which found that fluoxetine did not appear to alter the plasma methadone levels of patients treated for cocaine dependence.[2,3] However, the plasma samples for 7 of the 9 patients in the first study[1] were subsequently analysed again to measure the (*S*)- and (*R*)-enantiomers of methadone separately. This analysis revealed that fluoxetine 20 mg daily modestly increased the levels-to-dose ratio of the active (*R*)-methadone (by 33%) without significantly changing either the total or inactive (*S*)-methadone level-to-dose ratios.[4] Moreover, a patient on methadone developed opioid toxicity when given ciprofloxacin and fluoxetine, see 'Opioids; Methadone + Ciprofloxacin', p.114.

(b) Fluvoxamine

Five patients on maintenance treatment with methadone were additionally given fluvoxamine. Two of them had an increase of about 20% in the methadone plasma/dose ratio, while the other 3 showed 40 to 100% rises. One of them developed asthenia, marked drowsiness and nausea, which disappeared when both drug dosages were reduced.[5] A subsequent analysis of the enantiomers of methadone revealed that fluvoxamine increased levels of both (*R*)- and (*S*)-methadone.[4] A report describes one patient who was unable to maintain adequate methadone levels, despite a daily dosage of 200 mg, and experienced withdrawal symptoms until fluvoxamine was added.[6] Another patient on methadone 70 mg daily and diazepam 2 mg twice daily was admitted to hospital with an acute exacerbation of asthma and intractable cough 3 weeks after additionally starting fluvoxamine 100 mg daily. Blood gas measurements indicated severe hypoxaemia and hypercapnia. The symptoms resolved when the methadone dose was reduced to 50 mg daily and diazepam was gradually withdrawn, at which point methadone levels fell by about 23% (from 262 to 202 nanograms/ml).[7]

(c) Paroxetine

Paroxetine 20 mg daily increased steady-state methadone levels by 35% in 10 patients on methadone maintenance. Both (*R*)- and (*S*)-methadone levels were increased in the 8 patients who were extensive metabolisers of the cytochrome P450 isoenzyme CYP2D6 (see 'Genetic factors', (p.4)), but in the 2 patients who were poor metabolisers, only the (*S*)-methadone levels were increased. Apart from one patient who reported feeling high during the first night after starting paroxetine, no symptoms of overmedication or toxicity were noted.[8]

(d) Sertraline

A placebo-controlled study in 31 depressed methadone-maintained patients found that sertraline significantly increased the methadone plasma level/dose ratio by 26% while patients on placebo showed a 16% decrease after 6 weeks treatment, but by 12 weeks ratios had shifted towards baseline values. Adverse effects were similar in both groups.[9]

Mechanism

Fluvoxamine, and to a lesser extent fluoxetine, paroxetine, and sertraline, can inhibit the liver metabolism of the methadone (possibly by the cytochrome P450 isoenzymes CYP3A4,[10] CYP2D6,[10,11] and/or CYP1A2[4]) thereby allowing it to accumulate in the body.

Importance and management

Information is limited, but it indicates that the effects of starting or stopping fluvoxamine should be monitored in patients on methadone, being alert for the need to adjust the methadone dosage. Although the increase in methadone levels with sertraline and paroxetine, and possibly also fluoxetine, is unlikely to have clinical effects in most patients, the possibility should be borne in mind. Caution is warranted, particularly if other inhibitors of hepatic enzymes are also being used as the effects may be additive.

1. Bertschy G, Eap CB, Powell K, Baumann P. Fluoxetine addition to methadone in addicts: pharmacokinetic aspects. *Ther Drug Monit* (1996) 18, 570–2.
2. Batki SL, Manfredi LB, Jacob P, Jones RT. Fluoxetine for cocaine dependence in methadone maintenance: quantitative plasma and urine cocaine-benzoylecgonine concentrations. *J Clin Psychopharmacol* (1993) 13, 243–50.
3. Baño MD, Agujetas M, M, López ML, Tena T, Rodríguez A. Lora-Tamayo C, Guillén JL. Eficacia de la fluoxetina (FX) en el tratamiento de la adicción a cocaína en pacientes en mantenimiento con metadona y su interacción en los niveles plasmáticos. *Actas Esp Psiquiatr* (1999) 27, 321–4.
4. Eap CB, Bertschy G, Powell K, Baumann P. Fluvoxamine and fluoxetine do not interact in the same way with the metabolism of the enantiomers of methadone. *J Clin Psychopharmacol* (1997) 17, 113–17.
5. Bertschy G, Baumann P, Eap CB, Baettig D. Probable metabolic interaction between methadone and fluvoxamine in addict patients. *Ther Drug Monit* (1994) 16, 42–5.
6. DeMaria PA, Serota RD. A therapeutic use of the methadone fluvoxamine drug interaction. *J Addict Dis* (1999) 18, 5–12.
7. Alderman CP, Frith PA. Fluvoxamine-methadone interaction. *Aust N Z J Psychiatry* (1999) 33, 99–101.
8. Begré S, von Bardeleben U, Ladewig D, Jaquet-Rochat S, Cosendai-Savary L, Golay KP, Kosel M, Baumann P, Eap CB. Paroxetine increases steady-state concentrations of (R)-methadone in CYP2D6 extensive but not poor metabolizers. *J Clin Psychopharmacol* (2002) 22, 211–15.
9. Hamilton SP, Nunes EV, Janal M, Weber L. The effect of sertraline on methadone plasma levels in methadone-maintenance patients. *Am J Addict* (2000) 9, 63–9.
10. Iribarne C, Picart D, Dreano Y, Berthou F. In vitro interactions between fluoxetine or fluvoxamine and methadone or buprenorphine. *Fundam Clin Pharmacol* (1998) 12, 194–9.
11. Wang J-S, DeVane CL. Involvement of CYP3A4, CYP2C8, and CYP2D6 in the metabolism of (*R*)- and (*S*)-methadone in vitro. *Drug Metab Dispos* (2003) 31, 742–7.

Opioids; Methadone + Urinary acidifiers or alkalinisers

Urinary methadone clearance is increased if the urine is made acid (e.g. by giving ammonium chloride) and reduced if it is made alkaline (e.g. by giving sodium bicarbonate).

Clinical evidence

A study in patients on methadone found that the urinary clearance in those with urinary pHs of less than 6 was greater than those with higher urinary pHs.[1] When the urinary pH of one subject was lowered from 6.2 to 5.5, the loss of unchanged methadone in the urine was nearly doubled.[2]

A pharmacokinetic study in 5 healthy subjects given 10-mg intramuscular doses of methadone found that the plasma half-life was 19.5 hours when the urine was made acidic (pH 5.2) with **ammonium chloride** compared with 42.1 hours when the urine was made alkaline (pH 7.8) with **sodium bicarbonate**. The clearance of the methadone fell from 134 to 91.9 ml/minute when the urine was changed from acidic to alkaline.[3]

Mechanism

Methadone is eliminated from the body both by liver metabolism and excretion of unchanged methadone in the urine. Above pH 6 the urinary excretion is less important, but with urinary pH below 6 the half-life becomes dependent on both excretion (30%) and metabolism (70%).[2-4] Methadone is a weak base (pKa 8.4) so that in acidic urine little of the drug is in the un-ionised form and little is reabsorbed by simple passive diffusion. On the other hand, in alkaline solution most of the drug is in the un-ionised form, which is readily reabsorbed by the kidney tubules, and little is lost in the urine.

Importance and management

An established interaction, but of uncertain importance. Be alert for any evidence of reduced methadone effects in patients whose urine becomes acidic because they are taking large doses of ammonium chloride. Lowering the urinary pH to 5 with ammonium chloride to increase the clearance can also be used to treat toxicity. Theoretically, urinary alkalinisers such as sodium bicarbonate and **acetazolamide** may increase the effect of methadone.

1. Bellward GD, Warren PM, Howald W, Axelson JE, Abbott FS. Methadone maintenance: effect of urinary pH on renal clearance in chronic high and low doses. *Clin Pharmacol Ther* (1977) 22, 92–9.
2. Inturrisi CE, Verebely K. Disposition of methadone in man after a single oral dose. *Clin Pharmacol Ther* (1972) 13, 923–30.
3. Nilsson M-I, Widerlöv E, Meresaar U, Änggård E. Effect of urinary pH on the disposition of methadone in man. *Eur J Clin Pharmacol* (1982) 22, 337–42.
4. Baselt RC, Casarett LJ. Urinary excretion of methadone in man. *Clin Pharmacol Ther* (1972) 13, 64–70.

Opioids; Morphine + Food

Food increases the bioavailability of oral morphine solution and produces a sustained serum level.

Clinical evidence, mechanism, importance and management

Twelve patients with chronic pain were given oral morphine hydrochloride 50 mg in 200 ml water either while fasting or after a **high-fat breakfast** (fried eggs and bacon, toast with butter, and milk). The maximum blood morphine concentrations and the time to achieve these concentrations were not significantly altered by the presence of the food, but the AUC was increased by 34% and blood morphine levels were maintained at higher levels over the period from 4 to 10 hours after being given the morphine.[1] The reasons are not understood. The inference to be drawn is that pain relief is likely to be increased if the morphine solution is given with food. This appears to be an advantageous interaction. More confirmatory study is needed. Consider also 'Opioids; Dextropropoxyphene (Propoxyphene) + Food', p.109.

1. Gourlay GK, Plummer JL, Cherry DA, Foate JA, Cousins MJ. Influence of a high-fat meal on the absorption of morphine from oral solutions. *Clin Pharmacol Ther* (1989) 46, 463–8.

Opioids; Morphine + Local anaesthetics

Chloroprocaine can reduce epidural morphine analgesia when compared with lidocaine. Lidocaine does not appear to increase respiratory depressant effects of morphine, and may have synergistic analgesic effects. However, one case of respiratory depression has been reported. Morphine given as an intravenous bolus does not alter lidocaine serum levels given as a continuous intravenous infusion.

Clinical evidence, mechanism, importance and management

(a) Chloroprocaine

Two studies[1,2] have found that chloroprocaine decreases the duration of epidural morphine analgesia (16 hours for chloroprocaine compared with 24 hours for lidocaine[1]). A third study showed that morphine requirements after caesarean section were much higher in women who had received chloroprocaine for epidural anaesthesia than in those receiving lidocaine.[3] The authors of one of the studies suggest that chloroprocaine should be avoided if epidural morphine therapy is used.[1]

(b) Lidocaine

A double-blind controlled study in 10 patients who were receiving continuous lidocaine infusions during suspected myocardial infarction found that a 10-mg intravenous morphine sulphate bolus did not significantly alter the steady-state serum levels of lidocaine.[4] In another study, giving lidocaine with extradural morphine did not increase the risk of respiratory depression associated with the morphine.[5] However, in one case, respiratory depression occurred within 5 minutes of giving intravenous lidocaine for an episode of ventricular tachycardia in a patient who had previously been given spinal opioids (fentanyl and morphine). Naloxone successfully reversed this.[6] Numerous studies in *animals* have shown that lidocaine and morphine have synergistic analgesic effects. Just one is cited here as an example.[7]

1. Eisenach JC, Schlairet TJ, Dobson CE, Hood DH. Effect of prior anesthetic solution on epidural morphine analgesia. *Anesth Analg* (1991) 73, 119–23.
2. Phan CQ, Azar I, Osborn IP, Lear E. The quality of epidural morphine analgesia following epidural anesthesia with chloroprocaine or chloroprocaine mixed with epinephrine for cesarean delivery. *Anesth Analg* (1988) 67, S171.
3. Karambelkar DJ, Ramanathan S. 2-Chloroprocaine antagonism of epidural morphine analgesia. *Acta Anaesthesiol Scand* (1997) 41, 774–8.
4. Vacek JL, Wilson DB, Hurwitz A, Gollub SB, Dunn MI. The effect of morphine sulfate on serum lidocaine levels. *Clin Res* (1988) 36, 325A.
5. Saito Y, Sakura S, Kaneko M, Kosaka Y. Interaction of extradural morphine and lignocaine on ventilatory response. *Br J Anaesth* (1995) 75, 394–8.
6. Jensen E, Nader ND. Potentiation of narcosis after intravenous lidocaine in a patient given spinal opioids. *Anesth Analg* (1999) 89, 758–9.
7. Maves TJ, Gebhart GF. Antinociceptive synergy between intrathecal morphine and lidocaine during visceral and somatic nociception in the rat. *Anesthesiology* (1992) 76, 91–9.

Opioids; Morphine + Metoclopramide

Metoclopramide increases the rate of absorption of oral morphine and increases its rate of onset and sedative effects.

Clinical evidence

A single 10-mg dose of oral metoclopramide given to 10 patients before surgery markedly increased the extent and speed of sedation due to a 20-mg oral dose of modified-release morphine (*MST Continus Tablets*) in the first 1.5 hours after the dose. The time to peak plasma levels of morphine was almost halved, but peak plasma morphine levels and the total absorption remained unaltered.[1]

Mechanism

Metoclopramide increases the rate of gastric emptying so that the rate of morphine absorption from the small intestine is increased. An alternative idea is that both drugs act additively on opiate receptors to increase sedation.[1]

Importance and management

An established interaction that can be usefully exploited in anaesthetic practice, but the increased sedation may also represent a problem if the morphine is being given long-term. Compare 'Opioids; Butorphanol + Metoclopramide', p.108.

1. Manara AR, Shelly MP, Quinn K, Park GR. The effect of metoclopramide on the absorption of oral controlled release morphine. *Br J Clin Pharmacol* (1988) 25, 518–21.

Opioids; Morphine + Miscellaneous

Some preliminary evidence suggests that antidepressants, antipsychotics, NSAIDs and thiethylperazine may increase the myoclonus caused by high doses of morphine.

Clinical evidence, mechanism, importance and management

In 19 patients with malignant disease on high doses of morphine (daily doses of 500 mg or more orally or 250 mg or more parenterally), an analysis was made of the relationship between myoclonus and the use of supplemental drugs. In the 12 patients with myoclonus, 8 patients were taking antidepressants (**amitriptyline**, **doxepin**) or antipsychotics (**chlorpromazine**, **haloperidol**) compared to none of 6 patients without myoclonus. In addition, there was a higher use of NSAIDs (**indometacin**, **naproxen**, **piroxicam**, **aspirin**) and an antiemetic (**thiethylperazine**).[1] The reasons are not understood, and the findings of this paper have been questioned.[2] Supplemental drugs are very commonly used with opioids such as morphine in the treatment of cancer pain. See also 'Opioids; Morphine + NSAIDs', and 'Opioids; Morphine + Tricyclic antidepressants', below.

1. Potter JM, Reid DB, Shaw RJ, Hackett P, Hickman PE. Myoclonus associated with treatment with high doses of morphine: the role of supplemental drugs. *BMJ* (1989) 299, 150–3.
2. Quinn N. Myoclonus associated with high doses of morphine. *BMJ* (1989) 299, 683–4.

Opioids; Morphine + NSAIDs

Ketoprofen reduced morphine-associated respiratory depression, and did not alter morphine pharmacokinetics. Similarly, diclofenac did not alter morphine pharmacokinetics in one study. However, in another, diclofenac slightly increased respiratory depression despite reducing morphine use, possibly because of persistent levels of an active metabolite of morphine.

Clinical evidence, mechanism, importance and management

An infusion of **ketoprofen** 1.5 mg/kg with morphine 100 micrograms/kg reduced the respiratory depression associated with morphine alone in 11 healthy subjects. There was no change in plasma morphine levels.[1] Another study in 6 patients found that intramuscular **diclofenac** 75 mg twice daily for 5 days did not affect the half-life and AUC of oral morphine solution.[2]

However, in contrast to these reports, a study in 7 patients on the first postoperative day after spinal surgery found that, although **diclofenac** 100 mg rectally reduced patient-controlled morphine consumption by 20%, respiratory rates were significantly lower after the **diclofenac**, and minimal at about 200 minutes. Levels of an active metabolite, morphine-6-glucuronide did not significantly decrease until 420 minutes.[3]

NSAIDs are frequently used with opioids because of their lack of respiratory depression and opioid-sparing effects. However, this study demonstrates that there may be a risk of respiratory depression and other adverse effects due to persistently high levels of morphine-6-glucuronide for a number of hours after receiving an NSAID. During this time period, patients should be more closely monitored.[3]

For mention of the suggestion that NSAIDs may increase the incidence of myoclonus with high-dose morphine, see 'Opioids; Morphine + Miscellaneous', above.

1. Moren J, Francois T, Blanloeil Y, Pinaud M. The effects of a nonsteroidal antiinflammatory drug (ketoprofen) on morphine respiratory depression: a double-blind, randomized study in volunteers. *Anesth Analg* (1997) 85, 400–5.
2. De Conno F, Ripamonti C, Bianchi M, Ventafridda V, Panerai AE. Diclofenac does not modify morphine bioavailability in cancer patients. *Pain* (1992) 48, 401–2.
3. Tighe KE, Webb AM, Hobbs GJ. Persistently high plasma morphine-6-glucuronide levels despite decreased hourly patient-controlled analgesia morphine use after single-dose diclofenac: potential for opioid-related toxicity. *Anesth Analg* (1999) 88, 1137–42.

Opioids; Morphine + Quinidine

Quinidine appears to increase the oral absorption of morphine, and so increases its effects, but does not significantly alter intravenous morphine-induced miosis.

Clinical evidence, mechanism, importance and management

Quinidine sulfate 600 mg, given one hour before intravenous morphine sulfate 150 micrograms/kg, did not alter morphine-induced miosis in healthy subjects. However, the same dose of quinidine before oral morphine sulfate 30 mg (with ondansetron as an antiemetic) increased morphine-induced miosis by 55%. This increase was considered proportionate to the increase in morphine AUC (60%) and maximum level (88%). There was no change in morphine elimination half-life.[1] Similarly, in another study in healthy subjects, quinidine 800 mg, given one hour before intravenous morphine 7.5 mg did not alter the respiratory depressant nor mitotic effects of morphine, and there was no change in plasma morphine or morphine glucuronide levels.[2]

It was suggested that quinidine inhibits the intestinal drug efflux pump P-glycoprotein and so allows an increase in oral morphine absorption.[1] In addition, the effects on miosis suggest that quinidine has no effect on the brain distribution of morphine. It was concluded that, assuming quinidine is an inhibitor of brain P-glycoprotein, P-glycoprotein is not important for brain access of morphine.[1,2]

The clinical importance of these findings remains to be determined, but it appears that quinidine may increase the effects of orally administered morphine.

1. Kharasch ED, Hoffer C, Whittington D, Sheffels. Role of P-glycoprotein in the intestinal absorption and clinical effects of morphine. *Clin Pharmacol Ther* (2003) 74, 543–54.
2. Skarke S, Jarrar M, Erb K, Schmidt H, Geisslinger G, Lotsch J. Respiratory and miotic effects of morphine in healthy volunteers when P-glycoprotein is blocked by quinidine. *Clin Pharmacol Ther* (2003) 74, 303–11.

Opioids; Morphine + Secobarbital

Secobarbital increases the respiratory depressant effects of morphine.

Clinical evidence, mechanism, importance and management

In 30 healthy subjects it was found that both intravenous secobarbital and intravenous morphine depressed respiration when given alone, and a much greater and more prolonged respiratory depression occurred when they were given together.[1] The combination should be used with caution. Consider also 'Opioids; Pethidine (Meperidine) + Barbiturates', p.121.

1. Zsigmond EK, Flynn K. Effect of secobarbital and morphine on arterial blood gases in healthy human volunteers. *J Clin Pharmacol* (1993) 33, 453–7.

Opioids; Morphine + Tricyclic antidepressants

The bioavailability and the degree of analgesia of oral morphine is increased by clomipramine, desipramine and possibly amitriptyline. In some circumstances this may be a useful interaction. Consider also 'Opioids + Tricyclic antidepressants; Amitriptyline', p.106.

Clinical evidence, mechanism, importance and management

Clomipramine or **amitriptyline** in doses of 20 or 50 mg daily increased the AUC of oral morphine by 28% to 111% in 24 patients being treated for cancer pain. The half-life of morphine was also prolonged.[1] A previous study[2] found that **desipramine**, but not **amitriptyline**, increased and prolonged morphine analgesia, and a later study by the same group confirmed the value of **desipramine**.[3] The reasons are not understood. The increased analgesia may be due not only to the increased serum levels of morphine, but possibly also to some alteration in the way the morphine affects its receptors. In some circumstances this may be a useful interaction, but the possibility of increased morphine toxicity should also be borne in mind. Whether other tricyclic antidepressants behave similarly is uncertain. Note that makers' prescribing information for opioid analgesics generally include the information that CNS effects are expected to be increased when used with other CNS depressant drugs such as tricyclic antidepressants, see also 'Opioids + Tricyclic antidepressants; Amitriptyline', p.106.

For mention of the suggestion that antidepressants and antipsychotics may increase the incidence of myoclonus with high-dose morphine, see 'Opioids; Morphine + Miscellaneous', p.120.

1. Ventafridda V, Ripamonti C, De Conno F, Bianchi M, Pazzuconi F, Panerai AE. Antidepressants increase bioavailability of morphine in cancer patients. *Lancet* (1987) i, 1204.
2. Levine JD, Gordon NC, Smith R, McBryde R. Desipramine enhances opiate postoperative analgesia. *Pain* (1986) 27, 45–9.
3. Gordon NC, Heller PH, Gear RW, Levine JD. Temporal factors in the enhancement of morphine analgesia by desipramine. *Pain* (1993) 53, 273–6.

Opioids; Pethidine (Meperidine) + Aciclovir

An isolated report describes pethidine toxicity associated with the use of high dose aciclovir.

Clinical evidence, mechanism, importance and management

A man with Hodgkin's disease was treated with high-dose intravenous aciclovir for localised herpes zoster, and with intramuscular pethidine, and oral methadone and carbidopa-levodopa. On the second day he experienced nausea, vomiting and confusion, and later dysarthria, lethargy and ataxia. Despite vigorous treatment he later died. It was concluded that some of the adverse effects were due to pethidine toxicity arising from norpethidine accumulation, associated with renal impairment due to the aciclovir.[1]

1. Johnson R, Douglas J, Corey L, Krasney H. Adverse effects with acyclovir and meperidine. *Ann Intern Med* (1985) 103, 962–3.

Opioids; Pethidine (Meperidine) + Barbiturates

A single case report describes greatly increased sedation with severe CNS toxicity in a woman given pethidine after receiving phenobarbital for two weeks. The analgesic effects of pethidine can be reduced by barbiturates.

Clinical evidence

(a) Increased pethidine toxicity

A woman whose pain had been satisfactorily controlled with pethidine without particular CNS depression, showed prolonged sedation with severe CNS toxicity when she was given pethidine after being treated with **phenobarbital** 30 mg four times daily for 2 weeks, as anticonvulsant therapy.[1]

(b) Pethidine effects reduced

Studies in women undergoing dilatation and curettage found that **thiopental** and **pentobarbital** increased their sensitivity to pain, and opposed the analgesic effects of pethidine.[2] This confirmed the findings of previous studies.[3] A marked anti-analgesic effect has been seen for up to 5 hours after high doses (6 to 10 mg/kg) of **thiopental**.[2] This anti-analgesic effect also occurred with **phenobarbital**.[2]

Mechanism

Studies suggest that phenobarbital stimulates the liver enzymes concerned with the metabolism (*N*-demethylation) of pethidine so that the production of its more toxic metabolite (norpethidine) is increased. The toxicity seen appears to be the combined effects of this compound and the directly sedative effects of the barbiturate.[1,4]

Importance and management

There is only one report of toxicity, but the metabolic changes described under 'Mechanism' were seen in other patients and subjects. The general clinical importance is uncertain but concurrent use should be undertaken with care. It has also been suggested that if the pethidine is continued but the barbiturate suddenly withdrawn, the toxic concentrations of norpethidine might lead to convulsions in the absence of an anticonvulsant.[1] Whether other barbiturates behave similarly is not clear, but it is possible. More study is needed to confirm these possibilities. Be aware that the barbiturates reduce analgesia. The metabolic product of pethidine is a less effective analgesic than the parent compound. Consider also 'Opioids; Morphine + Secobarbital', p.120.

1. Stambaugh JE, Wainer IW, Hemphill DM, Schwartz I. A potentially toxic drug interaction between pethidine (meperidine) and phenobarbitone. *Lancet* (1977) i, 398–9.
2. Dundee JW. Alterations in response to somatic pain associated with anaesthesia. II. The effect of thiopentone and pentobarbitone. *Br J Anaesth* (1960) 32, 407–14.
3. Clutton-Brock J. Some pain threshold studies with particular reference to thiopentone. *Anaesthesia* (1960) 15, 71–2.
4. Stambaugh JE, Wainer IW, Schwartz I. The effect of phenobarbital on the metabolism of meperidine in normal volunteers. *J Clin Pharmacol* (1978) 18, 482–90.

Opioids; Pethidine (Meperidine) + Furazolidone

On the basis of *animal* experiments it has been suggested that if pethidine and furazolidone are used concurrently, a serious hyperpyrexic reaction may occur similar to that seen with the antidepressant MAOIs. This has yet to be confirmed.

Clinical evidence, mechanism, importance and management

Fatal hyperpyrexia followed the injection of pethidine in *rabbits* given oral furazolidone for 4 days.[1] On the basis of this observation, linked with the known MAO-inhibitory properties of furazolidone in humans (see 'Furazolidone + Sympathomimetics', p.144) and the well-documented MAOI/pethidine interaction (see 'MAOIs + Opioids, p.869), there would seem to be the possibility of some risk if these two drugs are used together. However, there do not appear to be any clinical reports of this interaction. One such interaction has occurred between 'furazolidone and amitriptyline', (p.1004).

1. Eltayeb IB, and Osman OH. Furazolidone-pethidine interactions in rabbits. *Br J Pharmacol* (1975) 55, 497–501.

Opioids; Pethidine (Meperidine) + Phenothiazines

Pethidine and chlorpromazine can be used together for increased analgesia and for premedication before anaesthesia, but increased respiratory depression, sedation, CNS toxicity and hypotension can also occur. Other phenothiazines such as levomepromazine, promethazine, prochlorperazine, propiomazine and thioridazine may also interact to cause some of these effects.

Clinical evidence

Chlorpromazine 25 mg/70 kg body-weight given alone had no consistent effect on respiratory function in 6 healthy subjects but the respiratory depression produced by pethidine 100 mg/70 kg body-weight was exacerbated when the two drugs were given together. One subject showed marked respiratory depression, beginning about 30 minutes after receiving both drugs and lasting 2 hours.[1] No change in the pharmacokinetics of pethidine was found when **chlorpromazine** was given in a single-dose study in healthy subjects, but the excretion of the metabolites of pethidine was increased. The symptoms of light-headedness, dry mouth and lethargy were significantly increased and 4 subjects experienced such marked debilitation that they required assistance to continue the study. Systolic and diastolic blood pressures were also reduced.[2]

Studies with other phenothiazines have shown that **promethazine**[3] prolongs the anaesthetic action of pethidine (consider also 'Opioids + Promethazine', p.104). **Promethazine** with **pentobarbital**,[4] **propiomazine**[5,6] and **levomepromazine**[7] can all increase its respiratory depressant effects, but the effects of **prochlorperazine**[8] on respiration were not statistically significant. A 12-year-old patient on long-term **thioridazine** 50 mg twice daily, given premedication with pethidine, diphenhydramine and glycopyrrolate, was very lethargic after surgery and stopped breathing. He responded to naloxone.[9] Increased respiratory depression has also been seen with **hydroxyzine** [not a phenothiazine] with opioids in one study,[6] but not in two others.[10,11]

Mechanism

There is evidence that chlorpromazine can increase the activity of the liver microsomal enzymes so that the metabolism of pethidine to norpethidine and norpethidinic acid are increased. These metabolites are toxic and probably account for the lethargy and hypotension seen in one study.[2] The effects of the phenothiazines on pethidine-induced respiratory depression may be related.

Importance and management

Lower doses of pethidine can be used if chlorpromazine is given,[12] but concurrent use is clearly not without its problems. A marked increase in respiratory depression can occur in some susceptible individuals.[1] The authors of one study[2] suggest that the risks of using the combination of pethidine with chlorpromazine outweighs the advantages and so their use as combination analgesics should probably be discontinued.

Information about other adverse interactions with pethidine and phenothiazines seems to be very limited: the interaction with thioridazine seems to be the only one reported.[9] Increased analgesia may occur but it may be accompanied by increased respiratory depression,[3,5] which is undesirable in patients with existing respiratory insufficiency.

1. Lambertsen CJ, Wendel H, Longenhagen JB. The separate and combined respiratory effects of chlorpromazine and meperidine in normal men controlled at 46 mmHg alveolar pCO_2. *J Pharmacol Exp Ther* (1961) 131, 381–93.
2. Stambaugh JE, Wainer IW. Drug interaction: meperidine and chlorpromazine, a toxic combination. *J Clin Pharmacol* (1981) 21, 140–6.
3. Keèri-Szàntò M. The mode of action of promethazine in potentiating narcotic drugs. *Br J Anaesth* (1974) 46, 918–24.
4. Pierce JA, Garofalvo ML. Preoperative medication and its effect on blood gases. *JAMA* (1965) 194, 487.
5. Hoffman JC, Smith TC. The respiratory effects of meperidine and propiomazine in man. *Anesthesiology* (1970) 32, 325–31.
6. Reier CE, Johnstone RE. Respiratory depression: narcotic versus narcotic-tranquillizer combinations. *Anesth Analg* (1970) 49, 119–124.
7. Zsigmond EK, Flynn K. The effect of methotrimeprazine on arterial blood gases in human volunteers. *J Clin Pharmacol* (1988) 28, 1033–7.
8. Steen SN, Yates M. The effects of benzquinamide and prochlorperazine, separately and combined, on the human respiratory center. *Anesthesiology* (1972) 36, 519–20.
9. Grothe DR, Ereshefsky L, Jann MW, Fidone GS. Clinical implications of the neuroleptic-opioid interaction. *Drug Intell Clin Pharm* (1986) 20, 75–7.
10. Zsigmond EK, Flynn K, Shively JG. Effect of hydroxyzine and meperidine on arterial blood gases in healthy human volunteers. *J Clin Pharmacol* (1989) 29, 85–90.
11. Zsigmond EK, Flynn K, Shively JG. Effect of hydroxyzine and meperidine on arterial blood gases in patients with chronic obstructive pulmonary disease. *Int J Clin Pharmacol Ther Toxicol* (1993) 31, 124–9.
12. Sadove MS, Levin MJ, Rose RF, Schwartz L, Witt FW. Chlorpromazine and narcotics in the management of pain of malignant lesions. *JAMA* (1954) 155, 626–8.

Opioids; Pethidine (Meperidine) + Phenytoin

An isolated report describes pethidine toxicity in a man taking phenytoin. A pharmacokinetic study confirms that phenytoin increases the production of the toxic metabolite of pethidine.

Clinical evidence

A 61-year-old man who was addicted to pethidine, taking 5 to 10 g weekly, is reported to have developed repeated seizures and myoclonus when he also took phenytoin. The problem resolved when both drugs were stopped.[1]

It is known that phenytoin increases the production of norpethidine, the metabolic product of pethidine that is believed to be responsible for the neurotoxicity of pethidine (seizures, myoclonus, tremors etc). A study[2] in healthy subjects found that phenytoin 300 mg daily for 9 days decreased the elimination half-life of pethidine (100 mg orally and 50 mg intravenously) from 6.4 to 4.3 hours, and the systemic clearance increased by 27%. Phenytoin is a well recognised and potent enzyme inducing agent.

This seems to be the only report[1] of an adverse interaction between phenytoin and pethidine so its general importance is uncertain. Bear it in mind if there is an unexpected response to treatment. Since the study cited[2] found that pethidine given orally produced more of the toxic metabolite (norpethidine) than when given intravenously, it may be preferable to give pethidine intravenously in patients taking phenytoin, or use an alternative opioid.

1. Hochman MS. Meperidine-associated myoclonus and seizures in long-term hemodialysis patients. *Ann Neurol* (1983) 14, 593.
2. Pond SM, Kretschzmar KM. Effect of phenytoin on meperidine clearance and normeperidine formation. *Clin Pharmacol Ther* (1981) 30, 680–6.

Opioids; Tramadol + Carbamazepine

The plasma levels of tramadol are reduced by carbamazepine, and the analgesic efficacy would be expected to be reduced.

Clinical evidence, mechanism, importance and management

An unpublished study by the makers found that the maximum plasma levels and the elimination half-life of a single 50-mg dose of tramadol were reduced by 50% by carbamazepine 400 mg twice daily for 9 days.[1] It is likely that carbamazepine increases the metabolism of tramadol. On the basis of this study the makers say that the analgesic effectiveness of tramadol[2] and its duration of action would be expected to be reduced.[1,3] Monitor efficacy if the two drugs are required.

1. GD Searle. Personal Communication, November 1994.
2. Ultram (Tramadol). Ortho-McNeil Pharmaceutical Inc. US Prescribing information, May 2004.
3. Zydol SR (Tramadol). Grünenthal Ltd. UK Summary of product characteristics, February 2005.

Opioids; Tramadol + MAOIs

The serotonin syndrome developed in one patient on iproniazid and tramadol, and delirium in another given tramadol shortly after stopping phenelzine. A fatal case of possible serotonin syndrome has been seen with tramadol, moclobemide and clomipramine. See also 'MAOIs + Opioids', p.869.

Clinical evidence, mechanism, importance and management

The makers of tramadol contraindicated its use with the MAOIs[1,2] on the basis that it is an opioid agonist, like pethidine (meperidine). This may mean the serotonin syndrome could develop (see 'MAOIs + Opioids', p.869). This prediction was confirmed by a report[3] of the development of the serotonin syndrome (myoclonus, tremor, sweating, hyperreflexia, tachycardia) in a patient on **iproniazid** when tramadol was added to his drug regimen. When the tramadol was stopped the patient recovered within 48 hours. Another single case report describes the development of severe delirium in a patient within 3 days of stopping long term treatment with **phenelzine** 45 mg daily and starting intramuscular tramadol 100 mg three times daily. The patient became anxious and confused, and developed visual hallucinations and persecutory ideation. The symptoms disappeared within 48 hours of stopping the tramadol.[4] Another report suggests that tramadol may have contributed to the development of a fatal serotonin syndrome in a patient abusing tramadol, **moclobemide** and clomipramine.[5]

This demonstrates that there are sound practical and theoretical reasons for patients on MAOIs to avoid tramadol. Note that the serotonin syndrome has also occurred with 'tramadol and SSRIs', (p.123).

1. Zydol SR (Tramadol). Grünenthal Ltd. UK Summary of product characteristics, February 2005.
2. Ultram (Tramadol). Ortho-McNeil Pharmaceutical Inc. US Prescribing information, May 2004.
3. de Larquier A, Vial T, Bréjoux G, Descotes J. Syndrome sérotoninergique lors de l'association tramadol et iproniazide. *Therapie* (1999) 54, 767–8.
4. Calvisi V, Ansseau M. Confusion mentale liée à l'administration de tramadol chez une patiente sous IMAO. *Rev Med Liege* (1999) 54, 912–3.
5. Hernandez AF, Montero MN, Pla A, Villanueva E. Fatal moclobemide overdose or death caused by serotonin syndrome? *J Forensic Sci* (1995) 40, 128–30.

Opioids; Tramadol + Quinidine

The analgesic effects of tramadol are not affected by quinidine.

Clinical evidence, mechanism, importance and management

A double-blind placebo controlled study in 12 healthy subjects found that when they were given tramadol 100 mg with and without quinidine 50 mg, the quinidine had virtually no effect on the analgesic effects of tramadol but it inhibited its effect on pupil size.[1] There was about a 25% increase in the tramadol AUC and maximum level.[2] Tramadol is partially metabolised to the active metabolite *O*-desmethyltramadol (which affects opioid receptors), by the cytochrome P450 isoenzyme CYP2D6, and it is this enzyme that is inhibited by quinidine. Blockade of the production of this metabolite appears to have little effect on the analgesic effect of tramadol, (which may also involve non-opioid mechanisms).[1] No special precautions are needed. See also 'Opioids; Codeine and related drugs + Quinidine', p.108.

1. Collart L, Luthy C, Dayer P. Multimodel analgesic effect of tramadol. *Clin Pharmacol Ther* (1993) 53, 223.
2. Tramadol. Pliva Pharma Ltd. UK Summary of product characteristics, June 2003.

Opioids; Tramadol + SSRIs

Six reports describe the development of the serotonin syndrome in patients on fluoxetine, paroxetine or sertraline when tramadol was given. Another patient developed hallucinations with tramadol and paroxetine. Tramadol should be used with caution with SSRIs because of the possible increased risk of seizures.

Clinical evidence

(a) Seizures

The UK Committee on Safety of Medicines has publicised 27 reports of convulsions and one of worsening epilepsy with tramadol, a reporting rate of 1 in 7000 patients. Some of the patients were given doses well in excess of those recommended, and some were taking SSRIs (5 patients) or 'tricyclic antidepressants', (below), both of which are known to reduce the convulsive threshold.[1]

(b) Serotonin syndrome

(i) Fluoxetine. A woman who had been taking fluoxetine 20 mg daily for 3 years developed what was eventually diagnosed as the serotonin syndrome. A month previously she had started to take tramadol 50 mg four times daily, increased after a fortnight to 100 mg four times daily. Ten days before hospitalisation she had developed a tremor of the right hand and face, and in hospital she showed agitation, marked facial blepharospasm, some sweating and pyrexia, and stuttering. The symptoms began to subside 7 days after both drugs were stopped, and after 2 months she had recovered fully.[2]

(ii) Paroxetine. A man who had been taking paroxetine 20 mg daily for 4 months without problems developed shivering, diaphoresis and myoclonus and became subcomatose within 12 hours of taking tramadol 100 mg. This was diagnosed as the serotonin syndrome. Tramadol was stopped, the paroxetine dosage halved and he became conscious within a day. The other symptoms gradually disappeared over the next week.[3] A 78-year-old woman taking paroxetine 20 mg daily developed nausea, diaphoresis and irritability 3 days after starting tramadol 50 mg three times a day. The next day she developed muscular weakness and confusion, and was found to have a temperature of 100.8°F and a pulse rate of 110 bpm. She recovered when the drugs were withdrawn. Similar symptoms but without an increased temperature occurred in another elderly woman on paroxetine 10 mg daily within 2 days of starting tramadol 50 mg four times daily. Both women were later able to continue on the paroxetine alone without problems.[4]

A tetraparetic patient with chronic pain developed nightmares and hallucinations 56 days after starting treatment with tramadol, paroxetine and dosulepin, which only stopped when the drugs were withdrawn.[5]

(iii) Sertraline. A 42-year-old woman was admitted to intensive care with atypical chest pain, sinus tachycardia, confusion, psychosis, sundowning [increased agitation, activity and negative behaviours, which happen late in the day or evening], agitation, diaphoresis and tremor. Medications on admission were orciprenaline (metaproterenol), pravastatin, triamcinolone by inhalation, chlorzoxazone, nabumetone, theophylline, naphazoline ophthalmic solution, omeprazole, paracetamol, terfenadine, sertraline and tramadol. She was diagnosed as having the serotonin syndrome, attributed to an increase in the dosage of tramadol (from 150 mg daily to 300 mg daily in increments of 50 mg every 2 to 3 days), and an increased sertraline dosage [original amounts not stated but 100 mg daily when the adverse events developed]. The tramadol had been started 3 weeks previously and she had been taking the sertraline for a year.[6]

An 88-year-old woman taking sertraline 50 mg daily (later increased to 100 mg daily), as well as several other medications (propafenone, furosemide, spironolactone, enoxaparin sodium, omeprazole, domperidone, paracetamol and bromazepam) was given dextropropoxyphene/paracetamol and tramadol 200 mg daily increased to 400 mg daily for pain relief after a fracture. Ten days after starting tramadol she became confused, with alterations in cognitive function, tremor, problems with co-ordination and muscle weakness. The serotonin syndrome was suspected and therefore sertraline was withdrawn over a period of 2 days, the dose of tramadol was reduced from 400 to 200 mg daily, and the patient recovered over a period of about 2 weeks.[7]

Mechanism

SSRIs can reduce the seizure threshold, and tramadol may increase this effect. The serotonin syndrome seems to develop unpredictably in a few patients given two or more serotonergic drugs (in this case, tramadol and SSRIs). See 'Additive or synergistic interactions', (p.9) for a general discussion of the serotonin syndrome.

Importance and management

Because of the possible increased risk of seizures, tramadol should be used with caution in patients on drugs such as the SSRIs, which can lower the seizure threshold.[8] The six, possibly seven, cases seem to be the only reports of the serotonin syndrome or other reactions due to an interaction between an SSRI and tramadol, and they need to be set in the wider context of apparently uneventful and advantageous use in other patients[9,10]. There would therefore seem to be little reason for totally avoiding the concurrent use of the SSRIs and tramadol but it would clearly be prudent to monitor the outcome closely.

1. Committee on Safety of Medicines/Medicines Control Agency. In focus–tramadol. *Current Problems* (1996) 22, 11.
2. Kesavan S, Sobala GM. Serotonin syndrome with fluoxetine plus tramadol. *J R Soc Med* (1999) 92, 474–5.
3. Egberts ACG, ter Borgh J, Brodie-Meijer CCE. Serotonin syndrome attributed to tramadol addition to paroxetine therapy. *Int Clin Psychopharmacol* (1997) 12, 181–182.
4. Lantz MS, Buchalter EN, Giambanco V. Serotonin syndrome following the administration of tramadol with paroxetine. *Int J Geriatr Psychiatry* (1998) 13, 343–5.
5. Devulder J, De Laat M, Dumoulin K, Renson A, Rolly G. Nightmares and hallucinations after long term intake of tramadol combined with antidepressants. *Acta Clin Belg* (1996) 51, 184–6.
6. Mason BJ, Blackburn KH. Possible serotonin syndrome associated with tramadol and sertraline coadministration. *Ann Pharmacother* (1997) 31, 175–7.
7. Sauget D, Franco PS, Amaniou M, Mazere J, Dantoine T. Possible syndrome sérotoninergique induit par l'association de tramadol à de la sertraline chez une femme âgée. *Therapie* (2002) 57, 309–10.
8. Zydol SR (Tramadol). Grünenthal Ltd. UK Summary of product characteristics, February 2005.
9. Fanelli J, Montgomery C. Use of the analgesic tramadol in antidepressant potentiation. *Psychopharmacol Bull* (1996) 32, 442.
10. Barkin RL. Alternative dosing for tramadol aids effectiveness. *Formulary* (1995) 30, 542–3.

Opioids; Tramadol + Tricyclic antidepressants

Tramadol should be used with caution with tricyclic antidepressants because of the possible risk of seizures. A fatal case of possible serotonin syndrome has been seen with tramadol, moclobemide and clomipramine.

Clinical evidence, mechanism, importance and management

The UK Committee on Safety of Medicines has publicised 27 reports of convulsions and one of worsening epilepsy with tramadol, a reporting rate of 1 in 7000 patients. Some of the patients were given doses well in excess of those recommended, and 8 patients were also taking tricyclic antidepressants, which are known to reduce the convulsive threshold. For this reason tramadol should be used with caution with tricyclic antidepressants.[1-3]

Another report suggests that tramadol may have contributed to the development of a fatal serotonin syndrome in a patient abusing tramadol, moclobemide and **clomipramine**.[4]

1. Committee on Safety of Medicines/Medicines Control Agency. In focus—tramadol. *Current Problems* (1996) 22, 11.
2. Zydol SR (Tramadol). Grünenthal Ltd. UK Summary of product characteristics, February 2005.
3. Ultram (Tramadol). Ortho-McNeil Pharmaceutical Inc. US Prescribing information, May 2004.
4. Hernandez AF, Montero MN, Pla A, Villanueva E. Fatal moclobemide overdose or death caused by serotonin syndrome? *J Forensic Sci* (1995) 40, 128–30.

Paracetamol (Acetaminophen) + Anticholinergics

Propantheline reduced the rate, but not the extent, of absorption of paracetamol. This would be expected to reduce the rate of onset of analgesia. Other anticholinergic drugs that delay gastric

emptying would be expected to interact similarly. In one case, the diphenhydramine component of a paracetamol product delayed paracetamol absorption after an overdose, and complicated the evaluation of the risk of toxicity.

Clinical evidence, mechanism, importance and management

Propantheline 30 mg intravenously delayed the peak serum levels of paracetamol (acetaminophen) 1.5 g in 6 convalescent patients from about 1 hours to 3 hours. Peak concentrations were lowered by about one-third, but the total amount of paracetamol absorbed was unchanged.[1] The reason is that **propantheline** is an anticholinergic drug that slows the rate at which the stomach empties, so that the rate of absorption in the gut is reduced. The practical consequence of this is likely to be that rapid pain relief with single-doses of paracetamol may be delayed and reduced by anticholinergics (see 'Table 16.1', (p.500), and 'Table 16.2', (p.502) for a list) but this needs clinical confirmation. If the paracetamol is being taken in repeated doses over extended periods this seems unlikely to be an important interaction because the total amount absorbed is unchanged.

A case has been described where the **diphenhydramine** component of a paracetamol product (*Tylenol PM*) taken in overdose (paracetamol 7.5 g and **diphenhydramine** 375 mg) delayed the absorption of paracetamol, so that the peak paracetamol level did not occur until 8 hours after ingestion, compared with the usual maximum of 2 hours.[2] In this situation there is a danger that early paracetamol levels could incorrectly be assessed. Therefore, when assessing paracetamol overdoses, it is important to consider whether any concurrent drugs could delay the absorption of paracetamol.

1. Nimmo J, Heading RC, Tothill P, Prescott LF. Pharmacological modification of gastric emptying: effects of propantheline and metoclopramide on paracetamol absorption. *BMJ* (1973) 1, 587–9.
2. Tsang WO, Nadroo AM. An unusual case of acetaminophen overdose. *Pediatr Emerg Care* (1999) 15, 344–6.

Paracetamol (Acetaminophen) + Anticonvulsants

The metabolism of paracetamol is increased in patients taking enzyme-inducing anticonvulsants (carbamazepine, phenytoin, phenobarbital, primidone). Isolated reports describe unexpected hepatotoxicity in patients on phenobarbital, phenytoin, or carbamazepine after taking paracetamol. Paracetamol modestly increases the loss of lamotrigine from the body but appears not to affect phenytoin or carbamazepine.

Clinical evidence

(a) Effect on paracetamol (acetaminophen)

(i) Pharmacokinetic studies. The AUC of oral paracetamol 1 g was found to be 40% lower (and when given intravenously, 31% lower) in 6 epileptic subjects than in 6 healthy subjects. Five of the epileptics were taking at least two of the following drugs: **carbamazepine**, **phenobarbital**, **primidone**, **phenytoin**. One was taking **phenytoin** alone.[1] Similar findings (a 38% decrease in AUC) were reported in another study in 13 patients on these anticonvulsants and 2 patients on rifampicin. In these patients, the amount of glucuronide, but not sulfate, metabolites of paracetamol were higher than controls, but the potentially hepatotoxic metabolite (assessed by mercapturic acid and cysteine conjugates) was not raised.[2] Similar changes in paracetamol metabolites were reported in Chinese patients on **phenytoin** alone. However, those on **carbamazepine** alone had no difference in paracetamol metabolites when compared with control subjects.[3] Other studies have also reported a greater rate of paracetamol glucuronidation and unchanged sulfation in patients on **phenytoin** alone[4] and patients on **phenytoin** and/or **carbamazepine**.[5] In contrast, this latter study also found an increase in clearance of the glutathione-derived conjugates (mercapturic and cysteine conjugates), which may indicate an increased risk of paracetamol hepatotoxicity.[5]

(ii) Paracetamol-induced hepatotoxicity. An epileptic woman on **phenobarbital** 100 mg daily developed hepatitis after taking paracetamol 1 g daily for 3 months for headaches. Within 2 weeks of stopping the paracetamol her serum transaminase levels had fallen within the normal range, which implied drug-induced liver damage.[6] Another patient on **phenobarbital** developed liver and kidney toxicity after taking only 9 g of paracetamol over 48 hours.[7] **Phenobarbital** also appeared to have increased the toxic effects of paracetamol in an adolescent who took an overdose of both drugs, which resulted in fatal hepatic encephalopathy.[8]
Other case reports describe unexpected paracetamol hepatotoxicity in two patients on **phenytoin**,[9,10] two patients on **carbamazepine**,[11,12] and a patient on **phenytoin** and **primidone**.[13] Another analysis of patients with paracetamol-induced fulminant hepatic failure suggested that mortality was higher in the group of patients on anticonvulsants (including **phenytoin**, **phenobarbital**, **carbamazepine**, **primidone** and **valproate** alone or in combination).[14]

(b) Effect on anticonvulsants

The serum levels of **phenytoin** and **carbamazepine** in 10 epileptics were not significantly affected by paracetamol 1.5 g daily for 3 days.[15]

A study in 8 healthy subjects found that paracetamol 2.7 g daily reduced the AUC of a 300-mg dose of **lamotrigine** by 20% and reduced its half-life by 15%.[16]

Mechanism

The increased paracetamol clearance is due to the well-recognised enzyme inducing effects of the anticonvulsants, which increase its metabolism (glucuronidation and oxidation) and loss from the body. It has been suggested that this could result in an increase in the production of the hepatotoxic metabolites of paracetamol. If this then exceeds the normal glutathione binding capacity, liver damage may occur (see 'paracetamol', (p.72)). This depends on which isoenzymes are important in producing this metabolite. Some consider that the available evidence indicates that the cytochrome P450 isoenzyme CYP2E1 is the primary enzyme.[17] Therefore, since the above enzyme-inducing anticonvulsants do not induce this isoenzyme, some consider the few possible cases described merely represent idiosyncratic effects.[17]

It seems possible that paracetamol increases the metabolism of the lamotrigine.

Importance and management

Information is limited. The clinical importance of these interactions is not established and further study is needed. Paracetamol is possibly a less effective analgesic in patients taking the interacting anticonvulsants. Some believe that the evidence indicates that the risk of liver damage after overdose is increased, and they suggest that patients on enzyme-inducing anticonvulsants should be treated with antidotes at lower plasma levels of paracetamol.[9,11,13] In addition, some suggest that therapeutic doses of paracetamol should be used with caution in patients on these drugs.[10,14] Conversely, others consider that therapeutic doses of paracetamol are not associated with an increased risk of toxicity when used with enzyme-inducers. Moreover, phenytoin, by increasing glucuronidation, may actually be hepato-protective.[17] The differences stem from different understandings of which isoenzyme(s) are important in the production of the hepatotoxic metabolite of paracetamol[10,17] (see Mechanism, above).

It is unlikely that the interaction between lamotrigine and paracetamol is of practical importance, but this needs confirmation.

1. Perucca E, Richens A. Paracetamol disposition in normal subjects and in patients treated with antiepileptic drugs. *Br J Clin Pharmacol* (1979) 7, 201–6.
2. Prescott LF, Critchley JAJH, Balali-Mood M, Pentland B. Effects of microsomal enzyme induction on paracetamol metabolism in man. *Br J Clin Pharmacol* (1981) 12, 149–53.
3. Tomlinson B, Young RP, Ng MCY, Anderson PJ, Kay R, Critchley JAJH. Selective liver enzyme induction by carbamazepine and phenytoin in Chinese epileptics. *Eur J Clin Pharmacol* (1996) 50, 411–15.
4. Bock KW, Wiltfang J, Blume R, Ullrich D, Bircher J. Paracetamol as a test drug to determine glucuronide formation in man. Effects of inducers and of smoking. *Eur J Clin Pharmacol* (1987) 31, 677–83.
5. Miners JO, Attwood J, Birkett DJ. Determinants of acetaminophen metabolism: effect of inducers and inhibitors of drug metabolism on acetaminophen's metabolic pathways. *Clin Pharmacol Ther* (1984) 35, 480–6.
6. Pirotte JH. Apparent potentiation by phenobarbital of hepatotoxicity from small doses of acetaminophen. *Ann Intern Med* (1984) 101, 403.
7. Marsepoil T, Mahassani B, Roudiak N, Sebbah JL, Caillard G. Potentialisation de la toxicité hépatique et rénale du paracétamol par le phénobarbital. *JEUR* (1989) 2, 118–20.
8. Wilson JT, Kasantikul V, Harbison R, Martin D. Death in an adolescent following an overdose of acetaminophen and phenobarbital. *Am J Dis Child* (1978) 132, 466–73.
9. McClements BM, Hyland M, Callender ME. Management of paracetamol poisoning complicated by enzyme induction due to alcohol or drugs. *Lancet* (1990) 335, 1526.
10. Brackett CC, Bloch JD. Phenytoin as a possible cause of acetaminophen hepatotoxicity: case report and review of the literature. *Pharmacotherapy* (2000) 20, 229–33.
11. Smith JAE, Hine ID, Beck P, Routledge PA. Paracetamol toxicity: is enzyme-induction important? *Hum Toxicol* (1986) 5, 383–5.
12. Young CR, Mazure CM. Fulminant hepatic failure from acetaminophen in an anorexic patient treated with carbamazepine. *J Clin Psychiatry* (1998) 59, 622.
13. Minton NA, Henry JA, Frankel RJ. Fatal paracetamol poisoning in an epileptic. *Hum Toxicol* (1988) 7, 33–4.

14. Bray GP, Harrison PM, O'Grady JG, Tredger JM, Williams R. Long-term anticonvulsant therapy worsens outcome in paracetamol-induced fulminant hepatic failure. *Hum Exp Toxicol* (1992) 11, 265–70.
15. Neuvonen PJ, Lehtovaara R, Bardy A, Elomaa E. Antipyretic analgesics in patients on antiepileptic drug therapy. *Eur J Clin Pharmacol* (1979) 15, 263–8.
16. Depot M, Powell JR, Messenheimer JA, Cloutier G, Dalton MJ. Kinetic effects of multiple oral doses of acetaminophen on a single oral dose of lamotrigine. *Clin Pharmacol Ther* (1990) 48, 346–55.
17. Rumack BH. Acetaminophen hepatotoxicity: the first 35 years. *J Toxicol Clin Toxicol* (2002) 40, 3–20.

Paracetamol (Acetaminophen) + Caffeine

Caffeine has been variously reported to increase, decrease, and have no effect on the absorption of paracetamol.

Clinical evidence, mechanism, importance and management

Caffeine citrate 120 mg increased the AUC of a single 500-mg dose of paracetamol in 10 healthy subjects by 29%, increased the maximum plasma levels by 15% and decreased the total body clearance by 32%. The decrease in time to maximum level and increase in absorption rate did not reach statistical significance.[1] However, in another study, although caffeine slightly increased the rate of absorption of paracetamol, it had no effect on the extent of absorption.[2] Moreover, a third study states that caffeine decreased plasma paracetamol levels and AUC and increased paracetamol elimination in healthy men.[3] Caffeine is commonly included in paracetamol preparations as an analgesic adjuvant. Its potential benefit and the mechanisms behind its possible effects remain unclear.

1. Iqbal N, Ahmad B, Janbaz KH, Gilani A-UH, Niazi SK. The effect of caffeine on the pharmacokinetics of acetaminophen in man. *Biopharm Drug Dispos* (1995) 16, 481–7.
2. Tukker JJ, Sitsen JMA, Gusdorf CF. Bioavailability of paracetamol after oral administration to healthy volunteers. Influence of caffeine on rate and extent of absorption. *Pharm Weekbl (Sci)* (1986) 8, 239–43.
3. Rainska-Giezek T. Influence of caffeine on toxicity and pharmacokinetics of paracetamol [Article in Polish]. *Ann Acad Med Stetin* (1995) 41, 69–85.

Paracetamol (Acetaminophen) + Colestyramine

The absorption of paracetamol may possibly be reduced if colestyramine is given at the same time, but the reduction in absorption is small if colestyramine is given an hour later.

Clinical evidence

When 4 healthy subjects took colestyramine 12 g and paracetamol (acetaminophen) 2 g together, the absorption of the paracetamol was reduced by 60% (range 30 to 98%) at 2 hours, but the results were said not to be statistically significant. When the colestyramine was given 1 hour after the paracetamol, the absorption was reduced by only 16%.[1]

Mechanism

Colestyramine reduces absorption, presumably because it binds with the paracetamol in the gut. Separating the dosages minimises mixing in the gut.

Importance and management

Although information is limited, it suggests that colestyramine should not be given within 1 hour of paracetamol if maximal analgesia is to be achieved. It is normally recommended that other drugs are given 1 hour before or 4 to 6 hours after colestyramine.

1. Dordoni B, Willson RA, Thompson RPH, Williams R. Reduction of absorption of paracetamol by activated charcoal and cholestyramine: a possible therapeutic measure. *BMJ* (1973) 3, 86–7.

Paracetamol (Acetaminophen) + Disulfiram

Disulfiram had no important effect on the metabolism of paracetamol in one study, but decreased the production of the glutathione (hepatotoxic) metabolites in another.

Clinical evidence, mechanism, importance and management

After taking disulfiram 200 mg daily for 5 days, the clearance of a single 500-mg intravenous dose of paracetamol was slightly reduced (by about 10%) in 5 healthy subjects without liver disease and 5 others with alcoholic liver cirrhosis. The fractional clearance of paracetamol to its glucuronide, sulfate and glutathione metabolites was not altered.[1] In contrast, another study found that pretreatment of healthy subjects with a single 500-mg dose of disulfiram 10 hours before a single 500-mg dose of paracetamol reduced the recovery of glutathione metabolites (a measure of the production of the hepatotoxic metabolite, see 'paracetamol', (p.72)) by 69%.[2]

Disulfiram is an inhibitor of the cytochrome P450 isoenzyme CYP2E1, which is involved in the metabolism of paracetamol. Previously, the authors of the first study[1] had shown that in *rats*, high doses of disulfiram protected against the hepatotoxicity of paracetamol. Therefore, it was suggested that disulfiram might be useful in reducing the risks of paracetamol overdose. However, the authors of the first study concluded that disulfiram at doses used clinically is unlikely to have any beneficial (or adverse) effect on paracetamol metabolism.[1] In contrast, the authors of the second study consider that disulfiram may be useful in reducing the formation of the hepatotoxic metabolite of paracetamol in some situations.[2] Further study is needed.

1. Poulson HE, Ranek L, Jørgensen L. The influence of disulfiram on acetaminophen metabolism in man. *Xenobiotica* (1991) 21, 243–9.
2. Manyike PT, Kharasch ED, Kalhorn TF, Slattery JT. Contribution of CYP2E1 and CYP3A to acetaminophen reactive metabolite formation. *Clin Pharmacol Ther* (2000) 67, 275–82.

Paracetamol (Acetaminophen) + H_2-blockers

Cimetidine, nizatidine, and ranitidine do not appear to alter the pharmacokinetics of paracetamol to a clinically relevant extent.

Clinical evidence

(a) Cimetidine

Cimetidine (given as a single 200-mg dose or as 1 g daily in divided doses for 7 days) had no statistically significant effect on the pharmacokinetics of a single 750-mg dose of paracetamol in 4 healthy subjects.[1] Similarly, in another study, a single 800-mg dose of cimetidine given 1 hour before paracetamol 1 g had no effect on paracetamol half-life or plasma clearance, and no effect on urinary excretion of its principal metabolites (glucuronide, sulfate, mercapturate) in 10 healthy subjects.[2] Furthermore, the pharmacokinetics of a single 1-g dose of paracetamol were not altered by 2 months of treatment with cimetidine 400 mg twice daily in 10 patients. The only difference in urinary metabolites was a modest 37% decrease in paracetamol mercapturate (indicating a reduction in the hepatotoxic metabolite).[2] Other studies have shown that cimetidine does not alter the clearance[3-5] or metabolic pathways of paracetamol.[3,5]

In contrast, one study reported that cimetidine 300 mg every 6 hours decreased the fractional clearance of the oxidised metabolites (mercapturate and cysteine conjugates) of paracetamol in healthy subjects.[6] Another study showed that a single 400-mg dose of cimetidine given 1 hour before paracetamol 1 g in fasting subjects delayed the absorption of paracetamol (for instance, there was a 37% reduction in peak salivary level and a 63% increase in time to peak level). [Note that the effect on extent of absorption (AUC) was not reported.] This effect was not seen when the two drugs were given simultaneously.[7]

(b) Nizatidine

Nizatidine 300 mg given to 5 healthy subjects with paracetamol 1 g modestly increased the paracetamol AUC in the first 3 hours by 25%. Over this time period, there was also a nonsignificant 4% reduction in formation of paracetamol glucuronide, but this did reach statistical significance at 30 and 45 minutes. Nizatidine 150 mg had a similar, but smaller, effect.[8]

(c) Ranitidine

In one study, ranitidine 300 mg twice daily for 4 days had no effect on the clearance and half-life of single, intravenous and oral doses of paracetamol 1 g in 8 healthy subjects. In addition, there was no difference in the urinary excretion of paracetamol metabolites. In this study, ranitidine was given one hour before paracetamol.[9,10] Another study reported similar findings when ranitidine 300 mg was given 1 hour before paracetamol 1 g. However, when the two drugs were given simultaneously, there was a change in paracetamol pharmacokinetics. The 0 to 3-hour AUC of paracetamol was increased by 63%, and there was a 35% decrease in the 0 to 3-hour AUC of paracetamol glucuronide, but no change occurred in sulfate levels.[11] An isolated case describes a man who noted his urine was dark 3 weeks after starting ranitidine 150 mg twice daily and paracetamol 1.3 to 2 g daily. He was found to have raised liver enzyme values (alkaline phosphatase 708 units/l; AST 196 mIU/ml), which returned to normal on discontinuing ranitidine.[12]

Mechanism

Cimetidine may inhibit the oxidative metabolism of paracetamol by cytochrome P450 isoenzymes, resulting in a reduction in the hepatotoxic metabolite, see 'paracetamol', (p.72). It was suggested that cimetidine delayed paracetamol absorption by reducing gastric emptying.[7] Nizatidine may cause a minor inhibition of glucuronyltransferases.[8] Ranitidine may also inhibit paracetamol glucuronyltransferases when given simultaneously, but this was not seen when given one hour apart.

Importance and management

Any changes in the pharmacokinetics of paracetamol with these H_2-blockers appear to be clinically unimportant. Thus, no special precaution would seem to be necessary when paracetamol is used with cimetidine, nizatidine or ranitidine. The effect of cimetidine on the oxidative metabolism of paracetamol has been investigated as a means of reducing paracetamol hepatotoxicity. However, it appears that cimetidine is not effective for this purpose.[13] The possibility that single-dose cimetidine can delay the absorption of paracetamol requires confirmation, and any effect on efficacy assessed.

1. Chen MM, Lee CS. Cimetidine-acetaminophen interaction in humans. *J Clin Pharmacol* (1985) 25, 227–9.
2. Vendemiale G, Altomare E, Trizio T, Leandro G, Manghisi OG, Albano O. Effect of acute and chronic cimetidine administration on acetaminophen metabolism in humans. *Am J Gastroenterol* (1987) 82, 1031–4.
3. Slattery JT, McRorie TI, Reynolds R, Kalhorn TF, Kharasch ED, Eddy AC. Lack of effect of cimetidine on acetaminophen disposition in humans. *Clin Pharmacol Ther* (1989) 46, 591–7.
4. Abernethy DR, Greenblatt DJ, Divoll M, Ameer B, Shader RI. Differential effect of cimetidine on drug oxidation (antipyrine and diazepam) *vs* conjugation (acetaminophen and lorazepam): prevention of acetaminophen toxicity by cimetidine. *J Pharmacol Exp Ther* (1983) 224, 508–13.
5. Miners JO, Attwood J, Birkett DJ. Determinants of acetaminophen metabolism: effect of inducers and inhibitors of drug metabolism on acetaminophen's metabolic pathways. *Clin Pharmacol Ther* (1984) 35, 480–6.
6. Mitchell MC, Schenker S, Speeg KV. Selective inhibition of acetaminophen oxidation and toxicity by cimetidine and other histamine H_2-receptor antagonists in vivo and in vitro in rat and in man. *J Clin Invest* (1984) 73, 383–91.
7. Garba M, Odunola MT, Ahmed BH. Effect of study protocol on the interactions between cimetidine and paracetamol in man. *Eur J Drug Metab Pharmacokinet* (1999) 24, 159–62.
8. Itoh H, Nagano T, Takeyama M. Effect of nizatidine on paracetamol and its metabolites in human plasma. *J Pharm Pharmacol* (2002) 54, 869–73.
9. Thomas M, Michael MF, Andrew P, Scully N. A study to investigate the effects of ranitidine on the metabolic disposition of paracetamol in man. *Br J Clin Pharmacol* (1988) 25, 671P.
10. Jack D, Thomas M, Skidmore IF. Ranitidine and paracetamol metabolism. *Lancet* (1985) ii, 1067.
11. Itoh H, Nagano T, Hayashi T, Takeyama M. Ranitidine increases bioavailability of acetaminophen by inhibiting the first-pass glucuronidation in man. *Pharm Pharmacol Commun* (2000) 6, 495–500.
12. Bredfeldt JE, von Huene C. Ranitidine, acetaminophen, and hepatotoxicity. *Ann Intern Med* (1984) 101, 719.
13. Kaufenberg AJ, Shepherd MF. Role of cimetidine in the treatment of acetaminophen poisoning. *Am J Health-Syst Pharm* (1998) 55, 1516–19.

Paracetamol (Acetaminophen) + HRT or Oral contraceptives

Paracetamol clearance is increased in women taking oral contraceptives, although the clinical relevance of this is uncertain. Paracetamol also increases the absorption of ethinylestradiol from the gut by about 20%. HRT appears not to interact with paracetamol.

Clinical evidence

(a) Effect of oral contraceptives or HRT on paracetamol

In 7 healthy women taking combined oral contraceptives (containing **ethinylestradiol**), the plasma clearance of a single 1.5-g dose of paracetamol was 64% higher and the elimination half-life 30% lower than in 7 healthy women not taking oral contraceptives. The fractional clearance by glucuronidation and of the cysteine conjugate increased, but that of sulfation and the mercapturic acid conjugate were unchanged.[1] Similarly, other studies have found higher paracetamol clearances of 30 to 49%, and corresponding lower half-lives, in women on oral contraceptives, when compared with control subjects.[2-4]

One study found that the pharmacokinetics of single 650-mg intravenous doses of paracetamol did not differ between women who had taken **conjugated oestrogens** for at least 3 months and control women.[5]

(b) Effect of paracetamol on oral contraceptives

A single 1-g oral dose of paracetamol increased the AUC of **ethinylestradiol** by 22% in 6 healthy women, and decreased the AUC of ethinylestradiol sulfate by 41%. Plasma levels of **levonorgestrel** were not affected.[6]

Mechanism

The evidence suggests that oral contraceptives increase the metabolism (both oxidation and glucuronidation) of paracetamol by the liver so that it is cleared from the body more quickly.[3] The increased absorption of the ethinylestradiol probably occurs because the paracetamol reduces its metabolism by the gut wall during absorption.[6] It has been suggested that the differences between the effects of oral contraceptives and conjugated oestrogens on paracetamol may be attributable to the influence of progestogens on glucuronide and sulphate conjugation.[5] This needs confirmation.

Importance and management

The modest pharmacokinetic interaction of the oral contraceptives on paracetamol appears to be established, but its clinical importance has not been directly studied. The clinical importance of the modest increased ethinylestradiol absorption is also uncertain, but likely to be minor. HRT appears not to interact with paracetamol.

1. Mitchell MC, Hanew T, Meredith CG, Schenker S. Effects of oral contraceptive steroids on acetaminophen metabolism and elimination. *Clin Pharmacol Ther* (1983) 34, 48–53.
2. Abernethy DR, Divoll M, Ochs HR, Ameer B, Greenblatt DJ. Increased metabolic clearance of acetaminophen with oral contraceptive use. *Obstet Gynecol* (1982) 60, 338–41.
3. Miners JO, Attwood J, Birkett DJ. Influence of sex and oral contraceptive steroids on paracetamol metabolism. *Br J Clin Pharmacol* (1983) 16, 503–9.
4. Mucklow JC, Fraser HS, Bulpitt CJ, Kahn C, Mould G, Dollery CT. Environmental factors affecting paracetamol metabolism in London factory and office workers. *Br J Clin Pharmacol* (1980) 10, 67–74.
5. Scavone JM, Greenblatt DJ, Blyden GT, Luna BG, Harmatz JS. Acetaminophen pharmacokinetics in women receiving conjugated estrogen. *Eur J Clin Pharmacol* (1990) 38, 97–8.
6. Rogers SM, Back DJ, Stevenson PJ, Grimmer SFM, Orme ML'E. Paracetamol interaction with oral contraceptive steroids: increased plasma concentration of ethinyloestradiol. *Br J Clin Pharmacol* (1987) 23, 721–5.

Paracetamol (Acetaminophen) + Isoniazid

A number of reports suggest that the toxicity of paracetamol may be increased by isoniazid so that normal daily analgesic dosages (4 g) may not be safe in some individuals. Pharmacokinetic studies suggest that isoniazid usually inhibits the metabolism of paracetamol, but that metabolism to toxic metabolites may be induced shortly after stopping isoniazid, or late in the isoniazid dose-interval in fast acetylators of isoniazid.

Clinical evidence

A 21-year-old woman who had been taking isoniazid 300 mg for 6 months took 3.25 g of paracetamol for abdominal cramping. Within about 6 hours she developed marked evidence of liver damage (prolonged prothrombin time, elevated ammonia, transaminases, hyperbilirubinaemia).[1]

A young woman on isoniazid who had ingested up to 11.5 g paracetamol in a suicide gesture, developed life-threatening hepatic and renal toxicity despite the fact that her serum paracetamol levels 13 hours later were only 15 micromol/l (toxicity normally associated with levels above 26 micromol/l).[2]

Three other cases were reported in patients who had taken only 2 to 6 g paracetamol daily and were also taking isoniazid, rifampicin and pyrazinamide.[3] Three other possible cases of this toxic interaction have been described.[4]

However, in a pharmacokinetic study in 10 healthy subjects of both slow and fast acetylator status, isoniazid 300 mg daily for 7 days modestly decreased the total clearance of a single 500-mg dose of paracetamol by 15%. Moreover, the clearance of paracetamol to oxidative metabolites was *decreased*.[5] Similarly, in a further study in 10 healthy slow acetylators of isoniazid, the formation of paracetamol thioether metabolites and oxidate metabolites was reduced by 63% and 49% respectively by isoniazid 300 mg daily. However, one day after stopping isoniazid, the formation of thioether metabolites was *increased* by 56%, and this returned to pretreatment values 3 days after the discontinuation of isoniazid.[6] In yet another study in patients on isoniazid prophylaxis, paracetamol, given simultaneously with the daily isoniazid dose inhibited the formation clearance of paracetamol to *N*-acetyl-*p*-benzoquinone imine (NAPQI) by 57%, but when the paracetamol was taken 12 hours after the isoniazid, there was no difference in NAPQI clearance. When the results were analysed by acetylator status, it appeared that the NAPQI clearance was *increased* in fast acetylators taking paracetamol 12 hours after the isoniazid dose.[7]

Mechanism

Not established. A possible reason is that isoniazid induces the cytochrome P450 isoenzyme CYP2E1 by stabilisation.[8] This means that while the isoniazid is still present, the metabolism of substrates such as paracetamol is inhibited. However, when isoniazid levels drop sufficiently (as may be the case late in the dosing interval in fast acetylators), metabolism may be induced resulting in a greater proportion of the paracetamol being converted into toxic metabolites than would normally occur.[7]

Importance and management

Information is limited, but it would now seem prudent to warn patients taking isoniazid to limit their use of paracetamol because it seems that some individuals risk possible paracetamol-induced liver toxicity, even with normal recommended doses. Pharmacokinetic studies suggest that it is possible that the risk is greatest shortly after stopping isoniazid. The risk may also be higher if paracetamol is taken late in the isoniazid dosing interval, particularly in fast acetylators of isoniazid. More study is needed to clarify the situation.

1. Crippin JS. Acetaminophen hepatotoxicity: potentiation by isoniazid. *Am J Gastroenterol* (1993) 88, 590–2.
2. Murphy R, Swartz R, Watkins P B. Severe acetaminophen toxicity in a patient receiving isoniazid. *Ann Intern Med* (1990) 113, 799–800.
3. Nolan CM, Sandblom RE, Thummel KE, Slattery JT, Nelson SD. Hepatotoxicity associated with acetaminophen usage in patients receiving multiple drug therapy for tuberculosis. *Chest* (1994) 105, 408–11.
4. Moulding TS, Redeker AG, Kanel GC. Acetaminophen, isoniazid, and hepatic toxicity. *Ann Intern Med* (1991) 114, 431.
5. Epstein MM, Nelson SD, Slattery JT, Kalhorn TF, Wall RA, Wright JM. Inhibition of the metabolism of paracetamol by isoniazid. *Br J Clin Pharmacol* (1991) 31, 139–42.
6. Zand R, Nelson SD, Slattery JT, Thummel KE, Kalhorn TF, Adams SP, Wright JM. Inhibition and induction of cytochrome P4502E1-catalyzed oxidation by isoniazid in humans. *Clin Pharmacol Ther* (1993) 54, 142–9.
7. Chien JY, Peter RM, Nolan CM, Wartell C, Slattery JT, Nelson SD, Carithers RL, Thummel KE. Influence of polymorphic N-acetyltransferase phenotype on the inhibition and induction of acetaminophen bioactivation with long-term isoniazid. *Clin Pharmacol Ther* (1997) 61, 24–34.
8. Chien JY, Thummel KE, Slattery JT. Pharmacokinetic consequences of induction of CYP2E1 by ligand stabilization. *Drug Metab Dispos* (1997) 25, 1165–75.

Paracetamol (Acetaminophen) + Kakkonto

Single-dose studies in healthy subjects found that kakkonto did not affect the pharmacokinetics of paracetamol, but *animal* studies found increased paracetamol levels.

Clinical evidence, mechanism, importance and management

A study in 6 healthy subjects found that 5 g of Kakkonto extract, a Chinese herbal medicine containing extracts of *Puerariae*, *Ephedrae*, *Zingiberis*, *Cinnamomi*, *Glycyrrhizae*, *Paeoniae* and *Zizphi* spp. had no effects on the pharmacokinetics of a single 12-mg/kg dose of paracetamol. A further study in 19 healthy subjects found that 1.25 g of Kakkonto had no effect on the pharmacokinetics of paracetamol 150 mg (from a preparation also containing salicylamide, caffeine and promethazine methylene disalicylate). Because in *animal* studies high doses of Kakkonto for 7 days were found to significantly increase serum levels of paracetamol, the authors concluded that further investigations were required to assess safety and efficacy of concurrent use.[1]

1. Qi J, Toyoshima A, Honda Y, Mineshita S. Pharmacokinetic study on acetaminophen: interaction with a Chinese medicine. *J Med Dent Sci* (1997) 44, 31–5.

Paracetamol (Acetaminophen) + Metoclopramide

Metoclopramide increases the rate of absorption of paracetamol and raises its maximum plasma levels.

Clinical evidence, mechanism, importance and management

Intravenous metoclopramide 10 mg increased the peak plasma levels of a single 1.5 g dose of paracetamol by 64% in 5 healthy subjects (slow absorbers of paracetamol), and increased its rate of absorption (peak levels reached in 48 instead of 120 minutes), but the total amount absorbed remained virtually unaltered.[1] Oral metoclopramide also increases the rate of paracetamol absorption,[2] probably because the rate of gastric emptying is increased. This interaction is exploited in *Paramax* (a proprietary oral preparation containing both drugs) to increase the effectiveness and onset of analgesia for the treatment of migraine. This is obviously an advantageous interaction in this situation.

1. Nimmo J, Heading RC, Tothill P, Prescott LF. Pharmacological modification of gastric emptying: effects of propantheline and metoclopramide on paracetamol absorption. *BMJ* (1973) 1, 587–9.
2. Crome P, Kimber GR, Wainscott G, Widdop B. The effect of the simultaneous administration of oral metoclopramide on the absorption of paracetamol in healthy volunteers. *Br J Clin Pharmacol* (1981) 11, 430P–431P.

Paracetamol (Acetaminophen) + Opioids

Pethidine, pentazocine and diamorphine delay gastric emptying so that the rate of absorption of paracetamol given orally is reduced. There is no pharmacokinetic interaction between codeine and paracetamol, but the combination may not always result in increased analgesia.

Clinical evidence

(a) Codeine

Paracetamol 1 g every 8 hours for 7 doses had no effect on the pharmacokinetics of codeine and its metabolites after a single 30-mg oral dose of codeine phosphate in 6 healthy subjects.[1] Similarly in other studies, codeine had no effect on the pharmacokinetics of paracetamol.[2,3] Paracetamol and codeine are often combined because the combination is more effective than either drug given alone. However, note that not all studies have found this. For example, in one clinical study of surgical removal of impacted third molar teeth, there was no difference in analgesic efficacy between patients given paracetamol alone (800 mg given 3, 6 and 9 hours after surgery, then 400 mg four times daily for 2 days) and those given the same dose of paracetamol with the addition of codeine phosphate 30 mg. Moreover, patients given codeine experienced more adverse effects (nausea, dizziness, drowsiness).[4]

(b) Diamorphine, pethidine and pentazocine

The absorption of a single 20-mg/kg dose of paracetamol in 8 healthy subjects given 30 minutes after an intramuscular injection of either pethidine 150 mg or diamorphine 10 mg was markedly delayed and reduced. Peak plasma paracetamol levels were reduced by 31% and 74%, respectively, and delayed from 22 minutes to 114 and 142 minutes, respectively.[5] This interaction was also observed by the same study group in women in labour who had been given pethidine, diamorphine or pentazocine.[6]

Mechanism, importance and management

The underlying mechanism of these interactions is that the opiate analgesics delay gastric emptying so that the rate of absorption of paracetamol is reduced, but the total amount absorbed is not affected. These were largely investigational studies, where paracetamol was used as a measure of gastric emptying, and any clinical relevance has not been determined. Reducing the rate of paracetamol absorption would be expected to reduce the onset of analgesic effect, but this is unlikely to be clinically relevant in patients who have recently received these potent opioids. See also (a) above.

1. Somogyi A, Bochner F, Chen ZR. Lack of effect of paracetamol on the pharmacokinetics and metabolism of codeine in man. *Eur J Clin Pharmacol* (1991) 41, 279–82.

2. Bajorek P, Widdop B, Volans G. Lack of inhibition of paracetamol absorption by codeine. *Br J Clin Pharmacol* (1978) 5, 346–8.
3. Sonne J, Poulsen HE, Loft S, Døssing M, Vollmer-Larsen A, Simonsen K, Thyssen H, Lundstrøm K. Therapeutic doses of codeine have no effect on acetaminophen clearance or metabolism. *Eur J Clin Pharmacol* (1988) 35, 109–11.
4. Skjelbred P, Løkken P. Codeine added to paracetamol induced adverse effects but did not increase analgesia. *Br J Clin Pharmacol* (1982) 14, 539–43.
5. Nimmo WS, Heading RC, Wilson J, Tothill P, Prescott LF. Inhibition of gastric emptying and drug absorption by narcotic analgesics. *Br J Clin Pharmacol* (1975) 2, 509–13.
6. Nimmo WS, Wilson J, Prescott LF. Narcotic analgesics and delayed gastric emptying during labour. *Lancet* (1975) i, 890–3.

Paracetamol (Acetaminophen) + Probenecid

Probenecid reduces the clearance of paracetamol from the body.

Clinical evidence, mechanism, importance and management

A metabolic study in 10 healthy subjects found that the clearance of paracetamol 1.5 g was almost halved (from 6.23 to 3.42 ml/minute) when taken 1 hour after probenecid 1 g. The amount of unchanged paracetamol in the urine stayed the same, but the amount of paracetamol glucuronide fell sharply.[1] Another study in 11 subjects also found that while taking probenecid 500 mg every 6 hours the clearance of a 650-mg intravenous dose of paracetamol was almost halved (from 5.05 to 2.72 ml/min/kg). The urinary excretion of the glucuronide metabolite was decreased by 68% and the excretion of the sulfate metabolite increased by 49%.[2] These studies suggest that probenecid inhibits paracetamol glucuronidation, possibly by inhibiting glucuronyltransferase. See also 'paracetamol', (p.72). The practical consequences of this interaction are uncertain but there seem to be no adverse reports.

1. Kamali F. The effect of probenecid on paracetamol metabolism and pharmacokinetics. *Eur J Clin Pharmacol* (1993) 45, 551–3.
2. Abernethy DR, Greenblatt DJ, Ameer B, Shader RI. Probenecid impairment of acetaminophen and lorazepam clearance: direct inhibition of ether glucuronide formation. *J Pharmacol Exp Ther* (1985) 234, 345–9.

Paracetamol (Acetaminophen) or Phenacetin + Proton pump inhibitors

Lansoprazole modestly increased the rate, but not the extent, of absorption of paracetamol solution. Omeprazole had no effect on the metabolism of phenacetin or paracetamol.

Clinical evidence

(a) Lansoprazole

In a study in 6 healthy subjects, lansoprazole 30 mg once daily for 3 days increased the peak level of paracetamol (given as a single 1-g dose in solution) by 43% and this occurred in half the time (about 17.5 versus 35 minutes). However, lansoprazole had no effect on the AUC and elimination half-life of paracetamol.[1]

(b) Omeprazole

Omeprazole 20 mg daily for 8 days had no effect on the pharmacokinetics of phenacetin, or paracetamol derived from phenacetin, in 10 healthy subjects, except that the peak plasma phenacetin level was higher during omeprazole treatment. There was no change in the metabolism (oxidative and conjugative) of phenacetin or derived paracetamol.[2] In another study, omeprazole 40 mg daily for 7 days had no effect on the formation of thioether metabolites of paracetamol in 5 rapid and 5 slow metabolisers of (*S*)-mephenytoin.[3]

Mechanism

Lansoprazole may increase the absorption of paracetamol by indirectly increasing the rate of release of gastric liquid.[1] Phenacetin is metabolised to paracetamol by the cytochrome P450 isoenzyme CYP1A2, and it has been suggested that omeprazole can induce CYP1A2, and possibly increase the formation of hepatotoxic metabolites of paracetamol. However, the findings here suggest that omeprazole has no important effect on CYP1A2, or on phenacetin or paracetamol metabolism.

Importance and management

The findings from these studies suggest that neither lansoprazole nor omeprazole cause any clinically important changes in the pharmacokinetics of paracetamol. No special precautions appear to be needed on concurrent use.

1. Sanaka M, Kuyama Y, Mineshita S, Qi J, Hanada Y, Enatsu I, Tanaka H, Makino H, Yamanaka M. Pharmacokinetic interaction between acetaminophen and lansoprazole. *J Clin Gastroenterol* (1999) 29, 56–8.
2. Xiaodong S, Gatti G, Bartoli A, Cipolla G, Crema F, Perucca E. Omeprazole does not enhance the metabolism of phenacetin, a marker of CYP1A2 activity, in healthy volunteers. *Ther Drug Monit* (1994) 16, 248–50.
3. Sarich T, Kalhorn T, Magee S, Al-Sayegh F, Adams S, Slattery J, Goldstein J, Nelson S, Wright J. The effect of omeprazole pretreatment on acetaminophen metabolism in rapid and slow metabolizers of *S*-mephenytoin. *Clin Pharmacol Ther* (1997) 62, 21–8.

Paracetamol (Acetaminophen) + Rifampicin (Rifampin)

Rifampicin increases the loss of paracetamol from the body.

Clinical evidence, mechanism, importance and management

The metabolite to paracetamol ratio for glucuronides was twice as high in 10 patients treated with rifampicin 600 mg daily than in 14 healthy control subjects. In contrast the ratio for sulfates did not differ between the two groups.[1] In a crossover study in healthy subjects, rifampicin 600 mg daily for 1 week, given before paracetamol 500 mg, had no effect on the formation of *N*-acetyl-*p*-benzoquinone imine (NAPQI) or the recovery of thiol metabolites formed by conjugation of NAPQI with glutathione.[2] These data suggest that rifampicin induces the glucuronidation of paracetamol and increases its loss from the body, but that it does not increase the formation of hepatotoxic metabolites of 'paracetamol', (p.72). The clinical importance of these findings awaits further study, but they suggest that rifampicin may reduce the efficacy of paracetamol.

1. Bock KW, Wiltfang J, Blume R, Ullrich D, Bircher J. Paracetamol as a test drug to determine glucuronide formation in man. Effects of inducers and of smoking. *Eur J Clin Pharmacol* (1987) 31, 677–83.
2. Manyike PT, Kharasch ED, Kalhorn TF, Slattery JT. Contribution of CYP2E1 and CYP3A to acetaminophen reactive metabolite formation. *Clin Pharmacol Ther* (2000) 67, 275–82.

Paracetamol (Acetaminophen) + Sucralfate

No change in the bioavailability of paracetamol 1 g was found in 6 healthy subjects given sucralfate 1 g, using salivary paracetamol levels over 4 hours as a measure.[1]

1. Kamali F, Fry JR, Smart HL, Bell GD. A double-blind placebo-controlled study to examine effects of sucralfate on paracetamol absorption. *Br J Clin Pharmacol* (1985) 19, 113–14.

Paracetamol (Acetaminophen) + Sulfinpyrazone

Sulfinpyrazone modestly increases the loss of paracetamol from the body.

Clinical evidence, mechanism, importance and management

Sulfinpyrazone 200 mg every 6 hours for one week increased the clearance of a single 1-g dose of paracetamol by 23% in 12 healthy subjects. There was a 26% increase in metabolic clearance of the glucuronide conjugate, and a 43% increase in the glutathione-derived conjugates (indicating an increased production of the hepatotoxic metabolite), but no change in sulfation.[1] It has been suggested that, as a result, the risk of liver damage may be increased after overdosage and perhaps during prolonged consumption,[1] (see also 'paracetamol', (p.72)) but there seem to be no adverse reports. The clinical importance of these findings awaits further study.

1. Miners JO, Attwood J, Birkett DJ. Determinants of acetaminophen metabolism: effect of inducers and inhibitors of drug metabolism on acetaminophen's metabolic pathways. *Clin Pharmacol Ther* (1984) 35, 480–6.

Paracetamol (Acetaminophen) + Tobacco smoking

Heavy, but not moderate, smoking may increase the metabolism of paracetamol. There is some evidence that smokers are at risk of a poorer outcome after paracetamol overdose.

Clinical evidence, mechanism, importance and management

There was no difference in the clearance of a single 1-g dose of paracetamol in 6 healthy smokers (more than 15 cigarettes per day) and 6 healthy nonsmokers in one study, and no difference in the paracetamol metabolites.[1] Similarly, another study found no difference in the pharmacokinetics of a single 650-mg intravenous dose of paracetamol in 14 healthy smokers (range 8 to 35 cigarettes per day) and 15 nonsmokers.[2] In contrast, in another study, the metabolite to paracetamol ratio for glucuronides was 83% higher in 9 heavy smokers (about 40 cigarettes daily) than in 14 healthy nonsmokers. However, it was not higher in moderate smokers (about 10 cigarettes daily).[3]

A retrospective survey of patients treated for single-dose paracetamol poisoning found that there was a much higher proportion of smokers than in the general population (70% versus 31%). Moreover, smoking was independently associated with an increased risk of hepatic encephalopathy (odds ratio 2.68) and death (odds ratio 3.64) following paracetamol overdose.[4]

No interaction is established, but the above studies suggest that heavy smoking may increase the metabolism of paracetamol. The retrospective survey also suggests that smoking is associated with a poorer outcome after paracetamol overdose. Further study is needed.

1. Miners JO, Attwood J, Birkett DJ. Determinants of acetaminophen metabolism: effect of inducers and inhibitors of drug metabolism on acetaminophen's metabolic pathways. *Clin Pharmacol Ther* (1984) 35, 480–6.
2. Scavone JM, Greenblatt DJ, LeDuc BW, Blyden GT, Luna BG, Harmatz JS. Differential effect of cigarette smoking on antipyrine oxidation versus acetaminophen conjugation. *Pharmacology* (1990) 40, 77–84.
3. Bock KW, Wiltfang J, Blume R, Ullrich D, Bircher J. Paracetamol as a test drug to determine glucuronide formation in man. Effects of inducers and of smoking. *Eur J Clin Pharmacol* (1987) 31, 677–83.
4. Schmidt LE, Dalhoff K. The impact of current tobacco use on the outcome of paracetamol poisoning. *Aliment Pharmacol Ther* (2003) 18, 979–85.

6

Anthelmintics, antifungals and antiprotozoals

'Table 6.1' lists the drugs covered in this section by therapeutic group. If the anti-infective is the affecting drug, the interaction is dealt with elsewhere. Also note that some anti-infectives have actions against more than one type of organism (e.g. bacteria and protozoa) and so may be covered in other sections.

Table 6.1 Anthelmintics, antifungals and antiprotozoals

Anthelmintics	Albendazole, Diethylcarbamazine, Ivermectin, Levamisole, Mebendazole, Metrifonate (Metriphonate), Niclosamide, Piperazine, Praziquantel, Pyrantel, Tiabendazole (Thiabendazole), Tetrachlorethylene
Antifungals	Anidulafungin, Amphotericin B, Amorolfine, Caspofungin, Clotrimazole, Econazole, Fenticonazole, Fluconazole, Flucytosine, Fosfomycin, Griseofulvin, Isoconazole, Itraconazole, Ketoconazole, Miconazole, Nystatin, Terbinafine, Tioconazole, Voriconazole
Antimalarials	Atovaquone, Chloroquine, Halofantrine, Hydroxychloroquine, Mefloquine, Mepacrine, Pamaquine, Primaquine, Proguanil, Pyrimethamine, Quinine, Sulfadoxine
Antiprotozoals	Clioquinol, Diloxanide furoate, Furazolidone

Albendazole or Mebendazole + Anticonvulsants

Phenytoin, carbamazepine and phenobarbital lower the plasma levels of albendazole and mebendazole, and therefore might reduce their efficacy for systemic infections. Valproate does not lower plasma mebendazole levels.

Clinical evidence

(a) Albendazole

A study in 32 patients with intraparenchymatous neurocysticercosis treated with either **phenytoin** 200 to 300 mg daily (9 patients), **carbamazepine** 600 to 1200 mg daily (9 patients), or **phenobarbital** 100 to 300 mg daily (5 patients) all for at least 3 months, and a control group consisting of 9 patients who did not receive any anticonvulsants, were given albendazole 7.5 mg/kg every 12 hours for 8 days. The AUCs for (+)-albendazole sulfoxide were 66%, 49%, and 61% lower than the control group for the **phenytoin**, **carbamazepine**, and **phenobarbital** groups respectively. The maximum plasma levels of (+)-albendazole sulfoxide were 50 to 63% lower and the half lives about 3 to 4 hours shorter. The AUCs, peak plasma levels and half-life of (–)-albendazole sulfoxide were similarly reduced by the anticonvulsants.[1]

(b) Mebendazole

A retrospective analysis found that patients with echinococcosis treated with mebendazole and taking **phenytoin** or **carbamazepine** tended to have lower plasma mebendazole levels than those not on these anticonvulsants.[2] **Valproic acid** tended to increase mebendazole levels, and some patients had a clinically important rise in mebendazole levels when they were switched from **phenytoin** or **carbamazepine** to **valproic acid**.[2]

Mechanism

Phenytoin, carbamazepine and phenobarbital appear to induce the oxidative metabolism of albendazole by the cytochrome P450 isoenzyme CYP3A to roughly the same extent, resulting in significantly reduced levels of albendazole sulfoxide. Phenytoin, and to a lesser extent carbamazepine, may also induce the metabolism of albendazole sulfone by CYP2C. Mebendazole is similarly affected.

Importance and management

These pharmacokinetic interactions are established, and are likely to be clinically important when these anthelmintics are used to treat systemic worm infections. For these infections it may be necessary to increase the albendazole and mebendazole dosage in patients on phenytoin, carbamazepine or phenobarbital. Monitor the outcome of concurrent use. The interactions are of no importance when these anthelmintics are used for intestinal worm infections (where their action is a local effect on the worms in the gut), which is the most common use of mebendazole in particular.

1. Lanchote L, Garcia FS, Dreossi SAC, Takayanagui OM. Pharmacokinetic interaction between albendazole sulfoxide enantiomers and antiepileptic drugs in patients with neurocysticercosis. *Ther Drug Monit* (2002) 24, 338–45.
2. Luder PJ, Siffert B, Witassek F, Meister F, Bircher J. Treatment of hydatid disease with high oral doses of mebendazole. Long-term follow-up of plasma mebendazole levels and drug interactions. *Eur J Clin Pharmacol* (1986) 31, 443–8.

Albendazole or Mebendazole + Cimetidine

Cimetidine raises serum mebendazole levels, and prolongs the half-life of albendazole sulfoxide, and might increase the effectiveness of these anthelmintics against systemic infection.

Clinical evidence

(a) Albendazole

A study in 6 healthy subjects given albendazole 20 mg/kg and cimetidine 10 mg/kg twice daily found that cimetidine decreased the maximum plasma level of albendazole sulfoxide by 52% (not statistically significant) and significantly inhibited the metabolism of albendazole sulfoxide as indicated by an increase in its elimination half-life from 7.4 to 19 hours. Cimetidine also reduced inter-individual variability in plasma albendazole levels.[1] Another study in patients with cystic echinococcosis given albendazole 20 mg/kg daily for three 4-week courses separated by intervals of 10 days found that levels of the active metabolite albendazole sulfoxide were higher in bile and hydatid cyst fluid in 7 patients who also received cimetidine 10 mg/kg daily. The therapeutic benefit of the combined treatment was reported to be greater than that with albendazole alone.[2] Cimetidine also appears to reduce the bioavailability of albendazole given with 'grapefruit juice', (p.132).

(b) Mebendazole

A study in 8 patients (5 with peptic ulcers and 3 with hydatid cysts) taking mebendazole 1.5 g three times daily found that cimetidine 400 mg three times daily for 30 days raised the maximum plasma mebendazole levels by 48%. The previously unresponsive hepatic hydatid cysts resolved totally.[3] However, a previous study had found smaller increases in serum mebendazole levels with cimetidine 1 g daily in divided doses, which were considered too small to be clinically useful.[4]

Mechanism

It is suggested that the interaction is caused by the enzyme inhibitory actions of cimetidine reducing the metabolism of albendazole and mebendazole.[1,3] Cimetidine may also have an effect on albendazole absorption by reducing gastric acidity.[1]

Importance and management

These pharmacokinetic interactions would appear to be established, but their clinical relevance is uncertain. Increased efficacy has been shown in some studies for systemic worm infections. There would seem to be no reason for avoiding concurrent use, but increased monitoring for efficacy and toxicity might be prudent.

1. Schipper HG, Koopmans RP, Nagy J, Butter JJ, Kager PA, Van Boxtel CJ. Effect of dose increase or cimetidine co-administration on albendazole bioavailability. *Am J Trop Med Hyg* (2000) 63, 270–3.
2. Wen H, Zhang HW, Muhmut M, Zou PF, New RRC, Craig PS. Initial observation on albendazole in combination with cimetidine for the treatment of human cystic echinococcosis. *Ann Trop Med Parasitol* (1994) 88, 49–52.
3. Bekhti A, Pirotte J. Cimetidine increases serum mebendazole concentrations. Implications for treatment of hepatic hydatid cysts. *Br J Clin Pharmacol* (1987) 24, 390–2.
4. Luder PJ, Siffert B, Witassek F, Meister F, Bircher J. Treatment of hydatid disease with high oral doses of mebendazole. Long-term follow-up of plasma mebendazole levels and drug interactions. *Eur J Clin Pharmacol* (1986) 31, 443–8.

Albendazole or Praziquantel + Corticosteroids

The continuous use of dexamethasone can reduce serum praziquantel levels by 50%, which might reduce its efficacy in systemic worm infections. Conversely, dexamethasone can raise levels of albendazole sulfoxide by 50%, which might increase its efficacy in systemic worm infections.

Clinical evidence

(a) Albendazole

In one study albendazole 15 mg/kg daily in three divided doses was given to 8 patients with cysticercosis. The plasma levels of the active metabolite of albendazole (albendazole sulfoxide) were found to be increased by about 50% by the use of **dexamethasone** 8 mg every 8 hours.[1] Another study did not detect significantly increased maximum plasma levels of albendazole sulfoxide, but the AUC was increased twofold, and there was a decrease in its clearance.[2]

(b) Praziquantel

Eight patients with parenchymal brain cysticercosis treated with praziquantel 50 mg/kg divided into three doses every 8 hours had a 50% reduction in steady-state serum levels, from 3.13 to 1.55 micrograms/ml when given **dexamethasone** 8 mg every 8 hours.[3]

Mechanism

Uncertain. Dexamethasone is an inducer of the cytochrome P450 isoenzyme CYP3A4, and might therefore be expected to reduce levels of both praziquantel and albendazole, so the finding with albendazole is unexpected. Dexamethasone appears not to alter the rate of formation of albendazole sulfoxide, but decreases its elimination.[2]

Importance and management

Information about praziquantel and albendazole seems to be limited but the interaction would appear to be established. Just how much it affects the outcome of treatment for systemic worm infections such as cysticercosis is unknown because the optimum praziquantel and albendazole levels are still uncertain. The authors of the reports suggest that dexamethasone should not be given continuously with praziquantel but only used transiently for the treatment of inflammatory reactions to praziquantel treatment. Conversely it would appear that albendazole can be given concurrently with dexamethasone without compromising treatment, and combined use may actually be beneficial.[4] Intravenous **methylprednisolone** has also been used for acute corticosteroid therapy with these anthelmintics, and oral **prednisone** has been used long-term to prevent further tissue damage associated with inflammation[4,5] but the effect of these corticosteroids on plasma levels of the anthelmintics appears not to have been studied.

The interaction with dexamethasone is of no importance when praziquantel is used for intestinal worm infections (where its action is a local effect on the worms in the gut).

1. Jung H, Hurtado M, Tulio Medina M, Sanchez M, Sotelo J. Dexamethasone increases plasma levels of albendazole. *J Neurol* (1990) 237, 279–80.
2. Takayanagui OM, Lanchote VL, Marques MPC, Bonato PS. Therapy for neurocysticercosis: pharmacokinetic interaction of albendazole sulfoxide with dexamethasone. *Ther Drug Monit* (1997) 19, 51–5.
3. Vazquez ML, Jung H, Sotelo J. Plasma levels of praziquantel decrease when dexamethasone is given simultaneously. *Neurology* (1987) 37, 1561–2.
4. Sotelo J, Jung H. Pharmacokinetic optimisation of the treatment of neurocysticercosis. *Clin Pharmacokinet* (1998) 34, 503–15.
5. Silva LCS, Maciel PE, Ribas JGR, Souza-Pereira SR, Antunes CM, Lambertucci JR. Treatment of schistosomal myeloradiculopathy with praziquantel and corticosteroids and evaluation by magnetic resonance imaging: a longitudinal study. *Clin Infect Dis* (2004) 39, 1618–24.

Albendazole + Food

Giving albendazole with a fatty meal markedly increases its absorption.

Clinical evidence, mechanism, importance and management

A study in Sudanese men found that giving a single 400-mg dose of albendazole with a meal resulted in a 7.9-fold higher level of the active metabolite, albendazole sulfoxide, than when albendazole was given in the fasted state.[1] Similarly, a further study in healthy subjects found that when albendazole 10 mg/kg was given with a fatty meal, rather than with water, the peak plasma levels of the active metabolite were increased by more than sixfold and the half-life was 8.8 hours and 8.2 hours with water and fatty meal respectively.[2] Albendazole absorption is poor, and if it is being used for systemic infections, it is advisable to take it with a meal.

1. Homeida M, Leahy W, Copeland S, Ali MMM, Harron DWG. Pharmacokinetic interaction between praziquantel and albendazole in Sudanese men. *Ann Trop Med Parasitol* (1994) 88, 551–9.
2. Nagy J, Schipper HG, Koopmans RP, Butter JJ, Van Boxtel CJ, Kager PA. Effect of grapefruit juice or cimetidine coadministration on albendazole bioavailability. *Am J Trop Med Hyg* (2002) 66, 260–3.

Albendazole + Grapefruit juice

Grapefruit juice increases the absorption of albendazole.

Clinical evidence, mechanism, importance and management

Grapefruit juice increased albendazole sulfoxide levels by about threefold and shortened its half-life by 46%.[1] However, when albendazole was given with grapefruit juice and cimetidine the peak plasma level was reduced from 760 to 410 micrograms/l.

It was suggested that the metabolism of albendazole by the cytochrome isoenzyme CYP3A4 in the intestinal mucosa is inhibited by grapefruit juice and that cimetidine decreased albendazole bioavailability.[1] (See also 'Albendazole or Mebendazole + Cimetidine', p.131.) The clinical relevance of the change with grapefruit juice is uncertain. For systemic infections, increased absorption might be beneficial, but the decrease in half-life might be detrimental.

1. Nagy J, Schipper HG, Koopmans RP, Butter JJ, Van Boxtel CJ, Kager PA. Effect of grapefruit juice or cimetidine coadministration on albendazole bioavailability. *Am J Trop Med Hyg* (2002) 66, 260–3.

Albendazole + Ivermectin

No pharmacokinetic interaction occurs between albendazole and ivermectin.

Clinical evidence, mechanism, importance and management

In a double-blind placebo-controlled study, 42 patients with onchocerciasis were given single doses of either ivermectin 200 micrograms/kg, albendazole 400 mg or both drugs together. There was no significant pharmacokinetic interaction, and although the combination seemed to offer no advantage over ivermectin alone for the treatment on onchocerciasis, the combination appeared safe. No dosage adjustments would be required during concurrent use.[1]

1. Awadzi K, Edwards G, Duke BOL, Opoku NO, Attah SK, Addy ET, Ardrey AE, Quarty BT. The co-administration of ivermectin and albendazole— safety, pharmacokinetics and efficacy against *Onchocerca volvulus*. *Ann Trop Med Parasitol* (2003) 97, 165–78.

Albendazole + Levamisole

Levamisole may markedly decrease the bioavailability of albendazole. Albendazole has no clinically significant effects on levamisole pharmacokinetics.

Clinical evidence, mechanism, importance and management

A study in 28 healthy subjects given levamisole 2.5 mg/kg alone or with albendazole 400 mg found that albendazole produced a modest reduction in the AUC but no other pharmacokinetic parameters of levamisole were affected. However, the AUC of albendazole sulfoxide was 75% lower when given with levamisole than historical values in subjects who had received levamisole alone.[1] An associated study in 44 patients found that levamisole with or without albendazole was not effective against *Onchocerca volvulus* infections. Both treatments caused a similar number of adverse effects.[1] The clinical relevance of these findings is unclear, but they suggest that caution is needed during combined use for systemic worm infections.

1. Awadzi K, Edwards G, Opoku NO, Ardrey AE, Favager S, Addy ET, Attah SK, Yamuah LK, Quartey BT. The safety, tolerability and pharmacokinetics of levamisole alone, levamisole plus ivermectin, and levamisole plus albendazole, and their efficacy against *Onchocerca volvulus*. *Ann Trop Med Parasitol* (2004) 98, 595–614.

Amphotericin B + Azoles

There is some clinical evidence that amphotericin B with either itraconazole, ketoconazole or miconazole may possibly be less effective than amphotericin B alone, and the adverse effects may be greater.

Clinical evidence

Studies in a few patients and *in vitro* experiments suggest that the antifungal effects of amphotericin B and **miconazole** used together may be antagonistic, and not additive as might be expected.[1,2] In another study, 4 out of 6 patients did not respond to amphotericin B treatment while also taking **ketoconazole**, whereas treatment was successful in 6 others, 5 of whom had stopped taking either prophylactic **miconazole** or **ketoconazole**. The authors suggested that the numbers are too small to draw any definite conclusions, but antagonism is certainly a possibility.[3] A comparative study in patients found that those on **itraconazole** and amphotericin B had serum **itraconazole** levels of less than 1 microgram/ml, whereas those on **itraconazole** alone had serum **itraconazole** levels of 3.75 micrograms/ml, which suggests that the amphotericin B actually reduces the **itraconazole** levels.[4] There are numerous *in vitro* and *animal* studies of the potential interaction of azoles with amphotericin B, which show conflicting results from antagonism to additive or synergistic effects, some of which have been the subject of a review.[5]

A retrospective study of **itraconazole** use found that 11 of 12 leukaemic patients given amphotericin B and **itraconazole** had raised liver enzymes. These abnormalities resolved in 7 patients when the amphotericin B was discontinued. **Itraconazole** alone, given to another 8 patients did not cause liver enzyme abnormalities, even though it was used in high doses.[6]

Mechanism

Uncertain. In theory, combinations of polyene antifungals such as amphotericin B that bind to ergosterol in fungal cell membranes and azoles which inhibit the synthesis of ergosterol would be expected to exert antagonistic effects.[5,7,8] *In vitro* studies with *Candida albicans* found that azole exposure may allow the generation of cells that are unaffected by subsequent exposure to amphotericin B. The degree of resistance appears to depend on concentration and the azole involved, with itraconazole causing more resistance than **fluconazole**.[9] Resistance of *Candida* spp. to amphotericin B appears to depend on the duration of pre-exposure to **fluconazole** and is also greater when amphotericin B is subsequently used in combination with **fluconazole** rather than alone.[8,10] Resistance may also depend on the organism involved and its sensitivity to azoles.[11,12] Amphotericin B has only rarely been associated with adverse effects on the liver and increases in liver enzymes may occur in patients treated with itraconazole.

Importance and management

Despite extensive *in vitro* and *animal* data, it is not entirely clear whether or not azoles inhibit the efficacy of amphotericin B.[7,13,14] Until more is known it may be better to avoid concurrent use, or the outcome should be very well monitored, being alert for a reduced antifungal response, or increasing liver enzyme values.[6] A valuable review has been written on this topic.[5]

1. Schacter LP, Owellen RJ, Rathbun HK, Buchanan B. Antagonism between miconazole and amphotericin B. *Lancet* (1976) ii, 318.
2. Cosgrove RF, Beezer AE, Miles RJ. In vitro studies of amphotericin B in combination with the imidazole antifungal compounds clotrimazole and miconazole. *J Infect Dis* (1978) 138, 681–5.
3. Meunier-Carpentier F, Cruciani M, Klastersky J. Oral prophylaxis with miconazole or ketoconazole of invasive fungal disease in neutropenic cancer patients. *Eur J Cancer Clin Oncol* (1983) 19, 43–8.
4. Pennick GJ, McGough DA, Barchiesi F, Rinaldi MG. Concomitant therapy with amphotericin B and itraconazole: Does this combination affect the serum concentration of itraconazole? *Intersci Conf Antimicrob Agents Chemother* (1994) 34, 39.
5. Sugar AM. Use of amphotericin B with azole antifungal drugs: what are we doing? *Antimicrob Agents Chemother* (1995) 39, 1907–12.
6. Persat F, Schwartzbrod PE, Troncy J, Timour Q, Maul A, Piens MA, Picot S. Abnormalities in liver enzymes during simultaneous therapy with itraconazole and amphotericin B in leukaemic patients. *J Antimicrob Chemother* (2000) 45, 928–30.
7. Pahls S, Schaffner A. *Aspergillus fumigatus* pneumonia in neutropenic patients receiving fluconazole for infection due to *Candida* species: is amphotericin B combined with fluconazole the appropriate answer? *Clin Infect Dis* (1994) 18, 484–5.
8. Ernst EJ, Klepser ME, Pfaller MA. In vitro interaction of fluconazole and amphotericin B administered sequentially against *Candida albicans*: effect of concentration and exposure time. *Diagn Microbiol Infect Dis* (1998) 32, 205–10.
9. Vazquez JA, Arganoza MT, Vaishampayan JK, Akins RA. In vitro interaction between amphotericin B and azoles in Candida albicans. *Antimicrob Agents Chemother* (1996) 40, 2511–16.
10. Louie A, Kaw P, Banerjee P, Liu W, Chen G, Miller MH. Impact of order of initiation of fluconazole and amphotericin B in sequential or combination therapy on killing of Candida albicans in vitro and in rabbit model of endocarditis and pyelonephritis. *Antimicrob Agents Chemother* (2001) 45, 485–10.
11. Louie A, Banerjee P, Drusano GL, Shayegani M, Miller MH. Interaction between fluconazole and amphotericin B in mice with systemic infection due to fluconazole-susceptible or –resistant strains of Candida albicans. *Antimicrob Agents Chemother* (1999) 43, 2841–7.
12. LeMonte AM, Washum KE, Smedema ML, Schnizlein-Bick C, Kohler SM, Wheat LJ. Amphotericin B combined with itraconazole or fluconazole for treatment of histoplasmosis. *J Infect Dis* (2000) 182, 545–50.
13. Meis JF, Donnelly JP, Hoogkamp-Korstanje JA, De Pauw BE. Reply. *Clin Infect Dis* (1994) 18, 485–6.
14. Scheven M, Scheven M-L. Interaction between azoles and amphotericin B in the treatment of candidiasis. *Clin Infect Dis* (1995) 20, 1079.

Amphotericin B + Corticosteroids

Amphotericin B and corticosteroids can cause both potassium loss and salt and water retention, which can have adverse effects on cardiac function.

Clinical evidence

Four patients treated with amphotericin B and **hydrocortisone** 25 to 40 mg daily developed cardiac enlargement and congestive heart failure. The cardiac size decreased and the failure disappeared within 2 weeks of stopping the **hydrocortisone**. The amphotericin B was continued successfully with the addition of potassium supplements.[1]

Mechanism

Amphotericin B causes potassium to be lost in the urine. Hydrocortisone can cause potassium to be lost and salt and water to be retained and occasional instances of hypernatraemia with amphotericin B have also been seen. Working in concert these could account for the hypokalaemic cardiopathy and the circulatory overload that was seen.

Importance and management

Information is limited but the interaction would seem to be established. Monitor electrolytes (especially potassium, which should be closely monitored in any patient on amphotericin B) and fluid balance if amphotericin B is given with corticosteroids. The elderly would seem to be particularly at risk.

1. Chung D-K, Koenig MG. Reversible cardiac enlargement during treatment with amphotericin B and hydrocortisone. Report of three cases. *Am Rev Respir Dis* (1971) 103, 831–41.

Amphotericin B + Low salt diet

The renal toxicity of amphotericin B can be associated with sodium depletion. When the sodium is replaced the renal function improves.[1,2]

1. Feeley J, Heidemann H, Gerkens J, Roberts LJ, Branch RA. Sodium depletion enhances nephrotoxicity of amphotericin B. *Lancet* (1981) i, 1422–3.
2. Heidemann HT, Gerkens JF, Spickard WA, Jackson EK, Branch RA. Amphotericin B nephrotoxicity in humans decreased by salt repletion. *Am J Med* (1983) 75, 476–81.

Amphotericin B + Pentamidine

There is evidence that acute renal failure may develop in patients on amphotericin if they are also given parenteral pentamidine.

Clinical evidence, mechanism, importance and management

A retrospective study between 1985 and 1988 identified 101 patients with AIDS who had been treated with amphotericin B for various systemic mycoses. The patients were given amphotericin 0.6 to 0.8 mg/kg daily for 7 to 10 days, followed by three times a week dosing for about 9 weeks. Nine patients were concurrently treated for *Pneumocystis carinii* pneumonia, but only the 4 who had been given pentamidine parenterally developed acute and rapid reversible renal failure. No renal failure was seen in 2 others given pentamidine by inhalation or 3 given intravenous co-trimoxazole.[1] In all 4 cases, renal function returned to normal when the drugs were withdrawn. The reason for the kidney damage appears to be the additive nephrotoxic effects of both drugs. The reason no toxicity occurred when the pentamidine was given by inhalation is probably because the serum levels achieved were low. The authors of the study advise caution if both drugs are used. More study is needed.

1. Antoniskis D, Larsen RA. Acute, rapidly progressive renal failure with simultaneous use of amphotericin B and pentamidine. *Antimicrob Agents Chemother* (1990) 34, 470–2.

Amphotericin B + Potassium-depleting diuretics

Amphotericin B may cause hypokalaemia. Loop diuretics or thiazides and related diuretics increase the risk of hypokalaemia when given with amphotericin.[1]

1. Ambisome (Amphotericin B). Gilead Sciences International Ltd. UK Summary of product characteristics, September 2004.

Amphotericin B + Sucralfate

An *in vitro* study with amphotericin B found that it became markedly and irreversibly bound to sucralfate at the pH values found in the gut. This suggests that efficacy for intestinal candidiasis or gut decontamination might be decreased.

Clinical evidence, mechanism, importance and management

To simulate what might happen in the gut, amphotericin B 25 mg/l was mixed with sucralfate 500 mg in 40 ml of water at pH 3.5 and allowed to stand for 90 minutes at 25°C. Analysis of the solution found that the amphotericin B concentration fell rapidly and progressively over 90 minutes to about 20%. When the pH of the mixture was then raised to about 6.5 to 7 for 90 minutes, there was no change in the concentration of amphotericin B, suggesting that the interaction was irreversible.[1] The reason for this change is not known, but the suggestion is that sucralfate forms insoluble chelates with amphotericin B.[1]

It is not known how important this interaction is likely to be in practice, but the efficacy of amphotericin B for intestinal candidiasis or gut decontamination may be decreased. Separating the dosages might not be effective in some postoperative patients because their gastric function may not return to normal for up to 5 days, and some sucralfate might still be present when the next dose is given.[1] More study is needed to find out whether this interaction is clinically important, but in the meanwhile it would seem prudent to monitor concurrent use carefully, being alert for any evidence of reduced effects.

1. Feron B, Adair CG, Gorman SP, McClurg B. Interaction of sucralfate with antibiotics used for selective decontamination of the gastrointestinal tract. *Am J Hosp Pharm* (1993) 50, 2550–3.

Anidulafungin + Miscellaneous

A pharmacokinetic analysis of anidulafungin in 225 patients with serious fungal infections suggested that cytochrome P450 isoenzyme inhibitors, substrates, or inducers, including rifampicin, did not affect the clearance of anidulafungin.[1]

1. Dowell J, Knebel W, Ludden T, Stogniew M, Krause D, Henkel T. Population pharmacokinetic analysis of anidulafungin, an echinocandin antifungal. *J Clin Pharmacol* (2004) 44, 590–8.

Antimalarials + Antacids or Antidiarrhoeals

The absorption of chloroquine is moderately reduced by magnesium trisilicate and kaolin. The absorption of proguanil is more markedly reduced by magnesium trisilicate. Magnesium carbonate halved the maximum plasma levels of halofantrine. *In vitro* studies suggest that pyrimethamine may be affected like chloroquine.

Clinical evidence

(a) Chloroquine or Pyrimethamine

Six healthy subjects were given chloroquine phosphate 1 g (equivalent to 620 mg of chloroquine base) with either **magnesium trisilicate** 1 g or **kaolin** 1 g after an overnight fast. The **magnesium trisilicate** reduced the AUC of the chloroquine by 18.2% and the **kaolin** reduced it by 28.6%.[1]

Related *in vitro* studies by the same authors using segments of *rat* intestine found that the absorption of chloroquine and pyrimethamine respectively were decreased as follows: **magnesium trisilicate** (31.3 and 37.5%), **kaolin** (46.5 and 49.9%), **calcium carbonate** (52.8 and 31.5%), and **gerdiga** (36.1 and 38.0%). **Gerdiga** is a clay containing hydrated silicates with sodium and potassium carbonates and bicarbonates. It is used as an antacid and is similar to **attapulgite**.[2]

(b) Halofantrine

Magnesium carbonate was shown *in vitro* to adsorb more halofantrine than **aluminium hydroxide** or **magnesium trisilicate** antacid preparations so its *in vivo* effects on halofantrine pharmacokinetics were studied in 7 healthy subjects. **Magnesium carbonate** 1 g did not affect the bioavailability of halofantrine 500 mg. However, the clinical efficacy of halofantrine is thought to be related to the maximum plasma concentration, which was almost halved by the **magnesium carbonate**. The active metabolite of halofantrine, which is equally potent was similarly affected and so it would seem inadvisable to give halofantrine with **magnesium carbonate**.[3]

(c) Proguanil

The bioavailability of a 200-mg dose of proguanil was reduced by almost two-thirds in 8 healthy subjects given **magnesium trisilicate**.[4]

Mechanism

These antacid and antidiarrhoeal compounds adsorb chloroquine and proguanil[4] thereby reducing the amount available for absorption by the gut. Pyrimethamine appears to be similarly affected.[2] Dissolution of chloroquine from tablets may also be delayed by adsorbent antacids.[5]

Importance and management

The interactions between chloroquine and magnesium trisilicate, chloroquine and kaolin, halofantrine and magnesium carbonate, and proguanil and magnesium trisilicate, are established, but their clinical importance does not seem to have been assessed. The antimalarial effects of proguanil would be expected to be reduced much more than those of chloroquine. One way to minimise the interaction is to separate the dosages of the antimalarials and magnesium trisilicate or kaolin as much as possible (2 to 3 hours) to reduce admixture in the gut. There do not appear to be any studies to see if other antacids behave similarly. There does not seem to be any direct clinical evidence that the pyrimethamine effects are reduced by antacids but its *in vitro* absorption pattern in *animal* studies is similar to chloroquine.[2]

1. McElnay JC, Mukhtar HA, D'Arcy PF, Temple DJ, Collier PS. The effect of magnesium trisilicate and kaolin on the *in vivo* absorption of chloroquine. *J Trop Med Hyg* (1982) 85, 159–63.
2. McElnay JC, Mukhtar HA, D'Arcy PF, Temple DJ. *In vitro* experiments on chloroquine and pyrimethamine absorption in the presence of antacid constituents of kaolin. *J Trop Med Hyg* (1982) 85, 153–8.
3. Aideloje SO, Onyeji CO, Ugwu NC. Altered pharmacokinetics of halofantrine by an antacid, magnesium carbonate. *Eur J Pharm Biopharm* (1998) 46, 299–303.
4. Onyeji CO, Babalola CP. The effect of magnesium trisilicate on proguanil absorption. *Int J Pharmaceutics* (1993) 100, 249–52.
5. Iwuagwu MA, Aloko KS. Adsorption of paracetamol and chloroquine phosphate by some antacids. *J Pharm Pharmacol* (1992) 44, 655–8.

Atovaquone + Miscellaneous

Preliminary evidence suggests that of the drugs currently studied only metoclopramide and tetracycline causes any marked changes (decreases) in the atovaquone serum levels. Atovaquone appears not to interact with phenytoin.

Clinical evidence, mechanism, importance and management

An analysis of 191 patients with AIDS, given atovaquone as part of efficacy studies found that when normalised for plasma albumin, bodyweight, and the absence of other drugs, the expected steady-state plasma levels of atovaquone were 14.8 micrograms/ml. Steady-state atovaquone plasma levels achieved in the presence of other drugs were examined in an attempt to identify possible interactions. **Fluconazole** and **prednisone** were associated with increases of 2.5 and 2.3 micrograms/ml respectively, whereas **paracetamol** (**acetaminophen**), **aciclovir**, **opioids**, **antidiarrhoeals**, **cephalosporins**, **benzodiazepines** and **laxatives** were associated with decreases of greater than 3.4 micrograms/ml. **Metoclopramide** was associated with a decrease of 7.2 micrograms/ml. **'Zidovudine'**, (p.605), **U plasma binders** [not defined], **erythromycin**, **clofazimine**, **antacids**, **clotrimazole**, **NSAIDs**, **ketoconazole**, **hydroxyzine**, **megestrol**, **antiemetics** (other than **metoclopramide**), **other systemic steroids**, and **H_2-blockers** were not associated with any change in steady-state atovaquone serum levels. **Zidovudine**, **U plasma binders**, **erythromycin** and **clofazimine** were represented by fewer than 5 subjects.[1,2]

The maker notes that **tetracycline** may reduce plasma levels of atovaquone by about 40%.[3] An *in vitro* study found that **doxycycline** potentiated the antimalarial activity of atovaquone,[4] but there appears to be no information on the effect **doxycycline** has on the absorption of atovaquone.

A single dose study in 12 healthy subjects found that atovaquone does not affect the pharmacokinetics of **phenytoin**, and it was concluded that a clinically important pharmacokinetic interaction is unlikely.[5]

The kind of analysis described above[1,2] provides only the very broadest indication that interactions might or might not occur between atovaquone and these drugs, but it highlights the need to be vigilant if an apparently interacting drug is used concurrently. Only the changes caused by **metoclopramide** and **tetracycline** seem likely to have any potential clinical importance and the makers recommend caution in their use with atovaquone.[2,3] If an antiemetic is required in patients on atovaquone, it has been suggested that **metoclopramide** should only be given if other antiemetics are unavailable,[3] and that parasitaemia should be closely monitored.[6] It is also suggested that parasitaemia should be closely monitored in patients on atovaquone and **tetracycline**.[3,6]

1. Sadler BM, Blum MR. Relationship between steady-state plasma concentrations of atovaquone (C_{ss}) and the use of various concomitant medications in AIDS patients with *Pneumocystis carinii* pneumonia. *IXth Int Conf AIDS & IVth STD World Congr, Berlin* (1993) June 6–11. 504.
2. Wellvone (Atovaquone). GlaxoSmithKline. UK Summary of product characteristics, May 2004.
3. Malarone (Atovaquone/Proguanil hydrochloride). GlaxoSmithKline. US Prescribing information, March 2005.
4. Yeo AET, Edstein MD, Shanks GD, Rieckmann KH. Potentiation of the antimalarial activity of atovaquone by doxycycline against *Plasmodium falciparum* in vitro. *Parasitol Res* (1997) 83, 489–91.
5. Davis JD, Dixon R, Khan AZ, Toon S, Rolan PE, Posner J. Atovaquone has no effect on the pharmacokinetics of phenytoin in healthy male volunteers. *Br J Clin Pharmacol* (1996) 42, 246–8.
6. Malarone (Atovaquone/proguanil hydrochloride). GlaxoSmithKline. UK Summary of product characteristics, March 2005.

Atovaquone + Rifampicin (Rifampin) or Rifabutin

Rifampicin reduces serum atovaquone levels whereas atovaquone raises serum rifampicin levels. No clinically relevant interaction appears to occur between atovaquone and rifabutin.

Clinical evidence

A steady-state study in 13 HIV+ patients found that atovaquone 750 mg twice daily given with rifampicin 600 mg four times daily resulted in a more than 50% reduction in the atovaquone AUC and serum levels, but a more than 30% rise in rifampicin AUC and serum levels.[1]

A study in 24 healthy subjects given atovaquone 750 mg twice daily found that rifabutin 300 mg daily caused a small (34%) decrease in the AUC of the atovaquone and a small decrease in the rifabutin levels, but the authors of the report suggest that no dosage adjustment is needed.[2]

Mechanism

Uncertain. Evidence from 6-beta-hydroxycortisol studies suggest that rifampicin, as expected, acts as an enzyme inducer thereby increasing the metabolism of the atovaquone, but just why atovaquone increases the serum levels of rifampicin is not known.[1]

Importance and management

Information is limited but the interactions appear to be established. Their clinical importance is unknown, but it seems highly likely that the efficacy of atovaquone will be reduced in the presence of rifampicin. More study is needed.

1. Sadler BM, Caldwell P, Scott JD, Rogers M, Blum MR. Drug interaction between rifampin and atovaquone (Mepron®) in HIV+ asymptomatic volunteers. *Intersci Conf Antimicrob Agents Chemother* (1995) 35, 7.
2. Gillotin C, Grandpierre I, Sadler BM. Pharmacokinetic interaction between atovaquone (ATVQ) suspension and rifabutin (RFB). *Clin Pharmacol Ther* (1998) 63, 229.

Atovaquone/Proguanil + Artesunate

Artesunate does not appear to affect the pharmacokinetics of atovaquone/proguanil.

Clinical evidence, mechanism, importance and management

In a study to assess the effect of artesunate on the pharmacokinetics of atovaquone/proguanil, a single dose of atovaquone/proguanil 1 g/400 mg was given to 12 healthy subjects with and without artesunate 250 mg. No change was noted in the pharmacokinetics of either atovaquone or proguanil and no unexpected adverse events were seen.[1] Although artesunate does not therefore appear to interact with atovaquone/proguanil, this needs confirmation in a multiple-dose study.

1. van Vugt M, Edstein MD, Proux S, Lay K, Ooh M, Looareesuwan S, White NJ, Nosten F. Absence of an interaction between artesunate and atovaquone – proguanil. *Eur J Clin Pharmacol* (1999) 55, 469–74.

Azoles + Antacids, H_2-blockers or Sucralfate

The gastrointestinal absorption of ketoconazole is markedly reduced by antacids, cimetidine and ranitidine, whereas sucralfate has a smaller effect. The absorption of itraconazole is reduced (possibly halved) by H_2-blockers, but the absorption of fluconazole appears not be to significantly affected by antacids, cimetidine, ranitidine or sucralfate. The absorption of posaconazole is not affected by antacids but is reduced by about 40% by cimetidine. The absorption of voriconazole is not significantly affected by cimetidine or ranitidine.

Clinical evidence

(a) Fluconazole

Maalox forte (**aluminium/magnesium hydroxide**) 20 ml did not affect the absorption of a single 100-mg dose of fluconazole in 14 healthy subjects.[1] The 48-hour AUC of fluconazole 100 mg was reduced by only 13% when it was given to 6 healthy subjects with a single 400-mg dose of **cimetidine**.[2] Two other studies found that **cimetidine**[3] and **famotidine**[4] did not affect fluconazole absorption. Sucralfate 2 g was found to have no significant effect on the pharmacokinetics of a single 200-mg dose of fluconazole in 10 healthy subjects, confirming the results of an *in vitro* study.[5]

(b) Itraconazole

Twelve healthy subjects were given **cimetidine** 400 mg twice daily or **ranitidine** 150 mg twice daily for 3 days before and after a single 200-mg dose of itraconazole. The AUC and maximum serum levels of the itraconazole were reduced, but not significantly. The largest changes were 20% reductions in the AUC and maximum serum levels with **ranitidine**.[6] In contrast, another study in 30 healthy subjects found that **ranitidine** 150 mg twice daily for 3 days reduced the AUC of a single 200-mg dose of itraconazole by 44%, and reduced the maximum serum levels by 52%.[7] A study of the bioavailability of itraconazole in 12 lung transplant patients also given **ranitidine** 150 mg twice daily and an **antacid** four times daily found that the serum levels of itraconazole were highly variable. However, satisfactory levels were achieved in all patients, even though some needed their doses of itraconazole increased from 200 to 400 mg daily.[8]

Famotidine 40 mg was found to reduce the serum levels of a 200-mg dose of itraconazole by about 50% in 12 healthy subjects.[4] **Famotidine** 20 mg twice daily was given with itraconazole 200 mg daily for 10 days to 16 patients undergoing chemotherapy for haematological malignancies. The minimum plasma levels of itraconazole were reduced by about 39%, and 8 patients did not achieve the levels considered necessary to protect neutropenic patients from fungal infections.[9]

A study in 8 healthy subjects found that itraconazole 200 mg twice daily for 3 days increased the AUC of intravenous **cimetidine** (loading dose 0.2 mg/kg followed by an infusion of 36 mg/hour for 4 hours) by 25%.[10]

(c) Ketoconazole

A haemodialysis patient did not respond to treatment with ketoconazole 200 mg daily while on **cimetidine**, **sodium bicarbonate** 2 g daily and **aluminium oxide** 2.5 g daily. Only when the ketoconazole dosage was increased to 200 mg four times daily did her serum levels rise. A later study in 3 healthy subjects found that when ketoconazole 200 mg was taken 2 hours after **cimetidine** 400 mg, the absorption was considerably reduced (AUC reduced by about 60%). When this was repeated with **sodium bicarbonate** 500 mg in addition, the absorption was reduced by about 95%. In contrast, when this was repeated once more but with the ketoconazole in an acidic solution, the absorption was increased by about 50%.[11]

Another study[3] in 24 healthy subjects found that intravenous **cimetidine** titrated to give a gastric pH of 6 or more reduced the absorption of ketoconazole by 95%. A study[12] in 6 healthy subjects found that **ranitidine** 150 mg given 2 hours before ketoconazole 400 mg reduced its AUC by about 95%. Sucralfate 1 g caused a smaller reduction of about 20%.[12] Another study found that sucralfate 1 g reduced the AUC and maximum serum levels of a single 100-mg dose of ketoconazole by about 25%, but no significant changes were seen when the ketoconazole was given 2 hours after the sucralfate.[13] A study in 4 patients found that the concurrent use of *Maalox* reduced the absorption of ketoconazole but this was not statistically significant.[14] An anecdotal report suggested that giving ketoconazole 2 hours before a stomatitis cocktail containing *Maalox* seemed to prevent the cocktail reducing its effectiveness.[15]

(d) Posaconazole

A study in 12 healthy subjects found that *Mylanta* (**aluminium/magnesium hydroxide**) 20 ml did not significantly affect the bioavailability of a single 200-mg dose of posaconazole, either when taken with food or when fasting.[16] In a placebo-controlled study in 12 healthy subjects **cimetidine** 400 mg every 12 hours given with posaconazole 200 mg once daily for 10 days reduced the AUC and maximum plasma levels of posaconazole by about 40%.[17]

(e) Voriconazole

A study in 12 healthy subjects found that **cimetidine** 400 mg twice daily given with voriconazole 200 mg twice daily increased the maximum plasma levels and AUC of voriconazole by about 20%, but this is not considered sufficient to warrant a dosage adjustment.[18] **Ranitidine** 150 mg twice daily had no significant effect on the AUC and maximum plasma levels of voriconazole.[18]

Mechanism

Ketoconazole is a poorly soluble base, which must be transformed by the acid in the stomach into the soluble hydrochloride salt. Agents that reduce gastric acidity, such as H_2-blockers or antacids, raise the pH in the stomach so that the dissolution of the ketoconazole and its absorption are reduced. Conversely, anything that increases the gastric acidity increases the dissolution and the absorption.[14,19] There is also *in vitro* evidence that an electrostatic interaction occurs between ketoconazole and sucralfate to form an ion pair that cannot pass through the gut wall.[20] The absorption of itraconazole is also affected by changes in gastric pH, but fluconazole is minimally affected. The increase in cimetidine levels in the presence of itraconazole may be due to inhibition of P-glycoprotein mediated renal tubular secretion of cimetidine.[10]

Importance and management

The interactions with ketoconazole are clinically important but not extensively documented. Advise patients to take antacids or sucralfate, not less than 2 to 3 hours before or after the ketoconazole so that absorption can take place with minimal changes in the pH of the gastric contents.[11] Monitor the effects to confirm that the ketoconazole is effective. Sucralfate would be expected to interact much more moderately than the other drugs.

The situation with itraconazole is not entirely clear, but some reduction in its absorption apparently occurs and it would therefore be prudent to confirm that it remains effective in the presence of H_2-blockers and possibly antacids. It has been suggested[7] that the reduction in bioavailability due to H_2-blockers can be minimised by giving itraconazole and ketoconazole with an acidic drink such as *'Coca-cola'*, (p.137).

Antacids do not significantly affect posaconazole levels but its bioavailability appears to be reduced by cimetidine.

Fluconazole only interacts to a small and clinically irrelevant extent with H_2-blockers and is therefore a possible alternative to ketoconazole and itraconazole. It is not expected to be affected by antacids and does not interact with sucralfate.

No special precautions seem necessary if voriconazole is used with any of the H_2-blockers.

1. Thorpe JE, Baker N, Bromet-Petit M. Effect of oral antacid administration on the pharmacokinetics of oral fluconazole. *Antimicrob Agents Chemother* (1990) 34, 2032–3.
2. Lazar JD, Wilner KD. Drug interactions with fluconazole. *Rev Infect Dis* (1990) 12 (Suppl 3), S327–S333.
3. Blum RA, D'Andrea DT, Florentino BM, Wilton JH, Hilligoss DM, Gardner MJ, Henry EB, Goldstein H, Schentag JJ. Increased gastric pH and the bioavailability of fluconazole and ketoconazole. *Ann Intern Med* (1991) 114, 755–7.
4. Lim SG, Sawyerr AM, Hudson M, Sercombe J, Pounder RE. Short report: The absorption of fluconazole and itraconazole under conditions of low intragastric acidity. *Aliment Pharmacol Ther* (1993) 7, 317–21.
5. Carver PL, Hoeschele JD, Partipilo L, Kauffman CA, Mercer BT, Pecoraro VL. Fluconazole: a model compound for in vitro and in vivo interactions with sucralfate. *Pharmacotherapy* (1994) 14, 347.
6. Stein AG, Daneshmend TK, Warnock DW, Bhaskar N, Burke J, Hawkey CJ. The effects of H_2-receptor antagonists on the pharmacokinetics of itraconazole, a new oral antifungal. *Br J Clin Pharmacol* (1989) 27, 105P–106P.
7. Lange D, Pavao JH, Wu J, Klausner M. Effect of a cola beverage on the bioavailability of itraconazole in the presence of H_2 blockers. *J Clin Pharmacol* (1997) 37, 535–40.
8. PattersonTF, Peters J, Levine SM, Anzueto A, Bryan CL, Sako EY, LaWayne Miller O, Calhoon JH, Rinaldi MG. Systemic availability of itraconazole in lung transplantation. *Antimicrob Agents Chemother* (1996) 40, 2217–20.
9. Kanda Y, Kami M, Matsuyama T, Mitani K, Chiba S, Yazaki Y, Hirai H. Plasma concentration of itraconazole in patients receiving chemotherapy for hematological malignancies: the effect of famotidine on the absorption of itraconazole. *Hematol Oncol* (1998) 16, 33–7.
10. Karyekar CS, Eddington ND, Briglia A, Gubbins PO, Dowling TC. Renal interaction between itraconazole and cimetidine. *J Clin Pharmacol* (2004) 44, 919–27.
11. Van der Meer JWM, Keuning JJ, Scheijgrond HW, Heykants J, Van Cutsem J, Brugmans J. The influence of gastric acidity on the bio-availability of ketoconazole. *J Antimicrob Chemother* (1980) 6, 552–4.
12. Piscitelli SC, Goss TF, Wilton JH, D'Andrea DT, Goldstein H, Schentag JJ. Effects of ranitidine and sucralfate on ketoconazole bioavailability. *Antimicrob Agents Chemother* (1991) 35, 1765–71.
13. Carver PL, Berardi RR, Knapp MJ, Rider JM, Kauffman CA, Bradley SF, Atassi M. In vivo interaction of ketoconazole and sucralfate in healthy volunteers. *Antimicrob Agents Chemother* (1994) 38, 326–9.
14. Brass C, Galgiani JN, Blaschke TF, Defelice R, O'Reilly RA, Stevens DA. Disposition of ketoconazole, an oral antifungal, in humans. *Antimicrob Agents Chemother* (1982) 21, 151–8.
15. Franklin MG. Nizoral and stomatitis cocktails may not mix. *Oncol Nurs Forum* (1991) 18, 1417.
16. Courtney R, Radwanski E, Lim J, Laughlin M. Pharmacokinetics of posaconazole coadministered with antacid in fasting or nonfasting healthy men. *Antimicrob Agents Chemother* (2004) 48, 804–8.
17. Courtney R, Wexler D, Statkevich P, Lim J, Batra V, Laughlin M. Effect of cimetidine on the pharmacokinetics of posaconazole in healthy volunteers. *Intersci Conf Antimicrob Agents Chemother* (2002) 42, 29.
18. Purkins L, Wood N, Kleinermans D, Nichols D. Histamine H_2-receptor antagonists have no clinically significant effect on the steady-state pharmacokinetics of voriconazole. *Br J Clin Pharmacol* (2003) 56, 51–5.
19. Sutherland C, Murphy JE, Schleifer NH. The effects of two gastric acidifying agents on the pharmacokinetics of ketoconazole. 18th Annual Midyear Clinical Meeting of the American Society of Hospital Pharmacists, Atlanta, Georgia, Dec 4–8, 1983, 141.
20. Hoeschele JD, Roy AK, Pecoraro VL, Carver PL. In vitro analysis of the interaction between sucralfate and ketoconazole. *Antimicrob Agents Chemother* (1994) 38, 319–25.

Azoles + Anticonvulsants

Phenytoin causes a very marked fall in serum itraconazole levels, thereby reducing or abolishing its antifungal effects. Phenobarbital and carbamazepine appear to interact similarly. Four patients had reduced serum ketoconazole levels and reduced antifungal effects while taking phenytoin. Two were also taking phenobarbital. Phenytoin reduces voriconazole levels and voriconazole increases phenytoin levels; dose adjustments are advised. Carbamazepine and phenobarbital may reduce voriconazole levels. For the effects of the azoles on the anticonvulsants see 'phenytoin', (p.365), and 'carbamazepine', (p.341).

Clinical evidence

(a) Itraconazole

After taking oral **phenytoin** 300 mg daily for 15 days, the AUC of a single 200-mg dose of itraconazole was reduced more than 90% to 13 healthy subjects. The half-life of itraconazole fell from 22.3 to 3.8 hours. A parallel study[1] in another group found that itraconazole 200 mg for 15 days increased the **phenytoin** AUC by 10.3%.

Two patients on **phenytoin** and two on **phenytoin** with **carbamazepine** either did not respond to treatment with itraconazole 400 mg daily for aspergillosis, coccidioidomycosis or cryptococcosis, or suffered a relapse. All of them had undetectable or substantially reduced serum itraconazole levels compared with other patients on itraconazole alone.[2] Two other patients also had very low serum itraconazole serum levels while taking **phenytoin** and **phenobarbital**.[3]

The serum levels of itraconazole 200 mg daily were very low (0.01 to 0.03 mg/l, therapeutic range 0.25 to 2 mg/l) in a patient taking **phenobarbital**. Two months after stopping the **phenobarbital** they were higher (0.15 mg/l), but still below the therapeutic range, apparently because **carbamazepine** had been recently started. However, 2 months later itraconazole serum levels were undetectable. **Carbamazepine** was stopped, and 3 weeks later the itraconazole serum levels were 0.36 mg/l.[4]

(b) Ketoconazole

A man being treated for coccidioidal meningitis with ketoconazole 400 mg daily relapsed when he was given **phenytoin** 300 mg daily. A pharmacokinetic study found that his peak serum ketoconazole levels and AUC were reduced compared with the values seen before the **phenytoin** was started. Even though the ketoconazole dose was increased to 600 mg, and later 1200 mg his serum levels remained low compared with other patients taking only 400 or 600 mg of ketoconazole.[5]

Coccidioidomycosis progressed in another patient on **phenytoin** despite the use of ketoconazole.[2] Low serum ketoconazole levels were seen in one patient[6] taking **phenytoin** and **phenobarbital**. Serum phenytoin levels are not affected by 'ketoconazole', (p.365).

(c) Voriconazole

Studies in healthy subjects found that **phenytoin** 300 mg daily decreased the maximum serum levels and AUC of voriconazole by 49 and 69% respectively. Also, voriconazole 400 mg twice daily increased the maximum serum levels and AUC of **phenytoin** 300 mg daily by 67 and 81% respectively.[7] Similarly, because **carbamazepine** and **phenobarbital** are potent inducers of cytochrome P450 isoenzymes they are also predicted to significantly reduce voriconazole levels.[8,9]

Mechanism

It seems almost certain that these anticonvulsants can increase the metabolism and clearance of azole antifungals by induction of the cytochrome P450 isoenzymes, thereby reducing azole serum levels and effects. At high doses voriconazole may increase levels of phenytoin by inhibition of the cytochrome P450 isoenzyme CYP2C9.[9]

Importance and management

The interaction between phenytoin and itraconazole is established, clinically important and its incidence appears to be high. Because such a marked fall in itraconazole levels occurs, it is difficult to predict by how much its dosage should be increased, for which reason the authors of one report advise using another antifungal instead.[1] The small rise in serum phenytoin levels caused by itraconazole is unlikely to be clinically important. The interactions of itraconazole with carbamazepine and phenobarbital are relatively poorly documented and their incidence is unknown, but if itraconazole is given to patients taking these anticonvulsants, be alert for the need to increase the itraconazole dosage. More study is needed.

Information on the interaction between ketoconazole and phenytoin or phenobarbital appears to be limited to these reports, but be alert for any signs of a reduced antifungal response in any patient also given phenytoin and or phenobarbital. It may be necessary to increase the dosage of the ketoconazole.

The interaction between phenytoin and voriconazole is established. The UK makers say that concurrent use of voriconazole and phenytoin should be avoided unless the benefits outweigh the risks.[8] If used together, they recommend careful monitoring of phenytoin levels and adverse effects, and doubling the dose of oral voriconazole (from 200 to 400 mg twice daily and from 100 mg to 200 mg orally, twice daily in patients less than 40 kg) or increasing the dose of intravenous voriconazole (from 4 to 5 mg/kg twice daily).[8,9] The makers contraindicate the concurrent use of carbamazepine and phenobarbital with voriconazole.[8,9] In the US the makers extend this contraindication to all long-acting barbiturates.[9] For mention of reduced phenytoin levels with fluconazole and miconazole, see 'Phenytoin + Azoles' p.365 and for increased carbamazepine levels with fluconazole, ketoconazole and miconazole, see 'Carbamazepine + Azoles', p.341.

1. Ducharme MP, Slaughter RL, Warbasse LH, Chandrasekar PH, Van der Velde V, Mannens G, Edwards DJ. Itraconazole and hydroxyitraconazole serum concentrations are reduced more than tenfold by phenytoin. *Clin Pharmacol Ther* (1995) 58, 617–24.
2. Tucker RM, Denning DW, Hanson LH, Rinaldi MG, Graybill JR, Sharkey PK, Pappagianis D, Stevens DA. Interaction of azoles with rifampin, phenytoin, and carbamazepine: in vitro and clinical observations. *Clin Infect Dis* (1992) 14, 165–74.
3. Hay RJ, Clayton YM, Moore MK, Midgely G. An evaluation of itraconazole in the management of onychomycosis. *Br J Dermatol* (1988) 119, 359–66.
4. Bonay M, Jonville-Bera AP, Diot P, Lemarie E, Lavandier M, Autret E. Possible interaction between phenobarbital, carbamazepine and itraconazole. *Drug Safety* (1993) 9, 309–11.
5. Brass C, Galgiani JN, Blaschke TF, Defelice R, O'Reilly RA, Stevens DA. Disposition of ketoconazole, an oral antifungal, in humans. *Antimicrob Agents Chemother* (1982) 21, 151–8.
6. Stockley RJ, Daneshmend TK, Bredow MT, Warnock DW, Richardson MD, Slade RR. Ketoconazole pharmacokinetics during chronic dosing in adults with haematological malignancy. *Eur J Clin Microbiol* (1986) 5, 513–17.
7. Purkins L, Wood N, Ghahramani P, Love ER, Eve MD, Fielding A. Coadministration of voriconazole and phenytoin: pharmacokinetic interaction, safety, and toleration. *Br J Clin Pharmacol* (2003) 56, 37–44.
8. VFEND (Voriconazole). Pfizer Ltd. UK Summary of product characteristics, March 2005.
9. VFEND (Voriconazole). Pfizer Inc. US Prescribing information, March 2005.

Azoles + Antineoplastics

Preliminary evidence suggests that the pharmacokinetics of fluconazole are less likely to be affected by antineoplastics than itraconazole, and it may therefore be the drug of choice for treating fungal infections in patients receiving chemotherapy.

Clinical evidence, mechanism, importance and management

A study in 10 leukaemic patients (AML and ALL) found that the pharmacokinetics of **fluconazole** 100 mg were not affected by 15 days of chemotherapy. The drugs used were **daunorubicin**, **cytarabine**, **vincristine**, **prednisone**, **asparaginase** and **idarubicin**, either alone or in combination. In contrast, a parallel study in another 10 leukaemic patients suggested that there may be some changes in the pharmacokinetics of **itraconazole** in individual patients. There was no consistent pattern of changes in the AUCs for these patients. The scatter was wide, and some AUCs were raised while others were lowered. The drugs used were as before.[1]

On the basis of these findings the authors of the report suggest that because of the apparent risk of over- or underdosage with **itraconazole** in these patients, **fluconazole** may be the more reliable choice for the prevention and treatment of candidiasis in the presence of these drugs.[1] It needs to be emphasised that these results were derived from only a relatively small number of patients, taking different combinations of drugs, so that the conclusions should only be regarded Of the antineoplastics listed above, only vincristine appears to have been studied for how it is affected by 'itraconazole', (p.496). Azole antifungals may alter the metabolism of a number of antineoplastics that are substrates of cytochrome P450 isoenzymes, and where data is available, this is covered under the affected drug.

1. Lazo de la Vega S, Volkow P, Yeates RA, Pfaff G. Administration of the antimycotic agents fluconazole and itraconazole to leukaemia patients: a comparative pharmacokinetic study. *Drugs Exp Clin Res* (1994) 20, 69–75.

Azoles + Cola drinks

Some cola drinks can lower the stomach pH in patients with achlorhydria or hypochlorhydria, which improves the bioavailability of itraconazole and ketoconazole. Normally a useful interaction but good monitoring is needed to ensure that the azole serum levels do not become excessive.

Clinical evidence

Eight healthy subjects were given **itraconazole** 100 mg with either 325 ml of water or *Coca-Cola* (pH 2.5). Their peak serum **itraconazole** levels were more than doubled by the *Coca-Cola* and the AUC was increased by 80%. Two of the subjects did not show this effect.[1]

Another study in 18 fasted AIDS patients who absorbed **itraconazole** poorly, found that the absorption was restored to that of fasted healthy subjects when the **itraconazole** was given with a cola drink.[2] A study in 30 healthy subjects compared the bioavailability of **itraconazole** alone or after ranitidine, both with and without a cola drink. Ranitidine reduced the absorption of **itraconazole** but this effect was countered by the cola drink.[3] Yet another study used omeprazole to raise the pH and *Coca-Cola Classic* to lower it. Absorption was greatest when **ketoconazole** was given alone, and least when given with omeprazole. However, *Coca-Cola* increased the absorption of **ketoconazole** in the presence of omeprazole.[4]

Mechanism

Itraconazole and ketoconazole are poorly soluble bases, which must be transformed by the acid in the stomach into a soluble hydrochloride salt. Therefore any clinical condition that reduces gastric acidity (or any drug that raises stomach pH, see 'H2-blockers', (p.135) and 'proton pump inhibitors', (p.138)) can reduce the dissolution and the absorption of these antifungals. Acidic drinks, which lower the pH, can increase the absorption.

Importance and management

The interactions of itraconazole and ketoconazole with Cola drinks that lower the gastric pH are established. The interaction can be exploited to improve the absorption of these antifungals in patients with achlorhydria or hypochlorhydria, and those taking gastric acid suppressants (see 'H2-blockers', (p.135) and 'proton pump inhibitors', (p.138)), but some caution is needed to ensure that serum levels do not rise excessively, which could lead to toxicity.

Coca-Cola Classic, Pepsi and ***Canada Dry Ginger Ale*** can be used because they can achieve stomach pH values of less than 3, but none of the other beverages examined in one study produced such a low pH. The authors suggest that these would be less effective, although they were not actually studied. They included ***Diet Coca-Cola***, ***Diet Pepsi***, ***Diet 7-Up***, ***Diet Canada Dry Ginger Ale***, ***Diet Canada Dry Orange juice***, ***7-Up*** and ***Canada Dry Orange juice***.[4]

1. Jaruratanasirikul S, Kleepkaew A. Influence of an acidic beverage (Coca-Cola) on absorption of itraconazole. *Eur J Clin Pharmacol* (1997) 52, 235–7.

2. Hardin J, Lange D, Heykants J, Ding C, Van de Velde V, Slusser C, Klausner M. The effect of co-administration of a cola beverage on the bioavailability of itraconazole in AIDS patients. *Intersci Conf Antimicrob Agents Chemother* (1995) 35, 6.
3. Lange D, Pavao JH, Wu J, Klausner M. Effect of cola beverage on the bioavailability of itraconazole in the presence of H_2 blockers. *J Clin Pharmacol* (1997) 37, 535–40.
4. Chin TWF, Leob M, Fong IW. Effects of an acidic beverage (Coca-Cola) on absorption of ketoconazole. *Antimicrob Agents Chemother* (1995) 39, 1671–5.

Azoles + Food

Itraconazole capsules should be taken with or after food to improve absorption, whereas itraconazole solution should be taken before food. The makers advise taking ketoconazole with food, but the background evidence supporting this is confusing and contradictory. Food does not appear to affect the bioavailability of fluconazole but increases that of posaconazole. The availability of voriconazole is modestly reduced by food.

Clinical evidence

(a) Fluconazole

A study in 12 healthy subjects found that food had no therapeutically relevant effect on the pharmacokinetics of fluconazole.[1]

(b) Itraconazole

A study in 24 patients with superficial dermatophyte, *Candida albicans* and pityriasis versicolor infections given itraconazole 50 or 100 mg daily found that taking the drug with or after breakfast produced higher serum levels and gave much better treatment results than taking it before breakfast.[2] A later study found that the relative bioavailability of itraconazole was 54% on an empty stomach, 86% after a light meal and 100% after a full meal.[1] Similar results were found in other studies.[3,4]

In contrast, studies with itraconazole oral solution give different results. A study in 30 healthy males given itraconazole solution 200 mg daily, either on an empty stomach or with a standard breakfast, found that the bioavailability was 29% higher when itraconazole was taken in the fasted state.[5]

In another study of 20 HIV+ patients, **glutamic acid** 1360 mg, given to acidify the stomach, either with or without food did not enhance itraconazole absorption.[3]

(c) Ketoconazole

One study found that the AUC and peak serum concentrations of a single 200-mg dose of ketoconazole were reduced by about 40% (from 14.4 to 8.6 micrograms/hour/ml and from 4.1 to 2.3 micrograms/ml respectively) when given to 10 healthy subjects after a standardised meal.[6] Another study found that high carbohydrate and fat diets tended to reduce the rate, but not the overall amount of ketoconazole absorbed.[7] A third study found that the absorption of single 200- or 800-mg doses of ketoconazole in 8 healthy subjects was not altered when it was taken after a standardised breakfast although the peak serum levels were delayed. The absorption of single 400- and 600-mg doses were somewhat increased by food.[8]

(d) Posaconazole

A study in 24 healthy subjects found that the maximum plasma levels and AUC of a single 400-mg dose of posaconazole oral suspension were increased 3.4- and 2.6-fold respectively when given with a **nutritional supplement** (*Boost Plus*) rather than in the fasting state.[9] In a further study in 20 healthy subjects, single 200-mg doses of posaconazole (as oral suspension) were given with either a high-fat meal, a non-fat breakfast or after a 10-hour fast. The AUC of the suspension was increased fourfold when given with a high-fat meal, and 2.7-fold when given with a non-fat breakfast rather than after fasting.[10]

(e) Voriconazole

In a study 12 healthy subjects were given voriconazole 200 mg twice daily either with food or in the fasted state (2 hours before or after food). Food delayed the oral absorption of voriconazole by about 1 hour and reduced the AUC by 22%.[11]

Mechanism

Not understood.

Importance and management

There appears to be no relevant interaction between food and fluconazole. Itraconazole absorption from capsule formulation is best with or after food, whereas absorption form the acidic solution appears to be better before food. Similarly, posaconazole absorption is improved by food. A confusing and conflicting picture is presented by the studies with ketoconazole. However the makers of ketoconazole say that the absorption of ketoconazole is maximal when it is taken during a meal, as it depends on stomach acidity and it should therefore always be taken with meals.[12] The makers of voriconazole recommend that it should be taken at least 1 hour before or at least 1 hour after a meal.[13,14]

1. Zimmermann T, Yeates RA, Laufen H, Pfaff G, Wildfeuer A. Influence of concomitant food intake on the oral absorption of two triazole antifungal agents, itraconazole and fluconazole. *Eur J Clin Pharmacol* (1994) 46, 147–150.
2. Wishart JM. The influence of food on the pharmacokinetics of itraconazole in patients with superficial fungal infection. *J Am Acad Dermatol* (1987) 17, 220–3.
3. Carver P, Welage L, Kauffman C. The effect of food and gastric pH on the oral bioavailability of itraconazole in HIV+ patients. *Intersci Conf Antimicrob Agents Chemother* (1996) 36, 6.
4. Barone JA, Koh JG, Bierman RH, Colaizzi JL, Swanson KA, Gaffar MC, Moskovitz BL, Mechlinski W, Van De Velde V. Food interaction and steady-state pharmacokinetics of itraconazole capsules in healthy male volunteers. *Antimicrob Agents Chemother* (1993) 37, 778–84.
5. Barone JA, Moskovitz BL, Guarnieri J, Hassell AE, Colaizzi JL, Bierman RH, Jessen L. Food interaction and steady-state pharmacokinetics of itraconazole oral solution in healthy volunteers. *Pharmacotherapy* (1998) 18, 295–301.
6. Männistö PT, Mäntylä R, Nykänen S, Lamminsivu U, Ottoila P. Impairing effect of food on ketoconazole absorption. *Antimicrob Agents Chemother* (1982) 21, 730–33.
7. Lelawongs P, Barone JA, Colaizzi JL, Hsuan ATM, Mechlinski W, Legendre R, Guarnieri J. Effect of food and gastric acidity on absorption of orally administered ketoconazole. *Clin Pharm* (1988) 7, 228–35.
8. Daneshmend TK, Warnock DW, Ene MD, Johnson EM, Potten MR, Richardson MD, Williamson PJ. Influence of food on the pharmacokinetics of ketoconazole. *Antimicrob Agents Chemother* (1984) 25, 1–3.
9. Courtney R, Sansone A, Calzetta A, Martinho M, Laughlin. The effect of a nutritional supplement (Boost Plus) on the oral bioavailability of posaconazole. *Intersci Conf Antimicrob Agents Chemother* (2003) 43, 33.
10. Courtney R, Wexler D, Radwanski E, Lim J, Laughlin M. Effect of food on the relative bioavailability of two oral formulations of posaconazole in healthy adults. *Br J Clin Pharmacol* (2004) 57, 218–22.
11. Purkins L, Wood N, Kleinermans D, Greenhalgh K, Nichols D. Effect of food on the pharmacokinetics of multiple-dose oral voriconazole. *Br J Clin Pharmacol* (2003) 56 (Suppl 1) 17–23.
12. Nizoral (Ketoconazole). Janssen-Cilag Ltd. UK Summary of product characteristics, May 2001.
13. VFEND (Voriconazole). Pfizer Ltd. UK Summary of product characteristics, March 2005.
14. VFEND (Voriconazole). Pfizer Inc. US Prescribing information, March 2005.

Azoles + Proton pump inhibitors

Omeprazole and rabeprazole reduce the bioavailability of ketoconazole markedly and modestly respectively. Other proton pump inhibitors are expected to behave similarly. Omeprazole also markedly reduced the absorption of itraconazole capsules, but not the oral solution. The bioavailabilities of fluconazole and voriconazole are not significantly affected by omeprazole. Omeprazole levels are increased by ketoconazole, and markedly increased by fluconazole and voriconazole.

Clinical evidence

(a) Esomeprazole

One study found that after taking esomeprazole 20 or 40 mg for 5 days the gastric pH of patients remained above 4 for a mean time of 13 and 17 hours respectively.[1] The makers therefore suggest that this might reduce the absorption of some drugs such as itraconazole and ketoconazole, which depend on a low pH for optimal dissolution and absorption.[1]

(b) Omeprazole

(i) Fluconazole. A study in 12 healthy subjects found that omeprazole 20 mg daily for 7 days did not affect the pharmacokinetics of a single 100-mg dose of fluconazole.[2] In another study in 18 healthy subjects, fluconazole 100 mg daily for 5 days increased the peak plasma levels and AUC of a single 20-mg dose of omeprazole by 2.4- and 6.3-fold respectively.[3]

(ii) Itraconazole. Itraconazole 200 mg [capsule formulation] was given to 11 healthy subjects after 14 days pre-treatment with omeprazole 40 mg daily. The AUC and maximum serum level of itraconazole were both reduced by about 65%.[4] Another study in 15 healthy subjects found that omeprazole 40 mg daily did not significantly affect the pharmacokinetics of single 400-mg doses of itraconazole or its metabolite hydroxyitraconazole when given as an oral solution. However, there was large interpatient variation in mean serum levels.[5]

(iii) Ketoconazole. A three-way crossover study in 9 healthy subjects found that omeprazole 60 mg reduced the AUC of ketoconazole 200 mg by about 80%.[6] Another study was carried out in 10 healthy subjects (both 'extensive' and 'poor' metabolisers) to find the extent to which cytochrome P450 isoenzyme CYP3A4 is involved in the metabolism (sulfoxidation) of omeprazole. This revealed that ketoconazole 100 to 200 mg a known inhibitor of CYP3A4, reduced the formation of the omeprazole sulfone in both groups, and doubled the serum omeprazole levels in the poor metabolisers.[7]

(iv) Voriconazole. A study in 18 healthy subjects found that omeprazole 40 mg daily for 7 days increased the maximum plasma levels and AUC of voriconazole by 15 and 41% respectively.[8] However, voriconazole 200 mg twice daily increased the maximum plasma levels and AUC of omeprazole 40 mg once daily by about twofold and fourfold respectively.[9]

(c) Rabeprazole

In a randomised placebo-controlled study 18 healthy subjects were given ketoconazole 400 mg before and after taking rabeprazole 20 mg daily or a placebo for 7 days. Significant decreases in the ketoconazole AUC and maximum serum levels were found,[10] representing about a 30% reduction in its bioavailability.[11] There was no evidence that ketoconazole affected rabeprazole metabolism.

Mechanism

Ketoconazole and itraconazole are poorly soluble bases, which must be transformed by the acid in the stomach into the soluble hydrochloride salt. Agents that reduce gastric secretions, such as proton pump inhibitors, 'H_2-blockers or antacids', (p.135), raise the pH in the stomach so that the dissolution and absorption of drugs such as itraconazole or ketoconazole are reduced. Conversely, anything that increases the gastric acidity increases their dissolution and absorption.[6]

Fluconazole and voriconazole is almost certainly cause a rise in omeprazole levels by inhibiting its metabolism by the cytochrome P450 isoenzymes CYP219 and CYP3A4. Inhibition of CYP3A4 alone by ketoconazole causes a less marked rise in omeprazole levels. Itraconazole would be expected to interact similarly to ketoconazole.

Importance and management

The interaction between ketoconazole and omeprazole appears to be established and of clinical importance. Direct evidence seems to be limited to this study but other drugs that raise the gastric pH have a similar effect (see 'Azoles + Antacids, H_2-blockers or Sucralfate', p.135). Such a large reduction in the absorption of ketoconazole would be expected to result in the failure of treatment. Separating the dosages of the two drugs is unlikely to be the answer because the effect of omeprazole is so prolonged. An alternative would simply be to monitor for any inadequate response to ketoconazole if omeprazole or esomeprazole is also given and to raise the dosage if necessary. However, bear in mind that ketoconazole can double omeprazole levels, although the clinical relevance of this is uncertain. Giving ketoconazole with an acidic drink such as 'Cola', (p.137) appears to minimise the interaction.[6]

The interaction between ketoconazole and rabeprazole is also established but the reduction in the bioavailability is only moderate (30%) and it may be possible to accommodate this by raising the antifungal dosage.

There seem to be no reports about ketoconazole and other proton pump inhibitors (pantoprazole, lansoprazole) but they are also expected to interact to reduce the bioavailability of the ketoconazole, but the extent is not known.

The interaction between itraconazole and omeprazole also appears to be established, but it appears that this can be minimised by using an oral itraconazole solution. As with ketoconazole, giving itraconazole with an acidic drink such as Cola would minimise the interaction. Monitor patients on itraconazole if either omeprazole or esomeprazole is also given and increase the antifungal dose if necessary. The effect of itraconazole on omeprazole is unknown, but it might be expected to increase omeprazole levels similarly to ketoconazole.

The interaction between voriconazole and omeprazole is established. No adjustment to the dose of voriconazole is required with concurrent omeprazole.[9,12] The clinical importance if the rise in serum omeprazole levels caused by voriconazole is not established, but the makers recommend that the omeprazole dose be halved.[9,12]

Fluconazole is not affected by omeprazole, and is unlikely to be affected by other proton pump inhibitors. However, fluconazole markedly increases omeprazole levels. The clinical relevance of these changes is uncertain, but not likely to be important for single-dose fluconazole regimens. More study is needed to establish whether it is advisable to reduce the omeprazole dose in those given both drugs longer-term.

1. Nexium (Esomeprazole). AstraZeneca UK Ltd. UK Summary of product characteristics, October 2004.
2. Zimmermann T, Yeates RA, Riedel K-D, Lach P, Laufen H. The influence of gastric pH on the pharmacokinetics of fluconazole: the effect of omeprazole. *Int J Clin Pharmacol Ther* (1994) 32, 491–6.
3. Kang BC, Yang CQ, Cho HK, Suh OK, Shin WG. Influence of fluconazole on the pharmacokinetics of omeprazole in healthy volunteers. *Biopharm Drug Dispos* (2002) 23, 77–81.
4. Jaruratanasirikul S, Sriwiriyajan S. Effect of omeprazole on the pharmacokinetics of itraconazole. *Eur J Clin Pharmacol* (1998) 54, 159–61.
5. Johnson MD, Hamilton CD, Drew RH, Sanders LL, Pennick GJ, Perfect JR. A randomized comparative study to determine the effect of omeprazole on the peak serum concentration of itraconazole oral solution. *J Antimicrob Chemother* (2003) 51, 453–7.
6. Chin TWF, Leob M, Fong IW. Effects of an acidic beverage (Coca-Cola) on absorption of ketoconazole. *Antimicrob Agents Chemother* (1995) 39, 1671–5.
7. Böttiger Y, Tybring G, Götharson E, Bertilsson L. Inhibition of the sulfoxidation of omeprazole by ketoconazole in poor and extensive metabolizers of S-mephenytoin. *Clin Pharmacol Ther* (1997) 62, 384–91.
8. Wood N, Tan K, Purkins L, Layton G, Hamlin J, Kleinermans D, Nichols D. Effect of omeprazole on the steady-state pharmacokinetics of voriconazole. *Br J Clin Pharmacol* (2003) 56, 56–61.
9. VFEND (Voriconazole). Pfizer Inc. US Prescribing information, March 2005.
10. Humphries TJ, Nardi RV, Spera AC, Lazar JD, Laurent AL, Spanyers SA. Coadministration of rabeprazole sodium (E3810) and ketoconazole results in a predictable interaction with ketoconazole. *Gastroenterology* (1996) 110 (Suppl), A138.
11. Personal communication. Eisai Corporation of North America, October 1996.
12. VFEND (Voriconazole). Pfizer Ltd. UK Summary of product characteristics, March 2005.

Azoles; Fenticonazole + Miscellaneous

Fenticonazole in the form of pessaries is absorbed very poorly from the vagina so that the risk of an interaction with other drugs given systemically is small.

Clinical evidence, mechanism, importance and management

A study in 14 women (5 of them healthy, 4 with relapsing vulvovaginal candidiasis, and 5 with cervico-carcinoma) found that the systemic absorption of fenticonazole nitrate from a single 1 g pessary was very small indeed. The amount absorbed, based on the amount recovered from the urine and faeces over 5 days ranged from 0.58 to 1.81% of the original dose.[1] The risk of a clinically relevant interaction with other drugs that may be present in the body would therefore seem to be very small. None appears to have been reported.

1. Upjohn Limited. Personal communication, May 1995.

Azoles; Fluconazole + Hydrochlorothiazide

A very brief report describes a 40% increase in fluconazole serum levels in a small group of healthy subjects when they were given hydrochlorothiazide.[1] However it is suggested that no change in the fluconazole dosage is needed.[1]

1. Grant SM, Clissold SP. Fluconazole. A review of its pharmacodynamic and pharmacokinetic properties, and therapeutic potential in superficial and systemic mycoses. *Drugs* (1990) 39, 877–916.

Azoles; Fluconazole + Rifamycins

Although rifampicin causes only a modest increase in the loss of fluconazole from the body, the reduction in its effects may possibly be clinically important. Fluconazole does not appear to affect rifampicin pharmacokinetics. There is an isolated report of hypercalcaemia in a patient taking both fluconazole and rifampicin. Rifabutin levels are increased by fluconazole, which carries an increased risk of uveitis.

Clinical evidence

(a) Rifampicin (Rifampin)

Rifampicin 600 mg daily for 19 days reduced the AUC of a single 200-mg dose of fluconazole by 23% and decreased the half-life by 19% in a study in healthy subjects.[1]

A study in two groups of 12 patients with AIDS found that the AUC and peak plasma level of fluconazole 400 mg daily given for cryptococcal meningitis were reduced by 22% and 17% by rifampicin 600 mg daily when compared with the group not given rifampicin. The elimination rate constant of fluconazole was increased by 39% and the elimination half life was reduced by 28%. There were no significant changes in clinical outcome although the subsequent use of a lower prophylactic dose of fluconazole 200 mg with rifampicin was found to result in levels of fluconazole below the MIC of the infecting organism.[2] Also, 3 patients with AIDS being treated for cryptococcal meningitis with fluconazole 400 mg daily relapsed when rifampicin was added.[3] Another undetailed report says that one of 5 patients on fluconazole needed an increased dosage or a replacement antifungal when given rifampicin.[4]

A study in 11 AIDS patients with cryptococcal meningitis found that fluconazole 200 mg twice daily for 14 days had no effect on the pharmacokinetics of rifampicin 300 mg daily.[5] Five AIDS patients with tuberculosis taking rifampicin and fluconazole had normal rifampicin levels compared with 14 similar patients taking rifampicin alone but in both groups rifampicin levels were only about 28% of that predicted.[6]

There is also an isolated report of severe hypercalcaemia attributed to the use of rifampicin and fluconazole in a patient with tuberculosis and pneumocystosis.[7]

(b) Rifabutin (Ansamycin)

Twelve HIV+ patients were given zidovudine 500 mg daily from day 1 to 44, fluconazole 200 mg daily from days 3 to 30 and rifabutin 300 mg daily from days 17 to 44. Rifabutin did not significantly affect the pharmacokinetics of fluconazole,[8] but fluconazole increased the AUC of rifabutin by 82%, and the AUC of the rifabutin metabolite LM565 was increased by 216%.[8] There is some evidence that fluconazole increases the prophylactic efficacy of rifabutin against *M. avium* complex disease, although there was also an increase in incidence of leucopenia.[9] Uveitis developed in 6 HIV+ patients on rifabutin 450 to 600 mg daily and fluconazole. Of these, 5 were also taking clarithromycin,[10] which is also known to increase rifabutin levels, see 'Macrolides + Rifamycins', p.217. Uveitis has been attributed to the concurrent use of rifabutin and fluconazole in other reports.[11,12]

Mechanism

Rifampicin increases the metabolism of the fluconazole by the liver, thereby increasing its loss from the body.[1] However, fluconazole (unlike ketoconazole) is mainly excreted unchanged in the urine so that changes in its metabolism would not be expected to have a marked effect. Fluconazole apparently increases the rifabutin levels by inhibiting its metabolism. The absorption of antitubercular drugs may be reduced in patients with AIDS and an increase in rifampicin levels may be due to increased absorption in the presence of fluconazole.[6]

Importance and management

Information is limited but the interaction between rifampicin and fluconazole appears to be established and of clinical importance. Although rifampicin has only a relatively small effect on fluconazole (compared with its considerable effects on 'ketoconazole', (p.141)), the cases of relapse cited above[3] and the need for an increased dosage[4] indicate that this interaction can be clinically important. Monitor concurrent use and increase the fluconazole dosage if necessary. One study suggests a 30% increase in fluconazole dose may be considered for serious infections during concurrent rifampicin therapy. This may be especially important during prophylaxis of cryptococcal meningitis with lower doses of fluconazole such as 200 mg daily.[2]

The interaction between rifabutin and fluconazole is established, the general picture being that concurrent use can be advantageous but because of the increased risk of uveitis, the UK Committee on Safety of Medicines says that full consideration should be given to reducing the dosage of rifabutin to 300 mg daily. The rifabutin should be stopped if uveitis develops and the patient referred to an ophthalmologist.[13] A later review suggests this 300 mg dose is associated with a reduced risk of uveitis and maintains efficacy.[14]

1. Apseloff G, Hilligoss M, Gardner MJ, Henry EB, Inskeep PB, Gerber N, Lazar JD. Induction of fluconazole metabolism by rifampin: *in vivo* study in humans. *J Clin Pharmacol* (1991) 31, 358–61.
2. Panomvana Na Ayudhya D, Thanompuangseree N, Tansuphaswadikul S. Effect of rifampicin on the pharmacokinetics of fluconazole in patients with AIDS. *Clin Pharmacokinet* (2004) 43, 725–32.
3. Coker RJ, Tomlinson DR, Parkin J, Harris JRW, Pinching AJ. Interaction between fluconazole and rifampicin. *BMJ* (1990) 301, 818.
4. Tett S, Carey D, Lee H-S. Drug interactions with fluconazole. *Med J Aust* (1992) 156, 365.
5. Jaruratanasirikul S, Kleepaew A. Lack of effect of fluconazole on the pharmacokinetics of rifampicin in AIDS patients. *J Antimicrob Chemother* (1996) 38, 877–80.
6. Peloquin CA, Nitta AT, Burman WJ, Brudney KF, Miranda-Massari JR, McGuinness ME, Berning SE, Gerena GT. Low antituberculosis drug concentrations in patients with AIDS. *Ann Pharmacother* (1996) 30, 919–25.
7. Bani-Sadr F, Hoff J, Chiffoleau A, Allavena C, Raffi F. Hypercalcémie sévère chez une patiente traitée par fluconazole et rifampicine. *Presse Med* (1998) 27, 860.
8. Trapnell CB, Narang PK, Li R, Lavelle JP. Increased plasma rifabutin levels with concomitant fluconazole therapy in HIV-infected patients. *Ann Intern Med* (1996) 124, 573–6.
9. Narang PK, Trapnell CB, Schoenfelder JR, Lavelle JP, Bianchine JR. Fluconazole and enhanced effect of rifabutin prophylaxis. *N Engl J Med* (1994) 330, 1316–17.
10. Becker K, Schimkat M, Jablonowski H, Häussinger D. Anterior uveitis associated with rifabutin medication in AIDS patients. *Infection* (1996) 24, 34–6.
11. Fuller JD, Stanfield LED, Craven DE. Rifabutin prophylaxis and uveitis. *N Engl J Med* (1994) 330, 1315–16.
12. Kelleher P, Helbert M, Sweeney J, Anderson J, Parkin J, Pinching A. Uveitis associated with rifabutin and macrolide therapy for *Mycobacterium avium intracellulare* infections in AIDS patients. *Genitourin Med* (1996) 72, 419–21.
13. Committee on Safety of Medicines/Medicines Control Agency. Stop Press: Rifabutin (Mycobutin) — uveitis. *Current Problems* (1994) 20, 4.
14. Committee on the Safety of Medicines/Medicines Control Agency. Revised indications and drug interactions of rifabutin. *Current Problems* (1997) 23, 14.

Azoles; Itraconazole + Grapefruit juice

Grapefruit juice impairs the absorption of itraconazole, but the clinical significance of this is unknown.

Clinical evidence, mechanism, importance and management

As grapefruit juice is an inhibitor of intestinal cytochrome P450 isoenzyme CYP3A4, the major enzyme involved in itraconazole metabolism, a study[1] was conducted to see if it could be used to enhance itraconazole absorption. Either 240 ml of double strength grapefruit juice or 240 ml water were given with, and 2 hours after a single 200-mg dose of itraconazole. When given with grapefruit juice, the AUC of itraconazole unexpectedly decreased, on average by 43% (range 81% reduction to 105% increase). The results were in line with decreased absorption, rather than altered metabolism and so the authors suggest that grapefruit juice may impair the absorption of itraconazole either by affecting P-glycoprotein or lowering the duodenal pH. However, another study found that grapefruit juice had no effect on itraconazole pharmacokinetics.[2] The clinical significance of these results is not known, but it would seem prudent to avoid concurrent use until more information is available. More study is needed.

1. Penzak SR, Gubbins PO, Gurley BJ, Wang P-L, Saccente M. Grapefruit juice decreases the systemic availability of itraconazole capsules in healthy volunteers. *Ther Drug Monit* (1999) 21, 304–309.
2. Kawakami M, Suzuki K, Ishizuka T, Hidaka T, Matsuki Y, Nakumara H. Effect of grapefruit juice on pharmacokinetics of itraconazole in healthy subjects. *Int J Clin Pharmacol Ther* (1998) 36, 306–308.

Azoles; Itraconazole + Rifamycins

Rifabutin reduces the plasma levels of itraconazole. An isolated report describes increased serum rifabutin levels associated with uveitis in a man given itraconazole. Rifampicin very markedly reduces serum itraconazole evels. This can reduce or abolish the antifungal effects of the itraconazole, possibly depending on the infection being treated.

Clinical evidence

(a) Rifabutin

(i) Itraconazole serum levels reduced. In a three period study, 6 HIV+ patients were given itraconazole 200 mg daily for 14 days, rifabutin 300 mg daily for 10 days, and then both drugs for 14 days. It was found that the rifabutin reduced the peak plasma levels of the itraconazole by 71% and reduced its AUC by 74%.[1]

(ii) Rifabutin serum levels raised. A 49-year-old HIV+ man on rifabutin 300 mg daily was started on itraconazole 600 mg daily. Because of low plasma levels after 3 weeks the itraconazole dose was increased to 900 mg daily. A week later the patient developed anterior uveitis. It was found that the itraconazole trough serum levels were normal but rifabutin trough serum levels were raised to 153 nanograms/ml (expected to be less than 50 nanograms/ml after 24 hours). Rifabutin was stopped and the uveitis was treated. Symptoms resolved after 5 days.[2]

(b) Rifampicin (Rifampin)

A patient on antitubercular treatment including rifampicin 600 mg and isoniazid 300 mg daily was additionally started on itraconazole 200 mg daily. After 2 weeks his serum itraconazole levels were negligible (0.011 mg/l). Even when the dosage was doubled the levels only reached a maximum of 0.056 mg/l. When the antitubercular drugs were stopped his serum itraconazole level was 3.23 mg/l with a 300 mg daily dose, and 2.35 to 2.6 mg/l with a 200 mg daily dose.[3]

A later study in 8 other patients confirmed that itraconazole levels were reduced by rifampicin but the clinical outcome depended on the mycosis being treated. Four out of 5 patients responded to treatment for a *Cryptococcus neoformans* infection, despite undetectable itraconazole levels, apparently because there is synergy between the two drugs. In contrast, 2 patients with coccidioidomycosis failed to respond, and 2 others with cryptococcosis suffered a relapse or persistence of seborrhoeic dermatitis (possibly due to *M. furfur*) while taking both drugs.[4] In a patient with AIDS the serum levels of itraconazole 400 to 600 mg daily were undetectable in the presence of rifampicin, and took 3 to 5 days to recover after the rifampicin was stopped.[5] Undetectable itraconazole levels occurred in another patient given rifampicin who was treated for histoplasmosis.[6] A study found that the AUC of itraconazole was reduced to 20% after 6 healthy subjects took rifampicin 600 mg daily for 3 days.[7] Very markedly reduced serum itraconazole levels (undetectable in some instances) have been seen in other healthy subjects and AIDS patients when given rifampicin.[8]

Mechanism

The suggested reason is that rifabutin and rifampicin increase the metabolism of the itraconazole by the liver, and hasten its loss from the body. Itraconazole inhibits the metabolism of rifabutin so that its serum levels rise, thereby precipitating uveitis.

Importance and management

Information on the interaction between itraconazole and rifabutin is very limited but monitor for reduced antifungal activity, raising the itraconazole dosage as necessary, and watch for increased rifabutin levels and toxicity (in particular uveitis). More study is needed to confirm and to assess the general importance of this interaction.

The interaction between itraconazole and rifampicin is established and clinically important. Monitor the effects of concurrent use, being alert for the need to increase the itraconazole dosage. The effect on serum itraconazole levels can be very marked indeed. The clinical importance of this interaction can apparently depend on the mycosis being treated.

1. Smith JA, Hardin TC, Patterson TF, Rinaldi MG, Graybill JR. Rifabutin (RIF) decreases itraconazole (ITRA) plasma levels in patients with HIV-infection. Am Soc Microbiol 2nd Nat Conf. Human retroviruses and related infections. Washington DC, Jan 29—Feb 2 1995, 77.
2. Lefort A, Launay O, Carbon C. Uveitis associated with rifabutin prophylaxis and itraconazole therapy. *Ann Intern Med* (1996) 125, 939–40.
3. Blomley M, Teare EL, de Belder A, Thway Y, Weston M. Itraconazole and anti-tuberculosis drugs. *Lancet* (1990) ii, 1255.
4. Tucker RM, Denning DW, Hanson LH, Rinaldi MG, Graybill JR, Sharkey PK, Pappagianis D, Stevens DA. Interaction of azoles with rifampin, phenytoin and carbamazepine: *in vitro* and clinical observations. *Clin Infect Dis* (1992) 14, 165–74.
5. Drayton J, Dickinson G, Rinaldi MG. Coadministration of rifampin and itraconazole leads to undetectable levels of serum itraconazole. *Clin Infect Dis* (1994) 18, 266.
6. Hecht FM, Wheat J, Korzun AH, Hafner R, Skahan KJ, Larsen R, Limjoco MT, Simpson M, Schneider D, Keefer MC, Clark R, Lai KK, Jacobsen JM, Squires K, Bartlett JA, Powderly W. Itraconazole maintenance treatment for histoplasmosis in AIDS: a prospective, multicenter trial. *J Acquir Immune Defic Syndr Hum Retrovirol* (1997) 16, 100–107.
7. Fromtling RA, ed. Recent Trends in the Discovery, Development and Evaluation of Antifungal Agents. SA: JR Prous Science Publishers, 1987 p 223–49.
8. Jaruratanasirikul S, Sriwiriyajan S. Effect of rifampicin on the pharmacokinetics of itraconazole in normal volunteers and AIDS patients. *Eur J Clin Pharmacol* (1998) 54, 155–8.

Azoles; Ketoconazole + Rifampicin (Rifampin) and/or Isoniazid

The serum levels of ketoconazole can be reduced by 50 to 90% by rifampicin and/or isoniazid. Serum rifampicin levels can also be halved by ketoconazole, but are possibly unaffected if the drugs are given 12 hours apart.

Clinical evidence

(a) Effect on serum ketoconazole levels

The serum levels of ketoconazole 200 mg daily were roughly halved by rifampicin 600 mg in one patient. After 5 months of concurrent use with rifampicin and isoniazid 300 mg daily, there was a ninefold decrease in peak serum levels and the AUC was reduced by nearly 90%.[1]

A study in a 3-year-old child who had responded poorly to treatment found that peak serum ketoconazole levels and AUC were reduced by about 65 to 80% by rifampicin and/or isoniazid. The interaction also occurred when the dosages were separated by 12 hours. When all three drugs were given together the ketoconazole serum levels were undetectable.[2] Other reports confirm these reports.[3-9]

(b) Effect on serum rifampicin levels

The rifampicin serum levels of a child were roughly halved by ketoconazole, but when the rifampicin was given 12 hours after the ketoconazole, the serum levels of rifampicin remained unaffected. Other studies also show a reduction in rifampicin levels caused by ketoconazole.[5,7,9] but one found no reduction in rifampicin levels.[6]

Mechanism

It seems probable that rifampicin reduces the serum levels of ketoconazole by increasing its rate of metabolism within the liver, thereby hastening its clearance from the body. Just how isoniazid interacts is uncertain. It is suggested that ketoconazole impairs the absorption of rifampicin from the gut.

Importance and management

The interactions between ketoconazole and rifampicin appear to be established and of clinical importance, but there is very much less information about the interaction with isoniazid. The effects on rifampicin can apparently be avoided by giving the ketoconazole at a different time (12 hours apart seems to be effective) but this does not solve the problem of the effects on ketoconazole. The dosage of at least one of the drugs will need to be increased to achieve both good antitubercular and antifungal responses. Concurrent use should be well monitored and dosage increases made if necessary.

1. Brass C, Galgiani JN, Blaschke TF, Defelice R, O'Reilly RA, Stevens DA. Disposition of ketoconazole, an oral antifungal, in humans. *Antimicrob Agents Chemother* (1982) 21, 151–8.
2. Engelhard D, Stutman HR,Marks MI. Interaction of ketoconazole with rifampin and isoniazid. *N Engl J Med* (1984) 311, 1681–3.
3. Drouhet E, Dupont B. Laboratory and clinical assessment of ketoconazole in deep-seated mycoses. *Am J Med* (1983) 74, 30–47.
4. Meunie F. Serum fungistatic and fungicidal activity in volunteers receiving antifungal agents. *Eur J Clin Microbiol* (1986) 5, 103–9.
5. Doble N, Hykin P, Shaw R, Keal EE. Pulmonary mycobacterium tuberculosis in acquired immune deficiency syndrome. *BMJ* (1985) 291, 849–50.
6. Doble H, Shaw R, Rowland-Hill C, Lush M, Warnock DW, Keal EE. Pharmacokinetic study of the interaction between rifampicin and ketoconazole. *J Antimicrob Chemother* (1988) 21, 633–5.
7. Abadie-Kemmerly S, Pankey GA, Dalvisio JR. Failure of ketoconazole treatment of *Blastomyces dermatidis* due to interaction of isoniazid and rifampin. *Ann Intern Med* (1988) 109, 844–5.
8. Tucker RM, Denning DW, Hanson LH, Rinaldi MG, Graybill JR, Sharkey PK, Pappagianis D, Stevens DA. Interaction of azoles with rifampin, phenytoin and carbamazepine: in vitro and clinical observations. *Clin Infect Dis* (1992) 14, 165–74.
9. Pilheu JA, Galati MR, Yunis AS, De Salvo MC, Negroni R, Garcia Fernandez JC, Mingolla L, Rubio MC, Masana M, Acevedo C. Interaccion farmacocinetica entre ketoconazol, isoniacida y rifampicina. *Medicina (B Aires)* (1989) 49, 43–7.

Azoles; Voriconazole + Rifamycins

Voriconazole is contraindicated with rifampicin. Rifabutin decreases voriconazole levels and voriconazole increases the levels of rifabutin.

Clinical evidence, mechanism, importance and management

(a) Rifabutin

Rifabutin 300 mg daily decreased the AUC and maximum plasma levels of voriconazole 200 mg twice daily by 69 and 78% respectively. Increasing the dose of voriconazole to 350 mg twice daily in the presence of rifabutin gave an AUC 68% of that achieved with voriconazole 200 mg twice daily alone while maximum plasma levels were more or less the same.[1] These effects are due to rifabutin inhibiting the cytochrome P450 isoenzyme CYP3A4, which is involved in the metabolism of voriconazole. However, voriconazole also inhibits CYP3A4, and at a dose of

400 mg twice daily, it increased the maximum plasma level and AUC of rifabutin 300 mg twice daily by 195 and 331% respectively. The makers in the US therefore say that the combination is contraindicated.[2] However, the UK makers permit concurrent use if the benefits outweigh the risks.[1] If used together, it is recommended that the dose of voriconazole be increased from 200 mg twice daily to 350 mg twice daily (and from 100 to 200 mg twice daily in patients under 40 kg). The intravenous dose should also be increased from 4 to 5 mg/kg twice daily. Importantly, the makers advise careful monitoring for rifabutin adverse effects (e.g. check full blood counts, monitor for uveitis).[1]

(b) Rifampicin

Rifampicin is a more potent inhibitor of CYP3A4 than rifabutin. Rifampicin[1] 600 mg once daily decreased the maximum plasma levels and AUC of voriconazole 200 mg twice daily by about 95%. Even doubling the dose of voriconazole did not give adequate exposure.[2] The makers of voriconazole therefore contraindicate concurrent use of rifampicin.[1,2]

1. VFEND (Voriconazole). Pfizer Ltd. UK Summary of product characteristics, March 2005.
2. VFEND (Voriconazole). Pfizer Inc. US Prescribing information, March 2005.

Caspofungin + Miscellaneous

As raised liver enzymes occur when caspofungin is used with ciclosporin the makers suggest that the combination should only be used if the benefits of treatment outweigh the risks. Caspofungin modestly reduces the levels of 'tacrolimus', (p.821). Carbamazepine, dexamethasone, efavirenz, nevirapine, phenytoin or rifampicin may all induce the metabolism of caspofungin and reduce its levels. Caspofungin appears not to interact with amphotericin B, itraconazole, mycophenolate or nelfinavir.

Clinical evidence, mechanism, importance and management

(a) Ciclosporin

The makers report that in two clinical studies single-dose ciclosporin increased the AUC of caspofungin by 35% and caused increases in AST and ALT of up to threefold. The liver enzymes returned to normal on discontinuation of both drugs, and during concurrent use the levels of ciclosporin were not affected.[1-3] The makers advise that ciclosporin and caspofungin should only be used together if the benefits outweigh the risks of treatment and that if they are used, close monitoring of liver enzymes is recommended.[1,2]

(b) Rifampicin (Rifampin) and other enzyme inducing agents

When started simultaneously, rifampicin increased the trough levels and AUC of caspofungin by 170 and 60% respectively. However, after 2 weeks the AUC had returned to normal and the trough levels of caspofungin were 30% lower than in patients not receiving rifampicin. The makers say that consideration should be given to increasing the dose of caspofungin from 50 to 70 mg daily in patients taking rifampicin.[1,2] Caspofungin appears not to alter the pharmacokinetics of rifampicin.[1]

On the basis of the interaction with rifampicin the makers suggest considering increasing the dose of caspofungin from 50 to 70 mg daily if it is used with **carbamazepine**, **dexamethasone**, **efavirenz**, **nevirapine** or **phenytoin**, all of which can induce cytochrome P450 enzymes.[1,2]

(c) Tacrolimus

For mention that caspofungin reduces the levels of tacrolimus see 'Tacrolimus + Caspofungin', p.821.

(d) Non-interacting drugs

Caspofungin 70 mg on day 1 and 50 mg for the next 13 days did not alter the pharmacokinetics of **itraconazole** 200 mg daily.[4] The pharmacokinetics of caspofungin were also unaltered. Similarly the makers of caspofungin say there are no interactions between caspofungin and **amphotericin B**, **mycophenolate** or **nelfinavir**.[1,2]

1. Cancidas (Caspofungin acetate). Merck Sharp & Dohme Ltd. UK Summary of product characteristics, October 2004.
2. Cancidas (Caspofungin acetate). Merck & Co., Inc. US Prescribing information, February 2005.
3. Sable CA, Nguyen B-YT, Chodakewitz JA, DiNubile MJ. Safety and tolerability of caspofungin acetate in the treatment of fungal infections. *Transpl Infect Dis* (2002) 4, 25–30.
4. Stone JA, McCrea JB, Wickersham PJ, Holland SD, Deutsch PJ, Bi S, Cicero T, Greenberg H, Waldman SA. A phase I study of caspofungin evaluating the potential for drug interactions with itraconazole, the effect of gender and the use of a loading dose regimen. *Intersci Conf Antimicrob Agents Chemother* (2000) 40, 26.

Chloroquine + Colestyramine

Colestyramine can reduce the absorption of chloroquine, but the clinical importance of this is uncertain.

Clinical evidence, mechanism, importance and management

Colestyramine 4 g reduced the absorption of chloroquine 10 mg/kg by about 30% in 5 children aged 6 to 13. Considerable individual differences were seen.[1] This reduced absorption is consistent with the way colestyramine interacts with other drugs by binding to them in the gut. The clinical importance is uncertain but separating the dosages is effective in reducing the effects of this interaction with other drugs. It is generally advised that other drugs are given 1 hour before or 4 to 6 hours after colestyramine.

1. Gendrel D, Verdier F, Richard-Lenoble D, Nardou M. Interaction entre cholestyramine et chloroquine. *Arch Fr Pediatr* (1990) 47, 387–8.

Chloroquine + H_2-blockers

Cimetidine reduces the metabolism and clearance of chloroquine, but the clinical importance of this is uncertain. Ranitidine appears not to interact.

Clinical evidence, mechanism, importance and management

Cimetidine 400 mg daily for 4 days approximately halved the clearance of a single 600-mg dose of chloroquine base in 10 healthy subjects. The elimination half-life was prolonged from 3.11 to 4.62 days.[1] It was suggested that these effects occurred because **cimetidine** inhibits the metabolism of chloroquine by the liver, thereby reducing its loss from the body. The clinical importance of this interaction is uncertain, but it would seem prudent to be alert for any signs of chloroquine toxicity during concurrent use. A similar study by the same authors found that **ranitidine** does not interact with chloroquine.[2]

1. Ette EI, Brown-Awala EA, Essien EE. Chloroquine elimination in humans: effect of low-dose cimetidine. *J Clin Pharmacol* (1987) 27, 813–16.
2. Ette EI, Brown-Awala EA, Essien EE. Effect of ranitidine on chloroquine disposition. *Drug Intell Clin Pharm* (1987) 21, 732–4.

Chloroquine + Imipramine

No pharmacokinetic interaction was seen in 6 healthy subjects given single doses of chloroquine 300 mg and imipramine 50 mg.[1] However, see also 'Drugs that prolong the QT interval + Other drugs that prolong the QT interval', p.170.

1. Onyeji CO, Toriola TA, Ogunbona FA. Lack of pharmacokinetic interaction between chloroquine and imipramine. *Ther Drug Monit* (1993) 15, 43–6.

Chloroquine + Promethazine

Promethazine appears to increase the blood levels of intramuscular chloroquine and its metabolites.

Clinical evidence, mechanism, importance and management

A study in healthy subjects found that intramuscular promethazine hydrochloride 25 mg, given with intramuscular chloroquine phosphate 200 mg increased the AUC of chloroquine and its metabolites by 85%. This may be due to promethazine enhancing absorption of chloroquine from the injection site or displacing it and its metabolites from binding sites in the blood. The initial rate of excretion of chloroquine and the total drug excreted within 3 hours was unaffected by concurrent promethazine.[1] The increased bioavailability of chloroquine may improve its therapeutic effects but could also increase toxicity. *In vitro* and *animal* studies suggest the combination may be effective in the treatment of uncomplicated chloroquine-resistant malaria.[2,3] More study is needed. For mention that chloroquine may increase chlorpromazine levels, see 'Phenothiazines + Antimalarials', p.568.

1. Ehiemua AO, Komolafe OO, Oyedeji GA, Olamijulo SK. Effect of promethazine on the metabolism of chloroquine. *Eur J Drug Metab Pharmacokinet* (1988) 13, 15–17.
2. Oduola OO, Happi TC, Gbotosho GO, Ogundahunsi OAT, Falade CO, Akinboye DO, Sowunmi A, Oduola AMJ. Plasmodium berghei: efficacy and safety of combinations of chloroquine and promethazine in chloroquine resistant infections in gravid mice. *Afr J Med Med Sci* (2004) 33, 77–81.
3. Oduola AMJ, Sowunmi A, Milhous WK, Brewer TG, Kyle DE, Gerena L, Rossan RN, Salako LA, Schuster BG. *In vitro* and *in vivo* reversal of chloroquine resistance in *Plasmodium falciparum* with promethazine. *Am J Trop Med Hyg* (1998) 58, 625–9.

Diethylcarbamazine + Urinary acidifiers or alkalinisers

Urinary alkalinisers can reduce the loss of diethylcarbamazine in the urine, whereas urinary acidifiers can increase the loss. The clinical importance of this is unknown.

Clinical evidence

Two studies, one in healthy subjects[1] and the other in patients with onchocerciasis,[2] found that making the urine alkaline with **sodium bicarbonate** markedly increased the retention of the diethylcarbamazine in the body. The urinary excretion of a 50-mg dose of diethylcarbamazine was 62.3% and its elimination half-life 4 hours when the urine was made acidic (pH less than 5.5) by giving ammonium chloride, compared with 5.1% and 9.6 hours respectively when the urine was made alkaline (pH more than 7.5) using sodium bicarbonate.[1]

Mechanism

In alkaline urine most of the diethylcarbamazine is non-ionised and is therefore easily reabsorbed in the kidney by simple diffusion through the lipid membrane. However, the conclusion was reached that in practice there is no advantage in making the urine alkaline in order to be able to use smaller doses of diethylcarbamazine because the severity of the adverse reactions (the Mazzotti reaction) is not reduced, and the microfilarial counts at the end of a month are not significantly different.[2]

Importance and management

The clinical importance of any unsought for changes in the urinary pH brought about by the use of other drugs during diethylcarbamazine treatment has not been assessed, but be aware that its pharmacokinetics and possibly the severity of its adverse effects can be changed.

1. Edwards G, Breckenridge AM, Adjepon-Yamoah KK, Orme M L'E, Ward SA. The effect of variations in urinary pH on the pharmacokinetics of diethylcarbamazine. *Br J Clin Pharmacol* (1981) 12, 807–12.
2. Awadzi K, Adjepon-Yamoah KK, Edwards G, Orme M L'E, Breckenridge AM, Gilles HM. The effect of moderate urine alkalinisation on low dose diethylcarbamazine therapy in patients with onchocerciasis. *Br J Clin Pharmacol* (1986) 21, 669–76.

Flucytosine + Antacids

Aluminium/magnesium hydroxide delays the absorption of flucytosine from the gut, but the total amount absorbed remains unaffected.[1]

1. Cutler RE, Blair AD, Kelly MR. Flucytosine kinetics in subjects with normal and impaired renal function. *Clin Pharmacol Ther* (1978) 24, 333–42.

Flucytosine + Cytarabine

Some very limited evidence suggests that cytarabine may oppose the antifungal effects of flucytosine.

Clinical evidence, mechanism, importance and management

A man with Hodgkin's disease treated for cryptococcal meningitis with flucytosine 100 mg/kg daily had a fall in his flucytosine serum and CSF levels from a range of 30 to 40 mg/l down to undetectable levels when given cytarabine intravenously. When the cytarabine was replaced by procarbazine, the flucytosine levels returned to their former values. *In vitro* tests found that cytarabine 1 mg/l completely abolished the activity of flucytosine against the patient's strain of Cryptococcus, even in levels up to 50 mg/l, whereas procarbazine did not.[1] In another study in a patient with acute myeloid leukaemia it was found that the predose flucytosine level fell from 65 to 42 mg/l and the postdose flucytosine level fell from and 80 to 53 mg/l when cytarabine and daunorubicin were given. These levels were still with in the therapeutic range.[2] The drop in levels was attributed to an improvement in renal function rather than antagonism between the two drugs.[2] In an *in vitro* study the antifungal effects of flucytosine against 14 out of 16 wild isolates of cryptococcus were not changed in the presence of cytarabine. In the remaining two patients, an increase in effect was seen in one and a decrease was seen the other.[2]

The evidence for this interaction is therefore very limited indeed and its general clinical importance remains uncertain, but the makers warn against concurrent use. It has been suggested that if both drugs are used, the flucytosine should be given 3 hours or more after the cytarabine, by which time its serum levels will have fallen.[3]

1. Holt RJ. Clinical problems with 5-fluorocytosine. *Mykosen* (1978) 21, 363–9.
2. Wingfield HJ. Absence of fungistatic antagonism between flucytosine and cytarabine *in vitro* and *in vivo*. *J Antimicrob Chemother* (1987) 20, 523–7.
3. Pfizer Limited. Personal communication, February 1988.

Flucytosine + Other antifungals

The combination of flucytosine with amphotericin B may be more effective than flucytosine alone, but toxicity may also occur. The combination of flucytosine and fluconazole was found advantageous in two patients, and *in vitro* studies suggest the combination of flucytosine and other azole antifungals or caspofungin may be more effective than flucytosine alone.

Clinical evidence, mechanism, importance and management

The combined use of flucytosine and **amphotericin B** is more effective than flucytosine alone in the treatment of cryptococcal meningitis, but **amphotericin B** can cause deterioration in renal function, which may result in raised flucytosine blood levels and a possible increase in flucytosine toxicity. Nevertheless combined use is thought to be useful.[1]

Two patients with invasive *Candida* infections with urinary-tract involvement were treated with **fluconazole**, but subsequent *in vitro* tests found **fluconazole** resistance. Flucytosine was added and the combination of drugs eradicated the fungal infections and the patients' renal function improved.[2] *In vitro* studies found the antifungal effects of the combination were additive.[2] Other *in vitro* studies found combinations of **fluconazole**, **itraconazole**, **voriconazole**, **amphotericin B** or **caspofungin** with flucytosine to be more effective than flucytosine alone against 60 to 80% of isolates of *Cryptococcus neoformans*. Killing curves showed indifferent interactions between the **azoles** and flucytosine and synergy between **amphotericin B** and flucytosine.[3] Another *in vitro* study and an *animal* study found that the combination of **posaconazole** and flucytosine was significantly more effective against *C. neoformans* than either drug alone.[4]

1. Bennett JE, Dismukes WE, Duma RJ, Medoff G, Sande MA, Gallis H, Leonard J, Fields BT, Bradshaw M, Haywood H, McGee ZA, Cate TR, Cobbs CG, Warner JF, Alling DW. A comparison of amphotericin B alone and combined with flucytosine in the treatment of cryptoccal meningitis. *N Engl J Med* (1979) 301, 126–31.
2. Girmenia C, Venditti M, Martino P. Fluconazole in combination with flucytosine in the treatment of fluconazole-resistant *Candida* infections. *Diagn Microbiol Infect Dis* (2003) 46, 227–31.
3. Schwarz P, Dromer F, Lortholary O, Dannaoui E. In vitro interaction of flucytosine with conventional and new antifungals against *Cryptococcus neoformans* clinical isolates. *Antimicrob Agents Chemother* (2003) 47, 3361–4.
4. Barchiesi F, Schimizzi AM, Najvar LK, Bocanegra R, Caselli F, Di Cesare S, Giannini D, Di Francesco LF, Giacometti A, Carle F, Scalise G, Graybill JR. Interactions of posaconazole and flucytosine against *Cryptococcus neoformans*. *Antimicrob Agents Chemother* (2001) 45, 1355–9.

Furazolidone + Omeprazole

Omeprazole modestly reduces the serum levels of furazolidone.

Clinical evidence, mechanism, importance and management

A study in 18 healthy subjects found that omeprazole 20 mg twice daily for 5 days reduced the peak serum level of a single 200-mg dose of furazolidone by about 30%. Omeprazole may alter the bioavailability of furazolidone by reducing its dissolution or increasing its degradation before it reached the intestine and/or induce the first-pass metabolism of furazolidone.[1] The clinical relevance of this modest change is uncertain.

1. Calafatti SA, Ortiz RAM, Deguer M, Martinez M, Pedrazzoli J. Effect of acid secretion blockade by omeprazole on the relative bioavailability of orally administered furazolidone in healthy volunteers. *Br J Clin Pharmacol* (2001) 52, 205–9.

Furazolidone + Sympathomimetics

After 5 to 10 days' use furazolidone has MAO-inhibitory activity about equivalent to that of the antidepressant and antihypertensive MAOIs. The concurrent use of furazolidone with sympathomimetic amines possessing indirect activity (amfetamines, phenylpropanolamine, ephedrine, etc.) or with tyramine-rich foods and drinks may be expected to result in a potentially serious rise in blood pressure, although direct evidence of accidental adverse reactions of this kind does not seem to have been reported. The pressor effects of noradrenaline (norepinephrine) are unchanged.

Clinical evidence

After 6 days' treatment with furazolidone 400 mg daily, the pressor responses to **tyramine** or **dexamfetamine** in 4 hypertensive patients had increased two to threefold, and after 13 days by about tenfold. These responses were about the same as those found in 2 other patients on **pargyline**.[1] The MAO-inhibitory activity of furazolidone was confirmed by measurements taken on jejunal specimens. The pressor effects of **noradrenaline** (**norepinephrine**) were unchanged by furazolidone.[1]

Mechanism

The MAO-inhibitory activity of furazolidone is not immediate and may in fact be due to a metabolite of furazolidone.[2] It develops gradually so that after 5 to 10 days' use, indirectly-acting sympathomimetics will interact with furazolidone in the same way as they do in the presence of other MAOIs.[3,4] More details of the mechanisms of this interaction are to be found elsewhere. See 'MAOIs + Tyramine-rich foods', p.876 and 'MAOIs + Sympathomimetics; Indirectly-acting', p.872.

Importance and management

The MAO-inhibitory activity of furazolidone after 5 to 10 days' use is established, but reports of hypertensive crises either with sympathomimetics or tyramine-containing foods or drinks appear to be lacking. Notwithstanding, it would seem prudent to warn patients given furazolidone not to take any of the drugs, foods or drinks that are prohibited to those on antidepressant or antihypertensive MAOIs. See the appropriate monographs on MAOIs for more detailed lists of these drugs, foods and drinks. No adverse interaction would be expected with noradrenaline (norepinephrine).

1. Pettinger WA, Oates JA. Supersensitivity to tyramine during monoamine oxidase inhibition in man. Mechanism at the level of the adrenergic neurone. *Clin Pharmacol Ther* (1968) 9, 341–4.
2. Stern IJ, Hollifield RD, Wilk S, Buzard JA. The anti-monoamine oxidase effects of furazolidone. *J Pharmacol Exp Ther* (1967) 156, 492–9.
3. Pettinger WA, Soyangco FG, Oates JA. Monoamine-oxidase inhibition by furazolidone in man. *Clin Res* (1966) 14, 258.
4. Pettinger WA, Soyangco FG, Oates JA. Inhibition of monoamine oxidase in man by furazolidone. *Clin Pharmacol Ther* (1968) 9, 442–7.

Griseofulvin + Food

The absorption of griseofulvin is markedly increased if it is taken with a high-fat meal.

Clinical evidence, mechanism, importance and management

A study in 5 healthy subjects found that the rate and extent of absorption of griseofulvin 125 mg was significantly enhanced if it was given with a fatty meal rather than in the fasting state.[1] Other studies similarly found the absorption of griseofulvin was about doubled when it was taken with a high-fat meal.[2,3] A further study in 12 healthy subjects found that the higher the fat content of the meal the higher the bioavailability of griseofulvin.[4] The extent of the effect of food on griseofulvin bioavailability may also depend of the product formulation.[5] One report suggested that giving griseofulvin with food tends to reduce the differences in the bioavailability of griseofulvin from micronised and ultramicronised tablets.[6] Enhanced absorption was also found with a formulation of griseofulvin in a **corn oil** emulsion, when compared with tablets or an aqueous suspension.[7]

This interaction is established and of clinical importance. The maker notes that griseofulvin should be given after meals, otherwise absorption is likely to be inadequate.[8]

1. Khalafalla N, Elgholmy ZA, Khalil SA. Influence of a high fat diet on GI absorption of griseofulvin tablets in man. *Pharmazie* (1981) 36, 692–3.
2. Crounse RG. Human pharmacology of griseofulvin: the effect of fat intake on gastrointestinal absorption. *J Invest Dermatol* (1961) 37, 529–33.
3. Crounse RG. Effective use of griseofulvin. *Arch Dermatol* (1963) 87, 176–8.
4. Ogunbona FA, Smith IF, Olawoye OS. Fat contents of meals and bioavailability of griseofulvin in man. *J Pharm Pharmacol* (1985) 37, 283–4.
5. Aoyagi N, Ogata H, Kaniwa N, Ejima A. Effect of food on the bioavailability of griseofulvin from microsize and PEG ultramicrosize (GRIS-PEG) plain tablets. *J Pharmacobiodyn* (1982) 4, 120–4.
6. Bijanzadeh M, Mahmoudian M, Salehian P, Khazainia T, Eshghi L, Khosravy A. The bioavailability of griseofulvin from microsized and ultramicrosized tablets in nonfasting volunteers. *Indian J Physiol Pharmacol* (1990) 34, 157–61.
7. Bates TR, Sequeria JA. Bioavailability of micronized griseofulvin from corn oil-in-water emulsion, aqueous suspension, and commercial tablet dosage forms in humans. *J Pharm Sci* (1975) 64, 793–7.
8. Grisovin (Griseofulvin). GlaxoSmithKline UK. UK Summary of product characteristics, July 2004.

Griseofulvin + Phenobarbital

The antifungal effects of griseofulvin can be reduced or even abolished by phenobarbital.

Clinical evidence

Two epileptic children taking phenobarbital 40 mg daily did not respond to long-term treatment for tinea capitis with griseofulvin 125 mg three times daily until the barbiturate was withdrawn.[1]

Five other patients (3 also taking phenytoin) similarly failed to respond to griseofulvin while taking phenobarbital.[2-4] Two studies, in a total of 14 healthy subjects, found that phenobarbital 30 mg three times daily reduced the serum levels of oral griseofulvin by about a third[5] and the absorption was reduced from 58.1% without phenobarbital to 40.6% in the presence of phenobarbital.[6]

Mechanism

Not fully understood. Initially it was thought that the phenobarbital increased the metabolism and clearance of the griseofulvin,[7] but it has also been suggested that it reduces the absorption of griseofulvin from the gut.[6] One idea is that the phenobarbital increases peristalsis so that the opportunity for absorption is diminished.[6] Another suggestion is that the phenobarbital forms a complex with the griseofulvin, which makes an already poorly soluble drug even less soluble, and therefore less readily absorbed.[8] A further suggestion is that phenobarbital may reduce the level of intestinal bile salts, which in turn may reduce the solubility and absorption of griseofulvin.[9]

Importance and management

An established interaction of clinical importance, although the evidence seems to be limited to the reports cited. If the barbiturate must be given, it has been suggested that the griseofulvin should be given in divided doses three times a day to give it a better chance of being absorbed,[6] although divided doses were used when the interaction occurred in one of the reports.[1] The effect of increasing the dosage of griseofulvin appears not to have been studied. An alternative, where possible, is to exchange the phenobarbital for a non-interacting anticonvulsant such as sodium valproate. This proved to be successful in one of the cases cited.[1]

1. Beurey J, Weber M, Vignaud J-M. Traitement des teignes microsporiques. Interférence métabolique entre phénobarbital et griséofulvine. *Ann Dermatol Venereol* (1982) 109, 567–70.
2. Lorenc E. A new factor in griseofulvin treatment failures. *Mo Med* (1967) 64, 32–3.
3. Stepanova ZV, Sheklakova AA. Liuminal kak prichina neudachi griseoful'vinoterapii bol'nogo mikrospoviei. *Vestn Dermatol Venerol* (1975) 12, 63–5.
4. Hay RJ, Clayton YM, Moore MK, Midgely G. An evaluation of itraconazole in the management of onychomycosis. *Br J Dermatol* (1988) 119, 359–66.
5. Busfield D, Child KJ, Atkinson RM, Tomich EG. An effect of phenobarbitone on blood-levels of griseofulvin in man. *Lancet* (1963) ii, 1042–3.
6. Riegelman S, Rowland M, Epstein WL. Griseofulvin-phenobarbital interaction in man. *JAMA* (1970) 213, 426–31.
7. Busfield D, Child KJ, Tomich EG. An effect of phenobarbitone on griseofulvin metabolism in the rat. *Br J Pharmacol* (1964) 22, 137–42.

8. Abougela IKA, Bigford DJ, McCorquodale I, Grant DJW. Complex formation and other physico-chemical interactions between griseofulvin and phenobarbitone. *J Pharm Pharmacol* (1976) 28, 44P.
9. Jamali F, Axelson JE. Griseofulvin–phenobarbital interaction: a formulation-dependent phenomenon. *J Pharm Sci* (1978) 67, 466–70.

Halofantrine + Miscellaneous

The UK Committee on Safety of Medicines recommends that halofantrine should not be used with other drugs that can prolong the QT interval because of the risk of cardiac arrhythmias. Some drugs (diltiazem, erythromycin, ketoconazole, mefloquine, pyrimethamine/sulfadoxine, quinine, quinidine, tetracycline) may increase plasma levels and possibly the toxicity of halofantrine by inhibition of its metabolism or elimination. Fatty food and grapefruit juice have a similar effect.

Clinical evidence, mechanism, importance and management

(a) Cytochrome P450 isoenzyme CYP3A4 inhibitors

A study in *animals* found that **ketoconazole** roughly doubled the AUC of halofantrine and inhibited its metabolism to the equipotent metabolite, desbutylhalofantrine.[1] In *in vitro* studies, **ketoconazole** markedly inhibited the metabolism of halofantrine by CYP3A4.[2,3] It has been suggested that the rise in halofantrine levels could reasonably be expected to increase toxicity.[2,3] Other CYP3A4 inhibitors, **diltiazem** and **erythromycin**, also inhibited the metabolism of halofantrine, and might do so clinically.[3] Further study is needed of these potential pharmacokinetic interactions. **Mefloquine**, **quinine** and **quinidine** may also inhibit the metabolism of halofantrine by CYP3A4, see (b) below.

(b) Drugs that prolong the QT interval

Halofantrine, in therapeutic doses, can prolong the QT interval in the majority of patients, causing ventricular arrhythmias in a very small number. The effect is increased if halofantrine is taken with **fatty foods** because of the markedly increased absorption, see (d) below. By 1993, worldwide, 14 cases of cardiac arrhythmias had been reported and 8 patients were known to have died. In order to reduce the likelihood of arrhythmias, the UK Committee on Safety of Medicines now advises that halofantrine should not be taken with **meals**, or with certain other drugs that may induce arrhythmias. They list **chloroquine**, **mefloquine** and **quinine**, **tricyclic antidepressants**, **antipsychotics**, **certain antiarrhythmic agents**, **terfenadine** and **astemizole**, as well as drugs causing electrolyte disturbances.[4] Although not listed, it would seem prudent to avoid other drugs that prolong the QT interval. For a list, see 'Table 7.3', (p.169)'.

A study into the enzyme inhibitory actions of **chloroquine** given with halofantrine found that both drugs inhibited the cytochrome P450 isoenzyme CYP2D6.[5] Similarly, **quinidine** and **quinine** have been shown *in vitro* to inhibit the metabolism of halofantrine by CYP3A4, and so may increase halofantrine levels, which could reasonably be expected to increase toxicity.[2,3] *Animal* studies found that although **mefloquine** alone did not significantly alter the QTc interval, it enhanced the effects of halofantrine by increasing blood levels.[6] The makers of **mefloquine** considers that this effect is clinically significant, and contraindicates concurrent or subsequent halofantrine therapy.[7,8]

(c) Food

A study in 6 healthy subjects found that the maximum plasma levels and AUC of a single 250-mg dose of halofantrine were increased by about 6.6-fold and 2.9-fold respectively when given with a **fatty meal** rather than in a fasting state. The AUC of the metabolite desbutylhalofantrine was also increased.[10] *Animal* data suggest that **fats** may reduce the presystemic metabolism of halofantrine.[1] Because this is likely to increase the risk of halofantrine-induced arrhythmias, halofantrine should not be taken with **meals**.

(d) Grapefruit juice or Orange juice

A crossover study in 12 healthy subjects given halofantrine 500 mg with 250 ml of either water, orange juice or grapefruit juice (standard strength), found that grapefruit juice increased the AUC and peak plasma levels of halofantrine by 2.8-fold and 3.2-fold respectively. The QTc interval increased from 17 to 31 milliseconds, which increases the risk of arrhythmias. Orange juice did not affect the pharmacokinetics or pharmacodynamics of halofantrine.[11] These data suggest that grapefruit juice should be avoided by patients on halofantrine.[11]

(e) Pyrimethamine/Sulfadoxine (Fansidar)

A preliminary clinical study suggests that *Fansidar* (**pyrimethamine** and **sulfadoxine**) may raise the AUC and peak plasma levels of halofantrine, which could lead to an increased incidence of arrhythmias,[9] see also (b) above.

(f) Tetracyclines

A study in 8 healthy subjects found that tetracycline 500 mg twice daily for 7 days increased the maximum plasma levels, AUC and elimination half life of a single 500-mg dose of halofantrine by 146%, 99%, and 73% respectively. Increases in the major metabolite of halofantrine also occurred in the presence of tetracycline.[12] In addition, *in vitro* studies found that **doxycycline** does not inhibit the metabolism of halofantrine.[2] Therefore an interaction based on inhibition of halofantrine metabolism is unlikely, but as both halofantrine and tetracycline are excreted into the bile, competition for this elimination route may result in increased plasma levels. There may be an increased risk of halofantrine toxicity if it is used with higher doses of tetracycline.[12]

1. Khoo S-M, Porter CJH, Edwards GA, Charman WN. Metabolism of halofantrine to its equipotent metabolite, desbutylhalofantrine, is decreased when orally administered with ketoconazole. *J Pharm Sci* (1998) 87, 1538–41.
2. Baune B, Furlan V, Taburet AM, Farinotti R. Effect of selected antimalarial drugs and inhibitors of cytochrome P-450 3A4 on halofantrine metabolism by human liver microsomes. *Drug Metab Dispos* (1999) 27, 565–8.
3. Baune B, Flinois JP, Furlan V, Gimenez F, Taburet AM, Becquemont L, Farinotti R. Halofantrine metabolism in microsomes in man: major role of CYP 3A4 and CYP 3A5. *J Pharm Pharmacol* (1999) 51, 419–26.
4. Committee on Safety of Medicines/Medicines Control Agency. Cardiac arrhythmias with halofantrine (Halfan). *Current Problems* (1994) 20, 6.
5. Simooya OO, Sijumbil G, Lennard MS, Tucker GT. Halofantrine and chloroquine inhibit CYP2D6 activity in healthy Zambians. *Br J Clin Pharmacol* (1998) 45, 315–17.
6. Lightbrown ID, Lambert JP, Edwards G, Coker SJ. Potentiation of halofantrine-induced QTc prolongation by mefloquine: correlation with blood concentrations of halofantrine. *Br J Pharmacol* (2001) 132, 197–204.
7. Lariam (Mefloquine hydrochloride). Roche Products Ltd. UK Summary of product characteristics, February 2005.
8. Lariam (Mefloquine hydrochloride). Roche Pharmaceuticals. US Prescribing information, May 2004.
9. Hombhanje FW. Effect of a single dose of Fansidar™ on the pharmacokinetics of halofantrine in healthy volunteers: a preliminary report. *Br J Clin Pharmacol* (2000) 49, 283–4.
10. Milton K, Edwards G, Ward SA, Orme ML'E, Breckenridge AM. Pharmacokinetics of halofantrine in man: effects of food and dose size. *Br J Clin Pharmacol* (1989) 28, 71–7.
11. Charbit B, Becquemont L, Lepère B, Peytavin G, Funck-Brentano C. Pharmacokinetic and pharmacodynamic interaction between grapefruit juice and halofantrine. *Clin Pharmacol Ther* (2002) 72, 514–23.
12. Bassi PU, Onyeji CO, Ukponmwan OE. Effects of tetracycline on the pharmacokinetics of halofantrine in healthy volunteers. *Br J Clin Pharmacol* (2004) 58, 52–5.

Hydroxychloroquine + Rifampicin (Rifampin)

The control of discoid lupus with hydroxychloroquine in a woman was rapidly lost when rifampicin was started. Control was regained when the hydroxychloroquine dosage was doubled.

Clinical evidence, mechanism, importance and management

A woman with discoid lupus, stable on hydroxychloroquine 200 mg daily, was also given rifampicin, isoniazid and pyrazinamide for tuberculosis. Within 1 to 2 weeks the discoid lupus flared-up again but it rapidly responded when the hydroxychloroquine dosage was doubled. The reason for this reaction is not known for certain but the authors of the report suggest that the rifampicin (a recognised and potent cytochrome P450 enzyme-inducing agent) increased the metabolism and clearance of the hydroxychloroquine so that it was no longer effective.[1] It is already known that discoid lupus flare-ups can occur within 2 weeks of stopping hydroxychloroquine,[2] which gives support to this suggested mechanism. Neither isoniazid nor pyrazinamide is likely to have been responsible for what happened.

This seems to be the first and only report of this interaction, but what happened is consistent with the way rifampicin interacts with many other drugs. If rifampicin is added to hydroxychloroquine, the outcome should be well monitored. Be alert for the need to increase the hydroxychloroquine dosage.

1. Harvey CJ, Bateman NT, Lloyd ME, Hughes GRV. Influence of rifampicin on hydroxychloroquine. *Clin Exp Rheumatol* (1995) 13, 536.
2. The Canadian Hydroxychloroquine Study Group. A randomized study of the effect of withdrawing hydroxychloroquine sulfate in systemic lupus erythematosus. *N Engl J Med* (1991) 324, 150–4.

Hydroxyquinoline + Zinc oxide

The presence of zinc oxide inhibits the therapeutic effects of 8-hydroxyquinoline in ointments.

Clinical evidence

The observation that a patient had an allergic reaction to 8-hydroxyquinoline in ointments with a paraffin base, but not a zinc oxide base, prompted further study of a possible incompatibility. The subsequent study in 13 patients confirmed that zinc oxide reduces the eczematogenic (allergic) properties of the 8-hydroxyquinoline. However, it also inhibits its antibacterial and antimycotic effects, and appears to stimulate the growth of *Candida albicans*.[1]

Mechanism

It seems almost certain that the zinc ions form chelates with 8-hydroxyquinoline, which have little or no antibacterial properties.[1,2]

Importance and management

The documentation is limited but the reaction appears to be established. There is no point in using zinc oxide to reduce the allergic properties of the 8-hydroxyquinoline if, at the same time, the therapeutic effects disappear.

1. Fischer T. On 8-hydroxyquinoline-zinc oxide incompatibility. *Dermatologica* (1974) 149, 129–35.
2. Albert A, Rubbo SD, Goldacre RJ, Balfour BG. The influence of chemical constitution on antibacterial activity. Part III: A study of 8-hydroxyquinoline (oxine) and related compounds. *Br J Exp Pathol* (1947) 28, 69–87.

Ivermectin + Levamisole

Levamisole may markedly increase the bioavailability of ivermectin. Ivermectin does not alter the pharmacokinetics of levamisole.

Clinical evidence, mechanism, importance and management

A study in 28 healthy subjects given levamisole 2.5 mg/kg alone or with ivermectin 200 micrograms/kg found that ivermectin had no effect on the AUC or maximum level of levamisole. However, the AUC of ivermectin was twofold higher when given with levamisole compared with historical values in subjects who had received ivermectin alone.[1] An associated study in 44 patients with *Onchocerca volvulus* infections found that levamisole given with ivermectin was neither macrofilaricidal nor more effective against microfilariae and adult worms than ivermectin alone. In addition, patients receiving ivermectin and levamisole had a higher incidence of pruritus, arthralgia and fever than those on ivermectin alone.[1] Caution is recommended with combined use.

1. Awadzi K, Edwards G, Opoku NO, Ardrey AE, Favager S, Addy ET, Attah SK, Yamuah LK, Quartey BT. The safety, tolerability and pharmacokinetics of levamisole alone, levamisole plus ivermectin, and levamisole plus albendazole, and their efficacy against *Onchocerca volvulus*. *Ann Trop Med Parasitol* (2004) 98, 595–614.

Ivermectin + Orange juice

Orange juice modestly reduces the bioavailability of ivermectin.

Clinical evidence, mechanism, importance and management

A study in 16 healthy subjects found that the AUC and peak plasma levels of a single 150-micrograms/kg dose of ivermectin were reduced by 36% and 39% respectively when the ivermectin was given with orange juice (750 ml over 4 hours) rather than with water. The mechanism for the reduced bioavailability is not known but it does not seem related to P-glycoprotein activity.[1] The clinical relevance of these changes is uncertain.

1. Vanapalli SR, Chen Y, Ellingrod VL, Kitzman D, Lee Y, Hohl RJ, Fleckenstein L. Orange juice decreases the oral bioavailability of ivermectin in healthy volunteers. *Clin Pharmacol Ther* (2003) 73, P94.

Levamisole + Miscellaneous

There is some evidence that levamisole can increase the effects of phenytoin, and that a disulfiram-like reaction can occur with alcohol.

Clinical evidence, mechanism, importance and management

The product information for levamisole describes an increase in the plasma levels of **phenytoin** due to fluorouracil with levamisole, and a disulfiram-like reaction with **alcohol**.[1] The general importance of these interactions is uncertain, but bear them in mind when prescribing levamisole.

1. Ergamisol (Levamisole). Janssen Pharmaceutica Inc. US Prescribing information, August 1999.

Lumefantrine + Mefloquine

The levels of lumefantrine (as co-artemether) are reduced by mefloquine pretreatment, but the changes are not thought to be clinically significant.

Clinical evidence, mechanism, importance and management

In a study, 6 doses of co-artemether (artemether 80 mg/lumefantrine 480 mg) were given over 60 hours to 42 healthy subjects, starting 12 hours after a short course of mefloquine (3 doses totalling 1 g given over 12 hours). The pharmacokinetics of the mefloquine and the artemether were unaffected by sequential use, but the lumefantrine maximum plasma concentrations and AUC were reduced by 29% and 41% respectively. However, given that the plasma levels of lumefantrine are usually highly variable, these changes were not thought large enough to affect the efficacy of treatment.[1]

In another study these drugs in combination were found not to affect the QT interval, and levels were also considered adequate for treatment.[2]

However, the maker of co-artemether notes that prolongation of the QT interval was seen in about 5% of patients in clinical trials (although they say this could be disease related). They state that, due to the limited data on safety and efficacy, co-artemether should not be given concurrently with any other antimalarial agent.[3] Consider also 'Mefloquine + Other antimalarials', p.147.

1. Lefèvre G, Bindschedler M, Ezzet F, Schaeffer N, Meyer I, Thomsen MS. Pharmacokinetic interaction trial between co-artemether and mefloquine. *Eur J Pharm Sci* (2000) 10, 141–51.
2. Bindschedler M, Lefèvre G, Ezzet F, Schaeffer N, Meyer I, Thomsen MS. Cardiac effects of co-artemether (artemether/lumefantrine) and mefloquine given alone or in combination to healthy volunteers. *Eur J Clin Pharmacol* (2000) 56, 375–81.
3. Riamet (Artemether/Lumefantrine). Novartis Pharmaceuticals UK Ltd. UK Summary of product characteristics, June 2002.

Mefloquine + Ampicillin

Ampicillin modestly increases the plasma levels of mefloquine, and reduces its half-life.

Clinical evidence, mechanism, importance and management

In a study, 8 healthy subjects were given ampicillin 250 mg four times daily for 5 days and a single 750-mg dose of mefloquine on day 2. The maximum plasma level and 0 to 5-day AUC of mefloquine were increased by 34% and 49% respectively, although the AUC from time zero to infinity was not significantly increased. The half-life and volume of distribution of mefloquine were reduced from 17.7 to 15.3 days and by 27% respectively in the presence of ampicillin. No increase in adverse events was seen.

The effects may be due to an increase in mefloquine bioavailability and a reduction in its enterohepatic recycling.[1]

The clinical relevance of these changes is uncertain, but the authors consider that the changes in elimination are unlikely to be clinically significant, since these occur after the resolution of infection.[1]

1. Karbwang J, Na Bangchang K, Back DJ, Bunnag D. Effect of ampicillin on mefloquine pharmacokinetics in Thai males. *Eur J Clin Pharmacol* (1991) 40, 631–3.

Mefloquine + Cardioactive drugs

Mefloquine might prolong the QT interval, and an isolated report describes cardiopulmonary arrest in one patient also taking propranolol. The WHO have issued a warning about the concurrent use of mefloquine with antiarrhythmics, beta-blockers, calcium-channel blockers, antihistamines, phenothiazines, and some related antimalarials. Mefloquine should not be used with halofantrine, because of a clinically significant lengthening of the QT interval.

Clinical evidence, mechanism, importance and management

The WHO[1] warn that the concurrent use of mefloquine with **antiarrhythmics**, **beta-blockers**, **calcium channel blockers**, **antihistamines** including H_1-histamine antagonists and **phenothiazines** might contribute to the prolongation of the QT_c interval but do not specifically contraindicate, the use of mefloquine.[1] It is also suggested that mefloquine and related drugs (e.g. **quinine** or **quinidine**) should only be given together under close medical supervision because of possible additive cardiotoxicity.[1] The makers of mefloquine also give this warning, pointing out that the interaction is theoretical, and that clinically significant QTc prolongation has not been found with mefloquine alone.[2,3] Apart from **quinine**, where two studies found minor QTc prolongation (see 'Mefloquine + Other antimalarials', p.147), no formal studies on the possible adverse effects of combining any of the above drugs with mefloquine seem to have been done. One 1990 review briefly mentions a single case of cardiopulmonary arrest in a patient on **propranolol** when a single dose of mefloquine was given.[4]

It remains to be confirmed whether the effects of mefloquine and these other drugs on cardiac function are normally additive, and whether the outcome is clinically important. However, until more is known it would seem prudent to err on the side of caution and to follow this cautionary advice. Drugs that prolong the QT interval, are listed in 'Table 7.1', (p.156). There is also a theoretical interaction with QT-prolonging 'quinolones' (p.148). The makers note that a clinically important lengthening of the QT interval has been seen [in *animals*] when halofantrine is used after **mefloquine**,[2,3] possibly halofantrine levels are raised by 'mefloquine', (p.145).

1. WHO. International travel and health. Geneva: WHO, 2005. Available at http://www.who.int/ith/en (accessed 30/06/05).
2. Lariam (Mefloquine hydrochloride). Roche Products Ltd. UK Summary of product characteristics, February 2005.
3. Lariam (Mefloquine hydrochloride). Roche Pharmaceuticals. US Prescribing information, May 2004.
4. Anon. Mefloquine for malaria. *Med Lett Drugs Ther* (1990) 31, 13–14.

Mefloquine + Cimetidine

Mefloquine levels are modestly increased and its elimination is reduced by the concurrent use of cimetidine, but the clinical importance of this is uncertain.

Clinical evidence, mechanism, importance and management

A single 500-mg dose of mefloquine was given to 10 healthy subjects before and after they took cimetidine 400 mg twice daily for 28 days. The cimetidine had no effect on the mefloquine serum levels or on its AUC, but its half-life increased by 50% (from 9.6 to 14.4 days) and the oral clearance decreased by almost 40%.[1] In another study mefloquine was given to 6 healthy subjects and to 6 patients with peptic ulcers before and after cimetidine 400 mg twice daily for 3 days. Cimetidine increased maximum plasma levels of mefloquine by about 42% and 20% and increased the AUC by about 37% and 32% in the healthy subjects and patients with ulcers respectively. The elimination half-life was increased but not to a significant extent.[2] The probable reason is that cimetidine (a recognised enzyme inhibitor) reduces the metabolism of the mefloquine by the liver so that plasma levels are increased and it is lost from the body more slowly. The clinical importance of this is uncertain, but to be on the safe side prescribers should be alert for any evidence of increased mefloquine adverse effects (dizziness, nausea, vomiting, abdominal pain) and psychiatric or neurological reactions during concurrent use. The UK Committee on Safety of Medicines say that patients should be informed about the adverse effects of mefloquine and they should seek medical advice if necessary before the next dose is due.[3]

1. Sunbhanichi M, Ridtitid W, Wongnawa M, Akesiripong S, Chamnongchob P. Effect of cimetidine on an oral single-dose mefloquine pharmacokinetics in humans. *Asia Pac J Pharmacol* (1997) 12, 51–5.
2. Kolawole JA, Mustapha A, Abdu-Aguye I, Ochekpe N. Mefloquine pharmacokinetics in healthy subjects and in peptic ulcer patients after cimetidine administration. *Eur J Drug Metab Pharmacokinet* (2000) 25, 165–70.
3. Committee on Safety of Medicines/Medicines Control Agency. Mefloquine (Lariam) and neuropsychiatric reactions. *Current Problems* (1996) 22, 6.

Mefloquine + Metoclopramide

Although metoclopramide increases the rate of absorption of a single-dose of mefloquine and increases its peak blood levels, its adverse effects are possibly reduced.

Clinical evidence, mechanism, importance and management

When metoclopramide 10 mg was taken 15 minutes before a single 750-mg dose of mefloquine, the absorption half-life of the mefloquine in 7 healthy subjects was reduced from 3.2 to 2.4 hours and the peak blood levels were raised by 31%. However, although the rate of absorption was increased, the total amount absorbed was unchanged. A possible reason for these changes is that the metoclopramide increases the gastric emptying so that the mefloquine reaches the small intestine more quickly, which would increase the rate of absorption. Despite these changes, the toxicity of mefloquine (dizziness, nausea, vomiting, abdominal pain) was noted to be reduced.[1] It is not clear what the outcome of chronic use might be, but it would be prudent to monitor the outcome closely. More study is needed.

1. Bangchang KN, Karbwang J, Bunnag D, Harinasuta T, Back DJ. The effect of metoclopramide on mefloquine pharmacokinetics. *Br J Clin Pharmacol* (1991) 32, 640–1.

Mefloquine + Other antimalarials

Primaquine can increase both the serum levels and adverse effects of mefloquine. Mefloquine serum levels may possibly be increased by quinine. In theory there is an increased risk of convulsions if mefloquine is given with quinine or chloroquine. Conflicting reports suggest that artemisinin derivatives may either reduce mefloquine levels or not adversely affect the pharmacokinetics of mefloquine, but the antimalarial activity may be improved.

Clinical evidence, mechanism, importance and management

(a) Artemisinin derivatives

A study in 20 patients with acute uncomplicated falciparum malaria given mefloquine 750 mg followed after 6 hours by 500 mg found that levels of mefloquine were reduced by 27% and its clearance rate increased 2.6-fold when the doses of mefloquine were given 6 and 12 hours after **artesunate** 200 mg. However, the patients who received the combination had shorter fever clearance and parasite clearance times than those given mefloquine alone, but the cure rate was lower for combined treatment than for mefloquine alone (66% versus 75%). To prevent the pharmacokinetic interaction resulting in a reduction in its efficacy, mefloquine should be given when **artesunate** and its metabolites have cleared the circulation (the authors suggest possibly 24 hours after a dose). This would minimise the pharmacokinetic interaction and allow the pharmacodynamic interaction to predominate. This could result in a synergistic effect due to the rapid clearance of parasites by **artesunate** and the full schizontocidal effect of the slower acting mefloquine.[1] Another study in 27 similar patients found that the AUC of a single dose of mefloquine 750 mg was reduced by 27% when given 24 hours after a single dose of **artemether** 300 mg. However, the addition of **artemether** improved the clinical efficacy.[2]

In a single-dose three-way crossover study, 10 healthy subjects were given either mefloquine 750 mg, **dihydroartemisinin** 300 mg or both drugs together. The pharmacokinetics of the drugs were unchanged on concurrent use, except for the rate of absorption of mefloquine, which was increased. Also the activity against *Plasmodium falciparum* was synergistic, rather than additive.[3] Another study in patients with falciparum malaria found no significant pharmacokinetic interaction between artemisinin and mefloquine. In this study, patients received mefloquine 750 mg alone or artemisinin 500 mg daily for 3 days with a single 750-mg dose of mefloquine either on day 1 or day 4. There was no difference in overall efficacy between treatments, although those treated with artemisinin together with mefloquine on the first day of treatment had the fastest parasite clearance rates.[4] For mention that the sequential use of mefloquine and **artemether**/lumefantrine did not alter mefloquine or artemether pharmacokinetics, see 'Lumefantrine + Mefloquine', p.146.

(b) Primaquine

A randomised crossover study in 14 healthy subjects given mefloquine 1 g found that the addition of primaquine 15 or 30 mg raised the peak serum levels of mefloquine by 48%, from 1.64 to 2.42 micrograms/ml and by 29%, from 2.52 to 3.24 micrograms/ml respectively. Those taking the larger dose of primaquine had a transient increase in peak primaquine serum levels, and its conversion to its inactive carboxyl metabolite also increased. Significant CNS symptoms were also experienced by those taking the larger dose of primaquine.[5] *In vitro* studies suggest that primaquine is a potent inhibitor of mefloquine metabolism.[6] However, these results contrast with a single dose study in 8 healthy subjects given mefloquine 750 mg and primaquine 45 mg in which no increased adverse effects attributable to concurrent use were seen.[7] The clinical significance of this interaction is uncertain, but combined used may increase the mefloquine adverse effects.

(c) Quinine

Mefloquine 750 mg was given to 7 healthy subjects either alone, or followed 24 hours later by quinine 600 mg. The combination did not affect the pharmacokinetics of either drug, but the number of adverse effects and the period of prolongation of the QT interval was greater with the combination, although no symptomatic cardiotoxicity was seen.[8] This absence of a change in pharmacokinetics is contrary to earlier *in vitro* data and unpublished clinical observations,[6] which suggested that quinine may inhibit the metabolism of mefloquine, thereby raising its serum levels. Another study in 13 patients with uncomplicated falciparum malaria given quinine dihydrochloride 10 mg/kg as a one-hour infusion and simultaneous oral mefloquine 15 mg/kg found no evidence of a pharmacokinetic interaction but postural hypotension was common. The QTc interval was prolonged by 12% although a clinically significant cardiovascular interaction was not reported.[9] The makers of mefloquine say that it should not be given with quinine or related compounds (e.g. **quinidine**, **chloroquine**) since this could increase the risk of ECG abnormalities and convulsions. They suggest that patients treated initially for 2 to 3 days with quinine given intravenously should delay mefloquine until at least 12 hours after the last dosing of quinine to largely prevent interactions leading to adverse events.[10,11] However, there seem to be no documented adverse reports of this interaction leading to convulsions. Consider also 'Mefloquine + Cardioactive drugs' p.147.

1. Karbwang J, Na Bangchang K, Thanavibul A, Back DJ, Bunnag D, Harinasuta T. Pharmacokinetics of mefloquine alone or in combination with artesunate. *Bull WHO* (1994) 72, 83–7.
2. Na-Bangchang K, Karbwang J, Molunto P, Banmairuroi V, Thanavibul A. Pharmacokinetics of mefloquine, when given alone and in combination with artemether, in patients with uncomplicated falciparum malaria. *Fundam Clin Pharmacol* (1995) 9, 576–82.
3. Na-Bangchang K, Tippawangkosol P, Thanavibul A, Ubalee R, Karbwang J. Pharmacokinetic and pharmacodynamic interactions of mefloquine and dihydroartemisinin. *Int J Clin Pharmacol Res* (1999) 19, 9–17.
4. Svensson USH, Alin MH, Karlsson MO, Bergqvist Y, Ashton M. Population pharmacokinetic and pharmacodynamic modelling of artemisinin and mefloquine enantiomers in patients with falciparum malaria. *Eur J Clin Pharmacol* (2002) 58, 339–51.
5. Macleod CM, Trenholme GM, Nora MV, Bartley EA, Frischer H. Interaction of primaquine with mefloquine in healthy males. *Intersci Conf Antimicrob Agents Chemother* (1990) 30, 213.
6. Na Bangchang K, Karbwang J, Back DJ. Mefloquine metabolism by human liver microsomes. Effect of other antimalarial drugs. *Biochem Pharmacol* (1992) 43, 1957–61.
7. Karbwang J, Na Bangchang K, Thanavibul A, Back DJ, Bunnag D. Pharmacokinetics of mefloquine in the presence of primaquine. *Eur J Clin Pharmacol* (1992) 42, 559–60.
8. Na-Bangchang K, Tan-Ariya P, Thanavibul A, Reingchainam S, Shrestha SB, Karbwang J. Pharmacokinetic and pharmacodynamic interactions of mefloquine and quinine. *Int J Clin Pharmacol Res* (1999) 19, 73–82.
9. Supanaranond W, Suputtamongkol Y, Davis TME, Pukrittayakamee S, Teja-Isavadharm P, Webster HK, White NJ. Lack of a significant adverse cardiovascular effect of combined quinine and mefloquine therapy for uncomplicated malaria. *Trans R Soc Trop Med Hyg* (1997) 91, 694–6.
10. Lariam (Mefloquine hydrochloride). Roche Products Ltd. UK Summary of product characteristics, February 2005.
11. Lariam (Mefloquine hydrochloride). Roche Pharmaceuticals. US Prescribing information, May 2004.

Mefloquine + Quinolones

Three non-epileptic patients had convulsions when they were treated for fever with mefloquine and a quinolone. Also, some quinolones, such as moxifloxacin, prolong the QT interval and concurrent use with mefloquine might theoretically result in additive effects.

Clinical evidence, mechanism, importance and management

(a) Convulsions

A large scale survey in India of the adverse effects of mefloquine identified 3 cases of convulsions out of a total of 150 patients also treated with **ciprofloxacin**, **ofloxacin** or **sparfloxacin**. All 3 patients were not epileptic, and had no family history of epilepsy. All were being treated for fever, which was due to *Plasmodium vivax* in one case, *P. falciparum* in the second, and was not established in the third. None of the patients had severe or complicated malaria. The **ofloxacin** was given 2 days before the mefloquine, and the other two quinolones were given together with the mefloquine.[1] The reason for the seizures is not known, but seizures are among the recognised adverse effects of both mefloquine and these quinolones. These adverse, apparently additive, adverse effects are rare, but prescribers should be aware of the potential increased risk of convulsions when prescribing these drugs together.

(b) Prolongation of the QT interval

Gatifloxacin, **moxifloxacin**, and **sparfloxacin** may cause clinically relevant prolongation of the QT interval. Although mefloquine alone has not been shown to cause a clinically relevant lengthening of the QT interval, caution has still been recommended when it is combined with some other drugs that prolong the QT interval, see 'Mefloquine + Cardioactive drugs', p.147, and it may be prudent to extend this caution to these fluoroquinolones. The makers of **moxifloxacin** note that an additive effect on QT prolongation between **moxifloxacin** and antimalarials cannot be excluded, and therefore contraindicates concurrent use.[2]

1. Mangalvedhekar SS, Gogtay NJ, Wagh VR, Waran MS, Mane D, Kshirsager NA. Convulsions in non-epileptics due to mefloquine-fluoroquinolone co-administration. *Natl Med J India* (2000) 13, 47.
2. Avelox (Moxifloxacin). Bayer plc. UK Summary of product characteristics, April 2005.

Mefloquine + Rifampicin (Rifampin)

Rifampicin significantly reduces the plasma concentrations of mefloquine.

Clinical evidence, mechanism, importance and management

Mefloquine 500 mg was given to 7 healthy subjects after 7 days of pretreatment with rifampicin 600 mg daily. The maximum plasma level of mefloquine decreased by 19% and the AUC decreased by 68%. Rifampicin, a potent enzyme-inducer, increases the metabolism of mefloquine by the cytochrome P450 isoenzyme CYP3A4 in the liver and gut wall. The authors suggest that simultaneous use of rifampicin and mefloquine should be avoided to prevent treatment failure and the risk of *Plasmodium falciparum* resistance to mefloquine.[1]

1. Ridtitid W, Wongnawa M, Mahattanatrakul W, Chaipol P, Sunbhanich M. Effect of rifampicin on plasma concentrations of mefloquine in healthy volunteers. *J Pharm Pharmacol* (2000) 52, 1265–9.

Mefloquine + Tetracycline

Mefloquine serum levels are modestly increased by tetracycline.

Clinical evidence, mechanism, importance and management

The maximum serum levels of mefloquine following a single 750-mg dose were increased by 38% (from 1.16 to 1.6 mg/ml) in 20 healthy Thai men who took tetracycline 250 mg four times daily for a week. The AUC was increased by 30% and the half-life reduced from 19.3 to 14.4 days, without evidence of any increase in adverse effects. The suggested reason for the increased mefloquine levels is that its enterohepatic recycling is reduced because of competition for biliary excretion.[1] The authors of the report conclude that concurrent use may be valuable for treating multi-drug resistant falciparum malaria because higher mefloquine levels are associated with a more effective response. However, more study is needed to confirm these findings. There seems to be no reason for avoiding concurrent use.

1. Karbwang J, Bangchang KN, Back DJ, Bunnag D, Rooney W. Effect of tetracycline on mefloquine pharmacokinetics in Thai males. *Eur J Clin Pharmacol* (1992) 43, 567–9.

Mefloquine + Typhoid vaccine; Oral

Mefloquine and oral attenuated live typhoid vaccine should not be given at the same time.

Clinical evidence, mechanism, importance and management

Mefloquine may attenuate immunisation with oral typhoid vaccine. As mefloquine is rapidly absorbed it has been suggested that by 8 hours after a dose, the levels of mefloquine will be insufficient to inhibit live oral typhoid vaccine.[1] The makers of mefloquine say that immunisation with vaccines like oral typhoid should be completed at least 3 days before the first dose of mefloquine.[2,3] The UK Department of Health agree that the 3-day gap is preferable, but they also say that mefloquine could be given 12 hours before or after vaccination with oral typhoid vaccine.[4] It would therefore seem advisable to separate administration by 3 days where possible, bearing in mind that a 12-hour gap may be sufficient in more urgent cases.

1. Cryz SJ. Post-marketing experience with live oral Ty21a vaccine. *Lancet* (1993) 341, 49–50.
2. Lariam (Mefloquine hydrochloride). Roche Products Ltd. UK Summary of product characteristics, February 2005.
3. Lariam (Mefloquine hydrochloride). Roche Pharmaceuticals. US Prescribing information, May 2004.
4. HMSO. *Immunisation Against Infectious Disease* (1996) 247.

Pamaquine or Primaquine + Mepacrine (Quinacrine)

Mepacrine elevates serum levels of pamaquine. Theoretically primaquine would be expected to interact similarly, but there do not seem to be any reports confirming or disproving this.

Clinical evidence, mechanism, importance and management

Patients given pamaquine, a predecessor of primaquine almost identical in structure, had grossly elevated pamaquine serum levels when they were concurrently treated with mepacrine.[1,2] The probable reason is that the mepacrine occupies binding sites in the body normally also used by the pamaquine and, as a result, the serum levels become very high. On theoretical grounds primaquine might be expected to interact with mepacrine similarly, but there seem to be no reports confirming that a clinically important interaction actually takes place.

1. Zubrod CG, Kennedy TJ, Shannon JA. Studies on the chemotherapy of the human malarias. VIII. The physiological disposition of pamaquine. *J Clin Invest* (1948) 27 (Suppl), 114–120.
2. Earle DP, Bigelow FS, Zubrod CG, Kane CA. Studies on the chemotherapy of the human malarias. IX. Effect of pamaquine on the blood cells of man. *J Clin Invest* (1948) 27, (Suppl), 121–9.

Piperazine + Chlorpromazine

An isolated case of convulsions in a child was attributed to the use of chlorpromazine followed by piperazine.

Clinical evidence, mechanism, importance and management

A child given piperazine for pin worms developed convulsions when treated with chlorpromazine several days later.[1] In a subsequent *animal* study using chlorpromazine 4.5 or 10 mg/kg, many of the *animals* died from respiratory arrest after severe clonic convulsions.[1] However, a later study did not confirm these findings[2] and it is by no means certain whether the adverse reaction in the child was due to an interaction or not. Given that both drugs may cause convulsions, there is probably enough evidence to warrant caution if they are used concurrently.

1. Boulos BM, Davis LE. Hazard of simultaneous administration of phenothiazine and piperazine. *N Engl J Med* (1969) 280, 1245–6.
2. Armbrecht BH. Reaction between piperazine and chlorpromazine. *N Engl J Med* (1970) 282, 1490–1.

Praziquantel + Albendazole or Food

Food, but not albendazole, increases the bioavailability of praziquantel. Praziquantel markedly increases the bioavailability of albendazole in fasted subjects, but much less so when given with a meal. None of these changes appears to have adverse consequences.

Clinical evidence, mechanism, importance and management

(a) Albendazole

A study in 21 children treated for giardiasis with a single 400-mg dose of albendazole either alone or with a single 20-mg/kg dose of praziquantel found that the pharmacokinetics of albendazole were not significantly affected by praziquantel when the drugs were given with 200 ml of **milk**, one hour after **breakfast**. There were wide inter-individual variations in the plasma levels and AUC of the active metabolite albendazole sulfoxide, but these were similar whether albendazole was given alone or with praziquantel.[1]

In contrast, in a study in Sudanese men the AUC of albendazole sulfoxide increased 4.5-fold when a single 400-mg dose of **albendazole** was given with praziquantel 40 mg/kg in fasting subjects. However, this difference was much less marked (only a 1.5-fold increase) when the drugs were given with food.[2] The reasons for these changes and their practical consequences are not known, but the increases in albendazole sulfoxide levels seemed not to cause any problems.[3] If both drugs are given with food, as may be advisable, see 'Albendazole + Food', p.132, any interaction is modest. On the basis of these studies there do not seem to be any obvious reasons why the concurrent use of these two drugs should be avoided.

(b) Food or grapefruit juice

A study found that the maximum plasma levels and AUC of a single 1.8-g dose of praziquantel were increased by 243% and 180% when it was given following a high-fat diet and by 515% and 271% after a high-carbohydrate diet respectively.[3] In another study in healthy Sudanese men, when praziquantel was given with food the AUC was 2.6-fold higher than when it was given in the fasted state.[2]

A further study in patients with neurocystercosis found that treatment with a short regimen of praziquantel 25 mg/kg for 3 doses every 2 hours with a high-carbohydrate diet, which increased plasma levels of praziquantel, provided an adequate clinical alternative to the traditional regimen of 50 mg/kg daily in divided doses for 15 days.[4] Of 6 patients receiving praziquantel with food, the clinical cure rate was 83% compared with only 50% in 6 patients receiving praziquantel while fasting.[4]

In another study by the same authors the maximum plasma level of a single 1.8-g dose of praziquantel was increased by about 63% and the AUC by 90% when given with 250 ml of **grapefruit juice** rather than with water.[5]

On the basis of the above studies, if praziquantel is used for systemic worm infections, administration with **food** is advisable.

1. Pengsaa K, Na-Bangchang K, Limkittikul K, Kabkaew K, Lapphra K, Sirivichayakul C, Wisetsing P, Pojjaroen-Anant C, Chanthavanich P, Subchareon A. Pharmacokinetic investigation of albendazole and praziquantel in Thai children infected with *Giardia intestinalis*. *Ann Trop Med Parasitol* (2004) 98, 349–57.
2. Homeida M, Leahy W, Copeland S, Ali MMM, Harron DWG. Pharmacokinetic interaction between praziquantel and albendazole in Sudanese men. *Ann Trop Med Parasitol* (1994) 88, 551–9.
3. Castro N, Medina R, Sotelo J, Jung H. Bioavailability of praziquantel increases with concomitant administration of food. *Antimicrob Agents Chemother* (2000) 44, 2903–4.
4. Castro N, González-Esquivel DF, López M, Jung H. Análisis comparativo de la influencia de los alimentos y la cimetidina en los niveles plasmáticos de prazicuantel. *Rev Invest Clin* (2003) 55, 655–61.
5. Castro N, Jung H, Medina R, González-Esquivel D, Lopez M, Sotelo J. Interaction between grapefruit juice and praziquantel in humans. *Antimicrob Agents Chemother* (2002) 46, 1614–16.

Praziquantel + Anticonvulsants and/or Cimetidine

Phenytoin and carbamazepine markedly reduce the serum levels of praziquantel and neurocysticercosis treatment failures may occur as a result. A case report suggests that the addition of cimetidine may control this interaction. Cimetidine alone can double the serum levels of praziquantel, and may improve its efficacy in neurocysticercosis.

Clinical evidence

(a) Carbamazepine or Phenytoin

A comparative study of patients on chronic anticonvulsant treatment with phenytoin, or carbamazepine, and healthy subjects (10 in each group) given single 25-mg/kg oral doses of praziquantel, found that phenytoin and carbamazepine reduced the AUC of the praziquantel by about 74% and 90% respectively when compared to the controls, and the maximum serum levels by 76% and 92% respectively.[1]

(b) Cimetidine

A randomised crossover study in 8 healthy subjects given three 25-mg/kg oral doses of praziquantel at 2-hourly intervals found that cimetidine 400 mg given 1 hour before each dose of praziquantel roughly doubled the praziquantel serum levels and AUC.[2,3] A further study in patients with neurocystercosis found that this short regimen of praziquantel with cimetidine (which increased plasma levels of praziquantel by about threefold), had similar efficacy to the traditional regimen of 50 mg/kg daily in divided doses for 15 days.[4] Of 6 patients receiving praziquantel with cimetidine, the clinical cure rate was 83% compared with only 50% in 6 patients receiving praziquantel while fasting.[4]

(c) Phenytoin/Phenobarbital and Cimetidine

A patient with neurocysticercosis taking phenytoin and phenobarbital for a seizure disorder and also on dexamethasone, repeatedly had no response to praziquantel until cimetidine 400 mg 4 times daily was added. His serum praziquantel levels then more than doubled (maximum serum levels raised from 350 to 826 nanograms/ml) and the AUC rose about fourfold, and became similar to that found in normal controls taking praziquantel alone. The patient responded to the praziquantel, but only slowly.[5]

Mechanism

Not established, but the probable reason is that these anticonvulsants and dexamethasone have enzyme inducing effects and can therefore increase the metabolism and loss of praziquantel by the liver, hastening its loss from the body. The cimetidine (a potent enzyme inhibitor) appears to oppose this effect.

Importance and management

Direct information appears to be limited to the reports cited, but the interactions appear to be established. When treating systemic worm infections such as neurocysticercosis some authors advise increasing the praziquantel dosage from 25 to 50 mg/kg if potent enzyme inducers such as carbamazepine or phenytoin are being used, in order to reduce the risk of treatment failure.[1] An alternative might be to add cimetidine. However, the authors of another study[5] were not sure whether the improvement they saw was in fact due to the cimetidine or simply part of the natural history of the disease. It is clear that cimetidine alone can markedly increase praziquantel levels, and the authors say that concurrent use can reduce treatment for neurocysticercosis from 2 weeks to 1 day.[2,4]

The interaction with anticonvulsants is of no importance when praziquantel is used for intestinal worm infections (where its action is a local effect on the worms in the gut).

1. Bittencourt PRM, Gracia CM, Martins R, Fernandes AG, Diekmann HW, Jung W. Phenytoin and carbamazepine decrease oral bioavailability of praziquantel. *Neurology* (1992) 42, 492–6.
2. Jung H, Medina R, Castro N, Corona T, Sotelo J. Pharmacokinetic study of praziquantel administered alone and in combination with cimetidine in a single-day therapeutic regimen. *Antimicrob Agents Chemother* (1997) 41, 1256–9.
3. Castro N, Gonzàlez-Esquivel D, Medina R, Sotelo J, Jung H. The influence of cimetidine on plasma levels of praziquantel after a single day therapeutic regimen. *Proc West Pharmacol Soc* (1997) 40, 33–4.
4. Castro N, González-Esquivel DF, López M, Jung H. Análisis comparativo de la influencia de los alimentos y la cimetidina en los niveles plasmáticos de prazicuantel. *Rev Invest Clin* (2003) 55, 655–61.
5. Dachman WD, Adubofour KO, Bikin DS, Johnson CH, Mullin PD, Winograd M. Cimetidine-induced rise in praziquantel levels in a patient with neurocysticercosis being treated with anticonvulsants. *J Infect Dis* (1994) 169, 689–91.

Praziquantel + Chloroquine

Chloroquine reduces the bioavailability of praziquantel, which would be expected to reduce its efficacy in systemic worm infections such as schistosomiasis.

Clinical evidence, mechanism, importance and management

A single 40-mg/kg oral dose of praziquantel was given to 8 healthy subjects alone, and 2 hours after chloroquine 600 mg. The chloroquine reduced the praziquantel AUC by 65% and reduced the maximum serum levels by 59%. The reasons are not understood. There were large individual variations and one subject was not affected. The effect of this interaction could be that some patients will not achieve high enough serum praziquantel levels to treat systemic worm infections such as schistosomiasis. After taking the chloroquine, the praziquantel serum levels of 4 out of the 8 subjects did not reach the threshold of 0.3 micrograms/ml for about 6 hours (which is required to effectively kill schistosomes), compared with only 2 of 8 during the control period.

The authors conclude that an increased dosage of praziquantel should be considered if chloroquine is given (they do not suggest how much), particularly in anyone who does not respond to initial treatment with praziquantel.[1] More study of this interaction is needed. The interaction is of no importance when praziquantel is used for intestinal worm infections (where its action is a local effect on the worms in the gut).

1. Masimirembwa CM, Naik YS, Hasler JA. The effect of chloroquine on the pharmacokinetics and metabolism of praziquantel in rats and in humans. *Biopharm Drug Dispos* (1994) 15, 33–43.

Proguanil + Cimetidine or Omeprazole

There is some evidence that omeprazole and cimetidine can moderately reduce the production of the active metabolite of proguanil, but the clinical relevance of this is unknown.

Clinical evidence

(a) Cimetidine

In one study, 4 patients with peptic ulcer disease and 6 healthy subjects were given a single 200-mg dose of proguanil on the last day of a 3-day course of cimetidine 400 mg twice daily. In both groups the half-life and AUC of proguanil were significantly increased, but only the healthy subjects had an increase (89%) in the maximum serum concentration. In both groups these pharmacokinetic changes resulted in lower levels of the active metabolite, cycloguanil.[1] This decrease in cycloguanil supported the findings of an earlier study, which had found a 30% decrease in the urinary recovery of cycloguanil when proguanil and cimetidine were given together.[2]

(b) Omeprazole

In a steady-state study in 12 healthy subjects taking proguanil 200 mg daily it was found that omeprazole 20 mg daily roughly halved the AUC of the active metabolite, cycloguanil.[3] However, another study found that omeprazole 20 mg had no effect on the urinary recovery of cycloguanil (or proguanil) following a single 200-mg dose of proguanil.[2]

Mechanism

Cimetidine and omeprazole increase the gastric pH, which may lead to an increase in the absorption of proguanil. Cimetidine[1,2] and omeprazole[3] are also thought to inhibit the metabolism of proguanil, due to their effects on cytochrome P450 isoenzyme CYP2C19.

Importance and management

The differences between the healthy subjects and patients with peptic ulcer disease seen in one study may have been because the disease itself alters the effects of the cimetidine in some way.[1] Patients with peptic ulcer disease are also likely to have an increased gastric pH, which will lead to altered proguanil absorption. The clinical relevance of all these findings is still unclear, although the implication is that decreased cycloguanil levels may lead to inadequate malaria prophylaxis. More study is needed.

1. Kolawole JA, Mustapha A, Abdul-Aguye I, Ochekpe N, Taylor RB. Effects of cimetidine on the pharmacokinetics of proguanil in healthy subjects and in peptic ulcer patients. *J Pharm Biomed Anal* (1999) 20, 737–43.
2. Somogyi AA, Reinhard HA, Bochner F. Effects of omeprazole and cimetidine on the urinary metabolic ratio of proguanil in healthy volunteers. *Eur J Clin Pharmacol* (1996) 50, 417–19.
3. Funck-Bretano C, Becquemont L, Leneveu A, Roux A, Jaillon P, Beaune P. Inhibition by omeprazole of proguanil metabolism: mechanism of the interaction *in vitro* and prediction of *in vivo* results from the *in vitro* experiments. *J Pharmacol Exp Ther* (1997) 280, 730–8.

Proguanil + Fluvoxamine

The conversion of proguanil to its active metabolite is inhibited by fluvoxamine in 'extensive metabolisers'. The clinical relevance of this is uncertain.

Clinical evidence

Twelve healthy subjects, 6 of whom were extensive metabolisers (i.e. who had the cytochrome P450 isoenzyme CYP2C19) and 6 were poor metabolisers (i.e. lacking/reduced CYP2C19 isoenzyme), were given proguanil 200 mg daily for 8 days. This was followed by fluvoxamine 100 mg for 8 days, to which a single 200-mg dose of proguanil was added, on day 6.

In the group of extensive metabolisers it was found that the fluvoxamine reduced the total clearance of the proguanil by about 40%. The partial clearance of proguanil via its two metabolites was reduced, by 85% for cycloguanil and by 89% for 4-chlorophenylbiguanide. The concentrations of these two metabolites in the plasma were hardly detectable while fluvoxamine was being taken. No interaction occurred in the poor metabolisers.[1]

Mechanism

Proguanil, which is a prodrug, is metabolised to its active metabolite, cycloguanil, in the body by the cytochrome P450 isoenzyme CYP2C19. This isoenzyme is inhibited by fluvoxamine in fast metabolisers so that the proguanil does not become activated.[2]

Importance and management

Information appears to be limited to the studies cited, the purpose of which was to confirm that fluvoxamine is an inhibitor of the cytochrome P450 isoenzyme CYP2C19. However, they also demonstrate that proguanil, which is a prodrug, will not be effectively converted into its active form in patients who are extensive metabolisers if fluvoxamine is being taken concurrently, making them effectively poor metabolisers. There are as yet no reports of treatment failures due to this interaction, but if the activity of proguanil is virtually abolished by fluvoxamine, as the authors suggest,[2] then proguanil would also be expected to be ineffective in the proportion of the population that are poor metabolisers. More study is needed.

1. Jeppesen U, Rasmussen BB, Brøsen K. Fluvoxamine inhibits the CYP2C19-catalyzed bioactivation of chloroguanide. *Clin Pharmacol Ther* (1997) 62, 279–86.
2. Rasmussen BB, Nielsen TL, Brøsen K. Fluvoxamine inhibits the CYP2C19-catalysed metabolism of proguanil in vitro. *Eur J Clin Pharmacol* (1998) 54, 735–40.

Proguanil + Other antimalarials

Chloroquine appears to almost double the incidence of mouth ulcers in those taking proguanil prophylactically. There appears to be no clinically relevant pharmacokinetic interaction between atovaquone and proguanil. See also 'Atovaquone/Proguanil + Artesunate', p.135.

Clinical evidence, mechanism, importance and management

(a) Atovaquone

Atovaquone did not affect the pharmacokinetics of proguanil in a comparative study of 4 patients taking proguanil 200 mg twice daily for 3 days and 12 patients taking proguanil 200 mg twice daily with atovaquone 500 mg twice daily for 3 days.[1] Similar results were seen in 18 healthy subjects given proguanil 400 mg daily with atovaquone 1 g daily for 3 days.[2]

In contrast, in a longer study 13 healthy subjects were given a single 250/100-mg dose of atovaquone/proguanil (*Malarone*) then after an interval of one week they were given daily doses for 13 days. There was no change in the AUC of atovaquone from single dose to steady state, indicating that accumulation did not occur. However, the AUC of proguanil was modestly increased at steady state, and the AUC of the active metabolite cycloguanil was modestly decreased, in the 9 subjects who were extensive metaboliser phenotypes for the cytochrome P450 isoenzyme CYP2C19 (see 'Genetic factors', (p.4)). It was suggested that atovaquone may have inhibited the production of cycloguanil by CYP3A4. However, since this study had no arm with each drug alone, it is impossible to determine whether these changes in pharmacokinetics were due to an interaction or not.[3]

A pharmacokinetic interaction is not established, and is anyway of little clinical relevance, since the efficacy of the combination product for malaria prophylaxis up to 12 weeks is established. The enhanced activity of the combination may, in part, be due to proguanil lowering the effective concentration at which atovaquone collapses the mitochondrial potential in malaria parasites.[4]

(b) Chloroquine

Following the observation that mouth ulcers appeared to be common in those taking prophylactic antimalarials, an extensive study was undertaken in 628 servicemen in Belize. Of those on proguanil 200 mg daily, 24% developed mouth ulcers, and in those additionally taking chloroquine 150 to 300 mg base weekly 37% developed mouth ulcers. The incidence of diarrhoea was also increased from 63% among those who did not develop ulcers to 83% in those that did develop ulcers (any treatment). The reasons are not understood. The authors of the study suggest that these two drugs should not be given together unnecessarily for prophylaxis against *Plasmodium falciparum*.[5]

1. Edstein MD, Looareesuwan S, Viravan C, Kyle DE. Pharmacokinetics of proguanil in malaria patients treated with proguanil plus atovaquone. *Southeast Asian J Trop Med Public Health* (1996) 27, 216–20.
2. Gillotin C, Mamet JP, Veronese L. Lack of pharmacokinetic interaction between atovaquone and proguanil. *Eur J Clin Pharmacol* (1999) 55, 311–15.
3. Thapar MM, Ashton M, Lindegardh N, Bergqvist Y, Nivelius S, Johansson I, Bjorkman A. Time-dependent pharmacokinetics and drug metabolism of atovaquone plus proguanil (Malarone) when taken as chemoprophylaxis. *Eur J Clin Pharmacol* (2002) 58, 19–27.
4. Srivastava IK, Vaidya AB. A mechanism for the synergistic antimalarial action of atovaquone and proguanil. *Antimicrob Agents Chemother* (1999) 43, 1334–9.
5. Drysdale SF, Phillips-Howard PA, Behrens RH. Proguanil, chloroquine, and mouth ulcers. *Lancet* (1990) 1, 164.

Pyrantel + Piperazine

Piperazine opposes the anthelmintic actions of pyrantel.

Clinical evidence, mechanism, importance and management

Pyrantel acts as an anthelmintic because it depolarises the neuromuscular junctions of some intestinal nematodes causing the worms to contract. This paralyses the worms so that they are dislodged by peristalsis and expelled in the faeces. Piperazine also paralyses nematodes but it does so by causing hyperpolarisation of the neuromuscular junctions. These two pharmacological actions oppose one another, as was shown in two *in vitro* pharmacological studies. Strips of whole *Ascaris lumbricoides,* which contracted when exposed to pyrantel failed to do so when also exposed to piperazine.[1] Parallel electrophysiological studies using *Ascaris* cells confirmed that the depolarisation due to pyrantel (which causes the paralysis) was opposed by piperazine.[1]

In practical terms this means that piperazine does not add to the anthelmintic effect of pyrantel on *Ascaris* as might be expected, but opposes it. For this reason it is usually recommended that concurrent use should be avoided, but direct clinical evidence confirming that combined use is ineffective seems to be lacking. It seems reasonable to extrapolate the results of these studies on *Ascaris lumbricoides* (roundworm) to the other gastrointestinal parasites for which pyrantel is used, i.e. *Enterobius vermicularis* (threadworm or pinworm), *Ancylostoma duodenale*, *Necator americanus* (hookworm) and *Trichostrongylus* spp. However, no one seems to have studied this.

1. Aubry ML, Cowell P, Davey MJ, Shevde S. Aspects of the pharmacology of a new anthelmintic: pyrantel. *Br J Pharmacol* (1970) 38, 332–44.

Pyrimethamine + Artemether

Artemether raises pyrimethamine plasma levels, but this does not appear to cause an increase in adverse effects.

Clinical evidence, mechanism, importance and management

In a three-way single-dose crossover study, 8 healthy subjects were given either artemether 300 mg, pyrimethamine 100 mg or both drugs together. Although there was large inter-individual variation in the pharmacokinetics of pyrimethamine, its maximum plasma levels were significantly raised, by 44%. As there was no corresponding increase in adverse effects the authors suggest that the interaction may be of benefit.[1] More study is warranted to confirm this result.

1. Tan-ariya P, Na-Bangchang K, Ubalee R, Thanavibul A, Thipawangkosol P, Karbwang J. Pharmacokinetic interaction or artemether and pyrimethamine in healthy male Thais. *Southeast Asian J Trop Med Public Health* (1998) 29, 18–23.

Pyrimethamine + Co-trimoxazole or Sulfonamides

Serious pancytopenia and megaloblastic anaemia have been described in patients given pyrimethamine and either co-trimoxazole or other sulfonamides.

Clinical evidence

A woman taking pyrimethamine 50 mg weekly as malaria prophylaxis, developed petechial haemorrhages and widespread bruising within 10 days of starting to take co-trimoxazole (trimethoprim 320 mg with sulfamethoxazole 800 mg) daily for a urinary-tract infection. She was found to have gross megaloblastic changes and pancytopenia in addition to being obviously pale and ill. After withdrawal of the two drugs she responded rapidly to hydroxocobalamin and folic acid, and a change to chloroquine for malaria prophylaxis.[1]

Similar cases have been described in other patients taking pyrimethamine with co-trimoxazole[2-4] or **sulfafurazole** (**sulfisoxazole**),[5] or other sulfonamides.[6]

Mechanism

Uncertain, but a reasonable surmise can be made. Pyrimethamine and trimethoprim are both 2,4 diamino-pyrimidines and both selectively inhibit the actions of the enzyme dihydrofolate reductase, which is concerned with the eventual synthesis of the nucleic acids needed for the production of new cells. The sulfonamides inhibit another part of the same synthetic chain. The adverse reactions seen would seem to reflect a gross depression of the normal folate metabolism caused by the combined actions of both drugs. Megaloblastic anaemia and pancytopenia are among the adverse reactions of pyrimethamine and, more rarely, of co-trimoxazole taken alone. In theory this should not occur but in practice it clearly does so occasionally.

Importance and management

Information seems to be limited to the reports cited, but the interaction appears to be established. Its incidence is unknown. Concurrent use need not be avoided but caution should be used in prescribing the combination, especially in the presence of other drugs or disease states that may predispose to folate deficiency.

1. Fleming AF, Warrell DA, Dickmeiss H. Co-trimoxazole and the blood. *Lancet* (1974) ii, 284–5.
2. Ansdell VE, Wright SG, Hutchinson DBA. Megaloblastic anaæmia associated with combined pyrimethamine and co-trimoxazole administration. *Lancet* (1976) ii, 1257.
3. Malfatti S, Piccini A. Anemia megaloblastica pancitopenica in corso di trattamento con pirimetamina, trimethoprim e sulfametossazolo. *Haematologica* (1976) 61, 349–57.
4. Borgstein A, Tozer RA. Infectious mononucleosis and megaloblastic anaemia associated with Daraprim and Bactrim. *Cent Afr J Med* (1974) 20, 185.
5. Waxman S, Herbert V. Mechanism of pyrimethamine-induced megaloblastosis in human bone marrow. *N Engl J Med* (1969) 280, 1316–19.
6. Weißbach G. Auswirkungen kombinierter Behandlung der kindlichen Toxoplasmose mit Pyrimethamin (Daraprim) und Sulfonamiden auf Blut und Knochenmark. *Z Arztl Fortbild (Berl)* (1965) 59, 10–22.

Pyrimethamine/Sulfadoxine (*Fansidar*) + Iron compounds

Iron compounds possibly delay the eradication of the malaria parasite by pyrimethamine/sulfadoxine (*Fansidar*).

Clinical evidence, mechanism, importance and management

Because malarial infection is associated with anaemia, the effect of iron supplements given with antimalarial treatment was investigated in 222 children under 5 years old who had sought treatment for malaria. The children were divided into 3 groups, and all were given pyrimethamine 12.5 to 25 mg plus sulfadoxine 250 to 500 mg *(Fansidar)* as a single dose. One group then received no **ferrous sulfate**, another was given **ferrous sulfate** weekly and the third group was given **ferrous sulfate** daily. **Ferrous sulfate** was given as a 1.2% solution at a dose of 2 ml/kg. It was found that the iron therapy enhanced the haematological recovery of patients but appeared to prolong their parasitaemia, although the difference was not statistically significant. The authors quote evidence that this trend has been seen elsewhere, and suggest that iron supplements should be delayed until the malarial infection has been cleared, especially as effective treatment of malaria often also treats the anaemia, independent of iron supplementation.[1]

1. Nwanyanwu OC, Ziba C, Kazembe PN, Gamadzi G, Gondwe J, Redd SC. The effect of oral iron therapy during treatment for *Plasmodium falciparum* malaria with sulphadoxine-pyrimethamine on Malawian children under 5 years of age. *Ann Trop Med Parasitol* (1996) 90, 589–95.

Pyrimethamine/Sulfadoxine (*Fansidar*) + Zidovudine

A study in patients with AIDS found that zidovudine 250 mg four times daily did not adversely affect the prevention of toxoplasma encephalitis with *Fansidar* (pyrimethamine/sulfadoxine), one tablet twice weekly for up to 8 months.[1]

1. Eljaschewitsch J, Schürmann D, Pohle HD, Ruf B. Zidovudine does not antagonize Fansidar in preventing toxoplasma encephalitis in HIV infected patients. 7th International Conference on AIDS; Science Challenging AIDS, Florence, Italy, 1991. Abstract W.B.2334.

Quinine + Co-artemether

No clinically significant pharmacokinetic interaction appears to occur between quinine and co-artemether. Prolongation of the QTc interval by quinine may be enhanced by co-artemether.

Clinical evidence, mechanism, importance and management

In a double-blind placebo-controlled study in healthy subjects, co-artemether (**artemether** 80 mg with **lumefantrine** 480 mg) was given to 14 subjects for 6 doses at 0, 8, 24, 36, and 60 hours followed 2 hours after the last dose by intravenous quinine 10 mg/kg (to a maximum of 600 mg) over 2 hours. Other groups of 14 subjects received either co-artemether placebo with quinine, or co-artemether with quinine placebo. The pharmacokinetics of lumefantrine and quinine were unaffected by combined use but the AUC and plasma levels of **artemether** and **dihydroartemisinin** appeared to be lower when co-artemether was given with quinine. However, the levels prior to quinine use in this group were also lower and the reduction in the presence of quinine was not considered clinically significant. The transient prolongation of QTc interval noted with quinine (average and peak increases of 3 and 6 milliseconds respectively) was slightly greater when quinine was given after co-artemether (average and peak increases 7 and 15 milliseconds respectively).[1] Both quinine and artemether are known to prolong the QT interval. In general, it is advised that the concurrent use of drugs that prolong the QT interval should be avoided (see also 'Drugs that prolong the QT interval + Other drugs that prolong the QT interval', p.170). However, the authors of this study considered that the modest increased risk of QTc prolongation was outweighed by the potential benefit of the combined treatment in complicated or multidrug-resistant falciparum malaria.[1] If the combination is used, careful cardiac monitoring is recommended.

1. Lefèvre G, Carpenter P, Souppart C, Schmidli H, Martin JM, Lane A, Ward C, Amakye D. Interaction trial between artemether-lumefantrine (Riamet®) and quinine in healthy subjects. *J Clin Pharmacol* (2002) 42, 1147–58.

Quinine + Miscellaneous

Quinine clearance is reduced by cimetidine, but not ranitidine. Urinary alkalinisers can increase the retention of quinine in man, and antacids can reduce the absorption in *animals*. None of these interactions appears to be of general clinical importance. Doxycycline, colestyramine and isoniazid do not appear to alter the pharmacokinetics of quinine. Tetracycline increased quinine levels and improved efficacy. Rifampicin induces the metabolism of quinine and may result in subtherapeutic quinine levels.

Clinical evidence, mechanism, importance and management

(a) Antacids

Aluminium/magnesium hydroxide gel reduces the absorption of quinine from the gut of *rats* and reduces blood quinine levels by 50 to 70%.[1] The reason appears to be that **aluminium hydroxide** slows gastric emptying, which reduces absorption, and **magnesium hydroxide** also forms an insoluble precipitate with quinine. However, there seem to be no clinical reports of a reduction in the therapeutic effectiveness of quinine due to the concurrent use of antacids.

(b) Colestyramine

Colestyramine 8 g did not alter the pharmacokinetics of quinine 600 mg, given concurrently to 8 healthy subjects. The authors warn that this lack of interaction may have been because only single doses were used, and suggest continuing to separate the administration of the two drugs until a lack of interaction is demonstrated in a multiple dose study.[2]

(c) H_2-blockers

Cimetidine 200 mg three times daily and 400 mg at night for a week reduced the clearance of quinine in 6 healthy subjects by 27% while its half-life was increased by 49%, from 7.6 to 11.3 hours, and the AUC was increased by 42%. Peak levels were unchanged. No interaction was seen when **cimetidine** was replaced by **ranitidine** 150 mg twice daily.[3] The probable reason is that **cimetidine** (a recognised enzyme inhibitor) reduces the metabolism of the quinine by the liver so that it is lost from the body more slowly, whereas **ranitidine** does not. The clinical importance of this is uncertain, but prescribers should be alert for any evidence of quinine toxicity during concurrent use.

(d) Isoniazid

A study in 9 healthy subjects found that the clearance of a single 600-mg dose of quinine sulfate was not significantly affected by pretreatment with isoniazid 300 mg daily for a week.[4]

(e) Rifampicin (Rifampin)

A study in 9 healthy subjects found that the clearance of quinine after a single 600-mg dose of quinine sulfate was increased more than sixfold by pretreatment with rifampicin 600 mg daily for 2 weeks. The elimination half-life of quinine was decreased from about 11 hours to 5.5 hours.[4]

A report describes a patient with myotonia controlled with quinine, whose symptoms worsened within 3 weeks of starting to take rifampicin for the treatment of tuberculosis. Peak quinine levels were found to be low, but rose again when the rifampicin was stopped. Control of the myotonia was regained 6 weeks later.[5]

The effect of adding rifampicin to quinine therapy was investigated in patients with uncomplicated falciparum malaria. They were treated with quinine sulfate 10 mg/kg three times daily either alone (30 patients) or with rifampicin 15 mg/kg daily (29 patients) for 7 days. Peak plasma levels of quinine during monotherapy were attained within 2 days of treatment and remained within the therapeutic range for the 7-day treatment period. Levels of quinine's main metabolite 3-hydroxyquinine followed a similar pattern. In patients treated with quinine and rifampicin, quinine was more extensively metabolised and quinine levels were sharply reduced after the second day of treatment to below therapeutic levels. Acute malaria reduces the metabolic clearance of quinine (by a reduction in hepatic mixed function oxidase activity, mainly by the cytochrome P450 isoenzyme CYP3A4) and recovery is associated with a sharp decline in quinine levels. Rifampicin induces the cytochrome P450 isoenzymes and this probably more than countered their inhibition during acute malaria and resulted in increased metabolism of quinine. Although patients who received rifampicin with quinine had shorter parasite clearance times than those who received quinine alone, suggesting rifampicin may enhance quinine's antimalarial activity, recrudescence rates were 5 times higher suggesting increased resistance. The authors suggest that rifampicin should not be given with quinine for the treatment of malaria. Patients receiving rifampicin who also require quinine for malaria may need increased doses of quinine.[6]

(f) Tetracyclines

The pharmacokinetics of intravenous quinine were found to be unchanged by intravenous **doxycycline** when two groups of 13 patients with acute falciparum malaria were compared,[7] although *in vitro*, **doxycycline** appears to be a potent inhibitor of quinine metabolism.[8] No special precautions would seem to be necessary on concurrent use.

A study in patients with acute falciparum malaria found that quinine levels were about doubled in those treated with quinine 600 mg every 8 hours with **tetracycline** 250 mg every 6 hours compared to those treated with quinine alone. Quinine levels were above the MIC for malaria with the combination but not for quinine alone. Two of 8 patients treated with quinine alone had malaria recrudescence compared with none of 8 patients receiving the combination.[9] *In vitro* **tetracycline** is also a potent inhibitor of quinine metabolism.[8] The authors considered that this pharmacokinetic interaction might be part of the explanation why the combination was more effective.[9]

(g) Urinary alkalinisers and acidifiers

The excretion of unchanged quinine is virtually halved (from 17.4 to 8.9%) if the urine is alkalinised. The reason is that in alkaline urine more of the quinine exists in the non-ionised (lipid soluble) form which is more easily reabsorbed by the kidney tubules.[10] However, there seem to be no reports of adverse effects arising from changes in excretion due to this interaction and no special precautions seem to be necessary.

1. Hurwitz A. The effects of antacids on gastrointestinal drug absorption. II. Effect of sulfadiazine and quinine. *J Pharmacol Exp Ther* (1971) 179, 485–9.
2. Ridtitid W, Wongnawa M, Kleekaew A, Mahatthanatrakul W, Sunbhanich M. Cholestyramine does not significantly decrease the bioavailability of quinine in healthy volunteers. *Asia Pac J Pharmacol* (1998) 13, 123–7.
3. Wanwimolruk S, Sunbhanich M, Pongmarutai M and Patamasucon P. Effects of cimetidine and ranitidine on the pharmacokinetics of quinine. *Br J Clin Pharmacol* (1986) 22, 346–50.
4. Wanwimolruk S, Kang W, Coville PF, Viriyayudhakorn S, Thitiarchakul S. Marked enhancement by rifampicin and lack of effect of isoniazid on the elimination of quinine in man. *Br J Clin Pharmacol* (1995) 40, 87–91.
5. Osborn JE, Pettit MJ, Graham P. Interaction between rifampicin and quinine: case report. *Pharm J* (1989) 243, 704.
6. Pukrittayakamee S, Prakongpan S, Wanwimolruk S, Clemens R, Looareesuwan S, White NJ. Adverse effect of rifampin on quinine efficacy in uncomplicated falciparum malaria. *Antimicrob Agents Chemother* (2003) 47, 1509–13.
7. Couet W, Laroche R, Floch JJ, Istin B, Fourtillan JB, Sauniere JF. Pharmacokinetics of quinine and doxycycline in patients with acute falciparum malaria: a study in Africa. *Ther Drug Monit* (1991) 13, 496–501.
8. Zhao X-J, Ishizaki T. A further interaction study of quinine with clinically important drugs by human liver microsomes: determinations of inhibition constant (K_i) and type of inhibition. *Eur J Drug Metab Pharmacokinet* (1999) 24, 272–8.
9. Karbwang J, Molunto P, Bunnag D, Harinasuta T. Plasma quinine levels in patients with falciparum malaria given alone or in combination with tetracycline with or without primaquine. *Southeast Asian J Trop Med Public Health* (1991) 22, 72–6.
10. Haag HB, Larson PS and Schwartz JJ. The effect of urinary pH on the elimination of quinine in man. *J Pharmacol Exp Ther* (1943) 79, 136–9.

Quinine + Tobacco smoking

Smokers clear quinine from the body much more quickly than non-smokers. The clinical importance of this is as yet uncertain.

Clinical evidence

A comparative study in 10 smokers (averaging 17 cigarettes daily) and 10 non-smokers given a single 600-mg dose of quinine sulphate found that the quinine AUC was reduced by 44%, the clearance was increased by 77% and the half-life was shortened (7.5 vs 12 hours), when compared to the non-smokers.[1]

Mechanism

The reason appears to be that tobacco smoke contains polycyclic aromatic compounds and other substances, which are potent inducers of the liver enzymes that metabolise quinine. As a result the quinine is metabolised and cleared from the body more quickly. It is not yet clear which cytochrome P450 isoenzymes are affected. Smoking induces CYP1A, but the formation of the major metabolite of quinine, 3-hydroxyquinine is catalysed by CYP3A, which suggests that other metabolic pathways of quinine are affected by smoking.[2]

Importance and management

Information seems to be limited but the interaction would appear to be established. These results suggest that heavy smokers may need an increased dosage to control malaria but more study is needed to confirm the clinical importance of this interaction.

1. Wanwimolruk S, Wong SM, Coville PF, Viriyayudhakorn S, Thitiarchakul S. Cigarette smoking enhances the elimination of quinine. *Br J Clin Pharmacol* (1993) 36, 610–14.
2. Wanwimolruk S, Wong S-M, Zhang H, Coville PF, Walker RJ. Metabolism of quinine in man: identification of a major metabolite, and effects of smoking and rifampicin pretreatment. *J Pharm Pharmacol* (1995) 47, 957–63.

Terbinafine + Miscellaneous

The serum levels of terbinafine are reduced by rifampicin. Terbinafine causes a small, usually clinically unimportant fall in ciclosporin serum levels. Two isolated reports describe increases in the serum levels of imipramine and nortriptyline. Terbinafine is reported not interact to a clinically relevant extent with astemizole, cimetidine, midazolam, nifedipine, oral contraceptives, ranitidine, terfenadine, tolbutamide or triazolam.

Clinical evidence, mechanism, importance and management

(a) Antihistamines

In a large scale post-marketing survey of 25,884 patients on terbinafine, over 40% were taking at least one other drug. From amongst this group, an unknown number of patients were taking **astemizole** or **terfenadine**. No adverse interactions were reported.[1] A cross-over study in 26 healthy subjects given terbinafine 250 mg daily or placebo and **terfenadine** 60 mg twice daily for 7 days found that terbinafine reduced the trough levels of terfenadine acid metabolite by about 20% on the last day of concurrent use. Other **terfenadine** acid metabolite pharmacokinetic parameters were not affected. The AUC and peak and trough plasma levels of terbinafine were increased by about 16%, 6.6%, and 22%, respectively after 7 days of concurrent use. Although the incidence of ECG abnormalities was not significantly higher in any group, a significant prolongation of the QT interval (by 10%) was found in those receiving **terfenadine** either alone or with terbinafine. Concurrent use was well-tolerated and it was concluded that terbinafine could safely be given with **terfenadine**.[2]

(b) Benzodiazepines

Terbinafine 250 mg daily for 4 days had no effect on the pharmacokinetics of a single 7.5-mg dose of **midazolam**[3] or a single 250-microgram dose of **triazolam**[4] in 12 healthy subjects. The performance of a number of psychomotor tests was unaffected by concurrent use. No special precautions would seem to be necessary.

(c) Ciclosporin

After taking terbinafine 250 mg daily for 6 to 7 days the mean AUC of a single 300-mg dose of ciclosporin in was decreased by 13% and the maximum blood concentration was reduced by 14% in 20 healthy subjects. It was suggested that as *Sandimmun* was used in the study, inter- and intra-individual variations in ciclosporin absorption caused these differences rather than any drug interaction.[5,6] Another study in 11 patients with kidney, heart or lung transplants found that terbinafine 250 mg daily for 12 weeks caused a small but clinically irrelevant decrease in serum ciclosporin levels.[7] Four renal transplant patients on ciclosporin were given terbinafine 250 mg daily for fungal skin and nail infections. Ciclosporin levels were reduced during concurrent treatment in all patients. However, in 3 of the patients ciclosporin levels remained within the therapeutic range and therefore no dose adjustment was made. One patient required an increase in ciclosporin dose to maintain levels within the therapeutic range, and then a reduction in dose on stopping terbinafine.[8] These studies broadly confirm previous *in vitro* work with human liver microsomal enzymes, which found that terbinafine either does not inhibit ciclosporin metabolism or only causes modest inhibition.[9-11] In general, the changes in the pharmacokinetics of ciclosporin appear to be clinically unimportant. However, patients whose ciclosporin levels are at the lower end of the therapeutic range should be closely monitored if they are given terbinafine.[8]

(d) Ethinylestradiol

An *in vitro* study in human livers found that terbinafine did not alter the pharmacokinetics of ethinylestradiol.[9] However, the makers of terbinafine note that menstrual disturbances have occurred in patients on both oral contraceptives and terbinafine.[12] In a post-marketing survey which included 314 patients taking both oral contraceptives and terbinafine the rate of menstrual disorders was within the rate reported for patients on oral contraceptives alone.[13]

(e) H_2-blockers

Cimetidine 400 mg twice daily for 5 days increased the AUC of a single 250-mg dose of terbinafine in 12 healthy subjects by 34% and reduced its clearance by 30%.[14] The likely reason is that **cimetidine** (a known enzyme inhibitor) reduces the metabolism of the terbinafine by the liver so that it is cleared from the body more slowly. However, it seems that this modest increase in the serum levels of terbinafine is of little or no clinical relevance, because in a large scale post-marketing survey (of patients taking terbinafine) no interactions were reported in patients taking terbinafine with **cimetidine** or **ranitidine** [number unknown].[1] No special precautions would appear to be necessary.

(f) Antidiabetics

On the basis of studies with human liver microsomes,[9] the makers of terbinafine suggest that an interaction with **tolbutamide** is unlikely.[12] This is supported by a large scale post-marketing survey, which identified no interaction in patients taking terbinafine with **tolbutamide** [number unknown].[1] In a 154 patient subgroup of this survey no additional risk was noted due to concurrent oral antidiabetics and terbinafine.[13]

(g) Nifedipine

A study in 12 healthy subjects found no alteration in the pharmacokinetics of nifedipine 30 mg (as *Procardia XL*) when given with terbinafine 250 mg.[15]

(h) Other antifungals

An *in vitro* study designed to assess the efficacy of combination antifungal therapy, found that terbinafine, in combination with **amphotericin B**, **fluconazole** or **itraconazole**, enhanced the activity of the antifungals against *Candida albicans*. The authors conclude that this enhanced activity is likely to be reflected in clinical practice, but this has not yet been assessed and so further investigation is needed.[16]

(i) Rifampicin (Rifampin)

In 12 subjects rifampicin 600 mg daily for 6 days halved the AUC of terbinafine and about doubled its clearance.[14] Rifampicin is a potent enzyme inducer, which increases the metabolism and loss from the body of many drugs. Be alert, therefore, for the need to increase the dosage of terbinafine if rifampicin is given.

(j) Tricyclic antidepressants

A 51-year-old man who had been on lithium carbonate and varying doses of **imipramine** 150 to 200 mg daily for 10 years was additionally started on oral terbinafine 250 mg daily for onychomycosis. About a week later he complained of dizziness, muscle twitching and excessive mouth dryness. His serum **imipramine** levels, measured 5 days later, had risen to 530 nanograms/ml from his usual range of 100 to 200 nanograms/ml. Within 10 days of reducing his daily **imipramine** dose from 200 to 75 mg daily, his serum levels had fallen to 229 nanograms/ml. His liver function was normal.[17] Another isolated report describes a marked increase in the serum levels of **nortriptyline** (about doubled) accompanied by evidence of toxicity (fatigue, vertigo, loss of energy and appetite, and falls) in a 74-year-old man taking **nortriptyline** 125 mg daily within 14 days of starting terbinafine 250 mg daily. His symptoms responded to a dose reduction to 75 mg daily. His serum levels were similarly elevated when he was later re-challenged with terbinafine. His liver function was normal.[18]

This seems to be the first and only report of an adverse terbinafine/tricyclic antidepressant interaction so that there would seem to be little reason for avoiding concurrent use, but be aware of this interaction in the case of an unexpected response to treatment.

1. Hall M, Monka C, Krupp P, O'Sullivan D. Safety of oral terbinafine. Results of a postmarketing surveillance study in 25 884 patients. *Arch Dermatol* (1997) 133, 1213–19.

2. Robbins B, Chang C-T, Cramer JA, Garreffa S, Hafkin B, Hunt TL, Meligeni J. Safe coadministration of terbinafine and terfenadine: a placebo-controlled crossover study of pharmacokinetic and pharmacodynamic interactions in healthy volunteers. *Clin Pharmacol Ther* (1996) 59, 275–83.
3. Ahonen J, Olkkola KT, Neuvonen PJ. Effect of itraconazole and terbinafine on the pharmacokinetics and pharmacodynamics of midazolam in healthy volunteers. *Br J Clin Pharmacol* (1995) 40, 270–2.
4. Varhe A, Olkkola KT, Neuvonen PJ. Fluconazole, but not terbinafine, enhances the effects of triazolam by inhibiting its metabolism. *Br J Clin Pharmacol* (1996) 41, 319–23.
5. Long CC, Hill SA, Thomas RC, Holt DW, Finlay AY. The effect of terbinafine on the pharmacokinetics of cyclosporin in vivo. *Skin Pharmacol* (1992) 5, 200–1.
6. Long CC, Hill SA, Thomas RC, Johnston A, Smith SG, Kendall F, Finlay AY. Effect of terbinafine on the pharmacokinetics of cyclosporin in humans. *J Invest Dermatol* (1994) 102, 740–3.
7. Jensen P, Lehne G, Fauchald P, Simonsen S. Effect of oral terbinafine treatment on cyclosporin pharmacokinetics in organ transplant recipients with dermatophyte nail infection. *Acta Derm Venereol (Stockh)* (1996) 76, 280–1.
8. Lo ACY, Lui S-L, Lo W-K, Chan DTM, Cheng IKP. The interaction of terbinafine and cyclosporine A in renal transplant patients. *Br J Clin Pharmacol* (1997) 43, 340–1.
9. Back DJ, Stevenson P, Tjia JF. Comparative effects of two antimycotic agents, ketoconazole and terbinafine, on the metabolism of tolbutamide, ethinyloestradiol, cyclosporin and ethoxycoumarin by human liver microsomes *in vitro*. *Br J Clin Pharmacol* (1989) 28, 166–70.
10. Shah IA, Whiting PH, Omar G, Ormerod AD, Burke MD. The effects of retinoids and terbinafine on the human hepatic microsomal metabolism of cyclosporin. *Br J Dermatol* (1993) 129, 395–8.
11. Back DJ, Tjia JF, Abel SM. Azoles, allylamines and drug metabolism. *Br J Dermatol* (1992) 126 (Suppl 39), 14–18.
12. Lamisil (Terbinafine). Novartis Pharmaceuticals UK Ltd. UK Summary of product characteristics, December 2004.
13. O'Sullivan DP, Needham CA, Bangs A, Atkin K, Kendall FD. Postmarketing surveillance of oral terbinafine in the UK: report of a large cohort study. *Br J Clin Pharmacol* (1996) 42, 559–65.
14. Jensen JC. Pharmacokinetics of Lamisil® in humans. *J Dermatol Treat* (1990) 1 (Suppl 2), 15–18.
15. Cramer JA, Robbins B, Barbeito R, Bedman TC, Dreisbach A, Meligeni JA. Lamisil®: interaction study with a sustained release nifedipine formulation. *Pharm Res* (1996) 13 (9 Suppl), S436.
16. Barchiesi F, Falconi Di Francesco L, Compagnucci P, Arzeni D, Giacometti A, Scalise G. In-vitro interaction of terbinafine with amphotericin B, fluconazole and itraconazole against clinical isolates of *Candida albicans*. *J Antimicrob Chemother* (1998) 41, 59–65.
17. Teitelbaum ML, Pearson VE. Imipramine toxicity and terbinafine. *Am J Psychiatry* (2001) 158, 2086.
18. van der Kuy P-HM, Hooymans PM, Verkaaik AJB. Nortriptyline intoxication induced by terbinafine. *BMJ* (1998) 316, 441.

7

Antiarrhythmics

This section is concerned with the class I antiarrhythmic agents, which also possess some local anaesthetic properties, and with class III antiarrhythmic agents. The drugs covered in this section are listed in 'Table 7.1', (below). Antiarrhythmic agents that fall into other classes are dealt with under beta-blockers, digitalis glycosides, and calcium channel blockers. Some antiarrhythmics that do not fit into the Vaughan Williams classification are also included in this section (e.g. adenosine). Interactions in which the antiarrhythmic drug is the affecting agent, rather than the drug whose activity is altered, are dealt with elsewhere. Consult the Index for a full listing.

Predicting interactions between two antiarrhythmics

It is difficult to know exactly what is likely to happen if two antiarrhythmics are used together. The hope is always that a combination will work better than just one drug, and many drug trials have confirmed that hope, but sometimes the combinations are unsafe. Predicting unsafe combina-

Table 7.1 Antiarrhythmic agents

Generic names	*Proprietary names*
Adenosine	Adenocard, Adenocor, Adenoject, Adenoscan, Adenyl, Adrekar, Ampecyclal, Atepadene, Atepodin, Euritsin, Krenosin, Krenosine
Ajmaline	Gilurytmal
Amiodarone	Aldarone, Amiobol, Amiobeta, Amiocar, Amiod, Amiodacore, Amiodar, Amiodarex, Amiodura, Amiogamma, Amiohexal, Amiokordin, Amirone, Amyben, Ancoron, Angiodarona, Angoron, Angoten, Angyton, Aratac, Asulblan, Atlansil, Braxan, Cardinorm, Cor Mio, Cordarex, Cordarone, Cordarone X, Cornaron, Coronovo, Diodarone, Escodarone, Eurythmic, Forken, Hexarone, Miocoron, Miodarid, Miodaron, Miodrone, Miotenk, Pacerone, Procor, Ritmocardyl, Rivodarone, Sedacoron, Tachydaron, Trangorex
Aprindine	Fiboran
Bretylium	Bretylate, Bretylol
Cibenzoline (Cifenline)	Cibenol, Cipralan, Exacor
Diprafenone	
Disopyramide	Dicorantil, Dicorynan, Dimodan, Dirytmin, Diso-Duriles, Disomet, Durbis, Isorythm, Norpace, Palpitin-PP, Ritmodan, Ritmoforine, Rythmical, Rythmodan, Rythmodul
Dofetilide	Tikosyn
Encainide	
Flecainide	Almarytm, Apocard, Aristocor, Diondel, Flecaine, Flecatab, Tambocor
Ibutilide	Corvert
Lidocaine (Lignocaine)	Basicaina, Dentaliv, Dentipatch, Dilocaine, Dimecaina, Docaine, Dube, Duo-Trach Kit, Dynexan, Ecocain, Emla, Emlapatch, Endogel Esteril, Esracain, Eutecaina, Gelcain, Gelicain, Gesicain, Gobbicaina, Indican, Larjancaina, Laryng-O-Jet, Licain, LidaMantle, Lident Adrenalina, Lident Andrenor, Lidesthesin, Lidial, Lidocabbott, Lidocadren, Lidocalm, Lidocation, Lidocaton, Lidodan, Lidogel, Lidogeyer, Lido-Hyal, Lidoject, Lidojet, Lidomol, Lidonostrum, Lidosen, Lidospray, Lido Spray, Lidoston, Lidrian, Lignospan, Lignostab-A, Lincaina, Linisol, L-M-X4, Luan, Mesocaine, Muco-Anestyl, Nene Dent, Neo-Lidocaton, Neo-Sinedol, Neo-Xylestesin, Nervocaine, Nurocain, Octocaine, Odontalg, Ortodermina, Pisacaina, Rapidocaine, Regiocaina, Remicaine, Rowo-629, Sedagul, Xilo-Mynol, Xilonibsa, Xylanaest, Xylesine, Xylestesin, Xylocain, Xylocaina, Xylocaine, Xylocitin, Xyloneural, Xylonor, Xylotox
Lorcainide	
Mexiletine	Mexilen, Mexitil, Mexitilen, Myovek, Ritalmex
Moracizine (Moricizine)	Ethmozine
Pirmenol	
Procainamide	Biocoryl, Procamide, Procan, Procanbid, Pronestyl
Propafenone	Arythmol, Asonacor, Cuxafenon, Fenorit, Homopafen, Nistaken, Norfenon, Normorytmin, Profex, Propamerck, Rhythmocor, Ritmocor, Ritmonorm, Rythmex, Rythmol, Rythmonopm, Rytmogenat, Rytmonorm, Rytmonorma, Rytmo-Puren
Quinidine	Biquin, Cardioquin, Chinteina, Chordichin, Kinidin, Kinidine, Kinidine Durules, Kiniduron, Longachin, Longacor, Naticardina, Natisedina, Quini, Quinicardine, Quinidex, Quiniduran, Quinimax, Ritmocor, Ydroquinidine, Ydroquinidine Cooper
Tocainide	Xylotocan

tions is difficult, but there are some very broad general rules that can be applied if the general pharmacology of the drugs is understood.

If drugs with similar effects are used together, whether they act on the myocardium itself or on the conducting tissues, the total effect is likely to be increased (additive). The classification of the antiarrhythmics in 'Table 7.2', (below) helps to predict what is likely to happen, but remember that the classification is not rigid so drugs in one class can share some characteristics with others. Here are some examples:

(a) Combinations of antiarrhythmics from the same class

The drugs in class Ia can prolong the QT interval so combining drugs from this class would be expected to show an increased effect on the QT interval. This prolongation carries the risk of causing torsade de pointes arrhythmias (see the monograph, 'Drugs that prolong the QT interval + Other drugs that prolong the QT interval', p.170). It would also be expected that the negative inotropic effects of quinidine would be additive with procainamide or any of the other drugs within Class Ia. For safety therefore it is sometimes considered best to avoid drugs that fall into the same subclass or only to use them together with caution.

(b) Combinations of antiarrhythmics from different classes

Class III antiarrhythmics such as amiodarone can also prolong the QT interval, so they would also be expected to interact with drugs in other classes that do the same, namely class Ia drugs (see 'Drugs that prolong the QT interval + Other drugs that prolong the QT interval', p.170). Verapamil comes into class IV and has negative inotropic effects, so it can interact with other drugs with similar effects, such as the beta-blockers, which fall into class III. For safety you should always look at the whole drug profile and take care with any two drugs, from any class, that share a common pharmacological action.

Table 7.2 Modified Vaughan Williams classification of the oral antiarrhythmic drugs

Class I: Membrane stabilising drugs
(a) Quinidine, Procainamide, Disopyramide, Tiracizine
(b) Lidocaine (Lignocaine), Mexiletine, Tocainide, Phenytoin
(c) Diprafenone, Encainide, Flecainide, Propafenone
Difficult to classify – Moracizine
Class II: Beta-blockers
Propranolol, Atenolol
Class III: Inhibitors of depolarisation
Amiodarone, Bretylium, Dofetilide, Ibutilide, Sotalol
Class IV: Calcium channel blockers
Verapamil, Diltiazem

Adenosine + Dipyridamole

Dipyridamole markedly reduces the bolus dose of adenosine necessary to convert supraventricular tachycardia to sinus rhythm (by about fourfold). Profound bradycardia occurred in one patient on dipyridamole given adenosine infusion for myocardial stress testing.

Clinical evidence

(a) Adenosine bolus for supraventricular tachycardia

Adenosine by rapid intravenous bolus (10 to 200 micrograms/kg in stepwise doses) was found to restore sinus rhythm in 10 of 14 episodes of tachycardia in 7 patients with supraventricular tachycardia (SVT). The mean dose was 8.8 mg compared with only 1 mg in two patients also taking oral dipyridamole.[1] Another study in 6 patients found that dipyridamole (560 microgram/kg intravenous bolus, followed by a continuous infusion of 5 micrograms/kg/minute) reduced the minimum effective bolus dose of intravenous adenosine required to stop the SVT from 68 to 17 micrograms/kg in 5 patients. In the other patient, dipyridamole alone stopped the SVT.[2]

Other studies in healthy subjects have clearly shown that dipyridamole reduced the dose of adenosine required to produce an equivalent cardiovascular effect by fourfold[3] or six- to sixteenfold.[4] A brief report describes a woman on dipyridamole (dosage not stated) with paroxysmal SVT who lost ventricular activity for 18 seconds when given adenosine 6 mg intravenously.[5] Another report describes 3 of 4 patients who had heart block of 3, 9 and 21-second duration respectively when given adenosine 3 to 6 mg by central venous bolus. The patient with the most profound heart block was also being treated with dipyridamole, which was thought to have contributed to the reaction.[6]

(b) Adenosine infusion for myocardial stress testing

A 79-year-old woman on a combination of low-dose aspirin and extended-release dipyridamole *(Aggrenox)* became profoundly bradycardic (36 bpm), dizzy and almost fainted 2 minutes after the start of an adenosine infusion for radionuclide myocardial imaging. Adenosine was stopped, and she recovered within 2 minutes. The last dose of *Aggrenox* had been taken 12 hours previously.[7] However, note that bradycardia is a rare adverse effect of adenosine.[8,9]

Mechanism

Not fully understood. Part of the explanation is that dipyridamole increases plasma levels of endogenous adenosine by inhibiting its uptake into cells.[2,4,10]

Importance and management

An established interaction.

(a) Patients will need much less adenosine to treat arrhythmias while taking dipyridamole. Initial dosage reductions of adenosine of twofold[5] or fourfold[2] have been suggested. The UK makers actually advise the avoidance of adenosine in patients on dipyridamole. If it must be used for supraventricular tachycardia in a patient on dipyridamole, they recommend that the adenosine dose should be reduced about fourfold.[8]

(b) The UK makers advise the avoidance of adenosine in patients on dipyridamole. If adenosine is considered necessary for myocardial imaging in a patient on dipyridamole, they suggest that the dipyridamole should be stopped 24 hours before, or the dose of adenosine should be greatly reduced.[9] This may be insufficient for extended-release dipyridamole preparations—the authors of the above report recommend several days.[7] Xanthines, such as intravenous aminophylline, may be used to terminate persistent adverse effects of adenosine infusion given for myocardial imaging.[9] Consider also 'Adenosine + Xanthines', below.

1. Watt AH, Bernard MS, Webster J, Passani SL, Stephens MR, Routledge PA. Intravenous adenosine in the treatment of supraventricular tachycardia: a dose-ranging study and interaction with dipyridamole. *Br J Clin Pharmacol* (1986) 21, 227–30.
2. Lerman BB, Wesley RC, Belardinelli L. Electrophysiologic effects of dipyridamole on atrioventricular nodal conduction and supraventricular tachycardia. Role of endogenous adenosine. *Circulation* (1989) 80, 1536–43.
3. Biaggioni I, Onrot J, Hollister AS, Robertson D. Cardiovascular effects of adenosine infusion in man and their modulation by dipyridamole. *Life Sci* (1986) 39, 2229–36.
4. Conradson T-BG, Dixon CMS, Clarke B, Barnes PJ. Cardiovascular effects of infused adenosine in man: potentiation by dipyridamole. *Acta Physiol Scand* (1987) 129, 387–91.
5. Mader TJ. Adenosine: adverse interactions. *Ann Emerg Med* (1992) 21, 453.
6. McCollam PL, Uber WE, Van Bakel AB. Adenosine-related ventricular asystole. *Ann Intern Med* (1993) 118, 315–16.
7. Littmann L, Anderson JD, Monroe MH. Adenosine and Aggrenox: a hazardous combination. *Ann Intern Med* (2002) 137, W1.
8. Adenocor (Adenosine). Sanofi Synthelabo. UK Summary of product characteristics, March 2004.
9. Adenoscan (Adenosine). Sanofi Synthelabo. UK Summary of product characteristics, February 2003.
10. German DC, Kredich NM, Bjornsson TD. Oral dipyridamole increases plasma adenosine levels in human beings. *Clin Pharmacol Ther* (1989) 45, 80–4.

Adenosine + Nicotine

Nicotine appears to enhance the effects of adenosine, but the clinical relevance of this is unclear.

Clinical evidence, mechanism, importance and management

Nicotine chewing gum 2 mg (approximately equal to 1 cigarette) increased the circulatory effects of a 70 microgram/kg/minute adenosine infusion in 10 healthy subjects. The increase in heart rate due to nicotine (5.5 bpm) was further increased to 14.9 bpm by the adenosine. The diastolic blood pressure rise due to nicotine (7 mmHg) was reduced to 1.1 mmHg by the adenosine.[1] In another study, nicotine chewing gum 2 mg increased chest pain and the duration of AV block when given with intravenous bolus doses of adenosine in 7 healthy subjects.[2] What this means in practical terms is uncertain, but be aware that the effects of adenosine may be modified to some extent by nicotine-containing products (**tobacco smoking**, **nicotine gum**, etc).

1. Smits P, Eijsbouts A, Thien T. Nicotine enhances the circulatory effects of adenosine in human beings. *Clin Pharmacol Ther* (1989) 46, 272–8.
2. Sylvén C, Beerman B, Kaijser L, Jonzon B. Nicotine enhances angina pectoris-like chest pain and atrioventricular blockade provoked by intravenous bolus of adenosine in healthy volunteers. *J Cardiovasc Pharmacol* (1990) 16, 962–5.

Adenosine + Xanthines

Caffeine and theophylline can inhibit the effects of adenosine infusions used in conjunction with radionuclide myocardial imaging. Xanthines should be withheld 12 to 24 hours prior to the procedure or they will interfere with test results. Aminophylline has been used to terminate persistent adverse effects of adenosine infusions. Adenosine may still be effective for terminating supraventricular tachycardia in patients on xanthines.

Clinical evidence

(a) Adenosine bolus for supraventricular tachycardia

It is usually considered that adenosine bolus for the termination of paroxysmal supraventricular tachycardia will be ineffective in patients on xanthines. However, one case describes a man on **theophylline** (serum level 8 nanograms/ml) in whom adenosine 9 mg terminated supraventricular tachycardia. Two previous adenosine doses, one of 3 mg and one of 6 mg had not been effective.[1] Another report found that higher adenosine doses (400 to 800 micrograms/kg; usual dose 50 to 200 micrograms/kg) were required to revert supraventricular tachycardia in a preterm infant on **theophylline**.[2]

(b) Adenosine infusion

Experimental studies in healthy subjects, on the way xanthine drugs possibly interact with adenosine, have shown that **caffeine** and **theophylline** (but not **enprofylline**) reduced the increased heart rate and the changes in blood pressure caused by infusions of adenosine,[3-6] and attenuated adenosine-induced vasodilatation.[7,8] **Theophylline** also attenuated adenosine-induced respiratory effects and chest pain.[5,6] Similarly, an adenosine infusion antagonised the haemodynamic effects of a single-dose of **theophylline** in healthy subjects, but did not reduce the metabolic effects (reductions in plasma potassium and magnesium).[5]

Mechanism

Caffeine and theophylline have an antagonistic effect on adenosine receptors.[9] They appear to have opposite effects on the circulatory system: caffeine and theophylline cause vasoconstriction whereas adenosine infusion generally causes vasodilatation.[3] Consequently their concurrent use is likely to result in an interaction.

Importance and management

(a) Adenosine bolus injection for the termination of paroxysmal supraventricular tachycardia may still be effective in patients on xanthines. The usual dose schedule should be followed. However, note that adenosine has induced bronchospasm. The US makers[10,11] state that adenosine preparations, whether used for supraventricular tachycardia or myocardial imaging, should be avoided in patients with asthma, and used cautiously in those with obstructive pulmonary disease. The UK makers give similar recommendations for the product used for supraventricular tachycardia[12] but are more cautious for diagnostic imaging[13] and contraindicate the use of adenosine in both asthma and obstructive pulmonary disease. Whether adenosine bolus can stop theophylline-induced supraventricular tachycardia appears not to have been studied.

(b) The makers of adenosine state that theophylline, aminophylline and other xanthines should be avoided for 24 hours before using an adenosine infusion for radionuclide myocardial imaging, and that xanthine-containing drinks (tea, coffee, chocolate, '*Coke*' etc.) should be avoided for at least 12 hours before imaging.[13] In a recent study in 70 patients, measurable caffeine serum levels were found in 74% of patients after 12 hours of self-reported abstention from caffeine-containing products. Patients with caffeine serum levels of at least 2.9 mg/l had significantly fewer stress symptoms (chest tightness, chest pain, headache, dyspnoea, nausea, dizziness) than those with lower serum levels. The authors suggest that a 12-hour abstention from caffeine-containing products may be insufficient, and could result in false-negative results.[14] Xanthines, such as intravenous aminophylline, may be used to terminate persistent adverse effects of adenosine infusion given for myocardial imaging.[13]

1. Giagounidis AAN, Schäfer S, Klein RM, Aul C, Strauer BE. Adenosine is worth trying in patients with paroxysmal supraventricular tachycardia on chronic theophylline medication. *Eur J Med Res* (1998) 3, 380–2.
2. Berul CI. Higher adenosine dosage required for supraventricular tachycardia in infants treated with theophylline. *Clin Pediatr (Phila)* (1993) 32, 167–8.
3. Smits P, Schouten J, Thien T. Cardiovascular effects of two xanthines and the relation to adenosine antagonism. *Clin Pharmacol Ther* (1989) 45, 593–9.
4. Smits P, Boekema P, De Abreu R, Thien T, van 't Laar A. Evidence for an antagonism between caffeine and adenosine in the human cardiovascular system. *J Cardiovasc Pharmacol* (1987) 10, 136–43.
5. Minton NA, Henry JA. Pharmacodynamic interactions between infused adenosine and oral theophylline. *Hum Exp Toxicol* (1991) 10, 411–18.
6. Maxwell DL, Fuller RW, Conradson T-B, Dixon CMS, Aber V, Hughes JMB, Barnes PJ. Contrasting effects of two xanthines, theophylline and enprofylline, on the cardio-respiratory stimulation of infused adenosine in man. *Acta Physiol Scand* (1987) 131, 459–65.
7. Taddei S, Pedrinelli R, Salvetti A. Theophylline is an antagonist of adenosine in human forearm arterioles. *Am J Hypertens* (1991) 4, 256–9.
8. Smits P, Lenders JWM, Thien T. Caffeine and theophylline attenuate adenosine-induced vasodilation in humans. *Clin Pharmacol Ther* (1990) 48, 410–18.
9. Fredholm BB. On the mechanism of action of theophylline and caffeine. *Acta Med Scand* (1985) 217, 149–53.
10. Adenocard (Adenosine). Fujisawa Healthcare Inc. US Prescribing information, August 2003.
11. Adenoscan (Adenosine). Fujisawa Healthcare Inc. US Prescribing information, September 2000.
12. Adenocor (Adenosine). Sanofi Synthelabo. UK Summary of product characteristics, March 2004.
13. Adenoscan (Adenosine). Sanofi Synthelabo. UK Summary of product characteristics, February 2003.
14. Majd-Ardekani J, Clowes P, Menash-Bonsu V, Nunan TO. Time for abstention from caffeine before an adenosine myocardial perfusion scan. *Nucl Med Commun* (2000) 21, 361–4.

Ajmaline + Miscellaneous

An isolated report describes cardiac failure in a patient given ajmaline and lidocaine. Quinidine causes a very considerable increase in the plasma levels of ajmaline, and phenobarbital appears to cause a marked reduction.

Clinical evidence, mechanism, importance and management

A woman showed marked aggravation of cardiac failure when treated with ajmaline orally and **lidocaine** intravenously for repeated ventricular tachycardias.[1]

A study[2] in 4 healthy subjects found that if a single 200-mg oral dose of **quinidine** was given with a single 50-mg oral dose of ajmaline, the AUC of ajmaline was increased 10- to 30-fold and the maximal plasma concentrations increased from 18 to 141 nanograms/ml. Another single-dose study in 5 healthy subjects found that the metabolism of ajmaline was inhibited by **quinidine**, possibly because the quinidine becomes competitively bound to the enzymes that metabolise ajmaline.[3]

The clearance of intravenous ajmaline was almost twice as high in 3 patients receiving **phenobarbital** when compared with 5 patients who were not. Therefore the clinical effects of ajmaline would be expected to be markedly diminished in those taking phenobarbital.[4]

The clinical importance of all of these interactions is uncertain but concurrent use should be well monitored.

1. Bleifeld W. Side effects of antiarrhythmics. *Naunyn Schmiedebergs Arch Pharmacol* (1971) 269, 282–97.
2. Hori R, Okumura K, Inui K-I, Yasuhara M, Yamada K, Sakurai T, Kawai C. Quinidine-induced rise in ajmaline plasma concentration. *J Pharm Pharmacol* (1984) 36, 202–4.
3. Köppel C, Tenczer J, Arndt I. Metabolic disposition of ajmaline. *Eur J Drug Metab Pharmacokinet* (1989) 14, 309–16.
4. Köppel C, Wagemann A, Martens F. Pharmacokinetics and antiarrhythmic efficacy of intravenous ajmaline in ventricular arrhythmia of acute onset. *Eur J Drug Metab Pharmacokinet* (1989) 14, 161–7.

Amiodarone + Anaesthetics, general

There is some evidence that the presence of amiodarone possibly increases the risk of complications (atropine-resistant bradycardia, hypotension, decreased cardiac output) during general anaesthesia.

Clinical evidence

(a) Evidence for complications

Several case reports[1-3] and two studies[4,5] suggest that severe intra-operative complications (atropine-resistant bradycardia, myocardial depression, hypotension) may occur in patients receiving amiodarone. One of these reports, a comparative retrospective review of patients (16 receiving amiodarone 300 to 800 mg daily and 30 controls) having operations under anaesthesia (mainly open-heart surgery), showed that the incidence of slow nodal rhythm, complete heart block or pacemaker dependency rose from 17% in controls to 66% in amiodarone-treated patients. Intra-aortic balloon pump augmentation (reflecting poor cardiac output) was 50% in the amiodarone group compared with 7% in the control group, and a state of low systemic vascular resistance with normal to high cardiac output occurred in 13% of the amiodarone-treated patients, but none of the controls. Overall there were 3 fatalities; all of these patients had received amiodarone and had been on cardiopulmonary bypass during surgery. **Fentanyl** was used for all of the patients, often combined with **diazepam**, and sometimes also **isoflurane**, **enflurane** or **halothane**.[4] Another study of 37 patients receiving amiodarone (mean dose about 250 mg daily) found no problems in 8 undergoing non-cardiac surgery. Of the 29 undergoing cardiac surgery, 52% had postoperative arrhythmias and 24% required a pacemaker, which was not considered exceptional for the type of surgery. However, one patient having coronary artery bypass surgery had fatal vasoplegia (a hypotensive syndrome), which was considered amiodarone-related. This occurred shortly after he was taken off of cardio-pulmonary bypass. Anaesthesia in all patients was **fentanyl**-based.[5] It was suggested in one case report that serious hypotension in two patients on amiodarone undergoing surgery may have been further compounded by **ACE inhibitor** therapy.[3] For the interactions of ACE inhibitors and anaesthetics see 'Anaesthetics, general + Antihypertensives', p.883.

(b) Evidence for no complications

The preliminary report of one study in 21 patients taking amiodarone (mean dose 538 mg daily) and undergoing defibrillator implantation suggested that haemodynamic changes during surgery were not significantly different from those in matched controls not taking amiodarone.[6] Similarly, another study found no difference in haemodynamic status or pacemaker dependency between patients on short-term amiodarone and a control group during valve replacement surgery with **thiopental-fentanyl** anaesthesia. The amiodarone group received 600 mg daily for 1 week then 400 mg daily for 2 weeks prior to surgery.[7] In a double-blind trial, there was no significant difference in haemodynamic instability during **fentanyl-isoflurane** anaesthesia between patients randomised to receive short-term amiodarone (3.4 g over 5 days or 2.2 g over 24 hours) or placebo before cardiac surgery. In this study, haemodynamic instability was assessed by fluid balance, use of dopamine or other vasopressor agents, and use of a phosphodiesterase inhibitor or intra-aortic balloon pump.[8]

Mechanism

In vitro and *in vivo* studies in *animals* suggest that amiodarone has additive cardiodepressant and vasodilator effects with volatile anaesthetics such as halothane, enflurane and isoflurane.[2,9]

Importance and management

The assessment of this interaction is complicated by the problem of conducting studies in anaesthesia, most being retrospective and using matched controls. The only randomised study used short-term amiodarone to assess its safety if used for prevention of post-operative atrial fibrillation, and its findings may not be relevant to patients on long-term amiodarone therapy.[8] It appears that potentially severe complications may occur in some patients taking amiodarone undergoing general anaesthesia, including bradycardia unresponsive to atropine, hypotension, conduction disturbances, and decreased cardiac output. Anaesthetists should take particular care in patients on amiodarone undergoing surgery on cardiopulmonary bypass.[10] Amiodarone persists in the body for many weeks, which usually means it cannot be withdraw before surgery, especially if there are risks in delaying surgery,[5] or the amiodarone is being used for serious arrhythmias.[10]

1. Gallagher JD, Lieberman RW, Meranze J, Spielman SR, Ellison N. Amiodarone-induced complications during coronary artery surgery. *Anesthesiology* (1981) 55, 186–8.
2. MacKinnon G, Landymore R, Marble A. Should oral amiodarone be used for sustained ventricular tachycardia in patients requiring open-heart surgery? *Can J Surg* (1983) 26, 355–7.
3. Mackay JH, Walker IA, Bethune DW. Amiodarone and anaesthesia: concurrent therapy with ACE inhibitors—an additional cause for concern? *Can J Anaesth* (1991) 38, 687.
4. Liberman BA, Teasdale SJ. Anaesthesia and amiodarone. *Can Anaesth Soc J* (1985) 32, 629–38.
5. Van Dyck M, Baele P, Rennotte MT, Matta A, Dion R, Kestens-Servaye Y. Should amiodarone be discontinued before cardiac surgery? *Acta Anaesthesiol Belg* (1988) 39, 3–10.
6. Elliott PL, Schauble JF, Rogers MC, Reid PR. Risk of decompensation during anesthesia in presence of amiodarone. *Circulation* (1983) 68 (Suppl 3), 280.
7. Chassard D, George M, Guiraud M, Lehot JJ, Bastien O, Hercule C, Villard J, Estanove S. Relationship between preoperative amiodarone treatment and complications observed during anaesthesia for valvular cardiac surgery. *Can J Anaesth* (1990) 37, 251–4.
8. White CM, Dunn A, Tsikouris J, Waberski W, Felton K, Freeman-Bosco L, Giri S, Kluger J. An assessment of the safety of short-term amiodarone therapy in cardiac surgical patients with fentanyl-isoflurane anesthesia. *Anesth Analg* (1999) 89, 585–9.
9. Rooney RT, Marijic J, Stommel KA, Bosnjak ZJ, Aggarwai A, Kampine JP, Stowe DF. Additive cardiac depression by volatile anesthetics in isolated hearts after chronic amiodarone treatment. *Anesth Analg* (1995) 80, 917–24.
10. Teasdale S, Downar E. Amiodarone and anaesthesia. *Can J Anaesth* (1990) 37, 151–5.

Amiodarone + Beta-blockers

Hypotension, bradycardia, ventricular fibrillation and asystole have been seen in a few patients given amiodarone with propranolol, metoprolol or sotalol (for sotalol, see also 'Drugs that prolong the QT interval + Other drugs that prolong the QT interval', p.170). However, analysis of clinical trials suggests that the combination can be beneficial.

Clinical evidence

A 64-year-old woman was treated for hypertrophic cardiomyopathy with amiodarone 1200 mg daily and **atenolol** 50 mg daily. Five days later the **atenolol** was replaced by **metoprolol** 100 mg daily. Within 3 hours she complained of dizziness, weakness and blurred vision. On examination she was found to be pale and sweating with a pulse rate of 20 bpm. Her systolic blood pressure was 60 mmHg. Atropine 2 mg did not produce chronotropic or haemodynamic improvement. She responded to isoprenaline (isoproterenol).[1] Severe hypotension has been reported in another patient on **sotalol** when given intravenous amiodarone (total dose 250 mg).[2] Another report describes cardiac arrest in one patient on amiodarone, and severe bradycardia and ventricular fibrillation (requiring defibrillation) in another, within 1.5 and 2 hours of starting to take **propranolol**.[3]

In contrast to the above case reports, an analysis of data from two large clinical trials of the use of amiodarone for post-myocardial infarction arrhythmias found that the combination of beta-blockers (unnamed) and amiodarone was beneficial (reduced cardiac deaths, arrhythmic deaths and resuscitated cardiac arrest) compared with either drug alone, or neither drug.[4] Similarly, in the analysis of another trial in ischaemic heart failure, the benefits of the beta-blocker **carvedilol** were still apparent in those patients already receiving amiodarone, and the combination was not associated with a greater incidence of adverse effects (worsened heart failure, hypotension/dizziness, bradycardia/atrioventricular block) than either drug alone.[5]

Mechanism

Not understood. The clinical picture is that of excessive beta-blockade, and additive pharmacodynamic effects are possible. The time course of the interaction makes it unlikely that amiodarone affected the hepatic metabolism of propranolol and metoprolol, although a pharmacokinetic interaction based on altered volume of distribution (due to protein binding changes) has been suggested.[1] Increased bradycardia and other ECG changes have been seen with amiodarone and practolol.[6]

Importance and management

The isolated reports of adverse reactions cited here (they seem to be the only ones so far documented) emphasise the need for caution when amiodarone is used with beta-blockers. The makers of amiodarone recommend that the combination should not be used[7] or used with caution[8] because potentiation of negative chronotropic properties and conduction slowing effects may occur. However, the concurrent use of beta-blockers and amiodarone is not uncommon and may be therapeutically useful. The authors of one of the analyses suggest that post-myocardial infarction, if possible, beta-blockers should be continued in patients for whom amiodarone is indicated.[4] See also 'Drugs that prolong the QT interval + Other drugs that prolong the QT interval', p.170, which deals with the possible risks of using amiodarone and sotalol.

1. Leor J, Levartowsky D, Sharon C, Farfel Z. Amiodarone and β-adrenergic blockers: an interaction with metoprolol but not with atenolol. *Am Heart J* (1988) 116, 206–7.
2. Warren R, Vohra J, Hunt D, Hamer A. Serious interactions of sotalol with amiodarone and flecainide. *Med J Aust* (1990) 152, 277.
3. Derrida JP, Ollagnier J, Benaim R, Haiat R, Chiche P. Amiodarone et propranolol; une association dangereuse? *Nouv Presse Med* (1979) 8, 1429.
4. Boutitie F, Boissel J-P, Connolly SJ, Camm AJ, Cairns JA, Julian DG, Gent M, Janse MJ, Dorian P, Frangin G. Amiodarone interaction with β-blockers: analysis of the merged EMIAT (European Myocardial Infarct Amiodarone Trial) and CAMIAT (Canadian Amiodarone Myocardial Infarction Trial) databases. *Circulation* (1999) 99, 2268–75.
5. Krum H, Shusterman N, MacMahon S, Sharpe N. Efficacy and safety of carvedilol in patients with chronic heart failure receiving concomitant amiodarone therapy. *J Card Fail* (1998) 4, 281–8.
6. Antonelli G, Cristallo E, Cesario S, Calabrese P. Modificazioni elettrocardiografiche indotte dalla somministrazione di amiodarone associato a practololo. *Boll Soc Ital Cardiol* (1973) 18, 236–42.
7. Cordarone X (Amiodarone hydrochloride). Sanofi Synthelabo. UK Summary of product characteristics, May 2004.
8. Cordarone (Amiodarone hydrochloride). Wyeth Laboratories. US Prescribing information, April 2004.

Amiodarone + Calcium channel blockers

Increased cardiac depressant effects would be expected if amiodarone is used with diltiazem or verapamil. One case of sinus arrest and serious hypotension has been reported in a woman on diltiazem when given amiodarone.

Clinical evidence, mechanism, importance and management

A woman with compensated congestive heart failure, paroxysmal atrial fibrillation and ventricular arrhythmias was treated with furosemide and **diltiazem** 90 mg six-hourly. Four days after starting additional treatment with amiodarone, 600 mg 12-hourly, she developed sinus arrest and a life-threatening low cardiac output state (systolic blood pressure 80 mmHg) with oliguria. **Diltiazem** and amiodarone were stopped and she was treated with pressor drugs and ventricular pacing. She had previously had no problems on **diltiazem** or **verapamil** alone, and later she did well on amiodarone 400 mg daily without **diltiazem.** The reason for this reaction is thought to be the additive effects of both drugs on myocardial contractility, and on sinus and atrioventricular nodal function.[1] Before this isolated case report was published, another author predicted this interaction with **diltiazem** or **verapamil** on theoretical grounds and warned of the risks if dysfunction of the sinus node, such as bradycardia or sick sinus syndrome is suspected, or if partial AV block exists.[2] The makers state that amiodarone should not be used[3] or used with caution[4] with certain calcium channel blockers (**diltiazem**, **verapamil**) because potentiation of negative chronotropic properties and conduction slowing effects may occur. Note that **diltiazem** has been used for rate control in patients developing postoperative atrial fibrillation despite the use of prophylactic amiodarone.[5] There do not appear to be any reports of adverse effects attributed to the use of amiodarone with the dihydropyridine class of calcium channel blockers (e.g. **nifedipine**), which typically have little or no negative inotropic activity at usual doses.

1. Lee TH, Friedman PL, Goldman L, Stone PH, Antman EM. Sinus arrest and hypotension with combined amiodarone-diltiazem therapy. *Am Heart J* (1985) 109, 163–4.
2. Marcus FI. Drug interactions with amiodarone. *Am Heart J* (1983) 106, 924–30.
3. Cordarone X (Amiodarone hydrochloride). Sanofi Synthelabo. UK Summary of product characteristics, May 2004.
4. Cordarone (Amiodarone hydrochloride). Wyeth Laboratories. US Prescribing information, April 2004.
5. Kim MH, Rachwal W, McHale C, Bruckman D, Decena BF, Russman P, Morady F, Eagle KA. Effect of amiodarone ± diltiazem ± beta blocker on frequency of atrial fibrillation, length of hospitalization, and hospital costs after coronary artery bypass grafting. *Am J Cardiol* (2002) 89, 1126–28.

Amiodarone + Cimetidine

Cimetidine possibly causes a modest rise in the serum levels of amiodarone in some patients.

Clinical evidence, mechanism, importance and management

The preliminary report of one study notes that the mean amiodarone serum levels of 12 patients on long-term treatment 200 mg twice daily rose by an average of 38%, from 1.4 to 1.93 micrograms/ml, when given cimetidine 1200 mg daily for a week. The desethyl-amiodarone levels rose by 54%. However, these increases were not statistically significant, and only 8 of the 12 patients showed any rise.[1] It is possible that cimetidine may inhibit the metabolism of amiodarone. Information seems to be limited to this study but this interaction may be clinically important in some patients. Monitor the effects when cimetidine is started, being alert for amiodarone adverse effects. Remember that amiodarone is lost from the body very slowly (half-life 25 to 100 days) so that the results of the one-week study cited here may possibly not adequately reflect the magnitude of this interaction. There does not appear to have been anything further published on this.

1. Hogan C, Landau S, Tepper D and Somberg J. Cimetidine-amiodarone interaction. *J Clin Pharmacol* (1988) 28, 909.

Amiodarone + Colestyramine

Colestyramine appears to reduce the serum levels of amiodarone.

Clinical evidence

When four doses of colestyramine 4 g were given to 11 patients at 1-hour intervals starting 1.5 hours after a single 400-mg dose of amiodarone, the serum amiodarone levels 7.5 hours later were reduced by about 50%.[1] In a further study, the amiodarone half-life was shorter (23.5, 29 and 32 days) in 3 patients given colestyramine 4 g daily after discontinuing long-term amiodarone compared with that in 8 patients discontinuing amiodarone and not given colestyramine (35 to 58 days).[1]

Mechanism

This interaction probably occurs because colestyramine binds with amiodarone in the gut, thereby reducing its absorption, and it may also affect the enterohepatic recirculation of amiodarone.[1] This is consistent with the way colestyramine interacts with other drugs.

Importance and management

Information is very limited but a reduced response to amiodarone may be expected. Separating the dosages to avoid admixture in the gut would reduce or prevent any effects on absorption from the gut, but not the effects due to reduced enterohepatic recirculation. Monitor the effects closely and consider an alternative to colestyramine, or raise the amiodarone dosage if necessary.

1. Nitsch J, Lüderitz B. Beschleunigte elimination von Amiodaron durch Colestyramin. *Dtsch Med Wochenschr* (1986) 111, 1241–4.

Amiodarone + Disopyramide

The risk of QT interval prolongation and torsade de pointes is increased if amiodarone is used with disopyramide.

Clinical evidence

A brief report describes 2 patients who developed torsade de pointes during the concurrent use of amiodarone and disopyramide. Their QT intervals became markedly prolonged to somewhere between 500 and 600 milliseconds.[1] In another study, 2 patients who had been taking disopyramide 300 mg daily for a number of months developed prolonged QT intervals of 640 and 680 milliseconds (increased from 450 and 390 milliseconds respectively) and torsade de pointes 2 and 5 days respectively after starting amiodarone 800 mg daily.[2]

Mechanism

Amiodarone is a class III antiarrhythmic and can prolong the QT interval. Disopyramide is in class Ia and also prolongs the QT interval. Their additive effects can result in the development of torsade de pointes arrhythmias.

Importance and management

An established and potentially serious interaction. In general, class Ia antiarrhythmics such as disopyramide (see 'Table 7.2', (p.157)) should be avoided or used with great caution with amiodarone because of their additive effects in delaying conduction. The makers of amiodarone contraindicate[3] or urge caution[4] with its use with class Ia antiarrhythmics. However, one early report also described the successful and apparently safe use of amiodarone 100 to 600 mg daily with disopyramide 300 to 500 mg daily,[5] although the results on long-term follow-up were not reported in all cases. See also 'Drugs that prolong the QT interval + Other drugs that prolong the QT interval', p.170, and for the interactions of other class Ia antiarrhythmics see 'Procainamide + Amiodarone', p.182, and 'Quinidine + Amiodarone', p.187.

1. Tartini R, Kappenberger L, Steinbrunn W. Gefährliche Interaktionen zwischen Amiodaron und Antiarrhythmika der Klass I. *Schweiz Med Wochenschr* (1982) 112, 1585–7.
2. Keren A, Tzivoni D, Gavish D, Levi J, Gottlieb S, Benhorin J, Stern S. Etiology, warning signs and therapy of Torsade de Pointes. *Circulation* (1981) 64, 1167–74.
3. Cordarone X (Amiodarone hydrochloride). Sanofi Synthelabo. UK Summary of product characteristics, May 2004.
4. Cordarone (Amiodarone hydrochloride). Wyeth Laboratories. US Prescribing information, April 2004.
5. James MA, Papouchado M, Vann Jonec J. Combined therapy with disopyramide and amiodarone: a report of 11 cases. *Int J Cardiol* (1986) 13, 248–52.

Amiodarone + Grapefruit juice

Grapefruit juice inhibits the metabolism of amiodarone.

Clinical evidence, mechanism, importance and management

Eleven healthy subjects were given a single 17-mg/kg dose of amiodarone on two occasions, once with water and once with grapefruit juice (300 ml taken three times on the same day). Grapefruit juice completely inhibited the metabolism of amiodarone to its major metabolite *N*-desethylamiodarone (N-DEA) and increased the amiodarone AUC by 50% and the peak serum level by 84%. The effect of amiodarone on the PR and QTc intervals was *decreased*.[1] Grapefruit juice inhibits cytochrome P450 isoenzyme CYP3A4, thus inhibiting the formation of N-DEA.

This interaction appears to be established, but its clinical consequences remain to be determined. N-DEA is known to be active, so this could possibly result in decreased activity.[1] In addition, high amiodarone concentrations may increase toxicity.[1] Conversely, a reduction in QT prolongation is potentially beneficial.[1] Further study is needed. In the meantime, it may be prudent to suggest to patients that they avoid grapefruit juice.

1. Libersa CC, Brique SA, Motte KB, Caron JF, Guédon-Moreau LM, Humbert L, Vincent A, Devos P, Lhermitte MA. Dramatic inhibition of amiodarone metabolism induced by grapefruit juice. *Br J Clin Pharmacol* (2000) 49, 373–8.

Amiodarone + Lithium

Hypothyroidism developed very rapidly in two patients on amiodarone when lithium was added.

Clinical evidence, mechanism, importance and management

A patient on amiodarone 400 mg daily for more than a year developed acute manic depression. He was started on 600 mg of lithium (salt unknown) daily, but within 2 weeks he developed clinical signs of hypothyroidism, which was confirmed by clinical tests. He made a complete recovery within 3 weeks of stopping the amiodarone while continuing the lithium.[1] Similarly, another patient on amiodarone rapidly developed hypothyroidism when additionally given lithium (dose and salt unknown), which resolved when the amiodarone was stopped.[1] Both lithium and amiodarone on their own can cause hypothyroidism, (Note that amiodarone can also cause hyperthyroidism). In these two cases the effects appear to have been additive, and very rapid.

These two cases appear to be the first and only reports of this interaction. Its general importance is therefore still uncertain, but it would be prudent to be extra vigilant for any signs of hypothyroidism (lethargy, weakness, depression, weight gain, hoarseness) in any patient when given both drugs.

More study is needed. Note that lithium has been tried for the treatment of amiodarone-induced hyperthyroidism,[2] and regular monitoring of thyroid status is recommended throughout amiodarone treatment.[3,4]

Lithium therapy has rarely been associated with cardiac QT prolongation, and consequently the UK maker of amiodarone contraindicates its combined use.[3] See also 'Drugs that prolong the QT interval + Other drugs that prolong the QT interval', p.170.

1. Ahmad S. Sudden hypothyroidism and amiodarone-lithium combination: an interaction. *Cardiovasc Drugs Ther* (1995) 9, 827–8.
2. Dickstein G, Shechner C, Adawi F, Kaplan J, Baron E, Ish-Shalom S. Lithium treatment in amiodarone-induced thyrotoxicosis. *Am J Med* (1997) 102, 454–8.
3. Cordarone X (Amiodarone hydrochloride). Sanofi Synthelabo. UK Summary of product characteristics, May 2004.
4. Cordarone (Amiodarone hydrochloride). Wyeth Laboratories. US Prescribing information, April 2004.

Amiodarone + Macrolides

Torsade de pointes occurred in a man on amiodarone when given intravenous erythromycin. QT prolongation occurred in another patient when azithromycin was added to established amiodarone therapy.

Clinical evidence, mechanism, importance and management

A 76-year-old man on amiodarone 200 mg daily had a prolonged QT interval and a syncopal episode with torsade de pointes 24 hours after starting a course of intravenous **erythromycin lactobionate**. This occurred on rechallenge.[1] Marked QT prolongation and increased QT dispersion occurred when **azithromycin** was started in a patient on long-term amiodarone therapy, and resolved when it was stopped.[2]

Amiodarone alone is well known to be able to prolong the QT interval and increase the risk of torsade de pointes. Of the macrolides, *intravenous* **erythromycin** is known to prolong the QT interval, and there is also some evidence that **clarithromycin** may prolong the QT interval.[3] Amiodarone and these macrolides may therefore have additive effects on the QT interval.

In general the concurrent use of two or more drugs that prolong the QT interval should be avoided, because this increases the risk of torsade de pointes arrhythmias (see also 'Drugs that prolong the QT interval + Other drugs that prolong the QT interval', p.170). For this reason, the UK maker of amiodarone contraindicates the concurrent use of *intravenous* **erythromycin**.[4] The authors of the above report suggest that the combination of **azithromycin** and amiodarone should be used with caution,[2] and this should probably also apply to **clarithromycin** until more is known.

1. Nattel S, Ranger S, Talajic M, Lemery R, Roy D. Erythromycin-induced long QT syndrome: concordance with quinidine and underlying cellular electrophysiologic mechanism. *Am J Med* (1990) 89, 235–8.
2. Samarendra P, Kumari S, Evans SJ, Sacchi TJ, Navarro V. QT prolongation associated with azithromycin/amiodarone combination. *Pacing Clin Electrophysiol* (2001) 24, 1572–4.
3. Lee KL, Man-Hong J, Tang SC, Tai Y-T. QT-prolongation and torsades de pointes associated with clarithromycin. *Am J Med* (1998) 104, 395–6.
4. Cordarone X (Amiodarone hydrochloride). Sanofi Synthelabo. UK Summary of product characteristics, May 2004.

Amiodarone + Oxygen

High-dose oxygen may increase the risks of amiodarone-induced postoperative adult respiratory distress syndrome.

Clinical evidence, mechanism, importance and management

Postoperative adult respiratory distress syndrome has been reported in patients on amiodarone who received 100% oxygen ventilation during surgery.[1,2] Increased pulmonary toxicity (pulmonary oedema) with the combination of amiodarone and 100% oxygen has been confirmed in *mice*.[3] The UK maker of amiodarone suggests caution in patients receiving high-dose oxygen therapy.[4] Others have suggested that the concentration of oxygen should be maintained at the lowest possible level consistent with adequate oxygenation.[3]

1. Saussine M, Colson P, Alauzen M, Mary H. Postoperative acute respiratory distress syndrome. A complication of amiodarone associated with 100 percent oxygen ventilation. *Chest* (1992) 102, 980–1.
2. Duke PK, Ramsay MAE, Herndon JC, Swygert TH, Cook AO. Acute oxygen induced amiodarone pulmonary toxicity after general anaesthesia. *Anesthesiology* (1991) 75, A228.
3. Donica SK, Paulsen AW, Simpson BR, Ramsay MAE, Saunders CT, Swygert TH, Tappe J. Danger of amiodarone therapy and elevated inspired oxygen concentrations in mice. *Am J Cardiol* (1996) 77, 109–10.
4. Cordarone X (Amiodarone hydrochloride). Sanofi Synthelabo. UK Summary of product characteristics, May 2004.

Amiodarone + Protease inhibitors

A case of enhanced serum levels of amiodarone during concomitant indinavir administration has been reported. Nelfinavir, ritonavir and, possibly, saquinavir are predicted to act similarly.

Clinical evidence

A patient on amiodarone 200 mg daily was additionally given zidovudine, lamivudine, and **indinavir** for 4 weeks, as post HIV-exposure prophylaxis after a needlestick injury. Amiodarone serum levels increased, from 0.9 mg/l before antiretroviral prophylaxis, to 1.3 mg/l during therapy, and gradually decreased to 0.8 mg/l during the 77 days after stopping prophylaxis. Although the reference range for amiodarone levels is not established, these levels were not outside those usually considered to achieve good antiarrhythmic control.[1]

Mechanism

HIV-protease inhibitors such as **indinavir** are metabolised by cytochrome P450 enzymes and pharmacokinetic interactions are therefore possible. It was considered that the increase in serum amiodarone in this case was due to decreased metabolism of amiodarone, although no decrease in the serum levels of desethylamiodarone were observed.[1]

Importance and management

Although in the case cited the interaction was not clinically relevant, the authors considered that it could be in patients with higher initial amiodarone levels. They recommend monitoring amiodarone therapy if indinavir is coadministered.[1] Based on theoretical considerations, the makers of **nelfinavir** and **ritonavir** predict that these HIV-protease inhibitors will inhibit the metabolism of amiodarone, and advise against concurrent use.[2,3] **Saquinavir** may possibly also interact.[4]

1. Lohman JJHM, Reichert LJM, Degen LPM. Antiretroviral therapy increases serum concentrations of amiodarone. *Ann Pharmacother* (1999) 33, 645–6.
2. Norvir (Ritonavir). Abbott Laboratories Ltd. UK Summary of product characteristics, January 2005.
3. Viracept (Nelfinavir mesilate). Roche Products Ltd. UK Summary of product characteristics, June 2005.
4. Fortovase (Saquinavir). Roche Products Ltd. UK Summary of product characteristics, January 2005.

Amiodarone + Quinolones

Torsade de pointes has been reported in two patients taking amiodarone and levofloxacin. An increased risk of this arrhythmia would also be expected if amiodarone is used with gatifloxacin, moxifloxacin, or sparfloxacin.

Clinical evidence, mechanism, importance and management

Torsade de pointes arrhythmia occurred in a patient taking **levofloxacin** and amiodarone.[1] The same authors subsequently encountered a second case of this reaction.[2] Four cases of torsade de pointes were noted in patients taking amiodarone and a quinolone (unspecified) in an analysis of cases of torsade de pointes associated with quinolones on the Adverse Events Reporting System database (there were 37 cases identified, and 19 occurred in patients also taking other drugs known to prolong the QT interval).[3]

Amiodarone is well known to prolong the QT interval and increase the risk of torsade de pointes. Of the quinolones used clinically, **gatifloxacin**, **moxifloxacin**, and **sparfloxacin** are known to prolong the QT interval (see 'Table 7.3', (p.169)). There is also evidence that **levofloxacin** may prolong the QT interval.[2,3]

In general the concurrent use of two or more drugs that prolong the QT interval should be avoided, because this increases the risk of torsade de pointes arrhythmias (see also 'Drugs that prolong the QT interval + Other drugs that prolong the QT interval', p.170). The above quinolones should probably be avoided in patients on amiodarone. **Ciprofloxacin** appears to have less effect on the QT interval.[3]

1. Iannini PB, Kramer H, Circiumaru I, Byazrova E, Doddamani S. QTc prolongation associated with levofloxacin. *Intersci Conf Antimicrob Agents Chemother* (2000) 40, 477.
2. Iannini P. Quinolone-induced QT interval prolongation: a not-so-unexpected class effect. *J Antimicrob Chemother* (2001) 47, 893–4.
3. Frothingham R. Rates of torsades de pointes associated with ciprofloxacin, ofloxacin, levofloxacin, gatifloxacin, and moxifloxacin. *Pharmacotherapy* (2001) 21, 1468–72.

Amiodarone + Rifampicin (Rifampin)

An isolated case report suggests that rifampicin may decrease serum levels of amiodarone and its metabolite *N*-desethylamiodarone.

Clinical evidence, mechanism, importance and management

A woman with congenital heart disease and atrial and ventricular arrhythmias managed by an implanted cardioverter defibrillator, epicardial pacing and amiodarone 400 mg daily, experienced deterioration in the control of her condition. She developed palpitations and experienced a shock from the defibrillator. Her amiodarone serum levels were 40% lower than 2 months previously, and her *N*-desethylamiodarone levels were undetectable. It was noted that 5 weeks earlier rifampicin 600 mg daily had been started to treat an infection of the pacing system. The amiodarone dose was doubled, but the palpitations continued. Amiodarone and *N*-desethylamiodarone levels increased after rifampicin was discontinued.[1] Rifampicin is a potent enzyme inducing agent and it may have increased the metabolism and clearance of amiodarone. This case suggests that combined use of amiodarone and rifampicin should be well monitored.

1. Zarembski DG, Fischer SA, Santucci PA, Porter MT, Costanzo MR, Trohman RG. Impact of rifampin on serum amiodarone concentrations in a patient with congenital heart disease. *Pharmacotherapy* (1999) 19, 249–51.

Amiodarone + Sertraline

In an isolated report, a slight to moderate rise in plasma amiodarone levels has been attributed to the concurrent use of sertraline.

Clinical evidence, mechanism, importance and management

A depressed patient on amiodarone 200 mg twice daily had his concurrent treatment with carbamazepine 200 mg twice daily and sertraline 100 mg daily stopped, just before ECT treatment. After 4 days it was noted that his plasma amiodarone levels had fallen by nearly 20%. The authors of the report drew the conclusion that while taking all three drugs, the amiodarone levels had become slightly raised due to the enzyme inhibitory effects of the sertraline, despite the potential enzyme-inducing activity of the carbamazepine.[1] The patient showed no changes in his cardiac status while on the reduced amiodarone levels, suggesting that this interaction (if such it is) is of limited clinical importance. However it may be worth considering an antidepressant with low affinity for cytochrome P450 isoenzyme CYP3A4 such as paroxetine or venlafaxine if concurrent use is required with amiodarone.[1]

1. DeVane CL, Gill HS, Markowitz JS, Carson WH. Awareness of potential drug interactions may aid avoidance. *Ther Drug Monit* (1997) 19, 366–7.

Amiodarone + Trazodone

An isolated report describes the development of torsade de pointes when a woman on amiodarone was given trazodone.

Clinical evidence, mechanism, importance and management

A 74-year-old woman with a pacemaker, taking nifedipine, furosemide, aspirin and amiodarone 200 mg daily, began to have dizzy spells but no loss of consciousness soon after starting trazodone (initially 50 mg and eventually 150 mg daily by the end of 2 weeks). Both the amiodarone and trazodone were stopped when she was hospitalised. She showed prolonged QT, QTc and JTc intervals on the ECG and recurrent episodes of torsade de pointes arrhythmia, which were controlled by increasing the ventricular pacing rate. The QTc and other ECG intervals shortened and she was later discharged on amiodarone without the trazodone, with an ECG similar to that seen 4 months before hospitalisation.[1] No general conclusions can be drawn from this apparent interaction, but prescribers should be aware of this case. The makers note that trazodone does have the potential to be arrhythmogenic.[2] See also, 'Drugs that prolong the QT interval + Other drugs that prolong the QT interval', p.170.

1. Mazur A, Strasberg B, Kusniec J, Sclarovsky S. QT prolongation and polymorphous ventricular tachycardia association with trazodone-amiodarone combination. *Int J Cardiol* (1995) 52, 27–9.
2. Molipaxin (Trazodone). Hoechst Marion Roussel Ltd. UK Summary of product characteristics, May 2002.

Aprindine + Amiodarone

Serum aprindine levels can be increased by the concurrent use of amiodarone. Toxicity may occur unless the dosage is reduced.

Clinical evidence, mechanism, importance and management

The serum aprindine levels of two patients rose, accompanied by signs of toxicity (nausea, ataxia, etc.), when they were additionally treated with amiodarone. One of them, taking aprindine 100 mg daily, showed a progressive rise in trough serum levels from 2.3 to 3.5 mg/l over a 5-week period, when given 1200 mg and later 600 mg of amiodarone daily. Even when the aprindine dosage was reduced, serum levels remained higher than before amiodarone was started.[1] The authors say that those given both drugs generally need less aprindine than those on aprindine alone. This interaction has been briefly reported elsewhere.[2] Its mechanism is not understood. Monitor the effects of concurrent use and reduce the dosage of aprindine as necessary.

1. Southworth W, Friday KJ, Ruffy R. Possible amiodarone-aprindine interaction. *Am Heart J* (1982) 104, 323.
2. Zhang Z, Wang G, Wang H, Zhang J. Effect of amiodarone on the plasma concentration of aprindine [Abstract 115: 197745u in Chemical Abstracts (1991) 115, 22]. *Zhongguo Yao Xue Za Zhi* (1991) 26, 156–9.

Bretylium + Sympathomimetics

The pressor effects of noradrenaline (norepinephrine) and adrenaline (epinephrine) are increased in the presence of bretylium. Amfetamine and protriptyline antagonised the blood pressure lowering effect of bretylium.

Clinical evidence

(a) Amfetamine

A single 25-mg dose of amfetamine caused a rise in blood pressure in 6 of 7 patients with hypertension satisfactorily controlled by bretylium 600 mg to 4 g daily.[1]

(b) Noradrenaline (norepinephrine) or Adrenaline (epinephrine)

A dose of bretylium sufficient to produce postural hypotension enhanced the pressor effect of noradrenaline in 4 healthy subjects. A similar effect was shown with adrenaline.[2]

(c) Protriptyline

An experimental study has shown that protriptyline can return the blood pressure to normal in patients taking bretylium, without reducing its antiarrhythmic efficacy.[3]

Mechanism

Animal studies have shown that bretylium reduces blood pressure via its blocking effects on adrenergic neurones similar to guanethidine.[4,5] Bretylium therefore enhances the effects of directly-acting sympathomimetics such as noradrenaline, and is antagonised by drugs with indirect sympathomimetic activity such as the amfetamines and tricyclic antidepressants.

Importance and management

Although documentation is limited, based on the known pharmacology of bretylium, these interactions would appear to be established. The use of bretylium is now limited to the short-term control of ventricular arrhythmias. In this situation, if directly-acting sympathomimetics such as noradrenaline are required to reverse bretylium-induced hypotension, this should be undertaken with caution since their effects may be enhanced.

Bretylium is no longer used for the treatment of hypertension, therefore the interactions with amfetamines and tricyclics described above are unlikely to be of much clinical relevance.

1. Wilson R, Long C. Action of bretylium antagonised by amphetamine. *Lancet* (1960) ii, 262.
2. Laurence DR, Nagle RE. The interaction of bretylium with pressor agents. *Lancet* (1961) i, 593–4.
3. Woosley RL, Reele SB, Roden DM, Nies AS, Oates JA. Pharmacological reversal of hypotensive effect complicating antiarrhythmic therapy with bretylium. *Clin Pharmacol Ther* (1982) 32, 313–21.
4. Day MD. Effect of sympathomimetic amines on the blocking action of guanethidine, bretylium and xylocholine. *Br J Pharmacol* (1962) 18, 421–39.
5. Boura ALA, Green AF. Comparison of bretylium and guanethidine: tolerance and effects on adrenergic nerve function and responses to sympathomimetic amines. *Br J Pharmacol* (1962) 19, 13–41.

Cibenzoline (Cifenline) + H_2-blockers

Cimetidine increases the plasma levels of cibenzoline, but ranitidine does not interact.

Clinical evidence, mechanism, importance and management

Cimetidine 1200 mg daily raised the maximum plasma levels of single 160-mg doses of cibenzoline in 12 healthy subjects by 27%, increased the AUC by 44%, and prolonged its half-life by 30%. **Ranitidine** 300 mg daily had no effect.[1] The probable reason is that **cimetidine**, an enzyme inhibitor, reduces the metabolism of the cibenzoline by the liver, whereas **ranitidine**, which has little enzyme inhibiting effects, does not. The clinical importance of this interaction is not known but be alert for increased cibenzoline effects.

1. Massarella JW, Defeo TM, Liguori J, Passe S, Aogaichi K. The effects of cimetidine and ranitidine on the pharmacokinetics of cifenline. *Br J Clin Pharmacol* (1991) 31, 481–3.

Disopyramide + Antacids

There is some inconclusive evidence that aluminium phosphate may possibly cause a small reduction in the absorption of disopyramide.

Clinical evidence, mechanism, importance and management

A single 11-g dose of an **aluminium phosphate** antacid had no statistically significant effect on the pharmacokinetics of a single 200-mg oral dose of disopyramide in 10 patients. However the antacid appeared to reduce the absorption of disopyramide to some extent in individual subjects.[1] The clinical importance of this interaction is uncertain, but probably small.

1. Albin H, Vincon G, Bertolaso D, Dangoumau J. Influence du phosphate d'aluminium sur la biodisponibilité de la procaïnamide et du disopyramide. *Therapie* (1981) 36, 541–6.

Disopyramide + Beta-blockers

Severe bradycardia has been described after the use of disopyramide with beta-blockers including practolol (3 cases, 1 fatal) pindolol (1 fatal) and metoprolol (1 case). Another patient given disopyramide and intravenous sotalol developed asystole (see also 'Drugs that prolong the QT interval + Other drugs that prolong the QT interval', p.170). Atenolol modestly decreased disopyramide clearance in one study. Oral propranolol and disopyramide have been combined without any increase in negative inotropic effects or pharmacokinetic changes in healthy subjects.

Clinical evidence

Two patients with supraventricular tachycardia (180 bpm) were treated, firstly with intravenous **practolol** (20 and 10 mg respectively) and shortly afterwards with disopyramide (150 and 80 mg respectively). The first patient rapidly developed sinus bradycardia of 25 bpm, lost consciousness and became profoundly hypotensive. He failed to respond to 600 micrograms of atropine, but later his heart rate increased to 60 bpm while a temporary pacemaker was being inserted.[1] He was successfully treated with disopyramide 150 mg alone for a later episode of tachycardia. The second patient also developed severe bradycardia and asystole, despite the use of atropine. He was resuscitated with adrenaline (epinephrine) but later died.[1]

Severe bradycardia has been reported in another patient, similarly treated with intravenous **practolol** and then disopyramide.[2] One other patient has been described who developed severe bradycardia and died when treated for supraventricular tachycardia with **pindolol** 5 mg and disopyramide 250 mg (both orally).[3] Another patient on oral disopyramide 250 mg twice daily developed asystole when given a total of 60 mg of intravenous **sotalol**.[4]

A patient with hypertrophic obstructive cardiomyopathy and paroxysmal atrial fibrillation on disopyramide 450 mg daily developed hypotension, bradycardia and cardiac conduction disturbances 5 days after starting **metoprolol** 50 mg daily.[5]

Atenolol 100 mg daily has been shown to increase the serum disopyramide steady-state levels from 3.46 to 4.25 micrograms/ml and reduce the clearance of disopyramide by 16% (from 1.9 to 1.59 ml/kg/minute) in healthy subjects and patients with ischaemic heart disease.[6] None of the subjects developed any adverse reactions or symptoms of heart failure, apart from one of the subjects who showed transient first degree heart block.[6]

In contrast, studies in healthy subjects have shown that the negative inotropic effect was no greater when oral **propranolol** and disopyramide were used concurrently,[7] nor were the pharmacokinetics of either drug affected.[8]

Mechanism

Not understood. Both disopyramide and the beta-blockers can depress the contractility and conductivity of the heart muscle.

Importance and management

The general clinical importance of this interaction is uncertain. A clear risk seems to exist in patients who are treated with disopyramide and practolol or sotalol given intravenously. Considerable caution should be exercised in these patients. More study is needed to find out what contributes to the development of this potentially serious interaction. The makers of disopyramide suggest that the combination of disopyramide and beta-blockers should generally be avoided, except in the case of life-threatening arrhythmias unresponsive to a single agent.[9,10]

The UK makers of sotalol also warn that both sotalol and disopyramide can prolong the QT interval, which may therefore increase the risk of torsade de pointes arrhythmia if both are used together.[11] The US makers recommend that this combination should be avoided.[12] See also 'Drugs that prolong the QT interval + Other drugs that prolong the QT interval', p.170.

1. Cumming AD, Robertson C. Interaction between disopyramide and practolol. *BMJ* (1979) 2, 1264.
2. Gelipter D, Hazell M. Interaction between disopyramide and practolol. *BMJ* (1980) 1, 52.
3. Pedersen C, Josephsen P, Lindvig K. Interaktion mellem disopyramid og pindolol efter oral indgift. *Ugeskr Laeger* (1983) 145, 3266.
4. Bystedt T, Vitols S. Sotalol-disopyramid ledde till asystoli. *Lakartidningen* (1994) 91, 2241.
5. Pernat A, Pohar B, Horvat M, Heart conduction disturbances and cardiovascular collapse after disopyramide and low-dose metoprolol in a patient with hypertrophic obstructive cardiomyopathy. *J Electrocardiol* (1997) 30, 341–4.
6. Bonde J, Bødtker S, Angelo HR, Svendsen TL, Kampmann JP. Atenolol inhibits the elimination of disopyramide. *Eur J Clin Pharmacol* (1986) 28, 41–3.
7. Cathcart-Rake WF, Coker JE, Atkins FL, Huffman DH, Hassanein KM, Shen DD, Azarnoff DL. The effect of concurrent oral administration of propranolol and disopyramide on cardiac function in healthy men. *Circulation* (1980) 61, 938–45.
8. Karim A, Nissen C, Azarnoff DL. Clinical pharmacokinetics of disopyramide. *J Pharmacokinet Biopharm* (1982) 10, 465–94.
9. Dirythmin (Disopyramide). AstraZeneca UK Ltd. UK Summary of product characteristics. January 2002.
10. Norpace (Disopyramide). Pharmacia. US Prescribing information, September 2001.
11. Beta-Cardone (Sotalol). Celltech Pharmaceuticals Ltd. UK Summary of product characteristics, December 2003.
12. Betapace (Sotalol). Berlex Laboratories. US Prescribing information, November 2001.

Disopyramide + H_2-blockers

A single-dose study has shown that cimetidine can slightly increase the serum levels of oral disopyramide. Cimetidine did not affect the pharmacokinetics of intravenous disopyramide. Ranitidine appears not to interact.

Clinical evidence, mechanism, importance and management

Cimetidine 400 mg twice daily by mouth for 14 days did not alter the pharmacokinetics of a single 150-mg intravenous dose of disopyramide in 7 healthy subjects.[1] Another study in 6 healthy subjects showed that a single 400-mg dose of **cimetidine** increased the AUC of a single 300-mg oral dose of disopyramide by 8.5% and increased the maximum serum levels by 18.5%, but did not significantly affect the metabolism of disopyramide. **Ranitidine** 150 mg was found not to interact significantly.[2] The reasons are not known, but the authors of the report suggest that **cimetidine** may have increased disopyramide absorption.[2] Cimetidine is only a weak inhibitor of disopyramide metabolism *in vitro*.[3] The changes described are unlikely to be clinically important, but this should probably be confirmed in a more clinically realistic situation, using multiple oral doses of both drugs.

1. Bonde J, Pedersen LE, Nygaard E, Ramsing T, Angelo HR, Kampmann JP. Stereoselective pharmacokinetics of disopyramide and interaction with cimetidine. *Br J Clin Pharmacol* (1991) 31, 708–10.
2. Jou M-J, Huang S-C, Kiang F-M, Lai M-Y, Chao P-DL. Comparison of the effects of cimetidine and ranitidine on the pharmacokinetics of disopyramide in man. *J Pharm Pharmacol* (1997) 49, 1072–5.
3. Echuzen H, Kawasaki H, Chiba K, Tani M. Ishizaki T. A potent inhibitory effect of erythromycin and other macrolide antibiotics on the mono-N-dealkylation metabolism of disopyramide with human liver microsomes. *J Pharmacol Exp Ther* (1993) 264, 1425–31.

Disopyramide + Macrolides

The serum disopyramide levels of two patients rose when they were given erythromycin and QT prolongation and cardiac arrhythmias developed. Another patient given both drugs developed heart block. One patient developed ventricular fibrillation and two patients developed torsade de pointes when given clarithromycin with disopyramide. Two other patients developed severe hypoglycaemia. Ventricular fibrillation occurred in a patient treated with azithromycin and disopyramide. See also 'Drugs that prolong the QT interval + Other drugs that prolong the QT interval', p.170.

Clinical evidence

(a) Azithromycin

A patient on disopyramide 150 mg three times daily developed ventricular tachycardia requiring cardioversion 11 days after starting azithromycin 250 mg daily.[1] Her disopyramide level was found to have risen from 2.6 to 11.1 micrograms/ml.

(b) Clarithromycin

A 74-year-old woman who had been taking disopyramide 200 mg twice daily for 7 years collapsed with ventricular fibrillation 6 days after starting to take omeprazole 40 mg, metronidazole 800 mg and clarithromycin 500 mg daily. After successful resuscitation, her QTc interval, which had never previously been above 440 milliseconds, was found to have risen to 625 milliseconds. Her disopyramide plasma level was also elevated (4.6 micrograms/ml) and the half-life was markedly prolonged (40 hours). The QTc interval normalised as her plasma disopyramide levels fell.[2] A 76-year old woman on disopyramide developed torsades de pointes when given clarithromycin 200 mg twice daily. Hypokalaemia (potassium 2.8 mmol/l) probably contributed to this case.[3]

An episode of torsades de pointes occurred in another elderly woman on disopyramide 5 days after starting clarithromycin 250 mg twice daily.[4]

A haemodialysis patient, receiving disopyramide 50 mg daily because of paroxysmal atrial fibrillation, was hospitalised with hypoglycaemic coma after additional treatment with clarithromycin 600 mg daily. Serum disopyramide levels increased from 1.5 to 8 micrograms/ml during treatment with clarithromycin. QT and QTc intervals were prolonged, but torsade de pointes did not occur.[5] Hypoglycaemic coma during concomitant disopyramide and clarithromycin treatment has also been reported in another patient.[6]

(c) Erythromycin

A woman with ventricular ectopy taking disopyramide (300 mg alternating with 150 mg six-hourly) developed new arrhythmias (ventricular asystoles and later torsade de pointes) within 36 hours of starting erythromycin lactobionate 1 g intravenously 6-hourly, and cefamandole. Her QTc interval had increased from 390 to 600 milliseconds and her serum disopyramide level was found to be 16 micromol/l. The problem resolved when the disopyramide was stopped and bretylium given, but it returned when the disopyramide was restarted. It resolved again when the erythromycin was stopped.[7] Another patient with ventricular tachycardia, well controlled over 5 years with disopyramide 200 mg four times daily, developed polymorphic ventricular tachycardia within a few days of starting erythromycin base 500 mg four times daily. His QTc interval had increased from 430 to 630 milliseconds and serum disopyramide levels were found to be elevated at 30 micromol/l. The problem resolved when both drugs were withdrawn and antiarrhythmics given.[7] Heart block is said to have developed in another patient treated with both drugs.[8]

Mechanism

Not fully established. An *in vitro* study using human liver microsomes indicated that erythromycin inhibits the metabolism (mono-*N*-dealkylation) of disopyramide which, *in vivo*, would be expected to reduce its loss from the body and increase its serum levels.[9] Clarithromycin and azithromycin probably do the same. The increased serum levels of disopyramide can result in adverse effects such as QT prolongation and torsade de pointes, and may result in enhanced insulin secretion and hypoglycaemia.[5,6] Both intravenous erythromycin[10] and clarithromycin[11] alone have been associated with prolongation of the QT interval and torsade de pointes. Therefore, disopyramide and macrolides may have additive effects on the QT interval in addition to the pharmacokinetic interaction.

Importance and management

An established interaction, although it is probably rare. Even so the effects of concurrent use should be well monitored if azithromycin, clarithromycin or erythromycin is added to disopyramide, being alert for the development of raised plasma disopyramide levels and prolongation of the QT interval. Some of the makers of disopyramide recommend[12,13] avoiding the combination of disopyramide and macrolides that inhibit cytochrome P450 isoenzyme CYP3A, and this would certainly be prudent in situations where close monitoring is not possible. Although direct clinical information is lacking, *in vitro* studies with human liver microsomes[9] indicate that **josamycin** is likely to interact similarly, and **telithromycin** (an erythromycin derivative) might also be expected to interact in the same way.[14] See also 'Drugs that prolong the QT interval + Other drugs that prolong the QT interval', p.170.

1. Granowitz EV, Tabor KJ, Kirchhoffer JB. Potentially fatal interaction between azithromycin and disopyramide. *Pacing Clin Electrophysiol* (2000) 23, 1433–5.

2. Paar D, Terjung B, Sauerbruch T. Life-threatening interaction between clarithromycin and disopyramide. *Lancet* (1997) 349, 326–7.
3. Hayashi Y, Ikeda U, Hashimoto T, Watanabe T, Mitsuhashi T, Shimada K. Torsade de pointes ventricular tachycardia induced by clarithromycin and disopyramide in the presence of hypokalaemia. *Pacing Clin Electrophysiol* (1999) 22, 672–4.
4. Choudhury L, Grais IM, Passman RS. Torsade de pointes due to drug interaction between disopyramide and clarithromycin. *Heart Dis* (1999) 1, 206–7.
5. Iida H, Morita T, Suzuki E, Iwasawa K, Toyo-oka T, Nakajima T. Hypoglycemia induced by interaction between clarithromycin and disopyramide. *Jpn Heart J* (1999) 40, 91–6.
6. Morlet-Barla N, Narbonne H, Vialettes B. Hypoglycémie grave et récidivante secondaire á l'interaction disopyramide-clarithromicine. *Presse Med* (2000) 29, 1351.
7. Ragosta M, Weihl AC, Rosenfeld LE. Potentially fatal interaction between erythromycin and disopyramide. *Am J Med* (1989) 86, 465–6.
8. Beeley L, Cunningham H, Carmichael A, Brennan A. *Bulletin of the West Midlands Centre for Adverse Drug Reaction Reporting* (1992) 35, 13.
9. Echizen H, Kawasaki H, Chiba K, Tani M. Ishizaki T. A potent inhibitory effect of erythromycin and other macrolide antibiotics on the mono-N-dealkylation metabolism of disopyramide with human liver microsomes. *J Pharmacol Exp Ther* (1993) 264, 1425–31.
10. Gitler B, Berger LS, Buffa SD. Torsades de pointes induced by erythromycin. *Chest* (1994) 105, 368–72.
11. Lee KL, Jim M-H, Tang SC, Tai Y-T. QT-prolongation and torsades de pointes associated with clarithromycin. *Am J Med* (1998) 104, 395–6.
12. Rythmodan (Disopyramide). Borg Medicare. UK Summary of product characteristics, January 2001.
13. Dirythmin (Disopyramide). AstraZeneca UK Ltd. UK Summary of product characteristics, January 2002.
14. Ketek (Telithromycin). Aventis Pharma Ltd. UK Summary of product characteristics, January 2004.

Disopyramide + Phenobarbital

Serum disopyramide levels are reduced by the concurrent use of phenobarbital.

Clinical evidence

After taking phenobarbital 100 mg daily for 21 days, the half-life and AUC of a single 200-mg dose of disopyramide were reduced by about 35%. The apparent metabolic clearance more than doubled, and the fraction recovered in urine as metabolite increased. Sixteen healthy subjects took part in the study and no significant differences were seen between those who smoked and those who did not.[1]

Mechanism

It seems probable that phenobarbital (a known enzyme inducing agent) increases the metabolism of disopyramide by the liver, and thereby increases its loss from the body.

Importance and management

This interaction appears to be established, but its clinical importance is uncertain. The extent to which it would reduce the control of arrhythmias by disopyramide in patients is unknown, but monitor the effects and the serum levels of disopyramide if phenobarbital is added or withdrawn. Some makers[2,3] of disopyramide recommend avoiding using it in combination with inducers of cytochrome P450 isoenzyme CYP3A, such as phenobarbital. Other barbiturates would be expected to interact similarly.

1. Kapil RP, Axelson JE, Mansfield IL, Edwards DJ, McErlane B, Mason MA, Lalka D, Kerr CR. Disopyramide pharmacokinetics and metabolism: effect of inducers. *Br J Clin Pharmacol* (1987) 24, 781–91.
2. Rythmodan (Disopyramide). Borg Medicare. UK Summary of product characteristics, January 2001.
3. Dirythmin (Disopyramide). AstraZeneca UK Ltd. UK Summary of product characteristics, January 2002.

Disopyramide + Phenytoin

Serum disopyramide levels are reduced by the concurrent use of phenytoin and may fall below therapeutic concentrations. Loss of arrhythmic control may occur.

Clinical evidence

Eight patients with ventricular tachycardia treated with disopyramide 600 to 2000 mg daily showed a 54% fall in their serum disopyramide levels (from a mean of 3.99 to 1.82 micrograms/ml) when concurrently treated with phenytoin 200 to 600 mg daily for a week. Two of the patients who responded to disopyramide and underwent Holter monitoring showed a 53- and 2000-fold increase in ventricular premature beat frequency as a result of this interaction.[1]

In other reports, 3 patients who had low levels of disopyramide and high levels of its metabolite were noted to be taking phenytoin,[2] and one patient receiving both drugs required an unusually high dose of disopyramide.[3] A marked fall in serum disopyramide levels (75% in one case) was seen in 2 patients after taking phenytoin 300 to 400 mg daily for up to two weeks.[4] Pharmacokinetic studies[3,5] in a total of 12 healthy subjects confirm this interaction. In addition, one healthy epileptic taking phenytoin had about a 50% lower disopyramide AUC and elimination half-life than control subjects.[5]

Mechanism

Phenytoin, which is a known enzyme-inducing agent, increases the metabolism of the disopyramide by the liver. Although, the major metabolite (*N*-dealkyldisopyramide) also possesses antiarrhythmic activity the net effect is a reduction in arrhythmic control.[1]

Importance and management

An established interaction of clinical importance. Some loss of arrhythmic control can occur during concurrent use. Disopyramide adverse effects and the antiarrhythmic response should be well monitored. An increase in the dosage of disopyramide may be necessary. The interaction appears to resolve fully within two weeks of withdrawing the phenytoin.

1. Matos JA, Fisher JD, Kim SG. Disopyramide-phenytoin interaction. *Clin Res* (1981) 29, 655A.
2. Aitio M-L, Vuorenmaa T. Enhanced metabolism and diminished efficacy of disopyramide by enzyme induction? *Br J Clin Pharmacol* (1980) 9, 149–152.
3. Nightingale J, Nappi JM. Effect of phenytoin on serum disopyramide concentrations. *Clin Pharm* (1987) 6, 46–50.
4. Kessler JM, Keys PW, Stafford RW. Disopyramide and phenytoin interaction. *Clin Pharm* (1982) 1, 263–4.
5. Aitio M-L, Mansury L, Tala E, Haataja M, Aitio A. The effect of enzyme induction on the metabolism of disopyramide in man. *Br J Clin Pharmacol* (1981) 11, 279–85.

Disopyramide + Quinidine

Disopyramide serum levels may be slightly raised by quinidine. Both drugs prolong the QT interval, and this may be additive on combined use.

Clinical evidence, mechanism, importance and management

After taking quinidine 200 mg four times a day, the peak serum levels of disopyramide, given as a single 150-mg dose to 16 healthy subjects, were raised by 20% from 2.68 to 3.23 micrograms/ml, and by 14% when given long-term, as 150 mg four times a day. Serum quinidine levels were decreased by 26%. However, there was no change in the half-life of either drug. Both quinidine and disopyramide caused a slight lengthening of the QTc interval, and when quinidine was added to disopyramide therapy additional lengthening of the QT interval occurred. The frequency of adverse effects such as dry mouth, blurred vision, urine retention and nausea were also somewhat increased.[1] The mechanism of the effect on serum levels is not understood. The anticholinergic adverse effects of disopyramide may be increased. Disopyramide and quinidine are both class Ia antiarrhythmics that prolong the QT interval, and, in general, such combinations should be avoided (see also 'Drugs that prolong the QT interval + Other drugs that prolong the QT interval', p.170).

1. Baker BJ, Gammill J, Massengill J, Schubert E, Karin A, Doherty JE. Concurrent use of quinidine and disopyramide: evaluation of serum concentrations and electrocardiographic effects. *Am Heart J* (1983) 105, 12–15.

Disopyramide + Rifampicin (Rifampin)

The plasma levels of disopyramide can be reduced by the concurrent use of rifampicin.

Clinical evidence

After taking rifampicin for 14 days the plasma levels of disopyramide were approximately halved in 11 patients with tuberculosis who had taken single 200- or 300-mg doses of disopyramide.[1] The disopyramide AUC was reduced by about two-thirds and the half-life was reduced from 5.9 to 3.25 hours by rifampicin. A woman who had been receiving rifampicin for 2 weeks initially had subtherapeutic serum levels of disopyramide of 0.9 micromol/l when first started on 100 mg 8-hourly. The dosage of disopyramide was increased to 300 mg 8-hourly, and the rifampicin was discontinued. Three days after discontinuing rifampicin the disopyramide level was 3.6 micromol/l and after 5 days it was 8.1 micromol/l. The patient was eventually maintained on disopyramide 250 mg 8-hourly.[2]

Mechanism

The most probable explanation is that rifampicin (a well known enzyme inducer) increases the metabolism of the disopyramide by the liver so that it is cleared from the body much more quickly.

Importance and management

Information seems to be limited to these studies, but they indicate that the dosage of disopyramide will need to be increased in most patients taking rifampicin.

1. Aitio M-L, Mansury L, Tala E, Haataja M, Aitio A. The effect of enzyme induction on the metabolism of disopyramide in man. *Br J Clin Pharmacol* (1981) 11, 279–85.
2. Staum JM. Enzyme induction: rifampin-disopyramide interaction. *DICP Ann Pharmacother* (1990) 24, 701–3.

Disopyramide + Verapamil

Profound hypotension and collapse has occurred in a small number of patients on verapamil who were given disopyramide.

Clinical evidence, mechanism, importance and management

A group of clinicians who had used single 400-mg oral doses of disopyramide successfully and with few side-effects for reverting acute supraventricular arrhythmias, reported 5 cases of profound hypotension and collapse. Three of the patients developed severe epigastric pain. All 5 had previous myocardial disease and/or were taking myocardial depressants — beta-blockers or verapamil in small quantities (not specified).[1]

On the basis of this report, and on reports of studies in *animals*,[2] and from the known risks associated with the concurrent use of beta-blockers (see 'Disopyramide + Beta-blockers', p.164), the makers warn about combining disopyramide and other drugs [such as verapamil] that may have additive negative inotropic effects.[3,4] However, they do point out that in some specific circumstances the combination may be beneficial.[3] They note that severe hypotension caused by disopyramide has usually been associated with cardiomyopathy or uncompensated congestive heart failure.[3,4]

1. Manolas EG, Hunt D, Dowling JT, Luxton M, Vohra J. Collapse after oral administration of disopyramide. *Med J Aust* (1979) 1, 20.
2. Lee JT, Davy J-M, Kates RE. Evaluation of combined administration of verapamil and disopyramide in dogs. *J Cardiovasc Pharmacol* (1985) 7, 501–7.
3. Rythmodan (Disopyramide). Borg Medicare. UK Summary of product characteristics, January 2001.
4. Dirythmin (Disopyramide). AstraZeneca UK Ltd. UK Summary of product characteristics, January 2002.

Dofetilide + Antacids

Antacids (aluminium/magnesium hydroxide) appear not to interact with dofetilide.

Clinical evidence, mechanism, importance and management

A study in 12 healthy subjects found that pre-treatment with **aluminium/magnesium hydroxide** *(Maalox)* 30 ml (10, 2 and 0.5 hours before dofetilide) did not affect the pharmacokinetics of a single 500-microgram dose of dofetilide, nor the dofetilide-induced change in QTc interval.[1] No special precautions appear to be necessary.

1. Vincent J, Gardner MJ, Baris B, Willavize SA. Concurrent administration of omeprazole and antacid does not alter the pharmacokinetics and pharmacodynamic of dofetilide in healthy subjects. *Clin Pharmacol Ther* (1996) 59, 182.

Dofetilide + Diuretics

Hydrochlorothiazide and hydrochlorothiazide/triamterene modestly increased dofetilide plasma levels, and caused a marked increase in the QT interval.

Clinical evidence

The maker notes that the concurrent use of dofetilide 500 micrograms twice daily with **hydrochlorothiazide** 50 mg daily for 7 days increased the dofetilide AUC by 14% and increased the QTc interval by 47.6 milliseconds.[1] Similar results were seen with the same dose of dofetilide combined with **hydrochlorothiazide/triamterene** 50/100 mg daily (18% increase in AUC, and 38.1 millisecond increase in QTc).[1]

Mechanism

Triamterene might be expected to increase dofetilide plasma levels by competing for its renal tubular secretion (see 'Dofetilide + Miscellaneous', p.168), but the effect of its combination with hydrochlorothiazide was no greater than with hydrochlorothiazide alone. Why hydrochlorothiazide should increase dofetilide levels is unclear. An increase in dofetilide levels would be expected to increase the QT interval, but the increase seen here was much greater than expected by the change in plasma levels. The maker suggests that a reduction in serum potassium could have contributed to the extent of QT prolongation.[1] This makes sense for hydrochlorothiazide (a potassium-depleting diuretic), but the combination with triamterene (a potassium-sparing diuretic) might therefore have been expected to have less effect on the QT interval.

Importance and management

On the basis of the above findings, the maker contraindicates the use of dofetilide with **hydrochlorothiazide** alone or in combination with **triamterene**.[2] Given the increase in QT interval, a risk factor for torsade de pointes arrhythmia, this appears a prudent precaution. Further study is needed. Any diuretic that depletes serum potassium might be expected to increase the risk of QT prolongation and torsade de pointes with dofetilide, and serum potassium should be monitored.[2]

1. Pfizer Global Pharmaceuticals. Personal Communication, June 2004.
2. Tikosyn (Dofetilide). Pfizer Labs. US Prescribing information, March 2004.

Dofetilide + H_2-blockers

Cimetidine markedly increases plasma dofetilide levels, and hence increases dofetilide-induced QT prolongation and the risk of torsade de pointes arrhythmias. Its combined use with dofetilide should be avoided. Dofetilide appears not to interact with ranitidine.

Clinical evidence

A placebo-controlled study in 24 healthy subjects indicated that **cimetidine** 400 mg twice daily given with dofetilide 500 micrograms twice daily for 7 days significantly decreased the renal clearance of dofetilide by 44%, and increased its AUC by 58% and peak blood levels by 50%, without significantly altering the QTc interval.[1] In a further study it was found that **cimetidine** 100 mg twice daily (over-the-counter dose) or 400 mg twice daily (a common prescription dose) for 4 days reduced the renal clearance of a single 500-microgram dose of dofetilide by 13 and 33%, respectively. In addition, the respective **cimetidine** doses increased the QTc interval by 22 and 33%. Conversely, **ranitidine** 150 mg twice daily did not significantly affect the pharmacokinetics or pharmacodynamics of dofetilide.[2]

Mechanism

At least 50% of a dofetilide dose is eliminated unchanged in the urine by an active renal tubular secretion mechanism.[3,4] Drugs that inhibit this mechanism, such as cimetidine, increase dofetilide plasma levels.[2,3] There is a linear relationship between plasma dofetilide concentrations and prolongation of the QT interval, which increases the risk of torsade de pointes arrhythmias.[3]

Importance and management

An established interaction. Because of the likely increased risk of torsade de pointes, the maker contraindicates the use of cimetidine in patients on dofetilide. This would seem to be a prudent precaution. This applies equally to cimetidine at over-the-counter doses, and patients on dofetilide should be warned to avoid this. No special precautions appear to be necessary with ranitidine. Note that 'omeprazole', (below) and 'antacids', (below) also appear not to interact.

1. Vincent J, Gardner MJ, Apseloff G, Baris B, Willavize S, Friedman HL. Cimetidine inhibits renal elimination of dofetilide without altering QTc activity on multiple dosing in healthy subjects. *Clin Pharmacol Ther* (1998) 63, 210.
2. Abel S, Nichols DJ, Brearly CJ, Eve MD. Effect of cimetidine and ranitidine on pharmacokinetics and pharmacodynamics of a single dose of dofetilide. *Br J Clin Pharmacol* (2000) 49, 64–71.
3. Tikosyn (Dofetilide). Pfizer Labs. US prescribing information, March 2004.
4. Rasmussen HS, Allen MJ, Blackburn KJ, Butrous GS, Dalrymple HW. Dofetilide, a novel class III antiarrhythmic agent. *J Cardiovasc Pharmacol* (1992) 20 (Suppl 2), S96–S105.

Dofetilide + Ketoconazole

Ketoconazole markedly increases the plasma levels of dofetilide. This is likely to be associated with an increased risk of dofetilide-induced QT prolongation and torsade de pointes.

Clinical evidence, mechanism, importance and management

The maker of dofetilide notes that ketoconazole 400 mg daily administered concurrently with dofetilide 500 micrograms twice daily for 7 days increased the dofetilide peak levels by 53% in men and 97% in women, and the AUC by 41% in men and 69% in women.[1] Ketoconazole decreased the renal clearance of dofetilide by 31.3% and the nonrenal clearance by 40.3%, resulting in a reduction in total clearance of 34.7%.[2]

Mechanism

Ketoconazole may inhibit the active renal tubular secretion mechanism by which dofetilide is eliminated, so reducing its loss from the body (see also 'Dofetilide + H_2-blockers', p.167).[1,2] Ketoconazole also inhibits the metabolism of dofetilide[2] by the cytochrome P450 isoenzyme CYP3A4. Both these mechanisms contribute to the increase in dofetilide plasma levels. There is a linear relationship between plasma dofetilide concentrations and prolongation of the QT interval, which increases the risk for torsade de pointes.[1]

Importance and management

An established interaction. Because of the likely increased risk of torsade de pointes, the maker contraindicates the use of ketoconazole in patients on dofetilide. This would seem to be a prudent precaution.

1. Tikosyn (Dofetilide). Pfizer Labs. US prescribing information, March 2004.
2. Tikosyn (Dofetilide). Pfizer US Pharmaceuticals. Product monograph, March 2002. Available at http:// http://www.tikosyn.com/pdf/prodmonograph.pdf (accessed 6 May 2004).

Dofetilide + Miscellaneous

The maker cautions about the use of various drugs that may have the potential to increase dofetilide plasma levels, so increasing the risk of QT prolongation and arrhythmias. Use with other drugs that prolong the QT interval should be avoided.

Clinical evidence, mechanism, importance and management

(a) Inhibitors/substrates for renal secretion

At least 50% of a dofetilide dose is eliminated unchanged in the urine by an active renal tubular secretion mechanism.[1,2] Some drugs that inhibit this mechanism have been shown to increase dofetilide plasma levels (e.g. see 'Dofetilide + H_2-blockers', p.167). The maker contraindicates their concurrent use since there is a linear relationship between plasma dofetilide concentrations and prolongation of the QT interval, which is a risk factor for torsade de pointes arrhythmias.[1] The maker also contraindicates the use of other drugs that inhibit the renal mechanism by which dofetilide is eliminated, such as **prochlorperazine** and **megestrol**,[1] although these have not been directly studied. Furthermore, the maker suggests[1] that there is a potential for dofetilide plasma levels to be increased by other drugs undergoing active renal secretion (e.g. **amiloride, metformin** and **triamterene**), but this needs confirmation in direct studies (see also 'Dofetilide + Diuretics', p.167). Until then, these drugs should be used cautiously with dofetilide.

(b) Inhibitors of hepatic metabolism

Dofetilide is also partially metabolised by the liver, primarily by cytochrome P450 isoenzyme CYP3A4.[3] The maker suggests[1] that there is a potential for dofetilide plasma levels to be increased by inhibitors of cytochrome P450 isoenzyme CYP3A4, and this has been shown for 'ketoconazole', (p.168). They recommend caution with other CYP3A4 inhibitors.

(c) Other drugs that prolong the QT interval

Dofetilide is a class III antiarrhythmic that prolongs the QT interval and can cause torsade de pointes arrhythmia. In general, use of two or more drugs that prolong the QT interval should be avoided. See also 'Drugs that prolong the QT interval + Other drugs that prolong the QT interval', p.170.

1. Tikosyn (Dofetilide). Pfizer Labs. US prescribing information, March 2004.
2. Rasmussen HS, Allen MJ, Blackburn KJ, Butrous GS, Dalrymple HW. Dofetilide, a novel class III antiarrhythmic agent. *J Cardiovasc Pharmacol* (1992) 20 (Suppl 2), S96–S105.
3. Walker DK, Alabaster CT, Congrave GS, Hargreaves MB, Hyland R, Jones BC, Reed LJ, Smith DA. Significance of metabolism in the disposition and action of the antidysrhythmic drug, dofetilide. *In vitro* studies and correlation with *in vivo* data. *Drug Metab Dispos* (1996) 24, 447–55.

Dofetilide + Omeprazole

Omeprazole appears not to interact with dofetilide.

Clinical evidence, mechanism, importance and management

A study in 12 healthy subjects found that pre-treatment with omeprazole 40 mg (10 or 2 hours before dofetilide) did not affect the pharmacokinetics of a single 500-microgram dose of dofetilide nor the dofetilide-induced change in QTc interval.[1] No special precautions appear to be necessary.

1. Vincent J, Gardner MJ, Baris B, Willavize SA. Concurrent administration of omeprazole and antacid does not alter the pharmacokinetics and pharmacodynamic of dofetilide in healthy subjects. *Clin Pharmacol Ther* (1996) 59, 182.

Dofetilide + Phenytoin

There does not appear to be any interaction between dofetilide and phenytoin.

Clinical evidence, mechanism, importance and management

In one study, 24 healthy subjects were stabilised on phenytoin to achieve steady-state plasma levels of 8 to 20 micrograms/ml and then either dofetilide 500 micrograms twice daily or placebo was given. No changes in phenytoin pharmacokinetics or cardiac effects were seen.[1] Another study by the same researchers in 24 subjects given dofetilide 500 micrograms 12-hourly found that the concurrent use of phenytoin 300 mg daily did not have a clinically important effect on either the pharmacokinetics of the dofetilide or on its cardiovascular pharmacodynamics (QTc, PR, QRS, RR intervals).[2]

These findings confirm those of an *in vitro* study[3] showing that dofetilide did not inhibit the cytochrome P450 isoenzyme CYP2C9, thus suggesting that dofetilide is unlikely to affect the metabolism of phenytoin. In addition, phenytoin is unlikely to affect the metabolism of dofetilide, since dofetilide is primarily metabolised by cytochrome P450 isoenzyme CYP3A4.[3] No special precautions appear to be necessary.

1. Vincent J, Gardner M, Scavone J, Ashton H, Willavize S, Friedman HL. The effect of dofetilide on the steady-state PK and cardiac effects of phenytoin in healthy subjects. *Clin Pharmacol Ther* (1997) 61, 233.
2. Gardner MJ, Ashton HM, Willavize SA, Friedman HL, Vincent J. The effects of phenytoin on the steady-state PK and PD of dofetilide in healthy subjects. *Clin Pharmacol Ther* (1997) 61, 205.
3. Walker DK, Alabaster CT, Congrave GS, Hargreaves MB, Hyland R, Jones BC, Reed LJ, Smith DA. Significance of metabolism in the disposition and action of the antidysrhythmic drug, dofetilide. *In vitro* studies and correlation with *in vivo* data. *Drug Metab Dispos* (1996) 24, 447–55.

Dofetilide + Theophylline

There does not appear to be any interaction between theophylline and dofetilide.

Clinical evidence, mechanism, importance and management

Studies in healthy subjects found that the concurrent use of theophylline 450 mg every 12 hours and dofetilide 500 micrograms every 12 hours did not alter the steady-state pharmacokinetics of either drug.[1,2] In addition, the increase in the QTc interval was no greater with the combination than with dofetilide alone.[1] No special precautions appear to be necessary.

1. Gardner MJ, Ashton HM, Willavize SA, Vincent J. The effects of concomitant dofetilide therapy on the pharmacokinetics and pharmacodynamics of theophylline. *Clin Pharmacol Ther* (1996) 59, 181.
2. Gardner MJ, Ashton HM, Willavize SA, Vincent J. The effects of orally administered theophylline on the pharmacokinetics and pharmacodynamics of dofetilide. *Clin Pharmacol Ther* (1996) 59, 182.

Table 7.3 Drugs causing QT prolongation and torsade de pointes

Drug class	*Drugs*	*Refs*
Antiarrhythmics	Class Ia (e.g. Disopyramide, Procainamide, Quinidine) Class III (e.g. Amiodarone, Dofetilide,* Ibutilide,* Sotalol*)	1–4, 6
Antibacterials	Macrolides: Clarithromycin, Erythromycin (intravenous), Spiramycin Quinolones: Gatifloxacin, Grepafloxacin,* Moxifloxacin, Sparfloxacin	2–4, 6, 7
Antimalarials	Artemether, Chloroquine, Halofantrine,* Quinine	1–4
Antiprotozoals	Pentamidine (intravenous)	2–4
Antivirals	Amantadine overdose	4
Antidepressants	Maprotiline overdose, Tricyclics (e.g. Amitriptyline, Desipramine, Imipramine)	2–4
Antihistamines	Astemizole,* Terfenadine* (usually when metabolism inhibited)	1–4, 6
Antipsychotics	Chlorpromazine, Droperidol,* Haloperidol, Lithium toxicity, Mesoridazine,* Pimozide,* Sertindole,* Thioridazine*	1–5
Miscellaneous	Cloral hydrate in overdosage, Bepridil, Cisapride* (usually when metabolism inhibited), Ketanserin, Levactymethadol, Organophosphates (poisoning), Probucol, Suxamethonium (Succinylcholine), Tacrolimus, Tamoxifen, Vasopressin	2–4, 6

* indicates drug suspended/restricted in some countries because of this effect.
This list is not exhaustive.

1. Committee on Safety of Medicines/Medicines Control Agency. Drug-induced prolongation of the QT interval. *Current Problems* (1996) 22, 2.
2. Thomas SHL. Drugs, QT interval abnormalities and ventricular arrhythmias. *Adverse Drug React Toxicol Rev* (1994) 13, 77–102.
3. De Ponti F, Poluzzi E, Montanaro N. QT-interval prolongation by non-cardiac drugs: lessons to be learned from recent experience. *Eur J Clin Pharmacol* (2000) 56, 1–18.
4. Haverkamp W, Breithardt G, Camm AJ, Janse MJ, Rosen MR, Antzelevitch C, Escande D, Franz M, Malik M, Moss A, Shah R. The potential for QT prolongation and pro-arrhythmia by non-anti-arrhythmic drugs: clinical and regulatory implications. Report on a policy conference of the European Society of Cardiology. *Cardiovasc Res* (2000) 47, 219–33.
5. Glassman AH, Bigger JT. Antipsychotic drugs: prolonged QTc interval, torsade de pointes, and sudden death. *Am J Psychiatry* (2001) 158, 1774–82.
6. Bednar MM, Harrigan EP, Anziano RJ, Camm AJ, Ruskin JN. The QT interval. *Prog Cardiovasc Dis* (2001) 43 (Suppl 1): 1–45.
7. Shaffer D, Singer S, Korvick J, Honig P. Concomitant risk factors in reports of torsade de pointes associated with macrolide use: review of the United States Food and Drug Administration Adverse Event Reporting System. *Clin Infect Dis* (2002) 35, 197–200.

Dofetilide + Trimethoprim

Trimethoprim markedly increases the plasma levels of dofetilide. This is likely to be associated with an increased risk of dofetilide-induced QT prolongation and torsade de pointes.

Clinical evidence, mechanism, importance and management

The maker of dofetilide notes that trimethoprim 160 mg (in combination with **sulfamethoxazole** 800 mg) twice daily administered concurrently with dofetilide 500 micrograms twice daily for 4 days increased dofetilide peak levels by 93% and AUC by 103%.[1] Trimethoprim inhibits the active renal tubular secretion mechanism by which dofetilide is eliminated, so reducing its loss from the body (see also 'Dofetilide + H_2-blockers', p.167). There is a linear relationship between plasma dofetilide concentrations and prolongation of the QT interval, which increases the risk of torsade de pointes arrhythmia.[1] For this reason, the maker contraindicates the use of trimethoprim in patients on dofetilide. This would seem to be a prudent precaution.

1. Tikosyn (Dofetilide). Pfizer Labs. US prescribing information, March 2004.

Dofetilide + Verapamil

Verapamil transiently increases dofetilide plasma levels and QTc prolongation, and has been associated with an increased risk of torsade de pointes. Its combined use with dofetilide is contraindicated.

Clinical evidence

A study in 12 healthy subjects found that concurrent administration of verapamil 80 mg three times daily and dofetilide 500 micrograms twice daily for 3 days caused a 42% increase in the peak plasma levels of dofetilide from 2.4 to 3.43 nanograms/ml. There was an increase in the 0 to 4 hour AUC from 7.4 to 9.3 nanograms.hour/ml, which was associated with a transient simultaneous increase in QTc of 20 milliseconds for dofetilide alone and 26 milliseconds for the combination. However, the 0 to 8 hour AUC was not significantly different.[1] The maker notes that an analysis of clinical trial data for dofetilide revealed a higher occurrence of torsade de pointes when verapamil was used with dofetilide.[2]

Mechanism

Verapamil is postulated to interact with dofetilide by increasing the rate of absorption of dofetilide by increasing hepatic blood flow.[1] There is a linear relationship between plasma dofetilide concentrations and prolongation of the QT interval, which is a risk factor for torsade de pointes.[2]

Importance and management

The concomitant use of verapamil with dofetilide appears to be associated with a transient increase in dofetilide plasma concentrations, and an increased risk of torsade de pointes. For this reason, the combination is contraindicated.

1. Johnson BF, Cheng SL, Venitz J. Transient kinetic and dynamic interactions between verapamil and dofetilide, a class III antiarrhythmic. *J Clin Pharmacol* (2001) 41, 1248–56.
2. Tikosyn (Dofetilide). Pfizer Labs. US prescribing information, March 2004.

Drugs that prolong the QT interval + Drugs that lower potassium levels

The combined use of drugs that can cause hypokalaemia (e.g. amphotericin, corticosteroids, thiazide and loop diuretics, and stimulant laxatives) and drugs that prolong the QT interval (e.g. class Ia and class III antiarrhythmics–see 'Table 7.3', (above)) should be well monitored because hypokalaemia increases the risk of torsade de pointes arrhythmias. There appear to be only a few re-

ports of this interaction, for example, see 'Beta-blockers; Sotalol + Potassium-depleting drugs', p.646.

Drugs that prolong the QT interval + Other drugs that prolong the QT interval

The consensus of opinion is that the concurrent use of two or more drugs that prolong the QT interval should be avoided because of the risk of additive effects, leading to the possible development of serious and potentially life-threatening torsade de pointes cardiac arrhythmia.

Clinical evidence, mechanism, importance and management

If the QT interval on the ECG becomes excessively prolonged, ventricular arrhythmias can develop, in particular a type of polymorphic tachycardia known as 'torsade de pointes'. On the ECG this arrhythmia can appear as an intermittent series of rapid spikes during which the heart fails to pump effectively, the blood pressure falls and the patient will feel dizzy and may possibly lose consciousness. Usually the condition is self-limiting but it may progress and degenerate into ventricular fibrillation, which can cause sudden death.

There are a number of reasons why QT interval prolongation can occur. These include congenital conditions, cardiac disease and some metabolic disturbances (hypokalaemia, hypomagnesaemia), but probably the most important cause is the use of various drugs including some antiarrhythmics, antipsychotics, antihistamines, antimalarials and others. These drugs all appear to cause this effect by blocking the rapid component of the delayed rectifier (repolarisation) potassium channel.

It is thought that torsade de pointes arrhythmia is unlikely to develop until the corrected QT (QTc) interval exceeds 500 milliseconds, but this is not an exact figure and the risks are uncertain and unpredictable. Because of these uncertainties, many drug manufacturers and regulatory agencies now contraindicate the concurrent use of drugs known to prolong the QT interval, and a 'blanket' warning is often issued because the QT prolonging effects of the drugs are expected to be additive. The extent of the drug-induced prolongation usually depends on the dosage of the drug and the particular drugs in question.

'Table 7.3', (p.169) is a list of drugs (derived from the sources indicated[1-6]) that are known to prolong the QT interval and cause torsade de pointes. Note that this list is not exhaustive of all the drugs that have ever been reported to be associated with QT interval prolongation and torsade de pointes. For some of the drugs listed, QT prolongation is a fairly frequent effect when the drug is used alone, and it is well accepted that use of these drugs requires careful monitoring (e.g. a number of the antiarrhythmics). For other drugs, QT prolongation is rare, but because of the relatively benign indications for these drugs, the risk-benefit ratio is considered poor, and use of these drugs has been severely restricted or discontinued (e.g. astemizole, terfenadine, cisapride). For others there is less clear evidence of the risk of QT prolongation (e.g. cloral hydrate, lithium, tacrolimus, tamoxifen, tricyclic antidepressants). Specific reports of additive QT prolonging effects with or without torsade de pointes are covered in individual monographs. See the Index.

Drugs that do not themselves prolong the QT interval, but potentiate the effect of drugs that do (e.g. by pharmacokinetic mechanisms, or lowering serum potassium) are not included in 'Table 7.3', (p.169). The interactions of these drugs (e.g. azole antifungals with cisapride, astemizole, or terfenadine, and potassium-depleting diuretics with sotalol) are dealt with in individual monographs. See the Index. However, note that some drugs, for example the macrolide antibacterials, may cause QT prolongation by dual mechanisms—they appear to have both the intrinsic ability to prolong the QT interval, and they may inhibit the metabolism of drug that prolong the QT interval.[7]

1. Committee on Safety of Medicines/Medicines Control Agency. Drug-induced prolongation of the QT interval. *Current Problems* (1996) 22, 2.
2. Thomas SHL. Drugs, QT interval abnormalities and ventricular arrhythmias. *Adverse Drug React Toxicol Rev* (1994) 13, 77–102.
3. De Ponti F, Poluzzi E, Montanaro N. QT-interval prolongation by non-cardiac drugs: lessons to be learned from recent experience. *Eur J Clin Pharmacol* (2000) 56, 1–18.
4. Haverkamp W, Breithardt G, Camm AJ, Janse MJ, Rosen MR, Antzelevitch C, Escande D, Franz M, Malik M, Moss A, Shah R. The potential for QT prolongation and pro-arrhythmia by non-anti-arrhythmic drugs: clinical and regulatory implications – Report on a policy conference of the European Society of Cardiology. *Cardiovasc Res* (2000) 47, 219–33.
5. Glassman AH, Bigger JT. Antipsychotic drugs: prolonged QTc interval, torsade de pointes, and sudden death. *Am J Psychiatry* (2001) 158, 1774–82.
6. Bednar MM, Harrigan EP, Anziano RJ, Camm AJ, Ruskin JN. The QT interval. *Prog Cardiovasc Dis* (2001) 43 (Suppl 1), 1–45.
7. Shaffer D, Singer S, Korvick J, Honig P. Concomitant risk factors in reports of torsades de pointes associated with macrolide use: review of the United States Food and Drug Administration Adverse Event Reporting System. *Clin Infect Dis* (2002) 35, 197–200.

Flecainide + Amiodarone

Serum flecainide levels are increased by amiodarone. The flecainide dosage should be reduced by between one-third and one-half. An isolated report describes torsade de pointes in a patient on amiodarone when given flecainide.

Clinical evidence

Seven patients on oral flecainide 200 to 500 mg daily were given reduced doses when amiodarone was added (1200 mg daily for 10 to 14 days as a loading dose, later reduced to 600 mg daily) because it was observed that the trough plasma levels of flecainide were increased by about 50%. The flecainide dosage was reduced by one-third (averaging a reduction from 325 to 225 mg daily) to keep the flecainide levels constant. Observations in two patients suggest that the interaction begins soon after the amiodarone is added, and it takes two weeks or more to develop fully.[1]

Other authors have reported this interaction, and suggest reducing the flecainide dosage by between one-third to one-half when amiodarone is added.[2-5] Another study found that amiodarone raised steady-state flecainide plasma levels by 37% in extensive metabolisers, and 55% in poor metabolisers, of dextromethorphan (a probe drug for cytochrome P450 isoenzyme CYP2D6 activity).[6] In a later report of this study the authors concluded that these differences were not clinically important, and that CYP2D6 phenotype does not affect the extent of the flecainide-amiodarone interaction.[7] An isolated report describes torsade de pointes in a patient on amiodarone when given flecainide.[8]

Mechanism

Amiodarone inhibits the cytochrome P450 isoenzyme CYP2D6, so that the flecainide is metabolised by the liver more slowly. Amiodarone also inhibits CYP2D6-independent mechanisms of flecainide elimination.[7]

Importance and management

An established interaction, but the documentation is limited. Reduce the flecainide dosage by one-third to one-half if amiodarone is added.[1-5,7] The makers of flecainide recommend a 50% reduction in dose if amiodarone is given, and that adverse effects and plasma flecainide levels should be monitored.[9,10] There seems to be no need to treat extensive metabolisers differently from poor metabolisers.[7] Remember that the interaction may take two weeks or more to develop fully, and also that amiodarone is cleared from the body exceptionally slowly so that this interaction may persist for some weeks after it has been withdrawn.

1. Shea P, Lal R, Kim SS, Schechtman K, Ruffy R. Flecainide and amiodarone interaction. *J Am Coll Cardiol* (1986) 7, 1127–30.
2. Leclercq JF, Coumel P. La flécaïnide: un nouvel antiarythmique. *Arch Mal Coeur* (1983) 76, 1218–29.
3. Fontaine G, Frank R, Tonet JL. Association amiodarone-flécaïnide dans le traitement des troubles du rythme ventriculaires graves. *Arch Mal Coeur* (1984) 77, 1421.
4. Leclercq JF, Coumel P. Association amiodarone-flécaïnide dans le traitement des troubles du rythme ventriculaires graves. Résponse. *Arch Mal Coeur* (1984) 77, 1421–2.
5. Leclercq JF, Denjoy I, Mentré F, Coumel P. Flecainide acetate dose-concentration relationship in cardiac arrhythmias: influence of heart failure and amiodarone. *Cardiovasc Drugs Ther* (1990) 4, 1161–65.
6. Funck-Brentano C, Kroemer HK, Becquemont L, Bühl K, Eichelbaum M, Jaillon P. The interaction between amiodarone and flecainide is genetically determined. *Circulation* (1992) 86, (Suppl I), I–720.
7. Funck-Brentano C, Becquemont L, Kroemer HK, Bühl K, Knebel NG, Eichelbaum M, Jaillon P. Variable disposition kinetics and electrocardiographic effects of flecainide during repeated dosing in humans: contribution of genetic factors, dose-dependent clearance, and interaction with amiodarone. *Clin Pharmacol Ther* (1994) 55, 256–69.
8. Andrivet P, Beaslay V, Canh VD. Torsades de pointe with flecainide-amiodarone therapy. *Intensive Care Med* (1990) 16, 342–3.
9. Tambocor (Flecainide). 3M Health Care Ltd. UK Summary of product characteristics, July 2003.
10. Tambocor (Flecainide). 3M Pharmaceuticals. US Prescribing information, June 1998.

Flecainide + Antacids or Food

The absorption of flecainide is not significantly altered if taken with food or an aluminium hydroxide antacid in adults, but it may possibly be reduced by milk in infants.

Clinical evidence, mechanism, importance and management

Neither food nor three 15-ml doses of *Aldrox* (280 mg **aluminium hydroxide** per 5 ml) had any significant effect on the rate or extent of absorption of a single 200-mg dose of flecainide in healthy adult subjects.[1] No special precautions seem necessary if they are taken together.

A premature baby being treated for refractory atrio-ventricular tachycardia with high doses of flecainide (40 mg/kg daily or 25 mg six-hourly) developed flecainide toxicity (seen as ventricular tachycardia) when his **milk feed** was replaced by **5% dextrose**. His serum flecainide levels approximately doubled, the conclusion being that the **milk** had reduced the absorption.[2] **Milk**-fed infants on high doses may therefore possibly need a reduced flecainide dosage if **milk** is reduced or stopped. Monitor the effects.

1. Tjandra-Maga TB, Verbesselt R, Van Hecken A, Mullie A, De Schepper PJ. Flecainide: single and multiple oral dose kinetics, absolute bioavailability and effect of food and antacid in man. *Br J Clin Pharmacol* (1986) 22, 309–16.
2. Russell GAB, Martin RP. Flecainide toxicity. *Arch Dis Child* (1989) 64, 860–2.

Flecainide + Anticonvulsants

Limited data suggest phenytoin or phenobarbital may modestly increase flecainide clearance, but this may not be clinically important.

Clinical evidence, mechanism, importance and management

Preliminary findings of a controlled study in 6 epileptic patients on **phenytoin** or **phenobarbital** showed that the pharmacokinetics of a single 2-mg/kg intravenous dose of flecainide were not statistically different from those in a group of 7 healthy subjects. A 25 to 30% shorter flecainide half-life and urine clearance of unchanged drug was noted. The authors[1] say that this change may not require any adjustment in the flecainide dosage.

1. Pentikäinen PJ, Halinen MO, Hiepakorpi S, Chang SF, Conard GJ, McQuinn RL. Pharmacokinetics of flecainide in patients receiving enzyme inducers. *Acta Pharmacol Toxicol (Copenh)* (1986) 59 (Suppl 5), 91.

Flecainide + Beta-blockers

For mention of the possible additive cardiac depressant effects, see 'Beta-blockers + Flecainide', p.634.

Flecainide + Cimetidine

Cimetidine can increase flecainide plasma levels.

Clinical evidence

After taking cimetidine 1 g daily for a week, the AUC of a single 200-mg dose of flecainide was increased by 28% in 8 healthy volunteers. The fraction of flecainide excreted unchanged in the urine was increased by 20%, but the total renal clearance was not altered.[1] In another study, cimetidine 1 g for 5 days almost doubled the plasma flecainide levels measured 2 hours after the morning dose in 11 patients taking flecainide 200 mg daily.[2]

Mechanism

Uncertain, but it is thought that the cimetidine reduces the hepatic metabolism of flecainide.[1,2]

Importance and management

An established but not extensively documented interaction. The clinical importance appears not to have been assessed, but be alert for the need to reduce the flecainide dosage if cimetidine is added. Caution is recommended in patients with impaired renal function, as the interaction is likely to be enhanced.[1]

1. Tjandra-Maga TB, Van Hecken A, Van Melle P, Verbesselt R, De Schepper PJ. Altered pharmacokinetics of oral flecainide by cimetidine. *Br J Clin Pharmacol* (1986) 22, 108–110.
2. Nitsch J, Köhler U, Neyses L, Lüderitz B. Flecainid-Plasmakonzentraionen bei Hemmung des hepatischen Metabolismus durch Cimetidin. *Klin Wochenschr* (1987) 65 (Suppl IX), 250.

Flecainide + Colestyramine

An isolated report describes reduced plasma flecainide levels in a patient given colestyramine. Studies in other subjects failed to demonstrate any interaction.

Clinical evidence, mechanism, importance and management

A patient taking flecainide 100 mg twice daily had unusually low trough plasma levels (100 nanograms/ml) while taking colestyramine. When he stopped taking the colestyramine 4 g three times daily his plasma flecainide levels rose. However a later study in 3 healthy subjects given flecainide 100 mg once daily and colestyramine 4 g three times daily, found little or no evidence of an interaction (steady-state flecainide levels of 63.1 and 59.1 nanograms/ml without and with colestyramine respectively). *In vitro* studies also failed to demonstrate any binding between flecainide and colestyramine that might result in reduced absorption from the gut.[1] The authors however postulate that the citric acid contained in the colestyramine formulation might have altered the urinary pH, which could have increased the renal clearance of the flecainide.[1]

Information seems to be limited to this preliminary report. Its general importance seems to be minor, nevertheless the outcome of concurrent use should be monitored so that any unusual cases can be identified.

1. Stein H, Hoppe U. Is there an interaction between flecainide and cholestyramine? *Naunyn Schmiedebergs Arch Pharmacol* (1989) 339 (Suppl), R114.

Flecainide + Quinidine or Quinine

Quinidine and quinine cause a modest reduction in the loss of flecainide from the body.

Clinical evidence, mechanism, importance and management

(a) Quinidine

A single 50-mg oral dose of quinidine given the night before a single 150-mg intravenous dose of flecainide decreased the flecainide clearance by 23% in 6 healthy subjects. The flecainide half-life was increased by 22% and its AUC by 28%.[1] In another study, 5 patients who were extensive metabolisers of the cytochrome P450 isoenzyme CYP2D6 and on chronic flecainide treatment were given quinidine 50 mg six-hourly for 5 days. The plasma levels and clearance of S-(+)-flecainide were unchanged, but plasma levels of R-(–)-flecainide increased by approximately 15% and its clearance reduced by 15%. The effects of the flecainide were slightly but not significantly increased.[2] Quinidine inhibits CYP2D6, which is concerned with the metabolism of flecainide. The clinical importance of this interaction is uncertain, but it is probably minor.

(b) Quinine

Three 500-mg doses of quinine administered over 24 hours increased the AUC of a single 150-mg intravenous infusion of flecainide (given over 30 minutes) by 21% (from 196 to 237 micrograms.minute/ml) and reduced the systemic clearance by 16.5% (from 9.1 to 7.6 ml/minute.kg) in 10 healthy subjects. Renal clearance remained unchanged. The increases in the PR and QRS intervals caused by flecainide were slightly, but not significantly, increased by quinine.[3] The evidence suggests that quinine reduces the metabolism of flecainide.[3] The clinical importance of this interaction is uncertain but a slight increase in the serum levels of flecainide would be expected, accompanied by some, probably minor, changes in its effects.

1. Munafo A, Buclin T, Tuto D, Biollaz J. The effect of a low dose of quinidine on the disposition of flecainide in healthy volunteers. *Eur J Clin Pharmacol* (1992) 43, 441–3.

2. Birgersdotter UM, Wong W, Turgeon J, Roden DM. Stereoselective genetically-determined interaction between chronic flecainide and quinidine in patients with arrhythmias. *Br J Clin Pharmacol* (1992) 33, 275–80.
3. Munafo A, Reymond-Michel G, Biollaz J. Altered flecainide disposition in healthy volunteers taking quinine. *Eur J Clin Pharmacol* (1990) 38, 269–73.

Flecainide + Tobacco smoking

Tobacco smokers need larger doses of flecainide than non-smokers to achieve the same therapeutic effects.

Clinical evidence

Prompted by the chance observation that smokers appeared to have a reduced pharmacodynamic response to flecainide than non-smokers, a meta-analysis[1] was undertaken of the findings of 7 premarketing pharmacokinetic studies and 5 multicentre efficacy trials in which flecainide had been studied and in which the smoking habits of the subjects/patients had been also been recorded. In the pharmacokinetic studies, the clearance of flecainide was found to be approximately 50% higher in smokers than in non-smokers. In the efficacy studies, average clinically effective flecainide doses were found to be 338 mg daily for smokers and 288 mg daily for non-smokers, while trough plasma concentrations of flecainide were 1.74 and 2.18 nanograms/ml per mg dose for the smokers and non-smokers, respectively. This confirmed that smokers needed higher doses of flecainide to achieve the same steady-state serum levels.[1]

Mechanism

The probable reason is that some components of the tobacco smoke stimulate the cytochrome P450 enzymes in the liver concerned with the *O*-dealkylation of flecainide, so that it is cleared from the body more quickly.[1]

Importance and management

An established interaction. Smokers seem likely to need higher doses of flecainide than non-smokers, but the way in which this interaction was identified suggests that in practice no specific action needs to be taken to accommodate it.

1. Holtzman JL, Weeks CE, Kvam DC, Berry DA, Mottonen L, Ekholm BP, Chang SF, Conard GJ. Identification of drug interactions by meta-analysis of premarketing trials: The effect of smoking on the pharmacokinetic and dosage requirements for flecainide acetate. *Clin Pharmacol Ther* (1989) 46, 1–8.

Flecainide + Urinary acidifiers and alkalinisers

The loss of flecainide is increased if the urine is made acidic (e.g. with ammonium chloride) and reduced if the urine is made alkaline (e.g. with sodium bicarbonate). The clinical importance of these changes is not known.

Clinical evidence

Six healthy subjects were given single 300-mg oral doses of flecainide on two occasions: once after taking **ammonium chloride** 1 g orally every 3 hours, and 2 g at bedtime, for a total of 21 hours to make the urine acidic (pH range 4.4 to 5.4): and the second after taking 4 g **sodium bicarbonate** every 4 hours for a total of 21 hours (including night periods) to make the urine alkaline (pH range 7.4 to 8.3). Over the next 32 hours, 44.7% of unchanged flecainide appeared in the acidic urine, but only 7.4% in alkaline urine.[1] This compares with 25% found by other researchers when urinary pH was not controlled.[1] A later similar study from the same research group broadly confirmed these findings; the elimination half-life of the flecainide was 10.7 hours in acidic urine and 17.6 hours in alkaline urine.[2] Another study also confirmed the effect of urinary pH on the excretion of flecainide, and found that the fluid load and the urinary flow rate had little effect on flecainide excretion.[3]

Mechanism

In alkaline urine at pH 8, much of the flecainide exists in the kidney tubules in the non-ionised form (non-ionised fraction 0.04), which is therefore more readily reabsorbed. In acidic urine at pH 5 more exists in the ionised form (non-ionised fraction 0.0001), which is less readily reabsorbed and is therefore lost in the urine.[3]

Importance and management

Established interactions, but their clinical importance is still uncertain. The effects of these changes on the subsequent control of arrhythmias by flecainide in patients seem not to have been studied, but the outcome should be well monitored if patients are given drugs that alter urinary pH to a significant extent (such as ammonium chloride, sodium bicarbonate). Large doses of some antacids may possibly do the same, but nobody seems to have studied this.

1. Muhiddin KA, Johnston A, Turner P. The influence of urinary pH on flecainide excretion and its serum pharmacokinetics. *Br J Clin Pharmacol* (1984) 17, 447–51.
2. Johnston A, Warrington S, Turner P. Flecainide pharmacokinetics in healthy volunteers: the influence of urinary pH. *Br J Clin Pharmacol* (1985) 20, 333–8.
3. Hertrampf R, Gundert-Remy U, Beckmann J, Hoppe U, Elsäßer W, Stein H. Elimination of flecainide as a function of urinary flow rate and pH. *Eur J Clin Pharmacol* (1991) 41, 61–3.

Flecainide + Verapamil

Although flecainide and verapamil have been used together successfully, serious and potentially life-threatening cardiogenic shock and asystole have been seen in a few patients, because the cardiac depressant effects of the two drugs can be additive.

Clinical evidence

A man with triple coronary vessel disease and on flecainide 200 mg daily for recurrent ventricular tachycardia, developed severe cardiogenic shock within two days of increasing the flecainide dosage to 300 mg daily and one day of starting verapamil 80 mg daily. His blood pressure fell to 60/40 mmHg and he had an idioventricular rhythm of 88 bpm.[1] Another patient with atrial flutter and fibrillation was treated with digitalis and verapamil 120 mg three times daily. He was additionally given flecainide 150 mg daily for 10 days, but three days after the dosage was raised to 200 mg daily he fainted, and later developed severe bradycardia (15 bpm) and asystoles of up to 14 seconds. He later died.[1]

Another report describes atrioventricular block in a patient with a pacemaker when treated with digoxin, flecainide and verapamil.[2]

Two earlier studies in patients[3] and healthy subjects[4] had found that the pharmacokinetics of flecainide and verapamil were only minimally affected by concurrent use, but the PR interval was increased by both drugs and additive depressant effects were seen on heart contractility and AV conduction. No serious adverse responses occurred.

Mechanism

Flecainide and verapamil have little or no effects on the kinetics of each other,[3,4] but they can apparently have additive depressant effects on the heart (negative inotropic and chronotropic) in both patients and healthy subjects.[1,3,4] Verapamil alone[5,6] and flecainide alone[7,8] have been responsible for asystole and cardiogenic shock in a few patients. In the cases cited above[1-3] the cardiac depressant effects were particularly serious because the patients already had compromised cardiac function.

Importance and management

An established interaction, but the incidence of serious adverse effects is probably not great. The additive cardiac depressant effects are probably of little importance in many patients, but may represent 'the last straw' in a few who have seriously compromised cardiac function. The authors of the reports cited[1] advise careful monitoring if both drugs are used and emphasise the potential hazards of combining Class Ic antiarrhythmics and verapamil. See also 'Beta-blockers + Flecainide', p.634.

1. Buss J, Lasserre JJ, Heene DL. Asystole and cardiogenic shock due to combined treatment with verapamil and flecainide. *Lancet* (1992) 340, 546.
2. Tworek DA, Nazari J, Ezri M, Bauman JL. Interference by antiarrhythmic agents with function of electrical cardiac devices. *Clin Pharm* (1992) 11, 48–56.
3. Landau S, Hogan C, Butler B, Somberg J. The combined administration of verapamil and flecainide. *J Clin Pharmacol* (1988) 28, 909.
4. Holtzman JL, Finley D, Mottonen L, Berry DA, Ekholm BP, Kvam DC, McQuinn RL, Miller AM. The pharmacodynamic and pharmacokinetic interaction between single doses of flecainide acetate and verapamil: Effects on cardiac function and drug clearance. *Clin Pharmacol Ther* (1989) 46, 26–32.
5. Perrot B, Danchin N, De La Chaise AT. Verapamil: a cause of sudden death in a patient with hypertrophic cardiomyopathy. *Br Heart J* (1984) 51, 532–4.
6. Cohen IL, Fein A, Nabi A. Reversal of cardiogenic shock and asystole in a septic patient with hypertrophic cardiomyopathy on verapamil. *Crit Care Med* (1990) 18, 775–6.

7. Forbes WP, Hee TT, Mohiuddin SM, Hillman DE. Flecainide-induced cardiogenic shock. *Chest* (1988) 94, 1121.
8. Echt DS, Liebson PR, Mitchell LB, Peters RW, Obias-Manno D, Barker AH, Arensberg D, Baker A, Friedman L, Greene HL, Huther ML, Richardson DW, CAST investigators. Mortality and morbidity in patients receiving encainide, flecainide or placebo. *N Engl J Med* (1991) 324, 781–8.

Ibutilide + Amiodarone

Concurrent use of ibutilide and amiodarone would be expected to further prolong the QT interval and increase the risk of torsade de pointes, but one report describes their successful use for cardioversion.

Clinical evidence, mechanism, importance and management

When intravenous ibutilide 2 mg was used for cardioversion of atrial fibrillation or flutter in 70 patients on long-term amiodarone the QT interval was further prolonged (from 371 to 479 milliseconds). However, only one patient had an episode of nonsustained torsade de pointes. Ibutilide was effective within 30 minutes of infusion in 39% of patients with atrial flutter, and 54% of patients with fibrillation.[1] Both amiodarone and ibutilide are class III antiarrhythmics and prolong the QT interval, with the consequent risk of torsade de pointes. The maker recommends that they should not be used concurrently[2] (see also 'Drugs that prolong the QT interval + Other drugs that prolong the QT interval', p.170). However, the authors of the above report suggest that ibutilide may be useful for cardioversion in those already on amiodarone. Combined use should be very well monitored.

1. Glatter K, Yang Y, Chatterjee K, Modin G, Cheng J, Kayser S, Scheinman MM. Chemical cardioversion of atrial fibrillation or flutter with ibutilide in patients receiving amiodarone therapy. *Circulation* (2001) 103, 253–7.
2. Corvert (Ibutilide fumarate). Pharmacia & Upjohn. US Prescribing information. July 2002.

Ibutilide + Calcium channel blockers

Calcium channel blockers (predominantly non-dihydropyridine type) have not altered the safety or efficacy of ibutilide in clinical trials.

Clinical evidence, mechanism, importance and management

Retrospective analysis of three clinical trials showed that calcium channel blockers did not alter the ECG effects (QT prolongation) or the efficacy of ibutilide. In these three studies, 68 of the 130 patients on ibutilide were taking calcium channel blockers. The report did not specify which calcium channel blockers were used, except to say that only 12 of the 68 (19%) were taking a dihydropyridine-type.[1]

In vitro studies have shown that **nifedipine** (a dihydropyridine) attenuated the effects of ibutilide.[2] The findings of the above report[1] suggest that this may not be clinically important. However, since so few patients were taking a dihydropyridine, an effect specific to dihydropyridines cannot be excluded. Further study is needed.

1. Wood MA, Gilligan DM, Brown-Mahoney C, Nematzadeh F, Stambler BS, Ellenbogen KA. Clinical and electrophysiologic effects of calcium channel blockers in patients receiving ibutilide. *Am Heart J* (2002) 143, 176–80.
2. Lee KS, Lee EW. Ionic mechanism of ibutilide in human atrium: evidence for a drug-induced Na^+ current through a nifedipine inhibited inward channel. *J Pharmacol Exp Ther* (1998) 286, 9–22.

Ibutilide + Class Ic antiarrhythmics

Some evidence suggests that pretreatment with propafenone or flecainide attenuates the increase in QT interval seen with ibutilide without affecting efficacy.

Clinical evidence, mechanism, importance and management

The increase in QTc interval after intravenous ibutilide 2 mg was less in 6 patients treated with **propafenone** (5 patients) or **flecainide** (1 patient) than in 85 other patients who had received ibutilide alone (34 versus 65 milliseconds). The effect appeared to be dose-related, with higher propafenone doses causing the largest attenuation in the ibutilide-induced QT prolongation. The efficacy of ibutilide was unaltered.[1] Ibutilide, a class III antiarrhythmic, is well known to increase the QT interval, so increasing the risk of torsade de pointes arrhythmia. Class Ic antiarrhythmics such as **propafenone** and **flecainide** generally shorten the QT interval. It is possible that class Ic agents may usefully attenuate the risk of torsade de pointes with ibutilide,[1] but further study is needed.

1. Reiffel JA, Blitzer M. The actions of ibutilide and class Ic drugs on the slow sodium channel: new insights regarding individual pharmacologic effects elucidated through combination therapies. *J Cardiovasc Pharmacol Ther* (2000) 5, 177–81.

Ibutilide + Miscellaneous

Ibutilide can prolong the QT interval, therefore caution has been advised about the concurrent use of other drugs that can do the same. Ibutilide is reported not to interact with beta-blockers or digoxin.

Clinical evidence, mechanism, importance and management

No specific drug interaction studies appear to have been undertaken with ibutilide, which is a class III antiarrhythmic, but because it can prolong the QT interval it has been recommended that other drugs that can do the same should be administered with caution, because of the potential additive effects.[1] The maker of ibutilide specifically recommends that **class Ia** and other **class III antiarrhythmics** should not be given within 4 hours of an ibutilide infusion (but see also, 'Ibutilide + Amiodarone', above).[2] The concern is that a prolongation of the QT interval is associated with an increased risk of torsade de pointes arrhythmia, which is potentially life threatening. See also 'Drugs that prolong the QT interval + Other drugs that prolong the QT interval', p.170.

The concurrent use of **beta-blockers** and **digoxin** during clinical trials is reported not to affect the safety or efficacy of ibutilide.[1,2] Ibutilide is said not to affect cytochrome P450 isoenzymes CYP3A4 or CYP2D6 so that metabolic interactions with drugs affected by these enzymes would not be expected.[1] Study is needed to confirm all of these predictions and findings.

1. Cropp JS, Antal EG, Talbert RL. Ibutilide: a new Class III antiarrhythmic agent. *Pharmacotherapy* (1997) 17, 1–9.
2. Corvert (Ibutilide fumarate). Pharmacia & Upjohn. US Prescribing information. July 2002.

Lidocaine + Amiodarone

Isolated reports describe a seizure in one man on lidocaine about two days after starting to take amiodarone, and sinoatrial arrest in another man with sick sinus syndrome who was given both drugs. There is conflicting evidence as to whether or not amiodarone affects the pharmacokinetics of lidocaine.

Clinical evidence

(a) Effects on lidocaine levels, seizure

An elderly man taking digoxin, enalapril, amitriptyline and temazepam was treated for monomorphic ventricular tachycardia, firstly with procainamide, later replaced by a 2-mg/minute infusion of lidocaine, to which oral amiodarone 600 mg twice daily was added. After 12 hours his lidocaine level was 5.4 mg/l (therapeutic levels 1.5 to 5 mg/l), but 53 hours later he developed a seizure and his lidocaine level was found to have risen to 12.6 mg/l. A tomography brain scan showed no abnormalities that could have caused the seizure and it was therefore attributed to the toxic lidocaine levels.[1] Six patients with symptomatic cardiac arrhythmias took part in a two-phase study. Initially, lidocaine 1 mg/kg was given intravenously over 2 minutes. In phase I, loading doses of amiodarone 500 mg daily for 6 days were given, followed by the same lidocaine dose. After 19 to 21 days, when the total cumulative amiodarone dose was 13 g, the same lidocaine dose was given again (phase II). The lidocaine AUC increased by about 20% and the systemic clearance decreased by about 20%. The elimination half-life and distribution volume at steady-state were unchanged. The pharmacokinetic parameters of lidocaine in phase II were the same as those in phase I, indicating that the interaction occurs early in the loading phase of amiodarone administration.[2] This is in contrast to an earlier study, in which the pharmacokinetics of a bolus dose of lidocaine 1 mg/kg over 2 minutes were not altered in 10 patients after taking amiodarone 200 to 400 mg daily (following an loading dose of 800 or 1200 mg) for 4 to 5 weeks.[3]

(b) Sinoatrial arrest

An elderly man with long standing brady-tachycardia was successfully treated for atrial flutter firstly with a temporary pacemaker (later withdrawn) and 600 mg amiodarone daily. Ten days later, and 25 minutes after a permanent pacemaker was inserted under local anaesthesia with 15 ml of 2% lidocaine when the brachiocephalic vein was exposed, severe sinus bradycardia and long sinoatrial arrest developed. He was effectively treated with atropine plus isoprenaline, and cardiac massage.[4]

Mechanism

(a). An *in vitro* study has demonstrated that amiodarone may inhibit lidocaine metabolism competitively and *vice versa*. The interaction *in vivo* may be due to inhibition of the cytochrome P450 isoenzyme CYP3A4 by amiodarone and/or its main metabolite desethylamiodarone.[3] CYP3A4 is partially involved in the metabolism of lidocaine.

(b). The authors of the report suggest a synergistic depression by both drugs of the sinus node.

Importance and management

Evidence of a pharmacokinetic interaction between lidocaine and amiodarone is conflicting. However, the two reports of adverse interactions and the study in patients with arrhythmias illustrate the importance of good monitoring if both drugs are used.

1. Siegmund JB, Wilson JH, Imhoff TE. Amiodarone interaction with lidocaine. *J Cardiovasc Pharmacol* (1993) 21, 513–5.
2. Ha HR, Candinas R, Steiger B, Meyer UA, Follath F. Interactions between amiodarone and lidocaine. *J Cardiovasc Pharmacol* (1996) 28, 533–9.
3. Nattel S, Talajic M, Beaudoin D, Matthews C, Roy D. Absence of pharmacokinetic interaction between amiodarone and lidocaine. *Am J Cardiol* (1994) 73, 92–4.
4. Keidar S, Grenadier E, Palant A. Sinoatrial arrest due to lidocaine injection in sick sinus syndrome during amiodarone administration. *Am Heart J* (1982) 104, 1384–5.

Lidocaine + Barbiturates

Plasma lidocaine levels following slow intravenous injection may be modestly lower in patients who are taking barbiturates.

Clinical evidence

A single 2-mg/kg dose of lidocaine was administered by slow intravenous injection (rate about 100 mg over 15 minutes) to 7 epileptic patients, firstly while taking their usual antiepileptic drugs and sedatives (including phenytoin, barbiturates, phenothiazines, benzodiazepines) and secondly after taking only **phenobarbital** 300 mg daily for 4 weeks. The same lidocaine dose was also administered to 6 control subjects who had not received any drugs. Plasma lidocaine levels were 10 to 25% higher after **phenobarbital** treatment alone in the patients with epilepsy. When compared with the levels in the 6 control subjects, plasma lidocaine levels were somewhat lower in the patients, and this was statistically significant at 30 and 60 minutes (18 and 29% lower).[1]

Mechanism

Not fully understood. One suggestion is that the barbiturates increase the activity of the liver microsomal enzymes, thereby increasing the rate of metabolism of the lidocaine.[1]

Importance and management

Direct information is very limited. It may be necessary to increase the dosage of lidocaine to achieve the desired therapeutic response in patients on phenobarbital or other barbiturates.

1. Heinonen J, Takki S, Jarho L. Plasma lidocaine levels in patients treated with potential inducers of microsomal enzymes. *Acta Anaesthesiol Scand* (1970) 14, 89–95.

Lidocaine + Beta-blockers

The plasma levels of lidocaine can be increased by the concurrent use of propranolol. Isolated cases of toxicity attributed to this interaction have been reported. Nadolol possibly interacts similarly, but there is uncertainty about metoprolol. Atenolol and pindolol appear not to interact, but the need for an increased loading dosage of lidocaine in the presence of penbutolol has been suggested.

Clinical evidence

(a) Atenolol

A study with oral atenolol 50 mg daily found that it did not affect the clearance of lidocaine.[1]

(b) Metoprolol

In 6 healthy subjects metoprolol 100 mg twice daily for 2 days did not affect the pharmacokinetics of a single intravenous dose of lidocaine.[2] Similarly, another study in 7 healthy subjects failed to find any changes in the pharmacokinetics of a single oral or intravenous dose of lidocaine after one weeks' treatment with metoprolol 100 mg 12-hourly.[1] In contrast, another study found that the clearance of a single intravenous dose of lidocaine was reduced by 31% by one day's pretreatment with metoprolol 50 mg six-hourly.[3]

(c) Nadolol

A study in 6 healthy subjects receiving 30-hour infusions of lidocaine at a rate of 2 mg/minute showed that 3 days' pretreatment with nadolol 160 mg daily raised the steady-state plasma lidocaine levels by 28% (from 2.1 to 2.7 micrograms/ml) and reduced the plasma clearance by 17% (from 1030 to 850 ml/min).[4]

(d) Penbutolol

In 7 healthy subjects, penbutolol 60 mg daily significantly increased the volume of distribution of a single 100-mg intravenous dose of lidocaine, thus prolonging its elimination half-life. However, the reduction in clearance of lidocaine did not reach significance.[5]

(e) Pindolol

A study with intravenous pindolol 23 micrograms/kg found that it did not affect the clearance of lidocaine.[6]

(f) Propranolol

A study in 6 healthy subjects receiving 30-hour infusions of lidocaine at a rate of 2 mg/minute showed that 3 days' pretreatment with propranolol 80 mg eight-hourly raised the steady-state plasma lidocaine levels by 19% (from 2.1 to 2.5 micrograms/ml) and reduced the plasma clearance by 16% (1030 to 866 ml/min).[4] Other similar studies have found a 22.5 to 30% increase in steady-state serum lidocaine levels and a 14.7 to 46% fall in plasma clearance due to the concurrent use of propranolol.[3,6,7] Two cases of lidocaine toxicity attributed to a lidocaine-propranolol interaction were revealed by a search[8] of the FDA adverse drug reaction file in 1981. A further case of lidocaine toxicity (seizures) has been described in a man on propranolol after accidental *oral* ingestion of lidocaine for oesophageal anaesthesia. High serum levels of lidocaine were detected.[9]

(g) Unnamed beta-blockers

A matched study in 51 cardiac patients on a variety of beta-blockers (including **propranolol, metoprolol, timolol, pindolol**) found no significant differences in either total or free concentrations of lidocaine, but there was a trend towards an increase in the adverse effects of lidocaine (bradycardias) with concurrent beta-blocker treatment.[10]

Mechanism

Not fully agreed. There is some debate about whether the increased serum lidocaine levels largely occur because of the decreased cardiac output caused by the beta-blockers, which decreases the flow of blood through the liver thereby reducing the metabolism of the lidocaine,[4] or because of direct liver enzyme inhibition.[11] There may also be a pharmacodynamic interaction, with an increased risk of myocardial depression.[10]

Importance and management

The lidocaine/propranolol interaction is established and of clinical importance. Monitor the effects of concurrent use and reduce the lidocaine dosage if necessary to avoid toxicity. The situation with other beta-blockers is less clear. Nadolol appears to interact like propranolol, but it is uncertain whether metoprolol interacts or not. Atenolol and pindolol are reported not to interact pharmacokinetically. It has been suggested that a higher loading dose (but not a higher maintenance dose) of lidocaine may be needed if penbutolol is used.[5] The suggestion has been made that a significant pharmacokinetic interaction is only likely to occur with non-selective beta-blockers without intrinsic sympathomimetic activity[11] e.g. nadolol or propranolol. Until the situation is better defined it would be prudent to monitor the effects of concurrent use with any beta-blocker.

Note that local anaesthetic preparations of lidocaine often contain adrenaline (epinephrine), which may interact with beta-blockers, see 'Beta-blockers + Sympathomimetics; Directly-acting', p.643.

1. Miners JO, Wing LMH, Lillywhite KJ, Smith KJ. Failure of 'therapeutic' doses of β-adrenoceptor antagonists to alter the disposition of tolbutamide and lignocaine. *Br J Clin Pharmacol* (1984) 18, 853–60.
2. Jordö L, Johnsson G, Lundborg P, Regårdh C-G. Pharmacokinetics of lidocaine in healthy individuals pretreated with multiple dose of metoprolol. *Int J Clin Pharmacol Ther Toxicol* (1984) 22, 312–15.
3. Conrad KA, Byers JM, Finley PR, Burnham L. Lidocaine elimination: effects of metoprolol and of propranolol. *Clin Pharmacol Ther* (1983) 33, 133–8.
4. Schneck DW, Luderer JR, Davis D, Vary J. Effects of nadolol and propranolol on plasma lidocaine clearance. *Clin Pharmacol Ther* (1984) 36, 584–7.
5. Ochs HR, Skanderra D, Abernethy DR, Greenblatt DJ. Effect of penbutolol on lidocaine kinetics. *Arzneimittelforschung* (1983) 33, 1680–1.
6. Svendsen TL, Tangø M, Waldorff S, Steiness E, Trap-Jensen J. Effects of propranolol and pindolol on plasma lignocaine clearance in man. *Br J Clin Pharmacol* (1982) 13, 223S–226S.
7. Ochs HR, Carstens G, Greenblatt DJ. Reduction in lidocaine clearance during continuous infusion and by co administration of propranolol. *N Engl J Med* (1980) 303, 373–7.
8. Graham CF, Turner WM, Jones JK. Lidocaine-propranolol interactions. *N Engl J Med* (1981) 304, 1301.
9. Parish RC, Moore RT, Gotz VP. Seizures following oral lidocaine for esophageal anesthesia. *Drug Intell Clin Pharm* (1985) 19, 199–201.
10. Wyse DG, Kellen J, Tam Y, Rademaker AW. Increased efficacy and toxicity of lidocaine in patients on beta-blockers. *Int J Cardiol* (1988) 21, 59–70.
11. Bax NDS, Tucker GT, Lennard MS, Woods HF. The impairment of lignocaine clearance by propranolol—major contribution from enzyme inhibition. *Br J Clin Pharmacol* (1985) 19, 597–603.

Lidocaine + Cocaine

Limited evidence suggests lidocaine use in patients with cocaine-associated myocardial infarction is not associated with significant toxicity.

Clinical evidence, mechanism, importance and management

A retrospective study, covering a 6-year period in 29 hospitals, identified 29 patients (27 available for review) who received lidocaine for prophylaxis or treatment of cocaine-associated myocardial infarction. No patient exhibited bradycardia, sustained ventricular tachycardia or ventricular fibrillation, and no patients died.[1]

Both lidocaine and cocaine exhibit class I antiarrhythmic effects and are proconvulsants. Lidocaine may potentiate the cardiac and CNS side-effects of cocaine. Therefore the use of lidocaine for cocaine-associated myocardial infarction is controversial. The lack of adverse effects in this study may have been due to delays of more than 5 hours between last exposure to cocaine and lidocaine therapy. The authors concluded that the cautious use of lidocaine does not appear to be contraindicated in patients with cocaine-associated myocardial infarction who require antiarrhythmic therapy. However, extra care should be taken in patients who receive lidocaine shortly after cocaine.[1]

1. Shih RD, Hollander JE, Burstein JL, Nelson LS, Hoffman RS, Quick AM. Clinical safety of lidocaine in patients with cocaine-associated myocardial infarction. *Ann Emerg Med* (1995) 26, 702–6.

Lidocaine + Dextromethorphan

Lidocaine does not inhibit the activity of cytochrome P450 isoenzyme CYP2D6 and is therefore unlikely to interact with drugs that are metabolised by this isoenzyme.

Clinical evidence, mechanism, importance and management

Although *in vitro* data suggested that lidocaine inhibited oxidative metabolism reactions mediated by the cytochrome P450 isoenzyme CYP2D6, a later *in vivo* study in 16 patients found that, while being given an infusion of lidocaine (serum level range 3.2 to 55.9 micromol/l), the metabolism of a single 30-mg dose of dextromethorphan remained unchanged. All of the patients were of the extensive metaboliser phenotype. Since dextromethorphan is a well-established marker of CYP2D6 activity, it was concluded that lidocaine is unlikely to interact with drugs that are extensively metabolised by this isoenzyme.[1]

1. Bartoli A, Gatt G, Chimienti M, Corbellini D, Perrucca E. Does lidocaine affect oxidative dextromethorphan metabolism «in vivo»? *G Ital Chim Clin* (1993/4) 18, 125–9.

Lidocaine + Disopyramide

Laboratory studies show that disopyramide can increase the levels of unbound lidocaine, but whether in practice their combined effects have a clinically important cardiac depressant effect is not known.

Clinical evidence, mechanism, importance and management

An *in vitro* study using serum taken from 9 patients receiving lidocaine for severe ventricular arrhythmias showed that there was an average 20% increase in its free (unbound) fraction when disopyramide in a concentration of 14.7 micromol/l was added.[1] This appears to occur because disopyramide can displace lidocaine from its binding sites on plasma proteins (alpha-1-acid glycoprotein).

The importance of this possible displacement interaction in clinical practice is uncertain. The suggestion made by the authors[1] is that, although lidocaine has only a minor cardiac depressant effect, a transient 20% increase in levels of free and active lidocaine plus the negative inotropic effects of the disopyramide might possibly be hazardous in patients with reduced cardiac function.

1. Bonde J, Jensen NM, Burgaard P, Angelo HR, Graudal N, Kampmann JP, Pedersen LE. Displacement of lidocaine from human plasma proteins by disopyramide. *Pharmacol Toxicol* (1987) 60, 151–5.

Lidocaine + Erythromycin

Erythromycin may markedly increase plasma levels of oral lidocaine, but causes only a minor increase after intravenous lidocaine.

Clinical evidence

Nine healthy subjects were given erythromycin 500 mg three times daily or placebo daily for 4 days, in a randomised double-blind crossover study. Erythromycin increased the AUC and peak plasma levels of a single 1-mg/kg *oral* dose of lidocaine by 50 and 40% respectively. Erythromycin also markedly increased the AUC of the metabolite of lidocaine, monoethylglycinexylidide (MEGX) by 60%.[1] In a similar study,[2] erythromycin had no effect on the AUC or peak plasma level of a single 1.5-mg/kg intravenous dose of lidocaine, but still increased the AUC of MEGX by 70%. In yet another study, erythromycin ethylsuccinate 600 mg three times daily for 5 doses had a minor effect on the pharmacokinetics of a single 1-mg/kg intravenous dose of lidocaine (an 18% decrease in clearance), and caused a 33% increase in the AUC of MEGX. There was no difference in the results from the 10 healthy subjects and the 20 patients with biopsy proven cirrhosis.[3]

Mechanism

Erythromycin is an inhibitor of the cytochrome P450 isoenzyme CYP3A4, the isoenzyme partially involved in the metabolism of lidocaine. Erythromycin appears to markedly reduce the first-pass metabolism of orally administered lidocaine so that its plasma levels rise.[1] The increase in MEGX could be due to either an increase in the production of this metabolite, or the inhibition of its further metabolism.

Importance and management

Information seems limited, and since lidocaine is not usually given orally the practical importance is minor. However, lidocaine is used for oro-pharyngeal topical anaesthesia, and there have been cases of toxicity after accidental ingestion. Thus, in a patient on erythromycin, the toxicity of *oral* lidocaine may be markedly increased. Further study is required to assess the significance of the increase in MEGX during prolonged intravenous lidocaine infusions.

1. Isohanni MH, Neuvonen PJ, Olkkola KT. Effect of erythromycin and itraconazole on the pharmacokinetics of oral lignocaine. *Pharmacol Toxicol* (1999) 84, 143–6.
2. Isohanni MH, Neuvonen PJ, Palkama VJ, Olkkola KT. Effect of erythromycin and itraconazole on the pharmacokinetics of intravenous lignocaine. *Eur J Clin Pharmacol* (1998) 54, 561–5.
3. Orlando R, Piccoli P, De Martin S, Padrini R, Palatini P. Effect of the CYP3A4 inhibitor erythromycin on the pharmacokinetics of lignocaine and its pharmacologically active metabolites in subjects with normal and impaired liver function. *Br J Clin Pharmacol* (2003) 55, 86–93.

Lidocaine + H_2-blockers

Cimetidine modestly reduces the clearance of lidocaine and raises its serum levels in some patients. Lidocaine toxicity may occur if the dosage is not reduced. Ranitidine appears to interact minimally. See also 'Anaesthetics, local + H_2-blockers', p.896.

Clinical evidence

(a) Cimetidine in cardiac patients

In one study, 15 patients were given a 1-mg/kg loading dose of lidocaine intravenously followed by a continuous infusion of 2 or 3 mg/minute over 26 hours. At 6 hours they were started on cimetidine (initial dose 300 mg intravenously, then 300 mg six-hourly by mouth). After 26 hours (20 hours after cimetidine) the serum levels of lidocaine were 30% higher (5.6 micrograms/ml) than in a control group of 6 patients (4.3 micrograms/ml). The most substantial rise in levels occurred in the first 6 hours after cimetidine administration. Six patients developed toxic serum levels (over 5 micrograms/ml) and two (with levels of 10 and 11 micrograms/ml) experienced lethargy and confusion attributed to lidocaine toxicity, which disappeared when the lidocaine was stopped.[1]

A study in patients with suspected myocardial infarction given two 300-mg oral doses of cimetidine 4 hours apart, starting 11 to 20 hours after a 2 mg/minute infusion of lidocaine began, showed that total lidocaine serum levels had risen by 28%, and unbound levels by 18%, 24 hours after the initial cimetidine dose. In three of these patients whose diagnosis of myocardial infarction was subsequently confirmed, rises in total and unbound lidocaine serum levels of 24% and 9% occurred by 24 hours.[2] In contrast, a study in six patients with suspected myocardial infarction given lidocaine infusions, followed later by a cimetidine infusion, failed to find a significant increase in the plasma accumulation of lidocaine.[3]

An 89-year-old man with congestive heart failure taking cimetidine had two seizures 10 to 15 minutes after accidental *oral* ingestion of lidocaine solution for oesophageal anaesthesia. He had a high serum lidocaine level of 7.8 micrograms/ml.[4]

(b) Cimetidine in healthy subjects

A rise in peak serum lidocaine levels of 50% after intravenous administration was seen in a study in 6 healthy subjects given cimetidine 300 mg six-hourly for a day. Systemic clearance fell by about 25% (from 766 to 576 ml/minute) and 5 of the 6 experienced toxicity (light-headedness, paraesthesia).[5] Similarly, another study in healthy subjects taking cimetidine 1.2 g daily showed a 30% fall in lidocaine clearance after intravenous administration.[6] In contrast, in another study, cimetidine 1.2 g daily caused only an 18% fall in lidocaine clearance after intravenous administration, which did not reach statistical significance.[7] Similarly, oral cimetidine 300 mg four times daily caused a 15% reduction in intravenous lidocaine clearance under both single-dose and steady-state conditions, but this was not statistically significant. In this study, the effect of intravenous cimetidine 300 mg four times daily was less than that of the oral cimetidine.[8]

Cimetidine pretreatment increased the *oral* bioavailability of lidocaine by 35% in healthy subjects, and reduced the apparent oral clearance by 42%.[9] A study in healthy subjects showed that 2 days of cimetidine pretreatment increased the AUC of lidocaine by 52% after aerosol application of lidocaine 120 mg (12 sprays of *Xylocaine* 10%) to the oropharynx.[10]

(c) Ranitidine in healthy subjects

A study in 10 healthy subjects given 150 mg ranitidine twice daily for 5 days showed that it increased the systemic clearance of lidocaine by 9%, but did not alter the oral clearance.[11] Two other studies in healthy subjects given ranitidine 150 mg twice daily for one to 2 days found no change in the clearance of lidocaine given intravenously.[7,12]

Mechanism

Not established. It seems possible that the metabolism of the lidocaine is reduced both by a fall in blood flow to the liver and by direct inhibition of the activity of the liver microsomal enzymes. As a result its clearance is reduced and its serum levels rise.

Importance and management

The lidocaine/cimetidine interaction is well studied but controversial. It is confused by the differences between the studies (healthy subjects, patients with different diseases, different modes of drug administration, etc). A fall in the clearance of lidocaine (15% or more) and a resultant rise in the serum levels should be looked for if cimetidine is used, but a clinically significant alteration may not occur in every patient. It may possibly be of less importance in patients following a myocardial infarction because of the increased amounts of alpha-1-acid glycoprotein which alter the levels of bound and free lidocaine.[2] Monitor all patients closely for evidence of toxicity and check serum lidocaine levels regularly. A reduced infusion rate may be needed. Ranitidine would appear to be a suitable alternative to cimetidine. See also 'Anaesthetics, local + H_2-blockers', p.896.

1. Knapp AB, Maguire W, Keren G, Karmen A, Levitt B, Miura DS, Somberg JC. The cimetidine-lidocaine interaction. *Ann Intern Med* (1983) 98, 174–7.
2. Berk SI, Gal P, Bauman JL, Douglas JB, McCue JD, Powell JR. The effect of oral cimetidine on total and unbound serum lidocaine concentrations in patients with suspected myocardial infarction. *Int J Cardiol* (1987) 14, 91–4.
3. Patterson JH, Foster J, Powell JR, Cross R, Wargin W, Clark JL. Influence of a continuous cimetidine infusion on lidocaine plasma concentrations in patients. *J Clin Pharmacol* (1985) 25, 607–9.
4. Parish RC, Moore RT, Gotz VP. Seizures following oral lidocaine for esophageal anesthesia. *Drug Intell Clin Pharm* (1985) 19, 199–201.
5. Feely J, Wilkinson GR, McAllister CB, Wood AJJ. Increased toxicity and reduced clearance of lidocaine by cimetidine. *Ann Intern Med* (1982) 96, 592–4.
6. Bauer LA, Edwards WAD, Randolph FP, Blouin RA. Cimetidine-induced decrease in lidocaine metabolism. *Am Heart J* (1984) 108, 413–15.
7. Jackson JE, Bentley JB, Glass SJ, Fukui T, Gandolfi AJ, Plachetka JR. Effects of histamine-2 receptor blockade on lidocaine kinetics. *Clin Pharmacol Ther* (1985) 37, 544–8.
8. Powell JR, Foster J, Patterson JH, Cross R, Wargin W. Effect of duration of lidocaine infusion and route of cimetidine administration on lidocaine pharmacokinetics. *Clin Pharm* (1986) 5, 993–8.
9. Wing LMH, Miners JO, Birkett DJ, Foenander T, Lillywhite K, Wanwimolruk S. Lidocaine disposition—sex differences and effects of cimetidine. *Clin Pharmacol Ther* (1984) 35, 695–701.
10. Parish RC, Gotz VP, Lopez LM, Mehta JL, Curry SH. Serum lidocaine concentrations following application to the oropharynx: effects of cimetidine. *Ther Drug Monit* (1987) 9, 292–7.
11. Robson RA, Wing LMH, Miners JO, Lillywhite KJ, Birkett DJ. The effect of ranitidine on the disposition of lignocaine. *Br J Clin Pharmacol* (1985) 20, 170–3.
12. Feely J, Guy E. Lack of effect of ranitidine on the disposition of lignocaine. *Br J Clin Pharmacol* (1983) 15, 378–9.

Lidocaine + Itraconazole

Itraconazole may markedly increase plasma levels of lidocaine after oral administration, but not after intravenous administration.

Clinical evidence

Nine healthy subjects were given either itraconazole 200 mg once daily or placebo for 4 days, in a randomised double-blind crossover study. Itraconazole increased the AUC and peak plasma levels of a single 1-mg/kg oral dose of lidocaine by 75 and 55% respectively. Itraconazole did not affect the concentration of the lidocaine metabolite, monoethylglycinexylidide (MEGX).[1] In a similar study, itraconazole had no effect on the AUC and peak plasma levels of lidocaine or MEGX after a single 1.5-mg/kg intravenous dose of lidocaine.[2]

Mechanism

Itraconazole is an inhibitor of cytochrome P450 isoenzyme CYP3A4, which is partially involved in the metabolism of lidocaine. Itraconazole appears to markedly reduce the first-pass metabolism of orally administered lidocaine so that its plasma levels rise.[1]

Importance and management

Information seems to be limited, and since lidocaine is not usually given orally the practical importance is minor. However, lidocaine is used for oro-pharyngeal topical anaesthesia, and there have been cases of toxicity after accidental ingestion. In patients on itraconazole, the toxicity of oral lidocaine may be markedly increased.

1. Isohanni MH, Neuvonen PJ, Olkkola KT. Effect of erythromycin and itraconazole on the pharmacokinetics of oral lignocaine. *Pharmacol Toxicol* (1999) 84, 143–6.
2. Isohanni MH, Neuvonen PJ, Palkama VJ, Olkkola KT. Effect of erythromycin and itraconazole on the pharmacokinetics of intravenous lignocaine. *Eur J Clin Pharmacol* (1998) 54, 561–5.

Lidocaine + Mexiletine

Mexiletine may increase the toxicity of lidocaine.

Clinical evidence, mechanism, importance and management

Lidocaine CNS toxicity occurred within one hour of administration of a total of 600 mg of oral lidocaine in a patient with cardiomyopathy who was receiving mexiletine 300 mg twice daily. Her lidocaine concentration was raised at 26.9 micrograms/ml.[1] Similarly, involuntary motion and muscular stiffness occurred in a man treated with oral mexiletine and an intravenous infusion of lidocaine for one day.[2] Studies in *animals* have shown that the concurrent use of mexiletine and intravenous lidocaine resulted in a decrease in total clearance of lidocaine and an increase in plasma levels. It appeared that this was due to mexiletine displacing the tissue binding of lidocaine and reducing its distribution.[3] Mexiletine is an oral lidocaine analogue, so it is perhaps not surprising the two drugs may interact. The combination should be used with caution, especially during the initial stages of treatment. Where possible, lidocaine levels should be closely monitored.

1. Geraets DR, Scott SD, Ballew KA. Toxicity potential of oral lidocaine in a patient receiving mexiletine. *Ann Pharmacother* (1992) 26, 1380–1.
2. Christie JM, Valdes C, Markowsky SJ. Neurotoxicity of lidocaine combined with mexiletine. *Anesth Analg* (1993) 77, 1291–4.
3. Maeda Y, Funakoshi S, Nakamura M, Fukuzawa M, Kugaya Y, Yamasaki M, Tsukiai S, Murakami T, Takano M. Possible mechanism for pharmacokinetic interaction between lidocaine and mexiletine. *Clin Pharmacol Ther* (2002) 71, 389–97.

Lidocaine + Omeprazole

Omeprazole does not appear to alter the pharmacokinetics of lidocaine.

Clinical evidence, mechanism, importance and management

Omeprazole 40 mg daily for one week did not affect the AUC or half-life of lidocaine or its metabolite methylglycinexylidine when a single 1-mg/kg intravenous dose of lidocaine was given to 10 healthy subjects.[1] This study suggests that no special precautions are required during concurrent use.

1. Noble DW, Bannister J, Lamont M, Andersson T, Scott DB. The effect of oral omeprazole on the disposition of lignocaine. *Anaesthesia* (1994) 49, 497–500.

Lidocaine + Phenytoin

The incidence of central toxic side-effects may be increased following the concurrent intravenous infusion of lidocaine and phenytoin. Sinoatrial arrest has been reported in one patient. In patients taking phenytoin, serum lidocaine levels may be slightly reduced when given intravenously, but markedly reduced if given orally.

Clinical evidence

(a) Cardiac depression and increased side-effects

A study in 5 patients with suspected myocardial infarction given lidocaine 0.5 to 3 mg/minute intravenously for at least 24 hours, followed by additional intravenous injections or infusions of phenytoin, showed that plasma levels of both drugs remained unchanged but the incidence of adverse effects (vertigo, nausea, nystagmus, diplopia, impaired hearing) were unusually high.[1]

Sinoatrial arrest occurred in a man with heart block following a suspected myocardial infarction, after he received lidocaine 1 mg/kg given intravenously over 1 minute, followed 3 minutes later by phenytoin 250 mg given over 5 minutes. The patient lost consciousness and his blood pressure could not be measured, but he responded to 200 micrograms of isoprenaline (isoproterenol).[2]

(b) Serum lidocaine levels

In the study described above,[1] intravenous phenytoin had no effect on plasma lidocaine levels during continuous infusion. However, in another study, lidocaine 2 mg/kg was given intravenously to 7 epileptic patients taking their usual anticonvulsants (including phenytoin, barbiturates, phenothiazines, benzodiazepines), and to 6 control subjects. Plasma lidocaine levels were 27 and 43% lower in the epileptic patients at 30 and 60 minutes.[3] Another study found that the clearance of intravenous lidocaine was slightly greater in patients taking anticonvulsants than in healthy subjects (850 compared with 770 ml/minute) but this difference was not statistically significant.[4] Other studies in epileptic patients and healthy subjects have shown that when taking phenytoin the bioavailability of *oral* lidocaine was halved.[4,5]

Mechanism

(a). Phenytoin and lidocaine appear to have additive cardiac depressant actions.

(b). The reduced lidocaine serum levels is possibly due to liver enzyme induction; when lidocaine is given orally the marked reduction in levels results from the stimulation of hepatic first-pass metabolism by phenytoin.[4,5] In addition, patients taking anticonvulsants including phenytoin had higher plasma concentrations of alpha-1-acid glycoprotein, which may result in a lower free fraction of lidocaine in the plasma.[6]

Importance and management

Information is limited and the importance of this interaction is not well established. (a) The case of sinoatrial arrest emphasises the need to exercise caution when giving two drugs that have cardiac depressant actions. (b) The reduction in serum lidocaine levels after intravenous administration in patients taking anticonvulsants, including phenytoin, is small and appears not to be of any clinical significance. Since lidocaine is not usually given orally, the practical importance of the marked reduction in bioavailability would also seem to be small.

1. Karlsson E, Collste P, Rawlins MD. Plasma levels of lidocaine during combined treatment with phenytoin and procainamide. *Eur J Clin Pharmacol* (1974) 7, 455–9.
2. Wood RA. Sinoatrial arrest: an interaction between phenytoin and lignocaine. *BMJ* (1971) i, 645.
3. Heinonen J, Takki S, Jarho L. Plasma lidocaine levels in patients treated with potential inducers of microsomal enzymes. *Acta Anaesthesiol Scand* (1970) 14, 89–95.
4. Perucca E, Richens A. Reduction of oral bioavailability of lignocaine by induction of first pass metabolism in epileptic patients. *Br J Clin Pharmacol* (1979) 8, 21–31.
5. Perucca E, Hedges A, Makki KA, Richens A. A comparative study of antipyrine and lignocaine disposition in normal subjects and in patients treated with enzyme-inducing drugs. *Br J Clin Pharmacol* (1980) 10, 491–7.
6. Routledge PA, Stargel WW, Finn AL, Barchowsky A, Shand DG. Lignocaine disposition in blood in epilepsy. *Br J Clin Pharmacol* (1981) 12, 663–6.

Lidocaine + Procainamide

An isolated case of delirium has been described in a patient given lidocaine and procainamide.

Clinical evidence, mechanism, importance and management

A man with paroxysmal tachycardia, treated with oral procainamide 1 g five-hourly and increasing doses of lidocaine by intravenous infusion (550 mg within 3.5 hours), became restless, noisy and delirious when given a further 250 mg intravenous dose of procainamide.[1] The symptoms disappeared within 20 minutes of discontinuing the lidocaine. The reason is not understood but the symptoms suggest that the neurotoxic effects of the two drugs might be additive. Other studies in patients have shown that lidocaine plasma levels are unaffected by intravenous or oral procainamide.[2]

1. Ilyas M, Owens D, Kvasnicka G. Delirium induced by a combination of anti-arrhythmic drugs. *Lancet* (1969) ii, 1368–9.
2. Karlsson E, Collste P, Rawlins MD. Plasma levels of lidocaine during combined treatment with phenytoin and procainamide. *Eur J Clin Pharmacol* (1974) 7, 455–9.

Lidocaine + Propafenone

Propafenone has minimal effects on the pharmacokinetics of lidocaine, but the severity and duration of the CNS adverse effects are increased.

Clinical evidence, mechanism, importance and management

Twelve healthy subjects, who had been taking 225 mg propafenone 8-hourly for 4 days, were given a continuous infusion of lidocaine

2 mg/kg/hour for 22 hours. The AUC of the lidocaine was increased by 7% (from 76.3 to 81.7 micrograms.h/ml) and the clearance was reduced by 7% (from 10.27 to 9.53 ml/min/kg) by the propafenone. One poor metaboliser of propafenone showed an increase in lidocaine clearance. Increases in the PR and QRS intervals of 10 to 20% were also seen. Combined use increased the severity and duration of adverse effects (lightheadedness, dizziness, paraesthesia, lethargy, somnolence). One subject withdrew from the study as a result.[1] In another study, combined infusion of lidocaine (100 mg bolus then a 2 mg/minute infusion) and propafenone (1 or 2 mg/kg) produced a minor additional negative inotropic effect (which was not statistically significant) and reversed the prolongation in atrial and ventricular refractoriness produced by propafenone alone.[2]

There would therefore appear to be no marked or important pharmacokinetic interaction between these two drugs, but the increased CNS side-effects may be poorly tolerated by some individuals, and cardiac depressant effects may be additive.

1. Ujhelyi MR, O'Rangers EA, Fan C, Kluger J, Pharand C, Chow MSS. The pharmacokinetic and pharmacodynamic interaction between propafenone and lidocaine. *Clin Pharmacol Ther* (1993) 53, 38–48.
2. Feld GK, Nademanee K, Singh BN, Kirsten E. Hemodynamic and electrophysiologic effects of combined infusion of lidocaine and propafenone in humans. *J Clin Pharmacol* (1987) 27, 52–9.

Lidocaine + Rifampicin (Rifampin)

Serum lidocaine levels may be reduced to a minor extent by rifampicin.

Clinical evidence, mechanism, importance and management

Rifampicin 600 mg daily for 6 days increased the clearance of lidocaine by 15% in 10 healthy subjects after they were given a single 50-mg intravenous dose. In addition, plasma concentrations of the lidocaine metabolite monoethylglycinexylidide (MEGX) increased by 34%, although this did not reach statistical significance.[1] Using cultured human hepatocytes it was found that rifampicin increases the metabolism of lidocaine, probably because the rifampicin induces the cytochrome P450 isoenzyme CYP3A4, which is partially concerned with the metabolism of lidocaine to MEGX.[2] These modest changes in lidocaine pharmacokinetics are unlikely to be of much importance, particularly as the lidocaine dose is usually titrated to effect.

1. Reichel C, Skodra T, Nacke A, Spengler U, Sauerbruch T. The lignocaine metabolite (MEGX) liver function test and P-450 induction in humans. *Br J Clin Pharmacol* (1998) 46, 535–9.
2. Li AP, Rasmussen A, Xu L, Kaminski DL. Rifampicin induction of lidocaine metabolism in cultured human hepatocytes. *J Pharmacol Exp Ther* (1995) 274, 673–7.

Lidocaine + Tobacco smoking

Smoking reduces the bioavailability of oral but not intravenous lidocaine.

Clinical evidence, mechanism, importance and management

A study in healthy subjects found that the bioavailability of oral lidocaine was markedly reduced in smokers (AUCs of 15.2 and 47.9 in smokers and non-smokers respectively) but when given intravenously only moderate changes were seen.[1] The reason for the changes is probably due to liver enzyme induction caused by components of tobacco smoke. With oral lidocaine this could result in increased first-pass hepatic clearance. In the case of intravenous lidocaine, first-pass clearance is bypassed, and the enzyme induction was opposed by a smoking-related decrease in hepatic flow. In practical terms this interaction is unlikely to be of much importance because lidocaine is usually titrated to the needs of the patient.

1. Huet P-M, Lelorier J. Effects of smoking and chronic hepatitis B on lidocaine and indocyanine green kinetics. *Clin Pharmacol Ther* (1980) 28, 208–15.

Lidocaine + Tocainide

A report describes a tonic-clonic seizure that occurred in a man during the period when his treatment for arrhythmia with lidocaine was being changed to tocainide.

Clinical evidence, mechanism, importance and management

An elderly man treated with furosemide and co-trimoxazole experienced a tonic-clonic seizure while his treatment with lidocaine was being changed to tocainide, although the serum levels of both antiarrhythmics remained within their therapeutic ranges. The patient became progressively agitated and disorientated about 2 hours after taking the second of two 600 mg (six-hourly) oral doses of tocainide while still receiving lidocaine 2 mg/minute intravenously, and about 1 hour later he had the seizure. The patient subsequently tolerated each drug separately, at concentrations similar to those that preceded the seizure, without problems.[1] A study in *animals*[2] showed that tocainide reduced the lidocaine serum levels at which seizures occurred by about 45%. The maker notes that concomitant use of lidocaine and tocainide may cause an increased incidence of adverse effects, including CNS adverse reactions such as seizure, since the two drugs have similar pharmacodynamic effects.[3] Great care must therefore be exercised if tocainide is given during lidocaine administration.

1. Forrence E, Covinsky JO, Mullen C. A seizure induced by concurrent lidocaine-tocainide therapy — Is it just a case of additive toxicity? *Drug Intell Clin Pharm* (1986) 20, 56–9.
2. Schuster MR, Paris PM, Kaplan RM, Stewart RD. Effect on the seizure threshold in dogs of tocainide/lidocaine administration. *Ann Emerg Med* (1987) 16, 749–51.
3. Tonocard (Tocainide). AstraZeneca. US prescribing information, September 2000.

Mexiletine + Amiodarone

Amiodarone does not affect the clearance of mexiletine. The concurrent use of mexiletine and amiodarone can be clinically useful.

Clinical evidence, mechanism, importance and management

The clearance of mexiletine in 10 patients did not differ before and after 1, 3 and 5 months concurrent use of amiodarone. In addition, the clearance of mexiletine did not differ between these patients and 155 other patients not on amiodarone.[1]

Torsade de pointes has been described in a patient taking amiodarone and mexiletine (a class Ib antiarrhythmic).[2] The makers of mexiletine say that this seems to be an isolated case.[3]

Class Ib antiarrhythmics are usually associated with shortening of the QT interval, and could therefore be expected to reduce the QT prolongation and risk of torsade de pointes seen with amiodarone alone (for examples of this effect of mexiletine see also 'Mexiletine + Beta-blockers', p.179 and 'Mexiletine + Quinidine', p.180. However, note that the UK makers of mexiletine[4] say that it may exacerbate arrhythmias [as all antiarrhythmics may], but also that it may be used concurrently with amiodarone. The two drugs have been used together successfully.[5,6]

1. Yonezawa E, Matsumoto K, Ueno K, Tachibana M, Hashimoto H, Komamura K, Kamakura S, Miyatake K, Tanaka K. Lack of interaction between amiodarone and mexiletine in cardiac arrhythmia patients. *J Clin Pharmacol* (2002) 42, 342–6.
2. Tartini R, Kappenberger L, Steinbrunn W. Gefährliche Interaktionen zwischen Amiodaron und Antiarrhythmika der Klasse I. *Schweiz Med Wochenschr* (1982) 112, 1585–7.
3. Boehringer Ingelheim. Personal Communication, July 1995.
4. Mexitil (Mexiletine). Boehringer Ingelheim Ltd. UK Summary of product characteristics, October 1999.
5. Waleffe A, Mary-Rabine L, Legrand V, Demoulin JC, Kulbertus HE. Combined mexiletine and amiodarone treatment of refractory recurrent ventricular tachycardia. *Am Heart J* (1980) 100, 788–93.
6. Hoffmann A, Follath F, Burckhardt D. Safe treatment of resistant ventricular arrhythmias with a combination of amiodarone and quinidine or mexiletine. *Lancet* (1983) i, 704–5.

Mexiletine + Antacids, Atropine or Metoclopramide

The absorption of mexiletine is slowed by almasilate and atropine and hastened by metoclopramide, but the extent of the absorption is unaltered.

Clinical evidence, mechanism, importance and management

Oral administration of the antacid almasilate (*Gelusil*) one hour before a single 400-mg dose of mexiletine resulted in a slight delay in absorption (time to maximum concentration prolonged from 1.7 to 2.9 hours), but had no effect on the extent of absorption in healthy subjects.[1]

A study in 8 healthy subjects found that a single 600-microgram dose of intravenous atropine reduced, and 10 mg of intravenous metoclopramide hastened, the rate of absorption of single 400-mg oral doses of mexiletine, but the mexiletine AUC remained unaffected. Intravenous metoclopramide tended to reverse the effect of diamorphine on plasma mexiletine levels in one clinical trial[2] (see also 'Mexiletine + Opioids', below).

Since the achievement of steady-state mexiletine levels depends on the extent of absorption, not on its rate, it seems very unlikely that these drugs will affect the antiarrhythmic effects of mexiletine during chronic dosing.[3] However, these drugs may cause variations in the antiarrhythmic effects of initial oral mexiletine doses, which may be a problem if rapid control of the arrhythmia is essential. In general, no special precautions would appear necessary.

1. Herzog P, Holtermüller KH, Kasper W, Meinertz T, Trenk D, Jähnchen E. Absorption of mexiletine after treatment with gastric antacids. *Br J Clin Pharmacol* (1982) 14, 746–7.
2. Smyllie HC, Doar JW, Head CD, Leggett RJ. A trial of intravenous and oral mexiletine in acute myocardial infarction. *Eur J Clin Pharmacol* (1984) 26, 537–42.
3. Wing LMH, Meffin PJ, Grygiel JJ, Smith KJ, Birkett DJ. The effect of metoclopramide and atropine on the absorption of orally administered mexiletine. *Br J Clin Pharmacol* (1980) 9, 505–9.

Mexiletine + Beta-blockers

The concurrent use of mexiletine and beta-blockers can be clinically useful. Mexiletine may reduce the QT prolonging effects of sotalol.

Clinical evidence, mechanism, importance and management

A study in 4 patients showed that a combination of mexiletine and **propranolol** 240 mg daily was more effective in blocking ventricular premature depolarisation (VPD) and ventricular tachycardia than mexiletine alone, and did not increase adverse effects. Plasma mexiletine concentrations were not changed significantly by **propranolol**.[1] Similar efficacy was reported for **metoprolol** with mexiletine.[2] Success in decreasing VPDs was noted in 30% of 44 patients taking mexiletine plus a beta-blocker (unspecified) compared with only 14% of 185 subjects taking mexiletine alone.[3] The UK makers of mexiletine state that it may be used concurrently with beta-blockers.[4]

A study in *animals* showed that mexiletine reduced the QT prolonging effect of **sotalol** and reduced the risk of torsade de pointes.[5]

1. Leahey EB, Heissenbuttel RH, Giardina E-GV, Bigger JT. Combined mexiletine and propranolol treatment of refractory ventricular tachycardia. *BMJ* (1980) 281, 357–8.
2. Ravid S, Lampert S, Graboys TB. Effect of the combination of low-dose mexiletine and metoprolol on ventricular arrhythmia. *Clin Cardiol* (1991) 14, 951–5.
3. Bigger JT. The interaction of mexiletine with other cardiovascular drugs. *Am Heart J* (1984) 107, 1079–85.
4. Mexitil (Mexiletine). Boehringer Ingelheim Ltd. UK Summary of product characteristics, October 1999.
5. Chézalveil-Guilbert F, Davy J-M, Poirier J-M, Weissenburger J. Mexiletine antagonizes effects of sotalol on QT interval duration and its proarrhythmic effects in a canine model of torsade de pointes. *J Am Coll Cardiol* (1995) 26, 787–92.

Mexiletine + Ciprofloxacin

Ciprofloxacin slightly reduces the clearance of mexiletine.

Clinical evidence, mechanism, importance and management

Preliminary results of a study in healthy subjects showed that the oral clearance of mexiletine was reduced by about 7 to 15% when a single dose was given on day 3 of a 5-day course of ciprofloxacin 750 mg twice daily. This was due to a decrease in the metabolic clearance of mexiletine, presumed to be because of ciprofloxacin-induced inhibition of the cytochrome P450 isoenzyme CYP1A2, which is involved in the metabolism of mexiletine.[1] It is unlikely that changes of this magnitude would be clinically relevant, but further study is needed to confirm this.

1. Labbé L, Lefez C, Gilbert M, O'Hara G, Turgeon J. Ciprofloxacin (CIPRO) decreases mexiletine (MEX) clearance in smokers and non-smokers. *Clin Pharmacol Ther* (1995) 57, 210.

Mexiletine + Fluconazole

Fluconazole does not interact pharmacokinetically with mexiletine.

Clinical evidence, mechanism, importance and management

Six healthy subjects were given single 200-mg doses of mexiletine before and after taking fluconazole 200 mg daily for 7 days. Two of the subjects were given fluconazole 400 mg daily for a further 7 days. No significant changes in the pharmacokinetics of mexiletine were seen.[1] The clinical outcome of concurrent use in patients was not examined, but there appear to be no adverse reports in the literature. No special precautions appear to be necessary if these drugs are used concurrently.

1. Ueno K, Yamaguchi R, Tanaka K, Sakaguchi M, Morishima Y, Yamauchi K, Iwai A. Lack of a kinetic interaction between fluconazole and mexiletine. *Eur J Clin Pharmacol* (1996) 50, 129–31.

Mexiletine + H_2-blockers

No adverse interaction occurs if mexiletine and cimetidine or ranitidine are given concurrently. Cimetidine can reduce the gastric side-effects of mexiletine.

Clinical evidence, mechanism, importance and management

The peak and trough plasma mexiletine levels of 11 patients were unaltered when they were given **cimetidine** 1.2 g daily for a week, and the frequency and severity of the ventricular arrhythmias for which they were receiving treatment remained unchanged. Moreover the gastric side-effects of mexiletine were reduced in half of the patients.[1] This study in patients confirms the findings of two other studies using **cimetidine** or **ranitidine** in healthy subjects.[2,3] There would seem to be no problems associated with giving these drugs concurrently, and some advantages.

1. Klein AL, Sami MH. Usefulness and safety of cimetidine in patients receiving mexiletine for ventricular arrhythmia. *Am Heart J* (1985) 109, 1281–6.
2. Klein A, Sami M, Selinger K. Mexiletine kinetics in healthy subjects taking cimetidine. *Clin Pharmacol Ther* (1985) 37, 669–73.
3. Brockmeyer NH, Breithaupt H, Ferdinand W, von Hattingberg M, Ohnhaus EE. Kinetics of oral and intravenous mexiletine: lack of effect of cimetidine and ranitidine. *Eur J Clin Pharmacol* (1989) 36, 375–8.

Mexiletine + Omeprazole

Omeprazole does not appear to interact pharmacokinetically with mexiletine.

Clinical evidence, mechanism, importance and management

A crossover study in 9 healthy Japanese men found that when they were given mexiletine 200 mg after taking omeprazole 40 mg daily for 8 days, the mexiletine serum concentrations and its AUCs remained unchanged. It was concluded that omeprazole does not affect the metabolism of mexiletine,[1] and no special precautions would seem to be needed if these drugs are used concurrently.

1. Kusumoto M, Ueno K, Tanaka K, Takeda K, Mashimo K, Kameda T, Fujimura Y, Shibakawa M. Lack of pharmacokinetic interaction between mexiletine and omeprazole. *Ann Pharmacother* (1998) 32, 182–4.

Mexiletine + Opioids

The absorption of mexiletine is reduced in patients following a myocardial infarction, and very markedly reduced and delayed if diamorphine or morphine is used concurrently. A higher loading dose may be needed if oral mexiletine is required as an antiarrhythmic agent during the first few hours following a myocardial infarction.

Clinical evidence

A pharmacokinetic study showed that the mean plasma levels of mexiletine (400 mg orally followed by 200 mg 2 hours later) in the first 3 hours were more than 50% lower in 6 patients who had suffered a myocardial infarction and who had been given **diamorphine** 5 to 10 mg or **morphine** 10 to 15 mg than in 4 patients who had not been given opioids. In addition, the 0 to 8 hour AUC was 38.6% lower in those who had received opioids.[1]

In a further study about the prophylactic use of mexiletine, the same authors found that plasma mexiletine levels 3 hours after the first oral dose were 31% lower in 10 patients who had received opioids than in 6 patients who had not. These patients were from a subset who were subsequently shown not to have had a myocardial infarction.[1] In another similar trial of mexiletine in acute myocardial infarction, use of **diamorphine** was associated with low plasma mexiletine levels at 3 hours, and possible reduced efficacy of mexiletine. In this study, pretreatment with intravenous metoclopramide tended to reduce the effect of **diamorphine** on mexiletine absorption,[2] although this was not noted in the above study.[1]

Mechanism

The reduced absorption of mexiletine would seem to result from inhibition of gastric emptying by the opioids. Other mechanisms probably contribute to its delayed clearance.

Importance and management

An established interaction although information is limited. The delay and reduction in the absorption would seem to limit the value of oral mexiletine during the first few hours after a myocardial infarction, particularly if opioid analgesics are used. The maker suggests that a higher loading dose of oral mexiletine may be preferable in this situation. Alternatively, an intravenous dose of mexiletine may be given. In addition, they note that it may be necessary to titrate the dose against therapeutic effects and adverse effects.[3]

1. Pottage A, Campbell RWF, Achuff SC, Murray A, Julian DC, Prescott LF. The absorption of oral mexiletine in coronary care patients. *Eur J Clin Pharmacol* (1978) 13, 393–9.
2. Smyllie HC, Doar JW, Head CD, Leggett RJ. A trial of intravenous and oral mexiletine in acute myocardial infarction. *Eur J Clin Pharmacol* (1984) 26, 537–42.
3. Mexitil (Mexiletine). Boehringer Ingelheim Ltd. UK Summary of product characteristics, October 1999.

Mexiletine + Phenytoin

Plasma mexiletine levels are reduced by the concurrent use of phenytoin. An increase in the dosage may be necessary.

Clinical evidence

The observation that 3 patients had unusually low plasma mexiletine levels while taking phenytoin prompted a pharmacokinetic study in 6 healthy subjects. After taking 300 mg phenytoin daily for a week, the mean mexiletine AUC and half-life following single 400-mg doses were reduced by an average of about 50% (AUC reduced from 17.7 to 8 micrograms/ml/h; half-life reduced from 17.2 to 8.4 hours).[1]

Mechanism

The most likely explanation is that phenytoin, a potent liver enzyme-inducing agent, particularly of the cytochrome P450 isoenzyme CYP1A2, by which mexiletine is metabolised, increases the metabolism and clearance of mexiletine from the body.

Importance and management

Information seems to be limited to this report[1] but the interaction appears to be established. It seems likely that the fall in mexiletine levels will be clinically important in some individuals. Monitor the plasma mexiletine levels and raise the dosage if necessary.

1. Begg EJ, Chinwah PM, Webb C, Day RO, Wade DN. Enhanced metabolism of mexiletine after phenytoin administration. *Br J Clin Pharmacol* (1982) 14, 219–23.

Mexiletine + Propafenone

Propafenone raises mexiletine serum levels in extensive metabolisers of the cytochrome P450 isoenzyme CYP2D6.

Clinical evidence, mechanism, importance and management

In one study in healthy subjects, propafenone reduced mexiletine clearance and increased plasma mexiletine concentrations in those subjects with extensive cytochrome P450 isoenzyme CYP2D6 activity, but had no effect in those of the poor metaboliser phenotype. The pharmacokinetics of mexiletine in extensive metabolisers after propafenone treatment became the same as those in poor metabolisers.[1] Mexiletine did not affect propafenone pharmacokinetics.[1] In this study, overall changes in ECG parameters were minor during concurrent administration of mexiletine and propafenone.[1] Propafenone is an inhibitor of CYP2D6, and inhibits the metabolism of mexiletine by this pathway.[1] Although the use of the combination was not associated with significant ECG changes, the potentiation of drug effects could predispose to proarrhythmias in patients with ischaemic heart disease. The authors suggest that slow dose titration of the combination may decrease the risk of adverse effects.[1] The UK maker[2] notes that it may be necessary to reduce the dose of mexiletine when used concurrently with drugs causing inhibition of hepatic enzymes, especially CYP1A2 and CYP2D6.

1. Labbé L, O'Hara G, Lefebvre M, Lessard É, Gilbert M, Adedoyin A, Champagne J, Hamelin B, Turgeon J. Pharmacokinetic and pharmacodynamic interaction between mexiletine and propafenone in human beings. *Clin Pharmacol Ther* (2000) 68, 44–57.
2. Mexitil (Mexiletine). Boehringer Ingelheim Ltd. UK Summary of product characteristics, October 1999.

Mexiletine + Quinidine

The concurrent use of mexiletine and quinidine can be clinically useful. Mexiletine limited the quinidine-induced increase in QT interval. Quinidine raises mexiletine serum levels in extensive metabolisers of cytochrome P450 isoenzyme CYP2D6.

Clinical evidence, mechanism, importance and management

Mexiletine and quinidine given concurrently were reported to be more effective than either drug alone, and the incidence of adverse effects was reduced. Mexiletine limited the quinidine-induced increase in QT interval.[1] A study in *animals* concluded the benefit of combined use may be due to prolonged refractoriness and conduction time in the peri-infarct zone.[2] Two studies[3,4] in healthy subjects have shown that quinidine reduced the metabolism and excretion of mexiletine in extensive metabolisers of the cytochrome P450 isoenzyme CYP2D6 (total clearance reduced by 24%[4]), but not poor metabolisers. Quinidine is an inhibitor of CYP2D6, and inhibits the metabolism of mexiletine by this pathway. Thus, a pharmacokinetic mechanism may also contribute to the increased efficacy of the combination.[4] The UK makers of mexiletine state that it may be used concurrently with quinidine.[5] They also note that it may be necessary to reduce the dose of mexiletine when used concurrently with drugs causing inhibition of hepatic enzymes, in particularly the cytochrome P450 isoenzymes CYP1A2 and CYP2D6.[5]

1. Duff HJ, Roden D, Primm RK, Oates JA, Woosley RL. Mexiletine in the treatment of resistant ventricular arrhythmias: enhancement of efficacy and reduction of dose-related side effects by combination with quinidine. *Circulation* (1983) 67, 1124–8.
2. Duff HJ, Rahmberg M, Sheldon RS. Role of quinidine in the mexiletine-quinidine interaction: electrophysiologic correlates of enhanced antiarrhythmic efficacy. *J Cardiovasc Pharmacol* (1990) 16, 685–92.
3. Broly F, Vandamme N, Caron J, Libersa C, Lhermitte M. Single-dose quinidine treatment inhibits mexiletine oxidation in extensive metabolizers of debrisoquine. *Life Sci* (1991) 48, PL-123–128.
4. Turgeon J, Fiset C, Giguère R, Gilbert M, Moerike K, Rouleau JR, Kroemer HK, Eichelbaum M, Grech-Bélanger O, Bélanger PM. Influence of debrisoquine phenotype and of quinidine on mexiletine disposition in man. *J Pharmacol Exp Ther* (1991) 259, 789–98.
5. Mexitil (Mexiletine). Boehringer Ingelheim Ltd. UK Summary of product characteristics, October 1999.

Mexiletine + Rifampicin (Rifampin)

The clearance of mexiletine is increased by the concurrent use of rifampicin. An increase in the dosage of mexiletine may be necessary.

Clinical evidence, mechanism, importance and management

After taking rifampicin 600 mg daily for 10 days, the half-life of a single 400-mg dose of mexiletine was reduced by 40% (from 8.5 to 5 hours) and the AUC fell by 39% in 8 healthy subjects.[1] The probable reason is that the rifampicin (a known, potent enzyme-inducing agent) increases the metabolism and clearance of the mexiletine. It seems likely that the mexiletine dosage will need to be increased during concurrent use. Monitor concurrent use well.

1. Pentikäinen PJ, Koivula IH, Hiltunen HA. Effect of rifampicin treatment on the kinetics of mexiletine. *Eur J Clin Pharmacol* (1982) 23, 261–6.

Mexiletine + SSRIs

Fluvoxamine markedly increases the AUC of mexiletine. Fluoxetine might also be expected to interact, albeit by a different mechanism.

Clinical evidence, mechanism, importance and management

Fluvoxamine 50 mg twice daily for 7 days increased the AUC of a single 200-mg dose of mexiletine by 55%, and decreased the clearance by 37% in 6 healthy subjects.[1] It is likely that **fluvoxamine** decreases the metabolism of mexiletine by inhibiting the cytochrome P450 isoenzyme CYP1A2, which is partially responsible for the metabolism of mexiletine.[1] The large changes in mexiletine AUC suggest that concurrent therapy should be well monitored.

Mexiletine is also metabolised by CYP2D6 (e.g. see 'Mexiletine + Propafenone', p.180). Of the SSRIs, **fluoxetine** is a known inhibitor of CYP2D6, and it has been suggested that the concurrent use of mexiletine and **fluoxetine** should be undertaken with caution (see 'SSRIs; Fluoxetine + Miscellaneous', p.988).

The UK makers note that it may be necessary to reduce the dose of mexiletine when used concurrently with drugs causing inhibition of hepatic enzymes, in particular the cytochrome P450 isoenzymes CYP1A2 and CYP2D6,[2] which is consistent with the proposed mechanism of the interaction.

1. Kusumoto M, Ueno K, Oda A, Takeda K, Mashimo K, Takaya K, Fujimura Y, Nishihori T, Tanaka K. Effect of fluvoxamine on the pharmacokinetics of mexiletine in healthy Japanese men. *Clin Pharmacol Ther* (2001) 69, 104–7.
2. Mexitil (Mexiletine). Boehringer Ingelheim Ltd. UK Summary of product characteristics, October 1999.

Mexiletine + Urinary acidifiers and alkalinisers

Large changes in urinary pH caused by the concurrent use of acidifying or alkalinising drugs can have a marked effect on the plasma levels of mexiletine in some patients.

Clinical evidence

In 4 healthy subjects, a single 200-mg intravenous dose of mexiletine was given, once when the urine was acidic (pH 5) after administration of **ammonium chloride**, and once when the urine was alkaline (pH 8) after administration of **sodium bicarbonate**. The plasma elimination half-life was significantly shorter when the urine was acidic (2.8 hours) compared with when it was alkaline (8.6 hours). In addition, the percentage of mexiletine excreted unchanged in the urine was 57.5% when acidic and just 0.6% when alkaline.[1] Similar results were found in another study.[2] A further study in patients with uncontrolled urine pH (range 5.04 to 7.86) given mexiletine orally for 5 days found that the plasma concentration of mexiletine correlated with urine pH. In addition, it was predicted that a normal variation in pH could cause more than a 50% variation in plasma mexiletine levels.[3] A later comprehensive pharmacokinetic study in 5 healthy subjects confirmed that renal clearance of mexiletine was 4 ml/minute in alkaline urine (pH 8) compared with 168 ml/minute in acidic urine (pH 5.2). In two subjects, this resulted in an increase in plasma concentrations of 61% and 96%, but in the other three the increase was less than 20%. Non-renal clearance (metabolic clearance) increased in the three subjects with little change in plasma concentrations, but did not in the two with marked changes.[4]

Mechanism

Mexiletine is a basic drug, and undergoes greater reabsorption by the kidneys when in the non-ionised form in alkaline urine. Mexiletine is also extensively cleared from the body by liver metabolism and only about 10% is excreted unchanged in the urine at physiological pH, although this is variable. Any changes in the renal clearance of mexiletine that occur as a result of urinary pH changes might therefore be expected to be compensated by an increase in metabolic clearance, but this does not seem to occur in all patients.[4]

Importance and management

Although changes in urinary pH can affect the amount of mexiletine lost in the urine, the effect of diet or the concurrent use of alkalinisers (sodium bicarbonate, **acetazolamide**) or acidifiers (ammonium chloride etc.) on the plasma concentrations of mexiletine does not appear to be predictable. There appear to be no reports of adverse interactions but concurrent use should be monitored. The UK maker of mexiletine recommends that the concomitant use of drugs that markedly acidify or alkalinise the urine should be avoided.[5]

1. Kiddie MA, Kaye CM, Turner P, Shaw TRD. The influence of urinary pH on the elimination of mexiletine. *Br J Clin Pharmacol* (1974) 1, 229–32.
2. Beckett AH, Chidomere EC. The distribution, metabolism and excretion of mexiletine in man. *Postgrad Med J* (1977) 53 (Suppl 1), 60–6.
3. Johnston A, Burgess CD, Warrington SJ, Wadsworth J, Hamer NAJ. The effect of spontaneous changes in urinary pH on mexiletine plasma concentrations and excretion during chronic administration to healthy volunteers. *Br J Clin Pharmacol* (1979) 8, 349–52.
4. Mitchell BG, Clements JA, Pottage A, Prescott LF. Mexiletine disposition: individual variation in response to urine acidification and alkalinisation. *Br J Clin Pharmacol* (1983) 16, 281–4.
5. Mexitil (Mexiletine). Boehringer Ingelheim Ltd. UK Summary of product characteristics, October 1999.

Moracizine + Beta-blockers

Moracizine appears not to interact adversely with propranolol.

Clinical evidence, mechanism, importance and management

The efficacy and tolerability of the combination of **propranolol** and moracizine was compared with either drug alone in patients with ventricular arrhythmias in controlled trials. The combination was well tolerated, with no evidence of any adverse interactions, nor any beneficial interactions. However, the dose of propranolol used was fairly low at 120 mg daily.[1,2] Further study is needed.

1. Pratt CM, Butman SM, Young JB, Knoll M, English LD. Antiarrhythmic efficacy of Ethmozine® (moricizine HCl) compared with disopyramide and propranolol. *Am J Cardiol* (1987) 60, 52F–58F.
2. Butman SM, Knoll ML, Gardin JM. Comparison of ethmozine to propranolol and the combination for ventricular arrhythmias. *Am J Cardiol* (1987) 60, 603–7.

Moracizine + Cimetidine

Cimetidine increases the plasma levels of moracizine but the clinical importance of this is uncertain.

Clinical evidence, mechanism, importance and management

After taking cimetidine 300 mg four times daily for 7 days, the clearance of a single 500-mg dose of moracizine in 8 healthy subjects was halved and both its half-life and the AUC were increased by 39%. It is believed that this is because the cimetidine reduces moracizine metabolism by the liver.[1] Despite the increase in plasma moracizine levels, the PR and QRS intervals were not further prolonged. One possible explanation (so it is postulated) is that some of the metabolites of moracizine, whose production is inhibited by cimetidine, could also be pharmacologically active. Concurrent use should be well monitored, but measuring plasma moracizine levels may be of limited value because of the potential effects of the moracizine metabolites.

1. Biollaz J, Shaheen O, Wood AJJ. Cimetidine inhibition of ethmozine metabolism. *Clin Pharmacol Ther* (1985) 37, 665–8.

Moracizine + Diltiazem

A pharmacokinetic interaction occurs between moracizine and diltiazem resulting in increased systemic availability of moracizine and decreased systemic availability of diltiazem.

Clinical evidence, mechanism, importance and management

After 16 healthy subjects took both diltiazem 60 mg and moracizine 250 mg every 8 hours for 7 days, the maximum plasma concentration of moracizine was increased by 89%, the AUC by 121%, and clearance was decreased by 54%. In contrast, the maximum plasma concentration and AUC of diltiazem decreased by 36% and clearance was increased by 52%.

The AUCs for the diltiazem metabolites were not significantly affected. No clinically significant changes in ECG parameters were see with the combination. However, the frequency of adverse events (e.g. headache, dizziness, paraesthesia) was greater with concomitant administration (76%) than with either drug alone (54 and 45% for moracizine and diltiazem respectively).[1] Diltiazem probably inhibits the hepatic metabolism of moracizine while moracizine increases that of diltiazem. The clinical significance of this interaction is not known. However, particular caution is advised if diltiazem and moracizine are given concurrently, in light of the increase in adverse events. Dose adjustments may also be required to obtain optimum therapeutic responses.[1]

1. Shum L, Pieniaszek HJ, Robinson CA, Davidson AF, Widner PJ, Benedek IH, Flamenbaum W. Pharmacokinetic interactions of moricizine and diltiazem in healthy volunteers. *J Clin Pharmacol* (1996) 36, 1161–8.

Pirmenol + Cimetidine

Cimetidine 300 mg four times daily for 8 days had no significant effect on the pharmacokinetics of single 150-mg oral doses of pirmenol in 8 healthy subjects.[1] No clinically important interaction would therefore be expected in patients given both drugs.

1. Stringer KA, Lebsack ME, Cetnarowski-Cropp AB, Goldfarb AL, Radulovic LL, Bockbrader HN, Chang T, Sedman AJ. Effect of cimetidine administration on the pharmacokinetics of pirmenol. *J Clin Pharmacol* (1992) 32, 91–4.

Pirmenol + Rifampicin (Rifampin)

Rifampicin markedly increases the loss of pirmenol from the body. A reduction in its antiarrhythmic effects is likely to occur.

Clinical evidence, mechanism, importance and management

Treatment with rifampicin 600 mg daily for 14 days markedly affected the pharmacokinetics of a single 150-mg dose of pirmenol in 12 healthy subjects.[1] The apparent plasma clearance increased sevenfold and the AUC decreased by 83%.[1] The probable reason is that rifampicin increases the hepatic metabolism of pirmenol. Monitor well and anticipate the need to increase the dosage of pirmenol if rifampicin is used concurrently.

1. Stringer KA, Cetnarowski AB, Goldfarb AB, Lebsack ME, Chang TS, Sedman AJ. Enhanced pirmenol elimination by rifampin. *J Clin Pharmacol* (1988) 28, 1094–7.

Procainamide + Amiodarone

The QT interval prolonging effects are increased when procainamide and amiodarone are used together, therefore the combination should generally be avoided. Serum procainamide levels are increased by about 60% and *N*-acetylprocainamide levels by about 30% if amiodarone is given concurrently. If the combination is used, the dosage of procainamide will need to be reduced to avoid toxicity.

Clinical evidence

Twelve patients were stabilised on procainamide (2 to 6 g daily, or about 900 mg six-hourly). When concurrently treated with amiodarone (600 mg loading dose 12-hourly for 5 to 7 days, then 600 mg daily) their mean serum procainamide levels rose by 57% (from 6.8 to 10.6 micrograms/ml) and their serum levels of the metabolite *N*-acetylprocainamide (NAPA) rose by 32% (from 6.9 to 9.1 micrograms/ml). Procainamide levels increased by more than 3 micrograms/ml in 6 patients. The increases usually occurred within 24 hours, but in other patients occurred as late as 4 or 5 days. Toxicity was seen in two patients. Despite lowering the procainamide dosages by 20%, serum procainamide levels were still higher (at 7.7 micrograms/ml) than before the amiodarone was started.[1]

In another study, intravenous procainamide was administered once before (at a mean dose of 13 mg/kg), and once during (at a 30% reduced dose—mean 9.2 mg/kg) administration of amiodarone 1600 mg daily for 7 to 14 days. Amiodarone decreased the clearance of procainamide by 23% and increased its elimination half-life by 38%. Both drugs prolonged the QRS and QTc intervals, and the extent of prolongation was significantly greater with the combination than either drug alone.[2]

Mechanism

The mechanism behind the pharmacokinetic interaction is not understood. The QT prolonging effects of the two drugs would be expected to be additive.

Importance and management

Information appears to be limited to these studies, but the pharmacokinetic/pharmacodynamic interaction would seem to be established and clinically important. The use of amiodarone with procainamide further prolongs the QTc interval, which can increase the risk of torsade de pointes. Therefore, the combination should generally be avoided. Whereas the UK makers of amiodarone contraindicate its use with class Ia antiarrhythmics such as procainamide[3], the US makers of amiodarone recommend that such combined therapy should be reserved for life-threatening ventricular arrhythmias incompletely responsive to either agent alone and recommend that the procainamide dosage should be reduced by one-third.[4] See also 'Drugs that prolong the QT interval + Other drugs that prolong the QT interval', p.170. The pharmacokinetic component has a high incidence (11 out of 12 in the report cited), and develops rapidly. Therefore, if the two drugs are considered essential, the dosage of procainamide may need to be reduced by 20 to 50%, and serum levels should be monitored and patients observed for adverse effects.[1,2]

1. Saal AK, Werner JA, Greene HL, Sears GK, Graham EL. Effect of amiodarone on serum quinidine and procainamide levels. *Am J Cardiol* (1984) 53, 1264–7.
2. Windle J, Prystowsky EN, Miles WM, Heger JJ. Pharmacokinetic and electrophysiologic interactions of amiodarone and procainamide. *Clin Pharmacol Ther* (1987) 41, 603–10.
3. Cordarone X (Amiodarone hydrochloride). Sanofi Synthelabo. UK Summary of product characteristics, May 2004.
4. Cordarone (Amiodarone hydrochloride). Wyeth Laboratories. US Prescribing information, April 2004.

Procainamide + Antacids or Antidiarrhoeals

There is some inconclusive evidence that aluminium phosphate may possibly cause a small reduction in the absorption of procainamide. Kaolin-pectin appears to reduce the bioavailability of procainamide.

Clinical evidence, mechanism, importance and management

A single 11-g dose of an **aluminium phosphate** antacid modestly reduced the AUC of a single 750-mg oral dose of procainamide by 14.6%.[1] The clinical importance of this interaction is uncertain, but probably small.

Kaolin-pectin was found to reduce the peak saliva concentrations and AUC of a single 250-mg dose of procainamide by about 30% in 4 healthy subjects. **Kaolin-pectin** and a variety of antacids (***Pepto-bismol***, ***Simeco***, and **magnesium trisilicate**) absorbed procainamide *in vitro*.[2] The clinical importance of this is uncertain.

1. Albin H, Vincon G, Bertolaso D, Dangoumau J. Influence du phosphate d'aluminium sur la biodisponibilité de la procaïnamide et du disopyramide. *Therapie* (1981) 36, 541–6.
2. Al-Shora HI, Moustafa MA, Niazy EM, Gaber M, Gouda MW. Interactions of procainamide, verapamil, guanethidine and hydralazine with adsorbent antacids and antidiarrhoeal mixtures. *Int J Pharmaceutics* (1988) 47, 209–13.

Procainamide + Beta-blockers

The pharmacokinetics of procainamide are little changed by either propranolol or metoprolol. Both sotalol and procainamide have QT-interval prolonging effects, which may be additive if they are used together.

Clinical evidence, mechanism, importance and management

Preliminary results of a study in 6 healthy subjects found that long-term treatment with **propranolol** (period and dosage not stated) increased the procainamide half-life from 1.71 to 2.66 hours and reduced the plasma clearance by 16%.[1] However a later study in 8 healthy subjects showed that the pharmacokinetics of a single 500-mg dose of procainamide were only slightly altered by the concurrent use of either **propranolol** 80 mg three times daily or **metoprolol** 100 mg twice daily. The procainamide half-life increased from 1.9 to 2.2 hours with **propranolol** and to 2.3 hours with **metoprolol**, but no significant changes in total clearance occurred. No changes in the AUC of the metabolite *N*-acetylprocainamide were seen.[2] It seems unlikely that a clinically important adverse interaction normally occurs between these drugs.

A clinical study describes the successful use of procainamide with **sotalol**.[3] However, both **sotalol** and procainamide can prolong the QT interval, and there may be an increased the risk of torsade de pointes arrhythmia if they are used together. See also 'Drugs that prolong the QT interval + Other drugs that prolong the QT interval', p.170.

1. Weidler DJ, Garg DC, Jallad NS, McFarland MA. The effect of long-term propranolol administration on the pharmacokinetics of procainamide in humans. *Clin Pharmacol Ther* (1981) 29, 289.
2. Ochs HR, Carstens G, Roberts G-M, Greenblatt DJ. Metoprolol or propranolol does not alter the kinetics of procainamide. *J Cardiovasc Pharmacol* (1983) 5, 392–5.
3. Dorian P, Newman D, Berman N, Hardy J, Mitchell J. Sotalol and type IA drugs in combination prevent recurrence of sustained ventricular tachycardia. *J Am Coll Cardiol* (1993) 22, 106–13.

Procainamide + H_2-blockers

Serum procainamide levels can be increased if cimetidine is given concurrently and toxicity may develop, particularly in those who have a reduced renal clearance such as the elderly. Ranitidine and famotidine appear to interact only minimally or not at all.

Clinical evidence

(a) Cimetidine

In one study, 36 elderly patients (65 to 90 years old) on sustained-release oral procainamide 6-hourly showed rises in mean steady-state serum levels of procainamide and its metabolite *N*-acetylprocainamide of 55 and 36% respectively after taking cimetidine 300 mg 6-hourly for 3 days. This was tolerated in 24 of them without side-effects (serum procainamide and *N*-acetylprocainamide less than 12 and less than 15 mg/l respectively) but the other 12 had some adverse effects (nausea, weakness, malaise PR interval increases of less than 20%), which was dealt with by stopping one or both drugs.[1] Another report describes an elderly man who developed procainamide toxicity when given cimetidine 1200 mg daily. His procainamide dosage was roughly halved (from 937.5 to 500 mg every 6 hours) to bring his serum procainamide and *N*-acetylprocainamide levels into the accepted therapeutic range.[2]

Four studies in healthy subjects have found that cimetidine increased the procainamide AUC by 24 to 43%, and decreased the renal clearance by 31 to 40%,[3-6] these changes occurring even with single doses of cimetidine.[5] A steady-state procainamide serum level increase of 43% has been seen following cimetidine 1200 mg daily.[6]

(b) Famotidine

Famotidine 40 mg daily for 5 days did not affect the pharmacokinetics or pharmacodynamics of a single 5-mg/kg intravenous dose of procainamide in 8 healthy subjects.[7]

(c) Ranitidine

One study[8] found that ranitidine 150 mg twice daily for one day reduced the absorption of procainamide from the gut by 10% and reduced its renal excretion by 19%, increasing the procainamide and *N*-acetylprocainamide AUC by about 14%. However, no change in the steady-state pharmacokinetics of procainamide was found with ranitidine 150 mg twice daily in another study, except that ranitidine delayed the time to maximum plasma concentration (from 1.4 to 2.7 hours).[6] In a further study, ranitidine 150 mg twice daily for 4 days caused no significant changes in the mean pharmacokinetics of oral procainamide 1 g in 13 healthy subjects. However, it appeared that subjects had either a modest 20% increase or decrease in procainamide clearance, with the direction of change related to their baseline procainamide clearance; the higher the baseline clearance the greater the decrease caused by ranitidine.[9]

Mechanism

Procainamide levels in the body are increased because cimetidine reduces its renal excretion by about one-third or more, but the precise mechanism is uncertain. One suggestion is that it interferes with the active secretion of procainamide by the kidney tubules.[3,4]

Importance and management

The procainamide/cimetidine interaction is established. Concurrent use should be undertaken with care because the safety margin of procainamide is low. Reduce the procainamide dosage as necessary. This is particularly important in the elderly because they have a reduced ability to clear both drugs. Ranitidine and famotidine appear not to interact to a clinically important extent, but it should be appreciated that what is known is based on studies in healthy subjects rather than patients.

1. Bauer LA, Black D, Gensler A. Procainamide-cimetidine drug interaction in elderly male patients. *J Am Geriatr Soc* (1990) 38, 467–9.
2. Higbee MD, Wood JS, Mead RA. Case report. Procainamide-cimetidine interaction. A potential toxic interaction in the elderly. *J Am Geriatr Soc* (1984) 32, 162–4.
3. Somogyi A, McLean A, Heinzow B. Cimetidine-procainamide pharmacokinetic interaction in man: evidence of competition for tubular secretion of basic drugs. *Eur J Clin Pharmacol* (1983) 25, 339–45.
4. Christian CD, Meredith CG, Speeg KV. Cimetidine inhibits renal procainamide clearance. *Clin Pharmacol Ther* (1984) 36, 221–7.
5. Lai MY, Jiang FM, Chung CH, Chen HC, Chao PDL. Dose dependent effect of cimetidine on procainamide disposition in man. *Int J Clin Pharmacol Ther Toxicol* (1988) 26, 118–21.
6. Rodvold KA, Paloucek FP, Jung D, Gallastegui J. Interaction of steady-state procainamide with H_2-receptor antagonists cimetidine and ranitidine. *Ther Drug Monit* (1987) 9, 378–83.
7. Klotz U, Arvela P, Rosenkranz B. Famotidine, a new H_2-receptor antagonist, does not affect hepatic elimination of diazepam or tubular secretion of procainamide. *Eur J Clin Pharmacol* (1985) 28, 671–5.
8. Somogyi A, Bochner F. Dose and concentration dependent effect of ranitidine on procainamide disposition and renal clearance in man. *Br J Clin Pharmacol* (1984) 18, 175–81.
9. Rocci ML, Kosoglou T, Ferguson RK, Vlasses PH. Ranitidine-induced changes in the renal and hepatic clearances of procainamide are correlated. *J Pharmacol Exp Ther* (1989) 248; 923–8.

Procainamide + Para-aminobenzoic acid (PABA)

A single case report found that para-aminobenzoic acid (PABA) increased the serum levels of procainamide and reduced the production and serum levels of the procainamide metabolite *N*-acetylprocainamide. In contrast, a later pharmacokinetic study in healthy subjects found that PABA had no effect on serum procainamide and increased serum *N*-acetylprocainamide.

Clinical evidence, mechanism, importance and management

A 61-year-old man who had sustained ventricular tachycardia, which failed to respond adequately to oral procainamide, was found to be a rapid acetylator of procainamide so that the serum levels of the procainamide metabolite (*N*-acetylprocainamide) were particularly high when compared with the procainamide levels. When he was additionally given 1.5 g of para-aminobenzoic acid (PABA) six-hourly for 30 hours to suppress the production of this metabolite, the serum level of procainamide increased, that of *N*-acetylprocainamide decreased, and control of his arrhythmia improved.[1] However, a later study in 10 healthy subjects, who were also fast acetylators, found that PABA did not significantly affect the pharmacokinetics of procainamide. In addition, although PABA inhibited the production of *N*-acetylprocainamide, it also inhibited renal excretion, so that the AUC and elimination half-life were increased. This suggests that PABA may in fact not be useful for increasing the efficacy and safety of procainamide.[2]

These contradictory findings are difficult to explain, but neither report suggests that concurrent use need be avoided.

1. Nylen ES, Cohen AI, Wish MH, Lima JL, Finkelstein JD. Reduced acetylation of procainamide by para-aminobenzoic acid. *J Am Coll Cardiol* (1986) 7, 185–7.
2. Tisdale JE, Rudis MI, Padhi ID, Svensson CK, Webb CR, Borzak S, Ware JA, Krepostman A, Zarowitz BJ. Inhibition of N-acetylation of procainamide by para-aminobenzoic acid in humans. *J Clin Pharmacol* (1995) 35, 902–10.

Procainamide + Probenecid

Probenecid appears not to interact with procainamide. The pharmacokinetics of a single 750-mg intravenous dose of procainamide and its effects on the QT interval were not altered by prior administration of probenecid 2 g in 6 healthy subjects.[1] No special precautions appear to be necessary.

1. Lam YWF, Boyd RA, Chin SK, Chang D, Giacomini KM. Effect of probenecid on the pharmacokinetics and pharmacodynamics of procainamide. *J Clin Pharmacol* (1991) 31, 429–32.

Procainamide + Quinidine

A single case report describes a marked increase in the plasma procainamide levels of a patient when he was concurrently treated with quinidine. The combination prolongs the QT interval, and should generally be avoided because of the increased risk of torsade de pointes.

Clinical evidence

A man with sustained ventricular tachycardia on high-dose intravenous procainamide 2 g eight-hourly showed a 70% increase from 9.1 to 15.4 nanograms/ml in his steady-state plasma procainamide levels when concurrently treated with quinidine gluconate 324 mg eight-hourly. The procainamide half-life increased from 3.7 to 7.2 hours and its clearance fell from 27 to 16 l/hour. His QTc interval increased from 648 to 678 milliseconds.[1] In another study in patients with ventricular arrhythmias, quinidine was combined with procainamide. The doses were adjusted based in part on the QT interval. The QTc interval was longer with the combination (499 milliseconds) than each drug alone (quinidine 470 milliseconds, procainamide 460 milliseconds) despite using reduced doses in the combination (mean quinidine dose reduced by 28%; procainamide by 32%).[2]

Mechanism

It has been suggested that the quinidine interferes with one or more of renal pathways by which procainamide is cleared from the body.[1]

Importance and management

Information on the possible pharmacokinetic interaction seems to be limited to this report. Both quinidine and procainamide are class Ia antiarrhythmics and prolong the QT interval, an effect that is increased with the combination. Such combinations should generally be avoided because of the increased risk of torsade de pointes. See also 'Drugs that prolong the QT interval + Other drugs that prolong the QT interval', p.170.

1. Hughes B, Dyer JE, Schwartz AB. Increased procainamide plasma concentrations caused by quinidine: a new drug interaction. *Am Heart J* (1987) 114, 908–9.
2. Kim SG, Seiden SW, Matos JA, Waspe LE, Fisher JD. Combination of procainamide and quinidine for better tolerance and additive effects for ventricular arrhythmias. *Am J Cardiol* (1985) 56, 84–8.

Procainamide + Quinolones

Ofloxacin causes a moderate increase in the serum levels of procainamide but the ECG appears to be unaltered in studies in healthy subjects. An increased risk of torsade de pointes would be expected if procainamide is used with gatifloxacin, moxifloxacin, or sparfloxacin, and possibly levofloxacin.

Clinical evidence, mechanism, importance and management

Nine healthy subjects were given a single 1-g oral dose of procainamide alone then again with the fifth dose of **ofloxacin** (400 mg given twice daily for five doses). The AUC of procainamide was increased 27% by the **ofloxacin**, the maximum plasma levels were increased by 21% (from 4.8 to 5.8 micrograms/l) and the total clearance was reduced by 22%,[1] whereas the pharmacokinetics of the active metabolite of procainamide (*N*-acetylprocainamide) were not significantly altered. The probable reason for the interaction is that the **ofloxacin** inhibits the secretion of unchanged procainamide by the kidney tubules. Despite the pharmacokinetic changes, no ECG changes were detected. These results suggest that **ofloxacin** interacts to a modest extent with procainamide, and that it might be prudent to monitor the outcome if both drugs are given together in patients.

One case of torsade de pointes was noted in a patient taking procainamide and a quinolone (unspecified) concurrently in an analysis of cases of torsade de pointes associated with quinolones on the FDA Adverse Events Reporting System database (there were 37 cases identified, and 19 occurred in patients also taking other drugs known to prolong the QT interval).[2]

Some quinolones can prolong the QT interval, and would be expected to increase the risk of torsade de pointes arrhythmias when used with procainamide. Of the quinolones used clinically, **gatifloxacin, moxifloxacin,** and **sparfloxacin** are known to prolong the QT interval (see 'Table 7.3', (p.169)). There is also evidence that **levofloxacin** may prolong the QT interval (see 'Amiodarone + Quinolones', p.163). These fluoroquinolones should probably be avoided in patients on procainamide (see also 'Drugs that prolong the QT interval + Other drugs that prolong the QT interval', p.170).

1. Martin DE, Shen J, Griener J, Raasch R, Patterson JH, Cascio W. Effects of ofloxacin on the pharmacokinetics and pharmacodynamics of procainamide. *J Clin Pharmacol* (1996) 36, 85–91.
2. Frothingham R. Rates of torsades de pointes associated with ciprofloxacin, ofloxacin, levofloxacin, gatifloxacin, and moxifloxacin. *Pharmacotherapy* (2001) 21, 1468–72.

Procainamide + Sucralfate

Sucralfate appears not to affect the absorption of procainamide.

Clinical evidence, mechanism, importance and management

In 4 healthy subjects sucralfate 1 g taken 30 minutes before a single 250-mg dose of procainamide reduced the mean maximum salivary level of procainamide by 5.3%, but did not significantly affect either the AUC or the rate of absorption.[1] These results suggest that a clinically significant interaction is unlikely.

1. Turkistani AAA, Gaber M, Al-Meshal MA, Al-Shora HI, Gouda MW. Effect of sucralfate on procainamide absorption. *Int J Pharmaceutics* (1990) 59, R1–R3.

Procainamide + Trimethoprim

Trimethoprim causes a marked increase in the plasma levels of procainamide and its active metabolite, *N*-acetylprocainamide, which increases the risk of toxicity.

Clinical evidence

Eight healthy subjects were given procainamide 500 mg six-hourly for three days. The concurrent use of trimethoprim 200 mg daily increased the 0 to 12 hour AUC of procainamide by 63% and of its active metabolite, *N*-acetylprocainamide (NAPA), by 51%. The renal clearance of procainamide decreased by 47% and that of NAPA by 13%. The QTc prolonging effects of procainamide were increased to a significant, but slight, extent by trimethoprim.[1] Another study found that trimethoprim 200 mg daily reduced the renal clearance of a single 1-g dose of procainamide by 45% and of NAPA by 26%. The QTc interval was increased from 400 to 430 milliseconds.[2]

Mechanism

Trimethoprim decreases the losses in the urine of both procainamide and its active metabolite by competing for active tubular secretion. It may also cause a small increase in the conversion of procainamide to *N*-acetylprocainamide.[1]

Importance and management

An established interaction but its documentation is limited. The need to reduce the procainamide dosage should be anticipated if trimethoprim is given to patients already controlled on procainamide. In practice the effects may be greater than the studies cited suggest because the elderly lose procainamide through the kidneys more slowly than young healthy subjects. Remember too that the daily dosage of trimethoprim in **co-trimoxazole** (trimethoprim 160 mg + sulfamethoxazole 800 mg) may equal or exceed the dosages used in the studies cited.

1. Kosoglou T, Rocci ML, Vlasses PH. Trimethoprim alters the disposition of procainamide and N-acetylprocainamide. *Clin Pharmacol Ther* (1988) 44, 467–77.
2. Vlasses PH, Kosoglou T, Chase SL, Greenspon AJ, Lottes S, Andress E, Ferguson RK, Rocci ML. Trimethoprim inhibition of the renal clearance of procainamide and N-acetylprocainamide. *Arch Intern Med* (1989) 149, 1350–3.

Propafenone + Barbiturates

Phenobarbital increases the loss of propafenone from the body, and reduces its serum levels.

Clinical evidence, mechanism, importance and management

In a preliminary report of a study in 7 non-smoking subjects who were fast metabolisers of propafenone, **phenobarbital** 100 mg daily for 3 weeks reduced the peak serum propafenone level (following a single 300-mg dose) by 26 to 87% and the AUC by 10 to 89%. The intrinsic clearance increased by 11 to 84%. The results in a further 4 heavy smokers were similar.[1] The probable reason is that **phenobarbital** (a potent stimulator of liver enzymes) increases the metabolism of the propafenone and its loss from the body. The clinical importance of this awaits assessment, but check that propafenone remains effective if **phenobarbital** is added, and that toxicity does not occur if it is stopped. If the suggested mechanism is correct, other barbiturates would be expected to interact similarly.

1. Chan GL-Y, Axelson JE, Kerr CR. The effect of phenobarbital on the pharmacokinetics of propafenone in man. *Pharm Res* (1988) 5, S153.

Propafenone + Cimetidine

Cimetidine appears to interact minimally with propafenone.

Clinical evidence, mechanism, importance and management

A study in 12 healthy subjects (10 extensive metabolisers and 2 poor metabolisers of propafenone) given 225 mg propafenone eight-hourly showed that the concurrent use of cimetidine 400 mg eight-hourly caused some changes in the pharmacokinetics and pharmacodynamics of the propafenone, with wide intersubject variability. Raised mean peak and steady-state plasma levels were seen (24 and 22%, respectively), but these did not reach statistical significance. A slight increase in the QRS duration also occurred.[1] However, none of the changes were considered clinically important.

1. Pritchett ELC, Smith WM, Kirsten EB. Pharmacokinetic and pharmacodynamic interactions of propafenone and cimetidine. *J Clin Pharmacol* (1988) 28, 619–24.

Propafenone + Erythromycin

Limited evidence suggests erythromycin may inhibit the metabolism of propafenone.

Clinical evidence, mechanism, importance and management

The preliminary results of a study in 12 healthy subjects given a single 300-mg dose of propafenone with or without erythromycin 250 mg showed that the increase in propafenone AUC with erythromycin was greater in those with lower cytochrome P450 isoenzyme CYP2D6 activity. It was suggested[1] that low CYP2D6 activity shifts propafenone metabolism to the CYP3A4/1A2-mediated *N*-depropylpropafenone pathway increasing the interaction with erythromycin, which is an inhibitor of CYP3A4. This appears to be the only documentation of a possible interaction with erythromycin and its clinical significance is not certain. More study is needed.

1. Munoz CE, Ito S, Bend JR, Tesoro A, Freeman D, Spence JD, Bailey DG. Propafenone interaction with CYP3A4 inhibitors in man. *Clin Pharmacol Ther* (1997) 61, 154.

Propafenone + Grapefruit juice

Limited evidence suggests grapefruit juice may inhibit the metabolism of propafenone.

Clinical evidence, mechanism, importance and management

Preliminary results of a study in 12 healthy subjects given a single 300-mg dose of propafenone with or without 250 ml of grapefruit juice showed that the increase in propafenone AUC with grapefruit juice was greater in those with lower cytochrome P450 isoenzyme CYP2D6 activity. It was suggested[1] that in the presence of low CYP2D6 activity a greater proportion of propafenone is eliminated by metabolism by CYP3A4 and CYP1A2 and the effect of grapefruit juice is increased since it is an inhibitor of CYP3A4. The clinical significance of this finding is not certain. Further study is needed

1. Munoz CE, Ito S, Bend JR, Tesoro A, Freeman D, Spence JD, Bailey DG. Propafenone interaction with CYP3A4 inhibitors in man. *Clin Pharmacol Ther* (1997) 61, 154.

Propafenone + Ketoconazole

An isolated case report describes a man taking propafenone who had convulsions 2 days after taking a dose of ketoconazole. Limited evidence suggests ketoconazole may inhibit the metabolism of propafenone.

Clinical evidence

A man who had been taking captopril and hydrochlorothiazide for 6 years and propafenone 300 mg daily for 4 years, without problems and without any history of convulsive episodes, experienced a tonic-clonic seizure while watching television. It was later found that he had started to take two capsules of ketoconazole daily two days previously for the treatment of a candidal infection.[1] The preliminary results of another study in 12 healthy subjects given a single 300-mg dose of propafenone with or without ketoconazole 200 mg showed that the increase in propafenone AUC with ketoconazole was greater in those with lower cytochrome P450 isoenzyme CYP2D6 activity.[2]

Mechanism

The authors of the case report postulate that the ketoconazole may have inhibited the metabolism of the propafenone so that this patient, in effect, may have developed an overdose.[1] However, convulsions with propafenone are rare.[3] Ketoconazole is an inhibitor of the cytochrome P450 isoenzyme CYP3A4, by which propafenone is metabolised to *N*-depropylpropafenone. Propafenone is also extensively metabolised by CYP2D6 to 5-hydroxypropafenone but it was suggested that if CYP2D6 activity is low, propafenone metabolism may be shifted to the CYP3A4 pathway increasing the possibility of an interaction with ketoconazole.[2]

Importance and management

The general importance of this interaction is uncertain. As of 1996, there had been no other cases reported to the maker of propafenone.[3] The more recent data suggest that an interaction can occur, and it would seem prudent to monitor concurrent use. More study is needed. There seems to be nothing documented about the effects of other azole antifungals.

1. Duvelleroy Hommet C, Jonville-Bera AP, Autret A, Saudeau D, Autret E, Fauchier JP. Une crise convulsive chez un patient traité par propafénone et kétoconazole. *Therapie* (1995) 50, 164–5.
2. Munoz CE, Ito S, Bend JR, Tesoro A, Freeman D, Spence JD, Bailey DG. Propafenone interaction with CYP3A4 inhibitors in man. *Clin Pharmacol Ther* (1997) 61, 154.
3. Knoll Ltd. Personal communication, February 1996.

Propafenone + Quinidine

Quinidine doubles the plasma levels of propafenone and halves the levels of its active metabolite in those with high levels of the cytochrome P450 isoenzyme CYP2D6. This interaction has been utilised clinically.

Clinical evidence

Nine patients on propafenone for frequent isolated ventricular ectopic beats, firstly had their dosage reduced to 150 mg eight-hourly and then 4 days later the steady-state pharmacokinetics of propafenone were determined at this new dose. Quinidine was then added at a dose of 50 mg eight-hourly, and after a further 4 days the steady-state plasma propafenone levels in 7 patients with high levels of the cytochrome P450 isoenzyme CYP2D6 ('extensive' metabolisers) had more than doubled from 408 to 1100 nanograms/ml, and 5-hydroxypropafenone concentrations had approximately halved, but the ECG intervals and arrhythmia frequency were unaltered. The steady-state plasma propafenone levels remained unchanged in the other two patients with low levels of CYP2D6 ('poor' metabolisers).[1] The same research group conducted a similar study in healthy subjects, which confirmed that quinidine increased the plasma levels of propafenone in 'extensive' but not 'poor' metabolisers. In addition, it was found that quinidine increased the extent of the beta-blockade caused by the propafenone in 'extensive' metabolisers to approach that seen in 'poor' metabolisers.[2] Another study has shown that the inhibition of propafenone metabolism by low-dose quinidine also occurs in Chinese as well as Caucasian patients.[3] [CYP2D6 shows pronounced interethnic differences in expression.] A further study showed that combining low-dose quinidine (150 mg daily) with standard dose propafenone in patients with atrial fibrillation resulted in a similar control of the arrhythmia as increasing the propafenone dose, but caused less gastrointestinal adverse effects.[4]

Mechanism

Quinidine inhibits the CYP2D6-dependent 5-hydroxylation of propafenone by the liver in those who are 'extensive' metabolisers so that it is cleared more slowly. Its plasma levels are doubled as a result, but the overall antiarrhythmic effects remain effectively unchanged, possibly because the production of its active antiarrhythmic metabolite (5-hydroxypropafenone) is simultaneously halved.[1] Quinidine increases the beta-blocking effects of propafenone in extensive metabolisers because only the parent drug, and not the metabolites, has beta-blocking activity.[2]

Importance and management

Quinidine appears to raise propafenone levels, and may also affect the beta-blocking properties of propafenone in some patients. In one study the concurrent use of propafenone and quinidine was said to have an effect similar to increasing the propafenone dose.[4] The importance of CYP2D6 metaboliser status is unclear, and more study is needed to clarify this.

1. Funck-Brentano C, Kroemer HK, Pavlou H, Woosley RL, Roden DM. Genetically-determined interaction between propafenone and low dose quinidine: role of active metabolites in modulating net drug effect. *Br J Clin Pharmacol* (1989) 27, 435–44.
2. Mörike K, Roden D. Quinidine-enhanced β-blockade during treatment with propafenone in extensive metabolizer human subjects. *Clin Pharmacol Ther* (1994) 55, 28–34.
3. Fan C, Tang M, Lau C-P, Chow M. The effect of quinidine on propafenone metabolism in Chinese patients. *Clin Invest Med* (1998) (Suppl) S12.
4. Lau C-P, Chow MSS, Tse H-F, Tang M-O, Fan C. Control of paroxysmal atrial fibrillation recurrence using combined administration of propafenone and quinidine. *Am J Cardiol* (2000) 86, 1327–32.

Propafenone + Rifampicin (Rifampin)

Propafenone serum levels and therapeutic effects can be markedly reduced by concurrent use of rifampicin.

Clinical evidence

A man successfully treated with propafenone showed marked falls in his plasma propafenone levels from 993 to 176 nanograms/ml within 12 days of starting to take rifampicin 450 mg twice daily. Levels of the two active metabolites of propafenone, 5-hydroxypropafenone and *N*-depropylpropafenone, changed from 195 to 64 nanograms/ml and from 110 to 192 nanograms/ml respectively. His arrhythmias returned but 2 weeks after stopping the rifampicin his arrhythmias had disappeared and the propafenone and its 5-hydroxy and *N*-depropyl metabolites had returned to acceptable levels (1411, 78 and 158 nanograms/ml respectively).[1] In a study in young healthy subjects, rifampicin 600 mg daily for 9 days reduced the bioavailability of a single 300-mg oral dose of propafenone from 30 to 10% in those with high levels of the cytochrome P450 isoenzyme CYP2D6 ('extensive' metabolisers), and from 81 to 48% in those with low levels of CYP2D6 ('poor' metabolisers). QRS prolongation decreased during enzyme induction. In contrast, in this study, rifampicin had no substantial effect on the pharmacokinetics of propafenone given intravenously.[2] Similar findings were reported in a further study by the same research group in healthy elderly subjects.[3]

Mechanism

Rifampicin induces the CYP3A4/1A2-mediated metabolism and phase II glucuronidation of propafenone. The effect of rifampicin on gastrointestinal clearance of propafenone was greater than that of its hepatic clearance. Rifampicin had no effect on CYP2D6-mediated metabolism of propafenone (the usual main metabolic route in 'extensive' metabolisers).[2,3]

Importance and management

An established and clinically relevant metabolic drug interaction. The dosage of oral propafenone will need increasing during concurrent use of rifampicin.[3] Alternatively, if possible, the authors of the case report[1] advise the use of another antibacterial because of the probable difficulty in adjusting the propafenone dosage.

1. Castel JM, Cappiello E, Leopaldi D, Latini R. Rifampicin lowers plasma concentrations of propafenone and its antiarrhythmic effect. *Br J Clin Pharmacol* (1990) 30, 155–6.
2. Dilger K, Greiner B, Fromm MF, Hofmann U, Kroemer HK, Eichelbaum M. Consequences of rifampicin treatment on propafenone disposition in extensive and poor metabolizers of CYP2D6. *Pharmacogenetics* (1999) 9, 551–9.
3. Dilger K, Hofmann U, Klotz U. Enzyme induction in the elderly: Effect of rifampin on the pharmacokinetics and pharmacodynamics of propafenone. *Clin Pharmacol Ther* (2000) 67, 512–20.

Propafenone + SSRIs

Fluoxetine markedly inhibits the metabolism (5-hydroxylation) of propafenone, and paroxetine would also be expected to behave similarly, but the clinical consequences of this are unknown. Fluvoxamine would be expected to inhibit the metabolism of propafenone by *N*-dealkylation. Sertraline and citalopram would not be expected to interact.

Clinical evidence, mechanism, importance and management

Fluoxetine 20 mg daily for 10 days decreased the oral clearance of a single 400-mg oral dose of propafenone by 34% for both the *R*- and *S*-enantiomers in healthy subjects. The peak plasma concentrations increased by 39% for *S*-propafenone and by 71% for *R*-propafenone. However, there were no differences in the changes to the PR and QRS intervals.[1] **Fluoxetine** is an inhibitor of the cytochrome P450 isoenzyme CYP2D6, which is responsible for the metabolism of propafenone to its primary active metabolite 5-hydroxypropafenone (see also mechanism under 'Propafenone + Quinidine', p.185). *In vitro* data have shown that, of the SSRIs, **fluoxetine** is the most potent inhibitor of propafenone 5-hydroxylation, and that **paroxetine** would also be expected to interact.[2] As with 'quinidine', (p.185), inhibition of 5-hydroxylation would be expected to increase the beta-blocking effects of propafenone.[2] Until more is known, it would be prudent to use caution when giving fluoxetine or paroxetine with propafenone. **Sertraline** and **citalopram** did not interact in vitro.[2]

Although **fluvoxamine** had no effect on propafenone 5-hydroxylation in vitro,[2] it did inhibit propafenone *N*-dealkylation[2] via its inhibitory effects on the cytochrome P450 isoenzyme CYP1A2. This isoenzyme has only a minor role in the metabolism of propafenone, but it may assume greater importance in those who have low levels of CYP2D6 ('poor' metabolisers).[2] Further study is needed.

1. Cai WM, Chen B, Zhou Y, Zhang YD. Fluoxetine impairs the CYP2D6-mediated metabolism of propafenone enantiomers in healthy Chinese volunteers. *Clin Pharmacol Ther* (1999) 66, 516–21.
2. Hemeryck A, De Vriendt C, Belpaire FM. Effect of selective serotonin reuptake inhibitors on the oxidative metabolism of propafenone: *in vitro* studies using human liver microsomes. *J Clin Psychopharmacol* (2000) 20, 428–34.

Quinidine + Amiloride

A single study has shown that the antiarrhythmic activity of quinidine can be opposed by amiloride.

Clinical evidence

A study in 10 patients with inducible sustained ventricular tachycardia was carried out to see whether a beneficial interaction occurred between quinidine and amiloride. Patients were given oral quinidine until their trough serum levels reached 10 micromol/l, or the maximum well-tolerated dose was reached. After electrophysiological studies had been done, oral amiloride was added at a dosage of 5 mg twice daily, increased up to 10 mg twice daily (if serum potassium levels remained normal) for 3 days. The electrophysiological studies were then repeated. Unexpectedly, 7 of the 10 patients demonstrated adverse responses while taking both drugs. Three developed sustained ventricular tachycardia and 3 others had somatic adverse effects (hypotension, nausea, diarrhoea), which prevented further studies being carried out. One patient had 12 episodes of sustained ventricular tachycardia while taking both drugs. Amiloride had no effect on quinidine levels.[1]

Mechanism

Not understood. The combination of quinidine and amiloride increased the QRS interval, but did not prolong the QT interval more than quinidine alone.

Importance and management

So far the evidence seems to be limited to this single study but it suggests that amiloride can oppose the antiarrhythmic activity of quinidine. The full clinical implications of this interaction are not yet known, but it would now clearly be prudent to monitor concurrent use very closely to confirm that the quinidine continues to be effective if amiloride is present.

1. Wang L, Sheldon RS, Mitchell B, Wyse DG, Gillis AM, Chiamvimonvat N, Duff HJ. Amiloride-quinidine interaction: adverse outcomes. *Clin Pharmacol Ther* (1994) 56, 659–67.

Quinidine + Amiodarone

The QT interval prolonging effects of quinidine and amiodarone are increased when they are used together, and torsade de pointes has occurred. Therefore the combination should generally be avoided. However, if the combination is used, reduce the quinidine dosage appropriately to avoid quinidine toxicity since serum quinidine levels can be increased by the concurrent use of amiodarone.

Clinical evidence

Eleven patients were stabilised on quinidine (daily doses of 1200 to 4200 mg). When concurrently treated with amiodarone (600 mg loading dose 12-hourly for 5 to 7 days, then 600 mg daily) their mean serum quinidine levels rose by an average of 32%, from 4.4 to 5.8 micrograms/ml and 3 of them had a substantial increase of 2 micrograms/ml. Signs of toxicity (diarrhoea, nausea, vomiting, hypotension) were seen in some, and the quinidine dosage was reduced in 9 of the patients by an average of 37%. Even so, the quinidine serum levels were still higher at 5.2 micrograms/ml than before the amiodarone was started.[1]

A test in a healthy subject showed that 3 days after amiodarone 600 mg was added to quinidine 1200 mg daily, the serum quinidine levels doubled and the relative QT interval was prolonged from 1 (no drugs) to 1.2 (quinidine alone) to 1.4 (quinidine plus amiodarone).[2] This report also described two patients with minor cardiac arrhythmias who developed QT prolongation and torsade de pointes when given both drugs.[2] A Russian study of the use of the combination in atrial fibrillation reported that one of 52 patients had a 50% increase in the QT interval resulting in torsade de pointes and subsequently ventricular fibrillation, which required repeated defibrillation over 6 hours.[3] A 76-year-old man on quinidine and amiodarone had a number of episodes of loss of consciousness, and subsequently QT prolongation and torsade de pointes, which stopped when the quinidine was discontinued.[4]

Mechanism

The mechanism behind the pharmacokinetic interaction is not understood. The QT prolonging effects of the two drugs would be expected to be additive.

Importance and management

An established and clinically important pharmacokinetic and pharmacodynamic interaction. The use of amiodarone with quinidine further prolongs the QT interval and increases the risk of torsade de pointes. Therefore, the combination should generally be avoided. The UK makers of amiodarone contraindicate its use with class Ia antiarrhythmics such as quinidine.[5] See also 'Drugs that prolong the QT interval + Other drugs that prolong the QT interval', p.170. The pharmacokinetic component appears to occur in most patients, and to develop rapidly. The US makers[6] of amiodarone consider such combination therapy should be reserved for life-threatening ventricular arrhythmias incompletely responsive to either agent alone and recommend that the dose of quinidine should be reduced by one-third. Others suggest that if the two drugs are considered essential, the dosage of quinidine should be reduced by about 30 to 50% and the serum levels should be monitored.[1] The ECG should also be monitored for evidence of changes in the QT interval when combined therapy is started or stopped.[7] Successful and uneventful concurrent use has been described in a report of 4 patients on quinidine (dose not stated) and amiodarone 200 mg five times weekly.[8] Another describes the successful use of a short course of quinidine to convert chronic atrial fibrillation to sinus rhythm in 9 of 15 patients on long-term amiodarone therapy. Patients were hospitalised and continuously monitored: no proarrhythmias occurred and the QT interval remained within acceptable limits.[9]

1. Saal AK, Werner JA, Greene HL, Sears GK, Graham EL. Effect of amiodarone on serum quinidine and procainamide levels. *Am J Cardiol* (1984) 53, 1265–7.
2. Tartini R, Kappenberger L, Steinbrunn W, Meyer UA. Dangerous interaction between amiodarone and quinidine. *Lancet* (1982) i, 1327–9.
3. Lipnitsky TN, Dorogan AV, Randin AG, Kotsuta GI. Clinical efficacy and potential hazards from combined cordarone-and-chinidine treatment in patients with atrial fibrillation (in Russian). *Klin Med (Mosk)* (1992) 70, 31–4.
4. Nattel S, Ranger S, Talajic M, Lemery R, Roy D. Erythromycin-induced long QT syndrome: concordance with quinidine and underlying cellular electrophysiologic mechanism. *Am J Med* (1990) 89, 235–8.
5. Cordarone X (Amiodarone hydrochloride). Sanofi Synthelabo. UK Summary of product characteristics, May 2004.
6. Cordarone (Amiodarone hydrochloride). Wyeth Laboratories. US Prescribing information, April 2004.
7. Kinidin Durules (Quinidine). AstraZeneca UK Ltd. UK Summary of product characteristics, June 2002.
8. Hoffmann A, Follath F, Burckhardt D. Safe treatment of resistant ventricular arrhythmias with a combination of amiodarone and quinidine or mexiletine. *Lancet* (1983) i, 704–5.
9. Kerin NZ, Ansari-Leesar M, Faitel K, Narala C, Frumin H, Cohen A. The effectiveness and safety of the simultaneous administration of quinidine and amiodarone in the conversion of chronic atrial fibrillation. *Am Heart J* (1993) 125, 1017–21.

Quinidine + Antacids or Urinary alkalinizers

Large rises in urinary pH due to the concurrent use of some antacids, diuretics or alkaline salts can cause the retention of quinidine, which could lead to quinidine toxicity, but there seems to be only one case on record of an adverse interaction (with *Mylanta*—magnesium and aluminium hydroxide). Aluminium hydroxide appears not to interact.

Clinical evidence

The renal clearance of oral quinidine in 4 subjects taking 200 mg six-hourly was reduced by an average of 50% (from 53 to 26 ml/minute) when their urine was made alkaline (i.e. changed from pH 6–7 to pH 7–8) with **sodium bicarbonate** and **acetazolamide** 500 mg twice daily. Below pH 6 their urinary quinidine level averaged 115 mg/l, whereas when urinary pH values rose above 7.5 the average quinidine level fell to 13 mg/l. The quinidine urinary excretion rate decreased from 103 to 31 micrograms/minute. In 6 other subjects the rise in serum quinidine levels was reflected in a prolongation of the QT interval. Raising the urinary pH from about 6 to 7.5 in one individual increased serum quinidine levels from about 1.6 to 2.6 micrograms/ml.[1]

A patient on quinidine who took eight *Mylanta* tablets daily (**aluminium hydroxide** gel 200 mg, **magnesium hydroxide** 200 mg and simeticone 20 mg) for a week and a little over 1 litre of fruit juice (orange and grapefruit) each day developed a threefold increase in serum quinidine levels (from 8 to 25 mg/l) and toxicity [but see Importance and management below]. In 6 healthy subjects, this dose of *Mylanta* for 3 days produced consistently alkaline urine in 4 subjects, and in 5 subjects when combined with fruit juice.[2]

In 4 healthy subjects, 30 ml of **aluminium hydroxide** gel *(Amphogel)* administered with, and one hour after, a single 200-mg dose of quinidine sulphate had no effect on serum quinidine levels, AUC or excretion (urine pH ranged from 5 to 6.2).[3] Two similar single-dose studies in healthy subjects found that the absorption and elimination of 400 mg of quinidine sulphate[4] or 648 mg of quinidine gluconate[5] was unaffected by 30 ml **aluminium hydroxide** gel, although the change in quinidine AUC did vary from a decrease of 18% to an increase of 35% in one study.[5] Urinary pH was unaffected in both studies.[4,5]

Mechanism

Quinidine is excreted unchanged in the urine. In acid urine much of the quinidine excreted by the kidney tubules is in the ionised (lipid-insoluble) form, which is unable to diffuse freely back into the cells and so is lost in the urine. In alkaline urine more of the quinidine is in the non-ionised (lipid-soluble) form, which freely diffuses back into the cells and is retained. In this way the pH of the urine determines how much quinidine is lost or retained and thereby governs the serum levels. *In vitro* data suggest changes in pH and adsorption effects within the gut due to antacids could also affect the absorption of quinidine.[6,7]

Importance and management

An established interaction, but with the exception of the one isolated case cited,[2] there seem to be no reports of problems in patients given quinidine and antacids or urinary alkalinizers. However, in this case quinidine was given with grapefruit juice, which may potentially have had an effect of its own, see 'Quinidine + Grapefruit juice', p.191. Nevertheless you should monitor the effects if drugs that can markedly change urinary pH are started or stopped. Reduce the quinidine dosage as necessary.

It is difficult to predict which antacids, if any, are likely to increase the serum levels of quinidine. As noted above, aluminium hydroxide gel and magnesium hydroxide (*Mylanta*) alkalinizes urine and can interact. Similarly, magnesium and aluminium hydroxide (*Maalox*) can raise the urinary pH by about 0.9 and could possibly interact.[8] Magnesium hydroxide (*Milk of magnesia*) and **calcium carbonate-glycine** (*Titralac*) in normal doses raise the urinary pH by about 0.5, so that a smaller effect is likely.[8] Aluminium hydroxide gel (*Amphogel*) and **dihydroxyaluminium glycinate** (*Robalate*) are reported to have no effect on urinary pH,[8] and the studies above confirm aluminium hydroxide gel does not generally interact.

1. Gerhardt RE, Knouss RF, Thyrum PT, Luchi RJ, Morris JJ. Quinidine excretion in aciduria and alkaluria. *Ann Intern Med* (1969) 71, 927–33.
2. Zinn MB. Quinidine intoxication from alkali ingestion. *Tex Med* (1970) 66, 64–6.
3. Romankiewicz JA, Reidenberg M, Drayer D, Franklin JE. The noninterference of aluminium hydroxide gel with quinidine sulfate absorption: an approach to control quinidine-induced diarrhea. *Am Heart J* (1978) 96, 518–20.
4. Ace LN, Jaffe JM, Kunka RL. Effect of food and antacid on quinidine bioavailability. *Biopharm Drug Dispos* (1983) 4, 183–90.
5. Mauro VF, Mauro LS, Fraker TD, Temesy-Armos PN, Somani P. Effect of aluminium hydroxide gel on quinidine gluconate absorption. *Ann Pharmacother* (1990) 24, 252–4.
6. Remon JP, Van Severen R, Braeckman P. Interaction entre antiarythmiques, antiacides et antidiarrhéiques. III. Influence d'antacides et d'antidiarrhéiques sur la réabsorption in vitro de sels de quinidine. *Pharm Acta Helv* (1979) 54, 19–22.
7. Moustafa MA, Al-Shora HI, Gaber M, Gouda MW. Decreased bioavailability of quinidine sulphate due to interactions with adsorbent antacids and antidiarrhoeal mixtures. *Int J Pharmaceutics* (1987) 34, 207–11.
8. Gibaldi M, Grundhofer B, Levy G. Effect of antacids on pH of urine. *Clin Pharmacol Ther* (1974) 16, 520–5.

Quinidine + Anticonvulsants

Serum quinidine levels can be reduced by the concurrent use of phenytoin, phenobarbital or primidone. Loss of arrhythmia control is possible if the quinidine dosage is not increased.

Clinical evidence

A man on long-term **primidone** 500 mg daily was started on quinidine 300 mg four-hourly, but only attained a plasma quinidine level of 0.8 micrograms/ml with an estimated half-life of 5 hours. When **primidone** was discontinued, quinidine levels rose to 2.4 micrograms/ml with a half-life of 12 hours. **Phenobarbital** 90 mg daily was then started, and the quinidine level fell to 1.6 micrograms/ml with a half-life of 7.6 hours. In another case, a woman required doses of quinidine sulfate of up to 800 mg four-hourly to achieve therapeutic levels while taking **phenytoin**. When the **phenytoin** was stopped, quinidine toxicity occurred, and the dose was eventually halved. Further study was then made in 4 healthy subjects. After 4 weeks treatment with either **phenytoin** (in dosages adjusted to give 10 to 20 micrograms/ml) or **phenobarbital**, the elimination half-life of a single 300-mg dose of quinidine sulphate was reduced by about 50% and the total AUC by about 60%.[1]

Similar results were found with **phenytoin** in another study in 3 healthy subjects.[2] Other cases have also been reported with **phenytoin, primidone, pentobarbital** and **phenobarbital**.[3-6] In one case, quinidine levels fell by 44% when **phenytoin** was added to quinidine therapy in a patient with recurrent ventricular tachycardia.[3] Quinidine levels increased from a mean of 0.8 to 2.2 micrograms/ml 15 days after **pentobarbital** was discontinued in another report.[4] Interestingly, in this case the patient was also on **digoxin**, and stopping phenobarbital precipitated **digoxin** toxicity by causing an increase in quinidine levels.

A 3-year-old child on both **phenobarbital** and **phenytoin** required 300 mg of quinidine 4-hourly to achieve therapeutic serum quinidine levels, and had an estimated quinidine half-life of only 1.4 hours.[5] Difficulty in achieving adequate serum quinidine levels was also reported in a woman on **phenytoin** and **primidone**. Her quinidine half-life was 2.7 hours, approximately half that usually seen in adults.[6]

Quinidine 200 mg had no effect on the metabolism (4-hydroxylation) of **mephenytoin** 100 mg in 10 healthy subjects.[7]

Mechanism

The evidence suggests that phenytoin, primidone or phenobarbital (all known enzyme-inducing agents) increase the metabolism by the liver of the quinidine and increase its loss from the body.[2]

Importance and management

Established interactions of clinical importance although the documentation is limited. The concurrent use of phenytoin, primidone, phenobarbital or any other barbiturate need not be avoided, but be alert for the need to increase the quinidine dosage. If the anticonvulsants are withdrawn the quinidine dosage may need to be reduced to avoid quinidine toxicity. Where possible, quinidine serum levels should be monitored.

1. Data JL, Wilkinson GR, Nies AS. Interaction of quinidine with anticonvulsant drugs. *N Engl J Med* (1976) 294, 699–702.
2. Russo ME, Russo J, Smith RA, Pershing LK. The effect of phenytoin on quinidine pharmacokinetics. *Drug Intell Clin Pharm* (1982) 16, 480.
3. Urbano AM. Phenytoin-quinidine interaction in a patient with recurrent ventricular tachyarrhythmias. *N Engl J Med* (1983) 308, 225.
4. Chapron DJ, Mumford D, Pitegoff GI. Apparent quinidine-induced digoxin toxicity after withdrawal of pentobarbital. A case of sequential drug interactions. *Arch Intern Med* (1979) 139, 363–5.
5. Rodgers GC, Blackman MS. Quinidine interaction with anticonvulsants. *Drug Intell Clin Pharm* (1983) 17, 819–20.
6. Kroboth FJ, Kroboth PD, Logan T. Phenytoin-theophylline-quinidine interaction. *N Engl J Med* (1983) 308, 725.
7. Schellens JHM, Ghabrial H, van der Wart HHF, Bakker EN, Wilkinson GR, Breimer DD. Differential effects of quinidine on the disposition of nifedipine, sparteine and mephenytoin in humans. *Clin Pharmacol Ther* (1991) 50, 520–8.

Quinidine + Aspirin

A patient and two healthy subjects given quinidine and aspirin showed a two- to threefold increase in bleeding times. The patient developed petechiae and gastrointestinal bleeding.

Clinical evidence, mechanism, importance and management

A patient with a prolonged history of paroxysmal atrial tachycardia was given quinidine 800 mg daily and aspirin 325 mg twice daily. After a week he showed generalised petechiae and blood in his faeces. His prothrombin and partial prothrombin times were normal but the template bleeding time was more than 35 minutes (normal 2 to 10 minutes). Further study in two healthy subjects showed that quinidine 975 mg daily given alone for 5 days and aspirin 650 mg three times a day given alone for 5 days prolonged bleeding times by 125% and 163% respectively; given together for 5 days the bleeding times were prolonged by 288%.[1] The underlying mechanism is not totally understood but it is believed to be the outcome of the additive effects of two drugs, both of which can reduce platelet aggregation,[1] although with quinidine this antiplatelet effect usually only occurs as the result of a hypersensitivity reaction.

This seems to be the only study of this adverse interaction, and its general importance is uncertain. It may be prudent to monitor concurrent use to check that bleeding does not occur.

1. Lawson D, Mehta J, Mehta P, Lipman BC, Imperi GA. Cumulative effects of quinidine and aspirin on bleeding time and platelet α_2-adrenoceptors: potential mechanism of bleeding diathesis in patients receiving this combination. *J Lab Clin Med* (1986) 108, 581–6.

Quinidine + Calcium channel blockers

A few patients have shown increased serum quinidine levels when stopping nifedipine, but others have shown no interaction and one study even suggests that quinidine serum levels may be slightly raised by nifedipine. Nifedipine levels may be modestly raised by quinidine. Verapamil reduces the clearance of quinidine and in

one patient the serum quinidine levels doubled and quinidine toxicity developed. Acute hypotension has also been seen in three patients on quinidine when given verapamil intravenously. Felodipine and nisoldipine appear not to interact, and the situation with diltiazem is unclear.

Clinical evidence

(a) Diltiazem

A study in 10 healthy subjects given quinidine 600 mg twice daily and diltiazem 120 mg daily for 7 days showed that the pharmacokinetics of neither drug was affected by the presence of the other.[1] These findings contrast with another crossover study in 12 healthy subjects given single-doses of diltiazem 60 mg or quinidine 200 mg alone, then after pretreatment with quinidine 100 mg twice daily or diltiazem 90 mg twice daily for 5 doses, respectively. The pharmacokinetics of diltiazem were unaffected by quinidine, but the AUC of quinidine was increased by 51% by diltiazem.[2] When quinidine was given after diltiazem pretreatment, there were significant increases in QTc and PR intervals, and a significant decrease in heart rate and diastolic blood pressure. Pretreatment with quinidine did not significantly alter the effects of diltiazem.[2]

(b) Felodipine

Felodipine 10 mg daily for 3 days was found to have no clinically significant effect on the pharmacokinetics or haemodynamic and ECG effects of a single 400-mg dose of quinidine in 12 healthy subjects. Felodipine did cause a modest 22% decrease in the AUC of the quinidine metabolite 3-hydroxyquinidine.[3]

(c) Nifedipine

(i) Quinidine serum levels. Two patients taking quinidine sulphate 300 or 400 mg six-hourly and nifedipine 10 or 20 mg six or eight-hourly showed a doubling of their serum quinidine levels (from a range of 2 to 2.5 up to 4.6 micrograms/ml and from 1.6 to 1.8 up to 3.5 micrograms/ml respectively) when the nifedipine was withdrawn. The increased serum quinidine levels were reflected in a prolongation of the QT_c interval. However, the first patient had demonstrated no change in quinidine levels when nifedipine was initially added to his existing quinidine therapy. In addition, 4 other patients failed to demonstrate this interaction.[4] Two other reports[5,6] describe a similar response: the quinidine serum level doubled in one patient when the nifedipine was stopped,[5] and in the other it was found difficult to achieve adequate serum quinidine levels when nifedipine was added, even when the quinidine dosage was increased threefold. When the nifedipine was withdrawn, the quinidine levels rose once again.[6] A study in 12 patients found no significant change in serum quinidine levels in the group as a whole when given nifedipine, but one patient showed a 41% decrease in quinidine levels.[7] Two other studies in healthy subjects found that the quinidine AUC was unchanged by nifedipine.[3,8] A further study in 12 healthy subjects found that the AUC of a single 200 mg oral dose of quinidine sulphate was increased 16% by 20 mg oral nifedipine, its clearance was reduced by 14% and the maximum serum level was raised almost 20%. These modest changes were not considered clinically relevant.[9]

(ii) Nifedipine serum levels. The nifedipine AUC in 10 healthy subjects was increased 37% when also given quinidine sulphate 200 mg eight-hourly, and heart rates were significantly increased. Quinidine levels were unchanged.[8] Another study found that quinidine had a modest inhibitory effect on the metabolism of nifedipine (half-life prolonged by 40%).[10] A further study in 12 healthy subjects found that the AUC of a single 20-mg oral dose of nifedipine was increased 16% by oral quinidine 200 mg and its clearance was reduced by 17%, but these modest changes were not considered clinically relevant.[9]

(d) Nisoldipine

An open crossover study in 20 healthy subjects found that nisoldipine 20 mg had no effect on the bioavailability of 648 mg of quinidine gluconate.[11]

(e) Verapamil

After taking verapamil 80 mg three times daily for 3 days, the clearance of a single 400-mg dose of quinidine sulphate in 6 healthy subjects was decreased by 32% and the half-life was increased by 35% from 6.87 to 9.29 hours.[12]

A patient given quinidine gluconate 648 mg six-hourly showed an increase in serum quinidine levels from 2.6 to 5.7 micrograms/ml when given verapamil 80 mg eight-hourly for a week. He became dizzy and had blurred vision and was found to have atrioventricular block (heart rate 38 bpm) and a systolic blood pressure of 50 mmHg. In a subsequent study in this patient it was found that the verapamil halved the quinidine clearance and almost doubled the serum half-life.[13]

Three other patients given quinidine orally showed marked hypotension when given intravenous verapamil 2.5 or 5 mg (blood pressure fall from 130/70 to 80/50 mmHg, systolic pressure fall from 140 to 85 mmHg and a mean arterial pressure fall from 100 to 60 mmHg, in the 3 patients respectively). In two of the patients, after quinidine was discontinued the same dose of verapamil did not cause a drop in blood pressure.[14]

Mechanism

Suggestions for how nifedipine could alter quinidine levels include changes in cardiovascular haemodynamics,[4] and effects on metabolism.[7] Quinidine probably inhibits nifedipine metabolism by the cytochrome P450 isoenzyme CYP3A4.[10] The quinidine/verapamil interaction is probably due to an inhibitory effect of verapamil on the metabolism of quinidine (inhibition of cytochrome P450 isoenzyme CYP3A).[12,15] The marked hypotension observed may be related to the antagonistic effects of the two drugs on catecholamine-induced alpha-receptor induced vasoconstriction.[14]

Importance and management

The results of studies of the quinidine/nifedipine interaction are inconsistent and contradictory, so that the outcome of concurrent use is uncertain. Monitor the response, being alert for the need to modify the dosage. More study of this interaction is needed. Quinidine appears to increase nifedipine levels, but the importance of this is uncertain.

What is known about the quinidine/verapamil interaction suggests that a reduction in the dosage of the quinidine may be needed to avoid toxicity. If the verapamil is given intravenously, use with caution and be alert for evidence of acute hypotension. Monitor the effects of concurrent use closely. There is actually a fixed dose preparation containing verapamil and quinidine (*Cordichin*) available in Germany, which is used for the management of atrial fibrillation. No interaction apparently occurs between quinidine and felodipine or nisoldipine. The situation with diltiazem is as yet uncertain but be alert for the need to reduce the quinidine dosage.

1. Matera MG, De Santis D, Vacca C, Fici F, Romano AR, Marrazzo R, Marmo E. Quinidine-diltiazem: pharmacokinetic interaction in humans. *Curr Ther Res* (1986) 40, 653–6.
2. Laganière S, Davies RF, Carignan G, Foris K, Goernert L, Carrier K, Pereira C, McGilveray I. Pharmacokinetic and pharmacodynamic interactions between diltiazem and quinidine. *Clin Pharmacol Ther* (1996) 60, 255–64.
3. Bailey DG, Freeman DJ, Melendez LJ, Kreeft JH, Edgar B, Carruthers SG. Quinidine interaction with nifedipine and felodipine: pharmacokinetic and pharmacodynamic evaluation. *Clin Pharmacol Ther* (1993) 53, 354–9.
4. Farringer JA, Green JA, O'Rourke RA, Linn WA, Clementi WA. Nifedipine-induced alterations in serum quinidine concentrations. *Am Heart J* (1984) 108, 1570–2.
5. Van Lith RM, Appleby DH. Quinidine-nifedipine interaction. *Drug Intell Clin Pharm* (1985) 19, 829–31.
6. Green JA, Clementi WA, Porter C, Stigelman W. Nifedipine-quinidine interaction. *Clin Pharm* (1983) 2, 461–5.
7. Munger MA, Jarvis RC, Nair R, Kasmer RJ, Nara AR, Urbancic A, Green JA. Elucidation of the nifedipine-quinidine interaction. *Clin Pharmacol Ther* (1989) 45, 411–16.
8. Bowles SK, Reeves RA, Cardozo L, Edwards DJ. Evaluation of the pharmacokinetic and pharmacodynamic interaction between quinidine and nifedipine. *J Clin Pharmacol* (1993) 33, 727–31.
9. Hippius M, Henschel L, Sigusch H, Tepper J, Brendel E. Hoffmann A. Pharmacokinetic interactions of nifedipine and quinidine. *Pharmazie* (1995) 50 613–16.
10. Schellens JHM, Ghabrial H, van der Wart HHF, Bakker EN, Wilkinson GR, Breimer DD. Differential effects of quinidine on the disposition of nifedipine, sparteine and mephenytoin in humans. *Clin Pharmacol Ther* (1991) 50, 520–8.
11. Schall R, Müller FO, Groenewoud G, Hundt HKL, Luus HG, Van Dyk M, Van Schalkwyk AMC. Investigation of a possible pharmacokinetic interaction between nisoldipine and quinidine in healthy volunteers. *Drug Invest* (1994) 8, 162–170.
12. Edwards DJ, Lavoie R, Beckman H, Blevins R, Rubenfire M. The effect of coadministration of verapamil on the pharmacokinetics and metabolism of quinidine. *Clin Pharmacol Ther* (1987) 41, 68–73.
13. Trohman RG, Estes DM, Castellanos A, Palomo AR, Myerburg RJ, Kessler KM. Increased quinidine plasma concentrations during administration of verapamil; a new quinidine-verapamil interaction. *Am J Cardiol* (1986) 57, 706–7.
14. Maisel AS, Motulsky HJ, Insel PA. Hypotension after quinidine plus verapamil. Possible additive competition at alpha-adrenergic receptors. *N Engl J Med* (1985) 312, 167–70.
15. Kroemer HK, Gautier J-C, Beaune P, Henderson C, Wolf CR, Eichelbaum M. Identification of P450 enzymes involved in metabolism of verapamil in humans. *Naunyn Schmiedebergs Arch Pharmacol* (1993) 348, 332–7.

Quinidine + Colesevelam

Colesevelam does not alter the pharmacokinetics of quinidine.

Clinical evidence, mechanism, importance and management

A single 4.5-g dose of colesevelam had no significant effect on the pharmacokinetics of a single 324-mg dose of quinidine in 25 healthy subjects.[1] This suggests that colesevelam does not reduce the absorption of quinidine. No special precautions appear to be needed during concurrent use.

1. Donovan JM, Stypinski D, Stiles MR, Olson TA, Burke SK. Drug interactions with colesevelam hydrochloride, a novel, potent lipid-lowering agent. *Cardiovasc Drugs Ther* (2000) 14, 681–90.

Quinidine + Co-phenotrope (Atropine/Diphenoxylate)

Co-phenotrope slightly reduced the rate, but not extent, of absorption of single doses of quinidine.

Clinical evidence, mechanism, importance and management

In one study, 8 healthy subjects were given a single 300-mg dose of quinidine sulphate alone and after taking two tablets of co-phenotrope (atropine sulphate 25 micrograms, diphenoxylate 2.5 mg; *Lomotil*) at midnight on the evening before and another two tablets the next morning an hour before the quinidine.[1] It was found that the maximum plasma quinidine levels were reduced by 21% from 2.1 to 1.65 micrograms/ml by the co-phenotrope, the time to maximum level was prolonged from 0.89 to 1.21 hours, and there was a slight increase in elimination half-life from 5.7 to 6.8 hours. While these results were statistically significant, the changes were relatively small and it seems doubtful if they are clinically relevant, particularly as the extent of absorption was unchanged. However it needs to be emphasised that because the quinidine formulation used was an immediate-release preparation, these results may not necessarily apply to sustained-release preparations, and also may not apply if multiple doses of quinidine are used.

1. Ponzillo JJ, Scavone JM, Paone RP, Lewis GP, Rayment CM, Fitzsimmons WE. Effect of diphenoxylate with atropine sulfate on the bioavailability of quinidine sulfate in healthy subjects. *Clin Pharm* (1988) 7, 139–42.

Quinidine + Diazepam

A single dose study suggests that diazepam does not affect the pharmacokinetics of quinidine.

Clinical evidence, mechanism, importance and management

A comparative study in 8 healthy subjects showed that the pharmacokinetics of a single 250-mg dose of quinidine sulphate was unaltered by a single 10-mg dose of diazepam.[1] This suggests that no interaction between these drugs is likely but it needs confirmation by further studies using multiple doses of both drugs.

1. Rao BR, Rambhau D. Absence of a pharmacokinetic interaction between quinidine and diazepam. *Drug Metabol Drug Interact* (1995) 12, 45–51.

Quinidine + Diclofenac

Diclofenac inhibits the metabolism of quinidine by *N*-oxidation but does not affect other pharmacokinetic parameters. *In vitro* and *animal* data suggest that quinidine may increase the metabolism of diclofenac.

Clinical evidence, mechanism, importance and management

In an open study, 6 healthy subjects were given a single 200-mg dose of quinidine sulphate before and on day 5 of a 6-day course of diclofenac 100 mg daily. Concomitant administration of diclofenac reduced the *N*-oxidation of quinidine by 33%, but no other pharmacokinetic changes were found.[1] Diclofenac is a substrate for, and therefore a possible competitive inhibitor of the cytochrome P450 isoenzyme CYP2C9. These results suggest CYP2C9 does not appear to have a major role in quinidine metabolism,[1] and so clinically relevant changes in quinidine pharmacokinetics with diclofenac would seem unlikely.

A study in *monkeys* found that plasma levels of diclofenac were approximately halved when diclofenac was given with quinidine (both by portal vein infusion).[2] *In vitro* study[3] has shown that quinidine stimulates the metabolism of diclofenac to its 5-hydroxylated derivative, via its effects on CYP3A4. Further study is required to assess the clinical relevance of these findings.

1. Damkier P, Hansen LL, Brøsen K. Effect of diclofenac, disulfiram, itraconazole, grapefruit juice and erythromycin on the pharmacokinetics of quinidine. *Br J Clin Pharmacol* (1999) 48, 829–38.
2. Tang W, Stearns RA, Kwei GY, Iliff SA, Miller RR, Egan MA, Yu NX, Dean DC, Kumar S, Shou M, Lin JH, Baillie TA. Interaction of diclofenac and quinidine in monkeys: stimulation of diclofenac metabolism. *J Pharmacol Exp Ther* (1999) 291, 1068–74.
3. Ngui JS, Tang W, Stearns RA, Shou M, Miller RR, Zhang Y, Lin JH, Baillie TA. Cytochrome P450 3A4-mediated interaction of diclofenac and quinidine. *Drug Metab Dispos* (2000) 28, 1043–50.

Quinidine + Disulfiram

Disulfiram does not affect the pharmacokinetics of quinidine.

Clinical evidence, mechanism, importance and management

In an open study, 6 healthy subjects were given a single 200-mg dose of quinidine sulphate before and on day 5 of a 6-day course of disulfiram 200 mg daily. There were no changes in quinidine pharmacokinetics during disulfiram administration.[1] Disulfiram is thought to be an inhibitor of the cytochrome P450 isoenzyme CYP2E1, but this isoenzyme does not appear to have a major role in quinidine metabolism.[1] Clinically relevant pharmacokinetic interactions between quinidine and disulfiram therefore seem unlikely. Concurrent use need not be avoided.

1. Damkier P, Hansen LL, Brøsen K. Effect of diclofenac, disulfiram, itraconazole, grapefruit juice and erythromycin on the pharmacokinetics of quinidine. *Br J Clin Pharmacol* (1999) 48, 829–38.

Quinidine + Erythromycin

Erythromycin can increase quinidine levels and cause a small further increase in the QT_c interval. An isolated report describes a moderate rise in serum quinidine levels in an elderly man attributed to the concurrent use of intravenous erythromycin, which was possibly a factor in an episode of torsade de pointes. Another isolated report describes the development of torsade de pointes arrhythmia in a very old man when given quinidine and erythromycin orally. See also 'Drugs that prolong the QT interval + Other drugs that prolong the QT interval', p.170.

Clinical evidence

A 74-year-old man with a history of cardiac disease (coronary artery bypass graft surgery, ventricular tachycardia) treated with quinidine sulphate 200 mg six-hourly and several other drugs (mexiletine, hydralazine, dipyridamole, aspirin and paracetamol (acetaminophen)), was hospitalised with suspected implantable cardioverter defibrillator infection. Within two days of starting to take erythromycin lactobionate 500 mg six-hourly and ceftriaxone 1 g daily, both given intravenously, his trough serum quinidine levels had risen by about one-third from about 2.8 to 4.2 mg/l. On day seven metronidazole 500 mg 8-hourly was added and the erythromycin dosage was doubled, and the patient experienced an episode of torsade de pointes. By day 12 his serum quinidine levels had further risen to 5.8 mg/l, whereupon the quinidine dosage was reduced by 25%. Because an interaction between quinidine and erythromycin had by then been suspected, the antibacterials were replaced by doxycycline and ciprofloxacin. By day 21 the quinidine serum levels had fallen to their former levels. The patient had a prolonged QTc interval of 504 milliseconds on admission, and this did not change.[1]

A 95-year-old man developed QT interval prolongation, torsade de pointes arrhythmia and subsequent cardiac arrest when given quinidine and erythromycin, both orally.[2]

Preliminary results of a randomised, placebo-controlled crossover study in 12 subjects found that when given a single 400-mg dose of quinidine after taking erythromycin 500 mg three times daily by mouth or a placebo for 5 days, the total QT_c AUC was significantly prolonged by about 6% from 10279 to 10878 millisecond.h during the erythromycin phase.[3] In a parallel study by the same group, peak levels of quinidine were increased by 39%, from 587 to 816 nanograms/ml, and the AUC by 62%, from 326 to 528 mg.min/ml, by day 5 of the erythromycin phase. Peak levels of the main metabolite of quinidine, 3-hydroxyquinidine, were significantly reduced.[4] Another study in 6 healthy subjects found that oral erythromycin 250 mg four times daily for 6 days reduced the total clearance of a single 200-mg dose of quinidine sulphate by 34% and increased its maximum serum concentration by 39%.[5]

Mechanism

Not fully understood, but erythromycin inhibits the metabolism of quinidine,[4] possibly by inhibition of cytochrome P450 isoenzyme CYP3A4,[5] thereby reducing its clearance from the body and increasing its effects. There are also a number of cases on record of prolongation of the QT interval and torsade de pointes associated with the use of intravenous erythromycin alone.[6] Therefore, quinidine and erythromycin may have additive effects on the QT interval in addition to the pharmacokinetic interaction.

Importance and management

Information about this interaction appears to be limited to these reports, but it would appear to be established. If erythromycin is essential in a patient taking quinidine, the effects of concurrent use should be well monitored, being alert for the development of raised plasma quinidine levels and prolongation of the QT interval (see also 'Drugs that prolong the QT interval + Other drugs that prolong the QT interval', p.170). There seems to be nothing documented about any other quinidine/macrolide antibacterial interactions.

1. Spinler SA, Cheng JWM, Kindwall KE, Charland SL. Possible inhibition of hepatic metabolism of quinidine by erythromycin. *Clin Pharmacol Ther* (1995) 57, 89–94.
2. Lin JC, Quasny HA. QT prolongation and development of torsades de pointes with the concomitant administration of oral erythromycin base and quinidine. *Pharmacotherapy* (1997) 17, 626–30.
3. Stanford RH, Geraets DR, Lee H-C, Min DI. Effect of oral erythromycin on quinidine pharmacodynamics in healthy volunteers. *Pharmacotherapy* (1997) 17, 1111.
4. Stanford RH, Park JM, Geraets Dr, Min DI, Lee H-C. Effect of oral erythromycin on quinidine pharmacokinetics in healthy volunteers. *Pharmacotherapy* (1998) 18, 426–7.
5. Damkier P, Hansen LL, Brøsen K. Effect of diclofenac, disulfiram, itraconazole, grapefruit juice and erythromycin on the pharmacokinetics of quinidine. *Br J Clin Pharmacol* (1999) 48, 829–38.
6. Gitler B, Berger LS, Buffa SD. Torsades de pointes induced by erythromycin. *Chest* (1994) 105, 368–72.

Quinidine + Fluvoxamine

Fluvoxamine appears to inhibit the metabolism and clearance of quinidine.

Clinical evidence, mechanism, importance and management

Six healthy subjects were given a single 250-mg dose of quinidine sulphate before and on day 5 of a 6-day course of fluvoxamine 100 mg daily.[1] The total apparent oral clearance of quinidine was reduced by 29%, and *N*-oxidation and 3-hydroxylation were reduced by 33 and 44% respectively. Renal clearance and elimination half-life were unchanged. It was concluded that fluvoxamine inhibited the metabolism of quinidine by the cytochrome P450 isoenzyme CYP3A4, although a role for CYP1A2 and CYP2C19 was not excluded. The clinical relevance of these findings is unclear. However, it would seem prudent to monitor the concurrent use of quinidine with fluvoxamine. More study is needed to assess the effect of multiple dosing and to establish the clinical significance of this interaction.

1. Damkier P, Hansen LL, Brøsen K. Effect of fluvoxamine on the pharmacokinetics of quinidine. *Eur J Clin Pharmacol* (1999) 55, 451–6.

Quinidine + Grapefruit juice

Grapefruit juice delays the absorption of quinidine and reduces its metabolism to some extent, but no clinically relevant adverse interaction seems to occur.

Clinical evidence, mechanism, importance and management

In one study, 12 healthy subjects were given quinidine sulphate 400 mg orally on two occasions, once with 240 ml of water and once with grapefruit juice. The pharmacokinetics of the quinidine were unchanged, except that its absorption was delayed (the time to reach maximum plasma concentrations was doubled from 1.6 to 3.3 hours), for reasons that are not understood. The AUC of its metabolite (3-hydroxyquinidine) was decreased by one-third, suggesting that the grapefruit juice inhibits the metabolism of the quinidine.[1] No important changes in the QTc interval were seen.[1] Similarly, another study in 6 healthy subjects found the total clearance of a single 200-mg dose of quinidine sulphate was reduced by 15% by 250 ml of grapefruit juice, with no change in maximum level. There was a small reduction in metabolite formation suggesting only minor inhibition of metabolism.[2] Grapefruit is known to inhibit the cytochrome P450 isoenzyme CYP3A4, which is involved with the metabolism of quinidine, so it seems likely that any interaction would occur via this pathway.[1,2] These studies suggest that it is not necessary for patients on quinidine to avoid grapefruit juice.

1. Min DI, Ku Y-M, Geraets DR, Lee H-c. Effect of grapefruit juice on the pharmacokinetics and pharmacodynamics of quinidine in healthy volunteers. *J Clin Pharmacol* (1996) 36, 469–76.
2. Damkier P, Hansen LL, Brøsen K. Effect of diclofenac, disulfiram, itraconazole, grapefruit juice and erythromycin on the pharmacokinetics of quinidine. *Br J Clin Pharmacol* (1999) 48, 829–38.

Quinidine + H_2-blockers

Quinidine serum levels can rise and toxicity may develop in some patients when concurrently treated with cimetidine. An isolated case of ventricular bigeminy (a form of arrhythmia) occurred in a patient on quinidine and ranitidine.

Clinical evidence

Cimetidine 1.2 g daily for 7 days prolonged the elimination half-life of a single 400-mg dose of quinidine sulphate by 55%, from 5.8 to 9 hours, and decreased its clearance by 37% in 6 healthy subjects. Peak plasma levels were raised by 21%. These changes were reflected in ECG changes, with 51% and 28% increases in the mean areas under the QT and QT_c time curves, respectively, but these were said not to be statistically significant.[1]

A later study, prompted by the observation of two patients who developed toxic quinidine levels when given **cimetidine**, found essentially the same. The AUC and half-life of quinidine were increased by 14.5 and 22.6% respectively, and the clearance was decreased by 25% by cimetidine 1.2 g daily in healthy subjects.[2] A further study in 4 healthy subjects found that **cimetidine** 1.2 g daily for 5 days prolonged the elimination half-life of quinidine by 54% and decreased its total clearance by 36%.[3,4] **Cimetidine** prolonged the QT interval by 30% more than quinidine's effect alone.[4] A case report describes marked increases in both quinidine and digitoxin concentrations in a woman also given **cimetidine**.[5] Similarly, quinidine levels increased by up to 50%, without causing any adverse effects, in a man on quinidine who was given cimetidine.[6]

Ventricular bigeminy (a form of arrhythmia) occurred in a man on quinidine when given **ranitidine**. His serum quinidine levels remained unchanged.[7]

Mechanism

It was originally suggested that the cimetidine inhibits the metabolism of the quinidine by the liver so that it is cleared more slowly.[2] However, further data suggest that cimetidine successfully competes with quinidine for its excretion by the kidneys.[8]

Importance and management

The quinidine/cimetidine interaction is established and of clinical importance. The incidence is unknown. Be alert for changes in the response to quinidine if cimetidine is started or stopped. Ideally the quinidine serum levels should be monitored and the dosage reduced as necessary. Reductions of 25% (oral) and 35% (intravenous) have been suggested.[3] Those at greatest risk are likely to be patients with impaired renal function, patients with impaired liver function, the elderly, and those with serum quinidine levels already at the top end of the therapeutic range.[2] The situation with ranitidine is uncertain.

1. Hardy BG, Zador IT, Golden L, Lalka D, Schentag JJ. Effect of cimetidine on the pharmacokinetics and pharmacodynamics of quinidine. *Am J Cardiol* (1983) 52, 172–5.
2. Kolb KW, Garnett WR, Small RE, Vetrovec GW, Kline BJ, Fox T. Effect of cimetidine on quinidine clearance. *Ther Drug Monit* (1984) 6, 306–12.
3. MacKichan JJ, Boudoulas H, Schaal SF. Effect of cimetidine on quinidine bioavailability. *Biopharm Drug Dispos* (1989) 10, 121–5.
4. Boudoulas H, MacKichan JJ, Schaal SF. Effect of cimetidine on the pharmacodynamics of quinidine. *Med Sci Res* (1988) 16, 713–14.
5. Polish LB, Branch RA, Fitzgerald GA. Digitoxin-quinidine interaction: potentiation during administration of cimetidine. *South Med J* (1981) 74, 633–4.
6. Farringer JA, McWay-Hess K, Clementi WA. Cimetidine–quinidine interaction. *Clin Pharm* (1984) 3, 81–3.
7. Iliopoulou A, Kontogiannis D, Tsoutsos D, Moulopoulos S. Quinidine-ranitidine adverse reaction. *Eur Heart J* (1986) 7, 360.
8. Hardy BG, Schentag JJ. Lack of effect of cimetidine on the metabolism of quinidine: effect on renal clearance. *Int J Clin Pharmacol Ther Toxicol* (1988) 26, 388–91.

Quinidine + Itraconazole

Itraconazole increases the plasma levels of quinidine.

Clinical evidence

In a double-blind, randomised, two-phase crossover study, 9 healthy subjects were given a single 100-mg dose of quinidine sulphate on day 4 of a four-day course of either itraconazole 200 mg daily or a placebo. The itraconazole caused a 1.6-fold increase in the peak plasma quinidine levels, a 2.4-fold increase in its AUC, a 1.6-fold increase in its elimination half-life and a 50% decrease in its renal clearance.[1] Similarly, another study in 6 healthy subjects found that itraconazole 100 mg daily for 6 days reduced the total clearance of a single 200-mg dose of quinidine sulphate by 61%, increased its elimination half-life by 35%, and decreased its renal clearance by 60%.[2]

Mechanism

The most likely explanation is that the itraconazole not only inhibits the metabolism of the quinidine by cytochrome P450 isoenzyme CYP3A4 in the gut wall and liver, but possibly also inhibits the active secretion of quinidine by the kidney tubules.[1,2]

Importance and management

Direct information appears to be limited to these studies, but the evidence suggests that this interaction is clinically important. What happens is consistent with the way itraconazole interacts with other drugs. If larger doses of itraconazole were to be used and for longer periods, it seems likely that the effects would be even greater. The concurrent use of these drugs should therefore be well monitored and the dosage of quinidine reduced accordingly. More study is needed. Consider also 'Quinidine + Ketoconazole', below.

1. Kaukonen K-M, Olkkola KT, Neuvonen PJ. Itraconazole increases plasma concentrations of quinidine. *Clin Pharmacol Ther* (1997) 62, 510–17.
2. Damkier P, Hansen LL, Brøsen K. Effect of diclofenac, disulfiram, itraconazole, grapefruit juice and erythromycin on the pharmacokinetics of quinidine. *Br J Clin Pharmacol* (1999) 48, 829–38.

Quinidine + Kaolin-pectin

There is some evidence that kaolin-pectin can reduce the absorption of quinidine and lower its serum levels.

Clinical evidence, mechanism, importance and management

When 4 patients were given 30 ml of kaolin-pectin (*Kaopectate*), after a single 100-mg oral dose of quinidine, the maximal salivary quinidine concentration was reduced by 54% and the AUC by 58%, without any effect on absorption rate.[1] There is a correlation between salivary and serum concentrations after a single (but not repeated) doses of quinidine.[2] This is consistent with *in vitro* data showing quinidine is adsorbed onto kaolin,[3] pectin,[3] and kaolin-pectin.[1] Documentation appears to be limited to these two studies, but be alert for the need to increase the quinidine dosage if kaolin-pectin is used concurrently.

1. Moustafa MA, Al-Shora HI, Gaber M, Gouda MW. Decreased bioavailability of quinidine sulphate due to interactions with adsorbent antacids and antidiarrhoeal mixtures. *Int J Pharmaceutics* (1987) 34, 207–11.
2. Narang PK, Carliner NH, Fisher ML, Crouthamel WG. Quinidine saliva concentrations: absence of correlation with serum concentrations at steady state. *Clin Pharmacol Ther* (1983) 34, 695–702.
3. Bucci AJ, Myre SA, Tan HSI, Shenouda LS. In vitro interaction of quinidine with kaolin and pectin. *J Pharm Sci* (1981) 70, 999–1002.

Quinidine + Ketoconazole

An isolated report describes a temporary marked increase in plasma quinidine levels in man when he was additionally treated with ketoconazole.

Clinical evidence, mechanism, importance and management

An elderly man with chronic atrial fibrillation, treated with quinidine sulphate 300 mg four times daily, was additionally given ketoconazole 200 mg daily for candidal oesophagitis after antineoplastic therapy. Within 7 days his plasma quinidine levels had risen from a range of 1.4 to 2.7 mg/l up to 6.9 mg/l (normal range 2 to 5 mg/l) but he showed no evidence of toxicity. The elimination half-life of quinidine was found to be 25 hours (normal values in healthy subjects 6 to 7 hours). The quinidine dosage was reduced to 200 mg twice daily, but it needed to be increased to the former dose by the end of a month, even though ketoconazole was continued at the same dosage. The reasons for this reaction are not understood, but may be that the ketoconazole initially inhibits the metabolism of quinidine, causing the plasma levels to rise, and then later induces the metabolism of quinidine, causing the levels to fall..[1] This is an isolated case so that its general importance is uncertain, but it draws attention to the need to monitor plasma quinidine levels patients given ketoconazole. See also 'Quinidine + Itraconazole', above.

1. McNulty RM, Lazor JA, Sketch M. Transient increase in plasma quinidine concentrations during ketoconazole-quinidine therapy. *Clin Pharm* (1989) 8, 222–5.

Quinidine + Laxatives

Quinidine plasma levels can be reduced by the concurrent use of the anthraquinone laxative senna.

Clinical evidence, mechanism, importance and management

A study in 7 patients with cardiac arrhythmias taking quinidine bisulfate 500 mg 12-hourly showed that concurrent use of the anthraquinone laxative **senna** (***Liquedepur***) reduced plasma quinidine levels, measured 12 hours after the last dose of quinidine, by about 25%.[1] This might be of clinical importance in patients whose plasma levels are barely adequate to control their arrhythmia.

1. Guckenbiehl W, Gilfrich HJ, Just H. Einfluß von Laxantien und Metoclopramid auf die Chindin-Plasmakonzentration während Langzeittherapie bei Patienten mit Herzrhythmusstörugen. *Med Welt* (1976) 27, 1273–6.

Quinidine + Lidocaine

A single case report describes a man on quinidine who had sinoatrial arrest when he was given lidocaine.

Clinical evidence, mechanism, importance and management

A man with Parkinson's disease was given quinidine 300 mg six-hourly for the control of ventricular ectopic beats. After receiving two doses he was given lidocaine as well, initially as a bolus of 80 mg, followed by an infusion of 4 mg/minute because persistent premature ventricular beats developed. Within 2.5 hours the patient complained of dizziness and weakness, and was found to have sinus bradycardia, sinoatrial arrest and atrioventricular escape rhythm. Normal sinus rhythm resumed when the lidocaine was stopped. Whether quinidine was a contributing factor in this reaction is uncertain.[1] However, this case emphasises the need to exercise caution when giving two drugs that have cardiac depressant actions.

1. Jeresaty RM, Kahn AH, Landry AB. Sinoatrial arrest due to lidocaine in a patient receiving quinidine. *Chest* (1972) 61, 683–5.

Quinidine + Metoclopramide

Metoclopramide slightly reduced the absorption of quinidine from a sustained-release formulation in one study, but modestly increased quinidine levels in another.

Clinical evidence

A study of this interaction was prompted by the case of a patient on sustained-release quinidine (*Quinidex*) whose arrhythmia failed to be controlled when metoclopramide was added. In a crossover study, 9 healthy subjects were given either metoclopramide 10 mg six-hourly for 24 hours before, and 48 hours after, a single 600- or 900-mg oral dose of quinidine sulphate or quinidine alone. It was found that metoclopramide caused a mean 10% decrease in the AUC of quinidine, although two subjects had decreases of 22.5 and 28.1%. The elimination rate constant was unaffected.[1] Another study in patients taking a sustained-release formulation of quinidine bisulphate 500 mg 12-hourly found that metoclopramide 10 mg three times daily increased the mean plasma levels measured 3.5 hours after the last dose of quinidine by almost 20%, from 1.6 to 1.9 micrograms/ml, and at 12 hours by about 16%, from 2.4 to 2.8 micrograms/ml.[2]

Mechanism

Not understood. Metoclopramide alters both the gastric emptying time and gastrointestinal motility, which can affect quinidine absorption.

Importance and management

Direct information seems to be limited to these studies using different quinidine preparations. Since the outcome of concurrent use is uncertain, the effects should be well monitored.

1. Yuen GJ, Hansten PD, Collins J. Effect of metoclopramide on the absorption of an oral sustained-release quinidine product. *Clin Pharm* (1987) 6, 722–5.
2. Guckenbiehl W, Gilfrich HJ, Just H. Einfluß von Laxantien und Metoclopramid auf die Chindin-Plasmakonzentration während Langzeittherapie bei Patienten mit Herzrhythmusstörugen. *Med Welt* (1976) 27, 1273–6.

Quinidine + Omeprazole

Omeprazole does not appear to alter the pharmacokinetics of quinidine, nor its QT-interval prolonging effect.

Clinical evidence, mechanism, importance and management

Omeprazole 40 mg daily for one week had no effect on the pharmacokinetics of a single 400-mg dose of quinidine in 8 healthy subjects. In addition, the corrected QT interval was not significantly changed.[1] There would not appear to be the need for any special precautions during concurrent use.

1. Ching MS, Elliott SL, Stead CK, Murdoch RT, Devenish-Meares S, Morgan DJ, Smallwood RA. Quinidine single dose pharmacokinetics and pharmacodynamics are unaltered by omeprazole. *Aliment Pharmacol Ther* (1991) 5, 523-31

Quinidine + Quinolones

Ciprofloxacin normally appears not to interact with quinidine to a clinically relevant extent. An increased risk of torsade de pointes might be expected if quinidine is used with gatifloxacin, moxifloxacin, or sparfloxacin, and possibly levofloxacin.

Clinical evidence, mechanism, importance and management

The pharmacokinetics of a single 400-mg oral dose of quinidine sulphate and QRS and QTc prolongation were not significantly changed in 7 healthy subjects after they took **ciprofloxacin** 750 mg daily for 6 days. The decrease in clearance ranged from a decrease of 10% to an increase of 20%, with a mean 1% increase, which is unlikely to be clinically relevant.[1] However an isolated case report describes a woman who started taking quinidine gluconate 324 mg eight-hourly while she was on **ciprofloxacin** and metronidazole. Her first trough serum quinidine levels was raised a little above normal at 6.3 micrograms/ml compared with the normal range of 2 to 5 micrograms/ml, without evidence of toxicity. Quinidine therapy was continued unchanged, and her next trough serum quinidine level was only 2.3 micrograms/ml, 3 days after finishing the course of antibacterials. This was tentatively attributed to the possible enzyme inhibitory effects of **ciprofloxacin** and metronidazole. This case is far from clear so that no firm conclusions can be reached.[2] There would seem to be little reason for avoiding concurrent use.

Some quinolones can prolong the QT interval, and would be expected to increase the risk of torsade de pointes arrhythmias when used with quinidine. Of the quinolones used clinically, **gatifloxacin, moxifloxacin,** and **sparfloxacin** are known to prolong the QT interval (see 'Table 7.3', (p.169)). There is also evidence that **levofloxacin** may prolong the QT interval (see 'Amiodarone + Quinolones', p.163). These quinolones should probably be avoided in patients on quinidine (see also 'Drugs that prolong the QT interval + Other drugs that prolong the QT interval', p.170).

1. Bleske BE, Carver PL, Annesley TM, Bleske JRM, Morady F. The effect of ciprofloxacin on the pharmacokinetic and ECG parameters of quinidine. *J Clin Pharmacol* (1990) 30, 911–15.
2. Cooke CE, Sklar GE, Nappi JM. Possible pharmacokinetic interaction with quinidine: ciprofloxacin or metronidazole? *Ann Pharmacother* (1996) 30, 364–6.

Quinidine + Rifamycins

The serum levels of quinidine and its therapeutic effects can be markedly reduced by the concurrent use of rifampicin.

Clinical evidence

It was noted that the control of ventricular arrhythmia deteriorated in a patient on quinidine sulphate 800 mg daily within a week of starting to take **rifampicin** 600 mg daily. His serum quinidine level fell from 4 to 0.5 micrograms/ml, and remained low despite doubling the quinidine dose to 1600 mg daily. The rifampicin was discontinued, and quinidine levels gradually increased over a week. Some signs of quinidine toxicity then occurred, and the quinidine dose was reduced back to 800 mg daily.[1] Further study in 4 healthy subjects showed that treatment with **rifampicin** 600 mg daily for 7 days reduced the mean half-life of a single 6-mg/kg oral dose of quinidine sulphate by about 62% (from 6.1 to 2.3 hours) and the AUC by 83%.[2] Similar findings were reported in 4 other subjects receiving the same dose of quinidine intravenously.[2]

Another case report describes a patient who did not achieve adequate serum quinidine levels despite large daily doses of up to 3200 mg of quinidine while taking **rifampicin**. When the **rifampicin** was stopped, ultimately, a reduced quinidine dosage of 1800 mg daily achieved a serum level of 2 micrograms/ml, reflecting a 44% decrease in dose and a 43% increase in level.[3] In a further case, a 'double interaction' was seen in a patient on quinidine and digoxin when given **rifampicin**: the quinidine levels fell, resulting in a fall in digoxin levels.[4]

Mechanism

Rifampicin is a potent enzyme-inducing agent which markedly increases the metabolism of the quinidine by 3-hydroxylation and N-oxidation, thereby increasing its loss from the body and reducing its effects.[5] It has been suggested that two of the quinidine metabolites (3-hydroxyquinidine and 2-oxoquinidinone) may be active, which might, to some extent, offset the effects of this interaction.[4]

Importance and management

An established and clinically important interaction, although documentation is limited. The dosage of quinidine will need to be increased if rifampicin is given concurrently. Monitor the serum levels. Doubling the dose may not be enough.[2,4] An equivalent dosage reduction will be needed if the rifampicin is stopped. There does not seem to be any information regarding the other rifamycins, **rifabutin** (a weak enzyme inducer) and **rifapentine** (a moderate enzyme inducer). However, the makers and the CSM in the UK warn that rifabutin may possibly reduce the effects of a number of drugs, including quinidine.[6,7]

1. Ahmad D, Mathur P, Ahuja S, Henderson R, Carruthers G. Rifampicin-quinidine interaction. *Br J Dis Chest* (1979) 73, 409–11.
2. Twum-Barima Y, Carruthers SG. Quinidine-rifampin interaction. *N Engl J Med* (1981) 304, 1466–9.
3. Schwartz A, Brown JR. Quinidine-rifampin interaction. *Am Heart J* (1984) 107, 789–90.
4. Bussey HI, Merritt GJ, Hill EG. The influence of rifampin on quinidine and digoxin. *Arch Intern Med* (1984) 144, 1021–3.

5. Damkier P, Hansen LL, Brøsen K. Rifampicin treatment greatly increases the apparent oral clearance of quinidine. *Pharmacol Toxicol* (1999) 85, 257–62.
6. Mycobutin (Rifabutin). Pharmacia Ltd. UK Summary of product characteristics, January 2003.
7. Committee on the Safety of Medicines/Medicines Control Agency. Revised indication and drug interactions of rifabutin. *Current Problems* (1997) 23, 14.

Quinidine + Sucralfate

An isolated report describes a marked reduction in serum quinidine levels in a patient attributed to the concurrent use of sucralfate.

Clinical evidence, mechanism, importance and management

An elderly woman on warfarin, digoxin, sustained-release quinidine and sucralfate was found to have subtherapeutic levels of all three even though the dosages were separated from the sucralfate by 2 hours (serum quinidine level 0.31 micromol/l). On hospitalisation, a variety of other medications were then started for chest pain (glyceryl trinitrate, diltiazem, pethidine, promethazine), and on day 4 the sucralfate was stopped. On day 5, her serum quinidine level was 5.55 micromol/l.[1] The patient denied noncompliance, and the suggestion was that sucralfate can bind with quinidine within the gut and reduce its absorption. However, a study in *dogs* found sucralfate did not alter quinidine bioavailability.[2] This isolated case report is of doubtful general importance.

1. Rey AM, Gums JG. Altered absorption of digoxin, sustained-release quinidine, and warfarin with sucralfate administration. *DICP Ann Pharmacother* (1991) 25, 745–6.
2. Lacz JP, Groschang AG, Geising DH, Browne RK. The effect of sucralfate on drug absorption in dogs. *Gastroenterology* (1982) 82, 1108.

Tocainide + Antacids or Urinary alkalinizers

Raising the pH of the urine (e.g. with concurrent use of some antacids, diuretics or alkaline salts) can modestly reduce the loss of tocainide from the body.

Clinical evidence

Preliminary findings of a study showed that when 5 healthy subjects took 30 ml of an **unnamed antacid** four times a day for 48 hours before and 58 hours after a single 600-mg dose of tocainide, the urinary pH rose from 5.9 to 6.9, the total clearance fell by 28%, the peak serum levels fell by 19% from 4.2 to 3.4 micrograms/ml, the AUC rose by 33% and the half-life was prolonged from 13.2 to 15.4 hours.[1]

Mechanism

Tocainide is a weak base so that its loss in the urine will be affected by the pH of the urine. Alkalinization of the urine increases the number of unionised molecules available for passive reabsorption, thereby reducing the urinary loss and raising the serum levels.

Importance and management

An established interaction of uncertain but probably limited clinical importance. There seem to be no reports of adverse reactions in patients as a result of this interaction, but be alert for any evidence of increased tocainide effects if other drugs are given that can raise the urinary pH significantly (e.g. **sodium bicarbonate** and **acetazolamide**). Reduce the tocainide dosage if necessary. Of the antacids, **magnesium** and **aluminium hydroxide** (*Maalox*) can raise urinary pH by about 0.9 whereas **magnesium hydroxide** (*Milk of magnesia*) and **calcium carbonate-glycine** (*Titralac*) in normal doses raise the pH by about 0.5.[2] **Aluminium hydroxide** (*Amphogel*) and **dihydroxyaluminium glycinate** (*Robalate*) are reported to have no effect on urinary pH.[2]

1. Meneilly GP, Scavone JM, Meneilly GS, Wei JY. Tocainide: pharmacokinetic alterations during antacid-induced urinary alkalinization. *Clin Pharmacol Ther* (1987) 41, 178.
2. Gibaldi M, Grundhofer B, Levy G. Effect of antacids on pH of urine. *Clin Pharmacol Ther* (1974) 16, 520–5.

Tocainide + H_2-blockers

There is some evidence that cimetidine can reduce the bioavailability and serum levels of tocainide, but ranitidine appears not to interact.

Clinical evidence, mechanism, importance and management

In a preliminary report of a study, four days of treatment with **cimetidine** (dose not stated) in 11 healthy subjects had a small effect on the pharmacokinetics of tocainide 500 mg given intravenously over 15 minutes (half-life increased, clearance decreased), which was not considered clinically important.[1] In another study, **cimetidine** 1200 mg daily for two days reduced the AUC of a single 400-mg oral dose of tocainide in 7 healthy subjects by about one-third. The peak serum levels were also reduced, from 2.81 to 1.7 micrograms/ml, but no changes in the half-life or renal clearance occurred.[2] The reasons for this, and its clinical importance are uncertain, but be alert for evidence of a reduced response to tocainide in the presence of **cimetidine**. **Ranitidine** 150 mg twice daily has been found not to interact.[2]

1. Price BA, Holmes GI, Antonello J, Yeh KC, Demetriades J, Irvin JD, McMahon FG. Intravenous tocainide (T) maintains safe therapeutic levels when administered concomitantly with cimetidine (C). *Clin Pharmacol Ther* (1987), 41, 237.
2. North DS, Mattern AL, Kapil RP, Lalonde RL. The effect of histamine-2 receptor antagonists on tocainide pharmacokinetics. *J Clin Pharmacol* (1988) 28, 640–3.

Tocainide + Phenobarbital

Phenobarbital does not appear to alter the pharmacokinetics of tocainide.

Clinical evidence, mechanism, importance and management

Phenobarbital 100 mg daily for 15 days did not alter the AUC of tocainide after a single 600-mg dose in 6 healthy subjects. In addition, the percentage of the dose excreted unchanged in the urine and as the glucuronide metabolite did not differ.[1] Phenobarbital at this dosage does not appear to alter the metabolism of tocainide. No special precautions appear to be necessary.

1. Elvin AT, Lalka D, Stoeckel K, du Souich P, Axelson JE, Golden LH, McLean AJ. Tocainide kinetics and metabolism: effects of phenobarbital and substrates of glucuronyl transferase. *Clin Pharmacol Ther* (1980) 28, 652–8.

Tocainide + Rifampicin (Rifampin)

The loss of tocainide from the body is increased by the concurrent use of rifampicin.

Clinical evidence, mechanism, importance and management

The AUC of a single 600-mg oral dose of tocainide was reduced by almost 30% (from 76.8 to 55 mg.h/l) and the half-life was also reduced by about 30%, from 13.2 to 9.4 hours, in 8 healthy subjects given rifampicin 300 mg twice daily for 5 days.[1]

This response is consistent with the well-recognised enzyme inducing effects of rifampicin. Information is limited to this single dose study, but the interaction would seem to be established and may be of clinical importance. Monitor any patients given rifampicin for evidence of reduced tocainide serum levels and reduced effects. Increase the dosage as necessary. Reduce the tocainide dosage if the rifampicin is withdrawn. More study is needed.

1. Rice TL, Patterson JH, Celestin C, Foster JR, Powell JR. Influence of rifampin on tocainide pharmacokinetics in humans. *Clin Pharm* (1989) 8, 200–205.

8

Antibacterials

Many of the interactions of the antibacterial drugs will be found elsewhere in this publication as they deal with the effects of antibacterial drugs on other drugs. Some of the macrolides and the quinolones are potent enzyme inhibitors; the macrolides exert their effects on the cytochrome P450 isoenzyme CYP3A4, whereas the quinolones affect CYP1A2. Rifampicin is a potent non-specific enzyme inducer. These interactions will be found in the section appropriate to the drug being affected.

Many of the interactions covered in this section concern absorption interactions, such as the ability of the tetracyclines and quinolones to chelate with divalent cations. More information on the mechanism of these interactions can be found in 'Drug absorption interactions', (p.3).

Many monographs concern the use of multiple antibacterials. One of the great difficulties with these interactions is the often poor correlation between *in vitro* and *in vivo* studies, so that it is difficult to get a thoroughly reliable indication of how antibacterial drugs will behave together in clinical practice. Two antibacterials may actually be less effective than one on its own, because, in theory, the effects of a bactericidal drug, which requires actively dividing cells for it to be effective, may be reduced by a bacteriostatic drug. However, in practice this seems to be less important than might be supposed and there are relatively few well-authenticated clinical examples.

The antibacterials covered in this section are listed in 'Table 8.1', (below).

Table 8.1 Antibacterials

Aminoglycosides	Amikacin, Astromicin, Dibekacin, Dihydrostreptomycin, Framycetin, Gentamicin, Isepamicin, Kanamycin, Micronomicin, Neomycin, Netilmicin, Paromomycin, Sisomicin, Streptomycin, Tobramycin
Antituberculars, Antileprotics and related derivatives	Aminosalicylic acid (PAS), Capreomycin, Clofazimine, Cycloserine, Dapsone, Ethambutol, Ethionamide, Isoniazid, Methaniazide, Protionamide, Pyrazinamide, Rifabutin, Rifampicin (Rifampin), Rifamycin, Rifapentine, Rifaximin
Carbapenems	Biapenem, Ertapenem, Faropenem, Imipenem, Meropenem, Panipenem
Cephalosporins	Cefaclor, Cefadroxil, Cefalexin, Cefaloglycin, Cefaloridine, Cefalotin, Cefamandole, Cefapirin, Cefatrizine, Cefazolin, Cefbuperazone, Cefcapene, Cefdinir, Cefditoren, Cefepime, Cefetamet, Cefixime, Cefmenoxime, Cefmetazole, Cefminox, Cefodizime, Cefonicid, Cefoperazone, Ceforanide, Cefoselis, Cefotaxime, Cefotetan, Cefotiam, Cefoxitin, Cefpirome, Cefpodoxime, Cefpiramide, Cefpirome, Cefpodoxime, Cefprozil, Cefradine, Cefsulodin, Ceftazidime, Cefteram, Ceftezole, Ceftibuten, Ceftizoxime, Ceftriaxone, Cefuroxime, Flomoxef, Latamoxef
Macrolides	Azithromycin, Clarithromycin, Dirithromycin, Erythromycin, Flurithromycin, Josamycin, Midecamycin, Rokitomycin, Roxithromycin, Spiramycin, Telithromycin, Troleandomycin
Penicillins	Amoxicillin (Amoxycillin), Ampicillin, Azidocillin, Azlocillin, Bacampicillin, Benzylpenicillin (Penicillin G), Carbenicillin, Carindacillin, Ciclacillin, Clometocillin, Cloxacillin, Dicloxacillin, Flucloxacillin, Mecillinam, Meticillin, Mezlocillin, Nafcillin, Oxacillin, Phenethicillin, Phenoxymethylpenicillin (Penicillin V), Piperacillin, Pivampicillin, Pivmecillinam, Procaine benzylpenicillin (Procaine penicillin), Propicillin, Sulbenicillin, Sultamicin, Temocillin, Ticarcillin
Polypeptides	Bacitracin, Colistimethate sodium, Colistin, Polymyxin B, Teicoplanin, Vancomycin
Quinolones	Alatrofloxacin, Cinoxacin, Ciprofloxacin, Enoxacin, Fleroxacin, Flumequine, Gatifloxacin, Gemifloxacin, Grepafloxacin, Levofloxacin, Lomefloxacin, Moxifloxacin, Nadifloxacin, Nalidixic acid, Norfloxacin, Ofloxacin, Oxolinic Acid, Pazufloxacin, Pefloxacin, Pipemidic Acid, Piromidic Acid, Rosoxacin, Rufloxacin, Sparfloxacin, Temafloxacin, Tosufloxacin, Trovafloxacin
Sulfonamides	Co-trimoxazole, Phthalylsulfathiazole, Sulfadiazine, Sulfadimidine (Sulfamethazine), Sulfafurazole (Sulfisoxazole), Sulfaguanidine, Sulfamerazine, Sulfamethizole, Sulfamethoxazole, Sulfalene (Sulfametopyrazine), Sulfametoxypyridazine, Sulfametrole, Sulphapyridine, Sulfathiazole, Sulfisomidine
Tetracyclines	Chlortetracyline, Demeclocycline, Doxycycline, Lymecycline, Methacycline, Minocycline, Oxytetracycline, Rolitetracycline, Tetracycline
Miscellaneous	Aztreonam, Carumonam, Cilastatin, Chloramphenicol, Clindamycin, Fusidic acid, Lincomycin, Loracarbef, Methenamine, Mupirocin, Nitrofurantoin, Novobiocin, Pristinamycin, Quinopristin/Dalfopristin, Spectinomycin, Trimethoprim, Virginiamycin

Aminoglycosides + Amphotericin B

Nephrotoxicity or raised gentamicin or amikacin levels attributed to amphotericin have been described in a number of patients.

Clinical evidence, mechanism, importance and management

The renal function of 4 patients given moderate doses of **gentamicin** deteriorated when they were given amphotericin B. Both drugs are known to be nephrotoxic and it is suggested, on the basis of what was seen, that combined use may have had additive nephrotoxic effects.[1] A further retrospective analysis found that the use of **amikacin** tended to increase amphotericin B-related nephrotoxicity.[2]

Another study found that **amikacin** or **gentamicin** clearance was impaired in 12 of 17 children given amphotericin B. Serum creatinine increased by 50% or more in 3 of them, but there was no significant increase in creatinine levels in 7 others. As a result, the aminoglycoside dose was decreased or the dose interval lengthened in 7 children.[3]

Aminoglycosides are generally considered to be nephrotoxic and avoidance of use with other nephrotoxic drugs (such as amphotericin B) is generally recommended. However, concurrent use may be essential. Renal function and drug levels should be routinely monitored during aminoglycoside therapy, and it may be prudent to increase monitoring if they are used with amphotericin.

1. Churchill DN, Seely J. Nephrotoxicity associated with combined gentamicin-amphotericin B therapy. *Nephron* (1977) 19, 176–181.
2. Harbath S, Pestotnik SL, Lloyd JF, Burke JP, Samore MH. The epidemiology of nephrotoxicity associated with conventional amphotericin B therapy. *Am J Med* (2001) 111, 528–34.
3. Goren MP, Viar MJ, Shenep JL, Wright RK, Baker DK, Kalwinsky DK. Monitoring serum aminoglycoside concentrations in children with amphotericin B nephrotoxicity. *Pediatr Infect Dis J* (1988) 7, 698–703.

Aminoglycosides + Cephalosporins

The nephrotoxic effects of gentamicin and tobramycin can be increased by cefalotin. This may possibly also occur with other aminoglycosides. On the whole cephalosporins appear not to interact adversely with aminoglycosides.

Clinical evidence

A randomised double-blind trial[1] in patients with sepsis showed the following incidence of definite nephrotoxicity;

- **gentamicin** with **cefalotin** 30.4% (7 of 23 patients),
- **tobramycin** with **cefalotin** 20.8% (5 of 24),
- **gentamicin** with **methicillin** 10% (2 of 20),
- **tobramycin** with **methicillin** 4.3% (1 of 23).

A very considerable number of studies and case reports confirm an increase in the incidence of nephrotoxicity when **gentamicin**[2-10] or **tobramycin**[11,12] are used with **cefalotin**. However, some other studies have found no increase in nephrotoxicity with the combination.[13-15] Acute renal failure has also been reported in a patient given **gentamicin** and **cefaloridine**,[16] and hypokalaemia has also been described in patients taking cytotoxic drugs for leukaemia when they were given **gentamicin** and **cefalexin**.[17]

No adverse interactions have been reported between;

- **amikacin** and **cefepime**[18]
- **gentamicin** and **cefuroxime**[19]
- **tobramycin** and **cefuroxime**,[20] **cefotaxime**,[21] or **ceftazidime**[22]

Mechanism

Uncertain. The nephrotoxic effects of gentamicin and tobramycin are well documented and it appears that these effects can be additive with cefalotin in some patients. Doses that are well tolerated separately can be nephrotoxic when given together.[9]

Importance and management

The gentamicin/cefalotin interaction is very well documented and potentially serious, but there is less information about tobramycin with cefalotin. The risk of nephrotoxicity is probably greatest if high doses of antibacterial are used in those with some existing renal impairment. One study suggests that short courses of treatment are sometimes justified[10] but renal function should be very closely monitored and dosages kept to a minimum. The combination of gentamicin or tobramycin and cefalotin is probably best avoided in high risk patients wherever possible. Whether other aminoglycosides interact similarly is uncertain, but the possibility should be borne in mind. Other cephalosporins appear not to interact.

1. Wade JC, Smith CR, Petty BG, Lipsky JJ, Conrad G, Ellner J, Lietman PS. Cephalothin plus an aminoglycoside is more nephrotoxic than methicillin plus an aminoglycoside. *Lancet* (1978) ii, 604–6.
2. Opitz A, Herrman I, von Harrath D, Schaefer K. Akute niereninsuffizienz nach Gentamycin-Cephalosporin-Kombinationstherapie. *Med Welt* (1971) 22, 434–8.
3. Plager JE. Association of renal injury with combined cephalothin-gentamicin therapy among patients severely ill with malignant disease. *Cancer* (1976) 37, 1937–43.
4. The EORTC International Antimicrobial Therapy Project Group. Three antibiotic regimens in the treatment of infection in febrile granulocytopenic patients with cancer. *J Infect Dis* (1978) 137, 14–29.
5. Kleinknecht D, Ganeval D, Droz D. Acute renal failure after high doses of gentamicin and cephalothin. *Lancet* (1973) i, 1129.
6. Bobrow SN, Jaffe E, Young RC. Anuria and acute tubular necrosis associated with gentamicin and cephalothin. *JAMA* (1972) 222, 1546–7.
7. Fillastre JP, Laumonier R, Humbert G, Dubois D, Metayer J, Delpech A, Leroy J, Robert M. Acute renal failure associated with combined gentamicin and cephalothin therapy. *BMJ* (1973) 2, 396–7.
8. Cabanillas F, Burgos RC, Rodríguez RC, Baldizón C. Nephrotoxicity of combined cephalothin-gentamicin regimen. *Arch Intern Med* (1975) 135, 850–52.
9. Tvedegaard E. Interaction between gentamicin and cephalothin as cause of acute renal failure. *Lancet* (1976) ii, 581.
10. Hansen MM, Kaaber K. Nephrotoxicity in combined cephalothin and gentamicin therapy. *Acta Med Scand* (1977) 201, 463–7.
11. Tobias JS, Whitehouse JM, Wrigley PFM. Severe renal dysfunction after tobramycin/cephalothin therapy. *Lancet* (1976) i, 425.
12. Klastersky J, Hensgens C, Debusscher L. Empiric therapy for cancer patients: comparative study of ticarcillin-tobramycin, ticarcillin-cephalothin, and cephalothin-tobramycin. *Antimicrob Agents Chemother* (1975) 7, 640–45.
13. Fanning WL, Gump D, Jick H. Gentamicin- and cephalothin-associated rises in blood urea nitrogen. *Antimicrob Agents Chemother* (1976) 10, 80–82.
14. Stille W, Arndt I. Argumente gegen eine Nephrotoxizität von cephalothin und gentamycin. *Med Welt* (1972) 23, 1603–1605.
15. Wellwood JM, Simpson PM, Tighe JR, Thompson AE. Evidence of gentamicin nephrotoxicity in patients with renal allografts. *BMJ* (1975) 3, 278–81.
16. Zazgornik J, Schmidt P, Lugscheider R, Kopsa H. Akutes Nierenversagen bei kombinierter Cephaloridin-Gentamycin-Therapie. *Wien Klin Wochenschr* (1973) 85, 839–41.
17. Young GP, Sullivan J, Hurley A. Hypokalaæmia due to gentamicin/cephalexin in leukaemia. *Lancet* (1973) ii, 855.
18. Barbhaiya RH, Knupp CA, Pfeffer M, Pittman KA. Lack of pharmacokinetic interaction between cefepime and amikacin in humans. *Antimicrob Agents Chemother* (1992) 36, 1382–6.
19. Cockram CS, Richards P, Bax RP. The safety of cefuroxime and gentamicin in patients with reduced renal function. *Curr Med Res Opin* (1980) 6, 398–403.
20. Trollfors B, Alestig K, Rödjer S, Sandberg T, Westin J. Renal function in patients treated with tobramycin-cefuroxime or tobramycin-penicillin G. *J Antimicrob Chemother* (1983) 12, 641–5.
21. Kuhlmann J, Seidel G, Richter E, Grötsch H. Tobramycin nephrotoxicity: failure of cefotaxime to potentiate injury in patient. *Naunyn Schmiedebergs Arch Pharmacol* (1981) 316 (Suppl), R80.
22. Aronoff GR, Brier RA, Sloan RS, Brier ME. Interactions of ceftazidime and tobramycin in patients with normal and impaired renal function. *Antimicrob Agents Chemother* (1990) 34, 1139–42.

Aminoglycosides + Clindamycin

Three cases of acute renal failure have been tentatively attributed to the use of gentamicin with clindamycin, but it seems unlikely that this is a common problem.

Clinical evidence, mechanism, importance and management

Acute renal failure has been reported in 3 patients with normal renal function when they were given **gentamicin** 3.9 to 4.9 mg/kg daily and clindamycin 0.9 to 1.8 mg/kg daily for 13 to 18 days. They recovered within 3 to 5 days of discontinuing the antibacterials[1] but in one patient acute renal failure only developed after the clindamycin was stopped. The reasons for the renal failure are not known, but given the long courses of **gentamicin** involved, the possibility that renal impairment occurred as an adverse effect of the aminoglycoside alone cannot be excluded.

Clindamycin with an aminoglycoside seems to be a fairly common antibacterial combination, especially following abdominal trauma. Given the scarcity of reports about nephrotoxicity with this combination it seems likely that treatment is without nephrotoxic risks above and beyond that seen with an aminoglycoside alone.

As renal function should be routinely monitored during the use of aminoglycosides, no additional precautions should be necessary if clindamycin is also given.

The combination of **tobramycin** and clindamycin is reported not to be nephrotoxic.[2]

1. Butkus DE, de Torrente A, Terman DS. Renal failure following gentamicin in combination with clindamycin. Gentamicin nephrotoxicity. *Nephron* (1976) 17, 307–13.

2. Gillett P, Wise R, Melikian V, Falk R. Tobramycin/cephalothin nephrotoxicity. *Lancet* (1976) i, 547.

Aminoglycosides + Indometacin

There are conflicting reports as to whether or not serum gentamicin and amikacin levels are raised by indometacin in premature infants.

Clinical evidence

(a) Amikacin

A study in 10 preterm infants on amikacin, with gestational ages ranging from 25 to 34 weeks, showed that the use of indometacin 200 micrograms/kg, every 8 hours, for up to 3 doses caused a rise in the serum levels of amikacin. Trough and peak levels of amikacin were raised by 28 and 17% respectively.[1]

(b) Gentamicin

A study in 10 preterm infants on gentamicin, with gestational ages ranging from 25 to 34 weeks, showed that the use of indometacin 200 micrograms/kg, every 8 hours, for up to 3 doses caused a rise in the serum levels of gentamicin. Trough and peak levels of gentamicin were raised by 48 and 33% respectively.[1] A later study[2] confirmed that indometacin (200 then 100 then 100 micrograms/kg given intravenously at 0, 12 and 36 hours respectively) decreased the clearance of doses of gentamicin 3 mg/kg daily by 23%, from 35 to 27 ml/hour, in preterm infants weighing less than 1250 g.

In contrast, 8 out of 13 infants showed no increase in serum gentamicin levels when given indometacin 200 to 250 micrograms/kg every 12 hours for 3 doses. Four showed slight to moderate rises and one had a substantial rise.[3] In another study no significant changes in serum gentamicin levels were seen in 31 preterm newborns given parenteral indometacin 200 micrograms/kg every 12 hours for 3 doses.[4]

Mechanism

Aminoglycosides are excreted by renal filtration, which can be inhibited by indometacin. This may result in the retention of the aminoglycoside.

Importance and management

Information seems to be limited to these conflicting studies, although supporting evidence comes from the fact that indometacin also causes the retention of digoxin in premature infants. The authors of one of the studies[3] suggest that the different results may be because aminoglycoside serum levels were lower in their study before the indometacin was given, and also because they measured the new steady-state levels after 40 to 60 hours instead of 24 hours. Whatever the explanation, concurrent use should be very closely monitored because toxicity is associated with raised aminoglycoside serum levels. It has been suggested that the aminoglycoside dosage should be reduced before giving indometacin and the serum levels and renal function well monitored during concurrent use.[1] Other aminoglycosides possibly behave similarly. This interaction does not seem to have been studied in adults.

1. Zarfin Y, Koren G, Maresky D, Perlman M, MacLeod S. Possible indomethacin-aminoglycoside interaction in preterm infants. *J Pediatr* (1985) 106, 511–13.

2. Dean RP, Domanico RS, Covert RF. Prophylactic indomethacin alters gentamicin pharmacokinetics in preterm infants <1250 grams. *Pediatr Res* (1994) 35, 83A.

3. Jerome M, Davis JC. The effects of indomethacin on gentamicin serum levels. *Proc West Pharmacol Soc* (1987) 30, 85–7.

4. Grylack LJ, Scanlon JW. Interaction of indomethacin (I) and gentamicin (G) in preterm newborns. *Pediatr Res* (1988) 23, 409A.

Aminoglycosides + Loop diuretics

The concurrent use of aminoglycosides and etacrynic acid should be avoided because their damaging actions on the ear can be additive. Intravenous use of etacrynic acid and renal impairment are additional causative factors. Even sequential use may not be safe. Bumetanide and piretanide have been shown to interact similarly in *animals*. Although some patients have developed nephrotoxicity and/or ototoxicity while taking furosemide and an aminoglycoside, it has not been established that the damage resulted from an interaction.

Clinical evidence

(a) Bumetanide

There seem to be no clinical reports of an interaction between aminoglycosides and bumetanide, but ototoxicity has been described in *animals* given **kanamycin** and bumetanide.[1,2]

(b) Etacrynic acid

Four patients with renal impairment became permanently deaf after treatment with intramuscular **kanamycin** 1 to 1.5 g and intravenous etacrynic acid 50 to 150 mg. One patient also received **streptomycin**, and another also received oral **neomycin**. Deafness took between 30 minutes and almost 2 weeks to develop. In some cases deafness developed despite the doses being given on separate days, and in all cases it appeared irreversible.[3] A patient on **gentamicin** rapidly developed deafness when furosemide was replaced by intravenous etacrynic acid.[4]

There are other reports describing temporary, partial or total permanent deafness as a result of giving intravenous etacrynic acid with **gentamicin**,[5] intramuscular **kanamycin**,[5-7] oral **neomycin**,[8] or **streptomycin**[6,9] This interaction has been extensively demonstrated in *animals*.

(c) Furosemide

An analysis of 3 prospective, controlled, randomised, double-blind trials showed that aminoglycosides (**amikacin**, **gentamicin**, **tobramycin**) and furosemide did not increase either aminoglycoside-induced nephrotoxicity, or ototoxicity. Nephrotoxicity developed in 20% (10 of 50 patients) given furosemide and 17% (38 of 222) not given furosemide. Auditory toxicity developed in 22% (5 of 23) given furosemide and 24% (28 of 119) not given furosemide.[4]

A clinical study evaluating a possible interaction found that furosemide increased aminoglycoside-induced renal damage,[10] whereas two other clinical studies found no interaction.[11,12] There are clinical reports claiming that concurrent use results in ototoxicity, but usually only small numbers of patients were involved and control groups were not included.[13-16] A retrospective study of neonates suggested the possibility of increased ototoxicity but no firm conclusions could be drawn.[17] Studies in patients and healthy subjects have shown that furosemide reduces the renal clearance of **gentamicin**[18,19] and can cause a rise in both serum **gentamicin**[19] and **tobramycin** levels.[20] Ototoxicity has been described in *animals* given **kanamycin** and furosemide.[1,2]

(d) Piretanide

There seem to be no clinical reports of an interaction between aminoglycosides and piretanide, but ototoxicity has been described in *animals* given **kanamycin** and piretanide.[21]

Mechanism

Aminoglycosides or etacrynic acid alone can damage the ear and cause deafness, the site of action of the aminoglycosides being the hair cell and that of etacrynic acid the stria vascularis. Other loop diuretics can similarly damage hearing.

Animal studies have shown that intramuscular neomycin can cause a fivefold increase in the concentration of etacrynate in cochlear tissues, and it is possible that the aminoglycoside has some effect on the tissues, which allows the etacrynic acid to penetrate more easily.[22] Similar results have been found with gentamicin.[23]

Importance and management

The interaction between etacrynic acid and aminoglycoside is well established and well documented. The concurrent or sequential use of etacrynic acid with parenteral aminoglycosides should be avoided because permanent deafness may result. Patients with renal impairment seem to be particularly at risk, most likely because the drugs are less rapidly cleared. Most of the reports describe deafness after intravenous use, but it has also been seen when etacrynic acid is given orally alone.[9] If it is deemed absolutely necessary to use etacrynic acid and intravenous aminoglycosides, minimal doses should be used and the effects on hearing should be monitored continuously. Not every aminoglycoside has been implicated, but their ototoxicity is clearly established and they may be expected to interact in a similar way. For this reason the same precautions should be used.

Although there is ample evidence of an adverse interaction between furosemide and aminoglycosides in *animals*,[2,24] the weight of clinical evidence suggests that furosemide does not normally increase either the nephrotoxicity or ototoxicity of the aminoglycosides. Nevertheless as there is still some uncertainty about the safety of concurrent use it would be prudent to monitor for any evidence of changes in aminoglycoside serum levels, and renal or hearing impairment. The authors of the major study cited[4] suggest that an interaction may possibly exist if high dose infusions of furosemide are used. The same precautions would seem to be appropriate with bumetanide and piretanide. Note that it is generally advised that aminoglycosides should not be used with other drugs that may cause ototoxicity or nephrotoxicity, such as etacrynic acid and furosemide.

1. Ohtani I, Ohtsuki K, Omata T, Ouchi J, Saito T. Interaction of bumetanide and kanamycin. *ORL J Otorhinolaryngol Relat Spec* (1978) 40, 216–25.
2. Brummett RE, Bendrick T, Himes D. Comparative ototoxicity of bumetanide and furosemide when used in combination with kanamycin. *J Clin Pharmacol* (1981) 21, 628–36.
3. Johnson AH, Hamilton CH. Kanamycin ototoxicity — possible potentiation by other drugs. *South Med J* (1970) 63, 511–13.
4. Smith CR, Lietman PS. Effect of furosemide on aminoglycoside-induced nephrotoxicity and auditory toxicity in humans. *Antimicrob Agents Chemother* (1983) 23, 133–7.
5. Meriwether WD, Mangi RJ, Serpick AA. Deafness following standard intravenous dose of ethacrynic acid. *JAMA* (1971) 216, 795–8.
6. Mathog RH, Klein WJ. Ototoxicity of ethacrynic acid and aminoglycoside antibiotics in uremia. *N Engl J Med* (1969) 280, 1223–4.
7. Ng PSY, Conley CE, Ing TS. Deafness after ethacrynic acid. *Lancet* (1969) i, 673–4.
8. Matz GJ, Beal DD, Krames L. Ototoxicity of ethacrynic acid. Demonstrated in a human temporal bone. *Arch Otolaryngol* (1969) 90, 152–5.
9. Schneider WJ, Becker EL. Acute transient hearing loss after ethacrynic acid therapy. *Arch Intern Med* (1966) 117, 715–17.
10. Prince RA, Ling MH, Hepler CD, Rainville EC, Kealey GP, Donta ST, LeFrock JL, Kowalsky SF. Factors associated with creatinine clearance changes following gentamicin therapy. *Am J Hosp Pharm* (1980) 37, 1489–95.
11. Bygbjerg IC, Møller R. Gentamicin-induced nephropathy. *Scand J Infect Dis* (1976) 8, 203–8.
12. Smith CR, Maxwell RR, Edwards CQ, Rogers JF, Lietman PS. Nephrotoxicity induced by gentamicin and amikacin. *Johns Hopkins Med J* (1978) 142, 85–90.
13. Gallagher KL, Jones JK. Furosemide-induced ototoxicity. *Ann Intern Med* (1979) 91, 744–5.
14. Noël P, Levy V-G. Toxicité rénale de l'association gentamicine-furosémide. Une observation. *Nouv Presse Med* (1978) 7, 351–3.
15. Brown CB, Ogg CS, Cameron JS, Bewick M. High dose frusemide in acute reversible intrinsic renal failure. A preliminary communication. *Scott Med J* (1974) 19, 35–9.
16. Thomsen J, Bech P, Szpirt W. Otological symptoms in chronic renal failure. The possible role of aminoglycoside-furosemide interaction. *Arch Otorhinolaryngol* (1976) 214, 71–9.
17. Salamy A, Eldredge L, Tooley WH. Neonatal status and hearing loss in high-risk infants. *J Pediatr* (1989) 114, 847–52.
18. Lawson DH, Tilstone WJ, Semple PF. Furosemide interactions: studies in normal volunteers. *Clin Res* (1976) 24, 3.
19. Lawson DH, Tilstone WJ, Gray JMB, Srivastava PK. Effect of furosemide on the pharmacokinetics of gentamicin in patients. *J Clin Pharmacol* (1982) 22, 254–8.
20. Kaka JS, Lyman C, Kilarski DJ. Tobramycin-furosemide interaction. *Drug Intell Clin Pharm* (1984) 18, 235–8.
21. Brummett RE. Ototoxicity resulting from the combined administration of potent diuretics and other agents: in 'Ototoxic side effects of diuretics' (ed by Klinke R, Lahn W, Querfurth H, Scholtholt J). *Scand Audiol* (1981) (Suppl 14), 215–24.
22. Orsulakova A, Schacht J. A biochemical mechanism of the ototoxic interaction between neomycin and ethacrynic acid. *Acta Otolaryngol* (1982) 93, 43–8.
23. Tran Ba Huy P, Meulemans A, Manuel C, Sterkers O, Wassef M. Critical appraisal of the experimental studies on the ototoxic interaction between ethacrynic acid and aminoglycoside antibiotics. A pharmacokinetical standpoint: in 'Ototoxic side effects of diuretics' (ed by Klinke R, Lahn W, Querfurth H, Scholtholt J). *Scand Audiol* (1981) (Suppl 14), 225–32.
24. Ohtani I, Ohtsuki K, Omata T, Ouchi J, Saito T. Potentiation and its mechanism of cochlear damage resulting from furosemide and aminoglycoside antibiotics. *ORL J Otorhinolaryngol Relat Spec* (1978) 40, 53–63.

Aminoglycosides + Magnesium compounds

A neonate with elevated serum magnesium levels had a respiratory arrest when given gentamicin.

Clinical evidence

An infant born to a woman whose pre-eclampsia had been treated with magnesium sulphate was found to have muscle weakness and a serum magnesium concentration of 1.77 mmol/l. The neonate was given ampicillin 100 mg/kg intravenously and **gentamicin** 2.5 mg/kg intramuscularly every 12 hours, starting 12 hours after birth. Soon after the second dose of **gentamicin** she stopped breathing and needed intubation. The **gentamicin** was stopped and the child improved.[1] *Animal* studies confirmed this interaction.[1]

Mechanism

Magnesium ions and the aminoglycosides have neuromuscular blocking activity, which can be additive (see also 'Neuromuscular blockers + Magnesium compounds', p.910 and 'Neuromuscular blockers + Aminoglycosides', p.898). In the case cited here it seems that it was enough to block the actions of the respiratory muscles.

Importance and management

Direct information about this interaction is very limited, but it is well supported by the recognised pharmacological actions of magnesium and the aminoglycosides, and their interactions with conventional neuromuscular blockers. The aminoglycosides as a group should be avoided in hypermagnesaemic infants needing antibacterial treatment. If this is not possible, the effects on respiration should be closely monitored.

1. L'Hommedieu CS, Nicholas D, Armes DA, Jones P, Nelson T, Pickering LK. Potentiation of magnesium sulfate-induced neuromuscular weakness by gentamicin, tobramycin and amikacin. *J Pediatr* (1983) 102, 629–31.

Aminoglycosides + Miconazole

A report describes a reduction in serum tobramycin levels due to miconazole.

Clinical evidence, mechanism, importance and management

Intravenous miconazole significantly lowered the peak serum **tobramycin** levels from 9.1 to 6.7 micrograms/ml in 9 patients undergoing bone marrow transplantation. Six of them needed **tobramycin** dosage adjustments.[1] Miconazole was stopped in 4 patients, and **tobramycin** pharmacokinetic parameters returned to normal 4 to 8 days later. The reasons for this interaction are not understood. Although the use of **tobramycin** should be well monitored it would be prudent to increase the frequency in patients also given miconazole. There does not appear to be any information on other aminoglycosides and azole antifungals.

1. Hatfield SM, Crane LR, Duman K, Karanes C, Kiel RJ. Miconazole-induced alteration in tobramycin pharmacokinetics. *Clin Pharm* (1986) 5, 415–19.

Aminoglycosides + Penicillins or Carbapenems

A reduction in serum aminoglycoside levels can occur if aminoglycosides and penicillins are given together to patients with severe renal impairment. Netilmicin and piperacillin appear to be the only documented non-interacting combination. No interaction of importance appears to occur with intravenous aminoglycoside and penicillins in those with normal renal function or between aminoglycosides and carbapenems. The serum levels of oral phenoxymethylpenicillin can be halved by oral neomycin.

Clinical evidence

A. Intravenous or intramuscular aminoglycosides

(a) With carbapenems

The suspicion that the low **tobramycin** levels of one patient might have been due to an interaction with **imipenem/cilastatin** was not confirmed in a later *in vitro* study.[1] It has also been suggested that the nephrotoxic effects of **imipenem** and the **aminoglycosides** might possibly be additive but this awaits confirmation.[2] The pharmacokinetics of neither **tobramycin** nor **biapenem** were found to be altered when given concurrently to 12 healthy subjects.[3] No inactivation occurred in an *in vitro* assessment of these two drugs in urine.[4]

(b) With penicillins in patients with renal impairment

A study in 6 patients with renal failure requiring dialysis, who were receiving intravenous **carbenicillin** 8 to 15 g daily in 3 to 6 divided doses, showed that the presence of the penicillin prevented the achievement of serum **gentamicin** levels above 4 micrograms/ml even though **gentamicin** doses of 1.2 to 2.1 mg/kg per day were given. When the **carbenicillin** was stopped, serum **gentamicin** levels rose.[5] The same interaction is described in another similar patient.[6]

Other reports similarly describe unusually low **gentamicin** levels in patients with impaired renal function, given **carbenicillin**,[7-10] **piperacillin**,[11] or **ticarcillin**,[8,10,12] and in patients given **tobramycin** with **carbenicillin**,[5] **piperacillin**[13] or **ticarcillin**.[14] The half-life of **gentamicin** has been reported to be reduced by **carbenicillin** or **piperacillin** by about a half or a third.[8,11,15]

Piperacillin 4 g 12-hourly did not affect the pharmacokinetics of **netilmicin** 2 mg/kg in 3 patients receiving long-term haemodialysis, whereas **piperacillin** doubled the clearance of **tobramycin** 2 mg/kg, and reduced its half-life from 73 to 22 hours.[16] A patient showed a reduction in the half-life of **tobramycin** from an expected 70 hours to 10.5 hours after being given **piperacillin**.[17]

(c) With penicillins in patients with normal renal function

A patient with normal renal function was given **gentamicin** 80 mg intravenously, with and without **carbenicillin** 4 g. The serum **gentamicin** concentration profiles in both cases were very similar.[7]

No interaction was seen in 10 patients given **tobramycin** with **piperacillin**,[18] and another 10 healthy subjects given once daily **gentamicin** with **piperacillin/tazobactam**.[19] Only minimal pharmacokinetic changes were seen in 9 healthy subjects given **tobramycin** with **piperacillin/tazobactam**,[20] and 18 cystic fibrosis patients (adults and children) given **tobramycin** with **ticarcillin**.[21]

B. Oral aminoglycosides

The serum concentrations of a 250-mg oral dose of **phenoxymethylpenicillin** were reduced by more than 50% in 5 healthy subjects after they took **neomycin** 3 g four times daily for 7 days. Normal penicillin pharmacokinetics were not seen until 6 days after the **neomycin** was withdrawn.[22]

Mechanism

In vitro, the amino groups on the aminoglycosides and the beta-lactam ring on the penicillins interact chemically to form biologically inactive amides.[23] It has been suggested that this reaction may also occur in the plasma, causing a drop in the levels of active antibacterial.[15] The interaction occurs in those with poor renal function as the drugs persist in the plasma for longer, allowing a greater time for inactivation. This therefore means the drug is lost more rapidly than has been accounted for by the renal function, and consequently lower than expected levels of the antibacterial.

In the case of phenoxymethylpenicillin, the levels are probably lowered because oral neomycin can cause a reversible malabsorption syndrome (histologically similar to nontropical sprue).

Importance and management

The interaction between parenteral aminoglycosides and penicillins seems only to occur in patients with renal impairment. In those cases where concurrent use is thought necessary, it has been recommended that the penicillin dosage should be adjusted according to renal function and the serum levels of both antibacterials closely monitored.[5] However, note that one author[6] points out that antibacterial inactivation can continue in the assay sample, and suggests that rapid assay is necessary.

There would seem to be no reason for avoiding concurrent use in patients with normal renal function because no significant *in vivo* inactivation appears to occur. Moreover there is good clinical evidence that concurrent use is valuable, especially in the treatment of Pseudomonas infections.[7,24]

Evidence for the oral neomycin/penicillin interaction seems limited to this one report and its clinical significance is unclear. It seems possible that oral **kanamycin** and **paromomycin** might interact similarly, but this needs confirmation.

1. Ariano RE, Kassum DA, Meatherall RC, Patrick WD. Lack of in vitro inactivation of tobramycin by imipenem/cilastatin. *Ann Pharmacother* (1992) 26, 1075–7.
2. Albrecht LM, Rybak MJ. Combination imipenem-aminoglycoside therapy. *Drug Intell Clin Pharm* (1986) 20, 506.
3. Muralidharan G, Buice R, Depuis E, Carver A, Friederici D, Kinchelow T, Kinzig M, Kuye O, Sorgel F, Yacobi A, Mayer P. Pharmacokinetics of biapenem with and without tobramycin in healthy volunteers. *Pharm Res* (1993) 10 (10 Suppl), S-396.
4. Muralidharan G, Carver A, Mayer P. Lack of in vitro inactivation of tobramycin by biapenem in human urine. *Pharm Res* (1994) 11 (10 Suppl), S-398.
5. Weibert R, Keane W, Shapiro F. Carbenicillin inactivation of aminoglycosides in patients with severe renal failure. *Trans Am Soc Artif Intern Organs* (1976) 22, 439–43.
6. Russo ME. Penicillin-aminoglycoside inactivation: another possible mechanism of interaction. *Am J Hosp Pharm* (1980) 37, 702–4.
7. Eykyn S, Phillips I, Ridley M. Gentamicin plus carbenicillin. *Lancet* (1971) i, 545–6.
8. Davies M, Morgan JR, Anand C. Interactions of carbenicillin and ticarcillin with gentamicin. *Antimicrob Agents Chemother* (1975) 7, 431–4.
9. Weibert RT, Keane WF. Carbenicillin-gentamicin interaction in acute renal failure. *Am J Hosp Pharm* (1977) 34, 1137–9.
10. Kradjan WA, Burger R. In vivo inactivation of gentamicin by carbenicillin and ticarcillin. *Arch Intern Med* (1980) 140, 1668–70.
11. Thompson MIB, Russo ME, Saxon BJ, Atkin-Thor E, Matsen JM. Gentamicin inactivation by piperacillin or carbenicillin in patients with end-stage renal disease. *Antimicrob Agents Chemother* (1982) 21, 268–73.
12. Chow MSS, Quintiliani R, Nightingale CH. In Vivo inactivation of tobramycin by ticarcillin. *JAMA* (1982) 247, 658–9.
13. Uber WE, Brundage RC, White RL, Brundage DM, Bromley HR. In vivo inactivation of tobramycin by piperacillin. *Ann Pharmacother* (1991) 25, 357–9.
14. Chow MSS, Quintiliani R, Nightingale CH. In vivo inactivation of tobramycin by ticarcillin. A case report. *JAMA* (1982) 247, 658–59.
15. Riff LJ, Jackson GG. Laboratory and clinical conditions for gentamicin activation by carbenicillin. *Arch Intern Med* (1972) 130, 887–91.
16. Matzke GR, Halstenson CE, Heim KL, Abraham PA, Keane WF. Netilmicin disposition is not altered by concomitant piperacillin administration. *Clin Pharmacol Ther* (1985) 41, 210.
17. Uber WE, Brundage RC, White RL, Brundage DM, Bromley HR. In vivo inactivation of tobramycin by piperacillin. *DICP Ann Pharmacother* (1991) 25, 357–9.
18. Lau A, Lee M, Flascha S, Prasad R, Sharifi R. Effect of piperacillin on tobramycin pharmacokinetics in patients with normal renal function. *Antimicrob Agents Chemother* (1983) 24, 533–7.
19. Hitt CM, Patel KB, Nicolau DP, Zhu Z, Nightingale CH. Influence of piperacillin-tazobactam on pharmacokinetics of gentamicin given once daily. *Am J Health-Syst Pharm* (1997) 54, 2704–8.
20. Lathia C, Sia L, Lanc R, Greene D, Kuye O, Batra V, Yacobi A, Faulkner R. Pharmacokinetics of piperacillin/tazobactam IV with and without tobramycin IV in healthy adult male volunteers. *Pharm Res* (1991) 8, (10 Suppl), S-303.
21. Roberts GW, Nation RL, Jarvinen AO, Martin AJ. An *in vivo* assessment of the tobramycin/ticarcillin interaction in cystic fibrosis patients. *Br J Clin Pharmacol* (1993) 36, 372–5.
22. Cheng SH, White A. Effect of orally administered neomycin on the absorption of penicillin V. *N Engl J Med* (1962) 267, 1296–7.
23. Perényi T, Graber H, Arr M. Über die Wechselwirkung der Penizilline und Aminoglykosid-Antibiotika. *Int J Clin Pharmacol Ther Toxicol* (1974) 10, 50–5.
24. Kluge RM, Standiford HC, Tatem B, Young VM, Schimpff SC, Greene WH, Calia FM, Hornick RB. The carbenicillin-gentamicin combination against *Pseudomonas aeruginosa*. Correlation of effect with gentamicin sensitivity. *Ann Intern Med* (1974) 81, 584–7.

Aminoglycosides + Polygeline (*Haemaccel*)

The incidence of acute renal failure appears to be increased in cardiac surgical patients given polygeline (*Haemaccel*) with gentamicin.

Clinical evidence

The observation of a differing incidence of acute renal failure in patients undergoing coronary artery bypass surgery in two similar units, prompted a retrospective review of patient records. This showed that the only management differences were related to antibacterial prophylaxis and the bypass prime content (i.e. the solution used to prime the cardiopulmonary bypass circuit).

Acute renal failure was defined as a more than 50% rise in serum creatinine on the first postoperative day in those patients whose creatinine was also greater than 120 micromol/l.

Four groups of patients were identified, and the incidence of renal failure was as follows:

- Group A (polygeline plus **gentamicin** and flucloxacillin) 31% (28 of 91 patients);
- Group B (polygeline plus cefalotin)12% (9 of 72 patients);
- Group C (crystalloid plus **gentamicin** and flucloxacillin) 7% (4 of 57 patients);
- Group D (crystalloid plus cefalotin) 2% (1 of 47 patients).

Polygeline (*Haemaccel*) 1 litre, which is a urea linked gelatine colloid with a calcium concentration of 6.25 micromol/l, was used for groups A and B, with crystalloid - Hartmann's solution or Ringer's injection (calcium concentration 2 mmol/l) to make up the rest of the prime volume of 2 litres. Groups C and D received only crystalloid (no polygeline) in the prime. Albumin 100 ml was used in groups B and D.[1]

Mechanism

Not fully understood. It is thought that the relatively high calcium content of the polygeline may have potentiated gentamicin-associated nephrotoxicity. Hypercalcaemia has been shown in *animals* to increase aminoglycoside-induced nephrotoxicity.[2]

Importance and management

Information appears to be limited to this clinical study and *animal* studies, but the evidence available suggests that a clinically important adverse interaction occurs between these drugs. The incidence of acute renal failure in cardiac surgery patients is normally about 3 to 5%[3] which is low compared with the 31% shown by those on polygeline and gentamicin. The authors of the study advise avoidance of these two drugs. More study is needed.

1. Schneider M, Valentine S, Clarke GM, Newman MAJ, Peakcock J. Acute renal failure in cardiac surgical patients potentiated by gentamicin and calcium. *Anaesth Intensive Care* (1996) 24, 647–50.
2. Elliott WC, Patchin DS, Jones DB. Effect of parathyroid hormone activity on gentamicin nephrotoxicity. *J Lab Clin Med* (1987) 109, 48–54.
3. Hilberman M, Myers BD, Carrie BJ, Derby G, Jamison RL, Stinson EB. Acute renal failure following cardiac surgery. *J Thorac Cardiovasc Surg* (1979) 77, 880–8.

Aminoglycosides + Vancomycin

The nephrotoxicity of aminoglycosides appears to be potentiated by vancomycin.

Clinical evidence, mechanism, importance and management

A retrospective review of 105 patients who had received an aminoglycoside with vancomycin for at least 5 days found that nephrotoxicity occurred in 27% of the patients. Of these, 6 had no other identifiable cause for nephrotoxicity.[1] A study assessing the risks factors for nephrotoxicity with aminoglycosides (**tobramycin** and **gentamicin**) enrolled 1489 patients, 157 of whom developed clinical nephrotoxicity. Of these patients 118 had no immediately identifiable cause (such as acute renal failure) and further evaluation of other risk factors found that the concurrent use of vancomycin significantly increased the risk of nephrotoxicity.[2]

A number of other studies,[3-9] including those where patients have had individualised pharmacokinetic monitoring,[3] and those using both once daily and multiple daily dosing,[4] have all found that vancomycin independently increases the risk of nephrotoxicity in patients on aminoglycosides. In one meta-analysis of 8 trials, the incidence of nephrotoxicity with the combination was 4.3% greater than with aminoglycosides alone and 13.3% greater than with vancomycin alone.[8]

Risk factors are said to include vancomycin peak and trough levels,[1,6] aminoglycoside trough levels,[1,3,6] decreased albumin,[2] male gender,[1-3] advanced age,[1-3] length of treatment,[1-3] liver disease or ascites,[1,2] as well as a large number of other disease states (such as leukaemia,[2] peritonitis[1] or neutropenia),[1] although their significance in practice has been questioned.[2]

Concurrent use of these antibacterials is therapeutically useful, but the risk of increased nephrotoxicity should be borne in mind. Therapeutic drug monitoring and regular assessment of renal function is warranted.

1. Pauly DJ, Musa DM, Lestico MR, Lindstrom MJ, Hetsko CM. Risk of nephrotoxicity with combination vancomycin-aminoglycoside antibiotic therapy. *Pharmacotherapy* (1990) 10, 378–82.
2. Bertino JS, Booker LA, Franck PA, Jenkins PL, Franck KR, Nafziger AN. Incidence of and significant risk factors for aminoglycoside-associated nephrotoxicity in patients doses by using individualised pharmacokinetic monitoring. *J Infect Dis* (1993) 167, 173–9.
3. Streetman DS, Nafziger AN, Destache CJ, Bertino JS. Individualized pharmacokinetic monitoring results in less aminoglycoside-associated nephrotoxicity and fewer associated costs. *Pharmacotherapy* (2001) 21, 443–51.
4. Rybak MJ, Abate BJ, Kang SL, Ruffing MJ, Lerner SA, Drusano GL. Prospective evaluation on the effect of an aminoglycoside dosing regimen on rates of observed nephrotoxicity and ototoxicity. *Antimicrob Agents Chemother* (1999) 43, 1549–55.
5. Farber BF, Moellering RC. Retrospective study of the toxicity of preparations of vancomycin from 1974 to 1981. *Antimicrob Agents Chemother* (1983) 23, 138–41.
6. Cimino MA, Rotstein C, Slaughter RL, Emrich LJ. Relationship of serum antibiotic concentrations to nephrotoxicity in cancer patients receiving concurrent aminoglycoside and vancomycin therapy. *Am J Med* (1987) 83, 1091–7.
7. Rybak MJ, Frankowski JJ, Edwards DJ, Albrecht LM. Alanine aminopeptidase and β_2-microglobulin excretion in patients receiving vancomycin and gentamicin. *Antimicrob Agents Chemother* (1987) 31, 1461–4
8. Goetz MB, Sayers J. Nephrotoxicity of vancomycin and aminoglycoside therapy separately and in combination. *J Antimicrob Chemother* (1993) 32, 325–34.
9. Rybak MJ, Albrecht LM, Boike SC, Chandrasekar PH. Nephrotoxicity of vancomycin, alone and with an aminoglycoside. *J Antimicrob Chemother* (1990) 25, 679–87.

Aminoglycosides + Verapamil

Verapamil appears to protect the kidney from damage caused by gentamicin.

Clinical evidence, mechanism, importance and management

In a comparative study, 9 healthy subjects were given **gentamicin** alone (2 mg/kg loading dose, followed by doses every 8 hours to achieve a peak concentration of 5.5 mg/l and a trough concentration of 0.5 mg/l), and 6 other subjects were given the same dosage of **gentamicin** with sustained-release verapamil 180 mg twice daily. The **gentamicin** AUCs of the two groups were virtually the same but the 24-hour urinary excretion of alanine aminopeptidase (AAP) was modestly reduced, by 18%, in the group given verapamil. The reduction in AAP excretion was particularly marked during the first 6 days.[1] The significance of urinary AAP is that this enzyme is found primarily in the brush border membranes of the proximal renal tubules, and its excretion is an early and sensitive marker of renal damage. Thus it seems that verapamil may modestly protect the kidneys from damage by **gentamicin**, but using a drug as potentially toxic as verapamil to provide this protection, when the risks of renal toxicity can be minimised by carefully controlling the **gentamicin** dosage, is unwarranted. Information about other aminoglycosides and other calcium channel blockers seems to be lacking.

1. Kazierad DJ, Wojcik GJ, Nix DE, Goldfarb AL, Schentag JJ. The effect of verapamil on the nephrotoxic potential of gentamicin as measured by urinary enzyme excretion in healthy volunteers. *J Clin Pharmacol* (1995) 35, 196–201.

Aminoglycosides; Tobramycin + Sucralfate

An *in vitro* study with tobramycin found that it became markedly and irreversibly bound to sucralfate at the pH values found in the gut. This suggests that the efficacy of tobramycin in gut decontamination might be decreased.

Clinical evidence, mechanism, importance and management

To simulate what might happen in the gut, tobramycin 50 mg/ml was mixed with sucralfate 500 mg in 40 ml of water at pH 3.5 and allowed to stand for 90 minutes at 25°C. Analysis of the solution showed that the tobramycin concentration fell rapidly and progressively over 90 minutes to about 1%. When the pH of the mixture was then raised to 6.5 to 7 for 90 minutes, there was no change in the concentration of tobramycin, suggesting that the interaction was irreversible.[1] The reason for this change is not known, but the suggestion is that sucralfate forms insoluble chelates with tobramycin.[1]

It is not known how important this interaction is likely to be in practice, but the efficacy of tobramycin in gut decontamination may be decreased. Separating the dosages might not be effective in some postoperative patients because their gastric function may not return to normal for up to 5 days, and some sucralfate might still be present when the next dose is given.[1] More study is needed to find out whether this interaction is clinically important, but in the meanwhile it would seem prudent to monitor concurrent use carefully, being alert for any evidence of reduced effects.

1. Feron B, Adair CG, Gorman SP, McClurg B. Interaction of sucralfate with antibiotics used for selective decontamination of the gastrointestinal tract. *Am J Hosp Pharm* (1993) 50, 2550–3.

Aminosalicylic acid + Diphenhydramine

Diphenhydramine can cause a small reduction in the absorption of aminosalicylic acid from the gut.

Clinical evidence, mechanism, importance and management

A study in 9 healthy subjects[1] showed that diphenhydramine 50 mg injected intramuscularly 10 minutes before a 2-g oral dose of aminosalicylic acid, reduced the mean peak serum aminosalicylic acid levels by about 15%. The possible reason is that diphenhydramine reduces peristalsis in the gut, which in some way reduces aminosalicylic acid absorption. The extent to which diphenhydramine or any other anticholinergic drug diminishes the therapeutic response to long-term treatment with aminosalicylic acid is uncertain, but it is probably small.

1. Lavigne J-G, Marchand C. Inhibition of the gastrointestinal absorption of p-aminosalicylate (PAS) in rats and humans by diphenhydramine. *Clin Pharmacol Ther* (1973) 14, 404–12.

Aminosalicylic acid + Probenecid

The serum levels of aminosalicylic acid can be raised up to fourfold by probenecid.

Clinical evidence, mechanism, importance and management

When probenecid 500 mg six-hourly was given to 7 patients the serum levels produced by aminosalicylic acid 4 g were increased by as much as fourfold.[1] Similar results are described in another report.[2]

The reasons are uncertain but it seems probable that probenecid successfully competes with aminosalicylic acid for active excretion by the kidney tubules, which results in the increased aminosalicylic acid levels.

The documentation of this interaction is limited but it appears to be established. Such large increases in serum aminosalicylic acid levels would be expected to lead to toxicity. It also seems possible that the dosage of aminosalicylic acid could be reduced without losing the required therapeutic response. This needs confirmation. Monitoring aminosalicylic acid levels, where possible, would probably be useful. Concurrent use should be undertaken with caution.

1. Boger WP, Pitts FW. Influence of *p*-(Di-n-propylsulfamyl)-benzoic acid, 'Benemid' on para-aminosalicylic acid (PAS) plasma concentrations. *Am Rev Tuberc* (1950) 61, 862–7.
2. Carr DT, Karlson AG, Bridge EV. Concentration of PAS and tuberculostatic potency of serum after administration of PAS with and without Benemid. *Proc Staff Meet Mayo Clin* (1952) 27, 209–15.

Antibacterials + Immunoglobulins

One *animal* study found that for severe infections antibacterials were less effective in the presence of high-dose immunoglobulin, but this was not seen in less severe infections. The clinical relevance of this is uncertain.

Clinical evidence, mechanism, importance and management

A study in an *animal* model of severe group B streptococcal infection found the following mortalities: 100% with immunoglobulin 2 g/kg alone, 51% with **benzylpenicillin** 200 mg/kg alone, and 88% with immunoglobulin and **benzylpenicillin**. A smaller dose of immunoglobulin 0.5 g/kg was not associated with an increase in mortality.[1] Not dissimilar results were found when the penicillin was replaced by **ceftriaxone**.[1] In another study using a 1000-fold smaller inoculum of group B streptococci, there was no difference in mortality between **benzylpenicillin** 200 mg/kg daily alone and **benzylpenicillin** with immunoglobulin 0.25 to 2 g/kg, and there was some evidence of a lower incidence of bacteraemia with the combination.[1,2]

Immunoglobulins are used with antibacterials in the successful prevention of infections in clinical practice, and no special precautions appear to be needed in this situation. However, their clinical use for treating established infection is unclear, and the above findings suggest some caution is warranted.

1. Kim KS. High-dose intravenous immune globulin impairs antibacterial activity of antibiotics. *J Allergy Clin Immunol* (1989) 84, 579–88.
2. Kim KS. Efficacy of human immunoglobulin and penicillin G in treatment of experimental group B streptococcal infection. *Pediatr Res* (1987) 21, 289–92.

Cephalosporins + Antacids

No clinically significant interactions appear to occur between an aluminium/magnesium hydroxide antacid and cefaclor AF, cefalexin, cefetamet pivoxil, cefixime or cefprozil; between *Alka-Seltzer* and cefixime; or between ceftibuten and *Mylanta*. Antacids reduce the bioavailability of cefpodoxime proxetil.

Clinical evidence, mechanism, importance and management

(a) Cefaclor

A study of cefaclor AF (a formulation with a slow rate of release) found that an **aluminium/magnesium hydroxide** antacid (*Maalox*) given one hour after the cefaclor AF to fed subjects reduced the AUC by 18%.[1] This reduction is small and unlikely to be clinically important.

(b) Cefalexin

An **aluminium/magnesium hydroxide** antacid (*Maalox*) given as 8 doses of 10 ml on day one and 2 doses on day 2, had only small and therapeutically unimportant effects on the pharmacokinetics of cefalexin 1 g.[2]

(c) Cefetamet pivoxil

Cefetamet pivoxil 1 g was given to 18 healthy subjects after breakfast with or without 80 ml of an **aluminium/magnesium hydroxide** antacid (*Maalox 70*) given the evening before, 2 hours before, and after breakfast. The pharmacokinetics of the cefetamet were unaffected by the antacid.[3]

(d) Cefixime

An **aluminium/magnesium hydroxide** antacid (*Maalox*) and ***Alka-Seltzer*** (aspirin, calcium phosphate, citric acid and **sodium bicarbonate**) do not significantly affect the absorption of cefixime,[4,5]

(e) Cefpodoxime proxetil

A study in 10 healthy subjects showed that 10 ml of an **aluminium/magnesium hydroxide** antacid (*Maalox*) reduced the bioavailability of cefpodoxime proxetil by about 40%. This was considered to be due to reduced dissolution at increased gastric pH values.[6] These results confirm the findings of a previous study with **sodium bicarbonate** and **aluminium hydroxide**.[7] It has been recommended that cefpodoxime is given at least 2 hours after antacids.[6]

(f) Cefprozil

An **aluminium/magnesium hydroxide** antacid (*Maalox*) does not affect the bioavailability of cefprozil.[8]

(g) Ceftibuten

In 18 healthy subjects, 60 ml of an antacid containing **aluminium/magnesium hydroxide** plus **simethicone** (*Mylanta II*) was found not to affect the pharmacokinetics of ceftibuten 400 mg.[9]

1. Satterwhite JH, Cerimele BJ, Coleman DL, Hatcher BL, Kisicki J, DeSante KA. Pharmacokinetics of cefaclor AF: effects of age, antacids and H_2-receptor antagonists. *Postgrad Med J* (1992) 68 (Suppl 3), S3–S9.
2. Deppermann K-M, Lode H, Höffken G, Tschink G, Kalz C, Koeppe P. Influence of ranitidine, pirenzepine, and aluminum magnesium hydroxide on the bioavailability of various antibiotics, including amoxicillin, cephalexin, doxycycline and amoxicillin-clavulanic acid. *Antimicrob Agents Chemother* (1989) 33, 1901–1907.
3. Blouin RA, Kneer J, Ambros RJ, Stoeckel K. Influence of antacid and ranitidine on the pharmacokinetics of oral cefetamet pivoxil. *Antimicrob Agents Chemother* (1990) 34, 1744–8.
4. Petitjean O, Brion N, Tod M, Montagne A, Nicolas P. Étude de l'interaction pharmacocinétique entre le céfixime et deux antiacides. Résultats préliminaires. *Presse Med* (1989) 18, 1596–8.
5. Healy DP, Sahai JV, Sterling LP, Racht EM. Influence of an antacid containing aluminum and magnesium on the pharmacokinetics of cefixime. *Antimicrob Agents Chemother* (1989) 33, 1994–7.
6. Saathoff N, Lode H, Neider K, Depperman KM, Borner K, Koeppe P. Pharmacokinetics of cefpodoxime proxetil and interactions with an antacid and an H_2 receptor antagonist. *Antimicrob Agents Chemother* (1992) 36, 796–800.
7. Hughes GS, Heald DL, Barker KB, Patel RK, Spillers CR, Watts KC, Batts DH, Euler AR. The effects of gastric pH and food on the pharmacokinetics of a new oral cephalosporin, cefpodoxime proxetil. *Clin Pharmacol Ther* (1989) 46, 674–85.
8. Shyu WC, Wilber RB, Pittman KA, Barbhaiya RH. Effect of antacid on the bioavailability of cefprozil. *Antimicrob Agents Chemother* (1992) 36, 962–5.
9. Radwanski E, Nomeir A, Cutler D, Affrime M, Lin C-C. Pharmacokinetic drug interaction study: administration of ceftibuten concurrently with the antacid Mylanta double-strength liquid or with ranitidine. *Am J Ther* (1998) 5, 67–72.

Cephalosporins + Calcium channel blockers

Nifedipine increases the serum levels of cefixime but this is unlikely to be clinically important. Neither nifedipine nor diltiazem affect the pharmacokinetics of cefpodoxime proxetil.

Clinical evidence, mechanism, importance and management

The AUC and peak serum levels of a single 200-mg dose of **cefixime** was increased by about 70% and 50% respectively in 8 healthy subjects when **cefixime** was taken 30 minutes after a 20-mg dose of **nifedipine**. The rate of absorption was also increased. No adverse responses were seen. One suggested reason for this interaction is that the **nifedipine** increases the absorption of the **cefixime** by affecting the carrier system across the epithelial wall of the gut.[1] It seems doubtful if this increased **cefixime** bioavailability is clinically important (the combination was well-tolerated) and no particular precautions would seem to be necessary on concurrent use.

The pharmacokinetics of a single 200-mg dose of **cefpodoxime proxetil** were found to be unchanged by single doses of either 60 mg of **diltiazem** or 20 mg of **nifedipine** in 12 healthy subjects.[2] No special precautions would seem necessary during concurrent use.

Information about other cephalosporins and calcium channel blockers seems to be lacking, but there seems to be no particular reason to suspect an interaction.

1. Duverne C, Bouten A, Deslandes A, Westphal J-F, Trouvin J-H, Farinotti R, Carbon C. Modification of cefixime bioavailability by nifedipine in humans: involvement of the dipeptide carrier system. *Antimicrob Agents Chemother* (1992) 36, 2462–7.
2. Deslandes A, Camus F, Lacroix C, Carbon C, Farinotti R. Effects of nifedipine and diltiazem on pharmacokinetics of cefpodoxime following its oral administration. *Antimicrob Agents Chemother* (1996) 40, 2879–81.

Cephalosporins + Colestyramine

Colestyramine binds with cefadroxil and cefalexin in the gut, which delays their absorption. The importance of this is probably small.

Clinical evidence

The peak serum levels of a 500-mg oral dose of **cefadroxil** were reduced and delayed in 4 subjects when it was taken with 10 g of colestyramine, but the total amount absorbed was not affected.[1] Similar results were found in a study involving **cefalexin** and colestyramine.[2]

Mechanism

Colestyramine is an ion-exchange resin, which binds with these two cephalosporins in the gut. This prevents the early and rapid absorption of the antibacterial, but as the colestyramine/cephalosporin complex passes along the gastrointestinal tract, the antibacterial is progressively released and eventually virtually all of it becomes available for absorption.[1]

Importance and management

Direct information seems to be limited to the studies cited. The clinical significance is uncertain, but as the total amount of antibacterial absorbed is not reduced this interaction is probably of little importance. This needs confirmation. Information about other cephalosporins seems to be lacking.

1. Marino EL, Vicente MT and Dominguez-Gil A. Influence of cholestyramine on the pharmacokinetic parameters of cefadroxil after simultaneous administration. *Int J Pharmaceutics* (1983) 16, 23–30.
2. Parsons RL, Paddock GM. Absorption of two antibacterial drugs, cephalexin and co-trimoxazole, in malabsorption syndromes. *J Antimicrob Chemother* (1975) 1 (Suppl), 59–67.

Cephalosporins + Furosemide

The nephrotoxic effects of cefaloridine and possibly cefalotin or cefacetrile appear to be increased by furosemide. Cefradine brain levels are reduced by furosemide. No important interactions appear to occur between furosemide and either cefoxitin, ceftazidime or ceftriaxone.

Clinical evidence

(a) Nephrotoxicity

Nine out of 36 patients who developed acute renal failure while taking **cefaloridine** had also been treated with a diuretic, furosemide being used in 7 cases. Other factors such as age and dosage may also have been involved. The authors of this report related their observations to previous *animal* studies, which showed that potent diuretics such as furosemide and etacrynic acid enhanced the incidence and extent of tubular necrosis.[1] Several other reports describe nephrotoxicity in patients given both **cefaloridine** and furosemide.[2-4] There is a question mark hanging over **cefalotin** and **cefacetrile** because *animal* studies found an increase in nephrotoxicity,[5,6] and there is a single report describing nephrotoxicity in one patient on **cefalotin** and furosemide.[2] **Cefoxitin** seems to be relatively free of nephrotoxicity alone or with furosemide.[7]

(b) Changes in serum levels and clearance

A clinical study[8] showed that furosemide 80 mg increased the serum half-life of **cefaloridine** by 25%, and in another study **cefaloridine** clearance was reduced.[9] A further study found that brain concentrations of **cefradine** are markedly reduced by furosemide.[10] In a study in 6 healthy subjects, furosemide 40 mg, given 1 hour before a 1-g intramuscular dose of **ceftazidime**, raised the serum **ceftazidime** levels by about 20 to 40% over 8 hours and increased the AUC by 28%. Furosemide given 3 hours before **ceftazidime** had much smaller effects.[11] **Ceftriaxone** does not appear to interfere with the diuretic effects of furosemide.[12]

Mechanism

Cefaloridine is nephrotoxic, but why this should be increased by furosemide is not understood. It may possibly be related to a reduction in its clearance.[9]

Importance and management

The cefaloridine/furosemide interaction is not well-established, but there is enough evidence to suggest that concurrent use should be undertaken with care. Age and/or renal impairment may possibly be predisposing factors. Renal function should be checked frequently. A pharmacokinetic study suggests that the development of this adverse interaction may possibly depend on the time relationship of drug use, and it has been recommended that furosemide should be avoided for 3 or 4 hours before the cefaloridine.[13]

Although the makers of ceftazidime issue a caution about the use of high doses of cephalosporins with other nephrotoxic drugs, they say that clinical experience has not shown this to be a problem with ceftazidime at the recommended doses.[14] The rest of the information about other cephalosporins and furosemide is fairly sparse. Most appear not to interact adversely, with a few possible exceptions, namely cefalotin (nephrotoxicity in a single case[2] and *animal* studies[5]) and cephacetrile (nephrotoxicity in *animal* studies[6]). Care is clearly prudent with these two cephalosporins.

1. Dodds MG, Foord RD. Enhancement by potent diuretics of renal tubular necrosis induced by cephaloridine. *Br J Pharmacol* (1970) 4, 227–36.
2. Simpson IJ. Nephrotoxicity and acute renal failure associated with cephalothin and cephaloridine. *N Z Med J* (1971) 74, 312–15.
3. Kleinknecht D, Jungers P, Fillastre J-P. Nephrotoxicity of cephaloridine. *Ann Intern Med* (1974) 80, 421–2.
4. Lawson DH, Macadam RF, Singh H, Gavras H, Linton AL. The nephrotoxicity of cephaloridine. *Postgrad Med J* (1970) 46 (Suppl), 36–9.
5. Lawson DH, Macadam RF, Singh H, Gavras H, Hartz S, Turnbull D, Linton AL. Effect of furosemide on antibiotic-induced renal damage in rats. *J Infect Dis* (1972) 126, 593–600.
6. Luscombe DK, Nichols PJ. Possible interaction between cephacetrile and frusemide in rabbits and rats. *J Antimicrob Chemother* (1975) 1, 67–77.
7. Trollfors B, Norrby R, Kristianson K, Nilsson NJ. Effects on renal function of treatment with cefoxitin alone or in combination with furosemide. *Scand J Infect Dis* (1978) (Suppl), 13, 73–7.
8. Norrby R, Stenqvist K, Elgefors B. Interaction between cephaloridine and furosemide in man. *Scand J Infect Dis* (1976) 8, 209–212.
9. Tilstone WJ, Semple PF, Lawson DH, Boyle JA. Effects of furosemide on glomerular filtration rate and clearance of practolol, digoxin, cephaloridine and gentamicin. *Clin Pharmacol Ther* (1977) 22, 389–94.
10. Adam D, Jacoby W, Raff WK. Beeinflussung der Antibiotika-Konzentration im Gewebe durch ein Saluretikum. *Klin Wochenschr* (1978) 56, 247–51.
11. Chrysos G, Gargalianos P, Lelekis M, Stefanou J, Kosmidis J. Pharmacokinetic interactions of ceftazidime and frusemide. *J Chemother* (1995) 7 (Suppl 4), 107–10.
12. Korn A, Eichler HG, Gasic S. A drug interaction study of ceftriaxone and frusemide in healthy volunteers. *Int J Clin Pharmacol Ther Toxicol* (1986) 24, 262–4.
13. Kosmidis J, Polyzos A, Daikos GK. Pharmacokinetic interactions between cephalosporins and furosemide are influenced by administration time relationships. *Curr Chemother Infect Dis, 11th Int Congr Chemother* (1979 and 1980) 673–5.
14. Fortum for injection (Ceftazidime). GlaxoSmithKline UK. UK Summary of product characteristics, February 2003.

Cephalosporins + H_2-blockers

Ranitidine and famotidine reduce the bioavailability of cefpodoxime proxetil. Ranitidine with sodium bicarbonate reduces the bioavailability of cefuroxime axetil, but not to an important extent if taken with food. No clinically significant pharmacokinetic interactions appear to occur between cefaclor AF and cimetidine, and between cefetamet pivoxil, cefalexin or ceftibuten and ranitidine.

Clinical evidence

(a) Cefaclor

A study of cefaclor AF (a formulation with a slow rate of release) found that **cimetidine** 800 mg taken the night before reduced its maximum serum concentration by 12%.[1]

(b) Cefalexin

Ranitidine 150 mg for 3 doses had only small and therapeutically unimportant effects on the pharmacokinetics of cefalexin 1 g.[2]

(c) Cefetamet pivoxil

Ranitidine 150 mg twice daily for 4 days did not affect the pharmacokinetics of cefetamet pivoxil 1 g given to 18 healthy subjects after breakfast.[3]

(d) Cefpodoxime proxetil

A study in 10 healthy fasted subjects showed that **famotidine** 40 mg reduced the bioavailability of cefpodoxime proxetil by about 40%.[4] This confirms the findings of a previous study with **ranitidine**.[5]

(e) Ceftibuten

Ranitidine 150 mg 12-hourly for 3 days raised the maximum serum levels and AUC of ceftibuten by 23% and 16% respectively in 18 healthy subjects. However these values lie within the normal ranges seen in healthy subjects and no dosage adjustment is thought to be needed.[6]

(f) Cefuroxime axetil

Ranitidine 300 mg with sodium bicarbonate 4 g reduced the AUC of cefuroxime axetil 1 g by 43% when given to fasted subjects. However, when cefuroxime was given after food, its bioavailability was higher, and minimally affected by **ranitidine** plus sodium bicarbonate (10% reduction in AUC) .[7]

Mechanism

The reduction in the bioavailability of some of the cephalosporins is thought to be due to reduced dissolution at increased gastric pH values.[4]

Importance and management

In most cases the interactions between the cephalosporins and H_2-blockers are not clinically significant. The clinical importance of the interaction with cefpodoxime has not been studied, but the maker recommends that cefpodoxime is given at least 2 hours before H_2-blockers.[8] As it is thought that a change in gastric pH is responsible for this interaction it would seem likely that **proton pump inhibitors** will interact similarly.

As long as cefuroxime is taken with food (as is recommended[9]), any interaction is minimal.

1. Satterwhite JH, Cerimele BJ, Coleman DL, Hatcher BL, Kisicki J, DeSante KA. Pharmacokinetics of cefaclor AF: effects of age, antacids and H_2-receptor antagonists. *Postgrad Med J* (1992) 68 (Suppl 3), S3–S9.
2. Deppermann K-M, Lode H, Höffken G, Tschink G, Kalz C, Koeppe P. Influence of ranitidine, pirenzepine, and aluminum magnesium hydroxide on the bioavailability of various antibiotics, including amoxicillin, cephalexin, doxycycline and amoxicillin-clavulanic acid. *Antimicrob Agents Chemother* (1989) 33, 1901–1907.
3. Blouin RA, Kneer J, Ambros RJ, Stoeckel K. Influence of antacid and ranitidine on the pharmacokinetics of oral cefetamet pivoxil. *Antimicrob Agents Chemother* (1990) 34, 1744–8.
4. Saathoff N, Lode H, Neider K, Depperman KM, Borner K, Koeppe P. Pharmacokinetics of cefpodoxime proxetil and interactions with an antacid and an H_2 receptor antagonist. *Antimicrob Agents Chemother* (1992) 36, 796–800.
5. Hughes GS, Heald DL, Barker KB, Patel RK, Spillers CR, Watts KC, Batts DH, Euler AR. The effects of gastric pH and food on the pharmacokinetics of a new oral cephalosporin, cefpodoxime proxetil. *Clin Pharmacol Ther* (1989) 46, 674–85.
6. Radwanski E, Nomeir A, Cutler D, Affrime M, Lin C-C. Pharmacokinetic drug interaction study: administration of ceftibuten concurrently with the antacid Mylanta double-strength liquid or with ranitidine. *Am J Ther* (1998) 5, 67–72.
7. Sommers De K, Van Wyk M, Moncrieff J, Schoeman HS. Influence of food and reduced gastric acidity on the bioavailability of bacampicillin and cefuroxime axetil. *Br J Clin Pharmacol* (1984) 18, 535–9.
8. Orelox Tablets (Cefpodoxime). Aventis Pharma Ltd. UK Summary of product characteristics, April 2002.
9. Zinnat Tablets (Cefuroxime axetil). GlaxoSmithKline UK. UK Summary of product characteristics, January 2003.

Cephalosporins + Miscellaneous

The pharmacokinetics of cefprozil are minimally affected by propantheline and metoclopramide,[1] and the pharmacokinetics of cefpodoxime proxetil are minimally affected by acetylcysteine.[2] Pirenzepine (50 mg for 4 doses) had only small and therapeutically unimportant effects on the pharmacokinetics of 1 g of cefalexin.[3] None of these interactions is likely to be clinically important. The clearance of ceftazidime is significantly reduced by indometacin in neonates, and dosage adjustments are likely to be necessary.[4]

1. Shukla UA, Pittman KA, Barbhaiya RH. Pharmacokinetic interactions of cefprozil with food, propantheline, metoclopramide, and probenecid in healthy volunteers. *J Clin Pharmacol* (1992) 32, 725–31.
2. Kees F, Wellenhofer M, Bröhl K, Grobecker H. Bioavailability of cefpodoxime proxetil with co-administered acetylcysteine. *Arzneimittelforschung* (1996) 46, 435–8.
3. Deppermann K-M, Lode H, Höffken G, Tschink G, Kalz C, Koeppe P. Influence of ranitidine, pirenzepine, and aluminum magnesium hydroxide on the bioavailability of various antibiotics, including amoxicillin, cephalexin, doxycycline and amoxicillin-clavulanic acid. *Antimicrob Agents Chemother* (1989) 33, 1901–1907.
4. van den Anker JN, Hop WCJ, Schoemaker RC, Van der Heijden BJ, Neijens HJ, De Groot R. Ceftazidime pharmacokinetics in preterm infants: effect of postnatal age and postnatal exposure to indomethacin. *Br J Clin Pharmacol* (1995) 40, 439–43.

Cephalosporins + Probenecid

The serum levels of many cephalosporins are raised by probenecid. This may possibly increase the risk of nephrotoxicity with some cephalosporins such as cefaloridine and cefalotin.

Clinical evidence

Ten healthy subjects given a single 500-mg oral dose of **cefradine** or **cefaclor** developed markedly raised serum antibacterial concentrations when given probenecid (500-mg doses taken 25, 13 and 2 hours before the antibacterial). Peak serum levels of the antibacterial were very roughly doubled.[1] Similar results were obtained in another study in healthy subjects given **cefradine** by mouth or intramuscularly.[2]

The following cephalosporins interact with probenecid similarly, but not identically, the overall picture being that their clearance is reduced, their serum levels are raised and sometimes their half-lives are prolonged. A review[3] identified the interaction with **cefadroxil**, **cefazedone**, **cefmenoxime**, **cefonicid**, **cefotaxime**, **cefradine**, and **cefaclor**, and other studies have reported an interaction with **cefalotin**,[4] **cefacetrile**,[5] **cefalexin**,[6] **cefamandole**,[7] **cefazolin**,[8-10] **cefmetazole**[11] **cefoxitin**,[12-14] **cefprozil**,[15] **ceftizoxime**,[16] **cefuroxime**,[17] **cefaloglycin**[18] and **cefaloridine**.[19]

Probenecid is reported to have no significant effect on the pharmacokinetics of **ceforanide**,[20] **ceftazidime**,[3] **ceftriaxone**[21] and **latamoxef**.[3]

Mechanism

Probenecid inhibits the excretion of most cephalosporins by the kidney tubules by successfully competing for the excretory mechanisms. A fuller explanation of this mechanism is set out in 'Drug excretion interactions', (p.7). Thus the cephalosporin is retained in the body and its serum levels rise. The extent of the rise cannot always be fully accounted for by this mechanism alone and it is suggested that some change in tissue distribution may sometimes have a part to play.[1]

Importance and management

An extremely well-documented interaction. Only a few representative references are listed below to save space, but the details of many are well described in a review paper.[3] The serum levels of many (but not all) cephalosporins will be higher if probenecid is given, but no special precautions are normally needed. The interaction has been used clinically. Elevated serum levels of some cephalosporins, in particular cefaloridine and cefalotin, might possibly increase the risk of nephrotoxicity.

1. Welling PG, Dean S, Selen A, Kendall MJ, Wise R. Probenecid: an unexplained effect on cephalosporin pharmacology. *Br J Clin Pharmacol* (1979) 8, 491–5.
2. Mischler TW, Sugerman AA, Willard DA, Brannick LJ, Neiss ES. Influence of probenecid and food on the bioavailability of cephradine in normal male subjects. *J Clin Pharmacol* (1974) 14, 604–11.
3. Brown GR. Cephalosporin-probenecid drug interactions. *Clin Pharmacokinet* (1993) 24, 289–300.
4. Tuano SB, Brodie JL, Kirby WMM. Cephaloridine versus cephalothin: relation of the kidney to blood level differences after parenteral administration. *Antimicrob Agents Chemother* (1966) 6, 101–6.
5. Wise R, Reeves DS. Pharmacological studies on cephacetrile in human volunteers. *Curr Med Res Opin* (1974) 2, 249–55.
6. Taylor WA, Holloway WJ. Cephalexin in the treatment of gonorrhea. *Int J Clin Pharmacol Ther Toxicol* (1972) 6, 7–9.
7. Griffith RS, Black HR, Brier GL, Wolny JD. Effect of probenecid on the blood levels and urinary excretion of cefamandole. *Antimicrob Agents Chemother* (1977) 11, 809–12.
8. Duncan WC. Treatment of gonorrhea with cefazolin plus probenecid. *J Infect Dis* (1974) 130, 398–401.
9. Brown G, Zemcov SJV, Clarke AM. Effect of probenecid on cefazolin serum concentrations. *J Antimicrob Chemother* (1993) 31, 1009–1011.
10. Spina SP, Dillon EC. Effect of chronic probenecid therapy on cefazolin serum concentrations. *Ann Pharmacother* (2003) 37, 621–4.
11. Ko H, Cathcart KS, Griffith DL, Peters GR, Adams WJ. Pharmacokinetics of intravenously administered cefmetazole and cefoxitin and effects of probenecid on cefmetazole elimination. *Antimicrob Agents Chemother* (1989) 33, 356–61.
12. Bint AJ, Reeves DS, Holt HA. Effect of probenecid on serum cefoxitin concentrations. *J Antimicrob Chemother* (1977) 3, 627–8.
13. Reeves DS, Bullock DW, Bywater MJ, Holt HA, White LO, Thornhill DP. The effect of probenecid on the pharmacokinetics and distribution of cefoxitin in healthy volunteers. *Br J Clin Pharmacol* (1981) 11, 353–9.

14. Vlasses PH, Holbrook AM, Schrogie JJ, Rogers JD, Ferguson RK, Abrams WB. Effect of orally administered probenecid on the pharmacokinetics of cefoxitin. *Antimicrob Agents Chemother* (1980) 17, 847–55.
15. Shukla UA, Pittman KA, Barbhaiya RH. Pharmacokinetic interactions of cefprozil with food, propantheline, metoclopramide, and probenecid in healthy volunteers. *J Clin Pharmacol* (1992) 32, 725–31.
16. LeBel M, Paone RP, Lewis GP. Effect of probenecid on the pharmacokinetics of ceftizoxime. *J Antimicrob Chemother* (1983) 12, 147–55.
17. Garton AM, Rennie RP, Gilpin J, Marrelli M, Shafran SD. Comparison of dose doubling with probenecid for sustaining serum cefuroxime levels. *J Antimicrob Chemother* (1997) 40, 903–6.
18. Applestein JM, Crosby EB, Johnson WD, Kaye D. In-vitro antimicrobial activity and human pharmacology of cephaloglycin. *Appl Microbiol* (1968) 16, 1006–10.
19. Kaplan KS, Reisberg BE, Weinstein L. Cephaloridine: antimicrobial activity and pharmacologic behaviour. *Am J Med Sci* (1967) 253, 667–74.
20. Jovanovich JF, Saravolatz LD, Burch K, Pohlod DJ. Failure of probenecid to alter the pharmacokinetics of ceforanide. *Antimicrob Agents Chemother* (1981) 20, 530–2.
21. Stoeckel K, Trueb V, Dubach UC, McNamara PJ. Effect of probenecid on the elimination and protein binding of ceftriaxone. *Eur J Clin Pharmacol* (1988) 34, 151–6.

Cephalosporins; Cefalotin + Colistin

Renal failure has been attributed to the concurrent use of cefalotin and colistin.

Clinical evidence, mechanism, importance and management

Four patients developed acute renal failure, which appeared to be reversible, during treatment with colistin. Three were given cefalotin concurrently and the fourth had previously been treated with this antibacterial.[1] An increase in renal toxicity associated with concurrent use has been described in another report.[2] The reason for this reaction is not known. What is known suggests that renal function should be closely monitored if these antibacterials are given concurrently or sequentially.

1. Adler S, Segal DP. Nonoliguric renal failure secondary to sodium colistimethate: a report of four cases. *Am J Med Sci* (1971) 262, 109–14.
2. Koch-Weser J, Sidel VW, Federman EB, Kanarek P, Finer DC, Eaton AE. Adverse effects of sodium colistimethate. Manifestations and specific reaction rates during 317 courses of therapy. *Ann Intern Med* (1970) 72, 857–68.

Cephalosporins; Cefdinir + Iron compounds

Ferrous sulphate markedly reduces the absorption of cefdinir.

Clinical evidence

When 6 healthy subjects were given **ferrous sulphate** (1050 mg *Fero-Gradumet*, sustained release, equivalent to 210 mg elemental iron) with cefdinir 200 mg the AUC of the cefdinir was reduced by 93%. When the **ferrous sulphate** was taken 3 hours after the cefdinir, the absorption of the cefdinir remained unchanged for 3 hours and then rapidly fell, the total AUC over 12 hours being reduced by 36%.[1]

Mechanism

It is believed that the ferrous sulphate chelates with the cefdinir in the gut to produce a poorly absorbed complex.

Importance and management

An established interaction of clinical importance. Avoid ferrous sulphate and other iron compounds while taking cefdinir. It is not yet known how far apart these drugs must be separated to avoid this interaction, but 3 hours improves the situation considerably even if it does not totally solve it. There is no information to suggest that other cephalosporins interact in this way.

1. Ueno K, Tanaka K, Tsujimura K, Morishima Y, Iwashige H, Yamazaki K, Nakata I. Impairment of cefdinir absorption by iron ion. *Clin Pharmacol Ther* (1993) 54, 473–5.

Cephalosporins; Cefotaxime + Mezlocillin

Mezlocillin reduces the loss of cefotaxime from the body in subjects with normal renal function.

Clinical evidence, mechanism, importance and management

When cefotaxime 30 mg/kg and mezlocillin 50 mg/kg were infused together over 30 minutes in 8 healthy subjects, the pharmacokinetics of the mezlocillin were unchanged but the clearance of the cefotaxime was reduced by about 40%. However, in a series of 5 patients with end-stage renal-disease no significant decrease in cefotaxime clearance was seen when these antibacterials were given together. The clinical significance of this interaction is uncertain.[1]

1. Rodondi LC, Flaherty JF, Schoenfeld P, Barriere SL, Gambertoglio JG. Influence of coadministration on the pharmacokinetics of mezlocillin and cefotaxime in healthy volunteers and in patients with renal failure. *Clin Pharmacol Ther* (1989) 45, 527–34.

Cephalosporins; Cefotaxime + Phenobarbital

A marked increase in serious skin reactions has been seen in children given cefotaxime and high-dose phenobarbital.

Clinical evidence, mechanism, importance and management

A 30-month study observed a very marked increase in drug-induced reactions in children in intensive care who were treated with high-dose phenobarbital and beta-lactam antibacterials, mainly cefotaxime. Twenty-four out of 49 children developed drug-induced reactions, which were mainly exanthematous skin reactions.[1] The reasons are not known.

1. Harder S, Schneider W, Bae ZU, Bock U, Zielen S. Unerwünschte Arzneimittelreaktionen bei gleichzeitiger Gabe von hochdosiertem Phenobarbital und Betalaktam-Antibiotika. *Klin Padiatr* (1990) 202, 404–7.

Chloramphenicol + Cimetidine

Isolated reports describe fatal aplastic anaemia in two patients given intravenous chloramphenicol and cimetidine.

Clinical evidence, mechanism, importance and management

Pancytopenia and aplastic anaemia developed in a man on cimetidine 1200 mg daily, within 18 days of being given intravenous chloramphenicol 1 g 6-hourly. It proved to be fatal.[1] Another patient, similarly treated, developed fatal aplastic anaemia after 19 days.[2] A drug interaction with cimetidine was suspected because the onset of pancytopenia was more rapid than in previous cases where chloramphenicol alone induced aplastic anaemia. A possible reason is that the bone marrow depressant effects of the two drugs were additive. There are at least 8 other cases of aplastic anaemia following the use of parenteral chloramphenicol in the absence of cimetidine.[2] The general importance of these observations is uncertain, but the authors of one of the reports suggest that these drugs should be used together with caution.

1. Farber BF, Brody JP. Rapid development of aplastic anemia after intravenous chloramphenicol and cimetidine therapy. *South Med J* (1981) 74, 1257–8.
2. West BC, DeVault GA, Clement JC, Williams DM. Aplastic anemia associated with parenteral chloramphenicol: review of 10 cases, including the second case of possible increased risk with cimetidine. *Rev Infect Dis* (1988) 10, 1048–51.

Chloramphenicol + Dapsone

Dapsone does not significantly affect the pharmacokinetics of oral chloramphenicol.

Clinical evidence, mechanism, importance and management

A comparison of the pharmacokinetics of oral chloramphenicol in 8 healthy subjects and 8 patients with uncomplicated lepromatous leprosy found that the half-life of a single 500-mg dose of chloramphenicol was prolonged from 4.3 to 6.4 hours in patients with leprosy possibly due to changes in liver function. The elimination half-life of chloramphenicol was further increased, to about 8 hours, after treatment with dapsone 100 mg daily for 8 days. However, this latter increase was not significant. The AUC of chloramphenicol was increased by about 40% in patients with leprosy when compared with healthy subjects (both groups given chloramphenicol alone), but this increase was not statistically significant. Although there was no clinically significant interaction between dapsone and chloramphenicol, the disposition of chloramphenicol may be altered in leprosy.[1]

1. Garg SK, Kumar B, Shukla VK, Bakaya V, Lal R, Kaur S. Pharmacokinetics of aspirin and chloramphenicol in normal and leprotic patients before and after dapsone therapy. *Int J Clin Pharmacol* (1988) 26, 204–5.

Chloramphenicol + Other antibacterials

Antagonism between chloramphenicol and other antibacterials has been described in a case of staphylococcal endocarditis, in bacterial meningitis in a large group of patients, and in an infant. In contrast, no antagonism and even additive antibacterial effects have been described in other infections. Chloramphenicol levels have been markedly lowered by rifampicin (rifampin) in 4 children.

Clinical evidence

(a) Antibacterial antagonism

A study in 264 patients (adults, and children over two months) with acute bacterial meningitis showed that when they were given **ampicillin** 150 mg/kg daily alone, the case-fatality ratio was 4.3% compared with 10.5% on a combination of **ampicillin**, chloramphenicol 100 mg/kg daily up to 4 g and **streptomycin** 40 mg/kg daily up to 2 g. The neurological sequelae (hemiparesis, deafness, cranial nerve palsies) were also markedly increased by the combined use of these drugs.[1]

Antibacterial antagonism was clearly seen in an 10-week-old infant with *Salmonella enteritidis* meningitis, who was treated with chloramphenicol and **ceftazidime**.[2]

However, in contrast a report claims that antibacterial antagonism was not seen in 65 of 66 patients given chloramphenicol and **benzylpenicillin** for bronchitis or bronchopneumonia.[3] **Ampicillin** with chloramphenicol is more effective than chloramphenicol alone in the treatment of typhoid,[4] and in a study of 700 patients, **procaine benzylpenicillin** with chloramphenicol was shown to be more effective than chloramphenicol alone in the treatment of gonorrhoea (failure rates of 1.8% compared with 8.5%).[5]

(b) Pharmacokinetic interactions

In a study on premature and full-term neonates, infants and small children, it was found that the presence of **penicillin** markedly raised the serum concentrations of chloramphenicol.[6]

Two children, aged 2 and 5, with *Haemophilus influenzae* meningitis, were given chloramphenicol 100 mg/kg/day in four divided doses by infusion over 30 minutes. Within 3 days of starting **rifampicin (rifampin)** 20 mg/kg/day their peak serum chloramphenicol levels were reduced by 86 and 64% respectively, and only returned to the therapeutic range when the chloramphenicol dosage was increased to 125 mg/kg/day.[7]

Two other children, of 5 and 18 months, with *Haemophilus influenzae* infections, are also reported to have shown reductions of 75% and 94% respectively in serum chloramphenicol levels when given **rifampicin** 20 mg/kg daily for 4 days. These reductions occurred despite 20 to 25% increases in the chloramphenicol dosage.[8]

Mechanism

By no means fully understood. Chloramphenicol inhibits bacterial protein synthesis and can change an actively growing bacterial colony into a static one. Thus the effects of a bactericide, such as penicillin, which interferes with cell wall synthesis, are blunted, and the death of the organism occurs more slowly. This would seem to explain the antagonism seen with some organisms.

It is thought that rifampicin, a potent enzyme inducing agent, markedly increases the metabolism of the chloramphenicol by the liver, thereby lowering its serum levels.[7,8]

Importance and management

Proven cases of antibacterial antagonism of chloramphenicol in patients seem to be few in number, and there is insufficient evidence to impose a general prohibition, because, depending on the organism, penicillins and chloramphenicol have been used together with clear advantage.[4,5]

So far only four cases of an interaction between rifampicin and chloramphenicol appear to have been reported. However, the evidence is of good quality and in line with the way rifampicin interacts with other drugs, so this interaction should be taken seriously. There is a risk that serum chloramphenicol levels will become subtherapeutic. The authors of the second report point out that raising the chloramphenicol dosage may possibly expose the patient to a greater risk of bone marrow aplasia. They suggest delaying rifampicin prophylaxis in patients with invasive *Haemophilus influenzae* infections until the end of chloramphenicol treatment.

1. Mathies AW, Leedom JM, Ivler D, Wehrle PF, Portnoy B. Antibiotic antagonism in bacterial meningitis. *Antimicrob Agents Chemother* (1967) 7, 218–24.
2. French GL, Ling TKW, Davies DP, Leung DTY. Antagonism of ceftazidime by chloramphenicol in vitro and in vivo during treatment of gram negative meningitis. *BMJ* (1985) 291, 636–7.
3. Ardalan P. Zur Frage des Antagonismus von Penicillin und Chloramphenicolus klinischer Sicht. *Prax Pneumol* (1969) 23, 772–6.
4. De Ritis R, Giammanco G, Manzillo G. Chloramphenicol combined with ampicillin in treatment of typhoid. *BMJ* (1972) 4, 17–18.
5. Gjessing HC, Ödegaard K. Oral chloramphenicol alone and with intramuscular procaine penicillin in the treatment of gonorrhoea. *Br J Vener Dis* (1967) 43, 133–6.
6. Windorfer A, Pringsheim W. Studies on the concentrations of chloramphenicol in the serum and cerebrospinal fluid of neonates, infants and small children. *Eur J Pediatr* (1977) 124, 129–38.
7. Prober CG. Effect of rifampin on chloramphenicol levels. *N Engl J Med* (1985) 312, 788–9.
8. Kelly HW, Couch RC, Davis RL, Cushing AH, Knott R. Interaction of chloramphenicol and rifampin. *J Pediatr* (1988) 112, 817–20.

Chloramphenicol + Paracetamol (Acetaminophen)

Although there is limited evidence to suggest that paracetamol may affect chloramphenicol pharmacokinetics its validity has been criticised. Evidence of a clinically relevant interaction appears to be lacking.

Clinical evidence, mechanism, importance and management

Two studies report alterations in the pharmacokinetics of chloramphenicol by paracetamol. The first was conducted in 6 adults in intensive care after an observation that the half-life of chloramphenicol was prolonged by paracetamol in children with kwashiorkor. The addition of 100 mg of intravenous paracetamol increased the half-life of chloramphenicol in the adults from 3.25 to 15 hours.[1] However, this study has been criticised because of potential errors in the method used to calculate the half life,[2] the unusual doses and routes of administration used,[2,3] and because the pharmacokinetics of the chloramphenicol with and without paracetamol were calculated at different times after the administration of chloramphenicol.[4] It has also been pointed out that malnutrition (e.g. kwashiorkor) can increase the elimination rate and AUC of chloramphenicol independently of paracetamol.[2]

The second study demonstrated a different interaction, in that the clearance of chloramphenicol was *increased* and the half-life *reduced*.[5] This study has also been criticised as it does not account for the fact that chloramphenicol clearance increases over the duration of a treatment course, which suggests that the changes seen in the pharmacokinetics of chloramphenicol may be independent of the paracetamol.[6] The authors later admit this as a possibility.[7]

Three other studies have failed to confirm the existence of a pharmacokinetic interaction between chloramphenicol and paracetamol.[2-4]

The clinical significance of these reports is unclear, and clinical evidence of toxicity or treatment failure of chloramphenicol appears to be lacking. It would seem prudent to remain aware of the potential for interaction, especially in malnourished patients, but routine monitoring would appear unnecessary without further evidence.

1. Buchanan N, Moodley GP. Interaction between chloramphenicol and paracetamol. *BMJ* (1979) 2, 307–308.
2. Kearns GL, Bocchini JA, Brown RD, Cotter DL, Wilson JT. Absence of a pharmacokinetic interaction between chloramphenicol and acetaminophen in children. *J Pediatr* (1985) 107, 134–9.
3. Rajpurohit R, Krishnaswamy K. Lack of effect of paracetamol on the pharmacokinetics of chloramphenicol in adult human subjects. *Indian J Pharm* (1984) 16, 124–8.
4. Stein CM, Thornhill DP, Neill P, Nyazema NZ. Lack of effect of paracetamol on the pharmacokinetics of chloramphenicol. *Br J Clin Pharmacol* (1989) 27, 262–4.
5. Spika JS, Davis DJ, Martin SR, Beharry K, Rex J, Aranda JV. Interaction between chloramphenicol and acetaminophen. *Arch Dis Child* (1986) 61, 1121–4.
6. Choonara IA. Interaction between chloramphenicol and acetaminophen. *Arch Dis Child* (1987) 62, 319.
7. Spika JS, Aranda JV. Interaction between chloramphenicol and acetaminophen. *Arch Dis Child* (1987) 62, 1087–8.

Chloramphenicol + Phenobarbital

Studies in children show that phenobarbital can markedly reduce serum chloramphenicol levels. There is a single report, in one adult, of markedly increased serum phenobarbital levels caused by chloramphenicol.

Clinical evidence

(a) Decreased serum chloramphenicol concentrations

A study in a group of infants and children (1 month to 12 years) on chloramphenicol 25 mg/kg 6-hourly found that 6 of them, also on phenobarbital, had reduced serum chloramphenicol levels compared with 17 controls. The peak levels were lowered by 34%, from 25.3 to 16.6 micrograms/ml), and the trough levels were lowered by 44%, from 13.4 to 7.5 micrograms/ml).[1] Two children aged 3 and 7 months were treated for *H. influenzae* meningitis with chloramphenicol 100 mg/kg daily, initially intravenously, and later orally. The chloramphenicol levels halved over the first 2 days of treatment, while the children were receiving phenobarbital 10 mg/kg/day to prevent convulsions. One child had serum chloramphenicol levels of only 5 micrograms/ml when the initial doses used were expected to give levels of 15 to 25 micrograms/ml.[2]

Another study confirmed that this interaction occurred in 20 neonates, but no statistically significant effect was confirmed in 40 infants.[3] Decreased chloramphenicol levels have been described in a single case report of a child who was also being treated with phenytoin and phenobarbital. The serum chloramphenicol levels were 35.1 micrograms/ml prior to the anticonvulsants, 19.1 micrograms/ml after 2 days of phenytoin and 13.2 micrograms/ml a month after the addition of phenobarbital.[4] For more information on the interaction of chloramphenicol with phenytoin see 'Phenytoin + Chloramphenicol', p.366.

(b) Increased serum phenobarbital concentrations

A man admitted to hospital on numerous occasions for pulmonary complications associated with cystic fibrosis, had average serum phenobarbital concentrations of 33 micrograms/ml while taking phenobarbital 200 mg daily and chloramphenicol 600 mg six-hourly by mouth. One week after the antibacterial was withdrawn, his serum phenobarbital levels were 24 micrograms/ml even though the phenobarbital dosage was increased from 200 to 300 mg daily.[5]

Mechanism

Phenobarbital is a potent liver enzyme inducing agent, which can increase the metabolism and clearance of chloramphenicol (clearly demonstrated in *rats*[6]), so that its serum levels fall and its effects are reduced. Chloramphenicol has the opposite effect and inhibits the metabolism of the phenobarbital (also demonstrated in *animals*[7]) so that the effects of the barbiturate are increased.

Importance and management

This interaction appears to be established. The documentation is limited but what happened is consistent with the recognised enzyme inducing actions of phenobarbital and the inhibitory actions of chloramphenicol. Concurrent use should be well monitored to ensure that chloramphenicol serum levels are adequate, and that phenobarbital levels do not become too high. Make appropriate dosage adjustments as necessary. Sodium valproate has little or no enzyme-inducing activity and may be a suitable anticonvulsant alternative for phenobarbital in some cases.[8]

1. Krasinski K, Kusmiesz H, Nelson JD. Pharmacologic interactions among chloramphenicol, phenytoin and phenobarbital. *Pediatr Infect Dis* (1982) 1, 232–5.
2. Bloxham RA, Durbin GM, Johnson T, Winterborn MH. Chloramphenicol and phenobarbitone—a drug interaction. *Arch Dis Child* (1979) 54, 76–7.
3. Windorfer A, Pringsheim W. Studies on the concentrations of chloramphenicol in the serum and cerebrospinal fluid of neonates, infants, and small children. *Eur J Pediatr* (1977) 124, 129–38.
4. Powell DA, Nahata MC, Durrell DC, Glazer JP, Hilty MD. Interactions among chloramphenicol, phenytoin, and phenobarbital in a pediatric patient. *J Pediatr* (1981) 98, 1001–1003.
5. Koup JR, Gibaldi M, McNamara P, Hilligoss DM, Colburn WA, Bruck E. Interaction of chloramphenicol with phenytoin and phenobarbital. Case report. *Clin Pharmacol Ther* (1978) 24, 571–5.
6. Bella DD, Ferrari V, Marca G,Bonanomi L. Chloramphenicol metabolism in the phenobarbital-induced rat. Comparison with thiamphenicol. *Biochem Pharmacol* (1968) 17, 2381–90.
7. Adams HR. Prolonged barbiturate anesthesia by chloramphenicol in laboratory animals. *J Am Vet Med Assoc* (1970) 157, 1908–13.
8. Oxley J, Hedges A, Makki KA, Monks A, Richens A. Lack of hepatic enzyme inducing effect of sodium valproate. *Br J Clin Pharmacol* (1979) 8, 189–90.

Clindamycin or Lincomycin + Food or Drinks

The serum levels of lincomycin are markedly reduced (by up to two-thirds) if taken in the presence of food, but clindamycin is not significantly affected. Cyclamate sweeteners can also reduce the absorption of lincomycin.

Clinical evidence

The mean peak serum levels of a single 500-mg oral dose of lincomycin in 10 healthy subjects were about 3 micrograms/ml when taken 4 hours before breakfast, 2 micrograms/ml when taken 1 hour before breakfast, and less than 1 microgram/ml when taken after breakfast. The mean total amounts of lincomycin recovered from the urine were 40.4, 23.8 and 8.9 mg respectively.[1]

Reduced serum lincomycin levels due to the presence of food have been described in other reports,[2,3] but the absorption of clindamycin is not affected.[3,4]

Sodium cyclamate, an artificial sweetener found in diet foods, drinks and some pharmaceuticals, can also markedly reduce the absorption of lincomycin. The AUC of lincomycin 500 mg was reduced by about 75% by 1 Molar equivalent of **sodium cyclamate** [said to be an amount equal to only part of a bottle of diet drink, but exact quantity not stated].[5]

Mechanism

Not understood.

Importance and management

The food interaction with lincomycin is well established and of clinical importance. Lincomycin should not be taken with food or within several hours of eating a meal if adequate serum levels are to be achieved. An alternative is clindamycin, a synthetic derivative of lincomycin, which has the same antibacterial spectrum but the absorption of which is not affected by the presence of food.

1. McCall CE, Steigbigel NH, Finland M. Lincomycin: activity *in vitro* and absorption and excretion in normal young men. *Am J Med Sci* (1967) 254, 144–55.
2. Kaplan K, Chew WH, Weinstein L. Microbiological, pharmacological and clinical studies of lincomycin. *Am J Med Sci* (1965) 250, 137–46.
3. McGehee RF, Smith CB, Wilcox C, Finland M. Comparative studies of antibacterial activity in vitro and absorption and excretion of lincomycin and clinimycin. *Am J Med Sci* (1968) 256, 279–92.
4. Wagner JG, Novak E, Patel NC, Chidester CG, Lummis WL. Absorption, excretion and half-life of clinimycin in normal adult males. *Am J Med Sci* (1968) 256, 25–37.
5. Wagner JG. Aspects of pharmacokinetics and biopharmaceutics in relation to drug activity. *Am J Pharm Sci Support Public Health* (1969) 141, 5–20.

Clindamycin or Lincomycin + Kaolin

Kaolin-containing antidiarrhoeal preparations can markedly reduce the absorption of lincomycin. This can be avoided by giving the lincomycin two hours after the kaolin. The rate but not the extent of clindamycin absorption is altered by kaolin-pectin. However, note that diarrhoea is often an indication that these antibacterials should be withdrawn.

Clinical evidence

About 85 ml of *Kaopectate* (kaolin-pectin) reduced the absorption of lincomycin 500 mg by about 90% in 8 healthy subjects. Giving the *Kaopectate* 2 hours before the antibacterial had little or no effect on its absorption, whereas when *Kaopectate* was given 2 hours after lincomycin, the absorption was reduced by about 50%. The absorption rate of clindamycin is markedly prolonged by kaolin, but the extent of its absorption remains unaffected.[1]

Mechanism

It seems probable that the lincomycin becomes adsorbed onto the kaolin, thereby reducing its bioavailability. The kaolin also coats the lining of the gut and acts as a physical barrier to absorption.[2]

Importance and management

Information seems to be limited to this study, but the lincomycin-kaolin interaction appears to be established and of clinical importance. For good absorption and a good antibacterial response separate their administration as much as possible, ideally giving the kaolin 2 hours before the antibacterial. Clindamycin appears to be a suitable alternative to lincomycin.

However, note that marked diarrhoea is an indication that lincomycin or clindamycin should be stopped immediately. This is because it may be a sign of pseudomembraneous colitis, which can be fatal.

1. Albert KS, DeSante KA, Welch RD, DiSanto AR. Pharmacokinetic evaluation of a drug interaction between kaolin-pectin and clindamycin. *J Pharm Sci* (1978) 67, 1579–82.
2. Wagner JG. Design and data analysis of biopharmaceutical studies in man. *Can J Pharm Sci* (1966) 1, 55–68.

Colistin + Sucralfate

An *in vitro* study with colistin sulphate found that it became markedly and irreversibly bound to sucralfate at the pH values found in the gut. This suggests that efficacy for gut decontamination or gastrointestinal infections might be decreased.

Clinical evidence, mechanism, importance and management

To simulate what might happen in the gut, colistin sulphate 50 mg/l was mixed with sucralfate 500 mg in 40 ml of water at pH 3.5 and allowed to stand for 90 minutes at 25°C. Analysis of the solution showed that the colistin concentration fell rapidly and progressively over 90 minutes to about 40%. When the pH of the mixture was then raised to 6.5 to 7 for 90 minutes, there was no change in the concentration of colistin, suggesting that the interaction was irreversible.[1] The reason for this change is not known, but the suggestion is that sucralfate forms insoluble chelates with colistin.[1]

It is not known how important this interaction is likely to be in practice, but the efficacy of colistin in gut decontamination and gut infections may be decreased. Separating the dosages might not be effective in some postoperative patients because their gastric function may not return to normal for up to 5 days, and some sucralfate might still be present when the next dose is given.[1] More study is needed to find out whether this interaction is clinically important, but in the meanwhile it would seem prudent to monitor concurrent use carefully, being alert for any evidence of reduced effects.

1. Feron B, Adair CG, Gorman SP, McClurg B. Interaction of sucralfate with antibiotics used for selective decontamination of the gastrointestinal tract. *Am J Hosp Pharm* (1993) 50, 2550–3.

Co-trimoxazole + Azithromycin

Azithromycin does not alter the pharmacokinetics of co-trimoxazole.

Clinical evidence, mechanism, importance and management

A study in 12 healthy subjects given **co-trimoxazole** (trimethoprim and sulfamethoxazole) 960 mg daily for 7 days found that a single 1200-mg dose of azithromycin given on day 7 did not alter the pharmacokinetics of either trimethoprim or sulfamethoxazole to a clinically relevant extent.[1]

1. Amsden GW, Foulds G, Thakker K. Pharmacokinetic study of azithromycin with fluconazole and cotrimoxazole (trimethoprim-sulfamethoxazole) in healthy volunteers. *Clin Drug Invest* (2000) 20, 135–42.

Co-trimoxazole + Cimetidine

Cimetidine has no significant effect on the pharmacokinetics of co-trimoxazole.

Clinical evidence, mechanism, importance and management

In a placebo controlled study, 6 healthy subjects were given cimetidine 400 mg every 6 hours for 6 days, with a single 960-mg dose of co-trimoxazole (trimethoprim + sulfamethoxazole) on day 6. Although trimethoprim levels were consistently slightly higher in the presence of cimetidine, they were not significantly different. Cimetidine had no effect on the pharmacokinetics sulphamethoxazole.[1]

1. Rogers HJ, James CA, Morrison PJ and Bradbrook ID. Effect of cimetidine on oral absorption of ampicillin and co-trimoxazole. *J Antimicrob Chemother* (1980) 6, 297–300.

Co-trimoxazole + Kaolin-pectin

Kaolin-pectin can cause a small but probably clinically unimportant reduction in serum trimethoprim levels, and has no effect on sulfamethoxazole pharmacokinetics.

Clinical evidence, mechanism, importance and management

Co-trimoxazole suspension (trimethoprim 160 mg with sulfamethoxazole 800 mg) was given to 8 healthy subjects, with and without 20 ml of kaolin-pectin suspension. The kaolin-pectin reduced the AUC and the maximum serum levels of the trimethoprim by about 12% and 20% respectively. Changes in the sulfamethoxazole pharmacokinetics were not significant.[1] The probable reason for this reduction in AUC is that trimethoprim is adsorbed onto the kaolin-pectin, which reduces the amount available for absorption. However, the reductions are small and unlikely to be clinically relevant.

1. Gupta KC, Desai NK, Satoskar RS, Gupta C, Goswami SN. Effect of pectin and kaolin on bioavailability of co-trimoxazole suspension. *Int J Clin Pharmacol Ther Toxicol* (1987) 25, 320–1.

Co-trimoxazole + Prilocaine/Lidocaine cream

Methaemoglobinaemia developed in a baby treated with co-trimoxazole when *Emla* (prilocaine/lidocaine) cream was applied to his skin.

Clinical evidence, mechanism, importance and management

A 12-week-old child, on co-trimoxazole for 2 months for pyelitis, was treated with 5 g of *Emla* cream (prilocaine 25 mg and lidocaine 25 mg per gram) applied to the back of his hands and the cubital regions. Unfortunately his operation was delayed, and 5 hours later, just before the operation began, his skin was noted to be pale and his lips had a brownish cyanotic colour. This was found to be due to the presence of 28% methaemoglobin (reference range: less than 3%).[1] The authors of the report suggest that the prilocaine together with the sulfamethoxazole (both known to be able to cause methaemoglobin formation) suppressed the activity of two enzymes (NADH-dehydrogenase and NADP-diaphorase), which normally keep blood levels of methaemoglobin to a minimum.[1] A study in 20 children[2] confirmed that *Emla* cream can increase methaemoglobin levels, although levels decreased in 6 of them. The maximum increase was 1.2% (from 0.7 to 1.9%), and the highest value was 2%. Another study showed similar small increases in methaemoglobin levels, and found that these remained elevated after 24 hours. The authors concluded that daily application may lead to accumulation, and a greater risk of toxicity.[3]

The case report appears to be unusual, but it has been suggested that there may be a special risk of methaemoglobinaemia with *Emla* in children with pre-existing anaemia, reduced renal excretion of the metabolites of prilocaine, or the concurrent use of sulphonamides.[3] It would seem prudent to keep *Emla* contact time to a minimum in these patients.

1. Jakobson B, Nilsson A. Methemoglobinemia associated with a prilocaine-lidocaine cream and trimethoprim-sulphamethoxazole. A case report. *Acta Anaesthesiol Scand* (1985) 29, 453–55.
2. Engberg G, Danielson K, Henneberg S, Nilsson A. Plasma concentrations of prilocaine and lidocaine and methaemoglobin formation in infants after epicutaneous application of a 5% lidocaine-prilocaine cream (Emla). *Acta Anaesthesiol Scand* (1987) 31, 624–8.
3. Frayling IM, Addison GM, Chattergee K, Meakin G. Methaemoglobinaemia in children treated with prilocaine-lignocaine cream. *BMJ* (1990) 301, 153–4.

Co-trimoxazole or Trimethoprim + Rifamycins

The pharmacokinetics of trimethoprim and sulfamethoxazole are not significantly affected by rifabutin, and probably not by rifampicin (rifampin). However, a significant reduction in co-trimoxazole levels and a decrease in prophylactic efficacy has been

seen in HIV+ patients. Limited evidence suggests that co-trimoxazole can increase rifampicin serum levels. Trimethoprim does not affect the pharmacokinetics of rifampicin.

Clinical evidence, mechanism, importance and management

(a) Rifabutin

Twelve HIV+ patients taking co-trimoxazole (sulfamethoxazole and trimethoprim) [strength not stated] twice daily for 7 days were additionally given rifabutin 300 mg daily for a further 14 days. The sulfamethoxazole component remained unaffected but the trimethoprim AUC was decreased by 22%. This small reduction is not expected to be clinically significant.[1]

(b) Rifampicin (Rifampin)

No significant pharmacokinetic interaction seems to occur when healthy subjects are given trimethoprim 240 mg daily with rifampicin 900 mg daily (both in divided doses). After 4 to 5 days, less trimethoprim is recovered in the urine as more is metabolised prior to excretion due to the enzyme inducing activity of rifampicin, but this does not appear to be of clinical importance.[2,3] Another study also reports the lack of a significant pharmacokinetic interaction between trimethoprim and rifampicin.[4]

However, a case-control study of the efficacy of co-trimoxazole in preventing toxoplasmosis in HIV+ patients found a link between rifampicin use and co-trimoxazole failure,[5] which prompted the authors to conduct a pharmacokinetic study. When rifampicin 600 mg daily was given to 10 HIV+ patients with co-trimoxazole 960 mg daily, it was found that the AUCs of trimethoprim and sulfamethoxazole were reduced by 56% and 28% respectively. These changes are sufficient to reduce the efficacy of co-trimoxazole treatment.[6] It would therefore seem prudent to consider this interaction when giving rifampicin to HIV+ patients taking co-trimoxazole prophylaxis.

In one study 15 patients with tuberculosis, who had taken rifampicin 450 mg daily for at least 15 days, were given co-trimoxazole (trimethoprim 320 mg and sulfamethoxazole 800 mg 12-hourly) for 5 to 10 days. Rifampicin levels were measured at 5 time points over 6 hours before and during co-trimoxazole treatment. At 4 and 6 hours, rifampicin levels were significantly higher (27 and 56%, respectively) during co-trimoxazole treatment, but peak levels were only increased by about 18%. Concurrent use did not result in any increase in adverse effects over the study period.[7]

1. Lee BL, Lampiris H, Colborn DC, Lewis RC, Narang PK, Sullam P. The effect of rifabutin (RBT) on the pharmacokinetics (PK) of trimethoprim-sulfamethoxazole (TMP-SMX) in HIV-infected patients. *Intersci Conf Antimicrob Agents Chemother* (1995) 35, 7.
2. Buniva G, Palminteri R, Berti M. Kinetics of a rifampicin-trimethoprim combination. *Int J Clin Pharmacol Biopharm* (1979) 17, 256–9.
3. Emmerson AM, Grüneberg RN, Johnson ES. The pharmacokinetics in man of a combination of rifampicin and trimethoprim. *J Antimicrob Chemother* (1978) 4, 523–31.
4. Acocella G, Scotti R. Kinetic studies on the combination rifampicin-trimethoprim in man. *J Antimicrob Chemother* (1976) 2, 271–77.
5. Ribera E, Fernandez-Sola A, Juste C, Rovira A, Romero FJ, Armandas-Gil L, Ruiz I, Ocaña I, Pahissa A. Comparison of high and low doses of trimethoprim-sulfamethoxazole for primary prevention of toxoplasmic encephalitis in human immunodeficiency virus-infected patients. *Clin Infect Dis* (1999) 29, 1461–6.
6. Ribera E, Pou L, Fernandez-Sola A, Campos F, Lopez RM, Ocaña I, Ruiz I, Pahissa A. Rifampin reduces concentrations of trimethoprim and sulfamethoxazole in serum in human immunodeficiency virus infected patients. *Antimicrob Agents Chemother* (2001) 45, 3238–41.
7. Bhatia RS, Uppal R, Malhi R, Behera D, Jindal SK. Drug interaction between rifampicin and co-trimoxazole in patients with tuberculosis. *Hum Exp Toxicol* (1991) 10, 419–21.

Co-trimoxazole + Salbutamol (Albuterol)

Salbutamol reduces the rate but increases the extent of sulfamethoxazole absorption.

Clinical evidence, mechanism, importance and management

Oral salbutamol 4 mg four times daily for 2 weeks had no effect on most of the pharmacokinetics of a single 400-mg oral dose of sulfamethoxazole (in co-trimoxazole) given to 6 healthy subjects. However, the absorption rate constant was reduced by about 40% and the extent of absorption over 72 hours was increased by 22.6%.[1] A possible reason is that salbutamol stimulates the beta-receptors in the gut, causing relaxation, which allows an increased contact time and therefore increased absorption of sulfamethoxazole.[1] The clinical significance of this interaction is unknown, but it seems unlikely to be of importance. No interaction would be expected with inhaled salbutamol.

1. Adebayo GI, Ogundipe TO. Effects of salbutamol on the absorption and disposition of sulphamethoxazole in adult volunteers. *Eur J Drug Metab Pharmacokinet* (1989) 14, 57–60.

Cycloserine + Isoniazid

The adverse CNS effects of cycloserine are increased by isoniazid.

Clinical evidence, mechanism, importance and management

In a report about the concurrent use of cycloserine and isoniazid, both an increase and a decrease in serum cycloserine levels were apparently caused by isoniazid, but the mean level was not significantly changed. Only one out of 11 patients on cycloserine alone developed adverse effects (drowsiness, dizziness, unstable gait), but when isoniazid was added, 9 of the 11 developed these effects.[1] The makers recommend monitoring for these adverse effects and adjusting the doses as necessary to manage them.[2]

1. Mattila MJ, Nieminen E, Tiitinen H. Serum levels, urinary excretion, and side-effects of cycloserine in the presence of isoniazid and p-aminosalicylic acid. *Scand J Respir Dis* (1969) 50, 291–300.
2. Cycloserine. King Pharmaceuticals Ltd. UK Summary of product characteristics, March 2001.

Dapsone + Antacids

The absorption of dapsone is unaltered by an antacid containing hydrated aluminium hydroxide, magnesium hydroxide and simeticone.

Clinical evidence, mechanism, importance and management

A study to see whether changes in gastric pH might affect the absorption of dapsone found that when a single 100-mg dose of dapsone was taken with the second of 11 doses of *Mylanta II* (**hydrated aluminium hydroxide**, **magnesium hydroxide** and **simeticone**), given every hour, the absorption of the dapsone remained unchanged. The mean gastric pH rose from 2.3 before using the antacid, to 4.5 or higher while taking dapsone and antacid.[1] No special precautions would therefore seem to be needed if *Mylanta* is used, nor any other similar antacid. See also 'NRTIs + Dapsone', p.594.

1. Breen GA, Brocavich JM, Etzel JV, Shah V, Schaefer P, Forlenza S. Evaluation of effects of altered gastric pH on absorption of dapsone in healthy volunteers. *Antimicrob Agents Chemother* (1994) 38, 2227–9.

Dapsone + Clarithromycin

Clarithromycin does not alter the metabolism of dapsone.

Clinical evidence, mechanism, importance and management

A study in 12 healthy subjects given single 100-mg doses of dapsone before and after taking clarithromycin 1 g twice daily for 10 days, found that the clearance of dapsone was unchanged. Of equal importance was finding that the AUC of the *N*-hydroxylation metabolite of dapsone, which appears to be responsible for the haematological toxicity (methaemoglobinaemia), was also unchanged.[1]

In another study, 11 HIV+ patients were given dapsone 100 mg daily then clarithromycin 500 mg twice daily for 2 weeks. Clarithromycin had no effect on dapsone clearance or the production of the hydroxylamine metabolite of dapsone.[2]

These results suggest that the cytochrome P450 isoenzyme CYP3A4, which is inhibited by clarithromycin, is not involved in dapsone metabolism.[2]

Clarithromycin would not therefore be expected to alter the toxicity of dapsone, and no special precautions are required during concurrent use.

1. Occhipinti DJ, Choi A, Deyo K, Danziger LH, Fischer JH. Influence of rifampin and clarithromycin on dapsone (D) disposition and methemoglobin concentrations. *Clin Pharmacol Ther* (1995) 57, 163.
2. Winter HR, Trapnell CB, Slattery JT, Jacobson M, Greenspan DL, Hooton TM, Unadkat JD. The effect of clarithromycin, fluconazole, and rifabutin on dapsone hydroxylamine formation in individuals with human immunodeficiency virus infection (AACTG 283). *Clin Pharmacol Ther* (2004) 76, 579–87.

Dapsone + Clofazimine

Dapsone can reduce the anti-inflammatory effects of clofazimine but clofazimine does not affect the pharmacokinetics of dapsone.

Clinical evidence, mechanism, importance and management

Fourteen out of 16 patients with severe recurrent erythema nodosum leprosum (ENL) failed to respond adequately when given dapsone and clofazimine and needed additional therapy with corticosteroids. When the dapsone was stopped the patients responded to clofazimine alone, and in some instances they were controlled on smaller doses.[1] Further evidence of this interaction comes from a laboratory study, which suggests that the actions of clofazimine may be related to its ability to inhibit neutrophil migration (resulting in decreased numbers of neutrophils in areas of inflammation), whereas dapsone can have the opposite effect.[1] Although the information is very limited, it would seem prudent to avoid concurrent use in the treatment of ENL. The authors of this report[1] are at great pains to emphasise that what they describe only relates to the effects of dapsone on the anti-inflammatory effects of clofazimine, and not to the beneficial effects of combined use when treating drug-resistant *Mycobacterium leprae*.

A study in patients taking clofazimine and dapsone[2] and 4 other studies in patients on isoniazid or rifampicin as well as clofazimine and dapsone suggest that clofazimine does not affect the pharmacokinetics of dapsone.[3-6] Conversely, one earlier study[7] found that clofazimine transiently increased the renal excretion of dapsone in 9 of 17 patients with leprosy who had recently discontinued dapsone.

1. Imkamp FMJH, Anderson R, Gatner EMS. Possible incompatibility of dapsone with clofazimine in the treatment of patients with erythema nodosum leprosum. *Lepr Rev* (1982) 53, 148–9.
2. George J, Balakrishnan S, Bhatia VN. Drug interaction during multidrug regimens for treatment of leprosy. *Indian J Med Res* (1988) 87, 151–6.
3. Venkatesan K, Mathur A, Girdhar BK, Bharadwaj VP. The effect of clofazimine on the pharmacokinetics of rifampicin and dapsone in leprosy. *J Antimicrob Chemother* (1986) 18, 715–18.
4. Pieters FAJM, Woonink F, Zuidema J. Influence of once-monthly rifampicin and daily clofazimine on the pharmacokinetics of dapsone in leprosy patients in Nigeria. *Eur J Clin Pharmacol* (1988) 34, 73–6.
5. Venkatesan K, Bharadwaj VP, Ramu R, Desikan KV. Study on drug interactions. *Lepr India* (1980) 52, 229–35.
6. Balakrishnan S, Seshadri PS. Drug interactions— the influence of rifampicin and clofazimine on the urinary excretion of DDS. *Lepr India* (1981) 53, 17–22.
7. Grabosz JAJ, Wheate HW. Effect of clofazimine on the urinary excretion of DDS (Dapsone). *Int J Lepr* (1975) 43, 61–2.

Dapsone + Fluconazole

Fluconazole decreases the production of the toxic metabolite of dapsone, and might therefore reduce the incidence of adverse reactions to dapsone.

Clinical evidence, mechanism, importance and management

Twelve HIV+ patients were given dapsone 100 mg daily for 2 weeks and then in random order either fluconazole 200 mg daily, rifabutin 300 mg daily or fluconazole with rifabutin, each for 2 weeks. Dapsone pharmacokinetics were unaffected by fluconazole. However, fluconazole inhibited the production of the *N*-hydroxylamine metabolite of dapsone (AUC, urinary recovery, and formation clearance reduced by 48%, 53%, and 55% respectively).[1] Fluconazole attenuated the inductive effect of rifabutin on hydroxylamine formation clearance, but only partially attenuated its effect on dapsone, see 'Dapsone + Rifamycins', p.210.

Hydroxylamine is assumed to be responsible for the haematological toxicity of dapsone (methaemoglobinaemia). The findings of this study suggest that the production of this metabolite is mediated via the cytochrome P450 isoenzyme CYP2C9, which fluconazole inhibits.

On the basis of these results, fluconazole would not be expected to alter the efficacy of dapsone, but might reduce its toxicity. Further study is needed to assess this potential.

1. Winter HR, Trapnell CB, Slattery JT, Jacobson M, Greenspan DL, Hooton TM, Unadkat JD. The effect of clarithromycin, fluconazole, and rifabutin on dapsone hydroxylamine formation in individuals with human immunodeficiency virus infection (AACTG 283). *Clin Pharmacol Ther* (2004) 76, 579–87.

Dapsone + H_2-blockers or Omeprazole

Cimetidine raises serum dapsone levels, and may reduce methaemoglobinaemia due to dapsone. Cimetidine, ranitidine and omeprazole do not appear to affect the outcome of dapsone prophylaxis against Pneumocystis pneumonia.

Clinical evidence, mechanism, importance and management

The AUC of a single 100-mg dose of dapsone was increased by 40% in 7 healthy subjects after they took **cimetidine** 400 mg three times daily for 3 days.[1] The probable reason is that the **cimetidine** (a known enzyme inhibitor) inhibits the metabolism of the dapsone by the liver. This might be expected to increase the risk of haematological adverse effects of dapsone by raising its serum levels, but the **cimetidine** also apparently markedly reduces the production of the metabolite dapsone hydroxylamine (the AUC fell by more than half). Dapsone hydroxylamine appears to be responsible for the methaemoglobinaemia and haemolysis that may occur with dapsone treatment.[1] These findings were later confirmed in 6 patients on long-term dapsone 75 to 350 mg daily who were given **cimetidine** 1.2 g daily for 2 weeks. Steady-state serum dapsone levels rose by about 47%, accompanied by a fall in serum methaemoglobin levels from 7.1 to 5.2% (normal range < 2%), in the first week.[2] Similar findings were reported in a further 3-month study in 8 patients.[3] However, a sustained decrease in methaemoglobin was not seen, with levels returning to baseline at week 12, despite the continuance of the **cimetidine**.[3] Another report on a small number of patients, comparing those treated with **cimetidine**, **ranitidine** or **omeprazole** with those not, found no difference in the outcome of dapsone prophylaxis for Pneumocystis pneumonia in HIV+ patients.[4] More study is needed to confirm these findings.

1. Coleman MD, Scott AK, Breckenridge AM, Park BK. The use of cimetidine as a selective inhibitor of dapsone *N*-hydroxylation in man. *Br J Clin Pharmacol* (1990) 30, 761–7.
2. Coleman MD, Rhodes LE, Scott AK, Verbov JL, Friedmann PS, Breckenridge AM, Park BK. The use of cimetidine to reduce dapsone-dependent methaemoglobinaemia in dermatitis herpetiformis patients. *Br J Clin Pharmacol* (1992) 34, 244–9.
3. Rhodes LE, Tingle MD, Park BK, Chu P, Verbov JL, Friedmann PS. Cimetidine improves the therapeutic/toxic ratio of dapsone in patients on chronic dapsone therapy. *Br J Dermatol* (1995) 132, 257–62.
4. Huengsberg M, Castelino S, Sherrard J, O'Farrell N, Bingham J. Does drug interaction cause failure of PCP prophylaxis with dapsone? *Lancet* (1993) 341, 48.

Dapsone + Probenecid

The serum levels of dapsone can be markedly raised by probenecid.

Clinical evidence

Twelve patients with quiescent tuberculoid leprosy were given dapsone 300 mg with probenecid 500 mg, and 5 hours later another 300-mg dose of dapsone. At 4 hours, the dapsone serum levels were raised about 50%. The urinary excretion of dapsone and its metabolites were reduced.[1]

Mechanism

Not fully examined. It seems probable that the probenecid inhibits the renal excretion of dapsone by the kidney.

Importance and management

The documentation is very limited. It is likely that the probenecid will raise the serum levels of dapsone given long-term. The importance of this is uncertain, but the extent of the rise and the evidence that the haematological toxicity of dapsone may be related to dapsone levels[2] suggests that it may well have some clinical importance. This needs confirmation.

1. Goodwin CS, Sparell G. Inhibition of dapsone excretion by probenecid. *Lancet* (1969) ii, 884–5.
2. Ellard GA, Gammon PT, Savin JA, Tan RS-H. Dapsone acetylation in dermatitis herpetiformis. *Br J Dermatol* (1974) 90, 441–4.

Dapsone + Proguanil

No pharmacokinetic interaction appears to occur between dapsone and proguanil, and they have been successfully used together for protection against malaria.

Clinical evidence, mechanism, importance and management

A comparative study in 6 healthy subjects found that proguanil 200 mg daily had no effect on the pharmacokinetics of dapsone 10 mg daily, nor on its principal metabolite, monoacetyldapsone. However, the authors of this report are ultra-cautious because, despite this lack of a pharmacokinetic interaction at these dosages, they say that increased dapsone toxicity cannot be ruled out.[1] Dapsone 25 mg was successfully used with proguanil 200 mg daily for malarial prophylaxis in the Vietnam war,[2] and the same regimen, but with the dapsone dosage every third day was successful as prophylaxis against proguanil-resistant falciparum malaria in Papua New Guinea.[1] Moreover, a different dosage (dapsone 4 or 12.5 mg with proguanil 200 mg daily), was well tolerated over a period of 80 days when used as malaria prophylaxis in Thailand.[3]

1. Edstein MD, Rieckmann KH. Lack of effect of proguanil on the pharmacokinetics of dapsone in healthy volunteers. *Chemotherapy* (1993) 39, 235–41.
2. Black RH. Malaria in the Australian army in South Vietnam. Successful use of a proguanil-dapsone combination for chemoprophylaxis of chloroquine-resistant falciparum malaria. *Med J Aust* (1973) 1, 1265–70.
3. Shanks GD, Edstein MD, Suriyamongkol V, Timsaad S, Webster HK. Malaria prophylaxis using proguanil/dapsone combinations on the Thai-Cambodian border. *Am J Trop Med Hyg* (1992) 46, 643–8.

Dapsone + Rifamycins

Rifampicin increases the excretion of dapsone, lowers its serum levels and increases the risk of toxicity (methaemoglobinaemia). Similarly, rifabutin increases the clearance of dapsone, and may also increase its toxicity.

Clinical evidence

(a) Rifabutin

Twelve HIV+ patients were given dapsone 100 mg daily for 2 weeks and then in random order either rifabutin 300 mg daily, fluconazole 200 mg daily, or fluconazole with rifabutin, each for 2 weeks. Rifabutin alone increased the clearance of dapsone by 67%. When combined with fluconazole, rifabutin increased the clearance of dapsone by 38%, which shows that fluconazole partially attenuated the enzyme-inducing effects of rifabutin. Rifabutin did not affect the AUC of the hydroxylamine metabolite of dapsone, or its excretion, but it increased the formation clearance of dapsone by 92%. Concurrent fluconazole inhibited most of the enzyme-inducing effects of rifabutin on hydroxylamine clearance.[1]

(b) Rifampicin (Rifampin)

A study in 7 patients with leprosy given single doses of dapsone 100 mg and rifampicin 600 mg, alone or together, found that while the pharmacokinetics of rifampicin were not significantly changed by dapsone, the half-life of the dapsone was roughly halved and the AUC was reduced by about 20%.[2] This confirms previous studies in patients given both drugs for several days, which found reduced dapsone serum levels and an increased urinary excretion.[3-5] Another study in 12 healthy subjects given a single 100-mg dose of dapsone before and after taking rifampicin 600 mg daily for 10 days, found that the clearance of the dapsone was considerably increased (from 2.01 to 7.17 litres/hour). Of equal importance was finding that the production of the *N*-hydroxylation metabolite of dapsone, which appears to be responsible for the haematological toxicity (methaemoglobinaemia), was markedly increased. The 24-hour AUC of methaemoglobin was increased by more than 60%.[6]

Mechanism

Rifampicin and rifabutin increase the metabolism and loss of dapsone from the body. Rifampicin also increases the blood levels of the toxic hydroxylamine metabolite of dapsone. Similarly, rifabutin increased the formation of this metabolite, although increases in the AUC were not seen.

Importance and management

The interaction between dapsone and rifampicin is established but of uncertain clinical importance. Concurrent use should be well monitored to confirm that treatment is effective. It may be necessary to raise the dosage of dapsone. It has been pointed out that there is the risk of treatment failures for *Pneumocystis carinii* pneumonia as well as for leprosy.[7] Also be alert for any evidence of methaemoglobinaemia.

Although there is less information, rifabutin appears to interact similarly to rifampicin. When dapsone is given with rifabutin, the dosage of dapsone may need to be increased, but this may increase exposure to the potentially toxic hydroxylamine metabolite.[1]

1. Winter HR, Trapnell CB, Slattery JT, Jacobson M, Greenspan DL, Hooton TM, Unadkat JD. The effect of clarithromycin, fluconazole, and rifabutin on dapsone hydroxylamine formation in individuals with human immunodeficiency virus infection (AACTG 283). *Clin Pharmacol Ther* (2004) 76, 579–87.
2. Krishna DR, Appa Rao AVN, Ramanakar TV, Prabhakar MC. Pharmacokinetic interaction between dapsone and rifampicin in leprosy patients. *Drug Dev Ind Pharm* (1986) 12, 443–59.
3. Balakrishnan S, Seshadri PS. Drug interactions – the influence of rifampicin and clofazimine on the urinary excretion of DDS. *Lepr India* (1981) 53, 17–22.
4. Peters JH, Murray JF, Gordon GR, Gelber RH, Laing ABG, Waters MFR. Effect of rifampin on the disposition of dapsone in Malaysian leprosy patients. *Fedn Proc* (1977) 36, 996.
5. George J, Balakrishnan S, Bhatia VN. Drug interaction during multidrug regimens for treatment of leprosy. *Indian J Med Res* (1988) 87, 151–6.
6. Occhipinti DJ, Choi A, Deyo K, Danziger LH, Fischer JH. Influence of rifampin and clarithromycin on dapsone (D) disposition and methemoglobin concentrations. *Clin Pharmacol Ther* (1995) 57, 163.
7. Jorde UP, Horowitz HW, Wormser GP. Significance of drug interactions with rifampin in *Pneumocystis carinii* pneumonia prophylaxis. *Arch Intern Med* (1992) 152, 2348.

Dapsone + Trimethoprim

The serum levels of both drugs are possibly raised by concurrent use. Both increased efficacy and dapsone toxicity have been seen.

Clinical evidence

Eighteen patients with AIDS, treated for Pneumocystis pneumonia (PCP) and taking dapsone 100 mg daily, were compared with 30 other patients taking dapsone and trimethoprim 20 mg/kg daily. The trimethoprim raised dapsone levels by 40%, from 1.5 to 2.1 micrograms/ml, at 7 days (steady-state). Dapsone toxicity (methaemoglobinaemia) was also increased.[1]

Trimethoprim plasma levels were 48.4% higher in the 30 patients also taking dapsone when compared with another group of 30 patients given co-trimoxazole (trimethoprim with sulfamethoxazole), but the incidence of toxicity was higher in the co-trimoxazole group.[1] However, a later study by the same authors in 8 asymptomatic HIV+ patients given dapsone 100 mg daily and trimethoprim 200 mg every 12 hours found that the steady-state pharmacokinetics of each drug was unaffected by the other, although the single dose pharmacokinetics showed higher serum levels than at steady state for both drugs.[2]

Mechanism

Not understood. Dapsone and trimethoprim appear to have mutually inhibitory effects on clearance.

Importance and management

Information is limited. The difference between the results of the two studies may be because the first was carried out on AIDS patients with PCP and the second on asymptomatic HIV+ patients whose drug metabolism may possibly be different. Concurrent use appears to be an effective form of treatment, but be alert for evidence of increased dapsone toxicity (methaemoglobinaemia).

1. Lee BL, Medina I, Benowitz NL, Jacob P, Wofsy CB, Mills J. Dapsone, trimethoprim, and sulfamethoxazole plasma levels during treatment of pneumocystis pneumonia in patients with acquired immunodeficiency syndrome (AIDS). *Ann Intern Med* (1989) 110, 606–11.
2. Lee BL, Safrin S, Makrides V, Gambertoglio JG. Zidovudine, trimethoprim, and dapsone pharmacokinetic interactions in patients with human immunodeficiency virus infection. *Antimicrob Agents Chemother* (1996) 40, 1231–6.

Dapsone + Ursodeoxycholic acid (Ursodiol)

A single case suggests that the effectiveness of dapsone in the treatment of dermatitis herpetiformis may be reduced by ursodeoxycholic acid.

Clinical evidence, mechanism, importance and management

A 61-year-old man taking dapsone 50 mg daily for dermatitis herpetiformis was started on ursodeoxycholic acid 450 mg twice daily for cholecystitis. Two weeks later the dermatitis herpetiformis worsened and the dose of dapsone was increased to 150 mg daily. However, his condition did not improve, so ursodeoxycholic acid was stopped and as his condition improved the dapsone was reduced to 100 mg, and then 50 mg daily. Two months later ursodeoxycholic acid was restarted and there was again an exacerbation of the dermatitis herpetiformis.[1] The general importance of this isolated report is unknown, but bear this interaction in mind when using both drugs.

1. Stroubou E, Dawn G, Forsyth A. Ursodeoxycholic acid causing exacerbation of dermatitis herpetiformis. *J Am Acad Dermatol* (2001) 45, 319–20.

Ethambutol + Antacids

Aluminium hydroxide and aluminium/magnesium hydroxide can cause a small, and probably clinically unimportant, reduction in the absorption of ethambutol in some patients.

Clinical evidence, mechanism, importance and management

A study in 13 patients with tuberculosis, given a single 50-mg/kg dose of ethambutol, showed that when they were also given three 1.5-g doses of **aluminium hydroxide gel** (at the same time and 15 and 30 minutes later) their peak serum ethambutol levels were delayed and reduced. The average urinary excretion of ethambutol over a 10-hour period was reduced about 15%, but there were marked variations between individual patients. Some showed no interaction, and others showed increased absorption.[1] No interaction was seen in 6 healthy subjects similarly treated.[1] A further study in 14 healthy subjects[2] found that 30 ml of an **aluminium/magnesium hydroxide** antacid decreased the AUC and maximum serum levels of a 25-mg/kg dose of ethambutol by 10% and 29% respectively.[2]

Just why this interaction occurs is not understood, but **aluminium hydroxide** can affect gastric emptying. The reduction in absorption is generally small and variable, and it seems doubtful if it will have a significant effect on the treatment of tuberculosis. However, the authors of the second study suggest avoiding giving antacid at the same time as ethambutol,[2] and the US prescribing information states that **aluminium hydroxide** containing antacids should not be taken until 4 hours after a dose of ethambutol.[3]

1. Mattila MJ, Linnoila M, Seppälä T, Koskinen R. Effect of aluminium hydroxide and glycopyrrhonium on the absorption of ethambutol and alcohol in man. *Br J Clin Pharmacol* (1978) 5, 161–6.
2. Peloquin CA, Bulpitt AE, Jaresko GS, Jelliffe RW, Childs JM, Nix DE. Pharmacokinetics of ethambutol under fasting conditions, with food, and with antacids. *Antimicrob Agents Chemother* (1999) 43, 568–72.
3. Myambutol (Ethambutol). Dura Pharmaceuticals. US Prescribing information, November 2003.

Ethambutol + Food

The pharmacokinetics of ethambutol given with a high-fat breakfast were only slightly different to its pharmacokinetics when it is given in the fasting state.[1] Therefore ethambutol may be given without regard to meals.

1. Peloquin CA, Bulpitt AE, Jaresko GS, Jelliffe RW, Childs JM, Nix DE. Pharmacokinetics of ethambutol under fasting conditions, with food, and with antacids. *Antimicrob Agents Chemother* (1999) 43, 568–72.

Ethambutol + Rifabutin

Rifabutin does not appear to affect the pharmacokinetics of ethambutol.

Clinical evidence, mechanism, importance and management

Ten healthy subjects were given a single 1200-mg dose of ethambutol before and after taking rifabutin 300 mg daily for a week. No clinically relevant changes in the pharmacokinetics of ethambutol were seen. Five of the subjects experienced moderate to severe chills, and one had transient thrombocytopenia.[1] However, these reactions are unlikely to have been due to an interaction. No special precautions would appear to be necessary during concurrent use.

1. Breda M, Benedetti MS, Bani M, Pellizzoni C, Poggesi I, Brianceschi G, Rocchetti M, Dolfi L, Sassella D, Rimoldi R. Effect of rifabutin on ethambutol pharmacokinetics in healthy volunteers. *Pharmacol Res* (1999) 40, 351–6.

Ethionamide + Miscellaneous

A study in 12 healthy subjects found that the bioavailability of a single 500-mg dose of ethionamide was not significantly affected by food, orange juice or antacids when compared to bioavailability under fasting conditions. It was suggested that ethionamide may be given with food if tolerance is a problem.[1]

1. Auclair B, Nix DE, Adam RD, James GT, Peloquin CA. Pharmacokinetics of ethionamide administered under fasting conditions or with orange juice, food, or antacids. *Antimicrob Agents Chemother* (2001) 45, 810–4.

Fosfomycin + Miscellaneous

Cimetidine does not affect the pharmacokinetics of fosfomycin. Metoclopramide reduces fosfomycin bioavailability but the evidence suggests that this probably does not affect the control of urinary tract infections.

Clinical evidence, mechanism, importance and management

Metoclopramide 20 mg given to 9 healthy subjects 30 minutes before fosfomycin 50 mg/kg reduced the peak serum levels of fosfomycin by 42% and reduced the AUC by 27%. The reason seems to be that the **metoclopramide** speeds the transit through the gut, so that less time is available for good absorption. However, despite these reductions the urinary concentrations of fosfomycin remained above the minimum levels required for common urinary pathogens for at least 36 hours after the dose.[1] This suggests that the interaction is unlikely to be clinically important.

Two 400-mg doses of **cimetidine** given to 9 healthy subjects the night before and 30 minutes before fosfomycin 50 mg/kg had almost no effect on the pharmacokinetics of fosfomycin trometamol.

1. Bergan T, Mastropaolo G, Di Mario F, Naccarato R. Pharmacokinetics of fosfomycin and influence of cimetidine and metoclopramide on the bioavailability of fosfomycin trometamol. New Trends in Urinary Tract Infections (eds Neu and Williams) Int Symp Rome 1987, pp 157–66. Published in 1988.

Isoniazid + Aminosalicylic acid

Isoniazid serum levels are raised by aminosalicylic acid.

Clinical evidence, mechanism, importance and management

A study showed that aminosalicylic acid significantly increased the serum level and half-life of isoniazid, due, it is suggested, to the inhibition of isoniazid metabolism by aminosalicylic acid. The effect was most marked among the 'fast' acetylators (see 'Genetic factors', (p.4)) of isoniazid.[1] No precise figures were stated. There seem to be no reports of isoniazid toxicity arising from this interaction, but the makers of isoniazid warn that adverse effects are more likely.[2]

1. Boman G, Borgå O, Hanngren Å, Malmborg A-S, Sjöqvist F. Pharmacokinetic interactions between the tuberculostatics rifampicin, para-aminosalicylic acid and isoniazid. *Acta Pharmacol Toxicol (Copenh)* (1970) 28 (Suppl 1), 15.
2. Isoniazid. Celltech Manufacturing Services Ltd. UK Summary of product characteristics, November 2001.

Isoniazid + Antacids

The absorption of isoniazid from the gut is modestly reduced by aluminium hydroxide, less so by magaldrate, and not by affected by aluminium/magnesium hydroxide tablets or didanosine chewable tablets.

Clinical evidence

Aluminium hydroxide (*Amphojel*) 45 ml was given to 10 patients with tuberculosis at 6, 7 and 8 am, followed immediately by isoniazid and any other medication they were receiving. The serum isoniazid levels at 1 hour were decreased, and peak serum concentrations occurring between 1 and 2 hours after ingestion were reduced by about 16% (or when adjusted for different dosages, by 25%).[1] The effect of **magaldrate (hydrated magnesium aluminate)** was less,[1] and in another well-controlled study **aluminium/magnesium hydroxide** *(Mylanta)* had no effect.[2]

Didanosine chewable tablets contain antacids (aluminium/magnesium hydroxide) in the formulation, but it has been shown that they do not affect the bioavailability of isoniazid.[3]

Mechanism

Aluminium hydroxide delays gastric emptying (in man[4] and in *rats*[5]), causing retention of the isoniazid in the stomach. Since isoniazid is largely absorbed from the intestine, this explains the slight decrease in serum isoniazid concentrations. Aluminium hydroxide also appears to inhibit absorption as well.

Importance and management

Information on this interaction is limited, and it is not established. The clinical importance of the modest reductions in isoniazid levels in one study is uncertain, but likely to be small. However, aluminium/magnesium hydroxide did not interact, and neither did didanosine chewable tablets.

1. Hurwitz A, Schlozman DL. Effects of antacids on gastrointestinal absorption of isoniazid in rat and man. *Am Rev Respir Dis* (1974) 109, 41–7.
2. Peloquin CA, Namdar S, Dodge AA, Nix DE. Pharmacokinetics of isoniazid under fasting conditions, with food, and with antacids. *Int J Tuberc Lung Dis* (1999) 3, 703–710.
3. Gallicano K, Sahai J, Zaror-Behrens G, Pakuts A. Effect of antacids in didanosine tablet on bioavailability of isoniazid. *Antimicrob Agents Chemother* (1994) 38, 894–7.
4. Vats TS, Hurwitz A, Robinson RG, Herrin W. Effects of antacids on gastric emptying in children. *Pediatr Res* (1973) 7, 340.
5. Hava M, Hurwitz A. The relaxing effect of aluminium and lanthanum on rat and human gastric smooth muscle in vitro. *Eur J Pharmacol* (1973) 22, 156–61.

Isoniazid + Corticosteroids

Prednisolone can lower serum isoniazid levels, but this may not be clinically important.

Clinical evidence, mechanism, importance and management

Isoniazid 10 mg/kg daily was given to 26 patients with tuberculosis. The 13 slow acetylators of isoniazid (see 'Genetic factors', (p.4)) showed a 23% fall in plasma isoniazid levels when they were given **prednisolone** 20 mg, while the 13 fast acetylators showed a 38% fall over 8.5 hours. The reasons are not understood but changes in the metabolism, and/or the excretion of the isoniazid by the kidney are possibilities. Despite these changes, the response to treatment was excellent.[1] In another group of 49 patients, both slow and fast acetylators of isoniazid, the additional use of rifampicin 12 mg/kg largely counteracted the isoniazid-lowering effects of the **prednisolone**.[1]

None of these interactions were of clinical importance, but the authors point out that if the dosage of isoniazid had been lower, its effects might have been reduced. Be aware of the possibility of a reduced response during concurrent use, and raise the isoniazid dosage if necessary. There seems to be no information about other corticosteroids.

1. Sarma GR, Kailasam S, Nair NGK, Narayana ASL, Tripathy SP. Effect of prednisolone and rifampin on isoniazid metabolism in slow and rapid inactivators of isoniazid. *Antimicrob Agents Chemother* (1980) 18, 661–6.

Isoniazid + Disulfiram

In most patients, the concurrent use of isoniazid and disulfiram is uneventful, but difficulties in co-ordination, with changes in mental status, behaviour, and drowsiness have been reported in a small number of patients taking disulfiram and isoniazid.

Clinical evidence

Seven patients with tuberculosis who had been taking isoniazid for at least 30 days, without problems, experienced adverse reactions within 2 to 8 days of starting to take disulfiram 500 mg daily. Among the symptoms were dizziness, disorientation, a staggering gait, insomnia, irritability and querulous behaviour, listlessness and lethargy. One patient became hypomanic. Most of them were also taking chlordiazepoxide, and other drugs included aminosalicylic acid, streptomycin and phenobarbital. The adverse reactions decreased or disappeared when the disulfiram was either reduced to 250 or 125 mg daily, or withdrawn. These 7 patients represented less than a third of those who received both drugs.[1] As disulfiram is known to inhibit the metabolism of chlordiazepoxide,[2] another 4 patients were given only isoniazid and disulfiram. Although their reaction was not as severe, all 4 showed drowsiness and depression.[1]

In contrast, another report describes the concurrent use of both drugs, without problems, in 200 patients.[3] Another patient taking disulfiram with isoniazid and rifampicin (rifampin) also did not experience any problems.[4]

Mechanism

Not understood. One idea is that some kind of synergy occurs between the two drugs because both can produce similar adverse effects if given in high doses. The authors of one report[1] speculate that isoniazid and disulfiram together inhibit two of three biochemical pathways concerned with the metabolism of dopamine. This leaves a third pathway open, catalysed by COMT (catechol-*O*-methyl transferase), which produces a number of methylated products of dopamine. These methylated products may possibly have been responsible for the mental and physical reactions seen.

Importance and management

Information about this interaction appears to be limited to the reports cited. Its incidence is uncertain but apparently quite small. Two-thirds of this particular group, and at least 200 other patients showed no interaction. It would seem therefore that concurrent use need not be avoided, but the response should be monitored. If marked changes in mental status occur, or there is unsteady gait, the makers recommend that the disulfiram should be withdrawn.[5]

1. Whittington HG, Grey L. Possible interaction between disulfiram and isoniazid. *Am J Psychiatry* (1969) 125, 1725–9.
2. Antabuse (Disulfiram). Dumex Ltd. UK Summary of product characteristics, August 1999.
3. McNichol RW, Ewing JA, Faiman MD, eds. Disulfiram (Antabuse), a unique medical aid to sobriety: history, pharmacology, research, clinical use. Springfield Ill: Thomas; 1987 p. 47–90.
4. Rothstein E. Rifampin with disulfiram. *JAMA* (1972) 219, 1216.
5. Antabuse (Disulfiram). Odyssey Pharmaceuticals Inc. US Prescribing information, September, 2001.

Isoniazid + Ethambutol

Ethambutol does not appear to affect serum isoniazid levels. However, it seems that the optic neuropathy caused by ethambutol may be increased by isoniazid.

Clinical evidence, mechanism, importance and management

The mean serum levels of a 300-mg dose of isoniazid were not significantly changed in 10 patients with tuberculosis when they were given a single 20-mg/kg dose of ethambutol.[1] The possible effects of concurrent use over a period of time were not studied. However, there is some evidence that the optic neuropathy caused by ethambutol may be increased by isoniazid, and any effects resolve more slowly after the use of isoniazid.[2-5]

1. Singhal KC, Varshney DP, Rathi R, Kishore K, Varshney SC. Serum concentration of isoniazid administered with and without ethambutol in pulmonary tuberculosis patients. *Indian J Med Res* (1986) 83, 360–2.
2. Renard G, Morax PV. Nevrite optique au cours des traitements antituberculeux. *Ann Ocul (Paris)* (1977) 210, 53–61.
3. Karmon G, Savir H, Zevin D, Levi J. Bilateral optic neuropathy due to combined ethambutol and isoniazid treatment. *Ann Ophthalmol* (1979) 11, 1013–17.
4. Garret CR. Optic neuritis in a patient on ethambutol and isoniazid evaluated by visual evoked potentials: Case report. *Mil Med* (1985) 150, 43–6.
5. Jimenez-Lucho VE, del Busto R, Odel J. Isoniazid and ethambutol as a cause of optic neuropathy. *Eur J Respir Dis* (1987) 71, 42–5.

Isoniazid + Fluconazole

Fluconazole does not appear to affect the pharmacokinetics of isoniazid.

Clinical evidence, mechanism, importance and management

A double blind crossover study in 16 healthy subjects (8 'fast' and 8 'slow' acetylators of isoniazid, see 'Genetic factors', (p.4)) found that fluconazole 400 mg daily for a week had no clinically significant effect on the pharmacokinetics of isoniazid.[1] No special precautions would appear necessary during concurrent use.

1. Buss DC, Routledge PA, Hutchings A, Brammer KW, Thorpe JE. The effect of fluconazole on the acetylation of isoniazid. *Hum Exp Toxicol* (1991) 10, 85–6.

Isoniazid + Food

The absorption of isoniazid is reduced by food. See also 'Isoniazid + Food; Cheese or Fish', below, for toxic reactions between isoniazid and specific foods.

Clinical evidence

The mean peak serum levels of isoniazid 10 mg/kg in 9 healthy subjects were delayed and reduced by 79% when isoniazid was given with **breakfast** rather than when fasting. The AUC was reduced by 43%.[1] In another study in 14 healthy subjects given isoniazid with a **full fat breakfast**, the maximum serum levels of isoniazid were decreased by 51%, the absorption was delayed, and the AUC was decreased by 12%.[2] Similar results have been found in another study.[3]

Mechanism

Uncertain. Food delays gastric emptying so that absorption further along the gut is also delayed, but the reduction in absorption is not understood.

Importance and management

Information is limited but the interaction seems to be established. For maximum absorption isoniazid should be taken without food, hence the maker's guidance to take it at least 30 minutes before or 2 hours after food.[4]

1. Melander A, Danielson K, Hanson A, Jansson L, Rerup C, Scherstén B, Thulin T, Wåhlin E. Reduction of isoniazid bioavailability in normal men by concomitant intake of food. *Acta Med Scand* (1976) 200, 93–7.
2. Peloquin CA, Namdar S, Dodge AA, Nix DE. Pharmacokinetics of isoniazid under fasting conditions, with food, and with antacids. *Int J Tuberc Lung Dis* (1999) 3, 703–710.
3. Männisto P, Mäntylä R, Klinge R, Nykänen S, Koponen A, Lamminsivu U. Influence of various diets on the bioavailability of isoniazid. *J Antimicrob Chemother* (1982) 10, 427–34.
4. Isoniazid. Celltech Manufacturing Services Ltd. UK Summary of product characteristics, November 2001.

Isoniazid + Food; Cheese or Fish

Patients taking isoniazid who eat some foods, particularly fish from the scombroid family (tuna, mackerel, salmon) that are not fresh, may experience an exaggerated histamine poisoning reaction. Cheese has also been implicated in this reaction, but the adverse effects may be due to the weak MAOI effects of isoniazid rather than histamine poisoning.

Clinical evidence

Three months after starting to take isoniazid 300 mg daily, a woman experienced a series of unpleasant reactions 10 to 30 minutes after eating cheese. These reactions included chills, headache (sometimes severe), itching of the face and scalp, slight diarrhoea, flushing of the face (and on one occasion the whole body), variable and mild tachycardia and a bursting sensation in the head. Blood pressure measurements showed only a modest rise (from her normal level of 95/65 to 110/80 mmHg). No physical or biochemical abnormalities were found.[1]

Headache, dizziness, blurred vision, tachycardia, flushing and itching of the skin, redness of the eyes, burning sensation of the body, difficulty in breathing, abdominal colic, diarrhoea, vomiting, sweating and wheezing have all been described in other patients on isoniazid after eating cheese.[2-6] Certain tropical fish, including **tuna** (**skipjack** or **bonito** — ***Katsuwanus pelamis***),[7-11] ***Sardinella (Amblygaster) sirm***,[12] ***Rastrigella kanagurta***[13] and others[14] are also implicated. There are a few hundred cases of this reaction on record.

Mechanism

The reaction appears to be an exaggeration of the histamine poisoning that can occur after eating some foods, such as members of the scombroid family of fish (tuna, mackerel, salmon, etc), if they are not fresh and adequately refrigerated. These fish (and some cheeses) have a high histidine content and under poor storage circumstances the histine is decarboxylated by bacteria to produce unusually large amounts of histamine. Normally this is inactivated by histaminase in the body, but isoniazid is a potent inhibitor of this enzyme, which means that the histamine is absorbed largely unchanged and histamine poisoning develops.[15] Histamine survives all but very prolonged cooking. Tuna fish can contain 180 to 500 mg histamine per 100 g, other types of fish may contain as little as 0.5 to 7.5 mg.[10]

Alternatively, it has been suggested that the cases of reactions to cheese are caused by tyramine content and the weak MAOI properties of isoniazid. See 'MAOIs + Tyramine-rich foods', p.876 for more details of the mechanism of this interaction.

Importance and management

An established interaction of clinical importance. With the exception of one patient who appeared to have had a cerebrovascular accident,[9] the reactions experienced by the others were unpleasant and alarming but usually not serious nor life-threatening. They required little or no treatment, although 'scombroid poisoning' in the absence of isoniazid is sometimes more serious. Two reports say that treatment with antihistamines can be effective.[10,14] Isoniazid has been in use since 1956 and there is little need to now introduce any general dietary restrictions, but if any of these reactions is experienced, examine the patient's diet and advise the avoidance of any probable offending foodstuffs. Very mature cheese and fish of the scombroid family (tuna, mackerel, salmon and other varieties of dark meat fish) that are not fresh are to be treated with suspicion, but there is no way that the likely histamine or tyramine content of food can be assessed without undertaking a detailed analysis. See 'Table 30.3', (p.877) and 'Table 30.4', (p.877) for a list of tyramine rich foods and drinks.

1. Smith CK, Durack DT. Isoniazid and reaction to cheese. *Ann Intern Med* (1978) 88, 520–1.
2. Uragoda CG, Lodha SC. Histamine intoxication in a tuberculous patient after ingestion of cheese. *Tubercle* (1979) 60, 59–61.
3. Lejonc JL, Gusmini D, Brochard P. Isoniazid and reaction to cheese. *Ann Intern Med* (1979) 91, 793.
4. Hauser MJ, Baier H. Interactions of isoniazid with foods. *Drug Intell Clin Pharm* (1982) 16, 617–18.
5. Toutoungi M, Carroll R, Dick P. Isoniazide (INH) and tyramine-rich food. *Chest* (1986) 89 (Suppl 6), 540S.
6. Carvalho ACC, Manfrin M, Gore RP, Capone S, Scalvini A, Armellini A, Giovine T, Carosi G, Matteelli A. Reaction to cheese during TB treatment. *Thorax* (2004) 59, 635.
7. Uragoda CG, Kottegoda SR. Adverse reactions to isoniazid on ingestion of fish with a high histamine content. *Tubercle* (1977) 58, 83–9.
8. Uragoda CG. Histamine poisoning in tuberculous patients after ingestion of tuna fish. *Am Rev Respir Dis* (1980) 121, 157–9.
9. Senanayake N, Vyravanathan S, Kanagasuriyam S. Cerebrovascular accident after a 'skipjack' reaction in a patient taking isoniazid. *BMJ* (1978) 2, 1127–8.
10. Senanayake N, Vyravanathan S. Histamine reactions due to ingestion of tuna fish (*Thunnus argentivittatus*) in patients on antituberculosis therapy. *Toxicon* (1981) 19, 184–5.
11. Morinaga S, Kawasaki A, Hirata H, Suzuki S, Mizushima Y. Histamine poisoning after ingestion of spoiled raw tuna in a patient taking isoniazid. *Intern Med* (1997) 36, 198–200.
12. Uragoda CG. Histamine poisoning in tuberculous patients on ingestion of tropical fish. *J Trop Med Hyg* (1978) 81, 243–5.
13. Uragoda CG. Histamine intoxication with isoniazid and a species of fish. *Ceylon Med J* (1978) 23, 109–10.
14. Diao Y *et al*. Histamine like reaction in tuberculosis patients taking fishes containing much of histamine under treatment with isoniazid in 277 cases. *Zhonghua Jie He He Hu Xi Xi Ji Bing Za Zhi* (1986) 9, 267–9, 317–18.
15. O'Sullivan TL. Drug-food interaction with isoniazid resembling anaphylaxis. *Ann Pharmacother* (1997) 31, 928–9.

Isoniazid + H_2-blockers

Pharmacokinetic evidence suggests that neither cimetidine nor ranitidine interact with isoniazid.

Clinical evidence, mechanism, importance and management

Cimetidine 400 mg or **ranitidine** 300 mg, three times a day, for three days had no effect on the pharmacokinetics of a single 10-mg/kg dose of isoniazid in 13 healthy subjects. Neither the absorption nor the metabolism of isoniazid were changed.[1] No special precautions would appear to be necessary on concurrent use.

1. Paulsen O, Höglund P, Nilsson L-G, Gredeby H. No interaction between H_2 blockers and isoniazid. *Eur J Respir Dis* (1986) 68, 286–90.

Isoniazid + Laxatives

Sodium sulfate and castor oil used as laxatives can cause a modest but probably clinically unimportant reduction in isoniazid absorption.

Clinical evidence, mechanism, importance and management

In an experimental study of the possible effects of laxatives on isoniazid absorption, healthy subjects were given 10 to 20 g of oral **sodium sulfate** and 20 g of **castor oil** (doses sufficient to provoke diarrhoea). Absorption, measured by the amount of isoniazid excreted in the urine, was decreased by 50% with **castor oil** and 41% with **sodium sulfate** at 4 hours. However, serum levels of isoniazid were relatively unchanged. The overall picture was that while these laxatives can alter the pattern of absorption, they do not seriously impair the total amount of drug absorbed.[1]

1. Mattila MJ, Takki S, Jussila J. Effect of sodium sulphate and castor oil on drug absorption from the human intestine. *Ann Clin Res* (1974) 6, 19–24.

Isoniazid + Pethidine (Meperidine)

An isolated case report describes hypotension and lethargy in a patient after he was given isoniazid and pethidine.

Clinical evidence, mechanism, importance and management

A patient became lethargic and his blood pressure fell from 124/68 to 84/50 mmHg within 20 minutes of being given pethidine 75 mg intramuscularly. An hour before, he had been given isoniazid. There was no evidence of fever or cardiac arrhythmias, and his serum electrolytes, glucose levels and blood gases were normal. His blood pressure returned to normal over the next 3 hours. He had previously had both pethidine and isoniazid separately without incident. He was subsequently treated with intravenous morphine sulphate, 4 mg every 2 to 4 hours uneventfully.[1] The authors of the report attribute this reaction to the MAO-inhibitory properties of the isoniazid and equate it with the severe and potentially fatal 'MAOI-pethidine interaction', (p.869), but in reality this reaction was mild and lacked many of the characteristics of the more serious reaction. Moreover, isoniazid possesses only mild MAO-inhibitory properties and does not normally interact to the same extent as the potent antidepressant and antihypertensive MAOIs.

There is too little evidence to advise against concurrent use, but bear this interaction in mind in the case of an unexpected response to treatment.

1. Gannon R, Pearsall W, Rowley R. Isoniazid, meperidine, and hypotension. *Ann Intern Med* (1983) 99, 415.

Isoniazid + Propranolol

Propranolol causes a small reduction in the clearance of isoniazid, which seems unlikely to be of much practical importance.

Clinical evidence, mechanism, importance and management

The clearance of a single 600-mg intravenous dose of isoniazid was reduced by 21%, from 16.4 to 13 l/h, in 6 healthy subjects after they took propranolol 40 mg three times daily for 3 days.[1] It is suggested that propranolol reduces the clearance of isoniazid by inhibiting its metabolism (acetylation) by the liver.[1] However, as the increase in isoniazid levels is likely to be only modest this interaction is probably of little clinical importance.

1. Santoso B. Impairment of isoniazid clearance by propranolol. *Int J Clin Pharmacol Ther Toxicol* (1985) 23, 134–6.

Isoniazid + Rifamycins

The concurrent use of a rifamycin and isoniazid is common and therapeutically valuable, but there is evidence that the incidence of hepatotoxicity may be increased, particularly in slow acetylators of isoniazid. No pharmacokinetic interaction occurs between rifampicin and isoniazid, and rifabutin does not alter the pharmacokinetics of isoniazid.

Clinical evidence, mechanism, importance and management

(a) Rifabutin

Rifabutin 300 mg given daily for 7 days to 6 healthy subjects had no significant effect on the pharmacokinetics of a single 300-mg dose of isoniazid or its metabolite acetylisoniazid. Two of the 6 subjects were rapid acetylators of isoniazid[1] (see 'Genetic factors', (p.4)).

Although both drugs have been effectively used together in the treatment of tuberculosis, it is not clear whether concurrent use increases the incidence of hepatotoxicity, as occurs with isoniazid and rifampicin (see below). However, as regular monitoring of liver function is required for both isoniazid and rifabutin, no additional monitoring seems necessary on concurrent use. The maker of rifabutin notes that haematological reactions of rifabutin could be increased by isoniazid, but, again, as regular monitoring of white blood cell and platelet counts is advised,[2] no additional monitoring seems necessary.

(b) Rifampicin (Rifampin)

Studies have shown that the serum levels and half lives of both drugs are not significantly affected by concurrent use,[3-6] even in those with hepatic impairment.[6] There was also no difference between rapid and slow acetylators of isoniazid,[4] (see 'Genetic factors', (p.4)). However, there is some evidence that the incidence and severity of hepatotoxicity rises if both drugs are given together.[7] Reports from India suggest that the incidence can be as high as 8 to 10%, while much lower figures of 2 to 3% are reported in the US.[8] There is certainly one case report that appears to prove that hepatotoxicity can arise rapidly from the use of both drugs. The patient tolerated both drugs individually, but hepatotoxicity reappeared on concurrent use.[9] Increased isoniazid hepatotoxicity caused by rifampicin has been demonstrated *in vitro*.[10]

The reasons for the hepatotoxicity are not fully understood but rifampicin or isoniazid alone can cause liver damage by their own toxic action. One suggestion is that the rifampicin alters the metabolism of isoniazid, resulting in the formation of hydrazine, which is a proven hepatotoxic agent.[8,9,11] Higher plasma levels of hydrazine are said to occur in slow acetylators of isoniazid,[8] but one study failed to confirm that this is so.[12] There has certainly been one fatality caused by this combination.[13] The makers of rifampicin advise that caution is particularly needed in patients with impaired liver function, the elderly, malnourished patients, and children under two years of age. After baseline LFTs, further tests are only needed if fever, vomiting, or jaundice occur, or if the patient deteriorates.[14] However, the makers of isoniazid suggest that liver function tests should be reviewed regularly in patients on combined treatment.[15]

1. Breda M, Painezzola E, Benedetti MS, Efthymiopoulos C, Carpentieri M, Sassella D, Rimoldi R. A study of the effects of rifabutin on isoniazid pharmacokinetics and metabolism in healthy volunteers. *Drug Metabol Drug Interact* (1993) 10, 323–40.
2. Mycobutin (Rifabutin). Pharmacia Ltd. UK Summary of product characteristics, January 2003.
3. Boman G. Serum concentration and half-life of rifampicin after simultaneous oral administration of aminosalicylic acid or isoniazid. *Eur J Clin Pharmacol* (1974) 7, 217–25.
4. Sarma GR, Kailasam S, Nair NGK, Narayana ASL, Tripathy SP. Effect of prednisolone and rifampin on isoniazid metabolism in slow and rapid inactivators of isoniazid. *Antimicrob Agents Chemother* (1980) 18, 661–6.
5. Venho VMK, Koskinen R. The effect of pyrazinamide, rifampicin and cycloserine on the blood levels and urinary excretion of isoniazid. *Ann Clin Res* (1971) 3, 277–80.
6. Acocella G, Bonollo L, Garimoldi M, Mainardi M, Tenconi LT. Kinetics of rifampicin and isoniazid administered alone and in combination to normal subjects and patients with liver disease. *Gut* (1972) 13, 47–53.
7. Steele MA, Burk RF, DesPrez RM. Toxic hepatitis with isoniazid and rifampin. A meta-analysis. *Chest* (1991) 99, 465–71.
8. Gangadharam PRJ. Isoniazid, rifampin and hepatotoxicity. *Am Rev Respir Dis* (1986) 133, 963–5.
9. Askgaard DS, Wilcke T, Døssing M. Hepatotoxicity caused by the combined action of isoniazid and rifampicin. *Thorax* (1995) 50, 213–14.
10. Nicod L, Viollon C, Regnier A, Jacqueson A, Richert L. Rifampicin and isoniazid increase acetaminophen and isoniazid cytotoxicity in human HepG2 hepatoma cells. *Hum Exp Toxicol* (1997) 16(1), 28–34.
11. Pessayre D, Bentata M, Degott C, Nouel O, Miguet J-P, Rueff B, Benhamou J-P. Isoniazid-rifampin fulminant hepatitis. A possible consequence of the enhancement of isoniazid hepatotoxicity by enzyme induction. *Gastroenterology* (1977) 72, 284–9.
12. Jenner PJ, Ellard GA. Isoniazid-related hepatotoxicity: a study of the effect of rifampicin administration on the metabolism of acetylisoniazid in man. *Tubercle* (1989) 70, 93–101.

13. Lenders JWM, Bartelink AKM, van Herwaarden CLA, van Haelst UJGM, van Tongeren JHM. Dodelijke levercelnecrose na kort durende toediening van isoniazide en rifampicine aan een patiënt die reeds werd behandeld met anti-epileptica. *Ned Tijdschr Geneeskd* (1983) 127, 420–3.
14. Rifadin (Rifampicin), Aventis Pharma Ltd. UK Summary of product characteristics, February 2000.
15. Isoniazid. Celltech Manufacturing Services Ltd. UK Summary of product characteristics, November 2001.

Isoniazid + SSRIs or related antidepressants

No important interaction appears to occur between isoniazid and the SSRIs or nefazodone. Adverse reactions have been seen during concurrent use but they are thought unlikely to have been due to an interaction.

Clinical evidence

Two HIV+ patients on **fluoxetine** 20 mg daily were also started on isoniazid. One of them tolerated the use of both drugs, but the other developed vomiting and diarrhoea, and after 10 days the **fluoxetine** was stopped. Another HIV+ patient on isoniazid, who had previously suffered nausea and vomiting 2 days after his dosage of **moclobemide** was increased, later tolerated the use of isoniazid and **fluoxetine** without adverse effects. The authors of this report were doubtful whether any of the adverse effects seen could be attributed to an interaction between isoniazid and moclobemide.[1]

A woman who had been hospitalised for serious depression was started on **nefazodone** 300 mg daily. A few days later she began to also take isoniazid 300 mg daily, and was later discharged on an increased **nefazodone** dose of 400 mg daily. She was reported to have had no problems while taking both drugs over a 5 month period.[2]

A woman with tuberculosis taking isoniazid 300 mg daily presented with depression and was additionally given **sertraline** 50 mg daily, later raised to 150 mg daily, without problems. She responded well and was reported to have taken both drugs together for 8 months without problems.[2]

Mechanism, importance and management

Direct information about the concurrent use of isoniazid and SSRIs seems to be limited, but the reports cited here and the absence of any other reports of adverse reactions would suggest that the combination of isoniazid and these SSRIs is normally without problems.

In theory isoniazid could interact with the SSRIs[3] because it has some weak MAO inhibitory activity. However, isoniazid rarely interacts like the MAOIs. This is because isoniazid seems to lack activity on mitochondrial MAO even though it has activity on plasma MAO. Therefore no adverse MAOI/SSRI interaction would usually be expected.

1. Judd FK, Mijch AM, Cockram A, Norman TR. Isoniazid and antidepressants: is there cause for concern? *Int Clin Psychopharmacol* (1994) 9, 123–5.
2. Malek-Ahmadi P, Chavez M, Contreras SA. Coadministration of isoniazid and antidepressant drugs. *J Clin Psychiatry* (1996) 57, 550.
3. Evans ME, Kortas KJ. Potential interaction between isoniazid and selective serotonin-reuptake inhibitors. *Am J Health-Syst Pharm* (1995) 52, 2135–6.

Linezolid + Antidepressants

The serotonin syndrome has been reported with linezolid and the SSRIs or venlafaxine. The serotonin syndrome is also predicted to occur when linezolid is used with tricyclic antidepressants.

Clinical evidence

(a) SSRIs

In an analysis of phase III studies, changes in vital signs did not differ between patients given linezolid and comparator drugs (i.e. antibiotics) when either were used with drugs that can interact with MAOIs, including unnamed SSRIs.[1,2] One patient on **fluoxetine** had a transient episode of asymptomatic hypertension after one dose of linezolid, but since this patient had no other symptoms of serotonin syndrome, it was not considered an interaction.[2] However, a case report describes an 85-year-old woman taking **citalopram** who developed tremor, confusion, dysarthria, hyperreflexia, agitation and restlessness after linezolid was started. **Citalopram** was stopped and the symptoms resolved over 72 hours.[3] There are several other case reports of this interaction between linezolid and SSRIs[4-7] including **citalopram**,[4,5] **sertraline**[5,6] and **paroxetine**.[7]

(b) Tricyclics

In an analysis of phase III studies, changes in vital signs did not differ between patients given linezolid and comparator drugs (i.e. antibiotics) when either were used with drugs that can interact with MAOIs including unnamed cyclic antidepressants.[1,2]

(c) Venlafaxine

An 85-year-old man taking venlafaxine 150 mg daily was started on ciprofloxacin, rifampicin and linezolid 600 mg twice daily for a hip prosthesis infection. After 20 days he was found to be confused and disorientated, and four days later he was also drowsy, and suffering myoclonic jerks. Linezolid and venlafaxine were stopped and the symptoms resolved over 2 days.[8]

Mechanism

Not fully understood. Linezolid is a weak MAOI inhibitor, and serotonin syndrome with MAOI inhibitors and 'SSRIs', (p.984), 'tricyclics', (p.873) and 'venlafaxine', (p.1007) is well described.

Importance and management

Information on the reaction between linezolid and the SSRIs or venlafaxine appears to be limited, but what is known suggests that the interaction is probably rare. The makers of linezolid say that patients on SSRIs and tricyclic antidepressants should have their blood pressure monitored and be closely observed if given linezolid. They say that if this is not possible, concurrent use should be avoided.[9] If linezolid is used with a drug with serotonergic actions it would seem prudent to monitor for symptoms of the serotonin syndrome, which may take several weeks to manifest. See 'The serotonin syndrome', (p.9).

1. Hartman CS, Leach TS, Todd WM, Hafkin B. Lack of drug-interaction with combination of linezolid and monoamine oxidase inhibitor-interacting medications. *Pharmacotherapy* (2000) 20, 1230.
2. Rubinstein E, Isturiz R, Standiford HC, Smith LG, Oliphant TH, Cammarata S, Hafkin B, Le V, Remington J. *Antimicrob Agents Chemother* (2003) 47, 1824–31.
3. Tahir N. Serotonin syndrome as a consequence of drug-resistant infections: an interaction between linezolid and citalopram. *J Am Med Dir Assoc* (2004) 5, 111–13.
4. Bernard L, Stern R, Lew D, Hoffmeyer P. Serotonin syndrome after concomitant treatment with linezolid and citalopram. *Clin Infect Dis* (2003) 36, 1197.
5. Hachem RY, Hicks K, Huen A, Raad I. Myelosuppression and serotonin syndrome associated with concurrent use of linezolid and selective serotonin reuptake inhibitors in bone marrow transplant recipients. *Clin Infect Dis* (2003) 37, 37: e8–e11.
6. Lavery S, Ravi H, McDaniel WW, Pushkin YR. Linezolid and serotonin syndrome. *Psychosomatics* (2001) 42, 432–4.
7. Wigen CL, Goetz MB. Serotonin syndrome and linezolid. *Clin Infect Dis* (2002) 34, 1651–2.
8. Jones SL, Athan E, O'Brien D. Serotonin syndrome due to co-administration of linezolid and venlafaxine. *J Antimicrob Chemother* (2004) 54, 289–90.
9. Zyvox (Linezolid). Pharmacia Ltd. UK Summary of product characteristics, November 2004.

Linezolid + Aztreonam

The pharmacokinetics of intravenous aztreonam 1000 mg and intravenous linezolid 375 mg were not affected when they were given together in a single-dose study in healthy subjects. Therefore dose alterations are not needed on concurrent use.[1]

1. Sisson TL, Jungbluth GL, Hopkins NK. A pharmacokinetic evaluation of concomitant administration of linezolid and aztreonam. *J Clin Pharmacol* (1999) 39, 1277–82.

Linezolid + Dextromethorphan

There is no important pharmacokinetic interaction between linezolid and dextromethorphan but one case of concurrent use resulted in the serotonin syndrome.

Clinical evidence, mechanism, importance and management

In a study in 14 healthy subjects, two 20-mg doses of dextromethorphan given 4 hours apart, before and during the use of linezolid 600 mg every 12 hours, had no effect on linezolid pharmacokinetics. The AUC and maximum level of the dextromethorphan metabolite, dextrorphan was decreased by 30%, but this was not considered sufficient to warrant any dosing alterations. There was no evidence of the serotonin syndrome, as measured by changes in body temperature, alertness and mental performance.[1] However, the makers say that there is one case where the concurrent use of linezolid and dextromethorphan resulted in the serotonin syndrome.[2] Linezolid has mild reversible MAOI activity, and the serotonin syndrome has been described when dextromethorphan was taken by patients also taking antidepressant MAOIs, see 'MAOIs + Dextromethorphan', p.865. If concurrent use of linezolid and dextromethorphan is considered necessary, it would therefore be prudent to monitor for 'symptoms of the serotonin syndrome', (p.9).

1. Hendershot PE, Antal EJ, Welshman IR, Batts DH, Hopkins NK. Linezolid: pharmacokinetic and pharmacodynamic evaluation of coadministration with pseudoephedrine HCl, phenylpropanolamine HCl, and dextromethorphan HBr. *J Clin Pharmacol* (2001) 41, 563–72.
2. Zyvox (Linezolid). Pharmacia Ltd. UK Summary of product characteristics, November 2004.

Linezolid + Sympathomimetics

Because of its weak MAO-inhibitory properties, the makers of linezolid caution its use with directly and indirectly-acting sympathomimetics (such as adrenergic bronchodilators, phenylpropanolamine, pseudoephedrine, adrenaline (epinephrine), noradrenaline (norepinephrine), dopamine and dobutamine). Hypertensive effects were additive in one study of linezolid with phenylpropanolamine or pseudoephedrine.

Clinical evidence

In a placebo controlled study, 14 healthy patients were given two 60-mg doses of **pseudoephedrine** or two 25-mg doses of **phenylpropanolamine** 4 hours apart, with and without linezolid. The mean maximum blood pressure rise was 11 mmHg with placebo, 15 mmHg with linezolid and placebo, 18 mmHg with **pseudoephedrine** alone and 14 mmHg with **phenylpropanolamine** alone. When the subjects were given linezolid plus **pseudoephedrine** the rise was 32 mmHg, which was similar to the 38 mmHg rise seen with linezolid plus **phenylpropanolamine**. However, these rises were transient, resolving in about 2 hours. No effects were seen on linezolid pharmacokinetics.[1]

Mechanism

Linezolid acts as a weak MAO-inhibitor, which allows the accumulation of some noradrenaline at adrenergic nerve endings associated with arterial blood vessels. Pseudoephedrine and phenylpropanolamine, both indirectly-acting sympathomimetics, can release these above-normal amounts of noradrenaline resulting in blood vessel constriction and a rise in blood pressure.

Importance and management

The makers caution the use of directly and indirectly acting sympathomimetics (including adrenergic bronchodilators, pseudoephedrine, phenylpropanolamine, adrenaline (epinephrine), noradrenaline (norepinephrine), dopamine, dobutamine) with linezolid unless there are facilities available for close observation of the patient and monitoring of blood pressure. Some indirectly-acting sympathomimetics occur in cough and cold remedies, which can be bought without prescription. To keep in line with the makers caution, patients should be told to avoid these preparations. However, it should be said that the evidence available indicates that blood pressure rises are unlikely to be of the hypertensive crisis proportions seen with the antidepressant MAOIs. Consider also 'MAOIs + Sympathomimetics; Indirectly-acting', p.872.

1. Hendershot PE, Antal EJ, Welshman IR, Batts DH, Hopkins NK. Linezolid: pharmacokinetic and pharmacodynamic evaluation of coadministration with pseudoephedrine HCl, phenylpropanolamine HCl, and dextromethorphan HBr. *J Clin Pharmacol* (2001) 41, 563–72.

Loracarbef + Probenecid

Probenecid increases the half-life of loracarbef by about 50% but the clinical importance of this is unknown.[1]

1. Force RW, Nahata MC. Loracarbef: a new orally administered carbacephem antibiotic. *Ann Pharmacother* (1993) 27, 321–9.

Macrolides + Antacids

Aluminium/magnesium hydroxide antacids may reduce the peak levels of azithromycin, and administration should be separated. *Mylanta* can prolong the absorption of erythromycin, but this is unlikely to be clinically important. Aluminium/magnesium hydroxide antacids do not appear to significantly alter the pharmacokinetics of clarithromycin, roxithromycin or telithromycin.

Clinical evidence, mechanism, importance and management

The peak serum levels, but not the total absorption, of **azithromycin** was reduced in 10 healthy subjects by 30 ml *Maalox* (**aluminium/magnesium hydroxide**).[1] It is suggested therefore that **azithromycin** should not be given at the same time as antacids, but should be taken at least 1 hour before or 2 hours after.[2,3]

Mylanta (**aluminium/magnesium hydroxide**, **dimeticone**) 30 ml given to 8 healthy subjects had no significant effect on the AUC, peak serum concentration, or time to peak serum concentration of **erythromycin stearate** 500 mg, but the mean elimination rate constant was more than doubled. It was suggested that the effect on elimination may be due to a possible prolonging of absorption, although the reason for this is unclear.[4] The clinical relevance of this is uncertain, but likely to be small.

Aluminium/magnesium hydroxide antacids are reported not to affect the pharmacokinetics of **clarithromycin**,[5] **roxithromycin**,[6] or **telithromycin**.[7,8]

1. Foulds G, Hilligoss DM, Henry EB, Gerber N. The effects of an antacid or cimetidine on the serum concentrations of azithromycin. *J Clin Pharmacol* (1991) 31, 164–7.
2. Hopkins S. Clinical toleration and safety of azithromycin. *Am J Med* (1991) 91 (Suppl 3A), 40S–45S.
3. Zithromax (Azithromycin). Pfizer Ltd. UK Summary of product characteristics, July 2004.
4. Yamreudeewong W, Scavone JM, Paone RP, Lewis GP. Effect of antacid coadministration on the bioavailability of erythromycin stearate. *Clin Pharm* (1989) 8, 352–4.
5. Zündorf H, Wischmann L, Fassenbender M, Lode H, Borner K, Koeppe P. Pharmacokinetics of clarithromycin and possible interaction with H_2 blockers and antacids. *Intersci Conf Antimicrob Agents Chemother* (1991) 31, 185.
6. Boeckh M, Lode H, Höffken G, Daeschlein S, Koeppe P. Pharmacokinetics of roxithromycin and influence of H_2-blockers and antacids on gastrointestinal absorption. *Eur J Clin Microbiol Infect Dis* (1992) 11, 465–8.
7. Ketek (Telithromycin). Aventis Pharmaceuticals Inc. US Prescribing information, June 2004.
8. Ketek (Telithromycin). Aventis Pharma Ltd. UK Summary of product characteristics, January 2004.

Macrolides + Azoles

Fluconazole causes a small to moderate increase in the plasma levels of clarithromycin, which is unlikely to be of clinical importance. Clarithromycin can almost double the serum levels of itraconazole. The pharmacokinetics of azithromycin do not appear to be affected by fluconazole, and erythromycin and azithromycin did not affect the pharmacokinetics of voriconazole.

Clinical evidence, mechanism, importance and management

(a) Azithromycin

Single doses of **fluconazole** 800 mg and azithromycin 1200 mg were given to 18 healthy subjects alone and together without any significant change in the pharmacokinetics of either drug.[1]

In healthy subjects, azithromycin 500 mg once daily for 3 days had no significant effect on the AUC and maximum plasma levels of **voriconazole** 200 mg twice daily.[2,3] **Voriconazole** is mainly metabolised by cytochrome P450 isoenzymes CYP2C19 and CYP2C9 and to a lesser extent by CYP3A4. Azithromycin, is not expected to interact with **voriconazole**.[4] The effect of **voriconazole** on azithromycin levels has not been studied.[2]

(b) Clarithromycin

Twenty healthy subjects were given clarithromycin 500 mg twice daily for 8 days. **Fluconazole** 400 mg daily was added on day 5, followed by 200 mg daily on days 6 to 8. The **fluconazole** increased the minimum plasma levels of the clarithromycin by 33% and the 0 to 12-hour AUC by 18%.[5] These relatively small changes in the pharmacokinetics of clarithromycin are almost certainly of little or no clinical importance.

A study in 8 AIDS patients taking **itraconazole** 200 mg daily found that when clarithromycin 500 mg twice daily was also given, for 14 days, the maximum serum levels and the AUC of the **itraconazole** were increased by 90% and 92% respectively.[6] Both clarithromycin and **itraconazole** are known to compete for the hepatic cytochrome P450 isoenzyme CYP3A4 and it is therefore probable that this leads to a reduction in the clearance of **itraconazole** from the body. This report does not comment on the outcome of this almost twofold increase in **itraconazole** levels, but it would seem prudent to be alert for the need to reduce its dosage. More study is needed.

(c) Erythromycin

In healthy subjects, erythromycin 1 g twice daily for 7 days had no significant effect on the AUC and maximum plasma levels of **voriconazole** 200 mg twice daily.[2,3] **Voriconazole** is mainly metabolised by the cytochrome P450 isoenzymes CYP2C19 and CYP2C9 and to a lesser extent by CYP3A4. Erythromycin is not expected to interact with **voriconazole**.[4] The effect of **voriconazole** on erythromycin levels has not been studied.[2]

1. Amsden GW, Foulds G, Thakker K. Pharmacokinetic study of azithromycin with fluconazole and cotrimoxazole (trimethoprim-sulfamethoxazole) in healthy volunteers. *Clin Drug Invest* (2000) 20, 135–42.
2. VFEND (Voriconazole). Pfizer Inc. US Prescribing information, March 2005.
3. Purkins L, Wood N, Ghahramani P, Kleinermans D, Layton G, Nichols. No clinically significant effect of erythromycin or azithromycin on the pharmacokinetics of voriconazole in healthy male volunteers. *Br J Clin Pharmacol* (2003) 56, 30–6.
4. VFEND (Voriconazole). Pfizer Ltd. UK Summary of product characteristics, March 2005.
5. Gustavson LE, Shi H, Palmer RN, Siepman NC, Craft JC. Drug interaction between clarithromycin and fluconazole in healthy subjects. *Clin Pharmacol Ther* (1996) 59, 185.
6. Hardin TC, Summers KS, Rinaldi MG, Sharkey PK. Evaluation of the pharmacokinetic interaction between itraconazole and clarithromycin following chronic oral dosing in HIV-infected patients. *Pharmacotherapy* (1997) 17, 195.

Macrolides + H_2-blockers

Cimetidine doubled the serum levels of erythromycin in one single-dose study. A single case report describes reversible deafness attributed to this interaction. No clinically significant interaction appears to occur when cimetidine is given with azithromycin or clarithromycin, or when ranitidine is given with clarithromycin, roxithromycin or telithromycin.

Clinical evidence

(a) Cimetidine

A 64-year-old woman was admitted to hospital with cough, dyspnoea and pleuritic pain and was found to have atypical pneumonia and renal impairment. All her antihypertensive treatment (methyldopa, propranolol, co-amilofruse) was stopped, due to hypotension, and her treatment for duodenal ulcer was changed from ranitidine 150 mg twice daily to cimetidine 400 mg at night. She was then started on amoxicillin 500 mg three times daily and **erythromycin** stearate 1 g four times daily. Two days later she complained of 'fuzzy hearing' and audiometry showed a bilateral hearing loss. The **erythromycin** was stopped and her hearing returned to normal after 5 days.[1]

A study of this possible interaction in 8 healthy subjects found that cimetidine 400 mg twice daily increased the AUC of a single 250-mg dose of **erythromycin** by 73%. Maximum serum **erythromycin** levels were doubled.[1]

The pharmacokinetics of **azithromycin** were not affected by a single 800-mg dose of cimetidine in one study,[2] and although cimetidine prolongs the absorption of **clarithromycin**, this is unlikely to be of significance.[3]

(b) Ranitidine

Ranitidine is reported not to affect the pharmacokinetics of **clarithromycin**,[4] **roxithromycin**[5] or **telithromycin**.[6,7]

Mechanism

Cimetidine is known to inhibit the *N*-demethylation of erythromycin so that it is metabolised and cleared from the body more slowly and its serum levels rise. Deafness is known to be one of the adverse effects of erythromycin,[1] which usually occurs with high-doses or intravenous therapy, and was probably exacerbated by renal impairment[4] in the patient described above.

Importance and management

Clinical information about an interaction between cimetidine and erythromycin seems to be limited to this case and the associated single-dose study. The makers[8] say that reversible hearing loss has been reported with erythromycin alone, usually in doses (greater than 4 g daily)[9] and usually by the intravenous route,[9] and in patients with renal impairment.[8] Most UK makers do not include this interaction in their product information, and evidence for an interaction seems limited. If deafness were to occur, the management would seem to be similar (withdraw the erythromycin) regardless of whether or not cimetidine was present, so no additional precautions seem necessary.

There is evidence that azithromycin and clarithromycin do not interact, and ranitidine does not interact with clarithromycin, roxithromycin or telithromycin. No interaction would be expected with other non-enzyme inducing H_2-blockers.

1. Mogford N, Pallett A, George C. Erythromycin deafness and cimetidine treatment. *BMJ* (1994) 309, 1620.
2. Foulds G, Hilligoss DM, Henry EB, Gerber N. The effects of an antacid or cimetidine on the serum concentrations of azithromycin. *J Clin Pharmacol* (1991) 31, 164–7.
3. Amsden GW, Cheng KL, Peloquin CA, Nafziger AN. Oral cimetidine prolongs clarithromycin absorption. *Antimicrob Agents Chemother* (1998) 42, 1578–80.
4. Zündorf H, Wischmann L, Fassenbender M, Lode H, Borner K, Koeppe P. Pharmacokinetics of clarithromycin and possible interaction with H_2 blockers and antacids. *Intersci Conf Antimicrob Agents Chemother* (1991) 31, 185.
5. Boeckh M, Lode H, Höffken G, Daeschlein S, Koeppe P. Pharmacokinetics of roxithromycin and influence of H_2-blockers and antacids on gastrointestinal absorption. *Eur J Clin Microbiol Infect Dis* (1992) 11, 465–8.
6. Ketek (Telithromycin). Aventis Pharmaceuticals Inc. US Prescribing information, June 2004.
7. Ketek (Telithromycin). Aventis Pharma Ltd. UK Summary of product characteristics, January 2004.
8. PCE (Erythromycin particles in tablets). Abbott Laboratories. US Prescribing information, May 1997.
9. Erymax Capsules (Erythromycin). Zeneus Pharma Ltd. UK Summary of product characteristics, November 2003.

Macrolides + Penicillins

There is some *in vitro* evidence that antagonism may occur between erythromycin (a bacteriostatic agent) and penicillins (bactericidal agents) against staphylococci[1] and *Streptococcus pneumoniae*.[2] However, another study has suggested that this *in vitro* antagonism against *S. pneumoniae* between 'penicillin' and erythromycin is minimal and dependent on the interpretative criteria applied.[3] Clinical evidence for this interaction is apparently lacking, and the combination is generally used successfully for pneumonia.[4] In the UK, the combination of amoxicillin and erythromycin or another macrolide (e.g. azithromycin or clarithromycin) is recommended by the BNF for uncomplicated community-acquired pneumonia, if atypical pathogens are suspected.[5]

1. Manten A. Synergism and antagonism between antibiotic mixtures containing erythromycin. *Antibiot Chemother* (1954) 4, 1228–33.
2. Johansen HK, Jensen TG, Dessau RB, Lundgren B, Frimodt-Møller N. Antagonism between penicillin and erythromycin against Streptococcus pneumoniae in vitro and in vivo. *J Antimicrob Chemother* (2000) 46, 973–80.
3. Deshpande LM, Jones RN. Antagonism between penicillin and erythromycin against Streptococcus pneumoniae: Does it exist? *Diagn Microbiol Infect Dis* (2003) 46, 223–5.
4. Feldman C. Clinical relevance of antimicrobial resistance in the management of pneumococcal community-acquired pneumonia. *J Lab Clin Med* (2004) 143, 269–83.
5. British National Formulary. 49th ed. London: The British Medical Association and The Pharmaceutical Press, 2005, p. 265.

Macrolides + Rifamycins

Rifabutin and azithromycin seem not to affect the serum levels of each other, but a very high incidence of neutropenia was seen in one study of the combination. Both rifabutin and rifampicin markedly reduce the serum levels of clarithromycin. Clarithromycin increases the serum levels of rifabutin and there is an increased risk of uveitis and neutropenia. Rifampicin (rifampin) greatly reduces telithromycin levels and concurrent use is not recommended. Cholestatic jaundice has been attributed to the use of troleandomycin with rifampicin.

Clinical evidence

(a) Rifabutin

(i) Neutropenia. A study in 12 healthy subjects was designed to investigate the safety and possible interactions between rifabutin 300 mg daily and **azithromycin** 250 mg daily or **clarithromycin** 500 mg twice daily, for a course of 14 days. The subjects were matched against 18 healthy controls

who received either of the macrolides or rifabutin alone. The study had to be abandoned after 10 days because 14 patients developed neutropenia; 2 taking rifabutin alone, and all 12 of those on rifabutin with a macrolide. Eight subjects developed a fever, 5 required colony simulating factors, and 3 required hospitalisation.[1]

(ii) Pharmacokinetics. In a study[2] investigating a possible regimen for the prophylaxis of *Mycobacterium avium* complex (MAC) disease, 12 HIV+ patients were started on **clarithromycin** 500 mg daily, to which rifabutin 300 mg daily was added on day 15. By day 42 the **clarithromycin** AUC had fallen by 44%, and levels of the metabolite, 14-hydroxyclarithromycin, had risen by 57%. A related study[2] in 14 patients given **clarithromycin** 500 mg 12-hourly and rifabutin 300 mg daily found that after 28 days the AUC of the rifabutin had increased by 99%, and that of the active metabolite 25-*O*-desacetyl-rifabutin had increased by 375%. Another group of patients with lung disease due to MAC were treated with **clarithromycin** 500 mg twice daily. When rifabutin 600 mg was added the levels fell by 63% (from 5.4 to 2 micrograms/ml).[3] Limited information from a randomised study in healthy subjects similarly suggested that **clarithromycin** markedly increased levels of rifabutin and 25-*O*-desacetyl-rifabutin, and that rifabutin increased 14-hydroxyclarithromycin levels. However, there was no apparent pharmacokinetic interaction between **azithromycin** and rifabutin.[1]

(iii) Uveitis or arthralgias. Uveitis, and in some cases pseudojaundice, aphthous stomatitis and an arthralgia syndrome have been described in patients treated with both **clarithromycin** 1 to 2 g daily and rifabutin 300 to 600 mg daily.[4-7]

One report describes 5 HIV+ patients who developed uveitis 6 weeks to 9 months after starting treatment with rifabutin 450 to 600 mg, **clarithromycin** 1.5 to 2 g and fluconazole 100 to 400 mg daily. One further patient who developed uveitis was taking rifabutin and **clarithromycin**, but not fluconazole.[5]

In a study of 68 HIV+ patients taking a variety of treatments for MAC, 10 developed uveitis within 27 to 370 days. All of these 10 patients had been given **clarithromycin** 1 to 2 g daily and rifabutin 300 to 600 mg daily. A further episode of uveitis occurred in a patient on rifabutin and ethambutol. Many patients were also taking fluconazole (which can interact with 'rifamycins', (p.139)), but this showed no statistical association with the development of uveitis, perhaps because many of the patients were only taking 50 mg daily. Further statistical analysis showed the risk of uveitis was greater with rifabutin plus **clarithromycin** than rifabutin alone, or rifabutin with other anti-MAC treatments.[6] None of the 8 patients taking rifabutin and **azithromycin** 500 mg daily developed uveitis.[6]

Other cases of uveitis have been reported in patients on rifabutin, fluconazole, and **azithromycin** 1200 mg weekly but they have been attributed to an interaction between rifabutin and fluconazole.[8] See 'Azoles; Fluconazole + Rifamycins', p.139.

(b) Rifampicin (Rifampin)

Patients with lung disease due to MAC were treated with **clarithromycin** 500 mg twice daily. When rifampicin 600 mg daily was added, the mean serum levels of **clarithromycin** fell by almost 90% (from 5.4 to 0.7 micrograms/ml).[3]

The maker notes that rifampicin reduced the AUC and maximum serum levels of **telithromycin** by 86 and 79% respectively.[9]

Two cases of cholestatic jaundice have been reported in patients treated with both rifampicin and **troleandomycin**.[10,11]

Mechanism

Both rifabutin and rifampicin are known enzyme inducing agents, which can increase the metabolism of other drugs by the liver, thereby reducing their serum levels. Rifampicin is recognised as being the more potent inducer. The reason for the uveitis is not known, but based on *animal* studies it has been suggested that it is associated with effective treatment of MAC and is due to release of a mycobacterial protein, rather than a toxic effect of the drugs.[12] The hepatotoxicity seen with rifampicin and troleandomycin is probably due to additive effects as both drugs are known to be hepatotoxic.

Importance and management

Direct information appears to be limited to these reports but the interactions would appear to be established. The pharmacokinetic interactions with clarithromycin are certainly consistent with the way these rifamycins interact with other drugs. What is not entirely clear is whether these interactions results in treatment failures because of the potentially subtherapeutic clarithromycin serum levels. However, the efficacy of rifabutin and clarithromycin for MAC infection is established, although not without risk (see uveitis below). Because of the lack of information, be alert for evidence of reduced efficacy if clarithromycin and rifampicin are used.

Information regarding neutropenia with macrolides and rifamycins is very limited but what is known suggests that white cell counts should be monitored closely if rifabutin is used with azithromycin or clarithromycin. Rifabutin is known to cause polyarthritis on rare occasions, but in conjunction with clarithromycin it appears to happen at much lower doses.[7] Careful monitoring is necessary. The UK Committee on Safety of Medicines (CSM) has also warned about the need to be aware of the increased risk of uveitis with clarithromycin and rifabutin[13] and of the raised rifabutin levels. If uveitis occurs the CSM recommends that rifabutin should be stopped and the patient should be referred to an ophthalmologist.[13] Because of the increased risk of uveitis the CSM says that consideration should be given to reducing the dosage of rifabutin to 300 mg daily in the presence of macrolides.[13] Later review suggests this dose is associated with a reduced risk of uveitis and maintains efficacy.[14]

Due to a pharmacokinetic interaction the UK makers recommend that telithromycin should not be given during and for 2 weeks after the use of rifampicin.[9]

1. Apseloff G, Foulds G, LaBoy-Goral L, Willavize S, Vincent J. Comparison of azithromycin and clarithromycin in their interactions with rifabutin in healthy volunteers. *J Clin Pharmacol* (1998) 38, 830–5.
2. Hafner R, Bethel J, Power M, Landry B, Banach M, Mole L, Standiford HC, Follansbee S, Kumar P, Raasch R, Cohn D, Mushatt D, Drusano G. Tolerance and pharmacokinetic interactions of rifabutin and clarithromycin in human immunodeficiency virus-infected volunteers. *Antimicrob Agents Chemother* (1998) 42, 631–9.
3. Wallace RJ, Brown BA, Griffith DE, Girard W, Tanaka K. Reduced serum levels of clarithromycin in patients treated with multidrug regimens including rifampin or rifabutin for *Mycobacterium avium-M. intracellulare* infection. *J Infect Dis* (1995) 171, 747–50.
4. Shafren SD, Deschênes J, Miller M, Phillips P, Toma E. Uveitis and pseudojaundice during a regimen of clarithromycin, rifabutin, and ethambutol. *N Engl J Med* (1994) 330, 438–9.
5. Becker K, Schimkat M, Jablonowski H, Häussinger D. Anterior uveitis associated with rifabutin medication in AIDS patients. *Infection* (1996) 24, 34–6.
6. Kelleher P, Helbert M, Sweeney J, Anderson J, Parkin J, Pinching A. Uveitis associated with rifabutin and macrolide therapy for *Mycobacterium avium intracellulare* infections in AIDS patients. *Genitourin Med* (1996) 72, 419–21.
7. Le Gars L, Collon T, Picard O, Kaplan G, Berenbaum F. Polyarthralgia-arthritis syndrome induced by low doses of rifabutin. *J Rheumatol* (1999) 26, 1201–2.
8. Havlir D, Torriani F, Dubé M. Uveitis associated with rifabutin prophylaxis. *Ann Intern Med* (1994) 121, 510–12.
9. Ketek (Telithromycin). Aventis Pharma Ltd. UK Summary of product characteristics, January 2004.
10. Piette F, Peyrard P. Ictère bénin médicamenteux lors d'un traitement associant rifampicine-triacétyloléandomycine. *Nouv Presse Med* (1979) 8, 368–9.
11. Givaudan JF, Gamby T, Privat Y. Ictère cholestatique après association rifampicine-troléandomycine: une nouvelle observation. *Nouv Presse Med* (1979) 8, 2357.
12. Opremcak EM, Cynamon M. Uveitogenic activity of rifabutin and clarithromycin in the *Mycobacterium avium*-infected beige mice. Am Soc Microbiol 2nd Nat Conf. Human retroviruses and related infections. Washington DC, Jan 29—Feb 2 1995, 74.
13. Committee on the Safety of Medicines. Rifabutin (Mycobutin) – uveitis. *Current Problems* (1994) 20, 4.
14. Committee on Safety of Medicines/Medicines Control Agency. Revised indications and drug interactions of rifabutin. *Current Problems* (1997) 23, 14.

Macrolides; Azithromycin + Miscellaneous

Azithromycin appears not to interact pharmacokinetically with methylprednisolone. In clinical trials, no interactions were noted with a number of other drugs used for analgesia, anxiety, arthritis, asthma, hypnosis or sedation. Food appears to halve azithromycin absorption from the capsule formulation, but does not alter the AUC of tablets or suspension.

Clinical evidence, mechanism, importance and management

A review by the makers briefly mentions that azithromycin did not interact pharmacokinetically with **methylprednisolone**.[1] Safety data from phase II and III clinical studies showed that concurrent treatment occurred with **bronchodilators**, **analgesics**, **hypnotics/sedatives/anxiolytics** or **anti-arthritic drugs** (none of them specifically named) in 45% of patients, with no interaction problems encountered.[1]

A review by the makers briefly mentions that **food** reduced the absorption of azithromycin by about half.[1] It is suggested therefore that azithromycin *capsules* should not be given at the same time as food, but should be taken at least 1 hour before or 2 hours after a **meal**.[1,2] However, the US prescribing information states that a **high-fat meal** increased the maximum levels of azithromycin *tablets* by 23%, and had no effect on the AUC.[3] Similarly, **food** increased the maximum levels of azithromycin *suspension* by 56%, without altering the AUC.[3] Azithromycin suspension[2,3] and tablets[3] may therefore be taken without regard to **food**.

1. Hopkins S. Clinical toleration and safety of azithromycin. *Am J Med* (1991) 91 (Suppl 3A), 40S–45S.
2. Zithromax (Azithromycin). Pfizer Ltd. UK Summary of product characteristics, July 2004.
3. Zithromax (Azithromycin). Pfizer Laboratories. US Prescribing information, January 2004.

Macrolides; Erythromycin + Sucralfate

Sucralfate appears not to affect the pharmacokinetics of erythromycin.

Clinical evidence, mechanism, importance and management

The pharmacokinetics (elimination rate constant, half-life, AUC) of a single 400-mg dose of erythromycin ethylsuccinate were not significantly altered by a single 1-g dose of sucralfate in 6 healthy subjects. It was concluded that the therapeutic effects of erythromycin are unlikely to be affected by concurrent use.[1]

1. Miller LG, Prichard JG, White CA, Vytla B, Feldman S, Bowman RC. Effect of concurrent sucralfate administration on the absorption of erythromycin. *J Clin Pharmacol* (1990) 30, 39–44.

Macrolides; Erythromycin + Urinary acidifiers or alkalinisers

In the treatment of urinary tract infections, the antibacterial activity of erythromycin is maximal in alkaline urine and minimal in acidic urine.

Clinical evidence

Urine taken from 7 subjects receiving erythromycin 1 g every 8 hours, was tested against 5 genera of Gram-negative bacilli (*Escherichia coli*, *Klebsiella pneumoniae*, *P. mirabilis*, *Ps. aeruginosa* and *Serratia* sp.) both before and after treatment with **acetazolamide** or **sodium bicarbonate**, given to alkalinise the urine. A direct correlation was found between the activity of the antibacterial and the pH of the urine. In general, acidic urine had little or no antibacterial activity, whereas alkalinised urine had activity.[1]

Clinical studies have confirmed the increased antibacterial effectiveness of erythromycin in the treatment of bacteriuria when the urine is made alkaline.[2,3]

Mechanism

The pH of the urine does not apparently affect the way the kidney handles the antibacterial (most of it is excreted actively rather than passively) but it does have a direct influence on the way the antibacterial affects the micro-organisms. Mechanisms suggested include effects on bacterial cell receptors, the induction of active transport mechanisms on bacterial cell walls, and changes in ionisation of the antibacterial, which enables it to enter the bacterial cell more effectively.

Importance and management

An established interaction, which can be exploited. Should erythromycin be used to treat urinary tract infections its efficacy can be maximised by making the urine alkaline (for example with acetazolamide or sodium bicarbonate). Treatment with urinary acidifiers will minimise the activity of the erythromycin for urinary tract infections and should be avoided. There is no evidence that the efficacy of erythromycin in other infections is affected by urinary acidifiers or alkalinisers.

1. Sabath LD, Gerstein DA, Loder PB, Finland M. Excretion of erythromycin and its enhanced activity in urine against gram-negative bacilli with alkalinization. *J Lab Clin Med* (1968) 72, 916–23.
2. Zinner SH, Sabath LD, Casey JI, Finland M. Erythromycin and alkalinisation of the urine in the treatment of urinary-tract infections due to gram-negative bacilli. *Lancet* (1971) i, 1267–8.
3. Zinner SH, Sabath LD, Casey JI, Finland M. Erythromycin plus alkalinization in treatment of urinary infections. *Antimicrob Agents Chemother* (1969) 9, 413–16.

Meropenem + Probenecid

Probenecid increases the serum levels of meropenem.

Clinical evidence, mechanism, importance and management

Probenecid (1 g given orally 2 hours before meropenem and 500 mg given orally 1.5 hours after meropenem) increased the AUC of meropenem 500 mg by 43% in 6 healthy subjects.[1] Another study found that probenecid (1.5 g in divided doses the day before and 500 mg one hour before meropenem) increased the AUC of meropenem 1 g in 6 healthy subjects by up to 55% and increased its half-life by 33% (from 0.98 to 1.3 hours).[2] In both studies the serum levels of meropenem were modestly increased. This is possibly because meropenem and probenecid compete for active kidney tubular secretion.[3,4] The makers say that because the potency and duration of meropenem are adequate without probenecid, they do not recommend concurrent use.[3,4]

1. Ishida Y, Matsumoto F, Sakai O, Yoshida M, Shiba K. The pharmacokinetic study of meropenem: effect of probenecid and hemodialysis. *J Chemother* (1993) 5 (Suppl 1), 124–6.
2. Bax RP, Bastain W, Featherstone A, Wilkinson DM, Hutchison M, Haworth SJ. The pharmacokinetics of meropenem in volunteers. *J Antimicrob Chemother* (1989) 24 (Suppl A), 311–20.
3. Meronem (Meropenem). AstraZeneca UK Ltd. UK Summary of product characteristics, January 2004.
4. Merrem (Meropenem). AstraZeneca. US Prescribing information, January 2004.

Methenamine + Miscellaneous

Urinary alkalinizers (e.g. potassium or sodium citrate) and those antacids that can raise the urinary pH above 5.5 should not be used during treatment with methenamine because they inhibit its activation. If some of the older less-soluble sulfonamides are used with methenamine there is the risk of kidney damage due to crystalluria at low urinary pH values.

Clinical evidence, mechanism, importance and management

Methenamine and methenamine mandelate are only effective as urinary antiseptics if the pH is about 5.5 or lower, when formaldehyde is released. This is normally achieved by giving urinary acidifiers such as ammonium chloride, ascorbic acid[1,2] or sodium acid phosphate. In the case of methenamine hippurate, the acidification of the urine is achieved by the presence of hippuric acid. The concurrent use of substances that raise the urinary pH such as **acetazolamide**, **sodium bicarbonate**, **potassium** or **sodium citrate** is clearly contraindicated. **Potassium citrate mixture BPC** has been shown to raise the pH by more than 1 at normal therapeutic doses, thereby making the urine sufficiently alkaline to interfere with the activation of methenamine to formaldehyde.[3] Some **antacids** (containing magnesium, aluminium or calcium as well as sodium bicarbonate mentioned above) can also cause a significant rise in the pH of the urine.[4]

1. Strom JG, Jun HW. Effect of urine pH and ascorbic acid on the rate of conversion of methenamine to formaldehyde. *Biopharm Drug Dispos* (1993) 14, 61–9.
2. Nahata MC, Cummins BA, McLeod DC, Schondelmeyer SW, Butler R. Effect of urinary acidifiers on formaldehyde concentration and efficacy with methenamine therapy. *Eur J Clin Pharmacol* (1982) 22, 281–4.
3. Lipton JH. Incompatibility between sulfamethizole and methenamine mandelate. *N Engl J Med* (1963) 268, 92.
4. Blondheim SH, Alkan WJ, Brunner D, eds. Frontiers of Internal Medicine. 1974. Basel: Karger; 1975 p. 404–8.

Metronidazole + Antacids, Colestyramine or Kaolin-pectin

The absorption of metronidazole is unaffected by kaolin-pectin, but it is slightly reduced by an aluminium hydroxide antacid and colestyramine, although not to a clinically relevant extent.

Clinical evidence, mechanism, importance and management

The bioavailability of a single 500-mg dose of metronidazole in 5 healthy subjects was not significantly changed by 30 ml of a kaolin-pectin antidiarrhoeal mixture. However, a 14.5% reduction in metronidazole bioavailability occurred with 30 ml of an **aluminium hydroxide/simeticone** suspension, and a 21.3% reduction occurred with a single 4-g dose of colestyramine.[1] The clinical importance of these reductions is probably small, and no special precautions seem necessary.

1. Molokhia AM, Al-Rahman S. Effect of concomitant oral administration of some adsorbing drugs on the bioavailability of metronidazole. *Drug Dev Ind Pharm* (1987) 13, 1229–37.

Metronidazole + Barbiturates

Phenobarbital markedly increases the metabolism of metronidazole and treatment failure has been reported in both adults and children. Dose increases are likely to be necessary.

Clinical evidence

A woman with vaginal trichomoniasis was given metronidazole on several occasions over the course of a year, but the infection flared up again as soon as it was stopped. When it was realised that she was also taking **phenobarbital** 100 mg daily, the metronidazole dosage was doubled to 500 mg three times daily, and she was cured after a 7-day course.[1] A pharmacokinetic study found that the clearance of metronidazole was increased (half-life 3.5 hours compared with the normal 8 to 9 hours).[1]

A retrospective study in children who had not responded to metronidazole for giardiasis or amoebiasis found that 80% of them had been on long-term **phenobarbital**. In a prospective study in 36 children the normal recommended metronidazole dosage had to be increased approximately threefold to 60 mg/kg to achieve a cure. The half-life of metronidazole in 15 other children on **phenobarbital** was found to be 3.5 hours compared with the normal 8 to 9 hours.[2]

Other studies in patients with Crohn's disease and healthy subjects showed that **phenobarbital** reduced the metronidazole AUC by about a third,[3] and increased the clearance of metronidazole 1.5-fold.[4]

Mechanism

Phenobarbital is a known, potent liver enzyme-inducing agent, which increases the metabolism and loss of metronidazole from the body.

Importance and management

An established and clinically important interaction. Monitor the effects of concurrent use and anticipate the need to increase the metronidazole dosage two to threefold if phenobarbital is given concurrently. All of the barbiturates are potent liver enzyme inducing agents and would therefore be expected to interact similarly.

1. Mead PB, Gibson M, Schentag JJ, Ziemniak JA. Possible alteration of metronidazole metabolism by phenobarbital. *N Engl J Med* (1982) 306, 1490.
2. Gupte S. Phenobarbital and metabolism of metronidazole. *N Engl J Med* (1983) 308, 529.
3. Eradiri O, Jamali F, Thomson ABR. Interaction of metronidazole with phenobarbital, cimetidine, prednisone, and sulfasalazine in Crohn's disease. *Biopharm Drug Dispos* (1988) 9, 219–27.
4. Loft S, Sonne J, Poulsen HE, Petersen KT, Jørgensen BG, Døssing M. Inhibition and induction of metronidazole and antipyrine metabolism. *Eur J Clin Pharmacol* (1987) 32, 35–41.

Metronidazole + Chloroquine

An isolated report describes acute dystonia in one patient, which was attributed to an interaction between metronidazole and chloroquine.

Clinical evidence, mechanism, importance and management

A patient was given a 7-day course of metronidazole and ampicillin, following a laparoscopic investigation. She developed acute dystonic reactions (facial grimacing, coarse tremors, and an inability to maintain posture) on day 6, within 10 minutes of being given chloroquine phosphate (equivalent to 200 mg of base) and intramuscular promethazine 25 mg. The dystonic symptoms started to subside within 15 minutes of being given diazepam 5 mg intravenously, and had completely resolved within 2 hours.[1]

The authors of the report attribute the dystonia to an interaction between metronidazole and chloroquine as she had taken both drugs alone without adverse effect. However, they do not fully assess the possible contribution of promethazine, which is known to cause dystonias. It is therefore possible that the reaction seen was an adverse effect of the **promethazine**, or perhaps even an interaction between **promethazine** and chloroquine. No general recommendations can be made from this single report.

1. Achumba JI, Ette EI, Thomas WOA, Essien EE. Chloroquine-induced acute dystonic reactions in the presence of metronidazole. *Drug Intell Clin Pharm* (1988) 22, 308–10.

Metronidazole or Tinidazole + Cimetidine

Cimetidine reduces the metabolism of tinidazole, and possibly also metronidazole, but this is probably not clinically important.

Clinical evidence

(a) Metronidazole

The half-life of a 400-mg intravenous dose of metronidazole was increased from 6.2 to 7.9 hours in 6 healthy subjects after they took cimetidine 400 mg twice daily for 6 days. The total plasma clearance was reduced by almost 30%.[1] However, in another study in 6 patients with Crohn's disease, cimetidine 600 mg twice daily for 7 days was found not to affect either the AUC or the half-life of metronidazole,[2] and no evidence of an interaction was found in a further study in 6 healthy subjects.[3]

(b) Tinidazole

Cimetidine 400 mg twice daily given to 6 healthy subjects for 7 days raised the peak serum levels of a single 600-mg dose of tinidazole by 21%, increased the 24-hour AUC by 40% and increased the half-life by 47%, from 7.66 to 11.23 hours.[4]

Mechanism

Cimetidine is a well known enzyme-inhibiting drug, which probably inhibits the metabolism of the metronidazole and tinidazole by the liver.

Importance and management

The modest changes in the pharmacokinetics of tinidazole with cimetidine seem unlikely to be clinically significant, but bear them in mind in the case of an unexpected response to treatment. The interaction between metronidazole and cimetidine is not established, but any changes in metronidazole pharmacokinetics were modest and unlikely to be important.

1. Gugler R, Jensen JC. Interaction between cimetidine and metronidazole. *N Engl J Med* (1983) 309, 1518–19.
2. Eradiri O, Jamali F, Thomson ABR. Interaction of metronidazole with phenobarbital, cimetidine, prednisone, and sulfasalazine in Crohn's disease. *Biopharm Drug Dispos* (1988) 9, 219–27.
3. Loft S, Døssing M, Sonne J, Dalhof K, Bjerrum K, Poulsen HE. Lack of effect of cimetidine on the pharmacokinetics and metabolism of a single oral dose of metronidazole. *Eur J Clin Pharmacol* (1988) 35, 65–8.
4. Patel RB, Shah GF, Raval JD, Gandhi TP, Gilbert RN. The effect of cimetidine and rifampicin on tinidazole kinetics in healthy human volunteers. *Indian Drugs* (1986) 23, 338–41.

Metronidazole + Diosmin

Diosmin reduces the metabolism of metronidazole to some extent, but the clinical importance of this is probably small.

Clinical evidence, mechanism, importance and management

A single 800-mg dose of metronidazole was given to 12 healthy subjects following 9 days of treatment with diosmin 500 mg daily. The metronidazole AUC and maximum plasma concentrations were raised by 27 and 25% respectively.[1] This interaction is thought to occur because of an inhibitory effect of diosmin on metronidazole metabolism by hepatic enzymes and P-glycoprotein.

Other drugs that raise metronidazole levels by a similar amount (e.g. 'cimetidine' (above)) are not considered to have clinically significant interactions with metronidazole, therefore no clinically significant interaction is likely to occur on the concurrent use of metronidazole and diosmin.

1. Rajnarayana K, Reddy MS, Krishna DR. Diosmin pretreatment affects bioavailability of metronidazole. *Eur J Clin Pharmacol* (2003) 58, 803–807.

Metronidazole + Disulfiram

Acute psychoses and confusion can be caused by the concurrent use of metronidazole and disulfiram.

Clinical evidence, mechanism, importance and management

In a double-blind study in 58 hospitalised chronic alcoholics on disulfiram, 29 were also given metronidazole 750 mg daily for a month, then 250 mg daily thereafter. Six of the 29 subjects in the group receiving metronidazole developed acute psychoses or confusion. Five of the 6 had paranoid delusions and in 3 visual and auditory hallucinations were also seen. The symptoms persisted for 2 to 3 days after the drugs were withdrawn, but disappeared at the end of a fortnight and did not reappear when disulfiram alone was restarted.[1] Similar reactions have been described in two other reports.[2,3]

The reason for this interaction is not understood, but it appears to be established. Concurrent use should be avoided or very well monitored.

1. Rothstein E, Clancy DD. Toxicity of disulfiram combined with metronidazole. *N Engl J Med* (1969) 280, 1006–7.
2. Goodhue WW. Disulfiram-metronidazole (well-identified) toxicity. *N Engl J Med* (1969) 280, 1482–3.
3. Scher JM. Psychotic reaction to disulfiram. *JAMA* (1967) 201,1051.

Metronidazole + Prednisone

Prednisone modestly increases the loss of metronidazole from the body.

Clinical evidence, mechanism, importance and management

The AUC of metronidazole 250 mg twice daily was reduced by 31% by prednisone 10 mg twice daily for 6 days in 6 patients with Crohn's disease, probably because prednisone induces the metabolism of metronidazole by liver-enzymes.[1]

Information appears to be limited to this report and the interaction is probably of only limited clinical importance, although the occasional patient may be affected. Information about other corticosteroids is lacking.

1. Eradiri O, Jamali F, Thomson ABR. Interaction of metronidazole with phenobarbital, cimetidine, prednisone, and sulfasalazine in Crohn's disease. *Biopharm Drug Dispos* (1988) 9, 219–27.

Metronidazole or Tinidazole + Rifampicin (Rifampin)

Rifampicin modestly increases the clearance of metronidazole and tinidazole but the clinical importance of this is uncertain.

Clinical evidence

(a) Metronidazole

Intravenous metronidazole 500 mg or 1 g was given to 10 healthy subjects before and after taking rifampicin 450 mg daily for 7 days. The rifampicin reduced the metronidazole AUC by 33% and increased its clearance by 44%. Results were the same with both metronidazole doses.[1]

(b) Tinidazole

After 6 healthy subjects took rifampicin 600 mg daily for 7 days the peak serum levels of a single 600-mg dose of tinidazole were reduced by 22%, the 24-hour AUC was reduced by 30% and the half-life was reduced by 27% (from 7.66 to 5.6 hours).[2]

Mechanism

This interaction almost certainly occurs because rifampicin (a well-recognised and potent enzyme inducer) increases the metabolism of metronidazole and tinidazole by the liver.

Importance and management

The clinical significance of these interactions appear not to have been studied. Other drugs that cause a 30% reduction in metronidazole levels (e.g. 'prednisone' (above)) have not been shown to have any clinically significant interaction, and there do not appear to be reports of one with rifampicin. Rifampicin is known to act synergistically with metronidazole,[3] so it may be that any reduction in levels is offset by enhanced antimicrobial activity. Tinidazole acts very much like metronidazole, and therefore a clinically significant interaction between rifampicin and either of these drugs seems unlikely.

1. Djojosaputro M, Mustofa SS, Donatus IA, Santoso B. The effects of doses and pre-treatment with rifampicin on the elimination kinetics of metronidazole. *Eur J Pharmacol* (1990) 183, 1870–1.
2. Patel RB, Shah GF, Raval JD, Gandhi TP, Gilbert RN. The effect of cimetidine and rifampicin on tinidazole kinetics in healthy human volunteers. *Indian Drugs* (1986) 23, 338–41.
3. Metronidazole tablets 500 mg. Dumex Ltd. UK Summary of product characteristics, August 1999.

Metronidazole + Silymarin

Silymarin (the active constituent of milk thistle) modestly reduces metronidazole levels, but the clinical significance of this is unclear.

Clinical evidence, mechanism, importance and management

Silymarin 140 mg daily was given to 12 healthy subjects for 9 days, with metronidazole 400 mg three times daily on days 7 to 10. Silymarin reduced the AUC of metronidazole and hydroxymetronidazole (a major active metabolite) by 28% and the maximum serum levels by 29 and 20% respectively. The authors suggest that silymarin causes these pharmacokinetic changes by inducing P-glycoprotein and the cytochrome P450 isoenzyme CYP3A4, both of which are involved in the metabolism of metronidazole.[1] The clinical significance of this interaction is unclear, but other drugs that cause a 30% reduction in metronidazole levels (e.g. 'prednisone' (p.221)) have not been shown to have any clinically significant interaction.

1. Rajnarayana K, Reddy MS, Vidyasagar J, Krishna DR. Study on the influence of silymarin pretreatment on metabolism and disposition of metronidazole. *Arzneimittelforschung* (2004) 54, 109–113.

Metronidazole + Sucralfate

Sucralfate does not alter the pharmacokinetics of metronidazole.

Clinical evidence, mechanism, importance and management

Because oral triple therapy using sucralfate instead of bismuth to eradicate *H. pylori* has yielded inconsistent results, a 5-day study was undertaken in 14 healthy subjects to investigate whether sucralfate interacts with metronidazole. It was found that sucralfate 2 g twice daily had no effect on the pharmacokinetics of a single 400-mg dose of metronidazole.[1] No special precautions therefore appear necessary on concurrent use.

1. Amaral Moraes ME, De Almeida Pierossi M, Moraes MO, Bezerra FF, Ferreira De Silva CM, Dias HB, Muscará MN, De Nucci G, Pedrazzoli J. Short-term sucralfate administration does not alter the absorption of metronidazole in healthy male volunteers. *Int J Clin Pharmacol Ther* (1996) 34, 433–7.

Nitrofurantoin + Antacids

Magnesium trisilicate reduces the absorption of nitrofurantoin, but the clinical significance of this is unknown. Aluminium hydroxide is reported not to interact. Whether other antacids interact adversely is uncertain.

Clinical evidence

Magnesium trisilicate 5 g in 150 ml of water reduced the absorption of a single 100-g oral dose of nitrofurantoin in 6 healthy subjects by more than 50%. The time during which the concentration of nitrofurantoin in the urine was at, or above 32 micrograms/ml (a level stated to be the minimum inhibitory concentration) was also reduced.[1] The amounts of nitrofurantoin adsorbed by other antacids in *in vitro* tests were as follows: **magnesium trisilicate** and **charcoal** 99%, **bismuth subcarbonate** and **talc** 50 to 53%, **kaolin** 31%, **magnesium oxide** 27%, **aluminium hydroxide** 2.5% and **calcium carbonate** 0%.[1]

A crossover study in 6 healthy subjects confirmed that **aluminium hydroxide gel** does not affect the absorption of nitrofurantoin from the gut (as measured by its excretion into the urine).[2] Another study in 10 healthy subjects found that an antacid containing **aluminium hydroxide**, **magnesium carbonate** and **magnesium hydroxide** reduced the absorption of nitrofurantoin by 22%.[3]

Mechanism

Antacids can, to a greater or lesser extent, adsorb nitrofurantoin onto their surfaces, as a result less is available for absorption by the gut and for excretion into the urine.

Importance and management

Information appears to be limited to these reports. There seems to be nothing in the literature confirming that a clinically important nitrofurantoin/antacid interaction occurs. One reviewer offers the opinion that common antacid preparations are unlikely to interact with nitrofurantoin.[4]

It is not yet known whether magnesium trisilicate significantly reduces the antibacterial effectiveness of nitrofurantoin but the response should be monitored. While it is known that the antibacterial action of nitrofurantoin is increased by drugs that acidify the urine (so that reduced actions would be expected if the urine were made more alkaline by antacids) this again does not seem to have been confirmed. The results of the *in vitro* studies suggest that the possible effects of the other antacids are quite small, and aluminium hydroxide is reported not to interact.

1. Naggar VF, Khalil SA. Effect of magnesium trisilicate on nitrofurantoin absorption. *Clin Pharmacol Ther* (1979) 25, 857–63.
2. Jaffe JM, Hamilton B, Jeffers S. Nitrofurantoin-antacid interaction. *Drug Intell Clin Pharm* (1976) 10, 419–20.
3. Männistö P. The effect of crystal size, gastric content and emptying rate on the absorption of nitrofurantoin in healthy human volunteers. *Int J Clin Pharmacol Biopharm* (1978) 16, 223–8.
4. D'Arcy PF. Nitrofurantoin. *Drug Intell Clin Pharm* (1985) 19, 540–7.

Nitrofurantoin + Anticholinergics or Diphenoxylate

Diphenoxylate and anticholinergic drugs such as propantheline can double the absorption of nitrofurantoin in some patients, but the clinical importance of this is uncertain.

Clinical evidence, mechanism, importance and management

Propantheline 30 mg given 45 minutes before nitrofurantoin approximately doubled the absorption of nitrofurantoin 100 mg (as measured by the urinary excretion) in 6 healthy subjects.[1] In another study, 2 out of 6 men similarly showed that diphenoxylate 200 mg daily for 3 days nearly doubled nitrofurantoin absorption.[2] **Atropine** 500 micrograms given subcutaneously 30 minutes before a single 100-mg dose of nitrofurantoin had little effect on the bioavailability of nitrofurantoin, but the absorption and excretion into the urine was delayed.[3]

It was suggested that the reduced gut motility caused by these drugs allows the nitrofurantoin to dissolve more completely so that it is absorbed by the gut more easily. Whether this is of any clinical importance is uncertain but it could possibly increase the incidence of dose-related adverse reactions. So far there appear to be no reports of any problems arising from concurrent use.

1. Jaffe JM. Effect of propantheline on nitrofurantoin absorption. *J Pharm Sci* (1975) 64, 1729–30.
2. Callahan M, Bullock FJ, Braun J, Yesair DW. Pharmacodynamics of drug interactions with diphenoxylate (Lomotil®). *Fedn Proc* (1974) 33, 513.
3. Männistö P. The effect of crystal size, gastric content and emptying rate on the absorption of nitrofurantoin in healthy human volunteers. *Int J Clin Pharmacol Biopharm* (1978) 16, 223–8.

Nitrofurantoin + Antigout drugs

On theoretical grounds the efficacy and toxicity of nitrofurantoin may possibly be increased by probenecid or sulfinpyrazone.

Clinical evidence, mechanism, importance and management

A study of the way the kidneys handle nitrofurantoin found that **sulfinpyrazone** 2.5 mg/kg given intravenously reduced the secretion of nitrofurantoin by the kidney tubules by about 50%.[1] This reduction would be expected to reduce its urinary antibacterial efficacy, and the higher serum levels might lead to increased systemic toxicity, but there do not seem to be any reports confirming or denying that this represents a real problem in practice. The same situation would also seem likely with **probenecid**, but there do not appear to be any reports confirming this interaction.

The clinical importance of both of these interactions is therefore uncertain, but it would seem prudent to be alert for any evidence of reduced antibacterial efficacy and increased systemic toxicity if either of these uricosuric agents is used with nitrofurantoin.

1. Schirmeister J, Stefani F, Willmann H, Hallauer W. Renal handling of nitrofurantoin in man. *Antimicrob Agents Chemother* (1965) 5, 223–6.

Nitrofurantoin + Azoles

An isolated case indicates hepatic and pulmonary toxicity may occur if nitrofurantoin is given with fluconazole, but not with itraconazole.

Clinical evidence, mechanism, importance and management

A 73-year-old man on nitrofurantoin 50 mg daily for 5 years was given **fluconazole** 150 mg weekly for onychomycosis. At the start of treatment with **fluconazole** his hepatic enzyme levels were slightly raised and 3 weeks later were increased more than twofold. Two months after starting **fluconazole** the patient's hepatic enzyme levels had increased fivefold and he had fatigue, dyspnoea on exertion, pleuritic pain, burning tracheal pain and a cough. Bilateral pulmonary disease was confirmed by chest X-rays, and pulmonary function tests suggested nitrofurantoin toxicity. Both **fluconazole** and nitrofurantoin were discontinued, and hepatic and lung function gradually improved.[1]

Either **fluconazole** or nitrofurantoin could have caused the liver toxicity. However, it was considered that both the lung and liver toxicity may have been due to an interaction between nitrofurantoin and **fluconazole**, possibly due to increased nitrofurantoin concentrations resulting from competition with **fluconazole** for renal tubular secretion.

Some 2 years earlier the patient had received pulse **itraconazole** (less than 1% excreted in the urine as active drug) with nitrofurantoin without raised lever enzymes or any other adverse effects.[1]

Information appears to be limited to this report, but bear it in mind in the event of unexpected toxicity to treatment. More study is needed.

1. Linnebur SA, Parnes BL. Pulmonary and hepatic toxicity due to nitrofurantoin and fluconazole treatment. *Ann Pharmacother* (2004) 38, 612–6.

Nitrofurantoin + Metoclopramide

Metoclopramide reduces the absorption of nitrofurantoin.

Clinical evidence, mechanism, importance and management

The urinary excretion of nitrofurantoin was approximately halved in 10 healthy subjects when they were given nitrofurantoin 100 mg after pretreatment with a 10-mg intramuscular dose of metoclopramide and 10 mg orally half an hour before.[1]

It is thought that metoclopramide increases the gastric emptying rate, thus decreasing nitrofurantoin absorption. The practical importance of this is uncertain because there seem to be no reports describing problems.

1. Männistö P. The effect of crystal size, gastric content and emptying rate on the absorption of nitrofurantoin in healthy human volunteers. *Int J Clin Pharmacol Biopharm* (1978) 16, 223–8.

Nitroxoline + Antacids

There is *in vitro* evidence that divalent ions such as magnesium and calcium can reduce the antibacterial effects of nitroxoline, but it is not known whether clinically important interactions occur.

Clinical evidence, mechanism, importance and management

The antibacterial effects of nitroxoline have been found to be reduced *in vitro* by **magnesium** and **calcium** ions because it can form chelates with them.[1] What is not known is whether in clinical practice nitroxoline would interact significantly with these ions in antacids, and whether this would result in inadequate urine concentrations (nitroxoline is mainly used for urinary-tract infections). In the absence of any direct clinical information it would however seem prudent to monitor concurrent use for any evidence that its antibacterial effects are reduced.

1. Pelletier C, Prognon P, Bourlioux P. Roles of divalent cations and pH in mechanism of action of nitroxoline against *Escherichia coli* strains. *Antimicrob Agents Chemother* (1995) 707–13.

Novobiocin + Rifampicin (Rifampin)

Rifampicin reduces the half-life of novobiocin but this is unlikely to be of clinical significance.

Clinical evidence, mechanism, importance and management

When 10 healthy subjects were given novobiocin 1 g daily for 13 days with rifampicin 600 mg daily, the novobiocin half-life was reduced from 5.85 to 2.66 hours and the AUC was reduced by almost 50%. However, the plasma novobiocin levels were not significantly altered and the trough serum levels remained in excess of the MIC for 90% of the strains of MRSA tested. No significant changes in the rifampicin pharmacokinetics were seen.[1] No special precautions would therefore seem to be necessary during concurrent use.

1. Drusano GL, Townsend RJ, Walsh TJ, Forrest A, Antal EJ, Standiford HC. Steady-state serum pharmacokinetics of novobiocin and rifampin alone and in combination. *Antimicrob Agents Chemother* (1986) 30, 42–5.

Penicillins + Allopurinol

The incidence of skin rashes among those taking either ampicillin or amoxicillin is increased by allopurinol.

Clinical evidence

A retrospective search through the records of 1324 patients, 67 of whom were taking allopurinol and **ampicillin**, showed that 15 of them (22%) developed a skin rash compared with 94 (7.5%) of the rest not taking allopurinol.[1] The types of rash were not defined. Another study found that 35 out of 252 patients (13.9%) taking allopurinol and **ampicillin** developed a rash, compared with 251 out of 4434 (5.9%) taking **ampicillin** alone.[2] A parallel study revealed that 8 out of 36 patients (22%) on **amoxicillin** and allopurinol developed a rash, whereas only 52 out of 887 (5.9%) did so on **amoxicillin** alone.[2]

A case report describes a patient who developed erythema multiforme shortly after starting **amoxicillin** and allopurinol and who was found to have both allopurinol hypersensitivity and type IV amoxicillin hypersensitivity.[3]

In contrast, one study did not find that the incidence of penicillin-related rashes was increased by allopurinol, and the authors suggested that this contrasting finding may be because exposure to penicillins was shorter in their study.[4]

Mechanism

Not understood. One suggestion is that the hyperuricaemia was responsible.[1] Another is that hyperuricaemic individuals may possibly have an altered immunological reactivity.[5]

Importance and management

An established interaction of limited importance. There would seem to be no strong reason for avoiding concurrent use, but prescribers should recognise that the development of a rash is by no means unusual. Whether this also occurs with penicillins other than ampicillin or amoxicillin is uncertain, and does not seem to have been reported.

1. Boston Collaborative Drug Surveillance Programme. Excess of ampicillin rashes associated with allopurinol or hyperuricemia. *N Engl J Med* (1972) 286, 505–7.
2. Jick H, Porter JB. Potentiation of ampicillin skin reactions by allopurinol or hyperuricemia. *J Clin Pharmacol* (1981) 21, 456–8.
3. Pérez A, Cabrerizo S, de Barrio M, Díaz MP, Herrero T, Tornero P, Baeza ML. Erythema-multiforme-like eruption from amoxicillin and allopurinol. *Contact Dermatitis* (2001) 44, 113–14.
4. Sonntag MR, Zoppi M, Fritschy D, Maibach R, Stocker F, Sollberger J, Buchli W, Hess T, Hoigné R. Exantheme unter haufig angewandten Antibiotika und antibakteriellen Chemotherepeutika (Penicilline, speziell Aminopenicilline, Cephalosporine und Cotrimoxazol) sowie Allopurinol. *Schweiz Med Wochenschr* (1986) 116, 142–5.
5. Fessel WJ. Immunological reactivity in hyperuricemia. *N Engl J Med* (1972) 286, 1218.

Penicillins + Antacids

Aluminium/magnesium hydroxide and aluminium hydroxide do not significantly affect the bioavailability of amoxicillin or amoxicillin with clavulanic acid (co-amoxiclav).

Clinical evidence, mechanism, importance and management

The pharmacokinetics of **amoxicillin** 1 g, and both amoxicillin and clavulanic acid (given as **co-amoxiclav** 625 mg), were not significantly altered by 10 doses of **aluminium/magnesium hydroxide** (*Maalox*) 10 ml, with the last dose given 30 minutes before **amoxicillin**.[1] Another study found that four 40-mg doses of **aluminium hydroxide** (*Aludrox*) given at 20 minute intervals had no effect on the pharmacokinetics of either amoxicillin or clavulanic acid (given as **co-amoxiclav** 750 mg with the second dose of antacid).[2]

There would seem to be no reason for avoiding the concurrent use of antacids and **amoxicillin** or **co-amoxiclav**.

1. Deppermann K-M, Lode H, Höffken G, Tschink G, Kalz C, Koeppe P. Influence of ranitidine, pirenzepine, and aluminium magnesium hydroxide on the bioavailability of various antibacterials, including amoxicillin, cephalexin, doxycycline, and amoxicillin-clavulanic acid. *Antimicrob Agents Chemother* (1989) 33, 1901–7.
2. Staniforth DH, Clarke HL, Horton R, Jackson D, Lau D. Augmentin bioavailability following cimetidine, aluminum hydroxide and milk. *Int J Clin Pharmacol Ther Toxicol* (1985) 23, 145–7.

Penicillins + Chloroquine

Chloroquine reduces the absorption of ampicillin, but bacampicillin is not affected.

Clinical evidence

Chloroquine 1 g reduced the absorption (as measured by excretion in the urine) of a single 1-g dose of oral **ampicillin** by about a third (from 29 to 19%) in 7 healthy subjects.[1] Another study by the same author demonstrated that the absorption of **ampicillin** from **bacampicillin** tablets was unaffected by chloroquine.[2]

Mechanism

A possible reason for the reduction in absorption is that the chloroquine irritates the gut so that the ampicillin is moved through more quickly, thereby reducing the time for absorption.

Importance and management

Information appears to be limited to the studies cited, which used large doses of chloroquine (1 g) when compared with those usually used for malarial prophylaxis (300 mg base weekly) or for rheumatic diseases (150 mg daily). The reduction in the ampicillin absorption is also only moderate (about a third). The general clinical importance of this interaction is therefore uncertain. However one report suggests separating the dosing by not less than 2 hours.[1] An alternative would be to use bacampicillin (an ampicillin pro-drug) the bioavailability of which is not affected by chloroquine.[2] More study is needed to confirm and evaluate the importance of this interaction.

1. Ali HM. Reduced ampicillin bioavailability following oral coadministration with chloroquine. *J Antimicrob Chemother* (1985) 15, 781–4.
2. Ali HM. The effect of Sudanese food and chloroquine on the bioavailability of ampicillin from bacampicillin tablets. *Int J Pharmaceutics* (1981) 9, 185–90.

Penicillins + Food

Dietary fibre can cause a small reduction in the absorption of amoxicillin, but this is unlikely to be clinically significant. Food reduces the absorption of oral ampicillin, but parenteral and enteral nutrition do not affect intravenous ampicillin levels. The pharmacokinetics of amoxicillin, bacampicillin and co-amoxiclav do not seem to be significantly affected by food.

Clinical evidence, mechanism, importance and management

(a) Dietary fibre

The AUC of a single 500-mg oral dose of **amoxicillin** was found to be 12.17 micrograms/ml per hour in 10 healthy subjects on a low fibre diet (7.8 g of insoluble fibre daily) but only 9.65 micrograms/ml per hour when they ate a high fibre diet (36.2 g of insoluble fibre daily); a difference of about 20%. Peak serum levels were the same and occurred at 3 hours.[1] The clinical relevance of these changes is likely to be minimal.

(b) Enteral and parenteral feeds

A single 250-mg intravenous dose of **ampicillin** was given to 7 healthy subjects 2 hours into a 12-hour infusion of parenteral nutrition or 4 hours after an enteral meal. The parenteral nutrition was of two types, one without amino acids, calcium and phosphorus, both without lipids, and of similar calorific content and volume to the enteral feed. None of the three regimens altered the pharmacokinetics of intravenous **ampicillin**.[2] Note that the **ampicillin** was given in a separate limb to the parenteral nutrition.

(c) Food

(i) Amoxicillin and co-amoxiclav. A standard breakfast had no effect on the AUC of a single 500-mg dose of amoxicillin in 16 healthy subjects.[3] Similarly, a crossover study in 18 healthy subjects given co-amoxiclav (amoxicillin 500 mg with **clavulanic acid** 250 mg), either 2 hours before or with a fried breakfast, found that the breakfast had no significant effect on the pharmacokinetics of amoxicillin or **clavulanic acid**. Moreover, a further study in 43 healthy subjects found that taking co-amoxiclav with food tended to minimise the incidence (but not the severity) of gastrointestinal adverse effects (watery stools, nausea and vomiting).[4] It would therefore be beneficial to take co-amoxiclav with a meal.

(ii) Ampicillin. A standard breakfast reduced the AUC of a single 500-mg dose of ampicillin by 31% in 16 healthy subjects.[3] It is recommended that ampicillin is taken one hour before food or on an empty stomach to optimise absorption.

(iii) Bacampicillin. The AUC of ampicillin was assessed when 6 healthy subjects took a 1600-mg dose of bacampicillin either 35 minutes after breakfast or 2 hours before breakfast. The AUC was 26% lower with the post-breakfast dose, but this difference was not statistically significant.[5] On the basis of other work that also suggests that no important interaction occurs with food,[6,7] the makers say that bacampicillin can be given without regard to time of food intake.

(d) Milk

Co-amoxiclav (**amoxicillin** 500 mg with **clavulanic acid** 250 mg) was given to 16 healthy subjects at the same time as the second of four 200-ml glasses of milk (taken at 20 minute intervals). Although the bioavailability of the **amoxicillin** and **clavulanic acid** tended to be decreased, and the time to peak levels delayed, the changes did not reach statistical significance.[8] No special precautions would seem to be necessary.

1. Lutz M, Espinoza J, Arancibia A, Araya M, Pacheco I, Brunser O. Effect of structured dietary fiber on bioavailability of amoxicillin. *Clin Pharmacol Ther* (1987) 42, 220–4.
2. Koo WWK, Ke J, Tam YK, Finegan BA, Marriage B. Pharmacokinetics of ampicillin during parenteral nutrition. *J Parenter Enteral Nutr* (1990) 14, 279–82.
3. Eshelman FN, Spyker DA. Pharmacokinetics of amoxicillin and ampicillin: crossover study of the effect of food. *Antimicrob Agents Chemother* (1978) 14, 539–43.
4. Staniforth DH, Lillystone RJ, Jackson D. Effect of food on the bioavailability and tolerance of clavulanic acid/amoxycillin combination. *J Antimicrob Chemother* (1982) 10, 131–9.
5. Sommers DK, van Wyk M, Moncrieff J, Schoeman HS. Influence of food and reduced gastric acidity on the bioavailability of bacampicillin and cefuroxime axetil. *Br J Clin Pharmacol* (1984) 18, 535–9.
6. Magni L, Sjöberg B, Sjövall J, Wessman J. Clinical pharmacological studies with bacampicillin. *Chemotherapy* (1976) 5, 109–114.
7. Ali HM. The effect of Sudanese food and chloroquine on the bioavailability of ampicillin from bacampicillin tablets. *Int J Pharmaceutics* (1981) 9, 185–90.
8. Staniforth DH, Clarke HL, Horton R, Jackson D, Lau D. Augmentin bioavailability following cimetidine, aluminium hydroxide and milk. *Int J Clin Pharmacol Ther Toxicol* (1985) 23, 154–7.

Penicillins + Guar gum

Guar gum causes a small reduction in the absorption of phenoxymethylpenicillin (penicillin V).

Clinical evidence, mechanism, importance and management

Guar gum 5 g (*Guarem*, 95% guar gum) reduced the absorption of a single 1980-mg dose of **phenoxymethylpenicillin** (penicillin V) in 10 healthy subjects. Peak serum penicillin levels were reduced by 25% and the 0 to 6-hour AUC was reduced by 28%.[1] The reasons are not understood.

The clinical significance of this interaction is uncertain, but the reduction in serum levels is only small. It would clearly only be important if the reduced amount of penicillin absorbed was inadequate to control infection, and for this reason the makers suggest giving penicillin an hour before the guar gum if it is important to establish maximum serum levels.[2] The effect of guar gum on other penicillins seems not to have been studied.

1. Huupponen R, Seppälä P, Iisalo E. Effect of guar gum, a fibre preparation, on digoxin and penicillin absorption in man. *Eur J Clin Pharmacol* (1984) 26, 279–81.
2. Guarem granules (Guar gum). Rybar Laboratories Ltd. UK Summary of product characteristics, March 2001.

Penicillins + H_2-blockers

Cimetidine does not adversely affect the bioavailability of ampicillin or co-amoxiclav, but the bioavailability of oral benzylpenicillin may be increased in some subjects. Ranitidine does not affect the pharmacokinetics of amoxicillin, but may possibly reduce the bioavailability of bacampicillin.

Clinical evidence, mechanism, importance and management

(a) Amoxicillin and co-amoxiclav

Cimetidine 200 mg, given three times daily the day before and with a single 200-mg dose of co-amoxiclav (amoxicillin with clavulanic acid), had no significant effect on the bioavailability of amoxicillin or clavulanic acid.[1] Another study found that **ranitidine** (300 mg given the day before and 150 mg given with the antibacterial) had no effect on the pharmacokinetics of a single 1-g dose of amoxicillin.[2]

(b) Ampicillin

The pharmacokinetics of ampicillin were unchanged in a placebo controlled study in which 6 healthy subjects were given **cimetidine** 400 mg 6-hourly for 6 days, with a single 500-mg dose of ampicillin on day 6.[3]

(c) Bacampicillin

One small study suggested that when bacampicillin was given with **ranitidine** 300 mg and **sodium bicarbonate** 4 g, the AUC was reduced by 78% when the drugs were given with breakfast and by 55% when the drugs were given without food.[4] However, these results have been criticised because the study only included 6 subjects and because of differences in methodology between compared groups.[5] The findings remain unconfirmed, and their clinical significance is uncertain.

(d) Benzylpenicillin

A study using a 600-mg *oral* dose of benzylpenicillin found that **cimetidine** raised the benzylpenicillin serum levels by about 3-fold in one subject, but did not significantly affect benzylpenicillin levels in another 4 subjects.[5] The clinical significance of these findings is unclear, especially as benzylpenicillin is more usually given parenterally.

1. Staniforth DH, Clarke HL, Horton R, Jackson D, Lau D. Augmentin bioavailability following cimetidine, aluminum hydroxide and milk. *Int J Clin Pharmacol Ther Toxicol* (1985) 23, 145–7.
2. Deppermann K-M, Lode H, Höffken G, Tschink G, Kalz C, Koeppe P. Influence of ranitidine, pirenzepine, and aluminium magnesium hydroxide on the bioavailability of various antibiotics, including amoxicillin, cephalexin, doxycycline, and amoxicillin-clavulanic acid. *Antimicrob Agents Chemother* (1989) 33, 1901–7.
3. Rogers HJ, James CA, Morrison PJ and Bradbrook ID. Effect of cimetidine on oral absorption of ampicillin and co-trimoxazole. *J Antimicrob Chemother* (1980) 6, 297–300.
4. Sommers DK, van Wyk M, Moncrieff J, Schoeman HS. Influence of food and reduced gastric acidity on the bioavailability of bacampicillin and cefuroxime axetil. *Br J Clin Pharmacol* (1984) 18, 535–9.
5. Fairfax AJ, Adam J and Pagan FS. Effect of cimetidine on absorption of oral benzylpenicillin. *BMJ* (1977) 2, 820.

Penicillins + Khat (Catha)

Chewing khat reduces the absorption of ampicillin and, to a lesser extent, amoxicillin, but the effects are minimal 2 hours after khat chewing stops.

Clinical evidence, mechanism, importance and management

A study in 8 healthy Yemeni male subjects found that chewing khat reduced the absorption of oral **ampicillin** from the gut.[1] When the **ampicillin** 500 mg was taken with 250 ml water 2 hours before or just before khat chewing started, or midway through a 4 hour chewing session, the amounts of unchanged **ampicillin** in the urine fell by 46, 41 and 49% respectively. Even when **ampicillin** was taken 2 hours after a chewing session had stopped, the amount of drug excreted unchanged in the urine fell by 12%. A parallel series of studies with **amoxicillin** 500 mg found much smaller reductions. The equivalent reductions were 14, 9, 22 and 13%. A similar study found that chewing khat resulted in variable reduction in the bioavailability of **amoxicillin** 500 mg, which was maximal (22%) when it was given midway during the 4-hour chewing period.[2]

The reasons for this interaction are not known, but the authors of the reports suggest that tannins from the khat might form insoluble and non-absorbable complexes with these penicillins, and possibly also directly reduce the way the gut absorbs them.[1]

Khat (the leaves and stem tips of *Catha edulis*) is chewed in some African and Arabian countries for its stimulatory properties. The authors of one of the studies concluded that both **ampicillin** and **amoxicillin** should be taken 2 hours after khat chewing to ensure that maximum absorption occurs.[1]

1. Attef OA, Abdul-Azem A, Hassan MA. Effect of Khat chewing on the bioavailability of ampicillin and amoxycillin. *J Antimicrob Chemother* (1997) 39, 523–5.
2. Abdel Ghani YM, Etman MA, Nada AH. Effect of khat chewing on the absorption of orally administered amoxycillin. *Acta Pharm* (1999) 49, 43–50.

Penicillins + Miscellaneous

Aspirin, indometacin, phenylbutazone, sulfaphenazole and sulfinpyrazone prolong the half-life of benzylpenicillin whereas chlorothiazide, sulfamethizole and sulfamethoxypyridazine do not. Some sulphonamides reduce oxacillin blood levels. Pirenzepine does not affect the pharmacokinetics of amoxicillin.

Clinical evidence, mechanism, importance and management

Studies in patients given different drugs for 5 to 7 days showed the following increases in the half-life of **benzylpenicillin**: **aspirin** 63%, **indometacin** 22%, **phenylbutazone** 139%, **sulfaphenazole** 44% and **sulfinpyrazone** 65%. It seems likely that competition between these drugs and **benzylpenicillin** for excretion by the kidney tubules caused these increases. Changes in the half-life with **chlorothiazide**, **sulfamethizole** and **sulfamethoxypyridazine** were not significant.[1]

In healthy subjects, **sulfamethoxypyridazine** 3 g given 8 hours before a 1-g dose of oral **oxacillin** reduced the 6-hour urinary recovery by 55%. **Sulfaethidole** 3.9 g given 3 hours before the **oxacillin** reduced the 6-hour urinary recovery by 42%.[2]

Pirenzepine 50 mg given three times daily on the day before and with a single 1-g dose of **amoxicillin** had no significant effect on the pharmacokinetics of the antibacterial.[3]

None of the interactions listed appears to be adverse, and no particular precautions would seem necessary during concurrent use of these drugs and the penicillins. The importance of the interaction between **oxacillin** and the sulphonamides is uncertain, but it can easily be avoided by choosing alternative drugs.

1. Kampmann J, Hansen JM, Siersboek-Nielsen K, Laursen H. Effect of some drugs on penicillin half-life in blood. *Clin Pharmacol Ther* (1972) 13, 516–19.
2. Kunin CM. Clinical pharmacology of the new penicillins. II. Effect of drugs which interfere with binding to serum proteins. *Clin Pharmacol Ther* (1966) 7, 180–88.
3. Deppermann K-M, Lode H, Höffken G, Tschink G, Kalz C, Koeppe P. Influence of ranitidine, pirenzepine, and aluminium magnesium hydroxide on the bioavailability of various antibiotics, including amoxicillin, cephalexin, doxycycline, and amoxicillin-clavulanic acid. *Antimicrob Agents Chemother* (1989) 33, 1901–7.

Penicillins + Nifedipine

Nifedipine increases the absorption of amoxicillin from the gut but this is unlikely to be clinically important. Nafcillin increases the clearance of nifedipine, but the clinical significance of this is unclear.

Clinical evidence, mechanism, importance and management

(a) Amoxicillin

When amoxicillin 1 g was given half-an-hour after a nifedipine 20-mg capsule, the peak serum amoxicillin levels in 8 healthy subjects were raised by 33%, the bioavailability was raised by 21% and the absorption rate was raised by 70%.[1] The authors speculate that the uptake of amoxicillin through the gut wall is increased by nifedipine in some way.[1] There would seem to be no good reason for avoiding concurrent use.

(b) Nafcillin

In a randomised placebo-controlled crossover study, 9 healthy subjects were given a single 10-mg nifedipine capsule after a 5-day course of nafcillin 500 mg four times daily. The nifedipine AUC was decreased by 63% and the clearance was increased by 145%, but the effect of these changes on nifedipine pharmacodynamics was not assessed. It was suggested that nafcillin is an inducer of cytochrome P450 isoenzymes, and increased the metabolism of nifedipine.[2] The clinical significance of these changes is unclear.

1. Westphal J-F, Trouvin J-H, Deslandes A, Carbon C. Nifedipine enhances amoxicillin absorption kinetics and bioavailability in humans. *J Pharmacol Exp Ther* (1990) 255, 312–17.
2. Lang CC, Jamal SK, Mohamed Z, Mustafa MR, Mustafa AM, Lee TC. Evidence of an interaction between nifedipine and nafcillin in humans. *Br J Clin Pharmacol* (2003) 55, 588–90.

Penicillins + Probenecid

Probenecid reduces the excretion of the penicillins.

Clinical evidence

(a) Amoxicillin

Amoxicillin 3 g twice daily plus placebo, amoxicillin 1 g twice daily plus probenecid 1 g twice daily, and amoxicillin 1 g twice daily plus probenecid 500 mg four times daily were given to 6 patients to treat bronchiectasis. The maximum serum concentration and half-life of both high- and low-dose amoxicillin were similar, but in the regimens containing probenecid the clearance of amoxicillin dropped to one-third of the level of that seen with amoxicillin alone.[1]

(b) Nafcillin

A study in 5 healthy subjects given 500 mg of intravenous nafcillin sodium with probenecid, 1 g given orally the previous night and 1 g given 2 hours prior to the antibacterial, showed that the urinary recovery of nafcillin dropped from 30% to 17% and its AUC was approximately doubled.[2]

(c) Piperacillin/Tazobactam

Probenecid 1 g given 1 hour before a single infusion of piperacillin 3 g/tazobactam 375 mg in 10 healthy subjects caused a decrease of about 25% in the clearance of both components. The half-life of tazobactam was increased by 72%.[3]

(d) Ticarcillin

Probenecid, either 500 mg twice daily, 1 g daily, or 2 g daily was added to ticarcillin 3 g four-hourly, which was being given to treat infections in adult cystic fibrosis patients. In all cases the clearance of ticarcillin was reduced: to 72.7% with the 500-mg dose regimen, to 67.5% with the 1-g dose regimen and to 57.3% with the 2-g dose regimen.[4]

Mechanism

In each case the penicillin competes with the probenecid for excretion by the kidney tubules, although with the nafcillin, non-renal clearance may also play a part.

Importance and management

In the case of amoxicillin, nafcillin and ticarcillin the effects are of clinical significance. In the case of the ticarcillin study the authors suggest that a 12-hourly dosing regimen could be used if probenecid is given concurrently, which has implications for home treatment. With piperacillin/tazobactam the changes were not thought to provide any benefit in terms of dose reduction or alteration of the dosage interval.

1. Allen MB, Fitzpatrick RW, Barratt A, Cole RB. The use of probenecid to increase the serum amoxycillin levels in patients with bronchiectasis. *Respir Med* (1990) 84, 143–6.
2. Waller ES, Sharanevych MA, Yakatan GJ. The effect of probenecid on nafcillin disposition. *J Clin Pharmacol* (1982) 22, 482–9.
3. Ganes D, Batra V, Faulkner R, Greene D, Haynes J, Kuye O, Ruffner A, Shin K, Tonelli A, Yacobi A. Effect of probenecid on the pharmacokinetics of piperacillin and tazobactam in healthy volunteers. *Pharm Res* (1991) 8 (10 Suppl), S-299.
4. Corvaia L, Li SC, Ioannides-Demos LL, Bowes G, Spicer WJ, Spelman DW, Tong N, McLean AJ. A prospective study of the effects of oral probenecid on the pharmacokinetics of intravenous ticarcillin in patients with cystic fibrosis. *J Antimicrob Chemother* (1992) 30, 875–8.

Penicillins + Tetracyclines

Tetracyclines can reduce the effectiveness of penicillins in the treatment of pneumococcal meningitis and probably scarlet fever. It is uncertain whether a similar interaction occurs with other infections. This interaction may possibly be important only with those infections where a rapid kill is essential.

Clinical evidence

When **chlortetracycline** originally became available it was tested as a potential treatment for meningitis. In patients with pneumococcal meningitis it was shown that penicillin one million units, intramuscularly every 2 hours was more effective than the same regimen of penicillin with **chlortetracycline** 500 mg intravenously every 6 hours. Out of 43 patients given penicillin alone, 70% recovered compared with only 20% in another group of 14 essentially similar patients who had received both antibacterials.[1]

Another report about the treatment of pneumococcal meningitis with penicillin and tetracyclines (**chlortetracycline**, **oxytetracycline**, tetracycline) confirmed that the mortality was much lower in those given only penicillin, rather than the combination of penicillin and a tetracycline.[2] In the treatment of scarlet fever (Group A beta-haemolytic streptococci), no difference was seen in the initial response to treatment with penicillin and tetracycline or penicillin alone, but spontaneous re-infection occurred more frequently in those who had received penicillin and **chlortetracycline**.[3]

Mechanism

The generally accepted explanation is that bactericides such as penicillin, which inhibits bacterial cell wall synthesis, require cells to be actively growing and dividing to be maximally effective, a situation that will not occur in the presence of bacteriostatic antibacterials, such as the tetracyclines.

Importance and management

An established and apparently important interaction when treating pneumococcal meningitis (although this combination has largely been superseded), and probably scarlet fever as well. The documentation seems to be limited to the reports cited. Concurrent use should be avoided in these infections, but the importance of this interaction with other infections is uncertain. It has not been shown to occur when treating pneumococcal pneumonia.[4] It has been suggested that antagonism, if it occurs, may only be significant when it is essential to kill bacteria rapidly,[4] i.e. in serious infections such as meningitis. Any penicillin and any tetracycline would be expected to behave in this way.

Note, macrolides, which are also bacteriostatic would be expected to attenuate the action of penicillins, but this does not seem to occur in practice. See 'Macrolides + Penicillins', p.217.

1. Lepper MH, Dowling HF. Treatment of pneumococcic meningitis with penicillin compared with penicillin plus aureomycin: studies including observations on an apparent antagonism between penicillin and aureomycin. *Arch Intern Med* (1951) 88, 489–94.
2. Olsson RA, Kirby JC, Romansky MJ. Pneumococcal meningitis in the adult. Clinical, therapeutic and prognostic aspects in forty-three patients. *Ann Intern Med* (1961) 55, 545–9.
3. Strom J. The question of antagonism between penicillin and chlortetracycline, illustrated by therapeutical experiments in Scarlatina. *Antibiotic Med* (1955) 1,6–12.
4. Ahern JJ, Kirby WMM. Lack of interference of aureomycin in treatment of pneumoccic pneumonia. *Arch Intern Med* (1953) 91, 197–203.

Penicillins; Amoxicillin + Amiloride

Amiloride can cause a small, probably clinically unimportant, reduction in the absorption of amoxicillin.

Clinical evidence, mechanism, importance and management

When 8 healthy subjects were given amiloride 10 mg followed 2 hours later by a single 1-g oral dose of amoxicillin, the bioavailability and maximum serum levels of amoxicillin were reduced by 27 and 25% respectively, and the time to reach maximum levels was delayed from 1 hour to 1.56 hours. When amoxicillin was given intravenously its bioavailability was unchanged by amiloride.[1] It is thought that the absorption of beta lactams like amoxicillin depends on a dipeptide carrier system in the cells (brush border membrane) lining the intestine. This system depends on the existence of a pH gradient between the outside and inside of the cells, which is maintained by a Na-H exchanger. As this exchanger is inhibited by amiloride the reduced absorption would seem to be explained.

This reported reduction in the absorption of the amoxicillin is only small and unlikely to have very much clinical relevance, but this needs confirmation. There seems to be no information about other penicillins.

1. Westphal JF, Jehl F, Brogard JM, Carbon C. Amoxicillin intestinal absorption reduction by amiloride: possible role of the Na(+)-H(+) exchanger. *Clin Pharmacol Ther* (1995) 57, 257–64.

Penicillins; Piperacillin/tazobactam + Vancomycin

Vancomycin does not interact to a clinically relevant extent with piperacillin/tazobactam.

Clinical evidence, mechanism, importance and management

A three-way, randomised crossover study in 9 healthy subjects found that infusions of vancomycin 500 mg and piperacillin 3 g with tazobactam 375 mg had little or no effect on the pharmacokinetics of any of the antibacterials, except that the piperacillin AUC was slightly raised, by about 7%. It was concluded that no dosage adjustments are needed if these drugs are given together.[1]

1. Vechlekar D, Sia L, Lanc R, Kuye O, Yacobi A, Faulkner R. Pharmacokinetics of piperacillin/tazobactam (Pip/Taz) IV with and without vancomycin IV in healthy adult male volunteers. *Pharm Res* (1992) 9 (10 Suppl), S-322.

Penicillins; Pivampicillin + Miscellaneous

On theoretical grounds the makers of pivampicillin advise the avoidance of sodium valproate because of the increased risk of carnitine deficiency. Antacids may reduce the absorption of the hydrochloride salt of pivampicillin.

Clinical evidence, mechanism, importance and management

Pivampicillin is a prodrug of ampicillin which, following absorption, is hydrolysed to release ampicillin, pivalic acid and formaldehyde. One of the potential problems of this drug is that the pivalic acid can react with carnitine to form pivaloyl-carnitine, which is excreted in the urine, and so the body can become depleted of carnitine. Carnitine deficiency manifests as muscle weakness and cardiomyopathy.

The risks of carnitine deficiency due to pivampicillin (or pivmecillinam, which similarly releases pivalic acid) seem to be small in healthy adults, but the makers of pivampicillin issue a warning about long-term or frequently repeated treatment.[1] They also advise the avoidance of **valproic acid** or **valproate**[1] because they too can cause an increased carnitine loss from the body (for reasons that are not well understood).[2] However, there seem to be no reports of carnitine deficiency in patients that have resulted from the additive effects of pivampicillin and **valproic acid** or **valproate**, so that the risk as yet appears to be only theoretical.

The UK makers[1] used to recommend that, because antacids may decrease pivampicillin absorption, concurrent use should be avoided. This warning relates to a hydrochloride salt formulation, which needs acidic conditions for optimal absorption, whereas the basic salt formulation should not be affected by any pH change.[3]

1. Pondocillin (Pivampicillin). Leo Laboratories Ltd. ABPI Compendium of Datasheets and Summaries of Product Characteristics, 1998–99, 625–6.
2. Melegh B, Kerner J, Jaszai V, Bieber LL. Differential excretion of xenobiotic acyl-esters of carnitine due to administration of pivampicillin and valproate. *Biochem Med Metab Biol* (1990) 43, 30–8.
3. Leo Laboratories Limited. Personal communication, March 1995.

Protionamide + Other antituberculars

Protionamide appears to be very hepatotoxic and this is possibly increased by the concurrent use of rifampicin or rifandin. Protionamide does not affect the pharmacokinetics of either dapsone or rifampicin.

Clinical evidence

In a study of 39 patients with leprosy, 39% became jaundiced after 24 to 120 days' treatment with **dapsone** 100 mg daily, protionamide 300 mg daily and **rifandin** [isopiperazinylrifamycin SV] 300 to 600 mg monthly. Laboratory evidence of liver damage occurred in a total of 56% of patients and despite the withdrawal of the drugs from all the patients, 2 of them died.[1] All the patients except two had taken **dapsone** before, alone, for 3 to 227 months without reported problems.[1] In another group of leprosy patients, 22% (11 of 50) had liver damage after treatment with **dapsone** 100 mg and protionamide 300 mg daily, with **rifampicin** 900 mg, protionamide 500 mg and **clofazimine** 300 mg monthly for 30 to 50 days. One patient died.[1] Most of the patients recovered within 30 to 60 days after withdrawing the treatment.

Jaundice, liver damage and deaths have occurred in other leprosy patients given **rifampicin** and protionamide or **ethionamide**.[2-4] Protionamide does not affect the pharmacokinetics of either **dapsone** or **rifampicin**.[5]

Mechanism

Although not certain, it seems probable that the liver damage was primarily caused by the protionamide, possibly exacerbated by the rifampicin or the rifandin.

Importance and management

This serious and potentially life-threatening hepatotoxic reaction to protionamide is established, but the part played by the other drugs, particularly the rifampicin, is uncertain. Strictly speaking this may not be an interaction. If protionamide is given the liver function should be very closely monitored in order to detect toxicity as soon as possible.

1. Baohong J, Jiakun C, Chenmin W, Guang X. Hepatotoxicity of combined therapy with rifampicin and daily prothionamide for leprosy. *Lepr Rev* (1984) 55, 283–9.
2. Lesobre R, Ruffino J, Teyssier L, Achard F, Brefort G. Les ictères au cours du traitement par la rifampicine. *Rev Tuberc Pneumol (Paris)* (1969) 33, 393–403.
3. Report of the Third Meeting of the Scientific Working Group on Chemotherapy of Leprosy (THELEP) of the UNDP/World Bank/WHO Special Programme for Research and Training in Tropical Diseases. *Int J Lepr* (1981) 49, 431–6.
4. Cartel J-L, Millan J, Guelpa-Lauras C-C, Grosset JH. Hepatitis in leprosy patients treated by a daily combination of dapsone, rifampin, and a thioamide. *Int J Lepr* (1983) 51, 461–5.
5. Mathur A, Venkatesan K, Girdhar BK, Bharadwaj VP, Girdhar A, Bagga AK. A study of drug interactions in leprosy — 1. Effect of simultaneous administration of prothionamide on metabolic disposition of rifampicin and dapsone. *Lepr Rev* (1986) 57, 33–7.

Pyrazinamide + Antacids

An aluminium/magnesium hydroxide antacid had no important effect on the absorption of pyrazinamide.

Clinical evidence, mechanism, importance and management

In 14 healthy subjects 30 ml of *Mylanta* (**aluminium/magnesium hydroxide**) given 9 hours before, with, and after a single 30-mg/kg dose of pyrazinamide decreased the time to peak absorption by 17%, but had no effect on other pharmacokinetics parameters.[1] This change is not clinically important.

1. Peloquin CA, Bulpitt AE, Jaresko GS, Jelliffe RW, James GT, Nix DE. Pharmacokinetics of pyrazinamide under fasting conditions, with food, and with antacids. *Pharmacotherapy* (1998) 18, 1205–11.

Pyrazinamide + Antigout drugs

Allopurinol is unlikely to be effective against pyrazinamide-induced hyperuricaemia, and may exacerbate the situation. The uricosuric effects of probenecid are reduced by pyrazinamide. The makers of pyrazinamide say that it is contraindicated in hyperuricaemia and should be stopped if gouty arthritis develops.

Clinical evidence, mechanism, importance and management

(a) Allopurinol

It is thought that pyrazinamide is hydrolysed in the body to pyrazinoic acid, which appears to be responsible for the hyperuricaemic effect of pyrazinamide. Pyrazinoic acid is oxidised by the enzyme xanthine oxidase to 5-hydroxypyrazoic acid.[1] Since allopurinol is an inhibitor of xanthine oxidase, its presence increases pyrazinoic acid concentrations[2] thereby probably worsening the pyrazinamide-induced hyperuricaemia.[3] Allopurinol would therefore appear to be unsuitable for treating pyrazinamide-induced hyperuricaemia.

In addition it should be pointed out that the makers of pyrazinamide warn that hyperuricaemia is a contraindication for its use, and that if hyperuricaemia accompanied by acute gouty arthritis occurs during treatment, the pyrazinamide should be stopped and not restarted. They also say that pyrazinamide should not be given unless regular uric acid determinations can be made.[4]

(b) Probenecid

The interactions of probenecid and pyrazinamide and their effects on the excretion of uric acid are complex and intertwined. Probenecid increases the secretion of uric acid into the urine, apparently by inhibiting its reabsorption from the kidney tubules.[5] Pyrazinamide on the other hand decreases the secretion of uric acid into the urine by a third to a half,[6] resulting in a rise in the serum levels of urate in the blood, thereby causing hyperuricaemia.[6,7] The result of using probenecid and pyrazinamide together is not however merely the simple sum of these two effects. This is because pyrazinamide additionally decreases the metabolism of the probenecid so that the uricosuric effects of probenecid are prolonged, and the effect of pyrazinamide is reduced. Also, probenecid inhibits the secretion of pyrazinamide, increasing its effects.[8]

The likely overall effect is that if probenecid were to be used to treat the hyperuricaemia caused by pyrazinamide, the normal uricosuric effects of probenecid would be diminished, and larger doses would be required. However, see (a) allopurinol above, for advice relating to hyperuricaemia caused by pyrazinamide.

1. Weiner IM, Tinker JP. Pharmacology of pyrazinamide: metabolic and renal function studies related to the mechanism of drug-induced urate retention. *J Pharmacol Exp Ther* (1972) 180, 411–34.
2. Lacroix C, Guyonnaud C, Chaou M, Duwoos H, Lafont O. Interaction between allopurinol and pyrazinamide. *Eur Respir J* (1988) 807–11.
3. Urban T, Maquarre E, Housset C, Chouaid C, Devin E, Lebeau B. Hypersensibilité à l'allopurinol. Une cause possible d'hépatite et d'éruption cutanéo-muqueuse chez un patient sous antituberculeux. *Rev Mal Respir* (1995) 12, 314–16.
4. Zinamide (Pyrazinamide). Merck Sharp & Dohme. UK Summary of product characteristics, January 1998.
5. Meisel AD, Diamond HS. Mechanism of probenecid-induced uricosuria: inhibition of reabsorption of secreted urate. *Arthritis Rheum* (1977) 20, 128.
6. Cullen JH, LeVine M, Fiore JM. Studies of hyperuricemia produced by pyrazinamide. *Am J Med* (1957) 23, 587–95.
7. Shapiro M, Hyde L. Hyperuricemia due to pyrazinamide. *Am J Med* (1957) 23, 596–9.
8. Yü T-F, Perel J, Berger L, Roboz J, Israili ZH, Dayton PG. The effect of the interaction of pyrazinamide and probenecid on urinary uric acid excretion in man. *Am J Med* (1977) 63, 723–8.

Pyrazinamide + Food

Food reduces the rate but not the extent of absorption of pyrazinamide.

Clinical evidence, mechanism, importance and management

A single 30-mg/kg dose of pyrazinamide taken with a **high-fat breakfast** approximately doubled the time to peak absorption in 14 subjects but had no effect on other pharmacokinetics parameters.[1] It would therefore seem that pyrazinamide may be taken without regard to meals.

1. Peloquin CA, Bulpitt AE, Jaresko GS, Jelliffe RW, James GT, Nix DE. Pharmacokinetics of pyrazinamide under fasting conditions, with food, and with antacids. *Pharmacotherapy* (1998) 18, 1205–11.

Quinolones + Antacids or Calcium compounds

The serum levels of many of the quinolone antibacterials can be reduced by aluminium and magnesium antacids. Calcium compounds interact to a lesser extent, and bismuth compounds only minimally. Separating administration by 2 to 6 hours where significant interactions occur reduces admixture in the gut and can minimise the effects. The details are shown in 'Table 8.2', (p.228).

Clinical evidence

There is a wealth of information about the interaction between quinolones and antacids and for simplicity this is summarised in 'Table 8.2', (p.228). This table shows what happens to the maximum serum levels (C_{max}) and

Table 8.2 Quinolone antibacterial/antacid interactions

Quinolone (mg:time[a])	Antacid or other coadministered drug	C_{max} (μg/ml) alone	C_{max} (μg/ml) with	Relative bioavailability (%)[b]	Refs
Ciprofloxacin					
250	$Mg(OH)_2$ + $Al(OH)_3$	3.69	<1.25	NR	1
500	$Mg(OH)_2$ + $Al(OH)_3$	2.6	0.88	NR	2
500: +24 h	$Mg(OH)_2$ + $Al(OH)_3$	1.7	0.1	NR	3
500: +24 h	$Mg(OH)_2$ + $Al(OH)_3$	1.9	0.13	9.5	4
750: –2 h	$Mg(OH)_2$ + $Al(OH)_3$	3.01	3.96	107.0	5
+0.08 h		3.42	0.68	15.1	
+2 h		3.42	0.88	23.2	
+4 h		3.01	2.62	70.0	
+6 h		2.63	2.64	108.5	
750: +0.08 h	$Al(OH)_3$	3.2	0.6	15.0	6
750	$Al(OH)_3$	2.3	0.8	NR	7
200	$Al(OH)_3$	1.3	0.2	12.0	8
250	$CaCO_3$	3.69	3.42 (ns)	NR	1
500	$CaCO_3$	1.53	1.37 (ns)	94.0 (ns)	9
500	$CaCO_3$	2.9	1.8	58.8	10
750: 0.08 h	$CaCO_3$	3.2	1.7	64.5	6
500: +2 h	$CaCO_3$	1.25	1.44	102.4	11
500	$CaCO_3$	2.9	1.8	58.9	12
500	Mg citrate	2.4	0.6	21.0	13
500	Bismuth salicylate (subsalicylate)	3.8	2.9	83.8	14
750	Bismuth salicylate (subsalicylate)	2.95	2.57	87.0	15
500	Tripotassium dicitratobismuthate			100	13
Enoxacin					
200	$Al(OH)_3$	2.26	0.46	15.4	16
400: +0.5 h	$Mg(OH)_2$ + $Al(OH)_3$	3.17	0.95	26.8	17
+2 h		3.17	1.95	52.3	
+8 h		3.17	2.88	82.7	
200	$Al(OH)_3$	2.3	0.5	15.8	8
Fleroxacin					
200	$Al(OH)_3$	2.4	1.8	82.8	8
Gatifloxacin					
200	$Al(OH)_3$	1.71	0.75	45.9	18
400	$Mg(OH)_2$ + $Al(OH)_3$	3.8	1.2	35.6	19
400: –2 h		3.8	2.1	57.9	
+2 h		3.4	3.3	82.5	
+4 h		3.4	3.5 (ns)	100.0 (ns)	
Gemifloxacin					
320	$CaCO_3$	1.13	0.9	77	20
320: –2 h		1.13	1.13	93	
+2 h		1.11	1.01	90	
Grepafloxacin					
200	$Al(OH)_3$	NR	NR	60.0	21
Levofloxacin					
100	$Al(OH)_3$	1.82	0.64	56.3	22
100	$Al(OH)_3$	1.8	0.6	54.8	8
100	MgO	1.82	1.13	78.2	22
100	$CaCO_3$	1.45	1.12	96.7	22
Lomefloxacin					
200	$Mg(OH)_2$ + $Al(OH)_3$	1.91	1.03	59.2	23
200	$Al(OH)_3$	2.2	1.0	65.2	8
NR: +2 h	$Mg(OH)_2$ + $Al(OH)_3$	2.85	2.67 (ns)	88.2	24
–2 h		2.85	2.16	80.4	
–4 h		2.85	2.67 (ns)	90.1	
400	$Mg(OH)_2$ + $Al(OH)_3$	3.25	1.31	52.1	25
400: +12 h		3.25	3.66 (ns)		
–4 h		3.25	3.69 (ns)		
400	$CaCO_3$	4.72	4.08	97.9 (ns)	26

Continued

Table 8.2 Quinolone antibacterial/antacid interactions *(continued)*

Quinolone (mg:time[a])	*Antacid or other coadministered drug*	*C_{max} (μg/ml)*		*Relative bioavailability (%)[b]*	*Refs*
		alone	*with*		
Moxifloxacin					
400	$Mg(OH)_2 + Al(OH)_3$	2.57	1.0	74.0	27
400	$CaCO_3$	2.71	2.29	97.6	28
Norfloxacin					
200	$Al(OH)_3$	1.45	< 0.01	2.7	16
400: +0.08 h	$Mg(OH)_2 + Al(OH)_3$	1.64	0.08	9.0 (based on urinary recovery)	29
−2 h		1.64	1.25	81.3	
200	$Al(OH)_3$	1.5	< 0.10	3.0	8
400	$Al(OH)_3$	1.51	1.09	71.2 (from saliva)	30
400	Mg trisilicate	1.51	0.43	19.3 (from saliva)	30
400	$CaCO_3$	1.64	0.56	37.5	29
400	$CaCO_3$	1.51	1.08	52.8 (from saliva)	30
400	Bismuth salicylate (subsalicylate)			89.7 (ns)	31
400	Sodium bicarbonate	1.40	1.47	104.9 (ns)	30
Ofloxacin					
200	$Al(OH)_3$	3.23	1.31	52.1	16
200	$Al(PO)_4$			93.1 (ns)	32
200	$MgO + Al(OH)_3$	1.97	1.10	62.0	33
200: +24 h	$Mg(OH)_2 + Al(OH)_3$	2.6	0.7	30.8	4
400: +2 h	$Mg(OH)_2 + Al(OH)_3$	3.7	2.6	79.2	34
−2 h		3.7	3.8 (ns)	101.9 (ns)	
+24 h		3.7	3.5 (ns)	95.3 (ns)	
600	$Mg(OH)_2 + Al(OH)_3$	8.11	6.13	NR	35
200	$Al(OH)_3$	3.2	1.3	52.1	8
400: +2 h	$CaCO_3$	3.2	3.3 (ns)	103.6 (ns)	34
−2 h		3.2	3.3 (ns)	97.9 (ns)	
+24 h		3.2	3.5 (ns)	95.9 (ns)	
Pefloxacin					
400	$Mg(OH)_2 + Al(OH)_3$	5.14	1.95	44.2	36
400	$Mg(OH)_2 + Al(OH)_3$	3.95	1.25	NR	37
400	$Mg(OH)_2 + Al(OH)_3$	5.1	2.0	45.7	38
Rufloxacin					
400: +0.08 h	$Mg(OH)_2 + Al(OH)_3$	3.74	2.12	59.7	39
−4 h		3.74	3.97 (ns)	84.7	39
Sparfloxacin					
400: −2 h	$Mg(OH)_2 + Al(OH)_3$	1.09	0.77	74.4	40
+2 h		1.09	0.95	82.4	
+4 h		1.09	1.17	93.4	
200	$Al(OH)_3$	0.865	0.683	64.9	8, 41
Tosufloxacin					
150	$Al(OH)_3$	0.3	0.1	29.2	8
Trovafloxacin					
300: −2 h	$Mg(OH)_2 + Al(OH)_3$	2.8	2.5	71.7	42
+0.5 h		2.8	1.1	33.7	

[a]*Time interval between intake of quinolone and the other agent: – and + indicate that the quinolone was administered before and after, respectively, intake of the other agent.*
[b]*Calculated from AUC data.*
NR = not reported; h = hour; ns = not significant

1. Fleming LW, Moreland TA, Stewart WK, Scott AC. Ciprofloxacin and antacids. *Lancet* (1986) ii, 294.
2. Preheim LC, Cuevas TA, Roccaforte JS, Mellencamp MA, Bittner MJ. Ciprofloxacin and antacids. *Lancet* (1986) ii, 48.
3. Höffken G, Borner K, Glatzel PD, Koeppe P, Lode H. Reduced enteral absorption of ciprofloxacin in the presence of antacids. *Eur J Clin Microbiol* (1985) 4, 345.
4. Höffken G, Lode H, Wiley R, Glatzel TD, Sievers D, Olschewski T, Borner K, Koeppe T. Pharmacokinetics and bioavailability of ciprofloxacin and ofloxacin: effect of food and antacid intake. *Rev Infect Dis* (1988) 10 (Suppl 1), S138–S139.
5. Nix DE, Watson WA, Lener ME, Frost RW, Krol G, Goldstein H, Lettieri J, Schentag JJ. Effects of aluminum and magnesium antacids and ranitidine on the absorption of ciprofloxacin. *Clin Pharmacol Ther* (1989) 46, 700–705.

Continued

Table 8.2 Quinolone antibacterial/antacid interactions *(continued)*

6. Frost RW, Lettieri JT, Noe A, Shamblen EC, Lasseter K. Effect of aluminum hydroxide and calcium carbonate antacids on ciprofloxacin bioavailability. *Clin Pharmacol Ther* (1989) 45, 165.7.Golper TA, Hartstein AI, Morthland VH, Christensen JM. Effects of antacids and dialysate dwell times on multiple-dose pharmacokinetics of oral ciprofloxacin in patients on continuous ambulatory peritoneal dialysis. *Antimicrob Agents Chemother* (1987) 31, 1787–90.
8. Shiba K, Sakamoto M, Nakazawa Y, Sakai O. Effect of antacid on absorption and excretion of new quinolones. *Drugs* (1995) 49 (Suppl 2), 360–1.9.Lomaestro BM, Bailie GR. Effect of multiple staggered doses of calcium on the bioavailability of ciprofloxacin. *Ann Pharmacother* (1993) 27, 1325–8.
10. Sahai J, Healey DP, Stotka J, Polk RE. The influence of chronic administration of calcium carbonate on the bioavailability of oral ciprofloxacin. *Br J Clin Pharmacol* (1993) 35, 302–4.
11. Lomaestro BM, Bailie GR. Effect of staggered dose of calcium on the bioavailability of ciprofloxacin. *Antimicrob Agents Chemother* (1991) 35, 1004–1007.
12. Sahai J, Healy D, Stotka J, Polk R. Influence of chronic administration of calcium (CA) on the bioavailability (BA) of oral ciprofloxacin (CIP). *Intersci Conf Antimicrob Agents Chemother* (1989) 29, 136.
13. Brouwers JRBJ, van der Kam HJ, Sijtsma J, Proost JH. Important reduction of ciprofloxacin absorption by sucralfate and magnesium citrate solution. *Drug Invest* (1990) 2, 197–9.
14. Sahai J, Oliveras L, Garber G. Effect of bismuth subsalicylate (Peptobismol. PB) on ciprofloxacin (C) absorption: a preliminary investigation. *17th Int Congr Chemother*, June 1991, Berlin, Abstract 414.
15. Rambout L, Sahai J, Gallicano K, Oliveras L, Garber G. Effect of bismuth subsalicylate on ciprofloxacin bioavailability. *Antimicrob Agents Chemother* (1994) 38, 2187–90.
16. Shiba K, Saito A, Miyahara T, Tachizawa H, Fujimoto T. Effect of aluminium hydroxide, an antacid, on the pharmacokinetics of new quinolones in humans. *Proc 15th Int Congr Chemother*, Istanbul 1987, 168–9.
17. Grasela TH, Schentag JJ, Sedman AJ, Wilton JH, Thomas DJ, Schultz RW, Lebsack ME, Kinkel AW. Inhibition of enoxacin absorption by antacids or ranitidine. *Antimicrob Agents Chemother* (1989) 33, 615–17.
18. Shiba K, Kusajima H, Momo K. The effects of aluminium hydroxide, cimetidine, ferrous sulfate, green tea and milk on pharmacokinetics of gatifloxacin in healthy humans. *J Antimicrob Chemother* (1999) 44 (Suppl A), 141.
19. Lober S, Ziege S, Rau M, Schreiber G, Mignot A, Koeppe P, Lode H. Pharmacokinetics of gatifloxacin and interaction with an antacid containing aluminum and magnesium. *Antimicrob Agents Chemother* (1999) 43, 1067–71.
20. Pletz MW, Petzold P, Allen A, Burkhardt O, Lode H. Effect of calcium carbonate on bioavailability of orally administered gemifloxacin. *Antimicrob Agents Chemother* (2003) 47, 2158–60.
21. Koneru B, Bramer S, Bricmont P, Maroli A, Shiba K. Effect of food, gastric pH and co-administration of antacid, cimetidine and probenecid on the oral pharmacokinetics of the broad spectrum antimicrobial agent grepafloxacin. *Pharm Res* (1996) 13 (9 Suppl), S414.
22. Shiba K, Sakai O, Shimada J, Okazaki O, Aoki H, Hakusui H. Effects of antacids, ferrous sulfate, and ranitidine on absorption of DR-3355 in humans. *Antimicrob Agents Chemother* (1992) 36, 2270–4.
23. Shimada J, Shiba K, Oguma T, Miwa H, Yoshimura Y, Nishikawa T, Okabayashi Y, Kitagawa T, Yamamoto S. Effect of antacid on absorption of the quinolone lomefloxacin. *Antimicrob Agents Chemother* (1992) 36, 1219–24.
24. Forster T, Blouin R. The effect of antacid timing on lomefloxacin bioavailability. *Intersci Conf Antimicrob Agents Chemother* (1989) 29, 318.
25. Kunka RL, Wong YY, Lyon JL. Effect of antacid on the pharmacokinetics of lemofloxacin. *Pharm Res* (1988) 5 (Suppl), S-165.
26. Lehto P, Kivistö KT. Different effects of products containing metal ions on the absorption of lomefloxacin. *Clin Pharmacol Ther* (1994) 56, 477–82.
27. Stass H, Böttcher M-F, Ochmann K. Evaluation of the influence of antacids and H_2 antagonists on the absorption of moxifloxacin after oral administration of a 400-mg dose to healthy volunteers. *Clin Pharmacokinet* (2001) 40 (Suppl 1), 39–48.
28. Stass H, Kubitza D. Profile of moxifloxacin drug interactions. *Clin Infect Dis* (2001) 32, (Suppl 1), S47–S50.
29. Nix DE, Wilton JH, Ronald B, Distlerath L, Williams VC, Norman A. Inhibition of norfloxacin absorption by antacids. *Antimicrob Agents Chemother* (1990) 34, 432–5.
30. Okhamafe AO, Akerele JO, Chukuka CS. Pharmacokinetic interactions of norfloxacin with some metallic medicinal agents. *Int J Pharmaceutics* (1991) 68, 11–18.
31. Campbell NRC, Kara M, Hasinoff BB, Haddara WM, McKay DW. Norfloxacin interaction with antacids and minerals. *Br J Clin Pharmacol* (1992) 33, 115–16.
32. Martínez Carbaga M, Sánchez Navarro A, Colino Gandarillas CI, Domínguez-Gil A. Effects of two cations on gastrointestinal absorption of ofloxacin. *Antimicrob Agents Chemother* (1991) 35, 2102–5.
33. Shiba K, Yoshida M, Kachi M, Shimada J, Saito A, Sakai N. Effects of peptic ulcer-healing drugs on the pharmacokinetics of new quinolone (OFLX). *17th Int Congr Chemother*, June 1991, Berlin, Abstract 415.
34. Flor S, Guay DRP, Opsahl JA, Tack K, Matzke GR. Effects of magnesium-aluminum hydroxide and calcium carbonate antacids on bioavailability of ofloxacin. *Antimicrob Agents Chemother* (1990) 34, 2436–8.
35. Maesen FPV, Davies BI, Geraedts WH, Sumajow CA. Ofloxacin and antacids. *J Antimicrob Chemother* (1987) 19, 848–50.
36. Metz R, Jaehde U, Sörgel F, Wiesemann H, Gottschalk B, Stephan U, Schunack W. Pharmacokinetic interactions and non-interactions of pefloxacin. *Proc 15th Int Congr Chemother*, Istanbul, 1987, 997–9.
37. Vinceneux P, Weber P, Gaudin H, Boussougant Y. Diminution de l'absorption de la péfloxacine par les pansements gastriques. *Presse Med* (1986) 15, 1826.
38. Jaehde U, Sörgel F, Stephan U, Schunack W. Effect of an antacid containing magnesium and aluminum on absorption, metabolism and mechanism of renal elimination of pefloxacin in humans. *Antimicrob Agents Chemother* (1994) 38, 1129–33.
39. Lazzaroni M, Imbimbo BP, Bargiggia S, Sangaletti O, Dal Bo L, Broccali G, Bianchi Porro G. Effects of magnesium-aluminum hydroxide antacid on absorption of rufloxacin. *Antimicrob Agents Chemother* (1993) 37, 2212–16.
40. Wilson J, Johnson RD, Caille G, Talbot G, Dorr MB, Heald D. The effect of staggered dosing of Maalox® on the oral bioavailability of sparfloxacin. *Pharm Res* (1994) 11 (10 Suppl), S-429.
41. Shimada J, Saito A, Shiba K, Hojo T, Kaji M, Hori S, Yoshida M, Sakai O. Pharmacokinetics and clinical studies on sparfloxacin. *Chemotherapy (Tokyo)* (1991) 39 (Suppl 4), 234–44.
42. Teng R, Dogolo LC, Willavize SA, Freidman HL, Vincent J. Effect of Maalox and omeprazole on the bioavailability of trovafloxacin. *J Antimicrob Chemother* (1997) 39 (Suppl B), 93–7.

the relative bioavailabilities (%) when the quinolones listed have been given at the same time as antacids, and when separated by time intervals (e.g. −2 h; two hours before the quinolone).

Mechanism

It is believed that certain of the quinolone functional groups (3-carboxyl and 4-oxo) form insoluble chelates with aluminium and magnesium ions within the gut, which reduces their absorption.[1-3] The stability of the chelate formed seems to be an important factor in determining the degree of interaction.[3] See also 'Quinolones + Iron or Zinc compounds', p.235).

Importance and management

The interaction between quinolones and antacids are generally well documented, well established and, depending on the particular quinolone and antacid concerned, of clinical importance. The risk is that the serum levels of the antibacterial may fall below minimally inhibitory concentrations (i.e. become subtherapeutic, particularly against organisms such as staphylococci and *Ps. aeruginosa*[4]), resulting in treatment failures.[5] The overall picture is that the aluminium/magnesium antacids interact to a greater extent than the calcium compounds, and bismuth compounds hardly at all.

(a) Aluminium/magnesium antacids

'Table 8.2', (p.228) shows that the aluminium/magnesium antacids can greatly reduce the bioavailabilities of the quinolones. Separating their administration to reduce the admixture of the two drugs in the gut minimises the interaction, a very broad rule-of-thumb being that the quinolones should be taken at least 2 hours before and not less than 4 to 6 hours after the antacid.[1,6-11] The only obvious exception is **fleroxacin**, which appears to interact minimally.

(b) Bismuth compounds

As can be seen from 'Table 8.2', (p.228), bismuth compounds have little or no effect on the bioavailability of **ciprofloxacin**. Information about other quinolones appears to be lacking. However, using **ciprofloxacin** as a guide it would seem that any interaction is likely only to be of minimal clinical importance, and no action appears to be necessary.

(c) Calcium compounds

Information about the interactions with calcium carbonate is more limited than with the aluminium/magnesium antacids, but 'Table 8.2', (p.228) shows that the bioavailabilities of **ciprofloxacin** and **norfloxacin** can be reduced, and to a lesser extent **gemifloxacin**. These reductions are less than those seen with the aluminium/magnesium antacids, but using **ciprofloxacin** as a guide[12,13] a very broad rule-of-thumb would be to separate the drug administration by about 2 hours to minimise this interaction. This is clearly not necessary with **levofloxacin**,[14] **lomefloxacin**,[15] **moxifloxacin**[16] or **ofloxacin**,[17] nor probably with some of the other quinolones that have yet to be studied, but in the absence of direct information a 2-hour separation errs on the side of caution.

(d) Sodium antacids

Sodium bicarbonate does not interact significantly with **norfloxacin**[18] but information about other quinolones appears to be lacking. However, bear in mind that in the case of **ciprofloxacin** an excessive rise in urinary pH [which can be caused by antacids like sodium bicarbonate] may possibly result in urinary crystalluria and kidney damage.[19]

Possible alternatives to the antacids, which do not appear to interact with the quinolones, include the 'H_2-blockers' (p.234) and the 'proton pump inhibitors', (p.738).

1. Nix DE, Watson WA, Lener ME, Frost RW, Krol G, Goldstein H, Lettieri J, Schentag JJ. Effects of aluminum and magnesium antacids and ranitidine on the absorption of ciprofloxacin. *Clin Pharmacol Ther* (1989) 46, 700–705.
2. Shimada J, Shiba K, Oguma T, Miwa H, Yoshimura Y, Nishikawa T, Okabayashi Y, Kitagawa T, Yamamoto S. Effect of antacid on absorption of the quinolone lomefloxacin. *Antimicrob Agents Chemother* (1992) 36, 1219–24.
3. Mizuki Y, Fujiwara I, Yamaguchi T. Pharmacokinetic interactions related to the chemical structures of fluoroquinolones. *J Antimicrob Chemother* (1996) 37 (Suppl), A41–A55.
4. Preheim LC, Cuevas TA, Roccaforte JS, Mellencamp MA, Bittner MJ. Ciprofloxacin and antacids. *Lancet* (1986) ii, 48.
5. Noyes M, Polk RE. Norfloxacin and absorption of magnesium-aluminium. *Ann Intern Med* (1988) 109, 168–9.
6. Grasela TH, Schentag JJ, Sedman AJ, Wilton JH, Thomas DJ, Schultz RW, Lebsack ME, Kinkel AW. Inhibition of enoxacin absorption by antacids or ranitidine. *Antimicrob Agents Chemother* (1989) 33, 615–17.
7. Nix DE, Wilton JH, Ronald B, Distlerath L, Williams VC, Norman A. Inhibition of norfloxacin absorption by antacids. *Antimicrob Agents Chemother* (1990) 34, 432–5.
8. Forster T, Blouin R. The effect of antacid timing on lomefloxacin bioavailability. *Intersci Conf Antimicrob Agents Chemother* (1989) 29, 318.
9. Wilson J, Johnson RD, Caille G, Talbot G, Dorr MB, Heald D. The effect of staggered dosing of Maalox® on the oral bioavailability of sparfloxacin. *Pharm Res* (1994) 11 (10 Suppl), S-429.
10. Lober S, Ziege S, Rau M, Schreiber G, Mignot A, Koeppe P, Lode H. Pharmacokinetics of gatifloxacin and interaction with an antacid containing aluminum and magnesium. *Antimicrob Agents Chemother* (1999) 43, 1067–71.
11. Misiak P, Toothaker R, Lebsack M, Sedman A, Colburn W. The effect of dosing-time intervals on the potential pharmacokinetic interaction between oral enoxacin and oral antacid. *Intersci Conf Antimicrob Agents Chemother* (1988) 28, 367.
12. Lomaestro BM, Bailie GR. Effect of staggered dose of calcium on the bioavailability of ciprofloxacin. *Antimicrob Agents Chemother* (1991) 35, 1004–1007.
13. Lomaestro BM, Bailie GR. Effect of multiple staggered doses of calcium on the bioavailability of ciprofloxacin. *Ann Pharmacother* (1993) 27, 1325–8.
14. Shiba K, Sakai O, Shimada J, Okazaki O, Aoki H, Hakusui H. Effects of antacids, ferrous sulfate, and ranitidine on absorption of DR-3355 in humans. *Antimicrob Agents Chemother* (1992) 36, 2270–4.
15. Lehto P, Kivistö KT. Different effects of products containing metal ions on the absorption of lomefloxacin. *Clin Pharmacol Ther* (1994) 56, 477–82.
16. Stass H, Kubitza D. Profile of moxifloxacin drug interactions. *Clin Infect Dis* (2001) 32, (Suppl 1), S47–S50.
17. Sánchez Navarro A, Martínez Cabarga M, Dominguez-Gil Hurlé A. Comparative study of the influence of Ca^{2+} on absorption parameters of ciprofloxacin and ofloxacin. *J Antimicrob Chemother* (1994) 34, 119–25.
18. Okhamafe AO, Akerele JO, Chukuka CS. Pharmacokinetic interactions of norfloxacin with some metallic medicinal agents. *Int J Pharmaceutics* (1991) 68, 11–18.
19. Ciproxin tablets (Ciprofloxacin hydrochloride). Bayer plc. UK Summary of product characteristics, June 2003.

Quinolones + Antineoplastics

The absorption of ciprofloxacin and ofloxacin can be reduced by some cytotoxic antineoplastics but this is unlikely to be clinically significant.

Clinical evidence

(a) Ciprofloxacin

Six patients with newly diagnosed haematological malignancies (5 with acute myeloid leukaemia and one with non-Hodgkin's lymphoma) were treated with ciprofloxacin 500 mg twice daily to control possible neutropenic infections. It was found that after 13 days of chemotherapy their mean maximum serum ciprofloxacin levels had fallen by 46%, from 3.7 to 2 mg/l and the 0 to 4-hour AUC was reduced by 47%. There were large individual differences between the patients. The cytotoxic agents used were **cyclophosphamide**, **cytarabine**, **daunorubicin**, **doxorubicin**, **mitoxantrone** and **vincristine**.[1]

(b) Ofloxacin

Ten patients with non-Hodgkin's lymphoma, hairy cell leukaemia or acute myeloid leukaemia were given ofloxacin 400 mg at breakfast time for antibacterial prophylaxis during neutropenia. Blood samples were taken 3 days before chemotherapy began and 2 to 3, 5 to 7 and 8 to 10 days afterwards. The maximum serum ofloxacin levels were reduced by 18% two to three days after the chemotherapy but none of the other pharmacokinetic measurements were changed by the cytotoxic treatment. The serum levels had returned to normal by days 5 to 7. At all times serum levels exceeded the expected MICs of the gram-negative potential pathogens. The cytotoxic agents used were **cyclophosphamide**, **cytarabine**, **doxorubicin**, **etoposide**, **ifosfamide** (with mesna), **vincristine**, and prednisolone.[2]

Mechanism

Uncertain. The interaction seems to result from a reduction in absorption of the quinolones by the small intestine, possibly related to the damaging effect these antineoplastics have on the rapidly dividing cells of the intestinal mucosa.

Importance and management

Direct information is limited, but these reports are consistent with the way cytotoxic antineoplastics can reduce the absorption of some other drugs. The authors of both reports suggest that these changes are probably clinically unimportant, because the serum levels of achieved are likely to be sufficient to treat most infections. If the suggested mechanism of interaction is correct, no interaction should occur if quinolones are given parenterally. Nothing appears to be documented about any of the other quinolones.

1. Johnson EJ, MacGowan AP, Potter MN, Stockley RJ, White LO, Slade RR, Reeves DS. Reduced absorption of oral ciprofloxacin after chemotherapy for haematological malignancy. *J Antimicrob Chemother* (1990) 25, 837–42.

2. Brown NM, White LO, Blundell EL, Chown SR, Slade RR, MacGowan AP, Reeves DS. Absorption of oral ofloxacin after cytotoxic chemotherapy for haematological malignancy. *J Antimicrob Chemother* (1993) 32, 117–22.

Table 8.3 Herbs contained in some Chinese herbal remedies[1,2]

Herb (plant part)	Amounts of herbs in the medicines (mg/2.5 g)				
	Hotyu-ekki-to	Rikkunshi-to	Juzen-taiho-to	Sho-saiko-to	Sairei-to
Atractylodis lanceae (rhizome)	278	248	175		125
Ginseng (root)	278	248	175	188	125
Glycyrrhizae (root)	104	662	688	125	83
Aurantii nobilis (pericarp)	139	124			
Zizyphi (fruit)	139	124		188	125
Zingiberis (rhizome)	635	631		63	42
Astragali (root)	278		175		
Angelicae (root)	208		175		
Bupleuri (root)	139			438	292
Cimicifugae (rhizome)	669				
Hoelen		248	175		125
Pinelliae (tuber)		248		313	208
Cinnamomi (cortex)			175		83
Rehmanniae (root)			175		
Paeoniae (root)			175		
Cnidii (rhizome)			175		
Scutellariae (root)				188	125
Alismatis (rhizome)					208
Polyporus					125

1. Hasegawa T, Yamaki K, Nadai M, Muraoka I, Wang L, Takagi K, Nabeshima T. Lack of effect of Chinese medicines on bioavailability of ofloxacin in healthy volunteers. *Int J Clin Pharmacol Ther* (1994) 32, 57-61.
2. Hasegawa T, Yamaki K-I, Muraoka I, Nadai M, Takagi K, Nabeshima T. Effects of traditional Chinese medicines on pharmacokinetics of levofloxacin. *Antimicrob Agents Chemother* (1995) 39, 2135-7.

Quinolones + Chinese herbal medicines

Sho-saiko-to, Rikkunshi-to and Sairei-to do not interact with ofloxacin, and Hotyu-ekki-to, Rikkunshi-to and Juzen-taiho-to do not interact with levofloxacin.

Clinical evidence, mechanism, importance and management

The bioavailability and urinary recovery of a single 200-mg oral dose of **ofloxacin** were not significantly altered in 7 healthy subjects when taken with any of three Chinese herbal medicines (**Sho-saiko-to, Rikkunshi-to** or **Sairei-to**).[1] The bioavailability and renal excretion of a single 200-mg oral dose of **levofloxacin** was not affected in 8 healthy subjects given single 2.5-g doses of **Hotyu-ekki-to, Rikkunshi-to** or **Juzen-taiho-to**.[2] There would therefore seem to be no reason for avoiding concurrent use. Information about other quinolones is lacking. The ingredients of three of these herbal medicines are detailed in 'Table 8.3', (above).

1. Hasegawa T, Yamaki K, Nadai M, Muraoka I, Wang L, Takagi K, Nabeshima T. Lack of effect of Chinese medicines on bioavailability of ofloxacin in healthy volunteers. *Int J Clin Pharmacol Ther* (1994) 32, 57–61.
2. Hasegawa T, Yamaki K-I, Muraoka I, Nadai M, Takagi K, Nabeshima T. Effects of traditional Chinese medicines on pharmacokinetics of levofloxacin. *Antimicrob Agents Chemother* (1995) 39, 2135–7.

Quinolones + Dairy products

Dairy products reduce the bioavailability of ciprofloxacin and norfloxacin, and to a minor extent, gatifloxacin, but not enoxacin, lomefloxacin, ofloxacin and probably not fleroxacin.

Clinical evidence

(a) Ciprofloxacin

A study in 7 healthy subjects given a single 500-mg dose of ciprofloxacin found that 300 ml of **milk** or **yoghurt** reduced the peak plasma levels by 36% and 47%, and the AUC by 33% and 36% respectively.[1] **Milk** (300 ml) reduced the AUC of ciprofloxacin 500 mg by about 30%.[2]

(b) Enoxacin

A study found that **milk** and a standard breakfast had no effect on enoxacin absorption.[3]

(c) Fleroxacin

In a study, a **fat and liquid calcium meal** had no clinically significant effect on the pharmacokinetics of fleroxacin.[4] In another study, **milk** had no effect on fleroxacin pharmacokinetics.[2]

(d) Gatifloxacin

In one study 200 ml of **milk** reduced the AUC of gatifloxacin 200 mg by about 15%.[5]

(e) Lomefloxacin

Milk had no effect on the pharmacokinetics of lomefloxacin.[6]

(f) Norfloxacin

A study found that 300 ml of **milk** or **yoghurt** reduced the absorption and the peak plasma levels of a single 200-mg dose of norfloxacin by roughly 50%.[7]

(g) Ofloxacin

A study in 21 healthy subjects found that 8 oz (about 250 ml) of **milk** had no clinically significant effects on the absorption of 300 mg of ofloxacin.[8] Another study confirmed the lack of a significant interaction between ofloxacin and both **milk** and **yoghurt**.[9]

Mechanism

The proposed reason for these changes is that the calcium in milk and yoghurt or other dairy products combines with the ciprofloxacin and norfloxacin to produce insoluble chelates. Compare also 'Quinolones + Antacids or Calcium compounds', p.227.

Importance and management

The effect of these changes to ciprofloxacin and norfloxacin pharmacokinetics on the control of infection is uncertain but until the situation is clear patients should be advised not to take these dairy products within 1 to 2 hours of either ciprofloxacin or norfloxacin to prevent admixture in the gut. The slight reduction in gatifloxacin levels is probably not clinically relevant.

The quinolones that do not interact significantly would appear to be enoxacin, lomefloxacin, ofloxacin and probably fleroxacin. They may provide a useful alternative to the interacting quinolones.

1. Neuvonen PJ, Kivistö KT, Lehto P. Interference of dairy products with the absorption of ciprofloxacin. *Clin Pharmacol Ther* (1991) 50, 498–502.
2. Hoogkamer JFW, Kleinbloesem CH. The effect of milk consumption on the pharmacokinetics of fleroxacin and ciprofloxacin in healthy volunteers. *Drugs* (1995) 49 (Suppl 2), 346–8.
3. Lehto P, Kivistö KT. Effects of milk and food on the absorption of enoxacin. *Br J Clin Pharmacol* (1995) 39, 194–6.
4. Bertino JS, Nafziger AN, Wong M, Stragand L, Puleo C. Effects of a fat- and calcium-rich breakfast on pharmacokinetics of fleroxacin administered in single and multiple doses. *Antimicrob Agents Chemother* (1994) 38, 499–503.
5. Shiba K, Kusajima H, Momo K. The effects of aluminium hydroxide, cimetidine, ferrous sulfate, green tea and milk on pharmacokinetics of gatifloxacin in healthy humans. *J Antimicrob Chemother* (1999) 44 (Suppl A), 141.

6. Lehto PL, Kivistö KT. Different effects of products containing metal ions on the absorption of lomefloxacin. *Clin Pharmacol Ther* (1994) 56, 477–82.
7. Kivistö KT, Ojala-Karlsson P, Neuvonen PJ. Inhibition of norfloxacin absorption by dairy products. *Antimicrob Agents Chemother* (1992) 36, 489–91.
8. Dudley MN, Marchbanks CR, Flor SC, Beals B. The effect of food or milk on the absorption kinetics of ofloxacin. *Eur J Clin Pharmacol* (1991) 41, 569–71.
9. Neuvonen PJ, Kivistö KT. Milk and yoghurt do not impair the absorption ofofloxacin. *Br J Clin Pharmacol* (1992) 33, 346–8.

Quinolones + Didanosine

An extremely marked reduction in the serum levels of ciprofloxacin occurs if it is given at the same time as didanosine tablets, because of an interaction with the antacid buffers in the didanosine formulation. Taking the ciprofloxacin 2 hours before or 6 hours after didanosine tablets minimises this interaction. Didanosine enteric-coated capsules do not interact with ciprofloxacin.

Clinical evidence

When 12 healthy subjects were given **ciprofloxacin** 750 mg with two didanosine placebo tablets (i.e. all of the antacid additives but no didanosine), the **ciprofloxacin** AUC and maximum serum levels were reduced by 98% and 93% respectively.[1] The antacids in this formulation were dihydroxyaluminium sodium carbonate and magnesium hydroxide.

Other studies have looked at the effect of separating the administration times. When 16 HIV+ patients were given **ciprofloxacin** 1500 mg daily 2 hours before didanosine tablets, the **ciprofloxacin** AUC was reduced by only 26%.[2] Another study in just one subject found that when **ciprofloxacin** 500 mg was given 2 hours after taking two didanosine placebo tablets the **ciprofloxacin** serum levels were reduced below minimal inhibitory concentrations, but giving the **ciprofloxacin** 2 hours before the didanosine placebo tablets resulted in normal blood levels.[3]

The maker notes that the newer didanosine enteric-coated capsule formulation (which contains no antacids) does not interact with **ciprofloxacin**.[4]

Mechanism

Didanosine is extremely acid labile at pH values below 3, so one of the formulations contains buffering agents (dihydroxyaluminium sodium carbonate and magnesium hydroxide) to keep the pH as high as possible to minimise the acid-induced hydrolysis. Ciprofloxacin forms insoluble non-absorbable chelates with these metallic ions in the buffer so that its bioavailability is markedly reduced. See also 'Quinolones + Antacids or Calcium compounds', p.227.

Importance and management

Direct information is limited to these reports but the didanosine tablet/ciprofloxacin interaction appears to be clinically important. Such drastic reductions in serum ciprofloxacin levels mean that minimal inhibitory concentrations are unlikely to be achieved. Ciprofloxacin should be given at least 2 hours before or 6 hours after didanosine tablets (see 'Quinolones + Antacids or Calcium compounds', p.227). Other quinolone antibacterials that interact with antacids are also expected to interact with didanosine tablets, but so far reports are lacking. Didanosine enteric-coated capsules do not interact.

1. Sahai J, Gallicano K, Oliveras L, Khaliq S, Hawley-Foss N, Garber G. Cations in the didanosine tablet reduce ciprofloxacin bioavailability. *Clin Pharmacol Ther* (1993) 53, 292–7.
2. Knupp CA, Barbhaiya RH. A multiple-dose pharmacokinetic interaction study between didanosine (Videx®) and ciprofloxacin (Cipro®) in male subjects seropositive for HIV but asymptomatic. *Biopharm Drug Dispos* (1997) 18, 65–77.
3. Sahai J. Avoiding the ciprofloxacin-didanosine interaction. *Ann Intern Med* (1995) 123, 394–5.
4. Videx EC (Didanosine). Bristol-Myers Squibb Pharmaceuticals Ltd. UK Summary of product characteristics, March 2005.

Quinolones + Enteral feeds or Food

The absorption of ciprofloxacin can be reduced by enteral feeds such as *Ensure, Jevity, Osmolite, Pulmocare* and *Sustacal*. The interaction with ofloxacin is much smaller and probably of little clinical importance. Apart from 'dairy products' (p.232), most foods delay but do not reduce the absorption of ciprofloxacin, enoxacin, gemifloxacin, lomefloxacin, ofloxacin or sparfloxacin. Calcium-fortified orange juice significantly reduces the absorption of ciprofloxacin, but not gatifloxacin or levofloxacin.

Clinical evidence

A. Enteral feeds

(a) Ciprofloxacin

The oral bioavailability of ciprofloxacin 750 mg was reduced by 28% and the mean maximum serum ciprofloxacin levels were reduced by 48% when it was given to 13 fasted subjects with ***Ensure***. In this study the subjects were given 120 ml of the study liquid (***Ensure*** or water) and this was repeated at 30-minute intervals for 5 doses. The ciprofloxacin was crushed and mixed with the second dose of the study liquid and the cup rinsed with another 60 ml of the study liquid.[1]

Other enteral feeds given orally (***Osmolite, Pulmocare*** and ***Resource***) similarly reduced the bioavailability and maximum serum levels of ciprofloxacin by about one-quarter to one-third in two other studies.[2,3] One comparative study found that ***Ensure*** reduced the AUC of ciprofloxacin by 40.2% in men but by only 14.5% in women.[4]

Ciprofloxacin bioavailability was reduced by 53% and 67% by ***Jevity*** or ***Sustacal*** when given via gastrostomy or jejunostomy tubes in a study of 26 hospitalised patients. Despite this, the serum levels achieved with gastrostomy tubes were roughly equivalent to those seen in subjects taking tablets orally.[5] In another study in patients given ***Jevity*** or ***Osmolite***, the 4 patients with a nasoduodenal tube achieved a ciprofloxacin AUC that was about double that seen in the 3 patients with a nasogastric tube or a gastrostomy.[6] In contrast, in another study in healthy subjects, there was no difference in the bioavailability of ciprofloxacin when it was given alone or when it was given with ***Osmolite*** via a nasogastric tube.[7]

(b) Ofloxacin

The oral bioavailability of **ofloxacin** 400 mg was reduced by 10% when given to 13 healthy subjects with ***Ensure***. The mean maximum serum **ofloxacin** levels were reduced by 36%. The same procedure as described in (a) was followed.[1] Only small reductions in the AUCs of **ofloxacin** were seen in another study (10.5% in men, 13.2% in women) with ***Ensure***.[4]

B. Food

Food delayed the absorption of **ciprofloxacin** and **ofloxacin** in 10 subjects, but their bioavailabilities remained unchanged.[8] Other studies suggest that a delay occurs with the absorption of **ofloxacin**[9] and **lomefloxacin**[10] but the bioavailability is unchanged. Food also has no effect on the absorption of **enoxacin**, but high carbohydrate meals delayed the peak serum levels by almost an hour.[11] No clinically significant effect was seen on the pharmacokinetics of **gemifloxacin** 320 mg or 640 mg[12] or **sparfloxacin** 200 mg[13] when they were given to healthy subjects with high fat or standard meals, although the absorption of **sparfloxacin** was slightly delayed.

C. Calcium-fortified foods

Calcium-fortified orange juice decreased the AUC of **ciprofloxacin** by 38% and the maximum plasma level by 41%, when compared to water.[14] However, the AUC of **gatifloxacin** was reduced by only 12% when given with calcium-fortified orange juice.[15] Similarly, in two studies, orange juice, calcium-fortified orange juice,[16] or a breakfast of calcium-fortified orange juice and cereal with or without milk[17] were found to decrease the bioavailability of **levofloxacin**. However, the **levofloxacin** AUC was decreased by less than 16%, an amount that rarely proves to be clinically significant.

Mechanism

The quinolone antibacterials can form insoluble chelates with divalent ions, which reduces their absorption from the gut. Enteral feeds such as those used above contain at least two divalent ions, calcium and magnesium. See also 'Quinolones + Antacids or Calcium compounds', p.227, 'Quinolones + Iron or Zinc compounds', p.235. The differences seen in men and women are possibly due to a slower gastric emptying rate in men, which increases the exposure of the quinolone to the enteral feed.[4]

Importance and management

The interaction between ciprofloxacin and enteral feeds is established. No treatment failures have been reported but it is expected to be clinically important. For example, if patients on enteral feeds were to be switched from parenteral to oral ciprofloxacin, there could be a significant reduction in serum ciprofloxacin levels. Be alert for any evidence that ciprofloxacin is less effective and raise the dosage as necessary. The interaction between ofloxacin and enteral feeds is much smaller and probably not clinically important but this needs confirmation. There are no specific reports about other quinolones but you should be alert for this interaction with any of them. Apart from 'dairy products' (p.232), quinolones can be given with food without any decrease in levels. However, calcium-fortified foods may cause significant interactions with ciprofloxacin.

1. Mueller BA, Brierton DG, Abel SR, Bowman L. Effect of enteral feeding with *Ensure* on oral bioavailabilities of ofloxacin and ciprofloxacin. *Antimicrob Agents Chemother* (1994) 38, 2101–5.
2. Noer BL, Angaran DM. The effect of enteral feedings on ciprofloxacin pharmacokinetics. *Pharmacotherapy* (1990) 10, 254.
3. Piccolo ML, Toossi Z, Goldman M. Effect of coadministration of a nutritional supplement on ciprofloxacin absorption. *Am J Hosp Pharm* (1994) 51, 2697–9.
4. Sowinski KM, Abel SR, Clark WR, Mueller BA. Effect of gender on relative oral bioavailability of ciprofloxacin and ofloxacin when administered with an enteral feeding product. *Pharmacotherapy* (1997) 17, 1112.
5. Healy DP, Brodbeck MC, Clendening CE. Ciprofloxacin absorption is impaired in patients given enteral feedings orally and via gastrostomy and jejunostomy tubes. *Antimicrob Agents Chemother* (1996) 40, 6–10.
6. Yuk JH, Nightingale CH, Quintiliani R, Yeston NS, Orlando R, Dobkin ED, Kambe JC, Sweeney KR, Buonpane EA. Absorption of ciprofloxacin administered through a nasogastric tube or a nasoduodenal tube in volunteers and patients receiving enteral nutrition. *Diagn Microbiol Infect Dis* (1990) 13, 99–102.
7. Yuk JH, Nightingale CH, Sweeney KR, Quintiliani R, Lettieri JT, Frost RW. Relative bioavailability in healthy volunteers of ciprofloxacin administered through a nasogastric tube with and without enteral feeding. *Antimicrob Agents Chemother* (1989) 33, 1118–20.
8. Höffken G, Lode H, Wiley R, Glatzel TD, Sievers D, Olschewski T, Borner K, Koeppe T. Pharmacokinetics and bioavailability of ciprofloxacin and ofloxacin: effect of food and antacid intake. *Rev Infect Dis* (1988) 10 (Suppl 1), S138–S139.
9. Dudley MN, Marchbanks CR, Flor SC, Beals B. The effect of food or milk on the absorption kinetics of ofloxacin. *Eur J Clin Pharmacol* (1991) 41, 569–71.
10. Hooper WD, Dickinson RG, Eadie MJ. Effect of food on absorption of lomefloxacin. *Antimicrob Agents Chemother* (1990) 34, 1797–9.
11. Somogyi AA, Bochner F, Keal JA, Rolan PE, Smith M. Effect of food on enoxacin absorption. *Antimicrob Agents Chemother* (1987) 31, 638–9.
12. Allen A, Bygate E, Clark D, Lewis A, Pay V. The effect of food on the bioavailability of oral gemifloxacin in healthy volunteers. *Int J Antimicrob Agents* (2000) 16, 45–50.
13. Johnson RD, Dorr MB, Hunt TL, Jensen BK, Talbot GH. Effects of food on the pharmacokinetics of sparfloxacin. *Clin Ther* (1999) 21, 982–91.
14. Neuhofel AL, Wilton JH, Victory JM, Hejmanowski LG, Amsden GW. Lack of bioequivalence of ciprofloxacin when administered with calcium-fortified orange juice: a new twist on an old interaction. *J Clin Pharmacol* (2002) 42, 461–6.
15. Wallace AW, Victory JM, Amsden GW. Lack of bioequivalence of gatifloxacin when coadministered with calcium-fortified orange juice in healthy volunteers. *J Clin Pharmacol* (2003) 43, 92–6.
16. Wallace AW, Victory JM, Amsden GW. Lack of bioequivalence when levofloxacin and calcium-fortified orange juice are co-administered to healthy volunteers. *J Clin Pharmacol* (2003) 43, 539–44.
17. Amsden GW, Whitaker A-M. Johnson PW. Lack of bioequivalence of levofloxacin when coadministered with a mineral-fortified breakfast of juice and cereal. *J Clin Pharmacol* (2003) 43, 990–95.

Quinolones + H_2-blockers

Cimetidine can increase the serum levels of some quinolones (intravenous enoxacin or fleroxacin and oral clinafloxacin or pefloxacin), famotidine can reduce the serum levels of norfloxacin, and ranitidine can reduce the absorption of enoxacin. None of these interactions appear to be clinically important.

Clinical evidence and mechanism

(a) Ciprofloxacin

Neither **cimetidine**[1,2] nor **ranitidine**[3,4] appear to have a clinically important effect on the pharmacokinetics of ciprofloxacin.

(b) Clinafloxacin

Cimetidine 300 mg four times daily for 4 days increased the maximum serum levels of clinafloxacin by 15% and increased its AUC by 44%.[5]

(c) Enoxacin

The plasma levels of a 400-mg intravenous dose of enoxacin were higher when **cimetidine** 300 mg four times daily was given concurrently. Renal clearance and systemic clearance were reduced by 26% and 20% respectively, and the elimination half-life was increased by 30%.[6]

In one study **ranitidine** 150 mg twice daily did not affect the pharmacokinetics of a single 400-mg intravenous dose of enoxacin.[6] However, in another, **ranitidine** 50 mg given intravenously 2 hours before a single 400-mg oral dose of enoxacin reduced the absorption by 26 to 40%,[7,8] which seemed to be related to changes in gastric pH caused by the **ranitidine**.[8]

(d) Fleroxacin

Cimetidine decreased the total clearance of fleroxacin by about 25%, without much effect on renal clearance, and increased its elimination half-life by 32%.[9]

(e) Gatifloxacin

Cimetidine does not alter the pharmacokinetics of gatifloxacin.[10]

(f) Grepafloxacin

Cimetidine does not alter the pharmacokinetics of grepafloxacin.[11] Similarly, intravenous **famotidine** in a dose of up to 40 mg had no effect on the pharmacokinetics of a 400-mg dose of grepafloxacin.[12]

(g) Levofloxacin

Cimetidine reduced the clearance of levofloxacin by about 25% and increased its AUC by almost 30%,[13] whereas **ranitidine** did not affect the pharmacokinetics of levofloxacin.[14]

(h) Lomefloxacin

Ranitidine does not affect the pharmacokinetics of lomefloxacin.[15-17]

(i) Moxifloxacin

Ranitidine does not affect the pharmacokinetics of moxifloxacin.[18]

(j) Norfloxacin

Famotidine given 8 hours before norfloxacin significantly reduced its maximum serum concentrations in 6 healthy subjects, but the AUC and urinary recovery rate were unchanged.[19]

(k) Ofloxacin

Cimetidine does not alter the pharmacokinetics of ofloxacin.[20]

(l) Pefloxacin

Cimetidine increased the AUC of intravenous pefloxacin by about 40%. It increased the half-life from 10.3 to 15.3 hours and the clearance was reduced by almost by 30%.[21]

(m) Sparfloxacin

Cimetidine does not alter the pharmacokinetics of sparfloxacin.[22]

Importance and management

Although the pharmacokinetic changes seen in some of these studies are moderate, none has been shown to affect the outcome of treatment and they are probably only of minor clinical relevance.

1. Ludwig E, Graber H, Székely É, Csiba A. Metabolic interactions of ciprofloxacin. *Diagn Microbiol Infect Dis* (1990) 13, 135–41.
2. Prince RA, Liou W-S, Kasik JE. Effect of cimetidine on ciprofloxacin pharmacokinetics. *Pharmacotherapy* (1990) 10, 233.
3. Höffken G, Lode H, Wiley R, Glatzel TD, Sievers D, Olschewski T, Borner K, Koeppe T. Pharmacokinetics and bioavailability of ciprofloxacin and ofloxacin: effect of food and antacid intake. *Rev Infect Dis* (1988) 10 (Suppl 1), S138–9
4. Nix DE, Watson WA, Lener ME, Frost RW, Krol G, Goldstein H, Letterei J, Schentag JJ. Effects of aluminum and magnesium antacids and ranitidine on the absorption of ciprofloxacin. *Clin Pharmacol Ther* (1989) 46, 700–5.
5. Randinitis EJ, Koup JR, Bron NJ, Hounslow NJ, Rausch G, Abel R, Vassos AB, Sedman AJ. Drug interaction studies with clinafloxacin and probenecid, cimetidine, phenytoin and warfarin. *Drugs* (1999) 58 (Suppl 2), 254–5.
6. Misiak PM, Eldon MA, Toothaker RD, Sedman AJ. Effects of oral cimetidine or ranitidine on the pharmacokinetics of intravenous enoxacin. *J Clin Pharmacol* (1993) 33, 53–6.
7. Grasela TH, Schentag JJ, Sedman AJ, Wilton JH, Thomas DJ, Schultz RW, Lebsack ME, Kinkel AW. Inhibition of enoxacin absorption by antacids or ranitidine. *Antimicrob Agents Chemother* (1989) 33, 615–17.
8. Lebsack ME, Nix D, Ryerson B, Toothaker RD, Welage L, Norman AM, Schentag JJ, Sedman AJ. Effect of gastric acidity on enoxacin absorption. *Clin Pharmacol Ther* (1992) 52, 252–6.
9. Portmann R. Influence of cimetidine on fleroxacin pharmacokinetics. *Drugs* (1993) 45 (Suppl 3), 471.
10. Shiba K, Kusajima H, Momo K. The effects of aluminium hydroxide, cimetidine, ferrous sulfate, green tea and milk on pharmacokinetics of gatifloxacin in healthy humans. *J Antimicrob Chemother* (1999) 44 (Suppl A), 141.
11. Koneru B, Bramer S, Bricmont P, Maroli A, Shiba K. Effect of food, gastric pH and co-administration of antacid, cimetidine and probenecid on the oral pharmacokinetics of the broad spectrum antimicrobial agent grepafloxacin. *Pharm Res* (1996) 13 (9 Suppl), S414.
12. Efthymiopoulos C, Bramer SL, Maroli A. Effect of food and gastric pH on the bioavailability of grepafloxacin. *Clin Pharmacokinet* (1997) 33 (Suppl 1), 18–24.
13. Gaitonde MD, Mendes P, House ESA, Lehr KH. The effects of cimetidine and probenecid on the pharmacokinetics of levofloxacin (LFLX). *Intersci Conf Antimicrob Agents Chemother* (1995) 35, 8.
14. Shiba K, Sakai O, Shimada J, Okazaki O, Aoki H, Hakusui H. Effects of antacids, ferrous sulphate, and ranitidine on absorption of DR-3355 in humans. *Antimicrob Agents Chemother* (1992) 36, 2270–4.
15. Nix D, Schentag J. Lomefloxacin (L) absorption kinetics when administered with ranitidine (R) and sucralfate (S). *Intersci Conf Antimicrob Agents Chemother* (1989) 29, 317.
16. Sudoh T, Fujimura A, Harada K, Sunaga K, Ohmori M, Sakamoto K, Kumagai Y. Effect of ranitidine on renal clearance of lomefloxacin (LFLX). *Jpn J Pharmacol* (1995) 67 (Suppl 1), 165P.
17. Sudoh T, Fujimura A, Harada K, Sunaga K, Ohmori M, Sakamoto K. Effect of ranitidine on renal clearance of lomefloxacin. *Eur J Clin Pharmacol* (1996) 51, 95–8.

18. Stass H, Böttcher M-F, Ochmann K. Evaluation of the influence of antacids and H_2 antagonists on the absorption of moxifloxacin after oral administration of a 400-mg dose to healthy volunteers. *Clin Pharmacokinet* (2001) 40 (Suppl 1), 39–48.
19. Shimada J, Hori S. Effect of antiulcer drugs on gastrointestinal absorption of norfloxacin. *Chemotherapy (Tokyo)* (1992) 40, 1141–7.
20. Shiba K, Yoshida M, Kachi M, Shimada J, Saito A, Sakai N. Effects of peptic ulcer-healing drugs on the pharmacokinetics of new quinolone (OFLX). 17th International Congress on Chemotherapy, Berlin, June 1991. Abstract 415.
21. Sörgel F, Mahr G, Koch HU, Stephan U, Wiesemann HG, Malter U. Effects of cimetidine on the pharmacokinetics of pefloxacin in healthy volunteers. *Rev Infect Dis* (1988) 10 (Suppl 1), S137.
22. Gries JM, Honorato J, Taburet AM, Alvarez MP, Sadaba B, Azanza JR, Singlas E. Cimetidine does not alter sparfloxacin pharmacokinetics. *Int J Clin Pharmacol Ther* (1995) 33, 585–7.

Quinolones + Iron or Zinc compounds

Ferrous fumarate, gluconate, sulfate and other iron compounds can reduce the absorption of ciprofloxacin, gatifloxacin, levofloxacin, norfloxacin, ofloxacin and sparfloxacin from the gut. Serum levels of the antibacterial may become subtherapeutic as a result. Limited evidence suggests that fleroxacin is not affected and lomefloxacin is only minimally affected. Gemifloxacin does not appear to interact when given 2 hours before or 3 hours after ferrous sulfate. No interaction appears to occur with iron-ovotransferrin. Zinc appears to interact like iron.

Clinical evidence

(a) Ciprofloxacin

The absorption of ciprofloxacin is markedly reduced by iron and zinc compounds. Several studies have clearly demonstrated reductions in the AUC and maximum serum levels of 30 to 90% with **ferrous fumarate**,[1] **ferrous gluconate**,[2] **ferrous sulfate**,[2-6] **iron-glycine sulfate**,[7] ***Centrum Forte***[2] (a multi-mineral preparation containing iron, magnesium, zinc, calcium, copper and manganese) and with ***Stresstabs 600-with-zinc***[5] (a multivitamin-with-zinc preparation). However **iron-ovotransferrin** has been found to have no significant effect on the absorption of ciprofloxacin.[8]

(b) Fleroxacin

A study in 12 subjects found that **ferrous sulfate** (equivalent to 100 mg of elemental iron) had no significant effect on the pharmacokinetics of fleroxacin.[9]

(c) Gatifloxacin

A study in 6 healthy subjects found that **ferrous sulfate** 160 mg given with gatifloxacin 200 mg caused a decrease in the maximum serum levels and AUC of gatifloxacin of 49 and 29% respectively.[10]

(d) Gemifloxacin

Gemifloxacin 320 mg was given either 2 hours after or 3 hours before **ferrous sulfate** 325 mg in a study in 27 healthy subjects. The pharmacokinetics of gemifloxacin were not significantly altered in either case.[11]

(e) Levofloxacin

Ferrous sulfate has been found to reduce the bioavailability of levofloxacin by 79%.[12]

(f) Lomefloxacin

When lomefloxacin 400 mg was given with **ferrous sulfate** (equivalent to 100 mg of elemental iron), the lomefloxacin maximum serum levels were reduced by about 28% and the AUC by about 14%.[13]

(g) Norfloxacin

Ferrous sulfate reduced the AUC and maximum serum levels of a single 400-mg dose of norfloxacin in 8 healthy subjects by 73 and 75% respectively.[6] **Ferrous sulfate** caused a 51% reduction in the norfloxacin AUC in another study,[14,15] and a 97% reduction in bioavailability in a further single dose study.[16] The same authors also found that both **ferrous sulfate** and **zinc sulfate** reduced the urinary recovery of norfloxacin by 55 and 56% respectively.[17]

(h) Ofloxacin

Ferrous sulfate (equivalent to 100 mg of elemental iron) reduced the AUC and maximum serum levels of single 400-mg dose of ofloxacin by 25% and 36% respectively in 8 healthy subjects.[6] An 11% decrease in absorption was seen when 9 healthy subjects were given ofloxacin 200 mg with **ferrous sulfate** 1050 mg.[18] Elemental iron 200 mg (in the form of an **iron-glycine-sulfate** complex) reduced the bioavailability of ofloxacin 400 mg by 36% in 12 healthy subjects.[7]

(i) Sparfloxacin

In a single dose study in 6 subjects, 525 mg of **ferrous sulfate** (equivalent to 170 mg of elemental iron) reduced the AUC of sparfloxacin 200 mg by 27%.[14,15]

Mechanism

It is believed that the quinolones form a complex with iron and zinc (by chelation between the metal ion and the 4-oxo and adjacent carboxyl groups) which is less easily absorbed by the gut. However, a study in *rats* using oral iron and intravenous ciprofloxacin suggested that the interaction may not be entirely confined to the gut.[19] This needs further study. Iron-ovotransferrin differs from other iron preparations in being able to combine directly with the transferrin receptors of intestinal cells, and appears to release little iron into the gut to interact with the quinolones.

Importance and management

The interactions between the quinolones and iron compounds are established and would appear to be of clinical importance because the serum antibacterial levels can become subtherapeutic. In descending order the extent of the interaction appears to be: norfloxacin, levofloxacin, ciprofloxacin, gatifloxacin, ofloxacin/sparfloxacin, then least affected, lomefloxacin.

None of these quinolones should be taken at the same time as any iron preparation that contains substantial amounts of iron (e.g. ferrous sulfate, ferrous gluconate, ferrous fumarate, iron-glycine sulfate). Since the quinolones are rapidly absorbed, taking them 2 hours before the iron should minimise the risk of admixture in the gut and largely avoid this interaction. Information about other quinolones seems to be lacking but the same precautions should be taken with all of them except fleroxacin, which appears not to interact, and lomefloxacin, which seems to interact only minimally.

Iron-ovotransferrin does not interact with ciprofloxacin and is not expected to interact with any of the quinolones (see 'Mechanism') but this awaits confirmation.

There seems to be very little data about the interactions between zinc compounds and quinolones, but zinc appears to interact like iron and therefore the same precautions suggested for iron should be followed.

1. Brouwers JRBJ, Van der Kam HJ, Sijtsma J, Proost JH. Decreased ciprofloxacin absorption with concomitant administration of ferrous fumarate. *Pharm Weekbl (Sci)* (1990) 12, 182–3.
2. Kara M, Hasinoff BB, McKay DW, Campbell NRC. Clinical and chemical interactions between iron preparations and ciprofloxacin. *Br J Clin Pharmacol* (1991) 31, 257–61.
3. Polk RE. Effect of ferrous sulfate and multivitamins with zinc on the absorption of ciprofloxacin in normal volunteers. *Intersci Conf Antimicrob Agents Chemother* (1989) 29, 136.
4. Le Pennec MP, Kitzis MD, Terdjman M, Foubard S, Garbarz E, Hanania G. Possible interaction of ciprofloxacin with ferrous sulphate. *J Antimicrob Chemother* (1990) 25, 184–5.
5. Polk RE, Healy DP, Sahai J, Drwal L, Racht E. Effect of ferrous sulfate and multivitamins with zinc on absorption of ciprofloxacin in normal volunteers. *Antimicrob Agents Chemother* (1989) 33, 1841–4.
6. Lehto P, Kivistö KT, Neuvonen PJ. The effect of ferrous sulphate on the absorption of norfloxacin, ciprofloxacin and ofloxacin. *Br J Clin Pharmacol* (1994) 37, 82–5.
7. Lode H, Stuhlert P, Deppermann KH, Mainz D, Borner K, Kotvas K, Koeppe P. Pharmacokinetic interactions between oral ciprofloxacin (CIP)/ofloxacin (OFL) and ferro-salts. *Intersci Conf Antimicrob Agents Chemother* (1989) 29,136.
8. Pazzucconi F, Barbi S, Baldassarre D, Colombo N, Dorigotti F, Sirtori CR. Iron-ovotransferrin preparation does not interfere with ciprofloxacin absorption. *Clin Pharmacol Ther* (1996) 59, 418–22.
9. Sörgel F, Naber KG, Kinzig M, Frank A, Birner B. Effect of ferrous sulfate on fleroxacin analyzed by the confidence interval (CI) approach. *Pharm Res* (1995) 12 (9 Suppl), S-422.
10. Shiba K, Kusajima H, Momo K. The effects of aluminium hydroxide, cimetidine, ferrous sulfate, green tea and milk on pharmacokinetics of gatifloxacin in healthy humans. *J Antimicrob Chemother* (1999) 44 (Suppl A), 141.
11. Allen A, Bygate E, Faessel H, Isaac L, Lewis A. The effect of ferrous sulphate and sucralfate on the bioavailability of oral gemifloxacin in healthy volunteers. *Int J Antimicrob Agents* (2000) 15, 283–9.
12. Shiba K, Okazaki O, Aoki H, Sakai O, Shimada J. Inhibition of DR-3355 absorption by metal ions. *Intersci Conf Antimicrob Agents Chemother* (1991) 31, 198.
13. Lehto P, Kivistö KT. Different effects of products containing metal ions on the absorption of lomefloxacin. *Clin Pharmacol Ther* (1994) 56, 477–82.
14. Kanemitsu K, Hori S, Yanagawa A, Shimada J. Effect of ferrous sulfate on the pharmacokinetics of sparfloxacin. *Chemotherapy* (1994) 42, 6–13.
15. Kanemitsu K, Hori S, Yanagawa A, Shimada J. Effect of ferrous sulfate on the absorption of sparfloxacin in healthy volunteers and rats. *Drugs* (1995) 49 (Suppl 2), 352–6.
16. Okhamafe AO, Akerele JO, Chukuka CS. Pharmacokinetic interactions of norfloxacin with some metallic medicinal agents. *Int J Pharmaceutics* (1991) 68, 11–18.
17. Campbell NRC, Kara M, Hasinoff BB, Haddara WM, McKay DW. Norfloxacin interaction with antacids and minerals. *Br J Clin Pharmacol* (1992) 33, 115–16.
18. Martínez Cabarga M, Sánchez Navarro A, Colino Gandarillas CI, Domínguez-Gil A. Effects of two cations on gastrointestinal absorption of ofloxacin. *Antimicrob Agents Chemother* (1991) 35, 2102–5.
19. Wong PY, Zhu M, Li RC. Pharmacokinetic and pharmacodynamic interactions between intravenous ciprofloxacin and oral ferrous sulfate. *J Chemother* (2000) 12, 286–93.

Quinolones + NSAIDs

A number of cases of convulsions have been seen in Japanese patients given fenbufen with enoxacin, and there is also one possible case involving ofloxacin. Use of these particular drugs together should be avoided. Normally no interaction seems to occur with most quinolones and NSAIDs, except where there is a predisposition to convulsive episodes. Isolated cases of convulsions or other neurological toxicity or skin eruptions have been seen with ciprofloxacin combined with indometacin, mefenamic acid or naproxen. These appear to be very rare events.

Clinical evidence

(a) Ciprofloxacin

As of 1995 the maker of ciprofloxacin had, on record, two confirmed spontaneous reports of convulsions in patients on ciprofloxacin and an NSAID, one with **mefenamic acid** and the other with **naproxen**.[1] These appear to be the only medically validated reports of ciprofloxacin/NSAID reactions by 1995.[1]

A woman on **chloroquine** 250 mg and **naproxen** 1 g daily developed dizziness, anxiety and tremors within a week of starting ciprofloxacin 1 g daily. The symptoms largely resolved when the **chloroquine** was stopped; it was not known if she also stopped the naproxen. Two months after **chloroquine** was discontinued, while she was still taking ciprofloxacin, **indometacin** was started. This time she developed pain in her feet and became extremely tired. The pain partially subsided and the fatigue vanished when the ciprofloxacin was stopped. Later she was found to have some axonal demyelination, compatible with drug-induced polyneuropathy.[2]

A study in 8 healthy subjects found that the pharmacokinetics of ciprofloxacin were unaffected by 3 days' treatment with **fenbufen**.[3] Another study found that combined single doses of ciprofloxacin and **fenbufen** in 12 healthy subjects produced no evidence, using EEG recordings, of increased CNS excitatory effects.[4]

(b) Enoxacin

A total of 17 Japanese patients have been identified, with apparently no previous history of seizures, who in the 1986 to 1987 period developed convulsions when treated with **fenbufen** 400 to 1200 mg daily and enoxacin 200 to 800 mg.[5] Two case reports of this interaction have been published.[6,7] An 87-year-old Japanese woman on enoxacin 200 mg also had convulsions when given a single 50-mg intravenous dose of **flurbiprofen**.[8]

(c) Ofloxacin

One patient on **fenbufen** 800 mg had involuntary movements of the neck and upper extremities after taking ofloxacin 600 mg.[5] The pharmacokinetics of ofloxacin 200 mg twice daily were unchanged by **ketoprofen** 100 mg daily for 3 days in 10 healthy subjects.[9] The incidence of psychotic adverse effects (euphoria, hysteria, psychosis) in 151 patients on ofloxacin were not increased by the concurrent use of NSAIDs (**aspirin, diclofenac, indometacin, dipyrone**).[10]

(d) Pefloxacin

The pharmacokinetics of pefloxacin 400 mg twice daily were not affected by **ketoprofen** 100 mg daily for 3 days in 10 healthy subjects.[9]

(e) Sparfloxacin

A single case report describes drug eruptions (erythematous papules) attributed to sparfloxacin hypersensitivity induced by **mefenamic acid** in a 62-year-old woman.[11]

Mechanism

Not fully understood. Convulsions have occurred in a few patients taking quinolones alone, some of whom were epileptics and some of whom were not (see 'Anticonvulsants + Quinolones', p.337). Experiments in *mice* have shown that quinolones competitively inhibit the binding of gamma-amino butyric acid (GABA) to its receptors.[12] GABA is an inhibitory transmitter in the CNS, which is believed to be involved in the control of convulsive activity. Enoxacin and fenbufen are known to affect the GABA receptor site in the hippocampus and frontal cortex of *mice*, which is associated with convulsive activity.[13] It could be that, if and when an interaction occurs, the NSAID simply lowers the amount of quinolone needed to precipitate convulsions in already susceptible individuals.

Importance and management

The interaction between enoxacin and fenbufen is established, but it seems to be uncommon. Nevertheless, it would seem prudent to avoid fenbufen with enoxacin. There are very many alternatives.

Reports of adverse interactions between other quinolones and NSAIDs are extremely rare. The general warning about convulsions with quinolones and NSAIDs issued by the CSM[14] seems to be an extrapolation from the interaction between enoxacin and fenbufen, and from some *animal* experiments, to cover all quinolones and all NSAIDs. In addition to the data cited above, an epidemiological study of 856 users of quinolones (ciprofloxacin, enoxacin, nalidixic acid) and a range of NSAIDs found no cases of convulsions.[15] The overall picture would therefore seem to be that although a potential for interaction exists, the risk is very small indeed and normally there would seem to be little reason for most patients on quinolones to avoid NSAIDs. Epileptic patients are a possible exception (see 'Anticonvulsants + Quinolones', p.337).

1. Bomford J. Ciprofloxacin. *Pharm J* (1995) 255, 674.
2. Rollof J, Vinge E. Neurological adverse effects during concomitant treatment with ciprofloxacin, NSAIDS, and chloroquine: possible drug interaction. *Ann Pharmacother* (1993) 27, 1058–9.
3. Kamali F. Lack of a pharmacokinetic interaction between ciprofloxacin and fenbufen. *J Clin Pharm Ther* (1994) 19, 257–9.
4. Kamali F, Ashton CH, Marsh VR, Cox J. Is there a pharmacodynamic interaction between ciprofloxacin and fenbufen? *Br J Clin Pharmacol* (1997) 43, 545P–546P.
5. Lederle. Data on file. Personal Communication, December 1995.
6. Takeo G, Shibuya N, Motomura M, Kanazawa H, Shishido H. A new DNA gyrase inhibitor induces convulsions: a case report and animal experiments. *Chemotherapy (Tokyo)* (1989) 37, 1154–9.
7. Morita H, Maemura K, Sakai Y, Kaneda Y. A case with convulsion, loss of consciousness and subsequent acute renal failure caused by enoxacin and fenbufen. *Nippon Naika Gakkai Zasshi* (1988) 77, 744–5.
8. Mizuno J, Takumi Z, Kaneko A, Tsutsui T, Tsutsui T, Zushi N, Machida K. Convulsion following the combination of single preoperative oral administration of enoxacine and single postoperative intravenous administration of flurbiprofen axetil. *Jpn J Anesthesiol* (2001) 50, 425–8.
9. Fillastre JP, Leroy A, Borsa-Lebas F, Etienne I, Gy C, Humbert G. Effects of ketoprofen (NSAID) on the pharmacokinetics of pefloxacin and ofloxacin in healthy volunteers. *Drugs Exp Clin Res* (1992) 18, 487–92.
10. Jüngst G, Weidmann E, Breitstadt A, Huppertz E. Does ofloxacin interact with NSAIDs to cause psychotic side effects? 17th International Congress on Chemotherapy, Berlin, June 23–8, 1991. Abstract 412.
11. Oiso N, Taniguchi S, Goto Y, Hisa T, Mizuno N, Mochida K, Hamada T, Yorifuji T. A case of drug eruption due to sparfloxacin (SPFX) and mefenamic acid. *Skin Res* (1995) 37, 321–7.
12. Hori S, Shimada J, Saito A, Matsuda M, Miyahara T. Comparison of the inhibitory effects of new quinolones on γ-aminobutyric acid receptor binding in the presence of antiinflammatory drugs. *Rev Infect Dis* (1989) 11 (Suppl 5), S1397–S1398.
13. Motomura M, Kataoka Y, Takeo G, Shibayama K, Ohishi K, Nakamura T, Niwa M, Tsujihata M, Nagataki S. Hippocampus and frontal cortex are the potential mediatory sites for convulsions induced by new quinolones and non-steroidal anti-inflammatory drugs. *Int J Clin Pharmacol Ther Toxicol* (1991) 29, 223–7.
14. Committee on Safety of Medicines. Convulsions due to quinolone antimicrobial agents. *Current Problems* (1991) 32, 2.
15. Mannino S, Garcia-Rodriguez LA, Jick SS. NSAIDs, quinolones and convulsions: an epidemiological approach. *Post Marketing Surveillance* (1992) 6, 119–28.

Quinolones + Opioids

Morphine modestly reduces the AUC of trovafloxacin, but this is not considered clinically significant. Trovafloxacin did not alter the effects or pharmacokinetics of morphine. Oxycodone does not appear to significantly affect the pharmacokinetics of either levofloxacin or gatifloxacin. It has been suggested that opiates decrease oral ciprofloxacin levels, but good evidence for this appears to be lacking.

Clinical evidence, mechanism, importance and management

(a) Ciprofloxacin

In one non-randomised study[1] the levels of oral ciprofloxacin were only 1.3 mg/l in the presence of intramuscular **papaveretum**, compared to 3.22 mg/l in a control group not receiving **papaveretum**. The authors say that this means the peak ciprofloxacin levels in the **papaveretum** group would not reach the MIC of a number of gut pathogens. They name *Bacteroides fragilis*, but it should be noted that the levels of the control group also did not reach the MIC of this organism, and *Enterococcus faecalis*, many strains of which are only moderately susceptible to ciprofloxacin anyway. Further, the **papaveretum** group in this study had only 4 patients, and, as the authors note, the control group was not matched.[1] Based on this rather slim evidence, the makers of ciprofloxacin state that the use of ciprofloxacin tablets is not recommended with opiate premedicants due to the risks of inadequate ciprofloxacin levels.[2,3] This advice is also given by the makers of **morphine** sulphate,[4] and was added at the request of the UK Medicines and Healthcare Regulatory Agency.[5]

(b) Gatifloxacin

In 12 healthy subjects, the pharmacokinetics of gatifloxacin 400 mg were not significantly altered by 4-hourly doses of **oxycodone** 5 mg.[6]

(c) Levofloxacin

In 8 healthy subjects, the pharmacokinetics of oral levofloxacin 500 mg were not significantly altered by 4-hourly doses of **oxycodone** 5 mg.[7]

(d) Trovafloxacin

An intravenous infusion of **morphine** 150 micrograms/kg given with oral trovafloxacin 200 mg to 18 healthy subjects caused a 36% reduction in the trovafloxacin AUC and a 46% reduction in the maximum serum levels. These levels were considered sufficient for prophylaxis of infection, and remained above the MICs of the most likely organisms to cause post-surgical infections. The bioavailability and effects of **morphine** were not significantly changed by trovafloxacin.[8]

1. Morran C, McArdle C, Petitt L, Sleigh D, Gemmell C, Hichens M, Felmingham D, Tillotson G. Brief report: pharmacokinetics of orally administered ciprofloxacin in abdominal surgery. *Am J Med* (1989) 87, (Suppl 5A), 86S–88S.
2. Ciproxin tablets (Ciprofloxacin hydrochloride). Bayer plc. UK Summary of product characteristics, June 2003.
3. Bayer Health Care. Personal Communication, September 2003.
4. Morphine sulphate injection. Celltech Pharmaceuticals Ltd. UK Summary of product characteristics, March 2003.
5. Celltech Pharmaceutical Ltd. Personal Communication, August 2003.
6. Grant EM, Nicolau DP, Nightingale C, Quintiliani R. Minimal interaction between gatifloxacin and oxycodone. *J Clin Pharmacol* (2002) 42, 928–32.
7. Grant EM, Zhong MK, Fitzgerald JF, Nicolau DP, Nightingale C, Quintiliani R. Lack of interaction between levofloxacin and oxycodone: pharmacokinetics and drug disposition. *J Clin Pharmacol* (2001) 41, 206–9.
8. Vincent J, Hunt T, Teng R, Robarge L, Willavize SA, Friedman HL. The pharmacokinetic effects of coadministration of morphine and trovafloxacin in healthy subjects. *Am J Surg* (1998) 176 (Suppl 6A), 32S–38S.

Quinolones + Other antibacterials

Rifampicin (rifampin) appears not to have a clinically important effect on ciprofloxacin, fleroxacin, pefloxacin and possibly grepafloxacin. Azlocillin reduces the clearance of ciprofloxacin. Piperacillin, ceftazidime and tobramycin appear not to affect the pharmacokinetics of pefloxacin, nor amoxicillin the absorption of ofloxacin. There was no pharmacokinetic interaction between pefloxacin and amikacin. Clindamycin appears not to affect the pharmacokinetics of ciprofloxacin but it may antagonise its effects on *S. aureus*. *In vitro* studies have demonstrated antagonistic antibacterial effects when nitrofurantoin and nalidixic acid are used together, and other quinolones are also said to antagonise the effects of nitrofurantoin. Cefotaxime appears not to interact with ofloxacin.

Clinical evidence, mechanism, importance and management

(a) Aminoglycosides

A study found that a single 100-mg intravenous dose of **tobramycin** had no effect on the pharmacokinetics of **pefloxacin**, and **pefloxacin** did affect the pharmacokinetics of **tobramycin**.[1] Similarly no pharmacokinetic interaction was found between **pefloxacin** and **amikacin**.[2]

(b) Cephalosporins

A study found that a single 2-g intravenous doses of **ceftazidime** had no effect on the pharmacokinetics of **pefloxacin**, and **pefloxacin** did affect the pharmacokinetics of **ceftazidime**.[1]

In a study of 11 healthy subjects, the pharmacokinetics of **cefotaxime** and **ofloxacin** were similar, whether given alone or in combination, and the antimicrobial effect of the combination was additive for *S. aureus*, *S. pneumoniae*, *E. cloacae* and *K. pneumoniae*, but not against *P. aeruginosa*.[3]

(c) Clindamycin

One study found that the pharmacokinetics of intravenous **ciprofloxacin** 200 mg were not affected by intravenous clindamycin 600 mg and there is evidence that combined use may possibly enhance the antibacterial activity, particularly against *S. aureus* and *S. pneumoniae*.[4] However, another study found that the serum bactericidal activity of **ciprofloxacin** against *S. aureus* was completely antagonised by clindamycin, if the strains were susceptible to the latter.[5]

(d) Macrolides

A study designed to assess the potential interaction between **trovafloxacin** and **azithromycin** found no significant alteration in the pharmacokinetics of either drug.[6]

(e) Metronidazole

A study found that a single 400-mg oral dose of metronidazole had no effect on the pharmacokinetics of **pefloxacin**, and similarly **pefloxacin** did not affect the pharmacokinetics of metronidazole.[1]

Similarly no interaction was found between **ciprofloxacin** or **ofloxacin** (both 200 mg intravenously) and metronidazole 500 mg intravenously,[7] and metronidazole with **ciprofloxacin** orally.[8]

A further study, investigating the use of metronidazole 500 mg intravenously and **ciprofloxacin** 200 mg intravenously, also did not find any significant pharmacokinetic changes, although metronidazole reduced the **ciprofloxacin** volume of distribution by 20%.[4] This is not expected to be clinically significant.

(f) Nitrofurantoin

The antibacterial activity of nalidixic acid can be attenuated by sub-inhibitory concentrations of nitrofurantoin. In 44 out of 53 strains of *Escherichia coli*, *Salmonella* and *Proteus*, antagonism was shown.[9] Another study confirmed these findings.[10] Whether this similarly occurs if both antibacterials are given to patients is uncertain, but the advice that concurrent use should be avoided when treating urinary tract infections seems sound.[9] Other quinolone antibacterials and nitrofurantoin are also said to be antagonistic and some standard reference books state that they should not be used together.[11]

(g) Penicillins

A single-dose study in 6 healthy subjects found that intravenous **azlocillin** 60 mg/kg reduced the clearance of intravenous **ciprofloxacin** 4 mg/kg by 35%. The pharmacokinetics of **azlocillin** were not affected.[12]

Another study found that a single 4-g intravenous dose of **piperacillin** and **pefloxacin** 400 mg caused no significant alteration in the pharmacokinetics of either drug.[1]

The absorption of **ofloxacin** 400 mg was not altered by **amoxicillin** 3 g in 6 healthy subjects.[13]

In another study in 12 healthy subjects, the serum bacterial activity of **ciprofloxacin** plus **piperacillin** against a variety of organisms was found to be additive, rather than antagonistic or synergistic despite the fact that the clearance of **ciprofloxacin** was reduced by 24%.[14]

(h) Rifampicin (Rifampin)

Ciprofloxacin 750 mg and **rifampicin** 300 mg, both given every 12 hours for 2 weeks, did not significantly affect the pharmacokinetics of either drug in 12 elderly patients (aged 67 to 95).[15] This is confirmed by other pharmacokinetic studies, one of which also reported that combined use provided excellent serum bactericidal activity against *S. aureus* strains, although activity was modestly lower than **rifampicin** alone.[5,16,17]

A study in 8 healthy subjects found that **rifampicin** 900 mg daily for 10 days decreased the half-life and 0 to 12-hour AUC of **pefloxacin** 400 mg twice daily by about 30%, due to a 35% increase in total plasma clearance.[18] Despite these changes the serum **pefloxacin** levels still remained well above the minimal inhibitory concentrations (0.50 mg/l) for 90% of strains of methicillin-sensitive *S. aureus* and *S. epidermis*.[18]

Another study in 13 healthy subjects found that **rifampicin** 600 mg daily for a week increased the clearance of **fleroxacin** 400 mg daily by 15%. However, the **fleroxacin** levels remained above the MIC_{90} of methicillin-sensitive strains of *S. aureus* and *S. epidermis* for at least 24 hours.[19] No special precautions would seem necessary if rifampicin is given with any of these quinolones.

1. Metz R, Jaehde U, Wiesemann H, Gottschalk B, Stephan U, Schunack W. Pharmacokinetic interactions and non-interactions of pefloxacin. Proc 15th Int Congr Chemother, Istanbul, 1987, 997–9.
2. Sultan E, Richard C, Pezzano M, Auzepy P, Singlas E. Pharmacokinetics of pefloxacin and amikacin administered simultaneously to intensive care patients. *Eur J Clin Pharmacol* (1988) 34, 637–43.
3. Nix DE, Wilton JH, Hyatt J, Thomas J, Strenkoski-Nix LC, Forrest A, Schentag JJ. Pharmacodynamic modeling of the in vivo interaction between cefotaxime and ofloxacin by using serum ultrafiltrate inhibitory titers. *Antimicrob Agents Chemother* (1997) 41, 1108–14.
4. Deppermann K-M, Boeckh M, Grineisen S, Shokry F, Borner K, Koeppe P, Krasemann C, Wagner J, Lode H. Brief report: combination effects of ciprofloxacin, clindamycin, and metronidazole intravenously in volunteers. *Am J Med* (1989) 87 (Suppl 5A), 46S–48S.

5. Weinstein MP, Deeter RG, Swanson KA, Gross JS. Crossover assessment of serum bactericidal activity and pharmacokinetics of ciprofloxacin alone and in combination in healthy elderly volunteers. *Antimicrob Agents Chemother* (1991) 35, 2352–8.
6. Foulds G, Cohen MJ, Geffken A, Willavize S, Hunt T. Coadministration of azithromycin 1-g packet does not affect the bioavailability of trovafloxacin. *Intersci Conf Antimicrob Agents Chemother* (1998) 38, 31.
7. Boeckh M, Grineisen S, Shokry F, Koeppe P, Borner K, Krasemann C, Lode H. Pharmacokinetics and serum bactericidal activity (SBA) of ciprofloxacin (CIP) and ofloxacin (OFL) alone and in combination with metronidazole (METRO) or clindamycin (CLINDA). *Intersci Conf Antimicrob Agents Chemother* (1988) 28, 246.
8. Ludwig E, Graber H, Székely É, Csiba A. Metabolic interactions of ciprofloxacin. *Diagn Microbiol Infect Dis* (1990) 13, 135–41.
9. Stille W and Ostner KH. Antagonismus Nitrofurantoin-Nalidixinsaure. *Klin Wochenschr* (1966) 44, 155–6.
10. Piguet D. L'action inhibitrice de la nitrofurantoïne sur le pouvoir bactériostatique *in vitro* de l'acide nalidixique. *Ann Inst Pasteur (Paris)* (1969) 116, 43–8.
11. Sweetman SC, editor. Martindale: The complete drug reference. 34th ed. London: Pharmaceutical Press; 2005 p. 238.
12. Barriere SL, Catlin DH, Orlando PL, Noe A, Frost RW. Alteration in the pharmacokinetic disposition of ciprofloxacin by simultaneous administration of azlocillin. *Antimicrob Agents Chemother* (1990) 34, 823–6.
13. Paintaud G, Alván G, Hellgren U, Nilsson-Ehle I. Lack of effect of amoxycillin on the absorption of ofloxacin. *Eur J Clin Pharmacol* (1993) 44, 207–9.
14. Strenkoski-Nix LC, Forrest A, Schentag JJ, Nix DE. Pharmacodynamic interactions of ciprofloxacin, piperacillin, and piperacillin/tazobactam in healthy volunteers. *J Clin Pharmacol* (1998) 38, 1063–71.
15. Chandler MHH, Toler SM, Rapp RP, Muder RR, Korvick JA. Multiple-dose pharmacokinetics of concurrent oral ciprofloxacin and rifampin therapy in elderly patients. *Antimicrob Agents Chemother* (1990) 34, 442–7.
16. Polk RE. Drug-drug interactions with ciprofloxacin and other fluoroquinolones. *Am J Med* (1989) 87 (Suppl 5A), 76S–81S.
17. Jhaj R, Roy A, Uppal R, Behera D. Influence of ciprofloxacin on pharmacokinetics of rifampin. *Curr Ther Res* (1997) 58, 260–5.
18. Humbert G, Brumpt I, Montay G, Le Liboux A, Frydman A, Borsa-Lebas F, Moore N. Influence of rifampin on the pharmacokinetics of pefloxacin. *Clin Pharmacol Ther* (1991) 50, 682–7.
19. Schrenzel J, Dayer P, Leemann T, Weidekamm E, Portmann R, Lew DP. Influence of rifampin on fleroxacin pharmacokinetics. *Antimicrob Agents Chemother* (1993) 37, 2132–8.

Quinolones + Pirenzepine

Four doses of pirenzepine 50 mg delayed the absorption of ciprofloxacin and ofloxacin in 10 healthy subjects, but their bioavailabilities remained unchanged.[1] The delayed absorption is unlikely to be of clinical significance.

1. Höffken G, Lode H, Wiley R, Glatzel TD, Sievers D, Olschewski T, Borner K, Koeppe T. Pharmacokinetics and bioavailability of ciprofloxacin and ofloxacin: effect of food and antacid intake. *Rev Infect Dis* (1988) 10 (Suppl 1), S138–S139.

Quinolones + Probenecid

Probenecid increases the serum levels and/or decreases the urinary excretion of cinoxacin, ciprofloxacin, clinafloxacin, enoxacin, fleroxacin, levofloxacin, nalidixic acid and norfloxacin. The clinical importance of these changes is uncertain, but is seems likely they will only be important in the presence of other drugs that also affect renal excretion. Grepafloxacin, moxifloxacin, sparfloxacin, and probably ofloxacin, appear not to interact with probenecid.

Clinical evidence

(a) Cinoxacin

A study in 6 healthy subjects found that probenecid 500 mg three times daily roughly doubled the serum levels of a 3-hour intravenous infusion of cinoxacin. The renal clearance of cinoxacin was also reduced from 68 to 46% during and for the 4 hours after the infusion.[1]

(b) Ciprofloxacin

In one study, probenecid 1 g, given 30 minutes before ciprofloxacin 500 mg, was found to reduce the renal clearance of ciprofloxacin by up to 50%. Other pharmacokinetic parameters (maximum serum levels, AUC) were unchanged and no accumulation of ciprofloxacin appeared to occur, probably due to an increase in extra-renal elimination.[2]

Another study found that the renal clearance of ciprofloxacin was reduced by 64% by probenecid. However, in contrast to the other study cited, the AUC of ciprofloxacin was increased by 74% and the AUC of its 2-aminoethylamino metabolite by 234%. As a consequence, levels of ciprofloxacin in tears, sweat and saliva were also increased, but probenecid had no direct effect on ciprofloxacin distribution into these fluids.[3]

(c) Clinafloxacin

Probenecid 1 g, given 1 hour before a single 400-mg dose of clinafloxacin, reduced the total and renal clearance of clinafloxacin by 24 and 36% respectively, raised the AUC by 32% and increased the elimination half-life from 6.3 to 7 hours.[4]

(d) Enoxacin

In one subject, the renal clearance of enoxacin 600 mg was approximately halved, and the half-life increased from 3.5 to 4.5 hours by a single 2.5-g dose of probenecid.[5]

(e) Fleroxacin

A study in 6 healthy subjects given a single 200-mg dose of fleroxacin, followed by 500 mg of probenecid 0.5, 12, 24 and 36 hours later, found that the fleroxacin AUC was increased by 37%, the maximum serum levels were slightly but not significantly increased, and the fleroxacin urinary excretion was decreased by 22%.[6] Another study found that probenecid increased the AUC of fleroxacin 400 mg by 26% (not statistically significant), but it had no effect on fleroxacin urinary excretion.[7]

(f) Grepafloxacin

A study in 32 healthy subjects found that probenecid had no effect on the pharmacokinetics of a single 200-mg dose of grepafloxacin.[8] Probenecid similarly had no significant effect on grepafloxacin pharmacokinetics in another 6 healthy subjects.[9]

(g) Levofloxacin

A study in 12 healthy subjects found that although probenecid reduced the renal clearance of a single 500-mg oral dose of levofloxacin by about a third and increased its AUC and half-life by similar amounts. The 72-hour urinary levofloxacin excretion was unaltered.[10]

(h) Moxifloxacin

A study in 12 healthy subjects found that probenecid had no clinically significant effects on the pharmacokinetics of a single 400-mg dose of moxifloxacin.[11]

(i) Nalidixic acid

Two volunteers, acting as their own controls, took nalidixic acid 500 mg with and without probenecid 500 mg. The peak serum levels of nalidixic acid were unaffected at 2 hours, but at 8 hours the levels were increased threefold by the probenecid.[12]

Another study in 5 women with urinary tract infections treated with nalidixic acid showed that probenecid increased the maximum serum nalidixic acid levels and AUC by 43% and 74% respectively.[13]

(j) Norfloxacin

The mean 12-hour urinary recovery of norfloxacin 200 mg was reduced to about half in 5 subjects when they were given probenecid 1 g. Norfloxacin serum concentrations were unaffected.[14]

(k) Ofloxacin

A study in 8 healthy subjects found that probenecid 500 mg increased the AUC of a single 200-mg dose of ofloxacin by 16% and decreased the total body clearance by 14%. Other pharmacokinetic parameters were not significantly affected.[15]

(l) Sparfloxacin

Probenecid 1.5 g did not significantly affect the clearance, the AUC or the half-life of sparfloxacin 200 mg in 6 healthy subjects.[16]

Mechanism

The likely explanation is that probenecid successfully competes with some quinolones for tubular excretion, so that their renal elimination is reduced. Some quinolones are more dependent on glomerular filtration (e.g. grepafloxacin)[9] than tubular excretion for elimination, and thus are unaffected by competition for tubular excretion.[7]

Importance and management

Established interactions, but their clinical importance seems not to have been assessed. There appears to be no reason for avoiding concurrent use.

The increased levels and decreased renal excretion of clinafloxacin caused by probenecid are not considered large enough to warrant dosage adjustment,[4] and most of the changes seen with the other quinolones were of a similar magnitude. However, caution has been advised in the presence of other drugs that may compete for renal excretion (such as some penicillins or cephalosporins).[3,4] Grepafloxacin, moxifloxacin, sparfloxacin, and probably ofloxacin, appear not to interact.

1. Rodriguez N, Madsen PO, Welling PG. Influence of probenecid on serum levels and urinary excretion of cinoxacin. *Antimicrob Agents Chemother* (1979) 15, 465–69.
2. Wingender W, Beerman D, Förster D, Graefe K-H, Kuhlmann J. Interactions of ciprofloxacin with food intake and drugs. *Curr Clin Pract Ser* (1986) 34, 136–40.
3. Jaehde U, Sörgel F, Reiter A, Sigl G, Naber KG, Schunack W. Effect of probenecid on the distribution and elimination of ciprofloxacin in humans. *Clin Pharmacol Ther* (1995) 58, 532–41.
4. Randinitis EJ, Koup JR, Bron NJ, Hounslow NJ, Rausch G, Abel R, Vassos AB, Sedman AJ. Drug interaction studies with clinafloxacin and probenecid, cimetidine, phenytoin and warfarin. *Drugs* (1999) 58 (Suppl 2), 254–5.
5. Wijnands WJA, Vree TB, Baars AM, van Herwaarden CLA. Pharmacokinetics of enoxacin and its penetration into bronchial secretions and lung tissue. *J Antimicrob Chemother* (1988) 21 (Suppl B), 67–77.
6. Shiba K, Saito A, Shimada J, Hori S, Kaji M, Miyahara T, Kusajima H, Kaneko S, Saito S, Uchida H. Interactions of fleroxacin with dried aluminium hydroxide gel and probenecid. *Rev Infect Dis* (1989) 11 (Suppl 5), S1097–S1098.
7. Weidekamm E, Portmann R, Suter K, Partos C, Dell D, Lücker PW. Single- and multiple dose pharmacokinetics of fleroxacin, a trifluorinated quinolone, in humans. *Antimicrob Agents Chemother* (1987) 31, 1909–14.
8. Koneru B, Bramer S, Bricmont P, Maroli A, Shiba K. Effect of food, gastric pH and co-administration of antacid, cimetidine and probenecid on the oral pharmacokinetics of the broad spectrum antimicrobial agent grepafloxacin. *Pharm Res* (1996) 13 (9 Suppl), S414.
9. Shiba K, Yoshida M, Hori S, Shimada J, Saito A, Sakai O. Pharmacokinetic interaction of OPC-17116 with probenecid in healthy volunteers. *Intersci Conf Antimicrob Agents Chemother* (1991) 31, 346.
10. Gaitonde MD, Mendes P, House ESA, Lehr KH. The effects of cimetidine and probenecid on the pharmacokinetics of levofloxacin (LVFX). *Intersci Conf Antimicrob Agents Chemother* (1995) 35, 8.
11. Stass H, Sachse R. Effect of probenecid on the kinetics of a single oral 400-mg dose of moxifloxacin in healthy male volunteers. *Clin Pharmacokinet* (2001) 40 (Suppl 1), 71–76.
12. Dash H, Mills J. Severe metabolic acidosis associated with nalidixic acid overdose. *Ann Intern Med* (1976) 84, 570–1.
13. Ferry N, Cuisinaud G, Pozet N, Zech PY, Sassard J. Influence du probénécide sur la pharmacocinétique de l'acide nalidixique. *Therapie* (1982) 37, 645–9.
14. Shimada J, Yamaji T, Ueda Y, Uchida H, Kusajima H, Irikura T. Mechanism of renal excretion of AM-715, a new quinolonecarboxylic acid derivative, in rabbits, dogs, and humans. *Antimicrob Agents Chemother* (1983) 23, 1–7.
15. Nataraj B, Rao Mamidi NVS, Krishna DR. Probenecid affects the pharmacokinetics of ofloxacin in healthy volunteers. *Clin Drug Invest* (1998) 16, 259–62.
16. Shimada J, Saito A, Shiba K, Hojo T, Kaji M, Hori S, Yoshida M, Sakai O. Pharmacokinetics and clinical studies of sparfloxacin. *Chemotherapy (Tokyo)* (1991) 39 (Suppl 4), 234–44.

Quinolones + Sucralfate

Sucralfate causes a marked reduction in the absorption of ciprofloxacin, enoxacin, gemifloxacin, lomefloxacin, moxifloxacin, ofloxacin, norfloxacin and sparfloxacin, but only a modest reduction in fleroxacin levels. The interaction is very much reduced or does not occur if the sucralfate is given 2 to 6 hours after the quinolone.

Clinical evidence

(a) Ciprofloxacin

Sucralfate 1 g four times daily reduced the AUC and maximum serum concentration of ciprofloxacin 500 mg by 88% and 90% respectively in 8 healthy subjects.[1]

A patient given sucralfate 1 g four times daily had serum ciprofloxacin levels which were 85 to 90% lower than 5 other patients who were not taking sucralfate.[2] A single dose study found a 96% reduction in the AUC of ciprofloxacin following a 2-g dose of sucralfate.[3] A study in 12 healthy subjects found that a 1-g dose of sucralfate given 6 and 2 hours before a single 750-mg dose of ciprofloxacin, reduced the ciprofloxacin AUC by about 30%. Three of the subjects showed little or no changes in AUC but a decrease of more than 50% was seen in 4 others.[4] A related study in 12 healthy subjects found that the bioavailability of ciprofloxacin 750 mg was reduced by 7%, 20% and 95% respectively when sucralfate was given 6 hours before, 2 hours before or at the same time as the ciprofloxacin.[5] Oral sucralfate does not alter the effects of ciprofloxacin on aerobic bacteria in the gut.[6]

(b) Enoxacin

In 8 healthy subjects the bioavailability of enoxacin 400 mg was reduced by 54% and 88% when sucralfate 1 g was given 2 hours before or with the enoxacin. When sucralfate was given 2 hours after the enoxacin the bioavailability was not affected.[7]

(c) Fleroxacin

The bioavailability of fleroxacin 400 mg was reduced by 24% in 20 healthy subjects taking sucralfate 1 g 6-hourly.[8]

(d) Gemifloxacin

Gemifloxacin 320 mg was given either 3 hours before or 2 hours after sucralfate 2 g in a study in 27 healthy subjects. The pharmacokinetics of gemifloxacin were not significantly altered when sucralfate was given after the gemifloxacin, probably due to its rapid absorption. However, when sucralfate was given 3 hours before gemifloxacin, the AUC and maximum plasma levels were decreased by 53% and 69% respectively.[9]

(e) Levofloxacin

The pharmacokinetics of levofloxacin are unaffected by sucralfate taken 2 hours after the quinolone.[10]

(f) Lomefloxacin

A study in 12 subjects found that when lomefloxacin 400 mg was given 2 hours after sucralfate 1 g the lomefloxacin AUC and maximum serum concentration was reduced by about 25% and 30% respectively.[11] Another study in 8 healthy subjects found that when lomefloxacin 400 mg was given with sucralfate 1 g, the lomefloxacin AUC was reduced by 51%.[12]

(g) Moxifloxacin

In 12 healthy subjects a total of five doses of sucralfate 1 g, given at the same time and 5, 10, 15 and 24 hours after a single 400-mg dose of moxifloxacin, reduced the AUC and maximum serum concentration of moxifloxacin by 40% and 29% respectively.[13]

(h) Norfloxacin

A study in 8 healthy subjects found that sucralfate 1 g four times daily reduced the AUC of a single 400-mg dose of norfloxacin by 98%, when taken with the sucralfate, and by 42% when taken 2 hours after the sucralfate.[14] Another study found a reduction of 91% in the AUC of norfloxacin 400 mg when it was taken with sucralfate 1 g, but no reduction when it was taken 2 hours before sucralfate.[15]

(i) Ofloxacin

A single dose study found that sucralfate [dose not stated] reduced the maximum serum levels and AUC of a single 200-mg dose of ofloxacin by about two-thirds.[16] Another study found a reduction of 61% when ofloxacin 400 mg was taken with sucralfate 1 g, but no reduction when the ofloxacin was taken 2 hours before sucralfate.[15] Food reduced the extent of the interaction but it was still marked.[17]

(j) Sparfloxacin

In a study in 15 healthy subjects sucralfate 1 g four times daily reduced the maximum serum levels, the AUC and the relative bioavailability of sparfloxacin 400 mg daily by 39, 47 and 44% respectively.[18] In a study assessing staggered dosing of sucralfate 1.5 g on the pharmacokinetics of sparfloxacin 300 mg, the AUC was unaffected when sucralfate was given 4 hours after the quinolone, but was decreased by 34% when given 2 hours before, and 51% when given at the same time as sucralfate.[19]

Mechanism

The aluminium hydroxide component of sucralfate (about 200 mg in each gram) forms an insoluble chelate between the cation and the 4-keto and 3-carboxyl groups of the quinolone, which reduces its absorption. See 'Quinolones + Antacids or Calcium compounds', p.227 for more on this mechanism.

Importance and management

Established and clinically important interactions. Because it seems probable that serum ciprofloxacin, enoxacin, gemifloxacin, levofloxacin, lomefloxacin, moxifloxacin, ofloxacin, norfloxacin and sparfloxacin levels will be reduced to subtherapeutic concentrations if given with the sucralfate, separate the dosages as much as possible (by 2 hours or more), giving the quinolone first. The study with moxifloxacin suggested that sucralfate should not be given for 2 hours before or 4 hours after the quinolone, but more study is needed to confirm both these findings and the effectiveness of separating the dosages. The interaction with fleroxacin is only modest (bioavailability reduced by 24%) and probably not clinically important, but some separation of the dosages may reduce the interaction further. This needs confirmation. **Pefloxacin** also interacts with antacids containing aluminium hydroxide (see 'Quinolones + Antacids or Calcium compounds', p.227) and is therefore likely to interact with sucralfate. The

'H_2-blockers' (p.234) and 'proton pump inhibitors', (p.738) do not interact and may therefore be alternatives to sucralfate in many situations.

1. Garrelts JC, Godley PJ, Peterie JD, Gerlach EH, Yakshe CC. Sucralfate significantly reduces ciprofloxacin concentrations in serum. *Antimicrob Agents Chemother* (1990) 34, 931–3.
2. Yuk JH, Nightingale CN, Quintiliani R. Ciprofloxacin levels when receiving sucralfate. *JAMA* (1989) 262, 901.
3. Brouwers JRBJ, Van Der Kam HJ, Sijtsma J, Proost JH. Important reduction of ciprofloxacin absorption by sucralfate and magnesium citrate solution. *Drug Invest* (1990) 2, 197–9.
4. Nix DE, Watson WA, Handy L, Frost RW, Rescott DL, Goldstein HR. The effect of sucralfate pretreatment on the pharmacokinetics of ciprofloxacin. *Pharmacotherapy* (1989) 9, 377–80.
5. Van Slooten AD, Nix DE, Wilton JH, Love JH, Spivey JM, Goldstein HR. Combined use of ciprofloxacin and sucralfate. *DICP Ann Pharmacother* (1991) 25, 578–82.
6. Krueger WA, Ruckdeschel G, Unertl K. Influence of intravenously administered ciprofloxacin on aerobic intestinal microflora and fecal drug levels when administered simultaneously with sucralfate. *Antimicrob Agents Chemother* (1997) 41, 1725–30.
7. Ryerson B, Toothaker R, Schleyer I, Sedman A, Colburn W. Effect of sucralfate on enoxacin pharmacokinetics. *Intersci Conf Antimicrob Agents Chemother* (1989) 29, 136.
8. Lubowski TJ, Nightingale CH, Sweeney K, Quintiliani R. Effect of sucralfate on pharmacokinetics of fleroxacin in healthy volunteers. *Antimicrob Agents Chemother* (1992) 36, 2758–60.
9. Allen A, Bygate E, Faessel H, Isaac L, Lewis A. The effect of ferrous sulphate and sucralfate on the bioavailability of oral gemifloxacin in healthy volunteers. *Int J Antimicrob Agents* (2000) 15, 283–9.
10. Lee L-J, Hafkin B, Lee I-D, Hoh J, Dix R. Effect of food and sucralfate on a single oral dose of 500 milligrams of levofloxacin in healthy subjects. *Antimicrob Agents Chemother* (1997) 41, 2196–2200.
11. Nix D, Schentag J. Lomefloxacin (L) absorption kinetics when administered with ranitidine (R) and sucralfate (S). *Intersci Conf Antimicrob Agents Chemother* (1989) 29, 317.
12. Lehto P, Kivistö KT. Different effects of products containing metal ions on the absorption of lomefloxacin. *Clin Pharmacol Ther* (1994) 56, 477–82.
13. Stass H, Schühly U, Möller J-G, Delesen H. Effects of sucralfate on the oral bioavailability of moxifloxacin, a novel 8-methoxyfluoroquinolone, in healthy volunteers. *Clin Pharmacokinet* (2001) 40 (Suppl 1), 49–55.
14. Parpia SH, Nix DE, Hejmanowski LG, Goldstein HR, Witton JH, Schentag JJ. Sucralfate reduces the gastrointestinal absorption of norfloxacin. *Antimicrob Agents Chemother* (1989) 33, 99–102.
15. Lehto P, Kvistö KT. Effect of sucralfate on absorption of norfloxacin and ofloxacin. *Antimicrob Agents Chemother* (1994) 38, 248–51.
16. Shiba K, Yoshida M, Kachi M, Shimada J, Saito A, Sakai N. Effects of peptic ulcer-healing drugs on the pharmacokinetics of new quinolone (OFLX). 17th Int Congr Chemother, June 1991, Berlin, Abstract 415.
17. Kawakami J, Matsuse T, Kotaki H, Seino T, Fukuchi Y, Orimo H, Sawada Y, Iga T. The effect of food on the interaction of ofloxacin with sucralfate in healthy volunteers. *Eur J Clin Pharmacol* (1994) 47, 67–9.
18. Zix JA, Geerdes-Fenge HF, Rau M, Vöckler J, Borner K, Koeppe P, Lode H. Pharmacokinetics of sparfloxacin and interaction with cisapride and sucralfate. *Antimicrob Agents Chemother* (1997) 41, 1668–1672.
19. Kamberi M, Nakashima H, Ogawa K, Oda N, Nakano S. The effect of staggered dosing of sucralfate on oral bioavailability of sparfloxacin. *Br J Clin Pharmacol* (2000) 49, 98–103.

Quinolones; Ciprofloxacin + Pancreatic enzymes

The pharmacokinetics of ciprofloxacin are not affected by pancreatic enzyme supplements.

Clinical evidence, mechanism, importance and management

Six patients with cystic fibrosis, chronically infected with *P. aeruginosa* and treated with a range of drugs including ceftazidime, tobramycin, ticarcillin and salbutamol, demonstrated no significant changes in the pharmacokinetics of a single 250-mg dose of ciprofloxacin when given standard doses of pancreatic enzymes (seven *Pancrease* capsules).[1] No special precautions would seem to be necessary during concurrent use.

1. Mack G, Cooper PJ, Buchanan N. Effects of enzyme supplementation on oral absorption of ciprofloxacin in patients with cystic fibrosis. *Antimicrob Agents Chemother* (1991) 35, 1484–5.

Quinolones; Ciprofloxacin + Ursodeoxycholic acid (Ursodiol)

An isolated report describes a reduction in serum ciprofloxacin levels in a patient treated with ursodeoxycholic acid.

Clinical evidence, mechanism, importance and management

A man with metastatic colon cancer had unusually low serum levels of ciprofloxacin following oral dosing; his only other medication was ursodeoxycholic acid 300 mg twice daily for gallstones. Despite the low antibacterial serum levels the bacteraemia cleared. Several months later when he was readmitted to hospital, both drugs were again given, initially staggered, and then later together. When taken together the AUC of the ciprofloxacin was reduced by 50%.[1] The reason for this interaction is not understood.

This seems to be the first and only report of an interaction between a quinolone and ursodeoxycholic acid and its importance is uncertain. More study is needed to establish this interaction, its importance, and its mechanism.

1. Belliveau PP, Nightingale CH, Quintiliani R, Maderazo EG. Reduction in serum concentrations of ciprofloxacin after administration of ursodiol to a patient with hepatobiliary disease. *Clin Infect Dis* (1994) 19, 354–5.

Quinolones; Lomefloxacin + Furosemide

Furosemide causes a small, almost certainly unimportant, rise in the serum levels of lomefloxacin. The pharmacokinetics and diuretic effects of the furosemide are not changed.

Clinical evidence, mechanism, importance and management

A study in 8 healthy subjects found that when a single 200-mg dose of lomefloxacin was taken with furosemide 40 mg, the AUC of lomefloxacin was increased by 12%. The maximum serum levels and the half-life were also increased, but not to a statistically significant extent.[1] The suggested reason for the interaction is that there is some competition between the two drugs for excretion by the kidney tubules. No significant changes were seen in the pharmacokinetics of the furosemide nor in its diuretic effects.[1] The small rise in the serum levels of lomefloxacin is almost certainly too small to be important and there would seem to be no reason for avoiding concurrent use. Information about other quinolone antibacterials appears to be lacking.

1. Sudoh T, Fujimura A, Shiga T, Sasaki M, Harada K, Tateishi T, Ohashi K, Ebihara A. Renal clearance of lomefloxacin is decreased by furosemide. *Eur J Clin Pharmacol* (1994) 46, 267–9.

Quinolones; Ofloxacin + Cetraxate

A single-dose study found that cetraxate [dose not stated] did not affect the pharmacokinetics of a single 200-mg dose of ofloxacin.[1] No special precautions would seem to be necessary on concurrent use.

1. Shiba K, Yoshida M, Kachi M, Shimada J, Saito A, Sakai N. Effects of peptic ulcer-healing drugs on the pharmacokinetics of new quinolone (OFLX). 17th Int Congr Chemother, June 1991, Berlin, Abstract 415.

Rifampicin (Rifampin) + Aminosalicylic acid

The serum levels of rifampicin are approximately halved if aminosalicylic acid granules containing bentonite are given.

Clinical evidence

The serum rifampicin levels of 30 patients with tuberculosis given rifampicin 10 mg/kg were reduced by more than 50%, from 6.06 to 2.91 micrograms/ml, at 2 hours by aminosalicylate.[1,2] Later studies in 6 healthy subjects showed that this interaction was not due to the aminosalicylic acid itself but to the **bentonite**, which was the main excipient of the granules.[3] The rifampicin AUC was statistically unchanged in the presence of sodium aminosalicylate tablets (no **bentonite**), whereas it was reduced by more than 37% in the presence of **bentonite** from aminosalicylate granules.[3]

Other studies confirm this marked reduction in serum rifampicin levels in the presence of **bentonite** in aminosalicylic acid granules.[4]

Mechanism

The bentonite excipient in the aminosalicylic acid granules adsorbs the rifampicin onto its surface so that much less is available for absorption, which results in reduced serum levels.[3] Bentonite is a naturally occurring mineral (montmorillonite) consisting largely of hydrate aluminium silicate, and is similar to kaolin.

Importance and management

A well documented and clinically important interaction. Separating the administration of the two drugs by 8 to 12 hours to prevent their mixing in the gut has been suggested as an effective way to prevent this interaction.[1] An alternative is to give aminosalicylic acid preparations that do not contain bentonite.

1. Boman G, Hanngren Å, Malmborg A-S, Borgå O, Sjöqvist F. Drug Interaction: decreased serum concentrations of rifampicin when given with P.A.S. *Lancet* (1971) i, 800.
2. Boman G, Borgå O, Hanngren Å, Malmborg A-S and Sjöqvist F. Pharmacokinetic interactions between the tuberculostatics rifampicin, para-aminosalicylic acid and isoniazid. *Acta Pharmacol Toxicol (Copenh)* (1970) 28 (Suppl 1), 15.
3. Boman G, Lundgren P, Stjernström G. Mechanism of the inhibitory effect of PAS granules on the absorption of rifampicin: adsorption of rifampicin by an excipient, bentonite. *Eur J Clin Pharmacol* (1975) 8, 293–9.
4. Boman G. Serum concentration and half-life of rifampicin after simultaneous oral administration of aminosalicylic acid or isoniazid. *Eur J Clin Pharmacol* (1974) 7, 217–25.

Rifampicin (Rifampin) + Antacids

The absorption of rifampicin can be reduced up to about a third by antacids, but the clinical importance of this is uncertain.

Clinical evidence

When 5 healthy subjects took a single 600-mg dose of rifampicin with various antacids and 200 ml of water the absorption of rifampicin was reduced. The antacids caused a fall in the urinary excretion of rifampicin as follows: 15 or 30 ml of **aluminium hydroxide gel** 29 to 31%; 2 or 4 g of **magnesium trisilicate** 31 to 36%; and 2 g of **sodium bicarbonate** 21%.[1]

Three groups of 15 patients with tuberculosis were given a single oral dose of rifampicin 10 to 12 mg/kg, isoniazid 300 mg and ethambutol 20 mg/kg either alone or with 4 teaspoonfuls of antacid. A 'significant number' of patients had peak rifampicin concentrations below 6.5 micrograms/ml (serum level quoted as necessary to achieve adequate lung concentrations) in the group receiving *Aludrox* (**aluminium hydroxide**), but no significant effect was noted in the group receiving *Gelusil* (**aluminium hydroxide** plus **magnesium trisilicate**).[2] However, in a further study in 14 healthy subjects, 30 ml of *Mylanta* (**aluminium/magnesium hydroxide**) 9 hours before, with and after rifampicin had no effect on rifampicin pharmacokinetics.[3]

Mechanism

It has been suggested that the rise in stomach pH caused by these antacids reduces the dissolution of the rifampicin and thereby inhibits its absorption. In addition, aluminium ions may form less soluble chelates with rifampicin, and magnesium trisilicate can adsorb rifampicin, both of which would also be expected to reduce bioavailability.[1]

Importance and management

Direct information seems to be limited to these reports. No one seems to have assessed the effects of 20 to 35% reductions in absorption on rifampicin treatment, but if antacids are given it would be prudent to be alert for any evidence that treatment is less effective than expected. The US makers of rifampicin advise giving rifampicin 1 hour before antacids.[4] More study is needed.

1. Khalil SAH, El-Khordagui LK, El-Gholmy ZA. Effect of antacids on oral absorption of rifampicin. *Int J Pharmaceutics* (1984) 20, 99–106.
2. Gupta PR, Mehta YR, Gupta ML, Sharma TN, Jain D, Gupta RB. Rifampicin-aluminium antacid interaction. *J Assoc Physicians India* (1988) 36, 363–4.
3. Peloquin CA, Namdar R, Singleton MD, Nix DE. Pharmacokinetics of rifampin under fasting conditions, with food, and with antacids. *Chest* (1999) 115, 12–18.
4. Rifadin (Rifampicin). Product information. *Physicians Desk Reference* (2005) 59, 736.

Rifampicin (Rifampin) + Clofazimine

There is no pharmacokinetic interaction between rifampicin and clofazimine.

Clinical evidence, mechanism, importance and management

Clofazimine 100 mg daily, given to 15 patients with leprosy taking rifampicin 600 mg daily and dapsone 100 mg daily, had no effect on the pharmacokinetics of rifampicin.[1] A single-dose study similarly found that the bioavailability of clofazimine remained unaltered when rifampicin was given, although a reduction in the rate of absorption was seen.[2] No special precautions would seem to be necessary on concurrent use.

1. Venkatesan K, Mathur A, Girdhar BK, Bharadwaj VP. The effect of clofazimine on the pharmacokinetics of rifampicin and dapsone in leprosy. *J Antimicrob Chemother* (1986) 18, 715–18.
2. Mehta J, Gandhi IS, Sane SB, Wamburkar MN. Effect of clofazimine and dapsone on rifampicin (Lositril) pharmacokinetics in multibacillary and paucibacillary leprosy cases. *Indian J Lepr* (1985) 57, 297–310.

Rifampicin (Rifampin) + Food

Food delays and reduces the absorption of rifampicin from the gut.

Clinical evidence

The absorption of a single 10-mg/kg dose of rifampicin was reduced when it was given to 6 healthy subjects with a **standard Indian breakfast** (125 g wheat, 10 g visible fat, 350 g vegetables). The AUC after 8 hours was reduced by 26% and the peak plasma levels were prolonged (from 11.84 micrograms/ml at 2 hours to 8.35 micrograms/ml at 4 hours) and reduced by about 30%.[1] In another study, a **high-fat breakfast** reduced the maximum serum level of rifampicin 600 mg by 36% and delayed the absorption, but the AUC was not significantly altered.[2]

Mechanism

Not understood.

Importance and management

An established interaction. Rifampicin should be taken on an empty stomach (at least 30 minutes before a meal, or 2 hours after a meal) to ensure rapid and complete absorption.

1. Polasa K, Krishnaswamy K. Effect of food on bioavailability of rifampicin. *J Clin Pharmacol* (1983) 23, 433–7.
2. Peloquin CA, Namdar R, Singleton MD, Nix DE. Pharmacokinetics of rifampin under fasting conditions, with food, and with antacids. *Chest* (1999) 155, 12–18.

Rifampicin (Rifampin) + Phenobarbital

Phenobarbital possibly modestly increases the clearance of rifampicin. The effect of rifampicin on phenobarbital levels is unknown, but note that rifampicin markedly increased the clearance of another barbiturate hexobarbital, used as a marker of drug metabolism.

Clinical evidence

In one study, the serum levels of rifampicin were reduced by 20 to 40% in 12 of 15 patients taking phenobarbital 100 mg daily.[1] In another study, although phenobarbital 100 mg daily for 7 days reduced the mean half-life of a single 600-mg dose of rifampicin by 15%, this was not statistically significant. However, in a further 5 patients with cirrhosis of the liver, phenobarbital did reduce the half-life of rifampicin by a mean of 2.2 hours.[2]

The effect of rifampicin on phenobarbital levels does not appear to have been studied, but rifampicin markedly increased the clearance of another barbiturate **hexobarbital**, used as a marker of drug metabolism.[3-6]

Mechanism

Both rifampicin and phenobarbital are potent liver enzyme inducing agents. The outcome of their effects when combined is not clear.

Importance and management

The documentation for this interaction is very limited, and the outcome of concurrent use is unclear. Concurrent use need not be avoided, but be alert for a reduced response to both drugs.

1. de Rautlin de la Roy Y, Beauchant G, Breuil K, Patte F. Diminution du taux sérique de rifampicine par le phénobarbital. *Presse Med* (1971) 79, 350.
2. Acocella G, Bonollo L, Mainardi M, Margaroli P, Nicolis FB. Kinetic studies on rifampicin. III. Effect of phenobarbital on the half-life of the antibiotic. *Tijdschr Gastroenterol* (1974) 17, 151–8.

3. Breimer DD, Zilly W, Richter E. Influence of rifampicin on drug metabolism: differences between hexobarbital and antipyrine. *Clin Pharmacol Ther* (1977) 21, 470–81.
4. Zilly W, Breimer DD, Richter E. Induction of drug metabolism in man after rifampicin treatment measured by increased hexobarbital and tolbutamide clearance. *Eur J Clin Pharmacol* (1975) 9, 219–27.
5. Zilly W, Breimer DD, Richter E. Stimulation of drug metabolism by rifampicin in patients with cirrhosis or cholestasis measured by increased hexobarbital and tolbutamide clearance. *Eur J Clin Pharmacol* (1977) 11, 287–93.
6. Smith DA, Chandler MHH, Shedlofsky SI, Wedlund PJ, Blouin RA. Age-dependent stereoselective increase in the oral clearance of hexobarbitone isomers caused by rifampicin. *Br J Clin Pharmacol* (1991) 32, 735–9.

Rifampicin (Rifampin) + Probenecid

Probenecid increased rifampicin levels in one study, but not in another.

Clinical evidence, mechanism, importance and management

A study in 6 healthy subjects given probenecid 2 g before and after a single 300-mg dose of rifampicin found that mean peak serum rifampicin levels were raised by 86%. At 4, 6 and 9 hours after the dose the percentage increases were 118, 90 and 102% respectively.[1] However, subsequent studies in patients taking either rifampicin 600 mg daily, or rifampicin 300 mg daily with probenecid 2 g taken 30 minutes earlier, showed that the probenecid group achieved serum rifampicin levels that were only about half those achieved by those on rifampicin 600 mg, suggesting no interaction occurred.[2] The reasons for these discordant results are not understood, although it has been suggested that erratic rifampicin absorption may have played a part.[2] The interaction is not proven, but it seems possible that some patients will experience a rise in rifampicin levels. Monitor concurrent use carefully for rifampicin adverse effects.

1. Kenwright S, Levi AJ. Impairment of hepatic uptake of rifamycin antibiotics by probenecid, and its therapeutic implications. *Lancet* (1973) ii, 1401–5.
2. Fallon RJ, Lees AW, Allan GW, Smith J, Tyrrell WF. Probenecid and rifampicin serum levels. *Lancet* (1975) ii, 792–4.

Rifampicin (Rifampin) + Ranitidine

Ranitidine appears not to interact with rifampicin.

Clinical evidence, mechanism, importance and management

In a controlled study, 112 patients with pulmonary tuberculosis were treated in 2 groups, one with a daily regimen of rifampicin 10 mg/kg, isoniazid 300 mg and ethambutol 20 mg/kg and ranitidine 150 mg twice daily, and the other with the same regimen without ranitidine. The pharmacokinetics of rifampicin (as measured by the total and unchanged urinary excretion) were not affected by ranitidine. No changes occurred in the incidence of adverse hepatic reactions, while gastrointestinal reactions were reduced.[1] There would seem to be no reason for avoiding the concurrent use of these drugs.

1. Purohit SD, Johri SC, Gupta PR, Mehta YR, Bhatnagar M. Ranitidine-rifampicin interaction. *J Assoc Physicians India* (1992) 40, 308–10.

Sodium fusidate + Colestyramine

***In vitro* studies have shown that colestyramine can bind with sodium fusidate in the gut, thereby reducing its activity,[1] but whether this also occurs clinically awaits confirmation. It is generally recommended that other drugs are given 1 hour before or 4 to 6 hours after colestyramine.**

1. Johns WH, Bates TR. Drug-cholestyramine interactions. I: Physicochemical factors affecting *in vitro* binding of sodium fusidate to cholestyramine. *J Pharm Sci* (1972) 61, 730–5.

Sulfonamides + Local anaesthetics

The para-aminobenzoic acid (PABA) derived from certain local anaesthetics can reduce the effects of the sulphonamides and allow the development of local and even generalised infections. However, it should be noted that the limited evidence for this interaction is from the 1940s.

Clinical evidence

Four patients on sulphonamides developed local infections in areas where **procaine** had been injected before diagnostic taps for meningitis, or draining procedures in empyema. Extensive cellulitis of the lumbar region occurred in one case, and abscesses appeared at the puncture sites in another. However, it should be noted that lumbar punctures were being done at least daily and up to four times a day in the 3 patients with meningitis.[1]

An *in vitro* study demonstrated that the amount of **procaine** in pleural fluid after anaesthesia for thoracentesis was sufficient to inhibit the antibacterial activity of 0.005% **sulphapyridine** against type III pneumococci.[2] Other studies in *animals* confirm that antagonism can occur both *in vitro*[3-5] and *in vivo*[6] with local anaesthetics that are hydrolysed to **PABA**.

Mechanism

The ester type of local anaesthetic is hydrolysed within the body to produce PABA. Sulfonamides work by inhibiting bacterial DNA synthesis by competitively inhibiting folate production. The PABA competes with the sulfonamides, so higher PABA concentrations effectively dilute the effects of the sulfonamides.

Importance and management

Clinical examples of this interaction seem to be few and of poor quality (note that the patients were given repeated lumbar punctures, up to four times daily in some instances). It should also be noted that the supporting evidence (human, *animal* and *in vitro* studies) dates back to the mid-1940s with nothing more recent apparently on record. Local anaesthetics of the ester type that are hydrolysed to PABA (e.g. tetracaine, procaine, benzocaine) present the greatest risk of a reaction, whereas those of the amide type (bupivacaine, cinchocaine, lidocaine, mepivacaine and prilocaine) would not be expected to interact adversely. The evidence seems to be too slim to preclude concurrent use of these drugs, but it is perhaps worth considering this interaction if high or repeated doses of the local anaesthetic are used. However, high doses or prolonged use of these ester-type anaesthetics are best avoided given their toxicity when used in this manner.

1. Peterson OL, Finland M. Sulfonamide inhibiting action of procaine. *Am J Med Sci* (1944) 207, 166–75.
2. Boroff DA, Cooper A, Bullowa JGM. Inhibition of sulfapyridine by procaine in chest fluids after procaine anesthesia. *Proc Soc Exp Biol Med* (1941) 47,182–3.
3. Casten D, Fried JJ, Hallman FA. Inhibitory effect of procaine on the bacteriostatic activity of sulfathiazole. *Surg Gynecol Obstet* (1943) 76, 726–8.
4. Powell HM, Krahl ME, Clowes GHA. Inhibition of chemotherapeutic action of sulfapyridine by local anesthetics. *J Indiana State Med Assoc* (1942) 35, 62–3.
5. Walker BS, Derow MA. The antagonism of local anesthetics against the sulfonamides. *Am J Med Sci* (1945) 210, 585–8.
6. Pfeiffer CC, Grant CW. The procaine-sulfonamide antagonism: an evaluation of local anesthetics for use with sulfonamide therapy. *Anesthesiology* (1944) 5, 605–14.

Sulfonamides; Sulfafurazole (Sulfisoxazole) + Laxatives

Sodium sulphate and castor oil used as laxatives can cause a modest but probably clinically unimportant reduction in sulfafurazole absorption.

Clinical evidence, mechanism, importance and management

In an experimental study of the possible effects of laxatives on the absorption of sulfafurazole, healthy subjects were given 10 to 20 g of oral **sodium sulphate** and 20 g of **castor oil** (doses sufficient to provoke diarrhoea). Absorption, measured by the amount of sulfafurazole excreted in the urine, was decreased by 50% with **castor oil**, and by 33% with **sodium sulphate** at 4 hours. However, serum levels of the drugs were relatively unchanged. The overall picture was that while these laxatives can alter the pattern of absorption, they do not seriously impair the total amount of drug absorbed.[1]

1. Mattila MJ, Takki S, Jussila J. Effect of sodium sulphate and castor oil on drug absorption from the human intestine. *Ann Clin Res* (1974) 6, 19–24.

Tetracyclines + Antacids

The serum levels and therefore the therapeutic effectiveness of the tetracyclines can be markedly reduced or even abolished by antacids containing aluminium, bismuth, calcium or magnesium. Other antacids, such as sodium bicarbonate, may also reduce the bioavailability of some tetracyclines. Even intravenous doxycycline levels can be reduced by antacids.

Clinical evidence

(a) Aluminium-containing antacids

A study in 5 patients and 6 healthy subjects found that within 48 hours of starting to take 2 teaspoonfuls of aluminium hydroxide gel (*Amphogel*) every 6 hours with **chlortetracycline** 500 mg the serum levels of the antibacterial were reduced by 80 to 90%. One patient had a recurrence of her urinary tract infection, which only subsided when the antacid was withdrawn, and one patient maintained **chlortetracycline** levels despite antacid treatment.[1] Similar results were obtained in other studies.[2,3]

Further studies have shown similar interactions with other tetracyclines:

- 30 ml of aluminium hydroxide reduced **oxytetracycline** serum levels by more than 50%,[3]
- 20 ml of aluminium hydroxide caused a 75% reduction in **demeclocycline** serum levels,[4]
- 15 ml of aluminium hydroxide caused a 100% reduction in serum **doxycycline** levels,[5,6]
- 30 ml of aluminium/**magnesium** hydroxide (*Maalox*) caused a 90% reduction in **tetracycline** serum levels.[7]

Intravenous doxycycline also appears to be affected. The mean serum levels of an intravenous dose of **doxycycline** were found to be reduced by 36% when 30 ml of aluminium hydroxide was taken four times daily, for 2 days before and after the antibacterial.[8]

(b) Bismuth-containing antacids

Bismuth subsalicylate reduces the absorption of **tetracycline** by 34%[9] and reduces the maximum serum levels of **doxycycline** by 50%.[10] It has been suggested the excipient *Veegum* (**magnesium** aluminium silicate) in some bismuth subsalicylate formulations enhances the effects on tetracyclines.[11] Bismuth carbonate similarly interacts with the tetracyclines *in vitro*.[12]

(c) Calcium-containing antacids

There seem to be no direct clinical studies with calcium-containing antacids, but a clinically important interaction seems almost a certainty, based on *in vitro* studies with calcium carbonate,[12] calcium in milk, (see 'Tetracyclines + Food or Drinks', p.244), dicalcium phosphate,[13] and calcium as an excipient in tetracycline capsules.[14]

(d) Magnesium-containing antacids

Magnesium sulphate certainly interacts with **tetracycline**, but in the only clinical study available[15] the amount of magnesium was much higher than would normally be found in the usual dose of antacid.

(e) Sodium-containing antacids

Sodium bicarbonate 2 g reduced the absorption of a 250-mg capsule of **tetracycline** by 50% in 8 subjects. If however **tetracycline** was dissolved before administration, the absorption was unaffected by the sodium bicarbonate.[16] Another study stated that sodium bicarbonate 2 g had an insignificant effect on **tetracycline** absorption.[7]

Mechanism

The tetracyclines bind with aluminium, bismuth, calcium, magnesium and other metallic ions to form compounds (chelates), which are much less soluble and therefore much less readily absorbed by the gut.[17] Because doxycycline undergoes enterohepatic recirculation, even intravenous doxycycline is affected, although less so than oral. It has also been suggested that the antacids reduce gastric pH and thereby decrease the absorption of tetracyclines,[16] but studies demonstrating the lack of a significant interaction with 'H_2-blockers', (p.245) suggest that this is not the case. The reduced absorption with bismuth compounds may be because they adsorb tetracyclines.[9] The interaction of some tetracycline preparations with sodium bicarbonate is unexplained.

Importance and management

Extremely well-documented, and well-established interactions. Their clinical importance depends on how much the serum tetracycline levels are lowered, but with normal antacid dosages the reductions cited above (50 to 100%) are large enough to mean that many organisms will not be exposed to minimum inhibitory concentrations (MIC) of antibacterial. As a general rule none of the aluminium, bismuth, calcium or magnesium-containing antacids should be given at the same time as the tetracycline antibacterials. If they must be used, separate the dosages by 2 to 3 hours or more to prevent their admixture in the gut. This also applies to **quinapril** formulations containing substantial quantities of magnesium (such as *Accupro*), although the interaction is less pronounced (see 'Tetracyclines + Quinapril', p.246), and is also predicted to occur with **didanosine** tablets formulated with antacids.[18]

Patients should be warned about taking any antacids and indigestion preparations that they may have purchased without a prescription.

Instead of using antacids to minimise the gastric irritant effects of the tetracyclines it is usually recommended that tetracyclines are taken after food, however it is not entirely clear how much this affects their absorption (see 'Tetracyclines + Food or Drinks', p.244). H_2-blockers may be suitable alternatives to antacids in some situations, see 'Tetracyclines + H_2-blockers', p.245.

1. Waisbren BA, Hueckel JS. Reduced absorption of aureomycin caused by aluminum hydroxide gel (*Amphojel*). *Proc Soc Exp Biol Med* (1950) 73, 73–4.
2. Seed JC, Wilson CE. The effect of aluminum hydroxide on serum aureomycin concentrations after simultaneous oral administration. *Bull Johns Hopkins Hosp* (1950) 86, 415–8.
3. Michel JC, Sayer RJ, Kirby WMM. Effect of food and antacids on blood levels of aureomycin and terramycin. *J Lab Clin Med* (1950) 36, 632–4.
4. Scheiner J, Altemeier WA. Experimental study of factors inhibiting absorption and effective therapeutic levels of declomycin. *Surg Gynecol Obstet* (1962) 114, 9–14.
5. Rosenblatt JE, Barrett JE, Brodie JL, Kirby WMM. Comparison of in vitro activity and clinical pharmacology of doxycycline with other tetracyclines. *Antimicrob Agents Chemother* (1966) 6, 134–41.
6. Deppermann K-M, Lode H, Höffken G, Tschink G, Kalz C, Koeppe P. Influence of ranitidine, pirenzepine, and aluminum magnesium hydroxide on the bioavailability of various antibiotics, including amoxicillin, cephalexin, doxycycline, and amoxicillin-clavulanic acid. *Antimicrob Agents Chemother* (1989) 33, 1901–7.
7. Garty M, Hurwitz A. Effect of cimetidine and antacids on gastrointestinal absorption of tetracycline. *Clin Pharmacol Ther* (1980) 28, 203–7.
8. Nguyen VX, Nix DE, Gillikin S, Schentag JJ. Effect of oral antacid administration on the pharmacokinetics of intravenous doxycycline. *Antimicrob Agents Chemother* (1989) 33, 434–6.
9. Albert KS, Welch RD, De Sante KA, Disanto AR. Decreased tetracycline bioavailability caused by a bismuth subsalicylate antidiarrheal mixture. *J Pharm Sci* (1979) 68, 586–8.
10. Ericsson CD, Feldman S, Pickering LK, Cleary TG. Influence of subsalicylate bismuth on absorption of doxycycline. *JAMA* (1982) 247, 2266–7.
11. Healy DP, Dansereau RJ, Dunn AB, Clendening CE, Mounts AW, Deepe GS. Reduced tetracycline bioavailability caused by magnesium aluminum silicate in liquid formulations of bismuth subsalicylate. *Ann Pharmacother* (1997) 31, 1460–4.
12. Christensen EKJ, Kerckhoffs HPM, Huizinga T. De invloed van antacida op de afgifte in vitro van tetracycline hydrochloride. *Pharm Weekbl* (1967) 102, 463–73.
13. Boger WP, Gavin JJ. An evaluation of tetracycline preparations. *N Engl J Med* (1959) 261, 827–32.
14. Sweeney WM, Hardy SM, Dornbush AC, Ruegsegger JM. Absorption of tetracycline in human beings as affected by certain excipients. *Antibiotic Med Clin Ther* (1957) 4, 642–56.
15. Harcourt RS, Hamburger M. The effect of magnesium sulfate in lowering tetracycline blood levels. *J Lab Clin Med* (1957) 50, 464–8.
16. Barr WH, Adir J, Garrettson L. Decrease of tetracycline absorption in man by sodium bicarbonate. *Clin Pharmacol Ther* (1971) 12, 779–84.
17. Albert A, Rees CW. Avidity of the tetracyclines for the cations of metals. *Nature* (1956) 177, 433–4.
18. Videx Tablets (Didanosine). Bristol-Myers Squibb Pharmaceuticals Ltd. UK summary of product characteristics, December 2004

Tetracyclines + Anticonvulsants

The serum levels of doxycycline are reduced and may fall below the accepted minimum inhibitory concentration in patients on long-term treatment with barbiturates, phenytoin or carbamazepine. Other tetracyclines do not appear to be affected.

Clinical evidence

A study in 14 patients taking **phenytoin** 200 to 500 mg daily, **carbamazepine** 300 to 1000 mg daily, or both, found that the half-life of **doxycycline** was approximately halved from 15.1 hours in patients not taking anticonvulsants, to 7.2 hours in patients on **phenytoin**, 8.4 hours in patients on **carbamazepine**, and 7.4 hours in patients on both drugs.[1]

Similar results were found in 16 other patients taking various combinations of **phenytoin**, **carbamazepine**, **primidone** or **phenobarbital**. The serum **doxycycline** levels of almost all of them fell below 0.5 micrograms/ml during the 12 to 24 hour period following their last dose of **doxycycline** 100 mg. **Tetracycline**, **methacycline**, **oxytetracy-**

cline, **demeclocycline** and **chlortetracycline** levels were not significantly affected by these anticonvulsants.[2] Other studies confirm this interaction between some **barbiturates** (**amobarbital**, **pentobarbital**, **phenobarbital**) and **doxycycline**.[3,4]

Mechanism

Uncertain. These anticonvulsants are known enzyme-inducing agents and it seems probable that they increase the metabolism of the doxycycline by the liver, thereby increasing its clearance from the body.

Importance and management

The interactions between doxycycline and the enzyme-inducing anticonvulsants are established, but the clinical significance of the reduction in levels does not seem to have been studied. Serum doxycycline levels below 0.5 micrograms/ml are less than the minimum inhibitory concentration (MIC) quoted by the authors, so that it seems likely that the antibacterial will be less effective. To accommodate this potential problem it has been suggested that the doxycycline dosage could be doubled.[2] Alternatively any of the tetracyclines that are reported not to be affected by these anticonvulsants (tetracycline, methacycline, oxytetracycline, demeclocycline and chlortetracycline) may provide a suitable alternative.[2]

1. Penttilä O, Neuvonen PJ, Aho K, Lehtovaara R. Interaction between doxycycline and some antiepileptic drugs. *BMJ* (1974) 2, 470–2.
2. Neuvonen PJ, Penttilä O, Lehtovaara R, Aho K. Effect of antiepileptic drugs on the elimination of various tetracycline derivatives. *Eur J Clin Pharmacol* (1975) 9, 147–54.
3. Neuvonen PJ, Penttilä O. Interaction between doxycycline and barbiturates. *BMJ* (1974) 1, 535–6.
4. Alestig K. Studies on the intestinal excretion of doxycycline. *Scand J Infect Dis* (1974) 6, 265–71.

Tetracyclines + Colestipol

Colestipol can reduce the absorption of tetracycline by about a half. Information about other tetracyclines is lacking but it seems likely that they will interact similarly.

Clinical evidence

Colestipol 30 g taken either in 180 ml of water or orange juice reduced the absorption of a single 500-mg dose of oral **tetracycline** in 9 healthy subjects by 54 to 56%, as measured by recovery in the urine.[1]

Mechanism

Colestipol binds to bile acids in the gut and can also bind with some drugs, thereby reducing their availability for absorption. An *in vitro* study found a 30% binding with tetracycline.[2] The presence of citrate ions in the orange juice, which can also bind to colestipol, appears not to have a marked effect on the binding of the tetracycline.

Importance and management

An established interaction. Direct information seems to be limited to the report cited, but it is consistent with the way colestipol interacts with other drugs. In practice up to 30 g of colestipol is given in divided doses, and tetracycline 250 to 500-mg is given 6-hourly. As other drugs need to be given 1 hour before or 4 hours after colestipol it is difficult to avoid some mixing in the gut, without imposing quite a complicated dosing schedule. It seems very probable that a clinically important interaction will occur, but by how much the efficacy of tetracycline is affected seems not to have been determined. Tell patients to separate the dosages as much as possible. Monitor the outcome well. Information about other tetracyclines is lacking but it also seems likely that they will interact similarly, but those that can be given less often may prove easier to administer.

1. Friedman H, Greenblatt DJ, LeDuc BW. Impaired absorption of tetracycline by colestipol is not reversed by orange juice. *J Clin Pharmacol* (1989) 29, 748–51.
2. Ko H, Royer ME. *In vitro* binding of drugs to colestipol hydrochloride. *J Pharm Sci* (1974) 63, 1914–20.

Tetracyclines + Diuretics

It has been recommended by some that the concurrent use of tetracyclines and diuretics should be avoided because of their association with rises in blood urea nitrogen levels.

Clinical evidence, mechanism, importance and management

A retrospective study of patient records as part of the Boston Collaborative Drug Surveillance Program showed that an association existed between tetracycline use with diuretics [not named] and rises in blood urea nitrogen (BUN) levels.[1] Both diuretics and tetracyclines are known to cause rises in BUN levels.[2] It was suggested that tetracyclines should be avoided in patients on diuretics when alternative antibacterials could be substituted.[1] However, the results of this study have been much criticised as the authors could not exclude physician bias,[1,2] they did not define what was meant by 'clinically significant rise in BUN',[2] they did not state whether or not this rise affected the patients,[2] they did not measure creatinine levels[3] and they did not specify which diuretics were involved.[2] The patients most affected also had the highest levels of BUN before starting tetracyclines. Tetracyclines alone are known to cause rises in BUN, especially where a degree of renal impairment exists, although it has been suggested that **doxycycline** is less prone to this effect.[4] It would seem that tetracyclines and diuretics may be used together safely, although it would be wise to give thought to the patient's renal function.

1. Boston Collaborative Drug Surveillance Program. Tetracycline and drug-attributed rises in blood urea nitrogen. *JAMA* (1972) 220, 377–9.
2. Tannenberg AM. Tetracyclines and rises in urea nitrogen. *JAMA* (1972) 221, 713.
3. Dijkhuis HJPM, van Meurs AJ. Tetracycline and BUN level. *JAMA* (1973) 223, 441.
4. Alexander MR. Tetracyclines and rises in urea nitrogen. *JAMA* (1972) 221, 713–14.

Tetracyclines + Food or Drinks

The calcium in food can complex with tetracycline to reduce its absorption. This is particularly notable with dairy products, which can reduce the absorption of the tetracyclines by up to 80%, thereby reducing or even abolishing their therapeutic effects. Doxycycline and minocycline are less affected by dairy products (25 to 30% reduction). Orange juice and coffee do not interact with tetracycline.

Clinical evidence, mechanism, importance and management

(a) Dairy products

(i) Demeclocycline. The serum levels of a 300-mg dose of demeclocycline were 70 to 80% lower in 4 subjects given dairy products compared to those who took it with a meal containing no dairy products. The dairy products used were either 8 oz (about 250 ml) of **fresh pasteurized milk**, 8 oz of **buttermilk** or 4 oz of **cottage cheese**.[1]

(ii) Doxycycline. The serum doxycycline levels were reduced by 20%, from 1.79 to 1.45 micrograms/ml, 2 hours after a single 100-mg oral dose was taken with 240 ml of **milk**.[2] Another study in 9 healthy subjects found a 30% reduction in the absorption, and a 24% reduction in peak serum levels of doxycycline 200 mg when it was taken with 300 ml of **fresh milk**.[3] However, two other studies suggest that the absorption of 200 mg of doxycycline is unaffected by milk,[4,5] although in one the half-life was almost halved and the clearance increased.[5]

(iii) Methacycline. In one study a reduction in absorption of around 63% was seen in subjects given methacycline 300 mg with 300 ml of **milk**.[4]

(iv) Minocycline. About 180 ml (6 oz) of **homogenised milk** reduced the absorption of minocycline 100 mg by 27% in one study.[6]

(v) Oxytetracycline. In one study a reduction in absorption of around 64% was seen in subjects given oxytetracycline 500 mg with 300 ml of **milk**.[4]

(vi) Tetracycline. About 180 ml (6 oz) of **homogenised milk** reduced the absorption of tetracycline hydrochloride 250 mg by 65% in one study.[6] In another study the absorption of tetracycline 500 mg was reduced by about 50% by 300 ml of **milk**.[4]

(b) Other calcium containing foods or drinks

A study in 9 healthy subjects found that 200 ml of **orange juice** or **coffee** [milk content, if any, unstated] did not significantly affect the bioavailability of a single 250-mg dose of **tetracycline**. This is despite the fact that **orange juice** contains 35 to 70 mg calcium per 100 ml.[7]

Tetracycline 250 mg was given to 9 healthy subjects with 200 ml of water on a empty stomach. The **tetracycline** bioavailability was compared with its administration after taking a **standard meal** (two slices of bread, ham, tomato, and water, containing 145 mg calcium) and a **Mexican meal** (two tortillas, beans, two eggs, tomato and water, containing 235 mg calcium). The cumulative amounts of **tetracycline** excreted in the urine at 72 hours were about 151 mg (fasting), 90 mg (**standard meal**) and 68 mg (**Mexican meal**).[8] The absorption of a 300-mg dose of **demeclocycline** was not affected when it was given with a meal not containing dairy products,[1] and **doxycycline** seems to be minimally affected by food not containing dairy products.[2]

Mechanism

The tetracyclines have a strong affinity for the calcium ions that are found in abundance in dairy products and some foodstuffs. The tetracycline/calcium chelates formed are much less readily absorbed from the gastrointestinal tract and as a result the serum levels achieved are much lower. Some tetracyclines have a lesser tendency to form chelates, which explains why their serum levels are reduced to a smaller extent than other tetracyclines.[9]

Orange juice appears not to interact, despite its calcium content, because at the relevant pH values in the gut, the calcium is bound to components within the orange juice (citric, tartaric and ascorbic acids) and is not free to combine with the tetracycline.[7]

Importance and management

Well documented and very well established interactions of clinical importance. Reductions in serum tetracycline levels of 50 to 80% caused by calcium-rich foods are so large that their antibacterial effects may be reduced or even abolished. For this reason tetracyclines should not be taken with milk or dairy products such as yoghurt or cheese. Separate the ingestion of these foods and tetracycline as much as possible. In the case of iron, which interacts by the same mechanism, 2 to 3 hours is enough. Doxycycline[3,10] and minocycline[6] are not affected as much by dairy products (reductions of about 25 to 30%) and in this respect have some advantages over other tetracyclines.

With regard to meals, which often contain calcium, it is usual to recommend that tetracyclines are taken 1 hour before or 2 hours after food, to minimise admixture in the gut and thereby reduce the effects of the interaction. The separation is something of a compromise, because food can help to minimise the gastric irritant effects of the tetracyclines.

1. Scheiner J, Altemeier WA. Experimental study of factors inhibiting absorption and effective therapeutic levels of declomycin. *Surg Gynecol Obstet* (1962) 114, 9–14.
2. Rosenblatt JE, Barrett JE, Brodie JL, Kirby WMM. Comparison of in vitro activity and clinical pharmacology of doxycycline with other tetracyclines. *Antimicrob Agents Chemother* (1966) 6, 134–41.
3. Meyer FP, Specht H, Quednow B, Walther H. Influence of milk on bioavailability of doxycycline — new aspects. *Infection* (1989) 17, 245–6.
4. Matilla MJ, Neuvonen PJ, Gothoni G, Hackman CR. Interference of iron preparations and milk with the absorption of tetracyclines. *Int Congr Ser* (1972) 254, 128–33.
5. Saux M-C, Mosser J, Pontagnier H, Leng B. Pharmacokinetic study of doxycycline polyphosphate after simultaneous ingestion of milk. *Eur J Drug Metab Pharmacokinet* (1983) 8, 43–9.
6. Leyden JJ. Absorption of minocycline hydrochloride and tetracycline hydrochloride. Effect of food, milk, and iron. *J Am Acad Dermatol* (1985) 12, 308–12.
7. Jung H, Rivera O, Reguero MT, Rodríguez JM, Moreno-Esparza R. Influence of liquids (coffee and orange juice) on the bioavailability of tetracycline. *Biopharm Drug Dispos* (1990) 11, 729–34.
8. Cook HJ, Mundo CR, Fonseca L, Gasque L, Moreno-Esparza R. Influence of the diet on bioavailability of tetracycline. *Biopharm Drug Dispos* (1993) 14, 549–53.
9. Albert A, Rees CW. Avidity of the tetracyclines for the cations of metals. *Nature* (1956) 177, 433–4.
10. Siewert M, Blume H, Stenzhorn G, Kieferndorf U, Lenhard G. Zur Qualitätsbeurteilung von doxycyclinhaltigen ertigarzneimitteln. 3. Mitteilung: Vergleichende Bioverfügbarkeitsstudie unter Berücksichtigung einer Einnahme mit Milch. *Pharm Ztg* (1990) 3, 96–102.

Tetracyclines + H_2-blockers

Cimetidine reduces the absorption of tetracycline but does not appear to affect its serum levels. Ranitidine seems not to affect the bioavailability of doxycycline. Information about other tetracyclines and H_2-blockers is lacking, but there would seem to be no reason to suspect that they will interact.

Clinical evidence, mechanism, importance and management

A study in 5 subjects found that **cimetidine** 200 mg three times daily and 400 mg at bedtime of 3 days reduced the absorption of a single 500-mg dose of a **tetracycline** capsule by about 30%, but had no effect when the **tetracycline** was given as a solution.[1] However, when **tetracycline** as either a tablet or suspension was given to 6 subjects with **cimetidine** 1200 mg daily for 6 days, no changes in the serum levels of **tetracycline** were seen.[2] Similar results were found in another study.[3]

In 10 healthy subjects, the bioavailability of **doxycycline** 200 mg was not altered by three 150-mg doses of **ranitidine**.[4]

No special precautions would seem necessary with either combination. Information about other tetracyclines seems to be lacking, but there would seem to be no reason to suspect that they will interact.

1. Cole JJ, Charles BG, Ravenscroft PJ. Interaction of cimetidine with tetracycline absorption. *Lancet* (1980) ii, 536.
2. Fisher P, House F, Inns P, Morrison PJ, Rogers HJ, Bradbrook ID. Effect of cimetidine on the absorption of orally administered tetracycline. *Br J Clin Pharmacol* (1980) 9, 153–8.
3. Garty M, Hurwitz A. Effect of cimetidine and antacids on gastrointestinal absorption of tetracycline. *Clin Pharmacol Ther* (1980) 28, 203–7.
4. Deppermann K-M, Lode H, Höffken G, Tschink G, Kalz C, Koeppe P. Influence of ranitidine, pirenzepine, and aluminum magnesium hydroxide on the bioavailability of various antibiotics, including amoxicillin, cephalexin, doxycycline, and amoxicillin-clavulanic acid. *Antimicrob Agents Chemother* (1989) 33, 1901–7.

Tetracyclines + Iron compounds

The absorption of both the tetracyclines and iron compounds is markedly reduced by concurrent use, leading to reduced serum levels of the tetracyclines. Their therapeutic effectiveness may be reduced or even abolished.

Clinical evidence

(a) Effect of iron on absorption of the tetracyclines

An investigation in 10 healthy subjects given single oral doses of tetracyclines showed that **ferrous sulfate** 200 mg decreased the serum antibacterial levels as follows: **doxycycline** 200 mg, 80 to 90%; **methacycline** 300 mg, 80 to 85%; **oxytetracycline** 500 mg, 50 to 60% and **tetracycline** 500 mg, 40 to 50%.[1] Another study in 2 groups of 8 healthy subjects found that **ferrous sulfate** 300 mg reduced the absorption of **tetracycline** and **minocycline** by 81% and 77% respectively.[2]

Other studies found that in some instances iron caused the tetracycline serum levels to fall below minimum bacterial inhibitory concentrations (MIC).[3,4] If the iron was given 3 hours before or 2 hours after most tetracyclines the serum levels were not significantly reduced.[3-5] However, even when the iron was given up to 11 hours after **doxycycline**, serum concentrations were still lowered by 20 to 45%.[5] In contrast to this, another study found that four doses of **ferrous sulfate** (equivalent to 80 mg of elemental iron) starting 11.5 hours after doxycycline did not affect the absorption of a 200-mg dose of **doxycycline**, and only reduced the AUC of a 100-mg dose of **doxycycline** by 17%.[6]

(b) Effect of tetracyclines on the absorption of iron

When **ferrous sulfate** 250 mg (equivalent to 50 mg of elemental iron) was given with **tetracycline** 500 mg, the absorption of iron was reduced by up to 78% in healthy subjects, and up to 65% in those with depleted iron stores.[7,8]

Mechanism

The tetracyclines have a strong affinity for iron and form poorly soluble tetracycline-iron chelates, which are much less readily absorbed by the gut, and as a result the serum tetracycline levels achieved are much lower.[9,10] There is also less free iron available for absorption. Separating the administration of the two prevents their admixture.[3,4] However, doxycycline undergoes enterohepatic recycling, which could affect any attempt to keep the iron and antibacterial apart, although the significance of the enterohepatic recycling has been said to be minimal.[6] Even when given intravenously the half-life of doxycycline is reduced.[5] The different extent to which iron salts interact with the tetracyclines appears to be a reflection of their ability to liberate ferrous and ferric ions, which are free to combine with the tetracycline.[11]

Importance and management

The interactions between the tetracyclines and iron compounds are well-documented, well-established, and of clinical importance. The 30 to 90% reductions in serum tetracycline levels that are caused by iron are so large that tetracycline levels may fall below the MIC.[4] However, the extent of the reductions depends on a number of factors.

- *the particular tetracycline used:* tetracycline and oxytetracycline in the study cited above were affected the least.[1]
- *the time-interval between the administration of the two drugs:* giving the iron 3 hours before or 2 to 3 hours after the antibacterial is satisfactory with tetracycline itself,[3] but one study found that even 11 hours was inadequate for doxycycline.
- *the particular iron preparation used:* with tetracycline the reduction in serum levels with ferrous sulfate was 80 to 90%, with **ferrous fumarate**, **succinate** and **gluconate**, 70 to 80%; with **ferrous tartrate**, 50%; and with **ferrous sodium edetate**, 30%. This was with doses containing equivalent amounts of elemental iron.[11]

The interaction can therefore be accommodated by separating the dosages as much as possible. It would also seem logical to choose one of the iron preparations causing minimal interference, but it seems unlikely that there will be a clinically significant difference between those that are commonly available (i.e. sulfate, fumarate and gluconate).

Only tetracycline, oxytetracycline, methacycline, minocycline and doxycycline have been shown to interact with iron, but it seems reasonable to expect that the other tetracyclines will behave in a similar way.

1. Neuvonen PJ, Gothoni G, Hackman R, Björksten K. Interference of iron with the absorption of tetracyclines in man. *BMJ* (1970) 4, 532–4.
2. Leyden JJ. Absorption of minocycline hydrochloride and tetracycline hydrochloride. Effect of food, milk, and iron. *J Am Acad Dermatol* (1985) 12, 308–12.
3. Mattila MJ, Neuvonen PJ, Gothoni G, Hackman CR. Interference of iron preparations and milk with the absorption of tetracyclines. Excerpta Medica Int Congr Series No. *254* (1972). Toxicological problems of drug combinations, 128–33.
4. Gothoni G, Neuvonen PJ, Mattila M, Hackman R. Iron-tetracycline interaction: effect of time interval between the drugs. *Acta Med Scand* (1972) 191, 409–11.
5. Neuvonen PJ, Penttilä O. Effect of oral ferrous sulphate on the half-life of doxycycline in man. *Eur J Clin Pharmacol* (1974) 7, 361–3.
6. Venho VMK, Salonen RO, Mattila MJ. Modification of the pharmacokinetics of doxycyline in man by ferrous sulphate or charcoal. *Eur J Clin Pharmacol* (1978) 14, 277–80.
7. Heinrich HC, Oppitz KH, Gabbe EE. Hemmung der Eisenabsorption beim Menschen durch Tetracyclin. *Klin Wochenschr* (1974) 52, 493–8.
8. Heinrich HC, Oppitz KH. Tetracycline inhibits iron absorption in man. *Naturwissenschaften* (1973) 60, 524–5.
9. Albert A, Rees CW. Avidity of the tetracyclines for the cations of metals. *Nature* (1956) 177, 433–4.
10. Albert A, Rees C. Incompatibility of aluminium hydroxide and certain antibiotics. *BMJ* (1955) 2, 1027–8.
11. Neuvonen PJ, Turakka H. Inhibitory effect of various iron salts on the absorption of tetracycline in man. *Eur J Clin Pharmacol* (1974) 7, 357–60.

Tetracyclines + Kaolin-pectin

Kaolin-pectin reduces the absorption of tetracycline by about 50%.

Clinical evidence, mechanism, importance and management

Healthy subjects were given **tetracycline** 250 mg as a solution or as a capsule, with and without 30 ml of kaolin-pectin (*Kaopectate*). The absorption of both formulations was reduced by about 50% by the kaolin-pectin. Even when the kaolin-pectin was given 2 hours before or after the **tetracycline**, the drug absorption was still reduced by about 20%.[1] A likely reason for this interaction is that **tetracycline** becomes adsorbed onto the kaolin-pectin so that less is available for absorption.

If these two drugs are given together, consider separating the dosages by at least 2 hours to minimise admixture in the gut. It may even then be necessary to increase the **tetracycline** dosage. Information about other tetracyclines is lacking, but be alert for them to interact similarly.

1. Gouda MW. Effect of an antidiarrhoeal mixture on the bioavailability of tetracycline. *Int J Pharmaceutics* (1993) 89, 75–7.

Tetracyclines + Metoclopramide

Metoclopramide 20 mg was found to double the rate of absorption and slightly reduce the maximum serum levels of a single 500-mg dose of tetracycline in 4 patients.[1] This appears to be of little clinical importance.

1. Nimmo J. The influence of metoclopramide on drug absorption. *Postgrad Med J* (1973) 49 (July Suppl), 25–8.

Tetracyclines + Quinapril

The absorption of oral tetracycline is reduced by the magnesium carbonate excipient in the Parke Davis quinapril formulation.

Clinical evidence

The Parke Davis formulation of quinapril (*Accupro*) also contains **magnesium carbonate** (250 mg in a 40 mg quinapril capsule, 47 mg in a 5 mg capsule). A pharmacokinetic study in 12 healthy subjects of the potential interaction between the **magnesium carbonate** in these capsules and **tetracycline** found that single doses of both of these formulations of quinapril markedly reduced the **tetracycline** absorption. The 5 mg and 40 mg quinapril capsules reduced the **tetracycline** AUC by 28% and 37% respectively, and the maximum serum levels were reduced by 25% and 34% respectively.[1]

Mechanism

The reason for these reductions is that the magnesium carbonate and the tetracycline form a less soluble chelate in the gut which is less well absorbed (see 'Tetracyclines + Antacids', p.243).

Importance and management

An established interaction but the extent of the reduction is only moderate and its clinical importance is uncertain. However, the authors of the study recommend that the concurrent use of this formulation of quinapril and tetracycline should be avoided.[1] This is repeated by the makers.[2] Other tetracyclines would be expected to behave similarly. One possible way to accommodate this interaction (as with the tetracycline/antacid interaction) is to separate the dosages as much as possible (by about 2 to 3 hours) to minimise admixture in the gut.

1. Parke Davis Ltd. Effect of magnesium-containing quinapril tablets on the single-dose pharmacokinetics of tetracycline in healthy volunteers, protocol 906-237. Data on file, Report RR 764–00872.
2. Accupro (Quinapril). Pfizer Ltd. UK Summary of product characteristics, June 2004.

Tetracyclines + Sucralfate

On theoretical grounds the absorption of tetracycline may possibly be reduced by sucralfate, but clinical confirmation of this appears to be lacking.

Clinical evidence, mechanism, importance and management

The makers of sucralfate, point out that it may reduce the bioavailability of **tetracycline**, probably because the two become bound together in the gut, thereby reducing absorption. It is suggested that they should be given 2 hours apart to minimise their admixture in the gut.[1] However, there do not appear to be any clinical reports in the literature confirming this potential interaction so it has yet to be shown to be clinically relevant.

1. Antepsin (Sucralfate). Chugai Pharma UK Ltd. UK Summary of product characteristics, January 2004.

Tetracyclines + Thiomersal

Patients being treated with tetracyclines who use contact lens solutions containing thiomersal may experience an inflammatory ocular reaction.

Clinical evidence, mechanism, importance and management

The observation that 2 patients had ocular reactions (red eye, irritation, blepharitis) when they used a 0.004% thiomersal-containing contact lens solution while taking a tetracycline, prompted further study of this interaction. A questionnaire revealed another 9 similar cases that suddenly began shortly after patients who had used thiomersal containing solutions for 6 months without problem started to take a tetracycline. In each case the reaction cleared when the thiomersal or the tetracycline was stopped. The same reaction was also clearly demonstrated in *rabbits*.[1] The reasons are not understood. It would seem prudent to avoid the concurrent use of these compounds.

1. Crook TG, Freeman JJ. Reactions induced by the concurrent use of thimerosal and tetracycline. *Am J Optom Physiol Opt* (1983) 60, 759–61.

Tetracyclines + Zinc compounds

The absorption of tetracycline can be reduced by as much as 50% if zinc sulphate is taken concurrently. Separating their administration as much as possible minimises the effects of this interaction. Doxycycline interacts minimally with zinc.

Clinical evidence

When **tetracycline** 500 mg was given to 7 subjects either alone or with zinc sulfate 200 mg (equivalent to 45 mg of elemental zinc) the **tetracycline** serum concentrations and AUC were reduced by about 30 to 40%.[1] This study was repeated with **doxycycline** 200 mg and zinc, but **doxycycline** absorption was not affected.[1] A reduction in **tetracycline** absorption of more than 50% has been seen in other studies when zinc was given concurrently.[2,3]

Tetracycline appears to cause minimal reductions in zinc concentrations.[2]

Mechanism

Zinc (like iron, calcium, magnesium and aluminium) forms a relatively stable and poorly absorbed chelate with tetracycline in the gut, which results in a reduction in the amount of antibacterial available for absorption.[4,5]

Importance and management

An established and moderately well documented interaction of clinical importance. Separate the administration of tetracycline and zinc compounds as much as possible to minimise admixture in the gut. In the case of 'iron', (p.245), which interacts by the same mechanism, 2 to 3 hours is usually enough. Alternatively it would seem that doxycycline is less affected, so it may be a useful alternative.[1] Other tetracyclines would be expected to interact like tetracycline itself, but this needs confirmation. The small reduction in serum zinc concentrations is likely to be of little practical importance.[2]

1. Penttilä O, Hurme H, Neuvonen PJ. Effect of zinc sulphate on the absorption of tetracycline and doxycycline in man. *Eur J Clin Pharmacol* (1975) 9, 131–4.
2. Andersson K-E, Bratt L, Dencker H, Kamme C, Lanner E. Inhibition of tetracycline absorption by zinc. *Eur J Clin Pharmacol* (1976) 10, 59–62.
3. Mapp RK, McCarthy TJ. The effect of zinc sulphate and of bicitropeptide on tetracycline absorption. *S Afr Med J* (1976) 50, 1829–30.
4. Albert A, Rees CW. Avidity of the tetracyclines for the cations of metals. *Nature* (1956) 177, 433–4.
5. Doluisio JT, Martin AN. Metal complexation of the tetracycline hydrochlorides. *J Med Chem* (1963) 16, 16.

Tetracyclines; Doxycycline + Dimeticone

A study in 8 healthy subjects found that dimeticone 2.25 g did not alter the bioavailability of a single 200-mg dose of doxycycline.[1]

1. Bistue C, Perez P, Becquart D, Vinçon G, Albin H. Effet du diméticone sur la biodisponibilité de la doxycycline. *Therapie* (1987) 42, 13–16.

Tetracyclines; Doxycycline + Rifampicin (Rifampin)

Some patients show a marked fall in serum doxycycline levels if given rifampicin. Treatment failure may result.

Clinical evidence

Rifampicin 10 mg/kg daily caused a considerable reduction in the serum levels of doxycycline 200 mg daily in 7 patients. The reduction was very marked in 4 patients but not significant in the other 3 patients. A mean reduction of 36% (from 14.18 to 9.11 hours) occurred in the doxycycline half-life, a 106% increase occurred in clearance and a 54% reduction in the AUC was seen.[1,2]

Five patients with brucellosis on doxycycline 200 mg daily had a reduction in the doxycycline half-life from 14.52 to 7.99 hours when treated with rifampicin 200 mg daily.[3]

Another study of 20 patients treated for brucellosis found that the mean AUC of doxycycline was nearly 60% lower when given with rifampicin as opposed to streptomycin. There were no treatment failures in the patients taking doxycycline and streptomycin, but 2 treatment failures occurred in the 10 patients taking doxycycline and rifampicin.[4]

A meta-analysis of 6 trials involving 544 patients with brucellosis found a significantly higher numbers of relapses and lower numbers of initial cures with doxycycline and rifampicin than with doxycycline and streptomycin.[5]

Mechanism

Not established, but it seems almost certain that the rifampicin (a known potent enzyme inducing agent) increases the metabolism of the doxycycline thereby increasing its loss from the body.

Importance and management

The doxycycline/rifampicin interaction is established and of clinical importance. Monitor the effects of concurrent use and increase the doxycycline dosage as necessary. No clinically important adverse interaction appears to occur between doxycycline and streptomycin.

1. Garraffo R, Dellamonica P, Fournier JP, Lapalus P, Bernard E, Beziau H, Chichmanian RM. Effet de la rifampicine sur la pharmacocinétique de la doxycycline. *Pathol Biol (Paris)* (1987) 35, 746–9.
2. Garraffo R, Dellamonica P, Fourniuer JP, Lapalus P, Bernard E. The effect of rifampicin on the pharmacokinetics of doxycycline. *Infection* (1988) 16, 297–8.
3. Bessard G, Stahl JP, Dubois F, Gaillat J, Micoud M. Modification de la pharmacocinetique de la doxycycline par l'administration de rifampicine chez l'homme. *Med Mal Infect* (1983) 13, 138–41.
4. Colmenero JD, Fernández-Gallardo LC, Agúndez JAG, Sedeño J, Benítez J, Valverde E. Possible implications of doxycycline-rifampin interaction for the treatment of brucellosis. *Antimicrob Agents Chemother* (1994) 38, 2798–2802.
5. Solera J, Martínez-Alfaro J, Sáez L. Metaánalisis sobre la eficacia de la combinación de rifampicina y doxiciclina en el tratamiento de la brucelosis humana. *Med Clin (Barc)* (1994) 102, 731–8.

Tetracyclines; Minocycline + Ethinylestradiol

There is some evidence that ethinylestradiol may accentuate the facial pigmentation that can be caused by minocycline.

Clinical evidence

Two teenage sisters, taking minocycline 50 mg four times daily for 14 days then 50 mg twice daily thereafter for severe acne vulgaris, developed dark-brown pigmentation in their acne scars when they took *Dianette* (cyproterone acetate and ethinylestradiol) for about 15 months.[1] The type of pigmentation was not identified because they both declined to have a biopsy, but in other cases it has been found to consist of haemosiderin, iron, melanin and a metabolic degradation product of minocycline.[1] Two other reports describe facial pigmentation in other patients on minocycline, two of whom were taking oral contraceptives containing ethinylestradiol.[2,3] Other young women who have developed minocycline pigmentation may also have been taking **oral contraceptives** because they fall into the right age-group, but this is not specifically stated in any of the reports.

Mechanism

Not understood. It seems possible that the facial pigmentation (melasma, chloasma) that can occur with oral contraceptives may have been additive with the effects of the minocycline.[1]

Importance and management

Evidence is very limited but it has been suggested that everyone on long-term minocycline treatment should be well screened for the development of pigmentation, particularly if they are taking other drugs such as the oral contraceptives that are known to induce hyperpigmentation.[1] Remember also that very rarely contraceptive failure has been associated with the use of minocycline and other tetracyclines, see 'Oral contraceptives + Antibacterials; Tetracyclines', p.750.

1. Eedy DJ, Burrows D. Minocycline-induced pigmentation occurring in two sisters. *Clin Exp Dermatol* (1991) 16, 55–7.
2. Ridgeway HA, Sonnex TS, Kennedy CTC. et al. Hyperpigmentation associated with oral minocycline. *Br J Dermatol* (1982) 107, 95–102.
3. Prigent F, Cavelier-Balloy B, Tollenaere C, Civatte J. Pigmentation cutanée induite par la minocycline: deux cas. *Ann Dermatol Venereol* (1986) 113, 227–33.

Tetracyclines; Minocycline + Phenothiazines

An isolated report describes black galactorrhoea in a woman treated with minocycline, perphenazine, amitriptyline and diphenhydramine.

Clinical evidence, mechanism, importance and management

A woman taking minocycline 100 mg twice daily for 4 years to control pustulocystic acne, and also taking **perphenazine**, amitriptyline and diphenhydramine, developed irregular darkly pigmented macules in the areas of acne scarring and later began to produce droplets of darkly coloured milk. The milk was found to contain macrophages filled with positive iron-staining particles, assumed to be haemosiderin. The situation resolved when the drugs were withdrawn; the galactorrhoea within a week and the skin staining over 6 months.[1] Galactorrhoea is a known adverse effect of the phenothiazines and is due to an elevation of serum prolactin levels caused by the blockade of dopamine receptors in the hypothalamus. The dark colour appeared to be an adverse effect of the **minocycline**, which can cause haemosiderin to be deposited in cells, and in this instance to be scavenged by the macrophages that were then secreted in the milk.

1. Basler RSW, Lynch PJ. Black galactorrhoea as a consequence of minocycline and phenothiazine therapy. *Arch Dermatol* (1985) 121, 417–18.

Trimethoprim + Food or Guar gum

Guar gum and food can modestly reduce the absorption of trimethoprim suspension.

Clinical evidence, mechanism, importance and management

A study over a 24-hour period, in 12 healthy subjects given a single 3-mg/kg oral dose of a trimethoprim suspension, showed that the mean peak serum levels were reduced by food and by food given with 5 g of guar gum by 21% and 15% respectively. Food, both with guar gum and alone, reduced the AUC of trimethoprim by about 22%.[1] The greatest individual reductions in peak serum levels and AUC were 44% and 36% with food, and 48% and 38% with food and guar gum.[1] The reasons are not understood but it may be due to adsorption of the trimethoprim onto the food and guar gum.

The clinical importance of this interaction is uncertain but a marked reduction in absorption can occur in some individuals. However, trimethoprim is generally taken without regard to food, so this interaction would not appear to be significant in most patients.

1. Hoppu K, Tuomisto J, Koskimies O and Simell O. Food and guar decrease absorption of trimethoprim. *Eur J Clin Pharmacol* (1987) 32, 427–9.

Vancomycin + Colestyramine

Colestyramine may bind with vancomycin in the gut.

Clinical evidence, mechanism, importance and management

Colestyramine binds with vancomycin within the gut, thereby reducing its biological activity (about tenfold according to *in vitro* studies). The combination of vancomycin and colestyramine used to be used in antibiotic-associated colitis (now no longer recommended) and to overcome this interaction it was suggested that a vancomycin dosage of 2 g daily should be used, and that administration of the vancomycin and colestyramine should be separated as much as possible to minimise their admixture in the gut.[1] It is usually recommended that other drugs should be taken 1 hour before or 4 to 6 hours after colestyramine.

1. Taylor NS, Bartlett JG. Binding of *Clostridium difficile* cytotoxin and vancomycin by anion-exchange resins. *J Infect Dis* (1980) 141, 92–7.

Vancomycin + Dobutamine, Dopamine and Furosemide

There is some evidence that dobutamine, dopamine and furosemide can markedly reduce vancomycin serum levels in patients in intensive care following cardiac surgery.

Clinical evidence, mechanism, importance and management

A retrospective evaluation of the records of 18 critically ill patients in intensive care units following cardiac surgery, suggested that drugs with important haemodynamic effects (dopamine, dobutamine, furosemide) may lower the serum levels of vancomycin. It was noted that withdrawal of the interacting drugs was followed by an increase of in the minimum steady-state serum levels of vancomycin, from 8.79 mg/l to 13.3 mg/l, despite no major changes in body weight or estimated renal clearance. This resulted in a mean dose reduction of 4.26 mg/kg/day.

It is suggested that this interaction occurs because these drugs increase cardiac output, which increases the renal clearance of vancomycin, and therefore reduces its serum levels.[1] The clinical implication is that in this particular situation creatinine clearance is a less good predictor of vancomycin clearance and consequently dose. Good therapeutic drug monitoring is needed to ensure that serum vancomycin levels are optimal. More confirmatory study is needed.

1. Pea F, Porreca L, Baraldo M, Furlanut M. High vancomycin dosage regimens required by intensive care unit patients cotreated with drugs to improve haemodynamics following cardiac surgical procedures. *J Antimicrob Chemother* (2000) 45, 329–35.

Vancomycin + Indometacin

Indometacin reduces the renal clearance of vancomycin in premature neonates. This interaction appears not to have been studied in adults.

Clinical evidence, mechanism, importance and management

The half-life of vancomycin 15 to 20 mg/kg given intravenously over 1 hour was found to be 24.6 hours in 6 premature neonates with patent ductus arteriosus given indometacin, compared with only 7 hours in 5 other premature neonates without patent ductus arteriosus who were not given indometacin.[1] The reason is uncertain but it seems possible that the indometacin reduces the clearance of the vancomycin by the kidneys. The authors of this report suggest that the usual vancomycin maintenance dosage should be halved if indometacin is also being used. If vancomycin therapeutic drug monitoring is possible it would be advisable to take levels and adjust the vancomycin dose accordingly. It is not known whether indometacin has the same effect on vancomycin in adults.

1. Spivey JM, Gal P. Vancomycin pharmacokinetics in neonates. *Am J Dis Child* (1986) 140, 859.

Vancomycin + Nephrotoxic or Ototoxic drugs

The risk of nephrotoxicity and ototoxicity with vancomycin may possibly be increased if it is given with other drugs with similar toxic effects.

Clinical evidence, mechanism, importance and management

Vancomycin is both potentially nephrotoxic and ototoxic, and its makers therefore suggest that it should be used with particular care, or avoided in patients with renal impairment or deafness.[1] They also advise the avoidance of other drugs that have nephrotoxic potential, because the effects could be additive. They list **amphotericin B**, **aminoglycosides**, **bacitracin**, **colistin**, **polymyxin B**, **viomycin** and **cisplatin**. They also list **etacrynic acid** and **furosemide** as potentially aggravating ototoxicity.

The monograph 'Aminoglycosides + Vancomycin', p.200 outlines some of the evidence that additive nephrotoxicity can occur with the **aminoglycosides**, but there seems to be no direct evidence about the other drugs. Even so, the general warning issued by the makers to monitor carefully is a reasonable precaution.

1. Vancomycin. Mayne Pharma plc. UK Summary of product characteristics, December 2003.

Vancomycin + Theophylline

Theophylline appears not to interact with vancomycin in infants.

Clinical evidence, mechanism, importance and management

Five premature infants (mean gestational age of 25 weeks and weighing 1.1 kg) were treated with theophylline (serum levels of 6.6 mg/l) for apnoea of prematurity. It was found that the pharmacokinetics of vancomycin 20 mg/kg at 12 to 18 hour intervals given for suspected sepsis were unchanged by the presence of the theophylline, when compared with previously published data on the pharmacokinetics of vancomycin in neonates.[1] There seems to be no other clinical reports about vancomycin with theophylline, and nothing to suggest that vancomycin has any effect on the serum levels of theophylline.

1. Ilagan NB, MacDonald JL, Liang K-C, Womack SJ. Vancomycin pharmacokinetics in low birth weight preterm neonates on therapeutic doses of theophylline. *Pediatr Res* (1996) 39, 74A.

9

Anticholinesterases

The anticholinesterase drugs (or cholinesterase inhibitors) can be classified as **centrally acting, reversible** inhibitors such as tacrine (used in the treatment of Alzheimer's disease), **reversible** inhibitors with **poor CNS penetration**, such as neostigmine (used in the treatment of myasthenia gravis), or **irreversible** inhibitors, such as ecothiopate and metrifonate. Organophosphorus compounds such as insecticides are also cholinesterase inhibitors. It is these first two groups, the centrally acting anticholinesterases and the reversible anticholinesterases that form the basis of this section, and these are listed in 'Table 9.1', (below). Interactions where the anticholinesterases are affecting other drugs are covered elsewhere in the publication.

Due to their differing pharmacokinetic characteristics, the centrally acting anticholinesterases have slightly different interaction profiles, although they share a number of common pharmacodynamic interactions. Tacrine[1] is metabolised by the cytochrome P450 isoenzyme CYP1A2, and so interacts with fluvoxamine, a potent inhibitor of this isoenzyme, whereas there is no evidence as yet to suggest the other centrally acting anticholinesterases do. On the other hand, donepezil[1] and galantamine[1] are metabolised by the cytochrome P450 isoenzymes CYP3A4 and CYP2D6, and so they may interact with ketoconazole and quinidine, respectively, whereas tacrine would not be expected to do so. Rivastigmine,[1] which is metabolised by conjugation, seems relatively free of *pharmacokinetic* interactions. Consideration of concurrent drug use would therefore seem to be an important factor in the choice of centrally acting cholinesterase inhibitor.

1. Jann MW, Shirley KL, Small GW. Clinical pharmacokinetics and pharmacodynamics of cholinesterase inhibitors. *Clin Pharmacokinet* (2002) 719–39.

Table 9.1 Anticholinesterase drugs

Centrally-acting reversible inhibitors used principally for Alzheimer's disease	*Reversible inhibitors with poor CNS penetration used principally for myasthenia gravis*
Donepezil	Ambenonium
Galantamine	Distigmine
Rivastigmine	Edrophonium
Tacrine	Neostigmine
	Pyridostigmine (also used for glaucoma)

Anticholinesterases + Antimalarials

On theoretical grounds, the neuromuscular blocking effects occasionally seen with chloroquine and quinine might be expected to worsen the symptoms of myasthenia gravis, and oppose the effects of anticholinesterases used in its treatment.

Clinical evidence, mechanism, importance and management

Quinine and **chloroquine**[1-4] can very occasionally cause muscular weakness similar to that seen in myasthenia gravis, and rarely this neuromuscular blocking effect has been seen to be additive with the effects of conventional neuromuscular blockers (see 'Neuromuscular blockers + Chloroquine or Quinine', p.905).

One patient developed a myasthenic syndrome within a week of starting to take 300 mg of **chloroquine** daily. This was controllable with **edrophonium**, but recurred on re-challenge, and then disappeared within a few days of stopping the **chloroquine**.[2]

There seem to be no cases on record of myasthenic patients who have shown increased muscular weakness when given either of these antimalarial drugs, so the risk is still uncertain, but be alert for evidence of worsening myasthenia if either drug is used. It has been suggested that **quinine** should be avoided by myasthenics as it may aggravate their condition.[5] Strictly speaking this is a drug-disease rather than a drug-drug interaction.

1. De Bleecker J, De Reuck J, Quatacker J, Meire F. Persisting chloroquine-induced myasthenia? *Acta Clin Belg* (1991) 46, 401–6.
2. Robberecht W, Bednarik J, Bourgeois P, van Hees J, Carton H. Myasthenic syndrome caused by direct effect of chloroquine on neuromuscular junction. *Arch Neurol* (1989) 46, 464–8.
3. Sghirlanzoni A, Mantegazza R, Mora M, Pareyson D, Cornelio F. Chloroquine myopathy and myasthenia-like syndrome. *Muscle Nerve* (1988) 11, 114–19.
4. Pichon P, Soichot P, Loche D, Chapelon M. Syndrome myasthenique induit par une intoxication a la choroquine: une forme clinique inhabituelle confirmee par une atteinte oculaire. *Bull Soc Ophtalmol Fr* (1984) 84, 219–22.
5. Sweetman SC, editor. Martindale: The complete drug reference. 34th ed. London: Pharmaceutical Press; 2005 p. 441.

Anticholinesterases + Miscellaneous

Acetazolamide, ampicillin, aspirin, chlorpromazine, dipyridamole, erythromycin, imipenem/cilastatin, ketoprofen, lithium carbonate, methocarbamol, procainamide, propafenone and quinidine have all been implicated in unmasking myasthenia gravis or worsening the muscular weakness of one or more patients with the disease. Penicillamine, phenytoin and trimethadione have been associated with the development of myasthenia. Theoretically any of these drugs may oppose the effects of anticholinesterases used in the treatment of myasthenia gravis, and some should probably be avoided.

Clinical evidence, mechanism, importance and management

Acetazolamide 500 mg intravenously, was observed to worsen the muscular weakness of patients with myasthenia gravis taking anticholinesterase drugs. This increasing weakness has been shown in an electromyographic study in 7 patients given **acetazolamide** followed by **edrophonium chloride** 5 mg, and also in an isolated *animal* nerve-muscle preparation.[1] A patient well maintained on **distigmine bromide** experienced an aggravation of his myasthenic symptoms on two occasions when additionally given **dipyridamole** 75 mg three times daily.[2] **Ampicillin**,[3] **aspirin**,[4] **chlorpromazine**,[5] **erythromycin**,[6] **imipenem/cilastatin**,[7] **ketoprofen**,[4] **lithium carbonate**,[8] **methocarbamol**,[9] **procainamide**,[10,11] **propafenone**[12] and **quinidine**[11,13-15] have also been observed to increase the muscular weakness in one or more patients with myasthenia gravis, or to unmask the disease. **Phenytoin**,[16] **trimethadione**,[17] **penicillamine**,[18-20] and possibly also the **tricyclic antidepressants**,[20] have been associated with the development of myasthenia in a few patients. The mechanisms of most of these interactions are not understood.

The evidence for many of these interactions is very sparse indeed, and in some instances they are simply rare and isolated cases. It would therefore be wrong to exaggerate their importance, but it would nevertheless be prudent to be alert for any evidence of worsening myasthenia if any of the drugs listed is added to established treatment. However, the exceptions to this are **chlorpromazine** and other **phenothiazines**, **methocarbamol**, **procainamide**, and **propafenone**, which should generally be avoided in patients with myasthenia gravis, and **erythromycin**, **lithium** and **quinidine**, which are known to aggravate myasthenia gravis and should be used with caution. Strictly speaking these are drug-disease rather than drug-drug interactions.

1. Carmignani M, Scoppetta C, Ranelletti OF, Tonali P. Adverse interaction between acetazolamide and anticholinesterase drugs at the normal and myasthenic neuromuscular junction level. *Int J Clin Pharmacol Ther Toxicol* (1984) 22, 140–4.
2. Haddad M, Zelikovski A, Reiss R. Dipyridamole counteracting distigmine in a myasthenic patient. *IRCS Med Sci* (1986) 14, 297.
3. Argov Z, Brenner T, Abramsky O. Ampicillin may aggravate clinical and experimental myasthenia gravis. *Arch Neurol* (1986) 43, 255–6.
4. McDowell IFW, McConnell JB. Cholinergic crisis in myasthenia gravis precipitated by ketoprofen. *BMJ* (1985) 291, 1094.
5. McQuillen MP, Gross M, Johns RJ. Chlorpromazine-induced weakness in myasthenia gravis. *Arch Neurol* (1963) 8, 286–90.
6. Absher JR, Bale JF. Aggravation of myasthenia gravis by erythromycin. *J Pediatr* (1991) 119, 155–6.
7. O'Riordan J, Javed M, Doherty C, Hutchinson M. Worsening of myasthenia gravis on treatment with imipenem/cilastatin. *J Neurol Neurosurg Psychiatry* (1994) 57, 383.
8. Neil JF, Himmelhoch JM, Licata SM. Emergence of myasthenia gravis during treatment with lithium carbonate. *Arch Gen Psychiatry* (1976) 33, 1090–2.
9. Podrizki A. Methocarbamol and myasthenia gravis. *JAMA* (1968) 205, 938.
10. Drachman DA, Skom JH. Procainamide - a hazard in myasthenia gravis. *Arch Neurol* (1965) 13, 316–20.
11. Kornfeld P, Horowitz SH, Genkins G, Papatestas AE. Myasthenia gravis unmasked by antiarrhythmic agents. *Mt Sinai J Med* (1976) 43, 10–14.
12. Committee on Safety of Medicines. Respiratory and neuromuscular effects of propafenone. *Current Problems* (1990) 29, 4.
13. Aviado DM, Salem H. Drug action, reaction, and interaction. I. Quinidine for cardiac arrhythmias. *J Clin Pharmacol* (1975) 15, 477–85.
14. Stoffer SS, Chandler JH. Quinidine-induced exacerbation of myasthenia gravis in patient with Graves' disease. *Arch Intern Med* (1980) 140, 283–4.
15. Weisman SJ. Masked myasthenia gravis. *JAMA* (1949) 141, 917–18.
16. Brumlik J, Jacobs RS. Myasthenia gravis associated with diphenylhydantoin therapy for epilepsy. *Can J Neurol Sci* (1974) 1, 127–9.
17. Booker HE, Chun RWM, Sanguino M. Myasthenia gravis syndrome associated with trimethadione. *JAMA* (1970) 212, 2262–3.
18. Vincent A, Newsom-Davis J, Martin V. Anti-acetylcholine receptor antibodies in D-penicillamine-associated myasthenia gravis. *Lancet* (1978) i, 1254.
19. Masters CL, Dawkins RL, Zilko PJ, Simpson JA, Leedman RJ, Lindstrom J. Penicillamine-associated myasthenia gravis, antiacetylcholine receptor and antistriational antibodies. *Am J Med* (1977) 63, 689–94.
20. Ferro J, Susano R, Gómez C, de Quirós FB. Miastenia inducida por penicilamina: ¿existe interacción con los antidepresivos tricíclicos? *Rev Clin Esp* (1993) 192, 358–9.

Anticholinesterases + Other Anticholinesterases, Cholinergics or Anticholinergics

The effects of centrally acting anticholinesterases are expected to be additive with those of other anticholinesterases and cholinergics. The effects of the centrally acting anticholinesterases are expected to oppose the actions of drugs with anticholinergic effects and in turn to be opposed by anticholinergics.

Clinical evidence, mechanism, importance and management

The effects of **centrally acting anticholinesterases** may be expected to be additive with those of other **anticholinesterases** (**neostigmine**, **pyridostigmine**, etc.). The actions are also expected to be additive with directly-acting **cholinergic** drugs (e.g. **bethanechol**, **carbachol**, **pilocarpine**).[1-4]

Anticholinesterases are expected to oppose the actions of drugs with **anticholinergic** (antimuscarinic) effects (see 'Table 16.2', (p.502)). This could be a disadvantage if the drug were being used for its anticholinergic activity (for example in the treatment of Parkinson's disease, see 'Levodopa + Tacrine', p.512), but it might be useful if the anticholinergic effect is simply an unwanted side-effect. Similarly, **anticholinesterases** are expected to affect the action of drugs altering the nicotinic actions of acetylcholine. For example, **neostigmine** is used to reverse the action of competitive neuromuscular blockers, and the centrally-acting anticholinesterase **tacrine** has also been shown to have this effect, see 'Neuromuscular blockers + Anticholinesterases', p.899. Conversely, **anticholinesterases** (including **tacrine**, and theoretically other centrally acting anticholinesterases)[1-4] prolong the effects of depolarising neuromuscular blockers such as suxamethonium, see 'Neuromuscular blockers + Anticholinesterases', p.899. The effects of the **anticholinesterases** may also be opposed by **anticholinergics** and drugs with anticholinergic (antimuscarinic) effects (see 'Table 16.2', (p.502), and also 'Anticholinesterases + Miscellaneous', above).

The predicted interaction between centrally acting anticholinesterases and other anticholinesterases is illustrated by the case of an 85-year-old woman taking **donepezil**, who developed prolonged neuromuscular blockade after the administration of **neostigmine** to reverse the effects of pancuronium (she had also received suxamethonium). This patient probably had atypical pseudocholinesterase activity, and the authors suggest the interaction may not be clinically relevant in patients with normal enzyme activity.[5]

Cases of other interactions have also been described. Two patients taking **donepezil** and one taking **rivastigmine** were additionally given **tolterodine** (an anticholinergic). One patient (on **donepezil**) developed confusion, while the other two developed delusional states. This is the opposite effect to the predicted interaction (where the anticholinesterase inhibitor may be expected to oppose the anticholinergic effects of tolterodine). The authors suggest that the combination causes 'cholinergic neurogenic hypersensitivity' similar to that seen as a withdrawal reaction to anticholinesterases.[6]

All of these interactions, additive or antagonistic, are in theory possible, but whether most of them are of real practical importance awaits confirmation. It would certainly be prudent to monitor the concurrent use of any of these potentially interacting groups of drugs.

1. Aricept (Donepezil hydrochloride). Eisai Ltd. UK Summary of product characteristics, January 2002.
2. Reminyl (Galantamine hydrobromide). Shire Pharmaceuticals Ltd. UK Summary of product characteristics, November 2004.
3. Exelon (Rivastigmine). Novartis Pharmaceuticals UK Ltd. UK Summary of product characteristics, June 2003.
4. Cognex (Tacrine). Product Information. Physicians Desk Reference, 2002, p 1351–5.
5. Sprung J, Castellani WJ, Srinivasan V, Udayashankar S. The effects of donepezil and neostigmine in a patient with unusual pseudocholinesterase activity. *Anesth Analg* (1998) 87, 1203–5.
6. Edwards KR, O'Connor JT. Risk of delirium with concomitant use of tolterodine and acetylcholinesterase inhibitors. *J Am Geriatr Soc* (2002) 50, 1165–6.

Anticholinesterases + Quinolones

Three reports describe a worsening of the symptoms of myasthenia gravis in one patient given norfloxacin, and two patients given ciprofloxacin.

Clinical evidence

A woman with myasthenia gravis on **pyridostigmine** 360 mg and prednisone 20 mg daily, was started on **norfloxacin** 400 mg twice daily for a urinary tract infection. Over the next 4 hours she progressively developed double vision, weakness of the neck and proximal muscles of the arms and legs, dysphagia, weakness of the chest wall muscles, and shortness of breath. She complained of increasing fatigue and shortness of breath with each subsequent dose. It was necessary to double the **pyridostigmine** dosage to control the symptoms. The problems vanished within 2 days of stopping the **norfloxacin**. Re-challenge with 400 mg of **norfloxacin** 6 months later in the absence of the prednisone produced essentially the same response.[1]

Another woman with myasthenia gravis controlled with 180 mg of **pyridostigmine** 4 to 6 hourly, intravenous cyclophosphamide and prednisone, developed shortness of breath and weakness of limb and neck muscles within 8 hours of starting to take **ciprofloxacin** 750 mg twice daily for a respiratory tract infection. Initially, the symptoms were tolerable when the **ciprofloxacin** dose was reduced to 500 mg twice daily. However, after briefly increasing the dose back to 750 mg twice daily, it was found necessary to continue to reduce the **ciprofloxacin** dose and eventually to stop it altogether because of worsening myasthenia gravis. Improvement occurred once the **ciprofloxacin** was stopped.[2] Another report describes a man who developed myasthenic symptoms (severe dysphagia, dysarthria and ptosis) within 48 hours of starting to take **ciprofloxacin** 250 mg twice daily, which was later relieved by **edrophonium** and **pyridostigmine**. He appeared to have had mild undiagnosed myasthenia for several months.[3]

Mechanism

Not understood. The inference to be drawn is that these quinolones have sufficient neuromuscular blocking activity in some myasthenic patients to oppose the actions of anticholinesterases.

Importance and management

Information seems to be limited to these three reports. It would be prudent to monitor the effects of ciprofloxacin and norfloxacin in any patient with myasthenia gravis, although the general importance of these interactions in myasthenic patients is not known. There seems to be no information about any of the other quinolones.

1. Rauser EH, Ariano RE, Anderson BA. Exacerbation of myasthenia gravis by norfloxacin. *DICP Ann Pharmacother* (1990) 24, 207–8.
2. Moore B, Safani M, Keesey J. Possible exacerbation of myasthenia gravis by ciprofloxacin. *Lancet* (1988) 1, 882.
3. Mumford CJ, Ginsberg L. Ciprofloxacin and myasthenia gravis. *BMJ* (1990) 301, 818.

Anticholinesterases; Centrally acting + Cimetidine

Cimetidine possibly increases the effects and side-effects of tacrine. Cimetidine does not appear to interact pharmacokinetically with donepezil to a clinically relevant extent.

Clinical evidence, mechanism, importance and management

(a) Tacrine

The clearance of a single 40-mg dose of tacrine was decreased by 30%, and the AUC and maximum level increased by about 35% in 11 healthy subjects when they were given cimetidine 300 mg four times daily for 2 days.[1] The makers of tacrine also say that cimetidine increases the AUC and the maximum plasma level of tacrine by 64 and 54% respectively.[2] The reason is not known, but it seems probable that the cimetidine (a well-recognised liver enzyme inhibitor) reduces the metabolism of the tacrine by the cytochrome P450 isoenzyme CYP1A2 (see also 'Anticholinesterase drugs', (p.250)).[1] An increase in the effects and possibly side-effects of tacrine (nausea, vomiting, diarrhoea) seems possible. One patient in the study mentioned[1] had to be withdrawn due to nausea and vomiting, but none of the other 11 subjects particularly suffered from side-effects. More study is needed to find out whether this interaction is generally clinically important. If the suggested mechanism of interaction is correct, the other H_2-blockers would not be expected to interact. Tacrine also increases the secretion of gastric acid but it is not clear whether this would oppose the actions of H_2-blockers.

(b) Donepezil

In one study, donepezil 5 mg daily was given to 18 healthy subjects with cimetidine 800 mg daily. It was found that after a week of concurrent use the maximum serum levels and AUC of donepezil were increased by 13% and 10% respectively. Donepezil had no effect on the pharmacokinetics of cimetidine.[3] None of the increases in donepezil levels were considered to be clinically relevant.[3]

1. Forgue ST, Reece PA, Sedman AJ, deVries TM. Inhibition of tacrine oral clearance by cimetidine. *Clin Pharmacol Ther* (1996) 59, 444–9.
2. Cognex (Tacrine). First Horizon Pharmaceutical™ Corp. US Prescribing information, January 2002.
3. Tiseo PJ, Perdomo CA, Friedhoff LT. Concurrent administration of donepezil HCl and cimetidine: assessment of pharmacokinetic changes following single and multiple doses. *Br J Clin Pharmacol* (1998) 46 (Suppl 1), 25–29.

Anticholinesterases; Centrally acting + Ketoconazole

Ketoconazole modestly increases the levels of donepezil and galantamine. Other potent inhibitors of the cytochrome P450 isoenzyme CYP3A4 are predicted to do the same.

Clinical evidence, mechanism, importance and management

(a) Donepezil

Donepezil 5 mg daily was given to 18 healthy subjects with ketoconazole 200 mg daily, which is a specific and potent inhibitor of the cytochrome P450 isoenzyme CYP3A4. After a week of concurrent use, the maximum serum levels and AUC of donepezil were increased by 26.8% and 26.5% respectively. Donepezil had no effect on the pharmacokinetics of ketoconazole.[1] None of the increases in donepezil levels were considered to be clinically relevant, and the authors suggest that no dose modifications will be required with ketoconazole or other CYP3A4 inhibitors.[1] However, the maker recommends that such drug combinations should be used with care.[2]

(b) Galantamine

The maker notes that ketoconazole increased the bioavailability of galantamine by 30%, probably as a result of CYP3A4 inhibition. They therefore predict that ketoconazole (and other potent CYP3A4 inhibitors such as ritonavir) may increase the incidence of nausea and vomiting with galantamine, and suggest that, based on tolerability, a decrease in the maintenance dose be considered.[3] Whether this is in fact necessary in practice remains to be established.

1. Tiseo PJ, Perdomo CA, Friedhoff LT. Concurrent administration of donepezil HCl and ketoconazole: assessment of pharmacokinetic changes following single and multiple doses. *Br J Clin Pharmacol* (1998) 46 (Suppl 1), 30–34.
2. Aricept (Donepezil hydrochloride). Eisai Ltd. UK Summary of product characteristics, January 2002.
3. Reminyl (Galantamine hydrobromide). Shire Pharmaceuticals Ltd. UK Summary of product characteristics, November 2004.

Anticholinesterases; Centrally acting + Memantine

An *in vitro* study in *rats* suggested that memantine does not attenuate the anticholinesterase effects of tacrine, galantamine or donepezil at therapeutic concentrations.[1]

1. Wenk GL, Quack G, Moebius H-J, Danysz W. No interaction of memantine with anticholinesterase inhibitors approved for clinical use. *Life Sci* (2000) 66, 1079–83.

Anticholinesterases; Centrally acting + Quinidine

Quinidine does not affect the metabolism of tacrine, but is predicted to inhibit the metabolism of donepezil and galantamine.

Clinical evidence, mechanism, importance and management

(a) Donepezil

In vitro study has shown that **quinidine** inhibits donepezil metabolism, and, as no clinical information is available, the maker suggests care with the combination.[1]

(b) Galantamine

Quinidine, like paroxetine, is an inhibitor of the cytochrome P450 isoenzyme CYP2D6, an enzyme involved in the metabolism of galantamine. Paroxetine has been shown to increase galantamine levels see 'Anticholinesterases; Centrally acting + SSRIs', below and therefore quinidine is predicted to do the same. Consequently the makers of galantamine suggest that concurrent treatment with **quinidine** may result in increased cholinergic side effects, and, if this occurs, a reduction in the maintenance dose of galantamine can be considered.[2]

(c) Tacrine

Quinidine 83 mg eight-hourly did not affect the clearance of a single 40-mg dose of tacrine in 11 healthy subjects.[3] Since **quinidine** inhibits the cytochrome P450 isoenzyme CYP2D6 in the liver, it may be concluded that CYP2D6 does not have an important role to play in the metabolism of tacrine and therefore that other drugs that inhibit this enzyme are unlikely to interact with tacrine by this means.

1. Aricept (Donepezil hydrochloride). Eisai Ltd. UK Summary of product characteristics, January 2002.
2. Reminyl (Galantamine hydrobromide). Shire Pharmaceuticals Ltd. UK Summary of product characteristics, November 2004.
3. deVries TM, O'Connor-Semmes RL, Guttendorf RJ, Reece PA, Posvar EL, Sedman AJ, Koup JR, Forgue ST. Effect of cimetidine and low-dose quinidine on tacrine pharmacokinetics in humans. *Pharm Res* (1993) 10 (10 Suppl), S-337.

Anticholinesterases; Centrally acting + SSRIs

Fluvoxamine markedly increases the levels of tacrine, and increases its cholinergic side-effects, whereas fluoxetine, paroxetine, and sertraline are not expected to interact. Paroxetine modestly increases the bioavailability of galantamine. Two cases suggest an interaction between paroxetine and donepezil; fluoxetine is predicted to interact similarly. Rivastigmine and fluoxetine appear not to interact.

Clinical evidence, mechanism, importance and management

(a) Donepezil

Two case reports suggest that donepezil and **paroxetine** may interact, in one case with an increase in gastrointestinal side effects, and the other with increased CNS effects. This was thought to be due to inhibition of the cytochrome P450 isoenzyme CYP2D6, an enzyme involved in the metabolism of donepezil, by **paroxetine**.[1] The maker predicts that **fluoxetine** could also inhibit the metabolism of donepezil, and until more information is available, they suggest caution with concurrent use of donepezil and CYP2D6 inhibitors.[2]

(b) Galantamine

The maker notes that interaction studies have shown that **paroxetine** increases the bioavailability of galantamine by about 40%, because it is a potent inhibitor of the cytochrome P450 isoenzyme CYP2D6. They therefore warn about the increased risk of galantamine side-effects (in particular nausea and vomiting) if **paroxetine** is added. If these side-effects develop or worsen, the makers suggest a reduction in the galantamine dosage.[3] The makers also predict that other SSRIs that are potent inhibitors of CYP2D6 may interact similarly, and they list **fluoxetine** and **fluvoxamine**,[3] although it should be noted that **fluvoxamine** is only a weak inhibitor of CYP2D6. Thus far there appear to be no reports of adverse reactions with any of these drugs.

(c) Rivastigmine

The makers of rivastigmine report that in studies in healthy subjects no pharmacokinetic interactions were seen between rivastigmine and **fluoxetine**.[4] No special precautions appear necessary.

(d) Tacrine

Fluvoxamine is an inhibitor of cytochrome P450 isoenzyme CYP1A2, an enzyme responsible for the metabolism of tacrine. *In vitro* study showed that **fluvoxamine** is a potent inhibitor of tacrine metabolism, and it was therefore predicted that **fluvoxamine** could possibly 'dramatically' increase tacrine plasma levels in patients.[5] This prediction was confirmed in a placebo-controlled study, in 13 healthy subjects, who showed an eightfold increase in the mean AUC of a single 40-mg dose of tacrine after taking **fluvoxamine** 100 mg for 6 days. A very large increase in the AUC of the hydroxylated metabolites of tacrine, and an eightfold fall in clearance of tacrine itself was also seen. No subjects had any adverse effects when they took tacrine after placebo, but 5 had side effects (nausea, vomiting, sweating, and diarrhoea) when they took tacrine after fluvoxamine.[6] Another pilot study in one individual found that the total clearance of tacrine was reduced about tenfold and its half-life increased tenfold by **fluvoxamine** 100 mg daily.[7] A further study by the same authors found that the clearance of tacrine was reduced by about 85% in 18 healthy subjects taking either 50 or 100 mg of **fluvoxamine**.[8] It is likely that standard doses of tacrine with **fluvoxamine** will be poorly tolerated because of cholinergic adverse effects, and a decrease in tacrine dose would be necessary.[8] Alternatively, use of other SSRIs such as **fluoxetine, paroxetine**, or **sertraline** may be considered, since these are unlikely to inhibit tacrine metabolism (they are only weak inhibitors of CYP1A2).

1. Carrier L. Donepezil and paroxetine: possible drug interaction. *J Am Geriatr Soc* (1999) 47, 1037.
2. Aricept (Donepezil hydrochloride). Eisai Ltd. UK Summary of product characteristics, January 2002.
3. Reminyl (Galantamine hydrobromide). Shire Pharmaceuticals Ltd. UK Summary of product characteristics, November 2004.
4. Exelon (Rivastigmine). Novartis Pharmaceuticals UK Ltd. UK Summary of product characteristics, June 2003.
5. Becquemont L, Le Bot MA, Riche C, Beaune P. Influence of fluvoxamine on tacrine metabolism in vitro: potential implication for the hepatotoxicity in vivo. *Fundam Clin Pharmacol* (1996) 10, 156–7.
6. Becquemont L, Ragueneau I, Le Bot MA, Riche C, Funck-Brentano C, Jaillon P. Influence of the CYP1A2 inhibitor fluvoxamine on tacrine pharmacokinetics in humans. *Clin Pharmacol Ther* (1997) 61, 619–27.
7. Larsen JT, Hansen LL, Brøsen K. Tacrine-fluvoxamine interaction study in healthy volunteers. *Eur J Clin Pharmacol* (1997) 52 (Suppl), A136.
8. Larsen JT, Hansen LL, Spigset O, Brøsen K. Fluvoxamine is a potent inhibitor of tacrine metabolism in vivo. *Eur J Clin Pharmacol* (1999) 55, 375–82.

Tacrine + Enoxacin

Enoxacin possibly increases the effects and side-effects of tacrine.

Clinical evidence, mechanism, importance and management

In vitro studies with human and *rat* liver microsomes found that enoxacin, a specific inhibitor of the cytochrome P450 isoenzyme CYP1A2, significantly inhibited all known routes by which tacrine is metabolised.[1] A reasonable conclusion to be drawn from this is that the effects and side effects of tacrine would be increased by enoxacin, but this interaction does not appear to have been studied in patients or healthy subjects. The same study also suggested that enoxacin possibly inhibits the production of the hepatotoxic metabolites of tacrine.[1]

Other quinolones vary in the extent to which they inhibit CYP1A2 (see 'Theophylline + Quinolones', p.951), so that any interaction with other quinolones would be expected to reflect this variation.

1. Madden S, Woolf TF, Pool WF, Park BK. An investigation into the formation of stable, protein-reactive and cytotoxic metabolites from tacrine *in vitro*. Studies with human and rat liver microsomes. *Biochem Pharmacol* (1993) 46, 13–20.

Tacrine + Haloperidol

Two isolated reports describe severe parkinsonism following the concurrent use of haloperidol and tacrine.

Clinical evidence, mechanism, importance and management

An isolated report describes an 87-year-old man with dementia, who was started on haloperidol 5 mg daily for symptoms of agitation and paranoia. Doses of greater than 5 mg were noted to cause extrapyramidal symptoms. After 10 days, tacrine 10 mg four times daily was added. Within 72 hours he developed severe parkinsonian symptoms, which resolved within 8 hours of stopping both drugs.[1] Another isolated report describes a woman on haloperidol 10 mg daily who similarly developed a disabling parkinsonian syndrome within a week of starting tacrine 10 mg four times daily.[2] One possible reason is that the haloperidol blocked the dopamine receptors in striatum, thereby increasing striatal acetylcholine activity, which was further increased by the tacrine.[1] It is not clear whether other patients given other dopamine receptor blocking drugs and tacrine would similarly show this reaction.

1. McSwain ML, Forman LM. Severe parkinsonian symptom development on combination treatment with tacrine and haloperidol. *J Clin Psychopharmacol* (1995) 15, 284.
2. Maany I. Adverse interaction of tacrine and haloperidol. *Am J Psychiatry* (1996) 153, 1504.

Tacrine + HRT

There is evidence that HRT treatment can almost double the serum levels of tacrine.

Clinical evidence, mechanism, importance and management

Following the observation that **HRT** appeared to increase the response of postmenopausal Alzheimer's patients to tacrine, a study was undertaken in 10 healthy women who were given either once-daily **HRT** (2 mg **estradiol** + 0.25 mg **levonorgestrel**) or a placebo in a randomised crossover study. On day 10 of the **HRT** treatment, they were also given a single 40-mg dose of tacrine. It was found that the mean tacrine AUC was increased by 60% by the **HRT**, the mean peak serum level was increased 46% and the clearance reduced by 31%. The AUC of one individual was increased threefold. The reason for these changes is thought to be that the **HRT** reduces the metabolism of the tacrine to its main metabolite (1-hydroxytacrine) by cytochrome P450 isoenzyme CYP1A2.[1]

The importance of this interaction is still uncertain, but increased tacrine levels would be expected to increase its adverse effects. Be alert therefore for the need to use a smaller tacrine dose (about half?) in patients given **HRT**. More study of this interaction is needed.

1. Laine K, Palovaara S, Tapanainen P, Manninen P. Plasma tacrine concentrations are significantly increased by concomitant hormone replacement therapy. *Clin Pharmacol Ther* (1999) 66, 602–8.

Tacrine + Ibuprofen

An isolated report describes delirium in a woman taking tacrine when ibuprofen was added.

Clinical evidence, mechanism, importance and management

A 71-year-old diabetic woman with probable Alzheimer's disease developed delirium while taking tacrine 40 mg four times daily. The symptoms included delusions, hallucinations, and fluctuating awareness. She was also bradycardic, diaphoretic and dizzy.[1] She was eventually stabilised on tacrine 20 mg four times daily, and continued this for 8 months without problems, but became delirious again 2 weeks after starting to take ibuprofen 600 mg daily. The delirium resolved when both drugs were withdrawn. The reasons for this reaction are unknown. This is the first and only report of this apparent interaction and its general importance is probably small, but consider it as a possible cause if delirium occurs in a patient taking both drugs.

1. Hooten WM, Pearlson G. Delirium caused by tacrine and ibuprofen interaction. *Am J Psychiatry* (1996) 153, 842.

Tacrine + Tobacco smoking

Smoking tobacco reduces the serum levels of tacrine.

Clinical evidence, mechanism, importance and management

A comparative study in 7 tobacco smokers and 4 non-smokers found that after taking single 40-mg doses of tacrine the AUC of the tacrine in the smokers was about 10% of that in the non-smokers. The elimination half-life in the smokers was also reduced, to about two-thirds of that in non-smokers. The reason is thought to be that some of the components of tobacco smoke increase the activity of the cytochrome P450 isoenzyme CYP1A2 in the liver, so that the metabolism of the tacrine is markedly increased.[1] In practical terms this means that smokers are likely to need larger doses of tacrine than non-smokers, although this needs confirmation in multiple dose studies.

1. Welty D, Pool W, Woolf T, Posvar E, Sedman A. The effect of smoking on the pharmacokinetics and metabolism of Cognex® in healthy volunteers. *Pharm Res* (1993) 10 (10 Suppl), S-334.

10

Anticoagulants

The blood clotting process

When blood is lost or clotting is initiated in some other way, a complex cascade of biochemical reactions is set in motion, which ends in the formation of a network or clot of insoluble protein threads enmeshing the blood cells. These threads are produced by the polymerization of the molecules of fibrinogen (a soluble protein present in the plasma) into threads of insoluble fibrin. The penultimate step in the chain of reactions requires the presence of an enzyme, thrombin, which is produced from its precursor prothrombin, already present in the plasma. 'Figure 10.1', (below) is a highly simplified diagram to illustrate the final stages of this cascade of reactions.

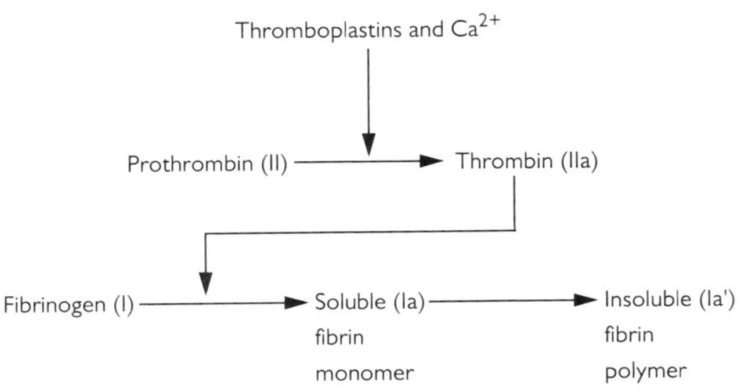

Fig. 10.1 A highly simplified flow diagram of the final stages of the blood clotting process.

Mode of action of the anticoagulants

The oral anticoagulants (see 'Table 10.1', (p.256)) extend the time taken for blood to clot and are also said to inhibit the pathological formation of blood clots within blood vessels by reducing the plasma concentrations of a number of components necessary for the cascade to proceed; namely factors VII, IX, X and II (prothrombin). The parts played by three of these four clotting factors are not shown in the simplified diagram illustrated but they are essential for the production of the thromboplastins (i.e. the substances that covert prothrombin to thrombin).

The synthesis of normal amounts of the four clotting factors takes place within the liver, with vitamin K as one of the essential ingredients, but in the presence of an oral anticoagulant, the rate of synthesis is reduced. One of the early theories to explain why this happens was based on the observed resemblance between the molecular shapes of vitamin K and the oral anticoagulants. It was suggested that the molecules were sufficiently similar for the anticoagulant to take part in the biochemical reactions by which the clotting factors are synthesised, but sufficiently dissimilar to prevent the completion of these reactions. The term 'competitive antagonist' is used to describe this situation because vitamin K and the oral anticoagulants compete to take part in the reactions, their relative concentrations being among the factors that determine the 'winner'. This theory is now known to be too simple, but the basic principle of a concentration competition between the two types of molecules remains perfectly valid. A reduction in the concentrations and activity of all four clotting factors is embraced by the portmanteau term 'hypoprothrombinaemia'.

Coagulation tests

During anticoagulant therapy it is usual to reduce the levels of prothrombin and factors VII, IX and X to those that give protection against intravascular clotting, without running the risk of excessive depression, which leads to bleeding. To achieve this each patient is individually titrated with doses of anticoagulant until the desired response is attained, a procedure that normally takes several days because the oral anticoagulants do not act directly on the blood clotting factors already in circulation, but on the rate of synthesis of new factors by the liver. The successful titration is determined by one of a number of different but closely related laboratory tests, see 'Table 10.2', (p.256).

(a) Prothrombin time

The prothrombin time test (PT, Pro-Time, tissue factor induced coagulation time) is the most common method employed in clinical situations. It measures the time taken for a fibrin clot to form in a citrated plasma sample containing calcium ions and tissue thromboplastin. The PT is usually reported as the International Normalised Ratio (INR) or the Quick Value.

(i) International normalised ratio (INR). The INR was adopted by the WHO in 1982 to standardise (using the International Sensitivity Index) oral anticoagulant therapy to take into account the sensitivities of the different thromboplastins (see prothrombin time) used in laboratories across the world. The formula for calculating the INR is as follows:

$$\text{INR} = \left(\frac{\text{patient's prothrombin time in seconds}}{\text{mean normal prothrombin time in seconds}}\right)^{\text{ISI}}$$

The PT values obtained from the patient's sample are compared to a control, and this gives the INR. The higher the INR, the higher the PT value so if the patient's ratio is 2, this means the PT (and therefore clotting) is twice as long as the normal plasma. The British Corrected Ratio is essentially the same, but was calculated to a standard British thromboplastin.

(ii) Quick Value. The Quick Value is expressed as a percentage; the lower the value, the longer the blood takes to coagulate. Therefore as the Quick Value increases, the corresponding INR value gets smaller and vice versa.

(b) Activated partial thromboplastin time

The activated partial thromboplastin time (aPTT) is the second most common method for monitoring anticoagulant therapy, measuring all the clotting factors in the intrinsic pathway as opposed to the PT test, which measures the extrinsic pathway.

(c) Other methods of assessing clotting

Other tests used, which in some instances offer more sensitivity to specific aspects of therapy, include the prothrombin-proconvertin ratio (PP), the thrombotest, the thrombin clotting time test (TCT, activated clotting time, activated coagulation time), the platelet count and the bleeding time test. The use of the most appropriate test will depend on the situation and the desired result.

Table 10.1 Anticoagulants

Generic names	Proprietary names
Oral anticoagulants	
Coumarins	
Acenocoumarol	Acenox, Acitrom, Coarol, Isquelium, Mini-sintrom, Neo-Sintrom, Sinthrome, Sintrom, Sintrom Mitis
Dicoumarol	
Ethyl biscoumacetate	Pelentan, Pelentanettae
Phenprocoumon	Falithrom, Marcoumar, Marcumar, marcuphen, Phenpro, Phenprogamma
Tioclomarol	
Warfarin potassium and sodium	Aldocumar, Befarin, Circuvit, Coumadin, Coumadine, Jantoven, Lawarin, Maforan, Marevan, Orfarin, Panwarfin, Tedicumar, Uniwarfin, Varfine, Waran, Warf, Warfant
Indanediones	
Anisindione	
Bromindione	
Diphenadione	
Phenindione	Dindevan
Parenteral anticoagulants	
Heparin	Ateroclar, Beparine, Calcihep, Calciparin, Calciparina, Calciparine, Calparine, Canusal, Cervep, Clarisco, Croneparina, Demovarin, Disebrin, Disotron, Ecabil, Ecafast, Ecasolv, Emoklar, Epacalcica, Eparical, Eparinlider, Eparinovis, Eparven, Epsoclar, Epsodilave, Flusolv, Gelparine, Hep Lok, Hepaflex, Hepa-Gel, Hepalean, Hepalean-Lok, Heparibene, Hepa-Salbe, Hepasol Lipogel, HepaSpray, Hepathromb, Hepathrombin, Hepflush, Hep-Lock, Hepsal, Heptar, Inhepar, Isoclar, Lioton, Lipohep, Liquemin, Liquemin N, Liquemine, Menaven, Mica, Minihep, Monoparin, Multiparin, Parinix, Perivar Venensalbe, Pharepa, Proparin, Pump-Hep, Reoflus, Riveparin, Serianon, Sobrius, Sodiparin, Sosefluss, Sportino, Thrombareduct, Thrombophob, Thrombophob-S, Trombex, Trombofob, Trombolisin, Uniparin, Venalitan, Venoruton Emulgel, Venoruton Heparin, Vetren, Viatromb, Zepac
Dalteparin	Boxol, Fragmin, Fragmine, Ligofragmin
Enoxaparin	Clexane, Decipar, Klexane, Lovenox
Lepirudin	Refludan, Refludin
Tinzaparin	Innohep

Anticoagulant interactions

Therapeutically desirable prothrombin levels can be upset by a number of factors including diet, disease and the use of other drugs. In the case of drugs, either the addition or the withdrawal may upset the balance in a patient already well stabilised on an anticoagulant. Some drugs increase the activity of the anticoagulants and can cause bleeding if the dosage of the anticoagulant is not reduced appropriately. Others reduce the activity and return the prothrombin time to normal. Both situations are serious and may be fatal, although excessive hypoprothrombinaemia manifests itself more obviously and immediately as bleeding and is usually regarded as the more serious.

Bleeding and its treatment

When prothrombin times become excessive, bleeding can occur. In order of decreasing frequency the bleeding shows itself as ecchymoses, blood in the urine, uterine bleeding, black faeces, bruising, nose-bleeding, haematoma, gum bleeding, coughing and vomiting blood.

The British Society for Haematology has given advice on the appropriate course of action if bleeding occurs in patients taking anticoagulants, and this is readily available in summarised form in the British National Formulary.

Table 10.2 Coagulation tests

Test	Normal range	Therapeutic/diagnostic range
Activated partial thromboplastin time	20 to 39 seconds after reagents added	1.5 to 2.5 x control
Bleeding time	1 to 9 minutes depending on method used	Critical value greater than 15 minutes
International normalised ratio	0.9 to 1.2	2 to 4 depending on indication for anticoagulation
Plasma thrombin time test	10 to 15 seconds	Greater than 15 seconds
Prothrombin–proconvertin ratio	70 to 130%	10 to 30%
Prothrombin time	10 to 15 seconds	1 to 2 x control
Quick value	70 to 130%	10 to 20%
Thrombin clotting time	70 to 120 seconds	150 to 600 seconds depending on indication for anticoagulation
Thrombotest	100%	10 to 20%

Anticoagulants + ACE inhibitors

With the exception of a single, isolated and unexplained case of haemorrhage attributed to an interaction between acenocoumarol and fosinopril, no other ACE inhibitor has so far been shown to interact significantly with an oral anticoagulant.

Clinical evidence, mechanism, importance and management

Benazepril 20 mg daily has been found not affect the plasma levels of either **warfarin** or **acenocoumarol**. The anticoagulant activity of **acenocoumarol** was not altered, but the effects of **warfarin** were slightly reduced, but not by enough to be clinically important.[1]

Cilazapril 2.5 mg daily for 3 weeks had no effect on the thrombotest times or coagulation factors II, VII and X in 28 patients on long-term **acenocoumarol** or **phenprocoumon** treatment.[2]

Enalapril 20 mg for 5 days did not affect the anticoagulant effects of **warfarin** 2.5 to 7.5 mg daily.[3]

In 10 healthy subjects **moexipril** 15 mg daily for 6 days did not affect the pharmacokinetics or pharmacodynamics of single 50-mg doses of **warfarin**.[4] **Ramipril** 5 mg daily for 7 days in 8 healthy subjects had no effect on the pharmacokinetics or anticoagulant effects of **phenprocoumon**.[5] **Ramipril** 5 mg daily for 3 weeks had no effect on the anticoagulant effects of **acenocoumarol** or **phenprocoumon** in groups of 10 subjects.[6]

Temocapril 20 mg daily for 2 weeks had no effect on the pharmacokinetics or pharmacodynamics of **warfarin** in 24 healthy subjects.[7] The absence of an interaction between **warfarin** and **temocapril** was confirmed in another study.[8]

In a study in 19 healthy subjects[9] **trandolapril** 2 mg daily for 13 days did not affect the pharmacodynamics of a single 25-mg dose of **warfarin** given on day 8.

Contrasting with all this evidence, there is a single, unexplained and isolated case of haemorrhage attributed to an interaction between **acenocoumarol** and **fosinopril**.[10] There seems to be no other evidence that **fosinopril** normally interacts with the oral anticoagulants and so this interaction is unlikely to be of general significance.

No special precautions would therefore seem necessary if any of these anticoagulants and ACE inhibitors are used concurrently. There appears to be nothing documented about any of the other anticoagulants and ACE inhibitors but it seems unlikely that a clinically relevant interaction will occur between any of them.

1. Van Hecken A, De Lepeleire I, Verbesselt R, Arnout J, Angehrn J, Youngberg C, De Schepper PJ. Effect of benazepril, a converting enzyme inhibitor, on plasma levels and activity of acenocoumarol and warfarin. *Int J Clin Pharmacol Res* (1988) 8, 315–19.
2. Boeijinga JK, Breimer DD, Kraay CJ, Kleinbloesem CH. Absence of interaction between the ACE inhibitor cilazapril and coumarin derivatives in elderly patients on long term oral anticoagulants. *Br J Clin Pharmacol* (1992) 33, 553P.
3. Gomez HJ, Cirillo VJ, Irvin JD. Enalapril: a review of human pharmacology. *Drugs* (1985) 30 (Suppl 1), 13–24.
4. Van Hecken A, Verbesselt R, Depré M, Tjandramaga TB, Angehrn J, Cawello W, De Schepper PJ. Moexipril does not alter the pharmacokinetics of pharmacodynamics of warfarin. *Eur J Clin Pharmacol* (1993) 45, 291–3.
5. Verho M, Malerczyk V, Grötsch H, Zenbil I. Absence of interaction between ramipril, a new ACE-inhibitor, and phenprocoumon, an anticoagulant agent. *Pharmatherapeutica* (1989) 5, 392–9.
6. Boeijinga JK, Matroos AW, van Maarschalkerweerd MW, Jeletich-Bastiaanse A, Breimer DD. No interaction shown between ramipril and coumarine derivatives. *Curr Ther Res* (1988) 44, 902–8.
7. Siepmann M, Kirch W, Kleinbloesem CH. Non-interaction of temocapril, an ACE-inhibitor, with warfarin. *Clin Pharmacol Ther* (1996) 59, 214.
8. Lankhaar G, Eckenberger P, Ouwerkerk MJA, Dingemanse J. Pharmacokinetic-pharmacodynamic investigation of a possible interaction between steady-state temocapril and warfarin in healthy subjects. *Clin Drug Invest* (1999) 17, 399–405.
9. Meyer BH, Muller FO, Badenhorst PN, Luus HG, De La Rey N. Multiple doses of trandolapril do not affect warfarin pharmacodynamics. *S Afr Med J* (1995) 85, 768–70.
10. de Tomás ME, Sáez L, Beltrán S, Gato A. Probable interacción farmacológica entre fosinopril y acenocumarol. *Med Clin (Barc)* (1997) 108, 757.

Anticoagulants + Alcohol

The effects of the oral anticoagulants are unlikely to be changed in those with normal liver function who drink small or moderate amounts of alcohol, but heavy drinkers or patients with some liver disease may show considerable fluctuations in their prothrombin times when they drink alcohol.

Clinical evidence

(a) Patients and subjects free from liver disease

The daily consumption of 1 pint (about 560 ml or 56.4 g ethanol) of Californian white table wine for a 3-week period at meal times by 8 subjects anticoagulated with **warfarin**, was found to have no significant effects on either the serum **warfarin** levels or the anticoagulant response.[1]

Other studies in both patients and healthy subjects on either **warfarin** or **phenprocoumon** have very clearly confirmed the absence of an interaction with alcohol.[1-4] In one study the subjects were given almost 600 ml of a table wine (12% alcohol) or 300 ml of a fortified wine (20% alcohol) without adverse effects on coagulation.[4]

(b) Chronic alcoholics or those with liver disease

In one study, 15 alcoholics who had been drinking heavily (250 g ethanol or more daily) for at least 3 months were given a single 40-mg dose of **warfarin**. The half-life of **warfarin** was reduced from 41.1 to 26.5 hours confirming the results of a previous study, but surprisingly, a comparison of the prothrombin times with those of healthy subjects showed no differences.[5]

Other reports have shown that prothrombin times and **warfarin** levels of those with liver cirrhosis and other liver dysfunction can rise markedly after they have been binge drinking, but restabilise soon after the drinking stops.[3,6]

Mechanism

It seems probable that, as in *rats*,[7] continuous heavy drinking stimulates the hepatic enzymes concerned with the metabolism of warfarin, leading to its more rapid elimination.[5,8] As a result the half-life shortens. The fluctuations in prothrombin times in those with liver dysfunction[3,6] may possibly occur because sudden large amounts of alcohol exacerbate the general dysfunction of the liver and this affects the way it metabolises warfarin. It may also change the ability of the liver to synthesise clotting factors.[9]

Importance and management

The absence of an interaction between warfarin or phenprocoumon and alcohol in those free from liver disease is well documented and well established. It appears to be quite safe for patients on oral anticoagulants to drink small or moderate amounts of alcohol. Even much less conservative amounts (up to 8 oz/250 ml of spirits[2] or a pint of wine[1]) do not create problems with the anticoagulant control, so that there appears to be a good margin of safety even for the less than abstemious. Only warfarin and phenprocoumon have been investigated but other anticoagulants are expected to behave similarly. On the other hand those who drink heavily may possibly need above-average doses of the anticoagulant, while those with liver damage who continue to drink may experience marked fluctuations in their prothrombin times. This typically occurs in alcoholics following weekend binge drinking. It would seem prudent to avoid anticoagulation in this type of patient unless they can abstain from drinking.

1. O'Reilly RA. Lack of effect of mealtime wine on the hypoprothrombinemia of oral anticoagulants. *Am J Med Sci* (1979) 277, 189–94.
2. Waris E. Effect of ethyl alcohol on some coagulation factors in man during anticoagulant therapy. *Ann Med Exp Biol Fenn* (1963) 41, 45–53.
3. Udall JA. Drug interference with warfarin therapy. *Clin Med* (1970) 77, 20–25.
4. O'Reilly RA. Lack of effect of fortified wine ingested during fasting and anticoagulant therapy. *Arch Intern Med* (1981) 141, 458–9.
5. Kater RMH, Roggin G, Tobon F, Zieve P, Iber FL. Increased rate of clearance of drugs from the circulation of alcoholics. *Am J Med Sci* (1969) 258, 35–9.
6. Breckenridge A, Orme M. Clinical implications of enzyme induction. *Ann N Y Acad Sci* (1971) 179, 421–31.
7. Rubin E, Hutterer F, Lieber CS. Ethanol increases hepatic smooth endoplasmic reticulum and drug-metabolizing enzymes. *Science* (1968) 159, 1469–70.
8. Kater RMH, Carruli N, Iber FL. Differences in the rate of ethanol metabolism in recently drinking alcoholic and nondrinking subjects. *Am J Clin Nutr* (1969) 22, 1608–17.
9. Riedler G. Einfluß des Alkohols auf die Antikoagulantientherapie. *Thromb Diath Haemorrh* (1966) 16, 613–35.

Anticoagulants + Allopurinol

Most patients on oral anticoagulants given allopurinol do not develop an adverse interaction, but because excessive hypoprothrombinaemia and bleeding can occur quite unpredictably in a few individuals it is important to monitor the initial anticoagulant response.

Clinical evidence

An extensive multi-hospital study[1] of the adverse effects of allopurinol identified 3 patients who had developed excessive anticoagulation while taking **warfarin** and allopurinol. One of them developed extensive intrapulmonary haemorrhage and had a prothrombin time of 71 seconds.

A sharp increase in prothrombin time was seen in a very elderly woman on **warfarin** when given allopurinol.[2] Two patients on long-term treatment with **phenprocoumon** developed prolonged bleeding times, with haematuria in one of them, when they started to take allopurinol.[3] A man on **warfarin** had a 42% increase in his prothrombin ratio after taking allopurinol 100 mg for 2 days.[4] Allopurinol 2.5 mg/kg twice daily for 14 days increased the mean half-life of a single dose of **dicoumarol** in 6 healthy subjects from 51 to 153 hours,[5] whereas 1 of 3 other subjects showed an increase from 13 to 17 hours.[6] The disposition of **warfarin** remained unaltered.[6] No change was seen in the prothrombin ratios of 2 patients on **warfarin** who took allopurinol for 3 weeks,[7] whereas one out of 6 subjects taking allopurinol for a month had a 30% reduction in the elimination of **warfarin**.[7]

Mechanism

It has been suggested that, as in *rats*, allopurinol inhibits the metabolism of the anticoagulants by the liver, thereby prolonging their effects and half-lives.[4-6] There is a wide individual variability in the effects of allopurinol on drug metabolism in man,[7] so that only a few individuals are affected.

Importance and management

An established, clinically important but very uncommon interaction. Since it is impossible to predict who is likely to be affected, consider monitoring the prothrombin times of any patient on an anticoagulant when allopurinol is first added. The interaction has only been reported with warfarin, phenprocoumon and dicoumarol, but it would be prudent to apply the same precautions with any coumarin.

1. McInnes GT, Lawson DH, Jick H. Acute adverse reactions attributed to allopurinol in hospitalised patients. *Ann Rheum Dis* (1981) 40, 245–9.
2. Self TH, Evans WE, Ferguson T. Drug enhancement of warfarin activity. *Lancet* (1975) ii, 557–8.
3. Jähnchen E, Meinertz T, Gilfrich HJ. Interaction of allopurinol with phenprocoumon in man. *Klin Wochenschr* (1977) 55, 759–61.
4. Barry M, Feeley J. Allopurinol influences aminophenazone elimination. *Clin Pharmacokinet* (1990) 19, 167–9.
5. Vesell ES, Passananti GT, Greene FE. Impairment of drug metabolism in man by allopurinol and nortriptyline. *N Engl J Med* (1970) 283, 1484–8.
6. Pond SM, Graham GG, Wade DN, Sudlow G. The effects of allopurinol and clofibrate on the elimination of coumarin anticoagulants in man. *Aust N Z J Med* (1975) 5, 324–8.
7. Rawlins MD, Smith SE. Influence of allopurinol on drug metabolism in man. *Br J Pharmacol* (1973) 48, 693–8.

Anticoagulants + Alpha blockers

No significant interaction appears to occur with acenocoumarol and tamsulosin, or alfuzosin and warfarin. Doxazosin is said not to interact with anticoagulants.

Clinical evidence, mechanism, importance and management

A double-blind, placebo-controlled, crossover study in 15 healthy subjects found that **tamsulosin** [dose not stated] had no effect on the pharmacokinetics or anticoagulant effects of a single dose of **acenocoumarol**.[1] There would therefore appear to be no reason for taking special precautions if these drugs are used concurrently.

The UK makers of alfuzosin report that no pharmacodynamic or pharmacokinetic interaction was observed in healthy subjects given **alfuzosin** with **warfarin**,[2] and the US makers report that **alfuzosin** 5 mg twice daily did not affect the pharmacological response to a single 25-mg dose of **warfarin**.[3] The UK maker of **doxazosin** says that no adverse drug interaction has been observed with **anticoagulants**.[4]

1. Rolan P, Clarke C, Mullins F, Terpstra IJ. Assessment of potential effects of tamsulosin (Omnic®) on the pharmacokinetics and pharmacodynamics of nicoumalone; are there interactions between tamsulosin (Omnic®) and nicoumalone? *J Urol (Baltimore)* (1999) 161 (4 Suppl), 235.
2. Xatral (Alfuzosin). Sanofi-Aventis. UK Summary of product characteristics, March 2003.
3. Uroxatral (Alfuzosin). Sanofi-Synthelabo Inc. US Prescribing information, June 2003.
4. Cardura (Doxazosin). Pfizer Ltd. UK Summary of product characteristics, May 2003.

Anticoagulants + Aminoglycosides

If the intake of vitamin K is normal, no clinically significant interaction occurs between the coumarins and neomycin, kanamycin or paromomycin. No interaction of any importance is likely with other parenteral aminoglycosides.

Clinical evidence

Six out of 10 patients on **warfarin** who were given **neomycin** 2 g daily over a three-week period showed a gradual increase in their prothrombin times averaging 5.6 seconds.[1] The author of this report also describes another study in 10 patients taking **warfarin** given **neomycin** 4 g daily that produced essentially similar results.[2]

A small increase in the effects of an unnamed anticoagulant was seen in 2 patients given **neomycin** with bacitracin, one patient on **streptomycin** 500 mg twice daily, and 2 patients on **streptomycin** 500 mg twice daily with 1 million units of penicillin daily.[3] No interaction was found in other long-term studies of **neomycin** with **warfarin**,[4,5] or **paromomycin** with **warfarin** or **dicoumarol**.[5]

Mechanism

Not understood. One idea is that these antibacterials increase the anticoagulant effects by diminishing the bacterial population in the gut, thereby reducing their production of vitamin K. However, this incorrectly supposes that the gut bacteria are normally an essential source of the vitamin.[5] Another suggestion is that these antibacterials decrease the vitamin K absorption as part of a general antibacterial-induced malabsorption syndrome.[6]

Importance and management

A sparsely documented interaction but common experience seems to confirm that normally no interaction of any significance occurs. Concurrent use need not be avoided. Occasionally vitamin K deficiency and/or spontaneous bleeding[7,8] is seen after the prolonged use of gut-sterilising antibacterials, a totally inadequate diet, starvation or some other condition in which the intake of vitamin K is very limited. Under these circumstances the effects of the oral anticoagulants would be expected to be significantly increased and appropriate precautions should be taken. Only warfarin and dicoumarol feature in the reports cited but it seems probable that the other coumarins will behave similarly. There is nothing to suggest that an adverse interaction occurs between the oral anticoagulants and parenteral aminoglycosides.

1. Udall JA. Drug interference with warfarin therapy. *Clin Med* (1970) 77, 20–25.
2. Udall JA. Human sources and absorption of vitamin K in relation to anticoagulation stability. *JAMA* (1965) 194, 107–9.
3. Magid E. Tolerance to anticoagulants during antibiotic therapy. *Scand J Clin Lab Invest* (1962) 14, 565–6.
4. Schade RWB, van't Laar A, Majoor CLH, Jansen AP. A comparative study of the effects of cholestyramine and neomycin in the treatment of type II hyperlipoproteinaemia. *Acta Med Scand* (1976) 199, 175–80.
5. Messinger WJ, Samet CM. The effect of a bowel sterilizing antibiotic on blood coagulation mechanisms. The anti-cholesterol effect of paromomycin. *Angiology* (1965) 16, 29–36.
6. Faloon WW, Paes IC, Woolfolk D, Nankin H, Wallace K, Haro EN. Effect of neomycin and kanamycin upon intestinal absorption. *Ann N Y Acad Sci* (1966) 132, 879–87.
7. Haden HT. Vitamin K deficiency associated with prolonged antibiotic administration. *Arch Intern Med* (1957) 100, 986–8.
8. Frick PG, Riedler G, Brögli H. Dose response and minimal daily requirement for vitamin K in man. *J Appl Physiol* (1967) 23, 387–9.

Anticoagulants + Aminosalicylic acid and/or Isoniazid

A report attributes bleeding in a patient on warfarin to the use of isoniazid. Another report describes a markedly increased anticoagulant response in a patient on warfarin who was given aminosalicylic acid and isoniazid.

Clinical evidence

A man on **warfarin** taking isoniazid 300 mg daily began to bleed (haematuria, bleeding gums) within 10 days of accidentally doubling his dosage of isoniazid. His prothrombin time had increased from about 26 to 53 seconds.[1]

Another patient taking digoxin, potassium chloride, docusate, diazepam and **warfarin**, was additionally given aminosalicylic acid 12 g, isoniazid 300 mg and pyridoxine 100 mg daily. His prothrombin time increased from 18 to 130 seconds over 20 days but no signs of haemorrhage were seen.[2]

Mechanism

Not understood. The small depressant effect which aminosalicylic acid has on prothrombin formation in man is unlikely to have been responsible. Isoniazid can increase the anticoagulant effects of dicoumarol in *dogs*[3] but not of warfarin in *rabbits*.[4] Two patients on isoniazid, aminosalicylic acid and streptomycin (but not taking anticoagulants) developed haemorrhage attributed to the anticoagulant effects of isoniazid.[5] It seems possible that isoniazid may inhibit the metabolism of the anticoagulants, but this needs confirmation.

Importance and management

The interactions of warfarin with isoniazid and aminosalicylic acid are not established. Concurrent use need not be avoided, but prescribers should be aware of these cases.

1. Rosenthal AR, Self TH, Baker ED, Linden RA. Interaction of isoniazid and warfarin. *JAMA* (1977) 238, 2177.
2. Self TH. Interaction of warfarin and aminosalicylic acid. *JAMA* (1973) 223, 1285.
3. Eade NR, McLeod PJ, MacLeod SM. Potentiation of bishydroxycoumarin in dogs by isoniazid and p-aminosalicylic acid. *Am Rev Respir Dis* (1971) 103, 792–9.
4. Kiblawi SS, Jay SJ, Bang NU, Rowe HM. Influence of isoniazid on the anticoagulant effect of warfarin. *Clin Ther* (1979) 2, 235–9.
5. Castell FA. Accion anticoagulante de la isoniazida. *Enferm Torax* (1969) 18, 153–62.

Anticoagulants + Amiodarone

The anticoagulant effects of warfarin, phenprocoumon and acenocoumarol are increased by amiodarone and bleeding may occur if the dosage of the anticoagulant is not reduced appropriately. The onset of this interaction may be slow, and may persist long after the amiodarone has been withdrawn. Amiodarone-induced thyrotoxicosis may affect the prothrombin time.

Clinical evidence

Five out of 9 patients who were well stabilised on **warfarin** showed signs of bleeding (4 had microscopic haematuria and one had diffuse ecchymoses) within 3 to 4 weeks of starting to take amiodarone [dosage not stated]. All 9 had increases in their prothrombin times averaging 21 seconds. It was necessary to decrease the **warfarin** dosage by an average of a third (range 16 to 45%) to return their prothrombin times to the therapeutic range. The effects of amiodarone persisted for 6 to 16 weeks in 4 of the patients from whom it was withdrawn.[1]

A prolongation in prothrombin times and/or bleeding has been described in other patients on **warfarin** given amiodarone 200 to 800 mg daily.[2-12] Amiodarone similarly interacts with **phenprocoumon**[13] and **acenocoumarol**.[14-20]

The INR of a patient stabilised on **warfarin** and amiodarone was noted to increase from about 2 to 5.5 after he developed amiodarone-induced thyrotoxicosis.[21]

Mechanism

Experimental evidence suggests that amiodarone inhibits the cytochrome P450 isoenzyme CYP2C9[22], and isoenzyme CYP3A4 (enzymes concerned with the metabolism of *(S)*- and *(R)*-warfarin, respectively),[23] which leads to an increase in warfarin levels and effects. There is also evidence to suggest that desethylamiodarone, the active metabolite of amiodarone, is a more potent inhibitor of these isoenzymes and an inhibitor of isoenzyme CYP1A2, which is also concerned with the metabolism of (*R*)-warfarin.[24]

Warfarin interferes with the activation of clotting factors II, VII, IX and X. In thyrotoxicosis the metabolic clearance of some of these factors is increased and the concentration of factor II is reduced. As a result less warfarin would be required to prolong the prothrombin time.[21]

Importance and management

A well documented, established and clinically important interaction. It appears to occur in most patients.[1,4,10,25] The dosage of warfarin and phenprocoumon should be reduced by one-third to two-thirds[1,7,10,13,26] if amiodarone is added to established anticoagulant treatment. Average warfarin dose reductions of 25% for amiodarone 100 mg daily, 30 to 35% for amiodarone 200 mg daily, 35% for amiodarone 300 mg daily, 40 to 50% for amiodarone 400 mg daily, and 65% for amiodarone 600 mg daily and above have been suggested.[7,27] The dosage of acenocoumarol should be reduced by between about 30 and 50%.[14,15,20] Some of these suggested reductions are very broad generalisations and individual patients may need more or less.[20,28]

The interaction begins to develop within 2 weeks and may persist for many weeks after the withdrawal of the amiodarone because up to one-third of the amiodarone may still be present a month after treatment has ceased.[29] Prothrombin times should be very closely monitored both during and following treatment. One study advises weekly monitoring for the first 4 weeks,[10] the importance of which was underlined by a case report of a patient who bled more than 2 weeks after it was thought that stability had been achieved.[11]

In patients stabilised on warfarin and amiodarone, the possibility of amiodarone-induced thyrotoxicosis should be considered if an abrupt increase in prothrombin time occurs.[21]

It would seem prudent to assume that other coumarin anticoagulants interact similarly, but so far there is no direct evidence that they do so.

1. Martinowitz U, Rabinovici J, Goldfarb D, Many A, Bank H. Interaction between warfarin sodium and amiodarone. *N Engl J Med* (1981) 304, 671–2.
2. Rees A, Dalal JJ, Reid PG, Henderson AH, Lewis MJ. Dangers of amiodarone and anticoagulant treatment. *BMJ* (1981) 282, 1756–7.
3. Serlin MJ, Sibeon RG, Green GJ. Dangers of amiodarone and anticoagulant treatment. *BMJ* (1981) 283, 58.
4. Hamer A, Peter T, Mandel WJ, Scheinman MM, Weiss D. The potentiation of warfarin anticoagulation by amiodarone. *Circulation* (1982) 65, 1025–29.
5. McGovern B, Garan H, Kelly E, Ruskin JN. Adverse reactions during treatment with amiodarone hydrochloride. *BMJ* (1983) 287, 175–80.
6. Raeder EA, Podrid PJ, Lown B. Side effects and complications of amiodarone therapy. *Am Heart J* (1985) 109, 975–83.
7. Almog S, Shafran N, Halkin H, Weiss P, Farfel Z, Martinowitz U, Bank H. Mechanism of warfarin potentiation by amiodarone: dose- and concentration-dependent inhibition of warfarin elimination. *Eur J Clin Pharmacol* (1985) 28, 257–261.
8. Watt AH, Stephens MR, Buss DC, Routledge PA. Amiodarone reduces plasma warfarin clearance in man. *Br J Clin Pharmacol* (1985) 20, 707–9.
9. O'Reilly RA, Trager WF, Rettie AE, Goulart DA. Interaction of amiodarone with racemic warfarin and its separate enantiomorphs in humans. *Clin Pharmacol Ther* (1987) 42, 290–4.
10. Kerin NZ, Blevins RD, Goldman L, Faitel K, Rubenfire M. The incidence, magnitude, and time course of the amiodarone-warfarin interaction. *Arch Intern Med* (1988) 148, 1779–81.
11. Cheung B, Lam FM, Kumana CR. Insidiously evolving, occult drug interaction involving warfarin and amiodarone. *BMJ* (1996) 312, 107–8.
12. Chan TYK. Drug interactions as a cause of overanticoagulation and bleedings in Chinese patients receiving warfarin. *Int J Clin Pharmacol Ther* (1998) 36, 403–5.
13. Broekmans AW, Meyboom RHB. Bijwerkingen van geneesmiddelen. Potentiëring van het cumarine-effect door amiodaron (Cordarone). *Ned Tijdschr Geneeskd* (1982) 126, 1415–17.
14. Caraco Y, Chajek-Shaul T. The incidence and clinical significance of amiodarone and acenocoumarol interaction. *Thromb Haemost* (1989) 62, 906–8.
15. Arboix M, Frati ME, Laporte J-R. The potentiation of acenocoumarol anticoagulant effect by amiodarone. *Br J Clin Pharmacol* (1984) 18, 355–60.
16. El Allaf D, Sprynger M, Carlier J. Potentiation of the action of oral anticoagulants by amiodarone. *Acta Clin Belg* (1984) 39, 306–8.
17. Richard C, Riou B, Fournier C, Rimailho A, Auzépy P. Depression of vitamin K-dependent coagulation by amiodarone. *Circulation* (1983) 68 (Suppl III), 278.
18. Richard C, Riou B, Berdeaux A, Forunier C, Khayat D, Rimailho A, Giudicelli JF, Auzépy P. Prospective study of the potentiation of acenocoumarol by amiodarone. *Eur J Clin Pharmacol* (1985) 28, 625–9.
19. Pini M, Manotti C, Quintavalla R. Interaction between amiodarone and acenocoumarin. *Thromb Haemost* (1985) 54, 549.
20. Fondevila C, Meschengieser S, Lazzari MA. Amiodarone potentiates acenocoumarin. *Thromb Res* (1988) 53, 203–8.
21. Woeber KA, Warner I. Potentiation of warfarin sodium by amiodarone-induced thyrotoxicosis. *West J Med* (1999) 170, 49–51.
22. Heimark LD, Wienkers L, Kunze K, Gibaldi M, Eddy AC, Trager WF, O'Reilly RA, Goulart DA. The mechanism of the interaction between amiodarone and warfarin in humans. *Clin Pharmacol Ther* (1992) 51, 398–407.
23. Kaminsky LS, Zhang Z-Y. Human P450 metabolism of warfarin. *Pharmacol Ther* (1997) 73, 67–74.
24. Naganuma M, Shiga T, Nishikata K, Tsuchiya T, Kasaniki H, Fujii E. Role of desethylamiodarone in the anticoagulant effect of concurrent amiodarone and warfarin therapy. *J Cardiovasc Pharmacol Ther* (2001) 6, 363–7.
25. Kerin N, Blevins R, Goldman L, Faitel K, Rubenfire M. The amiodarone-warfarin interaction: incidence, time course and clinical significance. *J Am Coll Cardiol* (1986) 7, 91A.
26. Watt AH, Stephens MR, Buss DC, Routledge PA. Amiodarone reduces plasma warfarin clearance in man. *Br J Clin Pharmacol* (1985) 20, 707–9.
27. Sanoski CA, Bauman JL. Clincal observations with the amiodarone/warfarin interaction: dosing relationships with long-term therapy. *Chest* (2002) 121, 19–23.
28. Fondevila C, Meschengieser S, Lazzari M. Amiodarone-acenocoumarin interaction. *Thromb Haemost* (1991) 65, 328.
29. Broekhuysen J, Laruel R, Sion R. Recherches dans la série des benzofurannes. XXXVII. Étude comparée du transit et du métabolisme de l'amiodarone chez diverses espèces animales et chez l'homme. *Arch Int Pharmacodyn Ther* (1969) 177, 340–59.

Anticoagulants + Anabolic steroids and related sex hormones

Increased anticoagulant effects and bleeding has been seen in patients on a number of oral anticoagulants given with anabolic steroids or related drugs (e.g. danazol, testosterone). Bleeding may occur if the anticoagulant dosage is not reduced appropriately.

Clinical evidence

Six patients stabilised on **warfarin** or **phenindione** were started on **oxymetholone** 15 mg daily. One patient developed extensive subcutaneous bleeding and another had haematuria. After 30 days on **oxymetholone** all 6 patients had thrombotests of less than 5%, which returned to the therapeutic range within a few days of its withdrawal.[1]

Similarly increased anticoagulant effects and bleeding have been described in studies and case reports involving:

- **acenocoumarol** with **oxymetholone**,[2]
- **bromindione** with **methandienone**,[3]
- **dicoumarol** with **norethandrolone**[4] or **stanozolol**,[5]
- **phenindione** with **methandienone**[6] or **ethylestrenol**,[7]
- **phenprocoumon** with **methyltestosterone**,[8]
- **warfarin** with **danazol**,[9-12] **oxymetholone**,[3,13,14] **methandienone**[3,6,15,16] or **stanozolol**.[17-20]

One report says that 3 patients on **warfarin** given *Sustanon* (containing four combined esters of **testosterone**) developed no changes in their anticoagulant requirements,[14] whereas another report describes a woman who showed a 78% and a 65% increase in prothrombin times on two occasions when using a 2% **testosterone propionate** vaginal ointment twice daily. A 25% reduction in **warfarin** dosage was needed.[21]

Mechanism

Not understood. Various theories have been put forward including increased metabolic destruction or decreased synthesis of the blood clotting factors;[4,6] reduced levels of plasma triglycerides, which might reduce vitamin-K availability (though this is disputed);[3,15] increased concentrations of the anticoagulant at the receptor site; or increased receptor affinity.

Importance and management

Well documented, well established and clinically important interactions that develop rapidly, possibly within 2 to 3 days. Most, if not all, patients are affected.[1,4] If concurrent use cannot be avoided, the dosage of the anticoagulant should be appropriately reduced. One-third to one-quarter of the original dosage of acenocoumarol was needed in one patient given oxymetholone,[2] but the size of the reduction with other steroids is uncertain. With danazol, one recommendation is that the initial dosage of anticoagulant[10] should be halved. After withdrawal of the interacting drug the anticoagulant dosage will need to be increased.

It seems probable that all the anticoagulants will interact with any 17-alkyl substituted steroid such as fluoxymesterone and oxandrolone, but as yet there is no direct evidence that they do so. The situation with testosterone and other non 17-alkylated steroids is not clear (see cases cited above).[14,21]

1. Longridge RGM, Gillam PMS, Barton GMG. Decreased anticoagulant tolerance with oxymetholone. *Lancet* (1971) ii, 90.
2. de Oya JC, del Río A, Noya M, Villeneuva A. Decreased anticoagulant tolerance with oxymetholone in paroxysmal nocturnal hæmoglobinuria. *Lancet* (1971) ii, 259.
3. Murakami M, Odake K, Matsuda T, Onchi K, Umeda T, Nishino T. Effects of anabolic steroids on anticoagulant requirements. *Jpn Circ J* (1965) 29, 243–50.
4. Schrogie JJ, Solomon HM. The anticoagulant response to bishydroxycoumarin. II. The effect of d-thyroxine, clofibrate, and norethandrolone. *Clin Pharmacol Ther* (1967) 8, 70–7.
5. Howard CW, Hanson SG, Wahed MA. Anabolic steroids and anticoagulants. *BMJ* (1977) 1, 1659–60.
6. Pyörälä K, Kekki M. Decreased anticoagulant tolerance during methandrostenolone therapy. *Scand J Clin Lab Invest* (1963) 15, 367–74.
7. Vere DW, Fearnley GR. Suspected interaction between phenindione and ethylœstrenol. *Lancet* (1968) ii, 281.
8. Husted S, Andreasen F, Foged L. Increased sensitivity to phenprocoumon during methyltestosterone therapy. *Eur J Clin Pharmacol* (1976) 10, 209–16.
9. Goulbourne IA, Macleod DAD. An interaction between danazol and warfarin. Case report. *Br J Obstet Gynaecol* (1981) 88, 950–1.
10. Small M, Peterkin M, Lowe GDO, McCune G, Thomson JA. Danazol and oral anticoagulants. *Scott Med J* (1982) 27, 331–2.
11. Meeks ML, Mahaffey KW, Katz MD. Danazol increases the anticoagulant effect of warfarin. *Ann Pharmacother* (1992) 26, 641–2.
12. Booth CD. A drug interaction between danazol and warfarin. *Pharm J* (1993) 250, 439.
13. Robinson BHB, Hawkins JB, Ellis JE, Moore-Robinson M. Decreased anticoagulant tolerance with oxymetholone. *Lancet* (1971) i, 1356.
14. Edwards MS, Curtis JR. Decreased anticoagulant tolerance with oxymetholone. *Lancet* (1971) ii, 221.
15. Dresdale FC, Hayes JC. Potential dangers in the combined use of methandrostenolone and sodium warfarin. *J Med Soc New Jers* (1967) 64, 609–12.
16. McLaughlin GE, McCarty DJ, Segal BL. Hemarthrosis complicating anticoagulant therapy. Report of three cases. *JAMA* (1966) 196, 1020–1.
17. Acomb C, Shaw PW. A significant interaction between warfarin and stanozolol. *Pharm J* (1985) 234, 73–4.
18. Cleverly CR. Personal communication, March 1987.
19. Shaw PW, Smith AM. Possible interaction of warfarin and stanozolol. *Clin Pharm* (1987) 6, 500–2.
20. Elwin C-E, Törngren M. Samtidigt intag av warfarin och stanozolol orsak till blödningar hos patienten. *Lakartidningen* (1988) 85, 3290.
21. Lorentz SM, Weibert RT. Potentiation of warfarin anticoagulation by topical testosterone ointment. *Clin Pharm* (1985) 4, 332–4.

Anticoagulants + Angiotensin II receptor antagonists

None of the angiotensin II receptor antagonists appear to interact to a clinically relevant extent with warfarin.

Clinical evidence, mechanism, importance and management

(a) Candesartan

Candesartan cilexetil 16 mg daily for 10 days reduced the trough serum levels of **warfarin** by 7%, but this had no effect on prothrombin times.[1]

(b) Eprosartan

No clinically relevant changes in anticoagulation occurred in 18 healthy subjects on **warfarin** with INRs between 1.3 and 1.6 when they were given eprosartan 300 mg twice daily for 7 days.[2]

(c) Irbesartan

Warfarin 2.5 to 10 mg daily was given to 16 healthy subjects for 2 weeks, with irbesartan 300 mg or a placebo daily for a further week. There was no evidence of any pharmacokinetic or pharmacodynamic interactions.[3]

(d) Losartan

In a two-period placebo-controlled, randomised crossover study, 10 healthy subjects were given losartan 100 mg daily for 13 days with a single 30-mg oral dose of **warfarin** on day 7. The pharmacokinetics of **warfarin** (both *R*- and *S*-enantiomers) and its anticoagulant effects were not altered. Losartan, given alone for a week, also had no effect on prothrombin times.[4]

(e) Telmisartan

Telmisartan 120 mg daily for 10 days was given to 12 healthy subjects stabilised on **warfarin**, with INRs between 1.2 and 1.8. A small statistically significant decrease in the mean trough plasma **warfarin** concentrations occurred but the anticoagulation remained unchanged.[5]

(f) Valsartan

Warfarin 10 mg daily for 3 days had no effect on the pharmacokinetics of a single 160-mg dose of valsartan in 12 healthy subjects. Valsartan caused a small increase in prothrombin time of about 12%, which was not considered clinically important. No dosage adjustment of either drug is required on concurrent use.[6,7]

1. Jonkman JHG, van Lier JJ, van Heiningen PNM, Lins R, Sennewald R, Högemann A. Pharmacokinetic drug interaction studies with candesartan cilexetil. *J Hum Hypertens* (1997) 11 (Suppl 2), S31–S35.
2. Kazierad DJ, Martin DE, Ilson B, Boike S, Zariffa N, Forrest A, Jorkasky DK. Eprosartan does not affect the pharmacodynamics of warfarin. *J Clin Pharmacol* (1998) 38, 649–53.
3. Mangold B, Gielsdorf W, Marino MR. Irbesartan does not affect the steady-state pharmacodynamics and pharmacokinetics of warfarin. *Eur J Clin Pharmacol* (1999) 55, 593–8.
4. Kong A-N T, Tomasko P, Waldman SA, Osborne B, Deutsch PJ, Goldberg MR, Bjornsson TD. Losartan does not affect the pharmacokinetics and pharmacodynamics of warfarin. *J Clin Pharmacol* (1995) 35, 1008–15.
5. Stangier J, Su C-APF, Hendriks MGC, van Lier JJ, Sollie FAE, Oosterhuis B, Jonkman JHG. Steady-state pharmacodynamics and pharmacokinetics of warfarin in the presence and absence of telmisartan in healthy male volunteers. *J Clin Pharmacol* (2000) 40, 1331–7.
6. Novartis Pharmaceuticals Ltd. Data on file, Protocol 40.
7. Knight H, Flesch G, Prasad P, Lloyd P, Douglas J. Lack of pharmacokinetic and pharmacodynamic interaction between valsartan and warfarin. *J Hypertens* (2000) 18 (Suppl 4), S89.

Anticoagulants + Antacids

There is some evidence that the absorption of dicoumarol may be increased by magnesium hydroxide and the absorption of warfarin by magnesium trisilicate, but there is no direct evidence that this is clinically important. Aluminium hydroxide does not interact with either warfarin or dicoumarol, and magnesium hydroxide does not interact with warfarin.

Clinical evidence

(a) Dicoumarol

Magnesium hydroxide (*Milk of Magnesia*) 15 ml taken with and 3 hours after dicoumarol was found to raise the plasma levels and AUC of dicoumarol 75% and 50% respectively in 6 healthy subjects. No interaction occurred with **aluminium hydroxide**.[1]

(b) Warfarin

Aluminium/magnesium hydroxide (*Maalox*) 30 ml given with and for four 2-hourly doses after warfarin had no effect on the plasma warfarin levels or on the anticoagulant response of 6 subjects.[2]

No interaction occurs with warfarin and **aluminium hydroxide** (*Amphogel*),[1] but an *in vitro* study suggests that the absorption of warfarin may be increased by **magnesium trisilicate**.[3]

Mechanism

It is suggested that dicoumarol forms a more readily absorbed chelate with magnesium so that its effects are increased.[1,4]

Importance and management

No special precautions need be taken if aluminium or magnesium hydroxide antacids are given to patients on warfarin, or if aluminium hydroxide is given to those on dicoumarol. Choosing these antacids avoids the possibility of an adverse interaction. Despite the evidence from the studies cited, there seems to be no direct clinical evidence of any important adverse interaction between any anticoagulant and an antacid.

1. Ambre JJ, Fischer LJ. Effect of coadministration of aluminum and magnesium hydroxides on absorption of anticoagulants in man. *Clin Pharmacol Ther* (1973) 14, 231–7.
2. Robinson DS, Benjamin DM, McCormack JJ. Interaction of warfarin and nonsystemic gastrointestinal drugs. *Clin Pharmacol Ther* (1971) 12, 491–5.
3. McElnay JC, Harron DWG, D'Arcy PF, Collier PS. Interaction of warfarin with antacid constituents. *BMJ* (1978) 2, 1166.
4. Akers MJ, Lach JL, Fischer LJ. Alterations in the absorption of dicoumarol by various excipient materials. *J Pharm Sci* (1973) 62, 391–5.

Anticoagulants + Anticholinesterases; Centrally acting

Warfarin does not appear to interact adversely with donepezil, galantamine, rivastigmine or tacrine.

Clinical evidence, mechanism, importance and management

A study in 10 patients taking **warfarin** found that the addition of **tacrine** 20 mg four times daily for 5 days had no significant effect on prothrombin times.[1] In an open-label crossover study, 12 healthy men were given **donepezil** 10 mg daily for 19 days with a single 25-mg dose of **warfarin** on day 14. It was found that the pharmacokinetics of ***(R)***- and ***(S)*-warfarin** and the prothrombin times were unchanged by the presence of the **donepezil**, and vital signs, ECG and laboratory tests were unaltered.[2] The makers of **galantamine**[3,4] and **rivastigmine**[5,6] also say that no interactions have been noted with **warfarin**.

1. Reece PA, Garnett WR, Rock WL, Taylor JR, Underwood B, Sedman AJ, Rajagopalan R. Lack of effect of tacrine administration on the anticoagulant activity of warfarin. *J Clin Pharmacol* (1995) 35, 526–8.
2. Tiseo PJ, Foley K, Friedhoff LT. The effect of multiple doses of donepezil hydrochloride on the pharmacokinetic and pharmacodynamic profile of warfarin. *Br J Clin Pharmacol* (1998) 46 (Suppl 1), 45–50.
3. Reminyl (Galantamine hydrobromide). Shire Pharmaceuticals Ltd. UK Summary of product characteristics, November 2004.
4. Reminyl (Galantamine hydrobromide). Janssen. US Prescribing information, March 2005.
5. Exelon (Rivastigmine). Novartis Pharmaceuticals UK Ltd. UK Summary of product characteristics, June 2003.
6. Exelon (Rivastigmine). Novartis. US Prescribing information, October 2004.

Anticoagulants + Antidiabetics

Although isolated cases of interactions (raised prothrombin times, bleeding or hypoglycaemia) have been seen in patients on sulphonylureas and anticoagulants in general no important interaction appears to occur. The exception may be dicoumarol with tolbutamide, which has resulted in diabetic coma and several cases of serious bleeding.

Clinical evidence

(a) Acenocoumarol

A woman with normal renal function had an increase in the half-life of **chlorpropamide** to 88 hours (normally about 36 hours) when she took acenocoumarol.[1]

(b) Dicoumarol

The observation of severe hypoglycaemia in a patient on **chlorpropamide** and dicoumarol prompted further study in 3 other patients and 2 non-diabetics. Dicoumarol doubled the serum **chlorpropamide** levels within 3 to 4 days and also more than doubled the half-life.[2]

A retrospective study of 24 patients given dicoumarol suggested that **insulin** did not alter its anticoagulant effects.[3] However, what is not clear is whether this study would have revealed an interaction because the patients were already taking the antidiabetic and would have been routinely stabilised on the anticoagulant.

Dicoumarol has been shown to increase the serum levels of **tolbutamide**, prolong its half-life (more than threefold), and reduce blood sugar levels in both diabetics[4] and healthy subjects.[4,5] This may become excessive in a few patients and coma has been described.[4,6-8] Two patients on dicoumarol had marked increases in prothrombin times (a rise from 33 to 60 seconds) within 2 days of starting **tolbutamide** but no bleeding occurred. Increases were seen in 3 other patients who took **tolbutamide** and dicoumarol simultaneously.[9] Another patient on dicoumarol had a similar increase in his prothrombin time and bled (haematuria, purpura) within 5 days of starting **tolbutamide**.[7] The half-life of dicoumarol was approximately halved in 2 out of 4 healthy subjects given **tolbutamide**, but the hypoprothrombinaemic effects were unchanged.[10] However, a retrospective study on 15 patients found no evidence that the anticoagulant effects of dicoumarol were altered by **tolbutamide**[3] but the form of the study may possibly have obscured evidence of an interaction. No change in overall anticoagulant control was seen in another study.[11]

(c) Phenindione

Phenindione does not affect the half-life of **tolbutamide**.[4]

(d) Phenprocoumon

Phenprocoumon has been found to cause a slight increase in the half-life of **glibornuride**,[12] but the pharmacokinetics of **glibenclamide**[13] and the hypoglycaemic effects of **tolbutamide** remained unchanged.[13]

The plasma levels and half-life of single doses of phenprocoumon did not differ between patients with type 2 diabetes treated with diet alone, **insulin**, **tolbutamide**, or **glibornuride** or between elderly or young non-diabetic subjects. Similarly the efficacy of phenprocoumon was the same in the diabetics as in the elderly non-diabetic subjects, but was less effective in healthy young subjects.[14]

(e) Warfarin

A retrospective study of 54 patients given warfarin suggested that **insulin** did not alter its anticoagulant effects; similarly **tolbutamide** is said not to have altered the anticoagulant effects of warfarin in 42 patients.[3] However, what is not clear is whether this study would have revealed an interaction because the patients were already taking the hypoglycaemic agent and would have been routinely stabilised on the anticoagulant. A study in healthy subjects found that only minor, clinically unimportant changes in the prothrombin times occurred in response to single 25-mg doses of warfarin when **glimepiride** 4 mg daily was given.[15] Three isolated reports describe increased warfarin effects (serious in one instance) in 2 patients given **glibenclamide**,[16,17] and another given **tolbutamide**.[18]

Mechanism

Dicoumarol appears to increase the effects of tolbutamide by inhibiting its metabolism by the liver.[4,5] This may also be true for chlorpropamide.[2] The increase in the anticoagulant effects of dicoumarol by tolbutamide may in part be due to a plasma protein binding interaction. In the case of phenprocoumon there seem to be several different mutually opposing processes going on which cancel each other out and produce a 'silent' interaction.[11] There is no clear explanation for most of these interactions.

Importance and management

Information is patchy and very incomplete. Dicoumarol with tolbutamide has been most thoroughly investigated and the interaction is clinically important. Increased hypoglycaemic effects may be expected if dicoumarol is given to patients taking tolbutamide and there is a risk of coma. If tolbutamide is given to those taking dicoumarol an increase in prothrombin times and possibly bleeding may occur. Avoid concurrent use unless the outcome can be well monitored and dosage adjustments made. The same precautions should be taken with dicoumarol and chlorpropamide, but information is limited to one study.[2]

Other interactions are limited to isolated cases and are therefore of doubtful general significance.

1. Petitpierrre B, Perrin L, Rudhardt M, Herrera A, Fabre J. Behaviour of chlorpropamide in renal insufficiency and under the effect of associated drug therapy. *Int J Clin Pharmacol* (1972) 6, 120–4.
2. Kristensen M, Hansen JM. Accumulation of chlorpropamide caused by dicoumarol. *Acta Med Scand* (1968) 183, 83–6.
3. Poucher RL, Vecchio TJ. Absence of tolbutamide effect on anticoagulant therapy. *JAMA* (1966) 197, 1069–70.
4. Kristensen M, Hansen JM. Potentiation of the tolbutamide effect by dicoumarol. *Diabetes* (1967) 16, 211–14.
5. Solomon HM, Schrogie JJ. Effect of phenyramidol and bishydroxycoumarin on the metabolism of tolbutamide in human subjects. *Metabolism* (1967) 16, 1029–33.
6. Spurny OM, Wolf JW, Devins GS. Protracted tolbutamide-induced hypoglycemia. *Arch Intern Med* (1965) 115, 53–6.
7. Schwartz JF. Tolbutamide-induced hypoglycemia in Parkinson's disease. A case report. *JAMA* (1961) 176, 106–9.
8. Fontana G, Addarii F, Peta G. Su di un caso di coma ipoglicemico in corso di terapia con tolbutamide e dicumaroli. *G Clin Med* (1968) 49, 849–58.
9. Chaplin H, Cassell M. Studies on the possible relationship of tolbutamide to dicumarol in anticoagulant therapy. *Am J Med Sci* (1958) 235, 706–15.
10. Jähnchen E, Gilfrich HJ, Groth U, Meinertz T. Pharmacokinetic analysis of the dicumarol-tolbutamide interaction in man. *Naunyn Schmiedebergs Arch Pharmacol* (1975) 287 (Suppl), R88.
11. Jähnchen E, Meinertz T, Gilfrich H-J, Groth U. Pharmacokinetic analysis of the interaction between dicoumarol and tolbutamide in man. *Eur J Clin Pharmacol* (1976) 10, 349–56.
12. Eckhardt W, Rudolph R, Sauer H, Schubert WR, Undeutsch D. Zur pharmakologischen Interferenz von Glibornurid mit Sulfaphenazol, Phenylbutazon und phenprocoumon beim Menschen. *Arzneimittelforschung* (1972) 22, 2212–19.
13. Schulz E, Schmidt FH. Über den Einfluss von Sulphaphenazol, Phenylbutazon und Phenprocumarol auf die Elimination von Glibenclamid beim Menschen. *Verh Dtsch Ges Inn Med* (1970) 76, 435–8.
14. Heine P, Kewitz H, Wiegboldt K-A. The influence of hypoglycaemic sulphonylureas on elimination and efficacy of phenprocoumon following a single oral dose in diabetic patients. *Eur J Clin Pharmacol* (1976) 10, 31–6.
15. Schaaf LJ, Sisson TA, Dietz AJ, Viveash DM, Oliver LK, Knuth DW, Carel BJ. Influence of multiple dose glimepiride on the pharmacokinetics and pharmacodynamics of racemic warfarin in healthy volunteers. *Pharm Res* (1994) 11 (10 Suppl), S-359.
16. Beeley L, Stewart P, Hickey FM. *Bulletin of the West Midlands Centre for Adverse Drug Reaction Reporting* (1988) 26, 27.
17. Jassal SV. Drug points. *BMJ* (1991) 303, 789.
18. Beeley L, Magee P, Hickey FN. *Bulletin of the West Midlands Centre for Adverse Drug Reaction Reporting* (1990) 30, 32.

Anticoagulants + Antidiabetics; Alpha glucosidase inhibitors

Acarbose, miglitol and voglibose do not usually appear to interact with warfarin, although there are a few cases of reduced or increased INRs in patients given warfarin and acarbose.

Clinical evidence, mechanism, importance and management

(a) Acarbose

In a double-blind, placebo-controlled study, 24 patients on **warfarin** with stable INRs between 1.8 and 3.6 were given either a placebo for 4 weeks or acarbose 100 mg three times daily for 2 weeks and then 200 mg three times daily for a further 2 weeks. Their INRs, prothrombin times and partial prothrombin times were not altered to any significant extent by the acarbose.[1]

However, there are 3 isolated case reports of apparent interactions between **warfarin** and acarbose. A 66-year-old man taking fosinopril, hydrochlorothiazide, diphenhydramine, insulin, glipizide and **warfarin** was additionally started on acarbose to improve the control of his diabetes. Four days before starting acarbose his INR was 3.09, but after 2 weeks (25 mg acarbose daily for week 1 and then 50 mg daily for week 2) his INR had risen to 4.85. The **warfarin** was temporarily stopped, then it was reintroduced at a lower dosage, and finally the acarbose was withdrawn, resulting in an INR of 2.84. No bleeding was seen.[2] The maker has on record 2 other cases of patients on **warfarin** whose INRs were reduced when acarbose was added. One of them stopped taking the acarbose, whereupon her INR returned to its previous value. The other patient needed an increased **warfarin** dosage.[1]

The picture presented by these reports and the absence of any others is that usually no interaction occurs, but in isolated cases some changes in **warfarin** requirements occur. Bear this interaction in mind if anticoagulant control alters in a patient on acarbose. Information about other anticoagulants appears to be lacking.

(b) Miglitol

In a double-blind, randomised placebo-controlled study 24 healthy subjects were given miglitol 100 mg three times daily for 7 days, with a single 25-mg oral dose of **warfarin** on day 4. Neither the pharmacokinetics nor the pharmacodynamics of ***(R)****- or* ***(S)*****-warfarin** were affected by the miglitol,[3] and there would therefore seem to be no reason for avoiding concurrent use. Information about other anticoagulants is lacking.

(c) Voglibose

Twelve healthy male subjects were given individually adjusted doses of **warfarin** to give Quick values of 30 to 40%, and then from day 11 to 15 they were also given voglibose 5 mg three times daily. It was found that the voglibose had no effect on the pharmacokinetics of the **warfarin** nor on its anticoagulant effects.[4] No special precautions would therefore appear to be needed if these two drugs are used concurrently.

1. Bayer. Personal communication, December 1997.
2. Morreale AP, Janetzky K. Probable interaction of warfarin and acarbose. *Am J Health-Syst Pharm* (1997) 54, 1551–2.
3. Schall R, Müller FO, Hundt HKL, Duursema L, Groenewoud G, Middle MV. Study of the effect of miglitol on the pharmacokinetics and pharmacodynamics of warfarin in healthy males. *Arzneimittelforschung* (1996) 46, 41–6.
4. Fuder H, Kleist P, Birkel M, Ehrlich A, Emeklibas S, Maslak W, Stridde E, Wetzelsberger N, Wieckhorst G, Lücker PW. The α-glucosidase inhibitor voglibose (AO-128) does not change pharmacodynamics or pharmacokinetics of warfarin. *Eur J Clin Pharmacol* (1997) 53, 153–7.

Anticoagulants + Antidiabetics; Biguanides

One patient needed an increase in her phenprocoumon dose when she was given metformin, and there is some evidence that metformin increases the metabolism of phenprocoumon. Two patients on warfarin had serious bleeds after taking metformin or phenformin. However, these interactions are isolated and seem unlikely to be of general importance.

Clinical evidence

(a) Phenprocoumon

The observation that a woman diabetic needed more phenprocoumon while taking **metformin** prompted further study in 13 patients with type 2 diabetes. It was found that those taking **metformin** 1.1 to 3 g daily were less well anticoagulated than those taking only 400 mg to 1 g, even though the phenprocoumon dosage was slightly higher in those on **metformin** 1.1 to 3 g.[1] In one study the half-life of phenprocoumon was reduced about one-third (from 123 to 85 hours) while taking **metformin** 1.7 g daily.[1]

(b) Warfarin

An elderly woman on warfarin 5 mg daily and **metformin** 1 g twice daily developed fatigue, epistaxis, haematuria and gingival bleeding, with an INR of 16.9, which was treated with vitamin K. The following morning, she was given **metformin**, then she was found to have a retroperitoneal haematoma and bilateral perinephric blood with obstruction of both renal collecting systems. Over the next 8 hours, she developed progressive metabolic acidosis and suffered a cardiopulmonary arrest. Her **metformin** level was 7.3 micrograms/ml (therapeutic range 1 to 2 micrograms/ml). It was suggested that **metformin** accumulation occurred because of renal insufficiency caused by bleeding secondary to the excessive effects of warfarin. This then resulted in metabolic acidosis.[2] **Metformin** should be withheld when there are signs of renal impairment. Haematuria occurred in a patient on warfarin 3 months after **phenformin** was started. Her prothrombin values were normal.[3] The **phenformin** may have increased fibrinolysis to the point where it was additive with the effects of the warfarin.

Mechanism

Metformin possibly reduces the effects of phenprocoumon by altering blood flow to the liver and interfering with the enterohepatic circulation.

Importance and management

The information appears to be limited to these reports, which are mainly isolated case reports. In general no interaction would be expected between metformin and warfarin. A small increase in the dosage of phenprocoumon may be necessary if metformin is given.

1. Ohnhaus EE, Berger W, Duckert F, Oesch F. The influence of dimethylbiguanide on phenprocoumon elimination and its mode of action. *Klin Wochenschr* (1983) 61, 851–8.
2. Schier JG, Hoffman RS, Nelson LS. Metformin-induced acidosis due to a warfarin adverse drug event. *Ann Pharmacother* (2003) 37, 1145.
3. Hamblin TJ. Interaction between warfarin and phenformin. *Lancet* (1971) ii, 1323.

Anticoagulants + Antidiabetics; Nateglinide or Repaglinide

Nateglinide and repaglinide do not appear to interact with warfarin.

Clinical evidence, mechanism, importance and management

(a) Nateglinide

In a randomised double-blind study 11 healthy subjects were given nateglinide 120 mg three times daily for 5 days, with a single 10-mg dose of **acenocoumarol** on day 3. Nateglinide had no effect on the tolerability, pharmacokinetics or anticoagulant activity of **acenocoumarol**.[1]

In another study 12 healthy subjects were given a single 30-mg dose of **warfarin** on the second day of 4 days' treatment with nateglinide 120 mg three times daily. No pharmacokinetic or pharmacodynamic interaction was noted.[2] The makers say that no protein binding interaction occurs between nateglinide and **warfarin** and that nateglinide does not interact with **warfarin**.[3,4]

No dosage adjustments are therefore necessary if either acenocoumarol or warfarin is taken with nateglinide.

(b) Repaglinide

A double-blind, placebo controlled study in 28 healthy subjects found that repaglinide does not affect the anticoagulant effects of **warfarin**.[5] No special precautions would therefore appear necessary on concurrent use.

1. Sunkara G, Bigler H, Wang Y, Smith H, Prasad P, McLeod J, Ligueros-Saylan M. The effect of nateglinide on the pharmacokinetics and pharmacodynamics of acenocoumarol. *Curr Med Res Opin* (2004) 20, 41–8.
2. Anderson DM, Shelley S, Crick N, Buraglio M. No effect of the novel antidiabetic agent nateglinide on the pharmacokinetics and anticoagulant properties of warfarin in healthy volunteers. *J Clin Pharmacol* (2002) 42, 1358–65.
3. Starlix (Nateglinide). Novartis Pharmaceuticals UK Ltd. UK Summary of product characteristics, August 2004.
4. Starlix (Nateglinide). Novartis Pharmaceuticals Corporation. US Prescribing information, January 2004.
5. Rosenberg M, Strange P, Cohen A. Assessment of pharmacokinetic (PKP and pharmacodynamic (PD) interaction between warfarin and repaglinide. *Diabetes* (1999) 48 (Suppl 1), A356.

Anticoagulants + Antidiabetics; Pioglitazone or Rosiglitazone

Pioglitazone and rosiglitazone do not affect warfarin pharmacokinetics and pioglitazone does not affect phenprocoumon pharmacokinetics.

Clinical evidence, mechanism, importance and management

(a) Pioglitazone

Co-administration of pioglitazone 45 mg daily with **warfarin** did not alter the steady-state pharmacokinetics of **warfarin** and there was no significant change in prothrombin time.[1,2] Similar results were noted with **phenprocoumon**.[2]

(b) Rosiglitazone

Rosiglitazone has been found to have no clinically relevant effect on the steady-state levels of **warfarin**.[3]

1. Actos (Pioglitazone hydrochloride). Takeda Ltd. US Prescribing information, August 2004.
2. Kortboyer JM, Eckland DJA. Pioglitazone has low potential for drug interactions. *Diabetologia* (1999) 42 (Suppl 1), A228.
3. Avandia (Rosiglitazone maleate). GlaxoSmithKline. US Prescribing information, March 2005.

Anticoagulants + Antihistamines

The anticoagulant effects of acenocoumarol may be reduced by loratadine, ebastine, or cetirizine. An isolated report describes bleeding and a markedly raised INR in an elderly man on acenocoumarol and cetirizine.

Clinical evidence, mechanism, importance and management

A review of patients treated with **acenocoumarol** and **loratadine**, **ebastine**, or **cetirizine** found that INRs were decreased during concurrent use and temporary increases in the anticoagulant dosage were required.[1]

In contrast, there is a case report of an 88-year-old man taking **acenocoumarol** for a deep vein thrombosis who developed acute and severe epistaxis after a fall within 3 days of starting to take **cetirizine** 10 mg daily for allergic rhinitis.[2] His INR was found to have risen from 1.5 to 14. The **cetirizine** concentration may have been particularly high because of some renal impairment, resulting in **acenocoumarol** displacement from its plasma protein binding sites and increased effects, although this mechanism on its own is now largely discredited as an explanation for interactions between anticoagulants and highly bound drugs.

Information is limited, and given the widespread use of these drugs any consistent clinically significant interaction would be expected to have come to light by now. No specific precautions seem necessary if these drugs are given in combination, but bear the interaction in mind in the case of an unexpected response to treatment.

1. García Callejo FJ, Velert Vila MM, Marco Sanz M, Fernández Julián EN. Empleo simultáneo de antihistamínicos H_1 y anticoagulantes orales. *Acta Otorrinolaringol Esp* (2001) 52, 442–5.
2. Berod T, Mathiot I. Probable interaction between cetirizine and acenocoumarol. *Ann Pharmacother* (1997) 31, 122.

Anticoagulants + Antineoplastics

A number of case reports describe an increase in the effects of warfarin, accompanied by bleeding in some cases, caused by antineoplastic regimens containing broxuridine, capecitabine, carboplatin, chlormethine, cyclophosphamide, doxorubicin, etoposide, 5-fluorouracil, ftorafur, gemcitabine, ifosfamide with mesna, methotrexate, procarbazine, sulofenur, tegafur with uracil, vincristine and vindesine. Capecitabine is reported to increase the anticoagulant effects of phenprocoumon and warfarin in some patients.

A decrease in the effects of warfarin has been seen with regimens containing azathioprine, cyclophosphamide, mercaptopurine and mitotane, a decrease in the effects of phenprocoumon has been seen with azathioprine and a decrease in the effects of acenocoumarol has been seen with mercaptopurine.

Clinical evidence

(a) Anticoagulant effects increased

The INR of a man on **warfarin** increased from a baseline range of 1.15 to 2.11 up to 12.6 within 16 days of a first course of chemotherapy with **carboplatin** and **etoposide**.[1]

A man on **warfarin** showed a progressive rise in prothrombin times when given a continuous infusion of **fluorouracil**.[2] Three out of 25 patients developed blood loss from the gut when treated with **warfarin** and rapid intravenous **fluorouracil**, which was controlled by giving a transfusion and stopping the **warfarin**.[3] A man developed a prolonged prothrombin time with epistaxis, haematemesis, haematuria and haematochezia attributed to an interaction between **warfarin** and **fluorouracil**.[4]

The INR of an elderly man on **warfarin** increased from 3 to almost 40 after he was given **fluorouracil** and **levamisole** for 4 weeks, and he again demonstrated increased **warfarin** effects when rechallenged with **fluorouracil**.[5] A 60-year-old woman on **warfarin** had an increase in her prothrombin time from a range of 13.6 to 19.7 seconds up to 22.6 seconds ten days after completing the first cycle of **levamisole** and **fluorouracil**. Eight days later after completing a 3-day course of **levamisole** she developed gross haematuria and was found to have a prothrombin time greater than 40 seconds.[6]

A number of other patients have been described who similarly showed increased INRs and/or needed **warfarin** dosage reductions while receiving **fluorouracil**.[7-10] A study found that 24 of 70 patients with cancer treated with continuous infusions of **fluorouracil** and also given **warfarin** 1 mg daily as prophylaxis against central venous catheter-associated thrombosis had INR abnormalities. Epistaxis and haematuria occurred in 6 of the patients.[11]

Increased INRs and bleeding (haemoptysis) were also seen in a patient on **warfarin** when treated with *Orzel* (**uracil/ftorafur** in a 4:1 molar ratio). **Ftorafur** is a pro-drug of **fluorouracil**. This patient needed a 63% reduction in the warfarin dosage.[12] *Uftoral* (**tegafur/uracil**) is another prodrug of **fluorouracil** and the makers say that marked elevations in prothrombin times and INRs have been reported in patients on **warfarin** when *Uftoral* was added.[13]

A woman stabilised on **warfarin** developed an iliopsoas [muscle] haematoma 3 weeks after starting treatment with **cyclophosphamide**, **methotrexate**, **fluorouracil**, **vincristine** and prednisone.[14] The prothrombin times of 2 women on **warfarin** approximately doubled, accompanied by bleeding, on day 15 of each cycle of adjuvant treatment with **CMF** (**cyclophosphamide**, **methotrexate** and **fluorouracil**).[15] The INR of a woman on **warfarin** rose from below 2.8 up to a range of 4.15 to 10 by day 23 of her first cycle of **CMF**.[16]

A 63-year-old man needed a reduction in his weekly **warfarin** dosage from 59.23 mg to 50.75 mg in order to keep his INR at about 2.5 while receiving 2 cycles of **gemcitabine**. When the **gemcitabine** treatment was finished his **warfarin** dosage had to be increased again.[17] The makers have information on 4 cases of suspected interactions between **gemcitabine** and **warfarin**, one with **phenprocoumon** and one involving **heparin** (reported by December 2000).[18] Based on 724 reports of the concurrent use of **gemcitabine** and **anticoagulants**,[18] they suggest the incidence of the suspected interaction as 0.8%.

Another elderly man on **warfarin** showed a marked increase in prothrombin times (prolongation of 8 to 15 seconds) on two occasions when he took **etoposide** 500 mg and **vindesine** 5 mg.[19] The prothrombin times of an elderly man given **warfarin** increased by 50 to 100% in the middle of three cycles of treatment with ProMace-Mopp (**cyclophosphamide**, **doxorubicin**, **etoposide**, **chlormethine**, **vincristine**, **procarbazine**, **methotrexate** and prednisone), and he developed a subconjunctival haemorrhage during the first cycle.[15] Three patients on **warfarin** showed a marked and very rapid increase in their INRs when they took **ifosfamide** with **mesna**.[20] Three patients developed a marked increase in prothrombin times while receiving **warfarin** and **sulofenur**.[21]

A man on **warfarin** with grade III anaplastic astrocytoma was given intravenous **broxuridine** as a radiosensitiser. His prothrombin times were unaffected by the first course of **broxuridine** 1400 mg daily for 4 days, but became more prolonged with successive courses, and after the fourth course his prothrombin time reached about 45 seconds, which was treated with 10 mg of vitamin K. Warfarin was stopped after a significant increase also took place with a fifth cycle of **broxuridine** 990 mg daily.[22]

A marked elevation in INR and prothrombin time occurred in 2 patients on warfarin after they received **capecitabine** (a prodrug of fluorouracil) 2000 mg/m^2 daily in divided doses (given for 2 weeks followed by a one week rest period). In both patients there was gastrointestinal bleeding, which developed after two cycles of **capecitabine** treatment.[23]

The makers of **capecitabine** report that changes in coagulation parameters and/or bleeding have been seen in a few patients on anticoagulants such as **warfarin** and **phenprocoumon** within several days or months of adding **capecitabine**. In one case it occurred a month after the **capecitabine** had been stopped. The reasons for the interaction are not understood, but what has been seen is consistent with reports of increased warfarin effects seen with another 5-fluorouracil prodrug containing **uracil** and **ftorafur** (*Orzel*) and with 5-fluorouracil itself (see above). On the basis of these clinical observations the makers say that prothrombin times or INR should be regularly monitored in patients taking capecitabine with these and other **coumarin oral anticoagulants**.[24] The incidence of this interaction is not known.

(b) Anticoagulant effects decreased

A survey of 103 patients with antiphospholipid syndrome found that **azathioprine** appeared to increase **warfarin** requirements.[25] A woman who was resistant to **warfarin**, needing 14 to 17 mg daily while taking **azathioprine**, began to bleed (epistaxes, haematemesis) when the **azathioprine** was stopped. She was restabilised on **warfarin** 5 mg daily.[26] Reduced **warfarin** effects were seen in 2 other patients taking **azathioprine**,[27,28] one of whom had a marked fall in serum **warfarin** levels during **azathioprine** treatment.[28] Two women with systemic lupus erythematosus on **phenprocoumon**[29] and a third on **warfarin**[30] had marked falls in their INRs during treatment with **azathioprine**, and another woman needed an almost 4-fold increase in the dose of **warfarin** when she was given **azathioprine**.[31] A man well stabilised on **warfarin** showed a marked reduction in his anticoagulant response on two occasions when treated with **mercaptopurine**, but no changes occurred when given **busulfan**, **cyclophosphamide**, **cytarabine**, **hydroxycarbamide**, **mitobronitol**, **demecolcine** or **melphalan**.[32] A woman needed a marked increase in her dosage of **acenocoumarol**, from 21 to 70 mg weekly, when she was given **mercaptopurine** 100 mg daily.[33] A woman on **warfarin** showed a marked rise in prothrombin times when her treatment with **cyclophosphamide** was withdrawn.[34] The anticoagulant effects of **warfarin** were progressively reduced in a woman taking **mitotane**.[35] Later this effect began to reverse.

Mechanism, importance and management

Not well understood. Mercaptopurine appears to increase the synthesis or activation of prothrombin[36]. Fluorouracil may inhibit the cytochrome P450 isoenzyme CYP2C9 in the liver, and consequently reduce warfarin metabolism. It may also have a direct effect on the gastrointestinal tract, which could affect warfarin or vitamin K absorption.[10] In the case of capecitabine it has been suggested that metabolic intermediates may be inhibitors of P450 isoenzymes.[23]

It is not even possible in some cases to identify precisely the drug (or drugs) responsible. In the case of patients given fluorouracil and warfarin[5,6] some of the changes were probably due to fluorouracil but the levamisole may have had some part to play because the makers refer to reports of increased prothrombin times with warfarin and levamisole.[37] The absence of problems in many studies using warfarin as an adjunct to chemotherapy[38,39] and the small number of reports describing difficulties suggest that many of these interactions may be uncommon events. The concurrent use of most of these drugs need not be avoided but there is clearly a need to be aware that antineoplastic regimens, particularly involving gemcitabine or fluorouracil and its prodrugs can increase the response to anticoagulants. It would also be prudent to note that mercaptopurine and azathioprine may decrease the anticoagulant response. The anticoagulant dosages may need adjustment. It has been suggested that subcutaneous heparin should be given rather than warfarin to patients on sulofenur.[21] Information about other anticoagulants appears to be lacking.

1. Le AT, Hasson NK, Lum BL. Enhancement of warfarin response in a patient receiving etoposide and carboplatin chemotherapy. *Ann Pharmacother* (1997) 31, 1006–8.
2. Wajima T, Mukhopadhyay P. Possible interactions between warfarin and 5-fluorouracil. *Am J Hematol* (1992) 40, 238.
3. Chlebowski RT, Gota CH, Chann KK, Weiner JM, Block JB, Batemen JR. Clinical and pharmacokinetic effects of combined warfarin and 5-fluorouracil in advanced colon cancer. *Cancer Res* (1982) 42, 4827–30.
4. Brown MC. Multisite mucous membrane bleeding due to a possible interaction between warfarin and 5-fluorouracil. *Pharmacotherapy* (1997) 17, 631–3.
5. Scarfe MA, Israel MK. Possible drug interaction between warfarin and combination of levamisole and fluorouracil. *Ann Pharmacother* (1994) 28, 464–7.
6. Wehbe TW, Warth JA. A case of bleeding requiring hospitalisation that was likely caused by an interaction between warfarin and levamisole. *Clin Pharmacol Ther* (1996) 59, 360–2.
7. Brown MC. An adverse interaction between warfarin and 5-fluorouracil; a case report and review of the literature. *Chemotherapy* (1999) 45, 392–5.
8. Kolesar JM, Johnson CL, Freeberg BL, Berlin JD, Schiller JH. Warfarin-5-FU interaction – a consecutive case series. *Pharmacotherapy* (1999) 19, 1445–9.
9. Aki Z, Kotiloğlu G, Özyilkan Ö. A patient with a prolonged prothrombin time due to an adverse interaction between 5-fluorouracil and warfarin. *Am J Gastroenterol* (2000) 95, 1093–4.
10. Carabino J, Wang F. International normalized ratio fluctuation with warfarin-fluorouracil therapy. *Am J Health-Syst Pharm* (2002), 59, 875.
11. Masci G, Zucali PA, Sarina B, Magagnoli M, Castagna L, Fallini M, Carnaghi C, Santoro A. Adverse interactions between continuous infusion of 5-fluorouracil (5-FU) based chemotherapy and warfarin inducing prothrombin time abnormalities. *Haemostasis* (2001) 31 (Suppl1), 101–2.
12. Karwal MW, Schlueter AJ, Arnold MM, Davis RT. Presumed drug interaction between Orzel® and warfarin. *Blood* (1999) 94 (10 Suppl 1, part 2), 106b.
13. Uftoral (Tegafur/uracil). Bristol-Myers Squibb Pharmaceuticals. UK Summary of product characteristics, January 2001.
14. Booth BW, Weiss RB. Venous thrombosis during adjuvant chemotherapy. *N Engl J Med* (1981) 305, 170.
15. Seifter EJ, Brooks BJ, Urba WJ. Possible interactions between warfarin and antineoplastic drugs. *Cancer Treat Rep* (1985) 69, 244–5.
16. Malacarne P, Maestri A. Possible interactions between antiblastic agents and warfarin inducing prothrombin time abnormalities. *Recenti Prog Med* (1996) 87, 135.
17. Kinikar SA, Kolesar JM. Identification of a gemcitabine-warfarin interaction. *Pharmacotherapy* (1999) 19, 1331–3.

18. Kilgour-Christie J, Czarnecki A. Gemcitabine and the interaction with anticoagulants. *Lancet Oncol* (2002) 3, 460.
19. Ward K, Bitran JD. Warfarin, etoposide, and vindesine interactions. *Cancer Treat Rep* (1984) 68, 817–18.
20. Hall G, Lind MJ, Huang M, Moore A, Gane A, Roberts JT, Cantwell BMJ. Intravenous infusions of ifosfamide/mesna and perturbation of warfarin anticoagulant control. *Postgrad Med J* (1990) 66, 860–1.
21. Fossella FV, Lippman SM, Seitz DE, Alberts DS, Taylor CW, Wiltshaw E, Hardy J, O'Brien M, Haynes TR, Wolen RL. Hypoprothrombinemia from coadministration of sulofenur (LY 186641) and warfarin: report of three cases. *Invest New Drugs* (1991) 9, 357–9.
22. Oster SE, Lawrence HJ. Potentiation of anticoagulant effect of coumadin by 5-bromo-2′-deoxyuridine (BUDR). *Cancer Chemother Pharmacol* (1988) 22, 181.
23. Sitki Copur M, Ledakis P, Bolton M, Morse AK, Werner T, Norvell M, Muhvic J, Chu E. An adverse interaction between warfarin and capecitabine: a case report and review of the literature. *Clin Colorectal Cancer* (2001) 3, 182–4.
24. Xeloda (Capecitabine). Roche Products Ltd. UK Summary of product characteristics, March 2005.
25. Khamashta MA, Cuadrado MJ, Mujic F, Taub N, Hunt BJ, Hughes GRV. Effect of azathioprine on the anticoagulant activity of warfarin in patients with the antiphospholipid syndrome. *Lupus* (1998) 7 (Suppl 2), S227.
26. Singleton JD, Conyers L. Warfarin and azathioprine: an important drug interaction. *Am J Med* (1992) 92, 217.
27. Rivier G, Khamashta MA, Hughes GRV. Warfarin and azathioprine: a drug interaction does exist. *Am J Med* (1993) 95, 342.
28. Rotenberg M, Levy Y, Shoenfeld Y, Almog S, Ezra D. Effect of azathioprine on the anticoagulant activity of warfarin. *Ann Pharmacother* (2000) 34, 120–2.
29. Jeppesen U, Rasmussen JM, Brøsen K. Clinically important interaction between azathioprine (Imurel) and phenprocoumon (Marcoumar). *Eur J Clin Pharmacol* (1997) 52, 503–4.
30. Walker J, Mendelson H, McClure A Smith MD. Warfarin and azathioprine: clinically significant drug interaction. *J Rheumatol* (2002) 29, 398–9.
31. Havrda DE, Rathbun S, Scheid D. A case report of warfarin resistance due to azathioprine and review of the literature. *Pharmacotherapy* (2001) 21, 355–7.
32. Spiers ASD, Mibashan RS. Increased warfarin requirement during mercaptopurine therapy: a new drug interaction. *Lancet* (1974) ii, 221–2.
33. Fernádez MA, Regadera A, Aznar J. Acenocoumarol and 6-mercaptopurine: an important drug interaction. *Haematologica* (1999) 84, 664–5.
34. Tashima CK. Cyclophosphamide effect on coumarin anticoagulation. *South Med J* (1979) 72, 633–4.
35. Cuddy PG, Loftus LS. Influence of mitotane on the hypoprothrombinemic effect of warfarin. *South Med J* (1986) 79, 387–8.
36. Martini A, Jähnchen E. Studies in rats on the mechanisms by which 6-mercaptopurine inhibits the anticoagulant effect of warfarin. *J Pharmacol Exp Ther* (1977) 201, 547–53.
37. Ergamisol (Levamisole). Product information. *Physicians Desk Reference* (2002) 1789–91.
38. Zacharski LR, Henderson WG, Rickles FR, Forman WB, Cornell CJ, Forcier RJ, Edwards RL, Headley E, Kim S-H, O'Donnell JR, O'Dell R, Tornyos K, Kwaan HC. Effect of warfarin anticoagulation on survival in carcinoma of the lung, colon, head and neck, and prostate. *Cancer* (1984) 53, 2046–52.
39. Zacharski LR, Henderson WG, Rickles FR, Forman WB, Cornell CJ, Forcier RJ, Edwards R, Headley E, Kim S-H, O'Donnell JR, O'Dell R, Tornyos K, Kwaan HC. Effect of warfarin on survival in small cell carcinoma of the lung. *JAMA* (1981) 245, 831–5.

Anticoagulants + Aprepitant

Aprepitant modestly reduces warfarin levels and slightly decreases the INR in healthy subjects.

Clinical evidence, mechanism, importance and management

Healthy subjects were stabilised on **warfarin** and then given aprepitant 125 mg on day one, then 80 mg daily on days 2 and 3. On day 3, there was no change in **warfarin** levels. However, by day 8 (5 days after stopping aprepitant) there was a 34% decrease in ***(S)*-warfarin** levels, and a 14% decrease in INR.[1,2]

Aprepitant is an inducer of the cytochrome P450 isoenzyme CYP2C9, by which ***(S)*-warfarin** is metabolised. The maker recommends that, in patients on **warfarin**, the INR should be monitored closely for 2 weeks, particularly at 7 to 10 days,[2] after each 3-day course of aprepitant,[1,2] and this seems a prudent precaution.

1. Emend (Aprepitant). Merck Sharp & Dohme Ltd. UK Summary of product characteristics, April 2005.
2. Emend (Aprepitant). Merck & Co., Inc. US Prescribing information, March 2005.

Anticoagulants + Aromatase inhibitors

The anticoagulant effects of warfarin and acenocoumarol can be reduced by aminoglutethimide. The extent of the reduction appears to be related to the aminoglutethimide dosage. Anastrozole and letrozole do not appear to interact with warfarin.

Clinical evidence

(a) Aminoglutethimide

A study in patients on warfarin who were treated for breast cancer with aminoglutethimide found that a low dose aminoglutethimide regimen (125 mg twice daily) increased the clearance of **warfarin** by 41.2% whereas a high-dose regimen (250 mg four times daily) increased the clearance by 90.8%. The effects of the interaction had developed fully by 14 days. Both isomers of **warfarin** were equally affected.[1]

Two patients needed a three to fourfold increase in **warfarin** dosage while taking aminoglutethimide 250 mg four times a day.[2] The increased requirement persisted for 2 weeks after the aminoglutethimide was stopped, and then declined. Brief mention of the need to take greatly increased doses of **warfarin** while on aminoglutethimide is reported elsewhere.[3] Three patients on **acenocoumarol** needed a doubled dosage to maintain adequate anticoagulation while taking aminoglutethimide 250 mg four times daily for 3 to 4 weeks.[4]

(b) Anastrozole

A randomised, double-blind, placebo-controlled, two-way crossover study in 16 healthy subjects found that anastrozole (7 mg loading dose followed by 1 mg daily for a further 10 days) had no effect on the pharmacokinetics or pharmacodynamics of **warfarin**.[5]

(c) Letrozole

The makers report that no clinically significant interaction occurs between letrozole and **warfarin**.[6]

Mechanism

Uncertain. The most likely explanation is that aminoglutethimide, like glutethimide, stimulates the activity of the liver enzymes concerned with the metabolism of the anticoagulants, thereby increasing their loss from the body. Alternatively, it has been suggested that aminoglutethimide may affect blood steroid levels, which in turn might affect coagulation.[2]

Importance and management

An established and clinically important interaction. Monitor the effects of adding aminoglutethimide to patients already on warfarin or acenocoumarol and increase the anticoagulant dosage as necessary. Up to four times the dosage may be needed. The extent of the effects would appear to be related to the dosage of aminoglutethimide used. Monitor the INR and reduce the anticoagulant dosage accordingly if aminoglutethimide is withdrawn. Information about other coumarins is lacking but it would be prudent to apply the same precautions with any of them.

1. Lønning PE, Ueland PM, Kvinnsland S. The influence of a graded dose schedule of aminoglutethimide on the disposition of the optical enantiomers of warfarin in patients with breast cancer. *Cancer Chemother Pharmacol* (1986) 17, 177–81.
2. Lønning PE, Kvinnsland S, Jahren G. Aminoglutethimide and warfarin. A new important drug interaction. *Cancer Chemother Pharmacol* (1984) 12, 10–12.
3. Murray RML, Pitt P, Jerums G. Medical adrenalectomy with aminoglutethimide in the management of advanced breast cancer. *Med J Aust* (1981) 1, 179–81.
4. Bruning PF, Bonfrèr JGM. Aminoglutethimide and oral anticoagulant therapy. *Lancet* (1983) ii, 582.
5. Yates RA, Wong J, Seiberling M, Merz M, März W, Nauck M. The effect of anastrozole on the single-dose pharmacokinetics and anticoagulant activity of warfarin in healthy volunteers. *Br J Clin Pharmacol* (2001) 51, 429–35.
6. Femara (Letrozole). Novartis Pharmaceuticals UK Ltd. UK Summary of product characteristics, September 2004.

Anticoagulants + Ascorbic acid (Vitamin C)

Although two isolated cases have been reported in which the effects of warfarin were reduced by ascorbic acid, four controlled studies with large numbers of patients failed to demonstrate any interaction.

Clinical evidence

The prothrombin time of a woman, stabilised on **warfarin** 7.5 mg daily, who began to take regular amounts of ascorbic acid [dose not stated], fell steadily from 23 seconds, to 19, 17 and then 14 seconds with no response to an increase in the dosage of **warfarin** to 10, 15 and finally 20 mg daily. The prothrombin time returned to 28 seconds within 2 days of stopping the ascorbic acid.[1] A woman who had been taking ascorbic acid 16 g daily proved to be unusually resistant to the actions of **warfarin** and required 25 mg daily before a significant increase in prothrombin times was achieved.[2]

In contrast, no changes in the effects of **warfarin** were seen in a total of 119 patients given ascorbic acid; 1 g daily for a fortnight,[3] an unstated dose for 10 weeks,[4] up to 4 g daily for 2 weeks,[5] or 3 to 10 g daily for 1 or

2 weeks.[6] In this last study a mean fall of 17.5% in total plasma **warfarin** concentrations was seen.

Mechanism

Not understood. One *animal* study has demonstrated this interaction[7] and others have not,[8,9] but none of them has provided any definite clues about why it ever occurs. One suggestion is that high doses of ascorbic acid can cause diarrhoea, which might prevent adequate absorption of the anticoagulant.

Importance and management

Well controlled clinical studies in large numbers of patients on warfarin have failed to confirm this interaction, even using very large doses of ascorbic acid (up to 10 g daily). There is no good reason for avoiding the concurrent use. Information about other anticoagulants is lacking, but it seems likely that they will behave similarly. However check on any patient particularly resistant to the warfarin to confirm that ascorbic acid is not being taken.

1. Rosenthal G. Interaction of ascorbic acid and warfarin. *JAMA* (1971) 215, 1671.
2. Smith EC, Skalski RJ, Johnson GC, Rossi GV. Interaction of ascorbic acid and warfarin. *JAMA* (1972) 221, 1166.
3. Hume R, Johnstone JMS, Weyers E. Interaction of ascorbic acid and warfarin. *JAMA* (1972) 219, 1479.
4. Dedichen J. The effect of ascorbic acid given to patients on chronic anticoagulant therapy. *Boll Soc Ital Cardiol* (1973) 18, 690–2.
5. Blakely JA. Interaction of warfarin and ascorbic acid. 1st Florence Conference on Haemostasis and Thrombosis, May 1977. Abstracts p 99.
6. Feetam CL, Leach RH, Meynell MJ. Lack of a clinically important interaction between warfarin and ascorbic acid. *Toxicol Appl Pharmacol* (1975) 31, 544–7.
7. Sigell LT, Flessa HC. Drug interactions with anticoagulants. *JAMA* (1970) 214, 2035–8.
8. Weintraub M, Griner PF. Warfarin and ascorbic acid: lack of evidence for a drug interaction. *Toxicol Appl Pharmacol* (1974) 28, 53–6.
9. Deckert FW. Ascorbic acid and warfarin. *JAMA* (1973) 223, 440.

Anticoagulants + Aspirin or Salicylates

Aspirin 500 mg daily increases the likelihood of bleeding 3 to 5 times in those taking anticoagulants, it damages the stomach wall, prolongs bleeding times and in daily doses of 2 to 4 g it can increase prothrombin times. Low-dose aspirin (75 to 100 mg daily) seems to be safer, and some large scale studies have concluded that the overall benefits of concurrent use may outweigh the risks in certain patient groups. Increased warfarin effects have been seen when methyl salicylate or trolamine salicylate were used on the skin.

Clinical evidence

(a) Analgesic-dose aspirin

A study in 534 patients with artificial heart valves found that three times as many had bleeding episodes requiring blood transfusion or hospitalisation among those on aspirin 500 mg daily (14%) and **warfarin** compared to those on **warfarin** alone (5%). Bleeding was mainly gastrointestinal or cerebral. All of those with intracerebral bleeding died.[1]

This finding broadly confirms two other studies in a total of 270 patients in whom bleeding was found to be about five times more common if aspirin 500 mg to 1 g daily was given with an anticoagulant than if the anticoagulant was given alone.[2,3] A further study found that aspirin 1 g daily increased the bleeding episodes in those on **un-named anticoagulants** from 4.7 to 13.9 per 100 patients per year.[4] A 20% incidence of severe upper gastrointestinal bleeding was seen in a study of 138 coronary stent patients given heparin or **warfarin** with 325 mg aspirin daily. Ten of the patients needed a blood transfusion.[5] A study of 75 patients taking **acenocoumarol** and aspirin reported serious bleeding in 2.7% and mild bleeding in 33% but no fatalities.[6] Other studies in patients taking **dicoumarol**, **acenocoumarol** or **warfarin** found that aspirin 2 to 4 g daily increased the anticoagulant effects. The anticoagulant dosage could be reduced about 30%.[7,8] However another study found that adding aspirin 3 g daily to **warfarin** had no effect on prothrombin times.[9]

(b) Antiplatelet-dose aspirin

Low-dose aspirin (75 mg daily) doubles the normal blood loss from the gastric mucosa but it still remains very small (compared with the 14-fold increase with 2.4 g of aspirin daily) and **warfarin** does not increase it.[10] Only minor episodes of bleeding (nose bleeds, bruising) occur with low dose aspirin and low intensity **warfarin** (INR 1.5).[11] Another study using aspirin 100 mg daily found that although there was some increase in bleeding, the risk was more than offset by the overall reduction in mortality.[12]

A meta-analysis of four studies involving almost 900 patients carried out between 1976 and 1993 concluded that the combined use of oral anticoagulants and aspirin (100 to 500 mg daily) significantly reduced mortality and embolic complications in patients with prosthetic heart valves, although this was partly offset by some increase in major bleeding episodes. Nevertheless the overall picture was that the benefits possibly outweighed the problems.[13] Another very large scale study comparing **warfarin** alone (INRs 2.5 to 4.2) with warfarin plus aspirin 150 mg daily (INRs 2.2 to 2.8) found that the aspirin group showed a higher incidence of minor bleeding (2.9% compared with 1.4%) but the incidence of serious and fatal bleeding was the same in the two groups.[14] Yet another study found no differences in bleeding rates in stroke patients given heparin and/or **warfarin** with or without aspirin.[15] Another study in 677 patients compared **warfarin sodium** 1.25 mg daily alone, **warfarin sodium** 1.25 mg daily with aspirin 300 mg daily, aspirin 300 mg daily, and adjusted dose **warfarin** for stroke prevention in atrial fibrillation.[16] Significant adverse effects were not found.[16]

(c) Topical salicylates

Methyl salicylate, in the form of gels, oil, or ointment applied to the skin, has been found to increase the effects of **warfarin**. Bleeding and bruising and/or raised INRs have been seen with both high[17-19] and low doses[20] of **methyl salicylate**. One report[21] described the possible additive effects of **methyl salicylate oil** (*Kwan Loong Medicated Oil*) and a decoction of *'Danshen'* (the root of *Salvia miltiorrhiza*) on the response to **warfarin** (see also 'Anticoagulants + Herbal medicines; Danshen', p.285. A raised prothrombin time has also been reported with topical **trolamine salicylate**.[19]

Mechanism

Aspirin has a direct irritant effect on the stomach lining and can cause gastrointestinal bleeding. It also decreases platelet aggregation and prolongs bleeding times, all of which would seem to account for some of the bleeding episodes described.[2,3] In addition, large doses (2 to 4 g daily) of aspirin alone are known to have a direct hypoprothrombinaemic effect, which are reversible by vitamin K.[22-24] The effects of the aspirin can be additive with the effects of the anticoagulant. Methyl and trolamine salicylates can also interact because they are absorbed through the skin.

Importance and management

The interaction of aspirin and warfarin at high doses is well documented and clinically important, for which reason it is usual to avoid normal analgesic and anti-inflammatory doses while taking any anticoagulant, although only dicoumarol, acenocoumarol (nicoumalone) and warfarin appear to have been investigated. Patients should be told that many non-prescription analgesic, antipyretic, cold and influenza preparations may contain substantial amounts of aspirin. Warn them that it may be listed as acetylsalicylic acid. Paracetamol is a safer analgesic substitute (but not entirely without problems – see 'Anticoagulants + Paracetamol (Acetaminophen)', p.303.

Low-dose aspirin used for its platelet anti-aggregant effects appears to interact to a lesser extent, and where problems are seen it still appears that the benefits of use outweigh the risks, in certain patient groups.

Some of the other salicylates are less irritant and have a smaller effect on platelet function than aspirin so that, on theoretical grounds, the avoidance of concurrent use may be less important. Remember too that topical methyl salicylate and trolamine salicylate can also interact.

1. Chesebro JH, Fuster V, Elveback LR, McGoon DC, Pluth JR, Puga FJ, Wallace RB, Danielson GK, Orszulak TA, Piehler JM, Schaff HV. Trial of combined warfarin plus dipyridamole or aspirin therapy in prosthetic heart valve replacement: danger of aspirin compared with dipyridamole. *Am J Cardiol* (1983) 51, 1537–41.
2. Altman R, Boullon F, Rouvier J, Rada R, de la Fuente L, Favaloro R. Aspirin and prophylaxis of thromboembolic complications in patients with substitute heart valves. *J Thorac Cardiovasc Surg* (1976) 72, 127–9.
3. Dale J, Myhre E, Storstein O, Stormorken H, Efskind L. Prevention of arterial thromboembolism with acetylsalicylic acid. A controlled clinical study in patients with aortic ball valves. *Am Heart J* (1977) 94, 101–111.
4. Dale J, Myhre E, Loew D. Bleeding during acetylsalicylic acid and anticoagulant therapy in patients with reduced platelet reactivity after aortic valve replacement. *Am Heart J* (1980) 99, 746–52.

5. Younossi ZM, Strum WB, Cloutier D, Teirstein PS, Schatz RA. Upper GI bleeding in post-coronary stent patients following aspirin and anticoagulant treatment. *Gastroenterology* (1995) 108 (4 Suppl), A265.
6. Sámóczi M, Farkas A, Sipos E, Tarján J. Acenocoumarol és acetylsalicylsav együttes alkalmazásának szövődmenyei szívinfarktus után és instabil anginában. *Orv Hetil* (1995) 136, 177–9.
7. Watson RM, Pierson RN. Effect of anticoagulant therapy upon aspirin-induced gastrointestinal bleeding. *Circulation* (1961) 24, 613–16.
8. O'Reilly RA, Sahud MA, Aggeler PM. Impact of aspirin and chlorthalidone on the pharmacodynamics of oral anticoagulants drugs in man. *Ann N Y Acad Sci* (1971) 179, 173–86.
9. Udall JA. Drug interference with warfarin therapy. *Am J Cardiol* (1969) 23, 143.
10. Prichard PJ, Kitchingman GK, Walt RP, Daneshmend TK, Hawkey CJ. Human gastric mucosal bleeding induced by low dose aspirin, but not warfarin. *BMJ* (1989) 298, 493–6.
11. Meade TW, Roderick PJ, Brennan PJ, Wilkes HC, Kelleher CC. Extra-cranial bleeding and other symptoms due to low dose aspirin and low intensity oral anticoagulation. *Thromb Haemost* (1992) 68, 1–6.
12. Turpie AGG, Gent M, Laupacis A, Latour Y, Gunstensen J, Basile F, Klimek M, Hirsh J. A comparison of aspirin with placebo in patients treated with warfarin after heart-valve replacement. *N Engl J Med* (1993) 329, 524–9.
13. Fiore L, Brophy M, Deykin D, Cappelleri J, Lau J. The efficacy and safety of the addition of aspirin in patients treated with oral anticoagulants after heart valve replacement: a meta-analysis. *Blood* (1993) 82 (10 Suppl 1), 409a.
14. Hurlen M, Erikssen J, Smith P, Arnesen H, Rollag A. Comparison of bleeding complications of warfarin and warfarin plus acetylsalicylic acid: a study in 3166 outpatients. *J Intern Med* (1994) 236, 299–304.
15. Fagan SC, Kertland HR, Tietjen GE. Safety of combination aspirin and anticoagulation in acute ischemic stroke. *Ann Pharmacother* (1994) 28, 441–3.
16. Gulløv AL, Koefoed BG, Petersen P, Pedersen TS, Andersen ED, Godtfredsen J, Boysen G. Fixed minidose warfarin and aspirin alone and in combination vs adjusted-dose warfarin for stroke prevention in atrial fibrillation. Second Copenhagen atrial fibrillation, aspirin, and anticoagulant study. *Arch Intern Med* (1998) 158, 1513–21.
17. Chow WH, Cheung KL, Ling HM, See T. Potentiation of warfarin anticoagulation by topical methylsalicylate ointment. *J R Soc Med* (1989) 82, 501–2.
18. Yip ASB, Chow WH, Tai YT, Cheung KL. Adverse effect of topical methylsalicylate ointment on warfarin anticoagulation: an unrecognized potential hazard. *Postgrad Med J* (1990) 66, 367–9.
19. Littleton F. Warfarin and topical salicylates. *JAMA* (1990) 263, 2888.
20. Joss JD, LeBlond RF. Potentiation of warfarin anticoagulation associated with topical methyl salicylate. *Ann Pharmacother* (2000) 34, 729–33.
21. Tam LS, Chan TYK, Leung WK, Critchley JAJH. Warfarin interactions with Chinese traditional medicines: danshen and methyl salicylate medicated oil. *Aust N Z J Med* (1995) 25, 258.
22. Shapiro S. Studies on prothrombin. VI. The effect of synthetic vitamin K on the prothrombinopenia induced by salicylate in man. *JAMA* (1944) 125, 546–8.
23. Quick AJ, Clesceri L. Influence of acetylsalicylic acid and salicylamide on the coagulation of blood. *J Pharmacol Exp Ther* (1960) 128, 95–8.
24. Park BK, Leck JB. On the mechanism of salicylate-induced hypoprothrombinaemia. *J Pharm Pharmacol* (1981) 33, 25–8.

Anticoagulants + Azoles; Fluconazole

The anticoagulant effects of warfarin are increased by fluconazole and bleeding has been seen. Acenocoumarol appears to interact similarly.

Clinical evidence

(a) Acenocoumarol

A patient on acenocoumarol suffered an intracranial haemorrhage (prothrombin time 170 seconds) 5 days after starting to take fluconazole 200 mg daily.[1]

(b) Warfarin

When fluconazole 100 mg daily was given to 7 patients on warfarin the prothrombin time was increased on average by 15.8 seconds on day one, 18.9 seconds on day 5, and 21.9 seconds on day 8. The fluconazole was stopped early in 3 of the patients due to high prothrombin times, but none exceeded an increase of 9.7 seconds and no bleeding occurred.[2]

A crossover study in 13 healthy subjects given fluconazole 200 mg daily for 7 days and then a single 15-mg dose of warfarin found that the changes in the prothrombin time curve over 168 hours were increased by about 10 to 13% in 12 subjects, and doubled in one other. This last subject was given vitamin K.[3] Fluconazole 400 mg daily for a week increased the prothrombin time AUC following a single dose of pseudoracemic warfarin in 6 subjects by 44%.[4] Increased prothrombin times and INRs have been reported in a number of other patients and subjects on warfarin when treated with fluconazole.[5-13] Several patients bled.[5,9,11-13]

Mechanism

In vitro studies using human liver microsomes clearly demonstrate that fluconazole inhibits the cytochrome P450 isoenzymes CYP2C9, CYP3A4 and possibly others, which are the major enzymes involved in the metabolism of warfarin.[14] *In vivo* this results in the accumulation of warfarin and in an increase in its effects, possibly leading to bleeding.[15]

Importance and management

An established and clinically important interaction. If fluconazole is added to treatment with warfarin or acenocoumarol the prothrombin times should be very well monitored and the anticoagulant dosage reduced as necessary. On the basis of pharmacokinetic studies it has been predicted that the warfarin dosage may need to be reduced by about 20% when using fluconazole 50 mg daily, ranging to a reduction of about 70% when using fluconazole 600 mg daily.[16] However, remember that individual variations between patients can be considerable. There seems to be no information about other anticoagulants.

1. Isalska BJ, Stanbridge TN. Fluconazole in the treatment of candidal prosthetic valve endocarditis. *BMJ* (1988) 297, 178–9.
2. Crussell-Porter LL, Rindone JP, Ford MA, Jaskar DW. Low-dose fluconazole therapy potentiates the hypoprothrombinemic response of warfarin sodium. *Arch Intern Med* (1993) 153, 102–4.
3. Lazar JD, Wilner KD. Drug interactions with fluconazole. *Rev Infect Dis* (1990) 12 (Suppl 3), S327–S333.
4. Black DJ, Gidal BE, Seaton TL, McDonnell ND, Kunze KL, Evans JS, Bauwens JE, Petersdorf SH, Trager WF. An evaluation of the effect of fluconazole on the stereoselective metabolism of warfarin (W). *Clin Pharmacol Ther* (1992) 51, 184.
5. Seaton TL, Celum CL, Black DJ. Possible potentiation of warfarin by fluconazole. *DICP Ann Pharmacother* (1990) 24, 1177–8.
6. Tett S, Carey D, Lee H-S. Drug interactions with fluconazole. *Med J Aust* (1992) 156, 365.
7. Beeley L, Cunningham H, Brennan A. *Bulletin of the West Midlands Centre for Adverse Drug Reaction Reporting* (1993) 36, 17.
8. Rieth H, Sauerbrey N. Interaktionsstudien mit Fluconazol, einem neuen Triazolantimykotikum. *Wien Med Wochenschr* (1989) 139, 370–4.
9. Kerr HD. Case report: potentiation of warfarin by fluconazole. *Am J Med Sci* (1993) 305, 164–5.
10. Gericke KR. Possible interaction between warfarin and fluconazole. *Pharmacotherapy* (1993) 13, 508–9.
11. Baciewicz AM, Menke JJ, Bokar JA, Baud EB. Fluconazole-warfarin interaction. *Ann Pharmacother* (1994) 28, 1111.
12. Mootha VV, Schluter ML, Das A. Intraocular hemorrhages due to warfarin-fluconazole drug interaction in a patient with presumed *Candida* endophthalmitis. *Arch Ophthalmol* (2002) 120, 94–5.
13. Allison EJ, McKinney TJ, Langenberg JN. Spinal epidural haematoma as a result of warfarin/fluconazole drug interaction. *Eur J Emerg Med* (2002) 9, 175–7.
14. Kunze KL, Wienkers LC, Thummel KE, Trager WF. Warfarin-fluconazole I. Inhibition of the human cytochrome P450–dependent metablism of warfarin by fluconazole: *in vitro* studies. *Drug Metab Dispos* (1996) 24, 414–21.
15. Black DJ, Kunze KL, Wienkers LC, Gidal BE. Seaton TL, McDonnell ND, Evans JS, Bauwens JE, Trager WF. Warfarin-fluconazole II. A metabolically based drug interaction: *in vivo* studies. *Drug Metab Dispos* (1996) 24, 422–8.
16. Kunze KL, Trager WF. Warfarin-fluconazole III. A rational approach to management of a metabolically based drug interaction. *Drug Metab Dispos* (1996) 24, 429–35.

Anticoagulants + Azoles; Itraconazole

An isolated report describes a very marked increase in the anticoagulant effects of warfarin, accompanied by bruising and bleeding, in a patient given itraconazole.

Clinical evidence, mechanism, importance and management

A woman stabilised on **warfarin** 5 mg daily and also taking ipratropium bromide, salbutamol, budesonide, quinine sulphate and omeprazole, was additionally started on itraconazole 200 mg twice daily for oral candidiasis caused by the inhaled steroid. Within 4 days she developed generalised bleeding and recurrent nose bleeds. Her INR had risen to more than 8. The **warfarin** and itraconazole were stopped, but next day she had to be admitted to hospital for intractable bleeding and increased bruising, for which she was treated with fresh frozen plasma. Two days later when the bleeding had stopped and her INR had returned to 2.4, she was restarted on **warfarin** and later restabilised on her original dosage.[1] The reasons for this reaction are not understood but it is possible that the itraconazole inhibited the metabolism of the **warfarin**. The quinine and the omeprazole may also have had some minor part to play in what happened.

This seems to be the first and only report of this interaction so that its general importance is uncertain. Warn patients to seek informed advice if any unexplained bruising or bleeding occurs. Information about other anticoagulants is lacking.

1. Yeh J, Soo S-C, Summerton C, Richardson C. Potentiation of action of warfarin by itraconazole. *BMJ* (1990) 301, 669.

Anticoagulants + Azoles; Ketoconazole

Three elderly patients showed an increase in the anticoagulant effects of warfarin when given ketoconazole.

Clinical evidence

An elderly woman, stabilised on **warfarin** for 3 years, complained of spontaneous bruising 3 weeks after starting a course of ketoconazole 200 mg twice daily. Her British Comparative Ratio was found to have risen from 1.9 to 5.4. Her liver function was normal. She was restabilised on her previous **warfarin** dosage 3 weeks after the ketoconazole was withdrawn.[1]

The UK Committee on Safety of Medicines has a report of an 84-year-old man taking **warfarin** whose British Comparative Ratio rose to 4.8 when he was given ketoconazole, and fell to 1.4 when it was withdrawn.[1] The makers of ketoconazole also have a report of an elderly man on **warfarin** whose prothrombin time rose from a range of 34 to 39 seconds to over 60 seconds when he was given ketoconazole 400 mg daily.[2] In contrast, 2 subjects showed no changes in their anticoagulant response to **warfarin** when they were given ketoconazole 200 mg daily over a 3-week period.[3]

Mechanism

Uncertain. It has been suggested[4] that in humans, as in *rats*,[5] ketoconazole may inhibit liver enzymes concerned with the metabolism of warfarin so that its effects are increased. It is perhaps noteworthy that all of the cases involved elderly patients whose liver function may already have been poor.

Importance and management

Information about this interaction seems to be limited to the reports cited. Its general importance and incidence is therefore uncertain, but it is probably quite small. However, it would now seem prudent to monitor the anticoagulant response of any patient when first given both drugs, particularly the elderly, to ensure that excessive anticoagulation does not occur. Information about other anticoagulants is lacking.

1. Smith AG, Potentiation of oral anticoagulants by ketoconazole. *BMJ* (1984) 288, 188–9.
2. Janssen Pharmaceutical Limited. Personal communication, April 1986.
3. Stevens DA, Stiller RL, Williams PL, Sugar AM. Experience with ketoconazole in three major manifestations of progressive coccidioidomycosis. *Am J Med* (1983) 74, 58–63.
4. Simpson JG, Cunningham C, Whiting P. Potentiation of oral anticoagulants by ketoconazole. *BMJ* (1984) 288, 646.
5. Niemegeers CJE, Levron JC, Awouters F, Janssen PAJ. Inhibition and induction of microsomal enzymes in the rat. A comparative study of four antimycotics: miconazole, econazole, clotrimazole and ketoconazole. *Arch Int Pharmacodyn Ther* (1981) 251, 26–38.

Anticoagulants + Azoles; Miconazole

The anticoagulant effects of acenocoumarol, ethyl biscoumacetate, fluindione, phenindione, phenprocoumon, tioclomarol and warfarin can be markedly increased if miconazole is given orally, and bleeding can occur. The interaction can occur with buccal gel formulations and has also been seen in some women using intravaginal miconazole, and in one elderly man using a miconazole cream on his skin.

Clinical evidence

(a) Oral dose forms

Two patients with prosthetic heart valves on **warfarin** developed haemorrhagic complications within 10 days of starting miconazole 250 g four times a day. One of them developed blood blisters and bruised easily. Her prothrombin time ratio had risen from under 3 to about 16. The other patient had a prothrombin time ratio of 23.4. He developed two haematomas soon after both drugs were withdrawn. Both patients were subsequently restabilised in the absence of miconazole on their former doses of **warfarin**.[1]

The Centres de Pharmacovigilance Hospitaliere in Bordeaux have on record 5 cases where miconazole (in doses of 500 mg daily, where stated) was responsible for a marked increase in prothrombin times and/or bleeding (haematomas, haematuria, gastrointestinal bleeding) in patients taking **acenocoumarol** (2 cases), **ethyl biscoumacetate** (1 case), **tioclomarol** (1 case) and **phenindione** (1 case).[2] Other cases and reports of this interaction have been described elsewhere involving **acenocoumarol, phenprocoumon** and **warfarin**.[2-9]

(b) Topical or local dose forms

The New Zealand Centre for Adverse Reactions Monitoring reported 5 patients on **warfarin** whose INRs rose from normal values to between 7.5 and 18 within 7 to 15 days of starting to use miconazole oral gel.[10] Other reports confirm that this interaction takes place between **acenocoumarol**,[11-14] **fluindione**,[15] or **warfarin**[16-21] and miconazole oral gel.

The Netherlands Pharmacovigilance Foundation LAREB reported 2 elderly women patients on **acenocoumarol** whose INRs rose sharply and rapidly when given a 3-day course of 400-mg miconazole pessaries.[22] Another report describes the development of ecchymoses and an INR of about 9.78 in a 55-year-old woman on **warfarin** on the third day of using 200-mg miconazole pessaries. She had increased INRs on two subsequent occasions attributed to this interaction.[23] Yet another report describes haemorrhage of the kidney in a 52-year old woman on **warfarin** after she used vaginal miconazole for 12 days.[24] An 80-year-old man stabilised on long term **warfarin** had a rise in his INR to 21.4 after using a miconazole cream for 2 weeks for a fungal infection in his groin. He showed no evidence of bruising or bleeding.[25]

Mechanism

There is evidence that miconazole inhibits the metabolism of both *(S)*- and *(R)*-warfarin by the liver by inhibiting the cytochrome P450 isoenzyme CYP2C9, with (*S*)-warfarin being inhibited to a greater extent than (*R*)-warfarin.[7] Absorption of miconazole from the gut, or very unusually from the vagina in some post-menopausal women (see also comments below) and even exceptionally through the skin, can result in increased anticoagulant effects.

Importance and management

A very well established and potentially serious interaction of clinical importance. Many of the reports are about warfarin but most of the common oral anticoagulants in current use have been implicated. In some cases the bleeding has taken 7 to 15 days to develop,[1,2,8] whereas others have bled within only 3 days.[4,23] Raised INRs have been seen even sooner. Miconazole tablets should therefore not be given to patients on any oral anticoagulant unless the prothrombin times can be closely monitored and suitable dosage reductions made. Two reports indicate that halving the dose may be sufficient[2,5] but in some instances the reduction needed may be much greater. One patient required an increase in her acenocoumarol dosage from 2 mg twice weekly to 3 to 4 mg daily when she stopped miconazole.[3] The authors of an epidemiological study similarly recommend frequent monitoring of the INR in patients on coumarins during the early stages of additional treatment with antifungals, but they also suggest that the concurrent use of miconazole and coumarins should be discouraged.[26]

The interaction can also occur with miconazole oral gel because much of it is swallowed. Patients have bled or showed prolonged prothrombin times as a result of this interaction.[6,8,11-17,19,20]

An interaction with intravaginal miconazole would not normally be expected because its systemic absorption is usually very low (less than 2%) in healthy women of child-bearing age.[27] However, the reports cited above[22-24] show that significant absorption can apparently occur in a few patients with particular conditions (possibly in postmenopausal women with inflamed vaginal tissue), which allows an interaction to occur. Appropriate monitoring is therefore needed even with this route of administration in potentially at-risk women. Topical miconazole would also not be expected to interact, but the single report cited shows that sometimes it can.[25]

Nystatin is a possible alternative antifungal, which would not be expected to interact with the oral anticoagulants due to its low oral absorption.

1. Watson PG, Lochan RG, Redding VJ. Drug interaction with coumarin derivative anticoagulants. *BMJ* (1982) 285, 1044–5
2. Loupi E, Descotes J, Lery N, Evreux J C. Interactions medicamenteuses et miconazole. *Therapie* (1982) 37, 437–41
3. Anon. New possibilities in the treatment of systemic mycoses. Reports on the experimental and clinical evaluation of miconazole. Round table discussion and Chairman's summing up. *Proc R Soc Med* (1977), 70 (Suppl 1), 51–4.
4. Ponge T, Barrier J, Spreux A, Guillou B, Larousse C, Grolleau JY. Potentialisation des effets de l'acénocoumarol par le miconazole. *Therapie* (1982) 37, 221–2.
5. Goenen M, Reynaert M, Jaumin P, Chalant CH, Tremouroux J. A case of candida albicans endocarditis three years after an aortic valve replacement. *J Cardiovasc Surg* (1977) 18, 391–6.
6. Beeley L, Magee P, Hickey FM. *Bulletin of the West Midlands Centre for Adverse Drug Reaction Reporting* (1989) 29, 33.
7. O'Reilly RA, Goulart DA, Kunze KL, Neal J, Gibaldi M, Eddy AC, Trager WF. Mechanisms of the stereoselective interaction between miconazole and racemic warfarin in human subjects. *Clin Pharmacol Ther* (1992) 51, 656–67.
8. Bailey GM, Magee P, Hickey FM, Beeley L. Miconazole and warfarin interaction. *Pharm J* (1989) 242, 183.

9. Marco M, Guy AJ. Retroperitoneal haematoma and small bowel intramural haematoma caused by warfarin and miconazole interaction. *Int J Oral Maxillofac Surg* (1997) 27, 485.
10. Pillans P, Woods DJ. Interaction between miconazole oral gel (Daktarin) and warfarin. *N Z Med J* (1996) 109, 346.
11. Ducroix JP, Smail A, Sevenet F, Andrejak M, Baillet J. Hématome oesophagien secondaire à une potentialisation des effets de l'acénocoumarol par le gel buccal de miconazole. *Rev Med Interne* (1989) 10, 557–9.
12. Marotel C, Cerisay D, Vasseur P, Rouvier B, Chabanne JP. Potentialisation des effets de l'acénocoumarol par le gel buccal de miconazole. *Presse Med* (1986) 15, 1684–5.
13. Gutierrez MA, Olalla I, Muruzábal MJ, Ortín M, Peralta FG. Miconazole oral gel enhances acenocoumarol anticoagulant activity. Report of three cases. *Eur J Clin Pharmacol* (1997) 52 (Suppl), A132.
14. Ortín M, Olalla JI, Muruzábal MJ, Peralta FG, Gutiérrez MA. Miconazole oral gel enhances acenocoumarol anticoagulant activity: a report of three cases. *Ann Pharmacother* (1999) 33, 175–77.
15. Ponge T, Rapp MJ, Fruneau P, Ponge A, Wassen-Hove L, Larousse C, Cottin S. Interaction médicamenteuse impliquant le miconazole en gel et la fluindione. *Therapie* (1987) 42, 412–13.
16. Colquhoun MC, Daly M, Stewart P, Beeley L. Interaction between warfarin and miconazole oral gel. *Lancet* (1987) i, 695–6.
17. Shenfield GM, Page M. Potentiation of warfarin action by miconazole oral gel. *Aust N Z J Med* (1991) 21, 928.
18. Ariyaratnam S, Thakker NS, Sloan P, Thornhill MH. Potentiation of warfarin anticoagulant activity by miconazole oral gel. *BMJ* (1997) 314, 349.
19. Evans J, Orme DS, Sedgwick ML, Youngs GR. Treating oral candidiasis: potentially fatal. *Br Dent J* (1997) 182, 452.
20. Pemberton MN, Sloan P, Ariyaratnam S, Thakker NS, Thornhill MH. Derangement of warfarin anticoagulation by miconazole oral gel. *Br Dent J* (1998) 184, 68–9.
21. Øgard CG, Vestergaad H. Interaktion mellem warfarin og oral miconazol-gel. *Ugeskr Laeger* (2000) 162, 5511.
22. Lansdorp D, Bressers HPHM, Dekens-Konter JAM, Meyboom RHB. Potentiation of acenocoumarol during vaginal administration of miconazole. *Br J Clin Pharmacol* (1999) 47, 225–6.
23. Thirion DJ, Zanetti LAF. Potentiation of warfarin's hypoprothrombinemic effect with miconazole vaginal suppositories. *Pharmacotherapy* (2000) 20, 98–9.
24. Anon. Miconazole-warfarin interaction: increased INR. *Can Med Assoc J* (2001) 165, 81.
25. Devaraj A, O'Beirne JPO, Veasey R, Dunk AA. Interaction between warfarin and topical miconazole cream. *BMJ* (2002) 325, 77.
26. Visser LE, Penning-van Beest FJA, Kasbergen AAH, De Smet PAGM, Vulto AG, Hofman A, Stricker BHC. Overanticoagulation associated with combined use of antifungal agents and coumarin anticoagulants. *Clin Pharmacol Ther* (2002) 71, 496–502.
27. Daneshmend TK. Systemic absorption of miconazole from the vagina. *J Antimicrob Chemother* (1986) 18, 507–11.

Anticoagulants + Azoles; Voriconazole

Voriconazole increases the effects of warfarin.

Clinical evidence

The makers of voriconazole say that because the coumarins (**phenprocoumon**, **acenocoumarol** and **warfarin**) are substrates of the cytochrome P450 isoenzymes CYP3A4 and CYP2C9 their plasma levels may be raised by voriconazole, an inhibitor of these isoenzymes.[1,2] When a single 30-mg dose of **warfarin** was given to healthy subjects with voriconazole 300 mg twice daily, the prothrombin time was about doubled.[3] The makers therefore advise close monitoring of the prothrombin time in any patient on an oral anticoagulant who is given voriconazole. Dose adjustments of the anticoagulant should be made accordingly.[1,2]

1. VFEND (Voriconazole). Pfizer Ltd. UK Summary of product characteristics, March 2005.
2. VFEND (Voriconazole). Pfizer Ltd. US Prescribing information, March 2005.
3. Purkins L, Wood N, Kleinermans D, Nichols D. Voriconazole potentiates warfarin-induced prothrombin time prolongation. *Br J Clin Pharmacol* (2003) 56 (Suppl 1), 24–9.

Anticoagulants + Aztreonam

Aztreonam occasionally causes a prolongation in prothrombin times, which in theory might possibly be additive with the effects of conventional anticoagulants.

Clinical evidence, mechanism, importance and management

A few patients on aztreonam (with cefoperazone in one report[1]) developed prolonged prothrombin times, which were either self-limiting,[2,3] or which responded to vitamin K treatment.[1] In three studies 1 to 10% of patients experienced this effect.[2-4] The partial thromboplastin time is also increased. There seem to be no confirmed adverse reports about patients taking oral anticoagulants and aztreonam together, but it seems possible that their hypoprothrombinaemic effects might be additive. If you add aztreonam to an established regimen with **warfarin** or any other anticoagulant, be alert for any evidence of otherwise unexplained bruising or bleeding.

1. Bodey G, Reuben A, Elting L, Kantarjian H, Keating M, Hagemeister F, Koller C, Velasquez W, Papadopoulos N. Comparison of two schedules of cefoperazone plus aztreonam in the treatment of neutropenic patients with fever. *Eur J Clin Microbiol Infect Dis* (1991) 10, 551–8.
2. Rusconi F, Assael BM, Boccazzi A, Colombo R, Crossignani RM, Garlaschi L, Rancilio L. Aztreonam in the treatment of severe urinary tract infections in pediatric patients. *Antimicrob Agents Chemother* (1986) 30, 310–14.
3. Giamarellou H, Galanakis N, Dendrinos CH, Kanellakopoulou K, Petrikkos G, Koratzanis G, Daikos GK. Clinical experience with aztreonam in a variety of gram-negative infections. *Chemioterapia* (1985) 4 (Suppl 1), 75–80.
4. Giamerellou H, Koratzanis G, Kanellakopoulou K, Galanakis N, Papoulias G, El Messidi M, Daikos G. Aztreonam versus cefamandole in the treatment of urinary tract infections. *Chemioterapia* (1984) 3, 127–31.

Anticoagulants + Barbiturates

The effects of the anticoagulants are reduced by the barbiturates. Full therapeutic anticoagulation may only be achieved by raising the anticoagulant dosage about 30 to 60%. If the barbiturate is later withdrawn, the anticoagulant dosage should be reduced to avoid the risk of bleeding. Primidone is metabolised to phenobarbital and is expected to interact similarly.

Clinical evidence

Two examples from many:

A study in 16 patients on long-term **warfarin** treatment showed that when they were also given **phenobarbital** 2 mg/kg their average daily **warfarin** requirements rose over a 4-week period by 25% (from 5.7 to 7.1 mg daily).[1]

An investigation on 12 patients taking either **warfarin** or **phenprocoumon** demonstrated that **secbutabarbital sodium**, 15 mg four times daily for the first week and 30 mg four times daily for the next two weeks, increased their anticoagulant requirements by 35 to 60%, reaching a maximum after 4 to 5 weeks.[2]

This interaction has been described between:

- **acenocoumarol** and **pentobarbital**[3] and **heptabarb**;[4]
- **dicoumarol** and **aprobarbitone**,[5] **heptabarb**,[4,6] **phenobarbital**,[7-9] **secobarbital**,[10] and **vinbarbital**;[5]
- **ethyl biscoumacetate** and **amobarbital**,[11] **heptabarb**,[4,11] **pentobarbital**,[12] **phenobarbital**,[11] and **secobarbital**;[11]
- **phenprocoumon** and **secbutobarbital**;[2]
- **warfarin** and **amobarbital**,[13-16] **butobarbital**,[17] **heptabarb**,[18,19] **phenobarbital**,[20-23] **secobarbital**[13,14,16,23-25] and **secbutobarbital**.[2]

Mechanism

Studies in man and *animals*[14,18,20,22,25] clearly show that the barbiturates are potent liver enzyme inducing agents, which increase the metabolism and clearance of the anticoagulants from the body. They may also reduce the absorption of dicoumarol from the gut.[6]

Importance and management

The interactions between the anticoagulants and barbiturates are clinically important and very well documented. The reduced anticoagulant effects expose the patient to the risk of thrombus formation if the dosage is not increased appropriately. A very large number of anticoagulant/barbiturate pairs have been found to interact and the others may be expected to behave similarly. The barbiturates interact less with *(R)*-warfarin than *(S)*-warfarin, but in practice *R*-warfarin appears to have little advantage over the usual racemic mixture.[26,27]

The reduction in the anticoagulant effects begins within a week, sometimes within 2 to 4 days, reaching a maximum after about 3 weeks, and it may still be evident up to 6 weeks after stopping the barbiturate.[2] Patients' responses can vary considerably. Stable anticoagulant control can be re-established[15] in the presence of the barbiturate by increasing the anticoagulant dosage by about 30 to 60%.[1,2,9,21] Care must be taken not to withdraw the barbiturate without also reducing the anticoagulant dosage, otherwise bleeding will occur.[1,15,21] Alternative non-interacting drugs that are now considered more appropriate sedatives than the barbiturates include nitrazepam, diazepam, and flurazepam. See 'Anticoagulants + Benzodiazepines or related drugs', p.271.

Primidone is metabolised in the body to phenobarbital and is therefore expected to interact like phenobarbital, although there seem to be no reports of interactions with anticoagulants. Notwithstanding it would be prudent to be alert for reduced anticoagulant effects if primidone is given concurrently.

1. Robinson DS, MacDonald MG. The effect of phenobarbital administration on the control of coagulation achieved during warfarin therapy in man. *J Pharmacol Exp Ther* (1966) 153, 250–3.
2. Antlitz AM, Tolentino M, Kosai MF. Effect of butabarbital on orally administered anticoagulants. *Curr Ther Res* (1968) 10, 70–3.
3. Kroon C, de Boer A, Hoogkamer JFW, Schoemaker HC, vd Meer FJM, Edelbroek PM, Cohen AF. Detection of drug interactions with single dose acenocoumarol: new screening method? *Int J Clin Pharmacol Ther Toxicol* (1990) 28, 355–60.
4. Dayton PG, Tarcan Y, Chenkin T, Weiner M. The influence of barbiturates on coumarin plasma levels and prothrombin response. *J Clin Invest* (1961) 40, 1797–1802.
5. Johansson S-A. Apparent resistance to oral anticoagulant therapy and influence of hypnotics on some coagulation factors. *Acta Med Scand* (1968) 184, 297–300.
6. Aggeler PM, O'Reilly RA. Effect of heptabarbital on the response to bishydroxycoumarin in man. *J Lab Clin Med* (1969) 74, 229–38.
7. Corn M, Rockett JF. Inhibition of bishydroxycoumarin activity by phenobarbital. *Med Ann Dist Columbia* (1965) 34, 578–9, 588.
8. Cucinell SA, Conney AH, Sansur M, Burns JJ. Drug interactions in man. I. Lowering effect of phenobarbital on plasma levels of bishydroxycoumarin (Dicumarol) and diphenylhydantoin (Dilantin). *Clin Pharmacol Ther* (1965) 6, 420–9.
9. Goss JE, Dickhaus DW. Increased bishydroxycoumarin requirements in patients receiving phenobarbital. *N Engl J Med* (1965) 273, 1094–5.
10. Cucinell SA, Odessky L, Weiss M, Dayton PG. The effect of chloral hydrate on bishydroxycoumarin metabolism. A fatal outcome. *JAMA* (1966) 197, 144–6.
11. Avellaneda M. Interferencia de los barbituricos en la accion del Tromexan. *Medicina (B Aires)* (1955) 15, 109–15.
12. Reverchon F, Sapir M. Constatation clinique d'un antagonisme entre barbituriques et anticoagulants. *Presse Med* (1961) 69, 1570–1.
13. Breckenridge A, Orme M. Clinical implications of enzyme induction. *Ann N Y Acad Sci* (1971) 179, 421–31.
14. Robinson DS, Sylwester D. Interaction of commonly prescribed drugs and warfarin. *Ann Intern Med* (1970) 72, 853–6.
15. Williams JRB, Griffin JP, Parkins A. Effect of concomitantly administered drugs on the control of long term anticoagulant therapy. *Q J Med* (1976) 45, 63–73.
16. Whitfield JB, Moss DW, Neale G, Orme M, Breckenridge A. Changes in plasma γ-glutamyl transpeptidase activity associated with alterations in drug metabolism in man. *BMJ* (1973) 1, 316–18.
17. Macgregor AG, Petrie JC and Wood RA. Therapeutic conferences. Drug interaction. *BMJ* (1971) 1, 389–91.
18. Levy G, O'Reilly RA, Aggeler PM, Keech GM. Pharmacokinetic analysis of the effect of barbiturate on the anticoagulant action of warfarin in man. *Clin Pharmacol Ther* (1970) 11, 372–7.
19. O'Reilly RA, Aggeler PM. Effect of barbiturates on oral anticoagulants in man. *Clin Res* (1969) 17, 153.
20. MacDonald MG, Robinson DS, Sylwester D, Jaffe JJ. The effects of phenobarbital, chloral betaine, and glutethimide administration on warfarin plasma levels and hypoprothrombinemic responses in man. *Clin Pharmacol Ther* (1969) 10, 80–4.
21. MacDonald MG, Robinson DS. Clinical observations of possible barbiturate interference with anticoagulation. *JAMA* (1968) 204, 97–100.
22. Corn M. Effect of phenobarbital and glutethimide on biological half-life of warfarin. *Thromb Diath Haemorrh* (1966) 16, 606–12.
23. Udall JA. Clinical implications of warfarin interactions with five sedatives. *Am J Cardiol* (1975) 35, 67–71.
24. Feuer DJ, Wilson WR, Ambre JJ. Duration of effect of secobarbital on the anticoagulant effect and metabolism of warfarin. *Pharmacologist* (1974) 16, 195.
25. Breckenridge A, Orme ML'E, Davies L, Thorgeirsson SS, Davies DS. Dose-dependent enzyme induction. *Clin Pharmacol Ther* (1973) 14, 514–20.
26. Orme M, Breckenridge A. Enantiomers of warfarin and phenobarbital. *N Engl J Med* (1976) 295, 1482.
27. O'Reilly RA, Trager WF, Motley CH, Howald W. Interaction of secobarbital with warfarin pseudoracemates. *Clin Pharmacol Ther* (1980) 28, 187–95.

Anticoagulants + Benfluorex

Benfluorex does not alter the anticoagulant effects of phenprocoumon.

Clinical evidence, mechanism, importance and management

No significant changes occurred in the prothrombin times of 22 patients on **phenprocoumon** when they were given benfluorex 150 mg three times daily for 9 weeks, when compared with equivalent periods before and after while not taking benfluorex.[1] There seems to be no information about other anticoagulants.

1. De Witte P, Brems HM. Co-administration of benfluorex with oral anticoagulant therapy. *Curr Med Res Opin* (1980) 6, 478–80.

Anticoagulants + Benzbromarone

The anticoagulant effects of warfarin are increased by benzbromarone and bleeding has been seen. Acenocoumarol, ethyl biscoumacetate and phenindione are said not to interact but the information available is very limited.

Clinical evidence

The observation that 2 patients bled (haematuria, gastrointestinal bleeding) when given **warfarin** and benzbromarone for gout, prompted a more detailed study in 7 other patients. The thrombotest values of these 7 averaged 24.7% while taking both **warfarin** and benzbromarone (average dosage 57.1 mg daily), but when the benzbromarone was stopped for a week they rose to 47.3%. On restarting the benzbromarone the thrombotest values decreased to 30.3%. The Factor II activity parallelled the thrombotest values. The total plasma **warfarin** levels were reduced during the period that benzbromarone was stopped.[1] Another later controlled study found that benzbromarone reduced the **warfarin** requirements of 13 patients by 36% (from 3.9 to 2.5 mg daily).[2] These two studies confirm observations on other patients with prosthetic valve replacements who showed haemorrhagic tendencies when given both drugs.[1]

In contrast it has been claimed that no increases in the anticoagulant effects of **acenocoumarol**, **ethyl biscoumacetate** or **phenindione** were seen in a few patients given benzbromarone.[3]

Mechanism

Benzbromarone selectively inhibits the metabolism of *(S)*-warfarin so that its loss from the body is reduced and its effects are increased. The metabolism of the *(R)*-warfarin remains unchanged.[2]

Importance and management

The interaction between warfarin and benzbromarone is established and clinically important. If benzbromarone is added to warfarin monitor prothrombin times and be alert for the need to reduce the dosage by about one-third to prevent over-anticoagulation. Information about other anticoagulants is very limited but what is known suggests that acenocoumarol, ethyl biscoumacetate, and phenindione do not interact. More study is needed.

1. Shimodaira H, Takahashi K, Kano K, Matsumoto Y, Uchida Y, Kudo T. Enhancement of anticoagulant action by warfarin-benzbromarone interaction. *J Clin Pharmacol* (1996) 36, 168–74.
2. Takahashi H, Sato T, Shimoyama Y, Shioda N, Shimizu T, Kubo S, Tamura N, Tainaka H, Yasumori T, Echizen H. Potentiation of anticoagulant effect of warfarin caused by enantioselective metabolic inhibition by the uricosuric agent benzbromarone. *Clin Pharmacol Ther* (1999) 66, 569–81.
3. Masbernard A. Quoted as personal communication (1977) by Heel RC, Brogden RN, Speight TM, Avery GS. Benzbromarone: a review of its pharmacological properties and therapeutic use in gout and hyperuricaemia. *Drugs* (1977) 14, 349–66.

Anticoagulants + Benziodarone

The anticoagulant effects of acenocoumarol, ethyl biscoumacetate, diphenadione and warfarin are increased by benziodarone. The dosage of anticoagulant should be reduced appropriately. Clorindione, dicoumarol and indandione do not interact, but the situation with phenprocoumon is not clear.

Clinical evidence

Benziodarone 200 mg three times a day was given to 90 patients on anticoagulants for 2 days, with 100 mg three times a day thereafter. To maintain constant prothrombin-proconvertin percentages the anticoagulant dosages were reduced as follows: **ethyl biscoumacetate** 17% (9 patients), **diphenadione** 42% (8 patients), **acenocoumarol** 25% (7 patients) and **warfarin** 46% (15 patients). No changes were needed in those taking **clorindione** (5 patients), **dicoumarol** (9 patients), **phenindione** (10 patients) or **phenprocoumon** (8 patients). A parallel study in 12 healthy subjects also found that benziodarone increased the effects of **warfarin**.[1]

The absence of an interaction with **dicoumarol** was also found in a previous study.[2] In another study benziodarone 300 to 600 mg daily increased the anticoagulant effects of **phenprocoumon** in 9 out of 29 patients and the ecchymoses observed were larger and more frequent.[3] The metabolism of **ethyl biscoumacetate** appears to be increased by benziodarone.[3]

Mechanism

Not understood. Benziodarone alone has no definite effect on the activity of prothrombin or factors VII, IX or X.

Importance and management

Information appears to be limited to the studies cited, but the interaction would seem to be established. The dosages of the interacting anticoagulants and possibly of phenprocoumon should be reduced appropriately to prevent bleeding. No particular precautions are necessary with the non-interacting anticoagulants.

1. Pyörälä K, Ikkala E, Siltanen P. Benziodarone (Amplivix®) and anticoagulant therapy. *Acta Med Scand* (1963) 173, 385–9.
2. Gillot P. Valeur therapeutique du L. 2329 dans l'angine de poitrine. *Acta Cardiol* (1959) 14, 494–515.
3. Verstraete M, Vermylen J, Claeys H. Dissimilar effect of two anti-anginal drugs belonging to the benzofuran group on the action of coumarin derivatives. *Arch Int Pharmacodyn Ther* (1968) 176, 33–41.

Anticoagulants + Benzodiazepines or related drugs

The anticoagulant effects of warfarin are not affected by chlordiazepoxide, diazepam, flurazepam, or nitrazepam. The effects of phenprocoumon are not affected by nitrazepam or oxazepam, nor those of ethyl biscoumacetate by chlordiazepoxide. An interaction between any oral anticoagulant and a benzodiazepine is unlikely, but there are three unexplained and unconfirmed cases of increased or decreased anticoagulant responses, which were attributed to an interaction.

Clinical evidence

A number of studies on a very large number of patients given anticoagulants and benzodiazepines for extended periods have found no interaction between **warfarin** and **chlordiazepoxide**,[1-5] **diazepam**,[1,4,5] **flurazepam**,[6] or **nitrazepam**,[1,4,7] **zaleplon**,[8,9] **zolpidem**;[10] between **ethyl biscoumacetate** and **chlordiazepoxide**;[11] and between **phenprocoumon** and **oxazepam**[12] or **nitrazepam**.[13]

However, there are three discordant reports. A patient on **warfarin** showed an increased anticoagulant response when given **diazepam**.[14] A patient on **dicoumarol** developed multiple ecchymoses and a prothrombin time of 53 seconds within a fortnight of starting to take **diazepam** 5 mg four times daily.[15] And a patient showed a fall in serum **warfarin** levels and in the anticoagulant response when given **chlordiazepoxide**.[7] It is by no means certain that these responses were due to an interaction.

Mechanism

The three discordant reports are not understood. Enzyme induction is a possible explanation in one case.[7] because increases in the urinary excretion of 6-beta-hydroxycortisol (a marker of enzyme induction) have been described during chlordiazepoxide use.[1,7]

Importance and management

The weight of evidence and common experience shows that the benzodiazepines do not normally interact with the anticoagulants. Not all of the anticoagulant/benzodiazepine pairs have been examined, but none of them would be expected to interact.

1. Orme M, Breckenridge A, Brooks RV. Interactions of benzodiazepines with warfarin. *BMJ* (1972) 3, 611–14.
2. Lackner H, Hunt VE. The effect of Librium on hemostasis. *Am J Med Sci* (1968) 256, 368–72.
3. Robinson DS, Sylwester D. Interaction of commonly prescribed drugs and warfarin. *Ann Intern Med* (1970) 72, 853–6.
4. Garattini S, Mussini E, Randall LO, eds. The Benzodiazepines. New York: Raven Press; 1973 p. 647–54.
5. Solomon HM, Barakat MJ, Ashley CJ. Mechanisms of drug interaction. *JAMA* (1971) 216, 1997–9.
6. Garattini S, Mussini E, Randall LO, eds. The Benzodiazepines. New York: Raven Press; 1973 p. 641–6.
7. Breckenridge A, Orme M. Clinical implications of enzyme induction. *Ann N Y Acad Sci* (1971) 179, 421–31.
8. Darwish M. Overview of drug interaction studies with zaleplon. Poster presented at 13th Annual Meeting of Associated Professional Sleep Studies (APSS), Orlando, Florida, June 23rd, 1999.
9. Darwish M. Analysis of potential drug interactions with zaleplon. *J Am Geriatr Soc* (1999) 47, S62.
10. Sauvanet JP, Langer SZ, Morselli PL, eds. Imidazopyridines in Sleep Disorders. New York: Raven Press; 1988 p. 165–73.
11. van Dam FE, Gribnau-Overkamp MJH. The effect of some sedatives (phenobarbital, glutethimide, chlordiazepoxide, chloral hydrate) on the rate of disappearance of ethyl biscoumacetate from the plasma. *Folia Med Neerl* (1967) 10, 141–5.
12. Schneider J, Kamm G. Beeinflußt Oxazepam (Adumbran®) die Antikoagulanzientherapie mit Phenprocoumon? *Med Klin* (1978) 73, 153–6.
13. Bieger R, De Jonge H, Loeliger EA. Influence of nitrazepam on oral anticoagulation with phenprocoumon. *Clin Pharmacol Ther* (1972) 13, 361–5.
14. McQueen EG. New Zealand Committee on Adverse Drug Reactions: Ninth Annual Report 1974. *N Z Med J* (1974) 80, 305–11.
15. Taylor PJ. Hemorrhage while on anticoagulant therapy precipitated by drug interaction. *Ariz Med* (1967) 24, 697–9.

Anticoagulants + Benzydamine

Benzydamine does not alter the anticoagulant effects of phenprocoumon.

Clinical evidence, mechanism, importance and management

The anticoagulant response to **phenprocoumon** was not significantly changed in 10 patients who took benzydamine 50 mg three times daily for 2 weeks, although there was some evidence of an increase in blood levels of the anticoagulant.[1] No particular precautions would seem necessary during concurrent use. Information about other anticoagulants is lacking.

1. Duckert F, Widmer LK, Madar G. Gleichzeitige Behandlung mit oralen Antikoagulantien und Benzydamin. *Schweiz Med Wochenschr* (1974) 104, 1069–71.

Anticoagulants + Beta-blockers

The effects of the oral anticoagulants are not normally affected by the beta-blockers although one or two isolated and unexplained cases have been reported.

Clinical evidence, mechanism, importance and management

No clinically important interactions were seen between

- **acenocoumarol** and **atenolol** or **metoprolol**[1]
- **phenprocoumon** and **pindolol**[2]
- **warfarin** and **acebutolol**,[3] **atenolol**,[1,4] **betaxolol**,[5] **bisoprolol**,[6] **esmolol**,[7] **metoprolol**,[1,4] or **propranolol**[4]

Carvedilol is also reported not to alter the *in vitro* protein binding of **warfarin**.[8]

In contrast, a 15% rise in the steady state plasma **warfarin** levels of 6 healthy subjects was seen when they took **propranolol** 80 mg twice daily,[9] but while this was statistically significant it is unlikely to be clinically relevant. A transient increase in **phenprocoumon** levels was seen in single dose studies in healthy subjects given **metoprolol**,[10] but no significant effects occurred when they were given **atenolol**[10] or **carvedilol**.[11,12]

A patient on **warfarin** showed a marked rise in his British Corrected Ratio when given **propranolol**.[13] Haemorrhagic tendencies without any changes in Quick time or any other impairment of coagulation has been described in three patients on **phenindione** and **propranolol**.[14]

Overall, these findings confirm the general clinical experience that the effects of the oral anticoagulants are not normally affected by beta-blockers. No special precautions are needed on concurrent use.

1. Mantero F, Procidano M, Vicariotto MA , Girolami A. Effect of atenolol and metoprolol on the anticoagulant activity of acenocoumarin. *Br J Clin Pharmacol* (1984) 17, 94S–96S.
2. Vinazzer H. Effect of the beta-receptor blocking agent Visken® on the action of coumarin. *Int J Clin Pharmacol* (1975) 12, 458–60.
3. Ryan JR. Clinical pharmacology of acebutolol. *Am Heart J* (1985) 109, 1131–6.
4. Bax NDS, Lennard MS, Tucker GT, Woods HF, Porter NR, Malia RG, Preston FE. The effect of β-adrenoceptor antagonists on the pharmacokinetics and pharmacodynamics of warfarin after a single dose. *Br J Clin Pharmacol* (1984) 17, 553–7.
5. Thiercelin JF, Warrington SJ, Thenot JP, Orofiamma B. Lack of interaction of betaxolol on warfarin induced hypocoagulability. In Proc 2nd Eur. Cong Biopharm Pharmacokinet. Vol III: Clinical Pharmacokinetics (published by Imprimerie de l'Université de Clermont Ferrand, 1984) edited by Aiache JM and Hirtz J, pp 73–80.
6. Warrington SJ, Johnston A, Lewis Y, Murphy M. Bisoprolol: studies of potential interactions with theophylline and warfarin in healthy volunteers. *J Cardiovasc Pharmacol* (1990) 16 (Suppl 5), S164–S168.
7. Lowenthal DT, Porter RS, Saris SD, Bies CM, Slegowski MB, Staudacher A. Clinical pharmacology, pharmacodynamics and interactions with esmolol. *Am J Cardiol* (1985) 56, 14F–17F.
8. Data on file, database on carvedilol, SmithKline Beecham, quoted by Ruffolo RR, Boyle DA, Venuti RP, Lukas MA. Carvedilol (Kredex®): a novel multiple action cardiovascular agent. *Drugs Today* (1991) 27, 465–92.
9. Scott AK, Park BK, Breckenridge AM. Interaction between warfarin and propranolol. *Br J Clin Pharmacol* (1984) 17, 86S.
10. Spahn H, Kirch W, Mutschler E, Ohnhaus EE, Kitteringham NR, Lögering HJ, Paar D. Pharmacokinetic and pharmacodynamic interactions between phenprocoumon and atenolol or metoprolol. *Br J Clin Pharmacol* (1984) 17, 97S–102S.
11. Caspary S, Merz P-G, Brei R, Harder S. Interaction profile of carvedilol: investigations with digitoxin and phenprocoumon. *Int J Clin Pharmacol Ther Toxicol* (1992) 30, 537–8.

12. Harder S, Brei R, Caspary S, Merz PG. Lack of a pharmacokinetic interaction between carvedilol and digitoxin or phenprocoumon. *Eur J Clin Pharmacol* (1993) 44, 583–6.
13. Bax NDS, Lennard MS, Al-Asady S, Deacon CS, Tucker GT, Woods HF. Inhibition of drug metabolism by β-adrenoceptor antagonists. *Drugs* (1983) 25 (Suppl 2), 121–6.
14. Neilson GH, Seldon WA. Propranolol in angina pectoris. *Med J Aust* (1969) 1, 856–57.

Anticoagulants + Bicalutamide

The suggestion that bicalutamide might interact with warfarin appears to be based largely on questionable theoretical considerations.

Clinical evidence, mechanism, importance and management

The makers say[1] that *in vitro* studies show that bicalutamide can displace **warfarin** from its protein binding sites. They therefore recommended close monitoring of the prothrombin time. It used to be thought that the displacement of **warfarin** from its protein binding sites by other drugs normally resulted in clinically important interactions, but that is now known to rarely be true (see 'Protein-binding interactions', (p.3)). The makers say that they do not know of any reports of an interaction between **warfarin** and bicalutamide, apart from an isolated case of a raised INR in one patient on **warfarin** who had taken bicalutamide 150 mg, but no causal link with bicalutamide was established.[2] There would therefore seem little reason at the moment to believe that bicalutamide in normal doses interacts with **warfarin**, but until more is known it would seem prudent to remain aware of the possibility if it is started.

1. Casodex (Bicalutamide). AstraZeneca UK Ltd. UK Summary of product characteristics, January 2004.
2. Zeneca. Personal Communication, October 1995.

Anticoagulants + Bile-acid binding resins

The anticoagulant effects of phenprocoumon and warfarin can be reduced by colestyramine. An isolated and unexplained report describes a paradoxical increase in the effects of warfarin. No important interaction occurs between phenprocoumon or warfarin and colestipol.

Clinical evidence

(a) Colestipol

Phenprocoumon plasma levels and the prothrombin response were unaffected in 4 healthy subjects when they were given colestipol 8 g at the same time.[1] In another study colestipol 10 g did not cause any changes in the absorption of a single 10-mg dose of **warfarin.**[2]

(b) Colestyramine

Ten subjects were treated for one-week periods either with **warfarin** alone or **warfarin** with colestyramine 8 g given three times a day. With **warfarin** alone peak plasma levels reached 5.6 micrograms/ml and prothrombin times were prolonged by 11 seconds. With colestyramine given 30 minutes before the **warfarin**, peak levels were reduced to 2.7 micrograms/ml and the prothrombin times were prolonged by 8 seconds, whereas when the colestyramine was given 6 hours before the **warfarin**, peak levels reached 4.7 micrograms/ml and prothrombin times were again prolonged by 11 seconds.[3]

Comparable results have been found in other studies using single doses of **warfarin** or **phenprocoumon.**[4,5]

An isolated and unexplained report describes a very marked increase in the effects of **warfarin** (prothrombin time 78.9 seconds) in a very elderly patient with multiple pathologies when given colestyramine.[6]

Mechanism

Colestyramine binds to bile acids within the gut and also to coumarin anticoagulants, thereby preventing their absorption.[4,5,7-9] As both warfarin and phenprocoumon undergo enterohepatic recycling, continuous further contact with the colestyramine can occur.[10,11] Colestyramine also reduces the absorption of fat-soluble vitamins such as vitamin K so that it can have some direct hypoprothrombinaemic effects of its own.[12,13] This may to some extent offset the full effects of its interaction with anticoagulants. Colestipol on the other hand appears not to bind to any great extent at the pH values in the gut.[1] The paradoxical increase in the effects of warfarin in the isolated case cited above remains unexplained.[6]

Importance and management

The phenprocoumon or warfarin and colestyramine interactions are established, but their magnitude and clinical importance is still uncertain. If concurrent use is thought necessary, prothrombin times should be monitored and the dosage of the anticoagulant increased appropriately. Giving the colestyramine 3 to 6 hours after the anticoagulant has been shown to minimise the effects of this interaction,[3,14] and it is a standard recommendation that other drugs should be given 1 hour before or 4 to 6 hours after colestyramine. Information about other anticoagulants is lacking but as colestyramine interacts with dicoumarol and ethyl biscoumacetate in *animals*[9] it would be prudent to expect all coumarins to interact similarly.

No special precautions appear necessary if warfarin or phenprocoumon and colestipol are given concurrently. There seems to be no information about other anticoagulants.

1. Harvengt C, Desager JP. Effects of colestipol, a new bile acid sequestrant, on the absorption of phenprocoumon in man. *Eur J Clin Pharmacol* (1973) 6, 19–21.
2. Heel RC, Brogden RN, Pakes GE, Speight TM, Avery GS. Colestipol: a review of its pharmacological properties and therapeutic effects in patients with hypercholesterolaemia. *Drugs* (1980) 19, 161–80.
3. Kuentzel WP, Brunk SF. Cholestyramine-warfarin interaction in man. *Clin Res* (1970) 18, 594.
4. Robinson DS, Benjamin DM, McCormack JJ. Interaction of warfarin and nonsystemic gastrointestinal drugs. *Clin Pharmacol Ther* (1971) 12, 491–5.
5. Hahn KJ, Eiden W, Schettle M, Hahn M, Walter E, Weber E. Effect of cholestyramine on the gastrointestinal absorption of phenprocoumon and acetylosalicylic acid in man. *Eur J Clin Pharmacol* (1972) 4, 142–5.
6. Lawlor DP, Hyers TM. Extreme prolongation of the prothrombin time in a patient receiving warfarin and cholestyramine. *Cardiovasc Rev Rep* (1993) April, 72–4.
7. Benjamin D, Robinson DS, McCormack J. Cholestyramine binding of warfarin in man and in vitro. *Clin Res* (1970) 18, 336.
8. Gallo DG, Bailey KR, Sheffner AL. The interaction between cholestyramine and drugs. *Proc Soc Exp Biol Med* (1965) 120, 60–5.
9. Tembo AV, Bates TR. Impairment by cholestyramine of dicumarol and tromexan absorption in rats: a potential drug interaction. *J Pharmacol Exp Ther* (1974) 191, 53–9.
10. Jähnchen E, Meinertz T, Gilfrich H-J, Kersting F, Groth U. Enhanced elimination of warfarin during treatment with cholestyramine. *Br J Clin Pharmacol* (1978) 5, 437–40.
11. Meinertz T, Gilfrich H-J, Groth U, Jonen HG, Jähnchen E. Interruption of the enterohepatic circulation of phenprocoumon by cholestyramine. *Clin Pharmacol Ther* (1977) 21, 731–5.
12. Casdorph HR. Safe uses of cholestyramine. *Ann Intern Med* (1970) 72, 759.
13. Gross L, Brotman M. Hypoprothrombinemia and hemorrhage associated with cholestyramine therapy. *Ann Intern Med* (1970) 72, 95–6.
14. Cali TJ. Combined therapy with cholestyramine and warfarin. *Am J Pharm Sci Support Public Health* (1975) 147, 166–9.

Anticoagulants + Bosentan

Bosentan may reduce the anticoagulant effects of warfarin.

Clinical evidence

In a double-blind randomised placebo-controlled crossover study, 12 healthy subjects were given bosentan 500 mg twice daily or placebo for 10 days, with a single 26-mg dose of **warfarin** given on day 6. Bosentan reduced the AUC of ***(R)*-warfarin** by 38% and of ***(S)*-warfarin** by 29%. A significant decrease in the anticoagulant effects of **warfarin** was also noted, with a 23% reduction in prothrombin time occurring with bosentan.[1]

One case highlights the clinical significance of this interaction. A 35-year-old woman on **warfarin** with a stable INR of 2 to 3 over three months was started on bosentan 62.5 mg twice daily. After 10 days her INR was 1.7, and remained at this level over the next 4 weeks, despite an increase in her weekly **warfarin** dose from 27.5 to 40 mg. The bosentan dose was then increased to the maintenance dose of 125 mg twice daily, and two further weekly increases in **warfarin** dose made. The INR was then high (3.2 to 4.1) for 3 weeks, before she was finally stabilised on **warfarin** 45 mg each week.[2]

However, the maker of bosentan notes that clinical experience of concurrent use of bosentan with **warfarin** did not result in clinically relevant changes in the INR or **warfarin** dose. There was no difference in the frequency of **warfarin** dose changes (due to INR changes or adverse effects) between bosentan or placebo recipients.[3]

Mechanism

It has been suggested that bosentan induces both cytochrome P450 isoenzymes CYP3A4 and CYP2C9, which are involved in the metabolism of *(S)*- and *(R)*-warfarin respectively.[1]

Importance and management

Both the reports suggest that a clinically significant interaction between warfarin and bosentan is possible, although exactly how frequently this may occur is unclear, since it was not detected in clinical trials. However, the INR should be closely monitored in any patient on warfarin during the period that bosentan is started or stopped, or if the dose is altered.[3]

1. Weber C, Banken L, Birnboeck H, Schulz R. Effect of the endothelin-receptor antagonist bosentan on the pharmacokinetics and pharmacodynamics of warfarin. *J Clin Pharmacol* (1999) 39, 847–54.
2. Murphey LM, Hood EH. Bosentan and warfarin interaction. *Ann Pharmacother* (2003) 37, 1028–31.
3. Tracleer (Bosentan monohydrate). Actelion Pharmaceuticals UK. UK Summary of product characteristics, September 2004.

Anticoagulants + Bucolome

Bucolome increases the anticoagulant effects of warfarin.

Clinical evidence

A study in Japanese patients on **warfarin** found that the addition of bucolome 300 mg daily in 21 patients increased their INRs 1.5-fold (despite a 58% **warfarin** dosage reduction) when compared with another group of 34 patients on **warfarin** not receiving bucolome.[1] In another 7-day study, 25 Japanese patients with heart disease on **warfarin** and bucolome 300 mg daily were compared with another control group of 30 taking **warfarin** alone. It was found that bucolome had no effect on the serum levels of ***(R)*-warfarin** but both the serum levels of ***(S)*-warfarin** and the prothrombin times rose. These changes were complete within 7 days.[2]

Mechanism

In vitro studies show that the buculome can inhibit the metabolism of the more potent enantiomer *(S)*-warfarin by the cytochrome P450 isoenzyme CYP2C9, thereby reducing its clearance and increasing its effects.[1]

Importance and management

Information appears to be limited to the reports cited here but the interaction would seem to be established and clinically important. Monitor the INR closely. A reduced warfarin dosage (the study cited above suggests a 30 to 60% reduction)[2] is likely to be needed if both drugs are used concurrently to avoid excessive anticoagulation and possible bleeding. Information about other anticoagulants is lacking.

1. Takahashi H, Kashima T, Kimura S, Murata N, Takaba T, Iwade K, Abe T, Tainaka H, Yasumori T, Echizen H. Pharmacokinetic interaction between warfarin and a uricosuric agent, bucolome: application of in vitro approaches to predicting in vivo reduction of (S)-warfarin clearance. *Drug Metab Dispos* (1999) 27, 1179–86.
2. Matsumoto K, Ishida S, Ueno K, Hashimoto H, Takada M, Tanaka K, Kamakura S, Miyatake K, Shibakawa M. The stereoselective effects of bucolome on the pharmacokinetics and pharmacodynamics of racemic warfarin. *J Clin Pharmacol* (2001) 41, 459–64.

Anticoagulants + Calcium channel blockers

Amlodipine, diltiazem and felodipine appear not to significantly affect the anticoagulant effects of warfarin.

Clinical evidence, mechanism, importance and management

The makers say that studies in healthy subjects have shown that **amlodipine** does not significantly alter the effect of **warfarin** on prothrombin times.[1,2] **Felodipine** 10 mg daily for 14 days was found not to alter the anticoagulant effects of **warfarin** in healthy subjects.[3]

In another study, 11 healthy men were given racemic **warfarin**, and eight were given ***(R)*-warfarin**, both as a single 1.5-mg/kg intravenous dose, while 10 were given ***(S)*-warfarin** as a single 0.75-mg/kg intravenous dose. After taking **diltiazem** 120 mg three times a day for 4 days before and 9 days after the dose of **warfarin** the clearance of ***(R)*-warfarin** was decreased by about 20% but the more potent ***(S)*-warfarin** remained unaffected. The total anticoagulant response remained unchanged.[4] Two other studies found that **diltiazem** 30 mg three times daily for a week caused no clinically relevant changes in the anticoagulant effects of **warfarin** in 20 healthy subjects.[5]

No special precautions would therefore seem to be necessary during concurrent use of any of these anticoagulants and calcium channel blockers. Information about other anticoagulants and other calcium channel blockers appears to be lacking, but the absence of adverse reports about these very widely used drugs suggests that concurrent use is normally uneventful.

1. Istin (Amlodipine besilate). Pfizer Ltd. UK Summary of product characteristics, April 2005.
2. Norvasc (Amlodipine). Pfizer Labs. US Prescribing information, January 2005.
3. Grind M, Murphy M, Warrington S, Åberg J. Method for studying drug-warfarin interactions. *Clin Pharmacol Ther* (1993) 54, 381–7.
4. Abernethy DR, Kaminsky LS, Dickinson TH. Selective inhibition of warfarin metabolism by diltiazem in humans. *J Pharmacol Exp Ther* (1991) 257, 411–15.
5. Stoysich AM, Lucas BD, Mohiuddin SM, Hilleman DE. Further elucidation of pharmacokinetic interaction between diltiazem and warfarin. *Int J Clin Pharmacol Ther* (1996) 34, 56–60.

Anticoagulants + Carbamazepine or Oxcarbazepine

The anticoagulant effects of warfarin can be markedly reduced by carbamazepine but oxcarbazepine appears not to interact significantly. Carbamazepine reduced the anticoagulant effects of phenprocoumon in two patients.

Clinical evidence

(a) Carbamazepine

(i) Phenprocoumon. A man in his mid-twenties developed multiple thrombotic episodes due to hereditary resistance to activated protein C. Because of cerebral embolic strokes he developed epileptic seizures and was started on carbamazepine 400 mg daily, followed 6 days later by phenprocoumon. It was found that relatively large doses (8 mg daily) had to be given to achieve adequate anticoagulation (prothrombin time ratio of 50 to 60%) until the carbamazepine was withdrawn, whereupon the phenprocoumon dosage could be reduced to 1.5 mg daily with a prothrombin time ratio of 30 to 40%.[1] Another patient on phenprocoumon showed a dramatic increase in his prothrombin time ratio when he was given carbamazepine. The values returned to normal when the carbamazepine was stopped.[2]

(ii) Warfarin. Two patients on warfarin given carbamazepine (200 mg daily for the first week, 400 mg daily for the second and 600 mg for the third) showed a fall of about 50% in serum warfarin levels, and sharp rises in their prothrombin-proconvertin percentages.[3] The half-life of warfarin in three other patients fell by 53, 11 and 60% respectively when they were similarly treated.[3]

This interaction has been described in 6 other reports.[4-8] One of them describes a patient stabilised on warfarin and carbamazepine who developed widespread dermal ecchymoses and a prothrombin time of 70 seconds, a week after stopping the carbamazepine. She was restabilised on approximately half the dose of warfarin in the absence of the carbamazepine.[8]

(b) Oxcarbazepine

A study in 10 healthy subjects on warfarin found that oxcarbazepine 450 mg twice daily for a week increased the Quick values from 41 to only 46%.[9] A very similar study by the same workers found a change in Quick values from 36.6 to 38.1% due to oxcarbazepine.[10]

Mechanism

Uncertain, but the available evidence suggests that carbamazepine increases the metabolism of warfarin by the liver, thereby increasing its loss from the body and reducing its effects.[3,4] This may also possibly explain the phenprocoumon interaction. Oxcarbazepine on the other hand has relatively little enzyme inducing activity.

Importance and management

The interaction between warfarin and carbamazepine is moderately well documented, established and clinically important. The incidence is uncertain but monitor the anticoagulant response if carbamazepine is added to established treatment with warfarin and anticipate the need to double the dosage. Oxcarbazepine appears to be a relatively non-interacting alternative.

Information about an interaction between phenprocoumon and carbamazepine seems to be limited to the two reports cited. Nevertheless it would be prudent to monitor concurrent use in any patient, being alert for the need to increase the phenprocoumon dosage. The same precautions would seem sensible with any other coumarin but information appears to be lacking.

1. Böttcher T, Buchmann J, Zettl U-K, Benecke R. Carbamazepine-phenprocoumon interaction. *Eur Neurol* (1997) 38, 132–3.
2. Schlienger R, Kurmann M, Drewe J, Müller-Spahn F, Seifritz E. Inhibition of phenprocoumon anticoagulation by carbamazepine. *Eur Neuropsychopharmacol* (2000) 10, 219–21.
3. Hansen JM, Siersbæk-Nielsen K, Skovsted L. Carbamazepine-induced acceleration of diphenylhydantoin and warfarin metabolism in man. *Clin Pharmacol Ther* (1971) 12, 539–43.
4. Ross JRY, Beeley L. Interaction between carbamazepine and warfarin. *BMJ* (1980) 1, 1415–16.
5. Kendall AG, Boivin M. Warfarin-carbamazepine interaction. *Ann Intern Med* (1981) 94, 280.
6. Massey EW. Effect of carbamazepine on Coumadin metabolism. *Ann Neurol* (1983) 13, 691–2.
7. Beeley L, Stewart P, Hickey FM. *Bulletin of the West Midlands Centre for Adverse Drug Reaction Reporting* (1988) 26, 18.
8. Denbow CE, Fraser HS. Clinically significant hemorrhage due to warfarin-carbamazepine interaction. *South Med J* (1990) 83, 981.
9. Krämer G, Tettenborn B, Klosterkov-Jensen P, Stoll K-D. Oxcarbazepine-warfarin drug interaction study in healthy volunteers. *Epilepsia* (1991) 32 (Suppl 1), 70.
10. Krämer G, Tettenborn B, Klosterkov Jensen P, Menge GP, Stoll KD. Oxcarbazepine does not affect the anticoagulant activity of warfarin. *Epilepsia* (1992) 33, 1145–8.

Anticoagulants + Carbon tetrachloride

A single case report describes an increase in the anticoagulant effects of dicoumarol in a patient who accidentally drank some carbon tetrachloride.

Clinical evidence, mechanism, importance and management

A patient, well stabilised on **dicoumarol**, accidentally drank 0.1 ml of carbon tetrachloride. The next day his prothrombin time had risen to 41 seconds (prothrombin activity fall from 18 to 10%). These values were about the same next day although the **dicoumarol** had been withdrawn, and marked hypoprothrombinaemia persisted for another 5 days.[1]

The probable reason for this reaction is that carbon tetrachloride is very toxic to the liver, the changed anticoagulant response being a manifestation of this. Carbon tetrachloride, once used as an anthelmintic in man, is no longer used in human medicine, but is still employed as an industrial solvent and degreasing agent. On theoretical grounds it would seem possible for anticoagulated patients exposed to substantial amounts of the vapour to experience this interaction but this has not been reported.

1. Luton EF. Carbon tetrachloride exposure during anticoagulant therapy. Dangerous enhancement of hypoprothrombinemic effect. *JAMA* (1965) 194, 1386–7.

Anticoagulants + Carnitine

An isolated report describes gastrointestinal bleeding and a marked increase in the anticoagulant effects of acenocoumarol in a patient given L-carnitine.

Clinical evidence, mechanism, importance and management

A woman who had taken **acenocoumarol** for 17 years because of aortic and mitral prosthetic valves, was admitted to hospital with melaena within 5 days of starting to take 1 g of L-carnitine daily. Her INR had risen from 2.1 to 7. Endoscopy and colonoscopy revealed diffuse bleeding from superficial erosions in the gut. She was discharged 10 days later on the same dose of **acenocoumarol** with an INR of 2.1 without the carnitine.[1] The reason for this apparent interaction is not known.

This seems to the first and only recorded case of an interaction between an oral anticoagulant and carnitine, but it would now be prudent to bear this interaction in mind if carnitine is added to a stable regimen with any oral anticoagulant, being alert for an increased response.

1. Martinez E, Domingo P, Roca-Cusachs A. Potentiation of acenocoumarol action by L-carnitine. *J Intern Med* (1993) 233, 94.

Anticoagulants + Cephalosporins or Vancomycin

Most cephalosporins do not interact with oral anticoagulants, but those with an *N*-methylthiotetrazole side-chain and some others can occasionally cause enough hypoprothrombinaemia for bleeding to occur when they are used alone. These effects could therefore be additive with those of conventional anticoagulants. Vancomycin possibly causes a small increase in the effects of warfarin.

Clinical evidence

A study of this interaction was prompted by 2 patients who developed unusually high prothrombin times, with bleeding in one case, when they were given **warfarin** and **cefamandole**. Sixty other patients undergoing heart valve replacement surgery were given antibacterials prophylactically before the chest incision was made, and at six-hourly intervals thereafter for about 72 hours. The 44 patients given **cefamandole** 2 g showed a much greater anticoagulant response than the 16 patients given **vancomycin** 500 mg.[1] In a later study by the same workers, after 3 days of concurrent use with **warfarin** the prothrombin times as a percentage of activity were as follows: **cefamandole** 29%, **cefazolin** 38%, **vancomycin** 51%, suggesting that **cefamandole** had a much greater effect on anticoagulant response than **vancomycin**.[2]

Serious bleeding following the use of **cefamandole** (in the absence of an anticoagulant) has been described in 3 out of 37 patients in another report,[3] and a further report highlights a further 16 cases.[4]

Other cephalosporins that have been reported to cause hypoprothrombinaemia when used alone include **cefoperazone**,[5-9] **cefotetan**,[10] **cefoxitin**,[11] **ceftriaxone**,[12] **cefalotin**,[13] **cefazolin**,[14-16] and **latamoxef**.[11,17] Extended prothrombin times are also said to occur with **cefaloridine**.[18]

Cefixime has also been implicated in a handful of cases of bleeding and/or increased INRs in patients taking **warfarin** or **phenindione**, but the evidence is inconclusive.[19] A 'Drug Analysis Print' from the UK Committee on Safety of Medicines covering the period 1979 to 1997 very briefly records raised INRs in three patients on **acenocoumarol**, **warfarin** or an unknown anticoagulant when given **cefaclor**. When set against the extensive use of **cefaclor** over almost 30 years, these interactions are clearly very rare indeed.[20]

Severe haemorrhage has been reported in 3 patients on **acenocoumarol** when they took **cefotiam**. One developed an abdominal haematoma and an INR of 10.4 within 2 days. Another had gastrointestinal bleeding and melaena after one day's use. The third died from intracranial haemorrhage on the day she started **cefotiam**.[21] A study in 9 patients on **warfarin** failed to find a clinically relevant interaction with **cefonicid**.[22] A later study identified 9 patients on **acenocoumarol** who had increased INRs within 3 to 8 days of being given **cefonicid**. They needed a reduction in the anticoagulant dosage of about one-third to one-half.[23] A patient on **acenocoumarol** bled after being additionally given **cefonicid**.[24]

Mechanism

Cephalosporins with an *N*-methylthiotetrazole side-chain can, like the oral anticoagulants, act as vitamin K antagonists to reduce the production of some blood clotting factors. They can therefore cause bleeding on their own and worsen the risk of bleeding by simple addition if given with conventional anticoagulants. In addition, some of them may also inhibit platelet function.[25] Ceftriaxone seems to act similarly although it has an *N*-methylthio*triazine* ring instead.

Importance and management

Most cephalosporins do not normally cause bleeding or interact with the oral anticoagulants. In contrast, cefaclor, cefaloridine, cefalotin, cefazolin, cefixime, cefonicid, cefoperazone, cefotetan, cefotiam, cefoxitin, ceftriaxone, cefamandole and latamoxef have all sometimes caused bleeding alone or in the presence of an anticoagulant. The incidence is very variable: in some instances only isolated cases have been reported whereas a 15% bleeding rate was found in one study with latamoxef alone, 22% in another, but only 8% with cefoxitin alone.[11,26] Patients most at risk seem to be those whose intake of vitamin K is restricted (poor diet, malabsorption syndromes, etc.) and those with renal failure. The use of an anticoagulant represents just another factor that may precipitate bleeding.

A possible solution to the problem is to use a non-interacting cephalosporin. Alternatively you should monitor the outcome closely, particularly in the early stages of treatment, adjusting the anticoagulant dosage if necessary. Excessive hypoprothrombinaemia can be controlled with vitamin K.

A number of cephalosporins that also possess the *N*-methylthiotetrazole side-chain are expected to behave similarly, but have not so far been reported to do so. These include **cefazaflur**, **cefmenoxime**, **cefmetazole**,

cefminox, **ceforanide** and **cefpiramide**. The situation with cefixime is still uncertain.[19]

The study[1] cited above, in which surgical patients were given warfarin with either a cephalosporin or vancomycin, indicates that vancomycin interacts with warfarin but the increase in prothrombin times seems not to be large. There seem to be no reports of problems with vancomycin and warfarin or any other anticoagulant.

1. Angaran DM, Dias VC, Arom KV, Northrup WF, Kersten TE, Lindsay WG, Nicoloff DM. The influence of prophylactic antibiotics on the warfarin anticoagulation response in the postoperative prosthetic cardiac valve patient. *Ann Surg* (1984) 199, 107–111.
2. Angaran DM, Dias VC, Arom KV, Northrup WF, Kersten TG, Lindsay WG, Nicoloff DM. The comparative influence of prophylactic antibiotics on the prothrombin response to warfarin in the postoperative prosthetic cardiac valve patient. *Ann Surg* (1987) 206, 155–61.
3. Hooper CA, Haney BB, Stone HH. Gastrointestinal bleeding due to vitamin K deficiency in patients on parenteral cefamandole. *Lancet* (1980) i, 39–40.
4. Rymer W, Greenlaw CW. Hypoprothrombinemia associated with cefamandole. *Drug Intell Clin Pharm* (1980) 14, 780–3.
5. Meisel S. Hypoprothrombinemia due to cefoperazone. *Drug Intell Clin Pharm* (1984) 18, 316.
6. Cristiano P. Hypoprothrombinemia associated with cefoperazone treatment. *Drug Intell Clin Pharm* (1984) 18, 314–16.
7. Osborne JC. Hypoprothrombinemia and bleeding due to cefoperazone. *Ann Intern Med* (1985) 102, 721–2.
8. Freedy HR, Cetnarowski AB, Lumish RM, Schafer FJ. Cefoperazone-induced coagulopathy. *Drug Intell Clin Pharm* (1986) 20, 281–3.
9. Andrassy K, Koderisch J, Fritz S, Bechtold H, Sonntag H. Alteration of hemostasis associated with cefoperazone treatment. *Infection* (1986) 14, 27–31.
10. Conjura A, Bell W, Lipsky JJ. Cefotetan and hypoprothrombinemia. *Ann Intern Med* (1988) 108, 643.
11. Brown RB, Klar J, Lemeshow S, Teres D, Pastides H, Sands M. Enhanced bleeding with cefoxitin or moxalactam. Statistical analysis within a defined population of 1493 patients. *Arch Intern Med* (1986) 146, 2159–64.
12. Haubenstock A, Schmidt P, Zazgornik J, Balcke P, Kopsa H. Hypoprothrombinaemic bleeding associated with ceftriaxone. *Lancet* (1983) i, 1215–16.
13. Natelson EA, Brown CH, Bradshaw MW, Alfrey CP, Williams TW. Influence of cephalosporin antibiotics on blood coagulation and platelet function. *Antimicrob Agents Chemother* (1976) 9, 91–3.
14. Lerner PI, Lubin A. Coagulopathy with cefazolin in uremia. *N Engl J Med* (1974) 290, 1324.
15. Khaleeli M, Giorgio AJ. Defective platelet function after cephalosporin administration. *Blood* (1976) 48, 971.
16. Dupuis LL, Paton TW, Suttie JW, Thiessen JJ, Rachlis A. Cefazolin-induced coagulopathy. *Clin Pharmacol Ther* (1984) 35, 237.
17. Beeley L, Beadle R and Lawrence R. *Bulletin of the West Midlands Centre for Adverse Drug Reaction Reporting* (1984) 19, 15.
18. Council on Drugs (American Medical Association). Evaluation of a new antibacterial agent, cephaloridine (Loridine). *JAMA* (1968) 206, 1289–90.
19. Lederle Laboratories. Personal communication, December 1995.
20. Distaclor (Cefaclor). Dista Products Ltd. UK Summary of product characteristics, May 1999.
21. Gras-Champel V, Sauvé L, Perault MC, Laine P, Gouello JP, Decocq G, Masson H, Touzard M, Andréjak M. Association cefotiam et acenocoumarol: a propos de 3 cas d'hémorragies. *Therapie* (1998) 53, 191.
22. Angaran DM, Tschida VH, Copa AK. Effect of cefonicid (CN) on prothrombin time (PT) in outpatients (OP) receiving warfarin (W) therapy. *Pharmacotherapy* (1988) 8, 120.
23. Puente Garcia M, Bécares Martínez FJ, Merlo Arroyo J, García Sánchez G, García Díaz B, Cervero Jiménez M. Potenciación del efecto anticoagulante del acenocoumarol por cefonicid. *Rev Clin Esp* (1999) 199, 620–1.
24. Riancho JA, Olmos JM, Sedano C. Life-threatening bleeding in a patient being treated with cefonicid. *Ann Intern Med* (1995) 123, 472–3.
25. Bang NU, Tessler SS, Heidenreich RO, Marks CA, Mattler LE. Effects of moxalactam on blood coagulation and platelet function. *Rev Infect Dis* (1982) 4 (Suppl), S546–S554.
26. Morris DL. Fabricius PJ, Ambrose NS, Scammell B, Burdon DW, Keighley MRB. A high incidence of bleeding is observed in a trial to determine whether addition of metronidazole is neeeded with latamoxef for prophylaxis in colorectal surgery. *J Hosp Infect* (1984) 5, 398–408.

Anticoagulants + Chloramphenicol

There is some limited evidence that the anticoagulant effects of acenocoumarol and dicoumarol can be increased by oral chloramphenicol. An isolated report attributes a marked INR rise in a patient on warfarin to the use of chloramphenicol eye drops.

Clinical evidence

A study in 4 patients showed that the half-life of **dicoumarol** was increased on average from 8 to 25 hours when they were given chloramphenicol 2 g daily for 5 to 8 days.[1]

Three out of 9 patients taking an unnamed anticoagulant showed a fall in their prothrombin-proconvertin values from a range of 10 to 30% down to less than 6% when given chloramphenicol 1 to 2 g daily for 4 to 6 days. One patient showed a smaller reduction.[2] There is another report of an increased anticoagulant response involving **acenocoumarol** and chloramphenicol.[3]

An isolated report describes an 83-year-old woman on **warfarin** who showed a rise in her INR to about 8.9 from a normal range of 1.9 to 2.8 within 2 weeks of starting to use eye drops containing chloramphenicol 5 mg/ml, dexamethasone sodium phosphate 1 mg/ml and tetrahydrozoline hydrochloride 0.25 mg/ml. She used one drop in each eye four times daily.[4] Hypoprothrombinaemia and bleeding have also been described in patients on chloramphenicol in the absence of an anticoagulant.[5,6]

Mechanism

Uncertain. One suggestion is that the chloramphenicol inhibits the liver enzymes concerned with the metabolism of the anticoagulants so that their effects are prolonged and increased.[4] Another is that the antibacterial diminishes the gut bacteria thereby decreasing a source of vitamin K, but it is doubtful if these bacteria are normally an important source of the vitamin except in exceptional cases where dietary levels are very inadequate.[7] A third suggestion is that chloramphenicol blocks production of prothrombin by the liver.[5]

Importance and management

The documentation for the interaction between anticoagulants and oral chloramphenicol interaction is very sparse and poor (the best being the report about dicoumarol) so that this interaction is by no means adequately established. There would therefore appear to be little reason for avoiding concurrent use, but for complete safety it might be prudent to monitor prothrombin times if oral chloramphenicol is started in patients taking any anticoagulant, being alert for the need to reduce the anticoagulant dosage.

The report about an apparent warfarin/topical chloramphenicol interaction is very surprising because the amount of chloramphenicol absorbed from eye drops is relatively small and because, despite the very widespread use of warfarin and chloramphenicol for very many years, this report appears to be the only one implicating warfarin and chloramphenicol in any form. This suggests that any such interaction is very unlikely indeed, however the ultracautious may wish to monitor the outcome if topical chloramphenicol is used.

1. Christensen LK, Skovsted L. Inhibition of drug metabolism by chloramphenicol. *Lancet* (1969) ii, 1397–9.
2. Magid E. Tolerance to anticoagulants during antibiotic therapy. *Scand J Clin Lab Invest* (1962) 14, 565–6.
3. Johnson R, David A, Chartier Y. Clinical experience with G-23350 (Sintrom). *Can Med Assoc J* (1957) 77, 756–61.
4. Leone R, Ghiotto E, Conforti A, Velo G. Potential interaction between warfarin and ocular chloramphenicol. *Ann Pharmacother* (1999) 33, 114.
5. Klippel AP, Pitsinger B. Hypoprothrombinemia secondary to antibiotic therapy and manifested by massive gastrointestinal hemorrhage. *Arch Surg* (1968) 96, 266–8.
6. Matsaniotis N, Messaritakis J, Vlachou C. Hypoprothrombinaemic bleeding in infants associated with diarrhoea and antibiotics. *Arch Dis Child* (1970) 45, 586–7.
7. Udall JA. Human sources and absorption of vitamin K in relation to anticoagulation stability. *JAMA* (1965), 194, 107–9.

Anticoagulants + Cilostazol

Cilostazol does not appear to interact to a clinically relevant extent with warfarin.

Clinical evidence, mechanism, importance and management

A randomised, double-blind, two-way crossover study in 15 healthy subjects found that cilostazol 100 mg twice daily for 7 or 13 days did not alter the pharmacokinetics of a single 25-mg dose of warfarin. Prothrombin times, aPTT time and Ivy bleeding time were unaffected.[1] This suggests that no interaction is likely during concurrent use.

1. Millakaarjun S, Bramer SL. Effect of cilostazol on the pharmacokinetics and pharmacodynamics of warfarin. *Clin Pharmacokinet* (1999) 37 (Suppl 2), 79–86.

Anticoagulants + Clindamycin

An isolated report describes bleeding and a markedly increased INR in a woman on warfarin tentatively attributed to an interaction with clindamycin.

Clinical evidence, mechanism, importance and management

A 47-year-old woman with multiple medical problems receiving **warfarin** (and also taking azathioprine, captopril, furosemide, insulin, captopril, prednisone, levothyroxine, valproic acid and zolpidem) had all her teeth removed under general anaesthetic. Sixteen days later she needed a dental abscess drained and was started on oral clindamycin 300 mg four times daily with ibuprofen 600 mg for any discomfort. On day 17 she needed a suture to stop some bleeding and her INR was found to be 3.5. By day 20 she had developed more severe oral bleeding, which needed emergency room treatment. Her INR was found to have risen to 13 and her haematocrit to 18%. She was treated successfully with a blood transfusion and vitamin K.[1]

This appears to be an isolated case, from which no general conclusions should be drawn because the whole picture is so obscure and uncertain. This woman had a history of rheumatic fever, an artificial heart valve, hypertension, diabetes, arthritis, autoimmune haemolytic anaemia, a major and several minor strokes, peptic ulceration, hypothyroidism, renal vein thrombosis, a single kidney, seizures, systemic lupus erythematosus and some liver impairment.

1. Aldous JA, Olson CJ. Managing patients on warfarin therapy: a case report. *Spec Care Dentist* (2001) 21, 109–112.

Anticoagulants + Cloral and derivatives

The anticoagulant effects of warfarin are transiently increased by cloral hydrate, but this is normally of little or no clinical importance. Cloral betaine and triclofos may be expected to behave similarly.

Clinical evidence

A retrospective study on patients just starting **warfarin** showed that while the same loading doses of **warfarin** were given to 67 patients and 32 patients treated with **cloral hydrate**, the **warfarin** requirements of the **cloral** group during the first 4 days fell by about one-third, but rose again to control requirements by the fifth day.[1]

A study in 10 patients and 4 healthy subjects taking **warfarin** showed that when they were given **cloral hydrate** 1 g each night, there was a minor, clinically unimportant and short-lived increase in the prothrombin times of 5 of them during the first few days of concurrent use, but no change in the overall long-term anticoagulant control occurred.[2]

Similar results have been described in other studies on large numbers of patients taking **warfarin** and **cloral hydrate**[3-8] or **triclofos**.[9] **Cloral betaine** appears to behave similarly.[10] An isolated and by no means fully explained case of fatal hypoprothrombinaemia in a patient on **dicoumarol** who was given **cloral hydrate** for 10 days, later replaced by secobarbital, has been reported.[11] Another patient on **dicoumarol** showed a reduction in prothrombin times with **cloral hydrate**.[11]

Mechanism

Cloral hydrate is mainly metabolised to trichloroacetic acid, which then successfully competes with warfarin for its binding sites on plasma proteins.[6] As a result, free and active molecules of warfarin flood are displaced into plasma water and the effects of the warfarin are increased. But this is only short-lived because the warfarin molecules become exposed to metabolism by the liver, so the warfarin level is reduced.

Importance and management

The interaction between warfarin and cloral hydrate is well documented and well understood, but normally of little or no clinical importance. There is very good evidence that concurrent use need not be avoided.[1-8] However, the ultracautious might wish to keep an eye on the anticoagulant response during the first 4 to 5 days, just to make sure it does not become excessive. It is not certain whether other anticoagulants behave in the same way because the evidence is sparse, indirect and inconclusive,[11,12] but what is known suggests that the coumarins probably do.

Triclofos and cloral betaine appear to behave like cloral hydrate. Dichloralphenazone on the other hand interacts quite differently (see 'Anticoagulants + Dichloralphenazone', p.277).

1. Boston Collaborative Drug Surveillance Program. Interaction between chloral hydrate and warfarin. *N Engl J Med* (1972) 286, 53–5.
2. Udall JA. Warfarin-chloral hydrate interaction. Pharmacological activity and significance. *Ann Intern Med* (1974) 81, 341–4.
3. Griner PF, Raisz LG, Rickles FR, Wiesner PJ, Odoroff CL. Chloral hydrate and warfarin interaction: clinical significance? *Ann Intern Med* (1971) 74, 540–3.
4. Udall JA. Clinical implications of warfarin interactions with five sedatives. *Am J Cardiol* (1975) 35, 67–71.
5. Udall JA. Warfarin interactions with chloral hydrate and glutethimide. *Curr Ther Res* (1975) 17, 67–74.
6. Sellers EM, Koch-Weser J. Kinetics and clinical importance of displacement of warfarin from albumin by acidic drugs. *Ann N Y Acad Sci* (1971) 179, 213–25.
7. Breckenridge A, Orme ML'E, Thorgeirsson S, Davies DS, Brooks RV. Drug interactions with warfarin: studies with dichloralphenazone, chloral hydrate and phenazone (antipyrine). *Clin Sci* (1971) 40, 351–64.
8. Breckenridge A, Orme M. Clinical implications of enzyme induction. *Ann N Y Acad Sci* (1971) 179, 421–31.
9. Sellers EM, Lang M, Koch-Weser J, Colman RW. Enhancement of warfarin-induced hypoprothrombinemia by triclofos. *Clin Pharmacol Ther* (1972) 13, 911–15.
10. MacDonald MG, Robinson DS, Sylwester D, Jaffe JJ. The effects of phenobarbital, chloral betaine, and glutethimide administration on warfarin plasma levels and hypoprothrombinemic responses in man. *Clin Pharmacol Ther* (1969) 10, 80–4.
11. Cucinell SA, Odessky L, Weiss M, Dayton PG. The effect of chloral hydrate on bishydroxycoumarin metabolism. A fatal outcome. *JAMA* (1966) 197, 144–6.
12. van Dam FE, Gribnau-Overkamp MJH. The effect of some sedatives (phenobarbital, glutethimide, chlordiazepoxide, chloral hydrate) on the rate of disappearance of ethyl biscoumacetate from the plasma. *Folia Med Neerl* (1967) 10, 141–5.

Anticoagulants + Corticosteroids or Corticotropin

Only small increases or decreases in anticoagulation normally occur when oral anticoagulants and low-to-moderate doses of corticosteroids or corticotrophin are used, but one patient on ethyl biscoumacetate bled severely when given corticotropin. Other patients have shown very marked prothrombin time increases when given high-dose corticosteroids.

Clinical evidence

(a) Increased anticoagulant effects

Ten out of 14 patients on long-term treatment with either **dicoumarol** or **phenindione** showed a small but definite increase in their anticoagulant responses when they were treated with corticotropin for 4 to 9 days.[1] A patient stable on **ethyl biscoumacetate** began to bleed severely from the gut and urinary tract within 3 days of starting treatment with intravenous corticotropin 10 mg twice daily.[2] A sharp increase in the INR on a patient with APS (antiphospholipid syndrome) occurred after **methylprednisolone** was added to treatment with an unnamed oral anticoagulant,[3] and this prompted a controlled study in 10 patients, 5 on **fluindione** or **acenocoumarol** and 5 without an anticoagulant. It was found that pulse high-dose intravenous **methylprednisolone** increased the mean INR of those taking an anticoagulant from a baseline of 2.75 to 8.04. **Methylprednisolone** alone did not increase the prothrombin time.[4] Two patients on **warfarin** are also reported to have shown significant prolongations in their prothrombin times when given high-dose corticosteroids (**methylprednisolone, dexamethasone**) for the treatment of multiple sclerosis.[5]

(b) Decreased anticoagulant effects

A study in 24 patients anticoagulated for several days with **dicoumarol** showed that 2 hours after receiving **prednisone** 10 mg their silicone coagulation time had decreased from 28 to 24 minutes, and 2 hours later was down to 22 minutes.[6]

A decrease in the anticoagulant effects of **ethyl biscoumacetate** is described in 2 patients given corticotropin and **cortisone**.[7]

Mechanism

Not understood. Corticosteroids can increase the coagulability of the blood in the absence of anticoagulants,[8,9] and increased effects have been described in *animals*.[2] It has been suggested that methylprednisolone may inhibit the metabolism of anticoagulants.[4]

Importance and management

The interaction with low to moderate doses of corticosteroids is by no means well established and is very poorly documented. Very few serious reports seem to have been reported in the last 30 years suggesting that problems are rare. The most constructive thing that can be said is that if either corticotropin (corticotrophin, ACTH) or any corticosteroid is given to patients taking anticoagulants, be aware that an interaction can very rarely occur, but it is impossible to predict whether any dosage adjustments will be upward or downward.

The situation with high dose methylprednisolone or dexamethasone is clearly different. Although the evidence is limited, marked INR increases have been reported and INRs should be closely monitored (daily has been recommended[4]) if these or other high-dose corticosteroids are added to established treatment with any oral anticoagulant. More study is needed.

1. Hellem AJ, Solem JH. The influence of ACTH on prothrombin-proconvertin values in blood during treatment with dicumarol and phenylindandione. *Acta Med Scand* (1954) 150, 389–93.
2. van Cauwenberge H, Jacques LB. Haemorrhagic effect of ACTH with anticoagulants. *Can Med Assoc J* (1958) 79, 536–40.
3. Costedoat-Chalumeau N, Amoura Z, Wechsler B, Ankri A, Piette J-C. Implications of interaction between vitamin K antagonists and high-dose intravenous methylprednisolone in the APS. *J Autoimmun* (2000) 15, A22.
4. Costedoat-Chalumeau N, Amoura Z, Aymard G, Sevin O, Wechsler B, Cacoub P, Huong Du, Le Th, Diquet B, Ankri A, Piette J-C. Potentiation of vitamin K antagonists by high-dose intravenous methylprednisolone. *Ann Intern Med* (2000) 132, 631–5.
5. Kaufman M. Treatment of multiple sclerosis with high-dose corticosteroids may prolong the prothrombin time to dangerous levels in patients taking warfarin. *Multiple Sclerosis* (1997) 3, 248–9.
6. Menczel J, Dreyfuss F. Effect of prednisone on blood coagulation time in patients on dicumarol therapy. *J Lab Clin Med* (1960) 56, 14–20.
7. Chatterjea JB, Salomon L. Antagonistic effects of A.C.T.H. and cortisone on the anticoagulant activity of ethyl biscoumacetate. *BMJ* (1954) 2, 790–2.
8. Cosgriff SW, Diefenbach AF, Vogt W. Hypercoagulability of the blood associated with ACTH and cortisone therapy. *Am J Med* (1950) 9, 752–6.
9. Ozsoylu S, Strauss HS, Diamond LK. Effects of corticosteroids on coagulation of the blood. *Nature* (1962) 195, 1214–15.

Anticoagulants + Cranberry juice

Four patients showed an increase in the anticoagulant effects of warfarin after drinking cranberry juice. One showed a very marked increase and died from a haemorrhage. Another showed an INR reduction.

Clinical evidence, mechanism, importance and management

The adverse reactions register, compiled by the UK Committee on Safety of Medicines and the UK Medicines and Healthcare products Regulatory Agency over the period 1999 to 2003, contains 5 reports suggesting an interaction between **warfarin** and cranberry juice (*Vaccinium macrocarpon*). The most serious case involved a man on **warfarin** whose INR markedly increased (INR greater than 50) 6 weeks after starting to drink cranberry juice. He died from gastrointestinal and pericardial haemorrhages. Less marked INR increases (not specified) were seen in two other patients, one of whom was restabilized on a lower **warfarin** dosage, while the other regained normal INR values after stopping cranberry juice. A further patient showed unstable INRs while in the final case the INR was seen to fall.[1]

The reasons for this interaction are not known, but a suggested possible reason is that one or more of the constituents of cranberry juice (possibly flavonoids, which are known to inhibit cytochrome P450 activity[2]) might have inhibited the metabolism of **warfarin** by the cytochrome isoenzyme CYP2C9, thereby reducing its clearance from the body and increasing its effects.[1]

The incidence and general clinical importance of this interaction is unknown but the current recommendation of the CSM/MHRA is that patients on **warfarin** should now limit or avoid drinking cranberry juice.[1] Information about the possible effects of cranberry juice on other oral anticoagulants is lacking.

1. Committee on the Safety of Medicines/Medicines and Healthcare products Regulatory Agency. Possible interaction between warfarin and cranberry juice. *Current Problems* (2003) 29, 8.
2. Hodek P, Trefil P, Stiborova M. Flavonoids-potent and versatile biologically active compounds interacting with cytochromes P450. *Chem Biol Interact* (2002) 139, 1–21.

Anticoagulants + Dextropropoxyphene (Propoxyphene)

Seven patients on warfarin have shown a marked increase in prothrombin times and/or bleeding when given co-proxamol but the interaction seems to be very uncommon.

Clinical evidence

(a) Co-proxamol

A man on **warfarin** 6 mg daily developed marked haematuria within 6 days of starting to take two tablets of co-proxamol three times a day. His plasma **warfarin** levels had risen by one-third (from 1.8 to 2.4 micrograms/ml).[1] A woman stable for 6 weeks on **warfarin** developed gross haematuria 11 hours after starting co-proxamol. She had taken 6 tablets of co-proxamol over a 6-hour period. Her prothrombin time increased from about 30 to 40 seconds up to 130 seconds.[1]

This interaction has been seen in 5 other patients on **warfarin**.[2-6] The prothrombin time of one of them rose from 28 to 44 seconds up to 80 seconds within 3 days of substituting paracetamol with two tablets of co-proxamol four times a day.[3] Another developed a prothrombin time of more than 50 seconds after taking 30 tablets of *Darvocet-N 100* (dextropropoxyphene 100 mg, paracetamol 650 mg) and possibly an unknown amount of ibuprofen over a 3-day period. Increased **warfarin** effects leading to severe retroperitoneal haemorrhage have also been briefly reported in a patient taking co-proxamol. In this case methocarbamol may have been a contributory factor.[5]

(b) Dextropropoxyphene

A double-blind study in 23 patients anticoagulated with un-named coumarol derivatives and given dextropropoxyphene 450 mg daily for 15 days did not show any change in prothrombin times.[7]

Mechanism

Not understood. It seems possible that dextropropoxyphene inhibits or competes with the liver enzymes concerned with the metabolic clearance of warfarin, thereby prolonging and increasing its effects. There is also the possibility that the paracetamol component had some part to play (see also 'Anticoagulants + Paracetamol (Acetaminophen)', p.303. But just why only a few individuals are affected is not clear.

Importance and management

Information about this interaction is very sparse and seems to be limited to the reports cited. This suggests that only a few patients are likely to develop this interaction with warfarin and c-proxamol or dextropropoxyphene, but it is not possible to predict who will be affected. Concurrent use need not be avoided but it would be prudent initially to monitor the effects of adding these drugs to warfarin, because the occasional patient may show a marked response.

1. Orme M, Breckenridge A, Cook P. Warfarin and Distalgesic interaction. *BMJ* (1976) i, 200.
2. Jones RV. Warfarin and Distalgesic interaction. *BMJ* (1976) i, 460.
3. Smith R, Prudden D, Hawkes C. Propoxyphene and warfarin interaction. *Drug Intell Clin Pharm* (1984) 18, 822.
4. Justice JL, Kline SS. Analgesics and warfarin. A case that brings up questions and cautions. *Postgrad Med* (1988) 83, 217-8, 220.
5. Beeley L, Magee P, Hickey FN. *Bulletin of the West Midlands Centre for Adverse Drug Reaction Reporting* (1990) 30, 20.
6. Pilszek FH, Moloney D, Sewell JR. Case report: increased anticoagulant effect of warfarin in patient taking a small dose of co-proxamol. Personal communication, 1994.
7. Franchimont P, Heynen G. Comparative study of ibuprofen and dextropropoxyphene in scapulo-humeral periarthritis following myocardial infarction. 13th International Congress of Rheumatol, Kyoto, Japan. 30th Sept–6th Oct 1973.

Anticoagulants + Dichloralphenazone

The anticoagulant effects of warfarin are reduced by dichloralphenazone.

Clinical evidence

Five patients on long-term **warfarin** given dichloralphenazone 1.3 g each night for 30 days had a reduction of about 50% (range 20.2 to 68.5%) in plasma **warfarin** levels and a fall in the anticoagulant response during the last 14 days of concurrent use. Another patient given dichloralphenazone 1.3 g nightly for a month had a 70% fall in plasma **warfarin** levels and a thrombotest percentage rise from 9 to 55%. These values returned to normal when the hypnotic was withdrawn.[1,2]

Mechanism

The phenazone (antipyrine) component of the hypnotic is a potent liver enzyme inducing agent, which increases the metabolism and clearance of the warfarin, thereby reducing its effects.[1,2] The effects of the chloral appear to be minimal (see 'Anticoagulants + Cloral and derivatives', p.276).

Importance and management

Information is limited, but it appears to be an established and clinically important interaction, probably affecting most patients. The dosage of warfarin will need to be increased to accommodate this interaction. The 'benzodiazepines', (p.271) may be useful non-interacting alternatives to dichloralphenazone. If the dosage of warfarin has been disturbed by using dichloralphenazone, it may take up to a month for it to restabilise. There does not appear to be any information about other anticoagulants.

1. Breckenridge A, Orme ML'E, Thorgeirsson S, Davies DS, Brooks RV. Drug interaction with warfarin: studies with dichloralphenazone, chloral hydrate and phenazone (antipyrine). *Clin Sci* (1971) 40, 351–64.
2. Breckenridge A, Orme M. Clinical implications of enzyme induction. *Ann N Y Acad Sci* (1971) 179, 421–31.

Anticoagulants + Dipyridamole

Mild bleeding can sometimes occur if anticoagulants are given with dipyridamole, although prothrombin times remain stable and well within the therapeutic range.

Clinical evidence

Thirty patients with glomerulonephritis stabilised on either **warfarin** (28 patients) or **phenindione** (2 patients) showed no significant changes in prothrombin times when they were given dipyridamole in doses increased from 100 mg daily up to a maximum of 400 mg daily over about a month. Twelve to 19 days after starting dipyridamole, 3 patients with normal renal function developed mild bleeding (epistaxis, bruising, haematuria), which resolved when either drug was withdrawn or the dosage reduced.[1]

Another report states that prothrombin ratios remain unaltered when dipyridamole is given with **warfarin**, and claims that there is no risk of bleeding.[2] No bleeding problems were described in a study of the value of the combined use of warfarin and **dipyridamole** 300 mg daily in patients with heart valve replacements.[3]

Mechanism

Uncertain. A reduction in platelet adhesiveness or aggregation induced by the dipyridamole may have been responsible.[1]

Importance and management

Information seems to be very limited. Since bleeding can sometimes occur even when prothrombin values are within the therapeutic range, some caution is appropriate. Only warfarin and phenindione have been implicated, but it would be sensible to apply the same precautions with any anticoagulant.

1. Kalowski S, Kincaid-Smith P. Interaction of dipyridamole with anticoagulants in the treatment of glomerulonephritis. *Med J Aust* (1973) 2, 164–6.
2. Donaldson DR, Sreeharan N, Crow MJ, Rajah SM. Assessment of the interaction of warfarin with aspirin and dipyridamole. *Thromb Haemost* (1982) 47, 77.
3. Kawazoe K, Fujita T, Manabe H. Dipyridamole combined with anticoagulant in prevention of early postoperative thromboembolism after cardiac valve replacement. *Thromb Res* (1991) (Suppl 12), 27–33.

Anticoagulants + Disopyramide

The anticoagulant effects of warfarin are reduced to some extent by disopyramide in some patients, but there are two reports of patients who needed less warfarin while taking disopyramide.

Clinical evidence

(a) Reduced warfarin effects

A study in 10 patients with recent atrial fibrillation maintained on **warfarin** and with a British Corrected Ratio of 2 to 3, found that disopyramide increased the clearance of **warfarin** by 21%.[1] Another study found that 2 out of 3 patients needed a **warfarin** dosage increase of about 10% when they were given disopyramide 200 mg three times daily for atrial fibrillation.[2]

(b) Increased warfarin effects

A report describes a patient who, following a myocardial infarction, was given **warfarin** 3 mg daily and disopyramide 100 mg six-hourly with digoxin, furosemide and potassium supplements. When the disopyramide was withdrawn his **warfarin** requirements doubled over a nine-day period.[3] An increased response to **warfarin** has been seen in another patient given disopyramide.[4]

Mechanism

Unknown. One idea is that when the disopyramide controls fibrillation, changes occur in cardiac output and in the flow of blood through the liver, which might have an effect on the synthesis of the blood clotting factors.[2,5] But the discordant response in the two patients remains unexplained.

Importance and management

Very poorly documented and not established. The outcome of concurrent use is uncertain. Bear this interaction in mind in the case of an unexpected response to warfarin.

1. Woo KS, Chan K, Pun CO. The mechanisms of warfarin-disopyramide interaction. *Circulation* (1987) 76 (Suppl 4), IV-520.
2. Sylvén C, Anderson P. Evidence that disopyramide does not interact with warfarin. *BMJ* (1983) 286, 1181.
3. Haworth E, Burroughs AK. Disopyramide and warfarin interaction. *BMJ* (1977) 2, 866–7.
4. Marshall J. Personal communication, 1987.
5. Ryll C, Davis LJ. Warfarin-disopyramide interaction? *Drug Intell Clin Pharm* (1979) 13, 260.

Anticoagulants + Disulfiram

The anticoagulant effects of warfarin are increased by disulfiram.

Clinical evidence

Haemorrhage in a patient given **warfarin** and disulfiram prompted a study of this interaction.[1] Disulfiram 500 mg daily was given to 8 healthy subjects anticoagulated with **warfarin** for 21 days. The plasma **warfarin** levels of 7 of the subjects rose by an average of 20% and their prothrombin activity fell from about 34% to 24% of normal.[2]

Other experiments with single doses of **warfarin** confirm these results,[2] and the interaction has been described in another report.[3]

Mechanism

Not fully understood. The suggestion[2] that disulfiram inhibits the liver enzymes concerned with the metabolism of warfarin has not been confirmed by later studies.[4] It is now postulated[4] that disulfiram may chelate with the metal ions necessary for the production of active thrombin from prothrombin, thereby augmenting the actions of warfarin.

Importance and management

An established interaction, although direct information about patients is very limited. What is known suggests that most individuals will demonstrate this interaction. If concurrent use is thought appropriate, the effects of warfarin should be monitored and suitable dosage adjustments made when adding or withdrawing disulfiram. Care should be taken when starting warfarin in patients already on disulfiram, and consideration should be given to using a smaller loading dose.

1. Rothstein E. Warfarin effect enhanced by disulfiram. *JAMA* (1968) 206, 1574–5.
2. O'Reilly RA. Interaction of sodium warfarin and disulfiram (Antabuse®) in man. *Ann Intern Med* (1973) 78, 73–6.
3. Rothstein E. Warfarin effect enhanced by disulfiram (Antabuse). *JAMA* (1972) 221, 1052–3.
4. O'Reilly RA. Dynamic interaction between disulfiram and separated enantiomorphs of racemic warfarin. *Clin Pharmacol Ther* (1981) 29, 332–6.

Anticoagulants + Ditazole

Ditazole does not alter the anticoagulant effects of acenocoumarol.

Clinical evidence, mechanism, importance and management

Fifty patients with artificial heart valves taking **acenocoumarol** showed no changes in their prothrombin times while taking ditazole 800 mg daily.[1] No special precautions are needed. There seems to be no information about other anticoagulants.

1. Jacovella G, Milazzotto F. Ricerca di interazioni fra ditazolo e anticoagulanti in portatori di protesi valvolari intracardiache. *Clin Ter* (1977) 80, 425–31.

Anticoagulants + Diuretics

Bumetanide, chlortalidone, chlorothiazide, furosemide, torasemide and spironolactone have been shown either not to interact or to cause only a small reduction in the effects of the anticoagulants of minimal or no clinical importance, and in general diuretics don't appear to interact with anticoagulants. The possible exceptions are etacrynic acid and tienilic acid, which on rare occasions has caused a marked increase in the effects of warfarin.

Clinical evidence

(a) Bumetanide

A study in 10 healthy subjects showed that their response to a single 0.8-mg/kg dose of **warfarin** were unaffected by bumetanide 1 mg daily for 14 days.[1] This confirms a previous study in 5 healthy subjects given **warfarin** and bumetanide 2 mg daily.[2]

(b) Chlortalidone

Six healthy subjects given a single 1.5-mg/kg dose of **warfarin** showed reduced hypoprothrombinaemia (prothrombin activity reduced from 77 to 58 units) when they were also given chlortalidone 100 mg daily, although the plasma **warfarin** levels remained unaltered.[3] Similarly, reduced anticoagulant effects have been described when chlortalidone was given with **phenprocoumon**, but no significant effects were seen on the activity of **acenocoumarol**.[4]

(c) Chlorothiazide

A study in 8 healthy subjects given single 40 to 60-mg oral doses of **warfarin** and chlorothiazide 1 g daily showed that the mean half-life of the anticoagulant was increased from 39 to 44 hours but the prothrombin time was only decreased by 0.3 seconds.[5]

(d) Etacrynic acid

A case report describes a marked increase in the anticoagulant effects of **warfarin** in a woman with hypoalbuminaemia on two occasions when they were given 50 to 300 mg doses of etacrynic acid.[6] A therapeutically significant interaction between **warfarin** and etacrynic acid is reported elsewhere, but no details are given.[7]

(e) Furosemide

A study in 6 healthy subjects found that plasma levels, half-lives and prothrombin times in response to a 50-mg oral dose of **warfarin** were not significantly altered by the presence of furosemide 80 mg daily.[2] A 28% decrease in the INR of one patient on **warfarin** was seen when furosemide was given, attributed to volume depletion caused by the diuretic.[8] A pharmacokinetic study in 17 healthy subjects found that furosemide 40 mg twice daily had no effect on the pharmacokinetics of single 0.22-mg/kg oral doses of **phenprocoumon**.[9] Another study in 46 patients with congestive heart failure found that furosemide 40 mg or torasemide 20 mg daily for 8 days did not alter the anticoagulant effects of **phenprocoumon**.[10]

(f) Spironolactone

A study in 9 healthy subjects given a single 1.5-mg/kg dose of **warfarin** found that spironolactone 50 mg four times daily for 8 days reduced the prothrombin time (expressed as a percentage of the control activity with **warfarin** alone) from 100 to 76%. Plasma **warfarin** levels remained unchanged.[11]

(g) Tienilic acid

Two patients taking **ethyl biscoumacetate** began to bleed spontaneously (haematuria, ecchymoses of the legs and gastrointestinal bleeding) when they started to take tienilic acid 250 mg daily. The thrombotest percentage of one of them was found to have fallen by 10%.[12] Increased anticoagulant effects and/or bleeding, beginning within a few days, have been described in patients or subjects given tienilic acid while taking **ethyl biscoumacetate**,[13,14] **acenocoumarol**[15] or **warfarin**.[13,16,17]

(h) Torasemide

A study in 46 patients with congestive heart failure found that furosemide 40 mg or torasemide 20 mg daily for 8 days did not alter the anticoagulant effects of **phenprocoumon**.[10]

Mechanism

It has been suggested that the diuresis induced by chlortalidone, furosemide and spironolactone reduces plasma water, which leads to a concentration of the blood clotting factors.[3,8,11] Etacrynic acid can displace warfarin from its plasma protein binding sites,[18] and it was originally thought that other diuretics also interacted by drug displacement.[12,19,20] Only 3% of total plasma warfarin is in the free active form, thus a small displacement could result in marked enhancement of activity,[6] but it is almost certain that this, on its own, does not explain the interaction described.[7] Tienilic acid reduces the metabolism of *S*-warfarin (but not *R*-warfarin) thereby prolonging its stay in the body and increasing its effects.[17]

Importance and management

The documentation relating to diuretics in general (other than tienilic acid) is very limited and seems to be confined to the reports cited here, most of which are single dose studies. The evidence suggests that these diuretics either do not interact at all with the anticoagulants, or only to an extent which is of little clinical relevance. This is in general agreement with common experience. No special precautions normally seem to be necessary, except possibly with etacrynic acid where it might be prudent to monitor the outcome particularly in those with hypoalbuminaemia or renal impairment.

The anticoagulant/tienilic acid interaction is established and of clinical importance. The incidence is uncertain. Concurrent use should be avoided. If that is not possible, prothrombin times should be closely monitored and the anticoagulant dosage reduced as necessary. There seems to be no information about other anticoagulants not specifically cited here but it would be prudent to assume that they will interact with tienilic acid similarly. Tienilic acid has been withdrawn in many countries because of its hepatotoxicity.

1. Nipper H, Kirby S, Iber FL. The effect of bumetanide on the serum disappearance of warfarin sodium. *J Clin Pharmacol* (1981) 21, 654–6.
2. Nilsson CM, Horton ES, Robinson DS. The effect of furosemide and bumetanide on warfarin metabolism and anticoagulant response. *J Clin Pharmacol* (1978) 18, 91–4.
3. O'Reilly RA, Sahud MA, Aggeler PM. Impact of aspirin and chlorthalidone on the pharmacodynamics of oral anticoagulant drugs in man. *Ann N Y Acad Sci* (1971) 179, 173–86.
4. Vinazzer H. Die Beeinflussung der Antikoagulantientherapie durch ein Diuretikum. *Wien Z Inn Med* (1963) 44, 323–7.
5. Robinson DS, Sylwester D. Interaction of commonly prescribed drugs and warfarin. *Ann Intern Med* (1970) 72, 853–6.
6. Petrick RJ, Kronacher N, Alcena V. Interaction between warfarin and ethacrynic acid. *JAMA* (1975) 231, 843–4.
7. Koch-Weser J. Hemorrhagic reactions and drug interactions in 500 warfarin-treated patients. *Clin Pharmacol Ther* (1973) 14, 139.
8. Laizure SC, Madlock L, Cyr M, Self T. Decreased hypoprothrombinemic effect of warfarin associated with furosemide. *Ther Drug Monit* (1997) 19, 361–3.
9. Mönig H, Böhm M, Ohnhaus EE, Kirch W. The effects of frusemide and probenecid on the pharmacokinetics of phenprocoumon. *Eur J Clin Pharmacol* (1990) 39, 261–5.
10. Piesche L, Bölke T. Comparative clinical trial investigating possible interactions of torasemide (20 mg o.d.) or furosemide (40 mg o.d.) with phenprocoumon in patients with congestive heart failure. 4th International Congress on Diuretics, Boca Raton, Florida Oct 11–16th 1992. Eds. Puschett JB, Greenberg A. *Int Congr Ser 1023* (1993) 267–70.
11. O'Reilly RA. Spironolactone and warfarin interaction. *Clin Pharmacol Ther* (1980) 27, 198–201.
12. Detilleux M, Caquet R, Laroche C. Potentialisation de l'effet des anticoagulants comariniques par un nouveaux diurétique, l'acide tiénilique. *Nouv Presse Med* (1976) 5, 2395.
13. Prandota J, Pankow-Prandota L. Klinicznie znamienna interakcja nowego leku moczopednego kwasu tienylowego z lekami przeciwzakrzepowymi pochodnymi kumaryny. *Przegl Lek* (1982) 39, 385–8.
14. Portier H, Destaing F, Chauve L. Potentialisation de l'effet des anticoagulants coumariniques par l'acide tiénilique: une nouvelle observation. *Nouv Presse Med* (1977) 6, 468.
15. Grand A, Drouin B, Arche G-J. Potentialisation de l'action anticoagulante des anti-vitamines K par l'acide tiénilique. *Nouv Presse Med* (1977) 6, 2691.
16. McLain DA, Garriga FJ, Kantor OS. Adverse reactions associated with ticrynafen use. *JAMA* (1980) 243, 763–4.
17. O'Reilly RA. Ticrynafen-racemic warfarin interaction: hepatotoxic or stereoselective? *Clin Pharmacol Ther* (1982) 32, 356–61.
18. Sellers EM, Koch-Weser J. Kinetics and clinical importance of displacement of warfarin from albumin by acidic drugs. *Ann N Y Acad Sci* (1971) 179, 213–25.
19. Slattery JT, Levy G. Ticrynafen effect on warfarin protein binding in human serum. *J Pharm Sci* (1979) 68, 393.
20. Prandota J, Albengres E, Tillement JP. Effect of tienilic acid (Diflurex) on the binding of warfarin ^{14}C to human plasma proteins. *Int J Clin Pharmacol Ther Toxicol* (1980) 18, 158–62.

Anticoagulants + Dofetilide

The prothrombin time response to a single 40-mg dose of warfarin was found to be unchanged when given to 14 healthy subjects on day 5 of an 8-day course of dofetilide 750 micrograms twice daily.[1]

1. Nichols DJ, Dalrymple I, Newgreen MW, Kleinermans D. The effect of dofetilide on pharmacodynamics of warfarin and pharmacokinetics of digoxin. *Eur Heart J* (1999) 20 (Abstr Suppl), 586.

Anticoagulants + Ethchlorvynol

The anticoagulant effects of dicoumarol and warfarin are reduced by ethchlorvynol.

Clinical evidence

Six patients on **dicoumarol** showed a rise in their Quick index from 38 to 55% while taking ethchlorvynol 1 g daily over an 18-day period. One patient on **dicoumarol** became over-anticoagulated and developed haematuria on two occasions when the ethchlorvynol was withdrawn for periods of 6 days and 4 days.[1] A marked reduction in the anticoagulant effects of **warfarin** occurred in another patient given ethchlorvynol.[2]

Mechanism

Uncertain. The idea that ethchlorvynol increases the metabolism of the anticoagulants by the liver has not been confirmed by studies in *dogs* and *rats*.[3]

Importance and management

Information is very sparse and limited to dicoumarol and warfarin, but the interaction seems to be established. Be alert for other coumarins to behave similarly. Anticipate the need to alter the anticoagulant dosage if ethchlorvynol is started or stopped. The benzodiazepines may be a useful non-interacting alternative, see 'Anticoagulants + Benzodiazepines or related drugs', p.271.

1. Johansson S-A. Apparent resistance to oral anticoagulant therapy and influence of hypnotics on some coagulation factors. *Acta Med Scand* (1968) 184, 297–300.
2. Cullen SI and Catalano PM. Griseofulvin-warfarin antagonism. *JAMA* (1967) 199, 582–3.
3. Martin YC. The effect of ethchlorvynol on the drug-metabolizing enzymes of rats and dogs. *Biochem Pharmacol* (1967) 16, 2041–4.

Anticoagulants + Ezetimibe

No clinically significant interaction appears to occur between ezetimibe and warfarin.

Clinical evidence, mechanism, importance and management

In a two-way crossover study 12 healthy subjects were given ezetimibe 10 mg or placebo daily for 11 days, with a single 25-mg dose of **warfarin** on day 7. The pharmacokinetics and pharmacodynamics (prothrombin time) of **warfarin** were not significantly altered by ezetimibe. In addition, the pharmacokinetics of ezetimibe were similar to those previously seen with the drug alone.[1] No additional precautions therefore seem necessary on concurrent use.

1. Bauer KS, Kosoglou T, Statkevich P, Calzetta A, Maxwell SE, Patrick JE, Batra V. Ezetimibe does not affect the pharmacokinetics or pharmacodynamics of warfarin. *Clin Pharmacol Ther* (2001) 69, P5.

Anticoagulants + Felbamate

An isolated case report describes a marked increase in the effects of warfarin, which were attributed to felbamate.

Clinical evidence, mechanism, importance and management

A 62-year-old man with a seizure disorder who was receiving **warfarin** had his antiepileptic treatment with carbamazepine, phenobarbital and sodium valproate discontinued and replaced by felbamate 2.4 g daily and later 3.2 g daily. Within 14 days his INR had risen from a normal range of 2.5 to 3.5 up to 7.8. After stopping and later restarting the **warfarin** his INR rose within about another 14 days to 18.2. He was eventually restabilised on about half his former **warfarin** dosage. The authors of the report suggest that the withdrawal of the carbamazepine and phenobarbital was an unlikely reason for this reaction because no increases in **warfarin** dosage had been needed when they were started. Suspicion therefore falls on the felbamate, but it is clearly difficult to be sure that the withdrawal of the anticonvulsants did not have some part to play. Just why felbamate should interact like this is not known, but it is suggested that it inhibits the metabolism of the **warfarin**.[1] A letter commenting on this report favours the idea that what occurred was in fact due to the withdrawal of the carbamazepine and phenobarbital.[2]

The general importance of this interaction (if such it is) is uncertain, but it would seem prudent be aware of this interaction if felbamate is started or stopped in any patient, being alert for the need to adjust the **warfarin** dosage. More study is needed.

1. Tisdel KA, Israel DS, Kolb KW. Warfarin-felbamate interaction: first report. *Ann Pharmacother* (1994) 28, 805.
2. Glue P, Banfield CR, Colucci RD, Perhach JL. Comment: warfarin-felbamate interaction. *Ann Pharmacother* (1994) 28, 1412–13.

Anticoagulants + Fenyramidol

The anticoagulant effects of warfarin, dicoumarol and phenindione are increased by fenyramidol and bleeding has been seen.

Clinical evidence

Two patients on **warfarin** showed a marked increase in their prothrombin times when given fenyramidol 400 mg two to four times daily. One of them bled. Further study on 8 other patients taking **warfarin**, **dicoumarol**, or **phenindione** showed that a marked increase in their prothrombin times occurred within 3 to 7 days of starting to take fenyramidol 0.8 to 1.6 g daily. No marked change occurred in a patient on **phenprocoumon**, but he only took the fenyramidol for three days.[1]

Mechanism

Studies in man, *mice* and *rabbits* suggest that fenyramidol inhibits the metabolism of dicoumarol so that it is cleared from the body more slowly and its effects are thereby increased and prolonged.[2]

Importance and management

An established interaction although the documentation is very limited. Monitor prothrombin times and reduce the anticoagulant dosage as necessary to avoid bleeding. Anticoagulants other than those cited may be expected to behave similarly. The failure to demonstrate an interaction with phenprocoumon may have been because the fenyramidol was given for such a short time.

1. Carter SA. Potentiation of the effect of orally administered anticoagulants by phenyramidol hydrochloride. *N Engl J Med* (1965) 273, 423–6.
2. Solomon HM, Schrogie JJ. The effect of phenyramidol on the metabolism of bishydroxycoumarin. *J Pharmacol Exp Ther* (1966) 154, 660–6.

Anticoagulants + Fibrates

The fibrates increase the effects of oral anticoagulants. This has been reported with: bezafibrate and acenocoumarol, phenprocoumon or warfarin; ciprofibrate and warfarin; clofibrate and dicoumarol, phenindione or warfarin; fenofibrate and acenocoumarol or warfarin, and with gemfibrozil and warfarin. There have been fatalities.

Clinical evidence

(a) Bezafibrate

A study in 15 patients with hyperlipidaemia on **phenprocoumon** found that it was necessary to reduce the anticoagulant dosage by 20% when they were given bezafibrate 450 mg daily, and by 33% when they were given bezafibrate 600 mg daily.[1] In another study in 22 patients taking bezafibrate 400 mg daily the dosage of **acenocoumarol** had to be reduced by 20% to maintain a constant INR.[2] Severe hypoprothrombinaemia and gastrointestinal bleeding occurred in a patient (with hypoalbuminaemia due to nephrotic syndrome and chronic renal failure) on **acenocoumarol** when bezafibrate was added.[3] A woman had an increased response to **warfarin** while she was taking bezafibrate, and a man had a reduced response to **warfarin** when he stopped taking bezafibrate.[4]

(b) Ciprofibrate

In a two-way randomised placebo-controlled crossover study 12 young healthy men were given a single 25-mg dose of racemic **warfarin** on day 21 of a 26-day course of ciprofibrate 100 mg daily. The ciprofibrate increased the anticoagulant response to warfarin by 50% and caused a 28% decrease in the apparent intrinsic clearance of ***(S)*-warfarin**, which is the more active enantiomer.[5]

(c) Clofibrate

A study in three hospitals, of 47 patients taking either **phenindione** or **warfarin**, showed that when they were given clofibrate it was necessary to reduce the dosages of the anticoagulants. Nine out of 14 in Belfast needed a 30% reduction and 14 out of 18 in Johannesburg also needed a reduction. Ten out of 15 in Edinburgh needed a 33% reduction and 5 of them bled.[6]

This interaction has been confirmed in other studies in considerable numbers of patients anticoagulated with **warfarin**,[7-12] **phenindione**[13-15] or **dicoumarol**.[16] Bleeding has been described frequently, and death due to haemorrhage has occurred in at least two cases.[10,15]

(d) Fenofibrate

Two patients on **acenocoumarol** needed a 30% reduction in their dosage to maintain the same prothrombin time when they were given fenofibrate 200 mg in the morning and 100 mg in the evening.[17]

A patient on **warfarin** showed a rise in his INR to 8.5 (from a previous range of 2 to 2.5) within a week of starting to take fenofibrate 200 mg daily. His INR later restabilised when the **warfarin** dosage was reduced by 27%. Another patient on **warfarin** similarly showed a marked INR rise from a range of 2.8 to 3.5 up to 5.6 within 10 days of starting to take fenofibrate [dosage not stated].[18] Six patients taking unnamed **coumarins** needed an average dosage reduction of 12% (range 0 to 21%) when treated with fenofibrate.[19] Yet another patient on **warfarin** bled, and was found to have an INR of 18 when his gemfibrozil was replaced by fenofibrate.[20] In another study it was found that fenofibrate increased the effects of unnamed anticoagulants in 4 patients by about one-third.[21] A patient on an unnamed anticoagulant developed haematuria when treated with fenofibrate.[22]

(e) Gemfibrozil

A brief report describes bleeding ('menstrual cycle prolonged and lots of blood clots') and much higher prothrombin times [values not given] two weeks after a woman on **warfarin** started to take gemfibrozil 1200 mg daily in divided doses. Halving the **warfarin** dosage resolved the problem.[23] A patient stabilised on **warfarin** developed severe hypoprothrombinaemia and bleeding 4 weeks after starting gemfibrozil.[24]

Mechanism

Uncertain. Clofibrate can displace warfarin from its plasma protein binding sites,[5,25-27] but this does not adequately explain the interaction. Another suggestion is that the fibrates increase the affinity of the anticoagulant for the receptor sites or possibly alter their metabolism.[1,5,16]

Importance and management

The interactions of clofibrate with dicoumarol, phenindione and warfarin are established, clinically important and potentially serious. Severe bleeding (fatal in some instances) has been seen. The incidence of the interaction is reported to be between 20 and 100%,[7] but it would be prudent to assume that all patients will be affected. Dosage reductions of one-third to one-half may be needed to avoid the risk of bleeding. Monitor the INR and adjust the dose accordingly. Information about other oral anticoagulants is lacking but it would be prudent to assume that they will interact with clofibrate in a similar way.

Less is known about fenofibrate and even less about bezafibrate, ciprofibrate and gemfibrozil but it would be prudent to follow the same precautions suggested for ciprofibrate if any of them is used with any oral anticoagulant.

1. Zimmermann R, Ehlers W, Walter E, Hoffrichter A, Lang PD, Andrassy K, Schlierf G. The effect of bezafibrate on the fibrinolytic enzyme system and the drug interaction with racemic phenprocoumon. *Atherosclerosis* (1978) 29, 477–85.
2. Manotti C, Quintavalla R, Pini M, Tomasini G, Vargiu G, Dettori AG. Interazione farmacologica tra bezafibrato in formulazione retard ed acenocoumarolo. Studio clinico. *G Arterioscler* (1991) 16, 49–52.
3. Blum A, Seligmann H, Livneh A, Ezra D. Severe gastrointestinal bleeding induced by a probable hydroxycoumarin-bezafibrate interaction. *Isr J Med Sci* (1992) 28, 47–9.
4. Beringer TRO. Warfarin potentiation with bezafibrate. *Postgrad Med J* (1997) 73, 657–8.
5. Sanofi Withrop Ltd. Personal communication, December 1997.
6. Oliver MF, Roberts SD, Hayes D, Pantridge JF, Suzman MM, Bersohn I. Effect of Atromid and ethyl chlorophenoxyisobutyrate on anticoagulant requirements. *Lancet* (1963) i, 143–4.
7. Udall JA. Drug interference with warfarin therapy. *Clin Med* (1970) 77, 20–5.
8. Eastham RD. Warfarin dosage, clofibrate, and age of patient. *BMJ* (1973) ii, 554.
9. Roberts SD, Pantridge JF. Effect of Atromid on requirements of warfarin. *J Atheroscler Res* (1963) 3, 655–7.
10. Solomon RB, Rosner F. Massive hemorrhage and death during treatment with clofibrate and warfarin. *N Y State J Med* (1973) 73, 2002.
11. Bjornsson TD, Meffin PJ, Blaschke TF. Interaction of clofibrate with the optical enantiomorphs of warfarin. *Pharmacologist* (1976) 18, 207.
12. Counihan TB, Keelan P. Atromid in high cholesterol states. *J Atheroscler Res* (1963) 3, 580–3.
13. Williams GEO, Meynell MJ, Gaddie R. Atromid and anticoagulant therapy. *J Atheroscler Res* (1963) 3, 658–70.
14. Rogen AS, Ferguson JC. Clinical observations on patients treated with Atromid and anticoagulants. *J Atheroscler Res* (1963) 3, 671–6.
15. Rogen AS, Ferguson JC. Effect of Atromid on anticoagulant requirements. *Lancet* (1963) i, 272.
16. Schrogie JJ, Solomon HM. The anticoagulant response to bishydroxycoumarin. II. The effect of d-thyroxine, clofibrate, and norethandrolone. *Clin Pharmacol Ther* (1967) 8, 70–7.
17. Harvengt C, Heller F, Desager JP. Hypolipidemic and hypouricemic action of fenofibrate in various types of hyperlipoproteinemias. *Artery* (1980) 7, 73–82.
18. Ascah KJ, Rock GA, Wells PS. Interaction between fenofibrate and warfarin. *Ann Pharmacother* (1998) 32, 765–8.
19. Stähelin HB, Seiler W, Pult N. Erfahrungen mit dem Lipidsenker Procetofen (Lipanthyl®). *Schweiz Rundsch Med Prax* (1979) 68, 24–8.
20. Aldridge MA, Ito MK. Fenofibrate and warfarin interaction. *Pharmacotherapy* (2001) 21, 886–9.
21. Raynaud P. Un nouvel hypolipidemiant: le procetofene. *Rev Med Tours* (1977) 11, 325–30.
22. Lauwers PL. Effect of procetofene on blood lipids of subjects with essential hyperlipidaemia. *Curr Ther Res* (1979) 26, 30–8.
23. Ahmad S. Gemfibrozil interaction with warfarin sodium (Coumadin). *Chest* (1990) 98, 1041–2.
24. Rindone JP, Keng HC. Gemfibrozil-warfarin interaction resulting in profound hypoprothrombinemia. *Chest* (1998) 114, 641–2.
25. Solomon HM, Schrogie JJ, Williams D. The displacement of phenylbutazone-C^{14} and warfarin-C^{14} from human albumin by various drugs and fatty acids. *Biochem Pharmacol* (1968) 17, 143–51.
26. Solomon HM, Schrogie JJ. The effect of various drugs on the binding of warfarin-^{14}C to human albumin. *Biochem Pharmacol* (1967) 16, 1219–26.
27. Bjornsson TD, Meffin PJ, Swezey S, Blaschke TF. Clofibrate displaces warfarin from plasma proteins in man: an example of a pure displacement interaction. *J Pharmacol Exp Ther* (1979) 210, 316–21.

Anticoagulants + Fish oils

The makers of *Omacor* (omega-3-acid ethyl esters) say that because high-dose treatment (4 capsules daily) causes a moderate increase in bleeding time, patients on anticoagulant therapy should be monitored, and the dose of anticoagulant adjusted as necessary.[1]

1. Omacor (Omega-3-acid ethyl esters). Solvay Healthcare Ltd. UK Summary of product characteristics, March 2004.

Anticoagulants + Flupirtine

Flupirtine does not interact with phenprocoumon.

Clinical evidence, mechanism, importance and management

Twelve healthy subjects showed no significant changes in the plasma levels of **phenprocoumon** 1.5 mg daily when they were given flupirtine 100 mg three times daily for 14 days. The prothrombin times were also not significantly changed.[1] There would therefore seem to be no reason for taking special precautions if these drugs are given concurrently. Information about other oral anticoagulants seems to be lacking.

1. Harder S, Thürmann P, Hermann R, Weller S, Mayer M. Effects of flupirtine coadministration on phenprocoumon plasma concentrations and prothrombin time. *Int J Clin Pharmacol Ther* (1994) 32, 577–581.

Anticoagulants + Flutamide

Flutamide can increase the anticoagulant effects of warfarin.

Clinical evidence

Five patients with prostatic cancer receiving **warfarin** showed increases in their prothrombin times when given flutamide. For example, one patient needed reductions in his **warfarin** dosage from 35 to 22.5 mg weekly over a 2-month period. Another showed a prothrombin time rise from 15 to 37 seconds within 4 days of starting flutamide 750 mg daily.[1]

Information is very limited but the interaction would seem to be established. Monitor prothrombin times if flutamide is given to patients on **warfarin**, reducing the dosage when necessary. Nothing seems to be known about the effects on other anticoagulants.

1. Schering-Plough Ltd. Personal communication, March 1990.

Anticoagulants + Food or Drinks

The rate of absorption of dicoumarol can be increased by food. Grapefruit juice is reported not to affect acenocoumarol but it may possibly cause a modest INR rise in a few individuals on warfarin. Two reports describe antagonism of the effects of warfarin by ice-cream, and another report attributes an increase in prothrombin time to the use of aspartame. Avocado, soybean protein and soybean oil and other intravenous lipids may also reduce the effects of warfarin. See also 'Anticoagulants + Alcohol', p.257, and 'Anticoagulants + Natto', p.294. Foods known to interact due to their vitamin K content are discussed in 'Anticoagulants + Vitamin K', p.321.

Clinical evidence

(a) Grapefruit juice

No clinically important interaction was detected when 12 healthy subjects were given a single 10-mg oral dose of **acenocoumarol** and 150 ml of grapefruit juice or placebo.[1,2] Another two-way crossover study in 24 patients found that while taking 250 ml of grapefruit juice over a 4-week period the frequency of the **warfarin** dosage adjustments needed by the group as a whole was the same as when taking the placebo (orange juice), but 4 individuals showed a clinically significant, progressive and sustained 12 to 25% decrease in the **warfarin** dose/INR ratio.[3]

(b) Foods

(i) Dicoumarol. A study in 10 healthy subjects showed that the peak serum concentrations of a single 250-mg dose of dicoumarol, were increased on average by 85% by food. Two subjects showed increases of 242 and 206%.[4]

(ii) Warfarin. A very brief report states that a patient on warfarin had a raised prothrombin time, possibly due to the use of **aspartame**.[5] Two women on warfarin had falls in their INRs (from 2.5 to 1.7 and from 2.7 to 1.6 respectively) when they started to eat **avocado** 100 g daily, or 200 g of **avocado** on two consecutive days. Their INRs climbed again when the **avocado** was stopped.[6]

A woman taking warfarin 22.5 mg daily did not have the expected prolongation of her prothrombin times. It was then discovered that she took the warfarin in the evening and she always ate **ice cream** before going to bed. When the warfarin was taken in the mornings, the prothrombin times increased.[7] Another patient's warfarin requirements almost doubled when she started to eat very large quantities of **ice cream** (1 litre each evening). The effect was not seen when she ate normal amounts of **ice cream**. She took the warfarin at 6 pm and the **ice cream** at about 10 pm.[8]

A study in 10 patients with hypercholesterolaemia found that two weeks' treatment with a **soy-protein** cholesterol-lowering diet caused a marked reduction (Quick time increase of 114%) in the anticoagulant effects of warfarin.[9] 'Warfarin resistance' was seen in two other patients, one when given a constant intravenous infusion of **soybean oil emulsion** (*Intralipid*),[10] and the other when given an emulsified infusion of propofol containing 10% **soybean oil**, and later when given 20% *Liposyn II*.[11]

Mechanism

Not understood. One suggestion for the interaction between food and dicoumarol[4] is that food may cause prolonged retention of dicoumarol in the upper part of the gut, leading to increased tablet dissolution and increased absorption. Soy protein possibly increases the activity of vitamin K at its liver receptors, thereby reducing the effects of warfarin. Avocado contains too little vitamin K (8 micrograms/100 g) for it to affect warfarin by competitive inhibition. The patients who showed some evidence of an interaction between grapefruit juice and warfarin may possibly have had an increased susceptibility to the inhibitory effects of grapefruit juice on the activity of the cytochrome P450 isoenzyme CYP3A4 in the gut.[3]

Importance and management

None of these interactions is very well documented but they clearly demonstrate that some foods and drinks, and particularly intravenous lipid preparations, can affect the response to the oral anticoagulants and may account for the otherwise unexplained fluctuations or changes in the anticoagulant response which some patients show. There is not enough evidence to suggest that any of these foods, drinks or preparations should be avoided unless serious problems develop.

1. van Rooij J, van der Meer FJM, Schoemaker HC, Cohen AF. Comparison of the effect of grapefruit juice and cimetidine on pharmacokinetics and anticoagulant effect of a single dose of acenocoumarol. *Br J Clin Pharmacol* (1993) 35, 548P.
2. van der Meer FJM. Personal communication, April 1994.
3. Dresser GK, Munoz C, Cruikshank M, Kovacs M, Spence JD. Grapefruit juice-warfarin interaction in anticoagulated patients. *Clin Pharmacol Ther* (1999) 65, 193.
4. Melander A, Wåhlin E. Enhancement of dicoumarol bioavailability by concomitant food intake. *Eur J Clin Pharmacol* (1978) 14, 441–4.
5. Beeley L, Beadle F, Lawrence R. *Bulletin of the West Midlands Centre for Adverse Drug Reaction Reporting* (1984) 19, 9.
6. Blickstein D, Shaklai M, Inbal A. Warfarin antagonism by avocado. *Lancet* (1991) 337, 914–15.
7. Simon LS, Likes KE. Hypoprothrombinemic response due to ice cream. *Drug Intell Clin Pharm* (1978) 12, 121–2.
8. Blackshaw CA, Watson VA. Interaction between warfarin and ice cream. *Pharm J* (1990) 244, 318.
9. Gaddi A, Sangiorgi Z, Ciarrocchi A, Braiato A, Descovich GC. Hypocholesterolemic soy protein diet and resistance to warfarin therapy. *Curr Ther Res* (1989) 45, 1006–10.
10. Lutomski DM, Palascak JE, Bower RH. Warfarin resistance associated with intravenous lipid administration. *J Parenter Enteral Nutr* (1987) 11, 316–18.
11. MacLaren R, Wachsman BA, Swift DK, Kuhl DA. Warfarin resistance associated with intravenous lipid administration: discussion of propofol and review of the literature. *Pharmacotherapy* (1997) 17, 1331–7.

Anticoagulants + Glucagon

The anticoagulant effects of warfarin are rapidly and markedly increased by glucagon in large doses, and bleeding can occur.

Clinical evidence

Eight out of 9 patients on **warfarin** showed a marked increase in its anticoagulant effects (prothrombin times of 30 to 50 seconds or more) when they were given glucagon 62 to 362 mg over 3 to 8 days. Three of them bled. This interaction did not occur in 11 other patients given a total of less than 30 mg of glucagon over 1 to 2 days.[1]

Mechanism

Unknown. Changes in the production of blood clotting factors and an increase in the affinity of warfarin for its site of action have been proposed.[1] A study in *guinea pigs* using acenocoumarol suggested that changes in warfarin metabolism or its absorption from the gut are not responsible.[2]

Importance and management

This appears to be an established interaction of clinical importance, although direct information is limited to the report cited.[1] Its authors recommend that if glucagon 25 mg per day or more is given for two or more days, the dosage of warfarin should be reduced in anticipation of the interaction, and prothrombin times closely monitored.[1] Information about other anticoagulants is lacking, but it would be prudent to assume that all coumarins will interact similarly.

1. Koch-Weser J. Potentiation by glucagon of the hypoprothrombinemic action of warfarin. *Ann Intern Med* (1970) 72, 331—5.
2. Weiner M, Moses D. The effect of glucagon and insulin on the prothrombin response to coumarin anticoagulants. *Proc Soc Exp Biol Med* (1968) 127, 761–3.

Anticoagulants + Glucosamine ± Chondroitin

A couple of reports suggest that glucosamine with or without chondroitin may increase the INR in patients on warfarin. In contrast, one case of a decreased INR has been reported with glucosamine and acenocoumarol.

Clinical evidence, mechanism, importance and management

A 69-year-old man stabilised on **warfarin** 47.5 mg weekly had an increase in his INR from 2.58 to 4.52 four weeks after starting to take 6 capsules of *Cosamin DS* (glucosamine hydrochloride 500 mg, sodium chondroitin sulfate 400 mg, manganese ascorbate per capsule) daily. His **warfarin** dose was reduced to 40 mg weekly, and his INR returned to the target range of 2 to 3 (INR 2.15) with continued *Cosamin DS* therapy.[1] A comment on this report noted that this is twice the usual dose of glucosamine.[2] The Canadian Adverse Drug Reaction Monitoring Program (CADRMP) briefly reported that an increase in INR had been noted when glucosamine was given to patients on **warfarin**, and that INR values decreased when glucosamine was stopped.[3]

In contrast, a 71-year-old stabilised on **acenocoumarol** 15 mg weekly had a decrease in his INR to 1.6 after taking glucosamine sulfate (*Xicil*) 1500 mg daily for 10 days. The glucosamine was stopped and the INR reached 2.1. When the glucosamine was restarted with an increase in **acenocoumarol** dose to 17 mg weekly, the INR only reached 1.9. The glucosamine was eventually stopped.[4]

There do not appear to have been any controlled studies of the pharmacodynamic or pharmacokinetic effects of glucosamine supplements on oral anticoagulants. The cases described suggest it would be prudent to monitor the INR more closely if glucosamine is started. If a patient shows an unexpected change in INR, bear in mind the possibility of self-medication with supplements such as glucosamine.

1. Rozenfeld V, Crain JL, Callahan AK. Possible augmentation of warfarin effect by glucosamine–chondroitin. *Am J Health-Syst Pharm* (2004) 61, 306–7.
2. Scott GN. Interaction of warfarin with glucosamine—chondroitin. *Am J Health-Syst Pharm* (2004) 61, 1186.
3. Canadian Adverse Drug Reaction Monitoring Program. Communiqué. Warfarin and glucosamine: interaction. *Can Adverse Drug React News* (2001) 11 (Apr), 8.
4. Garrote García M, Iglesias Piñeiro MJ, Martín Álvarez R, Pérez González J. Interacción farmacológica del sulfato de glucosamina con acenocumarol. *Aten Primaria* (2004) 33, 162–4.

Anticoagulants + Glutethimide

The anticoagulant effects of warfarin and ethyl biscoumacetate can be decreased by glutethimide.

Clinical evidence

Ten subjects on **warfarin**, with average prothrombin times of 18.8 seconds, had a mean reduction of 2.7 seconds in their prothrombin times after they took glutethimide 500 mg daily for 4 weeks.[1] Similar results are published elsewhere by the same author.[2] Other studies have shown that up to 1 g of glutethimide daily for 1 to 3 weeks reduces the half-life of **warfarin** by between one-third to one-half.[3,4] An unexplained report describes a paradoxical increase in prothrombin times and haemorrhage in a patient on **warfarin** who took 3.5 g of glutethimide over a 5-day period.[5]

Glutethimide 500 or 750 mg daily for 10 days has been shown to reduce the half-life of **ethyl biscoumacetate** by about one-third,[6,7] whereas in contrast, an early study in 25 patients on **ethyl biscoumacetate** found no evidence of an interaction.[8]

Mechanism

Glutethimide is a liver enzyme inducing agent, which increases the metabolism and clearance of the anticoagulants from the body, thereby reducing their effects.[1-4,6,7] There is no obvious explanation for the reports finding no interaction or increased effects.

Importance and management

The interaction of glutethimide with warfarin is established, while the interaction with ethyl biscoumacetate is uncertain. Information about both interactions is limited and there seems to be nothing documented about any other anticoagulant. However, it would be prudent to monitor the effect of adding glutethimide to patients taking any oral anticoagulant, being alert for the need to increase the anticoagulant dosage. Other interactions due to enzyme induction can take several weeks to develop fully and persist after withdrawal, so good monitoring and dosage adjustment should continue until anticoagulant stability has been achieved. The benzodiazepines may be a useful non-interacting alternative, see 'Anticoagulants + Benzodiazepines or related drugs', p.271.

1. Udall JA. Clinical implications of warfarin interactions with five sedatives. *Am J Cardiol* (1975) 35, 67–71.
2. Udall JA. Warfarin interactions with chloral hydrate and glutethimide. *Curr Ther Res* (1975) 17, 67–74.
3. Corn M. Effect of phenobarbital and glutethimide on biological half-life of warfarin. *Thromb Diath Haemorrh* (1966) 16, 606–12.
4. MacDonald MG, Robinson DS, Sylwester D, Jaffe JJ. The effects of phenobarbital, chloral betaine, and glutethimide administration on warfarin plasma levels and hypoprothrombinemic responses in man. *Clin Pharmacol Ther* (1969) 10, 80–4.
5. Taylor PJ. Hemorrhage while on anticoagulant therapy precipitated by drug interaction. *Ariz Med* (1967) 24, 697–9.
6. van Dam FE, Gribnau-Overkamp MJH. The effect of some sedatives (phenobarbital, glutethimide, chlordiazepoxide, chloral hydrate) on the rate of disappearance of ethyl biscoumacetate from the plasma. *Folia Med Neerl* (1967) 10, 141–5.
7. van Dam FE, Overkamp M, Haanen C. The interaction of drugs. *Lancet* (1966) ii, 1027.
8. Grilli H. Glutethimida y tiempo de protrombina. Su aplicación en la terapéutica anticoagulante. *Prensa Med Argent* (1959) 46, 2867–9.

Anticoagulants + Griseofulvin

The anticoagulant effects of warfarin can be reduced by griseofulvin in some but not all patients.

Clinical evidence

The anticoagulant effects of **warfarin** were markedly reduced in both of 2 patients and in 1 of 2 healthy individuals when they were given griseofulvin 1 to 2 g daily in divided doses. The other healthy subject showed no interaction, even when the griseofulvin dosage was raised to 4 g daily for 2 weeks.[1]

In another study[2] only 4 out of 10 patients on **warfarin** had decreased anticoagulant effects after taking griseofulvin 1 g daily in divided doses for 2 weeks.[2] The average reduction in prothrombin time was 4.2 seconds. A very brief report describes a coagulation defect in a patient on **warfarin** and griseofulvin.[3] Yet another report describes decreased anticoagulant effects in a man, which took 12 weeks to develop fully.[4] He eventually needed a 41% increase in his daily dose of **warfarin**.

Mechanism

Not understood. It has been suggested that the griseofulvin acts as a liver enzyme inducer, which increases the metabolism of the warfarin, thereby reducing its effects.[1,4]

Importance and management

An established interaction but not well documented. It affects some but not all patients. Because of its unpredictability, the prothrombin times of all patients on warfarin who are given griseofulvin should be monitored, and suitable warfarin dosage increases made as necessary. Information about other anticoagulants is lacking.

1. Cullen SI, Catalano PM. Griseofulvin-warfarin antagonism. *JAMA* (1967) 199, 582–3.
2. Udall JA. Drug interference with warfarin therapy. *Clin Med* (1970) 77, 20–5.
3. McQueen EG. New Zealand Committee on Adverse Drug Reactions: 14th Annual Report 1979. *N Z Med J* (1980) 91, 226–9.
4. Okino K, Weibert RT. Warfarin-griseofulvin interaction. *Drug Intell Clin Pharm* (1986) 20, 291–3.

Anticoagulants + H_2-blockers

The anticoagulant effects of warfarin can be increased by cimetidine. Severe bleeding has occurred in a few patients but some show no interaction at all. Acenocoumarol and phenindione seem to interact similarly but phenprocoumon appears not to be affected. Famotidine, nizatidine, ranitidine and roxatidine normally appear to be non-interacting alternative H_2-blockers but bleeding has been reported in a handful of cases.

Clinical evidence

(a) Cimetidine

A very brief report in 1978, published as a letter by the makers of cimetidine, stated that at that time they were aware of 17 cases worldwide, indicating that cimetidine 1 g daily could cause a prothrombin time rise of about 20% in those stabilised on **warfarin**.[1]

A number of studies and case reports have confirmed this interaction with **warfarin**.[2-9] Plasma **warfarin** levels are reported to rise by 25 to 80%, and prothrombin times can be increased by more than 30 seconds. Severe bleeding (haematuria, internal haemorrhages) and very prolonged prothrombin times have been seen in few patients.[2,4,6,7,9] However, one study found that only 7 out of 14 patients actually demonstrated this interaction,[10] and another study in 27 patients found that although the AUC of **warfarin** was increased by 21 to 39% and the clearance fell by 22 to 28%, prothrombin times only increased by 2 to 2.6 seconds.[11] A pharmacokinetic study in 6 healthy subjects found that cimetidine did not affect

***(S)*-warfarin** but increased the plasma levels of ***(R)*-warfarin**, but the overall clinical effect was minimal.[12] **Acenocoumarol**[13] and **phenindione**[3] appear to interact with cimetidine like **warfarin**, but **phenprocoumon** does not seem to interact.[14]

(b) Famotidine

A study in 8 healthy subjects taking doses of **warfarin** titrated to prolong the prothrombin time by 2 to 5 seconds (mean dose 4 mg daily) showed that 7 days' treatment with famotidine 40 mg did not affect prothrombin times, thrombotest coagulation times or steady-state plasma **warfarin** levels.[15] No changes in prothrombin times were seen in 3 patients on **acenocoumarol** or **fluindione** when they were given famotidine.[16] However, in another report 2 patients on **warfarin** are said to have had prolonged prothrombin times and bled when they took famotidine.[17]

(c) Nizatidine

Nizatidine 300 mg daily for 2 weeks had no significant effect on the prothrombin times, kaolin-cephalin clotting times, the activity of factors II, VII, XI and X, or on their steady-state serum **warfarin** levels in 7 healthy subjects on warfarin.[18] This lack of an effect of nizatidine is consistent with its lack of enzyme inhibitory activity, and thus its similarity to ranitidine rather than cimetidine.[19] No particular precautions appear to be necessary during concurrent use, although an isolated case of bleeding, associated with markedly prolonged prothrombin times, has been seen.[17]

(d) Ranitidine

Ranitidine 200 mg twice daily for 2 weeks had no effect on **warfarin** concentrations or on prothrombin times in 5 healthy subjects.[20] In another study in 11 healthy subjects it was found that ranitidine 150 mg twice daily for 3 days had no effect on the pharmacodynamics or pharmacokinetics of a single dose of **warfarin**.[8] In contrast, a third study in 5 subjects reported that ranitidine 150 mg twice daily for a week reduced the clearance of a single dose of **warfarin** by almost 30%, but the half-life was not significantly changed and prothrombin times were not measured.[21] Ranitidine 750 mg daily given to 2 subjects was reported to have reduced the **warfarin** clearance by more than 50%.[21] A number of aspects of this last study are open to question and the clinical relevance of the results is doubtful.[22] In an isolated case ranitidine 300 mg twice daily, but not 150 mg twice daily, appeared to have been the cause of hypoprothrombinaemia and bleeding in a patient on **warfarin**.[23]

(e) Roxatidine

Roxatidine 150 mg daily for 4 days had no effect on the pharmacokinetics of **warfarin** or the prothrombin ratio in 12 healthy subjects.[24]

Mechanism

Cimetidine binds with the cytochrome P450 isoenzymes and inhibits oxidative metabolism in the liver. Although cimetidine is considered to be a general inhibitor, it exhibits a degree of specificity for certain isoenzymes such as CYP1A2 and CYP2C19. Thus cimetidine can inhibit the liver enzymes concerned with the metabolism (phase one hydroxylation) and clearance of warfarin, which results in prolonged and increased effects.[25] This also appears to be true for acenocoumarol and phenindione, but not phenprocoumon, which is metabolised by different enzymes using another biochemical pathway (phase two glucuronidation).[14] The warfarin/cimetidine interaction has been found to be stereoselective, that is to say the cimetidine interacts with the *(R)*-isomer but not with the *(S)*-isomer.[12,26-28] The other H_2-blockers normally do not act as enzyme inhibitors.

Importance and management

The interaction between warfarin and cimetidine is well documented, well established and clinically important but for reasons that are not understood many patients (probably up to 50% or even more) may not develop this interaction. Because of this unpredictability and to avoid bleeding with certainty the response should be monitored well in every patient when cimetidine is first added, being alert for the need to reduce the warfarin dosage. The onset of the interaction appears rapid; effects have been seen within days,[2,7] and even as early as 24 hours.[10] Acenocoumarol and phenindione are reported to interact similarly, and perhaps more rapidly,[3] but the documentation is much more limited. Expect other anticoagulants to behave in the same way, with the possible exception of phenprocoumon.

Famotidine, nizatidine, ranitidine and roxatidine normally appear not to interact with oral anticoagulants although note that in rare cases extension of prothrombin times and bleeding have been seen.

1. Flind AC. Cimetidine and oral anticoagulants. *Lancet* (1978) ii, 1054.
2. Silver BA, Bell WR. Cimetidine potentiation of the hypoprothrombinemic effect of warfarin. *Ann Intern Med* (1979) 90, 348–9.
3. Serlin MJ, Sibeon RG, Mossman S, Breckenridge AM, Williams JRB, Atwood JL, Willoughby JMT. Cimetidine: interaction with oral anticoagulants in man. *Lancet* (1979) ii, 317–19.
4. Hetzel D, Birkett D, Miners J. Cimetidine interaction with warfarin. *Lancet* (1979) ii, 639.
5. Breckenridge AM, Challiner M, Mossman S, Park BK, Serlin MJ, Sibeon RG, Williams JRB, Willoughby JMT. Cimetidine increases the action of warfarin in man. *Br J Clin Pharmacol* (1979) 8, 392P–393P.
6. Wallin BA, Jacknowitz A, Raich PC. Cimetidine and effect of warfarin. *Ann Intern Med* (1979) 90, 993.
7. Kerley B, Ali M. Cimetidine potentiation of warfarin action. *Can Med Assoc J* (1982) 126, 116.
8. O'Reilly RA. Comparative interaction of cimetidine and ranitidine with racemic warfarin in man. *Arch Intern Med* (1984) 144, 989–91.
9. Devanesen S. Prolongation of prothrombin time with cimetidine. *Med J Aust* (1981) 1, 537.
10. Bell WR, Anderson KC, Noe DA, Silver BA. Reduction in the plasma clearance rate of warfarin induced by cimetidine. *Arch Intern Med* (1986) 146, 2325–8.
11. Sax MJ, Randolph WC, Peace KE, Chretien S, Frank WO, Braverman AJ, Gray DR, McCree LC, Wyle F, Jackson BJ, Beg MA, Young MD. Effect of two cimetidine regimens on prothrombin time and warfarin pharmacokinetics during long-term warfarin therapy. *Clin Pharm* (1987) 6, 492–5.
12. Niopas I, Toon S, Aarons L, Rowland M. The effect of cimetidine on the steady-state pharmacokinetics and pharmacodynamics of warfarin in humans. *Eur J Clin Pharmacol* (1999) 55, 399–404.
13. van Rooij J, van der Meer FJM, Schoemaker HC, Cohen AF. Comparison of the effect of grapefruit juice and cimetidine on pharmacokinetics and anticoagulant effect of a single dose of acenocoumarol. *Br J Clin Pharmacol* (1993) 35, 548P.
14. Harenberg J, Staiger C, de Vries JX, Walter E, Weber E, Zimmermann R. Cimetidine does not increase the anticoagulant effect of phenprocoumon. *Br J Clin Pharmacol* (1982) 14, 292–3.
15. De Lepeleire I, van Hecken A, Verbesselt R, Tjandra-Maga TB, Buntinx A, Distlerath L, De Schepper PJ. Lack of interaction between famotidine and warfarin. *Int J Clin Pharmacol Res* (1990) 10, 167–71.
16. Chichmanian RM, Mignot G, Spreux A, Jean-Girard C, Hofliger P. Tolérance de la famotidine. Étude due réseau médecins sentinelles en pharmacovigilance. *Therapie* (1992) 47, 239–43.
17. Shinn AF. Unrecognized drug interactions with famotidine and nizatidine. *Arch Intern Med* (1991) 151, 810, 814.
18. Cournot A, Berlin I, Sallord JC, Singlas E. Lack of interaction between nizatidine and warfarin during chronic administration. *J Clin Pharmacol* (1988) 28, 1120–2.
19. Callaghan JT, Nyhart EH. Drug interactions between H_2-blockers and theophylline (T) or warfarin (W). *Pharmacologist* (1988) 30, A14.
20. Serlin MJ, Sibeon RG, Breckenridge AM. Lack of effect of ranitidine on warfarin action. *Br J Clin Pharmacol* (1981) 12, 791–4.
21. Desmond PV, Mashford ML, Harman PJ, Morphett BJ, Breen KJ, Wang YM. Decreased oral warfarin clearance after ranitidine and cimetidine. *Clin Pharmacol Ther* (1984) 35, 338–41.
22. Fischer J. Ranitidine and warfarin interaction. *Drug Intell Clin Pharm* (1985) 19, 664–5.
23. Baciewicz AM, Morgan PJ. Ranitidine-warfarin interaction. *Ann Intern Med* (1990) 112, 76–7.
24. Bender W, Brockmeier D. Pharmacokinetic characteristics of roxatadine. *J Clin Gastroenterol* (1989) 11 (Suppl 1), S6–S19.
25. Henry DA, MacDonald IA, Kitchingman G, Bell GD, Langman MJS. Cimetidine and ranitidine: comparison of effects on hepatic drug metabolism. *BMJ* (1980) 281, 775–7.
26. Choonara IA, Cholerton S, Haynes BP, Breckenridge AM, Park BK. Stereoselective interaction between the R enantiomer of warfarin and cimetidine. *Br J Clin Pharmacol* (1986) 21, 271–77.
27. Toon S, Hopkins KJ, Garstang FM, Diquet B, Gill TS, Rowland M. The warfarin-cimetidine interaction: stereochemical considerations. *Br J Clin Pharmacol* (1986) 21, 245–6.
28. Niopas I, Toon S, Rowland M. Further insight into the stereoselective interaction between warfarin and cimetidine in man. *Br J Clin Pharmacol* (1991) 32, 508–11.

Anticoagulants + Haloperidol

A single case report describes a marked reduction in the anticoagulant effects of phenindione caused by haloperidol.

Clinical evidence, mechanism, importance and management

A man stabilised on **phenindione** 50 mg daily was given haloperidol by injection (5 mg every 8 hours for 24 hours) followed by 3 mg twice daily by mouth. Adequate anticoagulation was not achieved even when the **phenindione** dosage was increased to 150 mg. When the haloperidol dosage was halved, the necessary dose of anticoagulant was reduced to 100 mg, and only when the haloperidol was withdrawn was it possible to achieve adequate anticoagulation with the original dosage.[1] The reasons for this are not understood. The general importance of this interaction is probably small and concurrent use need not be avoided, but prescribers should be aware of this case.

1. Oakley DP, Lautch H. Haloperidol and anticoagulant treatment. *Lancet* (1963) ii, 1231.

Anticoagulants + Heparinoids

An isolated case report describes bleeding in a patient on acenocoumarol after using a heparinoid-impregnated bandage. Some of the normal tests of anticoagulation are unreliable for a few hours after giving danaparoid to patients already on acenocoumarol.

Clinical evidence, mechanism, importance and management

A man who was well stabilised on **acenocoumarol** and also taking metoprolol, dipyridamole and isosorbide dinitrate began to bleed within about 3 days of starting to use a medicated bandage on an inflamed lesion on his hand, probably caused by a mosquito bite. His prothrombin percentage was found to have fallen to less than 10%. The bandage was impregnated with a semi-synthetic heparinoid compound based on **xylane acid polysulphate** [possibly pentosan polysulphate].[1] It would appear that enough of the heparinoid had been absorbed through his skin to increase his anticoagulation to the point where he began to bleed. This case is unusual but it illustrates the need to keep a close watch on patients who are given a range of drugs, some of which can potentially cause bleeding.

A study in 6 healthy subjects on **acenocoumarol** (steady-state thrombotest values of 10 to 15%), found that a single intravenous bolus injection of 3250 anti-Xa units of **danaparoid** prolonged the prothrombin time, activated partial thromboplastin time and Stypven time more than would have been expected by the simple addition of the effects of both drugs. These effects were seen for up to 1 hour. The thrombotest was affected for up to 5 hours.[2] The results of these clinical tests may therefore be unreliable during these periods.

1. Potel G, Maulaz B, Pabœuf C, Touze MD, Baron D. Potentialisation de l'acénocoumarol après application cutanée d'un héparinoide semi-synthétique. *Therapie* (1989) 44, 67–8.
2. Stiekema JCJ, de Boer A, Danhof M, Kroon C, Broekmans AW, van Dinther TG, Voerman J, Breimer DD. Interaction of the combined medication with the new low-molecular-weight heparinoid lomoparan® (Org 10172) and acenocoumarol. *Haemostasis* (1990) 20,136–46.

Anticoagulants + Herbal medicines; Boldo or Fenugreek

A report describes a woman on warfarin whose INR rose modestly when she began to take boldo and fenugreek.

Clinical evidence, mechanism, importance and management

A woman on **warfarin** for atrial fibrillation whose INRs normally fell within the range 2 to 3 showed a modest rise in her INR to 3.4, apparently due to the use of 10 drops of boldo after meals and one capsule of fenugreek before meals, to help her liver. A week after stopping these two herbal medicines her INR had fallen to 2.6. When she restarted them, her INR rose to 3.1 after a week and to 3.4 after 2 weeks. Her INR was later restabilised in the normal range in the presence of these two medicines by reducing the **warfarin** dosage by 15%.[1] The mechanism of this apparent interaction remains unknown, and it is not known whether both herbs or just one was responsible for what happened. Boldo comes from *Peumas boldus* and fenugreek from *Trigonelle foenum-graecum*, neither of which is recognised as having either anticoagulant or antiplatelet activity.

This patient showed no undesirable reactions (e.g. bruising or bleeding), but this case serves to draw attention to the possibility of an interaction in other patients on anticoagulants if these herbal medicines are taken concurrently.

1. Lambert JP, Cormier A. Potential interaction between warfarin and boldo-fenugreek. *Pharmacotherapy* (2001) 21, 509–12.

Anticoagulants + Herbal medicines; Curbicin

The INRs of two patients increased after taking Curbicin. One of them was also taking warfarin.

Clinical evidence, mechanism, importance and management

A 73-year-old man who was taking 3 tablets of Curbicin daily was found to have an INR of 2.1 (normal 0.9 to 1.2) despite no anticoagulant treatment. His INR improved (1.3 to 1.4) when he was given vitamin K, but did not normalize (to 1) until a week after stopping the Curbicin. Another patient on **warfarin** and simvastatin, with a stable INR of around 2.4, showed an increase in his INR to 3.4 within 6 days of starting to take 5 tablets of Curbicin daily. Within a week of stopping the Curbicin, his INR had fallen to its previous value. Curbicin is a herbal remedy used for micturition problems, and contains extracts from the fruit of *Serenoa repens* and the seed of *Cucurbita pepo*.[1]

The authors of this report suggest that what happened was possibly due to the presence of vitamin E in the Curbicin preparation (each tablet also contains 10 mg), but vitamin E does not normally affect INRs (see 'Anticoagulants + Vitamin E', p.321). The clinical significance of this interaction is unknown, but bear it in mind in the case of an unexpected response to treatment.

1. Yue, Q-Y, Jansson K. Herbal drug Curbicin and anticoagulant effect with and without warfarin: possibly related to the vitamin E component. *J Am Geriatr Soc* (2001) 49, 838.

Anticoagulants + Herbal medicines; Danshen

Two case reports and some other evidence indicates that *Danshen*, a Chinese herbal remedy, can increase the effects of warfarin resulting in bleeding.

Clinical evidence

A woman who had undergone venous mitral valve valvuloplasty and who was taking furosemide, digoxin and **warfarin**, began additionally to take *Danshen* (the root of *Salvia miltiorrhiza*) every other day for intermittent influenza-like symptoms. After about a month she was hospitalised with malaise, breathlessness and fever and was found to be both very anaemic and over-anticoagulated (prothrombin time greater than 60 seconds, INR greater than 5.62). The anaemia was attributed to occult gastrointestinal bleeding and the over-anticoagulation to an interaction with the *Danshen*. She was later restabilised on the **warfarin** in the absence of the *Danshen* with an INR of 2.5, and within 4 months her haemoglobin levels were normal.[1]

Another report describes a man on **warfarin**, digoxin, captopril and frusemide with an INR of about 3, who developed chest pain and breathlessness about 2 weeks after starting to take *Danshen*. He was found to have a massive pleural effusion, which was later drained of blood, and an INR of more than 8.4. He was later discharged on his usual dose of **warfarin** with an INR stable at 3, in the absence of the *Danshen*.[2]

Mechanism

Not fully understood. Studies in *rats* show that *Danshen* can increase the bioavailability of both *(R)*- and *(S)*-warfarin thereby increasing its effects.[3]

It may affect haemostasis by inhibiting platelet aggregation and by interfering with extrinsic coagulation, and it also has antithrombin III-like activity and can promote fibrinolytic activity. Acting in concert these activities might be expected to result in bleeding complications.

Importance and management

Clinical information appears to be limited to these two case reports and one other, which also involved 'methyl salicylate', (p.266), which is also known to increase the effects of warfarin. This interaction is therefore not very well established but there is enough evidence to suggest that normally *Danshen* should be avoided by patients on warfarin (although with very careful monitoring and warfarin dosage adjustments safe concurrent use might be possible). More study is needed. Information about other oral anticoagulants is lacking but, given the proposed mechanism of interaction, it would seem sensible to take the same precautions if using any of them.

1. Yu CM, Chan JCN, Sanderson JE. Chinese herbs and warfarin potentiation by 'Danshen'. *J Intern Med* (1997) 241, 337–9.
2. Izzat MB, Yim APC, El-Zufari MH. A taste of Chinese medicine. *Ann Thorac Surg* (1998) 66, 941–2.
3. Lo ACT, Chan K, Yeung JHK, Woo KS. The effects of Danshen (*Salvia miltiorrhiza*) on pharmacokinetics and dynamics of warfarin in rats. *Eur J Drug Metab Pharmacokinet* (1992) 17, 257–62.

Anticoagulants + Herbal medicines; Dong quai (*Angelica sinensis*)

Two case reports describe a very marked increase in the anticoagulant effects of warfarin when dong quai was added.

Clinical evidence, mechanism, importance and management

A 46-year-old African-American woman with atrial fibrillation taking **warfarin** showed a greater than twofold increase in her prothrombin time and INR after taking dong quai for 4 weeks. The prothrombin time and INR were back to normal 4 weeks after stopping the dong quai.[1] Another woman who had been taking **warfarin** for 10 years developed widespread bruising and an INR of 10, a month after starting to take dong quai.[2]

The reasons are not understood but dong quai is known to consist of natural coumarin derivatives, which may possibly have anticoagulant properties and inhibit platelet aggregation.

These seem to be only reports of this apparent interaction, but patients on **warfarin** should be warned of the potential risks of also taking dong quai. For safety dong qaui should be avoided unless the effects on anticoagulation can be monitored. More study is needed. Information about other anticoagulants is lacking.

1. Page RL, Lawrence JD. Potentiation of warfarin by dong quai. *Pharmacotherapy* (1999) 19, 870–6.
2. Ellis GR, Stephens MR. Untitled report. *BMJ* (1999) 319, 650.

Anticoagulants + Herbal medicines; Garlic

Isolated reports described increases in the anticoagulant effects of warfarin in patients taking medicinal garlic.

Clinical evidence

The INR of a patient stabilised on **warfarin** more than doubled and haematuria occurred 8 weeks after the patient started to take three *Höfels garlic pearles* daily. The situation resolved when the garlic was stopped. The INR rose on a later occasion while the patient was taking two *Kwai* garlic tablets daily. The INR of another patient was also more than doubled by six *Kwai* garlic tablets daily.[1,2] One review of the use of alternative and complementary medicines in 156 patients on **warfarin** found that 10% were also taking garlic, without any apparent increased risk or bleeding or raised INRs.[3]

Mechanism

Garlic has been associated with decreased platelet aggregation, which has on two documented occasions led to spontaneous bleeding in the absence of an anticoagulant.[4,5] The interaction may therefore probably occur as a result of additive anticoagulant effects.

Importance and management

Information about an adverse interaction between warfarin and garlic seems to be limited to these reports from one author. Bearing in mind the wide-spread use of garlic and garlic products, and the information from the review,[3] it seems most unlikely that garlic usually has any generally important interaction with anticoagulants.

1. Sunter W. Warfarin and garlic. *Pharm J* (1991) 246, 722.
2. Sunter W. Personal communication, July 1991.
3. Shalansky S, Neall E, Lo M, Abd-Elmessih E, Vickars L, Lynd L. The impact of complementary and alternative medicine use on warfarin-related adverse outcomes. *Pharmacotherapy* (2002) 22, 1345.
4. German K, Kumar U, Blackford HN. Garlic and the risk of TURP bleeding. *Br J Urol* (1995) 76, 518.
5. Rose KD, Croissant PD, Parliament CF, Levin MP. Spontaneous spinal epidural hematoma with associated platelet dysfunction from excessive garlic ingestion: a case report. *Neurosurgery* (1990) 26, 880–2.

Anticoagulants + Herbal medicines; Ginger

Despite some claims that ginger can interact with warfarin, there seems to be no clinical evidence to support this suggestion.

Clinical evidence, mechanism, importance and management

Ginger (*Zingiber Officinale*) is sometimes listed as a herb that interacts with **warfarin**,[1,2] but there do not appear to be any clinical reports of such an interaction. No reports were also found by two authors who undertook a comprehensive literature search using MEDLINE and a whole range of abstracting services (International Bibliographic Information on Dietary Supplements, International Pharmaceutical Abstracts, Reactions, Natural Medicines Comprehensive Database, German Commission E Monographs, The Review of Natural Products, Drug Interaction Facts, AltMedDex, Drug Therapy Screening System).[3] A randomised crossover study in 12 healthy subjects found that ginger did not affect either the pharmacokinetics or pharmacodynamics of a single 25-mg dose of **warfarin**.[4]

There is a case report suggesting that ginger can inhibit platelet aggregation but other studies failed to confirm this effect, and the evidence to date suggests that there is no real substance to the idea that an interaction can take place between **warfarin** and ginger.

1. Argento A, Tiraferri E, Marzaloni M. Anticoagulanti orali e piante medicinali. Una interazione emergente. *Ann Ital Med Int* (2000) 15, 139–43
2. Braun L. Herb-drug interaction guide. *Aust Fam Physician* (2001) 30, 473–6.
3. Vaes LPJ, Chyka PA. Interactions of warfarin with garlic, ginger, ginkgo, or ginseng: nature of the evidence. *Ann Pharmacother* (2000) 34, 1478–82.
4. Jiang X, Williams KM, Liauw WS, Ammit AJ, Roufogalis BD, Duke CC, Day RO, McLachlan AJ. Effect of ginkgo and ginger on the pharmacokinetics and pharmacodynamics of warfarin in healthy subjects. *Br J Clin Pharmacol* (2005) 59, 425–32.

Anticoagulants + Herbal medicines; Ginkgo biloba

An isolated report describes intracerebral haemorrhage associated with the use of *Ginkgo biloba* and warfarin. Other evidence suggests that no interaction occurs.

Clinical evidence, mechanism, importance and management

A report describes an intracerebral haemorrhage in an elderly woman within 2 months of starting *Ginkgo biloba*. Her prothrombin time was found to be 16.9 and her PTT 35.5 seconds. She had been on **warfarin** uneventfully for 5 years.[1] The author of the report speculated that both drugs may have contributed towards the haemorrhage, but no interaction is established.

A short report notes 6 cases of bleeding associated with the use of ginkgo biloba extract (EGb 761) with one also linked to concurrent **warfarin**.[2] A subsequent study in 12 healthy subjects found that EGb 761 120 mg daily for 4 weeks did not significantly alter coagulation parameters including platelet counts, INR, bleeding time and clotting time,[2] and another study in healthy subject similarly found that ginkgo biloba did not affect either the pharmacokinetics or pharmacodynamics of **warfarin**.[3] A retrospective review of clinical cases also found no evidence of altered haemostasis. However, in *animal* studies it was found that the AUC of **warfarin** was decreased by 23.4% during EGb 761 administration. The prothrombin time was also reduced by EGb 761.[2]

The evidence from these reports is far too slim to forbid patients taking **warfarin** to avoid *Ginkgo biloba* but they should be told to monitor for early signs of bruising or bleeding and seek informed professional advice if any bleeding problems arise.

1. Matthews MK. Association of *Ginkgo biloba* with intracerebral hemorrhage. *Neurology* (1998) 50, 1933.
2. Lai C-F, Chang C-C, Fu C-H, Chen C-M. Evaluation of the interaction between warfarin and ginkgo biloba extract. *Pharmacotherapy* (2002) 22, 1326.
3. Jiang X, Williams KM, Liauw WS, Ammit AJ, Roufogalis BD, Duke CC, Day RO, McLachlan AJ. Effect of ginkgo and ginger on the pharmacokinetics and pharmacodynamics of warfarin in healthy subjects. *Br J Clin Pharmacol* (2005) 59, 425–32.

Anticoagulants + Herbal medicines; Ginseng

Information is conflicting. A case report and a study suggest that a decrease in anticoagulant effect may be expected, but in theory increased bleeding is also possible.

Clinical evidence, mechanism, importance and management

A man on long-term **warfarin** because of a heart valve prosthesis and diltiazem, glyceryl trinitrate and salsalate had a fall in his INR from 3.1 to 1.5 within 2 weeks of starting to take ginseng capsules (*Ginsana*) three times daily. This preparation contains 100 mg of standardised concentrated ginseng in each capsule. Within 2 weeks of stopping the ginseng his INR had risen again to 3.3.[1] Apart from the ginseng there was no other identifiable cause for this reaction, the mechanism of which is not clear. A later study in *rats* failed to find any evidence of an interaction between **warfarin** and ginseng.[2] However, a study in 20 healthy subjects stabilised on **warfarin** found that the INR of 12 patients also given American ginseng 1 g twice daily for 3 weeks was reduced by 0.16 compared with a non-significant reduction of 0.02 in 8 patients given **warfarin** and placebo.[3]

The authors of the study suggest that all patients prescribed **warfarin** should be asked about the use of ginseng, but a letter in reply to this study notes that there is more than one type of ginseng available and so the results of this study cannot be generalised.[4]

In contrast there have been handful of reports of spontaneous bleeding in patients using ginseng preparations in the absence of an anticoagulant,[5,6] and Panax ginseng has been found to contain antiplatelet components.[7] Until further information becomes available it would seem prudent to be alert for the possible effects of using ginseng in patients taking anticoagulants. Both decreases in INR and an increase in bleeding seem possible.

1. Janetzky K, Morreale AP. Probable interaction between warfarin and ginseng. *Am J Health-Syst Pharm* (1997) 54, 692–3.
2. Zhu M, Chan KW, Ng LS, Chang Q, Chang S, Li RC. Possible influences of ginseng on the pharmacokinetics and pharmacodynamics of warfarin in rats. *J Pharm Pharmacol* (1999) 51, 175–80.
3. Yuan C-S, Wei G, Dey L, Karrison T, Nahlik L, Maleckar S, Kasza K, Ang-Lee M, Moss J. Brief communication: American ginseng reduces warfarin's effect in healthy patients. *Ann Intern Med* (2004) 141, 23–27.
4. Plotnikoff GA, McKenna D, Watanabe K, Blumenthal M. *Ann Intern Med* (2004) 141, 893–4.
5. Hopkins MP, Androff L, Benninghoff AS. Ginseng face cream and unexplained vaginal bleeding. *Am J Obstet Gynecol* (1988) 159, 1121–2.
6. Greenspan EM. Ginseng and vaginal bleeding. *JAMA* (1983) 249, 2018.
7. Kuo S-C, Teng C-M, Leed J-C, Ko F-N, Chen S-C, Wu T-S. Antiplatelet components in Panax ginseng. *Planta Med* (1990) 56, 164–7.

Anticoagulants + Herbal medicines; Kangen-Karyu

Kangen-Karyu inhibits the metabolism of warfarin, but only in doses much higher than those recommended therapeutically.

Clinical evidence, mechanism, importance and management

A study in *animals* showed that high doses of Kangen-Karyu (a mixture of **peony root**, **cnidium rhizome**, **safflower**, **cyperus rhizome**, **saussurea root** and the root of ***Salvia miltiorrhiza***) 2 g/kg twice daily inhibited the metabolism and elimination of single doses of **warfarin** and prolonged bleeding time. There was no interaction at a lower dose of 500 mg/kg, so that a clinical interaction is unlikely at the recommended dose of 90 mg/kg of Kangen-Karyu daily.[1] Kangen-Karyu contains antiplatelet components so it is possible that the occasional patient may experience a pharmacodynamic interaction. The evidence is too slim to forbid patients taking warfarin to avoid Kangen-Karyu but careful monitoring is advised.

1. Makino T, Wakushima H, Okamoto T, Okukubo Y, Deguchi Y, Kano Y. Pharmacokinetic interactions between warfarin and *kangen-karyu*, a Chinese traditional herbal medicine, and their synergistic action. *J Ethnopharmacol* (2002) 82, 35–40.

Anticoagulants + Herbal medicines; Lycium barbarum

Isolated reports described an increase in the anticoagulant effects of warfarin in a patient taking a herbal tea made from *Lycium barbarum* L.

Clinical evidence, mechanism, importance and management

A 61-year-old Chinese woman stabilised on **warfarin** (INRs normally 2 to 3) showed an unexpected rise in her INR to 4.1 during a routine monthly check. No bleeding was seen. She was also taking atenolol, benazepril, digoxin and fluvastatin. It was found that 4 days before visiting the clinic she had started to take 3 or 4 glasses (about 6 oz) daily of a Chinese herbal tea made from the fruits of *Lycium barbarum* L (also known as Chinese wolfberry, gou qi zi, Fructus Lycii Chinensis, or *Lycium chinense*) to treat blurred vision caused by a sore eye. The authors of the report say that this herbal remedy is used to combat yin deficiences. When the herbal treatment was stopped, her INRs rapidly returned to normal. Later *in vitro* studies showed that an infusion of *Lycium barbarum* L caused some inhibition of the cytochrome P450 isoenzyme CYP2C9 but this was apparently too weak to explain why this interaction occurred.[1] So far this is an isolated case but it draws attention to the possibility of problems with this herbal remedy in other patients.

1. Lam AY, Elmer GW, Mohutsky M. Possible interaction between warfarin and *Lycium barbarum*. *Ann Pharmacother* (2001) 35, 1199–1201.

Anticoagulants + Herbal medicines; Melilot

Increased anticoagulation was seen in a patient on acenocoumarol after using a melilot-containing topical cream.

Clinical evidence, mechanism, importance and management

A 66-year-old on **acenocoumarol**, levothyroxine and prazepam showed an increase in her INR after massaging a proprietary topical cream (*Cyclo 3*) containing melilot and *ruscus aculeatus* on her legs three times daily. On the first occasion her INR rose from about 2 to 5.8 after 7 days' use, and on a later occasion it rose to 4.6 after 10 days' use.[1]

A woman with unexplained abnormal menstrual bleeding was found to have a prothrombin time of 53 seconds, and laboratory tests showed that her blood clotting factors were abnormally low. When given parenteral vitamin K her prothrombin time rapidly returned to normal (suggesting that she was taking a vitamin K antagonist of some kind). She strongly denied taking any anticoagulant drugs, but it was eventually discovered that she had been drinking large quantities of a herbal tea containing among other ingredients tonka beans, melilot and sweet woodruff, all of which contain natural coumarins that can be converted into anticoagulants by moulds.[2] The anticoagulant effects of these compounds may possibly have been increased by the paracetamol (acetaminophen) and dextropropoxyphene (propoxyphene) that she was also taking.

These cases are isolated but they show that herbal preparations of this kind can affect anticoagulation. No prescribed anticoagulant drug was being used by the second patient, but it demonstrates the potential anticoagulant effect of herbal remedies. In the first case, absorption through the skin was enough to upset the anticoagulant control.

1. Chiffoleau A, Huguenin H, Veyrac G, Argaiz V, Dupe D, Kayser M, Bourin M, Jolliet P. Interaction entre mélilot et acénocoumarol ? (mélilot-*ruscus aculeatus*). *Therapie* (2001) 56, 321–7.
2. Hogan RP. Hemorrhagic diathesis caused by drinking an herbal tea. *JAMA* (1983) 249, 2679–80.

Anticoagulants + Herbal medicines; St John's wort (*Hypericum perforatum*)

St John's wort can cause a moderate reduction in the anticoagulant effects of phenprocoumon and warfarin. An isolated and unconfirmed report also describes a reduced anticoagulant effect in one patient on phenprocoumon.

Clinical evidence

(a) Phenprocoumon

A randomised, single blind placebo-controlled crossover study[1] in 10 healthy men found that 900 mg of St John's wort extract (*LI 160*, *Lichtwer Pharma*) daily for 11 days reduced the AUC of a single 12-mg dose of phenprocoumon by 17.4%. There is also a case report about a 75-year old woman on phenprocoumon who showed a reduced anticoagulant response (a rise in the Quick value) 2 months after starting to take St John's wort.[2]

(b) Warfarin

The Swedish Medical Products Agency received 7 case reports over the 1998 to 1999 period of patients stabilised on warfarin who showed decreased INRs when St John's wort was added. Their INRs fell from the normal therapeutic range of about 2 to 4 to about 1.5. Two patients are described who needed warfarin dosage increases of 6.6% and 15% when St John's wort was added. The INRs of 4 of the patients returned to their former values when the St John's wort was stopped.[3]

Mechanism

Not known, but it is suggested that the St John's wort increases the metabolism and clearance of the anticoagulants[1,3] possibly by induction of cytochrome P450 isoenzyme CYP2C9, or it inhibits its absorption from the gut.[1] Just why one patient showed a paradoxical increase in anticoagulant effects is not known.

Importance and management

Information seems to be limited to these brief reports, the picture being that these interactions are of moderate clinical importance. It would be prudent to monitor the INRs of patients on phenprocoumon, warfarin or any other coumarin if they start taking St John's wort, being alert for the need to raise the anticoagulant the dosage. The two patients described above needed warfarin increases of 6.6 and 15%. The advice of the CSM in the UK is to check the INR, stop St John's wort and then adjust the anticoagulant dosage as necessary.[4] More study is needed.

1. Maurer A, Johne A, Bauer S, Brockmöller J, Donath F, Roots I, Langheinrich M, Hübner W-D. Interaction of St John's wort extract with phenprocoumon. *Eur J Clin Pharmacol* (1999) 55, A22.
2. Bon S, Hartmann, Kuhn M. Johanniskraut: Ein Enzyminduktor? *Schweiz Apothekerzeitung* (1999) 16, 535–6.
3. Yue Q-Y, Bergquist C, Gerdén B. Safety of St John's wort *(Hypericum perforatum). Lancet* (2000) 355, 576–7.
4. Committee on Safety of Medicines. Message from Professor A Breckenridge, Chairman, Committee on Safety of Medicines, and Fact Sheet for Health Care Professionals, February 2000. Available from http://medicines.mhra.gov.uk/aboutagency/regframework/csm/csmhome.htm

Anticoagulants + Herbicides

An isolated report describes a marked increase in the anticoagulant effects of acenocoumarol with bleeding caused by use of a herbicide.

Clinical evidence, mechanism, importance and management

A 55-year-old patient with mitral and aortic prostheses, stabilised on **acenocoumarol** 2 mg daily and with a normal thrombotest of 6 to 7% (INR 3.6 to 4.2), was hospitalised because of severe and uncontrollable gum bleeding. He responded when given a transfusion of fresh plasma. The cause of the marked increase in the anticoagulant effects of the **acenocoumarol** was eventually identified as almost certainly being due to the use of a herbicide (*SATURN-S*) containing **thiobencarb** and **molinate** (two thiocarbamates), which the patient was using to spray his rice crop. The **thiobencarb** can be absorbed through the skin and the **molinate** by inhalation. Just how these two compounds interact with **acenocoumarol** is not known but the authors of the report suggest the possibility that these herbicides may have inhibited the metabolism of the anticoagulant, thereby increasing its effects. The patient was later restabilised on his former dose of **acenocoumarol**.[1]

This seems to be the first and only report of this interaction but it highlights one of the possible risks of using chemical sprays (herbicides, pesticides etc), which have never been formally tested for their potential to interact with drugs.

1. Fernández MA, Aznar J. Potenciación del efecto anticoagulante del acenocumarol por un herbicida. *Rev Iberoamer Tromb Hemostasia* (1988) 1, 40–1.

Anticoagulants + Hydrocodone

The anticoagulant effects of warfarin have been shown to be increased by hydrocodone in a patient and in a healthy subject.

Clinical evidence, mechanism, importance and management

A patient, well stabilised on **warfarin** (and also taking digoxin, propranolol, clofibrate and spironolactone) showed a rise in his prothrombin time of about 2 to 3 times his control value when he began to take *Tussionex* (hydrocodone with phenyltoloxamine) for a chronic cough. When the cough syrup was discontinued, his prothrombin time fell again. In a subsequent study in a healthy subject the equivalent dosage of hydrocodone increased the elimination half-life of **warfarin** from 30 to 42 hours.[1] The reason is not known, but be aware of this interaction in the case or an unexpected increase in the response to warfarin.

1. Azarnoff DL. Drug interactions: the potential for adverse effects. *Drug Inf J* (1972) 6, 19–25.

Anticoagulants + Influenza vaccines

The concurrent use of warfarin and influenza vaccine is usually safe and uneventful, but there are reports of bleeding in a handful of patients (life-threatening in one case) attributed to an interaction. Acenocoumarol also does not normally interact.

Clinical evidence

(a) Evidence of no interaction

After vaccination with 1982/3 trivalent influenza vaccines, types A and B, the prothrombin times of 21 men on long-term **warfarin** treatment were not significantly altered.[1]

Other studies in a total of 94 male and female patients[2-5] found no evidence of an adverse interaction between **warfarin** and influenza vaccine, although a small increase in the prothrombin ratio (from 1.68 to 1.81) was seen in one study[4] and a small prothrombin time decrease in another.[5] No interaction was seen in other studies in 4 healthy subjects[6] or in 40 residents in nursing homes.[7,8] One case of gross but transient haematuria occurred, but it was not possible to link this firmly with the vaccination.[7] Trivalent influenza vaccine has also been shown not to affect anticoagulation with **acenocoumarol**.[9,10]

(b) Evidence of an interaction

A very brief report describes a patient on long-term **warfarin** treatment who had serious bleeding, which was almost fatal, after receiving a 'flu shot'. No further details are given.[11] An elderly man on long-term **warfarin** treatment developed bleeding (haematemesis and melaena) within 10 days of influenza vaccination. His prothrombin time was found to be 36 seconds.[12] A subsequent study in 8 patients showed that influenza vaccination (with trivalent types A and B) prolonged their prothrombin times by 40%, but no signs of bleeding were seen.[12] Another patient on **warfarin** showed INR increases on two successive years when vaccinated against influenza.[13]

Mechanism

Not understood. One suggestion is that when an interaction occurs the synthesis of the blood clotting factors is altered.[12] There is no evidence that the vaccine changes the metabolism of the warfarin,[12] although the metabolism of aminopyrine (used as an indicator of changes in metabolism) is reduced.[14]

Importance and management

A well-investigated interaction. The weight of evidence shows that influenza vaccination in those taking warfarin is normally safe and uneventful, nevertheless it would be prudent to be on the alert because very occasionally and unpredictably bleeding may occur. Acenocoumarol appears to behave like warfarin. Information about other anticoagulants is lacking.

1. Lipsky BA, Pecoraro RE, Roben NJ, de Blaquiere P, Delaney CJ. Influenza vaccination and warfarin anticoagulation. *Ann Intern Med* (1984) 100, 835–7.
2. Gomolin IH, Chapron DJ, Luhan PA. Effects of influenza virus vaccine on theophylline and warfarin clearance in institutionalized elderly. *J Am Geriatr Soc* (1984) 32 (April Suppl), S21.
3. Gomolin IH, Chapron DJ, Luhan PA. Lack of effect of influenza vaccine on theophylline levels and warfarin anticoagulation in the elderly. *J Am Geriatr Soc* (1985) 33, 269–72.
4. Weibert RT, Lorentz SM, Norcross WA, Klauber MR, Jagger PI. Effect of influenza vaccine in patients receiving long-term warfarin therapy. *Clin Pharm* (1986) 5, 499–503.
5. Bussey HI, Saklad JJ. Effect of influenza vaccine on chronic warfarin therapy. *Drug Intell Clin Pharm* (1988) 22, 198–201.
6. Scott AK, Cannon J, Breckenridge AM. Lack of effect of influenza vaccination on warfarin in healthy volunteers. *Br J Clin Pharmacol* (1985) 19, 144P–145P.
7. Patriarca PA, Kendal AP, Stricof RL, Weber JA, Meissner MK, Dateno B. Influenza vaccination and warfarin or theophylline toxicity in nursing-home residents. *N Engl J Med* (1983) 308, 1601–2.
8. Gomolin IH. Lack of effect of influenza vaccine on warfarin anticoagulation in the elderly. *Can Med Assoc J* (1986) 135, 39–41.
9. Souto JC, Oliver A, Montserrat I, Mateo J, Sureda A, Fontcuberta J. Lack of effect of influenza vaccine on anticoagulation by acenocoumarol. *Ann Pharmacother* (1993) 27, 365–8.
10. Souto JC, Garí M, Borrell M, Fontcuberta J. Ausencia de interacción entre los anticoagulantes orales y la vacuna antigripal. *Med Clin (Barc)* (1993) 101, 637.
11. Sumner HW, Holtzman JL, McClain CJ. Drug-induced liver disease. *Geriatrics* (1981) 36, 83–96.
12. Kramer P, Tsuru M, Cook CE, McClain CJ, Holtzman JL. Effect of influenza vaccine on warfarin anticoagulation. *Clin Pharmacol Ther* (1984) 35, 416–18.
13. Beeley L, Cunningham H, Carmichael A, Brennan A. *Bulletin of the West Midlands Centre for Adverse Drug Reaction Reporting* (1991), 33, 19.
14. Kramer P, McClain CJ. Depression of aminopyrine metabolism by influenza vaccine. *N Engl J Med* (1981) 305, 1262–4.

Anticoagulants + Insecticides

A patient showed a marked increase in his response to acenocoumarol when exposed to insecticides containing ivermectin and methidathion. Another patient was resistant to the effects of warfarin after very heavy exposure to a toxaphene/lindane insecticide.

Clinical evidence

(a) Acenocoumarol

A farmer in Spain, normally well stabilised on acenocoumarol and amiodarone, had marked rises in his INR, from 3.5 up to 7.9, requiring a reduction in his anticoagulant dosage (from 12 to 8 mg weekly), which occurred during the summer months. It was then discovered that he was using insecticides containing **ivermectin** and an organophosphate, **methidathion** on his trees without any protective clothing. No bleeding occurred.[1]

(b) Warfarin

A rancher in the USA, who was on warfarin, showed a very marked reduction in his anticoagulant response after dusting his sheep with an insecticide containing 5% **toxaphene** (**camphechlor**) and 1% **lindane** (**gamma-benzene hexachloride**). Over a 2-year period he showed periods of considerable 'warfarin resistance', which were linked to the use of this insecticide. Normally 7.5 mg of warfarin daily maintained his prothrombin time in the therapeutic range, but after exposure to the insecticide even 15 mg daily failed to have any effect at all.[2] The dusting was done by putting the insecticide in a sack and hitting the sheep with it in an enclosed barn.[2]

Mechanism

The interaction between acenocoumarol and ivermectin with methidathion is not understood. Ivermectin used for onchocerciasis normally has no effect on prothrombin times when used alone,[3,4] but two unexplained cases of prolonged prothrombin times associated with the development of haematomas have been reported.[5] Methidathion is an organophosphate. Lindane and other chlorinated hydrocarbon insecticides are known liver enzyme inducing agents,[6] which increase the metabolism and clearance of the warfarin, thereby reducing or even abolishing its effects.

Importance and management

Information about these interactions appears to be limited to these isolated case reports. Neither interaction is well established and neither would appear not to be of general clinical importance. The chlorinated hydrocarbon insecticides have been withdrawn from general use in most countries so that the possibility of an interaction with any anticoagulant is now very small. No other cases of an interaction between an anticoagulant and ivermectin, whether used as an insecticide or for the treatment of onchocerciasis, appear to have been reported.

As a general rule farm workers and others should use proper protection (gloves, masks, protective clothing) if they are exposed to substantial amounts of any insecticide, because they can be both directly toxic and can also apparently interact with some prescribed drugs, including the anticoagulants, even if only very rarely.

1. Fernandéz MA, Ballasteros S, Aznar J. Oral anticoagulants and insecticides. *Thromb Haemost* (1998) 80, 724.
2. Jeffery WH, Ahlin TA, Goren C, Hardy WR. Loss of warfarin effect after occupational insecticide exposure. *JAMA* (1976) 236, 2881–2.
3. Richards FO, McNeeley MB, Bryan RT, Eberhard ML, McNeeley DF, Lammie PJ, Spencer HC. Ivermectin and prothrombin time. *Lancet* (1989) i, 1139–40.
4. Pacque MC, Munoz B, White AT, Williams PN, Greene BM, Taylor HR. Ivermectin and prothrombin time. *Lancet* (1989) i, 1140.
5. Homeida MMA, Bagi IA, Ghalib HW, El Sheikh H, Ismail A, Yousif MA, Sulieman S, Ali HM, Bennett JL, Williams J. Prolongation of prothrombin time with ivermectin. *Lancet* (1988) i, 1346–7.
6. Kolmodin B, Azarnoff DL, Sjöqvist F. Effect of environmental factors on drug metabolism: Decreased plasma half-life of antipyrine in workers exposed to chlorinated hydrocarbon insecticides. *Clin Pharmacol Ther* (1969) 10, 638–42.

Anticoagulants + Interferons

Preliminary evidence indicates that the effects of acenocoumarol and warfarin may be increased by interferons.

Clinical evidence

A woman on long-term **warfarin** 2.5 to 3.5 mg daily had a prothrombin time rise from 16.7 to 20.4 seconds after receiving 6 million units of interferon-alfa daily for 10 days, then three times a week. Her serum **warfarin** levels rose from about 0.8 to 5.2 micrograms/ml. She responded to a reduction in the **warfarin** dosage to 2 mg daily. The authors of the report also say that they have seen 4 other patients on **warfarin** who needed a dosage reduction when given interferon, two of them while taking interferon beta and the other two while taking interferon alfa-2b.[1] A woman on **acenocoumarol** 1 and 2 mg on alternate days had gingival bleeding and a thrombotest change from 35% to 19% within 6 weeks of starting treatment with 3 million units of interferon-alpha 2b three times weekly. Her thrombotest percentages stabilised between 25 and 40% when the **acenocoumarol** dosage was reduced to 1 mg daily. The extent of the anticoagulation decreased (thrombotest 69%) when the interferon was reduced to twice weekly.[2]

Mechanism

Not understood. The authors of both reports postulate that interferon reduces the metabolism of the anticoagulants by the liver, thereby reducing their clearance and increasing their effects.[1,2]

Importance and management

These reports seem to be the only ones to describe this interaction so the interaction is not yet well established. However it would seem prudent to monitor the effects if interferon is added to acenocoumarol or warfarin, reducing the dosage if necessary. Information about other anticoagulants is lacking, but the same precautions would be appropriate with any of them.

1. Adachi Y, Yokoyama Y, Nanno T, Yamamoto T. Potentation of warfarin by interferon. *BMJ* (1995) 311, 292.
2. Serratrice J, Durand J-M, Morange S. Interferon-alpha 2b interaction with acenocoumarol. *Am J Hematol* (1998) 57, 89–92.

Anticoagulants + Laxatives, Liquid paraffin or Psyllium

The theoretical possibility that laxatives or liquid paraffin might affect the response to oral anticoagulants appears to be unconfirmed. Psyllium (ispaghula) has been shown not to affect either the absorption or the anticoagulant effects of warfarin.

Clinical evidence, mechanism, importance and management

A study in 6 healthy subjects showed that psyllium, given as a 14-g dose of colloid (*Metamucil*) in a small amount of water with a single 40-mg dose of **warfarin**, and three further doses of psyllium at 2-hourly intervals thereafter, did not affect either the absorption or the anticoagulant effects of the **warfarin**.[1] In theory, laxatives and liquid paraffin (mineral oil), which shorten the transit time along the gut, might be expected to decrease the absorption of both vitamin K and the oral anticoagulants. Liquid paraffin might also be expected to impair the absorption of the lipid-soluble vitamin, but despite warnings in various books, reviews and lists of drug interactions, there appears to be no direct evidence, as yet, that this is an interaction of any practical importance.

1. Robinson DS, Benjamin DM, McCormack JJ. Interaction of warfarin and nonsystemic gastrointestinal drugs. *Clin Pharmacol Ther* (1971) 12, 491–5.

Anticoagulants + Leflunomide

Leflunomide appears to raise the INR of patients taking warfarin.

Clinical evidence, mechanism, importance and management

A short report describes a patient on **warfarin** whose INR rose from 2.5 to over 6, resulting in a hospital admission, after she took three 100-mg doses of leflunomide.[1]

Another report describes a patient on **warfarin** who developed haematuria following two 100-mg doses of leflunomide. His INR was found to have risen from 3.4 to over 11, and **warfarin** was discontinued. The haematuria spontaneously resolved, but as the INR remained elevated for the next 2 days he was given 1 mg of vitamin K, which brought his INR down to 1.9. He was later stabilised on warfarin 1 mg daily with a leflunomide maintenance dose of 20 mg daily.[2]

The authors of this report say that at that time [2002] the UK Committee on Safety of Medicines had received over 300 reports of leflunomide raising the INRs of patients on **warfarin**, so these reports appear to be just the tip of the iceberg. The makers advise caution if the combination is used, and it would seem prudent to monitor the INR of any patient taking **warfarin** who is started on leflunomide.

1. Mason JP. Warfarin and leflunomide. *Pharm J* (2000) 265, 267.
2. Lim V, Pande I. Leflunomide can potentiate the anticoagulant effect of warfarin. *BMJ* (2002) 325, 1333.

Anticoagulants + Levetiracetam

Levetiracetam appears not to interact adversely with warfarin.

Clinical evidence, mechanism, importance and management

A randomised double-blind placebo-controlled trial in 42 healthy subjects given **warfarin** found that levetiracetam 1 g twice daily had no significant effect on the pharmacokinetics of either drug and the INRs were not significantly altered.[1] No special precautions are therefore needed.

1. Ragueneau-Majlessi I, Levy RH, Meyerhoff C. Lack of effect of repeated administration of levetiracetam on the pharmacodynamic and pharmacokinetic profiles of warfarin. *Epilepsy Res* (2001) 47, 55–63.

Anticoagulants + Linezolid

Linezolid 600 mg twice daily was given to 13 healthy subjects for 5 days followed by a single 25-mg dose of warfarin. The pharmacokinetics of warfarin and the INR were unchanged.[1]

1. Azie NE, Stalker DJ, Jungbluth GL, Sisson T, Adams G. Effect of linezolid on CYP2C9 using racemic warfarin (W) as a probe. *Clin Pharmacol Ther* (2001) 69, 21.

Anticoagulants + Lysine clonixinate (Clonixin)

Lysine clonixinate does not alter the anticoagulant effects of phenprocoumon.

Clinical evidence, mechanism, importance and management

An open, randomised, crossover study in 12 healthy men found that the pharmacokinetics and the anticoagulant activity of a single 18-mg dose of **phenprocoumon** were unchanged by **lysine clonixinate** 125 mg, given five times daily for 3 days before and for 13 days after the **phenprocoumon**.[1] No special precautions would therefore seem to be required if these two drugs are taken concurrently. Although remember most NSAIDs, which can cause some gastrointestinal bleeding, affect platelet function, and sometimes unpredictably interfere with anticoagulant effects.

1. Russmann S, Dilger K, Trenk D, Nagyivanyi P, Jänchen E. Effect of lysine clonixate on the pharmacokinetics and anticoagulant activity of phenprocoumon. *Arzneimittelforschung* (2001) 51, 891–895.

Anticoagulants + Macrolides

A marked increase in the effects of warfarin and bleeding has been seen in a small number of patients given azithromycin, clarithromycin, erythromycin, or roxithromycin but most patients are unlikely to develop a clinically important interaction. This interaction has also been seen in a few patients on acenocoumarol or phenprocoumon and either clarithromycin, erythromycin, or roxithromycin. In healthy subjects, midecamycin diacetate appears not to interact with acenocoumarol, and dirithromycin does not appear to interact with warfarin.

Clinical evidence

(a) Azithromycin

(i) Warfarin. A very large scale study found no evidence that azithromycin 1.5 g daily for 5 days had any effect on the prothrombin time response to single doses of warfarin given to a subset of patients.[1] A retrospective study of 26 patients on warfarin found no evidence that treatment with azithromycin had any effect on their INRs.[2] A study in healthy subjects found that azithromycin did not alter the anticoagulant effects of single 15-mg doses of warfarin.[3]

A 41-year-old woman on haemodialysis and taking warfarin was given a short course of azithromycin 500 mg on day 1, reduced to 250 mg daily for the next 4 days. Three days after finishing the azithromycin the woman's INR was found to have risen to 4.88 from her normal range of 1.5 to 2.7.[4]

A 53-year-old man who had been taking warfarin for several years following a mitral valve replacement (INR 2 to 2.8), was hospitalised a couple of days after starting to cough up blood and blood-streaked mucus. He had finished a 5-day course of azithromycin 2 days previously. His prothrombin time was found to have risen to 106 seconds. The warfarin was stopped and phytomenadione given, but he later died following a cardiac arrest.[5]

A 71-year old woman stabilised on warfarin with INRs between 2.5 and 3.5 developed an INR of 15.16 a day after she finished a 5-day course of azithromycin.[6]

The makers of azithromycin are quoted as having 26 reports of a potential interaction between warfarin and azithromycin on their records.[6] The reports included increased or prolonged PT and increased INRs (18 cases), haemorrhage not otherwise specified (6), blood in stools (1) and decreased PT (1). The makers of warfarin has received fewer than 15 such reports,[6] most of which involved increase in INR or PT. The makers[7] say that 2 unconfirmed cases of a possible interaction have been reported to the UK Medicines Control Agency, and 2 other cases have been reported from Australia.[8]

(b) Clarithromycin

(i) Acenocoumarol. The INR of a 75-year-old woman on long-term treatment with acenocoumarol rose from 2.1 to 9 within a week of starting to take clarithromycin 250 mg twice daily.[9] Five patients on acenocoumarol had a mean increase in their INRs from about 2.5 to 5.5 when they were treated with clarithromycin.[10] The largest increase was from 1.95 to 7.01.

(ii) Phenprocoumon. A 70-year-old woman on long-term phenprocoumon developed a marked increase in prothrombin times, but no bleeding, within 4 days of starting to take clarithromycin 500 mg daily. The phenprocoumon was stopped and phytomenadione given. When the antibacterial was withdrawn she was restabilised on the original dosage of phenprocoumon.[11]

(iii) Warfarin. Another patient developed prothrombin times in the high twenties within a week of starting to take clarithromycin 1 g daily and his warfarin dosage was accordingly halved. When the clarithromycin was stopped and the warfarin dosage was raised to its usual dose his prothrombin times returned to their former values. A man on warfarin with INRs in the range of 1.6 to 4 developed an INR of almost 17 within 17 days of starting to take clarithromycin 500 mg twice daily.[12]

Other patients have been found to have INRs of 5.6 and 90.3 five days after starting clarithromycin,[13] and of 7.3 within 12 days of starting clarithromycin.[14] A further 2 patients on warfarin developed haematuria[15] and had a suprachoroidal haemorrhage[16] after being given clarithromycin. The makers of clarithromycin have a number of individual case reports on record describing patients worldwide on warfarin who have shown elevated prothrombin times (sometimes accompanied by serious bleeding) when they were treated with clarithromycin.[15] In 1992 the UK Committee on Safety of Medicines notified prescribers in the UK of a case of a woman taking warfarin for mitral valve disease who suffered a fatal cerebrovascular bleed 3 days after starting to take clarithromycin.[17] Her INR was above 10.

(c) Dirithromycin

(i) Warfarin. The pharmacokinetic and pharmacodynamics of single 0.5-mg/kg oral doses of warfarin in 15 healthy subjects were not altered by dirithromycin 500 mg daily for 5 days.[18]

(d) Erythromycin

(i) Acenocoumarol. Haemorrhage occurred in a patient on acenocoumarol treated with erythromycin.[19] Another patient on acenocoumarol showed a rise in INR from a range of 3 to 4.5 up to 15 within a week of starting to take erythromycin ethylsuccinate 1.5 g daily but no bleeding was seen.[20]

(ii) Warfarin. An elderly woman on warfarin, digoxin, hydrochlorothiazide and quinidine developed haematuria and bruising within a week of starting to take erythromycin stearate 500 mg four times daily. Her prothrombin time had risen to 64 seconds.[21] At least 8 other cases of bleeding and/or hypoprothrombinaemia have been described in patients on warfarin when given erythromycin (as ethylsuccinate, stearate, estolate, lactobionate or base).[22-28]

There is also a case report of sulphonamide-induced bullous haemorrhagic eruption in a patient on co-trimoxazole, in which the haemorrhagic component may have been due to a interaction between warfarin and erythromycin.[29]

A study in 12 healthy subjects found that the clearance of a single dose of warfarin was reduced by an average of 14% (range 0 to about 30%) after taking erythromycin 250 mg every 6 hours for 8 days.[30] Erythromycin caused only a small increase in the effects of warfarin in another study in 8 patients.[31] A single-dose study with warfarin in 15 healthy subjects found that 5 days' treatment with erythromycin 250 mg four times daily increased the AUC of *(S)*-warfarin by 11.2% and of *(R)*-warfarin by 11.9%. The INR increased by 10.2%.[32]

(e) Midecamycin diacetate

(i) Acenocoumarol. The pharmacokinetics of a single oral dose of acenocoumarol were not significantly changed in 6 healthy subjects after they took midecamycin diacetate 800 mg twice daily for 4 days.[33]

(f) Roxithromycin

(i) Acenocoumarol. A 79-year-old man on long-term acenocoumarol treatment developed a large abdominal wall haematoma shortly after starting to take roxithromycin 150 mg twice daily for a lung infection.[34] His INR had risen to 5.9.

(ii) Phenprocoumon. A 75-year-old man taking phenprocoumon chronically developed a marked increase in prothrombin times but no bleeding when given roxithromycin. The phenprocoumon was stopped and phytomenadione given. When the antibacterial was withdrawn he was restabilised on the original dosage of phenprocoumon.[11]

(iii) Warfarin. Roxithromycin 150 mg twice daily for 2 weeks had no significant effect on the thrombotest percentages of 21 healthy subjects given enough warfarin to maintain the values at 10 to 20%. Serum roxithromycin levels also remained unchanged.[35] However, during the 1992 to 1995 period The Centre for Adverse Reactions Monitoring of New Zealand (CARM) received 7 reports of a possible interaction with roxithromycin resulting in increased warfarin effects, and, during the same period, the Adverse Drug Reactions Advisory Committee of Australia (ADRAC) received 9 similar reports.[36]

(g) Telithromycin

(i) Warfarin. A 73-year-old man taking warfarin for a metallic valve replacement was started on telithromycin 800 mg daily for 5 days for a cough. On the last day of treatment he developed haemoptysis and was found to have an INR of 11. His INR 10 days before telithromycin was started was 3.1. The telithromycin was stopped and he was subsequently restabilised on warfarin.[37]

Mechanism

Erythromycin (and many of the macrolides) are known inhibitors of the cytochrome P450 isoenzymes, and it is therefore suggested that the metabolism of warfarin is reduced and its effects are thereby increased.[30] One study in patients taking acenocoumarol or phenprocoumon, found that clarithromycin significantly increased the risk of over-anticoagulation only during the first 3 days of combined use, which may be explained by enzyme inhibition resulting in reduced anticoagulant clearance.[38] It is not clear why only some individuals are affected. Compared to erythromycin, roxithromycin has only a weak effect on cytochrome P450 enzymes and interaction with warfarin has not been found in healthy subjects. However, clinically significant interactions may occur in severely ill, elderly, or compromised patients.[36] The mechanism for an interaction with azithromycin, which does not undergo hepatic metabolism, is not understood.[6,8]

Importance and management

An established and unpredictable interaction. Reports of problems with erythromycin, clarithromycin, roxithromycin and telithromycin suggest that the clinical relevance in most patients is very limited, but in a few patients the effects are apparently considerable. Normally no interaction occurs with azithromycin, but because very occasionally and unpredictably the effects of warfarin are increased, all patients should be well monitored when first given azithromycin, bearing in mind that because of azithromycin's long half-life the interaction may possibly not become apparent until a couple of days after a short course (i.e. 5 days) of azithromycin has been stopped. These precautions are in line with the maker's recommendations.[3]

Similarly, concurrent use of warfarin with clarithromycin, erythromycin, roxithromycin or telithromycin need not be avoided but it would be prudent initially to monitor the effects closely, especially in those who clear warfarin and other anticoagulants slowly and who therefore only need low doses. The elderly in particular would seem to fall into this higher risk category. Reports of interactions between these macrolide antibacterials and anticoagulants other than warfarin are limited, but the same precautions would seem advisable with any coumarin. Information about midecamycin diacetate and dirithromycin is very sparse. Studies in healthy subjects indicate a lack of an interaction between these drugs and anticoagulants, but until this has been confirmed in clinical practice, it would be prudent to apply the same precautions recommended for other macrolides.

1. Hopkins S. Clinical toleration and safety of azithromycin. *Am J Med* (1991) 91 (Suppl 3A), 40S–45S.
2. Beckey NP, Parra D, Colon A. Retrospective evaluation of a potential interaction between azithromycin and warfarin in patients stabilized on warfarin. *Pharmacotherapy* (2000) 20, 1055–9.
3. Zithromax (Azithromycin). Pfizer Ltd. UK Summary of product characteristics, July 2004.
4. Lane G. Increased hypoprothrombinemic effect of warfarin possibly induced by azithromycin. *Ann Pharmacother* (1996) 30, 884–5.
5. Woldtveldt BR, Cahoon CL, Bradley LA, Miller SJ. Possible increased anticoagulation effect of warfarin induced by azithromycin. *Ann Pharmacother* (1998) 32, 269–70.
6. Foster DR, Milan NL. Potential interaction between azithromycin and warfarin. *Pharmacotherapy* (1999) 19, 902–8.
7. Pfizer Limited. Personal Communication, December 1998.
8. Wiese MD, Cosh DG. Raised INR with concurrent warfarin and azithromycin. *Aust J Hosp Pharm* (1999) 29, 159–161.
9. Grau E, Real E, Pastor E. Interaction between clarithromycin and oral anticoagulants. *Ann Pharmacother* (1996) 30, 1495–6.
10. Sánchez B, Muruzábal MJ, Peralta G, Santiago G, Castilla A, Aguilera JP, Arjona R. Clarithromycin-oral anticoagulants interaction. Report of five cases. *Clin Drug Invest* (1997) 13, 220–2.
11. Meyboom RHB, Heere FJ, Egberts ACG, Lastdrager CJ. Vermoedelijke potentiëring van fenprocoumon door claritromycine en roxitromycine. *Ned Tijdschr Geneeskd* (1996) 140, 375–7.
12. Recker MW, Kier KL. Potential interaction between clarithromycin and warfarin. *Ann Pharmacother* (1997) 31, 996–8.
13. Oberg KC. Delayed elevation of international normalized ratio with concurrent clarithromycin and warfarin therapy. *Pharmacotherapy* (1998) 18, 386–91.
14. Gooderham MJ, Bolli P, Fernandez PG. Concomitant digoxin toxicity and warfarin interaction in a patient receiving clarithromycin. *Ann Pharmacother* (1999) 33, 796–9.
15. Abbott Laboratories. Data on file, February 1995.
16. Dandekar SS, Laidlaw DAH. Suprachoroidal haemorrhage after addition of clarithromycin. *J R Soc Med* (2001) 94, 583–4.
17. Committee on Safety of Medicines. Reminders: interaction between macrolide antibiotics and warfarin. *Current Problems* (1992) 35, 4.
18. Ellsworth A, Horn JR, Wilkinson W, Black DJ, Church L, Sides GD, Harris J, Cullen PD. An evaluation of the effect of dirithromycin (D) and erythromycin (E) on the pharmacokinetics and pharmacodynamics of warfarin (W). *Intersci Conf Antimicrob Agents Chemother* (1995) 35, 9.
19. Grau E, Fontcuberta J, Félez J. Erythromycin-oral anticoagulants interaction. *Arch Intern Med* (1986) 146, 1639.
20. Grau E, Real E, Pastor E. Macrolides and oral anticoagulants: a dangerous association. *Acta Haematol (Basel)* (1999) 102, 113–14.
21. Bartle WR. Possible warfarin-erythromycin interaction. *Arch Intern Med* (1980) 140, 985–7.
22. Schwartz JI, Bachmann KA. Erythromycin-warfarin interaction. Arch Intern Med (1984) 144, 2094.22. Husserl FE. Erythromycin-warfarin interaction. *Arch Intern Med* (1983) 143, 1831, 1836
23. Sato RI, Gray DR, Brown SE. Warfarin interaction with erythromycin. *Arch Intern Med* (1984) 144, 2413–14.
24. Friedman HS, Bonventre MV. Erythromycin-induced digoxin toxicity. *Chest* (1982) 82, 202.
25. Hassell D, Utt JK. Suspected interaction: warfarin and erythromycin. *South Med J* (1985) 78, 1015–16.
26. Bussey HI, Knodel LC, Boyle DA. Warfarin-erythromycin interaction. *Arch Intern Med* (1985) 145, 1736–7.
27. O'Donnell D. Antibiotic-induced potentiation of oral anticoagulant agents. *Med J Aust* (1989) 150, 163–4.
28. Schwartz J, Bachmann K, Perigo E. Interaction between warfarin and erythromycin. *South Med J* (1983) 76, 91–3.
29. Wolf R, Elman M, Brenner S. Sulfonamide-induced bullous hemorrhagic eruption in a patient with low prothrombin time. *Isr J Med Sci* (1992), 28, 88204.
30. Bachmann K, Schwartz JI, Forney R, Frogameni A, Jauregui LE. The effect of erythromycin on the disposition kinetics of warfarin. *Pharmacology* (1984) 28, 171–6.

31. Weibert RT, Lorentz SM, Townsend RJ, Cook CE, Klauber MR, Jagger PI. Effect of erythromycin in patients receiving long-term warfarin therapy. *Clin Pharm* (1989) 8, 210–14.
32. Ellsworth A, Horn JR, Wilkinson W, Black DJ, Church L, Sides GD, Harris J, Cullen PD. An evaluation of the effect of dirithromycin (D) and erythromycin (E) on the pharmacokinetics and pharmacodynamics of warfarin (W). *Intersci Conf Antimicrob Agents Chemother* (1995) 35, 9.
33. Couet W, Istin B, Decourt JP, Ingrand I, Girault J, Fourtillan JB. Lack of effect of ponsinomycin on the pharmacokinetics of nicoumalone enantiomers. *Br J Clin Pharmacol* (1990) 30, 616–20.
34. Chassany O, Logeart I, Choulika S, Caulin C. Hématome pariétal abdominal lors d'un traitement associant acénocoumarol et roxithromycine. *Presse Med* (1998) 27, 1103.
35. Paulsen O, Nilsson L-G, Saint-Salvi B, Manuel C, Lunell E. No effect of roxithromycin on pharmacokinetic or pharmacodynamic properties of warfarin and its enantiomers. *Pharmacol Toxicol* (1988) 63, 215–20.
36. Ghose K, Ashton J, Rohan A. Possible interaction of roxithromycin with warfarin; updated review of ADR reports. *Clin Drug Invest* (1995) 10, 302–9.
37. Kolilekas L, Anagnostopoulos GK, Lampaditis I, Eleftheriadis I. Potential interaction between telithromycin and warfarin. *Ann Pharmacother* (2004) 38, 1424–7.
38. Visser LE, Penning-van Beest FJA, Kasbergen AAH, De Smet PAGM, Vulto AG, Hofman A, Stricker BHC. Overanticoagulation associated with combined use of antibacterial drugs and acenocoumarol or phenprocoumon anticoagulants. *Thromb Haemost* (2002) 88, 705–10.

Anticoagulants + Mango fruit (*Mangifera indica*)

There is evidence that eating mango fruit can moderately increase the anticoagulant effects of warfarin. None of the patients in whom this interaction was seen showed any evidence of bleeding.

Clinical evidence, mechanism, importance and management

A study in 13 patients on **warfarin** found that eating mango fruit (*Mangifera indica*) increased their INRs by an average of 38% (from 2.79 to 3.85) but no bleeding occurred. No other explanation for the increased INRs could be identified. The patients were reported to have eaten 1 to 6 mangos daily for 2 days to 1 month before attending the anticoagulant clinic. When mango was identified as a possible cause for their increased INRs, the patients were told to stop eating mango, whereupon their mean INR fell within 2 weeks, by almost 18%. When 2 of the patients whose mean INRs had originally risen by 13% were later rechallenged with mango (rather less than before), their mean INR rose by 9%.[1]

The reason for this apparent interaction is not known but the authors of the report speculate about the possible role of vitamin A (reported to be 8061 units in an average sized mango of 130 g, without seed). In practical terms this increase in INR would not seem to represent a serious problem, because none of the patients studied showed any evidence of bleeding although one patient's INR rose to 5.1 (a 54% increase). There appear to be no other reports in the literature of an interaction between mango and **warfarin**, nor of interactions between mango or any other oral anticoagulant. More study of this interaction is needed but at the present time there insufficient reason to suggest that patients on **warfarin** should avoid mango fruit.

1. Monterrey-Rodríguez J, Feliú JF, Rivera-Miranda GC. Interaction between warfarin and mango fruit. *Ann Pharmacother* (2002) 36, 940–1.

Anticoagulants + MAOIs

The theoretical possibility that MAOIs might increase the effects of the oral anticoagulants has not been confirmed. Moclobemide does not interact with phenprocoumon nor brofaromine with warfarin.

Clinical evidence, mechanism, importance and management

A number of studies[1-4] have shown that the MAOIs can increase the effects of some oral anticoagulants in *animals*, but reports of this interaction in man are lacking and no special precautions seem to be necessary. A study in healthy subjects found that **moclobemide** 200 mg three times daily for 7 days had no effect on the anticoagulant effects of **phenprocoumon**.[5,6] Another study in 12 healthy subjects also found no evidence that **brofaromine** alters the anticoagulant effects of **warfarin**.[7]

1. Fumarola D, De Rinaldis P. Ricerche sperimentali sugli inibitori della mono-aminossidasi. Influenza della nialamide sulla attività degli anticoagulanti indiretti. *Haematologica* (1964) 49, 1248–66.
2. Reber K, Studer A. Beeinflussung der Wirkung einiger indirekter Antikoagulantien durch Monoaminoxydase-Hemmer. *Thromb Diath Haemorrh* (1965) 14, 83–7.
3. de Nicola P, Fumarola D, de Rinaldis P. Beeinflussung der gerinnungshemmenden Wirkung der indirekten Antikoagulantien durch die MAO-Inhibitoren. *Thromb Diath Haemorrh* (1964) 12 (Suppl), 125–7.
4. Hrdina P, Rusnáková M, Kovalčík V. Changes of hypoprothrombinaemic activity of indirect anticoagulants after MAO inhibitors and reserpine. *Biochem Pharmacol* (1953) 12 (Suppl), 241.
5. Zimmer R, Gieschke R, Fischbach R, Gasic S. Interaction studies with moclobemide. *Acta Psychiatr Scand* (1990) (Suppl 360), 84–6.
6. Amrein R, Güntert TW, Dingemanse J, Lorscheid T, Stabl M, Schmid-Burgk W. Interactions of moclobemide with concomitantly administered medication: evidence from pharmacological and clinical studies. *Psychopharmacology (Berl)* (1992) 106, S24–S31.
7. Harding SR, Conly J, Lawrin-Workewych M, D'Souza J. A study of the interaction between brofaromine and warfarin in healthy volunteers. *Clin Invest Med* (1992) 15 (Suppl), A18.

Anticoagulants + Meprobamate

The anticoagulant effects of warfarin are not altered to a clinically relevant extent by meprobamate.

Clinical evidence, mechanism, importance and management

Meprobamate 400 mg four times daily was given to 9 men stabilised on **warfarin** for 2 weeks. Three of them showed a small increase in prothrombin times, five a small decrease and one remained unaffected.[1] In a placebo-controlled study in 17 patients on **warfarin**, the 8 patients who were also given meprobamate 2400 mg daily for 4 weeks showed only a small clinically unimportant reduction in prothrombin times.[2] Similar results were found in another study.[3] No particular precautions would therefore seem to be needed if meprobamate is added to established treatment with **warfarin**.

1. Udall JA. Warfarin therapy not influenced by meprobamate. A controlled study in nine men. *Curr Ther Res* (1970) 12, 724–8.
2. Gould L, Michael A, Fisch S, Gomprecht RF. Prothrombin levels maintained with meprobamate and warfarin. A controlled study. *JAMA* (1972) 220, 1460–2.
3. deCarolis PP, Gelfand ML. Effect of tranquilizers on prothrombin time response to coumarin. *J Clin Pharmacol* (1975) 15, 557.

Anticoagulants + Meptazinol

The anticoagulant effects of warfarin are not altered by meptazinol.

Clinical evidence, mechanism, importance and management

Meptazinol 200 mg four times daily for 7 days had no significant effect on the prothrombin indexes of 6 elderly patients on **warfarin** (about 5 mg daily).[1] No special precautions seem to be necessary. Information about other anticoagulants is lacking.

1. Ryd-Kjellen E, Alm A. Effect of meptazinol on chronic anticoagulant therapy. *Hum Toxicol* (1986) 5, 101–2.

Anticoagulants + Mesalazine (Mesalamine)

A single case report describes reduced warfarin effects in a patient when given mesalazine.

Clinical evidence

A woman on **warfarin** 5 mg daily, with INRs between 2 and 3, was started on mesalazine 800 mg three times daily for the treatment of a caecal ulcer. Four weeks later she presented in hospital with left leg pain, which was diagnosed as an acute popliteal vein thrombosis, and at the same time it was found that her prothrombin time and INR had fallen to 11.3 seconds and 0.9 respectively. The patient was treated with intravenous heparin. Over the next 10 days INRs of up to 1.7 were achieved by increasing the doses of **warfarin** up to 10 mg daily, but a satisfactory INR of 2.1 was only reached when the mesalazine was stopped. The report says that serum **warfarin** levels were not detectable during the use of mesalazine.[1]

Mechanism

Not understood.

Importance and management

This appears to be the first and only report of an interaction between warfarin and mesalazine, which suggests that it is unlikely to be of general importance. Information about other oral anticoagulants is lacking. See also 'Anticoagulants + Sulfasalazine', p.314.

1. Marinella MA. Mesalamine and warfarin therapy resulting in decreased warfarin effect. *Ann Pharmacother* (1998) 32, 841–2.

Anticoagulants + Methaqualone

Methaqualone may cause a very small and clinically unimportant reduction in the anticoagulant effects of warfarin.

Clinical evidence, mechanism, importance and management

The average prothrombin times of 10 patients on **warfarin** were 20.9 seconds before, 20.4 seconds during, and 19.6 seconds after taking methaqualone 300 mg at bedtime for 4 weeks.[1] The plasma **warfarin** levels of another patient were unaffected by methaqualone, although there was some evidence that enzyme induction had occurred.[2] Methaqualone has some enzyme-inducing effects so that any small changes in prothrombin times reflect a limited increase in the metabolism and clearance of **warfarin**, but these appear to be too small to matter.[2,3] No special precautions seem to be necessary.

1. Udall JA. Clinical implications of warfarin interactions with five sedatives. *Am J Cardiol* (1975) 35, 67–71.
2. Whitfield JB, Moss DW, Neale G, Orme M, Breckenridge A. Changes in plasma γ-glutamyl transpeptidase activity associated with alterations in drug metabolism in man. *BMJ* (1973) 1, 316–18.
3. Nayak RK, Smyth RD, Chamberlain AP, Polk A, DeLong AF, Herczeg T, Chemburkar PB, Joslin RS, Reavey-Cantwell NH. Methaqualone pharmacokinetics after single- and multiple-dose administration in man. *J Pharmacokinet Biopharm* (1974) 2, 107–21.

Anticoagulants + Methylphenidate

Methylphenidate appears not to interact with ethyl biscoumacetate.

Clinical evidence, importance and management

One study found that in 4 healthy subjects the half-life of single doses of **ethyl biscoumacetate** was approximately doubled after they took methylphenidate 20 mg daily for 3 to 5 days, due, it was suggested, to the enzyme inhibitory effects of the methylphenidate.[1] However, a later double blind study in 12 subjects failed to confirm this interaction.[2] The clinical significance of the prolonged half life is unknown, but given the lack of an interaction in the other study it seems likely to be small. There does not seem to be any information about other anticoagulants.

1. Garrettson LK, Perel JM, Dayton PG. Methylphenidate interaction with both anticonvulsants and ethyl biscoumacetate. *JAMA* (1969) 207, 2053–6.
2. Hague DE, Smith ME, Ryan JR, McMahon FG. The effect of methylphenidate and prolintane on the metabolism of ethyl biscoumacetate. *Clin Pharmacol Ther* (1971) 12, 259–62.

Anticoagulants + Metoclopramide

Metoclopramide causes a small change in the pharmacokinetics of phenprocoumon, but no important changes in the anticoagulant effects seem to occur.

Clinical evidence, mechanism, importance and management

Four days' treatment with metoclopramide 30 mg daily reduced the AUC of a single dose of **phenprocoumon** in 12 healthy subjects by 16%, but no significant changes were seen in the anticoagulant effects.[1] There seems to be no other information about **phenprocoumon** or any other anticoagulant.

1. Wesermeyer D, Mönig H, Gaska T, Masuch S, Seiler KU, Huss H, Bruhn HD. Der Einfluß von Cisaprid und Metoclopramid auf die Bioverfügbarkeit von Phenprocoumon. *Hamostaseologie* (1991) 11, 95–102.

Anticoagulants + Metrifonate

Metrifonate appears not to interact with warfarin.

Clinical evidence, mechanism, importance and management

A double-blind, placebo-controlled crossover study in 14 healthy subjects found that metrifonate 50 mg daily for 8 days did not change the pharmacokinetics and pharmacodynamics of a single 25-mg dose of **warfarin** given on day 4. Plasma **warfarin** levels and prothrombin times remained unchanged.[1] This suggests that no special precautions are needed if these two drugs are used concurrently. Information about other anticoagulants is lacking.

1. Heinig R, Kitchin N, Rolan P. Disposition of a single dose of warfarin in healthy individuals after pretreatment with metrifonate. *Clin Drug Invest* (1999) 18, 151–9.

Anticoagulants + Metronidazole

The anticoagulant effects of warfarin are markedly increased by metronidazole and bleeding has been seen.

Clinical evidence

Metronidazole 250 mg three times daily for a week increased the half-life of **warfarin** by about one-third (from 35 to 46 hours) in 8 healthy subjects. The anticoagulant effects of ***(S)*-warfarin** were virtually doubled and the half-life increased by 60%, but the response to ***(R)*-warfarin** was only affected in one subject.[1]

Bleeding has been seen in 2 patients taking **warfarin** and metronidazole.[2,3] One of them had severe pain in one leg, ecchymoses and haemorrhage of both legs, and an increase in her prothrombin time from 17 to 19 seconds to 147 seconds within 17 days of starting the metronidazole.[2]

Mechanism

Metronidazole appears to inhibit the activity of the enzymes responsible for the metabolism (ring oxidation) of the *(S)*-warfarin, but not the *(R)*-warfarin.[1] As a result the racemate with the more potent activity is retained within the body, and its actions are increased and prolonged.

Importance and management

An established and clinically important interaction, although the documentation is small. Monitor the INR when both drugs are used and adjust the warfarin dose accordingly. Nothing seems to be documented about other anticoagulants but it would be prudent to expect the coumarins to behave similarly, although some indirect evidence suggests that no interaction occurs with **phenprocoumon**.[4]

1. O'Reilly RA. The stereoselective interaction of warfarin and metronidazole in man. *N Engl J Med* (1976) 295, 354–7.
2. Kazmier FJ. A significant interaction between metronidazole and warfarin. *Mayo Clin Proc* (1976) 51, 782–4.
3. Dean RP, Talbert RL. Bleeding associated with concurrent warfarin and metronidazole therapy. *Drug Intell Clin Pharm* (1980) 14, 864–6.
4. Staiger C, Wang NS, de Vries J, Weber E. Untersuchungen zur Wirkung von Metronidazol auf den Phenazon-Metabolismus. *Arzneimittelforschung* (1984) 34, 89–91.

Anticoagulants + Misoprostol

A reduction in the anticoagulant effects of acenocoumarol has been attributed to the use of misoprostol in one patient.

Clinical evidence, mechanism, importance and management

A 39-year-old woman on **acenocoumarol**, celiprolol, triamterene, cyclothiazide, pravastatin and diosmin had a rise in her prothrombin levels from 0.3 to 1 within 8 days of starting diclofenac and misoprostol 400 micrograms daily. A day after these two drugs had been withdrawn her prothrombin level had fallen to 0.67, and after another 3 days to 0.32.[1] The reasons for this reaction is not known, but suspicion falls on the misoprostol because diclofenac, if and when it interacts with anticoagulants, increases rather than reduces their effects (see 'Anticoagulants + NSAIDs; Miscellaneous', p.298). But just why misoprostol should cause these changes is not clear.

This is an isolated case, complicated by the presence of a number of other drugs, nevertheless bear it in mind if misoprostol is added to established treatment with any anticoagulant. More study is needed.

1. Martin MP, Jonville-Bera AP, Bera F, Caillard X, Autret E. Interaction entre le misoprostol et l'acénocoumarol. *Presse Med* (1995) 24, 195.

Anticoagulants + Montelukast

Montelukast does not affect the pharmacokinetics of warfarin.

Clinical evidence, mechanism, importance and management

In a double-blind placebo-controlled randomised study, 12 healthy subjects were given oral montelukast 10 mg for 12 days and a single 30-mg dose of **warfarin** on day 7. It was found that the pharmacokinetics of the **warfarin** were virtually unchanged by the montelukast, and prothrombin times and INRs were not significantly altered.[1] No special precautions are needed if both drugs are used concurrently.

1. Van Hecken A, Depre M, Verbesselt R, Wynants K, De Lepeleire I, Arnoudt J, Wong PH, Freeman A, Holland S, Gertz B, De Schepper PJ. Effect of montelukast on the pharmacokinetics and pharmacodynamics of warfarin in healthy subjects. *J Clin Pharmacol* (1999) 39, 495–500.

Anticoagulants + Moracizine

An isolated report describes bleeding in a patient on warfarin when given moracizine, but most patients do not seem to be affected.

Clinical evidence

The prothrombin time of a woman on **warfarin**, digoxin, captopril and prednisone rose from a range of 15 to 20 seconds up to 41 seconds within 4 days of starting moracizine 300 mg three times daily. She bled (haematemesis, haematuria), but responded rapidly to withdrawal of the **warfarin** and moracizine, and the administration of phytomenadione.[1]

This report contrasts with two others in which moracizine 250 mg every 8 hours for 14 days caused little or no change in the pharmacokinetics of single 25-mg doses of **warfarin** in 12 healthy subjects. There was only a slight decrease in the **warfarin** elimination half-life, from 37.6 to 34.2 hours and no change in prothrombin times.[2,3] No significant changes in **warfarin** dosage requirements were needed in 34 patients after moracizine was started.[2]

Mechanism

Not understood.

Importance and management

Information appears to be limited to these reports. Although most patients seem unlikely to be affected, it would be prudent to bear this interaction in mind when prescribing both drugs. As yet information about other anticoagulants does not appear to be available.

1. Serpa MD, Cossolias J, McGreevy MJ. Moricizine-warfarin: a possible interaction. *Ann Pharmacother* (1992) 26, 127.
2. Siddoway LA, Schwartz SL, Barbey JT, Woosley RL. Clinical pharmacokinetics of moricizine. *Am J Cardiol* (1990) 65, 21D–25D.
3. Benedek IH, King S-YP, Powell RJ, Agra AM, Schary WL, Pieniaszek HJ. Effect of moricizine on the pharmacokinetics and pharmacodynamics of warfarin in healthy volunteers. *J Clin Pharmacol* (1992) 32, 558–63.

Anticoagulants + Natto

Natto, a Japanese food made from fermented soya bean, can reduce the effects of warfarin.

Clinical evidence

A retrospective study of 10 patients on **warfarin**, who had received heart valve replacements, found that eating natto caused the thrombotest values to rise from a range of 12 to 29% up to a range of 33 to 100%. The extent of the rise appeared to be related to the amount eaten. The thrombotest values fell again when the natto was stopped. A healthy subject on **warfarin**, with a thrombotest value of 40%, showed no changes 5 hours after eating 100 g of natto, but demonstrated a rise to 86% 24 hours later and to 90% 48 hours later.[1] Similar rises were seen in *animals*.[1]

Mechanism

Not fully established. Natto does not appear to contain significant amounts of vitamin K, but there is evidence that after ingestion, the activity of *Bacillus natto* on the natto in the gut causes a marked increase in the synthesis and subsequent absorption of vitamin K.[1] This would oppose the actions of the warfarin (see 'Anticoagulants + Vitamin K', p.321).

Importance and management

Information appears to be limited to this study[1] and a previous one by the same author.[2] However, the interaction appears to be established. Patients on warfarin should be advised to avoid natto. Other oral anticoagulants would be expected to be similarly affected (assuming that the proposed mechanism of interaction is correct).

1. Kudo T. Warfarin antagonism of natto and increase in serum vitamin K by intake of natto. *Artery* (1990) 17, 189–201.
2. Kudo T, Uchibori Y, Astumi K, Numao K, Miura M, Shigara M, Hashimoto A. Antagonism of natto in anticoagulant therapy. *Igaku No Ayumi* (1978) 104, 36–8.

Anticoagulants + Nevirapine

Three cases suggest that warfarin requirements are approximately doubled by nevirapine.

Clinical evidence, mechanism, importance and management

A man taking **warfarin** 2.5 mg daily (INR 2.1 to 2.4) needed a doubled **warfarin** dose when his treatment with zidovudine and didanosine was replaced by stavudine, lamivudine and nevirapine. A few days later when his treatment was again changed (to stavudine, lamivudine and saquinavir) his original **warfarin** dosage was found to be adequate. Another patient was resistant to doses of **warfarin** of up to 17 mg daily while taking zidovudine, lamivudine and nevirapine, but he responded to **warfarin** 5 mg daily when the nevirapine was withdrawn. The warfarin dosage had to be raised to 12 mg daily when nevirapine was restarted. Yet another patient showed resistance to **warfarin** while taking nevirapine.[1]

The reasons for this interaction are not known but it is suggested that nevirapine possibly induces the enzymes concerned with the metabolism of the **warfarin** so that it is cleared from the body more quickly. Information seems to be limited to these three cases, but it would now be prudent to monitor prothrombin times and INRs in any patient if **warfarin** and nevirapine are used concurrently, being alert for the need to increase the **warfarin** dosage (possibly twofold). Information about other oral anticoagulants seems to be lacking.

1. Dionisio D, Mininni S, Bartolozzi D, Esperti F, Vivarelli A, Leoncini F. Need for increased dose of warfarin in HIV patients taking nevirapine. *AIDS* (2001) 15, 277–8.

Anticoagulants + NSAIDs; Acemetacin or Oxametacin

The anticoagulant effects of warfarin and acenocoumarol can be increased by oxametacin. Acemetacin does not interact with phenprocoumon.

Clinical evidence, mechanism, importance and management

Oxametacin 100 mg three times a day for 14 days reduced the thrombotest percentages of 12 anticoagulated patients (11 on **warfarin** and one on **acenocoumarol**) from 11.2 to 7.8%. Four of the patients needed a reduction in their anticoagulant dosage or its withdrawal.[1] Concurrent use should be monitored, reducing the anticoagulant dosage if necessary. Direct information about other anticoagulants is lacking, but it seems possible other coumarins may interact similarly. Apply the same precautions. A study in 20 patients on **phenprocoumon** found no interaction with acemetacin 60 mg three times daily.[2]

1. Baele G, Rasquin K, Barbier F. Effects of oxametacin on coumarin anticoagulation and on platelet function in humans. *Arzneimittelforschung* (1983) 33, 149–52.
2. Hess H, Koeppen R. Kontrollierte Doppelblindestudie zur Frage einer möglichen Interferenz von Acemetacin mit einer laufenden Antikoagulanzien-Therapie. *Arzneimittelforschung* (1980) 30, 1421–3.

Anticoagulants + NSAIDs; Azapropazone

The anticoagulant effects of warfarin are markedly increased by azapropazone. The makers contraindicate concurrent use.

Clinical evidence

A woman on digoxin, furosemide, spironolactone, allopurinol, and **warfarin** (prothrombin ratio 2.8) developed haematemesis within 4 days of starting to take azapropazone 300 mg four times a day. Her prothrombin ratio was found to have risen to 15.7. Subsequent gastroscopic examination revealed a benign ulcer, the presumed site of the bleeding.[1]

At least 12 other patients are reported to have developed this interaction. Bruising or bleeding (melaena, epistaxis, haematuria) and prolonged prothrombin times have occurred within a few days of starting azapropazone.[2-7] Three patients died.[4-6] Another patient on **warfarin** and azapropazone, diclofenac and co-proxamol showed an increase in prothrombin time.[8]

Mechanism

Not understood. Azapropazone displaces warfarin from its plasma protein binding sites[9-11] thereby increasing the amount of free and pharmacologically active molecules, but it is almost certain that this alone does not fully account for the clinical effects reported. Changes in the metabolism of warfarin are probably mainly responsible.

Importance and management

The interaction between warfarin and azapropazone is established and clinically important. The incidence is uncertain. Because of the risk of serious bleeding the makers of azapropazone say that it should not be used with warfarin or any other anticoagulant.[12]

1. Powell-Jackson PR. Interaction between azapropazone and warfarin. *BMJ* (1977) 1, 1193–4.
2. Green AE, Hort JF, Korn HET, Leach H. Potentiation of warfarin by azapropazone. *BMJ* (1977) 1, 1532.
3. Beeley L. *Bulletin of the West Midlands Adverse Drug Reaction Study Group* (1980), 10.
4. Anon. Interactions. Doctors warned on warfarin dangers. *Pharm J* (1983) 230, 676.
5. Win N, Mitchell DC, Jones PAE, French EA. Azapropazone and warfarin. *BMJ* (1991) 302, 969–70.
6. Beeley L, Cunningham H, Carmichael A, Brennan A. *Bulletin of the West Midlands Centre for Adverse Drug Reaction Reporting* (1991) 33, 19.
7. Beeley L, Magee P, Hickey FM. *Bulletin of the West Midlands Centre for Adverse Drug Reaction Reporting* (1989) 28, 34.
8. Beeley L, Stewart P, Hickey FL. *Bulletin of the West Midlands Centre for Adverse Drug Reaction Reporting* (1988) 27, 27.
9. McElnay JC, D'Arcy PF. Interaction between azapropazone and warfarin. *BMJ* (1977) 2, 773–4.
10. McElnay JC, D'Arcy PF. The effect of azapropazone on the binding of warfarin to human serum proteins. *J Pharm Pharmacol* (1978) 30 (Suppl), 73P.
11. McElnay JC, D'Arcy PF. Interaction between azapropazone and warfarin. *Experientia* (1978) 34, 1320–1.
12. Rhuemox (Azapropazone dihydrate). Goldshield Pharmaceuticals Ltd. UK Summary of product characteristics, February 2000.

Anticoagulants + NSAIDs; Cyclooxygenase-2 inhibitors

There is evidence that celecoxib, rofecoxib, parecoxib and valdecoxib do not normally interact with warfarin. However, raised INRs accompanied by bleeding, particularly in the elderly, have been attributed to the use of warfarin and celecoxib or rofecoxib, and fluindione with rofecoxib. Etoricoxib causes a small increase in INR when taken with warfarin.

Clinical evidence

(a) Celecoxib

In a placebo-controlled study **warfarin** 2.5 to 5 mg daily was given to 24 healthy subjects to produce a stable prothrombin time of 1.2 to 1.7 times their pretreatment values for at least 3 consecutive days. They were then given celecoxib 200 mg twice daily for a week. It was found that the pharmacokinetics of both the *(S)*- and *(R)*-enantiomers of **warfarin** and the prothrombin times were unchanged by the presence of the celecoxib.[1]

However, in contrast, a report describes an 88-year-old woman on **warfarin** who had a rise in her INR when celecoxib 200 mg daily was started. After several **warfarin** dosage adjustments she was later restabilised on a 25% lower **warfarin** dose.[2] There is a similar report of a 77-year old patient who required a 10% decrease in **warfarin** dosage to maintain her target INR when celecoxib 100 mg twice daily was also given.[3] Other reports describe at least 6 patients on **warfarin** who had INR increases (of 77 to 114%)[4] during concurrent treatment with celecoxib. Two patients had bruising and epistaxis or haemoptysis, which required treatment with phytomenadione.[4,5] The makers also report that bleeding events have been reported with this combination, predominantly in the elderly.[6]

(b) Etoricoxib

Studies in healthy subjects on **warfarin** found that etoricoxib 120 mg daily caused an increase of about 13% in INR,[7] which is unlikely to be clinically relevant.

(c) Parecoxib

A study in 18 healthy subjects found that pretreatment with 40 mg of intravenous parecoxib twice daily for 6 days produced no clinically or statistically significant differences in their coagulation parameters (PT, aPPT and platelet counts) when compared with **heparin** alone (a 36-hour infusion of 10 to 14 units/kg). Use of these drugs together was well tolerated.[8]

A study in 12 healthy adults on **warfarin** found that additional treatment with 10 mg of intravenous parecoxib twice daily for 7 days had no significant effects on prothrombin times when compared with 13 control subjects given **warfarin** and a placebo. Parecoxib did not affect the pharmacokinetics of ***(S)***- or ***(R)*-warfarin**.[9] Valdecoxib would be expected to interact similarly.[10]

(d) Rofecoxib

In a single-dose study,[11] the INRs of 12 healthy subjects given 50-mg doses of rofecoxib and 30 mg of **warfarin** were increased by about 11%. In a steady-state study 15 healthy subjects were given **warfarin** 5 mg daily to produce a stable prothrombin time of 1.4 to 1.7 for at least 3 consecutive days. They were then additionally given rofecoxib 25 mg or placebo daily for 3 weeks. It was found that INRs were increased by 8%. Rofecoxib had no effect on the pharmacokinetics of the more potent ***(S)*-warfarin** enantiomer, but the AUC of ***(R)*-warfarin** was increased by about 40% in both the single dose and steady-state studies.[11] Such changes are probably not clinically important in most patients.

However, there are reports of an increase in INR in two elderly patients taking **warfarin** and rofecoxib. The INRs were raised, in one case from less than 3 to 4.1 within a month of starting rofecoxib 12.5 mg daily, and in the other case from 3.2 to 4.6 within 2 days of starting rofecoxib. The INRs decreased when **warfarin** dosage was reduced.[4] The makers note there have been isolated reports of increases in INR in patients taking rofecoxib and either **warfarin** or **fluindione**.[12]

Mechanism, importance and management

The interaction with these cyclooxygenase-2 (COX-2) inhibitors is clinically significant but apparently rare. For example, of the 4 million prescriptions for celecoxib dispensed over the 18-month period from December 1998, about 1% were estimated to be for patients who would have been on warfarin,[6] and only a handful of cases have been reported. However, the makers recommend that anticoagulant activity should be monitored in patients taking warfarin or other anticoagulants particularly in the first few days after initiating or changing the dose of COX-2 inhibitor, but given the number of reported cases of a problem this seems very cautious. Some monitoring is certainly appropriate because all NSAIDS can irritate the gastrointestinal tract and cause bleeding.

1. Karim A, Tolbert D, Piergies A, Hubbard RC, Harper K, Wallemark C-B, Slater M, Geis GS. Celecoxib does not significantly alter the pharmacokinetics or hypoprothrombinemic effect of warfarin in healthy subjects. *J Clin Pharmacol* (2000) 40, 655–63.
2. Haase KK, Rojas-Fernandez CH, Lane L, Frank DA. Potential interaction between celecoxib and warfarin. *Ann Pharmacother* (2000) 34, 666–7.
3. O'Donnell DC, Hooper JS. Increased international normalized ratio in a patient taking warfarin and celecoxib. *J Pharm Technol* (2001), 17, 3–5.
4. Stading JA, Skrabal MZ, Faulkner MA. Seven cases of interaction between warfarin and cyclooxygenase-2 inhibitors. *Am J Health-Syst Pharm* (2001) 58, 2076–80.
5. Mersfedler TL, Stewart LR. Warfarin and celecoxib interaction. *Ann Pharmacother* (2000) 34, 325–7.
6. FDA MedWatch Program, May 1999. Available at: http://www.fda.gov/medwatch/safety/1999/celebr.htm (accessed 07/09/05).
7. Arcoxia (Etoricoxib). Merck Sharp & Dohme Ltd. UK Summary of product characteristics, May 2005.
8. Noveck RJ, Kuss ME, Qian J, North J, Hubbard RC. Parecoxib sodium, an injectable COX-2 specific inhibitor, does not affect heparin-regulated blood coagulation parameters. *Reg Anesth Pain Med* (2001) 26 (Suppl), 20.

9. Karim A, Bradford D, Qian J, Hubbard R. The COX-2-specific inhibitor parecoxib sodium does not affect warfarin pharmacokinetic and pharmacodynamic parameters. American College of Emergency Physicians. Scientific Assembly, Chicago, Illinois, 15-18 October 2001. Abstract 130.
10. Bextra (Valdecoxib). Pfizer Inc. US Prescribing information, November 2004.
11. Schwartz JI, Bugianesi KJ, Ebel DL, De Smet M, Haesen R, Larson PJ, Ko A, Verbesselt R, Hunt TL, Lins R, Lens S, Porras AG, Dieck J, Keymeulen B, Gertz BJ. The effect of rofecoxib on the pharmacodynamics and pharmacokinetics of warfarin. *Clin Pharmacol Ther* (2000) 68, 626–36.
12. Vioxx (Rofecoxib). Merck Sharp & Dohme Ltd. UK Summary of product characteristics, August 2003.

Anticoagulants + NSAIDs; Diflunisal

There is limited evidence that diflunisal can increase the anticoagulant effects of acenocoumarol and possibly warfarin, but phenprocoumon appears not to be affected.

Clinical evidence

The total plasma **warfarin** levels of 5 healthy subjects fell by about a third (from 741 to 533 nanograms/ml) when they were given diflunisal 500 mg twice daily for 2 weeks. Also, unbound **warfarin** increased from 1.02 to 1.34%, but the anticoagulant response was unaffected. When the diflunisal was withdrawn the anticoagulant response was reduced.[1] Another report very briefly describes an increased INR when a patient on **warfarin** was given diflunisal.[2]

A brief report states that 3 out of 6 subjects on **acenocoumarol** had significant increases in prothrombin times, but no interaction was seen in 2 subjects on **phenprocoumon**, when they were given diflunisal 750 mg daily.[3]

Mechanism

Uncertain. Diflunisal can displace warfarin from its plasma protein binding sites but this on its own is almost certainly not the full explanation.[1] The fall in anticoagulant response when diflunisal was stopped is possibly linked to a difference in the rates that total and unbound plasma warfarin returned to their original levels.[1]

Importance and management

This interaction is neither well defined nor well documented. Its importance is uncertain. However, the reports cited and the makers literature suggest that an increased anticoagulant effect should be looked for if diflunisal is added to established treatment with any anticoagulant. A decreased effect would be expected if diflunisal is withdrawn. Phenprocoumon is possibly an exception and appears not to interact. The risk of bleeding (because of changes in platelet activity or gastrointestinal irritation) appears to be less than with analgesic doses of aspirin.

1. Serlin MJ, Mossman S, Sibeon RG, Tempero KF, Breckenridge AM. Interaction between diflunisal and warfarin. *Clin Pharmacol Ther* (1980) 28, 493–8.
2. Beeley L, Cunningham H, Carmichael A, Brennan A. *Bulletin of the West Midlands Centre for Adverse Drug Reaction Reporting* (1992) 35, 51.
3. Tempero KF, Cirillo VJ, Steelman SL. Diflunisal: a review of pharmacokinetic and pharmacodynamic properties, drug interactions, and special tolerability studies in humans. *Br J Clin Pharmacol* (1977) 4, 31S–36S.

Anticoagulants + NSAIDs; Etodolac

Etodolac appears not to interact significantly with warfarin.

Clinical evidence, mechanism, importance and management

Warfarin 20 mg on day 1, 10 mg on days 2 and 3 and etodolac 200 mg every 12 hours were given to 18 healthy subjects in a three-period crossover study, each period lasting 2.5 days. Although the median peak serum levels of the **warfarin** fell by 19% and the median total clearance rose by 13% in the presence of etodolac, the prothrombin time response remained unchanged.[1] Another study in 16 healthy subjects given **warfarin** 20 mg on day 1, 10 mg on days 2 and 3 with and without etodolac 200 mg every 12 hours found some small changes in the pharmacokinetics of **warfarin** but its effects were unchanged. The pharmacokinetics of etodolac were unaffected by **warfarin**.[2]

There would therefore seem to be no reason for avoiding concurrent use although it would be prudent to monitor the response, because all NSAIDs have some effect on platelet activity. There seems to be nothing documented about other anticoagulants.

1. Ermer JC, Hicks DR, Wheeler SC, Kraml M, Jusko WJ. Concomitant etodolac affects neither the unbound clearance nor the pharmacologic effect of warfarin. *Clin Pharmacol Ther* (1994) 55, 305–16.
2. Zvaifler N. A review of the antiarthritic efficacy and safety of etodolac. *Clin Rheumatol* (1989) 8 (Suppl 1), 43–53.

Anticoagulants + NSAIDs; Feprazone

The anticoagulant effects of warfarin are increased by feprazone, which can lead to bleeding.

Clinical evidence

Five patients on long-term **warfarin** treatment showed a mean prothrombin time rise from 29 to 38 seconds after 5 days' treatment with feprazone 200 mg twice daily, despite a 40% reduction in the **warfarin** dosage (from 5 to 3 mg daily). Four days after withdrawal of the feprazone, their prothrombin times were almost back to their usual levels.[1]

Mechanism

Unknown. Feprazone is highly bound to plasma proteins so that some displacement from plasma protein binding sites can occur, but this alone almost certainly does not explain this interaction.

Importance and management

Although information is limited to the study cited, the interaction would appear to be established. Concurrent use should be avoided to prevent bleeding. If that is not possible, the anticoagulant response should be closely monitored and suitable reductions made to the warfarin dosage. Other coumarins may be expected to behave similarly.

1. Chierichetti S, Bianchi G, Cerri B. Comparison of feprazone and phenylbutazone interaction with warfarin in man. *Curr Ther Res* (1975) 18, 568–72.

Anticoagulants + NSAIDs; Floctafenine or Glafenine

The anticoagulant effects of acenocoumarol are increased by floctafenine and those of phenprocoumon are increased by floctafenine and glafenine. No interaction occurs with acenocoumarol, ethyl biscoumacetate or 'indanedione'.

Clinical evidence, mechanism, importance and management

(a) Floctafenine

A double-blind study in 20 patients on **acenocoumarol** or **phenprocoumon** and given either floctafenine or placebo showed that floctafenine 200 mg four times daily prolonged their thrombotest times by an average of about one-third,[1] even though the anticoagulant dosage of some of the patients was reduced. The reasons are not understood. The effects of concurrent use should be monitored and the anticoagulant dosage reduced as necessary. Information about other anticoagulants is lacking.

(b) Glafenine

A double-blind study in 20 patients stabilised on **phenprocoumon** and given either glafenine or placebo showed that a significant increase in thrombotest times occurred within a week of starting to take glafenine 200 mg three times daily.[2] Another report states that 5 out of 7 patients needed an anticoagulant dosage reduction while taking glafenine.[3] The reason is not understood. Monitor the effects of concurrent use and reduce the anticoagulant dosage appropriately. Ten patients on **acenocoumarol**, **ethyl biscoumacetate** or '**indanedione**' showed no changes in their anticoagulant response when given glafenine 800 mg daily over a 4-week period.[4]

1. Boeijinga JK, van de Broeke RN, Jochemsen R, Breimer DD, Hoogslag MA, Jeletich-Bastiaanse A. De invloed van floctafenine (Idalon) op antistollingsbehandeling met coumarinederivaten. *Ned Tijdschr Geneeskd* (1981) 125, 1931–5.

2. Boeijinga JK, van der Vijgh WJF. Double blind study of the effect of glafenine (Glifanan®) on oral anticoagulant therapy with phenprocoumon (Marcumar®). *Eur J Clin Pharmacol* (1977) 12, 291–6.
3. Boeijinga JK, Bing GT, van der Meer J. De invloed van glafenine (Glifanan) op antistollingsbehandeling met coumarinederivaten. *Ned Tijdschr Geneeskd* (1974) 118, 1895–8.
4. Raby C. Recherches sur une éventuelle potentialisation de l'action des anticoagulants de synthèse par la glafénine. *Therapie* (1977) 32, 293–9.

Anticoagulants + NSAIDs; Indometacin

The anticoagulant effects of acenocoumarol, phenprocoumon and warfarin are not normally affected by indometacin. However, some caution is still necessary because indometacin can irritate the gut, and in a handful of cases bleeding, attributed to an interaction, has been reported.

Clinical evidence

In a placebo-controlled double-blind study indometacin 100 mg daily for 5 days had no effect on the anticoagulant effects of **warfarin** in 8 healthy subjects.[1] When 19 healthy subjects took either indometacin 25 mg four times daily or placebo for 11 days, neither the anticoagulant effects nor the half-life of single doses of **warfarin** were affected by indometacin.[1]

Other studies in healthy subjects and patients anticoagulated with **acenocoumarol**[2] or **phenprocoumon**[3-5] similarly showed that the anticoagulant effects were not changed by indometacin.

In contrast, a handful of somewhat equivocal reports describe possible interactions in patients taking **warfarin**.[6-11] One patient was also taking allopurinol, which is known to occasionally interact with anticoagulants.[11] The report involving allopurinol has also been criticised, as the INR was raised by less than 0.2, which could be explained by the general fluctuations in INR that are commonly seen.[12] In one report the patient was taking indometacin before the warfarin was started, and a very large loading dose was given, so the reaction cannot clearly be attributed to an interaction.[9] Two further reports give no details of the interaction.[7,10]

Mechanism

None. Indometacin reduces platelet aggregation and thereby prolongs bleeding when it occurs.

Importance and management

It is well established that indometacin does not normally alter the anticoagulant effects acenocoumarol, phenprocoumon or warfarin. Concurrent use need not be avoided but caution is still appropriate, firstly because indometacin, like other NSAIDs, can cause gastrointestinal irritation, ulceration and bleeding, which may be prolonged, and secondly because the handful of cases of unexplained and unconfirmed possible interactions cannot be dismissed entirely.

1. Vesell ES, Passananti GT, Johnson AO. Failure of indomethacin and warfarin to interact in normal human volunteers. *J Clin Pharmacol* (1975) 15, 486–95.
2. Gáspárdy G, Bálint G, Gáspárdy G. Wirkung der Kombination Indomethacin und Syncumar (Acenocumarol) auf den Prothrombinspiegel im Blutplasma. *Z Rheumaforsch* (1967) 26, 332–5.
3. Müller G, Zollinger W. The influence of indomethacin on blood coagulation, particularly with regard to the interference with anticoagulant treatment. Die Entzundung-Grundlagen und Pharmakologische Beeinflussung. International Symposium on Inflammation. Freiburg, Breisgau, May 4–6, 1966. *Heister R and Hofmann HF (eds), Urban and Schwarzenburg, Munich* (1966).
4. Frost H, Hess H. Concomitant administration of indomethacin and anticoagulants. Die Entzundung-Grundlagen und Pharmakologische Beeinflussung. International Symposium on Inflammation. Freiburg, Breisgau, May 4–6, 1966. *Heister R and Hofmann HF (eds), Urban and Schwarzenburg, Munich* (1966).
5. Muller KH, Herrmann K. Is simultaneous therapy with anticoagulants and indomethacin feasible? *Med Welt* (1966) 17, 1553–4.
6. Chan TYK. Prolongation of prothrombin time with the use of indomethacin and warfarin. *Br J Clin Pract* (1997) 51, 177–8.
7. Koch-Weser J. Haemorrhagic reactions and drug interactions in 500 warfarin-treated patients. *Clin Pharmacol Ther* (1973) 14, 139.
8. McQueen EG. New Zealand Committee on Adverse Reactions: fourteenth annual report 1979. *N Z Med J* (1980) 91, 226–9.
9. Self TH, Soloway MS, Vaughn D. Possible interaction of indomethacin and warfarin. *Drug Intell Clin Pharm* (1978) 12, 580–1.
10. Beeley L, Stewart P. *Bulletin of the West Midlands Centre for Adverse Drug Reaction Reporting* (1987) 25, 28.
11. Chan TYK, Lui SF, Chung SY, Luk S, Critchley JAJH. Adverse interaction between warfarin and indomethacin. *Drug Safety* (1994) 10, 267–9.
12. Day R, Quinn D. Adverse interaction between warfarin and indomethacin. *Drug Safety* (1994) 11, 213–14.

Anticoagulants + NSAIDs; Ketorolac

Ketorolac appears not to interact with warfarin, but it may possibly cause serious gastrointestinal bleeding and is considered by the UK Committee on Safety of Medicines and its makers as contraindicated in patients taking anticoagulants. Bleeding time may be prolonged by concurrent dalteparin and ketorolac, but intramuscular ketorolac and subcutaneous enoxaparin appear not to interact adversely.

Clinical evidence

(a) Low-molecular-weight heparins

A study in healthy subjects indicated that giving ketorolac with **dalteparin** resulted in prolongation of bleeding time.[1] However, a study in hip replacement patients given subcutaneous **enoxaparin** 40 mg once daily found that there were no significant differences in intra-operative blood loss, post-operative drainage, transfusion requirements, bruising, wound oozing, and leg swelling between 34 patients given intramuscular ketorolac 30 mg and 26 patients given un-named opioids.[2]

(b) Warfarin

After taking ketorolac 10 mg four times daily for 6 days, no major changes occurred in the pharmacokinetics of ***(R)-*** or ***(S)-warfarin***, nor in the pharmacokinetic profile of a single 25-mg dose of racemic **warfarin** in 12 healthy subjects.[3] This suggests that ketorolac is normally unlikely to affect the anticoagulant response of patients taking **warfarin** chronically. However, the UK Committee on Safety of Medicines has had 5 reports of postoperative haemorrhage and four reports of gastrointestinal haemorrhage (one fatal) in patients taking ketorolac.[4]

Mechanism, importance and management

The UK Committee on Safety of Medicines and the makers say that ketorolac is contraindicated with anticoagulants, including **low doses of heparin**.[4,5]

1. Greer IA, Gibson JL, Young A, Johnstone J, Walker ID. Effect of ketorolac and low-molecular-weight heparin individually and in combination on haemostasis. *Blood Coag Fibrinol* (1999) 10, 367–73.
2. Weale AE, Warwick DJ, Durant N, Prothero D. Is there a clinically significant interaction between low molecular weight heparin and non-steroidal analgesics after total hip replacement? *Ann R Coll Surg Engl* (1995) 77, 35–7.
3. Toon S, Holt BL, Mullins FGP, Bullingham R, Aarons L, Rowland M. Investigations into the potential effects of multiple dose ketorolac on the pharmacokinetics and pharmacodynamics of racemic warfarin. *Br J Clin Pharmacol* (1990) 30, 743–50.
4. Committee on the Safety of Medicines/Medicines Control Agency. Ketorolac: new restrictions on dose and duration of treatment. *Current Problems* (1993) 19, 5–6.
5. Toradol (Ketorolac trometamol). Roche Products Ltd. UK Summary of product characteristics, October 2002.

Anticoagulants + NSAIDs; Meclofenamic acid or Mefenamic acid

The anticoagulant effects of warfarin are increased to some extent by meclofenamic acid and a moderate reduction in the warfarin dosage may be needed. One small study found that mefenamic acid did not interact significantly with warfarin.

Clinical evidence

(a) Meclofenamic acid

After taking sodium meclofenamate 200 to 300 mg daily for 7 days, the average dose of **warfarin** required by 7 patients fell from 6.5 to 4.25 mg daily, and by the end of 4 weeks it was 5.5 mg (a 16% reduction with a 0 to 25% range).[1]

(b) Mefenamic acid

After taking mefenamic acid 500 mg four times daily for a week the mean prothrombin concentrations of 12 healthy subjects on **warfarin** fell by about 3.5%.[2] Microscopic haematuria was seen in 3 of them, but no overt haemorrhage. Their prothrombin concentrations were 15 to 25% of normal, well within the accepted anticoagulant range.

Mechanism

Uncertain. Mefenamic acid can displace warfarin from its plasma protein binding sites,[3-5] and *in vitro* studies have shown that therapeutic concentrations (equivalent to 4 g daily) can increase the unbound and active warfarin concentrations by 140 to 340%,[3,4] but this interaction mechanism alone is only likely to have a transient effect.

Importance and management

The interaction between warfarin and meclofenamic acid is established but of only moderate clinical importance. A small reduction in warfarin dosage may be needed. Mefenamic acid appears not to interact significantly, but bear in mind this was only one small study. Note that both of these NSAIDs may irritate the gut and affect platelet function. There seems to be no information about other anticoagulants.

1. Baragar FD, Smith TC. Drug interaction studies with sodium meclofenamate (Meclomen®). *Curr Ther Res* (1978) 23 (April Suppl), S51–S59.
2. Holmes EL. Pharmacology of the fenamates: IV. Toleration by normal human subjects. *Ann Phys Med* (1966) 9 (Suppl), 36–49.
3. Sellers EM, Koch-Weser J. Displacement of warfarin from human albumin by diazoxide and ethacrynic, mefenamic and nalidixic acids. *Clin Pharmacol Ther* (1970) 11, 524–9.
4. Sellers EM, Koch-Weser J. Kinetics and clinical importance of displacement of warfarin from albumin by acidic drugs. *Ann N Y Acad Sci* (1971) 179, 213–25.
5. McElnay JC, D'Arcy PFD. Displacement of albumin-bound warfarin by anti-inflammatory agents *in vitro*. *J Pharm Pharmacol* (1980) 32, 709–11.

Anticoagulants + NSAIDs; Metamizole sodium (Dipyrone)

One report claims that metamizole sodium does not interact with phenprocoumon or ethyl biscoumacetate, whereas another describes a rapid but transient increase in the effects of ethyl biscoumacetate.

Clinical evidence, mechanism, importance and management

Metamizole sodium 1 g daily did not alter the anticoagulant effects of either **phenprocoumon** (5 subjects) or **ethyl biscoumacetate** (6 subjects).[1] Another report describes a short-lived but rapid increase (within 4 hours) in the effects of **ethyl biscoumacetate** caused by metamizole sodium.[2] The reasons are not understood. Metamizole sodium causes blood dyscrasias including agranulocytosis so that the advisability of its use is uncertain.

1. Badian M, Le Normand Y, Rupp W, Zapf R. There is no interaction between dipyrone (metamizol) and the anticoagulants, phenprocoumon and ethylbiscoumacetate, in normal caucasian subjects. *Int J Pharmaceutics* (1984) 18, 9–15.
2. Mehvar SR, Jamali F. Dipyrone-ethylbiscoumacetate interaction in man. *Indian J Pharm* (1981) 7, 293–9.

Anticoagulants + NSAIDs; Miscellaneous

No interaction normally occurs with normal doses of ibuprofen and probably diclofenac, fenbufen, indoprofen, ketoprofen, naproxen, oxaprozin, pirprofen and tolmetin, but isolated cases of raised INRs have been described with diclofenac, ibuprofen, ketoprofen, tiaprofenic acid and tolmetin. The effects of the anticoagulants can be increased by flurbiprofen in a few patients and they may bleed. All NSAIDs cause some gastrointestinal irritation and possible bleeding, and should be used with care in patients taking oral anticoagulants.

Clinical evidence

(a) Diclofenac

A study in 29 patients showed that diclofenac 100 mg daily does not alter the anticoagulant effects of **acenocoumarol**.[1] Other studies similarly confirm that diclofenac does not interact with either **acenocoumarol**, **phenprocoumon** or **warfarin**.[2-5] However, an unexplained case of pulmonary haemorrhage associated with a very prolonged prothrombin time has been described in a patient on **acenocoumarol** within 10 days of starting diclofenac.[6] Another report states that the INR of a patient on **warfarin** rose following the use of diclofenac.[7] A Chinese patient on **warfarin** developed an INR of 4 within 4 days of using a 1% diclofenac topical gel for joint pain.[8] Note that Chinese patients are particularly sensitive to the anticoagulant effects of **warfarin**.

(b) Fenbufen

A study in 10 subjects on **warfarin** given either fenbufen 400 mg twice daily or placebo for a week showed that in the fenbufen-treated group prothrombin times were increased by 1.9 seconds within 2 days, and the serum **warfarin** levels fell by 14%.[9] These changes are unlikely to be clinically significant.

(c) Flurbiprofen

A small but significant fall in prothrombin times occurred in 19 patients on **phenprocoumon** when they were given flurbiprofen 150 mg daily. Two patients bled (haematuria, epistaxis, haemorrhoidal bleeding) and the prothrombin times of 3 patients fell below the therapeutic range. The authors concluded that concurrent use is compatible with anticoagulation, but suggested good monitoring in the early stages.[10]

Two patients on **acenocoumarol** had a rise in thrombotest times and bled (haematuria, melaena, haematomas) within 2 to 3 days of starting to take **flurbiprofen** 150 to 300 mg daily.[11]

(d) Ibuprofen

Studies with 19 patients[12,13] and 24 patients[14] on **phenprocoumon**; 36 healthy subjects,[15] 50 patients and 30 subjects[16] on **warfarin**; and a further 40 patients[17] on **dicoumarol derivatives** found that the effects of these anticoagulants were not altered by ibuprofen 600 mg to 2.4 g daily for 7 to 14 days. However, one study in 20 patients taking **warfarin** showed that ibuprofen 600 mg three times daily prolonged bleeding times (4 cases above the normal range) and microscopic haematuria and haematoma were seen.[18] A raised INR occurred in one patient on **warfarin** who used topical ibuprofen,[7] and subclinical bleeding with a raised INR occurred in a 74-year-old woman with multiple medical problems taking **warfarin** when she was given ibuprofen.[19]

(e) Indoprofen

A study in 18 patients on **warfarin** given indoprofen 600 mg daily for 7 days found that no changes occurred in any of the blood coagulation measurements made.[20]

(f) Ketoprofen

A study in 15 healthy subjects stabilised on **warfarin** found that ketoprofen 100 mg twice daily for 7 days had no effect on their prothrombin times or coagulation cascade parameters, and there was no evidence of bleeding.[21] This contrasts with an isolated case of bleeding in a patient on **warfarin** (prothrombin time increased from 18 to 41 seconds) a week after starting ketoprofen 25 mg three times daily.[22]

(g) Naproxen

A study in 10 healthy subjects showed that 17 days' treatment with naproxen 375 mg twice daily did not alter the pharmacokinetics of a single dose of **warfarin**, or its anticoagulant effects.[23] Similar results were found in another study.[24] A further study in patients on **phenprocoumon** showed that naproxen 250 mg twice daily transiently increased the anticoagulant effects and caused an unimportant change in primary bleeding time.[25]

(h) Oxaprozin

A study in 10 healthy subjects stabilised on **warfarin** for an average of 15 days showed that oxaprozin 1200 mg daily for 7 days did not significantly alter their prothrombin times.[26]

(i) Pirprofen

A study in 18 patients on long-term treatment with **phenprocoumon** found that bleeding time was prolonged by 50% while they were taking pirprofen 200 mg three times daily.[27]

(j) Tiaprofenic acid

A study in 6 healthy subjects on **phenprocoumon** found that the anticoagulant effects and the pharmacokinetic profiles of both drugs remained unchanged when they took tiaprofenic acid daily for 2 days.[28] This study is also published elsewhere.[29] No significant interaction occurred in 9 patients on **acenocoumarol** given tiaprofenic acid 200 mg three times daily for 2 weeks, but in 4 patients a 'rebound' rise in prothrombin percentages occurred following its withdrawal.[30] However, an elderly man on **acenocoumarol** had severe epistaxis and bruising 4 to 6 weeks after starting to take tiaprofenic acid 300 mg twice daily. His prothrombin time had risen to 129 seconds.[31]

(k) Tolmetin

In a placebo-controlled study no changes in prothrombin times occurred in 15 healthy subjects on **warfarin** when they took tolmetin 400 mg three times daily over a 3-week period.[32] Similarly, no changes in prothrombin times occurred in 15 patients on **phenprocoumon** when they were given tolmetin 200 mg four times daily for 10 days.[33] Bleeding times were reported to be slightly altered, though not to a clinically relevant extent.[33] Bleeding times were not significantly altered in healthy subjects given **acenocoumarol** and tolmetin 400 mg twice daily.[34] However, there is a single unexplained case report of a diabetic patient on insulin, digoxin, theophylline, ferrous sulfate, furosemide and sodium polystyrene sulfonate who bled after taking three 400-mg doses of tolmetin. His prothrombin time had risen from a range of 15 to 22 seconds up to 70 seconds.[35] The makers of tolmetin and the US Food and Drug Administration also have 10 other cases on record.[35,36] However, the makers of tolmetin point out that over a 10-year period about 10 million patients have received tolmetin, so that the risk of an interaction appears to be very small indeed.[36]

Mechanism

Drug displacement and enzyme inhibition do not seem to explain the interaction of flurbiprofen.[10] Most of the phenylalkanoic acid derivatives can displace the anticoagulants from plasma protein binding sites to some extent, but this mechanism on its own is rarely, if ever, responsible for clinically important drug interactions.

Importance and management

It is well established that no adverse interaction normally occurs between ibuprofen and either warfarin or phenprocoumon, (although isolated and unexplained cases of bleeding or raised INRs have occurred but only very rarely). Other anticoagulants would be expected to behave similarly. The absence of a clinically relevant interaction also appears to be true for indoprofen, fenbufen, ketoprofen, naproxen, and oxaprozin, although the documentation is more limited. However, a few patients have bled when given diclofenac, flurbiprofen or tolmetin. There also seems to be a slight possibility of an interaction with tiaprofenic acid or pirprofen.

Some care is still needed with every NSAID because, to a greater or lesser extent, they irritate the stomach lining, which can result in gastrointestinal bleeding, which will be more severe in anticoagulated patients. Some have effects on platelet activity, which can affect bleeding times. One very extensive study found an almost 13-fold increase in the risk of developing haemorrhagic peptic ulcer disease in elderly patients taking oral anticoagulants and NSAIDs.[37]

1. Michot F, Ajdacic K, Glaus L. A double-blind clinical trial to determine if an interaction exists between diclofenac sodium and the oral anticoagulant acenocoumarol (nicoumalone). *J Int Med Res* (1975) 3, 153–7.
2. Wagenhäuser F. Research findings with a new, non-steroidal antirheumatic agent. *Scand J Rheumatol* (1975) 4 (Suppl 8), S05–S01.
3. Krzywanek HJ, Breddin K. Beeinflußt Diclofenac die orale Antikoagulantientherapie und die Plättchenaggregation? *Med Welt* (1977) 28, 1843–5.
4. Breddin K (1975) Cited as personal communication in Michot F, Ajdacic K, Glaus L. A double-blind clinical trial to determine if an interaction exists between diclofenac sodium and the oral anticoagulant acenocoumarol (nicoumalone). *J Int Med Res* (1975) 3, 153–7.
5. Fitzgerald DE, Russell JG. Voltarol and warfarin, an interaction? In Current Themes in Rheumatology, Chiswell RJ and Birdwood GFB (Eds). Cambridge Medical Publications p 26–7.
6. Cuadrado Gómez LM, Palau Beato E, Pérez Venegas J, Pérez Moro E. Hemorragia pulmonar debido a la interacción de acenocoumarina y diclofenac sódico. *Rev Clin Esp* (1987) 181, 227–8.
7. Beeley L, Cunningham H, Carmichael AE, Brennan A. *Bulletin of the West Midlands Centre for Adverse Drug Reaction Reporting* (1992), 35, 18.
8. Chan TYK. Drug interactions as a cause of overanticoagulation and bleedings in Chinese patients receiving warfarin. *Int J Clin Pharmacol Ther* (1998) 36, 403–5.
9. Savitsky JP, Terzakis T, Bina P, Chiccarelli F, Haynes J. Fenbufen-warfarin interaction in healthy volunteers. *Clin Pharmacol Ther* (1980) 27, 284.
10. Marbet GA, Duckert F, Walter M, Six P, Airenne H. Interaction study between phenprocoumon and flurbiprofen. *Curr Med Res Opin* (1977) 5, 26–31.
11. Stricker BHC, Delhez JL. Interaction between flurbiprofen and coumarins. *BMJ* (1982) 285, 812–13.
12. Thilo D, Nyman F, Duckert F. A study of the effects of the anti-rheumatic drug ibuprofen (Brufen) on patients being treated with the oral anti-coagulant phenprocoumon (Marcoumar). *J Int Med Res* (1974) 2, 276–8.
13. Duckert F. The absence of effect of the antirheumatic drug ibuprofen on oral anticoagulation with phenprocoumon. *Curr Med Res Opin* (1975) 3, 556–7.
14. Boekhout-Mussert MJ, Loeliger EA. Influence of ibuprofen on oral anti-coagulation with phenprocoumon. *J Int Med Res* (1974) 2, 279–83.
15. Penner JA, Abbrecht PH. Lack of interaction between ibuprofen and warfarin. *Curr Ther Res* (1975) 18, 862–71.
16. Goncalves L. Influence of ibuprofen on haemostasis in patients on anticoagulant therapy. *J Int Med Res* (1973) 1, 180–3.
17. Marini U, Cecchi A, Venturino M. Mancanza di interazione tra ibuprofen lisinato e anticoagulanti orali. *Clin Ter* (1985) 112, 25–9.
18. Schulman S, Henriksson K. Interaction of ibuprofen and warfarin on primary haemostasis. *Br J Rheumatol* (1989) 28, 46–9.
19. Ernst ME, Buys LM. Reevaluating the safety of concurrent warfarin and ibuprofen. *J Pharm Technol* (1997) 13, 244–7.
20. Jacono A, Caso P, Gualtieri S, Raucci D, Bianchi A, Vigorito C, Bergamini N, Iadevaia V. Clinical study of the possible interactions between indoprofen and oral anticoagulants. *Eur J Rheumatol Inflamm* (1981) 4, 32–5.
21. Mieszczak C, Winther K. Lack of interaction of ketoprofen with warfarin. *Eur J Clin Pharmacol* (1993) 44, 205–6.
22. Flessner MF, Knight H. Prolongation of prothrombin time and severe gastrointestinal bleeding associated with combined use of warfarin and ketoprofen. *JAMA* (1988) 259, 353.
23. Slattery JT, Levy G, Jain A, McMahon FG. Effect of naproxen on the kinetics of elimination and anticoagulant activity of a single dose of warfarin. *Clin Pharmacol Ther* (1979) 25, 51–60.
24. Jain A, McMahon FG, Slattery JT, Levy G. Effect of naproxen on the steady-state serum concentration and anticoagulant activity of warfarin. *Clin Pharmacol Ther* (1979) 25, 61–6.
25. Angelkort B. Zum einfluß von Naproxen auf die thrombozytäre Blutstillung und die Antikoagulantien-Behandlung mit Phenprocoumon. *Fortschr Med* (1978) 96, 1249–52.
26. Davis LJ, Kayser SR, Hubscher J, Williams RL. Effect of oxaprozin on the steady-state anticoagulant activity of warfarin. *Clin Pharm* (1984) 3, 295–7.
27. Marbet GA, Duckert F, Schönenberger PM. Eine Untersuchung über Wechselwirkungen zwischen Pirprofen und Phenprocoumon. *Fortschr Med* (1985) 103, 207–9.
28. Dürr J, Pfeiffer MH, Wetzelsberger K, Lücker PW. Untersuchung zur Frage einer Interaktion von Tiaprofensäure und Phenprocoumon. *Arzneimittelforschung* (1981) 31, 2163–7.
29. Lücker PW, Penth B, Wetzelsberger K. Pharmacokinetic interaction between tiaprofenic acid and several other compounds for chronic use. *Rheumatology (Oxford)* (1982) 7, 99–106.
30. Meurice J. Interaction of tiaprofenic acid and acenocoumarol. *Rheumatology (Oxford)* (1982) 7, 111–17.
31. Whittaker SJ, Jackson CW, Whorwell PJ. A severe, potentially fatal, interaction between tiaprofenic acid and nicoumalone. *Br J Clin Pract* (1986) 40, 440.
32. Whitsett TL, Barry JP, Czerwinski AW, Hall WH, Hampton JW. Tolmetin and warfarin: a clinical investigation to determine if interaction exists. In 'Tolmetin, A New Non-steroidal Anti-Inflammatory Agent.' Ward JR (ed). Proceedings of a Symposium, Washington DC, April 1975, Excerpta Medica, Amsterdam, New York, p. 160–7.
33. Rüst O, Biland L, Thilo D, Nyman D, Duckert F. Prüfung des Antirheumatikums Tolmetin auf Interaktionen mit oralen Antikoagulantien. *Schweiz Med Wochenschr* (1975) 105, 752–3.
34. Malbach E. Über die Beeinflussung der Blutungszeit durch Tolectin. *Schweiz Rundsch Med Prax* (1978) 67, 161–3.
35. Koren JF, Cochran DL, Janes RL. Tolmetin-warfarin interaction. *Am J Med* (1987) 82, 1278–9.
36. Santopolo AC. Tolmetin-warfarin interaction. *Am J Med* (1987) 82, 1279–80.
37. Shorr RI, Ray WA, Daugherty JR, Griffin MR. Concurrent use of nonsteroidal anti-inflammatory drugs and oral anticoagulants places elderly persons at high risk for hemorrhagic peptic ulcer disease. *Arch Intern Med* (1993) 153, 1665–70.

Anticoagulants + NSAIDs; Nabumetone

Nabumetone normally does not interact with acenocoumarol or warfarin, but an isolated report describes a raised INR and haemarthrosis in one patient on warfarin attributed to an interaction with nabumetone.

Clinical evidence, mechanism, importance and management

Nabumetone has been found not to affect significantly the anticoagulant effects of **warfarin** in either healthy subjects[1] or patients,[2,3] moreover it also appears not to affect bleeding time, platelet aggregation or prothrombin times in the absence of an anticoagulant.[4] However, an isolated and unexplained report describes an increased INR and haemarthrosis in a patient on **warfarin** a week after nabumetone was added.[5] Another clinical study in osteoarthritis patients also found that nabumetone did not affect the anticoagulant effects of **acenocoumarol**.[6,7] However if anticoagulants are used concurrently, bear in mind that nabumetone can irritate the gut and thereby increase the risk of gastrointestinal bleeding so that good monitoring would be a prudent precaution. Information about other anticoagulants seems to be lacking.

1. Fitzgerald DE. Double blind study to establish whether there is any interaction between nabumetone and warfarin in healthy adult male volunteers. *Roy Soc Med Int Congr Symp* (1985) Series 69, 47–53.
2. Hilleman DE, Mohiuddin SM, Lucas BD. Nonsteroidal antiinflammatory drug use in patients receiving warfarin: emphasis on nabumetone. *Am J Med* (1993) 95 (Suppl 2A), 30S–34S.
3. Hilleman DE, Mohiuddin SM, Lucas BD. Hypoprothrombinemic effect of nabumetone in warfarin-treated patients. *Pharmacotherapy* (1993) 13, 270–1.
4. Al Balla S, Al Momen AK, Al Arfaj H, Al Sugair S, Gader AMA. Interaction between nabumetone — a new non-steroidal anti-inflammatory drug — and the haemostatic system ex vivo. *Haemostasis* (1990) 20, 270–5.
5. Dennis VC, Thomas BK, Hanlon JE. Potentiation of oral anticoagulation and hemarthrosis associated with nabumetone. *Pharmacotherapy* (2000) 20, 234–9.
6. Pardo A, García-Losa M, Fernández-Pavón A, del Castillo S, Pascual-García T, García-Méndez E, Dal-Ré R. A placebo-controlled study of interaction between nabumetone and acenocoumarol. *Br J Clin Pharmacol* (1999) 47, 441–4.
7. Pardo A, Garcia-Losa M, Fernández-Pavón, A, Del Castillo S, Pascual T, García-Méndez E, Dal-Ré R. Drug interaction with acenocoumarol: nabumetone not different from placebo. *Methods Find Exp Clin Pharmacol* (1998) 20 (Suppl A), 69.

Anticoagulants + NSAIDs; Nimesulide

Good monitoring has been suggested if nimesulide is added to warfarin.

Clinical evidence, mechanism, importance and management

A pilot study in 6 patients stabilised on **acenocoumarol** found that a single 100-mg dose of nimesulide did not affect the clotting mechanisms, although the platelet aggregating response to adenosine diphosphate, adrenaline (epinephrine) and collagen were reduced for 2 to 4 hours.[1] Ten patients on **warfarin** 5 mg daily had no significant changes in their prothrombin times, partial thromboplastin time or bleeding times when they were given nimesulide 100 mg twice daily for a week.[2] However since a few patients showed some increased anticoagulant effects, good monitoring has been recommended.[1]

1. Perucca E. Drug interactions with nimesulide. *Drugs* (1993) 46 (Suppl 1), 79–82.
2. Auteri A, Bruni F, Blardi P, Di Renzo M, Pasqui AL, Saletti M, Verzuri MS, Scaricabarozzi I, Vargiu G, Di Perri T. Clinical study on pharmacological interaction between nimesulide and warfarin. *Int J Clin Pharmacol Res* (1991) 11, 267–70.

Anticoagulants + NSAIDs; Oxicam derivatives

Piroxicam can increase the effects of warfarin and acenocoumarol and bleeding may occur. Lornoxicam can increase the anticoagulant effects of warfarin, and possibly phenprocoumon, but it appears not to interact with acenocoumarol. Studies have indicated that meloxicam does not interact with warfarin, and that tenoxicam does not interact with warfarin or phenprocoumon. It should however be noted that cases of interactions have been reported with other NSAIDs, where studies had previously found that no interaction occurred.

Clinical evidence

(a) Lornoxicam

An open crossover study in 6 healthy subjects found that lornoxicam 8 mg twice daily had no effect on the pharmacokinetics or the anticoagulant activity of **acenocoumarol** 10 mg.[1]

An open crossover study in 6 healthy subjects given a single 9-mg dose of **phenprocoumon** found that lornoxicam increased the bioavailabilities of ***(S)***- and ***(R)*-phenprocoumon** by 14 and 6% respectively, and decreased their clearances by 15 and 6%. Statistically significant reductions in the activities of factors II and VII were seen.[2] Lornoxicam 4 mg twice daily was given to 12 healthy subjects for 5 days, then **warfarin** was added until a stable prothrombin time, averaging about 23.6 seconds, was achieved. The period to achieve this varied from 9 to 24 days, depending on the subject. The **warfarin** was continued but the lornoxicam withdrawn, whereupon the mean prothrombin time fell to 19.5 seconds, the INR fell from 1.48 to 1.23 and the serum **warfarin** levels fell by 25%.[3]

(b) Meloxicam

Meloxicam 15 mg daily for 7 days did not significantly affect the pharmacokinetics of **warfarin** or INR values[4] in a group of 13 healthy subjects stabilised at INRs of 1.2 to 1.8.

(c) Piroxicam

A man stabilised on **warfarin** had a fall in his prothrombin time from a range of 1.7 to 1.9 times his control value to 1.3 when he stopped taking piroxicam 20 mg daily. The prothrombin times rose and fell when he restarted and then stopped the piroxicam.[5] Another patient on **warfarin** showed an increase in his prothrombin time when piroxicam 20 mg daily was started, and a decrease when it was then stopped.[6] The INR of 2 Chinese patients rose to 4.5 after they were treated with piroxicam 20 mg daily and 0.5% topical piroxicam gel. One of them showed bruises over the legs within 3 days.[7] Note that Chinese patients are more sensitive to the anticoagulant effects of **warfarin** than some other races.

A woman who spread **warfarin** rat poison with her bare hands developed intracerebral bleeding, possibly exacerbated by the piroxicam she was taking.[8]

Piroxicam 20 mg daily increased the effects of **acenocoumarol** in 4 out of 11 subjects, 3 being considered mild and one being significant.[9] An increased prothrombin ratio has been seen in another patient.[10] A further patient on **acenocoumarol** developed gastrointestinal bleeding 3 days after starting to take piroxicam 20 mg daily. His INR rose from 2.2 to 6.5.[11] A single dose clinical study found that piroxicam 40 mg caused major changes in the pharmacokinetics of racemic **acenocoumarol**. The AUC of the more active ***(R)*-isomer** of **acenocoumarol** was found to be increased by 47% and its maximum plasma levels were increased by 28%.[12]

(d) Tenoxicam

Single-dose and steady-state studies in a total of 16 healthy subjects found that tenoxicam 20 mg daily for 14 days had no significant effect on the anticoagulant effects of **warfarin** or on bleeding times.[13] This report also mentions case studies in a small number of patients and healthy subjects, which similarly found that tenoxicam had no significant effect on the anticoagulant effects of **phenprocoumon**.[13]

Mechanism

What is known suggests that piroxicam and lornoxicam inhibit the metabolism of these anticoagulants by the liver, thereby increasing their anticoagulant effects.[12] In addition NSAIDs have antiplatelet effects, which can prolong bleeding if it occurs.

Importance and management

The interactions of piroxicam with acenocoumarol and warfarin are established but the documentation is only moderate. Concurrent use need not be avoided but monitor the outcome well and anticipate the need to reduce the anticoagulant dosage. Remember that to varying degrees, all NSAIDs can cause gastrointestinal irritation and reduce platelet aggregation, which can worsen any bleeding event.

Lornoxicam, meloxicam and tenoxicam, appear to interact less frequently, if at all, but note that case reports of interactions have been seen with NSAIDs found not to interact in studies. It is therefore worth bearing this interaction in mind if any of these oxicam derivatives are given with coumarins.

1. Masche UP, Rentsch KM, von Felten A, Meier PJ, Fattinger KE. No clinically relevant effect of lornoxicam intake on acenocoumarol pharmacokinetics and pharmacodynamics. *Eur J Clin Pharmacol* (1999) 54, 865–8.
2. Masche UP, Rentsch KM, von Felten A, Meier PJ, Fattinger KE. Opposite effects of lornoxicam co-administration on phenprocoumon pharmacokinetics and pharmacodynamics. *Eur J Clin Pharmacol* (1999) 54, 857–64.
3. Ravic M, Johnston A, Turner P, Ferber HP. A study of the interaction between lornoxicam and warfarin in healthy volunteers. *Hum Exp Toxicol* (1990) 9, 413–14.
4. Türck D, Su CAPF, Heinzel G, Busch U, Bluhmki E, Hoffmann J. Lack of interaction between meloxicam and warfarin in healthy volunteers. *Eur J Clin Pharmacol* (1997) 51, 421–5.
5. Rhodes RS, Rhodes PJ, Klein C, Sintek CD. A warfarin-piroxicam drug interaction. *Drug Intell Clin Pharm* (1985) 19, 556–8.
6. Mallet L, Cooper JW. Prolongation of prothrombin time with the use of piroxicam and warfarin. *Can J Hosp Pharm* (1991) 44, 93–4.
7. Chan TYK. Drug interactions as a cause of overanticoagulation and bleedings in Chinese patients receiving warfarin. *Int J Clin Pharmacol Ther* (1998) 36, 403–5.
8. Abell TL, Merigian KS, Lee JM, Holbert JM, McCall JW. Cutaneous exposure to warfarin-like anticoagulant causing an intracerebral hemorrhage: a case report. *Clin Toxicol* (1994) 32, 69–73.
9. Jacotot B. Interaction of piroxicam with oral anticoagulants. 9th European Congress of Rheumatology, Wiesbaden, September 1979, pp 46–47.
10. Beeley L, Stewart P. *Bulletin of the West Midlands Centre for Adverse Drug Reaction Reporting* (1987) 25, 28.
11. Desprez D, Blanc P, Larrey D, Michel H. Hémorragie digestive favorisée par une hypocoagulation excessive due à une interaction médicamenteuse piroxicam — antagoniste de la vitamine K. *Gastroenterol Clin Biol* (1992) 16, 906–7.
12. Bonnabry P, Desmeules J, Rudaz S, Leemann T, Veuthey J-L, Dayer P. Stereoselective interaction between piroxicam and acenocoumarol. *Br J Clin Pharmacol* (1996) 41, 525–30.
13. Eichler H-G, Jung M, Kyrle PA, Rotter M, Korn A. Absence of interaction between tenoxicam and warfarin. *Eur J Clin Pharmacol* (1992) 42, 227–9.

Anticoagulants + NSAIDs; Oxyphenbutazone

The anticoagulant effects of warfarin are markedly increased by oxyphenbutazone, which can lead to serious bleeding.

Clinical evidence, mechanism, importance and management

A man on **warfarin** developed gross haematuria within 9 days of starting to take oxyphenbutazone 400 mg daily. His prothrombin time had increased to 68 seconds.[1] Two similar cases have been described elsewhere.[2,3] A clinical study has also shown that oxyphenbutazone slows the clearance of **dicoumarol**.[4]

Oxyphenbutazone is the major metabolite of phenylbutazone and it seems likely that the explanation for the anticoagulant/phenylbutazone interaction equally applies to oxyphenbutazone (see 'Anticoagulants + NSAIDs; Phenylbutazone', p.301). Direct evidence of this interaction seems to be limited to the reports cited here, but it would appear to be established and of clinical importance. It would be prudent to avoid concurrent use where possible or apply all the precautions suggested for phenylbutazone.

1. Taylor PJ. Hemorrhage while on anticoagulant therapy precipitated by drug interaction. *Ariz Med* (1967) 24, 697–9.

2. Hobbs CB, Miller AL, Thornley JH. Potentiation of anticoagulant therapy by oxyphenylbutazone (a probable case). *Postgrad Med J* (1965) 41, 563–5.
3. Fox SL. Potentiation of anticoagulants caused by pyrazole compounds. *JAMA* (1964) 188, 320–1.
4. Weiner M, Siddiqui AA, Bostanci N, Dayton PG. Drug interactions: the effect of combined administration on the half-life of coumarin and pyrazolone drugs in man. *Fedn Proc* (1965) 24, 153.

Anticoagulants + NSAIDs; Phenylbutazone

The anticoagulant effects of warfarin are markedly increased by phenylbutazone. Concurrent use should be avoided because serious bleeding can occur. Bleeding has been seen in patients on phenindione or phenprocoumon when given phenylbutazone, but successful concurrent use has been achieved with both phenprocoumon and acenocoumarol apparently because the anticoagulant dosage was carefully reduced.

Clinical evidence

A man, stabilised on **warfarin** following mitral valve replacement, was later given **phenylbutazone** for back pain by his general practitioner. On admission to hospital a week later he had epistaxis, and his face, legs and arms had begun to swell. He showed extensive bruising of the jaw, elbow and calves, some evidence of gastrointestinal bleeding, and a prothrombin time of 89 seconds. Two similar cases are also reported.[1] A man, hospitalised following a myocardial infarction, was given a single 600-mg dose of **phenylbutazone**. Next day, when coagulation studies were done, his prothrombin time was 12 seconds and he was given **warfarin** 40 mg to initiate anticoagulant therapy. Within 48 hours he developed massive gastrointestinal bleeding and was found to have a prothrombin time exceeding 100 seconds.[2] However, note that it is unusual to initiate warfarin in such a high dose.

There are numerous other reports of this interaction with phenylbutazone involving **warfarin**,[3-9] **phenprocoumon**[10,11] and **acenocoumarol**.[12] A single unconfirmed report describes this interaction in two patients taking **phenindione**.[13]

Mechanism

Phenylbutazone inhibits the metabolism of *(S)*-warfarin (the more potent of the two warfarin isomers) so that it is cleared from the body more slowly and its effects are increased and prolonged.[14,15] Phenylbutazone also very effectively displaces the anticoagulants from their plasma protein binding sites, thereby increasing the concentrations of free and active anticoagulant molecules in plasma water,[3,16-20] but the importance of this latter mechanism is probably small.

Importance and management

The interaction between warfarin and phenylbutazone is very well established and clinically important. Serious bleeding can occur and concurrent use should be avoided. Much less is known about phenindione with phenylbutazone but it is probably equally unsafe.[13] Direct evidence of a serious interaction with phenprocoumon seems to be limited to two reports, and there is some evidence (from one paper published in 1957) that successful and apparently uneventful concurrent use is possible, presumably because in the case cited the response and the anticoagulant dosages were carefully controlled.[21] However, the practicalities of such close monitoring outside of a study are unclear. One study found that 25% less acenocoumarol was needed in patients given phenylbutazone.[12] Information about other anticoagulants is lacking, but until there is clear evidence to the contrary, expect them to behave like warfarin. Remember too that phenylbutazone affects platelet aggregation and can cause gastrointestinal bleeding, whether an anticoagulant is present or not. It would seem advisable to use an alternative NSAID that interacts to a lesser extent, such as ibuprofen or naproxen, although it should be noted that no NSAID is entirely free from interactions with anticoagulants.

1. Bull J, Mackinnon J. Phenylbutazone and anticoagulant control. *Practitioner* (1975) 215, 767–9.
2. Robinson DS. The application of basic principles of drug interaction to clinical practice. *J Urol (Baltimore)* (1975) 113, 100–7.
3. Aggeler PM, O'Reilly RA, Leong I, Kowitz PE. Potentiation of anticoagulant effect of warfarin by phenylbutazone. *N Engl J Med* (1967) 276, 496–501.
4. Udall JA. Drug interference with warfarin therapy. *Clin Med* (1970) 77, 20–5.
5. McLaughlin GE, McCarty DJ, Segal BL. Hemarthrosis complicating anticoagulant therapy. Report of three cases. *JAMA* (1966) 196, 1020–1.
6. Hoffbrand BI, Kininmonth DA. Potentiation of anticoagulants. *BMJ* (1967) 2, 838–9.
7. Eisen MJ. Combined effect of sodium warfarin and phenylbutazone. *JAMA* (1964) 189, 64–5.
8. Schary WL, Lewis RJ, Rowland M. Warfarin-phenylbutazone interaction in man: a long-term multiple-dose study. *Res Commun Chem Pathol Pharmacol* (1975) 10, 663–72.
9. Chierichetti S, Bianchi G, Cerri B. Comparison of feprazone and phenylbutazone interaction with warfarin in man. *Curr Ther Res* (1975) 18, 568–72.
10. Sigg A, Pestalozzi H, Clauss A, Koller F. Verstärkung der Antikoagulantienwirkung durch Butazolidin. *Schweiz Med Wochenschr* (1956) 42, 1194–5.
11. O'Reilly RA. Phenylbutazone and sulfinpyrazone interaction with oral anticoagulant phenproumon. *Arch Intern Med* (1982) 142, 1634–7.
12. Guggisberg W, Montigel C. Erfahrungen mit kombinierter Butazolidin-Sintrom-Prophylaxe und Butazolidin-prophylaxe thromboembolischer Erkrangungen. *Ther Umsch* (1958) 15, 227.
13. Kindermann A. Vaskuläres Allergid nach Butalidon und Gefahren kombinierter Anwendung mit Athrombon (Phenylindandion). *Dermatol Wochenschr* (1961) 143, 172–8.
14. Lewis RJ, Trager WF, Chan KK, Breckenridge A, Orme M, Rowland M, Schary W. Warfarin. Stereochemical aspects of its metabolism and the interaction with phenylbutazone. *J Clin Invest* (1974) 53, 1607–17.
15. O'Reilly RA, Trager WF, Motley CH, Howald W. Stereoselective interaction of phenylbutazone with [$^{12}C/^{13}C$] warfarin pseudoracemates in man. *J Clin Invest* (1980) 65, 746–53.
16. O'Reilly RA. The binding of sodium warfarin to plasma albumin and its displacement by phenylbutazone. *Ann N Y Acad Sci* (1973) 226, 293–308.
17. Seiler K, Duckert F. Properties of 3-(1-phenyl-propyl)-4-oxycoumarin (Marcoumar®) in the plasma when tested in normal cases under the influence of drugs. *Thromb Diath Haemorrh* (1968) 19, 389–96.
18. Tillement J-P, Zini R, Mattei C, Singlas E. Effect of phenylbutazone on the binding of vitamin K antagonists to albumin. *Eur J Clin Pharmacol* (1973) 6, 15–18.
19. Solomon HM, Schrogie JJ. The effect of various drugs on the binding of warfarin-^{14}C to human albumin. *Biochem Pharmacol* (1967) 16, 1219–26.
20. O'Reilly RA. Interaction of several coumarin compounds with human and canine plasma albumin. *Mol Pharmacol* (1971) 7, 209–18.
21. Kaufmann P. Vergleich zwischen einer Thromboembolieprophylaxe mit Antikoagulantien und mit Butazolidin. *Schweiz Med Wochenschr* (1957) 87 (Suppl 24), 755–9.

Anticoagulants + NSAIDs; Proquazone

The anticoagulant effects of phenprocoumon are not affected by proquazone.

Clinical evidence, mechanism, importance and management

Proquazone 300 mg three times daily or placebo for 14 days had no effect on the plasma levels of factors II, VII, X, or prothrombin times or platelet aggregation of 20 patients on phenprocoumon.[1]

1. Vinazzer H. On the interaction between the anti-inflammatory substance proquazone (RU 43-715) and phenprocoumone. *Int J Clin Pharmacol Biopharm* (1977) 15, 214–16.

Anticoagulants + NSAIDs; Sulindac

Five patients have shown a marked increase in the anticoagulant effects of warfarin when given sulindac (two of them bled), but it seems probable that only the occasional patient will develop this interaction.

Clinical evidence

A patient on **warfarin**, ferrous sulphate, phenobarbital and sulfasalazine showed a marked increase in his prothrombin times (more than three times the control value) after taking sulindac 200 mg daily for 5 days.[1,2] There are 4 similar cases of this interaction on record.[3-6] Two of the patients bled, one of whom did so after taking only three 100-mg doses of sulindac (but note, this patient was also on flurbiprofen).[3,5]

In contrast, studies in healthy subjects on **warfarin**[6] or patients on **phenprocoumon**[7] and given sulindac did not demonstrate this interaction.

Mechanism

Not understood. In one patient renal impairment may have caused sulindac accumulation, which in turn may have affected warfarin pharmacokinetics. More study is needed.

Importance and management

An established but uncommon and unpredictable interaction affecting only the occasional patient.[3,6] Monitor the effects if sulindac is added to warfarin or any other anticoagulant, bearing in mind that all NSAIDs can irritate the gastric mucosa, affect platelet activity and cause gastrointestinal bleeding.

1. Beeley L. *Bulletin of the West Midlands Centre for Adverse Drug Reaction Reporting* (1978) No. 6.
2. Beeley L, Baker S. Personal communication, 1978.
3. Ross JRY, Beeley L. Sulindac, prothrombin time, and anticoagulants. *Lancet* (1979) ii, 1075.

4. Carter SA. Potential effect of sulindac on response of prothrombin-time to oral anticoagulants. *Lancet* (1979) ii, 698–9.
5. McQueen EG. New Zealand Committee on Adverse Drug Reactions. 17th Annual Report 1982. *N Z Med J* (1983) 96, 95–9.
6. Loftin JP, Vesell ES. Interaction between sulindac and warfarin: different results in normal subjects and in an unusual patient with a potassium-losing renal tubular defect. *J Clin Pharmacol* (1979) 19, 733–42.
7. Schenk H, Klein G, Haralambus J, Goebel R. Coumarintherapie unter dem antirheumaticum sulindac. *Z Rheumatol* (1980) 39, 102–8.

Anticoagulants + NSAIDs; Tolfenamic acid

Tolfenamic acid has a small, clinically irrelevant effect on bleeding time when given alone,[1,2] but it is not entirely clear whether it is safe with anticoagulants or not. To be on the safe side the makers suggest good monitoring during concurrent use.[2]

1. Vapaatalo H, Österman T, Tokola O, Tokola R. Acute effects of tolfenamic acid on hemostatic functions and arachidonic acid metabolism. *Curr Ther Res* (1986) 39, 250–9.
2. Thames Laboratories. Personal communication, November 1996.

Anticoagulants + Olanzapine

No clinically significant interaction occurs between olanzapine and warfarin.

Clinical evidence, mechanism, importance and management

In a three-way randomised crossover study, 15 healthy subjects were given olanzapine 10 mg, **warfarin** 20 mg or both drugs together as single doses. No significant changes were seen in the pharmacokinetics of either drug, and the adverse effects of the olanzapine and the anticoagulant effects of the **warfarin** were unchanged.[1] No additional precautions seem necessary on concurrent use.

1. Maya JF, Callaghan JT, Bergstrom RF, Cerimele BJ, Kassahun K, Nyhart EH, Brater DC. Olanzapine and warfarin drug interaction. *Clin Pharmacol Ther* (1997) 61, 182.

Anticoagulants + Oral contraceptives and related sex hormones

The anticoagulant effects of dicoumarol and phenprocoumon can be decreased, and those of acenocoumarol increased by oral contraceptives. High dose medroxyprogesterone acetate and megestrol prolong the half-life of warfarin. An isolated report describes a marked INR increase in a woman on warfarin when she was given emergency contraception with levonorgestrel. A report describes a woman who needed more acenocoumarol when her HRT treatment with oral conjugated oestrogens was changed to transdermal estradiol.

Clinical evidence

(a) Acenocoumarol

A survey on 12 patients taking acenocoumarol showed that while taking oral contraceptives, over an average of 2 years their anticoagulant dosage requirements were reduced by about 20%. Even then they were anticoagulated to a higher degree (prothrombin ratio of 1.67 compared with 1.5) than with the anticoagulant alone. The contraceptives used were *Neogynona*, *Microgynon*, *Eugynon* (**ethinylestradiol** with **levonorgestrel**) or *Topasel* (intramuscular **estradiol enantate** with **algestone**).[1]

A postmenopausal 53-year-old woman needed an increase in her daily dose of acenocoumarol from 2 to 3.5 mg when her **HRT** was changed from **oral conjugated oestrogens** 0.625 mg daily to **transdermal estradiol** 50 micrograms daily. When the oral **HRT** was restarted, her acenocoumarol requirements returned to their former levels.[2]

(b) Dicoumarol

A study in 4 healthy subjects given single 150- or 200-mg doses of dicoumarol on day 17 of a 20-day course of *Enovid* (**noretynodrel** and **mestranol**) showed that the anticoagulant effects were decreased in 3 of the 4 subjects, although the dicoumarol half-life remained unaltered.[3]

(c) Phenprocoumon

A controlled study in 14 women showed that in the 7 taking combined oral contraceptives the clearance of a single 0.22-mg/kg dose of phenprocoumon was increased by 20% compared to that in the 7 not taking oral contraceptives.[4]

(d) Unnamed anticoagulants

Megestrol is reported to increase bleeding times with unnamed anticoagulants in a very brief report about one patient.[5]

(e) Warfarin

A 39-year-old woman with familial type 1 antithrombin deficiency and a history of extensive deep vein thrombosis and pulmonary embolism, taking warfarin, was given **levonorgestrel** for emergency contraception. Within 3 days her INR had risen from 2.1 to 8.1. No bleeding occurred. Her INR returned to normal after stopping the warfarin for 2 days.[6]

Single 0.3-mg/kg doses of warfarin were given to 4 patients before and after 5 weeks of treatment with oral **medroxyprogesterone acetate** 500 mg twice daily or **megestrol** 160 mg daily. The half-life of warfarin was increased by 71% and the clearance decreased by 35%.[7]

A bulletin includes a brief mention of an increased INR with vaginal bleeding and multiple bruising in a woman on warfarin and **gestrinone**.[8]

Mechanism

Not understood. The oral contraceptives increase plasma levels of some blood clotting factors (particularly factor X and fibrinogen) and reduce levels of antithrombin III.[9] They can apparently increase the metabolism (glucuronidation) of phenprocoumon.[4,10] The authors of the report about levonorgestrel suggest that it might have displaced the warfarin from its binding sites thereby increasing its activity,[6] although this mechanism is now generally discounted.

Importance and management

Direct information seems to be limited to these reports. Oral contraceptives are normally contraindicated in those with thromboembolic disorders but if they must be used, be alert for any changes in the anticoagulant response if an oral contraceptive is started or stopped. One study suggests that the progestogen-only contraceptives may not affect the coagulability of the blood as much as the oestrogen/progestogen combined contraceptives, but whether this is reflected in an absence of an interaction with the oral anticoagulants is not documented.[11] However, it would be prudent to monitor prothrombin times in patients on warfarin given high doses of certain progestogens (such as medroxyprogesterone acetate), being alert for any increased warfarin effects.

The report about the apparent interaction between warfarin and levonorgestrel seems thus far to be isolated so that its general importance is unknown. Information about HRT or estrogens and anticoagulants appears to be limited to the report cited, but be alert for any changes in anticoagulant requirements if the route of administration is changed.

1. de Teresa E, Vera A, Ortigosa J, Alonso Pulpon L, Puente Arus A, de Artaza M. Interaction between anticoagulants and contraceptives: an unsuspected finding. *BMJ* (1979) 2, 1260–1.
2. Cotton F, Sorlin P, Corvilain B, Fockedey J-M, Capel P. Interference with oral anticoagulant treatment by oestrogen - influence of oestrogen administration route. *Thromb Haemost* (1999) 81, 471–2
3. Schrogie JJ, Solomon HM, Zieve PD. Effect of oral contraceptives on vitamin K-dependent clotting activity. *Clin Pharmacol Ther* (1967) 8, 670–5.
4. Mönig H, Baese C, Heidemann HT, Ohnhaus EE, Schulte HM. Effect of oral contraceptive steroids on the pharmacokinetics of phenprocoumon. *Br J Clin Pharmacol* (1990) 30, 115–18.
5. Beeley L, Stewart P, Hickey FM. *Bulletin of the West Midlands Centre for Adverse Drug Reaction Reporting* (1988) 27, 24.
6. Ellison J, Thomson AJ, Greer IA, Walker ID. Apparent interaction between warfarin and levonorgestrel used for emergency contraception. *BMJ* (2000) 321, 1382.
7. Lundgren S, Kvinnsland S, Utaaker E, Bakke O, Ueland PM. Effect of oral high-dose progestins on the disposition of antipyrine, digitoxin, and warfarin in patients with advanced breast cancer. *Cancer Chemother Pharmacol* (1986) 18, 270–5.
8. Beeley L, Cunningham H, Carmichael A, Brennan A. *Bulletin of the West Midlands Centre for Adverse Drug Reaction Reporting* (1992) 35, 18.
9. Robinson GE, Burren T, Mackie IJ, Bounds W, Walshe K, Faint R, Guillebaud J, Machin SJ. Changes in haemostasis after stopping the combined contraceptive pill: implications for major surgery. *BMJ* (1991) 302, 269–71.
10. Mönig H, Baese C, Heidemann HT, Schulte HM. The use of oral contraceptive steroids affects the pharmacokinetics of phenprocoumon. *Acta Endocrinol (Copenh)* (1989) 120 (Suppl), 180–1.
11. Poller L, Thomson JM, Tabiowo A, Priest CM. Progesterone oral contraception and blood coagulation. *BMJ* (1969) 1, 554–6.

Anticoagulants + Orlistat

One patient on warfarin developed an increased INR after taking orlistat. In contrast, a study in healthy subjects found no interaction.

Clinical evidence, mechanism, importance and management

In a placebo-controlled, randomised and two-way crossover study, 12 healthy subjects were given orlistat 120 mg three times daily for 16 days, with a single 30-mg dose of **warfarin** on day 11. The pharmacokinetics and pharmacodynamics of the **warfarin** were not altered by the orlistat, and the absorption of vitamin K from regular diets was not affected.[1]

However, in contrast to this, a 66-year-old man stabilised on **warfarin** for 2.5 years who was started on orlistat 120 mg three times daily for weight reduction had an increase in his INR, from less than 3, to 4.7 within 18 days. **Warfarin** was withdrawn and he was restabilised on approximately two-thirds of the previous dose. It was suggested that orlistat may have reduced the absorption of water soluble vitamins including vitamin K, and that a change to a lower fat diet associated with the use of orlistat may also have contributed to changes in the balance between vitamin K and **warfarin** in this patient.[2]

The US makers says that no pharmacokinetic interaction has been seen between warfarin and orlistat, but in clinical studies fluctuating anticoagulation was noted.[3] Close monitoring has been recommended by some for the first 4 weeks of concurrent use.[2] The UK maker also recommends monitoring, with all anticoagulants.[4] Given that changes in diet are known to affect warfarin levels (see 'Anticoagulants + Food or Drinks', p.282) this seems prudent.

1. Zhi J, Melia AT, Guerciolini R, Koss-Twardy SG, Passe SM, Rakhit A, Sadowski JA. The effect of orlistat on the pharmacokinetics and pharmacodynamics of warfarin in healthy volunteers. *J Clin Pharmacol* (1996) 36, 659–666.
2. MacWalter RS, Fraser HW, Armstrong KM. Orlistat enhances warfarin effect. *Ann Pharmacother* (2003) 37, 510–12.
3. Xenical (Orlistat). Roche Laboratories Inc. US Prescribing information, January 2005.
4. Xenical (Orlistat). Roche Products Ltd. UK Summary of product characteristics, June 2005.

Anticoagulants + Oxaceprol

An isolated report describes a marked fall in the response to fluindione in a patient given oxaceprol.

Clinical evidence, mechanism, importance and management

A 77-year-old woman with hypertension and atrial fibrillation, treated with propafenone, furosemide, enalapril and fluindione 15 mg daily, was additionally started on **oxaceprol** 300 mg daily. Within 2 days her Quick Time had risen from 26 to 57% and by the end of the week to 65%. When the **oxaceprol** was withdrawn, her Quick Time returned to its previous values of 23 to 30%.[1] The mechanism is not understood. The general importance of this interaction is not known but bear it in mind when prescribing **oxaceprol** and fluindione. Be alert for the need to modify the anticoagulant dosage.

1. Bannwarth B, Tréchot P, Mathieu J, Froment J, Netter P. Interaction oxacéprol-fluindione. *Therapie* (1990) 45, 162–3.

Anticoagulants + Paracetamol (Acetaminophen)

The anticoagulant effects of acenocoumarol, anisindione, dicoumarol, phenprocoumon and warfarin are normally not affected, or only slightly increased by small occasional doses of paracetamol, but larger doses taken regularly for longer periods may have a greater effect. There is evidence from large-scale studies that concurrent use increases the incidence of upper gastrointestinal bleeding.

Clinical evidence

(a) Prothrombin times unchanged

Ten patients on **warfarin** showed no changes in their prothrombin times when given paracetamol 3.25 g daily for 2 weeks.[1] A further study in 10 patients given **warfarin** or **phenprocoumon** found that two 650-mg doses of paracetamol similarly had no effect on prothrombin times measured over the following 48 hours.[2]

The pharmacokinetics and prothrombin time of a single 20-mg dose of **warfarin** was not significantly altered in 20 healthy subjects who took paracetamol 4 g daily for 2 weeks.[3]

(b) Prothrombin times increased

The prothrombin times of 50 patients taking **anisindione**, **dicoumarol**, **phenprocoumon** or **warfarin** were increased by an average of 3.6 seconds after they took paracetamol 650 mg four times daily for 2 weeks.[4] Paracetamol 2 g daily for 3 weeks increased the thrombotest times of 10 patients on coumarin anticoagulants (6 on **phenprocoumon** and 4 on **acenocoumarol**) by about 20%. The anticoagulant dosage was reduced in 5 out of the 10 patients and in one of the 10 control patients.[5] Fifteen healthy subjects, given enough **warfarin** to increase their prothrombin time ratios by 1.35 to 1.5 times control, were additionally given paracetamol 4 g daily for 2 weeks. The prothrombin time ratios of 7 subjects rose by more than 20% (to greater than 1.75) compared with one subject taking placebo, and by more than 33% (to greater than 2) in 5 others. The increases were seen from about day 7 and were maximal after 12.5 days.[6]

A man on **acenocoumarol** 2 mg daily and paracetamol 1 to 2 g daily for about 6 months had a stable INR of about 2.5, which decreased to 1.6 within 13 days of stopping paracetamol. The INR rose to 2 within about a week of re-starting paracetamol.[7] The INR of a woman on **warfarin** rose to 7.5, and she developed a retroperitoneal haematoma after taking 8 to 10 tablets (4 to 5 g) of paracetamol over a period of 4 days.[8] A report describes bleeding (haematuria, gum bleeding) in a woman on **warfarin** after she took about 1.6 g of paracetamol daily for 10 days in a compound paracetamol and codeine preparation. Her prothrombin time rose to 96 seconds.[9] This case is also reported elsewhere.[10] Another report describes bleeding from the gums, bruising and increased INRs (up to 12) in a woman on **warfarin** after taking 14 g of paracetamol (in co-dydramol) over 7 days on one occasion, and 14 g of paracetamol as *Tylex* over 8 days on another.[11] A 74-year-old man stabilised on **warfarin** for 4 years experienced an increased in his INR to 4 after taking paracetamol. Subsequently paracetamol 1 g four times daily for 3 days produced an increase in his INR from 2.3 to 6.4 on day 4. During the following 6 months he occasionally took paracetamol (up to 2 g weekly) and his INR was maintained in the therapeutic range on **warfarin** 5 mg daily without adjustment.[12] A retrospective study[13] of the factors that increased the risk of excessive anticoagulation with **warfarin** found that taking paracetamol 9.1 g or more weekly increased by tenfold the odds of having an INR greater than 6. The increases occurred in a dose-dependent manner.[13] A very large-scale study in Denmark found that the incidence of hospitalisation for upper gastrointestinal bleeding in patients on **warfarin** or **phenprocoumon** rose from a standard incidence ratio of 2.8 to 4.4 when paracetamol was also taken.[14]

Consider also 'Anticoagulants + Dextropropoxyphene (Propoxyphene)', p.277 because paracetamol is a component of co-proxamol, which is discussed in this monograph.

Mechanism

Not fully understood. Paracetamol is mainly metabolised by glucuronidation and sulfation,[15,16] but the cytochrome P450 isoenzymes CYP1A2, CYP3A4 and CYP2E1 metabolise up to 15% of paracetamol under normal conditions.[15] *R*-warfarin is mainly metabolised by CYP3A4 and CYP1A2.[15,16] It has been suggested that in conditions such as ageing, hypoxia or hypertension, the isoenzymes play a more important part in paracetamol metabolism. Consequently paracetamol may then compete with the metabolism of *R*-warfarin to a sufficient degree to provoke an interaction.[16] However, as the *S*-warfarin enantiomer has significantly greater anticoagulant activity than the *R*-warfarin enantiomer, interactions with *R*-warfarin are considered by some to be of questionable significance.[16]

Importance and management

An established interaction although there are unexplained inconsistencies in the evidence. Clinical evidence and common experience indicates that occasional small doses of paracetamol (acetaminophen) (said to be no more than about 2.5 to 3 g weekly[13]) are unlikely to cause important INR rises in patients on oral anticoagulants, but there is evidence that if larger amounts are taken the risk of getting INRs above 6 steadily rises in a dose-dependent manner, and only 1.3 g daily for a week may increase the risks up to tenfold.[13] This means that if more than occasional doses are taken for longer than a few days,[17] and because of a high degree of interpatient variability and unpredictability[15] there is some risk that occasional patients will develop raised INRs. However, the study[13] suggesting a dose-dependent paracetamol interaction with anticoagulants has been criticised, because other factors, such as normal dose fluctuations, other interacting medication, diet and concurrent illness (diarrhoea, fever, malignancy) may also be involved,[18-22] and an increase in monitoring is unnecessary.[21] However, the authors of the study considered that even in the presence of other factors the link between paracetamol intake and raised INR was significant.[23]

Anticoagulants other than those specifically cited above would be expected to interact similarly. Paracetamol is generally safer than aspirin as an analgesic in the presence of an anticoagulant because it does not affect platelets or cause gastric bleeding.

1. Udall JA. Drug interference with warfarin therapy. *Clin Med* (1970) 77, 20–5.
2. Antlitz AM, Awalt LF. A double blind study of acetaminophen used in conjunction with oral anticoagulant therapy. *Curr Ther Res* (1969) 11, 360–1.
3. Kwan D, Bartle WR, Walker SE. The effects of acetaminophen on pharmacokinetics and pharmacodynamics of warfarin. *J Clin Pharmacol* (1999) 39, 68–75.
4. Antlitz AM, Mead JA ,Tolentino MA. Potentiation of oral anticoagulant therapy by acetaminophen. *Curr Ther Res* (1968) 10, 501–7.
5. Boeijinga JK, Boerstra EE, Ris P, Breimer DD, Jeletich-Bastiaanse A. De invloed van paracetamol op antistollingsbehandeling met coumarinederivaten. *Pharm Weekbl* (1983) 118, 209–12.
6. Rubin RN, Mentzer RL, Budzynski AZ. Potentiation of anticoagulant effect of warfarin by acetaminophen (Tylenol[R]). *Clin Res* (1984) 32, 698A.
7. Bagheri H, Bernhard NB, Montastruc JL. Potentiation of acenocoumarol anticoagulant effect by acetaminophen. *Ann Pharmacother* (1999) 33, 506.
8. Andrews FJ. Retroperitoneal haematoma after paracetamol increased anticoagulation. *Emerg Med J* (2002) 19. 84–5.
9. Kwan D, Bartle WR. Drug interactions with warfarin. *Med J Aust* (1993) 158, 574.
10. Bartle WR, Blakely JA. Potentiation of warfarin anticoagulation by acetaminophen. *JAMA* (1991) 265, 1260.
11. Fitzmaurice DA, Murray JA. Potentiation of anticoagulant effect of warfarin. *Postgrad Med J* (1997) 73, 439–40.
12. Gebauer MG, Nyfort-Hansen K, Henschke PJ, Gallus AS. Warfarin and acetaminophen interaction. *Pharmacotherapy* (2003) 23, 109–112.
13. Hylek EM, Heiman H, Skates SJ, Sheehan MA, Singer DE. Acetaminophen and other risk factors for excessive warfarin anticoagulation. *JAMA* (1998) 279, 657–62
14. Johnsen SP, Sorensen HT, Mellemkjoer L, Blot WJ, Nielsen GL, McLaughlin JK, Olsen JH. Hospitalisation for upper gastrointestinal bleeding associated with the use of oral anticoagulants. *Thromb Haemost* (2001) 86, 563–8.
15. Shek KLA, Chan L-N, Nutescu E. Warfarin-acetaminophen drug interaction revisited. *Pharmacotherapy* (1999) 19, 1153-8.
16. Lehmann DF. Enzymatic shunting: resolving the acetaminophen-warfarin controversy. *Pharmacotherapy* (2000) 20, 1464-8.
17. Bell WR. Acetaminophen and warfarin: an undesirable synergy. *JAMA* (1998) 279, 702–3.
18. Estrada C. Acetaminophen and risk factors for excess anticoagulation with warfarin. *JAMA* (1998) 280, 695.
19. Gray CD. Acetaminophen and risk factors for excess anticoagulation with warfarin. *JAMA* (1998) 280, 695.
20. Amato MG, Bussey H, Farnett L, Lyons R. Acetaminophen and risk factors for excess anticoagulation with warfarin. *JAMA* (1998) 280, 695–6.
21. Riser J, Gilroy C, Hudson P, McCay L, Willis TA. Acetaminophen and risk factors for excess anticoagulation with warfarin. *JAMA* (1998) 280, 696.
22. Eliason BC, Larson W. Acetaminophen and risk factors for excess anticoagulation with warfarin. *JAMA* (1998) 280, 696–7.
23. Hylek EM. Acetaminophen and risk factors for excess anticoagulation with warfarin. *JAMA* (1998) 280, 697.

Anticoagulants + Penicillins

The effects of the oral anticoagulants are not normally altered by the penicillins but isolated cases of increased prothrombin times and/or bleeding have been seen in patients given amoxicillin, ampicillin/flucloxacillin, benzylpenicillin, co-amoxiclav, or talampicillin. Carbenicillin in the absence of an anticoagulant can prolong prothrombin times. In contrast, a handful of cases of reduced warfarin effects have been seen with dicloxacillin and nafcillin, and possibly with amoxicillin.

Clinical evidence

(a) Increased anticoagulant effects

A woman on **acenocoumarol** developed bruising and an increased INR of 7.1 within a week of starting **amoxicillin** 500 mg 8-hourly.[1] Another patient stabilised on **warfarin** had an increased INR and haematuria about 2.5 weeks after completion of a 7-day course of **co-amoxiclav** (amoxicillin with clavulanic acid).[2] The results of a case control study suggest that **co-amoxiclav** may increase the risk of an INR of greater than 6 in patients stabilised on either **acenocoumarol** or **phenprocoumon**.[3] A population-based cohort study involving patients treated with either **acenocoumarol** or **phenprocoumon** found that the risk of over-anticoagulation (INR greater than or equal to 6) was increased by **amoxicillin** (adjusted relative risk 8 and 22.4 respectively).[4] The increased risk was observed in the early stages of concurrent use but was greater after 4 or more days treatment. However, the risk was much lower when **amoxicillin** was combined with an enzyme inhibitor [no details given].[4]

The prothrombin time of a patient on **warfarin** was increased by treatment with **ampicillin** and **flucloxacillin**,[5] and both bleeding (haematuria, epistaxis) and an increase in the prothrombin ratio has been described in a patient on **warfarin** given **talampicillin**.[6] Hypoprothrombinaemia has been described in one patient on **warfarin** given intravenous **benzylpenicillin** 24 million units daily.[7] **Benzylpenicillin** is also known to be able to increase bleeding times and cause bleeding in the absence of an anticoagulant.[8] Increases in bleeding times, bleeding,[9-13] and extended prothrombin times[12,13] have been described with **carbenicillin** in the absence of an anticoagulant. **Ampicillin**, **methicillin** and **ticarcillin** are also reported to prolong bleeding times,[14-16] and in theory might also increase the effects of the oral anticoagulants, but reports of such interactions seem to be lacking (except with **ampicillin** and **flucloxacillin** mentioned above).

(b) Decreased anticoagulant effects

The prothrombin time of a patient stabilised on **warfarin** fell from a range of 20 to 25 seconds down to 14 to 17 seconds (despite a doubling of the **warfarin** dosage) when given **nafcillin** 2 g every 4 hours intravenously.[17] A few months after the **nafcillin** was discontinued, the half-life of the **warfarin** was found to have risen from 11 to 44 hours. Ten other cases of this 'warfarin resistance' with high dose **nafcillin** have been reported.[18-23] Seven days' treatment with **dicloxacillin** 500 mg four times daily reduced the mean prothrombin times of 7 patients on **warfarin** by 1.9 seconds. One patient showed a 5.6 second reduction.[24] Another patient on **warfarin** showed a 17% fall in prothrombin times within 4 to 5 days of starting **dicloxacillin** 500 mg four times daily, and 7 other patients out of 26 similarly treated were also identified as having shown a 17% reduction in prothrombin times.[25] Yet another case involving **dicloxacillin** is described elsewhere.[22] A very brief report states that **amoxicillin** caused an unspecified decrease in prothrombin times in 5 patients but, by implication, it was small and of limited clinical importance.[26]

Mechanism

Not understood. The nafcillin-warfarin interaction is possibly due to increases in the metabolism of warfarin by the liver. Changes in bleeding times caused by the other penicillins appear to result from changes in antithrombin III activity, blood platelet changes, and alterations in the fibrinogen to fibrin conversion. Dicloxacillin possibly reduces serum warfarin levels.[25]

Importance and management

Documented reports of interactions between oral anticoagulants and penicillins are relatively rare, bearing in mind how frequently these drugs are used, so that the broad picture is that no clinically relevant interaction normally occurs with most penicillins. This lack of interaction was supported by a fairly limited clinical study,[27] although other studies suggest that patients taking either acenocoumarol, phenprocoumon, or warfarin may risk over-anticoagulation with amoxicillin or co-amoxiclav and recommend increased monitoring[2,4] or if possible, even avoidance of this combination.[3] Other possible exceptions are warfarin with dicloxacillin and particularly high dose nafcillin, which may possibly call for an increased warfarin dosage in some patients.

Even though the general picture is of no interaction some individual physicians say that they have seen changes with otherwise normally non-interacting penicillins. The British National Formulary say that experience in anticoagulant clinics suggests that the INR can be altered by courses of broad-spectrum antibacterials such as ampicillin, even though studies do not demonstrate an interaction.[28] For this reason concurrent use should be monitored so that the very occasional and unpredictable cases (increases or decreases in the anticoagulant effects) can be identified and handled accordingly.

1. Soto J, Sacristan JA, Alsar MJ, Fernandez-Viadero C, Verduga R. Probable acenocoumarol-amoxycillin interaction. *Acta Haematol (Basel)* (1993) 90, 195–7.
2. Davydov L, Yermolnik M, Cuni LJ. Warfarin and amoxicillin/clavulanate drug interaction. *Ann Pharmacother* (2003) 37, 367–70.

3. Penning-van Beest FJA, van Meegen E, Rosendaal FR, Stricker BH. Drug interactions as a cause of overanticoagulation on phenprocoumon or acenocoumarol predominantly concern antibacterial drugs. *Clin Pharmacol Ther* (2001) 69, 451–457.
4. Visser LE, Penning-van Beest FJA, Kasbergen AAH, De Smet PAGM, Vulto AG, Hofman A, Stricker BHC. Overanticoagulation associated with combined use of antibacterial drugs and acenocoumarol or phenprocoumon anticoagulants. *Thromb Haemost* (2002) 88, 705–10.
5. Beeley L, Stewart P. *Bulletin of the West Midlands Centre for Adverse Drug Reaction Reporting* (1987) 25, 21.
6. Beeley L, Daly M. *Bulletin of the West Midlands Centre for Adverse Drug Reaction Reporting* (1986) 23, 13.
7. Brown MA, Korchinski ED, Miller DR. Interaction of penicillin-G and warfarin? *Can J Hosp Pharm* (1979) 32, 18–19.
8. Roberts PL. High-dose penicillin and bleeding. *Ann Intern Med* (1974) 81, 267–8.
9. Brown CH, Natelson EA, Bradshaw MW, Williams TW, Alfrey CP. The hemostatic defect produced by carbenicillin. *N Engl J Med* (1974) 291, 265–70.
10. McClure PD, Casserly JG, Monsier C, Crozier D. Carbenicillin-induced bleeding disorder. *Lancet* (1970) ii, 1307–8.
11. Waisbren BA, Evani SV, Ziebert AP. Carbenicillin and bleeding. *JAMA* (1971) 217, 1243.
12. Yudis M, Mahood WH, Maxwell R. Bleeding problems with carbenicillin. *Lancet* (1972) ii, 599.
13. Lurie A, Ogilvie M, Townsend R, Gold C, Meyers AM, Goldberg B. Carbenicillin-induced coagulopathy. *Lancet* (1970) i, 1114–15.
14. Andrassy K, Ritz E, Weisschedel E. Bleeding after carbenicillin administration. *N Engl J Med* (1975) 292, 109.
15. Brown CH, Bradshaw MW, Natelson EA, Alfrey CP, Williams TW. Defective platelet function following the administration of penicillin compounds. *Blood* (1976) 47, 949–56.
16. Brown CH, Natelson EA, Bradshaw MW, Alfrey CP, Williams TW. Study of the effects of ticarcillin on blood coagulation and platelet function. *Antimicrob Agents Chemother* (1975) 7, 652–7.
17. Qureshi GD, Reinders TP, Somori GJ, Evans HJ. Warfarin resistance with nafcillin therapy. *Ann Intern Med* (1984) 100, 527–9.
18. Fraser GL, Miller M, Kane K. Warfarin resistance associated with nafcillin therapy. *Am J Med* (1989) 87, 237–8.
19. Davis RL, Berman W, Wernly JA, Kelly HW. Warfarin-nafcillin interaction. *J Pediatr* (1991) 118, 300–3.
20. Shovick VA, Rihn TL. Decreased hypoprothrombinemic response to warfarin secondary to the warfarin-nafcillin interaction. *DICP Ann Pharmacother* (1991) 25, 598–9.
21. Heilker GM, Fowler JW, Self TH. Possible nafcillin-warfarin interaction. *Arch Intern Med* (1994) 154, 822–4.
22. Taylor AT, Pritchard DC, Goldstein AO, Fletcher JL. Continuation of warfarin-nafcillin interaction during dicloxacillin therapy. *J Fam Pract* (1994) 39, 182–5.
23. Baciewicz AM, Heugel AM, Rose PG. Probable nafcillin-warfarin interaction. *J Pharm Technol* (1999) 15, 5–7.
24. Krstenansky PM, Jones WN, Garewal HS. Effect of dicloxacillin sodium on the hypoprothrombinemic response to warfarin sodium. *Clin Pharm* (1987) 6, 804–6.
25. Mailloux AT, Gidal BE, Sorkness CA. Potential interaction between warfarin and dicloxacillin. *Ann Pharmacother* (1996) 30, 1402–7.
26. Radley AS, Hall J. Interactions. *Pharm J* (1992) 249, 81.
27. Pharmacy Anticoagulant Clinic Study Group. A multicentre survey of antibiotics on the INR of anticoagulated patients. *Pharm J* (1996) 257 (Pharmacy Practice Suppl), R30.
28. British National Formulary. 49th ed. London: The British Medical Association and The Pharmaceutical Press; 2005. p. 669

Anticoagulants + Pentoxifylline

The anticoagulant effects of phenprocoumon were not significantly altered by pentoxifylline in one study, but serious bleeding has been seen with pentoxifylline alone and in the presence of acenocoumarol.

Clinical evidence, mechanism, importance and management

The anticoagulant effects of **phenprocoumon** were slightly but not significantly altered by pentoxifylline 400 mg four times daily for 27 days in 10 patients.[1] Conversely, another report describes 3 major haemorrhagic problems (2 fatal cerebral, 1 gastrointestinal bleeding) in a group of patients taking **acenocoumarol** with pentoxifylline 400 mg three times daily for the treatment of intermittent claudication. However, it should be noted that one case of cerebral haemorrhage (resulting in hemiplegia) and another of haematuria with epistaxis occurred in the group treated with **acenocoumarol** alone.[2] Yet another report describes acute gastrointestinal bleeding in a woman after being given pentoxifylline 400 mg three times daily for 2 days, in the absence of an anticoagulant,[3] clearly indicating that bleeding may not necessarily be the result of an interaction, but may be associated with antiplatelet effects and gastritis due to pentoxifylline.

Since there is some risk of bleeding, possibly serious, with pentoxifylline, it would be prudent to monitor its use, whether an anticoagulant is present or not. It has been suggested that the combination should be avoided because of the potential for a pharmacodynamic interaction.[2]

1. Ingerslev J, Mouritzen C, Stenbjerg S. Pentoxifylline does not interfere with stable coumarin anticoagulant therapy: a clinical study. *Pharmatherapeutica* (1986) 4, 595–600.
2. Dettori AG, Pini M, Moratti A, Paolicelli M, Basevi P, Qintavalla R, Manotti C, Di Lecce C and The APIC Study Group. Acenocoumarol and pentoxifylline in intermittent claudication. A controlled clinical study. *Angiology* (1989) 40, 237–48.
3. Oren R, Yishar U, Lysy J, Livshitz T, Ligumsky M. Pentoxifylline-induced gastrointestinal bleeding. *DICP Ann Pharmacother* (1991) 25, 315–16.

Anticoagulants + Phenazone (Antipyrine)

The anticoagulant effects of warfarin are reduced by phenazone.

Clinical evidence

The plasma **warfarin** concentrations were halved (from 2.93 to 1.41 micrograms/ml) and the anticoagulant effects accordingly reduced after 5 patients took **phenazone** 600 mg daily for 50 days.[1] The thrombotest percentage of one patient rose from 5 to 50%. In an associated study it was found that **phenazone** 600 mg daily for 30 days caused falls in the **warfarin** half-lives from 47 to 27 hours and from 69 to 39 hours respectively in 2 patients.[1,2]

Mechanism

Phenazone is an enzyme inducing agent, which increases the metabolism and clearance of warfarin from the body, thereby reducing its effects.[1,2]

Importance and management

An established interaction. The effects of concurrent use should be monitored and the dosage of warfarin increased appropriately. Other anticoagulants may be expected to behave similarly.

1. Breckenridge A, Orme M. Clinical implications of enzyme induction. *Ann N Y Acad Sci* (1971) 179, 421–31.
2. Breckenridge A, Orme ML'E, Thorgeirsson S, Davies DS, Brooks RV. Drug interactions with warfarin: studies with dichloralphenazone, chloral hydrate and phenazone (antipyrine). *Clin Sci* (1971) 40, 351–64.

Anticoagulants + Phenothiazines

Chlorpromazine does not interact significantly with acenocoumarol.

Clinical evidence, mechanism, importance and management

Although **chlorpromazine** 40 to 100 mg is said to have slightly sensitised 2 out of 8 patients to the effects of **acenocoumarol**[1] and is reported to increase its anticoagulant effects in *animals*,[2] there is nothing to suggest that special precautions are needed during concurrent use in man. No important interactions appear to occur between any of the oral anticoagulants and phenothiazines.

1. Johnson R, David A, Chartier Y. Clinical experience with G-23350 (Sintrom). *Can Med Assoc J* (1957) 77, 756–61.
2. Weiner M. Effect of centrally active drugs on the action of coumarin anticoagulants. *Nature* (1966) 212, 1599–1600.

Anticoagulants + Picotamide

Picotamide does not alter the anticoagulant effects of warfarin.

Clinical evidence, mechanism, importance and management

Picotamide 300 mg three times daily for 10 days had no effect on the anticoagulant effects of **warfarin** in 10 patients with aortic or mitral valve prostheses.[1] No special precautions would seem necessary. There seems to be no information about other anticoagulants.

1. Parise P, Gresele P, Viola E, Ruina A, Migliacci R, Nenci GG. La picotamide non interferisce con l'attività antiacoagulante del warfarin in pazienti portatori di protesi valvolari cardiache. *Clin Ter* (1990) 135, 479–82.

Anticoagulants + Piracetam

A single case report describes a woman on warfarin who began to bleed within a month of starting to take piracetam.

Clinical evidence, mechanism, importance and management

A woman patient on regular treatment with **warfarin**, insulin, levothyroxine and digoxin complained of menorrhagia at a routine follow up. Investigations revealed that her British Corrected Ratio had risen to 4.1 (normal range 2.3 to 2.8), and that one month previously she had started to take piracetam 200 mg three times daily. Within 2 days of withdrawing both the **warfarin** and piracetam her BCR had fallen to 2.07.[1] The reason for this apparent interaction is not known. There is far too little evidence to forbid concurrent use, but be alert for this reaction if both drugs are used.

1. Pan HYM, Ng RP. The effect of Nootropil in a patient on warfarin. *Eur J Clin Pharmacol* (1983) 24, 711.

Anticoagulants + Pirmenol

The anticoagulant effects of warfarin are not changed by pirmenol.

Clinical evidence, mechanism, importance and management

The prothrombin time response to a single 25-mg dose of **warfarin** was reduced by 0.2 to 1.3 seconds in an experimental study in 12 healthy subjects who had taken **pirmenol** 150 mg twice daily for 7 days.[1] This suggested that some changes in the dosage of **warfarin** might be required in practice, but a later study found that the prothrombin times of 10 patients on **warfarin** were not significantly changed when they were given oral **pirmenol** 150 mg twice daily for 14 days.[2] No special precautions would therefore seem to be necessary. There seems to be no information about other anticoagulants.

1. Janiczek N, Bockbrader HN, Lebsack ME, Sedman AJ, Chang T. Effect of pirmenol (CI-845) on prothrombin (PT) time following concomitant administration of pirmenol and warfarin to healthy volunteers. *Pharm Res* (1988) 5, S-155.
2. Stringer KA, Switzer DF, Abadier R, Lebsack ME, Sedman A, Chrymko M. The effect of pirmenol administration on the anti-coagulant activity of warfarin. *J Clin Pharmacol* (1991) 31, 607–10.

Anticoagulants + Probenecid

Some preliminary evidence suggests that probenecid increases the clearance of phenprocoumon. The anticoagulant effects would be expected to be decreased.

Clinical evidence, mechanism, importance and management

Probenecid 500 mg four times daily for 7 days reduced the AUC of a single 0.22-mg/kg dose of phenprocoumon by 47% in 9 healthy subjects.[1] The reasons are not understood, but one possibility is that while probenecid inhibits the glucuronidation of phenprocoumon (its normal route of metabolism) it may also increase the formation of hydroxylated metabolites so that its overall loss is increased.[1] This study suggests that, in the presence of probenecid, the dosage of phenprocoumon may need to be increased, but this awaits formal clinical confirmation in patients. There seems to be nothing documented about other anticoagulants.

1. Mönig H, Böhm M, Ohnhaus EE, Kirch W. The effects of frusemide and probenecid on the pharmacokinetics of phenprocoumon. *Eur J Clin Pharmacol* (1990) 39, 261–5.

Anticoagulants + Proguanil

An isolated report describes bleeding in a patient on warfarin after she took proguanil for about 5 weeks.

Clinical importance, mechanism, importance and management

A woman stabilised on **warfarin** developed haematuria, bruising and abdominal and flank discomfort about 5 weeks after starting to take proguanil 200 mg daily. Her prothrombin ratio was found to be 8.6. Within 12 hours of being treated with fresh frozen plasma and vitamin K her prothrombin ratio had fallen to 2.3. The mechanism of this interaction is unknown.[1] Its general importance is uncertain.

1. Armstrong G, Beg MF, Scahill S. Warfarin potentiated by proguanil. *BMJ* (1991) 303, 789.

Anticoagulants + Prolintane

The anticoagulant effects of ethyl biscoumacetate are not affected by prolintane.

Clinical evidence, mechanism, importance and management

The responses to single 20-mg/kg doses of **ethyl biscoumacetate** were examined in 12 healthy subjects before and after 4 days' treatment with prolintane 20 mg daily. The mean half-life of the anticoagulant and prothrombin times remained unchanged.[1] There would seem to be no reason for avoiding concurrent use.

1. Hague DE, Smith ME, Ryan JR, McMahon FG. The effect of methylphenidate and prolintane on the metabolism of ethyl biscoumacetate. *Clin Pharmacol Ther* (1971) 12, 259–62.

Anticoagulants + Propafenone

The anticoagulant effects of warfarin and possibly fluindione and phenprocoumon are increased by propafenone.

Clinical evidence

The mean steady-state plasma levels of 8 healthy subjects taking **warfarin** 5 mg daily rose by 38% (from 0.98 to 1.36 micrograms/ml) after they took propafenone 225 mg three times daily for a week. Five of the 8 showed a distinct prothrombin time increase. The average rise in prothrombin time of the whole group was about 7 seconds, which was considered to be clinically significant.[1] Two further reports describe marked increases in the anticoagulant effects of **fluindione** and **phenprocoumon** in 2 patients treated with propafenone.[2,3]

Mechanism

Propafenone may reduce the metabolism and loss from the body of these anticoagulants, thereby increasing their effects.

Importance and management

Information seems to be limited to these reports but they show that prothrombin times should be well monitored if propafenone is given to patients on fluindione, warfarin or phenprocoumon. The anticoagulant dosage should be reduced where necessary. It would be prudent to apply the same precautions with any other anticoagulant.

1. Kates RE, Yee Y-G, Kirsten EB. Interaction between warfarin and propafenone in healthy volunteer subjects. *Clin Pharmacol Ther* (1987) 42, 305–11.
2. Körst HA, Brandes J-W, Littmann K-P. Cave: Propafenon potenziert Wirkung von oralen Antikoagulantien. *Med Klin* (1981) 76, 349–50.
3. Welsch M, Heitz C, Stephan D, Imbs JL. Potentialisation de l'effet anticoagulant de la fluindione par la propafénone. *Therapie* (1991) 46, 254–5.

Anticoagulants + Protease inhibitors

Ritonavir has been predicted to raise warfarin levels and INRs. This was confirmed by one case report whereas two others found entirely the opposite. One of these latter reports also suggests that indinavir might cause a moderate reduction in anticoagulation. There is also a report of a marked reduction in anticoagulation in a patient on acenocoumarol associated with concurrent ritonavir or nelfinavir. An isolated report describes a gradual INR rise in an elderly patient on warfarin when he was given saquinavir.

Clinical evidence

(a) Acenocoumarol

A 46-year-old HIV+ man with mitraortic valve replacements stabilised on acenocoumarol (INR 2.5 to 3.5) for 5 years and treated with zidovudine and didanosine for 17 months was found to have a dramatic decrease in INR when his drug regimen was changed to stavudine, lamivudine and **ritonavir** 600 mg twice daily. Increasing the acenocoumarol dosage over 5 days from an average of 24 mg to over 70 mg failed to increase the INR to target levels. The INR returned to previous levels within 4 days of withdrawal of **ritonavir**, and the acenocoumarol dosage could be reduced to 3 mg daily. The patient was subsequently given **nelfinavir** and a similar, though less dramatic interaction occurred: while taking **nelfinavir** an INR of 2.5 was achieved with a 210% increase in acenocoumarol dose.[1]

(b) Warfarin effects increased

(i) Ritonavir. A man with deep vein thrombosis on warfarin 10 mg daily (INRs 2.4 to 3) had his treatment for HIV changed from efavirenz and abacavir to ritonavir, **nelfinavir** and *Combivir* (zidovudine/lamivudine). Within 5 days his INR had risen to 10.4 without any sign of bleeding. It proved difficult to achieve acceptable and steady INRs both while in hospital and after discharge, but eventually it was discovered that the patient could not tolerate liquid ritonavir because of nausea and vomiting, so that he had sometimes skipped or lowered the ritonavir dose or even refused to take it. On the occasions where no ritonavir or low-dose ritonavir was taken, the INRs had been low, whereas when he took the full dose of ritonavir the INRs were high.[2]

(ii) Saquinavir. A 73-year-old man who was HIV+ and who had been on warfarin, co-trimoxazole, nizatidine, stavudine and lamivudine for 7 months was started on saquinavir 600 mg three times daily. His INR, which had been stable at around 2 for five months, rose to about 2.5 after 4 weeks, and to about 4.2 after 8 weeks, which the author of the report attributed to an interaction with the saquinavir. The situation was solved by reducing the warfarin dosage by 20%.[3]

(c) Warfarin effects reduced

A 50-year-old HIV+ man, stabilised on warfarin (prothrombin complex activity (PCA) range of 20 to 35%), was additionally started on **indinavir** 800 mg 8-hourly, but it had to be withdrawn after 12 days because of a generalised skin rash. It was then found that the **indinavir** had caused a moderate reduction in his level of anticoagulation. Ten and 25 days after **indinavir** was stopped his PCA was 53% and 43% respectively. The warfarin dosage was increased to 6.25 and 7.5 mg on alternate days for one week, during which time a PCA of 34% was achieved, and he was then subsequently given warfarin 6.25 mg daily. At this point **ritonavir** (escalating doses up to 600 mg 12 hourly) was started and 20 days later his PCA was 62%. The warfarin dosage was then increased to 8.75 mg daily and 24 days later a satisfactory PCA of 33% was achieved.[4]

The INR of a 27-year-old woman with HIV and taking warfarin fell when she was additionally given **ritonavir**, clarithromycin and zidovudine. It was necessary almost to double the warfarin dosage to maintain satisfactory INRs. Three months later when the **ritonavir** was withdrawn, her INR more than tripled within a week. Her final warfarin maintenance dose was half of that needed before the **ritonavir** was started, and a quarter of the dose needed just before she stopped the **ritonavir**. This case was complicated by the use or withdrawal of a number of other drugs (co-trimoxazole, rifabutin, an oral contraceptive, megestrol), which can also interact with warfarin.[5]

Mechanism

The increase in the anticoagulant effects is consistent with the makers prediction that warfarin levels are expected to be increased by the inhibitory effects of ritonavir on the metabolism of warfarin, leading to increased warfarin effects. *In vitro* and *in vivo* studies have shown that ritonavir is a potent inhibitor of cytochrome P450 isoenzymes CYP3A4 and to a lesser extent CYP2C9, enzymes that are concerned with the metabolism of warfarin.

However, other cases suggest that warfarin effects are decreased. Ritonavir acts as an inducer of the isoenzyme CYP1A2 and is a substrate for CYP2C9. In these cases it would seem that the enzyme inducing effects of competition for metabolism predominated, resulting in increased metabolism of warfarin and acenocoumarol.

Importance and management

The interaction between warfarin and ritonavir is not established, but until more is known it would be prudent to monitor the prothrombin times and INRs of any patient if ritonavir is added, being alert for the need to modify the warfarin dosage. Information about an interaction between warfarin and indinavir so far seems to be limited to the report cited, but the same precautions suggested for ritonavir would be appropriate. Information about other coumarin anticoagulants is lacking but the same precautions would seem sensible.

1. Libre JM, Romeu J, López E, Sirera G. Severe interaction between ritonavir and acenocoumarol. *Ann Pharmacother* (2002) 36, 621–3.
2. Newshan G, Tsang P. Ritonavir and warfarin interaction. *AIDS* (1999) 13, 1788–9.
3. Darlington MR. Hypoprothrombinemia during concomitant therapy with warfarin and saquinavir. *Ann Pharmacother* (1997) 31, 647.
4. Gatti G, Alessandrini A, Camera M, Di Biagnio A, Bassetti M, Rizzo F. Influence of indinavir and ritonavir on warfarin anticoagulant activity. *AIDS* (1998) 12, 825–6.
5. Knoell KR, Young TM, Cousins ES. Potential interaction involving warfarin and ritonavir. *Ann Pharmacother* (1998) 32, 1299–1302.

Anticoagulants + Proton pump inhibitors

Raised INRs and/or bleeding has been seen in patients on warfarin and esomeprazole, lansoprazole or omeprazole, and acenocoumarol and omeprazole, but on the whole the proton pump inhibitors do not appear to have any clinically significant interactions with these anticoagulants. Omeprazole is said to have raised the prothrombin time of a patient on heparin.

Clinical evidence

(a) Esomeprazole

The makers say that esomeprazole has been shown not to have any clinically relevant effects on the pharmacokinetics of **warfarin**, but a few cases of raised INRs have been seen in practice.[1]

(b) Lansoprazole

A study in 24 subjects found that **lansoprazole** 60 mg daily for 9 days had no effect on the pharmacokinetics of either ***(S)***- or ***(R)*-warfarin**, and no significant changes were seen in their prothrombin times.[2]

In contrast the makers of lansoprazole have in their records two reports of possible interactions. An elderly patient on **warfarin** with an aortic valve replacement developed an INR of 7 when lansoprazole was added. Despite a **warfarin** dosage adjustment he had a gastrointestinal haemorrhage, a myocardial infarction and died after 3 weeks. Another man on **warfarin** (as well as amiodarone, furosemide and lisinopril) became confused, had hallucinations and developed an increased INR [value not known] when given lansoprazole. The lansoprazole was stopped after 4 days, and he then recovered. However, it is uncertain whether this was an interaction or whether he had taken an incorrect **warfarin** dosage because of his confusion.[3]

(c) Omeprazole

A comparative retrospective study of 118 patients given **acenocoumarol** with omeprazole and 299 patients on **acenocoumarol** without omeprazole (matched for age and sex), found no evidence that an interaction occurs.[4] In a placebo-controlled study 8 healthy subjects were given omeprazole 40 mg daily for 3 days with a single 10-mg dose of acenocoumarol on day 2. Omeprazole had no effect on the pharmacokinetics or anticoagulant effects of the **acenocoumarol**.[5]

In contrast, an isolated case report describes a 78-year-old woman stabilised on **acenocoumarol** for 60 days who developed gross haematuria within 5 days of starting omeprazole 20 mg daily. Her INR had risen from under 3 to 5.7 but when the omeprazole was stopped the INR fell.[6]

An isolated report very briefly describes a decrease in the prothrombin time of a patient treated with **heparin** and omeprazole. No details are given.[7]

A small but statistically significant decrease in the mean thrombotest percentage, from 21.1 to 18.7%, occurred in 21 patients on warfarin when they took omeprazole 20 mg daily for 2 weeks. ***(S)*-warfarin** serum levels remained unchanged but a small 12% rise in ***(R)*-warfarin** levels was seen.[8] No changes in coagulation times or thrombotest values occurred in 28 patients anticoagulated with **warfarin** given omeprazole 20 mg daily for 3 weeks. ***(S)*-warfarin** levels were unchanged while a 9.5% increase in ***(R)*-warfarin** levels occurred.[9]

In contrast, a man stabilised on **warfarin** 5 mg daily developed widespread bruising and haematuria 2 weeks after starting to take omeprazole 20 mg daily. His prothrombin time was found to have risen to 48 seconds. He was later restabilised on omeprazole 20 mg daily with the **warfarin** dosage reduced to 2 mg daily.[10]

(d) Pantoprazole

In 26 healthy subjects pantoprazole 40 mg daily caused no change in the response to a single 25-mg dose of **warfarin**. The pharmacokinetics of ***(R)***- and ***(S)*- warfarin** were unaltered and no changes in the pharmacodynamics of the **warfarin** (prothrombin time, factor VII) were seen.[11] No change in the responses to **phenprocoumon**, either pharmacokinetic or pharmacodynamic was seen in 16 healthy subjects when they were additionally given pantoprazole 40 mg daily for 5 days.[12]

(e) Rabeprazole

In a placebo-controlled study a single 0.75-mg/kg dose of **warfarin** was given to 21 patients before and after rabeprazole 20 mg daily for 7 days. No significant changes in prothrombin times or in the pharmacokinetics of ***(R)***- or ***(S)***- **warfarin** were seen.[13]

Mechanism

It seems possible that proton pump inhibitors cause a slight to moderate inhibition of the metabolism of oral anticoagulants by the liver in a stereoselective manner, but just why only a few patients should show such marked effects is not known. In one case[5] it has been suggested that the interaction occurred because the patient was a 'poor metaboliser', (p.4).

Importance and management

On the whole the evidence for an interaction between oral anticoagulants and proton pump inhibitors is poor, but it is clear that occasionally and unpredictably bleeding does occur with esomeprazole, lansoprazole and omeprazole. The makers of esomeprazole cite studies where no interaction occurred but on the basis of a few case reports of raised INRs with occasional bleeding recommend monitoring all patients.[1] This seems a cautious approach. The US makers suggest that some patients may need to be monitored[14] but it is not clear how these patients can be identified. When prescribing esomeprazole, lansoprazole and omeprazole to patients on warfarin it would seem prudent to bear in mind that rarely bleeding can occur. No adverse interaction would be expected with rabeprazole or pantoprazole.The general importance of the single report of an interaction between heparin and omeprazole is uncertain but it seems likely to be small.

1. Nexium (Esomeprazole). AstraZeneca UK Ltd. UK Summary of product characteristics, October 2004.
2. Cavanaugh JH, Winters EP, Cohen A, Locke CS, Braeckman R. Lack of effect of lansoprazole on steady state warfarin metabolism. *Gastroenterology* (1991) 100, A40.
3. Wyeth. Personal communication, January 1998.
4. Vreeburg EM, De Vlaam-Schluter GM, Trienekens PH, Snel P, Tytgat GNJ. Lack of effect of omeprazole on oral acenocoumarol anticoagulant therapy. *Scand J Gastroenterol* (1997) 32, 991–4.
5. de Hoon JNJM, Thijssen HHW, Beysens AJMM, Van Bortel LMAB. No effect of short-term omeprazole intake on acenocoumarol pharmacokinetics and pharmacodynamics. *Br J Clin Pharmacol* (1997) 44, 399–401.
6. García B, Lacambra C, Garrote F, García-Plaza I, Solis J. Possible potentiation of anticoagulant effect of acenocoumarol by omeprazole. *Pharm World Sci* (1994) 16, 231–2.
7. Beeley L, Cunningham H, Brennan A. *Bulletin of the West Midlands Centre for Adverse Drug Reaction Reporting* (1993) 36, 9.
8. Sutfin T, Balmer K, Boström H, Eriksson S, Höglund P, Paulsen O. Stereoselective interaction of omeprazole with warfarin in healthy men. *Ther Drug Monit* (1989) 11, 176–84.
9. Unge P, Svedberg L-E, Nordgren A, Blom H, Andersson T, Lagerström P-O, Idström J-P. A study of the interaction of omeprazole and warfarin in anticoagulated patients. *Br J Clin Pharmacol* (1992) 34, 509–12.
10. Ahmad S. Omeprazole-warfarin interaction. *South Med J* (1991) 84, 674–5.
11. Duursema L, Müller FO, Schall R, Middle MV, Hundt HKL, Groenewoud G, Steinijans VW, Bliesath H. Lack of effect of pantoprazole on the pharmacodynamics and pharmacokinetics of warfarin. *Br J Clin Pharmacol* (1995) 39, 700–703.
12. Ehrlich A, Fuder H, Hartmann M, Wieckhorst G, Timmer W, Huber R, Birkel M, Bliesath H, Steinijans VW, Wurst W, Lücker PW. Lack of pharmacokinetic and pharmacodynamic interaction between pantoprazole and phenprocoumon in man. *Eur J Clin Pharmacol* (1996) 51, 277–281.
13. Humphries TJ, Nardi RV, Spera AC, Lazar JD, Laurent AL, Spanyers SA. Coadministration of rabeprazole sodium (E3810) does not affect the pharmacokinetics of anhydrous theophylline or warfarin. *Gastroenterology* (1996) 110 (Suppl), A138.
14. Nexium (Esomeprazole). AstraZeneca. US Prescribing information, June 2005.

Anticoagulants + Quetiapine

A case report describes a woman on warfarin who developed a raised INR when quetiapine was added.

Clinical evidence, mechanism, importance and management

A 71-year old woman on long-term treatment with **warfarin**, phenytoin and benztropine had her **warfarin** dosage slightly reduced (from 20 to 19.5 mg weekly) because her INR was moderately raised (from 1.6 to 2.6). After 8 days her treatment with olanzapine was changed to quetiapine 200 mg daily. Two weeks later she was found to have an INR of 9.2. The quetiapine was stopped and she was given two doses of vitamin K by injection. The only clinical symptoms seen were a small amount of bleeding from the injection site and a bruise on the hand. She was eventually later restabilised on phenytoin, olanzapine and **warfarin** 17.5 mg weekly with an INR of 1.6.

The reasons for this apparent interaction are not known but the authors suggest that the quetiapine may have inhibited the metabolism of the **warfarin** (possibly by competitive inhibition of the cytochrome P450 isoenzymes CYP3A4 and CYP2C9), thereby increasing its effects. They also suggest that the phenytoin may have had some part to play.[1] This is only an isolated case but bear it in mind in the case of an unexpected response to concurrent use.

1. Rogers T, de Leon J, Atcher D. Possible interaction between warfarin and quetiapine. *J Clin Psychopharmacol* (1999) 19, 382–3.

Anticoagulants + Quinidine

The anticoagulant effects of warfarin can be increased (bleeding has been seen), decreased or remain unaltered when quinidine is given. A decrease in the effects of dicoumarol has also been reported.

Clinical evidence

(a) Anticoagulant effects increased

Three patients stabilised on **warfarin**, with prothrombin levels within the range of 15 to 25%, began to bleed within 7 to 10 days of starting to take quinidine 800 to 1200 mg daily. Their prothrombin levels were found to have fallen to 6 to 8%. Bleeding ceased when the warfarin was withdrawn.[1]

There are other reports of haemorrhage associated with the concurrent use of **warfarin** and quinidine.[2,3]

(b) Anticoagulant effects decreased

Four patients on **warfarin** or **dicoumarol** needed dosage increases of 8 to 24% to maintain adequate anticoagulation while receiving quinidine 400 mg three times daily.[4]

(c) Anticoagulant effects unaltered

Ten patients on long-term treatment with **warfarin** 2.5 to 12.5 mg daily showed no significant alteration in their prothrombin times when given quinidine 200 mg four times daily for 2 weeks.[5-7] Another 8 patients are also reported not to have shown an interaction.[8]

Mechanism

Quinidine can depress the synthesis of the vitamin-K dependent blood clotting factors and has a direct hypoprothrombinaemic effect of its own.[3] This would account for its additive effects with warfarin,[2] but does not explain why it can apparently also have antagonistic effects.[4]

Importance and management

Since increases (with subsequent bleeding) and decreases in the effects of warfarin, as well as the absence of an interaction have been described, the outcome adding quinidine is clearly very uncertain. It would therefore be prudent to monitor the effects of quinidine closely to ensure that prothrombin times remain within the therapeutic range. The same precautions should apply with all the other anticoagulants, although nothing seems to be documented about any but dicoumarol, cited above.[4]

1. Koch-Weser J. Quinidine-induced hypoprothrombinemic hemorrhage in patients on chronic warfarin therapy. *Ann Intern Med* (1968) 68, 511–17.
2. Gazzaniga AB, Stewart DR. Possible quinidine-induced hemorrhage in a patient on warfarin sodium. *N Engl J Med* (1969) 280, 711–12.
3. Beaumont JL, Tarrit A. Les accidents hémorrhagiques survenus au cours de 1500 traitements anticoagulants. *Sang* (1955) 26, 680–94.
4. Sylvén C, Anderson P. Evidence that disopyramide does not interact with warfarin. *BMJ* (1983) 286, 1181.
5. Udall JA. Quinidine and hypoprothrombinemia. *Ann Intern Med* (1968) 69, 403–4.
6. Udall JA. Drug interference with warfarin therapy. *Am J Cardiol* (1969) 23, 143.
7. Udall JA. Drug interference with warfarin therapy. *Clin Med* (1970) 77, 20–5.
8. Jones FL. More on quinidine induced hypoprothrombinaemia. *Ann Intern Med* (1986) 69, 1074.

Anticoagulants + Quinine

Normally no clinically significant interaction occurs but isolated reports describe increased warfarin effects in two women who drank large amounts of quinine-containing tonic water, and increased phenprocoumon effects and bleeding in a man.

Clinical evidence

A woman on **warfarin** needed a dosage reduction from 6 to 4 mg daily when she started to drink 1 to 1.5 litres of tonic water containing quinine each day. Her **warfarin** requirements rose again when the tonic water was stopped. Another woman needed a **warfarin** dosage reduction from 4 to 2 mg daily when she started to drink over 2 litres of tonic water daily. They were probably taking about 80 to 180 mg of quinine daily.[1] A patient on long-term **phenprocoumon** treatment repeatedly developed extensive haematuria within 24 hours of drinking 1 litre of Indian tonic water containing 30 mg of quinine.[2]

Mechanism

Not understood. Two studies[3,4] using the Page method[5] to measure prothrombin times showed that marked increases of up to 12 seconds could occur when 330-mg doses of quinine were given in the absence of an anticoagulant, but other studies[4,6] using the conventional Quick method found that the prothrombin times were only prolonged by up to 2.1 seconds. The changes in prothrombin times could be completely reversed by vitamin K (menadiol sodium diphosphate),[3,4] which suggests that quinine, like the oral anticoagulants, is a competitive inhibitor of vitamin K. The increase in prothrombin times and their decrease in response to vitamin K took several days, which is consistent with a pharmacological action involving changes in the synthesis by the liver of blood clotting factors.

Importance and management

Common experience would seem to confirm that any increase in the effects of oral anticoagulants is normally very small and of little or no clinical importance. Concurrent use need not be avoided, however the isolated cases cited show that very exceptionally much larger changes and even bleeding can occur even with doses as small as 30 mg.

1. Clark DJ. Clinical curio: warfarin and tonic water. *BMJ* (1983) 286, 1258.
2. Iven H, Lerche L, Kaschube M. Influence of quinine and quinidine on the pharmacokinetics of phenprocoumon in rat and man. *Eur J Pharmacol* (1990) 183, 662.
3. Pirk LA, Engelberg R. Hypoprothrombinemic action of quinine sulfate. *JAMA* (1945) 128, 1093–5.
4. Pirk LA, Engelberg R. Hypoprothrombinemic action of quinine sulfate. *Am J Med Sci* (1947) 213, 593–7.
5. Page RC, de Beer EJ, Orr ML. Prothrombin studies using Russell viper venom. II. Relation of clotting time to prothrombin concentration in human plasma. *J Lab Clin Med* (1941) 27, 197–201.
6. Quick AJ. Effect of synthetic vitamin K and quinine sulfate on the prothrombin level. *J Lab Clin Med* (1946) 31, 79–84.

Anticoagulants + Quinolones

The quinolone antibacterials normally appear not to increase the effects of anticoagulants in most patients, but increased effects and even bleeding have been seen quite unpredictably in some patients on warfarin when given gatifloxacin, levofloxacin, nalidixic acid, norfloxacin, ofloxacin or particularly ciprofloxacin; or while taking acenocoumarol when given nalidixic acid, norfloxacin or pefloxacin, or phenprocoumon with norfloxacin. A very small and probably clinically irrelevant increase in INR has been seen in patients on warfarin given clinafloxacin.

Clinical evidence

(a) Ciprofloxacin

No clinically relevant effects on **warfarin** anticoagulation were seen in studies in a total of 25 patients given ciprofloxacin 500 mg twice daily for 7 or 10 days,[1,2] or in 36 patients given ciprofloxacin 750 mg twice daily for 12 days.[3]

In contrast, there are many scattered reports where ciprofloxacin has apparently been responsible for increased prothrombin times and/or bleeding in patients on **warfarin.** The FDA has a total of 64 such cases over the 10 year period 1987 to 1997 on its Spontaneous Reporting System database. Those cases where details were available plus an additional 2 cases showed that the median prothrombin time was 38 seconds, the INR 10, and the mean time when the problem was identified was 5.5 days. Hospitalisation was reported in 15 cases, bleeding in 25 cases and death in one case.[4] There are a number of other individual case reports describing moderate to marked increases in prothrombin times and/or bleeding in patients on **warfarin** associated with taking ciprofloxacin.[5-11]

(b) Clinafloxacin

Clinafloxacin 200 mg twice daily for 14 days had no effect on the steady-state ***(S)*-warfarin** levels in healthy subjects but the levels of the less active enantiomer ***(R)*-warfarin** were increased 32% and the mean INR was increased by 13%. The reason is not known but the authors of the report attributed it to changes in gut flora caused by the clinafloxacin.[12]

(c) Enoxacin

Enoxacin 400 mg twice daily did not affect the pharmacokinetics of ***(S)*-warfarin** in 6 healthy subjects, whereas the clearance of ***(R)*-warfarin** was decreased from 0.22 to 0.15 l/hour and its elimination half-life was prolonged from 36.8 to 52.2 hours. The overall anticoagulant response to the **warfarin** was unaltered.[13] Another report about one patient is in agreement with these findings.[14]

(d) Fleroxacin

The pharmacokinetics, prothrombin time and factor VII clotting time of single 25-mg doses of **warfarin** were unaffected in 12 healthy subjects after taking fleroxacin 400 mg daily for 9 days.[15]

(e) Gatifloxacin

A review of 94 patients on **warfarin**, given antibacterials for community-acquired pneumonia, found that 55% of the 40 patients treated with gatifloxacin had INRs greater than 3 during or within 48 hours of starting gatifloxacin, compared with 37% of 54 patients treated with other antibacterials (ceftriaxone or azithromycin). In the gatifloxacin group 38% needed a **warfarin** dose adjustment, compared with 18% of patients on other antibacterials.[16]

(f) Gemifloxacin

A double-blind, randomised, placebo controlled study found that healthy subjects on fixed doses of **warfarin** and with INRs in the range of 1.3 to 1.8 had no INR changes when they were given gemifloxacin 320 mg daily for 7 days.[17]

(g) Levofloxacin

Levofloxacin 500 mg twice daily for 6 days had no effect on the pharmacokinetics or pharmacodynamics of ***(R)*-** and ***(S)*-warfarin** in 15 healthy subjects given single 30-mg oral doses.[18] However, two elderly patients on **warfarin** were found to have increases in their INRs to 5.7 and to 7.9 shortly after stopping levofloxacin 500 mg daily.[19] Six other cases of increased INR have been reported in patients stabilised on **warfarin** who were given courses of levofloxacin 500 mg daily for 5 to 10 days;[20,21] epistaxis occurred in one patient.[21]

(h) Nalidixic acid

A patient, well stabilised on **warfarin** (prothrombin ratio 2), developed a purpuric rash and bruising within 6 days of starting nalidixic acid 500 mg four times daily. Her prothrombin time had risen to 45 seconds (prothrombin ratio 3.46).[22] Another patient, previously well controlled on **warfarin**, developed a prothrombin time of 60 seconds 10 days after starting nalidixic acid 1 g three times daily.[23] The INR of an 84-year-old woman on **warfarin** rose from 1.9 to 9.6 when nalidixic acid was added.[24] Yet another patient on **acenocoumarol** developed hypoprothrombinaemia after receiving nalidixic acid 1 g daily.[25]

(i) Norfloxacin

Six days' treatment with norfloxacin 400 mg twice daily was found not to alter either the pharmacokinetics or anticoagulant effects of single 30-mg doses of **warfarin** in 10 healthy subjects.[26]

In contrast, a 91-year-old woman on **warfarin** and digoxin developed a brain haemorrhage within 11 days of starting to take norfloxacin [precise dose not stated]. Her prothrombin times had risen from 21.6 to 36.5 seconds. The makers of norfloxacin are said to have other reports of an interaction between warfarin and norfloxacin but no details are given.[27] In a population-based cohort study, patients treated with **acenocoumarol** or **phenprocoumon** were found to have an increased risk of over-anticoagulation (INR greater than or equal to 6) during norfloxacin treatment. The risk was greatest during the first 3 days of treatment.[28]

(j) Ofloxacin

Ofloxacin 200 mg daily for week did not significantly affect the prothrombin times of 7 subjects on **phenprocoumon**.[29] However, a woman with a mitral valve replacement treated with digoxin, furosemide, spironolactone, verapamil and **warfarin** 5 mg daily, showed a marked increase in her INR (from 2.5 to 4.4) within 2 days of starting to take ofloxacin 200 mg three times daily.[30] Two days later her INR had risen to 5.8. Another patient on **warfarin** developed gross haematuria and a prothrombin time of 78 seconds 5 days after starting to take ofloxacin 400 mg twice daily.[31]

(k) Pefloxacin

A patient showed a marked increase in the effects of **acenocoumarol** (Quick time reduced from 26% to less than 5%) within 5 days of starting to take pefloxacin 800 mg daily and rifampicin 1200 mg daily.[32] Rifampicin is an enzyme inducer, which normally causes a reduction in the effects of the anticoagulants, which would suggest that the pefloxacin was responsible for this reaction.

(l) Trovafloxacin

Healthy subjects stabilised on **warfarin** with INRs in the range of 1.3 to 1.7 were additionally given trovafloxacin 200 mg daily for 7 days. No changes in the pharmacokinetics of either ***(S)*- or *(R)*-warfarin** occurred and no significant changes in mean INRs were seen.[33]

Mechanism

Uncertain. It is not clear what other factors might have been responsible in those cases where the effects of the anticoagulants were increased. Infection rather than the antibacterial used to treat it may be responsible for increased INRs. However, one study that controlled for infection indicated this is not the case and that an interaction between the quinolone and anticoagulant probably occurs.[16] *In vitro* experiments[34,35] have shown that nalidixic acid can displace warfarin from its binding sites on human plasma albumin, but this mechanism on its own is almost certainly not the full explanation. In a single-dose study enoxacin was shown to inhibit the metabolism of the less potent *(R)*-warfarin isomer, without affecting the anticoagulant response.[13] This effect may become important if accumulation of the *(R)*-warfarin isomer (which is cleared slowly) occurred during prolonged dosing.[2] It has also been suggested that ofloxacin may suppress vitamin K-producing gut bacteria with resultant potentiation of anticoagulant effects.[30]

Importance and management

The extent of the documentation is variable depending on the quinolone in question but generally moderate. The overall picture is that no adverse interaction normally occurs between these quinolones and oral anticoagulants, but rarely and unpredictably increased anticoagulant effects and even bleeding can occur with some of them. It is difficult to know whether the relatively large number of cases seen with ciprofloxacin are because this quinolone interacts more frequently than the others or whether the figure is boosted by the very widespread use of ciprofloxacin. Whatever the answer, there is no need to avoid using any of the quinolones with oral anticoagulants but it would be prudent to monitor the effects when any quinolone antibacterial is first added to treatment with any coumarin so that any problems can be quickly identified. So far there appears to be no information about any of the other quinolones or oral anticoagulants not cited here.

1. Rindone JP, Keuey CL, Jones WN, Garewal HS. Hypoprothrombinemic effect of warfarin not influenced by ciprofloxacin. *Clin Pharm* (1991) 10, 136–8.
2. Bianco TM, Bussey HI, Farnett LE, Linn WD, Roush MK, Wong YWJ. Potential warfarin-ciprofloxacin interaction in patients receiving long-term anticoagulation. *Pharmacotherapy* (1992) 12, 435–9.
3. Israel DS, Stotka J, Rock W, Sintek CD, Kamada AK, Klein C, Swaim WR, Pluhar RE, Toscano JP, Lettieri JT, Heller AH, Polk RE. Effect of ciprofloxacin on the pharmacokinetics and pharmacodynamics of warfarin. *Clin Infect Dis* (1996) 22, 251–6.
4. Ellis RJ, Mayo MS, Bodensteiner DM. Ciprofloxacin-warfarin coagulopathy: a case series. *Am J Hematol* (2000) 63, 28–31.
5. Mott FE, Murphy S, Hunt V. Ciprofloxacin and warfarin. *Ann Intern Med* (1989) 111, 542–3.
6. Linville D, Emory C, Graves L. Ciprofloxacin and warfarin interaction. *Am J Med* (1991) 90, 765.
7. Beeley L, Cunningham H, Carmichael A, Brennan A. *Bulletin of the West Midlands Centre for Adverse Drug Reaction Reporting* (1991), 33, 36.
8. Kamada AK. Possible interaction between ciprofloxacin and warfarin. *DICP Ann Pharmacother* (1990) 24, 27–8.
9. Johnson KC, Joe RH, Self TH. Drug interaction. *J Fam Pract* (1991) 33, 338.
10. Renzi R, Finkbeiner S. Ciprofloxacin interaction with warfarin: a potentially dangerous side-effect. *Am J Emerg Med* (1991) 9, 551–2.
11. Dugoni-Kramer BM. Ciprofloxacin-warfarin interaction. *DICP Ann Pharmacother* (1991) 25, 1397.
12. Randinitis EJ, Koup JR, Bron NJ, Hounslow NJ, Rausch G, Abel R, Vassos AB, Sedman AJ. Drug interaction studies with clinafloxacin and probenecid, cimetidine, phenytoin and warfarin. *Drugs* (1999) 58 (Suppl 2), 254–5.
13. Toon S, Hopkins KJ, Garstang FM, Aarons L, Sedman A, Rowland M. Enoxacin-warfarin interaction: pharmacokinetic and stereochemical aspects. *Clin Pharmacol Ther* (1987) 42, 33–41.
14. McLeod AD, Burgess C. Drug interaction between warfarin and enoxacin. *N Z Med J* (1988) 101, 216.
15. Holazo AA, Soni PP, Kachevsky V, Min BH, Townsend L, Patel IH. Fleroxacin-warfarin interaction in humans. *Intersci Conf Antimicrob Agents Chemother* (1990) 30, 253.
16. Artymowicz RJ, Cino BJ, Rossi JG, Walker JL, Moore S. Possible interaction between gatifloxacin and warfarin. *Am J Health-Syst Pharm* (2002) 59 1205–6.
17. Davy M, Bird N, Rost KL, Fuder H. Lack of effect of gemifloxacin on the steady-state pharmacodynamics of warfarin in healthy volunteers. *Chemotherapy* (1999) 45, 491–5.
18. Liao S, Palmer M, Fowler C, Nayak RK. Absence of an effect of levofloxacin on warfarin pharmacokinetics and anticoagulation in male volunteers. *J Clin Pharmacol* (1996) 36, 1072–7.
19. Ravnan SL, Locke C. Levofloxacin and warfarin interaction. *Pharmacotherapy* (2001) 21, 884–5.
20. Gheno G, Cinetto L. Levofloxacin-warfarin interaction. *Eur J Clin Pharmacol* (2001) 57, 427.
21. Jones CB, Fugate SE. Levofloxacin and warfarin interaction. *Ann Pharmacother* (2002) 36, 1554–7.
22. Hoffbrand BI. Interaction of nalidixic acid and warfarin. *BMJ* (1974) 2, 666.
23. Leor J, Levartowsky D, Sharon C. Interaction between nalidixic acid and warfarin. *Ann Intern Med* (1987) 107, 601.
24. Gulløv AL, Koefoed BG, Petersen P. Interaktion mellem warfarin og nalidixinsyre. *Ugeskr Laeger* (1996) 158, 5174–5.
25. Potasman I, Bassan H. Nicoumalone and nalidixic acid interaction. *Ann Intern Med* (1980) 92, 571.
26. Rocci ML, Vlasses PH, Distlerath LM, Gregg MH, Wheeler SC, Zing W, Bjornsson TD. Norfloxacin does not alter warfarin's disposition or anticoagulant effect. *J Clin Pharmacol* (1990) 30, 728–32.
27. Linville T, Matanin D. Norfloxacin and warfarin. *Ann Intern Med* (1989) 110, 751–2.
28. Visser LE, Penning-van Beest FJA, Kasbergen AAH, De Smet PAGM, Vulto AG, Hofman A, Stricker BHC. Overanticoagulation associated with combined use of antibacterial drugs and acenocoumarol or phenprocoumon anticoagulants. *Thromb Haemost* (2002) 88, 705–10.
29. Verho M, Malerczyk V, Rosenkranz B, Grötsch H. Absence of interaction between ofloxacin and phenprocoumon. *Curr Med Res Opin* (1987) 10, 474–9.
30. Leor J, Matetzki S. Ofloxacin and warfarin. *Ann Intern Med* (1988) 109, 761.
31. Baciewicz AM, Ashar BH, Locke TW. Interaction of ofloxacin and warfarin. *Ann Intern Med* (1993) 119, 1223.
32. Pertek JP, Helmer J, Vivin P, Kipper R. Potentialisation d'une antivitamine K par l'association péfloxacine-rifampicine. *Ann Fr Anesth Reanim* (1986) 5, 320–1.
33. Teng R, Apseloffl G, Vincent J, Pelletier SM, Willavize SA, Friedman JL. Effect of trovafloxacin (CP-99,219) on the pharmacokinetics and pharmacodynamics of warfarin in healthy male subjects. *Intersci Conf Antimicrob Agents Chemother* (1996) 36, A2.
34. Sellers EM, Koch-Weser J. Kinetics and clinical importance of displacement of warfarin from albumin by acidic drugs. *Ann N Y Acad Sci* (1971) 179, 213–25.
35. Sellers EM, Koch-Weser J. Displacement of warfarin from human albumin by diazoxide and ethacrynic, mefenamic, and nalidixic acids. *Clin Pharmacol Ther* (1970) 11, 524–9.

Anticoagulants + Raloxifene

A small and slow decrease in prothrombin times may occur when raloxifene is given with warfarin and possibly other anticoagulants.

Clinical evidence, mechanism, importance and management

A single-dose study found that when raloxifene 120 mg was given with and a single 20-mg dose of **warfarin** the pharmacokinetics of both drugs were not altered.[1] However, because modest decreases in prothrombin times have been seen, which may develop over several weeks, the makers recommend that prothrombin times should be checked. They extend this recommendation to cover the use of other coumarins.[2]

1. Miller JW, Skerjanec A, Knadler MP, Ghosh A, Allerheiligen SRB. Divergent effects of raloxifene HCl on the pharmacokinetics and pharmacodynamics of warfarin. *Pharm Res* (2001) 18, 1024–8.
2. Evista (Raloxifene). Eli Lilly and Company Ltd. UK Summary of product characteristics, July 2003.

Anticoagulants + Retinoids

A single case report describes reduced warfarin effects in a patient given etretinate. Acitretin does not significantly alter the anticoagulant effects of phenprocoumon.

Clinical evidence

(a) Phenprocoumon

Acitretin 50 mg daily for 10 days slightly increased the Quick test of 10 healthy subjects on phenprocoumon from 22 to 24%, and the corresponding INR value decreased from 2.91 to 2.71. However, these changes were not considered to be significant.[1]

(b) Warfarin

A man with T-cell lymphoma who had recently been given chemotherapy (cyclophosphamide, doxorubicin, vincristine and prednisolone) was anticoagulated with warfarin after developing a pulmonary embolism. After he started **etretinate** 40 mg daily it was found necessary to increase his warfarin dosage from 7 to 10 mg daily. His liver function tests were normal.[2] This report is complicated as the patients was also taking co-proxamol, tolbutamide and cimetidine, which have been reported to interact with warfarin.

Mechanism

Not understood. It has been suggested that etretinate may increase the rate of metabolism of warfarin.[2]

Importance and management

Information appears to be limited to these reports. Consideration could be given to monitoring the INR if patients are given warfarin and etretinate, but this seems over-cautious given that all the evidence for an interaction comes from one case report. No special precautions seem necessary if acitretin is given to patients on phenprocoumon but the outcome should be monitored. There seems to be no information about other anticoagulants.

1. Hartmann D, Mosberg H, Weber W. Lack of effect of acitretin on the hypoprothrombinemic action of phenprocoumon in healthy volunteers. *Dermatologica* (1989) 178, 33–6.
2. Ostlere LS, Langtry JAA, Jones S, Staughton RCD. Reduced therapeutic effect of warfarin caused by etretinate. *Br J Dermatol* (1991) 124, 505–10.

Anticoagulants + Rifamycins

The anticoagulant effects of acenocoumarol, phenprocoumon and warfarin are markedly reduced by rifampicin (rifampin).

Clinical evidence

The dosage of **acenocoumarol** needed to be markedly increased to maintain the Quick value within the therapeutic range in 18 patients who were given rifampicin 450 mg twice daily for 7 days.[1] There are numerous reports and studies of this interaction involving a considerable number of patients and subjects on **acenocoumarol**,[2] **phenprocoumon**[3,4] or **warfarin**.[5-15]

Mechanism

Rifampicin is a potent liver enzyme inducing agent, which increases the metabolism and clearance of the anticoagulants from the body, thereby reducing their effects.[14] Other mechanisms may also be involved.[12] One study found that the serum levels of warfarin and the prothrombin response were approximately halved.[6]

Importance and management

The interaction between rifampicin and the coumarins is very well documented, clinically important, and occurs in most patients. A marked reduction in the anticoagulant effects may be expected within 5 to 7 days of starting the rifampicin,[1,5] persisting for one,[1,5] three,[3,8,12] or even five[15] weeks after the rifampicin has been withdrawn. With warfarin there is evidence that the dosage may need to be doubled[5] or even tripled[9] to accommodate this interaction, and reduced by an equivalent amount following withdrawal of the rifampicin.[5,8,12] In one patient increases in warfarin dosage from 5 to 25 mg daily were required to attain a therapeutic INR during long-term rifampicin therapy. A gradual dose reduction over 4 to 5 weeks was required when rifampicin was discontinued.[15] Warfarin dose titrations should be carried out with close monitoring. There does not seem to be any information regarding the other rifamycins, **rifabutin** (a weak enzyme inducer) and **rifapentine** (a moderate enzyme inducer). However, the makers and the UK Committee on Safety of Medicines warn that rifabutin may possibly reduce the effects of a number of drugs, including oral anticoagulants.[16,17]

1. Michot F, Bürgi M, Büttner J. Rimactan (Rifampizin) und Antikoagulantientherapie. *Schweiz Med Wochenschr* (1970) 100, 583–4.
2. Sennwald G. Etude de l'influence de la rifampicine sur l'effet anticoagulant de l'acénocoumarol. *Rev Med Suisse Romande* (1974) 94, 945–54.
3. Boekhout-Mussert RJ, Bieger R, van Brummelen A, Lemkes HHPJ. Inhibition by rifampin of the anticoagulant effect of phenprocoumon. *JAMA* (1974) 229, 1903–4.
4. Ohnhaus EE, Kampschulte J, Mönig H. Effect of propranolol and rifampicin on liver blood flow and phenoprocoumon elimination. *Acta Pharmacol Toxicol (Copenh)* (1986) 59 (Suppl 4), 92.
5. Romankiewicz JA, Ehrman M. Rifampin and warfarin: a drug interaction. *Ann Intern Med* (1975) 82, 224–5.
6. O'Reilly RA. Interaction of sodium warfarin and rifampin. Studies in man. *Ann Intern Med* (1974) 81, 337–40.
7. O'Reilly RA. Interaction of rifampin and warfarin in man. *Clin Res* (1973) 21, 207.
8. Self TH, Mann RB. Interaction of rifampicin and warfarin. *Chest* (1975) 67, 490–1.
9. Fox P. Warfarin-rifampicin interaction. *Med J Aust* (1982) 1, 60.
10. O'Reilly RA. Interaction of chronic daily warfarin therapy and rifampin. *Ann Intern Med* (1975) 83, 506–8.
11. Beeley L, Daly M, Stewart P. *Bulletin of the West Midlands Centre for Adverse Drug Reaction Reporting* (1987) 24, 23.
12. Almog S, Martinowitz U, Halkin H, Bank HZ, Farfel Z. Complex interaction of rifampin and warfarin. *South Med J* (1988) 81, 1304–6.
13. Casner PR. Inability to attain oral anticoagulation: warfarin-rifampin interaction revisited. *South Med J* (1996) 89, 1200–3.
14. Heimark LD, Gibaldi M, Trager WF, O'Reilly RA, Goulart DA. The mechanism of the warfarin-rifampicin drug interaction in humans. *Clin Pharmacol Ther* (1987) 42, 388–94.
15. Lee CR, Thrasher KA. Difficulties in anticoagulation management during coadministration of warfarin and rifampin. *Pharmacotherapy* (2001) 21, 1240–6.
16. Mycobutin (Rifabutin). Pharmacia Ltd. UK Summary of product characteristics, January 2003.
17. Committee on the Safety of Medicines/Medicines Control Agency. Revised indication and drug interactions of rifabutin. *Current Problems* (1997) 23, 14.

Anticoagulants + Sodium valproate

Sodium valproate appears not to interact with the oral anticoagulants to a clinically relevant extent.

Clinical evidence, mechanism, importance and management

The makers of sodium valproate recommend caution with vitamin K dependent anticoagulants because sodium valproate may displace them from protein binding sites.[1] There is certainly some *in vitro* evidence that the serum binding of **warfarin** is decreased by sodium valproate so that free **warfarin** levels rise,[2-4] by 32% according to one study.[3] Linked with this last study is a report of a woman on **warfarin** whose prothrombin time and INR were briefly raised when sodium valproate was added.[3] Numerous dosage adjustments were needed to keep the INR therapeutic, but ultimately she was discharged on the same warfarin dose as before the sodium valproate was started.[3] It may be that, as with the interaction between warfarin and 'cloral hydrate', (p.276), any interaction occurs only transiently when the sodium valproate is added, and the situation rapidly restabilises without any real need to adjust the **warfarin** dosage. There seem to be no other reports of problems associated with concurrent use nor any other direct evidence that an interaction of clinical importance normally occurs. A report about one patient found that sodium valproate did not alter the anticoagulant effects of **phenprocoumon**.[5]

The makers also point out that sodium valproate inhibits the second stage of platelet aggregation, and that a reversible prolongation of bleeding times and thrombocytopenia has been reported with doses above those recommended.[1] But there seems to be little reason for particular precautions when using sodium valproate, over and above those normally taken with the oral anticoagulants.

1. Epilim (Sodium valproate). Sanofi-Aventis. UK Summary of product characteristics, March 2004.
2. Urien S, Albengres E, Tillement J-P. Serum protein binding of valproic acid in healthy subjects and in patients with liver disease. *Int J Clin Pharmacol Ther Toxicol* (1981) 19, 319–25.
3. Guthrie SK, Stoysich AM, Bader G, Hilleman DE. Hypothesized interaction between valproic acid and warfarin. *J Clin Psychopharmacol* (1995) 15, 138–9.
4. Panjehshahin MR, Bowmer CJ, Yates MS. Effect of valproic acid, its unsaturated metabolites and some structurally related fatty acids on the binding of warfarin and dansylsarcosine to human albumin. *Biochem Pharmacol* (1991) 41, 1227–33.
5. Schlienger R, Kurmann M, Drewe J, Müller-Spahn F, Seifritz E. Inhibition of phenprocoumon anticoagulation by carbamazepine. *Eur Neuropsychopharmacol* (2000) 10, 219–21.

Anticoagulants + SSRIs

Warfarin plasma levels can be increased by fluvoxamine and raised INRs have been seen in several cases. Isolated reports describe raised INRs and/or haemorrhage in patients taking acenocoumarol with citalopram or paroxetine, and warfarin with fluoxetine or paroxetine.

Clinical evidence and mechanism

(a) Citalopram

A 63-year-old patient treated with **acenocoumarol** 18 mg per week for deep vein thrombosis developed spontaneous gingival haemorrhage 10 days after starting citalopram 20 mg daily for depression. Her INR had increased from its usual value of 1.8 to greater than 15. She was treated with 2 units of blood and citalopram was withdrawn. Her INR was reduced to 1.95 within 5 days and she was able to continue on **acenocoumarol** 18 mg per week.[1] The reasons for the interaction are not clear.

A study in 12 healthy subjects given a single 25-mg oral dose of **warfa-**

rin either alone or on day 15 of a 21-day course of citalopram 40 mg daily, found that the pharmacokinetics of both ***(R)*- and *(S)*-warfarin** remained unchanged in the presence of the citalopram, but the maximum prothrombin time was increased by 1.6 seconds. This was considered to be clinically irrelevant.[2]

(b) Fluoxetine

Fluoxetine 30 mg given to healthy subjects as a single dose or daily for 8 days had no effect on the pharmacokinetics or the anticoagulant effects of a single 20-mg dose of **warfarin**.[3] The half-life of **warfarin** was not significantly changed in 3 subjects by either a single 30-mg dose of fluoxetine given 3 hours before the **warfarin**, or by fluoxetine 30 mg daily for a week.[4] Six patients anticoagulated with **warfarin** showed no significant changes in their prothrombin times while taking fluoxetine 20 mg daily for 21 days.[5]

In contrast, the INR of a man on **warfarin**, amiodarone, furosemide, digoxin, ciprofloxacin and levothyroxine rose sharply from a range of 1.8 to 2.3 up to 14.9 within 5 days of starting fluoxetine 30 mg daily. The INR of another man with metastatic carcinoma on **warfarin**, dexamethasone, bisacodyl and lactulose rose from a range of 2.5 to 3.5 up to 15.5 within 2 weeks of starting fluoxetine 20 mg daily. He showed microscopic haematuria but no bleeding. Other reports describe an abdominal haematoma,[6] cerebral haemorrhage,[7] severe bruising[8] and prolonged prothrombin times of INRs in patients given fluoxetine while taking **warfarin**.[9,10] The UK Committee on Safety of Medicines is also said to have 4 other similar cases on record.[11] Bowel haemorrhage has been reported in a patient on acenocoumarol given fluoxetine, but this was complicated by the presence of mefenamic acid.[12,13]

(c) Fluvoxamine

Fluvoxamine can increase plasma **warfarin** levels by about 65% and raised INRs have been seen.[14] A worldwide literature search by the makers of fluvoxamine identified only 11 reported interactions between **warfarin** and fluvoxamine by 1995, all with clinical signs that included prolonged prothrombin times.[15] An 80-year-old woman on **warfarin**, digoxin and colchicine developed an elevated INR within a week of starting to take fluvoxamine. Both the **warfarin** and fluvoxamine were stopped but her INR only stabilised 2 weeks after the fluvoxamine was withdrawn.[16] Another report describes a 79-year-old woman admitted to hospital because of suicidal thoughts. She was on **warfarin** (INR 1.6 to 1.8) and citalopram 10 mg at night and other medications included paracetamol with dextropropoxyphene. On the third day in hospital the citalopram dose was increased to 30 mg at bedtime and after 2 days it was discontinued and fluvoxamine 50 mg daily was started to treat depression and possibly obsessive thoughts. Within 4 days the patient's INR had increased to 3.7. Fluvoxamine was replaced with venlafaxine and **warfarin** was omitted for 1 day. The INR gradually decreased to the normal range over about 7 days.[17] A further isolated report describes a woman anticoagulated for 4 years on **fluindione** whose INR rose to 7.13 (from a normal value of about 2.5) within 13 days of starting to take fluvoxamine 100 mg daily. She had received fluoxetine, dosulepin and lorazepam for 15 days before fluvoxamine was started.[11]

(d) Paroxetine

Paroxetine 30 mg daily, given to healthy subjects with **warfarin** 5 mg daily, did not significantly increase their mean prothrombin times, but mild, clinically significant bleeding was seen in 5 out of 27 subjects. Two withdrew from the study because of increased prothrombin times, and another because of haematuria. The disposition of the **warfarin** and the paroxetine remained unchanged.[18] A brief report describes 4 patients on **warfarin** whose INR was said to have increased by an average of 3 points (increases of nearly 100% in some cases) associated with the use of paroxetine and sertraline.[19]

A single case report[20] describes severe bleeding (abdominal haematoma) in a patient on **acenocoumarol** and paroxetine when given phenytoin, but it is by no means clear whether the paroxetine had any part to play in what happened (see 'Phenytoin + Anticoagulants', p.361).

(e) Sertraline

After taking sertraline in increasing doses up to 200 mg daily for 22 days, the prothrombin time AUC in response to a single 0.75-mg/kg dose of **warfarin** in 6 healthy subjects was increased by 7.9%. This was statistically significant, but regarded as too small to be clinically relevant.[21] A brief report describes 4 patients on **warfarin** whose INR was said to have increased by an average of 3 points (increases of nearly 100% in some cases) associated with the use of paroxetine and sertraline.[19]

Importance and management

The general picture appears to be that very occasionally and unpredictably a interaction can occurs between the SSRIs and anticoagulants. However, studies have not demonstrated a consistent interaction, perhaps with the exception of fluvoxamine and warfarin. Concurrent use need not be avoided but the response should be monitored when fluvoxamine is first added, being alert for the need to decrease the anticoagulant dosage.

Definitive information about other anticoagulants and SSRIs seems to be lacking. Note that bruising and bleeding have been reported with fluoxetine alone.[22,23] Consider monitoring the INR if both drugs are given but note only a few patients appear to have demonstrated this interaction.

1. Borrás-Blasco J, Marco-Garbayo JL, Bosca-Sanleon B, Navarro-Ruiz A. Probable interaction between citalopram and acenocoumarol. *Ann Pharmacother* (2002) 36, 345.
2. Priskorn M, Sidhu JS, Larsen F, Davis JD, Khan AZ, Rolan PE. Investigation of multiple dose citalopram on the pharmacokinetics and pharmacodynamics of racemic warfarin. *Br J Clin Pharmacol* (1997) 44, 199–202.
3. Lemberger L, Bergstrom RF, Wolen RL, Farid NA, Enas GG, Aronoff GR. Fluoxetine: clinical pharmacology and physiologic disposition. *J Clin Psychiatry* (1985) 46, 14–19.
4. Rowe H, Carmichael R, Lemberger L. The effect of fluoxetine on warfarin metabolism in the rat and man. *Life Sci* (1978) 23, 807–12.
5. Ford MA, Anderson ML, Rindone JP, Jaskar DW. Lack of effect of fluoxetine on the hypoprothrombinemic response of warfarin. *J Clin Psychopharmacol* (1997) 17, 110–12.
6. Hanger HC, Thomas F. Fluoxetine and warfarin interactions. *N Z Med J* (1995), 108, 157.
7. Dent LA, Orrock MW. Warfarin-fluoxetine and diazepam-fluoxetine interaction. *Pharmacotherapy* (1997) 17, 170–2.
8. Claire RJ, Servis ME, Cram DL. Potential interaction between warfarin sodium and fluoxetine. *Am J Psychiatry* (1991) 148, 1604.
9. Woolfrey S, Gammack NS, Dewar MS, Brown PJE. Fluoxetine-warfarin interaction. *BMJ* (1993) 307, 241.
10. Wu J-R, Li P-YY, Yang Y-HK. Concurrent use of fluoxetine and warfarin prolongs prothrombin time: a retrospective survey. *Pharmacotherapy* (1997) 17, 1080.
11. Nezelof S, Vandel P, Bonin B. Fluvoxamine interaction with fluindione: a case report. *Therapie* (1997) 52, 608–9.
12. Beeley L, Magee P, Hickey FN. *Bulletin of the West Midlands Centre for Adverse Drug Reaction Reporting* (1990) 30, 32.
13. Dista Products Limited. Personal communication, May 1990.
14. Benfield P, Ward A. Fluvoxamine. A review of its pharmacodynamic and pharmacokinetic properties, and therapeutic efficacy in depressive illness. *Drugs* (1986) 32, 313–34.
15. Wagner W, Vause EW. Fluvoxamine. A review of global drug-drug interaction data. *Clin Pharmacokinet* (1995) 29 (Suppl 1), 26–32.
16. Yap KB, Low ST. Interaction of fluvoxamine with warfarin in an elderly woman. *Singapore Med J* (1999) 40, 480–2.
17. Limke KK, Shelton AR, Elliott ES. Fluvoxamine interaction with warfarin. *Ann Pharmacother* (2002) 36, 1890–2.
18. Bannister SJ, Houser VP, Hulse JD, Kisicki JC, Rasmussen JGC. Evaluation of the potential for interactions of paroxetine with diazepam, cimetidine, warfarin, and digoxin. *Acta Psychiatr Scand* (1989) 80 (Suppl 350), 102–6.
19. Askinazi C. SSRI treatment of depression with comorbid cardiac disease. *Am J Psychiatry* (1996) 153, 135–6.
20. Abad-Santos F, Carcas AJ, Capitán CF, Frias J. Case report. Retroperitoneal haematoma in a patient treated with acenocoumarol, phenytoin and paroxetine. *Clin Lab Haematol* (1995) 17, 195–7.
21. Apseloff G, Wilner KD, Gerber N, Tremaine LM. Effect of sertraline on protein binding of warfarin. *Clin Pharmacokinet* (1997) 32 (Suppl 1), 37–42.
22. Aranth J, Lindberg C. Bleeding, a side effect of fluoxetine. *Am J Psychiatry* (1992) 149, 412.
23. Yaryura-Tobias JA, Kirschen H, Ninan P, Mosberg HJ. Fluoxetine and bleeding in obsessive-compulsive disorder. *Am J Psychiatry* (1991) 148, 949.

Anticoagulants + Statins

The anticoagulant effects of warfarin can be increased by fluvastatin and lovastatin in some patients. Simvastatin normally causes only a small, clinically irrelevant increase in the anticoagulant effects of warfarin. Simvastatin caused more marked effects in one patient on warfarin and another on acenocoumarol. There is an isolated report of rhabdomyolysis in a patient on simvastatin when warfarin was given. Atorvastatin and pravastatin appear not to interact with warfarin, but an isolated case of bleeding has been seen in a patient taking fluindione and pravastatin.

Clinical evidence

(a) Atorvastatin

A study in 12 patients chronically treated with **warfarin** found that the addition of atorvastatin 80 mg daily for 2 weeks caused only a slight fall of about 1.7 seconds in prothrombin times for the first few days.[1]

(b) Fluvastatin

The makers say that *in vitro* protein binding studies found no interaction at therapeutic concentrations, but note that there have been cases of increased prothrombin times in patients on fluvastatin given **coumarin derivatives**.[2]

An anticoagulant clinic study identified 3 patients out of a group of 42 on **warfarin** who, when given fluvastatin 20 mg daily, showed a moderate INR rise (from 3 to 4.8, from 2.18 to 3.54, and from 3.31 to 4.45) over a 5 to 6-week period, necessitating a 10 to 14% reduction in their **warfarin** dosages. No bleeding occurred. One of these subjects experienced another rise in INR, needing a further dosage reduction, when the fluvastatin was increased to 40 mg daily.[3] Another anticoagulant clinic identified 3 patients on **warfarin** who similarly showed this interaction within 1 to 2 weeks of starting fluvastatin 20 mg daily. One of them showed evidence of rectal bleeding. **Warfarin** dosages were reduced to bring their INRs into an acceptable range.[4]

(c) Lovastatin

The prothrombin times of 2 patients on **warfarin** were approximately doubled, from 18 to 24 seconds up to 42 to 48 seconds within 10 to 21 days of starting to take lovastatin 20 mg daily. One developed minor rectal bleeding and the other had haematuria and epistaxes. The problem rapidly resolved when the **warfarin** dosage was reduced from 5 to 2 mg daily.[5] A prothrombin time increase, from 15 to 24 seconds, occurred in another patient on **warfarin** after taking lovastatin 20 mg daily for 2 weeks.[6]

The makers of lovastatin have 10 other reports of bleeding and/or increased prothrombin times in patients on **warfarin** given lovastatin, but no details are given.[7,8] A study in 8 patients on **warfarin** found that lovastatin 40 mg daily for 7 days increased the INR by 17%.[9]

(d) Pravastatin

A woman with atrial fibrillation on **fluindione** and with an INR between 2.5 and 3.5, developed haematuria within 5 days of starting pravastatin 10 mg daily. Her INR had risen to 10.2. Treatment was stopped and her INR then fell to 3.8 within 72 hours.[10]

Ten healthy subjects were given pravastatin 20 mg alone twice daily for three-and-a-half days, **warfarin** 5 mg alone twice daily for 6 days, and then both pravastatin and **warfarin** together for 6 days. The **warfarin** did not alter the pharmacokinetics of pravastatin, nor were the anticoagulant effects or the plasma protein binding of the **warfarin** significantly changed.[11] Pravastatin 20 mg daily for 7 days had no effect on the INRs of 8 patients on **warfarin**.[9] No interaction was seen in another 46 patients on **warfarin** and pravastatin.[12]

(e) Simvastatin

Twenty-three patients anticoagulated with **warfarin** had a mean increase in INR of 0.8 with simvastatin daily 20 or 40 mg. No **warfarin** dose changes were needed and no problems with anticoagulation occurred.[13] The UK makers of *Zocor* (simvastatin)[14] say that simvastatin 20 to 40 mg daily modestly potentiates the effect of **coumarin anticoagulants**, with INRs increased from a baseline of 1.7 to 1.8 and from 2.6 to 3.4 in subjects and patients respectively. A patient on **warfarin** with type III hyperlipoproteinaemia showed no changes in her INR over 20 weeks when treated with simvastatin 20 mg daily.[15] A study in 46 patients on **warfarin** found that when their treatment for hyperlipidaemia was changed from pravastatin to simvastatin, no important **warfarin** dosage changes were needed and no unusual bleeding was seen.[12]

In contrast a single very brief case report notes a raised INR in one patient given simvastatin and **warfarin**.[16] Another single report describes a patient on **acenocoumarol** whose INR rose from a range of 2 to 3.5 up to 9 within 3 weeks of starting to take simvastatin 20 mg daily.[17]

An isolated report[18] describes rhabdomyolysis with acute renal failure in a 82-year-old man on simvastatin 20 mg daily within 7 days of starting warfarin 5 mg daily; his INR was raised to 4.3.

Mechanism

Unknown. The cytochrome P450 isoenzyme CYP2C9 is of the most important isoenzyme in the metabolism of warfarin, although CYP1A2 and CYP3A4 do have some relevance.[19] Fluvastatin is also primarily metabolised by CYP2C9, but it appears that this statin interacts with warfarin only occasionally. It may be that because warfarin has multiple routes of metabolism that other isoenzymes can 'pick up' warfarin metabolism if competition for metabolism occurs. Interactions may therefore only occur if other confounding factors are present. See 'Lipid-regulating drugs' (p.827) for a further discussion on the metabolism of statins.

Importance and management

The clinical evidence is that only some patients can develop this interaction, particularly those on fluvastatin, or lovastatin, and possibly those on simvastatin. It has been suggested that, in order to identify these individuals, it would be prudent to monitor the early stages of concurrent use in all patients, or if the dosage of statin is changed, being alert for the need to adjust the anticoagulant dosage. The makers of **rosuvastatin**[20] also recommend monitoring if they are used concurrently with warfarin. However, this interaction has only been clinically significant in a handful of patients, so monitoring every patient may be over-cautious. Information about anticoagulants other than acenocoumarol and warfarin is generally lacking.

1. Stern R, Abel R, Gibson GL, Besserer J. Atorvastatin does not alter the anticoagulant activity of warfarin. *J Clin Pharmacol* (1997) 37, 1062–4.
2. Lescol (Fluvastatin). Novartis Pharmaceuticals UK Ltd. UK Summary of product characteristics, December 2000.
3. Trilli LE, Kelley CL, Aspinall SL, Kroner BA. Potential interaction between warfarin and fluvastatin. *Ann Pharmacother* (1996) 30, 1399–1402.
4. Kline SS, Harrell C. Potential warfarin-fluvastatin interaction. *Ann Pharmacother* (1997) 31, 790.
5. Ahmad S. Lovastatin. Warfarin interaction. *Arch Intern Med* (1990) 150, 2407.
6. Hoffman HS. The interaction of lovastatin and warfarin. *Conn Med* (1992) 56, 107.
7. Tobert JA, Shear CL, Chremos AN, Mantell GE. Clinical experience with lovastatin. *Am J Cardiol* (1990) 65, 23F–26F.
8. Tobert JA. Efficacy and long-term adverse effect pattern of lovastatin. *Am J Cardiol* (1988) 62, 28J–34J.
9. O'Rangers EA, Ford M, Hershey A. The effect of HMG-coA reductase inhibitors on the anticoagulant response to warfarin. *Pharmacotherapy* (1994) 14, 349.
10. Trenque T, Choisy H, Germain M-L. Pravastatin: interaction with oral anticoagulant? *BMJ* (1996) 312, 886.
11. Light RT, Pan HY, Glaess SR, Bakry D (ER Squibb). A report on the pharmacokinetic and pharmacodynamic interaction of pravastatin and warfarin in healthy male volunteers. Data on file, (Protocol No 27, 201-59), 1988.
12. Lin JC, Ito MK, Stolley SN, Morreale AP, Marcus DB. The effect of converting from pravastatin to simvastatin on the pharmacodynamics of warfarin. *J Clin Pharmacol* (1999) 39, 86–90.
13. Keech A, Collins R, MacMahon S, Armitage J, Lawson A, Wallendszus K, Fatemian M, Kearney E, Lyon V, Mindell J, Mount J, Painter R, Parish S, Slavin B, Sleight P, Youngman L, Peto R. Three-year follow-up of the Oxford cholesterol study: assessment of the efficacy and safety of simvastatin in preparation for a large mortality study. *Eur Heart J* (1994) 15, 255–69.
14. Zocor (Simvastatin). Merck Sharp & Dohme Ltd. UK Summary of product characteristics, July 2004.
15. Gaw A, Wosornu D. Simvastatin during warfarin therapy in hyperlipoproteinaemia. *Lancet* (1992) 340, 979–80.
16. Beeley L, Cunningham H, Carmichael AE, Brennan A. Bulletin of the West Midlands Centre for Adverse Drug Reaction Reporting, July 1991, p 19.
17. Grau E, Perella M, Pastor E. Simvastatin-oral anticoagulant interaction. *Lancet* (1996) 347, 405–6.
18. Mogyorósi A, Bradley B, Showalter A, Schubert ML. Rhabdomyolysis and acute renal failure due to combination therapy with simvastatin and warfarin. *J Intern Med* (1999) 246, 599–602.
19. Shek KLA, Chan L-N, Nutescu E. Warfarin-acetaminophen drug interaction revisited. *Pharmacotherapy* (1999) 19, 1153–8.
20. Crestor (Rosuvastatin calcium). AstraZeneca UK Ltd. UK Summary of product characteristics, February 2005.

Anticoagulants + Sucralfate

Four case reports describe a marked reduction in the effects of warfarin in four patients given sucralfate. Other evidence suggests that this interaction is uncommon.

Clinical evidence

A man on multiple therapy (digoxin, furosemide, chlorpropamide, potassium chloride) had serum **warfarin** levels that were about two-thirds lower when he was given sucralfate. When the sucralfate was withdrawn, his serum **warfarin** levels rose to their former levels accompanied by a prolongation of prothrombin times.[1] Another patient's prothrombin times remained subtherapeutic in the presence of sucralfate, despite **warfarin** doses of up to 17.5 mg daily. When the sucralfate was stopped his prothrombin time rose to 1.5 times the control, even though the **warfarin** dose was reduced to 10 mg daily.[2] Two other patients showed reduced responses to **warfarin** while taking sucralfate.[3,4]

In contrast, an open crossover study in 8 elderly patients taking **warfarin** found that their anticoagulant response and serum **warfarin** levels remained unchanged while taking sucralfate 1 g three times a day over a 2-week period.[5] No interaction was found between **warfarin** and sucralfate in another study.[6]

Mechanism

Unknown. It is suggested that the sucralfate may possibly adsorb the warfarin so that its bioavailability is reduced.[2]

Importance and management

The documentation appears to be limited to the reports cited. Any interaction would therefore seem to be uncommon. Concurrent use need not be avoided but bear this interaction in mind if a patient has a reduced anticoagulant response to warfarin. Information about other anticoagulants is lacking, but it would seem prudent to take the same precautions. Ranitidine and other H_2-blockers apart from cimetidine may be useful alternatives in some cases (see 'Anticoagulants + H_2-blockers', p.283).

1. Mungall D, Talbert RL, Phillips C, Jaffe D, Ludden TM. Sucralfate and warfarin. *Ann Intern Med* (1983) 98, 557.
2. Braverman SE, Marino MT. Sucralfate-warfarin interaction. *Drug Intell Clin Pharm* (1988) 22, 913.
3. Rey AM, Gums JG. Altered absorption of digoxin, sustained-release quinidine, and warfarin with sucralfate absorption. *DICP Ann Pharmacother* (1991) 25, 745–6.
4. Parrish RH, Waller B, Gondalia BG. Sucralfate-warfarin interaction. *Ann Pharmacother* (1992) 26, 1015–16.
5. Neuvonen PJ, Jaakkola A, Tötterman J, Penttilä O. Clinically significant sucralfate-warfarin interaction is not likely. *Br J Clin Pharmacol* (1985) 20, 178–80.
6. Talbert RL, Dalmady-Israel C, Bussey HI, Crawford MH, Ludden TM. Effect of sucralfate on plasma warfarin concentration in patients requiring chronic warfarin therapy. *Drug Intell Clin Pharm* (1985) 19, 456–7.

Anticoagulants + Sucrose polyesters

Sucrose polyesters (*Olestra, Olean*) do not interact with warfarin.

Clinical evidence, mechanism, importance and management

A randomised, double-blind, placebo-controlled study in 40 patients found that sucrose polyester 12 g daily for 2 weeks had no significant effect on the anticoagulant effects of **warfarin**. The sucrose polyester was contained in *Pringles Original Flavor Fat Free Potato Crisps with Olean* and the patients took 1.5 servings daily.[1] Sucrose polyesters, are non-absorbable, non-calorific fat replacements. It has been concluded that sucrose polyesters are unlikely to reduce the absorption of oral drugs in general.[2]

1. Beckey NP, Korman LB, Parra D. Effect of the moderate consumption of olestra in patients receiving long-term warfarin therapy. *Pharmacotherapy* (1999) 19, 1075–9.
2. Goldman P. Olestra: assessing its potential to interact with drugs in the gastrointestinal tract. *Clin Pharmacol Ther* (1997) 61, 613–18.

Anticoagulants + Sulfasalazine

An isolated case report describes a marked reduction in the response to warfarin when sulfasalazine was started.

Clinical evidence, mechanism, importance and management

A 37-year-old woman on long-term **warfarin** 30 mg weekly (and also taking beclometasone, salbutamol, aspirin, azathioprine, ethinyloestradiol/norgestrel) had her treatment for arthritis and ulcerative colitis changed from 5-aminosalicylic acid to sulfasalazine 1 g four times daily. The day after the change her INR was found to be subtherapeutic (1.5 compared with the usual 2 to 3) and she needed numerous increases in the **warfarin** doses over the next 6 weeks, eventually needing **warfarin** 75 mg weekly before acceptable INRs were achieved. During this period she developed a new deep vein thrombosis. When the sulfasalazine was later stopped and the 5-aminosalicylate restarted, her **warfarin** dosage requirements dropped to 45 mg weekly.[1]

This is an unexplained and isolated case, and its validity has been debated.[2,3] There are no other reports in the literature and this possible interaction seems unlikely to be of general importance. Nevertheless prescribers should be aware of it if sulfasalazine is added to **warfarin** treatment. Information about other oral anticoagulants is lacking. See also 'Anticoagulants + Mesalazine (Mesalamine)', p.292.

1. Teefy AM, Martin JE, Kovacs MJ. Warfarin resistance due to sulfasalazine. *Ann Pharmacother* (2000) 34, 1265–8.
2. Sherman JJ. Comment: other factors should be considered in a possible warfarin and sulfasalazine interaction. *Ann Pharmacother* (2001) 35, 506.
3. Kovacs MJ, Teefy AM. Comment: other factors should be considered in a possible warfarin and sulfasalazine interaction. Author's reply. *Ann Pharmacother* (2001) 35, 506.

Anticoagulants + Sulfinpyrazone

The anticoagulant effects of warfarin and acenocoumarol are markedly increased by sulfinpyrazone and serious bleeding has occurred. Phenprocoumon does not interact significantly.

Clinical evidence

The prothrombin ratios of 5 patients on **warfarin** rose rapidly over 2 to 3 days after sulfinpyrazone 200 mg every 6 hours was added. The average **warfarin** requirements fell by 46% and 2 patients needed vitamin K to combat the excessive hypoprothrombinaemia. When the sulfinpyrazone was withdrawn, the **warfarin** requirements returned to their former levels within 1 to 2 weeks.[1]

This interaction has been described in numerous studies and case reports in those taking **warfarin**[2-11] and **acenocoumarol**.[12] Severe bleeding occurred in some instances. An increased anticoagulant effect of **warfarin** followed by an unexplained reduced effect has been described in one report.[6] In a trial using **acenocoumarol** it was found possible to reduce the anticoagulant dosage by an average of 20% while taking sulfinpyrazone 800 mg daily.[12] **Phenprocoumon** is reported not to interact.[13,14]

Mechanism

Some early *in vitro* evidence[15] suggested that plasma protein binding displacement might explain this interaction, but more recent clinical studies[1,16-18] indicate that sulfinpyrazone also inhibits the metabolism of the anticoagulants (the more potent *(S)*-isomer in the case of warfarin) so that the anticoagulant is cleared from the body more slowly and its effects are increased and prolonged.

Importance and management

A well established interaction of clinical importance. If sulfinpyrazone is added, the prothrombin time should be well monitored and suitable anticoagulant dosage reductions made. Halving the dosage of warfarin[1,11,19] and reducing the acenocoumarol dosage by one-fifth[12] has proven to be adequate in patients taking sulfinpyrazone 600 to 800 mg daily. Phenprocoumon is reported not to interact. It has been recommended that because of the difficulties of monitoring this interaction and of making the necessary dosage adjustments, concurrent use should not be undertaken unless the patient is hospitalised.[3]

1. Miners JO, Foenander T, Wanwimolruk S, Gallus AS, Birkett DJ. Interaction of sulphinpyrazone with warfarin. *Eur J Clin Pharmacol* (1982) 22, 327–31.
2. Weiss M. Potentiation of coumarin effect by sulfinpyrazone. *Lancet* (1979) i, 609.
3. Mattingly D, Bradley M, Selley PJ. Hazards of sulphinpyrazone. *BMJ* (1978) 2, 1786–9.
4. Davis JW, Johns LE. Possible interaction of sulfinpyrazone with coumarins. *N Engl J Med* (1978) 299, 955.
5. Bailey RR, Reddy J. Potentiation of warfarin action by sulphinpyrazone. *Lancet* (1980) i, 254.
6. Nenci GG, Agnelli G, Berrettini M. Biphasic sulphinpyrazone-warfarin interaction. *BMJ* (1981) 282, 1361–2.
7. Gallus A, Birkett D. Sulphinpyrazone and warfarin: a probable drug interaction. *Lancet* (1980) i, 535–6.
8. Jamil A, Reid JM, Messer M. Interaction between sulphinpyrazone and warfarin. *Chest* (1981) 79, 375.
9. Girolami A, Schivazappa L, Fabris F, Randi ML. Biphasic sulphinpyrazone-warfarin interaction. *BMJ* (1981) 283, 1338.
10. Thompson PL, Serjeant C. Potentially serious interaction of warfarin with sulphinpyrazone. *Med J Aust* (1981) 1, 41.
11. Girolami A, Fabris F, Casonato A, Randi ML. Potentiation of anticoagulant response to warfarin by sulphinpyrazone: a double-blind study in patients with prosthetic heart valves. *Clin Lab Haematol* (1982) 4, 23–6.
12. Michot F, Holt NF, Fontanilles F. Über die Beeinflussung der gerinnungshemmenden Wirkung von Acenocoumarol durch Sulfinpyrazon. *Schweiz Med Wochenschr* (1981) 111, 255–60.
13. O'Reilly RA. Phenylbutazone and sulphinpyrazone interaction with oral anticoagulant phenprocoumon. *Arch Intern Med* (1982) 142, 1634–7.
14. Heimark LD, Toon S, Gibaldi M, Trager WF, O'Reilly RA, Goulart DA. The effect of sulfinpyrazone on the disposition of pseudoracemic phenprocoumon in humans. *Clin Pharmacol Ther* (1987) 42, 312–19.
15. Seiler K, Duckert F. Properties of 3-(1-phenyl-propyl)-4-oxycoumarin (Marcoumar®) in the plasma when tested in normal cases and under the influence of drugs. *Thromb Diath Haemorrh* (1968) 19, 389–96.
16. O'Reilly RA, Goulart DA. Comparative interaction of sulfinpyrazone and phenylbutazone with racemic warfarin: alteration *in vivo* of free fraction of plasma albumin. *J Pharmacol Exp Ther* (1981) 219, 691–4.
17. O'Reilly RA. Stereoselective interaction of sulfinpyrazone with racemic warfarin and its separated enantiomorphs in man. *Circulation* (1982) 65, 202–7.
18. Toon S, Low LK, Gibaldi M, Trager WF, O'Reilly RA, Motley CH, Goulart DA. The warfarin-sulfinpyrazone interaction: stereochemical considerations. *Clin Pharmacol Ther* (1986) 39, 15–24.
19. Tulloch JA, Marr TCK. Sulphinpyrazone and warfarin after myocardial infarction. *BMJ* (1979) ii, 133.

Anticoagulants + Sulfonamides

The anticoagulant effects of warfarin, acenocoumarol, and phenprocoumon are increased by co-trimoxazole (sulfamethoxazole with trimethoprim). Bleeding may occur if the anticoagulant dosage is not reduced appropriately. Phenindione does not interact

with co-trimoxazole. There is also evidence that sulfaphenazole, sulfafurazole and sulfamethizole may interact like co-trimoxazole.

Clinical evidence

(a) Co-trimoxazole (Sulfamethoxazole with trimethoprim)

Six out of 20 patients taking **warfarin** showed an increase in their prothrombin ratios within 2 to 6 days of starting to take two tablets of co-trimoxazole 960 mg twice daily.[1] One patient bled and needed to be given vitamin K. The **warfarin** was temporarily withdrawn from 2 patients and the dosage was reduced in one patient to control excessive hypoprothrombinaemia.[1]

An increase in the effects of **warfarin** caused by co-trimoxazole has been described in numerous other reports.[2-17] In some cases bleeding occurred. A population based cohort study[18] in patients treated with **acenocoumarol** or **phenprocoumon** found that co-trimoxazole was associated with an increased risk of over-anticoagulation (INR greater than or equal to 6); the adjusted relative risk of over anticoagulation was noted to be 20.1, and the greatest risk was after 4 days of concurrent use. **Phenindione** is reported not to interact.[19]

(b) Sulfafurazole (Sulfisoxazole)

A man taking digitalis, diuretics, antacids and **warfarin** was later started on sulfafurazole 500 mg six-hourly. After 9 days his prothrombin time had risen from 20 to 28 seconds, and after 14 days he bled (haematuria, haemoptysis, gum bleeding). His prothrombin time had risen to 60 seconds.[20]

Two other patients bled and demonstrated prolonged prothrombin times when given **warfarin** and sulfafurazole.[21]

(c) Sulfamethizole

The half-life of **warfarin** was increased by over 40% (from 65 to 93 hours) in 2 patients after taking sulfamethizole 1 g four times daily for a week.[22]

(d) Sulfaphenazole

Sixteen patients given single oral doses of **phenindione** and sulfaphenazole 500 mg had prothrombin time increases after 24 hours of 16.8 seconds compared with 10.3 seconds in 12 other patients who took **phenindione** alone.[23]

Mechanism

Not fully understood. Plasma protein binding displacement can occur,[24,25] but on its own it does not provide an adequate explanation. It may be relevant in the elderly, in whom plasma protein binding decreases.[18] Sulfonamides can drastically reduce the intestinal bacterial synthesis of vitamin K, but this is not normally an essential source of the vitamin unless dietary sources are exceptionally low.[26]

Evidence suggesting that the metabolism of the anticoagulants is decreased appears not to be fully established.[22] Sulfamethoxazole and acenocoumarol are both metabolised by the CYP2C9 P450 isoenzyme,[18] and has been shown that co-trimoxazole largely affects the metabolism of the more potent (*S*)-warfarin.[13]

Importance and management

The interaction between co-trimoxazole and anticoagulants is well documented and well established. The incidence appears to be high. If bleeding is to be avoided the INR should be well monitored and the warfarin, acenocoumarol, or phenprocoumon dosage should be reduced. Phenindione is said not to interact.

The other interactions are poorly documented. However, it would seem prudent to follow the precautions suggested for co-trimoxazole if any sulfonamide is given with an oral anticoagulant.

1. Hassall C, Feetam CL, Leach RH, Meynell MJ. Potentiation of warfarin by co-trimoxazole. *Lancet* (1975) ii, 1155–6.
2. Barnett DB, Hancock BW. Anticoagulant resistance: an unusual case. *BMJ* (1975) 1, 608–9.
3. O'Reilly RA, Motley CH. Racemic warfarin and trimethoprim-sulfamethoxazole interaction in humans. *Ann Intern Med* (1979) 91, 34–6.
4. Hassal C, Feetam CL, Leach RH, Meynell MJ. Potentiation of warfarin by co-trimoxazole. *BMJ* (1975) 2, 684.
5. Tilstone WJ, Gray JMB, Nimmo-Smith RH, Lawson DH. Interaction between warfarin and sulphamethoxazole. *Postgrad Med J* (1977) 53, 388–90.
6. Kaufman JM, Fauver HE. Potentiation of warfarin by trimethoprim-sulfamethoxazole. *Urology* (1980) 16, 601–3.
7. Beeley L, Ballantine N, Beadle F. *Bulletin of the West Midlands Centre for Adverse Drug Reaction Reporting* (1983) 16, 7.
8. McQueen EG. New Zealand Committee on Adverse Drug Reactions. 17th Annual Report 1982. *N Z Med J* (1983) 96, 95–9.
9. Greenlaw CW. Drug interaction between co-trimoxazole and warfarin. *Am J Hosp Pharm* (1979) 36, 1155.
10. Errick JK, Keys PW. Co-trimoxazole and warfarin: case report of an interaction. *Am J Hosp Pharm* (1979) 35, 1399–1401.
11. O'Donnell D. Antibiotic-induced potentiation of oral anticoagulant agents. *Med J Aust* (1989) 150, 163–4.
12. Keys PW. Drug interaction between co-trimoxazole and warfarin. *Am J Hosp Pharm* (1979) 36, 1155–6.
13. O'Reilly RA. Stereoselective interaction of trimethoprim-sulfamethoxazole with the separated enantiomorphs of racemic warfarin in man. *N Engl J Med* (1980) 302, 33–5.
14. Wolf R, Elman M, Brenner S. Sulfonamide-induced bullous hemorrhagic eruption in a patient with low prothrombin time. *Isr J Med Sci* (1992) 28, 882–4.
15. Erichsen C, Sndenaa K, Sreide JA, Andersen E, Tysvœr A. Spontaneous liver hematomas induced by anti-coagulation therapy. A case report and review of the literature. *Hepatogastroenterology* (1993) 40, 402–6.
16. Cook DE, Ponte CD. Suspected trimethoprim/sulfamethoxazole-induced hypoprothrombinemia. *J Fam Pract* (1994) 39, 589–91.
17. Chafin CC, Ritter BA, James A, Self TH. Hospital admission due to warfarin potentiation by TMP-SMX. *Nurse Pract* (2000) 25, 73–75.
18. Visser LE, Penning-van Beest FJA, Kasbergen AAH, De Smet PAGM, Vulto AG, Hofman A, Stricker BHC. Overanticoagulation associated with combined use of antibacterial drugs and acenocoumarol or phenprocoumon anticoagulants. *Thromb Haemost* (2002) 88, 705–10.
19. De Swiet J. Potentiation of warfarin by co-trimoxazole. *BMJ* (1975) 3, 491.
20. Self TH, Evans W, Ferguson T. Interaction of sulfisoxazole and warfarin. *Circulation* (1975) 52, 528.
21. Sioris LJ, Weibert RT, Pentel PR. Potentiation of warfarin anticoagulation by sulfisoxazole. *Arch Intern Med* (1980) 140, 546–7.
22. Lumholtz B, Siersbaek-Nielsen K, Skovsted L, Kampmann J, Hansen JM. Sulphamethizole-induced inhibition of diphenylhydantoin, tolbutamide and warfarin metabolism. *Clin Pharmacol Ther* (1975) 17, 731.
23. Varma DR, Gupta RK, Gupta S, Sharma KK. Prothrombin response to phenindione during hypoalbuminaemia. *Br J Clin Pharmacol* (1975) 2, 467–8.
24. Seiler K, Duckert F. Properties of 3-(1-phenyl-propyl)-4-oxycoumarin (Marcoumar®) in the plasma when tested in normal cases and under the influence of drugs. *Thromb Diath Haemorrh* (1968) 19, 389–96.
25. Solomon HM, Schrogie JJ. The effect of various drugs on the binding of warfarin-^{14}C to human albumin. *Biochem Pharmacol* (1967) 16, 1219–26.
26. Udall JA. Human sources and absorption of vitamin K in relation to anticoagulation stability. *JAMA* (1965) 194, 107–9.

Anticoagulants + Tamoxifen or Toremifene

The anticoagulant effects of acenocoumarol and warfarin are markedly increased by tamoxifen and bleeding has been seen. Toremifene may interact similarly.

Clinical evidence

(a) Tamoxifen

A woman on **warfarin** needed a dosage reduction from 5 to 1 mg daily to keep her prothrombin time within the range of 20 to 25 seconds when given tamoxifen 40 mg daily. A retrospective study of the records of 5 other patients on tamoxifen revealed that 2 had shown marked increases in prothrombin times, and bleeding, shortly after starting **warfarin**. The other 3 needed **warfarin** doses that were about one-third of those taken by other patients not on tamoxifen.[1]

This confirms the first report of this interaction in a woman on **warfarin** who developed haematemesis, abdominal pain and haematuria 6 weeks after starting tamoxifen 10 mg twice daily. Her prothrombin time had risen from 39 to 206 seconds. She was restabilised on a little over half the **warfarin** dosage while continuing to take the tamoxifen.[2] The Aberdeen Hospitals Drug File has on record 22 patients given both drugs. Of these, 17 had no problems, but 2 developed grossly elevated British Comparative Ratios and 3 haemorrhaged.[3] The makers of tamoxifen have another report of this interaction on their files.[2] A woman on **acenocoumarol** died after a massive brain haemorrhage about 3 weeks after starting to take tamoxifen 20 mg daily.[4]

(b) Toremifene

The makers of toremifene warn about the possibility of increased bleeding if it is given with **warfarin**-type anticoagulants, because it is known that other anti-oestrogens (e.g. tamoxifen) have shown this interaction. However, as yet, there is no direct clinical evidence that an interaction occurs.[5,6]

Mechanism

Uncertain. It seems possible that these drugs compete for the same metabolising systems in the liver, the result being that the loss of the anticoagulant is reduced and its effects are increased and prolonged.

Importance and management

An established and clinically important interaction, which apparently affects some but not all patients. Monitor the effects closely if tamoxifen is added to treatment with warfarin or acenocoumarol and reduce the dosage as necessary. The reports cited here indicate a reduction of between one-half to two-thirds for warfarin but some patients may need much larger reductions. The dosage reduction needed for acenocoumarol is not known. The dosage will need to be increased if the tamoxifen is later withdrawn. The authors of one of the reports[1] postulate that the anti-tumour effects of the tamoxifen may also possibly be reduced. This needs further study. The effect of tamoxifen on other anticoagulants is uncertain but be alert for the same interaction to occur.

1. Tenni P, Lalich DL, Byrne MJ. Life threatening interaction between tamoxifen and warfarin. *BMJ* (1989) 298, 93.
2. Lodwick R, McConkey B, Brown AM, Beeley L. Life threatening interaction between tamoxifen and warfarin. *BMJ* (1987) 295, 1141.
3. Ritchie LD, Grant SMT. Tamoxifen-warfarin interaction: the Aberdeen hospitals drug file. *BMJ* (1989) 298, 1253.
4. Gustovic P, Baldin B, Tricoire MJ, Chichmanian RM. Interaction tamoxifène-acénocoumarol. Une interaction potentiellement dangereuse. *Therapie* (1994) 49, 55–6.
5. Fareston (Toremifene). Orion Pharma UK Ltd. UK Summary of product characteristics, May 2001.
6. Orion Pharma UK Ltd. Personal communication, August 1996.

Anticoagulants + Teicoplanin

An isolated case report describes a marked reduction in the effects of warfarin, which was attributed to teicoplanin.

Clinical evidence, mechanism, importance and management

A 60-year-old woman on digoxin, furosemide and **warfarin** (INR 3.5 to 5) developed a fever after mitral valve replacement surgery and was given rifampicin 450 mg twice daily and teicoplanin 400 mg twice daily. Within 3 days her INR began to fall and by day 6 the anticoagulant effect was completely lost. Despite progressive **warfarin** increases to 10, 15 and 20 mg daily, her INR stayed between 1.2 and 1.6, even when the rifampicin was stopped, and remained low for a further 20 days at which point the teicoplanin was also stopped.[1]

Some of this resistance to **warfarin** was undoubtedly due to the rifampicin (a known and potent inducer of **warfarin** metabolism) but as the INRs remained depressed for a further 20 days after rifampicin was withdrawn the authors suggest that the teicoplanin had its own part to play. However, rifampicin has been shown is several cases to have effects on warfarin for 3 or more weeks after its withdrawal (see 'Anticoagulants + Rifamycins' p.311), so an interaction with teicoplanin would seem doubtful.

1. Agosta FG, Liberato NL, Chiofalo F. Warfarin resistance induced by teicoplanin. *Haematologica* (1997) 82, 637–40.

Anticoagulants + Terbinafine

Terbinafine does not normally interact with warfarin, but two isolated case describe reduced and increased anticoagulation respectively.

Clinical evidence

A randomised, double-blind, placebo-controlled study in 16 healthy subjects, given terbinafine 250 mg or a placebo daily for 14 days, found that the pharmacokinetics and anticoagulant effects of a single 30-mg oral dose of **warfarin** given on day 8 remained unchanged.[1] A large scale post-marketing surveillance study involving 9879 patients treated with terbinafine identified a total of 26 who had also been given **warfarin**.[2] Only 4 showed any adverse effects, none of which suggested an interaction with terfenadine.[3] Other *in vivo* and *in vitro* studies (see 'Mechanism') provide further evidence that no interaction would be expected.[4,5]

In contrast, an isolated report describes a 68-year-old woman on long term **warfarin** treatment whose INR fell from 2.1 to 1.1 within a month of starting a 3-month course of treatment with terbinafine 250 mg daily for tinea unguium. It was necessary to raise her **warfarin** dosage from 5.5 mg daily to a range of 7.5 to 8 mg daily while taking the terbinafine, and to reduce it stepwise to 5.5 mg over the 4 weeks after the terbinafine was stopped.[6] Another isolated case report describes and elderly woman on **warfarin** and cimetidine who developed gastrointestinal bleeding about a month after starting to take terbinafine.[7]

Mechanism

Normally none. *In vivo* studies with antipyrine show that terbinafine has little or no effect as an enzyme inducer, and this is confirmed by *in vitro* studies using human liver microsomes.[4,5] The isolated cases are not understood.

Importance and management

Normally no interaction occurs between warfarin and terbinafine, while the two isolated cases cited are rarities, and unexplained. There appears therefore to be no reason for avoiding concurrent use, but bear these cases in mind if terbinafine is given to patients on warfarin. Information about other anticoagulants is lacking.

1. Guerret M, Francheteau P, Hubert M. Evaluation of effects of terbinafine on single oral dose pharmacokinetics and anticoagulant actions of warfarin in healthy volunteers. *Pharmacotherapy* (1997) 17, 767–73.
2. O'Sullivan DP, Needham CA, Bangs A, Atkin K, Kendall FD. Postmarketing surveillance of oral terbinafine in the UK; report of a large cohort study. *Br J Pharmacol* (1996) 42, 559–65.
3. Novartis. Personal communication, February 1998.
4. Back DJ, Tjia JF. Comparative effects of the antimycotic drugs ketoconazole, fluconazole, itraconazole and terbinafine on the metabolism of cyclosporin by human liver microsomes. *Br J Clin Pharmacol* (1991) 32, 624–6.
5. Seyffer R, Eichelbaum M, Jensen JC, Klotz U. Antipyrine metabolism is not affected by terbinafine, a new antifungal agent. *Eur J Clin Pharmacol* (1989) 37, 3231–3.
6. Warwick JA, Corrall RJ. Serious interaction between warfarin and oral terbinafine. *BMJ* (1998) 316, 440.
7. Gupta AK, Ross GS. Interaction between terbinafine and warfarin. *Dermatology* (1998) 196, 266–7.

Anticoagulants + Tetracyclic or Tricyclic antidepressants

Amitriptyline and possibly other tricyclics can cause unpredictable increases or decreases in prothrombin times which can make stable anticoagulation difficult. Maprotiline and mianserin do not usually interact, but isolated cases have been reported with both mianserin and lofepramine.

Clinical evidence

A study[1,2] in 6 healthy subjects given **nortriptyline** 200 micrograms/kg three times daily for 8 days indicated that the mean half-life of **dicoumarol** was increased from 35 to 106 hours. A later study similarly found that **amitriptyline** 40 mg daily and **nortriptyline** 25 mg every 8 hours significantly decreased the half-life of **dicoumarol** but failed to find a consistent effect.[3] A similar study in healthy subjects found that neither **amitriptyline** nor **nortriptyline** affected the plasma half-life of **warfarin**.[3]

Three reports have noted that the control of anticoagulation may be more difficult in patients taking **amitriptyline** and other tricyclic antidepressants.[4-6] One of them found that **amitriptyline** caused unpredictable and 'massive fluctuations' in prothrombin times (increases and decreases) in 7 patients given **phenprocoumon**, which made it difficult to establish stable anticoagulation when compared with 7 other patients not taking amitriptyline.[7]

Another very brief report suggests the possibility of increased **warfarin** effects in a patient given **lofepramine**.[8]

The anticoagulant effects of **acenocoumarol** in 20 patients was shown to be unaffected by **maprotiline** 50 mg three times daily,[9] and in 60 patients the effects of **phenprocoumon** were not affected by **mianserin** 30 to 60 mg daily.[10] A single case report describes a man on **warfarin** whose prothrombin time rose from 20 to 25 seconds after taking **mian_serin** 10 mg daily for 7 days.[11] However, a man on **acenocoumarol** and amiodarone needed an increase in his **acenocoumarol** dosage when given **mianserin**.[12]

Mechanism

Not understood. One suggestion is that the tricyclic antidepressants inhibit the metabolism of the anticoagulant (seen in *animals* with nortriptyline or amitriptyline and warfarin,[13] but not with desipramine and acenocoumarol[14]). Another idea is that the tricyclics slow gastrointestinal motility thereby increasing the time available for the dissolution and absorption of dicoumarol.

Importance and management

Information about interactions between anticoagulants and tricyclic antidepressant is limited, patchy and inconclusive, but some difficulty in maintaining stable anticoagulation seems possible. Maprotiline and mianserin do not usually interact. There is insufficient evidence to recommend that all patients have their INR measured, but it would at least seem prudent to bear this interaction in mind when prescribing anticoagulants and tricyclic or tetracyclic antidepressants.

1. Vesell ES, Passananti GT, Greene FE. Impairment of drug metabolism in man by allopurinol and nortriptyline. *N Engl J Med* (1970) 283, 1484–8.
2. Vesell ES, Passananti GT, Aurori KC. Anomalous results of studies on drug interaction in man. *Pharmacology* (1975) 13, 101–111.
3. Pond SM, Graham GG, Birkett DJ, Wade DN. Effects of tricyclic antidepressants on drug metabolism. *Clin Pharmacol Ther* (1975) 18, 191–9.
4. Koch-Weser J. Hemorrhagic reactions and drug interactions in 500 warfarin-treated patients. *Clin Pharmacol Ther* (1973) 14, 139.
5. Williams JRB, Griffin JP, Parkins A. Effect of concomitantly administered drugs on the control of long term anticoagulant therapy. *Q J Med* (1976) 45, 63.
6. Hampel H, Berger C, Müller-Spahn F. Modified anticoagulant potency in an amitriptyline-treated patient? *Acta Haematol (Basel)* (1996) 96, 178–80.
7. Hampel H, Berger C, Kuss H-J, Müller-Spahn F. Unstable anticoagulation in the course of amitriptyline treatment. *Pharmacopsychiatry* (1996) 29, 33–7.
8. Beeley L, Stewart P, Hickey FM. *Bulletin of the West Midlands Centre for Adverse Drug Reaction Reporting* (1988) 26, 21.
9. Michot F, Glaus K, Jack DB, Theobald W. Antikoagulatorische Wirkung von Sintrom® und Konzentration von Ludiomil® im Blut bei gleichzeitiger Verabreichung beider Präparate. *Med Klin* (1975) 70, 626–9.
10. Kopera H, Schenk H, Stulemeijer S. Phenprocoumon requirement, whole blood coagulation time, bleeding time and plasma γ-GT in patients receiving mianserin. *Eur J Clin Pharmacol* (1978) 13, 351–6.
11. Warwick HMC, Mindham RHS. Concomitant administration of mianserin and warfarin. *Br J Psychiatry* (1983) 143, 308.
12. Baettig D, Tillement J-P, Baumann P. Interaction between mianserin and acenocoumarin: a single case study. *Int J Clin Pharmacol Ther* (1994) 32, 165–7.
13. Loomis CW, Racz WJ. Drug interactions of amitriptyline and nortriptyline with warfarin in the rat. *Res Commun Chem Pathol Pharmacol* (1980) 30, 41–58.
14. Weiner M. Effect of centrally active drugs on the action of coumarin anticoagulants. *Nature* (1966) 212, 1599–1600.

Anticoagulants + Tetracyclines

The effects of the anticoagulants are not usually altered to a clinically relevant extent by treatment with tetracycline antibacterials, but a few patients have shown increases in anticoagulant effect and a handful have bled.

Clinical evidence

(a) Chlortetracycline

Six out of 9 patients on an unnamed anticoagulant had a fall in their prothrombin-proconvertin concentration from a range of 10 to 30% to less than 6% when treated with chlortetracycline 250 mg four times a day for 4 days.[1]

(b) Doxycycline

A woman on **warfarin** developed menorrhagia after taking doxycycline 100 mg twice daily for 10 days.[2] Two patients on **acenocoumarol** or **warfarin** developed markedly increased prothrombin ratios with bruising, haematomas and bleeding when treated with doxycycline.[3] Another patient with multiple medical problems, taking **warfarin** and a range of drugs (alendronate, atorvastatin, salbutamol, diltiazem, fluticasone) developed peritoneal bleeding and an INR of 7.2 (previously 2.6) 6 days after starting doxycycline 100 mg twice daily.[4] In a population-based cohort study in patients on **acenocoumarol** or **phenprocoumon**, doxycycline was found to increase the risk of over-anticoagulation (INR greater than or equal to 6). The risks were greatest after 4 or more days of concurrent use.[5]

(c) Tetracycline

One patient out of 20 on **dicoumarol** bled when given tetracycline.[6] A patient on **warfarin** showed a marked increase in INR (from about 2 to 7.7) 6 weeks after starting to take tetracycline 250 mg four times daily, with INR changes over the following months, which broadly paralleled the decreases in the tetracycline dosage.[7] An increased anticoagulant effect is briefly mentioned in two other reports.[8,9] A patient on **warfarin** bled (right temporal lobe haematoma) and had an extended prothrombin time a week after starting to take tetracycline and nystatin.[10] Another patient on **warfarin** also bled (epistaxis, haematemesis, melaena) 3 weeks after starting to take tetracycline and nystatin.[10] A clinical study in 9 patients on **warfarin** found an estimated 0.53 increase in the INR in the presence of unnamed tetracyclines.[11]

Mechanism

Not understood. Tetracyclines in the absence of anticoagulants can reduce prothrombin activity,[12,13] and both hypoprothrombinaemia and bleeding have been described.[14,15] It seems possible that very occasionally the anticoagulant and the tetracycline have additive hypoprothrombinaemic effects. The idea that antibacterials can diminish the intestinal flora of the gut thereby depleting the body of an essential source of vitamin K has been shown to be incorrect, apart from exceptional cases where normal dietary sources are extremely low.[16,17]

Importance and management

A relatively sparsely documented interaction, bearing in mind that the tetracyclines have been in very wide-spread use for many years. It can therefore reasonably be concluded that normally any changes are of little clinical relevance. As a few patients have unpredictably shown increased anticoagulant effects and even bleeding, bear this interaction in mind when a tetracycline is first added to established anticoagulant treatment.

1. Magid E. Tolerance to anticoagulants during antibiotic therapy. *Scand J Clin Lab Invest* (1962) 14, 565–6.
2. Westfall LK, Mintzer DL, Wiser TH. Potentiation of warfarin by tetracycline. *Am J Hosp Pharm* (1980) 37, 1620, 1625.
3. Caraco Y, Rubinow A. Enhanced anticoagulant effect of coumarin derivatives induced by doxycycline coadministration. *Ann Pharmacother* (1992) 26, 1084–6.
4. Baciewicz AM, Bal BS. Bleeding associated with doxycycline and warfarin treatment. *Arch Intern Med* (2001) 161, 1231.
5. Visser LE, Penning-van Beest FJA, Kasbergen AAH, De Smet PAGM, Vulto AG, Hofman A, Stricker BHC. Overanticoagulation associated with combined use of antibacterial drugs and acenocoumarol or phenprocoumon anticoagulants. *Thromb Haemost* (2002) 88, 705–10.
6. Chiavazza F, Merialdi A. Sulle interferenze fra dicumarolo e antibiotici. *Minerva Ginecol* (1973) 25, 630–1.
7. Danos EA. Apparent potentiation of warfarin activity by tetracycline. *Clin Pharm* (1992) 11, 806–8.
8. Wright IS. The pathogenesis and treatment of thrombosis. *Circulation* (1952) 5, 161–88.
9. Scarrone LA, Beck DF, Wright IS. A comparative evaluation of Tromexan and dicumarol in the treatment of thromboembolic conditions — based on experience with 514 patients. *Circulation* (1952) 6, 489–514.
10. O'Donnell D. Antibiotic-induced potentiation of oral anticoagulant agents. *Med J Aust* (1989) 150, 163–4.
11. Pharmacy Anticoagulant Clinic Study Group. A multicentre survey of antibiotics on the INR of anticoagulated patients. *Pharm J* (1996) 257 (Pharmacy Practice Suppl), R30.
12. Searcy RL, Craig RG, Foreman JA, Bergqvist LM. Blood clotting anomalies associated with intensive tetracycline therapy. *Clin Res* (1964) 12, 230.
13. Searcy RL, Simms NM, Foreman JA, Bergquist LM. Evaluation of the blood-clotting mechanism in tetracycline-treated patients. *Antimicrob Agents Chemother* (1964) 4, 179–83.
14. Rios JF. Hemorrhagic diathesis induced by antimicrobials. *JAMA* (1968) 205, 142.
15. Kippel AP, Pitsinger B. Hypoprothrombinemia secondary to antibiotic therapy and manifested by massive gastrointestinal hemorrhage. *Arch Surg* (1968) 96, 266–8.
16. Udall JA. Human sources and absorption of vitamin K in relation to anticoagulation stability. *JAMA* (1965) 194, 107–9.
17. Pineo GF, Gallus AS, Hirsh J. Unexpected vitamin K deficiency in hospitalized patients. *Can Med Assoc J* (1973) 109, 880–3.

Anticoagulants + Thyroid or Antithyroid compounds

The anticoagulant effects of acenocoumarol, dicoumarol, phenindione, and warfarin are increased by thyroid compounds and bleeding has been seen. A reduction in the anticoagulant effects may be expected if antithyroid compounds are used. This is largely due to alteration of thyroid function, rather than a direct drug-drug interaction.

Clinical evidence

Hypothyroid patients are relatively resistant to the effects of the oral anticoagulants and need larger doses than hyperthyroid patients who are relatively sensitive.[1-5] Drug-induced changes in thyroid status (even in those who are euthyroid but who are taking dextrothyroxine for hypercholesterolaemia) will alter the response to the oral anticoagulants.

(a) Thyroid compounds

A patient with myxoedema required a gradual reduction in his dosage of **phenindione** from 200 to 75 mg daily as his thyroid status was restored by the administration of **liothyronine**.[6] Seven out of 11 euthyroid patients on **warfarin** showed lengthening prothrombin times and needed a weekly dosage reduction of **warfarin** (by 2.5 mg to 30 mg) during the first 4 weeks of treatment with **dextrothyroxine** 4 to 8 mg daily for hypercholesterolaemia. One patient bled.[7] Hypoprothrombinaemia and bleeding have been described in 2 patients on **warfarin** when their **thyroid** replacement therapy was started or increased.[8] Similar responses have been described in other reports and studies involving **warfarin**,[5,9-11] **dicoumarol**[12] or **acenocoumarol**.[6]

(b) Antithyroid compounds

A hyperthyroid patient on **warfarin** showed a marked increase in his prothrombin times on two occasions when his treatment with **thiamazole** was stopped and he became hyperthyroid again.[1]

Mechanism

In hypothyroid patients the catabolism (destruction) of the blood clotting factors (II, VII, IX and X) is low and this tends to cancel, to some extent, the effects of the anticoagulants, which reduce blood clotting factor synthesis. Conversely, in hyperthyroid patients in whom the catabolism is increased, the net result is an increase in the effects of the anticoagulants.[13] It has also been suggested that the thyroid hormones may increase the affinity of the anticoagulants for its receptor sites.[9,14]

Importance and management

A well documented and clinically important interaction occurs if oral anticoagulants and thyroid compounds are taken concurrently.

Hypothyroid patients taking an anticoagulant who are subsequently treated with thyroid hormones as replacement therapy will need a downward adjustment of the anticoagulant dosage as treatment proceeds if excessive hypoprothrombinaemia and bleeding are to be avoided. Some adjustment may be necessary with euthyroid (normal) patients given dextrothyroxine for hypercholesterolaemia. All of the oral anticoagulants may be expected to behave similarly.

As the thyroid status of hyperthyroid patients returns to normal by the use of antithyroid drugs (e.g. **carbimazole**, thiamazole, **propylthiouracil**) an increase in the anticoagulant requirements would be expected. Propylthiouracil in the absence of an anticoagulant has very occasionally been reported to cause hypoprothrombinaemia and bleeding.[15,16]

1. Vagenakis AG, Cote R, Miller ME, Braverman LE, Stohlman F. Enhancement of warfarin-induced hypoprothrombinemia by thyrotoxicosis. *Johns Hopkins Med J* (1972) 131, 69–73.
2. Self TH, Straughn AB, Weisburst MR. Effect of hyperthyroidism on hypoprothrombinemic response to warfarin. *Am J Hosp Pharm* (1976) 33, 387–9.
3. McIntosh TJ, Brunk SF, Kölln I. Increased sensitivity to warfarin in thyrotoxicosis. *J Clin Invest* (1970) 49, 63a–64a.
4. Rice AJ, McIntosh TJ, Fouts JR, Brunk SF, Wilson WR. Decreased sensitivity to warfarin in patients with myxedema. *Am J Med Sci* (1971) 262, 211–15.
5. Chute JP, Dahut WL, Shakir KM, Georgiadis MS, Frame JN. Enhancement of warfarin induced hypoprothrombinemia by hyperthyroidism. *Blood* (1994) 84 (10 Suppl 1), 674a.
6. Walters MB. The relationship between thyroid function and anticoagulant therapy. *Am J Cardiol* (1963) 11, 112–14.
7. Owens JC, Neeley WB, Owen WR. Effect of sodium dextrothyroxine in patients receiving anticoagulants. *N Engl J Med* (1962) 266, 76–9.
8. Hansten PD. Oral anticoagulants and drugs which alter thyroid function. *Drug Intell Clin Pharm* (1980) 14, 331–4.
9. Solomon HM, Schrogie JJ. Change in receptor site affinity: a proposed explanation for the potentiating effect of d-thyroxine on the anticoagulant response to warfarin. *Clin Pharmacol Ther* (1967) 8, 797–9.
10. Winters WL, Soloff LA. Observations on sodium d-thyroxine as a hypocholesterolemic agent in persons with hypercholesterolemia with and without ischemic heart disease. *Am J Med Sci* (1962) 243, 458–69.
11. Costigan DC, Freedman MH, Ehrlich RM. Potentiation of oral anticoagulant effect by L-thyroxine. *Clin Pediatr (Phila)* (1984) 23, 172–4.
12. Jones RJ, Cohen L. Sodium dextro-thyroxine in coronary disease and hypercholesterolemia. *Circulation* (1961) 24, 164–70.
13. Loeliger EA, van der Esch B, Mattern MJ, Hemker HC. The biological disappearance rate of prothrombin, factors VII, IX and X from plasma in hypothyroidism, hyperthyroidism and during fever. *Thromb Diath Haemorrh* (1964) 10, 267–77.
14. Schrogie JJ, Solomon HM. The anticoagulant response to bishydroxycoumarin. II. The effect of d-thyroxine, clofibrate and norethandrolone. *Clin Pharmacol Ther* (1967) 8, 70–7.
15. D'Angelo G, Le Gresley LP. Severe hypoprothrombinæmia after propylthiouracil therapy. *Can Med Assoc J* (1959) 81, 479–81.
16. Gotta AW, Sullivan CA, Seaman J, Jean-Gilles B. Prolonged intraoperative bleeding caused by propylthiouracil-induced hypoprothrombinemia. *Anesthesiology* (1972) 37, 562–3.

Anticoagulants + Tiabendazole

An isolated case report describes a marked increase in the anticoagulant effects of acenocoumarol in a patient given tiabendazole.

Clinical evidence, mechanism, importance and management

An increase in the anticoagulant effects of **acenocoumarol** occurred in a patient with nephrotic syndrome undergoing dialysis, who was given tiabendazole 8 g daily for 3 days.[1] His INR rose from 2.9 to more than 5. The reasons are not understood, nor is the general importance of this interaction known. There seem to be no other reports.

1. Henri P, Mosquet B, Hurault de Ligny B, Lacotte J, Cardinau E, Moulin M, Ryckelinck JP. Imputation d'une hypocoagulabilité à l'interaction tiabendazole-acénocoumarol. *Therapie* (1993) 48, 500–501.

Anticoagulants + Tibolone

On theoretical grounds the makers of tibolone suggest that it may possibly increase the effects of anticoagulants.

Clinical evidence, mechanism, importance and management

A study in 60 post-menopausal women given tibolone 2.5 mg daily or placebo for 12 weeks found no changes in coagulation (prothrombin time, clotting factors VII, VIII, X), but some changes in fibrinolysis (lower fibrinogen levels, higher antithrombin III, plasminogen and fibrin plate fibrinolytic activity values).[1] Because of this increased fibrinolytic activity, the makers say that the sensitivity of patients to anticoagulants may be enhanced during tibolone therapy.[2] There seem to be no studies or case reports about concurrent use, but until more is known it would seem prudent to monitor the effects if tibolone is added to established anticoagulant treatment.

1. Cortes-Prieto J. Coagulation and fibrinolysis in post-menopausal women treated with Org OD 14. *Maturitas* (1987) Suppl 1, 67–72.
2. Livial (Tibolone). Organon Laboratories Ltd. UK Summary of product characteristics, December 2003.

Anticoagulants + Ticlopidine

The anticoagulant effects of acenocoumarol are modestly reduced by ticlopidine, but the anticoagulant effects of warfarin are unchanged. The makers of ticlopidine strongly advise avoiding the concurrent use of other anticoagulants because of the possible increased bleeding risks. There is some evidence that liver damage may occur in a small number of patients given warfarin and ticlopidine.

Clinical evidence

(a) Acenocoumarol

A retrospective study of 36 patients with heart valve prostheses found that when they took ticlopidine 250 mg daily, 29 of them needed a mean 13% increase in acenocoumarol dosage from 15.5 to 17.5 mg weekly, accompanied by a small INR rise from 3.05 to 3.13. One patient needed a dosage increase from 14 to 22 mg weekly. INR changes were detectable with a week of starting the ticlopidine.[1]

(b) Warfarin

Ticlopidine 250 mg twice daily for 2 weeks given to 9 men on long-term warfarin increased the mean *(R)*-warfarin levels by 25.7% but did not change *(S)*-warfarin levels or their INRs.[2] *(R)*-warfarin is the much less active of the two enantiomers.

A Japanese study found evidence that warfarin and ticlopidine together can very occasionally cause cholestatic liver injury and severe jaundice. Four out of 132 patients (3%) given both drugs after cardiovascular surgery demonstrated hepatotoxicity.[3]

Mechanism

Not understood. It seems possible that ticlopidine inhibits the metabolism of *(R)*-warfarin, but just why concurrent use very occasionally causes liver injury is not known. The interaction with acenocoumarol is not understood.

Importance and management

Information seems to be limited to the reports cited. A small to moderate increase in the acenocoumarol dosage may be needed if ticlopidine is added, but none seems to be necessary with warfarin, although it might be prudent to monitor for any evidence of liver damage if both drugs are used. There appears to be no information about other anticoagulants. However, the makers of ticlopidine[4] strongly advise the avoidance of ticlopidine with any anticoagulant because of the increased risk of bleeding (a combination of anticoagulant and platelet anti-aggregant activity). If both drugs are essential the makers recommend monitoring the clinical outcome and aPTT.

1. Salar A, Domenech P, Martínez F. Ticlopidine antagonizes acenocoumarol treatment. *Thromb Haemost* (1997) 77, 223–4.
2. Gidal BE, Sorkness CA, McGill KA, larson R, Levine RR. Evaluation of a potential enantioselective interaction between ticlopidine and warfarin in chronically anticoagulated patients. *Ther Drug Monit* (1995) 27, 33–8.
3. Takase K, Fujioka H, Ogasawara M, Aonuma H, Tameda Y, Nakano T, Kosaka Y. Drug-induced hepatitis during combination therapy of warfarin potassium and ticlopidine hydrochloride. *Mie Med J* (1990) 40, 27–32.
4. Ticlid (Ticlopidine). Sanofi-Synthelabo. UK Summary of product characteristics, May 2000.

Anticoagulants + Tobacco smoking

Tobacco smoking slightly reduces the response to warfarin, but this appears not be clinically relevant in most patients.

Clinical evidence, mechanism, importance and management

When 9 smokers who normally smoked at least one pack daily (size unknown) stopped smoking, they showed a 13% increase in their average steady-state **warfarin** levels, a 13% decrease in **warfarin** clearance and a 23% increase in the **warfarin** half-life but no changes in prothrombin times.[1] An 80-year-old man on **warfarin** had a steady rise in his INR (from a range of 2 to 2.8 up to 3.7) over a 3-month period when he gave up smoking. No bleeding occurred.[2]

These changes appear to occur because some of the components of tobacco smoke act as liver enzyme inducing agents, which cause a small increase in the metabolism of the **warfarin**. When smoking stops, the enzymes are therefore no longer stimulated, the metabolism of the **warfarin** falls slightly and its effects are correspondingly slightly increased. A later retrospective study of 200 patients who had undergone cardiac valve replacement found no statistically significant differences between the **warfarin** dosage requirements of non-smokers, light smokers (20 or less cigarettes daily) or heavy smokers (greater than 20 cigarettes daily).[3]

The overall picture seems to be that smoking (or giving up smoking) only has a slight to moderate effect on the response to **warfarin**, and only the occasional patient will need a small dosage alteration. This should easily be detected in the course of routine INR checks. Information about other anticoagulants seems to be lacking.

1. Bachmann K, Shapiro R, Fulton R, Carroll FT, Sullivan TJ. Smoking and warfarin disposition. *Clin Pharmacol Ther* (1979) 25, 309–15.
2. Colucci VJ. Increase in international normalized ratio associated with smoking cessation. *Ann Pharmacother* (2001) 35, 385–6.
3. Weiner B, Faraci PA, Fayad R, Swanson L. Warfarin dosage following prosthetic valve replacement: effect of smoking history. *Drug Intell Clin Pharm* (1984) 18, 904–6.

Anticoagulants + Tolterodine

Tolterodine does not normally appear to interact with warfarin but two cases of raised INRs have been reported.

Clinical evidence, mechanism, importance and management

The UK makers report that clinical studies have shown that no interactions occur between tolterodine and **warfarin**,[1] and the US makers[2] report that tolterodine 2 mg twice daily for 7 days did not affect the pharmacokinetics of a single 25-mg dose of warfarin given on day 4. However, a report describes two patients on stable doses **warfarin** who showed elevated INRs 2 weeks after tolterodine was started. Their INRs fell again when the tolterodine was stopped.[3] Additional monitoring would seem over-cautious on the basis of these two cases, but bear the interaction in mind in the case of an unexpected response to warfarin. Information about other anticoagulants appears to be lacking.

1. Detrusitol (Tolterodine). Pharmacia Ltd. UK Summary of product characteristics, October 2004.
2. Detrol (Tolterodine). Pharmacia & Upjohn Company. US Prescribing information, July 2003.
3. Colucci VJ, Rivey MP. Tolterodine-warfarin drug interaction. *Ann Pharmacother* (1999) 33, 1173–6.

Anticoagulants + Tramadol

Tramadol has been reported to increase the anticoagulant effects of warfarin and phenprocoumon in a few patients.

Clinical evidence, mechanism, importance and management

A brief report describes 5 elderly patients (ages 71 to 84), anticoagulated with **warfarin** or **phenprocoumon** and on a range of other drugs, who showed clinically important rises in INRs (up to threefold) a few days after starting to take tramadol. One of the patients bled. In some of the cases it was possible to manage the situation by reducing the anticoagulant dosage.[1]

A 61-year old woman with a mitral valve replacement on **warfarin** developed ecchymoses about 2 weeks after starting tramadol 50 mg 6-hourly. Her prothrombin time was found to have risen to 39.6 seconds and her INR was 10.6. These values returned to normal when the tramadol was withdrawn and the **warfarin** temporarily stopped.[2] Another patient on **warfarin** developed a prothrombin time of 27.8 seconds, an INR of 7.31 and some bleeding about 5 weeks after starting tramadol 150 mg daily.[3] Two further patients on **phenprocoumon** developed raised INRs (5 and 8.5 respectively) shortly after starting tramadol 50 to 100 mg four times daily, but this report is complicated by use of paracetamol (acetaminophen) 4 g daily, which can also, rarely, interact with coumarin anticoagulants.[4]

In contrast, the mean INR values of 19 patients anticoagulated with **phenprocoumon** were unchanged when they were given tramadol 50 mg three times daily for a week,[5,6] but one patient had an INR rise from 4 to 7.5, and another from a just under 5 to 6. The reasons for this interaction, when it occurs, are not understood.

These reports clearly show that some patients on anticoagulants may develop clinically important INR rises and even bleeding when given tramadol. The incidence is not known but because the interaction is unpredictable it would now be prudent to consider monitoring prothrombin times in any patient on anticoagulants when tramadol is first added, being alert for the need to reduce the anticoagulant dosage. Information about anticoagulants other than **warfarin** and **phenprocoumon** is lacking. More study is needed.

1. Jensen K. Interaktion mellem tramadol og orale antikoagulantia. *Ugeskr Laeger* (1997) 159, 785–6.
2. Sabbe JR, Sims PJ, Sims MH. Tramadol-warfarin interaction. *Pharmacotherapy* (1998) 18, 871–3.
3. Scher ML, Huntington NH, Vitillo JA. Potential interaction between tramadol and warfarin. *Ann Pharmacother* (1997) 31, 646–7.
4. Madsen H, Rasmussen JM, Brøsen K. Interaction between tramadol and phenprocoumon. *Lancet* (1997) 350, 637.
5. Boeijinga JK, van Meegen E. Pharmacodynamic/-kinetic influence of tramadol on the anticoagulant coumarin derivative phenprocoumon in patients. Data on file, Searle 1997.
6. Boeijinga JK, van Meegen E, van den Ende R, Schook CE, Cohen AF. Is there interaction between tramadol and phenprocoumon? *Lancet* (1997) 350, 1552.

Anticoagulants + Trazodone

A handful of case reports describe a moderate reduction in the anticoagulant effects of warfarin caused by trazodone, whereas one small formal study found no interaction.

Clinical evidence, mechanism, importance and management

A woman needed an increase in her **warfarin** dose, from 6.4 to 7.5 mg, when she was given trazodone 300 mg daily, in order to maintain her prothrombin time at 20 seconds. Her **warfarin** requirements fell when the trazodone was later withdrawn.[1] A retrospective chart review identified 3 other patients whose INRs also fell when trazodone was added to treatment with **warfarin** but no adverse effects were seen. One of the patients needed a 25% increase in the **warfarin** dosage.[2] The reasons for this reaction are not understood. In contrast, 6 anticoagulated patients on **heparin** or **warfarin** or other **coumarin anticoagulants** showed no significant changes in prothrombin times when given trazodone 75 mg daily.[3]

The incidence of this interaction is unknown. All the evidence suggests that it is uncommon but because quite unpredictably the occasional patient may show an interaction, be aware of this interaction in all patients on **warfarin** if trazodone is started or stopped, and adjust the dosage if necessary. The interaction can occur within a few days. Information about other anticoagulants seems to be lacking.

1. Hardy J-L, Sirois A. Reduction of prothrombin and partial thromboplastin times with trazodone. *Can Med Assoc J* (1986) 135, 1372.
2. Small NL, Giamonna KA. Interaction between warfarin and trazodone. *Ann Pharmacother* (2000) 34, 734–6.
3. Cozzolino G, Pazzaglia I, De Gaetano V, Macri M. Clinical investigation on the possible interaction between anti-coagulants and a new psychotropic drug (Trazodone). *Clin Eur* (1972) 11, 593.

Anticoagulants + Trimethoprim

Trimethoprim can cause a small increase in the effects of warfarin, which appears to be of little or no clinical importance.

Clinical evidence, mechanism, importance and management

Some books, charts and reviews of interactions say that trimethoprim interacts with the oral anticoagulants to increase their effects, the implication being that it is clinically important, However, there appears to only one published study of this interaction, which identified 12 patients on **warfarin** who showed a small INR increase of about 0.36 when given trimethoprim, but this was not statistically significant.[1] Nor is It likely to be significant when set in the context of expected fluctuations in the INR. There do not appear to be any other reports, and none describing real clinical problems during concurrent use (except when combined with sulfamethoxazole in 'co-trimoxazole', (p.314)). A literature search undertaken in 1992 by the makers of trimethoprim similarly failed to find any reports of a clinically important interaction between trimethoprim and anticoagulants.[2] This relative silence in the literature would therefore suggest that in practice any interaction, if it occurs, is of only minor importance, and the anticoagulant dosage probably needs little or no adjustment.

1. Pharmacy Anticoagulant Clinic Study Group. A multicentre survey of antibiotics on the INR of anticoagulated patients. *Pharm J* (1996) 257 (Pharmacy Practice Suppl), R30.
2. Bristol-Myers Squibb Pharmaceuticals Ltd. Personal Communication, January 1997.

Anticoagulants + Ubidecarenone (Coenzyme Q10)

The anticoagulant effects of warfarin are reported to have been reduced in four patients by ubidecarenone, but only transiently increased or not affected in others.

Clinical evidence, mechanism, importance and management

Two patients on **warfarin** had INR reductions from about 2.5 to 1.4 after taking ubidecarenone 30 mg daily for 2 weeks. The INRs rapidly returned to normal when the ubidecarenone was stopped. Another patient on **warfarin** similarly showed INR falls on two occasions while taking ubidecarenone,[1] and another patient showed a reduced response to **warfarin** while taking ubidecarenone, but responded normally when it was stopped.[2]

In contrast 1 of 2 other patients taking ubidecarenone to treat alopecia caused by long-term **warfarin** treatment showed a transient INR *increase* when ubidecarenone was started.[3] The reasons for these INR changes is not known but it may be that ubidecarenone has some vitamin K-like activity. There is evidence from *animal* studies that ubidecarenone may alter the metabolism of both enantiomers of **warfarin**.[4] However, a study in patients stabilised on long-term **warfarin** found that ubidecarenone 100 mg daily did not alter the response to **warfarin**.[5]

Direct information seems to be conflicting and limited to these reports, but they act as a useful warning about the possibility of an interaction. Bear this interaction in mind if ubidecarenone is added to established **warfarin** treatment. Information about other oral anticoagulants is lacking.

1. Spigset O. Reduced effect of warfarin caused by ubidecarenone. *Lancet* (1994) 344, 1372–3.
2. Landbo C, Almdal TP. Interaction mellem warfarin og coenzym Q10. *Ugeskr Laeger* (1998) 160, 3226–7.
3. Nagao T, Ibayashi S, Fujii K, Sugimori H, Sadoshima S, Fujishima M. Treatment of warfarin-induced hair loss with ubidecarenone. *Lancet* (1995) 346, 1104–5.
4. Zhou S, Chan E. Effect of ubidearenone on warfarin anticoagulation and pharmacokinetics of warfarin enantiomers in rats. *Drug Metabol Drug Interact* (2001) 18, 99–122.
5. Engelsen J, Nielsen JD, Winther K. Effect of coenzyme Q_{10} and ginkgo biloba on warfarin dosage in stable, long-term warfarin treated outpatients. A randomised, double blind, placebo-crossover trial. *Thromb Haemost* (2002) 87, 1075–6.

Anticoagulants + Venlafaxine

A handful of reports describe increased INRs and bleeding in patients on warfarin and venlafaxine.

Clinical evidence, mechanism, importance and management

The possible interactions of **warfarin** or other anticoagulants with venlafaxine do not appear to have been studied, but the makers have on record a handful of case reports indicating that the effects of **warfarin** are occasionally increased by venlafaxine. These reports describe increased prothrombin times, raised INRs and bleeding (haematuria, gastrointestinal bleeding, melaena, haemarthrosis) in patients on **warfarin** who had also been treated with venlafaxine.[1] Just why these adverse interactions should have occurred is not understood, especially as no pharmacokinetic interaction is thought likely. From this it is not unreasonable to conclude that venlafaxine is normally unlikely to affect the metabolism of **warfarin**, but there are certainly other possible mechanisms of interaction. To be on the safe side, because an interaction can apparently occur very occasionally and unpredictably, it would be prudent to monitor prothrombin times if venlafaxine is started or stopped by patients taking any oral anticoagulant so that any problems can be quickly identified and dealt with. More study is needed.

1. Wyeth Laboratories. Personal communication, May 2000.

Anticoagulants + Viloxazine

The anticoagulant effects of acenocoumarol and fluindione are increased by viloxazine.

Clinical evidence

An 82-year-old woman with angina, hypertension and atrial fibrillation, who was taking **acenocoumarol**, molsidomine and flunitrazepam, had a rise in her INR from 3.3 to 7.9 when she started to take viloxazine [dose not stated] for depression. Five days after stopping the viloxazine her INR had fallen to 2.6. This report also briefly describes 3 other cases where viloxazine caused an increase in the anticoagulant effects of **acenocoumarol** and **fluindione**.[1]

Mechanism

Not understood. The authors of the report suggest that viloxazine possibly inhibits cytochrome P450 within the liver, resulting in a reduction in the metabolism and loss of the anticoagulants from the body.[1]

Importance and management

Information seems to be limited to this report so that its general importance is uncertain. Be alert for the need to reduce the dosage of acenocoumarol and fluindione if viloxazine is added to established anticoagulant treatment. Take the same precautions with any of the other oral anticoagulants but so far there seems to be no direct evidence that they interact.

1. Chiffoleau A, Delavaud P, Spreux A, Fialip J, Kergueris MF, Chichmanian RM, Lavarenne J, Bourin M, Larousse C. Existe-t-il une interaction métabolique entre la viloxazine et les antivitamines K? *Therapie* (1993) 48, 492–3.

Anticoagulants + Vinpocetine

Preliminary evidence suggests that the anticoagulant effects of warfarin may possibly be reduced to a small extent by vinpocetine.

Clinical evidence, mechanism, importance and management

A study in 18 healthy subjects compared the effects of single 25-mg doses of warfarin before and while taking vinpocetine 10 mg three times daily.[1] A small reduction in the anticoagulant effects occurred, but more study is needed to find out whether this is clinically important. Be aware of the small potential for interaction on concurrent use.

1. Hitzenberger G, Sommer W, Grandt R. Influence of vinpocetine on warfarin-induced inhibition of coagulation. *Int J Clin Pharmacol Ther Toxicol* (1990) 28, 323–8.

Anticoagulants + Vitamin E

The anticoagulant effects of warfarin normally appear to be unchanged by vitamin E, although there is an isolated case of bleeding attributed to concurrent use. The effects of dicoumarol may possibly be reduced by vitamin E.

Clinical evidence

(a) Warfarin effects unchanged

A double-blind placebo controlled study in 25 patients on warfarin found that 800 or 1200 units of vitamin E daily for a month caused no clinically relevant changes in their prothrombin times and INRs.[1] Another study in 12 anticoagulated patients also found that the anticoagulant effects of warfarin were unchanged by 100 or 400 units of vitamin E daily for 4 weeks.[2]

(b) Warfarin effects increased

A patient on warfarin (and also taking digoxin, furosemide, clofibrate, potassium chloride and phenytoin, later substituted by quinidine and later by procainamide) began to bleed, apparently as a result of taking 1200 units of vitamin E daily over a 2-month period. His prothrombin time was found to be 36 seconds. A later study in this patient showed that 800 units of vitamin E daily reduced his blood clotting factor levels and caused bleeding.[3]

(c) Dicoumarol effects reduced

A study on 3 healthy subjects found that 42 units of vitamin E daily for a month reduced the response to a single dose of dicoumarol after 36 hours from 52 to 33%.[4]

Mechanism

Not understood. The suggested explanations are that vitamin E interferes with the activity of vitamin K in producing the blood clotting factors,[3] and increases in the dietary requirements of vitamin K.[5,6]

Importance and management

Information is limited but the evidence suggests that most patients on warfarin are unlikely to have problems if given even quite large daily doses (up to 1200 units) of vitamin E, nevertheless the isolated case cited here shows that occasionally and unpredictably the warfarin effects can be changed. It has been recommended that prothrombin times should be monitored when vitamin E is first added (within 1 to 2 weeks has been recommended).[1] The same precautions could be applied to dicoumarol as well. However, as only one case has been reported with each of these anticoagulants this does seem somewhat over-cautious. Information about other oral anticoagulants is lacking.

1. Kim JM, White RH. Effect of vitamin E on the anticoagulant response to warfarin. *Am J Cardiol* (1996) 77, 545–6.
2. Corrigan JJ, Ulfers LL. Effect of vitamin E on prothrombin levels in warfarin-induced vitamin K deficiency. *Am J Clin Nutr* (1981) 34, 1701–5.
3. Corrigan JJ, Marcus FI. Coagulopathy associated with vitamin E ingestion. *JAMA* (1974) 230, 1300–1.
4. Schrogie JJ. Coagulopathy and fat-soluble vitamins. *JAMA* (1975) 232, 19.
5. Anon. Vitamin K, vitamin E and the coumarin drugs. *Nutr Rev* (1982) 40, 180–2.
6. Anon. Megavitamin E supplementation and vitamin K-dependent carboxylation. *Nutr Rev* (1983) 41, 268–70.

Anticoagulants + Vitamin K

The effects of the anticoagulants can be reduced or abolished by vitamin K. This can be used as an effective antidote for anticoagulant overdosage, but unintentional and unwanted antagonism has occurred in patients after taking some proprietary chilblain preparations, health foods, food supplements, enteral feeds or exceptionally large amounts of some green vegetables, seaweed, or green tea, which can contain significant amounts of vitamin K. See also 'Anticoagulants + Food or Drinks', p.282 and 'Anticoagulants + Natto', p.294.

Table 10.3 Vitamin K content of some meat and vegetables

Foods	Vitamin K content (microgram/100 g)
Turnip greens	650
Beetroot	650
Broccoli	200
Cabbage	125
Green beans	14
Lettuce	129
Liver, pig	25
Liver, beef	92
Potatoes	3
Spinach	89

Data from:
1. Olson RE. Vitamin K. In: Modern nutrition in health and disease. Goodhart RS and Shils ME (eds.) Lea and Febiger, Philadelphia (1980) p. 170–80.
2. Chow WH, Chow TC, Tse TM, Tai YT, Lee WT. Anticoagulation instability with life-treatening complication after dietary modification. *Postgrad Med J* (1990) 66, 855–7.

Clinical evidence

(a) Enteral feeds

Anticoagulant antagonism has been described in patients on **warfarin** taking liquid dietary supplements such as ***Ensure***,[1-5] ***Ensure-Plus***,[6-8] ***Isocal***,[9] ***Nutrilite 330***[10] and ***Osmolite***.[3,11-13] Reformulation to reduce the vitamin K content appears not to have completely solved the problem,[8] but a preparation with only traces of vitamin K, ***Meritene***, was found not to interact.[3]

(b) Green vegetables

A reduction in the effects of **dicoumarol**, **acenocoumarol** and **warfarin** (described as 'warfarin resistance') has been seen in those whose diets contained large amounts of green vegetables (up to about 500 g daily)[14-16] such as **spinach**,[17,18] **brussels sprouts**,[19] or **broccoli**,[16,18,20] which are rich in vitamin K. A formal study of the effects of vitamin K-rich vegetables (**brussels sprouts**, **broccoli**, **lettuce**, **spinach**) clearly demonstrated a disturbance of the control of anticoagulation in 37 patients on **warfarin**.[21]

(c) Vitamin K substances

A woman on **acenocoumarol** showed a fall in her British Corrected Ratio to 1.2 (normal range 1.8 to 3) within two days of starting to take an OTC chilblain preparation (*Gon*) containing **acetomenaphthone** 10 mg per tablet. She took a total of 50 mg of vitamin K over 48 hours.[22] A patient who required 15 to 17.5 mg of **warfarin** daily to maintain an INR of about 3 was found to be taking vitamin K as part of a dietary vitamin supplement. When he stopped taking the vitamin K, his **warfarin** dose could be reduced to 10.5 to12.5 mg daily.[23]

(d) Miscellaneous vitamin-K containing foods

A patient on **warfarin** showed a fall in his INR from a range of 3.2 to 3.79 down to 1.37, which was attributed to the ingestion of very large quantities of **green tea** (about 2 to 4 litres) each day for a week.[24]

A reduction in the effects of, **acenocoumarol** and **warfarin** has been seen in those whose diets contained large amounts of **liver**,[20,25] (1 kg per week), which is rich in vitamin K.

A patient on **warfarin** following a mitral valve replacement had, on two occasions, reduced INRs of 1.6 and 1.8 (usual range 2 to 3) within 24 hours of ingesting sushi with **seaweed** (***asakusa-nori***). It was estimated that she had consumed only about 45 micrograms of **phytomenadione**, but because her vitamin stores may have been low, this amount could have accounted for a large percentage of her vitamin K intake or stores.[26]

Mechanism

The oral anticoagulants compete with the normal supply of vitamin K from the gut to reduce the synthesis of blood clotting factors by the liver. If this supply is boosted by an unusually large intake of vitamin K, the competition swings in favour of the vitamin and the synthesis of the blood clotting factors begins to return to normal. As a result the prothrombin time also begins to fall to its normal value. Brussels sprouts increase the metabolism of warfarin to a small extent, which would also decrease its effects.[19] There is also some evidence that a physicochemical interaction (possibly binding to protein) may possibly occur between warfarin and enteral foods in the gut.[13,27]

Importance and management

A very well established, well documented and clinically important interaction expected to occur with every oral anticoagulant because they have a common mode of action. The drug intake and diet of any patient who shows 'warfarin resistance' should be investigated for the possibility of this interaction. It can be accommodated either by increasing the anticoagulant dosage, or by reducing the intake of vitamin K. In one case separating the administration of the warfarin and an enteral feed by 3 hours or more was effective.[13] However, patients on vitamin K-rich diets should not change their eating habits without at the same time reducing the anticoagulant dosage, because excessive anticoagulation and bleeding may occur.[20] It is estimated that a normal Western diet contains 300 to 500 micrograms of vitamin K daily. The minimum daily requirement is about 1 micrograms/kg and in the US has been determined to be 120 micrograms for adult men and 90 micrograms daily for adult women. 'Table 10.3', (p.321), gives the vitamin K content of some foods. Other tables listing the vitamin K content of the enteral feeds have been published,[3,9,10,12,28] but the situation is continually changing as manufacturers reformulate their products, in some instances to accommodate the problem of this interaction.

1. O'Reilly RA, Rytand DA. 'Resistance' to warfarin due to unrecognized vitamin K supplementation. *N Engl J Med* (1980) 303, 160–1.
2. Westfall LK. An unrecognized cause of warfarin resistance. *Drug Intell Clin Pharm* (1981) 15, 131.
3. Howard PA, Hannaman KN. Warfarin resistance linked to enteral nutrition products. *J Am Diet Assoc* (1985) 85, 713–15.
4. Bridgen MI. When bleeding complicates oral anticoagulant therapy. *Postgrad Med* (1995) 98, 153–68.
5. Lee M, Schwartz RN, Sharifi R. Warfarin resistance and vitamin K. *Ann Intern Med* (1981) 94, 140–1.
6. Zallman JA, Lee DP, Jeffrey PL. Liquid nutrition as a cause of warfarin resistance. *Am J Hosp Pharm* (1981) 38, 1174.
7. Michaelson R, Kempin SJ, Navia B, Gold JWM. Inhibition of the hypoprothrombinemic effect of warfarin (Coumadin®) by Ensure-Plus, a dietary supplement. *Clin Bull* (1980) 10, 171–2.
8. Griffith LD, Olvey SE, Triplett WC, Stotter Cuddy ML. Increasing prothrombin times in a warfarin-treated patient upon withdrawal of Ensure Plus. *Crit Care Med* (1982) 10, 799–800.
9. Watson AJM, Pegg M, Green JRB. Enteral feeds may antagonise warfarin. *BMJ* (1984) 288, 557.
10. Oren B, Shvartzman P. Unsuspected source of vitamin K in patients treated with anticoagulants: a case report. *Fam Pract* (1989) 6, 151–2.
11. Lader EW, Yang L, Clarke A. Warfarin dosage and vitamin K in Osmolite. *Ann Intern Med* (1980) 93, 373–4.
12. Parr MD, Record KE, Griffith GL, Zeok JV, Todd EP. Effect of enteral nutrition on warfarin therapy. *Clin Pharm* (1982) 1, 274–6.
13. Petretich DA. Reversal of Osmolite-warfarin interaction by changing warfarin administration time. *Clin Pharm* (1990) 9, 93.
14. Anon. Leafy vegetables in diet alter prothrombin time in patients taking anticoagulant drugs. *JAMA* (1964) 187, 27.
15. Qureshi GD, Reinders P, Swint JJ, Slate MB. Acquired warfarin resistance and weight-reducing diet. *Arch Intern Med* (1981) 141, 507–9.
16. Kempin SJ. Warfarin resistance caused by broccoli. *N Engl J Med* (1983) 308, 1229–30.
17. Udall JA, Krock LB. A modified method of anticoagulant therapy. *Curr Ther Res* (1968) 10, 207–11.
18. Karlson B, Leijd B, Hellström A. On the influence of vitamin K-rich vegetables and wine on the effectiveness of warfarin treatment. *Acta Med Scand* (1986) 220, 347–50.
19. Ovesen L, Lyduch S, Idorn ML. The effect of a diet rich in brussel sprouts on warfarin pharmacokinetics. *Eur J Clin Pharmacol* (1988) 33, 521–3.
20. Chow WH, Chow TC, Tse TM, Tai YT, Lee WT. Anticoagulation instability with life-threatening complication after dietary modification. *Postgrad Med J* (1990) 66, 855–7.
21. Pedersen FM, Hamberg O, Hess K, Ovesen L. The effect of dietary vitamin K on warfarin-induced anticoagulation. *J Intern Med* (1991) 229, 517–20.
22. Heald GE, Poller L. Anticoagulants and treatment for chilblains. *BMJ* (1974) 1, 455.
23. Eliason BC, Larson W. Acetaminophen and risk factors for excess anticoagulation with warfarin. *JAMA* (1998) 280, 696–7.
24. Taylor JR, Wilt VM. Probable antagonism of warfarin by green tea. *Ann Pharmacother* (1999) 33, 426–8.
25. Kalra PA, Cooklin M, Wood G, O'Shea GM, Holmes AM. Dietary modification as a cause of anticoagulation instability. *Lancet* (1988) ii, 803.
26. Bartle WR, Madorin P, Ferland G. Seaweed, vitamin K, and warfarin. *Am J Health-Syst Pharm* (2001) 58, 2300.
27. Allen JB, Penrod LE, Vickery WE. Warfarin resistance and enteral feedings: an in vitro study. *Arch Phys Med Rehabil* (1991) 72, 832.
28. Kutsop JJ. Update on vitamin K_1 content of enteral products. *Am J Hosp Pharm* (1984) 41, 1762.

Anticoagulants + Zafirlukast

Zafirlukast increases the anticoagulant effects of warfarin and bleeding has been seen.

Clinical evidence

In a placebo-controlled study 16 healthy subjects taking zafirlukast 80 mg twice daily for 10 days were given a single 25-mg dose of racemic **warfarin** on day 5. The mean AUC of the ***(S)*-warfarin** was increased by 63% and the half life by 36%, but the pharmacokinetics of the ***(R)*-warfarin** were not significantly changed. The mean prothrombin time increased by 35%.[1]

An 85-year-old woman on **warfarin**, salbutamol (albuterol), diltiazem, digoxin, furosemide and potassium was admitted to hospital with various cardiac-related problems and bleeding (epistaxis, melaena, multiple bruising), which was attributed to the use of zafirlukast 20 mg twice daily. Her INR had risen from 1.1 (measured 6 months previously) to 4.5. The report does not say how long she had been taking the both drugs together.[2]

Mechanism

The reason for the interaction is thought to be that the zafirlukast inhibits cytochrome P450 isoenzyme CYP2C9, which is concerned with the metabolism of *(S)*-warfarin, and as a result its serum levels and its effects are increased.[1,3]

Importance and management

Information appears to be limited to these reports but the interaction would seem to be established. If zafirlukast is given to patients stabilised on warfarin, monitor prothrombin times well and be alert for the need to reduce the warfarin dosage to avoid over-anticoagulation. Information about other oral anticoagulants is lacking but phenprocoumon would not be expected to interact in this way because it is metabolised differently (mainly by conjugation to a glucuronide), but this needs confirmation.

1. Suttle AB, Vargo DL, Wilkinson LA, Birmingham BK, Lasseter K. Effect of zafirlukast on the pharmacokinetics of R- and S-warfarin in healthy men. *Clin Pharmacol Ther* (1997) 61, 186.
2. Morkunas A, Graeme K. Zafirlukast-warfarin drug interaction with gastrointestinal bleeding. *J Toxicol Clin Toxicol* (1997) 35, 501.
3. Accolate (Zafirlukast). AstraZeneca UK Ltd. UK Summary of product characteristics, December 2004.

Anticoagulants + Zileuton

Zileuton slightly increases the anticoagulant effects of warfarin but the clinical significance of this is unclear.

Clinical evidence

In a placebo-controlled study zileuton 600 mg 6-hourly was given to 24 healthy subjects who had been titrated with racemic **warfarin** to achieve prothrombin times of 14 to 18 seconds for one week. The zileuton had no effect on the pharmacokinetics of ***(S)*-warfarin**, but the ***(R)*-warfarin** plasma levels rose, and its clearance fell by 15%. The mean prothrombin times in the mornings before taking the **warfarin** rose from 17.5 to 19.8 seconds, and in the evenings, 12 hours later, they rose from 17.1 to 19.1 seconds. The corresponding changes in the placebo group were from 18.1 to 18.8 seconds and 17.3 to 17.5 seconds.[1]

Mechanism

Not yet established but it seems likely that the zileuton inhibits the metabolism of the *(R)*-warfarin, probably by the cytochrome P450 isoenzyme CYP1A2, causing it to accumulate, thereby increasing its effects.

Clinical importance and management

Information seems to be limited to this study, but the interaction appears to be established. The clinical significance of a 2 to 3 second rise in prothrombin times is unclear, but it seems likely to be small. Information about other anticoagulants is lacking.

1. Awni WM, Hussein Z, Granneman GR, Patterson KJ, Dube LM, Cavanaugh JH. Pharmacodynamic and stereoselective pharmacokinetic interactions between zileuton and warfarin in humans. *Clin Pharmacokinet* (1995) 29 (Suppl 2), 67–76.

Anticoagulants + Zomepirac

The anticoagulant effects of warfarin were unaltered in 16 healthy subjects given zomepirac 150 mg four times daily.[1] No

special precautions would therefore seem to be necessary on concurrent use.

1. Minn FL, Zinny MA. Zomepirac and warfarin: a clinical study to determine if interaction exists. *J Clin Pharmacol* (1980) 20 (5-6 part 2), 418–21.

Drotrecogin alfa + Miscellaneous

Drotrecogin alfa has antithrombotic, and profibrinolytic activity. It inactivates factors Va and VIIIa and so indirectly decreases prothrombin production.[1] The makers of drotrecogin alfa therefore contraindicate its use with heparin (at more than 15 units/kg/hour). They also say that drotrecogin alfa should only be used in patients who have received thrombolytics in the last 3 days, or oral anticoagulants, aspirin or platelet inhibitors within 7 days, if the benefits outweigh the risks.[2]

1. McCoy C, Matthews SJ. Drotrecogin alfa (recombinant human activated protein C) for the treatment of severe sepsis. *Clin Ther* (2003) 25, 396–421.

2. Xigris (Drotrecogin alfa). Eli Lilly and Company Ltd. UK Summary of product characteristics, July 2005.

Fondaparinux + Antiplatelet drugs or NSAIDs

Neither aspirin nor piroxicam altered the pharmacokinetics of fondaparinux, and there was no significant change in bleeding time. Nevertheless, the maker recommends close monitoring if antiplatelet drugs or NSAIDs are used with fondaparinux.

Clinical evidence, mechanism, importance and management

A single 975-mg dose of **aspirin** given on day 4 of an 8-day course of subcutaneous fondaparinux 10 mg daily had no effect on fondaparinux pharmacokinetics in 16 healthy subjects. The increase in bleeding time with fondaparinux and **aspirin** was greater than with **aspirin** alone, but this was not statistically significant. **Aspirin** had no effect on the small prolongation of aPTT seen with fondaparinux.[1]

In another study, **piroxicam** 20 mg daily for 10 days was given to 12 healthy subjects with fondaparinux 10 mg daily starting on day 7. Both drugs were also given alone. **Piroxicam** had no effect on fondaparinux pharmacokinetics, and had no effect on the small prolongation of aPTT seen with fondaparinux. There was no difference in bleeding time between the treatments.[1]

Despite the lack of adverse findings in the above studies, the UK the makers of fondaparinux say that antiplatelet drugs (**aspirin**, **dipyridamole**, **sulfinpyrazone**, **ticlopidine** or **clopidogrel**) and NSAIDs should be used with caution. They recommend that if concurrent use is essential, close monitoring is necessary.[2]

1. Ollier C, Faaij RA, Santoni A, Duvauchelle T, van Haard PMM, Schoemaker RC, Cohen AF, de Greef R, Burggraaf J. Absence of interaction of fondaparinux sodium with aspirin and piroxicam in healthy male volunteers. *Clin Pharmacokinet* (2002) 41 (Suppl 2), 31–37.

2. Arixtra (Fondaparinux sodium). GlaxoSmithKline UK. UK Summary of product characteristics, January 2005.

Fondaparinux + Miscellaneous

In the UK, the maker recommends avoiding other drugs that may enhance the risk of haemorrhage with fondaparinux. They specifically name, desirudin, fibrinolytic agents, GP IIb/IIIa receptor antagonists, heparin, heparinoids and low molecular weight heparins.[1] See also 'warfarin', (below), and 'antiplatelet drugs and NSAIDs', (above).

1. Arixtra (Fondaparinux sodium). GlaxoSmithKline UK. UK Summary of product characteristics, January 2005.

Fondaparinux + Warfarin

Warfarin did not alter the pharmacokinetics of fondaparinux, and fondaparinux did not alter the effect of warfarin on prothrombin time.

Clinical evidence, mechanism, importance and management

Subcutaneous fondaparinux 4 mg was given daily for 5 days to 12 healthy subjects, with warfarin 15 mg given on day 4 and 10 mg on day 5 in a placebo controlled study. Warfarin had no effect on fondaparinux pharmacokinetics. In addition, the effect of warfarin on prothrombin time was not altered by fondaparinux. The authors concluded that the prothrombin time (INR) can still be used to monitor the effect of oral anticoagulants during the switch from fondaparinux to oral anticoagulants.[1]

1. Faaij RA, Burggraaf J, Schoemaker RC, van Amsterdam RGM, Cohen AF. Absence of an interaction between the synthetic pentasaccharide fondaparinux and oral warfarin. *Br J Clin Pharmacol* (2002) 54, 304–8.

Heparin + Miscellaneous

Changes in the protein binding of diazepam, propranolol, quinidine and verapamil caused by heparin do not appear to be of clinical importance. Patients who smoke may possibly need fractionally more heparin than non-smokers.

Clinical evidence, mechanism, importance and management

A number of studies have found that heparin reduces the plasma protein binding of several drugs including **diazepam**,[1,2] **propranolol**,[1] **quinidine**[3] and **verapamil**[4] in man and in *animals*. For example, 3 patients on oral **propranolol** and 5 patients given intramuscular **diazepam** 10 mg were given 3000 units of heparin just before cardiac catheterization. Five minutes after the heparin was given, the free fraction of **diazepam** was found to have risen fourfold (from 1.8 to 7.9%) while the free levels had risen from 2 to 8.4 nanograms/ml. The free fraction of the **propranolol** rose from 7.4 to 12.5% and the free levels rose from 1.7 to 2.7 nanograms/ml.[1]

The postulated reason for these changes is that the heparin displaces these drugs from their binding sites on the plasma albumins with additionally some changes in free fatty acid levels. It was also suggested that these changes in protein binding might possibly have some clinical consequences. For example, there could, theoretically, be sudden increases in sedation or respiratory depression because of the rapid increase in the active (free) fraction of **diazepam**.

However, these changes are unlikely to be of clinical importance (see 'Protein binding interactions', (p.3)). One study even suggested that the heparin-induced protein binding changes are an artefact of the study methods used,[5] and this would seem to be supported by an experimental study, which found that heparin did not have any effect on the beta-blockade caused by **propranolol**.[6] Moreover there seem to be no other reports confirming that these interactions are of real clinical importance. No special precautions would seem to be necessary.

A study of the factors affecting the sensitivity of individuals to heparin found that its half-life in **smokers** was 0.62 hours compared with 0.97 hours in non-smokers. The dosage requirements of the smokers were slightly increased (18.8 compared with 16 units/hour per lean body weight).[7] These differences would seem to be too small to be of much practical importance.

1. Wood AJJ, Robertson D, Robertson RM, Wilkinson GR, Wood M. Elevated plasma free drug concentrations of propranolol and diazepam during cardiac catheterization. *Circulation* (1980) 62, 1119–22.

2. Routledge PA, Kitchell BB, Bjornsson TD, Skinnner T, Linnoila M, Shand DG. Diazepam and *N*-desmethyldiazepam redistribution after heparin. *Clin Pharmacol Ther* (1980) 27, 528–32.

3. Kessler KM, Leech RC, Spann JF. Blood collection techniques, heparin and quinidine protein binding. *Clin Pharmacol Ther* (1979) 25, 204–10.

4. Keefe DL, Yee Y-G, Kates RE. Verapamil protein binding in patients and normal subjects. *Clin Pharmacol Ther* (1981) 29, 21–6.

5. Brown JE, Kitchell BB, Bjornsson TD, Shand DG. The artifactual nature of heparin-induced drug protein-binding alterations. *Clin Pharmacol Ther* (1981) 30, 636–43.

6. DeLeve LD, Piafsky KM. Lack of heparin effect on propranolol-induced β-adrenoceptor blockade. *Clin Pharmacol Ther* (1982) 31, 216.

7. Cipolle RJ, Seifert RD, Neilan BA, Zaske DE, Haus E. Heparin kinetics: variables related to disposition and dosage. *Clin Pharmacol Ther* (1981) 29, 387–93.

Heparin + Nitrates

Some studies claim that the effects of heparin are reduced by the concurrent infusion of nitrates, but others have failed to confirm this interaction.

Clinical evidence

(a) Heparin effects reduced

While receiving intravenous **glyceryl trinitrate**, 7 patients with coronary artery disease needed an increased dose of intravenous heparin to achieve satisfactory aPTT ratios of 1.5 to 2.5. When the **glyceryl trinitrate** was stopped 6 out of the 8 showed a marked increase in aPTT values to 3.5. One patient had transient haematuria.[1]

This study confirms a previous report, the authors of which attributed this response to an interaction with the propylene glycol diluent of the **glyceryl trinitrate** infusion.[2] However it still occurred when **glyceryl trinitrate** was given without propylene glycol.[1] The PTT of 27 patients given heparin was more than halved (from 130 to about 60 seconds) when additionally given **glyceryl trinitrate** 2 to 5 mg/hour intravenously. The heparin levels measured in 9 patients were unchanged. The PTT rose again when the **glyceryl trinitrate** was stopped.[3,4] The PTT in 8 out of 10 patients treated with heparin was reduced by **glyceryl trinitrate** 2 to 5 mg/hour.[5] Yet another study found that concurrent use had no effect at 2 hours, but heparin levels were reduced by 56% at 4 hours, and the aPTT ratio was accordingly lower.[6] Reduced heparin effects have been described in other studies.[7,8]

(b) Heparin effects unchanged

A study in 10 patients following angioplasty found no significant aPTT changes over a 30 minute period following the addition of intravenous **glyceryl trinitrate** (41 to 240 micrograms/ml) to infusions of heparin.[9] A 60-minute infusion of **glyceryl trinitrate** 5 mg in eight healthy subjects had no effect on the aPTT or prothrombin time following a 5000 unit intravenous injection of heparin.[10] A further study in 24 patients failed to find any effects on aPTT in 17 of the patients on heparin given infusions of **glyceryl trinitrate** 1 to 5 mg or **isosorbide dinitrate**, and only 3 had increases of more than 17 seconds when the nitrate was stopped.[11] A 100 micrograms/minute infusion of **glyceryl trinitrate** did not alter the anticoagulant effect of a 40 units/kg bolus of heparin in 7 healthy subjects.[12] Several other reports have found no interaction, or questioned the existence of an interaction, between heparin and glyceryl trinitrate[13-18] or isosorbide dinitrate[17] infusions.

A comparative study in 15 patients treated with intravenous heparin and **molsidomine** 2 mg found that **molsidomine** had no effect the PTT due to the heparin.[4]

Mechanism

Not understood. One study suggests that what occurs is related to a glyceryl trinitrate-induced antithrombin III abnormality, and is apparent at doses above 350 micrograms/minute.[7] Others say that heparin levels are lowered.[6,8]

Importance and management

The discord between these reports is not understood. Given that heparin is routinely monitored, it is likely that if any interaction occurs, it will be rapidly detected and compensated for. However, do bear in mind that the dose of heparin may need to be increased if glyceryl trinitrate is added, or reduced if glyceryl trinitrate is withdrawn. No special precautions would appear to be needed if heparin is given with molsidomine.

1. Habbab MA, Haft JI. Heparin resistance induced by intravenous nitroglycerin. A word of caution when both drugs are used concomitantly. *Arch Intern Med* (1987) 147, 857–60.
2. Col J, Col-Debeys C, Lavenne-Pardonge E, Meert P, Hericks L, Broze MC, Moriau M. Propylene glycol-induced heparin resistance during nitroglycerin infusion. *Am Heart J* (1985) 110, 171–3.
3. Pizzulli L, Nitsch J, Lüderitz B. Hemmung der Heparinwirkung durch Glyceroltrinitrat. *Dtsch Med Wochenschr* (1988) 113, 1837–40.
4. Wiemer M, Pizzulli L, Reichert H, Lüderitz B. Gibt es eine Wechselwirkung zwischen Heparin und Moldisomin?. *Med Klin* (1994) 89, 45–6.
5. Dascalov TN, Chaushev AG, Petrov AB, Stancheva LG, Stanachcova SD, Ivanov AA. Nitroglycerin inhibition of the heparin effect in acute myocardial infarction patients. *Eur Heart J* (1990) 11 (Abstract Suppl), 321.
6. Brack MJ, Gershlick AH. Nitrate infusion even in low dose decreases the anticoagulant effect of heparin through a direct effect on heparin levels. *Eur Heart J* (1991) 12 (Abstract Suppl), 80.
7. Becker RC, Corrao JM, Bovill EG, Gore JM, Baker SP, Miller ML, Lucas FV, Alpert JA. Intravenous nitroglycerin-induced heparin resistance: a qualitative antithrombin III abnormality. *Am Heart J* (1990) 119, 1254–61.
8. Brack MJ, More RS, Hubner PJB, Gerschlick AH. The effect of low dose nitroglycerine on plasma heparin concentrations and activated partial thromboplastin times. *Blood Coag Fibrinol* (1993) 4, 183–6.
9. Lepor NE, Amin DK, Berberian L, Shah PK. Does nitroglycerin induce heparin resistance? *Clin Cardiol* (1989) 12, 432–4.
10. Bode V, Welzel D, Franz G, Polensky U. Absence of drug interaction between heparin and nitroglycerin. *Arch Intern Med* (1990) 150, 2117–19.
11. Pye M, Olroyd KG, Conkie J, Hutton I, Cobbe SM. Is there an interaction between IV nitrate therapy and heparin anticoagulation? A clinical and in vitro study. *Eur Heart J* (1991) 12 (Abstract Suppl), 80.
12. Schoenenberger RA, Ménat L, Weiss P, Marbet GA, Ritz R. Absence of nitroglycerin-induced heparin resistance in healthy volunteers. *Eur Heart J* (1992) 13, 411–14.
13. Gonzalez ER, Jones HD, Graham S, Elswick RK. Assessment of the drug interaction between intravenous nitroglycerin and heparin. *Ann Pharmacother* (1992) 26, 1512–14.
14. Day MW, Absher RK. We don't observe the same heparin-nitroglycerin reactions. *Crit Care Nurse* (1992) 12, 18.
15. Reich DL, Hammerschlag BC, Rand JH, Perucho-Powell MH, Thys DM. Modest doses of nitroglycerin do not interfere with beef lung heparin anticoagulation in patients taking nitrates. *J Cardiothorac Vasc Anesth* (1992) 6, 677–9
16. Nottestad SY, Mascette AM. Nitroglycerin-induced resistance: absence of interaction at clinically relevant doses. *Mil Med* (1994) 159, 569–71.
17. Bechtold H, Kleist P, Landgraf K, Möser K. Einfluß einer niedrigdosierten intravenösen Nitrattherpie auf die antikagulatorische Wirkung von Heparin. *Med Klin* (1994) 89, 360–6.
18. Berk SI, Grunwald A, Pal S, Bodenheimer MM. Effect of intravenous nitroglycerin on heparin dosage requirements in coronary artery disease. *Am J Cardiol* (1993) 72, 393–6.

Heparin and related drugs + Other drugs affecting coagulation

One report suggests that aprotinin decreases the effects of heparin, but this is complicated by the presence of protamine. Another suggests anticoagulation is harder to achieve in the presence of streptokinase. Additive effects on coagulation occur when heparin is given with aspirin or dextrans.

Clinical evidence, mechanism, importance and management

(a) Aprotinin + Heparin

One report suggested that patients who had been treated with aprotinin needed considerably more heparin than usual. It was suggested that this occurred because the aprotinin has an effect on antithrombin III.[1] However, a later report pointed out that the more likely reason was that these aprotinin-treated patients had also been given protamine, which would oppose the effects of the heparin.[2]

(b) Aspirin + Heparin

Eight out of 12 patients developed serious bleeding when treated with heparin 5000 units subcutaneously every 12 hours and aspirin 600 mg twice daily. Haematomas of the hip and thigh occurred in 3 patients, bleeding through the wound in 4, and uterine bleeding in the other patient.[3]

An epidemiological study, which included 302 patients on heparin and aspirin revealed that the incidence of bleeding was almost 2.5 times that which was seen in patients not given aspirin.[4] Other reports confirm this.[5,6]

(c) Aspirin + Reviparin

A study in 9 healthy subjects indicated that bleeding time may be prolonged by combined aspirin and reviparin, but not to a clinically significant extent.[7]

(d) Dextrans + Heparin

A study in 9 patients with peripheral vascular disease given 500 ml of dextran showed that the mean clotting time 1 hour after an infusion of 10 000 units of heparin was increased from 36 to 69 minutes. Dextran alone had no effect, but the mean clotting time after 5000 units of heparin with dextran was almost the same as after 10 000 units of heparin alone.[8,9] This study would seem to support two other reports of an increase in the incidence of bleeding in those given both heparin and dextran 70.[10,11] Uneventful concurrent use[12,13] has been described with dextran 40.

(e) Streptokinase + Heparin

Fifty patients given streptokinase 750 000 to 1 500 000 units for acute myocardial infarction needed about 24% more heparin (37 755 compared with 30 294 units daily) in order to achieve the desired aPTT than other patients who had not had streptokinase. Even then their aPTTs were 15% lower. Anticoagulation was also delayed by 2 days. The reasons are not understood. On the basis of this study, anticipate the need to use higher heparin doses and to make more frequent dosage adjustments if streptokinase has been given.[14] These patients also needed more warfarin (+12%) but this value was not statistically significant.[14] More study is needed.

1. Fisher AR, Bailey CR, Shannon CN, Wielogorski AK. Heparin resistance after aprotinin. *Lancet* (1992) 340, 1230–1.
2. Hunt BJ, Murkin JM. Heparin resistance after aprotinin. *Lancet* (1993) 341, 126.
3. Yett HS, Skillman JJ, Salzman EW. The hazards of aspirin plus heparin. *N Engl J Med* (1978) 298, 1092.
4. Walker AM, Jick H. Predictors of bleeding during heparin therapy. *JAMA* (1980) 244, 1209–12.
5. Heiden D, Rodvien R, Mielke CH. Heparin bleeding, platelet dysfunction, and aspirin. *JAMA* (1981) 246, 330–1.
6. Younossi ZM, Strum WB, Cloutier D, Teirstein PS, Schatz RA. Upper GI bleeding in post-coronary stent patients following aspirin and anticoagulant treatment. *Gastroenterology* (1995) 108 (4 Suppl), A265.
7. Klinkhardt U, Breddin HK, Esslinger HU, Haas S, Kalatzis A, Harder S. Interaction between the LMWH reviparin and aspirin in healthy volunteers. *Br J Clin Pharmacol* (2000) 49, 337–41.
8. Atik M. Potentiation of heparin by dextran and its clinical implication. *Thromb Haemost* (1977) 38, 275.
9. Atik M. Personal communication, April 1980.
10. Bloom WL, Brewer SS. The independent yet synergistic effects of heparin and dextran. *Acta Chir Scand* (1968) 387 (Suppl), 53–7.
11. Morrison ND, Stephenson CBS, Maclean D, Stanhope JM. Deep vein thrombosis after femoropopliteal bypass grafting with observations on the incidence of complications following the use of dextran 70. *N Z Med J* (1976) 84, 233–6.
12. Schöndorf TH, Weber U. Prevention of deep vein thrombosis in orthopedic surgery with the combination of low dose heparin plus either dihydroergotamine or dextran. *Scand J Haematol* (1980) 36 (Suppl), 126–40.
13. Serjeant JCB. Mesenteric embolus treated with low-molecular weight dextran. *Lancet* (1965) i, 139–40.
14. Zagher D, Maaravi Y, Matzner Y, Gilon D, Gotsman MS, Weiss AT. Partial resistance to anticoagulation after streptokinase treatment for acute myocardial infarction. *Am J Cardiol* (1990) 66, 28–30.

Heparin + Probenecid

An isolated case report from the 1950s suggests that the effects of heparin may be possibly increased by probenecid and bleeding may occur.

Clinical evidence, mechanism, importance and management

In 1950 (but not reported until 1975) a woman with subacute bacterial endocarditis was treated with probenecid orally and penicillin by intravenous drip, which was kept open with minimal doses of heparin. After a total of about 20 000 units of heparin had been given over a 3-week period, increasing epistaxes developed and the clotting time was found to be 24 minutes (normal 5 to 6 minutes). This was controlled with protamine.[1] However, no reports of this interaction appear to have been made subsequently. This interaction seems unlikely to be of general significance.

1. Sanchez G. Enhancement of heparin effect by probenecid. *N Engl J Med* (1975) 292, 48.

Thrombin inhibitors + Erythromycin

Erythromycin increases the AUC of melagatran, the active metabolite of ximelagatran, and causes a small additional effect on coagulation parameters. Erythromycin has no effect on the pharmacokinetics or activity of argatroban.

Clinical evidence, mechanism, importance and management

(a) Argatroban

In 10 healthy subjects, erythromycin 500 mg four times daily was given for 7 days with a single 5-hour intravenous infusion of argatroban 1 microgram/kg per minute given before erythromycin and on day 6. Erythromycin had no effect on the pharmacokinetics of argatroban, and had no effect on the argatroban-induced prolongation of aPTT.[1] No special precautions are likely to be required on concurrent use of argatroban and erythromycin or other inhibitors of the cytochrome P450 isoenzyme CYP3A4 (for a list, see 'Table 1.4', (p.6)).

(b) Ximelagatran

In 16 healthy subjects, erythromycin 500 mg three times daily was given for 5 days with a single 36-mg oral dose of ximelagatran given before erythromycin and on day 5. Erythromycin increased the AUC of melagatran (the active metabolite of ximelagatran) 1.8-fold, and the maximum plasma level by 1.7-fold. This resulted in a small increase in peak aPTT from 41 to 44 seconds.[2]

The mechanism of this interaction is unknown. Ximelagatran is not metabolised by cytochrome P450 isoenzymes, so the known inhibitory effect of erythromycin on CYP3A4 is not thought to be the mechanism.

The findings of a pharmacokinetic interaction with a small pharmacodynamic effect indicate that further study is needed. Until more is known, it would certainly be prudent to be cautious when ximelagatran is used in patients on erythromycin, although note that the pharmacodynamic effect was small and all patients tolerated the combination well.[2]

1. Tran JQ, Di Cicco RA, Sheth SB, Tucci M, Peng L, Jorkasky DK, Hursting MJ, Benincosa LJ. Assessment of the potential pharmacokinetic and pharmacodynamic interactions between erythromycin and argatroban. *J Clin Pharmacol* (1999) 39, 513–19.
2. Dorani H, Schützer K, Sarich TC, Wall U, Ohlsson L, Eriksson UG. Effect of erythromycin on the pharmacokinetics and pharmacodynamics or the oral direct thrombin inhibitor ximelagatran and its active form melagatran. *Clin Pharmacol Ther* (2004) 75, P78.

Thrombin inhibitors + Other drugs affecting coagulation

Use of argatroban with warfarin and related drugs has an effect on the measurement of INR, and this needs to be adjusted. No interaction occurred between argatroban and aspirin. Aspirin did not alter the pharmacokinetics of melagatran, the active metabolite of ximelagatran, or its effects on the aPTT, but the combination had additive effects on bleeding time. There was no pharmacodynamic interaction between bivalirudin and aspirin, ticlopidine, clopidogrel, abciximab, eptifibatide or tirofiban. The makers warn of the increased bleeding risks if argatroban, bivalirudin or lepirudin are used with other drugs affecting coagulation.

Clinical evidence, mechanism, importance and management

(a) Argatroban

In 12 healthy subjects, argatroban 1.25 micrograms/kg per minute was given for 100 hours, with a single 7.5-mg dose of **warfarin** given at hour 4. Neither drug affected the pharmacokinetics of the other. The single dose of warfarin in this study did not add to the anticoagulant effect of argatroban.[1] However, a previous study found that the INR and prothrombin time were increased when **warfarin** (7.5 mg on day one, then 3 to 6 mg for 9 days) was used with argatroban (1 to 4 micrograms/kg per minute for 5 hours daily for 11 days), but without any additional effect on vitamin K-dependent factor Xa activity.[2] A similar finding was reported in a study using **acenocoumarol** or **phenprocoumon** and argatroban.[3] This means that the INR reading needs to be corrected before it can be used as a clinical indicator of coagulation status when **warfarin** or other vitamin-K antagonists are used with argatroban. The maker provides detailed information on how this should be done while switching from argatroban to **warfarin**.[4]

The maker notes that no pharmacokinetic or pharmacodynamic interaction has been detected between argatroban and **aspirin**, but warns that the use of argatroban with antiplatelet drugs may increase the risk of bleeding, as may concurrent use of other drugs affecting coagulation.[4]

(b) Bivalirudin

The UK makers say that no pharmacodynamic interactions were detected when bivalirudin was used with platelet inhibitors, including **aspirin**, **ticlopidine**, **clopidogrel**, **abciximab**, **eptifibatide**, or **tirofiban**.[5] They recommend regular monitoring of haemostasis when bivalirudin is used with platelet inhibitors or other anticoagulants.[5] Bivalirudin can be started 30 minutes after stopping **heparin**, but 8 hours should be left after stopping a **low-molecular weight heparin**.[5]

(c) Lepirudin

The makers of lepirudin say that no formal interaction studies have been done but they reasonably warn that the concurrent use of lepirudin and other thrombolytics (they name **alteplase** and **streptokinase**) may increase the risk of bleeding complications and considerably enhance the effect of lepirudin on the aPTT. They also warn about the increased risks of bleeding if coumarin derivatives (**warfarin** and other **oral anticoagulants**), **clopidogrel**, **ticlopidine**, **abciximab**, **eptifibatide** or **tirofiban** are used concurrently. Their recommendation[6,7] for exchanging lepirudin treatment with an **oral anticoagulant** is to reduce the lepirudin dosage gradually to reach an aPTT ratio just above 1.5 before beginning the **oral anticoagulant**, and to stop the lepirudin as soon as the INR reaches the target range.

(d) Ximelagatran

In young healthy subjects, **aspirin** 450 mg the day before, and 150 mg just before melagatran had no effect on the pharmacokinetics of intravenous melagatran 4.12 mg. In addition, **aspirin** did not alter the increases seen in aPTT or activated clotting time seen with melagatran. Both **aspirin** and melagatran increased bleeding time, and the increase with the combination was additive.[8]

1. Brown PM, Hursting MJ. Lack of pharmacokinetic interactions between argatroban and warfarin. *Am J Health-Syst Pharm* (2002) 59, 2078–83.
2. Sheth SB, DiCicco RA, Hursting MJ, Montague T, Jorkasky DK. Interpreting the international normalized ratio (INR) in individuals receiving argatroban and warfarin. *Thromb Haemost* (2001) 85, 435–40. Erratum *ibid.* 86, 727.
3. Harder S, Graff J, Klinkhardt U, von Hentig N, Walenga JM, Watanabe H, Osakabe M, Breddin HK. Transition from argatroban to oral anticoagulation with phenprocoumon or acenocoumarol: effects on prothrombin time, activated partial thromboplastin time, and Ecarin clotting time. *Thromb Haemost* (2004) 91, 1137–45.
4. Argatroban. GlaxoSmithKline. US Prescribing information, April 2005.
5. Angiox (Bivalirudin). Nycomed. UK Summary of product characteristics, September 2004.
6. Refludan (Lepirudin). Hoechst Marion Roussel Ltd. UK Summary of product characteristics, December 2004.
7. Refludan (Lepirudin). Berlex. US Prescribing information, December 2004.
8. Fager G, Cullberg M, Eriksson-Lepkowska M, Frison L, Eriksson UG. Pharmacokinetics and pharmacodynamics of melagatran, the active form of the oral direct thrombin inhibitor ximelagatran, are not influenced by acetylsalicylic acid. *Eur J Clin Pharmacol* (2003) 59, 283–9.

Thrombin inhibitors; Argatroban + Lidocaine

There was no pharmacokinetic interaction between argatroban and lidocaine, and no further change in coagulation parameters on combined use.

Clinical evidence, mechanism, importance and management

In 12 healthy subjects, lidocaine 2 mg/kg per hour was infused for 16 hours (after a loading dose of 1.5 mg/kg over 10 minutes) alone then in combination with intravenous argatroban 1.5 micrograms/kg per minute for 16 hours. Lidocaine had no effect on the pharmacokinetics of argatroban, and argatroban had no effect on lidocaine pharmacokinetics. Lidocaine did not alter the effect of argatroban on aPTT.[1]

No special precautions appear likely to be necessary on concurrent use of lidocaine and argatroban.

1. Inglis AML, Sheth SB, Hursting MJ, Tenero DM, Graham AM, DiCicco RA. Investigation of the interaction between argatroban and acetaminophen, lidocaine, or digoxin. *Am J Health-Syst Pharm* (2002) 59, 1257–66.

Thrombin inhibitors; Argatroban + Paracetamol (Acetaminophen)

There was no pharmacokinetic interaction between argatroban and paracetamol, and no further change in coagulation parameters on combined use.

Clinical evidence, mechanism, importance and management

In 11 healthy subjects, paracetamol 1 g every 6 hours for 5 doses had no effect on the pharmacokinetics of a 19-hour infusion of argatroban 1.5 micrograms/kg per minute, started with the second dose of paracetamol. In addition, argatroban had no effect on paracetamol pharmacokinetics. Paracetamol did not alter the effect of argatroban on aPTT.[1]

No special precautions appear necessary on concurrent use of paracetamol and argatroban.

1. Inglis AML, Sheth SB, Hursting MJ, Tenero DM, Graham AM, DiCicco RA. Investigation of the interaction between argatroban and acetaminophen, lidocaine, or digoxin. *Am J Health-Syst Pharm* (2002) 59, 1257–66.

Thrombin inhibitors; Ximelagatran + Amiodarone

The concurrent use of amiodarone and ximelagatran caused a slight increase in the AUC of melagatran and a slight decrease in the AUC of amiodarone, but the clinical relevance of this is unknown.

Clinical evidence, mechanism, importance and management

In a placebo-controlled study in 26 healthy subjects, ximelagatran 36 mg was given every 12 hours for 8 days with a single 600-mg dose of amiodarone on day 4. With combined use there was a slight 21% increase in the AUC of melagatran (the active metabolite of ximelagatran), and a slight 15% decrease in the AUC of amiodarone. Amiodarone did not alter the effect of melagatran on aPTT.[1]

The mechanism of this interaction is unknown. The pharmacokinetic changes seen were not considered to be clinically relevant. Nevertheless, further study is needed to confirm that these small pharmacokinetic changes are not greater after longer-term amiodarone use, and to check their clinical relevance.

1. Teng R, Sarich TC, Eriksson UG, Hamer JE, Gillette S, Schützer KM, Carlson GF, Knowey PR. A pharmacokinetic study of the combined administration of amiodarone and ximelagatran, an oral direct thrombin inhibitor. *J Clin Pharmacol* (2004) 44, 1063–71.

Thrombin inhibitors; Ximelagatran + Atorvastatin

No pharmacokinetic interaction occurs between ximelagatran and atorvastatin, and concurrent use does not change coagulation status.

Clinical evidence, mechanism, importance and management

In 15 healthy subjects, ximelagatran 36 mg twice daily was given for 5 days with a single 40-mg dose of atorvastatin on day 4. There was no change in the pharmacokinetics of either drug or their active metabolites. Atorvastatin did not alter the effect of melagatran on aPTT.[1]

No special precautions are expected to be needed if ximelagatran is used in patients on atorvastatin.

1. Sarich TC, Schützer K-M, Dorani H, Wall U, Kalies I, Ohlsson L, Eriksson UG. No pharmacokinetic or pharmacodynamic interaction between atorvastatin and the oral direct thrombin inhibitor ximelagatran. *J Clin Pharmacol* (2004) 44, 928–34.

Thrombin inhibitors; Ximelagatran + Miscellaneous

No pharmacokinetic interaction appears to occur between ximelagatran and diazepam, diclofenac or nifedipine. This suggests that ximelagatran has no clinically relevant effect on drugs that are substrates for the cytochrome P450 isoenzymes CYP2C9, CYP2C19, and CYP3A4. There was no pharmacodynamic interaction between diclofenac and ximelagatran.

Clinical evidence, mechanism, importance and management

(a) Diazepam

In 24 healthy subjects, ximelagatran 24 mg twice daily was given for 8 days with a single 100-microgram/kg intravenous dose of diazepam given on day 3. There was no change in the pharmacokinetics of either drug or of N-desmethyl-diazepam.[1]

Metabolism of diazepam to *N*-desmethyl-diazepam occurs via the cytochrome P450 isoenzyme CYP2C19, and *in vitro* studies had shown that melagatran was a weak inhibitor of this isoenzyme (up to 35%)[1] However, the lack of a pharmacokinetic interaction with diazepam suggests that no clinically relevant interaction occurs, and is also unlikely with other CYP2C19 substrates[1] (for a list see 'Table 1.3', (p.6)).

(b) Diclofenac

In a single-dose study in 24 healthy subjects, simultaneous administration of ximelagatran 24 mg and enteric-coated diclofenac 50 mg caused no change in the pharmacokinetics of either drug. In this study, there was also no additional effect of the combination on activated partial thromboplastin time or capillary bleeding time, suggesting that no pharmacodynamic interaction occurs.[1]

Diclofenac is a substrate for the cytochrome P450 isoenzyme CYP2C9, and *in vitro* study has shown that ximelagatran and melagatran are weak inhibitors of this isoenzyme (up to 36%).[1] However, the lack of a pharmacokinetic interaction with diclofenac suggests that no clinically relevant interaction occurs, and is also unlikely with other CYP2C9 substrates[1] (for a list see 'Table 1.3', (p.6)).

(c) Nifedipine

In a single-dose study in 34 healthy subjects, giving ximelagatran 24 mg four hours after slow-release nifedipine 60 mg caused no change in the pharmacokinetics of either drug.[1]

Nifedipine is a substrate for the cytochrome P450 isoenzyme CYP3A4, and *in vitro* studies had shown that ximelagatran metabolites might be weak inhibitors of this isoenzyme.[1] However, the lack of a pharmacokinetic interaction with nifedipine suggests that no clinically relevant interaction occurs, and is also unlikely with other CYP3A4 substrates[1] (for a list see 'Table 1.4', (p.6)).

1. Bredberg E, Andersson TB, Frison L, Thuresson A, Johansson S, Eriksson-Lepkowska M, Larsson M, Eriksson UG. Ximelagatran, an oral direct thrombin inhibitor, has a low potential for cytochrome P450-mediated drug-drug interactions. *Clin Pharmacokinet* (2003) 42, 765–77.

11

Anticonvulsants

The anticonvulsant drugs listed in 'Table 11.1', (p.329) find their major application in the treatment of various kinds of epilepsy, although some of them are also used for other conditions. The list is not exhaustive, but it contains most of the anticonvulsant drugs that are discussed either in this section or elsewhere in the publication.

Drug interactions

The drugs used as anticonvulsants are a disparate group, and their interactions need to be considered individually.

The older anticonvulsants carbamazepine and phenytoin have established ranges of therapeutic plasma levels and these are typically fairly narrow. Modest changes in plasma levels may therefore be clinically important.

(a) Carbamazepine or oxcarbazepine

Carbamazepine is extensively metabolised by the cytochrome P450 isoenzyme CYP3A4 to the active 10,11-epoxide metabolite, which is then further metabolised. Concurrent use of CYP3A4 inhibitors or inducers may therefore lead to toxicity or reduced efficacy. However, importantly, carbamazepine also induces CYP3A4 and so induces its own metabolism (autoinduction). Because of this, it is important that drug interaction studies are multiple-dose and carried out at steady state. Auto-induction also means that moderate inducers of CYP3A4 may have less effect on steady-state carbamazepine levels than expected. Oxcarbazepine is a derivative of carbamazepine, but has a lesser effect on CYP3A4. However, both carbamazepine and oxcarbazepine can act as inhibitors of CYP2C19, which shows genetic polymorphism. See 'Phenytoin + Carbamazepine', p.366.

(b) Phenobarbital

Phenobarbital is an inducer of a wide range of cytochrome P450 isoenzymes, and may increase the metabolism of a variety of drugs. It may, itself, also be affected by some enzyme inducers or inhibitors, although these interactions are less established.

(c) Phenytoin

Phenytoin is extensively metabolised by hydroxylation, principally by CYP2C9, although CYP2C19 also plays a role. These isoenzymes show genetic polymorphism, (see 'Genetic factors', (p.4)) and CYP2C19 may assume a greater role in individuals who have a poor metaboliser phenotype of CYP2C9. The concurrent use of inhibitors of CYP2C9, and sometimes also CYP2C19, can lead to phenytoin toxicity. In addition, phenytoin metabolism is saturable (it shows nonlinear pharmacokinetics), therefore, small changes in metabolism or phenytoin dose can result in marked changes in plasma levels. Moreover, phenytoin is highly protein bound, and drugs that alter its protein binding may alter its levels. Although protein binding interactions are usually not clinically relevant (unless metabolism is also inhibited, see 'Phenytoin + Sodium valproate', p.373), they can be important in interpreting drug levels.

(d) Valproate

Valproate undergoes glucuronidation and β-oxidation, and possibly also some metabolism via CYP2C isoenzymes. It can therefore undergo drug interactions via a variety of mechanisms. It acts as an inhibitor of glucuronidation and so may affect other drugs that undergo glucuronidation. Valproate also has nonlinear pharmacokinetics due to saturation of plasma protein binding, and so may interact with drugs that alter its protein binding.

(e) Newer anticonvulsants

Of the newer anticonvulsants, both felbamate and topiramate are weak inducers of CYP3A4. They may also inhibit CYP2C19. They are also themselves partially metabolised by the cytochrome P450 isoenzyme system, so may have their metabolism altered by other drugs such as the older enzyme-inducing anticonvulsants.

Gabapentin, lamotrigine, levetiracetam, tiagabine, vigabatrin and zonisamide do not appear to act as inhibitors or inducers of cytochrome P450 isoenzymes, and so appear to cause less drug interactions than the older anticonvulsants. Moreover, gabapentin, levetiracetam, and vigabatrin do not appear to be metabolised by the cytochrome P450 system, so appear to be little affected by drug interactions. Tiagabine and zonisamide are metabolised by the cytochrome P450 system, so may have their metabolism altered by other drugs such as the older enzyme-inducing anticonvulsants. Lamotrigine is metabolised by glucuronidation, and may be affected by inhibitors (e.g. valproate) or inducers (e.g. the older enzyme-inducing anticonvulsants) of this process. Lamotrigine may also act as an inducer of glucuronidation.

Table 11.1 Anticonvulsant drugs

Generic names	*Proprietary names*
Acetazolamide	Acetadiazol, Azomid, Carbinib, Defiltran, Diacarb, Diamox, Diluran, Diuramid, Edemox, Glaupax, Huma-Zolamide, Odemin, Uramox, Zolamox
Carbamazepine	Actinerval, Antafit, Arbil, Azepal, Bioneuryl, Bioreunil, Biston, Carba, Carbabeta, Carbactol Retard, Carbadura, Carbaflux, Carbagamma, Carbagen, Carbagramon, Carbalan, Carbamat, Carbatol, Carbatrol, Carbaval, Carbazene, Carbazep, Carbazina, Carbi, Carbium, Carmapine, Carmazin, Carpin, Carpine, Carzepine, Cizetol, Clostedal, CMP, Conformal, Convulsan, CP-Carba, Degranol, Deleptin, Epimaz, Epitol, Eposal, Equetro, espa-lepsin, Finlepsin, Fitzecalm, Fokalepsin, Gericarb, Hermolepsin, Mapezine, Mazetol, Neugeron, Neurotol, Neurotop, Novo-Carbamaz, Panitol, Sirtal, Stazepine, Taver, Tegretal, Tegretard, Tegretol, Tegrex, Tegrezin, Tegrital, Temporol, Teril, Timonil, Trimonil, Uni Carbamaz, Volutol, Zeptol
Ethosuximide	Emeside, Petinimid, Petnidan, Suxilep, Suxinutin, Zarondan, Zarontin
Ethylphenacemide (Pheneturide)	
Felbamate	Felbamyl, Felbatol, Taloxa
Fosphenytoin	Cerebyx, Cereneu, Prodilantin, Pro-Epanutin
Gabapentin	Dineurin, Gabamox, Gabarone, Gabatal, Gabatur, Gantin, Geabatan, Neuril, Neurontin, Neurostil, Normatol, Nupentin , Pendine, Progresse
Lamotrigine	Crisomet, Elmendos, Labileno, Lafigin, Lamepil, Lametec, Lamictal, Lamictin, Lamitor, Lamitrin, Lamodex, Lamogine, Neurium, Plexxo, Tradox
Levetiracetam	Keppra, Kepra
Mesuximide	Celontin, Petinutin
Methylphenobarbital	Mebaral
Oxcarbazepine	Alox, Apydan, Atoxecar, Auram, Aurene, Oxcarb, Oxcazen, Oxicodal, Oxrate, Timox, Tolep, Trileptal, Trileptin
Paraldehyde	Paral
Phenobarbital	Alepsal, Aparoxal, Aphenylbarbit, Barbitron, Bialminal, Comizial, Edhanol, Fenemal, Fenocris, Gardenal, Gardenale, Gratusminal, Kaneuron, Lethyl, Lumidrops, Luminal, Luminale, Luminaletas, Luminalette, Luminaletten, Luminalettes, Menobarb, Phenaemal, Phenaemaletten, Phenetone, Phenotal, Sevenal, Sevenaletta, Unifenobarb
Phenytoin	Aurantin, Biodan, Dantalin, Di-Hydan, Dilantin, Dintoina, Diphantoine, Diphedan, Ditoin, Ditomed, Epamin, Epanutin, Epelin, Epilan-D, Epilantine, Epinat, Epsolin, Eptoin, Etoina, Fenantoin, Fenidantoin S, Fenigramon, Fenital, Fenitenk, Feniton, Fenitron, Hidantal, Hidantina, Hidantoina, Hydantin, Lehydan, Lotoquis Simple, Neosidantoina, Nuctane, Opliphon, Phenhydan, Phenytek, Sinergina, Sodanton
Primidone	Cyral, Epidona, Liskantin, Mylepsinum, Mysoline, Prysoline, Resimatil, Sertan
Progabide	
Remacemide	
Retigabine	
Sodium valproate (Valproic acid)	Absenor, Atemperator, Convulex, Convulsofin, Criam, Delepsine, Depacon, Depakene, Depakin, Depakin Chrono, Depakine, Depakine Chrono, Depakine Crono, Depakote, Depalept, Depalept Chrono, Depamag, Deprakine, Deprakine Depot, Diplexil, Diplexil-R, Diproex, Encorate Chrono, Epiject, Epilex, Epilim, Epilim Chrono, Epival, Ergenyl, Ergenyl Chrono, Espa-Valept, Everiden, Exibral, Leptilan, Logical, Micropakine, Neuractin, Orfiril, Orlept, Pimiken, Tekaval, Valcote, Valnar, Valopin, Valpakine, Valparin, Valporal, Valprene, Valpro, Valpro Beta, Valprodura, Valproflux, Valprolept, Valprosid, Valrate CR, Valtec
Stiripentol	Diacomit
Sulthiame	
Tiagabine	Gabatril, Gabitril
Topiramate	Epitomax, Topamac, Topamate, Topamax, Topimax, Toprel
Valpromide	Depamide
Vigabatrin	Sabril, Sabrilan, Sabrilex
Zonisamide	Excegran, Zonegran

Anticonvulsants + Acetazolamide

Severe osteomalacia and rickets have been seen in a few patients on phenytoin, phenobarbital and primidone when they were concurrently treated with acetazolamide. A marked reduction in serum primidone levels with a loss in seizure control, rises in serum carbamazepine levels with toxicity, and rises in phenytoin levels have also been described in a very small number of patients given acetazolamide.

Clinical evidence

(a) Osteomalacia

Severe osteomalacia developed in 2 women on **phenytoin** or **primidone** and **phenobarbital** while they were taking acetazolamide 750 mg daily, despite a normal intake of calcium. When the acetazolamide was withdrawn, the hyperchloraemic acidosis found in both patients abated and their high urinary excretion of calcium fell by 50%.[1,2]

Similar cases have been described in 3 children on **phenytoin** and **primidone** with **phenobarbital** and/or metharbital,[3] who developed rickets.

(b) Reduced serum primidone levels

A patient on primidone showed an increased seizure-frequency and a virtual absence of primidone (or phenobarbital) in the serum when treated with acetazolamide 250 mg daily. Primidone levels rose when the acetazolamide was withdrawn, probably due to improved absorption. A subsequent study in 2 other patients found that acetazolamide had a small effect on the primidone in one, and no effect in the other.[4]

(c) Increased serum carbamazepine levels

A 9-year-old girl and two teenage boys, all of them on the highest dosages of carbamazepine tolerable without adverse effects, developed signs of toxicity after taking acetazolamide 250 to 750 mg daily. Their serum carbamazepine levels were found to have increased by about 25 to 50%. In one instance toxicity appeared within 48 hours.[5]

The seizure control of 54 children with grand mal and temporal lobe epilepsy was improved when acetazolamide 10 mg/kg daily was added to carbamazepine. Serum carbamazepine levels rose by 1 to 6 mg/l in 60% of the 33 patients sampled. Adverse effects developed in 10 children, and in 8 children this was within 1 to 10 days of starting the acetazolamide. The adverse effects responded to a reduction in the carbamazepine dosage.[6]

(d) Increased serum phenytoin levels

When acetazolamide was added to phenytoin treatment in 6 children, 5 of them had an increase in the phenytoin level (range 20% to 132%, representing an increase of 3 to 12.5 mg/l), and one had a slight decrease (20% or 3 mg/l) [values estimated from figure].[7]

Mechanism

Uncertain. Mild osteomalacia induced by anticonvulsants is a recognised phenomenon[8] (see also 'Vitamin D substances + Phenytoin', p.1041). It seems that this is exaggerated by acetazolamide, which increases urinary calcium excretion, possibly by causing systemic acidosis, which results from the reduced absorption of bicarbonate by the kidney. The changes in the anticonvulsant levels are not understood.

Importance and management

The documentation of all of these interactions is very limited, and their incidence is uncertain. Concurrent use should be monitored for the possible development of osteomalacia or altered anticonvulsant levels and steps taken to accommodate them. Withdraw the acetazolamide if necessary, or adjust the dosage of anticonvulsants appropriately. In the case of the children with rickets[3] the acetazolamide was withdrawn and high doses of vitamin D was given. It seems possible that other carbonic anhydrase inhibitors may behave like acetazolamide.

1. Mallette LE. Anticonvulsants, acetazolamide and osteomalacia. *N Engl J Med* (1975) 292, 668.
2. Mallette LE. Acetazolamide-accelerated anticonvulsant osteomalacia. *Arch Intern Med* (1977) 137, 1013–17.
3. Matsuda I, Takekoshi Y, Shida N, Fujieda K, Nagai B, Arashima S, Anakura M, Oka Y. Renal tubular acidosis and skeletal demineralization in patients on long-term anticonvulsant therapy. *J Pediatr* (1975) 87, 202–5.
4. Syversen GB, Morgan JP, Weintraub M, Myers GJ. Acetazolamide-induced interference with primidone absorption. *Arch Neurol* (1977) 34, 80–4.
5. McBride MC. Serum carbamazepine levels are increased by acetazolamide. *Ann Neurol* (1984) 16, 393.
6. Forsythe WI, Owens JR, Toothill C. Effectiveness of acetazolamide in the treatment of carbamazepine-resistant epilepsy in children. *Dev Med Child Neurol* (1981) 23, 761–9.
7. Norell E, Lilienbeg G, Gamstorp I. Systematic determination of the serum phenytoin level as an aid in the management of children with epilepsy. *Eur Neurol* (1975) 13, 232–44.
8. Anast CS. Anticonvulsant drugs and calcium metabolism. *N Engl J Med* (1975) 292, 567–8.

Anticonvulsants + Aciclovir

An isolated report describes a marked reduction in serum phenytoin and sodium valproate levels in a child given aciclovir. Seizure frequency increased.

Clinical evidence, mechanism, importance and management

A 7-year-old boy with epilepsy on **phenytoin, sodium valproate** and nitrazepam was started on oral aciclovir 1 g daily for 6 days. After 4 days his trough serum **phenytoin** levels had fallen from 17 to 5 micrograms/ml, and his trough **sodium valproate** levels from 32 to 22 micrograms/ml. When the aciclovir was stopped, the serum levels of both anticonvulsants rose, over 3 to 6 days. During the period when the anticonvulsant levels were restabilising, the seizure frequency markedly increased and his EEG worsened. The reason for this apparent interaction is not known, but the authors of the report suggest that the aciclovir may possibly have reduced the absorption of the anticonvulsants, in some way not understood.[1]

This appears to be the first and only report of an interaction between these drugs. Its general clinical importance is not known, but it would now seem prudent to be alert to the possibility of this interaction in any patient on either anticonvulsant if aciclovir is given. More study is needed.

1. Parmeggiani A, Riva R, Posar A, Rossi PG. Possible interaction between acyclovir and antiepileptic treatment. *Ther Drug Monit* (1995) 17, 312–15.

Anticonvulsants + Antineoplastics

Carbamazepine, phenytoin and sodium valproate serum levels can be reduced by several antineoplastic drug regimens and seizures can occur if the anticonvulsant dosages are not raised appropriately. In contrast, phenytoin toxicity has occurred with fluorouracil and fluorouracil prodrugs such as capecitabine, doxifluridine and tegafur. The effects of many antineoplastics are reduced or changed by enzyme-inducing anticonvulsants.

Clinical evidence

(a) Anticonvulsant levels reduced

A retrospective study reviewed the effects of 3 or more cycles of 72 hours of **carmustine** and **cisplatin** chemotherapy on the **phenytoin** levels of patients with brain tumours. Patients who vomited because of the chemotherapy were excluded, leaving 19 patients for assessment. A **phenytoin** dose increase was required in three-quarters of patients, which was, on average, 40% of the original dose (range 20 to 100%). The effect on **phenytoin** levels persisted after the chemotherapy had finished, with levels returning to normal 2 to 3 weeks later.[1]

There are many other case reports of a variety of types of chemotherapy having a similar effect on **phenytoin** levels.[2-9] Two reports also describe reduced **carbamazepine** levels,[5,6] and three reports describe reduced **valproate** levels.[5,10,11] Two reports suggest that **phenobarbital** levels are not affected.[3,4] See 'Table 11.2', (p.331) for details. For mention of a case of reduced efficacy of **phenytoin** with tegafur/uracil/folinic acid, see below.

(b) Anticonvulsant levels raised

Three patients with malignant brain tumours developed acute **phenytoin** toxicity associated with raised serum **phenytoin** levels when they were treated with ***UFT*** (**uracil** and **tegafur**, a prodrug of **fluorouracil**).[12] Another case of **phenytoin** toxicity has been reported with ***UFT***.[13] **Phenytoin** toxicity was also seen in a woman treated with combination therapy that included the fluorouracil prodrug **doxifluridine**.[14] Similarly, **phenytoin** toxicity has occurred in a patient given **capecitabine** (another prodrug of **fluorouracil**).[15] Although in the first report,[12] no interaction occurred in one of the patients when the ***UFT*** was replaced by **fluorouracil**, cases of **phenytoin** toxicity in 3 patients on **fluorouracil** with **folinic acid** have subsequently been reported.[15,16] Conversely, another report

Table 11.2 Cases of reduced anticonvulsant levels during antineoplastic therapy

Anticonvulsant	*Antineoplastic*	*Malignancy*	*Outcome*	*Refs*
Phenytoin	Cisplatin Vinblastine Bleomycin	Metastatic germ cell tumour	Estimated phenytoin level 15 micrograms/ml, but level only reached 2 micrograms/ml. Patient fitted.	1
Phenytoin Primidone	Cisplatin Vinblastine Bleomycin	Metastatic embryonal cell cancer	Phenytoin 800 mg daily gave a level of 15 micrograms/ml whilst on chemotherapy. After chemotherapy the same dose produced a toxic level of 42.8 micrograms/ml. Phenobarbital levels unaffected.	2
Phenytoin Phenobarbital	Vinblastine Carmustine Methotrexate	Lung cancer with brain metastases	Phenytoin levels fell from 9.4 to 5.6 micrograms/ml 24 h after vinblastine. Patient fitted. Phenytoin levels returned to normal 2 weeks after chemotherapy. Phenobarbital levels unaffected.	3
Phenytoin Carbamazepine Sodium valproate	Doxorubicin Cisplatin Cyclophosphamide Altretamine	Papillary adenocarcinoma of the ovaries	Seizures occurred 2 to 3 days after starting chemotherapy. All drug levels dropped to one-third or lower. Doses increased to compensate, which led to phentoin toxicity when the chemotherapy finished.	4
Phenytoin	Carboplatin	Small cell lung cancer with brain metastases	Phenytoin level dropped from 9.7 to 4.6 micrograms/ml 10 days into chemotherapy, resulting in seizures. Phenytoin dose had to be increased by 35% to achieve a level of 10.7 micrograms/ml.	5
Phenytoin	Dacarbazine Carmustine Cisplatin Tamoxifen	Malignant melanoma with brain metastases	Phenytoin level of only 2.5 micrograms/ml despite a loading 1 g dose and a daily dose of 500 mg phenytoin.	6
Phenytoin followed by Carbamazepine	Vincristine Cytarabine Hydroxycarbamide Duanorubicin Methotrexate Tioguanine Cyclophosphamide Carmustine	Stage IV T-cell lymphoma	Phenytoin failed to reach therapeutic levels and so was substituted with carbamazepine. Chemotherapy caused carbamazepine levels to drop below therapeutic levels resulting in seizures. Increasing the dose from 30 to 50 mg/kg/day prevented subtherapeutic levels.	7
Phenytoin	Methotrexate 6-Mercaptopurine Vincristine	Acute lymphoblastic leukaemia	Phenytoin levels dropped from 19.8 micrograms/ml on the day before chemotherapy to 3.6 micrograms/ml on the 6th day of chemotherapy.	8
Sodium valproate	Methotrexate (high dose)	Acute lymphoblastic leukaemia	A child had a seizure a few hours after methotrexate. Serum valproate levels reduced by 75%. The valproate dose was increased by 50% and clonazepam added.	9
Sodium valproate	Methotrexate Cytarabine Nimustine (by CSF perfusion)	Glioblastoma	CSF valproic acid levels reduced by 70% during the perfusion, but returned to normal levels within 7 hours.	10

1. Sylvester RK, Lewis FB, Caldwell KC, Lobell M, Perri R, Sawchuk RA. Impaired phenytoin bioavailability secondary to cisplatinum, vinblastine, and bleomycin. *Ther Drug Monit* (1984) 6, 302–5.
2. Fincham RW, Schottelius DD. Case report. Decreased phenytoin levels in antineoplastic therapy. *Ther Drug Monit* (1979) 1, 277–83.
3. Bollini P, Riva R, Albani F, Ida N, Cacciari L, Bollini C, Baruzzi A. Decreased phenytoin level during antineoplastic therapy: a case report. *Epilepsia* (1983) 24, 75–8.
4. Neef C, de Voogd-van der Straaten I. An interaction between cytostatic and anticonvulsant drugs. *Clin Pharmacol Ther* (1988) 43, 372–5.
5. Dofferhoff ASM, Berensen HH, Naalt Jvd, Haaxma-Reiche H, Smit EF, Postmus PE. Decreased phenytoin level after carboplatin treatment. *Am J Med* (1990) 89, 247–8.
6. Gattis WA, May DB. Possible interaction involving phenytoin, dexamethasone, and antineoplastic agents: a case report and review. Ann Pharmacother (1996) 30, 520–6.
7. Nahum MP, Ben Arush MW, Robinson E. Reduced plasma carbamazepine level during chemotherapy in a child with malignant lymphoma. *Acta Paediatr Scand* (1990) 79, 873–5.
8. Jarosinski PF, Moscow JA, Alexander MS, Lesko LJ, Balis FM, Poplack DG. Altered phenytoin clearance during intensive treatment for acute lymphoblastic leukemia. *J Pediatr* (1988) 112, 996–9.
9. Schrøder H, Østergaard JR. Interference of high-dose methotrexate in the metabolism of valproate? *Pediatr Hematol Oncol* (1994) 11, 445–9.
10. Morikawa N, Mori T, Abe T, Kawashima H, Takeyama M, Hori S. Pharmacokinetics of cytosine arabinoside, methotrexate, nimustine and valproic acid in cerebrospinal fluid during cerebrospinal fluid perfusion chemotherapy. *Biol Pharm Bull* (2000) 23, 784–7.

describes lack of **phenytoin** efficacy in a patient on ***UFT*** with **folinic acid**, attributed to the effect of the **folinic acid** on **phenytoin** levels[17] (see 'Anticonvulsants + Folic acid', p.335).

(c) Antineoplastic effects reduced or altered

See 'Anthracyclines; Doxorubicin + Barbiturates', p.451, 'Busulfan + Phenytoin', p.456, 'Cyclophosphamide or Ifosfamide + Barbiturates', p.459, 'Cyclophosphamide or Ifosfamide + Phenytoin', p.463, 'Etoposide + Anticonvulsants', p.465, 'Imatinib + Miscellaneous', p.471, 'Irinotecan + Anticonvulsants', p.472, 'Methotrexate + Anticonvulsants', p.477, 'Procarbazine + Anticonvulsants', p.486, 'Streptozocin + Phenytoin', p.487, 'Taxanes; Paclitaxel + Anticonvulsants', p.491, 'Teniposide + Anticonvulsants', p.492, 'Topotecan + Phenytoin', p.494, 'Toremifene + Anticonvulsants', p.495.

Mechanism

Not fully understood, but a suggested reason for the fall in serum anticonvulsant levels is that these antineoplastics damage the intestinal wall, which reduces the absorption of the anticonvulsants. Other mechanisms may also have some part to play. The raised serum phenytoin levels possibly occur because the liver metabolism of the phenytoin is reduced by these antineoplastics. Changes in plasma protein binding may also have been involved.

Importance and management

Information is scattered and incomplete. However, it appears that both altered anticonvulsant levels and altered antineoplastic levels can occur, possibly leading to loss of efficacy or toxicity. Where possible, it may be prudent to avoid concurrent use of enzyme-inducing anticonvulsants and antineoplastics. If this is not possible, serum anticonvulsant levels should be closely monitored during treatment with any of these antineoplastics, making dosage adjustments as necessary, and the efficacy of the antineoplastics should also be closely monitored.

1. Grossman SA, Sheidler VR, Gilbert MR. Decreased phenytoin levels in patients receiving chemotherapy. *Am J Med* (1989) 87, 505–10.
2. Sylvester RK, Lewis FB, Caldwell KC, Lobell M, Perri R, Sawchuk RA. Impaired phenytoin bioavailability secondary to cisplatinum, vinblastine, and bleomycin. *Ther Drug Monit* (1984) 6, 302–5.
3. Fincham RW, Schottelius DD. Case report. Decreased phenytoin levels in antineoplastic therapy. *Ther Drug Monit* (1979) 1, 277–83.
4. Bollini P, Riva R, Albani F, Ida N, Cacciari L, Bollini C, Baruzzi A. Decreased phenytoin level during antineoplastic therapy: a case report. *Epilepsia* (1983) 24, 75–8.
5. Neef C, de Voogd-van der Straaten I. An interaction between cytostatic and anticonvulsant drugs. *Clin Pharmacol Ther* (1988) 43, 372–5.
6. Nahum MP, Ben Arush MW, Robinson E. Reduced plasma carbamazepine level during chemotherapy in a child with malignant lymphoma. *Acta Paediatr Scand* (1990) 79, 873–5.
7. Jarosinski PF, Moscow JA, Alexander MS, Lesko LJ, Balis FM, Poplack DG. Altered phenytoin clearance during intensive treatment for acute lymphoblastic leukemia. *J Pediatr* (1988) 112, 996–9.
8. Dofferhoff ASM, Berensen HH, Naalt Jvd, Haaxma-Reiche H, Smit EF, Postmus PE. Decreased phenytoin level after carboplatin treatment. *Am J Med* (1990) 89, 247–8.
9. Gattis WA, May DB. Possible interaction involving phenytoin, dexamethasone, and antineoplastic agents: a case report and review. *Ann Pharmacother* (1996) 30, 520–6.
10. Schrøder H, Østergaard JR. Interference of high-dose methotrexate in the metabolism of valproate? *Pediatr Hematol Oncol* (1994) 11, 445–9.
11. Morikawa N, Mori T, Abe T, Kawashima H, Takeyama M, Hori S. Pharmacokinetics of cytosine arabinoside, methotrexate, nimustine and valproic acid in cerebrospinal fluid during cerebrospinal fluid perfusion chemotherapy. *Biol Pharm Bull* (2000) 23, 784–7.
12. Wakisaka S, Shimauchi M, Kaji Y, Nonaka A, Kinoshita K. Acute phenytoin intoxication associated with the antineoplastic agent UFT. *Fukuoka Igaku Zasshi* (1990) 81, 192–6.
13. Errea-Abad JM, González-Igual J, Eito-Cativiela JL, Gastón-Añaños J. Intoxicación aguda por fenitoína debida a interacción col el derivado fluoropirimidínico. *Rev Neurol* (1998) 27, 1066–7.
14. Konishi H, Morita K, Minouchi T, Nakajima M, Matsuda M, Yamaji A. Probable metabolic interaction of doxifluridine with phenytoin. *Ann Pharmacother* (2002) 36, 831–4.
15. Brickell K, Parter D, Thompson P. Phenytoin toxicity due to fluoropyrimidines (5FU/capecitabine): three case reports. *Br J Cancer* (2003) 89, 615–16.
16. Gilbar PJ, Brodribb TR. Phenytoin and fluorouracil interaction. *Ann Pharmacother* (2001) 35, 1367–70.
17. Veldhorst-Janssen NML, Boersma HH, de Krom MCTFM, van Rijswijk REN. Oral tegafur/folinic acid chemotherapy decreases phenytoin efficacy. *Br J Cancer* (2004) 90, 745.

Anticonvulsants + Ayurvedic medicines

A case report, and an *animal* study, indicate that an anticonvulsant Ayurvedic herbal preparation, SRC (Shankhapushpi), can markedly reduce serum phenytoin levels, leading to an increased seizure frequency if the phenytoin dosage is not raised. Phenobarbital levels appear to be unchanged. Liv-52 increased carbamazepine levels in an *animal* study.

Clinical evidence

(a) Liv.52

A study in *monkeys* found that Liv.52 syrup increased the AUC and elimination half-life of **carbamazepine** by about 50% when both drugs were given for 14 days. This change was not seen in a single-dose study.[1]

(b) Shankhapushpi (SRC)

An epileptic man on **phenobarbital** 120 mg daily and **phenytoin** 500 mg daily developed an increased seizure frequency when Shankhapushpi (*SRC*) three times a day was added. His serum **phenytoin** levels were found to have fallen from 18.2 to 9.3 micrograms/ml whereas his **phenobarbital** levels were little changed. When the *SRC* was stopped the **phenytoin** serum levels climbed to 30.3 micrograms/ml, and toxicity was seen. A reduction in the dose of **phenytoin** to 400 mg daily resulted in levels of 16.2 micrograms/ml. Another possible case was reported.[2,3]

Subsequent studies in *rats* found that *SRC* reduces the serum levels of **phenytoin** by about half.[4] These pharmacokinetic effects were only seen after multiple doses, not single doses of **phenytoin**. A pharmacodynamic interaction, resulting in reduced antiepileptic activity was also noted.[2,4,5]

Mechanism

Not understood. Liv-52 may decrease the metabolism of carbamazepine.[1] There is evidence from *animal* studies that *SRC* may affect the pharmacokinetics of the phenytoin and possibly its pharmacodynamics as well,[2,4] thereby reducing its anticonvulsant activity. It is also suggested that one of the ingredients of *SRC* may have some anticonvulsant activity.[4]

Importance and management

Information about these interactions appears to be limited to these reports. Although the data for Liv-52 is from an *animal* study, the findings suggest that caution is required when combining this with carbamazepine, being alert for signs of toxicity. It may be prudent to monitor carbamazepine levels. Liv-52 is prepared from *Capparis spinosa, Phyllanthus amarus, Tamarix gallica, Achillea millefolium, Terminalia arjuna, Cassia occidentalis, Cichorium intybus,* and *Solanum nigrum*.

Shankhapushpi (SRC) is given because it has some anticonvulsant activity (demonstrated in *animal* studies[4,5]), but there is little point in combining it with phenytoin if the outcome is a fall in serum phenytoin levels, accompanied by an increase in fit-frequency. For this reason concurrent use should be avoided. *SRC* is a syrup prepared from *Convolvulus pluricaulis* leaves, *Nardostachys jatamansi* rhizomes, *Onosma bracteatum* leaves and flowers and the whole plant of *Centella asiatica, Nepeta hindostana* and *Nepeta elliptica*.[4] The first two of these plants appear to contain compounds with anticonvulsant activity.[6,7] Phenobarbital possibly does not interact.

It has been suggested that adulteration of traditional medicines with various anticonvulsants[8,9] may be an unexpected factor in these interactions.

1. Dixit RK, Kumar N, Garg SK, Bhargava VK. Effect of Liv-52 an ayurvedic preparation on the pharmacokinetic profile of carbamazepine in monkeys. *Indian J Physiol Pharmacol* (2001) 45, 378–80.
2. Kshirsagar NA, Personal communication 1991.
3. Kshirsagar NA, Dalvi SS, Joshi MV, Sharma SS, Sant HM, Shah PU, Chandra RS. Phenytoin and ayurvedic preparation – clinically important interaction in epileptic patients. *J Assoc Physicians India* (1992) 40, 354–5.
4. Dandekar UP, Chandra RS, Dalvi SS, Joshi MV, Gokhale PC, Sharma AV, Shah PU, Kshirsagar NA. Analysis of a clinically important interaction between phenytoin and Shankhapushpi, an Ayurvedic preparation. *J Ethnopharmacol* (1992) 35, 285–8.
5. Kshirsagar NA, Chandra RS, Dandekar UP, Dalvi SS, Sharma AV, Joshi MV, Gokhale PC, Shah PU. Investigation of a novel clinically important interaction between phenytoin and Ayurvedic preparation. *Eur J Pharmacol* (1990) 183, 519.
6. Sharma VN, Barar FSK, Khanna NK, Mahawar MM. Some pharmacological actions of *convolvulus pluricaulis* chois — an Indian indigenous herb. *Indian J Med Res* (1965) 53, 871–6.
7. Arora RB. In: Nardostachys jatamansi: a chemical, pharmacological and clinical appraisal. Pharmacological actions of Jatamansi. *Indian Council of Medical Research Publications, Delhi* (1965), 136.
8. Bharucha NE. Co-prescription of conventional and 'alternative' medicines. *J R Coll Physicians Lond* (1999) 33, 285.
9. Gogtay NJ, Dalvi SS, Rane CT, Pawar HS, Narayana RV, Shah PU, Kshirsagar NA. A story of "ayurvedic" tablets and misled epileptic patients. *J Assoc Physicians India* (1999) 47, 1116.

Anticonvulsants + Calcium carbimide or Disulfiram

Phenytoin serum levels are markedly and rapidly increased by the concurrent use of disulfiram. Phenytoin toxicity can develop. There is evidence that phenobarbital and carbamazepine are not

affected by disulfiram, and that phenytoin is not affected by calcium carbimide.

Clinical evidence

The serum **phenytoin** levels of 4 patients on long-term treatment rose by 100 to 500% over a 9-day period when they also took disulfiram 400 mg daily. **Phenytoin** levels were still rising even 3 to 4 days after the disulfiram was withdrawn. Levels had still not returned to normal 14 days after the disulfiram was withdrawn. Two patients developed signs of mild **phenytoin** toxicity.[1] In a follow-up study in two of the patients, one of them developed ataxia and both had a rise in serum **phenytoin** levels, of 25 and 50% respectively, during 5 days of disulfiram treatment.[2]

Disulfiram increased the half-life of **phenytoin** from 11 to 19 hours in 10 healthy subjects.[3] There are also other case reports describing this interaction.[4-7]

Phenobarbital levels (from **primidone** in 3 patients and **phenobarbital** in one patient) fluctuated by about 10% when disulfiram was given for 9 days.[1,2]

Carbamazepine also appears not to interact with disulfiram. Signs of toxicity disappeared in a patient when **phenytoin** was replaced by **carbamazepine**,[6] and the observation that disulfiram does not interact with **carbamazepine** was confirmed in a study of 5 epileptic, non-alcoholic patients.[8]

A study in 4 patients found that calcium carbimide 50 mg daily for a week followed by 100 mg for 2 weeks had no effect on serum **phenytoin** levels.[2]

Mechanism

Disulfiram inhibits the liver enzymes concerned with the metabolism of phenytoin (possibly the cytochrome P450 isoenzyme CYP2C9) thereby prolonging its stay in the body and resulting in a rise in its serum levels, to toxic concentrations in some instances. One study concluded that the inhibition was non-competitive.[7]

Importance and management

The interaction between phenytoin and disulfiram is established, moderately well documented, clinically important and potentially serious. It seems to occur in most patients and develops rapidly. Recovery may take 2 to 3 weeks after the disulfiram is withdrawn. It has been suggested that the dosage of phenytoin could be reduced to accommodate the interaction, but it may be difficult to maintain the balance required. Monitor very closely if both drugs are given.[2]

Non-interacting anticonvulsants include phenobarbital or carbamazepine.

Unlike disulfiram, calcium carbimide appears not to interact.

1. Olesen OV. Disulfiramum (Antabuse®) as inhibitor of phenytoin metabolism. *Acta Pharmacol Toxicol (Copenh)* (1966) 24, 317–22.
2. Olesen OV. The influence of disulfiram and calcium carbimide on the serum diphenylhydantoin excretion of HPPH in the urine. *Arch Neurol* (1967) 16, 642–4.
3. Svendsen TL, Kristensen MB, Hansen JM, Skovsted L. The influence of disulfiram on the half-life and metabolic clearance rate of diphenylhydantoin and tolbutamide in man. *Eur J Clin Pharmacol* (1976) 9, 439–41.
4. Kiørboe E. Phenytoin intoxication during treatment with Antabuse®. *Epilepsia* (1966) 7, 246–9.
5. Kiørboe E. Antabus som årsag til forgiftning med fenytoin. *Ugeskr Laeger* (1966) 128, 1531–6.
6. Dry J, Pradalier A. Intoxication par la phénytoïne au cours d'une association thérapeutique avec le disulfirame. *Therapie* (1973) 28, 799–802.
7. Taylor JW, Alexander B, Lyon LW. Mathematical analysis of a phenytoin-disulfiram interaction. *Am J Hosp Pharm* (1981) 38, 93–5.
8. Krag B, Dam M, Angelo H, Christensen JM. Influence of disulfiram on the serum concentration of carbamazepine in patients with epilepsy. *Acta Neurol Scand* (1981) 63, 395–8.

Anticonvulsants + Calcium channel blockers

(A) Anticonvulsant effects: both diltiazem and verapamil can increase serum carbamazepine levels causing toxicity. Diltiazem can also increase serum phenytoin levels. A single case report describes phenytoin toxicity with nifedipine but, like amlodipine, usually it appears not to interact. A single case report describes neurological toxicity in a patient on phenytoin and carbamazepine given isradipine.

(B) Calcium channel blocker effects altered: the serum levels of felodipine and nimodipine are very markedly reduced by carbamazepine, phenobarbital and phenytoin, but felodipine levels are only modestly reduced by oxcarbazepine. Verapamil levels may also be very much reduced by phenobarbital and phenytoin. Phenytoin reduces nisoldipine levels. Nimodipine levels are raised by sodium valproate.

Clinical evidence

(A) Anticonvulsant effects

(a) Carbamazepine + Diltiazem

An epileptic patient on carbamazepine 400 mg in the morning and 600 mg in the evening developed signs of toxicity (dizziness, nausea, ataxia and diplopia) within 2 days of starting to take diltiazem 60 mg three times daily. His serum carbamazepine levels had risen by about 40% to 21 mg/l, but fell once again when the diltiazem was stopped. No interaction occurred when the diltiazem was replaced by **nifedipine** 20 mg three times daily.[1] Other case reports describe carbamazepine toxicity and a rise in serum levels of up to fourfold in a total of 10 patients also given diltiazem.[2-6] One patient required a 62% reduction in the carbamazepine dose.[2] Another patient had a marked fall in serum carbamazepine levels of 54% when diltiazem was stopped.[7]

(b) Carbamazepine + Isradipine

A man on carbamazepine and phenytoin developed neurological toxicity while on isradipine, which was attributed to an interaction between the phenytoin and isradipine.[8] However, although carbamazepine levels remained within normal limits, a commentator suggested that an interaction between carbamazepine and isradipine was plausible.[9]

(c) Carbamazepine + Nifedipine

Nifedipine 20 mg twice daily for 2 weeks did not affect the steady-state concentrations of carbamazepine in 12 epileptic patients.[10] Similarly, a retrospective study of 5 patients suggested that nifedipine does not usually cause raised carbamazepine levels or toxicity.[4] A man had a marked rise in serum carbamazepine levels when nifedipine was replaced by **diltiazem**. When **diltiazem** was replaced by **amlodipine**, his carbamazepine levels returned to normal, suggesting that neither nifedipine nor **amlodipine** interact with carbamazepine.[11] Another patient had no change in carbamazepine levels when given nifedipine.[1]

(d) Carbamazepine + Verapamil

Carbamazepine toxicity developed in 6 epileptic patients within 36 to 96 hours of starting verapamil 120 mg three times daily. The symptoms disappeared when the verapamil was withdrawn. Total carbamazepine serum levels had risen by 46% (a 33% rise in free plasma carbamazepine concentrations). Rechallenge of two of the patients who only showed mild toxicity with a lower dose of verapamil 120 mg twice a day caused a similar rise in serum verapamil levels, again with mild toxicity. This report also describes another patient with elevated serum carbamazepine levels while also taking verapamil.[12]

Carbamazepine toxicity is described in 3 other patients, again caused by verapamil.[13,14] The verapamil was successfully replaced by **nifedipine** in one patient.[13]

(e) Oxcarbazepine + Verapamil

Oxcarbazepine 450 mg twice daily was given to 10 healthy subjects who were then additionally given verapamil 120 mg twice daily for 5 days. The AUC of the monohydroxy derivative of the oxcarbazepine (the active metabolite) fell by about 20% but oxcarbazepine levels were unaltered.[15]

(f) Phenytoin + Diltiazem

Elevated serum phenytoin levels and signs of toxicity developed in 2 out of 14 patients on phenytoin when they were given diltiazem.[4] A patient taking 250 mg phenytoin twice daily developed signs of toxicity within 2 weeks of starting diltiazem 240 mg every 8 hours.[16]

(g) Phenytoin + Isradipine

A man on carbamazepine and phenytoin developed neurological toxicity while on isradipine, which the authors attributed to a pharmacokinetic or pharmacodynamic interaction between the phenytoin and isradipine.[8] However, a commentator considered that an interaction between the carbamazepine and isradipine was more plausible.[9]

(h) Phenytoin + Nifedipine

An isolated report describes phenytoin toxicity in a man on phenytoin, 3 weeks after he started to take nifedipine 30 mg daily. His serum phenytoin level was 30.4 micrograms/ml. The nifedipine was stopped, and over the next 2 weeks his serum phenytoin levels fell to 10.5 micrograms/ml. A further 2 weeks later all the symptoms had resolved.[17] However, a retrospective study of 8 patients suggested that nifedipine does not usually interact.[4]

(B) Calcium channel blocker effects altered

(a) Felodipine

After taking felodipine 10 mg daily for 4 days, 10 epileptics on **carbamazepine**, **phenytoin**, **phenobarbital**, or **carbamazepine** with **phenytoin**, had markedly reduced serum felodipine levels (peak levels of 1.6 nanomol/l compared with 8.9 nanomol/l in 12 control subjects). The felodipine bioavailability was reduced to 6.6%.[18] Another study in 8 subjects found that the AUC of felodipine was reduced by only 28% by **oxcarbazepine** 600 to 900 mg daily for a week.[19]

(b) Nifedipine

A study in 12 epileptics on long-term treatment with **carbamazepine** found that the AUC of nifedipine 20 mg was only 22% of the values seen in 12 healthy subjects not taking **carbamazepine**.[10]

After taking **phenobarbital** 100 mg daily for 2 weeks the clearance of a single 20-mg dose of nifedipine in a 'cocktail' also containing sparteine, mephenytoin and antipyrine was increased almost threefold in 15 healthy subjects. The nifedipine AUC was reduced by about 60%.[20]

(c) Nimodipine

A study in 8 epileptic patients on long-term treatment with **phenobarbital**, **carbamazepine** with **phenobarbital**, **carbamazepine** with **clobazam**, or **carbamazepine** with **phenytoin** found that the AUC of a single 60-mg oral dose of nimodipine was only about 15% of that obtained from a group of healthy subjects. In another group of epileptic patients on **sodium valproate**, the AUC of nimodipine was about 50% higher than in the control group.[21]

(d) Nisoldipine

Twelve epileptic patients on long-term **phenytoin** treatment and 12 healthy subjects were given single 40- or 20-mg doses of nisoldipine. The mean nisoldipine AUCs (normalised for a 20-mg dose) were 1.6 micrograms/l per hour for the epileptics, and 15.2 micrograms/l per hour for the healthy subjects.[22] The authors of this study predict that **carbamazepine** and **phenobarbital** will interact similarly, because they, like **phenytoin**, induce the cytochrome P450 isoenzyme CYP3A4. However, this needs confirmatory clinical studies.

(e) Verapamil

A study in 7 healthy subjects found **phenobarbital** 100 mg daily for 3 weeks increased the clearance of verapamil 80 mg every 6 hours fourfold and reduced the bioavailability fivefold.[23]

A woman on **phenytoin** given verapamil had persistently subnormal serum verapamil levels (less than 50 nanograms/ml) despite increases in the verapamil dosage from 80 mg twice daily to 160 mg three times daily. When the **phenytoin** was stopped, her serum verapamil levels rose to the expected concentrations.[24]

Mechanism

It would appear that diltiazem and verapamil inhibit the metabolism of carbamazepine by the cytochrome P450 isoenzyme CYP3A4, thereby reducing its loss from the body and increasing serum levels. Diltiazem may also inhibit the metabolism of phenytoin. In contrast, the anticonvulsants are well recognised as enzyme inducers, which can increase the metabolism of the calcium channel blockers by the liver, resulting in a very rapid loss from the body.

Importance and management

(A) Anticonvulsant and toxic effects increased

Information about the effects of calcium channel blockers on anticonvulsants is limited, but what is known indicates that if verapamil or diltiazem are given with carbamazepine, or diltiazem is given with phenytoin, the anticonvulsant dosage may possibly need to be reduced to avoid toxicity. A 50% reduction in the dose of carbamazepine has been suggested if diltiazem is to be used.[5] Nifedipine and amlodipine normally appear to be non-interacting alternatives, but there is an isolated case of a nifedipine interaction with phenytoin. There is also an isolated case of possible carbamazepine or phenytoin toxicity with isradipine. Oxcarbazepine appears to be a non-interacting alternative for carbamazepine. There appears to be no information about the effects of calcium channel blockers on other anticonvulsants.

(B) Calcium channel blocker effects altered

Carbamazepine, phenobarbital and phenytoin markedly reduce felodipine and nimodipine levels, and both phenobarbital and phenytoin can have the same effect on verapamil, and possibly nifedipine. Nisoldipine levels are reduced by phenytoin, and are predicted to be reduced by carbamazepine and phenobarbital. A considerable increase in the dosage of these calcium channel blockers will probably be needed in epileptic patients taking these drugs, but oxcarbazepine has only a moderate effect. The nimodipine dosage may need to be reduced with sodium valproate. There is no direct information of interactions with other calcium channel blockers, but be alert for evidence of reduced effects with others metabolised in a similar way.

1. Brodie MJ, Macphee GJA. Carbamazepine neurotoxicity precipitated by diltiazem. *BMJ* (1986) 292, 1170–1.
2. Eimer M, Carter BL. Elevated serum carbamazepine concentrations following diltiazem initiation. *Drug Intell Clin Pharm* (1987) 21, 340–2.
3. Ahmad S. Diltiazem-carbamazepine interaction. *Am Heart J* (1990) 120, 1485.
4. Bahls FH, Ozuna J, Ritchie DE. Interactions between calcium channel blockers and the anticonvulsants carbamazepine and phenytoin. *Neurology* (1991) 41, 740–2.
5. Shaughnessy AF, Mosley MR. Elevated carbamazepine levels associated with diltiazem use. *Neurology* (1992) 42, 937–8.
6. Maoz E, Grossman E, Thaler M, Rosenthal T. Carbamazepine neurotoxic reaction after administration of diltiazem. *Arch Intern Med* (1992) 152, 2503–4.
7. Gadde K, Calabrese JR. Diltiazem effect on carbamazepine levels in manic depression. *J Clin Psychopharmacol* (1990) 10, 378–9.
8. Cachat F, Tufro A. Phenytoin/isradipine interaction causing severe neurologic toxicity. *Ann Pharmacother* (2002) 36: 1399–1402.
9. Hauben M. Comment: phenytoin/isradipine interaction causing severe neurologic toxicity. *Ann Pharmacother* (2002) 36: 1974–5.
10. Routledge PA, Soryal I, Eve MD, Williams J, Richens A, Hall R. Reduced bioavailability of nifedipine in patients with epilepsy receiving anticonvulsants. *Br J Clin Pharmacol* (1998) 45, 196P.
11. Cuadrado A, Sánchez MB, Peralta G, González M, Verdejo A, Amat G, Bravo J,Fdez Cortizo MJ, Adín J, De Cos MA, Mediavilla A, Armijo JA. Carbamazepine-amlodipine: a free interaction association? *Methods Find Exp Clin Pharmacol* (1996) 18 (Suppl C), 65.
12. Macphee GJA, McInnes GT, Thompson GG, Brodie MJ. Verapamil potentiates carbamazepine neurotoxicity: a clinically important inhibitory interaction. *Lancet* (1986) i, 700–3.
13. Beattie B, Biller J, Mehlhaus B, Murray M. Verapamil-induced carbamazepine neurotoxicity. *Eur Neurol* (1988) 28, 104–5.
14. Price WA, DiMarzio LR. Verapamil-carbamazepine neurotoxicity. *J Clin Psychiatry* (1988) 49, 80.
15. Krämer G, Tettenborn B, Flesch G. Oxcarbazepine-verapamil drug interaction in healthy volunteers. *Epilepsia* (1991) 32 (Suppl 1), 70–1.
16. Clarke WR, Horn JR, Kawabori I, Gurtel S. Potentially serious drug interactions secondary to high-dose diltiazem used in the treatment of pulmonary hypertension. *Pharmacotherapy* (1993) 13, 402–5.
17. Ahmad S. Nifedipine-phenytoin interaction. *J Am Coll Cardiol* (1984) 3, 1582.
18. Capewell S, Freestone S, Critchley JAJH, Pottage A, Prescott LF. Reduced felodipine bioavailability in patients taking anticonvulsants. *Lancet* (1988) ii, 480–2.
19. Zaccara G, Gangemi PF, Bendoni L, Menge GP, Schwabe S, Monza GC. Influence of single and repeated doses of oxcarbazepine on the pharmacokinetic profile of felodipine. *Ther Drug Monit* (1993) 15, 39–42.
20. Schellens JHM, van der Wart JHF, Brugman M, Breimer DD. Influence of enzyme induction and inhibition on the oxidation of nifedipine, sparteine, mephenytoin and antipyrine in humans assessed by a cocktail study design. *J Pharmacol Exp Ther* (1989) 249, 638–45.
21. Tartara A, Galimberti CA, Manni R, Parietti L, Zucca C, Baasch H, Caresia L, Mück W, Barzaghi N, Gatti G, Perucca E. Differential effects of valproic acid and enzyme-inducing anticonvulsants on nimodipine pharmacokinetics in epileptic patients. *Br J Clin Pharmacol* (1991) 32, 335–40.
22. Michelucci R, Cipolla G, Passarelli D, Gatti G, Ochan M, Heinig R, Tassinari CA, Perucca E. Reduced plasma nisoldipine concentrations in phenytoin-treated patients with epilepsy. *Epilepsia* (1996) 37, 1107–10.
23. Rutledge DR, Pieper JA, Sirmans SM, Mirvis DM. Verapamil disposition after phenobarbital treatment. *Clin Pharmacol Ther* (1987) 41, 245.
24. Woodcock BG, Kirsten R, Nelson K, Rietbrock S, Hopf R, Kaltenbach M. A reduction in verapamil concentrations with phenytoin. *N Engl J Med* (1991) 325, 1179.

Anticonvulsants + Chinese herbal medicines

Paeoniae Radix had no effect on the pharmacokinetics of valproic acid. *Animal* studies suggest that Sho-saiko-to may reduce the absorption of carbamazepine.

Clinical evidence

(a) Carbamazepine

In *animals,* pretreatment with **Sho-saiko-to** did not affect the metabolism of carbamazepine, but simultaneous use reduced gastrointestinal absorption. **Sho-saiko-to** is a powder produced from a water extract of 7 herbs: Bupleuri root, Pinelliae tubers, Scutellariae root, Zizyphi fruit, Ginseng root, Glycyrrhizae root and Zingiberis rhizome.[1]

(b) Valproic acid

The pharmacokinetics of a single 200-mg dose of valproic acid were unaffected by 1.2 g of a powder extract of **Paeoniae Radix** daily for 7 days had no effect on in 6 healthy subjects. **Paeoniae Radix** is the dried root of *Paeonia lactiflora*.[2]

Mechanism

Sho-saiko-to delays gastric emptying, and so may delay or reduce gastrointestinal absorption of other drugs.

Importance and management

Traditional Chinese herbal medicines are commonly used alongside conventional Western drugs, but little is known about potential interactions. There appears to be no pharmacokinetic interaction between Paeoniae Radix and valproate. Sho-saiko-to may have the potential to reduce carbamazepine absorption, but this requires confirmation in humans. Note that adulteration of Chinese medicines with various anticonvulsants may lead to unexpected toxicity.[3]

1. Ohnishi N, Okada K, Yoshioka M, Kuroda K, Nagasawa K, Takara K, Yokoyama T. Studies on interactions between traditional herbal and Western medicines. V. Effects of Sho-saiko-to (Xiao-Cai-hu-Tang) on the pharmacokinetics of carbamazepine in rats. *Biol Pharm Bull* (2002) 25, 1461–6.
2. Chen LC, Chou MH, Lin MF, Yang LL. Lack of pharmacokinetic interaction between valproic acid and a traditional Chinese medicine, Paeoniae Radix, in healthy volunteers. *J Clin Pharm Ther* (2000) 25, 453–9.
3. Lau KK, Lai CK, Chan AYM. Phenytoin poisoning after using Chinese proprietary medicines. *Hum Exp Toxicol* (2000) 19, 385–6.

Anticonvulsants + Dextromethorphan

Dextromethorphan appears not to affect the serum levels of carbamazepine or phenytoin.

Clinical evidence, mechanism, importance and management

A double-blind crossover study in epileptic patients with severe complex partial seizures, 5 on **carbamazepine** and 4 on **phenytoin**, found that dextromethorphan 120 mg daily in liquid form (*Delsym*) over 3 months had no effect on the serum anticonvulsant levels. There was a non-significant alteration in the complex partial seizure and tonic-clonic seizure frequency.[1]

1. Fisher RS, Cysyk BJ, Lesser RP, Pontecorvo MJ, Ferkany JT, Schwerdt PR, Hart J, Gordon B. Dextromethorphan for treatment of complex partial seizures. *Neurology* (1990) 40, 547–9.

Anticonvulsants + Dextropropoxyphene (Propoxyphene)

Carbamazepine serum levels can be raised by dextropropoxyphene. Toxicity may develop unless suitable dosage reductions are made. A trivial or only modest rise in serum phenytoin or phenobarbital levels may occur so that the development of toxicity is unlikely in most patients. Oxcarbazepine appears not to interact with dextropropoxyphene.

Clinical evidence

(a) Carbamazepine

The observation of toxicity (headache, dizziness, ataxia, nausea, tiredness) in patients taking both carbamazepine and dextropropoxyphene prompted further study. Five carbamazepine-treated patients given dextropropoxyphene 65 mg three times daily had a mean rise in serum carbamazepine levels of 65%, and 3 showed evidence of carbamazepine toxicity. Carbamazepine levels were not taken in a further 2 patients because they withdrew after 2 days of treatment due to adverse effects.[1,2] In a further study a 66% rise in carbamazepine levels was seen after 6 days' treatment with dextropropoxyphene.[3]

Carbamazepine toxicity due to this interaction is reported elsewhere,[4-7] and rises in trough serum carbamazepine levels of 69% to 600% have been described.[8] A study in the elderly compared groups of patients taking either carbamazepine or dextropropoxyphene alone, with patients on both drugs (21 subjects). The carbamazepine dose was about a third lower in those receiving combined treatment, yet the mean serum carbamazepine levels were still 25% higher than in the patients not taking dextropropoxyphene. The prevalence of adverse effects was also higher in patients on both drugs.[9]

(b) Oxcarbazepine

Dextropropoxyphene 65 mg three times daily for 7 days did not affect the steady-state levels of the active metabolite of oxcarbazepine in 7 patients with epilepsy or trigeminal neuralgia.[10]

(c) Phenobarbital

An average rise in the serum phenobarbital levels of 20% was seen in 4 epileptic patients after they took dextropropoxyphene 65 mg three times a day for a week.[3]

(d) Phenytoin

Only a very small rise in serum phenytoin levels occurred in 6 patients who were also given dextropropoxyphene 65 mg three times daily for 6 to 13 days.[3] In contrast, a review briefly mentions one patient who developed toxic serum phenytoin levels while taking dextropropoxyphene in doses of up to 600 mg daily on an as-required basis.[11]

Mechanism

Uncertain. It is suggested that dextropropoxyphene inhibits the metabolism of carbamazepine by the liver, leading to its accumulation in the body.[1,2] This may also be true to a lesser extent for phenobarbital.

Importance and management

The interaction between carbamazepine and dextropropoxyphene is very well established and clinically important. If concurrent use is necessary reduce the dosage of carbamazepine appropriately to prevent the development of toxicity. In many cases it may be simpler to use a non-interacting analgesic, although the occasional single dose of dextropropoxyphene probably does not matter. The concurrent use of dextropropoxyphene and either phenytoin or phenobarbital need not be avoided, but since rises in the serum levels of both anticonvulsants can occur it would be prudent to monitor the outcome. It is probably sufficient just to monitor for increased adverse effects. No special precautions seem necessary with oxcarbazepine.

1. Dam M, Christiansen J. Interaction of propoxyphene with carbamazepine. *Lancet* (1977) ii, 509.
2. Dam M, Kristensen CB, Hansen BS, Christiansen J. Interaction between carbamazepine and propoxyphene in man. *Acta Neurol Scand* (1977) 56, 603–7.
3. Hansen BS, Dam M, Brandt J, Hvidberg EF, Angelo H, Christensen JM, Lous P. Influence of dextropropoxyphene on steady state serum levels and protein binding of three anti-epileptic drugs in man. *Acta Neurol Scand* (1980) 61, 357–67.
4. Yu YL, Huang CY, Chin D, Woo E, Chang CM. Interaction between carbamazepine and dextropropoxyphene. *Postgrad Med J* (1986) 62, 231–3.
5. Kubacka RT, Ferrante JA. Carbamazepine-propoxyphene interaction. *Clin Pharm* (1983) 2, 104.
6. Risinger MW. Carbamazepine toxicity with concurrent use of propoxyphene: a report of five cases. *Neurology* (1987) 37 (Suppl 1), 87.
7. Allen S. Cerebellar dysfunction following dextropropoxyphene-induced carbamazepine toxicity. *Postgrad Med J* (1994) 70, 764.
8. Oles KS, Mirza W, Penry JK. Catastrophic neurologic signs due to drug interaction: Tegretol and Darvon. *Surg Neurol* (1989) 32, 144–51.
9. Bergendal L, Friberg A, Schaffrath AM, Holmdahl M, Landahl S. The clinical relevance of the interaction between carbamazepine and dextropropoxyphene in elderly patients in Gothenburg, Sweden. *Eur J Clin Pharmacol* (1997) 53, 203–6.
10. Mogensen PH, Jorgensen L, Boas J, Dam M, Vesterager A, Flesch G, Jensen PK. Effects of dextropropoxyphene on the steady-state kinetics of oxcarbazepine and its metabolites. *Acta Neurol Scand* (1992) 85, 14–17.
11. Kutt H. Biochemical and genetic factors regulating Dilantin metabolism in man. *Ann N Y Acad Sci* (1971) 179, 704–22.

Anticonvulsants + Folic acid

If folic acid supplements are given to treat folate deficiency, which can be caused by the use of anticonvulsants (phenytoin, phenobarbital, primidone and possibly pheneturide), the serum anticonvulsant levels may fall, leading to decreased seizure control in some patients.

Clinical evidence

A study in 50 folate-deficient epileptics (taking **phenytoin**, **phenobarbital** and **primidone** in various combinations) found that after one months' treatment with folic acid 5 mg daily, the serum **phenytoin** levels of one group of 10 patients had fallen from 20 to 10 micrograms/ml. In another group of patients taking folic acid 15 mg daily the levels of **phenytoin** fell from 14 to 11 micrograms/ml. Only one patient (in the 5-mg folic acid group) had a marked increase in seizure frequency and severity. No alterations were seen in the **phenobarbital** levels.[1]

Another long-term study was conducted in 26 patients with folic acid deficiency (serum folate less than 5 nanograms/ml), and treated with two or more drugs (**phenytoin**, **phenobarbital**, **primidone**). The mental state of 22 of them (as shown by increased alertness, concentration, sociability etc) improved to a variable degree when they were given folic acid 5 mg three times daily. However, the frequency and severity of seizures in 13 patients (50%) increased to such an extent that the vitamin had to be withdrawn from 9 of them.[2]

Similar results, both of increased seizure activity and decreased serum folate levels, have been described in other studies and reports in patients on **phenytoin**, **phenobarbital**, **primidone** and **pheneturide**.[3-6]

Mechanism

Patients on anticonvulsants may have subnormal serum folic acid levels, and frequencies of 27 to 76% have been reported for phenobarbital, primidone, and phenytoin alone or in various combinations.[7] One possible explanation is that this is due to the enzyme-inducing characteristics of these anticonvulsants, which makes excessive demands on folate for the synthesis of the enzymes concerned with drug metabolism. Ultimately drug metabolism becomes limited by the lack of folate, and patients may also develop a reduction in their general mental health[2] and even frank megaloblastic anaemia.[7,8] If folic acid is then given to treat this deficiency, the metabolism of the anticonvulsant increases once again,[9] resulting in a reduction in serum anticonvulsant levels, which in some instances may become so low that seizure control is partially or totally lost.

Importance and management

A very well documented and clinically important interaction (only a few references are listed here). Reductions in serum phenytoin levels of 16 to 50% after taking 5 to 15 mg folic acid daily for 2 to 4 weeks have been described.[1,3,10] The incidence is uncertain. If folic acid supplements are given to folate-deficient epileptics taking phenytoin, phenobarbital, primidone and possibly pheneturide, their serum anticonvulsant levels should be well monitored so that suitable dosage increases can be made.

1. Baylis EM, Crowley JM, Preece JM, Sylvester PE, Marks V. Influence of folic acid on blood-phenytoin levels. *Lancet* (1971) i, 62–4.
2. Reynolds EH. Effects of folic acid on the mental state and fit-frequency of drug-treated epileptic patients. *Lancet* (1967) i, 1086–9.
3. Strauss RG, Bernstein R. Folic acid and Dilantin antagonism in pregnancy. *Obstet Gynecol* (1974) 44, 345–8.
4. Latham AN, Millbank L, Richens A, Rowe DJF. Liver enzyme induction by anticonvulsant drugs, and its relationship to disturbed calcium and folic acid metabolism. *J Clin Pharmacol* (1973) 13, 337–42.
5. Berg MJ, Fincham RW, Ebert BE, Schottelius DD. Phenytoin pharmacokinetics: before and after folic acid administration. *Epilepsia* (1992) 33, 712–20.
6. Seligmann H, Potasman I, Weller B, Schwartz M, Prokocimer M. Phenytoin-folic acid interaction: a lesson to be learned. *Clin Neuropharmacol* (1999) 5, 268–72.
7. Davis RE, Woodliff HJ. Folic acid deficiency in patients receiving anticonvulsant drugs. *Med J Aust* (1971) 2, 1070–2.
8. Ryan GMS, Forshaw JWB. Megaloblastic anaemia due to phenytoin sodium. *BMJ* (1955) 11, 242–3.
9. Berg MJ, Fischer LJ, Rivey MP, Vern BA, Lantz RK, Schottelius DD. Phenytoin and folic acid interaction: a preliminary report. *Ther Drug Monit* (1983) 5, 389–94.
10. Furlanut M, Benetello P, Avogaro A, Dainese R. Effects of folic acid on phenytoin kinetics in healthy subjects. *Clin Pharmacol Ther* (1978) 24, 294–7.

Anticonvulsants + Isotretinoin

A study in one patient found that isotretinoin modestly reduced the serum levels of both carbamazepine and its active metabolite. Another study found that isotretinoin does not affect phenytoin levels.

Clinical evidence, mechanism, importance and management

(a) Carbamazepine

The carbamazepine AUC in an epileptic patient taking carbamazepine 600 mg daily was reduced by 11% while taking isotretinoin 500 micrograms/kg daily, and by 24% when taking 1 mg/kg daily. The AUC of carbamazepine-epoxide (the active metabolite of carbamazepine) was reduced by 21 and 44% by the small and large doses of isotretinoin respectively. The patient had no adverse effects, but the author of the report suggests that concurrent use should be monitored.[1]

(b) Phenytoin

A study in 7 healthy subjects taking phenytoin 300 mg daily found that the addition of isotretinoin 40 mg twice daily for 11 days had no effect on the steady-state pharmacokinetics of phenytoin.[2] No special precautions would seem to be needed if these drugs are given concurrently.

1. Marsden JR. Effect of isotretinoin on carbamazepine pharmacokinetics. *Br J Dermatol* (1988) 119, 403–4.
2. Oo C, Barsanti F, Zhang R. Lack of effect of isotretinoin on the pharmacokinetics of phenytoin at steady-state. *Pharm Res* (1997) 14 (11 Suppl), S-561.

Anticonvulsants + Mefloquine

A woman whose epilepsy was controlled on sodium valproate developed convulsions when given mefloquine. Note that mefloquine is normally contraindicated in epilepsy.

Clinical evidence, mechanism, importance and management

An isolated report describes a 20-year-old woman, with a 7-year history of epilepsy (bilateral myoclonus and generalised tonic-clonic seizures) treated with **sodium valproate** 1.3 g daily, who developed tonic-clonic seizures 8 hours after taking the second of 3 prophylactic doses of mefloquine 250 mg.[1] It is not clear whether this resulted from a drug-drug or a drug-disease interaction. The makers of mefloquine advise its avoidance in those with a history of convulsions as it may increase the risk of convulsions. In these patients mefloquine should be used only for curative treatment if compelling reasons exist.[2]

1. Besser R, Krämer G. Verdacht auf anfallfördernde Wirkung von Mefloquin (Lariam®). *Nervenarzt* (1991) 62, 760–1.
2. Lariam (Mefloquine hydrochloride). Roche Products Ltd. UK Summary of product characteristics, February 2005.

Anticonvulsants + Methylphenidate

Although two small studies found that methylphenidate did not alter phenytoin levels raised serum phenytoin levels and phenytoin toxicity have been seen in three patients given methylphenidate. One of the patients also had raised serum primidone and phenobarbital levels. Two children on valproic acid developed severe dyskinesia and bruxism when given methylphenidate.

Clinical evidence

A 5-year-old hyperkinetic epileptic boy taking **phenytoin** 8.9 mg/kg and **primidone** 17.7 mg/kg daily, developed ataxia without nystagmus when he was also given methylphenidate 40 mg daily. Serum levels of both the anticonvulsants were found to be at toxic concentrations and only began to fall when the methylphenidate dosage was reduced.[1]

A further case of **phenytoin** toxicity occurred in another child given methylphenidate.[2] Only one other case has been seen, but this patient was later rechallenged with the two drugs and **phenytoin** toxicity was not seen.[3]

Conversely, this interaction has not been seen in clinical studies and observations of 3 healthy subjects[3] and more than 11 patients[4] taking **phenytoin** and methylphenidate.

Two children on **valproic acid** rapidly developed severe dyskinesia and bruxism after the first and second dose of methylphenidate, respectively.[5]

Mechanism

Not fully understood. The suggestion is that methylphenidate acts as an enzyme inhibitor, slowing the metabolism of the phenytoin by the liver and leading to its accumulation in those individuals whose drug metabolising system is virtually saturated by phenytoin. Valproate appears to potentiate the effects of methylphenidate, possibly by a pharmacokinetic mechanism, or because of additive dopaminergic effects.[5]

Importance and management

These appear to be the only reports, and any interaction is not established. Concurrent use of phenytoin need not be avoided but be alert for any evidence of toxicity, particularly if the phenytoin dosage is high. Similarly, caution is warranted if methylphenidate is started in a child on valproate.

The authors of the report advise clinical observation while the dose of methylphenidate is being established.[5]

1. Garrettson LK, Perel JM, Dayton PG. Methylphenidate interaction with both anticonvulsants and ethyl biscoumacetate. A new action of methylphenidate. *JAMA* (1969) 207, 2053–6.
2. Ghofrani M. Possible phenytoin-methylphenidate interaction. *Dev Med Child Neurol* (1988) 30, 267–8.
3. Mirkin BL, Wright F. Drug interactions: effect of methylphenidate on the disposition of diphenylhydantoin in man. *Neurology* (1971) 21, 1123–8.
4. Kupferberg HJ, Jeffery W, Hunninghake DB. Effect of methylphenidate on plasma anticonvulsant levels. *Clin Pharmacol Ther* (1972) 13, 201–4.
5. Gara L, Roberts W. Adverse response to methylphenidate in combination with valproic acid. *J Child Adolesc Psychopharmacol* (2000) 10, 39–43.

Anticonvulsants + Oxiracetam

The half-life of oxiracetam was shorter in 4 patients on carbamazepine and valproate or clobazam, but oxiracetam did not affect the serum levels of sodium valproate, carbamazepine or clobazam.

Clinical evidence, mechanism, importance and management

Oxiracetam 800 mg twice daily for 14 days did not affect the serum levels of **sodium valproate**, **carbamazepine**, or **clobazam** and their metabolites in 3 epileptics on **carbamazepine** and **valproate** and one on **carbamazepine** and **clobazam**.[1] However, it was noted that the oxiracetam half-life was shorter (2.8 to 7.56 hours)[1] than in a previous study (5.6 to 11.7 hours) in healthy subjects who had been given oxiracetam 2 g.[2] The clinical relevance of this is uncertain, but the authors suggest that it may be necessary to raise the oxiracetam dosage or give it more frequently in the presence of these drugs.[1]

1. van Wieringen A, Meijer JWA, van Emde Boas W, Vermeij TAC. Pilot study to determine the interaction of oxiracetam with antiepileptic drugs. *Clin Pharmacokinet* (1990) 18, 332–8.
2. Perucca E, Albrici A, Gatti G, Spalluto R, Visconti M, Crema A. Pharmacokinetics of oxiracetam following intravenous and oral administration in healthy volunteers. *Eur J Drug Metab Pharmacokinet* (1984) 9, 267–74.

Anticonvulsants + Quinine

Preliminary evidence suggests that the effects of carbamazepine and phenobarbital may be increased by quinine, possibly leading to toxicity. Phenytoin appears not to be affected.

Clinical evidence, mechanism, importance and management

Single doses of **carbamazepine** 200 mg, **phenobarbital** 120 mg or **phenytoin** 200 mg were given to 3 groups of 6 healthy subjects with and without a single 600-mg dose of quinine sulphate. The AUC and peak plasma level of **carbamazepine** and **phenobarbital** were increased by 104% and 57%, and by 81% and 53% respectively. **Phenytoin** was not significantly affected. The reasons are not known but the authors suggest that quinine inhibits the metabolism of **carbamazepine** and **phenobarbital** (but not **phenytoin**) by the liver, so that they are lost from the body more slowly.[1] In an earlier study, **phenobarbital** 125 mg daily for 4 days caused only a small reduction in the plasma half-life of quinine in 2 healthy subjects.[2]

Information seems to be limited to these studies. The importance of these interactions awaits assessment in a clinically realistic situation (i.e. in patients taking multiple doses) but in the meantime it would seem prudent to monitor the effects of **carbamazepine** or **phenobarbital** for evidence of increased effects and possible toxicity if quinine is added. **Phenytoin** appears not to interact.

1. Amabeoku GJ, Chikuni O, Akino C, Mutetwa S. Pharmacokinetic interaction of single doses of quinine and carbamazepine, phenobarbitone and phenytoin in healthy volunteers. *East Afr Med J* (1993) 70, 90–3.
2. Saggers VH, Hariratnajothi N, McLean AEM. The effect of diet and phenobarbitone on quinine metabolism in the rat and in man. *Biochem Pharmacol* (1970) 19, 499–503.

Anticonvulsants + Quinolones

Ciprofloxacin did not significantly alter phenytoin levels in two studies, but some individuals have shown a marked fall in serum phenytoin levels when ciprofloxacin was started, whereas one showed a rise. Seizures have also been reported with the combination. Phenytoin levels may slightly rise if clinafloxacin is given. Enoxacin did not alter phenytoin levels. Quinolones alone very occasionally cause convulsions, therefore they should be used with caution in patients with epilepsy.

Clinical evidence

(a) Ciprofloxacin

In a study in 4 healthy subjects of the effect of ciprofloxacin on **phenytoin** levels, there was no difference in the pharmacokinetics of **phenytoin** 200 mg daily when given with ciprofloxacin 500 mg twice daily. However, one of the 4 subjects experienced a 30% decrease in the **phenytoin** maximum serum levels when ciprofloxacin was added.[1] In another study in 7 patients on **phenytoin**, ciprofloxacin 500 mg twice daily for 10 days caused no significant change in **phenytoin** levels, although there was a tendency for an increase (mean 24% rise).[2] Four case reports describe falls of 50% or more in **phenytoin** serum levels when ciprofloxacin was added, accompanied by seizures in 3 instances.[3-6] Another report describes unexpectedly low **phenytoin** levels after a loading dose in a woman on ciprofloxacin.[7] Conversely, **phenytoin** levels rose in an elderly woman, possibly as a result of taking ciprofloxacin.[8] In one report, blood levels of **phenytoin** and **valproic acid** were not affected by ciprofloxacin although a seizure occurred on the fourth day of therapy.[9] Other cases describe seizures in patients on **phenytoin** when given ciprofloxacin, but with little or no information on **phenytoin** levels.[10]

(b) Clinafloxacin

Phenytoin 300 mg daily was given to healthy subjects for 10 days, then clinafloxacin 400 mg twice daily was added for a further 2 weeks. The maximum serum **phenytoin** levels rose by 18%, from 6.74 to 7.95 mg/l, the AUC rose by 20% and the clearance fell by 17%.[11]

(c) Enoxacin

In a study in healthy subjects, enoxacin did not appear to alter **phenytoin** serum levels, nor were multiple-dose serum enoxacin levels significantly altered by **phenytoin**.[12]

Mechanism

Fluoroquinolones alone rarely cause convulsions both in patients with and without a history of seizures. The mechanism for the effect of ciprofloxacin on phenytoin levels is unknown, and is unlikely to be due to effects on hepatic metabolism or oral absorption.[13,14] However, ciprofloxacin decreased phenytoin levels in an *animal* study, and a suggested reason for this was increased urinary excretion.[15]

Importance and management

The known potential for quinolones to induce seizures suggests that these antibacterials should either be avoided in epileptics, or only used when the benefits of treatment outweigh the potential risks of seizures. Some of the reactions seem to be disease/drug interactions rather than drug/drug interactions, the usual outcome being that the control of epilepsy is worsened. However, it appears that ciprofloxacin may also alter (usually decrease) phenytoin levels, and if this combination is used, phenytoin levels should be closely monitored. Clinafloxacin may cause a small increase in phenytoin levels, and phenytoin levels should be closely monitored. Enoxacin appears not to alter phenytoin levels.

1. Job ML, Arn SK, Strom JG, Jacobs NF, D'Souza MJ. Effect of ciprofloxacin on the pharmacokinetics of multiple-dose phenytoin serum concentrations. *Ther Drug Monit* (1994) 16, 427–31.
2. Schroeder D, Frye J, Alldredge B, Messing R, Flaherty J. Effect of ciprofloxacin on serum phenytoin concentrations in epileptic patients. *Pharmacotherapy* (1991) 11, 275.
3. Dillard ML, Fink RM, Parkerson R. Ciprofloxacin-phenytoin interaction. *Ann Pharmacother* (1992) 26, 263.
4. Pollak PT, Slayter KL. Hazards of doubling phenytoin dose in the face of an unrecognized interaction with ciprofloxacin. *Ann Pharmacother* (1997) 31, 61–4.
5. Brouwers PJ, DeBoer LE, Guchelaar H-J. Ciprofloxacin-phenytoin interaction. *Ann Pharmacother* (1997) 31, 498.
6. Otero M-J, Morán D, Valverde M-P. Interaction between phenytoin and ciprofloxacin. *Ann Pharmacother* (1999) 33, 251–2.
7. McLeod R, Trinkle R. Comment: unexpectedly low phenytoin concentration in a patient receiving ciprofloxacin. *Ann Pharmacother* (1998) 32, 1110–11.
8. Hull RL. Possible phenytoin-ciprofloxacin interaction. *Ann Pharmacother* (1993) 27, 1283.
9. Slavich IL, Gleffe R, Haas EJ. Grand mal epileptic seizures during ciprofloxacin therapy. *JAMA* (1989) 261, 558–9.
10. Anon. Risk of seizures from concomitant use of ciprofloxacin and phenytoin in patients with epilepsy. *Can Med Assoc J* (1998) 158, 104–5.

11. Randinitis EJ, Koup JR, Bron NJ, Hounslow NJ, Rausch G, Abel R, Vassos AB, Sedman AJ. Drug interaction studies with clinafloxacin and probenecid, cimetidine, phenytoin and warfarin. *Drugs* (1999) 58 (Suppl 2), 254–5.
12. Thomas D, Humphrey G, Kinkel A, Sedman A, Rowland M, Toon S, Aarons L, Hopkins K. A study to evaluate the potential pharmacokinetic interaction between oral enoxacin (ENX) and oral phenytoin (PHE). *Pharm Res* (1986) 3 (Suppl), 99S.
13. Pollak PT, Slayter KL. Comment: ciprofloxacin-phenytoin interaction. *Ann Pharmacother* (1997) 31, 1549–50.
14. Brouwers PJ, de Boer LE, Guchelaar H-J. Comment: ciprofloxacin-phenytoin interaction. *Ann Pharmacother* (1997) 31, 1550.
15. al-Humayyd MS. Ciprofloxacin decreases plasma phenytoin concentrations in the rat. *Eur J Drug Metab Pharmacokinet* (1997) 22, 35–9.

Anticonvulsants + St John's wort *(Hypericum perforatum)*

St John's wort modestly increased the clearance of single-dose carbamazepine, but had no effect on multiple-dose carbamazepine. St John's wort is predicted to reduce the blood levels of phenytoin and phenobarbital, but this awaits clinical confirmation.

Clinical evidence, mechanism, importance and management

In a multiple-dose study, St John's wort had no effect on the pharmacokinetics of **carbamazepine** or its 10,11-epoxide metabolite in 8 healthy subjects. In this study, subjects took **carbamazepine** 200 mg increased to 400 mg daily alone for 20 days, then concurrently with St John's wort 300 mg (standardised to 0.3% hypericin) three times daily for 14 days.[1] In contrast, the AUC of a single 400-mg dose of **carbamazepine** was reduced by 21% after St John's wort 300 mg three times daily for 14 days was given, and the AUC of the 10,11-epoxide metabolite increased by 26%.[2]

St John's wort is a known enzyme inducer, and the results with single-dose **carbamazepine** are as predicted. However, **carbamazepine** is also an enzyme inducer, and induces its own metabolism (autoinduction). It is suggested that St John's wort is not sufficiently potent an inducer to further induce **carbamazepine** metabolism when autoinduction has occurred.[1]

The lack of effect of St John's wort on multiple-dose **carbamazepine** pharmacokinetics, and the modest effect on single-dose pharmacokinetics suggest that the potential for a clinically important interaction is minimal. Nevertheless, it may be prudent to monitor **carbamazepine** levels on concurrent use to confirm this. Prior to the publication of the above reports, the UK Committee on Safety of Medicines had advised that patients taking a number of drugs including the anticonvulsants **carbamazepine**, **phenytoin** and **phenobarbital** should not take St John's wort.[3] This advice was based on predicted pharmacokinetic interactions. In the light of the above studies, this advice no longer applies to **carbamazepine**, but until more is known, it should probably still apply to **phenytoin** and **phenobarbital**.

1. Burstein AH, Horton RL, Dunn T, Alfaro RM, Piscitelli SC, Theodore W. Lack of effect of St John's wort on carbamazepine pharmacokinetics in healthy volunteers. *Clin Pharmacol Ther* (2000) 68, 605–12.
2. Burstein AH, Piscitelli SC, Alfaro RM, Theodore W. Effect of St John's wort on carbamazepine single-dose pharmacokinetics. *Epilepsia* (2001) 42 (Suppl 7), 253.
3. Committee on the Safety of Medicines (UK). Message from Professor A Breckenridge (Chairman of CSM) and Fact Sheet for Health Care Professionals, 29th February 2000.

Anticonvulsants + Tamoxifen

Some preliminary evidence suggests that high-dose tamoxifen can cause the serum levels of phenytoin to rise, causing toxicity. Carbamazepine may possibly not interact. Phenytoin may lower tamoxifen levels.

Clinical evidence, mechanism, importance and management

A man who had undergone an operation 10 years previously for a brain tumour and had since remained seizure-free on **phenytoin** 200 mg twice daily began to have breakthrough seizures. It was established that his brain tumour had recurred and so tamoxifen was started as experimental treatment. The dose of tamoxifen was slowly titrated to 200 mg daily over a 6-week period. He continued to receive **phenytoin** and was also given **carbamazepine** as his seizures were not controlled, but when the maximum dosage of tamoxifen (200 mg daily) was reached he began to develop symptoms of **phenytoin** toxicity with a serum level of 28 micrograms/ml. The toxicity disappeared and the **phenytoin** levels decreased when the **phenytoin** dosage was reduced. The **carbamazepine** serum levels remained unchanged throughout.[1]

The authors of this report say that other patients of theirs similarly treated with tamoxifen also developed **phenytoin** toxicity, which disappeared when the **phenytoin** dosage was reduced by 15 to 20%. Another study of the pharmacokinetics of high dose tamoxifen in patients with brain tumours found that the mean tamoxifen levels in 15 patients on **phenytoin** were about 60% lower than in patients not taking **phenytoin**, although this did not reach statistical significance due to high inter-patient variability.[2] The reasons for these possible interactions are not known, but it could be that tamoxifen and **phenytoin** both compete for the same metabolising enzymes.

The evidence for this interaction is very slim indeed and it may possibly only occur with high dose tamoxifen. Consider monitoring **phenytoin** levels if high-dose tamoxifen is added and monitor the efficacy of the tamoxifen. More study is needed.

1. Rabinowicz AL, Hinton DR, Dyck P, Couldwell WT. High-dose tamoxifen in treatment of brain tumors: interaction with antiepileptic drugs. *Epilepsia* (1995) 36, 513–15.
2. Ducharme J, Fried K, Shenouda G, Leyland-Jones B, Wainer IW. Tamoxifen metabolic patterns within a glioma patient population treated with high-dose tamoxifen. *Br J Clin Pharmacol* (1997) 43: 189–93.

Anticonvulsants + Terbinafine

An isolated report describes the development of fatal toxic epidermal necrolysis shortly after a patient on long-term phenobarbital and carbamazepine started to take terbinafine.

Clinical evidence, mechanism, importance and management

An isolated report describes a 26-year-old woman with cerebral palsy who had been taking **phenobarbital** 15 mg with **carbamazepine** 400 mg daily for 12 years to control epilepsy, and who developed fatal toxic epidermal necrolysis 2 weeks after starting oral terbinafine 250 mg daily for tinea corporis. The reasons are not understood, but the authors point out that all three drugs can cause adverse skin reactions (erythema multiforme) and suggest that some synergism may have occurred.[1] It is uncertain whether this was a true interaction or a terbinafine adverse effect, but prescribers should be aware of this case if these drugs are used together.

1. White SI, Bowen-Jones D. Toxic epidermal necrolysis induced by terbinafine in a patient on long-term anti-epileptics. *Br J Dermatol* (1996) 134, 188–9.

Anticonvulsants + Terfenadine

Carbamazepine toxicity, attributed to the use of terfenadine, has been described in one case report but the interaction is not established. Terfenadine does not alter the pharmacokinetics of phenytoin.

Clinical evidence, mechanism, importance and management

(a) Carbamazepine

A 18-year-old woman taking carbamazepine after treatment for brain metastases, developed confusion, disorientation, visual hallucinations, nausea and ataxia shortly after starting terfenadine 60 mg twice daily for rhinitis. The symptoms were interpreted as carbamazepine toxicity. However, her total carbamazepine serum levels of 8.9 mg/l were within the normal range. An interaction due to protein binding displacement was suspected and measurement of free carbamazepine revealed levels of 6 mg/l, almost three times the upper limit of normal. All the symptoms disappeared when the terfenadine was stopped. The authors speculate that the terfenadine had displaced the carbamazepine from its plasma protein binding sites, thereby increasing the levels of free and active carbamazepine.[1] The report is very brief and does not say whether any other drugs were being taken concurrently, so that this interaction is not established.

(b) Phenytoin

A 1-day and a 2-week course of terfenadine 60 mg twice daily had no effect on the pharmacokinetics of phenytoin in 12 patients with epilepsy.[2] No special precautions are needed if both drugs are used.

1. Hirschfeld S, Jarosinski P. Drug interaction of terfenadine and carbamazepine. *Ann Intern Med* (1993) 118, 907–8.
2. Coniglio AA, Garnett WR, Pellock JH, Tsidonis O, Hepler CD, Serafin R, Small RE, Driscoll SM, Karnes HT. Effect of acute and chronic terfenadine on free and total serum phenytoin concentrations in epileptic patients. *Epilepsia* (1989) 30, 611–16.

Anticonvulsants + Tobacco smoking

Smoking appears to have no important effect on the serum levels of phenytoin, phenobarbital or carbamazepine.

Clinical evidence, mechanism, importance and management

A comparative study in 88 epileptic patients taking anticonvulsants (**phenobarbital**, **phenytoin** and **carbamazepine** alone or in combination) found that although smoking had a tendency to lower the steady-state serum concentrations of these drugs, a statistically significant effect on the concentration–dose ratios was only found in the **phenobarbital**-treated patients.[1] In another study in healthy subjects, there was no difference in the pharmacokinetics of a single 60-mg dose of **phenobarbital** between smokers and non-smokers.[2] In practical terms smoking appears to have only a negligible effect on the serum levels of these anticonvulsants and epileptics who smoke are unlikely to need higher doses than non-smokers.

1. Benetello P, Furlanut M, Pasqui L, Carmillo L, Perlotto N, Testa G. Absence of effect of cigarette smoking on serum concentrations of some anticonvulsants in epileptic patients. *Clin Pharmacokinet* (1987) 12, 302–4.
2. Mirfazaelian A, Jahanzad F, Tabatabaei-far M, Farsam H, Mahmoudian M. Effect of smoking on single dose pharmacokinetics of phenobarbital. *Biopharm Drug Dispos* (2001) 22, 403–6.

Anticonvulsants + Viloxazine

Viloxazine can cause a marked rise in serum carbamazepine levels and toxicity has been seen. Viloxazine can also raise serum phenytoin to toxic levels, but appears not to alter oxcarbazepine levels.

Clinical evidence

(a) Carbamazepine

The serum carbamazepine levels of 7 patients rose by 50%, from 8.1 to 12.1 micrograms/ml, after they took viloxazine 100 mg three times daily for 3 weeks.[1] Signs of mild toxicity (dizziness, ataxia, fatigue, drowsiness) developed in 5 of them. These symptoms disappeared and the serum carbamazepine levels fell when the viloxazine was withdrawn.[1] Another report found a 2.5-fold increase in serum carbamazepine levels in one patient within 2 weeks of adding viloxazine 300 mg daily.[2] Another report found an average 55% rise in plasma carbamazepine levels and toxicity in 4 of the 7 patients studied.[3] Yet another patient developed choreoathetosis and increased serum carbamazepine levels, which was attributed to the addition of viloxazine.[4] In one study, the pharmacokinetics of a single dose of viloxazine were reported to be unaffected by carbamazepine,[5] but in the case report cited above, which was at steady state, the viloxazine levels were found to be reduced.[2]

(b) Oxcarbazepine

In 6 patients with simple or partial seizures the steady-state serum levels of oxcarbazepine (average dose 1500 mg daily) were unaffected by the addition of viloxazine 100 mg twice daily for 10 days. No adverse effects were seen.[6]

(c) Phenytoin

The serum phenytoin levels of 10 epileptic patients rose by 37%, from 18.8 to 25.7 micrograms/ml over the 3 weeks following the addition of viloxazine 150 to 300 mg daily. The rise ranged from 7 to 94%. Signs of toxicity (ataxia, nystagmus) developed in 4 of the patients 12 to 16 days after starting the viloxazine. Their serum phenytoin levels had risen to between 32.3 and 41 micrograms/ml.[7] The symptoms disappeared and phenytoin levels fell when the viloxazine was withdrawn.[7] The pharmacokinetics of viloxazine were unaffected by phenytoin.[5]

Mechanism

Uncertain. What is known suggests that viloxazine inhibits the metabolism of some anticonvulsants, thereby reducing their clearance from the body and raising their serum levels.

Importance and management

Information seems to be limited to the reports cited. If concurrent use is undertaken, both serum carbamazepine and phenytoin levels should be monitored closely and suitable dosage reductions made as necessary to avoid possible toxicity. No special precautions seem necessary with oxcarbazepine.

1. Pisani F, Narbone MC, Fazio A, Crisafulli P, Primerano G, Amendola D'Angostino A, Oteri G, Di Perri R. Effect of viloxazine on serum carbamazepine levels in epileptic patients. *Epilepsia* (1984) 25, 482–5.
2. Odou P, Geronimi-Ferret D, Degen P, Robert H. Viloxazine-carbamazépine. Double interaction dangereuse? A propos d'un cas. *J Pharm Clin* (1996) 15, 157–60.
3. Pisani F, Fazio A, Oteri G, Perucca E, Russo M, Trio R, Pisani B, Di Perri R. Carbamazepine-viloxazine interaction in patients with epilepsy. *J Neurol Neurosurg Psychiatry* (1986) 49, 1142–5.
4. Mosquet B, Starace J, Madelaine S, Simon JY, Lacotte J, Moulin M. Syndrome choréo-athétosique sous carbamazépine et viloxazine. *Therapie* (1994) 49, 513–14.
5. Pisani F, Fazio A, Spina E, Artesi C, Pisani B, Russo M, Trio R, Perucca E. Pharmacokinetics of the antidepressant drug viloxazine in normal subjects and in epileptic patients receiving chronic anticonvulsant treatment. *Psychopharmacology (Berl)* (1986) 90, 295–8.
6. Pisani F, Fazio A, Oteri G, Artesi C, Xiao B, Perucca E, Di Perri R. Effects of the antidepressant drug viloxazine on oxcarbazepine and its hydroxylated metabolites in patients with epilepsy. *Acta Neurol Scand* (1994) 90, 130–2.
7. Pisani F, Fazio A, Artesi C, Russo M, Trio R, Oteri G, Perucca E, Di Perri R. Elevation of plasma phenytoin by viloxazine in epileptic patients: a clinically significant interaction. *J Neurol Neurosurg Psychiatry* (1992) 55, 126–7.

Anticonvulsants + Vitamin B substances

High daily doses of pyridoxine can cause 35% reductions in phenytoin levels and 50% reductions in phenobarbital levels in some patients. Some evidence suggests that high doses of nicotinamide reduce the conversion of primidone to phenobarbital, and increase carbamazepine levels.

Clinical evidence

(a) Nicotinamide

Nicotinamide 41 to 178 mg/kg daily increased the levels of **primidone** and decreased the levels of **primidone**-derived phenobarbital in 3 children. Although two of the children had refractory seizures, seizure frequency decreased while on nicotinamide. Two of the children on **carbamazepine** had increases in their **carbamazepine** levels.[1]

(b) Pyridoxine

Pyridoxine 200 mg daily for 4 weeks reduced the **phenobarbital** serum levels of 5 epileptics by about 50%. Reductions in serum **phenytoin** levels of about 35% (range 17 to 70%) were also seen when patients were given pyridoxine 80 to 400 mg daily for 2 to 4 weeks. However, no interaction occurred in a number of other patients taking these drugs.[2]

Mechanism

It is suggested that the pyridoxine increases and nicotinamide decreases the activity of the liver enzymes concerned with the metabolism of these anticonvulsants.[1,2]

Importance and management

Information seems to be limited, but what is known suggests that concurrent use should be monitored if large doses of pyridoxine or nicotinamide are used, being alert for the need to modify the anticonvulsant dosage. It seems unlikely that small doses (as in multivitamin preparations) will interact to any great extent.

1. Bourgeois BF, Dodson WE, Ferrendelli JA. Interactions between primidone, carbamazepine, and nicotinamide. *Neurology* (1982) 32, 1122–26.
2. Hansson O, Sillanpaa M. Pyridoxine and serum concentration of phenytoin and phenobarbitone. *Lancet* (1976) i, 256.

Carbamazepine + Allopurinol

There is some evidence that high-dose allopurinol (15 mg/kg or 600 mg daily) can gradually raise serum carbamazepine levels by about a third. It appears that allopurinol 300 mg daily has no effect on carbamazepine levels.

Clinical evidence

In a 6-month study, 7 epileptic patients on anticonvulsants, which included carbamazepine, were also given allopurinol 100 mg three times daily for 3 months then 200 mg three times daily for 3 months. The mean trough steady-state serum carbamazepine levels of 6 of the patients rose by 30% or more and the carbamazepine clearance fell by 32% during the second 3-month period. A reduction in the carbamazepine dosage was needed in 3 patients because of the symptoms that developed.[1] Similarly, in another study add-on allopurinol 10 mg/kg increased to 15 mg/kg daily for 12 weeks increased carbamazepine levels by 29% in 11 patients on anticonvulsants including carbamazepine.[2] Conversely, in another add-on study, allopurinol (150 mg daily in those less than 20 kg, and 300 mg daily for other patients) for 4 months had no effect on carbamazepine levels in 53 patients on anticonvulsants including carbamazepine.[3]

Mechanism

Uncertain. A possible explanation is that allopurinol can act as a liver enzyme inhibitor, which reduces the metabolism and clearance of other drugs by the liver.

Importance and management

Information is limited to these studies, but be alert for the need to reduce the dosage of carbamazepine if high doses of allopurinol are used long-term. This interaction apparently takes several weeks or even months to develop fully. More study is needed.

1. Mikati M, Erba G, Skouteli H, Gadia C. Pharmacokinetic study of allopurinol in resistant epilepsy: evidence for significant drug interactions. *Neurology* (1990) 40 (Suppl 1), 138.
2. Coppola G, Pascotto A. Double-blind, placebo-controlled, cross-over trial of allopurinol as add-on therapy in childhood refractory epilepsy. *Brain Dev* (1996) 18, 50–2.
3. Zagnoni PG, Bianchi A, Zolo P, Canger R, Cornaggia C, D'Alessandro P, DeMarco P, Pisani F, Gianelli M, Verzé L, Viani F, Zaccara G. Allopurinol as add-on therapy in refractory epilepsy: a double-blind placebo-controlled randomized study. *Epilepsia* (1994) 35, 107–12.

Carbamazepine + Amiodarone

Carbamazepine pharmacokinetics appear not to be affected by amiodarone.

Clinical evidence, mechanism, importance and management

A single 400-mg dose of carbamazepine was given to 9 patients with cardiac disease (premature ventricular contractions, supraventricular tachycardia, sinus arrhythmia) before and after they took amiodarone 200 mg twice daily for a month. The pharmacokinetics of carbamazepine were found to be unchanged by the amiodarone treatment. This certainly suggests that no clinically important interaction occurs, but it needs confirmation in patients who are treated with both drugs long term. The authors postulate that a higher amiodarone dose may inhibit the metabolism of the carbamazepine by the liver.[1]

1. Leite SAO, Leite PJM, Rocha GA, Routledge PA, Bittencourt PRM. Carbamazepine kinetics in cardiac patients before and during amiodarone. *Arq Neuropsiquiatr* (1994) 52, 210–15.

Carbamazepine + Antipsychotics

An increase in the serum levels of carbamazepine or its epoxide metabolite has been reported in patients given loxapine, haloperidol, quetiapine, risperidone or chlorpromazine with amoxapine. Toxicity has occurred. Thioridazine appears not to raise carbamazepine-epoxide levels. Isolated cases of Stevens-Johnson syndrome have occurred in patients taking antipsychotics with carbamazepine. Carbamazepine may reduce levels of many of the antipsychotics. A case of neuroleptic malignant syndrome had been described in a patient on antipsychotics and carbamazepine. See also 'Antipsychotics + Anticonvulsants', p.530.

Clinical evidence, mechanism, importance and management

(a) Raised carbamazepine or carbamazepine-epoxide levels

Two patients, one on **loxapine** 500 mg daily and the other on **chlorpromazine** 350 mg and **amoxapine** 300 mg daily, developed toxicity (ataxia, nausea, anxiety) when given carbamazepine 600 to 900 mg daily, even though their serum carbamazepine levels were low to normal.[1] In another case, neurotoxicity (ataxia, lethargy, visual disturbances) developed in a man given carbamazepine and **loxapine**.[2] In all 3 cases, the toxicity appeared to be due to elevated carbamazepine-epoxide levels (the metabolite of carbamazepine).[1,2] The problem resolved when the carbamazepine dosages were reduced. Raised carbamazepine-epoxide levels have also been reported in 2 patients after they were given **quetiapine**, with toxicity in one of the patients.[3] **Risperidone** 1 mg daily for 2 weeks raised carbamazepine levels by about 20% in 8 patients.[4] Raised serum carbamazepine levels have also been seen with **'haloperidol'**, (p.530).

It is relatively well documented that carbamazepine can reduce the levels of many of the antipsychotics (discussed in individual monographs elsewhere). The above reports show that the effect of the antipsychotic on carbamazepine should also be considered. The levels of both carbamazepine and its metabolite should be monitored if toxicity develops.

(b) No changes to carbamazepine-epoxide levels

Thioridazine 100 to 200 mg daily was found to have no effect on the steady-state levels of carbamazepine or carbamazepine-epoxide in 8 epileptic patients,[5] and also carbamazepine had no significant effect on **thioridazine** serum levels in 6 patients.[6]

(c) Stevens-Johnson syndrome

Three patients on various antipsychotics (**fluphenazine**, **haloperidol**, **trifluoperazine**, **chlorpromazine**) developed Stevens-Johnson syndrome within 8 to 14 days of starting to take carbamazepine. All 3 had erythema multiforme skin lesions and involvement of at least two mucous membranes. After treatment, all 3 were restarted on all their previous drugs, except carbamazepine, without problems.[7] Another case has been reported in a patient on carbamazepine, **lithium carbonate**, **haloperidol** and **trihexyphenidyl**.[8] A few other cases have been reported.[9] The reasons are not understood. Stevens-Johnson syndrome with carbamazepine alone is rare, and the risk appears to be mostly confined to the first 8 weeks of treatment.[10] It may be more common in patients being treated for conditions other than epilepsy.[11] It is not possible to say whether the concurrent use of antipsychotics increases the risk of its development, but until more is known it would be prudent to monitor the outcome, particularly during the first 2 weeks of combined use. More study is needed.

(d) Neuroleptic malignant syndrome

A 54-year old man living in a psychiatric hospital, who had been on long-term **haloperidol**, **levomepromazine**, **sultopride**, and metixene was started on carbamazepine 400 mg daily for impulsive behaviour. The following day he became unstable on his feet, and after 3 days could no longer walk by himself. He had a fever of 40°C, muscle rigidity, diaphoresis, and serum creatine phosphokinase was elevated to 923 units/l. He was diagnosed as having neuroleptic malignant syndrome (NMS), and recovered after body cooling and administration of fluids, with symptoms resolving over 12 days. Before carbamazepine treatment, his **haloperidol** level was 19 nanograms/ml and after 3 days of carbamazepine it was reduced at 10.9 nanograms/ml.[12]

Carbamazepine alone is not associated with NMS. It was suggested that carbamazepine may have reduced levels of the anticholinergic antipsychotics (**levomepromazine** and **sultopride**), resulting in cholinergic rebound, and inducing NMS.[12] The general applicability of this case is unknown, but bear it in mind if NMS occurs in a patient on antipsychotics given carbamazepine.

1. Pitterle ME, Collins DM. Carbamazepine-10,11-epoxide evaluation associated with coadministration of loxitane or amoxapine. *Epilepsia* (1988) 29, 654.
2. Collins DM, Gidal BE, Pitterle ME. Potential interaction between carbamazepine and loxapine: case report and retrospective review. *Ann Pharmacother* (1993) 27, 1180–3.
3. Fitzgerald BJ, Okos AJ. Elevation of carbamazepine-10,11-epoxide by quetiapine. *Pharmacotherapy* (2002) 22, 1500–503.
4. Mula M, Monaco F. Carbamazepine–risperidone interactions in patients with epilepsy. *Clin Neuropharmacol* (2002) 25, 97–100.
5. Spina E, Amendola D'Agostino AM, Ioculano MP, Oteri G, Fazio A, Pisani F. No effect of thioridazine on plasma concentrations of carbamazepine and its active metabolite carbamazepine-10,11-epoxide. *Ther Drug Monit* (1990) 12, 511–13.
6. Tiihonen J, Vartiainen H, Hakola P. Carbamazepine-induced changes in plasma levels of neuroleptics. *Pharmacopsychiatry* (1995) 28, 26–8.

7. Wong KE. Stevens-Johnson Syndrome in neuroleptic-carbamazepine combination. *Singapore Med J* (1990) 31, 432–3.
8. Fawcett RG. Erythema multiforme major in a patient treated with carbamazepine. *J Clin Psychiatry* (1987) 48, 416–17.
9. Wong KE. Stevens-Johnson syndrome in neuroleptic-carbamazepine combination. *Singapore Med J* (1990) 31, 432–3.
10. Rzany B, Coreia O, Kelly JP, Naldi L, Auquier A, Stern R. Risk of Stevens-Johnson syndrome and toxic epidermal necrolysis during the first weeks of antiepileptic therapy: a case-control study. *Lancet* (1999) 353, 2190–4.
11. Dhar S, Todi SK. Are carbamazepine-induced Stevens-Johnson syndrome and toxic epidermal necrolysis more common in nonepileptic patients? *Dermatology* (1999) 199, 194.
12. Nisijima K, Kusakabe Y, Ohtuka K, Ishiguro T. Addition of carbamazepine to long-term treatment with neuroleptics may induce neuroleptic malignant syndrome. *Biol Psychiatry* (1998) 44, 930–1.

Carbamazepine + Aspirin or NSAIDs

Carbamazepine levels are unaffected by aspirin or tolfenamic acid.

Clinical evidence, mechanism, importance and management

No changes in carbamazepine serum levels were seen in 10 patients who took aspirin 1.5 g daily for 3 days.[1] It would appear that no precautions are necessary if aspirin is used in patients on carbamazepine.

Tolfenamic acid 300 mg for 3 days had no significant effect on the serum levels of carbamazepine in 11 patients.[1] No special precautions seem necessary if these drugs are taken concurrently.

1. Neuvonen PJ, Lehtovaara R, Bardy A, Elomaa E. Antipyretic analgesics in patients on antiepileptic drug therapy. *Eur J Clin Pharmacol* (1979) 15, 263–8.

Carbamazepine + Azoles

Ketoconazole causes a small to moderate rise in serum carbamazepine levels. A marked rise in carbamazepine levels has been seen in two patients on fluconazole, with toxicity in one. Adverse effects have been seen in another patient when carbamazepine was used concurrently with miconazole. Carbamazepine may reduce the levels of 'itraconazole', (p.136), and is predicted to greatly lower the levels of 'voriconazole', (p.136).

Clinical evidence

(a) Fluconazole

A 33-year-old man who was stabilised on carbamazepine for seizures became extremely lethargic after taking fluconazole 150 mg for 3 days. His carbamazepine level was found to have risen from 11.1 to 24.5 micrograms/ml. Symptoms resolved when both drugs were stopped, and carbamazepine was later re-introduced without problem.[1] Another well-documented case report describes a threefold increase in carbamazepine levels after 10 days' concurrent use of fluconazole 400 mg daily (without any signs of toxicity).[2]

(b) Ketoconazole

A study in 8 patients with epilepsy taking carbamazepine found that the addition of oral ketoconazole 200 mg daily for 10 days increased their serum carbamazepine levels by 28.6% (from 5.6 to 7.2 micrograms/ml) whereas the carbamazepine-epoxide levels were unchanged. When the ketoconazole was stopped the serum carbamazepine levels returned to their former levels.[3]

(c) Miconazole

A patient on long-term treatment with carbamazepine 400 mg daily developed malaise, myoclonia and tremor within 3 days of being given oral miconazole 1125 mg. The same reaction occurred on each subsequent occasion when the patient was again given miconazole. These toxic effects disappeared when the miconazole was withdrawn.[4]

Mechanism

The reason for the carbamazepine serum level rise is thought to be that the azole antifungals inhibit the cytochrome P450 isoenzyme CYP3A4 to varying degrees, and this isoenzyme is concerned with the metabolism of carbamazepine.

Importance and management

The rise in carbamazepine serum levels seen in the studies with ketoconazole is only moderate, but the case reports with fluconazole and miconazole indicate that larger, potentially more serious interactions are possible. It would seem prudent to monitor the outcome of adding azole antifungals to established carbamazepine treatment, being alert for any evidence of increased carbamazepine adverse effects. Note also that carbamazepine may reduce the levels of azole antifungals: a marked reduction in itraconazole levels has been reported, see 'Azoles + Anticonvulsants', p.136.

1. Nair DR, Morris HH. Potential fluconazole-induced carbamazepine toxicity. *Ann Pharmacother* (1999) 33, 790–2.
2. Finch CK, Green CA, Self TH. Fluconazole-carbamazepine interaction. *South Med J* (2002) 95, 1099–1100.
3. Spina E, Arena D, Scordo MG, Fazio A, Pisani F, Perucca E. Elevation of plasma carbamazepine concentrations by ketoconazole in patients with epilepsy. *Ther Drug Monit* (1997) 19, 535–8.
4. Loupi E, Descotes J, Lery N, Evreux JC. Interactions medicamenteuses et miconazole. A propos de 10 observations. *Therapie* (1982) 37, 437–41.

Carbamazepine + Colestyramine or Colestipol

Colestipol causes a minor reduction in the absorption of carbamazepine, which is unlikely to be clinically significant. Colestyramine does not appear to interact.

Clinical evidence, mechanism, importance and management

Colestyramine 8 g did not affect the absorption of carbamazepine 400 mg in 6 healthy subjects, whereas colestipol 10 g reduced it by 10%. Both colestyramine and colestipol were given as a single dose 5 minutes after the carbamazepine.[1] This small reduction is unlikely to be clinically important.

1. Neuvonen PJ, Kivistö K, Hirvisalo EL. Effects of resins and activated charcoal on the absorption of digoxin, carbamazepine and frusemide. *Br J Clin Pharmacol* (1988) 25, 229–33.

Carbamazepine + Danazol

Serum carbamazepine levels can be doubled by danazol and carbamazepine toxicity may occur.

Clinical evidence

The serum carbamazepine levels of 6 epileptics approximately doubled within 7 to 30 days of taking danazol 400 to 600 mg daily. Acute carbamazepine toxicity (dizziness, drowsiness, blurred vision, ataxia, nausea) was experienced by 5 out of the 6 patients.[1]

Other reports similarly describe rises in serum carbamazepine levels of 50 to 100% (with toxicity seen in some instances) when danazol was added.[2-4]

Mechanism

Danazol inhibits the metabolism (by the epoxide-trans-diol pathway) of carbamazepine by the liver, thereby reducing its loss from the body.[2,5] During danazol treatment the clearance of carbamazepine has been found to be reduced by 60%, and the half-life more than doubled.[2]

Importance and management

An established and clinically important interaction. If concurrent use is necessary carbamazepine serum levels should be monitored and the dosage reduced as necessary.

1. Zeilinski JJ, Lichten EM, Haidukewych D. Clinically significant danazol-carbamazepine interaction. *Ther Drug Monit* (1987) 9, 24–7.
2. Krämer G, Theisohn M, von Unruh GE, Eichelbaum M. Carbamazepine-danazol drug interaction: its mechanism examined by a stable isotope technique. *Ther Drug Monit* (1986) 8, 387–92.
3. Hayden M, Buchanan N. Danazol-carbamazepine interaction. *Med J Aust* (1991) 155, 851.
4. Nelson MV. Interaction of danazol and carbamazepine. *Am J Psychiatry* (1988) 145, 768–9.
5. Krämer G, Besser R, Theisohn M, Eichelbaum M. Carbamazepine-danazol drug interaction: mechanism and therapeutic usefulness. *Acta Neurol Scand* (1984) 70, 249.

Carbamazepine + Diuretics

Two patients on carbamazepine developed hyponatraemia when given hydrochlorothiazide or furosemide. Another developed hyponatraemia on carbamazepine, hydrochlorothiazide and paroxetine.

Clinical evidence, mechanism, importance and management

Two epileptic patients developed symptomatic hyponatraemia while on carbamazepine, one while taking **hydrochlorothiazide** and the other while taking **furosemide**.[1] Another case has been described in a patient on carbamazepine given **hydrochlorothiazide** and paroxetine.[2] The reasons are uncertain but all these drugs can cause sodium to be lost from the body. This seems to be an uncommon interaction, but be aware that it can occur.

For mention of a few cases of increased carbamazepine levels with the diuretic acetazolamide, see 'Anticonvulsants + Acetazolamide', p.330.

1. Yassa R, Nastase C, Camille Y, Henderson M, Belzile L, Beland F. Carbamazepine, diuretics and hyponatremia: a possible interaction. *J Clin Psychiatry* (1987) 48, 281–3.
2. Kalksma R, Leemhuis MP. Hyponatriëmie bij gebruik van thiazidediuretica: let op combinaties van geneesmiddelen die dit effect versterken. *Ned Tijdschr Geneeskd* (2002) 146, 1521–5.

Carbamazepine + Felbamate

Felbamate modestly reduces serum carbamazepine levels but increases serum levels of the active metabolite, carbamazepine-epoxide. Felbamate levels may fall. The importance of these changes is uncertain but it is likely to be small.

Clinical evidence

The serum carbamazepine levels of 22 patients, with doses adjusted to keep levels in the range of 4 to 12 micrograms/ml, fell by 25% (range 10 to 42%) when they were given felbamate 3 g daily. The decrease occurred within a week, reaching a plateau after 2 to 4 weeks, and returning to the original levels within 2 to 3 weeks of stopping the felbamate.[1] Other studies in epileptics have found reductions in carbamazepine levels of between 18 and 31% when felbamate was given.[2-7] Some of these studies also found that the serum levels of the active carbamazepine metabolite carbamazepine-epoxide rose by 33% to 57%.[1,4,5]

Carbamazepine increased the clearance of felbamate by up to 49%.[8-10]

Mechanism

Not established. Felbamate does not induce the cytochrome P450 isoenzyme CYP3A4-mediated metabolism of carbamazepine, but appears to cause heteroactivation of CYP3A4.[11]

Importance and management

This interaction is established, but its clinical importance is uncertain because the modest fall in serum carbamazepine levels would seem to be offset by the rise in levels of its metabolite, carbamazepine-epoxide, which also has anticonvulsant activity. However, monitor carbamazepine levels carefully, reducing the dose as necessary, and be alert for any changes in the anticonvulsant control. The importance of the increased felbamate clearance is uncertain. More study is needed.

1. Albani F, Theodore WH, Washington P, Devinsky O, Bromfield E, Porter RJ, Nice FJ. Effect of Felbamate on plasma levels of carbamazepine and its metabolites. *Epilepsia* (1991) 32, 130–2.
2. Fuerst RH, Graves NM, Leppik IE, Remmel RP, Rosenfeld WE, Sierzant TL. A preliminary report on alteration of carbamazepine and phenytoin metabolism by felbamate. *Drug Intell Clin Pharm* (1986) 20, 465–6.
3. Fuerst RH, Graves NM, Leppik IE, Brundage RC, Holmes GB, Remmel RP. Felbamate increases phenytoin but decreases carbamazepine concentrations. *Epilepsia* (1988) 29, 488–91.
4. Howard JR, Dix RK, Shumaker RC, Perhach JL. The effect of felbamate on carbamazepine pharmacokinetics. *Epilepsia* (1992) 33 (Suppl 3), 84–5.
5. Wagner ML, Remmel RP, Graves NM, Leppik IE. Effect of felbamate on carbamazepine and its major metabolites. *Clin Pharmacol Ther* (1993) 53, 536–43.
6. Theodore WH, Raubertas RF, Porter RJ, Nice F, Devinsky O, Reeves P, Bromfield E, Ito B, Balish M. Felbamate: a clinical trial for complex partial seizures. *Epilepsia* (1991) 32, 392–7.
7. Leppik IE, Dreifuss FE, Pledger GW, Graves NM, Santilli N, Drury I, Tsay JY, Jacobs MP, Bertram E, Cereghino JJ, Cooper G, Sahlroot JT, Sheridan P, Ashworth M, Lee SI, Sierzant TL. Felbamate for partial seizures: results of a controlled clinical trial. *Neurology* (1991) 41, 1785–9.
8. Wagner ML, Graves NM, Marienau K, Holmes GB, Remmel RP, Leppik IE. Discontinuation of phenytoin and carbamazepine in patients receiving felbamate. *Epilepsia* (1991) 32, 398–406.
9. Kelley MT, Walson PD, Cox S, Dusci LJ. Population pharmacokinetics of felbamate in children. *Ther Drug Monit* (1997) 19, 29–36.
10. Banfield CR, Zhu G-RR, Jen JF, Jensen PK, Schumaker RC, Perhach JL Affrime MB, Glue P. The effect of age on the apparent clearance of felbamate: a retrospective analysis using nonlinear mixed-effects modeling. *Ther Drug Monit* (1996) 18, 19–29.
11. Egnell A-C, Houston B, Boyer S. In vivo CYP3A4 heteroactivation is a possible mechanism for the drug interaction between felbamate and carbamazepine. *J Pharmacol Exp Ther* (2003) 305, 1251–62.

Carbamazepine + Gemfibrozil

Two patients with hyperlipoproteinaemia had raised carbamazepine serum levels after additionally taking gemfibrozil.

Clinical evidence, mechanism, importance and management

Two patients stabilised on carbamazepine and treated for type IV hyperlipoproteinaemia with gemfibrozil had rises in their serum carbamazepine levels. One patient had a rise from 8.8 to 11.4 micrograms/ml within 4 days of starting gemfibrozil 300 mg daily, while a rise from 8.3 to 13.7 micrograms/ml was found in the other patient 3 months after gemfibrozil 300 mg twice daily was started.[1] The suggested reason is that the clearance of carbamazepine is increased in those with elevated cholesterol and total lipids. Thus, when the condition is treated with gemfibrozil, the clearance becomes more normal, which results in a rise in the serum carbamazepine levels.[2] The clinical importance of this interaction is uncertain but be alert for any evidence of carbamazepine toxicity if gemfibrozil is added.

1. Denio L, Drake ME, Pakalnis A. Gemfibrozil-carbamazepine interaction in epileptic patients. *Epilepsia* (1988) 29, 654.
2. Wichlinski LM, Sieradzki E, Gruchala M. Correlation between the total cholesterol serum concentration data and carbamazepine steady-state blood levels in humans. *Drug Intell Clin Pharm* (1983) 17, 812–14.

Carbamazepine + Grapefruit juice

Grapefruit juice increases carbamazepine levels. A case of possible carbamazepine toxicity has been seen in a man on carbamazepine after he started to eat grapefruit.

Clinical evidence, mechanism, importance and management

A 58-year-old man, taking carbamazepine 1 g daily for epilepsy developed visual disturbances with diplopia, and was found to have a carbamazepine level of 11 micrograms/ml (therapeutic range 4 to 10 micrograms/ml). Previous levels had not exceeded 5.4 micrograms/ml. The patient said that one month previously he had started to eat one whole grapefruit each day. The levels restabilised at 5.1 micrograms/ml after the carbamazepine dose was reduced to 800 mg daily.[1]

A randomised crossover study in 10 epileptic patients on carbamazepine 200 mg three times daily found that a single dose of grapefruit juice 300 ml increased the plasma levels and AUC of carbamazepine by about 40%.[2]

Mechanism

The cytochrome P450 isoenzyme CYP3A4 is the main enzyme involved in the metabolism of carbamazepine.[3] Components of grapefruit juice are known to inhibit CYP3A4, which in this case would lead to a reduction in the metabolism of carbamazepine, and therefore an increase in levels.[1,2,4]

Importance and management

Although the information is sparse, the interaction has been predicted, demonstrated in a study, and has also occurred in practice. The authors of the study,[2] suggest that grapefruit juice should be avoided in patients taking carbamazepine. In the case report,[1] the patient continued to eat grapefruit, and this was successfully managed by a reduction in the carbamazepine dose. However, it should be noted that intake of a set amount of grapefruit would need to be maintained for this approach to work. The makers advise carbamazepine dosage adjustment and monitoring of carbamazepine levels in patients on agents that may raise carbamazepine levels, such as grapefruit juice.[3] If monitoring is not practical, or regular intake of grapefruit is not desired, it would seem prudent to avoid grapefruit/grapefruit juice.

What is of particular interest in the case cited is that the interaction apparently occurred with whole grapefruit, which is not usually considered to be a problem, although it is known that the fruit content of possible active components (e.g. flavonoids) do vary considerably. The juice (as opposed to the whole fruit) more commonly interacts, as the juicing process can increase the flavonoid content.[4]

1. Bonin B, Vandel P, Vandel S, Kantelip JP. Effect of grapefruit intake on carbamazepine bioavailability: a case report. *Therapie* (2001) 56, 69–71.
2. Garg SK, Kumar N, Bhargava VK, Prabhakar SK. Effect of grapefruit juice on carbamazepine bioavailability in patients with epilepsy. *Clin Pharmacol Ther* (1998) 64, 286–8.
3. Tegretol chewtabs and tablets (Carbamazepine). Cephalon UK Ltd. UK Summary of product characteristics, January 2003.
4. Ameer B, Weintraub RA. Drug interactions with grapefruit juice. *Clin Pharmacokinet* (1997) 33, 103–21.

Carbamazepine or Oxcarbazepine + H_2-blockers

The serum levels of those on long-term carbamazepine may transiently increase, possibly accompanied by an increase in adverse effects, for the first few days after starting to take cimetidine, but these adverse effects rapidly disappear. This does not occur with oxcarbazepine. Ranitidine appears not to interact with carbamazepine.

Clinical evidence

(a) Carbamazepine

The steady-state carbamazepine levels of 8 healthy subjects on carbamazepine 300 mg twice daily were increased by 17% within 2 days of them starting **cimetidine** 400 mg three times daily. Adverse effects occurred in 6 patients, but after 7 days' treatment the carbamazepine levels had fallen again and the adverse effects disappeared.[1]

Conversely, the steady-state carbamazepine levels of 7 epileptic patients on chronic treatment remained unaltered when they were given **cimetidine** 1 g daily for a week.[2] Another study also showed a lack of an interaction in 11 epileptic patients.[3] However, an 89-year-old woman developed symptoms of carbamazepine toxicity within 2 days of starting to take **cimetidine** 400 mg daily, and had a rise in serum carbamazepine levels, which fell when the **cimetidine** was withdrawn.[4] The effects of **cimetidine** may be additive with those of isoniazid, see 'Carbamazepine + Isoniazid or Rifampicin (Rifampin)', below.

The results of these studies in patients and subjects taking carbamazepine long term differ from single-dose studies and short-term studies in healthy subjects. For example, a 33% rise in serum carbamazepine levels,[5] a 20% fall in clearance[6] and a 26% increase in the AUC[7] have been reported, which would indicate potential for a clinically significant interaction (see 'Mechanism' below).

In 8 healthy subjects **ranitidine** 300 mg daily did not affect the pharmacokinetics of a single 600-mg dose of carbamazepine.[8]

(b) Oxcarbazepine

No changes in the pharmacokinetics of a single 600-mg oral dose of oxcarbazepine were seen in 8 healthy subjects who took **cimetidine** 400 mg twice daily for 7 days.[9]

Mechanism

Not fully understood. It is thought that cimetidine can inhibit the activity of the liver enzymes concerned with the metabolism of carbamazepine, resulting in its reduced clearance from the body, but the effect is short-lived because the auto-inducing effects of the carbamazepine oppose it. This would possibly explain why the single-dose and short-term studies in healthy subjects suggest that a clinically important interaction could occur, but in practice the combination causes few problems in patients on long-term treatment.

Importance and management

The interaction between carbamazepine and cimetidine is established but of minimal importance. Patients on long-term treatment with carbamazepine should be warned that for the first few days after starting to take cimetidine they may possibly experience some increase in carbamazepine adverse effects (nausea, headache, dizziness, fatigue, drowsiness, ataxia, an inability to concentrate, a bitter taste). However, because the serum levels are only transiently increased, these effects normally subside and disappear by the end of a week. **Ranitidine** appears to be a non-interacting alternative to cimetidine. Oxcarbazepine appears not to interact with cimetidine.

1. Dalton MJ, Powell JR, Messenheimer JA, Clark J. Cimetidine and carbamazepine: a complex drug interaction. *Epilepsia* (1986) 27, 553–8.
2. Sonne J, Lühdorf K, Larsen NE and Andreasen PB. Lack of interaction between cimetidine and carbamazepine. *Acta Neurol Scand* (1983) 68, 253–6.
3. Levine M, Jones MW, Sheppard I. Differential effect of cimetidine on serum concentrations of carbamazepine and phenytoin. *Neurology* (1985) 35, 562–5.
4. Telerman-Topet N, Duret ME, Coërs C. Cimetidine interaction with carbamazepine. *Ann Intern Med* (1981) 94, 544.
5. Macphee GJA, Thompson GG, Scobie G, Agnew E, Park BK, Murray T, McColl KEL, Brodie MJ. Effects of cimetidine on carbamazepine auto- and hetero-induction in man. *Br J Clin Pharmacol* (1984) 18, 411–19.
6. Webster LK, Mihaly GW, Jones DB, Smallwood RA, Phillips JA, Vajda FJ. Effect of cimetidine and ranitidine on carbamazepine and sodium valproate pharmacokinetics. *Eur J Clin Pharmacol* (1984) 27, 341–3.
7. Dalton MJ, Powell JR, Messenheimer JA. The influence of cimetidine on single-dose carbamazepine pharmacokinetics. *Epilepsia* (1985) 26, 127–30.
8. Dalton MJ, Powell JR, Messenheimer JA. Ranitidine does not alter single-dose carbamazepine pharmacokinetics in healthy adults. *Drug Intell Clin Pharm* (1985) 19, 941–4.
9. Keränen T, Jolkkonen J, Klosterskov-Jensen P, Menge GP. Oxcarbazepine does not interact with cimetidine in healthy volunteers. *Acta Neurol Scand* (1992) 85, 239–42.

Carbamazepine + Influenza vaccines

Carbamazepine levels rose modestly 14 days after influenza vaccination in one study. A case report describes carbamazepine toxicity and markedly increased carbamazepine levels in a teenager 13 days after influenza vaccination.

Clinical evidence, mechanism, importance and management

The serum carbamazepine levels of 20 children rose by 47% from 6.17 to 9.04 micrograms/ml 14 days after they were given 0.5 ml of influenza vaccine USP, types A and B, whole virus (Squibb). Levels remained elevated on day 28.[1] A teenager on carbamazepine 400 mg in the morning and 600 mg at night and gabapentin 600 mg three times daily developed signs of carbamazepine toxicity (unsteady, lethargic, slurred speech) 13 days after influenza vaccination (*Fluzone,* Aventis Pasteur). Her serum carbamazepine level was 27.5 micrograms/ml (previous levels 8.2 to 12.4 micrograms/ml), and she required intubation and maintenance on a ventilator for 19 hours. A urine drug screen was positive for tricyclic antidepressants and cocaine, but it was eventually concluded that these were likely to represent false-positive results.[2]

The suggested reason for the interaction is the vaccine inhibits the liver enzymes concerned with the metabolism of carbamazepine, thereby reducing its loss from the body. Information is very limited. The moderate increase in serum carbamazepine levels seen in the first study is unlikely to have much clinical relevance. However, the case report of markedly increased carbamazepine levels introduces a note of caution. Further study is needed.

1. Jann MW, Fidone GS. Effect of influenza vaccine on serum anticonvulsant concentrations. *Clin Pharm* (1986) 5, 817–20.
2. Robertson WC. Carbamazepine toxicity after influenza vaccination. *Pediatr Neurol* (2002) 26, 61–3.

Carbamazepine + Isoniazid or Rifampicin (Rifampin)

Carbamazepine serum levels are markedly and very rapidly increased by isoniazid and toxicity can occur. Rifampicin has been reported both to augment and negate the interaction between carbamazepine and isoniazid. Limited evidence suggests that carbamazepine may potentiate isoniazid hepatotoxicity.

Clinical evidence

Disorientation, listlessness, aggression, lethargy and, in one case, extreme drowsiness developed in 10 out of 13 patients stabilised on carbamazepine when they were given isoniazid 200 mg daily. Serum carbamazepine levels were measured in 3 of the patients and they were found to have risen above the normal therapeutic range [initial level not stated].[1]

Carbamazepine toxicity, associated with marked rises in serum carbamazepine levels, has been described in other reports.[2-6] Some of the patients were also taking sodium valproate, which does not seem to be implicated in the interaction, and in one case cimetidine, which was thought to have potentiated the interaction.[6] See also 'Carbamazepine or Oxcarbazepine + H_2-blockers', p.343.

One report describes carbamazepine toxicity in a patient given isoniazid, but only when rifampicin was present as well. Usually the enzyme-inducing effects of rifampicin would be expected to counteract any enzyme inhibition by isoniazid, so this report is somewhat inexplicable.[7] Conversely, a case of reduced carbamazepine levels in a woman given rifampicin and isoniazid has been described, with reduced carbamazepine efficacy (symptoms of hypomania).[8]

Isoniazid hepatotoxicity has occurred in a 74-year-old woman[9] and a 10-year-old boy[10] on carbamazepine shortly after treatment with isoniazid, rifampicin, ethambutol, with or without pyrazinamide, was started.

Mechanism

It seems probable that isoniazid inhibits the activity of the cytochrome P450 isoenzyme CYP3A4, which is concerned with the metabolism of carbamazepine, so that it accumulates in the body.[11] Rifampicin is a potent enzyme inducer, and would be expected to negate the effects of isoniazid, and to further induce the metabolism of carbamazepine compared with carbamazepine alone. This is supported by one report, but not another.

Importance and management

The documentation is limited, but a clinically important and potentially serious interaction is established between isoniazid and carbamazepine. Toxicity can develop quickly (within 1 to 5 days) and also seems to disappear quickly if the isoniazid is withdrawn. Concurrent use should not be undertaken unless the effects can be closely monitored and suitable downward dosage adjustments made (a reduction to between one-half or one-third was effective in 3 patients[1]). It seems probable that those who are 'slow' metabolisers of isoniazid may show this interaction more quickly and to a greater extent than fast metabolisers.[2]

The effect of concurrent rifampicin on the interaction between isoniazid and carbamazepine is unclear. One report showed negation of the interaction, whereas another showed potential augmentation. Limited evidence suggests that carbamazepine may potentiate isoniazid hepatotoxicity.

1. Valsalan VC, Cooper GL. Carbamazepine intoxication caused by interaction with isoniazid. *BMJ* (1982) 285, 261–2.
2. Wright JM, Stokes EF, Sweeney VP. Isoniazid-induced carbamazepine toxicity and vice versa: a double drug interaction. *N Engl J Med* (1982) 307, 1325–7.
3. Block SH. Carbamazepine-isoniazid interaction. *Pediatrics* (1982) 69, 494–5.
4. Poo Argüelles P, Samarra Riera JM, Gairí Tahull JM, Vernet Bori A. Interacción carbamacepina-tuberculostáticos. *Med Clin (Barc)* (1984) 83, 867–8.
5. Beeley L, Ballantine N. *Bulletin of the West Midlands Centre for Adverse Drug Reaction Reporting* (1981) 13, 8.
6. García B, Zaborras E, Areas V, Obeso G, Jiménez I, de Juana P, Bermejo T. Interaction between isoniazid and carbamazepine potentiated by cimetidine. *Ann Pharmacother* (1992) 26, 841–2.
7. Fleenor ME, Harden JW, Curtis G. Interaction between carbamazepine and antituberculous agents. *Chest* (1991) 99, 1554.
8. Zolezzi M, Antituberculosis agents and carbamazepine. *Am J Psychiatry* (2002) 159, 874.
9. Barbare JC, Lallement PY, Vorhauer W, Veyssier P. Hépatotoxicité de l'isoniazide: influence de la carbamazépine? *Gastroenterol Clin Biol* (1986) 10, 523–4.
10. Berkowitz FE, Henderson SL, Fajman N, Schoen B, Naughton M. Acute liver failure caused by isoniazid in a child receiving carbamazepine. *Int J Tuberc Lung Dis* (1998) 2, 603–6.
11. Desta Z, Soukhova NV, Flockhart DA. Inhibition of cytochrome P450 (CYP450) isoforms by isoniazid: potent inhibition of CYP2C19 and CYP3A. *Antimicrob Agents Chemother* (2001) 45, 384–92.

Carbamazepine + Lamotrigine

Most studies have found that lamotrigine has no effect on the pharmacokinetics of carbamazepine or its epoxide metabolite. However, some studies have found that lamotrigine raises the serum levels of carbamazepine-epoxide. Carbamazepine reduces lamotrigine levels. Toxicity has been seen irrespective of changes in levels.

Clinical evidence

(a) Evidence of changes in carbamazepine metabolism

The addition of lamotrigine increased the serum levels of carbamazepine-epoxide, the active metabolite of carbamazepine, in 3 epileptic patients, but carbamazepine levels remained unchanged. One of the patients had carbamazepine-epoxide serum levels of 2 to 2.2 micrograms/ml while taking carbamazepine 1.1 g daily. The levels rose to 4.7 to 8.7 micrograms/ml when lamotrigine was added. Symptoms of toxicity occurred in 2 patients (dizziness, double vision, sleepiness, nausea).[1] In another study in 9 patients, the addition of lamotrigine 200 mg increased the mean serum carbamazepine-epoxide levels by 45%. Toxicity was seen in 4 patients (dizziness, nausea, diplopia).[2] Cerebellar toxicity (nausea, vertigo, nystagmus, ataxia) developed in 8 out of 9 patients on subtoxic and just-tolerated doses of carbamazepine when lamotrigine was added. Analysis showed that in all 8 cases at least one of the levels of carbamazepine, carbamazepine-epoxide or lamotrigine had become unusually high, but the authors concluded the interaction was likely to be pharmacodynamic rather than pharmacokinetic.[3]

(b) Evidence of no changes in carbamazepine metabolism

The studies cited in (a) contrast with others that found no pharmacokinetic effects. No changes in carbamazepine levels were seen in two clinical studies,[4,5] and another pharmacokinetic study found that lamotrigine 200 to 300 mg daily had no effect on the disposition of a single dose of oral carbamazepine-epoxide.[6] Another study in 47 patients on carbamazepine, to which lamotrigine was added, found no significant changes in carbamazepine or carbamazepine-epoxide levels. Despite this 9 cases of diplopia or dizziness were recorded, predominantly in those whose carbamazepine levels were already high before the lamotrigine was added, although even these 9 patients had no change in carbamazepine or carbamazepine-epoxide levels.[7] A further well-designed study in healthy subjects found that lamotrigine 100 mg twice daily for a week had no effect on the pharmacokinetics of carbamazepine or carbamazepine-epoxide after a single 200-mg dose of carbamazepine.[8] Similarly, lamotrigine had no effect on mean carbamazepine levels, and actually decreased mean carbamazepine-epoxide levels by 23% in a study in 14 children. Two children developed diplopia, which was unrelated to drug levels, but responded to a reduction in lamotrigine dose in one, and a reduction in carbamazepine dose in the other.[9]

(c) Reduced lamotrigine levels

In a retrospective study, the lamotrigine serum concentration-to-dose ratio was much lower in patients also taking carbamazepine than in those on lamotrigine monotherapy (0.38 versus 0.84).[10] Other studies have reported similar findings.[11,12] In another study, mean increases in lamotrigine levels of about 60% occurred in patients on lamotrigine and carbamazepine when the carbamazepine was withdrawn.[13] Similarly, a case report describes a rapid increase in lamotrigine levels when carbamazepine was withdrawn.[14]

Mechanism

The apparent contradiction between the results described in (a) and (b) is not understood. One suggestion to account for the toxic symptoms seen in some patients is that it occurs at the site of action (a pharmacodynamic interaction) rather than because lamotrigine increases the carbamazepine-epoxide serum levels.[3,7] Carbamazepine may induce the glucuronidation of lamotrigine.

Importance and management

Overall lamotrigine does not appear to significantly alter carbamazepine levels. However, toxicity has occurred, therefore patients should be well monitored if lamotrigine is added, and the carbamazepine dose reduced if CNS adverse effects occur. Carbamazepine induces the metabolism of lamotrigine, and the recommended starting dose and long-term maintenance dose of lamotrigine in patients already taking carbamazepine is twice that of patients on lamotrigine monotherapy.[15] However, if they are also taking valproate in addition to carbamazepine, the lamotrigine dose should be reduced.[15] See 'Lamotrigine + Sodium valproate', p.354.

1. Graves NM, Ritter FJ, Wagner ML, Floren KL, Alexander BJ, Campbell JI, Leppik IE. Effect of lamotrigine on carbamazepine epoxide concentrations. *Epilepsia* (1991) 32 (Suppl 3), 13.
2. Warner T, Patsalos PN, Prevett M, Elyas AA, Duncan JS. Lamotrigine-induced carbamazepine toxicity: an interaction with carbamazepine-10,11-epoxide. *Epilepsy Res* (1992) 11, 147–50.
3. Wolf P. Lamotrigine: preliminary clinical observations on pharmacokinetics and interactions with traditional antiepileptic drugs. *J Epilepsy* (1992) 5, 73–9.
4. Jawad S, Richens A, Goodwin G, Yuen WC. Controlled trial of lamotrigine (Lamictal) for refractory partial seizures. *Epilepsia* (1989) 30, 356–63.
5. Eriksson A-S, Hoppu K, Nergårdh A, Boreus L. Pharmacokinetic interactions between lamotrigine and other antiepileptic drugs in children with intractable epilepsy. *Epilepsia* (1996) 37, 769–73.
6. Pisani F, Xiao B, Fazio A, Spina E, Perucca E, Tomson T. Single dose pharmacokinetics of carbamazepine-10,11-epoxide in patients on lamotrigine monotherapy. *Epilepsy Res* (1994) 19, 245–8.
7. Besag FMC, Berry DJ, Pool F, Newbery JE, Subel B. Carbamazepine toxicity with lamotrigine: a pharmacokinetic or pharmacodynamic interaction? *Epilepsia* (1998) 39, 183–7.

8. Malminiemi K, Keränen T, Kerttula T, Moilanen E, Ylitalo P. Effects of short-term lamotrigine treatment on pharmacokinetics of carbamazepine. *Int J Clin Pharmacol Ther* (2000) 38, 540–5.
9. Eriksson A-S, Boreus LO. No increase in carbamazepione-10,11-epoxide during addition of lamotrigine treatment in children. *Ther Drug Monit* (1997) 19, 499–501.
10. Armijo JA, Bravo J, Cuadrado A, Herranz JL. Lamotrigine serum concentration-to-dose ratio: influence of age and concomitant antiepileptic drugs and dosage implications. *Ther Drug Monit* (1999) 21, 182–190.
11. Böttiger Y, Svensson J-O, Ståhle L. Lamotrigine drug interactions in a TDM material. *Ther Drug Monit* (1999) 21, 171–4.
12. May TW, Rambeck B, Jürgens U. Influence of oxcarbazepine and methsuximide on lamotrigine concentrations in epileptic patients with and without valproic acid comedication: results of a retrospective study. *Ther Drug Monit* (1999) 21, 175–81.
13. Anderson GD, Gidal BE, Messenheimer J, Gilliam FG. Time course of lamotrigine de-induction: impact of step-wise withdrawal of carbamazepine or phenytoin. *Epilepsy Res* (2002) 49, 211–17.
14. Koch HJ, Szecsey A, Vogel M. Clinically relevant reduction of lamotrigine concentrations by carbamazepine. *Eur Psychiatry* (2003) 18, 42.
15. Lamictal (Lamotrigine). GlaxoSmithKline UK. UK Summary of product characteristics, June 2005.

Carbamazepine + Macrolides

Carbamazepine serum levels are markedly and rapidly increased by erythromycin or troleandomycin, and to a lesser extent clarithromycin. Toxicity can often develop within 1 to 3 days. Flurithromycin, josamycin and midecamycin acetate appear not to interact to a clinically relevant extent, and azithromycin and roxithromycin not at all. Telithromycin is predicted to interact.

Clinical evidence

(a) Azithromycin

Azithromycin 500 mg once daily for 3 days had no effect on the pharmacokinetics of carbamazepine 200 mg twice daily or its active metabolite in healthy subjects.[1]

(b) Clarithromycin

A pharmacokinetic study[2] in healthy subjects found that clarithromycin 500 mg every 12 hours for 5 days increased the AUC of a single 400-mg dose of carbamazepine by 26%. A retrospective study of 5 epileptic patients found that when they were given clarithromycin [dosage not stated] their serum carbamazepine levels rose by 20 to 50% within 3 to 5 days, despite 30 to 40% reductions in the carbamazepine dosage in 4 of them. Carbamazepine levels in the toxic range were seen in 3 of them, and their carbamazepine dosages were then even further reduced.[3] A number of case reports have described carbamazepine toxicity following the addition of clarithromycin in adults,[4-6] and children.[7,8] Two other epileptic patients had marked rises in serum carbamazepine levels when they were given clarithromycin 500 mg three times daily and omeprazole.[9] It is not clear whether the omeprazole also had some part to play.[10,11] See also 'Carbamazepine + Proton pump inhibitors', p.347).

(c) Erythromycin

An 8-year-old girl on phenobarbital 50 mg and carbamazepine 800 mg daily was given 500 mg, then later 1 g of erythromycin daily. Within 2 days she began to experience balancing difficulties and ataxia, which were eventually attributed to carbamazepine toxicity. Her serum carbamazepine levels were found to have risen from a little below 10 micrograms/ml to over 25 micrograms/ml (therapeutic range 2 to 10 micrograms/ml). The levels rapidly returned to normal after carbamazepine was withheld for 24 hours and the erythromycin stopped.[12]

A study in 7 healthy subjects confirmed that erythromycin can cause significant increases in carbamazepine levels,[13] and a study in 8 healthy subjects found that the clearance of carbamazepine is reduced by an average of 20% (range 5 to 41%) by erythromycin 1 g daily for 5 days.[14]

Marked rises in serum carbamazepine levels (up to fivefold in some cases) and/or toxicity (including cases of hepatorenal failure and AV block as well as more typical signs of carbamazepine toxicity) have been described in over 30 cases involving both children and adults. Symptoms commonly began within 24 to 72 hours of starting erythromycin, although in some cases it was as early as 8 hours. In most cases toxicity resolved within 3 to 5 days of stopping the erythromycin.[7,15-33]

(d) Flurithromycin

Flurithromycin 500 mg three times daily for a week increased the AUC of a single 400-mg dose of carbamazepine by about 20% and moderately reduced the production of carbamazepine-epoxide in healthy subjects.[34]

(e) Josamycin

Josamycin 2 g daily for a week reduced the clearance of carbamazepine by about 20% in healthy subjects and in patients.[35,36]

(f) Midecamycin acetate

A single dose study in 14 subjects found that after taking midecamycin acetate 800 mg twice daily for 8 days the AUC of a single 200-mg dose of carbamazepine was increased by 15%, and the AUC of its active metabolite (10,11-epoxycarbamazepine) was reduced 26%.[37] Another study in patients on carbamazepine found that the addition of midecamycin acetate 600 mg twice daily caused a small increase in the trough serum levels of carbamazepine, and only an 11.6% increase in the AUC.[38]

(g) Roxithromycin

Roxithromycin 150 mg twice daily for 8 days did not affect the pharmacokinetics of a single 200-mg dose of carbamazepine.[39]

(h) Telithromycin

The maker predicts that carbamazepine will reduce the levels of telithromycin, with possible loss of efficacy, because carbamazepine induces the cytochrome P450 isoenzyme CYP3A4. Telithromycin is an inhibitor of CYP3A4, and may therefore raise carbamazepine levels.[40]

(i) Troleandomycin

Symptoms of carbamazepine toxicity (dizziness, nausea, vomiting, excessive drowsiness) developed in 8 epileptic patients on carbamazepine within 24 hours of starting to take troleandomycin. The only 2 patients available for examination showed a sharp rise in serum carbamazepine levels, from about 5 to 28 micrograms/ml over 3 days, and a rapid fall following withdrawal of the troleandomycin.[41,42]

Another report by the same authors describes a total of 17 similar cases of carbamazepine toxicity caused by troleandomycin.[15] Some of the patients had three or fourfold increases in serum carbamazepine levels. Another case has been described elsewhere.[12] In most instances the serum carbamazepine levels returned to normal within about 3 to 5 days of withdrawing the macrolide.[15]

Mechanism

It seems probable that clarithromycin, erythromycin and troleandomycin, and to a lesser extent some of the other macrolides, slow the rate of metabolism of the carbamazepine by the cytochrome P450 isoenzyme CYP3A4 so that the anticonvulsant accumulates within the body.[43,44] Telithromycin is predicted to interact similarly.[40]

Importance and management

The interaction between carbamazepine and troleandomycin is established, clinically important and potentially serious. The incidence is high. The rapidity of its development (within 24 hours in some cases) and the extent of the rise in serum carbamazepine levels suggest that it would be difficult to control carbamazepine levels by reducing the dosage. Concurrent use should probably be avoided.

The interaction between carbamazepine and erythromycin is also very well documented, well established and of clinical importance. Concurrent use should be avoided unless the effects can be very closely monitored by measurement of serum carbamazepine levels and suitable dosage reductions made. Toxic symptoms (ataxia, vertigo, drowsiness, lethargy, confusion, diplopia) can develop within 24 hours, but serum carbamazepine levels can return to normal within 8 to 12 hours of withdrawing the antibacterial.[35]

The interaction between carbamazepine and clarithromycin is also established, clinically important and potentially serious. However, the extent of the interaction is less with clarithromycin than erythromycin or troleandomycin (i.e. the rise in carbamazepine levels is less).[45] It has been recommended that carbamazepine dosages should be reduced by 30 to 50% during treatment with clarithromycin, with monitoring within 3 to 5 days, and patients should be told to tell their doctor of any symptoms of toxicity (dizziness, diplopia, ataxia, mental confusion).

Analysis of the macrolide/carbamazepine interactions has shown that patients requiring high doses of carbamazepine to reach therapeutic levels are likely to have a greater rise in their carbamazepine levels.[45] The extent of the interactions is also correlated with the macrolide dose.[45]

Josamycin, flurithromycin and midecamycin acetate appear to be safer alternatives to either clarithromycin, erythromycin or troleandomycin, nevertheless a small or moderate reduction in the dosage of the carbamazepine may be needed, with subsequent good monitoring. Pharmacokinetic data suggest that azithromycin and roxithromycin do not interact. Telithromycin is predicted to interact, and the maker advises avoidance of the combination.[40]

1. Rapeport WG, Dewland PM, Muirhead DC, Forster PL. Lack of an interaction between azithromycin and carbamazepine. *Br J Clin Pharmacol* (1992) 33, 551P.
2. Richens A, Chu S-Y, Sennello LT, Sonders RC. Effect of multiple doses of clarithromycin (C) on the pharmacokinetics (Pks) of carbamazepine (Carb). *Intersci Conf Antimicrob Agents Chemother* (1990) 30, 213.
3. O'Connor NK, Fris J. Clarithromycin-carbamazepine interaction in a clinical setting. *J Am Board Fam Pract* (1994) 7, 489–92.
4. Albani F, Riva R, Baruzzi A. Clarithromycin-carbamazepine interaction: a case report. *Epilepsia* (1993) 34, 161–2.
5. Yasui N, Otani K, Kaneko S, Shimoyama R, Ohkubo T, Sugawara K. Carbamazepine toxicity induced by clarithromycin coadministration in psychiatric patients. *Int Clin Psychopharmacol* (1997) 12, 225–9.
6. Tatum WO, Gonzalez MA. Carbamazepine toxicity in an epileptic induced by clarithromycin. *Hosp Pharm* (1994) 29, 45–6.
7. Stafstrom CE, Nohria V, Loganbill H, Nahouraii R, Boustany R-M, DeLong GR. Erythromycin-induced carbamazepine toxicity: a continuing problem. *Arch Pediatr Adolesc Med* (1995) 149, 99–101.
8. Carmona Ibáñez G, Guevara Serrano J, Gisbert González S. Toxicidad de carbamacepina inducida por eritromicina. Un problema frencuente. *Farm Clin* (1996) 13, 698–700.
9. Metz DC, Getz HD. *Helicobacter pylori* gastritis therapy with omeprazole and clarithromycin increases serum carbamazepine levels. *Dig Dis Sci* (1995) 40, 912–15.
10. Dammann H-G. Therapy with omeprazole and clarithromycin increases serum carbamazepine levels in patients with *H.pylori* gastritis. *Dig Dis Sci* (1996) 41, 519.
11. Metz DC, Getz HD. Therapy with omeprazole and clarithromycin increases serum carbamazepine levels in patients with *H.pylori* gastritis. *Dig Dis Sci* (1996) 41, 519–20.
12. Amedee-Manesme O, Rey E, Brussieux J, Goutieres F, Aicardi J. Antibiotiques à ne jamais associer à la carbamazépine. *Arch Fr Pediatr* (1982) 39, 126.
13. Miles MV, Tennison MB. Erythromycin effects on multiple-dose carbamazepine kinetics. *Ther Drug Monit* (1989) 11, 47–52.
14. Wong YY, Ludden TM, Bell RD. Effect of erythromycin on carbamazepine kinetics. *Drug Intell Clin Pharm* (1982) 16, 484.
15. Mesdjian E, Dravet C, Cenraud B, Roger J. Carbamazepine intoxication due to triacetyloleandomycin administration in epileptic patients. *Epilepsia* (1980) 21, 489–96.
16. Straughan J. Erythromycin-carbamazepine interaction? *S Afr Med J* (1982) 61, 420–1.
17. Vajda FJE, Bladin PF. Carbamazepine-erythromycin-base interaction. *Med J Aust* (1984) 140, 81.
18. Hedrick R, Williams F, Morin R, Lamb WA, Cate JC. Carbamazepine-erythromycin interaction leading to carbamazepine toxicity in four epileptic children. *Ther Drug Monit* (1983) 5, 405–7.
19. Miller SL. The association of carbamazepine intoxication and erythromycin use. *Ann Neurol* (1985) 18, 413.
20. Berrettini WH. A case of erythromycin-induced carbamazepine toxicity. *J Clin Psychiatry* (1986) 47, 147.
21. Carranco E, Kareus J, Co S, Peak V, Al-Rajeh S. Carbamazepine toxicity induced by concurrent erythromycin therapy. *Arch Neurol* (1985) 42, 187–8.
22. Goulden KJ, Camfield P, Dooley JM, Fraser A, Meek DC, Renton KW, Tibbles JAR. Severe carbamazepine intoxication after coadministration of erythromycin. *J Pediatr* (1986) 109, 135–8.
23. Wroblewski BA, Singer WD, Whyte J. Carbamazepine-erythromycin interaction. Case studies and clinical significance. *JAMA* (1986) 255, 1165–7.
24. Kessler JM. Erythromycin-carbamazepine interaction. *S Afr Med J* (1985) 67, 1038.
25. Jaster PJ, Abbas D. Erythromycin-carbamazepine interaction. *Neurology* (1986) 36, 594–5.
26. Loiseau P, Guyot M, Pautrizel B, Vincon G, Albin H. Intoxication par la carbamazépine due à l'interaction carbamazépine-érythromycine. *Presse Med* (1985) 14, 162.
27. Zitelli BJ, Howrie DL, Altman H, Marcon TJ. Erythromycin-induced drug interactions. *Clin Pediatr (Phila)* (1987) 26, 117–19.
28. Goldhoorn PB, Hofstee N. Een interactie tussen erytromycine en carbamazepine. *Ned Tijdschr Geneeskd* (1989) 133, 1944.
29. Mitsch RA. Carbamazepine toxicity precipitated by intravenous erythromycin. *DICP Ann Pharmacother* (1989) 23, 878–9.
30. Macnab AJ, Robinson JL, Adderly RJ, D'Orsogna L. Heart block secondary to erythromycin-induced carbamazepine toxicity. *Pediatrics* (1987) 80, 951–3.
31. Woody RC, Kearns GL, Bolyard KJ. Carbamazepine intoxication following the use of erythromycin in children. *Pediatr Infect Dis J* (1987) 6, 578–9.
32. Mota CR, Carvalho C, Mota C, Ferreira P, Vilarinho A, Pereira E. Severe carbamazepine toxicity induced by concurrent erythromycin therapy. *Eur J Pediatr* (1996) 155, 345–8.
33. Viani F, Claris-Appiani A, Rossi LN, Giani M, Romeo A. Severe hepatorenal failure in a child receiving carbamazepine and erythromycin. *Eur J Pediatr* (1992) 151, 715–16.
34. Barzaghi N, Gatti G, Crema F, Faja A, Monteleone M, Amione C, Leone L, Perucca E. Effect of flurithromycin, a new macrolide antibiotic, on carbamazepine disposition in normal subjects. *Int J Clin Pharmacol Res* (1988) 8, 101–5.
35. Albin H, Vincon G, Pehourcq F, Dangoumau J. Influence de la josamycine sur la pharmacocinétique de la carbamazépine. *Therapie* (1982) 37, 151–6.
36. Vincon G, Albin H, Demotes-Mainard F, Guyot M, Brachet-Liermain A, Loiseau P. Pharmacokinetic interaction between carbamazepine and josamycin. Proc Eur Congr Biopharmaceutics Pharmacokinetics vol III: Clinical Pharmacokinetics. Edited by Aiache JM and Hirtz J. Published by Imprimerie de l'Universite de Clermont-Ferrand. *(1984) pp 270–6.* (1984) pp 270–6.
37. Couet W, Istin B, Ingrand I, Girault J, Fourtillan J-B. Effect of ponsinomycin on single-dose kinetics and metabolism of carbamazepine. *Ther Drug Monit* (1990) 12, 144–9.
38. Zagnoni PG, DeLuca M, Casini A. Carbamazepine-miocamycin interaction. *Epilepsia* (1991) 32 (Suppl 1), 28.
39. Saint-Salvi B, Tremblay D, Surjus A, Lefebvre MA. A study of the interaction of roxithromycin with theophylline and carbamazepine. *J Antimicrob Chemother* (1987) 20 (Suppl B), 121–9.
40. Ketek (Telithromycin). Aventis Pharma Ltd. UK Summary of product characteristics, January 2004.
41. Dravet C, Mesdjian E, Cenraud B, Roger J. Interaction between carbamazepine and triacetyloleandomycin. *Lancet* (1977) i, 810–11.
42. Dravet C, Mesdjian E, Cenraud B, Roger J. Interaction carbamazépine triacétyloléandomycine: une nouvelle interaction médicamenteuse? *Nouv Presse Med* (1977) 6, 467.
43. Pessayre D, Larrey D, Vitaux J, Breil P, Belghiti J, Benhamou J-P. Formation of an inactive cytochrome P-450 Fe(II)-metabolite complex after administration of troleandomycin in humans. *Biochem Pharmacol* (1982) 31, 1699–1704.
44. Levy RH, Johnson CM, Thummel KE, Kerr BM, Kroetz DL, Korzecwa KR, Gonzales FJ. Mechanism of the interaction between carbamazepine and erythromycin. *Epilepsia* (1993) 34 (Suppl 6), 37–8.
45. Pauwels O. Factors contributing to carbamazepine-macrolide interactions. *Pharmacol Res* (2002) 45, 291–8.

Carbamazepine + MAOIs

Phenelzine, moclobemide and tranylcypromine appear not to interact adversely with carbamazepine.

Clinical evidence, mechanism, importance and management

There appear to be no reports of adverse reactions during the concurrent use of MAOIs and carbamazepine. However, the makers of carbamazepine say that concurrent use should be avoided because of the close structural similarity between carbamazepine and the tricyclic antidepressants (and therefore the theoretical risk of an adverse interaction). Several reports describe successful use of carbamazepine and MAOIs, namely **tranylcypromine**,[1,2] **phenelzine**,[3] and **moclobemide**.[4] Bearing in mind that the MAOIs and the tricyclics can be given together under certain well controlled conditions (see 'MAOIs + Tricyclic antidepressants', p.873), the warning about the risks may possibly prove to be overcautious. As yet there seems to be no direct information about other MAOIs.

1. Lydiard RB, White D, Harvey B, Taylor A. Lack of pharmacokinetic interaction between tranylcypromine and carbamazepine. *J Clin Psychopharmacol* (1987) 7, 360.
2. Joffe RT, Post RM, Uhde TW. Lack of pharmacokinetic interaction of carbamazepine with tranylcypromine. *Arch Gen Psychiatry* (1985) 42, 738.
3. Yatham LN, Barry S, Mobayed M, Dinan TG. Is the carbamazepine-phenelzine combination safe? *Am J Psychiatry* (1990) 147, 367.
4. Amrein R, Güntert TW, Dingemanse J, Lorscheid T, Stabl M, Schmid-Burgk W. Interactions of moclobemide with concomitantly administered medication: evidence from pharmacological and clinical studies. *Psychopharmacology (Berl)* (1992) 106, S24–S31.

Carbamazepine + Metronidazole

Increased serum carbamazepine levels and toxicity have been seen in a patient also given metronidazole.

Clinical evidence, mechanism, importance and management

A woman on carbamazepine 1 g daily was additionally started on co-trimoxazole twice daily and metronidazole 250 g three times daily for diverticulitis. After 2 days the co-trimoxazole was stopped, she was changed to intravenous metronidazole 500 mg three times daily, and cefazolin 500 mg every 8 hours added. After 2 days she complained of diplopia, dizziness and nausea, and her serum carbamazepine levels were found to have risen from 9 to 14.3 micrograms/ml. A month later (presumably after the metronidazole had been withdrawn) her serum carbamazepine levels had fallen to 7.1 micrograms/ml. The reasons for this reaction are not understood.[1]

This appears to be the first and only report of an interaction between carbamazepine and metronidazole, so its general importance is uncertain. More study is needed.

1. Patterson BD. Possible interaction between metronidazole and carbamazepine. *Ann Pharmacother* (1994) 28, 1303–4.

Carbamazepine + Nefazodone

Five patients developed elevated serum carbamazepine levels and toxicity when nefazodone was added. A study in healthy subjects using lower carbamazepine doses found only modest increases in carbamazepine levels, and no evidence of toxicity when nefazodone was given. Carbamazepine markedly reduced nefazodone levels.

Clinical evidence

A patient on carbamazepine 1 g daily developed evidence of toxicity (light-headedness, ataxia) within 15 days of starting to take nefazodone (initially 100 mg twice daily increasing to 150 mg twice daily after a week). Her serum carbamazepine levels had risen from a range of 7 to 8.3 micrograms/ml up to 10.8 micrograms/ml. It was found necessary to reduce the carbamazepine dosage to 600 mg daily to eliminate these adverse effects and to achieve serum levels of 7.4 micrograms/ml.[1] In 4 other patients on carbamazepine 800 or 1000 mg daily the addition of nefazodone caused up to threefold rises in carbamazepine levels. The carbamazepine dose was reduced by 25 to 60%.[1,2] In a study in 12 healthy subjects no evidence of toxicity was seen when carbamazepine 200 mg twice daily was given with nefazodone 200 mg twice daily for 5 days. However, the levels of carbamazepine were slightly increased (23% increase in AUC) and the levels of nefazodone markedly decreased (93% decrease in AUC). The authors suggest that there may be a greater effect with higher doses of carbamazepine.[3]

Mechanism

Both drugs are metabolised by the cytochrome P450 isoenzyme CYP3A4, so it would seem that nefazodone can inhibit carbamazepine metabolism, while carbamazepine can induce nefazodone metabolism.

Importance and management

Information is limited, but it would seem prudent to monitor for signs of carbamazepine toxicity if nefazodone is added to established treatment, especially with doses of carbamazepine above 800 mg. The nefazodone dosage may need to be increased in the presence of carbamazepine, so be alert for a reduced effect. Further study is needed.

1. Ashton AK, Wolin RE. Nefazodone-induced carbamazepine toxicity. *Am J Psychiatry* (1996) 153, 733.
2. Roth L, Bertschy G. Nefazodone may inhibit the metabolism of carbamazepine: three case reports. *Eur Psychiatry* (2001) 16, 320–1.
3. Laroudie C, Salazar DE, Cosson J-P, Cheuvart B, Istin B, Girault J, Ingrand I, Decourt J-P. Carbamazepine-nefazodone interaction in healthy subjects. *J Clin Psychopharmacol* (2000) 20, 46–53.

Carbamazepine + Phenobarbital

Carbamazepine serum levels are reduced to some extent by phenobarbital, and carbamazepine-epoxide levels are raised. In children, phenobarbital clearance is decreased by carbamazepine.

Clinical evidence

A comparative study found that on average patients taking both carbamazepine and phenobarbital (44 patients) had carbamazepine serum levels that were 18% lower than those taking carbamazepine alone (43 patients).[1] Similar results were found in other studies in both adult and paediatric patients taking both drugs.[2,3] Levels of the active metabolite, carbamazepine-epoxide, were increased.[3,4]

In a prospective study the clearance of phenobarbital in 222 patients on monotherapy was compared to that in 63 patients who were also taking carbamazepine. During phenobarbital monotherapy, clearance was highest in the very young, decreased with increasing weight, and was lowest in adults. The pattern was similar for carbamazepine, except that clearance was decreased compared with that in monotherapy. Further, the effects of carbamazepine on phenobarbital clearance were maximal in young children (about 54%) and minimal in adults.[5]

Mechanism

Phenobarbital and carbamazepine are both known enzyme inducers, and may therefore increase each others metabolism.

Importance and management

An established interaction. It would be prudent to monitor phenobarbital levels in children also given carbamazepine as changes in clearance may affect dose requirements. The small fall in serum carbamazepine levels probably has little practical importance, especially since the metabolite carbamazepine-epoxide also has anticonvulsant activity. See also 'Carbamazepine + Primidone', below.

1. Christiansen J, Dam M. Influence of phenobarbital and diphenylhydantoin on plasma carbamazepine levels in patients with epilepsy. *Acta Neurol Scand* (1973) 49, 543–6.
2. Cereghino JJ, Brock JT, Van Meter JC, Penry JK, Smith LD, White BG. The efficacy of carbamazepine combinations in epilepsy. *Clin Pharmacol Ther* (1975) 18, 733–41.
3. Rane A, Höjer B, Wilson JT. Kinetics of carbamazepine and its 10,11-epoxide metabolite in children. *Clin Pharmacol Ther* (1976) 19, 276–83.
4. Dam M, Jensen A, Christiansen J. Plasma level and effect of carbamazepine in grand mal and psychomotor epilepsy. *Acta Neurol Scand* (1975) 75 (Suppl 51), 33–8.
5. Yukawa E, To H, Ohdo S, Higuchi S, Aoyama T. Detection of a drug-drug interaction on population-based phenobarbitone clearance using nonlinear mixed-effects modelling. *Eur J Clin Pharmacol* (1998) 54, 69–74.

Carbamazepine + Primidone

A single case report suggests that primidone can reduce the effects of carbamazepine. There is other evidence that carbamazepine may reduce primidone serum levels and increase derived phenobarbital levels.

Clinical evidence

The complex partial seizures of a 15-year-old boy were not controlled despite treatment with primidone 12 mg/kg daily in three divided doses and carbamazepine 10 mg/kg daily in three divided doses. Even when the carbamazepine dosage was increased to 20 and then to 30 mg/kg daily his serum carbamazepine levels only rose from 3.5 to 4 and then 4.8 micrograms/ml, and his seizures continued. When the primidone was gradually withdrawn his serum carbamazepine levels increased to 12 micrograms/ml and his seizures completely disappeared.[1]

An analysis of serum levels of anticonvulsants in children found that the serum levels of primidone tended to be lower in those also on carbamazepine, but no details were given.[2] Another study found that levels of phenobarbital derived from primidone were higher in patients also on carbamazepine plus phenytoin (42 micrograms/ml) than in those also on phenytoin and primidone (24.7 micrograms/ml) or primidone alone (9.9 micrograms/ml).[3] In a retrospective study, the plasma level to dose ratio for primidone was lower in patients also taking carbamazepine than in those on primidone alone, and the derived phenobarbital levels were higher.[4]

Mechanism

When the primidone was stopped in the single case cited, the clearance of the carbamazepine decreased by about 60%.[1] This is consistent with the known enzyme-inducing effects of primidone (converted in the body to phenobarbital) which can increase the metabolism of other drugs by the liver. Carbamazepine also appears to increase the metabolism of primidone to phenobarbital.

Importance and management

Direct information seems to be limited to these reports. It may be prudent to monitor combined treatment, and adjust doses if necessary. See also 'Carbamazepine + Phenobarbital', above.

1. Benetello P, Furlanut M. Primidone-carbamazepine interaction: clinical consequences. *Int J Clin Pharmacol Res* (1987) 7, 165–8.
2. Windorfer A, Sauer W. Drug interactions during anticonvulsant therapy in childhood: diphenylhydantoin, primidone, phenobarbitone, clonazepam, nitrazepam, carbamazepin and dipropylacetate. *Neuropadiatrie* (1977) 8, 29–41.
3. Callaghan N, Feeley M, Duggan F, O'Callaghan M, Seldrup J. The effect of anticonvulsant drugs which induce liver microsomal enzymes on derived and ingested phenobarbitone levels. *Acta Neurol Scand* (1977) 56, 1–6.
4. Battino D, Avanzini G, Bossi L, Croci D, Cusi C, Gomeni C, Moise A. Plasma levels of primidone and its metabolite phenobarbital: effect of age and associated therapy. *Ther Drug Monit* (1983) 5, 73–9.

Carbamazepine + Protease inhibitors

For mention that ritonavir can precipitate carbamazepine toxicity, and of the effect that carbamazepine has on protease inhibitors, see 'Protease inhibitors + Anticonvulsants; Carbamazepine', p.608.

Carbamazepine + Proton pump inhibitors

Omeprazole markedly raised the levels of a single dose of carbamazepine, but this did not occur with long-term carbamazepine treatment. Some anecdotal reports suggest that carbamazepine serum levels may possibly be reduced by lansoprazole. Pantoprazole did not affect the pharmacokinetics of carbamazepine.

Clinical evidence

(a) Lansoprazole

The makers of lansoprazole have on record 5 undetailed case reports of apparent interactions between lansoprazole and carbamazepine. One of them describes the development of carbamazepine toxicity when lansoprazole was added, but there is some doubt about this case because it is thought that the patient may have started to take higher doses of carbamazepine.

The other 4 cases are consistent in that carbamazepine levels fell shortly after lansoprazole was added and/or the control of seizures suddenly worsened. One patient had a fall in carbamazepine serum levels from 11.5 to 7.7 mg/l. The carbamazepine levels of another patient returned to normal when the lansoprazole was stopped.[1]

(b) Omeprazole

Omeprazole 20 mg daily for 14 days was found to increase the AUC of a single 400-mg dose of carbamazepine in 7 patients by 75%. The clearance was reduced by 40% and the elimination half-life was more than doubled (from 17.2 to 37.3 hours).[2] However, a retrospective study of the records of 10 patients on omeprazole 20 mg daily and continuous treatment with carbamazepine (rather than a single dose) found a non-significant reduction in carbamazepine serum levels.[3]

(c) Pantoprazole

Pantoprazole 40 mg daily for 5 days had no effect on the AUC of carbamazepine or carbamazepine epoxide after a single 400-mg dose of carbamazepine in healthy subjects.[4]

Mechanism

Omeprazole may inhibit the oxidative metabolism of single doses of carbamazepine. However, when carbamazepine is taken continuously it induces its own metabolism by the cytochrome P450 isoenzyme CYP3A4, thereby possibly opposing the effects of this interaction.[3]

Importance and management

It seems that in practice no clinically relevant interaction is likely to occur between omeprazole and carbamazepine. For lansoprazole, information seems to be limited to this handful of reports from which no broad general conclusions can be drawn, but they do suggest that this interaction should be considered if **lansoprazole** is added to established treatment with carbamazepine. Pantoprazole appears not to affect the pharmacokinetics of carbamazepine.

1. Wyeth (UK). Personal communication, September 2001.
2. Naidu MUR, Shoba J, Dixit VK, Kumar A, Kumar TR, Sekhar KR, Sekhar EC. Effect of multiple dose omeprazole on the pharmacokinetics of carbamazepine. *Drug Invest* (1994) 7, 8–12.
3. Böttiger Y, Bertilsson L. No effect on plasma carbamazepine concentration with concomitant omeprazole treatment. *Drug Invest* (1995) 9, 180–1.
4. Huber R, Bliesath H, Hartmann M, Steinijans VW, Koch H, Mascher H, Wurst W. Pantoprazole does not interact with the pharmacokinetics of carbamazepine. *Int J Clin Pharmacol Ther* (1998) 36, 521–4.

Carbamazepine + Sodium valproate

The serum levels of carbamazepine are usually only slightly affected by sodium valproate although a moderate to marked rise in the levels of its epoxide metabolite may occur. The carbamazepine dose may need to be reduced if symptoms of toxicity occur. Carbamazepine may reduce the serum levels of sodium valproate by 60% or more. Concurrent use may possibly increase the incidence of sodium valproate-induced hepatotoxicity.

Clinical evidence

(a) Carbamazepine and carbamazepine epoxide levels

A study in 7 adult epileptics who had been taking carbamazepine 8.3 to 13.3 mg/kg for more than 2 months found that their steady-state serum carbamazepine levels fell by an average of 24% (range 3 to 59%) over a 6-day period when they were given sodium valproate 1 g twice daily. The carbamazepine levels were reduced in 6 of the patients and remained unchanged in one. The levels of the active metabolite, carbamazepine-10,11-epoxide, increased by a mean of 38%, with small decreases or no change in 4 patients and 24 to 150% increases in the remaining 3 patients.[1,2]

Other reports state that falls,[3,4] no changes[3,5-7] and even a slight rise[4] in carbamazepine levels have been seen in some patients also given sodium valproate or valproic acid. The serum levels of carbamazepine-10,11-epoxide are reported to be increased by about 50 to 100%.[6,8,9] This active metabolite may cause the development of marked adverse effects such as blurred vision, dizziness, vomiting, tiredness and even nystagmus.[6-8,10] Acute psychosis, tentatively attributed to elevated epoxide levels, occurred in one patient when carbamazepine was added to sodium valproate treatment.[11]

(b) Serum sodium valproate levels reduced

A study on the pharmacokinetics of sodium valproate in 6 healthy subjects found that carbamazepine, 200 mg daily, over a 17-day period increased the sodium valproate clearance by 30%.[12]

Other reports have described reductions in serum sodium valproate levels of 34 to 38% when carbamazepine was added,[13,14] and rises of 50 to 65% when the carbamazepine was withdrawn.[15,16] The rise appears to reach a plateau after about 4 weeks.[16] A pharmacokinetic model has been devised to estimate valproate clearance when given with carbamazepine.[17]

(c) Increased sodium valproate-induced hepatotoxicity or neurological effects

Evidence from epidemiological studies suggests that the risk of fatal hepatotoxicity is higher when sodium valproate is given with other anticonvulsants than when it is given alone, especially in infants.[18,19] A single case report describes hepatocellular and cholestatic jaundice and a reversible Parkinsonian syndrome in a woman on sodium valproate when carbamazepine was added, which reversed when the carbamazepine was withdrawn. Levels of both drugs did not exceed the therapeutic range at any stage. The Parkinsonian syndrome was attributed to a drug interaction, whereas the hepatotoxicity was considered most likely to be due to the carbamazepine, although the valproate may have contributed.[20]

Mechanism

The evidence suggests that carbamazepine increases the metabolism of valproate, so that it is cleared from the body more quickly. However, the latter stages of carbamazepine metabolism appear to be inhibited by valproate. The levels of the metabolite carbamazepine-epoxide increase during concurrent use, probably by inhibition of its metabolism to carbamazepine-10,11-trans-diol,[21,22] by epoxide hydrolase. (Note that valproate is a weaker inhibitor of this enzyme than valpromide, see 'Carbamazepine + Valpromide', p.350). The trans-diol metabolite is then further converted by glucuronidation, and it seems that this step is also inhibited.[22] Carbamazepine may also possibly increase the formation of a minor but hepatotoxic metabolite of sodium valproate (2- propyl-4-pentenoic acid or 4-ene-VPA).[23]

Importance and management

Moderately well documented interactions, both of which seem to be established. Be alert for falls in the serum levels of valproate if carbamazepine is added, and rises if carbamazepine is withdrawn. A minor to modest fall in carbamazepine levels may occur, but there may be a moderate to marked rise in the active epoxide metabolite. Therefore, be alert for signs of toxicity, which may indicate high levels of carbamazepine-epoxide and a need to reduce the carbamazepine dose.

Sodium valproate has been associated with serious hepatotoxicity, especially in children aged less than 3 years, and this has been more common in those receiving other anticonvulsants. Sodium valproate monotherapy is to be preferred in this group.

1. Levy RH, Morselli PL, Bianchetti G, Guyot M, Brachet-Liermain A, Loiseau P. Interaction between valproic acid and carbamazepine in epileptic patients. Metabolism of Antiepileptic Drugs edited by RH Levy et al. *Raven Press, New York* (1984) 45–51.
2. Levy RH, Moreland TA, Morselli PL, Guyot M, Brachet-Liermain A, Loiseau P. Carbamazepine/valproic acid interaction in man and rhesus monkey. *Epilepsia* (1984) 25, 338–45.
3. Wilder BJ, Willmore LJ, Bruni J, Villarreal HJ. Valproic acid: interaction with other anticonvulsant drugs. *Neurology* (1978) 28, 892–6.
4. Varma R, Michos GA, Varma RS, Hoshino AY. Clinical trials of Depakene (valproic acid) coadministered with other anticonvulsants in epileptic patients. *Res Commun Psychol Psychiatr Behav* (1980) 5, 265–73.
5. Fowler GW. Effects of dipropylacetate on serum levels of anticonvulsants in children. *Proc West Pharmacol Soc* (1978) 21, 37–40.
6. Pisani F, Fazio A, Oteri G, Ruello C, Gitto C, Russo R, Perucca E. Sodium valproate and valpromide: differential interactions with carbamazepine in epileptic patients. *Epilepsia* (1986) 27, 548–52.
7. Sunaoshi W, Miura H, Takanashi S, Shira H, Hosoda N. Influence of concurrent administration of sodium valproate on the plasma concentrations of carbamazepine and its epoxide and diol metabolites. *Jpn J Psychiatry Neurol* (1991) 45, 474–7.
8. Kutt H, Solomon G, Peterson H, Dhar A, Caronna J. Accumulation of carbamazepine epoxide caused by valproate contributing to intoxication syndromes. *Neurology* (1985) 35 (Suppl 1), 286.

9. Liu H, Delgado MR. Improved therapeutic monitoring of drug interactions in epileptic children using carbamazepine polytherapy. *Ther Drug Monit* (1994) 16, 132–8.
10. Rambeck B, Sälke-Treumann A, May T, Boenigk HE. Valproic acid-induced carbamazepine-10,11-epoxide toxicity in children and adolescents. *Eur Neurol* (1990) 30, 79–83.
11. McKee RJW, Larkin JG, Brodie MJ. Acute psychosis with carbamazepine and sodium valproate. *Lancet* (1989) i, 167.
12. Bowdle TA, Levy RH, Cutler RE. Effects of carbamazepine on valproic acid kinetics in normal subjects. *Clin Pharmacol Ther* (1979) 26, 629–34.
13. Reunanen MI, Luoma P, Myllylä VV, Hokkanen E. Low serum valproic acid concentrations in epileptic patients on combination therapy. *Curr Ther Res* (1980) 28, 456–62.
14. May T, Rambeck B. Serum concentrations of valproic acid: influence of dose and comedication. *Ther Drug Monit* (1985) 7, 387–90.
15. Henriksen O, Johannessen SI. Clinical and pharmacokinetic observations on sodium valproate — a 5 year follow-up study in 100 children with epilepsy. *Acta Neurol Scand* (1982) 65, 504–23.
16. Jann MW, Fidone GS, Israel MK, Bonadero P. Increased valproate serum concentrations upon carbamazepine cessation. *Epilepsia* (1988) 29, 578–81.
17. Yukawa E, Honda T, Ohdo S, Higuchi S, Aoyama T. Detection of carbamazepine-induced changes in valproic acid relative clearance in man by simple pharmacokinetic screening. *J Pharm Pharmacol* (1997) 49, 751–6.
18. Dreifuss FE, Santilli N, Langer DH, Sweeney KP, Moline KA, Menander KB. Valproic acid fatalities: a retrospective review. *Neurology* (1987) 37, 379–85.
19. Dreifuss FE, Langer DH, Moline KA, Maxwell DE. Valproic acid hepatic fatalities. II. US experience since 1984. *Neurology* (1989) 39, 201–7.
20. Froomes PR, Stewart MR. A reversible Parkinsonian syndrome and hepatotoxicity following addition of carbamazepine to sodium valproate. *Aust N Z J Med* (1994) 24, 413–14.
21. Pisani F, Caputo M, Fazio A, Oteri G, Russo M, Spina E, Perucca E, Bertilsson L. Interaction of carbamazepine-10,11-epoxide, an active metabolite of carbamazepine, with valproate: a pharmacokinetic study. *Epilepsia* (1990) 31, 339–42.
22. Bernus I, Dickinson RG, Hooper WD, Eadie MJ. The mechanism of the carbamazepine-valproate interaction in humans. *Br J Clin Pharmacol* (1997) 44, 21–27.
23. Levy RH, Rettenmeier AW, Anderson GD, Wilensky AJ, Friel PN, Baillie TA, Acheampong A, Tor J, Guyot M, Loiseau P. Effects of polytherapy with phenytoin, carbamazepine, and stiripentol on formation of 4-ene-valproate, a hepatotoxic metabolite of valproic acid. *Clin Pharmacol Ther* (1990) 48, 225–35.

Carbamazepine + SSRIs

Some, but not all, reports indicate that carbamazepine serum levels can be increased by fluoxetine and fluvoxamine. Toxicity may develop. Sertraline normally appears not to affect carbamazepine, and citalopram and paroxetine do not. Citalopram, paroxetine and sertraline levels may be reduced by carbamazepine. Isolated cases of a Parkinson-like and serotonin syndrome have occurred with fluoxetine and carbamazepine, while an isolated case of pancytopenia has been reported with sertraline and carbamazepine. Consideration should be given to the fact that SSRIs have been known to cause seizures.

Clinical evidence

(a) Citalopram

Citalopram 40 mg daily for 2 weeks caused no change in the pharmacokinetics of carbamazepine 400 mg once daily in a study in 12 healthy subjects.[1] An approximate 30% decrease in citalopram levels occurred in 6 patients on citalopram 40 to 60 mg daily when they were given carbamazepine 200 to 400 mg daily for 4 weeks. Despite this decrease, the combination was considered clinically useful.[2] Similarly, two patients with epilepsy, major depression and panic disorder had increased citalopram levels (one had an improved antidepressant response, but the other patient experienced tremor and increased anxiety) when their treatment with carbamazepine was replaced by oxcarbazepine.[3]

(b) Fluoxetine

Two patients developed carbamazepine toxicity (diplopia, blurred vision, tremor, vertigo, nausea, tinnitus etc.) within 7 and 10 days of starting to take fluoxetine 20 mg daily. Their serum carbamazepine levels were found to have risen by about 33 and 60%. The problem was resolved in one of them by reducing the carbamazepine dosage from 1000 mg to 800 mg daily, and in the other by stopping the fluoxetine.[4] The effects seen in these cases are supported by a study in 6 healthy patients, where adding fluoxetine 20 mg daily to steady-state carbamazepine caused a rise in the AUC of carbamazepine and its active epoxide metabolite of about 25 to 50%.[5]

In contrast, fluoxetine 20 mg daily for 3 weeks was found to have no effect on the serum levels of carbamazepine or its active epoxide metabolite in 8 epileptic patients stabilised on carbamazepine.[6]

Aside from these pharmacokinetic changes two cases of parkinsonism have been seen within 3 and 9 days of adding fluoxetine to carbamazepine treatment. In both cases carbamazepine levels were unaffected.[7] A case of the serotonin syndrome (shivering, agitation, myoclonic-like leg contractions, diaphoresis etc.) has also been seen, in a woman on carbamazepine 200 mg daily and fluoxetine 20 mg daily.[8]

(c) Fluvoxamine

Increased serum levels and signs of carbamazepine toxicity (nausea, vomiting) were seen in 3 patients on long-term carbamazepine when the were additionally given fluvoxamine. The carbamazepine level almost doubled in one of them within 10 days of starting fluvoxamine 50 to 100 mg daily. The interaction was accommodated by reducing the carbamazepine dosage by 200 mg daily in all three (from 1000 to 800 mg in one of them, and from 800 to 600 mg daily in the other two).[9,10] An approximate doubling of carbamazepine levels has also been seen in other patients given fluvoxamine.[11-14]

In contrast, fluvoxamine 100 mg daily for 3 weeks was found to have no effect on the serum levels of carbamazepine or its active epoxide metabolite in 7 epileptic patients stabilised on carbamazepine.[6]

(d) Paroxetine

Sixteen days' treatment with paroxetine 30 mg daily in epileptics caused no changes in the plasma levels or therapeutic effects of carbamazepine. Steady-state paroxetine plasma levels were lower in those taking phenytoin (16 nanograms/ml) than in those on carbamazepine (27 nanograms/ml) or sodium valproate (73 nanograms/ml).[15]

(e) Sertraline

A double blind, placebo-controlled, parallel group study in 13 healthy subjects (7 on sertraline, 6 on placebo) found that sertraline 200 mg daily for 17 days had no effect on the pharmacokinetics of carbamazepine 200 mg twice daily, nor on the pharmacokinetics of carbamazepine-epoxide. In addition, sertraline did not potentiate the cognitive effects of carbamazepine.[16]

However, an isolated report describes a woman stabilised for 2 years on carbamazepine 600 mg and flecainide 100 mg daily, who had a rise in trough serum carbamazepine levels from 4.7 to 8.5 micrograms/ml within 4 weeks of starting sertraline 100 mg daily. After 3 months of treatment, carbamazepine levels were 11.9 micrograms/ml. At the same time she developed pancytopenia (interpreted as a toxic bone marrow reaction to the increased carbamazepine), which improved when the carbamazepine and sertraline were stopped.[17]

An isolated report describes a woman with schizoaffective disorder successfully treated for 3 years with haloperidol and carbamazepine who was additionally given sertraline 50 mg daily for depression. When she failed to respond, the sertraline dosage was progressively increased to 300 mg daily but her sertraline serum levels remained low (about 17 to 25% of those predicted). Another patient on carbamazepine similarly failed to respond to the addition of sertraline and had low sertraline levels.[18]

Mechanism

The evidence suggests that fluoxetine and fluvoxamine inhibit the metabolism of carbamazepine by the liver (presumably inhibition of the cytochrome P450 isoenzyme CYP3A4) so that its loss from the body is reduced, leading to a rise in its serum levels.[5,12]

Citalopram, sertraline and possibly paroxetine serum levels may be reduced because carbamazepine is an inducer of CYP3A4, which would increase its metabolism and clearance from the body. Oxcarbazepine appears not to interact.

Importance and management

Information for fluoxetine and fluvoxamine appears to be limited to these reports. It is not clear why they are inconsistent, but be alert for an increase in carbamazepine serum levels and toxicity if fluoxetine or fluvoxamine is added. The interaction appears rare. A literature search[19] by the makers of fluvoxamine only identified 8 cases of an interaction between fluvoxamine and carbamazepine up until 1995. However, because of the unpredictability of this interaction it would be prudent to monitor concurrent use, particularly in the early stages, so that any patient affected can be identified. Be alert for the need to reduce the carbamazepine dosage. The makers of fluoxetine suggest that carbamazepine should be started at or adjusted towards the lower end of the dosage range in those on fluoxetine. They additionally suggest caution if fluoxetine has been taken during the previous 5 weeks.[20]

Sertraline appears not affect carbamazepine, nevertheless there is one report of carbamazepine toxicity, and also a suggestion of reduced efficacy of sertraline. Monitor concurrent use.

Citalopram and paroxetine appear not to affect carbamazepine levels, but modestly reduced citalopram and paroxetine levels may occur. Monitor concurrent use.

Note that SSRIs may increase seizure frequency and should therefore be used with caution in patients with epilepsy, and avoided in those with unstable epilepsy.

1. Møller SE, Larsen F, Khan AZ, Rolan PE. Lack of effect of citalopram on the steady-state pharmacokinetics of carbamazepine in healthy male subjects. *J Clin Psychopharmacol* (2001) 21, 493–9.
2. Steinacher L, Vandel P, Zullino DF, Eap CB, Brawand-Amey M, Baumann P. Carbamazepine augmentation in depressive patients non-responding to citalopram: a pharmacokinetic and clinical pilot study. *Eur Neuropsychopharmacol* (2002) 12, 255–60.
3. Leinonen E, Lepola U, Koponen H. Substituting carbamazepine with oxcarbazepine increases citalopram levels. A report on two cases. *Pharmacopsychiatry* (1996) 29, 156–8.
4. Pearson HJ. Interaction of fluoxetine with carbamazepine. *J Clin Psychiatry* (1990) 51, 126.
5. Grimsley SR, Jann MW, Carter JG, D'Mello AP, D'Souza MJ. Increased carbamazepine plasma concentrations after fluoxetine coadministration. *Clin Pharmacol Ther* (1991) 50, 10–15.
6. Spina E, Avenoso A, Pollicino AM, Caputi AP, Fazio A, Pisani F. Carbamazepine coadministration with fluoxetine or fluvoxamine. *Ther Drug Monit* (1993) 15, 247–50.
7. Gernaat HBPE, van de Woude J, Touw DJ. Fluoxetine and parkinsonism in patients taking carbamazepine. *Am J Psychiatry* (1991) 148, 1604–5.
8. Dursun SM, Mathew VM, Reveley MA. Toxic serotonin syndrome after fluoxetine plus carbamazepine. *Lancet* (1993) 342, 442–3.
9. Fritze J, Unsorg B, Lanczik M. Interaction between carbamazepine and fluvoxamine. *Acta Psychiatr Scand* (1991) 84, 583–4.
10. Fritze J, Lanczik M. Pharmacokinetic interactions of carbamazepine and fluvoxamine. *Pharmacopsychiatry* (1993) 26, 153.
11. Bonnet P, Vandel S, Nezelof S, Sechter D, Bizouard P. Carbamazepine, fluvoxamine. Is there a pharmacokinetic interaction? *Therapie* (1992) 47, 165.
12. Martinelli V, Bocchetta A, Palmas AM, del Zompo M. An interaction between carbamazepine and fluvoxamine. *Br J Clin Pharmacol* (1993) 36, 615–16.
13. Debruille C, Robert H, Cottencin O, Regnaut N, Gignac C. Interaction carbamazépine/fluvoxamine: à propos de deux observations. *J Pharm Clin* (1994) 13, 128–30.
14. Cottencin O, Regnaut N, Thevenon Gignac C, Thomas P, Goudemand M, Debruille C, Robert H. Interaction carbamazepine-fluvoxamine sur le taux plasmatique de carbamazepine. *Encephale* (1995) 21, 141–5.
15. Andersen BB, Mikkelsen M, Versterager A, Dam M, Kristensen HB, Pedersen B, Lund J, Mengel H. No influence of the antidepressant paroxetine on carbamazepine, valproate and phenytoin. *Epilepsy Res* (1991) 10, 201–4.
16. Rapeport WG, Williams SA, Muirhead DC, Dewland PM, Tanner T, Wesnes K. Absence of a sertraline-mediated effect on the pharmacokinetics and pharmacodynamics of carbamazepine. *J Clin Psychiatry* (1996) 57 (Suppl 1), 20–3.
17. Joblin M, Ghose K. Possible interaction of sertraline with carbamazepine. *N Z Med J* (1994) 107, 43.
18. Khan A, Shad MU, Preskorn SH. Lack of sertraline efficacy probably due to an interaction with carbamazepine. *J Clin Psychiatry* (2000) 61, 526–7.
19. Wagner W, Vause EW. Fluvoxamine. A review of global drug-drug interaction data. *Clin Pharmacokinet* (1995) 29 (Suppl 1), 26–32.
20. Prozac (Fluoxetine). Eli Lilly and Company Ltd. UK Summary of product characteristics, September 2004.

Carbamazepine + Ticlopidine

One case report suggests that ticlopidine may have caused increased carbamazepine levels, with associated toxicity.

Clinical evidence, mechanism, importance and management

A 67-year-old man on carbamazepine 600 mg twice daily developed symptoms of carbamazepine toxicity (drowsiness, dizziness, ataxia) within a week of starting to take ticlopidine 250 mg twice daily. His carbamazepine level one week after starting the ticlopidine was 75 mol/l, but had been only 43 mol/l five weeks earlier. The carbamazepine dose was reduced to 500 mg twice daily, with resolution of symptoms, and producing a level of 53 mol/l one week later. After stopping the ticlopidine, carbamazepine levels fell to 42 mol/l. It was suggested that ticlopidine may interfere with carbamazepine metabolism.[1] However, carbamazepine is principally metabolised by the cytochrome P450 isoenzyme CYP3A4, and ticlopidine is not usually considered and inhibitor of this isoenzyme. This is the only report so far, and its general relevance is uncertain.

1. Brown RIG, Cooper TG. Ticlopidine-carbamazepine interaction in a coronary stent patient. *Can J Cardiol* (1997) 13, 853–4.

Carbamazepine + Trazodone

A single case report describes a moderate rise in serum carbamazepine levels in a patient when given trazodone. Carbamazepine may moderately decrease trazodone levels.

Clinical evidence, mechanism, importance and management

A 53-year-old man who had been taking carbamazepine 700 mg daily for 7 months (serum levels 7.2 and 7.9 mg/l) was started on trazodone 100 mg daily. Two months later his serum carbamazepine levels were 10 mg/l and the concentration/dose ratio had increased by about 26%, but no signs or symptoms of carbamazepine toxicity were seen. The reasons for this interaction are not known but the authors suggest that it might be because the trazodone inhibits the cytochrome P450 isoenzyme CYP3A4 resulting in a reduction in the metabolism of the carbamazepine.[1]

In 6 patients treated with trazodone 150 or 300 mg daily, the addition of carbamazepine 400 mg daily for 4 weeks decreased the plasma levels of trazodone by 24%, and of the active metabolite of trazodone by 40%.[2] However, the combination was considered clinically useful in three of the cases.[2]

This seems to be the first and only report of raised carbamazepine levels with trazodone, and its general importance is unknown. The rise was only moderate and in this case was clinically irrelevant, but a carbamazepine serum rise of 26% might possibly be of importance in those patients with serum levels already near the top end of the therapeutic range. The clinical importance of the moderate decrease in trazodone levels is uncertain. Nevertheless, monitoring would now seem to be appropriate in any patient given both drugs.

1. Romero AS, Delgado RG, Peña MF. Interaction between trazodone and carbamazepine. *Ann Pharmacother* (1999) 33, 1370.
2. Otani K, Ishida M, Kaneko S, Mihara K, Ohkubo T, Osanai T, Sugawara K. Effects of carbamazepine coadministration on plasma concentrations of trazodone and its active metabolite, *m*-chlorophenylpiperazine. *Ther Drug Monit* (1996) 18, 164–7.

Carbamazepine + Valnoctamide

Carbamazepine toxicity may develop if valnoctamide is taken concurrently.

Clinical evidence, mechanism, importance and management

A study in 6 epileptics on carbamazepine 800 to 1200 mg daily found that valnoctamide 200 mg three times daily for 7 days caused a 1.5 to 6.5-fold increase in the serum levels of carbamazepine-epoxide (an active metabolite). Clinical signs of carbamazepine toxicity (drowsiness, ataxia, nystagmus) were seen in 4 of them. One patient who was also taking phenytoin and one patient who was also taking phenobarbital had no changes in the serum levels of either of these anticonvulsants.[1] A further study in 6 healthy subjects found that valnoctamide 600 mg daily for 8 days increased the half-life of a single 100-mg dose of carbamazepine-epoxide threefold, from 6.7 to 19.7 hours, and decreased its oral clearance fourfold.[2]

Mechanism

Valnoctamide inhibits the enzyme epoxide hydrolase, which is concerned with the metabolism and elimination of carbamazepine and its active epoxide metabolite.[1,2]

Importance and management

Information is limited but the interaction appears to be established. Patients on carbamazepine who additionally take valnoctamide could rapidly develop carbamazepine toxicity because the metabolism of its major metabolite, carbamazepine-epoxide, is inhibited. This interaction is very similar to the interaction that occurs between carbamazepine and valpromide (an isomer of valnoctamide), see 'Carbamazepine + Valpromide', below. Valnoctamide should be avoided unless the carbamazepine dosage can be reduced appropriately.

1. Pisani F, Fazio A, Artesi C, Oteri G, Spina E, Tomson T, Perucca E. Impairment of carbamazepine-10,11-epoxide elimination by valnoctamide, a valpromide isomer, in healthy subjects. *Br J Clin Pharmacol* (1992) 34, 85–7.
2. Pisani F, Haj-Yehia A, Fazio A, Artesi C, Oteri G, Perucca E, Kroetz DL, Levy RH, Bialer M. Carbamazepine-valnoctamide interaction in epileptic patients: in vitro/in vivo correlation. *Epilepsia* (1993) 34, 954–9.

Carbamazepine + Valpromide

Carbamazepine toxicity can occur if valpromide is substituted for sodium valproate in patients taking carbamazepine. The serum levels of carbamazepine may not rise but the levels of its active metabolite, carbamazepine-epoxide, can be markedly increased. The dose of carbamazepine may need to be reduced.

Clinical evidence

Symptoms of carbamazepine toxicity developed in 5 out of 7 epileptic patients on carbamazepine when concurrent treatment with sodium valproate was replaced by valpromide, despite the fact that their serum carbamazepine levels did not increase.[1] The toxicity appeared to be connected with a fourfold increase in the serum levels of the metabolite of carbamazepine, carbamazepine-10,11-epoxide, which rose to 8.5 micrograms/ml.[1]

In another study in 6 epileptic patients the serum levels of carbamazepine-10,11-epoxide rose by 330% (range 110 to 864%) within a week of starting valpromide, and two of the patients developed confusion, dizziness and vomiting. The symptoms disappeared and serum carbamazepine-epoxide levels fell when the valpromide dosage was reduced by one-third.[2]

A study in healthy subjects given a single 100-mg oral dose of carbamazepine-epoxide confirmed that valpromide 300 mg twice daily for 8 days reduced carbamazepine-epoxide clearance by 73%, and increased peak levels by 62%.[3]

Mechanism

Valpromide reduces the metabolism by the liver of carbamazepine-epoxide, because it inhibits epoxide hydrolase.[4] Valpromide (an amide derivative of valproate) was about 100 times more potent an inhibitor of this enzyme than sodium valproate *in vitro*[5] and caused a threefold higher rise in epoxide levels than valproate in one study.[2] The carbamazepine-epoxide metabolite has anticonvulsant activity, but it may also cause toxicity if its serum levels become excessive.[2,6]

Importance and management

An established interaction. It is suggested that both carbamazepine and carbamazepine-epoxide serum levels should be monitored during concurrent use.[2] The dosages should be reduced appropriately if necessary. There is also some debate about whether this combination should be avoided, not only because of the risk of toxicity but also because inhibition of epoxide hydrolase may be undesirable.[1] This enzyme is possibly important for the detoxification of a number of teratogenic, mutagenic and carcinogenic epoxides.[1,2] More study is needed.

1. Meijer JWA, Binnie CD, Debets RMChr, Van Parys JAP and de Beer-Pawlikowski NKB. Possible hazard of valpromide-carbamazepine combination therapy in epilepsy. *Lancet* (1984) i, 802.
2. Pisani F, Fazio A, Oteri G, Ruello C, Gitto C, Russo R, Perucca E. Sodium valproate and valpromide: differential interactions with carbamazepine in epileptic patients. *Epilepsia* (1986) 27, 548–52.
3. Perucca E, Pisani F, Spina E, Oteri G, Fazio A, Bertilsson L. Effects of valpromide and viloxazine on the elimination of carbamazepine-10,11-epoxide, an active metabolite of carbamazepine. *Pharm Res* (1989) 21, 111–12.
4. Pisani F, Fazio A, Oteri G, Spina E, Perucca E and Bertilsson L. Effect of valpromide on the pharmacokinetics of carbamazepine-10,11-epoxide. *Br J Clin Pharmacol* (1988) 25, 611–13.
5. Kerr BM, Rettie AE, Eddy AC, Loiseau P, Guyot M, Wilensky AJ, Levy RH. Inhibition of human liver microsomal epoxide hydrolase by valproate and valpromide: in vitro/in vivo correlation. *Clin Pharmacol Ther* (1989) 46, 82–93. Erratum. ibid., 343.
6. Levy RH, Kerr BM, Loiseau P, Guyot M and Wilensky AJ. Inhibition of carbamazepine epoxide elimination by valpromide and valproic acid. *Epilepsia* (1986) 27, 592.

Carbamazepine + Vigabatrin

No change in carbamazepine levels usually occurs with vigabatrin, although one study has shown a modest increase, and one a modest decrease.

Clinical evidence

In an early clinical study, vigabatrin 2 to 3 g daily did not change the serum levels of carbamazepine in 12 patients.[1] Similarly, other studies found that carbamazepine levels were not significantly altered by the addition of vigabatrin.[2,3] However, in one study in which 59 patients on carbamazepine received vigabatrin, 34 patients had an increase in carbamazepine levels, 3 had no change, and 22 had a decrease, resulting in a mean overall increase of 6%, which was not significant.[4] Similarly, in another study 46 out of 66 patients had an increase in carbamazepine level of at least 10% (mean increase about 24%), and in 24 of these patients the carbamazepine level exceeded the therapeutic level.[5] In this study, the increase in carbamazepine level was greater the lower the initial carbamazepine level.[5] In contrast, one study in 15 patients reported a mean 18% decrease in carbamazepine levels when vigabatrin was added.[6]

Mechanism

Not understood.

Importance and management

The information is contradictory and no interaction is established. Because of the uncertainty, it would be prudent to monitor carbamazepine levels when vigabatrin is added or stopped, and the dose adjusted as required.

1. Tassinari CA, Michelucci R, Ambrosetto G, Salvi F. Double-blind study of vigabatrin in the treatment of drug-resistant epilepsy. *Arch Neurol* (1987) 44, 907–10.
2. Rimmer EM, Richens A. Interaction between vigabatrin and phenytoin. *Br J Clin Pharmacol* (1989) 27, 27S–33S.
3. Bernardina BD, Fontana E, Vigevano F, Fusco L, Torelli D, Galeone D, Buti D, Cianchetti C, Gnanasakthy A, Iudice A. Efficacy and tolerability of vigabatrin in children with refractory partial seizures: a single-blind dose-increasing study. *Epilepsia* (1995) 36, 687–91.
4. Browne TR, Mattson RH, Penry JK, Smith DB, Treiman DM, Wilder BJ, Ben-Menachem E, Napoliello MJ, Sherry KM, Szabo GK. Vigabatrin for refractory complex partial seizures: multicenter single-blind study with long-term follow up. *Neurology* (1987) 37, 184–9.
5. Jędrzejczak J, Dławichowska E, Owczarek K, Majkowski J. Effect of vigabatrin addition on carbamazepine blood serum levels in patients with epilepsy. *Epilepsy Res* (2000) 39, 115–20.
6. Sánchez-Alcaraz A, Quintana B, López E, Rodríguez I, Llopis P. Effect of vigabatrin on the pharmacokinetics of carbamazepine. *J Clin Pharm Ther* (2002) 27, 427–30.

Ethosuximide + Isoniazid

A single report describes a patient who developed psychotic behaviour and signs of ethosuximide toxicity when given isoniazid.

Clinical evidence, mechanism, importance and management

An epileptic patient, well controlled on ethosuximide and sodium valproate for 2 years, developed persistent hiccupping, nausea, vomiting, anorexia and insomnia within a week of starting to take isoniazid 300 mg daily. Psychotic behaviour gradually developed over the next 5 weeks and so the isoniazid was stopped. The appearance of these symptoms appeared to be related to the sharp rise in serum ethosuximide levels (from about 50 up to 198 micrograms/ml).[1] It is suggested that the isoniazid may have inhibited the metabolism of the ethosuximide, leading to accumulation and toxicity. The general importance of this case is uncertain.

1. van Wieringen A, Vrijlandt CM. Ethosuximide intoxication caused by interaction with isoniazid. *Neurology* (1983) 33, 1227–8.

Ethosuximide + Other anticonvulsants

Minor to modest falls in serum ethosuximide levels may occur if carbamazepine, primidone or phenytoin are also given, whereas methylphenobarbital or sodium valproate may cause a rise in ethosuximide levels. The effect of all these changes on seizure control is uncertain. Lamotrigine appears not to affect ethosuximide levels.

Ethosuximide is reported to have caused phenytoin toxicity in a few cases, and it appears that ethosuximide can reduce valproate serum levels.

Clinical evidence

(a) Barbiturates

In a retrospective analysis, the level to dose ratio of ethosuximide was 33% lower in 29 epileptic patients on ethosuximide and **primidone** than in 39 patients on ethosuximide alone.[1]

Similarly, in another study, which compared the pharmacokinetics of a single dose of ethosuximide in 10 epileptic patients on **phenobarbital**, phenytoin and/or carbamazepine with 12 healthy controls, the epileptic group had markedly shorter (about halved) ethosuximide half-lives.[2] Conversely, another report stated that ethosuximide levels tended to rise [amount not stated] when **methylphenobarbital** was used, but did not appear to be affected by **phenobarbital** or **primidone**.[3] Phenobarbital levels (from **primidone**) do not appear to be affected by ethosuximide.[4]

(b) Carbamazepine

A study in 6 healthy subjects taking ethosuximide 500 mg daily found that the mean serum levels of ethosuximide were reduced by 17%, from 32 to 27 mg/ml by carbamazepine 200 mg daily for 18 days. One individual had a 35% reduction in ethosuximide levels.[5] Another study, which compared

10 epileptic patients (taking enzyme-inducing antiepileptic drugs, including 4 taking carbamazepine) with 12 healthy controls found that the epileptic group had markedly shorter (about halved) ethosuximide half-lives.[2]

In contrast, the concurrent use of carbamazepine did not affect the correlation between ethosuximide dose and levels in another study.[3]

(c) Lamotrigine

Five children on ethosuximide and various other anticonvulsants had no change in their serum ethosuximide levels when lamotrigine was also given.[6]

(d) Phenytoin

A study compared the pharmacokinetics of a single dose of ethosuximide in 10 epileptic patients on phenobarbital, phenytoin and/or carbamazepine with 12 healthy controls. The epileptic group had markedly shorter (about halved) ethosuximide half-lives.[2] In contrast, the concurrent use of phenytoin did not affect the correlation between ethosuximide levels and dose in another study.[3]

Three cases have occurred in which ethosuximide appeared to have been responsible for increasing phenytoin levels,[7-9] leading to the development of phenytoin toxicity in 2 patients.[8,9]

(e) Sodium valproate

Four out of 5 patients taking ethosuximide (average dose 27 mg/kg) had an increase of about 50%, from 73 to 112 micrograms/ml, in serum levels within 3 weeks of starting to take sodium valproate (adjusted to the maximum tolerated dose). Sedation occurred and ethosuximide dose reductions were necessary.[10] In a single-dose study in 6 healthy subjects, 9 days' treatment with sodium valproate was reported to have increased the ethosuximide half-life and reduced the clearance by 15%.[11] However, other studies have described no changes[12,13] or even lower serum ethosuximide levels (level to dose ratio reduced by 36%).[1]

One study in 13 children found that ethosuximide can lower valproate serum levels. In the presence of ethosuximide the valproate serum levels were lower than with valproate alone (87 versus 120 micrograms/ml). After stopping ethosuximide the valproate levels rose by about 40% and when combined they fell by about 27%.[14]

Mechanism

The most probable explanation for the fall in ethosuximide levels is that the carbamazepine and the other enzyme inducing anticonvulsants increase the metabolism and clearance of ethosuximide, which is known to be metabolised by the cytochrome P450 isoenzyme CYP3A.[2]

Importance and management

The concurrent use of anticonvulsants is common and often advantageous. Information on these interactions is sparse and even contradictory and their clinical importance is uncertain. Nevertheless, good monitoring would clearly be appropriate if these drugs are used with ethosuximide to monitor for potential toxicity and to ensure adequate seizure control.

1. Battino D, Cusi C, Franceschetti S, Moise A, Spina S, Avanzini G. Ethosuximide plasma concentrations: influence of age and associated concomitant therapy. *Clin Pharmacokinet* (1982) 7, 176–80.
2. Giaccone M, Bartoli A, Gatti G, Marchiselli R, Pisani F, Latella MA, Perucca E. Effect of enzyme inducing anticonvulsants on ethosuximide pharmacokinetics in epileptic patients. *Br J Clin Pharmacol* (1996) 41, 575–9.
3. Smith GA, McKauge L, Dubetz D, Tyrer JH, Eadie MJ. Factors influencing plasma concentrations of ethosuximide. *Clin Pharmacokinet* (1979) 4, 38–52.
4. Schmidt D. The effect of phenytoin and ethosuximide on primidone metabolism in patients with epilepsy. *J Neurol* (1975) 209, 115–23.
5. Warren JW, Benmaman JD, Wannamaker BB, Levy RH. Kinetics of a carbamazepine-ethosuximide interaction. *Clin Pharmacol Ther* (1980) 28, 646–51.
6. Eriksson A-S, Hoppu K, Nergårdh A, Boreus L. Pharmacokinetic interactions between lamotrigine and other antiepileptic drugs in children with intractable epilepsy. *Epilepsia* (1996) 37, 769–73.
7. Lander CM, Eadie MJ, Tyrer JH. Interactions between anticonvulsants. *Proc Aust Assoc Neurol* (1975) 12, 111–16.
8. Dawson GW, Brown HW, Clark BG. Serum phenytoin after ethosuximide. *Ann Neurol* (1978) 4, 583–4.
9. Frantzen E, Hansen JM, Hansen OE, Kristensen M. Phenytoin (Dilantin) intoxication. *Acta Neurol Scand* (1967) 43, 440–6.
10. Mattson RH, Cramer JA. Valproic acid and ethosuximide interaction. *Ann Neurol* (1980) 7, 583–4.
11. Pisani F, Narbone MC, Trunfio C, Fazio A, La Rosa G, Oteri G, Di Perri R. Valproic acid-ethosuximide interaction: a pharmacokinetic study. *Epilepsia* (1984) 25, 229–33.
12. Fowler GW. Effect of dipropylacetate on serum levels of anticonvulsants in children. *Proc West Pharmacol Soc* (1978) 21, 37–40.
13. Bauer LA, Harris C, Wilensky AJ, Raisys VA, Levy RH. Ethosuximide kinetics: possible interaction with valproic acid. *Clin Pharmacol Ther* (1982) 31, 741–5.
14. Sälke-Kellermann RA, May T, Boenigk HE. Influence of ethosuximide on valproic acid serum concentrations. *Epilepsy Res* (1997) 26, 345–349.

Felbamate + Antacids

An aluminium/magnesium hydroxide-containing antacid had no effect on the absorption of felbamate.

Clinical evidence, mechanism, importance and management

Felbamate 2.4 g daily was given to 9 epileptic women for 2 weeks. For a third week the felbamate was taken with an antacid containing **aluminium/magnesium hydroxide** (*Maalox Plus*). No significant changes in the serum levels or AUC were seen.[1] No special precautions would seem to be needed if felbamate is taken with this or any other similar antacid.

1. Sachdeo RC, Narang-Sachdeo SK, Howard JR, Dix RK, Shumaker RC, Perhach JL, Rosenberg A. Effect of antacid on the absorption of felbamate in subjects with epilepsy. *Epilepsia* (1993) 34 (Suppl 6), 79–80.

Felbamate + Erythromycin

Erythromycin does not alter felbamate pharmacokinetics.

Clinical evidence, mechanism, importance and management

In a randomised two-period crossover study, 12 epileptics were given felbamate 3 g or 3.6 g daily, either alone or with erythromycin 333 mg every 8 hours for 10 days. The pharmacokinetics of felbamate were unchanged by erythromycin.[1] There would therefore seem no reason for avoiding erythromycin in patients taking felbamate.

1. Sachdeo RJ, Narang-Sachdeo SK, Montgomery PA, Shumaker RC, Perhach JL, Lyness WH, Rosenberg A. Evaluation of the potential interaction between felbamate and erythromycin in patients with epilepsy. *J Clin Pharmacol* (1998) 38, 184–90.

Felbamate + Gabapentin

There is some evidence that the half-life of felbamate may be prolonged by gabapentin.

Clinical evidence, mechanism, importance and management

In a retrospective examination of clinical data from patients taking felbamate, its half-life was found to be 24 hours in 40 patients taking felbamate alone, whereas in 18 other patients also taking gabapentin (including 7 taking a third drug), the half-life was extended to 32.7 hours.[1] The practical clinical importance of this is uncertain but be alert for the need to reduce the felbamate dosage. More study is needed.

1. Hussein G, Troupin AS, Montouris G. Gabapentin interaction with felbamate. *Neurology* (1996) 47, 1106.

Fosphenytoin + Miscellaneous

Fosphenytoin is a prodrug of phenytoin, which is rapidly and completely hydrolysed to phenytoin in the body. It is predicted to interact with other drugs in the same way as phenytoin.[1,2] No drugs are known to interfere with the conversion of fosphenytoin to phenytoin.[2]

1. Fierro LS, Savulich DH, Benezra DA. Safety of fosphenytoin sodium. *Am J Health-Syst Pharm* (1996) 53, 2707–12.
2. Pro-Epanutin (Fosphenytoin sodium). Parke Davis. UK Summary of product characteristics, April 2004.

Gabapentin + Antacids

Aluminium/magnesium hydroxide slightly reduces the absorption of gabapentin.

Clinical evidence, mechanism, importance and management

An **aluminium/magnesium hydroxide** antacid (*Maalox TC*) reduced the bioavailability of gabapentin 400 mg by about 20% when given either at the same time or 2 hours afterwards. When the antacid was given 2 hours before, the bioavailability was reduced by about 10%.[1] These small changes are unlikely to be of clinical importance. However, the maker does recommend that gabapentin is taken about 2 hours after **aluminium/magnesium-containing antacids**.[2]

1. Busch JA, Radulovic LL, Bockbrader HN, Underwood BA, Sedman AJ, Chang T. Effect of *Maalox TC®* on single-dose pharmacokinetics of gabapentin capsules in healthy subjects. *Pharm Res* (1992) 9 (10 Suppl), S-315.
2. Neurontin (Gabapentin). Parke Davis. UK Summary of product characteristics, January 2004.

Gabapentin + Cimetidine

A brief report notes that cimetidine decreased the renal clearance of gabapentin by 12%, which was not expected to be clinically important. No study details were given.[1]

1. Busch JA, Bockbrader HN, Randinitis EJ, Chang T, Welling PG, Reece PA, Underwood B, Sedman AJ, Vollmer KO, Türck D. Lack of clinically significant drug interactions with Neurontin (Gabapentin). 20th International Epilepsy Congress. Oslo, Norway, July 1993. Abstract 013958.

Gabapentin + Food

Food, including protein and enteral feeds, does not have a clinically important effect on the absorption of gabapentin.

Clinical evidence, mechanism, importance and management

A high-protein meal (80 g total protein) increased the maximum serum levels of a single 800-mg dose of gabapentin by 36% in healthy subjects. The AUC was increased by 11%, which was not statistically significant. These findings were the opposite of those expected, since L-amino acids compete for gabapentin intestinal transport *in vitro*.[1]

In another single-dose study, the absorption of gabapentin capsules did not differ when opened and mixed with either **apple sauce** or **orange juice**, but tended to be higher (AUC increased by 26%) when mixed with a protein-containing option (**chocolate pudding**).[2] Similarly, no change in absorption was found when gabapentin syrup was mixed with tap water, **grape juice**, or an **enteral feed** (*Sustacal*), but a modest 31% increase in AUC was seen when it was mixed with **chocolate milk**.[3]

These small changes are unlikely to be of clinical importance, so it does not matter when gabapentin is taken in relation to food.

1. Gidal BE, Maly MM, Budde J, Lensmeyer GL, Pitterle ME, Jones JC. Effect of a high-protein meal on gabapentin pharmacokinetics. *Epilepsy Res* (1996) 23, 71–6.
2. Gidal BE, Maly MM, Kowalski JW, Rutecki PA, Pitterle ME, Cook DE. Gabapentin absorption: effect of mixing with foods of varying macronutrient composition. *Ann Pharmacother* (1998) 32, 405–9.
3. Parnell J, Sheth R, Limdi N, Gidal BE. Oral absorption of gabapentin syrup is not impaired by concomitant administration with various beverages or enteral nutrition supplement. *Epilepsia* (2001) 42 (Suppl 7), 91.

Gabapentin + Other anticonvulsants

Gabapentin does not normally affect the pharmacokinetics of carbamazepine, phenytoin, phenobarbital or sodium valproate, and no dosage adjustments are needed on concurrent use. However, isolated reports describe increased phenytoin levels and toxicity in two patients given gabapentin.

Clinical evidence, mechanism, importance and management

The pharmacokinetics of both **phenytoin** and gabapentin remained unchanged in 8 epileptics who were given gabapentin 400 mg three times daily for 8 days, in addition to their normal **phenytoin** treatment, which they had been taking for at least 2 months.[1] Other studies confirm that the steady-state pharmacokinetics of **phenytoin** are unaffected by gabapentin, and that the pharmacokinetics of gabapentin are similarly unaffected by **phenytoin**.[2,3] These reports contrast with an isolated report of a patient on **phenytoin**, **carbamazepine** and **clobazam** whose serum **phenytoin** levels increased three to fourfold, with symptoms of toxicity, on two occasions when given gabapentin 300 to 600 mg daily. **Carbamazepine** serum levels remained unchanged. The author suggests that this differing reaction may be because the patient was on more than one antiepileptic, unlike previous studies where only single drugs had been used.[4] However, another case of **phenytoin** toxicity possibly attributable to gabapentin has been described in a patient not on any other anticonvulsants.[5]

Gabapentin does not affect **phenobarbital** levels, nor is it affected by **phenobarbital**.[2,3,6] Other studies confirm that the steady-state pharmacokinetics of **carbamazepine** and **sodium valproate** are unaffected by gabapentin, and that the pharmacokinetics of gabapentin are similarly unaffected by these anticonvulsants.[2,3,7]

It would seem therefore that no dosage adjustments are normally needed if gabapentin is added to treatment with most of these anticonvulsants. However, if gabapentin is added to **phenytoin** it may be wise to bear the possibility of raised **phenytoin** levels in mind. For mention that gabapentin may prolong the half-life of **felbamate**, see 'Felbamate + Gabapentin', p.352. For mention of the lack of interaction between **levetiracetam** and gabapentin, see 'Levetiracetam + Other anticonvulsants', p.356

1. Anhut H, Leppik I, Schmidt B, Thomann P. Drug interaction study of the new anticonvulsant gabapentin with phenytoin in epileptic patients. *Naunyn Schmiedebergs Arch Pharmacol* (1988) 337 (Suppl), R127.
2. Brockbrader HN, Radulovic LL, Loewen G, Chang T, Welling PG, Reece PA, Underwood B, Sedman AJ. Lack of drug-drug interactions between Neurontin (gabapentin) and other antiepileptic drugs. 20th International Epilepsy Congress, Oslo, Norway. July 1993 (Abstract).
3. Richens A. Clinical pharmacokinetics of gabapentin.New Trends in Epilepsy Management: The Role of Gabapentin International Congress and Symposium Series No 198, Royal Society of Medicine Services, London, NY 1993, 41–6.
4. Tyndel F. Interaction of gabapentin with other antiepileptics. *Lancet* (1994) 343, 1363–4.
5. Sánchez-Romero A, Durán-Quintana JA, García-Delgado R, Margariot-Rangel C, Proveda-Andrés JL. Posible interacción gabapentina-fenitoína. *Rev Neurol* (2002) 34, 952–3.
6. Hooper WD, Kavanagh MC, Herkes GK, Eadie MJ. Lack of a pharmacokinetic interaction between phenobarbitone and gabapentin. *Br J Clin Pharmacol* (1991) 31, 171–4.
7. Radulovic LL, Wilder BJ, Leppik IE, Bockbrader HN, Chang T, Posvar EL, Sedman AJ, Uthman BM, Erdman GR. Lack of interaction of gabapentin with carbamazepine or valproate. *Epilepsia* (1994) 35, 155–61.

Gabapentin + Probenecid

A brief report notes that probenecid had no effect on the renal clearance of gabapentin. No study details were given.[1]

1. Busch JA, Bockbrader HN, Randinitis EJ, Chang T, Welling PG, Reece PA, Underwood B, Sedman AJ, Vollmer KO, Türck D. Lack of clinically significant drug interactions with Neurontin (Gabapentin). 20th International Epilepsy Congress. Oslo, Norway, July 1993. Abstract 013958.

Lamotrigine + Antituberculars

Rifampicin markedly increased the clearance of lamotrigine in a pharmacokinetic study. A case report has described a similar finding, and also included some limited evidence suggesting that isoniazid may inhibit lamotrigine metabolism.

Clinical evidence, mechanism, importance and management

Rifampicin 600 mg daily for 5 days increased the clearance of a single 25-mg dose of lamotrigine by 97% and decreased the AUC by 44% in 10 healthy subjects. The amount of lamotrigine glucuronide recovered in the urine was increased by 36%.[1] Similarly, a case report describes a 56 year-old woman taking lamotrigine 150 mg daily who had unexpectedly low serum lamotrigine levels of 1.3 mg/l after starting **rifampicin**, **isoniazid** and pyrazinamide. The lamotrigine dosage was therefore increased to 250 mg daily. After the antitubercular treatment was changed to **isoniazid** and ethambutol, the lamotrigine serum levels rose to 12.4 mg/l. No toxicity was seen.[2]

Mechanism

Rifampicin increases the loss of lamotrigine from the body, probably by inducing glucuronidation via UDP-glucuronyl transferases.[1] It was suggested that isoniazid may have inhibited lamotrigine metabolism.[2]

Importance and management

Information appears to be limited to these reports, but the interaction between lamotrigine and rifampicin would appear to be established. Be aware that rifampicin could reduce the efficacy of lamotrigine, and that increased lamotrigine doses are likely to be required.

The case report also raises the possibility of an interaction between lamotrigine and isoniazid. If isoniazid is added to or withdrawn from lamotrigine treatment, be alert for the need to adjust the lamotrigine dosage.

1. Ebert U, Thong NQ, Oertel R, Kirch W. Effects of rifampicin and cimetidine on pharmacokinetics and pharmacodynamics of lamotrigine in healthy subjects. *Eur J Clin Pharmacol* (2000) 56, 299–304.
2. Armijo JA, Sánchez B, Peralta FG, Cuadrado A, Leno C. Lamotrigine interaction with rifampicin and isoniazid. A case report. *Methods Find Exp Clin Pharmacol* (1996) 18 (Suppl C), 59.

Lamotrigine + Cimetidine

Cimetidine 400 mg twice daily for 5 days had no effect on the pharmacokinetics of a single 25-mg dose of lamotrigine in 10 healthy subjects. No change in lamotrigine dose appears to be needed during concurrent use.[1]

1. Ebert U, Thong NQ, Oertel R, Kirch W. Effects of rifampicin and cimetidine on pharmacokinetics and pharmacodynamics of lamotrigine in healthy subjects. *Eur J Clin Pharmacol* (2000) 56, 299–304.

Lamotrigine + Felbamate

Felbamate appears not to affect the pharmacokinetics of lamotrigine.

Clinical evidence, mechanism, importance and management

In 21 healthy subjects felbamate 1.2 g twice daily had minimal effects on the pharmacokinetics of lamotrigine 100 mg twice daily when they were given together for 10 days to. A 14% increase in the lamotrigine AUC was seen, which was not considered clinically relevant.[1] Similarly, there was no difference in lamotrigine pharmacokinetics between 6 patients receiving lamotrigine and felbamate and 5 patients on lamotrigine alone.[2] No change in lamotrigine dose is required when given with felbamate.

1. Colucci R, Glue P, Holt B, Banfield C, Reidenberg P, Meehan JW, Pai S, Nomeir A, Lim J, Lin C-C, Affrime MB. Effect of felbamate on the pharmacokinetics of lamotrigine. *J Clin Pharmacol* (1996) 36, 634–8.
2. Gidal BE, Kanner A, Maly M, Rutecki P, Lensmeyer GL. Lamotrigine pharmacokinetics in patients receiving felbamate. *Epilepsy Res* (1997) 27, 1–5.

Lamotrigine + Phenobarbital or Primidone

Phenobarbital has been associated with reduced lamotrigine serum levels. Phenobarbital and primidone levels were unchanged.

Clinical evidence, mechanism, importance and management

In a retrospective study, the lamotrigine serum concentration-to-dose ratio was lower in patients also taking phenobarbital than in those on lamotrigine monotherapy (0.52 versus 0.99).[1] Similar findings have been reported in another study.[2] No changes in the serum levels of phenobarbital or primidone were seen in a study in 12 patients when they were given lamotrigine 75 to 400 mg daily.[3]

Phenobarbital induces the metabolism of lamotrigine, and the recommended starting dose and long-term maintenance dose of lamotrigine in patients already taking phenobarbital or primidone is twice that of patients on lamotrigine monotherapy.[4] [However, note that if they are also taking valproate in addition to phenobarbital, the lamotrigine dose should be reduced.[4,5] See 'Lamotrigine + Sodium valproate', below.] The lamotrigine dosage may need to be reduced if phenobarbital is withdrawn.

1. May TW, Rambeck B, Jürgens U. Serum concentrations of lamotrigine in epileptic patients: the influence of dose and comedication. *Ther Drug Monit* (1996) 18, 523–31.
2. Armijo JA, Bravo J, Cuadrado A, Herranz JL. Lamotrigine serum concentration-to-dose ratio: influence of age and concomitant antiepileptic drugs and dosage implications. *Ther Drug Monit* (1999) 21, 182–190.
3. Jawad S, Richens A, Goodwin G, Yuen WC. Controlled trial of lamotrigine (Lamictal) for refractory partial seizures. *Epilepsia* (1989) 30, 356–63.
4. Lamictal (Lamotrigine). GlaxoSmithKline UK. UK Summary of product characteristics, June 2005.
5. Lamictal (Lamotrigine). GlaxoSmithKline. US Prescribing information, August 2004.

Lamotrigine + Phenytoin

Phenytoin has been associated with reduced lamotrigine serum levels. Lamotrigine has no effect on phenytoin levels.

Clinical evidence, mechanism, importance and management

In a retrospective study, the lamotrigine serum concentration-to-dose ratio was much lower in patients receiving concomitant phenytoin than in those on lamotrigine monotherapy (0.32 versus 0.98).[1] Other studies have reported similar findings.[2,3] In another study, the mean lamotrigine levels were approximately doubled in patients on lamotrigine and phenytoin when the phenytoin was withdrawn.[4] Phenytoin is a known hepatic enzyme inducer and this may have lead to an increased clearance of lamotrigine.

No changes in the serum level of phenytoin was seen in another study in patients given lamotrigine 75 to 400 mg daily.[5]

Phenytoin induces the metabolism of lamotrigine, and the recommended starting dose and long-term maintenance dose of lamotrigine in patients already taking phenytoin is twice that of patients on lamotrigine monotherapy.[6]

[However, note that if they are also taking valproate in addition to phenytoin, the lamotrigine dose should be reduced[6,7] – see 'Lamotrigine + Sodium valproate', below.] The lamotrigine dosage may need to be reduced if phenytoin is withdrawn.

1. May TW, Rambeck B, Jürgens U. Serum concentrations of lamotrigine in epileptic patients: the influence of dose and comedication. *Ther Drug Monit* (1996) 18, 523–31.
2. Armijo JA, Bravo J, Cuadrado A, Herranz JL. Lamotrigine serum concentration-to-dose ratio: influence of age and concomitant antiepileptic drugs and dosage implications. *Ther Drug Monit* (1999) 21, 182–190.
3. Böttiger Y, Svensson J-O, Ståhle L. Lamotrigine drug interactions in a TDM material. *Ther Drug Monit* (1999) 21, 171–4.
4. Anderson GD, Gidal BE, Messenheimer J, Gilliam FG. Time course of lamotrigine de-induction: impact of step-wise withdrawal of carbamazepine or phenytoin. *Epilepsy Res* (2002) 49, 211–17.
5. Jawad S, Richens A, Goodwin G, Yuen WC. Controlled trial of lamotrigine (Lamictal) for refractory partial seizures. *Epilepsia* (1989) 30, 356–63.
6. Lamictal (Lamotrigine). GlaxoSmithKline UK. UK Summary of product characteristics, June 2005.
7. Lamictal (Lamotrigine). GlaxoSmithKline. US Prescribing information, August 2004.

Lamotrigine + Sertraline

A report of two cases suggests that sertraline may increase lamotrigine levels and cause toxicity.

Clinical evidence, mechanism, importance and management

A patient's lamotrigine levels were found to have doubled and symptoms of toxicity were noted (confusion, cognitive impairment) 6 weeks after sertraline 25 mg daily was started.[1] The lamotrigine dose was halved, and the sertraline dose titrated to 50 mg daily. Symptoms of toxicity resolved, and the lamotrigine levels were 24% higher than before sertraline was started. In another patient on sertraline and lamotrigine with signs of lamotrigine toxicity, a 33% reduction in sertraline dose resulted in a halving of the lamotrigine level even though the lamotrigine dose was increased by 33%.

The authors suggest that sertraline may competitively inhibit the glucuronidation of lamotrigine. Evidence so far appears limited to this case report. In view of the increased risk of rash with increased lamotrigine levels (see also 'Lamotrigine + Sodium valproate', below), it may be prudent to monitor the combination. Further study is needed.

1. Kaufman KR, Gerner R. Lamotrigine toxicity secondary to sertraline. *Seizure* (1998) 7, 163–5.

Lamotrigine + Sodium valproate

The serum levels of lamotrigine can be markedly increased by sodium valproate. Concurrent use has been associated with skin rashes, tremor and other toxic reactions. The dose of lamotrigine should be halved when valproate is given. Small increases, decreases or no changes in sodium valproate levels have been seen with lamotrigine.

Clinical evidence

(a) Effects on lamotrigine levels

Sodium valproate 200 mg every 8 hours reduced the clearance of lamotrigine in 6 healthy subjects by 20%, and increased the AUC by 30%.[1] In another study in 18 healthy subjects receiving valproate 500 mg twice daily, the clearance of lamotrigine 50, 100 or 150 mg daily was also markedly reduced, and the half-life increased.[2] In a retrospective study, the lamotrigine serum concentration-to-dose ratio was markedly higher in patients also taking valproate than in those on lamotrigine monotherapy (3.57 versus 0.98). In patients also taking phenytoin, the effects of valproate on lamotrigine were offset (0.99 vs 0.98). However, the effects of valproate on lamotrigine were not completely offset by either carbamazepine or phenobarbital (1.67 or 1.8 versus 0.98).[3] Other studies have reported broadly similar findings.[4-6] Three studies have reported that the effect of valproate on lamotrigine was independent of the valproate dose or serum level (that is, it is maximal within the usual therapeutic dose range of valproate).[6-8] Another study has shown that the inhibition of lamotrigine clearance by valproate begins at very low valproate dosages (less than 125 mg daily), and is maximal at doses of about 500 mg daily.[9]

(b) Effects on valproate levels

In one study, 18 healthy subjects taking valproate 500 mg twice daily were also given lamotrigine 50, 100 or 150 mg daily. The lamotrigine caused a 25% decrease in valproate serum levels and a 25% increase in valproate oral clearance.[2] A study in 11 children on valproate and other antiepileptics noted that no clinically important changes in valproate serum levels occurred when lamotrigine was added.[10] A retrospective analysis found that lamotrigine was associated with only a 7% reduction in valproate levels.[11]

(c) Toxic reactions

(i) Tremor. Severe and disabling tremor (sometimes preventing them from feeding themselves) was seen in 3 patients when they were treated with lamotrigine and sodium valproate. The problem resolved when the dosages were reduced.[12] In a study of 13 adult patients, all developed upper limb tremor when given lamotrigine with sodium valproate, which could be minimised by reducing the dosage of either or both drugs.[13] Other studies have shown similar findings.[7,14,15]

(ii) Rash. In a survey of adult epileptics who had lamotrigine added to their therapy, 33 were also taking valproate. Of these, 10 patients (30%) developed a rash, whereas only 6 of the 70 (8%) not on valproate did so.[16] In another analysis of skin rash in patients on lamotrigine, 11 of 12 patients with serious rash were also taking sodium valproate, and all but one had a lamotrigine starting dose that is higher than currently recommended.[17] However, in another study in which patients on valproate were given lower initial doses of lamotrigine, there was no difference in incidence of rash in those on lamotrigine and valproate compared with those on lamotrigine and other anticonvulsants (13% versus 14.2%).[18] Another study successfully reintroduced lamotrigine in 3 patients, despite previous rashes.[19]

(iii) Other. Severe multiorgan dysfunction and disseminated intravascular coagulation was seen in 2 children when they took lamotrigine with sodium valproate.[20] Three patients on lamotrigine developed neurotoxicity (confusion, lethargy) after starting treatment with valproate (an intravenous bolus dose of valproic acid then oral therapy). Lamotrigine levels had risen by 2.9 to 6.9 times those before valproic acid.[14]
The formation of hepatotoxic metabolites of valproate was unaffected by lamotrigine.[2]

Mechanism

Not fully understood. It is thought that valproate reduces lamotrigine glucuronidation by competitive inhibition, which results in a decreased lamotrigine clearance.[1,2,21] Raised lamotrigine levels have been implicated in the development of rash.[18,22] Increased valproate clearance may be due to enzyme induction. Tremor may be the result of a pharmacodynamic interaction.[7,13]

Importance and management

A well documented interaction. Concurrent use can be therapeutically valuable, but the lamotrigine dosage should be reduced by about half when valproate is added to avoid possible toxicity (sedation, tremor, ataxia, fatigue, rash).[2,7-9,12,18,23] In patients already on valproate, the maker of lamotrigine recommends a lamotrigine starting dose that is half that of lamotrigine monotherapy, irrespective of whether they are also receiving enzyme-inducing anticonvulsants, and a very gradual dose-escalation rate.[24] The outcome should be very well monitored. The UK Committee on Safety of Medicines has suggested that the concurrent use of sodium valproate is one of the main risk factors for the development of serious skin reactions to lamotrigine, because it prolongs the half-life of lamotrigine.[22] Rashes are potentially serious and should be evaluated promptly.[18,24,25] The reports cited above[12,20] also suggest that sometimes other serious reactions (disabling tremor, multiorgan dysfunction) can occur.

1. Yuen AWC, Land G, Weatherley BC, Peck AW. Sodium valproate acutely inhibits lamotrigine metabolism. *Br J Clin Pharmacol* (1992) 33, 511–13.
2. Anderson GD, Yau MK, Gidal BE, Harris SJ, Levy RH, Lai AA, Wolf KB, Wargin WA, Dren AT. Bidirectional interaction of valproate and lamotrigine in healthy subjects. *Clin Pharmacol Ther* (1996) 60, 145–56.
3. May TW, Rambeck B, Jürgens U. Serum concentrations of lamotrigine in epileptic patients: the influence of dose and comedication. *Ther Drug Monit* (1996) 18, 523–31.
4. Armijo JA, Bravo J, Cuadrado A, Herranz JL. Lamotrigine serum concentration-to-dose ratio: influence of age and concomitant antiepileptic drugs and dosage implications. *Ther Drug Monit* (1999) 21, 182–190.
5. Böttiger Y, Svensson J-O, Ståhle L. Lamotrigine drug interactions in a TDM material. *Ther Drug Monit* (1999) 21, 171–4.
6. Gidal BE, Anderson GD, Rutecki PR, Shaw R, Lanning A. Lack of effect of valproate concentration on lamotrigine pharmacokinetics in developmentally disabled patients with epilepsy. *Epilepsy Res* (2000) 42, 23–31.
7. Kanner A, Frey M. Adding valproate to lamotrigine: a study of their pharmacokinetic interaction. *Neurology* (2000) 55, 588–91.
8. Decerce J, McJilton JS, Nadkarni MA, Ramsay RE. Lamotrigine-valproate interaction: relationship to the dose of valproate. *Epilepsia* (2000) 41(Suppl. 7), 220–1.
9. Gidal BE, Sheth R, Parnell J, Maloney K, Sale M. Evaluation of VPA dose and concentration effects on lamotrigine pharmacokinetics: implications for conversion to monotherapy. *Epilepsy Res* (2003) 57, 85–93.
10. Eriksson A-S, Hoppu K, Nergårdh A, Boreus L. Pharmacokinetic interactions between lamotrigine and other antiepileptic drugs in children with intractable epilepsy. *Epilepsia* (1996) 37, 769–73.
11. Mataringa M-I, May TW, Rambeck B. Does lamotrigine influence valproate concentrations? *Ther Drug Monit* (2002) 24, 631–6.
12. Reutens DC, Duncan JS, Patsalos PN. Disabling tremor after lamotrigine with sodium valproate. *Lancet* (1993) 342, 185–6.
13. Pisani F, Oteri G, Russo MF, Di Perri R, Perucca E, Richens A. The efficacy of valproate-lamotrigine comedication in refractory complex partial seizures: evidence for a pharmacodynamic interaction. *Epilepsia* (1999) 40, 1141–6.
14. Voudris K, Mastroyianni S, Skardoutsou A, Katsarou E, Mavrommatis P. Disabling tremor in epileptic children receiving sodium valproate after addition of lamotrigine. P2197. *Eur J Neurol* (2003) 10 (Suppl. 1), 180.
15. Burneo JG, Limdi N, Kuzniecky RI, Knowlton RC, Mendez M, Lawn N, Faught E, Welty TE, Prasad A. Neurotoxicity following addition of intravenous valproate to lamotrigine therapy. *Neurology* (2003) 60, 1991–2.
16. Li LM, Russo M, O'Donoghue MF, Duncan JS, Sander JWAS. Allergic skin rash and concomitant valproate therapy: evidence for an increased risk. *Arq Neuropsiquiatr* (1996) 54, 47–9.
17. Wong ICK, Mawer GE, Sander JWAS. Factors influencing the incidence of lamotrigine-related skin rash. *Ann Pharmacother* (1999) 33, 1037–42.
18. Faught E, Morris G, Jacobson M, French J, Harden C, Montouris G, Rosenfeld W. Adding lamotrigine to valproate: incidence of rash and other adverse effects. Postmarketing antiepileptic drug survey (PADS) Group. *Epilepsia* (1999) 40, 1135–40.
19. Tavernor SJ, Wong ICK, Newton R, Brown SW. Rechallenge with lamotrigine after initial rash. *Seizure* (1995) 4, 67–71.
20. Chattergoon DS, McGuigan M, Koren G, Hwang P, Ito S. Multiorgan dysfunction and disseminated intravascular coagulation in children receiving lamotrigine and valproic acid. *Neurology* (1997) 49, 1442–4.
21. Panayiotopoulos CP, Ferrie CD, Knott C, Robinson RO. Interaction of lamotrigine with sodium valproate. *Lancet* (1993) 341, 445.
22. Committee on the Safety of Medicines/Medicines Control Agency. *Current Problems* (1996) 22, 12.
23. Pisani F, Di Perri R, Perucca E, Richens A. Interaction of lamotrigine with sodium valproate. *Lancet* (1993) 341, 1224.
24. Lamictal (Lamotrigine). GlaxoSmithKline UK. UK Summary of product characteristics, June 2005.
25. Lamictal (Lamotrigine). GlaxoSmithKline. US Prescribing information, August 2004.

Lamotrigine + Topiramate

Topiramate appears not alter the pharmacokinetics of lamotrigine, although one study suggested that it reduced lamotrigine levels. Lamotrigine has no effect on topiramate levels.

Clinical evidence, mechanism, importance and management

In the preliminary report of one study, it was found that serum lamotrigine levels decreased by 40 to 50% in 4 of 7 patients on stable lamotrigine 350 to 800 mg daily when they were given topiramate, titrated to 800 mg daily.[1] In contrast, other authors reported that the addition of topiramate 75 to 800 mg daily had little effect on the steady state serum levels of lamotrigine 100 to 950 mg daily in 24 patients. The mean lamotrigine level before topiramate was 10.4 mg/l and during topiramate was 9.7 mg/l. Only 2 of the patients had reductions of greater than 30% (40% and 43%).[2] A further study by the same research group confirmed the lack of effect of topiramate on lamotrigine pharmacokinetics.[3] The authors of the second study[2] note that there is some evidence that peak-to-trough variations of as much as 30 to 40% can occur during lamotrigine therapy, and therefore timing of blood sampling might be a factor in the findings of the first study.[1]

Lamotrigine had no effect on topiramate pharmacokinetics in one study in 13 patients. The oral clearance of topiramate 400 mg daily was 2.6 l/hour when given alone, and 2.7 l/hour when given with lamotrigine, and the AUC and plasma levels of topiramate were also similar.[3]

The balance of the evidence suggests that there is no important pharmacokinetic interaction between topiramate and lamotrigine. No special precautions appear to be necessary during concurrent use.

1. Wnuk W, Volanski A, Foletti G. Topiramate decreases lamotrigin concentrations. *Ther Drug Monit* (1999) 21, 449.
2. Berry DJ, Besag FMC, Pool F, Natarajan J, Doose D. Lack of an effect of topiramate on lamotrigine serum concentrations. *Epilepsia* (2002) 43, 818–23.
3. Doose DR, Brodie MJ, Wilson EA, Chadwick D, Oxbury J, Berry DJ, Schwabe S, Bialer M. Topiramate and lamotrigine pharmacokinetics during repetitive monotherapy and combination therapy in epilepsy patients. *Epilepsia* (2003) 44, 917–22.

Levetiracetam + Other anticonvulsants

There is some evidence that the enzyme-inducing anticonvulsants such as carbamazepine, phenobarbital, phenytoin and primidone may modestly reduce levetiracetam levels, but this is not thought to be clinically relevant. Levetiracetam does not alter the levels of these anticonvulsants. However, some trials found modestly raised phenytoin levels, and there is also one report of 4 cases of possible carbamazepine toxicity. There appears to be no pharmacokinetic interaction between levetiracetam and gabapentin, lamotrigine, or sodium valproate.

Clinical evidence, mechanism, importance and management

(a) Carbamazepine

There is evidence from clinical trials that levetiracetam does not affect the serum levels of carbamazepine.[1-3] There is also some evidence that patients on enzyme-inducing anticonvulsants such as carbamazepine had modestly (24%) lower levetiracetam levels than those on other anticonvulsants, but this was not considered clinically relevant, see (d) below.[4] Similarly, another retrospective analysis of patient data found that the serum levetiracetam level to dose ratio was modestly lower in patients also receiving carbamazepine than those on monotherapy (0.32 versus 0.52).[5] However, one report describes 4 patients who experienced disabling symptoms compatible with carbamazepine toxicity when levetiracetam was added. The symptoms resolved after a decrease in carbamazepine dosage or withdrawal of levetiracetam. A pharmacodynamic interaction was suggested, because levels of carbamazepine and its epoxide metabolite were not affected.[6]

In general, there is no need to modify the dose of either carbamazepine or levetiracetam when used together. However, the report of possible toxicity suggests that some caution is warranted.

(b) Phenytoin

There is some evidence that patients on enzyme-inducing anticonvulsants such as phenytoin had modestly (24%) lower levetiracetam levels than those on other anticonvulsants, but this was not considered clinically relevant, see (d) below.[4] Similarly, another retrospective analysis of patient data found that the serum levetiracetam level-to-dose ratio was modestly lower in patients also receiving phenytoin than those on monotherapy (0.32 versus 0.52).[5]

There is also evidence from clinical trials that levetiracetam does not affect the serum levels of phenytoin.[1-3] Similarly, in another study, levetiracetam 1.5 g twice daily for 12 weeks had no effect on the steady-state pharmacokinetics of phenytoin in 6 subjects with epilepsy on stable doses of phenytoin.[7] However, in one clinical trial the addition of levetiracetam increased phenytoin levels by 27% to 52% in 4 patients. A further patient had a 75% increase in phenytoin levels [estimated from figure] and experienced signs of toxicity (sedation, ataxia) and required a reduction in phenytoin dose. Another patient with raised phenytoin levels [estimated 47%] had the dose of levetiracetam reduced.[8]

In general therefore, there is no need to modify the dose of either phenytoin or levetiracetam when they are used together. However, the report of raised phenytoin levels suggests that some caution is warranted.

(c) Sodium valproate

There was no difference in the pharmacokinetics of a single 1.5-g dose of levetiracetam when given to healthy subjects before or after sodium valproate 500 mg twice daily for 8 days. In addition, levetiracetam did not affect the pharmacokinetics of valproate.[9] In an analysis of clinical trial data, the AUC of levetiracetam in 57 patients on valproic acid was slightly (11%) higher than in 28 patients on anticonvulsants not thought to affect microsomal enzymes (gabapentin, lamotrigine, vigabatrin), but this was not thought to be clinically relevant.[4] In another retrospective analysis of patient data, the serum levetiracetam level-to-dose ratio was the same in patients also receiving valproic acid than those on monotherapy (0.53 versus 0.52).[5] There is also evidence from clinical trials that levetiracetam does not affect the serum levels of valproate.[3] There appears to be no need to adjust the doses of either sodium valproate or levetiracetam if these drugs are used together.

(d) Other anticonvulsants

The AUC of levetiracetam tended to be lower in 436 patients on enzyme-inducing anticonvulsants (**carbamazepine**, **phenobarbital**, **phenytoin**, **primidone**) than in 28 patients on anticonvulsants not thought to affect microsomal enzymes (**gabapentin**, **lamotrigine**, **vigabatrin**), but the difference was modest (24%).[4] Another retrospective analysis of patient data found that the serum levetiracetam level-to-dose ratio did not differ significantly between patients also receiving **lamotrigine** than those on monotherapy (0.45 versus 0.52), but was modestly lower in those on **oxcarbazepine** (0.34 versus 0.52).[5]

There is also evidence from clinical trials that levetiracetam does not affect the serum levels of **gabapentin**, **lamotrigine**, **phenobarbital**, or **primidone**.[1-3] In general therefore, no dosage adjustments would seem to be needed if levetiracetam is used as add-on therapy with any of these drugs.

1. Levetiracetam (Keppra). UCB Pharma Ltd. UK Summary of product characteristics, July 2004.
2. Patsalos PN. Pharmacokinetic profile of levetiracetam: towards ideal characteristics. *Pharmacol Ther* (2000) 85, 77–85.
3. Levetiracetam (Keppra). UCB Pharma Inc. US Prescribing information, November 2004.
4. Perucca E, Gidal BE, Baltès E. Effects of antiepileptic comedication on levetiracetam pharmacokinetics: a pooled analysis of data from randomized adjunctive therapy trials. *Epilepsy Res* (2003) 53, 47–56.
5. May TW, Rambeck B, Jürgens U. Serum concentrations of levetiracetam in epileptic patients: the influence of dose and co-medication. *Ther Drug Monit* (2003) 25, 690–9.
6. Sisodiya SM, Sander JWAS, Patsalos PN. Carbamazepine toxicity during combination therapy with levetiracetam: a pharmacodynamic interaction. *Epilepsy Res* (2002) 48, 217–19.
7. Browne TR, Szabo GK, Leppik IE, Josephs E, Paz J, Baltes E, Jensen CM. Absence of pharmacokinetic drug interaction of levetiracetam with phenytoin in patients with epilepsy determined by new technique. *J Clin Pharmacol* (2000) 40, 590–5.
8. Sharief MK, et al. Efficacy and tolerability study of ucb L059 in patients with refractory epilepsy. *J Epilepsy* (1996) 9, 106–12.
9. Coupez R, Nicolas J-M, Browne TR. Levetiracetam, a new antiepileptic agent: lack of in vitro and in vivo pharmacokinetic interaction with valproic acid. *Epilepsia* (2003) 44, 171–8.

Levetiracetam + Probenecid

Probenecid increased the plasma levels of an inactive metabolite of levetiracetam.

Clinical evidence, mechanism, importance and management

Probenecid 500 mg four times daily did not affect the renal excretion of levetiracetam. However, the renal excretion of its primary and pharmacologically inactive metabolite (ucb L057) was reduced by 61%, and plasma concentrations increased 2.5-fold,[1] although the maker says they remained low.[2] The clinical relevance of elevated levels of L057 is not known, therefore some have suggested caution is warranted.[1] The effect of levetiracetam on probenecid has not been studied.[2,3]

1. Patsalos PN. Pharmacokinetic profile of levetiracetam: towards ideal characteristics. *Pharmacol Ther* (2000) 85, 77–85.
2. Levetiracetam (Keppra). UCB Pharma Ltd. UK Summary of product characteristics, July 2004.
3. Levetiracetam (Keppra), UCB Pharma Inc. US Prescribing information, November 2004.

Mesuximide + Other anticonvulsants

Phenobarbital, phenytoin, and possibly felbamate increase the levels of the active metabolite of mesuximide. Mesuximide increases the serum levels of phenobarbital and phenytoin, and de-

creases the levels of lamotrigine, and to a lesser extent, sodium valproate.

Clinical evidence

(a) Felbamate

Three adolescent epileptics on mesuximide developed mild adverse effects within 3 days of starting to take felbamate, which became more serious by the end of a month (decreased appetite, nausea, weight loss, insomnia, dizziness, hiccups, slurred speech). During this time the levels of the metabolite normethsuximide rose by 26 and 46% in two patients respectively. The adverse effects disappeared and the normethsuximide levels fell when the mesuximide dosage was reduced. Other anticonvulsants being taken were carbamazepine, ethotoin and sodium valproate.[1]

(b) Lamotrigine

Lamotrigine levels were 53% lower (range 36 to 72%) while 6 patients were taking mesuximide when compared with lamotrigine levels before starting or after stopping mesuximide. In some patients deterioration in seizure control was seen while taking mesuximide, or improvement in seizure control occurred after mesuximide was stopped.[2] In another study, lamotrigine levels were about 70% lower in 13 patients on mesuximide than in 64 patients on lamotrigine monotherapy, when corrected for dose. [Note that in patients also on sodium valproate, the reduction caused by mesuximide was compensated for by the increase caused by valproate, see also 'Lamotrigine + Sodium valproate', p.354].[3]

(c) Phenobarbital or primidone

A study in hospitalised patients with petit mal epilepsy found that when mesuximide was given to 8 patients on phenobarbital and 13 patients on primidone, the mean serum levels of phenobarbital rose by 38 and 40% respectively. Dose reductions were needed in 50% and 62% of patients, respectively. It was also found that the concurrent use of phenobarbital increased the serum levels of the active anticonvulsant metabolite of mesuximide.[4]

(d) Phenytoin

Mesuximide was given to 17 patients on phenytoin, which resulted in a 78% rise in the phenytoin serum levels requiring dose reductions in about 30% of the patients. It was also found that the concurrent use of phenytoin increased the serum levels of the active anticonvulsant metabolite of mesuximide.[4]

(e) Sodium valproate

A retrospective analysis of serum valproate levels was carried out in 17 patients who started and/or stopped taking mesuximide and whose concurrent medication remained unaltered. In the 14 patients starting mesuximide, a mean decrease in valproate levels of 32% was seen. In the 8 patients who stopped mesuximide a 30% increase in valproate levels occurred.[5] [Note that the related drug, ethosuximide, has also been reported to lower valproate levels, see 'Ethosuximide + Other anticonvulsants', p.351.]

Mechanism

It has been suggested that phenobarbital, phenytoin and felbamate compete with mesuximide for the same metabolic mechanisms (hydroxylation) in the liver. As a result each one is metabolised more slowly and is therefore is lost from the body more slowly. Mesuximide appears to increase the loss of lamotrigine from the body (which is principally via glucuronidation), and also of valproate.

Importance and management

Information about these interactions is limited. Nevertheless, concurrent therapy should be monitored. Anticipate the need to reduce the dose of phenytoin, phenobarbital or primidone if mesuximide is given. It has been suggested that levels of normethsuximide should also be monitored.[4] Anticipate the need to reduce the dose of mesuximide if felbamate is added. The dose of lamotrigine may need to be increased if mesuximide is given. There is also some evidence that the dose of valproate may need to be increased.

1. Patrias J, Espe-Lillo J, Ritter FJ. Felbamate-methsuximide interaction. *Epilepsia* (1992) 33 (Suppl 3) 84.
2. Besag FM, Berry DJ, Pool F. Methsuximide lowers lamotrigine blood levels: a pharmacokinetic antiepileptic drug interaction. *Epilepsia* (2000) 41, 624–7.
3. May TW, Rambeck B, Jürgens U. Influence of oxcarbazepine and methsuximide on lamotrigine concentrations in epileptic patients with and without valproic acid comedication: results of a retrospective study. *Ther Drug Monit* (1999) 21, 175–81.
4. Rambeck B. Pharmacological interactions of mesuximide with phenobarbital and phenytoin in hospitalized epileptic patients. *Epilepsia* (1979) 20, 147–56.
5. Besag FMC, Berry DJ, Vasey M. Methsuximide reduces valproic acid serum levels. *Ther Drug Monit* (2001) 23, 694–7.

Oxcarbazepine + Erythromycin

Erythromycin does not appear to affect the pharmacokinetics of oxcarbazepine.

Clinical evidence, mechanism, importance and management

The pharmacokinetics of a single 600-mg dose of oxcarbazepine was unaffected by 7 days' treatment with erythromycin 500 mg twice daily in a study in 8 healthy subjects.[1] Erythromycin appears not to interact with oxcarbazepine, and no special precautions seem to be required during concurrent use.

1. Keränen T, Jolkkonen J, Jensen PK, Menge GP, Andersson P. Absence of interaction between oxcarbazepine and erythromycin. *Acta Neurol Scand* (1992) 86, 120–3.

Oxcarbazepine + Felbamate

Felbamate has no clinically relevant effect on the pharmacokinetics of oxcarbazepine, but the incidence of adverse effects is increased.

Clinical evidence, mechanism, importance and management

A double-blind randomised study in 8 healthy subjects found that oxcarbazepine 300 to 600 mg every 12 hours, given with felbamate 600 to 1200 mg every 12 hours for 10 days had no effect on the plasma levels of the major active metabolite of oxcarbazepine (monohydroxyoxcarbazepine). However, the levels of dihydroxycarbazepine (a minor, inactive metabolite) were reduced, and the maximum serum levels of oxcarbazepine were reduced, by about 20%. These changes were considered to be clinically irrelevant, however, the incidence of some adverse effects (dizziness, somnolence, nausea, diplopia) rose during concurrent use.[1]

1. Hulsman JARJ, Rentmeester TW, Banfield CR, Reidenberg P, Colucci RD, Meehan JW, Radwanski E, Mojaverian P, Lin C-C, Nezamis J, Affrime MB, Glue P. Effects of felbamate on the pharmacokinetics of the monohydroxy and dihydroxy metabolites of oxcarbazepine. *Clin Pharmacol Ther* (1995) 58, 383–9.

Oxcarbazepine + Other anticonvulsants

Oxcarbazepine appears not to affect the pharmacokinetics of carbamazepine, phenobarbital or sodium valproate to a clinically relevant extent, but modestly reduces lamotrigine levels. High doses of oxcarbazepine increase phenytoin levels, and a reduction in the phenytoin dose may be required. Phenytoin and phenobarbital can increase the loss of the active metabolite of oxcarbazepine, although this is probably not clinically relevant. Lamotrigine can increase levels of the active metabolite. See also 'Oxcarbazepine + Felbamate', above.

Clinical evidence

(a) Effects of oxcarbazepine on other anticonvulsants

A double-blind crossover comparison of oxcarbazepine and **carbamazepine** in 42 epileptics found that when **carbamazepine** was replaced by oxcarbazepine, the serum levels of **sodium valproate** rose by 32%, and the serum levels of **phenytoin** rose by 23%. In patients taking both **sodium valproate** and **phenytoin** together, oxcarbazepine caused a rise in the serum levels of 21% and 25% respectively. The trial extended over 12 weeks to establish steady-state levels.[1] Another study in 4 young epileptics (aged 13 to 17) found that the level to dose ratio of free **sodium valproate** rose when switched from **carbamazepine** to oxcarbazepine, with an increase in sodium valproate adverse effects, which resolved when the valproate dose was decreased.[2]

A later study in 35 epileptic patients found that oxcarbazepine 300 mg three times daily added to treatment with **carbamazepine**, **sodium valproate** or **phenytoin** for 3 weeks caused no clinically relevant changes in the pharmacokinetics of any of these anticonvulsants.[3] However, analysis of data from clinical trials found that oxcarbazepine decreased **carbamazepine** levels by about 15–22%, increased **phenobarbital** levels by about 14%, and at high doses increased **phenytoin** levels by up to 40%.[4,5] In another analysis, **lamotrigine** levels were about 34% lower in 14 patients on oxcarbazepine than in 64 patients on **lamotrigine** monotherapy, when corrected for dose. In this study, the effect of oxcarbazepine was less than that of **carbamazepine** (34% verses 47%).[6] Similarly, in another analysis, the addition of oxcarbazepine to **lamotrigine** reduced **lamotrigine** levels by 15 to 75%.[7]

(b) Effects of other anticonvulsants on oxcarbazepine

The pharmacokinetics of oxcarbazepine and its active metabolite (10-hydroxy-carbazepine) were not significantly affected by **sodium valproate**, but the AUCs of both were reduced by **phenobarbital**, by 43% and 25% respectively.[8] Similarly a study found that **phenytoin** caused a 29% reduction in the AUC of 10-hydroxy-carbazepine.[3] Another study found that the serum levels of the active metabolite 10-hydroxy-carbazepine were not affected by **phenobarbital** or **phenytoin** but the further conversion of the 10-hydroxy-carbazepine to *trans*-10,11-dihydroxy-10,11-dihydrocarbamazepine was increased.[9] Since the conversion to *trans*-10,11-dihydroxy-10,11-dihydrocarbamazepine is a minor step in the metabolism of 10-hydroxy-carbazepine, the overall antiepileptic action of oxcarbazepine is unlikely to be altered. Correspondingly, a study found that **phenytoin** 100 to 375 mg daily increased the clearance of the active oxcarbazepine metabolite by almost 40%.[10] The AUC of 10-hydroxy-carbazepine was also 40% lower in the presence of **carbamazepine**.[3] Similarly, **carbamazepine**, **phenobarbital**, and **phenytoin** were found to increase the apparent clearance of the 10-hydroxy metabolite of oxcarbazepine by 31 to 35% in a study in children.[11]

Conversely, a retrospective analysis found that 10-hydroxycarbamazepine levels to oxcarbazepine dose ratios were higher in 7 patients on concurrent **lamotrigine** than in those on oxcarbazepine monotherapy.[12]

Mechanism

Unlike carbamazepine, oxcarbazepine appears not to have marked enzyme-inducing properties so that it would not be expected to have as great an effect on the metabolism of other anticonvulsants. However, oxcarbazepine does appear to act as an inhibitor of cytochrome P450 isoenzyme CYP2C19 at high concentrations and therefore may raise phenytoin levels (see also 'Phenytoin + Carbamazepine', p.366 for more on this mechanism). Other anticonvulsants can increase the metabolism of the active metabolite of oxcarbazepine, 10-hydroxy-carbazepine. Lamotrigine appears to decrease it.

Importance and management

Information about the concurrent use of oxcarbazepine and other anticonvulsants is limited, but growing. The overall picture seems to be that, oxcarbazepine is a less potent enzyme inducer than carbamazepine, and therefore it does not markedly affect the serum levels of other anticonvulsants. If oxcarbazepine is substituted for carbamazepine, be aware that drug levels of some other anticonvulsants may rise. High oxcarbazepine doses may increase phenytoin levels, and the maker notes that a decrease in the phenytoin dose may be required.[4] The clinical relevance of the modest reductions in lamotrigine levels is uncertain. For mention of modestly reduced levetiracetam levels, see 'Levetiracetam + Other anticonvulsants', p.356.

Any changes in the pharmacokinetics of oxcarbazepine brought about by other anticonvulsants seem to be of minimal clinical relevance. However, the clinical relevance of the increase in the active metabolite 10-hydroxy-carbazepine with lamotrigine requires further study. In addition, there is the theoretical risk that 10-hydroxy-carbazepine levels might rise to toxic levels if carbamazepine or phenytoin were withdrawn.[3] For mention that there may be an increase in adverse effects if oxcarbazepine is used with felbamate, see 'Oxcarbazepine + Felbamate', p.357.

1. Houtkooper MA, Lammertsma A, Meyer JWA, Goedhart DM, Meinardi H, van Oorschot CAEH, Blom GF, Höppener RJEA, Hulsman JARJ. Oxcarbazepine (GP 47.680): a possible alternative to carbamazepine? *Epilepsia* (1987) 28, 693–8.
2. Battino D, Croci D, Granata T, Bernadi G, Monza G. Changes in unbound and total valproic acid concentrations after replacement of carbamazepine with oxcarbazepine. *Ther Drug Monit* (1992) 14, 376–9.
3. McKee PJW, Blacklaw J, Forrest G, Gillham RA, Walker SM, Connelly D, Brodie MJ. A double blind, placebo-controlled interaction study between oxcarbazepine and carbamazepine, sodium valproate and phenytoin in epileptic patients. *Br J Clin Pharmacol* (1994) 37, 27–32.
4. Trileptal (Oxcarbazepine). Novartis Pharmaceuticals UK Ltd. UK Summary of product characteristics. July 2005.
5. Hossain M, Sallas W, D'Souza J. Drug-drug interaction profile of oxcarbazepine in children and adults. *Neurology* (1999) 52 (Suppl 2), A525.
6. May TW, Rambeck B, Jürgens U. Influence of oxcarbazepine and methsuximide on lamotrigine concentrations in epileptic patients with and without valproic acid comedication: results of a retrospective study. *Ther Drug Monit* (1999) 21, 175–81.
7. Krämer G, Dorn T, Etter H. Oxcarbazepine: clinically relevant drug interaction with lamotrigine. *Epilepsia* (2003) 44 (Suppl 9), 95–6.
8. Tartara A, Galimberti CA, Manni R, Morini R, Limido G, Gatti G, Bartoli A, Strad G, Perucca E. The pharmacokinetics of oxcarbazepine and its active metabolite 10-hydroxy-carbazepine in healthy subjects and in epileptic patients taking phenobarbitone or valproic acid. *Br J Clin Pharmacol* (1993) 36, 366–8.
9. Kumps A, Wurth C. Oxcarbazepine disposition: preliminary observations in patients. *Biopharm Drug Dispos* (1990) 11, 365–70.
10. Arnoldussen W, Hulsman J, Rentmeester T. Interaction between oxcarbazepine and phenytoin. *Epilepsia* (1993) 34 (Suppl 6), 37.
11. Sallas WM, Milosavljev S, D'Souza J, Hossain M. Pharmacokinetic drug interactions in children taking oxcarbazepine. *Clin Pharmacol Ther* (2003) 74, 138–49.
12. Guénault N, Odou P, Robert H. Increase in dihydroxycarbamazepine serum levels in patients co-medicated with oxcarbazepine and lamotrigine. *Eur J Clin Pharmacol* (2003) 59, 781–2.

Paraldehyde + Disulfiram

***Animal* data suggest that disulfiram can increase paraldehyde levels and prolong its effect. There is a theoretical potential for a disulfiram reaction.**

Clinical evidence, mechanism, importance and management

It is thought that paraldehyde is depolymerised in the liver to acetaldehyde, and then oxidised by acetaldehyde dehydrogenase.[1] Since disulfiram inhibits this enzyme, concurrent use would be expected to result in the accumulation of acetaldehyde and result in a modified disulfiram reaction.[2] However, studies in *animals* given disulfiram and paraldehyde found increases in paraldehyde levels and hypnotic effect, with only small increases in acetaldehyde and no increase in toxicity.[2,3] In addition, there appear to be no reports of a disulfiram reaction in humans. Three cases of mental confusion have been reported in patients receiving disulfiram and paraldehyde.[4] Moreover, patients with liver disease are at greater risk of adverse effects of paraldehyde. Because of this increased risk of paraldehyde adverse effects with disulfiram and with liver disease, it may be prudent to avoid concurrent use.

1. Hitchcock P, Nelson EE. The metabolism of paraldehyde: II. *J Pharmacol Exp Ther* (1943) 79, 286–94.
2. Keplinger ML, Wells JA. Effect of Antabuse on the action of paraldehyde in mice and dogs. *Fedn Proc* (1956) 15, 445–6.
3. Keplinger ML, Wells JA. The effect of disulfiram on the action and metabolism of paraldehyde. *J Pharmacol Exp Ther* (1957), 119: 19–25.
4. Christie GL. Three cases of transient confusional psychosis in patients receiving con-current antabuse and paraldehyde therapy. *Med J Aust* (1956) May 12: 789–91.

Phenobarbital or Primidone + Allopurinol

Allopurinol appears not to alter phenobarbital levels, including those derived from primidone.

Clinical evidence, mechanism, importance and management

In a study of add-on therapy, allopurinol (150 mg daily in those less than 20 kg, and 300 mg daily for other patients) for 4 months, had no effect on phenobarbital levels in 46 patients on anticonvulsants including phenobarbital.[1] In another similar study, allopurinol 10 mg/kg increased to 15 mg/kg daily for 12 weeks had no effect on serum phenobarbital levels in 11 patients on primidone or phenobarbital with or without other anticonvulsants.[2] Therefore phenobarbital or primidone dosage alterations are unlikely to be required if allopurinol is used.

1. Zagnoni PG, Bianchi A, Zolo P, Canger R, Cornaggia C, D'Alessandro P, DeMarco P, Pisani F, Gianelli M, Verzé L, Viani F, Zaccara G. Allopurinol as add-on therapy in refractory epilepsy: a double-blind placebo-controlled randomized study. *Epilepsia* (1994) 35, 107–12.
2. Coppola G, Pascotto A. Double-blind, placebo-controlled, cross-over trial of allopurinol as add-on therapy in childhood refractory epilepsy. *Brain Dev* (1996) 18, 50–2.

Phenobarbital or Primidone + Felbamate

Felbamate causes a moderate increase in serum phenobarbital levels, which has resulted in phenobarbital toxicity.

Clinical evidence

When 24 healthy subjects on phenobarbital 100 mg daily were additionally given felbamate 1.2 g twice daily for 10 days, the AUC and the maximum serum levels of phenobarbital were raised by 22 and 24% respectively. Concurrent use was said to be safe and well tolerated.[1] A 30% increase in phenobarbital plasma concentrations was seen in another 19 patients on phenobarbital or primidone (which is metabolised to phenobarbital) when given felbamate (average dose 2458 mg daily).[2] A phenobarbital dosage reduction of about 30% was needed in another 6 patients when they started on felbamate.[3] A man on sodium valproate and phenobarbital had an almost 50% increase in phenobarbital serum levels over a 5-week period after felbamate 50 mg/kg was added, despite an initial phenobarbital dosage reduction from 230 mg to 200 mg daily. He was hospitalised because of increased lethargy, anorexia and ataxia and was eventually discharged on a phenobarbital dosage of 150 mg daily.[4]

It was noted that felbamate levels were lower in patients on phenobarbital than in historical control patients not on phenobarbital.[1] However, in a modelling study, phenobarbital apparently had little or no effect on the pharmacokinetics of felbamate.[5]

Mechanism

Not established. It seems possible that the felbamate may inhibit more than one pathway in the metabolism of the phenobarbital, resulting in a reduction in its loss from the body. The cytochrome P450 isoenzyme CYP2C19 may be involved.[1,6]

Importance and management

An established interaction. If felbamate is added to established treatment with phenobarbital or primidone, particularly in patients already taking substantial doses, monitor well for any evidence of increased adverse effects (drowsiness, lethargy, anorexia, ataxia) and reduce the dosages of the phenobarbital or primidone if necessary.

1. Reidenberg P, Glue P, Banfield CR, Colucci RD, Meehan JW, Radwanski E, Mojavarian P, Lin C-C, Nezamis J, Guillaume M, Affime MB. Effects of felbamate on the pharmacokinetics of phenobarbital. *Clin Pharmacol Ther* (1995) 58, 279–87.
2. Kerrick JM, Wolff DL, Risinger MW, Graves NM. Increased phenobarbital plasma concentrations after felbamate initiation. *Epilepsia* (1994) 35 (Suppl 8), 96.
3. Sachdeo RC, Padela MF. The effect of felbamate on phenobarbital serum concentrations. *Epilepsia* (1994) 35 (Suppl 8), 94.
4. Gidal BE, Zupanc ML. Potential pharmacokinetic interaction between felbamate and phenobarbital. *Ann Pharmacother* (1994) 28, 455–8.
5. Kelley MT, Walson PD, Cox S, Dusci LJ. Population pharmacokinetics of felbamate in children. *Ther Drug Monit* (1997) 19, 29–36.
6. Glue P, Banfield CR, Perhach JL, Mather GG, Racha JK, Levy RH. Pharmacokinetic interactions with felbamate. *Clin Pharmacokinet* (1997) 33, 214–24.

Phenobarbital + Influenza vaccines

Influenza vaccine can cause a moderate rise in serum phenobarbital levels.

Clinical evidence, mechanism, importance and management

Serum phenobarbital levels rose by about 30% in 11 out of 27 children when given 0.5 ml of a whole virus influenza vaccine USP, types A and B, (Squibb). Levels remained elevated 28 days after vaccination.[1]

It was suggested that the vaccine inhibits the liver enzymes concerned with the metabolism of phenobarbital, thereby reducing its loss from the body. Information is very limited but it seems unlikely that this moderate increase in serum phenobarbital levels will usually have much clinical relevance. Further study is needed.

1. Jann MW, Fidone GS. Effect of influenza vaccine on serum anticonvulsant concentrations. *Clin Pharm* (1986) 5, 817–20.

Phenobarbital + Sodium valproate

Serum phenobarbital levels can be increased by sodium valproate, which may result in excessive sedation and lethargy. A reduction in the dosage of the phenobarbital of between one-third and one-half may be needed. Small reductions in sodium valproate levels have also been reported. Combined use of phenobarbital and sodium valproate may cause an increase in serum liver enzymes.

Clinical evidence

A 6-month study in 11 epileptics on phenobarbital 90 to 400 mg daily found that when they were also given valproic acid 11.2 to 42.7 mg/kg daily sedation developed. On average the dosage of phenobarbital was reduced to 54% of the original dose with continued good seizure control. Another 2 patients who did not have their phenobarbital dose reduced had an increase in their phenobarbital levels of 12 and 48% when valproic acid was added.[1]

Another study found that sodium valproate 1.2 g daily raised serum phenobarbital levels in 20 patients by an average of 27%. Signs of toxicity occurred in 13 patients, but the dose only needed to be reduced in 3 patients.[2] This interaction has been described in numerous other reports, and dose reductions of the phenobarbital were almost always necessary to avoid excessive drowsiness.[3-17] In one study the rise in phenobarbital levels was much greater in children (over 100%) than in adults (about 50%).[18]

A reduction in sodium valproate levels of about 25% has also been reported, but the effect on seizure control was not mentioned.[19] A reduction in valproate levels caused by phenobarbital has also been reported elsewhere.[20]

The incidence of increased liver enzyme activity was found to be higher in 41 patients receiving phenobarbital with valproate than in 40 patients on valproate monotherapy (ALT 7.3% versus 0%). Use of phenytoin as well resulted in even greater increases (ALT 26.1% and AST 28.3% versus about 20%). However, the increases were mild and were not considered clinically important.[21]

Mechanism

The evidence indicates that sodium valproate inhibits three steps in the metabolism of phenobarbital by the liver, leading to its accumulation in the body. The inhibited steps are the formation of *p*-hydroxyphenobarbital by the cytochrome P450 isoenzyme CYP2C9,[22] the *N*-glucosidation of phenobarbital[23] and the *O*-glucuronidation of *p*-hydroxyphenobarbital.[23]

Importance and management

An extremely well documented and well established interaction of clinical importance. The incidence seems to be high. The effects of concurrent use should be well monitored and suitable phenobarbital dosage reductions made as necessary to avoid toxicity. The dosage may need to be reduced by a third to a half.[1] The significance of the modest reduction in sodium valproate levels is not clear, especially as valproate levels do not correlate well with efficacy of treatment. Sodium valproate has been associated with serious hepatotoxicity, especially in children aged less than 3 years, and this has been more common in those receiving other anticonvulsants. Sodium valproate monotherapy is to be preferred in this group.

1. Wilder BJ, Willmore LJ, Bruni J, Villarreal HJ. Valproic acid: interaction with other anticonvulsant drugs. *Neurology* (1978) 28, 892–6.
2. Richens A, Ahmad S. Controlled trial of sodium valproate in severe epilepsy. *BMJ* (1975) 4, 255–6.
3. Schobben F, van der Kleijn E and Gabreëls FJM. Pharmacokinetics of di-n-propylacetate in epileptic patients. *Eur J Clin Pharmacol* (1975) 8, 97–105.
4. Gram L, Wulff K, Rasmussen KE, Flachs H, Würtz-Jørgensen A, Sommerbeck KW, Løhren V. Valproate sodium: a controlled clinical trial including monitoring of drug levels. *Epilepsia* (1977) 18, 141–8.
5. Jeavons PM, Clark JE. Sodium valproate in treatment of epilepsy. *BMJ* (1974) 2, 584–6.
6. Völzke E, Doose H. Dipropylacetate (Dépakine®, Ergenyl®) in the treatment of epilepsy. *Epilepsia* (1973) 14, 185–93.
7. Millet Y, Sainty JM, Galland MC, Sidoine R, Jouglard J. Problèmes posés par l'association thérapeutique phénobarbital-dipropylacétate de sodium. A propos d'un cas. *Eur J Toxicol Environ Hyg* (1976) 9, 381–3.
8. Jeavons PM, Clark JE, Maheshwari MC. Treatment of generalized epilepsies of childhood and adolescence with sodium valproate ('Epilim'). *Dev Med Child Neurol* (1977) 19, 9–25.
9. Vakil SD, Critchley EMR, Phillips JC, Fahim Y, Haydock C, Cocks A, Dyer T. The effect of sodium valproate (Epilim) on phenytoin and phenobarbitone blood levels. Clinical and Pharmacological Aspects of Sodium Valproate (Epilim) in the Treatment of Epilepsy. Proceedings of a Symposium held at Nottingham University, September 1975, 75–7.

10. Scott DF, Boxer CM, Herzberg JL. A study of the hypnotic effects of Epilim and its possible interaction with phenobarbitone. Clinical and Pharmacological Aspects of Sodium Valproate (Epilim) in the Treatment of Epilepsy. Proceedings of a Symposium held at Nottingham University, September 1975, 155–7.
11. Richens A, Scoular IT, Ahmad S, Jordan BJ. Pharmacokinetics and efficacy of Epilim in patients receiving long-term therapy with other antiepileptic drugs. Clinical and Pharmacological Aspects of Sodium Valproate (Epilim) in the Treatment of Epilepsy. Proceedings of a Symposium held at Nottingham University, September 1975, 78–88.
12. Loiseau P, Orgogozo JM, Brachet-Liermain A, Morselli PL. Pharmacokinetic studies on the interaction between phenobarbital and valproic acid. In Adv Epileptol Proc Cong Int League Epilepsy 13th. Edited by Meinardi H and Rowan A. *(1977/8) p 261–5.* (1977/8) p 261–5.
13. Fowler GW. Effect of dipropylacetate on serum levels of anticonvulsants in children. *Proc West Pharmacol Soc* (1978) 21, 37–40.
14. Patel IH, Levy RH, Cutler RE. Phenobarbital-valproic acid interaction. *Clin Pharmacol Ther* (1980) 27, 515–21.
15. Coulter DL, Wu H, Allen RJ. Valproic acid therapy in childhood epilepsy. *JAMA* (1980) 244, 785–8.
16. Kapetanovic IM, Kupferberg HJ, Porter RJ, Theodore W, Schulman E, Penry JK. Mechanism of valproate-phenobarbital interaction in epileptic patients. *Clin Pharmacol Ther* (1981) 29, 480–6.
17. Yukara E, To H, Ohdo S, Higuchi S, Aoyama T. Detection of a drug-drug interaction on population based phenobarbitone clearance using nonlinear mixed-effects modeling. *Eur J Clin Pharmacol* (1998) 54, 69–74.
18. Fernandez de Gatta MR, Alonso Gonzalez AC, Garcia Sanchez MJ, Dominguez-Gil Hurle A, Santos Borbujo J, Monzon Corral L. Effect of sodium valproate on phenobarbital serum levels in children and adults. *Ther Drug Monit* (1986) 8, 416–20.
19. May T, Rambeck B. Serum concentrations of valproic acid: influence of dose and comedication. *Ther Drug Monit* (1985) 7, 387–90.
20. Meinardi H, Bongers E. Analytical data in connection with the clinical use of di-n-propylacetate. In Clinical Pharmacology of Antiepileptic Drugs, edited by Schneider H et al. *Springer-Verlag, NY and Berlin* (1975) 235–41.
21. Haidukewych D, John G. Chronic valproic acid and coantiepileptic drug therapy and incidence of increases in serum liver enzymes. *Ther Drug Monit* (1986) 8, 407–410.
22. Hurst SI, Hargreaves JA, Howald WN, Racha JK, Mather GG, Labroo R, Carlson SP, Levy RH. Enzymatic mechanism for the phenobarbital-valproate interaction. *Epilepsia* (1997) 38 (Suppl 8), 111–12.
23. Bernus I, Dickinson RG, Hooper WD, Eadie MJ. Inhibition of phenobarbitone *N*-glucosidation by valproate. *Br J Clin Pharmacol* (1994) 38, 411–16.

Phenobarbital + Troleandomycin

Troleandomycin caused a modest fall in the serum phenobarbital levels of one patient.

Clinical evidence, mechanism, importance and management

A patient on phenobarbital and carbamazepine had a modest fall in serum phenobarbital levels from about 40 to 31 micrograms/ml, and a rise in carbamazepine levels, when given troleandomycin.[1] The general importance of this single report is uncertain, but this modest change is probably of limited clinical importance. For a discussion of the rise in carbamazepine levels with troleandomycin, see 'Carbamazepine + Macrolides', p.345.

1. Dravet C, Mesdjian E, Cenraud B and Roger J. Interaction between carbamazepine and triacetyloleandomycin. *Lancet* (1977) i, 810.

Phenytoin + Allopurinol

A case report describes phenytoin toxicity in a boy given allopurinol. Another study found raised phenytoin levels in 2 of 18 patients given allopurinol.

Clinical evidence, mechanism, importance and management

A 13-year-old boy with Lesch-Nyhan syndrome who was taking phenobarbital, clonazepam, sodium valproate and phenytoin 200 mg daily became somnolent within 7 days of starting to take allopurinol 150 mg daily. His serum phenytoin levels were found to have increased from 7.5 to 20.8 micrograms/ml.[1] In another study, 2 patients had a marked increase in phenytoin levels when given allopurinol (150 mg daily in those less than 20 kg, and 300 mg daily for other patients) for 4 months, which in one case led to withdrawal from the study, and in the other to a phenytoin dosage reduction. However, 16 other patients had no change in phenytoin levels while on this dose of allopurinol.[2]

The reason for this reaction is not known. An *animal* study confirmed that 50 mg/kg, but not 20 mg/kg, of allopurinol reduced phenytoin elimination, but was unable to work out the mechanism.[3]

Although information is limited, it appears that allopurinol may raise phenytoin levels in a few patients. It would be prudent to monitor for phenytoin toxicity when allopurinol is added.

1. Yokochi K, Yokochi A, Chiba K, Ishizaki T. Phenytoin-allopurinol interaction: Michaelis-Menten kinetic parameters of phenytoin with and without allopurinol in a child with Lesch-Nyhan syndrome. *Ther Drug Monit* (1982) 4, 353–7.
2. Zagnoni PG, Bianchi A, Zolo P, Canger R, Cornaggia C, D'Alessandro P, DeMarco P, Pisani F, Gianelli M, Verzé L, Viani F, Zaccara G. Allopurinol as add-on therapy in refractory epilepsy: a double-blind placebo-controlled randomized study. *Epilepsia* (1994) 35, 107–12.
3. Ogiso T, Ito Y, Iwaki M, Tsunekawa K. Drug interaction between phenytoin and allopurinol. *J Pharmacobiodyn* (1990) 13, 36–43.

Phenytoin + Amiodarone

Serum phenytoin levels can be raised by amiodarone, markedly so in some individuals, and phenytoin toxicity may occur. Amiodarone serum levels are reduced by phenytoin.

Clinical evidence

(a) Phenytoin serum levels increased

Three patients had a marked rise in serum phenytoin levels 10 days to 4 weeks after being given amiodarone 400 to 1200 mg daily. One of them developed phenytoin toxicity (ataxia, lethargy, vertigo) within 4 weeks of starting to take amiodarone and had a serum phenytoin level of 40 micrograms/ml, representing a three to fourfold rise. Levels restabilised when the phenytoin dosage was withheld and then reduced from 300 to 200 mg daily. The serum phenytoin levels of the other 2 patients were approximately doubled by the amiodarone.[1]

A study in healthy subjects found that amiodarone 200 mg daily for 3 weeks increased the AUC of a single 5-mg/kg intravenous dose of phenytoin by 40%.[2] Another pharmacokinetic study found that amiodarone 200 mg daily for 6 weeks raised the AUC and steady-state peak serum levels of phenytoin by 40% and 33% respectively. Phenytoin 2 to 4 mg/kg daily was given orally for 14 days before and during the last 2 weeks of amiodarone therapy.[3] Other case reports describe 3 patients who had two to threefold rises in serum phenytoin levels and toxicity 2 to 6 weeks after starting amiodarone.[4-6]

(b) Amiodarone serum levels reduced

A study in 5 healthy subjects given amiodarone 200 mg daily found that over a 5-week period the serum amiodarone levels gradually increased. When phenytoin 3 to 4 mg/kg daily was added for a period of 2 weeks, the serum amiodarone levels fell to concentrations that were between about 50 and 65% of those predicted.[7]

Mechanism

Uncertain. It seems possible that amiodarone inhibits the liver enzymes concerned with the metabolism of phenytoin, resulting in a rise in its serum levels.[3] It seems unlikely that drug displacement from protein binding sites had a part to play as free and bound levels of phenytoin remained constant.[3]

Phenytoin is an enzyme-inducing agent that possibly increases the metabolism of the amiodarone by the liver.

Importance and management

Information seems to be limited to the reports cited, but both interactions appear to be clinically important. Concurrent use should not be undertaken unless the effects can be well monitored.

The phenytoin dosage should be reduced as necessary. A 25 to 30% reduction has been recommended for those taking 2 to 4 mg/kg daily, but it should be remembered that small alterations in phenytoin dose may result in a large change in phenytoin levels, as phenytoin kinetics are non-linear.[3,8,9] Note that the phenytoin levels in some individuals were doubled after only 10 days of concurrent use.[1] Amiodarone is cleared from the body very slowly so that this interaction will persist for weeks after its withdrawal. Continued monitoring is important. Be aware that ataxia due to phenytoin toxicity may be confused with amiodarone-induced ataxia.[1,5]

It is not clear whether the amiodarone dosage should be increased or not to accommodate this interaction because the metabolite of amiodarone (*N*-desethylamiodarone) also has important antiarrhythmic effects.[7]

1. McGovern B, Geer VR, LaRaia PJ, Garan H, Ruskin JN. Possible interaction between amiodarone and phenytoin. *Ann Intern Med* (1984) 101, 650–1.
2. Nolan PE, Marcus FI, Hoyer GL, Bliss M, Gear K. Pharmacokinetic interaction between intravenous phenytoin and amiodarone in healthy volunteers. *Clin Pharmacol Ther* (1989) 46, 43–50.
3. Nolan PE, Erstad BL, Hoyer GL, Bliss M, Gear K, Marcus FI. Steady-state interaction between amiodarone and phenytoin in normal subjects. *Am J Cardiol* (1990) 65, 1252–7.
4. Gore JM, Haffajee CI, Alpert JS. Interaction of amiodarone and diphenylhydantoin. *Am J Cardiol* (1984) 54, 1145.

5. Shackleford EJ, Watson FT. Amiodarone-phenytoin interaction. *Drug Intell Clin Pharm* (1987) 21, 921.
6. Ahmad S. Amiodarone and phenytoin: interaction. *J Am Geriatr Soc* (1995) 43, 1449–50
7. Nolan PE, Marcus FI, Karol MD, Hoyer GL, Gear K. Effect of phenytoin on the clinical pharmacokinetics of amiodarone. *J Clin Pharmacol* (1990) 30, 1112–19.
8. Nolan PE, Erstad BL, Hoyer GL, Bliss M, Gear K, Marcus FI. Interaction between amiodarone and phenytoin. *Am J Cardiol* (1991) 67, 328–9.
9. Duffal SB, McKenzie SK. Interaction between amiodarone and phenytoin. *Am J Cardiol* (1991) 67, 328.

Phenytoin + Antacids

Some, but not all studies have shown that antacids can reduce phenytoin serum levels and this may have been responsible for some loss of seizure control in a few patients, but usually no clinically important interaction occurs.

Clinical evidence

(a) Evidence of an interaction

A review briefly mentions that 3 patients taking phenytoin were found to have low serum phenytoin levels of 2 to 4 micrograms/ml when they were given phenytoin and unnamed antacids at the same time, but when the antacid administration was delayed by 2 to 3 hours the serum phenytoin levels rose two to threefold.[1]

A controlled study in 6 epileptics found that a **magnesium trisilicate** and **aluminium hydroxide** antacid (*Gelusil*) caused a 12% reduction in steady-state serum phenytoin levels, although seizure frequency was not affected.[2] Elsewhere, 2 epileptics are reported to have had inadequate seizure control, which coincided with the ingestion of **aluminium/magnesium hydroxide** antacids for dyspepsia.[3] The AUC of a single dose of phenytoin was reduced by about 25% in 8 healthy subjects given either **aluminium/magnesium hydroxide** or **calcium carbonate**.[4] Three of 6 healthy subjects given a **dimeticone**, **aluminium hydroxide** and **magnesium oxide** antacid (*Asilone*) had a reduction in the AUC of a single dose of phenytoin, but this did not reach statistical significance.[5]

(b) Evidence of no interaction

A study in 6 healthy subjects given **aluminium** or **magnesium hydroxide** failed to show any change in the rate or extent of absorption of a single dose of phenytoin,[3] and a similar study found **calcium carbonate** also had no effect on the absorption of phenytoin.[2] A study in 2 subjects found no alteration in the absorption of phenytoin due to a mixture of **aluminium/magnesium hydroxide** and **magnesium trisilicate**, or **calcium carbonate**.[6] In another study, no statistically significant decrease in absorption was seen in 6 healthy subjects given a **dimeticone**, **aluminium hydroxide** and **magnesium oxide** antacid (*Asilone*), although 3 patients did have a decrease[5] (see above).

Mechanism

Not understood. One suggestion is that diarrhoea and a general increase in peristalsis caused by some antacids may cause a reduction in phenytoin absorption. Another is that antacids may cause changes in gastric acid secretion, which could affect phenytoin solubility.

Importance and management

This possible interaction is fairly well documented, but the results are conflicting. In practice it appears not to be important in most patients, although some loss of seizure control has been seen to occur in a few. The interaction is unpredictable because it seems to depend on the individual patient and the antacid being taken. Concurrent use need not be avoided but if there is any hint that an epileptic patient is being affected, separation of the dosages by 2 to 3 hours may minimise the effects.

1. Pippinger L. Personal communication quoted by Kutt H in Interactions of antiepileptic drugs. *Epilepsia* (1975) 16, 393–402.
2. Kulshreshtha VK, Thomas M, Wadsworth J, Richens A. Interaction between phenytoin and antacids. *Br J Clin Pharmacol* (1978) 6, 177–9.
3. O'Brien LS, Orme ML'E, Breckenridge AM. Failure of antacids to alter the pharmacokinetics of phenytoin. *Br J Clin Pharmacol* (1978) 6, 176–7.
4. Carter BL, Garnett WR, Pellock JM, Stratton MA, Howell JR. Effect of antacids on phenytoin bioavailability. *Ther Drug Monit* (1981) 3, 333–40.
5. McElnay JC, Uprichard G, Collier PS. The effect of activated dimethicone and a proprietary antacid preparation containing this agent on the absorption of phenytoin. *Br J Clin Pharmacol* (1982) 13, 501–5.
6. Chapron DJ, Kramer PA, Mariano SL, Hohnadel DC. Effect of calcium and antacids on phenytoin bioavailability. *Arch Neurol* (1979) 36, 436–8.

Phenytoin + Anticoagulants

The serum levels of phenytoin can be increased by dicoumarol (toxicity seen) and phenprocoumon, but they are usually unchanged by warfarin and phenindione. However, a single case of phenytoin toxicity has been seen with warfarin. Phenytoin would be expected to reduce the anticoagulant effects of coumarin anticoagulants, and this has been demonstrated for dicoumarol. However, cases of increased effects of warfarin have been reported, and one study showed the effects of phenprocoumon were generally unaltered. A single case of severe bleeding has been described with acenocoumarol, paroxetine and phenytoin.

Clinical evidence

The reports of interactions between phenytoin and various anticoagulants are summarised in 'Table 11.3', (p.362), and discussed in further detail below.

(a) Acenocoumarol

A 68-year-old woman with a double mitral valve lesion, atrial fibrillation and hypertension, on digoxin and diuretics, was stabilised on acenocoumarol 17 mg per week in divided doses and paroxetine. Phenytoin 400 mg daily for 3 days then 300 mg daily was started because of a seizure, and 11 days later she developed ataxia, lethargy and nystagmus (free phenytoin levels of 12.5 micromol/l). At the same time her INR was found to have risen from a range of 2 to 4, up to 14.5 and a huge retroperitoneal haematoma was discovered. After appropriate treatment she was discharged on acenocoumarol 13 mg per week in divided doses and half the phenytoin dosage.[1]

(b) Dicoumarol

Phenytoin 300 mg daily was given to 6 subjects on dicoumarol 40 to 160 mg daily for a week. No significant changes in the prothrombin-proconvertin concentration occurred until 3 days after stopping the phenytoin. In the following 5 days it climbed from 20 to 50%, with an accompanying drop in the serum dicoumarol levels.[2] Four other subjects on dicoumarol 60 mg daily were also given phenytoin 300 mg daily for the first week of treatment, and then 100 mg daily for 5 more weeks. The prothrombin-proconvertin concentration had risen from 20 to 70% after 2 weeks of concurrent treatment, and only fell to previous levels 5.5 weeks after stopping the phenytoin.[2]

A study in 6 subjects taking phenytoin 300 mg daily found that when they were also given dicoumarol (doses adjusted to give prothrombin values of about 30%) their serum phenytoin levels rose on average by almost 10 micrograms/ml (126%) over 7 days.[3] In another study the half-life of phenytoin in 3 patients increased by about fivefold during dicoumarol treatment.[4]

A patient on dicoumarol developed phenytoin toxicity within a few days of starting to take phenytoin 300 mg daily (dose based on a weight of 62 kg). Phenytoin was withdrawn, and re-introduced at 200 mg daily, which gave satisfactory phenytoin levels.[5]

(c) Phenindione

A study in 4 patients on phenytoin 300 mg daily found that phenindione did not affect their serum phenytoin levels.[4]

(d) Phenprocoumon

An investigation in patients on long-term phenprocoumon treatment found that in the majority of cases phenytoin had no significant effect on either serum phenprocoumon levels or the anticoagulant control, although a few patients had a fall and others a rise in serum anticoagulant levels, with consequent decreased or increased effect.[6]

A study in 4 patients on phenytoin 300 mg daily found that when they were additionally given phenprocoumon their serum phenytoin levels rose from about 10 micrograms/ml to 14 micrograms/ml over 7 days.[4] The phenytoin half-life increased from 9.9 to 14 hours.

(e) Warfarin

The prothrombin time of a patient on warfarin increased from 21 to 32 seconds over a month when phenytoin 300 mg daily was given, despite a 22% reduction in the warfarin dosage. He was restabilised on the original warfarin dosage when the phenytoin was withdrawn. Six other reports describe this interaction.[7-12] One of them describes a patient who had an increased anticoagulant response to warfarin for the first 6 days after phenytoin was added. The anticoagulant effect then declined to less than the level seen before the addition of phenytoin.[10] Conversely, a population pharmacokinetic analysis reported that the clearance of warfarin was *increased* by 30% in 6 patients on phenytoin or phenobarbital.[13] However, the findings were not reported separately for the two drugs, and are therefore difficult to interpret (phenobarbital is a known inducer of warfarin clearance, see 'Anticoagulants + Barbiturates', p.269).

A study in 2 patients on phenytoin 300 mg daily found that their serum phenytoin levels were unaffected by warfarin given for 7 days, and the half-life of phenytoin in 4 other patients was unaffected.[4] However, a patient on phenytoin 300 mg daily developed symptoms of toxicity shortly after starting to take warfarin.[14] Another patient developed phenytoin toxicity 6 months after starting concurrent phenytoin and warfarin therapy.[12]

Mechanism

Multiple, complex and poorly understood. Dicoumarol and phenprocoumon (but not normally warfarin) appear to inhibit the metabolism of phenytoin by the liver, so that its loss from the body is reduced. Phenytoin is an inducer of cytochrome P450 isoenzyme CYP2C9, which is involved in metabolism of some of the coumarin anticoagulants. Phenytoin would therefore be expected to decrease the levels and effect of some coumarins, and this has been shown for dicoumarol. However, increased effects of warfarin have been noted, suggesting reduced metabolism of warfarin. Why this occurs is uncertain, but poor CYP2C9 metaboliser phenotype (see 'Genetic factors', (p.4)) may provide an explanation.[15] Phenytoin possibly also has a diverse depressant effect on the liver, which lowers blood clotting factor production.[16]

Importance and management

None of these interactions has been extensively studied nor are they well established, but what is known suggests that the use of dicoumarol with phenytoin should be avoided or monitored very closely. Serum phenytoin levels and anticoagulant control should be well monitored if acenocoumarol, phenprocoumon or warfarin is given with phenytoin. Dosage adjustments may be needed to accommodate any interactions. Information about other anticoagulants (apart from phenindione, which had no effect on phenytoin levels) appears to be lacking, but it would clearly be prudent to monitor the effects of concurrent use.

1. Abad-Santos F, Carcas AJ, F-Capitán C, Frias J. Case report. Retroperitoneal haematoma in a patient treated with acenocoumarol, phenytoin and paroxetine. *Clin Lab Haematol* (1995) 17, 195–7.
2. Hansen JM, Siersbæk-Nielsen K, Kristensen M, Skovsted L,Christensen LK. Effect of diphenylhydantoin on the metabolism of dicoumarol in man. *Acta Med Scand* (1971) 189, 15–19.
3. Hansen JM, Kristensen M, Skovsted L, Christensen LK. Dicoumarol-induced diphenylhydantoin intoxication. *Lancet* (1966) ii, 265–6.
4. Skovsted L, Kristensen M, Hansen JM, Siersbæk-Nielsen K. The effect of different oral anticoagulants on diphenylhydantoin (DPH) and tolbutamide metabolism. *Acta Med Scand* (1976) 199, 513–15.
5. Franzten E, Hansen JM, Hansen OE, Kristensen M. Phenytoin (Dilantin®) intoxication. *Acta Neurol Scand* (1967) 43, 440–6.
6. Chrishe HW, Tauchert M, Hilger HH. Effect of phenytoin on the metabolism of phenprocoumon. *Eur J Clin Invest* (1974) 4, 331.
7. Nappi JM. Warfarin and phenytoin interaction. *Ann Intern Med* (1979) 90, 852.
8. Koch-Weser J. Haemorrhagic reactions and drug interactions in 500 warfarin treated patients. *Clin Pharmacol Ther* (1973) 14, 139.
9. Taylor JW, Alexander B, Lyon LW. A comparative evaluation of oral anticoagulant-phenytoin interactions. *Drug Intell Clin Pharm* (1980) 14, 669–73.
10. Levine M, Sheppard I. Biphasic interaction of phenytoin with warfarin. *Clin Pharm* (1984) 3, 200–3.
11. Panegyres PK, Rischbieth RH. Fatal phenytoin warfarin interaction. *Postgrad Med J* (1991) 67, 98.
12. Meisheri YV. Simultaneous phenytoin and warfarin toxicity on chronic concomitant therapy. *J Assoc Physicians India* (1996) 44, 661–2.
13. Mungall DR, Ludden TM, Marshall J, Hawkins DW, Talbert RL, Crawford MH.. Population pharmacokinetics of racemic warfarin in adult patients. *J Pharmacokinet Biopharm* (1985) 13, 213–27.
14. Rothermich NO. Diphenylhydantoin intoxication. *Lancet* (1966) ii, 640.
15. Rettie AE, Haining RL, Bajpai M, Levy RH. A common genetic basis for idiosyncratic toxicity of warfarin and phenytoin. *Epilepsy Res* (1999) 35, 253–5.
16. Solomon GE, Hilgartner MW, Kutt H. Coagulation defects caused by diphenylhydantoin. *Neurology* (1972) 22, 1165–71.

Table 11.3 Summary of interactions between phenytoin and anticoagulants

Concurrent treatment with phenytoin and anticoagulant	*Effect on anticoagulant*	*Effect on serum phenytoin levels*
Dicoumarol	Reduced[1]	Markedly increased[10–12]
Phenprocoumon	Usually unchanged[2]	Increased[11]
Acenocoumarol	Single case of increase[3]	Uncertain
Warfarin	Increased[4–9] Single case of increase followed by decrease[7]	Usually unchanged[11] Increased in two cases[9,13]
Phenindione	Not documented	Usually unchanged[10,11]

1. Hansen JM, Siersbæk-Nielsen K, Kristensen M, Skovsted L, Christensen LK. Effect of diphenylhydantoin on the metabolism of dicoumarol in man. *Acta Med Scand* (1971) 189, 15–19.
2. Chrishe HW, Tauchert M, Hilger HH. Effect of phenytoin on the metabolism of phenprocoumon. *Eur J Clin Invest* (1974) 4, 331.
3. Abad-Santos F, Carcas AJ, F-Capitán C, Frias J. Case report. Retroperitoneal haematoma in a patient treated with acenocoumarol, phenytoin and paroxetine. *Clin Lab Haematol* (1995) 17, 195–7.
4. Nappi JM. Warfarin and phenytoin interaction. *Ann Intern Med* (1979) 90, 852.
5. Koch-Weser J. Haemorrhagic reactions and drug interactions in 500 warfarin treated patients. *Clin Pharmacol Ther* (1973) 14, 139.
6. Taylor JW, Alexander B, Lyon LW. A comparative evaluation of oral anticoagulant-phenytoin interactions. *Drug Intell Clin Pharm* (1980) 14, 669–73.
7. Levine M, Sheppard I. Biphasic interaction of phenytoin with warfarin. *Clin Pharm* (1984) 3, 200–3.
8. Panegyres PK, Rischbieth RH. Fatal phenytoin warfarin interaction. *Postgrad Med J* (1991) 67, 98.
9. Meisheri YV. Simultaneous phenytoin and warfarin toxicity on chronic concomitant therapy. *J Assoc Physicians India* (1996) 44, 661–2.
10. Hansen JM, Kristensen M, Skovsted L, Christensen LK. Dicoumarol-induced diphenylhydantoin intoxication. *Lancet* (1966) ii, 265-6.
11. Skovsted L, Kristensen M, Hansen JM, Siersbæk-Nielsen K. The effect of different oral anticoagulants on diphenylhydantoin (DPH) and tolbutamide metabolism. *Acta Med Scand* (1976) 199, 513–15.
12. Franzten E, Hansen JM, Hansen OE, Kristensen M. Phenytoin (Dilantin®) intoxication. *Acta Neurol Scand* (1967) 43, 440–6.
13. Rothermich NO. Diphenylhydantoin intoxication. *Lancet* (1966) ii, 640.

Phenytoin + Antidiabetics

Large and toxic doses of phenytoin have been observed to cause hyperglycaemia, but normal therapeutic doses do not usually affect the control of diabetes. Two isolated cases of phenytoin toxicity have been attributed to the use of tolazamide or tolbutamide.

Clinical evidence

(a) Response to hypoglycaemic agents

Phenytoin has been shown in a number of reports[1-6] to raise the blood sugar levels of both diabetics and non-diabetics. However, in all but one of the cases quoted here the phenytoin dosage was large (at least 8 mg/kg) or even in the toxic range (70 to 80 mg/kg). There is little evidence that a hyperglycaemic response to usual doses of phenytoin is normally large enough to interfere with the control of diabetes, either with diet alone or with conventional antidiabetic agents. In the case excepted above, where the patient received phenytoin 1.2 g in the 24 hours following status epilepticus, the situation was complicated by the use of many other drugs and by renal impairment.[2]

(b) Response to phenytoin

Tolbutamide 500 mg two or three times daily was given to 17 patients on phenytoin 100 to 400 mg daily.[7] The patients had a transient 45% rise in the amount of non-protein-bound phenytoin by day 2, which had disappeared by day 4. The introduction to this report briefly mentions a man given phenytoin and **tolazamide** who developed phenytoin toxicity, which disappeared when the **tolazamide** was replaced by **insulin**.[7] A woman previously successfully treated with phenytoin and **tolbutamide** developed toxicity on a later occasion when again given **tolbutamide**, but this time with twice the dose of phenytoin.[8]

Mechanism

Studies in *animals* and man[9-11] suggest that phenytoin-induced hyperglycaemia occurs because the release of insulin from the pancreas is impaired. This implies that no interaction is possible without functional pancreatic tissue. Just why the phenytoin appeared to interact with tolazamide and tolbutamide is uncertain, but it is possible that these antidiabetics competitively inhibit phenytoin hydroxylation[12] by the cytochrome P450 isoenzyme CYP2C9.[13]

Importance and management

The weight of evidence shows that no interaction of clinical importance normally occurs between phenytoin and the antidiabetic agents. No special precautions seem normally to be necessary.

1. Klein JP. Diphenylhydantoin intoxication associated with hyperglycaemia. *J Pediatr* (1966) 69, 463–5.
2. Goldberg EM, Sanbar SS. Hyperglycaemic, non-ketotic coma following administration of Dilantin (diphenylhydantoin). *Diabetes* (1969) 18, 101–6.
3. Peters BH, Samaan NA. Hyperglycaemia with relative hypoinsulinemia in diphenylhydantoin toxicity. *N Engl J Med* (1969) 281, 91–2.
4. Millichap JG. Hyperglycaemic effect of diphenylhydantoin. *N Engl J Med* (1969) 281, 447.
5. Fariss BL, Lutcher CL. Diphenylhydantoin-induced hyperglycaemia and impaired insulin release. *Diabetes* (1971) 20, 177–81.
6. Treasure T, Toseland PA. Hyperglycaemia due to phenytoin toxicity. *Arch Dis Child* (1971) 46, 563–4.
7. Wesseling H, Mols-Thürkow I. Interaction of diphenylhydantoin (DPH) and tolbutamide in man. *Eur J Clin Pharmacol* (1975) 8, 75–8.
8. Beech E, Mathur SVS, Harrold BP. Phenytoin toxicity produced by tolbutamide. *BMJ* (1988) 297, 1613–14.
9. Kizer JS, Vargas-Cordon M, Brendel K, Bressler R. The *in vitro* inhibition of insulin secretion by diphenylhydantoin. *J Clin Invest* (1970) 49, 1942–8.
10. Levin SR, Booker J, Smith DF, Grodsky M. Inhibition of insulin secretion by diphenylhydantoin in the isolated perfused pancreas. *J Clin Endocrinol Metab* (1970) 30, 400–1.
11. Malherbe C, Burrill KC, Levin SR, Karam JH, Forsham PH. Effect of diphenylhydantoin on insulin secretion in man. *N Engl J Med* (1972) 286, 339–42.
12. Wesseling H, Thurkow I and Mulder GJ. Effect of sulphonylureas (tolazamide, tolbutamide and chlorpropamide) on the metabolism of diphenylhydantoin in the rat. *Biochem Pharmacol* (1973) 22, 3033–40.
13. Tassaneeyakul W, Veronese ME, Birkett DJ, Doecke CJ, McManus ME, Sansom LN, Miners JO. Co-regulation of phenytoin and tolbutamide metabolism in humans. *Br J Clin Pharmacol* (1992) 34, 494–8.

Phenytoin + Antituberculars

Serum phenytoin levels are markedly reduced by rifampicin, but can be raised by isoniazid. Those who are slow 'metabolisers' of isoniazid may develop phenytoin toxicity if the dosage of phenytoin is not reduced appropriately. If rifampicin and isoniazid are given together, serum phenytoin levels may fall in patients who are fast acetylators of isoniazid, but may occasionally rise in those who are slow acetylators. Clofazimine may reduce serum phenytoin levels.

Clinical evidence

(a) Isoniazid

A study in 32 patients on phenytoin 300 mg daily found that within a week of starting to take isoniazid 300 mg daily and aminosalicylic acid 15 g daily, 6 of them had phenytoin levels almost 5 micrograms/ml higher than the rest of the group. On the following days when levels of these 6 patients rose above 20 micrograms/ml the typical signs of phenytoin toxicity were seen. All 6 had unusually high serum isoniazid levels and were identified as slow metabolisers of isoniazid.[1]

Rises in serum phenytoin levels and toxicity induced by the concurrent use of isoniazid has been described in numerous other reports[2-15] involving large numbers of patients, one of which describes a fatality.[8]

(b) Rifampicin

A study in 6 patients found that the clearance of intravenous phenytoin 100 mg doubled from 46.7 to 97.8 ml/minute after rifampicin 450 mg daily was taken for 2 weeks.[16]

A man on phenytoin 400 mg daily experienced a seizure 3 days after starting rifampicin 600 mg daily. His phenytoin level was low (5.1 micrograms/ml) so the rifampicin was stopped and the phenytoin dose increased to 500 mg daily. His level increased slowly over the next 2 weeks, eventually ranging between 16 and 25 micrograms/ml.[17] Another man on phenytoin needed a dosage reduction from 375 to 325 mg to keep his serum phenytoin levels within the therapeutic range when his treatment with rifampicin came to an end.[18]

(c) Rifampicin/Clofazimine

A man with AIDS taking a number of drugs (rifampicin, clofazimine, ciprofloxacin, ethambutol, clarithromycin, diphenoxylate, bismuth, octreotide, co-trimoxazole, amphotericin, 5-flucytosine, amikacin, zalcitabine) was also given phenytoin to control a right-sided seizure disorder. Despite taking phenytoin 1.6 mg daily, and a trial of intravenous treatment, his trough phenytoin plasma levels remained almost undetectable until the rifampicin was withdrawn, when they rose to 5 micrograms/ml with the oral dose. When the clofazimine was withdrawn the levels rose even further to 10 micrograms/ml.[19]

(d) Rifampicin/Isoniazid

A patient on phenytoin 300 mg daily developed progressive drowsiness (a sign of phenytoin toxicity) during the first week of starting treatment with isoniazid, rifampicin and ethambutol. His serum phenytoin levels rose to 46.1 micrograms/ml. He slowly recovered when the phenytoin was stopped, and he was later stabilised on only 200 mg of phenytoin daily. He proved to be a slow acetylator of isoniazid.[20] Another patient on phenytoin 300 mg daily was also started on isoniazid, rifampicin and ethambutol but, in anticipation of the response seen in the previous patient, his phenytoin dosage was reduced to 200 mg daily. Within 3 days he developed seizures because his serum phenytoin levels had fallen to only 8 micrograms/ml. He needed a daily dosage of 400 mg of phenytoin to keep the serum levels within the therapeutic range. He was a fast acetylator of isoniazid.[20]

The clearance of phenytoin was doubled in 14 patients given rifampicin 450 mg, isoniazid 300 mg and ethambutol 900 to 1200 mg daily for 2 weeks. No further changes occurred in the pharmacokinetics of phenytoin after 3 months of antitubercular treatment. In this study, the interaction was of a similar magnitude in both the 8 slow and the 6 fast acetylators.[16]

Mechanism

Rifampicin (a known potent liver enzyme-inducing agent) increases the metabolism and clearance of the phenytoin from the body so that a larger dose is needed to maintain adequate serum levels. Isoniazid inhibits the liver microsomal enzymes that metabolise phenytoin, and as a result the phenytoin accumulates and its serum levels rise.[21] Only those who are 'slow metabolisers' of isoniazid (this is genetically determined) normally attain blood levels of isoniazid that are sufficiently high to cause extensive inhibition of the phenytoin metabolism. 'Fast metabolisers' remove the isoniazid too quickly for this to occur. Thus some individuals will show a rapid rise in phenytoin levels, which eventually reaches toxic concentrations, whereas others will show only a relatively slow and unimportant rise to a plateau within, or only slightly above the therapeutic range.

If isoniazid and rifampicin are given together, the enzyme inhibitory effects of isoniazid may oppose the effects of rifampicin in those who are slow acetylators of isoniazid, but in those who are fast acetylators, the isoniazid will be cleared too quickly for it effectively to oppose the rifampicin effects. However, in one study isoniazid did not counter the effects of rifampicin in slow acetylators.[16]

The interaction involving clofazimine is not understood.

Importance and management

Direct information seems to be limited to these reports, but the interactions appear to be of clinical importance. Monitor the serum phenytoin levels and increase the dosage appropriately if rifampicin alone is started. Reduce the dosage if the rifampicin is stopped. If both rifampicin and isoniazid are given, the outcome may depend on the isoniazid acetylator status of the patient. Those who are fast acetylators will probably also need an increased phenytoin dosage. Those who are slow acetylators may need a smaller phenytoin dosage if toxicity is to be avoided. All patients should be monitored very closely as the outcome is unpredictable.

The interaction with phenytoin and isoniazid alone is well-documented, well-established, clinically important and potentially serious. About 50% of the population are slow or relatively slow metabolisers of isoniazid,[1] but not all of them develop serum phenytoin levels in the toxic range. The reports indicate that somewhere between 10 and 33% of patients are at risk.[1-4,10] This adverse interaction may take only a few days to develop fully in some patients, but several weeks in others. Therefore concurrent use should be very closely monitored, making suitable dosage reductions as necessary. One patient was reported to have had better seizure control with fewer adverse effects while taking both drugs than with phenytoin alone.[22]

Information about clofazimine seems to be limited to one report. Monitor concurrent use, anticipating the need to increase the phenytoin dosage.

1. Brennan RW, Dehejia H, Kutt H, Verebely K, McDowell F. Diphenylhydantoin intoxication attendant to slow inactivation of isoniazid. *Neurology* (1970) 20, 687–93.
2. Kutt H, Brennan R, Dehejia H, Verebely K. Diphenylhydantoin intoxication. A complication of isoniazid therapy. *Am Rev Respir Dis* (1970) 101, 377–84.
3. Murray FJ. Outbreak of unexpected reactions among epileptics taking isoniazid. *Am Rev Respir Dis* (1962) 86, 729–32.
4. Kutt H, Winters W, McDowell FH. Depression of parahydroxylation of diphenylhydantoin by antituberculosis chemotherapy. *Neurology* (1966) 16, 594–602.
5. Manigand G, Thieblot P, Deparis M. Accidents de la diphénylhydantoïne induits par les traitements antituberculeux. *Presse Med* (1971) 79, 815–16.
6. Beauvais P, Mercier D, Hanoteau J, Brissand H-E. Intoxication a la diphenylhydantoine induite par l'isoniazide. *Arch Fr Pediatr* (1973) 30, 541–6.
7. Johnson J. Epanutin and isoniazid interaction. *BMJ* (1975) 1, 152.
8. Johnson J, Freeman HL. Death due to isoniazid (INH) and phenytoin. *Br J Psychiatry* (1975) 129, 511.
9. Geering JM, Ruch W, Dettli L. Diphenylhydantoin-Intoxikation durch Diphenylhydantoin-Isoniazid-Interaktion. *Schweiz Med Wochenschr* (1974) 104, 1224–8.
10. Miller RR, Porter J, Greenblatt DJ. Clinical importance of the interaction of phenytoin and isoniazid. A report from the Boston Collaborative Drug Surveillance Program. *Chest* (1979) 75, 356–8.
11. Witmer DR, Ritschel WA. Phenytoin-isoniazid interaction: a kinetic approach to management. *Drug Intell Clin Pharm* (1984) 18, 483–6.
12. Perucca E and Richens A. Anticonvulsant drug interactions. In: Tyrer J (ed) The treatment of epilepsy. MTP Lancaster. *(1980) pp 95–128.* (1980) pp 95–128.
13. Sandyk R. Phenytoin toxicity induced by antituberculosis drugs. *S Afr Med J* (1982) 61, 382.
14. Yew WW, Lau KS, Ling MHM. Phenytoin toxicity in a patient with isoniazid-induced hepatitis. *Tubercle* (1991) 72, 309–10.
15. Walubo A, Aboo A. Phenytoin toxicity due to concomitant antituberculosis therapy. *S Afr Med J* (1995) 85, 1175–6.
16. Kay L, Kampmann JP, Svendsen TL, Vergman B, Hansen JEM, Skovsted L, Kristensen M. Influence of rifampicin and isoniazid on the kinetics of phenytoin. *Br J Clin Pharmacol* (1985) 20, 323–6.
17. Wagner JC, Slama TG. Rifampin-phenytoin drug interaction. *Drug Intell Clin Pharm* (1984) 18, 497.
18. Abajo FJ. Phenytoin interaction with rifampicin. *BMJ* (1988) 297, 1048.
19. Cone LA, Woodard DR, Simmons JC, Sonnenshein MA. Drug interactions in patients with AIDS. *Clin Infect Dis* (1992) 15, 1066–8.
20. O'Reilly D, Basran GS, Hourihan B, Macfarlane JT. Interaction between phenytoin and antituberculous drugs. *Thorax* (1987) 42, 736.
21. Desta Z, Soukhova NV, Flockhart DA. Inhibition of cytochrome P450 (CYP450) isoforms by isoniazid: potent inhibition of CYP2C19 and CYP3A. *Antimicrob Agents Chemother* (2001), 45, 384–92.
22. Thulasimnay M, Kela AK. Improvement of psychomotor epilepsy due to interaction of phenytoin-isoniazid. *Tubercle* (1984) 65, 229–30.

Phenytoin + Aspirin or NSAIDs

Serum phenytoin levels can be markedly increased by azapropazone and toxicity can develop rapidly. It is inadvisable for patients to take these drugs together. Phenytoin serum levels can also be increased by phenylbutazone and phenytoin toxicity may occur. It seems likely that oxyphenbutazone will interact similarly. Phenytoin toxicity has been seen in one patient on ibuprofen, although no pharmacokinetic interaction was seen in a study. Phenytoin toxicity occurred in a patient on celecoxib. High-dose aspirin can cause protein-binding displacement of phenytoin, but this does not usually seem to be clinically important. No clinically significant interaction occurs between phenytoin and bromfenac, etodolac or tolfenamic acid.

Clinical evidence, mechanism, importance and management

(a) Aspirin

It has been suggested that if a patient has been taking large quantities of aspirin, phenytoin is 'potentiated'.[1] This comment remains unconfirmed, although a study in 10 healthy subjects did find that aspirin 975 mg every 4 hours caused protein binding displacement of phenytoin, resulting in a 16% rise in free salivary phenytoin levels and a 24% decrease in serum levels. However, these changes were considered unlikely to be clinically significant, and aspirin doses of 325 and 650 mg every 4 hours had no appreciable effect on phenytoin.[2] Similar effects on protein binding displacement have been seen in other studies.[3-7] However, although the ratios of free and bound phenytoin may change, there does not appear to be a clinical effect, possibly because the extra free phenytoin is metabolised by the liver.[6] A study in 10 epileptics on phenytoin found that when they were given aspirin 500 mg three times daily for 3 days, no significant changes in serum phenytoin levels or anticonvulsant effects occurred.[8] The extremely common use of aspirin, and the almost total silence in the literature about an adverse interaction between phenytoin and aspirin implies that no special precautions are normally needed.

(b) Azapropazone

When a patient developed phenytoin toxicity within 2 weeks of starting azapropazone 600 mg twice daily, further study was made in 5 healthy subjects given phenytoin 125 to 250 mg daily. When they were additionally given azapropazone 600 mg twice daily, their mean serum phenytoin levels fell briefly from 5 to 3.7 micrograms/ml before rising steadily over the next 7 days to 10.5 micrograms/ml.[9,10] An extension of this study is described elsewhere.[11]

Another report describes phenytoin toxicity in a woman when fenclofenac was replaced by azapropazone 1.2 g daily.[12]

The most likely explanation is that azapropazone inhibits the liver enzymes concerned with the metabolism of phenytoin, resulting in its accumulation. It also seems possible that azapropazone displaces phenytoin from its plasma protein binding sites so that levels of unbound (and active) phenytoin are increased. Information seems to be limited to the reports cited, but it appears to be a clinically important interaction. The incidence is uncertain, but an interaction occurred in all 5 of the subjects in the study cited.[9,11] The makers state that azapropazone should not be given to patients taking phenytoin.

(c) Bromfenac

Twelve healthy subjects were given a 50-mg dose of oral bromfenac three times daily for 4 days and then phenytoin 300 to 330 mg for up to 14 days (to achieve stable levels), and then both drugs for 8 days. It was found that the peak phenytoin serum levels and AUC were increased by 9% and 11% respectively, while the bromfenac peak levels and AUC were reduced by 42%. The suggested reason for the reduction in bromfenac levels is that the phenytoin increases its metabolism by the liver.[13] In practical terms these results indicate that there is no need to adjust the dosage of phenytoin if bromfenac is added, nor any need to increase the bromfenac dosage unless there is any evidence that its efficacy is diminished.

(d) Celecoxib

An elderly woman on phenytoin 300 mg daily who had also been taking celecoxib for the past 6 months, developed signs of phenytoin toxicity. She was found to have a phenytoin level of 42 micrograms/ml, and a very slow rate of elimination.[14] It was thought that celecoxib may have competed with phenytoin for elimination via the cytochrome P450 isoenzyme CYP2C9. Further study is needed. Until then, it may be prudent to warn patients to monitor for signs of phenytoin toxicity if celecoxib is started, or monitor phenytoin levels.

(e) Etodolac

A three-way crossover study in 16 healthy subjects found that etodolac 200 mg every 12 hours for 3 days had no effect on the pharmacokinetics or the pharmacological effects of phenytoin (100 mg twice daily for 2 days, 100 mg on day three).[15] There would seem to be no reason for avoiding the concurrent use of these drugs.

(f) Ibuprofen

Studies in healthy subjects found that the pharmacokinetics of single 300- or 900-mg doses of phenytoin were not significantly altered by ibuprofen 300 or 400 mg every 6 hours.[16,17] However, a single report describes a woman stabilised on phenytoin 300 mg daily who developed phenytoin toxicity within a week of starting to take ibuprofen 400 mg four times daily.[18] Her serum phenytoin levels had risen to 101 mmol/l. The phenytoin was stopped for 3 days and the ibuprofen withdrawn, and within 10 days the phenytoin level had dropped to 68 mmol/l. The reasons for this interaction are not understood.

Both phenytoin and ibuprofen have been available for many years and this case seems to be the first and only report of an adverse interaction. No special precautions would normally seem to be necessary.

(g) Oxyphenbutazone or Phenylbutazone

Six epileptics on phenytoin 200 to 350 mg daily given phenylbutazone 100 mg three times daily had a mean fall in their phenytoin serum levels from 15 to 13 micrograms/ml over the first 3 days, after which the levels rose steadily to 19 micrograms/ml over the next 11 days. One patient developed symptoms of toxicity. His levels of free phenytoin more than doubled.[8] Another study found that phenylbutazone increased the steady-state half-life of phenytoin from 13.7 to 22 hours.

The predominant effect of phenylbutazone seems to be the inhibition of the enzymes concerned with the metabolism of phenytoin,[19] leading to its accumulation in the body and a rise in its serum levels. The initial transient fall may possibly be related in some way to the displacement by the phenylbutazone of the phenytoin from its plasma protein binding sites.[20] An established interaction, although the documentation is very limited. Monitor the outcome of adding phenylbutazone and reduce the phenytoin dosage as necessary. There is no direct evidence that oxyphenbutazone interacts like phenylbutazone, but since it is the main metabolic product of phenylbutazone in the body and has been shown to prolong the half-life of phenytoin in *animals*[21] it would be expected to interact similarly.

(h) Tolfenamic acid

Tolfenamic acid 300 mg for 3 days had no significant effect on the serum levels of phenytoin in 11 patients.[8] No special precautions seem necessary if these drugs are taken concurrently.

1. Toakley JG. Dilantin overdosage. *Med J Aust* (1968) 2, 640.
2. Leonard RF, Knott PJ, Rankin GO, Robinson DS, Melnick DE. Phenytoin-salicylate interaction. *Clin Pharmacol Ther* (1981) 29, 56–60.
3. Ehrnebo M, Odar-Cederlöf I. Distribution of pentobarbital and diphenylhydantoin between plasma and cells in blood: effect of salicylic acid, temperature and total drug concentration. *Eur J Clin Pharmacol* (1977) 11, 37–42.
4. Fraser DG, Ludden TM, Evens RP, Sutherland EW. Displacement of phenytoin from plasma binding sites by salicylate. *Clin Pharmacol Ther* (1980) 27, 165–9.
5. Paxton JW. Effects of aspirin on salivary and serum phenytoin kinetics in healthy subjects. *Clin Pharmacol Ther* (1980) 27, 170–8.
6. Olanow CW, Finn A, Prussak C. The effect of salicylate on phenytoin pharmacokinetics. *Trans Am Neurol Assoc* (1979) 104, 109–10.
7. Inoue F, Walsh RJ. Folate supplements and phenytoin-salicylate interaction. *Neurology* (1983) 33, 115–16.
8. Neuvonen PJ, Lehtovaara R, Bardy A, Elomaa E. Antipyretic analgesics in patients on antiepileptic drug therapy. *Eur J Clin Pharmacol* (1979) 15, 263–8.
9. Geaney DP, Carver JG, Aronson JK, Warlow CP. Interaction of azapropazone with phenytoin. *BMJ* (1982) 284, 1373.
10. Aronson JK, Hardman M, Reynolds DJM. ABC of monitoring drug therapy. Phenytoin. *BMJ* (1992) 305, 1215–18.
11. Geaney DP, Carver JG, Davies CL, Aronson JK. Pharmacokinetic investigation of the interaction of azapropazone with phenytoin. *Br J Clin Pharmacol* (1983) 15, 727–34.
12. Roberts CJC, Daneshmend TK, Macfarlane D, Dieppe PA. Anticonvulsant intoxication precipitated by azapropazone. *Postgrad Med J* (1981) 57, 191–2.
13. Gumbhir-Shah K, Cevallos WH, DeCleene SA, Korth-Bradley JM. Evaluation of pharmacokinetic interaction between bromfenac and phenytoin in healthy males. *J Clin Pharmacol* (1997) 37, 160–8.
14. Keeling KL, Jortani SA, Linder MW, Valdes R. Prolonged elimination half-life of phenytoin in an elderly patient also on celecoxib. *Clin Chem* (2002) 48 (Suppl.), A52–A53.
15. Zvaifler N. A review of the antiarthritic efficacy and safety of etodolac. *Clin Rheumatol* (1989) 8 (Suppl 1), 43–53.
16. Bachmann KA, Schwartz JI, Forney RB, Jauregui L, Sullivan TJ. Inability of ibuprofen to alter single dose phenytoin disposition. *Br J Clin Pharmacol* (1986) 21, 165–9.
17. Townsend RJ, Fraser DG, Scavone JM, Cox SR. The effects of ibuprofen on phenytoin pharmacokinetics. *Drug Intell Clin Pharm* (1985) 19, 447–8.
18. Sandyk R. Phenytoin toxicity induced by interaction with ibuprofen. *S Afr Med J* (1982) 62, 592.
19. Andreasen PB, Frøland A, Skovsted L, Andersen SA, Hague M. Diphenylhydantoin half-life in man and its inhibition by phenylbutazone: the role of genetic factors. *Acta Med Scand* (1973) 193, 561–4.
20. Lunde PKM, Rane A, Yaffe SJ, Lund L, Sjöqvist F. Plasma protein binding of diphenylhydantoin in man. Interaction with other drugs and the effect of temperature and plasma dilution. *Clin Pharmacol Ther* (1970) 11, 846–55.
21. Soda DM, Levy G. Inhibition of drug metabolism by hydroxylated metabolites: cross-inhibition and specificity. *J Pharm Sci* (1975) 64, 1928–31.

Phenytoin + Azoles

Phenytoin serum levels can rise rapidly if fluconazole is given and toxicity has been seen. Two reports describe phenytoin toxicity in two patients given miconazole. Voriconazole also increases phenytoin levels, but ketoconazole and itraconazole appear to have little effect.

Phenytoin markedly reduces itraconazole and voriconazole levels, and probably also ketoconazole levels. Fluconazole levels are not affected by phenytoin, although there is one report of reduced efficacy.

Clinical evidence

(a) Fluconazole

In a randomised placebo-controlled study, 10 subjects given phenytoin 200 mg daily for the last 3 days of a 14-day course of fluconazole 200 mg daily were compared with 10 other subjects on phenytoin alone. The fluconazole caused the phenytoin AUC to rise by 75%, and the trough phenytoin serum levels to rise by 128%. Phenytoin appeared not to affect fluconazole trough serum levels.[1] Two other studies reported similar findings.[2,3]

At least 7 cases of phenytoin toxicity caused by fluconazole have been documented.[4-7]

A brief report noted that 3 of 9 patients on fluconazole and phenytoin required an increase in fluconazole dose or the substitution of another antifungal due to a lack of efficacy. It was suggested that phenytoin may reduce fluconazole levels in some patients.[8] However, in the controlled studies cited above[1,3] the fluconazole serum levels were unaltered by phenytoin.

(b) Itraconazole

For mention that itraconazole caused a small (10%) increase in the AUC of phenytoin, and that phenytoin markedly reduced itraconazole levels, see 'Azoles + Anticonvulsants', p.136.

(c) Ketoconazole

A study in 9 healthy subjects found that ketoconazole 200 mg twice daily for 6 days did not significantly alter the 0 to 48-hour AUC of a single 250-mg dose of phenytoin.[2] For mention of the limited evidence that phenytoin may reduce ketoconazole levels, see 'Azoles + Anticonvulsants', p.136.

(d) Miconazole

An epileptic man, well controlled on phenytoin, developed symptoms of toxicity within a day of starting treatment with intravenous miconazole 500 mg every 8 hours and flucytosine. After a week of concurrent treatment his serum phenytoin levels had risen by 50%, from 29 to 43 micrograms/ml. He had some symptoms of very mild phenytoin toxicity even before the antifungal treatment was started.[9] Another patient developed symptoms of toxicity (nystagmus, ataxia) within 5 days of starting to take miconazole 500 mg daily. His serum phenytoin rose to 40.8 micrograms/ml. After discontinuation of the miconazole the same dose of phenytoin resulted in a level of 14.5 micrograms/ml.[10]

(e) Voriconazole

For mention that concurrent use of voriconazole and phenytoin decreases voriconazole levels and increases phenytoin levels, see 'Azoles + Anticonvulsants', p.136.

Mechanism

It has been suggested that fluconazole inhibits the cytochrome P450 isoenzymes responsible for phenytoin metabolism (CYP2C9 or CYP2C10).[2] Voriconazole and possibly miconazole probably act similarly, but ketoconazole and itraconazole do not. Phenytoin is an enzyme inducer, and appears to induce the metabolism of these azoles to varying degrees.

Importance and management

The increase in serum phenytoin levels with fluconazole is established and clinically important. Toxicity can develop within 2 to 7 days unless the phenytoin dosage is reduced. Monitor serum phenytoin levels closely and reduce the dosage appropriately. Also be alert for any evidence of reduced fluconazole effects. Evidence for increased phenytoin levels with miconazole is limited, even so it would be prudent to monitor serum phenytoin levels.

Ketoconazole and itraconazole probably do not have an important effect on phenytoin levels, but levels of these antifungals may be markedly reduced. An important interaction occurs between 'voriconazole and phenytoin', (p.136).

1. Blum RA, Wilton JH, Hilligoss DM, Gardner MJ, Henry EB, Harrison NJ, Schentag JJ. Effect of fluconazole on the disposition of phenytoin. *Clin Pharmacol Ther* (1991) 49, 420–5.
2. Touchette MA, Chandrasekar PH, Millad MA, Edwards DJ. Contrasting effects of fluconazole and ketoconazole on phenytoin and testosterone disposition in man. *Br J Clin Pharmacol* (1992) 34, 75–8.
3. Lazar JD, Wilner KD. Drug interactions with fluconazole. *Rev Infect Dis* (1990) 12 (Suppl 3), S327–S333.
4. Mitchell AS, Holland JT. Fluconazole and phenytoin: a predictable interaction. *BMJ* (1989) 298, 1315.
5. Howitt KM, Oziemski MA. Phenytoin toxicity induced by fluconazole. *Med J Aust* (1989) 151, 603–4.
6. Sugar AM. Quoted as Personal Communication by Grant SM, Clissold SP. Fluconazole. A review of its pharmacodynamic and pharmacokinetic properties, and therapeutic potential in superficial and system mycoses. *Drugs* (1990) 39, 877–916.
7. Cadle RM, Zenon GJ, Rodriguez-Barradas MC, Hamill RJ. Fluconazole-induced symptomatic phenytoin toxicity. *Ann Pharmacother* (1994) 28, 191–5.
8. Tett S, Carey D, Lee H-S. Drug interactions with fluconazole. *Med J Aust* (1992) 156, 365.
9. Rolan PE, Somogyi AA, Drew MJR, Cobain WG, South D, Bochner F. Phenytoin intoxication during treatment with parenteral miconazole. *BMJ* (1983) 287, 1760.
10. Loupi E, Descotes J, Lery N, Evreux JC. Interactions medicamenteuses et miconazole. A propos de 10 observations. *Therapie* (1982) 37, 437–41.

Phenytoin + Carbamazepine

Some reports describe rises in serum phenytoin levels, with toxicity, whereas others describe falls in phenytoin levels. Genetic polymorphism may be an explanation for the differences. Falls in carbamazepine serum levels, sometimes with rises in carbamazepine epoxide levels, have been described.

Clinical evidence

(a) Reduced serum phenytoin levels

Carbamazepine 600 mg daily for 4 to 14 days reduced the serum phenytoin levels of 3 out of 7 patients from 15 to 7 micrograms/ml, 18 to 12 micrograms/ml and 16 to 10 micrograms/ml respectively. Phenytoin serum levels rose again 10 days after withdrawal of the carbamazepine.[1]

Reduced serum phenytoin levels in patients given carbamazepine have been described in other reports.[2-5]

(b) Raised serum phenytoin levels

A study in 6 epileptics treated with phenytoin 350 to 600 mg daily found that the addition of carbamazepine 600 to 800 mg daily increased the phenytoin serum levels by 35%, increased its half-life by 41% and reduced its clearance by 36.5% over a 12-week period. Neurotoxicity increased by 204%, with additional symptoms of toxicity (sedation, ataxia, nystagmus, etc.) developing in 5 of the 6 patients. The phenytoin dosage remained unchanged throughout the period of the study.[6]

Other reports have also described increases in serum phenytoin levels,[7-12] which were as large as 81%, and even up to 100% in some cases.[8,10]

(c) Reduced serum carbamazepine levels

A series of multiple regression analyses on data from a large number of patients [the precise number is not clear from the report], showed that phenytoin reduced serum carbamazepine on average by 0.9 micrograms/ml for each 2 mg/kg of phenytoin taken each day.[7]

Reduced serum carbamazepine levels have been described in other studies and reports.[3,11,13-16] Two studies found that phenytoin markedly increased the levels of the active metabolite of carbamazepine, carbamazepine-10,11-epoxide.[17,18]

Mechanism

Not understood. Both carbamazepine and phenytoin are enzyme inducers, and might therefore be expected to decrease the metabolism of each other. However, more recently it has been shown that carbamazepine can inhibit the cytochrome P450 isoenzyme CYP2C19, which is one of the enzymes involved in phenytoin metabolism.[19] Carbamazepine might therefore cause increases in phenytoin levels by this mechanism. Moreover, CYP2C19 shows genetic polymorphism (see 'Genetic factors', (p.4)), so an interaction via this mechanism would not occur in all patients.

Importance and management

Phenytoin may decrease carbamazepine levels, but carbamazepine has variable effects on phenytoin levels, with both increases and decreases described. Monitor anticonvulsant levels during concurrent use (where possible including the active metabolite of carbamazepine, carbamazepine-epoxide) so that steps can be taken to avoid the development of toxicity or lack of efficacy. Not all patients appear to have an adverse interaction, and, at present, it does not seem possible to identify those potentially at risk. The risk of carbamazepine-induced water intoxication is reported to be reduced in patients concurrently taking phenytoin.[14]

1. Hansen JM, Siersbæk-Nielsen K, Skovsted L. Carbamazepine-induced acceleration of diphenylhydantoin and warfarin metabolism in man. *Clin Pharmacol Ther* (1971) 12, 539–43.
2. Cereghino JJ, Van Meter JC, Brock JT, Penry JK, Smith LD, White BG. Preliminary observations of serum carbamazepine concentration in epileptic patients. *Neurology* (1973) 23, 357–66.
3. Hooper WD, Dubetz DK, Eadie MJ, Tyrer JH. Preliminary observations on the clinical pharmacology of carbamazepine ('Tegretol'). *Proc Aust Assoc Neurol* (1974) 11, 189–98.
4. Lai M-L, Lin T-S, Huang JD. Effect of single- and multiple-dose carbamazepine on the pharmacokinetics of diphenylhydantoin. *Eur J Clin Pharmacol* (1992) 43, 201–3.
5. Windorfer A, Sauer W. Drug interactions during anticonvulsant therapy in childhood: diphenylhydantoin, primidone, phenobarbitone, clonazepam, nitrazepam, carbamazepin and dipropylacetate. *Neuropadiatrie* (1977) 8, 29–41.
6. Browne TR, Szabo GK, Evans JE, Evans BA, Greenblatt DJ, Mikati MA. Carbamazepine increases phenytoin serum concentration and reduces phenytoin clearance. *Neurology* (1988) 38, 1146–50.
7. Lander CM, Eadie MJ, Tyrer JH. Interactions between anticonvulsants. *Proc Aust Assoc Neurol* (1975) 12, 111–16.
8. Gratz ES, Theodore WH, Newmark ME, Kupferberg HJ, Porter RJ, Qu Z. Effect of carbamazepine on phenytoin clearance in patients with complex partial seizures. *Neurology* (1982) 32, A223.
9. Leppik IE, Pepin SM, Jacobi J, Miller KW. Effect of carbamazepine on the Michaelis-Menten parameters of phenytoin. In Metabolism of Antiepileptic Drugs (ed Levy RH et al) Raven Press, New York. *(1984) pp 217–22.* (1984) pp 217–22.
10. Zielinski JJ, Haidukewych D, Leheta BJ. Carbamazepine-phenytoin interaction: elevation of plasma phenytoin concentrations due to carbamazepine comedication. *Ther Drug Monit* (1985) 7, 51–3.
11. Hidano F, Obata N, Yahaba Y, Unno K, Fukui R. Drug interactions with phenytoin and carbamazepine. *Folia Psychiatr Neurol Jpn* (1983) 37, 342–4.
12. Zielinski JJ, Haidukewych D. Dual effects of carbamazepine-phenytoin interaction. *Ther Drug Monit* (1987) 9, 21–3.
13. Cereghino JJ, Brock JT, Van Meter JC, Penry JK, Smith LD, White BG. The efficacy of carbamazepine combinations in epilepsy. *Clin Pharmacol Ther* (1975) 18, 733–41.
14. Perucca E, Richens A. Reversal by phenytoin of carbamazepine-induced water intoxication: a pharmacokinetic interaction. *J Neurol Neurosurg Psychiatry* (1980) 43, 540–5.
15. Ramsay RE, McManus DQ, Guterman A, Briggle TV, Vazquez D, Perchalski R, Yost RA, Wong P. Carbamazepine metabolism in humans: effect of concurrent anticonvulsant therapy. *Ther Drug Monit* (1990) 12, 235–41.
16. Chapron DJ, LaPierre BA, Abou-Elkair M. Unmasking the significant enzyme-inducing effects of phenytoin on serum carbamazepine concentrations during phenytoin withdrawal. *Ann Pharmacother* (1993) 27, 708–11.
17. Hagiwara M, Takahashi R, Watabe M, Amanuma I, Kan R, Takahashi Y, Kumashiro H. Influence of phenytoin on metabolism of carbamazepine. *Neurosciences* (1989) 15, 303–9.
18. Dam M, Jensen A, Christiansen J. Plasma level and effect of carbamazepine in grand mal and psychomotor epilepsy. *Acta Neurol Scand* (1975) 75 (Suppl 51), 33–8.
19. Lakehal F, Wurden CJ, Kalhorn TF, Levy RH. Carbamazepine and oxcarbazepine decrease phenytoin metabolism through inhibition of CYP2C19. *Epilepsy Res* (2002) 52, 79–83.

Phenytoin + Chloramphenicol

Serum phenytoin levels can be raised by intravenous chloramphenicol and phenytoin toxicity may occur. Other evidence indicates that phenytoin may increase or decrease serum chloramphenicol levels in children.

Clinical evidence

(a) Serum phenytoin levels increased

A man on phenytoin 100 mg four times daily developed signs of toxicity within a week of also receiving intravenous chloramphenicol 1 g every 6 hours for 4 doses then 2 g every 6 hours. His serum phenytoin levels had risen by about threefold, from about 7 to 24 micrograms/ml.[1]

This interaction has been described in a number of other reports.[2-10] One study found that intravenous chloramphenicol more than doubled the half-life of phenytoin.[2] The AUC of phenytoin after a single intravenous dose of fosphenytoin was 23% higher (not significant) in children also given intravenous chloramphenicol when compared with those given intravenous cefotaxime. In addition, the phenytoin half-life was significantly prolonged by chloramphenicol (23.7 hours versus 15.5 hours).[11]

(b) Serum chloramphenicol levels reduced or increased

A child on a 6-week course of intravenous chloramphenicol 100 mg/kg daily in four divided doses had a reduction in peak and trough serum levels of 46 and 74% respectively within 2 days of beginning additional treatment with phenytoin 4 mg/kg daily. Levels were further reduced by 63 and 87% respectively by the addition of phenobarbital 4 mg/kg daily.[12] See also 'Chloramphenicol + Phenobarbital', p.206).

In contrast, 6 children (aged 1 month to 12 years) developed raised, toxic chloramphenicol levels while receiving phenytoin.[13]

Mechanism

It seems probable that chloramphenicol, a known enzyme inhibitor,[14] affects the liver enzymes concerned with the metabolism of phenytoin thereby reducing its rate of clearance from the body. The changes in the pharmacokinetics of chloramphenicol in children are not understood.

Importance and management

The rise in serum phenytoin levels with intravenous chloramphenicol in adults is well documented and clinically important. A two to fourfold rise can occur within a few days of starting concurrent treatment. Concurrent use should be avoided unless the effects can be closely monitored and appropriate phenytoin dosage reductions made as necessary. The use of a single prophylactic dose of phenytoin or fosphenytoin may be an exception to this.[11] It seems very doubtful if enough chloramphenicol is absorbed from eye drops or ointments for an interaction to occur, but this needs confirmation.

The general clinical importance of the changes in serum chloramphenicol-col levels in children is uncertain, but the effects of concurrent use should certainly be monitored. More study is needed.

1. Ballek RE, Reidenberg MM, Orr L. Inhibition of diphenylhydantoin metabolism by chloramphenicol. *Lancet* (1973) i, 150.
2. Christensen LK, Skovsted L. Inhibition of drug metabolism by chloramphenicol. *Lancet* (1969) ii, 1397–9.
3. Houghton GW, Richens A. Inhibition of phenytoin metabolism by other drugs used in epilepsy. *Int J Clin Pharmacol Biopharm* (1975) 12, 210–16.
4. Rose JQ, Choi HK, Schentag JJ, Kinkel WR, Jusko WJ. Intoxication caused by interaction of chloramphenicol and phenytoin. *JAMA* (1977) 237, 2630–1.
5. Koup JR, Gibaldi M, McNamara P, Hilligoss DM, Colburn WA, Bruck E. Interaction of chloramphenicol with phenytoin and phenobarbital. *Clin Pharmacol Ther* (1978) 24, 571–5.
6. Vincent FM, Mills L, Sullivan JK. Chloramphenicol-induced phenytoin intoxication. *Ann Neurol* (1978) 3, 469.
7. Harper JM, Yost RL, Stewart RB, Ciezkowski J. Phenytoin-chloramphenicol interaction. *Drug Intell Clin Pharm* (1979) 13, 425–9.
8. Greenlaw CW. Chloramphenicol-phenytoin drug interaction. *Drug Intell Clin Pharm* (1979) 13, 609–10.
9. Saltiel M, Stephens NM. Phenytoin-chloramphenicol interaction. *Drug Intell Clin Pharm* (1980) 14, 221.
10. Cosh DG, Rowett DS, Lee PC, McCarthy PJ. Case report — phenytoin therapy complicated by concurrent chloramphenicol and enteral nutrition. *Aust J Hosp Pharm* (1987) 17, 51–3.
11. Ogutu BR, Newton CRJC, Muchohi SN, Otieno GO, Kokwaro GO. Phenytoin pharmacokinetics and clinical effects in African children following fosphenytoin and chloramphenicol coadministration. *Br J Clin Pharmacol* (2002) 54, 635–42.
12. Powell DA, Nahata M, Durrell DC, Glazer JP and Hilty MD. Interactions among chloramphenicol, phenytoin and phenobarbitone in a pediatric patient. *J Pediatr* (1981) 98, 1001.
13. Krasinski K, Kusmiesz H, Nelson JD. Pharmacologic interactions among chloramphenicol, phenytoin and phenobarbital. *Pediatr Infect Dis* (1982) 1, 232–5.
14. Dixon RL, Fouts JR. Inhibition of microsomal drug metabolism pathway by chloramphenicol. *Biochem Pharmacol* (1962) 11, 715–20.

Phenytoin + Chlorphenamine

Phenytoin toxicity in two patients has been attributed to the concurrent use of chlorphenamine.

Clinical evidence, mechanism, importance and management

A week or so after starting to take chlorphenamine 4 mg three times daily, a woman on phenytoin and phenobarbital developed phenytoin toxicity with serum phenytoin levels of about 65 micrograms/ml. The toxic symptoms disappeared and phenytoin levels fell when the chlorphenamine was withdrawn.[1] Another woman on anticonvulsants, including phenytoin, developed slight grimacing of the face and involuntary jaw movements (but no speech slurring, ataxia or nystagmus) within 12 days of starting to take chlorphenamine 12 to 16 mg daily. Her serum phenytoin level had risen to 30 micrograms/ml but it fell when the chlorphenamine was withdrawn.[2]

The reason for these reactions is not clear but it has been suggested that chlorphenamine may have inhibited the metabolism of phenytoin by the liver. These are isolated cases, and their general relevance is uncertain.

1. Pugh RNH, Geddes AM, Yeoman WB. Interaction of phenytoin with chlorpheniramine. *Br J Clin Pharmacol* (1975) 2, 173–5.
2. Ahmad S, Laidlaw J, Houghton GW, Richens A. Involuntary movements caused by phenytoin intoxication in epileptic patients. *J Neurol Neurosurg Psychiatry* (1975) 38, 225–31.

Phenytoin + Colestyramine or Colestipol

Neither colestyramine nor colestipol affect the absorption of phenytoin from the gut.

Clinical evidence, mechanism, importance and management

Neither colestyramine 5 g nor colestipol 10 g had a significant effect on the absorption of a single 500-mg dose of phenytoin in 6 healthy subjects. The resins were given 2 minutes before and 6 and 12 hours after the phenytoin.[1] Another study in 6 healthy subjects found that colestyramine 4 g four times daily for 5 days had no significant effect on the extent of the absorption of a single 400-mg dose of phenytoin (given on day 3, two minutes after the colestyramine).[2] No special precautions would seem to be necessary if either of these drugs and phenytoin is taken concurrently.

1. Callaghan JT, Tsuru M, Holtzman JL, Hunninghshake DB. Effect of cholestyramine and colestipol on the absorption of phenytoin. *Eur J Clin Pharmacol* (1983) 24, 675–8.
2. Barzaghi N, Monteleone M, Amione C, Lecchini S, Perucca E, Frigo GM. Lack of effect of cholestyramine on phenytoin bioavailability. *J Clin Pharmacol* (1988) 28, 1112–14.

Phenytoin + Diazoxide

Three children and one adult had very marked reductions in serum phenytoin levels when diazoxide was given, and in one case seizure control was lost. There is some evidence that the effects of diazoxide may also be reduced.

Clinical evidence

A child receiving phenytoin 29 mg/kg daily and an adult receiving phenytoin 1 g daily were unable to achieve therapeutic phenytoin serum levels when given diazoxide. When the diazoxide was withdrawn, satisfactory serum phenytoin levels were achieved with dosages of only 6.6 mg/kg and 400 mg daily respectively. When diazoxide was restarted experimentally in the adult, the serum phenytoin was reduced over 4 days to undetectable levels, and seizures occurred.[1] Two other reports describe this interaction.[2,3] In addition it appears that the effects of the diazoxide can also be reduced.[2,4]

Mechanism

What is known suggests that diazoxide increases the metabolism and the clearance of phenytoin from the body.[1,2] The half-life of diazoxide is possibly reduced by phenytoin.[4]

Importance and management

Information is limited to these reports, but the interaction would appear to be established. Monitor the effects of concurrent use, being alert for the need to increase the phenytoin dosage. The clinical importance of the reduced diazoxide effects is uncertain.

1. Roe TF, Podosin RL, Blaskovics ME. Drug Interaction: diazoxide and diphenylhydantoin. *J Pediatr* (1975) 87, 480–4.
2. Petro DJ, Vannucci RC, Kulin HE. Diazoxide-diphenylhydantoin interaction. *J Pediatr* (1976) 89, 331–2.
3. Turck D, Largilliere C, Dupuis B, Farriaux JP. Interaction entre le diazoxide et la phénytoïne. *Presse Med* (1986) 15, 31.
4. Pruitt AW, Dayton PG, Patterson JH. Disposition of diazoxide in children. *Clin Pharmacol Ther* (1973) 14, 73–82.

Phenytoin + Dichloralphenazone

There is some evidence that serum phenytoin levels may be reduced by dichloralphenazone.

Clinical evidence, mechanism, importance and management

After taking dichloralphenazone 1.3 g each night for 13 nights the total body clearance of a single intravenous dose of phenytoin was doubled in 5 healthy subjects.[1] The phenazone component of dichloralphenazone is a known enzyme-inducer and the increased clearance of phenytoin is probably due to an enhancement of its metabolism by the liver. There seem to be no additional reports of adverse effects in patients given both drugs, so that the clinical importance of this interaction is uncertain. However, it would seem prudent to watch for a reduction in serum phenytoin levels if dichloralphenazone is added to established treatment with phenytoin.

1. Riddell JG, Salem SAM, McDevitt DG. Interaction between phenytoin and dichloralphenazone. *Br J Clin Pharmacol* (1980) 9, 118P.

Phenytoin + Felbamate

Felbamate causes a moderate increase in serum phenytoin levels, which may require 20 to 40% reductions in dose. Felbamate serum levels are reduced, but the importance of this is uncertain.

Clinical evidence

A pilot study in 4 patients noted that felbamate increased serum phenytoin levels.[1] Therefore, in a further study the phenytoin dose was automatically reduced by 20% when felbamate was given. Of 5 patients, one needed a slight increase in phenytoin dosage, whereas 2 others needed a further reduction in their phenytoin dosage.[2] In a later full report of this study, it was noted that phenytoin dosage decreases of 10 to 30% were required to maintain stable levels.[3] Another study in epileptic patients found that felbamate 1.2 g or 1.8 g daily increased the maximum serum phenytoin levels by 31% and 69%, respectively. Higher felbamate doses necessitated phenytoin dose reductions of 20 to 40%.[4]

Studies in children and adults have found that phenytoin increased the clearance of felbamate by about 40%,[5,6] and decreased maximum felbamate levels by 56 to 60% when compared with patients receiving monotherapy.[4] Another report says that felbamate clearance is reduced if the dosage of phenytoin is reduced.[7]

Mechanism

Uncertain but felbamate probably acts as a competitive inhibitor of phenytoin metabolism, thereby reducing its loss from the body and increasing its serum levels,[2,8] whereas phenytoin induces felbamate metabolism, thereby increasing its clearance.[7]

Importance and management

Established interactions. The phenytoin dosage may need to be reduced (a 20 to 40% reduction seems to be about right[2,4,8]) if felbamate is added, and to increase it if felbamate is withdrawn. The importance of the reduced felbamate levels is uncertain, but is probably less important because felbamate has a wide therapeutic range.[4]

1. Sheridan PH, Ashworth M, Milne K, White BG, Santilli N, Lothman EW, Dreifuss FE, Jacobs MP, Martinez P, Leppik IE. Open pilot study of felbamate (ADD 03055) in partial seizures. *Epilepsia* (1986) 27, 649.
2. Fuerst RH, Graves NM, Leppik IE, Remmel RP, Rosenfeld WE, Sierzant TL. A preliminary report on alteration of carbamazepine and phenytoin metabolism by felbamate. *Drug Intell Clin Pharm* (1986) 20, 465–6.
3. Leppik IE, Dreifuss FE, Pledger GW, Graves NM, Santilli N, Drury I, Tsay JY, Jacobs MP, Bertram E, Cereghino JJ, Cooper G, Sahlroot JT, Sheridan P, Ashworth M, Lee SI, Sierzant TL. Felbamate for partial seizures: results of a controlled clinical trial. *Neurology* (1991) 41, 1785–9.
4. Sachdeo R, Wagner M, Sachdeo S, Schumaker RC, Lyness WH, Rosenberg A, Ward D, Perhach JL. Coadministration of phenytoin and felbamate: evidence of additional phenytoin dose-reduction requirements based on pharmacokinetics and tolerability with increasing doses of felbamate. *Epilepsia* (1999) 40, 1122–8.
5. Kelley MT, Walson PD, Cox S, Dusci LJ. Population pharmacokinetics of felbamate in children. *Ther Drug Monit* (1997) 19, 29–36.
6. Banfield CR, Zhu G-RR, Jen JF, Jensen PK, Schumaker RC, Perhach JL Affrime MB, Glue P. The effect of age on the apparent clearance of felbamate: a retrospective analysis using nonlinear mixed-effects modeling. *Ther Drug Monit* (1996) 18, 19–29.
7. Wagner ML, Graves NM, Marienau K, Holmes GB, Remmel RP, Leppik IE. Discontinuation of phenytoin and carbamazepine in patients receiving felbamate. *Epilepsia* (1991) 32, 398–406.
8. Fuerst RH, Graves NM, Leppik IE, Brundage RC, Holmes GB, Remmel RP. Felbamate increases phenytoin but decreases carbamazepine concentrations. *Epilepsia* (1988) 29, 488–91.

Phenytoin + Food

The absorption of phenytoin can be affected by some foods. A very marked reduction in phenytoin absorption has been described when it was given with enteral feeds (e.g. *Isocal*, *Osmolite*), by nasogastric or jejunostomy tubes.

Clinical evidence

(a) Food by mouth

A study found that serum drug levels were lower than expected when phenytoin was disguised in **vanilla pudding** and given to mentally retarded children. However, when the phenytoin was mixed with **apple sauce**, 3 out of 10 patients developed serum phenytoin levels within the toxic range, and the mean levels were twice those seen when the tablets were mixed with the **vanilla pudding**.[1] An epileptic had a marked fall in his serum phenytoin levels accompanied by an increased seizure frequency when phenytoin was given at bedtime with 8 oz of a food supplement (***Ensure***).[2] Another patient had reduced phenytoin serum levels when phenytoin was given as an oral suspension with oral ***Fresubin liquid food concentrate***.[3] However, in contrast, a study in 10 healthy subjects found that when ***Ensure*** or ***Vivonex TEN*** was given every 4 hours for 24 hours, the absorption of a single 400-mg dose of phenytoin was unaffected.[4] The absorption of phenytoin as the acid in a micronised form (*Fenantoin*, ACO, Sweden) was faster and the peak serum levels were on average 40% higher when it was given after food.[5] One single dose study found that, when taken with a meal, the total absorption of phenytoin was not affected, although it was slightly delayed.[6]

(b) Food by nasogastric tube

A patient on phenytoin 300 mg daily who was being fed with ***Fortison*** through a nasogastric tube had a phenytoin serum level of only 1 mg/l. When phenytoin 420 mg was given diluted in water and separated from the food by 2 hours, a serum level of 6 mg/l was achieved.[7] This report describes a similar reaction in another patient.[7]

A study in 20 patients and 5 healthy subjects found that phenytoin absorption was reduced by about 70% when it was given by nasogastric tube with an **enteral feed** product (***Isocal***) at a rate of 100 to 125 ml/hour.[8] Other reports describe the same interaction in patients given ***Ensure***,[9] ***Isocal***,[10,11] or ***Osmolite***.[9,12-14]

(c) Food by jejunostomy tube

A woman with a history of seizures had acceptable serum phenytoin levels when phenytoin was given intravenously, but they fell from 19.1 micrograms/ml to less than 2.5 micrograms/ml when a comparable dose of phenytoin suspension was given in the presence of an **enteral feed** product (***Jevity***), administered by jejunostomy tube.[15]

Mechanism

Not fully resolved. Phenytoin can bind to some food substances, which reduces its absorption.[16,17] It can also become bound to the nasogastric tubing[18] and may also be poorly absorbed if the tubing empties into the duodenum rather than the stomach.[18] Delivery into the jejunum apparently makes matters even worse, because there is even less time for adequate absorption.[15]

Importance and management

Phenytoin is often taken orally with water or food to reduce gastric irritation. This normally appears not to have a marked effect on absorption, but the studies cited above show that some formulations and some foods can interact. If there are problems with the control of convulsions or evidence of toxicity, review how and when the patient is taking the phenytoin.

The interaction between phenytoin and enteral feeds given by nasogastric tube is well established and clinically important. The markedly reduced bioavailability has been successfully managed by giving the phenytoin diluted in water 2 hours after stopping the feed, flushing with 60 ml of water, and waiting another 2 hours before restarting the feed.[7,8] However, one limited study failed to confirm that this method is successful,[9] and some sources suggest waiting 6 hours after the phenytoin dose before restarting the feed.[10] Some increase in the phenytoin dosage may also be needed. Monitor concurrent use closely. The same problem can clearly also occur when enteral feeds are given by the jejunostomy tube but methods to manage this are not yet established.

1. Jann MW, Bean J, Fidone G. Interaction of dietary pudding with phenytoin. *Pediatrics* (1986) 78, 952–3.
2. Longe RL, Smith OB. Phenytoin interaction with an oral feeding results in loss of seizure control. *J Am Geriatr Soc* (1988) 36, 542–4.
3. Taylor DM, Massey CA, Willson WG, Dhillon S. Lowered serum phenytoin concentrations during therapy with liquid food concentrates. *Ann Pharmacother* (1993) 27, 369.
4. Marvel ME, Bertino JS. Comparative effects of an elemental and a complex enteral feeding formulation on the absorption of phenytoin suspension. *J Parenter Enteral Nutr* (1991) 15, 316–8.
5. Melander A, Brante G, Johansson Ö, Lindberg T, Wåhlin-Boll E. Influence of food on the absorption of phenytoin in man. *Eur J Clin Pharmacol* (1979) 15, 269–74.
6. Kennedy MC, Wade DN. The effect of food on the absorption of phenytoin. *Aust N Z J Med* (1982) 12, 258–61.
7. Summers VM, Grant R. Nasogastric feeding and phenytoin interaction. *Pharm J* (1989) 243, 181.
8. Bauer LA. Interference of oral phenytoin absorption by continuous nasogastric feedings. *Neurology* (1982) 32, 570–2.
9. Ozuna J, Friel P. Effect of enteral tube feeding on serum phenytoin levels. *J Neurosurg Nurs* (1984) 16, 289–91.
10. Pearce GA. Apparent inhibition of phenytoin absorption by an enteral nutrient formula. *Aust J Hosp Pharm* (1988) 18, 289–92.
11. Worden JP, Wood CA, Workman CH. Phenytoin and nasogastric feedings. *Neurology* (1984) 34, 132.
12. Hatton RC. Dietary interaction with phenytoin. *Clin Pharm* (1984) 3, 110–11.
13. Weinryb J, Cogen R. Interaction of nasogastric phenytoin and enteral feeding solution. *J Am Geriatr Soc* (1989) 37, 195–6.
14. Maynard GA, Jones KM, Guidry JR. Phenytoin absorption from tube feedings. *Arch Intern Med* (1987) 147, 1821.
15. Rodman DP, Stevenson TL, Ray TR. Phenytoin malabsorption after jejunostomy tube delivery. *Pharmacotherapy* (1995) 15, 801–5.
16. Millar SW, Strom JG. Stability of phenytoin in three enteral nutrient formulas. *Am J Hosp Pharm* (1988) 45, 2529–32.
17. Hooks MA, Longe RL, Taylor AT, Francisco GE. Recovery of phenytoin from an enteral nutrient formula. *Am J Hosp Pharm* (1986) 43, 685–8.
18. Fleisher D, Sheth N, Kou JH. Phenytoin interaction with enteral feedings administered through nasogastric tubes. *J Parenter Enteral Nutr* (1990) 14, 513–16.

Phenytoin + H_2-blockers

Phenytoin serum levels are raised by the use of cimetidine and toxicity has occurred. Limited evidence suggests that low (non-prescription) doses of cimetidine may not interact. Very rarely bone marrow depression develops on concurrent use. Famotidine, nizatidine and ranitidine do not normally interact with phenytoin but they appear to do so on rare occasions.

Clinical evidence

(a) Cimetidine

A 60% rise (from 5.7 to 9.1 micrograms/ml) was seen in the serum phenytoin levels of 9 patients when they were given cimetidine 200 mg three times daily and 400 mg at night for 3 weeks. The serum phenytoin level returned to its former levels within 2 weeks of stopping the cimetidine.[1]

This interaction has been described in many reports and studies involving patients[2-7] and healthy subjects.[8-11] Phenytoin toxicity has developed in some individuals. The extent of the rise in serum levels is very variable being quoted as 13 to 33% over about 6 days in one report[2] and 22 to 280% over 3 weeks in another.[4,12] There is some evidence that the effect may be dependent on cimetidine dose. One study found that the effect of cimetidine 2.4 g daily was greater than that of 1.2 g daily or 400 mg daily, which did not differ from each other.[9] In another study, the maximum non-prescription dose of cimetidine (200 mg twice daily for 2 weeks) had no effect on serum phenytoin levels in 9 patients stabilised on phenytoin.[13]

Severe and life-threatening agranulocytosis in 2 patients[14,15] and thrombocytopenia in 6 others[16-18] have been attributed to the concurrent use of phenytoin and cimetidine. Severe skin reactions have also been reported in 3 patients treated with phenytoin, cimetidine (with ranitidine as well in one), and dexamethasone after resection of brain tumours, which resolved on discontinuing phenytoin.[19] See also 'Corticosteroids + Phenytoin', p.808.

(b) Famotidine

A study in 10 subjects found that famotidine 40 mg daily for 7 days did not alter the pharmacokinetics of a single dose of phenytoin.[20] However, a single case report describes phenytoin toxicity and an almost doubled serum level (increase from 18 to 33 micrograms/ml) in a patient also given famotidine. This was managed by a reduction in the phenytoin dose.[21]

(c) Nizatidine

Nizatidine 150 mg twice daily for 9 doses had no effects on the pharmacokinetics of a single dose of phenytoin in 18 healthy subjects.[22]

(d) Ranitidine

A study in 4 patients found that ranitidine 150 mg twice daily for 2 weeks did not alter phenytoin levels.[4,12] Similarly, a double-blind crossover study in healthy subjects found that ranitidine 150 mg twice daily for 6 days had no significant effect on the steady state phenytoin levels.[23] However, one patient had a 40% increase in serum phenytoin levels over a month when ranitidine 150 mg twice daily was given,[24] and another also developed elevated serum phenytoin levels and signs of toxicity, which were attributed to the use of ranitidine.[25] Another patient developed a severe skin reaction when treated with phenytoin, ranitidine and dexamethasone after resection of a brain tumour, which resolved on discontinuing phenytoin.[19]

Mechanism

Cimetidine inhibits the activity of the liver enzymes concerned with the metabolism of phenytoin, thus allowing it to accumulate in the body and, in some instances, to reach toxic concentrations. Famotidine, nizatidine and ranitidine normally do not affect these enzymes. Agranulocytosis and thrombocytopenia are relatively rare manifestations of bone marrow depression caused by both phenytoin and the H_2-blockers.

Importance and management

The interaction between phenytoin and cimetidine is well documented and clinically important. It is not possible to identify individuals who will show the greatest response, but those with serum levels at the top end of the therapeutic range are most at risk. Do not give cimetidine to patients already taking phenytoin unless the serum levels can be monitored and suitable dosage reductions made as necessary. The results from one small study suggest that non-prescription doses of cimetidine may not interact.[13] Since there are only rare cases cited for famotidine, nizatidine, and ranitidine extra monitoring beyond that usually carried out in patients receiving phenytoin does not appear to be warranted but be alert for signs of phenytoin toxicity when these H_2-blockers are first added to established treatment with phenytoin.

1. Neuvonen PJ, Tokola R, Kaste M. Cimetidine-phenytoin interaction: effect on serum phenytoin concentration and antipyrine test. *Eur J Clin Pharmacol* (1981) 21, 215–20.
2. Hetzel DJ, Bochner F, Hallpike JF, Shearman DJC, Hann CS. Cimetidine interaction with phenytoin. *BMJ* (1981) 282, 1512.
3. Algozzine GJ, Stewart RB, Springer PK. Decreased clearance of phenytoin with cimetidine. *Ann Intern Med* (1981) 95, 244–5.
4. Watts RW, Hetzel DJ, Bochner F, Hallpike JF, Hann CS, Shearman DJC. Lack of interaction between ranitidine and phenytoin. *Br J Clin Pharmacol* (1983) 15, 499–500.
5. Phillips P, Hansky J. Phenytoin toxicity secondary to cimetidine administration. *Med J Aust* (1984) 141, 602.
6. Griffin JW, May JR, DiPiro JT. Drug interactions: theory versus practice. *Am J Med* (1984) 77 (Suppl 5B), 85–9.
7. Salem RB, Breland BD, Mishra SK, Jordan JE. Effect of cimetidine on phenytoin serum levels. *Epilepsia* (1983) 24, 284–8.
8. Iteogu MO, Murphy JE, Shleifer N, Davis R. Effect of cimetidine on single-dose phenytoin kinetics. *Clin Pharm* (1983) 2, 302–4.
9. Bartle WR, Walker SE, Shapero T. Dose-dependent effect of cimetidine on phenytoin kinetics. *Clin Pharmacol Ther* (1983) 33, 649–55.
10. Frigo GM, Lecchini S, Caravaggi M, Gatti G, Tonini M, D'Angelo L, Perucca E, Crema A. Reduction of phenytoin clearance caused by cimetidine. *Eur J Clin Pharmacol* (1983) 25, 135–7.
11. Hsieh Y-Y, Huang J-D, Lai M-L, Lin M-S, Liu R-T, Wan EC-J. The complexity of cimetidine-phenytoin interaction. *Taiwan Yi Xue Hui Za Zhi* (1986) 85, 395–402.
12. Hetzel DJ, Watts RW, Bochner F, Shearman DJC. Ranitidine, unlike cimetidine, does not interact with phenytoin. *Aust N Z J Med* (1983) 13, 324.
13. Rafi JA, Frazier LM, Driscoll-Bannister SM, O'Hara KA, Garnett WR, Pugh CB. Effect of over-the-counter cimetidine on phenytoin concentrations in patients with seizures. *Ann Pharmacother* (1999) 33, 769–74.
14. Sazie E, Jaffe JP. Severe granulocytopenia with cimetidine and phenytoin. *Ann Intern Med* (1980) 93, 151–2.
15. Al-Kawas FH, Lenes BA, Sacher RA. Cimetidine and agranulocytosis. *Ann Intern Med* (1979) 90, 992–3.
16. Wong YY, Lichtor T, Brown FD. Severe thrombocytopenia associated with phenytoin and cimetidine therapy. *Surg Neurol* (1985) 23, 169–72.
17. Yue CP, Mann KS, Chan KH. Severe thrombocytopenia due to combined cimetidine and phenytoin therapy. *Neurosurgery* (1987) 20, 963–5.
18. Arbiser JL, Goldstein AM, Gordon D. Thrombocytopenia following administration of phenytoin, dexamethasone and cimetidine: a case report and a potential mechanism. *J Intern Med* (1993) 234, 91–4.
19. Cohen AD, Reichental E, Halevy S. Phenytoin-induced severe cutaneous drug reactions: suspected interactions with corticosteroids and H2-blockers. *Isr Med Assoc J* (1999) 1, 95–7.
20. Sambol NC, Upton RA, Chremos AN, Lin ET, Williams RL. A comparison of the influence of famotidine and cimetidine on phenytoin elimination and hepatic blood flow. *Br J Clin Pharmacol* (1989) 27, 83–7.
21. Shinn AF. Unrecognized drug interactions with famotidine and nizatidine. *Arch Intern Med* (1991) 151, 810,814.
22. Bachmann KA, Sullivan TJ, Jauregui L, Reese JH, Miller K, Levine L. Absence of an inhibitory effect of omeprazole and nizatidine on phenytoin disposition, a marker of CYP2C activity. *Br J Clin Pharmacol* (1993) 36, 380–2.
23. Mukherjee S, Wicks JFC, Dixon JS, Richens A. Absence of a pharmacokinetic interaction between ranitidine and phenytoin. *Gastroenterology* (1996) 110 (Suppl), A202.
24. Bramhall D, Levine M. Possible interaction of ranitidine with phenytoin. *Drug Intell Clin Pharm* (1988) 22, 979–80.
25. Ted Tse CS, Akinwande KI, Biallowons K. Phenytoin concentration elevation subsequent to ranitidine administration. *Ann Pharmacother* (1993) 27, 1448–51.

Phenytoin + Immunoglobulins

An isolated report describes an epileptic patient on phenytoin who died, probably from hypersensitivity myocarditis, two days after receiving immunoglobulins for Guillain-Barré syndrome.

Clinical evidence, mechanism, importance and management

A man who had been taking phenytoin for 8 years was diagnosed as having Guillain-Barré syndrome for which intravenous immunoglobulin was started at 400 mg/kg daily. On day 2 the patient complained of abdominal pain, aching shoulders and backache. He subsequently developed hypotension and died, despite resuscitation attempts. A post-mortem suggested that he had died from hypersensitivity myocarditis, which the authors of the report suggest might have resulted from the long-term use of the phenytoin.[1] This hypersensitivity with phenytoin has been reported before.[2] Because this complication is so serious, the authors of this report suggest that leukocyte counts, in particular eosinophils, should be monitored if these two drugs are given concurrently.[1] The general importance of this alleged interaction is not known. However, note that subsequent to this report, intravenous immunoglobulin has successfully been used to treat a two cases of hypersensitivity syndrome to phenytoin,[3,4] one including eosinophilia.[3] Intravenous immunoglobulin alone has also been associated with causing myocarditis.[5]

1. Koehler PJ, Koudstaal J. Lethal hypersensitivity myocarditis associated with the use of intravenous gammaglobulin for Guillain-Barré syndrome, in combination with phenytoin. *J Neurol* (1996) 243, 366–7.
2. Fenoglio JJ, McAllister HA, Mullick FG. Drug related myocarditis.I. Hypersensitivity myocarditis. *Hum Pathol* (1981) 12, 900–7.
3. Scheuerman O, Nofech-Moses Y, Rachmel A, Ashkenazi S. Successful treatment of antiepileptic drug hypersensitivity syndrome with intravenous immune globulin. *Pediatrics* (2001) 107, E14.
4. Salzman MB, Smith EM. Phenytoin-induced thrombocytopenia treated with intravenous immune globulin. *J Pediatr Hematol Oncol* (1998) 20, 152–3.
5. Akhtar I, Bastani B. Acute renal failure and myocarditis associated with intravenous immunoglobulin therapy. *Ann Intern Med* (2003) 139, W65.

Phenytoin + Influenza vaccines

Influenza vaccine is reported to increase, decrease or to have no effect on phenytoin serum levels. The efficacy of the vaccine remains unchanged.

Clinical evidence

(a) Phenytoin levels

The serum phenytoin levels of 8 epileptic children were increased by about 50%, from 9.5 to 15.16 micrograms/ml, 7 days after they were given 0.5 ml of an influenza virus vaccine USP, types A and B, whole virus (Squibb). The phenytoin levels returned to baseline over the following 7 days.[1] Temporary rises in the serum phenytoin levels of 3 patients, apparently caused by influenza vaccination, are briefly described in another report.[2]

In contrast, another study in 16 patients given 0.5 ml of an inactivated whole-viron trivalent influenza vaccine found that 7 and 14 days later their mean serum phenytoin levels were not significantly altered, although 4 of them showed a trend towards raised levels. Subsequently, these 4 patients had serum phenytoin increases ranging from 46 to 170%, which returned to baseline between week 4 and 17 after immunisation.[3]

In yet another study, within 4 days of receiving 0.5 ml of a subviron, trivalent influenza vaccine, the serum phenytoin levels of 7 patients were reduced by 11 to 14%, which is unlikely to have much clinical significance.[4] A further study[5] measured both free and total phenytoin levels in 8 patients on stable phenytoin monotherapy. Two days after receiving 0.5 ml of a trivalent influenza vaccine, the total phenytoin level had increased by 10%, and this then returned to baseline levels by day 7. However, the free phenytoin level gradually decreased after vaccination to a maximum of 25% less at day 14.

(b) Vaccine efficacy

The efficacy of influenza vaccine is reported to be unchanged by phenytoin.[6]

Mechanism

Where an interaction occurs it is suggested that it may be due to the inhibitory effect of the vaccine on the liver enzymes concerned with the metabolism of the phenytoin, resulting in a reduced clearance from the body.[1]

Importance and management

The outcome of immunisation with influenza vaccine on phenytoin levels is uncertain. Concurrent use need not be avoided but it would be prudent to monitor the effects closely. Be aware that any alteration in levels may take a couple of weeks to develop and usually resolves spontaneously.

1. Jann MW, Fidone GS. Effect of influenza vaccine on serum anticonvulsant concentrations. *Clin Pharm* (1986) 5, 817–20.
2. Mooradian AD, Hernandez L, Tamai IC, Marshall C. Variability of serum phenytoin concentrations in nursing home patients. *Arch Intern Med* (1989) 149, 890–2.
3. Levine M, Jones MW, Gribble M. Increased serum phenytoin concentration following influenza vaccination. *Clin Pharm* (1984) 3, 505–9.
4. Sawchuk RJ, Rector TS, Fordice JJ, Leppik IE. Case report. Effect of influenza vaccination on plasma phenytoin concentrations. *Ther Drug Monit* (1979) 1, 285–8.
5. Smith CD, Bledsoe MA, Curran R, Green L, Lewis J. Effect of influenza vaccine on serum concentrations of total and free phenytoin. *Clin Pharm* (1988) 7, 828–32.
6. Levine M, Beattie BL, McLean DM, Corman D. Phenytoin therapy and immune response to influenza vaccine. *Clin Pharm* (1985) 4, 191–4.

Phenytoin + Loxapine

A single case report describes decreased serum phenytoin levels in a patient given loxapine.

Clinical evidence, mechanism, importance and management

The serum phenytoin levels of an epileptic were reduced by loxapine, and showed a marked rise when it was withdrawn.[1] The general importance of this is uncertain, but bear this interaction in mind, particularly as loxapine can lower the convulsive threshold. More study is needed.

1. Ryan GM, Matthews PA. Phenytoin metabolism stimulated by loxapine. *Drug Intell Clin Pharm* (1977) 11, 428.

Phenytoin + Macrolides

Erythromycin appears not to interact with phenytoin. Limited evidence suggests that clarithromycin may possibly raise serum phenytoin levels.

Clinical evidence

(a) Clarithromycin

A retrospective study of serum phenytoin levels in a group of 21 patients with AIDS and a large control group of 557 subjects suggested that the concurrent use of clarithromycin (a total of 22 samples from at least 10 patients) was associated with higher serum phenytoin levels. The concentration/dose ratio of the phenytoin was 1.6 without clarithromycin and 3.9 with clarithromycin.[1]

(b) Erythromycin

A single-dose study found that the mean clearance of phenytoin was unchanged by erythromycin 333 mg every 8 hours for 7 days in 8 healthy subjects. However, there were occasional large changes in phenytoin clearance.[2] Similarly, in another study erythromycin 250 mg every 6 hours for 7 days had no effect on the pharmacokinetics of a single-dose of phenytoin in 8 healthy subjects.[3]

Mechanism

Not known, but it could be that clarithromycin inhibits the metabolism of the phenytoin by the liver. An animal study found that erythromycin, clarithromycin, and **roxithromycin** reduced the metabolism and increased levels of phenytoin.[4]

Importance and management

This seems to be the first and only evidence that clarithromycin possibly interacts like this. More study is needed to clarify this situation. Erythromycin appears not to interact with phenytoin, but nevertheless caution has been recommended.[2]

1. Burger DM, Meenhorst PL, Mulder JW, Kraaijeveld CL, Koks CHW, Bult A, Beijnen JH. Therapeutic drug monitoring of phenytoin in patients with the acquired immunodeficiency syndrome. *Ther Drug Monit* (1994) 16, 616–20.
2. Bachmann K, Schwartz JI, Forney RB, Jauregui L. Single dose phenytoin clearance during erythromycin treatment. *Res Commun Chem Pathol Pharmacol* (1984) 46, 207–17.
3. Milne RW, Coulthard K, Nation RL, Penna AC, Roberts G, Sansom LN. Lack of effect of erythromycin on the pharmacokinetics of single oral doses of phenytoin. *Br J Clin Pharmacol* (1988) 26, 330–3.
4. Al-Humayyd MS. Pharmacokinetic interactions between erythromycin, clarithromycin, roxithromycin and phenytoin in the rat. *Chemotherapy* (1997) 43, 77–85.

Phenytoin + Metronidazole

One study found that the half-life of phenytoin was modestly prolonged by metronidazole, whereas another found no change in phenytoin pharmacokinetics. An anecdotal report describes a few patients who developed toxic phenytoin levels when given metronidazole.

Clinical evidence, mechanism, importance and management

A pharmacokinetic study[1] in 7 healthy subjects found that metronidazole 250 mg three times daily increased the half-life of a single 300-mg intravenous dose of phenytoin by about 40% (from 16 to 23 hours) and reduced the clearance by 15%. In contrast, another study in 5 healthy subjects found that the pharmacokinetics of a single 300-mg oral dose of phenytoin were unaffected by metronidazole 400 mg twice daily for 6 days.[2] An anecdotal report describes several patients [number not stated] who developed toxic phenytoin serum levels when given metronidazole.[3] These appear to be the only reports of this potential interaction, and the reason for their discordant findings is not clear. More study is needed.

1. Blyden GT, Scavone JM, Greenblatt DJ. Metronidazole impairs clearance of phenytoin but not of alprazolam or lorazepam. *J Clin Pharmacol* (1988) 28, 240–5.
2. Jensen JC, Gugler R. Interaction between metronidazole and drugs eliminated by oxidative metabolism. *Clin Pharmacol Ther* (1985) 37, 407–10.
3. Picard EH. Side effects of metronidazole. *Mayo Clin Proc* (1983) 58, 401.

Phenytoin + Nitrofurantoin

An isolated report describes a reduction in serum phenytoin levels and poor seizure control in a patient given nitrofurantoin.

Clinical evidence, mechanism, importance and management

A patient with seizures due to a brain tumour was treated with phenytoin 300 mg daily. He had a seizure within a day of starting additional treatment with nitrofurantoin 200 mg for a urinary tract infection and, despite a recent increase in the phenytoin dose to 350 mg, his serum phenytoin levels were found to be modestly reduced (from 36 to 30 micromol/l). They continued to fall to 25 micromol/l despite a further increase in the phenytoin dosage to 400 mg daily. When the nitrofurantoin was stopped he was restabilised on his original dosage of phenytoin. The reasons are not understood but, on the basis of a noted rise in serum gamma glutamyltransferase levels during the use of the nitrofurantoin, the authors speculate that it increased the metabolism of the phenytoin by the liver.[1] The general importance of this interaction is uncertain, but probably small.

1. Heipertz R, Pilz H. Interaction of nitrofurantoin with diphenylhydantoin. *J Neurol* (1978) 218, 297–301.

Phenytoin + Orlistat

Orlistat does not alter the pharmacokinetics of phenytoin.

Clinical evidence, mechanism, importance and management

In a placebo-controlled, randomised, two-day crossover study, 12 healthy subjects were given a single 300-mg dose of phenytoin or a placebo on day 4 of a 7-day course of orlistat 120 mg three times daily. The pharmacokinetics of phenytoin were unchanged by orlistat,[1] and no special precautions are therefore thought to be needed if these two drugs are given concurrently.

1. Melia AT, Mulligan TE, Zhi J. The effect of orlistat on the pharmacokinetics of phenytoin in healthy volunteers. *J Clin Pharmacol* (1996) 36, 654–8.

Phenytoin + Penicillins

An isolated case describes a marked reduction in serum phenytoin levels, resulting in seizures, which was attributed to the use of oxacillin.

Clinical evidence, mechanism, importance and management

An epileptic woman taking phenytoin 400 mg daily, hospitalised for second degree burns sustained during a generalised seizure, experienced brief clonic seizures and was found to have an marked reduction in serum phenytoin levels, from 16.3 to 3.5 micrograms/ml, which was attributed to the concurrent use of oral **oxacillin** 500 mg every 6 hours. The phenytoin dose was increased, but seizures continued and progressed to status epilepticus, and intravenous phenytoin was given. Doses of oral phenytoin of about 600 mg daily were required to maintain minimum therapeutic levels, sometimes with supplementation of small intravenous doses. Just before the **oxacillin** was withdrawn the serum phenytoin level was 22.3 micrograms/ml, but 6 months later it had risen to 39.9 micrograms/ml, and the phenytoin dose was reduced.[1] Other studies have shown that penicillins such as **oxacillin**, **cloxacillin** and **dicloxacillin** can displace phenytoin from plasma protein binding, decreasing total serum levels but increasing the free fraction of phenytoin. If anything, this would be predicted to increase phenytoin toxicity.[2,3] This seems to be only report of an adverse interaction between phenytoin and a penicillin. Its general importance is probably small.

1. Fincham RW, Wiley DE, Schottelius DD. Use of phenytoin levels in a case of status epilepticus. *Neurology* (1976) 26, 879–81.
2. Arimori K, Nakano M, Otagiri M, Uekama K. Effects of penicillins on binding of phenytoin to plasma proteins *in vitro* and *in vivo*. *Biopharm Drug Dispos* (1984) 5, 219–27.
3. Dasgupta A, Sperelakis A, Mason A, Dean R. Phenytoin-oxacillin interactions in normal and uremic sera. *Pharmacotherapy* (1997) 17, 375–8.

Phenytoin + Pheneturide

Phenytoin serum levels can be increased by about 50% by pheneturide.

Clinical evidence, mechanism, importance and management

In 9 patients the steady-state half-life of phenytoin was prolonged from 32 to 47 hours by pheneturide. Mean serum levels were raised by about 50% but fell rapidly over the 2 weeks after pheneturide was withdrawn.[1] This study confirms a previous report of this interaction.[2] The reason for this reaction is uncertain, but since the two drugs have a similar structure it is possible that they compete for the same metabolising enzymes in the liver, thereby resulting, at least initially, in a reduction in the metabolism of the phenytoin. If concurrent use is undertaken the outcome should be well monitored. Reduce the phenytoin dosage as necessary.

1. Houghton GW, Richens A. Inhibition of phenytoin metabolism by other drugs used in epilepsy. *Int J Clin Pharmacol Biopharm* (1975) 12, 210–16.
2. Hulsman JW, van Heycop Ten Ham MW and van Zijl CHW. Influence of ethylphenacemide on serum levels of other anticonvulsant drugs. *Epilepsia* (1970) 11, 207.

Phenytoin + Phenobarbital

The concurrent use of phenytoin and phenobarbital is normally advantageous and uneventful. Changes in serum phenytoin levels (often decreases but sometimes increases) can occur if phenobarbital is added, but seizure control is not usually affected. Phenytoin toxicity following phenobarbital withdrawal has been seen. Increased phenobarbital levels and possibly toxicity may result from the addition of phenytoin to phenobarbital treatment.

Clinical evidence

(a) Phenytoin treatment to which phenobarbital is added

A study in 10 epileptics treated with phenytoin 2.8 to 6.8 mg/kg daily found that while taking phenobarbital 1.1 to 2.5 mg/kg daily their serum phenytoin levels were reduced. Five patients had a mean reduction of about 65%, from 15.7 to 5.7 micrograms/ml. In most cases phenytoin levels rose again when the phenobarbital was withdrawn. In one patient this was so rapid and steep that he developed ataxia and a cerebellar syndrome with phenytoin levels of up to 60 micrograms/ml, despite a reduction in the phenytoin dosage.[1]

This reduction in phenytoin levels by phenobarbital has been described in other reports.[2-5] However, some of these also described a very transient and small rise[4] or no alteration[4,5] in serum phenytoin levels in individual patients. Three other studies have found that phenobarbital does not alter phenytoin levels.[6-8]

(b) Phenobarbital treatment to which phenytoin is added

Elevated serum phenobarbital levels occurred in epileptic children when they were also given phenytoin. In 5 patients the phenobarbital levels were approximately doubled. In some cases mild ataxia was seen but the relatively high barbiturate levels were well tolerated.[1] A long-term study in 6 adult epileptics found that when phenytoin was added to phenobarbital, the level/dose ratio of the phenobarbital gradually rose from an average of 8.66 to a maximum of 13.8 day/kg/l for one year, and then gradually fell again over the next 2 years.[9]

Mechanism

Phenobarbital can have a dual effect on phenytoin metabolism: it may cause enzyme induction, which results in a more rapid clearance of the phenytoin from the body, or with large doses it may inhibit metabolism by competing for enzyme systems. The total effect will depend on the balance between the two drugs. The reason for the elevation of serum phenobarbital levels is not fully understood.

Importance and management

Concurrent use can be therapeutically valuable. Changes in dosage or the addition or withdrawal of either drug need to be monitored to ensure that toxicity does not occur, or that seizure control is not worsened. The contradictory reports cited here do not provide a clear picture of what is likely to happen. See also 'Primidone + Phenytoin', p.378.

1. Morselli PL, Rizzo M, Garattini S. Interaction between phenobarbital and diphenylhydantoin in animals and in epileptic patients. *Ann N Y Acad Sci* (1971) 179, 88–107.
2. Cucinell SA, Conney AH, Sansur M, Burns JJ. Drug interactions in man. I. Lowering effect of phenobarbital on plasma levels of bishydroxycoumarin (Dicumarol) and diphenylhydantoin (Dilantin). *Clin Pharmacol Ther* (1965) 6, 420–9.
3. Buchanan RA, Heffelfinger JC, Weiss CF. The effect of phenobarbital on diphenylhydantoin metabolism in children. *Pediatrics* (1969) 43, 114–16.
4. Kutt H, Haynes J, Verebely K, McDowell F. The effect of phenobarbital on plasma diphenylhydantoin level and metabolism in man and rat liver microsomes. *Neurology* (1969) 19, 611–16.
5. Garrettson LK, Dayton PG. Disappearance of phenobarbital and diphenylhydantoin from serum of children. *Clin Pharmacol Ther* (1970) 11, 674–9.
6. Diamond WD, Buchanan RA. A clinical study of the effect of phenobarbital on diphenylhydantoin plasma levels. *J Clin Pharmacol* (1970) 10, 306–11.
7. Booker HE, Tormey A, Toussaint J. Concurrent administration of phenobarbital and diphenylhydantoin: lack of interference effect. *Neurology* (1971) 21, 383–5.
8. Browne TR, Szabo GK, Evans J, Evans BA, Greenblatt DJ, Mikati MA. Phenobarbital does not alter phenytoin steady-state serum concentration or pharmacokinetics. *Neurology* (1988) 38, 639–42.
9. Encinas MP, Santos Buelga D, Alonso González AC, García Sánchez MJ, Domínguez-Gil Hurlé A. Influence of length of treatment on the interaction between phenobarbital and phenytoin. *J Clin Pharm Ther* (1992) 17, 49–50.

Phenytoin + Phenothiazines

The serum levels of phenytoin can be raised or lowered by the use of chlorpromazine, prochlorperazine or thioridazine. Phenytoin may reduce levels of the active metabolite of thioridazine.

Clinical evidence

(a) Chlorpromazine

The serum phenytoin levels of a patient stabilised on phenytoin, primidone and sulthiame doubled after chlorpromazine 50 mg daily was taken for a month.[1] However, another 4 patients on of chlorpromazine 50 to 100 mg daily showed no interaction.[1] In another report, one out of 3 patients treated with phenytoin and phenobarbital had a fall in serum phenytoin levels when given chlorpromazine.[2] A further very brief report states that in rare instances chlorpromazine has been noted to impair phenytoin metabolism.[3]

In a large study in patients on phenytoin taking various phenothiazines (chlorpromazine, **thioridazine** or **mesoridazine**), phenytoin levels were decreased by 44% when phenothiazines were started, and by 33% when the phenothiazine dose was increased. A number of patients experienced an increased frequency of seizures. In patients who had these phenothiazines discontinued or the dosage decreased, phenytoin levels increased by 55% and 71%, respectively, and toxic levels occurred in some patients.[4]

(b) Prochlorperazine

A single very brief report states that in rare instances prochlorperazine has been noted to impair phenytoin metabolism.[3]

(c) Thioridazine

One out of 6 patients on phenytoin and phenobarbital had a marked rise in serum phenytoin levels when thioridazine was added, whereas 4 others had a fall.[2] Phenytoin toxicity has also been described in 2 patients after about 2 weeks of concurrent treatment with thioridazine.[5] A retrospective study in 27 patients on phenytoin found that when given thioridazine their serum phenytoin levels were increased by at least 4 micrograms/ml (4 patients), decreased by at least 4 micrograms/ml (2), or were unchanged (21).[6] Another retrospective study comparing 28 patients taking both phenytoin and thioridazine with patients taking either drug alone found no evidence that thioridazine increased the risk of phenytoin toxicity.[7] A further study found no changes in serum phenytoin or thioridazine levels in patients given both drugs, but serum levels of mesoridazine (the active metabolite of thioridazine) were reduced, suggesting higher doses of thioridazine may be necessary to achieve the same effect.[8] See also the study[4] in section (a), which found a decrease in phenytoin levels and an increase in seizure frequency with phenothiazines including thioridazine.

Mechanism

Uncertain. Phenothiazines such as thioridazine are inhibitors of the cytochrome P450 isoenzyme CYP2D6, and as such would not be expected to affect phenytoin metabolism.

Importance and management

A confusing situation as the results are inconsistent. The concurrent use of phenytoin and the phenothiazines cited need not be avoided, but it would be prudent to watch for any signs of changes in serum phenytoin levels that would affect anticonvulsant control. It is also worth remembering that phenothiazines may decrease the seizure threshold. In one study a trend towards increased seizure frequency was noted after phenothiazines were added, or doses increased.[4] Also note that phenytoin may reduce levels of some phenothiazines. Whether all phenothiazines interact similarly is uncertain.

1. Houghton GW, Richens A. Inhibition of phenytoin metabolism by other drugs used in epilepsy. *Int J Clin Pharmacol Biopharm* (1975) 12, 210–16.
2. Siris JH, Pippenger CE, Werner WL, Masland RL. Anticonvulsant drug-serum levels in psychiatric patients with seizure disorders. Effects of certain psychotropic drugs. *N Y State J Med* (1974) 74, 1554–6.
3. Kutt H, McDowell F. Management of epilepsy with diphenylhydantoin sodium. Dosage regulation for problem patients. *JAMA* (1968) 203, 969–72.
4. Haidukewych D, Rodin EA. Effect of phenothiazines on serum antiepileptic drug concentrations in psychiatric patients with seizure disorder. *Ther Drug Monit* (1985) 7, 401–4.
5. Vincent FM. Phenothiazine-induced phenytoin intoxication. *Ann Intern Med* (1980) 93, 56–7.
6. Sands CD, Robinson JD, Salem RB, Stewart RB, Muniz C. Effect of thioridazine on phenytoin serum concentration: a retrospective study. *Drug Intell Clin Pharm* (1987) 21, 267–72.
7. Gotz VP, Yost RL, Lamadrid ME, Buchanan CD. Evaluation of a potential interaction: thioridazine-phenytoin — negative findings. *Hosp Pharm* (1984) 19, 555–7.
8. Linnoila M, Viukari M, Vaisanen K, Auvinen J. Effect of anticonvulsants on plasma haloperidol and thioridazine levels. *Am J Psychiatry* (1980) 137, 819–21.

Phenytoin + Protease inhibitors

For discussion of the differing interactions between phenytoin and protease inhibitors, see 'Protease inhibitors + Anticonvulsants; Phenytoin', p.608.

Phenytoin + Proton pump inhibitors

A study in epileptic patients found that omeprazole 20 mg daily did not affect the serum levels of phenytoin, whereas earlier studies in healthy subjects suggested that phenytoin levels might be modestly raised by omeprazole 40 mg daily. A study with esomeprazole also suggests it may cause a minor rise in phenytoin levels. Lansoprazole does not normally interact with phenytoin, but an isolated case report of toxicity is tentatively attributed to an interaction. Pantoprazole and rabeprazole appear not to interact.

Clinical evidence

(a) Esomeprazole

Esomeprazole inhibits the cytochrome P450 isoenzyme CYP2C19 so that the plasma levels of drugs metabolised by this enzyme might be expected to be increased by concurrent use. This is true for phenytoin, which the makers say showed a 13% increase in trough plasma levels in patients given esomeprazole 40 mg.[1]

(b) Lansoprazole

Lansoprazole 60 mg daily for 7 days caused only a very small and clinically irrelevant rise (<3%) in the AUC of a single intravenous dose of phenytoin in a group of 12 healthy subjects.[2,3] In contrast the maker has an isolated report of the development of blurred vision, diarrhoea, muscle pain, dizziness, abdominal pain, salivary hypersecretion, increased sweating and incoordination in a man on phenytoin within a day of stopping sustained-release propranolol 80 mg and starting lansoprazole.[4] The phenytoin serum levels were not measured but the symptoms might possibly have been due to phenytoin toxicity, although it should be said that if an interaction with lansoprazole was responsible, it developed unusually quickly.

(c) Omeprazole

Omeprazole 20 mg daily for 3 weeks caused no changes in the mean steady-state serum phenytoin levels in 8 epileptic patients.[5] Four patients had unchanged levels, 2 had falls and 2 had rises, but none of them was adversely affected by the omeprazole treatment.[5]

After taking omeprazole 40 mg daily for 7 days the AUC of a single 300-mg dose of phenytoin was increased by 25% in 10 healthy subjects.[6] In another study the clearance of a 250-mg intravenous dose of phenytoin was reduced by 15% by omeprazole 40 mg given for 7 days.[7] A further study found that 3 doses of omeprazole 40 mg had no effect on the pharmacokinetics of a single dose of phenytoin.[8]

(d) Pantoprazole

In a randomised crossover study 24 healthy subjects found that pantoprazole 40 mg daily for 7 days did not alter the pharmacokinetics (AUC, maximum serum levels, half-life) of a single 300-mg dose of phenytoin.[9]

(e) Rabeprazole

A preliminary report, which gives no details, states that when rabeprazole was used with phenytoin, no significant changes in the pharmacokinetics of phenytoin were seen.[10]

Mechanism

Not understood. A possible explanation is that if the dosage of omeprazole is high enough, it may possibly reduce the metabolism of phenytoin by CYP2C19. However, CYP2C19 has only a minor role in phenytoin metabolism.[11] Esomeprazole may interact similarly. With lansoprazole, the overall picture is that it does not act as an enzyme inducer or inhibitor[12] (or it is only very weak) so that it would not be expected to interact with phenytoin to a clinically relevant extent (confirmed by the study cited above[2]). The same appears to be true for pantoprazole and rabeprazole.

Importance and management

Information is very limited but it seems that omeprazole 20 mg daily does not affect serum phenytoin levels, whereas 40 mg daily may possibly modestly increase them. The isolated report[4] of an interaction involving lansoprazole remains unexplained. No special precautions would normally seem necessary if lansoprazole or omeprazole is given with phenytoin, but until more is known it would be prudent to be aware of this possible interaction if concurrent use is necessary. Similarly, the makers of esomeprazole suggest concurrent use should be monitored,[1] although the elevation in levels seen in the study would not usually be expected to be clinically significant. More study is needed. No special precautions would seem to be necessary if rabeprazole or pantoprazole and phenytoin are given concurrently.

1. Nexium (Esomeprazole). AstraZeneca UK Ltd. UK Summary of product characteristics, October 2004.
2. Karol MD, Mukherji D, Cavanaugh JH. Lack of effect of concomitant multi-dose lansoprazole on single-dose phenytoin pharmacokinetics in subjects. *Gastroenterology* (1994) 106, A103.
3. Karol MD, Locke CS, Cavanaugh JH. Lack of a pharmacokinetic interaction between lansoprazole and intravenously administered phenytoin. *J Clin Pharmacol* (1999) 39, 1283–9.
4. Wyeth, personal communication, January 1998.
5. Andersson T, Lagerström P-O, Unge P. A study of the interaction between omeprazole and phenytoin in epileptic patients. *Ther Drug Monit* (1990) 12, 329–33.
6. Prichard PJ, Walt RP, Kitchingman GK, Somerville KW, Langman MJS, Williams J, Richens A. Oral phenytoin pharmacokinetics during omeprazole therapy. *Br J Clin Pharmacol* (1987) 24, 543–5.
7. Gugler R, Jensen JC. Omeprazole inhibits oxidative drug metabolism. *Gastroenterology* (1985) 89, 1235–41.
8. Bachmann KA, Sullivan TJ, Jauregui L, Reese JH, Miller K, Levine L. Absence of an inhibitory effect of omeprazole and nizatidine on phenytoin disposition, a marker of CYP2C activity. *Br J Clin Pharmacol* (1993) 36, 380–2.
9. Müller FO, Bliesath H, Middle MV, Hundt HKL, Hartmann M, Schall R, Steinijans VW, Huber R, Wurst W. Pantoprazole does not influence the pharmacokinetics of phenytoin in man. *Klin Pharmakol Akt* (1993) 4, 26.
10. Humphries TJ, Nardi RV, Lazar JD, Spanyers SA. Drug-drug interaction evaluation of rabeprazole sodium: a clean/expected slate? *Gut* (1996) 39 (Suppl 3), A47.
11. Giancarlo GM, Venkatakrishnan K, Granda BW, von Moltke LL, Greenblatt DJ. Relative contributions of CYP2C9 and 2C19 to phenytoin 4-hydroxylation in vitro: inhibition by sulfaphenazole, omeprazole, and ticlopidine. *Eur J Clin Pharmacol* (2001) 57, 31–36.
12. Cavanaugh JH, Park YK, Awni WM, Mukherjee DX, Karol MD, Granneman GR. Effect of lansoprazole on antipyrine and ICG pharmacokinetics. *Gastroenterology* (1991) 100, A40.

Phenytoin + Sodium valproate

The concurrent use of phenytoin and sodium valproate is common and usually uneventful. Initially total serum phenytoin levels may fall but this is offset by a rise in the levels of free (and active) phenytoin, which may very occasionally cause some toxicity. After continued use the total serum phenytoin levels rise once again, and there might be sustained increases in free phenytoin levels. There is also some very limited evidence that concurrent use possibly increases the incidence of sodium valproate hepatotoxicity.

Clinical evidence

(a) Phenytoin levels

A number of reports clearly show that total serum levels of phenytoin fall during the early concurrent use of sodium valproate, while the concentrations of free phenytoin rise.[1-5] In one report it was noted that within 4 to 7 days the total serum phenytoin levels had fallen from 19.4 to 14.6 micrograms/ml.[1] A study extending over a year in 8 patients taking phenytoin and sodium valproate found that by the end of 8 weeks the total serum phenytoin levels of 6 of them had fallen by almost as much as 50%, but had returned to their original levels in all but one patient by the end of the year.[6] Similar results were found in another study.[7] However, in a further study, some patients had a sustained increase in the free fraction of phenytoin.[4] Another regression analysis showed that sodium valproate increased the free fraction of phenytoin.[8] The occasional patient may have symptoms of phenytoin toxicity and the dosage may need to be reduced.[9] Delirium and an increased seizure frequency was seen in one patient on sodium valproate when given phenytoin.[10]

(b) Sodium valproate levels

Sodium valproate levels are reduced by the presence of phenytoin.[11,12] Sodium valproate levels increased by 30 to 200% when phenytoin was discontinued in 12 patients on combined therapy, allowing dosage reductions in 6. In these patients, there was no change in seizure control when phenytoin was stopped.[13]

(c) Toxicity to the liver

Epidemiological studies suggest that the risk of fatal hepatotoxicity is higher when sodium valproate is given as polytherapy with enzyme inducers such as phenytoin than when it is given as monotherapy, especially in infants.[14,15] Hence concurrent use apparently carries some small risk. For mention of raised liver enzymes with concurrent use of valproate, phenobarbital and phenytoin, see 'Phenobarbital + Sodium valproate', p.359.

Mechanism

The initial fall in total serum phenytoin levels appears to result from the displacement of phenytoin from its protein binding sites by sodium valproate,[1-5,10] the extent being subject to the diurnal variation in valproate levels.[16] This allows more of the unbound drug to be exposed to metabolism by the liver and the total phenytoin levels fall. After several weeks the metabolism of the phenytoin is inhibited by the valproate and its levels rise.[2,4] This may result in sustained elevation of free (active) phenytoin levels.[17] Phenytoin reduces sodium valproate levels, probably because it increases its metabolism by the liver. Because phenytoin is an enzyme inducer it may also possibly increase the formation of a minor but hepatotoxic metabolite of sodium valproate (2-propyl-4-pentenoic acid or 4-ene-VPA).[18]

Importance and management

An extremely well-documented interaction (only a selection of the references being listed here). Concurrent use is common and usually advantageous, the adverse effects of the interactions between the drugs usually being of only minor practical importance. However, the outcome should still be monitored. A few patients may experience mild toxicity if sodium valproate is started, but most patients on phenytoin do not need a dosage change. During the first few weeks total serum phenytoin levels may fall by 20 to 50%, but usually no increase in the dosage is needed, because it is balanced by an increase in the levels of free (active) phenytoin levels. In the following period, the total phenytoin levels may rise again. This may result in a sustained rise in free phenytoin levels.

When monitoring concurrent use it is important to understand fully the implications of changes in 'total' and 'free' or 'unbound' serum phenytoin concentrations. Where monitoring of free phenytoin levels is not available, various nomograms have been designed for predicting unbound phenytoin concentrations during the use of sodium valproate.[17,19] Bear in mind the evidence that the incidence of sodium valproate induced liver toxicity may be increased, especially in infants.

1. Mattson RH, Cramer JA, Williamson PD, Novelly RA. Valproic acid in epilepsy: clinical and pharmacological effects. *Ann Neurol* (1978) 3, 20–5.
2. Perucca E, Hebdige S, Frigo GM, Gatti G, Lecchini S, Crema A. Interaction between phenytoin and valproic acid: plasma protein binding and metabolic effects. *Clin Pharmacol Ther* (1980) 28, 779–89.
3. Tsanaclis LM, Allen J, Perucca E, Routledge PA, Richens A. Effect of valproate on free plasma phenytoin concentrations. *Br J Clin Pharmacol* (1984) 18, 17–20.
4. Bruni J, Gallo JM, Lee CS, Pershalski RJ, Wilder BJ. Interactions of valproic acid with phenytoin. *Neurology* (1980) 30, 1233–6.
5. Friel PN, Leal KW, Wilensky AJ. Valproic acid-phenytoin interaction. *Ther Drug Monit* (1979) 1, 243–8.
6. Bruni J, Wilder BJ, Willmore LJ, Barbour B. Valproic acid and plasma levels of phenytoin. *Neurology* (1979) 29, 904–5.
7. Vakil SD, Critchley EMR, Philips JC, Fahim Y, Haydock D, Cocks A, Dyer T. The effect of sodium valproate (Epilim) on phenytoin and phenobarbitone blood levels. In 'Clinical and Pharmacological Aspects of Sodium Valproate (Epilim) in the Treatment of Epilepsy'. Proceedings of a symposium held at Nottingham University, September 1975, MCS Consultants, England, p 75–7.
8. Mamiya K, Yukawa E, Matsumoto T, Aita C, Goto S. Synergistic effect of valproate coadministration and hypoalbuminemia on the serum-free phenytoin concentration in patients with severe motor and intellectual disabilities. *Clin Neuropharmacol* (2002) 25, 230–3.
9. Haigh D, Forsythe WI. The treatment of childhood epilepsy with sodium valproate. *Dev Med Child Neurol* (1975) 17, 743–8.
10. Tollefson GD. Delirium induced by the competitive interaction between phenytoin and dipropylacetate. *J Clin Psychopharmacol* (1981) 1, 154–8.
11. May T, Rambeck B. Serum concentrations of valproic acid: influence of dose and co-medication. *Ther Drug Monit* (1985) 7, 387–90.
12. Sackellares JC, Sato S, Dreifuss FE, Penry JK. Reduction of steady-state valproate levels by other antiepileptic drugs. *Epilepsia* (1981) 22, 437–41.
13. McNew CD, Michel NC, McCabe PH. Pharmacokinetic interaction between valproic acid and phenytoin: is combination of these drugs "rational" polypharmacy. *Epilepsia* (1998) 39 (Suppl 6), abstract 4.100.
14. Dreifuss FE, Santilli N, Langer DH, Sweeney KP, Moline KA, Menander KB. Valproic acid fatalities: a retrospective review. *Neurology* (1987) 37, 379–85.
15. Dreifuss FE, Langer DH, Moline KA, Maxwell JE. Valproic acid hepatic fatalities. II. US experience since 1984. *Neurology* (1989) 39, 201–7.
16. Riva R, Albani F, Contin M, Perucca E, Ambrosetto G, Gobbi G, Santucci M, Procaccianti G, Baruzzi A. Time-dependent interaction between phenytoin and valproic acid. *Neurology* (1985) 35, 510–15.
17. Kerrick JM, Wolff DL, Graves NM. Predicting unbound phenytoin concentrations in patients receiving valproic acid: a comparison of two predicting methods. *Ann Pharmacother* (1995) 29, 470–4.
18. Levy RH, Rettenmeier AW, Anderson GD, Wilensky AJ, Friel PN, Baillie TA, Acheampong A, Tor J, Guyot M, Loiseau P. Effects of polytherapy with phenytoin, carbamazepine, and stiripentol on formation of 4-ene-valproate, a hepatotoxic metabolite of valproic acid. *Clin Pharmacol Ther* (1990) 48, 225–35.
19. May TW, Rambeck B, Nothbaum N. Nomogram for the prediction of unbound phenytoin concentrations in patients on a combined treatment of phenytoin and valproic acid. *Eur Neurol* (1991) 31, 57–60.

Phenytoin + SSRIs

Phenytoin serum levels can be increased in some patients by fluoxetine and toxicity may occur. There are also isolated reports of phenytoin toxicity on concurrent use with fluvoxamine. Phenytoin and sertraline do not normally interact, but two patients have shown increased serum phenytoin levels. Note that SSRIs should be avoided in unstable epilepsy and used with care in other epileptics.

Clinical evidence

(a) Fluoxetine

A woman on phenytoin 370 mg, diazepam 4 mg and clonazepam 6 mg daily was started on fluoxetine 20 mg for depression.[1] Five days later her serum phenytoin levels had risen from 18 to 26.5 mg/l, and a further 9 days later to 30 mg/l, accompanied by signs of toxicity (tremor, headache, abnormal thinking, increased partial seizure activity). Seven days after stopping the phenytoin the serum levels had fallen to 22 mg/l.

Two other patients, on phenytoin 300 and 400 mg daily respectively, had marked rises in serum phenytoin levels (from 15 to 35 micrograms/ml and from 11.5 to 47 micrograms/ml), accompanied by signs of phenytoin toxicity, within 5 to 10 days of starting fluoxetine 20 or 40 mg daily. The problem resolved when the fluoxetine was stopped or the phenytoin dosage reduced.[2] Another patient only developed this interaction after taking fluoxetine for about 9 months.[3]

A review initiated by the US Food and Drug Administration and the makers of fluoxetine briefly describes another 23 anecdotal observations of suspected phenytoin/fluoxetine interactions (most of them incompletely documented). These suggest that a marked 1.5-fold increase in serum phenytoin levels, with accompanying toxicity, can occur within 1 to 42 days (mean onset time of 2 weeks) after starting fluoxetine.[4] Another case describes raised phenytoin levels with improved efficacy on starting fluoxetine, and reduced levels and possible loss of efficacy on stopping fluoxetine.[5] Conversely, a retrospective review of 7 patients on the combination found no cases of a drug interaction.[6]

(b) Fluvoxamine

About one month after starting to take fluvoxamine 50 mg daily, a woman on phenytoin 300 mg daily experienced ataxia and was found to have a threefold increase in phenytoin levels (from 16.6 to 49.1 micrograms/ml). Fluvoxamine was subsequently discontinued, and the phenytoin dose reduced, with gradual recovery.[7] Another report describes phenytoin toxicity (serum levels of 48 mg/l) in an 86-year-old woman after she took fluvoxamine 100 to 200 mg daily for 10 days.[8] However the fluvoxamine was started only 2 days after the phenytoin, in a dose of 200 mg twice daily, had been started, and the serum phenytoin levels were not checked until the toxicity had actually developed. Both drugs were then stopped and the phenytoin later successfully reinstated without the fluvoxamine. A worldwide analysis of data up to 1995 by the makers of fluvoxamine identified only 2 reported cases of drug-drug interactions (clinical symptoms only) between phenytoin and fluvoxamine.[9]

(c) Paroxetine

Sixteen days' treatment with paroxetine 30 mg daily in epileptics caused no changes in the plasma levels or therapeutic effects of phenytoin. Steady-state paroxetine plasma levels were lower in those taking phenytoin (16 nanograms/ml) than in those on carbamazepine (27 nanograms/ml) or sodium valproate (73 nanograms/ml).[10]

(d) Sertraline

A double-blind, randomised, placebo-controlled study in 30 healthy subjects taking phenytoin 100 mg three times daily, found that sertraline 50 to 200 mg daily did not affect the steady-state trough serum levels of phenytoin, nor was there any evidence that concurrent use impaired cognitive function.[11] However, another report describes 2 elderly patients whose serum phenytoin levels rose when they were given sertraline, but there was no evidence of toxicity. One of them had an almost fourfold rise in serum phenytoin levels whereas the other had a rise of only about one-third.[12]

Mechanism

An *in vitro* investigation found that fluoxetine and fluvoxamine inhibited the metabolism of phenytoin by the cytochrome P450 isoenzyme CYP2C9 in human liver tissue.[13] This would presumably lead to a rise in serum phenytoin levels. In this study, sertraline was a weaker inhibitor of CYP2C9, and was considered less likely to interact with phenytoin.[13] A similar study also suggested that the risk of interaction was greatest for fluoxetine, and less likely with sertraline and paroxetine.[14]

Importance and management

The interaction between phenytoin and fluoxetine appears to be established but its incidence is not known. Because of the unpredictable nature of this interaction, if fluoxetine is added to treatment with phenytoin in any patient be alert for the need to reduce the phenytoin dosage. Ideally the phenytoin serum levels should be monitored. Similarly, to be on the safe side you should monitor phenytoin levels when fluvoxamine is first added to treatment with phenytoin so that any patient affected can be identified. Although an interaction with sertraline appears less likely, be alert for any evidence of an increase in phenytoin adverse effects if sertraline is used with phenytoin. More study of these interactions is needed. Note that SSRIs should be avoided in patients with unstable epilepsy, and those with controlled epilepsy should be carefully monitored, because of the potential increased seizure risk.

1. Woods DJ, Coulter DM, Pillans P. Interaction of phenytoin and fluoxetine. *N Z Med J* (1994) 107, 19.
2. Jalil P. Toxic reaction following the combined administration of fluoxetine and phenytoin: two case reports. *J Neurol Neurosurg Psychiatry* (1992) 55, 412–13.
3. Darley J. Interaction between phenytoin and fluoxetine. *Seizure* (1994) 3, 151–2.
4. Shader RI, Greenblatt DJ, von Moltke LL. Fluoxetine inhibition of phenytoin metabolism. *J Clin Psychopharmacol* (1994) 14, 375–6.
5. Shad MU, Preskorn SH. Drug-drug interaction in reverse: possible loss of phenytoin efficacy as a result of fluoxetine discontinuation. *J Clin Psychopharmacol* (1999) 19, 471–2.
6. Bécares J, Puente M, De Juana P, García B, Bermego T. Fluoxetina y fenitoína: interacción o interpretación errónea de los niveles séricos? *Farm Clin* (1997) 14, 474–8.
7. Mamiya K, Kojima K, Yukawa E, Higuchi S, Ieiri I, Ninomiya H, Tashiro N. Case report. Phenytoin intoxication induced by fluvoxamine. *Ther Drug Monit* (2001) 23, 75–7.

8. Feldman D, Claudel B, Feldman F, Allilaire JF, Thuillier A. Cas clinique d'interaction médicamenteuse entre phénytoïne et fluvoxamine. *J Pharm Clin* (1995) 14, 296–7.
9. Wagner W, Vause EW. Fluvoxamine. A review of global drug-drug interaction data. *Clin Pharmacokinet* (1995) 29 (Suppl 1), 26–32.
10. Andersen BB, Mikkelsen M, Versterager A, Dam M, Kristensen HB, Pedersen B, Lund J, Mengel H. No influence of the antidepressant paroxetine on carbamazepine, valproate and phenytoin. *Epilepsy Res* (1991) 10, 201–4.
11. Rapeport WG, Muirhead DC, Williams SA, Cross M, Wesnes K. Absence of effect of sertraline on the pharmacokinetics and pharmacodynamics of phenytoin. *J Clin Psychiatry* (1996) 57 (Suppl 1), 24–8.
12. Haselberger MB, Freedman LS, Tolbert S. Elevated serum phenytoin concentrations associated with coadministration of sertraline. *J Clin Psychopharmacol* (1997) 17, 107–9.
13. Schmider J, Greenblatt DJ, von Moltke LL, Karsov D, Shader RI. Inhibition of CYP2C9 by selective serotonin reuptake inhibitors *in vitro*: studies of phenytoin *p*-hydroxylation. *Br J Clin Pharmacol* (1997) 44, 495–8.
14. Nelson MH, Birnbaum AK, Remmel RP. Inhibition of phenytoin hydroxylation in human liver microsomes by several selective serotonin re-uptake inhibitiors. *Epilepsy Res* (2001) 44, 71–82.

Phenytoin + Sucralfate

The absorption of single-dose phenytoin can be reduced by about 7 to 20% by sucralfate, but this was not seen in a multiple-dose study. The interaction is unlikely to be clinically relevant.

Clinical evidence

Sucralfate 1 g was found to reduce the absorption (measured over a 24-hour period) of a single 300-mg dose of phenytoin in 8 healthy subjects by 20%.[1] Peak serum phenytoin levels were also reduced, but this was said not to be statistically significant. Another single-dose study found a reduction in absorption of 7.7 to 9.5%.[2] However, sucralfate 1 g four times daily for 7 days had no effect on steady-state levels of phenytoin 5 to 7 mg/kg daily in 6 healthy subjects. The fourth daily dose of sucralfate was taken simultaneously with the daily phenytoin dose at bedtime. After 7 days, all phenytoin levels were within 15% of the baseline values (range, 6% decrease to 15% increase).[3]

Mechanism

Uncertain. Reduced bioavailability has been demonstrated in a single-dose study in *dogs* when the drugs were used simultaneously, and this did not occur if the phenytoin was given 2 hours after the sucralfate.[4]

Importance and management

Information is limited. The reduction in absorption shown in single-dose studies was quite small, and was not seen in a multiple-dose study, suggesting it is unlikely to be clinically relevant.

1. Smart HL, Somerville KW, Williams J, Richens A, Langman MJS. The effects of sucralfate upon phenytoin absorption in man. *Br J Clin Pharmacol* (1985) 20, 238–40.
2. Hall TG, Cuddy PG, Glass CJ, Melethil S. Effect of sucralfate on phenytoin bioavailability. *Drug Intell Clin Pharm* (1986) 20, 607–11.
3. Malli R, Jones WN, Rindone JP, Labadie EL. The effect of sucralfate on the steady-state serum concentrations of phenytoin. *Drug Metabol Drug Interact* (1989) 7, 287–93.
4. Lacz JP, Groschang AG, Giesing DH, Browne RK. The effect of sucralfate on drug absorption in dogs. *Gastroenterology* (1982) 82, 1108.

Phenytoin + Sulfinpyrazone

Some limited evidence indicates that phenytoin serum levels may be markedly increased by sulfinpyrazone.

Clinical evidence

A review of the drug interactions of sulfinpyrazone identified two studies that found interactions with phenytoin.[1] In the first, the serum phenytoin levels of 2 out of 5 patients on phenytoin 250 to 350 mg daily were doubled from about 10 micrograms/ml to 20 micrograms/ml within 11 days of starting to take sulfinpyrazone 800 mg daily. One of the remaining patients had a small increase in phenytoin levels, but the other two had no changes at all. When the sulfinpyrazone was withdrawn, the serum phenytoin concentrations fell to their former levels. The second was a clinical study in epileptic patients that found that sulfinpyrazone 800 mg daily for a week increased the phenytoin half-life from 10 to 16.5 hours and reduced the metabolic clearance from 59 to 32 ml/minute.

Mechanism

Uncertain. It seems probable that sulfinpyrazone inhibits the metabolism of the phenytoin by the liver, thereby allowing it to accumulate in the body and leading to a rise in its serum levels. Displacement of phenytoin from its plasma protein binding sites may also have a small part to play.

Importance and management

Information seems to be limited to these studies, which await confirmation. A similar interaction with phenytoin has been reported with phenylbutazone, which has a very close chemical relationship with sulfinpyrazone (see 'Phenytoin + Aspirin or NSAIDs', p.364). Thus what is known suggests that concurrent use should be monitored and suitable phenytoin dosage reductions made where necessary.

1. Pedersen AK, Jacobsen P, Kampmann JP, Hansen JM. Clinical pharmacokinetics and potentially important drug interactions of sulphinpyrazone. *Clin Pharmacokinet* (1982) 7, 42–56.

Phenytoin + Sulfonamides and/or Trimethoprim

Phenytoin serum levels can be raised by co-trimoxazole, sulfamethizole, sulfamethoxazole, sulfadiazine and trimethoprim. Phenytoin toxicity may develop in some cases. A single case of liver failure has been described in a patient treated with phenytoin and co-trimoxazole. Sulfamethoxypyridazine, and sulfafurazole (sulfisoxazole) are reported not to interact.

Clinical evidence

(a) Co-trimoxazole or Trimethoprim

A patient on phenytoin 400 mg daily developed signs of toxicity (ataxia, nystagmus, loss of balance) within 2 weeks of starting to take co-trimoxazole 960 mg twice daily. His serum levels were found to have risen to 152 micromol/l (normal range 40 to 80 micromol/l).[1]

A child on a stable regimen of phenytoin and sultiame developed phenytoin toxicity within 48 hours of starting co-trimoxazole. Toxicity resolved when treatment was changed to amoxicillin.[2] A clinical study found that co-trimoxazole and trimethoprim can increase the phenytoin half-life by 39% and 51%, and decrease the mean metabolic clearance by 27 and 30%, respectively.[3] Sulfamethoxazole alone had only a small effect on the half-life and did not affect the clearance of phenytoin.[3] A case report describes fatal acute hepatic failure in a 60-year-old woman 10 days after starting co-trimoxazole and 14 days after starting phenytoin.[4] This patient was also given cimetidine, which may raise phenytoin levels (see 'Phenytoin + H_2-blockers', p.369).

(b) Sulfadiazine

After taking sulfadiazine 4 g daily for a week, the half-life of a single intravenous dose of phenytoin was found to have increased by 80% in 8 patients. The mean metabolic clearance decreased by 45%.[3]

(c) Sulfamethizole

The development of phenytoin toxicity in a patient given sulfamethizole prompted a study of this interaction in 8 patients. After 7 days treatment with sulfamethizole 1 g four times daily the phenytoin half-life had lengthened from 11.8 to 19.6 hours. Of 4 further patients on long-term treatment, 3 had rises in serum phenytoin levels from 22 to 33 micrograms/ml, from 19 to 23 micrograms/ml and from 4 to 7 micrograms/ml respectively. The phenytoin levels of the fourth patient were not affected.[5,6]

Another single-dose study found that the half-life of phenytoin was increased and the mean metabolic clearance reduced by 36%.[3]

(d) Other sulfonamides

One week's pretreatment with **sulfamethoxypyridazine** or **sulfafurazole** did not significantly alter the pharmacokinetics of a single dose of phenytoin.[3]

Mechanism

The sulfonamides that interact appear to do so by inhibiting the metabolism of the phenytoin by the liver (possibly by the cytochrome P450 isoenzyme CYP2C9)[7], resulting in its accumulation in the body. This would also seem to be true for trimethoprim. Depletion of glucuronic acid by phenytoin may have increased the hepatotoxicity of co-trimoxazole.[4]

Importance and management

The documentation seems to be limited to the reports cited, but the interaction is established. Co-trimoxazole, sulfamethizole, sulfadiazine and trimethoprim can increase serum phenytoin levels. It probably occurs in most patients, but the small number of adverse reaction reports suggests that the risk of toxicity is small. It is clearly most likely in those with serum phenytoin levels at the top end of the range. If concurrent use is thought appropriate, the serum phenytoin levels should be closely monitored and the phenytoin dosage reduced if necessary. Alternatively, if appropriate, use a non-interacting sulfonamide (see (d) above). There seems to be no information about other sulfonamides but it would be prudent to be alert for this interaction with any of them.

1. Wilcox JB. Phenytoin intoxication and co-trimoxazole. *N Z Med J* (1981) 94, 235–6.
2. Gillman MA, Sandyk R. Phenytoin toxicity and co-trimoxazole. *Ann Intern Med* (1985) 102, 559.
3. Hansen JM, Kampmann JP, Siersbæk-Nielsen K, Lumholtz B, Arrøe M, Abildgaard U, Skovsted L. The effect of different sulfonamides on phenytoin metabolism in man. *Acta Med Scand* (1979) (Suppl 624), 106–10.
4. Ilario MJ-M, Ruiz JE, Axiotis CA. Acute fulminant hepatic failure in a woman treated with phenytoin and trimethoprim-sulfamethoxazole. *Arch Pathol Lab Med* (2000) 124, 1800–3.
5. Lumholtz B, Siersbaek-Nielsen K, Skovsted L, Kampmann J, Hansen JM. Sulfamethizole-induced inhibition of diphenylhydantoin, tolbutamide and warfarin metabolism. *Clin Pharmacol Ther* (1975) 17, 731–4.
6. Siersbaek-Nielsen K, Hansen JM, Skovsted L, Lumholtz B, Kampmann J. Sulphamethizole-induced inhibition of diphenylhydantoin and tolbutamide metabolism in man. *Clin Pharmacol Ther* (1973) 14, 148.
7. Giancarlo GM, Venkatakrishnan K, Granda BW, von Moltke LL, Greenblatt DJ. Relative contributions of CYP2C9 and 2C19 to phenytoin 4-hydroxylation in vitro: inhibition by sulfaphenazole, omeprazole, and ticlopidine. *Eur J Clin Pharmacol* (2001) 57, 31–36.

Phenytoin + Sultiame

Serum phenytoin levels can be approximately doubled by sultiame and phenytoin toxicity may occur.

Clinical evidence

The serum phenytoin levels in 6 out of 7 epileptic patients approximately doubled within about 5 to 25 days of starting to take sultiame 400 mg daily. All experienced an increase in adverse effects and definite phenytoin toxicity occurred in 2 of them. In most of the patients, phenytoin serum levels fell back to baseline over the 2 months following the withdrawal of sultiame.[1] All of the patients were also taking **phenobarbital** and greater variations in serum **phenobarbital** were seen, but this was not clinically significant.[1]

A number of other reports confirm this interaction,[2-8] some of which describe the development of phenytoin toxicity.

Mechanism

The evidence suggests that sultiame interferes with the metabolism of the phenytoin by the liver, leading to its accumulation in the body.

Importance and management

A reasonably well-documented, established and clinically important interaction. The incidence seems to be high. If sultiame is added to established treatment with phenytoin, increases in serum phenytoin levels of up to 75% or more may be expected.[3,7] Phenytoin serum levels should be closely monitored and appropriate dosage reductions made to prevent the development of toxicity. The changes in phenobarbital levels appear to be unimportant.

1. Olesen OV, Jensen ON, Drug-interaction between sulthiame (Ospolot (R)) and phenytoin in the treatment of epilepsy. *Dan Med Bull* (1969) 16, 154–8.
2. Houghton GW, Richens A. Inhibition of phenytoin metabolism by sulthiame. *Br J Pharmacol* (1973) 49, 157P–158P.
3. Houghton GW, Richens A. Inhibition of phenytoin metabolism by sulthiame in epileptic patients. *Br J Clin Pharmacol* (1974) 1, 59–66.
4. Richens A, Houghton GW. Phenytoin intoxication caused by sulthiame. *Lancet* (1973) ii, 1442–3.
5. Houghton GW, Richens A. Inhibition of phenytoin metabolism by other drugs used in epilepsy. *Int J Clin Pharmacol Biopharm* (1975) 12, 210–16.
6. Frantzen E, Mølholm Hansen J, Hansen OE, Kristensen M. Phenytoin (Dilantin®) intoxication. *Acta Neurol Scand* (1967) 43, 440–6.
7. Houghton GW, Richens A. Phenytoin intoxication induced by sulthiame in epileptic patients. *J Neurol Neurosurg Psychiatry* (1974) 37, 275–81.
8. Mølholm Hansen J, Kristensen M and Skovsted L. Sulthiame (Ospolot®) as inhibitor of diphenylhydantoin metabolism. *Epilepsia* (1968) 9, 17–22.

Phenytoin + Ticlopidine

Ticlopidine reduces the metabolism of phenytoin. A number of case reports describe patients who developed phenytoin toxicity when ticlopidine was added.

Clinical evidence

A 65-year-old man on phenytoin 200 mg daily and clobazam developed signs of phenytoin toxicity (vertigo, ataxia, somnolence) within a week of starting ticlopidine 250 mg daily. His serum phenytoin levels had risen from 18 mg/l to 34 mg/l. When the phenytoin dosage was reduced to 200 mg daily the toxic symptoms disappeared within a few days and his serum phenytoin levels fell to 18 mg/l. To test whether an interaction had occurred, the ticlopidine was stopped, whereupon the serum phenytoin levels fell within about 3 weeks to 8 mg/l, during which time the patient experienced his first seizure in 2 years. When the ticlopidine was restarted, his serum phenytoin levels rose again, within a month, to 19 mg/l.[1] A number of other case reports describe phenytoin toxicity within 2 to 6 weeks of starting ticlopidine 250 mg once or twice daily.[2-7] These were usually managed by reducing the phenytoin dose. One patient then experienced breakthrough seizures after the ticlopidine was stopped without increasing the phenytoin dose again.[6] One case in a patient also taking **phenobarbital** reported that no change in **phenobarbital** levels occurred.[4]

A study in 6 patients on phenytoin monotherapy found that ticlopidine 250 mg twice daily approximately halved the steady-state phenytoin clearance.[8]

Mechanism

The metabolism of phenytoin to 5-(4-hydroxyphenyl)-5-phenylhydantoin (HPPH) by the cytochrome P450 isoenzyme CYP2C19, and to a lesser extent by CYP2C9, in the liver is inhibited by ticlopidine.[1,3,4,9] Further metabolism of HPPH to dihydroxylated products is mediated mainly by CYP2C19 and may also be inhibited by ticlopidine.[9]

Importance and management

The interaction is established and clinically important, but its incidence is unknown. It would now be prudent to monitor serum phenytoin levels very closely in any patient if ticlopidine is added to established treatment, being alert for the need to reduce the phenytoin dosage. If ticlopidine is discontinued, the phenytoin dose may need to be increased.

1. Riva R, Cerullo A, Albani F, Baruzzi A. Ticlopidine impairs phenytoin clearance: a case report. *Neurology* (1996) 46, 1172–3.
2. Rindone JP, Bryan G. Phenytoin toxicity associated with ticlopidine administration. *Arch Intern Med* (1996) 156, 1113.
3. Privitera M, Welty TE. Acute phenytoin toxicity followed by seizure breakthrough from a ticlopidine-phenytoin interaction. *Arch Neurol* (1996) 53, 1191–2.
4. Donahue SR, Flockhart DA, Abernethy DR, Ko J-W. Ticlopidine inhibition of phenytoin metabolism mediated by potent inhibition of CYP2C19. *Clin Pharmacol Ther* (1997) 62, 572–7.
5. López-Ariztegui N, Ochoa M, Sánchez-Migallón, Nevado C, Martín M, Intoxicación aguda por fenitoína secundaria a interacción con ticlopidina. *Rev Neurol* (1998) 26, 1017–18.
6. Klaassen SL. Ticlopidine-induced phenytoin toxicity. *Ann Pharmacother* (1998) 32, 1295–8.
7. Dahm AEA, Brørs O. Fenytoinforgiftning forårsaket av interaksjon med tiklopidin. *Tidsskr Nor Laegeforen* (2002) 122, 278–80.
8. Donahue S, Flockhart DA, Abernethy DR. Ticlopidine inhibits phenytoin clearance. *Clin Pharmacol Ther* (1999) 66, 563–8.
9. Giancarlo GM, Venkatakrishnan K, Granda BW, von Moltke LL, Greenblatt DJ. Relative contributions of CYP2C9 and 2C19 to phenytoin 4-hydroxylation in vitro: inhibition by sulfaphenazole, omeprazole, and ticlopidine. *Eur J Clin Pharmacol* (2001) 57, 31–36.

Phenytoin + Tizanidine

An isolated report describes a modest increase in serum phenytoin levels caused by tizanidine.

Clinical evidence, mechanism, importance and management

An isolated report describes a 59-year-old man whose phenytoin levels rose by one-third, from about 75 to 101 micromol/l, and who experienced drowsiness within a week of starting tizanidine 6 mg daily. The phenytoin was stopped for 3 days and restarted at a reduced dose, but the drowsiness recurred in 3 weeks (phenytoin level 81 micromol/l). Therefore, the tizanidine was withdrawn.[1] The general importance of this interaction is unclear, but it would seem prudent to remain aware of this interaction in case of an unusual response to treatment.

1. Ueno K, Miyai K, Mitsuzane K. Phenytoin-tizanidine interaction. *DICP Ann Pharmacother* (1991) 25, 1273.

Phenytoin + Trazodone

An isolated case report describes phenytoin toxicity in a patient given trazodone.

Clinical evidence, mechanism, importance and management

A patient taking phenytoin 300 mg daily developed progressive signs of phenytoin toxicity after taking trazodone 500 mg daily for 4 months. His serum phenytoin levels had risen from 17.8 to 46 micrograms/ml.[1] Therapeutic phenytoin serum levels were restored by reducing the phenytoin dosage to 200 mg daily and the trazodone to 400 mg daily. The reasons for this apparent interaction are not understood, and nothing further appears to have been published on it. No general conclusions can be drawn.

1. Dorn JM. A case of phenytoin toxicity possibly precipitated by trazodone. *J Clin Psychiatry* (1986) 47, 89–90.

Phenytoin + Tricyclic antidepressants

Some very limited evidence suggests that imipramine can raise serum phenytoin levels but nortriptyline and amitriptyline appear not to do so. Phenytoin possibly reduces serum desipramine levels. The tricyclics also lower the convulsive threshold.

Clinical evidence

(a) Serum phenytoin levels increased or unchanged

The serum phenytoin levels of 2 patients rose over a 3-month period when they were given **imipramine** 75 mg daily. One of them had an increase in phenytoin levels from 30 to 60 micromol/l and developed mild toxicity (drowsiness and uncoordination). These signs disappeared and the phenytoin serum levels of both patients fell when the **imipramine** was withdrawn. One of them was also taking nitrazepam and clonazepam, and the other sodium valproate and carbamazepine, but were stable on these combinations before the addition of **imipramine**.[1]

Other studies have shown that **nortriptyline** 75 mg daily had an insignificant effect on the serum phenytoin levels of 5 patients,[2] and that **amitriptyline** had no effect on the elimination of phenytoin in 3 subjects.[3]

(b) Serum tricyclic antidepressant levels reduced

A report describes 2 patients who had low serum **desipramine** levels, despite taking standard dosages, while they were also taking phenytoin.[4]

Mechanism

One suggestion is that imipramine inhibits the metabolism of the phenytoin by the liver, which results in its accumulation in the body. *In vitro* study[5] has shown that the tricyclics can inhibit the cytochrome P450 isoenzyme CYP2C19, which usually has only a minor role in phenytoin metabolism (see 'Anticonvulsants', (p.328)). The reduced desipramine levels may be a result of enzyme induction by the phenytoin.

Importance and management

The documentation is very limited indeed and none of these interactions is adequately established. The results of the *in vitro* study suggest that the interaction may only assume importance in those who are deficient in CYP2C9, the enzyme usually responsible for phenytoin metabolism.[5] The tricyclic antidepressants as a group lower the seizure threshold,[6] which suggests extra care should be taken anyway, if deciding to use them in epileptic patients. If concurrent use is undertaken the effects should be very well monitored.

1. Perucca E, Richens A. Interaction between phenytoin and imipramine. *Br J Clin Pharmacol* (1977) 4, 485–6.
2. Houghton GW, Richens A. Inhibition of phenytoin metabolism by other drugs used in epilepsy. *Int J Clin Pharmacol Biopharm* (1975) 12, 210–16.
3. Pond SM, Graham GG, Birkett DJ, Wade DN. Effects of tricyclic antidepressants on drug metabolism. *Clin Pharmacol Ther* (1975) 18, 191–9.
4. Fogel BS, Haltzman S. Desipramine and phenytoin: a potential drug interaction of therapeutic relevance. *J Clin Psychiatry* (1987) 48, 387–8.
5. Shin J-G, Park J-Y, Kim M-J, Shon J-H, Yoon Y-R, Cha I-J, Lee S-S, Oh S-W, Kim S-W, Flockhart DA. Inhibitory effects of tricyclic antidepressants (TCAs) on human cytochrome P450 enzymes in vitro: mechanism of drug interaction between TCAs and phenytoin. *Drug Metab Dispos* (2002) 30, 1102–7.
6. Dallos V, Heathfield K. Iatrogenic epilepsy due to antidepressant drugs. *BMJ* (1969) 4, 80–2.

Phenytoin + Vigabatrin

Vigabatrin causes a small to moderate fall in serum phenytoin levels, which may require a dose increase in some patients.

Clinical evidence

In one early clinical study, the mean serum phenytoin levels in 19 patients were about 30% lower when they were given vigabatrin 2 to 3 g daily, and in 2 patients they fell below the therapeutic range. However, the change in phenytoin levels was not correlated with the change in seizure-frequency.[1] Another clinical study found that vigabatrin reduced the mean serum phenytoin levels by 20% in 53 patients; 41 patients had a decrease in phenytoin levels and 12 had an increase. In this study, some of the patients [number not stated] with decreased phenytoin levels had an increase in seizure frequency and required a phenytoin dosage increase.[2,3] In another analysis, the decrease in phenytoin levels did not occur until the fifth week of vigabatrin therapy.[4] Three other studies have shown roughly similar decreases in phenytoin levels with the addition of vigabatrin.[5-7]

Mechanism

Not understood. The decrease in phenytoin levels does not appear to be due to reduced metabolism or altered plasma protein binding.[4] Similarly, it is not due to altered bioavailability, since it occurred with intravenous phenytoin.[5]

Importance and management

The interaction between phenytoin and vigabatrin would appear to be established. Vigabatrin causes a modest decrease in phenytoin levels in some patients, which takes a number of weeks to become apparent. A small increase in the dosage of phenytoin may possibly be needed in some patients.

1. Tassinari CA, Michelucci R, Ambrosetto G, Salvi F. Double-blind study of vigabatrin in the treatment of drug-resistant epilepsy. *Arch Neurol* (1987) 44, 907–10.
2. Browne TR, Mattson RH, Penry JK, Smith DB, Treiman DM, Wilder BJ, Ben-Menachem E, Miketta RM, Sherry KM, Szabo GK. A multicentre study of vigabatrin for drug-resistant epilepsy. *Br J Clin Pharmacol* (1989) 95S–100S.
3. Browne TR, Mattson RH, Penry JK, Smith DB, Treiman DM, Wilder BJ, Ben-Menachem E, Napoliello MJ, Sherry KM, Szabo GK. Vigabatrin for refractory complex partial seizures: multicenter single-blind study with long-term follow up. *Neurology* (1987) 37, 184–9.
4. Rimmer EM, Richens A. Double-blind study of γ-vinyl GABA in patients with refractory epilepsy. *Lancet* (1984) i, 189–90.
5. Gatti G, Bartoli A, Marchiselli R, Michelucci R, Tassinari CA, Pisani F, Zaccara G, Timmings P, Richens A, Perucca E. Vigabatrin-induced decrease in serum phenytoin concentration does not involve a change in phenytoin bioavailability. *Br J Clin Pharmacol* (1993) 36, 603–6.
6. Rimmer EM, Richens A. Interaction between vigabatrin and phenytoin. *Br J Clin Pharmacol* (1989) 27, 27S–33S.
7. Bernardina BD, Fontana E, Vigevano F, Fusco L, Torelli D, Galeone D, Buti D, Cianchetti C, Gnanasakthy A, Iudice A. Efficacy and tolerability of vigabatrin in children with refractory partial seizures: a single-blind dose-increasing study. *Epilepsia* (1995) 36, 687–91.

Phenytoin + Zidovudine

Although one study found that zidovudine did not alter the pharmacokinetics of phenytoin, there is other evidence suggesting that some changes possibly occur, but these may be due to HIV infection.

Clinical evidence, mechanism, importance and management

Although there are said to have been 13 cases of a possible interaction between zidovudine and phenytoin, the details are not described in the report.[1] No significant changes in the pharmacokinetics of phenytoin 300 mg daily were seen in 12 asymptomatic HIV+ patients who were taking zidovudine 200 mg every 4 hours.[1] Another study found that the mean phenytoin dose was higher in HIV+ patients when compared to epileptic subjects without the virus, while the mean phenytoin levels in the HIV+

group were lower (i.e. a higher dose resulted in lower serum levels in HIV+ subjects). Zidovudine did not appear to affect the levels.[2,3] The current evidence would suggest that it is HIV infection, rather than zidovudine that affects phenytoin levels, but more study is needed to confirm this.

1. Sarver P, Lampkin TA, Dukes GE, Messenheimer JA, Kirby MG, Dalton MJ, Hak LJ. Effect of zidovudine on the pharmacokinetic disposition of phenytoin in HIV positive asymptomatic patients. *Pharmacotherapy* (1991) 11, 108–9.
2. Burger DW, Meerhorst PL, Koks CHW, Beijnen JH. Phenytoin (PH) monitoring in HIV (+) individuals: is there an interaction with zidovudine (ZDV)? 9th International Conference on AIDS & 5th World Congress on Sexually Transmitted Diseases, Berlin. June 6–11, 1993. Abstract PO-B31-2214.
3. Burger DM, Meenhorst PL, Mulder JW, Kraaijeveld CL, Koks CHW, Bult A, Beijnen JH. Therapeutic drug monitoring of phenytoin in patients with the acquired immunodeficiency syndrome. *Ther Drug Monit* (1994) 16, 616–20.

Phenytoin + Zileuton

The pharmacokinetics of phenytoin are unchanged by zileuton.

Clinical evidence, mechanism, importance and management

A controlled study in 20 healthy subjects found that the pharmacokinetics of a single 300-mg dose of phenytoin was unaltered by zileuton 600 mg every 6 hours for 5 days.[1] An *in vitro* study found that zileuton had little effect on the isoenzymes responsible for the metabolism of phenytoin.[2] These studies suggest that zileuton is unlikely to affect phenytoin levels in clinical use.

1. Samara E, Cavanaugh JH, Mukherjee D, Granneman GR. Lack of pharmacokinetic interaction between zileuton and phenytoin in humans. *Clin Pharmacokinet* (1995) 29 (Suppl 2), 84–91.
2. Lu P, Schrag ML, Slaughter DE, Raab CE, Shou M, Rodrigues AD. Mechanism-based inhibition of human liver microsomal cytochrome P450 1A2 by zileuton, a 5-lipoxygenase inhibitor. *Drug Metab Dispos* (2003) 31, 1352–60.

Piracetam + Other anticonvulsants

Piracetam does not appear to alter the levels of sodium valproate or primidone.

Clinical evidence, mechanism, importance and management

Add-on piracetam (2 to 4 g three times daily, increased to a maximum of 18 to 24 g daily) did not affect plasma levels of **sodium valproate** or **primidone** in patients with myoclonus. The exact number of patients on these drugs is unclear, since the report just states that 28 patients were being treated with **clonazepam**, **sodium valproate**, or **primidone**, alone or in combination.[1] Another similar report, briefly noted the same finding.[2] No special precautions appear to be required if piracetam is used with these anticonvulsants.

1. Obeso JA, Artieda J, Quinn N, Rothwell JC, Luquin MR, Vaamonde J, Marsden CD. Piracetam in the treatment of different types of myoclonus. *Clin Neuropharmacol* (1988) 11, 529–36.
2. Raychev I. Piracetam (pyramem) in the treatment of cortical myoclonus. *5th European Congress of Epileptology* (2002), Madrid.

Pregabalin + Miscellaneous

There appears to be no pharmacokinetic interaction between pregabalin and carbamazepine, lamotrigine, phenobarbital, phenytoin, topiramate, valproate, lorazepam, oxycodone or ethanol. However, the impairment of cognitive and gross motor function caused by oxycodone was additive with pregabalin, and pregabalin may potentiate the effects of ethanol and lorazepam.

Clinical evidence, mechanism, importance and management

(a) Alcohol or Lorazepam

The maker notes that there was no clinically relevant pharmacokinetic interaction between pregabalin and lorazepam or alcohol, and that concurrent use caused no clinically important effect on respiration. However, they note that pregabalin may potentiate the effects of lorazepam and alcohol.[1]

(b) Other anticonvulsants

Pregabalin 600 mg three times daily for 7 days was added to monotherapy with various anticonvulsants in patients with partial epilepsy. Pregabalin did not alter the steady-state levels of **phenytoin**, **carbamazepine**, **valproic acid** or **lamotrigine**. In addition, the steady-state pharmacokinetics of pregabalin were not different to those seen previously in healthy subjects on pregabalin alone, suggesting these drugs do not alter pregabalin pharmacokinetics.[2] Similarly, in population pharmacokinetic analyses of clinical studies, no important changes in the pharmacokinetics of **lamotrigine**, **phenobarbital**, **phenytoin**, **topiramate** or **valproate** were found when they were given with pregabalin, and the pharmacokinetics of pregabalin were unaffected by these drugs.[2]

(c) Oxycodone

The maker notes that there was no clinically relevant pharmacokinetic interaction between pregabalin and oxycodone, and that there was no clinically important effect on respiration. However, pregabalin appeared to cause an additive impairment in cognitive and gross motor function when given with oxycodone.[1] This suggests caution is warranted during combined use.

1. Lyrica (Pregabalin). Pfizer Ltd. UK Summary of product characteristics, July 2004.
2. Ben-Menachem E. Pregabalin pharmacology and its relevance to clinical practice. *Epilepsia* (2004) 45 (Suppl 6), 13–18.

Primidone + Isoniazid

A single case report describes elevated serum primidone levels and reduced phenobarbital levels during the concurrent use of primidone and isoniazid.

Clinical evidence, mechanism, importance and management

A patient on primidone had raised serum primidone levels and reduced serum phenobarbital levels due, it was found, to the concurrent use of isoniazid, which inhibited the metabolism of the primidone by the liver. The half-life of primidone rose from 8.7 to 14 hours while taking isoniazid and steady-state primidone levels rose by 83%. The importance of this interaction is uncertain but prescribers should be aware that it can occur if concurrent treatment is undertaken.[1]

1. Sutton G, Kupferberg HJ. Isoniazid as an inhibitor of primidone metabolism. *Neurology* (1975) 25, 1179–81.

Primidone + Miscellaneous

Primidone is substantially converted to phenobarbital within the body and it is therefore expected to interact with other drugs in the same way as phenobarbital. Some drugs may increase the conversion of primidone to phenobarbital.

Clinical evidence, mechanism, importance and management

Primidone is substantially converted to phenobarbital within the body. For example, a group of patients on long-term primidone without a barbiturate developed serum primidone levels of 9 micrograms/ml and serum phenobarbital levels of 31 micrograms/ml.[1] Primidone would therefore be expected to interact with other drugs in the same way as phenobarbital. Some enzyme-inducing drugs might increase the conversion of primidone to phenobarbital, and this has been demonstrated for 'phenytoin', (below), and 'carbamazepine', (p.347).

1. Booker HE, Hosokowa K, Burdette RD, Darcey B. A clinical study of serum primidone levels. *Epilepsia* (1970) 11, 395–402.

Primidone + Phenytoin

Primidone-derived serum phenobarbital levels are increased by phenytoin. This is normally an advantageous interaction, but phenobarbital toxicity occurs occasionally.

Clinical evidence

A study in 44 epileptic patients taking primidone and phenytoin found that their serum phenobarbital:primidone ratio was high (4.35) when compared with that in 15 other patients who were only taking primidone (1.05).[1] Similar results are described in other studies.[2-6] A few patients may develop barbiturate toxicity.[7]

An initial marked decrease in phenytoin levels, then an increase to half the initial phenytoin level, was seen in the first few weeks after withdrawing primidone in an infant. Derived phenobarbital levels before discontinuing the primidone were very high, associated with marked sedation.[8]

Mechanism

Phenytoin increases the metabolic conversion of primidone to phenobarbital, while possibly depressing the subsequent metabolic destruction (hydroxylation) of the phenobarbital. The net effect is a rise in phenobarbital levels.[9] Phenobarbital may increase or decrease phenytoin levels, see 'Phenytoin + Phenobarbital', p.371.

Importance and management

Well documented. This is normally an advantageous interaction since phenobarbital is itself an active anticonvulsant. However, it should be borne in mind that phenobarbital serum levels could sometimes reach toxic concentrations,[7] even if only a small dose of phenytoin is added. Changes in phenytoin levels may also occur (see 'Phenytoin + Phenobarbital', p.371).

1. Fincham RW, Schottelius DD, Sahs AL. The influence of diphenylhydantoin on primidone metabolism. *Arch Neurol* (1974) 30, 259–62.
2. Fincham RW, Schottelius DD, Sahs AL. The influence of diphenylhydantoin on primidone metabolism. *Trans Am Neurol Assoc* (1973) 98, 197–9.
3. Schmidt D. The effect of phenytoin and ethosuximide on primidone metabolism in patients with epilepsy. *J Neurol* (1975) 209, 115–23.
4. Reynolds EH, Fenton G, Fenwick P, Johnson AL, Laundy M. Interaction of phenytoin and primidone. *BMJ* (1975) 2, 594–5.
5. Callaghan N, Feeley M, Duggan F, O'Callaghan M, Seldrup J. The effect of anticonvulsant drugs which induce liver microsomal enzymes on derived and ingested phenobarbitone levels. *Acta Neurol Scand* (1977) 56, 1–6.
6. Battino D, Avanzini G, Bossi L, Croci D, Cusi C, Gomeni C, Moise A. Plasma levels of primidone and its metabolite phenobarbital: effect of age and associated therapy. *Ther Drug Monit* (1983) 5, 73–9.
7. Galdames D, Ortiz M, Saavedra I, Aguilera L. Interaccion fenitoina-primidona: intoxicacion por fenobarbital, en un adulto tratado con ambas drogas. *Rev Med Chil* (1980) 108, 716–20.
8. Wilson JT, Wilkinson GR. Chronic and severe phenobarbital intoxication in a child treated with primidone and diphenylhydantoin. *J Pediatr* (1973) 83, 484–9.
9. Porro MG, Kupferberg HJ, Porter RJ, Theodore WH, Newmark ME. Phenytoin: an inhibitor and inducer of primidone metabolism in an epileptic patient. *Br J Clin Pharmacol* (1982) 14, 294–7.

Primidone + Sodium valproate

Sodium valproate has been reported to cause increases, decreases, and no change in serum primidone levels. Primidone-derived phenobarbital levels appear to be increased by sodium valproate.

Clinical evidence

In a number of cases, patients taking primidone required a decrease in the primidone dosage after sodium valproate was added.[1-4] In 6 cases this was due to an increase in the primidone-derived phenobarbital level,[1] and in the other cases phenobarbital levels were not measured, but the dosage reduction was needed to overcome the sedation that occurred when the sodium valproate was added.[2-4] Primidone levels were not measured in any of these cases.[1-4] In two other studies, primidone levels either decreased,[5] or did not change when sodium valproate was added.[6] However, phenobarbital levels, where measured, had increased.[6]

In 7 children the serum levels of primidone 10 to 18 mg/kg daily rose two to threefold when sodium valproate [dosage not stated] was also given. After 1 to 3 months of continued therapy the serum primidone levels fell in 3 of the patients but persisted in one. Follow-up primidone levels were not taken in the other 3 patients, and no patient had phenobarbital levels measured.[7]

In contrast, in a further study, neither phenobarbital levels nor primidone levels were significantly altered when sodium valproate was added to treatment.[8]

Mechanism

It has been suggested that sodium valproate decreases the conversion of primidone to phenobarbital, and decreases the metabolism of phenobarbital (see also 'Phenobarbital + Sodium valproate', p.359). This would result in increased primidone and phenobarbital levels. However, increased renal clearance of primidone may occur, resulting in no overall change to the primidone levels. Depending on the balance between these various effects a variety of levels may result.[8] The results of one study suggest that proposed inhibition of primidone caused by sodium valproate may diminish over the first few months of concurrent use.[7]

Importance and management

There seems to be little consistency about the effect of sodium valproate on primidone levels. However, in the majority of cases phenobarbital levels seem to be raised (see also 'Phenobarbital + Sodium valproate', p.359). It would seem prudent not to measure primidone levels without corresponding phenobarbital levels. Monitor the patient for increased signs of sedation, which may be resolved by a reduction in the primidone dose.

1. Wilder BJ, Willmore LJ, Bruni J, Villarreal HJ. Valproic acid: interaction with other anticonvulsant drugs. *Neurology* (1978) 28, 892–6.
2. Haigh D, Forsythe WI. The treatment of childhood epilepsy with sodium valproate. *Dev Med Child Neurol* (1975) 17, 743–8.
3. Richens A, Ahmad S. Controlled trial of sodium valproate in severe epilepsy. *BMJ* (1975) 4, 255–6.
4. Völzke E, Doose H. Dipropylacetate (Dépakine®, Ergenyl®) in the treatment of epilepsy. *Epilepsia* (1973) 14, 185–93.
5. Varma R, Michos GA, Varma RS, Hoshino AY. Clinical trials of Depakene (valproic acid) coadministered with other anticonvulsants in epileptic patients. *Res Commun Psychol Psychiatr Behav* (1980) 5, 265–73.
6. Yukawa E, Higuchi S, Aoyama T. The effect of concurrent administration of sodium valproate on serum levels of primidone and its metabolite phenobarbital. *J Clin Pharm Ther* (1989) 14, 387–92.
7. Windorfer A, Sauer W, Gädeke R. Elevation of diphenylhydantoin and primidone serum concentration by addition of dipropylacetate, a new anticonvulsant drug. *Acta Paediatr Scand* (1975) 64, 771–2.
8. Bruni J. Valproic acid and plasma levels of primidone and derived phenobarbital. *Can J Neurol Sci* (1981) 8, 91–2.

Progabide + Other anticonvulsants

Serum phenytoin levels can rise if progabide is given, and a reduced phenytoin dosage may be required. Changes in the serum levels of carbamazepine, clonazepam, phenobarbital and sodium valproate caused by progabide and their effects on serum progabide levels appear to be only moderate or small.

Clinical evidence

(a) Phenytoin

Marked increases in serum phenytoin levels have been seen in a few patients also given progabide[1-4] while smaller changes have been described in some studies,[5,6] and negligible changes in others.[7]

In one study, 17 out of 26 epileptics needed a reduction in phenytoin dosage to keep the levels within 25% of the serum levels before progabide was given. Over half the patients needed a dose reduction within 4 weeks of starting concurrent treatment. Most of those needing a dosage reduction had a maximum increase in the serum level of 40% or more, which was sometimes accompanied by toxicity.[2,8] In a later report of this study, of a total of 32 epileptics taking carbamazepine plus phenytoin, 22 needed a reduction in phenytoin dosage to maintain serum levels within 25% when progabide was given. In addition, it appeared this effect on phenytoin serum levels continued for a while after progabide was withdrawn.[4]

(b) Other anticonvulsants

Information about other anticonvulsants is limited, but progabide is reported to minimally reduce,[1,9,10] minimally increase[1] or not to change **carbamazepine**[2,3,5-7] serum levels. An increase in the levels of the **epoxide** metabolite of **carbamazepine** of up to 24% has also been reported.[6,10] **Sodium valproate**,[3,5-7] and **clonazepam**[11] serum levels were not significantly affected by progabide. Progabide appears to cause a small increase in serum **phenobarbital** levels, which is of little clinical importance.[1,5-7]

Mechanism

Uncertain.

Importance and management

Some small to moderate changes in the serum levels of carbamazepine, phenobarbital, sodium valproate and clonazepam can apparently occur in the presence of progabide, but only the interaction with phenytoin appears to be clinically relevant. Be alert for the need to reduce the dosage of phenytoin if progabide is used concurrently. The minor effects of the antiepileptics on progabide levels are of unknown significance.

1. Schmidt D, Utech K. Progabide for refractory partial epilepsy: a controlled add-on trial. *Neurology* (1986) 36, 217–221.
2. Cloyd JC, Brundage RC, Leppik IE, Graves NM, Welty TE. Effect of progabide on serum phenytoin and carbamazepine concentrations: a preliminary report. In: LERS Monograph series, volume 3. Edited by Bartholini G et al. Epilepsy and GABA receptor agonists: basic and therapeutic research. Meeting, Paris, March 1984. Raven Press, New York. (1985) pp 271–8. ISBN: 0881671061
3. Crawford P, Chadwick D. A comparative study of progabide, valproate and placebo as add-on therapy in patients with refractory epilepsy. *J Neurol Neurosurg Psychiatry* (1986) 49, 1251–7.
4. Brundage RC, Cloyd JC, Leppik IE, Graves NM and Welty TE. Effect of progabide on serum phenytoin and carbamazepine concentrations. *Clin Neuropharmacol* (1987) 10, 545–54.
5. Bianchetti G, Thiercelin JF, Thenot JP, Feuerstein J, Lambert D, Rulliere R, Thebault JJ, Morselli PL. Effect of progabide on the pharmacokinetics of various antiepileptic drugs. *Neurology* (1984) 34 (Suppl 1), 213.
6. Bianchetti G, Padovani P, Thénot JP, Thiercelin JF, Morselli PL. Pharmacokinetic interactions of progabide with other antiepileptic drugs. *Epilepsia* (1987) 28, 68–73.
7. Thénot JP, Bianchetti G, Abriol C, Feuerstein J, Lambert D, Thébault JJ, Warrington SJ, Rowland M. Interactions between progabide and antiepileptic drugs. In: LERS Monograph series, volume 3. Edited by Bartholini G et al. Epilepsy and GABA receptor agonists: basic and therapeutic research. Meeting, Paris, March 1984. Raven Press, New York. (1985) pp 259–69. ISBN: 0881671061
8. Brundage RC, Leppik IE, Cloyd JC, Graves NM. Effect of progabide on phenytoin pharmacokinetics. *Epilepsia* (1984) 25, 656–7.
9. Dam M, Gram L, Philbert A, Hansen BS, Blatt Lyon B, Christensen JM, Angelo HR. Progabide: a controlled trial in partial epilepsy. *Epilepsia* (1983) 24, 127–34.
10. Graves NM, Fuerst RH, Cloyd JC, Brundage RC, Welty TE, Leppik IE. Progabide-induced changes in carbamazepine metabolism. *Epilepsia* (1988) 29, 775–80.
11. Warrington SJ, O'Brien C, Thiercelin JF, Orofiamma B and Morselli PL. Evaluation of pharmacodynamic interaction between progabide and clonazepam in healthy men. In: LERS Monograph series, volume 3. Edited by Bartholini G et al. Epilepsy and GABA receptor agonists: basic and therapeutic research. Meeting, Paris, March 1984. Raven Press, New York. (1985) pp 279–86. ISBN: 0881671061

Remacemide + Other anticonvulsants

Remacemide causes modest increases in carbamazepine and phenytoin serum levels. Carbamazepine, phenobarbital and phenytoin moderately reduce remacemide serum levels. Sodium valproate and lamotrigine do not appear to interact with remacemide.

Clinical evidence

(a) Carbamazepine

A group of 10 patients on carbamazepine were additionally given up to 300 mg of remacemide twice daily for 2 weeks. Small increases in carbamazepine minimum serum levels and AUC of 20% and of 22% respectively were found. No patients had symptoms of carbamazepine toxicity.[1] Another study of 11 patients on carbamazepine found that remacemide caused a similar 20 to 30% increase in the AUC of carbamazepine, again without signs of toxicity. No consistent changes in the AUC of the main metabolite of carbamazepine were seen.[2] Another study has reported a slight inhibitory effect of remacemide on carbamazepine metabolism, which is in line with these other findings.[3] One of these studies also reported that the AUC of remacemide was decreased by 40 to 50% and the AUC of its main metabolite by about 70% when compared with healthy subjects (presumably not taking carbamazepine).[2]

However, a further trial of the efficacy of remacemide and carbamazepine in combination found that about two-thirds of the 120 patients treated needed 14 to 50% reductions in their carbamazepine dose, to ensure levels remained in the therapeutic range.[4]

(b) Lamotrigine

There was no clinically relevant pharmacokinetic interaction between remacemide (200 mg daily increased to 200 mg three times daily) and lamotrigine (200 mg twice daily decreased to 100 mg daily) in healthy subjects.[5]

(c) Phenobarbital

Phenobarbital 30 mg daily increased to 90 mg daily increased the clearance of remacemide 200 mg twice daily by 67%, and slightly increased the plasma levels of phenobarbital (by 9%) in a study in healthy subjects.[6]

(d) Phenytoin

A group of 10 patients on phenytoin were additionally given up to 300 mg remacemide twice daily for 2 weeks. On average remacemide did not affect phenytoin pharmacokinetics but 5 patients had an increase in minimum serum levels of 30% or more. No patients had symptoms of phenytoin toxicity.[1] In another study 10 epileptics, who had been on phenytoin for at least 3 months, were given remacemide 300 mg twice daily for 12 days. Phenytoin maximum serum levels were increased by 13.7% and the AUC was raised by 11.5%. Average concentrations of remacemide and its main metabolite were around only 40 and 30% of those achieved in healthy volunteers taking remacemide alone, at the same dosage.[7] Another study reported a slight inhibitory effect of remacemide on phenytoin metabolism, which is in line with these other findings.[3]

(e) Sodium valproate

A group of 10 patients on sodium valproate were additionally given remacemide up to 300 mg twice daily for 14 days. The pharmacokinetics of sodium valproate remained unchanged.[1] Another study in 17 patients confirmed these findings,[8] and an earlier study by the same authors also noted no effect of remacemide on valproate metabolism.[3]

Mechanism

Not fully understood, but *in vitro* studies indicate that remacemide inhibits the cytochrome P450 isoenzyme CYP3A4 which *in vivo* would be expected to result in a reduction in the metabolism of the carbamazepine resulting in an increase in its serum levels. Remacemide appears to inhibit CYP2C9 to a lesser extent, which is reflected in a smaller interaction with phenytoin. Sodium valproate is metabolised by glucuronidation and is therefore unaffected.[1]

Carbamazepine and phenytoin also seem to increase the metabolism of the remacemide.[7]

Importance and management

Information is limited, but the interactions of remacemide with carbamazepine, phenobarbital and phenytoin appear to be established, but so far only the carbamazepine interaction seems to have been shown to be of clinical importance. Even so, until more experience has been gained, monitor the effects of concurrent use with phenytoin or phenobarbital. No interaction occurs between remacemide and sodium valproate or lamotrigine.

1. Riley RJ, Slee D, Martin CA, Webborn PJH, Wattam DG, Jones T, Logan CJ. *In vitro* evaluation of pharmacokinetic interactions between remacemide hydrochloride and established anticonvulsants. *Br J Clin Pharmacol* (1996) 41, 461P.
2. Leach JP, Blacklaw J, Stewart M, Jamieson V, Jones T, Oxley R, Richens A, Brodie MJ. Mutual pharmacokinetic interactions between remacemide hydrochloride and carbamazepine. *Epilepsia* (1995) 36 (Suppl 3), S163.
3. Leach JP, Blacklaw J, Stewart M, Jamieson V, Oxley R, Richens A, Brodie MJ. Interactions between remacemide and the established antiepileptic drugs. *Epilepsia* (1994) 35 (Suppl 7), 75.
4. Mawer GE, Jamieson V, Lucas SB, Wild JM. Adjustment of carbamazepine dose to offset the effects of the interaction with remacemide hydrochloride in a double-blind, multicentre, add-on drug trial (CR2237) in refractory epilepsy. *Epilepsia* (1999) 40, 190–6.
5. Blakey GE, Lockton JA, Rolan IP. The effect of lamotrigine on the disposition of remacemide hydrochloride. *Epilepsia* (1999) 40 (Suppl 2), 251.
6. Hooper WD, Eadie MJ, Blakey GE, Lockton JA, Manun'Ebo M. Evaluation of a pharmacokinetic interaction between remacemide hydrochloride and phenobarbitone in healthy males. *Br J Clin Pharmacol* (2001) 51, 249–55.
7. Leach JP, Girvan J, Jamieson V, Jones T, Richens A, Brodie MJ. Mutual interaction between remacemide hydrochloride and phenytoin. *Epilepsy Res* (1997) 26, 381–8.
8. Leach JP, Girvan J, Jamieson V, Jones T, Richens A, Brodie MJ. Lack of pharmacokinetic interaction between remacemide hydrochloride and sodium valproate in epileptic patients. *Seizure* (1997) 6, 179–84.

Retigabine + Other anticonvulsants

The clearance of retigabine is increased by carbamazepine and phenytoin, but not phenobarbital, topiramate, or valproate. Retigabine does not alter the pharmacokinetics of any of these drugs. There is a modest pharmacokinetic interaction between retigabine and lamotrigine.

Clinical evidence, mechanism, importance and management

(a) Enzyme-inducing anticonvulsants

The preliminary report of a study notes that the clearance of retigabine was increased [amount not stated] by **carbamazepine** and **phenytoin**, but that retigabine did not alter **carbamazepine** or **phenytoin** pharmacokinetics in patients with epilepsy.[1] This is consistent with the known enzyme-inducing properties of **carbamazepine** and **phenytoin**, and the fact that retigabine has not been shown to induce hepatic enzymes. In contrast, **phenobarbital** 90 mg daily did not affect the pharmacokinetics of retigabine 200 mg every 8 hours in a study in healthy subjects, and the pharmacokinetics of **phenobarbital** were not altered by retigabine.[2] The clinical relevance of the effect of **carbamazepine** and **phenytoin** on retigabine remains to be assessed. No dosage adjustments seem to be necessary with **phenobarbital**.

(b) Lamotrigine

Lamotrigine 25 mg daily for 5 days increased the AUC of a single 200-mg dose of retigabine by 15% and decreased the clearance by 13% in a study in 14 healthy subjects.[3] In another 15 subjects, retigabine 200 mg twice daily increased to 300 mg twice daily over 15 days decreased the AUC of a single 200-mg dose of lamotrigine by 18% and increased clearance by 22%. It was suggested that lamotrigine competes for renal elimination of retigabine, but the mechanism behind the decreased lamotrigine levels is unknown.[3] These modest changes are unlikely to be clinically important for most patients, but the authors suggest that the effects need to be assessed at the upper recommended dose ranges and so advise caution.

(c) Topiramate

The preliminary report of a study notes that the pharmacokinetics of retigabine and topiramate were not altered by concurrent use in patients with epilepsy.[1] No special dosing precautions are necessary.

(d) Valproate

The preliminary report of a study notes that the pharmacokinetics of retigabine and valproic acid were not altered by concurrent use in patients with epilepsy.[1] No special dosing precautions are necessary.

1. Sachdeo RC, Ferron GM, Partiot AM, Biton V, Rosenfeld WB, Porter RJ, Fritz T, Althouse S, Troy SM. An early determination of drug-drug interaction between valproic acid, phenytoin, carbamazepine or topiramate, and retigabine in epileptic patients. *Neurology* (2001) 56 (Suppl 3). A331–A332.
2. Ferron GM, Patat A, Parks V, Rolan P, Troy SM. Lack of pharmacokinetic interaction between retigabine and phenobarbitone at steady state in healthy subjects. *Br J Clin Pharmacol* (2003) 56, 39–45.
3. Hermann R, Knebel NG, Niebch G, Richards L, Borlak J, Locher M. Pharmacokinetic interaction between retigabine and lamotrigine in healthy subjects. *Eur J Clin Pharmacol* (2003) 58, 795–802.

Sodium valproate + Acarbose

An isolated case report describes reduced valproate levels in a patient given acarbose.

Clinical evidence, mechanism, importance and management

An epileptic patient on sodium valproate for 10 years had a 40% fall in his normally stable plasma levels from 67 to 40.5 micrograms/ml when acarbose was added. No other drugs were being taken. When the acarbose was stopped and then restarted, the valproate levels rose and then fell once again. The reason is not understood but the authors of the report suggest that the acarbose possibly reduces the absorption of valproate.[1] This is an isolated report and its general importance is unknown, but it would now be prudent to be alert for any evidence of reduced anticonvulsant effects if acarbose is added to valproate treatment.

1. Serrano JS, Jiménez CM, Serrano MI, Garrido H, Balboa B. May acarbose impair valproate bioavailability? *Methods Find Exp Clin Pharmacol* (1996) 18 (Suppl C), 98.

Sodium valproate + Allopurinol

Allopurinol appears not to alter valproate levels.

Clinical evidence, mechanism, importance and management

In a study of add-on therapy, allopurinol (150 mg daily in those less than 20 kg, and 300 mg daily for other patients for 4 months) had no effect on valproate levels in 28 patients on anticonvulsants including valproate.[1] In another similar study, allopurinol 10 mg/kg increased to 15 mg/kg daily for 12 weeks had no effect on serum valproate levels in 6 patients on anticonvulsants including valproate.[2] Therefore valproate dosage alterations are likely to be required if allopurinol is used.

1. Zagnoni PG, Bianchi A, Zolo P, Canger R, Cornaggia C, D'Alessandro P, DeMarco P, Pisani F, Gianelli M, Verzé L, Viani F, Zaccara G. Allopurinol as add-on therapy in refractory epilepsy: a double-blind placebo-controlled randomized study. *Epilepsia* (1994) 35, 107–12.
2. Coppola G, Pascotto A. Double-blind, placebo-controlled, cross-over trial of allopurinol as add-on therapy in childhood refractory epilepsy. *Brain Dev* (1996) 18, 50–2.

Sodium valproate + Antacids

The absorption of valproate was slightly, but not significantly, increased by an aluminium/magnesium hydroxide suspension but not by magnesium trisilicate or a calcium carbonate suspension.

Clinical evidence, mechanism, importance and management

The AUC of a single 500-mg dose of valproic acid, given 1 hour after breakfast, was increased by 12% (range 3 to 28%) in 7 healthy subjects given 62 ml of an **aluminium/magnesium hydroxide** suspension (*Maalox*) 1 hour and 3 hours after breakfast and at bedtime. Neither **magnesium trisilicate** suspension (*Trisogel*) nor **calcium carbonate** suspension (*Titralac*) had a significant effect on absorption.[1] No special precautions would seem necessary during concurrent use.

1. May CA, Garnett WR, Small RE, Pellock JM. Effects of three antacids on the bioavailability of valproic acid. *Clin Pharm* (1982) 1, 244–7.

Sodium valproate + Aspirin or NSAIDs

Sodium valproate toxicity developed in three patients given large and repeated doses of aspirin. Conversely, a slightly reduced valproate level was reported in one patient after taking ibuprofen. Modestly altered protein binding has been shown with sodium valproate and diflunisal or naproxen, but this appears unlikely to be clinically important.

Clinical evidence, mechanism, importance and management

(a) Aspirin

A 17-year-old girl taking sodium valproate 21 mg/kg daily was prescribed aspirin 18 mg/kg daily for lupus arthritis. Within a few days she developed a disabling tremor which disappeared when the aspirin was stopped. Total serum valproate levels were not significantly changed, but the free fraction fell from 24% to 14% when the aspirin was withdrawn. Similar toxic reactions (tremor, nystagmus, drowsiness, ataxia) were seen in 2 children, aged 6 and 4 years, given 12 and 20 mg/kg aspirin every 4 hours while taking sodium valproate.[1] One case report of fatal hyperammonaemia was speculated to have been induced by valproate, and the authors also considered that concurrent use of aspirin and 'cimetidine', (p.384) may have contributed.[2]

Aspirin displaces sodium valproate from its protein binding sites[3] and also alters its metabolism by the liver[4] so that the levels of free (and pharmacologically active) sodium valproate rise. This could temporarily increase both the therapeutic and toxic effects of the sodium valproate. However, there is evidence that increased hepatic elimination of sodium valproate counterbalances this effect.

Direct information seems to be limited to the studies cited. Clinically relevant interactions appear rare, probably because in most cases the effects of aspirin on free valproate levels cancel each other out. The combination need not necessarily be avoided, but it would seem prudent to be aware of this interaction if valproate and high-dose aspirin are used. More study is needed.

(b) Diflunisal

Diflunisal 250 mg twice daily for 7 days given with sodium valproate 200 mg twice daily caused a 20% increase in the unbound fraction of valproate in 7 healthy subjects. There was a 35% increase in the AUC of one of the oxidation metabolites of valproate, and a small decrease in the AUC of some of the diflunisal glucuronide metabolites. This was shown to be due to changes in renal clearance of these metabolites.[5] Whether any of these modest changes have any clinical relevance remains to be seen, but it appears unlikely.

(c) Ibuprofen

A 15-year-old boy was found to have a subtherapeutic valproate level (43 micrograms/ml) 3 days after starting to take ibuprofen 600 mg every 6 hours for post-fracture analgesia. The ibuprofen was stopped, and after one week the valproate levels were within the therapeutic range (60 micrograms/ml).[6] The general importance of this isolated case is unknown. More study is needed.

(d) Naproxen

A study in 6 healthy subjects found that naproxen 500 mg twice daily moderately decreased the AUC of valproate by 11% after a single 800-mg dose of sodium valproate.[7] Similarly, in another study, when naproxen 500 mg twice daily was given with sodium valproate 500 mg twice daily the AUC of valproate was decreased by 20% and the AUC of naproxen was increased by 7%. It is suggested that naproxen and sodium valproate displace each other from their protein binding sites.[7,8] The clinical relevance of these modest changes is uncertain, but is likely to be small.[7]

1. Goulden KJ, Dooley JM, Camfield PR, Fraser AD. Clinical valproate toxicity induced by acetylsalicylic acid. *Neurology* (1987) 37, 1392–4.
2. Ichikawa H, Amano T, Kawabata K, Kushiro M, Wada J, Nagake Y, Makino H. Fatal hyperammonemia in a patient with systemic lupus erythematosus. *Intern Med* (1998) 37, 700–3.
3. Orr JM, Abbott FS, Farrell K, Ferguson S, Sheppard I, Godolphin W. Interaction between valproic acid and aspirin in epileptic children: serum protein binding and metabolic effects. *Clin Pharmacol Ther* (1982) 31, 642–9.
4. Abbott FS, Kassam J, Orr JM, Farrell K. The effect of aspirin on valproic acid metabolism. *Clin Pharmacol Ther* (1986) 40, 94–100.
5. Addison RS, Parker-Scott SL, Eadie MJ, Hooper WD, Dickinson RG. Steady-state dispositions of valproate and diflunisal alone and coadministration to healthy volunteers. *Eur J Clin Pharmacol* (2000) 56, 715–21.
6. Mankin KP, Scanlon M. Side effect of ibuprofen and valproic acid. *Orthopedics* (1998) 21, 264, 270.
7. Grimaldi R, Lecchini S, Crema F, Perucca E. *In vivo* plasma protein binding interaction between valproic acid and naproxen. *Eur J Drug Metab Pharmacokinet* (1984) 9, 359–63.
8. Addison RS, Parker-Scott SL, Hooper WD, Eadie MJ, Dickinson RG. Effect of naproxen co-administration on valproate disposition. *Biopharm Drug Dispos* (2000) 21, 235–42.

Sodium valproate + Bile-acid binding resins

Colestyramine causes a very small reduction in the absorption of valproate. No interaction occurs if administration of the drugs is separated by 3 hours. Colesevelam does not interact.

Clinical evidence

(a) Colesevelam

Colesevelam 4.5 g had no effect on the pharmacokinetics of valproic acid 250 mg in a single-dose study in 26 healthy subjects.[1]

(b) Colestyramine

A single 250-mg dose of valproic acid was given to 6 healthy subjects either alone, at the same time as colestyramine 4 g twice daily, or with the colestyramine taken 3 hours after the valproic acid. The bioavailability of valproate taken alone and when separated from the colestyramine by 3 hours remained the same. When the valproate was taken at the same time as the colestyramine the valproate AUC fell by 15% and the maximum serum levels fell by 21%.[2,3]

Mechanism

Colestyramine is a ion-exchange resin intended to bind with bile acids in the gut, but it can also bind with drugs as well, leading to a reduction in their absorption. This apparently occurs to a limited extent with sodium valproate.

Importance and management

Direct information on colestyramine appears to be limited to this single study, but what happened is consistent with the way colestyramine interacts with a number of other drugs. The fall in the bioavailability is small and probably of very limited clinical importance, but the interaction can be totally avoided by separating the dosages by 3 hours so that admixture in the gut is minimised. Colesevelam does not interact.

1. Donovan JM, Stypinski D, Stiles MR, Olson TA, Burke SK. Drug interactions with colesevelam hydrochloride, a novel, potent lipid-lowering agent. *Cardiovasc Drugs Ther* (2000) 14, 681–90.
2. Pennell AT, Ravis WR, Malloy MJ, Sead A, Diskin C. Cholestyramine decreases valproic acid serum concentrations. *J Clin Pharmacol* (1992) 32, 755.
3. Malloy MJ, Ravis WR, Pennell AT, Diskin CJ. Effect of cholestyramine resin on single dose valproate pharmacokinetics. *Int J Clin Pharmacol Ther* (1996) 34, 208–11.

Sodium valproate + Carbapenems

Panipenem/betamipron dramatically reduced the valproate serum levels of 6 patients. Meropenem had a similar effect in 2 patients. Ertapenem is predicted to interact similarly.

Clinical evidence

(a) Meropenem

A report describes two cases of a drop in valproate levels in patients who were given meropenem and amikacin. The first patient had been maintained on intravenous valproate 1.2 to 1.6 g daily with valproate levels of between 50 and 100 mg/l. Two days after the addition of the antibacterials the levels had halved, and after three days of subtherapeutic levels, phenytoin was substituted for valproate. The other patient experienced a drop in valproate levels from 44 mg/l to 5 mg/l within 24 hours of being given meropenem, despite being given greater doses of valproic acid.[1]

(b) Panipenem

A report describes 3 cases of Japanese children on anticonvulsant therapy who had marked reductions in valproate serum levels while receiving panipenem/betamipron for serious chest infections.[2] An increased seizure-frequency occurred in 2 of the patients. In one case the serum valproate levels fell from 30.1 to 1.53 mg/l within 4 days of starting the antimicrobial treatment, and rose again when it was stopped. All 3 patients were also taking carbamazepine but its serum levels were unchanged by the panipenem/betamipron. In a further 3 cases, 60 to 100% reductions in valproate levels, occurring within 2 days of starting concurrent treatment have been reported. Increased seizure frequency occurred in 2 cases.[3]

Mechanism

Unknown, but the speed of the interaction is said to be inconsistent with enzyme induction, and accelerated renal excretion has been suggested.[1] Altered protein binding has been shown in *animal* and *in vitro* studies.[4]

Importance and management

Information appears to be limited to these reports but it would now be prudent to monitor the valproate levels in any patient given carbapenems, being alert for the need to increase the valproate dosage, or to use another antibacterial, or an alternative to valproate. Carbamazepine[2] and phenytoin[1] did not interact in the above reports. The makers of **ertapenem** have no reports of an interaction on their files,[5] but prudently warn about a possible interaction with valproate[6] because of warnings given about all carbapenems by the authors of these reports.

1. De Turck BJG, Diltoer MW, Cornelis PJWW, Maes V, Spapen HDM, Camu F, Huyghens LP. *J Antimicrob Chemother* (1998) 42, 563–4.
2. Nagai K, Shimizu T, Togo A, Takeya M, Yokomizo Y, Sakata Y, Matsuishi T, Kato H. Decrease in serum levels of valproic acid during treatment with a new carbapenem, panipenem/betamipron. *J Antimicrob Chemother* (1997) 39, 295–6.
3. Yamagata T, Momoi MY, Murai K, Ikematsu K, Suwa K, Sakamoto K, Fujimura A. Panipenem—Betamipron and decreases in serum valproic acid concentration. *Ther Drug Monit* (1998) 20, 396–400.
4. Hobara N, Hokama N, Ohshiro S, Kameya H, Sakanashi M. Possible mechanisms of low levels of plasma valproate concentration following simultaneous administration of sodium valproate and meropenem. *Biog Amines* (2003) 17, 409–20.
5. Merck Sharp & Dohme. Personal communication, September 2003.
6. Invanz (Ertapenem). Merck Sharp & Dohme Ltd. UK Summary of product characteristics, January 2004.

Sodium valproate + Chlorpromazine

Sodium valproate serum levels are slightly raised in patients given chlorpromazine, but this appears to be of minimal clinical importance. An isolated report describes severe hepatotoxicity on concurrent use.

Clinical evidence, mechanism, importance and management

The steady-state trough serum levels of valproate 400 mg daily rose by 22% when 6 patients were given chlorpromazine 100 to 300 mg daily. The half-life increased by 14% and the clearance fell by 14% (possibly due to some reduction in the metabolism by the liver)[1]. This interaction would normally seem to be of minimal importance. Severe hepatotoxicity occurred in another patient when given both drugs,[2] but remember that both drugs independently, can be hepatotoxic.

1. Ishizaki T, Chiba K, Saito M, Kobayashi K, Iizuka R. The effects of neuroleptics (haloperidol and chlorpromazine) on the pharmacokinetics of valproic acid in schizophrenic patients. *J Clin Psychopharmacol* (1984) 4, 254–61.
2. Bach N, Thung SN, Schaffner F, Tobias H. Exaggerated cholestasis and hepatic fibrosis following simultaneous administration of chlorpromazine and sodium valproate. *Dig Dis Sci* (1989) 34, 1303–7.

Sodium valproate + Erythromycin

Two isolated reports describe sodium valproate toxicity in a woman and a child given erythromycin. Another report describes vitamin K deficiency in a child given valproate and erythromycin.

Clinical evidence, mechanism, importance and management

A woman taking lithium and sodium valproate 3.5 g daily developed fatigue and walking difficulties a day after starting to take erythromycin 250 mg four times daily. Within a week she had also developed slurred speech, confusion, difficulty in concentrating and a worsening gait. Her serum valproate levels had risen from 88 mg/l (measured 2 months before) to 260 mg/l. She recovered within 24 hours of the valproate and erythromycin being withdrawn. Her serum lithium levels remained unchanged.[1] A child on sodium valproate had a threefold increase in serum valproate levels when treated with erythromycin 150 mg every 8 hours and aspirin 250 mg every 6 hours for 3 days.[2] These case reports contrast with another study in a 10-year-old boy taking valproic acid 375 mg twice daily who had only very small and clinically unimportant changes in the pharmacokinetics of valproate, consistent with inhibition of cytochrome P450 metabolism, when given erythromycin 250 mg four times daily.[3]

Another child on valproic acid developed a deficiency of prothrombin complex after treatment with erythromycin 300 mg three times daily. This resolved when the patient was treated with oral vitamin K. It was suggested that the effect was because of suppression of vitamin-K producing intestinal bacteria.[4]

The general relevance of these isolated reports is unclear, but probably small. Further study is needed.

1. Redington K, Wells C, Petito F. Erythromycin and valproate interaction. *Ann Intern Med* (1992) 116, 877–8.
2. Sanchez-Romero A, Pamirez IO. Interacción ácido valproico-eritromicina. *An Esp Pediatr* (1990) 32, 78–9.
3. Gopaul SV, Farrell K, Rakshi K, Abbott FS. A case study of erythromycin interaction with valproic acid. *Pharm Res* (1996) 13 (9 Suppl), S434.
4. Cordes I, Buchmann S, Scheffner D. Vitamin K-mangel unter Erythromycin. Beobachtung bei einem mit Valproat behandelten Jungen. *Monatsschr Kinderheilkd* (1990) 138, 85–7.

Sodium valproate + Felbamate

Felbamate can raise sodium valproate serum levels causing toxicity.

Clinical evidence

(a) Effect on sodium valproate

The average steady-state valproate serum levels in 7 epileptics were raised by 28%, from 66.9 to 85.4 micrograms/ml, by felbamate 1.2 g daily, and by 54%, from 66.9 to 103 micrograms/ml by felbamate 2.4 g daily. The AUC of valproate was raised by 28% and 54% by felbamate 1.2 and 2.4 g respectively.[1] Valproate clearance was correspondingly reduced by felbamate.[1] Similar effects were seen in another study.[2,3] It was suggested that in children the interaction may be more marked.[3] Many of the patients experienced nausea. Other toxic effects included lethargy, drowsiness, headaches, cognitive disturbances and low platelet counts.[1,2]

(b) Effect on felbamate

The clearance of felbamate was decreased 21% by sodium valproate in one study,[4] and another reported a significantly lower felbamate clearance in the presence of valproate.[5] Yet another study noted only a minimal effect of sodium valproate on felbamate clearance.[6]

Mechanism

Uncertain. Altered plasma protein binding of sodium valproate is unlikely to be important.[7] Felbamate may cause inhibition of the oxidative pathway of valproate metabolism.[8]

Importance and management

An established interaction. It may be necessary to reduce the sodium valproate dosage to avoid toxicity if felbamate is given. The authors of one report suggest a 30 to 50% reduction. It may also be necessary to reduce the felbamate dosage as well. Monitor concurrent use closely, particularly during the initial stages.

1. Wagner ML, Graves NM, Leppik IE, Remmel RP, Shumaker RC, Ward DL, Perhach JL. The effect of felbamate on valproic acid disposition. *Clin Pharmacol Ther* (1994) 56, 494–502.
2. Liu H, Delgado MR. Significant drug interaction between valproate and felbamate in epileptic children. *Epilepsia* (1995) 36 (Suppl 3), S160.
3. Delgado MR. Changes in valproic acid concentrations and dose/level ratios by felbamate coadministration in children. *Ann Neurol* (1994) 36, 538.
4. Kelley MT, Walson PD, Cox S, Dusci LJ. Population pharmacokinetics of felbamate in children. *Ther Drug Monit* (1997) 19, 29–36.
5. Wagner ML, Leppik IE, Graves NM, Remme RP, Campbell JI. Felbamate serum concentrations: effect of valproate, carbamazepine, phenytoin and phenobarbital. *Epilepsia* (1990) 31, 642.
6. Banfield CR, Zhu G-RR, Jen JF, Jensen PK, Schumaker RC, Perhach JL Affrime MB, Glue P. The effect of age on the apparent clearance of felbamate: a retrospective analysis using nonlinear mixed-effects modeling. *Ther Drug Monit* (1996) 18, 19–29.
7. Bernus I, Dickinson RG, Hooper WD, Franklin ME. Effect of felbamate on the plasma protein binding of valproate. *Clin Drug Invest* (1995) 10, 288–95.
8. Hooper WD, Franklin ME, Glue P, Banfield CR, Radwanski E, McLaughlin DB, McIntyre ME, Dickinson RG, Eadie MJ. Effect of felbamate on valproic acid disposition in healthy volunteers: inhibition of ß-oxidation. *Epilepsia* (1996) 37, 91–7.

Sodium valproate + Fluoxetine

Isolated reports describe marked increases or modest decreases in serum valproate levels in a small number of patients given fluoxetine. Valproate toxicity occurred in one patient.

Clinical evidence

A mentally retarded patient with an atypical bipolar disorder on semisodium valproate (divalproex sodium) 3 g daily had a rise in serum valproic acid levels from 93.5 to 152 mg/l within 2 weeks of starting to take fluoxetine 20 mg daily. The valproate dosage was reduced to 2.25 g daily and 2 weeks later the serum valproic acid levels had fallen to 113 mg/l. No adverse effects were seen.[1] Another woman developed elevated serum valproate levels (a rise from 78 to 126 mg/l) without any accompanying clinical symptoms within 1 month of starting to take fluoxetine 20 mg daily. Valproate levels fell again when the fluoxetine was stopped.[2] Similarly, a 17-year old on valproic acid and felbamate developed drowsiness and difficulty in being roused 2 weeks after starting fluoxetine 20 mg daily. His valproate level had increased to 141 micrograms/ml from a previous range of 100 to 110 micrograms/ml. His valproate dose was reduced by about 15%, and his consciousness improved.[3]

In contrast 2 cases of reduced valproate levels with fluoxetine have also been reported. In the first case, a 67-year-old woman taking valproic acid 2 g daily and fluoxetine 20 mg daily had a serum valproate level of 51.9 mg/l. This increased to 64.9 mg/l 9 days after fluoxetine was discontinued and fell to 32.6 mg/l 6 days after fluoxetine was re-started. In the second case, an 81-year-old woman was taking valproic acid 1 g with fluoxetine 20 mg daily and had serum valproate levels of 41.9 mg/l. The fluoxetine was stopped, and 6 days later valproate serum levels had risen to 56.2 mg/l. After re-introduction of fluoxetine her valproate levels fell to 45.6 mg/l.[4]

Mechanism

Not understood.

Importance and management

These reports are somewhat confusing and inconsistent, but the overall picture is that concurrent use need not be avoided, but that the outcome should probably be monitored. More study is needed.

1. Sovner R, Davis JM. A potential drug interaction between fluoxetine and valproic acid. *J Clin Psychopharmacol* (1991) 11, 389.
2. Lucena MI, Blanco E, Corrales MA, Berthier ML. Interaction of fluoxetine and valproic acid. *Am J Psychiatry* (1998) 155, 575.

3. Cruz-Flores S, Hayat GR, Mirza W. Valproic toxicity with fluoxetine therapy. Missouri Med 1995 Jun 92 (6) 296–7.
4. Droulers A, Bodak N, Oudjhani M, Lefevre des Noettes V, Bodak A. Decrease of valproic acid concentration in the blood when coprescribed with fluoxetine. *J Clin Psychopharmacol* (1997) 17, 139–40.

Sodium valproate + H_2-blockers

Ranitidine does not interact with sodium valproate, and cimetidine interacts only minimally.

Clinical evidence, mechanism, importance and management

The clearance of a single oral dose of sodium valproate was reduced in 6 patients by 2 to 17% after a 4-week course of **cimetidine**, but not by **ranitidine**.[1] It seems doubtful if the interaction between sodium valproate and **cimetidine** is of clinical importance. However, a case of fatal hyperammonaemia in a patient with systemic lupus erythematosus was speculated to have been induced by valproate, and the authors also considered that the concurrent use of **cimetidine** and aspirin (see 'Sodium valproate + Aspirin or NSAIDs', p.381) may have contributed.[2] The general importance of this case is unknown.

1. Webster LK, Mihaly GW, Jones DB, Smallwood RA, Phillips JA, Vajda FJ. Effect of cimetidine and ranitidine on carbamazepine and sodium valproate pharmacokinetics. *Eur J Clin Pharmacol* (1984) 27, 341–3.
2. Ichikawa H, Amano T, Kawabata K, Kushiro M, Wada J, Nagake Y, Makino H. Fatal hyperammonemia in a patient with systemic lupus erythematosus. *Intern Med* (1998) 37, 700–3.

Sodium valproate + Isoniazid

An isolated report describes the development of raised serum valproate levels and toxicity in a child concurrently treated with valproate and isoniazid. Another describes raised hepatic enzymes and drowsiness.

Clinical evidence, mechanism, importance and management

A 5-year-old girl with left partial seizures, successfully controlled on sodium valproate 600 mg daily and clonazepam for 7 months, developed signs of sodium valproate toxicity (drowsiness, asthenia) shortly after starting to take isoniazid 200 mg daily (because of a positive tuberculin reaction). Her serum valproate levels were found to have risen to around 121 to 139 mg/l (normal therapeutic range 50 to 100 mg/l).[1] Over the next few months various changes were made in her treatment, the most significant being a 62% reduction in the dosage of sodium valproate, needed to maintain satisfactory therapeutic levels. Later when the isoniazid was stopped her valproate levels fell below therapeutic levels and seizures recurred. It was then found necessary to increase the valproate to its former dosage. The suggested explanation is that the isoniazid inhibited the metabolism (oxidation) of the sodium valproate by the liver so that it accumulated. The child was found to be a very slow acetylator of isoniazid.[1]

Another child who had been treated with valproate for several years was started on isoniazid for the treatment of tuberculosis. At the same time, seizures recurred, and the valproate was stopped and primidone 750 mg daily started. Seven months later seizures persisted, and she was admitted to hospital. Liver enzyme values were normal. Valproate, 300 mg daily increased to 600 mg daily was added, and within 2 days she was vomiting and drowsy. After 5 days she had increased liver enzymes and her prothrombin time had fallen, so the valproate was stopped. Valproate levels were 81 micrograms/ml. It was speculated that the CNS effects and hepatic impairment were due to an interaction between the valproate and isoniazid.[2]

The general importance of these cases is uncertain, but bear them in mind in the event of an unexpected response to treatment.

1. Jonville AP, Gauchez AS, Autret E, Billard C, Barbier P, Nsabiyumva F, Breteau M. Interaction between isoniazid and valproate: a case of valproate overdosage. *Eur J Clin Pharmacol* (1991) 40, 197–8.
2. Dockweiler U. Isoniazid-induced valproic-acid toxicity, or vice versa. *Lancet* (1987) ii, 152.

Sodium valproate + Propranolol

One patient had a reduction in sodium valproate clearance when given propranolol, but 12 other patients had no changes.

Clinical evidence, mechanism, importance and management

An isolated report describes a 28% reduction in sodium valproate clearance in a patient given propranolol 40 mg, and a 35% reduction with propranolol 80 mg. However, 12 other patients on sodium valproate had no changes in clearance, serum levels or half-life when given propranolol 60 or 120 mg daily for 3 weeks.[1] This interaction would therefore not appear to be of general importance. No special precautions would seem necessary.

1. Nemire RE, Toledo CA, Ramsay RE. A pharmacokinetic study to determine the drug interaction between valproate and propranolol. *Pharmacotherapy* (1996) 16, 1059–62.

Sodium valproate + Theophylline

A study in 6 healthy subjects found that oral aminophylline 200 mg every 6 hours for 3 doses did not affect the pharmacokinetics of a single 400-mg dose of sodium valproate.[1]

1. Kulkarni C, Vaz J, David J, Joseph T. Aminophylline alters pharmacokinetics of carbamazepine but not that of sodium valproate — a single dose pharmacokinetic study in human volunteers. *Indian J Physiol Pharmacol* (1995) 39, 122–6.

Stiripentol + Other anticonvulsants

Stiripentol causes marked rises in the serum levels of carbamazepine, phenobarbital and phenytoin. Reduce their dosages to avoid the development of toxicity. Stiripentol causes only a small rise in the serum levels of sodium valproate and dosage adjustments are not needed.

Clinical evidence

Epileptic patients taking two or three anticonvulsants (**phenytoin**, **phenobarbital**, **carbamazepine**, **clobazam**, **primidone**, **nitrazepam**) were also given stiripentol, increasing from 600 mg to 2.4 g daily. All 5 patients on **phenytoin** had an average 37% reduction in the **phenytoin** clearance while taking stiripentol 1.2 g daily, and a 78% reduction while taking stiripentol 2.4 g daily. These changes in clearance were reflected in marked rises in the steady-state serum levels of **phenytoin**: for example the serum **phenytoin** levels of one patient rose from 14.4 to 27.4 mg/l over 30 days while he was taking stiripentol, despite a 50% reduction in his **phenytoin** dosage. **Phenytoin** toxicity was seen in another two subjects.[1] The clearance of **carbamazepine** in one subject fell by 39% with stiripentol 1.2 g daily and by 71% with stiripentol 2.4 g daily. **Phenobarbital** clearance in two subjects fell by about 30 to 40% with stiripentol 2.4 g daily.[1] Three other studies in adults and children confirmed that stiripentol reduces the clearance of **carbamazepine** by between about 50% and 65%,[2-4] and significantly increases carbamazepine levels.[5] Another study found that the formation of the active epoxide metabolite of **carbamazepine** was markedly reduced in children on **carbamazepine** given stiripentol.[6]

Sodium valproate 1 g daily was given to 8 subjects with or without stiripentol 1.2 g daily. The stiripentol caused a 14% increase in peak serum levels of the **valproate**.[7] In another 11 patients no adverse effects on motor, perceptual or attention tests were seen when stiripentol was combined with other antiepileptic drugs, but the doses of **phenobarbital**, **phenytoin** and **carbamazepine** were reduced before the combination was taken.[8]

Mechanism

Stiripentol inhibits the activity of various cytochrome P450 liver isoenzymes including CYP1A2, CYP2C9, CYP2C19, CYP2D6 and CYP3A4, some of which are concerned with the metabolism of other anticonvulsants. As a result the loss of the anticonvulsant from the body is reduced and the serum levels rise accordingly.[3,9] In the case of sodium valproate, cytochrome P450-mediated metabolism is only involved in minor valproate metabolic pathways and therefore only a small rise in serum levels occurs.[7] However, there is evidence that stiripentol may reduce the formation of a minor but hepatotoxic metabolite of sodium valproate (2-propyl-4-pentenoic acid or 4-ene-VPA).[10]

Importance and management

Established and clinically important interactions. The phenytoin, phenobarbital and carbamazepine dosages should be reduced to avoid the development of elevated serum levels and possible toxicity during the concurrent use of stiripentol. In the case of phenytoin, halving the dose may not be enough. One study[3] suggests that the carbamazepine dosage should be decreased incrementally over 7 to 10 days, beginning as soon as the stiripentol is started and, regardless of age, the maintenance dose of carbamazepine should aim to give serum levels of 5 to 10 micrograms/ml. Stiripentol causes only small changes in the serum levels of sodium valproate and dosage adjustments are unlikely to be needed with this combination.

1. Levy RH, Loiseau P, Guyot M, Blehaut HM, Tor J, Morland TA. Stiripentol kinetics in epilepsy: nonlinearity and interactions. *Clin Pharmacol Ther* (1984) 36, 661–9.
2. Levy RH, Kerr BM, Farwell J, Anderson GD, Martinez-Lage JM, Tor J. Carbamazepine/stiripentol interaction in adult and pediatric patients. *Epilepsia* (1989) 30, 701.
3. Kerr BM, Martinez-Lage JM, Viteri C, Tor J, Eddy AC, Levy RH. Carbamazepine dose requirements during stiripentol therapy: influence of cytochrome P-450 inhibition by stiripentol. *Epilepsia* (1991) 32, 267–74.
4. Levy RH, Martinez-Lage JM, Tor J, Blehaut H, Gonzalez I, Bainbridge B. Stiripentol level-dose relationship and interaction with carbamazepine in epileptic patients. *Epilepsia* (1985) 26, 544–5.
5. Tran A, Vauzelle-Kervroedan F, Rey E, Pons G. d'Athis P, Chiron C, Dulac O, Renard F, Olive G. Effect of stiripentol on carbamazepine plasma concentration and metabolism in epileptic children. *Eur J Clin Pharmacol* (1996) 50, 497–500.
6. Cazali N, Tran A, Treluyer JM, Rey E, d'Athis P, Vincent J, Pons G. Inhibitory effect of stiripentol on carbamazepine and saquinavir metabolism in human. *Br J Clin Pharmacol* (2003) 56, 526–36.
7. Levy RH, Loiseau P, Guyot M, Acheampong A, Tor J, Rettenmeier AW. Effects of stiripentol on valproate plasma level and metabolism. *Epilepsia* (1987) 28, 605.
8. Loiseau P, Strube E, Tor J, Levy RH, Dodrill C. Evaluation neuropsychologique et thérapeutique du stiripentol dans l'épilepsie. *Rev Neurol (Paris)* (1988) 144, 165–72.
9. Mather GG, Bishop FE, Trager WF, Kunze KK, Thummel KE, Shen DD, Roskos LK, Lepage F, Gillardin JM, Levy RH. Mechanisms of stiripentol interactions with carbamazepine and phenytoin. *Epilepsia* (1995) 36 (Suppl 3), S162.
10. Levy RH, Rettenmeier AW, Anderson GD, Wilensky AJ, Friel PN, Baillie TA, Acheampong A, Tor J, Guyot M, Loiseau P. Effects of polytherapy with phenytoin, carbamazepine, and stiripentol on formation of 4-ene-valproate, a hepatotoxic metabolite of valproic acid. *Clin Pharmacol Ther* (1990) 48, 225–35.

Tiagabine + Miscellaneous

The pharmacokinetics of tiagabine were not altered by cimetidine or erythromycin. No clinically relevant pharmacokinetic interactions occur between tiagabine and theophylline or warfarin.

Clinical evidence, mechanism, importance and management

Cimetidine 400 mg twice daily for 5 days increased the steady-state AUC of tiagabine 4 mg twice daily by just 5% in a study in 12 healthy subjects.[1,2] This change would not be clinically relevant.

Erythromycin 500 mg twice daily had no clinically relevant effect on the steady-state pharmacokinetics of tiagabine 4 mg twice daily in a study in 14 healthy subjects.[3] No dose adjustment would be required during concurrent use.

Multiple dose studies in healthy subjects have also excluded any clinically relevant pharmacokinetic interactions between tiagabine and **theophylline** or **warfarin** but no further study details were given.[1]

1. Mengel H, Jansen JA, Sommerville K, Jonkman JHG, Wesnes K, Cohen A, Carlson GF, Marshall R, Snel S, Dirach J, Kastberg H. Tiagabine: evaluation of the risk of interaction with theophylline, warfarin, digoxin, cimetidine, oral contraceptives, triazolam, or ethanol. *Epilepsia* (1995) 36 (Suppl 3), S160.
2. Snel S, Jonkman JHG, van Heiningen PNM, Jansen JA, Mengel HB. Tiagabine: evaluation of risk of interaction with cimetidine in healthy male volunteers. *Epilepsia* (1994) 35 (Suppl 7), 74.
3. Thomsen MS, Groes L, Agersø H, Kruse T. Lack of pharmacokinetic interaction between tiagabine and erythromycin. *J Clin Pharmacol* (1998) 38, 1051–6.

Tiagabine + Other anticonvulsants

Tiagabine serum levels are reduced by enzyme-inducing anticonvulsants (carbamazepine, phenytoin, phenobarbital and primidone). Tiagabine doses may need to be lower in patients *not* on these drugs. Tiagabine may cause a slight reduction in sodium valproate levels (not clinically relevant), but has no effect on carbamazepine, phenytoin or vigabatrin levels.

Clinical evidence, mechanism, importance and management

In an early clinical study, tiagabine was reported to have no significant effect on the plasma levels of **carbamazepine**, **phenytoin**, **valproate**, and **vigabatrin**.[1] Similarly, tiagabine (titrated from 8 mg up to a maximum of 48 mg daily over 18 days) did not alter the steady-state pharmacokinetics of **phenytoin** or **carbamazepine** in 12 patients with epilepsy.[2] However, in another similar study, it reduced the AUC of **valproate** by 10%, but this reduction is not expected to be clinically significant.[3]

A study in patients taking 1 to 3 other enzyme-inducing anticonvulsants (**phenobarbital**, **phenytoin**, **carbamazepine**, **primidone**) found that tiagabine half-lives were shorter (3.8 to 4.9 hours) when compared with historical values in healthy subjects taking only tiagabine (7.1 hours).[4] The makers say that the plasma concentrations of tiagabine may be reduced 1.5 to 3-fold by these enzyme-inducing anticonvulsants.[5] Based on this, they recommend that the initial maintenance dose of tiagabine in patients *not* on enzyme-inducing drugs should be lower (15 to 30 mg daily) than in those on these drugs (30 to 45 mg daily).[5]

1. Richens A, Chadwick DW, Duncan JS, Dam M, Gram L, Mikkelsen M, Morrow J, Mengel H, Shu V, McKelvy JF, Pierce MW. Adjunctive treatment of partial seizures with tiagabine: a placebo-controlled trial. *Epilepsy Res* (1995) 21, 37–42.
2. Gustavson LE, Cato A, Boellner SW, Cao GX, Qian JX, Guenther HJ, Sommerville KW. Lack of pharmacokinetic drug interactions between tiagabine and carbamazepine or phenytoin. *Am J Ther* (1998) 5, 9–16.
3. Gustavson LE, Sommerville KW, Boellner SW, Witt GF, Guenther HJ, Granneman GR. Lack of a clinically significant pharmacokinetic drug interaction between tiagabine and valproate. *Am J Ther* (1998) 5, 73–79.
4. So EL, Wolff D, Graves NM, Leppik IE, Cascino GD, Pixton GC, Gustavson LE. Pharmacokinetics of tiagabine as add-on therapy in patients taking enzyme-inducing drugs. *Epilepsy Res* (1995) 22, 221–6.
5. Gabitril (Tiagabine). Cephalon UK Ltd. UK Summary of product characteristics, November 2003.

Topiramate + Carbamazepine

Topiramate serum levels may be reduced by carbamazepine. Carbamazepine levels are not affected by topiramate, although one report suggests that toxicity seen on the addition of topiramate to maximum tolerated doses of carbamazepine may respond to a reduction in the carbamazepine dose.

Clinical evidence

(a) Carbamazepine levels

Topiramate titrated up to a maximum of 400 mg twice daily had no effect on the steady-state serum levels of carbamazepine 300 to 800 mg every 8 hours or on its main metabolite in a study in 12 epileptic patients.[1] An earlier study in epileptic patients also reported that topiramate does not affect the pharmacokinetics of carbamazepine.[2] In contrast, another report describes 2 patients on a maximum tolerated dose of carbamazepine who started treatment with topiramate and subsequently developed symptoms suggestive of carbamazepine toxicity. In both these cases, the symptoms resolved when the carbamazepine dose was reduced, and this enabled continued titration of the topiramate dose in one. A review of clinical experience found another 23 cases that fitted this pattern. Carbamazepine levels were not reported.[3]

(b) Topiramate levels

The topiramate serum levels and AUC were found to be about 40% lower in the presence of carbamazepine in a study in 12 epileptic patients.[1] A population pharmacokinetic study reported that patients on carbamazepine had 32% lower morning topiramate concentration than patients not on enzyme-inducing anticonvulsants.[4] In contrast, an earlier study reported that carbamazepine did not have a major effect on the pharmacokinetics of topiramate.[2]

Mechanism

Carbamazepine appears to induce the metabolism of topiramate. Topiramate would not be expected to affect the metabolism of carbamazepine since it does not affect the cytochrome P450 isoenzyme CYP3A4.[5]

Importance and management

Carbamazepine possibly results in a moderate reduction in topiramate serum levels, but this is probably of limited clinical importance. There is some evidence that toxicity seen on the addition of topiramate to maximum tolerated doses of carbamazepine may respond to a reduction in the carbamazepine dose.

1. Sachdeo RC, Sachdeo SK, Walker SA, Kramer LD, Nayak RK, Doose DR. Steady-state pharmacokinetics of topiramate and carbamazepine in patients with epilepsy during monotherapy and concomitant therapy. *Epilepsia* (1996) 37, 774–80.
2. Wilensky AJ, Ojemann LM, Chemelir T, Margul BL, Doose DR. Topiramate pharmacokinetics in epileptic patients receiving carbamazepine. *Epilepsia* (1989) 30, 645–6.
3. Mack CJ, Kuc S, Mulcrone SA, Pilley A, Grünewald RA. Interaction of topiramate with carbamazepine: two case reports and a review of clinical experience. *Seizure* (2002) 11, 464–7.
4. May TW, Jürges U. Serum concentrations of topiramate in epileptic patients: the influence of dose and comedication. *Epilepsia* (1999) 40 (Suppl 2), 249.
5. Levy RH, Bishop F, Streeter AJ, Trager WF, Kunze KL, Thummel KT, Mather GG. Explanation and prediction of drug interactions with topiramate using a CYP450 inhibition spectrum. *Epilepsia* (1995) 36 (Suppl 4), 47.

Topiramate + Phenobarbital or Primidone

Topiramate appears not to alter the pharmacokinetics of phenobarbital or primidone. Phenobarbital reduces topiramate levels.

Clinical evidence, mechanism, importance and management

A review of data from double blind, placebo-controlled studies found that over periods of 8 to 12 weeks the serum levels of phenobarbital or primidone in outpatients [number not stated] with partial seizures remained unchanged when they were also given topiramate.[1]

A population pharmacokinetic study reported that patients on phenobarbital had 31% lower morning topiramate concentration than patients not on enzyme-inducing anticonvulsants.[2] Another study that grouped carbamazepine, phenobarbital and phenytoin reported that patients on one or more of these drugs had 1.5-fold greater topiramate clearance than patients on lamotrigine or valproate.[3] Phenobarbital probably induces the metabolism of topiramate so reducing its levels.

When topiramate is added to existing therapy, its dose should be titrated to effect. If phenobarbital or primidone are withdrawn or added, be aware that the dose of topiramate may need adjustment.

1. Doose DR, Walker SA, Pledger G, Lim P, Reife RA. Evaluation of phenobarbital and primidone/phenobarbital (primidone's active metabolite) plasma concentrations during administration of add-on topiramate therapy in five multicenter, double-blind, placebo-controlled trials in outpatients with partial seizures. *Epilepsia* (1995) 36 (Suppl 3), S158.
2. May TW, Jürges U. Serum concentrations of topiramate in epileptic patients: the influence of dose and comedication. *Epilepsia* (1999) 40 (Suppl 2), 249.
3. Contin M, Riva R, Albani F, Avoni P, Baruzzi A. Topiramate therapeutic monitoring in patients with epilepsy: effect of concomitant antiepileptic drugs. *Ther Drug Monit* (2002) 24, 332–7.

Topiramate + Phenytoin

The serum levels of phenytoin in some patients are slightly raised by topiramate, and topiramate serum levels may be reduced by phenytoin.

Clinical evidence

Topiramate, titrated to a maximum of 400 mg twice daily, was given to 12 epileptics stabilised on phenytoin 260 to 600 mg daily. When the maximum tolerated dose of topiramate was reached, the phenytoin dose was then reduced, and in some cases subsequently discontinued. Topiramate clearance was assessed in 2 patients and was found to be increased two to threefold by phenytoin.[1] Similarly, a population pharmacokinetic study reported that patients on phenytoin had 50% lower morning topiramate concentrations than patients not on enzyme-inducing anticonvulsants.[2]

In the first study above, 3 of the 12 patients had a decrease in phenytoin clearance and an increase of 25 to 55% in phenytoin AUC with topiramate, but 9 had no changes.[1] This slight increase is said not to be clinically significant based on analyses from six add-on trials.[3]

Mechanism

An *in vitro* study using human liver microsomes found that topiramate does not inhibit most hepatic cytochrome P450 isoenzymes, except for CYP2C19 at high concentrations.[1] This isoenzyme plays a minor role in phenytoin metabolism, but it has been suggested this may become important at high doses of topiramate in patients who are poor CYP2C9 metabolisers.[1] Phenytoin appears to induce the metabolism of topiramate.

Importance and management

The interaction between topiramate and phenytoin appears to be established, and topiramate dose adjustments may be required when phenytoin therapy is added or discontinued. No reduction in the phenytoin dosage seems necessary in the majority of patients, but be aware that a few patients may have increased phenytoin levels, particularly at high topiramate doses. Monitor phenytoin levels.

1. Sachdeo RC, Sachdeo SK, Levy RH, Streeter AJ, Bishop FE, Kunze KL, Mather GG, Roskos LK, Shen DD, Thummel KE, Trager WF, Curtin CR, Doose DR, Gisclon LG, Bialer M. Topiramate and phenytoin pharmacokinetics during repetitive monotherapy and combination therapy to epileptic patients. *Epilepsia* (2002) 43: 691–6.
2. May TW, Jürges U. Serum concentrations of topiramate in epileptic patients: the influence of dose and comedication. *Epilepsia* (1999) 40 (Suppl, 2), 249.
3. Johannessen SI. Pharmacokinetics and interaction profile of topiramate: review and comparison with other newer antiepileptic drugs. *Epilepsia* (1997) 38 (Suppl 1), S18–S23.

Topiramate + Sodium valproate

There is no clinically relevant pharmacokinetic interaction between topiramate and sodium valproate.

Clinical evidence, mechanism, importance and management

In a study in 12 epileptic patients, the pharmacokinetics of both topiramate, titrated to 400 mg twice daily, and sodium valproate 1 to 4.5 g daily were slightly changed by concurrent use. The topiramate AUC was raised by about 18%, and the sodium valproate AUC was reduced by 11.3%, but these changes were not considered clinically relevant.[1] However, the proportion of various metabolites of valproate was altered by topiramate: metabolism to 4-ene-valproate (a putative hepatotoxin) and metabolism by oxidation increased, whereas conjugation decreased.[1] The clinical importance of these changes is uncertain. Similar changes have been see with other enzyme-inducing anticonvulsants (see Mechanism under 'Phenytoin + Sodium valproate', p.373). At present, there is nothing to suggest that dosage adjustments or special precautions are required during concurrent use.

1. Rosenfeld WE, Liao S, Kramer LD, Anderson G, Palmer M, Levy RH, Nayak RK. Comparison of the steady-state pharmacokinetics of topiramate and valproate in patients with epilepsy during monotherapy and concomitant therapy. *Epilepsia* (1997) 38, 324–33.

Valproate semisodium + Miscellaneous

Valproate semisodium (semisodium valproate, divalproex sodium) is a compound of sodium valproate and valproic acid in a 1:1 molar ratio. There is nothing to suggest that the interactions of this compound will be different to those seen with sodium valproate.

Vigabatrin + Clomipramine

An isolated case report describes mania in an epileptic patient on vigabatrin and clomipramine.

Clinical evidence, mechanism, importance and management

An isolated report describes an epileptic man on carbamazepine and clobazam who was started on clomipramine 35 mg daily for depression. About one month later, vigabatrin 2 g daily was added for better seizure control. After about a week, the patient then progressively showed signs of mania, requiring hospitalisation after about 10 weeks. The clomipramine was stopped, the vigabatrin continued (because of its efficacy), and haloperidol started. Within a week the patient's mood had stabilised. The authors of the report attributed the mania to an interaction between the vigabatrin and the clomipramine.[1] Note that both clomipramine and vigabatrin can cause psychiatric disorders including mania, and vigabatrin should be used with caution in patients with depression. No general conclusions can be based on this single report.

1. Sastre-Garau P, Thomas P, Beaussart M, Goudemand M. Accès maniaque consécutif à une association vigabatrin-clomipramine. *Encephale* (1993) 19, 351–2.

Vigabatrin + Felbamate

No clinically relevant pharmacokinetic interactions appear to occur between vigabatrin and felbamate.

Clinical evidence, mechanism, importance and management

In a study of 16 subjects, felbamate 2.4 g daily increased the AUC of vigabatrin 2 g daily by 13%, which is unlikely to be clinically significant. In a second study in a further 18 subjects, no changes were detected in felbamate pharmacokinetics.[1] There would therefore seem to be no reason for avoiding concurrent use.

1. Reidenberg P, Glue P, Banfield C, Colucci R, Meehan J, Rey E, Radwanski E, Nomeir A, Lim J, Lin C, Guillaume M, Affrime MB. Pharmacokinetic interaction studies between felbamate and vigabatrin. *Br J Clin Pharmacol* (1995) 40, 157–60.

Vigabatrin + Phenobarbital or Primidone

Vigabatrin causes a trivial decrease in phenobarbital and primidone levels. There is some evidence that phenobarbital may reduce the efficacy of vigabatrin in infantile spasms.

Clinical evidence

In an early clinical study, vigabatrin 2 to 3 g daily did not change the serum levels of phenobarbital in 26 patients.[1] Similarly, another study found that phenobarbital levels were not significantly altered by vigabatrin.[2] Another study found that vigabatrin caused serum level reductions of 7% with phenobarbital and 11% with primidone.[3,4]

There is some evidence that the efficacy of vigabatrin for infantile seizures may be reduced in those taking phenobarbital. The median time to response after starting vigabatrin was 3 days in 3 infants not on phenobarbital and 34 days in 6 patients on phenobarbital. Three patients did not respond to vigabatrin until after phenobarbital was withdrawn.[5]

Mechanism

Not understood.

Importance and management

There appears to be no change in phenobarbital levels with vigabatrin, but some suggestion that vigabatrin may be less effective for infantile spasms in the presence of phenobarbital. Bear this possibility in mind.

1. Tassinari CA, Michelucci R, Ambrosetto G, Salvi F. Double-blind study of vigabatrin in the treatment of drug-resistant epilepsy. *Arch Neurol* (1987) 44, 907–10.
2. Bernardina BD, Fontana E, Vigevano F, Fusco L, Torelli D, Galeone D, Buti D, Cianchetti C, Gnanasakthy A, Iudice A. Efficacy and tolerability of vigabatrin in children with refractory partial seizures: a single-blind dose-increasing study. *Epilepsia* (1995) 36, 687–91.
3. Browne TR, Mattson RH, Penry JK, Smith DB, Treiman DM, Wilder BJ, Ben-Menachem E, Miketta RM, Sherry KM, Szabo GK. A multicentre study of vigabatrin for drug-resistant epilepsy. *Br J Clin Pharmacol* (1989) 95S–100S.
4. Browne TR, Mattson RH, Penry JK, Smith DB, Treiman DM, Wilder BJ, Ben-Menachem E, Napoliello MJ, Sherry KM, Szabo GK. Vigabatrin for refractory complex partial seizures: multicenter single-blind study with long-term follow up. *Neurology* (1987) 37, 184–9.
5. Spence SJ, Nakagawa J, Sankar R, Shields WD. Phenobarbital interfers with the efficacy of vigabatrin in treating infantile spasms in patients with tuberous sclerosis. *Epilepsia* (2000) 41 (Suppl 7), 189.

Vigabatrin + Sodium valproate

No pharmacokinetic interaction appears to occur between vigabatrin and sodium valproate, but one retrospective study found a correlation between valproate level and vigabatrin levels corrected for dose.

Clinical evidence, mechanism, importance and management

Vigabatrin 40 to 80 mg/kg daily did not change the serum levels of sodium valproate in 11 children.[1] The combined use of vigabatrin and sodium valproate in 16 children with refractory epilepsy was found not to affect the steady-state serum levels of either drug and the combination reduced the frequency of seizures.[2] However, a retrospective analysis of serum samples from 53 patients found that the vigabatrin concentration-to-dose ratio was increased as the valproate trough steady state levels increased.[3] No dosage adjustments usually appear to be necessary on combined use, but further study is needed.

1. Bernardina BD, Fontana E, Vigevano F, Fusco L, Torelli D, Galeone D, Buti D, Cianchetti C, Gnanasakthy A, Iudice A. Efficacy and tolerability of vigabatrin in children with refractory partial seizures: a single-blind dose-increasing study. *Epilepsia* (1995) 36, 687–91.
2. Armijo JA, Arteaga R, Valdizán EM, Herranz JL. Coadministration of vigabatrin and valproate in children with refractory epilepsy. *Clin Neuropharmacol* (1992) 15, 459–69.
3. Armijo JA, Cuadrado A, Bravo J, Arteaga R. Vigabatrin serum concentration to dosage ratio: influence of age and associated antiepileptic drugs. *Ther Drug Monit* (1997) 19, 491–8

Zonisamide + Miscellaneous

Cimetidine does not alter zonisamide pharmacokinetics. Food has no effect on the absorption of zonisamide. A case of reduced zonisamide levels possibly caused by risperidone has been described.
Strong inhibitors of the cytochrome P450 isoenzyme CYP3A4 are predicted to modestly decrease zonisamide clearance.

Clinical evidence, mechanism, importance and management

(a) Cimetidine

When a single 300-mg oral dose of zonisamide was given to healthy subjects, it was found that cimetidine 300 mg four times daily for 13 days did not affect the zonisamide clearance, half-life, apparent volume of distribution or the amount of drug recovered from the urine. The drugs were well tolerated.[1,2] No special precautions would seem to be needed if both drugs are used.

(b) Food

There was no difference in the pharmacokinetics of a single 300- or 400-mg dose of zonisamide when given in the fasted state or after breakfast in a study in healthy subjects. Zonisamide may be taken without regard to the timing of meals.[3]

(c) Risperidone

A 57-year-old man on zonisamide was started on risperidone 2 mg daily, which was and gradually increased to 10 mg daily. About 2 months after starting the risperidone, the zonisamide level had fallen from 23.7 to 10.7 micrograms/ml. The risperidone was stopped, and the zonisamide level had slightly increased again to 12.4 micrograms/ml about one month later. It was suggested that a metabolic interaction occurred.[4] More study is needed.

(d) Cytochrome P450 isoenzyme CYP3A4 inhibitors

In vitro studies have shown that the cytochrome P450 isoenzyme CYP3A4 is the principal enzyme involved in the metabolism of zonisamide.[5] Based on *in vitro* data, it is predicted that **ketoconazole**, **ciclosporin**, **miconazole** and **fluconazole** may cause a modest to minor decrease in the clearance of zonisamide. Conversely, **itraconazole** and **triazolam** are not predicted to have an effect.[5] *In vitro* predictions do not always mirror what happens in clinical use, therefore, further study is needed.

1. Schentag JJ, Gengo FM, Wilton JH, Sedman AJ, Grasela TH, Brockbrader HN. Influence of phenobarbital, cimetidine, and renal disease on zonisamide kinetics. *Pharm Res* (1987) 4 (Suppl), S-79.
2. Groves L, Wallace J, Shellenberger K. Effect of cimetidine on zonisamide pharmacokinetics in healthy volunteers. *Epilepsia* (1998) 39 (Suppl 6), 191.
3. Shellenberger K, Wallace J, Groves L. Effect of food on pharmacokinetics of zonisamide in healthy volunteers. *Epilepsia* (1998) 39 (Suppl 6), 191.
4. Okumura K. Decrease in plasma zonisamide concentrations after coadministration of risperidone in a patient with schizophrenia receiving zonisamide therapy. *Int Clin Psychopharmacol* (1999) 14, 55.
5. Nakasa H, Nakamura H, Ono S, Tsutsui M, Kiuchi M, Ohmori S, Kitada M. Prediction of drug-drug interactions of zonisamide metabolism in humans from in vitro data. *Eur J Clin Pharmacol* (1998) 54, 177–83.

Zonisamide + Other anticonvulsants

Phenobarbital, phenytoin and carbamazepine can cause a small to moderate reduction in the serum levels of zonisamide, while lamotrigine may increase them. Clonazepam and valproate have no or little effect. Zonisamide shows variable effects (a modest decrease, an increase, or no effect) on carbamazepine serum levels, but has no important effect on lamotrigine, phenobarbital, prim-

idone or valproate levels. Most studies have also shown no effect on phenytoin levels, but two showed a modest increase.

Clinical evidence

(a) Carbamazepine

In one study the ratio of plasma level to zonisamide dose was 39% lower in 17 patients on concurrent carbamazepine than in 28 patients on zonisamide alone, suggesting carbamazepine modestly reduces zonisamide levels.[1] Similarly, in another study in 12 epileptic children taking zonisamide 8.6 to 13.6 mg/kg daily, carbamazepine 12.1 to 18.1 mg/kg daily reduced zonisamide plasma levels by about 35 to 37%.[2] In an early study in 2 groups of patients, one taking carbamazepine and the other phenytoin, it was noted that the zonisamide AUC following a single 400-mg dose was 40% higher in the carbamazepine group than the phenytoin group.[3] However, in the first study, the plasma concentration-to-dose ratio was the same in patients on carbamazepine as in those on phenytoin.[1] Therefore the comparative effects of carbamazepine and phenytoin on zonisamide levels are unclear.

In one study, the ratio of carbamazepine-10,11-epoxide (the major active metabolite of carbamazepine) to carbamazepine in the plasma was 50% lower in patients also taking zonisamide, suggesting that zonisamide reduces carbamazepine metabolism. However, the plasma concentration-to-dose ratio of carbamazepine was only 20% higher, which was not significant.[1] An early pilot study had noted a consistent rise in carbamazepine plasma levels following initiation of zonisamide therapy in 7 patients (range 26% to 270%).[4] The opposite effect was seen in a study of 16 paediatric patients in whom zonisamide reduced the ratio of carbamazepine serum levels to dose by up to 22% and increased the relative amount of its major metabolite in the serum by up to 100%, suggesting that zonisamide increases the metabolism of carbamazepine. However, the free fraction of carbamazepine remained unaltered.[5]

Contrasting with these three studies are three others that found no changes in the serum levels of carbamazepine or its metabolite when zonisamide was used.[2,6,7] A further study similarly found no change in the plasma level of carbamazepine in 41 patients given zonisamide as an add-on therapy (7.5 versus 7.4 micrograms/ml).[8]

(b) Clonazepam

In one study the ratio of plasma level to dose of zonisamide did not differ between 8 patients on concurrent clonazepam and 28 patients on zonisamide alone, suggesting clonazepam has no effect on zonisamide levels.[1]

(c) Lamotrigine

Zonisamide 100 mg daily increased to 200 mg twice daily did not alter the steady-state pharmacokinetics of lamotrigine in 18 patients.[9] However, in 2 patients stabilised on zonisamide 600 mg daily or 800 mg daily, the addition of lamotrigine (incremental doses up to 400 mg daily) caused about twofold increases in their zonisamide levels, with symptoms of toxicity that were maximal 40 to 60 minutes after taking a zonisamide dose.[10]

(d) Phenobarbital or primidone

In one study the ratio of plasma level to dose of zonisamide was 29% lower in 11 patients taking concurrent phenobarbital than in 28 patients on zonisamide alone, suggesting that phenobarbital reduces zonisamide levels.[1] Similarly, another study in healthy subjects found that pretreatment with phenobarbital increased the clearance of a single dose of zonisamide by about twofold.[11] A further study found no changes in the serum levels of phenobarbital or primidone in 34 and 13 patients, respectively, given zonisamide as an add-on therapy.[8]

(e) Phenytoin

In one study the ratio of plasma level to dose of zonisamide was 39% lower in 14 patients taking concurrent phenytoin than in 28 patients on zonisamide alone, suggesting phenytoin modestly reduces zonisamide levels.[1] In an early study in 2 groups of patients, one taking carbamazepine and the other phenytoin, it was noted that the zonisamide AUC following a single 400-mg dose was 40% higher in the carbamazepine group than the phenytoin group.[3] However, in the first study, the reduction in zonisamide level-to-dose ratio was the same for phenytoin as for carbamazepine.[1] Therefore the comparative effect of phenytoin and carbamazepine on zonisamide levels is unclear.

Zonisamide 300 to 600 mg daily did not affect the phenytoin serum levels in 10 patients.[6] Another study found that zonisamide did not affect the serum levels of phenytoin in 9 children.[12] A further study similarly found no change in the plasma level of phenytoin in 33 patients given zonisamide as an add-on therapy.[8] In contrast to these three studies, the preliminary results from 9 patients in another study showed that there was a 28% increase in the steady-state AUC of phenytoin when zonisamide 100 mg daily increased to 200 mg twice daily was added.[13] Similarly, in a population pharmacokinetic analysis, the clearance of phenytoin at a given dose was 14% lower and the serum level 16% higher in 39 patients also on zonisamide.[14]

(f) Sodium valproate

In one study the ratio of plasma level to dose of zonisamide was about 20% lower in 24 patients on concurrent valproate than in 28 on zonisamide alone, suggesting that valproate has little effect on zonisamide levels.[1]

Another study found that zonisamide did not affect the serum levels of sodium valproate in 12 children.[12] A further study similarly found no marked changes in the plasma level of valproic acid in 7 patients given zonisamide as an add-on therapy.[8] Similarly, the steady-state pharmacokinetics of valproate did not change when zonisamide 100 mg daily increased to 200 mg twice daily was added to the therapy of 16 patients.[15]

Mechanism

Uncertain. It seems possible that phenobarbital, phenytoin and carbamazepine can induce the metabolism of zonisamide thereby reducing its serum levels. The plasma protein binding of zonisamide is unaffected by other anticonvulsants (phenobarbital, phenytoin, carbamazepine, sodium valproate).[16]

Importance and management

None of these studies reported any major problems during concurrent use of zonisamide and these other antiepileptic drugs. Zonisamide serum levels are lower with phenobarbital, phenytoin and carbamazepine, and there is the possibility of carbamazepine or phenytoin level changes, so it would be prudent to monitor patients taking any of these combinations.

1. Shinoda M, Akita M, Hasegawa M, Hasegawa T, Nabeshima T. The necessity of adjusting the dosage of zonisamide when coadministered with other anti-epileptic drugs. *Biol Pharm Bull* (1996) 19, 1090–2.
2. Abo J, Miura H, Takanashi S, Shirai H, Sunaoshi W, Hosoda N, Abo K, Takei K. Drug interaction between zonisamide and carbamazepine: a pharmacokinetic study in children with cryptogenic localization-related epilepsies. *Epilepsia* (1995) 36 (Suppl 3), S162.
3. Ojemann LM, Shastri RA, Wilensky AJ, Friel PN, Levy RH, McLean JR, Buchanan RA. Comparative pharmacokinetics of zonisamide (CI-912) in epileptic patients on carbamazepine or phenytoin monotherapy. *Ther Drug Monit* (1986) 8, 293–6.
4. Sackellares JC, Donofrio PD, Wagner JG, Abou-Khalil B, Berent S, Aasved-Hoyt K. Pilot study of zonisamide (1,2-Benzisoxazole-3-methanesulfonamide) in patients with refractory partial seizures. *Epilepsia* (1985) 26, 206–11.
5. Minami T, Ieiri I, Ohtsubo K, Hirakawa Y, Ueda K, Higuchi S, Aoyama T. Influence of additional therapy with zonisamide (Excegran) on protein binding and metabolism of carbamazepine. *Epilepsia* (1994) 35, 1023–5.
6. Browne TR, Szabo GK, Kres J, Pylilo RJ. Drug interactions of zonisamide (CI–912) with phenytoin and carbamazepine. *J Clin Pharmacol* (1986) 26, 555.
7. Rosenfeld WE, Bergen D, Garnett W, Shah J, Floren LC, Gross J, Tupper R, Shellenberger K. Steady-state drug interaction study of zonisamide and carbamazepine in patients with epilepsy. *Neurology* (2001) 56 (Suppl 3), A336.
8. Schmidt D, Jacob R, Loiseau P, Deisenhammer E, Klinger D, Despland A, Egli M, Bauer G, Stenzel E, Blankenhorn V. Zonisamide for add-on treatment of refractory partial epilepsy: a European double-blind trial. *Epilepsy Res* (1993) 15, 67–73.
9. Brodie M, Wilson E, Smith D, Dunkley D, Shah J, Floren L, Shellenberger K. Steady-state drug interaction study of zonisamide and lamotrigine in epileptic patients. *Neurology* (2001) 56 (Suppl 3), A337.
10. McJilton J, DeToledo J, DeCerce J, Huda S, Abubakr A, Ramsay RE. Cotherapy of lamotrigine/zonisamide results in significant elevation of zonisamide levels. *Epilepsia* (1996) 37 (Suppl 5), 173.
11. Schentag JJ, Gengo FM, Wilton AJ, Sedman AJ, Grasela TH, Bockbrader HN. Influence of phenobarbital, cimetidine, and renal disease on zonisamide kinetics. *Pharm Res* (1987) 4 (Suppl), S-79.
12. Tasaki K, Minami T, Ieiri I, Ohtsubo K, Hirakawa Y, Ueda K, Higuchi S. Drug interactions of zonisamide with phenytoin and sodium valproate: serum concentrations and protein binding. *Brain Dev* (1995) 17, 182–5.
13. Garnett WR, Towne AR, Rosenfeld WE, Shah J, Floren LC, Gross J, Tupper R, Shellenberger K. Steady-state pharmacokinetic interaction study of zonisamide (Zonegran) and phenytoin in subjects with epilepsy. *Neurology* (2001) 56 (Suppl 3), A336.
14. Odani A, Hashimoto Y, Takayanagi K, Otsuki Y, Koue T, Takano M, Yasuhara M, Hattori H, Furusho K, Inui K-I. Population pharmacokinetics of phenytoin in Japanese patients with epilepsy: analysis with a dose-dependent clearance model. *Biol Pharm Bull* (1996) 19, 444–8.
15. Smith D, Brodie M, Dunkley D, Shah J, Floren L, Shellenberger K. Steady-state drug interaction study of zonisamide and sodium valproate in epileptic patients. *Neurology* (2001) 56 (Suppl 3), A338.
16. Kimura M, Tanaka N, Kimura Y, Miyake K, Kitaura T, Fukuchi H, Harada Y. Factors influencing serum concentration of zonisamide in epileptic patients. *Chem Pharm Bull (Tokyo)* (1992) 40, 193–5.

12

Antidiabetics

The antidiabetics are used to control diabetes mellitus, a disease in which there is total or partial failure of the beta-cells within the pancreas to secrete into the circulation enough insulin, one of the hormones concerned with the handling of glucose. In some cases there is evidence to show that the disease results from the presence of factors that oppose the activity of insulin.

With insufficient insulin, the body tissues are unable to take up and utilise the glucose which is in circulation in the blood. Because of this, the glucose, which is derived largely from the digestion of food and which would normally be removed and stored in tissues throughout the body, accumulates and boosts the glucose in the blood to such grossly elevated proportions that the kidney is unable to cope with such a load and glucose appears in the urine. Raised blood sugar levels (hyperglycaemia) with glucose and ketone bodies in the urine (glycosuria and ketonuria) are among the manifestations of a serious disturbance in the metabolic chemistry of the body which, if untreated, can lead to the development of diabetic coma and death.

There are two main types of diabetes: one develops early in life and occurs when the ability of the pancreas suddenly, and often almost totally, fails to produce insulin. The first is called type 1, juvenile or insulin-dependent diabetes (IDDM). The other form is type 2, maturity-onset or non-insulin dependent diabetes mellitus (NIDDM), which is most often seen in those over 40 years old. This occurs when the pancreas gradually loses the ability to produce insulin over a period of months or years. It is often associated with being over-weight and can sometimes be satisfactorily controlled simply by losing weight and adhering to an appropriate diet. A list of oral antidiabetics is given in 'Table 12.1', (p.390).

The modes of action of the antidiabetics

(a) Insulin

Insulin extracted from the pancreatic tissue of pigs and cattle is so similar to human insulin that it can be used as a replacement. However, human insulin, manufactured by genetically engineered micro-organisms, is more commonly used. Insulin is given by injection in order to bypass the enzymes of the gut, which would digest and destroy it like any other protein. There are now many formulations of insulin, some of them designed to delay absorption from the subcutaneous or intramuscular tissue into which the injection is made, so that repeated daily injections can be avoided, but all of them sooner or later release insulin into the circulation where it acts to replace or top-up the insulin from the human pancreas.

(b) Sulphonylureas and biguanides

The sulphonylurea and other sulphonamide-related compounds such as chlorpropamide and tolbutamide were the first synthetic compounds used in medicine as antidiabetics and have the advantage of being given by mouth. Among their actions they stimulate the remaining beta-cells of the pancreas to grow and secrete insulin which, with a restricted diet, controls blood sugar levels and permits normal metabolism to occur. Clearly they can only be effective in those diabetics whose pancreas still has the capacity to produce some insulin, so their use is confined to type 2 diabetes.

The mode of action of the biguanides, such as metformin, is obscure, but they do not stimulate the pancreas like the sulphonylureas to release insulin, but appear to facilitate the uptake and utilisation of glucose by the cells in some way. Their use is restricted to type 2 diabetes because they are not effective unless insulin is also present.

(c) Other oral antidiabetics

Acarbose and voglibose act against alpha glucosidases and specifically against sucrase in the gut to delay the digestion and absorption of monosaccharides from starch and sucrose. More recently introduced drug classes include the **thiazolidinediones** (e.g. rosiglitazone), which appear to increase the sensitivity of the receptors to insulin, and the **meglitinides** (e.g. repaglinide), which increases endogenous insulin secretion. Outside orthodox Western medicine, there are herbal preparations which are used to treat diabetes and which can be given by mouth. Blueberries were traditionally used by the Alpine peasants, and bitter gourd or karela *(Momordica charantia)* is an established part of herbal treatment in the Indian subcontinent and elsewhere. Traditional Chinese medicine also has herbal medicines for diabetes. As yet it is not known how these herbal medicines act and their efficacy awaits formal clinical evaluation.

(d) Interactions

The commonest interactions are those that result in a rise or fall in blood glucose levels, thereby disturbing the control of diabetes. These are detailed in this section. Other interactions where the antidiabetic drug is the affecting drug are described elsewhere.

Table 12.1 Oral antidiabetics

Generic names	*Proprietary names*
Alpha glucosidase inhibitors	
Acarbose	Acarbay, Asucrose, Glicobase, Glubose, Glucar, Glucobay, Glucor, Glumida, Prandase, Precose
Miglitol	Diastabol, Glyset, Mignar, Plumarol
Voglibose	Basen
Biguanides	
Buformin	Adebit, Silubin
Metformin	Adimet, Ammiformin, Anglucid, Apophage, Bigomet, Biocos, Clonarol, CP-Metform, Dabex, DBI AP, Deson, Desugar, Diabamyl, Diabemet, Diabesin, Diabetex, Diabetmin, Diabex, Diaformin, Dialon, Diamet, Dianben, Diaphage, Diformin, Dimefor, Emfor, Emnorm, espa-formin, Exermet, Fintaxim, Formin, Fortamet, Glafornil, Glifage, Glifortex, Glucaminol, Glucobon, Glucoformin, Glucohexal, Glucoles-500, Glucomerck, Glucomet, Glucomin, Glucono, Gluconormine, Glucophage, Glufor, Gluformin, Glumet, Gluzolyte, Glyciphage, Glycomet, Glyree M, Hipoglucin, Islotin, Juformin, Macromin, Maformin, Mediabet, ME-F, Meforal, Meformed, Meglucon, Melbin, Menarini-Metforal, Merckformin, Mescorit, Met, Metbay, Metfin, Metfirex, Metfogamma, Metfonorm, Metfor, Metforal, Metforem, Metfori, Metform, Metformax, Metfron, Metiguanide, Metlong, Metomin, Metrivin, Miformin, Novomet, Orabet, Oramet, Pocophage, Poli-Formin, Prophage, Riomet, Risidon, Serformin, Siamformet, Siofor, Stagid, Teutoformin, Thiabet, Walaphage, X-Met
Phenformin	Azucaps, Debeina, Debeone
Meglitinides	
Nateglinide	Glinate, Nateglin, Starlix, Starsis
Repaglinide	Gluconorm, NovoNorm, Prandin, Rapilin, Sestrine
Sulfonylureas	
Acetohexamide	Dymelor
Carbutamide	Glucidoral
Chlorpropamide	Copamide, Diabecontrol, Diabeedol, Diabemide, Diabiclor, Diabinese, Diabitex, Dibecon, Glicoben, Glicorp, Glycemin, Hypomide, Idle, Insogen, Propamide, Trane
Glibenclamide (Glyburide)	Abuglib, Aglucil, Bastiverit, Benclamin, Betanase, Bevoren, Biostin, BNIL, Clamiben, Clamide, Cytagon, Daonil, Daono, Debtan, Deroctyl, Diabefar, Diabemin, Diaben, Diabenol, DiaBeta, Diabexil, Diacare, Dia-Eptal, Dibelet, Diclanil, Diglexol, duraglucon N, Euglamin, Euglucan, Euglucon, Euglucon N, Euglusid, Gardoton, Gen-Glybe, Gilemal, Glemicid, Glib, gli-basan, Glibediab, Gliben, Glibenbeta, Glibenclamon, Glibendoc, Glibenhexal, Glibenil, Glibenorme, Gliben-Puren N, Glibenval, Glibesifar, Glibesyn, Glibetic, Glibexil, Glibic, Gliboral, Glib-ratiopharm, Glidanil, Glifarcal, Glikeyer, Glimel, Glimide, Glimidstada, Glinil, Glionil, Glitisol, Glitral, Gluben, Glucal, Glucobene, Glucolon, Gluconil, Glucostad, Glucoven, Glukovital, Gluzo, Glybovin, Glycomin, Glynase, Gon, Hemi-Daonil, Hexaglucon, Humedia, Jutaglucon, Lisaglucon, Locose, Maninil, Manoglucon, Melix, Micronase, Miglucan, Mini-Glynase, Nadib, Norboral, Norglicem, Normoglucon, Origlucon, Pira, Praeciglucon, Reglusan, Semi-Daonil, Semi-Euglucon, Semi-Euglucon N, Sugril, Uni Gliben, Xeltic
Glibornuride	Gluborid, Glutril
Gliclazide	Aglucide, Cadicon, CP-Gliz, Diabeside, Diabeton, Diabrezide, Diaclide, Diaglucide, Diaglyk, Diamaze, Diamexon, Diamicron, Diamitex, Dianid, Dianorm, Dianormax, Diaprel, Glicron, Glimicron, Gliza, Glizid, Glucocron, Glucomed, Glucozide, Gluctam, Glupozide, Glyade, Glycigon, Glycinorm, Glycon, Glycron, Glydiab, Glygard, Glyzide, Licla, Lycazid, Medoclazide, Melicron, Nidem, Reclide, Semi-Glycigon, Serviclazide, Suclear, Sun-Glizide, Unava, Uni Diamicron, Ziclin
Glimepiride	Amarel, Amaryl, Amarylle, Betaglim, Diaglim, Diapiride, Diapride, Dimirel, Endial, Euglim, Glemaz, Glimcip, Glimepil, Glimesec, Glimial, Glimiprex, Glimitab, Glimulin, Gluceride, Glucopirida, Glyree, Glyree M, Islopir, Roname, Solosa
Glipizide	Antidiab, Apamid, Beapizide, Diaglip, Diasef, Dibizide, Dipazide, Gipzide, Glez, Glibenese, Glide, Glipgen, Glipid, Glix, Glizide, Glucodiab, Glucolip, Gluco-Rite, Glucotrol, Glupitel, Glygen, Glynase, Glyzip, Luditec, Mediab, Melizid, Melizide, Mindiab, Minibit, Minidiab, Minodiab, Ozidia, Pezide, Sunglucon, Xiprine
Gliquidone	Glurenor, Glurenorm
Glisoxepide	
Glybuzole	
Glycyclamide	
Tolazamide	Tolinase
Tolbutamide	Arcosal, Bioglusil, Dabetil, Diatol, Diaval, Dirastan, Flusan, Ifumelus, Orabet, Orinase, Orinase Diagnostic, Orsinon, Rastinon, Tydadex
Sulfonamide-related compounds	
Glymidine	
Thiazolidienones	
Pioglitazone	Actos, Cereluc, Diabestat, Diaglit, Glita, Glizone, G-Tase, Opam, Pepar, P-Glitz, Pioglit, Piomed, Piosafe, Zactos
Rosiglitazone	Avandia, Glimide, Roglin, Rosicon

Acarbose + Miscellaneous

Charcoal and digestive enzyme preparations are expected to reduce the effects of acarbose. Neomycin may increase the efficacy and the gastrointestinal adverse effects of acarbose. There is some indirect evidence that acarbose with alcohol may increase the hepatotoxicity of paracetamol (acetaminophen). Ileus has been reported in a Japanese patient treated with acarbose and an anticholinergic drug.

Clinical evidence, mechanism, importance and management

(a) Anticholinergics

A 69-year-old man with a partial gastrectomy and type 2 diabetes, treated with insulin 24 units and acarbose 300 mg daily, was admitted to hospital with diabetic gangrene. After developing cold symptoms he was treated with *PL granules* (salicylamide, paracetamol, caffeine, **promethazine** methylene disalicylate). The next day he experienced sudden abdominal pain, nausea and vomiting, which was diagnosed as paralytic ileus. He was given intravenous fluids and piperacillin. Oral intake and acarbose were withheld and the ileus resolved after 2 days. The authors note that there are several reports of ileus developing in Japanese patients within 3 months of treatment with alpha glucosidase inhibitors such as acarbose. The risk seems to be increased with age, a history of abdominal surgery, and a Japanese diet (high in carbohydrates and fibre) rather than Western diet. However, in this case the patient had been taking acarbose for 15 months without problem and it is possible that the anticholinergic effects of **promethazine** in the *PL granules* may have contributed to the development of ileus.[1] The general clinical relevance of this case is uncertain. However, the authors consider that patients at risk should be monitored if treated with alpha glucosidase inhibitors, especially if the dose is increased or during concurrent therapy with anticholinergics.[1]

(b) Digestive enzyme preparations

The makers of acarbose reasonably suggest the avoidance of intestinal adsorbents (e.g. **charcoal**) or digestive enzyme preparations (such as **amylase**, **pancreatin**) because, theoretically these would be expected to reduce the effects of acarbose.[2]

(c) Neomycin

Neomycin alone can reduce postprandial blood glucose levels and may enhance the reduction in postprandial glucose levels associated with acarbose.[3] Neomycin 1 g three times daily increased the unpleasant gastrointestinal adverse effects (flatulence, cramps and diarrhoea) of acarbose 200 mg three times daily in 7 healthy subjects.[4] The makers suggest that if these adverse effects are severe the dosage of acarbose should be reduced.[2]

(d) Paracetamol

Studies in *rats* have found that acarbose alone or in combination with alcohol may potentiate the hepatotoxicity of paracetamol.[5] However, it is not known whether this has any clinical relevance.

1. Oba K, Kudo R, Yano M, Watanabe K, Ajiro Y, Okazaki K, Susuki T, Nakano H, Metori S. Ileus after administration of cold remedy in an elderly diabetic patient treated with acarbose. *J Nippon Med Sch* (2001) 68, 61–4.
2. Glucobay (Acarbose). Bayer plc. UK Summary of product characteristics, March 2004.
3. Bayer, Personal Communications, June-July 1993.
4. Lembcke B, Caspary WF, Fölsch UR, Creutzfeldt W. Influence of neomycin on postprandial metabolic changes and side effects of an α-glucosidehydrolase inhibitor (BAY g 5421). I. Effects on intestinal hydrogen gas production and flatulence. In Frontiers of Hormone Research, vol 7. The Entero-Insular Axis. Satellite Symposium to Xth IDF-Meeting, September 7–8, Göttingen 1979, p 294–5.
5. Wang P-Y, Kaneko T, Wang Y, Sato A. Acarbose alone or in combination with ethanol potentiates the hepatotoxicity of carbon tetrachloride and acetaminophen in rats. *Hepatology* (1999) 29, 161–5.

Antidiabetics + ACE inhibitors

The concurrent use of ACE inhibitors and antidiabetics normally appears to be uneventful but hypoglycaemia, marked in some instances, has occurred in a small number of diabetics taking insulin or sulphonylureas when treated with captopril, enalapril, lisinopril or perindopril. This has been attributed, but not proved, to be due to an interaction.

Clinical evidence

'Table 12.2', (p.392) and 'Table 12.3', (p.392) summarise the findings of studies in subjects taking both ACE inhibitors and antidiabetics.

A brief report states that spirapril does not have a pharmacokinetic interaction with glibenclamide,[1] but this does not exclude the possibility of an interaction, see Mechanism.

Mechanism

Not understood. An increase in glucose utilisation and increased insulin sensitivity have been suggested.[2,3] Other possibilities (e.g. altered kidney function) are discussed in a series of letters in *The Lancet*.[4-9] There is also an isolated report of persistent severe hypoglycaemia in a non-diabetic patient associated with both **captopril** and **ramipril** therapy.[10]

Importance and management

This interaction is not yet well established nor understood, and it remains the subject of considerable study and debate. However, some cases of severe hypoglycaemia have undoubtedly occurred due to the use of ACE inhibitors by diabetic patients. In practical terms this means that concurrent use need not be avoided but it would be prudent to warn all patients on insulin or oral antidiabetics who are just starting any ACE inhibitors (although only captopril, enalapril, lisinopril and perindopril have been implicated) that excessive hypoglycaemia has been seen very occasionally and unpredictably. The problem has been resolved in some patients by reducing the sulphonylurea dosage to a half or a quarter.[11,12] A false positive urine ketone test can also occur with captopril when using the alkaline-nitroprusside test (*Ketodiastix*).[13]

1. Grass P, Gerbeau C, Kutz K. Spirapril: pharmacokinetic properties and drug interactions. *Blood Press Suppl* (1994) 2, 7–13.
2. Ferriere M, Lachkar H, Richard J-L, Bringer J, Orsetti A, Mirouze J. Captopril and insulin sensitivity. *Ann Intern Med* (1985) 102, 134–5.
3. Girardin E, Vial T, Pham E, Evreux J-C. Hypoglycémies induites par les sulfamides hypoglycémiants. *Ann Med Interne (Paris)* (1992) 143, 11–17.
4. van Haeften TW. ACE inhibitors and hypoglycaemia. *Lancet* (1995) 346, 125.
5. Kong N, Bates A, Ryder REJ. ACE inhibitors and hypoglycaemia. *Lancet* (1995) 346, 125.
6. Feher MD, Amiel S. ACE inhibitors and hypoglycaemia. *Lancet* (1995) 346, 125–6.
7. Davie AP. ACE inhibitors and hypoglycaemia. *Lancet* (1995) 346, 126.
8. Wildenborg IHM, Veenstra J, van der Voort PHJ, Verdegaal WP, Silberbusch J. ACE inhibitors and hypoglycaemia. *Lancet* (1995) 346, 126.
9. Herings RMC, de Boer A, Stricker BHC, Leufkens HGM, Porsius AJ. ACE inhibitors and hypoglycaemia. *Lancet* (1995) 346, 126–7.
10. Elorriaga-Sánchez F, Corrales-Bobadilla H, Sosa-Trinidad E, Domínguez-Quezada B. Hipoglucemia severa secundaria a inhibidores de la enzima convertidora de angiotensina en ausencia de diabetes mellitus. Reporte de un caso. *Gac Med Mex* (2001) 137, 249–52.
11. Arauz-Pacheco C, Ramirez LC, Rios JM, Raskin P. Hypoglycemia induced by angiotensin-converting enzyme inhibitors in patients with non-insulin-dependent diabetes receiving sulfonylurea therapy. *Am J Med* (1990) 89, 811–13.
12. Ahmad S. Drug interaction induces hypoglycemia. *J Fam Pract* (1995) 40, 540–1.
13. Warren SE. False-positive urine ketone test with captopril. *N Engl J Med* (1980) 303, 1003–4.

Antidiabetics + Alcohol

Diabetics controlled on insulin, oral antidiabetics or diet alone need not abstain from alcohol, but they should drink only in moderation and accompanied by food. Alcohol makes the signs of hypoglycaemia less clear and delayed hypoglycaemia can occur. The CNS depressant effects of alcohol plus hypoglycaemia can make driving or the operation of dangerous machinery much more hazardous. A flushing reaction is common in patients on chlorpropamide who drink, but is rare with other sulphonylureas. Alcoholic patients may require above-average doses of tolbutamide.

Clinical evidence

(a) Antidiabetics, general

The blood glucose levels of diabetics may either be reduced or remain unchanged by alcohol. In one study, 2 out of 7 diabetics using **insulin** became severely hypoglycaemic after drinking the equivalent of about 3 measures of spirits.[1] In a hospital study over a 3-year period, 5 insulin-dependent diabetics were hospitalised with severe hypoglycaemia after binge-drinking. Two of them died without recovery from the initial coma and the other 3 suffered permanent damage to the nervous system.[2] In another study it was found that alcohol was involved in about 4% of hypoglycaemic episodes requiring hospitalisation.[3] In contrast to these alcohol-induced hypoglycaemic episodes, it was found in two other studies[4,5] that pure alcohol and dry wine had little effect on blood glucose

Table 12.2 Antidiabetic/ACE inhibitor interactions: evidence for no interaction

Patients	*ACE inhibitor*	*Antidiabetic*	*Notes*
8 cases	Captopril 37.5 mg/day	Insulin	No change to daily insulin requirements. No evidence of symptomatic hypoglycaemia[1]
38 cases	Captopril 50 to 100 mg/day or Enalapril 20 to 40 mg/day	Insulin or oral hypoglycaemics	Antidiabetic treatment unaltered, no evidence of unusual or unexplained hypoglycaemia.[2]
18 cases case control study	Enalapril 20 to 40 mg/day	Insulin	No change to daily insulin requirements. No evidence of unexplained hypoglycaemia[2]
428 patients randomised controlled trial	Lisinopril 10 to 20 mg/day or placebo	Insulin	No difference in the number of hypoglycaemic episodes between lisinopril and placebo recipients.[3]
22 cases case control study	Captopril or Enalapril	Insulin and oral hypoglycaemics	Data from Centres Regionaux de Pharmacovigilance in France used. No increased risk of hypoglycaemia detected.[4]

1. Winocour P, Waldek S, Anderson DC. Captopril and blood glucose. *Lancet* (1986) ii, 461.
2. Passa P, Marre M, Leblanc H. Enalapril, captopril and blood glucose. *Lancet* (1986) i, 1447.
3. The EUCLID study group. Randomized placebo-controlled trial of lisinopril in normotensive patients with insulin-dependent diabetes and normoalbuminuria or microalbuminuria. *Lancet* (1997) 349, 1787-92.
4. Moore N, Kreft-Jais C, Haramburu F, Noblet C, Andrjak M, Ollanngier M, Bégaud B. Reports of hypoglycaemia associated with the use of ACE inhibitors and other drugs: a case/non-case study in the French pharmacovigilance system database. *Br J Clin Pharmacol* (1997) 44, 513-8.

Table 12.3 Antidiabetic/ACE inhibitor interactions: evidence for an interaction

Patients	*ACE inhibitor*	*Antidiabetic*	*Notes*
1 case	Captopril 50 mg/day	Glibenclamide (glyburide) 10 mg/day Metformin 1700 mg/day	Blood glucose 2.2 mmol/L 24 hours after the addition of captopril.[1]
1 case	Captopril	Glibenclamide 10.5 mg/day Metformin 1700 mg/day	Blood glucose of 2.9 mmol/L 48 hours after starting captopril. Hypoglycaemic drugs stopped.[1]
3 cases	Captopril	Glibenclamide	Hypoglycaemia reported to a Spanish Regional Pharmacosurveillance centre.[2]
1 case	Captopril 12.5 mg/day	Glibenclamide 2.5 mg/day	Hypoglycaemia 7 hours after first dose, blood glucose 2.1 mmol/L, glibenclamide stopped.[3]
1 case	Captopril	Unspecified oral hypoglycaemic	Hypoglycaemia, oral hypoglycaemics withdrawn.[4]
5 cases	Captopril	Unspecified sulfonylureas	Hypoglycaemia reported to Centres Regionaux de Pharmacovigilance in France.[5]
3 cases case control study	Captopril	Unspecified oral hypoglycaemic	Risk of hypoglycaemia increased 3.1-fold.[6]
9 cases case control study	Captopril	Insulin	3.7-fold increase in the risk of hypoglycaemia.[6]
4 cases	Captopril	Insulin	Hypoglycaemia reported to a Spanish Regional Pharmacosurveillance centre[2]
3 cases	Captopril	Insulin	Unexplained hypoglycaemia.[4]
1 case	Enalapril 5 mg/day	Glibenclamide 5 mg/day	Hypoglycaemia, blood glucose 2.3 mmol/L. Dose of glibenclamide reduced to 2.5 mg/day.[3]
2 cases	Enalapril 5 mg/day	Glibenclamide 5 mg/day	Hypoglycaemic attacks, glibenclamide reduced to 1.25 mg/day.[7]
9 healthy subjects	Enalapril 5 mg/day	Glibenclamide 3.5 mg/day	Hypoglycaemic effects of glibenclamide enhanced.[8]
4 cases	Enalapril	Glibenclamide	Hypoglycaemia reported to a Spanish Regional Pharmacosurveillance centre.[2]
1 case	Enalapril	Gliclazide 80 mg/day	Hypoglycaemia when enalapril dose increased from 5 to 10 mg/day.[9]
4 cases	Enalapril	Unspecified sulfonylureas	Hypoglycaemia reported to Centres Regionaux de Pharmacovigilance in France.[5]
1 case	Enalapril	Unspecified sulfonylureas	Recurrent hypoglycaemia, sulfonylurea withdrawn.[10]
10 cases case control study	Enalapril	Unspecified sulfonylureas Insulin	2.4-fold increase in the risk of hypoglycaemia with sulfonylureas. However, no increased risk was seen in insulin users. In addition when all ACE inhibitors were considered together, no significant increase in risk was seen.[11]
2 cases case control study	Enalapril	Unspecified oral hypoglycaemic	Non-significant 5.4-fold increase in the risk of hypoglycaemia.[6]
3 cases case control study	Enalapril	Insulin	Non-significant 1.7-fold increase in the risk of hypoglycaemia.[6]
1 case	Enalapril	Insulin	Reduced insulin requirements.[10]

Continued

Table 12.3 Antidiabetic/ACE inhibitor interactions: evidence for an interaction *(continued)*

Patients	*ACE inhibitor*	*Antidiabetic*	*Notes*
11 cases	Enalapril	Insulin	Hypoglycaemia reported to a Spanish Regional Pharmacosurveillance centre.[2]
1 case	Lisinopril	Glibenclamide and metformin	Hypoglycaemia reported to a Spanish Regional Pharmacosurveillance centre.[2]
1 case	Lisinopril 10 mg/day	Gliclazide	Hypoglycaemia resolved on stopping gliclazide.[9]
1 case	Perindopril	Glibenclamide	Hypoglycaemia reported to a Spanish Regional Pharmacosurveillance centre.[2]
1 case	Ramipril 2.5 mg/day	Glibenclamide 5 mg/day Metformin 1700 mg/day	Patient also on naproxen, renal function deteriorated causing hypoglycaemia due to accumulation of oral hypoglycaemics.[12]
7 cases case control study	Unspecified ACE inhibitor	Insulin or oral hypoglycaemic agents	3.2-fold increase in the risk of hypoglycaemia leading to hospitalisation.[13]

1. Rett K, Wicklmayr M, Dietz GJ. Hypoglycemia in hypertensive diabetic patients treated with sulfonylureas, biguanides and captopril. *N Engl J Med* (1988) 319, 1609
2. Aguirre C, Ayani I, Rodriguez-Sasiain JM. Hypoglycaemia associated with angiotensin converting enzyme inhibitors. *Therapie* (1995) 50 (Suppl), 198.
3. Arauz-Pacheco C, Ramirez LC, Rios JM, Raskin P. Hypoglycemia induced by angiotensin-converting enzyme inhibitors in patients with non-insulin-dependent diabetes receiving sulfonylurea therapy. *Am J Med* (1990) 89, 811–13.
4. Ferriere M, Lachkar H, Richard J-L, Bringer J, Orsetti A, Mirouze J. Captopril and insulin sensitivity. *Ann Intern Med* (1985) 102, 134–5.
5. Girardin E, Vial T, Pham E, Evreux J-C. Hypoglycémies induites par les sulfamides hypoglycémiants. *Ann Med Interne (Paris)* (1992) 143, 11–17.
6. Herings RMC, de Boer A, Stricker BHC, Leufkens HGM, Porsius A. Hypoglycaemia associated with use of inhibitors of angiotensin converting enzyme. *Lancet* (1995) 345, 1195–8.
7. Ahmad S. Drug interaction induces hypoglycemia. *J Fam Pract* (1995) 40, 540–1.
8. Heise T, Hompesch BC, Flesch S, Rave K, Linkeschowa R, Heinemann L. Drug-interaction between enalapril and glibenclamide might lead to hypoglycaemia. *Diabetes* (1999) 48 (Suppl 1), A70–A71.
9. Veyre B, Ginon I, Vial T, Dragol F, Daumont M. Hypoglycémies par interférence entre un inhibiteur de l'enzyme de conversion et un sulfamide hypoglycémiant. *Presse Med* (1993) 22, 738.
10. McMurray J and Fraser DM. Captopril, enalapril and blood glucose. *Lancet* (1986) i, 1035.
11. Thamer M, Ray NF, Taylor T. Association between antihypertensive drug use and hypoglycemia: a case-control study of diabetic users of insulin or sulfonylureas. *Clin Ther* (1999) 21, 1387–1400.
12. Collin M, Mucklow JC. Drug interactions, renal impairment and hypoglycaemia in a patient with type II diabetes. *Br J Clin Pharmacol* (1999) 48, 134–7.
13. Morris AD, Boyle DIR, McMahon AD, Pearce H, Evans JMM, Newton RW, Jung RT, MacDonald TM, The DARTS/MEMO collaboration. ACE inhibitor use is associated with hospitalization for severe hypoglycaemia in patients with diabetes. *Diabetes Care* (1997) 20, 1363–7.

levels. An extensive study found that alcohol causes some deterioration in the metabolic control of elderly patients with type 2 diabetes (increased lipolysis, raised triglyceride levels, ketogenesis).[6]

(b) Sulphonylureas

About one-third of those on **chlorpropamide** who drink alcohol, even in quite small amounts, experience a warm, tingling or burning sensation of the face, and sometimes the neck and arms as well. It may also involve the conjunctivae. This can begin within 5 to 20 minutes of drinking, reaching a peak within 30 to 40 minutes, and may persist for 1 to 2 hours. Very occasionally headache occurs, and light-headedness, palpitations, wheezing and breathlessness have also been experienced.[7,8]

This disulfiram-like flushing reaction has been described in numerous reports (far too many to list here) involving large numbers of patients on **chlorpropamide**. These reports have been extensively reviewed.[7,9-11] A similar reaction can occur, but only very rarely, with other sulphonylureas including **carbutamide**,[12] **gliclazide**,[13] **glipizide**,[8] **glibenclamide** (**glyburide**),[8,14] **tolbutamide**,[15,16] **tolazamide**[17]. A comparative study showed that the mean half-life of **tolbutamide** in alcoholics was reduced by about one-third, from 384 to 232 minutes.[18] Alcohol is also reported to prolong but not increase the hypoglycaemic effects of **glipizide**.[19]

(c) Biguanides

A controlled study in 5 ketosis-resistant patients with type 2 diabetes taking **phenformin** 50 to 100 mg daily found that the equivalent of 3 oz whiskey markedly raised their blood lactate and lactate-pyruvate levels. Two of them had blood-lactate levels of more than 50 mg%, and one of these patients had previously experienced nausea, weakness and malaise while taking **phenformin** and alcohol.[20] The ingestion of alcohol is described in other reports as having preceded the onset of **phenformin**-induced lactic-acidosis.[21-23] Some patients have complained that alcohol tastes metallic.

(d) Rosiglitazone

An 8-week study in type 2 diabetics taking rosiglitazone 8 mg or a placebo daily found that 0.6 g/kg of alcohol taken with a meal did not have a clinically relevant effect on plasma glucose levels and no episodes of hypoglycaemia were seen.[24]

Mechanism

The exacerbation of hypoglycaemia by alcohol is not fully understood. However, it is known that if hypoglycaemia occurs when liver glycogen stores are low, the liver turns to the formation of new glucose from amino acids (neoglucogenesis). This neoglucogenesis is inhibited by the presence of alcohol so that the fall in blood glucose levels may not be prevented and a full-scale hypoglycaemic episode can result. The chlorpropamide-alcohol flush reaction, although extensively studied, is by no means fully understood. It seems to be related to the disulfiram-alcohol reaction, and is accompanied by a rise in blood-acetaldehyde levels (see also 'Alcohol + Disulfiram', p.50). It also appears to be genetically determined[8] and may involve both prostaglandins and endogenous opioids.[25] The decreased half-life of tolbutamide in alcoholics is probably due to the inducing effects of alcohol on liver microsomal enzymes.[18,26,27]

The reasons for the raised blood lactate levels seen during the concurrent use of phenformin and alcohol are not clear, but one suggestion is that it may possibly be related to the competitive demands for isoenzymes by the reactions that convert alcohol to acetaldehyde, and lactate to pyruvate.[20] A study in healthy subjects found that moderate alcohol consumption both improves insulin action, without affecting non-insulin mediated glucose uptake, and decreases lactate clearance. The increase in blood lactate with alcohol is therefore mainly due to inhibition of clearance. Alcohol did not appear to significantly affect beta-cell function.[28]

Importance and management

The documentation of the hypoglycaemic agent/alcohol interactions is surprisingly patchy (with the exception of chlorpropamide and alcohol) but they are of recognised clinical importance. The following contains the main recommendations of Diabetes UK (formerly The British Diabetic Association) based on a review of what is currently known:[29,30]

General comments

Most diabetics need not avoid alcohol totally, but they are advised not to exceed 2 drinks (for women) or 3 drinks (for men) daily. A drink (or unit) is defined in 'Table 3.2', (p.37). The intake of drinks with high-carbohydrate content (sweet sherries, sweet wines, most liqueurs, and low alcohol wines) should be limited. Diabetics should not drink on an empty stomach and they should know that the warning signs of hypoglycaemia may possibly be obscured by the effects of the alcohol. Driving or handling dangerous machinery should be avoided because the CNS depressant effects of alcohol plus hypoglycaemia can be particularly hazardous. Warn them of the risks of hypoglycaemia occurring several hours after drinking. Those with peripheral neuropathy should be told that alcohol may aggravate the condition and they should not have more than one drink daily. Provided drinking is restricted as suggested and drinks containing a lot of carbohydrate are avoided, there is no need to include the drink in the dietary allowance. However, diabetics on a weight-reducing diet should try to limit intake to the occasional drink and should include it in their daily calorie allowance.

Additional comments about the oral antidiabetics

The chlorpropamide-alcohol interaction (flushing reaction) is very well documented, but of minimal importance. It is a nuisance and possibly socially embarrassing but normally requires no treatment. Patients should be warned. The incidence is said to lie between 13 and 33%[31,32] although one study claims that it may be as low as 4%.[33] Since it can be provoked by quite small amounts of alcohol (half a glass of sherry or wine) it is virtually impossible for sensitive patients to avoid it if they drink. Most makers issue warnings about the possibility of this reaction with other sulphonylureas, but it is very rarely seen and can therefore almost always be avoided by replacing chlorpropamide with another sulphonylurea. Alcoholic subjects may need above-average doses of tolbutamide.

Metformin does not carry the same risk of lactic acidosis seen with phenformin and it is suggested in the paper[29] prepared for and approved by the British Diabetic Association that one or two drinks a day are unlikely to be harmful. However, the drug should not be given to alcoholic patients because of the possibility of liver damage.

1. Walsh CH, O'Sullivan DJ. Effect of moderate alcohol intake on control of diabetes. *Diabetes* (1974) 23, 440–2.
2. Arky RA, Veverbrants E, Abramson EA. Irreversible hypoglycemia. A complication of alcohol and insulin. *JAMA* (1968) 206, 575–8.
3. Potter J, Clarke P, Gale EAM, Dave SH, Tattersall RB. Insulin-induced hypoglycaemia in an accident and emergency department: the tip of an iceberg? *BMJ* (1982) 285, 1180–2.
4. McMonagle J, Felig P. Effects of ethanol ingestion on glucose tolerance and insulin secretion in normal and diabetic subjects. *Metabolism* (1975) 24, 625–32.
5. Lolli G, Balboni C, Ballatore C, Risoldi L, Carletti D, Silvestri L, Pacifici De Tommaso G. Wine in the diets of diabetic patients. *Q J Stud Alcohol* (1963) 24, 412–6.
6. Ben G, Gnudi L, Maran A, Gigante A, Duner E, Iori E, Tiengo A, Avogaro A. Effects of chronic alcohol intake on carbohydrate and lipid metabolism in subjects with type II (non-insulin dependent) diabetes. *Am J Med* (1991) 90, 70–6.
7. Johnston C, Wiles PG, Pyke DA. Chlorpropamide-alcohol flush: the case in favour. *Diabetologia* (1984) 26, 1–5.
8. Leslie RDG, Pyke DA. Chlorpropamide-alcohol flushing: a dominantly inherited trait associated with diabetes. *BMJ* (1978) 2, 1519.
9. Hillson RM, Hockaday TDR. Chlorpropamide-alcohol flush: a critical reappraisal. *Diabetologia* (1984) 26, 6–11.
10. Waldhäusl W. To flush or not to flush? Comments on the chlorpropamide-alcohol flush. *Diabetologia* (1984) 26, 12–14.
11. Groop L, Eriksson CJP, Huupponen R, Ylikarhi R, Pelkonen R. Roles of chlorpropamide, alcohol and acetaldehyde in determining the chlorpropamide-alcohol flush. *Diabetologia* (1984) 26, 34–38.
12. Signorelli S. Tolerance for alcohol in patients on chlorpropamide. *Ann N Y Acad Sci* (1959) 74, 900–903.
13. Conget JI, Vendrell J, Esmatjes E, Halperin I. Gliclazide alcohol flush. *Diabetes Care* (1989) 12, 44.
14. Stowers JM. Alcohol and glibenclamide. *BMJ* (1971) 3, 533.
15. Dolger H. Experience with the tolbutamide treatment of 500 cases of diabetes on an ambulatory basis. *Ann N Y Acad Sci* (1957) 71, 275.
16. Büttner H. Äthanolunverträglichkeit beim Menschen nach Sulfonylharnstoffen. *Dtsch Arch Klin Med* (1961) 207, 1–18.
17. McKendry JBR, Gfeller KF. Clinical experience with the oral antidiabetic compound tolazamide. *Can Med Assoc J* (1967) 96, 531–5.
18. Carulli N, Manenti F, Gallo M, Salvioli GF. Alcohol-drugs interaction in man: alcohol and tolbutamide. *Eur J Clin Invest* (1971) 1, 421–4.
19. Hartling SG, Faber OK, Wegmann M-L, Wahlin-Boll E and Melander A. Interaction of ethanol and glipizide in humans. *Diabetes Care* (1987) 10, 683–6.
20. Johnson HK, Waterhouse C. Relationship of alcohol and hyperlactatemia in diabetic subjects treated with phenformin. *Am J Med* (1968) 45, 98–104.
21. Davidson MB, Bozarth WR, Challoner DR, Goodner CJ. Phenformin hypoglycaemia and lactic acidosis. Report of an attempted suicide. *N Engl J Med* (1966) 275, 886–8.
22. Gottlieb A, Duberstein J, Geller A. Phenformin acidosis. *N Engl J Med* (1962) 267, 806.
23. Schaffalitzky de Muckadell OB, Koster A and Jensen SL. Fenformin-alkohol interaktion. *Ugeskr Laeger* (1973) 135, 925.
24. Culkin KT, Patterson SD, Jorkasky DK, Jorkasy DK, Freed MI. Rosiglitazone (RSG) does not increase the risk of alcohol-induced hypoglycemia in diet-treated type 2 diabetics. *Diabetes* (1999) 48 (Suppl 1), A350.
25. Johnston C, Wiles PG, Medbak S, Bowcock S, Cooke ED, Pyke DA and Rees LH. The role of endogenous opioids in the chlorpropamide alcohol flush. *Clin Endocrinol (Oxf)* (1984) 21, 489–97.
26. Kater RMH, Roggin G, Tobon F, Zieve P and Iber FL. Increased rate of clearance of drugs from the circulation of alcoholics. *Am J Med Sci* (1969) 258, 35.
27. Kater RMH, Tobon F and Iber FL. Increased rate of tolbutamide metabolism in alcoholic patients. *JAMA* (1969) 207, 363.
28. Avogaro A, Watanabe RM, Gottardo L, de Kreutzenberg S, Tiengo A, Pacini G. Glucose tolerance during moderate alcohol intake: insights on insulin action from glucose/lactate dynamics. *J Clin Endocrinol Metab* (2002) 87, 1233–8.
29. Connor H, Marks V. Alcohol and diabetes. A position paper prepared by the Nutrition Subcommittee of the British Diabetic Association's Medical Advisory Committee and approved by the Executive Council of the British Diabetic Association. *Hum Nutr Appl Nutr* (1985) 39A, 393–9.
30. Diabetes UK (formerly the British Diabetic Association). Care recommendation: alcohol. Available at http://www.diabetes.org.uk/infocentre/inform/alcohol.htm (accessed 23/06/05).
31. Fitzgerald MG, Gaddie R, Malins JM and O'Sullivan DJ. Alcohol sensitivity in diabetics receiving chlorpropamide. *Diabetes* (1962) 11, 40.
32. Daeppen JP, Hofstetter JR, Curchod B and Saudan Y. Traitment oral du diabete par un nouvel hypoglycemiant, le P 607 ou Diabinese. *Schweiz Med Wochenschr* (1959) 89, 817.
33. De Silva NE, Tunbridge WMG and Alberti KGMM. Low incidence of chlorpropamide-alcohol flushing in diet-treated, non-insulin-dependent diabetics. *Lancet* (1981) i, 128–31.

Antidiabetics + Alpha glucosidase inhibitors

Acarbose causes a moderate increase in the hypoglycaemic effects of insulin, the sulphonylureas and metformin. Miglitol causes a small reduction in serum glibenclamide levels, but blood glucose levels are reduced more than with glibenclamide alone or glibenclamide in combination with metformin. No significant pharmacokinetic interaction occurs between voglibose and glibenclamide (glyburide) or acarbose and rosiglitazone.

Clinical evidence, mechanism, importance and management

(a) Acarbose

The makers say that while acarbose does not cause hypoglycaemia when given alone, it may increase the hypoglycaemic effects of **insulin** and the **sulphonylureas**, for which reason it may be necessary to reduce their dosages. Monitor the outcome when acarbose is first given. Any hypoglycaemic episodes should be treated with glucose, not sucrose, because acarbose delays the digestion and absorption of disaccharides, but not monosaccharides.[1] A study in 6 healthy subjects found that acarbose 50 to 100 mg three times daily reduced the maximum serum levels and the 0 to 9-hour AUC of **metformin** 1 g by about 35%, but the 24-hour urinary excretion was unchanged.[2]

Another study in 19 diabetic patients given acarbose 50 or 100 mg three times daily and **metformin** 500 mg twice daily, also found that acarbose lowered **metformin** levels (AUC reduced 12 to 13%, maximum plasma levels reduced 17 to 20%). Nevertheless, the postprandial glucose levels at 3 hours were still reduced 15% more by the drug combination than by **metformin** alone.[3] There would therefore appear to be no reason for avoiding concurrent use.

A study in 16 healthy subjects found that acarbose 100 mg three times daily for a week slightly reduced the absorption of a single 8-mg oral dose of **rosiglitazone** (AUC reduced by 12%) but this was not considered to be clinically relevant.[4]

(b) Miglitol

In a randomised, double-blind, placebo controlled study, 28 patients with type 2 diabetes mellitus were given **glibenclamide** 2.5 mg twice daily with either miglitol 100 mg or a placebo three times daily for 2 days. It was found that the miglitol reduced the maximum plasma **glibenclamide** levels and its AUC by 16 and 19% respectively. Nevertheless, the average blood glucose levels were reduced more by the drug combination than by the **glibenclamide** alone. Over 5 hours there was a 15% greater reduction, and over 10 hours a 9% greater reduction.[5] Another study in patients with type 2 diabetes inadequately controlled by a combination of diet, **glibenclamide** and **metformin** found that the addition of miglitol improved glycaemic control.[6] There would therefore appear to be advantages in combining these drugs together.

(c) Voglibose

In a double-blind crossover trial, 12 healthy male subjects were given either voglibose 5 mg or a placebo three times daily for 8 days and a single 1.75-mg dose of **glibenclamide (glyburide)** on the morning of day 8, taken at the same time as the first dose of the voglibose or placebo. The voglibose had no effect on the pharmacokinetics of the **glibenclamide** and it was concluded that concurrent use is safe.[7]

1. Glucobay (Acarbose). Bayer plc. UK Summary of product characteristics, March 2004.
2. Scheen AJ, Fierra Alves de Magalhaes AC, Salvatore T, Lefebrve PJ. Reduction of the acute bioavailability of metformin by the α-glucosidase inhibitor acarbose in normal man. *Eur J Clin Invest* (1994) 24 (Suppl 3), 50–4.
3. Lettieri J, Liu MC, Sullivan JT, Heller AH. Pharmacokinetic (PK) and pharmacodynamic (PD) interaction between acarbose (A) and metformin (M) in diabetic (NIDDM) patients. *Clin Pharmacol Ther* (1998) 63, 155.
4. Miller AK, Inglis AM, Culkin KT, Jorkaksy DK, Freed MI. The effect of acarbose on the pharmacokinetics of rosiglitazone. *Eur J Clin Pharmacol* (2001) 57, 105–9.

5. Sullivan JT, Lettieri JT, Heller AH. Effects of miglitol on pharmacokinetics and pharmacodynamics of glyburide. *Clin Pharmacol Ther* (1998) 63, 155.
6. Standl E, Schernthaner G, Rybka J, Hanefeld M, Raptis SA, Naditch L. Improved glycaemic control with miglitol in inadequately-controlled type 2 diabetics. *Diabetes Res Clin Pract* (2001) 52, 205–13.
7. Kleist P, Ehrlich A, Suzuki Y, Timmer W, Wetzelsberger N, Lücker PW, Fuder H. Concomitant administration of the α-glucosidase inhibitor voglibose (AO-128) does not alter the pharmacokinetics of glibenclamide. *Eur J Clin Pharmacol* (1997) 53, 149–52.

Antidiabetics + Anabolic steroids

Nandrolone, methandienone, testosterone and stanozolol can enhance the blood sugar reducing effects of insulin.

Clinical evidence

In a study in 54 diabetics taking **nandrolone phenylpropionate** 25 mg weekly or **nandrolone decanoate** 50 mg given every three weeks by intramuscular injection, it was found necessary to reduce the insulin dosage by an average of 36% (reduction range 4 to 56 units) in about one-third of the patients.[1]

Other reports similarly describe an enhanced reduction in blood sugar levels in diabetics treated with insulin and **nandrolone**,[2,3] **methandienone**,[4] **testosterone propionate**[5] or **stanozolol**.[6] A reduction in blood sugar levels has also been seen in healthy subjects given **testosterone propionate**.[7] No changes were seen when **ethylestrenol** was used.[1,2]

Mechanism

Uncertain.

Importance and management

Established interactions but the total picture is incomplete because not all of the anabolic steroids appear to have been studied and they may not necessarily behave identically. A fall in the dosage requirements of insulin may be expected in many patients with the steroids cited. An average reduction of a third is reported.[1] Monitor concurrent use well being alert for the need to reduce the dosage of the antidiabetic agent.

1. Houtsmuller AJ. The therapeutic applications of anabolic steroids in ophthalmology: biochemical results. *Acta Endocrinol (Copenh)* (1961) 39 (Suppl 63), 154–74.
2. Dardenne U. The therapeutic applications of anabolic steroids in ophthalmology. *Acta Endocrinol (Copenh)* (1961) 39 (Suppl 63), 143–53.
3. Weissel W. Anaboles Hormon bei malignem oder kompliziertem Diabetes mellitus. *Wien Klin Wochenschr* (1962) 74, 234.
4. Landon J, Wynn V, Samols E, Bilkus D. The effect of anabolic steroids on blood sugar and plasma insulin levels in man. *Metabolism* (1963) 12, 924–35.
5. Veil WH, Lippross O. 'Unspezifische' wirkungen der Männlichen keimdrücenhormone. *Klin Wochenschr* (1938) 17, 655–8.
6. Pergola F. El estanozolol, nuevo anabolico. *Prensa Med Argent* (1962) 49, 274–90.
7. Talaat M, Habib YA, Habib M. The effect of testosterone on the carbohydrate metabolism in normal subjects. *Arch Int Pharmacodyn Ther* (1957) 111, 215–26.

Antidiabetics + Antacids

The rate of absorption of some antidiabetics is increased by some antacids, but there appear to be no reports of adverse responses in diabetic patients as a result of any of these interactions.

Clinical evidence

(a) Acarbose

A placebo-controlled study found that 10 ml of *Maalox 70* (**aluminium hydroxide/magnesium hydroxide**) had no effect on the blood glucose and insulin-lowering effects of acarbose 100 mg in 24 healthy subjects given a 75-g dose of sucrose. It was concluded that no special precautions are needed if this or similar antacids are used with acarbose.[1]

(b) Chlorpropamide

Magnesium hydroxide 850 mg increased the rate of absorption of chlorpropamide 250 mg in healthy subjects, but the insulin and glucose responses were unaffected.[2]

(c) Glibenclamide (Glyburide)

A single-dose study in healthy subjects found that **magnesium hydroxide** 850 mg had little effect on the rate or extent of absorption of a micronised glibenclamide preparation (*Semi-Euglucon*), but it caused a threefold increase in the peak plasma concentration and the bioavailability of a non-micronised preparation (*Gilemid*).[3] *Maalox* (**aluminium/magnesium hydroxide**) increased the AUC of a glibenclamide formulation (*Daonil*) by one-third, and its maximum serum level by 50%.[4]

Sodium bicarbonate 1 to 3 g very markedly increased the early bioavailability of non-micronised glibenclamide in healthy subjects, but its activity remained unaltered.[5]

(d) Glipizide

Sodium bicarbonate 3 g significantly increased the absorption of glipizide 5 mg and enhanced its effects to some extent, but the total absorption was unaltered.[6] The AUCs from 0 to 30 minutes, 1-hour and 2-hour were increased six-, four- and twofold, and the time to reach the peak serum level fell from 2.5 to 1 hours. **Aluminium hydroxide** 1 g did not appear to affect the absorption of glipizide 5 mg.[6] **Magnesium hydroxide** 850 mg also considerably increased the rate of absorption of glipizide 5 mg, the AUCs from 0 to 30 minutes and 1-hour being increased by 180 and 69%, respectively.[7]

(e) Tolbutamide

Magnesium hydroxide 850 mg increased the 0 to 1-hour and 2-hour AUCs of a single 500-mg dose of tolbutamide fivefold and 2.5-fold respectively in healthy subjects. The total AUC was unaffected. The maximum insulin response was increased fourfold and occurred about an hour earlier, and the glucose responses were also larger and occurred earlier.[2]

Mechanism

Uncertain. The small increase in gastric pH caused by these antacids possibly increases the solubility of these sulphonylureas and therefore increases their absorption.[8]

Importance and management

Although some interactions certainly occur in healthy subjects, their clinical importance in diabetics is uncertain. No reports of adverse reactions appear to have been published, but note that in patients on glipizide and sodium bicarbonate or magnesium hydroxide or tolbutamide and magnesium hydroxide may experience transient hypoglycaemia. If a problem does occur, separating the dosages as much as possible would probably minimise any effects. Giving glibenclamide half to one hour before the antacid has been suggested.[4]

1. Höpfner M, Durani B, Spengler M, Fölsch UR. Effect of acarbose and simultaneous antacid therapy on blood glucose. *Arzneimittelforschung* (1997) 47, 1108–1111.
2. Kivistö KT, Neuvonen PJ. Effect of magnesium hydroxide on the absorption and efficacy of tolbutamide and chlorpropamide. *Eur J Clin Pharmacol* (1992) 42, 675–80.
3. Neuvonen PJ, Kivistö KT. The effects of magnesium hydroxide on the absorption and efficacy of two glibenclamide preparations. *Br J Clin Pharmacol* (1991) 32, 215–20.
4. Zuccaro P, Pacifici R, Pichini S, Avico U, Federzoni G, Pini LA, Sternieri E. Influence of antacids on the bioavailability of glibenclamide. *Drugs Exp Clin Res* (1989) 15, 165–9.
5. Kivistö KT, Lehto P, Neuvonen PJ. The effects of different doses of sodium bicarbonate on the absorption and activity of non-micronized glibenclamide. *Int J Clin Pharmacol Ther Toxicol* (1993) 31, 236–40.
6. Kivistö KT, Neuvonen PJ. Differential effects of sodium bicarbonate and aluminium hydroxide on the absorption and activity of glipizide. *Eur J Clin Pharmacol* (1991) 40, 383–6.
7. Kivistö KT, Neuvonen PJ. Enhancement of absorption and effect of glipizide by magnesium hydroxide. *Clin Pharmacol Ther* (1991) 49, 39–43.
8. Lehto P, Laine K, Kivistö K, Neuvonen PJ. The effect of pH on the *in vitro* dissolution of sulfonylurea preparations — a mechanism for the antacid-sulfonylurea interaction? *Therapie* (1995) 50 (Suppl), 413.

Antidiabetics + Antimalarials

Patients, especially children or pregnant women, with falciparum malaria who have severe disease and/or are treated with quinine or quinidine may show very severe hypoglycaemia. The impact of this on the control of diabetes has yet to be determined. Other antimalarials appear to have lesser effects on blood glucose. Quinine very occasionally causes hypoglycaemia in non-diabetics treated for muscle cramps.

Clinical evidence, mechanism, importance and management

(a) Treatment of malaria

Hypoglycaemia is a complication of falciparum malaria, which occurs mainly in severe life-threatening disease,[1,2] in pregnant women[1] or children,[3,4] and in patients who are treated with **quinine** or **quinidine**.[2,4-7] The reasons are not fully understood but renal impairment and poor nutrition, may be contributing factors. In severe malaria, hypoglycaemia may increase as the patient's glucose production becomes insufficient for the host/parasite demand because in this situation glucose utilisation can be increased by 50%.[8]

Additionally, **quinine** reduces plasma glucose by stimulating the release of large amounts of **insulin** from the pancreas,[9] possibly associated with an increase in the sensitivity to **insulin** as the malaria improves,[10] although other factors may also be involved. A study in 32 patients with malaria found that their pre-treatment capillary glucose was below normal in 12.5% of cases. One hour after intravenous **quinine** was given, glucose levels in all patients fell by an average of 11.4% and after 6 hours a further fall of 20.5% was found in 75% of patients (with an increase at 6 hours in the remaining 25% of patients).[7] **Quinidine** has been shown to have a similar effect.[11] Whether these changes can also occur in patients with quinine- or quinidine-treated malaria and diabetes, despite their pancreatic beta cell impairment, seems not to have been studied, but any interpretation of disturbances in the control of the diabetes should take into account possible effects of these drugs. **Artemisinin derivatives** such as **artemether** may be associated with fewer episodes of hypoglycaemia than **quinine** in children with severe malaria.[4] **Chloroquine**, **amodiaquine** and **halofantrine** do not apparently stimulate the release of **insulin**.[11]

(b) Treatment of cramps

Quinine has also been responsible for hypoglycaemia in non-diabetic patients, one of whom was taking **quinine sulphate** 325 mg four times daily for leg muscle cramps.[12] Two other non-diabetic patients, one with congestive heart failure and the other with terminal cancer, similarly developed hypoglycaemia when given **quinine** for leg cramps.[13,14]

1. Chogle AR. Hypoglycaemia in falciparum malaria. *J Assoc Physicians India* (1998) 46, 921–2.
2. Metha SR, Joshi V, Lazar AI. Unusual acute and chronic complications of malaria. *J Assoc Physicians India* (1996) 44, 451-3.
3. Singh B, Choo KE, Ibrahim J, Johnston W, Davis TME. Non-radioisotopic glucose turnover in children with falciparum malaria end enteric fever. *Trans R Soc Trop Med Hyg* (1998) 92, 532–7.
4. Agbenyega T, Angus BJ, Bedu-Addo G, Baffoe-Bonnie B, Guyton T, Stacpoole PW, Krishna S. Glucose and lactate kinetics in children with severe malaria. *J Clin Endocrinol Metab* (2000) 85, 1569–76.
5. White NJ, Warrell DA, Chanthavanich P, Looareesuwan S, Warrell MJ, Krishna S, Williamson DH, Turner RC. Severe hypoglycemia and hyperinsulinemia in falciparum malaria. *N Engl J Med* (1983) 309, 61–6.
6. Looareesuwan S, Phillips RE, White NJ, Kietinun S, Karbwang J, Rackow C, Turner RC, Warrell DA. Quinine and severe falciparum malaria in late pregnancy. *Lancet* (1985) ii, 4–8.
7. Gupta GB, Varma S. Effect of intravenous quinine on capillary glucose levels in malaria. *J Assoc Physicians India* (2001) 49, 426–9.
8. Binh TQ, Davis TME, Johnston W, Thu LTA, Boston R, Danh PT, Anh TK. Glucose metabolism in severe malaria: minimal model analysis of the intravenous glucose tolerance test incorporating a stable glucose label. *Metabolism* (1997) 46, 1435–40.
9. Davis TME, Binh TQ, Thu LTA, Long TTA, Johnston W, Robertson K, Barrett PHR. Glucose and lactate turnover in adults with falciparum malaria: effect of complications and antimalarial therapy. *Trans R Soc Trop Med Hyg* (2002) 96, 411–17.
10. Davis TME, Pukrittayakamee S, Supanaranond W, Looareesuwan S, Krishna S, Nagachinta B, Turner RC, White NJ. Glucose metabolism in quinine-treated patients with uncomplicated falciparum malaria. *Clin Endocrinol (Oxf)* (1990) 33, 739–49.
11. Phillips RE, Looareesuwan S, White NJ, Chanthavanich P, Karbwang J, Supanaranond W, Turner RC, Warrell DA. Hypoglycaemia and antimalarial drugs: quinidine and release of insulin. *BMJ* (1986) 292, 1319–21.
12. Limburg PJ, Katz H, Grant CS, Service FJ. Quinine-induced hypoglycemia. *Ann Intern Med* (1993) 119, 218–19.
13. Harats N, Ackerman Z, Shalit M. Quinine-related hypoglycemia. *N Engl J Med* (1984) 310, 1331.
14. Jones RG, Sue-Ling HM, Kear C, Wiles PG, Quirke P. Severe symptomatic hypoglycaemia due to quinine therapy. *J R Soc Med* (1986) 79, 426–8.

Antidiabetics + Antineoplastics

Asparaginase sometimes induces temporary diabetes mellitus. It seems possible that some diabetics will need changes in the dose of their antidiabetic drugs. There is also evidence that the control of diabetes can be severely disturbed in patients given cyclophosphamide.

Clinical evidence and mechanism

(a) Asparaginase (Colaspase)

Three patients with acute lymphocytic leukaemia developed diabetes after treatment with asparaginase with or without corticosteroids. In two of them this occurred 2 and 4 days after a single dose of asparaginase, and in another patient it occurred 2 days after the fourth dose. Plasma insulin was undetectable. A normal insulin response returned in one patient after 23 days, whereas the other 2 showed a suboptimal response 2 weeks, and 9 months afterwards.[1] In another study, 5 out of 39 patients (3 adults, 2 children) developed hyperglycaemia and glycosuria after treatment with asparaginase. This responded to insulin, and blood sugar levels returned to normal in about 2 weeks.[2] In a retrospective analysis, it was found that about 10% of 421 children with leukaemia treated with asparaginase and prednisone developed hyperglycaemia, which resolved in all patients. A family history of diabetes and obesity were found to be risk factors.[3] Other cases have been described,[4-6] including one who, unusually, developed persistent hyperglycaemia and required long-term treatment with oral antidiabetics.[5] The reasons for this reaction are not understood but suggestions include inhibition of insulin synthesis,[7] direct damage to the islets of Langerhans,[1] and reduced insulin binding.[7] Hyperglycaemia can be caused by 'corticosteroids', see (p.402), and their combined use with asparaginase is probably a contributing factor.

(b) Capecitabine

There appear to be no reports of adverse interactions between antidiabetics and capecitabine, but it is reported that the control of diabetes mellitus may be affected by capecitabine for which reason the makers advise caution.[8]

(c) Cyclophosphamide

Acute hypoglycaemia has been described in 2 diabetic patients under treatment with **insulin** and **carbutamide** who were concurrently treated with cyclophosphamide.[9] Three cases of diabetes, apparently induced by the use of cyclophosphamide, have also been reported.[10] The reasons are not understood.

Importance and management

Strictly speaking probably none of these reactions is an interaction, but they serve to underline the importance of monitoring the diabetic control of patients receiving asparaginase, capecitabine or cyclophosphamide.

1. Gailani S, Nussbaum A, Ohnuma T, Freeman A. Diabetes in patients treated with asparaginase. *Clin Pharmacol Ther* (1971) 12, 487–90.
2. Ohnuma T, Holland JF, Freeman A, Sinks LF. Biochemical and pharmacological studies with asparaginase in man. *Cancer Res* (1970) 30, 2297–2305.
3. Pui C-H, Burghen GA, Bowman WP, Aur RJA. Risk factors for hyperglycemia in children with leukemia receiving L-asparaginase and prednisone. *J Pediatr* (1981) 99, 46–50.
4. Wang Y-J, Chu H-Y, Shu S-G, Chi C-S. Hyperglycemia induced by chemotherapeutic agents used in acute lymphoblastic leukemia; report of three cases. *Chin Med J* (1993) 51, 457–61.
5. Hsu Y-J, Chen Y-C, Ho C-L, Kao W-Y, Chao T-Y. Diabetic ketoacidosis and persistent hyperglycemia as long-term complications of L-asparaginase-induced pancreatitis. *Chin Med J* (2002) 65, 441–5.
6. Charan VD, Desai N, Singh AP, Choudhry VP. Diabetes mellitus and pancreatitis as a complication of L-asparaginase therapy. *Indian Pediatr* (1993) 30, 809–10.
7. Burghen G, Pui C-H, Yasuda K and Kitabchi AE. Decreased insulin binding and production: probable mechanism for hyperglycaemia due to therapy with prednisone (PRED) and l-asparaginase (ASP). *Pediatr Res* (1981) 15, 626.
8. Xeloda (Capecitabine). Roche Products Ltd. UK Summary of product characteristics, March 2005.
9. Krüger H-U. Blutzuckersenkende Wirkung von Cyclophosphamid bei Diabetikern. *Med Klin* (1966) 61, 1462–3. Roche Product Limited.
10. Pengelly CR. Diabetes mellitus and cyclophosphamide. *BMJ* (1965) i, 1312–13.

Antidiabetics + Antipsychotics

Chlorpromazine may raise blood sugar levels, particularly in daily doses of 100 mg or more, and disturb the control of diabetes. Clozapine, olanzapine and risperidone are associated with an increased risk of glucose intolerance.

Clinical evidence

(a) Phenothiazines and butyrophenones

A long-term study was undertaken over the period 1955 to 1966 in a large number of women treated for a year or longer with **chlorpromazine** 100 mg daily or more, or corresponding doses of **perphenazine**, **thioridazine**, **trifluoperazine**. This found that about 25% developed hyperglycaemia accompanied by glycosuria, compared with less than 9% in a control group who were not taking phenothiazines. Of those given a phenothiazine, about a quarter had complete remission of the symptoms when the drug was withdrawn or the dosage reduced. **Thioridazine** appeared to be less diabetogenic than the other phenothiazines used.[1]

There are other reports of this response to **chlorpromazine**.[2-11] However, in contrast one study in 850 patients suggests that **chlorpromazine** has no effect on blood sugar levels; 22 diabetic patients in the study had no significant changes in their blood sugar levels. Five patients developed diabetes, but this was believed to be due to factors other than **chlorpromazine** treatment.[12] **Chlorpromazine** 50 to 70 mg daily does not affect blood sugar levels significantly.[11] Further, the recent analysis discussed in

(b) below did not find an increased risk of glucose intolerance with **chlorpromazine** or **haloperidol**, and notes that the number of reports of glucose intolerance with these drugs has remained small.[13]

(b) Atypical antipsychotics

An analysis of reports of glucose intolerance in the adverse reaction database of the WHO Collaborating Centre for International Drug Monitoring found that **clozapine**, **olanzapine** and **risperidone** were associated with an increased risk of glucose intolerance. It is uncertain whether this is a dose-related effect. Additional risk factors with these antipsychotics were an underlying diabetic condition, weight increase, male gender, or the concurrent use of valproic acid, SSRIs or buspirone.[13]

Mechanism

Although some studies found that drugs such as chlorpromazine and haloperidol were not associated with glucose intolerance,[11,13] it seems that chlorpromazine can inhibit the release of insulin, and possibly cause adrenaline release from the adrenals, both of which could result in a rise in blood sugar levels. This may be a dose related effect.[11] Further, chlorpromazine may cause aggregation and inactivation of insulin by reduction of disulfide bonds.[14] Clozapine may induce insulin resistance and a compensatory increase in insulin secretion. Patients may develop diabetes if this compensatory increase is not achieved. Clozapine and olanzapine may cause weight gain and hypertriglyceridaemia.[13] Schizophrenia itself may be associated with an increased risk of hyperglycaemia.

Importance and management

A long-established reaction first recognised in the early 1950s. The incidence of hyperglycaemia with chlorpromazine in doses of 100 mg or more is about 25%. Increases in the dosage requirements of the antidiabetic should be anticipated during concurrent use.[1] Smaller chlorpromazine doses, of 50 to 70 mg daily do not appear to cause hyperglycaemia. There seems to be little clinical evidence that other phenothiazines or butyrophenones significantly disturb blood sugar levels in diabetics. The atypical antipsychotics, clozapine, olanzapine and risperidone appear to be associated with an increased risk of glucose intolerance and regular monitoring is recommended in the presence of additional risk factors for diabetes mellitus.[13]

1. Thonnard-Neumann E. Phenothiazines and diabetes in hospitalized women. *Am J Psychiatry* (1968) 124, 978–82.
2. Hiles BW. Hyperglycaemia and glycosuria following chlorpromazine therapy. *JAMA* (1956) 162, 1651.
3. Dobkin AB, Lamoureux L, Letienne R, Gilbert RGB. Some studies with Largactil. *Can Med Assoc J* (1954) 70, 626–8.
4. Célice J, Porcher P, Plas F, Hélie J, Peltier A. Action de la chlorpromazine sur la vésicule biliare et le clon droit. *Therapie* (1955) 10, 30–38.
5. Charatan FBE, Bartlett NG. The effect of chlorpromazine ('Largactil') on glucose tolerance. *J Ment Sci* (1955) 101, 351–3.
6. Cooperberg AA, Eidlow S. Haemolytic anaemia, jaundice and diabetes mellitus following chlorpromazine therapy. *Can Med Assoc J* (1956) 75, 746–9.
7. Blair D, Brady DM. Recent advances in the treatment of schizophrenia: group training and tranquillizers. *J Ment Sci* (1958) 104, 625–64.
8. Amidsen A. Diabetes mellitus as a side effect of treatment with tricyclic neuroleptics. *Acta Psychiatr Scand* (1964) 40 (Suppl 180), 411–14.
9. Arneson GA. Phenothiazine derivatives and glucose metabolism. *J Neuropsychiatr* (1964) 5, 181–5.
10. Korenyi C, Lowenstein B. Chlorpromazine induced diabetes. *Dis Nerv Syst* (1971) 29, 827–8.
11. Erle G, Basso M, Federspil G, Sicolo N, Scandellari C. Effect of chlorpromazine on blood glucose and plasma insulin in man. *Eur J Clin Pharmacol* (1977) 11, 15–18.
12. Schwarz L, Munoz R. Blood sugar levels in patients treated with chlorpromazine. *Am J Psychiatry* (1968) 125, 253–5.
13. Hedenmalm K, Hägg S, Ståhl M, Mortimer Ö, Spigset O. Glucose intolerance with atypical antipsychotics. *Drug Safety* (2002) 25, 1107–16.
14. Bhattacharyya J, Das KP. Aggregation of insulin by chlorpromazine. *Biochem Pharmacol* (2001) 62, 1293–7.

Antidiabetics + Azoles

Fluconazole normally appears not to affect the diabetic control of most patients taking sulphonylureas, but isolated reports describe hypoglycaemic coma in one patient on glipizide and hypoglycaemia and aggressive behaviour in a patient on gliclazide. There is some evidence that the hypoglycaemic effects of both glipizide and glibenclamide (glyburide) may be modestly increased. Fluconazole may cause marked increases in plasma levels of glimepiride.

Itraconazole also appears not to affect diabetic control in most patients, but there are reports of hypoglycaemia or hyperglycaemia associated with its use. Ketoconazole increases the hypoglycaemic effects of tolbutamide in healthy subjects and possibly increases the effects of pioglitazone. Posaconazole slightly enhanced the hypoglycaemic effects of glipizide in healthy subjects. Hypoglycaemia has been seen in few diabetics taking tolbutamide, glibenclamide or gliclazide when they were given miconazole. Clotrimazole used intravaginally appears not to interact.

Clinical evidence

A. Clotrimazole

A group of 15 postmenopausal diabetic women with vulvovaginal candidiasis taking either **gliclazide** or **glibenclamide** (**glyburide**) were treated with intravaginal **clotrimazole** 100 mg daily for 14 days. None of the patients developed symptoms of hypoglycaemia and their glycosylated haemoglobin and fructosamine concentrations were unchanged. No pharmacokinetic data were reported.[1]

B. Fluconazole

(a) Chlorpropamide

After taking fluconazole 100 mg daily for 7 days, the AUC of single 250-mg doses of chlorpropamide was increased by 28% in 18 healthy subjects but the maximum plasma levels and blood glucose levels were unchanged. There was no evidence of hypoglycaemia.[2]

(b) Glibenclamide (Glyburide)

After taking fluconazole 100 mg daily for 7 days, the AUC of a single 5-mg dose of glibenclamide was increased by 44% in 20 healthy subjects and maximum plasma levels rose by 19%. The change in blood glucose levels was not statistically significant but the number of subjects who had symptoms of hypoglycaemia increased.[3] In another study, a group of 14 postmenopausal diabetic women with vulvovaginal candidiasis taking either gliclazide or glibenclamide were treated with fluconazole 50 mg daily for 14 days. In contrast, none of the patients in this study developed symptoms of hypoglycaemia and their glycosylated haemoglobin and fructosamine concentrations were unchanged. No pharmacokinetic data were reported.[1]

(c) Gliclazide

A group of 14 postmenopausal diabetic women with vulvovaginal candidiasis taking either gliclazide or glibenclamide were treated with fluconazole 50 mg daily for 14 days. None of the patients developed symptoms of hypoglycaemia and their glycosylated haemoglobin and fructosamine concentrations were unchanged. No pharmacokinetic data were reported.[1]

However, a 56-year-old patient with HIV (antiretroviral treatment refused) and type 2 diabetes treated with gliclazide for 2 years was treated with fluconazole 50 mg daily for 2 weeks for oral candidiasis and prophylactic co-trimoxazole (sulfamethoxazole 400 mg and trimethoprim 80 mg daily). One week after the re-introduction of fluconazole at a higher dose of 200 mg daily he was hospitalised because of weakness and aggressive behaviour. His blood glucose was 2.2 mmol/l and gliclazide was stopped. He experienced brief loss of consciousness 2 days later while driving his car, but his condition then improved and neurological symptoms did not recur during 3 months follow-up without gliclazide treatment.[4] For the possible contribution of sulfamethoxazole to this interaction, see Mechanism, below.

(d) Glimepiride

A double-blind study in 12 healthy subjects found that fluconazole 400 mg on day one then 200 mg daily for a further 3 days increased the AUC and peak plasma level of a single 0.5-mg dose of glimepiride by about 2.5-fold and 1.5-fold respectively. Fluconazole increased the mean elimination half-life of glimepiride from 2 to 3.3 hours.[5]

(e) Glipizide

After taking fluconazole 100 mg daily for 7 days, the AUC of single 2.5-mg doses of glipizide was increased by 49% in 13 healthy subjects and their maximum serum levels rose by 17%. Although blood glucose levels went down the change was not statistically significant. However, the number of subjects who had symptoms suggestive of hypoglycaemia increased.[6]

A diabetic on glipizide 2.5 mg three times daily developed a hypoglycaemic coma within 4 days of starting to take fluconazole 200 mg daily. Her blood sugar levels had fallen to less than 1 g/l. She rapidly recovered when given glucose.[7]

(f) Nateglinide

In a randomised double-blind crossover study, 10 healthy subjects were given a single 30-mg dose of nateglinide on day 4 of a course of fluconazole (given as 400 mg on day one, then 200 mg daily). Fluconazole raised the AUC of nateglinide by 48% (range 20 to 73%) and increased the nateglinide half life from 1.6 to 1.9 hours. Despite these pharmacokinetic changes fluconazole did not potentiate the hypoglycaemic effects of nateglinide.[8] It was predicted that this interaction may occur with **miconazole**, but this needs confirmation.

(g) Tolbutamide

After taking a single 150-mg dose and a further 6 doses of fluconazole 100 mg daily, the AUC of a single 500-mg dose of tolbutamide were increased by about 50%, and the peak plasma levels were raised in 13 healthy subjects. The half-life of the tolbutamide was increased about 40%. Blood glucose levels remained unaltered and none of the subjects showed any evidence of hypoglycaemia.[9,10] However, the authors caution against extrapolating this finding to diabetic patients taking tolbutamide regularly.[9,10]

C. Itraconazole

Post-marketing surveillance over 10 years indicated that in most patients, itraconazole given with either **insulin** or **oral antidiabetics** did not affect diabetic control. However, there were 15 reports suggesting hyperglycaemia and 9 reports suggesting hypoglycaemia with itraconazole and antidiabetics.[11] In clinical trials only one of 189 diabetic patients experienced aggravated diabetes when given itraconazole.[11] The patient in question was also receiving ciclosporin for a renal transplant.

Itraconazole 200 mg then 100 mg twice daily for 3 days increased the AUC of a single 250-microgram dose of **repaglinide** by 40%.[12] However, no change was noted in blood glucose levels when compared with **repaglinide** alone.[12,13]

D. Ketoconazole

After an overnight fast and breakfast the next morning, 7 healthy subjects were given a single 500-mg dose of **tolbutamide** before and after taking ketoconazole 200 mg daily for a week. The ketoconazole increased the elimination half life of the **tolbutamide** more than threefold (from 3.7 to 12.3 hours) and increased its AUC by 77%. Blood glucose measurements showed that the ketoconazole increased the blood sugar lowering effects of the **tolbutamide** by about 10 to 15%, and 5 of the subjects experienced mild hypoglycaemic symptoms (weakness, sweating and a reeling sensation) at about 2 hours after the dose.[14]

Ketoconazole 200 mg for 5 days increased the AUC and maximum plasma levels of a single dose of **repaglinide** 2 mg by 15 and 8% respectively in healthy subjects.[13]

Although there appear to be no adverse reports of an interaction between **pioglitazone** and ketoconazole, the US prescribing information refers to a 7-day study in which ketoconazole inhibited the liver metabolism of pioglitazone.[15]

E. Miconazole

A diabetic patient taking **tolbutamide** was hospitalised with severe hypoglycaemia about 10 days after starting to take miconazole.[16] In 1983 the French Commission Nationale de Pharmacovigilance reported 6 cases of hypoglycaemia in diabetics on sulphonylureas within 2 to 6 days of beginning treatment with miconazole (5 with **gliclazide** and one with **glibenclamide (glyburide)**).[16] The same organisation report a further 8 cases in the 1985 to 1990 period but individual sulphonylureas were not named.[17] Three other cases (two with **gliclazide** and one with **glibenclamide**) are reported elsewhere, in patients given miconazole up to 750 mg daily.[18]

F. Posaconazole

A study in 12 healthy subjects found that posaconazole 400 mg twice daily for 10 days had no significant effects on the steady-state pharmacokinetics of **glipizide** 10 mg daily, but there was a small significant decrease in blood glucose levels following concurrent use. **Glipizide** did not affect the pharmacokinetics of posaconazole.[19]

Mechanism

Uncertain. When the plasma levels and effects of these hypoglycaemic agents are increased, a possible mechanism is that fluconazole or miconazole inhibits their metabolism by the liver causing them to accumulate and thereby increasing their effects. The hypoglycaemia in the patient on gliclazide (metabolised by the cytochrome P450 isoenzyme CYP2C9) and fluconazole, which inhibits isoenzyme CYP2C9, may have been enhanced by sulfamethoxazole, which also inhibits this isoenzyme.[4] The moderate pharmacokinetic changes seen when fluconazole is given with nateglinide are also though to be mediated by CYP2C9. The modest changes in repaglinide pharmacokinetics may be because repaglinide is metabolised by both CYP2C8 and CYP3A4, and one pathway may have the capacity to compensate if the other is inhibited.[20]

Importance and management

The almost total absence of adverse reports implies that fluconazole and itraconazole do not usually markedly disturb the control of diabetes in those taking sulphonylureas. For fluconazole the increased plasma levels of glipizide and glimepiride, and the single case of severe hypoglycaemia, as well as the hypoglycaemic symptoms shown by those on glibenclamide (glyburide) or gliclazide suggest that patients on these sulphonylureas in particular should be warned to be alert for any evidence of hypoglycaemia. However, there seems to be no reason for avoiding concurrent use. Note that in the study with nateglinide a sub-therapeutic dose was given to healthy subjects, so in clinical practice a greater hypoglycaemic effect may possibly occur. The effect of itraconazole on repaglinide could potentially be important so increased monitoring of glucose levels is advisable.

Information about ketoconazole appears to be limited to one study in healthy subjects. The reaction in diabetics is uncertain, but if ketoconazole is added to tolbutamide, patients should be warned to be alert for any evidence of increased hypoglycaemia. It may become necessary to reduce the tolbutamide dosage. Ketoconazole may also inhibit the metabolism of pioglitazone and more frequent blood glucose monitoring is recommended. The pharmacokinetic changes with ketoconazole and repaglinide are minor, and unlikely to be of any clinical relevance.

The interaction between miconazole and the sulphonylureas is established and clinically important, but of uncertain (but probably low) incidence. Concurrent use need not be avoided but it should be monitored and the dosage of the sulphonylurea reduced if necessary. Patients should be warned. Information about other sulphonylureas not cited is lacking but it seems possible that they may interact similarly with miconazole.

Information about intravaginal clotrimazole is very sparse, but it appears not to interact with gliclazide or glibenclamide (glyburide), and probably not with any of the other oral hypoglycaemic agents, not least because its absorption from the vagina is very small.

1. Rowe BR, Thorpe J, Barnett A. Safety of fluconazole in women taking oral hypoglycaemic agents. *Lancet* (1992) 339, 255–6.
2. Anon. A volunteer-blind, placebo-controlled study to assess potential interaction between fluconazole and chlorpropamide in healthy male volunteers. Protocol 238: Pfizer, data on file.
3. Anon. A volunteer-blind, placebo-controlled study to assess potential interaction between fluconazole and glibenclamide in healthy male volunteers. Protocol 236: Pfizer, data on file.
4. Abad S, Moachon L, Blanche P, Bavoux F, Sicard D, Salmon-Céron D. Possible interaction between gliclazide, fluconazole and sulfamethoxazole resulting in severe hypoglycaemia. *Br J Clin Pharmacol* (2001) 52, 456–7.
5. Niemi M, Backman JT, Neuvonen M, Laitila J, Neuvonen PJ, Kivistö KT. Effects of fluconazole and fluvoxamine on the pharmacokinetics and pharmacodynamics of glimepiride. *Clin Pharmacol Ther* (2001) 69, 194–200.
6. Anon. A volunteer-blind, placebo-controlled study to assess potential interaction between fluconazole and glipizide in healthy male volunteers. Protocol 237: Pfizer, data on file.
7. Fournier JP, Schneider S, Martinez P, Mahagne MH, Ducoeur S, Haffner M, Thiercelin D, Chichmanain RM, Bertrand F. Coma hypoglycémique chez une patiente traitée par glipizide et fluconazole: une possible interaction? *Therapie* (1992) 47, 446–7.
8. Niemi M, Neuvonen M, Juntti-Patinen L, Backman JT, Neuvonen PJ. Effect of fluconazole on the pharmacokinetics and pharmacodynamics of nateglinide. *Clin Pharmacol Ther* (2003) 74, 25–31.
9. Lazar JD, Wilner KD. Drug interactions with fluconazole. *Rev Infect Dis* (1990) 12 (Suppl 3), S327—S333.
10. Anon. A double-blind placebo-controlled study to assess the potential interaction between fluconazole and tolbutamide in healthy male volunteers. Pfizer, data on file.
11. Verspeelt J, Marynissen G, Gupta AK, De Doneker P. Safety of itraconazole in diabetic patients. *Dermatology* (1999) 198, 382–4.
12. Niemi M, Backman JT, Neuvonen M, Neuvonen PJ. Effects of gemfibrozil, itraconazole, and their combination on the pharmacokinetics and pharmacodynamics of repaglinide: potentially hazardous interaction between gemfibrozil and repaglinide. *Diabetologia* (2003) 46, 347–51.
13. Hatorp V, Hansen KT, Thomsen MS. Influence of drugs interacting with CYP3A4 on the pharmacokinetics, pharmacodynamics, and safety of the prandial glucose regulator repaglinide. *J Clin Pharmacol* (2003) 43, 649–60.
14. Krishnaiah YSR, Satyanarayana S, Visweswaram D. Interaction between tolbutamide and ketoconazole in healthy subjects. *Br J Clin Pharmacol* (1994) 37, 205–7.
15. Actos (Pioglitazone hydrochloride). Takeda Ltd. US Prescribing information, August 2004.
16. Meurice JC, Lecomte P, Renard JP, Girard JJ. Interaction miconazole et sulfamides hypoglycémiants. *Presse Med* (1983) 12, 1670.
17. Girardin E, Vial T, Pham E, Evreux J-C. Hypoglycémies induites par les sulfamides hypoglycémiants. *Ann Med Interne (Paris)* (1992) 143, 11–17.
18. Loupi E, Descotes J, Lery N, Evreux JC. Interactions médicamenteuses et miconazole. A propos de 10 observations. *Therapie* (1982) 37, 437–41.
19. Courtney R, Sansone A, Statkevich P, Martinho M, Laughlin M. Assessment of the pharmacokinetic (PK), pharmacodynamic (PD) interaction potential between posaconazole and glipizide in healthy volunteers. *Clin Pharmacol Ther* (2003) 73, P45.
20. Bidstrup TB, Bjørnsdottir I, Sidelmann UG, Thomsen MS, Hansen KT. CYP2C8 and CYP3A4 are the principal enzymes involved in the human in vitro biotransformation of the insulin secretagogue repaglinide. *Br J Clin Pharmacol* (2003) 56, 305–14.

Antidiabetics + Benzodiazepines

No adverse interaction normally occurs between antidiabetics and benzodiazepines, but an isolated case of hyperglycaemia has been seen in an insulin-treated patient with type 2 diabetes associated with the use of chlordiazepoxide. The effects of lorazepam were found to be increased in patients given beef/pork insulin rather than human insulin.

Clinical evidence, mechanism, importance and management

A woman with long-standing type 2 diabetes, stable on 45 units of **isophane insulin suspension** daily, had a rise in her mean fasting blood sugar from 220 to 380 mg/100 ml during a 3-week period while taking **chlordiazepoxide** 40 mg daily. Four other patients with type 2 diabetes, 2 diet-controlled and 2 on **tolbutamide**, had no changes in blood sugar levels while taking **chlordiazepoxide**.[1] In another study **diazepam** did not change the half-life of **chlorpropamide**.[2] A preliminary report in 8 healthy type 1 diabetics given **lorazepam** 2 mg suggested that while they were taking **human insulin** they were more alert and less impaired than when taking **beef/pork insulin**.[3]

There seems to be nothing in the literature to suggest that a clinically important adverse interaction normally takes place between the hypoglycaemic agents and the benzodiazepines. No special precautions would appear to be necessary.

1. Zumoff B, Hellman L. Aggravation of diabetic hyperglycemia by chlordiazepoxide. *JAMA* (1977) 237, 1960–1.
2. Petitpierre B, Perrin L, Rudhardt M, Herrera A, Fabre J. Behaviour of chlorpropamide in renal insufficiency and under the effect of associated drug therapy. *Int J Clin Pharmacol* (1972) 6, 120–4.
3. Dahlan AA, Vrbancic MI, Hogan TE, Woo D, Herman RI. Greater sedative response to lorazepam in patients with insulin-dependent diabetes mellitus while on treatment with beef/pork versus human insulin. *Clin Invest Med* (1993) 16 (4 Suppl), B18.

Antidiabetics + Beta-blockers

In diabetics using insulin, the normal recovery reaction (blood sugar rise) if hypoglycaemia occurs may be impaired to some extent by propranolol, but serious and severe hypoglycaemia and hypertension seem rare. Other beta-blockers normally interact to a lesser extent or not at all. The hypoglycaemic effects of the sulphonylureas may possibly be reduced by the beta-blockers. Whether insulin or the sulphonylureas are given, be aware that some of the familiar warning signs of hypoglycaemia (tachycardia, tremor) may not occur, although sweating may be increased.

Clinical evidence

(a) Insulin

(i) Hypoglycaemia. Although **propranolol** has occasionally been associated with spontaneous episodes of hypoglycaemia in non-diabetics,[1] and a number of studies in diabetic patients[2] and healthy subjects[3-6] have found that **propranolol** impairs the normal blood sugar rebound if blood sugar levels fall, there appear to be few reports of severe hypoglycaemia or coma in diabetics on **insulin** and **propranolol**. Marked hypoglycaemia and/or coma occurred in 5 diabetic patients on **insulin** due to the use of **propranolol**,[1,7,8] **pindolol**,[8] and **timolol** eye-drops.[9] Other contributory factors (fasting, haemodialysis, etc.) probably had some part to play.[8] **Metoprolol** interacts like **propranolol** but to a lesser extent,[3,5,10] whereas **acebutolol**,[2,5] **alprenolol**,[11] **atenolol**,[2,12,13] **oxprenolol**,[10] **penbutolol**,[6] **pindolol**[14] have been found to interact minimally or not at all. The situation with **pindolol** is therefore not clear. **Propranolol** (a vasoconstrictor) has also been found to reduce the rate of absorption of subcutaneous **insulin** by almost 50%, but the importance of this is uncertain.[15]

(ii) Hypertension. Marked increases in blood pressure and bradycardia may develop if hypoglycaemia occurs in diabetics on **insulin** and beta-blockers.[16] In one study in diabetics, insulin-induced hypoglycaemia resulted in blood pressure rises of 38.8/14.3 mmHg in those on **propranolol** 80 mg twice daily, 27.9/0 mmHg in those on **atenolol** 100 mg daily and in those on placebo the systolic blood pressure rose by 15.6 mmHg whereas the diastolic blood pressure fell by 9.2 mmHg.[17] In another study insulin-induced hypoglycaemia resulted in blood rises of 27/14 mmHg in those taking **alprenolol** 200 to 800 mg daily, but no rise occurred in those on **metoprolol** 100 to 400 mg daily.[18] A report describes a pressure rise to 258/144 mmHg in a patient having a hypoglycaemic episode within 2 days of starting **propranolol**.[7] Another patient on **metoprolol** 50 mg twice daily experienced a rise from 190/96 to 230/112 mmHg during a hypoglycaemic episode.[16]

(b) Oral antidiabetics

(i) Hyperglycaemia, hypoglycaemia or no interaction. The sulphonylurea-induced insulin-release from the pancreas can be inhibited by beta-blockers so that the hypoglycaemic effects are opposed to some extent. The effects of **glibenclamide (glyburide)**,[19] **chlorpropamide**[20] and **tolbutamide**[21] have been shown to be inhibited by **propranolol**. **Acebutolol** affects **glibenclamide** in the same way as **propranolol** but has fewer unwanted haemodynamic effects,[19] and has no effect on **tolbutamide**.[22] Two isolated cases of hypoglycaemia have been seen with **acebutolol**, in one patient taking **gliclazide** and the other taking **chlorpropamide**.[23] One study did not find an interaction between **tolbutamide** and either **propranolol** or **metoprolol**,[24] and another found no interaction between **betaxolol** and **glibenclamide** or **metformin**.[25] No pharmacokinetic interaction was seen in a study in healthy subjects given **glibenclamide** with **carvedilol**.[26] An isolated report describes hyperosmolar non-ketotic coma in a patient on **tolbutamide** and **propranolol**.[27] It is worth noting that the United Kingdom Prospective Diabetes Study Group (UKPDS) used **atenolol** 50 to 100 mg daily or captopril 25 to 50 mg twice daily as a first line agent in the control of raised blood pressure in diabetics on a range of antidiabetics. The number of patients experiencing hypoglycaemic attacks did not differ for the two antihypertensives, although weight gain was greater in the group treated with atenolol (3.4 kg for the **atenolol** group compared to 1.6 kg for the captopril group).[28] This would suggest that beta-blockers are generally useful in the treatment of diabetics.

Mechanism

One of the normal physiological responses to a fall in blood sugar levels is the mobilisation of glucose from the liver under the stimulation of adrenaline from the adrenals. This sugar mobilisation is blocked by non-selective beta-blockers (such as propranolol) so that recovery from hypoglycaemia is delayed and may even proceed into a full-scale episode in a hypoglycaemia-prone diabetic. Normally the adrenaline would also increase the heart rate, but with the beta-receptors in the heart already blocked this fails to occur. A rise in blood pressure occurs because the stimulant effects of adrenaline on the beta-2 receptors (vasodilation) are blocked leaving the alpha (vasoconstriction) effects unopposed. Non-selective beta-blockers can also block beta-2 receptors in the pancreas concerned with insulin-release, so that the effects of the sulphonylureas may be blocked.

Importance and management

Extremely well-studied interactions. Concurrent use can be uneventful but there are some risks.

Diabetics on insulin may have a prolonged or delayed recovery response to hypoglycaemia while on beta-blockers, but very severe hypoglycaemia and/or coma is rare. If hypoglycaemia occurs it may be accompanied by a sharp rise in blood pressure. The risk is greatest with propranolol and possibly other non-selective blockers and least with the cardio-selective blockers (e.g. atenolol, metoprolol, etc.). Monitor the effects of concurrent use well, avoid the non-selective blockers where possible, and check for any evidence that the insulin dosage needs some adjustment. Warn all patients that some of the normal premonitory signs of a hypoglycaemic attack may not appear, in particular tachycardia and tremors, whereas the hunger, irritability and nausea signs may be unaffected and sweating may even be increased.

Diabetics taking oral sulphonylureas rarely seem to have serious hypoglycaemic episodes caused by beta-blockers, and any reductions in the hypoglycaemic effects of the sulphonylureas normally appear to be of little clinical importance. The selective beta-blockers are probably safer than those that are non-selective. Nevertheless, always monitor concurrent use to confirm that diabetic control is well maintained, adjusting the dose of antidiabetic as necessary, and warn all patients (as above) that some of the premonitory signs of hypoglycaemia may not occur.

One experimental study indicated that no interaction occurred between betaxolol and metformin,[25] but direct information about other beta-blockers seems to be lacking.

There is also a hint from one report that the peripheral vasoconstrictive effects of non-selective beta-blockers and the poor peripheral circulation in diabetics could be additive,[7] which is another good reason for avoiding this type of beta-blocker in diabetics.

1. Kotler MN, Berman L, Rubenstein AH. Hypoglycaemia precipitated by propranolol. *Lancet* (1966) 2, 1389–90.
2. Deacon SP, Karunanayake A, Barnett D. Acebutolol, atenolol, and propranolol and metabolic responses to acute hypoglycaemia in diabetics. *BMJ* (1977) 2, 1255–7.
3. Davidson NM, Corrall RJM, Shaw TRD, French EB. Observations in man of hypoglycaemia during selective and non-selective beta-blockade. *Scott Med J* (1976) 22, 69–72.
4. Abramson EA, Arky RA, Woeber KA. Effects of propranolol on the hormonal and metabolic responses to insulin-induced hypoglycaemia. *Lancet* (1966) ii, 1386–9.
5. Newman RJ. Comparison of propranolol, metoprolol, and acebutolol on insulin-induced hypoglycaemia. *BMJ* (1976) 2, 447–9.
6. Sharma SD, Vakil BJ, Samuel MR, Chadha DR. Comparison of penbutolol and propranolol during insulin-induced hypoglycaemia. *Curr Ther Res* (1979) 26, 252–9.
7. McMurtry RJ. Propranolol, hypoglycemia, and hypertensive crisis. *Ann Intern Med* (1974) 80, 669–70.
8. Samii K, Ciancioni C, Rottembourg J, Bisseliches F, Jacobs C. Severe hypoglycaemia due to beta-blocking drugs in haemodialysis patients. *Lancet* (1976) i, 545–6.
9. Angelo-Nielsen K. Timolol topically and diabetes mellitus. *JAMA* (1980) 244, 2263.
10. Viberti GC, Stimmler M, Keen H. The effect of oxprenolol and metoprolol on the hypoglycaemic response to insulin in normals and insulin-dependent diabetics. *Diabetologia* (1978) 15, 278.
11. Eisalo A, Heino A, Munter J. The effect of alprenolol in elderly patients with raised blood pressure. *Acta Med Scand* (1974) (Suppl), 554, 23–31.
12. Deacon SP, Barnett D. Comparison of atenolol and propranolol during insulin-induced hypoglycaemia. *BMJ* (1976) 2, 272–3.
13. Waal-Manning HJ. Atenolol and three nonselective β-blockers in hypertension. *Clin Pharmacol Ther* (1979) 25, 8–18.
14. Patsch W, Patsch JR, Sailer S. Untersuchung zur Wirkung von Pindolol auf Kohlehydrat- und Fettstoffwechsel bei Diabetes Mellitus. *Int J Clin Pharmacol Biopharm* (1977) 15, 394–6.
15. Veenstra J, van der Hulst JP, Wildenborg IH, Njoo SF, Verdegaal WP, Silberbusch J. Effect of antihypertensive drugs on insulin absorption. *Diabetes Care* (1991) 14, 1089–92.
16. Shepherd AMM, Lin M-S, Keeton TK. Hypoglycemia-induced hypertension in a diabetic patient on metoprolol. *Ann Intern Med* (1981) 94, 357–8.
17. Ryan JR, Lacorte W, Jain A, McMahon FG. Response of diabetics treated with atenolol or propranolol to insulin-induced hypoglycaemia. *Drugs* (1983) 25 (Suppl), 256–7.
18. Östman J, Arner P, Haglund K, Juhlin-Dannfelt A, Nowak J, Wennlund A. Effect of metoprolol and alprenolol on the metabolic, hormonal, and haemodynamic response to insulin-induced hypoglycaemia in hypertensive, insulin-dependent diabetics. *Acta Med Scand* (1982) 211, 381–5.
19. Zaman R, Kendall MJ, Biggs PI. The effect of acebutolol and propranolol on the hypoglycaemic action of glibenclamide. *Br J Clin Pharmacol* (1982) 13, 507–12.
20. Holt RJ, Gaskins JD. Hyperglycaemia associated with propranolol and chlorpropamide coadministration. *Drug Intell Clin Pharm* (1981) 15, 599–600.
21. Massara F, Strumia E, Camanni F, Molinatti GM. Depressed tolbutamide-induced insulin response in subjects treated with propranolol. *Diabetologia* (1971) 7, 287–9.
22. Ryan JR. Clinical pharmacology of acebutolol. *Am Heart J* (1985) 109, 1131–6.
23. Girardin E, Vial T, Pham E, Evreux J-C. Hypoglycémies induites par les sulfamides hypoglycémiants. *Ann Med Interne (Paris)* (1992) 143, 11–17.
24. Tötterman KJ, Groop LC. No effect of propranolol and metoprolol on the tolbutamide-stimulated insulin-secretion in hypertensive diabetic and non-diabetic patients. *Ann Clin Res* (1982) 14, 190–3.
25. Sinclair AJ, Davies IB, Warrington SJ. Betaxolol and glucose-insulin relationships: studies in normal subjects taking glibenclamide or metformin. *Br J Clin Pharmacol* (1990) 30, 699–702.
26. Harder S, Merz PG, Rietbrock N. Lack of pharmacokinetic interaction between carvedilol and digitoxin, phenprocoumon or glibenclamide. *Cardiovasc Drugs Ther* (1993) 7 (Suppl 2), 447.
27. Podolsky S, Pattavina CG. Hyperosmolar nonketotic diabetic coma: a complication of propranolol therapy. *Metabolism* (1973) 22, 685–93.
28. UK Prospective Diabetes Study Group. Efficacy of atenolol and captopril in reducing risk of macrovascular and microvascular complications in type 2 diabetes: UKPDS 39. *BMJ* (1998) 317, 713–20.

Antidiabetics + Bile-acid binding resins

A report suggests that the hypocholesterolaemic effects of colestipol are unaffected in insulin-treated diabetics but they may be ineffective in those treated with phenformin and sulphonylureas. There is evidence that the absorption of glipizide may be reduced about 30% if it is taken at the same time as colestyramine. Tolbutamide is reported not to interact with colestyramine.

Clinical evidence

(a) Colestipol

The concurrent use of **phenformin** and a sulphonylurea (**chlorpropamide**, **tolbutamide** or **tolazamide**) inhibited the normal hypocholesterolaemic effects of the colestipol in 12 diabetics with elevated serum cholesterol levels. No such antagonism was seen in two patients with type 2 diabetes treated with **insulin**. The control of diabetes was not affected by the colestipol.[1]

(b) Colestyramine

Colestyramine 12 g daily for 6 days given to 8 healthy subjects taking **acarbose** 100 mg three times daily improved the reduction in postprandial insulin levels.[2] The mean serum insulin levels fell by 23% while taking both drugs, but showed a 'rebound' 31% increase above baseline when both were stopped.[2]

Colestyramine 8 g in 150 ml water reduced the absorption of a single 5-mg dose of **glipizide** in 6 healthy subjects by a mean of 29%. One subject had a 41% reduction. Peak serum levels were reduced by 33%. The 0 to 10-hour AUC was used to measure absorption.[3]

A single dose study indicated that colestyramine 8 g, given 2 minutes before and 6 and 12 hours after a 500-mg dose of **tolbutamide**, does not reduce the amount of **tolbutamide** absorbed, although the rate may be changed.[4]

Mechanism

Colestyramine is an anion-exchange resin, intended to bind to bile acids within the gut, but it can also bind with some acidic drugs thereby reducing the amount available for absorption.

Importance and management

Information about glipizide is limited to this single-dose study so that the clinical importance of the interaction is unknown, but it would seem prudent to monitor the effects of concurrent use in patients. It has been suggested[3] that the glipizide should be taken 1 to 2 hours before the colestyramine to minimise admixture in the gut, but this may only be partially effective because it is believed that glipizide undergoes some enterohepatic circulation (i.e. after absorption it is excreted in the bile and reabsorbed). The effect of colestyramine on other sulphonylureas is uncertain, with the exception of tolbutamide, which is reported not to interact. The clinical importance of the effects of colestyramine on acarbose in diabetics is uncertain.

The study with colestipol suggests that it may not be suitable for lowering the blood cholesterol levels of diabetics treated with chlorpropamide, tolbutamide, tolazamide or phenformin, but more study is needed to confirm these findings. Phenformin has been withdrawn from many countries because of severe, often fatal, lactic acidosis.

1. Bandisode MS, Boshell BR. Hypocholesterolemic activity of colestipol in diabetes. *Curr Ther Res* (1975) 18, 276–84.
2. Bayer, Personal Communications, June-July 1993.
3. Kivistö K T, Neuvonen P J. The effect of cholestyramine and activated charcoal on glipizide absorption. *Br J Clin Pharmacol* (1990) 30, 733–6.
4. Hunninghake D B, Pollack E. Effect of bile acid sequestering agents on the absorption of aspirin, tolbutamide and warfarin. *Fedn Proc* (1977) 35, 996.

Antidiabetics + Calcium channel blockers

Calcium channel blockers are known to have effects on insulin secretion and glucose regulation, but significant disturbances in the control of diabetes are uncommon. A report describes a patient whose diabetes worsened, requiring an increase in the dose of insulin when diltiazem was given, and a similar case has been seen in a patient on nifedipine. Hypoglycaemia occurred in a patient taking gliclazide and nicardipine.

Clinical evidence

(a) Dihydropyridines

A study in 20 patients with type 2 diabetes (5 on **metformin** and 15 diet-controlled) found that both **nifedipine** 10 mg every 8 hours and **nicardipine** 30 mg every 8 hours for 4 weeks did not affect either glucose tolerance tests or the control of the diabetes, but both systolic and diastolic blood pressures were reduced by 4 to 7 mmHg.[1] Another study in 8 non-diabetics and 8 type 2 diabetics (3 on **chlorpropamide**, one on **glipizide** and 4 on diet alone) found that the use of **nifedipine** 30 mg daily for a month did not significantly alter their glucose tolerance tests.[2] No important changes occurred in 6 type 2 diabetic patients taking **glibenclamide** (**glyburide**) when they were given nifedipine 20 to 60 mg daily for 12 to 25 weeks.[3] Another study in 6 type 2 diabetics found that single 20-mg doses of **nifedipine** had no effect on the pharmacokinetics or actions of **glipizide** 5 to 20 mg daily.[4] This confirms other studies with **nifedipine**[5] and **nicardipine**.[6] **Nitrendipine** 30 mg daily over a 5-year period was reported to have had no adverse effect on the control of diabetes in 14 elderly patients with type 2 diabetes using **insulin** or oral antidiabetic agents.[7] No clinically relevant interactions were found in 11 type 2 diabetics on **glibenclamide** while treated with **nimodipine**.[8] The makers of acarbose say that in a pilot study of a possible interaction with **nifedipine**, no significant or reproducible changes were seen in the plasma **nifedipine** profiles.[9,10]

A three-period cross-over open-label study in healthy subjects found that **nifedipine** 10 mg daily decreased the maximum plasma level of repaglinide 2 mg three times daily by 2.7% and increased the bioavailability of repaglinide by 11%, but this was not statistically significant. There was a higher incidence of adverse effects during concurrent use.[11]

However, there are other reports of a deterioration in glucose tolerance during the use of **nifedipine** in a total of 12 subjects with impaired glucose tolerance.[12,13] A further case report described a 30% increase in the insulin requirements of a diabetic man after he took **nifedipine** 60 mg daily.[14] One study found that **nifedipine** 10 mg increased the rate of absorption of subcutaneous **insulin** by about 50%.[15]

An isolated case of hypoglycaemia has been described in a patient on **gliclazide** when treated with **nicardipine**.[16]

Rosiglitazone 8 mg daily for 2 weeks was found to have no clinically relevant effect on the pharmacokinetics of **nifedipine** in 28 healthy subjects.[17]

(b) Diltiazem

A patient with type 1 diabetes developed worsening and intractable hyperglycaemia (mean serum glucose levels above 13 mmol/l) when given diltiazem 90 mg every 6 hours. Her **insulin** requirements dropped when the diltiazem was withdrawn. When she was started on diltiazem 30 mg every 6 hours her blood sugar levels were still high, but she needed less **insulin** than when taking the higher diltiazem dosage.[18]

A study in 12 healthy subjects found that diltiazem 60 mg three times daily had no effect on the secretion of insulin or glucagon, or on plasma glucose levels.[19]

A study in 8 healthy subjects found that a single 500-mg dose of **tolbutamide** had no effect on the serum levels of a single 60-mg dose of diltiazem. There was an increase of about 10% in the 0 to 24-hour AUC and maximum serum levels of **tolbutamide** in the presence of diltiazem but the hypoglycaemic effects of **tolbutamide** were not significantly changed.[20]

(c) Verapamil

A study in 23 type 2 diabetics, 7 of whom were taking **glibenclamide (glyburide)**, found that verapamil improved the response to an oral glucose tolerance test but did not increase the hypoglycaemic effects of the **glibenclamide**.[21] Two studies in type 2 diabetics found that verapamil improved the response to glucose tolerance tests,[22,23] but in one of the studies, no alterations in the hypoglycaemic effects of **glibenclamide** were found.[22] A study in healthy subjects found that verapamil raised serum **glibenclamide** levels but plasma glucose levels were unchanged.[24]

Mechanism

The changes that occur are not fully understood. Suggestions include: inhibition of insulin secretion by the calcium channel blockers and inhibition of glucagon secretion by glucose; changes in glucose uptake by liver and other cells; blood glucose rises following catecholamine release after vasodilation, and changes in glucose metabolism. In contrast, one study in non-diabetics suggested that long-acting nifedipine could improve insulin sensitivity.[25]

Importance and management

Very extensively studied, but many of the reports describe single-dose studies or multiple-dose studies in healthy subjects (only a few are cited here), which do not give a clear picture of what may be expected in diabetic patients. Those studies that have concentrated on diabetics indicate that the control of the diabetes is not usually adversely affected by calcium channel blockers although isolated cases with diltiazem, nicardipine and nifedipine have been reported.[14,16,18] No particular precautions normally seem to be necessary, nevertheless be alert for any signs of a worsening control of the diabetes. More study in diabetics is needed.

1. Collins WCJ, Cullen MJ, Feely J. Calcium channel blocker drugs and diabetic control. *Clin Pharmacol Ther* (1987) 42, 420–3.
2. Donnelly T, Harrower ADB. Effect of nifedipine on glucose tolerance and insulin secretion in diabetic and non-diabetic patients. *Curr Med Res Opin* (1980) 6, 690–3.
3. Kanatsuna T, Nakano K, Mori H, Kano Y, Nishioka H, Kajiyama S, Kitagawa Y, Yoshida T, Kondo M, Nakamura N, Aochi O. Effects of nifedipine on insulin secretion and glucose metabolism in rats and hypertensive type 2 (non-insulin dependent) diabetics. *Arzneimittelforschung* (1985) 35, 514–17.
4. Connacher AA, El Debani AH, Stevenson IH. A study of the influence of nifedipine on the disposition and hypoglycaemic action of glipizide. *Br J Clin Pharmacol* (1986) 22, 240 P.
5. Abadie E, Passa PH. Diabetogenic effects of nifedipine. *BMJ* (1984) 289, 438.
6. Sakata S, Miura K. Effect of nicardipine in a hypertensive patient with diabetes mellitus. *Clin Ther* (1984) 6, 600–2.
7. Trost BN, Weidmann P. 5 years of antihypertensive monotherapy with the calcium antagonist nitrendipine do not alter carbohydrate homeostasis in diabetic patients. *Diabetes Res Clin Pract* (1988) 5 (Suppl 1), S511.
8. Mück W, Heine PR, Breuel H-P, Niklaus H, Horkulak J, Ahr G. The effect of multiple oral dosing of nimodipine on glibenclamide pharmacodynamics and pharmacokinetics in elderly patients with type-2 diabetes mellitus. *Int J Clin Pharmacol Ther* (1995) 33, 89–94.
9. Bayer, Personal Communications, June-July 1993.
10. Glucobay (Acarbose). Bayer plc. UK Summary of product characteristics, March 2004.
11. Hatorp V, Hansen KT, Thomsen MS. Influence of drugs interacting with CYP3A4 on the pharmacokinetics, pharmacodynamics, and safety of the prandial glucose regulator repaglinide. *J Clin Pharmacol* (2003) 43, 649–60.
12. Guigliano D, Torella R, Cacciapuoti F, Gentile S, Verza M, Varricchio M. Impairment of insulin secretion in man by nifedipine. *Eur J Clin Pharmacol* (1980) 18, 395–8.
13. Bhatnagar SK, Amin MMA, Al-Yusuf AR. Diabetogenic effects of nifedipine. *BMJ* (1984) 289, 19.
14. Heyman SN, Heyman A, Halperin I. Diabetogenic effect of nifedipine. *DICP Ann Pharmacother* (1989) 23, 236–7.
15. Veenstra J, van der Hulst JP, Wildenborg IH, Njoo SF, Verdegaal WP, Silberbusch J. Effect of antihypertensive drugs on insulin absorption. *Diabetes Care* (1991) 14, 1089–92.
16. Girardin E, Vial T, Pham E, Evreux J-C. Hypoglycémies induites par les sulfamides hypoglycémiants. *Ann Med Interne (Paris)* (1992) 143, 11–17.
17. Harris RZ, Inglis AML, Miller AK, Thompson KA, Finnerty D, Patterson S, Jorkasky DK, Freed MI. Rosiglitazone has no clinically significant effect on nifedipine pharmacokinetics. *J Clin Pharmacol* (1999) 39, 1189–94.
18. Pershadsingh HA, Grant N, McDonald JM. Association of diltiazem therapy with increased insulin resistance in a patient with type I diabetes mellitus. *JAMA* (1987) 257, 930–1.
19. Segrestaa JM, Caulin C, Dahan R, Houlbert D, Thiercelin JF, Herman P, Sauvanet JP, Laurribaud J. Effect of diltiazem on plasma glucose, insulin and glucagon during an oral glucose tolerance test in healthy volunteers. *Eur J Clin Pharmacol* (1984) 26, 481–3.
20. Dixit AA, Rao YM. Pharmacokinetic interaction between diltiazem and tolbutamide. *Drug Metabol Drug Interact* (1999) 15, 269–77.
21. Röjdmark S, Andersson DEH. Influence of verapamil on human glucose tolerance. *Am J Cardiol* (1986) 57, 39D–43D.
22. Röjdmark S, Andersson DEH. Influence of verapamil on glucose tolerance. *Acta Med Scand* (1984) (Suppl), 681, 37–42.
23. Andersson DEH, Röjdmark S. Improvement of glucose tolerance by verapamil in patients with non-insulin-dependent diabetes mellitus. *Acta Med Scand* (1981) 210, 27–33.
24. Semple CG, Omile C, Buchanan KD, Beastall GH, Paterson KR. Effect of oral verapamil on glibenclamide stimulated insulin secretion. *Br J Clin Pharmacol* (1986) 22, 187–90.
25. Koyama Y, Kodama K, Suzuki M, Harano Y. Improvement of insulin sensitivity by a long-acting nifedipine preparation (nifedipine-CR) in patients with essential hypertension. *Am J Hypertens* (2002) 15, 927–31.

Antidiabetics + Cibenzoline (Cifenline)

Hypoglycaemia has been seen in a few patients taking cibenzoline alone, and in one case with gliclazide. The risk factors appear to be age, renal insufficiency, malnutrition and high dosage.

Clinical evidence, mechanism, importance and management

Cibenzoline occasionally and unpredictably causes hypoglycaemia, which may be severe. Marked hypoglycaemia was seen in an 67-year-old non-diabetic patient when cibenzoline was given.[1] A further case report describes hypoglycaemia in an 84-year-old, in whom age, renal impairment and/or malnutrition acted as facilitating factors.[2] The authors of this report noted that hypoglycaemia has been reported in another 20 cases, where the dose was not corrected for age and renal function.[2] A more recent report describes an elderly patient with type 2 diabetes controlled by diet who developed hypoglycaemia and associated dementia-like symptoms during treatment with low dose cibenzoline.[3] Hypoglycaemia also occurred in a 61-year-old patient with renal insufficiency taking **gliclazide**.[4]

The reasons are not understood. However, in a controlled study in patients with abnormal glucose tolerance and ventricular arrhythmias, cibenzoline exerted a hypoglycaemic effect by facilitating insulin secretion.[5]

This appears to be a drug-disease rather than a drug-drug interaction and diabetic patients do not seem to be more at risk than non-diabetics, but good monitoring is advisable if cibenzoline is given.

1. Hilleman DE, Mohiuddin SM, Ahmed IS, Dahl JM. Cibenzoline-induced hypoglycemia. *Drug Intell Clin Pharm* (1987) 21, 38–40.
2. Houdent C, Noblet C, Vandoren C, Levesque H, Morin C, Moore N, Courtois H, Wolf LM. Hypoglycémia induite par la cibenzoline chez le sujet âgè. *Rev Med Interne* (1991) 12, 143–5.
3. Sakane N, Onishi N, Katamura M, Sato H, Takamasu M, Yoshida T. Cifenline succinate and dementia in an elderly NIDDM patient. *Diabetes Care* (1998) 21, 320–1.
4. Girardin E, Vial T, Pham E, Evreux J-C. Hypoglycémies induites par les sulfamides hypoglycémiants. *Ann Med Interne (Paris)* (1992) 143, 11–17.
5. Saikawa T, Arita M, Yamaguchi K, Ito M. Hypoglycemic effect of cibenzoline in patients with abnormal glucose tolerance and frequent ventricular arrhythmias. *Cardiovasc Drugs Ther* (2000) 14, 665–9.

Antidiabetics + Clonidine

There is evidence that clonidine may possibly suppress the signs and symptoms of hypoglycaemia in diabetic patients. An isolated report describes marked hyperglycaemia in a child on insulin

when given clonidine. Clonidine premedication may decrease or increase the hyperglycaemic response to surgery.

Clinical evidence, mechanism, importance and management

(a) Non-diabetic patients

Studies in healthy subjects and patients with hypertension found that their normal response to hypoglycaemia (tachycardia, palpitations, perspiration) caused by a 0.1 unit/kg dose of **insulin** was markedly reduced when they were taking clonidine 450 to 900 micrograms daily.[1,2] The suggested reason is that clonidine depresses the output of the catecholamines (adrenaline, noradrenaline), which are secreted in an effort to raise blood sugar levels, and which are also responsible for these signs. It seems possible that clonidine will similarly suppress the signs and symptoms of hypoglycaemia that can occur in diabetics, but there seem to be no reports confirming this. A study in healthy subjects and non-diabetic patients also found that clonidine raises blood glucose levels, apparently by reducing **insulin** secretion.[3]

(b) Diabetic patients

A 9-year-old girl with type 1 diabetes stable on **insulin** 4 units daily, developed substantial hyperglycaemia and needed up to 56 units of **insulin** daily when she began to take clonidine 50 micrograms daily for Tourette's syndrome. When the clonidine was stopped, she had numerous hypoglycaemic episodes, and within a few days it was possible to reduce her daily dosage of **insulin** to 6 units.[4] The general importance of this interaction is uncertain, but this isolated case seems to be the only one where an obviously adverse response occurred.

(c) Hyperglycaemia during surgery

Forty patients with type 2 diabetes (controlled by diet alone, **sulphonylureas**, **biguanides**, or **insulin**), having eye surgery under general anaesthesia were given either clonidine 225 to 375 micrograms or flunitrazepam as premedication. In diabetic patients there is an increase in blood glucose during stress because of an increase in catecholamine release. Therefore the patients were also given continuous infusion of **insulin** to maintain blood glucose at 5.5 to 11.1 mmol/l. Clonidine decreased the **insulin** requirement because of improved blood glucose control due to inhibition of catecholamine release.[5] Contrasting results were found in a study in 16 non-diabetic women undergoing abdominal hysterectomy. Eight were given intravenous clonidine 1 microgram/kg and 8 control patients were given saline. Intraoperative plasma glucose levels were higher in the clonidine group and these patients also had lower insulin levels. The influence of clonidine on the surgical stress response appears to vary depending on the dose of clonidine and the type of surgery.[6] Thus, clonidine at about 4 micrograms/kg may attenuate the hyperglycaemic response to neurosurgical and non-abdominal procedures, but low dose clonidine accentuates the hyperglycaemic response to lower abdominal surgery that results from a decrease in plasma insulin.[5,6]

1. Hedeland H, Dymling J-F, Hökfelt B. The effect of insulin induced hypoglycaemia on plasma renin activity and urinary catecholamines before and following clonidine (Catapresan) in man. *Acta Endocrinol (Copenh)* (1972) 71, 321–30.
2. Hedeland H, Dymling J-F, Hökfelt B. Pharmacological inhibition of adrenaline secretion following insulin induced hypoglycaemia in man: the effect of Catapresan. *Acta Endocrinol (Copenh)* (1971) 67, 97–103.
3. Metz SA, Halter JB, Robertson RP. Induction of defective insulin secretion and impaired glucose tolerance by clonidine. Selective stimulation of metabolic alpha-adrenergic pathways. *Diabetes* (1978) 27, 554–62.
4. Mimouni-Bloch A, Mimouni M. Clonidine-induced hyperglycemia in a young diabetic girl. *Ann Pharmacother* (1993) 27, 980.
5. Belhoula M, Ciébiéra JP, De La Chapelle A, Boisseau N, Coeurveille D, Raucoules-Aimé M. Clonidine premedication improves metabolic control in type 2 diabetic patients during ophthalmic surgery. *Br J Anaesth* (2003) 90, 434–9.
6. Lattermann R, Schricker T, Georgieff M, Schreiber M. Low dose clonidine premedication accentuates the hyperglycaemic response to surgery. *Can J Anesth* (2001) 48, 755–9.

Antidiabetics + Corticosteroids

The blood sugar lowering effects of the antidiabetics are opposed by corticosteroids with glucocorticoid (hyperglycaemic) activity and significant hyperglycaemia has been seen.

Clinical evidence, mechanism, importance and management

Systemic corticosteroids with glucocorticoid activity can raise blood sugar levels and induce diabetes,[1] though this is rarely seen with topical corticosteroids.[2] This can oppose the blood sugar lowering effects of the antidiabetics used in the treatment of diabetes mellitus. For example, a disturbance of the control of diabetes is very briefly described in a patient treated with **insulin** and **hydrocortisone**.[3] A study in 5 patients with type 2 diabetes showed that a single 200-mg dose of **cortisone** modified their glucose tolerance curves while taking an unstated amount of **chlorpropamide**. The blood glucose levels of 4 of them rose (3 showed an initial fall), whereas in a previous test with **chlorpropamide** alone the blood sugar levels of 4 of them had fallen.[4] This almost certainly reflects a direct antagonism between the pharmacological effects of the two drugs, and this would seem to be confirmed by a study in healthy subjects which showed that another glucocorticoid, **prednisone**, had no significant effect on the metabolism or clearance of **tolbutamide**[5]

There are very few studies of this interaction, probably because the hyperglycaemic activity of the **corticosteroids** has been known for such a long time that the outcome of concurrent use is self-evident. A case-control study found that in patients treated with glucocorticoids, the relative risk for development of hyperglycaemia requiring treatment was 2.23 as compared with controls. Risk increased with increasing dose with an odds ratio of 1.77, 3.02, 5.82 and 10.34 for daily doses equivalent to 1 to 39 mg, 40 to 79 mg, 80 to 119 mg, and 120 mg or more of **hydrocortisone** respectively.[6]

The effects of corticosteroid treatment in diabetics should be closely monitored and the dosage of the antidiabetic raised as necessary. Antidiabetics are sometimes needed in non-diabetic patients taking **corticosteroids** to reduce blood sugar levels.

1. David DS, Cheigh JS, Braun DW, Fotino M, Stenzel KH, Rubin AL. HLA-A28 and steroid-induced diabetes in renal transplant patients. *JAMA* (1980) 243, 532–3.
2. Gomez EC, Frost P. Induction of glycosuria and hyperglycemia by topical corticosteroid therapy. *Arch Dermatol* (1976) 112, 1559–62.
3. Manchon ND, Bercoff E, Lemarchand P, Chassagne P, Senant J, Bourreille J. Fréquence et gravité des interactions médicamenteuses dan une population âgée: étude prospective concernant 639 malades. *Rev Med Interne* (1989) 10, 521–5.
4. Danowski TS, Mateer FM, Moses C. Cortisone enhancement of peripheral utilization of glucose and the effects of chlorpropamide. *Ann N Y Acad Sci* (1959) 74, 988–96.
5. Breimer DD, Zilly W, Richter E. Influence of corticosteroid on hexobarbital and tolbutamide disposition. *Clin Pharmacol Ther* (1978) 24, 208–12.
6. Gurwitz JH, Bohn RL, Glynn RJ, Monane M, Mogun H, Avorn J. Glucocorticoids and the risk for initiation of hypoglycaemic therapy. *Arch Intern Med* (1994) 154, 97–101.

Antidiabetics + Danazol

Danazol causes insulin resistance. Therefore, on theoretical grounds danazol would be expected to oppose the effects of antidiabetics, but the practical clinical importance of this is uncertain.

Clinical evidence, mechanism, importance and management

Danazol can disturb glucose metabolism. A study in 14 non-diabetic subjects found that 3 months' treatment with danazol 600 mg daily caused a mild but definite deterioration in glucose tolerance, associated with high insulin levels. Insulin resistance was also seen in 5 subjects on danazol when given intravenous **tolbutamide**.[1] Similarly, another study in 9 non-diabetic women found that danazol 600 mg daily raised insulin levels in response to glucose or intravenous **tolbutamide**.[2] A further study in 9 non-diabetic women also found that danazol caused a mild deterioration in glucose tolerance and a marked increase in the insulin response to glucose loading.[3] Other studies have found that danazol causes marked resistance to both insulin[4-6] and glucagon,[5,6] which could be due to receptor down-regulation resulting from hypersecretion of insulin and glucagon.[5,6]

There is also a report of danazol-associated type 1 diabetes in a patient with endometriosis who took danazol 400 mg twice daily for 8 weeks. The diabetes resolved on withdrawal of danazol, but the development of hyperglycaemia about 5 months later suggested a predisposition to diabetes.[7] However, it has been suggested that the patient probably had type 2 diabetes precipitated by danazol-induced insulin resistance, which would possibly have responded to dietary restriction. Danazol-associated hyperglucagonaemia may have exacerbated the symptoms.[8,9]

For these reasons the makers of danazol advise caution if danazol is given to diabetic patients.[10] Danazol would be expected to oppose the actions of antidiabetics to some extent, but there do not appear to be any studies assessing the clinical relevance of this.

1. Wynn V. Metabolic effects of danazol. *J Int Med Res* (1977) 5 (Suppl 3), 25–35.
2. Goettenberg N, Schlienger J L, Becmeur F, Dellenbach P. Traitement de l'endométriose pelvienne par le danazol. Incidence sur le métabolisme glucidique. *Nouv Presse Med* (1982) 11, 3703–6.
3. Vaughan-Williams C A, Shalet S M. Glucose tolerance and insulin resistance after danazol treatment. *J Obstet Gynaecol* (1989) 9, 229–32.

4. Matalliotakis I, Panidis D, Vlassis G, Neonaki M, Koumantakis E. Decreased sensitivity to insulin during treatment with danazol in women with endometriosis. *Clin Exp Obstet Gynecol* (1997) 24, 160–2.
5. Bruce R, Godsland I, Stevenson J, Devenport M, Borth F, Crook D, Ghatei M, Whitehead M, Wynn V. Danazol induces resistance to both insulin and glucagon in young women. *Clin Sci* (1992) 82, 211–17.
6. Kotzmann H, Linkesch M, Ludvik B, Clodi M, Luger A, Schernthaner G, Prager R, Klauser R. *Eur J Clin Invest* (1995) 25, 942–7.
7. Seifer DB, Freedman LN, Cavender JR, Baker RA. Insulin-dependent diabetes mellitus associated with danazol. *Am J Obstet Gynecol* (1990) 162, 474–5.
8. Williams G. Metabolic effects of danazol. *Am J Obstet Gynecol* (1991) 164, 933–4.
9. Seifer DB. Metabolic effects of danazol. *Am J Obstet Gynecol* (1991) 164, 934.
10. Danol (Danazol). Sanofi-Synthelabo. UK Summary of product characteristics, August 2004.

Antidiabetics + Dextropropoxyphene (Propoxyphene)

Dextropropoxyphene does not appear to interact pharmacokinetically with tolbutamide. Hypoglycaemia was seen in a patient on an unnamed sulphonylurea and co-proxamol, and has also been reported in non-diabetic patients given dextropropoxyphene alone.

Clinical evidence, mechanism, importance and management

After taking dextropropoxyphene 65 mg every 8 hours for 4 days, the clearance of a 500-mg intravenous dose of **tolbutamide** was not affected in 6 healthy subjects.[1] There is an isolated case of hypoglycaemia in a patient taking an unnamed sulphonylurea and co-proxamol (dextropropoxyphene with paracetamol (acetaminophen)).[2] There are also several reports of hypoglycaemia in non-diabetic patients taking dextropropoxyphene alone,[3-7] sometimes associated with renal failure,[3,4] advanced age,[5] or with high doses or overdose.[6] There would normally seem to be little reason for avoiding the concurrent use of antidiabetics and dextropropoxyphene, or for taking particular precautions.

1. Robson RA, Miners JO, Whitehead AG, Birkett DJ. Specificity of the inhibitory effect of dextropropoxyphene on oxidative drug metabolism in man: effects on theophylline and tolbutamide disposition. *Br J Clin Pharmacol* (1987) 23, 772–5.
2. Girardin E, Vial T, Pham E, Evreux J-C. Hypoglycémies induites par les sulfamides hypoglycémiants. *Ann Med Interne (Paris)* (1992) 143, 11–17.
3. Wiederholt IC, Genco M, Foley JM. Recurrent episodes of hypoglycemia induced by propoxyphene. *Neurology* (1967) 17, 703–6.
4. Almirall J, Montoliu J, Torras A, Revert L. Propoxyphene-induced hypoglycemia in a patient with chronic renal failure. *Nephron* (1989) 53, 273–5.
5. Laurent M, Gallinari C, Bonnin M, Soubrie C. Hypoglycémie sous dextropropoxyphène chez des grands vieillards. 7 observations. *Presse Med* (1991) 20, 1628.
6. Karunakara BP, Maiya PP, Hegde SR, Pradeep GCM. Accidental dextropropoxyphene poisoning. *Indian J Pediatr* (2003) 70, 357–8.
7. Santos Gil I, Junquera Crespo M, Sanz Sanz J, Lahulla Pastor F. Hipglucernia secundaria a ingestión de dextropropoxifeno en un paciente adicto a drogas. Med Clin (Barc) 1998, 110, 475–6.

Antidiabetics + Disopyramide

Disopyramide occasionally causes hypoglycaemia, which may be severe. Isolated reports describe severe hypoglycaemia when disopyramide was used in diabetic patients on gliclazide, or metformin and/or insulin.

Clinical evidence, mechanism, importance and management

Disopyramide occasionally and unpredictably causes hypoglycaemia, which may be severe.[1-7] The reasons are not fully understood, but *in vitro* studies suggest that disopyramide and its main metabolite may enhance insulin release from the pancreas.[8] There is a report of severe hypoglycaemia in an 82-year-old woman with diabetes treated with **gliclazide**, which occurred 6 months after she started disopyramide 300 mg daily.[9] A further case of hypoglycaemia associated with disopyramide therapy occurred in a 70-year-old woman who had been treated with **metformin** 500 mg twice daily and **insulin** 62 units daily. Within 3 months of starting disopyramide 250 mg twice daily her **insulin** dose was reduced to 24 units daily, she stopped taking **metformin** and was eating 'substantial snacks' to avoid hypoglycaemia.[10] **Insulin** requirement was markedly reduced in another patient with type 2 diabetes when disopyramide therapy was started.[11]

The makers note that patients at particular risk for hypoglycaemia are the elderly, the malnourished and diabetics, and that impaired renal function and impaired cardiac function may be predisposing factors.[12,13] They advise close monitoring of blood glucose levels[12,13] and withdrawal of disopyramide if problems arise.[12] This is not simply a problem for diabetics, but certainly within the context of diabetes the hypoglycaemic effects of disopyramide may possibly cause particular difficulties. Although not strictly an interaction, the concurrent use of disopyramide and antidiabetics should be well monitored because of the potential for severe hypoglycaemia, as the cases show.

1. Goldberg IJ, Brown LK, Rayfield EJ. Disopyramide (Norpace)-induced hypoglycemia. *Am J Med* (1980) 69, 463–6.
2. Quevdeo SF, Krauss DS, Chazan JA, Crisafulli FS, Kahn CB. Fasting hypoglycemia secondary to disopyramide therapy. Report of two cases. *JAMA* (1981) 245, 2424.
3. Strathman I, Schubert EN, Cohen A, Nitzberg DM. Hypoglycemia in patients receiving disopyramide phosphate. *Drug Intell Clin Pharm* (1983) 17, 635–8.
4. Semel JD, Wortham E, Karl DM. Fasting hypoglycemia associated with disopyramide. *Am Heart J* (1983) 106, 1160–1.
5. Seriès C. Hypoglycémie induite ou favorisée par le disopyramide. *Rev Med Interne* (1988) 9, 528–9.
6. Cacoub P, Deray G, Baumelou A, Grimaldi C, Soubrie C, Jacobs C. Disopyramide-induced hypoglycemia: case report and review of the literature. *Fundam Clin Pharmacol* (1989) 3, 527–35.
7. Stapleton JT, Gillman MW. Hypoglycemic coma due to disopyramide toxicity. *South Med J* (1983) 76, 1453.
8. Horie M, Mizuno N, Tsuji K, Haruna T, Ninomiya T, Ishida H, Seino Y, Sasayama S. Disopyramide and its metabolite enhance insulin release from clonal pancreatic β-cells by blocking K_{ATP} channels. *Cardiovasc Drugs Ther* (2001) 15, 31–9.
9. Wahl D, de Korwin JD, Paille F, Trechot P, Schmitt J. Hypoglycémie sévère probablement induite par le disopyramide chez un diabétique. *Therapie* (1988) 43, 321–2.
10. Reynolds RM, Walker JD. Hypoglycaemia induced by disopyramide in a patient with type 2 diabetes mellitus. *Diabet Med* (2001) 18, 1009–10.
11. Onada N, Kawagoe M, Shimizu M, Komori T, Takahashi C, Oomori Y, Hirata Y. A case of non-insulin dependent diabetes mellitus whose insulin requirement was markedly reduced after disopyramide treatment for arrhythmia. *Nippon Naika Gakkai Zasshi* (1989) 78, 820–5. [in Japanese]
12. Rythmodan (Disopyramide). Borg Medicare. UK Summary of product characteristics, January 2001.
13. Norpace (Disopyramide). Pharmacia. US Prescribing information, September 2001.

Antidiabetics + Disulfiram

Disulfiram appears not to affect the control of diabetes mellitus. No pharmacokinetic interaction occurs with tolbutamide and there appears to be no evidence that disulfiram interacts with any other antidiabetics.

Clinical evidence, mechanism, importance and management

The makers of disulfiram say that caution should be exercised if it is used in diabetics,[1] but a reviewer[2] who has given disulfiram to over 20 000 alcoholics says that he has prescribed disulfiram for several hundred patients with diabetes mellitus over 20 years without any apparent adverse effects and therefore any theoretical interaction is rarely, if ever, applicable to clinical practice. It would be reasonable to assume that many of these patients (probably most) were also taking **insulin** or one of the oral antidiabetics. There do not appear to be any reported cases in the literature of adverse interactions between disulfiram and any of the antidiabetics. Studies in 5 healthy subjects have shown that disulfiram (first day 400 mg three times; second day 400 mg; third and fourth days 200 mg daily) had no significant effect on the half-life or clearance of intravenous **tolbutamide** 500 mg.[3]

The conclusion to be drawn from all of this is that any reaction is very rare (if it ever occurs), and no special precautions would normally appear to be necessary.

1. Antabuse (Disulfiram). Dumex Ltd. UK Summary of product characteristics, August 1999.
2. McNichol RW, Ewing JA, Faiman MD, eds. Disulfiram (Antabuse): a unique medical aid to sobriety: history, pharmacology, research, clinical use. Springfield, Ill: Thomas; 1987 pp. 47–90.
3. Svendsen TL, Kristensen MB, Hansen JM, Skovsted L. The influence of disulfiram on the half life and metabolic clearance rate of diphenylhydantoin and tolbutamide in man. *Eur J Clin Pharmacol* (1976) 9, 439–41.

Antidiabetics + Diuretics; Cicletanine

Preliminary evidence suggests that cicletanine and tolbutamide do not interact adversely.

Clinical evidence, mechanism, importance and management

The hypoglycaemic responses of 10 healthy subjects were studied following an intravenous infusion of **tolbutamide** 3 mg/kg, 3 days before and one hour after the last dose of oral cicletanine 100 mg daily for a week.[1] No clinically relevant changes were seen. Note that, studies in *animals* and in non-diabetic hypertensive patients found that, at therapeutic doses, cicletanine did not affect glycoregulation.[2] The conclusion to be drawn is that cicletanine is unlikely to affect the control of diabetes in patients, but this needs confirmation from longer-term clinical studies.

1. Bayés MC, Barbanoj MJ, Vallès J, Torrent J, Obach R, Jané F. A drug interaction study between cicletanine and tolbutamide in healthy volunteers. *Eur J Clin Pharmacol* (1996) 50, 381–4.
2. Mashori GR, Tariq AR, Shahimi MM, Suhaimi H. The effects of cicletanine, a new antihypertensive agent on insulin release in rat isolated pancreas by the perfusion technique. *Singapore Med J* (1996) 37, 278–81.

Antidiabetics + Diuretics; Etacrynic acid

Etacrynic acid can raise blood sugar levels in diabetics, which opposes the effects of the antidiabetics to some extent. The clinical importance of this seems to be negligible.

Clinical evidence, mechanism, importance and management

A double-blind study in 24 hypertensive patients, one-third of whom were diabetics, found that daily treatment with etacrynic acid 200 mg over a 6-week period impaired their glucose tolerance and raised the blood sugar levels of the diabetics to the same extent as those diabetics and non-diabetics taking hydrochlorothiazide 200 mg daily.[1] In another study no change in carbohydrate metabolism was seen in 6 diabetics given etacrynic acid 150 mg daily for a week.[2]

Information is very limited indeed. Some impairment of the glucose tolerance may possibly occur, but there seems to be a lack of evidence in the literature to show that etacrynic acid has much effect on the control of diabetes in most patients. Even so it would be prudent to monitor the effects of concurrent use with antidiabetics.

1. Russell RP, Lindeman RD, Prescott LF. Metabolic and hypotensive effects of ethacrynic acid. Comparative study with hydrochlorothiazide. *JAMA* (1968) 205, 81–5.
2. Dige-Petersen H. Ethacrynic acid and carbohydrate metabolism. *Nord Med* (1966) 75, 123–5.

Antidiabetics + Diuretics; Furosemide

The control of diabetes is not usually disturbed by furosemide, although there are a few reports showing that it can sometimes raise blood sugar levels.

Clinical evidence, mechanism, importance and management

Although furosemide can elevate blood sugar levels[1] (but to a much lesser extent than the thiazide diuretics), worsen glucose tolerance[2] and occasionally cause glycosuria or even acute diabetes in individual patients,[3] the general picture is that the control of diabetes is not usually affected by the use of furosemide.[4] No clinically relevant changes in the control of diabetes were seen in a 3-month trial of 29 patients with type 2 diabetes taking furosemide 40 mg daily and an average of 7 mg **glibenclamide (glyburide)** daily.[5] It has been described[6] as the diuretic of choice for the diabetic patient. Even so, prescribers should be aware of its hyperglycaemic potential.

1. Hutcheon DE, Leonard G. Diuretic and antihypertensive action of frusemide. *J Clin Pharmacol* (1967) 7, 26–33.
2. Breckenridge A, Welborn TA, Dollery CT, Fraser R. Glucose tolerance in hypertensive patients on long-term diuretic therapy. *Lancet* (1967) i, 61–4.
3. Toivonen S, Mustala O. Diabetogenic action of frusemide. *BMJ* (1966) i, 920–21.
4. Bencomo L, Fyvolent J, Kahana S, Kahana L. Clinical experience with a new diuretic, furosemide. *Curr Ther Res* (1965) 7, 339–45.
5. Lehnert H, Schmitz H, Beyer J, Wilmbusse H, Piesche L. Controlled clinical trial investigating the influence of torasemide and furosemide on carbohydrate metabolism in patients with cardiac failure and concomitant type II diabetes. 4th Int Congr Diuretics, Boca Raton, Florida Oct 11–16th 1992. Eds. Puschett JB, Greenberrg A. *Int Congr Ser 1023* (1993), 271–4.
6. Malins JM. Diuretics in diabetes mellitus. *Practitioner* (1968) 201, 529.

Antidiabetics + Diuretics; Metolazone

An isolated report describes severe hypoglycaemia in a patient on glibenclamide (glyburide) shortly after starting treatment with metolazone.

Clinical evidence, mechanism, importance and management

A man with type 2 diabetes, stabilised on **glibenclamide (glyburide)** 10 mg daily and hospitalised for congestive heart failure, became clinically hypoglycaemic (blood glucose levels unmeasurable by *Labstix*) within 40 hours of starting metolazone 5 mg daily. He was treated with intravenous glucose. Although both **glibenclamide** and metolazone were stopped, he had 4 further hypoglycaemic episodes over the next 30 hours.[1] The reasons are not understood. *In vitro* studies failed to find any evidence that metolazone displaces **glibenclamide** from its protein binding sites, which might possibly have provided some explanation for what happened.[1] The general importance of this apparent interaction is not clear, but until more is known it would seem prudent to monitor the effects of concurrent use. More study is needed.

1. George S, McBurney A, Cole A. Possible protein binding displacement interaction between glibenclamide and metolazone. *Eur J Clin Pharmacol* (1990) 38, 93–5.

Antidiabetics + Diuretics; Thiazides or related diuretics

By raising blood sugar levels, the thiazide and related diuretics can reduce the effects of the antidiabetics and impair the control of diabetes. Hyponatraemia also occurs occasionally.

Clinical evidence

(a) Reduced hypoglycaemic effects

Chlorothiazide, the first of the thiazide diuretics, was found within a year of its introduction in 1958 to have hyperglycaemic effects.[1] Since then a very large number of reports have described hyperglycaemia, the precipitation of diabetes in prediabetics, and the disturbance of blood sugar control in diabetics on thiazides. One example from many:

A long-term study in 53 patients with type 2 diabetes found that **chlorothiazide** 500 mg or 1 g daily or **trichlormethiazide** 4 or 8 mg daily caused a mean rise in blood sugar levels from 120 to 140 mg%. Only 7 patients needed a change in their treatment: 4 required more of their oral drug, 2 an increase in **insulin** dose, and one was transferred from **tolbutamide** to **insulin**. The oral drug used included **tolbutamide**, **chlorpropamide**, **acetohexamide** and **phenformin**.[2]

A rise in blood sugar levels has been observed with **bendroflumethiazide**,[3,4] **benzthiazide**,[5] **hydrochlorothiazide** 100 to 300 mg daily,[3] and **chlortalidone** 50 to 100 mg daily.[6] A study in hypertensive patients found that **chlortalidone** 50 mg daily increased glucose and insulin levels, but **hydrochlorothiazide** 50 mg daily alone or as part of a potassium and/or magnesium conserving regimen did not.[7]

More recent data suggest that the effects of thiazides on blood glucose may be dose related. In a double-blind randomised study comparing the effects of 1.25 or 5 mg of **bendroflumethiazide** on blood glucose, the lower dose had no effects on insulin action, whereas when the higher dose was given, there was evidence of impaired glucose tolerance.[8] A review of the literature on **hydrochlorothiazide** similarly reports that low doses (6.25 to 12.5 mg) lack significant effects on blood glucose levels.[9]

(b) Hyponatraemia

A hospital report describes 8 cases of low serum sodium concentrations observed over a 5-year period in patients taking **chlorpropamide** and *Moduretic* (**hydrochlorothiazide** 50 mg with amiloride 5 mg).[10]

(c) Pharmacokinetics

A study in 12 healthy subjects given a single 25-mg dose of hydrochlorothiazide before and after taking **voglibose** 5 mg three times daily for 11 days found that the hydrochlorothiazide plasma levels were slightly increased by the **voglibose** (AUC increased 7.5%, maximum plasma levels increased 15%) but these were considered to be clinically irrelevant. The combination was well tolerated and adverse events were unchanged.[11]

Mechanism

Not understood. One study suggested that the hyperglycaemia is due to some inhibition of insulin release by the pancreas.[12] Another suggestion is that the peripheral action of insulin is affected in some way.[5,13] There is also evidence that the effects may be related in part to potassium depletion.[14] The hyponatraemia appears to be due to the additive sodium-losing effects of the chlorpropamide, thiazide and amiloride. Obese patients may be more sensitive to the effects of hydrochlorothiazide on insulin metabolism.[7]

Importance and management

The reduction in hypoglycaemic effect is extremely well documented (not all references are given here) but of only moderate practical importance. One study noted that none of the patients had a dramatic deterioration in their diabetic control. The incidence is said to lie between 10 and 30%.[2,15] Concurrent use of thiazides and antidiabetics need not be avoided, but the outcome should be monitored. There is evidence that the full effects may take many months to develop in some patients.[4] Most patients respond to a modest increase in the dosage of the antidiabetics, or to a change from an oral drug to insulin. The adverse hyperglycaemic effects can also be reversed significantly by the use of potassium supplements,[14] but this would not usually be an appropriate strategy for managing the interaction in practice. This interaction may be expected to occur with all thiazides and possibly related diuretics such as clopamide, clorexolone, metolazone, quinethazone, etc. This requires confirmation. However, see also 'Antidiabetics + Diuretics; Metolazone', p.404.

Hyponatraemia is a rare but recognised adverse effect of the thiazides and no additional precautions would therefore seem necessary.

1. Wilkins RW. New drugs for the treatment of hypertension. *Ann Intern Med* (1959) 50, 1–10.
2. Kansal PC, Buse J, Buse MG. Thiazide diuretics and control of diabetes mellitus. *South Med J* (1969) 62, 1374–9.
3. Goldner MG, Zarowitz H, Akgun S. Hyperglycemia and glycosuria due to thiazide derivatives administered in diabetes mellitus. *N Engl J Med* (1960) 262, 403–5.
4. Lewis PJ, Kohner EM, Petrie A, Dollery CT. Deterioration of glucose tolerance in hypertensive patients on prolonged diuretic treatment. *Lancet* (1976) i, 564–6.
5. Runyan JW. Influence of thiazide diuretics on carbohydrate metabolism in patients with mild diabetes. *N Engl J Med* (1962) 267, 541–3.
6. Carliner NH, Schelling J-L, Russell RP, Okun R, Davis M. Thiazide- and phthalimidine-induced hyperglycemia in hypertensive patients. *JAMA* (1965) 191, 535–40.
7. Siegel D, Saliba P, Haffner S. Glucose and insulin levels during diuretic therapy in hypertensive men. *Hypertension* (1994) 23, 688–94.
8. Harper R, Ennis CN, Sheridan B, Atkinson AB, Johnston GD, Bell PM. Effects of low dose versus conventional dose thiazide diuretic on insulin action in essential hypertension. *BMJ* (1994) 309, 226–30.
9. Neutel JM. Metabolic manifestations of low-dose diuretics. *Am J Med* (1996) 101 (Suppl 3A), 71S–82S.
10. Zalin AM, Hutchinson CE, Jong M, Matthews K. Hyponatraemia during treatment with chlorpropamide and Moduretic (amiloride plus hydrochlorothiazide). *BMJ* (1984) 289, 659.
11. Kleist P, Suzuki Y, Thomsen T, Möller M, Römer A, Hucke HP, Kurowski M, Eckl KM. Voglibose has no effect on the pharmacokinetics of hydrochlorothiazide. *Eur J Clin Pharmacol* (1998) 54, 273–4.
12. Fajans SS, Floyd JC, Knopf RF, Rull J, Guntsche EM, Conn JW. Benzothiadiazine suppression of insulin release from normal and abnormal islet tissue in man. *J Clin Invest* (1966) 45, 481–92.
13. Remenchik AP, Hoover C, Talso PJ. Insulin secretion by hypertensive patients receiving hydrochlorothiazide. *JAMA* (1970) 212, 869.
14. Rapoport MI, Hurd HF. Thiazide-induced glucose intolerance treated with potassium. *Arch Intern Med* (1964) 113, 405–8.
15. Wolff FW, Parmley WW, White K, Okun R. Drug-induced diabetes. Diabetogenic activity of long-term administration of benzothiadiazines. *JAMA* (1963) 185, 568–74.

Antidiabetics + Diuretics; Torasemide

No adverse interaction occurs if torasemide and glibenclamide (glyburide) are taken concurrently.

Clinical evidence, mechanism, importance and management

A three-month trial in 32 patients with congestive heart failure and type 2 diabetes mellitus on **glibenclamide (glyburide)** found that torasemide 5 mg daily caused a small but clinically insignificant fall in blood glucose levels.[1] There would seem to be no reason for avoiding torasemide in patients taking **glibenclamide**.

1. Lehnert H, Schmitz H, Beyer J, Wilmbusse H, Piesche L. Controlled clinical trial investigating the influence of torasemide and furosemide on carbohydrate metabolism in patients with cardiac failure and concomitant type II diabetes. 4th Int Congr Diuretics, Boca Raton, Florida Oct 11–16th 1992. Eds. Puschett JB, Greenberrg A. *Int Congr Ser 1023* (1993), 271–4.

Antidiabetics + Fenfluramine

Fenfluramine has inherent hypoglycaemic activity that can add to, or in some instances replace, the effects of conventional antidiabetic agents.

Clinical evidence, mechanism, importance and management

A study of the substitution of fenfluramine (initially 40 mg daily, increased to 120 mg daily) to a biguanide antidiabetic found that diabetes was equally well controlled by either drug in 4 of 6 patients.[1] The hypoglycaemic effects of fenfluramine are described elsewhere.[2,3] It seems that fenfluramine increases the uptake of glucose into skeletal muscle, thereby lowering blood glucose levels.[3,4]

This is a well established and, on the whole, an advantageous rather than an adverse reaction, but it would be prudent to check on the extent of the response if fenfluramine is added or withdrawn from the treatment being received by diabetics. However, note that fenfluramine was generally withdrawn in 1997 because its use was found to be associated with a high incidence of abnormal echocardiograms indicating abnormal functioning of heart valves.

1. Jackson WPU. Fenfluramine trials in a diabetic clinic. *S Afr Med J* (1971) 45 (Suppl), 29–30.
2. Turtle JR, Burgess JA. Hypoglycemic action of fenfluramine in diabetes mellitus. *Diabetes* (1973) 22, 858–67.
3. Dykes JRW. The effect of a low-calorie diet with and without fenfluramine, and fenfluramine alone on the glucose tolerance and insulin secretion of overweight non-diabetics. *Postgrad Med J* (1973) 49, 314–17.
4. Kirby MJ, Turner P. Effect of amphetamine, fenfluramine and norfenfluramine on glucose uptake into human isolated skeletal muscle. *Br J Clin Pharmacol* (1974) 1, 340P–341P.

Antidiabetics + Fibrates

The effects of the sulphonylureas can be enhanced by clofibrate in some patients and a reduction in the dosage of the antidiabetics may be necessary. Gemfibrozil has both increased and decreased dose requirements of various antidiabetics. Hypoglycaemia has been reported with bezafibrate, ciprofibrate and fenofibrate. The antidiuretic effects of clofibrate in the treatment of diabetes insipidus are opposed by glibenclamide (glyburide).

Clinical evidence, mechanism, importance and management

(a) Altered hypoglycaemic effects

(i) Bezafibrate. Three elderly patients with type 2 diabetes and mild renal dysfunction taking **glibenclamide** developed hypoglycaemia when given bezafibrate: one of them needed a 60% dosage reduction, another was given **tolbutamide** instead, and the third was able to stop both **glibenclamide** and **buformin**.[1] The French Centres Régionaux de Pharmacovigilance recorded 7 cases of hypoglycaemia during the period 1985 to 1990 in patients on unnamed sulphonylureas when given fibrates (one with bezafibrate).[2]

(ii) Ciprofibrate. The French Centres Régionaux de Pharmacovigilance recorded 7 cases of hypoglycaemia during the period 1985 to 1990 in patients on unnamed sulphonylureas when given fibrates (3 with ciprofibrate).[2]

(iii) Clofibrate. Over a 5-day period while taking clofibrate 2 g daily, the control of diabetes was improved in 6 out of 13 patients with type 2 diabetes on various unnamed sulphonylureas. Hypoglycaemia (blood glucose levels of 30 to 40 mg per 100 ml) was seen in 4 patients.[3] Other studies confirm that some, but not all, patients have a fall in blood glucose levels while taking clofibrate and the control of the diabetes can improve.[4-11] In one study[12] the half-life of **chlorpropamide** ranged from 40 to 62 hours in 5 subjects treated with clofibrate compared with a mean of about 36 hours in control subjects.

(iv) Fenofibrate. The French Centres Régionaux de Pharmacovigilance recorded 7 cases of hypoglycaemia during the period 1985 to 1990 in patients on unnamed sulphonylureas when given fibrates (3 with fenofibrate).[2]

(v) Gemfibrozil. Fasting blood glucose values decreased in 10, and increased in 4 of 14 diabetic patients on **insulin**, **acetohexamide**, **chlorpropamide** or **glipizide** who were given gemfibrozil, 800 mg daily initially, reduced later to 400 to 600 mg daily.[13] Another study found that of 20 patients, 9 required a slight increase in the dosage of **insulin** or sulphonylurea (**glibenclamide** or **chlorpropamide**), and one a decreased dosage, when treated with gemfibrozil 800 to 1600 mg daily.[14] A single report describes hypoglycaemia, which occurred in a diabetic on **glibenclamide** when gemfibrozil 1200 mg daily was started.[15] The **glibenclamide** dosage was reduced from 5 to 1.25 mg daily with satisfactory diabetic control. When the gemfibrozil was later stopped and restarted, the dosage of the **glibenclamide** had to be increased and then again reduced. A placebo-controlled study in 10 healthy subjects found that gemfibrozil 600 mg twice daily for 5 doses increased the AUC of a single 500-microgram dose of **glimepiride** by 23%, but there were no significant changes in serum insulin or blood glucose.[16]

In a randomised crossover study 12 healthy subjects were given gemfibrozil 600 mg twice daily for 3 days, with a 250-microgram dose of repaglinide on day 3. Gemfibrozil raised the AUC of repaglinide 8-fold and increased the plasma levels nearly 29-fold.[17] Itraconazole (which may interact, see 'Antidiabetics + Azoles', p.397), given with gemfibrozil and repaglinide further increased these effects. The hypoglycaemic effects of repaglinide were considerably enhanced and prolonged, both by gemfibrozil alone and in combination with itraconazole.[17]

(b) Reduced antidiuretic effects

Clofibrate 2 g daily reduced the volume of urine excreted by 2 patients with pituitary diabetes insipidus, but when **glibenclamide (glyburide)** was also given the volume increased once again. Without treatment they excreted 5.8 and 6.5 litres of urine daily, and this reduced to only 2.4 and 1.7 litres while taking **clofibrate**, whereas with **glibenclamide** and **clofibrate** they excreted 3.6 and 3.7 litres daily, respectively.[18]

Mechanism

Among the suggestions are the displacement of the sulphonylureas from their plasma protein binding sites,[6] alterations in their renal excretion,[12] and a decrease in insulin resistance.[5,19] Clofibrate has also been shown to have a hypoglycaemic action of its own which improves the glucose tolerance of diabetics.[11] It is thought that gemfibrozil inhibits the metabolism of repaglinide by the cytochrome P450 isoenzyme CYP2C8, and that inhibition of CYP3A4 by itraconazole further blocks repaglinide metabolism.[17] Gemfibrozil may also inhibit CYP2C9-mediated metabolism of glimepiride and other sulphonylureas such as glipizide, glibenclamide and gliclazide.[16] It seems possible that any or all of these mechanisms might contribute towards enhanced hypoglycaemia.

Importance and management

The interaction between the sulphonylureas and clofibrate is established and well documented. The incidence is uncertain, but what is known suggests that between about one-third and one-half of patients may be affected. Gemfibrozil has both increased and decreased antidiabetic dose requirements. Hypoglycaemia has been reported with bezafibrate, ciprofibrate and fenofibrate There would seem to be no good reason for avoiding the concurrent use of antidiabetics and fibrates, but be aware that the dosage of the antidiabetic may need adjustment. Patients should be warned that excessive hypoglycaemia occurs occasionally and unpredictably. Note that on the basis of the study,[17] and following five reports of serious hypoglycaemic episodes with gemfibrozil and repaglinide, the European Agency for the Evaluation of Medicinal Products decided to contraindicate concurrent use.[20]

Information about reduced diuretic effects is limited. It would seem prudent to avoid the concurrent use of drugs with actions that are antagonistic.

1. Ohsawa K, Koike N, Takamura T, Nagai Y, Kobayashi KI. Hypoglycaemic attacks after administration of bezafibrate in three cases of non-insulin dependent diabetes mellitus. *J Jpn Diabetes Soc* (1994) 37, 295–300.
2. Girardin E, Vial T, Pham E, Evreux J-C. Hypoglycémies induites par les sulfamides hypoglycémiants. *Ann Med Interne (Paris)* (1992) 143, 11–17.
3. Daubresse J-C, Luyckx AS, Lefebvre PJ. Potentiation of hypoglycemic effect of sulfonylureas by clofibrate. *N Engl J Med* (1976) 294, 613.
4. Jain AK, Ryan JR, McMahon FG. Potentiation of hypoglycemic effect of sulfonylureas by halofenate. *N Engl J Med* (1975) 293, 1283–6.
5. Ferrari C, Frezzati S, Testori GP, Bertazzoni A. Potentiation of hypoglycemic response to intravenous tolbutamide by clofibrate. *N Engl J Med* (1976) 294, 1184.
6. Jain AK, Ryan JR, McMahon FG. Potentiation of hypoglycemic effect of sulfonylureas by clofibrate. *N Engl J Med* (1976) 294, 613.
7. Daubresse J-C, Daigneux D, Bruwier M, Luyckx A, Lefebvre PJ. Clofibrate and diabetes control in patients treated with oral hypoglycaemic agents. *Br J Clin Pharmacol* (1979) 7, 599–603.
8. Miller RD. *Atromid* in the treatment of post-climacteric diabetes. *J Atheroscler Res* (1963) 3, 694–700.
9. Csögör SI, Bornemisza P. The effect of clofibrate (Atromid) on intravenous tolbutamide, oral and intravenous glucose tolerance tests. *Clin Trials J* (1977) 14, 15–19.
10. Herriott SC, Percy-Robb IW, Strong JA, Thomson CG. The effect of Atromid on serum cholesterol and glucose tolerance in diabetes mellitus. *J Atheroscler Res* (1963) 3, 679–88.
11. Barnett D, Craig JG, Robinson DS, Rogers MP. Effect of clofibrate on glucose tolerance in maturity-onset diabetes. *Br J Clin Pharmacol* (1977) 4, 455–8.
12. Petitpierre B, Perrin L, Rudhardt M, Herrera A, Fabre J. Behaviour of chlorpropamide in renal insufficiency and under the effect of associated drug therapy. *Int J Clin Pharmacol* (1972) 6, 120–4.
13. De Salcedo I, Gorringe JAL, Silva JL and Santos JA. Gemfibrozil in a group of diabetics. *Proc R Soc Med* (1976) 69 (Suppl 2), 64–70.
14. Konttinen A, Kuisma I, Ralli R, Pohjola S and Ojala K. The effect of gemfibrozil on serum lipids in diabetic patients. *Ann Clin Res* (1979) 11, 240–5.
15. Ahmad S. Gemfibrozil: interaction with glyburide. *South Med J* (1991) 84, 102.
16. Niemi M, Neuvonen PJ, Kivistö KT. Effect of gemfibrozil on the pharmacokinetics and pharmacodynamics of glimepiride. *Clin Pharmacol Ther* (2001) 70, 439–45.
17. Niemi M, Backman JT, Neuvonen M, Neuvonen PJ. Effects of gemfibrozil, itraconazole, and their combination on the pharmacokinetics and pharmacodynamics of repaglinide: potentially hazardous interaction between gemfibrozil and repaglinide. *Diabetologia* (2003) 46, 347–51.
18. Rado JP, Szende L, Marosi J, Juhos E, Sawinsky I and Tako J. Inhibition of the diuretic action of glibenclamide by clofibrate, carbamazepine and 1-deamino-8-D-arginine-vasopressin (DDAVP) in patients with pituitary diabetes insipidus. *Acta Diabetol Lat* (1974) 11, 179–97.
19. Ferrari C, Frezzati S, Romussi M, Bertazzoni A, Testori GP, Antonini S, Paracchi A. Effects of short-term clofibrate administration on glucose tolerance and insulin secretion in patients with chemical diabetes or hypertriglyceridemia. *Metabolism* (1977) 26, 129–39.
20. EMEA public statement on repaglinide (NovoNorm/Prandin): contraindication of concomitant use of repaglinide and gemfibrozil. Available at http://www.emea.eu.int/pdfs/human/press/pus/117003en.pdf (accessed 27/06/05).

Antidiabetics + Guanethidine and related drugs

Guanethidine has hypoglycaemic activity, which may possibly add to the effects of conventional antidiabetics. Soluble insulin may also exaggerate the hypotensive effects of debrisoquine.

Clinical evidence

(a) Debrisoquine

An man with type 1 diabetes taking debrisoquine 20 mg twice daily developed severe postural hypotension within an hour of using 28 units of a short-acting **insulin** (soluble insulin) plus 20 units of **isophane insulin**. He became dizzy and was found to have a standing blood pressure of 97/72 mmHg. The postural fall in systolic pressure was 65 mmHg. He had no evidence of hypoglycaemia and no hypotension when using 48 units of **isophane insulin**.[1] **Insulin** can cause hypotension but this is only seen in those with an impaired reflex control of blood pressure.[1]

(b) Guanethidine

A diabetic needed an **insulin** dose increase from 70 to 94 units daily when guanethidine was withdrawn.[2] A later study in 3 patients with type 2 diabetes found that guanethidine 50 to 90 mg daily caused a significant improvement in their glucose tolerance.[3] Two other reports also describe the hypoglycaemic effects of guanethidine.[4,5]

Mechanism

A suggested reason for the interaction between insulin and guanethidine is that guanethidine can impair the homoeostatic mechanism concerned with raising blood sugar levels, by affecting the release of catecholamines. The balance of the system thus impaired tends to be tipped in favour of a reduced blood sugar level, resulting in a reduced requirement for the antidiabetic. The interaction between debrisoquine and insulin is not understood.

Importance and management

Information about both of these interactions is very limited, and their general importance is uncertain. Check on the dosage requirements of the antidiabetic if guanethidine or related drugs (guanadrel, debrisoquine, etc.) are started or stopped. Also check patients given debrisoquine and insulin, particularly if they are taking vasodilators, to ensure that excessive hypotension does not develop.

1. Hume L. Potentiation of hypotensive effect of debrisoquine by insulin. *Diabet Med* (1985) 2, 390–1.
2. Gupta KK, Lillicrap CA. Guanethidine and diabetes. *BMJ* (1968) 2, 697–8.
3. Gupta KK. The anti-diabetic action of guanethidine. *Postgrad Med J* (1969) 45, 455–6.
4. Kansal PC, Buse J, Durling FC. Effect of guanethidine and reserpine on glucose tolerance. *Curr Ther Res* (1971) 13, 517–22.
5. Woeber KA, Arky R, Braverman LE. Reversal by guanethidine of abnormal oral glucose tolerance in thyrotoxicosis. *Lancet* (1966) i, 895–8.

Antidiabetics + Guar gum or Glucomannan

Guar gum appears not to affect the absorption of glipizide or one formulation of glibenclamide (glyburide). Although it reduces the absorption of metformin, it enhances its postprandial hypoglycaemic effect. Glucomannan appears to reduce the absorption of glibenclamide, but also enhanced its hypoglycaemic effect.

Clinical evidence, mechanism, importance and management

(a) Glucomannan

Glucomannan 3.9 g reduced the plasma levels of a single 2.5-mg dose of **glibenclamide (glyburide)** in 9 healthy subjects. Four samples taken over 30 to 150 minutes found that the plasma levels of **glibenclamide** were reduced by about 50%.[1] Despite this, plasma glucose levels were lower with the combination than with glibenclamide alone. Because plasma samples were not taken beyond 150 minutes, it is unclear what effect glucomannan has on the extent of glibenclamide absorption. The clinical relevance of these changes is unclear, but as with guar gum, they seem unlikely to be important.

(b) Guar gum

Guar gum granules (4.75 g guar gum) taken alone or 30 minutes later with breakfast did not significantly affect the absorption of a single 2.5-mg dose of **glipizide** in 10 healthy subjects.[2]

In one comparative study, guar gum was found to reduce the absorption of **glibenclamide (glyburide)** in one formulation *(Semi-Euglucon)* but not another newer formulation *(Semi-Euglucon-N)*,[3] possibly because the latter preparation is more rapidly and completely absorbed. Similarly, in a double-blind crossover study in 9 patients with type 2 diabetes, guar gum granules 5 g three times daily with meals did not significantly affect the absorption of **glibenclamide** 3.5 mg twice daily from the newer formulation.[4]

In a single-dose study, guar gum 10 g reduced the absorption rate of **metformin** 1.7 g and reduced the AUC by 39% in healthy subjects, but the total reduction in postprandial blood sugar levels was increased.[5]

It seems doubtful if any of these interactions has much, if any, clinical relevance because guar gum can improve the metabolic control and decrease serum lipids in patients with type 2 diabetes[4] and among its indications guar gum is used to reduce oral antidiabetic dosage levels.[6]

1. Shima K, Tanaka A, Ikegami H, Tabata M, Sawazaki N, Kumahara Y. Effect of dietary fiber, glucomannan, on absorption of sulfonylurea in man. *Horm Metab Res* (1983) 15, 1–3.
2. Huupponen R, Karhuvaara S, Seppälä P. Effect of guar gum on glipizide absorption in man. *Eur J Clin Pharmacol* (1985) 28, 717–9.
3. Neugebauer G, Akpan W, Abshagen U. Interaktion von Guar mit Glibenclamid und Bezafibrat. *Beitr Infusionther Klin Ernahr* (1983) 12, 40–7.
4. Uusitupa M, Södervik H, Silvasti M, Karttunen P. Effects of a gel forming dietary fiber, guar gum, on the absorption of glibenclamide and metabolic control and serum lipids in patients with non-insulin-dependent (type 2) diabetes. *Int J Clin Pharmacol Ther Toxicol* (1990) 28, 153–7.
5. Gin H, Orgerie MB, Aubertin J. The influence of guar gum on absorption of metformin from the gut in healthy volunteers. *Horm Metab Res* (1989) 21, 81–3.
6. Guarem granules (Guar gum). Rybar Laboratories Ltd. UK Summary of product characteristics, March 2001.

Antidiabetics + H_2-blockers

Marked changes in the control of diabetes in patients on sulphonylureas given either cimetidine or ranitidine seem to be unusual. Cimetidine also does not interact with repaglinide and ranitidine does not interact with pioglitazone or rosiglitazone. However, a possible exception is glipizide with cimetidine, and isolated cases of hypoglycaemia have been seen with gliclazide and cimetidine or glibenclamide (glyburide) and ranitidine. Cimetidine appears to reduce the clearance of metformin.

Clinical evidence

A. Studies in diabetic patients

(a) Gliclazide or Glibenclamide (Glyburide)

An elderly type 2 diabetic taking gliclazide 160 mg daily developed very low blood sugar levels (1 mmol/l) after starting to take **cimetidine** 800 mg daily.[1] Marked hypoglycaemia was seen in a patient on glibenclamide when treated with **ranitidine**,[2] and another report briefly describes hypoglycaemia in 2 patients on unnamed sulphonylureas given **cimetidine**.[3]

(b) Glipizide

Patients with type 2 diabetes were given **cimetidine** 400 mg 1 hour before taking a dose of glipizide (average dose 5.7 mg) and then 3 hours later they were given a standard meal with **cimetidine** 200 mg. The expected rise in blood sugar levels after the meal was reduced by 40% and in some of the patients it fell to less than 3 mmol/l.[4,5] Two studies in type 2 diabetics found that **ranitidine** 150 mg or 300 mg had no significant effects on the pharmacokinetics or the effects of glipizide, except that the absorption was delayed,[6,7] whereas a later study by the same group of workers found that the expected rise in blood sugar levels after a meal was reduced by 25%.[5]

B. Studies in healthy subjects

(a) Metformin

Cimetidine 800 mg daily was found to reduce the renal clearance of metformin in 7 healthy subjects by 27% and increase the AUC by 50%.[8]

(b) Pioglitazone

A study in healthy subjects indicated that the pharmacokinetics of pioglitazone 45 mg daily are not significantly affected by **ranitidine** 150 mg twice daily, and that pioglitazone does not affect the pharmacokinetics of **ranitidine**.[9]

(c) Repaglinide

An open label crossover trial in 14 healthy subjects found that **cimetidine** 400 mg twice daily had no effect on the pharmacokinetics of repaglinide 2 mg three times daily.[10]

(d) Rosiglitazone

A study found that pre-treatment with **ranitidine**, 150 mg twice daily for 4 days, had no effect on the pharmacokinetics of either single 4 mg oral or 2 mg intravenous doses of rosiglitazone.[11]

(e) Sulphonylureas

The pharmacokinetics of **tolbutamide** 250 mg daily for 4 days were not significantly changed in 7 subjects when **cimetidine** 800 mg daily was added for a further 4 days.[12] Other studies also found no pharmacokinetic interaction between **tolbutamide**[13,14] or **chlorpropamide**[15] and **cimetidine**, or between **tolbutamide** and **ranitidine**,[14] and the hypoglycaemic activities of **tolbutamide**, **chlorpropamide**, **glibenclamide** (**glyburide**) and **glipizide** remained unaltered by **cimetidine**.[16]

In contrast, in another study the AUC of **tolbutamide** was found to be increased by 20% and the elimination half-life decreased by 17% by **cimetidine** 1.2 g daily, but plasma glucose levels were not significantly changed. **Ranitidine** 300 mg had no effect.[17] A later study found effectively the same results.[18] Yet another study reported that the hypoglycaemic effects of **glibenclamide** were reduced by **cimetidine** and **ranitidine**.[19] No relevant interactions, either pharmacokinetic or pharmacodynamic, were seen in a study of **glimepiride** with either **cimetidine** or **ranitidine**.[20]

Mechanism

If an interaction occurs[17] it may be because the cimetidine inhibits the metabolism of the sulphonylurea by the liver, thereby increasing its effects. Cimetidine appears to inhibit the excretion of metformin by the kidneys.[8]

Importance and management

Information is limited and not easy to assess because of the differences between the sulphonylureas and repaglinide, or between healthy subjects and diabetics, but all the evidence cited here, as well as the relative paucity of adverse reports, suggests that most diabetics do not experience any marked changes in their diabetic control if given cimetidine. It has been suggested that the dosage of metformin may need to be reduced if cimetidine is used, bearing in mind the possibility of lactic acidosis if levels become too high.[8] Ranitidine normally appears not to interact with either the sulphonylureas, pioglitazone or rosiglitazone.

1. Archambeaud-Mouveroux F, Nouaille Y, Nadalon S, Treves R, Merle L. Interaction between gliclazide and cimetidine. *Eur J Clin Pharmacol* (1987) 31, 631.
2. Lee K, Mize R, Lowenstein SR. Glyburide-induced hypoglycaemia and ranitidine. *Ann Intern Med* (1987) 107, 261–2.
3. Girardin E, Vial T, Pham E, Evreux J-C. Hypoglycémies induites par les sulfamides hypoglycémiants. *Ann Med Interne (Paris)* (1992) 143, 11–17.
4. Feely J, Peden N. Enhanced sulphonylurea-induced hypoglycaemia with cimetidine. *Br J Clin Pharmacol* (1983) 15, 607P.
5. Feeley J, Collins WCJ, Cullen M, El Debani AH, MacWalter RS, Peden NR, Stevenson IH. Potentiation of the hypoglycaemic response to glipizide in diabetic patients by histamine H_2–receptor antagonists. *Br J Clin Pharmacol* (1993) 35, 321–3.
6. MacWalter RS, El Debani AH, Feeley J, Stevenson IH. Potentiation by ranitidine of the hypoglycaemic response to glipizide in diabetic patients. *Br J Clin Pharmacol* (1985) 19, 121P–122P.
7. Stevenson IH, El Debani AH, MacWalter RS. Glipizide pharmacokinetics and effect in diabetic patients given ranitidine. *Acta Pharmacol Toxicol (Copenh)* (1986) 59 (Suppl 4), 97.
8. Somogyi A, Stockley C, Keal J, Rolan P, Bochner F. Reduction of metformin renal tubular secretion by cimetidine in man. *Br J Clin Pharmacol* (1987) 23, 545–51.
9. Glazer NB, Sanes-Miller C. Pharmacokinetics of coadministration of pioglitazone with ranitidine. *Diabetes* (2001) 50 (suppl 2) A114.
10. Hatorp V, Thomsen MS. Drug interaction studies with repaglinide: repaglinide on digoxin or theophylline pharmacokinetics and cimetidine on repaglinide pharmacokinetics. *J Clin Pharmacol* (2000) 40, 184–92.
11. Freed MI, Miller A, Jorkasky DK, Dicicco RA. Rosiglitazone pharmacokinetics are not affected by coadministration of ranitidine. *Diabetes* (1998) 43 (Suppl 1), A353.
12. Stockley C, Keal J, Rolan P, Bochner F, Somogyi A. Lack of inhibition of tolbutamide hydroxylation by cimetidine in man. *Eur J Clin Pharmacol* (1986) 31, 235–7.

13. Dey NG, Castleden CM, Ward J, Cornhill J, McBurney A. The effect of cimetidine on tolbutamide kinetics. *Br J Clin Pharmacol* (1983) 16, 438–440.
14. Adebayo GI, Coker HAB. Lack of efficacy of cimetidine and ranitidine as inhibitors of tolbutamide metabolism. *Eur J Clin Pharmacol* (1988) 34, 653–6.
15. Shah GF, Ghandi TP, Patel PR, Patel MR, Gilbert RN, Shridhar PA. Tolbutamide and chlorpropamide kinetics in the presence of cimetidine in human volunteers. *Indian Drugs* (1985) 22, 455–8.
16. Shah GF, Ghandi TP, Patel PR, Patel MR, Gilbert RN, Shridhar PA. The effect of cimetidine on the hypoglycaemic activity of four commonly used sulphonylurea drugs. *Indian Drugs* (1985) 22, 570–2.
17. Cate EW, Rogers JF, Powell JR. Inhibition of tolbutamide elimination by cimetidine but not ranitidine. *J Clin Pharmacol* (1986) 26, 372–7.
18. Toon S, Holt BL, Mullins FGP, Khan A. Effects of cimetidine, ranitidine and omeprazole on tolbutamide pharmacokinetics. *J Pharm Pharmacol* (1995) 47, 85–88.
19. Kubacka RT, Antal EJ, Juhl RP. The paradoxical effect of cimetidine and ranitidine on glibenclamide pharmacokinetics and pharmacodynamics. *Br J Clin Pharmacol* (1987) 23, 743–51.
20. Schaaf LJ, Welshman IR, Viveash DM, Carel BJ. The effects of cimetidine and ranitidine on glimepiride pharmacokinetics and pharmacodynamics in normal subjects. *Pharm Res* (1994) 11 (10 Suppl), S-360.

Antidiabetics + HRT or Oral contraceptives

Some diabetics may require small increases or decreases in their dosage of antidiabetic while taking oral contraceptives or HRT, but it is unusual for the control of diabetes to be seriously disturbed.

Clinical evidence

(a) HRT

More than half of a group of 30 menopausal diabetics had abnormal glucose tolerance when given **noretynodrel** 5 mg with **mestranol** 75 micrograms, but the changes in their requirements of **insulin** or oral hypoglycaemic agent were rare and slight.[1]

(b) Oral contraceptives

There are numerous reports of the effect of contraceptive steroids on glucose tolerance in non-diabetics. More recent reports from studies using newer, low-dose oral contraceptives, support the suggestion that changes in glucose metabolism are minimal.[2] Problems with glucose metabolism seem very unlikely when the dose of oestrogen is less then 50 micrograms.[3] The progestogen in oral contraceptives may also be important.[3-5] Progestogens with androgenic properties, such as **norgestrel**, **levonorgestrel** and to a lesser extent **norethisterone**, may affect carbohydrate metabolism. **Etynodrel**, which has weak androgenic activity, was found to cause smaller reductions in glucose tolerance, and **noretynodrel** was found to have no effect.[3-5]

(i) Insulin. In one study in 179 diabetic women, 34% needed an increase and 7% needed a decrease in insulin dose when they were given a variety of oral contraceptives.[6] There are also a few scattered reports of individual diabetics who experienced a marked disturbance of their diabetic control when given an oral contraceptive, some of which were low dose.[7-10] However, in a study of 38 insulin-dependent diabetics it was found that progestogen-only and combined oral contraceptives had little effect on the control of diabetes,[11] and another report[12] about women taking *Orthonovin* (**norethisterone** with **mestranol**) stated that no insulin dose changes were necessary.

(ii) Pioglitazone. A randomised double-blind study in 35 healthy women given pioglitazone 45 mg once daily with either a combined oral contraceptive (**ethinylestradiol/norethisterone** 35 micrograms/1 mg) or placebo for 21 days found that pioglitazone does not affect systemic exposure to the oral contraceptive as measured by AUC.[13]

(iii) Repaglinide. A three-period cross-over open-label study in healthy subjects found that a combined oral contraceptive (**ethinylestradiol/levonorgestrel** 30/150 micrograms) increased the maximum plasma level of repaglinide 2 mg three times daily by 17% although the bioavailability of repaglinide was not altered.[14] Repaglinide did not significantly alter the bioavailability of **ethinylestradiol** or **levonorgestrel**.[14]

(iv) Rosiglitazone. Rosiglitazone 8 mg daily for the first two weeks of two cycles in 32 women taking an oral contraceptive (**ethinylestradiol/norethisterone** 35 micrograms/1 mg, *Ortho-Novum*) was found to have no effect on the pharmacokinetics of either steroid.[15]

Mechanism

Not understood. Many mechanisms have been considered including changes in cortisol secretion, alterations in tissue glucose utilisation, production of excessive amounts of growth hormone, and alterations in liver function.[16]

Importance and management

Moderately well documented. Concurrent use need not be avoided, but because some patients need a small adjustment in their dosage of antidiabetic (increases or decreases) and because very occasionally serious disturbances occur, the diabetic response should be monitored. Also bear in mind that the lowest-strength combined oral contraceptive preparations (20 micrograms oestrogen) are recommended for patients with risk factors for circulatory disease (such as diabetics), so the potential for interference with their diabetic control will be minimised if this recommendation is followed. The choice of progestogen may also be important, with levonorgestrel having the most detrimental effect.

Similarly, irrespective of control of diabetes, menopausal HRT should be used with caution in diabetes because of the increased risk of heart disease. See also 'Antidiabetics + Tibolone', p.418.

1. Cochran B and Pote WWH. C–19 nor-steroid effects on plasma lipid and diabetic control of postmenopausal women. *Diabetes* (1963) 12, 366.
2. Miccoli R, Orlandi MC, Fruzzetti F, Giampietro O, Melis G, Ricci C, Bertolotto A, Fioretti P, Navalesi R, Masoni A. Metabolic effects of three new low-dose pills: a six-month experience. *Contraception* (1989) 39, 643–52.
3. Spellacy WN. Carbohydrate metabolism during treatment with estrogen, progestogen, and low-dose oral contraceptives. *Am J Obstet Gynecol* (1982) 142, 732–4.
4. Perlman JA, Russell-Briefel R, Ezzati T, Lieberknecht G. Oral glucose tolerance and the potency of contraceptive progestins. *J Chron Dis* (1985) 38, 857–64.
5. Wynn V. Effect of duration of low-dose oral contraceptive administration on carbohydrate metabolism. *Am J Obstet Gynecol* (1982) 142, 739–46.
6. Zeller WJ, Brehm H, Schoffling K and Melzer H. Vertraglichkeit von hormonalen Ovulationshemmern bei Diabetikerinnen. *Arzneimittelforschung* (1974) 24, 351.
7. Kopera H, Dukes NG and Ijzerman GL. Critical evaluation of clinical data on *Lyndiol*. *Int J Fertil* (1964) 9, 69.
8. Peterson WF, Steel MW and Coyne RY. Analysis of the effect of ovulatory suppressants on glucose tolerance. *Am J Obstet Gynecol* (1966) 95, 484.
9. Reder JA and Tulgan H. Impairment of diabetic control by norethynodrel with mestranol. *N Y State J Med* (1967) 67, 1073.
10. Rennie NJ. Hyperglycaemic episodes in a young woman after taking levonorgestrel-containing oral contraceptives. *N Z Med J* (1994) 107, 440–1.
11. Rådberg T, Gustafson A, Skryten A and Karlsson K. Oral contraception in diabetic women. Diabetes control, serum and high density lipoprotein lipids during low-dose progestogen, combined oestrogen/progestogen and non-hormonal contraception. *Acta Endocrinol (Copenh)* (1981) 98, 246–51.
12. Tyler ET, Olsen HJ, Gotlib M, Levin M and Behne D. Long term usage of norethindrone with mestranol preparations in the control of human fertility. *Clin Med* (1964) 71, 997.
13. Karim A, Schwartz L, Perez A, Cao C. Lack of clinically significant drug interaction in the coadministration of pioglitazone with ethinyl estradiol and norethindrone. *Diabetes* (2003) 52 (suppl 1) A123.
14. Hatorp V, Hansen KT, Thomsen MS. Influence of drugs interacting with CYP3A4 on the pharmacokinetics, pharmacodynamics, and safety of the prandial glucose regulator repaglinide. *J Clin Pharmacol* (2003) 43, 649–60.
15. Inglis AML, Miller AK, Culkin KT, Finnerty D, Patterson SD, Jorkasky DK, Freed MI. Lack of effect of rosiglitazone on the pharmacokinetics of oral contraceptives in healthy female volunteers. *J Clin Pharmacol* (2001) 41, 683–90.
16. Spellacy WN. A review of carbohydrate metabolism and the oral contraceptives. *Am J Obstet Gynecol* (1969) 104, 448.

Antidiabetics + Isoniazid

Some reports state that isoniazid can raise blood sugar levels in diabetics, whereas one describes a fall. The outcome of concurrent use is uncertain.

Clinical evidence

A study in 6 diabetics taking **insulin** found that **isoniazid** 300 to 400 mg daily increased their fasting blood sugar levels by 40% (from an average of 255 to 357 mg%), and their glucose tolerance curves rose and returned to normal levels more slowly. After 6 days' treatment the average rise was only 20%. Two other patients needed an increased dosage of **insulin** while taking **isoniazid** 200 mg daily, but this was reduced again when the isoniazid was withdrawn.[1]

Another report describes glycosuria and the development of frank diabetes in 3 out of 50 patients given **isoniazid** 300 mg daily,[2] and hyperglycaemia has been seen in cases of **isoniazid** poisoning.[3]

In contrast, another study found that **isoniazid** had a hypoglycaemic effect in 6 out of 8 diabetics.[4] A 500-mg dose of **isoniazid** caused an 18% (range 5 to 34%) reduction in blood sugar levels after 4 hours; 3 g of **tolbutamide** caused a 28% (19 to 43%) reduction, and together they caused a 35% (17 to 57%) reduction. However, one patient had a 10% increase in blood sugar levels after taking **isoniazid**, a 41% decrease after **tolbutamide**, and a 30% decrease after taking both drugs. The diabetic-control of another patient was not affected by either drug.[4]

Mechanism

Not understood.

Importance and management

The major documentation for these reactions dates back to the 1950s, since when the literature has been virtually (and perhaps significantly) silent. The outcome of concurrent use is therefore somewhat uncertain. Nevertheless it would be prudent for diabetics given isoniazid to be monitored for changes in the control of the diabetes. Appropriate dosage adjustments of the antidiabetic should be made where necessary.

1. Luntz GRWN, Smith SG. Effect of isoniazid on carbohydrate metabolism in controls and diabetics. *BMJ* (1953) i, 296–9.
2. Dickson I. Glycosuria and diabetes mellitus following INAH therapy. *Med J Aust* (1962) i, 325–6.
3. Tovaryš A, Šiler Z. Diabetic syndrome and intoxication with INH. *Prakt Lekar (1968) 48, 286; quoted in Int Pharm Abstr* (1968) 5, 286.
4. Segarra FO, Sherman DS, Charif BS. Experiences with tolbutamide and chlorpropamide in tuberculous diabetic patients. *Ann N Y Acad Sci* (1959) 74, 656–61.

Antidiabetics + Karela (*Momordica charantia*)

The hypoglycaemic effects of chlorpropamide and other antidiabetics can be increased by karela.

Clinical evidence

A report of a diabetic who was poorly controlled on diet and **chlorpropamide**, but much better controlled when she also ate karela, provides evidence that the hypoglycaemic effects of karela and conventional oral antidiabetics can be additive.[1] Other studies have subsequently shown that karela produces a significant improvement in glucose tolerance in patients with type 2 diabetes, both when being treated with **chlorpropamide**, **tolbutamide**, **glibenclamide** or **glymidine**,[2] and when not.[3,4]

Hypoglycaemic coma and seizures occurred in 2 young non-diabetic children after they were given bitter melon (karela) tea.[5]

Mechanism

Karela (also known as bitter melon, bitter gourd, balsam pear, cundeamor) is the fruit of *Momordica charantia* which is indigenous to Asia and South America. The hypoglycaemic effects of karela may be due to its content of polypeptide P, a hypoglycaemic peptide,[6] also known as vegetable insulin (v-insulin).[7] This substance is effective when given subcutaneously,[7] but its oral activity is uncertain.[8] Other hypoglycaemic compounds isolated from karela include charantin (sterol glucoside mixture in the fruit) and vicine a pyrimidine nucleoside found in the seeds). Karela fruit may have both insulin-like effects and stimulate insulin secretion.[8]

Importance and management

Karela is available in the UK and elsewhere, and is used to flavour foods such as curries, and also used as a herbal medicine for the treatment of diabetes mellitus. Its hypoglycaemic activity is clearly established. Health professionals should therefore be aware that patients may possibly be using karela as well as more orthodox drugs to control their diabetes. Irregular consumption of karela as part of the diet could possibly contribute to unexplained fluctuations in diabetic control.

1. Aslam M, Stockley IH. Interaction between curry ingredient (karela) and drug (chlorpropamide). *Lancet* (1979) i, 607.
2. Leatherdale BA, Panesar KR, Singh G, Atkins TW, Bailey CJ, Bignell AHC. Improvement in glucose tolerance due to Momordica charantia (karela). *BMJ* (1981) 282, 1823–4.
3. Welihinda J, Karunanayake EH, Sheriff MHR, Jaysinghe KSA . Effect of *Momordica charantia* on the glucose tolerance in maturity onset diabetes. *J Ethnopharmacol* (1986) 17, 277–82.
4. Akhtar MS. Trial of Momordica Charantia Linn (Karela) powder in patients with maturity-onset diabetes. *J Pakistan Med Assoc* (1982) 32, 106–7.
5. Hulin A, Wavelet M, Desbordes JM. Intoxication aiguë par *Momordica charantia* (sorrossi). A propos de deux cas. *Sem Hop Paris* (1988) 64, 2847–8.
6. Khanna P, Jain SC, Panagariya A, Dixit VP. Hypoglycemic activity of polypeptide-p from a plant source. *J Nat Prod* (1981) 44, 648–55.
7. Baldwa VS, Bhandari CM, Pangaria A, Goyal RK. Clinical trial in patients with diabetes mellitus of an insulin-like compound obtained from plant source. *Ups J Med Sci* (1977) 82, 39–41.
8. Raman A, Lau C. Anti-diabetic properties and phytochemistry of *Momordica charantia* (Cucurbitaceae). *Phytomedicine* (1996) 2, 349–62.

Antidiabetics + Ketotifen

The concurrent use of sulphonylureas or biguanides and ketotifen appears to be well tolerated, but a fall in the number of platelets has been seen in one study in patients on biguanides while taking ketotifen. The clinical importance of this is uncertain.

Clinical evidence, mechanism, importance and management

A study in 30 hospitalised diabetics (10 on diet alone, 10 on unnamed **sulphonylureas**, 10 on unnamed **biguanides**) found that the concurrent use of ketotifen 4 mg daily for 14 days was generally well tolerated. However, those on **biguanides** had a significant decrease in platelet counts and 3 had a marked fall on day 14 to slightly below 100×10^9/l, which returned to normal after a few days.[1] This finding underlies the precaution issued by the makers of ketotifen,[2] that the combination should be avoided until this effect is explained. However, no other studies appear to have confirmed the fall in thrombocyte count so that its importance still remains uncertain.[3]

1. Doleček R. Ketotifen in the treatment of diabetics with various allergic conditions. *Pharmatherapeutica* (1981) 2, 568–74.
2. Zaditen (Ketotifen). Novartis Pharmaceuticals UK Ltd. UK Summary of product characteristics, November 2000.
3. Sandoz. Personal communication, 1991.

Antidiabetics + Lithium

Lithium can raise blood sugar levels and in some instances has been associated with the development of diabetes mellitus, but the association is unclear and there is little or no evidence that its use normally causes significant changes in diabetic control.

Clinical evidence, mechanism, importance and management

A study in 10 psychiatric patients found that lithium carbonate for 2 weeks raised their blood glucose levels and impaired their glucose tolerance.[1] There are also a few case reports of hyperglycaemia, impaired glucose tolerance and diabetes mellitus in patients treated with lithium.[2-4]

Although there appear to be no reports of disturbed diabetic control in diabetics treated with lithium (any marked effect might be expected to have been reported by now), it would seem prudent to bear this interaction in mind if lithium is added to the treatment being received by diabetic patients.

1. Shopsin B, Stern S, Gershon S. Altered carbohydrate metabolism during treatment with lithium carbonate. *Arch Gen Psychiatry* (1972) 26, 566–71.
2. Craig J, Abu-Saleh M, Smith B, Evans I. Diabetes mellitus in patients on lithium. *Lancet* (1977) ii, 1028.
3. Johnstone BB. Diabetes mellitus in patients on lithium. *Lancet* (1977) ii, 935.
4. Martinez-Maldonado M, Terrell J. Lithium carbonate-induced nephrogenic diabetes insipidus and glucose intolerance. *Arch Intern Med* (1973) 132, 881–4.

Antidiabetics + Macrolides

An isolated report describes severe liver damage with prolonged cholestasis in a patient on chlorpropamide after the concurrent use of erythromycin. Isolated cases of hypoglycaemia have been described in other patients on glibenclamide (glyburide) when given erythromycin or on glibenclamide or glipizide with clarithromycin. A study in healthy subjects found that hypoglycaemia may occur if tolbutamide and clarithromycin are given concurrently and another study suggests that clarithromycin may enhance the effects of repaglinide.

Clinical evidence, mechanism, importance and management

(a) Effects on the liver

A man with type 2 diabetes was treated with phenformin for 10 years. Four months after the phenformin was replaced by **chlorpropamide**, he was given **erythromycin ethylsuccinate** 1 g daily for 3 weeks for a respiratory infection. Two weeks later he complained of increasing fatigue and fever. A short episode of pruriginous skin rash was followed by the appearance of dark urine, jaundice and hepatomegaly. The picture over the next 2 years was that of profound cholestasis, complicated by steatorrhoea and marked hyperlipidaemia with disappearance of interlobular bile ducts. He died of ischaemic cardiomyopathy.[1] The reasons for this serious reaction are not understood, but the authors point out that liver damage occurs in a very small number of patients given sulphonylureas, such as **chlorpropamide**, and also with **erythromycin**. They suggest that there may have been an interaction between the two drugs.[1] No general conclusions can be drawn from this unusual case.

(b) Hypoglycaemia

Isolated cases of severe hypoglycaemia occurred in type 2 diabetic patients given **glibenclamide** and **clarithromycin** or **glipizide** and **clarithromycin**.[2] A further case occurred in a patient on **glibenclamide** and **erythromycin**,[3] but an earlier single-dose study in 12 patients with type 2 diabetes found that **erythromycin** had little effect on **glibenclamide** pharmacokinetics or on its hypoglycaemic effects.[4] The general importance of these isolated cases is uncertain, but some caution may be warranted with concurrent use in the elderly or those with renal impairment.[2]

A study in 9 healthy subjects found that **clarithromycin** 250 mg increased the rate of absorption of **tolbutamide** 500 mg by about 20% and increased its bioavailability by 26%. Hypoglycaemia, reported as uneasiness and giddiness, occurred on taking the combination.[5]

(c) Pharmacokinetic studies

Clarithromycin 250 mg given to healthy subjects increased the AUC and maximum plasma concentrations of **repaglinide** by 40 and 67% respectively. **Clarithromycin** may inhibit the metabolism of **repaglinide** by inhibition of cytochrome P450 isoenzyme CYP3A4. There was a similar corresponding rise in circulating insulin levels.[6] The effect of concurrent administration of these drugs should therefore be monitored.

1. Geubel AP, Nakad A, Rahier J, Dive C. Prolonged cholestasis and disappearance of interlobular bile ducts following chlorpropamide and erythromycin ethylsuccinate. Case of drug interaction? *Liver* (1988) 8, 350–3.
2. Bussing R, Gende A. Severe hypoglycemia from clarithromycin-sulfonylurea drug interaction. *Diabetes Care* (2002) 25, 1659–60.
3. Girardin E, Vial T, Pham E, Evreux J-C. Hypoglycémies induites par les sulfamides hypoglycémiants. *Ann Med Interne (Paris)* (1992) 143, 11–17.
4. Fleishaker JC, Phillips JP. Evaluation of a potential interaction between erythromycin and glyburide in diabetic volunteers. *J Clin Pharmacol* (1991) 31, 259–62.
5. Jayasagar G, Dixit AA, Kirshan V, Rao YM. Effect of clarithromycin on the pharmacokinetics of tolbutamide. *Drug Metabol Drug Interact* (2000) 16, 207–15.
6. Niemi M, Neuvonen PJ, Kivistö KT. The cytochrome P4503A4 inhibitor clarithromycin increases the plasma concentrations and effects of repaglinide. *Clin Pharmacol Ther* (2001) 70, 58–65.

Antidiabetics + MAOIs

The hypoglycaemic effects of insulin and the oral antidiabetics can be increased by MAOIs. This may improve the control of blood sugar levels in most diabetics, but in a few it may cause undesirable hypoglycaemia. Moclobemide appears not to interact.

Clinical evidence

(a) Moclobemide

No clinically relevant interaction was reported to occur between **glibenclamide (glyburide)** and **moclobemide**.[1] A study in healthy subjects on **glibenclamide** 2.5 mg daily found that **moclobemide** 200 mg three times daily for a week had no effect on glucose or **insulin** concentrations after oral glucose tolerance tests.[2] Clinical trials in 8 diabetics taking **glibenclamide (glyburide)**, **gliclazide**, **metformin** or **chlorpropamide** also found that **moclobemide** had no effect on blood glucose levels or any other evidence of an interaction.[2]

(b) Non-selective MAOIs

A diabetic patient experienced postural syncope and hypoglycaemia associated with the concurrent use of **mebanazine** and **insulin**, and required a reduction in insulin dose.[3] Other reports in diabetics showed that **mebanazine** increased the hypoglycaemic activity of **insulin, tolbutamide** and **chlorpropamide,** and improved diabetic control.[4-7]

Mechanism

Not fully understood. Mebanazine,[5] iproniazid,[8] isocarboxazid,[9] phenelzine,[5] and tranylcypromine[10] have all been shown to reduce blood glucose levels in the absence of conventional antidiabetics, possibly due to some direct action of the MAOI on the pancreas, which causes the release of insulin.[10] It would seem that this can be additive with the effects of the conventional hypoglycaemics.

Importance and management

The interaction of the non-selective MAOIs is an established interaction of only moderate clinical importance. It can benefit the control of diabetes in many patients, but some individuals may need a reduction in the dose of their antidiabetic to avoid excessive hypoglycaemia. The effects of concurrent use should be monitored.This interaction would seem possible with any antidiabetic/MAOI combination, but this requires confirmation.

No clinically important interaction seems to occur between antidiabetics and moclobemide.

1. Zimmer R, Gieschke R, Fischbach R, Gasic S. Interaction studies with moclobemide. *Acta Psychiatr Scand* (1990) (Suppl 360), 84–6.
2. Amrein R, Güntert TW, Dingemanse J, Lorscheid T, Stabl M, Schmid-Burgk W. Interactions of moclobemide with concomitantly administered medication: evidence from pharmacological and clinical studies. *Psychopharmacology (Berl)* (1992) 106, S24–S31.
3. Cooper AJ, Keddie KMG. Hypotensive collapse and hypoglycaemia after mebanazine-a monoamine oxidase inhibitor. *Lancet* (1964) i, 1133–5.
4. Wickström L, Pettersson K. Treatment of diabetics with monoamine-oxidase inhibitors. *Lancet* (1964) ii, 995–7.
5. Adnitt PI. Hypoglycemic action of monoamineoxidase inhibitors (MAOI's). *Diabetes* (1968) 17, 628–33.
6. Cooper AJ. The action of mebanazine, a mono amine oxidase inhibitor antidepressant drug in diabetes-part II. *Int J Neuropsychiatry* (1966) 2, 342–5.
7. Adnitt PI, Oleesky S, Schnieden H. The hypoglycaemic action of monoamineoxidase inhibitors (MAOI's). *Diabetologia* (1968) 4, 379.
8. Weiss J, Weiss S, Weiss B. Effects of iproniazid and similar compounds on the gastrointestinal tract. *Ann N Y Acad Sci* (1959) 80, 854–9.
9. van Praag HM, Leijnse B. The influence of some antidepressives of the hydrazine type on the glucose metabolism in depressed patients. *Clin Chim Acta* (1963) 8, 466–75.
10. Bressler R, Vargas-Cordon M, Lebovitz HE. Tranylcypromine: a potent insulin secretagogue and hypoglycemic agent. *Diabetes* (1968) 17, 617–24.

Antidiabetics + NSAIDs

No adverse interaction normally occurs between most NSAIDs and antidiabetics. However, there are isolated cases of hypoglycaemia in patients given fenclofenac with chlorpropamide and metformin, glibenclamide with diflunisal or ibuprofen and naproxen with glibenclamide and metformin. Another describes loss of diabetic control attributed to indometacin. Indobufen increases the effects of glipizide, and piroxicam increases the effects of glibenclamide. The risk of fluid retention with pioglitazone or rosiglitazone is increased by the NSAIDs.

Consider also 'azapropazone, phenylbutazone, and oxyphenbutazone', (p.412) and the 'salicylates', (p.415) for related drugs that do have adverse interactions with antidiabetics.

Clinical evidence

(a) Chlorpropamide

Ibuprofen 1.2 g daily had no significant effect on the blood sugar levels of type 2 diabetic patients taking chlorpropamide 62.5 to 375 mg daily.[1]

A woman whose type 2 diabetes was well controlled on chlorpropamide 500 mg and metformin 1.7 g daily, developed hypoglycaemia within 2 days of exchanging **flurbiprofen** 150 mg daily and **indometacin** 150 mg daily for **fenclofenac** 1.2 g daily. The hypoglycaemic agents were withdrawn the next day, but later in the evening she went into a hypoglycaemic coma. The reasons for this are not understood, but was attributed to a protein binding interaction between chlorpropamide and **fenclofenac**.[2] Conversely, another isolated report briefly describes hyperglycaemia with chlorpropamide possibly due to **indometacin**.[3]

(b) Glibenclamide

A study in 16 healthy subjects found that **ibuprofen** produced no significant changes in the pharmacokinetics of glibenclamide. However, **ibuprofen** with glibenclamide caused a greater hypoglycaemic effect than glibenclamide alone, but the clinical significance of this was uncertain.[4] A 72-year-old man with longstanding type 2 diabetes, well-controlled with glibenclamide 2.5 mg daily took a single 150-mg dose of **ibuprofen**, and 30 minutes later experienced severe nausea, sweating and palpitations, which were immediately relieved by taking sugar. The symptoms occurred again the next morning after a second dose of **ibuprofen** and after a further dose in the afternoon he became unconscious requiring intravenous glucose. **Ibuprofen** was withdrawn and there were no further episodes of hypoglycaemia. It was also noted that hypoglycaemia had not occurred when he had previously taken **aspirin**, **paracetamol** or **diclofenac**.[5]

No changes in the control of diabetes was seen in 20 patients with type 2 diabetes on glibenclamide when they were given **acemetacin** 60 mg three times daily.[6] The blood sugar levels of 12 diabetics taking glibenclamide 10 mg daily were unchanged by **bromfenac** 50 mg three times daily for 3 days, and the pharmacokinetics of glibenclamide were also unaltered.[7] The blood sugar levels of 12 diabetics with rheumatic diseases taking glibenclamide were unchanged by **diclofenac** 150 mg daily for 4 days,[8] but an isolated case of hypoglycaemia has been reported with **diflunisal**.[9] A case of severe hypoglycaemia in a diabetic patient was attributed to the accumulation of glibenclamide and metformin due to deterioration in renal function caused by the concurrent use of ramipril and **naproxen**.[10] Healthy subjects and type 2 diabetics had an increased hypoglycaemic response to glibenclamide (blood sugar levels down by 13 to 15%) when they were also given **piroxicam** 10 mg.[11] **Tenoxicam** 20 mg daily was found not to affect the glycoregulation of 8 healthy subjects given glibenclamide 2.5 mg daily.[12] No changes were seen in the blood sugar levels of 40 other diabetics on glibenclamide given either **tolmetin** 1.2 g or placebo daily for 5 days.[13] The makers of **valdecoxib** say that it has been found not to affect either the pharmacokinetics of glibenclamide nor its effects on insulin or blood glucose levels.[14,15] One study suggested that metamizole did not interact with glibenclamide,[16] and similarly etodolac did not affect diabetic control or the pharmacokinetics of glibenclamide.[17]

Lornoxicam 4 mg twice daily for 6 days had no effect on the pharmacokinetics of a single 5-mg dose of glibenclamide in 15 healthy subjects. The pharmacokinetics of lornoxicam also remained unchanged. However, concurrent use significantly increased plasma insulin levels (AUC 47%) and lowered serum glucose levels (8%), but this is probably not clinically important.[18]

Although a preliminary report suggested that nimesulide slightly increased the effects of glibenclamide,[19] a later study using various [unnamed] **sulphonylureas** failed to find that it affected fasting blood sugar levels or the glucose tolerance of diabetic patients.[19]

(c) Glibornuride

A study in healthy subjects found that **tenoxicam** 20 mg daily did not affect the pharmacokinetics of glibornuride nor the responses of plasma insulin and blood glucose to glibornuride.[20]

(d) Glipizide

Six healthy subjects had a rise in serum glipizide levels and a reduction in their blood sugar levels when they took **indobufen** 200 mg as a single dose and then twice daily for a 5 day period.[21] No important changes in blood sugar levels occurred in 24 type 2 diabetic patients on tolbutamide or glipizide when they took **indoprofen** 600 mg daily for 5 days.[22] A study found that although **indoprofen** (200 mg on day 1, then 600 mg daily on days 3 to 8) lowered the plasma levels of a single 5-mg dose of glipizide, the blood sugar levels remained unaffected.[23]

(e) Nateglinide

In a randomised crossover study, 18 healthy subjects were given modified-release **diclofenac** 75 mg on the same day as two 120-mg doses of nateglinide, given 4 hours apart. The pharmacokinetics of both drugs were unaltered by concurrent use.[24]

(f) Pioglitazone

The makers say that pioglitazone can cause fluid retention, which may exacerbate or precipitate heart failure. Because NSAIDs can also cause fluid retention, the makers issue a warning that concurrent use may possibly increase the risk of oedema.[25]

(g) Rosiglitazone

The makers say that rosiglitazone can cause fluid retention which may exacerbate or precipitate heart failure, particularly in those with limited cardiac reserve. Because NSAIDs can also cause fluid retention the makers therefore issue a warning that concurrent use may possibly increase the risk of oedema in these patients.[26]

(h) Tolbutamide

A brief report states that no changes in blood tolbutamide or in fasting blood glucose levels were seen in diabetics given **diflunisal** 375 mg twice daily.[27] The tolbutamide half-life, plasma levels, time-to-peak levels and AUC of 12 patients with type 2 diabetes were unaffected by **sulindac** 400 mg daily. An unimportant reduction in fasting blood sugar levels was seen.[28] **Naproxen** 375 mg every 12 hours had no effect on the pharmacokinetics or pharmacological effects of tolbutamide in 10 type 2 diabetics over 3 days.[29] The pharmacokinetics of a single 500-mg dose of tolbutamide were unaffected in 7 healthy subjects after they took **tenoxicam** 20 mg daily for 14 days, and blood glucose concentrations were not altered.[30] No important changes in blood sugar levels occurred in 24 type 2 diabetic patients on tolbutamide or **glipizide** when they were given **indoprofen** 600 mg daily for 5 days.[22] In other patients on tolbutamide it was found that **ibuprofen** lowered fasting blood sugar levels, but not below the normal lower limits.[31]

Mechanism

Normally none.

Importance and management

The reports briefly quoted here indicate that no adverse or clinically relevant interaction normally occurs between the oral antidiabetics and the NSAIDs cited. The general silence in the literature would seem to add confirmation, but some caution may be prudent with fenclofenac and indobufen. Also, caution is appropriate with pioglitazone or rosiglitazone and patients should be monitored for signs of heart failure. Adverse interactions can certainly occur between antidiabetics and azapropazone, phenylbutazone, oxyphenbutazone and the salicylates, see 'Antidiabetics + NSAIDs; Phenylbutazone and related drugs', p.412 and 'Antidiabetics + Salicylates', p.415.

1. Shah SJ, Bhandarkar SD, Satoskar RS. Drug interaction between chlorpropamide and non-steroidal anti-inflammatory drugs, ibuprofen and phenylbutazone. *Int J Clin Pharmacol Ther Toxicol* (1984) 22, 470–2.
2. Allen PA, Taylor RT. Fenclofenac and thyroid function tests. *BMJ* (1980) 281, 1642.
3. Beeley L, Beadle F, Elliott D. *Bulletin of the West Midlands Centre for Adverse Drug Reaction Reporting* (1985) 21, 19.
4. Kubacka RT, Antal EJ, Juhl RP, Welshman IR, Effects of aspirin and ibuprofen on the pharmacokinetics and pharmacodynamics of glyburide in healthy subjects. *Ann Pharmacother* (1996) 30, 20–26.
5. Sone H, Takahashi A, Yamada N. Ibuprofen-related hypoglycemia in a patient receiving sulfonylurea. *Ann Intern Med* (2001) 134, 344.
6. Haupt E, Hoppe FK, Rechziegler H, Zündorf P. Zur Frage der Interaktionen von nichtsteroidalen Antirheumatika mit oralen Antidiabetika: Acemetacin-Glibenclamid. *Z Rheumatology* (1987) 46, 170–3.
7. Boni JP, Cevallos WH, DeCleene S, Korth-Bradley JM. The influence of bromfenac on the pharmacokinetics and pharmacodynamic responses to glyburide in diabetic subjects. *Pharmacotherapy* (1997) 17, 783–90.
8. Chlud K. Untersuchungen zur Wechselwirkung von Diclofenac und Glibenclamid. *Z Rheumatol* (1976) 35, 377–82.
9. Girardin E, Vial T, Pham E, Evreux J-C. Hypoglycémies induites par les sulfamides hypoglycémiants. *Ann Med Interne (Paris)* (1992) 143, 11–17.
10. Collin M, Mucklow JC. Drug interactions, renal impairment and hypoglycaemia in a patient with type II diabetes. *Br J Clin Pharmacol* (1999) 48, 134–7.
11. Diwan PV, Sastry MSP, Satyanarayana NV. Potentiation of hypoglycemic response of glibenclamide by piroxicam in rats and humans. *Indian J Exp Biol* (1992) 30, 317–9.
12. Hartmann D, Korn A, Komjati M, Heinz G, Haefelfinger P, Defoin R, Waldhäusl WK. Lack of effect of tenoxicam on dynamic responses to concurrent oral doses of glucose and glibenclamide. *Br J Clin Pharmacol* (1990) 30, 245–52.
13. Chlud K, Kaik B. Clinical studies of the interaction between tolmetin and glibenclamide. *Int J Clin Pharmacol Biopharm* (1977) 15, 409–10.
14. Dynastat injection (Parecoxib sodium). Pharmacia Ltd. UK Summary of product characteristics, April 2004.
15. Bextra (Valdecoxib). Pharmacia Ltd. UK Summary of product characteristics, May 2004.
16. Haupt E, Hoppe FU, Bamberg E. Zur frage der Wecheslwirkugen von Analgetika und oralen Antidiabetika — Metamizol-Glibenclamid. *Med Welt* (1989) 40, 681–3.
17. Zvaifler N. A review of the antiarthritic efficacy and safety of etodolac. *Clin Rheumatol* (1989) 8 (Suppl 1), 43–53.
18. Ravic M, Johnston A, Turner P. Clinical pharmacological studies of some possible interactions of lornoxicam with other drugs. *Postgrad Med J* (1990) 66 (Suppl 4), S30–S34.
19. Perucca E. Drug interactions with nimesulide. *Drugs* (1993) 46 (Suppl 1), 79–82.
20. Stoeckel K, Trueb V, Dubach UC, Heintz RC, Ascalone V, Forgo I, Hennes U. Lack of effect of tenoxicam on glibornuride kinetics and response. *Br J Clin Pharmacol* (1985) 19, 249–54.
21. Elvander-Ståhl E, Melander A, Wåhlin-Boll E. Indobufen interacts with the sulphonylurea, glipizide, but not with the β-adrenergic receptor antagonists, propranolol and atenolol. *Br J Clin Pharmacol* (1984) 18, 773–8.
22. Pedrazzi F, Bommartini F, Freddo J, Emanueli A. A study of the possible interaction of indoprofen with hypoglycemic sulfonylureas in diabetic patients. *Eur J Rheumatol Inflamm* (1981) 4, 26–31.
23. Melander A, Wåhlin-Boll E. Interaction of glipizide and indoprofen. *Eur J Rheumatol Inflamm* (1981) 4, 22–5.
24. Anderson DM, Shelley S, Crick N, Buraglio M. A 3-way crossover study to evaluate the pharmacokinetic interaction between nateglinide and diclofenac in healthy volunteers. *Int J Clin Pharmacol Ther* (2002) 40, 457–64.
25. Actos (Pioglitazone hydrochloride). Takeda UK Ltd. UK Summary of product characteristics, February 2005.
26. Avandia (Rosiglitazone maleate). GlaxoSmithKline UK. UK Summary of product characteristics, January 2005.
27. McMahon FG, Ryan JR. Unpublished observations quoted in Tempero KF, Cirillo VJ, Steelman SL. Diflunisal: a review of the pharmacokinetic and pharmacodynamic properties, drug interactions, and special tolerability studies in humans. *Br J Clin Pharmacol* (1977) 4, 31S–36S.
28. Ryan JR, Jain AK, McMahon FG, Vargas R. On the question of an interaction between sulindac and tolbutamide in the control of diabetes. *Clin Pharmacol Ther* (1977) 21, 231–3.
29. Whiting B, Williams RL, Lorenzi M, Varady JC, Robins DS. Effect of naproxen on glucose metabolism and tolbutamide kinetics and dynamics in maturity onset diabetics. *Br J Clin Pharmacol* (1981) 11, 295–302.

30. Day RO, Geisslinger G, Paull P, Williams KM. The effect of tenoxicam on tolbutamide pharmacokinetics and glucose concentrations in healthy volunteers. *Int J Clin Pharmacol Ther* (1995) 33, 308–10.
31. Andersen LA. Ibuprofen and tolbutamide drug interaction study. *Br J Clin Pract* (1980) 34 (Suppl 6), 10–12.

Antidiabetics + NSAIDs; Phenylbutazone and related drugs

The hypoglycaemic effects of acetohexamide, chlorpropamide, carbutamide, glymidine, glibenclamide (glyburide) and tolbutamide can be increased by phenylbutazone. Severe hypoglycaemia has occurred in a few patients. Similarly, azapropazone can increase the effects of tolbutamide and cause severe hypoglycaemia. Oxyphenbutazone may be expected to behave similarly but not mofebutazone.

Clinical evidence

(a) Azapropazone

A woman whose diabetes was well controlled for 3 years with **tolbutamide** 500 mg twice daily, became confused and semi-comatose 4 days after starting to take azapropazone 900 mg daily. She complained of having felt agitated since starting the azapropazone, so it was withdrawn on suspicion of causing hypoglycaemia. Later that evening she became semi-comatose and was found to have a plasma glucose level of 2 mmol/l.[1] A subsequent study in 3 healthy subjects found that azapropazone 900 mg daily increased the plasma half-life of **tolbutamide** 500 mg threefold (from 7.7 to 25.2 hours) and reduced its clearance accordingly.[1] Acute hypoglycaemia occurred in another patient on **tolbutamide** 500 mg three times daily, 5.5 hours after a single 600-mg dose of azapropazone was taken.[2]

(b) Mofebutazone

Mofebutazone 900 mg daily has not been found to cause any clinically important changes in blood sugar control in patients on **glibenclamide**.[3]

(c) Oxyphenbutazone

Oxyphenbutazone has been found to alter[4] or raise **glymidine** levels[5] and **tolbutamide** levels.[6,7]

(d) Phenylbutazone

A man with type 2 diabetes taking **tolbutamide** experienced an acute hypoglycaemic episode 4 days after starting phenylbutazone 200 mg three times daily, although there was no change in his diet or in the dosage of **tolbutamide**. He was able to control the hypoglycaemia by eating a large bar of chocolate.[8]

There are numerous other case reports and studies of this interaction involving phenylbutazone with **acetohexamide**,[9] **carbutamide**,[10] **chlorpropamide**,[11-13] **glibenclamide (glyburide)**,[14] **glymidine**,[15] and **tolbutamide**,[12,16-22] some of which describe acute hypoglycaemic episodes.[9,11,12,17,19] Several of these interactions have been fatal.[12,22] There is a report suggesting that the interaction between **glibornuride** and phenylbutazone may not be clinically important.[23] In contrast to these reports, a single study describes a paradoxical rise in blood sugar levels in 3 African patients taking **tolbutamide** and phenylbutazone.[24] In addition to these reports there is some evidence that **tolbutamide** increases the metabolism of phenylbutazone by 42%,[21] but the extent to which this affects its therapeutic effects is uncertain.

Mechanism

Not fully resolved. Some evidence shows that phenylbutazone can inhibit the renal excretion of glibenclamide (glyburide),[14] tolbutamide,[18] and the active metabolite of acetohexamide[9] so that they are retained in the body longer and their hypoglycaemic effects are increased and prolonged. It has also been shown that phenylbutazone can inhibit the metabolism of the sulphonylureas[6,21] as well as causing their displacement from protein binding sites.[25] Azapropazone also possibly inhibits the metabolism of tolbutamide,[1] as well as maybe causing displacement from plasma protein binding sites.[2]

Importance and management

The interactions between the antidiabetics and phenylbutazone are well documented and potentially clinically important. Blood sugar levels may be lowered, but the number of reports of acute hypoglycaemic episodes seems to be small. Concurrent use should therefore be well monitored. A reduction in the dosage of the sulphonylurea may be necessary if excessive hypoglycaemia is to be avoided. Not all sulphonylureas have been shown to interact (glibornuride probably does not do so) but it would be prudent to assume that they all interact until there is good evidence to suggest otherwise. Oxyphenbutazone may be expected to interact similarly (it is a metabolite of phenylbutazone) but, unexpectedly, not mofebutazone.

The cases cited and the associated clinical study appear to be all that is on record about the interaction between tolbutamide and azapropazone and information about other sulphonylureas seems to be lacking, but the makers of azapropazone say that the concurrent use of sulphonylureas is not recommended.[26]

1. Andreasen PB, Simonsen K, Brocks K, Dimo B, Bouchelouche P. Hypoglycaemia induced by azapropazone-tolbutamide interaction. *Br J Clin Pharmacol* (1981) 12, 581–3.
2. Waller DG, Waller D. Hypoglycaemia due to azapropazone-tolbutamide interaction. *Br J Rheumatol* (1984) 23, 24–5.
3. Speders S. Mofebutazon — Prufung einer moglichen Interaktion mit Glibenclamid. *Fortschr Med* (1993) 111, 366–8.
4. Held H, Scheible G. Interaktion von Phenylbutazon und Oxyphenbutazon mit glymidine. *Arzneimittelforschung* (1981) 31, 1036–8.
5. Held H, Scheible G, von Olderhausen HF. Über Stoffwechsel und Interferenz von Arzneimitteln bei Gesunden und Leberkranken. *Tag Deut Ges Inn Med (Wiesbaden)* (1970) 76, 1153–7.
6. Pond SM, Birkett DJ, Wade DN. Mechanisms of inhibition of tolbutamide metabolism: Phenylbutazone, oxyphenbutazone, sulfaphenazole. *Clin Pharmacol Ther* (1977) 22, 573–9.
7. Kristensen M, Christensen LK. Drug induced changes of the blood glucose lowering effect of oral hypoglycaemic agents. *Acta Diabetol Lat* (1969) 6 (Suppl 1), 116–36.
8. Mahfouz M, Abdel-Maguid R, El-Dakhakhny M. Potentiation of the hypoglycaemic action of tolbutamide by different drugs. *Arzneimittelforschung* (1970) 20, 120–2.
9. Field JB, Ohta M, Boyle C, Remer A. Potentiation of acetohexamide hypoglycemia by phenylbutazone. *N Engl J Med* (1967) 277, 889–94.
10. Kaindl F, Kretschy A, Puxkandl H, Wutte J. Zur steigerung des Wirkundseffektes peroraler Antidiabetika durch Pyrazolonderivate. *Wien Klin Wochenschr* (1961) 73, 79–80.
11. Dalgas M, Christiansen I, Kjerulf K. Fenylbutazoninduceret hypoglykaemitilfaelde hos klorpropamidbehandlet diabetiker. *Ugeskr Laeger* (1965) 127, 834–6.
12. Schulz E. Schwere hypoglykämische Reaktionen nach den Sulfonylharnstoffen Tolbutamid, Carbutamid und Chlorpropamid. *Arch Klin Med* (1968) 214, 135–62.
13. Shah SJ, Bhandarkar SD, Satoskar RS. Drug interaction between chlorpropamide and non-steroidal anti-inflammatory drugs, ibuprofen and phenylbutazone. *Int J Clin Pharmacol Ther Toxicol* (1984) 22, 470–2.
14. Schulz E, Koch K, Schmidt FH. Ursachen der Potenzierung der hypoglykämischen Wirkung von Sulfonylharnstoff-derivaten durch Medikamente. II. Pharmakokinetik und Metabolismus von Glibenclamid (HN 419) in Gegenwart von Phenylbutazon. *Eur J Clin Pharmacol* (1971) 4, 32–7.
15. Held H, Kaminski B, von Olderhausen HF. Die beeinflussung der Elimination von Glycodiazin durch Leber-und Nierenfunktionsstorugen und durch eine Behandlung mit Phenylbutazon, Phenprocumarol und Doxycyclin. *Diabetologia* (1970) 6, 386–91.
16. Gulbrandsen R. Økt tolbutamid-effekt ved hjelp av fenylbutazon? *Tidsskr Nor Laegeforen* (1959) 79, 1127–8.
17. Tannenbaum H, Anderson LG, Soeldner JS. Phenylbutazone-tolbutamide drug interaction. *N Engl J Med* (1974) 290, 344.
18. Ober K-F. Mechanism of interaction of tolbutamide and phenylbutazone in diabetic patients. *Eur J Clin Pharmacol* (1974) 7, 291–4.
19. Dent LA, Jue SG. Tolbutamide-phenylbutazone interaction. *Drug Intell Clin Pharm* (1976) 10, 711.
20. Christensen LK, Hansen JM, Kristensen M. Sulphaphenazole-induced hypoglycaemic attacks in tolbutamide-treated diabetics. *Lancet* (1963) ii, 1298–1301.
21. Szita M, Gachályi B, Tornyossy M, Káldor A. Interaction of phenylbutazone and tolbutamide in man. *Int J Clin Pharmacol Ther Toxicol* (1990) 18, 378–80.
22. Slade IH, Iosefa RN. Fatal hypoglycemic coma from the use of tolbutamide in elderly patients: report of two cases. *J Am Geriatr Soc* (1967) 15, 948–50.
23. Eckhardt W, Rudolph R, Sauer H, Schubert WR, Undeutsch D. Zur pharmackologischen Interferenz von Glibornurid mit Sulfaphenazol, Phenylbutazon und Phenprocoumon beim Menschen. *Arzneimittelforschung* (1972) 22, 2212–19.
24. Owusu SK, Ocran K. Paradoxical behaviour of phenylbutazone in African diabetics. *Lancet* (1972) i, 440–41.
25. Hellman B. Potentiating effects of drugs on the binding of glibenclamide to pancreatic beta cells. *Metabolism* (1974) 23, 839–46.
26. Rheumox (Azapropazone dihydrate). Goldshield Pharmaceuticals Ltd. UK Summary of product characteristics, February 2000.

Antidiabetics + Octreotide

Octreotide has a hypoglycaemic effect so that the dosage of insulin used by diabetics can be reduced. It appears to have no benefits in those with intact insulin reserves (type 2 diabetes).

Clinical evidence

(a) Insulin

When 7 patients with type 1 diabetes with poor metabolic control were given octreotide 50 micrograms subcutaneously three times daily (at 8, 15 and 23 hours) or by continuous subcutaneous infusion, their blood glucose levels were about 50% lower than with **insulin** alone. The effects on blood glucose levels of the two modes of administration of octreotide were virtually the same.[1] Another study in 6 patients with type 1 diabetes also found that octreotide 50 micrograms before meals reduced their daily **insulin** requirements by about 50%,[2] and other studies confirm that octreotide behaves in this way.[3,4]

Eight obese type 2 diabetic patients whose diabetes was not controlled with oral antidiabetics and who needed **insulin** treatment, had no significant increases in blood glucose levels following a meal when they were given octreotide 25 micrograms.[5]

(b) Oral antidiabetics

Octreotide appears not to have a clinically relevant beneficial or harmful effect on the hypoglycaemic effects of oral antidiabetics such as **glibenclamide (glyburide)** in patients with type 2 diabetes, although some metabolic changes can occur.[6,7]

Mechanism

Octreotide is an analogue of the natural hormone somatostatin, and similarly acts as a hypoglycaemic because it inhibits the actions of glucagon and growth hormone (which raise blood glucose levels), and because it also delays the absorption of carbohydrate from the gut. However, somatostatin is also diabetogenic, because it suppresses insulin release. In type 1 diabetes, because there is no endogenous insulin, the hypoglycaemic effects predominate. In non-diabetics and type 2 diabetes, the actions may cancel out, or there may be poorer glycaemic control. Octreotide is thought to cause less suppression of insulin release than somatostatin, but this may still be important in those with insulin-secreting reserves.

Importance and management

The interaction between insulin and octreotide is established. There seem to be no reports of marked hypoglycaemia during concurrent use, but if both drugs are used, anticipate the need to reduce the insulin dosage. The studies cited above[1,2] suggest that about a 50% reduction is possible.

The makers of octreotide say that octreotide may also reduce the requirements of oral antidiabetics in patients with type 1 diabetes mellitus. However, there do not appear to be any studies on this. Conversely, they state that in patients with type 2 diabetes, octreotide may result in prandial *increases* in glycaemia,[8] but two clinical studies in patients with type 2 diabetes given glibenclamide (glyburide) did not show any deterioration (or benefit) in glycaemia.[6,7] While it would certainly be prudent to monitor the effects of giving octreotide with any of the oral hypoglycaemic agents, what is known so far suggests that no clinically relevant interaction is likely.

1. Di Mauro M, Le Moli R, Nicoletti F, Lunetta M. Effects of octreotide on the glycemic levels in insulin-dependent diabetic patients. Comparative study between administration through multiple subcutaneous injections and continuous subcutaneous infusion. *Diabetologia* (1993) 36 (Suppl 1), A138.
2. Rios MS, Navascues I, Saban J, Ordoñez A, Sevilla F, Del Pozo E. Somatostatin analog SMS 201–995 and insulin needs in insulin-dependent diabetic patients studied by means of an artificial pancreas. *J Clin Endocrinol Metab* (1986) 63, 1071–4.
3. Candrina R, Giustina G. Effect of a new long-acting somatostatin analogue (SMS 201–995) on glycemic and hormonal profiles in insulin-treated type II diabetic patients. *J Endocrinol Invest* (1988) 11, 501–7.
4. Hadjidakis DJ, Halvatsiotis PG, Ioannou YJ, Mavrokefalos PJ, Raptis SA. The effects of the somatostatin analogue SMS 201–995 on carbohydrate homeostasis of insulin-dependent diabetics as assessed by the artificial endocrine pancreas. *Diabetes Res Clin Pract* (1988) 5, 91–8.
5. Giustina A, Girelli A, Buffoli MG, Cimino A, Legati F, Valentini U, Giustina G. Low-dose octreotide is able to cause a maximal inhibition of the glycemic responses to a mixed meal in obese type 2 diabetic patients treated with insulin. *Diabetes Res Clin Pract* (1991) 14, 47–54.
6. Davies RR, Miller M, Turner SJ, Watson M, McGill A, Ørskov H, Alberti KGMM, Johnston DG. Effects of somatostatin analogue SMS 201–995 in non-insulin-dependent diabetes. *Clin Endocrinol (Oxf)* (1986) 25, 739–47.
7. Williams G, Füessl HS, Burrin JM, Chilvers E, Bloom SR. Postprandial glycaemic effects of a long-acting somatostatin analogue (octreotide) in non-insulin dependent diabetes mellitus. *Horm Metab Res* (1988) 20, 168–170.
8. Sandostatin (Octreotide). Novartis Pharmaceuticals UK Ltd. UK Summary of product characteristics, March 2004.

Antidiabetics + Orlistat

The concurrent use of either biguanides or sulphonylureas with orlistat seems safe and effective. The makers recommend avoiding the concurrent use of acarbose and orlistat.

Clinical evidence, mechanism, importance and management

(a) Acarbose

The makers of orlistat say that in the absence of pharmacokinetic studies the concurrent use with acarbose is not recommended.[1]

(b) Metformin

In a randomised study, 21 healthy subjects were given metformin 500 mg daily for 6 days, with or without orlistat 120 mg three times daily. Orlistat had no effect on the pharmacokinetics of metformin, and the combination was well-tolerated.[2]

(c) Sulphonylureas

A placebo-controlled study in 12 healthy subjects found that orlistat 80 mg three times daily for a little over 4 days had no effect on the pharmacokinetics of a single 5-mg oral dose of **glibenclamide (glyburide)** and the blood glucose lowering effects remained unchanged.[3] A later large scale 1-year clinical trial in which 139 patients took orlistat found that 43% of the obese patients with type 2 diabetes taking orlistat 120 mg three times daily were able to decrease their sulphonylurea dosage (**glibenclamide** or **glipizide**), and 11.7% of them were able to discontinue the sulphonylurea. The average dose decrease was 23% compared with 9% in the placebo group.[4] Clearly concurrent use can be advantageous.

1. Xenical (Orlistat). Roche Products Ltd. UK Summary of product characteristics, June 2005.
2. Zhi J, Moore R, Kanitra L, Mulligan TE. Pharmacokinetic evaluation of the possible interaction between selected concomitant medications and orlistat at steady state in healthy subjects. *J Clin Pharmacol* (2002) 42, 1011–19.
3. Zhi J, Melia AT, Koss-Twardy SG, Min B, Guerciolini R, Freundlich NL, Milla G, Patel IH. The influence of orlistat on the pharmacokinetics and pharmacodynamics of glyburide in healthy volunteers. *J Clin Pharmacol* (1995) 35, 521–5.
4. Hollander PA, Elbein SC, Hirsch IB, Kelley D, McGill J, Taylor T, Weiss SR, Crockett SE, Kaplan RA, Comstock J, Lucas CP, Lodewick PA, Canovatchel W, Chung J, Hauptman J. Role of orlistat in the treatment of obese patients with type 2 diabetes. A 1-year randomized double-blind study. *Diabetes Care* (1998) 21, 1288–94.

Antidiabetics + Phenylephrine

Insulin-dependent diabetics can develop elevated blood pressures if treated with phenylephrine eye-drops.

Clinical evidence, mechanism, importance and management

A comparative study of 14 **insulin**-dependent diabetics who over a period of 2 hours before ocular surgery were given phenylephrine 10% eye drops (a total of 4 doses of one or two drops), found that they had an average blood pressure rise of 34/17 mmHg, whereas another 176 non-diabetic patients similarly treated had no increases in blood pressure.[1] The reason for this pressor reaction is not understood but it would seem that enough phenylephrine is absorbed systemically to stimulate the adrenoceptors of the sympathetic system, which innervates the cardiovascular system. The concentration of phenylephrine in the plasma is a balance between the amount absorbed and rate at which it is then inactivated. The inactivation in diabetics can be reduced (due to sympathetic denervation) so that their phenylephrine levels may rise higher than they would in normal subjects. The authors of this report say that they readily controlled these hypertensive reactions with halothane and by neuroleptanalgesia accompanying regional block with anaesthesia standby. Strictly speaking this is not a drug interaction, but a drug-disease reaction. The mydriatic dosage of phenylephrine should be reduced in **insulin**-dependent diabetics but whether this is also true for non insulin-dependent diabetics is uncertain.

1. Kim JM, Stevenson CE and Mathewson HS. Hypertensive reactions to phenylephrine eyedrops in patients with sympathetic denervation. *Am J Ophthalmol* (1978) 85, 862–8.

Antidiabetics + Quinolones

Ciprofloxacin does not interact to a clinically relevant extent with glibenclamide (glyburide), but there are two isolated reports of severe hypoglycaemia in elderly patients. There is one report of severe hypoglycaemia in three elderly patients treated with gatifloxacin and either glibenclamide plus pioglitazone, glimepiride, or repaglinide. Levofloxacin appears not to interact with glibenclamide.

Clinical evidence, mechanism, importance and management

(a) Ciprofloxacin

A study in 12 patients with type 2 diabetes mellitus taking **glibenclamide (glyburide)** 10 mg in the morning, plus in some instances 5 mg in the evening, found that ciprofloxacin 1 g daily for a week caused rises in maximum serum **glibenclamide** levels of 20 to 30%, and a rise in the AUC of 25 to 36%. However, none of these changes were statistically significant, and more importantly blood glucose levels were not altered.[1]

However an elderly patient on **glibenclamide** 5 mg daily for over 2 years was found to be confused, with slurred speech and diaphoresis within a week of starting ciprofloxacin 250 mg twice daily, and was found to have serum **glibenclamide** level several times greater than that those normally seen.[2] She needed treatment with intravenous glucose to correct the hypoglycaemia. A further similar case in another elderly patient has been reported.[3]

(b) Gatifloxacin

In a study in patients with type 2 diabetics controlled by diet and exercise, gatifloxacin 400 mg daily for 10 days had no significant effect on glucose tolerance or most aspects of glucose homoeostasis, but did cause a brief increase in serum insulin levels.[4] In contrast, there is a report of 3 cases of hypoglycaemia in elderly type 2 diabetic patients given gatifloxacin. In one case, a patient on **glibenclamide** 5 mg daily and **pioglitazone** 30 mg daily experienced severe, persistent hypoglycaemia within an hour of the first dose of gatifloxacin 200 mg. It resolved on withdrawal of all three drugs and she had no further episodes of hypoglycaemia when **glibenclamide** and **pioglitazone** were restarted.[5] Another patient on **glimepiride** 2 mg before breakfast and 1 mg before dinner developed severe hypoglycaemia 12 hours after the first dose of intravenous gatifloxacin 400 mg. Both drugs were discontinued and **glimepiride** was later restarted without further hypoglycaemia.[5] A third patient on **repaglinide** 500 micrograms every 8 hours was additionally given gatifloxacin 400 mg daily for a urinary-tract infection. **Repaglinide** was discontinued 6 hours after the first dose of gatifloxacin because of the patient's lack of appetite. Two hours after the second dose of gatifloxacin, he had severe hypoglycaemia and also experienced a tonic-clonic seizure. Gatifloxacin was discontinued but hypoglycaemia persisted for 32 hours. **Repaglinide** therapy was restarted 4 days later without further hypoglycaemia.[5]

(c) Levofloxacin

A study in 24 healthy subjects found that levofloxacin had no effect on the pharmacokinetics of **glibenclamide** nor its effect on plasma glucose levels.[6]

Mechanism

Unknown. The authors of one report suggest that the ciprofloxacin may have inhibited the metabolism of the glibenclamide, thereby raising its serum levels.[2] This may possibly be exaggerated in elderly patients whose liver function may be reduced. The authors of the report with gatifloxacin attribute the hypoglycaemia to a direct effect of gatifloxacin on oral antidiabetics, and suggest it is not a quinolone class effect.[5]

Importance and management

The concurrent use of glibenclamide and ciprofloxacin need not be avoided, but when ciprofloxacin is first started it might be prudent to warn patients to be alert for any problems. It has been suggested that levofloxacin and ofloxacin should be considered as possible alternatives in elderly patients because they are minimally involved in liver metabolism.[2] Although there is only one report, the severity of the hypoglycaemia seen in the 3 patients treated with gatifloxacin and various antidiabetics suggests that caution is warranted when gatifloxacin is used in diabetics.

1. Ludwig E, Szekely E, Graber H, Csiba A. Study of interaction between oral ciprofloxacin and glibenclamide. *Eur J Clin Microbiol Infect Dis* (1991) 10 (Special issue) 378–9.
2. Roberge RJ, Kaplan R, Frank R, Fore C. Glyburide-ciprofloxacin interaction with resistant hypoglycaemia. *Ann Emerg Med* (2000) 36, 160–3.
3. Whitely MS, Worldling J, Patel S, Gibbs KB. Hypoglycaemia in a diabetic patient, associated with ciprofloxacin therapy. *Pract Diabetes* (1993) 10, 35.
4. Gajjar DA, LaCreta FP, Kollia GD, Stolz RR, Berger S, Smith WB, Swingle M, Grasela DM. Effect of multiple-dose gatifloxacin or ciprofloxacin on glucose homeostasis and insulin production in patients with noninsulin-dependent diabetes mellitus maintained with diet and exercise. *Pharmacotherapy* (2000) 20, 76S–86S.
5. Menzies DJ, Dorsainvil PA, Cunha BA, Johnson DH. Severe and persistent hypoglycemia due to gatifloxacin interaction with oral hypoglycaemic agents. *Am J Med* (2002) 113, 232–4.
6. Hoechst Marion Roussel, Personal Communication, March 1999.

Antidiabetics + Rifamycins

Rifampicin (rifampin) reduces the serum levels and blood-glucose lowering effects of tolbutamide, glymidine, gliclazide, chlorpropamide (single case) and glibenclamide (glyburide), and to a lesser extent glimepiride and glipizide.

Clinical evidence

(a) Chlorpropamide

A single case report describes a man with type 2 diabetes who needed an increase in his daily dosage of chlorpropamide from 250 to 400 mg daily when he was given **rifampicin** 600 mg daily. His serum chlorpropamide levels rose dramatically 12 months later when the **rifampicin** was withdrawn.[1]

(b) Glibenclamide (Glyburide)

A study in 29 type 2 diabetics, well-controlled on glibenclamide, found that when they were also given **rifampicin** 450 or 600 mg daily for 10 days, their blood sugar levels both fasting and after meals were raised. Glibenclamide dosage changes were needed in 15 out of 17 patients in whom the diabetes became uncontrolled. Their blood sugar levels normalised 6 days after stopping the **rifampicin**.[2] Another patient with type 2 diabetes had a marked rise in trough serum glibenclamide levels, from 40 to 200 nanograms/ml, when **rifampicin** was stopped, but no hypoglycaemia occurred.[3] A study in 10 healthy subjects found that treatment with **rifampicin** 600 mg daily for 5 days decreased the AUC and peak plasma level of a single 1.75-mg dose of glibenclamide given on day 6 by 39% and 22% respectively. The elimination half-life was shortened from 2 to 1.7 hours. The blood glucose decremental AUC and maximum reduction in blood glucose level were decreased by 44% and 36% respectively by **rifampicin**.[4]

(c) Gliclazide

A 65-year-old patient with type 2 diabetes treated by diet and gliclazide 80 mg daily for 2 years without problem was given **rifampicin** 450 mg daily, isoniazid, ethambutol and clarithromycin for an atypical mycobacteriosis. Fasting blood glucose levels became elevated requiring an increase in the dose of gliclazide to 120 mg then 160 mg daily. The plasma level of gliclazide on day 75 was 1.4 micrograms/ml, 2 hours after an 80-mg dose. When **rifampicin** was discontinued the gliclazide level increased to 4.7 micrograms/ml and the dose was reduced back to 80 mg daily.[5] A study in 9 healthy subjects found that treatment with **rifampicin** 600 mg for 6 days decreased the AUC of a single 80-mg dose of gliclazide given on day 7 by 70%, decreased the mean elimination half-life from 9.5 to 3.3 hours and increased the gliclazide oral clearance by about fourfold. The blood-glucose lowering effects of gliclazide were significantly reduced by **rifampicin**.[6]

(d) Glimepiride

A placebo-controlled study in 10 healthy subjects found that **rifampicin** 600 mg daily for 5 days decreased the AUC of a single 1-mg dose of glimepiride given on day 6 by 34%. **Rifampicin** reduced the elimination half-life of glimepiride by 25%. However, no significant differences in blood glucose were found between the **rifampicin** and placebo regimens.[7]

(e) Glipizide

A placebo-controlled study in 10 healthy subjects found **rifampicin** 600 mg daily for 5 days decreased the AUC of a single 2.5-mg dose of glipizide given on day 6 by 22%. The elimination half life was shortened from 3 to 1.9 hours by **rifampicin**. However, no significant differences in blood glucose concentrations were found.[4]

(f) Glymidine

In one study the half-life of glymidine was reduced by about one-third by the concurrent use of **rifampicin**.[8]

(g) Nateglinide

In a randomised crossover study, 10 healthy subjects were given a single 60-mg dose of nateglinide the day after a 5-day course of **rifampicin** 600 mg daily. **Rifampicin** reduced the 7-hour AUC of nateglinide by 24% (range 5 to 53%) and decreased the nateglinide half life from 1.6 to 1.3 hours. **Rifampicin** did not potentiate the hypoglycaemic effects of nateglinide.[9] However, because of the high degree of inter-subject variation, the authors suggest that the hypoglycaemic effects of nateglinide may be reduced in some subjects.[9]

(h) Repaglinide

In one study, **rifampicin** 600 mg daily for 7 days decreased the AUC of a single 4-mg dose of repaglinide by 31% and the mean maximum plasma concentration by 26% in healthy subjects.[10] Similarly, in another study,[11] pretreatment with **rifampicin** 600 mg daily for 5 days increased the AUC and maximum level of a single 500-microgram dose of repaglinide by 57% and 41% respectively. In this study, **rifampicin** reduced the blood glucose-lowering effect of repaglinide by 35%.

(i) Tolbutamide

After 4 weeks' treatment with **rifampicin** the half-life of tolbutamide in 9 diabetic patients with tuberculosis was reduced by 43%, and the serum concentrations measured at 6 hours were halved compared with other patients not taking **rifampicin.**[12] Similar results have been found in other studies in patients with cirrhosis or cholestasis,[13] in healthy subjects[14] and in other patients.[15]

Mechanism

Rifampicin is a potent inducer of the liver microsomal enzymes concerned with the metabolism of tolbutamide (cytochrome P450 isoenzyme CYP2C9), which hastens its clearance from the body, thereby reducing its effects.[12-14] The interaction between rifampicin and glibenclamide, glimepiride, glipizide, nateglinide and repaglinide is probably also due to induction of CYP2C9.[4-6,11] Induction of P-glycoprotein may also play a part.[4,6]

Importance and management

Information is limited, but the interactions of tolbutamide, glibenclamide (glyburide) and gliclazide with rifampicin appear to be established. Patients taking these sulphonylureas may need an increase in the dosage while taking rifampicin (possibly roughly doubled, but this needs confirmation). This also seems possibly true for glymidine and chlorpropamide, but the documentation about these two drugs is even more limited. The effect of rifampicin on the hypoglycaemic effects of glimepiride or glipizide may be of only limited clinical significance, but it should be noted that these were single-dose studies and it is possible that some effect may occur with multiple dosing. Caution is warranted. Similarly although the information regarding nateglinide and repaglinide is limited a significant interaction is possible, especially with repaglinide, and so an increase in blood glucose monitoring is warranted.

There does not seem to be any information regarding the other rifamycins, **rifabutin** (a weak enzyme inducer) and **rifapentine** (a moderate enzyme inducer). However, the makers and the UK Committee on Safety of Medicines warn that rifabutin may possibly reduce the effects of a number of drugs, including oral hypoglycaemics.[16,17]

1. Self TH, Morris T. Interaction of rifampin and chlorpropamide. *Chest* (1980) 77, 800–801.
2. Surekha V, Peter JV, Jeyaseelan L, Cherian AM. Drug interaction: rifampicin and glibenclamide. *Natl Med J India* (1997) 10, 11–12.
3. Self TH, Tsiu SJ, Fowler JW. Interaction of rifampin and glyburide. *Chest* (1989) 96, 1443–4.
4. Niemi M, Backman JT, Neuvonen M, Neuvonen PJ, Kivistö KT. Effects of rifampin on the pharmacokinetics and pharmacodynamics of glyburide and glipizide. *Clin Pharmacol Ther* (2001) 69, 400–6.
5. Kihara Y, Otsuki M. Interaction of gliclazide and rifampicin. *Diabetes Care* (2000) 23, 1204–5.
6. Park J-Y, Kim K-A, Park P-W, Park C-W, Shin J-G. Effect of rifampin on the pharmacokinetics and pharmacodynamics of gliclazide. *Clin Pharmacol Ther* (2003) 74, 334–40.
7. Niemi M, Kivistö KT, Backman JT, Neuvonen PJ. Effect of rifampicin on the pharmacokinetics and pharmacodynamics of glimepiride. *Br J Clin Pharmacol* (2000) 50, 591–5.
8. Held H, Schoene B, Laar HJ, Fleischmann R. Die Aktivität der Benzpyrenhydroxylase im Leberpunktat des Menschen in vitro und ihre Beziehung zur Eliminations-geschwindigkeit von Glycodiazin in vivo. *Verh Dtsch Ges Inn Med* (1974) 80, 501–3.
9. Niemi M, Backman JT, Neuvonen M, Neuvonen PJ. Effect of rifampicin on the pharmacokinetics and pharmacodynamics of nateglinide in healthy subjects. *Br J Clin Pharmacol* (2003) 56, 427–32.
10. Hatorp V, Hansen KT, Thomsen MS. Influence of drugs interacting with CYP3A4 on the pharmacokinetics, pharmacodynamics, and safety of the prandial glucose regulator repaglinide. *J Clin Pharmacol* (2003) 43, 649–60.
11. Niemi M, Backman JT, Neuvonen M, Neuvonen PJ, Kivistö KT. Rifampin decreases the plasma concentrations and effects of repaglinide. *Clin Pharmacol Ther* (2000) 68, 495–500.
12. Syvälahti EKG, Pihlajamäki KK, Iisalo EJ. Rifampicin and drug metabolism. *Lancet* (1974) 2, 232–3.
13. Zilly W, Breimer DD, Richter E. Stimulation of drug metabolism by rifampicin in patients with cirrhosis or cholestasis measured by increased hexobarbital and tolbutamide clearance. *Eur J Clin Pharmacol* (1977) 11, 287–93.
14. Zilly W, Breimer DD, Richter E. Induction of drug metabolism in man after rifampicin treatment measured by increased hexobarbital and tolbutamide clearance. *Eur J Clin Pharmacol* (1975) 9, 219–27.
15. Syvälahti E, Pihlajamäki K, Iisalo E. Effect of tuberculostatic agents on the response of serum growth hormone and immunoreactive insulin to intravenous tolbutamide, and on the half-life of tolbutamide. *Int J Clin Pharmacol Biopharm* (1976) 13, 83–9.
16. Mycobutin (Rifabutin). Pharmacia Ltd. UK Summary of product characteristics, January 2003.
17. Committee on the Safety of Medicines/Medicines Control Agency. Revised indication and drug interactions of rifabutin. *Current Problems* (1997) 23, 14.

Antidiabetics + Salicylates

Aspirin and other salicylates can lower blood sugar levels, but small analgesic doses do not normally have an adverse effect on patients taking antidiabetics. Larger doses of salicylates may have a more significant effect, and caution is warranted.

Clinical evidence

(a) Insulin

Twelve children with type 1 diabetes treated with insulin had a reduction in blood glucose levels averaging 15% (from 188 to 159 mg%) when they were additionally given either **aspirin** (patients under 27.2 kg given 1.2 g daily, patients over 27.2 kg given 2.4 g daily) for a week. No significant changes in insulin requirements were necessary.[1]

Eight patients on 12 to 48 units of insulin zinc suspension daily required no insulin when they were treated for 2 to 3 weeks with **aspirin** in doses of 3.5 to 7.5 g daily, which were large enough to give maximum therapeutic serum salicylate levels of 35 to 45 mg/dl. Six other patients were able to reduce their insulin requirements by between about 20 and 65%.[2]

(b) Chlorpropamide

The blood glucose-lowering effects of chlorpropamide and **sodium salicylate** were found to be additive in 5 healthy subjects. A further study in 6 healthy subjects found that chlorpropamide 100 mg given with **sodium salicylate** 1.5 g lowered blood sugar levels the same amount as either chlorpropamide 200 mg or **sodium salicylate** 3 g alone.[3]

The blood glucose levels of a patient on chlorpropamide 500 mg daily were lowered about two-thirds by **aspirin** in doses sufficient to give serum salicylate levels of 26 mg%.[4]

(c) Glibenclamide (Glyburide)

Sixteen healthy subjects took a single 5-mg dose of glibenclamide both before and on the fourth day of treatment with **aspirin** 975 mg four times daily for 4 days. It was found that the **aspirin** reduced the 0 to 4-hour AUC of the glibenclamide by 68% and reduced its mean peak serum levels by 35%. The effects of this on glucose tolerance tests and insulin responses were difficult to interpret, but there was no clear evidence that any clinically relevant changes occurred.[5]

Mechanism

It has been known for over 100 years that aspirin and salicylates have hypoglycaemic properties and in relatively large doses can be used on their own in the treatment of diabetes.[6-10] The simplest explanation for this interaction with antidiabetics is that the blood sugar lowering effects are additive,[3] but there is some evidence that other mechanisms may come into play.[10] In addition aspirin can raise serum chlorpropamide levels so that its effects are increased, possibly by interfering with renal tubular excretion.[4]

Importance and management

The interaction between the antidiabetics and salicylates is established but of limited importance. Considering the extremely wide use of aspirin it might reasonably be expected that any generally serious interaction would have come to light by now. The data available, coupled with the common experience of diabetics,[11] is that excessive and unwanted hypoglycaemia is very unlikely with small to moderate analgesic doses. Some downward readjustment of the dosage of the antidiabetic may be appropriate if large doses of salicylates are used. Information about other antidiabetics and salicylates appears to be lacking, but they are expected to behave similarly.

1. Kaye R, Athreya BH, Kunzman EE, Baker L. Antipyretics in patients with juvenile diabetes mellitus. *Am J Dis Child* (1966) 112, 52–5.
2. Reid J, Lightbody TD. The insulin equivalence of salicylate. *BMJ* (1959) i, 897–900.
3. Richardson T, Foster J, Mawer GE. Enhancement by sodium salicylate of the blood glucose lowering effect of chlorpropamide - drug interaction or summation of similar effects? *Br J Clin Pharmacol* (1986) 22, 43–48.
4. Stowers JM, Constable LW, Hunter RB. A clinical and pharmacological comparison of chlorpropamide and other sulfonylureas. *Ann N Y Acad Sci* (1959) 74, 689–95.

5. Kubacka RT, Antal EJ, Juhl RP, Welshman IR. Effects of aspirin and ibuprofen on the pharmacokinetics and pharmacodynamics of glyburide in healthy subjects. *Ann Pharmacother* (1996) 30, 20–6.
6. Gilgore SG, Rupp JJ. The long-term response of diabetes mellitus to salicylate therapy. Report of a case. *JAMA* (1962) 180, 65–6.
7. Reid J, Macdougall AI, Andrews MM. Aspirin and diabetes mellitus. *BMJ* (1957) 2, 1071–4.
8. Ebstein W. Zur Therapie des Diabetes mellitus, insbesondere über die Anwendung des salicylsauren Natron bei demselben. Berl Klin Wschr (1876) 13, 337–40.
9. Bartels K. Ueber die therapeutische Verwerthung der Salizylsäure und ihres Nastronsalzes in der inneren Medicin. Dtsch Med Wschr (1878) 4, 423–5.
10. Cattaneo AG, Caviezel F, Pozza G. Pharmacological interaction between tolbutamide and acetylsalicylic acid: study on insulin secretion in man. *Int J Clin Pharmacol Ther Toxicol* (1990) 28, 229–34.
11. Logie AW, Galloway DB, Petrie JC. Drug interactions and long-term antidiabetic therapy. *Br J Clin Pharmacol* (1976) 3, 1027–32.

Antidiabetics + SSRIs

SSRIs normally appear not to interact with antidiabetics, but isolated cases of hypoglycaemia have been reported.

Clinical evidence

(a) Fluoxetine

Although one study found that single, or multiple doses of fluoxetine for 8 days, did not affect the pharmacokinetics or the hypoglycaemic effects of **tolbutamide**1 g,[1] the makers of fluoxetine say that hypoglycaemia has been seen in diabetic patients when fluoxetine was started, and hyperglycaemia when it was stopped.[2] An **insulin**-dependent diabetic experienced symptoms of hypoglycaemia (nausea, tremor, sweating, anxiety, lightheadedness) after starting to take fluoxetine 20 mg each night. The symptoms disappeared when the fluoxetine was stopped and reappeared when it was restarted. However, blood sugar levels were found to be normal (9 to 11 mmol/l).[3]

(b) Fluvoxamine

A study in 14 healthy subjects given fluvoxamine 75 or 150 mg daily for 5 days, with a single 500-mg dose of **tolbutamide** on the third day, found that the clearance of **tolbutamide** and its metabolites (4-hydroxytolbutamide and carboxytolbutamide) were significantly decreased.[4]

A randomised, double-blind cross-over study in 12 healthy subjects given fluvoxamine 100 mg or placebo daily for 4 days, with a single 500-microgram dose of **glimepiride** on the fourth day, found the AUC of **glimepiride** was not significantly affected by fluvoxamine. Peak plasma levels of glimepiride were increased by 43% and the elimination half life was prolonged from 2 to 2.3 hours, but there was no significant change in the effects of **glimepiride** on blood glucose concentrations.[5]

(c) Sertraline

After taking sertraline 200 mg daily for 22 days the clearance of a single intravenous dose of **tolbutamide** was decreased by 16% in 25 healthy subjects.[6] In another study in 11 healthy subjects the pharmacokinetics of a single 5-mg dose of **glibenclamide** were found to be unaffected by sertraline taken in increasing doses up to 200 mg daily over 15 days. Blood glucose levels were also unchanged.[7] However, there is a report of a patient with schizoaffective disorder and type 2 diabetes who developed hypoglycaemia during treatment with sertraline, risperidone and **glibenclamide**.[8]

Mechanism

Fluvoxamine probably decreased the clearance of tolbutamide by inhibition of its metabolism by the cytochrome P450 isoenzyme CYP2C9. This mechanism may also partly explain the increase in plasma levels of glimepiride. However, as glimepiride AUC was not increased and the half-life was only slightly increased, the increase in plasma levels may also be due to an increased rate of glimepiride absorption by the SSRI.[4,5] The effects of other SSRIs may also be associated with enzyme inhibition.[8]

Importance and management

There would seem to be little reason for avoiding concurrent use of fluoxetine, fluvoxamine or sertraline with sulphonylureas, but until more is known it would seem prudent to monitor diabetic control. The makers of fluoxetine, **paroxetine** and sertraline warn that dosages of insulin or oral antidiabetics may need adjustment during concurrent use.[2,9-11]

1. Lemberger L, Bergstrom RF, Wolen RL, Farid NA, Enas GG, Aronoff GR. Fluoxetine: clinical pharmacology and physiologic disposition. *J Clin Psychiatry* (1985) 46, 14–19.
2. Prozac (Fluoxetine). Eli Lilly and Company Ltd. UK Summary of product characteristics, September 2004.
3. Lear J, Burden AC. Fluoxetine side-effects mimicking hypoglycaemia. *Lancet* (1992) 339, 1296.
4. Madsen H, Enggard TP, Hansen LL, Klitgaard NA, Brøsen K. Fluvoxamine inhibits the CYP2C9 catalysed biotransformation of tolbutamide. *Clin Pharmacol Ther* (2001) 69, 41–7.
5. Niemi M, Backman JT, Neuvonen M, Laitila J, Neuvonen PJ, Kivistö KT. Effects of fluconazole and fluvoxamine on the pharmacokinetics of glimepiride. *Clin Pharmacol Ther* (2001) 69, 194–200.
6. Tremaine LM, Wilner KD, Preskorn SH. A study of the potential effect of sertraline on the pharmacokinetics and protein binding of tolbutamide. *Clin Pharmacokinet* (1997) 32 (Suppl 1), 31–6.
7. Invicta Pharmaceuticals. A double blind placebo controlled, multiple dose study to assess potential interaction between oral sertraline (200 mg) and glibenclamide (5 mg) in healthy male volunteers. Data on file (Study 223), 1991.
8. Takhar J, Williamson P. Hypoglycemia associated with high doses of sertraline and sulphonylurea compound in a noninsulin-dependent diabetes mellitus patient. *Can J Clin Pharmacol* (1999)6, 12–4.
9. Lustral (Sertraline). Pfizer Ltd. UK Summary of product characteristics, December 2003.
10. Seroxat (Paroxetine). GlaxoSmithKline UK. UK Summary of product characteristics, April 2005.
11. Prozac (Fluoxetine). Eli Lilly and Company. US Prescribing information, January 2005.

Antidiabetics + Statins

No clinically relevant adverse interactions appear to have been reported between the statins and the sulphonylureas, between repaglinide and simvastatin or between pioglitazone and atorvastatin or simvastatin.

Clinical evidence

(a) Chlorpropamide

A study in 7 patients with type 2 diabetes and hypercholesterolaemia taking chlorpropamide 125 to 750 mg daily found that **lovastatin** 20 mg twice daily for 6 weeks reduced low-density lipoprotein cholesterol by 28%, total cholesterol by 24% and apolipoprotein B by 24%. The chlorpropamide plasma levels were unchanged, and the diabetic control remained unaltered.[1]

(b) Glibenclamide (Glyburide)

Groups of 16 healthy subjects on **fluvastatin** 40 mg or **simvastatin** 20 mg daily were given single 3.5-mg oral doses of glibenclamide on days 1, 8 and 15. The maximum plasma concentration and the AUC of the glibenclamide were increased by about 20% by the statins. The hypoglycaemic actions of the glibenclamide remained virtually unchanged by both **fluvastatin** and **simvastatin** in these subjects, and also when **fluvastatin** was tested in a group of 32 patients with type 2 diabetes.[2]

(c) Repaglinide

A three-period cross-over open-label study in healthy subjects found that **simvastatin** 20 mg daily increased the maximum plasma level of repaglinide 2 mg three times daily by 26%, although there was high variability and the mean bioavailability of repaglinide was increased by 8%. There was a higher incidence of adverse effects during concurrent use.[3]

(d) Thiazolidinediones

In a study in healthy subjects **pioglitazone** 45 mg daily did not significantly affect the pharmacokinetics of **simvastatin** 80 mg daily and concurrent use was well-tolerated.[4] Similarly, there was no pharmacokinetic interaction between pioglitazone 45 mg daily and **atorvastatin** 80 mg daily.[5]

There is some evidence that patients on thiazolidinediones (95% troglitazone) were more likely to have hepatotoxicity if taking **atorvastatin** than **simvastatin**.[6] However, **troglitazone** has now been withdrawn due to its hepatotoxic effects and the general importance of this to the other thiazolidinediones is probably small.

(e) Tolbutamide

A single 1-g oral dose of tolbutamide was given 16 healthy subjects on **fluvastatin** 40 mg and 16 healthy subjects on **simvastatin** 20 mg. The pharmacokinetics of the tolbutamide were affected only to a very minor extent, and the hypoglycaemic effects of the tolbutamide were unchanged.[2]

Mechanism

The small changes in the pharmacokinetics of glibenclamide caused by fluvastatin and simvastatin are not understood, but they do not appear to be clinically significant.

Importance and management

No special precautions appear to be needed by diabetic patients taking any of the pairs of drugs cited here, although the clinical significance of the small interaction between repaglinide and simvastatin is unclear and so an element of caution would seem prudent. Information about other sulphonylurea hypoglycaemic agents and statins seems not to be available.

1. Johnson BF, LaBelle P, Wilson J, Allan J, Zupkis RV, Ronca PD. Effects of lovastatin in diabetic patients treated with chlorpropamide. *Clin Pharmacol Ther* (1990) 48, 467–72.
2. Appel S, Rüfenacht T, Kalafsky G, Tetzloff W, Kallay Z, Hitzenberger G, Kutz K. Lack of interaction between fluvastatin and oral hypoglycemic agents in healthy subjects and in patients with non-insulin-dependent diabetes mellitus. *Am J Cardiol* (1995) 76, 29A–32A.
3. Hatorp V, Hansen KT, Thomsen MS. Influence of drugs interacting with CYP3A4 on the pharmacokinetics, pharmacodynamics, and safety of the prandial glucose regulator repaglinide. *J Clin Pharmacol* (2003) 43, 649–60.
4. Prueksaritanont T, Vega JM, Zhao J, Gagliano K, Kuznetsova O, Musser B, Amin RD, Liu L, Roadcap BA, Dilzer S, Lasseter KC, Rogers JD. Interactions between simvastatin and troglitazone or pioglitazone in healthy subjects. *J Clin Pharmacol* (2001) 41, 573–81.
5. Karim A, Schwartz L, Perez A, Chao C. Lack of clinically significant interaction in coadministration of pioglitazone and atorvastatin calcium. *Diabetes* (2003) 52 (suppl 1) A449.
6. Alsheikh-Ali AA, Abourjaily HM, Karas RH. Risk of adverse events with concomitant use of atorvastatin or simvastatin and glucose-lowering drugs (thiazolidinediones, metformin, sulfonylurea, insulin, acarbose). *Am J Cardiol* (2002) 89, 1308–10.

Antidiabetics + Sucralfate

Sucralfate appears not to affect the pharmacokinetics of chlorpropamide or rosiglitazone.

Clinical evidence, mechanism, importance and management

(a) Chlorpropamide

A two-way crossover study in 12 healthy subjects found that sucralfate 1 g four times daily, given 1 hour before meals, had no significant effect on the pharmacokinetics of a single 250-mg dose of chlorpropamide.[1] No additional precautions would therefore seem to be necessary on concurrent use.

(b) Rosiglitazone

A single-dose study found that sucralfate 2 g taken 45 minutes before rosiglitazone 8 mg had no significant effect on the pharmacokinetics of rosiglitazone. No special precautions are needed during concurrent use.[2]

1. Letendre PW, Carlson JD, Siefert RD, Dietz AJ, Dimmit D. Effect of sucralfate on the absorption and pharmacokinetics of chlorpropamide. *J Clin Pharmacol* (1986) 26, 622–5.
2. Rao MNVS, Mullangi R, Katneni K, Ravikanth B, Babu AP, Rani UP, Naidu MUR, Srinivas NR, Rajagopalan R. Lack of effect of sucralfate on the absorption and pharmacokinetics of rosiglitazone. *J Clin Pharmacol* (2002) 42, 670–5.

Antidiabetics + Sugar-containing pharmaceuticals

Some pharmaceutical preparations may contain sufficient amounts of sugar to affect the control of diabetes. Diabetics should be warned and advised of sugar-free alternatives where appropriate.

Clinical evidence, mechanism, importance and management

Pharmaceuticals, especially liquid formulations, may contain sugar in significant amounts. The extent to which the administration of preparations like these will affect the control of diabetes clearly depends upon the amounts ingested, but the problem is by no means merely theoretical. One report describes the loss of control in a woman with type 1 diabetes controlled with insulin given psyllium effervescent powder (*Metamucil* instant-mix) which contains sugar.[1]

The range of other sugar-containing preparations is far too extensive to be listed here. Because of concerns over sugar-containing medicines and dental caries, in children in particular, the number of sugar-free preparations has grown considerably over recent years. In the UK the British National Formulary and MIMS provide guidance as to which preparations are sugar-free. Diabetics should be warned about sugar-containing medicines, and given guidance about the terminology used in labelling. Sweetening agents of note to diabetics include: **invert sugar** (dextrose and fructose), **invert syrup** (67% w/w invert sugar), **syrup BP** (66% w/w sucrose), **glucose liquid** (dextrose content 10 to 20%), **glucose syrup** (33.3% liquid glucose in syrup) and **honey** (70 to 80% glucose and fructose).[2]

1. Catellani J, Collins RJ. Drug labelling. *Lancet* (1978) ii, 98.
2. Greenwood J. Sugar content of liquid prescription medicines. *Pharm J* (1989) 243, 553–7.

Antidiabetics + Sulfinpyrazone

Sulfinpyrazone has no effect on the insulin requirements of diabetics, nor does it affect the control of patients taking glibenclamide (glyburide). Increased hypoglycaemia might occur if sulfinpyrazone is given with tolbutamide, but as yet there appear to be no case reports of this interaction, nor of any adverse interactions with other antidiabetics.

Clinical evidence

(a) Glibenclamide (Glyburide)

A study in 19 type 2 diabetics taking glibenclamide found that sulfinpyrazone 800 mg daily did not affect diabetic control.[1]

(b) Insulin

A double-blind study over 12 months in 41 adult diabetics found that sulfinpyrazone 600 to 800 mg daily had no clinically significant effects on insulin requirements.[2]

(c) Tolbutamide

A detailed study of the pharmacokinetics of tolbutamide in 6 healthy subjects found that sulfinpyrazone 200 mg every 6 hours for a week, almost doubled the half-life of a 500-mg intravenous dose of tolbutamide, from 7.3 to 13.2 hours, and reduced the plasma clearance by 40%.[3]

Mechanism

The available evidence suggests that sulfinpyrazone inhibits the metabolism of tolbutamide by the liver.[3]

Importance and management

Information about an interaction between tolbutamide and sulfinpyrazone appears to be limited to the report cited. So far there appear to be no reports of adverse interactions in patients, but what is known suggests that increased and possibly excessive hypoglycaemia could occur if the dosage of tolbutamide is not reduced. Such an interaction has been described with phenylbutazone with which sulfinpyrazone has a close structural similarity (see 'Antidiabetics + NSAIDs; Phenylbutazone and related drugs', p.412). Patients should be warned if sulfinpyrazone is added to established treatment with tolbutamide. There seems to be nothing documented about any other clinically important interactions between antidiabetics and sulfinpyrazone.

1. Kritz H, Najemnik C, Irsigler K. Interaktionsstudie mit Sulfinpyrazon (Anturan) und Glibenclamid (Euglucon) bei Typ-II-Diabetikern. *Wien Med Wochenschr* (1983) 133, 237–43.
2. Pannebakker MAG, den Ottolander GJH, ten Pas JG. Insulin requirements in diabetic patients treated with sulphinpyrazone. *J Int Med Res* (1979) 7, 328–31.
3. Miners JO, Foenander T, Wanwimolruk S, Gallus AS, Birkett DJ. The effect of sulphinpyrazone on oxidative drug metabolism in man: inhibition of tolbutamide elimination. *Eur J Clin Pharmacol* (1982) 22, 321–6.

Antidiabetics + Tetracyclines

A few scattered reports indicate that the hypoglycaemic effects of insulin and the sulphonylureas may sometimes be increased by oxytetracycline, and limited evidence suggests that this may also occur with doxycycline. Phenformin-induced lactic acidosis may be precipitated by tetracyclines.

Clinical evidence

(a) Insulin

A poorly controlled diabetic needed a marked reduction in his insulin dosage from 208 to 64 units daily in order to control the hypoglycaemia that developed when **oxytetracycline** 250 mg four times daily was given. This reaction was also seen when the patient was given a second course of antibacterials, and in another patient.[1] A very brief report describes hypoglycaemia when a patient on insulin was given **doxycycline**.[2]

(b) Phenformin

There are now at least 6 cases on record of lactic-acidosis in patients on phenformin that were apparently precipitated by the concurrent use of tetracycline.[3-6]

(c) Sulphonylureas

Marked hypoglycaemia occurred in an elderly patient on **tolbutamide** when given **oxytetracycline**,[7] and the hypoglycaemic effects of **oxytetracycline** have also been demonstrated in *dogs*.[7] Another study in diabetic subjects similarly found that **oxytetracycline** can reduce blood sugar levels.[8] The half-life of **glymidine** in man has been found to be prolonged from 4.6 to 7.6 hours by **doxycycline**,[9] whereas a brief comment in another report suggests that **demeclocycline** and **doxycycline** may not affect **chlorpropamide**.[10]

Mechanism

Not understood.

Importance and management

Information about the interactions between the sulphonylureas or insulin and the tetracyclines is very limited indeed, and clinically important interactions appear to be very uncommon. Concurrent use need not be avoided, but be aware of this interaction in case of an unexpected response to treatment.

Phenformin was withdrawn in some countries because it was associated with a high incidence of lactic acidosis; where available, concurrent use with tetracyclines should be avoided. However, there is nothing to suggest that there is an increased risk if tetracyclines are given with metformin.

1. Miller JB. Hypoglycaemic effect of oxytetracycline. *BMJ* (1966) 2, 1007.
2. New Zealand Committee on Adverse Drug Reactions. Ninth Annual Report. *N Z Dent J* (1975) 71, 28–32.
3. Aro A, Korhonen T, Halinen M. Phenformin-induced lactic acidosis precipitated by tetracycline. *Lancet* (1978) 1, 673–4.
4. Tashima CK. Phenformin, tetracycline, and lactic acidosis. *BMJ* (1971) 4, 557–8.
5. Blumenthal SA, Streeten DHP. Phenformin-related lactic acidosis in a 30–year old man. *Ann Intern Med* (1976) 84, 55–6.
6. Phillips PJ, Pain RW. Phenformin, tetracycline and lactic acidosis. *Ann Intern Med* (1977) 86, 111.
7. Hiatt N, Bonorris G. Insulin response in pancreatectomized dogs treated with oxytetracycline. *Diabetes* (1970) 19, 307–10.
8. Sen S, Mukerjee AB. Hypoglycaemic action of oxytetracycline. A preliminary study. *J Indian Med Assoc* (1969) 52, 366–9.
9. Held H, Kaminski B, von Olderhausen HF. Die beeinflussung der Elimination von Glycodiazin durch Leber- und Nierenfunctionssorungen und durch eine Behandlung mit Phenylbutazon, Phenprocoumarol und Doxycyclin. *Diabetologia* (1970) 6, 386.
10. Petitpierre B, Perrin L, Rudhardt M, Herrera A, Fabre J. Behaviour of chlorpropamide in renal insufficiency and under the effect of associated drug therapy. *Int J Clin Pharmacol* (1972) 6, 120–24.

Antidiabetics + Thioctic acid

Thioctic acid is reported not to interact with acarbose, metformin or glibenclamide (glyburide).

Clinical evidence, mechanism, importance and management

A study in 24 healthy subjects given tablets containing thioctic acid 200 mg and **metformin** 500 mg found that the pharmacokinetics of the **metformin** were unchanged by the presence of the thioctic acid, and the authors of the report say that there was also no pharmacodynamic interaction.[1] The report gives very few details. A further study in 24 healthy subjects found that a single 600-mg dose of thioctic acid given with **glibenclamide** (**glyburide**) 3.5 mg did not result in any clinically relevant pharmacokinetic interaction, and thioctic acid did not alter the effect of **glibenclamide** on glucose and insulin levels.[2] A study in healthy subjects given **acarbose** and thioctic acid indicated that no clinically relevant pharmacokinetic interaction occurs between these drugs.[3]

No special precautions seem to be required if thioctic acid is given to patients on **acarbose**, **metformin** or **glibenclamide**.

1. Schug BS, Schneider E, Elze M, Fieger-Büschges H, Larsimont V, Popescu G, Molz KH, Blume HH, Hermann R. Study of pharmacokinetic interaction of thioctic acid and metformin. *Eur J Clin Pharmacol* (1997) 52 (Suppl), A140.
2. Gleiter CH, Schreeb KH, Freudenthaler S, Thomas M, Elze M, Fieger-Büschges H, Potthast H, Schneider E, Schug BS, Blume HH, Hermann R. Lack of interaction between thioctic acid, glibenclamide and acarbose. *Br J Clin Pharmacol* (1999) 48, 81–25.
3. Gleiter CH, Schreeb KH, Freudenthaler S, Thomas M, Elze M, Fieger-Bueschges H, Potthast H, Schneider E, Schug BS, Blume HH, Hermann R. Lack of interaction between thioctic acid, glibenclamide and acarbose. *Br J Clin Pharmacol* (1999) 48, 819–25.

Antidiabetics + Tibolone

Tibolone may slightly impair glucose tolerance and therefore possibly reduce the effects of antidiabetics.

Clinical evidence, mechanism, importance and management

One woman developed diabetes 14 weeks after starting tibolone 2.5 mg daily. However, she had a high normal fasting blood glucose before starting tibolone, and the diabetes did not resolve on withdrawing the drug.[1] The makers of tibolone noted that on their adverse drug event database they had only 3 cases of diabetes occurring during the use of tibolone, and 3 cases of aggravation of diabetes during its use, which they considered a very low number in relation to the extent of use of the drug.[2]

A metabolic study in 10 women with type 2 diabetes given tibolone 2.5 mg daily and treated with diet and oral antidiabetics found there were no changes in glycaemic control as measured by glycated haemoglobin levels.[3] Conversely, a longer 12-month study in 14 women with type 2 diabetes given tibolone found a slight deterioration in glycaemic control (serum fructosamine),[4] and an early study found that tibolone caused a slight decrease in glucose tolerance in non-diabetic patients.[5]

The makers of tibolone say that patients with diabetes should be closely supervised.[6,7] This seems to be a prudent precaution.

1. Konstantopoulos K, Adamides S. A case of diabetes following tibolone therapy. *Maturitas* (1994) 19, 77–8.
2. Atsma WJ. Is Livial diabetogenic? *Maturitas* (1994) 19, 239–40.
3. Feher MD, Cox A, Levy A, Mayne P, Lant AF. Short term blood pressure and metabolic effects of tibolone in postmenopausal women with non-insulin dependent diabetes. *Br J Obstet Gynaecol* (1996) 103, 281–3.
4. Prelevic GM, Beljic T, Balint-Peric L, Ginsburg J. Metabolic effects of tibolone in postmenopausal women with non-insulin dependent diabetes mellitus. *Maturitas* (1998) 28, 271–6.
5. Crona N, Silfverstolpe G, Samsioe G. A double-blind cross-over study on the effects of ORG OD14 compared to oestradiol valerate and placebo on lipid and carbohydrate metabolism in oophorectomized women. *Acta Endocrinol (Copenh)* (1983) 102, 451–5.
6. Livial (Tibolone). Organon Laboratories Ltd. UK Summary of product characteristics, December 2003.
7. Livial (Tibolone). Organon. US Prescribing information, May 2004.

Antidiabetics + Tobacco smoking

Diabetics who smoke need more insulin than non-smokers, and stopping smoking can improve glycaemic control in both type 1 and type 2 diabetics.

Clinical evidence, mechanism, importance and management

A study in 163 patients with type 1 diabetes found that, on average, the 114 who smoked needed 15 to 20% more **insulin** than the non-smokers, and up to 30% more if they smoked heavily.[1] Possible mechanisms include decreased absorption of insulin from the subcutaneous tissue because of peripheral vasoconstriction,[2] and a significant rise (40 to 120%) in the levels of the hormones that oppose the actions of **insulin**.[3]

In another study, glycaemic control (glycosylated haemoglobin) was modestly improved in 7 subjects with type 1 diabetes and 27 subjects with type 2 diabetes, one year after they had stopped smoking. This improved control was considered clinically significant.[4] In a study in patients with type 2 diabetes treated with diet alone or diet plus **sulphonylureas** with or without **metformin**, insulin resistance was higher in the 28 smokers than the 12 non-smokers.[5]

There are numerous other studies on the relationship between smoking and diabetes or insulin resistance in non-diabetics, and only a few are cited here as examples. Some studies have indicated that smoking could increase the risk of type 2 diabetes (relative risk of 2.6) and that tobacco use is associated with a low insulin response.[6] However, other studies suggest that a causal relationship between smoking and **insulin** resistance is unlikely,[7,8] although in one of the studies[8] exposure to environmental tobacco smoke was associated with lower insulin sensitivity.

Diabetics who smoke should be given all the help they need to stop smoking.

1. Madsbad S, McNair P, Christensen MS, Christiansen C, Faber OK, Binder C, Transbøl I. Influence of smoking on insulin requirement and metabolic status in diabetes mellitus. *Diabetes Care* (1980) 3, 41–3.
2. Klemp P, Staberg B, Madsbad S, Kølendorf K. Smoking reduces insulin absorption from subcutaneous tissue. *BMJ* (1982) 284, 237.
3. Helve E, Yki-Järvinen H, Koivisto VA. Smoking and insulin sensitivity in type I diabetes. *Diabetes Res Clin Pract* (1985) (Suppl 1), S232.
4. Gunton JE, Davies L, Wilmshurst E, Fulcher G, McElduff A. Cigarette smoking affects glycemic control in diabetes. *Diabetes Care* (2002) 25, 796–7.
5. Targher G, Alberiche M, Zenere MB, Bonadonna RC, Muggeo M, Bonora E. Cigarette smoking and insulin resistance in patients with noninsulin-dependent diabetes mellitus. *J Clin Endocrinol Metab* (1997) 82, 3619–24.
6. Persson P-G, Carlsson S, Svanström L, Östenson C-G, Efendic S, Grill V. Cigarette smoking, oral moist snuff use and glucose intolerance. *J Intern Med* (2000) 248, 103–110.
7. Wareham NJ, Ness EM, Byrne CD, Cox BD, Day NE, Hales CN. Cigarette smoking is not associated with hyperinsulinemia: evidence against a causal relationship between smoking and insulin resistance. *Metabolism* (1996) 45, 1551–6.
8. Henkin L, Zaccaro D, Haffner S, Karter A, Rewers M, Sholinsky P, Wagenknecht L. Cigarette smoking, environmental tobacco smoke exposure and insulin sensitivity: the Insulin Resistance Atherosclerosis Study. *Ann Epidemiol* (1999) 9, 290–6.

Antidiabetics + Tolrestat

Tolrestat does not affect the control of diabetes in patients using diet, glibenclamide (glyburide) or insulin.

Clinical evidence, mechanism, importance and management

In a randomised double-blind placebo-controlled crossover study, 46 patients using either **diet** alone, **glibenclamide** (**glyburide**) or **insulin** were also treated with tolrestat 400 mg daily for 7 days. The pharmacokinetics of the tolrestat and the **glibenclamide** (**glyburide**) were not significantly changed and the control of their diabetes was unaltered. Tolrestat did not alter glucose or insulin levels. On the basis of these findings it was concluded that diabetic patients using diet and these drugs do not need to adjust their diabetic treatment if given tolrestat.[1] Information about other antidiabetics is lacking.

1. Meng X, Parker V, Burghart P, DiLea C, Mallett S, Gonen B, Chiang S. Effects of tolrestat (T) on plasma glucose (G) levels in diet-, glyburide- and insulin-controlled (D, Gly and I) diabetics. *Clin Pharmacol Ther* (1995) 57, 154.

Antidiabetics + Tricyclic or Tetracyclic antidepressants

Interactions between antidiabetics and tricyclic or tetracyclic antidepressants appear to be rare, but four isolated cases of hypoglycaemia have been recorded in patients taking tolazamide and doxepin, chlorpropamide and nortriptyline, insulin and amitriptyline, or glibenclamide (glyburide) with phenformin and maprotiline. The control of diabetes appears to be unaffected by the use of mianserin.

Clinical evidence, mechanism, importance and management

A patient on **tolazamide** became hypoglycaemic 11 days after starting to take **doxepin** 250 mg daily; another on **chlorpropamide** (initially 25 mg increased to 75 mg daily) developed marked hypoglycaemia 3 days after starting **nortriptyline** 125 mg daily;[1] and a further patient on **insulin** developed violent and agitated behaviour (but no adrenergic symptoms) and hypoglycaemia when she started to take **amitriptyline** 25 mg at bedtime.[2] An elderly diabetic woman on **glibenclamide** (**glyburide**) and **phenformin** developed hypoglycaemia when given **maprotiline**.[3] The reasons are not understood. The patient on **doxepin** was eventually stabilised on a daily dose of **tolazamide** which was only 10% of that used before the **doxepin** was given.[1] The woman given **nortriptyline** stopped **chlorpropamide**,[1] and the woman given **maprotiline** was restabilised on half the dose of **glibenclamide** and **phenformin**.[3]

An earlier study suggested that no interaction was likely: **amitriptyline** 75 mg daily for 9 days did not affect the half-life of a single 500-mg dose of **tolbutamide** in 4 patients.[4]

Although there is some evidence of a change in glucose metabolism during treatment with **mianserin**,[5-7] the alteration failed to affect the control of diabetes in a study in 10 patients and there appear to be no reports of adverse effects caused by concurrent use.[6]

Apart from these isolated cases[1-3] the literature seems to be silent about interactions between these antidiabetics and the tricyclic or tetracyclic antidepressants. Bearing in mind the length of time these groups of drugs have been available, the risk of a clinically important interaction would seem to be very small, nevertheless bear this interaction in mind if increased hypoglycaemia occurs.

1. True BL, Perry PJ, Burns EA. Profound hypoglycemia with the addition of a tricyclic antidepressant to maintenance sulfonylurea therapy. *Am J Psychiatry* (1987) 144, 1220–1.
2. Sherman KE, Bornemann M. Amitriptyline and asymptomatic hypoglycemia. *Ann Intern Med* (1988) 109, 683–4.
3. Zogno MG, Tolfo L, Draghi E. Hypoglycemia caused by maprotiline in a patient taking oral antidiabetics. *Ann Pharmacother* (1994) 28, 406.
4. Pond SM, Graham GG, Birkett DJ, Wade DN. Effects of tricyclic antidepressants on drug metabolism. *Clin Pharmacol Ther* (1975) 18, 191–9.
5. Fell PJ, Quantock DC, van der Burg WJ. The human pharmacology of GB94–a new psychotropic agent. *Eur J Clin Pharmacol* (1973) 5, 166–73.
6. Peet M, Behagel H. Mianserin: a decade of scientific development. *Br J Clin Pharmacol* (1978) 5, 5S–9S.
7. Moonie L. Unpublished data quoted by Brogden RN, Heel RC, Speight TM, Avery GS. Mianserin: a review of its pharmacological properties and therapeutic efficacy in depressive illness. *Drugs* (1978) 16, 273–301.

Insulin + Naltrexone

The insulin requirements of a patient rose by about 30% during treatment with naltrexone.

Clinical evidence, mechanism, importance and management

A patient with type 1 diabetes was given naltrexone in an experimental study of the treatment of anorexia nervosa. During two periods of 5 days while given the naltrexone [dosage not stated], the blood glucose levels of the patient remained unchanged but the **insulin** dosage requirements rose from 52.8 and 61.4 units daily during the control periods to 71.4 and 76 units daily during the naltrexone periods (a rise of about 30%). The reason is not known but the authors of this report point out that this apparent interaction must have been on the actions of **insulin** rather than on its release because this patient had no endogenous insulin.[1]

The general clinical importance of this interaction is not known but it would be prudent to be alert for any evidence of increased **insulin** requirements if naltrexone is used in any patient.

1. Marrazzi MA, Jacober S, Luby ED. A naltrexone-induced increase in insulin requirement. *J Clin Psychopharmacol* (1994) 14, 363–5.

Metformin + Cefalexin

Cefalexin modestly increased serum levels of metformin in a single-dose study.

Clinical evidence, mechanism, importance and management

Twelve healthy subjects were given single 500-mg doses of metformin with either placebo or cefalexin 500 mg. The AUC and maximum serum levels of metformin were increased by 24% and 34% respectively by cefalexin. Renal clearance of metformin was reduced by 14% due to the inhibition by cefalexin of tubular secretion via the organic cation system.[1] The clinical relevance of these small changes is uncertain, but they could be greater with longer-term use. The authors recommend that patients receiving concurrent metformin and cefalexin should have metformin levels monitored or an alternative antibacterial to cefalexin should be considered.[1] However, based on the available evidence this seems somewhat overcautious.

1. Jayasagar G, Krishna Kumar M, Chandrasekhar K, Madhusudan Rao C, Madhusudan Rao Y. Effect of cephalexin on the pharmacokinetics of metformin in healthy human volunteers. *Drug Metabol Drug Interact* (2002) 19, 41–8.

Metformin + Iodinated contrast media

Intravascular administration of iodinated contrast media may cause renal failure, which could result in lactic acidosis in patients taking metformin.

Clinical evidence, mechanism, importance and management

Intravascular administration of iodinated contrast media to patients on metformin may result in lactic acidosis. However, the problem is reported to occur only if the contrast media causes renal failure and metformin use is continued. This is because metformin is mainly excreted by the kidneys and in renal failure toxic levels may accumulate.[1] A literature search identified 18 cases of lactic acidosis after the use of contrast media in patients on metformin.[2] Of these 18 cases, 14 or 15 were associated with pre-existing renal impairment and 2 cases with other contraindications to metformin (sepsis and cirrhosis). The remaining case was in an elderly woman with neurological disease.

The makers of metformin say that it should be stopped before, or at the time of giving the contrast media and not restarted until 48 hours later, and then only after renal function has been re-checked and found to be normal.[3] Guidelines issued by the Royal College of Radiologists are based on this statement and they say that referring clinicians should assess renal function before the test.[4] Similar guidelines have been issued by the European Society for Urogenital medicine.[5,6] However, some consider that metformin need not be stopped for 48 hours in those patients with normal renal function.[2]

1. Rasuli P, Hammond DI. Metformin and contrast media: where is the conflict? *Can Assoc Radiol J* (1998) 49, 161–6.
2. McCartney MM, Gilbert FJ, Murchison LE, Pearson D, McHardy K, Murray AD. Metformin and contrast media – a dangerous combination? *Clin Radiol* (1999) 54, 29–33.
3. Glucophage (Metformin hydrochloride). Merck Pharmaceuticals. UK Summary of product characteristics, October 2004.
4. The Royal College of Radiologists. Guidelines with regard to metformin-induced lactic acidosis and x-ray contrast medium agents. 19th March 1999. Available at: http://www.rcr.ac.uk/pubtop.asp?PublicationID=70 (accessed 03/02/05).
5. Morcos SK, Thomsen HS. European Society of Urogenital Radiology guidelines on administering contrast media. *Abdom Imaging* (2003) 28, 187–190.
6. Thomsen HS, Morcos SK. Contrast media and the kidney: European Society of Urogenital Radiology (ESUR) guidelines. *Br J Radiol* (2003) 76, 513–8.

Pioglitazone + Fexofenadine

A study in healthy subjects indicated that the pharmacokinetics of pioglitazone 45 mg daily are not significantly affected by fexofenadine 60 mg twice daily, and that pioglitazone does not affect the pharmacokinetics of fexofenadine.[1]

1. Robert M. Pharmacokinetics of coadministration of pioglitazone with fexofenadine. *Diabetes* (2001) 50 (Suppl 2), A443.

Pioglitazone or Rosiglitazone + Insulin

The UK makers contraindicate the use of pioglitazone and rosiglitazone with insulin but the US specifically indicate the combination.

Clinical evidence, mechanism, importance and management

(a) Pioglitazone

It has been noted that in patients on insulin the dose may need to be reduced by 10 to 25% if pioglitazone 15 or 30 mg daily is given.[1] In one 16-week study, pioglitazone with insulin was compared with insulin alone in 566 patients with long-standing diabetes and a high incidence of cardiovascular disorders. Four of the 379 patients treated with pioglitazone and insulin developed congestive heart failure compared with none of the 187 patients on insulin alone. Analysis of this study did not identify specific factors that predict this possible increased risk of congestive heart failure.[1] Pioglitazone alone may exacerbate or precipitate heart failure because it can cause fluid retention.[1,2] The combination of pioglitazone with insulin is licensed for use in the US,[1] however, in the UK, the combination is contraindicated because of the reports of cardiac failure.[2]

(b) Rosiglitazone

A study in poorly controlled type-2 diabetic patients using insulin twice daily found that the addition of rosiglitazone 2 or 4 mg twice daily for 26 weeks improved the control of their blood sugar levels and they needed less insulin.[3] However, it has also been found that there is a fourfold increase in the incidence of cardiac failure (2.5%) if both drugs are used and it is for this reason that the UK makers contraindicate rosiglitazone with insulin.[4] However, in the US rosiglitazone is specifically indicated for use with insulin.[5]

1. Actos (Pioglitazone hydrochloride). Takeda Ltd. US Prescribing information, August 2004.
2. Actos (Pioglitazone hydrochloride). Takeda UK Ltd. UK Summary of product characteristics, February 2005.
3. Raskin P, Dole JF, Rappaport EB. Rosiglitazone (RSG) improves glycemic control in poorly controlled, insulin-treated type 2 diabetes (T2D). *Diabetes* (1999) 48 (Suppl 1), A94.
4. Avandia (Rosiglitazone maleate). GlaxoSmithKline UK. UK Summary of product characteristics, January 2005.
5. Avandia (Rosiglitazone maleate). GlaxoSmithKline. US Prescribing information, March 2005.

Sulphonylureas + Allopurinol

Allopurinol caused an increase in the half-life of chlorpropamide, and a minor decrease in the half-life of tolbutamide but the effect of these changes on the hypoglycaemic response of patients is uncertain. Marked hypoglycaemia and coma occurred in one patient on gliclazide and allopurinol.

Clinical evidence

(a) Chlorpropamide

A brief report describes 6 patients given chlorpropamide with allopurinol. The half-life of chlorpropamide in one patient with gout and normal renal function exceeded 200 hours (normally 36 hours) after taking allopurinol for 10 days, and in 2 others the half-life was extended to 44 and 55 hours. The other 3 patients were given allopurinol for only 1 or 2 days and the half-life of chlorpropamide remained unaltered.[1]

(b) Gliclazide

Severe hypoglycaemia (1.6 mmol/l) and coma occurred in a patient with renal insufficiency taking gliclazide and allopurinol.[2] Hypoglycaemia has been seen in another patient taking both drugs, but enalapril and ranitidine were also involved.[2]

(c) Tolbutamide

Allopurinol 2.5 mg/kg twice daily for 15 days reduced the half-life of intravenous tolbutamide in 10 healthy subjects by 25%, from 360 to 267 minutes.[3,4]

Mechanism

Not understood. In the case of chlorpropamide it has been suggested that it possibly involves some competition for renal tubular mechanisms.[1]

Importance and management

Information is very limited. Only gliclazide has been implicated in severe hypoglycaemia and there seem to be no reports of either grossly enhanced hypoglycaemia with chlorpropamide, or reduced hypoglycaemia with tolbutamide. More study is needed to find out whether any of these interactions has general clinical importance, but it seems unlikely.

1. Petitpierre B, Perrin L, Rudhardt M, Herrera A, Fabre J. Behaviour of chlorpropamide in renal insufficiency and under the effect of associated drug therapy. *Int J Clin Pharmacol* (1972) 6, 120–4.
2. Girardin E, Vial T, Pham E, Evreux J-C. Hypoglycémies induites par les sulfamides hypoglycémiants. *Ann Med Interne (Paris)* (1992) 143, 11–17.
3. Gentile S, Porcellini M, Loguercio C, Foglia F, Coltorti M. Modificazioni della depurazione plasmatica di tolbutamide e rifamicina-SV indotte dal trattamento con allopurinolo in volontari sono. *Progr Med (Napoli)* (1979) 35, 637–42.
4. Gentile S, Porcellini M, Foglia F, Loguercio C, Coltorti M. Influenza di allopurinolo sull'emivita plasmatica di tolbutamide e rifamicina-SV in soggetti sani. *Boll Soc Ital Biol Sper* (1979) 55, 345–8.

Sulphonylureas + Angiotensin II receptor antagonists

Glibenclamide (glyburide) causes a small reduction in valsartan plasma levels, but this is unlikely to be of any clinical significance. No clinically relevant pharmacokinetic interactions occur between glibenclamide and candesartan cilexetil or telmisartan, or between tolbutamide and irbesartan. Glibenclamide does not alter the efficacy of eprosartan.

Clinical evidence and mechanism

A. Glibenclamide

(a) Candesartan

Glibenclamide 3.5 mg daily did not significantly affect the pharmacokinetics of candesartan 16 mg daily, both given for 7 days, although the maximum plasma concentration of candesartan was slightly increased by 12%. The pharmacokinetics of glibenclamide were not altered by the candesartan.[1]

(b) Eprosartan

Fifteen type 2 diabetes stabilised on glibenclamide 3.75 to 10 mg daily for at least 30 days had no changes in their 24-hour plasma glucose concentrations when additionally treated for a further 7 days with eprosartan 200 mg twice daily. Concurrent use was safe and well tolerated and it was concluded that there is no clinically relevant interaction between these two drugs.[2]

(c) Telmisartan

The maker of telmisartan notes that, in a pharmacokinetic study, no clinical significant interaction occurred with glibenclamide.[3]

(d) Valsartan

In a randomised, crossover study, 12 healthy subjects were given single oral doses of valsartan 160 mg and glibenclamide (glyburide) 1.75 mg alone and together.[4] Glibenclamide appeared to decrease the valsartan AUC by 16%, and the plasma concentrations of valsartan showed wide variations between subjects. The pharmacokinetics of glibenclamide were not affected.[4] The changes in valsartan pharmacokinetics seen with glibenclamide appear to have little or no clinical relevance.

B. Tolbutamide

(a) Irbesartan

A study in 18 healthy subjects given irbesartan 300 mg daily and tolbutamide 1 g daily, either alone or in combination, found that no clinically important pharmacokinetic interactions occurred.[5]

Importance and management

No special precautions would appear to be needed if candesartan, eprosartan, telmisartan or valsartan are given with glibenclamide, or if irbesartan is given with tolbutamide. However, further clinical study is needed. For reports of hypoglycaemia in diabetics given ACE inhibitors, see 'Antidiabetics + ACE inhibitors', p.391.

1. Jonkman JHG, van Lier JJ, van Heiningen PNM, Lins R, Sennewald R, Högemann A. Pharmacokinetic drug interaction studies with candesartan cilexetil. *J Hum Hypertens* (1997) 11 (Suppl 2), S31–S35.
2. Martin DE, DeCherney GS, Ilson BE, Jones BA, Boike SC, Freed MI, Jorasky DK. Eprosartan, an angiotensin II receptor antagonist, does not affect the pharmacodynamics of glyburide in patients with type II diabetes mellitus. *J Clin Pharmacol* (1997) 37, 155–9.
3. Micardis (Telmisartan). Boehringer Ingelheim Ltd. UK Summary of product characteristics, December 2004.
4. Novartis Pharmaceuticals Ltd. Data on file, Protocol 52.
5. Marino MR, Vachharajani NN. Drug interactions with irbesartan. *Clin Pharmacokinet* (2001) 40, 605–14.

Sulphonylureas + Aprepitant

Aprepitant slightly reduces tolbutamide levels.

Clinical evidence, mechanism, importance and management

In a study in 12 healthy subjects aprepitant 125 mg on day one, then 80 mg daily on days 2 and 3 decreased the AUC of a single 500-mg dose of **tolbutamide** given on day 4 by 23%, on day 8 by 28%, and on day 15 by 15% when compared to 12 subjects not given aprepitant.[1]

Aprepitant increases the metabolism of **tolbutamide** because it is an inducer of the cytochrome P450 isoenzyme CYP2C9.

The clinical relevance of these small changes has not been assessed, nevertheless the maker recommends caution.[2]

1. Shadle CR, Lee Y, Majumdar AK, Petty KJ, Gargano C, Bradstreet TE, Evans JK, Blum RA. Evaluation of potential inductive effects of aprepitant on cytochrome P450 3A4 and 2C9 activity. *J Clin Pharmacol* (2004) 44, 215–23.
2. Emend (Aprepitant). Merck Sharp & Dohme Ltd. UK Summary of product characteristics, April 2005.

Sulphonylureas + Chloramphenicol

The hypoglycaemic effects of tolbutamide and chlorpropamide can be increased by chloramphenicol and acute hypoglycaemia can occur.

Clinical evidence

A man taking chloramphenicol 2 g daily was started on **tolbutamide** 2 g daily. Three days later he had a typical hypoglycaemic collapse and was found to have serum **tolbutamide** levels three to fourfold higher than expected.[1]

Studies in diabetics have shown that chloramphenicol 2 g daily can increase the serum level and half-life of **tolbutamide** twofold and two to threefold respectively.[1,2] Blood sugar levels were reduced by about 25 to 30%.[2,3] Hypoglycaemia, acute in one case, developed in two other patients on **tolbutamide** given chloramphenicol.[4,5] in another study chloramphenicol 1 to 2 g daily caused an average twofold increase in the half-life of **chlorpropamide**.[6]

Mechanism

Chloramphenicol inhibits the liver enzymes concerned with the metabolism of tolbutamide, and probably chlorpropamide as well, leading to their accumulation in the body. This is reflected in prolonged half-lives, reduced blood sugar levels and occasionally acute hypoglycaemia.[1-4,6]

Importance and management

The interaction between tolbutamide and chloramphenicol is well established and of clinical importance. The incidence is uncertain, but an increased hypoglycaemic response should be expected if both drugs are given. The interaction between chlorpropamide and chloramphenicol is less well documented. Nevertheless, monitor concurrent use carefully and reduce the dosage of both sulphonylureas as necessary. Some patients may show a particularly exaggerated response. The makers of other sulphonylureas often list chloramphenicol as an interacting drug, based on its interactions with tolbutamide and chlorpropamide, but direct information of an interaction does not appear to be available. No interaction would be expected with chloramphenicol eye drops, because the systemic absorption is likely to be small, but this needs confirmation.

1. Christensen LK, Skovsted L. Inhibition of drug metabolism by chloramphenicol. *Lancet* (1969) ii, 1397–9.
2. Brunová E, Slabochová Z, Platilová H, Pavlík F, Grafnetterová J, Dvořáček K. Interaction of tolbutamide and chloramphenicol in diabetic patients. *Int J Clin Pharmacol Biopharm* (1977) 15, 7–12.
3. Brunová E, Slabochová Z, Platilová H. Influencing the effect of Dirastan (tolbutamide). Simultaneous administration of chloramphenicol in patients with diabetes and bacterial urinary tract inflammation. *Cas Lek Cesk* (1974) 113, 72–5.
4. Ziegelasch H-J. Extreme hypoglykämie unter kombinierter behandlung mit tolbutamid, n-1-butylbiguanidhydrochlorid und chloramphenikol. *Z Gesamte Inn Med* (1972) 27, 63–6.
5. Soeldner JS, Steinke J. Hypoglycemia in tolbutamide-treated diabetes. *JAMA* (1965) 193, 398–9.
6. Petitpierre B, Perrin L, Rudhardt M, Herrera A, Fabre J. Behaviour of chlorpropamide in renal insufficiency and under the effect of associated drug therapy. *Int J Clin Pharmacol* (1972) 6, 120–4.

Sulphonylureas + Heparin

Two isolated reports describe hypoglycaemia in a diabetic on glipizide and another on glibenclamide (glyburide), both attributed to concurrent treatment with heparin.

Clinical evidence, mechanism, importance and management

A diabetic, treated for 6 months with **glipizide** 5 mg daily with fair control, experienced recurring episodes of hypoglycaemia over a period of 4 days, after taking a routine 5-mg dose of **glipizide** while hospitalised for the treatment of a foot ulcer. It was suggested that this might possibly have been due to an interaction with subcutaneous heparin calcium 5000 units every 12 hours which, it is postulated, might have displaced the **glipizide** from its protein binding sites.[1] The patient was also treated with diamorphine. Another very brief report describes hypoglycaemia in a patient treated with **glibenclamide** (**glyburide**) and heparin.[2] No other information seems to be available. The general importance of these reports is unknown, but seems likely to be small.

1. McKillop G, Fallon M, Slater SD. Possible interaction between heparin and a sulphonylurea a cause of prolonged hypoglycaemia? *BMJ* (1986) 293, 1073.
2. Beeley L, Daly M, Stewart P. *Bulletin of the West Midlands Centre for Adverse Drug Reaction Reporting* (1987) 24, 24.

Sulphonylureas + Methysergide

A preliminary study indicates that methysergide may enhance the activity of tolbutamide.

Clinical evidence, mechanism, importance and management

Two days pretreatment with methysergide 2 mg every 6 hours increased the amount of insulin secreted in response to a 1-g intravenous dose of **tolbutamide** by almost 40% in 8 patients with type 2 diabetes.[1] Whether in practice the addition or withdrawal of methysergide adversely affects the control of diabetes is uncertain, but the possibility should be borne in mind.

1. Baldridge JA, Quickel KE, Feldman JM and Lebovitz HE. Potentiation of tolbutamide-mediated insulin release in adult onset diabetics by methysergide maleate. *Diabetes* (1974) 23, 21–4.

Sulphonylureas + Probenecid

The clearance of chlorpropamide is prolonged by probenecid, but the clinical importance of this is uncertain. Tolbutamide appears not to interact.

Clinical evidence, mechanism, importance and management

A study in 6 patients given single oral doses of **chlorpropamide** found that the concurrent use of probenecid 1 to 2 g daily increased the chlorpropamide half-life from about 36 to 50 hours.[1] It seems that the probenecid reduces the renal excretion of **chlorpropamide**. Another report in healthy subjects claimed that the half-life of **tolbutamide** was also prolonged by probenecid,[2] but this was not confirmed by a further controlled study.[3]

Information is very limited but it may possibly be necessary to reduce the dosage of **chlorpropamide** in the presence of probenecid. Information about other sulphonylureas appears to be lacking.

1. Petitpierre B, Perrin L, Rudhardt M, Herrera A, Fabre J. Behaviour of chlorpropamide in renal insufficiency and under the effect of associated drug therapy. *Int J Clin Pharmacol* (1972) 6, 120–4.
2. Stowers JM, Mahler RF, Hunter RB. Pharmacology and mode of action of the sulphonylureas in man. *Lancet* (1958) i, 278–83.
3. Brook R, Schrogie JJ, Solomon HM. Failure of probenecid to inhibit the rate of metabolism of tolbutamide in man. *Clin Pharmacol Ther* (1968) 9, 314–17.

Sulphonylureas + Sulfonamides

The hypoglycaemic effects of some of the sulphonylureas are increased by some, but not all, sulfonamides. Occasionally and unpredictably acute hypoglycaemia has occurred in individual patients. There appear to be no reports of adverse interaction between insulin and the sulfonamides. Co-trimoxazole alone may rarely cause hypoglycaemia.

Clinical evidence

'Table 12.4', (p.423) summarises the information on the interactions between sulphonylureas and sulfonamides. For a report of the combined use of co-trimoxazole and fluconazole causing hypoglygaemia with **gliclazide**, see 'Antidiabetics + Azoles', p.397.

Mechanism

Not fully understood. The sulfonamides may inhibit the metabolism of the sulphonylureas so that they accumulate in the body. In this way their serum levels and hypoglycaemic effects are enhanced.[1-4] There is also evidence that the sulphonamides can displace the sulphonylureas from their protein binding sites.[4] Hypoglycaemia induced by co-trimoxazole, in the absence of a conventional antidiabetic,[5-9] and sometimes associated with renal failure,[7] high dose of sulphonamide,[5,9] advanced age,[6,8] or malnutrition,[5] has been described.

Importance and management

Information is very patchy and incomplete. Most sulfonamides seem to have caused marked problems (acute hypoglycaemia) in only a few patients and serious interactions are uncommon. Firm predictions cannot be made about what will, or what will not, interact in individual patients, nor how clinically important the reaction may prove to be, but 'Table 12.4', (p.423) can be used as a broad guide. When a sulfonamide is first added to established treatment with a sulphonylurea, warn the patient that increased hypoglycaemia, sometimes excessive, is a possibility, but that problems appear to be uncommon or rare. It may be prudent to increase the frequency of blood glucose monitoring. In one study, co-trimoxazole did not appear to cause any significant changes in blood glucose or insulin concentrations in patients receiving **insulin**.[10] However, note that co-trimoxazole alone may rarely cause hypoglycaemia (see Mechanism above).

1. Lumholtz B, Siersbaek-Nielsen K, Skovsted L, Kampmann J, Hansen JM. Sulphamethizole-induced inhibition of diphenylhydantoin, tolbutamide, and warfarin metabolism. *Clin Pharmacol Ther* (1975) 17, 731–4.
2. Kristensen M, Christensen LK. Drug induced changes of the blood glucose lowering effect of oral hypoglycemic agents. *Acta Diabetol Lat* (1969) 6 (Suppl 1), 116–23.
3. Christensen LK, Hansen JM, Kristensen M. Sulphaphenazole-induced hypoglycaemic attacks in tolbutamide-treated diabetics. *Lancet* (1963) ii, 1298–1301.
4. Hellman B. Potentiating effects of drugs on the binding of glibenclamide to pancreatic beta cells. *Metabolism* (1974) 23, 839–46.
5. Hekimsoy Z, Biberoğlu S, Çömleçki A, Tarhan O, Mermut C, Biberoğlu K. Trimethoprim-sulfamethoxazole-induced hypoglycemia in a malnourished patient with severe infection. *Eur J Endocrinol* (1997) 136, 304–6.
6. Mathews WA, Manint JE, Kleiss J. Trimethoprim-sulfamethoxazole-induced hypoglycemia as a cause of altered mental status in an elderly patient. *J Am Board Fam Pract* (2000) 13, 211–12.
7. Lee AJ, Maddix DS. Trimethoprim/sulfamethoxazole-induced hypoglycemia in a patient with acute renal failure. *Ann Pharmacother* (1997) 31, 727–32.
8. Rutschmann OT, Wicki J, Micheli P, Kondo Oestreicher M, Guillermin Spahr ML, Droz M. Co-trimoxazole administration: a rare cause of hypoglycemia in elderly persons. *Schweiz Med Wochenschr* (1998) 128, 1171–4.
9. Johnson JA, Kappel JE, Sharif MN. Hypoglycemia secondary to trimethoprim/sulfamethoxazole administration in a renal transplant patient. *Ann Pharmacother* (1993) 27, 304–6.
10. Mihic M, Mautner LS, Feness JZ, Grant K. Effect of trimethoprim-sulfamethoxazole on blood insulin and glucose concentrations of diabetics. *Can Med Assoc J* (1975), 112, 80S–82S.

Sulphonylureas; Chlorpropamide + Urinary alkalinisers and acidifiers

On theoretical grounds the response to chlorpropamide may be decreased if the urine is made alkaline, and increased if urine is acidified. Metabolic interactions with chlorpropamide are likely to be more apparent when the urine is acidic, but so far no adverse interactions appear to have been reported.

Clinical evidence, mechanism, importance and management

A study in 6 healthy subjects given a 250-mg oral dose of chlorpropamide found that when the urine was made alkaline (pH 7.1 to 8.2) with **sodium bicarbonate**, the half-life of the chlorpropamide was reduced from 50 to 13 hours, and the 72-hour clearance was increased fourfold. In contrast, when the urine was acidified (pH 5.5 to 4.7) with **ammonium chloride**, the chlorpropamide half-life was increased from 50 to 69 hours and the 72-hour urinary clearance was decreased to 5%, and non-renal (i.e. metabolic) clearance predominated.[1] Another study found that the renal clearance of chlorpropamide was almost 100 times greater at pH 7 than at pH 5.[2] The reasons are that changes in urinary pH affect the ionisation of the chlorpropamide, and this affects the ability of the kidney to reabsorb it from the kidney filtrate (see more details under 'Drug excretion interactions', (p.7)). Thus, urinary pH determines the relative contribution of renal and metabolic clearance.

There appear to be no reports of adverse interactions between chlorpropamide and drugs that can alter urinary pH, but prescribers should be aware of the possibilities: a reduced response if the pH is raised significantly and renal clearance predominates (e.g. with **sodium bicarbonate**, **acetazolamide**, some **antacids**); an increased response if the pH is made

Table 12.4 Antidiabetic/sulfonamide interactions

Drugs	Information documented	Refs
Chlorpropamide		
+ sulfafurazole (sulfisoxazole)	1 case of acute hypoglycaemia	1
+ sulfadimidine	1 case of acute hypoglycaemia	2
+ co-trimoxazole	2 cases of acute hypoglycaemia	3, 4
Glibenclamide		
+ co-trimoxazole		
	In a large review of glibenclamide-associated hypoglycaemia 11% were also taking co-trimoxazole	5
	8 cases of hypoglycaemia	6, 7
	Stated to be no pharmacokinetic interaction	5, 8
Glibornuride		
+ sulfaphenazole	Stated to be no interaction	9
Gliclazide		
+ co-trimoxazole	4 cases of acute hypoglycaemia	7
Glipizide		
+ co-trimoxazole	1 case of acute hypoglycaemia	10
	1 study stating no interaction	11
Insulin		
+ co-trimoxazole	No significant changes in blood glucose or insulin concentrations	12
Tolbutamide		
+ co-trimoxazole	Clearance reduced 25%, half-life increased 30%	13
+ sulfafurazole (sulfisoxazole)	3 cases of severe hypoglycaemia	14, 15
	4 reports state no interaction	1, 16, 17
+ sulfamethizole	Half-life of tolbutamide increased 60%. Metabolic clearance reduced 40%	16, 18
+ sulfaphenazole	2 cases of severe hypoglycaemia	19
	Half-life of tolbutamide increased x4–6	17, 19, 20
+ sulfadiazine	Half-life of tolbutamide increased	20
+ sulfadimethoxine	Stated to be no interaction	16, 17, 19
+ sulfametoxypyridazine	Stated to be no interaction	16, 19
+ sulfamethoxazole	Clearance reduced 14%, half-life increased 20%	13
	5 cases of no interaction	17
Un-named sulfonylurea		
+ co-trimoxazole	1 case of acute hypoglycaemia	12

1. Tucker HSG, Hirsch JI. Sulfonamide-sulfonylurea interaction. *N Engl J Med* (1972) 286, 110–11.
2. Dall JLC, Conway H, McAlpine SG. Hypoglycaemia due to chlorpropamide. *Scott Med J* (1967) 12, 403–4.
3. Ek I. Långvarigt klorpropamidutöst hypoglykemitillstand Låkemedelsinteraktion? *Lakartidningen* (1974) 71, 2597–8.
4. Baciewicz AM, Swafford WB. Hypoglycemia induced by the interaction of chlorpropamide and co-trimoxazole. *Drug Intell Clin Pharm* (1984) 18, 309–10.
5. Sjöberg S, Wiholm BE, Gunnarsson R, Emilsson H, Thunberg E, Christenson I, Östman J. No evidence for pharmacokinetic interaction between glibenclamide and trimethoprim-sulfamethoxazole. *Diabetes Res Clin Pract* (1985) (Suppl 1), S522.
6. Asplund K, Wiholm B-E, Lithner F. Glibenclamide-associated hypoglycaemia: a report on 57 cases. *Diabetologia* (1983) 24, 412–7.
7. Girardin E, Vial T, Pham E, Evreux J-C. Hypoglycémies induites par les sulfamides hypoglycémiants. *Ann Med Interne (Paris)* (1992) 143, 11–17.
8. Sjöberg S, Wiholm BE, Gunnarsson R, Emilsson H, Thunberg E, Christenson I, Östman J. Lack of pharmacokinetic interaction between glibenclamide and trimethoprim-sulphamethoxazole. *Diabet Med* (1987) 4, 245–7.
9. Eckhardt W, Rudolph R, Sauer H, Schubert WR, Undeutsch D. Zur pharmakologischen Interferenz von Glibornurid mit Sulfaphenazol, Phenylbutazon und Phenprocoumon beim Menschen. *Arzneimittelforschung* (1972) 22, 2212–19.
10. Johnson JF, Dobmeier ME. Symptomatic hypoglycemia secondary to a glipizide-trimethoprim/sulfamethoxazole drug interaction. *DICP Ann Pharmacother* (1990) 24, 250–1.
11. Kradjan WA, Witt DM, Opheim KE, Wood FC. Lack of interaction between glipizide and co-trimoxazole. *J Clin Pharmacol* (1994) 34, 997-1002.
12. Mihic M, Mautner LS, Feness JZ, Grant K. Effect of trimethoprim-sulfamethoxazole on blood insulin and glucose concentrations of diabetics. *Can Med Assoc J* (1975), 112, 80S–82S.
13. Wing LMH, Miners JO. Cotrimoxazole as an inhibitor of oxidative drug metabolism: effects of trimethoprim and sulphamethoxazole separately and combined on tolbutamide disposition. *Br J Clin Pharmacol* (1985) 20, 482–5.
14. Soeldner JS, Steinke J. Hypoglycemia in tolbutamide-treated diabetes. *JAMA* (1965) 193, 148–9.
15. Robinson DS. The application of basic principles of drug interaction to clinical practice. *J Urol* (1975) 113, 100–107.
16. Siersbaek-Nielsen K, Møholm Hansen J, Skovsted L, Lumholtz B, Kampmann J. Sulfamethizole-induced inhibition of diphenylhydantoin and tolbutamide metabolism in man. *Clin Pharmacol Ther* (1973) 14, 148.
17. Dubach UC, Buckert A, Raaflaub J. Einfluss von Sulfonamiden auf die blutzuckersenkende Wirkung oraler Antidiabetica. *Schweiz Med Wochenschr* (1966) 96, 1483–6.
18. Lumholtz B, Siersbaek-Nielsen K, Skovsted L, Kampmann J, Hansen JM. Sulphamethizole-induced inhibition of diphenylhydantoin, tolbutamide, and warfarin metabolism. *Clin Pharmacol Ther* (1975) 17, 731–4.
19. Christensen LK, Hansen JM, Kristensen M. Sulphaphenazole-induced hypoglycaemic attacks in tolbutamide-treated diabetics. *Lancet* (1963) ii, 1298–1301.
20. Kristensen M, Christensen LK. Drug induced changes of the blood glucose lowering effect of oral hypoglycemic agents. *Acta Diabetol Lat* (1969) 6 (Suppl 1), 116–23.

more acid than usual and metabolic clearance predominates (e.g. with **ammonium chloride**). Perhaps more importantly, the effects of drugs that alter the hepatic clearance of chlorpropamide are likely to be more significant when its renal clearance is low (i.e. when the urine is acid).[2]

1. Neuvonen PJ, Kärkkäinen S. Effects of charcoal, sodium bicarbonate, and ammonium chloride on chlorpropamide kinetics. *Clin Pharmacol Ther* (1983) 33, 386–93.

2. Neuvonen PJ, Kärkkäinen S and Lehtovaara R. Pharmacokinetics of chlorpropamide in epileptic patients: effects of enzyme induction and urine pH on chlorpropamide elimination. *Eur J Clin Pharmacol* (1987) 32, 297–301.

Sulphonylureas; Glibenclamide (Glyburide) + Bosentan

There appears to be an increased risk of liver toxicity if bosentan is used with glibenclamide, and the combination should probably be avoided. Glibenclamide modestly reduces the plasma levels of bosentan, and bosentan reduces the plasma levels of glibenclamide.

Clinical evidence, mechanism, importance and management

In clinical trials, bosentan was noted to be associated with dose-related asymptomatic elevations in liver enzymes in some patients, and these elevations were higher in patients also receiving glibenclamide.[1] Study in *rats* confirmed that combined use of bosentan and glibenclamide caused increases in serum bile salt levels that were greater than with either drug alone.[1] In addition, *in vitro* study showed bosentan inhibits the bile salt export pump,[1] and glibenclamide also inhibits this pump. Because of the possibility that there may be a pharmacokinetic component to the interaction, the pharmacokinetics of both bosentan and glibenclamide were determined in a crossover study in 12 healthy subjects. However, glibenclamide actually reduced the maximum plasma levels and AUC of bosentan by 24 and 29% respectively, while bosentan reduced the maximum plasma levels and AUC of glibenclamide by 22 and 40% respectively. Two subjects had asymptomatic elevated liver enzyme levels while receiving the concurrent bosentan and glibenclamide.[2]

Based on the limited evidence available on the increased risk of liver toxicity, the maker of bosentan recommends that it should not be used with drugs that are inhibitors of the bile salt export pump such as glibenclamide. They suggest that an alternative antidiabetic treatment should be used.[3] The US makers contraindicate concurrent use because of the potential for raised liver enzymes.[4] This seems a sensible precaution. Note also that a decrease of 40% in the AUC of glibenclamide is possibly of clinical significance.[2]

1. Fattinger K, Funk C, Pantze M, Weber C, Reichen J, Stieger B, Meier PJ. The endothelin antagonist bosentan inhibits the canalicular bile salt export pump: a potential mechanism for hepatic adverse reactions. *Clin Pharmacol Ther* (2001) 69, 223–31.

2. van Giersbergen PLM, Treiber A, Clozel M, Bodin F, Dingemanse J. In vivo and in vitro studies exploring the pharmacokinetic interaction between bosentan, a dual endothelin receptor antagonist, and glyburide. *Clin Pharmacol Ther* (2002) 71, 252–62.

3. Tracleer (Bosentan monohydrate). Actelion Pharmaceuticals UK. UK Summary of product characteristics, September 2004.

4. Tracleer (Bosentan). Actelion Pharmaceuticals Ltd. US Prescribing information, November 2004.

Sulphonylureas; Glibenclamide (Glyburide) + Naftidrofuryl oxalate

There is one very brief report describing severe hypoglycaemia when glibenclamide was given with naftidrofuryl oxalate, possibly due to an interaction.[1] No details are given.

1. Beeley L, Magee P, Hickey FM. *Bulletin of the West Midlands Centre for Adverse Drug Reaction Reporting* (1990) 30, 17.

Sulphonylureas; Glibenclamide (Glyburide) + Pantoprazole

There is no pharmacokinetic interaction between glibenclamide and pantoprazole, and pantoprazole does not alter the glucose-lowering effect of glibenclamide.

Clinical evidence, mechanism, importance and management

Pantoprazole 40 mg daily or placebo were given to 20 healthy subjects for 5 days. On day 5 the subjects were additionally given 3.5 mg of a micronised preparation of glibenclamide. The pharmacokinetics of the glibenclamide and the pharmacodynamic profiles of glucose and insulin serum concentrations were not significantly altered, and the pharmacokinetics of pantoprazole were not affected. It was concluded that dosage changes of the micronised preparation of glibenclamide are not needed during treatment with pantoprazole.[1]

1. Walter-Sack IE, Bliesath H, Stötzer F, Huber R, Steinijans VW, Ding R, Mascher H, Wurst W. Lack of pharmacokinetic and pharmacodynamic interaction between pantoprazole and glibenclamide in humans. *Clin Drug Invest* (1998) 15, 253–60.

Sulphonylureas; Glibenclamide (Glyburide) + Vinpocetine

Vinpocetine does not interact with glibenclamide.

Clinical evidence, mechanism, importance and management

A study in 18 elderly patients with type 2 diabetes and symptoms of dementia, taking glibenclamide, found that 4 days' treatment with vinpocetine 10 mg three times daily did not affect either the pharmacokinetics of the glibenclamide or the control of blood glucose levels.[1] There would seem to be no reason for avoiding concurrent use.

1. Grandt R, Braun W, Schulz H-U, Lührmann B, Frercks H-J. Glibenclamide steady-state plasma levels during concomitant vinpocetine administration in type II diabetic patients. *Arzneimittelforschung* (1989) 39, 1451–4.

Sulphonylureas; Glymidine + Phenobarbital

A study in one subject found that the hypoglycaemic effects of glymidine were unaffected by phenobarbital.[1] No special precautions would appear necessary.

1. Gerhards E, Kolb KH, Schulze PE. Über 2-Benzolsulfonylamino- 5(ß-methoxy-äthoxy) pyrimidin (Glycodiazin). V. In vitro- und in vivo-Versuche zum Einfluß von Phenyläthylbarbitursäure (Luminal) auf den Stoffwechsel und die blutzuckersenkende Wirkung des Glycodiazins. *Naunyn Schmiedebergs Arch Pharmakol Exp Pathol* (1966) 255, 200–220.

13

Antihistamines

Antihistamines (histamine H_1-antagonists) vary in their interaction profiles, which can be broadly described by considering them as two groups.

The older antihistamines (e.g. chlorphenamine (chlorpheniramine), diphenhydramine and hydroxyzine) are also referred to as sedating antihistamines. As the name suggests they have the potential to cause additive sedative effects with other sedating drugs. This type of interaction is discussed elsewhere, see 'CNS depressants + CNS depressants', p.1017. The sedating antihistamines also tend to have anticholinergic (or more correctly antimuscarinic) side effects and so therefore may interact additively with other anticholinergic-type drugs. This is also discussed elsewhere, see 'Anticholinergics + Anticholinergics', p.501.

The newer (or non-sedating antihistamines) have a low potential to cause sedative effects. Nevertheless, sedation may occur on rare occasions and patients should be advised to be alert to the possibility of drowsiness if they have not taken the drug before. Any drowsiness is likely to become apparent after the first few doses, and would indicate that additive sedative effects with other sedating drugs might be expected. The antihistamines are listed, by sedative potential, in 'Table 13.1', below.

Important drug interactions occur with astemizole and terfenadine. Raised serum levels of these two antihistamines can lengthen the QT interval and therefore cause cardiac arrhythmias (torsade de pointes). Therefore, dangerous interactions may result when the metabolism of astemizole or terfenadine is reduced by other drugs, usually those that inhibit the cytochrome P450 isoenzyme CYP3A4. Such drugs include the macrolide antibacterials and azole antifungals. Adverse interactions are also predicted when astemizole or terfenadine are used with other drugs that may also prolong the QT interval (see 'Drugs that prolong the QT interval + Other drugs that prolong the QT interval', p.170). Due to these potentially fatal interactions, astemizole has largely been withdrawn from many countries, while terfenadine has been reclassified in the UK as a prescription-only medicine. Apart from possibly ebastine and mizolastine, none of the other non-sedating antihistamines has been clearly shown to be associated with torsade de pointes arrhythmias, therefore, even when pharmacokinetic interactions result in increased levels, these are unlikely to be clinically important.

Some other interactions with antihistamines are dealt with elsewhere. A complete listing is to be found in the Index.

Table 13.1 Antihistamines (classified by sedative potential)

Significantly sedating	*Sedating*	*Non-sedating*
Dimenhydrinate	Brompheniramine	Acrivastine
Diphenhydramine	Buclizine	Astemizole
Doxylamine	Chlorphenamine	Azatadine
Hydroxyzine	Cinnarizine	Cetirizine
Promethazine	Clemastine	Desloratidine
Trimeprazine	Clemizole	Ebastine
	Cyclizine	Fexofenadine
	Cyproheptadine	Levocetirizine
	Dexchlorpheniramine	Loratadine
	Mebhydrolin	Mizolastine
	Mequitazine	Terfenadine
	Pheniramine	
	Tripelennamine	
	Triprolidine	

Antihistamines + Azoles

Because some of the azole antifungals can raise the plasma levels of astemizole and terfenadine causing serious and even life-threatening arrhythmias the concurrent use of all azoles is contraindicated with these two antihistamines. The makers also contraindicate mizolastine and azole antifungals. An isolated case describes an arrhythmia in one patient given terfenadine and topical oxiconazole.

Azelastine, cetirizine, desloratadine, emedastine, fexofenadine, levocabastine and loratadine seem to be free from clinically significant interactions with azole antifungals, although in some cases their serum levels may be raised.

Clinical evidence

(a) Astemizole

(i) Itraconazole. Itraconazole 200 mg or a placebo were given to 12 healthy subjects twice daily for 14 days, with a single oral 10-mg dose of astemizole on day 11. The peak plasma astemizole levels were slightly but not significantly increased by the itraconazole, but the AUC was approximately doubled and the half-life was increased from 2.1 to 3.6 days. The QTc interval was unaltered.[1]

(ii) Ketoconazole. A 63-year old woman developed torsade de pointes arrhythmia and was found to have a prolonged QT interval after taking astemizole and ketoconazole. These two drugs were withdrawn and she was successfully treated with a temporary pacemaker, magnesium sulphate and lidocaine (lignocaine). She was later discharged with a normal ECG.[2]

(iii) Miconazole. An *in vitro* study using human liver microsomal enzymes and ^{14}C-labelled compounds found that miconazole inhibits the metabolism of astemizole. On the basis of the values obtained it has been predicted that a clinically relevant interaction could occur *in vivo*.[3]

(b) Azelastine

In a three-period open-label study 12 healthy subjects were given azelastine 4 mg 12-hourly for 14 days, followed by a further 7 days with either 200 mg of **ketoconazole** or a placebo, daily. None of the treatments caused any significant ECG changes. Other *in vitro* studies indicated that no pharmacokinetic interaction is likely to occur *in vivo* between azelastine and **ketoconazole**.[4]

(c) Cetirizine

Two studies in healthy subjects found that 400 mg of **ketoconazole** daily for 10 days had no significant effect on the pharmacokinetics of cetirizine 20 mg daily. The pharmacokinetics of **ketoconazole** were unchanged, and there was no evidence that the QT_c interval was significantly prolonged. Any effects on QT_c were small and inconsistent.[5]

(d) Desloratadine

A 10-day placebo-controlled study in 24 healthy subjects found that 200 mg of **ketoconazole** twice daily raised the AUC of desloratadine 7.5 mg daily 1.39-fold and the maximum serum levels 1.45-fold. There were no statistical or clinically relevant changes in the ventricular rate, QT, PR, QRS or QTc intervals.[6] Tests to find out if desloratadine affected the QTc interval[7] showed that, even when using 45 mg daily (i.e. nine times the normal recommended dose) for 10 days, no prolongation of the QTc interval occurs (unlike with astemizole and terfenadine).

(e) Emedastine

Emedastine 4 mg daily was given to 12 healthy subjects for 10 days, with the addition of **ketoconazole** 200 mg twice daily from days 6 to 10. **Ketoconazole** reduced the clearance of emedastine by 30%, and increased the AUC by 33%. The QTc intervals remained the same, and the combination was well tolerated.[8]

(f) Fexofenadine

In two steady-state studies 24 healthy subjects were given 120 mg of fexofenadine twice daily (twice the recommended dose) for a week. It was found that the concurrent use of 400 mg of **ketoconazole** once daily increased the maximum fexofenadine serum levels by 135%, and the 12-hour AUC by 164%. The reasons are not known, but increased absorption and decreased biliary secretion have been suggested.[9] Fexofenadine had no effect on the pharmacokinetics of **ketoconazole**.[10]

Of far more importance than any changes in drug pharmacokinetics was the finding that the concurrent use of ketoconazole and fexofenadine had no effect on the QTc interval and no adverse events occurred, which contrasts markedly with the potentially life-threatening interactions of ketoconazole with terfenadine. Fexofenadine (a metabolite of terfenadine), does not affect the QT interval even in overdose in man (and quite massive overdosage in *animals*).[9,10]

(g) Levocabastine

In a randomised crossover study, 37 subjects were given 200 micrograms of a levocabastine nasal spray twice daily for 13 doses, with a single 200-mg dose of **ketoconazole** on day 7. **Ketoconazole** had no apparent effect on the pharmacokinetics of levocabastine.[11]

(h) Loratadine

A single 20-mg dose of loratadine was given to 12 healthy subjects while they were taking either 200 mg of **ketoconazole** or a placebo twice daily for 8 days. The maximum serum loratadine levels and its AUC were increased two- to threefold.[12] Another study in 24 healthy subjects on 10 mg of loratadine daily found that the addition of 200 mg of **ketoconazole** twice daily for 10 days raised the serum levels of loratadine and its metabolite by 300% and 73% respectively. However, no clinically relevant changes in ECGs (in particular the QTc interval) were seen, and no syncope or sedation was reported.[13]

(i) Mizolastine

The makers say that mizolastine is contraindicated with **systemic imidazole antifungals**[14] because **ketoconazole** increases the plasma levels of mizolastine by about 50%.[15] The implication is that this will increase its prolonging effects on the QT interval, which may result in an increased risk of cardiac arrhythmias (in particular torsade de pointes).

(j) Terfenadine

(i) Fluconazole. Terfenadine 60 mg 12-hourly was given to 6 healthy subjects for 6 days. None of them showed any evidence of accumulating terfenadine when additionally given 200 mg fluconazole daily for a week, and no significant ECG changes were seen.[16] By January 1993 no clinically significant interactions between terfenadine and fluconazole had been reported to the FDA.[16] However, a study in a group of healthy subjects taking terfenadine 60 mg 12-hourly, demonstrated a 52% rise in the terfenadine AUC while the subjects were additionally taking fluconazole 800 mg daily for a week. An increased QT_c was also seen.[17]

(ii) Itraconazole. A 26-year-old woman taking 60 mg terfenadine twice daily began to have fainting episodes on the third evening after starting to take 100 mg of itraconazole twice daily for vaginitis. When admitted to hospital the next morning her ECG showed a QT interval of 580 milliseconds and her heart rate was 67 bpm. Several episodes of torsade de pointes were recorded, and she fainted during two of them. No arrhythmias were seen 20 hours after the last itraconazole dose. Her QT interval returned to normal after 3 days. She was found to have terfenadine levels of 28 nanograms/ml in the first sample of serum taken (normally less than 5 nanograms/ml) and she still had levels of 12 nanograms/ml about 60 hours after taking the last tablet.[18,19] Two other similar cases have been reported,[20,21] and the FDA has on record four well-documented cases of severe cardiac complications due to this interaction.[22] Studies in healthy subjects confirm that itraconazole increases the AUC of terfenadine by 30%, almost doubles its half-life (from 3.4 to 6.3 hours), and prolongs the QT_c interval.[22]

(iii) Ketoconazole. A 39-year-old woman taking 60 mg terfenadine twice daily developed a number of episodes of syncope and light-headedness, preceded by palpitations, dyspnoea and diaphoresis, within 2 days of starting to take 200 mg ketoconazole twice daily. ECG monitoring revealed torsade de pointes and a QT_c interval of 655 milliseconds. Her terfenadine serum levels were 57 nanograms/ml (expected levels were 10 nanograms/ml or less). Other drugs being taken were cefaclor (stopped 3 to 4 days before the problems started) and medroxyprogesterone acetate. She had taken terfenadine and cefaclor on two previous occasions in the absence of ketoconazole without problems.[23,24] Other cases of an interaction between terfenadine and ketoconazole have also been reported.[25,26] Ketoconazole 400 mg daily for a week markedly increased the serum levels of single 120-mg doses of terfenadine in 12 healthy subjects (a rise from less than 10 up to 27 nanograms/ml). The clearance of the active metabolite of terfenadine was reduced by about 30% and its half-life prolonged almost threefold.[27] ECGs in patients given both drugs showed a prolongation of 10 to 20 milliseconds in the corrected QT interval when

they were compared to ECGs from patients on ketoconazole alone.[28] Ketoconazole 200 mg 12-hourly for 6 days increased the QT interval in 6 healthy subjects taking 60 mg terfenadine 12-hourly from 416 to 490 milliseconds, and raised the plasma terfenadine levels of all of them. Terfenadine serum levels increased to 81 nanograms/ml in one individual. Due to significant ECG repolarisation changes, four subjects were withdrawn before the course of ketoconazole was completed.[29]

(iv) Oxiconazole. A 25-year-old woman complained of palpitations and chest pain radiating down her left arm, and was also found to be having frequent ventricular premature beats in a pattern of bigeminy. On questioning it turned out that she was taking terfenadine and using a topical antifungal agent containing oxiconazole for ringworm on her arm. Both were stopped and her symptoms disappeared the following week.[30]

Mechanism

In vitro studies have shown that ketoconazole inhibits the metabolism of astemizole.[31] Ketoconazole, and to a lesser extent itraconazole and miconazole,[3,31] appear to reduce the metabolism of terfenadine by inhibition of the cytochrome P450 isoenzyme CYP3A.[32-34] High serum levels of astemizole and terfenadine (but not its metabolites) cause a prolongation of the QT interval and may precipitate the development of torsade de pointes arrhythmia. This has been seen in young otherwise healthy individuals after astemizole overdosage.[35-37] The risk of cardiac arrhythmias with other non-sedating antihistamines appears to be non-existent or very much lower, so any pharmacokinetic interactions do not result in clinically relevant toxicity.

Importance and management

The astemizole/ketoconazole, terfenadine/itraconazole, and terfenadine/ketoconazole interactions are established and clinically important, although much of the evidence for them is indirect. Poor metabolisers of terfenadine (in whom even normal doses may result in higher than average levels of terfenadine) are likely to be at particular risk. The risk of an interaction with terfenadine or astemizole and other azole antifungals seems smaller. The incidence is probably low, but because of the potential severity and unpredictability of this interaction, the concurrent use of astemizole and terfenadine is contraindicated with azole antifungals in all patients. This is a recommendation of the makers[38,39] and the CSM in the UK.[40] Use with mizolastine is also contraindicated.[14]

The cardiac safety of high-dose loratadine has been demonstrated,[41] so no clinically relevant interaction is expected, even if a rise in the serum levels of loratadine results. Azelastine, cetirizine, desloratadine, fexofenadine, levocabastine and loratadine seem to be free from clinically significant interactions and so may therefore provide a suitable alternative if a non-sedating antihistamine is needed in a patient on azole antifungals. The situation with emedastine is less clear.

1. Lefebvre RA, Van Peer A, Woestenborghs R. Influence of itraconazole on the pharmacokinetics and electrocardiographic effects of astemizole. *Br J Clin Pharmacol* (1997) 43, 319–22.
2. Tsai W-C, Tsai L-M, Chen J-H. Combined use of astemizole and ketoconazole resulting in torsade de pointes. *J Formos Med Assoc* (1977) 96, 144–6.
3. Lavrijsen K, Heykants J. Interaction potential of miconazole with the metabolism of astemizole and desmethylastemizole in human liver microsomes. Data on file, Janssen Research Foundation, N 102975/1, December 1993.
4. Morganroth J, Lyness WH, Perhach JL, Mather GG, Harr JE, Trager WF, Levy RH, Rosenberg A. Lack of effect of azelastine and ketoconazole coadministration on electrocardiographic parameters in healthy volunteers. *J Clin Pharmacol* (1997) 37, 1065–72.
5. UCB Pharma. Personal communication, September 1994.
6. Banfield C, Herron JM, Keung A, Pahdi D, Affrime M. Desloratadine has no clinically relevant electrocardiographic or pharmacodynamic interactions with ketoconazole. *Clin Pharmacokinet* (2002) 41 (Suppl 1), 37–44.
7. Neoclarityn (Desloratadine). Schering-Plough Ltd. UK Summary of product characteristics, July 2002.
8. Herranz U, Rusca A, Assandri A. Emedastine-ketoconazole: pharmacokinetic and pharmacodynamic interactions in healthy volunteers. *Int J Clin Pharmacol Ther* (2001) 39, 102–109.
9. Telfast (Fexofenadine hydrochloride). Aventis Pharma Ltd. UK Summary of product characteristics, September 2004.
10. Allegra (Fexofenadine hydrochloride). Aventis Pharmaceuticals Inc. US Prescribing Information, May 2003.
11. Hassell AE, Zhou H, Lee P, Wiesinger B, Mechlinski W, Gruver M, Algeo S, West M, Moore LRC. Effect of ketoconazole on the pharmacokinetics of steady-state intranasal levocabastine in healthy male volunteers. *J Clin Pharmacol* (1996) 36, 847.
12. Van Peer A, Crabbé R, Woestenborghs R, Heykants J, Janssens M. Ketoconazole inhibits loratadine metabolism in man. *Allergy* (1993) 48 (Suppl 16), 34.
13. Kosoglou T, Salfi M, Lim JM, Batra VK, Cayen MN, Affrime MB. Evaluation of the pharmacokinetics and electrocardiographic pharmacodynamics of loratadine with concomitant administration of ketoconazole or cimetidine. *Br J Clin Pharmacol* (2000) 50, 581–9.
14. Mizollen (Mizolastine). Schwarz Pharma Ltd. UK Summary of product characteristics, October 2003.
15. Dubruc C, Gillet G, Chaufour S, Holt B, Jensen R, Maurel P, Thenot JP. Metabolic interaction studies of mizolastine with ketoconazole and erythromycin in rat, dog and man. *Clin Pharmacol Ther* (1998) 63, 228.
16. Honig PK, Wortham DC, Zamani K, Mullin JC, Conner DP, Cantilena LR. The effect of fluconazole on the steady-state pharmacokinetics and electrographic pharmacodynamics of terfenadine in humans. *Clin Pharmacol Ther* (1993) 53, 630–6.
17. Cantilena LR, Sorrels S, Wiley T, Wortham D. Fluconazole alters terfenadine pharmacokinetics and electrocardiographic pharmacodynamics. *Clin Pharmacol Ther* (1995) 57, 185.
18. Pohjola-Sintonen S, Viitasalo M, Toivonen L, Neuvonen P. Torsades de pointes after terfenadine-itraconazole interaction. *BMJ* (1993) 306, 186.
19. Pohjola-Sintonen S, Viitasalo M, Toivonen L, Neuvonen P. Itraconazole prevents terfenadine metabolism and increases risk of torsades de pointes ventricular tachycardia. *Eur J Clin Pharmacol* (1993) 45, 191–3.
20. Crane JK, Shih H-T. Syncope and cardiac arrhythmia due to an interaction between itraconazole and terfenadine. *Am J Med* (1993) 95, 445–6.
21. Romkes JH, Froger CL, Wever EFD, Westerhof PW. Wegrakingen tijdens simultaan gebruik van terfenadine en itraconazol. *Ned Tijdschr Geneeskd* (1997) 141, 950–3.
22. Honig PK, Wortham DC, Hull R, Zamani K, Smith JE, Cantilena LR. Itraconazole affects single-dose terfenadine pharmacokinetics and cardiac repolarization pharmacodynamics. *J Clin Pharmacol* (1993) 33, 1201–6.
23. Monahan BP, Ferguson CL, Killeavy ES, Lloyd BK, Troy J, Cantilena LR. Torsades de pointes occurring in association with terfenadine use. *JAMA* (1990) 264, 2788–90.
24. Cantilena LR, Ferguson CL, Monahan BP. Torsades de Pointes occurring in association with terfenadine use. *JAMA* (1991) 266, 2375–6.
25. Zimmermann M, Duruz H, Guinand O, Broccard O, Levy P, Lacatis D, Bloch A. Torsades de pointes after treatment with terfenadine and ketoconazole. *Eur Heart J* (1992) 13, 1002–3.
26. Peck CC, Temple R, Collins JM. Understanding consequences of concurrent therapies. *JAMA* (1993) 269, 1550–2.
27. Eller MG, Okerholm RA. Pharmacokinetic interaction between terfenadine and ketoconazole. *Clin Pharmacol Ther* (1991) 49, 130.
28. Mathews DR, McNutt B, Okerholm R, Flicker M, McBride G. Torsades de pointes occurring in association with terfenadine use. *JAMA* (1991) 266, 2375–6.
29. Honig PK, Wortham DC, Zamani K, Conner DP, Mullin JC, Cantilena LR. Terfenadine-ketoconazole interaction. Pharmacokinetic and electrocardiographic consequences. *JAMA* (1993) 269, 1513–18.
30. Griffith JS. Interaction between terfenadine and topical antifungal agents. *Am Fam Physician* (1995) 51, 1396–7.
31. Lavrijsen K, Van Houdt J, Meuldermans W, Janssens M, Heykants J. The interaction of ketoconazole, itraconazole and erythromycin with the in vitro metabolism of antihistamines in human liver microsomes. *Allergy* (1993) 48 (Suppl 16), 34.
32. Lavrijsen K, Van Houdt J, Meuldermans W, Janssens M, Heykants J. The interaction of ketoconazole, itraconazole and erythromycin with the in vitro metabolism of antihistamines in human liver microsomes. *Allergy* (1993) 48 (Suppl 16), 34.
33. Jurima-Romet M, Crawford K, Cyr T, Inaba T. Terfenadine metabolism in human liver. In vitro inhibition by macrolide antibiotics and azole antifungals. *Drug Metab Dispos* (1994) 22, 849–57.
34. von Moltke LL, Greenblatt DJ, Duan SX, Harmatz JS, Shader RI. *In vitro* prediction of the terfenadine-ketoconazole pharmacokinetic interaction. *J Clin Pharmacol* (1994) 34, 1222–7.
35. Snook J, Boothman-Burrell D, Watkins J, Colin-Jones D. Torsade de pointes ventricular tachycardia associated with astemizole overdose. *Br J Clin Pract* (1988) 42, 257–9.
36. Craft TM. Torsade de pointes after astemizole overdose. *BMJ* (1985) 292, 660.
37. Bishop RO, Gaudry PL. Prolonged Q-T interval following astemizole overdose. *Arch Emerg Med* (1989) 6, 63–5.
38. Hismanal (Astemizole). Janssen-Cilag Ltd. UK Summary of product characteristics, June 1998.
39. Triludan (Terfenadine). Hoechst Marion Roussel Ltd. UK Summary of product characteristics, October 1998.
40. Committee on Safety of Medicines. Ventricular arrhythmias due to terfenadine and astemizole. *Current Problems* (1992) 35, 1–2.
41. Affrime MB, Lorber R, Danzig M, Cuss F, Brannan MD. Three month evaluation of electrocardiographic effects of loratadine in humans. *J Allergy Clin Immunol* (1993) 91, 259.

Antihistamines + Benzodiazepines and related drugs

Benzodiazepines impair psychomotor performance, but neither ebastine nor mizolastine (both non-sedating antihistamines) further impaired this. Similarly diphenhydramine did not alter the effects of zaleplon. An enhanced sedative effect would be expected with known sedative antihistamines.

Clinical evidence

(a) Diphenhydramine

A randomised single dose 3-period crossover study in healthy subjects found that diphenhydramine 50 mg had no significant effect on the pharmacokinetics of single 10-mg doses of **zaleplon**, despite the fact diphenhydramine is a moderate inhibitor of aldehyde oxidase, the primary metabolic pathway of **zaleplon**.[1]

(b) Ebastine

Ebastine 20 mg daily was found not to impair the performance of a number of psychomotor tests in 12 healthy subjects, although body sway and flicker fusion tests were altered. When given with **diazepam** 15 mg, ebastine did not further impair performance compared with diazepam alone, and ebastine did not alter plasma **diazepam** levels.[2]

(c) Mizolastine

Mizolastine appears to lack sedative effects, and does not have a detrimental effect on psychomotor performance.[3] A single 2-mg oral dose of **lorazepam** was found to impair the performance of psychomotor tests in 16 healthy subjects, and caused some sedation and amnesia, but these effects were not changed while the subjects were also taking 10 mg mizolastine daily for 8 days.[3]

Mechanism, importance and management

A number of older antihistamines cause sedation, and this would be expected to be increased by some of the benzodiazepines by the simple addition of their CNS depressant effects. Non-sedating antihistamines would not be expected to have this effect (but see also 'Antihistamines', (p.425)), and this has been confirmed for ebastine and mizolastine.

1. Darwish M. Overview of drug interaction studies with zaleplon. Poster presented at 13th Annual Meeting of Associated Professional Sleep Studies (APSS), Orlando, Florida, June 23rd, 1999.
2. Mattila MJ, Aranko K, Kuitunen T. Diazepam effects on the performance of healthy subjects are not enhanced by treatment with the antihistamine ebastine. *Br J Clin Pharmacol* (1993) 35, 272–77.
3. Patat A, Perault MC, Vandel B, Ulliac N, Zieleniuk I, Rosenzweig P. Lack of interaction between a new antihistamine, mizolastine, and lorazepam on psychomotor performance and memory in healthy volunteers. *Br J Clin Pharmacol* (1995) 39, 31–8.

Antihistamines + Drugs that prolong the QT interval

Astemizole[1] and terfenadine[2] should generally not be used with other drugs that can also prolong the QT interval (see 'Drugs that prolong the QT interval + Other drugs that prolong the QT interval', p.170). However, there do not appear to be any reports of QT prolongation with astemizole or terfenadine attributed solely to additive effects with these drugs. The primary risk of QT prolongation with astemizole and terfenadine appears to be from drugs that significantly inhibit their metabolism (e.g. see 'Antihistamines + Azoles', p.426 and 'Antihistamines + Macrolides', p.429). Clinically relevant QT prolongation has not yet been shown conclusively for any of the other antihistamines, although the makers of mizolastine[3] still contraindicate its use with drugs that prolong the QT interval.

1. Hismanal (Astemizole). Janssen-Cilag Ltd. UK Summary of product characteristics, June 1998.
2. Histafen (Terfenadine). Approved Prescription Services Ltd. UK Summary of product characteristics, December 1999.
3. Mizollen (Mizolastine). Schwarz Pharma Ltd. UK Summary of product characteristics, October 2003.

Antihistamines + Grapefruit juice

Grapefruit juice causes terfenadine to accumulate in the body, increasing the risk of serious cardiotoxicity (prolongation of the QTc interval) and the possibility of torsade de pointes arrhythmia. The absorption of fexofenadine is modestly reduced by grapefruit juice but astemizole and desloratadine do not appear to interact.

Clinical evidence

(a) Astemizole

The steady-state pharmacokinetics of astemizole in 12 healthy subjects given astemizole 30 mg daily for 4 days, then 10 mg daily for the next 20 days, was unaffected by 800 ml of grapefruit juice given as 200 ml every four hours.[1]

(b) Desloratadine

The bioavailability of a single 5-mg dose of desloratadine was unaffected by 8 oz (240 ml) of grapefruit juice given three times daily for 2 days preceding the desloratadine and then 5 minutes before and 4 hours after the dose.[2]

(c) Fexofenadine

The AUC of fexofenadine 60 mg was reduced by 30% in 23 healthy subjects by 8 oz (240 ml) of grapefruit juice given three times daily for 2 days before the fexofenadine and then 5 minutes before and 4 hours after the dose.[2]

(d) Terfenadine

Terfenadine 60 mg was given to 6 healthy subjects 12-hourly for 7 days, after which 240 ml double-strength grapefruit juice 12-hourly was added, and taken simultaneously with the terfenadine, for a further 7 days. Terfenadine was only detectable in the plasma while taking the grapefruit juice. The mean QTc interval was found to have risen from 420 to 434 milliseconds,[3,4] which is not of a magnitude usually considered to be clinically significant. The effects were less pronounced in a further 6 subjects who took the grapefruit juice 2 hours after the terfenadine.[4] Several other reports confirm these pharmacokinetics findings, although not all demonstrated changes in the QTc interval.[5-7]

Mechanism

Not fully understood, but it seems likely that some component of the juice inhibits the metabolism of the terfenadine to its active metabolite (by cytochrome P450 isoenzyme CYP3A4), so that the parent drug accumulates.[6] Terfenadine, but not its metabolite, causes QTc prolongation. Increased QTc intervals are associated with the development of ventricular tachycardia and torsade de pointes cardiac arrhythmias, which are potentially life-threatening.

Fexofenadine is a substrate for P-glycoprotein, and organic anion transporting polypeptide (both of which affect fexofenadine uptake). These transporters are inhibited by grapefruit juice, so grapefruit juice may reduce fexofenadine levels by preventing its absorption.[8]

Importance and management

The terfenadine/grapefruit juice interaction is established and potentially clinically important, the toxic effects of which may possibly only affect a small subset of individuals. As of 1996 neither the FDA nor the CSM appeared to have reports of problems in patients that were attributable to the use of antihistamines and grapefruit juice,[5,9] although in 1997 the CSM had one report of a probable interaction with terfenadine.[10] Nevertheless because of the risk (however small) of serious cardiotoxicity it would be prudent for all patients on terfenadine to avoid grapefruit juice, and at least one maker includes grapefruit juice among the contraindications.[11]

The evidence from healthy subjects suggests that astemizole does not interact, but it is possible that individuals predisposed to cardiac conduction disorders are at risk. It would seem to be prudent to avoid grapefruit juice with astemizole wherever possible.

Desloratadine and fexofenadine appear to be safe alternatives, although further study is required to determine the clinical relevance, if any, of the modest reduction in fexofenadine bioavailability in the presence of grapefruit juice.

1. Janssen-Cilag Ltd, Data on file (Study AST-BEL-7 + Amendment) 1995.
2. Banfield C, Gupta S, Marino M, Lim J, Affrime M. Grapefruit juice reduces the bioavailability of fexofenadine but not desloratadine. *Clin Pharmacokinet* (2002) 41, 311–18.
3. Benton R, Honig P, Zamani K, Hewett RN, Cantilena LR, Woosley RL. Grapefruit juice alters terfenadine pharmacokinetics resulting in prolongation of the QTc. *Clin Pharmacol Ther* (1994) 55, 146.
4. Benton RE, Honig PK, Zamani K, Cantilena LR, Woosley RL. Grapefruit juice alters terfenadine pharmacokinetics, resulting in prolongation of repolarization on the electrocardiogram. *Clin Pharmacol Ther* (1996) 59, 383–8.
5. Honig PK, Wortham DC, Lazarev A, Cantilena LR. Grapefruit juice alters the systemic bioavailability and cardiac repolarization of terfenadine in poor metabolizers of terfenadine. *J Clin Pharmacol* (1996) 36, 345–51.
6. Clifford CP, Adams DA, Murray S, Taylor GW, Wilkins MR, Boobis AR, Davies DS. The cardiac effects of terfenadine after inhibition of its metabolism by grapefruit juice. *Eur J Clin Pharmacol* (1997) 52, 311–15.
7. Rau SE, Bend JR, Arnold JMO, Tran LT, Spence JD, Bailey DG. Grapefruit juice–terfenadine single-dose interaction: magnitude, mechanism, and relevance. *Clin Pharmacol Ther* (1997) 61, 401–9.
8. Dresser GK, Bailey DG, Leake BF, Schwarz UI, Dawson PA, Freeman DJ, Kim RB. Fruit juices inhibit organic anion transporting polypeptide–mediated drug uptake to decrease the oral availability of fexofenadine. *Clin Pharmacol Ther* (2002) 71, 11–20.
9. Committee on Safety of Medicines/Medicines Control Agency. Drug interactions with grapefruit juice. *Current Problems* (1997) 23, 2.
10. Anon. Grapefruit juice and terfenadine: the "final straw". *Pharm J* (1997) 258, 618.
11. Histafen (Terfenadine). Approved Prescription Services Ltd. UK Summary of product characteristics, December 1999.

Antihistamines + H_2-blockers

No pharmacokinetic interaction appears to occur between cimetidine and cetirizine, ebastine or terfenadine, or between ranitidine and terfenadine or chlorphenamine. However, an isolated case report describes torsade de pointes in one patient on terfena-

dine and cimetidine. Cimetidine moderately raises hydroxyzine levels and considerably raises loratadine levels, but this is not thought to be of clinical significance.

Clinical evidence

(a) Cetirizine

Patients with chronic urticaria were given 10 mg cetirizine before and after taking 600 mg **cimetidine** 12-hourly for 10 days. The pharmacokinetics of cetirizine were statistically unaltered and its effects remained unchanged.[1]

(b) Chlorphenamine

A study in healthy subjects found that the pharmacokinetics of a single 4-mg dose of racemic chlorphenamine were unaffected by 6 days' treatment with 75 mg **ranitidine** twice daily.[2]

(c) Ebastine

Cimetidine 400 mg three times daily was found to have no significant effect on the conversion of single 20-mg doses of ebastine to carebastine in 12 healthy subjects, nor was there any evidence of any sedation or other side effects.[3]

(d) Hydroxyzine

In one study, patients with chronic urticaria were given 25 mg hydroxyzine before and after taking 600 mg of **cimetidine** 12-hourly for 10 days. The **cimetidine** increased the AUC of hydroxyzine by 33% and also increased its suppression of the wheal and flare response (although this was not statistically significant).[1] A previous study found that **cimetidine** raised serum hydroxyzine levels.[4]

(e) Loratadine

Loratadine 10 mg and **cimetidine** 300 mg six-hourly were given alone and together to 24 healthy subjects for 10 days. The AUCs of loratadine and its metabolite were increased by 203% and 106% respectively, but the safety profile of the loratadine (clinical laboratory tests, vital signs and adverse events) were unchanged. Cardiac repolarisation and all other ECG measurements were unaltered, and no sedation or syncope were seen.[5] Similar results were found in another study.[6] Very high levels of loratadine do not appear to be associated with cardiac arrhythmias.[7]

(f) Terfenadine

Five days' treatment with 1200 mg of **cimetidine** had no effect on the pharmacokinetics of a single 120-mg dose of terfenadine in 12 healthy subjects.[8] Another study in two groups of 6 healthy subjects confirmed that 600 mg of **cimetidine** 12-hourly or 150 mg **ranitidine** 12-hourly had no effect on the pharmacokinetics of terfenadine 60 mg 12-hourly. No adverse ECG changes were seen.[9] However, an isolated case report describes a 63-year-old woman who had 8 episodes of syncope (later identified as being due to torsade de pointes) and a convulsion 2 days after starting 60 mg terfenadine twice daily and 400 mg **cimetidine** twice daily. She was also taking chlorphenamine and co-proxamol (paracetamol (acetaminophen) and dextropropoxyphene (propoxyphene)).[10]

Mechanism

Cimetidine is a non-specific enzyme inhibitor, but it would seem that in most cases, with the exception of loratadine, these enzyme inhibitory effects do not affect the metabolism of antihistamines.

Importance and management

There would seem to be no good reason for avoiding the concurrent use of either cetirizine, ebastine, hydroxyzine, or loratadine with cimetidine, or chlorphenamine with ranitidine, nor would any of the other H_2-blockers be expected to interact with any of these antihistamines.

The situation with terfenadine and cimetidine is not totally clear because of the isolated case report of toxicity cited here, but currently there is not enough evidence to advise against the use of these two drugs.

1. Simons FER, Sussman GL, Simons KJ. Effect of the H_2-antagonist cimetidine on the pharmacokinetics and pharmacodynamics of the H_1-antagonists hydroxyzine and cetirizine in patients with chronic urticaria. *J Allergy Clin Immunol* (1995) 95, 685–93.
2. Koch KM, O'Connor-Semmes RL, Davis IM, Yin Y. Stereoselective pharmacokinetics of chlorpheniramine and the effect of ranitidine. *J Pharm Sci* (1998) 87, 1097–1100.
3. van Rooij J, Schoemaker HC, Bruno R, Reinhoudt JF, Breimer DD, Cohen AF. Cimetidine does not influence the metabolism of the H_1-receptor antagonist ebastine to its active metabolite carebastine. *Br J Clin Pharmacol* (1993) 35, 661–3.
4. Salo OP, Kauppinen K, Männistö PT. Cimetidine increases the plasma concentration of hydroxyzine. *Acta Derm Venereol (Stockh)* (1986), 66, 349–50.
5. Brannan MD, Affrime MB, Reidenberg P, Radwanski E, Lin CC. Evaluation of the pharmacokinetics and electrocardiographic pharmacokinetics of loratadine with concomitant administration of cimetidine. *Pharmacotherapy* (1994) 14, 347.
6. Kosoglou T, Salfi M, Lim JM, Batra VK, Cayen MN, Affrime MB. Evaluation of the pharmacokinetics and electrocardiographic pharmacodynamics of loratadine with concomitant administration of ketoconazole or cimetidine. *Br J Clin Pharmacol* (2000) 50, 581–9.
7. Affrime MB, Lorber R, Danzig M, Cuss F, Brannan MD. Three month evaluation of electrocardiographic effects of loratadine in humans. *J Allergy Clin Immunol* (1993) 91, 259.
8. Eller MG, Okerhold RA. Effect of cimetidine on terfenadine and terfenadine metabolite pharmacokinetics. *Pharm Res* (1991) 8 (10 Suppl), S-297.
9. Honig PK, Wortham DC, Zamani K, Conner DP, Mullin JC, Cantilena LR. Effect of concomitant administration of cimetidine and ranitidine on the pharmacokinetics and electrocardiographic effects of terfenadine. *Eur J Clin Pharmacol* (1993) 45, 41–6.
10. Ng PW, Chan WK, Chan TYK. Torsade de pointes during concomitant use of terfenadine and cimetidine. *Aust N Z J Med* (1996) 26, 120–1.

Antihistamines + Macrolides

Erythromycin causes terfenadine and astemizole to accumulate in a few individuals, which can lead to life-threatening torsade de pointes arrhythmias. Other macrolides are believed to interact similarly, with the exception of azithromycin and possibly dirithromycin. The makers of mizolastine contraindicate erythromycin, although the evidence for an interaction is poor. There is a slight prolongation of the QT interval with ebastine/erythromycin, and there is an isolated case of torsade de pointes possibly due to spiramycin/mequitazine.

Azelastine, cetirizine, desloratadine, fexofenadine, levocabastine, and loratadine seem to be free of clinically relevant interactions with macrolides, although in some cases their serum levels may be raised.

Clinical evidence

(a) Astemizole

(i) Azithromycin. The makers of astemizole report that an *in vivo* study has shown that azithromycin had a negligible effect on the bioavailability of astemizole.[1]

(ii) Dirithromycin. A 10-day course of dirithromycin 500 mg daily or a placebo was given to 18 healthy subjects, and on day 4 they were additionally given a single 30-mg oral dose of astemizole. It was found that the pharmacokinetics of the major metabolite of astemizole (*N*-desmethylastemizole) were unchanged by the dirithromycin, whereas the astemizole clearance was reduced by 34%, the volume of distribution increased by 24% and the half-life extended from 25 to 45.9 hours. However, no changes in the mean QTc intervals were seen.[2]

(iii) Erythromycin. An 87-year-old woman collapsed suddenly in her kitchen 4 days after starting to take 10 mg of astemizole daily and a tablet of erythromycin (unknown strength) twice daily. An ECG showed her to be having multiple episodes of torsade de pointes arrhythmia, the longest of 17 seconds duration. Her QT_c was 720 milliseconds and she was mildly hypokalaemic. She was given a temporary pacemaker and when eventually discharged with a normal sinus rhythm, her QT_c had fallen to 475 milliseconds.[3]

(b) Azelastine

An, open-label, crossover study in 8 healthy subjects found that when 500 mg **erythromycin** three times daily was added to 4 mg azelastine twice daily for a week, no changes in the pharmacokinetics of the azelastine were seen, suggesting that azelastine is not metabolised by the cytochrome P450 isoenzyme CYP3A4, since erythromycin is a potent inhibitor of this isoenzyme. There were no adverse ECG changes when both drugs were given concurrently.[4]

(c) Cetirizine

Two studies in healthy subjects found that **erythromycin** 500 mg 8-hourly for 10 days had no significant effect on the pharmacokinetics of cetirizine 20 mg daily. The pharmacokinetics of erythromycin were unchanged, and there was no evidence that the QT_c interval was significantly prolonged. Any effects on QT_c were small and inconsistent.[5]

(d) Desloratadine

(i) Azithromycin. In a randomised placebo-controlled study, 18 healthy subjects were given desloratadine 5 mg daily for 7 days, with 500 mg azithromycin on day 3 followed by a further 4 days of azithromycin 250 mg

daily. When the results were compared with those from another 18 subjects given placebo it was found that azithromycin had only minor effects on the pharmacokinetics of desloratadine, and no ECG changes occurred.[6]

(ii) Erythromycin. A 10-day study in 24 healthy subjects found that 500 mg erythromycin 8-hourly raised the AUC of desloratadine 7.5 mg daily by 10% compared with a placebo, and the maximum serum levels were raised by 20%. There were no statistical or clinically relevant changes in the ventricular rate, QT, PR, QRS or QTc intervals.[7]

(e) Ebastine

A blinded crossover study in 30 healthy subjects taking 20 mg ebastine daily found that the concurrent use of **erythromycin** 2.4 g daily for 10 days more than doubled the maximum ebastine plasma levels from 8.5 to 18.6 nanograms/ml, and almost tripled the AUC. The maximum plasma levels of carebastine (the active metabolite of ebastine) were doubled, and the AUC was almost tripled. Ebastine alone increased the QTc interval by 6.1 milliseconds, **erythromycin** alone increased it by 8.9 milliseconds, and together they increased it by 19.6 milliseconds.[8]

(f) Fexofenadine

(i) Azithromycin. In a randomised placebo-controlled study, 18 healthy subjects were given fexofenadine 60 mg twice daily for 7 days, with 500 mg of azithromycin on day 3 followed by a further 4 days of azithromycin 250 mg daily. When the results were compared with those from another 18 subjects given placebo, it was found that azithromycin increased the fexofenadine serum levels and AUC by almost 70%. However, no significant differences were noted in the ECGs.[6]

(ii) Erythromycin. Two steady-state studies in 24 healthy subjects given 120 mg of fexofenadine twice daily (twice the recommended dose) for a week found that the concurrent use of 500 mg of erythromycin 8-hourly increased the maximum fexofenadine serum levels by 82%, and the 12-hour AUC by 109%. Fexofenadine had no effect on the pharmacokinetics of erythromycin.[9] Of far more importance than any change in drug pharmacokinetics was the finding that the concurrent use of these two drugs had no effect on the QTc interval and no adverse events occurred. Fexofenadine is a metabolite of terfenadine, which even in overdose does not affect the QT interval.[9,10]

(g) Levocabastine

Levocabastine 200 micrograms twice daily for 6 days, plus a single dose on day 7 was given to 38 healthy subjects in the form of a nasal spray. On day 7 they were also given a single oral dose of **erythromycin** 333 mg or a placebo. The **erythromycin** was found to have no effect on the steady-state serum levels of levocabastine.[11]

(h) Loratadine

(i) Clarithromycin. Loratadine 10 mg and clarithromycin 500 mg 12-hourly were given alone and together to 24 healthy subjects for 10 days. The AUCs of loratadine and its active metabolite were increased by 76% and 49% respectively, and the maximum serum levels were increased by 36% and 69% respectively. The maximum QTc interval was slightly increased (by 3%), but no QTc exceeded 439 milliseconds and there was no evidence that concurrent use caused any cardiotoxicity.[12]

(ii) Erythromycin. Loratadine 10 mg daily and erythromycin 500 mg 8-hourly were given alone and together to 24 healthy subjects for 10 days. The AUCs of loratadine and its active metabolite were increased by about 40%, but the ECGs showed no changes in the QTc interval or any evidence of cardiotoxicity.[13] A study of loratadine alone in 50 healthy subjects found that 40 mg of loratadine daily (four times the recommended dose) for 90 days caused no changes in the ECG measurements, no episodes of dizziness or syncope, and no arrhythmias.[14]

(i) Mequitazine

A 21-year-old woman with a congenital long QT syndrome had several syncopal attacks, one at least of which was caused by torsade de pointes. This was attributed to the concurrent use of mequitazine and **spiramycin** over a 2-day period. The problem resolved when the drugs were withdrawn.[15]

(j) Mizolastine

When **erythromycin** 1 g twice daily was taken by 12 healthy subjects with 10 mg mizolastine daily for a week, the maximum serum levels of the mizolastine were increased by 40% and its AUC was increased by 53%. More importantly no significant changes were seen in QT or QTc intervals when compared with the values seen before treatment.[16] A further study of mizolastine alone, showed that increasing the dosage of mizolastine fourfold (to 40 mg daily) over a week had no effect on any ECG parameters, including the QT interval, in a group of healthy subjects.[17]

(k) Terfenadine

(i) Azithromycin. No measurable plasma terfenadine was found in healthy subjects taking terfenadine 60 mg twice daily when given 250 mg azithromycin daily for 5 days,[18,19] nor were there any changes in the QT_c interval.[19]

(ii) Clarithromycin. Clarithromycin 500 mg twice daily for 7 days increased the mean AUC of the acid metabolite of terfenadine two to threefold in 6 healthy subjects who were taking 60 mg twice daily. Four of them had detectable terfenadine in their serum (normally undetectable).[18] Almost identical results were found in another study in 14 healthy subjects, two of whom had detectable plasma terfenadine levels.[20]

(iii) Dirithromycin. Terfenadine 60 mg twice daily was given to 6 healthy subjects for 8 days, after which dirithromycin 500 mg daily was added for a further 10 days. No terfenadine was detectable (i.e. the levels were less than 5 nanograms/ml) in 5 subjects throughout the study, but the remaining subject had a maximum of 8.1 nanograms/ml on terfenadine alone, and 7.2 nanograms/ml when the dirithromycin was added. Their mean QTc was 369 milliseconds on terfenadine alone and 367 milliseconds on terfenadine plus dirithromycin. No changes in the pharmacokinetics of the acid metabolite of terfenadine were seen.[21]

(iv) Erythromycin. A 18-year-old girl who was taking 60 mg of terfenadine twice daily and 250 mg of erythromycin 6-hourly, fainted while at school and, when later hospitalised, was seen to have repeated episodes of ventricular tachycardia and ventricular fibrillation requiring resuscitation. Later she was also noted to have torsade de pointes. Her QTc interval was found to be prolonged at 630 milliseconds. The drugs were withdrawn and 9 days later, after a period in intensive care she was discharged symptom free, with a normal QTc interval.[22]

Nine subjects on terfenadine 60 mg 12-hourly showed a 107% rise in the maximum serum levels of the acid metabolite of terfenadine, and a 170% rise in its AUC after additionally taking 500 mg of erythromycin three times daily for a week. Three of the 9 subjects accumulated terfenadine in their serum (normally undetectable). These 3 subjects showed an increase in the QT_c interval of 33 milliseconds on terfenadine alone, and 64 milliseconds on the combination, whereas the other patients had no statistically significant rise in QTc interval.[23] One subject showed pronounced notching of the T wave. Another study by the same research group confirmed that erythromycin increases the AUC of terfenadine and prolongs the QT interval.[18] These studies seem to contrast with yet another, which found that 1 g of erythromycin daily for 5 days had little effect on the serum levels of either terfenadine or its metabolite after taking a single 120-mg dose, and no additional prolongation of the QT interval occurred.[24,25] Another retrospective report found no documented cardiac adverse events in 92 patients who had received erythromycin and terfenadine.[26]

(v) Troleandomycin. The makers of terfenadine have on record a case of a woman with a history of aortic valve disease, who suffered an episode of torsade de pointes arrhythmia while taking troleandomycin. She had taken more than the maximum recommended dose of terfenadine.[27] Another woman taking 60 mg of terfenadine three times daily developed torsade de pointes arrhythmia and a prolonged QTc interval when troleandomycin 500 mg three times daily was added. She recovered when both were stopped, but again developed a significantly prolonged QTc interval when both were restarted.[28]

Mechanism

Some macrolides (particularly erythromycin and clarithromycin) appear to reduce the metabolism of terfenadine and astemizole by inhibition of the cytochrome P450 isoenzyme CYP3A.[29,30] In the case of terfenadine, metabolism is only inhibited in a small number of susceptible individuals[18,24] and therefore only a few show terfenadine serum rises. High serum levels of astemizole[31] (and even normal levels in some cases[32]) and high serum levels of terfenadine (which appears to have a quinidine-like action[33]) cause a prolongation of the QT interval and may precipitate the development of torsade de pointes arrhythmia. Loratadine metabolism is similarly affected by macrolides,[34-36] but high loratadine levels are not significantly toxic and so no arrhythmias result.[14] Dirithromycin and azithromycin appear not to inhibit the metabolism of terfenadine.[18,19,21] The increased levels of fexofenadine with erythromycin may be due to increased absorption and decreased biliary secretion.[10]

Importance and management

The interactions of terfenadine with erythromycin, clarithromycin, and troleandomycin; and astemizole with erythromycin are established, clinically important and potentially hazardous. In fact only erythromycin and troleandomycin have actually been directly implicated, but the prolongation of the QT_c interval which occurs with clarithromycin indicates that it is also unsafe, and there is indirect evidence that **josamycin** will interact similarly. From the reports above it does seem that only a very few individuals develop a clinically important adverse interaction with these macrolides, but identifying them in advance is not often practical.

Because of the unpredictability and potential severity of this interaction, the FDA,[26] the CSM[37] in the UK and the makers of terfenadine[38] and astemizole[1] now contraindicate macrolide antibacterials in anyone taking terfenadine or astemizole. The only exception to this is azithromycin with astemizole.[1] The makers of mizolastine also contraindicate the concurrent use of the macrolides,[39] despite the absence of any ECG changes seen with either mizolastine given alone in doses four times the usual, or when given with erythromycin. Cetirizine and loratadine appear to be suitable alternative non-sedating non-interacting antihistamines to use with macrolides. Although there is much less evidence, and this needs confirming, azelastine, desloratadine, fexofenadine, and levocabastine also seem to lack a significant interaction. The isolated case with mequitazine is unlikely to be of general importance, since this drug is not usually associated with causing ventricular arrhythmias. The clinical significance of the ebastine/erythromycin interaction needs further study.

1. Hismanal (Astemizole). Janssen-Cilag Ltd. UK Summary of product characteristics, June 1998.
2. Bachmann K, Sullivan TJ, Reese JH, Jauregui L, Miller K, Scott M, Stotka J, Harris J. A study of the interaction between dirithromycin and astemizole in healthy adults. *Am J Ther* (1997) 4, 73–9.
3. Goss JE, Ramo BW, Blake K. Torsades de pointes associated with astemizole (Hismanal) therapy. *Arch Intern Med* (1993) 153, 2705.
4. Sale M, Lyness W, Perhach J, Woosley R, Rosenberg A. Lack of effect of coadministration of erythromycin (ERY) with azelastine (AZ) on pharmacokinetic (PK) or ECG parameters. *Ann Allergy Asthma Immunol* (1996) 74, 91.
5. UCB Pharma. Personal communication, September 1994.
6. Gupta S, Banfield C, Kantesaria B, Marino M, Clement R, Affrime M, Batra V. Pharmacokinetic and safety profile of desloratadine and fexofenadine when coadministered with azithromycin: a randomized, placebo-controlled, parallel-group study. *Clin Ther* (2001) 23, 451–66.
7. Banfield C, Hunt T, Reyderman L, Statkevich P, Pahdi D, Affrime M. Lack of clinically relevant interaction between desloratadine and erythromycin. *Clin Pharmacokinet* (2002) 41 (Suppl 1), 29–35.
8. Gillen M, Pentikis H, Rhodes G, Chaikin P, Morganroth J. Pharmacokinetic (PK) and pharmacodynamic (PD) interaction of ebastine (EBA) and erythromycin (ERY). *Clin Invest Med* (1998) (Suppl), S20.
9. Allegra (Fexofenadine hydrochloride). Aventis Pharmaceuticals Inc. US Prescribing Information, May 2003.
10. Telfast (Fexofenadine hydrochloride). Aventis Pharma Ltd. UK Summary of product characteristics, September 2004.
11. Lee P, Zhou H, Hassell AE, Mechlinski W, Wiesinger B, Gruver M, Algeo S, Hunt T, Moore LRC. Effect of erythromycin on the pharmacokinetics of steady-state intranasal levocabastine in healthy male volunteers. *J Clin Pharmacol* (1996) 36, 847.
12. Carr RA, Edmonds A, Shi H, Locke CS, Gustavson LE, Craft JÇ, Harris SI, Palmer R. Steady-state pharmacokinetics and electrocardiographic pharmacodynamics of clarithromycin and loratadine after individual or concomitant administration. *Antimicrob Agents Chemother* (1998) 42, 1176–80.
13. Brannan MD, Reidenberg P, Radwanski E, Shneyer L, Lin C-C, Cayen MN, Affrime MB. Loratadine administered concomitantly with erythromycin: pharmacokinetic and electrocardiographic evaluations. *Clin Pharmacol Ther* (1995) 58, 269–78.
14. Affrime MB, Lorber R, Danzig M, Cuss F, Brannan MD. Three month evaluation of electrocardiographic effects of loratadine in humans. *J Allergy Clin Immunol* (1993) 91, 259.
15. Verdun F, Mansourati J, Jobic Y, Bouquin V, Munier S, Guillo P, Pagès Y, Boschat J, Blanc J-J. Torsades de pointes sous traitement par spiramycine et méquitazine. À propos d'un cas. *Arch Mal Coeur Vaiss* (1997) 90, 103–6.
16. Chaufour S, Holt B, Jensen R, Dubruc C, Deschamp C, Rosenzweig R. Interaction study between mizolastine, a new H_1 antihistamine, and erythromycin. *Clin Pharmacol Ther* (1998) 63, 214.
17. Chaufour S, Caplain H, Lilienthal N, L'Héritier C, Deschamps C, Rosenzweig P. Mizolastine, a new H_1 antagonist, does not affect the cardiac repolarisation in healthy volunteers. *Clin Pharmacol Ther* (1998) 63, 214.
18. Honig PK, Wortham DC, Zamani K, Cantilena LR. Comparison of the effect of the macrolide antibiotics erythromycin, clarithromycin and azithromycin on terfenadine steady-state pharmacokinetics and electrocardiographic parameters. *Drug Invest* (1994) 7, 148–56.
19. Harris S, Hilligoss DM, Colangelo PM, Eller M, Okerholm R. Azithromycin and terfenadine: lack of drug interaction. *Clin Pharmacol Ther* (1995) 58, 310–15.
20. Gustavson LE, Blahunka KS, Witt GF, Harris SI, Palmer RN. Evaluation of the pharmacokinetic drug interaction between terfenadine and clarithromycin. *Pharm Res* (1993) 10 (10 Suppl), S-311.
21. Goldberg MJ, Ring B, DeSante K, Cerimele B, Hatcher B, Sides G, Wrighton S. Effect of dirithromycin on human CYP3A *in vitro* and on pharmacokinetics and pharmacodynamics of terfenadine *in vivo*. *J Clin Pharmacol* (1996) 36, 1154–60.
22. Biglin KE, Faraon MS, Constance TD, Lieh-Lai M. Drug-induced torsades de pointes: a possible interaction of terfenadine and erythromycin. *Ann Pharmacother* (1994) 28, 282.
23. Honig PK, Woosley RL, Zamani K, Conner DP, Cantilena LR. Changes in the pharmacokinetics and electrocardiographic pharmacodynamics of terfenadine with concomitant administration of erythromycin. *Clin Pharmacol Ther* (1992) 52, 231–8.
24. Eller M, Russell T, Ruberg S, Okerholm R, McNutt B. Effect of erythromycin on terfenadine metabolite pharmacokinetics. *Clin Pharmacol Ther* (1993) 53, 161.
25. Mathews DR, McNutt B, Okerholm R, Flicker M, McBride G. Torsades de pointes occurring in association with terfenadine use. *JAMA* (1991) 266, 2375–6.
26. Schoenwetter WF, Kelloway JS, Lindgren D. A retrospective evaluation of potential cardiac side-effects induced by concurrent use of terfenadine and erythromycin. *J Allergy Clin Immunol* (1993) 91, 259.
27. Marion Merrell Dow. Personal Communication, August 1993.
28. Fournier P, Pacouret G, Charbonnier B. Une nouvelle cause de torsades de pointes: association terfénadine et troléandomycine. *Ann Cardiol Angeiol (Paris)* (1993) 42, 249–52.
29. Yun C-H, Okerholm RA, Guengerich FP. Oxidation of the antihistaminic drug terfenadine in human liver microsomes. Role of cytochrome P-450 3A(4) in *N*-dealkylation and C-hydroxylation. *Drug Metab Dispos* (1993) 21, 403–9.
30. Jurima-Romet M, Crawford K, Cyr T, Inaba T. Terfenadine metabolism in human liver. In vitro inhibition by macrolide antibiotics and azole antifungals. *Drug Metab Dispos* (1994) 22, 849–57.
31. Snook J, Boothman-Burrell D, Watkins J, Colin-Jones D. Torsade de pointes ventricular tachycardia associated with astemizole overdose. *Br J Clin Pract* (1988) 42, 257–9.
32. Simons FER, Kesselman MS, Giddins NG, Pelech AN, Simons KJ. Astemizole-induced torsade de pointes. *Lancet* (1988) ii, 624.
33. Woosley RL, Chen Y, Freiman JP. Mechanism of the cardiotoxic actions of terfenadine. *JAMA* (1993) 269, 1532–6.
34. Lavrijsen K, Van Houdt J, Meuldermans W, Janssens M, Heykants J. The interaction of ketoconazole, itraconazole and erythromycin with the in vitro metabolism of antihistamines in human liver microsomes. *Allergy* (1993) 48 (Suppl 16), 34.
35. Yumibe N, Huie K, Chen KJ, Clement RP, Cayen MN. Identification of human liver cytochrome P450s involved in the microsomal metabolism of the antihistaminic drug loratadine. *J Allergy Clin Immunol* (1994) 93, 234.
36. Brannan MD, Affrime MB, Radwanski E, Cayen MN, Banfield C. Effects of various cytochrome P450 inhibitors on the metabolism of loratadine. *Clin Pharmacol Ther* (1995) 57, 193.
37. Committee on Safety of Medicines. Ventricular arrhythmias due to terfenadine and astemizole. *Current Problems* (1992) 35, 1–2.
38. Histafen (Terfenadine). Approved Prescription Services Ltd. UK Summary of product characteristics, December 1999.
39. Mizollen (Mizolastine). Schwarz Pharma Ltd. UK Summary of product characteristics, October 2003.

Antihistamines + Nefazodone

Nefazodone inhibits the metabolism of terfenadine and thereby prolongs the QT interval. Unexpectedly, there is also evidence that it increases the QT interval with loratadine. *In vitro* evidence suggests nefazodone will also inhibit the metabolism of astemizole.

Clinical evidence, mechanism, importance and management

(a) Astemizole

The makers of nefazodone say that an *in vitro* study also suggests that nefazodone may increase astemizole levels, and so concurrent use is contraindicated.[1] This is a predicted interaction, the clinical importance of which awaits confirmation.[2]

(b) Loratadine

A randomised, placebo-controlled study in healthy subjects found that when they were given nefazodone 300 mg twice daily, with loratadine 20 mg once daily the loratadine AUC was increased by 39%. Similarly, the QTc interval was increased with the combination, but only by 21.6 milliseconds.[3] This finding is in direct contrast with a number of other studies that have found no QTc prolongation with high doses of loratadine alone (40 mg daily),[4] or when combined with drugs, such as ketoconazole (see 'Antihistamines + Azoles', p.426), that markedly increase its plasma levels.

(c) Terfenadine

In a randomised, placebo-controlled study, healthy subjects were given nefazodone 300 mg twice daily, terfenadine 60 mg twice daily or the combination. Nefazodone caused about a fivefold increase in terfenadine AUC, which was associated with a mean increase in the QTc interval of 42.4 milliseconds. This was considered to be clinically significant, increasing the risk of torsade de pointes arrhythmias.[3] Studies using human liver microsomes found that nefazodone is a moderately weak inhibitor of the *N*-dealkylation and *C*-hydroxylation of terfenadine.[5] Nefazodone is currently considered to be contraindicated with terfenadine,[1] and it has been suggested that this explains the lack of clinical reports.[5]

1. Robinson DS, Roberts DL, Smith JM, Stringfellow JC, Kaplita SB, Seminara JA, Marcus RN. The safety profile of nefazodone. *J Clin Psychiatry* (1996) 57 (Suppl 2), 31–8.
2. Hismanal (Astemizole). Janssen-Cilag Ltd. UK Summary of product characteristics, June 1998.
3. Abernethy DR, Barbey JT, Franc J, Brown KS, Feirrera I, Ford N, Salazar DE. Loratadine and terfenadine interaction with nefazodone; both antihistamines are associated with QTc prolongation. *Clin Pharmacol Ther* (2001) 69; 96–103.
4. Affrime MB, Lorber R, Danzig M, Cuss F, Brannan MD. Three month evaluation of electrocardiographic effects of loratadine in humans. *J Allergy Clin Immunol* (1993) 91, 259.
5. Jurima-Romet M, Wright M, Neigh S. Terfenadine-antidepressant interactions: an *in vitro* inhibition study using human liver microsomes. *Br J Clin Pharmacol* (1998) 45, 318–21.

Antihistamines + Oral contraceptives

The pharmacokinetics of doxylamine and diphenhydramine appear not to be altered by the concurrent use of oral contraceptives.

Clinical evidence, mechanism, importance and management

The pharmacokinetics of 25 mg of **doxylamine** in 13 subjects and the pharmacokinetics of 50 mg of **diphenhydramine** in 10 subjects were not significantly altered by the use of low dose combined oral contraceptives.[1] Cases of oral contraceptive failure have been attributed to the use of **doxylamine**, **chlorpheniramine**, and an unnamed antihistamine,[2] but these antihistamines were all used in conjunction with penicillins, which would seem to be a more likely cause of contraceptive failure (see 'Oral contraceptives + Antibacterials; Penicillins', p.746, for further information). Therefore no particular precautions would seem to be necessary during concurrent use.

1. Luna BG, Scavone JM, Greenblatt DJ. Doxylamine and diphenhydramine pharmacokinetics in women on low-dose estrogen oral contraceptives. *J Clin Pharmacol* (1989) 29, 257–60.
2. DeSano EA, Hurley SC. Possible interactions of antihistamines and antibiotics with oral contraceptive effectiveness. *Fertil Steril* (1982) 37, 853–4.

Antihistamines + Protease inhibitors

Nelfinavir markedly increases terfenadine levels. Other protease inhibitors are predicted to interact similarly.

Clinical evidence, mechanism, importance and management

Nelfinavir 750 mg 8-hourly for 5 days raised the levels of a single 60-mg dose of **terfenadine** from less than 5 nanograms/ml to a range of 5 to 15 nanograms/ml. The pharmacokinetics of **nelfinavir** were unaffected.[1] This rise in terfenadine levels is predicted to prolong the QT interval, and to increase the risk of torsade de pointes arrhythmias. Other protease inhibitors are predicted to interact similarly with **terfenadine**, and also with **astemizole**, and consequently these two antihistamines are generally contraindicated with protease inhibitors. Because of the seriousness of this reaction, and the fact that it is not possible to predict individuals who will be affected, this seems a sensible precaution.

1. Kerr B, Yuep G, Daniels R, Quart B, Kravcik S, Sahai J, Anderson R. Strategic approach to nelfinavir mesylate (NFV) drug interactions involving CYP3A metabolism. 6th European Conference on Clinical Aspects and Treatment of HIV-infection, Hamburg, October 11–15th 1997. Abstracts.

Antihistamines + SSRIs

Two isolated reports provide some evidence of cardiotoxicity attributed to the concurrent use of terfenadine and fluoxetine, although other evidence suggests an interaction is unlikely. Terfenadine and paroxetine or sertraline do not appear to interact. Nonetheless, the makers of astemizole and terfenadine contraindicate the concurrent use of SSRIs.

Clinical evidence

(a) Astemizole

The makers of astemizole contraindicate the concurrent use of SSRIs because there is a risk that they will inhibit its metabolism, leading to a rise in its serum levels, which could result in QT interval prolongation and the development of torsade de pointes arrhythmias.[1]

(b) Loratadine

Fluoxetine inhibits the cytochrome P450 isoenzymes CYP3A4 and CYP2D6, isoenzymes involved in the metabolism of loratadine. However, because of the safety of high-dose loratadine,[2] no clinically relevant interaction is expected, even if fluoxetine causes a rise in the serum levels of loratadine.

(c) Terfenadine

(i) Fluoxetine. A 41-year-old man with no previous history of heart disease awoke one night short of breath, with a sensation of his heart missing beats and beating irregularly. He also experienced orthostatic hypotension on a number of occasions. However, a later ECG showed a normal sinus rhythm. He was taking daily doses of terfenadine 120 mg, fluoxetine 20 mg (started a month previously), ibuprofen 2400 mg, misoprostol 400 micrograms, *Midrin* (paracetamol (acetaminophen), dichloralphenazone, isometheptene mucate) and ranitidine 300 mg. A few days after stopping the terfenadine, and 12 days after this episode, his cardiac rhythm as recorded by a 24-hour Holter monitor showed some minor abnormalities (intermittent sinus tachycardia, isolated premature beats) but nothing approaching the previous alarming episode.[3] A woman taking several drugs (topical aciclovir, beclometasone, pseudoephedrine, ibuprofen) showed a lengthened QT_c interval of 550 milliseconds two weeks after starting terfenadine and fluoxetine, but she remained asymptomatic. Within a week of stopping the terfenadine her QT_c interval had returned to normal.[4]
In contrast, 12 healthy subjects who were given a single 60-mg dose of terfenadine before and after taking 60 mg fluoxetine daily for 8 days showed no significant changes in the pharmacokinetics of terfenadine or its acid metabolite.[5] Other *in vitro* studies with human liver microsomal enzymes confirmed that fluoxetine has only a very slight inhibitory effect on the metabolism of terfenadine, which was considered to be clinically irrelevant.[6]

(ii) Paroxetine. A two-period crossover study in 11 healthy subjects given 60 mg of terfenadine twice daily found that the concurrent use of paroxetine 20 mg daily for 8 days had no effect on the AUC of terfenadine or the QTc interval. A small, clinically unimportant reduction in the levels of carboxyterfenadine was seen. It was concluded that there is no clinically relevant interaction between terfenadine and paroxetine.[7] *In vitro* studies with human liver microsomal enzymes confirmed that paroxetine has only a very slight inhibitory effect on the metabolism of terfenadine, which is considered to be clinically insignificant.[6]

(iii) Sertraline. Although the UK Committee on Safety of Medicines (CSM) in the UK initially stated that terfenadine should not be used with sertraline, the CSM subsequently reviewed the data and now consider that an interaction is unlikely.[8]

Mechanism

Not understood. An *in vitro* model study using human liver microsomal enzymes, which accurately predicted a large and potentially hazardous interaction between terfenadine and ketoconazole or itraconazole (now clinically proven–see 'Antihistamines + Azoles', p.426), found that six SSRIs (desmethylsertraline, fluoxetine, fluvoxamine, norfluoxetine, paroxetine, sertraline) at usual clinical doses were at least 20 times less potent than ketoconazole at inhibiting terfenadine metabolism.[6] This suggests that all of these SSRIs are very unlikely to interact with terfenadine clinically, although the authors of the study warn that if high doses of SSRIs are used (particularly fluoxetine) some caution is appropriate.[6] Astemizole is metabolised in part by the cytochrome P450 isoenzyme CYP2D6, which also metabolises the SSRIs, and therefore interactions involving this isoenzyme are possible.

Importance and management

The SSRI/terfenadine interaction is not adequately established, and there is little evidence regarding SSRI/astemizole interactions, although it is possible that the contraindication with astemizole has contributed to minimal usage of the combination and therefore a lack of reported interactions. In addition to fluoxetine and paroxetine, the makers of terfenadine list fluvoxamine and citalopram as drugs that are expected to increase terfenadine serum levels,[9] but direct evidence of this seems to be lacking. Nonetheless, the maker contraindicates the use of all these SSRIs with terfenadine.[9] Due to the severity of the potential interaction, it would appear prudent to use caution if terfenadine is used with any SSRI (excepting perhaps sertraline), and consider an alternative antihistamine (such as loratadine) wherever possible.

1. Hismanal (Astemizole). Janssen-Cilag Ltd. UK Summary of product characteristics, June 1998.

2. Affrime MB, Lorber R, Danzig M, Cuss F, Brannan MD. Three month evaluation of electrocardiographic effects of loratadine in humans. *J Allergy Clin Immunol* (1993) 91, 259.
3. Swims MP. Potential terfenadine-fluoxetine interaction. *Ann Pharmacother* (1993) 27, 1404–5.
4. Marchiando RJ, Cook MD, Jue SG. Probable terfenadine-fluoxetine-associated cardiac toxicity. *Ann Pharmacother* (1995) 29, 937–8.
5. Bergstrom RF, Goldberg MJ, Cerimele BJ, Hatcher BL. Assessment of the potential for a pharmacokinetic interaction between fluoxetine and terfenadine. *Clin Pharmacol Ther* (1997) 62, 643–51.
6. von Moltke LL, Greenblatt DJ, Duan SX, Harmatz JS, Wright CE, Shader RI. Inhibition of terfenadine metabolism *in vitro* by azole antifungal agents and by selective serotonin reuptake inhibitor antidepressants: relation to pharmacokinetic interactions *in vivo*. *J Clin Psychopharmacol* (1996) 16, 104–112.
7. Martin DE, Zussman BD, Everitt DE, Benincosa LJ, Etheredge RC, Jorkasky DK. Paroxetine does not affect the cardiac safety and pharmacokinetics of terfenadine in healthy adult men. *J Clin Psychopharmacol* (1997) 17, 451–9.
8. Committee on Safety of Medicines/Medicines Control Agency. Sertraline and terfenadine. *Current Problems* (1998) 24, 4.
9. Histafen (Terfenadine). Approved Prescription Services Ltd. UK Summary of product characteristics, December 1999.

Antihistamines; Astemizole + Quinine

Quinine causes a marked but transient increase in plasma astemizole levels, and to avoid the possible risk of cardiac arrhythmias the makers contraindicate this combination. There are 3 reports that appear to confirm that this is a clinically important interaction.

Clinical evidence

Astemizole 30 mg daily for 4 days followed by 10 mg daily for the next 20 days, was given to 12 healthy subjects. The steady-state pharmacokinetics of the astemizole were then examined after the subjects took 20 mg of quinine 4-hourly for 12 hours (a total of 80 mg quinine), and after a single 430-mg dose of quinine. The smaller dose of quinine caused only a slight increase in the maximum plasma astemizole levels and AUC, but the larger single quinine dose resulted in a transient threefold increase in both maximum plasma levels and AUC, especially of desmethylastemizole, the metabolite of astemizole.[1]

A patient on astemizole with slight hypomagnesaemia is reported to have experienced torsade de pointes arrhythmia after taking only a single dose of quinine sulphate.[2] The makers have on record two other case reports[3] of cardiac arrhythmias possibly attributable to an astemizole/quinine interaction.

Mechanism

Uncertain. One suggestion is that the interaction is not primarily due to inhibition of the metabolism of astemizole by the quinine, but rather to a transient quinine-induced displacement of both astemizole and its metabolite from its tissue binding sites.[1]

Importance and management

Information is very limited, but on the basis of the evidence cited above the makers of astemizole contraindicate the concurrent use of quinine in order to avoid the risk of cardiac arrhythmias.[4] The case report that is cited here confirms that this is a potentially clinically hazardous drug combination.[2]

The larger single dose of 430 mg of quinine used in the study approached the dosage used for the treatment of malaria, whereas the smaller dose of 80 mg was equivalent to the amount contained in 2 litres of a quinine-containing soft drink.[1] There would therefore appear to be no reason for those on astemizole to avoid moderate quantities of these quinine-containing drinks. See also 'Drugs that prolong the QT interval + Other drugs that prolong the QT interval', p.170.

1. Janssen-Cilag Ltd, Data on file (Study AST-BEL-7 + Amendment) 1995.
2. Martin ES, Rogalski K, Black JN. Quinine may trigger torsades de pointes during astemizole therapy. *Pacing Clin Electrophysiol* (1997) 20, 2024–5.
3. Janssen-Cilag Ltd. Personal Communication, May 1997.
4. Hismanal (Astemizole). Janssen-Cilag Ltd. UK Summary of product characteristics, June 1998.

Antihistamines; Cinnarizine + Phenylpropanolamine

Phenylpropanolamine 50 mg counteracted the mild sedation caused by cinnarizine 25 or 50 mg, and improved the performance of some skills related to driving in 12 healthy subjects.[1]

1. Savolainen K, Mattila MJ, Mattila ME. Actions and interactions of cinnarizine and phenylpropanolamine on human psychomotor performance. *Curr Ther Res* (1992) 52, 160–8.

Antihistamines; Fexofenadine + Rifampicin (Rifampin)

Rifampicin increases the oral clearance of fexofenadine, but the clinical significance of this is unclear.

Clinical evidence, mechanism, importance and management

A single 60-mg dose of fexofenadine was given to 24 healthy subjects 2 days before and on the last day of a 6-day course of rifampicin 600 mg daily. The oral clearance of fexofenadine was increased 1.3- to 5.3-fold, with no effect on renal clearance or half life. This was thought to be due to the effect of rifampicin on P-glycoprotein, which is involved in the uptake of fexofenadine.[1] The clinical significance of this interaction is unclear, but until more is known it would seem prudent to monitor the efficacy of fexofenadine if it is given in combination with rifampicin.

1. Hamman MA, Bruce MA, Haehner-Daniels BD, Hall SD. The effect of rifampin administration on the disposition of fexofenadine. *Clin Pharmacol Ther* (2001) 69, 114–21.

Antihistamines; Hydroxyzine + Drugs that prolong the QT interval

Hydroxyzine can cause ECG abnormalities in high doses. It has been suggested that its use with other drugs that can cause cardiac abnormalities might increase the likelihood of arrhythmias and sudden death.

Clinical evidence, mechanism, importance and management

A study in 25 elderly psychotic patients on hydroxyzine 300 mg daily over a 9-week period showed that ECG changes were mild, except for alteration in T waves, which were definite in 9 patients. In each case the T waves were lower in altitude, broadened and flattened and sometimes notched. The QT interval was usually prolonged. In a repeat of the study in a few patients, at least one given hydroxyzine 400 mg, gave similar results, the most pronounced change being a marked attenuation of cardiac repolarisation. On the basis of these observations the authors suggest that other drugs that cause ECG abnormalities might aggravate and exaggerate these hydroxyzine-induced changes and increase the risk of sudden death.[1] More study is needed to assess the practical importance of these potential interactions, especially with lower doses of hydroxyzine. See also 'Drugs that prolong the QT interval + Other drugs that prolong the QT interval', p.170 and 'Table 7.3', (p.169) for a list of drugs shown to prolong the QT interval.

1. Hollister LE. Hydroxyzine hydrochloride: possible adverse cardiac interactions. *Psychopharmacol Comm* (1975) 1, 61–5.

Antihistamines; Terfenadine + Atorvastatin

No interaction appears to occur between atorvastatin and terfenadine.

Clinical evidence, mechanism, importance and management

A group of healthy subjects were given a single dose of terfenadine on day 7 of a 9-day course of atorvastatin 80 mg daily. It was found that the atorvastatin caused some small to moderate changes in the pharmacokinetics of the terfenadine and fexofenadine (AUC +35% and −2% respectively, maximum serum levels 8% and –16% respectively), none of which reached statistical significance. More importantly there were no changes in the QTc interval, which indicates that atorvastatin does not increase the cardiotoxicity of the terfenadine.[1] There would therefore appear to be no reason for avoiding concurrent use.

1. Stern RH, Smithers JA, Olson SC. Atorvastatin does not produce a clinically significant effect on the pharmacokinetics of terfenadine. *J Clin Pharmacol* (1998) 38, 753–7.

Antihistamines; Terfenadine + Paracetamol (Acetaminophen)

An isolated report describes the development of torsade de pointes arrhythmia in an old man on very large doses of paracetamol (acetaminophen) and amitriptyline when he began to take terfenadine.

Clinical evidence, mechanism, importance and management

An 86-year-old man on **amitriptyline** 25 mg nightly, prednisone 3 mg daily and excessive amounts of paracetamol (acetaminophen) – up to 1 g two-hourly over a 6-month period – developed breathlessness and bradycardia shortly after starting to take 60 mg terfenadine twice daily. In hospital he became unconscious and was initially pulseless but recovered spontaneously. An ECG showed that he had AV block and a prolonged QT interval, which resulted in runs of self-limiting torsade de pointes arrhythmia.[1] The reasons for this reaction are not known, but a suggested explanation is that overdosage with paracetamol produced large amounts of a metabolite (*N*-acetyl-p-benzoquinoneimine). This metabolite could have inhibited the metabolism of the terfenadine by the cytochrome P450 isoenzyme CYP3A4, thereby resulting in terfenadine accumulation and the development of its cardiotoxic effects.[1] The **amitriptyline** may additionally have had some part to play because it can also (although rarely) cause torsade de pointes.

This is an isolated case and unlikely to be of general importance. There would seem to be little reason on the basis of this report for patients on terfenadine to avoid normal therapeutic doses of paracetamol (acetaminophen). There appear to be no other reports of this interaction.

1. Matsis PP, Easthorpe RN. Torsades de pointes ventricular tachycardia associated with terfenadine and paracetamol self medication. *N Z Med J* (1994) 107, 402–403.

Antihistamines; Terfenadine + Venlafaxine

Venlafaxine does not appear to significantly interact with terfenadine.

Clinical evidence, mechanism, importance and management

A study in 24 subjects given a single 120-mg oral dose of terfenadine before and after taking venlafaxine 75 mg every 12 hours for 9 days found that the pharmacokinetic profile of terfenadine was unchanged, although its acid metabolite concentrations were slightly decreased.[1] This study was undertaken to confirm that venlafaxine lacks inhibitory activity on the cytochrome P450 isoenzyme CYP3A4, but at the same time it also indicates that venlafaxine does not raise the serum levels of terfenadine, which are associated with serious cardiotoxicity. There would therefore seem to be no reason for avoiding concurrent use.

1. Amchin J, Zarycranski W, Taylor K. Venlafaxine's lack of CYP3A4 inhibition assessed by terfenadine metabolism. *Clin Pharmacol Ther* (1997) 61,179.

Antihistamines; Terfenadine + Zileuton

Zileuton modestly increases terfenadine levels.

Clinical evidence, mechanism, importance and management

Terfenadine 60 mg 12-hourly for 7 days was given to 15 healthy subjects with either 600 mg of zileuton 6-hourly or a placebo. The mean 12-hour AUC and the maximum plasma concentrations of terfenadine increased by 35% in the presence of zileuton, but the levels were still very low (less than 5 nanograms/ml). The maximum plasma concentration and AUC of carboxyterfenadine (a terfenadine metabolite) were increased by about 15% while concurrently taking the zileuton. ECG measurements showed that the addition of zileuton did not increase the QTc interval nor cause any other significant changes.[1] The authors concluded that the interaction was unlikely to be of clinical significance.[1] However, the makers of terfenadine currently contraindicate zileuton, on the basis that any drug that inhibits terfenadine metabolism may result in accumulation of terfenadine and prolongation of the QT interval with risk of life-threatening arrhythmias.[2] Because of the unpredictability of these interactions, this seems a sensible precaution.

1. Awni WM, Cavanaugh JH, Leese P, Kasier J, Cao G, Locke CS, Dube LM. The pharmacokinetic and pharmacodynamic interaction between zileuton and terfenadine. *Eur J Clin Pharmacol* (1997) 52, 49–54.
2. Histafen (Terfenadine). Approved Prescription Services Ltd. UK Summary of product characteristics, December 1999.

14

Antimigraine drugs

The drugs dealt with in this section are the ergot derivatives and the triptans (or more properly the serotonin 5-HT_1 agonists), whose main use is in the treatment of migraine. 'Table 14.1', (below) lists some of the drugs commonly used in migraine. Drugs such as propranolol, which are more commonly used in other conditions, are discussed elsewhere in the publication.

Although the triptans would be expected to share a number of pharmacodynamic drug interactions, due to their differing metabolic pathways they will not all necessarily share the same pharmacokinetic interactions. For example, sumatriptan, which is metabolised mainly by monoamine oxidase A, is unlikely to interact with macrolide antibacterials, which are inhibitors of the cytochrome P450 isoenzyme CYP3A4. However, eletriptan, which is metabolised by CYP3A4 and possibly CYP2D6 could potentially interact (see 'Triptans + Macrolides', p.440 for full details). Frovatriptan and zolmitriptan are substrates for CYP1A2, and are affected by CYP1A2 inhibitors such as fluvoxamine, but zolmitriptan also inhibits CYP1A2 and may therefore be expected to have additional interactions. Rizatriptan, which possibly inhibits CYP2D6 (all be it at levels 10 times those expected clinically), is also likely to interact differently. Naratriptan appears unlikely to undergo significant pharmacokinetic interactions since half the dose is excreted unchanged and the rest metabolised by a variety of isoenzymes.

Early in the development of triptans it was theorised that they might possibly add to the increased levels of serotonin caused by other serotonergic drugs, leading to excess serotonergic activity and increasing the risk of the serotonin syndrome. Therefore sumatriptan was contraindicated in patients taking SSRIs, MAOIs, and lithium, but note, there is little evidence that this occurs in practice. However, there is also a pharmacokinetic interaction with some 'triptans and MAOIs', (see (p.440) or 'SSRIs', (p.441).

The main problem with the use of the ergot derivatives is that of ergotism. Drug interactions may result in additive effects or cause raised levels of ergot derivatives, which may result in the symptoms of ergot poisoning. This may include severe circulatory problems e.g. the extremities may become numb, cold to the touch, tingle, and muscle pain may result. In extreme cases there may be no palpable pulse. Ultimately gangrene may develop, and amputation may be required. Chest pain can also occur, and in some cases myocardial infarction has been reported.

Table 14.1 Antimigraine drugs

Group	*Drugs*
Antihistamines	Flunarizine, Pizotifen
Beta blockers	Atenolol, Metoprolol, Nadolol, Propranolol, Timolol
Ergot derivatives	Co-dergocrine, Ergotamine, Dihydroergotamine, Methysergide
Triptans (Serotonin (5-HT_1) agonists)	Almotriptan, Eletriptan, Frovatriptan, Naratriptan, Rizatriptan, Sumatriptan, Zolmitriptan

Ergot derivatives + Antidepressants

Three isolated cases of the serotonin syndrome have been seen in patients on amitriptyline, paroxetine/imipramine, or sertraline when given dihydroergotamine.

Clinical evidence

A woman on **imipramine**, **paroxetine** and lithium, who had a 3-week continuous headache, was treated with 300 micrograms of dihydroergotamine intravenously. Within 5 minutes of a subsequent 500-microgram dose she developed dysarthria, dilated pupils, diaphoresis, diffuse weakness, and barely responded to commands. She was diffusely hyperreflexic and showed occasional myoclonic jerks. She recovered after 90 minutes.[1]

A woman with a history of migraine headaches responded well to **amitriptyline**, metoclopramide, and dihydroergotamine. Six weeks after the **amitriptyline** was replaced by **sertraline**, she was again successfully treated for acute migraine with 10 mg of intravenous metoclopramide and 1 mg of intravenous dihydroergotamine. However, 2 hours later she developed nausea, emesis, agitation, weakness, diaphoresis, salivation, chills, and fever. All of the symptoms subsided after 24 hours.[1]

A woman with a history of migraines (treated prophylactically with **amitriptyline** and propranolol) was admitted to hospital in status migrainosus. She was given 1 mg of dihydroergotamine, 10 mg of prochlorperazine and 10 mg of metoclopramide (all intravenously). Within 20 minutes she became diaphoretic, tachycardic, diffusely hyperreflexic, agitated, confused, and briefly lost consciousness twice. Diazepam 8 mg given intramuscularly calmed her agitation, and all the symptoms resolved after 6 hours. A year later she was given 6 mg of subcutaneous sumatriptan while taking **nortriptyline** daily with no ill effects.[1]

Mechanism

Not understood. All of these patients appeared to have developed the serotonin syndrome, which is thought to be due to hyperstimulation of 5-HT receptors in the brain. Dihydroergotamine is a 5-HT agonist while paroxetine and sertraline are both serotonin (5-HT) reuptake inhibitors, all of which might be expected to increase 5-HT concentrations in the CNS, and thereby increase receptor stimulation.

Importance and management

These appear to be isolated cases and not of general importance, nevertheless they illustrate the potential for the development of the serotonin syndrome in patients given multidrug regimens that affect 5-HT receptors. The syndrome is rare and it may (so it has been suggested[1]) sometimes be an idiosyncratic reaction.

1. Mathew NT, Tietjen GE, Lucker C. Serotonin syndrome complicating migraine pharmacotherapy. *Cephalalgia* (1996) 16, 323–7.

Ergot derivatives + Glyceryl trinitrate (Nitroglycerin)

The ergot derivatives such as dihydroergotamine would be expected to oppose the anti-anginal effects of glyceryl trinitrate.

Clinical evidence, mechanism, importance and management

There seem to be no clinical reports of adverse interactions between these drugs, but since **ergot** causes vasoconstriction and can provoke angina it would be expected to oppose the effects of glyceryl trinitrate when used as a vasodilator for the treatment of angina. Ergot derivatives are regarded as contraindicated in those with ischaemic heart disease. However, glyceryl trinitrate has also been shown to increase the bioavailability of **dihydroergotamine** (by up to 370% in one case) in subjects with orthostatic hypotension, which would increase its vasoconstrictor effects.[1] The clinical outcome of concurrent use is therefore uncertain. Monitor well if the decision is taken to use both drugs.

1. Bobik A, Jennings G, Skews H, Esler M, McLean A. Low oral bioavailability of dihydroergotamine and first-pass extraction in patients with orthostatic hypotension. *Clin Pharmacol Ther* (1981) 30, 673–9.

Ergot derivatives + Macrolides

Ergot toxicity can develop rapidly in patients on ergotamine or dihydroergotamine if they are given erythromycin or troleandomycin. Three possible cases of toxicity have occurred with clarithromycin, and another case has been reported with josamycin. Toxicity is predicted to occur with midecamycin. No cases of toxicity appear to have been described with spiramycin, and none would be expected. There is no direct information about azithromycin.

Clinical evidence

(a) Azithromycin

It has been suggested that **ergot alkaloids** should be avoided with azithromycin, because clinically important interactions have been seen between these drugs and other macrolide antibacterials related to azithromycin.[1-3] However, there seems so far to be no direct evidence of any adverse interactions between **ergot alkaloids** and azithromycin, and the US makers say that concurrent use can be undertaken with careful monitoring.[4]

(b) Clarithromycin

A woman of 59 took **ergotamine tartrate** 2 mg for a typical migraine headache. After 2 hours her tongue became swollen, painful and bluish in colour. She showed some hypertension (BP 200/110 mmHg) and her fingers and toes were cold and cyanotic (blue). She had taken this dose of **ergotamine** many times previously without problems, but on this occasion she was on the fifth day of a course of clarithromycin 500 mg twice daily. This adverse reaction was diagnosed as ergotism. Other evidence suggests that this patient may possibly have been unusually sensitive to vascular occlusion.[5] The authors of this report briefly quote another case, originating from the makers of clarithromycin, of a possible **dihydroergotamine**/clarithromycin interaction, although this was complicated by the concurrent use of other medications (not named) used in the management of AIDS.[5] A woman who had previously uneventfully taken *Cafergot* (**ergotamine tartrate** 1 mg, caffeine 100 mg) for migraine developed ergotism (leg pain, cold and cyanosed limbs, and impalpable pulses) within 3 days of starting to take clarithromycin (dosage not stated). The authors postulated that **smoking** and the use of **oxymetazoline** (both of which have vasoconstrictor effects) may also have had some part to play.[6]

(c) Erythromycin

A woman who had regularly and uneventfully taken *Migral* (**ergotamine tartrate** 2 mg, cyclizine hydrochloride 50 mg, caffeine 100 mg) on a number of previous occasions, took one tablet during a course of treatment with erythromycin 250 mg every 6 hours. Within 2 days she developed severe ischaemic pain in her arms and legs during exercise, with a burning sensation in her feet and hands. When admitted to hospital 10 days later, her extremities were cool and cyanosed. Her pulse could not be detected in the lower limbs.[7]

Eight other cases of acute ergotism are reported elsewhere[8-15] involving **ergotamine tartrate** or **dihydroergotamine** and additional treatment with erythromycin. The reaction has been reported to develop within a few hours,[11] but it may take several days to occur.[14] One case appeared to occur when the erythromycin was started 3 days after the last dose of **dihydroergotamine**.[9]

(d) Josamycin

An isolated report describes a woman of 33 who developed severe ischaemia of the legs within 3 days of starting to take josamycin 2 g daily and capsules containing **ergotamine tartrate** 300 micrograms. Her legs and feet were cold, white and painful, and most of her peripheral pulses were impalpable.[16]

(e) Midecamycin diacetate (miocamycin)

After taking 800 mg of midecamycin diacetate twice daily for 8 days, peak concentrations of **dihydroergotamine** following single 9-mg doses were raised 3 to 40-fold in 12 healthy subjects.[17]

(f) Troleandomycin

A woman of 40 who had been taking **dihydroergotamine**, 90 drops daily, for 3 years without problems, developed cramp in her legs within a few hours of starting to take troleandomycin 250 mg four times a day. Five days later she was admitted to hospital as an emergency, with severe ischaemia of her arms and legs. Her limbs were cold and all her peripheral pulses were impalpable.[18]

There are reports of several other patients who had taken normal doses of **ergotamine tartrate** or **dihydroergotamine** for months or years without problems, who then developed severe ergotism within hours or days of starting to take normal doses of troleandomycin.[19-26] Myocardial infarction developed in one individual.[27]

Mechanism

Erythromycin and troleandomycin are potent inhibitors of the cytochrome P450 isoenzyme CYP3A4, an enzyme involved in the metabolism of ergot derivatives.[28] Clarithromycin is also known to inhibit CYP3A4. As a result the ergot is poorly metabolised and accumulates in the body. This leads to increased vasoconstriction and ultimately ischaemia. **Spiramycin**, and josamycin normally do not inhibit CYP3A4 and are therefore not expected to interact,[28] although a case has been reported.[16]

Importance and management

The interactions of ergot derivatives with erythromycin and troleandomycin are well documented, well established, and clinically important, whereas information about clarithromycin appears to be confined to three possible cases. There are no adverse reports about midecamycin, but it is expected to interact similarly. The concurrent use of all of these macrolides and ergot derivatives should be avoided. Some of the cases cited were effectively treated with sodium nitroprusside or naftidrofuryl oxalate, with or without heparin.[5,9,11-13,24] Spiramycin, and josamycin would not be expected to interact because they do not inhibit CYP3A4. However, there is one unexplained and unconfirmed report of an interaction with josamycin.[16]

1. Hopkins S. Clinical toleration and safety of azithromycin. *Am J Med* (1991) 91 (Suppl 3A), 40S–45S.
2. Zithromax (Azithromycin). Pfizer Ltd. UK Summary of product characteristics, July 2004.
3. Lode H. The pharmacokinetics of azithromycin and their clinical significance. *Eur J Clin Microbiol Infect Dis* (1991) 10, 807–12.
4. Zithromax (Azithromycin). Pfizer Laboratories. US Prescribing information, January 2004.
5. Horowitz RS, Dart RC, Gomez HF. Clinical ergotism with lingual ischemia induced by a clarithromycin-ergotamine interaction. *Arch Intern Med* (1996) 156, 456–8.
6. Ausband SC, Goodman PE. An unusual case of clarithromycin associated ergotism. *J Emerg Med* (2001) 21, 411–13.
7. Francis H, Tyndall A, Webb J. Severe vascular spasm due to erythromycin-ergotamine interaction. *Clin Rheumatol* (1984) 3, 243–6.
8. Lagier G, Castot A, Riboulet G, Boesh C. Un cas d'ergotisme mineur semblant en rapport avec une potentialisation de l'ergotamine par l'éthylsuccinate d'érythromycine. *Therapie* (1979) 34, 515–21.
9. Neveux E, Lesgourgues B, Luton J-P, Guilhaume B, Bertagna, Picard J. Ergotisme aigu par association proprionate d'érythromycine-dihydroergotamine. *Nouv Presse Med* (1981) 10, 2830.
10. Collet AM, Moncharmont D, San Marco JL, Eissinger F, Pinot JJ, Laselve L. Ergotisme iatrogène: rôle de l'association tartrate d'ergotamine-propionate d'érythromycine. *Sem Hop Paris* (1982) 58, 1624–6.
11. Boucharlat J, Franco A, Carpentier P, Charignon Y, Denis B, Hommel M. Ergotisme en milieu psychiatrique par association D.H.E. propionate d'erythromycine. A propos d'une observation. *Ann Med Psychol (Paris)* (1980) 138, 292–6.
12. Leroy F, Asseman P, Pruvost P, Adnet P, Lacroix D, Thery C. Dihydroergotamine-erythromycin-induced ergotism. *Ann Intern Med* (1988) 109, 249.
13. Ghali R, De Léan J, Douville Y, Noël H-P, Labbé R. Erythromycin-associated ergotamine intoxication: arteriographic and electrophysiologic analysis of a rare cause of severe ischemia of the lower extremities and associated ischemic neuropathy. *Ann Vasc Surg* (1993) 7, 291–6.
14. Bird PA, Sturgess AD. Clinical ergotism with severe bilateral upper limb ischaemia precipitated by an erythromycin-ergotamine interaction. *Aust N Z J Med* (2000) 30, 635–6.
15. Karam B, Farah E, Ashoush R, Jebara V, Ghayad E. Ergotism precipitated by erythromycin: a rare case of vasospasm. *Eur J Vasc Endovasc Surg* (2000) 19, 96–8.
16. Grolleau JY, Martin M, de la Guerrande B, Barrier J, Peltier P. Ergotism aigu lors d'une association josamycine/tartrate d'ergotamine. *Therapie* (1981) 36, 319–21.
17. Couet W, Mathieu HP, Fourtillan JB. Effect of ponsinomycin on the pharmacokinetics of dihydroergotamine administered orally. *Fundam Clin Pharmacol* (1991) 5, 47–52.
18. Franco A, Bourlard P, Massot C, Lecoeur J, Guidicelli H, Bessard G. Ergotisme aigu par association dihdyroergotamine-triacétyloléandomycine. *Nouv Presse Med* (1978) 7, 205.
19. Lesca H, Ossard D, Reynier P. Les risques de l'association tri-acétyl-oléandomycine et tartrate d'ergotamine. *Nouv Presse Med* (1976) 5, 1832–3.
20. Hayton AC. Precipitation of acute ergotism by triacetyloleandomycin. *N Z Med J* (1969) 69, 42.
21. Dupuy JC, Lardy P, Seaulau P, Kervoelen P, Paulet J. Spasmes artériels systémiques. Tartrate d'ergotamine. *Arch Mal Coeur* (1979) 72, 86–91.
22. Bigorie B, Aimez P, Soria RJ, Samama F di Maria G, Guy-Grand B, Bour H. L'association triacétyl oléandomycin-tartrate d'ergotamine est-elle dangereuse? *Nouv Presse Med* (1975) 4, 2723–5.
23. Vayssairat M, Fiessinger J-N, Becquemin M-H, Housset E. Association dihydroergotamine et triacétyloléandomycine. Rôle dans une nécrose digitale iatrogène. *Nouv Presse Med* (1978) 7, 2077.
24. Matthews NT, Havill JH. Ergotism with therapeutic doses of ergotamine tartrate. *N Z Med J* (1979) 89, 476–7.
25. Chignier E, Riou R, Descotes J, Meunier P, Courpron P, Vignon G. Ergotisme iatrogène aigu par association médicamenteuse diagnostiqué par exploration non invasive (vélocimétrie à effet Doppler). *Nouv Presse Med* (1978) 7, 2478.
26. Bacourt F, Couffinhal J-C. Ischémie des membres par association dihydroergotamine-triacétyloléandomycine. Nouvelle observation. *Nouv Presse Med* (1978) 7, 1561.
27. Baudouy PY, Mellat M, Velleteau de Moulliac M. Infarctus du myocarde provoqué par l'association tartrate d'ergotamine-troléandomycine. *Rev Med Interne* (1988) 9, 420–2.
28. Pessayre D, Larrey D, Funck-Brentano C, Benhamou JP. Drug interactions and hepatitis produced by some macrolide antibiotics. *J Antimicrob Chemother* (1985) 16 (Suppl A), 181–94.

Ergot derivatives + Methysergide

The concurrent use of methysergide and other ergot derivatives can increase the risk of severe and persistent spasm of major arteries in some patients.

Clinical evidence

A man developed loss of temperature sensitivity over the right side of his face and arm, as well as vertigo, dysphagia and hoarseness 7 days after starting combined treatment with methysergide 2 mg three times daily and 500 micrograms of subcutaneous **ergotamine tartrate** at night. Continued use resulted in impaired pain, touch and temperature sensation over the right side of his face, shoulder and arm. Arteriography demonstrated left vertebral artery occlusion and right vertebral arterial spasm. These symptoms, apart from the loss of temperature sensitivity, resolved when the drugs were stopped.[1] Another man treated for cluster headaches with methysergide 2 mg, intramuscular **ergotamine tartrate** and pizotifen developed ischaemia of the right foot, with impalpable popliteal and pedal pulses. Arteriography showed that blood flow to the arteries of the right leg was reduced.[1]

Another report describes prolonged myocardial ischaemia in a patient with cluster headaches when a single 2-mg dose of **ergotamine tartrate** was added to methysergide 2 mg three times daily. Sublingual glyceryl trinitrate relieved the pain,[2] (but see also 'Ergot derivatives + Glyceryl trinitrate (Nitroglycerin)', p.436)

Mechanism

Cluster headaches are associated with abnormal dilatation of the carotid arteries, which can be constricted by ergot derivatives. In the cases cited it would seem that combined vasoconstrictor effects caused arterial spasm elsewhere in the body, resulting in serious tissue ischaemia. Parenteral ergotamine increases the risk of arterial spasm.

Importance and management

Direct information seems to be limited to these cases. Cardiovascular complications can occur with ergot derivatives given alone, but these cases suggest that their concurrent use may unpredictably increase the risk in some patients. Clearly they should be used together with great caution, or avoided.

1. Joyce DA, Gubbay SS. Arterial complications of migraine treatment with methysergide and parenteral ergotamine. *BMJ* (1982) 285, 260–1.
2. Galer BS, Lipton RB, Solomon S, Newman LC, Spierings ELH. Myocardial ischemia related to ergot alkaloids: a case report and literature review. *Headache* (1991) 31, 446–50.

Ergot derivatives + Protease inhibitors

A patient on indinavir rapidly developed ergotism after taking normal doses of ergotamine. At least six other patients on ritonavir also taking ergotamine have shown the same interaction. A patient on nelfinavir developed peripheral arterial vasoconstriction after taking ergotamine. Other ergot derivatives are predicted to interact similarly.

Clinical evidence

(a) Indinavir

An HIV+ man who had been taking lamivudine, stavudine, co-trimoxazole and indinavir (2400 mg daily) for more than a year was additionally prescribed *Gynergene caféiné* (1 mg **ergotamine tartrate** + 100 mg caffeine) for migraine. He took two doses on two consecutive days, and 5 days later presented in hospital with numbness and cyanosis of the toes of his left foot. The next day he complained of intermittent claudication of his left leg, and 6 days later was admitted to hospital because of worsening symptoms and night cramps. Examination showed a typical picture of ergotism, with vasospasm and reduced blood flow in the popliteal, tibial and femoral arteries. He was treated with heparin and buflomedil, and recovered after 3 days.[1]

(b) Nelfinavir

A 40-year-old HIV+ woman twice took **ergotamine** 2 mg for a migraine while also taking nelfinavir, zidovudine and lamivudine. On the first occasion she developed pain and cyanosis in her toes, and on the second occasion she developed cyanosis and oedema in her hands and feet, causing pain so severe that she was unable to walk. On both occasions peripheral arterial pulses were not palpable. Although she recovered spontaneously on both occasions, the authors caution concurrent use due to the extremely severe potential effects.[2]

(c) Ritonavir

A man of 63 with AIDS, who had taken 1 to 2 mg **ergotamine tartrate** daily for migraine headaches over the last 5 years, had his treatment with zidovudine, zalcitabine and co-trimoxazole changed to zidovudine, didanosine and ritonavir (600 mg 12 hourly). Within 10 days he developed paraesthesias, coldness, cyanosis and skin paleness of both arms, and when admitted to hospital his axillary, brachial, radial and ulnar pulses were found to be absent. An arterial doppler test showed the absence of blood flow in both his radial and ulnar arteries and he was diagnosed as having ergotism. The **ergotamine** and ritonavir were stopped, and he recovered when treated with prostaglandin E1 and calcium nadroparin.[3]

Another man, aged 31, taking 400 mg ritonavir twice daily (and also taking pizotifen, nelfinavir, stavudine, lamivudine, co-trimoxazole and venlafaxine) developed severe burning and numbness in both feet, and paraesthesias in his hands after taking 4 tablets, each containing **ergotamine** 1 mg and caffeine 100 mg, over 10 days. He was diagnosed as having ergotism. The drugs were stopped and he was treated effectively with intravenous alprostadil and heparin.[4] At least 4 other cases of ergotism have been reported in patients on ritonavir after taking ergot,[5-8] and one required surgical amputation of the toes.[6] The ergotism developed in two of the patients within a few hours of taking a single 1- or 2-mg dose of **ergotamine tartrate**,[5,7] and in the other two within about 4 to 15 days.[6,8] One was on a combination drug (0.3 mg **ergotamine tartrate**, 0.2 mg belladonna extract and 20 mg phenobarbital) twice daily for gastric discomfort,[6] and the other took up to 2 mg of **ergotamine** daily.[8]

Mechanism

Protease inhibitors reduce the metabolism of ergotamine by inhibiting the cytochrome P450 isoenzyme CYP3A4 to varying degrees. Therefore ergotamine levels are increased, which may result in toxicity. Ergotamine poisoning causes arterial spasm, which reduces and even shuts down the flow of blood in arteries.

Importance and management

Information appears to be limited to these reports, but what happened is consistent with the way other drugs that are potent inhibitors of CYP3A4 can interact with ergot derivatives (see 'Ergot derivatives + Macrolides', p.436). This interaction would appear to be established, and is clearly clinically important. It would now be prudent for any patient on indinavir or ritonavir, and probably nelfinavir to avoid the concurrent use of ergotamine or any other ergot derivative such as dihydroergotamine. Information about possible interactions between ergot derivatives and other protease inhibitors seems to be lacking. Even so to be on the safe side the makers of most of the other protease inhibitors contraindicate concurrent use.

1. Rosenthal E, Sala F, Chichmanian R-M, Batt M, Cassuto J-P. Ergotism related to concurrent administration of ergotamine tartrate and indinavir. *JAMA* (1999) 281, 987.
2. Mortier E, Pouchot J, Vinceneux P, Lalande M. Ergotism related to interaction between nelfinavir and ergotamine. *Am J Med* (2001) 110, 594.
3. Cabellero-Granada FJ, Vician P, Cordero E, Gómez-Vera MJ, de Nozal M, López-Cortés LF. Ergotism related to concurrent administration of ergotamine tartrate and ritonavir in an AIDS patient. *Antimicrob Agents Chemother* (1997), 41,1207.
4. Phan TG, Agaliotis D, White G, Britton WJ. Ischaemic peripheral neuritis secondary to ergotism associated with ritonavir therapy. *Med J Aust* (1999) 171, 502, 504.
5. Montero A, Giovannoni AG, Tvrde PL. Leg ischemia in a patient receiving ritonavir and ergotamine. *Ann Intern Med* (1999) 130, 329–30.
6. Liaudet L, Buclin T, Jaccard C, Eckert P. Severe ergotism associated with interaction between ritonavir and ergotamine. *BMJ* (1999) 318, 771.
7. Blanche P, Rigolet A, Gombert B, Ginsburg C, Salmon D, Sicard D. Ergotism related to a single dose of ergotamine tartrate in an AIDS patient treated with ritonavir. *Postgrad Med J* (1999) 75, 546–7.
8. Vila A, Mykietiuk A, Bonvehl, Temporiti E, Urueqa A, Herrera F. Clinical ergotism induced by ritonavir. *Scand J Infect Dis* (2001) 33, 788–9.

Ergot derivatives + Tetracyclines

Five patients taking ergotamine or dihydroergotamine developed ergotism when additionally treated with doxycycline or tetracycline.

Clinical evidence

A woman who had previously taken **ergotamine tartrate** successfully and uneventfully for 16 years, was treated with **doxycycline** and **dihydroergotamine** 30 drops three times a day. Five days later her hands and feet became cold and reddened, and she was diagnosed as having a mild form of ergotism.[1]

Other cases of ergotism, some of them more severe, have been described in one patient taking **ergotamine tartrate** and doxycycline,[2] and in 3 patients taking **tetracycline** containing preparations.[2-4]

Mechanism

Unknown. One suggestion is that these antibacterials may inhibit the activity of the liver enzymes concerned with the metabolism and clearance of ergotamine, thereby prolonging its stay in the body and enhancing its activity.[1] One of the patients had a history of alcoholism[2] and two of them were in their eighties,[4] so that their liver function may have already been reduced.

Importance and management

Information is very limited indeed. The incidence and general importance of this interaction is uncertain, but it would clearly be prudent to be on the alert for signs of ergotism in any patient given ergot derivatives and a tetracycline. Impairment of liver function may possibly be a contributory factor.

1. Amblard P, Reymond JL, Franco A, Beani JC, Carpentier P, Lemonnier D, Bessard G. Ergotisme. Forme mineure par association dihydroergotamine-chlorhydrate de doxycycline, étude capillaroscopique. *Nouv Presse Med* (1978) 7, 4148–9.
2. Dupuy JC, Lardy P, Seaulau P, Kervoelen P, Paulet J. Spasmes artériels systémiques. Tartrate d'ergotamine. *Arch Mal Coeur* (1979) 72, 86–91.
3. L'Yvonnet M, Boillot A, Jacquet AM, Barale F, Grandmottet P, Zurlinden B, Gillet JY. A propos d'un cas exceptionnel d'intoxication aigue par un dérivé de l'ergot de seigle. *Gynecologie* (1974) 25, 541–3.
4. Sibertin-Blanc M. Les dangers de l'ergotisme a propos de deux observations. *Arch Med Ouest* (1977) 9, 265–6.

Flunarizine + Anticonvulsants

Limited evidence suggests that anticonvulsants can reduce serum flunarizine levels.

Clinical evidence, mechanism, importance and management

A study found that flunarizine levels were lower in patients receiving multiple anticonvulsants than in those receiving only one anticonvulsant (statistically significant only for the 10 mg flunarizine dose). The anticonvulsants taken were **carbamazepine**, **phenytoin**, and **sodium valproate**. Flunarizine did not affect the serum levels of these other anticonvulsants.[1] There would seem to be no reason for avoiding concurrent use, but the outcome should be monitored.

1. Binnie CD, de Beukelaar F, Meijer JWA, Meinardi H, Overweg J, Wauquier A, van Wieringen A. Open dose-ranging trial of flunarizine as add-on therapy in epilepsy. *Epilepsia* (1985) 26, 424–8.

Triptans + Beta-blockers

No clinically important interaction occurs between most triptans and propranolol, but because the plasma levels of rizatriptan are almost doubled by propranolol the makers recommend a dosage reduction and a 2-hour dosage separation.

Clinical evidence, mechanism, importance and management

(a) Almotriptan

Twelve healthy subjects were given a single 12.5-mg dose of almotriptan following 7 days of **propranolol** 80 mg twice daily. Although some small changes were noted in the pharmacokinetics of almotriptan, these were not considered to be clinically significant and concurrent use of the combination was well tolerated.[1]

(b) Eletriptan

In an interaction study, 12 healthy subjects were given a single 80-mg dose of eletriptan following 7 days' pre-treatment with **propranolol** 80 mg twice daily. It was found that the eletriptan AUC was increased 1.3-fold and the half life increased from 4.9 to 5.2 hours. However, these changes were not considered to be clinically important. No significant blood pressure changes or any adverse events were seen when compared with taking eletriptan alone.[2]

The makers say that in clinical trials where eletriptan was taken with beta-blockers, no evidence of an interaction was seen.[3]

(c) Frovatriptan

A single 2.5-mg oral dose of frovatriptan was given to 12 healthy subjects after they had received 7 days' pre-treatment with **propranolol** 80 mg twice daily. The AUC and maximum levels of frovatriptan were increased by 25 and 23% respectively. However, no changes occurred in the ECGs and vital signs of the subjects, and so the pharmacokinetic interaction was not thought to be of clinical significance.[4]

(d) Naratriptan

The makers of naratriptan report that there is no evidence of interactions with **beta-blockers** (none specifically named)[5] so that there would appear to be no problems with the concurrent use of **propranolol** or with other beta-blockers.

(e) Rizatriptan

A series of double-blind placebo-controlled studies were conducted in a total of 51 patients who were given a single 10-mg dose of rizatriptan after 7 days treatment with **propranolol** 60 or 120 mg twice daily, **nadolol** 80 mg daily, **metoprolol** 100 mg daily or placebo.[6] **Nadolol** and **metoprolol** had no effect on the pharmacokinetics of rizatriptan. **Propranolol** however raised the AUC and the maximum plasma concentration of rizatriptan by 1.67 and 1.75-fold respectively. Adjusting the dose of **propranolol** and separating the administration by 2 hours had little effect on this interaction.[6] *In vitro* studies have shown that **propranolol** markedly inhibits the metabolism of rizatriptan, whereas **atenolol**, **nadolol** and **timolol** did not affect the metabolism of rizatriptan.[6] The makers recommend that a 5-mg dose of rizatriptan (rather than the more usual 10 mg) should be used in the presence of **propranolol**. They also state that administration should be separated by at least 2 hours,[7] although the rationale for this is less clear given the findings of the above study.[6] No reduction in the rizatriptan dosage would seem to be needed in the presence of **nadolol**, **metoprolol**, **atenolol** or **timolol**.

(f) Sumatriptan

No pharmacokinetic interaction occurs with sumatriptan 300 mg orally, and **propranolol** 80 mg twice daily for 7 days.[8]

(g) Zolmitriptan

In a double-blind, randomised, crossover study, 12 healthy subjects were given 160 mg of **propranolol** or a placebo daily for 7 days, and then on day 7 a single 10-mg oral dose of zolmitriptan. The **propranolol** increased the maximum serum levels and the AUC of the zolmitriptan by 56% and 37% respectively, and reduced the extent of its conversion to the active metabolite (183C91), probably due to inhibition of cytochrome P450. However, it was concluded that no clinically important changes in the therapeutic effects of zolmitriptan are likely, nor are any adjustments in its dosage needed.[9]

1. Fleishaker JC, Sisson TA, Carel BJ, Azie NE. Lack of pharmacokinetic interaction between the antimigraine compound, almotriptan, and propranolol in healthy volunteers. *Cephalalgia* (2001) 21, 61–65.
2. Milton KA, Tan L, Love R. The pharmacokinetic and pharmacodynamic interactions of oral eletriptan and propranolol in healthy volunteers. *Cephalalgia* (1998) 18, 412.
3. Relpax (Eletriptan). Pfizer Ltd. UK Summary of product characteristics, December 2003.
4. Buchan P, Ward C, Stewart AJ. The effect of propranolol on the pharmacokinetic and safety profiles of frovatriptan. *Headache* (1999) 39, 345.
5. Naramig (Naratriptan). GlaxoSmithKline UK. UK Summary of product characteristics, July 2004.
6. Goldberg MR, Sciberras D, De Smet M, Lowry R, Tomasko L, Lee Y, Olah TV, Zhao J, Vyas KP, Halpin R, Kari PH, James I. Influence of β-adrenoceptor antagonists on the pharmacokinetics of rizatriptan, a $5\text{-HT}_{1B/1D}$ agonist: differential effects of propranolol, nadolol and metoprolol. *Br J Clin Pharmacol* (2001) 52, 69–76.
7. Maxalt (Rizatriptan). Merck Sharp & Dohme Ltd. UK Summary of product characteristics, April 2003.
8. Scott AK, Walley T, Breckenridge AM, Lacey LF, Fowler PA. Lack of an interaction between propranolol and sumatriptan. *Br J Clin Pharmacol* (1991) 32, 581–4.
9. Peck RW, Seaber EJ, Dixon R, Gillotin CG, Weatherley BC, Layton G, Posner J. The interaction between propranolol and the novel antimigraine agent zolmitriptan (311C90). *Br J Clin Pharmacol* (1997) 44, 595–9.

Triptans + Ergot derivatives

Simultaneous use of the ergot derivatives is contraindicated with all the triptans because of the risk of additive vasoconstriction, although there is some evidence of safe use. Some of the makers of the triptans give recommendations for the number of hours that should be allowed between administration of triptans and ergot derivatives.

Clinical evidence

(a) Almotriptan

The makers of almotriptan say that no additive vasospastic effects were seen in a clinical trial in 12 healthy subjects given almotriptan and **ergotamine**.[1]

(b) Eletriptan

The makers report that when oral **ergotamine** with caffeine was given 1 hour and 2 hours after eletriptan, minor additive increases in blood pressure were seen.[2]

(c) Frovatriptan

In a randomised crossover study, 12 healthy subjects were given a single 5-mg dose of oral frovatriptan, a single 2-mg sublingual dose of **ergotamine**, or both drugs together. The **ergotamine** reduced the maximum levels and AUC of frovatriptan by about 25%. However, the frovatriptan had no effect on **ergotamine** pharmacokinetics, and no clinically significant changes in the haemodynamics or the ECGs of the subjects were noted.[3]

(d) Naratriptan

A study in 12 healthy subjects found that 1 mg of intramuscular **dihydroergotamine** reduced the AUC and the maximum serum levels of a single 2.5-mg dose of naratriptan by 15% and 20% respectively, but this was considered to be clinically irrelevant. Concurrent use was well tolerated and no clinically significant blood pressure, heart rate or ECG effects were seen.[4]

(e) Rizatriptan

Additive vasospastic effects were not observed in a pharmacodynamic study in 16 healthy subjects given oral rizatriptan and parenteral **ergotamine**.[5]

(f) Sumatriptan

A study in 38 migraine sufferers found that 1 mg of intravenous **dihydroergotamine** alone caused maximum increases in blood pressure of 13/9 mmHg, while 2 or 4 mg subcutaneous sumatriptan alone caused a smaller rise in blood pressure of 7/6 mmHg. When given together the blood pressure rises were no greater than with **dihydroergotamine** alone.[6] A clinical study of subcutaneous sumatriptan in patients on oral **dihydroergotamine** found that the adverse event profile of sumatriptan was not affected by concurrent use.[7] However, another pharmacodynamic study found that subcutaneous sumatriptan and intravenous **ergotamine** had additive vasoconstrictive effects (as assessed by decreases in toe-arm systolic blood pressure gradients).[8]

Myocardial infarction has been reported in a 43-year-old woman after she took two 2-mg doses of **methysergide** 12 hours apart, followed by sumatriptan 6 mg subcutaneously. Severe chest pain and tightness with breathlessness began 15 minutes later, and results of various tests were consistent with 'coronary spasm on an area of atherosclerosis'.[9]

(g) Zolmitriptan

In a randomised, double-blind, placebo-controlled study, 12 healthy subjects were given 5 mg of oral **dihydroergotamine** or a placebo twice daily for 10 days, and on day 10 they were also given oral zolmitriptan 10 mg (four times the usual dose). No significant changes in blood pressure, ECGs, or zolmitriptan pharmacokinetics were seen. Concurrent use was well tolerated.[10] Another randomised, double-blind, placebo-controlled trial in 12 healthy subjects studied the effects of oral zolmitriptan 20 mg (eight times the usual dose) when combined with oral **ergotamine** 2 mg (contained in *Cafergot* tablets, 1 mg **ergotamine** + 100 mg caffeine). Using a very detailed and thorough range of techniques, no clinically relevant cardiovascular changes were found, even at this large dose of zolmitriptan, and concurrent use was generally well tolerated. No important changes in the zolmitriptan pharmacokinetics were seen.[11]

Mechanism

Vasoconstriction is a well known adverse effect of ergot derivatives, and coronary vasoconstriction may also occur rarely with the triptans. (Note that in 1992, soon after the marketing of sumatriptan, the CSM in the UK had received 34 reports of pain or tightness in the chest caused by sumatriptan, possibly due to coronary vasoconstriction.[12]) It is therefore theoretically possible that the drugs may have additive vasoconstrictive effects, although there is little evidence of this in practice.

Importance and management

Due to the theoretical risk of additive vasoconstriction, and possible significant coronary vasoconstriction (see (f) sumatriptan above) ergot derivatives are considered contraindicated with triptans. The makers of sumatriptan say that ergotamine should not be given less than 6 hours after taking the triptan, and recommend that the triptan should not be taken less than 24 hours after taking ergotamine.[13] Similar recommendations are made by the makers of almotriptan,[1] rizatriptan,[5] and zolmitriptan,[14] whereas the makers of eletriptan,[2] and frovatriptan,[15] recommend that ergot derivatives are not given for a minimum of 24 hours (not just 6 hours) after these triptans.

1. Almogran (Almotriptan). Organon Laboratories Ltd. UK Summary of product characteristics, March 2005.
2. Relpax (Eletriptan). Pfizer Ltd. UK Summary of product characteristics, December 2003.
3. Buchan P, Ward C, Oliver SD. Lack of clinically significant interactions between frovatriptan and ergotamine. *Cephalalgia* (1999) 19, 364.
4. Kempsford RD, Nicholls B, Lam R, Wintermute S. A study to investigate the potential interaction of naratriptan and dihydroergotamine. 8th International Headache Congress, Amsterdam, June 1997.
5. Maxalt (Rizatriptan). Merck Sharp & Dohme Ltd. UK Summary of product characteristics, April 2003.
6. Fowler PA, Lacey LF, Thomas M, Keene ON, Tanner RJN, Baber NS. The clinical pharmacology, pharmacokinetics and metabolism of sumatriptan. *Eur Neurol* (1991) 31, 291–4.
7. Henry P, d'Allens H and the French Migraine Network Bordeaux-Lyon-Grenoble. Subcutaneous sumatriptan in the acute treatment of migraine in patients using dihydroergotamine as prophylaxis. *Headache* (1993) 33, 432–5.
8. Tfelt-Hansen P, Sperling B, Winter PDO'B. Transient additional effect of sumatriptan on ergotamine-induced constriction of peripheral arteries in man. *Clin Pharmacol Ther* (1992) 51, 149.
9. Liston H, Bennett L, Usher B, Nappi J. The association of the combination of sumatriptan and methysergide in myocardial infarction in a premenopausal woman. *Arch Intern Med* (1999) 159, 511–13.
10. Veronese L, Gillotin C, Marion-Gallois R, Weatherley BC, Thebault JJ, Guillaume M, Peck RW. Lack of interaction between oral dihydroergotamine and the novel antimigraine compound zolmitriptan in healthy volunteers. *Clin Drug Invest* (1997) 14, 217–20.
11. Dixon RM, Meire HB, Evans DH, Watt H, On N, Posner J, Rolan PE. Peripheral vascular effects and pharmacokinetics of the antimigraine compound, zolmitriptan, in combination with oral ergotamine in healthy volunteers. *Cephalalgia* (1997) 17, 639–46.
12. Committee on Safety of Medicines. Sumatriptan (Imigran) and chest pain. *Current Problems* (1992) 34, 2.
13. Imigran Radis (Sumatriptan succinate). GlaxoSmithKline UK. UK Summary of product characteristics, December 2004.
14. Zomig (Zolmitriptan). AstraZeneca UK Ltd. UK Summary of product characteristics, May 2004.
15. Migard (Frovatriptan). A. Menarini Pharma UK SRL. UK Summary of product characteristics, February 2005.

Triptans + Flunarizine

Flunarizine did not alter the pharmacokinetics or pharmacodynamics of sumatriptan in one study. Flunarizine does not appear to interact with eletriptan.

Clinical evidence, mechanism, importance and management

(a) Eletriptan

The maker notes that although no formal interaction studies have been carried out, there was no evidence of an interaction between eletriptan and flunarizine in clinical trials.[1]

(b) Sumatriptan

A double-blind study found that flunarizine 10 mg daily for 8 days had no effect on pharmacokinetics of single doses of sumatriptan, and the combination caused no significant changes in blood pressure, ECG or heart rate.[2]

1. Relpax (Eletriptan). Pfizer Ltd. UK Summary of product characteristics, December 2003.
2. Van Hecken AM, Depré M, De Schepper PJ, Fowler PA, Lacey LF, Durham JM. Lack of effect of flunarizine on the pharmacokinetics and pharmacodynamics of sumatriptan in healthy volunteers. *Br J Clin Pharmacol* (1992) 34, 82–4.

Triptans + Macrolides

Erythromycin markedly raises the plasma levels of eletriptan, but clarithromycin does not significantly alter the pharmacokinetics of sumatriptan.

Clinical evidence, mechanism, importance and management

(a) Eletriptan

A clinical pharmacokinetic study by the makers of eletriptan[1] found that **erythromycin** 1000 mg increased the maximum serum levels of eletriptan 2-fold, the AUC 3.6-fold and prolonged its half-life from 4.6 to 7.1 hours. Because of this, they contraindicate the concurrent use of **erythromycin** and eletriptan. Other drugs that are potent inhibitors of the cytochrome P450 isoenzyme CYP3A4, an enzyme involved in the metabolism of eletriptan, are predicted to raise serum eletriptan levels similarly. Such drugs include **clarithromycin** and **josamycin**.

(b) Sumatriptan

A study in which 24 healthy subjects were given 50 mg of sumatriptan on the morning of the fourth day of a course of **clarithromycin** 500 mg twice daily, found that **clarithromycin** did not significantly affect the pharmacokinetics of sumatriptan.[2]

1. Relpax (Eletriptan). Pfizer Ltd. UK Summary of product characteristics, June 2001.
2. Moore KHP, Leese PT, McNeal S, Gray P, O'Quinn S, Bye C, Sale M. The pharmacokinetics of sumatriptan when administered with clarithromycin in healthy volunteers. *Clin Ther* (2002) 24, 583–94.

Triptans + MAOIs

Moclobemide (an inhibitor of MAO-A) markedly inhibits the metabolism of rizatriptan, and approximately doubles the bioavailability of sumatriptan. The makers contraindicate these triptans with moclobemide and all MAOIs.
Moclobemide modestly inhibited the metabolism of zolmitriptan (a dosage adjustment is recommended) and almotriptan (this was not considered clinically relevant).
Non-selective MAOIs (e.g. phenelzine) are not expected to interact with eletriptan, frovatriptan, or naratriptan. Nevertheless, the maker of frovatriptan contraindicates the concurrent use of MAOIs, based on a theoretical increased risk of serotonin syndrome.
Selegiline (an inhibitor of MAO-B) does not interact with zolmitriptan, and would not be expected to interact with any of the other triptans.

Clinical evidence, mechanism, importance and management

(a) Almotriptan

A multiple dose study using **moclobemide** (a reversible and selective inhibitor of monoamine oxidase A) found that the AUC of almotriptan was increased by 37%, without any clinically relevant changes in maximum serum levels or half-life. No clinically significant interactions were seen.[1] These findings are consistent with the fact that less than half of a dose of almotriptan is metabolised by monoamine oxidase A,[1] and it would seem therefore that concurrent use need not be avoided. There appears to be no direct clinical information about the use of **non-selective MAOIs** but it seems unlikely that a clinically relevant interaction will occur. This needs confirmation.

(b) Eletriptan

The maker of eletriptan notes that it is not a substrate for monoamine oxidase, and therefore no interaction with MAOIs is expected. Because of this, they have not undertaken a formal interaction study.[2]

(c) Frovatriptan

The maker of frovatriptan notes that it is not a substrate for, or an inhibitor of, monoamine oxidase. Nevertheless, they say that a potential risk of serotonin syndrome or hypertension cannot be excluded when it is used with MAOIs, so concomitant use is not recommended[3] (but see also 'Antimigraine drugs', (p.435)). A study in 9 healthy subjects given a single 2.5-mg oral dose of frovatriptan following 7 days' pre-treatment with **moclobemide** 150 mg twice daily did not find any pharmacokinetic changes, or any changes in the vital signs and ECGs of the subjects. Therefore no adverse interaction would be expected on concurrent use.[4]

(d) Naratriptan

The maker of naratriptan notes that it is not a substrate for monoamine oxidase. Therefore interactions with MAOIs are not anticipated.[5]

(e) Rizatriptan

In a double blind, randomised, crossover trial, 12 healthy subjects were given **moclobemide** 150 mg or a placebo three times daily for 4 days, and then a single 10-mg dose of rizatriptan on day 4. The **moclobemide** increased the AUCs of rizatriptan and its active (but minor) metabolite by 2.2- and 5.3-fold respectively, and increased their maximum serum levels by 1.4- and 2.6-fold respectively. The reason appears to be that **moclobemide** is an inhibitor of MAO-A, which is the principal enzyme concerned with the metabolism of rizatriptan. Despite these rises, the concurrent use of these drugs was well tolerated and any adverse effects were mild and similar to those seen when rizatriptan was given with the placebo. However, because of the magnitude of the rises, the authors recommend avoiding the combination.[6] The makers of rizatriptan issue a 'blanket' contraindication covering all MAOIs, that covers the time during, and 2 weeks after stopping the MAOI, the stated reasons being that similar or greater rises in serum levels may be expected with irreversible non-selective MAOIs.[7]

(f) Sumatriptan

For eight days three groups of 14 subjects were given a placebo, **moclobemide** 150 mg three times daily, or **selegiline** 5 mg twice daily, and then on day 8 all of the subjects were also given 6 mg sumatriptan subcutaneously. No statistically significant differences in pulse rates or in blood pressures were seen between any of the groups following the injection of the sumatriptan, however the sumatriptan AUC of the **moclobemide**-treated group was approximately doubled (+ 129%), its clearance was reduced by 56% and its half-life increased by 52%. The pharmacokinetic changes seen in the **selegiline** group were not consistent. There were no differences in the adverse events experienced by any of the three groups.[8]

A patient taking 300 mg **moclobemide** three times daily showed no adverse effects when given 100 mg oral sumatriptan on six occasions.[9]

A comprehensive search of the literature and reports from proprietary manufacturers, identified published reports of 31 patients taking sumatriptan and MAOIs concurrently, but no adverse events were reported.[10]

The moclobemide/sumatriptan interaction appears to be established. The same interaction seems likely to occur with any of the other selective MAO-A inhibitors and with the non-selective MAOIs too, but not with the selective MAO-B inhibitors like selegiline. This needs confirmation. However, the increased sumatriptan bioavailability appears not to be clinically important because, in the study cited, those subjects on moclobemide did not experience any more adverse effects than those taking the selegiline or placebo. Despite this the makers of sumatriptan quite clearly say that the concurrent use of sumatriptan and MAOIs is contraindicated, and within 2 weeks of stopping an MAOI.[11]

(g) Zolmitriptan

In a series of 3-period, crossover, randomised studies, 12 healthy subjects were given **selegiline** 10 mg daily or **moclobemide** 150 mg twice daily for 7 days, and then on day 7 a single 10-mg oral dose of zolmitriptan.[12] It was found that the AUC of the zolmitriptan was increased by 26% by the **moclobemide**. A threefold increase in the AUC of the active metabolite also occurred.[13] It is likely that moclobemide inhibited the metabolism of zolmitriptan via monoamine oxidase A. Despite these increases, because of the good tolerability profile of zolmitriptan, no dosage reductions are thought to be needed if given with **moclobemide**, but a maximum intake of 5 mg in 24 hours is recommended by the makers.[13]

Selegiline on the other hand had no effect on the pharmacokinetics of zolmitriptan or its metabolites, apart from a small (7%) reduction in its renal clearance.[12] This finding was expected, since **selegiline** is specific for monoamine oxidase B (but note that this specificity is lost at higher doses). No special precautions would therefore seem to be necessary with **selegiline**.

1. Almogran (Almotriptan). Organon Laboratories Ltd. UK Summary of product characteristics, March 2005.
2. Relpax (Eletriptan). Pfizer Ltd. UK Summary of product characteristics, December 2003.
3. Migard (Frovatriptan). A. Menarini Pharma UK SRL. UK Summary of product characteristics, February 2005.
4. Buchan P, Ward C, Freestone S. Lack of interaction between frovatriptan and monoamine oxidase inhibitor. *Cephalalgia* (1999) 19, 364.
5. Naramig (Naratriptan). GlaxoSmithKline. UK Summary of product characteristics, July 2004.
6. van Haarst AD, van Gerven JMA, Cohen AF, De Smet M, Sterrett A, Birk KL, Fisher AL, De Puy ME, Goldberg MR, Musson DG. The effects of moclobemide on the pharmacokinetics of the 5-$HT_{1B/1D}$ agonist rizatriptan in healthy volunteers. *Br J Clin Pharmacol* (1999) 48, 190–96.
7. Maxalt (Rizatriptan). Merck Sharp & Dohme Ltd. UK Summary of product characteristics, April 2003.
8. Glaxo Pharmaceuticals UK Limited. A study to determine whether the pharmacokinetics, safety or tolerability of subcutaneously administered sumatriptan (6 mg) are altered by interaction with concurrent oral monoamine oxidase inhibitors. Data on file (Protocol C92–050), 1993.
9. Blier P, Bergeron R. The safety of concomitant use of sumatriptan and antidepressant treatments. *J Clin Psychopharmacol* (1995) 15, 106–9.
10. Gardner DM, Lynd LD. Sumatriptan contraindications and the serotonin syndrome. *Ann Pharmacother* (1998) 32, 33–38.
11. Imigran Radis (Sumatriptan succinate). GlaxoSmithKline UK. UK Summary of product characteristics, December 2004.
12. Rolan P. Potential drug interactions with the novel antimigraine compound zolmitriptan (Zomig™, 311C90). *Cephalalgia* (1997) 17 (Suppl 18), 21–7.
13. Zomig (Zolmitriptan). AstraZeneca UK Ltd. UK Summary of product characteristics, May 2004.

Triptans + Pizotifen

Pizotifen does not alter the pharmacokinetics or pharmacodynamics of sumatriptan or zolmitriptan. It seems unlikely that any of the other triptans will interact.

Clinical evidence

(a) Sumatriptan

Pizotifen 500 micrograms three times daily for 8 days in 14 healthy subjects was found to have no significant effect on the pharmacokinetics of sumatriptan. In addition, there were no significant changes in blood pressure or heart rate.[1]

(b) Zolmitriptan

A double-blind, randomised study was carried out in 12 healthy subjects who were given pizotifen 1.5 mg or a placebo once daily for 8 days, and then on day 8 they were also given oral zolmitriptan 10 mg. Pizotifen did not significantly alter the pharmacokinetics of zolmitriptan, and no clinically relevant changes in heart rates or ECGs or blood pressures were seen as a result of concurrent use.[2]

Mechanism, importance and management

Although the information is limited there would seem to be no reason for avoiding the concurrent use of both drugs nor any need to modify the dosages. On the basis of the information on sumatriptan and zolmitriptan it seems unlikely that any of the other triptans will interact.

1. Fowler PA, Lacey LF, Thomas M, Keene ON, Tanner RJN, Baber NS. The clinical pharmacology, pharmacokinetics and metabolism of sumatriptan. *Eur Neurol* (1991) 31, 291–4.
2. Seaber EJ, Gillotin C, Mohanlal R, Layton G, Posner J, Peck R. Lack of interaction between pizotifen and the novel antimigraine compound zolmitriptan in healthy volunteers. *Clin Drug Invest* (1997) 14, 221–5.

Triptans + SSRIs

The SSRIs normally appear not to interact with the triptans, but there are a few rare cases of dyskinesias with sumatriptan, and there is some evidence to suggest that the serotonin syndrome may occasionally develop. Fluvoxamine modestly inhibits the metabolism of frovatriptan, and may inhibit the metabolism of zolmitriptan.

Clinical evidence

(a) Almotriptan

Fluoxetine 60 mg daily was given to 14 healthy subjects for 8 days, with a single 12.5-mg dose of almotriptan on day 8. **Fluoxetine** raised the maximum plasma levels of almotriptan by about 18%, but the combination was well tolerated and caused no ECG changes, so no dose alterations were considered necessary by the authors.[1]

(b) Eletriptan

The maker notes that although no formal interaction studies have been carried out, there was no evidence of an interaction between eletriptan and **SSRIs** in clinical trials, and that **SSRIs** appeared unlikely to alter the pharmacokinetics of eletriptan.[2]

(c) Frovatriptan

Fluvoxamine has been shown to increase the blood levels of frovatriptan by 27 to 49%.[3] The maker recommends caution with concurrent use of frovatriptan and **fluvoxamine** or other SSRIs.[4]

(d) Naratriptan

The maker of naratriptan notes that there was no evidence of interactions with SSRIs.[5]

(e) Rizatriptan

A single 10-mg dose of rizatriptan was given to 12 healthy subjects after taking **paroxetine** 20 mg or a placebo daily for 14 days. The plasma levels of rizatriptan and its active metabolite were not altered by **paroxetine**, and no adverse effects were seen. Safety evaluations included blood pressure, heart rate, temperature and a visual analogue assessment of mood. There was no evidence of the serotonin syndrome.[6]

(f) Sumatriptan

A study in 11 healthy subjects found that 16 days' treatment with **paroxetine** 20 mg daily had no effect on the response to 6 mg of subcutaneous sumatriptan, as measured by prolactin levels. The sumatriptan levels remained unaltered, its cardiovascular effects were unchanged and no clinically significant adverse effects occurred.[7] Other studies report that the concurrent use of sumatriptan and SSRIs (**fluoxetine** 20 to 60 mg daily, **fluvoxamine** 200 mg daily, **paroxetine** 20 to 50 mg daily, **sertraline** 50 to 100 mg daily) was successful and uneventful.[8,9] No adverse effects have been noted in 148 other patients.[10]

However, in Canada, post-marketing surveillance of the voluntary reports received by the makers of **fluoxetine**, identified 2 cases that showed good evidence, and another 4 cases that showed some, but not strong evidence, of reactions consistent with the serotonin syndrome.[11] Other cases describe a decrease in the efficacy of sumatriptan with fluoxetine,[12] dyskinesias and dystonias with sumatriptan and paroxetine,[13] and twenty possible cases of the serotonin syndrome with sumatriptan and SSRIs.[10,14]

The makers of sumatriptan also say that they have rare post-marketing reports of weakness, hyperreflexia and incoordination following the use of sumatriptan and SSRIs.[15]

(g) Zolmitriptan

A two-period crossover, double-blind study in 20 subjects given **fluoxetine** 20 mg or a placebo daily for 28 days, with the addition of zolmitriptan 10 mg on day 28, found that the pharmacokinetics of zolmitriptan were unaffected by **fluoxetine**.[16] Only very slight changes were seen in the pharmacokinetics of its active metabolite.[16] **Sertraline**, **paroxetine**, and **citalopram** are also not expected to alter the pharmacokinetics of zolmitriptan. However, **fluvoxamine** is predicted to increase levels of zolmitriptan,[17] based on the known interaction with cimetidine (see 'Triptans; Zolmitriptan + Cimetidine', p.443).

Mechanism

Not understood.SSRIs increase the levels of 5-HT (serotonin) at post-synaptic receptors. In theory the triptans (5-HT_1 agonists) might possibly add to the effects of these increased levels of serotonin, but in practice it is questionable whether this is normally clinically relevant (see also 'Antimigraine drugs', (p.435)). Fluvoxamine probably inhibits the metabolism of frovatriptan[4] by cytochrome P450 isoenzyme CYP1A2, and is predicted to interact with zolmitriptan[17] by the same mechanism.

Importance and management

The weight of evidence suggests that the concurrent use of the triptans and SSRIs is normally uneventful, but adverse reactions do occur occasionally. The authors of some of the references above concluded that their findings do not imply that concurrent use should be avoided, but that caution and close monitoring should be used.[10,11] Since fluvoxamine is predicted to interact pharmacokinetically, the makers of zolmitriptan recommend a dosage reduction to a maximum of 5 mg in 24 hours when used with fluvoxamine.[17]

1. Fleishaker JC, Ryan KK, Carel BJ, Azie NE. Evaluation of the potential pharmacokinetic interaction between almotriptan and fluoxetine in healthy volunteers. *J Clin Pharmacol* (2001) 41, 217–23.
2. Relpax (Eletriptan). Pfizer Ltd. UK Summary of product characteristics, December 2003.
3. Wade A, Buchan P, Mant T, Ward C. Frovatriptan has no clinically significant interaction with fluvoxamine. *Cephalalgia* (2001) 21, 427.
4. Migard (Frovatriptan). A. Menarini Pharma UK SRL. UK Summary of product characteristics, February 2005.
5. Naramig (Naratriptan). GlaxoSmithKline UK. UK Summary of product characteristics, July 2004.
6. Goldberg MR, Lowry RC, Musson DG, Birk KL, Fisher A, DePuy ME, Shadle CR. Lack of pharmacokinetic and pharmacodynamic interaction between rizatriptan and paroxetine. *J Clin Pharmacol* (1999) 39, 192–9.
7. Wing Y-K, Clifford EM, Sheehan BD, Campling GM, Hockney RA, Cowen PJ. Paroxetine treatment and the prolactin response to sumatriptan. *Psychopharmacology (Berl)* (1996) 124, 377–9.
8. Blier P, Bergeron R. The safety of concomitant use of sumatriptan and antidepressant treatments. *J Clin Psychopharmacol* (1995) 15, 106–9.
9. Leung M. Lack of an interaction between sumatriptan and selective serotonin reuptake inhibitors. *Headache* (1995) 35, 488–9.
10. Gardner DM, Lynd LD. Sumatriptan contraindications and the serotonin syndrome. *Ann Pharmacother* (1998) 32, 33–8.
11. Joffe RT, Sokolov STH. Co-administration of fluoxetine and sumatriptan: the Canadian experience. *Acta Psychiatr Scand* (1997) 95, 551–2.
12. Szabo CP. Fluoxetine and sumatriptan: possibly a counterproductive combination. *J Clin Psychiatry* (1995) 56, 37–8.
13. Abraham JT, Brown R, Meltzer HY. Clozapine treatment of persistent paroxysmal dyskinesia associated with concomitant paroxetine and sumatriptan use. *Biol Psychiatry* (1997) 42, 144–6.
14. Mathew NT. Serotonin syndrome complicating migraine pharmacotherapy. *Cephalalgia* (1996) 16, 323–7.
15. GlaxoWellcome. Personal communication, August 1997.
16. Smith DA, Cleary EW, Watkins S, Huffman CS, Polvino WJ. Zolmitriptan (311C90) does not interact with fluoxetine in healthy volunteers. *Int J Clin Pharmacol Ther* (1998) 36, 301–5.
17. Zomig (Zolmitriptan). AstraZeneca UK Ltd. UK Summary of product characteristics, May 2004.

Triptans + St John's wort (*Hypericum perforatum*)

The UK CSM noted that pharmacodynamic (potentiation) interactions have been identified between triptans and St John's wort (*Hypericum perforatum*) leading to an increased risk of adverse effects. They suggest that patients on triptans should not take St John's wort preparations.[1]

1. Committee on Safety of Medicines/Medicines Control Agency. Reminder: St John's Wort (*Hypericum perforatum*) interactions. *Current Problems* (2000) 26, 6–7.

Triptans; Almotriptan + Verapamil

Verapamil inhibits almotriptan metabolism, but only to a small, clinically insignificant extent.

Clinical evidence, mechanism, importance and management

In a crossover study, 12 healthy subjects were given a single 12.5-mg dose of almotriptan, either alone or following a week of treatment with sustained-release verapamil 120 mg twice daily. The AUC and maximum plasma level of almotriptan were raised by 20.5 and 23.7% respectively by verapamil. However, the only effect this caused was a slight increase in systolic BP (8 mmHg) 2 hours after the dose. It was suggested that verapamil may inhibit the metabolism of almotriptan via the cytochrome P450 isoenzyme CYP3A4. The authors suggest that changes of this magnitude do not warrant dosage adjustments.[1]

1. Fleishaker JC, Sisson TA, Carel BJ, Azie NE. Pharmacokinetic interaction between verapamil and almotriptan in healthy volunteers. *Clin Pharmacol Ther* (2000) 67, 498–503.

Triptans; Eletriptan + Azoles

Ketoconazole markedly raises the plasma levels of eletriptan.

Clinical evidence, mechanism, importance and management

A clinical pharmacokinetic study by the makers of eletriptan found that **ketoconazole** 400 mg increased the maximum serum levels of eletriptan 2.7-fold, the AUC 5.9-fold and prolonged its half-life from 4.8 to

8.3 hours. Because of this, they say that **ketoconazole**, **itraconazole** and a number of other potent inhibitors of the cytochrome P450 isoenzyme CYP3A4, an enzyme involved in the metabolism of eletriptan, are predicted to raise serum eletriptan levels and should not be used with eletriptan.[1]

1. Relpax (Eletriptan). Pfizer Ltd. UK Summary of product characteristics, December 2003.

Triptans; Eletriptan + Protease inhibitors

The maker states that the concurrent use of eletriptan and ritonavir, indinavir, or nelfinavir should be avoided, because these protease inhibitors are inhibitors of the cytochrome P450 isoenzyme CYP3A4, an enzyme involved in the metabolism of eletriptan, and are therefore predicted to markedly increase levels of eletriptan.[1] This is based on the known interaction with 'erythromycin', (p.440) and 'ketoconazole' (see (p.442)).

1. Relpax (Eletriptan). Pfizer Ltd. UK Summary of product characteristics, December 2003.

Triptans; Sumatriptan + Butorphanol

Sumatriptan given by injection appears not to interact with butorphanol nasal spray, but if both drugs are given by nasal spray a significant pharmacokinetic interaction may occur.

Clinical evidence, mechanism, importance and management

No pharmacokinetic interactions or change in side effects were found to occur between single 1-mg doses of butorphanol tartrate nasal spray and a 6-mg subcutaneous dose of sumatriptan succinate in 24 healthy subjects. It was concluded that concurrent use during acute migraine attacks need not be avoided.[1]

In another study, 19 healthy subjects were given a 1-mg dose of butorphanol nasal spray either 1 or 30 minutes following a 20-mg dose of sumatriptan nasal spray. When butorphanol was given 1 minute after sumatriptan the AUC and maximum plasma levels of butorphanol were reduced by 28.6 and 38.3% respectively. When butorphanol was given 30 minutes after sumatriptan no significant pharmacokinetic interaction was noted. It was suggested that sumatriptan may cause a transient vasoconstriction of nasal blood vessels, leading to reduced butorphanol absorption. It would therefore seem wise to separate administration to ensure the full effects of butorphanol are achieved.[2]

1. Srinivas NR, Shyu WC, Upmalis D, Lee JS, Barbhaiya RH. Lack of pharmacokinetic interaction between butorphanol tartrate nasal spray and sumatriptan succinate. *J Clin Pharmacol* (1995) 35, 432–7.
2. Vachharajani NN, Shyu W-C, Nichola PS, Boulton DW. A pharmacokinetic interaction study between butorphanol and sumatriptan nasal sprays in healthy subjects: importance of the timing of butorphanol administration. *Cephalalgia* (2002) 22, 282–7.

Triptans; Sumatriptan + Loxapine

An isolated report describes a woman on loxapine who developed a severe dystonic reaction when given sumatriptan.

Clinical evidence, mechanism, importance and management

A woman was treated with loxapine 10 mg twice daily for psychotic target symptoms, benzatropine for the prophylaxis of extrapyramidal effects, carbamazepine for mood stabilisation, and *Fiorcet* (paracetamol (acetaminophen), caffeine, butalbital) for migraine headaches. Two days after the loxapine dosage was raised to 35 mg daily she was given a single 6-mg subcutaneous dose of sumatriptan for a migraine headache. Within 15 minutes she developed torticollis, which was treated with intramuscular benzatropine and intravenous diphenhydramine.

The authors of the report suggest that this reaction was possibly caused by the additive dystonic effects of the loxapine and sumatriptan, despite the presence of the benzatropine. Dystonia is not an uncommon extrapyramidal reaction associated with antipsychotics, and neck stiffness and dystonia are recognised adverse effects of sumatriptan, but of low incidence.[1] This seems to be the first and only report this apparent interaction, but the authors suggest good monitoring if both drugs are used concurrently.

1. Garcia G, Kaufman MB, Colucci RD. Dystonic reaction associated with sumatriptan. *Ann Pharmacother* (1994) 28, 1199.

Triptans; Sumatriptan + Naproxen

A study in 12 healthy subjects found that a single 500-mg dose of naproxen had no significant effect on the pharmacokinetics of a single 100-mg oral dose of sumatriptan.[1]

1. Srinivasu P, Rambhau D, Rao BR, Rao YM. Lack of pharmacokinetic interaction between sumatriptan and naproxen. *J Clin Pharmacol* (2000) 40, 99–104.

Triptans; Zolmitriptan + Cimetidine

Cimetidine raises the plasma levels of zolmitriptan.

Clinical evidence, mechanism, importance and management

The maker of zolmitriptan notes that the half-life of zolmitriptan was increased by 44% and the AUC by 48% when it was given after the administration of cimetidine. They suggest that this may be because of the inhibitory effect of cimetidine on cytochrome P450 isoenzyme CYP1A2, an enzyme involved in the metabolism of zolmitriptan. The maker recommends a zolmitriptan dose reduction to a maximum of 5 mg in 24 hours in patients on cimetidine.[1]

1. Zomig (Zolmitriptan). AstraZeneca UK Ltd. UK Summary of product characteristics, May 2004.

Triptans; Zolmitriptan + Metoclopramide

Metoclopramide does not interact pharmacokinetically with zolmitriptan.

Clinical evidence, mechanism, importance and management

In a randomised, crossover study, 15 healthy subjects were given single 10-mg doses of zolmitriptan alone or with 10 mg metoclopramide. Metoclopramide had no effect on the pharmacokinetics of zolmitriptan, so there would appear to be no reason for avoiding concurrent use of these two drugs.[1]

1. Seaber EJ, Ridout G, Layton G, Posner J, Peck RW. The novel anti-migraine zolmitriptan (Zomig 311C90) has no clinically significant interactions with paracetamol or metoclopramide. *Eur J Clin Pharmacol* (1997) 53, 229–34.

Triptans; Zolmitriptan + Paracetamol (Acetaminophen)

A pharmacokinetic interaction occurs between zolmitriptan and paracetamol, but this does not appear to be clinically significant.

Clinical evidence, mechanism, importance and management

In a randomised, crossover study, 15 healthy subjects were given single 10-mg doses of zolmitriptan, alone or with 1 g paracetamol. The paracetamol increased the zolmitriptan maximum plasma levels and AUC by 11%, while reducing its renal clearance by 9%. The paracetamol maximum plasma levels, AUC and half-life were reduced by 31%, 11% and 8% respectively.[1] These small changes were considered to be clinically irrelevant, and there would therefore appear to be no reason for avoiding concurrent use of these two drugs.

1. Seaber EJ, Ridout G, Layton G, Posner J, Peck RW. The novel anti-migraine zolmitriptan (Zomig 311C90) has no clinically significant interactions with paracetamol or metoclopramide. *Eur J Clin Pharmacol* (1997) 53, 229–34.

Triptans; Zolmitriptan + Quinolones

The maker recommends a dose reduction of zolmitriptan to a maximum of 5 mg in 24 hours in patient taking quinolone antibacterials such as ciprofloxacin. This is because these antibacterials are predicted to increase levels of zolmitriptan by inhibiting cytochrome P450 isoenzyme CYP1A2, an enzyme involved in the metabolism of zolmitriptan.[1] This is based on the known interaction with 'cimetidine', (p.443). Further study is needed.

1. Zomig (Zolmitriptan). AstraZeneca UK Ltd. UK Summary of product characteristics, May 2004.

15

Antineoplastics

The antineoplastic drugs (e.g. cytotoxics, cytostatics) are used in the treatment of malignant disease alone or in conjunction with radiotherapy, surgery or immunosuppressants. They also find application in the treatment of a number of autoimmune disorders such as rheumatoid arthritis and psoriasis, and a few are used with other immunosuppressant drugs (ciclosporin, corticosteroids) to prevent transplant rejection. These other drugs are dealt with under 'immunosuppressants', (p.767).

Of all the drugs discussed in this publication, the antineoplastic drugs are amongst the most toxic and have a low therapeutic index. This means that a quite small increase in their activity can lead to the development of serious and life-threatening toxicity. A list of the antineoplastic drugs that are featured in this section appears in 'Table 15.1', (below), grouped by their primary mechanism of action. This table also includes a number of hormone antagonists that are used in the treatment of cancer.

Unlike most of the other interaction monographs in this publication, some of the information on the antineoplastic drugs is derived from *animal* experiments and *in vitro* studies, so that confirmation of their clinical relevance is still needed. The reason for including these data is that the antineoplastic drugs as a group do not lend themselves readily to the kind of clinical studies that can be undertaken with many other drugs, and there would seem to be justification in this instance for including indirect evidence of this kind. The aim is not to make definite predictions, but to warn users of the interaction possibilities.

Table 15.1 Antineoplastics used in the treatment of cancer

Action	*Generic name*	*Proprietary names*
Alkylating agents, and drugs that appear to have an alkylating action		
Nitrosureas	Carmustine (BCNU)	Becenun, BiCNU, Carmubris, Gliadel, Nitrourean, Nitrumon
	Lomustine (CCNU)	Belustine, CCNU, Cecenu, CeeNU, Citostal, Prava
	Streptozocin (Streptozotocin)	Zanosar
Platinum derivatives	Carboplatin	Biocarbo, Blastocarb, Boplatex, B-Platin, Carboplat, Carbosin, Carbosol, Carboxtie, Cycloplatin, Emorzim, Ercar, Ifacap, Kemocarb, Megaplatin, Nealorin, Neocarbo, Novoplatinum, Omilipis, Oncocarb, Paraplatin, Paraplatine, Platicarb, Platinwas, Ribocarbo, Tecnocarb
	Cisplatin (CDDP)	Abiplatin, Astaplatin, Bioplatino, Blastolem, C-Platin, Cis-Gry, Cishexal, Cisplamol, Cisplatex, Cisplatyl, Citoplatino, Elvecis, Faulplatin, Kemoplat, Lederplatin, Neoplatin, Noveldexis, Placis, Platamine, Platiblastin, Platiblastin-S, Platidiam, Platinex, Platino II, Platinol, Platiran, Platistil, Platistin, Platistine, Platosin, Pronto Platamine, Sicatem, Tecnoplatin, Unistin
	Oxaliplatin	Crisapla, Dabenzol, Dacplat, Eloxatin, Eloxatine, Kebir, Metaplatin, Mitog, O-Plat, Oxaltie, Platenk, Platinostyl, Plusplatin, Uxalun, Xaliplat
Others	Altretamine (Hexamethylmelamine)	Hexalen, Hexastat
	Busulfan (Busulphan)	Busulfex, Busulivex, Myleran
	Chlorambucil	Chloraminophene, Leukeran, Linfolysin
	Chlormethine (Mustine)	Caryolysine, Mustargen, Onco-Cloramin
	Cyclophosphamide	Alkyloxan, Carloxan, Cyclan, Cycloblastin, Cyclostin, Cycloxan, Cytoxan, Endoxan, Endoxana, Genoxal, Genuxal, Ledoxina, Neosar, Procytox, Sendoxan
	Dacarbazine	Dacarb, Dacarbaziba, Dacatic, Deticene, Detilem, Detimedac, DTIC, DTIC-Dome, Fauldetic, Ifadac
	Estramustine	Cellmustin, Emcyt, Estracyt, Multosin, Prostamustin
	Ifosfamide	Asoifos, Cuantil, Duvaxan, Fentul, Holoxan, Holoxane, Ifex, Ifocris, Ifolem, Ifomida, Ifomixan, Ifoxan, IFO-cell, IFX, Mitoxana, Tronoxal
	Melphalan	Alkeran, Alkerana
	Temozolomide	Temodal, Temodar, Temoxol
	Thiotepa	Ledertepa, Onco Tiotepa, Thioplex

Continued

Table 15.1 Antineoplastics used in the treatment of cancer *(continued)*

Action	*Generic name*	*Proprietary names*
Antimetabolites		
Folate antagonists	Methotrexate (Amethopterin)	Abitrexate, Artrait, Biometrox, Biotrexate, Emthexat, Emthexate, Ervemin, Farmitrexat, Fauldexato, Ifamet, Lantarel, Ledertrexate, Maxtrex, Medsatrexate, Metex, Methoblastin, Metrexato, Miantrex, MTX, Neotrexate, Novatrex, O-trexat, Rheumatrex, Trexall, Trexan, Trixilem, Unitrexate, Xantromid
	Raltitrexed	Tomudex
Podophylotoxin derivatives	Etoposide	Celltop, Citodox, Eposido, Eposin, Epsidox, Etocris, ETO CS, Eto-Gry, Etomedac, Etopofos, Etopophos, Etopos, Etopul, Etosid, Etosin, Eunades, Euvaxon, Exitop, Fytosid, Kenazol, Labimion, Lastet, Neoplaxol, Nexvep, Onkoposid, Optasid, Percas, Riboposid, Toposar, Vepesid, Vepeside, VP-Gen
	Teniposide	VM 26, Vumon
Purine analogues	Azathioprine	Azafalk, Azahexal, Azamedac, Azamun, Azapress, Azasan, Azathiodura, Azatrilem, Azopi, Azoran, Colinsan, Immunoprin, Imuger, Imunen, Imuprin, Imuran, Imurek, Imurel, Thioprine, Transimune, Zytrim
	Cladribine	Intocel, Leustat, Leustatin, Leustatine, Litak
	Fludarabine	Beneflur, Fludara, Forclina
	Mercaptopurine	Puri-Nethol, Purinethol, Varimer
	Tioguanine (Thioguanine)	Lanvis, Tabloid, Tioguanina
Pyrimidine analogues		
	Capecitabine	Apecitab, Xeloda
	Carmofur	Mirafur
	Cytarabine (Cytosine arabinoside)	Alexan, Arabine, Aracytin, Aracytine, ARA-cell, Citab, Citagenin, Citaloxan, Cylocide, Cytarine, Cytosar, Cytosar-U, DepoCyt, DepoCyte, Erpalfa, Ifarab, Laracit, Medsara, Novutrax, Tabine, Udicil
	Fluorouracil (5-FU)	Adrucil, Carac, Cinco-Fu, Cinkef-U, Efudex, Efudix, Fivefluro, Fivoflu, Fluoroplex, Flurablastin, Fluracedyl, Fluracil, Fluroblastin, Fluroblastine, Flurox, Ifacil, Ifocid, Killit, O-fluor, Oncofu, Oncofluor, Ribofluor, Utoral
	Gemcitabine	Abine, Antoril, Gemcite, Gemtro, Gemzar
	Tegafur	Asofurtal, Citofur, Ftorafur, Ftoral, Ftoralon, UFT, Uftoral, Utefos
Mitotic inhibitors		
Vinca alkaloids	Vinblastine	Blastovin, Cellblastin, Cytoblastin, Ifabla, Lemblastine, Solblastin, Velban, Velbe, Xintoprost
	Vincristine	Biocrist, Cellcristin, Citomid, Cytocristin, Farmistin, Faulcris, Ifavin, Neocristin, Oncovin, Onkocristin, Tenocris, Vincasar PFS, Vinces, Vincizina, Vincresyex, Vincrisul, Vinracine
	Vindesine	Eldisin, Eldisine, Enison, Gesidine
	Vinorelbine	Filcrin, Navelbin, Navelbine, Neocitec, Norelbin, Sulcoline, Vilbine, Vilne, Vinarine, Vinelbine, Vinorgen
Taxanes	Docetaxel	Asdocel, Daxotel, Dolectran, Donataxel, Doxetal, Doxmil, Neocel, Plustaxano, Taxotere, Texot, Trazoteva, Trixotene
	Paclitaxel	Anzatax, Asotax, Biotaxel, Biotax, BrisTaxol, Britaxol, Clitaxel, Dalys, Drifen, Ifaxol, Intaxel, Magytax, Medixel, Onxol, Paclikebir, Paclitax, Pacliteva, Paklitaxfil, Panataxel, Parexel, Paxel, Paxene, Praxel, Taclipaxol, Tarvexol, Taxocris, Taxodiol, Taxol, Taycovit
Topoisomerase inhibitors	Irinotecan	Biotecan, Campto, Camptosar, CPT, Efixano, Irenax, Irinogen, Irinotel, Itoxaril, Kebirtecan, Pipetecan, Satigene, Sibudan, Tecnotecan, Trinotecan, Winol
	Topotecan	Asotecan, Hycamtin, Potekam, Tisogen, Topestin, Topokebir, Topotag, Topotel, TPT, Viatopin
	9-Aminocamptothecin	
Cytotoxic antibiotics		
Anthracyclines	Aclarubicin (Aclacinomycin A)	Aclacin, Aclaplastin
	Daunorubicin (Daunomycin, Rubidomycin)	Cerubidin, Cerubidine, Daunoblastin, Daunoblastina, Daunocin, DaunoXome, Daurocina, Maxiduano, Rubilem

Continued

Table 15.1 Antineoplastics used in the treatment of cancer *(continued)*

Action	*Generic name*	*Proprietary names*
	Doxorubicin (Adriamycin)	Adriblastin, Adriblastina, Adriblastine, Adrim, Adrimedac, Biorrub, Caelyx, Colhidrol, Daxotel, Dicladox, Doxil, Doxocris, Doxolem, Doxorbin, Doxorubin, DOXO-cell, Doxtie Farmiblastina, Fauldoxo, Flavicina, Ifadox, Myocet, Nagun, Neoxane, Pallagicin, Ranxas, Ribodoxo-L, Roxorin, Rubex
	Epirubicin	Crisabon, Cuatroepil, Ellence, Epi-cell, Epidoxo, Epifil, Epikebir, Epilem, EPR, Farmorubicin, Farmorrubicina, Farmorubicina, Farmorubicine, Pharmorubicin, Robanol, Rubifarm, Rubina
	Idarubicin	Idamycin, Idaralem, Zavedos
	Mitoxantrone (Mitozantrone)	Batinel, Formyxan, Genefadrone, Micraleve, Misotel, Mitoxal, Mitoxgen, Mitoxmar, Neotalem, Novantron, Novantrone, Oncotron, Onkotrone, Pralifan, Refador
Others	Bleomycin	Bileco, Blanoxan, Blenamax, Blenoxane, Bleo, Bleolem, Bleo-cell, Bleo-S, Bleocris, Blexit, Blio, Blocamicina, Bonar, Nikableomicina, Tecnomicina
	Dactinomycin	Ac-De, Cosmegen, Dacmozen, Lyovac Cosmegen
	Mitomycin	Ametycine, Asomutan, Crisofimina, Datisan, Ifamit, Maximiton, Metomit, Mitocin, Mitocin-C, Mitocyna, Mitokebir, Mitolem, Mito-medac, Mitonovag, Mitostat, Mitotie, Mitozytrex, Mixandex, Mutamycin, Mutamycine, Oncotaxina, Sintemicina, Vetio
	Plicamycin	Mithracin
Anti-androgens		
	Bicalutamide	Androxinon, Bicaprost, Bidrostat, Bosconar, Casodex, Cosudex, Gepeprostin, Imda, Liberprost, Lutamidal, Raffolutil
	Flutamide	Afluta, Androbloc, Androdor, Apimid, Asoflut, Biomida, Chimax, Dedile, Drogenil, Elbat, Etaconil, Euflex, Eulexin, Eulexine, Flucinom, Flucinome, Fluken, Flulem, Flumid, Fluprosin, Fluprost, Fluta, Flutabene, Flutacan, Flutamin, Flutan, Flutandrona, Flutaplex, Flutastad, Flutax, Flutepan, Flutol, Flutrax, FTDA, Fugerel, Grisetin, Olter, Oncosal, Palistop, Profamid, Prostacur, Prostadirex, Prostamid, Prostica, Prostogenat, Tafenil, Tecnoflut, Testotard, Tremexal, Virflutam
	Nilutamide	Anandron, Nilandron
Anti-oestrogens		
Oestrogen-receptor antagonists	Tamoxifen	Adifen, Apo-Tamox, Bilem, Bioxifeno, Crisafeno, Cryoxifeno, Defarol, Diemon, Ebefen, Farmifeno, Genox, Ginarson, Jenoxifen, Kessar, Ledertam, Mamofen, Neophedan, Nolgen, Nolvadex, Nomafen, Nourytam, Novofen, Oncotam, Ralsifen-X, Rolap, Sinmaren, Soltamox, Tadex, Tamax, Tamec, Tamexin, Tamifen, Tamizam, Tamofen, Tamofene, Tamokadin, Tamolem, Tamooex, Tamopham, Tamophar, Tamoplex, Tamosin, Tamox, Tamoxan, Tamoxasta, Tamoxen, Tamoxene, Tamoxi, Tamoximerck, Tamoxin, Tamoxis, Tamoxistad, Taxfeno, Taxofen, Taxus, Tecnotax, Trimetrox, Tuosomin, Virtamox, Zemide, Zitazonium, Zymoplex
	Toremifene	Fareston
Aromatase inhibitors	Aminoglutethimide	Cytadren, Orimeten, Orimetene
	Anastrozole	Arimidex, Asiolex, Distalene, Gondonar, Lezole, Pantestone, Trozolet, Trozolite
	Exemestane	Aromacin, Aromasil, Aromasin, Aromasine
	Formestane	Lentare, Lentaron
	Letrozole	Cendalon, Fecinole, Femar, Femara
Miscellaneous		
	Amsacrine	Amekrin, Amsa P-D, Amsidine, Amsidyl
	Asparaginase (Colaspase, crisantaspase, pegaspargase)	Elspar, Erwinase, Kidrolase, L-Asp, Laspar, Leunase, Oncaspar, Paronal
	Bexarotene	Targretin
	Hydroxycarbamide (Hydroxyurea)	Dacrodil, Droxia, Droxiurea, Hydrea, Hydrine, Litalir, Medroxyurea, Mylocel, Neodrea, Onco-Carbide, Syrea
	Imatinib	Gleevec, Glivec
	Mitotane	Lisodren, Lysodren
	Pentostatin	Nipent
	Procarbazine	Matulane, Natulan
	Trastuzumab	Herceptin

Altretamine (Hexamethylmelamine) + Antidepressants

Severe orthostatic hypotension has been described in patients concurrently treated with altretamine and either phenelzine, amitriptyline or imipramine.

Clinical evidence, mechanism, importance and management

Four patients experienced very severe orthostatic hypotension (described by the authors as potentially life-threatening) when concurrently treated with altretamine 150 to 250 mg/m^2 and either **phenelzine** 60 mg daily, **amitriptyline** 50 mg daily or **imipramine** 50 to 150 mg daily.[1] They experienced incapacitating dizziness, severe lightheadedness, and/or fainting within a few days of taking both drugs concurrently. Standing blood pressures as low as 50/30 and 60/40 mmHg were recorded. The reasons are not known. One of the patients had no problems when **imipramine** was replaced by **nortriptyline** 50 mg daily. One other patient who had also taken altretamine with antidepressants reported dizziness, while another noted nonspecific discomfort. The incidence of this interaction is unknown, but it is clear that the concurrent use of altretamine and **tricyclics** or **MAOIs** should be closely monitored.

1. Bruckner HW, Schleifer SJ. Orthostatic hypotension as a complication of hexamethylmelamine antidepressant interaction. *Cancer Treat Rep* (1983) 67, 516.

Altretamine (Hexamethylmelamine) + Pyridoxine (Vitamin B_6)

Pyridoxine reduced neurotoxicity associated with altretamine, but also reduced its effectiveness.

Clinical evidence, mechanism, importance and management

In a large randomised study in women with advanced ovarian cancer the neurotoxicity associated with altretamine and cisplatin chemotherapy was reduced by pyridoxine, but the response duration was also reduced.[1] In this study, cisplatin was given on day 1 (37.5 or 75 mg/m^2) and altretamine 200 mg/m^2 daily on days 8 to 21, and half the patients also received pyridoxine 100 mg three times daily on days 1 to 21. It is unclear how pyridoxine reduced the activity of this regimen, but the use of pyridoxine (vitamin B_6) should probably be avoided in patients on altretamine.

1. Wiernik PH, Yeap B, Vogel SE, Kaplan BH, Comis RL, Falkson G, Davis TE, Fazzini E, Cheuvart B, Horton J. Hexamethylmelamine and low or moderate dose cisplatin with or without pyridoxine for treatment of advanced ovarian carcinoma: a study of the Eastern Cooperative Oncology Group. *Cancer Invest* (1992) 10, 1–9.

9-Aminocamptothecin + Anticonvulsants

Anticonvulsants can lower the serum levels of 9-aminocamptothecin.

Clinical evidence, mechanism, importance and management

A study in 59 patients with glioblastoma multiforme or recurrent high grade astrocytomas found that the steady-state plasma levels of 9-aminocamptothecin were reduced to about one third in 29 of the patients concurrently taking anticonvulsants (**carbamazepine**, **phenobarbital**, **phenytoin**, **sodium valproate**). The incidence of myelosuppression was greater in those not taking anticonvulsants.[1] The reason for the reduced 9-aminocamptothecin levels is not known, but it seems likely that it was due to the enzyme inducing activity of **carbamazepine**, **phenobarbital** and **phenytoin**. These results suggest that higher than usual doses of 9-aminocamptothecin are possibly needed in the presence of enzyme-inducing anticonvulsants. For similar effects of anticonvulsants on related topoisomerase inhibitors, see 'Irinotecan + Anticonvulsants', p.472' and 'Topotecan + Phenytoin', p.494.

1. Grossman SA, Hochberg F, Fisher J, Chen T-L, Kim L, Gregory R, Grochow LB, Piantadosi S. Increased 9-aminocamptothecin dose requirements in patients on anticonvulsants. *Cancer Chemother Pharmacol* (1998) 42, 118–26.

Aminoglutethimide + Danazol

Danazol may reduce the efficacy of aminoglutethimide.

Clinical evidence, mechanism, importance and management

In a randomised clinical trial, the addition of danazol to aminoglutethimide in women with breast cancer, reduced the response rate compared with aminoglutethimide alone. It was found that danazol suppresses sex hormone binding globulin leading to increased free oestradiol, which counteracts the oestradiol suppressive effect of aminoglutethimide.[1] Danazol should probably not be combined with anti-oestrogenic treatments.

1. Dowsett M, Murray RML, Pitt P, Jeffcoate SL. Antagonism of aminoglutethimide and danazol in the suppression of serum free oestradiol in breast cancer patients. *Eur J Cancer Clin Oncol* (1985) 21, 1063–8.

Aminoglutethimide + Diuretics

A single case report describes hyponatraemia in a patient after 10 months treatment with both aminoglutethimide and bendroflumethiazide.

Clinical evidence, mechanism, importance and management

A woman who, for several years, had been taking four tablets daily of **bendroflumethiazide** 2.5 mg and **potassium chloride** 578 mg for hypertension and mild cardiac decompensation, was additionally treated with aminoglutethimide 1 g daily, and hydrocortisone 60 mg daily, for breast cancer. After 10 months treatment she was hospitalised with severe hyponatraemia, which resolved on withdrawal of all the drugs. No significant change in electrolytes occurred over 3 months when the aminoglutethimide and hydrocortisone were used alone, but serum sodium fell again when the diuretic was restarted. The serum sodium levels were subsequently maintained by the addition of fludrocortisone 100 micrograms daily.[1] The hyponatraemia was thought to be caused by the combined inhibitory effect of the aminoglutethimide on aldosterone production (which normally retains sodium in the body) and the sodium loss caused by the diuretic. Plasma electrolytes should be monitored when aminoglutethimide is used, and this would seem particularly important if it is given with any diuretic.

1. Bork E, Hansen M. Severe hyponatremia following simultaneous administration of aminoglutethimide and diuretics. *Cancer Treat Rep* (1986) 70, 689–90.

Anastrozole + Miscellaneous

Anastrozole does not appear to interact with aspirin, cimetidine, digoxin or oral hypoglycaemics. It also appears to have no effect on cytochrome P450 enzymes, so it is unlikely to interact with drugs that are affected by enzyme inducers or inhibitors.

Clinical evidence, mechanism, importance and management

A clinical study with **cimetidine** has shown that it does not affect the pharmacokinetics of anastrozole,[1] which suggests that anastrozole is unlikely to be affected by other drugs that inhibit cytochrome P450. Another clinical study showed that anastrozole does not affect the pharmacokinetics of **antipyrine** (**phenazone**),[2] so that it is unlikely to interact with those drugs which are known to be affected by enzyme inducers and inhibitors. The UK makers also say that in clinical trials there was no evidence of any interactions between anastrozole and commonly used drugs;[3] **aspirin**, **digoxin**, and **oral hypoglycaemic agents** were specifically mentioned in the early product information.[4]

1. Zeneca. Effect of cimetidine on anastrozole pharmacokinetics. Data on file, 1995.

2. Zeneca. Effect of anastrozole treatment on antipyrine pharmacokinetics in postmenopausal female volunteers. Data on file, 1995.
3. Arimidex (Anastrozole). AstraZeneca UK Ltd. UK Summary of product characteristics, July 2004.
4. Arimidex (Anastrozole) Monograph. Zeneca. September 1995.

Anthracyclines + Calcium channel blockers

Verapamil can increase the efficacy of doxorubicin in tissue culture systems and increase doxorubicin levels in patients. D-verapamil can alter the pharmacokinetics of epirubicin and possibly increase its bone marrow depressant effects. Consider also 'Calcium channel blockers + Antineoplastics', p.650.

Clinical evidence, mechanism, importance and management

(a) Doxorubicin

The efficacy of doxorubicin can be increased by **verapamil** and **nicardipine** in doxorubicin-resistant tissue culture systems,[1] while **nifedipine** has only minimal activity. A study in five patients with small cell lung cancer given doxorubicin, vincristine, etoposide and cyclophosphamide showed that when given **verapamil** 240 to 480 mg daily the AUC of the doxorubicin was doubled, peak serum levels were raised and the clearance was reduced. No increased toxicity was seen in this study.[2] However, although another study found no increase in noncardiac toxicities, **verapamil** caused an unacceptable degree of cardiac toxicity.[3] Be alert for this possibility if both drugs are used.

(b) Epirubicin

When used to reduce multidrug resistance in patients with advanced colorectal cancer treated with epirubicin, the **D-isomer of verapamil** appears to increase the bone marrow depressant toxicity of epirubicin.[4] Another study found that **D-verapamil** halved the AUC and half-life of epirubicin, and increased its clearance,[5] while yet another did not find these changes but found that the production of the metabolites of epirubicin was increased.[6] These changes should be taken into account if both drugs are used. More study is needed to evaluate the possible advantages and disadvantages of giving these drugs together.

1. Ramu A, Spanier R, Rahamimoff H, Fuks Z. Restoration of doxorubicin responsiveness in doxorubicin-resistant P388 murine leukaemia cells. *Br J Cancer* (1984) 50, 501–7.
2. Kerr DJ, Graham J, Cummings J, Morrison JG, Thompson GG, Brodie MJ, Kaye SB. The effect of verapamil on the pharmacokinetics of adriamycin. *Cancer Chemother Pharmacol* (1986) 18, 239–42.
3. Ozols RF, Cunnion RE, Klecker RW, Hamilton TC, Ostchega Y, Parrillo JE, Young RC. Verapamil and adriamycin in the treatment of drug-resistant ovarian cancer patients. *J Clin Oncol* (1987) 5, 641–7.
4. Kornek G, Despisch D, Kastner J, Schenk T, Locker G, Raderer M, Scheithauer W. A phase II study of D-verapamil (DVPM) plus doxorubicin in advanced colorectal cancer. *Ann Hematol* (1992) 56 (Suppl), 59.
5. Scheithauer W, Schenk T, Czejka M. Pharmacokinetic interaction between epirubicin and the multidrug resistance reverting agent D-verapamil. *Br J Cancer* (1993) 68, 8–9.
6. Mross K, Hamm K, Hossfeld DK. Effects of verapamil on the pharmacokinetics and metabolism of epirubicin. *Cancer Chemother Pharmacol* (1993) 31, 369–75.

Anthracyclines + Ciclosporin

High-dose ciclosporin increases the serum levels and the myelotoxicity of doxorubicin. An isolated report describes severe neurotoxicity and coma in a patient previously on ciclosporin who was given doxorubicin. Ciclosporin can similarly increase daunorubicin, epirubicin, idarubicin and mitoxantrone serum levels.

Clinical evidence

(a) Daunorubicin

Ciclosporin significantly reduced the frequency of resistance to induction therapy (31% versus 47%) and increased relapse-free and overall survival in a randomised trial in patients treated with daunorubicin. Ciclosporin recipients had higher steady-state serum concentrations of daunorubicin and its active metabolite daunorubicinol.[1]

(b) Doxorubicin

Eight patients with small cell lung cancer were given an initial course of doxorubicin (25 to 70 mg/m^2 over 1 hour) and a subsequent ciclosporin-modulated doxorubicin course (ciclosporin 6 mg/kg bolus, then 16 mg/kg daily for 2 days) for multidrug resistant tumour modulation. All of the patients were also given cyclophosphamide and vincristine. Ciclosporin increased the AUC of doxorubicin by 48%, and that of its active metabolite doxorubicinol by 443%. The myelotoxicity was increased by concurrent use: the leucocyte count fell by 84% after doxorubicin and by 91% after doxorubicin with ciclosporin. The platelet counts fell by 36% and a 73% respectively. The patients showed significant weight loss and severe myalgias.[2]

Three preliminary Phase I studies[3-5] are consistent with this report. In these studies, ciclosporin was found to increase the doxorubicin AUCs by 40 to 73%, and the doxorubicinol AUCs by 250 to 285%. However, no evidence of increased cardiotoxicity was found in a study of 23 patients given ciclosporin and doxorubicin.[6]

A cardiac transplant patient was given ciclosporin 2 mg/kg daily for 22 months. The ciclosporin was stopped and he was given doxorubicin 60 mg, vincristine 2 mg, cyclophosphamide 600 mg and prednisone 80 mg to treat Burkitt's lymphoma stage IVB. Eight hours later he developed disturbances of consciousness which lead to stage I coma, from which he spontaneously recovered 12 hours later. A week later a similar course of chemotherapy was started, and 10 to 15 minutes later he lost consciousness and generalised tonic clonic seizures progressively developed. He died 8 days later without recovering consciousness.[7]

(c) Epirubicin

There is preliminary evidence that ciclosporin can markedly increase the AUC of epirubicin (up to about fourfold) and increase the bone marrow suppression.[5] Ciclosporin did not increase the cardiotoxicity of epirubicin in 20 patients in one study.[6]

(d) Idarubicin

Concurrent use of ciclosporin and idarubicin increased the AUC of idarubicin and its active metabolite idarubicinol by 77% and 181% respectively in 9 patients, when compared with 11 patients receiving idarubicin alone.[8] Unacceptable toxicity occurred when idarubicin 9 or 12 mg/m^2 daily was combined with ciclosporin 16 mg/kg daily, when compared with idarubicin 12 mg/m^2 alone; 3 of 7 patients treated with the combination died. Increases in the AUC of idarubicin and idarubicinol produced by ciclosporin have also been reported elsewhere.[9]

(e) Mitoxantrone

The pharmacokinetics of mitoxantrone 10 mg/m^2 daily were compared with mitoxantrone 6 mg/m^2 (a 40% reduction in dose) plus high-dose ciclosporin in children. The ciclosporin recipients had a 42% reduction in mitoxantrone clearance, a 12% increase in mitoxantrone AUC, and similar toxicity.[10]

Mechanism

Uncertain. One reason may be that the ciclosporin affects the P-glycoprotein of the biliary tract so that the clearance of these anthracyclines in the bile is reduced. An additional reason may be that ciclosporin inhibits the metabolism of metabolites such as doxorubicinol so that they accumulate.[2] The increased levels of both would explain the increases in toxicity. It is not clear why such severe neurotoxicity was seen in one patient.

Importance and management

An established and clinically important interaction. Ciclosporin alters the pharmacokinetics of the anthracyclines resulting in increased serum levels. This pharmacokinetic interaction has complicated study into the value of using ciclosporin to modulate multidrug resistance in tumours and thereby improve the response to chemotherapy. In the case of anthracyclines and 'etoposide', (p.465), any benefit could just be attributed to dose intensification. Consequently, some have suggested reducing the dose of the anthracycline.[10] The use of high-dose ciclosporin for multidrug resistant tumour modulation remains experimental and should only be used in clinical trials. Concurrent use should be very well monitored. More study is needed to find out the possible effects of low-dose ciclosporin.

1. List AF, Kopecky KL, Willman CL, Head DR, Persons DL, Slovak ML, Dorr R, Karanes C, Hynes HE, Doroshow JH, Shurafa M, Appelbaum FR. Benefit of cyclosporine modulation of drug resistance in patients with poor-risk acute myeloid leukemia: a Southwest Oncology Group study. *Blood* (2001) 98, 3212–20.
2. Rushing DA, Raber SR, Rodvold KA, Piscitelli SC, Plank GS, Tewksbury DA. The effects of cyclosporine on the pharmacokinetics of doxorubicin in patients with small cell lung cancer. *Cancer* (1994) 74, 834–41.

3. Scheulen ME, Budach W, Skorzec M, Wiefelspütz JK, Seeber S. Influence of cyclosporin A on the pharmacokinetics and pharmacodynamics of doxorubicin. *Proc Am Assoc Cancer Res* (1993) 34, 213.
4. Bartlett NL, Lum BL, Fisher GA, Brophy NA, Ehsan MN, Halsey J, Sikic BI. Phase I trial of doxorubicin with cyclosporine as a modulator of multidrug resistance. *J Clin Oncol* (1994) 12, 835–42.
5. Eggert J, Scheulen ME, Schütte J, Budach W, Annweiler HM, Mengelkolch B, Skorzec M, Wiefelspütz J, Sack H, Seeber S. Influence of cyclosporin A on the pharmacokinetics and pharmacodynamics of doxorubicin and epirubicin. *Ann Hematol* (1994) 68, A26.
6. Eising EG, Gries P, Eggert J, Scheulen ME. Does the multi-drug resistance modulator cyclosporin A increase the cardiotoxicity of high-dose anthracycline chemotherapy. *Acta Oncol* (1997) 36, 735–40.
7. Barbui T, Rambaldi A, Parenzan L, Zucchelli M, Perico N, Remuzzi G. Neurological symptoms and coma associated with doxorubicin administration during chronic cyclosporin therapy. *Lancet* (1992) 339, 1421.
8. Pea F, Damiani D, Michieli M, Ermacora A, Baraldo M, Russo D, Fanin R, Baccarani M, Furlanut M. Multidrug resistance modulation in vivo: the effect of cyclosporin A alone or with dexverapamil on idarubicin pharmacokinetics in acute leukemia. *Eur J Clin Pharmacol* (1999) 55, 361–8.
9. Smeets M, Raymakers R, Muus P, Vierwinden G, Linssen P, Masereeuw R, de Witte T. Cyclosporin increases cellular idarubicin and idarubicinol concentrations in relapsed or refractory AML mainly due to reduced systemic clearance. *Leukemia* (2001) 15, 80–8.
10. Lacayo NJ, Lum BL, Becton DL, Weinstein H, Ravindranath Y, Chang MN, Bomgaars L, Lauer SJ, Sikic BI. Pharmacokinetic interactions of cyclosporine with etoposide and mitoxantrone in children with acute myeloid leukemia. *Leukemia* (2002) 16, 920–7.

Anthracyclines + Taxanes

Toxicity associated with combinations of paclitaxel with doxorubicin or epirubicin depends on the order of administration. The combination of doxorubicin and paclitaxel is more cardiotoxic than doxorubicin alone. Paclitaxel increases the levels of doxorubicin, and paclitaxel and docetaxel may affect the pharmacokinetics of epirubicin. Paclitaxel clearance was reduced by epirubicin in one study but unchanged in another. The pharmacokinetics of paclitaxel were unaltered by doxorubicin.

Clinical evidence

(a) Doxorubicin

Early studies in patients with breast cancer found a higher frequency of toxicity (particularly mucositis) when **paclitaxel** was given before doxorubicin (given as 24-hour and 48-hour infusions, respectively).[1] A subsequent study with similar effects revealed that doxorubicin clearance was reduced by a third if **paclitaxel** was given first.[2] In another study doxorubicin's peak plasma levels were increased when it was given by bolus injection 15 minutes after a 3-hour infusion of **paclitaxel**. The effect was non-linear and dependent on the dose of **paclitaxel**.[3] The same authors had already shown that this regimen produced a higher than expected incidence of cardiac toxicity.[4] Subsequent studies[5,6] have shown this schedule to result in unacceptable cardiotoxicity when the total cumulative doxorubicin dose exceeds 340 to 380 mg/m^2. However, when **paclitaxel** and doxorubicin were given together as a 3-hour infusion the levels of doxorubicin were lower than when it was given before **paclitaxel**,[3] and in another study the pharmacokinetics of each drug were found to be unchanged when they were given simultaneously as a 72-hour infusion.[7]

(b) Epirubicin

The pharmacokinetics of epirubicin were compared in 4 patients with breast cancer given intravenous epirubicin 90 mg/m^2 alone and 16 patients given the same dose followed immediately either by **paclitaxel** 175 mg/m^2 as a 3-hour infusion or **docetaxel** 70 mg/m^2 as a 1-hour infusion. No effect on epirubicin levels was detected, but the concentrations of epirubicin metabolites (epirubicinol and deoxydoxorubicinone) were increased by both **paclitaxel** and **docetaxel**.[8] In a subsequent study 21 patients were given the same regimen of epirubicin followed immediately by **paclitaxel** and 18 patients were given the drugs in the reverse order. Non-haematological toxicity was unaffected by the order of administration but when **paclitaxel** was given first the neutrophil and platelet nadir was lower and neutrophil recovery was slower. The AUC for epirubicin was also higher when **paclitaxel** was given first but the pharmacokinetics of **paclitaxel** were unaffected.[9] Exposure to **epirubicin** metabolites, but not epirubicin itself, was increased when it was given 15 minutes before a 3-hour infusion of **paclitaxel** when compared to a regimen using a 24-hour interval between the two drugs. In addition, the neutrophil nadir was lower, and clearance of **paclitaxel** was 30% slower with the former regimen, but cardiac toxicity was uncommon.[10] Conversely, a study of the combination of **docetaxel** and epirubicin did not find that the sequence of drug administration affected the pharmacokinetics of epirubicin, nor was there any difference in toxicity.[11] In another study, 16 patients with breast cancer had a transient but significant increase in epirubicin plasma levels during the subsequent infusion (after an interval of 1 hour) of **docetaxel** 75 mg/m^2, which was not seen if the **docetaxel** was given within 10 minutes of epirubicin.[12]

Mechanism

Studies in *mice* have found that the taxanes docetaxel and paclitaxel, and the vehicle used for paclitaxel *Cremophor*, may all modify the distribution and metabolism of doxorubicin increasing its levels in the heart, liver and kidneys. This may contribute to the cardiac toxicity seen during use with paclitaxel.[13] Similarly, *in vitro* studies in human myocardium showed that paclitaxel and docetaxel increased the conversion of doxorubicin to doxorubicinol, the metabolite that is thought to be responsible for cardiotoxicity.[14] In addition, *in vitro* studies have shown that the taxanes may reduce the biliary excretion of doxorubicin and epirubicin by inhibiting P-glycoprotein.[3]

Importance and management

The effect of paclitaxel on doxorubicin appears to be established. Various strategies have been suggested to reduce the cardiotoxicity of the combination. These include giving doxorubicin at least 24 hours before paclitaxel; reducing the cumulative dose of doxorubicin; or adding the cytoprotective drug dexrazoxane.[15] Epirubicin is considered less cardiotoxic than doxorubicin, and may be an alternative in some situations. However, it still appears preferable to give the anthracycline before the taxane. Docetaxel appears to have little clinically relevant effect on epirubicin, but this requires confirmation. Further study is needed on the optimum scheduling of anthracyclines and taxanes to maximise efficacy and minimise toxicity.

1. Sledge GW, Robert N, Sparano JA, Cogleigh M, Goldstein LJ, Neuberg D, Rowinsky E, Baughman C, McCaskill-Stevens W. Eastern Cooperative Oncology Group studies of paclitaxel and doxorubicin in advanced breast cancer. *Semin Oncol* (1995) 22, 105–8.
2. Holmes FA, Madden T, Newman RA, Valero V, Theriault RL, Fraschini G, Walters RS, Booser DJ, Buzdar AU, Willey J, Hortobagyi GN. Sequence-dependent alteration of doxorubicin pharmacokinetics by paclitaxel in a phase I study of paclitaxel and doxorubicin in patients with metastatic breast cancer. *J Clin Oncol* (1996) 14, 2713–21.
3. Gianni L, Viganò L, Locatelli A, Capri G, Giani A, Tarenzi E, Bonadonna G. Human pharmacokinetic characterization and in vitro study of the interaction between doxorubicin and paclitaxel in patients with breast cancer. *J Clin Oncol* (1997) 15, 1906–15.
4. Gianni L, Munzone E, Capri G, Fulfaro F, Tarenzi E, Villani F, Spreafico C, Laffranchi A, Caraceni A, Martini C, Stefanelli M, Valagussa P, Bonadonna G. Paclitaxel by 3-hour infusion in combination with bolus doxorubicin in women with untreated metastatic breast cancer: high antitumor efficacy and cardiac effects in a dose-finding and sequence-finding study. *J Clin Oncol* (1995) 13, 2688–99.
5. Gianni L, Dombernowsky P, Sledge G, Martin M, Amadori D, Arbuck SG, Ravdin P, Brown M, Messina M, Tuck D, Weil C, Winograd B. Cardiac function following combination therapy with paclitaxel and doxorubicin: an analysis of 657 women with advanced breast cancer. *Ann Oncol* (2001) 12, 1067–73.
6. Giordano SH, Booser DJ, Murray JL, Ibrahim NK, Rahman ZU, Valero V, Theriault RL, Rosales MF, Rivera E, Frye D, Ewer M, Ordonez NG, Buzdar AU, Hortobagyi GN. A detailed evaluation of cardiac toxicity: a phase II study of doxorubicin and one- or three-hour-infusion paclitaxel in patients with metastatic breast cancer. *Clin Cancer Res* (2002) 8, 3360–8.
7. Berg SL, Cowan KH, Balis FM, Fisherman JS, Denicoff AM, Hillig M, Poplack DG, O'Shaughnessy JA. Pharmacokinetics of Taxol and doxorubicin administered alone and in combination by continuous 72-hour infusion. *J Natl Cancer Inst* (1994) 86, 143–5.
8. Eposito M, Venturini M, Vannozzi MO, Tolino G, Lunardi G, Garrone O, Angiolini C, Viale M, Bergaglio M, Del Mastro L, Rosso R. Comparative effects of paclitaxel and docetaxel on the metabolism and pharmacokinetics of epirubicin in breast cancer patients. *J Clin Oncol* (1999) 17, 1132–40.
9. Venturini M, Lunardi G, Del Mastro L, Vannozzi MO, Tolino G, Numico G, Viale M, Pastrone I, Angiolini C, Bertelli G, Straneo M, Rosso R, Esposito M. Sequence effect of epirubicin and paclitaxel treatment on pharmacokinetics and toxicity. *J Clin Oncol* (2000) 18, 2116–25.
10. Grasselli G, Viganò L, Capri G, Locatelli A, Tarenzi E, Spreafico C, Bertuzzi A, Giani A, Materazzo C, Cresta S, Perotti A, Valagussa P, Gianni L. Clinical and pharmacologic study of the epirubicin and paclitaxel combination in women with metastatic breast cancer. *J Clin Oncol* (2001) 19, 2222–31.
11. Lunardi G, Venturini M, Vannozzi MO, Tolino G, Del Mastro L, Bighin C, Schettini G, Esposito M. Influence of alternate sequences of epirubicin and docetaxel on the pharmacokinetic behaviour of both drugs in advanced breast cancer. *Ann Oncol* (2002) 13, 280–5.
12. Ceruti M, Tagini V, Recalenda V, Arpicco S, Cattel L, Airoldi M, Bumma C. Docetaxel in combination with epirubicin in metastatic breast cancer: pharmacokinetic interactions. *Farmaco* (1999) 54, 733–9.
13. Colombo T, Parisi I, Zucchetti M, Sessa C, Goldhirsch A, D'Incalci M. Pharmacokinetic interactions of paclitaxel, docetaxel and their vehicles with doxorubicin. *Ann Oncol* (1999) 10, 391–5.
14. Minotti G, Saponiero A, Licata S, Menna P, Calafiore AM, Teodori G, Gianni L. Paclitaxel and docetaxel enhance the metabolism of doxorubicin to toxic species in human myocardium. *Clin Cancer Res* (2001) 7, 1511–15.
15. Sparano JA. Use of dexrazoxane and other strategies to prevent cardiomyopathy associated with doxorubicin-taxane combinations. *Semin Oncol* (1998) 25 (Suppl 10), 66–71.

Anthracyclines; Aclarubicin + Other antineoplastics

The bone marrow depressant effects of aclarubicin can be increased by previous treatment with nitrosoureas or mitomycin. Aclarubicin appears not to interact with cyclophosphamide, cytarabine, enocitabine (behenoyl cytarabine), fluorouracil, mercaptopurine, tioguanine or vincristine.

Clinical evidence, mechanism, importance and management

Myelosuppression is among the adverse effects of aclarubicin. The makers warn that the concurrent use of other drugs with similar myelosuppressant actions may be expected to have additive effects and dosage reductions should be considered.[1] Prior treatment with **nitrosoureas** (not specifically named) or **mitomycin** has been shown to increase the severity of the myelosuppression.[2,3]

Aclarubicin has been given in combination with **cyclophosphamide**, **cytarabine**, **enocitabine**, **fluorouracil**, **mercaptopurine**, **tioguanine** or **vincristine** without signs of an interaction.[1]

1. Aclarubicin. Medac GmbH. UK Summary of product characteristics, March 1998.
2. Van Echo DA, Whitacre MY, Aisner J, Applefeld MM, Wiernik PH. Phase I trial of aclacinomycin A. *Cancer Treat Rep* (1982) 66, 1127–32.
3. Bedikian AY, Karlin D, Stroehlein J, Valdivieso M, Korinek J, Bodey G. Phase II evaluation of aclacinomycin A (ACM-A, NSC208734) in patients with metastatic colorectal cancer. *Am J Clin Oncol* (1983) 6, 187–190.

Anthracyclines; Doxorubicin + Barbiturates

The effects of doxorubicin may be reduced by the concurrent use of barbiturates.

Clinical evidence, mechanism, importance and management

A comparative study in patients treated with doxorubicin showed that those concurrently taking barbiturates had a plasma clearance that was 50% higher than those who were not (318 compared with 202 ml/minute).[1] This clinical study is in agreement with previous studies in *mice*.[2] A possible explanation is that the barbiturate increases the metabolism of the doxorubicin. It seems possible that the dosage of doxorubicin will need to be increased in barbiturate-treated patients to achieve maximal therapeutic effects.

1. Riggs CE, Engel S, Wesley M, Wiernik PH, Bachur NR. Doxorubicin pharmacokinetics, prochlorperazine and barbiturate effects. *Clin Pharmacol Ther* (1982) 31, 263.
2. Reich SD, Bachur NR. Alterations in adriamycin efficacy by phenobarbital. *Cancer* (1976) 36, 3803–6.

Anthracyclines; Doxorubicin + Tamoxifen

Tamoxifen appears to have no significant effect on the pharmacokinetics of doxorubicin.

Clinical evidence, mechanism, importance and management

A pharmacokinetic study in patients with non-Hodgkin's lymphoma on CHOP (cyclophosphamide, vincristine, prednisone and doxorubicin 37.5 to 50 mg/m^2) found that the addition of tamoxifen 480 mg daily for 5 days had no significant effect on the AUC or total clearance of doxorubicin.[1] For the possible additive thromboembolic effect of doxorubicin and tamoxifen, see 'Antineoplastics + Tamoxifen', p.453.

1. El-Yazigi A, Berry J, Ezzat A, Wahab FA. Effect of tamoxifen on the pharmacokinetics of doxorubicin in patients with non-Hodgkin's lymphoma. *Ther Drug Monit* (1997) 19, 632–6.

Anthracyclines; Epirubicin + Cimetidine

Cimetidine can increase epirubicin serum levels.

Clinical evidence, mechanism, importance and management

In a study of 8 patients, cimetidine 400 mg twice daily increased the AUC of epirubicin by 50%. At the same time the AUCs of two metabolites of epirubicin, epirubicinol and 7-deoxydoxorubicinol aglycone, increased by 41 and 357% respectively. Liver blood flow also increased by 17%.[1] The mechanism is unknown. More study of this interaction is needed but be aware of the possibility of cimetidine increasing the exposure to epirubicin; monitor the patient closely and adjust epirubicin dosage if needed. Cimetidine can be bought over the counter in some countries so that patients may unwittingly increase the toxicity of epirubicin. Cimetidine has also increased the levels or toxicity of some other antineoplastics, see 'Nitrosoureas + Cimetidine', p.485, 'Cyclophosphamide + H$_2$-blockers', p.462 and 'Fluorouracil + H$_2$-blockers', p.469.

1. Murray LS, Jodrell DI, Morrison JG, Cook A, Kerr DJ, Whiting B, Kaye SB, Cassidy J. The effect of cimetidine on the pharmacokinetics of epirubicin in patients with advanced breast cancer: preliminary evidence of a potentially common drug interaction. *Clin Oncol* (1998) 10, 35–8.

Antineoplastics + Aprepitant

Aprepitant had no effect on the pharmacokinetics of a single dose of docetaxel. The activation of cyclophosphamide and thiotepa was slightly lower in patients receiving aprepitant, but not to a clinically relevant extent. However, the maker recommends caution with antineoplastics principally metabolised by the cytochrome P450 isoenzyme CYP3A4, particularly irinotecan, and also etoposide, vinorelbine, paclitaxel, ifosfamide, imatinib, vinblastine and vincristine.

Clinical evidence

(a) Cyclophosphamide

The rate of autoinduction of cyclophosphamide was 23% lower and exposure to the active metabolite 4-hydroxycyclophosphamide was 5% lower in 6 patients receiving aprepitant with a 4-day course of high-dose CTC (cyclophosphamide, thiotepa, carboplatin) when compared with 49 patients receiving high-dose CTC without aprepitant.[1]

(b) Docetaxel

Aprepitant 125 mg given one hour before docetaxel on day one, then 80 mg daily on days 2 and 3 had no effect on the pharmacokinetics of a single infusion of docetaxel 60 to 100 mg/m^2 in 10 cancer patients, and did not alter the toxicity profile. Each subject acted as their own control.[2]

(c) Thiotepa

The formation clearance of thiotepa was 33% lower and exposure to the active metabolite tepa was 20% lower in 6 patients receiving aprepitant with a 4-day course of high-dose CTC (cyclophosphamide, thiotepa, carboplatin) when compared with 49 patients receiving high-dose CTC without aprepitant.[1]

Mechanism

In the short-term, aprepitant is an inhibitor of the cytochrome P450 isoenzyme CYP3A4, and might therefore reduce the activation of antineoplastics activated by this isoenzyme (cyclophosphamide, thiotepa), or increase the toxicity of antineoplastics metabolised by this enzyme (docetaxel, irinotecan).

Importance and management

The UK maker of aprepitant recommends caution when it is used with chemotherapeutic agents that are metabolised by CYP3A4, particularly **irinotecan**, because of the possibility of increased toxicity with this drug.[3] They also mention that **etoposide**, **vinorelbine**, docetaxel and **paclitaxel**,[3,4] (and the US makers) **ifosfamide**, **imatinib**, **vinblastine** and **vincristine**,[4] were given without dosage adjustment for potential interactions, but as this was not a formal interaction study they recommend caution. However, with intravenous docetaxel, it appears that no important changes in pharmacokinetics occur, and therefore dosage adjustments are unlikely to be needed for this drug, and possibly also other intravenous antineoplastics metabolised by CYP3A4.[2] Similarly, the minor reductions in activation of cyclophosphamide and thiotepa were considered small compared to total variability, and therefore unlikely to be clinically important.

1. de Jonge ME, Huitaema AD, Holtkamp MJ, van Dam SM, Beijnen JH, Rodenhuis S. Aprepitant inhibits cyclophosphamide bioactivation and thiotepa metabolism. *Cancer Chemother Pharmacol* (2005) Apr 19, Epub.

2. Nygren P, Hande K, Petty KJ, Fedgchin M, van Dyck K, Majumdar A, Panebianco D, de Smet M, Ahmed T, Murphy MG, Gottesdiener KM, Cocquyt V, van Belle S. Lack of effect of aprepitant on the pharmacokinetics of docetaxel in cancer patients. *Cancer Chemother Pharmacol* (2005) 55, 609–16.
3. Emend (Aprepitant). Merck Sharp & Dohme Ltd. UK Summary of product characteristics, April 2005.
4. Emend (Aprepitant). Merck & Co., Inc. US Prescribing information, March 2005.

Antineoplastics + Colony stimulating factors

Because of the increased risk of myelosuppression, colony stimulating factors such as filgrastim, lenograstim, and molgramostim should not be given at the same time as myelosuppressive cytotoxic antineoplastics.

Clinical evidence, mechanism, importance and management

Colony stimulating factors such as filgrastim, lenograstim, and molgramostim promote the growth of myeloid cell lines. Since rapidly dividing myeloid cells have increased sensitivity to cytotoxic chemotherapy the manufacturers advise that these drugs should not be used from 24 hours before until 24 hours after cytotoxic chemotherapy.[1-3] In support of this, the maker of filgrastim notes that preliminary evidence confirmed that the severity of neutropenia could be exacerbated when patients were treated concurrently with fluorouracil and filgrastim.[2]

Note also that there is some evidence that colony stimulating factors may potentiate the pulmonary toxicity of 'bleomycin', (p.455) and 'cyclophosphamide', (p.461).

1. Granocyte (Lenograstim). Chugai Pharma UK Ltd. UK Summary of product characteristics, September 2004.
2. Neupogen (Filgrastim). Amgen Ltd. UK Summary of product characteristics, October 2001.
3. Leucomax (Molgramostim). Schering-Plough Ltd. UK Summary of product characteristics, June 2000.

Antineoplastics + Megestrol

There is some *in vitro* evidence that megestrol acetate may antagonise the antitumour activity of cisplatin. In one clinical study megestrol reduced response rates to etoposide/cisplatin but in another had no effect on response rates to alternating cycles of cyclophosphamide/doxorubicin/vincristine and etoposide/cisplatin.

Clinical evidence

A study in 243 patients with advanced small-cell lung cancer (SCLC) treated with **etoposide/cisplatin** found that those who also received megestrol acetate 800 mg daily had increased non-fluid body-weight and significantly less nausea and vomiting. Although the 1-year survival rate was similar in both groups those who received megestrol had a significantly worse response rate to cisplatin (68% compared with 80%) and a higher incidence of thromboembolic events. However the megestrol recipients did have poorer quality of life (a prognostic factor) at the beginning of the study and this may have influenced the findings.[1] In a similar study, megestrol acetate had no effect on response rates, symptom profile or overall survival in patients with SCLC receiving chemotherapy (alternating cycles of **cyclophosphamide/doxorubicin/vincristine** and **etoposide/cisplatin** for a maximum of 6 cycles). In this study, megestrol acetate was given at a dose of 160 mg three times daily for 8 days commencing 3 days before each cycle of chemotherapy.[2]

Mechanism

An *in vitro* study found that megestrol may antagonise the antineoplastic activity of cisplatin by upregulating cellular detoxification mechanisms.[3]

Importance and management

The authors of the first study suggest that megestrol acetate should not be used routinely at the time of chemotherapy.[1] Be aware that the use of megestrol may antagonise the antitumour activity of cisplatin. More study is needed.

1. Rowland KM, Loprinzi CL, Shaw EG, Maksymiuk AW, Kuross SA, Jung S-H, Kugler JW, Tschetter LK, Ghosh C, Schaefer PL, Owen D, Washburn JH, Webb TA, Mailliard JA, Jett JR. Randomized double-blind placebo-controlled trial of cisplatin and etoposide plus megestrol acetate/placebo in extensive-stage small-cell lung cancer: a North Central Cancer Treatment Group Study. *J Clin Oncol* (1996) 14, 135–41.
2. Wood L, Palmer M, Hewitt J, Urtasun R, Bruera E, Rapp E, Thaell JF. Results of a phase III, double-blind, placebo-controlled trial of megestrol acetate modulation of P-glycoprotein-mediated drug resistance in the first-line management of small-cell lung carcinoma. *Br J Cancer* (1998) 77, 627–31.
3. Pu Y-S, Cheng A-L, Chen J, Guan J-Y, Lu S-H, Lai M-K, Hsieh C-Y. Megestrol acetate antagonizes cisplatin cytotoxicity. *Anticancer Drugs* (1998) 9, 733–8.

Antineoplastics + Ondansetron

Some evidence suggests ondansetron may modestly affect the pharmacokinetics of cyclophosphamide and cisplatin but it does not appear to affect those of carmustine. Cisplatin and fluorouracil do not affect the pharmacokinetics of ondansetron.

Clinical evidence, mechanism, importance and management

The pharmacokinetics of high-dose **cyclophosphamide**, **cisplatin** and **carmustine** in 23 patients given ondansetron, lorazepam and diphenhydramine as antiemetics were compared with those in 129 patients who received prochlorperazine instead of ondansetron. It was found that the AUCs of **cyclophosphamide** and **cisplatin**, but not that of **carmustine**, were significantly lower (by 15% and 19% respectively) in the ondansetron group.[1] Similarly, in another study, the pharmacokinetics of antineoplastics were analysed in 54 patients with breast cancer who were receiving high-dose **cyclophosphamide**, **cisplatin** and **carmustine** with lorazepam and ondansetron with or without prochlorperazine and compared with 75 matched control patients whose antiemetic regimen had been prochlorperazine and lorazepam. In those given ondansetron the median AUC of **cyclophosphamide** was 17% lower, the **cisplatin** AUC was about 10% higher and the **carmustine** AUC was unchanged.[2] In contrast, a study in 10 patients who received intravenous **cyclophosphamide** 600 mg/m^2 and **epirubicin** 90 mg/m^2 and either oral ondansetron 16 mg or placebo found that the pharmacokinetic parameters of **cyclophosphamide** or its metabolite were not significantly altered by ondansetron although there was considerable variation between subjects. It was concluded that ondansetron can be safely co-administered with **cyclophosphamide**.[3] No significant changes in the pharmacokinetics of ondansetron occurred in 20 cancer patients on **cisplatin** 20 to 40 mg/m^2 and/or **fluorouracil** 1 g/m^2 for 5 days but the clearance was lower than in healthy subjects.[4]

Information seems to be limited to these studies, and the interaction is not established. The clinical relevance of these possible modest changes in AUC of cyclophosphamide (0 to 17% reduction) and cisplatin (19% reduction or 10% increase) remain to be determined.

1. Cagnoni PJ, Matthes S, Day TC, Bearman SI, Shpall EJ, Jones RB. Modification of the pharmacokinetics of high-dose cyclophosphamide and cisplatin by antiemetics. *Bone Marrow Transplant* (1999) 24, 1–4.
2. Gilbert CJ, Petros WP, Vredenburgh J, Hussein A, Ross M, Rubin P, Fehdrau R, Cavanaugh C, Berry D, McKinstry C, Peters WP. Pharmacokinetic interaction between ondansetron and cyclophosphamide during high-dose chemotherapy for breast cancer. *Cancer Chemother Pharmacol* (1998) 42, 497–503.
3. Lorenz C, Eickhoff C, Baumann F, Sehouli J, Preiss R, Schunack W, Jaehde U. Does ondansetron affect the metabolism of cyclophosphamide? *Int J Clin Pharmacol Ther* (2000) 38, 143–4.
4. Hsyu P-H, Bozigian HP, Pritchard JF, Kernodle A, Panella J, Hansen LA, Griffin RH. Effect of chemotherapy on the pharmacokinetics of oral ondansetron. *Pharm Res* (1991) 8 (Suppl 10), S-257.

Antineoplastics + Propofol

There are two isolated reports of severe pain occurring in patients given intravenous propofol via hand veins who had previously received intravenous chemotherapy.

Clinical evidence, mechanism, importance and management

Although pain on injection of propofol is well known one group of workers noted that on a number of occasions patients previously treated with intravenous chemotherapy had marked pain, both at the site of injection and up the arm, when given propofol for induction via hand veins.[1] This would seem to link with a report of a 15-year-old girl with acute lymphoblastic leukaemia who had been treated with several injections of **cyclophosphamide**, **methotrexate** and **vincristine** during the previous 6 months, and who was cannulated in her hand and infused with *Plasmalyte B*. An injection of 60 micrograms of fentanyl via this cannula was painful and 20 mg of lidocaine helped, but 20 mg of propofol caused extreme pain. A further 20 mg of lidocaine was given and the propofol administration was stopped, but the pain continued. The whole hand became blue and congested, and blood began to move backwards up the drip tubing. The venous congestion gradually subsided over the next 15 minutes.[2] The authors recommended that propofol should be avoided in patients who have recently had intravenous chemotherapeutic agents.[2] The general applicability of these reports remains to be determined. Use of propofol alone may cause pain and it should be noted that the makers of propofol recommend that local pain associated with propofol during the induction phase can be minimised by the use of the larger veins on the forearm and antecubital fossa.[3]

1. Whitlock JC, Nicol ME, Pattison J. Painful injection of propofol. *Anaesthesia* (1989) 44, 618.
2. Butt AD, James MFM. Venospasm due to propofol after chemotherapy. *S Afr Med J* (1990) 77, 168.
3. Diprivan (Propofol). AstraZeneca UK Ltd. UK Summary of product characteristics, February 2004.

Antineoplastics + Semaxanib

The combination of semaxanib, cisplatin and gemcitabine has caused an unexpectedly high incidence of thromboembolic events.

Clinical evidence, mechanism, importance and management

The pharmacokinetics of semaxanib (SU5416), **cisplatin** and **gemcitabine** were unaltered when given together in a phase I study but investigation of the combination was terminated after 8 of the 19 patients had thromboembolic events (transient ischaemic attacks, cerebrovascular accidents, deep vein thromboses). **Gemcitabine** 1250 mg/m^2 was given on day 1, immediately followed by **cisplatin** 80 mg/m^2, then semaxanib 85 mg/m^2 (escalated to 145 mg/m^2 in some patients). **Gemcitabine** then semaxanib were given on day 8, and semaxanib alone on days 4, 11, 15, and 18. The cycle was repeated every 3 weeks.[1] The incidence of thromboembolic events in this study (42%) was much higher than that seen with **cisplatin** and **gemcitabine** (0%) or semaxanib alone (2.2%), and was thought to be a result of the drug combination.[1] **Cisplatin** in particular, due to its effects on platelets and its vasoconstrictive effects, may be responsible.[2] Preliminary results of other studies of semaxanib with **fluorouracil**/folinic acid, **irinotecan/fluorouracil**/folinic acid, and **paclitaxel/carboplatin** did not report this complication.[3-5] The authors of the first study[1] caution against further clinical trials of antineoplastics with angiogenesis inhibitors such as semaxanib until the exact cause of the thromboembolic events has been elucidated.

1. Kuenen BC, Rosen L, Smit EF, Parson MRN, Levi M, Ruijter R, Huisman H, Kedde MA, Noordhuis P, van der Vijgh WJF, Peters GJ, Cropp GF, Scigalla P, Hoekman K, Pinedo HM, Giaccone G. Dose-finding and pharmacokinetic study of cisplatin, gemcitabine, and SU5416 in patients with solid tumors. *J Clin Oncol* (2002) 20, 1657–67.
2. Marx GM, Steer CB, Harper P, Pavlakis N, Rixe O, Khayat D. Unexpected serious toxicity with chemotherapy and antiangiogenic combinations: time to take stock. *J Clin Oncol* (2002) 20, 1446–8.
3. Rosen PJ, Amado R, Hecht JR, Chang D, Mulay M, Parson M Laxa B, Brown J, Cropp G, Hannah A, Rosen L. A phase I/II study of SU5416 in combination with 5-FU/leucovorin in patients with metastatic colorectal cancer. *Proc Am Soc Clin Oncol* (2000) 19, 3A.
4. Rothenberg ML, Berlin JD, Cropp GF, Fleischer AC, Schumaker RD, Hande KR, Culley A, Dorminy C, Donnelly E, Chen J, Schaaf L, Hannah AL. A phase I/II study of SU5416 in combination with irinotecan/5-FU/LV (IFL) in patients with metastatic colorectal cancer. *Proc Am Soc Clin Oncol* (2001) 20, 75A.
5. Rosen P, Kabbinavar F, Figlin RA, Parson M, Laxa B, Hernandez L, Mayers A, Cropp GF, Hannah AL, Rosen LS. A phase I/II trial and pharmacokinetic (PK) study of SU5416 in combination with paclitaxel/carboplatin. *Proc Am Soc Clin Oncol* (2001) 20, 98A.

Antineoplastics + Tamoxifen

Antineoplastics and tamoxifen are associated with an increased risk of thrombosis and there is the possibility that combined use may increase this risk further.

Clinical evidence, mechanism, importance and management

A retrospective analysis of data from various Eastern Cooperative Oncology Group studies, suggested that venous thromboembolic complications were more common in women treated concurrently with tamoxifen and adjuvant chemotherapy (**CMF**; **cyclophosphamide**, **methotrexate**, **fluorouracil**) than women given **CMF** alone (3.8% vs 0% in one study).[1] In another study of patients given tamoxifen 30 mg daily for 2 years the incidence of thromboembolic events was 2.6% compared with 13.6% in those also given 8 cycles of **CMF**. The authors of this study considered the rate of thromboembolic events with the combination to be higher than that usually seen with **CMF**, and hypothesised an interaction between tamoxifen and **CMF**.[2] In contrast, in another study, in the first 12 weeks of therapy, thrombosis occurred in 5 of 103 patients treated with tamoxifen and chemotherapy (**cyclophosphamide**, **methotrexate**, **fluorouracil**, **vincristine**, prednisone, **doxorubicin**) compared with 4 of 102 treated with the same chemotherapy alone, suggesting no significant contribution of the tamoxifen.[3]

Tamoxifen alone is known to carry a small risk of thromboembolic events when used for primary prevention of breast cancer.[4] Antineoplastic chemotherapy also increases the risk of thrombosis,[3] and cancer *per se* increases the risk, as does surgery for cancer.[5]

To what extent, if any, tamoxifen further increases the risk of thrombosis with antineoplastic therapy is unclear from the above studies. However, some authors recommend that serious consideration be given to the use of prophylactic anticoagulants if adjuvant CMF is used with tamoxifen in women with breast cancer,[2] and the UK makers endorse this.[6] This may be prudent with antineoplastic chemotherapy in any case.

1. Saphner T, Tormey DC, Gray R. Venous and arterial thrombosis in patients who received adjuvant therapy for breast cancer. *J Clin Oncol* (1991) 9, 286–94.
2. Pritchard KI, Paterson AHG, Paul NA, Zee B, Fine S, Pater J. Increased thromboembolic complications with concurrent tamoxifen and chemotherapy in a randomized trial of adjuvant therapy for women with breast cancer. National Cancer Institute of Canada Clinical Trials Group Breast Cancer Site Group. *J Clin Oncol* (1996) 14, 2731–7.
3. Levine MN, Gent M, Hirsh J, Arnold A, Goodyear MD, Hryniuk W, De Pauw S. The thrombogenic effect of anticancer drug therapy in women with stage II breast cancer. *N Engl J Med* (1988) 318; 404–7.
4. Fischer B, Constantino JP, Wickerham DL, Redmond CK, Kavanah M, Cronin WM, Vogel V, Robidoux A, Dimitrov N, Atkins J, Daly M, Wieand S, Tan-Chiu E, Ford L, Wolmark N. Tamoxifen for prevention of breast cancer: report of the National Surgical Adjuvant Breast and Bowel Project P-1 Study. *J Natl Cancer Inst* (1998) 90, 1371–88.
5. Rickles FR, Levine MN. Venous thromboembolism in malignancy and malignancy in venous thromboembolism. *Haemostasis* (1998) 28 (Suppl 3), 43–9.
6. Nolvadex (Tamoxifen). AstraZeneca UK Ltd. UK Summary of product characteristics, January 2004.

Antineoplastics + Vaccines

The immune response of the body is suppressed by cytotoxic antineoplastics. The effectiveness of vaccines may be poor and generalised infection may occur in patients immunised with live vaccines.

Clinical evidence, mechanism, importance and management

Since cytotoxic antineoplastics are immunosuppressant, they reduce the response of the body to immunisation. A study[1] in 53 patients with Hodgkin's disease showed that chemotherapy reduced the antibody response by 60% when measured 3 weeks after immunisation with a **pneumococcal vaccine**. The patients were treated with **chlormethine** (mechlorethamine**)**, **vincristine**, prednisone and **procarbazine**. A few of them also had **bleomycin**, **vinblastine** or **cyclophosphamide**. Subtotal radiotherapy reduced the response by a further 15%. The response to **influenza immunisation** in children with various malignancies was also markedly suppressed by chemotherapy. The regimen included prednisone and the cytotoxic drugs **mercaptopurine**, **methotrexate**, and **vincristine**. Some of them were also treated with **vincristine, dactinomycin** (actinomycin D) and **cyclophosphamide**.[2] In another study only 9 out of 17 children with leukaemia or other malignant diseases treated with **methotrexate, cyclophosphamide, mercaptopurine** and prednisone developed a significant response to immunisation with **inactivated measles vaccine**.[3] Furthermore, immunisation with **live vaccines** may result in a potentially life-threatening infection. For example, a woman taking **methotrexate** 15 mg once a month for psoriasis developed a generalised vaccinial infection after vaccination against **smallpox**.[4] Studies in *animals* given **smallpox vaccine** confirmed that they were more susceptible to infection if treated with **methotrexate, mercaptopurine** or **cyclophosphamide**.[5]

Extreme care should therefore be exercised when using live vaccines for immunisation of patients who are receiving cytotoxics or other immunosuppressant drugs (see also 'Corticosteroids + Vaccines; Live', p.811, and 'Immunosuppressants + Vaccines', p.812).

1. Siber GR, Weitzman SA, Aisenberg AC, Weinstein HJ, Schiffman G. Impaired antibody response to pneumococcal vaccine after treatment for Hodgkins disease. *N Engl J Med* (1978) 299, 442–8.
2. Gross PA, Lee H, Wolff JA, Hall CB, Minnefore AB, Lazicki ME. Influenza immunization in immunosuppressed children. *J Pediatr* (1978) 92, 30–5.
3. Stiehm ER, Ablin A, Kushner JH, Zoger S. Measles vaccination in patients on immunosuppressive drugs. *Am J Dis Child* (1966) 111, 191–4.
4. Allison J. Methotrexate and smallpox vaccination. *Lancet* (1968) ii, 1250.
5. Rosenbaum EH, Cohen RA, Glatstein HR. Vaccination of a patient receiving immunosuppressive therapy for lymphosarcoma. *JAMA* (1966) 198, 737–40.

Bexarotene + Miscellaneous

The makers say that gemfibrozil raises bexarotene plasma levels and should therefore be avoided. They warn about the theoretical possibility that inhibitors of the cytochrome P450 isoenzyme CYP3A4 (clarithromycin, erythromycin, grapefruit juice, itraconazole, ketoconazole, protease inhibitors) may possibly raise bexarotene levels, whereas CYP3A4 inducers (dexamethasone, phenytoin, phenobarbital, rifampicin (rifampin)) may possibly reduce them. They also suggest the possibility of reduced efficacy of oral contraceptives, and increased hypoglycaemic effects with insulin or oral hypoglycaemic agents. No interaction seems to occur with atorvastatin or levothyroxine.

Clinical evidence, mechanism, importance and management

No formal interaction studies appear to have been carried out, and most of drug interactions cited in this monograph are suggestions by the makers, based on theoretical considerations.[1,2]

(a) Effects of enzyme inducers and inhibitors

Because it is known that bexarotene is metabolised by the cytochrome P450 isoenzyme CYP3A4, the makers point out that there is a theoretical risk that compounds that inhibit CYP3A4 might increase bexarotene levels. They list **clarithromycin**, **erythromycin**, **itraconazole**, **ketoconazole**, **protease inhibitors** (none specifically named) and **grapefruit juice** as possible interacting drugs because of their known inhibitory effects on CYP3A4. They also list a number of known CYP3A4 inducers, namely **dexamethasone**, **phenytoin**, **phenobarbital** and **rifampicin** (**rifampin**), because they may theoretically increase the metabolism of bexarotene and reduce its levels.

The makers also say that because bexarotene can induce liver enzymes, it may theoretically increase the metabolism of other substances metabolised by CYP3A4 such as **tamoxifen** and the steroids in oral or other systemic **contraceptives**, thereby reducing both their serum levels and their efficacy. For this reason they advise the use of additional non-hormonal contraception (e.g. a barrier method) to avoid the risk of contraceptive failure. They point out that this is particularly important because if failure were to occur, the foetus might be exposed to the teratogenic effects of bexarotene.[1,2]

(b) Other possible drug interactions

The makers report that a population analysis of patients with cutaneous T-cell lymphoma found that the concurrent use of **gemfibrozil** substantially increased the plasma levels of bexarotene for reasons unknown; the US makers suggest inhibition of CYP3A4 by **gemfibrozil** may be partially responsible and that concurrent use is not recommended,[2] but note that fibrates are not generally recognised as inhibitors of this isoenzyme, see 'Lipid-regulating drugs', (p.827). However, under similar conditions, they say that bexarotene levels were not affected by **atorvastatin** or **levothyroxine**. Changes in thyroid function caused by bexarotene have been successfully treated with **thyroid hormone supplements**.[1,2]

The makers recommend that because bexarotene is related to **vitamin A**, any **vitamin A supplements** should be limited to 15,000 units or less daily to avoid potentially additive toxic effects. The makers additionally say that although no cases of hypoglycaemia have been seen, because of the known mode of action of bexarotene it should be used with caution if given with **insulin** or agents enhancing insulin secretion (e.g. **sulphonylureas**) or insulin sensitisers (e.g. **thiazolidinediones**).[1,2] For a list of these drugs see 'Table 12.1', (p.390).

1. Targretin (Bexarotene). Medeus Pharma Ltd. UK Summary of product characteristics, June 2002.
2. Targretin (Bexarotene). Ligand Pharmaceuticals. US Prescribing information, April 2003.

Bicalutamide + Phenazone (Antipyrine)

The results of an interaction study between bicalutamide and phenazone (antipyrine) suggest that bicalutamide is unlikely to interact with other drugs through enzyme induction.

Clinical evidence, mechanism, importance and management

The pharmacokinetics and metabolism of phenazone (largely used as an investigational marker drug of enzyme induction or inhibition) were studied in two groups of patients with prostate cancer before and after taking either bicalutamide 50 mg daily (7 patients) or 150 mg daily (11 patients) for 12 weeks. Small changes in the phenazone pharmacokinetics were found (half-life shorter by 16.3% with the 50 mg bicalutamide dosage, the AUC reduced by 18.6% with the 150 mg bicalutamide dosage). Nevertheless it was considered that bicalutamide does not significantly induce the liver enzymes responsible for the metabolism of phenazone and is therefore unlikely to interact with any other drugs by causing enzyme induction.[1]

1. Kaisary A, Klarskov P, McKillop D. Absence of hepatic enzyme induction in prostate cancer patients receiving 'Casodex' (bicalutamide). *Anticancer Drugs* (1996) 7, 54–9.

Bleomycin + Cisplatin

Cisplatin can increase the pulmonary toxicity of bleomycin by reducing its renal excretion. Digital ischaemia and arterial thrombosis have also been described.

Clinical evidence

Thirty patients with carcinoma of the cervix and 15 patients with germ cell tumours were given combination chemotherapy including bleomycin and cisplatin. Cisplatin was given by infusion on day 1, followed by bleomycin given intramuscularly every 12 hours for 4 days or by continuous infusion over 72 hours. Nine of the patients with normal renal function and no previous pulmonary disease developed serious pulmonary toxicity and 6 died from respiratory failure.[1]

In a study of 18 patients given both drugs for the treatment of disseminated testicular non-seminoma 2 patients developed pneumonitis and it was found that cisplatin-induced reduction in renal function was paralleled by an increase in bleomycin-induced pulmonary toxicity.[2] Similar findings were made in a much larger study of 54 patients by the same group.[3] A study in 2 children showed that the total plasma clearance of bleomycin was halved (from 39 to 18 ml/minute/m^2) when they were also treated with cisplatin in cumulative doses exceeding 300 mg/m^2. The renal clearance in one of them fell from 30 to 8.2 ml/minute/m^2 although there was no evidence of severe bleomycin toxicity in either child.[4] Two cases of fatal bleomycin toxicity have been described in patients with cisplatin-induced renal dysfunction.[5,6]

A case report describes arterial thrombosis associated with pathological vascular changes in the arteries of a man treated with cisplatin, bleomycin and etoposide.[7] Another man developed fatal thrombotic microangiopathy (characterised by microangiopathic haemolytic anaemia, thrombocytopenia, renal impairment), which was attributed to the use of bleomycin and cisplatin.[8]

In an earlier study, digital ischaemia occurred in 41% of patients treated with cisplatin, bleomycin and vinblastine compared with 21% of patients treated with only cisplatin and vinblastine.[9]

Mechanism

Excretion by the kidney accounts for almost half of the total body clearance of bleomycin. Cisplatin is nephrotoxic and reduces the glomerular filtration rate so that the clearance of bleomycin is reduced. The accumulating bleomycin apparently causes the pulmonary toxicity.

Importance and management

Pulmonary toxicity with bleomycin is an established reaction with a potentially serious, sometimes fatal, outcome. Concurrent use should be very closely monitored and renal function checked. One of the problems is that levels of creatinine may not accurately indicate the extent of renal damage, both during and after cisplatin treatment. The renal toxicity of cisplatin may also develop rapidly. Other toxic effects on the vascular system can also occur.

1. Rabinowits M, Souhami L, Gil RA, Andrade CAV, Paiva HC. Increased pulmonary toxicity with bleomycin and cisplatin chemotherapy combinations. *Am J Clin Oncol* (1990) 13, 132–8.
2. van Barneveld PWC, Sleijfer D Th, van der Mark Th W, Mulder NH, Donker AJM, Meijer S, Schraffordt Koops H, Sluiter HJ, Peset R. Influence of platinum-induced renal toxicity on bleomycin-induced pulmonary toxicity in patients with disseminated testicular carcinoma. *Oncology* (1984) 41, 4–7.

3. Sleijfer S, van der Mark TW, Schraffordt Koops H, Mulder NH. Enhanced effects of bleomycin on pulmonary function disturbances in patients with decreased renal function due to cisplatin. *Eur J Cancer* (1996) 32A, 550–2.
4. Yee GC, Crom WR, Champion JE, Brodeur GM, Evans WE. Cisplatin-induced changes in bleomycin elimination. *Cancer Treat Rep* (1983) 67, 587–9.
5. Bennett WM, Pastore L, Houghton DC. Fatal pulmonary bleomycin toxicity in cisplatin-induced acute renal failure. *Cancer Treat Rep* (1980) 64, 921–4.
6. Perry DJ, Weiss RB, Taylor HG. Enhanced bleomycin toxicity during acute renal failure. *Cancer Treat Rep* (1982) 66, 592–3.
7. Garstin IWH, Cooper GG, Hood JM. Arterial thrombosis after treatment with bleomycin and cisplatin. *BMJ* (1990) 300, 1018.
8. Fields SM, Lindley CM. Thrombotic microangiopathy associated with chemotherapy: case report and review of the literature. *DICP Ann Pharmacother* (1989) 23, 582–8.
9. Vogelzang NJ, Bosl GJ, Johnson K, Kennedy BJ. Raynaud's phenomenon : a common toxicity after combination chemotherapy for testicular cancer. *Ann Intern Med* (1981) 95, 288–92.

Bleomycin + Colony stimulating factors

The concurrent use of granulocyte colony stimulating factor or granulocyte-macrophage stimulating factor has been linked with an increased occurrence of bleomycin-induced pulmonary toxicity.

Clinical evidence, mechanism, importance and management

Pulmonary toxicity that developed at low cumulative bleomycin doses (70 to 130 units/m^2 in at least 3 of 5 patients given standard ABVD treatment was attributed by the author of the report to the synergistic action of concurrent treatment with **G-CSF** (granulocyte colony stimulating factor).[1] In another report 8 out of 40 patients with malignant non-Hodgkin's lymphoma given **G-CSF** developed drug-induced pneumonia. Three of these patients were treated with chemotherapy regimens including bleomycin (MACOB-B, COP-BLAM III), and all 3 died of respiratory failure. None of 35 other patients, similarly treated but without **G-CSF**, developed pneumonia.[2] Non-infectious interstitial pneumonitis developed in a patient given doxorubicin, cyclophosphamide, bleomycin, vinblastine, methotrexate and prednisone with **GM-CSF** (granulocyte macrophage colony stimulating factor).[3] Five further reports have identified a total of 23 other patients who developed bleomycin-pulmonary toxicity probably potentiated by **G-CSF** or **GM-CSF**, including at least 7 fatalities.[4-8]

In contrast, analysis of two placebo-controlled trials of the use of adjuvant **G-CSF** (**filgrastim** or **lenograstim**) with combination chemotherapy including bleomycin found no evidence of an increase in pulmonary complications. Overall 7 of 139 patients treated with placebo and 9 of 139 treated with the **G-CSF** had pulmonary complications possibly related to bleomycin.[9,10] Similarly, another retrospective analysis found that 34% of patients treated with bleomycin and **G-CSF** developed pulmonary toxicity compared with 33% of those treated with bleomycin alone.[11]

These interactions are not firmly established, but good pulmonary function monitoring appears to be advisable when colony stimulating factors are used with antineoplastics causing pulmonary toxicity such as bleomycin. If interstitial pneumonia occurs, the drugs should be discontinued and high-dose corticosteroids started immediately.[7] More study is needed. Consider also 'Cyclophosphamide + Colony stimulating factors', p.461.

1. Matthews JH. Pulmonary toxicity of ABVD chemotherapy and G-CSF in Hodgkin's disease: possible synergy. *Lancet* (1993) 342, 988.
2. Iki S, Yoshinaga K, Ohbayashi Y, Urabe A. Cytotoxic drug-induced pneumonia and possible augmentation by G-CSF — clinical attention. *Ann Hematol* (1993) 66, 217–18.
3. Philippe B, Couderc LJ, Balloul-Delclaux E, Janvier M, Caubarrere I. Pulmonary toxicity of chemotherapy and GM-CSF. *Respir Med* (1994) 88, 715.
4. Dirix LY, Schrijvers D, Druwè P, Van Den Brande J, Verhoeven D, Van Oosterom AT. Pulmonary toxicity and bleomycin. *Lancet* (1994) 344, 56.
5. Lei KIK, Leung WT, Johnson PJ. Serious pulmonary complications in patients receiving recombinant granulocyte colony-stimulating factor during BACOP chemotherapy for aggressive non-Hodgkin's lymphoma. *Br J Cancer* (1994) 70, 1009–13.
6. Katoh M, Shikoshi K, Takada M, Umeda M, Tsukahara T, Kitagawa S, Shirai T. Development of interstitial pneumonitis during treatment with granulocyte colony-stimulating factor. *Ann Hematol* (1993) 67, 201–2.
7. Niitsu N, Iki S, Muroi K, Motomura S, Murakami M, Takeyama H, Ohsaka A, Urabe A. Interstitial pneumonia in patients receiving granulocyte colony-stimulating factor during chemotherapy: survey in Japan 1991–96. *Br J Cancer* (1997) 76, 1661–6.
8. Couderc L-J, Stelianides S, Franchon I, Stern M, Epardeau B, Baumelou E, Caubarrere I, Hermine O. Pulmonary toxicity of chemotherapy and G/GM-CSF: a report of five cases. *Respir Med* (1999) 93, 65–8.
9. Bastion Y, Reyes F, Bosly A, Gisselbrecht C, Yver A, Gilles E, Maral J, Coiffier B. Possible toxicity with the association of G-CSF and bleomycin. *Lancet* (1994) 343, 1221–2.
10. Bastion Y, Coiffier B. Pulmonary toxicity of bleomycin: is G-CSF a risk factor? *Lancet* (1994) 344, 474.
11. Saxman SB, Nichols CR, Einhorn LH. Pulmonary toxicity in patients with advanced-stage germ cell tumors receiving bleomycin with and without granulocyte colony stimulating factor. *Chest* (1997) 111, 657–60.

Bleomycin + Oxygen

Serious and potentially fatal pulmonary toxicity can develop in patients treated with bleomycin who are exposed to conventional oxygen concentrations during anaesthesia.

Clinical evidence

Five patients treated with bleomycin, exposed to oxygen concentrations of 35 to 42% during and immediately following anaesthesia, developed a severe respiratory distress syndrome and died. Bleomycin-induced pneumonitis and lung fibrosis were diagnosed at post-mortem. Another group of 12 matched patients who underwent the same procedures but with lower oxygen concentrations (22 to 25%) had an uneventful postoperative course.[1]

Another comparative study[2] similarly demonstrated that adult respiratory distress syndrome (ARDS) in patients on bleomycin was reduced by a technique allowing the use of lower oxygen concentrations of 22 to 30%. Bleomycin-induced pulmonary toxicity apparently related to oxygen concentrations has also been described in other case reports.[3-6] Studies in *animals* have also confirmed that the severity of bleomycin-induced pulmonary toxicity is increased by oxygen.[7-9] However, in two other series of patients treated with bleomycin and undergoing surgery there was no obvious increase in pulmonary complications despite the use of usual concentrations of oxygen.[10,11]

Mechanism

Not understood. One suggestion is that bleomycin-injured lung tissue is less able to scavenge free oxygen radicals, which may be present, and damage occurs as a result.[3]

Importance and management

An established, well-documented, serious and potentially fatal interaction. It is advised that any patient on bleomycin undergoing general anaesthesia should have their inspired oxygen concentrations limited to less than 30% and the fluid replacement should be carefully monitored to minimise the crystalloid load. This is clearly very effective because one author has treated 700 patients following these guidelines without a single case of pulmonary failure.[12] It has also been suggested that reduced oxygen levels should be continued during the recovery period and at any time during hospitalisation.[3] If an oxygen concentration equal or greater than 30% has to be used, short term prophylactic corticosteroid administration should be considered. Intravenous corticosteroids should be given at once if bleomycin toxicity is suspected.[3]

1. Goldiner PL, Carlon CG, Cvitkovic E, Schweizer O, Howland WS. Factors influencing postoperative morbidity and mortality in patients treated with bleomycin. *BMJ* (1978) 1, 1664–7.
2. El-Baz N, Ivankovich AD, Faber LP, Logas WG. The incidence of bleomycin lung toxicity after anesthesia for pulmonary resection: a comparison between HFV and IPPV. *Anesthesiology* (1984) 61, A107.
3. Gilson AJ, Sahn SA. Reactivation of bleomycin lung toxicity following oxygen administration. A second response to corticosteroids. *Chest* (1985) 88, 304–6.
4. Cersosimo RJ, Matthews SJ, Hong WK. Bleomycin pneumonitis potentiated by oxygen administration. *Drug Intell Clin Pharm* (1985) 19, 921–3.
5. Hulbert JC, Grossman JE, Cummings KB. Risk factors of anesthesia and surgery in bleomycin-treated patients. *J Urol (Baltimore)* (1983) 130, 163–4.
6. Donohue JP, Rowland RG. Complications of retroperitoneal lymph node dissection. *J Urol (Baltimore)* (1981) 125, 338–40.
7. Toledo CH, Ross WE, Hood I, Block ER. Potentiation of bleomycin toxicity by oxygen. *Cancer Treat Rep* (1982) 66, 359–62.
8. Berend N. The effect of bleomycin and oxygen on rat lung. *Pathology* (1984) 16, 136–9.
9. Rinaldo J, Goldstein RH, Snider GL. Modification of oxygen toxicity after lung injury by bleomycin in hamsters. *Am Rev Respir Dis* (1982) 126, 1030–3.
10. Douglas MJ, Coppin CML. Bleomycin and subsequent anesthesia: a retrospective study at Vancouver General Hospital. *Can Anaesth Soc J* (1980) 27, 449–52.
11. Mandelbaum I, Williams SD, Einhorn LH. Aggressive surgical management of testicular carcinoma metastatic to lungs and mediastinum. *Ann Thorac Surg* (1980) 30, 224–9.
12. Goldiner PL. Editorial comment. *J Urol (Baltimore)* (1983) 130, 164.

Busulfan + Azoles

Itraconazole, but not fluconazole, modestly reduces the clearance of busulfan. There is some limited evidence that concurrent ketoconazole may increase the risk of hepatic veno-occlusive disease.

Clinical evidence, mechanism, importance and management

The pharmacokinetics of busulfan in 26 bone marrow transplant patients, who had received busulfan without concurrent antifungal therapy, were compared with those in 13 similar patients given busulfan with **itraconazole** and in 13 given busulfan with **fluconazole**. The busulfan clearance was decreased by 20% by **itraconazole** but not by the **fluconazole**,[1] probably because the **itraconazole** inhibits the metabolism of busulfan by the liver. The expected rise in serum busulfan levels is only likely to be moderate, but until more information is available it would be prudent to monitor for any signs of increased busulfan toxicity if **itraconazole** is used, but no special precautions seem to be needed with **fluconazole**. Concurrent **ketoconazole** has been identified as a possible risk factor for hepatic veno-occlusive disease after high-dose busulfan.[2] Further study is needed to confirm or refute this.

1. Buggia I, Zecca N, Alessandrino EP, Locatelli F, Rosti G, Bosi A, Pession A, Rotoli B, Majolino I, Dallorso A, Regazzi MB. Itraconazole can increase systemic exposure to busulfan in patients given bone marrow transplantation. *Anticancer Res* (1996) 16, 2083–8.
2. Méresse V, Hartmann O, Vassal G, Benhamou E, Valteau-Couanet D, Brugieres L, Lemerie J. Risk factors for hepatic veno-occlusive disease after high-dose busulfan-containing regimens followed by autologous bone marrow transplantation: a study in 136 children. *Bone Marrow Transplant* (1992) 10, 135–41.

Busulfan + Benzodiazepines

Diazepam and lorazepam appear not to alter busulfan pharmacokinetics.

Clinical evidence, mechanism, importance and management

In a study in patients receiving high-dose busulfan, no pharmacokinetic changes were seen in 8 patients given **diazepam**, apart from a steady decline in steady-state serum levels in just one.[1] Similarly, in another study, **lorazepam** did not alter the absorption and clearance of high-dose busulfan in children undergoing stem-cell transplantation.[2] Benzodiazepines may therefore be a suitable alternative to 'phenytoin', (below) for seizure prophylaxis during high-dose busulfan treatment.[2]

1. Hassan M, Öberg G, Björkholm M, Wallin I, Lindgren M. Influence of prophylactic anticonvulsant therapy on high-dose busulphan kinetics. *Cancer Chemother Pharmacol* (1993) 33, 181–6.
2. Chan KW, Mullen CA, Worth LL, Choroszy M, Koontz S, Tran H, Slopis J. Lorazepam for seizure prophylaxis during high-dose busulfan administration. *Bone Marrow Transplant* (2002) 29, 963–5.

Busulfan + Ketobemidone

Ketobemidone may increase plasma levels of busulfan.

Clinical evidence, mechanism, importance and management

A patient with acute myeloid leukaemia was started on a 4-day course of busulfan 1 mg/kg four times daily followed by cyclophosphamide for 2 days before bone marrow transplantation. At the time he was also receiving ketobemidone 1000 mg daily for a rectal fissure. Busulfan plasma levels after the first dose were elevated (AUC increased by about one-third). Later, when the dose of ketobemidone was reduced and morphine substituted, busulfan levels decreased.[1] The use of ketobemidone with high-dose busulfan is not recommended without monitoring. Dose adjustments may be required to prevent busulfan toxicity. An alternative analgesic should be considered.

1. Hassan M, Svensson J-O, Nilsson C, Hentschke P, AL-Shurbaji A, Aschan J, Ljungman P, Ringdén O. Ketobemidone may alter busulfan pharmacokinetics during high-dose therapy. *Ther Drug Monit* (2000) 22, 383–5.

Busulfan + Phenytoin

Phenytoin increases the loss of busulfan from the body and lowers its serum levels.

Clinical evidence, mechanism, importance and management

Seven patients given high-dose busulfan (1 mg/kg four times daily for 4 days) before bone marrow transplantation showed a 19% increase in clearance, a 16% lower AUC and a shorter half-life, reduced from 3.94 to 3.03 hours, while taking phenytoin 2.5 to 5 mg/kg daily. A continuous decline in the steady-state plasma levels of busulfan was also seen in 4 of the patients.[1]

It seems likely that the phenytoin (a well recognised enzyme inducer) increases the metabolism of the busulfan by the liver, thereby increasing its loss from the body. The authors of the study suggest that anticonvulsants with fewer enzyme-inducing properties than phenytoin should be used as prophylactic anticonvulsants if busulfan is used for bone marrow transplant pretreatment. Consider also 'Busulfan + Benzodiazepines', above.

1. Hassan M, Öberg G, Björkholm M, Wallin I, Lindgren M. Influence of prophylactic anticonvulsant therapy on high-dose busulphan kinetics. *Cancer Chemother Pharmacol* (1993) 33, 181–6.

Busulfan + Tioguanine

There is evidence that long-term concurrent use of busulfan and tioguanine increases the risk of nodular regenerative hyperplasia of the liver, portal hypertension and oesophageal varices.

Clinical evidence, mechanism, importance and management

Five patients on continuous busulfan 2 mg and tioguanine 80 mg five days weekly for chronic myeloid leukaemia (CML) developed oesophageal varices and abnormal liver function tests. Three of them had gastrointestinal haemorrhages and one died. Liver biopsy of 4 of the patients showed nodular regenerative hyperplasia, which was the cause of portal hypertension and varices.[1] A later analysis of the Medical Research Council trial comparing busulfan with busulfan and tioguanine in 675 patients with CML, revealed a total of 18 cases of portal hypertension and oesophageal varices (including 4 described in the first report[1]), all 18 of which occurred in patients receiving the combination. In addition, there was no survival advantage for the combination.[2] The risk of portal hypertension may be related to long-term use of tioguanine, or to its combination with busulfan. This drug combination should not be used for long-term maintenance therapy of CML.

1. Key NS, Kelly PMA, Emerson PM, Chapman RWG, Allan NC, McGee JO'D. Oesophageal varices associated with busulphan-thioguanine combination therapy for chronic myeloid leukaemia. *Lancet* (1987) 2, 1050–2.
2. Shepherd, PCA, Fooks J, Gray R, Allan NC. Thioguanine used in maintenance therapy of chronic myeloid leukaemia causes non-cirrhotic portal hypertension. *Br J Haematol* (1991) 79, 185–92.

Chlorambucil + Prednisone

A single report describes seizures in a patient possibly caused by co-administration of chlorambucil and prednisone.

Clinical evidence, mechanism, importance and management

A patient with non-Hodgkin's lymphoma experienced a syncopal episode with generalised tonic-clonic seizures 8 days after completing an initial 5-day course of treatment with chlorambucil 12 mg daily and prednisone 50 mg daily. The seizures were controlled with intravenous clonazepam. Four weeks later, on the third day of a second course, she again had generalised tonic-clonic seizures, which resolved spontaneously.

Chlorambucil-induced seizures have occurred in children with the nephrotic syndrome. Cases in adults usually involve high-dose chlorambucil or are in patients with a history of seizures. The seizures in this patient may have been due to the additive effects of both drugs in reducing the seizure threshold.[1]

Note that chlorambucil and prednisone or prednisolone have been widely used together.

1. Jourdan E, Topart D, Pinzani V, Jourdan J. Chlorambucil/prednisone-induced seizures in a patient with non-Hodgkin's lymphoma. *Am J Hematol* (2001) 67, 147.

Cisplatin + Aminoglycosides

The renal toxicity of cisplatin is potentiated by aminoglycoside antibacterials such as gentamicin and tobramycin. Extra care is required in patients treated with cisplatin requiring these antibacterials.

Clinical evidence

Early after the introduction of cisplatin it became apparent that aminoglycosides could increase the nephrotoxicity of this drug. In one report, 4 patients treated with cisplatin in dosages ranging from low to very high (eight doses of 0.5 mg/kg, one or two doses of 3 mg/kg or a single-dose of 5 mg/kg) and who were subsequently given **gentamicin** and cefalotin developed acute and fatal renal failure. Autopsy revealed extensive renal tubular necrosis.[1]

Two similar cases of severe renal toxicity attributed to the use of **gentamicin** and cefalotin after cisplatin are described elsewhere.[2,3] Another patient treated with cisplatin and **gentamicin** developed acute renal failure.[4] A further 3 patients treated with cisplatin then **gentamicin** or **tobramycin** had greater decreases in creatinine levels than 12 others receiving cisplatin alone.[4] A retrospective comparative study confirmed that the incidence of abnormal renal function was higher in patients who had received cisplatin and an aminoglycoside than in those who had received cisplatin alone (12 of 17 versus 19 of 50 patients respectively), but the renal insufficiency was described as usually mild and not clinically significant.[5] Similarly, a brief report stated that aminoglycoside use was associated with a greater decline in renal function in children receiving high-dose cisplatin therapy.[6] Conversely, in another study aminoglycosides were not found to be a significant factor in the development of renal dysfunction after administration of high-dose cisplatin-based therapy, and use of appropriate supportive care (hydration and mannitol diuresis) probably played a part in this.[7]

There is also evidence from a study in children to show that previous treatment with cisplatin is a risk factor for the delayed elimination of aminoglycosides (**gentamicin, amikacin, tobramycin**).[8]

Both cisplatin and the aminoglycosides can cause excessive loss of magnesium, and it has been suggested that combined use increases this loss.[9]

Mechanism

Cisplatin is nephrotoxic and it would appear that its damaging effects on the kidney are additive with the nephrotoxic effects of the aminoglycoside antibacterials. Enhanced renal toxicity and ototoxicity have been reported in *guinea pigs* concurrently treated with cisplatin and **kanamycin** for 2 weeks.[10] Prior exposure to cisplatin caused a significant decrease in gentamicin clearance in *rats*.[11]

Importance and management

An established and potentially serious interaction. However, aminoglycosides remain an important group of antibacterials for the empirical treatment of febrile neutropenia in patients receiving chemotherapy, including cisplatin-based regimens.[12] Good supportive care is required (e.g. pre and post-treatment hydration with mannitol diuresis), and renal function should be well monitored.

1. Gonzalez-Vitale JC, Hayes DM, Cvitkovic E, Sternberg SS. Acute renal failure after *cis*-Dichlorodiammineplatinum (II) and gentamicin-cephalothin therapies. *Cancer Treat Rep* (1978) 62, 693–8.
2. Salem PA, Jabboury KW, Khalil MF. Severe nephrotoxicity: a probable complication of cis-dichorodiammineplatinum (II) and cephalothin-gentamicin therapy. *Oncology* (1982) 39, 31–2.
3. Leite JBF, De Campelo Gentil F, Burchenal J, Marques A, Teixeira MIC, Abrão FA. Insuficiênza renal aguda após o uso de cis-diaminodicloroplatina, gentamicina e cefalosporina. *Rev Paul Med* (1981) 97, 75–7.
4. Dentino M, Luft FC, Yum MN, Williams SD, Einhorn LH. Long term effect of cis-diamminedichloride platinum (CDDP) on renal function and structure in man. *Cancer* (1978) 41, 1274–81.
5. Haas A, Anderson L, Lad T. The influence of aminoglycosides on the nephrotoxicity of *cis*-diamminedichloroplatinum in cancer patients. *J Infect Dis* (1983) 147, 363.
6. Pearson ADJ, Kohli M, Scott GW, Craft AW. Toxicity of high dose cisplatinum in children — the additive role of aminoglycosides. *Proc Am Assoc Cancer Res* (1987) 28, 221.
7. Cooper BW, Creger RJ, Soegiarso W, Mackay WL, Lazarus HM. Renal dysfunction during high-dose cisplatin therapy and autologous hematopoietic stem cell transplantation: effect of aminoglycoside therapy. *Am J Med* (1993) 94, 497–504.
8. Christensen ML, Stewart CF, Crom WR. Evaluation of aminoglycoside disposition in patients previously treated with cisplatin. *Ther Drug Monit* (1989) 11, 631–6.
9. Flombaum CD. Hypomagnesemia associated with cisplatin combination chemotherapy. *Arch Intern Med* (1984) 144, 2336–7.
10. Schweitzer VG, Hawkins JE, Lilly DJ, Litterst CJ, Abrams G, Davis JA, Christy M. Ototoxic and nephrotoxic effects of combined treatment with *cis*-diamminedichloroplatinum and kanamycin in the guinea pig. *Otolaryngol Head Neck Surg* (1984) 92, 38–49.
11. Engineer MS, Bodey GP, Newman RA, Ho DH. Effects of cisplatin-induced nephrotoxicity on gentamicin pharmacokinetics in rats. *Drug Metab Dispos* (1987) 15, 329–34.
12. Viscoli C. The evolution of the empirical management of fever and neutropenia in cancer patients. *J Antimicrob Chemother* (1998) 41 (Suppl D), 65–80.

Cisplatin + Antihypertensives

A single report describes the development of renal failure in a patient treated with furosemide, hydralazine, diazoxide and propranolol for hypertension occurring during cisplatin therapy. However, note that furosemide can be used to promote diuresis during cisplatin therapy to reduce the risk of nephrotoxicity. *Animal* studies show that the damaging effects of cisplatin on the ear can be markedly increased by the concurrent use of etacrynic acid or furosemide. In one retrospective analysis, this was not seen in patients.

Clinical evidence, mechanism, importance and management

(a) Nephrotoxicity

Three hours after receiving cisplatin intravenously (70 mg/m^2) a patient experienced severe nausea and vomiting and his blood pressure rose from 150/90 to 248/140 mmHg. This was treated with **furosemide** 40 mg intravenously, **hydralazine** 10 mg intramuscularly, **diazoxide** 300 mg intravenously and **propranolol** 20 mg orally twice daily for 2 days. Nine days later the patient showed evidence of renal failure, which resolved within 3 weeks. The patient was subsequently similarly treated on two occasions with cisplatin and again developed hypertension, but no treatment was given and there was no evidence of renal impairment.[1] The reasons for the renal impairment are not known, but a study in *rats*[2] indicate that kidney damage may possibly be related to the concentrations of cisplatin and that **furosemide** can increase cisplatin levels in the kidney. However, another study in patients showed that there was no difference in the toxicity or pharmacokinetics of cisplatin when **furosemide** was used to induce diuresis compared with mannitol.[3] Two other studies have also shown that **furosemide** does not alter cisplatin pharmacokinetics.[4,5]

Information seems to be limited to the case cited and its general clinical importance is uncertain. Although mannitol is by far the more usual drug used to induce diuresis during cisplatin therapy in order to reduce the risk of nephrotoxicity, **furosemide** may also be used for this indication.[6]

(b) Ototoxicity

Both cisplatin and loop diuretics such as **etacrynic acid** and **furosemide** given alone can be ototoxic in man. A study[7] in *guinea pigs* showed that when cisplatin 7 mg/kg or **etacrynic acid** 50 mg/kg were given alone their ototoxic effects were reversible, but when given together the damaging effects on the ear were profound, prolonged and possibly permanent. Similarly, while cisplatin-induced ototoxicity was potentiated by **furosemide** in *guinea pigs* in one study[8] in another this was only seen when a very high dose of **furosemide** was used.[9] In one small retrospective analysis of cancer patients, the risk of developing hearing loss after low-dose slow-infusion cisplatin did not correlate significantly with concurrent use of other ototoxic drugs such as **furosemide**.[10] Audiometric tests should be carried out when cisplatin is used anyway, and particularly when other ototoxic drugs are used concurrently.

1. Markman M, Trump DL. Nephrotoxicity with cisplatin and antihypertensive medications. *Ann Intern Med* (1982) 96, 257.
2. Pera MF, Zook BC, Harder HC. Effects of mannitol or furosemide diuresis on the nephrotoxicity and physiological disposition of *cis*-dichlorodiammineplatinum-(II) in rats. *Cancer Res* (1979) 39, 1269–79.
3. Ostrow S, Egorin MJ, Hahn D, Markus S, Aisner J, Chang P, LeRoy A, Bachur NR, Wiernik PH. High-dose cisplatin therapy using mannitol versus furosemide diuresis: comparative pharmacokinetics and toxicity. *Cancer Treat Rep* (1981) 65, 73–8.
4. Dumas M, d'Athis P, de Gislain C, Lautissier JL, Autissier N, Escousse A, Guerrin J. Influence of frusemide on cis-dichlorodiammineplatinum (II) pharmaco-kinetics. *Eur J Drug Metab Pharmacokinet* (1987) 12, 203–6.
5. Dumas M, de Gislain C, d'Athis P, Chadoint-Noudeau V, Escousse A, Guerrin J, Autissier N. Evaluation of the effect of furosemide on ultrafilterable platinum kinetics in patients treated with *cis*-diamminedichloroplatinium. *Cancer Chemother Pharmacol* (1989) 23, 37–40.
6. Numico G, Benasso M, Vannozzi MO, Merlano M, Rosso R, Viale M, Esposito M. Hydration regimen and hematological toxicity of a cisplatin-based chemotherapy regimen. Clinical observations and pharmacokinetic analysis. *Anticancer Res* (1998) 18, 1313–18.
7. Komune S, Snow JB. Potentiating effects of cisplatin and ethacrynic acid in ototoxicity. *Arch Otolaryngol* (1981) 107, 594–7.
8. McAlpine D, Johnstone BM. The ototoxic mechanism of cisplatin. *Hear Res* (1990) 47, 191–203.
9. Laurell G, Engström B. The combined effect of cisplatin and furosemide on hearing function in guinea pigs. *Hear Res* (1989) 38, 19–26.
10. Hallmark RJ, Snyder JM, Jusenius K, Tamimi HK. Factors influencing ototoxicity in ovarian cancer patients treated with Cis-platinum based chemotherapy. *Eur J Gynaecol Oncol* (1992) 13, 35–44.

Cisplatin + H_2-blockers

Cimetidine and ranitidine probably do not alter the renal clearance of cisplatin to a clinically relevant extent.

Clinical evidence, mechanism, importance and management

Some *animal* studies have shown that organic cations such as **cimetidine** and **ranitidine** may compete with the renal tubular transport of cisplatin and thus could be useful in reducing cisplatin nephrotoxicity.[1,2] However, in a study of 10 children receiving cisplatin, **ranitidine** had no effect on the total body disposition or renal clearance of cisplatin. This finding and further studies in *dogs* showed that cisplatin may not share transport systems with organic cations to a clinically relevant extent.[3] Although information is limited, it appears that there is no interaction between cisplatin and **cimetidine** or **ranitidine**. Note that **cimetidine** has increased the levels or toxicity of some other antineoplastics, see 'Nitrosoureas + Cimetidine', p.485, 'Cyclophosphamide + H_2-blockers', p.462, 'Anthracyclines; Epirubicin + Cimetidine', p.451, and 'Fluorouracil + H_2-blockers', p.469.

1. Klein J, Bentur Y, Cheung D, Moselhy G, Koren G. Renal handling of cisplatin: interactions with organic anions and cations in the dog. *Clin Invest Med* (1991) 14, 388–94.
2. Haragsim L, Zima T, Němeček K. Nephrotoxic effects of platinum cytostatics–preventive effects of nifedipine and cimetidine. *Sb Lek* (1994) 95, 173–83.
3. Ito S, Weitzman S, Klein J, Greenberg M, Lau R, Atanakovic G, Koren G. Lack of cisplatin-ranitidine kinetic interactions: *in vivo* study in children, and *in vitro* study using dog renal brush border membrane vesicles. *Life Sci* (1998) 62, PL387–PL392.

Cisplatin + Probenecid

On the basis of studies on *animals* it is uncertain whether the nephrotoxicity of cisplatin is increased or reduced by probenecid. The available clinical data suggest a reduction, but uncertainty remains.

Clinical evidence, mechanism, importance and management

In a randomised study in cancer patients, probenecid 2 to 4 g daily reduced the fractional clearance of free platinum after a single 60- to 100-mg/m^2 dose of cisplatin given as a 24-hour infusion, and no cases of renal impairment were seen.[1] Similarly, in a further phase I dose-escalation study no renal impairment was seen in patients given cisplatin at doses from 100 to 160 mg/m^2 when treated with probenecid 1 g six-hourly for 12 doses (beginning 24 hours before the cisplatin infusion, and continuing for 24 hours after).[2] An earlier study in *rats* suggested that giving probenecid before cisplatin reduced nephrotoxicity, as assessed by blood urea levels and serum creatinine.[3] Subsequently, a study in *dogs* has shown that probenecid decreased the renal clearance of free cisplatin,[4] and another in *mice* showed probenecid reduced the renal tubular damage seen with cisplatin alone.[5]

Conversely, some researchers have suggested that the combination of probenecid and cisplatin is potentially more toxic than cisplatin alone. They found that probenecid increased the fractional clearance of free platinum from cisplatin in *rats*, and that pretreatment with probenecid increased nephrotoxicity, as assessed by blood urea levels.[6] Other authors similarly reported that probenecid increased cisplatin clearance in *rats*.[7]

It is unclear why some *animal* studies show that probenecid increases cisplatin-induced nephrotoxicity whereas others show a decrease. Although the available clinical data suggests that there is a decrease, some uncertainty remains. The combination should be used with caution.

1. Jacobs C, Coleman CN, Rich L, Hirst K, Weiner MW. Inhibition of *cis*-diamminedichloroplatinum secretion by the human kidney with probenecid. *Cancer Res* (1984) 44, 3632–5.
2. Jacobs C, Kaubisch S, Halsey J, Lum BL, Gosland M, Coleman CN, Sikic BI. The use of probenecid as a chemoprotector against cisplatin nephrotoxicity. *Cancer* (1991) 67, 1518–24.
3. Ross DA, Gale GR. Reduction of the renal toxicity of *cis*-dichlorodiammineplatinum (II) by probenecid. *Cancer Treat Rep* (1979) 63, 781–7.
4. Klein J, Bentur Y, Cheung D, Moselhy G, Koren G. Renal handling of cisplatin: interactions with organic anions and cations in the dog. *Clin Invest Med* (1991) 14, 388–94.
5. Ban M, Hettich D, Huguet N. Nephrotoxicity mechanism of *cis*-platinum (II) diamine dichloride in mice. *Toxicol Lett* (1994) 71, 161–8.
6. Daley-Yates PT, McBrien DCH. Enhancement of cisplatin nephrotoxicity by probenecid. *Cancer Treat Rep* (1984) 68, 445–6.
7. Osman NM, Litterst CL. Effect of probenecid and *N'*-methylnicotinamide on renal handling of *cis*-dichlorodiammineplatinum-II in rats. *Cancer Lett* (1983) 19, 107–11.

Cyclophosphamide + Allopurinol

There is some evidence that the incidence of serious bone marrow depression caused by cyclophosphamide can be increased by the concurrent use of allopurinol, but this was not confirmed in a controlled study. Allopurinol may alter cyclophosphamide pharmacokinetics.

Clinical evidence

A retrospective epidemiological survey of patients in four hospitals who, over a 4-year period, had been treated with cyclophosphamide, showed that the incidence of serious bone marrow depression was 57.7% in 26 patients who had also received allopurinol, and 18.8% in 32 patients who had not.[1] A pharmacokinetic study in 9 patients with malignant disease and 2 healthy subjects showed that while taking allopurinol 600 mg daily the concentration of the cytotoxic metabolites of cyclophosphamide increased by an average of 37.5% (range 1.5 to 110%).[2] Another pharmacokinetic study reported that the half-life of cyclophosphamide was more than two-fold longer in 3 children also receiving allopurinol 300 mg/m^2 when compared with that in children not given allopurinol.[3] However, another study found that although allopurinol pretreatment increased the half-life of cyclophosphamide, the plasma alkylating activity and urinary metabolite and cyclophosphamide excretion were unchanged.[4] Moreover, a randomised controlled study,[5] designed as a follow-up to the survey cited above,[1] failed to confirm that allopurinol increased the toxicity of cyclophosphamide in 81 patients with Hodgkin's or non-Hodgkin's lymphoma. In this study, there was no difference in nadirs for white blood cells and platelets during 3 cycles of cyclophosphamide-containing chemotherapy between 44 patients receiving allopurinol and 37 patients not receiving allopurinol.

Mechanism

Not understood. Cyclophosphamide itself is inactive, but it is converted by the liver into cytotoxic metabolites.[6] Allopurinol or its metabolite oxypurinol may inhibit their renal excretion, or may alter hepatic metabolism.[2,3]

Importance and management

This interaction is not established with any certainty. The authors of the randomised study consider that, if necessary, allopurinol can be used safety with the chemotherapy regimens used for lymphomas to prevent hyperuricaemia.[5] However, the other data introduce a note of caution. Be alert for increased cyclophosphamide toxicity.

1. Boston Collaborative Drug Surveillance Programme. Allopurinol and cytotoxic drugs. Interaction in relation to bone marrow depression. *JAMA* (1974) 227, 1036–40.
2. Witten J, Frederiksen PL, Mouridsen HT. The pharmacokinetics of cyclophosphamide in man after treatment with allopurinol. *Acta Pharmacol Toxicol (Copenh)* (1980) 46, 392–4.
3. Yule SM, Boddy AV, Cole M, Price L, Wyllie R, Tasso MJ, Pearson ADJ, Idle JR. Cyclophosphamide pharmacokinetics in children. *Br J Clin Pharmacol* (1996) 41, 13–19.
4. Bagley CM, Bostick FW, DeVita VT. Clinical pharmacology of cyclophosphamide. *Cancer Res* (1973) 33, 226–33.
5. Stolbach L, Begg C, Bennett JM, Silverstein M, Falkson G, Harris DT, Glick J. Evaluation of bone marrow toxic reaction in patients treated with allopurinol. *JAMA* (1982) 247, 334–6.
6. Bagley CM, Bostick FW, DeVita VT. Clinical pharmacology of cyclophosphamide. *Cancer Res* (1973) 33, 226–33.

Cyclophosphamide + Amiodarone

Early-onset pulmonary toxicity occurred in a patient on amiodarone after high-dose cyclophosphamide.

Clinical evidence, mechanism, importance and management

A patient with dendritic cell carcinoma who had been treated with amiodarone for 18 months, and with 6 cycles of chemotherapy including cyclophosphamide over the last 12 months, was admitted to hospital with progressive shortness of breath 18 days after a single 4000-mg/m^2 dose of cyclophosphamide. He was found to have interstitial pneumonitis and a lung biopsy indicated drug-induced pulmonary toxicity. The patient's condition improved rapidly over the following 10 days with discontinuation of amiodarone and treatment with prednisolone 60 mg daily. Over the previous year he had also received vincristine, etoposide and prednisone, cisplatin, cytarabine and dexamethasone as part of his chemotherapy.[1]

Mechanism

Pulmonary toxicity may occur in about 10% of patients treated with amiodarone.[2,3] Pulmonary toxicity due to cyclophosphamide may occur between 1 to 6 months after exposure or occur as a more insidious form after about 6 months. The early onset of symptoms in this patient, just over 2 weeks after high-dose cyclophosphamide, suggests accelerated mechanisms of pulmonary toxicity. Both cyclophosphamide and amiodarone pulmonary toxicity appear to be enhanced by oxygen and the combination of cyclophosphamide with amiodarone may enhance oxidative stress and therefore pulmonary toxicity.

Importance and management

Although information seems to be limited to the single case report cited, the potential for both cyclophosphamide and amiodarone to cause pulmonary toxicity is established. Be alert to the possibility of enhanced pulmonary toxicity if these drugs are co-administered.

1. Bhagat R, Sporn TA, Long GD, Folz RJ. Amiodarone and cyclophosphamide: potential for enhanced lung toxicity. *Bone Marrow Transplant* (2001) 27, 1109–1111.
2. Martin WJ, Rosenow EC. Amiodarone pulmonary toxicity. Recognition and pathogenesis (Part 1). *Chest* (1988) 93, 1067–75.
3. Martin WJ, Rosenow EC. Amiodarone pulmonary toxicity. Recognition and pathogenesis (Part 2). *Chest* (1988) 93, 1242–8.

Cyclophosphamide + Azathioprine

A report describes liver damage in four patients given cyclophosphamide and who had previously been treated with azathioprine. However, another study showed that liver function improved when cyclophosphamide was substituted for azathioprine in 29 patients.

Clinical evidence, mechanism, importance and management

Four patients (two with systemic lupus erythematosus, one with Sjogren's syndrome, and one with Wegener's granulomatosis) developed liver injury when given cyclophosphamide and 3 of them had liver cell necrosis. All had previously been treated with azathioprine and 2 of them had received cyclophosphamide previously without apparent liver damage. It was suggested that azathioprine and cyclophosphamide may have interacted.[1] However, in a retrospective study of cardiac transplant recipients, substitution of cyclophosphamide for azathioprine was associated with improvement in liver function tests in 29 patients with suspected azathioprine-induced liver dysfunction.[2]

1. Shaunak S, Munro JM, Weinbren K, Walport MJ, Cox TM. Cyclophosphamide-induced liver necrosis: a possible interaction with azathioprine. *Q J Med* (1988) New Series 67, 309–17.
2. Wagoner LE, Olsen SL, Bristow MR, O'Connell JB, Taylor DO, Lappe DL, Renlund DG. Cyclophosphamide as an alternative to azathioprine in cardiac transplant recipients with suspected azathioprine-induced hepatotoxicity. *Transplantation* (1993) 56, 1415–18.

Cyclophosphamide or Ifosfamide + Azoles

Fluconazole and itraconazole inhibit the metabolism of cyclophosphamide. There is some evidence that, compared with fluconazole, itraconazole might increase cyclophosphamide toxicity. Ketoconazole inhibits the metabolism of ifosfamide. This did not improve the ratio of active to inactive/toxic metabolites, and the possibility remains that ifosfamide efficacy could be reduced.

Clinical evidence, mechanism, importance and management

(a) Cyclophosphamide

Twenty-two children with established cyclophosphamide metabolism profiles and who were not receiving other treatment known to affect drug metabolism were included in a retrospective case series investigation. The clearance of cyclophosphamide was reduced in 9 children who were given oral or intravenous **fluconazole** 5 mg/kg daily compared to the remaining 13 children who did not receive **fluconazole** (2.4 versus 4.2 litres/hour/m^2 respectively).[1] A study in patients given either intravenous or oral **fluconazole** 400 mg daily or **itraconazole** (either intravenous 200 mg daily or orally as 2.5 mg/kg three times daily) for prophylaxis after allogenic stem cell transplantation found that those given **itraconazole** developed higher bilirubin and creatinine levels in the first 20 days after transplantation than those given **fluconazole**. Highest values were in patients who received **itraconazole** with cyclophosphamide. In this study, analysis of cyclophosphamide pharmacokinetics in 9 **itraconazole** recipients and 140 **fluconazole** recipients revealed that **itraconazole** recipients had a 20% greater clearance of cyclophosphamide, leading to greater exposure to the active metabolite of cyclophosphamide, and its metabolites.[2]

Cyclophosphamide is oxidised to its active metabolite, 4-hydroxycyclophosphamide (HCY) by the cytochrome P450 isoenzymes CYP2B6, CYP3A4, CY2C9, and CYP2A6 and then undergoes further metabolism to produce several toxic metabolites. It is also metabolised by CYP3A4 to an inactive metabolite, deschloroethylcyclophosphamide (DCCP). **Itraconazole** is a more potent inhibitor of CYP3A4 than **fluconazole**, but unlike **itraconazole**, **fluconazole** can also inhibit CYP2C9. It has been suggested that **fluconazole** inhibition of CYP2C9 may decrease the formation of HCY and result in increased levels of DCCP and fewer toxic metabolites.[2] Further study is required to determine whether the inhibition of active metabolite formation by **fluconazole** reduces the therapeutic effect of cyclophosphamide.[1] Until more is known it may be prudent to encourage caution when azoles are used in patients on cyclophosphamide, other than therapies established in randomised clinical trials, being alert for unexpected toxicity or reduced efficacy.

(b) Ifosfamide

Eight patients undergoing chemotherapy were also given (for the first or second cycle of treatment) **ketoconazole** 200 mg twice daily for 4 days starting one day before treatment with ifosfamide. Concurrent treatment with **ketoconazole** modestly decreased the clearance of ifosfamide by 11%, increased the AUC by 14%, and increased urinary elimination by 26%. The fraction of ifosfamide metabolised to the inactive, neurotoxic, dechloroethylated metabolite was not affected, whereas the fraction metabolised to the active, hydroxylated metabolite was modestly decreased.[3]

Ketoconazole is an inhibitor of the cytochrome P450 isoenzyme CYP3A4, an enzyme that is involved in the production of active and inactive/toxic metabolites of ifosfamide (see also 'Cyclophosphamide or Ifosfamide + Barbiturates', below). In the clinical study cited, **ketoconazole** modestly decreased the proportion of ifosfamide undergoing activation. It was suggested that concurrent use should be avoided, since it might result in decreased ifosfamide efficacy,[3] although this remains to be shown.

1. Yule SM, Walker D, Cole M, Mcsorley L, Cholerton S, Daly AK, Pearson ADJ, Boddy AV. The effect of fluconazole on cyclophosphamide metabolism in children. *Drug Metab Dispos* (1999) 27, 417–21.
2. Marr KA, Leisenring W, Crippa F, Slattery JT, Corey L, Boeckh M, McDonald GB. Cyclophosphamide metabolism is affected by azole antifungals. *Blood* (2004) 103, 1557–9.
3. Kerbusch T, Jansen RLH, Mathôt RAA, Huitema ADR, Jansen M, van Rijswijk REN, Beijnen JH. Modulation of the cytochrome P450–mediated metabolism of ifosfamide by ketoconazole and rifampin. *Clin Pharmacol Ther* (2001) 70, 132–41.

Cyclophosphamide or Ifosfamide + Barbiturates

Evidence suggests that neither the toxicity nor the therapeutic effects of cyclophosphamide and ifosfamide are significantly altered by the concurrent use of barbiturates. However, an isolated report describes encephalopathy in a girl on phenobarbital when given the first dose of ifosfamide/mesna.

Clinical evidence

(a) Cyclophosphamide

Phenobarbital 180 mg daily in divided doses for 10 days increased the mean plasma levels of cyclophosphamide total metabolites by 50% in 4 patients and increased their rate of urinary excretion.[1] Similarly, another study in 11 patients reported that the peak level of normustard-like substances was 1.5 times higher after pretreatment with **phenobarbital**.[2] Similar changes in cyclophosphamide pharmacokinetics have been described in *animal* studies, and these have generally also shown that **phenobarbital** has no effect on the antitumour activity of cyclophosphamide[3] although some have shown a reduction.[4]

Cyclophosphamide was reported to inhibit the clearance and increase the effects of **pentobarbital** in a study in *rats*.[5] Another study reported that a patient on **phenobarbital** showed auto-induction of cyclophosphamide clearance with subsequent chemotherapy courses similar to that in patients not on **phenobarbital**.[6]

(b) Ifosfamide

A 15-year-old girl who had been taking **phenobarbital** for epilepsy since infancy developed confusion and gradually became unconscious 6 hours after being given a first dose of ifosfamide for metastatic rhabdomyosarcoma. Her chemotherapy regimen was ifosfamide 3 g/m^2, mesna 3.6 g/m^2, vincristine 2 mg and dactinomycin. An EEG revealed signs of severe diffuse encephalopathy. She remained unconscious for 24 hours but was asymptomatic after 48 hours.[7] In a pharmacokinetic study, **phenobarbital** 60 mg daily for 3 days had no effect on the pharmacokinetics of high-dose ifosfamide (4 g/m^2 over 1 hour each day for 3 days). The AUC for ifosfamide decreased from day one to day 3 irrespective of **phenobarbital** administration.[8]

Mechanism

Cyclophosphamide and ifosfamide are prodrugs that undergo hepatic metabolism, and it seems that they are able to induce their own metabolism. Cyclophosphamide appears to be hydroxylated by the cytochrome P450 subfamilies CYP2B and CYP2C, in particular, to form active metabolites, whereas ifosfamide appears to be principally hydroxylated by CYP3A. Both drugs also undergo dechloroethylation to produce inactive but neurotoxic metabolites, which can cause encephalopathy. For cyclophosphamide, this seems to be primarily catalysed by CYP3A, whereas for ifosfamide both CYP3A and CYP2B appear to be involved. Ifosfamide has a higher incidence of encephalopathy than cyclophosphamide.[9] Phenobarbital and other barbiturates are inducers of both CYP2B and CYP3A. Therefore, it is unlikely that barbiturates will generally alter the balance between dechloroethylation and hydroxylation for cyclophosphamide,[3] although there is some evidence from *animal* studies they may do so for ifosfamide.[10]

Importance and management

The relationship between the case of encephalopathy and the use of ifosfamide with phenobarbital is not established, but it serves to emphasise the need for particular caution and good monitoring if concurrent use is undertaken. More study is needed. Although barbiturates can cause an increase in the rate of metabolism of cyclophosphamide, this does not appear to alter the AUC and the efficacy of this drug.

1. Jao JY, Jusko WJ, Cohen JL. Phenobarbital effects on cyclophosphamide pharmacokinetics in man. *Cancer Res* (1972) 32, 2761–4.
2. Maezawa S, Ohira S, Sakauma M, Matsuoka S, Wakui A, Saito T. Effects of inducer of liver drug-metabolizing enzyme on blood level of active metabolites of cyclophosphamide in rats and in cancer patients. *Tohoku J Exp Med* (1981) 134, 45–53.
3. Yu LJ, Drewes P, Gustafsson K, Brain EGC, Hecht JED, Waxman DJ. In Vivo modulation of alternative pathways of P-450-catalyzed cyclophosphamide metabolism: impact on pharmacokinetics and antitumor activity. *J Pharmacol Exp Ther* (1999) 288, 928–37.
4. Alberts DS, van Daalen Wetters T. The effect of phenobarbital on cyclophosphamide antitumour activity. *Cancer Res* (1976) 36, 2785–9.
5. Donelli MG, Colombo T, Garattini S. Effect of cyclophosphamide on the activity and distribution of pentobarbital in rats. *Biochem Pharmacol* (1973) 22, 2609–14.
6. Chen T-L, Passos-Coelho JL, Noe DA, Kennedy MJ, Black KC, Colvin M, Grochow LB. Nonlinear pharmacokinetics of cyclophosphamide in patients with metastatic breast cancer receiving high-dose chemotherapy followed by autologous bone marrow transplantation. *Cancer Res* (1995) 55, 810–16. Erratum *ibid*., 1600.
7. Ghosn M, Carde P, Leclerq B, Flamant F, Friedman S, Droz JP, Hayat M. Ifosfamide/mesna related encephalopathy: a case report with a possible role of phenobarbital in enhancing neurotoxicity. *Bull Cancer* (1988) 75, 391–2.
8. Lokiec F, Santoni J, Weill S, Tubiana-Hulin M. Phenobarbital administration does not affect high-dose ifosfamide pharmacokinetics in humans. *Anticancer Drugs* (1996) 7, 893–6.
9. Goren MP, Wright RK, Pratt CB, Pell FE. Dechloroethylation of ifosfamide and neurotoxicity. *Lancet* (1986) ii, 1219–20.
10. Brain EGC, Yu LJ, Gustafsson K, Drewes P, Waxman DJ. Modulation of P450-dependent ifosfamide pharmacokinetics: a better understanding of drug activation in vivo. *Br J Cancer* (1998) 77, 1768–76.

Cyclophosphamide or Ifosfamide + Benzodiazepines

***Animal* studies suggest that the benzodiazepines may possibly increase the metabolic activation and the toxicity of high doses of cyclophosphamide and ifosfamide. However, diazepam did not alter the pharmacokinetics of high-dose cyclophosphamide in a clinical study. Note also that lorazepam is widely used for chemotherapy-induced nausea and vomiting.**

Clinical evidence, mechanism, importance and management

Studies in *mice* found that pretreatment with benzodiazepines (**chlordiazepoxide, diazepam, oxazepam**) increased the levels of active metabolites and the lethality of high-dose cyclophosphamide[1] and similarly increased the levels of active metabolites and enhanced the toxicity of high-dose ifosfamide.[2] However, a clinical study found that the prophylactic use of **diazepam** 5 mg daily as an anti-epileptic had no effect on the pharmacokinetics of very high-dose cyclophosphamide (60 mg/kg intravenously over 2 hours for 2 days) or its neurotoxic (dechloroethylated) metabolites in 3 patients receiving cyclophosphamide and busulfan before bone marrow transplantation.[3] In the *animal* studies, it was suggested that benzodiazepines may induce the liver enzymes concerned with the metabolism of cyclophosphamide and ifosfamide to its active cytotoxic products. There are very limited data on this potential interaction. The widespread use of the benzodiazepine **lorazepam** in anti-emetic regimens for chemotherapy-induced nausea and vomiting suggest that a significant increase in toxicity or alteration in efficacy of cyclophosphamide and ifosfamide does not occur clinically, but there do not appear to be any studies directly addressing this question.

1. Sasaki K-I, Furusawa S, Takayanagi G. Effects of chlordiazepoxide, diazepam and oxazepam on the antitumour activity, the lethality and the blood level of active metabolites of cyclophosphamide and cyclophosphamide oxidase activity in mice. *J Pharmacobiodyn* (1983) 6, 767–72.
2. Furusawa S, Fujimura T, Sasaki K, Takayanagi Y. Potentiation of ifosfamide toxicity by chlordiazepoxide, diazepam, and oxazepam. *Chem Pharm Bull (Tokyo)* (1989) 73, 3420–2.
3. Williams ML, Wainer IW, Embree L, Barnett M, Granvil CL, Ducharme MP. Enantioselective induction of cyclophosphamide metabolism by phenytoin. *Chirality* (1999) 11, 569–74.

Cyclophosphamide + Busulfan

Cyclophosphamide serum levels may be increased and those of its active metabolite decreased if given within 24 hours of busulfan treatment.

Clinical evidence, mechanism, importance and management

In one study, the ratio of the AUC of cyclophosphamide and that of its active metabolite hydroxycyclophosphamide was higher in patients also receiving phenytoin and busulfan than in those receiving irradiation.[1] In a similar study, 23 bone marrow transplant patients were pre-treated with busulfan 4 mg/kg/day for 4 days, followed by cyclophosphamide 60 mg/kg/day for 2 days. The interval between the last dose of busulfan and starting cyclophosphamide was 24 to 50 hours in 12 patients [group A] and 7 to 15 hours in the remaining 11 [group B]. Nine others pretreated with cyclophosphamide and total body irradiation acted as the controls. In group A the AUCs of cyclophosphamide and hydroxycyclophosphamide were similar to those in the controls but in group B the AUC of cyclophosphamide was more than doubled and the AUC of hydroxycyclophosphamide significantly lower (representing a reduced ratio of hydroxycyclophosphamide to cyclophosphamide). In addition group B had greater toxicity.[2] Busulfan may directly inhibit the hepatic activation of cyclophosphamide or may act indirectly by depleting glutathione. Phenytoin induces the metabolism of cyclophosphamide (see 'Cyclophosphamide or Ifosfamide + Phenytoin', p.463).

It seems therefore that if the cyclophosphamide is given at least 24 hours after the last busulfan dose, its serum levels will not be greatly affected, whereas if the interval is short, activation may be decreased and toxicity increased. Further study is required to determine the optimum timing to achieve maximum efficacy and minimum drug toxicity while taking into account other concurrent medication such as phenytoin.

1. Slattery JT, Kalhorn TF, McDonald GB, Lambert K, Buckner CD, Bensinger WI, Anasetti C, Appelbaum FR. Conditioning regimen-dependent disposition of cyclophosphamide and hydroxycyclophosphamide in human marrow transplantation patients. *J Clin Oncol* (1996) 14, 1484–94.
2. Hassan M, Ljungman P, Ringdén O, Hassan Z, Öberg G, Nilsson C, Békassy A, Bielenstein M, Abdel-Rehim M, Georén S, Astner L. The effect of busulphan on the pharmacokinetics of cyclophosphamide and its 4-hydroxy metabolite: time interval influence on the therapeutic efficacy and therapy-related toxicity. *Bone Marrow Transplant* (2000) 25, 915–24.

Cyclophosphamide + Chloramphenicol

Some limited evidence suggests that chloramphenicol may reduce the production of the active metabolites of cyclophosphamide. Whether this reduces its therapeutic efficacy remains to be determined.

Clinical evidence, mechanism, importance and management

Cyclophosphamide itself is inactive, but after administration it is metabolised to active alkylating metabolites. A study in *animals*[1] found that pretreatment with chloramphenicol reduced the effects of cyclophosphamide and reduced the production of active metabolites. Although another *animal* study also showed a reduction in lethality of cyclophosphamide with chloramphenicol, the immunosuppressive effect of cyclophosphamide was unchanged.[2] A study in 4 patients showed that chloramphenicol 1 g twice daily for 12 days prolonged the mean serum half-life of a single intravenous dose of cyclophosphamide from 7.5 to 11.5 hours, but the 28% reduction in the AUC of the metabolites did not reach significance.[3]

Chloramphenicol is an inhibitor of the cytochrome P450 isoenzyme subfamily CYP2B, which is partially responsible for the activation of cyclophosphamide. It therefore seems possible that a reduction in the activity of cyclophosphamide may occur, but the extent to which this affects treatment with cyclophosphamide is uncertain. Concurrent use need not be avoided, but be alert for evidence of a reduced response. More study is needed.

1. Dixon RL. Effect of chloramphenicol on the metabolism and lethality of cyclophosphamide in rats. *Proc Soc Exp Biol Med* (1968) 127, 1151–5.
2. Berenbaum MC, Cope WA, Double JA. The effect of microsomal enzyme inhibition on the immunosuppressive and toxic effects of cyclophosphamide. *Clin Exp Immunol* (1973) 14, 257–70.
3. Faber OK, Mouridsen HT, Skovsted L. The effect of chloramphenicol and sulphaphenazole on the biotransformation of cyclophosphamide in man. *Br J Clin Pharmacol* (1975) 2, 281–5.

Cyclophosphamide or Ifosfamide + Cisplatin

The renal toxicity of ifosfamide may be greater when used with cisplatin or in those who have had prior treatment with cisplatin. Ifosfamide may increase the hearing loss due to cisplatin.

Clinical evidence

(a) Nephrotoxicity

A comparative study in 36 children with malignant solid tumours on a range of drugs including some known to be potentially nephrotoxic (high dose methotrexate, aminoglycosides, cyclophosphamide), indicated that previous treatment with cisplatin increased their susceptibility to ifosfamide toxicity (neurotoxicity, severe leucopenia or acute tubular damage).[1] Similarly, in another study the cumulative cisplatin dose administered prior to high-dose ICE (ifosfamide, carboplatin, and etoposide) was found to be a strong risk factor for the development of nephrotoxicity.[2] The nephrotoxicity may not be reversible; 3 cases requiring long-term haemodialysis have been described.[3]

Other studies also suggested that concurrent use of ifosfamide with cisplatin appeared to increase nephrotoxicity; one showed an increase in depletion of phosphate reabsorption,[4] whereas the other showed increased microglobulin excretion.[5]

(b) Ototoxicity

A retrospective comparative study found that when ifosfamide was added to cisplatin, the hearing loss caused by cisplatin was exacerbated.[6]

Mechanism

Both cisplatin and ifosfamide are commonly associated with nephrotoxicity. It is thought that concurrent or possibly prior treatment with cisplatin damages the kidney tubules so that the clearance of the ifosfamide metabolites from the body is reduced and their toxic effects are thereby increased. Damaged kidney tubules may also be less capable of converting mesna to its active kidney-protecting form. The increase in the hearing loss is not understood.

Importance and management

These interactions appear to be established. The authors of the paper cited[1] point out that the majority of patients who develop toxicity have persistently high urinary NAG concentrations (*N*-acetyl-β-D-glucosaminidase, an enzyme released by renal tubular cells), even though serum creatinine levels remain within the acceptable range for ifosfamide treatment. They suggest that evidence of subclinical tubular damage should be sought for by monitoring the excretion of urinary NAG. Note that cisplatin and ifosfamide are widely used in combination, and the related drug cyclophosphamide is also routinely used with cisplatin. **Amifostine** may be useful in reducing the nephrotoxicity of this combination.[7] The authors who reported on hearing loss advise that serial audiograms are done in patients treated with both drugs.[6]

1. Goren MP, Wright RK, Pratt CB, Horowitz ME, Dodge RK, Viar MJ, Kovnar EH. Potentiation of ifosfamide neurotoxicity, hematotoxicity, and tubular nephrotoxicity by prior *cis*-diamminedichloroplatinum(II) therapy. *Cancer Res* (1987) 47, 1457–60.
2. Caglar K, Kinalp C, Arpaci F, Turan M, Saglam K, Ozturk B, Komurcu Ş, Yavuz I, Yenicesu M, Ozet A, Vural A. Cumulative prior dose of cisplatin as a cause of the nephrotoxicity of high-dose chemotherapy followed by autologous stem-cell transplantation. *Nephrol Dial Transplant* (2002) 17, 1931–5.
3. Martinez F, Deray G, Cacoub P, Beaufils H, Jacobs C. Ifosfamide nephrotoxicity: deleterious effect of previous cisplatin administration. *Lancet* (1996) 348, 1100–1.
4. Rossi R, Danzebrink S, Hillebrand D, Linnenbürger K, Ullrich K, Jürgens H. Ifosfamide-induced subclinical nephrotoxicity and its potentiation by cisplatinum. *Med Pediatr Oncol* (1994) 22, 27–32.
5. Hacke M, Schmoll H-J, Alt JM, Baumann K, Stolte H. Nephrotoxicity of *cis*-diamminedichloroplatinum with or without ifosfamide in cancer treatment. *Clin Physiol Biochem* (1983) 1, 17–26.
6. Meyer WH, Ayers D, McHaney VA, Roberson P, Pratt CB. Ifosfamide and exacerbation of cisplatin-induced hearing loss. *Lancet* (1993) 341, 754–5.
7. Hartmann JT, Fels LM, Knop S, Stolte H, Kanz L, Bokemeyer C. A randomized trial comparing the nephrotoxicity of cisplatin/ifosfamide-based combination chemotherapy with or without amifostine in patients with solid tumors. *Invest New Drugs* (2000) 18, 281–9.

Cyclophosphamide + Colony stimulating factors

Granulocyte colony-stimulating factor (G-CSF) has been associated with an increased occurrence of pulmonary toxicity when used with cyclophosphamide.

Clinical evidence, mechanism, importance and management

A 1-year-old boy with a neuroblastoma Evans stage III died of respiratory insufficiency following treatment with **filgrastim** (a **G-CSF**) and normal doses of cyclophosphamide and doxorubicin. The authors of the report suggest that the pulmonary toxicity of the cyclophosphamide (normally only seen with high cumulative doses) is potentiated by the **filgrastim**.[1] Six of 53 patients treated with CHOP (cyclophosphamide, doxorubicin, vincristine and prednisolone) and **G-CSF** developed pulmonary toxicity, which was considered a much higher incidence than usually seen with CHOP alone. The development of toxicity correlated with the mean peak leucocyte count.[2] Another 10 cases of interstitial pneumonitis have occurred with cyclophosphamide-based regimens (not including bleomycin or methotrexate) and **G-CSF**.[3,4] There is some evidence that the pulmonary toxicity of bleomycin might possibly also be increased by CSFs (see 'Bleomycin + Colony stimulating factors', p.455). These interactions are not firmly established, but good pulmonary function monitoring appears to be advisable when CSFs are used with antineoplastics causing pulmonary toxicity. If interstitial pneumonitis occurs, the drugs should be discontinued and high-dose corticosteroids started immediately.[2] More study is needed.

1. van Woensel JBM, Knoester H, Leeuw JA, van Aalderen WMC. Acute respiratory insufficiency during doxorubicin, cyclophosphamide, and G-CSF therapy. *Lancet* (1994) 344, 759–60.
2. Yokose N, Ogata K, Tamura H, An E, Nakamura K, Kamikubo K, Kudoh S, Dan K, Nomura T. Pulmonary toxicity after granulocyte colony-stimulating factor-combined chemotherapy for non-Hodgkin's lymphoma. *Br J Cancer* (1998) 77, 2286–90.
3. Niitsu N, Iki S, Muroi K, Motomura S, Murakami M, Takeyama H, Ohsaka A, Urabe A. Interstitial pneumonia in patients receiving granulocyte colony-stimulating factor during chemotherapy: survey in Japan 1991–96. *Br J Cancer* (1997) 76, 1661–6.
4. Hasegawa Y, Ninomiya J, Kamoshita M, Ohtani K, Kobayashi T, Kojima J, Nagasawa T, Abe T. Interstitial pneumonitis related to granulocyte colony-stimulating factor administration following chemotherapy for elderly patients with non-Hodgkin's lymphoma. *Intern Med* (1997) 36, 360–4.

Cyclophosphamide or Ifosfamide + Corticosteroids

There is limited and conflicting evidence on the effect of prednisone and prednisolone on the metabolic activation of cyclophosphamide. Synergistic increases in enzyme induction may occur with cyclophosphamide plus dexamethasone. Dexamethasone does not appear to alter ifosfamide metabolism.

Clinical evidence

(a) Dexamethasone

In an *in vitro* study it was noted that the combination of cyclophosphamide with dexamethasone resulted in a greater induction of the cytochrome P450 isoenzyme CYP3A4 than with cyclophosphamide alone—the extent of induction being dependent on baseline CYP3A4 activity.[1] In *rats*,[2] dexamethasone pretreatment increased the AUC of the inactive, neurotoxic, dechloroethylated metabolite of cyclophosphamide fourfold, and decreased the AUC of the active, hydroxylated metabolite by 60%. In an earlier study in patients on high-dose cyclophosphamide and dexamethasone for 2 days, total clearance of both cyclophosphamide and dexamethasone were higher on the second than the first day, with higher concentrations of cyclophosphamide metabolites.[3]

In *rats*, dexamethasone pretreatment had no net impact on the fraction of ifosfamide undergoing activation.[4] Similarly, in a clinical study, ifosfamide metabolism was no different when patients received dexamethasone 4 mg every 8 hours concurrently with ifosfamide for 3 days than when they received ifosfamide alone.[5]

(b) Prednisone or Prednisolone

In an early study, single doses of prednisone were shown to inhibit the metabolic activation of cyclophosphamide,[6,7] whereas another study briefly mentioned that massive single doses of prednisolone given just before cyclophosphamide did not inhibit cyclophosphamide metabolism.[8] Longer-term prednisone treatment (50 mg daily for 1 to 2 weeks) increased the rate of activation of cyclophosphamide in the first study.[6,7] Conversely, another study in 7 patients with systemic vasculitis given prednisone 1 mg/kg daily and cyclophosphamide 0.6 mg/m² intravenously every 3 weeks for 6 cycles found that, by the last cycle, the AUC of cyclophosphamide had significantly increased while that of its active metabolites had significantly decreased.[9]

Mechanism

Cyclophosphamide and ifosfamide are prodrugs that undergo hepatic metabolism to active and inactive/neurotoxic metabolites, and it appears they induce their own metabolism (see also 'Cyclophosphamide or Ifosfamide + Barbiturates', p.459). Corticosteroids are inducers of the cytochrome P450 isoenzymes CYP3A4. For cyclophosphamide, the CYP3A subfamily is thought to be principally involved in production of inactive/neurotoxic metabolites, whereas, for ifosfamide, CYP3A catalyses both the production of active and inactive/neurotoxic metabolites. On this basis, corticosteroids might be expected to decrease the efficacy and increase the neurotoxicity of cyclophosphamide (although this does not take account of autoinduction), whereas for ifosfamide they would not be expected to alter the balance between efficacy and toxicity.

Importance and management

The documentation is very limited. It appears that dexamethasone does not have any appreciable effect on the metabolism of ifosfamide. The information on cyclophosphamide is conflicting, and the clinical importance of any changes remains to be established. However, it should be noted that prednisone and prednisolone have a long established use as part of chemotherapy regimens including cyclophosphamide and are also often combined in various autoimmune diseases, and dexamethasone is widely used as an antiemetic with cancer chemotherapy.

1. Lindley C, Hamilton G, McCune JS, Faucette S, Shord SS, Hawke RL, Wang H, Gilbert D, Jolley S, Yan B, LeCluyse EL. The effect of cyclophosphamide with and without dexamethasone on cytochrome P450 3A4 and 2B6 in human hepatocytes. *Drug Metab Dispos* (2002) 30, 814–22.
2. Yu LJ, Drewes P, Gustafsson K, Brain EGC, Hecht JED, Waxman DJ. In vivo modulation of alternative pathways of P-450-catalyzed cyclophosphamide metabolism: impact on pharmacokinetics and antitumor activity. *J Pharmacol Exp Ther* (1999) 288, 928–37.
3. Moore MJ, Hardy RW, Thiessen JJ, Soldin SJ, Erlichman C. Rapid development of enhanced clearance after high-dose cyclophosphamide. *Clin Pharmacol Ther* (1988) 44, 622–8.
4. Brain EGC, Yu LJ, Gustafsson K, Drewes P, Waxman DJ. Modulation of P450-dependent ifosfamide pharmacokinetics: a better understanding of drug activation in vivo. *Br J Cancer* (1998) 77, 1768–76.
5. Singer JM, Hartley JM, Brennan C, Nicholson PW, Souhami RL. The pharmacokinetics and metabolism of ifosfamide during bolus and infusional administration: a randomized cross-over study. *Br J Cancer* (1998) 77, 978–84.
6. Faber OK, Mouridsen HT. Cyclophosphamide activation and corticosteroids. *N Engl J Med* (1974) 291, 211.
7. Faber OK, Mouridsen HT, Skovsted L. The biotransformation of cyclophosphamide in man: influence of prednisone. *Acta Pharmacol Toxicol (Copenh)* (1974) 35, 195–200.
8. Bagley CM, Bostick FW, DeVita VT. Clinical pharmacology of cyclophosphamide. *Cancer Res* (1973) 33, 226–33.
9. Belfayol-Pisanté L, Guillevin L, Tod M, Fauvelle F. Possible influence of prednisone on the pharmacokinetics of cyclophosphamide in systemic vasculitis. *Clin Drug Invest* (1999) 18, 225–31.

Cyclophosphamide + H_2-blockers

Ranitidine, and probably famotidine, appear not to increase the bone marrow toxicity of cyclophosphamide. *Animal* studies suggest that cimetidine might.

Clinical evidence, mechanism, importance and management

A study in 7 cancer patients found that although oral **ranitidine** 300 mg daily significantly prolonged the half-life and increased the AUC of intravenous cyclophosphamide 600 mg/m², it did not significantly affect the AUCs of the two major alkylating metabolites of cyclophosphamide, nor did it affect its bone marrow toxicity (leucopenia, granulocytopenia). The authors of the study conclude that **ranitidine** can safely be given with cyclophosphamide.[1] The same authors previously reported that **cimetidine**, when given with cyclophosphamide, increased the AUC of total alkylating metabolites of cyclophosphamide and resulted in greater toxicity to normal bone marrow, but increased survival of leukaemia-bearing *mice*.[2,3] Others have shown **cimetidine**, but not **famotidine**, to increase the toxicity of cyclophosphamide to normal bone marrow cells in *mice*.[4]

Cimetidine inhibits the cytochrome P450 isoenzyme CYP2C9, which has a minor role in the activation of cyclophosphamide (see 'Cyclophosphamide or Ifosfamide + Barbiturates', p.459). These results suggest that no special precautions are likely to be needed when **ranitidine** or **famotidine** are given with cyclophosphamide. The relevance of the findings with **cimetidine** are uncertain. **Cimetidine** has also increased the levels or toxicity of some other antineoplastics, see 'Nitrosoureas + Cimetidine', p.485, 'Anthracyclines; Epirubicin + Cimetidine', p.451, and 'Fluorouracil + H_2-blockers', p.469.

1. Alberts DS, Mason-Liddil N, Plezia PM, Roe DJ, Dorr RT, Struck RF, Phillips JG. Lack of ranitidine effects on cyclophosphamide bone marrow toxicity or metabolism: a placebo-controlled clinical trial. *J Natl Cancer Inst* (1991) 83, 1739–43.
2. Dorr RT, Alberts DS. Cimetidine enhancement of cyclophosphamide antitumour activity. *Br J Cancer* (1982) 45, 35–43.
3. Dorr RT, Soble MJ, Alberts DS. Interaction of cimetidine but not ranitidine with cyclophosphamide in mice. *Cancer Res* (1986) 46, 1795–9.
4. Lerza RA, Bogliolo GV, Mecoboni MP, Saviane AG, Pannacciulli IM. Effect of H2 antagonists cimetidine and famotidine on the hemotoxicity of cyclophosphamide. *Anticancer Res* (1988) 8, 1241–5.

Cyclophosphamide + Indometacin

A single case report describes acute water intoxication in a patient taking indometacin when given low-dose intravenous cyclophosphamide.

Clinical evidence, mechanism, importance and management

A patient with multiple myeloma on 50 mg indometacin 8-hourly, developed acute water intoxication and salt retention after being given a single bolus intravenous injection of cyclophosphamide 500 mg (less than 10 mg/kg). The reasons are not understood, but it is suggested that it was due to the additive or synergistic effects of the two drugs, since water intoxication had not been noted before with this low-dose of cyclophosphamide.[1] There do not appear to be any further reports/studies on this potential interaction but water intoxication has subsequently been reported with low-dose intravenous cyclophosphamide alone.[2] The evidence does not justify any special precautions when both drugs are used.

1. Webberley M J, Murray J A. Life-threatening acute hyponatraemia induced by low dose cyclophosphamide and indomethacin. *Postgrad Med J* (1989) 65, 950–2.
2. McCarron MO, Wright GD, Roberts SD. Water intoxication after low dose cyclophosphamide. *BMJ* (1995) 311, 292.

Cyclophosphamide + Metronidazole

A case report describes encephalopathy in a girl treated with cyclophosphamide and metronidazole.

Clinical evidence, mechanism, importance and management

After the fourth dose of pulse intravenous cyclophosphamide, a 9-year-old girl developed pancytopenia and gastrointestinal bleeding. She was then treated with metronidazole for presumptive *Clostridium difficile* colitis.

Within 6 hours she developed encephalopathy with seizures and visual hallucinations, requiring antipsychotic therapy. Metronidazole is thought to cause disulfiram-like reactions by inhibiting aldehyde dehydrogenase (see 'Alcohol + Metronidazole', p.58), and it was suggested that inhibition of this enzyme may cause accumulation of toxic metabolites of cyclophosphamide (see also 'Cyclophosphamide or Ifosfamide + Barbiturates', p.459).[1] This appears to be the only report of this potential interaction, and its general relevance is unclear. Further study is required.

1. Pinsk MN, Renton K, Crocker JFS, Acott PD. A proposed drug interaction leading to cyclophosphamide-induced encephalopathy. *Pediatr Res* (2002) 51, 437A.

Cyclophosphamide + Pentostatin

Acute and fatal cardiovascular collapse developed in two patients when pentostatin was added to high-dose cyclophosphamide treatment.

Clinical evidence, mechanism, importance and management

A clinical trial which was started to find out if pentostatin would improve the immunosuppressive effects of cyclophosphamide, carmustine and etoposide in bone marrow transplant patients was stopped when acute and fatal cardiovascular collapse developed in the first 2 patients. Both patients had been started on cyclophosphamide 800 mg/m^2 and etoposide 200 mg/m^2, both 12-hourly for 8 doses, and carmustine (BCNU) 112 mg/m^2 daily for 4 doses. On day 3 pentostatin 4 mg/m^2, given over 4 hours, was added. Within 8 to 18 hours after completion of chemotherapy both patients developed confusion, hypothermia, hypotension, respiratory distress, pulmonary oedema, and eventually fatal ventricular fibrillation within 45 to 120 min of the first symptoms. A later study in *rats* similarly found that pentostatin markedly increased the acute toxicity of cyclophosphamide. The reasons for this cardiotoxicity are not understood. Neither of the 2 patients had previously shown any evidence of cardiac abnormalities.[1] Other reports suggest that combining alkylating agents such as cyclophosphamide with nucleoside analogues such as pentostatin is still being investigated.[2,3]

Caution is required when the drugs are combined. More study is needed.

1. Gryn J, Gordon R, Bapat A, Goldman N, Goldberg J. Pentostatin increases the acute toxicity of high dose cyclophosphamide. *Bone Marrow Transplant* (1993) 12, 217–20.
2. Goodman M. Pentostatin (Nipent) and high-dose cyclophosphamide for the treatment of refractory autoimmune disorders. *Semin Oncol* (2000) 27 (Suppl 5), 67–71.
3. Weiss MA. A phase I and II study of pentostatin (Nipent) with cyclophosphamide for previously treated patients with chronic lymphocytic leukemia. *Semin Oncol* (2000) 27 (Suppl 5), 41–3.

Cyclophosphamide or Ifosfamide + Phenytoin

Phenytoin increases the metabolism of cyclophosphamide and ifosfamide, but the clinical relevance of this is uncertain. Both unchanged and increased efficacy have been suggested.

Clinical evidence

A child on phenytoin given ifosfamide and etoposide had a neurotoxic reaction. The plasma levels of the dechloroethylated metabolites of ifosfamide were subsequently found to be markedly altered compared with those previously seen in 14 other children receiving the same chemotherapy but not on phenytoin. The child recovered uneventfully after 3 days, and achieved clinical remission (she had not responded to first-line chemotherapy).[1] In a subsequent study, the use of prophylactic phenytoin increased the formation of *S*-dechloroethylated cyclophosphamide in 3 patients receiving cyclophosphamide and busulfan.[2] In yet another study, the ratio of the AUC of active hydroxycyclophosphamide to cyclophosphamide was higher in patients receiving phenytoin and busulfan than in those receiving irradiation.[3] It is likely that phenytoin was responsible for this effect since busulfan alone decreases cyclophosphamide metabolism (see 'Cyclophosphamide + Busulfan', p.460). In an earlier study, in patients receiving enzyme-inducing drugs (2 of whom received phenytoin), the peak plasma levels of alkylating metabolites were higher, but declined more rapidly, so that overall exposure was not different from those not on these drugs.[4] Another study reported that a patient on phenytoin had a high clearance rate for cyclophosphamide during her first chemotherapy course, and that autoinduction of cyclophosphamide clearance was not apparent during her second course.[5]

Mechanism

The alteration in the pattern of ifosfamide metabolites suggested that phenytoin had induced the activity of the cytochrome P450 isoenzyme CYP2B6, and to a lesser extent CYP3A4.[1] The pattern of increase in cyclophosphamide clearance is also consistent with induction of CYP2B and CYP3A.[2] See also 'Cyclophosphamide or Ifosfamide + Barbiturates', p.459.

Importance and management

That phenytoin alters the metabolism of cyclophosphamide and ifosfamide is not surprising, but the clinical importance of any changes remains to be established. The authors of the early study concluded that phenytoin was unlikely to have much effect on the antitumour and toxic effects of cyclophosphamide.[4] Conversely, the authors of the recent studies suggest that phenytoin may increase the therapeutic efficacy of cyclophosphamide and ifosfamide.[1,2] Further study is needed.

Note that reduced phenytoin levels and seizures have been reported in a patient on chemotherapy including cyclophosphamide, see 'Table 11.2', (p.331).

1. Ducharme MP, Bernstein ML, Granvil CP, Gehrcke B, Wainer IW. Phenytoin-induced alteration in the *N*-dechloroethylation of ifosfamide stereoisomers. *Cancer Chemother Pharmacol* (1997) 40, 531–3.
2. Williams ML, Wainer IW, Embree L, Barnett M, Granvil CL, Ducharme MP. Enantioselective induction of cyclophosphamide metabolism by phenytoin. *Chirality* (1999) 11, 569–74.
3. Slattery JT, Kalhorn TF, McDonald GB, Lambert K, Buckner CD, Bensinger WI, Anasetti C, Appelbaum FR. Conditioning regimen-dependent disposition of cyclophosphamide and hydroxycyclophosphamide in human marrow transplantation patients. *J Clin Oncol* (1996) 14, 1484–94.
4. Bagley CM, Bostick FW, DeVita VT. Clinical pharmacology of cyclophosphamide. *Cancer Res* (1973) 33, 226–33.
5. Chen T-L, Passos-Coelho JL, Noe DA, Kennedy MJ, Black KC, Colvin M, Grochow LB. Nonlinear pharmacokinetics of cyclophosphamide in patients with metastatic breast cancer receiving high-dose chemotherapy followed by autologous bone marrow transplantation. *Cancer Res* (1995) 55, 810–16. Erratum *ibid.*, 1600.

Cyclophosphamide or Ifosfamide + Rifampicin (Rifampin)

Rifampicin induced the metabolism of cyclophosphamide and ifosfamide. For ifosfamide, this did not improve the ratio of active to inactive/toxic metabolites, and the possibility remains that efficacy could be reduced.

Clinical evidence, mechanism, importance and management

In a clinical study, rifampicin increased the clearance of ifosfamide by about 100%. In this study, patients were given rifampicin 300 mg twice daily for 3 days before ifosfamide treatment and for 3 days concurrently for one cycle, then for another they were given the ifosfamide alone. The fraction of ifosfamide metabolised to the inactive, neurotoxic, dechloroethylated metabolite was increased, but elimination of this metabolite was also increased resulting in reduced exposure. The fraction metabolised to the active, hydroxylated metabolite, and its exposure, were not altered appreciably.[1]

An *in vitro* study in human liver cells showed that rifampicin was a potent inducer of the activation (hydroxylation) of cyclophosphamide and ifosfamide.[2]

Rifampicin is an inducer of the cytochrome P450 isoenzymes CYP3A4 and CYP2B6, which are involved in the metabolism of cyclophosphamide and ifosfamide (see also 'Cyclophosphamide or Ifosfamide + Barbiturates', p.459). In the clinical study cited,[1] rifampicin did not have a positive effect on the proportion of ifosfamide undergoing activation. In addition, since rifampicin increased metabolism overall, there is the possibility of decreased efficacy,[1] although this remains to be shown.

1. Kerbusch T, Jansen RLH, Mathôt RAA, Huitema ADR, Jansen M, van Rijswijk REN, Beijnen JH. Modulation of the cytochrome P450–mediated metabolism of ifosfamide by ketoconazole and rifampin. *Clin Pharmacol Ther* (2001) 70, 132–41.
2. Chang TKH, Yu L, Maurel P, Waxman DJ. Enhanced cyclophosphamide and ifosfamide activation in primary human hepatocyte cultures: response to cytochrome P-450 inducers and autoinduction by oxazaphosphorines. *Cancer Res* (1997) 57, 1946–54.

Cyclophosphamide + Sulfonamides

Some very limited evidence suggests that sulfaphenazole may modestly inhibit the metabolism of cyclophosphamide to its active metabolite, but the clinical importance of this is uncertain.

Clinical evidence, mechanism, importance and management

A study in 7 patients on a 50-mg dose of cyclophosphamide given **sulfaphenazole** 1 g twice daily for 9 to 14 days showed that the half-life of cyclophosphamide was unchanged in 3 patients, longer in 2 and shorter in the remaining 2 patients.[1] **Sulfaphenazole** and **sulfamethoxazole** are inhibitors of the cytochrome P450 isoenzyme CYP2C9, which shows genetic polymorphism (i.e. some people produce very little, while others produce larger quantities). This enzyme has a minor role in the metabolism (and therefore activation) of cyclophosphamide, and the extent of its involvement varies between patients. For example, and *in vitro* study showed that **sulfaphenazole** inhibited cyclophosphamide activation by 17 to 27% in one human liver sample, but insignificant inhibition occurred in two others.[2] Thus, sulfonamides such as **sulfaphenazole** and **sulfamethoxazole** may moderately inhibit the activation of cyclophosphamide in some patients, but the clinical relevance of this is uncertain. Note that **co-trimoxazole** is sometimes used for prophylaxis of infection in patients receiving chemotherapy. One study showed that this use did not *increase* the myelotoxicity of CAE (cyclophosphamide, doxorubicin, and etoposide).[3]

1. Faber OK, Mouridsen HT, Skovsted L. The effect of chloramphenicol and sulphaphenazole on the biotransformation of cyclophosphamide in man. *Br J Clin Pharmacol* (1975) 2, 281–5.
2. Roy P, Yu LJ, Crespi CL, Waxman DJ. Development of a substrate-activity based approach to identify the major human liver P-450 catalysts of cyclophosphamide and ifosfamide activation based on cDNA-expressed activities and liver microsomal P-450 profiles. *Drug Metab Dispos* (1999) 27, 655–66.
3. de Jongh CA, Wade JC, Finley RS, Joshi JH, Aisner J, Wiernik PH, Schimpff SC. Trimethoprim/sulfamethoxazole versus placebo: a double-blind comparison of infection prophylaxis in patients with small cell carcinoma of the lung. *J Clin Oncol* (1983) 1, 302–7.

Cyclophosphamide or Ifosfamide + Taxanes

The clearance of ifosfamide is higher when it is administered after docetaxel. This results in less toxicity, but the effect on efficacy is unknown. Ifosfamide did not alter the pharmacokinetics of docetaxel. The sequence of ifosfamide followed by paclitaxel was antagonistic *in vitro*.

Clinical evidence, mechanism, importance and management

(a) Docetaxel

The AUC of ifosfamide and of its metabolites were lower when ifosfamide was given immediately after docetaxel than when it was administered 24 hours before docetaxel, due to increased clearance. Docetaxel pharmacokinetics were unaltered by ifosfamide.[1] This supports the evidence that the maximum tolerated dose is greater when ifosfamide is administered after docetaxel.[2] The mechanism is unknown, but it has been suggested[3] that docetaxel may competitively inhibit the activation of ifosfamide by the cytochrome P450 isoenzyme CYP3A4. These results show that the toxicity, and possibly efficacy, of the combination are schedule dependent. More study is needed. Cyclophosphamide does not appear to alter docetaxel pharmacokinetics. For full details see also 'Taxanes + Cyclophosphamide', p.490.

(b) Paclitaxel

In vitro studies in human liver microsomes found that additive or synergistic cytotoxicity occurred when activated ifosfamide (hydroxyifosfamide) and paclitaxel were used together or when paclitaxel was used first followed by hydroxyifosfamide. In contrast pronounced antagonism was seen when hydroxyifosfamide was used before paclitaxel.[4] The mechanism is unknown. These results suggest that the scheduling of this combination may be important for efficacy. More study is needed. There is some evidence that toxicity associated with combinations of paclitaxel and cyclophosphamide is sequence-dependent. For full details see also 'Taxanes + Cyclophosphamide', p.490.

1. Schrijvers D, Pronk L, Highley M, Bruno R, Locci-Tonelli D, De Bruijn E, Van Oosterom AT, Verweij J. Pharmacokinetics of ifosfamide are changed by combination with docetaxel. *Am J Clin Oncol* (2000) 23, 358–63.
2. Pronk L, Schrijvers D, Schellens JHM, De Bruijn EA, Planting ASTh, Locci-Tonelli D, Groult V, Verweij J, Van Oosterom AT. Phase I study on docetaxel and ifosfamide in patients with advanced solid tumours. *Br J Cancer* (1998) 77, 153–8.
3. Ando Y. Possible metabolic interaction between docetaxel and ifosfamide. *Br J Cancer* (2000) 82, 497.
4. Vanhoefer U, Schleucher N, Klaassen U, Seeber S, Harstrick A. Ifosfamide-based drug combinations: preclinical evaluation of drug interactions and translation into the clinic. *Semin Oncol* (2000) 27 (Suppl 1), 8–13.

Cyclophosphamide + Thiotepa

Pretreatment with thiotepa may inhibit the metabolism of cyclophosphamide to its active metabolite and decrease both its efficacy and toxicity. Cyclophosphamide appears not to affect the metabolism of thiotepa.

Clinical evidence, mechanism, importance and management

(a) Effect on cyclophosphamide

The proportion of cyclophosphamide excreted unchanged in the urine (i.e. never metabolically activated) was found to be higher when cyclophosphamide was given as a 96-hour infusion with thiotepa and novobiocin than when administered alone. The authors suggested that the possibility that thiotepa inhibited the metabolism of cyclophosphamide should be investigated.[1] Later, other authors observed that the concentration of the active metabolite of cyclophosphamide, 4-hydroxycyclophosphamide, decreased sharply after thiotepa was given to 20 patients.[2] In a study to investigate this effect further, 3 patients were given high-dose cyclophosphamide 1000 or 1500 mg/m^2 as a 1-hour infusion, followed by carboplatin and thiotepa for 4 days. The order of infusion was reversed on one treatment day in each of 4 courses. Administration of thiotepa 1 hour before cyclophosphamide resulted in decreases in the peak plasma levels and AUC of 4-hydroxycyclophosphamide of 62% and 26% respectively, when compared with those when thiotepa was administered 1 hour after cyclophosphamide.[2] In human microsomes, thiotepa was found to inhibit the conversion of cyclophosphamide to hydroxycyclophosphamide.[2] These results suggest that thiotepa can decrease both the efficacy and toxicity of cyclophosphamide, and that the order of administration may be of critical importance. The authors question the practice of simultaneous infusion of cyclophosphamide and thiotepa.[2]

(b) Effect on thiotepa

In an *in vitro* study using human microsomes, cyclophosphamide had no effect on the metabolism of thiotepa to tepa by cytochrome P450 at therapeutic concentrations.[2,3]

1. Chen T-L, Passos-Coelho JL, Noe DA, Kennedy MJ, Black KC, Colvin M, Grochow LB. Nonlinear pharmacokinetics of cyclophosphamide in patients with metastatic breast cancer receiving high-dose chemotherapy followed by autologous bone marrow transplantation. *Cancer Res* (1995) 55, 810–16. Erratum ibid.,1600.
2. Huitema ADR, Kerbusch T, Tibben MM, Rodenhuis S, Beijnen JH. Reduction of cyclophosphamide bioactivation by thioTEPA: critical sequence-dependency in high-dose chemotherapy regimens. *Cancer Chemother Pharmacol* (2000) 46, 119–27.
3. Van Maanen MJ, Huitema ADR, Beijnen JH. Influence of co-medicated drugs on the biotransformation of thioTEPA to TEPA and thioTEPA-mercapturate. *Anticancer Res* (2000) 20, 1711–16.

Estramustine + Clodronate

Clodronate markedly increases serum levels of estramustine.

Clinical evidence, mechanism, importance and management

Estramustine bioavailability in 12 patients was increased by about 80% when clodronate 800 mg four times daily was given with estramustine 280 mg twice daily for 5 days. Clodronate serum levels and AUC were not changed by estramustine.[1] Documentation appears to be limited to this study. However, the efficacy and toxicity of estramustine should be monitored if clodronate is required concurrently. The effects of other bisphosphonates do not appear to have been studied.

1. Kylmälä T, Castrén-Kortekangas P, Seppänen J, Ylitalo P, Tammela TLJ. Effect of concomitant administration of clodronate and estramustine phosphate on their bioavailability in patients with metastasized prostate cancer. *Pharmacol Toxicol* (1996) 79, 157–60.

Estramustine + Food or Milk

The absorption of estramustine is reduced by milk and foods containing calcium.

Clinical evidence

A randomised three-way crossover study in 6 patients with prostate cancer showed that the absorption of single-doses of estramustine disodium (equivalent to 140 mg of estramustine) was reduced by 59% when taken with 200 ml of **milk**, and by 33% when taken with a standardised **breakfast** (2 pieces of white bread with margarine, ham, tomato, marmalade and water). Peak serum estramustine levels were reduced by 68 and 43% respectively.[1]

Mechanism

In vitro studies suggest that estramustine combines with calcium ions in milk and food to form a poorly-soluble complex that is not as well absorbed as the parent compound.[1]

Importance and management

An established interaction although the information is limited. The makers recommend that estramustine should be taken not less than 1 hour before or 2 hours after meals, and that it should not be taken with milk or milk products or calcium-rich foods.[2,3] If the suggested mechanism of interaction is correct, estramustine should also not be taken at the same time as **calcium-containing drugs** (e.g. some **antacids**).

1. Gunnarsson P O, Davidsson T, Andersson S-B, Backman C, Johansson S-Å. Impairment of estramustine phosphate absorption by concurrent intake of milk and food. *Eur J Clin Pharmacol* (1990) 38, 189–93.
2. Estracyt (Estramustine). Pharmacia Ltd. UK Summary of product characteristics, August 2003.
3. Emcyt (Estramustine). Pharmacia. US Prescribing information, March 2003.

Etoposide + Anticonvulsants

Etoposide clearance appears to be increased by phenobarbital or phenytoin, and this may result in reduced efficacy.

Clinical evidence, mechanism, importance and management

The clearance of etoposide was found to be highly variable in children given doses of 320 to 500 mg/m^2 over 6 hours on alternate days for a total of 3 doses. However, it was 77% higher in 7 children taking anticonvulsants (**phenobarbital**, **phenytoin** or both) than in 22 others not taking anticonvulsants.[1] In a retrospective survey, long-term anticonvulsant therapy (**phenytoin**, **phenobarbital**, **carbamazepine**, or a combination) was associated with worse event-free survival, and greater haematological and/or CNS relapse in children receiving chemotherapy for B-lineage acute lymphoblastic leukaemia. The authors considered that the increased clearance of etoposide induced by the anticonvulsants was a likely factor in these findings.[2] Be alert for the possible need to give larger doses of etoposide if these anticonvulsants are used. More study is needed.

1. Rodman JH, Murry DJ, Madden T, Santana VM. Altered etoposide pharmacokinetics and time to engraftment in pediatric patients undergoing autologous bone marrow transplantation. *J Clin Oncol* (1994) 12, 2390–7.
2. Relling MV, Pui C-H, Sandlund JT, Rivera GK, Hancock ML, Boyett JM, Schuetz EG, Evans WE. Adverse effect of anticonvulsants on efficacy of chemotherapy for acute lymphoblastic leukaemia. *Lancet* (2000) 356, 285–90.

Etoposide + Atovaquone

Concurrent use of atovaquone with etoposide may modestly increase exposure to etoposide catechol. The clinical relevance of this is unclear.

Clinical evidence, mechanism, importance and management

A study in 9 children with acute lymphoblastic leukaemia or non-Hodgkin's lymphoma found that the AUC of etoposide and its metabolite etoposide catechol were slightly increased by 8.6% and 28.4% respectively following atovaquone 45 mg/kg daily as compared with co-trimoxazole 150/750 mg/m^2 daily. The mechanism is unclear, but atovaquone may affect the metabolism of etoposide by cytochrome P450 isoenzyme CYP3A4 or its transport by P-glycoprotein.[1] The authors considered that an interaction with co-trimoxazole was unlikely, so used it as a control, however, ideally this requires confirmation. The relevance of the minor changes seen is unclear. However, the authors note that the risk of etoposide-related secondary acute myeloid leukaemia has been linked to minor changes in therapy, therefore, they advise caution if atovaquone is administered with etoposide, particularly if used with other substrates of CYP3A4 or P-glycoprotein.[1] They also say it may be possible to avoid the interaction by separating the administration by 1 to 2 days,[1] but this requires confirmation.

1. van de Poll MEC, Relling MV, Schuetz EG, Harrison PL, Hughes W, Flynn PM. The effect of atovaquone on etoposide pharmacokinetics in children with acute lymphoblastic leukemia. *Cancer Chemother Pharmacol* (2001),47, 467–72.

Etoposide + Carboplatin or Cisplatin

The clearance of etoposide may be modestly reduced by carboplatin and cisplatin, but this is probably unlikely to be clinically relevant.

Clinical evidence, mechanism, importance and management

(a) Carboplatin

In one study in 4 patients, the pharmacokinetics of etoposide did not differ when given alone or with carboplatin.[1] However, in another study of 14 young patients receiving etoposide and carboplatin the clearance of etoposide was lower than in previous reports in adults and children. They had been given an escalating dosage regimen starting with etoposide 960 mg/m^2, and increasing to 1200, and 1500 mg/m^2 given in three divided doses on alternate days, with carboplatin 400 to 700 mg/m^2 given on the other days, followed by autologous marrow rescue. The authors point out that the dose and the timing of carboplatin may be important determinants for any interaction.[2] In yet another study,[3] carboplatin did not affect the pharmacokinetics of etoposide during the first cycle of chemotherapy (etoposide was administered on days 1, 2 and 3, and carboplatin on day 2, and the AUC of etoposide was compared for days 1 and 2). However, during a second cycle of chemotherapy, the etoposide AUC was 8% higher on day 2 than day 1. These changes were considered unlikely to be clinically important.[3]

(b) Cisplatin

A study in 17 children with neuroblastoma found that when cisplatin 90 mg/m^2 intravenously was given immediately before etoposide, the clearance of etoposide 780 mg/m^2 fell by 20% and the serum levels rose. But after a cumulative dose of cisplatin of 360 mg/m^2 it had no effect on the clearance of etoposide.[4] In another study, cisplatin did not affect the pharmacokinetics of etoposide during the first cycle of chemotherapy (etoposide was administered on days 1, 2 and 3, and cisplatin on day 2, and the AUC of etoposide was compared for days 1 and 2). However, during a second cycle of chemotherapy, the etoposide AUC was 28% higher on day 3 than day 1. These changes were considered unlikely to be clinically important.[3]

1. Newell DR, Eeles RA, Gumbrell LA, Boxall FE, Horwich A, Calvert AH. Carboplatin and etoposide pharmacokinetics in patients with testicular teratoma. *Cancer Chemother Pharmacol* (1989) 23, 376–72.
2. Rodman JH, Murry DJ, Madden T, Santana VM. Altered etoposide pharmacokinetics and time to engraftment in pediatric patients undergoing autologous bone marrow transplantation. *J Clin Oncol* (1994) 12, 2390–7.
3. Thomas HD, Porter DJ, Bartelink I, Nobbs JR, Cole M, Elliott S, Newell DR, Calvert AH, Highley M, Boddy AV. Randomized cross-over clinical trial to study potential pharmacokinetics interactions between cisplatin or carboplatin and etoposide. *Br J Clin Pharmacol* (2002) 53, 83–91.
4. Relling MV, McLeod HL, Bowman LC, Santana VM. Etoposide pharmacokinetics and pharmacodynamics after acute and chronic exposure to cisplatin. *Clin Pharmacol Ther* (1994) 56, 503–11.

Etoposide + Ciclosporin

High-dose ciclosporin markedly raises etoposide serum levels and increases the suppression of white blood cell production. Severe toxicity has been reported in one patient.

Clinical evidence

In a comparative study 16 patients with multidrug resistant advanced cancer were given 20 paired courses of etoposide alone or with ciclosporin. Ciclosporin levels were measured at the end of a 2-hour infusion; ciclosporin levels of greater than 2000 nanograms/ml were defined as high-dose and those less than 2000 nanograms/ml as low-dose. High and low-dose ciclosporin increased the etoposide AUC by 80% and 50% respectively, decreased the total clearance by 38% and 28%, increased its half-life by 108 and 40%, reduced the leucocyte count nadir by 64% and 37% and altered the volume of distribution at steady state by 46% and 1.4%.[1] The patients were given 150 to 200 mg/m^2 of etoposide daily as a 2-hour intravenous infusion for 3 consecutive days and ciclosporin in doses ranging from 5 to 21 mg/kg daily as a 3-day continuous infusion.[1] In another study, the pharmacokinetics of etoposide 100 mg/m^2 daily were compared with etoposide 60 mg/m^2 (a 40% reduction in dose) plus high-dose ciclosporin in children. Despite the dose reduction, recipients of ciclosporin had a 71% reduction in etoposide clearance and a 47% increase in etoposide AUC, although toxicity was similar.[2]

The leukaemic cells in the bone marrow of a patient with acute T-lymphocyte leukaemia were totally cleared with ciclosporin 8.3 mg/kg orally twice daily and etoposide 100 to 300 mg daily for 2 to 5 days, but the adverse effects were severe (mental confusion, renal and hepatic toxicity). The patient died from respiratory failure precipitated by a chest infection.[3]

Mechanism

It is suggested that the ciclosporin decreases the metabolism of the etoposide by inhibiting its cytochrome P450 mediated metabolism[4] and inhibiting P-glycoprotein mediated efflux from the hepatocyte, as well as inhibiting some unknown non-renal clearance mechanism.[1] The total effect is to cause the retention of etoposide in the body, thereby increasing its effects.

Importance and management

An established interaction. Ciclosporin alters the pharmacokinetics of etoposide resulting in increased serum levels. This pharmacokinetic interaction has complicated the study of the value of using ciclosporin to modulate multidrug resistance in tumours to improve the response to chemotherapy. In the case of 'anthracyclines', (p.449) and etoposide, any benefit could just be attributed to dose intensification. Consequently, some have suggested reducing the dose of etoposide by 40% or 50%.[1,2] The use of high-dose ciclosporin for multidrug resistant tumour modulation remains experimental and should only be undertaken in clinical trials. Concurrent use should be very well monitored. More study is needed to find out the possible effects of low-dose ciclosporin.

1. Lum BL, Kaubisch S, Yahanda AM, Adler KM, Jew L, Ehsan MN, Brophy NA, Halsey J, Gosland MP, Sikic BI. Alteration of etoposide pharmacokinetics and pharmacodynamics by cyclosporine in a phase I trial to modulate multidrug resistance. *J Clin Oncol* (1992) 10, 1635–42.
2. Lacayo NJ, Lum BL, Becton DL, Weinstein H, Ravindranath Y, Chang MN, Bomgaars L, Lauer SJ, Sikic BI. Pharmacokinetic interactions of cyclosporine with etoposide and mitoxantrone in children with acute myeloid leukemia. *Leukemia* (2002) 16, 920–7.
3. Kloke O, Osieka R. Interaction of cyclosporin A with antineoplastic agents. *Klin Wochenschr* (1985) 63, 1081–2.
4. Kawashiro T, Yamashita K, Zhao X-J, Koyama E, Tani M, Chiba K, Ishizaki T. A study on the metabolism of etoposide and possible interaction with antitumor or supporting agents by human liver microsomes. *J Pharmacol Exp Ther* (1998) 386, 1294–1300.

Etoposide + CYP3A4 enzyme inhibitors

***In vitro* studies show that some inhibitors of the cytochrome P450 isoenzyme CYP3A4 may possibly increase the effects and toxicity of etoposide.**

Clinical evidence, mechanism, importance and management

In vitro studies using human liver microsomes show that **ketoconazole**, **prednisolone**, **troleandomycin**, **verapamil** and **vincristine** can inhibit the metabolism (3′-demethylation) of etoposide by cytochrome P450 isoenzyme CYP3A4. The implications of this are that concurrent use with these drugs might increase both the efficacy and the toxicity of etoposide.[1] There seems as yet to be no clinical confirmation that these potential interactions have clinical relevance, but good monitoring would be a prudent precaution.

1. Kawashiro T, Yamashita K, Zhao X-J, Koyama E, Tani M, Chiba K, Ishizaki T. A study on the metabolism of etoposide and possible interactions with antitumor or supporting agents by human liver microsomes. *J Pharmacol Exp Ther* (1998) 386, 1294–1300.

Etoposide + Food

The pharmacokinetics of etoposide in 8 patients with extensive small cell lung carcinoma given 100-mg oral doses were unaffected when taken with a full breakfast compared with the fasting state.[1]

1. Harvey VJ, Slevin ML, Joel SP, Johnston A, Wrigley PFM. The effect of food and concurrent chemotherapy on the bioavailability of oral etoposide. *Br J Cancer* (1985) 52, 363–7.

Etoposide + Other antineoplastics

Doxorubicin and cyclophosphamide have no clinically relevant effects on the pharmacokinetics of oral or intravenous etoposide. Methotrexate and procarbazine do not affect the pharmacokinetics of oral etoposide.

Clinical evidence, mechanism, importance and management

A pharmacokinetic study in 7 patients with small-cell lung cancer (SCLC) treated with **cyclophosphamide** 800 mg/m^2, **doxorubicin** 40 mg/m^2 and etoposide 100 mg/m^2 (all administered intravenously) found that the protein binding, metabolism and renal clearance of etoposide were unaffected by the other antineoplastics.[1] Similarly, another study found only modest changes in the pharmacokinetics of intravenous etoposide when given with **cyclophosphamide** and **doxorubicin** compared with use alone, and these were considered unlikely to be clinically relevant. Specifically, the AUC of etoposide was 9% higher and the clearance was 10% lower on day 1 of the CAE cycle (**cyclophosphamide**, **doxorubicin**, and etoposide) compared with days 2 and 3 (etoposide alone).[2] This is a commonly used regimen, and these data suggest there is no pharmacokinetic interaction.

Similarly, no changes in etoposide pharmacokinetics were seen when etoposide 100 mg was given orally immediately after oral **cyclophosphamide** 100 mg/m^2 and **methotrexate** 12.5 mg/m^2 in 8 patients with SCLC. In addition, no changes were seen when the same dose of oral etoposide was given 15 minutes after intravenous **doxorubicin** 35 mg/m^2 and oral **procarbazine** 60 mg/m.[2,3] Oral etoposide pharmacokinetics appear not to be affected by these concurrent antineoplastics.

For the lack of effect of platinum derivatives, see 'Etoposide + Carboplatin or Cisplatin', p.465.

1. Van Hoogenhuijze J, Lankelma J, Stam J, Pinedo HM. Unchanged pharmacokinetics of VP-16-213 (etoposide, NSC 141540) during concomitant administration of doxorubicin and cyclophosphamide. *Eur J Cancer Clin Oncol* (1987) 23, 807–11.
2. Busse D, Würthwein G, Hinske C, Hempel G, Fromm MF, Eichelbaum M, Kroemer HK, Busch FW. Pharmacokinetics of intravenous etoposide in patients with breast cancer: influence of dose escalation and cyclophosphamide and doxorubicin coadministration. *Naunyn Schmiedebergs Arch Pharmacol* (2002) 366, 218–25.
3. Harvey VJ, Slevin ML, Joel SP, Johnston A, Wrigley PFM. The effect of food and concurrent chemotherapy on the bioavailability of oral etoposide. *Br J Cancer* (1985) 52, 363–7.

Etoposide + St John's wort *(Hypericum perforatum)*

***In vitro* studies suggest that hypericin, a component of St John's wort may antagonise the effects of etoposide. It may also stimulate the hepatic metabolism of etoposide by the cytochrome P450 isoenzyme CYP3A4. Information is very limited but it seems that it would be prudent to avoid St John's wort in patients taking etoposide or related drugs.[1] More study is needed.**

1. Peebles KA, Baker RK, Kurz EU, Schneider BJ, Kroll DJ. Catalytic inhibition of human DNA topoisomerase IIα by hypericin, a naphthodianthrone from St. John's wort (*Hypericum perforatum*). *Biochem Pharmacol* (2001) 62, 1059–70.

Exemestane + CYP3A4 enzyme inducers and inhibitors

Ketoconazole appears not to interact with exemestane, whereas rifampicin reduces exemestane levels.

Clinical importance, mechanism, importance and management

The makers say that *in vitro* evidence shows that while exemestane is metabolised by both the cytochrome P450 isoenzyme CYP3A4 and aldoketoreductases, a clinical study found that **ketoconazole** (a specific inhibitor of CYP3A4) had no significant effects on the pharmacokinetics of exemestane. The makers therefore suggest that interactions with CYP3A4 enzyme inhibitors are unlikely.[1,2]

However, in an interaction study the potent enzyme inducer **rifampicin** reduced the AUC and maximum serum levels of exemestane by 54 and 41% respectively.

The makers therefore caution the use of exemestane with CYP3A4 inducers such as **carbamazepine**, **phenytoin** and **St John's wort**.[1,2] The clinical relevance of these potential interactions is unknown, but it would seem prudent to monitor the outcome of concurrent use to ensure exemestane efficacy.

1. Aromasin (Exemestane). Pharmacia Ltd. UK Summary of product characteristics, February 2003.
2. Aromasin (Exemestane). Pharmacia & Upjohn Company. US Prescribing information, March 2004.

Fludarabine + Dipyridamole

Dipyridamole may reduce the efficacy of fludarabine.

Clinical evidence, mechanism, importance and management

Because fludarabine phosphate is an analogue of adenine, the UK makers warn that drugs that are adenosine uptake inhibitors such as dipyridamole may prevent the uptake of fludarabine into cells and reduce its efficacy.[1,2] Dipyridamole should probably therefore be avoided in patients receiving fludarabine.

1. Schering Health Care Ltd. Personal communication, February 1995.
2. Fludara (Fludarabine). Schering Health Care Ltd. UK Summary of product characteristics, January 2003.

Fludarabine + Pentostatin

Fludarabine given with pentostatin can cause fatal pulmonary toxicity.

Clinical evidence, mechanism, importance and management

When fludarabine phosphate and pentostatin were used in the treatment of chronic lymphoid leukaemia, 4 out of 6 patients developed pulmonary toxicity consistent with interstitial pneumonitis, and 3 of them died.[1] Pentostatin should therefore not be used concurrently with fludarabine.[2,3]

1. Schering Health Care Ltd. Personal communication, February 1995.
2. Fludara (Fludarabine). Schering Health Care Ltd. UK Summary of product characteristics, January 2003.
3. Fludara (Fludarabine). Berlex. US Prescribing information, October 2003.

Fluorouracil + Allopurinol

Allopurinol has been studied as a modulator of the effects of fluorouracil, but has not gained an established clinical use in this setting.

Clinical evidence, mechanism, importance and management

Some early studies showed that allopurinol 300 mg two to four times daily allowed the usual maximum tolerated dose of fluorouracil to be increased by up to twofold.[1-3] The hope was that allopurinol would prove useful to decrease the toxicity and/or improve the activity of fluorouracil. However, most studies have shown no increase in response rates in colorectal cancer with allopurinol,[4,5] even when the fluorouracil dose was escalated,[2,4] and some have also shown no reduction in toxicity.[5-7] These are by no means all the studies, and are just cited as examples. Allopurinol mouthwash has also been investigated to reduce the incidence of stomatitis with fluorouracil. Some controlled studies have shown a benefit,[8] whereas others have not.[9] Allopurinol clearly modulates some of the effects of fluorouracil; however, this has not been shown to be obviously beneficial or harmful in the clinical setting.

1. Howell SB, Wung WE, Taetle R, Hussain F, Romine JS. Modulation of 5-fluorouracil toxicity by allopurinol in man. *Cancer* (1981) 48, 1281–9.
2. Fox RM, Woods RL, Tattersall MHN, Piper AA, Sampson D. Allopurinol modulation of fluorouracil toxicity. *Cancer Chemother Pharmacol* (1981) 5, 151–5.
3. Woolley PV, Ayoob MJ, Smith FP, Lokey JL, DeGreen P, Marantz A, Schein PS. A controlled trial of the effect of 4-hydroxypyrazolopyrimidine (allopurinol) on the toxicity of a single bolus dose of 5-fluorouracil. *J Clin Oncol* (1985) 3, 103–9.
4. Tsavaris N, Bacoyannis C, Milonakis N, Sarafidou M, Zamanis N, Magoulas D, Kosmidis P. Folinic acid plus high-dose 5-fluorouracil with allopurinol protection in the treatment of advanced colorectal carcinoma. *Eur J Cancer* (1990) 26, 1054–6.
5. Merimsky O, Inbar M, Chaitchik S. Treatment of advanced colorectal cancer by 5-fluorouracil–leucovorin combination with or without allopurinol: a prospective randomized study. *Anticancer Drugs* (1991) 2, 447–51.
6. Howell SB, Pfeifle CE, Wung WE. Effect of allopurinol on the toxicity of high-dose 5-fluorouracil administered by intermittent bolus injection. *Cancer* (1983) 51, 220–5.
7. Garewal H, Ahmann FR. Failure of allopurinol to provide clinically significant protection against the hematologic toxicity of a bolus 5-FU schedule. *Oncology* (1986) 43, 216–18.
8. Porta C, Moroni M, Nastasi G. Allopurinol mouthwashes in the treatment of 5-fluorouracil-induced stomatitis. *Am J Clin Oncol* (1994) 17, 246–7.
9. Loprinzi CL, Cianflone SG, Dose AM, Etzell PS, Burnham NL, Therneau TM, Hagen L, Gainey DK, Cross M, Athmann LM, Fischer T, O'Connell MJ. A controlled evaluation of an allopurinol mouthwash as prophylaxis against 5-fluorouracil–induced stomatitis. *Cancer* (1990) 65, 1879–82.

Fluorouracil + Aminoglycosides; Oral

Neomycin can delay the gastrointestinal absorption of fluorouracil, but the clinical importance of this is uncertain.

Clinical evidence, mechanism, importance and management

Some preliminary information from a study in 12 patients treated for metastatic adenocarcinoma showed that treatment with oral **neomycin** 500 mg four times daily for a week delayed the absorption of fluorouracil, but the effects were generally too small to reduce the therapeutic response, except possibly in one patient.[1] It seems probable that this interaction occurs because **neomycin** can induce a malabsorption syndrome. If **neomycin**, and most probably **paromomycin** or **kanamycin** are used in patients on fluorouracil, the possibility of this interaction should be borne in mind.

1. Bruckner HW, Creasey WA. The administration of 5-fluorouracil by mouth. *Cancer* (1974) 33, 14–18.

Fluorouracil + Cisplatin or Oxaliplatin

The addition of low-dose cisplatin to fluorouracil infusion markedly increased the toxicity in one study. Cardiotoxicity may possibly be increased with higher doses of cisplatin. Oxaliplatin appears to moderately raise fluorouracil levels, without increasing its toxicity.

Clinical evidence, mechanism, importance and management

(a) Cisplatin

The addition of low-dose cisplatin 20 mg/m^2 once a week to continuous ambulatory fluorouracil infusions of 300 mg/m^2 daily considerably increased the toxicity (nausea, vomiting, anorexia, diarrhoea, stomatitis, myelosuppression) in 18 patients with advanced cancers. More than half developed multiple toxicities, and severe toxicity occurred in two-thirds. Leucopenia occurred in 28% given both drugs whereas it is virtually nonexistent with fluorouracil alone. Toxicity requiring treatment interruption or dose reduction was seen in 55% of patients on fluorouracil alone, and this rose to 94% when given both drugs.[1] In another study, signs of cardiotoxicity (chest pain, ST-T wave changes, arrhythmias) were seen in 12 of 80 patients given fluorouracil with cisplatin for carcinoma of the head, neck, oesophagus and stomach.[2] Studies in humans and *rats* have shown that there is prolonged elevation of filterable platinum levels associated with concurrent use of cisplatin and fluorouracil.[3]

The combination of a platinum derivative and fluorouracil is widely used, but the optimum schedule to improve activity and reduce toxicity is not firmly established. In one study of bolus cisplatin and continuous infusion fluorouracil, modifying the dose of fluorouracil based on AUC reduced toxicity while still maintaining response rates.[4] In another study, cisplatin pharmacokinetics were said to be optimum when it was used as a continuous infusion with a continuous infusion of fluorouracil.[5] Further study is needed.

(b) Oxaliplatin

In one study, 28 patients with advanced or metastatic colorectal cancer were given fluorouracil alone, or immediately following an 85 mg/m^2 dose of oxaliplatin given over 2 hours. Oxaliplatin did not significantly affect the pharmacokinetics of fluorouracil (either 2 cycles of a 400 mg/m^2 bolus followed by a 46-hour infusion of 2400 mg/m^2 given to 10 patients, with pharmacokinetic sampling over 46 hours, or a single cycle of a 400 mg/m^2 bolus followed by 600 mg/m^2 over 22 hours given to 18 patients, with pharmacokinetic sampling over 22 hours).[6] However, in another study 29 patients with advanced colorectal cancer were given fluorouracil in a dose adjusted to give levels of between 2.5 and 3 mg/L (dose range 750 to 3500 mg/m^2 per week) either alone, or immediately following a 2-hour infusion of oxaliplatin 130 mg/m^2. In this study pharmacokinetic samples were taken on days 1, 8 and 15, and oxaliplatin raised the plasma levels of fluorouracil by about one-third, with the effect appearing to last for 15 days. Fluorouracil toxicity was not increased.[7]

The combination of fluorouracil and oxaliplatin is widely used, but one of the studies cited here suggest that the schedules could still be adjusted to optimise efficacy and minimise toxicity.[7]

1. Jeske J, Hansen RM, Libnoch JA, Anderson T. 5-Fluorouracil infusion and low-dose weekly cisplatin: an analysis of increased toxicity. *Am J Clin Oncol* (1990) 13, 485–8.
2. Jeremic B, Jevremovic S, Djuric L, Mijatovic L. Cardiotoxicity during chemotherapy treatment with 5-fluorouracil and cisplatin. *J Chemother* (1990) 2, 264–7.
3. Belliveau JF, Posner MR, Crabtree GW, Weitberg AB, Wiemann MC, Cummings FJ, O'Leary GP, Ingersoll E, Calabresi P. Clinical pharmacokinetics of 3-day continuous infusion cisplatin and daily bolus 5-fluorouracil. *Eur J Clin Pharmacol* (1991) 40, 115–17.
4. Fety R, Rolland F, Barberi-Heyob M, Hardouin A, Campion L, Conroy T, Merlin J-L, Riviére A, Perrocheau G, Etienne MC, Milano G. Clinical impact of pharmacokinetically-guided dose adaptation of 5-fluorouracil: results from a multicentric randomized trial in patients with locally advanced head and neck carcinomas. *Clin Cancer Res* (1998) 4, 2039–45.
5. Ikeda K, Terashima M, Kawamura H, Takiyama I, Koeda K, Takagane A, Sato N, Ishida K, Iwaya T, Maesawa C, Yoshinari H, Saito K. Pharmacokinetics of cisplatin in combined cisplatin and 5-fluorouracil therapy: a comparative study of three different schedules of cisplatin administration. *Jpn J Clin Oncol* (1998) 28, 168–75.
6. Joel SP, Papamichael D, Richards F, Davis T, Aslanis V, Chatelut E, Locke K, Slevin ML, Seymour MT. Lack of pharmacokinetic interaction between 5-fluorouracil and oxaliplatin. *Clin Pharmacol Ther* (2004) 76, 45–54.
7. Boisdron-Celle M, Craipeau MC, Brienza S, Delva R, Guérin-Meyer V, Cvitkovic E, Gamelin E. Influence of oxaliplatin on 5-fluorouracil plasma clearance and clinical consequences. *Cancer Chemother Pharmacol* (2002) 49, 235–43.

Fluorouracil + Dipyridamole

One study suggested that intravenous dipyridamole may reduce the steady-state plasma levels of fluorouracil, whereas others found oral dipyridamole caused no important changes in fluorouracil pharmacokinetics. Dipyridamole does not appear to improve the clinical response to fluorouracil.

Clinical evidence, mechanism, importance and management

Numerous preclinical studies found that dipyridamole enhanced the activity of fluorouracil, leading to its investigation as a biomodulating agent.[1] However, unexpectedly, in one phase I study of the combination, dipyridamole therapy was associated with lower steady state plasma level of fluorouracil suggesting an approximately 30% increase in total body clearance of fluorouracil or its volume of distribution.[2] In this study, 47 patients with advanced cancer were given fluorouracil in escalating doses ranging from 185 mg/m^2 daily to 3600 mg/m^2 daily with or without dipyridamole as a continuous infusion of 7.7 mg/kg/day for 72 hours.[2] In contrast, in a later randomised study, oral dipyridamole 75 mg three times daily for 5 days did not significantly alter the pharmacokinetic parameters of fluorouracil, except for prolonging the half-life and slightly increasing the dose-intensity; over 5 cycles the average dose of fluorouracil was 479 mg/m^2 alone, compared to 533 mg/m^2 in the presence of dipyridamole. In this study, orally administered dipyridamole did not improve the antineoplastic activity of fluorouracil and folinic acid.[3] Similarly, another clinical study found that oral dipyridamole did not significantly alter the pharmacokinetics of fluorouracil.[4] Thus, despite the promise of preclinical studies, the benefits of combining dipyridamole with fluorouracil have not yet been realised clinically.

1. Grem JL. Biochemical modulation of fluorouracil by dipyridamole: preclinical and clinical experience. *Semin Oncol* (1992) 19 (Suppl 3), 56–65.
2. Trump DL, Egorin MJ, Forrest A, Willson JKV, Remick S, Tutsch KD. Pharmacokinetic and pharmacodynamic analysis of fluorouracil during 72-hour continuous infusion with and without dipyridamole. *J Clin Oncol* (1991) 9, 2027–35.
3. Köhne C-H, Hiddemann W, Schüller J, Weiss J, Lohrmann H-P, Schmitz-Hüber U, Bodenstein H, Schöber C, Wilke H, Grem J, Schmoll H-J. Failure of orally administered dipyridamole to enhance the antineoplastic activity of fluorouracil in combination with leucovorin in patients with advanced colorectal cancer: a prospective randomized trial. *J Clin Oncol* (1995) 13, 1201–8.
4. Czejka MJ, Jäger W, Schüller J, Fogl U, Weiss C, Schernthaner G. Clinical pharmacokinetics of fluorouracil: influence of the biomodulating agents interferon, dipyridamole and folinic acid alone and in combination. *Arzneimittelforschung* (1993) 43, 387–90.

Fluorouracil + Folic acid

Two patients developed severe fluorouracil toxicity while taking multivitamin preparations containing folic acid.

Clinical evidence

A woman who underwent surgery for carcinoma of the rectum was treated a month later with intravenous fluorouracil 500 mg/m^2 daily for 5 days. At the end of this chemotherapy she was admitted to hospital with anorexia, severe mouth ulceration, bloody diarrhoea and vaginal bleeding, which was interpreted as fluorouracil toxicity. Her concurrent medication included folic acid 5 mg (in *Multi-B forte*) along with loperamide, sulfasalazine, vitamins B_{12} and K, and HRT. A month later, when treated again with fluorouracil but without the folic acid, her treatment was well tolerated and without toxicity. A man similarly treated with fluorouracil for colonic cancer was admitted 2 days later with severe mouth ulceration and bloody diarrhoea. He too was found to be taking a multivitamin preparation, containing folic acid 500 micrograms. Subsequent courses of fluorouracil at the same dosage but without the folic acid were well tolerated.[1]

Mechanism

It would seem that folic acid increases fluorouracil inhibition of thymidine formation which is important for DNA synthesis, and thereby increases fluorouracil toxicity.

Importance and management

Direct information seem to be limited to these two cases but the interaction would appear to be established. What happened is consistent with the way **folinic acid**, another source of folate, is used therapeutically to increase the potency of fluorouracil. Patients treated with fluorouracil should therefore not be given folic acid, and should be told to avoid multivitamin preparations containing folic acid to prevent the development of severe fluorouracil side-effects.

1. Mainwaring P, Grygiel JJ. Interaction of 5-fluorouracil with folates. *Aust N Z J Med* (1995) 25, 60.

Fluorouracil + Gemcitabine

Preliminary evidence suggests gemcitabine enhances systemic exposure to fluorouracil.

Clinical evidence, mechanism, importance and management

Pharmacokinetic analysis has shown that gemcitabine enhances systemic exposure to fluorouracil in patients with pancreatic carcinoma given folinic acid, fluorouracil, and gemcitabine.[1,2] In addition, *in vitro,* gemcitabine increases the accumulation of fluorouracil and its cytotoxicity.[1] Further study is needed.

1. Francini G, Correale P, Cetta F, Zuckermann M, Cerretani D, Micheli V, Bruni G, Clerici M, Pozzessere D, Petrioli R, Marsili S, Messinese S, Sabatino M, Giorgio G. Effects of gemcitabine on 5-fluorouracil activity, pharmacokinetics and pharmacodynamics in vitro and in cancer patients. *Gastroenterology* (2002) 122 (Suppl 1), A308.
2. Correale P, Cerretani D, Marsili S, Pozzessere D, Petrioli R, Messinese S, Sabatino M, Roviello F, Pinto E, Francini G, Giorgi G. Gemcitabine increases systemic 5-fluorouracil exposure in advanced cancer patients. *Eur J Cancer* (2003) 39, 1547–51.

Fluorouracil + H_2-blockers

Some data indicate that 4, but not 1 week, of treatment with cimetidine can markedly increase plasma fluorouracil levels. The combination may have increased activity in colorectal cancer.

Clinical evidence, mechanism, importance and management

A study in 6 patients with carcinoma treated with fluorouracil (15 mg/kg daily for 5 days, repeated every 4 weeks) showed that treatment with **cimetidine** 1 g daily for 4 weeks increased peak plasma fluorouracil concentrations by 74% and the AUC by 72% when fluorouracil was given orally. When fluorouracil was given intravenously the AUC was increased by 27% and the total body clearance was reduced by 28%. In this small group, no increased toxicity was noted. The pharmacokinetics of fluorouracil were unaltered by the use of **cimetidine** for only a week.[1] **Cimetidine** produced similar findings in *animal* studies but **ranitidine** had no effect.[2] It is suggested that **cimetidine** reduces the hepatic metabolism of fluorouracil.[1,2] At least two clinical trials have shown some benefit for combining fluorouracil and long-term **cimetidine** in treating colorectal cancer.[3,4] However, this benefit has been attributed to immunomodulation[3] or inhibition of adhesion,[4] rather than any pharmacokinetic interaction. Whatever the mechanism, it appears that **cimetidine** can increase the activity of fluorouracil. Concurrent treatment should be undertaken with care. **Cimetidine** can be bought over the counter in some countries so that patients may unwittingly increase the toxicity of fluorouracil. **Ranitidine**,[2] and probably other H_2-blockers, do not appear to interact.

1. Harvey VJ, Slevin ML, Dilloway MR, Clark PI, Johnston A, Lant AF. The influence of cimetidine on the pharmacokinetics of 5-fluorouracil. *Br J Clin Pharmacol* (1984) 18, 421–30.
2. Dilloway MR, Lant AF. Effect of H_2-receptor antagonists on the pharmacokinetics of 5-fluorouracil in the rat and monkey. *Biopharm Drug Dispos* (1991) 12, 17–28.
3. Links M, Clingan PR, Phadke K, O'Baugh J, Legge J, Adams WJ, Ross WB, Morris DL. A randomized trial of cimetidine with 5-fluorouracil and folinic acid in metastatic colorectal cancer. *Eur J Surg Oncol* (1995) 21, 523–5.
4. Matsumoto S, Imaeda Y, Umemoto S, Kobayashi K, Suzuki H, Okamoto T. Cimetidine increases survival of colorectal cancer patients with high levels of sialyl Lewis-X and sialyl Lewis-A epitope expression on tumour cells. *Br J Cancer* (2002) 86, 159–60.

Fluorouracil + Interferon alfa

Interferon alfa has increased plasma fluorouracil levels in some, but not other, studies. Despite some early promising data, interferon alfa does not appear to improve the response to fluorouracil in patients with colorectal cancer.

Clinical evidence, mechanism, importance and management

A pharmacokinetic study was completed in 26 patients with colorectal cancer given a 5-day continuous infusion of fluorouracil 750 mg/m^2 daily repeated in week 4 followed by a bolus intravenous injection of 750 mg/m^2 once a week with or without subcutaneous interferon alfa-2a (*Roferon*) 9 million units three times a week. There was considerable within-patient variation but no significant differences in steady-state plasma levels were found between the two groups.[1] Similarly, others have also reported no significant changes in fluorouracil pharmacokinetics when given with interferon alfa.[2,3] However, other studies[4-7] have found a significant increase in peak fluorouracil levels and AUC during co-administration with interferon alfa. Despite promising early preclinical and clinical data indicating that interferon may improve the response to fluorouracil, this has not yet been demonstrated in randomised trials.[8]

1. Pittman K, Perren T, Ward U, Primrose J, Slevin M, Patel N, Selby P. Pharmacokinetics of 5-fluorouracil in colorectal cancer patients receiving interferon. *Ann Oncol* (1993) 4, 515–6.
2. Seymour MT, Patel N, Johnston A, Joel SP, Slevin ML. Lack of effect of interferon α2a upon fluorouracil pharmacokinetics. *Br J Cancer* (1994) 70, 724–8.
3. Kim J, Zhi J, Satoh H, Koss-Twardy SG, Passe SM, Patel IH, Pazdur R. Pharmacokinetics of recombinant human interferon-α2a combined with 5-fluorouracil in patients with advanced colorectal carcinoma. *Anticancer Drugs* (1998) 9, 689–96.
4. Schüller J, Czejka MJ, Schernthaner G, Fogl U, Jäger W, Micksche M. Influence of interferon alfa-2b with or without folinic acid on pharmacokinetics of fluorouracil. *Semin Oncol* (1992) 19 (2 suppl 3) 93–7.
5. Grem JL, McAtee N, Murphy RF, Balis FM, Steinberg SM, Hamilton JM, Sorensen JM, Sartor O, Kramer BS, Goldstein LJ, Gay LM, Caubo KM, Goldspiel B, Allegra CJ. A pilot study of interferon alfa-2a in combination with fluorouracil plus high dose leucovorin in metastatic gastrointestinal carcinoma. *J Clin Oncol* (1991) 9, 1811–20.
6. Danhauser LL, Freimann JH, Gilchrist TL, Gutterman JU, Hunter CY, Yeomans AC, Markowitz AB. Phase I and plasma pharmacokinetic study of infusional fluorouracil combined with recombinant interferon alfa-2b in patients with advanced cancer. *J Clin Oncol* (1993) 11, 751–61.
7. Larsson P-A, Glimelius B, Jeppsson B, Jönsson P-E, Malmberg M, Gustavsson B, Carlsson G, Svedberg M. A pharmacokinetic study of 5-FU/leucovorin and alpha-interferon in advanced cancer. *Acta Oncol* (2000) 39, 59–63.
8. Makower D, Wadler S. Interferons as biomodulators of fluoropyrimidines in the treatment of colorectal cancer. *Semin Oncol* (1999) 26, 663–71.

Fluorouracil + Metronidazole or Misonidazole

The toxicity, but not the efficacy of fluorouracil, is increased by metronidazole and misonidazole.

Clinical evidence

A marked increase in fluorouracil toxicity was noted in 27 patients with metastatic colorectal cancer when they were given metronidazole 750 mg/m^2 intravenously one hour before fluorouracil 600 mg/m^2 intravenously 5 days per week once every 4 weeks. Granulocytopenia occurred in 74%, anaemia in 41%, stomatitis and oral ulceration in 34%, nausea and vomiting in 48% and thrombocytopenia in 19%.[1] A pharmacokinetic study in 10 patients showed that metronidazole reduced the clearance of fluorouracil by 27% over the 5-day period and increased the AUC by 34%. *In vitro* studies with human colon cancer cells failed to show any increased efficacy.[1]

Studies using another nitroimidazole, misonidazole, in patients with colorectal cancer also found an increased incidence and severity of gastrointestinal toxicity with concurrent use,[2,3] a slightly increased incidence of leucopenia[2] and a reduction in the clearance.[3]

Mechanism

Metronidazole reduces the clearance of fluorouracil, thereby increasing its toxic effects.

Importance and management

Information is limited but the fluorouracil/metronidazole interaction appears to be established. It was hoped that metronidazole or misonidazole (no longer in clinical use) might increase the efficacy of fluorouracil. However, the studies above show that the toxicity of fluorouracil is increased without an obvious increase in its therapeutic efficacy. Care should be taken if metronidazole is required for its antimicrobial effects in a patient on fluorouracil. Whether other nitroimidazoles (e.g. tinidazole) behave similarly appears not to have been studied.

1. Bardakji Z, Jolivet J, Langelier Y, Besner J-G, Ayoub J. 5-Fluorouracil-metronidazole combination therapy in metastatic colorectal cancer. *Cancer Chemother Pharmacol* (1986) 18, 140–44.
2. Spooner D, Bugden RD, Peckham MJ, Wist EA. The combination of 5-fluorouracil with misonidazole in patients with advanced colorectal cancer. *Int J Radiat Oncol Biol Phys* (1982) 8, 387–9.
3. McDermott BJ, Van den Berg HW, Martin WMC, Murphy RF. Pharmacokinetic rationale for the interaction of 5-fluorouracil and misonidazole in humans. *Br J Cancer* (1983) 48, 705–10.

Fluorouracil + Miscellaneous

The toxicity and efficacy of fluorouracil appear to be unaffected by chlorprothixene, cinnarizine, prochlorperazine, sodium pentobarbital, thiethylperazine and trimethobenzamide.

Clinical evidence, mechanism, importance and management

A retrospective analysis of studies in a total of 250 patients given fluorouracil for the treatment of gastrointestinal cancer found that the following drugs (studied for their possible antiemetic effects) did not cause any significant increase in toxicity or decrease in therapeutic effects when compared with a placebo: **chlorprothixene**, **cinnarizine**, **prochlorperazine**, **sodium pentobarbital**, **thiethylperazine**, **trimethobenzamide**.[1] No special precautions would seem necessary.

1. Moertel CG, Reitemeier RJ, Hahn RG. Effect of concomitant drug treatment on toxic and therapeutic activity of 5-fluorouracil (5-FU; NSC-19893). *Cancer Chemother Rep* (1972) 56, 245–7.

Fluorouracil prodrugs + Sorivudine

Marked and rapidly fatal toxicity, attributed to fluorouracil toxicity, has been seen in patients given tegafur or other fluorouracil prodrugs given with sorivudine. Fluorouracil is expected to interact similarly.

Clinical evidence, mechanism, importance and management

In 1993, the Japanese Ministry of Health reported that 15 Japanese patients with cancer and a viral disease died several days after being given a fluorouracil prodrug (e.g. **tegafur**) and sorivudine. Before death most of them developed severe toxicity including severe anorexia, marked damage to the bone marrow with decreases in white cell and platelet counts, and marked atrophy of the intestinal membrane with diarrhoea and loss of blood. Eight other patients given both drugs developed symptoms of severe toxicity.[1,2]

Mechanism

Sorivudine appears to be converted in the gut into a metabolite (BVU or bromovinyluracil) that is a potent inhibitor of dihydropyrimidine dehydrogenase (DPD), an enzyme involved in the metabolism of fluorouracil (derived from tegafur and other fluorouracil prodrugs).[1,3] There is some evidence that DPD activity is genetically determined, and that there are poor fluorouracil metabolisers with low DPD activity, who would be expected to be more susceptible to this interaction.[4]

Importance and management

Information appears to be limited to these reports but the interaction appears to be established and of clinical importance. The concurrent use of inhibitors of DPD (such as sorivudine and **brivudine**) and oral fluorouracil prodrugs such as **capecitabine**[5] and tegafur should be avoided. Note that sorivudine was withdrawn from the market following confirmation of this interaction.

1. Okuda H, Nishiyama T, Ogura Y, Nagayama S, Ikeda K, Yamaguchi S, Nakamura Y, Kawaguchi K, Watabe T. Lethal drug interactions of sorivudine, a new antiviral drug, with oral 5-fluorouracil prodrugs. *Drug Metab Dispos* (1997) 25, 270–3.
2. Diasio RB. Sorivudine and 5-fluorouracil; a clinically significant drug-drug interaction due to inhibition of dihydropyrimidine dehydrogenase. *Br J Clin Pharmacol* (1998) 46, 1–4.
3. Watabe T, Okuda H, Ogura K. Lethal drug interactions of the new antiviral, sorivudine, with anticancer prodrugs of 5-fluorouracil. *Yakugaku Zasshi* (1997) 117, 910–21. (In Japanese).
4. Watabe T, Ogura K, Nishiyama T. Molecular toxicological mechanism of the lethal interactions of the new antiviral drug, sorivudine, with 5-fluorouracil prodrugs and genetic deficiency of dihydropyrimidine dehydrogenase. *Yakugaku Zasshi* (2002) 122, 527–35. (In Japanese).
5. Xeloda (Capecitabine). Roche Products Ltd. UK Summary of product characteristics, March 2005.

Fluorouracil prodrugs; Capecitabine + Allopurinol

The activity of capecitabine is predicted to be decreased by allopurinol.

Clinical evidence, mechanism, importance and management

Capecitabine is a prodrug, which is activated by several enzymatic steps to produce active fluorouracil within the body. Because allopurinol is reported to modulate fluorouracil, with possible decreased efficacy (see 'Fluorouracil + Allopurinol', p.467), the UK makers of capecitabine say that allopurinol should be avoided.[1]

1. Xeloda (Capecitabine). Roche Products Ltd. UK Summary of product characteristics, March 2005.

Fluorouracil prodrugs; Capecitabine + Antacids

The absorption of capecitabine was not affected by an aluminium/magnesium hydroxide antacid.

Clinical evidence, mechanism, importance and management

A study in 12 patients on the effects of 20 ml of an **aluminium/magnesium hydroxide** antacid (*Maalox*) on the pharmacokinetics of a single 1250-mg/m^2 oral dose of capecitabine found that it caused a small increase in the plasma levels of capecitabine and one metabolite (5′-DFCR) but it had no effect on the other 3 major metabolites (5′DFUR, 5-FU and FBAL).[1] There would therefore seem to be no reason for taking special precautions if capecitabine and an antacid of this type are used concurrently.

1. Reigner B, Clive S, Cassidy J, Jodrell D, Schulz R, Goggin T, Banken L, Roos B, Utoh M, Mulligan T, Weidekamm E. Influence of the antacid Maalox on the pharmacokinetics of capecitabine in cancer patients. *Cancer Chemother Pharmacol* (1999) 43, 309–15.

Fluorouracil prodrugs; Capecitabine + Folinic acid

The maximum tolerated dose of capecitabine is decreased by folinic acid.

Clinical evidence, mechanism, importance and management

Studies in patients with refractory advanced cancer have shown that folinic acid 30 mg twice daily does not have a major effect on the pharmacokinetics of capecitabine.[1] However, the pharmacodynamics of capecitabine were affected as determined by the more frequent occurrence of dose-limiting gastrointestinal disorders or the hand-foot syndrome.[1] The UK makers say that the maximum tolerated capecitabine dose when used alone in the intermittent regimen is 3000 mg/m^2, but it is reduced to 2000 mg/m^2 if folinic acid 30 mg twice daily is added.[2]

1. Cassidy J, Dirix L, Bissett D, Reigner B, Griffin T, Allman D, Osterwalder B, Van Oosterom AT. A phase I study of capecitabine in combination with oral leucovorin in patients with intractable solid tumours. *Clin Cancer Res* (1998) 4, 2755–61.
2. Xeloda (Capecitabine). Roche Products Ltd. UK Summary of product characteristics, March 2005.

Fluorouracil prodrugs; Capecitabine + Interferon alfa

The maximum tolerated dose of capecitabine is decreased by interferon alfa.

Clinical evidence, mechanism, importance and management

The UK makers[1] say that the maximum tolerated capecitabine dose when used alone is 3000 mg/m^2, but when combined with interferon alfa-2a (3 million units/m^2 daily) the maximum tolerated dose is 2000 mg/m^2. Capecitabine is a prodrug of fluorouracil, which is thought to be modulated by interferon alfa. See also 'Fluorouracil + Interferon alfa', p.469.

1. Xeloda (Capecitabine). Roche Products Ltd. UK Summary of product characteristics, March 2005.

Fluorouracil prodrugs; Capecitabine + Taxanes

There are no clinically significant pharmacokinetic interactions between capecitabine and paclitaxel, and probably not between capecitabine and docetaxel, although more study is needed to establish this.

Clinical evidence, mechanism, importance and management

A study in patients with advanced solid tumours found that administration of the fluorouracil prodrug capecitabine with **docetaxel**, resulted in an almost twofold decrease in the maximum plasma concentration and AUC of fluorouracil. The authors suggest that more study is needed to assess the significance of this finding. Other pharmacokinetic parameters of capecitabine were not affected by co-administered **docetaxel**. The pharmacokinetics of **docetaxel** were not significantly affected by capecitabine or its metabolites.[1]

Another study in similar patients found that neither **paclitaxel** nor capecitabine significantly altered the pharmacokinetics of each other.[2]

1. Pronk LC, Vasey P, Sparreboom A, Reigner B, Planting AST, Gordon RJ, Osterwalder B, Verweij J. A phase I and pharmacokinetic study of the combination of capecitabine and docetaxel in patients with advanced solid tumours. *Br J Cancer* (2000) 83, 22–9.
2. Villalona-Calero MA, Weiss GR, Burris HA, Kraynak M, Rodrigues G, Drengler RL, Eckhardt SG, Reigner B, Moczygemba J, Burger HU, Griffin T, Von Hoff DD, Rowinsky EK. Phase I and pharmacokinetic study of the oral fluoropyrimidine capecitabine in combination with paclitaxel in patients with advanced solid malignancies. *J Clin Oncol* (1999) 17, 1915–25.

Gemcitabine + Anthracyclines

Gemcitabine, and doxorubicin or epirubicin, do not interact pharmacokinetically.

Clinical evidence, mechanism, importance and management

The pharmacokinetics of gemcitabine and **doxorubicin** did not differ when they were administered on the same day compared with when they were given alone in patients with breast cancer.[1] Similarly, gemcitabine pharmacokinetics were unchanged by concurrent use of **epirubicin** and paclitaxel in patients with breast cancer,[2] and gemcitabine did not alter the interaction between **epirubicin** and paclitaxel (see 'Anthracyclines + Taxanes', p.450).

1. Pérez-Manga G, Lluch A, Alba E, Moreno-Nogueira JA, Palomero M, García-Conde J, Khayat D, Rivelles N. Gemcitabine in combination with doxorubicin in advanced breast cancer: final results of a phase II pharmacokinetic trial. *J Clin Oncol* (2000) 18, 2545–52.
2. Conte PF, Gennari A, Donati S, Salvadori B, Baldini E, Bengala C, Pazzagli I, Orlandini C, Danesi R, Fogli S, Del Tacca M. Gemcitabine plus epirubicin plus taxol (GET) in advanced breast cancer: a phase II study. *Breast Cancer Res Treat* (2001) 68, 171–9.

Gemcitabine + Platinum derivatives

The toxicity and pharmacokinetics of gemcitabine combined with platinum drugs such as cisplatin is dependent upon the order in which they are given.

Clinical evidence, mechanism, importance and management

(a) Carboplatin

Gemcitabine 1000 mg/m^2 on days 1, 8, and 15 has been administered with carboplatin (maximum tolerated dose at AUC 5.2 mg/ml/minute) on day 1, in a monthly cycle. No difference was detected in toxicity or tolerated dose when the gemcitabine was administered before the carboplatin or in the reverse sequence.[1] However, subsequent authors reported that this same dose schedule, with carboplatin administered immediately after the gemcitabine, caused unexpected and severe thrombocytopenia, and could not be recommended.[2]

(b) Cisplatin

When gemcitabine was given 4 hours before or after cisplatin there were no major differences in the plasma pharmacokinetics of gemcitabine, deaminated gemcitabine and platinum. Similarly, cisplatin given 24 hours before gemcitabine did not significantly change gemcitabine and deaminated gemcitabine levels, although there was a trend towards an increased AUC of gemcitabine triphosphate.[3] Gemcitabine given 24 hours before cisplatin decreased the platinum AUC twofold,[3] and caused the least leucopenia of the schedules.[4] Anaemia, thrombocytopenia, nausea/vomiting and fatigue were not sequence dependent.[4] On the basis of these findings, the authors are further evaluating the schedule of cisplatin given 24 hours before gemcitabine.[3,4] Note that the combination of cisplatin and gemcitabine is commonly used for the treatment of various cancers, usually with the drugs given concurrently or sequentially on the same day.[5]

(c) Oxaliplatin

The pharmacokinetics of gemcitabine 800 to 1500 mg/m^2 and its main metabolite did not appear to be affected by oxaliplatin 70 to 100 mg/m^2 when oxaliplatin was given immediately after gemcitabine once every two weeks.[6]

1. Langer CJ, Claver P, Ozols RF. Gemcitabine and carboplatin in combination: phase I and phase II studies. *Semin Oncol* (1998) 25 (Suppl 9), 51–4.
2. Ng EW, Sandler AB, Robinson L, Einhorn LH. A phase II study of carboplatin plus gemcitabine in advanced non-small-cell lung cancer (NSCLC): a Hoosier Oncology Group study. *Am J Clin Oncol* (1999) 22, 550–3.
3. van Moorsel CJ, Kroep JR, Pinedo HM, Veerman G, Voorn DA, Postmus PE, Vermorken JB, van Groeningen CJ, van der Vijgh WJ, Peters GJ. Pharmacokinetic schedule finding study of the combination of gemcitabine and cisplatin in patients with solid tumors. *Ann Oncol* (1999) 10, 441–8.
4. Kroep JR, Peters GJ, van Moorsel CJA, Catik A, Vermorken JB, Pinedo HM, van Groeningen CJ. Gemcitabine-cisplatin: a schedule finding study. *Ann Oncol* (1999) 10, 1503–10.
5. Gemzar (Gemcitabine). Eli Lilly and Co Ltd. UK Summary of product characteristics. November 2004.
6. Faivre S, Le Chevalier T, Monnerat C, Lokiec F, Novello S, Taieb J, Pautier P, Lhommé C, Ruffié P, Kayitalire L, Armand J-P, Raymond E. Phase I-II and pharmacokinetic study of gemcitabine combined with oxaliplatin in patients with advanced non-small-cell lung cancer and ovarian carcinoma. *Ann Oncol* (2002) 13, 1479–89.

Gemcitabine + Taxanes

There does not appear to be any pharmacokinetic interaction between gemcitabine and paclitaxel. Gemcitabine distribution may be altered by docetaxel, but docetaxel pharmacokinetics are not affected.

Clinical evidence, mechanism, importance and management

(a) Docetaxel

In a study of gemcitabine and docetaxel, given on days 1 and 8 of a 21-day cycle, drug toxicity and pharmacokinetics were unaffected by the relative order of administration of gemcitabine and docetaxel.[1] However, in another study, it appeared that while docetaxel pharmacokinetics were unaffected the distribution of gemcitabine was altered by docetaxel, although there was no clear relationship between this and toxicity.[2]

(b) Paclitaxel

A study in 18 patients with non-small-cell lung cancer found that when given gemcitabine 1000 mg/m^2 on days 1 and 8 and paclitaxel 150 to 200 mg/m^2 on day one as a 3-hour infusion immediately before the gemcitabine, the plasma levels of gemcitabine and the AUC of its deaminated metabolite were unchanged, as was the AUC of paclitaxel. However, paclitaxel increased gemcitabine triphosphate levels, potentially improving efficacy.[3] In another study, no pharmacokinetic interactions were detected between gemcitabine and paclitaxel given once weekly, although gemcitabine showed saturation kinetics at higher doses.[4,5]

1. Bhargava P, Marshall JL, Fried K, Williams M, Lefebvre P, Dahut W, Hanfelt J, Gehan E, Figuera M, Hawkins MJ, Rizvi NA. Phase I and pharmacokinetic study of two sequences of gemcitabine and docetaxel administered weekly to patients with advanced cancer. *Cancer Chemother Pharmacol* (2001) 48, 95–103.
2. Dumez H, Louwerens M, Pawinsky A, Planting AST, de Jonge MJA, Van Oosterom AT, Highley M, Guetens G, Mantel M, De Boeck G, de Bruijn E, Verweij J. The impact of drug administration sequence and pharmacokinetic interaction in a phase I study of the combination of docetaxel and gemcitabine in patients with advanced solid tumors. *Anticancer Drugs* (2002) 13, 583–93.
3. Kroep JR, Giaccone G, Voorn DA, Smit EF, Beijnen JH, Rosing H, van Moorsel CJA, van Groeningen CJ, Postmus PE, Pinedo HM, Peters GJ. Gemcitabine and paclitaxel: pharmacokinetic and pharmacodynamic interactions in patients with non-small-cell lung cancer. *J Clin Oncol* (1999) 17, 2190–7.
4. De Pas T, de Braud F, Danesi R, Sessa C, Catania C, Curigliano G, Fogli S, del Tacca M, Zampino G, Sbanotto A, Rocca A, Cinieri S, Marrocco E, Milani A, Goldhirsch A. Phase I and pharmacologic study of weekly gemcitabine and paclitaxel in chemo-naïve patients with advanced non-small-cell lung cancer. *Ann Oncol* (2000) 11, 821–7.
5. Fogli S, Danesi R, De Braud F, De Pas T, Curigliano G, Giovannetti G, Del Tacca M. Drug distribution and pharmacokinetic/pharmacodynamic relationship of paclitaxel and gemcitabine in patients with non-small-cell lung cancer. *Ann Oncol* (2001) 12, 1553–9.

Imatinib + Miscellaneous

Ketoconazole raises serum imatinib levels; other cytochrome P450 isoenzyme CYP3A4 inhibitors are predicted to do the same. Rifampicin (rifampin) lowers serum imatinib levels; other CYP3A4 inducers are predicted to do the same. Imatinib increases serum simvastatin levels and is predicted to interact with other drugs whose metabolism is affected by CYP3A4 inhibition. Warnings have also been issued about warfarin. Based on *in vitro* studies, fluorouracil, paclitaxel and a number of other drugs are not expected to interact.

Clinical evidence, mechanism, importance and management

(a) Drugs that may raise imatinib serum levels

An open-label, randomised, crossover study in 14 healthy subjects found that the maximum serum levels and AUC of imatinib rose by 26 and 40% respectively when they were given single 400-mg doses of **ketoconazole** with single 200-mg doses of imatinib.[1] The reason is that **ketoconazole** is a potent inhibitor of the cytochrome P450 isoenzyme CYP3A4, which is involved in the metabolism of imatinib. As a result the metabolism and clearance of imatinib are reduced and its serum levels rise accordingly. The makers therefore advise caution with **ketoconazole** and with other CYP3A4 inhibitors (examples listed are **clarithromycin**, **erythromycin** and **itraconazole**),[2,3] but it is not entirely clear what action should be taken because information about excessive serum levels is very limited. The UK makers quote the case of a patient with myeloid blast crisis who inadvertently took 1200 mg imatinib for 6 days (the normal maximum is 800 mg). He showed elevations of serum creatinine, transaminases, bilirubin, and he developed ascites. He recovered within a week of stopping the imatinib and was later restarted on 400 mg daily.[2]

(b) Drugs that may lower imatinib serum levels

A study reported that pretreatment with **rifampicin** (**rifampin**) 600 mg decreased the maximum serum levels and AUC of a 400 mg dose of imatinib by 54 and 74% respectively.[2] No specific studies have been carried out with imatinib and other CYP3A4 inducing drugs, but the makers list **carbamazepine**, **dexamethasone**, **phenobarbital**, **phenytoin** and **St John's wort *(Hypericum perforatum)***, as enzyme inducers that are predicted to reduce imatinib serum levels. The makers therefore reasonably recommend caution, and suggest that concurrent use with potent enzyme inducing drugs should be avoided.[2,3] However, if this is not possible it would be prudent to monitor the outcome of concurrent use, and increase the imatinib dose as necessary. The makers have one case, from a clinical trial, of a likely interaction with **phenytoin**.[1]

(c) Drugs that may have their serum levels altered by imatinib

'**Simvastatin**', (p.843) levels are increased by imatinib probably due to the inhibitory effects of imatinib on the metabolism and clearance of **simvastatin** by the cytochrome P450 isoenzyme CYP3A4.[2,3] The makers name two other drugs, **pimozide** and **ciclosporin**, which are also predicted to show serum level rises with potentially serious consequences because of CYP3A4 inhibition. Other named groups of drugs that may also potentially show serum levels rises are the **triazolo-benzodiazepines** (e.g. **triazolam**, **midazolam**), **dihydropyridine calcium channel blockers** and **statins**.[2,3] However, note that the statins have varying metabolic routes, see 'Lipid-regulating drugs', (p.827).

The makers say that because **warfarin** is metabolised by CYP2C9, patients needing anticoagulation should be given low molecular weight or standard **heparin** instead. This recommendation is based on an observation in one patient[1] and on *in vitro* studies[2,3] that show that imatinib can inhibit CYP2C9. There seems to be no other evidence that a clinically relevant interaction is likely to occur. The makers also say that imatinib inhibits CYP2D6 and could therefore potentially increase the serum levels of drugs that are metabolised by this isoenzyme, but no specific *in vivo* studies of this interaction have been carried out.[2,3]

(d) Drugs that are not expected to interact with imatinib

In vitro studies showed no interference with the metabolism of **fluorouracil** by imatinib due to inhibition of the cytochrome P450 isoenzyme CYP2C8. Related studies showed some competitive inhibition of the metabolism of **paclitaxel**, but only at imatinib concentrations far higher than those expected in patients, and therefore the makers predict that no interaction is likely between imatinib and either of these two drugs. Other *in vitro* studies with CYP3A4 also suggest that **aciclovir**, **allopurinol**, **amphotericin B**, **cytarabine**, **hydroxycarbamide** (**hydroxyurea**), **norfloxacin** and **phenoxymethylpenicillin** (**penicillin V**) are unlikely to interact with imatinib.[2]

(e) Paracetamol (Acetaminophen)

During clinical trials of imatinib one patient regularly taking **paracetamol** for fever, died of acute liver failure after 11 days.[4] It is not known whether this was linked to the concurrent use of these two drugs. However the makers report that no interaction was noted during *in vitro* tests.[2,3] It seems likely that no interaction of note will normally occur.

1. Novartis Pharmaceuticals UK Limited. Personal communication, December 2001.
2. Glivec (Imatinib). Novartis Pharmaceuticals UK Ltd. UK Summary of product characteristics, May 2004.
3. Gleevec (Imatinib). Novartis Pharmaceuticals Corporation. US Prescribing information, July 2004.
4. Talpaz M, Silver RT, Druker B, Paquette R, Goldman JM, Reese SF, Capdeville R. A phase II study of STI 571 in adult patients with Philadelphia chromosome positive chronic myeloid leukaemia in accelerated phase. *Blood* (2000) 96 (Suppl 1), 469a.

Irinotecan + Anticonvulsants

A number of case reports suggest the clearance of irinotecan and its active metabolite SN-38 are increased by phenytoin. *Animal* data suggest that phenobarbital may increase, and sodium valproate decrease, the clearance of SN-38.

Clinical evidence, mechanism, importance and management

(a) Phenobarbital

Preclinical data from *rats*[1] indicate that phenobarbital may lead to a reduction in AUCs of irinotecan and its active metabolite SN-38. This is thought to be because phenobarbital induces the enzymes responsible for glucuronidation of SN-38. The clinical relevance of this remains to be determined.

(b) Phenytoin

A 14-year-old girl with glioblastoma was treated with irinotecan 20 to 60 mg/m^2 daily for 5 days on 2 consecutive weeks every 21 days for 2 cycles. During the first cycle she also received phenytoin 300 mg and dexamethasone 6 mg daily. Irinotecan clearance was increased 2.5-fold compared with that in other patients receiving irinotecan alone, and there was decreased exposure to irinotecan's active metabolite, SN-38. The effect on clearance decreased slowly over 8 days after stopping phenytoin.[2] Another patient on phenytoin and irinotecan was found to have much lower AUCs for irinotecan and SN-38 compared with data from patients not on phenytoin.[3] Similarly, a third patient had a threefold increase in irinotecan clearance and about a 60% reduction in the AUCs of irinotecan and SN-38 after starting phenytoin.[4] In a comparative study, the AUC of the lactone forms of irinotecan and SN-38 were 27% and 51% lower in 10 children on enzyme-inducing anticonvulsants (7 receiving phenytoin) than in 21 children not on these anticonvulsants.[5]

It is thought that phenytoin increases the metabolism of irinotecan to an inactive metabolite by inducing cytochrome P450 isoenzyme CYP3A, leading to decreased exposure to the active metabolite.[3]

The information is limited but serves to emphasise the need for caution and monitoring if irinotecan is administered with phenytoin, which may reduce the availability of its active metabolite. Note that phenytoin has also been shown to increase the clearance of a related topoisomerase inhibitors, topotecan (see 'Topotecan + Phenytoin', p.494) and 9-aminocamptothecin (see '9-Aminocamptothecin + Anticonvulsants', p.448).

(c) Valproate

Preclinical data from *rats*[1] suggests that sodium valproate increases the AUC of the active metabolite of irinotecan, SN-38. This is because valproate inhibits the subsequent glucuronidation of SN-38. The clinical relevance of this remains to be determined.

1. Gupta E, Wang X, Ramirez J, Ratain MJ. Modulation of the glucuronidation of SN-38, the active metabolite of irinotecan, by valproic acid and phenobarbital. *Cancer Chemother Pharmacol* (1997) 39, 440–4.
2. Radomski KM, Gajjar AJ, Kirstein MN, Ma MK, Wimmer P, Thompson SJ, Houghton PJ, Stewart CF. Irinotecan clearance is increased after concomitant administration of enzyme inducers in a patient with glioblastoma multiforme. *Pharmacotherapy* (2000) 20, 353.
3. Mathijssen RHJ, Sparreboom A, Dumez J, van Oosterom AT, de Bruijn EA. Altered irinotecan metabolism in a patient receiving phenytoin. *Anticancer Drugs* (2002) 13, 139–40.
4. Murry DJ, Cherrick I, Salama V, Berg S, Bernstein M, Kuttesch N, Blaney SM. Influence of phenytoin on the disposition of irinotecan: a case report. *J Pediatr Hematol Oncol* (2002) 24, 130–3.
5. Crews KR, Stewart CF, Jones-Wallace D, Thompson SJ, Houghton PJ, Heideman RL, Fouladi M, Bowers DC, Chintagumpala MM, Gajjar A. Altered irinotecan pharmacokinetics in pediatric high-grade glioma patients receiving enzyme-inducing anticonvulsant therapy. *Clin Cancer Res* (2002) 8, 2202–9.

Irinotecan + Fluorouracil

While some studies suggest administration of fluorouracil after irinotecan reduces the conversion of irinotecan to its active metabolite, others do not.

Clinical evidence, mechanism, importance and management

A study in 33 patients with metastatic colorectal cancer found that the toxicity and pharmacokinetics of irinotecan when used with fluorouracil depended upon the order of administration of the two drugs.[1] When irinotecan was given before fluorouracil, the AUC of SN-38, the major active irinotecan metabolite, was about 40% lower, and toxicity was lower. In this study, patients were randomised to receive a 60-minute infusion of irinotecan (150 mg/m^2 starting dose, escalated by 50 mg/m^2 increments) immediately before or after a 48-hour infusion of fluorouracil 3500 mg/m^2 modulated by folinic acid in cycle 1, then given in the reverse sequence in cycle 2. Similarly, in a study using historical controls, the AUC of SN-38 was about 28% lower and the AUC of irinotecan about 35% higher when irinotecan was given over 90 minutes immediately before a 7-day fluorouracil infusion, compared with irinotecan alone.[2] Similar findings were reported in a study in *rats*.[3] In contrast, another study found that fluorouracil did not substantially affect the metabolism of irinotecan to SN-38. The AUC of irinotecan and SN-38 did not differ between irinotecan alone, irinotecan immediately followed by folinic acid and fluorouracil, and irinotecan immediately after folinic acid and fluorouracil. In this study, irinotecan 100 to 150 mg/m^2 was given as a 90-minute infusion, and fluorouracil 210 to 500 mg/m^2 by rapid intravenous injection.[4] Similarly, preliminary reports from another research group found that the clearance of irinotecan did not differ when given one day before or one day after 5 daily bolus doses of fluorouracil.[5,6]

From these data it is unclear whether or not fluorouracil alters the pharmacokinetics of irinotecan. A key difference between the main studies is the use of bolus[4] or continuous infusion[1] fluorouracil. The combination is in established clinical usage, where the recommendation is to give irinotecan before fluorouracil/folinic acid.[7,8] This combination has been shown to be more effective than fluorouracil/folinic acid alone.[7,8] Whether this is the optimal schedule remains to be determined.

1. Falcone A, Di Paolo A, Masi G, Allegrini G, Danesi R, Lencioni M, Pfanner E, Comis S, Del Tacca M, Conte P. Sequence effect of irinotecan and fluorouracil treatment on pharmacokinetics and toxicity in chemotherapy-naive metastatic colorectal cancer patients. *J Clin Oncol* (2001) 19, 3456–62.
2. Sasaki Y, Ohtsu A, Shimada Y, Ono K, Saijo N. Simultaneous administration of CPT-11 and fluorouracil: alteration of the pharmacokinetics of CPT-11 and SN-38 in patients with advanced colorectal cancer. *J Natl Cancer Inst* (1994) 86 1096–8.
3. Umezawa T, Kiba T, Numata K, Saito T, Nakaoka M, Shintani S, Sekihara H. Comparisons of the pharmacokinetics and the leukopenia and thrombocytopenia grade after administration of irinotecan and 5-fluorouracil in combination to rats. *Anticancer Res* (2000) 20, 4235–42.
4. Salz LB, Kanowitz J, Kemeny NE, Schaaf L, Spriggs D, Staton BA, Berkery R, Steger C, Eng M, Dietz A, Locker P, Kelsen DP. Phase I clinical and pharmacokinetic study of irinotecan, fluorouracil, and leucovorin in patients with advanced solid tumors. *J Clin Oncol* (1996) 14, 2959–67.
5. Grossin F, Barbault H, Benhammouda A, Rixe O, Antoine E, Auclerc G, Weil M, Nizri D, Farabos C, Mignard D, Mahjoubi M, Khayat D, Bastian G. A phase I pharmacokinetics study of concomitant CPT-11 and 5FU combination. *Proc Am Assoc Cancer Res* (1996) 37, 168.
6. Benhammouda A, Bastian G, Rixe O, Antoine E, Gozy M, Auclerc G, Grossin F, Nizri D, Gil-Delgado M, Weil M, Bismuth H, Mignard DM, Mahjoubi M, Lenseigne S, Khayat D. A phase I pharmacokinetic study of CPT-11 and 5-FU combination. *Proc Am Soc Clin Oncol* (1997) 16. 202a
7. Campto (Irinotecan). Aventis Pharma Ltd. UK Summary of product characteristics, March 2003.
8. Camptosar (Irinotecan). Pharmacia & Upjohn Co. US Prescribing information, July 2004.

Irinotecan + Miscellaneous

Preclinical data suggest that vinorelbine and physostigmine may decrease the formation of the active metabolite of irinotecan, SN-38, and that ciclosporin may increase the exposure to SN-38.

Clinical evidence, mechanism, importance and management

In studies in human liver microsomes, **nifedipine**, **clonazepam**, **methylprednisolone**, **omeprazole**, and **vinorelbine** had significant effects on the metabolism of irinotecan. However, only the effect of **vinorelbine** occurred at a concentration considered clinically relevant.[1] Similarly, of various potential carboxylesterase inhibitors, only **physostigmine** was considered sufficiently potent to possibly inhibit irinotecan activation.[2] In a study in *rats*, **ciclosporin** increased the AUC of irinotecan and SN-38, probably by decreasing biliary excretion.[3] Further study is needed to assess the clinical relevance of these findings.

1. Charasson V, Haaz M-C, Robert J. Determination of drug interactions occurring with the metabolic pathways of irinotecan. *Drug Metab Dispos* (2002) 30, 731–3.
2. Slatter JG, Su P, Sams JP, Schaaf LJ, Wienkers LC. Bioactivation of the anticancer agent CPT-11 to SN-38 by human hepatic microsomal carboxylesterases and the *in vitro* assessment of potential drug interactions. *Drug Metab Dispos* (1997) 25, 1157–64.
3. Gupta E, Safa AR, Wang X, Ratain MJ. Pharmacokinetic modulation of irinotecan and metabolites by cyclosporin A. *Cancer Res* (1996) 56, 1309–14.

Irinotecan + Oxaliplatin

An isolated report suggests that the cholinergic toxicity associated with irinotecan may be enhanced by oxaliplatin.

Clinical evidence, mechanism, importance and management

One of 15 patients given irinotecan 80 mg/m^2 as a 1-hour infusion following an infusion of oxaliplatin 85 mg/m^2 over 2 hours experienced hypersalivation and abdominal pain, which was treated successfully with atropine. In this patient, symptoms did not recur during subsequent treatment with irinotecan alone, nor when drugs were separated by one day, but rechallenge with the original combined regimen produced cholinergic toxicity.[1] The combination of irinotecan with oxaliplatin did not alter the pharmacokinetics of either drug in one study[2] therefore it was suggested that the observed effects in the patient may have been due to a pharmacodynamic interaction.[3] It has been suggested that the cholinergic effects of irinotecan, which is a potent inhibitor of acetylcholinesterase,[4] may be enhanced by oxaliplatin, which may like other alkylating drugs also inhibit acetylcholinesterase.[3] The clinical relevance of this report is unknown. The combination of irinotecan and oxaliplatin has been extensively evaluated in clinical trials, and this appears to be the only report of this problem. However, it has been noted that the prophylactic use of atropine with irinotecan could mask any increased cholinergic toxicity.[3,5] Further study is needed.

1. Valencak J, Raderer M, Kornek GV, Henja MH, Scheithauer W. Irinotecan-related cholinergic syndrome induced by coadministration of oxaliplatin. *J Natl Cancer Inst* (1998) 90, 160.
2. Wasserman E, Cuvier C, Lokiec F, Goldwasser F, Kalla S, Méry-Mignard D, Ouldkaci M, Besmaine A, Dupont-André G, Mahjoubi M, Marty M, Misset JL, Cvitkovic E. Combination of oxaliplatin plus irinotecan in patients with gastrointestinal tumors: results of two independent phase I studies with pharmacokinetics. *J Clin Oncol* (1999) 17, 1751–9.
3. Dodds HM, Bishop JF, Rivory LP. More about: irinotecan-related cholinergic syndrome induced by coadministration of oxaliplatin. *J Natl Cancer Inst* (1999) 91, 91–2.
4. Dodds HM, Rivory LP. The mechanism of the inhibition of acetylcholinesterase by irinotecan (CPT-11)–a lead in explaining the cholinergic toxicity of CPT-11 and its time-course. *Proc Am Assoc Cancer Res* (1998) 39, 327.
5. Cvitkovic E, Marty M, Wasserman E, Cuvier C, Goldwasser F, Misset JL. Re: irinotecan-related cholinergic syndrome induced by coadministration of oxaliplatin. *J Natl Cancer Inst* (1998) 90, 1016–17.

Irinotecan + St John's wort (*Hypericum perforatum*)

St John's wort increases the metabolism of irinotecan, which may decrease its activity.

Clinical evidence

In a randomised crossover study St John's wort decreased the plasma levels of the active metabolite of irinotecan SN-38 by 42%. Myelosuppression was also reduced; with irinotecan alone the leucocyte and neutrophil counts decreased by 56 and 63% respectively, but in the presence of St John's wort the decreases were only 8.6 and 4.3% respectively. In this study, irinotecan was given as a single 350 mg/m^2 intravenous dose every 3 weeks, and during one cycle a St John's wort preparation was given three times daily, beginning 14 days before and stopping 4 days after the irinotecan.[1]

Mechanism

St John's wort induces the cytochrome P450 isoenzyme CYP3A4 and P-glycoprotein, which are both involved in the metabolism of irinotecan. The evidence suggests that St John's wort increases the metabolism of irinotecan to an unknown inactive metabolite, rather than the active SN-38, thereby reducing its effects.[1]

Importance and management

The evidence appears to be limited to this study. Irinotecan has a narrow therapeutic range, and the lower levels of SN-38 suggest that it's activity will be reduced in the presence of St John's wort. It would therefore seem sensible to warn patients who are about to receive irinotecan to avoid St John's wort. It seems likely that **topotecan**, a related drug that is also a substrate for CYP3A4, will be similarly affected, but evidence for this is currently lacking.

1. Mathijssen RHJ, Verweij J, de Bruijn P, Loos WJ, Sparreboom A. Effect of St John's wort on irinotecan metabolism. *J Natl Cancer Inst* (2002) 94, 1247–9.

Letrozole + Cimetidine

The pharmacokinetics of a single 2.5-mg dose of letrozole was unchanged by cimetidine 400 mg 12-hourly in 17 healthy subjects.[1]

1. Morgan JM, Palmisano M, Spencer S, Hirschhorn W, Piraino AJ, Rackley RJ, Choi L. Pharmacokinetic effect of cimetidine on a single 2.5-mg dose of letrozole in healthy subjects. *J Clin Pharmacol* (1996) 36, 852.

Letrozole + Miscellaneous

The UK makers report that in interaction clinical trials there was no evidence of clinically relevant interactions between letrozole and other commonly prescribed drugs (benzodiazepines such as diazepam, barbiturates, diclofenac, furosemide, ibuprofen, omeprazole, paracetamol (acetaminophen)).[1]

1. Femara (Letrozole). Novartis Pharmaceuticals UK Ltd. UK Summary of product characteristics, September 2004.

Lomustine + Theophylline

A single case report describes thrombocytopenia and bleeding attributed to the concurrent use of lomustine and theophylline.

Clinical evidence, mechanism, importance and management

An asthmatic woman taking theophylline and treated for medulloblastoma with lomustine, prednisone and vincristine, developed severe nose bleeding and thrombocytopenia three weeks after the third cycle of chemotherapy.[1] This was attributed to the concurrent use of lomustine and theophylline. The suggested explanation is that theophylline inhibited the activity of phosphodiesterase within the platelets, thereby increasing cyclic AMP levels and disrupting normal platelet function, which seems to be supported by an experimental study,[2] while lomustine causes thrombocytopenia. What is known is far too limited to act as more than a warning of the possibility of increased thrombocytopenia during the concurrent use of theophylline and lomustine.

1. Zeltzer PM, Feig SA. Theophylline-induced lomustine toxicity. *Lancet* (1979) ii, 960–1.
2. DeWys WD, Bathina S. Synergistic anti-tumour effect of cyclic AMP elevation (induced by theophylline) and cytotoxic drug treatment. *Proc Am Assoc Cancer Res* (1978) 19, 104.

Melphalan + Cimetidine

Cimetidine modestly reduces the bioavailability of melphalan.

Clinical evidence, mechanism, importance and management

A study in 8 patients with multiple myeloma or monoclonal gammopathy showed that pretreatment with cimetidine 1 g daily for 6 days reduced the bioavailability of a 10-mg oral dose of melphalan by 30%. The melphalan half-life was reduced from 1.94 to 1.57 hours. The interindividual variation in melphalan pharmacokinetics was high.[1] Note that, because of the variability in melphalan absorption, the dose of oral melphalan is usually cautiously increased until myelosuppression is seen, to ensure therapeutic levels. Therefore, this modest interaction with cimetidine is unlikely to have many clinical consequences.

1. Sviland L, Robinson A, Proctor SJ, Bateman DN. Interaction of cimetidine with oral melphalan. *Cancer Chemother Pharmacol* (1987) 20, 173–5.

Melphalan + Food

The absorption of oral melphalan can be reduced by food.

Clinical evidence, mechanism, importance and management

A study in 10 patients with multiple myeloma showed that the half-life of oral melphalan 5 mg/m^2 was unaffected when taken with a standardised **breakfast**, but the AUC was reduced by 39%. In one patient, no melphalan was detectable in the plasma when given with food. In 8 of the patients who had also been given intravenous melphalan at the same dose, the bioavailability of oral melphalan was calculated to be 85% (range 26% to 96%) when fasting and 58% (7% to 99%) when given with food. The authors recommend that melphalan should not be taken with food.[1] The maker notes that absorption after oral administration is highly variable, and that the dosage should be adjusted based on frequent monitoring of blood counts. They make no specific recommendations about intake in relation to food.[2,3]

1. Reece PA, Kotasek D, Morris RG, Dale BM, Sage RE. The effect of food on oral melphalan absorption. *Cancer Chemother Pharmacol* (1986) 16, 194–7.
2. Alkeran (Melphalan). GlaxoSmithKline. UK Summary of product characteristics, April 2003.
3. Alkeran (Melphalan). GlaxoSmithKline. US Prescribing information, May 2003.

Melphalan + Interferon alfa

Interferon alfa modestly decreases the AUC of melphalan, but melphalan cytotoxicity is possibly increased because of the interferon-induced fever. Clinical trials have shown disparate results for the value of combining interferon alfa with melphalan in multiple myeloma.

Clinical evidence, mechanism, importance and management

The AUC of melphalan 250 microgram/kg in 10 myeloma patients was reduced by 13% when it was given 5 hours after the administration of human interferon alfa (7 x 10^6 units/m^2) possibly due to the fever caused by the interferon.[1] The clinical importance of this is uncertain but the authors of the report suggest that despite this small reduction in the AUC, the cytotoxicity of the melphalan is increased by the fever. The use of interferon alfa with melphalan and prednisone in multiple myeloma showed some gain in survival in subsets of patients in one trial,[2] but no improvement in survival in two others,[3,4] and was associated with more adverse effects.[2-4]

1. Ehrsson H, Eksborg S, Wallin I, Österborg A, Mellstedt H. Oral melphalan pharmacokinetics: influence of interferon-induced fever. *Clin Pharmacol Ther* (1990) 47, 86–90.
2. Österborg A, Björkholm M, Björeman M, Brenning G, Carlson K, Celsing F, Gahrton G, Grimfors G, Gyllenhammar J, Hast R. Natural interferon-α in combination with melphalan/prednisone versus melphalan/prednisone in the treatment of multiple myeloma stages II and III: a randomized study from the Myeloma Group of Central Sweden. *Blood* (1993) 81, 1428–34.
3. Cooper MR, Dear K, McIntyre OR, Ozer H, Ellerton J, Canellos G, Bernhardt B, Duggan D, Faragher D, Schiffer C. A randomized clinical trial comparing melphalan/prednisone with or without interferon alfa-2b in newly diagnosed patients with multiple myeloma: a Cancer and Leukemia Group B study. *J Clin Oncol* (1993) 11, 155–60.
4. The Nordic Myeloma Study Group. Interferon-α 2b added to melphalan-prednisone for initial and maintenance therapy in multiple myeloma: a randomized, controlled trial. *Ann Intern Med* (1996) 124, 212–22.

Methotrexate + Amiodarone

An isolated case report tentatively attributes the development of methotrexate toxicity to additional treatment with amiodarone.

Clinical evidence, mechanism, importance and management

An elderly woman, whose psoriasis was effectively controlled for 2 years with methotrexate, developed ulceration of the psoriatic plaques within 2 weeks of starting treatment with amiodarone. The reason is not understood. A modest increase in her dosage of furosemide is a suggested contributory factor because it might have interfered with the excretion of the methotrexate.[1]

1. Reynolds NJ, Jones SK, Crossley J, Harman RRM. Methotrexate induced skin necrosis: a drug interaction with amiodarone? *BMJ* (1989) 299, 980–1.

Methotrexate + Amphotericin B

Amphotericin B may delay the clearance of methotrexate.

Clinical evidence, mechanism, importance and management

Two children had delayed clearance of methotrexate after pulse therapy (1 g/m^2 over 24 hours) while they were receiving amphotericin B. Methotrexate levels were about 300 to 500% higher 48 hours after methotrexate therapy when they were receiving amphotericin B compared with when they were not.[1] A history of heavy amphotericin B treatment (greater than

30 mg/kg) correlated with decreased methotrexate clearance in 24 children with relapsed leukaemia.[2] Amphotericin B may cause renal impairment, which can result in delayed methotrexate clearance. The adverse effects of methotrexate should be carefully monitored (e.g. patient reported symptoms, LFTs, blood counts) in patients on amphotericin B or those previously extensively treated with the drug. In patients on large doses of methotrexate (e.g. not the weekly doses given for conditions such as rheumatoid arthritis) the monitoring of methotrexate levels is recommended.

1. Parker RI, Mahan RM, Giugliano DA. Delayed methotrexate clearance during treatment with amphotericin B. *Pediatr Res* (2002) 51 (4 part 2), 258A.
2. Wall AM, Gajjar A, Link A, Mahmoud H, Pui C-H, Relling MV. Individualized methotrexate dosing in children with relapsed acute lymphoblastic leukemia. *Leukemia* (2000) 14, 221–5.

Methotrexate + Antibacterials; Aminoglycosides, oral

There is evidence that the gastrointestinal absorption of methotrexate can be reduced by paromomycin, neomycin and possibly other oral aminoglycosides, but increased by kanamycin.

Clinical evidence

A study in 10 patients with small cell bronchogenic carcinoma treated with methotrexate found that when additionally given a range of oral anti-infectives (**paromomycin**, vancomycin, polymyxin B, nystatin) the urinary recovery of methotrexate was reduced by over one-third (from 69 to 44%).[1] The **paromomycin** was believed to have been responsible. In another study the concurrent use of **neomycin** 500 mg four times a day for 3 days reduced the methotrexate AUC and the 72-hour cumulative excretion by 50%.[2] In contrast, the same report suggests that **kanamycin** can increase the absorption of methotrexate, but no details are given.

Mechanism

Paromomycin[3] and neomycin, in common with other oral aminoglycosides, can cause a malabsorption syndrome, which reduces drug absorption. Kanamycin may possibly be different because it causes less malabsorption. It also reduces the activity of the gut flora, which metabolise methotrexate so that more is available for absorption.

Importance and management

The documentation of these interactions is sparse, but it would seem prudent to be on the alert for a reduction in the response to methotrexate if patients are given oral aminoglycosides such as paromomycin or neomycin. An increased response may possibly occur with kanamycin. No interaction would be expected if aminoglycosides are given parenterally.

1. Cohen MH, Creaven PJ, Fossieck BE, Johnston AV, Williams CL. Effect of oral prophylactic broad spectrum nonabsorbable antibiotics on the gastrointestinal absorption of nutrients and methotrexate in small cell bronchogenic carcinoma patients. *Cancer* (1976) 38, 1556–9.
2. Shen DD, Azarnoff D. Clinical pharmacokinetics of methotrexate. *Clin Pharmacokinet* (1978) 3, 1–13.
3. Keusch GT, Troncale FJ, Buchanan RD. Malabsorption due to paromomycin. *Arch Intern Med* (1970) 125, 273–6.

Methotrexate + Antibacterials; Cefotiam

Pancytopenia and pseudomembraneous colitis occurred in a patient on low-dose methotrexate and loxoprofen who was given cefotiam.

Clinical evidence, mechanism, importance and management

An elderly woman who had been treated with low-dose methotrexate 5 mg weekly and loxoprofen for one month developed acute pyelonephritis. Intravenous cefotiam was started, and on day 7 she developed severe watery diarrhoea. Analysis showed pancytopenia and *Clostridium difficile* infection. Methotrexate and cefotiam were stopped, and vancomycin started, and the patient recovered.[1] It was suggested that the combination of the antineoplastic drug and antibacterial increased the risk of *Clostridium difficile* diarrhoea. In addition, the NSAID (see 'Methotrexate + NSAIDs or Paracetamol (Acetaminophen)', p.480) and renal impairment from the pyelonephritis could have contributed to the methotrexate toxicity.[1]

1. Nanke Y, Kotake S, Akama H, Tomii M, Kamatani N. Pancytopenia and colitis with *Clostridium difficile* in a rheumatoid arthritis patient taking methotrexate, antibiotics and non-steroidal anti-inflammatory drugs. *Clin Rheumatol* (2001) 20, 73–5.

Methotrexate + Antibacterials; Ciprofloxacin

A report describes methotrexate toxicity in two patients during concurrent treatment with ciprofloxacin.

Clinical evidence

When 2 patients with osteosarcoma treated with high-dose methotrexate 12 g/m^2 per course were treated with ciprofloxacin 500 mg twice daily, either during or 2 days before the start of the methotrexate course, methotrexate elimination was delayed, resulting in raised serum levels, severe cutaneous toxicity and renal failure. The first patient also had hepatic injury and haematological toxicity. Following increased folinic acid rescue, methotrexate levels normalised after several days. In earlier courses without ciprofloxacin in the first patient and subsequent courses in the second patient, methotrexate elimination was normal.[1] This preliminary report[1] has subsequently been published in full.[2,3]

Mechanism

Not fully understood. Ciprofloxacin may displace methotrexate from its plasma-protein binding sites resulting in a rise in levels of unbound methotrexate. Ciprofloxacin may also cause a decrease in renal clearance of methotrexate.

Importance and management

Information appears to be limited to one report, but it would seem prudent to monitor for raised methotrexate levels if concurrent use is necessary. More study is needed.

1. Dalle JH, Auvrignon A, Vassal G, Leverger G. Possible ciprofloxacin-methotrexate interaction: a report of 2 cases. *Intersci Conf Antimicrob Agents Chemother* (2000) 40, 477.
2. Dalle JH, Auvrignon A, Vassal G, Leverger G, Kalifa C. Interaction méthotrexate–ciprofloxacine: à propos de deux cas d'intoxication sévère. *Arch Pediatr* (2001) 8, 1078–81.
3. Dalle J-H, Auvrignon A, Vassal G, Leverger G. Interaction between methotrexate and ciprofloxacin. *J Pediatr Hematol Oncol* (2002) 24, 321–2.

Methotrexate + Antibacterials; Co-trimoxazole or Trimethoprim

Nine cases of severe bone marrow depression have been reported, two of them fatal, caused by the concurrent use of low-dose methotrexate and treatment doses of co-trimoxazole (sulfamethoxazole + trimethoprim) or trimethoprim. Pancytopenia has also been reported in a few patients treated with high-dose co-trimoxazole shortly after stopping methotrexate.

Clinical evidence

A 61-year-old patient with rheumatoid arthritis, taking methotrexate 7.5 mg once a week, developed generalised bone marrow hypoplasia over 2 months after a 10-day course of treatment with co-trimoxazole for a urinary tract infection. She had taken a total of 775 mg of methotrexate when the hypoplasia appeared.[1] Nine other cases of severe bone marrow depression, two of them fatal,[2,3] have been described in patients on low-dose weekly methotrexate when given co-trimoxazole[2,4-8] or trimethoprim[3,6,9] concurrently. Life-threatening complications (no details given) are said to have occurred in two other patients on low-dose methotrexate given **unnamed sulphonamides**.[10] A 10-year (1981 to 1991) regional survey in Ottawa identified co-trimoxazole as one of four factors associated with serious pancytopenia in patients taking low-dose methotrexate. The other factors were elevated BUN or creatinine levels, increased mean corpuscular volumes and increasing age.[11]

Three cases of severe pancytopenia, one of them fatal, have been reported in patients given high-dose co-trimoxazole for treating *Pneumocystis carinii* infection shortly after stopping low-dose methotrexate therapy.[12-14] A fatal case of severe agranulocytosis and toxic epidermal necrolysis occurred in a patient receiving co-trimoxazole for *Pneumocystis carinii* prophylaxis after high-dose methotrexate therapy.[15]

Mechanism

Not fully understood. Both drugs can suppress the activity of dihydrofolate reductase and it seems possible that they can act additively to produce folate deficiency, which could lead to some of the bone marrow changes seen. Another possible mechanism is that the drugs interact pharmacokinetically. An early study found that the concurrent use of co-trimoxazole had no effect on the pharmacokinetics of methotrexate in children.[16] However, another study reported that co-trimoxazole caused an increase in 'free' concentrations of methotrexate from about 37 to 52% while the renal clearance was more than halved.[17] This was calculated to increase the exposure to methotrexate by 66%.[17] Another sulphonamide, **sulfafurazole** (sulfisoxazole),[18] has been found to cause a small reduction in the clearance of methotrexate by the kidneys.

Importance and management

Information seems to be limited to the reports cited but the methotrexate/co-trimoxazole and methotrexate/trimethoprim interactions are established. Low-dose co-trimoxazole is commonly given to patients on methotrexate as prophylaxis of Pneumocystis carinii pneumonia without problem. This type of patient should be having regular blood monitoring as a matter of course. However, the situation with higher doses of either drug is potentially more hazardous. Some have recommended avoiding the combination. If both drugs must be used, the haematological picture should be very closely monitored because the outcome can be life-threatening.

1. Thomas MH, Gutterman LA. Methotrexate toxicity in a patient receiving trimethoprim-sulfamethoxazole. *J Rheumatol* (1986) 13, 440–1.
2. Groenendal H, Rampen FHJ. Methotrexate and trimethoprim-sulphamethoxazole — a potentially hazardous combination. *Clin Exp Dermatol* (1990) 15, 358–60.
3. Steuer A, Gumpel JM. Methotrexate and trimethoprim: a fatal interaction. *Br J Rheumatol* (1998) 37, 105–6.
4. Thevenet JP, Ristori JM, Cure H, Mizony MH, Bussiere JL. Pancytopénie au cours due traitement d'une polyarthrite rheumatoïde par méthotrexate après administration de triméthoprime-sulfaméthoxazole. *Presse Med* (1987) 16, 1487.
5. Maricic M, Davis M, Gall EP. Megaloblastic pancytopenia in a patient receiving concurrent methotrexate and trimethoprim-sulphamethoxazole treatment. *Arthritis Rheum* (1986) 29, 133–5.
6. Jeurissen ME, Boerbooms AM, van de Putte LB. Pancytopenia and methotrexate with trimethoprim-sulfamethoxazole. *Ann Intern Med* (1989) 111, 261.
7. Liddle BJ, Marsden JR. Drug interactions with methotrexate. *Br J Dermatol* (1989) 120, 582–3.
8. Govert JA, Patton S, Fine RL. Pancytopenia from using trimethoprim and methotrexate. *Ann Intern Med* (1992) 117, 877–8.
9. Ng HWK, Macfarlane AW, Graham RM, Verbov JL. Near fatal drug interactions with methotrexate given for psoriasis. *BMJ* (1987) 295, 752–3.
10. Zachariae H. Methotrexate and non-steroidal anti-inflammatory drugs. *Br J Dermatol* (1992) 126, 95.
11. Al-Awadhi A, Dale P, McKendry RJR. Pancytopenia associated with low dose methotrexate therapy. A regional survey. *J Rheumatol* (1993) 20, 1121–5.
12. Dan M, Shapira I. Possible role of methotrexate in trimethoprim- sulfamethoxazole-induced acute megaloblastic anemia. *Isr J Med Sci* (1984) 20, 262–3.
13. Kobrinsky NL, Ramsay NKC. Acute megaloblastic anemia induced by high-dose trimethoprim-sulfamethoxazole. *Ann Intern Med* (1981) 94, 780–1.
14. Chevrel G, Brantus JF, Sainte-Laudy, Miossec P. Allergic pancytopenia to trimethoprim-sulphamethoxazole for *Pneumocystis carinii* pneumonia following methotrexate treatment for rheumatoid arthritis. *Rheumatology (Oxford)* (1999) 38, 475–6.
15. Yang CH, Yang LJ, Jaing TH, Chan HL. Toxic epidermal necrolysis following combination of methotrexate and trimethoprim-sulfamethoxazole. *Int J Dermatol* (2000) 39, 621–3.
16. Beach BJ, Woods WG, Howell SB. Influence of co-trimoxazole on methotrexate pharmacokinetics in children with acute lymphoblastic leukemia. *Am J Pediatr Hematol Oncol* (1981) 3, 115–19.
17. Ferrazzini G, Klein J, Sulh H, Chung D, Griesbrecht E, Koren G. Interaction between trimethoprim-sulfamethoxazole and methotrexate in children with leukemia. *J Pediatr* (1990) 117, 823–6.
18. Liegler DG, Henderson ES, Hahn MA, Oliverio VT. The effect of organic acids on renal clearance of methotrexate in man. *Clin Pharmacol Ther* (1969) 10, 849–57.

Methotrexate + Antibacterials; Penicillins

Reduced clearance and acute methotrexate toxicity has been attributed to the concurrent use of various penicillins (amoxicillin, benzylpenicillin, carbenicillin, dicloxacillin, flucloxacillin, mezlocillin, oxacillin, penicillin, phenoxymethylpenicillin, piperacillin, ticarcillin) in a small number of case reports.

Clinical evidence

Four patients treated with methotrexate 15 to 60 mg/m² as an intravenous bolus and then 15 to 60 mg by infusion over 36 hours showed a marked reduction in methotrexate clearance when concurrently treated with different penicillins: with **penicillin** [sic] a 36% reduction; with **piperacillin** 67%; with **ticarcillin** 60%; and with **dicloxacillin** plus indometacin 93%. Prolonged folinic acid rescue was necessary.[1] A case of elevated methotrexate levels following **piperacillin** administration has also been described,[2] and acute methotrexate toxicity associated with increased serum levels developed in a 16-year-old when given **amoxicillin** 1 g six-hourly.[3] Increased methotrexate serum levels were seen in another patient when given **carbenicillin** 30 g daily.[4] A marked reduction in methotrexate clearance, accompanied by increased gastrointestinal toxicity, was seen in one patient when concurrently treated with **mezlocillin** 330 mg/kg daily.[5] A comparative study was prompted by the apparent development of methotrexate-induced pneumonitis in a patient given **flucloxacillin**. One of two groups of 10 patients with rheumatoid arthritis on methotrexate 5 to 15 mg weekly was also given **flucloxacillin** 500 mg four times daily. However, **flucloxacillin** had no clinically significant effect on the pharmacokinetics of methotrexate.[6] Five patients on low-dose methotrexate 7.5 to 12.5 mg weekly, for psoriasis or rheumatoid arthritis, developed neutropenia and thrombocytopenia when treated with penicillins (**amoxicillin** with or without clavulanic acid, **benzylpenicillin**, **flucloxacillin**, **piperacillin**). Three of the patients died and the other two required prolonged hospitalisation.[7] A patient on intravenous methotrexate 50 mg weekly, diethylstilbestrol (stilboestrol), prednisone and furosemide, developed severe toxicity within a week of starting **phenoxymethylpenicillin** 250 mg on alternate days.[8] In another case, administration of **oxacillin** 1 g 8-hourly starting 6 hours after high-dose methotrexate (15 g by intravenous infusion) resulted in a plasma methotrexate level that was 53 times higher than at the same time after a previous methotrexate cycle. Acute renal failure and aplastic anaemia occurred and the patient died.[9] A survey of the Wyeth/Lederle safety database in 1996 identified two additional unpublished cases of methotrexate toxicity (aplastic anaemia, thrombocytopenia, pneumonitis) in patients who had recently started penicillins.[10]

Mechanism

It is thought that weak acids such as the penicillins can possibly successfully compete with methotrexate in the kidney tubules for excretion so that the methotrexate is retained, thereby increasing its effects and its toxicity.[11] However, this was not demonstrated in the study of flucloxacillin above,[6] and the mechanism has been disputed.[12]

Importance and management

Information seems to be limited to the reports cited here, which would seem to indicate that serious interactions between methotrexate and penicillins are uncommon. It is not known why only a few patients have been affected and what other factors may have contributed, but the problem does not seem to be confined to patients on high-dose methotrexate. There is not enough evidence to forbid concurrent use (although some do advise against it[13]), but close monitoring is obviously advisable. One published recommendation is to carry out twice-weekly platelet and white cell counts for two weeks initially, with the measurement of methotrexate levels if toxicity is suspected. Folinic acid (leucovorin) rescue should be available.[7] For the general CSM guidelines on the use of methotrexate see 'Importance and management' in 'Methotrexate + NSAIDs or Paracetamol (Acetaminophen)', p.480.

1. Bloom EJ, Ignoffo RJ, Reis CA, Cadman E. Delayed clearance (CL) of methotrexate (MTX) associated with antibiotics and anti-inflammatory agents. *Clin Res* (1986) 34, 560A.
2. Yamamoto K, Sawada Y, Matsushita U, Moriwaki K, Bessho F, Iga T. Delayed elimination of methotrexate associated with piperacillin. *Ann Pharmacother* (1997) 31, 1261–2.
3. Ronchera CL, Hernández T, Peris JE, Torres F, Granero L, Jiménez NV, Plá JM. Pharmacokinetic interaction between high-dose methotrexate and amoxycillin. *Ther Drug Monit* (1993) 15, 375–9.
4. Gibson DL, Bleyer AW, Savitch JL. Carbenicillin potentiation of methotrexate plasma concentration during high dose methotrexate therapy. American Society of Hospital Pharmacists. Mid year clinical meeting abstracts, New Orleans, Dec 1981. p. 111.
5. Dean R, Nachman J, Lorenzana AN. Possible methotrexate-mezlocillin interaction. *Am J Pediatr Hematol Oncol* (1992) 14, 88–9.
6. Herrick AL, Grennan DM, Giriffen K, Aarons L, Gifford LA. Lack of interaction between flucloxacillin and methotrexate in patients with rheumatoid arthritis. *Br J Clin Pharmacol* (1996) 41, 223–7.
7. Mayall B, Poggi G, Parkin JD. Neutropenia due to low-dose methotrexate therapy for psoriasis and rheumatoid arthritis may be fatal. *Med J Aust* (1991) 155, 480–4.
8. Nierenberg DW, Mamelok RD. Toxic reaction to methotrexate in a patient receiving penicillin and furosemide: a possible interaction. *Arch Dermatol* (1983) 119, 449–50.
9. Titier K, Lagrange F, Péhourcq F, Moore N, Molimard M. Pharmacokinetic interaction between high-dose methotrexate and oxacillin. *Ther Drug Monit* (2002) 24, 570–2.
10. Wyeth/Lederle. Personal communication, July 1996.
11. Iven H, Brasch H. Influence of the antibiotics piperacillin, doxycycline, and tobramycin on the pharmacokinetics of methotrexate in rabbits. *Cancer Chemother Pharmacol* (1986) 17, 218–22.

12. Herrick AL, Grennan DM, Aarons L. Lack of interaction between methotrexate and penicillins. *Rheumatology (Oxford)* (1999) 38, 284–5.
13. Dawson JK, Abernethy VE, Lynch MP. Methotrexate and penicillin interaction. *Br J Rheumatol* (1998) 37, 807.

Methotrexate + Antibacterials; Pristinamycin

An isolated report describes severe methotrexate toxicity in a patient when treated with pristinamycin.

Clinical evidence

A 13-year-old boy with acute lymphoblastic leukaemia had a relapse and began a series of regimens with high-dose methotrexate in combination with other drugs including dexamethasone, mercaptopurine, vincristine, cytarabine and asparaginase, tioguanine (thioguanine) and ifosfamide. During a late cycle when he was also taking pristinamycin 2 g daily for a staphylococcal infection, the clearance of the methotrexate became markedly decreased (half-life prolonged from 6 to 203 hours). He developed severe methotrexate toxicity (oral mucositis, anusitis, balanitis, neutropenia and thrombocytopenia) and was given folinic acid rescue and haemodialysis.[1]

Mechanism

Not understood, but on the basis of experimental evidence the authors of the report excluded the possibilities of kidney impairment or reduction by the pristinamycin of liver metabolism.[1]

Importance and management

This appears to be the first and only report of an interaction between methotrexate and a macrolide antibacterial. Its general importance is unknown but the authors strongly advise the avoidance of pristinamycin in patients treated with methotrexate, and caution with other macrolides.[1]

1. Thyss A, Milano G, Renée N, Cassuto-Viguier E, Jambou P, Soler C. Severe interaction between methotrexate and a macrolide-like antibiotic. *J Natl Cancer Inst* (1993) 85, 582–3.

Methotrexate + Antibacterials; Tetracyclines

Two case reports describe the development of methotrexate toxicity in patients additionally given tetracycline or doxycycline.

Clinical evidence, mechanism, importance and management

A man being successfully and uneventfully treated for psoriasis with methotrexate 25 mg weekly was additionally started on **tetracycline** 500 mg four times daily for a mycoplasmal infection. Within 5 days he developed recurrent fever, ulcerative stomatitis and diarrhoea. His white cell count fell to 1000 and his platelet count to 30,000 (units not stated, previous counts not given), all signs of methotrexate toxicity. The problem resolved when the methotrexate was withdrawn, but the psoriasis returned.[1] A 17-year-old girl with osteosarcoma of the femur was given **doxycycline** 100 mg every 12 hours for an abscess in her left eye at the same time as her eleventh cycle of high-dose methotrexate with folinic acid rescue. Elevated plasma methotrexate levels were observed and she developed haematological toxicity and severe vomiting requiring antiemetics, continued folinic acid, a prolonged stay in hospital and postponement of her next dose of methotrexate. **Doxycycline** had not been taken during the first 10 cycles of methotrexate therapy and the pharmacokinetic changes and symptoms seen in the eleventh cycle were attributed to concurrent **doxycycline**.[2] This interaction has also been observed in *mice*,[3] but not *rabbits*.[4] Displacement of the methotrexate from its binding sites may be part of the explanation. There appears to be the only two clinical reports of this interaction on record. Concurrent use need not be avoided, but it should be well monitored.

1. Turck M. Successful psoriasis treatment then sudden 'cytotoxicity'. *Hosp Pract* (1984) 19, 175–6.
2. Tortajada-Ituren JJ, Ordovás-Baines JP, Llopis-Salvia P, Jiménez-Torres NV. High-dose methotrexate-doxycycline interaction. *Ann Pharmacother* (1999) 33, 804–8.
3. Dixon RL. The interaction between various drugs and methotrexate. *Toxicol Appl Pharmacol* (1968) 12, 308.
4. Iven H, Brasch H. Influence of the antibiotics piperacillin, doxycycline, and tobramycin on the pharmacokinetics of methotrexate in rabbits. *Cancer Chemother Pharmacol* (1986) 17, 218–22.

Methotrexate + Antibacterials; Vancomycin

Delayed excretion and toxicity was seen after high-dose methotrexate in two patients recently treated with vancomycin.

Clinical evidence, mechanism, importance and management

Two patients treated with a chemotherapy regimen containing high-dose methotrexate had delayed methotrexate excretion and methotrexate toxicity during a cycle soon after they had received vancomycin. Methotrexate levels took 170 to 231 hours to fall to 200 micromol/ml, and toxicity (mucositis) occurred. Subclinical renal impairment was found, which subsequently improved. In previous and subsequent cycles, where vancomycin was not given, serum methotrexate levels in both patients fell to 200 micromol/ml within 48 to 96 hours.[1] It was suggested that vancomycin caused subclinical nephrotoxicity, which resulted in delayed excretion of methotrexate, which is primarily renally excreted.[1] Vancomycin is commonly used in oncology patients with febrile neutropenia, and this appears to be the first report of this interaction. The authors suggest that it would be prudent to measure glomerular filtration rate before high-dose methotrexate administration in patients recently treated with vancomycin, to allow modification of the methotrexate dose if necessary.[1] Further study is needed.

1. Blum R, Seymour JF, Toner G. Significant impairment of high-dose methotrexate clearance following vancomycin administration in the absence of overt renal impairment. *Ann Oncol* (2002) 13, 327–30.

Methotrexate + Anticonvulsants

Anticonvulsant therapy appears to increase the clearance of methotrexate given as a 24-hour infusion, and is associated with lower efficacy of combination therapy for B-lineage leukaemia.

Clinical evidence, mechanism, importance and management

In a retrospective survey, long-term anticonvulsant therapy (**phenytoin, phenobarbital, carbamazepine**, or a combination) was associated with worse event-free survival, and greater haematological relapse and CNS relapse in children receiving chemotherapy for B-lineage acute lymphoblastic leukaemia. Faster clearance of high-dose methotrexate given as a 24-hour infusion was found in those receiving these anticonvulsants, but clearance of short 4 to 6-hour methotrexate infusions did not appear to be affected, neither was weekly low-dose methotrexate.[1] Further study is needed.

Note that reduced phenytoin and carbamazepine levels, but unaltered phenobarbital levels, have been reported in various case reports of patients receiving chemotherapy including methotrexate, see 'Table 11.2', (p.331).

1. Relling MV, Pui C-H, Sandlund JT, Rivera GK, Hancock ML, Boyett JM, Schuetz EG, Evans WE. Adverse effect of anticonvulsants on efficacy of chemotherapy for acute lymphoblastic leukaemia. *Lancet* (2000) 356, 285–90.

Methotrexate + Ascorbic acid (Vitamin C)

A study in a single patient showed that the urinary excretion of methotrexate was not significantly changed by the concurrent ingestion of large amounts of vitamin C.

Clinical evidence, mechanism, importance and management

Vitamin C 1 g three times daily was found to have no effect on the urinary excretion of methotrexate 45 mg given intravenously to a woman with breast cancer, despite the urine becoming more acidic at pH 5.9 (compare 'Methotrexate + Urinary alkalinisers', p.484). She was also receiving oral cyclophosphamide, propranolol, amitriptyline, perphenazine and prochlorperazine.[1] No special precautions appear to be necessary.

1. Sketris IS, Farmer PS, Fraser A. Effect of vitamin C on the excretion of methotrexate. *Cancer Treat Rep* (1984) 68, 446–7.

Methotrexate + Chloroquine or Hydroxychloroquine

Chloroquine caused a moderate reduction in the AUC of methotrexate in one study. Conversely, hydroxychloroquine caused a minor increase in methotrexate AUC in another study.

Clinical evidence, mechanism, importance and management

Eleven patients with rheumatoid arthritis taking regular weekly low doses of methotrexate 15 mg were studied after a single dose of methotrexate alone and after methotrexate plus chloroquine 250 mg. The chloroquine reduced the maximum plasma levels of the methotrexate by 20% and its AUC by 28%. The suggested reason is that the absorption of the methotrexate from the gut is reduced in some way.[1] These reductions would be expected to reduce both the toxicity and the efficacy of the methotrexate, but the clinical importance of this interaction awaits assessment.

In contrast, hydroxychloroquine 200 mg increased the AUC of methotrexate 15 mg by 52%, while still slightly decreasing the maximum methotrexate level (by 17%), in a randomised crossover study in 10 healthy subjects.[2] The authors considered that the increased AUC could explain the increased efficacy of the combination in rheumatoid arthritis, while the decreased maximum level could explain the reduction in acute liver toxicity.[2] Extra caution should be taken when using the combination. Further study is needed.

1. Seideman P, Albertioni F, Beck O, Eksborg S, Peterson C. Chloroquine reduces the bioavailability of methotrexate in patients with rheumatoid arthritis. A possible mechanism of reduced hepatotoxicity. *Arthritis Rheum* (1994) 37, 830–3.

2. Carmichael SJ, Beal J, Day RO, Tett SE. Combination therapy with methotrexate and hydroxychloroquine for rheumatoid arthritis increases exposure to methotrexate. *J Rheumatol* (2002) 29, 2077–83.

Methotrexate + Cisplatin

The risk of methotrexate toxicity appears to be markedly increased by previous treatment with cisplatin. Methotrexate levels should be monitored and folinic acid rescue therapy administered as necessary.

Clinical evidence, mechanism, importance and management

Six out of 106 patients developed clinical signs of methotrexate toxicity and died 6 to 13 days after receiving standard-dose methotrexate (20 to 50 mg/m²) in the absence of signs of renal dysfunction and despite having previously been treated with methotrexate without serious toxicity. All had received prior treatment with cisplatin. Four of the patients were regarded as good-risk (i.e. methotrexate toxicity was not considered likely as they did not have renal or hepatic impairment, and their general condition was good).[1] A study in children and adolescents suggested that those who had received a cumulative dose of cisplatin greater than 360 mg/m² showed delayed methotrexate clearance and a greater risk of methotrexate toxicity.[2] Similarly, a further report by the same authors in 14 patients on high-dose methotrexate[3] indicated that prior treatment with one course of cisplatin sharply increased the serum levels of methotrexate, particularly if the cumulative cisplatin dose exceeded 400 mg/m².

The picture is not totally clear but it seems possible that prior treatment with cisplatin causes kidney damage that may not necessarily be detectable with the usual creatinine clearance tests. The effect is to cause a marked reduction in the clearance of the methotrexate. The serum methotrexate levels of these patients should be closely monitored so that any delay in its clearance is detected early and folinic acid rescue therapy can be administered.[2] This appears to prevent serious toxicity.[1-3]

1. Haim N, Kedar A, Robinson E. Methotrexate-related deaths in patients previously treated with *cis*-diamminedichloride platinum. *Cancer Chemother Pharmacol* (1984) 13, 223–5.

2. Crom WR, Pratt CB, Green AA, Champion JE, Crom DB, Stewart CF, Evans WE. The effect of prior cisplatin therapy on the pharmacokinetics of high-dose methotrexate. *J Clin Oncol* (1984) 2, 655–61.

3. Crom WR, Teresi ME, Meyer WH, Green AA, Evans WE. The intrapatient effect of cisplatin therapy on the pharmacokinetics of high-dose methotrexate. *Drug Intell Clin Pharm* (1985) 19, 467.

Methotrexate + Colestyramine

The serum methotrexate levels of three patients given methotrexate by infusion were markedly reduced by the concurrent use of colestyramine.

Clinical evidence

An 11-year-old girl with osteosarcoma who developed colitis when treated with high-dose intravenous methotrexate, was subsequently treated with colestyramine 2 g six-hourly from 6 to 48 hours after the methotrexate. Serum methotrexate concentrations at 24 hours were approximately halved. A marked fall in serum methotrexate levels were seen in another patient similarly treated.[1] Colestyramine similarly reduced methotrexate levels in a case of toxicity in another patient.[2]

Mechanism

Methotrexate undergoes enterohepatic recirculation, that is to say it is excreted into the gut in the bile and re-absorbed further along the gut. If colestyramine is given orally, it can bind strongly to the methotrexate in the gut, thereby preventing its reabsorption and, as a result, the serum levels fall.[1,3]

Importance and management

The documentation seems to be limited. In the cases cited the colestyramine was deliberately used to reduce serum methotrexate levels, but in some circumstances it might represent an unwanted interaction. Since methotrexate is excreted into the gut in the bile, separating the oral dosages of the colestyramine and methotrexate may not necessarily prevent their coming into contact and interacting together. Monitor concurrent use.

1. Erttmann R, Landbeck G. Effect of oral cholestyramine on the elimination of high-dose methotrexate. *J Cancer Res Clin Oncol* (1985) 110, 48–50.
2. Shinozaki T, Watanabe H, Tomidokoro R, Yamamoto K, Horiuchi R, Takagishi K. Successful rescue by oral cholestyramine of a patient with methotrexate nephrotoxicity: nonrenal excretion of serum methotrexate. *Med Pediatr Oncol* (2000) 34, 226–8.
3. McAnena OJ, Ridge JA, Daly JM. Alteration of methotrexate metabolism in rats by administration of an elemental liquid diet. II. Reduced toxicity and improved survival using cholestyramine. *Cancer* (1987) 59, 1091–7.

Methotrexate + Corticosteroids

Methotrexate clearance may be modestly reduced by long-term prednisolone, but methotrexate does not alter prednisolone pharmacokinetics. Limited evidence suggests methotrexate may alter prednisone levels. Dexamethasone may increase the acute hepatotoxicity of high-dose methotrexate.

Clinical evidence, mechanism, importance and management

There is some evidence that **prednisolone** may reduce the clearance of methotrexate: patients on long-term **prednisolone** 15 mg daily had a 20% lower clearance of intramuscular methotrexate 10 mg and a 30% higher AUC than patients given **prednisolone** 15 mg daily for just 4 days before the methotrexate, or those not given corticosteroids.[1] In another study, methotrexate had no effect on **prednisolone** pharmacokinetics in 7 patients or **methylprednisolone** pharmacokinetics in one patient.[2] Preliminary findings of another study suggested that methotrexate may increase plasma methylprednisone levels after **prednisone**; in 2 of 4 patients given methotrexate, plasma methylprednisone levels remained stable despite a decrease in **prednisone** dose.[3] These findings require confirmation. Their clinical relevance is uncertain.

Dexamethasone may increase the acute hepatotoxicity of high-dose methotrexate. A retrospective comparison in children with brain tumours treated with methotrexate alone (24 patients) or with **dexamethasone** (33 patients), found that no serious brain oedema occurred in either of the groups and there were no differences in bone marrow toxicity or mucositis, but liver enzymes were significantly higher in the **dexamethasone** group indicating liver toxicity. AST levels were 76 compared with 19 units/l, and ALT levels were 140 compared with 39 units/l. This effect was not due to differences in serum methotrexate levels.[4] The authors recommend that **dexamethasone** should not be included in high-dose methotrexate protocols for children with brain tumours when they are not glucocorticoid dependent.[4]

1. Lafforgue P, Monjanel-Mouterde S, Durand A, Catalin J, Acquaviva PC. Is there an interaction between low doses of corticosteroids and methotrexate in patients with rheumatoid arthritis? A pharmacokinetic study in 33 patients. *J Rheumatol* (1993) 20, 263–7.
2. Glynn-Barnhart AM, Erzurum SC, Leff JA, Martin RJ, Cochran JE, Cott GR, Szefler SJ. Effect of low-dose methotrexate on the disposition of glucocorticoids and theophylline. *J Allergy Clin Immunol* (1991) 88, 180–6.
3. Sockin SM, Ostro MG, Goldman MA, Bloch KJ. The effect of methotrexate on plasma prednisolone levels in steroid dependent asthmatics. *J Allergy Clin Immunol* (1992) 89, 286.
4. Wolff JEA, Hauch H, Kühl J, Egeler RM, Jürgens H. Dexamethasone increases hepatotoxicity of MTX in children with brain tumours. *Anticancer Res* (1998) 18, 2895–9.

Methotrexate + Diuretics

Some very limited evidence suggests that triamterene may possibly increase the bone marrow suppressive effects of methotrexate. It seems doubtful if thiazides interact adversely.

Clinical evidence, mechanism, importance and management

A 57 year-old woman who had been treated for several years with daily doses of diclofenac 150 mg, atenolol 50 mg and **triamterene/hydrochlorothiazide** 50/25 mg, for rheumatoid arthritis and hypertension, was additionally started on methotrexate 5 mg weekly. After 2 months she was admitted to hospital with pancytopenia, extensive mucosal ulceration and renal impairment. The authors point out that **triamterene** is structurally similar to folate and has anti-folate activity, which may therefore have been additive with the effects of methotrexate,[1] but the diclofenac may also have contributed (see 'Methotrexate + NSAIDs or Paracetamol (Acetaminophen)', p.480). In 1998, the maker noted there were two other reports of pancytopenia in patients on methotrexate and **triamterene**, but again the patients were also taking NSAIDs.[2]

A study in 9 patients showed that neither **furosemide** nor **hydroflumethiazide** had any effect on the clearance of methotrexate in the urine.[3] However, a study in women with breast cancer, treated with methotrexate, cyclophosphamide and fluorouracil found that the concurrent use of a **thiazide diuretic** appeared to increase the myelosuppressant effects, but it is not clear which of the antineoplastics might have been affected.[4]

1. Richmond R, McRorie ER, Ogden DA, Lambert CM. Methotrexate and triamterene — a potentially fatal combination. *Ann Rheum Dis* (1997) 56, 209–10.
2. Wyeth/Lederle. Data on file, September 1998.
3. Kristensen LØ, Weismann K, Hutters L. Renal function and the rate of disappearance of methotrexate from serum. *Eur J Clin Pharmacol* (1975) 8, 439–44.
4. Orr LE. Potentiation of myelosuppression from cancer chemotherapy and thiazide diuretics. *Drug Intell Clin Pharm* (1981) 15, 967–70.

Methotrexate + Fluorouracil

Two patients on low-dose methotrexate had a toxic skin reaction when they started to use a cream containing fluorouracil. The activity of systemic treatment with methotrexate and fluorouracil are said to be dependent on the order in which the two drugs are given, but this does not appear to be important in the commonly used CMF regimen.

Clinical evidence, mechanism, importance and management

(a) Topical fluorouracil

Two patients with rheumatoid arthritis on low-dose methotrexate 7.5 to 12.5 mg weekly for 6 to 14 months were given 2% fluorouracil cream for actinic keratosis. Within 2 to 3 days both patients developed erythema, blister formation and necrosis. The cream was stopped and the lesions healed over the next 2 to 3 weeks.[1] It would seem that concurrent use should be avoided.

(b) Systemic fluorouracil

In vitro and *animal* data indicate that methotrexate and fluorouracil can be mutually antagonistic under certain conditions.[2-4] Other studies indicate that the sequence (methotrexate first)[5,6] is important for additive or synergistic activity. Note that the combination of cyclophosphamide, methotrexate and fluorouracil (CMF) has been the most commonly used adjuvant therapy in breast cancer, and the sequence of administration is said not to be important.[7]

1. Blackburn WD, Alarcón GS. Toxic response to topical fluorouracil in two rheumatoid arthritis patients receiving low dose weekly methotrexate. *Arthritis Rheum* (1990) 33, 303–4.
2. Tattersall MNH, Jackson RC, Connors TA, Harrap KR. Combination chemotherapy: the interaction of methotrexate and 5-fluorouracil. *Eur J Cancer* (1973) 9, 733–9.
3. Maugh TH. Cancer chemotherapy: an unexpected drug interaction. *Science* (1976) 194, 310.
4. Waxman S, Bruckner H. Antitumour drug interactions: additional data. *Science* (1976) 194, 672.
5. Bertino JR, Sawicki WL, Lindquist CA, Gupta VS. Schedule-dependent antitumor effects of methotrexate and 5-fluorouracil. *Cancer Res* (1977) 37, 327–8.
6. Brown I, Ward HWC. Therapeutic consequences of antitumour drug interactions: methotrexate and 5-fluorouracil in the chemotherapy of C3H mice with transplanted mammary adenocarcinoma. *Cancer Lett* (1978) 5, 291–7.
7. Summerhayes M, Daniels S, eds. Practical Chemotherapy: A Multidisciplinary Guide. 1st ed. UK: Radcliffe Medical Press; 2003 P. 91.

Methotrexate + Folic acid or Folinic acid

Folic acid or folinic acid are sometimes added to low-dose methotrexate treatment for rheumatoid arthritis or psoriasis to reduce adverse effects. Folinic acid is frequently used as an antidote to high-dose methotrexate in cancer therapy. Patients on methotrexate should avoid the inadvertent use of folates in multivitamin preparations.

Clinical evidence, mechanism, importance and management

Methotrexate acts as a folic acid antagonist by reversibly binding to the enzyme dihydrofolate reductase so blocking the conversion of folic acid to tetrahydrofolate. Therefore folic acid and folinic acid (a derivative of tetrahydrofolate) would be expected to interfere with the effects (toxic and therapeutic) of methotrexate.

Folic acid or folinic acid are commonly used to reduce the side effects of low-dose methotrexate treatment for rheumatoid arthritis and psoriasis, although the optimum doses and schedules to maximise tolerability and efficacy remain to be determined.

Similarly, folinic acid is used in conjunction with high-dose methotrexate therapy for various cancers to minimise toxicity, when it is typically started 24 hours after methotrexate administration (folinic acid or 'leucovorin' rescue). In this setting, the antidote effect is clearly influenced by the dose of folinate in relation to the dose of methotrexate, and the timing of folinate administration in relation to methotrexate administration.

Patients taking methotrexate for any indication should avoid the inadvertent/unsupervised use of folates, which are commonly found in multivitamin preparations.

Methotrexate + Food

Absorption of low-dose oral methotrexate appears not to be significantly affected by food.

Clinical evidence, mechanism, importance and management

The peak serum methotrexate levels (measured at 1.5 hours) of 10 children with lymphoblastic leukaemia, following an oral dose of 15 mg/m^2 were reduced by about 40% when taken with a **milky meal** (milk, cornflakes, sugar, white bread and butter). The 4-hour AUC was reduced by about 25%. A smaller reduction was seen after a '**citrus meal**' (orange juice, fresh orange, white bread, butter and jam).[1] However a 4-hour study is too short to assess the extent of the total absorption. Another study in 16 other children given methotrexate 8 to 22.7 mg/m^2 found that peak levels and AUC were not significantly affected if methotrexate was given before a meal.[2] Yet another study in 12 healthy subjects found that a **high fat-content breakfast** delayed the absorption of methotrexate 7.5 mg orally by about 30 minutes but the extent of the absorption was unchanged.[3] No special precautions appear to be necessary.

1. Pinkerton CR, Welshman SG, Glasgow JFT, Bridges JM. Can food influence the absorption of methotrexate in children with acute lymphoblastic leukaemia? *Lancet* (1980) 2, 944–6.
2. Madanat F, Awidi A, Shaheen O, Ottman S, Al-Turk W. Effects of food and gender on the pharmacokinetics of methotrexate in children. *Res Commun Chem Pathol Pharmacol* (1987) 55, 279–82.
3. Kozloski GD, De Vito JM, Kisicki JC, Johnson JB. The effect of food on the absorption of methotrexate sodium tablets in healthy volunteers. *Arthritis Rheum* (1992) 35, 761–4.

Methotrexate + Miscellaneous

Animal studies suggested that the toxicity of methotrexate might be increased by the use of chloramphenicol, aminosalicylic acid, sodium salicylate, sulfametoxypyridazine, tetracycline or tolbutamide, but confirmation of this in man has only been seen with the salicylates, sulphonamides and possibly tetracycline.

Clinical evidence, mechanism, importance and management

Some lists, reviews and books on interactions say that the drugs listed above interact with methotrexate, apparently based largely on the preliminary findings of a study in which male *mice* were treated for 5 days with each of 4 doses of methotrexate (1.53 to 12.25 mg/kg intravenously) and immediately afterwards with non-toxic intraperitoneal doses of the drugs listed. These drugs were said to decrease the lethal dose and/or decrease the survival time of the *mice*.[1] That is to say, the toxicity of the methotrexate was increased. The reasons are not understood, but it is suggested that displacement of the methotrexate from its plasma protein binding sites could result in a rise in the levels of unbound and active methotrexate, and in the case of **sodium salicylate** to a decrease in renal clearance.

These *animal* studies were done in 1968. Since then the clinical importance of the interaction with **salicylates** has been confirmed (see 'Methotrexate + NSAIDs or Paracetamol (Acetaminophen)', below); there are a few cases involving sulphonamides (**sulfamethoxazole** in the form of '**co-trimoxazole**', see (p.475)); and there are two isolated case report of an interaction with '**tetracyclines**', (p.477), but there appears to be no direct clinical evidence of interactions between methotrexate and **chloramphenicol** or **tolbutamide**. The results of *animal* experiments cannot be applied directly and uncritically to man and it now seems probable that some of these suggested or alleged interactions are more theoretical than real.

1. Dixon RL. The interaction between various drugs and methotrexate. *Toxicol Appl Pharmacol* (1968) 12, 308.

Methotrexate + Nitrous oxide

Methotrexate-induced stomatitis and other toxic effects may be increased by the use of nitrous oxide.

Clinical evidence, mechanism, importance and management

A study in which intravenous methotrexate, cyclophosphamide and fluorouracil (CMF) were used within 36 hours of mastectomy suggested that stomatitis may be caused by a toxic interaction between methotrexate and nitrous oxide used during anaesthesia. Stomatitis was much more common in those receiving CMF within 6 hours of surgery.[1-3] A possible reason is that the effects of methotrexate on tetrahydrofolate metabolism are increased by nitrous oxide, and this has been confirmed in *animals*.[4] It was found that the incidence of stomatitis, severe leucopenia, thrombocytopenia, and of severe systemic and local infections could be reduced by giving calcium folinate (leucovorin) and intravenous hydration.[2,3] Alternatively, the use of nitrous oxide shortly before methotrexate administration should be avoided.[4]

1. Ludwig Breast Cancer Study Group. Toxic effects of early adjuvant chemotherapy for breast cancer. *Lancet* (1983) ii, 542–4.
2. Goldhirsch A, Gelber RD, Tattersall MNH, Rudenstam C-M, Cavalli F. Methotrexate/nitrous-oxide toxic interaction in perioperative chemotherapy for early breast cancer. *Lancet* (1987) ii, 151.
3. Ludwig Breast Cancer Study Group. On the safety of perioperative adjuvant chemotherapy with cyclophosphamide, methotrexate and 5-fluorouracil in breast cancer. *Eur J Cancer Clin Oncol* (1988) 24, 1305–8.
4. Ermens AAM, Schoester M, Spijkers LJM, Lindemans J, Abels J. Toxicity of methotrexate in rats preexposed to nitrous oxide. *Cancer Res* (1989) 49, 6337–41.

Methotrexate + NSAIDs or Paracetamol (Acetaminophen)

Increased methotrexate toxicity, sometimes life-threatening, has been seen in few patients concurrently treated with some NSAIDs whereas other patients have been treated uneventfully. The pharmacokinetics of methotrexate can also be changed by some NSAIDs (aspirin, choline magnesium trisalicylate, etodolac, etoricoxib, ibuprofen, metamizole sodium, naproxen, rofecoxib, sodium salicylate, tolmetin). The development of toxicity may be dose related and the risk appears to be lowest in those taking low-dose methotrexate for psoriasis or rheumatoid arthritis with normal renal function.

Clinical evidence

(a) Aminophenazone

Megaloblastic pancytopenia occurred in a woman with rheumatoid arthritis given methotrexate 15 mg weekly and aminophenazone 1 to 1.5 g daily.[1]

(b) Aspirin and other salicylates

A study in 15 rheumatoid arthritis patients given a single 10-mg bolus dose of methotrexate, either with or without aspirin 975 mg four times daily, found that the methotrexate clearance was reduced by aspirin (systemic clearance about 16%, renal clearance of unbound methotrexate about 30%). Also the unbound fraction of methotrexate was higher in patients when taking aspirin. Despite these changes no acute toxicity was seen.[2] Another study found that aspirin did not affect the pharmacokinetics of methotrexate.[3] Yet another study found that, although aspirin did not alter the pharmacokinetics of methotrexate, it did increase the AUC of the metabolite 7-hydroxymethotrexate.[4]

A study in 4 patients found that the renal clearance of methotrexate was reduced by 35% by an infusion of **sodium salicylate** (2 g initially, then 33 mg/minute).[5] A further study found that **choline magnesium trisalicylate** reduced methotrexate clearance, compared with paracetamol (acetaminophen), by 24 to 41%, and increased the unbound fraction by 28%.[6]

Lethal pancytopenia in 2 patients given methotrexate and aspirin prompted a retrospective survey of the records of other patients treated with intra-arterial infusions of methotrexate 50 mg daily for 10 days for epidermoid carcinoma of the oral cavity. Six out of 7 who developed a rapid and serious pancytopenia were found to have had aspirin or other salicylates.[7] Similar results were found in studies on *mice*.[7] There are other case reports[8,9] of methotrexate toxicity in patients taking salicylates but whether a causal relationship exists is uncertain. It has been suggested that pneumonitis in patients on low-dose methotrexate may have resulted from the concurrent use of aspirin 4 to 5 g daily.[10]

See also the report about the comparative use of aspirin and other NSAIDs in section (v), below, on NSAIDs in general.

(c) Azapropazone

A woman given methotrexate 25 mg weekly for 4 years for psoriasis showed acute toxicity (oral and genital ulceration, bone marrow failure) shortly after starting to take azapropazone (reducing from a dose of 2.4 g on the first day, 1.8 g on the second day to 1.2 g daily for a week). She was also taking aspirin 300 mg daily.[11,12]

(d) Bromfenac

In a short-term study, 10 patients taking methotrexate weekly were given bromfenac 50 mg three times daily for 6 days. No significant changes were seen in either the pharmacokinetics of bromfenac, or methotrexate. However, the AUC of the major metabolite of methotrexate, 7-hydroxymethotrexate, was increased by 30% and its renal clearance was reduced by 16%. Eight of the patients had mild to moderate adverse effects and one patient had to withdraw because of moderate hypertension. No patient showed clinically important abnormal laboratory test results.[13] Note that systemic bromfenac has been withdrawn from the market because of reports of hepatic failure.

(e) Celecoxib

Fourteen female patients with rheumatoid arthritis taking methotrexate 5 to 20 mg weekly for at least 3 months were additionally given celecoxib 200 mg or a placebo twice daily for a week. It was found that the maximum serum levels of the methotrexate, its AUC, renal clearance and other pharmacokinetic parameters were unchanged by the celecoxib.[14] The authors note that, in clinical trials, celecoxib was taken in combination with low-dose methotrexate for up to 12 weeks by over 450 patients, and the incidence of adverse effects was similar to that in patients taking methotrexate with placebo.[14]

(f) Diclofenac

A study found that diclofenac 100 mg daily did not affect the pharmacokinetics of methotrexate,[3] however 5 patients on low-dose methotrexate

7.5 to 12.5 mg weekly for psoriasis or rheumatoid arthritis developed serious/fatal neutropenias. These cases probably involved other drug interactions, but diclofenac may have been an additional factor in two of them.[15] Other cases involving diclofenac are mentioned in the sections on indometacin (k) and ketoprofen (l).

(g) Etodolac

A pharmacokinetic study in patients with rheumatoid arthritis found that etodolac 600 mg daily did not affect the AUC of methotrexate, but duration of exposure was lengthened (mean residence time increased from 8.5 to 11.4 hours). No clinical toxicity was seen.[16]

(h) Etoricoxib

A study in patients taking methotrexate 7.5 to 20 mg weekly for rheumatoid arthritis found that the addition of etoricoxib 60, 90 or 120 mg daily had no effect on the methotrexate AUC or on its renal clearance. However, another similar study found that etoricoxib 120 mg daily increased the methotrexate AUC by 28% and reduced its clearance by 13%.[17]

(i) Flurbiprofen

A study in 6 patients taking low doses of methotrexate 10 to 25 mg weekly found no important changes in methotrexate levels when given flurbiprofen 100 mg three times daily.[18] In another study of 10 rheumatoid arthritis patients taking methotrexate 7.5 to 17.5 mg weekly and flurbiprofen 3 mg/kg daily, methotrexate oral and renal clearance were similarly unaffected by flurbiprofen.[19]

In contrast to these pharmacokinetic studies, a case report describes an elderly woman who had been taking methotrexate 2.5 mg three times a week for 3 years for rheumatoid arthritis, who developed haematemesis, neutropenia and thrombocytopenia (diagnosed as methotrexate toxicity) within 1 to 2 weeks of starting to take flurbiprofen 100 mg daily.[20]

(j) Ibuprofen

A study in 7 patients found that the clearance of methotrexate 7.5 to 15 mg orally was halved by ibuprofen 40 mg/kg/day when compared with paracetamol (acetaminophen).[21] In a related study the clearance was reduced by 40%.[6] Another study of 6 rheumatoid arthritis patients taking methotrexate 10 to 25 mg weekly found that ibuprofen 800 mg three times daily had no effect on methotrexate pharmacokinetics.[18] Similar findings have been reported by other workers.[3] A patient on methotrexate who was given ibuprofen required prolonged folinic acid rescue because the clearance of methotrexate had fallen by two-thirds.[22] Another patient on high-dose methotrexate (7.5 g/m^2) had severe methotrexate-induced nephrotoxicity and delayed excretion of methotrexate while taking ibuprofen 400 mg 4-hourly.[23] A report attributes pancytopenia and resulting *Pneumocystis carinii* pneumonia in a 16 year-old patient on methotrexate 5 to 10 mg weekly to the concurrent use of ibuprofen 600 mg twice daily (and also 1 mg prednisolone daily).[24]

(k) Indometacin

A child on methotrexate 7.5 mg/m^2 weekly for 9 months showed an AUC increase of 140% when given indometacin and **aspirin**.[25] Another study found that indometacin did not affect the pharmacokinetics of methotrexate.[3]

Two patients on sequential intermediate dose methotrexate and fluorouracil who were concurrently taking indometacin 75 to 100 mg daily died from acute drug toxicity, which the authors of the report attributed to indometacin-associated renal failure.[26] Another case of acute renal failure has been described,[27] but there were no cases of toxicity in 4 other patients on methotrexate given either paracetamol (acetaminophen) or indometacin.[9] An elderly woman died after a single 10-mg intramuscular dose of methotrexate while taking indometacin 50 mg daily rectally and **diclofenac** 100 mg daily intravenously.[28]

(l) Ketoprofen

In a study of 10 rheumatoid arthritis patients taking methotrexate 7.5 to 17.5 mg weekly and ketoprofen 3 mg/kg daily, the methotrexate oral and renal clearance and the fraction of methotrexate unbound were unaffected by ketoprofen.[19] Similarly, in another study in 18 rheumatoid arthritis patients who were given methotrexate 15 mg intravenously weekly, ketoprofen had no significant effect on the methotrexate AUC, half-life or clearance, or on those of its major metabolite 7-hydroxymethotrexate.[29] However, a retrospective study of 118 cycles of *high-dose* methotrexate treatment (800 to 8300 mg/m^2; mean 3200 mg/m^2) in 36 patients showed that 4 out the 9 patients who developed severe methotrexate toxicity had also taken ketoprofen 150 to 200 mg daily for 2 to 15 days. Three of them died. A marked and prolonged rise in serum methotrexate levels was observed. Another patient who showed toxicity had also been given **diclofenac** 150 mg in one day.[30] The authors of this report state that ketoprofen should not be given at the same time as high-dose methotrexate, but it may be safe to give it 12 to 24 hours after the methotrexate because 50% of the methotrexate is excreted by the kidneys within 6 to 12 hours. This was tried in two patients without ill-effects.[30]

(m) Meloxicam

Thirteen patients with rheumatoid arthritis were given intravenous methotrexate 15 mg before and after taking meloxicam 15 mg daily for a week. The pharmacokinetics of the methotrexate were unaffected by the meloxicam and no increase in toxicity was seen.[31]

(n) Metamizole sodium (Dipyrone)

A study in a patient with osteosarcoma showed that 4 g of metamizole sodium (dipyrone) daily more than doubled the methotrexate AUC during the first cycle of high dose methotrexate treatment.[32]

(o) Naproxen

Naproxen had no significant effect on the methotrexate AUC, half-life or clearance, or on those of its major metabolite 7-hydroxymethotrexate in 18 rheumatoid arthritis patients given methotrexate 15 mg intravenously weekly.[29] Other studies have found that naproxen did not affect the pharmacokinetics of methotrexate.[3] Another study in patients with rheumatoid arthritis with normal renal function found that no toxicity was caused by naproxen 500 mg twice daily with methotrexate 15 mg given orally or intravenously, nor was the methotrexate clearance altered.[33]

In contrast, a study found that the clearance of methotrexate was decreased by 22%[6,21] and two children on methotrexate for 1 and 2 years showed increases in the AUC of methotrexate of 22% and 71% when given naproxen with **aspirin** or **indometacin** respectively.[25] A further study in 9 children on methotrexate 0.22 to 1.02 mg/kg/week found that the clearance was increased in 4 children by more than 30% when naproxen 14.6 to 18.8 mg/kg was given daily. There was also a 30% or more change in the pharmacokinetics of naproxen in 6 of the patients, but as both increases and decreases in clearance occurred, the significance is uncertain.[34]

A woman died of gross methotrexate toxicity apparently exacerbated by the concurrent use of naproxen.[35] A report attributes pneumonitis in a patient on methotrexate 7.5 to 10 mg weekly to the concurrent use of naproxen (initially 1 g then 500 mg) daily.[36]

(p) Paracetamol (Acetaminophen)

Paracetamol (acetaminophen) appears not to interact with methotrexate, see the sections on aspirin (b), ibuprofen (j) and indometacin (k), above.

(q) Phenylbutazone

Two patients on methotrexate for psoriasis developed methotrexate toxicity and skin ulceration shortly after starting to take phenylbutazone 200 to 600 mg daily. One of them died from septicaemia following bone marrow depression.[37]

(r) Piroxicam

No effect on the pharmacokinetics of either free or bound methotrexate was seen in 20 rheumatoid arthritis patients taking methotrexate 10 mg weekly when they were given piroxicam 20 mg daily for at least 15 days.[38] In another study of 10 rheumatoid arthritis patients taking methotrexate 7.5 to 17.5 mg weekly and piroxicam 20 mg daily, methotrexate oral and renal clearance were similarly unaffected by piroxicam.[19]

(s) Rofecoxib

Rofecoxib 12.5 to 50 mg once daily had no effect on the AUC and renal clearance of methotrexate or 7-hydroxymethotrexate in 19 patients stabilised on methotrexate 7.5 to 20 mg once weekly.[39] However, the authors note that in previous evaluations (data on file), higher than therapeutic doses of rofecoxib (75 mg and 250 mg) were associated with a 23% and 40% increase in methotrexate AUC, and an 11% and 40% decrease in renal clearance, respectively.[39]

(t) Sulindac

Sulindac (mean dose 400 mg daily) had no effect on the pharmacokinetics of methotrexate after a single 10-mg/m^2 intravenous dose of, but it slightly increased the AUC of the 7-hydroxymethotrexate metabolite.[4]

(u) Tolmetin

Three children on methotrexate for between 6 months and 1 year showed increases in the AUC of methotrexate of 42%, and 18%, 25% when given tolmetin, and in the last two cases tolmetin with **aspirin**.[25]

(v) Valdecoxib or Parecoxib

Studies in patients with rheumatoid arthritis found that valdecoxib 40 mg twice daily of had no clinically significant effect on the plasma levels of methotrexate given weekly by the intramuscular route [dose not stated].[40,41] Even so the makers suggest that careful monitoring should be considered, probably because of the problems seen with other NSAIDs.

(w) NSAIDs in general

In a study of 34 rheumatoid arthritis patients taking methotrexate 5 or 10 mg/m^2 (to nearest 2.5 mg) weekly, 12 patients also took **aspirin** (average 4.5 g daily) and 22 took other NSAIDs. Twenty-one of the 34 also took prednisone. Toxicity, sometimes serious (5 patients withdrawn), was common but no clinical differences between **aspirin** or other NSAIDs with respect to this toxicity was seen during 12 months of therapy.[42]

A preliminary report of a study of 87 patients on long-term treatment with methotrexate (mean weekly dose 8.19 mg), most of whom were also taking unspecified NSAIDs, found that the majority (72%) experienced no untoward effects and in the rest they were only relatively mild.[43] Concurrent use of methotrexate and NSAIDs in more than 450 patients with psoriatic arthritis or rheumatoid arthritis was said to be without clinical interaction problems with NSAIDs.[44]

A literature review of methotrexate/NSAID interactions showed a lack of alteration of low-dose methotrexate pharmacokinetic parameters with NSAIDs with the exception of co-administered methotrexate and salicylates.[45]

In a review of the records of 315 rheumatoid arthritis patients taking low-dose methotrexate 13 patients had low platelet counts. The thrombocytopenia was believed to have resulted from an interaction with a NSAID or in some patients a multiple drug interaction. If multiple drug interactions were not involved, the authors found that if the NSAID was given on a separate day, or dosages spaced according to the NSAID half-life, therapy could be re-introduced avoiding the problems of thrombocytopenia.[46]

Mechanism

Methotrexate is largely cleared unchanged from the body by renal excretion. The NSAIDs as a group inhibit the synthesis of the prostaglandins (PGE_2) resulting in a fall in renal perfusion, which could lead to a rise in serum methotrexate levels, accompanied by increased toxicity. In addition, salicylates competitively inhibit the tubular secretion of methotrexate, which would further reduce its clearance.[5] NSAIDs can also cause renal impairment, which would allow the methotrexate to accumulate. The pyrazolone derivatives and related drugs (e.g. azapropazone, metamizole sodium, phenylbutazone, aminophenazone), in particular, can cause bone marrow depression, which could be additive with that of methotrexate. Protein binding displacement of methotrexate or its metabolite (7-hydroxymethotrexate) have also been suggested as possible additional mechanisms.[47,48] There is also some evidence that this metabolite is cleared more slowly in the presence of NSAIDs.[4]

Importance and management

The evidence presented here clearly shows that a few patients on methotrexate have developed very serious toxicity, apparently due to the concurrent use of NSAIDs (aspirin and other salicylates, aminophenazone, azapropazone, diclofenac, flurbiprofen, ibuprofen, indometacin, ketoprofen, naproxen and phenylbutazone) whereas many other patients have experienced no problems at all. There is also other evidence that the pharmacokinetics of the methotrexate are changed (in particular reduced clearance) by some NSAIDs (aspirin, choline magnesium trisalicylate, etodolac, ibuprofen, metamizole sodium, rofecoxib (at higher than therapeutic doses), sodium salicylate, tolmetin), which might be expected to increase its toxicity. Should all of these interacting NSAIDs therefore be totally avoided?

Because methotrexate alone is so potentially toxic, the advice of the Committee on the Safety of Medicines (CSM) in the UK is that any patient given methotrexate alone should have a full blood count and kidney and liver function tests before starting treatment. These should be repeated weekly until therapy is stabilised, and thereafter every 2 to 3 months. Patients should be told to report any sign or symptom suggestive of infection, particularly sore throat (which might possibly indicate that white cell counts have fallen) or dyspnoea or cough (suggestive of pulmonary toxicity).[49] The consensus of opinion seems to be that the risks are greatest with high-dose methotrexate (150 mg or more daily to treat neoplastic diseases) and in patients with impaired renal function, but less in those given low doses (5 to 25 mg weekly) for psoriasis or rheumatoid arthritis and with normal kidney function. The makers of methotrexate, the CSM and British National Formulary do not advise the avoidance of NSAIDs (except azapropazone and OTC aspirin and ibuprofen), even though their use is a recognised additional risk factor for toxicity. Instead their advice is that the methotrexate dosage should be well monitored, which implies that the precautions suggested above should be stepped up. Aminophenazone or metamizole sodium can cause agranulocytosis on their own (and they consequently have limited use) so their use with methotrexate should also be avoided.

Some of the NSAIDs cited here have not been reported to interact (celecoxib, meloxicam, piroxicam), and information about some other NSAIDs seems to be lacking, but the same general precautions indicated above should be followed with all NSAIDs just to be on the safe side.

1. Noskov SM. Megaloblastic pancytopenia in a female patient with rheumatoid arthritis given methotrexate and amidopyrine. *Ter Arkh* (1990) 62, 122–3.
2. Stewart CF, Fleming RA, Germain BF, Seleznick MJ, Evans WE. Aspirin alters methotrexate disposition in rheumatoid arthritis patients. *Arthritis Rheum* (1991) 34, 1514–20.
3. Iqbal MP, Baig JA, Ali AA, Niazi SK, Mehboobali N, Hussain MA. The effects of non-steroidal anti-inflammatory drugs on the disposition of methotrexate in patients with rheumatoid arthritis. *Biopharm Drug Dispos* (1998) 19, 163–7.
4. Furst DE, Herman RA, Koehnke R, Erickson N, Hash L, Riggs CE, Porras A, Veng-Pedersen P. Effect of aspirin and sulindac on methotrexate clearance. *J Pharm Sci* (1990) 79, 782–6.
5. Liegler DG, Henderson ES, Hahn MA, Oliverio VT. The effect of organic acids on renal clearance of methotrexate in man. *Clin Pharmacol Ther* (1969) 10, 849–57.
6. Tracy TS, Krohn K, Jones DR, Bradley JD, Hall SD, Brater DC. The effects of salicylate, ibuprofen, and naproxen on the disposition of methotrexate in patients with rheumatoid arthritis. *Eur J Clin Pharmacol* (1992) 42, 121–5.
7. Zuik M, Mandel MA. Methotrexate-salicylate interaction: a clinical and experimental study. *Surg Forum* (1975) 26, 567–9.
8. Dubin HV, Harrell ER. Liver disease associated with methotrexate treatment of psoriatic patients. *Arch Dermatol* (1970) 102, 498–503.
9. Baker H. Intermittent high dose oral methotrexate therapy in psoriasis. *Br J Dermatol* (1970) 82, 65–9.
10. Maier WP, Leon-Perez R, Miller SB. Pneumonitis during low-dose methotrexate therapy. *Arch Intern Med* (1986) 146, 602–3.
11. Daly HM, Scott GL, Boyle J, Roberts CJC. Methotrexate toxicity precipitated by azapropazone. *Br J Dermatol* (1986) 114, 733–35.
12. Burton JL. Drug interactions with methotrexate. *Br J Dermatol* (1991) 124, 300–1.
13. Gumbhir-Shah K, Cevallos WH, Decleene SA, Korth-Bradley JM. Lack of interaction between bromfenac and methotrexate in patients with rheumatoid arthritis. *J Rheumatol* (1996) 23, 984–9.
14. Karim A, Tolbert DS, Hunt TL, Hubbard RC, Harper KM, Geis GS. Celecoxib, a specific COX-2 inhibitor, has no significant effect on methotrexate pharmacokinetics in patients with rheumatoid arthritis. *J Rheumatol* (1999) 26, 2539–43.
15. Mayall B, Poggi G, Parkin JD. Neutropenia due to low-dose methotrexate therapy for psoriasis and rheumatoid arthritis may be fatal. *Med J Aust* (1991) 155, 480–4.
16. Anaya J-M, Fabre D, Bressolle F, Bologna C, Alric R, Cocciglio M, Dropsy R, Sany J. Effect of etodolac on methotrexate pharmacokinetics in patients with rheumatoid arthritis. *J Rheumatol* (1994) 21, 203–8.
17. Arcoxia (Etoricoxib). Merck Sharp & Dohme Ltd. UK Summary of product characteristics, May 2005.
18. Skeith KJ, Russell AS, Jamali F, Coates J, Friedman H. Lack of significant interaction between low dose methotrexate and ibuprofen or flurbiprofen in patients with arthritis. *J Rheumatol* (1990) 17, 1008–10.
19. Tracy TS, Worster T, Bradley JD, Greene PK, Brater DC. Methotrexate disposition following concomitant administration of ketoprofen, piroxicam and flurbiprofen in patients with rheumatoid arthritis. *Br J Clin Pharmacol* (1994) 37, 453–6.
20. Frenia ML, Long KS. Methotrexate and nonsteroidal antiinflammatory drug interactions. *Ann Pharmacother* (1992) 26, 234–7.
21. Tracy TS, Jones DR, Hall SD, Brater DC, Bradley JD, Krohn K. The effect of NSAIDs on methotrexate disposition in patients with rheumatoid arthritis. *Clin Pharmacol Ther* (1990) 47, 138.
22. Bloom EJ, Ignoffo RJ, Reis CA, Cadman E. Delayed clearance (CL) of methotrexate (MTX) associated with antibiotics and antiinflammatory agents. *Clin Res* (1986) 34, 560A.
23. Cassano WF. Serious methotrexate toxicity caused by interaction with ibuprofen. *Am J Pediatr Hematol Oncol* (1989) 11, 481–2.
24. Carmichael AJ, Ryatt KS. *Pneumocystis carinii* pneumonia following methotrexate. *Br J Dermatol* (1990) 122, 291.
25. Dupuis LL, Koren G, Shore A, Silverman ED, Laxer RM. Methotrexate-nonsteroidal antiinflammatory drug interaction in children with arthritis. *J Rheumatol* (1990) 17, 1469–73.
26. Ellison NM, Servi RJ. Acute renal failure and death following sequential intermediate-dose methotrexate and 5-FU: a possible adverse effect due to concomitant indomethacin administration. *Cancer Treat Rep* (1985) 69, 342–3.
27. Maiche AG. Acute renal failure due to concomitant action of methotrexate and indomethacin. *Lancet* (1986) i, 1390.
28. Gabrielli A, Leoni P, Danieli G. Methotrexate and non-steroidal anti-inflammatory drugs. *BMJ* (1987) 294, 776.
29. Christophidis N, Dawson TM, Angelis P, Ryan PFJ. A double-blind, randomised, placebo controlled pharmacokinetic and clinical study of the interaction of ketoprofen and naproxen with methotrexate in rheumatoid arthritis. *Arthritis Rheum* (1994) 37 (9 Suppl), S252.
30. Thyss A, Milano G, Kubar J, Namer M, Schneider M. Clinical and pharmacokinetic evidence of a life-threatening interaction between methotrexate and ketoprofen. *Lancet* (1986) i, 256–8.
31. Hübner G, Sander D, Degner FL, Türck D, Rau R. Lack of pharmacokinetic interaction of meloxicam with methotrexate in patients with rheumatoid arthritis. *J Rheumatol* (1997) 24, 845–51.
32. Hernández de la Figuera y Gómez T, Torres NVJ, Ronchera Oms CL, Ordovás Baines JP. Interacción farmacocinética entre metotrexato a altas dosis y dipirona. *Rev Farmacol Clin Exp* (1989) 6, 77–81.

33. Stewart CF, Fleming RA, Arkin CR, Evans WE. Coadministration of naproxen and low-dose methotrexate in patients with rheumatoid arthritis. *Clin Pharmacol Ther* (1990) 47, 540–6.
34. Wallace CA, Smith AL, Sherry DD. Pilot investigation of naproxen/methotrexate interaction in patients with juvenile rheumatoid arthritis. *J Rheumatol* (1993) 20, 1764–8.
35. Singh RR, Malaviya AN, Pandey JN, Guleria JS. Fatal interaction between methotrexate and naproxen. *Lancet* (1986) i, 1390.
36. Englebrecht JA, Calhoon SL, Scherrer JJ. Methotrexate pneumonitis after low-dose therapy for rheumatoid arthritis. *Arthritis Rheum* (1983) 26, 1275–8.
37. Adams JD, Hunter GA. Drug interaction in psoriasis. *Aust J Dermatol* (1976) 17, 39–40.
38. Combe B, Edno L, Lafforgue P, Bologna C, Bernard J-C, Acquaviva P, Sany J, Bressolle F. Total and free methotrexate pharmacokinetics, with and without piroxicam, in rheumatoid arthritis patients. *Br J Rheumatol* (1995) 34, 421–8.
39. Schwartz JI, Agrawal NGB, Wong PH, Bachmann KA, Porras AG, Miller JL, Ebel DL, Sack MR, Holmes GB, Redfern JS, Gertz BJ. Lack of pharmacokinetic interaction between rofecoxib and methotrexate in rheumatoid arthritis patients. *J Clin Pharmacol* (2001) 41, 1120–30.
40. Dynastat injection (Parecoxib sodium). Pharmacia Ltd. UK Summary of product characteristics, April 2004.
41. Bextra (Valdecoxib). Pharmacia Ltd. UK Summary of product characteristics, May 2004.
42. Rooney TW, Furst DE, Koehnke R, Burmeister L. Aspirin is not associated with more toxicity than other nonsteroidal antiinflammatory drugs in patients with rheumatoid arthritis treated with methotrexate. *J Rheumatol* (1993) 20, 1297–1302.
43. Wilke WS, Calabrese LH, Segal AM. Incidence of untoward reactions in patients with rheumatoid arthritis treated with methotrexate. *Arthritis Rheum* (1983) 26 (Suppl), S56.
44. Zachariae H. Methotrexate and non-steroidal anti-inflammatory drugs. *Br J Dermatol* (1992) 126, 95.
45. Carpentier N, Ratsimbazafy V, Bertin P, Vergne P, Bonnet C, Bannwarth B, Dehais J, Treves R.Interaction méthotrexate/anti-inflammatoires non stéroïdiens: importance de la dose. *J Pharm Clin* (1999) 18, 295–9.
46. Franck H, Rau R, Herborn G. Thrombocytopenia in patients with rheumatoid arthritis on long-term treatment with low dose methotrexate. *Clin Rheumatol* (1996) 15, 163–7.
47. Slørdal L, Sager G, Aarbakke J. Pharmacokinetic interactions with methotrexate: is 7-hydroxy-methotrexate the culprit? *Lancet* (1988) i, 591–2.
48. Parish RC, Johnson V. Effect of salicylate on plasma protein binding of methotrexate. *Clin Pharmacol Ther* (1996) 59, 162.
49. The Committee on Safety of Medicines/Medicines Control Agency. *Current Problems* (1997) 23, 12.

Methotrexate + Probenecid

Probenecid markedly increases serum methotrexate levels (three to fourfold). Dosage reductions are needed to avoid toxicity.

Clinical evidence

The concurrent use of probenecid 500 to 1000 mg and methotrexate 200 mg/m^2 as an intravenous bolus injection resulted in serum methotrexate levels in 4 patients that were more than four times higher than in 4 others who had not received probenecid (400 micrograms/l compared with 90 micrograms/l, measured 24-hours post-dose).[1]

A three to fourfold increase in serum methotrexate levels at 24 hours was seen in 4 patients given probenecid.[2] Pretreatment with probenecid (five 500-mg doses 6-hourly) doubled the serum methotrexate levels of another 4 patients.[3] Severe and life-threatening pancytopenia occurred in a woman on low-dose methotrexate 7.5 mg weekly for rheumatoid arthritis when given probenecid. She also had renal insufficiency, hypoalbuminaemia and was taking salsalate (a salicylic acid derivative).[4]

Mechanism

Probenecid inhibits the renal excretion of methotrexate in both *monkeys* and *rats*[5,6] and this probably also happens in man. Changes in the protein binding of methotrexate may also have some part to play.[7] The increased methotrexate levels increase the risk of serious bone marrow depression.

Importance and management

An established and clinically important interaction. A marked increase in both the therapeutic and toxic effects of methotrexate can occur, apparently even with low doses if other risk factors are present.[4] Anticipate the need to reduce the dosage of the methotrexate and monitor the effects well if probenecid is used concurrently, or avoid the combination.

There are some data from *animals* to suggest that, despite the rise in methotrexate levels, the clinically useful effects of the methotrexate may actually be reduced by the presence of probenecid.[8]

1. Aherne GW, Piall E, Marks V, Mould G, White WF. Prolongation and enhancement of serum methotrexate concentrations by probenecid. *BMJ* (1978) 1, 1097–99.
2. Howell SB, Olshen RA, Rice JA. Effect of probenecid on cerebrospinal fluid methotrexate kinetics. *Clin Pharmacol Ther* (1979) 26, 641–6.
3. Lilly MB, Omura GA. Clinical pharmacology of oral intermediate-dose methotrexate with or without probenecid. *Cancer Chemother Pharmacol* (1985) 15, 220–2.
4. Basin KS, Escalante A, Beardmore TD. Severe pancytopenia in a patient taking low dose methotrexate and probenecid. *J Rheumatol* (1991) 18, 609–10
5. Bourke RS, Chheda G, Bremer A, Watanabe O, Tower DB. Inhibition of renal tubular transport of methotrexate by probenecid. *Cancer Res* (1975) 35, 110–6.
6. Kates RE, Tozer TN, Sorby DL. Increased methotrexate toxicity due to concurrent probenecid administration. *Biochem Pharmacol* (1976) 25, 1485–8.
7. Paxton JW. Interaction of probenecid with the protein binding of methotrexate. *Pharmacology* (1984) 28, 86–9.
8. Gangji D, Ross WE, Bleyer WA, Poplack DG, Glaubiger DL. Probenecid inhibition of methotrexate cytotoxicity in mouse L1210 leukemia cells. *Cancer Treat Rep* (1984) 68, 521–5.

Methotrexate + Proton pump inhibitors

Two reports describe a reduction in the excretion of methotrexate in two patients treated with omeprazole. However, similar elevations in methotrexate levels in another patient treated with omeprazole were independent of omeprazole use. One patient had myalgia and elevated 7-hydroxymethotrexate levels when treated with methotrexate and pantoprazole.

Clinical evidence

(a) Omeprazole

A man with Hodgkin's disease developed osteosarcoma and was treated with cyclophosphamide, bleomycin, dactinomycin and methotrexate, followed by folinic acid rescue. He was also taking senna, levothyroxine, omeprazole, baclofen, aciclovir, ferrous sulfate and docusate sodium. During the first cycle of treatment his serum methotrexate levels remained elevated for several days, and suspicion fell on the omeprazole, which was stopped. The patient's serum methotrexate levels then fell rapidly, and during the following three cycles the methotrexate pharmacokinetics were normal.[1] An 11-year-old boy with osteoblastic osteosarcoma was given high-dose methotrexate 15 g as a 4-hour infusion. He was also given omeprazole 20 mg twice daily (for about one week prior to methotrexate), megestrol acetate, sucralfate and folinic acid rescue. Methotrexate elimination was delayed and so further folinic acid was given. When later cycles of methotrexate were given, with ranitidine instead of omeprazole, the elimination of methotrexate was normal. The elimination half-life of the initial phase after the first dose given with omeprazole was 65% longer when compared with that of the second dose without omeprazole.[2]

In contrast to these findings, a further case is reported in which a man with chondroblastic osteosarcoma, who had been taking omeprazole, was treated with high-dose methotrexate 20 g over 6 hours with hydration, urinary alkalinisation and, after 24 hours, folinic acid rescue. Folinic acid dose was adjusted in response to elevated methotrexate levels and omeprazole was stopped. A second dose of methotrexate 2 weeks later, this time without omeprazole, resulted in similar elevated methotrexate levels. Thus the elevated methotrexate levels in this patient could not be attributed to co-administered omeprazole.[3]

(b) Pantoprazole

Severe generalised myalgia occurred in a man on pantoprazole 20 mg daily after he received intramuscular methotrexate 15 mg weekly. The symptoms subsided and eventually disappeared when the pantoprazole was replaced with ranitidine. The symptoms reappeared in response to rechallenge with pantoprazole, and the AUC for 7-hydroxymethotrexate was found to be about 70% higher, although the AUC for methotrexate was unchanged.[4]

Mechanism

It was suggested that omeprazole may inhibit the activity of a hydrogen-ion dependent mechanism in the kidney on which methotrexate depends for its excretion, so that its loss is diminished.[1]

Additionally, it was postulated that the situation with **lansoprazole** may be similar, but that pantoprazole may differ since at about the pH found in the renal tubules (pH 5), pantoprazole is more slowly activated than omeprazole.[2] However, a case of an interaction with pantoprazole has also been reported.[4]

Importance and management

Information seems to be limited to these few reports and the picture they present is somewhat contradictory. Any changes in methotrexate kinetics are important in terms of the potential for increased toxicity. Further study is required to determine whether or not proton pump inhibitors affect methotrexate levels.

The authors of one report recommend that if omeprazole therapy is necessary for a patient about to receive methotrexate, then omeprazole should be discontinued 4 to 5 days before methotrexate administration.[2] The situation with other proton pump inhibitors may be similar. Ranitidine was found to be a suitable alternative in two of the cases.[2,4]

1. Reid T, Yuen A, Catolico M, Carlson RW. Impact of omeprazole on the plasma clearance of methotrexate. *Cancer Chemother Pharmacol* (1993) 33, 82–4.
2. Beorlegui B, Aldaz A, Ortega A, Aquerreta I, Sierrasesúmega L, Giráldez J. Potential interaction between methotrexate and omeprazole. *Ann Pharmacother* (2000) 34, 1024–7.
3. Whelan J, Hoare D, Leonard P. Omeprazole does not alter plasma methotrexate clearance. *Cancer Chemother Pharmacol* (1999) 44, 88–9.
4. Tröger U, Stötzel B, Martens-Lobenhoffer J, Gollnick H, Meyer FP. Severe myalgia from an interaction between treatments with pantoprazole and methotrexate. *BMJ* (2002) 324, 1497.

Methotrexate + Retinoids

Although concurrent use of methotrexate with etretinate can be successful, the incidence of severe liver toxicity appears to be considerably increased. The serum levels of methotrexate may be increased.

Clinical evidence

A man was given a 48-hour infusion of methotrexate 10 mg every week, for chronic discoid psoriasis but when he was also given **etretinate** 30 mg (0.05 mg/kg) daily his serum methotrexate levels almost doubled. Concentrations at 12 and 24 hours during the infusion were 0.11 mmol/l, compared with 0.07 and 0.05 mmol/l before the **etretinate**.[1] A later study in psoriatic patients found that those receiving **etretinate** had 38% higher maximum plasma levels of methotrexate, but no difference in clearance or elimination half-life (i.e. no methotrexate accumulation).[2]

Severe toxic hepatitis has been reported in a number of cases when both of these drugs were used.[3-5] It may take several months to develop.[5] In one clinic, signs of liver toxicity were seen in 2 out of 10 patients given both drugs, but none in another 531 patients given methotrexate alone or in 110 patients given **etretinate** alone.[3]

Mechanism

Not understood. The increased incidence of toxic hepatitis may possibly be related to the increased maximum methotrexate plasma levels.

Importance and management

Although methotrexate and etretinate have been used together with success for psoriasis,[6-8] the risk of severe drug-induced hepatitis seems to be very considerably increased. One author says that he has decided not to use this combination in future.[3] Concurrent use should clearly be undertaken with great care. Etretinate has been largely superseded by **acitretin** (a metabolite of etretinate, which has a shorter half-life) but some consider that the combination of methotrexate and **acitretin** should also be avoided.[9]

1. Harrison PV, Peat M, James R, Orrell D. Methotrexate and retinoids in combination for psoriasis. *Lancet* (1987) ii, 512.
2. Larsen FG, Nielsen-Kudsk F, Jakobsen P, Schrøder H, Kragballe K. Interaction of etretinate with methotrexate pharmacokinetics in psoriatic patients. *J Clin Pharmacol* (1990) 30, 802–7.
3. Zachariae H. Dangers of methotrexate/etretinate combination therapy. *Lancet* (1988) i, 422.
4. Zachariae H. Methotrexate and etretinate as concurrent therapies in the treatment of psoriasis. *Arch Dermatol* (1984) 120, 155.
5. Beck H-I, Foged EK. Toxic hepatitis due to combination therapy with methotrexate and etretinate in psoriasis. *Dermatologica* (1983) 167, 94–6.
6. Vanderveen EE, Ellis CN, Campbell JP, Case PC, Voorhees JJ. Methotrexate and etretinate as concurrent therapies in severe psoriasis. *Arch Dermatol* (1982) 118, 660–2.
7. Adams JD. Concurrent methotrexate and etretinate therapy for psoriasis. *Arch Dermatol* (1983) 119, 793.
8. Rosenbaum MM, Roenigk HH. Treatment of generalized pustular psoriasis with etretinate (Ro 10-9359) and methotrexate. *J Am Acad Dermatol* (1984) 10, 357–61.
9. van de Kerkhof PCM. Therapeutic strategies: rotational therapy and combinations. *Clin Exp Dermatol* (2001) 26, 356–61.

Methotrexate + Sulfasalazine

The pharmacokinetics of methotrexate are unaffected by sulfasalazine.

Clinical evidence, mechanism, importance and management

A study in 15 patients with rheumatoid arthritis found that when sulfasalazine 2000 mg was added to methotrexate 7.5 mg weekly, the pharmacokinetics of the methotrexate remained unchanged. Similarly, methotrexate did not alter the trough levels of sulfasalazine.[1] There seems to be no reason to avoid the concurrent use of sulfasalazine and methotrexate.

1. Haagsma CJ, Russel FGM, Vree TB, van Riel PLCM, van de Putte LBA. Combination of methotrexate and sulphasalazine in patients with rheumatoid arthritis: pharmacokinetic analysis and relationship to clinical response. *Br J Clin Pharmacol* (1996) 42, 195–200.

Methotrexate + Tacrolimus

No adverse interaction appears to occur between methotrexate and tacrolimus.

Clinical evidence, mechanism, importance and management

A study in 3 bone marrow transplant patients on tacrolimus 30 micrograms/kg/day found that low-dose methotrexate (15 mg/m^2 on day 1, and 10 mg/m^2 on days 3, 6 and 11) did not significantly affect clinical care and no interaction of clinical significance was seen.[1] A further study in 40 patients given methotrexate (15 mg/m^2 on day 1 followed by 10 mg/m^2 on days 3, 6 and 11 after a transplant) with 30 micrograms/kg of intravenous tacrolimus daily, similarly found no evidence of an adverse interaction.[2]

1. Dix S, Devine SM, Geller RB, Wingard JR. Re: severe interaction between methotrexate and a macrolide-like antibiotic. *J Natl Cancer Inst* (1995) 87, 1641–2.
2. Wingard JR, Nash RA, Ratanatharathorn V, Fay JW, Klein JL, Przepiorka D, Maher RM, Devine SM, Boswell G, Bekersky I, Fitzsimmons W. Lack of interaction between tacrolimus (FK506) and methotrexate in bone marrow transplant recipients. *Bone Marrow Transplant* (1997) 20, 49–51.

Methotrexate + Urinary alkalinisers

Alkalinisation increases the solubility of methotrexate in the urine and also increases its excretion.

Clinical evidence, mechanism, importance and management

Methotrexate is much more soluble in alkaline than in acid fluids, therefore urinary alkalinisers such as **sodium bicarbonate** and **acetazolamide** (and ample fluids) are often given to patients on high-dose methotrexate therapy to prevent the precipitation of methotrexate in the renal tubules, which would cause damage. However alkalinisation also increases the loss of methotrexate in the urine because at high pH values more of the drug exists in the ionised form, which is not readily reabsorbed by the tubules. This increased loss was clearly shown in about 70 patients in whom alkalinisation of the urine (to pH greater than 7) with **sodium bicarbonate** and hydration reduced the serum methotrexate concentrations at 48 hours by 73% and at 72 hours by 76%.[1] In this instance the interaction was being exploited therapeutically to avoid toxicity. This interaction has also been shown by others.[2] The possible consequences should be recognised if concurrent use is undertaken.

For the effects of acidic urine on methotrexate excretion see 'Methotrexate + Ascorbic acid (Vitamin C)', p.477.

1. Nirenberg A, Mosende C, Mehta BM, Gisolfi AL, Rosen G. High dose methotrexate with citrovorum factor rescue: predictive value of serum methotrexate concentrations and corrective measures to avert toxicity. *Cancer Treat Rep* (1977) 61, 779–83.
2. Sand TE, Jacobsen S. Effect of urine pH and flow on renal clearance of methotrexate. *Eur J Clin Pharmacol* (1981) 19, 453–6.

Mitomycin + Doxorubicin

An increased incidence of cardiotoxicity has been seen in patients treated with mitomycin who were previously or simultaneously given doxorubicin.

Clinical evidence, mechanism, importance and management

Fourteen out of 91 (15.3%) patients with advanced breast cancer who had previously failed to respond to doxorubicin developed congestive heart failure when later treated with a combination of mitomycin 20 mg/m^2 intravenously every 4 to 6 weeks and megestrol acetate 160 mg daily. None of them had any pre-existing heart disease. This compares with only 3 out of 89 (3.5%) of another group of patients who had received doxorubicin but no mitomycin. The maximum cumulative dose of doxorubicin was 450 mg/m^2 and all of the patients had also been given cyclophosphamide.

Some of them also received other drugs during the doxorubicin phase of treatment. These included fluorouracil, methotrexate, tegafur and vincristine. The heart failure developed slowly (mean time of 8.5 months) compared with those in the control group (1.5 months).[1]

Other studies have also suggested that the combination may increase cardiotoxicity.[2,3] In a randomised study, 2 of 39 patients treated with doxorubicin 45 mg/m^2 once every 3 weeks and mitomycin 10 mg/m^2 once every 6 weeks developed cardiomyopathy compared with none of 42 patients treated with doxorubicin 75 mg/m^2 once every 3 weeks alone.[4]

The reasons for this apparent synergistic cardiotoxicity are not understood, but it may be related to free radical generation. This interaction is not established with certainty. The authors of one report suggest that its incidence is probably less than 10%, and that it does not occur until a cumulative mitomycin dose of 30 mg/m^2 or more.[3] It may be prudent to monitor patients treated with mitomycin closely if they have previously received anthracycline drugs.[1] Note that the combination (FAM—fluorouracil, doxorubicin and mitomycin) has been widely used for gastric cancer.

1. Buzdar AU, Legha SS, Tashima CK, Hortobagyi GN, Yap HY, Krutchik AN, Luna MA, Blumenschein GR. Adriamycin and mitomycin C: possible synergistic cardiotoxicity. *Cancer Treat Rep* (1978) 62, 1005–8.
2. Villani F, Comazzi R, Lacaita G, Guindani A, Genitoni V, Volonterio A, Brambilla MC. Possible enhancement of the cardiotoxicity of doxorubicin when combined with mitomycin C. *Med Oncol Tumor Pharmacother* (1985) 2, 93–7.
3. Verweij J, Funke-Küpper AJ, Teule GJJ, Pinedo HM. A prospective study on the dose dependency of cardiotoxicity induced by mitomycin C. *Med Oncol Tumor Pharmacother* (1988) 5, 159–63.
4. Andersson M, Daugaard S, von der Maase H, Mouridsen HT. Doxorubicin versus mitomycin versus doxorubicin plus mitomycin in advanced breast cancer: a randomized study. *Cancer Treat Rep* (1986) 70, 1181–6.

Mitomycin + Fluorouracil

Serious and potentially life-threatening intravascular haemolysis and renal failure may develop rarely after long-term use of mitomycin and fluorouracil.

Clinical evidence, mechanism, importance and management

Two patients developed chronic haemolysis and progressive renal insufficiency after long-term treatment with mitomycin and fluorouracil following partial or total gastrectomy for gastric cancer. The haemolysis was exacerbated by blood transfusions. The authors of the report[1] say that these two cases are "... the extreme of a syndrome we are finding increasingly in our pretransfusion patients, after 6 months or more of maintenance therapy." A similar syndrome occurred in 2 other patients, one with gastric carcinoma and one without, when treated with these two drugs.[2,3] This severe and potentially fatal syndrome has also been seen with mitomycin alone.[4,5] Its incidence is not known, but note that a regimen of fluorouracil, doxorubicin and mitomycin (FAM) has been widely used in gastric cancer and there are only a few reports. The authors of one report suggest that the drugs should be stopped at the first sign of intravascular haemolysis, persistent proteinuria and rising serum-urea levels (two consecutive values above 8 mmol/l).[1] The syndrome has also occurred when tamoxifen was used after mitomycin, see 'Mitomycin + Tamoxifen', below.

1. Jones BG, Fielding JW, Newman CE, Howell A, Brookes VS. Intravascular haemolysis and renal impairment after blood transfusion in two patients on long-term 5-fluorouracil and mitomycin-C. *Lancet* (1980) i, 1275–7.
2. Krauss S, Sonoda T, Solomon A. Treatment of advanced gastrointestinal carcinoma with 5-fluorouracil and mitomycin C. *Cancer* (1979) 43, 1598–1603.
3. Lempert KD. Haemolysis and renal impairment syndrome in patients on 5-fluorouracil and mitomycin-C. *Lancet* (1980) ii, 369–70.
4. Rumpf KW, Reiger J, Lankisch PG, von Heyden HW, Nagel GA, Scheler F. Mitomycin-induced haemolysis and renal failure. *Lancet* (1980) ii, 1037–8.
5. Schiebe ME, Hoffmann W, Belka C, Bamberg M. Mitomycin C-related hemolytic uremic syndrome in cancer patients. *Anticancer Drugs* (1998) 9, 433–5.

Mitomycin + Furosemide

Furosemide does not interact pharmacokinetically with mitomycin.

Clinical evidence, mechanism, importance and management

A study in 5 patients with advanced solid tumours treated with mitomycin C 10 mg/m^2 showed that furosemide given as a 40 mg intravenous bolus either 120 or 200 minutes after the mitomycin had no effect on its pharmacokinetics.[1]

1. Verweij J, Kerpel-Fronius S, Stuurman M, de Vries J, Pinedo HM. Absence of interaction between furosemide and mitomycin C. *Cancer Chemother Pharmacol* (1987) 19, 84–6.

Mitomycin + Tamoxifen

Haemolytic anaemia, thrombocytopenia and renal dysfunction, leading to potentially fatal haemolytic uraemic syndrome, has occurred in a few patients given tamoxifen with, or shortly after, mitomycin.

Clinical evidence, mechanism, importance and management

After a woman with metastatic breast cancer who had previously had treatment with mitomycin/mitoxantrone/methotrexate, developed rapidly fatal acute renal failure 21 days after starting tamoxifen, a retrospective survey was undertaken of other patients who had also received all of these drugs.[1] Nine out of 94 (9.6%) patients developed anaemia, thrombocytopenia and renal dysfunction, compared with none in another group of 45 patients not given tamoxifen. One of the 9 died from renal failure. The doses used were mitomycin 7 mg/m^2 intravenously every 42 days for four courses; mitoxantrone 7 mg/m^2 and methotrexate 35 mg/m^2 intravenously every 21 days for eight courses; tamoxifen 20 mg orally daily.[1] A few other cases of haemolytic uraemic syndrome in patients on mitomycin and tamoxifen have been reported.[2-4]

The authors of the first study suggested that this haemolytic uraemic syndrome was due to a combination of subclinical endothelial damage induced by the mitomycin C, and the thrombotic effect on the platelets caused by the tamoxifen.[1] They advise the avoidance of tamoxifen with or shortly after mitomycin C unless carefully monitored. Erythropoietin may be useful in managing the syndrome.[4] This syndrome has also occurred rarely after mitomycin alone, or when combined with fluorouracil, see 'Mitomycin + Fluorouracil', above.

1. Montes A, Powles TJ, O'Brien MER, Ashley SE, Luckit J, Treleaven J. A toxic interaction between mitomycin C and tamoxifen causing the haemolytic uraemic syndrome. *Eur J Cancer* (1993) 29A, 1854–7.
2. Ellis PA, Luckitt J, Treleaven J, Smith IE. Haemolytic uraemic syndrome in a patient with lung cancer: further evidence for a toxic interaction between mitomycin-C and tamoxifen. *Clin Oncol (R Coll Radiol)* (1996) 8, 402–3.
3. Arola O, Aho H, Asola M, Kauppila M, Nikkanen V, Voipio-Pulkki LM. Hemolyyttis-ureeminen oireyhtymä-mitomysiinihoidon vakava komplikaatio. *Duodecim* (1997) 113, 1923–9.
4. O'Brien MER, Casey S, Treleaven J, Powles TJ. Use of erythropoietin in the management of the haemolytic uraemic syndrome induced by mitomycin C/tamoxifen. *Eur J Cancer* (1994) 30A, 894–5.

Mitotane + Spironolactone

An isolated report describes the inhibition of the effects of mitotane in Cushing's disease by spironolactone.

Clinical evidence, mechanism, importance and management

A woman with Cushing's disease treated with chlorpropamide, digoxin and furosemide was given spironolactone 50 mg four times daily to control hypokalaemia. She was additionally treated for 5 months with mitotane 3 g daily to control the elevated cortisol levels but without effect.[1] When an interaction was suspected (on the basis of *animal* studies[1]) it was decided to withdraw the spironolactone, whereupon severe nausea and profuse diarrhoea developed within 24 to 48 hours, suggesting mitotane toxicity. This subsided and then redeveloped when the mitotane was stopped and then restarted a week later. The mechanism of this apparent interaction is not understood. It would seem that mitotane can become ineffective in the management of Cushing's syndrome in the presence of spironolactone.

1. Wortsman J, Soler NG. Mitotane. Spironolactone antagonism in Cushing's syndrome. *JAMA* (1977) 238, 2527.

Nitrosoureas + Cimetidine

The bone marrow depressant effects of carmustine and lomustine are possibly increased by the concurrent use of cimetidine.

Clinical evidence

Nine patients treated with **carmustine** 80 mg/m^2 daily for 3 days, cimetidine 300 mg four times daily for 1 to 4 weeks, steroids, and cranial irradiation over 6 weeks, demonstrated marked leucopenia during the first cycle. Bone marrow aspirates confirmed the marked decrease in granulocytic elements in 2 patients. In comparison, 31 patients treated similarly, but without cimetidine, showed no significant white cell depression.[1,2]

Neutropenia was found in a man on regular cimetidine, phenytoin, phenobarbital, and dexamethasone, 53 days after receiving **lomustine** 120 mg and 16 days after receiving **lomustine** 160 mg. The cimetidine was discontinued and the neutropenia rapidly reversed within 14 days. The neutrophil nadir from the **lomustine** 160 mg dose occurred after a further 16 to 19 days and was much less severe.[3]

Mechanism

Studies in *animals* suggest that cimetidine impairs the clearance of carmustine.[4] Cimetidine has also increased the levels or toxicity of some other antineoplastics, see 'Cyclophosphamide + H_2-blockers', p.462, 'Anthracyclines; Epirubicin + Cimetidine', p.451, and 'Fluorouracil + H_2-blockers', p.469.

Importance and management

Information appears to be limited to the reports cited, but it seems to be an established reaction. Patients given both drugs should be closely monitored for changes in blood cell counts. Because of its immunomodulatory effects, cimetidine has been used as an adjunct to carmustine in the treatment of malignant melanoma, but this did not improve outcomes.[5]

1. Selker RG, Moore P, LoDolce D. Bone-marrow depression with cimetidine plus carmustine. *N Engl J Med* (1978) 299, 834.
2. Volkin RL, Shadduck RK, Winkelstein A, Zeigler ZR, Selker RG. Potentiation of carmustine-cranial irradiation-induced myelosuppression by cimetidine. *Arch Intern Med* (1982) 142, 243–5.
3. Hess WA, Kornblith PL. Combination of lomustine and cimetidine in the treatment of a patient with malignant glioblastoma: a case report. *Cancer Treat Rep* (1985) 69 , 733.
4. Dorr RT, Soble MJ. H_2-Antagonists and carmustine. *J Cancer Res Clin Oncol* (1989) 115, 41–6.
5. Morton RF, Creagan ET, Schaid DJ, Kardinal CG, McCormack GW, McHale MS, Wiesenfeld M. Phase II trial of recombinant leukocyte A interferon (IFN-α2A) plus 1,3-bis(2-chloroethyl)-1-nitrosourea (BCNU) and the combination cimetidine with BCNU in patients with disseminated malignant melanoma. *Am J Clin Oncol* (1991) 14, 152–5.

Pemetrexed + Miscellaneous

Aspirin and ibuprofen had little effect on pemetrexed clearance in patients with normal renal function, but they, and other short-acting NSAIDs, should be interrupted in patients with mild to moderate renal function. NSAIDs with longer half-lives such as piroxicam and rofecoxib should be interrupted in all patients. Caution is recommended with nephrotoxic drugs such as aminoglycosides, loop diuretics, and ciclosporin, and drugs that are secreted by the renal tubules, such as probenecid and penicillin.

Clinical evidence, mechanism, importance and management

(a) Cisplatin

The US makers state that there is no pharmacokinetic interaction between pemetrexed and cisplatin,[1] but there is the possibility that cisplatin-induced nephrotoxicity could decrease pemetrexed clearance and increase its toxicity.[2] However, it should be noted that the use of pemetrexed with cisplatin is indicated for mesothelioma.[1,2]

(b) Folic acid and vitamin B_{12}

Oral folic acid and intramuscular vitamin B_{12} has been reported to not alter the pharmacokinetics of pemetrexed and[1] because these vitamins were found to decrease pemetrexed toxicity, it is recommended that all patients receiving pemetrexed should receive folic acid and B_{12} supplements.[1,2]

(c) Nephrotoxic drugs

The makers consider that the concurrent use of nephrotoxic drugs and pemetrexed could potentially decrease the clearance of pemetrexed, and increase its toxicity.[1,2] In the UK, the maker specifically mentions **aminoglycosides**, **loop diuretics**, **platinum compounds** (see also (a) cisplatin above) and **ciclosporin**, and recommends caution with combined use, with, if necessary, close monitoring of creatinine clearance.[2]

(d) NSAIDs and aspirin

Aspirin 325 mg every 6 hours did not alter the pharmacokinetics of pemetrexed.[1] **Ibuprofen** 400 mg four times daily caused a slight 20% decrease in the clearance of pemetrexed, and increased its AUC by 20%.[1] The effects of higher doses of aspirin or ibuprofen are not known, but could be greater. Because of this, in patients with normal renal function, the maker recommends caution when pemetrexed is used with high doses of NSAIDs (e.g. **ibuprofen** greater than 1.6 g daily) or high-dose aspirin (greater than 1.3 g daily).[2] Moreover, in patients with mild to moderate renal impairment, the maker recommends that NSAIDs and higher dose aspirin be avoided for 2 days before, the day of, and for 2 days after pemetrexed administration.[1,2]

Because of the lack of data on pemetrexed clearance with NSAIDs with longer half-lives [e.g. **piroxicam**], the maker recommends that all patients taking these NSAIDs stop them for 5 days before pemetrexed, on the day, and for at least 2 days afterwards.[1,2]

(e) Probenecid and other drugs secreted by the renal tubules

It is possible that drugs that are also secreted by the renal tubules (e.g. probenecid, **penicillin**) could decrease the clearance of pemetrexed. For this reason, the maker recommends caution with combined use, with, if necessary, close monitoring of creatinine clearance.[2]

1. Alimta (Pemetrexed). Eli Lilly and Company. US Prescribing information, August 2004.
2. Alimta (Pemetrexed). Eli Lilly and Company Ltd. UK Summary of product characteristics, September 2004.

Procarbazine + Anticonvulsants

Anticonvulsant usage seems to increase the risk of procarbazine hypersensitivity reactions.

Clinical evidence, mechanism, importance and management

A study of the records of 83 patients with primary brain tumours who were treated with procarbazine between 1981 and 1996 showed that 20 of them had procarbazine hypersensitivity reactions. Of these 20, 95% had been treated with anticonvulsants compared with 71% of those not developing hypersensitivity. In addition, there was a significant dose-response association between the development of hypersensitivity reactions and the serum levels of the anticonvulsants used (**phenytoin**, **phenobarbital**, or **carbamazepine**, with or without **valproate**).[1] It was suggested that the enzyme-inducing anticonvulsants may increase the metabolism of procarbazine to metabolites causing hypersensitivity. This may also explain why the incidence of procarbazine-induced hypersensitivity is higher in patients with brain tumours, who commonly receive seizure-prophylaxis therapy.[1]

1. Lehmann DF, Hurteau TE, Newman N, Coyle TE. Anticonvulsant usage is associated with an increased risk of procarbazine hypersensitivity reactions in patients with brain tumours. *Clin Pharmacol Ther* (1997) 62, 225–9.

Procarbazine + Chlormethine (Mechlorethamine)

A report on two patients suggests that the concurrent use of high doses of procarbazine with chlormethine (mechlorethamine) may result in neurological toxicity.

Clinical evidence, mechanism, importance and management

Two patients with acute myelogenous leukaemia admitted to hospital for marrow transplantation and who were given *high doses* of procarbazine 12.5 and 15 mg/kg and chlormethine (mechlorethamine) 0.75 and 1 mg/kg on the same day became lethargic, somnolent and disorientated for about a week. Two other patients who received the same drugs on different days had no neurological complications. In addition, only one of 45 patients treated with high dose procarbazine alone had similar persistent lethargy. Although no interaction has been proved, the authors suggest that the chlormethine may have enhanced the neurotoxic effects of the procarbazine, and advise that it would be prudent to avoid high-dose administration of these drugs on the same day.[1] Note that lower doses of the combination have been widely used in the MOPP regimen without problems.

1. Weiss GB, Weiden PL, Thomas ED. Central nervous system disturbances after combined administration of procarbazine and mechlorethamine. *Cancer Treat Rep* (1977) 61, 1713–14.

Procarbazine + Miscellaneous

The effects of drugs that can cause CNS depression or lower blood pressure may possibly be increased by the presence of procarbazine.

Clinical evidence, mechanism, importance and management

(a) Antihypertensives

In one early clinical study, 4 of 48 patients developed postural hypotension when treated with procarbazine. In addition, another patient with hypertension (180/110 mmHg) had a progressive fall in blood pressure (to 110/80) while being treated with procarbazine.[1] Additive hypotensive effects may therefore be expected with the concurrent use of antihypertensives.

(b) CNS depressants

Procarbazine can cause CNS depression ranging from mild drowsiness to profound stupor. In early clinical trials, the incidence was variously reported as 8%, 14% and 31% (when combined with prochlorperazine, see also (c) below).[1-3] Additive CNS depression may therefore be expected if other drugs possessing CNS-depressant activity are given concurrently.

(c) Prochlorperazine

An isolated report describes an acute dystonic reaction (difficulty in speaking or moving, intermittent contractions of muscles on the left side of the neck) in a patient on procarbazine when given prochlorperazine.[4] Prochlorperazine was thought to have contributed to the sedative effects of procarbazine in one early clinical trial.[3]

1. Samuels ML, Leary WV, Alexanian R, Howe CD, Frei E. Clinical trials with N-isopropyl-á-(2-methylhydrazino)-p-toluamide hydrochloride in malignant lymphoma and other disseminated neoplasia. *Cancer* (1967) 20. 1187–94.
2. Stolinsky DC, Solomon J, Pugh RP, Stevens AR, Jacobs EM, Irwin LE, Wood DA, Steinfeld JL, Bateman JR. Clinical experience with procarbazine in Hodgkin's disease, reticulum cell sarcoma, and lymphosarcoma. *Cancer* (1970) 26, 984–90.
3. Brunner KW, Young CW. A methylhydrazine derivative in Hodgkin's disease and other malignant neoplasms: therapeutic and toxic effects studied in 51 patients. *Ann Intern Med* (1965) 63, 69–86.
4. Poster DS. Procarbazine-prochlorperazine interaction: an underreported phenomenon. *J Med* (1978) 9, 519–24.

Procarbazine + Tyramine-containing foods and Sympathomimetic amines

Despite warnings, it seems doubtful that the weak MAO-inhibitory properties of procarbazine can under normal circumstances cause a hypertensive reaction with tyramine or other sympathomimetic amines.

Clinical evidence, mechanism, importance and management

The makers say that procarbazine is a weak inhibitor of MAO and therefore predict that interactions with certain foods and drugs may occur in rare cases. This is apparently based on the results of *animal* experiments, which show that the monoamine oxidase inhibitory properties of procarbazine are weaker than pheniprazine.[1] There seem to be no formal reports of hypertensive reactions in patients on procarbazine who have eaten tyramine-containing foods (e.g. cheese) or after using indirectly-acting sympathomimetic amines (e.g. **phenylpropanolamine**, **amfetamines**, etc.). The only account traced is purely anecdotal and unconfirmed: "... I recall one patient who described vividly reactions to wine and chicken livers which had occurred while he was taking MOPP chemotherapy several years earlier. Since he had not been forewarned, the reactions had been a frightening experience."[2] A practical way to deal with this interaction problem has been suggested by a practitioner in an Oncology unit:[2] patients on procarbazine should ideally be given a list of the potentially interacting foodstuffs (see 'MAOIs + Tyramine-rich foods', p.876), with a warning about the nature of the possible reaction but also with the advice that it very rarely occurs. The foods may continue to be eaten, but patients should start with small quantities to ensure that they still agree with them. Those taking MOPP should also be told that any reaction is most likely to occur during the second week while on a 14-day course of treatment with procarbazine, and during the week following when not taking it.

1. De Vita VT, Hahn MA, Oliverio VT. Monoamine oxidase inhibition by a new carcinostatic agent. N-isopropyl-α-(2–methylhydrazino)-p-toluamide (MIH). *Proc Soc Exp Biol Med* (1965) 120, 561–5.
2. Maxwell MB. Reexamining the dietary restrictions with procarbazine (an MAOI). *Cancer Nurs* (1980) 3, 451–7.

Raltitrexed + Miscellaneous

On theoretical grounds the manufacturers say that folinic acid and folic acid may possibly interfere with the action of raltitrexed.

Clinical evidence, mechanism, importance and management

(a) Folinic acid, Folic acid

The antimetabolite, raltitrexed, is a folate analogue and is a potent and specific inhibitor of the enzyme thymidylate synthase. Inhibition of this enzyme ultimately interferes with the synthesis of deoxyribonucleic acid (DNA) leading to cell death. The intracellular polyglutamation of raltitrexed leads to the formation within cells of even more potent inhibitors of thymidylate synthase. Folate (methylene tetrahydrofolate) is a co-factor required by thymidylate synthase and therefore theoretically folinic acid or folic acid may interfere with the action of raltitrexed. Clinical interaction studies have not yet been undertaken to confirm these predicted interactions.[1]

(b) Warfarin, NSAIDs

The makers say that no specific clinical interaction studies have been conducted but a review of the clinical trial database did not reveal any evidence of interactions between raltitrexed and warfarin, NSAIDs or other drugs.[1]

1. Tomudex (Raltitrexed). AstraZeneca. UK Summary of product characteristics, October 2001.

Streptozocin + Phenytoin

A single case report indicates that phenytoin can reduce or abolish the effects of streptozocin.

Clinical evidence, mechanism, importance and management

A patient with an organic hypoglycaemic syndrome, due to a metastatic apud cell carcinoma of the pancreas, and who was treated with streptozocin 2 g daily together with phenytoin 400 mg daily for 4 days, failed to show the expected response until the phenytoin was withdrawn.[1] It would seem that the phenytoin inhibited the effects of the streptozocin by some mechanism as yet unknown. Although this is an isolated case report its authors recommend that concurrent use should be avoided.

1. Koranyi L, Gero L. Influence of diphenylhydantoin on the effect of streptozotocin. *BMJ* (1979) 1, 127.

Tamoxifen + Aromatase inhibitors

Aminoglutethimide, but not anastrozole or letrozole, markedly increases the loss of tamoxifen from the body and reduces its serum levels. Tamoxifen modestly reduces anastrozole and letrozole levels, but not aminoglutethimide levels.

Clinical evidence

(a) Effect on tamoxifen

When given **aminoglutethimide** 250 mg four times daily for 6 weeks the serum levels of tamoxifen 20 to 80 mg daily and most of its metabolites were markedly reduced in 6 menopausal women with breast cancer. The clearance of the tamoxifen was increased 222% and the tamoxifen AUC was reduced by 73% (range 56 to 80%).[1] Conversely, concurrent use of **anastrozole** 1 mg daily for 28 days did not affect the pharmacokinetics of tamoxifen in a double-blind, placebo-controlled study in 34 women with breast cancer who had been on tamoxifen 20 mg daily for at least 10 weeks.[2] Similarly, **letrozole** 2.5 mg daily had no effect on the pharmacokinetics of tamoxifen in 18 women on tamoxifen 20 mg daily.[3]

(b) Effect on aromatase inhibitors

The pharmacokinetics of **aminoglutethimide** 250 mg four times daily did not differ when being taken with tamoxifen 20 to 80 mg daily, compared with 6 weeks after tamoxifen was withdrawn.[1] **Letrozole** levels were reduced by 38% (range 0 to 70%) 6 weeks after tamoxifen 20 mg daily was added to **letrozole** 2.5 mg daily in 12 women. This reduction persisted after 4 to 8 months; however, the estradiol suppressant effects of **letrozole** did not appear to be affected.[4] Similarly, although the estradiol suppressant effects of **anastrozole** 1 mg daily did not appear to be affected by tamoxifen 20 mg daily in two studies,[2,5] in one of these studies, **anastrozole** levels where decreased by 27% by tamoxifen.[5]

Mechanism

It is likely that aminoglutethimide, an enzyme inducing agent, increases the metabolism of the tamoxifen by the liver, thereby increasing its loss from the body. It is not known how tamoxifen reduces anastrozole and letrozole levels, although it may be via enzyme induction.[4]

Importance and mechanism

Theoretically, the combination of an oestrogen antagonist such as tamoxifen and an aromatase inhibitor should provide additional benefit in the treatment of hormone-dependent cancers, however, no clinical trials have yet found this to be so. The pharmacokinetic interactions described above may partly explain this. It may be preferable to use these agents sequentially rather than concurrently.[4]

1. Lien EA, Anker G, Lønning PE, Solheim E, Ueland PM. Decreased serum concentrations of tamoxifen and its metabolites induced by aminoglutethimide. *Cancer Res* (1990) 50, 5851–7.
2. Dowsett M, Tobias JS, Howell A, Blackman GM, Welch H, King N, Ponzone R, von Euler M, Baum M. The effect of anastrozole on the pharmacokinetics of tamoxifen in post-menopausal women with early breast cancer. *Br J Cancer* (1999) 79, 311–15.
3. Ingle JN, Suman VJ, Johnson PA, Krook JE, Mailliard JA, Wheeler RH, Loprinzi CL, Perez EA, Jordan VC, Dowsett M. Evaluation of tamoxifen plus letrozole with assessment of pharmacokinetic interaction in postmenopausal women with metastatic breast cancer. *Clin Cancer Res* (1999) 5, 1642–9.
4. Dowsett M, Pfister C, Johnston SRD, Miles DW, Houston SJ, Verbeek JA, Gundacker H, Sioufi A, Smith IE. Impact of tamoxifen on the pharmacokinetics and endocrine effects of the aromatase inhibitor letrozole in postmenopausal women with breast cancer. *Clin Cancer Res* (1999) 5, 2238–43.
5. Dowsett M, on behalf of the ATAC Trialists' Group. Pharmacokinetics of 'Arimidex' and tamoxifen alone and in combination in the ATAC adjuvant breast cancer trial. *Breast Cancer Res Treat* (2000) 64, 64.

Tamoxifen and other anti-oestrogens + Herbal medicines

Indirect evidence hints at the possibility that some herbal medicines that possess oestrogenic activity may oppose the actions of anti-oestrogens such as tamoxifen used in the treatment of breast cancer.

Clinical evidence, mechanism, importance and management

A letter in the Medical Journal of Australia[1] draws attention to fact that some women with breast cancer on chemotherapy or hormone antagonists who develop menopausal symptoms have found relief from hot flushes by taking a Chinese herb '**dong quai**' (or '**danggui**' root), which has been identified as *Angelica sinensis*. A possible explanation is that this and some other herbs (**vitex berry (*Agnus castus*), hops flower (lupulus), ginseng root, black cohosh (cimicifuga)**) have significant oestrogen binding activity and physiological oestrogenic actions.[2] The concern expressed in the letter is that the oestrogenic activity of these herbs might directly stimulate breast cancer growth and oppose the actions of competitive oestrogen receptor antagonists such as tamoxifen. Consider also, 'Tamoxifen and other anti-oestrogens + HRT', below.

Although this is largely speculative at the moment, the writer of the letter suggests that such herbal medicines are undesirable in patients with breast cancer. In addition to tamoxifen, there are now a number of other drugs used for breast cancer that in one way or another reduce the stimulation of oestrogen receptors (**anastrozole**, **exemestane**, **letrozole**, **toremifene**). More study is needed.

1. Boyle FM. Adverse interaction of herbal medicine with breast cancer treatment. *Med J Aust* (1997) 167, 286.
2. Eagon CL, Elm MS, Teepe AG, Eagon PK. Medicinal botanicals: estrogenicity in rat uterus and liver. *Proc Am Assoc Cancer Res* (1997) 38, 293.

Tamoxifen and other anti-oestrogens + HRT

Contrary to expectations HRT may not increase the risk of recurrent breast cancer in women on tamoxifen. HRT is reported to oppose the blood lipid lowering effects of tamoxifen.

Clinical evidence, mechanism, importance and management

(a) Anti-oestrogenic effects

In a cohort study of the use of HRT in the management of menopausal symptoms in women treated for breast cancer, use of continuous combined HRT (an oestrogen plus a progestogen) was not associated with an increased risk of breast cancer recurrence in women on tamoxifen.[1] This is of interest since HRT might be expected to oppose the effects of anti-oestrogens such as tamoxifen in the treatment and prevention of breast cancer. For this reason, HRT and other oestrogens are often considered contraindicated in women on anti-oestrogens such as **anastrozole**,[2,3] **exemestane**,[4,5] **letrozole**, tamoxifen and **toremifene** (see also 'Tamoxifen and other anti-oestrogens + Herbal medicines', above). The cohort study described[1] suggests that there need not be a complete restriction on their concurrent use, but ideally randomised prospective studies are required to confirm this.

(b) Cardiovascular effects

A large-scale comparative study was undertaken over a 12-month period in groups of women taking tamoxifen alone, HRT alone, or tamoxifen plus transdermal HRT to see whether the cardiovascular risk factors (low-density lipoprotein cholesterol, high-density lipoprotein-cholesterol levels, platelet counts) were changed by concurrent use. It was found that the decrease in total and LDL-cholesterol levels due to the tamoxifen was unchanged in current HRT users, but reduced by two-thirds in women on tamoxifen who then started HRT.[6] It would therefore seem important to check the outcome of concurrent use. More study is needed.

1. Dew JE, Wren BG, Eden JA. Tamoxifen, hormone receptors, and hormone replacement therapy in women previously treated for breast cancer: a cohort study. *Climacteric* (2002) 5, 151–5.
2. Arimidex (Anastrozole). AstraZeneca UK Ltd. UK Summary of product characteristics, July 2004.
3. Arimidex (Anastrozole). AstraZeneca Pharmaceuticals LP. US Prescribing information, September 2002.
4. Aromasin (Exemestane). Pharmacia Ltd. UK Summary of product characteristics, February 2003.
5. Aromasin (Exemestane). Pharmacia & Upjohn Company. US Prescribing information, March 2004.
6. Decensi A, Robertson C, Rotmensz N, Severi G, Maisonneuve P, Sacchini V, Boyle P, Costa A, Veronesi U. Effect of tamoxifen and transdermal hormone replacement therapy on cardiovascular risk factors in a prevention trial. *Br J Cancer* (1998) 78, 572–8.

Tamoxifen + Medroxyprogesterone acetate

Medroxyprogesterone affects the metabolism of tamoxifen but the clinical importance of this is uncertain.

Clinical evidence, mechanism, importance and management

The addition of medroxyprogesterone acetate 500 mg twice daily only slightly reduced the tamoxifen serum levels over a 6 month period in 20 women with breast cancer given tamoxifen 20 mg twice daily, but considerably reduced the levels of the desmethyl metabolite of tamoxifen, presumably because of some effect on the metabolism of the tamoxifen by the liver.[1] The clinical importance of this interaction awaits assessment.

1. Reid AD, Horobin JM, Newman EL, Preece PE. Tamoxifen metabolism is altered by simultaneous administration of medroxyprogesterone acetate in breast cancer patients. *Breast Cancer Res Treat* (1992) 22, 153–6.

Tamoxifen + Rifampicin (Rifampin)

Rifampicin increased the metabolism of tamoxifen.

Clinical evidence, mechanism, importance and management

Rifampicin 600 mg daily for 5 days reduced the AUC of a single 80-mg dose of tamoxifen by 86%, the peak plasma levels by 55%, and the half-life by 44% in 10 healthy men. Similarly, the AUC of *N*-demethyltamoxifen was reduced by 62%.[1]

It is likely that rifampicin induces the metabolism of tamoxifen by the cytochrome P450 isoenzyme CYP3A4. These findings suggest that the efficacy of tamoxifen may be reduced by rifampicin. However, there is some *in vitro* evidence that tamoxifen and rifampicin have additive antineoplastic effects in pancreatic carcinoma cell lines.[2] Also, tamoxifen induces its own metabolism on long-term use.[3] Thus, further study is needed to assess the clinical impact of the long-term combined use of these drugs.

1. Kivistö KT, Villikka K, Nyman L, Anttila M, Neuvonen PJ. Tamoxifen and toremifene concentrations in plasma are greatly decreased by rifampin. *Clin Pharmacol Ther* (1998) 64, 648–54.
2. West CML, Reeves SJ, Brough W. Additive interaction between tamoxifen and rifampicin in human biliary tract carcinoma cells. *Cancer Lett* (1990) 55, 159–63.
3. Desai PB, Nallani SC, Sane RS, Moore LB, Goodwin BJ, Buckley DJ, Buckley AR. Induction of cytochrome P450 3A4 in primary human hepatocytes and activation of the human pregnane X receptor by tamoxifen and 4-hydroxytamoxifen. *Drug Metab Dispos* (2002) 30, 608–12.

Tamoxifen + SSRIs

Paroxetine reduces the metabolism of tamoxifen to one of its active metabolites. The clinical relevance of this is unknown, although one small case-control study found that inhibitors of the cytochrome P450 isoenzyme CYP2D6 such as the SSRIs did not increase recurrence of breast cancer in tamoxifen users.

Clinical evidence

Twelve women on tamoxifen 20 mg daily were also given **paroxetine** 10 mg daily for 4 weeks and plasma levels of tamoxifen and its metabolites were measured.[1] Before **paroxetine**, plasma levels of the 4-hydroxy-*N*-desmethyl-tamoxifen metabolite (endoxifen) were about 12 times higher than the 4-hydroxy-tamoxifen metabolite. **Paroxetine** reduced endoxifen levels by 56%, but those of *N*-desmethyl-tamoxifen, and 4-hydroxy-tamoxifen were unchanged. The reduction in endoxifen levels was greatest in those who were extensive metabolisers of the cytochrome P450 isoenzyme CYP2D6 (see 'Genetic factors', (p.4)). In a further study by the same research group, 80 women starting tamoxifen 20 mg daily had plasma levels of tamoxifen measured after 1 and 4 months of therapy.[2] These were then correlated with CYP2D6 metaboliser phenotype and concurrent use of CYP2D6 inhibitors (24 women were also taking these). In women who were CYP2D6 extensive metabolisers, use of CYP2D6 inhibitors was associated with a 58% lower endoxifen level, which was substantially lower in those on **paroxetine**, but only slightly reduced by venlafaxine, and intermediate in those on **sertraline**.[2]

However, a case-control study of 28 women on tamoxifen with recurrences of estrogen receptor positive breast cancer found that there was no difference in the number of women treated with CYP2D6 inhibitors (**fluoxetine**, **paroxetine**, **sertraline**) between cases and controls (women on tamoxifen with no recurrence). Similarly, there was no differences for CYP2C9 inhibitors (including **paroxetine** and **sertraline**).[3]

Mechanism

Endoxifen and 4-hydroxy-tamoxifen are more active antiestrogens than tamoxifen.[1] Tamoxifen is metabolised to 4-hydroxy-tamoxifen and *N*-desmethyl-tamoxifen principally by CYP3A,[1] although others have found that other isoenzymes are involved,[4], and to endoxifen by CYP2D6.[1] Of the SSRIs, paroxetine is the most potent inhibitor of CYP2D6. However, tamoxifen resistance may be more to do with altered estrogen receptor sensitivity than reduced levels of tamoxifen metabolites.[3]

Importance and management

Although information is limited, it is established that potent inhibitors of CYP2D6 such as paroxetine can alter the metabolism of tamoxifen to its active metabolites. However, the effect this has on the clinical efficacy of tamoxifen remains to be established. The one small case-control study suggests the effect is not great. At present, there is insufficient evidence to recommend caution when giving SSRIs with tamoxifen, but further study is clearly needed. Any interaction would apply equally to other CYP2D6 inhibitors, see 'Table 1.3', (p.6) for a list.

1. Stearns V, Johnson MD, Rae JM, Morocho A, Novielli A, Bhargava P, Hayes DF, Desta Z, Flockhart DA. Active tamoxifen metabolite plasma concentrations after coadministration of tamoxifen and the selective serotonin reuptake inhibitor paroxetine. *J Natl Cancer Inst* (2003) 95, 1758–64.
2. Jin Y, Desta Z, Stearns V, Ward B, Ho H, Lee K-H, Skaar T, Storniolo AM, Li L, Araba A, Blanchard R, Nguyen A, Ullmer L, Hayden J, Lemler S, Weinshilboum RM, Rae JM, Hayes DF, Flockhart DA. CYP2D6 genotype, antidepressant use, and tamoxifen metabolism during adjuvant breast cancer treatment. *J Natl Cancer Inst* (2005) 97, 30–9.
3. Lehmann D, Nelsen J, Ramanath V, Newman N, Duggan D, Smith A. Lack of attenuation in the antitumor effect of tamoxifen by chronic CYP isoform inhibition. *J Clin Pharmacol* (2004) 44, 861–5.
4. Coller JK, Krebsfaenger N, Klein K, Endrizzi K, Wolbold R, Lang T, Nüssler A, Neuhaus P, Zanger UM, Eichelbaum M, Mürdter TE. The influence of CYP2B6, CYP2C9 and CYP2D6 genotypes on the formation of the potent antioestrogen Z-4-hydroxy-tamoxifen in human liver. *Br J Clin Pharmacol* (2002) 54, 157–67.

Taxanes + Amifostine

Amifostine had no effect on docetaxel and paclitaxel pharmacokinetics, and appears not to reduce the toxicity of these taxanes.

Clinical evidence, mechanism, importance and management

In a randomised study, amifostine did not alter the response to, or the pharmacokinetics of, **paclitaxel**, neither did it protect against **paclitaxel**-related neurotoxicity or myelotoxicity.[1] Another study has confirmed that amifostine (750 mg/m^2 as a 15-minute infusion 30 minutes beforehand) had no effect on the pharmacokinetics of **paclitaxel** 135 to 200 mg/m^2 in 8 patients. Six of the patients were also taking epirubicin and cisplatin.[2] Although the preliminary findings of an earlier study had suggested that pre-treatment with amifostine reduced the AUC of **paclitaxel** by 29%,[3] the full report of this study concluded that amifostine had no clinically relevant effect on **paclitaxel** pharmacokinetics.[4]

Amifostine had no effect on the pharmacokinetics of **docetaxel,** nor did it reduce **docetaxel**-induced myelotoxicity.[5]

The finding in two of these studies[1,5] that the toxicity of taxanes was not reduced by amifostine does not support earlier *in vitro* data where amifostine protected normal tissue from **paclitaxel** toxicity.[6]

There appears to be no benefit or adverse consequences from administering amifostine with the taxanes.

1. Gelmon K, Eisenhauer E, Bryce C, Tolcher A, Mayer L, Tomlinson E, Zee B, Blackstein M, Tomiak E, Yau J, Batist G, Fisher B, Iglesias J. Randomized phase II study of high-dose paclitaxel with or without amifostine in patients with metastatic breast cancer. *J Clin Oncol* (1999) 17, 3038–47.
2. Van den Brande J, Nannan Panday VR, Hoekman K, Rosing H, Huijskes RVHP, Verheijen RHM, Beijnen JH, Vermorken JB. Pharmacologic study of paclitaxel administered with or without the cytoprotective agent amifostine, and given as a single agent or in combination with epirubicin and cisplatin in patients with advanced solid tumours. *Am J Clin Oncol* (2001) 24, 401–3.
3. Schüller J, Czejka M, Pietrzak C, Springer B, Wirth M, Schernthaner G. Influence of the cytoprotective agent amifostine (AMI) on pharmacokinetics (PK) of paclitaxel (PAC) and Taxotere® (TXT). *Proc Am Soc Clin Oncol* (1997) 16, 224a.
4. Czejka M, Schueller J, Eder I, Reznicek G, Kraule C, Zeleni U, Freitag R. Clinical pharmacokinetics and metabolism of paclitaxel after polychemotherapy with the cytoprotective agent amifostine. *Anticancer Res* (2000) 20, 3871–7.
5. Freyer G, Hennebert P, Awada A, Gil T, Kerger J, Selleslags J, Brassinne C, Piccart M, de Valeriola D. Influence of amifostine on the toxicity and pharmacokinetics of docetaxel in metastatic breast cancer patients: a pilot study. *Clin Cancer Res* (2002) 8, 95–102.
6. Taylor CW, Wang LM, List AF, Fernandes D, Paine-Murrieta GD, Johnson CS, Capizzi RL. Amifostine protects normal tissues from paclitaxel toxicity while cytotoxicity against tumour cells is maintained. *Eur J Cancer* (1997) 33, 1693–8.

Taxanes + Cisplatin or Carboplatin

The toxicity of the paclitaxel/cisplatin combination appears to be dependent on the order of administration, with more severe myelosuppression occurring if paclitaxel is given after cisplatin. There does not appear to be any sequence dependent interaction for the docetaxel/cisplatin combination. Paclitaxel may reduce the thrombocytopenia associated with carboplatin.

Clinical evidence, mechanism, importance and management

(a) Carboplatin

Several clinical trials have found that the severity of thrombocytopenia with the combination of **paclitaxel** and carboplatin was less than that expected with carboplatin alone.[1-5] This does not appear to be due to any changes in **carboplatin** pharmacokinetics. In one study, patients were given carboplatin as a 30-minute infusion, either alone or immediately following **paclitaxel** 175 mg/m^2 as a 3-hour infusion, and it was found that the pharmacokinetics of carboplatin were not significantly affected by **paclitaxel**.[6] Similarly, a pharmacokinetic interaction was not noted when **paclitaxel** and carboplatin were given in either order in another study.[1] Other studies found the AUC of carboplatin to be similar to that predicted, despite the presence of paclitaxel.[2,5] Although one study found the AUC of carboplatin to be about 12% lower in the presence of paclitaxel,[4] the same researchers also found that the AUC associated with a 50% decrease in platelet count increased from 34 to 57 micrograms/ml.h, which suggests a pharmacodynamic basis for the attenuated toxicity of the combination.[7] Other researchers also reported that the AUC of carboplatin causing a 50% reduction in platelets was about 6.3 mg/ml/minute when given with **paclitaxel** compared with historical data of 4 mg/ml/minute when given alone.[8] Although thrombocytopenia may be lower than expected, myelosuppression (in the form of neutropenia) is a dose-limiting toxicity of the combination of carboplatin and **paclitaxel**.[1-4]

(b) Cisplatin

Early studies of the combination of cisplatin and **paclitaxel** showed that the degree of myelosuppression was sequence dependent. When cisplatin was given first, a greater degree of myelosuppression was seen.[9] Pharmacokinetic studies suggest that sequence-dependent differences in myelosuppression may be due to a 25% reduction in **paclitaxel** clearance when cisplatin is given first.[9] For this reason, the makers recommend that **paclitaxel** is given before cisplatin.[10,11] There is also some evidence that myelosuppression is greater for the combination when **paclitaxel** is given over 24 hours as opposed to 3 hours.[10] When **paclitaxel** is given with cisplatin, neurotoxicity (peripheral neuropathy) is common,[10] and there is some evidence that this is more severe if the **paclitaxel** is given over 3 hours as opposed to over 24 hours.[12] In one study,[13] neurotoxicity was unexpectedly severe when **paclitaxel** alone was used in patients who had relapsed after treatment with cisplatin; however, this was not the case in another similar study.[14]

In contrast to **paclitaxel**, early studies did not reveal any obvious sequence dependent toxicity for the combination of **docetaxel** and cisplatin. In addition, cisplatin did not cause any significant changes **docetaxel** pharmacokinetics.[15]

1. Huizing MT, Giaccone G, van Warmerdam LJC, Rosing H, Bakker PJM, Vermorken JB, Postmus PE, van Zandwijk, Koolen MGJ, ten Bokkel Huinink, van der Vijgh WJF, Bierhorst FJ, Lai A, Dalesio O, Pinedo HM, Veenhof CHN, Beijnen JH. Pharmacokinetics of paclitaxel and carboplatin in a dose-escalating and dose-sequencing study in patients with non-small-cell lung cancer. *J Clin Oncol* (1997) 15, 317–29.
2. Bookman MA, McGuire WP, Kilpatrick D, Keenan E, Hogan WM, Johnson SW, O'Dwyer P, Rowinsky E, Gallion HH, Ozols RF. Carboplatin and paclitaxel in ovarian carcinoma: a phase I study of the Gynecologic Oncology Group. *J Clin Oncol* (1996) 14, 1895–902.
3. Huizing MT, van Warmerdam LJC, Rosing H, Schaefers MCW, Lai A, Helmerhorst TJM, Veenhof CHN, Birkhofer MJ, Rodenhuis S, Beijnen JH, ten Bokkel Huinink WW. Phase I and pharmacologic study of the combination paclitaxel and carboplatin as first-line chemotherapy in stage III and IV ovarian cancer. *J Clin Oncol* (1997) 15, 1953–64.
4. Belani CP, Kearns CM, Zuhowski EG, Erkmen K, Hiponia D, Zacharski D, Engstrom C, Ramanathan RK, Capozzoli MJ, Aisner J, Egorin MJ. Phase I trial, including pharmacokinetics and pharmacodynamic correlations, of combination paclitaxel and carboplatin in patients with metastatic non-small-cell lung cancer. *J Clin Oncol* (1999) 17, 676–84.
5. Siddiqui N, Boddy AV, Thomas HD, Bailey NP, Robson L, Lind MJ, Calvert AH. A clinical and pharmacokinetic study of the combination of carboplatin and paclitaxel for epithelial ovarian cancer. *Br J Cancer* (1997) 75, 287–94.
6. Obasaju CK, Johnson SW, Rogatko A, Kilpatrick D, Brennan JM, Hamilton TC, Ozols RF, O'Dwyer PJ, Gallo JM. Evaluation of carboplatin pharmacokinetics in the absence and presence of paclitaxel. *Clin Cancer Res* (1996) 2, 549–52.
7. Kearns CM, Belani CP, Erkmen K, Zuhowski M, Hiponia D, Ergstrom C, Ramanthan R, Trenn M, Aisner J, Ergorin MJ. Reduced platelet toxicity with combination carboplatin & paclitaxel: pharmacodynamic modulation of carboplatin associated thrombocytopenia. *Proc Am Soc Clin Oncol* (1995) 14, 170.
8. van Warmerdam LJC, Huizing MT, Giaccone G, Postmus PE, ten Bokkel Huinink WW, van Zandwijk N, Koolen MGJ, Helmerhorst TJM, van der Vijgh WJF, Veenhof CHN, Beijnen JH. Clinical pharmacology of carboplatin administered in combination with paclitaxel. *Semin Oncol* (1997) 24 (Suppl 2), S2-97–S2-104.
9. Rowkinsky EK, Gilbert M, McGuire WP, Noe DA, Grochow LB, Forastiere AA, Ettinger DS, Lubejko BG, Clarke B, Sartorius SE, Cornblath DR, Hendricks CB, Donehower RC. Sequences of taxol and cisplatin: a phase I and pharmacologic study. *J Clin Oncol* (1991) 9, 1692–1703.
10. Taxol (Paclitaxel). Bristol-Myers Squibb Pharmaceuticals Ltd. UK Summary of product characteristics, August 2004.
11. Taxol (Paclitaxel). Bristol-Myers Squibb Company. US Prescribing information, March 2003.
12. Connelly E, Markman M, Kennedy A, Webster K, Kulp B, Peterson G, Belinson J. Paclitaxel delivered as a 3-hr infusion with cisplatin in patients with gynecologic cancers: unexpected incidence of neurotoxicity. *Gynecol Oncol* (1996) 62, 166–8.
13. Cavaletti G, Bogliun G, Marzorati L, Zincone A, Marzola M, Colombo N, Tredici G. Peripheral neurotoxicity of taxol in patients previously treated with cisplatin. *Cancer* (1995) 75, 1141–50.
14. McGuire WP, Rowinsky EK, Rosenhein NB, Grumbine FC, Ettinger DS, Armstrong DK, Donehower RC. Taxol: a unique antineoplastic agent with significant activity in advanced ovarian epithelial neoplasms. *Ann Intern Med* (1989) 111, 273–9.
15. Pronk LC, Schellens JHM, Planting AST, van den Bent MJ, Hilkens PHE, van der Burg MEL, de Boer-Dennert M, Ma J, Blanc C, Harteveld M, Bruno R, Stoter G, Verweij J. Phase I and pharmacologic study of docetaxel and cisplatin in patients with advanced solid tumors. *J Clin Oncol* (1997) 15, 1071–9.

Taxanes + Cyclophosphamide

There is some evidence that the toxicity associated with combinations of paclitaxel and cyclophosphamide is dependent on the order of administration. Results of one study indicate that docetaxel pharmacokinetics are unaltered by cyclophosphamide.

Clinical evidence, mechanism, importance and management

(a) Docetaxel

The pharmacokinetics of docetaxel were not altered by pretreatment with an intravenous bolus dose of cyclophosphamide in a phase I study.[1]

(b) Paclitaxel

A study in patients given paclitaxel as a 24-hour infusion and cyclophosphamide as an infusion over 1 hour found that neutropenia and thrombocytopenia were more severe when paclitaxel preceded cyclophosphamide.[2] Similarly, in another study, concurrent use of a continuous 72-hour infusion of paclitaxel and a daily bolus of cyclophosphamide had acceptable toxicity. However, when the cyclophosphamide was given as a single intravenous dose after the end of the 72-hour paclitaxel infusion, severe haematological and gastrointestinal toxicity occurred.[3] Whether the clinical efficacy of this combination is also altered by the schedule and sequence has not been determined. See also 'Cyclophosphamide or Ifosfamide + Taxanes', p.464.

1. Vasey PA, Roché H, Bisset D, Terret C, Vernillet L, Riva A, Ramazeilles C, Azli N, Kaye SB, Twelves CJ. Phase I study of docetaxel in combination with cyclophosphamide as first-line chemotherapy for metastatic breast cancer. *Br J Cancer* (2002) 87, 1072–8.
2. Kennedy MJ, Zahurak ML, Donehower RC, Noe DA, Sartorius S, Chen T-L, Bowling K, Rowinsky EK. Phase I and pharmacologic study of sequences of paclitaxel and cyclophosphamide supported by granulocyte colony-stimulating factor in women with previously treated metastatic breast cancer. *J Clin Oncol* (1996) 14, 783–91.
3. Tolcher AW, Cowan KH, Noone MH, Denicoff AM, Kohler DR, Goldspiel BR, Barnes CS, McCabe M, Gossard MR, Zujewski J, O'Shaughnessy J. Phase I study of paclitaxel in combination with cyclophosphamide and granulocyte colony-stimulating factor in metastatic breast cancer patients. *J Clin Oncol* (1996) 14, 95–102.

Taxanes; Docetaxel + Miscellaneous

Based on *in vitro* studies, it is predicted that inhibitors of the CYP3A family of cytochrome P450 enzymes such as ciclosporin, erythromycin, ketoconazole, midazolam, orphenadrine, terfenadine and troleandomycin will increase docetaxel serum levels, whereas barbiturates are predicted to reduce them.

Clinical evidence, mechanism, importance and management

The makers[1,2] say that no formal clinical drug interaction studies have been carried out with docetaxel, but because it is known from *in vitro* studies that the metabolism of docetaxel is mainly mediated by the cytochrome P450 isoenzyme CYP3A family,[3] they say that drugs that are inhibitors of CYP3A might possibly increase its serum levels and increase its toxicity. Caution is advised. The drugs named are **ciclosporin**, **erythromycin**, **ketoconazole**, **terfenadine** and **troleandomycin**.[1,3] Other drugs that are known to inhibit docetaxel metabolism *in vitro* include **midazolam**, **testosterone** and **orphenadrine**, whereas **quinidine** (which affects CYP2D6), and **hexobarbital**, **mephenytoin** and **tolbutamide** (which affect CYP2C) have little or no effect.[4] *In vitro* testing of **cisplatin**, **diphenhydramine**, **doxorubicin**, **ranitidine**, **verapamil**, **vinblastine** and **vincristine** at concentrations usually recommended have been found not to modify docetaxel metabolism markedly.[4] Microsomes prepared from patients treated with **pentobarbital** and/or **phenobarbital** are reported to have stimulated docetaxel metabolism strikingly whereas those prepared from a patient taking **prednisone** did not.[4]

None of these drugs, with the exception of **pentobarbital**, **phenobarbital** and **prednisone**, appear to have been studied in patients, so that the clinical importance of these predicted interactions (and non-interactions) awaits formal clinical evaluation.

1. Taxotere (Docetaxel). Aventis Pharma Ltd. UK Summary of product characteristics, June 2004.
2. Taxotere (Docetaxel). Aventis Pharmaceuticals Inc. US Prescribing information, May 2004.
3. Clarke SJ, Rivory LP. Clinical pharmacokinetics of docetaxel. *Clin Pharmacokinet* (1999) 36, 99–114.
4. Royer I, Monsarrat B, Sonnier M, Wright M, Cresteil T. Metabolism of docetaxel by human cytochromes P450: Interactions with paclitaxel and other antineoplastic drugs. *Cancer Res* (1996) 56, 58–65.

Taxanes; Paclitaxel + Anticonvulsants

Enzyme-inducing anticonvulsants (phenytoin, carbamazepine, and phenobarbital) increase the clearance of paclitaxel and increase the maximum tolerated dose.

Clinical evidence, mechanism, importance and management

In a study in patients with glioblastoma multiforme the maximum tolerated dose (MTD) of paclitaxel was 43% higher in patients receiving anticonvulsants (**phenytoin**, **carbamazepine**, and **phenobarbital**) than in those not receiving them.[1] Another study in patients with recurrent malignant gliomas reported the same finding: a 50% increase in MTD coupled with a 104% increase in plasma clearance of paclitaxel in those on anticonvulsants. In addition, this study reported that the dose-limiting toxicity differed: central neurotoxicity in those on anticonvulsants and myelosuppression/gastrointestinal toxicity in those not.[2]

It is probable that enzyme-inducing anticonvulsants increase the metabolism of paclitaxel. It is likely that patients on these anticonvulsants will require an increase in paclitaxel dose. Further study is needed. Note that barbiturates are predicted to increase the metabolism of docetaxel, see 'Taxanes; Docetaxel + Miscellaneous', p.490.

1. Fetell MR, Grossman SA, Fisher JD, Erlanger B, Rowinsky E, Stockel J, Piantadosi S. Preirradiation paclitaxel in glioblastoma multiforme: efficacy, pharmacology, and drug interactions. New approaches to Brain Tumor Therapy Central Nervous System Consortium. *J Clin Oncol* (1997) 15, 3121–8.
2. Chang SM, Kuhn JG, Rizzo J, Robins HI, Schold SC, Spence AM, Berger MS, Mehta MP, Bozik ME, Pollack I, Gilbert M, Fulton C, Rankin C, Malec M, Prados MD. Phase I study of paclitaxel in patients with recurrent malignant glioma: a North American Brain Tumor Consortium report. *J Clin Oncol* (1998) 16, 2188–94.

Taxanes; Paclitaxel + Ciclosporin

Ciclosporin enhances plasma paclitaxel levels after *oral* administration.

Clinical evidence, mechanism, importance and management

Oral paclitaxel has poor bioavailability because of high affinity for P-glycoprotein in the gastrointestinal tract. Studies in *mice* have shown that the combination of ciclosporin with oral paclitaxel produced a tenfold increase in systemic exposure to paclitaxel. Plasma concentrations of paclitaxel were below therapeutic concentrations in 5 patients when they were given an oral dose (intravenous formulation) of paclitaxel 60 mg/m^2 followed by intravenous doses of 175 mg/m^2 for subsequent courses. However, therapeutic levels above 100 micromol/ml (a ninefold increase) were achieved in 9 patients who received the same regimen plus ciclosporin 15 mg/kg. The combination was well-tolerated, but further study is required to determine whether paclitaxel treatment via the oral route is as active as that by the intravenous route.[1]

1. Meerum Terwogt JM, Beijnen JH, ten Bokkel Huinink WW, Rosing H, Schellens JHM. Co-administration of cyclosporin enables oral therapy with paclitaxel. *Lancet* (1998) 352, 285.

Taxanes; Paclitaxel + Ketoconazole

Ketoconazole appears not to interact adversely with paclitaxel.

Clinical evidence, mechanism, importance and management

Women with ovarian cancer were treated with 3-hour infusions of paclitaxel 175 mg/m^2 once every 21 days. It was found that when single oral doses of ketoconazole were given 3 hours after or 3 hours before the paclitaxel, the serum levels of the paclitaxel and its principal metabolite (6-alpha-hydroxypaclitaxel) remained unchanged. These findings confirmed those of *in vitro* studies. The conclusion was reached that these two drugs can therefore be given together safely without any dosage adjustments.[1,2]

1. Jamis-Dow CA, Pearl ML, Watkins PB, Blake DS, Klecker RW, Collins JM. Predicting drug interactions in vivo from experiments in vitro: human studies with paclitaxel and ketoconazole. *Am J Clin Oncol* (1997) 20, 592–99.
2. Taxol (Paclitaxel). Bristol-Myers Squibb Pharmaceuticals Ltd. UK Summary of product characteristics, August 2004.

Taxanes; Paclitaxel + Miscellaneous

***In vitro* studies with human liver tissue suggest that no metabolic interactions are likely between paclitaxel and cimetidine, dexamethasone or diphenhydramine. *Cremophor* may inhibit intracellular uptake and metabolism of paclitaxel.**

Clinical evidence, mechanism, importance and management

(a) Cimetidine, Dexamethasone, Diphenhydramine

On the basis of an *in vitro* study using human liver slices and human liver microsomes it has been concluded that the metabolism of paclitaxel is unlikely to be altered by cimetidine, dexamethasone or diphenhydramine, all of which are frequently given to prevent the hypersensitivity reactions associated with paclitaxel or its vehicle, *Cremophor* (see b, below).[1] The UK makers say that paclitaxel clearance in patients is not affected by cimetidine premedication.[2]

(b) Cremophor (paclitaxel vehicle)

In vitro, *Cremophor* was found to inhibit the metabolism of paclitaxel in human liver microsomes,[1] which might be expected to increase its toxicity. This concentration may be achieved clinically in patients given paclitaxel.[3] This may be worth bearing in mind if other drugs formulated with *Cremophor* are given with paclitaxel.

(c) Methotrexate

An *in vitro* study on human bladder cancer cells found the antineoplastic effect of paclitaxel in combination with methotrexate was dependent on the order of exposure to the two drugs.[4]

1. Jamis-Dow CA, Klecker RW, Katki AG, Collins JM. Metabolism of taxol by humans and rat liver in vitro: a screen for drug interactions and interspecies differences. *Cancer Chemother Pharmacol* (1995) 36, 107–14.
2. Taxol (Paclitaxel). Bristol-Myers Squibb Pharmaceuticals Ltd. UK Summary of product characteristics, August 2004.
3. Rischin D, Webster LK, Millward MJ, Linahan BM, Toner GC, Woollett AM, Morton CG, Bishop JF. Cremophor pharmacokinetics in patients receiving 3-, 6-, and 24-hour infusions of paclitaxel. *J Natl Cancer Inst* (1996) 88, 1297–1301.
4. Cos J, Bellmunt J, Soler C, Ribas A, Lluis JM, Murio JE, Margarit C. Comparative study of sequential combinations of paclitaxel and methotrexate on a human bladder cancer cell line. *Cancer Invest* (2000) 18, 429–35.

Temozolomide + Miscellaneous

Valproic acid may reduce the clearance of temozolomide. Some other anticonvulsants, H_2-blockers, dexamethasone, prochlorperazine and ondansetron did not affect the clearance. Ranitidine did not affect the extent of absorption, but this was slightly reduced by food.

Clinical evidence, mechanism, importance and management

The maker notes that concurrent use of **carbamazepine**, **dexamethasone**, **H_2-blockers**, **ondansetron**, **phenobarbital**, **phenytoin** or **prochlorperazine** did not affect the clearance of temozolomide, based on an analysis of population pharmacokinetics from phase II trials.[1,2] However, **valproic acid** modestly reduced the clearance of temozolomide.[1,2]

Ranitidine 150 mg twice daily had no effect on the absorption or plasma pharmacokinetics of temozolomide, or that of its active metabolite in a study in 12 patients given temozolomide 150 mg/m^2 daily.[3] The maker notes that **food** slightly reduces the temozolomide AUC by 9% and maximum plasma concentration by 33%. They recommend that it be administered without **food**.[1,2]

1. Temodal (Temozolomide). Schering-Plough Ltd. UK Summary of product characteristics, February 2004.
2. Temodar (Temozolomide). Schering Corporation. US Prescribing information, February 2004.
3. Beale P, Judson I, Moore S, Statkevich P, Marco A, Cutler D, Reidenberg P, Brada M. Effect of gastric pH on the relative oral bioavailability and pharmacokinetics of temozolomide. *Cancer Chemother Pharmacol* (1999) 44, 389–94.

Teniposide + Anticonvulsants

Carbamazepine, phenytoin and phenobarbital markedly increase the clearance of teniposide. A reduction in its effects has been noted in B-lineage leukaemia.

Clinical evidence, mechanism, importance and management

The clearance of teniposide was increased two to threefold (from 13 to 32 ml/minute/m^2) in 6 children with acute lymphocytic leukaemia while taking **phenytoin** or **phenobarbital** concurrently.[1] Another patient showed a twofold increase in teniposide clearance when treated with **carbamazepine**.[1] In a retrospective survey, long-term anticonvulsant therapy (**phenytoin, phenobarbital, carbamazepine**, or a combination) was associated with worse event-free survival, and greater haematological relapse and CNS relapse in children receiving chemotherapy for B-lineage acute lymphoblastic leukaemia. In this study, faster clearance of teniposide was found in those receiving anticonvulsants.[2]

The most probable reason is that because these anticonvulsants are potent liver enzyme inducing agents they increase the metabolism of teniposide by the liver and thereby increase its loss from the body. The authors of these reports therefore conclude that an increased dosage of teniposide will be needed in the presence of these anticonvulsants to achieve systemic exposure to the drug comparable to that achievable in their absence.[1] Alternatives to enzyme-inducing anticonvulsants in patients requiring teniposide may be preferable.[2] More study is needed.

1. Baker DK, Relling MV, Pui C-H, Christensen ML, Evans WE, Rodman JH. Increased teniposide clearance with concomitant anticonvulsant therapy. *J Clin Oncol* (1992) 10, 311–5.
2. Relling MV, Pui C-H, Sandlund JT, Rivera GK, Hancock ML, Boyett JM, Schuetz EG, Evans WE. Adverse effect of anticonvulsants on efficacy of chemotherapy for acute lymphoblastic leukaemia. *Lancet* (2000) 356, 285–90.

Thiopurines + Allopurinol

The haematological effects of azathioprine and mercaptopurine are markedly increased by the concurrent use of allopurinol. The dosage of the antineoplastic drug should be reduced by two-thirds to three-quarters to minimise the risk of toxicity.

Clinical evidence

(a) Azathioprine

A patient on allopurinol 300 mg daily for gout was additionally given azathioprine 100 mg daily to treat autoimmune haemolytic anaemia. Within 10 weeks his platelet count fell from 236 to 45 x 10^1/l, his white cell count fell from 9.4 to 0.8 x 10^1/l and his haemoglobin concentration fell from 11.5 to 5.3 g/dl.[2]

A number of other reports similarly describe reversible bone marrow damage associated with anaemia, pancytopenia, leucocytopenia and thrombocytopenia in patients when concurrently treated with azathioprine and allopurinol.[1-9] One fatality has been described from neutropenia and septicaemia.[8] In a retrospective analysis of 24 patients who had received both azathioprine and allopurinol, 11 developed leucopenia, 7 moderate anaemia, and 5 thrombocytopenia. Only 14 of the patients had received a greater than two-thirds reduction in azathioprine dose when allopurinol was started, but even some of these patients still developed haematological toxicity.[10]

(b) Mercaptopurine

In early studies, allopurinol 200 to 300 mg reduced the effective dose of mercaptopurine approximately fourfold in 7 patients with chronic granulocytic leukaemia or variants.[11]

Profound pancytopenia developed in the first 3 of 13 children undergoing maintenance treatment with mercaptopurine 2.5 mg/kg daily and allopurinol 10 mg/kg daily, but when the mercaptopurine dosage was halved, toxicity was manageable in the remaining 9 children.[12] Severe leucopenia and thrombocytopenia occurred in another patient given allopurinol with standard dose mercaptopurine.[13]

A pharmacokinetic study found that allopurinol caused a fivefold increase the AUC and in peak plasma mercaptopurine concentrations when the mercaptopurine was given *orally*. The bioavailability increased from 12 to 59%.[14] This did not occur when the mercaptopurine was given *intravenously*.[14,15]

Mechanism

Azathioprine is firstly metabolised in the liver to mercaptopurine and then enzymatically oxidised in the liver and intestinal wall by xanthine oxidase to an inactive compound (6-thiouric acid), which is excreted. Allopurinol inhibits first-pass metabolism by xanthine oxidase so that the mercaptopurine accumulates, blood levels rise and its toxic effects develop (leucopenia, thrombocytopenia, etc.).

Importance and management

A well documented, well established, clinically important and potentially life-threatening interaction. The dosages of azathioprine and mercaptopurine should be reduced by about two-thirds or three-quarters when given orally to reduce the development of toxicity. Despite taking these precautions toxicity may still be seen[10] and very close haematological monitoring is advisable if concurrent administration is necessary. On the basis of two studies[14,15] it would seem that this precaution might not be necessary if mercaptopurine is given intravenously, but note that parenteral mercaptopurine is not routinely available.

1. Garcia-Ortiz RE, De Los Angeles Rodriguez M. Pancytopenia associated with the interaction of allopurinol and azathioprine. *J Pharm Technol* (1991) 7, 224–6.
2. Boyd IW. Allopurinol-azathioprine interaction. *J Intern Med* (1991) 229, 386.
3. Glogner P, Heni N. Panzytopenie nach Kombinationsbehandlung mit Allopurinol und Azathioprin. *Med Welt* (1976) 27, 1545–6.
4. Brooks RJ, Dorr RT, Durie BGM. Interaction of allopurinol with 6-mercaptopurine and azathioprine. *Biomedicine* (1982) 36, 217–22.
5. Klugkist H, Lincke HO. Panzytopenie unter Behandlung mit Azathioprin durch Interaktion mit Allopurinol bei Myasthenia gravis. *Akt Neurol* (1987) 14, 165–7.
6. Zazgornik J, Kopsa H, Schmidt P, Pils P, Kuschan K, Deutsch E. Increased danger of bone marrow damage in simultaneous azathioprine-allopurinol therapy. *Int J Clin Pharmacol Ther Toxicol* (1981) 19, 96–7.
7. Venkat Raman G, Sharman VL, Lee HA. Azathioprine and allopurinol: a potentially dangerous combination. *J Intern Med* (1990) 228, 69–71.
8. Adverse Drug Reactions Advisory Committee. Allopurinol and azathioprine. Fatal interaction. *Med J Aust* (1980) 2, 130.
9. Kennedy DT, Hayney MS, Lake KD. Azathioprine and allopurinol: the price of an avoidable drug interaction. *Ann Pharmacother* (1996) 30, 951–4.
10. Cummins D, Sekar M, Halil O, Banner N. Myelosuppression associated with azathioprine-allopurinol interaction after heart and lung transplantation. *Transplantation* (1996) 61, 1661–2.
11. Rundles RW, Wyngaarden JB, Hitchings GH, Elion GB, Silberman HR. Effects of xanthine oxidase inhibitor on thiopurine metabolism, hyperuricaemia and gout. *Trans Assoc Am Physicians* (1963) 76, 126–40.
12. Levine AS, Sharp HL, Mitchell J, Krivit W, Nesbit ME. Combination therapy with 6-mercaptopurine (NSC-755) and allopurinol (NSC-1390) during induction and maintenance of remission of acute leukaemia in children. *Cancer Chemother Rep* (1969) 53, 53–7.
13. Berns A, Rubenfeld S, Rymzo WI, and Calabro JJ. Hazard of combining allopurinol and thiopurine. *N Engl J Med* (1972) 286, 730–1.
14. Zimm S, Collins JM, O'Neill D, Chabner BA, Poplak DG. Inhibition of first-pass metabolism in cancer chemotherapy: interaction of 6-mercaptopurine and allopurinol. *Clin Pharmacol Ther* (1983) 34, 810–17.
15. Coffey JJ, White CA, Lesk AB, Rogers WI, Serpick AA. Effect of allopurinol on the pharmacokinetics of 6–mercaptopurine (NSC 755) in cancer patients. *Cancer Res* (1972) 32, 1283–9.

Thiopurines + 5-Aminosalicylates

The haematological toxicity of azathioprine and mercaptopurine may be increased by mesalazine, olsalazine or sulfasalazine. Balsalazide may be less likely to interact.

Clinical evidence

(a) Balsalazide

The frequency of clinically important neutropenia did not increase significantly in 10 patients with Crohn's disease on maintenance **azathioprine** or **mercaptopurine** when they were given balsalazide 6.75 g daily for 8 weeks, but significant increases in whole blood 6-thioguanine nucleotide concentrations were seen.[1]

(b) Mesalazine

A 13-year old boy with severe ulcerative pancolitis and cholangitis was being treated with prednisone 60 mg daily, ursodeoxycholic acid 15 mg/kg daily and mesalazine 25 mg/kg daily. When **azathioprine** 2 mg/kg daily was added in an attempt to reduce the prednisone dosage, he developed marked and prolonged **azathioprine** toxicity (severe pancytopenia), which was attributed to an interaction due to abnormally high, persistent levels of an azathioprine metabolite.[2] In another study, there was a trend towards an increased rate of clinically important neutropenia in 10 patients with Crohn's disease on maintenance **azathioprine** or **mercaptopurine** when they were given mesalazine 4 g daily for 8 weeks. One patient was withdrawn from the study after 6 weeks because of leucopenia. Significant increases in whole blood 6-thioguanine nucleotide concentrations were also seen.[1]

(c) Olsalazine

A case report describes a patient with Crohn's disease who had two separate episodes of bone marrow suppression while receiving **mercaptopurine** 50 to 75 mg daily and olsalazine 1000 to 1750 mg daily. It was found necessary to reduce the **mercaptopurine** dosage on the first occasion and to withdraw both drugs on the second.[3]

(d) Sulfasalazine

A decrease in leucocyte counts was seen in 4 patients on **azathioprine** (2.1 to 3.3 mg/kg daily) after the addition of sulfasalazine. This lasted several months in one patient, and was transitory in two. The fourth patient developed agranulocytosis after 4 days, which required treatment discontinuation. When the drugs were later resumed at a lower dose, no reduction in leucocyte counts occurred.[4] Another report describes 38 patients taking **azathioprine** (mean dose 92.8 mg) and sulfasalazine (mean dose 2.1 g) for rheumatoid or psoriatic arthritis. Some patients did well but in general the combination was poorly tolerated and only 45% continued after 6 months. Reasons for withdrawal included rash (3 patients), gastrointestinal upset (7), leucopenia (1) and nephrotic syndrome (1).[5] In another study, there was a trend towards an increased rate of clinically important neutropenia in 12 patients with Crohn's disease on maintenance **azathioprine** or **mercaptopurine** when they were given sulfasalazine 4 g daily for 8 weeks. One patient withdrew from the study after 6 weeks because of leucopenia. Significant increases in whole blood 6-thioguanine nucleotide concentrations were also found.[1]

Mechanism

The metabolism of azathioprine and mercaptopurine depends on *S*-methylation by thiopurine methyltransferase (TMPT) and oxidation by xanthine oxidase. An *in vitro* study using recombinant TMPT found that both sulfasalazine and its metabolites inhibit the activity of TMPT.[6] Therefore if these drugs are used together, the clearance of azathioprine and mercaptopurine may be reduced by the sulfasalazine, resulting in an increase in their toxicity (there is only a small margin between their therapeutic and toxic levels). About 11% of patients may be at particular risk because of genetic polymorphism whereby they have TMPT enzyme activity that is only half that of the rest of the population.[1,6] *In vitro* studies confirmed that mesalazine,[7] olsalazine and its metabolite olsalazine-*O*-sulphate[3,7] and balsalazide[7] are inhibitors of recombinant TPMT. In patients, increased levels of 6-thioguanine nucleotide are probably due to inhibition of TPMT.[1] It is suggested that the reported *in vitro* concentration (IC_{50}) of balsalazide required to halve the TPMT activity is about 1000 times higher than peak plasma levels after therapeutic doses and therefore an interaction is unlikely. Mesalazine and olsalazine peak levels may also be less than the IC_{50} concentrations, but peak plasma levels of sulfasalazine are close to IC_{50} concentrations.[8]

Importance and management

These reports underline the importance of taking particular care if azathioprine or mercaptopurine are used with balsalazide, mesalazine, olsalazine, or sulfasalazine. Balsalazide may be less likely to interact, but this requires confirmation.[1] Some have postulated that the interaction may actually benefit patients, as increased whole blood 6-thioguanine nucleotide or mild leucopenia is associated with a greater chance of remission in those treated with azathioprine or mercaptopurine.[1,9] Extra monitoring of white blood cell counts is required when starting therapy with the combination.[9] More study is needed.

1. Lowry PW, Franklin CL, Weaver AL, Szumlanski CL, Mays DC, Loftus EV, Tremaine WJ, Lipsky JJ, Weinshilboum RM, Sandborn WJ. Leucopenia resulting from a drug interaction between azathioprine or 6-mercaptopurine and mesalamine, sulphasalazine, or balsalazide. *Gut* (2001) 49, 656–64.
2. Chouraqui JP, Serre-Debeauvais F, Armari C, Savariau N. Azathioprine toxicity in a child with ulcerative colitis: interaction with mesalazine. *Gastroenterology* (1996) 110 (4 Suppl), A883.
3. Lewis LD, Benin A, Szumlanski CL, Otterness DM, Lennard L, Weinshilboum RM, Nierenberg DW. Olsalazine and 6-mercaptopurine-related bone marrow suppression: a possible drug-drug interaction. *Clin Pharmacol Ther* (1997) 62, 464–75.
4. Bliddal H, Helin P. Leucopenia in adult Still's disease during treatment with azathioprine and sulphasalazine. *Clin Rheumatol* (1987) 6, 244–50.
5. Helliwell PS. Combination therapy with sulphasalazine and azathioprine. *Br J Rheumatol* (1996) 35, 493–4.
6. Szumlanski CL, Weinshilboum RM. Sulphasalazine inhibition of thiopurine methyltransferase: possible mechanism for interaction with 6-mercaptopurine and azathioprine. *Br J Clin Pharmacol* (1995) 39, 456–9.
7. Lowry PW, Szumlanski CL, Weinshilboum RM, Sandborn WJ. Balsalazide and azathioprine or 6-mercaptopurine: evidence for a potentially serious drug interaction. *Gastroenterology* (1999) 116, 1505–6.
8. Green JRB. Balsalazide and azathioprine or 6-mercaptopurine. *Gastroenterology* (1999) 117, 1513–14.
9. Present DH. Interaction of 6-mercaptopurine and azathioprine with 5-aminosalicylic acid agents. *Gastroenterology* (2000) 119, 276–7.

Thiopurines; Azathioprine + Co-trimoxazole or Trimethoprim

There is some evidence that the risk of haematological toxicity may be increased in renal transplant patients taking azathioprine if they are treated with co-trimoxazole or trimethoprim, particularly if given for extended periods. However, other evidence suggests that the drugs may be used together safely, and the combination is commonly used in practice.

Clinical evidence

The observation that haematological toxicity often seemed to occur in renal transplant patients given azathioprine and co-trimoxazole, prompted a retrospective survey of the records of 40 patients. It was found that there was no difference in the incidence of thrombocytopenia and neutropenia in those given azathioprine alone or with co-trimoxazole (160 to 320 mg trimethoprim plus 800 to 1600 mg sulfamethoxazole daily) for a short time (6 to 16 days), but a significant increase occurred in the incidence and duration of these cytopenias if both drugs were given together for 22 days or more.[1]

A marked fall in white cell counts in renal transplant recipients during concurrent treatment with either co-trimoxazole (described as frequent) or trimethoprim (3 cases) has been reported elsewhere.[2] In one case the fall occurred within 5 days and was treated by temporarily withdrawing the azathioprine and reducing the trimethoprim dosage from 300 to 100 mg daily.[2]

Conversely, in an early trial, there was no difference in the incidence of leucopenia in renal transplant recipients whether treated with co-trimoxazole or other antibacterials.[3] Similarly, in 252 renal transplant patients given continuous prophylaxis with co-trimoxazole or **sulfafurazole** for 12 to 25 months, toxicity was minimal—leucopenia occurred only occasionally and was reversed by temporarily withholding azathioprine. This was needed in a similar number of patients with each antibacterial.[4] In another placebo-controlled study in cardiac transplant recipients on triple therapy including azathioprine, co-trimoxazole prophylaxis for 4 months did not alter total white blood cell counts–leucopenia did not occur and no change in azathioprine dose was required.[5]

Mechanism

Not understood. It seems possible that the bone marrow depressant effects of all three drugs may be additive. In addition in some patients, impaired renal function may allow co-trimoxazole levels to become elevated, and haemodialysis may deplete folate levels, which could exacerbate the antifolate effects of the co-trimoxazole. Trimethoprim has been shown to inhibit renal tubular creatinine secretion.[6]

Importance and management

Information appears to be limited and the interaction is not established. Although there is some evidence of increased risk of haematological toxicity in renal transplant patients taking azathioprine if they are treated with co-trimoxazole or trimethoprim, this has not been shown in all studies. Two of the early studies suggested that the incidence of leucopenia with co-trimoxazole was related to the time after transplantation, and it improved if the dose of azathioprine was decreased or temporarily suspended.[3,7] Prophylaxis with co-trimoxazole post-transplant is commonly used in some centres.

1. Bradley PP, Warden GD, Maxwell JG, Rothstein G. Neutropenia and thrombocytopenia in renal allograft recipients treated with trimethoprim-sulfamethoxazole. *Ann Intern Med* (1980) 93, 560–2.
2. Bailey RR. Leukopenia due to a trimethoprim-azathioprine interaction. *N Z Med J* (1984) 97, 739.
3. Hall CL. Co-trimoxazole and azathioprine: a safe combination. *BMJ* (1974) 4, 15–16.
4. Peters C, Peterson P, Marabella P, Simmons RL, Najarian JS. Continuous sulfa prophylaxis for urinary tract infection in renal transplant recipients. *Am J Surg* (1983) 146, 589–93.
5. Olsen SL, Renlund DG, O'Connell JB, Taylor DO, Lassetter JE, Eastburn TE, Hammond EH, Bristow MR. Prevention of *Pneumocystis carinii* pneumonia in cardiac transplant recipients by trimethoprim sulfamethoxazole. *Transplantation* (1993) 56, 359–62.

6. Berg KJ, Gjellestad A, Nordby G, Rootwelt K, Djoseland O, Fauchald P, Mehl A, Narverud J, Talseth T. Renal effects of trimethoprim in ciclosporin- and azathioprine-treated kidney-allografted patients. *Nephron* (1989) 53, 218–22.
7. Hulme B, Reeves DS. Leucopenia associated with trimethoprim-sulphamethoxazole after renal transplantation. *BMJ* (1971) 3, 610–12.

Thiopurines; Mercaptopurine + Doxorubicin

One study postulated that the hepatotoxicity of *intravenous* mercaptopurine can be increased by doxorubicin.

Clinical evidence, mechanism, importance and management

One report describes 11 patients who developed liver damage when treated with *intravenous* mercaptopurine 500 mg/m^2 daily on days 1 to 5 and doxorubicin 50 mg/m^2 on day 1. The frequency and severity of liver damage was greater than the authors had previously seen with mercaptopurine alone. They postulated that doxorubicin potentiated the hepatotoxicity of mercaptopurine.[1] Mercaptopurine is no longer used *intravenously*, and the dose given in this study is much higher than that currently used *orally*. The general applicability of this study is unknown.

1. Minow RA, Stern MH, Casey JH, Rodriguez V, Luna MA. Clinico-pathological correlation of liver damage in patients treated with 6-mercaptopurine and adriamycin. *Cancer* (1976) 38, 1524–8.

Thiopurines; Mercaptopurine + Food

Food may reduce and delay the absorption of mercaptopurine.

Clinical evidence

A study in 17 children with acute lymphoblastic leukaemia showed that the absorption of mercaptopurine 5 mg/m^2 was reduced if given 15 minutes after a standard **breakfast** of 250 ml of milk and 50 g biscuits, compared with absorption when fasting. The AUC was reduced by 26%, the maximum plasma concentration by 36%, and the time to maximum plasma concentration delayed from 1.2 to 2.3 hours.[1] Some individuals showed more marked effects than others; 11 subjects had a decrease, whereas 6 subjects had no change or a small increase.[1] Similarly, in another study in 7 children, peak plasma mercaptopurine levels were lower and were delayed when given with a **standard breakfast** compared with those after an overnight fast.[2] However, in a third study, mercaptopurine levels varied widely between individuals and there was no clear effect of food. Peak plasma concentrations were increased only 11% (range 67% decrease to 81% increase), and AUC by 3% (range 53% decrease to 86% increase) in the fasting state compared with after food in 10 children.[3]

Mechanism

Not understood. Delayed gastric emptying is a suggested reason.[1]

Importance and management

The documentation is limited, and the interaction is not established. Mercaptopurine levels vary widely, and it is not established whether food is a clear factor in this variation. Some have suggested that mercaptopurine should be taken before food to optimise its absorption,[2] whereas others do not consider the evidence sufficient to make a recommendation.[3]

1. Riccardi R, Balis FM, Ferrara P, Lasorella A, Poplak DG, Mastrangelo R. Influence of food intake on bioavailability of oral 6-mercaptopurine in children with acute lymphoblastic leukaemia. *J Pediatr Hematol Oncol* (1986) 3, 319–24.
2. Burton NK, Barnett MJ, Aherne GW, Evans J, Douglas I, Lister TA. The effect of food on the oral administration of 6-mercaptopurine. *Cancer Chemother Pharmacol* (1986) 18, 90–1.
3. Lönnerholm G, Kreuger A, Lindström B, Myrdal U. Oral mercaptopurine in childhood leukemia: influence of food intake on bioavailability. *Pediatr Hematol Oncol* (1989) 6, 105–12.

Thiopurines; Mercaptopurine + Methotrexate

Methotrexate can increase the bioavailability of mercaptopurine, but the contribution this makes to their synergistic action in leukaemia is unclear.

Clinical evidence, mechanism, importance and management

Oral low-dose methotrexate 20 mg/m^2 increased the AUC and peak plasma levels of mercaptopurine 75 mg/m^2 by 31% and 26% respectively in 14 children receiving maintenance therapy for leukaemia.[1] In another study, 10 children with acute lymphoblastic leukaemia in remission were treated with mercaptopurine 25 mg/m^2 daily and intravenous infusions of high-dose methotrexate 2 or 5 g/m^2 once every other week for consolidation therapy. It was found that methotrexate 2 or 5 g/m^2 increased the AUC of mercaptopurine by 69 and 93% respectively, and raised the maximum serum mercaptopurine levels by 108 and 121% respectively.[2] The reasons for this pharmacokinetic interaction are not understood, although it is thought that methotrexate is a xanthine oxidase inhibitor, and may therefore inhibit the metabolism of mercaptopurine.[1,2] The combination of methotrexate and mercaptopurine has an established place in the therapy of leukaemia and is known to be synergistic. These pharmacokinetic findings may be part of the explanation for this, although biochemical mechanisms may be more important.[3] The risk of relapse of leukaemia did not appear to be related to the pharmacokinetics of methotrexate or mercaptopurine, which showed considerable inter and intrapatient variability, in one study in children.[4]

1. Balis FM, Holcenberg JS, Zimm S, Tubergen D, Collins JM, Murphy RF, Gilchrist GS, Hammond D, Poplack DG. The effect of methotrexate on the bioavailability of oral 6-mercaptopurine. *Clin Pharmacol Ther* (1987) 41, 384–7.
2. Innocenti F, Danesi R, Di Paolo A, Loru B, Favre C, Nardi M, Bocci G, Nardini D, Macchia P, Del Tacca M. Clinical and experimental pharmacokinetic interaction between 6-mercaptopurine and methotrexate. *Cancer Chemother Pharmacol* (1996) 37, 409–14.
3. Giverhaug T, Loennechen T, Aarbakke J. The interaction of 6-mercaptopurine (6-MP) and methotrexate (MTX). *Gen Pharmacol* (1999) 33, 341–6.
4. Balis FM, Holcenberg JS, Poplack DG, Ge J, Sather HN, Murphy RF, Ames MM, Waskerwitz MJ, Tubergen DG, Zimm S, Gilchrist GS, Bleyer WA. Pharmacokinetics and pharmacodynamics of oral methotrexate and mercaptopurine in children with lower risk acute lymphoblastic leukemia: a joint Children's Cancer Group and Pediatric Oncology Branch study. *Blood* (1998) 92, 3569–77.

Topotecan + Amifostine

Amifostine did not significantly affect the pharmacokinetics of topotecan in 10 women with ovarian cancer when administered daily, prior to the topotecan dose, for 5 days.[1]

1. Zackrisson A-L, Malmström H, Peterson C. No evidence that amifostine influences the plasma pharmacokinetics of topotecan in ovarian cancer patients. *Eur J Clin Pharmacol* (2002) 58, 103–8.

Topotecan + Phenytoin

Phenytoin may possibly increase topotecan clearance.

Clinical evidence, mechanism, importance and management

A 5-year-old child with medulloblastoma received a course of topotecan, firstly with phenytoin and then without. Phenytoin increased the total topotecan clearance by 47%.[1] This suggests that an increased topotecan dosage may possibly be needed in the presence of phenytoin in other patients. For a similar effect of anticonvulsants on related topoisomerase inhibitors, see 'Irinotecan + Anticonvulsants', p.472 and '9-Aminocamptothecin + Anticonvulsants', p.448.

1. Zamboni WC, Gajjar AJ, Heideman RL, Beijnen JH, Rosing H, Houghton PJ, Stewart CF. Phenytoin alters the disposition of topotecan and N-desmethyl topotecan in a patient with medulloblastoma. *Clin Cancer Res* (1998) 4, 783–9.

Topotecan + Probenecid

In *mice*, probenecid markedly inhibited renal tubular secretion of topotecan, which led to an increase in topotecan systemic exposure.[1]

1. Zamboni WC, Houghton PJ, Johnson RK, Hulstein JL, Crom WR, Cheshire PJ, Hanna SK, Richmond LB, Luo X, Stewart CL. Probenecid alters topotecan systemic and renal disposition by inhibiting renal tubular secretion. *J Pharmacol Exp Ther* (1998) 284, 89–94.

Topotecan + Ranitidine

Ranitidine does not alter the pharmacokinetics of topotecan.

Clinical evidence, mechanism, importance and management

In 18 patients with solid tumours, the pharmacokinetics of topotecan (given in initial doses of 2.3 mg/m^2 daily for 5 days and repeated every 3 weeks) and its active metabolite topotecan lactone were not affected by prior administration of ranitidine 150 mg twice daily for 4 days. The rate of absorption was increased slightly (not statistically significant), and this was not considered clinically significant.[1] No special precautions would seem necessary if ranitidine or other drugs that increase gastric pH are given with oral topotecan.

1. Akhtar S, Beckman RA, Mould DR, Doyle E, Fields SZ, Wright J. Pretreatment with ranitidine does not reduce the bioavailability of orally administered topotecan. *Cancer Chemother Pharmacol* (2000) 46, 204–10.

Toremifene + Anticonvulsants

Carbamazepine, phenobarbital and possibly phenytoin can reduce the serum levels of toremifene.

Clinical evidence, mechanism, importance and management

A pharmacokinetic study of toremifene in two groups of 10 patients, a control group and a group of patients taking anticonvulsants, found that the AUC of a single 120-mg dose of toremifene and its half-life was approximately halved in the anticonvulsant group. The anticonvulsants used were **carbamazepine** alone (3 patients) or with clonazepam (3 patients), or **phenobarbital** alone (3 patients) or with **phenytoin** (1 patient). This interaction is thought to occur because these anticonvulsants induce the liver enzymes (almost certainly the cytochrome P450 isoenzyme CYP3A4) by which toremifene is metabolised, resulting in increased toremifene clearance.[1] The UK makers of toremifene have therefore reasonably suggested that the toremifene dosage may need to be doubled in the presence of these anticonvulsants.[2]

1. Anttila M, Laakso S, Nyländen P, Sotaniemi EA. Pharmacokinetics of the novel antiestrogenic agent toremifene in subjects with altered liver and kidney function. *Clin Pharmacol Ther* (1995) 57, 628–35.
2. Fareston (Toremifene). Orion Pharma UK Ltd. UK Summary of product characteristics, May 2001.

Toremifene + Miscellaneous

Based on theoretical considerations, the makers advise care when toremifene is given with thiazides and with inhibitors of the cytochrome P450 isoenzyme CYP3A such as erythromycin, ketoconazole, and troleandomycin.

Clinical evidence, mechanism, importance and management

In their prescribing information[1] the UK makers of toremifene have made a number of recommendations as follows: the metabolism of toremifene by the liver is mediated mainly by the cytochrome P450 isoenzymes CYP3A4 and CYP3A5 so it is suggested that drugs that can inhibit these enzymes (such as **erythromycin**, **troleandomycin**, **ketoconazole**) may possibly increase its effects; hypercalcaemia is a recognised side-effect of toremifene, and it is suggested that drugs such as the **thiazides**, which decrease renal calcium excretion, may increase the risk of hypercalcaemia. These warnings are based on indirect evidence and theoretical considerations so that their clinical importance awaits confirmation.

1. Fareston (Toremifene). Orion Pharma UK Ltd. UK Summary of product characteristics, May 2001.

Toremifene + Rifampicin (Rifampin)

Rifampicin increased the metabolism of toremifene, and might be expected to reduce its efficacy.

Clinical evidence, mechanism, importance and management

A study in 9 healthy men found that rifampicin 600 mg daily for 5 days reduced the AUC, peak plasma levels and half-life of a single 120-mg dose of toremifene by 87%, 55% and 44% respectively. Similarly, the AUC of *N*-demethyltoremifene was reduced by 80%.[1] Concomitant use of rifampicin may reduce the efficacy of toremifene.[1]

1. Kivistö KT, Villikka K, Nyman L, Anttila M, Neuvonen PJ. Tamoxifen and toremifene concentrations in plasma are greatly decreased by rifampin. *Clin Pharmacol Ther* (1998) 64, 648–54.

Tretinoin + Antifibrinolytics

The combination of tretinoin and antifibrinolytics such as tranexamic acid and aprotinin in acute promyelocytic leukaemia has been associated with fatal thrombotic complications.

Clinical evidence, mechanism, importance and management

In an analysis of 31 patients with acute promyelocytic leukaemia (APL) treated over a 7-year period, **tranexamic acid** 1 to 2 g daily for 6 days was given for prophylaxis of haemorrhage to 15 of 24 patients receiving tretinoin plus chemotherapy, 4 of 4 receiving tretinoin only and 2 of 3 receiving chemotherapy only. Seven of the patients treated with tretinoin died during the study period and 4 of them, who had received only the combination of tretinoin and **tranexamic acid**, died within 42 days (early deaths). Three of the early deaths were attributed to thrombotic complications.[1] Another earlier report describes a similar fatal case of thromboembolism in a patient treated with tretinoin and **tranexamic acid**,[2] and another in a patient treated with tretinoin and **aprotinin**.[3] Tretinoin alone causes a procoagulant tendency in APL, and this may be exacerbated by use of antifibrinolytics. Although antifibrinolytics and chemotherapy may be safely used concurrently in APL, combination of tretinoin and antifibrinolytics can cause fatal thrombotic complications and should be used with caution. The use of blood, platelets and plasma rather than **tranexamic acid** for prophylaxis of haemorrhage has been advocated for APL patients.[1]

1. Brown JE, Olujohungbe A, Chang J, Ryder WDJ, Chopra R, Scarffe JH. All-*trans* retinoic acid (ATRA) and tranexamic acid: a potentially fatal combination in acute promyelocytic leukaemia. *Br J Haematol* (2000) 110, 1010–12.
2. Hashimoto S, Koike T, Tatewaki W, Seki Y, Sato N, Azegami T, Tsukada N, Takahashi H, Kimura H, Ueno M, Arakawa M, Shibata A. fatal thromboembolism in acute promyelocytic leukemia during all-*trans* retinoic acid therapy combined with antifibrinolytic therapy for prophylaxis of hemorrhage. *Leukemia* (1994) 8, 1113–15.
3. Mahendra P, Keeling DM, Hood IM, Baglin TP, Marcus RE. Fatal thromboembolism in acute promyelocytic leukaemia treated with a combination of all-trans retinoic acid and aprotinin. *Clin Lab Haematol* (1996) 18, 51–2.

Tretinoin + Azoles

The metabolism of tretinoin can be inhibited by fluconazole. A case report describes tretinoin toxicity associated with concurrent fluconazole. Ketoconazole may interact similarly.

Clinical evidence, mechanism, importance and management

A 4-year-old boy with acute promyelocytic leukaemia was given induction chemotherapy consisting of cytarabine, daunorubicin and tretinoin 45 mg/m^2 daily in two divided doses. Febrile neutropenia was treated with meropenem and amphotericin B for periods up to day 20. On day 20 he was started on antifungal prophylaxis with **fluconazole** 100 mg daily. The next day he complained of headache and a week later he had headache, vomiting and papilloedema. His CT scan was normal. Pseudotumor cerebri was diagnosed and symptoms of increased intracranial pressure resolved within a day of stopping tretinoin. Restarting tretinoin on day 30 at 75% of the previous dose resulted in headache and vomiting, and the treatment was continued from day 35 with an even lower dose (30%), which caused headache but only one episode of vomiting. **Fluconazole** was stopped on day 41 and within 24 hours the patient had improved clinically with the headache and vomiting fully resolved. He was then able to tolerate the full dose of tretinoin without adverse effects.[1]

Fluconazole inhibits the cytochrome P450 isoenzymes CYP3A4 and CYP2C9, which are amongst those involved in the oxidative metabolism of tretinoin, and it was suggested that this resulted in increased plasma levels of tretinoin.[1] Another study has also shown that **fluconazole** may inhibit the ADPH-dependent cytochrome P450-mediated metabolism of tretinoin.[2] **Ketoconazole** may similarly affect the pharmacokinetics of tretinoin.[3]

Although it has been suggested that drugs such as **fluconazole** may be useful in overcoming clinical resistance to tretinoin,[2] it has also been suggested that the concurrent use of tretinoin with drugs that affect its metabolism should be avoided if possible, or patients should be carefully monitored.[1]

1. Vanier KL, Mattiussi AJ, Johnston DL. Interaction of all-trans-retinoic acid with fluconazole in acute promyelocytic leukaemia. *J Pediatr Hematol Oncol* (2003) 25, 403–4.
2. Schwartz EL, Hallam S, Gallagher RE, Wiernik PH. Inhibition of all-trans retinoic acid metabolism by fluconazole in vitro and in patients with acute promyelocytic leukaemia. *Biochem Pharmacol* (1995) 50, 923–8.
3. Rigas JR, Francis PA, Muindi JRF, Kris MG, Huselton C, DeGrazia F, Orazem JP, Young CW, Warrell RP. Constitutive variability in the pharmacokinetics of the natural retinoid, all-trans-retinoic acid, and its modulation by ketoconazole. *J Natl Cancer Inst* (1993) 85, 1921–6.

Vinca alkaloids + Azoles

Itraconazole can increase the toxicity of vincristine, and voriconazole may interact similarly.

Clinical evidence, mechanism, importance and management

Four out of 14 patients with ALL given induction chemotherapy with weekly injections of **vincristine** (with prednisone, daunorubicin and asparaginase) and antifungal prophylaxis with **itraconazole** 400 mg daily, developed severe and early **vincristine**-induced neurotoxicity (paraesthesia and muscle weakness of the hands and feet, paralytic ileus, mild laryngeal nerve paralysis). The degree and early onset of these neurotoxic reactions were unusual, and were all reversible except for mild paraesthesia in one patient. The complications were more serious than in a previous series of 460 patients previously treated with **vincristine** but without the **itraconazole** (29% compared to 6%).[1] Five children with ALL developed severe **vincristine** toxicity attributed to concurrent treatment with **itraconazole**. They were also receiving 'nifedipine', (p.498), which is known to reduce the clearance of **vincristine,** and which may have made things worse.[2] Severe **vincristine** neurotoxicity developed in two other children with ALL when they were also given **itraconazole**.[3] Other studies similarly indicate that greater **vincristine** toxicity may occur in patients given **itraconazole**.[2,4]

The reasons for this interaction are not understood, but among the suggestions are that the **itraconazole** inhibits the metabolism of **vincristine** by the cytochrome P450 enzyme system, so that it is cleared from the body less quickly.[1] Another possible explanation is that **itraconazole** inhibits the P-glycoprotein efflux pump,[1] and increased **vincristine** neurotoxicity may be the result of the inhibition of this pump in endothelial cells of the blood-brain barrier.[4]

The authors of one report[1] suggest that **itraconazole** should be avoided in patients on **vincristine**, and the makers of **vincristine** also issue a warning about the increased risks.[5]

The makers of **voriconazole** advise caution if it is given to patients treated with the vinca alkaloids (**vincristine** and **vinblastine** are named) because of the risk of neurotoxicity.[6,7]

For the possible effect of antineoplastic regimens containing **vincristine** on **itraconazole** and **fluconazole**, see 'Azoles + Antineoplastics', p.137.

1. Böhme A, Ganser A, Hoelzer D. Aggravation of vincristine-induced neurotoxicity by itraconazole in the treatment of adult ALL. *Ann Hematol* (1995) 71, 311–12.
2. Murphy JA, Ross LM, Gibson BES. Vincristine toxicity in five children with acute lymphoblastic leukaemia. *Lancet* (1995) 346, 443.
3. Ariffin H, Omar KZ, Ang EL, Shekhar K. Severe vincristine neurotoxicity with concomitant use of itraconazole. *J Paediatr Child Health* (2003) 39, 638–9.
4. Muenchow N, Janka G, Erttmann R, Looft G, Bielack S, Winkler K. Increased vincristine neurotoxicity during treatment with itraconazole in 3 pediatric patients with acute myelogenous leukaemia. *Blood* (1999) 94 (Suppl 1, part 2) 234b.
5. Vincristine sulphate. Mayne Pharma plc. UK Summary of product characteristics, February 2004.
6. VFEND (Voriconazole). Pfizer Ltd. UK Summary of product characteristics, March 2005.
7. VFEND (Voriconazole). Pfizer Inc. US Prescribing information, March 2005.

Vinca alkaloids + Macrolides

Erythromycin increased the toxicity of vinblastine in three patients. Clarithromycin possibly does not interact with vinca alkaloids.

Clinical evidence

Three patients with renal cell carcinoma given ciclosporin 10 or 13 mg/kg daily and **erythromycin** 333 mg three times daily or 250 mg four times daily for 3 days developed severe toxicity when treated with **vinblastine** 7 to 10 mg/m^2 on the third day. Ciclosporin was used as a modifier of multidrug resistance and **erythromycin** was given to achieve higher ciclosporin levels at a lower dose (see 'Ciclosporin + Antibacterials; Macrolides', p.773). To rule out increased ciclosporin toxicity, one patient was given **erythromycin** without ciclosporin but he still developed **vinblastine** toxicity (severe neutropenia, constipation, myositis, severe myalgia) typical of much higher doses of **vinblastine**. Of the other 2 patients, only negligible toxicity developed in one when he was later given **vinblastine** alone, and the other had received ciclosporin and **vinblastine** on two previous occasions without problems.[1] Other authors report that they have used **clarithromycin** with standard doses of vinca alkaloids in at least 6 patients without any evidence of increased toxicity.[2]

Mechanism

Uncertain, but erythromycin inhibits the cytochrome P450 isoenzyme CYP3A4, which is concerned with the metabolism of vinblastine.[3] This would be expected to reduce the metabolism of vinblastine resulting in an increase in its toxicity.

Importance and management

Information seems to be limited to this report. On the basis of their findings the authors suggest that erythromycin should be avoided at the time of vinblastine infusion.[1] Use with clarithromycin may be safe.[2] The UK maker of vinblastine, **vincristine** and **vindesine** has warned that caution should be exercised in patients taking any drugs known to inhibit the CYP3A subfamily because of the risk of an earlier onset and/or increased severity of side effects with these vinca alkaloids.[4-6] Note that itraconazole is known to increase the toxicity of vincristine, see 'Azoles + Antineoplastics', p.137.

1. Tobe SW, Siu LL, Jamal SA, Skorecki KL, Murphy GF, Warner E. Vinblastine and erythromycin: an unrecognized serious drug interaction. *Cancer Chemother Pharmacol* (1995) 35, 188–190.
2. Torresin A, Cassola G, Penco G, Crisalli MP, Piersantelli N. Vinca alkaloids and macrolides in human immunodeficiency virus-related malignancies: a safe association. *Cancer Chemother Pharmacol* (1996) 39, 176–7.
3. Zhour-Pan X-R, Sérée E, Zhou X-J, Placidi M, Maurel P, Barra Y, Rahmani R. Involvement of human liver cytochrome P450 3A in vinblastine metabolism: drug interactions. *Cancer Res* (1993) 53, 5121–6.
4. Velbe (Vinblastine). Eli Lilly and Company Ltd. UK Summary of product characteristics, July 1999.
5. Eldisine (Vindesine). Eli Lilly and Company Ltd. UK Summary of product characteristics, September 1998.
6. Vincristine sulphate. Mayne Pharma plc. UK Summary of product characteristics, February 2004.

Vinca alkaloids + Mitomycin

A syndrome of acute pulmonary toxicity, characterised by severe shortness of breath, can occur when vinblastine, vindesine or vinorelbine are used with mitomycin. Fatalities have occurred.

Clinical evidence, mechanism, importance and management

There are now numerous reports describing acute lung disease in patients treated with mitomycin and vinca alkaloids, which appears to be different to the chronic pulmonary fibrosis seen with mitomycin alone. Sudden onset of acute shortness of breath has been described shortly after administration of the vinca alkaloid as part of a vinca alkaloid/mitomycin regimen. Chest radiographs have shown diffuse lung damage characterised by interstitial infiltrates and pulmonary oedema. The acute syndrome has usually improved over 24 hours, although some patients have chronic respiratory impairment (60% in one series[1]). Fatalities have occurred.[2-4] The syndrome has been reported with mitomycin and **vinblastine,**[1-9] **vindesine**[1,8,10-12] and **vinorelbine**.[12-15] The incidence is reported to be about 3 to 6%.[1,7,12]

The potential hazards of combining these drugs should be recognised. In view of the unpredictability of the reaction, close observation of patients receiving this combination is recommended.[1,3] If the reaction occurs, supportive measures such as supplemental oxygen and mechanical ventilation may be needed. Corticosteroids are also often used in an attempt to treat the acute symptoms, and to possibly decrease the risk of chronic respiratory impairment.[1] In patients who have developed acute pulmonary toxicity, the use of both mitomycin and vinca alkaloids should subsequently be avoided.[1]

1. Rivera MP, Kris MG, Gralla RJ, White DA. Syndrome of acute dyspnea related to combined mitomycin plus vinca alkaloid chemotherapy. *Am J Clin Oncol* (1995) 18, 245–50.
2. Ozols RF, Hogan WM, Ostchega T, Young RC. MVP (mitomycin, vinblastine, progesterone): a second-line regimen in ovarian cancer with a high incidence of pulmonary toxicity. *Cancer Treat Rep* (1983) 67, 721–2.
3. Rao SX, Ramaswamy G, Levin M, McCravey JW. Fatal acute respiratory failure after vinblastine-mitomycin therapy in lung carcinoma. *Arch Intern Med* (1985) 145, 1905–7.
4. Ballen KK, Weiss ST. Fatal acute respiratory failure following vinblastine and mitomycin administration for breast cancer. *Am J Med Sci* (1988) 295, 558–60.
5. Israel RH, Olsen JP. Pulmonary edema associated with intravenous vinblastine. *JAMA* (1978) 240, 1585.
6. Konits PH, Aisner J, Sutherland JC, Wiernik PH. Possible pulmonary toxicity secondary to vinblastine. *Cancer* (1982) 50, 2771–4.
7. Hoelzer KL, Harrison BR, Luedke SW, Luedke DW. Vinblastine-associated pulmonary toxicity in patients receiving combination therapy with mitomycin and cisplatin. *Drug Intell Clin Pharm* (1986) 20, 287–9.
8. Kris MG, Pablo D, Gralla J, Burke MT, Prestifillippo J, Lewin D. Dyspnea following vinblastine or vindesine administration in patients receiving mitomycin plus vinca alkaloid combination therapy. *Cancer Treat Rep* (1984) 68, 1029–31.
9. Lagler U, Gattiker HH. Akute Dyspnoe nach intravenöser Gabe von Vinblastin/Mitomycin. *Schweiz Med Wochenschr* (1989) 119, 290–2.
10. Dyke RW. Acute bronchospasm after a vinca alkaloid in patients previously treated with mitomycin. *N Engl J Med* (1984) 310, 389.
11. Luedke D, McLaughlin TT, Daughaday C, Luedke S, Harrison B, Reed G, Martello O. Mitomycin C and vindesine associated pulmonary toxicity with variable clinical expression. *Cancer* (1985) 55, 542–5.
12. Thomas P, Pradal M, Le Caer H, Montcharmont D, Vervolet D, Kleisbauer JP. Bronchospasme aigu dû à l'association alcaloïde de la pervenche-mitomycine. *Rev Mal Respir* (1993) 10, 268–70.
13. Raderer M, Kornek G, Hejna M, Vorbeck F, Weinlaender G, Scheithauer W. Acute pulmonary toxicity associated with high-dose vinorelbine and mitomycin C. *Ann Oncol* (1996) 7, 973–5.
14. Rouzaud P, Estivals M, Pujazon MC, Carles P, Lauque D. Complications respiratoires de l'association vinorelbine-mitomycine. *Rev Mal Respir* (1999) 16, 81–4.
15. Uoshima N, Yoshioka K, Tegoshi J, Wada S, Fujiwara Y. Acute respiratory failure caused by vinorelbine tartrate in a patient with non-small cell lung cancer. *Intern Med* (2001) 40, 779–82.

Vinca alkaloids; Vinblastine + Bleomycin

The combination of vinblastine and bleomycin with or without cisplatin commonly causes Raynaud's phenomenon. Rarely, it also appears to cause serious life-threatening cardiovascular toxicity.

Clinical evidence, mechanism, importance and management

Five patients (aged 23 to 58) treated for germ cell tumours died from unexpected acute life-threatening vascular events (myocardial infarction, rectal infarction, cerebrovascular accident) following VBP therapy (vinblastine, bleomycin, cisplatin). A survey of the literature by the authors of this paper revealed 14 other cases of both acute and long-term cardiovascular problems (myocardial infarction, coronary heart disease, cerebrovascular accident) in patients given VBP therapy.[1]

Raynaud's phenomenon is common (one third to a half) in those treated with vinblastine and bleomycin or VBP,[2,3] and there is evidence that blood vessels are pathologically altered.[2] Cisplatin may contribute to the effect.[3] Analysis of late vascular toxicity after chemotherapy for testicular cancer revealed that the use of bleomycin with vinblastine and cisplatin (VBP regimen) carried a higher risk of Raynaud's phenomenon than bleomycin with etoposide and cisplatin (BEP regimen).[4]

The use of the VBP (PVB) regimen has largely been replaced by the BEP (PEB) regimen, because of its reduced toxicity.

1. Samuels BL, Vogelzang NJ, Kennedy BJ. Severe vascular toxicity associated with vinblastine, bleomycin and cisplatin chemotherapy. *Cancer Chemother Pharmacol* (1987) 19, 253–6.
2. Vogelzang NJ, Bosl GJ, Johnson K, Kennedy BJ. Raynaud's phenomenon: a common toxicity after combination chemotherapy for testicular cancer. *Ann Intern Med* (1981) 95, 288–92.
3. Hansen SW. Late-effects after treatment for germ-cell cancer with cisplatin, vinblastine, and bleomycin. *Dan Med Bull* (1992) 39, 391–9.
4. Berger CC, Bokemeyer C, Schneider M, Kuczyk MA, Schmoll H-J. Secondary Raynaud's phenomenon and other late vascular complications following chemotherapy for testicular cancer. *Eur J Cancer* (1995) 31A, 2229–38.

Vinca alkaloids; Vincristine + Anticonvulsants

Carbamazepine and phenytoin appear to reduce plasma levels of vincristine, and may reduce its efficacy. A number of case reports have described reduced phenytoin levels in patients on chemotherapy including vinca alkaloids.

Clinical evidence, mechanism, importance and management

The systemic clearance of vincristine 2 mg was 63% higher and the AUC was 43% lower in 9 patients receiving **carbamazepine** or **phenytoin** than in 6 patients not on anticonvulsants. In this study, patients were being treated with procarbazine, lomustine and vincristine for brain tumours.[1] In a retrospective survey, long-term anticonvulsant therapy (**phenytoin, phenobarbital, carbamazepine**, or a combination) was associated with worse event-free survival, and greater haematological relapse and CNS relapse in children receiving chemotherapy for B-lineage acute lymphoblastic leukaemia. The authors considered that the increased clearance of vincristine induced by the anticonvulsants was a likely factor in these findings.[2]

These enzyme-inducing anticonvulsants increase the metabolism of vincristine by the cytochrome P450 isoenzyme CYP3A4. However, *in vitro* studies have shown that **phenytoin** may potentiate the antineoplastic (antimitotic) effects of the vinca alkaloids.[3,4] Thus, further study is required to determine the overall effect of **phenytoin** on the efficacy and toxicity of vincristine and other **vinca alkaloids**. **Carbamazepine** would be expected to reduce the efficacy of vincristine.

Note that a number of case reports have described reduced **phenytoin** levels in patients on chemotherapy including **vinca alkaloids**, see 'Table 11.2', (p.331).

1. Villikka K, Kivistö KT, Mäenpää H, Joensuu H, Neuvonen PJ. Cytochrome P450-inducing antiepileptics increase the clearance of vincristine in patients with brain tumors. *Clin Pharmacol Ther* (1999) 66, 589–93.
2. Relling MV, Pui CH, Sandlund JT, Rivera GK, Hancock ML, Boyett JM, Schuetz EG, Evans WE. Adverse effect of anticonvulsants on efficacy of chemotherapy for acute lymphoblastic leukaemia. *Lancet* (2000) 356, 285–90.
3. Ganapathi R, Hercbergs A, Grabowski D, Ford J. Selective enhancement of vincristine cytotoxicity in multidrug-resistant tumor cells by dilantin (phenytoin). *Cancer Res* (1993) 53, 3262–5. Erratum *ibid.*, 6079.
4. Lobert S, Ingram JW, Correia JJ. Additivity of dilantin and vinblastine inhibitory effects on microtubule assembly. *Cancer Res* (1999) 59, 4816–22.

Vinca alkaloids; Vincristine + Asparaginase

An isolated case report suggests that vincristine neurotoxicity may possibly have been increased by subsequent asparaginase therapy.[1,2] The UK maker recommends that vincristine should be administered 12 to 24 hours before asparaginase.[3] Regimens including both drugs are commonly used in treating leukaemia.

1. Hildebrand J, Kenis Y. Vincristine neurotoxicity. *N Engl J Med* (1972) 287, 517.
2. Hildebrand J, Kenis Y. Additive toxicity of vincristine and other drugs for the peripheral nervous system. *Acta Neurol Belg* (1971) 71, 486–91.
3. Vincristine sulphate. Mayne Pharma plc. UK Summary of product characteristics, February 2004.

Vinca alkaloids; Vincristine + Isoniazid

Some limited evidence suggests that vincristine neurotoxicity may possibly be increased by the concurrent use of isoniazid.

Clinical evidence, mechanism, importance and management

An 85-year-old woman with Hodgkin's disease was given COPP/ABVD, alternating every 28 days. She started COPP (cyclophosphamide and 2 mg vincristine on day 1, procarbazine and prednisone days 1 to 14) and was additionally given isoniazid 300 mg daily as prophylaxis of tuberculosis. Five days after the start of this treatment she experienced tingling in her fingers and weakness in her legs, which was interpreted by the authors of this report as being vincristine toxicity brought about by the concurrent use of isoniazid (paraesthesia of the feet and/or hands being a recognised early manifestation of vincristine toxicity). Their reasoning was that such a small dosage of vincristine dosage on its own was unlikely to cause severe neurotoxicity of this kind, but it is not clear why isoniazid should apparently interact like this. The authors suggest that the age of this patient and her diabetes (well controlled) may have contributed to this increase in vincristine neurotoxicity.[1]

This report is consistent with another much earlier report of two patients who also developed peripheral neurotoxicity when treated with vincristine after the addition of isoniazid and pyridoxine, the cumulative doses of vincristine being 11 and 11.2 mg respectively,[2,3] and of a case of severe neurotoxicity with an overdose of isoniazid and high-dose vincristine.[4]

These reports appear to be the only ones implicating isoniazid in an increase in vincristine toxicity, but they serve to emphasise the importance of very close neurological supervision in anyone given both drugs.

1. Carrión C, Espinosa E, Herrero A, García B. Possible vincristine-isoniazid interaction. *Ann Pharmacother* (1995) 29, 201.
2. Hildebrand J, Kenis Y. Vincristine neurotoxicity. *N Engl J Med* (1972) 287, 517.
3. Hildebrand J, Kenis Y. Additive toxicity of vincristine and other drugs for the peripheral nervous system. *Acta Neurol Belg* (1971) 71, 486–91.
4. Frappaz D, Biron P, Biron E, Amrane A, Philip T, Brunat-Mentigny M. Toxicite neurologique severe (coma, convulsions, neuropathie motrice distale) secondaire a l'association d'une intoxication accidentelle a l'isoniazide (INH) et d'un protocole comportant de fortes doses de vincristine (VCR). *Pediatrie* (1984) 39, 133–40.

Vinca alkaloids; Vincristine + Itraconazole

Itraconazole enhances vincristine neurotoxicity. For a discussion, see 'Azoles + Antineoplastics', p.137.

Vinca alkaloids; Vincristine + Nifedipine

Nifedipine reduces the clearance of vincristine.

Clinical evidence, mechanism, importance and management

Nifedipine reduced the clearance of a single 2-mg intravenous dose of vincristine by 68%, and increased the AUC threefold in 12 patients when compared with 14 patients receiving vincristine alone. Nifedipine was given at a dose of 10 mg three times daily for 3 days before and 7 days after administration of vincristine. However, no important side effects were noted in either group of patients, suggesting that these pharmacokinetic changes did not markedly increase vincristine toxicity.[1] Increased vincristine-related neurotoxicity has been seen in a child on nifedipine and itraconazole (see 'Azoles + Antineoplastics', p.137). Further study is needed.

1. Fedeli L, Colozza M, Boschetti E, Sabalich I, Aristei C, Guerciolini R, Del Favero A, Rossetti R, Tonato M, Rambotti P, Davis S. Pharmacokinetics of vincristine in cancer patients treated with nifedipine. *Cancer* (1989) 64, 1805–11.

16

Antiparkinsonian and related drugs

The drugs in this section are considered together because their major therapeutic application is in the treatment of Parkinson's disease, although some of the related antimuscarinic (anticholinergic) drugs included here are also used for other conditions. Parkinson's disease is named after Dr James Parkinson who originally described the four main signs of the disease, namely rigidity, tremor, dystonias and dyskinesias (movement disorders). Similar symptoms may also be displayed as the unwanted side-effects of therapy with certain drugs.

The basic cause of the disease lies in the basal ganglia of the brain, particularly the striatum and the substantia nigra, where the normal balance between dopaminergic nerve fibres (those that use dopamine as the chemical transmitter) and cholinergic nerve fibres (those that use acetylcholine as the transmitter) is lost, because the dopaminergic fibres degenerate. As a result the cholinergic fibres end up in relative excess. Much of the treatment of Parkinson's disease is based on an attempt to redress the balance, and there are several groups of drugs that can be used to this end.

Levodopa can pass the blood-brain barrier (unlike dopamine), where it is converted into dopamine, and thus acts by 'topping up' the CNS dopaminergic system. Levodopa is most usually given with carbidopa or benserazide, which prevent the 'wasteful' peripheral metabolism of levodopa. This allows lower doses of levodopa to be given, which results in fewer side-effects.

Amantadine (and memantine) may augment dopaminergic activity in the brain.

Bromocriptine, cabergoline, pergolide, ropinirole and similar drugs act as dopamine agonists and so also have the effect of increasing dopaminergic activity in the brain.

Entacapone and tolcapone (now withdrawn in many countries) are both catechol-*O*-methyltransferase (COMT) inhibitors, and work by inhibiting the peripheral metabolism of levodopa by this enzyme.

Benzhexol, orphenadrine, procyclidine and other antimuscarinic drugs work by correcting the relative cholinergic excess.

In addition to the interactions discussed in this section, some of the drugs are involved in interactions that are described elsewhere. Selegiline is also discussed under Monoamine Oxidase Inhibitors, because, although it is a selective monoamine oxidase B inhibitor (and therefore enhances dopamine activity by preventing dopamine degradation), at higher doses it loses its selectivity and consequently acts like other MAOIs. Consult the Index for a full listing.

Table 16.1 Antiparkinsonian drugs

Generic Names	*Proprietary names*
Anticholinergics	
Benzatropine	Cogentin, Cogentinol, Phatropine
Biperiden	Akineton, Cinetol, Dekinet, Ipsatol, Kinex, Norakin N
Bornaprine	Sormodren
Caramiphen	
Chlorphenoxamine	Clorevan, Systral
Dexetimide	Tremblex
Diethazine	
Ethopropazine (Profenamine)	Parsitan
Ethybenztropine	
Metixene (Methixene)	Metixen, Tremaril, Tremarit, Tremoquil
Orphenadrine (Mephenamine)	Banflex, Biorphen, Disipal, Flexin, Flexoject, Flexon, Lysantin, Norflex, Orfenace, Orfenal
Procyclidine	Arpicolin, Kemadren, Kemadrin, Muscinil, Osnervan, Procyclid
Trihexyphenidyl (Benzhexol)	Aca, Acamed, Apo-Trihex, Artandyl, Artane, Broflex, B-Hex, Hipokinon, Pargitan, Parkinane, Parkopan, Partane, Peragit, Pozhexol, Tridyl, Triexidyl, Trihexy
Tropatepine	Lepticur
Other drugs possessing anticholinergic (antimuscarinic) activity are listed in Table 16.2, p.502	
Amantadine	Adekin, Aman, Amanta, Amantagamma, Amantan, Amixx, Atarin, A-Parkin, Cerebramed, Endantadine, Hofcomant, InfectoFlu, Infex, Lysovir, Mantadan, Mantadix, Mantidan, Noctal, Paritrel, Parkadina, PK-Merz, Profil, Symmetrel, Tregor, Virucid
Bromocriptine	Antiprotin, Bromed, Bromergon, Bromocrel, Bromohexal, Bromolactin, Bromopar, Bromo-Kin, Bromtine, Broptin, Cehapark, Crilem, Cryocriptina, Kirim, Kriptiser, Kripton, Medocriptine, Parilac, Parlodel, Pravidel, Serocryptin, Suplac, Umprel, Zolac
Levodopa (L-Dopa)	Dopaflex, Dopar, Larodopa, Levomet
Levodopa + Benserazide	Aktipar, Dopamed, Levobens, Levopar, PK-Levo, Madopar, Modopar, Prolopa
Levodopa + Carbidopa	Apo-Lovocarb, Atamet, Carbilev, Cloisone, Cronomet, Dopicar, Isicom, Kardopal, Kinson, Lemdopa, Levocarb, Levomed, Nacom, Nu-Levocarb, Racovel, Sinemet, Striaton
Pergolide	Celance, Nopar, Parkotil, Permax, Pharken
Piribedil	Trivastal, Trivastan
Pramipexole	Mirapex, Mirapexin, Sifrol
Selegiline	Amboneural, Amindan, Antiparkin, Apomex, Atapryl, Carbex, Clondepryl, Cognitiv, Deprenyl, Deprilan, Egibren, Eldepryl, Elegelin, Elepril, Julab, Jumex, Jumexal, Jumexil, Kinline, MAOtil, Movergan, Niar, Plurimen, Regepar, Sefmex, Selecim, Seledat, Selegam, Selegos, Selemerck, Selepark, Selgene, Selgimed, Seline, Tremorex, Zelapar

Amantadine + Co-trimoxazole

An elderly patient on amantadine developed acute mental confusion when given co-trimoxazole.

Clinical evidence, mechanism, importance and management

An 84-year-old man with parkinsonism, COPD and chronic atrial fibrillation, was treated with amantadine 100 mg twice daily and digoxin 125 micrograms daily for at least 2 years. Within 72 hours of starting co-trimoxazole (*Septra DS*) twice daily for bronchitis he became mentally confused, incoherent and combative. He also showed cogwheel rigidity and a resting tremor. Within 24 hours of stopping the amantadine and co-trimoxazole, the patient's mental status returned to normal.[1] The reasons for this reaction are not understood, but on the basis of *animal* studies, the authors suggest that the **trimethoprim** component of the co-trimoxazole may have competed with the amantadine for renal secretion. This resulted in an accumulation of amantadine and led to the toxic effects seen.[1] This interaction is more likely in the elderly because ageing results in a decrease in the clearance of these and many other drugs. However, it should be noted that both drugs can cause some mental confusion, and also that mental confusion is not an uncommon symptom of infection in the elderly.

This seems to be the only report of such an interaction, and there do not seem to be any reports involving trimethoprim, so the general importance of this interaction remains uncertain.

1. Speeg KV, Leighton JA, Maldonado AL. Case report: toxic delirium in a patient taking amantadine and trimethoprim-sulfamethoxazole. *Am J Med Sci* (1989) 298, 410–12.

Amantadine + Paracetamol (Acetaminophen)

No pharmacokinetic interaction apparently occurs with paracetamol and amantadine.

Clinical evidence, mechanism, importance and management

Paracetamol 650 mg was given to 5 healthy subjects following amantadine 200 mg daily for 42 days, and also after a single dose of amantadine. Although the apparent volume of distribution of paracetamol was very slightly larger on long-term amantadine administration no other pharmacokinetic parameters were altered. Therefore from this limited study it appears that no change in dose is necessary if these two drugs are given together.[1]

1. Aoki FY, Sitar DS. Effects of chronic amantadine hydrochloride ingestion on its and acetaminophen pharmacokinetics in young adults. *J Clin Pharmacol* (1992) 32, 24–7.

Amantadine + Phenylpropanolamine

The use of amantadine in a patient also taking phenylpropanolamine resulted in psychosis.

Clinical evidence, mechanism, importance and management

An isolated report describes the development of severe psychosis in a woman, within 7 to 8 days of starting 100 mg amantadine (frequency unclear but possibly twice daily) and phenylpropanolamine 80 mg daily. The reasons are not known, but both drugs alone, and in high doses sometimes cause psychosis, and concurrent use may enhance this effect.[1] Concurrent use need not be avoided, but remain aware of the potential for this interaction.

1. Stroe AE, Hall J, Amin F. Psychotic episode related to phenylpropanolamine and amantadine in a healthy female. *Gen Hosp Psychiatry* (1995) 17, 457–8.

Amantadine + Quinidine or Quinine

Quinidine and quinine can reduce the loss of amantadine in the urine. No problems have been seen, but amantadine toxicity is possible.

Clinical evidence, mechanism, importance and management

Single dose studies into the renal excretion of amantadine in human subjects found that quinine sulfate 200 mg and quinidine sulfate 200 mg reduced the renal clearance of oral amantadine 3 mg/kg by about 30%, but only in male subjects.[1] Whether long-term use of these drugs would therefore cause a clinically relevant rise in serum amantadine levels is uncertain. Be alert for any evidence of amantadine toxicity (e.g. headache, nausea, or dizziness) if either of these two drugs is used concurrently with amantadine.

1. Gaudry SE, Sitar DS, Smyth DD, McKenzie JK, Aoki FY. Gender and age as factors in the inhibition of renal clearance of amantadine by quinine and quinidine. *Clin Pharmacol Ther* (1993) 54, 23–7.

Amantadine + Thiazide diuretics

A patient has been described who developed amantadine toxicity when given hydrochlorothiazide-triamterene.

Clinical evidence

Amantadine toxicity (ataxia, agitation, hallucinations) developed in a patient within a week of starting to take two tablets of *Dyazide* (**hydrochlorothiazide** with **triamterene**) daily. The symptoms rapidly disappeared when all the drugs were withdrawn. In a later study this patient showed about a 50% rise in amantadine plasma levels (from 156 to 243 nanograms/ml) after taking the diuretic for 7 days.[1]

Mechanism

Uncertain. Amantadine is largely excreted unchanged in the urine and it seems probable that these diuretics reduce the renal clearance.[1]

Importance and management

Published information about an adverse interaction appears to be limited. There seems to be little reason for avoiding concurrent use, but bear this case in mind in the event of an unexpected response to treatment.

1. Wilson TW, Rajput AH. Amantadine–Dyazide interaction. *Can Med Assoc J* (1983) 129, 974–5.

Amantadine + Tobacco smoking

Amantadine does not appear to interact with tobacco smoking.

Clinical evidence, mechanism, importance and management

The elimination of a single 3-mg/kg dose of amantadine was compared between heavy smokers (20 or more cigarettes daily) and non-smokers.

Although a higher apparent volume of distribution was noted in the heavy smokers, renal and plasma clearances were unchanged, suggesting that no interaction of note occurs.[1]

1. Wong LTY, Sitar DS, Aoki FY. Chronic tobacco smoking and gender as variables affecting amantadine disposition in healthy subjects. *Br J Clin Pharmacol* (1995) 39, 81–4.

Anticholinergics + Anticholinergics

Additive anticholinergic (antimuscarinic) effects, both peripheral and central, can develop if drugs with anticholinergic effects are used together. The outcome may be harmful.

Clinical evidence, mechanism, importance and management

The anticholinergic (or more correctly antimuscarinic) effects of some drugs are exploited therapeutically. These include atropine, and drugs such as trihexyphenidyl (benzhexol) and benzatropine ('Table 16.1', (p.500)), which are used for the control of parkinsonian symptoms. Other drugs ('Table 16.2', (p.502)) may also possess some anticholinergic effects that are unwanted and troublesome, but usually not serious, unless they are worsened by the addition of another drug with similar properties.

The easily recognised and common peripheral anticholinergic effects are blurred vision, dry mouth, constipation, difficulty in urination, reduced sweating and tachycardia. Central effects include confusion, disorientation, visual hallucinations, agitation, irritability, delirium, memory problems, belligerence and even aggressiveness. Problems are most likely to arise with patients with particular physical conditions such as glaucoma, prostatic hypertrophy or constipation. It has been pointed out that these anticholinergic side-effects can mimic the effects of normal ageing.

'Table 16.1', (p.500) and 'Table 16.2', (below) list many of the drugs with anticholinergic effects, which may be expected to be additive if used together, but apart from some reports describing life-threatening reactions (see 'Antipsychotics + Anticholinergics', p.529) there are very few reports describing this simple additive interaction, probably because the outcome is so obvious. Many of these interactions are therefore 'theoretical' but their probability is high.

Some drugs with only minimal anticholinergic properties sometimes cause difficulties if given with other anticholinergics. A patient on **isopropamide iodide** developed urinary retention needing catheterisation, only when additionally given **trazodone** 75 mg daily, but not with either drug alone.[1] **Trazodone** is usually regarded as having minimal anticholinergic effects. Another case describes acute psychosis in an elderly woman taking **hyoscine** and **meclozine**, both of which have anticholinergic effects.[2]

If the central anticholinergic effects caused by the use of anticholinergic drugs are not clearly recognised for what they are, there is the risk that **antipsychotics** may be prescribed to treat them. Many **antipsychotics** also have anticholinergic side-effects so that matters are simply made worse. If the patient then demonstrates dystonias, akathisia, tremor and rigidity, even more anticholinergics may be added to control the extrapyramidal effects, which merely adds to the continuing downward cycle of drug-induced problems.

In addition to the obvious and very well recognised drugs with anticholinergic effects, a study of the 25 drugs most commonly prescribed for the elderly identified detectable anticholinergic activity (using an anticholinergic radioreceptor assay) in 14 of them, 9 of which (**codeine**, **digoxin**, **dipyridamole**, **isosorbide dinitrate**, **nifedipine**, **prednisolone**, **ranitidine**, **theophylline**, and **warfarin**) produced levels of anticholinergic activity that have been shown to cause significant impairment in tests of memory and attention in the elderly.[3] Thus the problem may not necessarily be confined to those drugs that have well recognised anticholinergic properties. See also 'Antipsychotics + Anticholinergics', p.529.

Table 16.2 Drugs with anticholinergic effects (main or adverse effects)

Drug group	*Individual drugs*
Antiarrhythmics	Disopyramide, Propafenone
Antiemetics	Cyclizine, Dimenhydrinate, Meclozine, Hyoscine (scopolamine)
Antihistamines	Brompheniramine, Chlorphenamine, Cyproheptadine, Diphenhydramine, Hydroxyzine, Triprolidine
Antiparkinson drugs (anticholinergics)	see Table 16.1, p.500
Antipsychotics	Chlorpromazine, Chlorprothixene, Clozapine, Loxapine, Perphenazine, Pimozide, Mesoridazine, Trifluoperazine, Thioridazine
Antispasmodics	Anisotropine, Atropine, Belladonna alkaloids, Dicycloverine (dicyclomine), Flavoxate, Hyoscine (scopolamine), Hyoscyamine, Isopropamide, Oxybutynin, Propantheline, Tolterodine
Antiulcer drugs	Clidinium, Hexocyclium, Isopropamide, Mepenzolate, Methanthelinium, Oxyphencyclimine, Pirenzepine, Tridihexethyl
Cycloplegic mydriatics	Atropine, Homatropine, Hyoscine (scopolamine), Cyclopentolate, Tropicamide
Muscle relaxants	Baclofen, Cyclobenzaprine, Orphenadrine
Peripheral vasodilator	Papaverine
Tricyclic and related antidepressants	Amitriptyline, Amoxapine, Clomipramine, Desipramine, Doxepin, Imipramine, Maprotiline, Protriptyline, Nortriptyline, Trimipramine

After Barkin RL, Stein ZLG. *South Med J* (1989) 82, 1547, and others.
The categorization is not exclusive; some of these drugs are used for a range of effects. There are many other anticholinergic drugs.

1. Chan CH, Ruskiewicz RJ. Anticholinergic side effects of trazodone combined with another pharmacologic agent. *Am J Psychiatry* (1990) 147, 533.
2. Osterholm RK, Camoriano JK. Transdermal scopolamine psychosis. *JAMA* (1982) 247, 3081.
3. Tune L, Carr S, Hoag E, Cooper T. Anticholinergic effects of drugs commonly prescribed for the elderly: potential means for assessing risk of delirium. *Am J Psychiatry* (1992) 149, 1393–4.

Anticholinergics + Areca (Betel nuts)

The control of the extrapyramidal (parkinsonian) side-effects of fluphenazine and flupenthixol with procyclidine was lost in two patients when they began to chew areca.

Clinical evidence

An Indian patient on depot fluphenazine (50 mg every three weeks) for schizophrenia, and with mild parkinsonian tremor controlled with **procyclidine** 5 mg twice daily, developed marked rigidity, bradykinesia and jaw tremor when he began to chew areca. The symptoms were so severe he could barely speak. When he stopped chewing the nuts his stiffness and abnormal movements disappeared. Another patient on depot flupenthixol developed marked stiffness, tremor and akathisia, despite taking up to 20 mg **procyclidine** daily, when he began to chew areca. The symptoms vanished within 4 days of stopping the areca.[1]

Mechanism

Areca contains arecoline, an alkaloid with cholinergic activity. It seems that the arecoline opposed the actions of the anticholinergic procyclidine that was being used to control the extrapyramidal side-effects of the two antipsychotics, thereby allowing these side-effects to re-emerge and worsen.

Importance and management

Direct information seems to be limited to this report but the interaction would seem to be established and clinically important. Patients taking anticholinergic drugs for the control of drug-induced extrapyramidal (parkinsonian) side-effects, or Parkinson's disease, should avoid areca. The authors of this report suggest that a dental inspection for the characteristic red stains of the areca may possibly provide a simple explanation for the sudden and otherwise mysterious deterioration in the symptoms of patients. Betel is traditionally chewed by those from the continent of Asia, and the East Indies. Symptoms seem to develop over a period of 2 weeks, and resolve fairly rapidly (within a week).

1. Deahl M. Betel nut-induced extrapyramidal syndrome: an unusual drug interaction. *Mov Disord* (1989) 4, 330–3.

Apomorphine + Miscellaneous

The hypotensive side-effects of apomorphine may possibly be increased by nitrates or alcohol. The concurrent use of other drugs used for erectile dysfunction or dopamine agonists or antagonists is not recommended. However, domperidone, and prochlorperazine are said not to interact when apomorphine is used for erectile dysfunction. There is evidence that ACE inhibitors, alpha blockers, antidepressants, anticonvulsants, beta-blockers, calcium channel blockers, and ondansetron do not interact adversely.

Clinical evidence, mechanism, importance and management

(a) Alcohol

The makers say that interaction studies in subjects given apomorphine (for erectile dysfunction) found that alcohol increased the incidence and extent of hypotension (one of the side-effects of apomorphine). They also point out that alcohol can diminish sexual performance.[1]

(b) Anticonvulsants, Antidepressants

The makers say that no studies about interactions between apomorphine and either anticonvulsants or antidepressants have been undertaken, but clinical experience in erectile dysfunction suggests that no interaction occurs.[1]

(c) Antiemetics

The small doses of apomorphine used for erectile dysfunction (2 to 3 mg) do not normally cause vomiting, but nausea does occur in about 7% of patients and the makers say that interaction studies and/or clinical experience show that **domperidone**, **ondansetron** or **prochlorperazine** may safely be given concurrently as antiemetics.[1] Studies with other antiemetics have not been carried out, so at the moment concurrent use is not recommended.[1]

Note that **prochlorperazine** should not be given if apomorphine is used for Parkinson's disease, as its dopamine antagonist actions can worsen the disease.

(d) Nitrates and antihypertensives

The makers report that in a group of 40 patients given 5 mg apomorphine (sublingually as for erectile dysfunction) and given nitrates (not specifically named), 4 patients experienced vasovagal symptoms and significant standing blood pressure decreases (i.e. they felt faint and dizzy). The dose used was slightly higher than the recommended 2- to 3-mg dose. On the basis of this study the makers suggest caution, which in practice means telling patients what may possibly happen and what to do (to lie down and raise their legs).[1] Parallel studies in patients taking **ACE inhibitors**, **alpha blockers**, **beta-blockers** or **calcium channel blockers** found no significant interactions.[1]

Probably because of the higher doses given for Parkinson's disease the makers suggest that in this case caution is advisable on concurrent use with any antihypertensive agent.[2]

(e) Other dopamine agonists or antagonists

The makers say that apomorphine should not be given with other centrally-acting dopamine agonists or antagonists[1,2] because potentially they may interact at dopamine receptors. Such drugs would include some **antipsychotics** but thus far clinical reports of problems seem to be lacking. However, see prochlorperazine in (c) above.

(f) Other drugs used for erectile dysfunction

The makers say that no formal studies have been done with a combination of apomorphine and other drugs used for erectile dysfunction but there seems to be no evidence of problems, nevertheless they do not recommend concurrent use.[1] The other drugs used for this condition would include **alprostadil**, **papaverine**, **phentolamine**, the **phosphodiesterase inhibitors**, and **thymoxamine**.

1. Uprima (Apomorphine). Abbott Laboratories Ltd. UK Summary of product characteristics, September 2004.
2. APO-go ampoules (Apomorphine). Britannia Pharmaceuticals Ltd. UK Summary of product characteristics, June 2002.

Apomorphine + Oral contraceptives

The sedative effects of apomorphine are decreased by the combined oral contraceptives.

Clinical evidence, mechanism, importance and management

A study[1] in a group of 9 women showed that the sedative effects of a single 5-micrograms/kg subcutaneous dose of apomorphine were decreased while taking a combined oral contraceptive (**ethinylestradiol** 30 micrograms, **levonorgestrel** 150 or 250 micrograms). The clinical importance of this is uncertain.

1. Chalmers JS, Fulli-Lemaire I, Cowen PJ. Effects of the contraceptive pill on sedative responses to clonidine and apomorphine in normal women. *Psychol Med* (1985) 15, 363–7.

Bromocriptine + Domperidone

Domperidone raises prolactin levels, sometimes causing galactorrhoea, gynaecomastia or mastalgia,[1,2] and may therefore be inappropriate for patients being treated with bromocriptine for its prolactin-lowering effect.

1. Cann PA, Read NW, Holdsworth CD. Oral domperidone: double blind comparison with placebo in irritable bowel syndrome. *Gut* (1983) 24, 1135–40.
2. Van der Steen M, Du Caju MVL, Van Acker KJ. Gynaecomastia in a male infant given domperidone. *Lancet* (1982) 2, 884–5.

Bromocriptine + Griseofulvin

Evidence from a single case, where bromocriptine was being used for acromegaly, suggests that its effects can be opposed by griseofulvin.

Clinical evidence, mechanism, importance and management

The effects of bromocriptine, used for the treatment of acromegaly, were abolished when a patient was given griseofulvin for the treatment of a fungal nail infection. When the griseofulvin was stopped, the bromocriptine was again effective.[1] The mechanism of this interaction and its general importance are unknown, but prescribers should be aware of it when treating patients with bromocriptine.

1. Schwinn G, Dirks H, McIntosh C, Köbberling J. Metabolic and clinical studies on patients with acromegaly treated with bromocriptine over 22 months. *Eur J Clin Invest* (1977) 7, 101–7.

Bromocriptine + Macrolides

Bromocriptine toxicity occurred in an elderly man additionally given josamycin and in an elderly woman additionally given erythromycin. Two reports found that erythromycin causes an increase in plasma bromocriptine levels.

Clinical evidence

(a) Erythromycin

Erythromycin estolate 250 mg four times daily for 4 days caused a marked change in the pharmacokinetics of a single 5-mg oral dose of bromocriptine in 5 healthy subjects. The peak plasma levels and the AUC of bromocriptine were raised by about 360% and 268%, respectively.[1]

Another report describes 2 women on levodopa/carbidopa and bromocriptine for parkinsonism, which was better controlled when erythromycin was added. Bromocriptine plasma levels were found to be 40 to 50% higher.[2] An elderly woman on levodopa and bromocriptine 15 mg developed psychotic symptoms when treated with erythromycin, which were attributed to bromocriptine toxicity.[3]

(b) Josamycin

An elderly man with Parkinson's disease, well-controlled for 10 months on daily treatment with levodopa/benserazide, bromocriptine 70 mg and domperidone, was additionally given josamycin 2 g daily for a respiratory infection. Shortly after the first dose he became drowsy with visual hallucinations, and began to show involuntary movements of his limbs, similar to the dystonic and dyskinetic movements seen in choreoathetosis. These adverse effects (interpreted as bromocriptine toxicity) disappeared within a few days of withdrawing the antibacterial.[4]

Mechanism

Bromocriptine undergoes extensive first pass metabolism. It has been suggested that erythromycin (and potentially other macrolides) inhibit this metabolism, thus significantly elevating bromocriptine plasma levels.[1]

Importance and management

Information seems to be limited to these reports. Concurrent use should be well monitored if either of these macrolides is added to bromocriptine treatment. Moderately increased bromocriptine levels may be therapeutically advantageous, but grossly elevated levels can be toxic. The authors of one report[1] suggest reducing the bromocriptine dose, while in another case the dose was reduced by 50% to avoid toxicity.[3] There seems to be no direct evidence about any other macrolides, but some of them certainly inhibit liver metabolism in the same way as erythromycin and josamycin, and have been shown to raise the levels of other similarly metabolised drugs.

1. Nelson MV, Berchou RC, Kareti D, LeWitt PA. Pharmacokinetic evaluation of erythromycin and caffeine administered with bromocriptine. *Clin Pharmacol Ther* (1990) 47, 694–7.
2. Sibley WA, Laguna JF. Enhancement of bromocriptine clinical effect and plasma levels with erythromycin. *Excerpta Med* (1981) 548, 329–30.
3. Alegre M, Noé E, Martínez Lage JM. Psicosis por interacción de eritromicina con bromocriptina en enfermedad de Parkinson. *Neurologia* (1997) 12, 429.
4. Montastruc JL, Rascol A. Traitement de la maladie de Parkinson par doses élevées de bromocriptine. Interaction possible avec la josamycine. *Presse Med* (1984) 13, 2267–8.

Bromocriptine + Sympathomimetics

A healthy woman taking bromocriptine developed very severe headache and marked hypertension after additionally taking phenylpropanolamine. Another woman developed seizures with cerebral vasospasm, and a third developed a severe headache, hypertension and severe cardiac dysfunction after additionally taking isometheptene. Yet another developed psychosis when pseudoephedrine was added.

Clinical evidence

Two healthy women who had given birth 3 to 4 days previously, developed severe headaches while taking bromocriptine 2.5 mg twice daily for milk suppression. After additionally taking three 65-mg doses of **isometheptene mucate**, the headache of one of them markedly worsened, and hypertension with life-threatening ventricular tachycardia and cardiac dysfunction developed. The other woman took two 75-mg doses of **phenylpropanolamine**, and developed grand mal seizures and cerebral vasospasm.[1]

A woman of 32 uneventfully took two 5-mg doses of bromocriptine for milk suppression following the birth of a child. Within 2 hours of taking a third dose with **phenylpropanolamine** 50 mg she awoke with a very severe headache and was found to have a blood pressure of 240/140 mmHg. She was given 5 mg of intramuscular morphine and her blood pressure became normal within 24 hours. Another 5-mg dose of bromocriptine taken 48 hours after the original dose of **phenylpropanolamine** had the same effect, but the blood pressure rise was less severe (160/120 mmHg).[2]

A woman who had recently given birth and who had taken bromocriptine 2.5 mg twice daily for 9 days without problems became psychotic shortly after starting **pseudoephedrine** 60 mg four times daily.[3]

Mechanism

Not understood. Severe hypertension occasionally occurs with both bromocriptine and phenylpropanolamine when given alone. Shortly after giving birth some individuals also show increased vascular reactivity, and it could be that all of these factors conspired together to cause these adverse effects.[2] Psychosis occasionally occurs after giving birth or on bromocriptine alone, so that the addition of pseudoephedrine may have been coincidental.[3]

Importance and management

Direct information seems to be limited to these four cases, but the severity of the reactions suggests that it might be prudent for other patients to avoid sympathomimetics like these while taking bromocriptine. More study is needed.

1. Kulig K, Moore LL, Kirk M, Smith D, Stallworth J, Rumack B. Bromocriptine-associated headache: possible life-threatening sympathomimetic interaction. *Obstet Gynecol* (1991) 78, 941–3.
2. Chan JCN, Critchley JAJH, Cockram CS. Postpartum hypertension, bromocriptine and phenylpropanolamine. *Drug Invest* (1994) 8, 254–6.
3. Reeves RR, Pinkofsky HB. Postpartum psychosis induced by bromocriptine and pseudoephedrine. *J Fam Pract* (1997) 45, 164–6.

Cabergoline + Miscellaneous

Dopamine antagonists (such as the phenothiazines) are expected to oppose the action of cabergoline. The makers also advise the avoidance of ergot derivatives and macrolides, which they suggest on theoretical grounds might interact. No significant pharmacokinetic interaction occurs between cabergoline and selegiline or levodopa.

Clinical evidence, mechanism, importance and management

Cabergoline acts by directly stimulating dopamine receptors (it is a D_2 agonist), which is why the makers suggest that dopamine antagonists (e.g. **phenothiazines**, **butyrophenones**, **thioxanthenes**, **metoclopramide**) should be avoided, because they would be expected to oppose its actions.[1] There is however no direct clinical evidence to confirm how important this is, but it is clearly a reasonable precaution to take.

Because cabergoline is an ergot derivative, the makers have looked at what happens if other **ergot derivatives** are used concurrently, but have so far found no evidence of changes in the efficacy or safety of cabergoline. Nevertheless they do not recommend their long-term concurrent use.[1] The makers also suggest, by analogy with other ergot derivatives (ergotamine, dihydroergotamine), that **macrolides** such as **erythromycin** should be avoided because of the risk that the cabergoline effects and adverse effects could be increased.[1] However, these theoretical interactions with cabergoline have yet to be shown to be of clinical importance. See also 'Ergot derivatives + Macrolides', p.436.

No pharmacokinetic interaction was found to occur between cabergoline 1 mg daily and **selegiline** 10 mg daily in a study covering a 22-day period in 6 subjects.[2] Similarly, **levodopa** did not cause a clinically significant change in the pharmacokinetics of cabergoline, when the combination was given to patients newly diagnosed with Parkinson's disease, or to those with fluctuating Parkinson's disease.[3]

1. Dostinex (Cabergoline). Pharmacia Ltd. UK Summary of product characteristics, February 2003.
2. Dostert P, Benedetti MS, Persiani S, La Croix R, Bosc M, Fiorentini F, Deffond D, Vernay D, Dordain G. Lack of pharmacokinetic interaction between the selective dopamine agonist cabergoline and the MAO-B inhibitor selegiline. *J Neural Transm* (1995) 45 (Suppl), 247–57.
3. Del Dotto P, Colzi A, Musatti E, Benedetti MS, Persiani S, Fariello R, Bonuccelli U. Clinical and pharmacokinetic evaluation of L-dopa and cabergoline cotreatment in Parkinson's disease. *Clin Neuropharmacol* (1997) 20, 455–65.

Entacapone + Ephedrine

A single case report describes severe hypertension in a patient given entacapone and ephedrine.

Clinical evidence, mechanism, importance and management

A woman of 76 with Parkinson's disease taking levodopa/carbidopa and entacapone 200 mg five times daily, was given 3 mg of ephedrine intravenously during cataract surgery to correct a low blood pressure of 85/35 mmHg. Her blood pressure immediately rose to 225/125 mmHg. The patient needed several doses of hydralazine over the following 140 minutes before her blood pressure returned to normal.[1] The authors believe that the marked rise in blood pressure was possibly because the entacapone inhibited catechol-O-methyl transferase so that the normal metabolism of ephedrine (and the catecholamines it releases at adrenergic nerve endings) was inhibited, which resulted in a gross exaggeration of their normal effects.[1]

1. Renfrew C, Dickson R, Schwab C. Severe hypertension following ephedrine administration in a patient receiving entacapone. *Anesthesiology* (2000) 93, 1562.

Entacapone + Imipramine

Entacapone and imipramine appear not to interact adversely.

Clinical evidence, mechanism, importance and management

In order to study the effects on haemodynamics, catecholamine metabolism, and tolerability of entacapone and imipramine, 12 healthy women were given entacapone 200 mg, imipramine 75 mg, a combination of the two drugs or a placebo in a single-dose crossover study. Although both drugs can impair the inactivation of catecholamines the study found no evidence that combined drug use had any relevant effect on haemodynamics or on free adrenaline (epinephrine) or noradrenaline (norepinephrine) plasma levels. The combination was well tolerated in all subjects.[1] There would appear to be no reason for avoiding concurrent use.

1. Illi A, Sundberg S, Ojala-Karlsson P, Scheinin M, Gordin A. Simultaneous inhibition of catecholamine-*O*-methylation by entacapone and neuronal uptake by imipramine: lack of interactions. *Eur J Clin Pharmacol* (1996) 51, 273–6.

Levodopa + Antacids

Antacids appear not to interact significantly with levodopa, although there is some evidence that antacids reduce the bioavailability of levodopa in modified release preparations.

Clinical evidence and mechanism

The small intestine is the major site of absorption for levodopa, and delayed gastric emptying appears to result in low plasma levodopa levels, probably because levodopa can be metabolised in the stomach.

One study showed that 15 ml of an **aluminium/magnesium hydroxide** antacid, given 30 minutes before levodopa, to a patient with a prolonged gastric emptying time, caused a threefold increase in levodopa serum levels, which was associated with a marked improvement in symptoms.[1] Another patients was able to reduce his levodopa dose when taking antacids, without affecting symptom control.[1] A further study showed that the maximum plasma concentration of levodopa was raised by 20% when 20 ml of an antacid was given before the levodopa.[2] However, when 8 patients (only 3 with Parkinson's disease) were given *Mylanta* (containing **aluminium/magnesium hydroxide** and simeticone), 30 minutes before, and/or with levodopa, only occasional increases in bioavailability were seen. One of the 3 patients with Parkinson's disease who had shown improved bioavailability while on antacids had his levodopa dose lowered and continued to take *Mylanta*, but the parkinsonian symptoms worsened and the levodopa was increased back to the original dose.[3] Another study, in 15 parkinsonian patients taking dopamine agonists (e.g. bromocriptine) and levodopa with carbidopa who were given six 30-ml doses of **aluminium hydroxide** daily, inferred that the antacid had no significant effect on levodopa bioavailability, because of the lack of clinical fluctuations in effect.[4] However, in a study using *Madopar HBS*, a sustained release preparation of levodopa and benserazide, the concurrent use of an unnamed antacid reduced the levodopa bioavailability by about one-third.[5] The makers of *Madopar* state in their SPCs that antacids reduce the bioavailability of levodopa from the modified release preparation, but not the standard preparation.[6,7]

Importance and management

The overall picture is that concurrent use need not be avoided with standard preparations, although some individuals may be affected so the outcome should be monitored. With modified release preparations it would seem advisable to avoid concurrent administration (1 to 2 hours is usually enough in other similar cases of interactions with antacids). Again, the outcome should be monitored.

1. Rivera-Calimlim L, Dujovne CA, Morgan JP, Lasagna L, Bianchine JR. Absorption and metabolism of L-dopa by the human stomach. *Eur J Clin Invest* (1971) 1, 313–20.
2. Pocelinko R, Thomas GB, Solomon HM. The effect of an antacid on the absorption and metabolism of levodopa. *Clin Pharmacol Ther* (1972) 13, 149.
3. Leon AS, Spiegel HE. The effect of antacid administration on the absorption and metabolism of levodopa. *J Clin Pharmacol* (1972) 12, 263–7.
4. Lau E, Waterman K, Glover R, Schulzer M, Calne DB. Effect of antacid on levodopa therapy. *Clin Neuropharmacol* (1986) 9, 477–9.
5. Malcolm SL, Allen JG, Bird H, Quinn NP, Marion MH, Marsden CD, O'Leary CG. Single-dose pharmacokinetics of Madopar HBS in patients and effect of food and antacid on the absorption of Madopar HBS in volunteers. *Eur Neurol* (1987) 27 (Suppl 1), 28–35.
6. Madopar CR (Levodopa/benserazide). Roche Products Ltd. UK Summary of product characteristics, December 2002.
7. Madopar (Levodopa/benserazide). Roche Products Ltd. UK Summary of product characteristics, December 2002.

Levodopa + Anticholinergics

Although anticholinergic drugs are very widely used in conjunction with levodopa, they may reduce the absorption of levodopa and reduce its therapeutic effects to some extent.

Clinical evidence

A study[1] in 6 healthy subjects and 6 patients with Parkinson's disease showed that the administration of **trihexyphenidyl** 2 mg twice daily for 3 days lowered the peak plasma levels of a 500-mg dose of levodopa by 42% in the healthy subjects and 17% in the patients, although the interaction was present in only about half of the subjects. The AUC was reduced in both groups by less than 20%.[1]

A study in 6 patients with Parkinson's disease found that **orphenadrine** caused a delay in levodopa absorption in one patient, and a reduction in levodopa absorption in two others.[2] Another study in 4 healthy subjects[3] showed that the concurrent use of **imipramine** 25 mg four times daily for 3 days reduced the peak plasma concentration of a single 500-mg dose of levodopa by about 50%. (See also 'Levodopa + Tricyclic antidepressants', p.513 for other non-anticholinergic interactions of the tricyclics.)

A patient who needed 7 g of levodopa daily while taking **homatropine** developed levodopa toxicity when the **homatropine** was withdrawn, and he was subsequently restabilised on only 4 g of levodopa daily.[4] This interaction between anticholinergics and levodopa is described in another report.[5]

Mechanism

The small intestine is the major site of absorption for levodopa. Delayed gastric emptying, which can be caused by anticholinergics, appears to result in low plasma levodopa levels, because the gastric mucosa has more time to metabolise the levodopa 'wastefully'. Therefore less is available for absorption.[6]

Importance and management

Anticholinergics are among the most commonly co-administered drugs with levodopa, and they are of established benefit. However, in some cases they have been shown to reduce levodopa efficacy. There is certainly no need to avoid concurrent use, but it would be prudent to be alert for any evidence of a reduced levodopa response if anticholinergics are added, or for levodopa toxicity if they are withdrawn.

1. Algeri S, Cerletti C, Curcio M, Morselli PL, Bonollo L, Buniva G, Minazzi M, Minoli G. Effect of anticholinergic drugs on gastro-intestinal absorption of L-dopa in rats and in man. *Eur J Pharmacol* (1976) 35, 293–9.
2. Contin M, Riva R, Martinelli P, Procaccianti G, Albani F, Baruzzi A. Combined levodopa-anticholinergic therapy in the treatment of Parkinson's disease. *Clin Neuropharmacol* (1991) 14, 148–55.
3. Morgan JP, Rivera-Calimlim L, Messiha F, Sundaresan PR, Trabert N. Imipramine-mediated interference with levodopa absorption from the gastrointestinal tract in man. *Neurology* (1975) 25, 1029–34.
4. Fermaglich J, O'Doherty DS. Effect of gastric motility on levodopa. *Dis Nerv Syst* (1972) 33, 624–5.
5. Birket-Smith E. Abnormal involuntary movements in relation to anticholinergics and levodopa therapy. *Acta Neurol Scand* (1975) 52, 158–60.
6. Rivera-Calimlim L, Dujovne CA, Morgan JP, Lasagna L, Bianchine JR. Absorption and metabolism of L-dopa by the human stomach. *Eur J Clin Invest* (1971) 1, 313–20.

Levodopa + Antiemetics

Domperidone can be used to prevent nausea and vomiting caused by levodopa. Other antiemetics that are generally considered useful include cyclizine and difenidol. Some of the effects of levodopa are increased by metoclopramide and other effects are opposed, and the outcome of concurrent use is uncertain. Phenothiazine antiemetics such as prochlorperazine are generally considered to be contraindicated in Parkinson's disease. See also 'Levodopa + Antipsychotics', p.506.

Clinical evidence, mechanism, importance and management

(a) Domperidone

Domperidone is a dopamine antagonist similar to metoclopramide, but domperidone can be used to control the nausea and vomiting associated with levodopa treatment of Parkinson's disease.[1] Since it acts on the dopamine receptors in the stomach wall, and unlike metoclopramide, it does not readily cross the blood-brain barrier, it does not appear to oppose the effects of levodopa within the brain, although some extrapyramidal symptoms have been observed. It may even slightly increase the bioavailability and effects of levodopa (by stimulating gastric emptying).[2]

(b) Metoclopramide

Metoclopramide is a dopamine antagonist that can cause extrapyramidal disturbances[3] (parkinsonian symptoms), especially in children.[4] On the other hand, metoclopramide stimulates gastric emptying, which can result in an increase in the bioavailability of levodopa.[5,6] The outcome of these two effects (enhanced extrapyramidal disturbances and increased bioavailability) is uncertain. However, if the use of alternative antiemetics is unsuitable and metoclopramide is used concurrently, it would seem prudent to monitor the outcome because its dopamine antagonist effects may aggravate Parkinson's disease.

(c) Phenothiazine antiemetics

Phenothiazines block the dopamine receptors in the brain and can therefore upset the balance between cholinergic and dopaminergic components within the striatum and substantia nigra. As a consequence they may not only induce the development of extrapyramidal (parkinsonian) symptoms, but they can aggravate parkinsonism and antagonise the effects of levodopa used in its treatment. See 'Levodopa + Antipsychotics', below. Phenothiazines, used in smaller doses as antiemetics, such as **prochlorperazine**,[7,8] can also behave in this way. For this reason drugs of this kind are generally regarded as contraindicated in patients with Parkinson's disease.

(d) Non-interacting antiemetics

Antiemetics that are generally considered useful in patients with Parkinson's disease include **cyclizine** and **difenidol**,[7] which do not affect dopamine, and **domperidone** as discussed above.

1. Bradbrook ID, Gillies HC, Morrison PJ, Rogers HJ. The effects of domperidone on the absorption of levodopa in normal subjects. *Eur J Clin Pharmacol* (1986) 29, 721–3.
2. Shindler JS, Finnerty GT, Towlson K, Dolan AL, Davies CL, Parkes JD. Domperidone and levodopa in Parkinson's disease. *Br J Clin Pharmacol* (1984) 18, 959–62.
3. Avorn J, Gurwitz JH, Bohn RL, Mogun H, Monane M, Walker A. Increased incidence of levodopa therapy following metoclopramide usage. *JAMA* (1995) 274, 1780–2.
4. Casteels-Van Daele M, Jaeken J, Van der Schueren P, Zimmerman A, Van den Bon P. Dystonic reactions in children caused by metoclopramide. *Arch Dis Child* (1970) 45, 130–3.
5. Berkowitz DM, McCallum RW. Interaction of levodopa and metoclopramide on gastric emptying. *Clin Pharmacol Ther* (1980) 27, 414–20.
6. Mearrick PT, Wade DN, Birkett DJ, Morris J. Metoclopramide, gastric emptying and L-dopa absorption. *Aust N Z J Med* (1974) 4, 144–8.
7. Duvoisin R.C. Diphenidol for levodopa induced nausea and vomiting. *JAMA* (1972) 221, 1408.
8. Campbell JB. Long-term treatment of Parkinson's disease with levodopa. *Neurology* (1970) 20, 18–22.

Levodopa + Antipsychotics

Phenothiazines and butyrophenones can oppose the effects of levodopa. The antipsychotic effects and extrapyramidal side-effects of the phenothiazines can be opposed by levodopa. See also 'Levodopa + Antiemetics', p.505.

Clinical evidence, mechanism, importance and management

Phenothiazines (e.g. chlorpromazine) and **butyrophenones** (e.g. haloperidol, droperidol) block the dopamine receptors in the brain and can therefore upset the balance between cholinergic and dopaminergic components within the striatum and substantia nigra. As a consequence they may not only induce the development of extrapyramidal (parkinsonian) symptoms, but they can aggravate parkinsonism and antagonise the effects of levodopa used in its treatment.[1-4] For this reason drugs of this kind are generally regarded as contraindicated in patients being treated for Parkinson's disease, or only used with great caution in carefully controlled conditions. The extrapyramidal symptoms that frequently occur with the **phenothiazines** have in the past been treated without much success with levodopa, however, the levodopa may also antagonise the antipsychotic effects of the **phenothiazines**.[5]

1. Duvoisin RC. Diphenidol for levodopa induced nausea and vomiting. *JAMA* (1972) 221, 1408.
2. Klawans HL, Weiner WJ. Attempted use of haloperidol in the treatment of L-dopa induced dyskinesias. *J Neurol Neurosurg Psychiatry* (1974) 37, 427–30.
3. Hunter KR, Stern GM, Laurence DR. Use of levodopa and other drugs. *Lancet* (1970) ii, 1283–5.
4. Lipper S. Psychosis in a patient on bromocriptine and levodopa with carbidopa. *Lancet* (1976) ii, 571–2.
5. Yaryura-Tobias JA, Wolpert A, Dana L, Merlis S. Action of L-dopa in drug induced extrapyramidalism. *Dis Nerv Syst* (1970) 1, 60–3.

Levodopa + Baclofen

Unpleasant side-effects (hallucinations, confusion, headache, nausea) and worsening of the symptoms of parkinsonism have occurred in patients on levodopa when given baclofen.

Clinical evidence

Twelve patients with parkinsonism on levodopa were additionally given baclofen. The eventual baclofen dosage was intended to be 90 mg daily, but the side-effects were considerable (visual hallucinations, a toxic confusional state, headaches, nausea) so that only 2 reached this dosage, and 2 patients withdrew because they could not tolerate these side-effects. The mean dosage for those who continued was 45 mg daily. Rigidity was aggravated by an average of 46% and functional capacity deteriorated by 21%.[1]

A patient with Parkinson's disease on *Sinemet* (levodopa/carbidopa), orphenadrine and diazepam became acutely confused, agitated, incontinent and hallucinated when given a third dose of baclofen (in all 15 mg). The baclofen was stopped, but on the following night she again hallucinated and became confused. The next day she was given two 2.5-mg doses of baclofen but she became anxious and hallucinated with paranoid ideas.[2]

Mechanism

Not understood. One suggestion is that the baclofen deranges the dopamine metabolism.[2] The toxicity seen appears to be an exaggeration of the known side-effects of baclofen.

Importance and management

Information appears to be limited to these reports, but they suggest that baclofen is probably best avoided, or at least used very cautiously, in patients taking levodopa.

1. Lees AJ, Shaw KM, Stern GM. Baclofen in Parkinson's disease. *J Neurol Neurosurg Psychiatry* (1978) 41, 707–8.
2. Skausig OB, Korsgaard S. Hallucinations and baclofen. *Lancet* (1977) 1, 1258.

Levodopa + Benzodiazepines and related drugs

On rare occasions it seems that the therapeutic effects of levodopa can be reduced by the concurrent use of chlordiazepoxide, diazepam or nitrazepam.

Clinical evidence

Various benzodiazepines (dose unstated) were given to 8 patients with Parkinson's disease in addition to their levodopa treatment. In 5 of the patients (3 on **chlordiazepoxide**, 1 on **nitrazepam**, 1 on **oxazepam**) no interactions were seen. However, the other 3 patients (1 on **diazepam**, 2 on **nitrazepam**) experienced transient disturbances in the control of their Parkinson's disease, which lasted up to 3 weeks in the case of the patient on **diazepam**.[1] Other cases of a reversible loss of control of Parkinson's disease have been seen in 3 patients on **diazepam**[2] and 4 patients on **chlordiazepoxide**.[3,4] In one further case, a patient on **chlordiazepoxide** experienced falls associated with a worsening of parkinsonian symptoms while on **chlordiazepoxide**. She recovered 5 days after the **chlordiazepoxide** was withdrawn.[5]

Mechanism

Not understood, although *animal* studies have shown that benzodiazepines can decrease the levels of dopamine in the striatum.[6]

Importance and management

Sleep disturbances are common in patients with Parkinson's disease. Given the widespread use of these drugs, any major or common interaction would be expected to have come to light by now. It would therefore seem that this interaction is fairly rare, and on the basis of one of the reports cited above, possibly only transient. There are reports about the successful use of benzodiazepines in patients on levodopa.[6,7] There is no need to avoid concurrent use, but be aware that the occasional patient may experience a worsening of symptoms, or perhaps a lack of response to levodopa. In one patient **hydroxyzine** was successfully substituted for chlordiazepoxide,[5] and so this may be a suitable non-interacting alternative.

1. Hunter KR, Stern GM, Laurence DR. Use of levodopa with other drugs. *Lancet* (1970) ii, 1283–5.
2. Wodak J, Gilligan BS, Veale JL, Dowty BJ. Review of 12 months' treatment with L-dopa in Parkinson's disease, with remarks on unusual side effects. *Med J Aust* (1972) 2, 1277–82.
3. Mackie L. Drug antagonism. *BMJ* (1971) 2, 651.
4. Schwarz GA, Fahn S. Newer medical treatments in parkinsonism. *Med Clin North Am* (1970) 54, 773–85.
5. Yosselson-Superstine S, Lipman AG. Chlordiazepoxide interaction with levodopa. *Ann Intern Med* (1982) 96, 259–60.
6. van de Vijver DAMC, Roos RAC, Jansen PAF, Porsius AJ, de Boer A. Influence of benzodiazepines on antiparkinsonian drug treatment in levodopa users. *Acta Neurol Scand* (2002) 105, 8–12.
7. Kales A, Ansel RD, Markham CH, Scharf MB, Tan T-L. Sleep in patients with Parkinson's disease and normal subjects prior to and following levodopa administration. *Clin Pharmacol Ther* (1971) 12, 397–406.

Levodopa + Beta-blockers

Concurrent use of levodopa and beta-blockers normally appears to be favourable, but the long-term effects of the elevated growth hormone levels are uncertain.

Clinical evidence, mechanism, importance and management

Most of the effects of combined use of levodopa and beta-blockers seem to be favourable, although additive hypotension can be a problem. Dopamine derived from levodopa stimulates beta-receptors in the heart, which can cause arrhythmias. These receptors are blocked by **propranolol**[1] and other beta-blockers. An enhancement of the effects of levodopa and a reduction in tremor has been described in 23 out of 25 patients taking **propranolol**,[2] but not in 9 patients taking **oxprenolol**,[3] or in other patients taking **propranolol**.[4] However, there is evidence that growth hormone levels are substantially raised by **propranolol**[5] or **practolol**[6] (now withdrawn due to fatal reactions) in conjunction with levodopa, but to what extent this might prove to be an adverse response during long-term treatment appears not to have been assessed.

1. Goldberg LI, Whitsett TL. Cardiovascular effects of levodopa. *Clin Pharmacol Ther* (1971) 12, 376–82.
2. Kissel P, Tridon P, André JM. Levodopa-propranolol therapy in parkinsonian tremor. *Lancet* (1974) ii, 403–4.
3. Sandler M, Fellows LE, Calne DB, Findley LJ. Oxprenolol and levodopa in parkinsonian patients. *Lancet* (1975) i, 168.
4. Marsden CD, Parkes JD, Rees JE. Propranolol in Parkinson's disease. *Lancet* (1974) ii, 410.
5. Camanni F, Massara F. Enhancement of levodopa-induced growth-hormone stimulation by propranolol. *Lancet* (1974) i, 942.
6. Lotti G, Delitala G, Masala A. Enhancement of levodopa-induced growth-hormone stimulation by practolol. *Lancet* (1974) 2, 1329.

Levodopa + Bromocriptine

A study suggests that bromocriptine can moderately alter levodopa levels, and an isolated report describes the development of the serotonin syndrome when levodopa/carbidopa was added to treatment with bromocriptine.

Clinical evidence

A study in 20 patients with Parkinson's disease found that overall there was no difference in plasma levodopa levels after the addition of bromocriptine to treatment, although some patients showed either significant elevations or significant reductions in levels. However, the only adverse clinical change found was an increase in dyskinesias in the patients with elevated levodopa levels.[1] An earlier study found no pharmacokinetic interaction between levodopa and bromocriptine, but it should be noted that this was a single-dose study and may not reflect long-term concurrent use.[2]

A patient with parkinsonism, who had been taking bromocriptine 60 mg daily for nearly 3 years, was additionally started on levodopa/carbidopa (250/25 mg daily increasing over a week to 750/75 mg) while the bromocriptine dose was reduced to 20 mg daily. On the seventh day he started shivering, and developed myoclonus of the trunk and limbs, hyperreflexia, patellar clonus, tremor, diaphoresis, anxiety, diarrhoea, tachycardia and had a temperature of 37.9°C with a blood pressure of 180/100 mmHg. Serotonin syndrome was suspected. The patient responded to treatment with the 5-HT antagonist methysergide.[3]

Mechanism

Not understood. The serotonin syndrome is thought to occur because of increased stimulation of the 5-HT receptors in the brainstem and spinal cord. A similar clinical picture is seen with neuroleptic malignant syndrome. A syndrome resembling neuroleptic malignant syndrome can occur when a dopamine agonist like bromocriptine is withdrawn abruptly.

Importance and management

Information is limited, but what is known suggests that concurrent use may result in dyskinesias in those patients where levodopa levels rise. Therefore if bromocriptine is added to levodopa treatment the outcome should be monitored to ensure overall control is improved. The serotonin syndrome described appears to be an isolated incident and not of general importance

1. Rabey JM, Schwartz M, Graff E, Harsat A, Vered Y. The influence of bromocriptine on the pharmacokinetics of levodopa in Parkinson's disease. *Clin Neuropharmacol* (1991) 14, 514–22.
2. Bentué-Ferrer D, Allain H, Reymann JM, Sabouraud O, Van den Driessche J. Lack of pharmacokinetic influence on levodopa by bromocriptine. *Clin Neuropharmacol* (1988) 11, 83–6.
3. Sandyk R. L-Dopa induced "serotonin syndrome" in a parkinsonian patient on bromocriptine. *J Clin Psychopharmacol* (1986) 6, 194–5.

Levodopa + Clonidine

Clonidine is reported to oppose the effects of levodopa.

Clinical evidence

A study in 2 patients taking levodopa with carbidopa found that concurrent treatment with clonidine (up to 1.5 mg daily for 10 to 24 days) caused a worsening of the parkinsonism (an exacerbation of rigidity and akinesia). The concurrent use of anticholinergic drugs reduced the effects of this interaction.[1]

Another report on 10 hypertensive and 3 normotensive patients with Parkinson's disease, 9 of them taking levodopa and 4 of them not, claimed that concurrent treatment with clonidine did not affect the control of the parkinsonism. However, 2 patients stopped taking the clonidine because of an increase in tremor and gait disturbance.[2]

Mechanism

Not understood. A suggestion is that the clonidine opposes the antiparkinson effects by stimulating alpha-receptors in the brain. Another idea is that the clonidine directly stimulates post-synaptic dopaminergic receptors.

Importance and management

Information seems to be limited to these reports. Be alert for a reduction in the control of the Parkinson's disease during concurrent use. The effects of this interaction appear to be reduced if anticholinergic drugs are also being used.[1]

1. Shoulson I, Chase TN. Clonidine and the anti-parkinsonian response to L-dopa or piribedil. *Neuropharmacology* (1976) 15, 25–7.
2. Tarsy D, Parkes JD, Marsden CD. Clonidine in Parkinson disease. *Arch Neurol* (1975) 32, 134–6.

Levodopa + Dacarbazine

An isolated report describes a reduction in the effects of levodopa caused by dacarbazine.

Clinical evidence, mechanism, importance and management

A patient who had been treated surgically for melanoma, continued to have intermittent dacarbazine treatment (200 mg intravenously daily) for sporadic positive melanuria. He later developed Parkinson's disease, and was started on levodopa. However, each time he was treated with dacarbazine he complained that the effects of the levodopa were reduced and his Schwab and England score (measures of activities of daily living) fell by as much as 25%. A subsequent double-blind study on the patient using a modified Columbia Score confirmed this.[1] The reasons are not understood, but since the serum dopamine levels remained unchanged it is suggested that competition between the two drugs at the blood-brain barrier may be the explanation.[1] Be alert for the need to modify treatment if dacarbazine is used concurrently.

1. Merello M, Esteguy M, Perazzo F, Leiguarda R. Impaired levodopa response in Parkinson's disease during melanoma therapy. *Clin Neuropharmacol* (1992) 15, 69–74.

Levodopa + Entacapone

Entacapone increases the plasma levels of levodopa, but this may be accompanied by an increase in levodopa side-effects.

Clinical evidence, mechanism, importance and management

Entacapone has been shown to increase the plasma levels and bioavailability of levodopa[1,2] and thus improve the clinical condition of patients with Parkinson's disease.[3] This improvement is mainly seen as a decrease in 'off' time. However, as levodopa levels are raised, there may be an accompanying increase in the side-effects of levodopa (e.g. dyskinesias).[4,5] The makers suggest that if entacapone is started, the dose of levodopa should be reduced by about 10 to 30% (within the first few days or weeks) to accommodate these potential adverse effects.[5]

1. Myllylä VV, Sotaniemi KA, Illi A, Suominen K, Keränen T. Effect of entacapone, a COMT inhibitor, on the pharmacokinetics of levodopa and on cardiovascular responses in patients with Parkinson's disease. *Eur J Clin Pharmacol* (1993) 45, 419–23.
2. Keränen T, Gordin A, Harjola V-P, Karlsson M, Korpela K, Pentikäinen PJ, Rita H, Seppälä L, Wikberg T. The effect of catechol-*O*-methyl transferase inhibition by entacapone on the pharmacokinetics and metabolism of levodopa in healthy volunteers. *Clin Neuropharmacol* (1993) 16, 145–56.
3. Heikkinen H, Nutt JG, LeWitt PA, Koller WC, Gordin A. The effects of different repeated doses of entacapone on the pharmacokinetics of L-dopa and on the clinical response to L-dopa in Parkinson's disease. *Clin Neuropharmacol* (2001) 24, 150–7.
4. Ruottinen HM, Rinne UK. Entacapone prolongs levodopa response in a one month double blind study in parkinsonian patients with levodopa related fluctuations. *J Neurol Neurosurg Psychiatry* (1996) 60, 36–40.
5. Comtess (Entacapone). Orion Pharma (UK) Ltd. UK Summary of product characteristics, March 2005.

Levodopa + Fluoxetine

The use of fluoxetine is often beneficial in parkinsonian patients on levodopa to treat the depression associated with the disease. However, sometimes parkinsonian symptoms are worsened.

Clinical evidence

Four patients on levodopa 375 to 990 mg daily, a dopamine decarboxylase inhibitor (drug and dose not stated) and amantadine (dose not stated), showed a deterioration in the control of their parkinsonism when additionally given fluoxetine 20 mg daily. The fluoxetine was withdrawn and their motor performance was restored. The antidepressant efficacy of fluoxetine was not found to be substantial in any of the 4 patients.[1] Another patient taking levodopa developed frequent hallucinations after the addition of fluoxetine. They resolved when the fluoxetine was withdrawn.[2] In a retrospective study of 23 parkinsonian patients who were given fluoxetine up to 40 mg daily, 20 patients showed no worsening of their parkinsonism but in 3 others experienced a worsening in their Parkinson's disease signs.[3]

Mechanism

Not understood. Extrapyramidal effects are rare but recognised side effects of fluoxetine.

Importance and management

Although the information is limited, it seems that in some cases parkinsonism can be worsened by fluoxetine. A study that found the combination was well-tolerated in 12 out of 14 subjects suggested that an interaction only occurs in susceptible individuals, but gave no clue as to which type of patient may be at risk.[4] Concurrent use is valuable and need not be avoided, but monitor the outcome and withdraw the fluoxetine if necessary.

1. Jansen Steur ENH. Increase of Parkinson disability after fluoxetine medication. *Neurology* (1993) 43, 211–13.
2. Lauterbach EC. Dopaminergic hallucinosis with fluoxetine in Parkinson's disease. *Am J Psychiatry* (1993) 150, 1750.
3. Caley CF, Friedman JH. Does fluoxetine exacerbate Parkinson's disease? *J Clin Psychiatry* (1992) 53, 278–282.
4. Montastruc J-L, Fabre N, Blin O, Senard J-M, Rascol O, Rascol A. Does fluoxetine aggravate Parkinson's disease? A pilot prospective study. *Mov Disord* (1995) 10, 355–6.

Levodopa + Food

The fluctuations in response to levodopa experienced by some patients may be due to timing of meals and the kind of diet, particularly the protein content, both of which can reduce the effects of levodopa. The effects of levodopa can be reduced by the amino acid methionine, and the blood levels of levodopa can be reduced by the amino acid tryptophan.

Clinical evidence

(a) Effects of meals

A study in patients with Parkinson's disease treated with levodopa showed that if taken with a meal, the mean absorption of the levodopa from the gut and the peak plasma levels were reduced by 27 and 29% respectively, and the peak plasma level was delayed by 34 minutes.[1] Another study showed that peak plasma levodopa levels were reduced if taken with food rather than when fasting.[2] A study in healthy subjects found that a **low protein meal** (protein 10.5 g) caused a small reduction in levodopa absorption when compared with the fasting state, but also found that a **high-protein meal** (protein 30.5 g) was no different to the fasting state.[3] Other studies have shown that a high daily intake of **protein** reduces the effects of levodopa, compared with a lower intake of **protein**.[4-6]

(b) Effects of amino acids

A study showed that the clinical response to a constant intravenous infusion of levodopa in 4 patients was unchanged by **glycine** and **lysine** but was reduced by **phenylalanine, leucine** and **isoleucine**, although the plasma levodopa levels remained unchanged.[1]

Fourteen patients treated with levodopa for Parkinson's disease were given a **low-methionine** diet (0.5 g daily) for a period of 8 days. Seven patients were given additional methionine (4.5 g daily), while the other 7 were given placebo. Five out of the 7 given **methionine** 4.5 g daily showed a definite worsening of the symptoms (gait, tremor, rigidity, etc.). The symptoms subsided when the **methionine** was withdrawn, although this took 7 to 10 days in one patient. Three out of the 7 given placebo (while on the low-methionine diet) showed some subjective improvement.[7]

The blood levels of levodopa were markedly reduced in normal healthy subjects when 500 mg levodopa was taken with 1 g of **tryptophan**.[8] The clinical importance of this was not assessed.

Mechanism

(a) Meals that delay gastric emptying allow the levodopa to be exposed to 'wasteful' peripheral metabolism in the gut, which reduces the amount available for absorption. In addition (b) some large neutral amino acids arising from the digestion of proteins can compete with levodopa for transport into the brain so that the therapeutic response may be reduced, whereas other amino acids do not have this effect.[1,3,5,9]

Importance and management

An established interaction, but unpredictable. Since the fluctuations in the response of patients to levodopa may be influenced by what is eaten and when, a change in the pattern of drug and food administration on a trial-and-error basis may be helpful. Multiple small doses of levodopa and distributing the intake of proteins may also diminish the effects of these interactions. Diets that conform to the recommended daily allowance of protein (said to be 800 mg/kg in this report) are reported to reduce this adverse drug-food interaction.[5]

The amino acid methionine is used therapeutically, and although information about its interaction with levodopa is very limited, it indicates that large doses of methionine should be avoided in patients being treated with levodopa.

1. Anon. Timing of meals may affect clinical response to levodopa. *Am Pharm* (1985) 25, 34–5.
2. Morgan JP, Bianchine JR, Spiegel HE, Nutley NJ, Rivera-Calimlim L, Hersey RM. Metabolism of levodopa in patients with Parkinson's disease. *Arch Neurol* (1971) 25, 39–44.
3. Robertson DRC, Higginson I, Macklin BS, Renwick AG, Waller DG, George CF. The influence of protein containing meals on the pharmacokinetics of levodopa in healthy volunteers. *Br J Clin Pharmacol* (1991) 31, 413–17.
4. Gillespie NG, Mena I, Cotzias GC, Bell MA. Diets affecting treatment of parkinsonism with levodopa. *J Am Diet Assoc* (1973) 62, 525–8.
5. Juncos JL, Fabbrini G, Mouradian MM, Serrati C, Chase TN. Dietary influences on the antiparkinsonian response to levodopa. *Arch Neurol* (1987) 44, 1003–1005.
6. Carter JH, Nutt JG, Woodward WR, Hatcher LF, Trotman TL. Amount and distribution of dietary protein affects clinical response to levodopa in Parkinson's disease. *Neurology* (1989) 39, 552–6.
7. Pearce LA, Waterbury LD. L-methionine: a possible levodopa antagonist. *Neurology* (1974) 24, 640–1.
8. Weitbrecht W-U, Weigel K. Der einfluß von L-tryptophan auf die L-dopa-resorption. *Dtsch Med Wochenschr* (1976) 101, 20–2.
9. Daniel PM, Moorhouse SR, Pratt OE. Do changes in blood levels of other aromatic aminoacids influence levodopa therapy? *Lancet* (1976) i, 95.

Levodopa + Iron compounds

Ferrous sulfate can reduce the bioavailability of levodopa and carbidopa, and may possibly reduce the control of Parkinson's disease.

Clinical evidence

A study in 9 patients with Parkinson's disease showed that a single 325-mg dose of **ferrous sulfate** reduced the AUC of levodopa by 30% and the AUC of carbidopa by more than 75%. There was a trend towards an increase in disability, suggesting a worsening of disease, but this did not reach statistical significance. Some, but not all of the patients showed some deterioration in the control of their disease[1]

In another study, 8 healthy subjects were given a single 250-mg dose of levodopa, with and without a single 325-mg dose of **ferrous sulfate**, and the plasma levodopa levels were measured for the following 6 hours. Peak plasma levodopa levels and the levodopa AUC were reduced by 55% (from 3.6 to 1.6 nmol/l) and the AUC was reduced by 51% (from 257 to 125 nmol.min/ml). Those subjects who had the highest peak levels and greatest absorption when given levodopa alone, showed the greatest reductions when additionally given **ferrous sulfate**.[2]

This interaction has also been demonstrated in *animal* studies.[3]

Mechanism

Ferrous iron rapidly oxidises to ferric iron at the pH values found in the gastrointestinal tract. Ferric iron binds strongly to carbidopa and levodopa to form chelation complexes that are poorly absorbed.[2,4]

Importance and management

Information appears to be limited to these single-dose and *in vitro* studies. The importance of this interaction in patients taking both drugs long-term awaits further study, but the extent of the reductions in absorption (30 to 50%) and the hint of worsening control[1] suggests that this interaction may be of clinical importance. Be alert for any evidence of this. Separating the administration of the iron as much as possible is likely to prove effective, as this appears to be an absorption interaction. More study is needed.

1. Campbell NRC, Rankine D, Goodridge AE, Hasinoff BB, Kara M. Sinemet-ferrous sulphate interaction in patients with Parkinson's disease. *Br J Clin Pharmacol* (1990) 30, 599–605.
2. Campbell NRC, Hasinoff B. Ferrous sulfate reduces levodopa bioavailability: chelation as a possible mechanism. *Clin Pharmacol Ther* (1989) 45, 220–5.
3. Campbell RRA, Hasinoff B, Chernenko G, Barrowman J, Campbell NRC. The effect of ferrous sulfate and pH on L-dopa absorption. *Can J Physiol Pharmacol* (1990) 68, 603–7.
4. Greene RJ, Hall AD, Hider RC. The interaction of orally administered iron with levodopa and methyldopa therapy. *J Pharm Pharmacol* (1990) 42, 502–4.

Levodopa + Isoniazid

There is evidence that isoniazid can reduce the control of Parkinson's disease with levodopa. Also an isolated case report describes hypertension, tachycardia, flushing and tremor in a patient attributed to concurrent use of levodopa and isoniazid.

Clinical evidence

Following the observation that levodopa-induced dyskinesias were reduced by isoniazid in one patient, a further study was made in 20 others. It was found that isoniazid (average dose 290 mg daily, range 100 to 800 mg daily) reduced the dyskinesias of 18 of the 20 patients. However, the reduction in dyskinesias was accompanied by an intolerable worsening of parkinsonism, shown by decreased mobility and greater 'off' periods. The reduction in mobility was so severe that the isoniazid had to be stopped immediately in several cases and was discontinued after an average of 5.2 weeks in all the patients. Control of parkinsonism was then restored.[1] Another patient similarly showed a deterioration in the control of parkinsonism within 1 to 2 weeks of starting isoniazid/rifampicin (*Rifinah*). When the antitubercular drugs were stopped, the patient's motor performance improved ('on' period lengthened by 75%), the levodopa AUC rose by 37%, its half-life doubled, while the maximum plasma levels fell by 33%.[2]

An isolated report describes a patient on levodopa who developed hypertension, agitation, tachycardia, flushing and severe non-parkinsonian tremor after starting to take isoniazid. He recovered when the isoniazid was stopped.[3]

Mechanism

Not understood. Metabolic studies in one patient suggest that isoniazid inhibits dopa-decarboxylase,[2] although other mechanisms have been proposed.[1,2] The isolated case of hypertension and tachycardia is also not understood, but it has been suggested that it may have been due to a weak monoamine oxidase inhibitory effect of the isoniazid metabolites.

Importance and management

Information seems to be limited to the reports cited. If concurrent use is thought to be necessary, be alert for any evidence of a reduction in the control of the parkinsonism, and be aware that drug treatment may need to be modified. One of the reports suggests that it may take 15 to 20 days or more for the deterioration in parkinsonian symptoms to occur.[1] More study is needed. The isolated case seems not to be of general importance.

1. Gershanik OS, Luquin MR, Scipioni O, Obeso JA. Isoniazid therapy in Parkinson's disease. *Mov Disord* (1988) 3, 133–9.
2. Wenning GK, O'Connell MT, Patsalos PN, Quinn NP. A clinical and pharmacokinetic case study of an interaction of levodopa and antituberculous therapy in Parkinson's disease. *Mov Disord* (1995) 10, 664–7.
3. Morgan JP. Isoniazid and levodopa. *Ann Intern Med* (1980) 92, 434.

Levodopa + Methyldopa

Methyldopa can increase the effects of levodopa and permit a reduction in the dosage in some patients, but it can also worsen dyskinesias in others. A small increase in the hypotensive actions of methyldopa may also occur.

Clinical evidence

(a) Effects on the response to levodopa

A double-blind crossover study in 10 patients with Parkinson's disease who had been taking levodopa for 12 to 40 months, showed that the optimum daily dose of levodopa fell by 68% when using the highest doses of methyldopa studied (1920 mg daily), and by 50% with methyldopa 800 mg daily.[1]

Other reports describe reductions in the levodopa dosage of up to 30%[2] and 70%[3] during concurrent treatment with methyldopa. Another report states that the control of Parkinson's disease in some patients improved during the concurrent use of methyldopa, but worsened the dyskinesias in others.[4] Methyldopa on its own can cause a reversible parkinsonian-like syndrome.[5-7]

(b) Effects on the response to methyldopa

A study in 18 patients with Parkinson's disease showed that combined use of levodopa and methyldopa lowered the blood pressure. The doses used did not affect the systolic blood pressure when given alone. Daily doses of 1 to 2.5 g of levodopa with 500 mg of methyldopa caused a 12/6 mmHg fall in blood pressure. No change in the control of the Parkinson's disease was seen, but the study lasted only a few days.[8]

Mechanism

Not understood.[9] (a) One idea is that the methyldopa inhibits the enzymic destruction of levodopa outside the brain so that more is available to exert its therapeutic effects. (b) The increased hypotension may simply be due to the additive effects of the two drugs.

Importance and management

Well documented, but the picture presented is a little confusing. Concurrent use need not be avoided but the outcome should be well monitored. The use of methyldopa may allow a reduction in the dosage of the levodopa (the reports cited[1-3] quote figures of between 30 and 70%) and may enhance the control of Parkinson's disease, but it should also be borne in mind that in some patients dyskinesias may be worsened. The increased hypotensive effects seem to be small, but they too should be checked.

1. Fermaglich J, Chase TN. Methyldopa or methyldopahydrazine as levodopa synergists. *Lancet* (1973) i, 1261–2.
2. Mones RJ. Evaluation of alpha methyl dopa and alpha methyl dopa hydrazine with L-dopa therapy. *N Y State J Med* (1974) 74, 47–51.

3. Fermaglich J, O'Doherty DS. Second generation of L-dopa therapy. *Neurology* (1971) 21, 408–9.
4. Sweet RD, Lee JE, McDowell FH. Methyldopa as an adjunct to levodopa treatment of Parkinson's disease. *Clin Pharmacol Ther* (1972) 13, 23–7.
5. Groden BM. Parkinsonism occurring with methyldopa treatment. *BMJ* (1963) 1, 1001.
6. Peaston MJT. Parkinsonism associated with alpha-methyldopa therapy. *BMJ* (1964) 2, 168.
7. Strang RR. Parkinsonism occurring during methyldopa therapy. *Can Med Assoc J* (1966) 95, 928–9.
8. Gibberd FB, Small E. Interaction between levodopa and methyldopa. *BMJ* (1973) 2, 90–1.
9. Smith SE. The pharmacological actions of 3,4-dihydroxyphenyl-α-methylalanine (α-methyldopa), an inhibitor of 5-hydroxytryptophan decarboxylase. *Br J Pharmacol* (1960) 15, 319–27.

Levodopa + Mirtazapine

An isolated report describes the development of serious psychosis attributed to a levodopa/mirtazapine interaction.

Clinical evidence, mechanism, importance and management

A 44-year-old woman treated with levodopa, pergolide, selegiline and memantine for Parkinson's disease, was additionally started on mirtazapine in increasing doses rising from 15 to 60 mg daily over 24 days, for depression, labile mood, anxiety, social withdrawal and sleep disturbance. She initially improved, but then major depression and psychosis developed, and on day 26 she attempted self-strangulation. She recovered when the mirtazapine, memantine and selegiline were stopped and low-dose clozapine started. The authors concluded that the reaction was attributable to dopamine-induced psychosis triggered by the addition of mirtazapine to levodopa.[1]

1. Normann C, Hesslinger B, Frauenknecht S, Berger M, Walden J. Psychosis during chronic levodopa therapy triggered by the new antidepressive drug mirtazapine. *Pharmacopsychiatry* (1997) 30, 263–5.

Levodopa or Whole broad beans + MAOIs

A rapid, serious and potentially life-threatening hypertensive reaction can occur in patients on non-selective, irreversible MAOIs if given levodopa or if they eat whole broad beans, which contain dopa in the pods. An interaction with compound levodopa preparations containing carbidopa or benserazide (*Sinemet, Madopar*) is unlikely. No serious hypertensive reaction has been reported to occur with selective MAO-A inhibitors such as moclobemide, and no serious acute interaction occurs with selegiline, a selective MAO-B inhibitor.

Clinical evidence

(a) Levodopa + Non-selective, irreversible MAOIs

A patient who had been taking **phenelzine** daily for 10 days was given 50 mg of levodopa by mouth. In just over an hour his blood pressure had risen from 135/90 to about 190/130 mmHg, and despite an intravenous injection of 5 mg phentolamine it continued to rise over the next 10 minutes to 200/135 mmHg, before falling after a further 4 mg injection of phentolamine. The following day the experiment was repeated with 25 mg of levodopa, but no blood pressure changes were seen. Three weeks after withdrawal of the **phenelzine** even 500 mg of levodopa had no hypertensive effect.[1]

Similar cases of severe and acute hypertension, accompanied in most instances by flushing, throbbing and pounding in the head, neck and chest, and light headedness have been described in other case reports and studies involving the concurrent use of levodopa with **pargyline**,[2] **nialamide**,[3] **tranylcypromine**,[4,5] **phenelzine**[6] and **isocarboxazid**.[1]

(b) Whole broad beans + Non-selective, irreversible MAOIs

A hypertensive reaction similar to the one described in (a) above can occur in patients taking non-selective, irreversible MAOIs who have eaten WHOLE broad beans (*Vicia faba*), that is to say the beans with pods, as the pods contain the dopa, and not the beans.[7] The reports of this interaction involved **pargyline**[8] and **phenelzine**.[9]

(c) Levodopa + Selective MAO-A inhibitors (Moclobemide)

A study in 12 healthy subjects given a single dose of *Madopar* (levodopa with benserazide) with moclobemide 200 mg twice daily found that nausea, vomiting and dizziness were increased, but no significant hypertensive reaction was seen.[10]

(d) Levodopa + Selective MAO-B inhibitors (Selegiline)

The combination of levodopa and selegiline has been very extensively used. No serious hypertensive reactions of the kind seen with non-selective MAOIs seem to occur. No adverse pharmacokinetic interactions have been reported,[11,12] and serious adverse interactions are said to be lacking.[13,14] Many studies have reported beneficial effects of this combination,[15-20] but one has suggested that it may result in increased mortality.[21] Urinary retention has also been suggested as being associated with this drug combination.[22]

Mechanism

Not fully understood. Levodopa is enzymically converted in the body, firstly to dopamine and then to noradrenaline, both of which are normally broken down by monoamine oxidase. But in the presence of an MAOI this breakdown is suppressed, which means that the total levels of dopamine and noradrenaline are increased. Precisely how this then leads to a sharp rise in blood pressure is not clear, but either dopamine or noradrenaline, or both, directly or indirectly stimulate the alpha-receptors of the cardiovascular system.

Importance and management

The interaction between the irreversible, older, non-selective MAOIs (listed in 'Table 30.1', (p.862)) and levodopa or whole broad beans is well documented, serious and potentially life-threatening. Patients should not be given levodopa during treatment with any of these MAOIs, nor for a period of 2 to 3 weeks after their withdrawal. The same precautions apply to the eating of WHOLE broad beans, the dopa being in the pods but not in the beans. This interaction is inhibited by the presence of dopa-decarboxylase inhibitors[4] such as carbidopa and benserazide (as in *Sinemet* and *Madopar*) so that a serious interaction is unlikely to occur with these preparations. Even so, the makers continue to list the MAOIs among their contraindications.

No important acute adverse interaction appears to occur between levodopa and moclobemide, but some side-effects can apparently occur.

No acute adverse interactions occur if levodopa and selegiline are given concurrently, but the makers say that on adding selegiline it is possible to reduce the dose of levodopa (about 30% is suggested).[23]

1. Hunter KR, Boakes AJ, Laurence DR, Stern GM. Monoamine oxidase inhibitors and L-dopa. *BMJ* (1970) 3, 388.
2. Hodge JV. Use of monoamine-oxidase inhibitors. *Lancet* (1965) i, 764–5.
3. Friend DG, Bell WR, Kline NS. The action of L-dihydroxyphenylalanine in patients receiving nialamide. *Clin Pharmacol Ther* (1965) 6, 362–6.
4. Teychenne PF, Calne DB, Lewis PJ, Findley LJ. Interactions of levodopa with inhibitors of monoamine oxidase and L-aromatic amino acid decarboxylase. *Clin Pharmacol Ther* (1975) 18, 273–7.
5. Sharpe J, Marquez-Julio A, Ashby P. Idiopathic orthostatic hypotension treated with levodopa and MAO inhibitor: a preliminary report. *Can Med Assoc J* (1972) 107, 296–300.
6. Kassirer JP, Kopelman RI. A modern medical Descartes. *Hosp Pract* (1987) 22, 17–25.
7. McGilchrist JM. Interactions with monoamine oxidase inhibitors. *BMJ* (1975) 3, 591–2.
8. Hodge JV, Nye ER, Emerson GW. Monoamine-oxidase inhibitors, broad beans, and hypertension. *Lancet* (1964) i, 1108.
9. Blomley DJ. Monoamine-oxidase inhibitors. *Lancet* (1964) ii, 1181–2.
10. Dingemanse J. An update of recent moclobemide interaction data. *Int Clin Psychopharmacol* (1993) 7, 167–80.
11. Roberts J, Waller DG, O'Shea N, Macklin BS, Renwick AG. The effect of selegiline on the peripheral pharmacokinetics of levodopa in young volunteers. *Br J Clin Pharmacol* (1995) 40, 404–6.
12. Cedarbaum JM, Silvestri M, Clark M, Harts A, Kutt H. L-Deprenyl, levodopa pharmacokinetics, and response fluctuations in Parkinson's disease. *Clin Neuropharmacol* (1990) 13, 29–35.
13. Birkmayer W, Riederer P, Ambrozi L, Youdim MBH. Implications of combined treatment with 'Madopar' and L-deprenil in Parkinson's disease. *Lancet* (1977) i, 439–43.
14. Elsworth JD, Glover V, Reynolds GP, Sandler M, Lees AJ, Phuapradit P, Shaw KM, Stern GM, Kumar P. Deprenyl administration in man: a selective monoamine oxidase B inhibitor without the 'cheese effect'. *Psychopharmacology (Berl)* (1978) 57, 33–8.
15. Shan DE, Yeh SI. An add-on study of selegiline to Madopar in the treatment of parkinsonian patients with dose-related fluctuations: comparison between Jumexal and Parkryl. *Zhonghua Yi Xue Za Zhi (Taipei)* (1996), 58, 264–8.
16. Brannan T, Yahr MD. Comparative-study of selegiline plus L-dopa–carbidopa versus L-dopa–carbidopa alone in the treatment of Parkinson's disease. *Ann Neurol* (1995) 37, 95–8.
17. Golbe LI, Lieberman AN, Muenter MD, Ahlslog JE, Gopinathan G, Neophytides AN, Foo SH, Duvoisin RC. Deprenyl in the treatment of symptom fluctuations in advanced Parkinson's disease. *Clin Neuropharmacol* (1988) 11, 45–55.
18. Presthus J, Berstad J, Lien K. Selegiline (l-deprenyl) and low-dose levodopa treatment of Parkinson's disease. *Acta Neurol Scand* (1987) 76, 200–3.
19. Birkmayer W, Birkmayer GD. Effect of (−)deprenyl in long-term treatment of Parkinson's disease. A 10-years experience. *J Neural Transm* (1986) 22 (Suppl), 219–25.
20. Birkmayer W, Knoll J, Riederer P, Youdim MBH, Hars V, Marton J. Increased life expectancy resulting from addition of L-deprenyl to Madopar® treatment in Parkinson's disease: a longterm study. *J Neural Transm* (1985) 64, 113–127.
21. Parkinson's Disease Research Group of the United Kingdom. Comparison of therapeutic effects and mortality data of levodopa and levodopa combined with selegiline in patients with early, mild Parkinson's disease. *BMJ* (1995) 311, 1602–7.

22. Waters CH. Side effects of selegiline (Eldepryl). *J Geriatr Psychiatry Neurol* (1992) 5, 31–34.
23. Eldepryl (Selegiline). Orion Pharma (UK) Ltd. UK Summary of product characteristics, October 2003.

Levodopa + Papaverine

There are case reports of a deterioration in the control of parkinsonism in patients treated with levodopa when given papaverine, but a controlled trial failed to confirm this interaction.

Clinical evidence

(a) Levodopa effects reduced

A woman with long-standing parkinsonism, well controlled on levodopa (with the later addition of carbidopa), began to show a steady worsening of her parkinsonism within a week of additionally starting papaverine 100 mg daily for cerebral vascular insufficiency. The deterioration continued until the papaverine was withdrawn. The normal response to levodopa returned within a week. Four other patients showed a similar response.[1]

Two other similar cases have been described in another report.[2]

(b) Levodopa effects unchanged

A double-blind crossover trial was carried out on 9 patients with parkinsonism being treated with levodopa (range 100 to 750 mg daily) plus a dopa-decarboxylase inhibitor. Two of them were also taking bromocriptine 40 mg daily and two trihexyphenidyl (benzhexol) 15 mg daily. No changes in the control of their disease were seen when they were concurrently treated with papaverine hydrochloride 150 mg daily for 3 weeks.[3]

Mechanism

Not understood. One suggestion is that papaverine blocks the dopamine receptors in the striatum of the brain, thereby inhibiting the effects of the levodopa.[1,4] Another is that papaverine may have a reserpine-like action on the vesicles of adrenergic neurones[1,5] (i.e. it depletes catecholamine stores).

Importance and management

Direct information seems to be limited to the reports cited. Concurrent use can apparently be uneventful, however, in the light of the reports of adverse interactions it would be prudent to monitor the outcome closely. Carefully controlled trials can provide a good picture of the general situation, but may not necessarily identify the occasional patient who may be affected by an interaction.

1. Duvoisin RC. Antagonism of levodopa by papaverine. *JAMA* (1975) 231, 845.
2. Posner DM. Antagonism of levodopa by papaverine. *JAMA* (1975) 233, 768.
3. Montastruc JL, Rascol O, Belin J, Ane M, Rascol A. Does papaverine interact with levodopa in Parkinson's disease? *Ann Neurol* (1987) 22, 558–9.
4. Gonzalez-Vegas JA. Antagonism of dopamine-mediated inhibition in the nigro-striatal pathway: a mode of action of some catatonia-inducing drugs. *Brain Res* (1974) 80, 219–28.
5. Cubeddu L, Weiner N. Relationship between a granular effect and exocytotic release of norepinephrine by nerve stimulation. *Pharmacologist* (1974) 16, 190.

Levodopa + Penicillamine

Penicillamine can raise plasma levodopa levels in a few patients. This may improve the control of the parkinsonism but the adverse effects of levodopa may also be increased.

Clinical evidence, mechanism, importance and management

A patient with Parkinson's disease had a 60% increase in their levodopa plasma levels after receiving penicillamine 600 mg daily. This resulted in improved control of symptoms but with an increase in dyskinesia. It was noted that this patient had slightly low serum copper and ceruloplasmin levels.[1] Another study also saw improvements in 2 patients with Parkinson's disease taking levodopa when they were additionally given penicillamine, but levodopa levels were apparently not measured. Again it was noted that the patients had slightly low copper and ceruloplasmin levels. In another 4 similar patients the effects of penicillamine seemed absent in the presence of normal copper and ceruloplasmin levels.[2] The authors of this report[2] attribute the improvement in parkinsonism to the copper chelating properties of penicillamine. However, the authors of the other report[1] suggest that as the effect of penicillamine would not be this rapid, penicillamine must be affecting levodopa pharmacokinetics.

This limited evidence suggests that the concurrent use of levodopa and penicillamine need not be avoided, and in some patients parkinsonian symptoms may be improved. However, if you give both drugs, monitor the effects as an increase in the adverse effects of levodopa is also possible.

1. Mizuta E, Kuno S. Effect of D-penicillamine on pharmacokinetics of levodopa in Parkinson's disease. *Clin Neuropharmacol* (1993) 16, 448–50.
2. Sato M, Yamane K, Oosawa Y, Tanaka H, Shirata A, Nagayama T, Maruyama S. Two cases of Parkinson's disease whose symptoms were markedly improved by D-penicillamine. A study with emphasis on cases displaying a slightly low level of serum copper and ceruloplasmin. *Neurol Ther Chiba* (1992) 9, 555–9.

Levodopa + Phenylbutazone

A single case report describes antagonism of the effects of levodopa by phenylbutazone.

Clinical evidence, mechanism, importance and management

A patient (who was very sensitive to levodopa) found that he was only able to prevent the involuntary movements of his tongue, jaw, neck and limbs caused by levodopa, by taking frequent small doses (125 mg). He was able to suppress the levodopa side-effects with phenylbutazone. However, the phenylbutazone also lessened the therapeutic effect of the levodopa.[1] The reason is not understood. This interaction has not been confirmed, and its general importance is not known.

1. Wodak J, Gilligan BS, Veale JL, Dowty BJ. Review of 12 months' treatment with L-dopa in Parkinson's disease, with remarks on unusual side effects. *Med J Aust* (1972) 2, 1277–82.

Levodopa + Phenytoin

The therapeutic effects of levodopa can be reduced or abolished by the concurrent use of phenytoin.

Clinical evidence, mechanism, importance and management

A study in 5 patients treated with levodopa 630 to 4600 mg (four also with 150 to 225 mg carbidopa daily) for Parkinson's disease, found that when they were additionally given phenytoin in doses of up to 500 mg daily for 5 to 19 days the levodopa-induced dyskinesias were relieved, but the beneficial effects of the levodopa on parkinsonism were also reduced or abolished. The patients became slow, rigidity re-emerged and some of them became unable to get out of a chair. Within 2 weeks of stopping the phenytoin, their parkinsonism was again well controlled by the levodopa.[1] Despite many suggestions, the mechanism of this interaction is not understood. Information seems to be limited to this study, nevertheless it would seem prudent, where possible, to monitor the concurrent use for any evidence of reduced levodopa efficacy.

1. Mendez JS, Cotzias GC, Mena I, Papavasiliou PS. Diphenylhydantoin blocking of levodopa effects. *Arch Neurol* (1975) 32, 44–6.

Levodopa + Pyridoxine (Vitamin B_6)

The effects of levodopa are reduced or abolished by the concurrent use of pyridoxine, but this interaction does not occur when levodopa is given in preparations with carbidopa or benserazide (e.g. *Sinemet, Madopar*).

Clinical evidence

(a) Levodopa

A study in 25 patients being treated with levodopa showed that if they were given high doses of pyridoxine (750 to 1000 mg daily), the effects of the levodopa were completely abolished within 3 to 4 days, and some reduction in the effects were evident within 24 hours. Daily doses of 50 to 100 mg of pyridoxine also reduced or abolished the effects of levodopa, and an increase in the signs and symptoms of parkinsonism occurred in 8 out of 10 patients taking only 5 to 10 mg of pyridoxine daily.[1]

The antagonism of the effects of levodopa by pyridoxine has been described in numerous other reports.[1-6]

(b) Levodopa/carbidopa

A study in 15 chronic levodopa-treated patients with Parkinson's disease found that when given single 250-mg doses of levodopa by mouth, the administration of pyridoxine 50 mg caused peak plasma levels of dopa to fall by approximately 70%. The concurrent administration of carbidopa 50 mg with levodopa 250 mg potentiated peak plasma dopa levels to 1300 nanograms/ml, however, the addition of pyridoxine to the levodopa/carbidopa combination did not significantly affect the plasma dopa levels.[6] The results from a subset of these patients have been reported elsewhere.[7] The absence of an interaction in the presence of a dopa-decarboxylase inhibitor is confirmed in another report.[8]

Mechanism

The conversion of levodopa to dopamine within the body requires the presence of pyridoxal-5-phosphate (derived from pyridoxine) as a co-factor. When dietary amounts of pyridoxine are high, the 'wasteful' peripheral metabolism of levodopa outside the brain is increased so that less is available for entry into the CNS, and its effects are reduced accordingly. Pyridoxine may also alter levodopa metabolism by Schiff-base formation. However, in the presence of dopa-decarboxylase inhibitors such as carbidopa or benserazide, this 'wasteful' peripheral metabolism of levodopa is reduced and much larger amounts are available for entry into the CNS, even if quite small doses are given. So even in the presence of large amounts of pyridoxine, the peripheral metabolism remains unaffected and the serum levels of levodopa are virtually unaltered.

Importance and management

A clinically important, well documented and well established interaction. Pyridoxine in doses as low as 5 mg daily can reduce the effects of levodopa and should therefore be avoided. Warn patients about proprietary pyridoxine-containing preparations. Some breakfast cereals are fortified with pyridoxine and other vitamins, but the amounts are usually too small to matter (e.g. a 30 g serving of Kellogg's Corn Flakes or Rice Krispies (UK preparations) contains only about 0.6 mg pyridoxine). There is no good clinical evidence to suggest that a low-pyridoxine diet is desirable, and indeed it may be harmful since the normal dietary requirements are about 2 mg daily.

The problem of this interaction can be totally solved by using levodopa/carbidopa or levodopa/benserazide preparations (e.g. *Sinemet* or *Madopar*), which are unaffected by pyridoxine.

1. Duvoisin RC, Yahr MD, Coté LD. Pyridoxine reversal of L-dopa effects in parkinsonism. *Trans Am Neurol Assoc* (1969) 94, 81–4.
2. Celesia GG, Barr AN. Psychosis and other psychiatric manifestations of levodopa therapy. *Arch Neurol* (1970) 23, 193–200.
3. Carter AB. Pyridoxine and parkinsonism. *BMJ* (1973) 4, 236.
4. Cotzias GC, Papavasiliou PS. Blocking the negative effects of pyridoxine on patients receiving levodopa. *JAMA* (1971) 215, 1504–5.
5. Leon AS, Spiegel HE, Thomas G, Abrams WB. Pyridoxine antagonism of levodopa in parkinsonism. *JAMA* (1971) 218, 1924–7.
6. Mars H. Levodopa, carbidopa, and pyridoxine in Parkinson disease: metabolic interactions. *Arch Neurol* (1974) 30, 444–7.
7. Mars H. Metabolic interactions of pyridoxine, levodopa, and carbidopa in Parkinson's disease. *Trans Am Neurol Assoc* (1973) 98, 241–5.
8. Papavasiliou PS, Cotzias GC, Düby SE, Steck AJ, Fehling C, Bell MA. Levodopa in parkinsonism: potentiation of central effects with a peripheral inhibitor. *N Engl J Med* (1972) 285, 8–14.

Levodopa + Rauwolfia alkaloids

The effects of levodopa are opposed by the concurrent use of rauwolfia alkaloids such as reserpine.

Clinical evidence, mechanism, importance and management

Reserpine and other rauwolfia alkaloids deplete the brain of monoamines, including dopamine, thereby reducing their effects.[1] This can lead to parkinsonian-like symptoms, and may oppose the actions of administered levodopa. There are not only sound pharmacological reasons for believing this to be an interaction of clinical importance, but a reduction in the antiparkinsonian activity of levodopa by **reserpine** has been observed.[2] The rauwolfia alkaloids should be avoided in patients with Parkinson's disease, whether or not they are taking levodopa.

1. Bianchine JR, Sunyapridakul L. Interactions between levodopa and other drugs: significance in the treatment of Parkinson's disease. *Drugs* (1973) 6, 364–88.
2. Yahr MD. Personal communication, February 1977.

Levodopa + Spiramycin

The plasma levels of levodopa with carbidopa are reduced by the concurrent use of spiramycin, thereby reducing its therapeutic effects.

Clinical evidence

The observation of a patient with Parkinson's disease on levodopa/carbidopa (*Sinemet*) who became less well-controlled when treated with spiramycin, prompted further study in 7 healthy subjects given 250 mg of levodopa with 25 mg of carbidopa. After taking spiramycin 1 g twice daily for 3 days, the AUC of the levodopa fell by 57%, while maximum plasma levels fell from 2162 to 1680 nanograms/ml (not significant). The relative bioavailability of levodopa was only 43%. The plasma levels of the carbidopa were barely detectable.[1]

Mechanism

Not fully established. In some way spiramycin markedly reduces the absorption of carbidopa, possibly by forming a non-absorbable complex in the gut or by accelerating its transit through the gut. As a result, not enough carbidopa is absorbed to inhibit the 'wasteful' peripheral metabolism of the levodopa, so that the effects of the levodopa are reduced.[1]

Importance and management

Information is very limited, but the interaction appears to be established and of clinical importance. If spiramycin is given, anticipate the need to increase the dosage of the levodopa/carbidopa preparation (approximately double the dose). It is not known whether other macrolide antibacterials behave in a similar way, or whether spiramycin affects levodopa/benserazide preparations. More study is needed.

1. Brion N, Kollenbach K, Marion MH, Grégoire A, Advenier C, Pays M. Effect of a macrolide (spiramycin) on the pharmacokinetics of L-dopa and carbidopa in healthy volunteers. *Clin Neuropharmacol* (1992) 15, 229–35.

Levodopa + Tacrine

A case report describes worsened parkinsonism in a patient given tacrine, which responded to levodopa. The effects of levodopa were opposed when the dose of tacrine was raised.

Clinical evidence

The mild parkinsonism of an elderly woman with Alzheimer's disease worsened, leading to severe tremor, stiffness and gait dysfunction within 2 weeks of doubling her tacrine dosage from 10 mg to 20 mg four times daily. She improved when levodopa/carbidopa was started, but the tremor returned when tacrine was increased to 30 mg four times daily. The symptoms disappeared when the tacrine dosage was reduced, back to 20 mg four times daily.[1]

Mechanism

Parkinsonism is due to an imbalance between two neurotransmitters, dopamine and acetylcholine, in the basal ganglia of the brain. Tacrine (a centrally acting anticholinesterase) increases the amount of acetylcholine in the brain, which in this case led to an exacerbation of the parkinsonian symptoms. Levodopa improves the situation by increasing the levels of dopamine, while the addition of more tacrine further increases the amounts of acetylcholine, which upsets the acetylcholine/dopamine balance, again exacerbating the parkinsonian symptoms.

Importance and management

Direct information seems to be limited to this single report, but it is consistent with the known pharmacology of both drugs and the biochemical pathology of Parkinson's disease. Be aware that if tacrine is given to any patient with parkinsonism, whether taking levodopa or any other anti-parkinson drug, the disease may possibly worsen. You may need to increase the anti-parkinson drug dosage and/or reduce the dosage of tacrine.

1. Ott BR, Lannon MC. Exacerbation of parkinsonism by tacrine. *Clin Neuropharmacol* (1992) 15, 322–5.

Levodopa + Tricyclic antidepressants

Concurrent use is usually uneventful although two unexplained hypertensive crises have occurred when imipramine or amitriptyline was used with *Sinemet*. See also 'Levodopa + Anticholinergics', p.505 for interactions due to the anticholinergic effects of tricyclic antidepressants.

Clinical evidence

A hypertensive crisis (blood pressure 210/110 mmHg) associated with agitation, tremor and generalised rigidity developed in a woman taking 6 tablets of *Sinemet* (levodopa 100 mg + 10 mg carbidopa) daily the day after she started to take 25 mg of **imipramine** three times daily. The imipramine was stopped and she recovered over the following 24 hours. The same reaction occurred again when she was later accidentally given 25 mg of **amitriptyline** three times daily.[1] A similar hypertensive reaction (a rise from 190/110 to 270/140 mmHg) occurred over 34 hours in another woman taking **amitriptyline** 20 mg at night when she was given half a tablet of *Sinemet* and 10 mg metoclopramide three times a day. This resolved when all three drugs were stopped.[2]

Mechanism

Not understood.

Importance and management

Information seems to be limited to these reports. Concurrent use is normally successful and uneventful.[3-5] However, be alert for the possibility of a hypertensive reaction, which resolves if the tricyclic antidepressant is withdrawn. See also 'Levodopa + Anticholinergics', p.505 for interactions due to the anticholinergic side effects of tricyclic antidepressants.

1. Edwards M. Adverse interaction of levodopa with tricyclic antidepressants. *Practitioner* (1982) 226, 1447 and 1449.
2. Rampton DS. Hypertensive crisis in a patient given Sinemet, metoclopramide, and amitriptyline. *BMJ* (1977) 3, 607–8.
3. Yahr MD. The treatment of Parkinsonism. Current concepts. *Med Clin North Am* (1972) 56, 1377–92.
4. Calne DB, Reid JL. Antiparkinsonian drugs: pharmacological and therapeutic aspects. *Drugs* (1972) 4, 49–74.
5. van Wieringen A, Wright J. Observations on patients with Parkinson's disease treated with L-dopa. I. Trial and evaluation of L-dopa therapy. *S Afr Med J* (1972) 46, 1262–6.

Lisuride + Miscellaneous

Neither erythromycin nor food interact to a clinically relevant extent with lisuride. Dopamine antagonists are expected to diminish the effects of lisuride, and lisuride may impair the effects of psychotropic drugs.

Clinical evidence, mechanism, importance and management

Twelve healthy subjects were given lisuride 200 micrograms orally or 50 micrograms as a 30 minute intravenous infusion after taking **erythromycin** (dose unknown) twice daily for 4 days. Another 30 healthy subjects were given lisuride 200 micrograms orally while fasting or with **food**. It was found that neither **erythromycin** nor **food** significantly modified either the pharmacokinetics or the pharmacodynamics of the lisuride.[1] There would therefore appear to be no reason for avoiding concurrent use.

Lisuride is a dopamine agonist, so the makers say that dopamine antagonists such as **haloperidol**, **sulpiride** and **metoclopramide** can weaken the effects of lisuride.[2] They also say that the concurrent use of lisuride may lessen the effects of some **psychotropic drugs**,[2] but there do not appear to be any reports of this interaction in the literature.

1. Gandon JM, Le Coz F, Kühne G, Hümpel M, Allain H. PK/PD interaction studies of lisuride with erythromycin and food in healthy volunteers. *Clin Pharmacol Ther* (1995) 57, 191.
2. Lisuride. Cambridge Laboratories Ltd. Summary of product characteristics, January 2001.

Piribedil + Clonidine

Clonidine is reported to oppose the effects of piribedil.

Clinical evidence, mechanism, importance and management

A study in 5 patients taking piribedil found that concurrent treatment with clonidine (up to 1.5 mg daily for 10 to 24 days) caused a worsening of the parkinsonism (an exacerbation of rigidity and akinesia). The concurrent use of anticholinergic drugs reduced the effects of this interaction.[1]

1. Shoulson I, Chase TN. Clonidine and the anti-parkinsonian response to L-dopa or piribedil. *Neuropharmacology* (1976) 15, 25–7.

Pramipexole + Miscellaneous

Cimetidine, probenecid and possibly amantadine reduce the clearance of pramipexole from the body. Pramipexole is not expected to interact with anticholinergic drugs, levodopa (although a dosage reduction may be needed), or selegiline, but it is cautioned in combination with antipsychotic drugs.

Clinical evidence, mechanism, importance and management

A study in 12 healthy subjects found that multiple doses of **cimetidine** reduced the clearance of a single 250-microgram dose of pramipexole by about 35% and increased its half-life by 40%.[1] The makers say that because **amantadine** and cimetidine are both eliminated by this route (i.e. via the renal cationic secretory transport system), reduced excretion of both drugs may occur.[2] Multiple doses of **probenecid** given to 12 healthy subjects reduced the clearance of a single 250-microgram dose of pramipexole by 10.3%.[1] The clinical significance of these interactions is uncertain, and as yet there appear to be no reports of any adverse interactions, however, the makers suggest a reduction of the pramipexole dose should be considered when amantadine or cimetidine are administered concurrently with pramipexole.

Although there is no pharmacokinetic interaction between pramipexole and **levodopa**, as pramipexole enhances the actions of **levodopa** the makers suggest reducing the dose of **levodopa** as the dose of pramipexole is increased.[2] The makers say that co-administration of **antipsychotics** should be avoided, presumably because their dopamine antagonist actions will antagonise the effect of pramipexole, a dopamine agonist. They also say that no pharmacokinetic interaction occurs with **selegiline**, and because pramipexole is largely unmetabolised it is unlikely to interact pharmacokinetically with **anticholinergics**.[2]

1. Wright CE, Lasher Sisson T, Ichhpurani AK, Peters GR. Influence of probenecid (PR) and cimetidine (C) on pramipexole (PX) pharmacokinetics. *Clin Pharmacol Ther* (1996) 59, 183.
2. Mirapexin (Pramipexole). Boehringer Ingelheim Ltd. UK Summary of product characteristics, March 2005.

Ropinirole + Miscellaneous

Ropinirole appears not to interact adversely with amantadine, levodopa, selegiline or trihexyphenidyl (benzhexol). Oestrogen may reduce the clearance of ropinirole. On theoretical grounds it is suggested that cimetidine, ciprofloxacin and fluvoxamine may increase the effects of ropinirole, and dopamine antagonists such as metoclopramide and sulpiride may reduce its effects. See also 'Theophylline + Ropinirole', p.953.

Clinical evidence, mechanism, importance and management

Trials with ropinirole carried out by the makers found no pharmacokinetic interactions between ropinirole and **levodopa** under steady-state conditions (using clinically relevant doses) that would call for large dosage adjustments of either drug. However, it is suggested that the dose of levodopa may be reduced gradually by around 20% in total.[1,2] **Amantadine**, **selegiline** and **trihexyphenidyl** were found not to have relevant effects on ropinirole.[2] During clinical trials no drugs or groups of drugs (the makers quote the **benzodiazepines**) had a clinically relevant effect on the clearance of oral ropinirole except **oestrogen** used in hormonal replacement therapy (**HRT**), which reduced the ropinirole clearance by one third. It is therefore suggested that a reduction in the ropinirole dosage may be needed if **HRT** is started, and an increase if it is withdrawn.[2]

In vitro studies show that the cytochrome P450 isoenzyme CYP1A2 is largely responsible for the metabolism of ropinirole, with a minor role being played by CYP3A. The potential therefore exists for the interaction with other drugs that either induce or inhibit CYP1A2. Given that in practice the doses of ropinirole are low and that *in vitro* evidence shows that it does not affect the activity of CYP1A2, it is thought that other drugs are more likely to affect ropinirole than vice versa.[2] The makers therefore suggest that concurrently used drugs such as **cimetidine**, **ciprofloxacin** and **fluvoxamine** may possibly increase the effects of ropinirole, calling for a reduction in its dosage if used concurrently.[1,2] Time alone will tell whether these largely theoretical predicted interactions are of practical importance or not, but good monitoring is advisable.

Ropinirole is a dopamine agonist, so the makers therefore reasonably suggest that antipsychotics and other drugs that act as central dopamine receptor antagonists (they name **sulpiride** and **metoclopramide**) should be avoided because they may reduce the effectiveness of ropinirole.[1] The practical importance of this also awaits confirmation.

1. Requip (Ropinirole). GlaxoSmithKline UK. UK Summary of product characteristics, August 2002.
2. SmithKline Beecham. Personal Communication, September 1996.

Selegiline + Antidepressants

A few cases of the serotonin syndrome and other serious CNS disturbances have been seen with selegiline and tricyclic antidepressants or SSRIs. One of the makers of selegiline contraindicates its use with any antidepressant drug, while another advises avoiding SSRIs and venlafaxine, and using caution with the tricyclics. See also 'MAOIs + MAOIs', p.867 for information on selegiline and MAOIs.

Clinical evidence

A. SSRIs

(a) Citalopram

A double-blind randomised study in 18 healthy subjects found no important pharmacokinetic or pharmacodynamic interactions between citalopram and selegiline. Healthy subjects were given 20 mg citalopram or a placebo daily for 10 days followed by 4 days with concurrent selegiline 10 mg daily. There was no evidence of changes in vital signs or in the frequency of adverse events, but the bioavailability of the selegiline was slightly reduced by about 30% in the presence of citalopram. The authors of this report concluded that no clinically relevant interaction occurred between selegiline and citalopram.[1]

(b) Fluoxetine

A woman with Parkinson's disease on selegiline, bromocriptine and levodopa/carbidopa was additionally started on fluoxetine 20 mg. Several days later she developed episodes of shivering and sweating in the mid-afternoon, which lasted several hours. Her hands became blue, cold and mottled and her blood pressure was elevated (200/120 mmHg). These episodes disappeared when both fluoxetine and selegiline were stopped, and did not reappear when the fluoxetine was restarted.[2]

Other similar patients have become hyperactive and apparently manic,[2] have developed ataxia,[3] or developed a tonic-clonic seizure and headache, flushes, palpitations, and a blood pressure of 250/130 mmHg (a pseudophaeochromocytoma syndrome),[4] all after the concurrent use of fluoxetine and selegiline. A possible serotonin syndrome has been described in another patient.[5] These reports contrast with a retrospective study of 23 patients with parkinsonism, who received both selegiline and fluoxetine without any serious side-effects occurring, although worsening confusion was noted in 5 patients.[6]

(c) Paroxetine

A retrospective study of patients with Parkinson's disease on selegiline 5 to 10 mg daily (and other antiparkinsonian drugs such as levodopa/carbidopa, bromocriptine, amantadine, pergolide, anticholinergics) noted that the addition of paroxetine 10 to 40 mg daily caused no adverse effects and the patients appeared to obtain overall benefit, including some improvement in parkinsonian symptoms.[7]

(d) Sertraline

A retrospective study of patients with Parkinson's disease on selegiline 5 to 10 mg daily (and other antiparkinsonian drugs such as levodopa/carbidopa, bromocriptine, amantadine, pergolide, anticholinergics) noted that the addition of sertraline 25 to 100 mg daily caused no adverse effects and the patients appeared to obtain overall benefit, including some improvement in parkinsonian symptoms.[7]

B. Tetracyclic antidepressants

There is an isolated case report of a man on selegiline, levodopa/carbidopa, lisuride, **maprotiline**, theophylline and ephedrine who developed hypertensive crises (blood pressure up to 300/150 mmHg), intense vasoconstriction, confusion, abdominal pain, sweating, and tachycardia (110 bpm) within 2 days of raising the doses of theophylline and ephedrine. All of the drugs were stopped, and the patient was treated with intravenous nicardipine. He recovered uneventfully. It is thought that this 'pseudophaeochromocytoma' was due to a selegiline/**maprotiline**/ephedrine interaction.[8]

C. Tricyclic antidepressants

Between 1989 and 1994 the FDA in the USA received 16 reports of adverse interactions between selegiline and tricyclic antidepressants, which were attributed to the serotonin syndrome. For this reason the US labelling for selegiline suggests that concurrent use should be avoided.[9]

One of the makers of selegiline in the UK issues a warning suggesting caution[10] and another maker issues a contraindication.[11] They very briefly describe severe CNS toxicity in one patient given selegiline and **amitriptyline** (hyperpyrexia and death), and in another given **protriptyline** (tremor, agitation, restlessness, followed by unresponsiveness and death).[10,11] A further report describes the serotonin syndrome in a woman given **nortriptyline** and selegiline concurrently.[12]

However, these warnings need to be balanced by other reports indicating that these reactions are uncommon. One study based on the findings of 45 investigators treating 4,568 patients with selegiline and antidepressants (not specifically named but possibly including the tricyclics) found that only 11 patients (0.24%) experienced symptoms considered to represent the serotonin syndrome, and only 2 patients (0.04%) experienced symptoms considered to be serious.[13] Another small retrospective study designed to evaluate the tolerability and efficacy of combining selegiline and tricyclic antidepressants (not specifically named) identified 28 patients who had taken both drugs.[9] In total, 17 patients definitely benefited and 6 patients possibly benefited from taking the combination. Another retrospective study of 25 occasions of combined tricyclic-selegiline use found no cases of the serotonin syndrome.[5]

D. Miscellaneous antidepressants

(a) Trazodone

A retrospective study of patients with Parkinson's disease on selegiline 5 to 10 mg daily (and other anti-parkinson drugs such as levodopa/carbidopa, bromocriptine, amantadine, pergolide, anticholinergics) noted that the addition of trazodone 25 to 150 mg daily caused no adverse effects and the patients appeared to obtain overall benefit, including some improvement in parkinsonian symptoms.[7]

(b) Venlafaxine

A man developed the serotonin syndrome 15 days after stopping selegiline 50 mg [daily] and within 30 minutes of starting venlafaxine 37.5 mg.[14]

Mechanism

Not fully understood. In some cases the symptoms seen appear to be consistent with the serotonin-syndrome, which is typified by CNS irritability, increased muscle tone, shivering, altered consciousness and myoclonus.

Importance and management

The situation with selegiline and fluoxetine is by no means clear cut, because they have been used together apparently safely and uneventfully in some patients,[6] and only a few of the cases cited above[2,5] seem to fit the serotonin syndrome. The makers of selegiline say that the addition of fluoxetine, paroxetine, sertraline or venlafaxine has resulted in a variety of adverse reactions including diaphoresis, flushing, ataxia, tremor, hyperthermia, hyper/hypotension, seizures, palpitation, dizziness and mental changes that include agitation, confusion and hallucinations progressing to delirium and coma, and they recommend that these drug combinations should be avoided.[10,11]

If the decision is made to combine selegiline and any of the tricyclic antidepressants, the outcome should be well monitored but the likelihood of problems seems to be small. Nevertheless, one of the makers of selegiline contraindicates tricyclic antidepressants with selegiline, and in fact contraindicates all antidepressant drug combinations.[11]

1. Laine K, Anttila M, Heinonen E, Helminen A, Huupponen R, Mäki-Ikola O, Reinikainen K, Scheinin M. Lack of adverse interactions between concomitantly administered selegiline and citalopram. *Clin Neuropharmacol* (1997) 20, 419–33.
2. Suchowersky O, deVries JD. Interaction of fluoxetine and selegiline. *Can J Psychiatry* (1990) 35, 571–2.
3. Jermain DM, Hughes PL, Follender AB. Potential fluoxetine-selegiline interaction. *Ann Pharmacother* (1992) 26, 1300.
4. Montastruc JL, Chamontin B, Senard JM, Tran MA, Rascol O, Llau ME, Rascol A. Pseudo-phaeochromocytoma in parkinsonian patient treated with fluoxetine plus selegiline. *Lancet* (1993) 341, 555.
5. Ritter JL, Alexander B. Retrospective study of selegiline-antidepressant drug interactions and a review of the literature. *Ann Clin Psychiatry* (1997) 9, 7–13.
6. Waters CH. Fluoxetine and selegiline — lack of significant interaction. *Can J Neurol Sci* (1994) 21, 259–61.
7. Toyama SC, Iacono RP. Is it safe to combine a selective serotonin reuptake inhibitor with selegiline? *Ann Pharmacother* (1994) 28, 405–6.
8. Lefebvre H, Noblet C, Moore N, Wolf LM. Pseudo-phaeochromocytoma after multiple drug interactions involving the selective monoamine oxidase inhibitor selegiline. *Clin Endocrinol (Oxf)* (1995) 42, 95–9.
9. Yu LJ, Zweig RM. Successful combination of selegiline and antidepressants in Parkinson's disease. *Neurology* (1996) 46 (2 Suppl), A374.
10. Eldepryl (Selegiline). Orion Pharma (UK) Ltd. UK Summary of product characteristics, October 2003.
11. Zelapar (Selegiline hydrochloride). Zeneus Pharma Ltd. UK Summary of product characteristics, February 2003.
12. Hinds NP, Hillier CEM, Wiles CM. Possible serotonin syndrome arising from an interaction between nortriptyline and selegiline in a lady with parkinsonism. *J Neurol* (2000) 247, 811.
13. Richard I, Kurlan R, Tanner C. Serotonin syndrome and the combined use of Deprenyl and an antidepressant in Parkinson's disease. *Neurology* (1996) 46 (2 Suppl), A374.
14. Gitlin MJ. Venlafaxine, monoamine oxidase inhibitors, and the serotonin syndrome. *J Clin Psychopharmacol* (1997) 17, 66–67.

Selegiline + Cocaine

Cocaine and selegiline appear not to interact adversely.

Clinical evidence, mechanism, importance and management

In a study to establish the safety of using selegiline to prevent relapse in cocaine addiction, 5 otherwise healthy intravenous cocaine users were given 0, 20 and 40 mg intravenous doses of cocaine one hour apart following treatment with selegiline 10 mg or placebo orally. The cocaine increased the heart rate, blood pressure, pupil diameter and subjective indices of euphoria as expected. However, the presence of selegiline reduced pupillary diameter, but did not alter the pupil dilation or other effects normally caused by cocaine. It was concluded that concurrent use is safe and unlikely to increase the reinforcing effects of cocaine.[1]

1. Haberny KA, Walsh SL, Ginn DH, Wilkins JN, Garner JE, Setoda D, Bigelow GE. Absence of acute cocaine interactions with the MAO-B inhibitor selegiline. *Drug Alcohol Depend* (1995) 39, 55–62.

Selegiline + Itraconazole

Itraconazole and selegiline appear not to interact.

Clinical evidence, mechanism, importance and management

In a randomised placebo-controlled crossover study, 12 healthy subjects were given selegiline 10 mg after taking itraconazole 200 mg daily for 4 days. Itraconazole did not have any significant effects on the pharmacokinetics of selegiline, although the AUC of desmethylselegiline, a primary metabolite, was increased by 11%. The pharmacokinetics of itraconazole were also unaffected. There would appear to be no reason for avoiding concurrent use.[1]

1. Kivistö KT, Wang J-S, Backman JT, Nyman L, Taavitsainen P, Anttila M, Neuvonen PJ. Selegiline pharmacokinetics are unaffected by the CYP3A4 inhibitor itraconazole. *Eur J Clin Pharmacol* (2001) 57, 37–42.

Tolcapone + Miscellaneous

No serious adverse interactions have been documented with tolcapone, but the makers contraindicate non-selective MAOIs and a combination of MAO-A and MAO-B inhibitors. They also issue a caution (on theoretical grounds) about the concurrent use of apomorphine, desipramine, dobutamine, adrenaline (epinephrine), isoprenaline (isoproterenol), maprotiline, alpha-methyldopa, venlafaxine and warfarin.

Clinical evidence, mechanism, importance and management

There do not appear to be any reports of serious adverse interactions between tolcapone and other drugs, but the makers[1,2] issue a number of cautionary warnings, largely based on the pharmacological and metabolic profile of tolcapone.

The makers contraindicate the use of non-selective MAOIs (e.g. **phenelzine**, **tranylcypromine**) and combinations of an MAO-A inhibitor (e.g. **moclobemide**) and an MAO-B inhibitor (**selegiline**), but **selegiline** alone is compatible with tolcapone provided not more than 10 mg daily is used.[1,2] Tolcapone does not affect the pharmacokinetics of **carbidopa**, but it increases the serum levels of **benserazide**. The benserazide levels remained within the usual range when 25 mg of benserazide was given, but were increased above the usual levels when 50 mg doses were given. The clinical significance of this is uncertain but the UK maker advises good monitoring for benserazide adverse effects.[1] Tolcapone inhibits the enzyme catechol-*O*-methyl transferase (COMT), which is concerned with the metabolism of drugs such as **apomorphine**, **adrenaline** (**epinephrine**), **dobutamine**, **isoprenaline** (**isoproterenol**) and **alpha-methyldopa**, for which reason the makers warn about the theoretical possibility of increased serum levels and related adverse effects of these drugs. Most of these combinations have not been specifically studied. However, no adverse interactions were seen in studies with **ephedrine**. Studies of tolcapone combined with **levodopa/carbidopa** and **desipramine** demonstrated no serious interactions (although the frequency of adverse events increased slightly).[1,2] Therefore the UK maker suggests that caution should be exercised with any drugs which are potent **noradrenaline** (**norepinephrine**), uptake inhibitors such as **desipramine**, **maprotiline** and **venlafaxine**.[1]

No pharmacokinetic interaction occurs between **tolbutamide** and tolcapone despite *in vitro* evidence that tolcapone inhibits the cytochrome P450 isoenzyme CYP2C9, and no interaction therefore seems likely with **warfarin**. Even so, because of the lack of experience, the makers advise good monitoring. Other *in vitro* studies have suggested that tolcapone is unlikely to interact with **caffeine**, **ciclosporin**, **midazolam**, **mephenytoin**, or **terfenadine**.

Tolcapone was withdrawn in Europe in November 1998 because of serious hepatic reactions,[3] but it has subsequently been selectively re-introduced.

1. Tasmar (Tolcapone). Valeant Pharmaceuticals Ltd. UK Summary of product characteristics, August 1997.
2. Tasmar (Tolcapone). Valeant Pharmaceuticals International. US Prescribing information, June 2004.
3. Committee on Safety of Medicines/Medicines Control Agency. Withdrawal of tolcapone (Tasmar). *Current Problems* (1999) 25, 2.

17

Antiplatelet drugs and thrombolytics

Platelets usually circulate in the plasma in an inactive form, but following injury to blood vessels they become activated and adhere to the site of injury. Platelet aggregation then occurs, which contributes to the haemostatic plug. Platelet aggregation involves the binding of fibrinogen with a glycoprotein IIb/IIIa receptor on the platelet surface. The activated platelets secrete substances such as adenosine diphosphate (ADP) and thromboxane A_2 that result in additional platelet aggregation and also cause vasoconstriction. Finally a number of platelet derived factors stimulate production of thrombin and hence fibrin through the coagulation cascade (see 'The blood clotting process', (p.255)). Opposing this process is the fibrinolysis pathway, which is initiated during clot formation by a number of mediators such as tissue plasminogen activator (tPA) and urokinase. These proteins convert plasminogen to plasmin, which in turn degrades fibrin, the main component of the clot.

Antiplatelet drugs (see 'Table 17.1', (p.517)) reduce platelet aggregation and are used to prevent thromboembolic events. They act through a wide range of mechanisms including:

- prevention of thromboxane A_2 synthesis or inhibition of thromboxane receptors e.g. aspirin inhibits platelet cyclo-oxygenase, preventing synthesis of thromboxane A_2
- interference with adenosine diphosphate mediated platelet activation e.g. thienopyridines; inhibition of adenosine reuptake e.g. dipyridamole; interference with adenosine metabolism by inhibiting cyclic adenosine monophosphate (cAMP) phosphodiesterase e.g. cilostazol
- interference in the final step in platelet aggregation by stopping fibrinogen binding with the glycoprotein IIb/IIIa receptor on the platelet surface

Therefore some antiplatelet drugs can have beneficial additive effects with other antiplatelet drugs that act via different mechanisms. Furthermore, other drugs such as dextrans, heparin, some prostaglandins and sulfinpyrazone also have some antiplatelet activity.

Thrombolytics (see 'Table 17.2', (p.517)) are used in the treatment of thromboembolic disorders. Thrombolytics activate plasminogen to form plasmin, which is a proteolytic enzyme that degrades fibrin and therefore produces dissolution of clots.

This section is primarily concerned with those interactions where the activities of antiplatelet drugs (except aspirin) or thrombolytics are changed by the presence of another drug. Interactions affecting aspirin are mainly covered under analgesics.

Table 17.1 Antiplatelet drugs

Generic names	*Proprietary names*
Adenosine reuptake inhibitors/Phosphodiesterase inhibitors	
Cilostazol	Artesol, Pletaal, Pletal, Pletoz, Stiloz, Trastocir, Zilast
Dipyridamole	Adezan, Aggrenox, Agremol, Atrombin, Cardoxin, Cleridium, Corosan, Curantyl N, Dipyrin, Maxicardil, Persantin, Persantine, Plato, Posanin, Pracem, Procardin, Pytazen, Trepol, Trompersantin, Vadinar
Cyclo-oxygenase inhibitors	
Aspirin	AAS, Acekapton, Acenterine, Acesal, Aceticil, Acetin, Acetosal, Acitab, Actorin, Acylpyrin, Adiro, Adprin-B, Aggrenox, Albyl minor, Albyl-E, Alcacyl instantanee, Alka-Seltzer, Analgesin, Angettes, Anopyrin, Antacsal, Antifebrin, Apo-Asa, Arthritis Pain Formula, ASA, Asaflow, Asaphen, ASA-ratio, Ascot, Ascriptin, ASL, Aspec, Aspegic, Aspent, Aspergum, Aspicalm, Aspicot, Aspidol, Aspiglicina, Aspilets, Aspiricor, Aspirin Cardio, Aspirin Protect, Aspirin with Stomach Guard, Aspirina, Aspirina 03, Aspirine, Aspirine Cardio, Aspirine pH8, Aspirine Protect, Aspirinetas, Aspirinetta, Aspirisucre, Aspisol, Asprimox, Aspro, ASS, Astrix, Bamyl, Bamyl S, Bayaspirina, Bayer Low Adult Strength, Bioplak, Buffered Pirin, Bufferin, Buffex, Caas, Cama Arthritis Pain Reliever, Caparin, Caprin, Cardegic, Cardioaspirin, Cardioaspirina, Cardioaspirine, Cardiosolupsan, Cardiprin, Cardirene, Cartia, Casprin, Catalgine, Cemirit, Cimaas, Claragine, Colfarit, Colsprin, Coraspir, Corplus, Decitriol, Delisprin, Desenfriolito, Disgren, Disperin, Dispril, Disprin, Disprin Direct, Disprina, Dolorosan, Dusil, Easprin, Ecasil, Ecoprin, Ecosprin, Ecotrin, Egicalm, Emotpin, Empirin, Enprin, Entrarin, Entrophen, Equate, Extra Strength Bayer Plus, Flectadol, Geniol AP, Geniol SC sin Cafeina, Geniolito, Genprin, Globoid, Glyprin, Godamed, Godasal, Halfprin, Hassapirin Puro, Herz ASS, HerzASS, Herzschutz ASS, Hipotermal, Hjerdyl, Hjertemagnyl, Idotyl, Inyesprin, Istopirin, Juridin, Jusprin, Kalmopyrin, Kardegic, Kardiren, Kilios, LAsprin, Lisaspin, Lowasa, Magnaprin, Magnecyl, Magnyl, Micropirin, Midolen, Migraspirina, Miniasal, Myoprin, Norwich Extra Strength, Novasen, Nuevapina, Nu-Seals, Okal, PostMI, Primaspan, Propirin, Pure Health, Regular Strength Bayer, Resprin, Rhonal, Rivasa, Salicil, Salimont, Salospir, Salycilina, Santasal N, Saspryl, Sedergine, Seferin, Solprin, Somalgin, Spren, St. Joseph Adult Chewable, Tevapirin, Therasa, Thrombace Neo, Thrombo AS, Thrombo ASS, Thrombostad, Tiatral 100 SR, Tiplac, Togal ASS, Togal Mono, Toldex, Tri-Buffered ASA, Tromalyt, Trombyl, Upsalgin-N, Upsarin, V-AS, Vincent's Powders, ZORprin
Indobufen	Ibustrin
Triflusal	Aflen, Disgren, Logrosal, Tecnosal, Triflux
Glycoprotein IIb/IIIa-receptor antagonists	
Abciximab	ReoPro
Eptifibatide	Integrilin
Lamifiban	
Tirofiban	Aggrastat, Aggrastet, Agrastat, Avastar
Thienopyridines	
Clopidogrel	Artevil, Cloflow, Clopact, Clopivas, Clopod, Iscover, Iscover , Nefazan, Noklot, Plavix
Ticlopidine	Agregamina, Anagregal, Anchostam-100, Anghostan-100, Antigreg, Aplaket, Aplatic, Apo-Tic, Ateroclar, Betlife, Cenpidine, Clox, Desiticlopidin, Dosier, Etfariol, Fluilast, Flupid, Fluxidin, Ipaton, Isaxion, Klodin, Klodipin, Movin, Neo Fulvigal, Neo-omnipen, Opidina, Opteron, Panaldine, Plaquetal, Plaquetil, Platigren, Ruxicolan, Siclot, Tacron, Tagren, Thrombodine, Ticlid, Ticlidil, Ticlo, Ticlobal, Ticlobest, Ticlodix, Ticlodone, Ticlop, Ticlopat, Ticlopid, Ticloproge, Tikleen, Tiklid, Tiklyd, Tikol, Tilodene, Tilopin, Tipidin, Tipidine, Trombenal, Trombopat, Tyklid, Viladil
Thromboxane receptor antagonist	
Picotamide	Plactidil
Miscellaneous	
Ditazole	Ageroplas, Fendazol
Trapidil	Rocornal, Travisco

Table 17.2 Thrombolytics

Generic names	*Proprietary names*
Alteplase (Recombinant Tissue-type Plasminogen Activator; rt-PA)	Actilyse, Activase, Cathflo
Anistreplase	Eminase
Defibrotide	Noravid, Prociclide
Monteplase	Cleactor
Nateplase	
Pamiteplase	
Reteplase	Rapilysin, Repilysin, Retavase
Streptokinase	Fibrokinase, Kabikinase, Streptase, Streptonase, Unitinase, Zykinase
Tenecteplase	Metalyse, TNKase
Urokinase	Abbokinase, Actosolv, Alfakinasi, Corase, Persolv Richter, Rheotromb, Solokinase, Ukidan, Urochinasi, Uronase, Uroquidan

Alteplase + Glyceryl trinitrate (Nitroglycerin)

Glyceryl trinitrate may reduce the thrombolytic efficacy of alteplase.

Clinical evidence, mechanism, importance and management

In a randomised study, 60 patients with acute anterior myocardial infarction were given intravenous alteplase 100 mg over 3 hours, as well as heparin and aspirin; in addition, 27 of the patients were also given intravenous glyceryl trinitrate 100 micrograms/minute for 8 hours. Patients receiving both alteplase and glyceryl trinitrate had signs of reperfusion less often (15 of 27; 56%) than the patients who received alteplase alone (25 of 33; 76%). Time to reperfusion was also longer in the combined-treatment group (37.8 versus 19.6 minutes) and the incidence of coronary artery re-occlusion was higher (53% versus 24%). Giving alteplase with glyceryl trinitrate produced plasma levels of tissue plasminogen activator (TPA) antigen that were about two-thirds lower than when alteplase was given alone.[1] Impaired thrombolysis has been found in another study[2] and also in an earlier study in *dogs*.[3]

It was postulated that the markedly reduced plasma TPA levels in patients given glyceryl trinitrate was due to an increase in the metabolism of alteplase as a result of increased hepatic blood flow.[1] However, an *in vitro* study found that glyceryl trinitrate enhanced the degradation of alteplase, and therefore a mechanism other than increased hepatic blood flow seems likely to be involved.[4] It has been suggested, that this interaction may not be clinically important,[5] and the current evidence is too sparse to suggest changing current practice.

1. Romeo F, Rosano GMC, Martuscelli E, De Luca F, Bianco C, Colistra C, Comito M, Cardona N, Miceli F, Rosano V, Mehta JL. Concurrent nitroglycerin administration reduces the efficacy of recombinant tissue-type plasminogen activator in patients with acute anterior wall myocardial infarction. *Am Heart J* (1995) 130, 692–7.
2. Nicolini FA, Ferrini D, Ottani F, Galvani M, Ronchi A, Behrens PH, Rusticali F, Mehta JL. Concurrent nitroglycerin therapy impairs tissue-type plasminogen activator-induced thrombolysis in patients with acute myocardial infarction. *Am J Cardiol* (1994) 74, 662–6.
3. Mehta JL, Nicolini FA, Nichols WW, Saldeen TGP. Concurrent nitroglycerin administration decreases thrombolytic potential of tissue-type plasminogen activator. *J Am Coll Cardiol* (1991) 17, 805–11.
4. White CM, Fan C, Chen BP, Kluger J, Chow MSS. Assessment of the drug interaction between alteplase and nitroglycerin: an in vitro study. *Pharmacotherapy* (2000) 20, 380–2.
5. Boehringer Ingelheim. Personal communication, March 1999.

Antiplatelet drugs + Antiplatelet drugs, Anticoagulants or Thrombolytics

Caution and careful monitoring is recommended when antiplatelet drugs are used with other drugs that affect haemostasis, such as other antiplatelet drugs, anticoagulants, or thrombolytics. The makers of clopidogrel recommend the avoidance of warfarin, although there is some evidence of safety. It is unclear whether the concurrent use of clopidogrel and cilostazol results in a prolonged bleeding time. Intravenous dipyridamole should not be given concurrently with oral dipyridamole. The risk of bleeding with glycoprotein IIb/IIIa antagonists may be increased by heparin and thrombolytics, but low-dose thrombolytic therapy appears less likely to cause a problem.
See also 'Antiplatelet drugs + Aspirin or other NSAIDs', p.519 and 'Streptokinase + Aspirin', p.524.

Clinical evidence, mechanism, importance and management

(a) Cilostazol

The concurrent use of cilostazol 150 mg twice daily and **clopidogrel** 75 mg daily for 5 days increased the AUC of cilostazol by only 9%, but increased the AUC of the dehydro metabolite of cilostazol by 24% (this metabolite has 3 to 4 times the potency of cilostazol in inhibiting platelet aggregation). No changes in platelet count, prothrombin time or aPTT were seen. However, **clopidogrel** alone prolonged bleeding time, and it was not possible to determine whether there was an additive effect with cilostazol.[1] The UK maker suggests caution if cilostazol is given with any drug that inhibits platelet aggregation, and say that consideration should be given to monitoring the bleeding time at intervals.[1] See also 'Anticoagulants + Cilostazol', p.275.

(b) Clopidogrel

The UK makers of clopidogrel state that the concurrent use of **warfarin** is not recommended because it may increase the intensity of bleedings;[2] the US makers recommend caution.[3] However, a randomised, double-blind, placebo-controlled study involving 43 patients who had been taking **warfarin** for at least 2 months found that the addition of clopidogrel 75 mg daily for 8 days had no effect on plasma **warfarin** levels or INRs. No bleeding occurred with clopidogrel and no serious adverse events were reported.[4]

A placebo-controlled study in 12 healthy subjects found that the dosage of **heparin** given over 4 days did not need modification when clopidogrel 75 mg daily was given, and the inhibitory effects of clopidogrel on platelet aggregation were unchanged on concurrent use.[5] However, the makers of clopidogrel say that a pharmacodynamic interaction between clopidogrel and **heparin** is possible, leading to increased risk of bleeding, and therefore concurrent use should be undertaken with caution.[2] They also report that in patients with recent myocardial infarction, the incidence of clinically significant bleeding with clopidogrel/**heparin/alteplase** is similar to that seen with aspirin/heparin/alteplase, but they say that the safety of clopidogrel with other thrombolytics has not been established and caution is required.[2]

As with other antiplatelet drugs, clopidogrel should be used with caution in patients who may be at risk of increased bleeding e.g. in surgery and in patients receiving **aspirin**, **heparin**, **glycoprotein IIb/IIIa inhibitors** (see *(d)* below) or thrombolytics. Monitor for any signs of bleeding including occult bleeding.[2]

(c) Glycoprotein IIb/IIIa antagonists

(i) Abciximab. Although the makers of abciximab recommend concurrent therapy with **heparin**, they also report that there is an increase in the incidence of bleeding.[6,7] In one study in patients with acute coronary syndromes without early revascularisation, the use of **low-molecular-weight heparin** was considered to be one of the factors that increased the risk of bleeding events with abciximab.[8]

Limited experience of abciximab in patients who have received thrombolytics suggests an increase in the risk of bleeding.[6,7] A retrospective analysis of 103 patients who presented with acute myocardial infarction and underwent angioplasty with adjunctive abciximab therapy, found that there was a significant increase in major bleeding complications when abciximab was used with full-dose **alteplase**. A major bleed occurred in 5 of 22 (23%) patients who underwent angioplasty within 15 hours of receiving thrombolytic therapy compared with 0 of 36 who underwent elective angioplasty more than 15 hours after fibrinolysis, and 1 of 45 (2%) without prior fibrinolysis.[9] However, the combination of abciximab with low-dose **reteplase** appeared not to result in the haemorrhagic complications associated with full-dose fibrinolytic therapy,[10] and no increase in bleeding complications were reported in studies using reduced-dose thrombolytic therapy with full-dose abciximab.[10,11]

The maker of abciximab recommends caution when it is used with other drugs that affect haemostasis, such as **heparin**, **warfarin**, thrombolytics and antiplatelet drugs other than aspirin, such as **dipyridamole** and **ticlopidine**.[6,7]

(ii) Eptifibatide. In an acute myocardial infarction study involving 181 patients, eptifibatide at the highest infusion rates studied (1.3 and 2 micrograms/kg per minute) appeared to increase the risk of bleeding when given with **streptokinase** 1.5 million units over 60 minutes. However, the makers state that data are limited on the use of eptifibatide in patients receiving thrombolytics, and in a percutaneous coronary intervention study or an acute myocardial infarction study there was no consistent evidence that eptifibatide increased the risk of major or minor bleeding associated with **alteplase**.[12,13]

The UK maker of eptifibatide reports that concurrent use with **warfarin** and **dipyridamole** did not appear to increase the risk of major and minor bleeding, and the use of **heparin** is recommended, but they warn that if eptifibatide is given with **heparin**, there must be careful monitoring including the aPTT.

Caution must be employed when eptifibatide is used with other drugs that affect haemostasis, including **clopidogrel**, **ticlopidine**, **dipyridamole**, **oral** anticoagulants or thrombolytics and concurrent or planned use of another **glycoprotein IIb/IIIa inhibitor** is contraindicated.[12,13]

(d) Ticlopidine

The UK makers of ticlopidine have stated that concurrent use with **heparins**, oral anticoagulants or antiplatelet drugs increases haemorrhagic risk, and therefore concurrent use requires close clinical and laboratory monitoring.[14]

See also, 'Anticoagulants + Ticlopidine', p.318.

1. Pletal (Cilostazol). Otsuka Pharmaceuticals (UK) Ltd. UK Summary of product characteristics, October 2002.
2. Plavix (Clopidogrel bisulfate). Sanofi-Aventis. UK Summary of product characteristics, January 2005.
3. Plavix (Clopidogrel bisulfate). Sanofi-Synthelabo. US Prescribing information, November 2004.
4. Lidell C, Svedberg L-E, Lindell P, Bandh S, Wallentin L. Absence of interaction between clopidogrel and warfarin in patients on long-term anticoagulation. *J Am Coll Cardiol* (2001) 37 (2 Suppl A), 314A.
5. Caplain H, D'Honneur G, Cariou R. Prolonged heparin administration during clopidogrel treatment in healthy subjects. *Semin Thromb Hemost* (1999) 25 (Suppl 2), 61–4.
6. ReoPro (Abciximab). Eli Lilly and Company Ltd. UK Summary of product characteristics, September 2004.
7. ReoPro (Abciximab). Centocor. US Prescribing information, November 2003.
8. Lenderink T, Boersma E, Ruzyllo W, Widimsky P, Ohman EM, Armstrong PW, Wallentin L, Simoons ML; GUSTO IV-ACS Investigators. Bleeding events with abciximab in acute coronary syndromes without early revascularization: an analysis of GUSTO IV-ACS. *Am Heart J* (2004) 147, 865–73.
9. Sundlof DW, Rerkpattanapitat P, Wongpraparut N, Pathi P, Kotler MN, Jacobs LE, Ledley GS, Yazdanfar S. Incidence of bleeding complications associated with *abciximab* use in conjunction with thrombolytic therapy in patients requiring percutaneous transluminal coronary angioplasty. *Am J Cardiol* (1999) 83, 1569 – 71.
10. Califf RM. Glycoprotein IIb/IIIa blockade and thrombolytics: early lessons from the SPEED and GUSTO IV trials. *Am Heart J* (1999) 138, S12–S15.
11. Gibson CM. Primary angioplasty compared with thrombolysis: new issues in the era of glycoprotein IIb/IIIa inhibition and intracoronary stenting. *Ann Intern Med* (1999) 130, 841–7.
12. Integrilin (Eptifibatide). GlaxoSmithKline. UK Summary of product characteristics, January 2005.
13. Integrilin (Eptifibatide). Millenium Pharmaceuticals Inc. US Prescribing information, June 2005.
14. Ticlid (Ticlopidine). Sanofi Synthelabo. UK Summary of product characteristics, May 2000.

Antiplatelet drugs + Aspirin or other NSAIDs

There is an increased risk of bleeding if clopidogrel is given with aspirin, but the use of low-dose aspirin and clopidogrel can be beneficial in some patients. The makers of clopidogrel warn about possible gastrointestinal bleeding if it is used with naproxen or other NSAIDs. Ticlopidine increases the antiaggregant effects of aspirin and there is an increased risk of bleeding if ticlopidine is given with aspirin or NSAIDs. Cilostazol appears not to interact to a clinically relevant extent with low-dose aspirin. Similarly, the addition of dipyridamole to aspirin does not appear to increase the incidence of bleeding.

See also 'Antiplatelet drugs + Antiplatelet drugs, Anticoagulants or Thrombolytics', p.518.

Clinical evidence, mechanism, importance and management

(a) Cilostazol + Aspirin

In a randomised, double-blind, placebo-controlled study involving 11 healthy subjects, cilostazol 100 mg twice daily given with aspirin 325 mg daily for 5 days increased the inhibition of ADP-induced platelet aggregation by 23 to 35% when compared with the use of cilostazol alone, but there were no statistically significant additive effects on arachidonic acid-induced platelet aggregation. In addition, no clinically relevant effects on prothrombin times, aPTT or bleeding times occurred when cilostazol was given with or without aspirin. There was a minor 22% increase in cilostazol AUC when given with aspirin.[1] The US makers report that in 8 randomised, placebo-controlled trials, in a total of 201 patients receiving cilostazol and aspirin, the incidence of bleeding was no greater than that seen with aspirin and placebo. The most frequent doses and mean duration of aspirin therapy were 75 to 81 mg daily for 137 days (107 patients) and 325 mg daily for 54 days (85 patients).[2] These studies suggest that no special precautions are needed if cilostazol is used concurrently with low-dose aspirin. The UK maker of cilostazol recommends that, when given with cilostazol, the daily dose of aspirin should not exceed 80 mg.[3]

(b) Clopidogrel + Aspirin

In a multicentre study involving 12 562 patients who had presented within 24 hours of onset of acute coronary syndromes, all patients received aspirin 75 to 325 mg daily for 3 to 12 months. Oral clopidogrel, 300 mg immediately, followed by 75 mg daily was also given to 6259 of the patients. There were significantly more patients with major bleeding in the clopidogrel and aspirin group compared with aspirin alone (3.7% versus 2.7%, respectively), and episodes of life-threatening bleeding occurred slightly more often (2.2% versus 1.8%, respectively; not statistically significant), but there was no excess of haemorrhagic strokes (0.1% versus 0.1%). However, clopidogrel with aspirin reduced the relative risk of cardiovascular death, myocardial infarction or stroke by about 20% compared with aspirin alone.[4]

The results of the MATCH (Management of Atherothrombosis with Clopidogrel in High-risk patients) trial in patients with recent (within the previous 3 months) transient ischaemic attack or ischaemic stroke, found no significant advantage in adding aspirin to clopidogrel for preventing a second ischaemic vascular event. However, the combination significantly increased the risk of serious and life-threatening haemorrhage. This randomised, double-blind study involved 7599 high-risk patients receiving clopidogrel 75 mg daily, who were additionally given aspirin 75 mg daily or placebo for 18 months; life-threatening bleedings were higher in the group receiving aspirin and clopidogrel versus clopidogrel alone (96 [2.6%] versus 49 [1.3%]).[5]

A study in 7 healthy subjects found that clopidogrel 75 mg and aspirin 150 mg daily for 2 days caused a significant 3.4-fold increase in bleeding time relative to baseline, and when the clopidogrel dose was increased to 300 mg there was a 5-fold increase in bleeding time.[6] Spontaneous haemarthrosis of the knee has been associated with aspirin and clopidogrel treatment in one patient.[7] A report of 2 cases of surgery complicated by bleeding associated with the combination of aspirin and clopidogrel. In both cases the bleeding was delayed in that it was not obvious until the end of surgery, causing unanticipated surgical re-exploration.[8] Further reports of increased perioperative bleeding in patients taking both aspirin and clopidogrel.[9,10]

The maker of clopidogrel warns that the concurrent use of clopidogrel and aspirin should be undertaken with caution because of the increased risk of bleeding, although the two drugs have been given together for up to one year. They recommend that, in patients on clopidogrel, the dose of aspirin should not be greater than 100 mg daily as higher doses are associated with higher bleeding risks.[11] It appears that the early use of the combination may be of benefit in certain patients with acute coronary syndromes, but because of the increased risk of bleeding, other patients such as stroke patients may be better treated with a single drug.[5,12] For surgery patients, it has been suggested that, if possible, combined clopidogrel and aspirin therapy should be discontinued about 5 days before surgery to minimise the risks of bleeding;[4,9,13] the maker says that if an antiplatelet effect is not necessary, clopidogrel should be discontinued 5 to 7 days prior to surgery.[11,14] However, this has to be balanced against the benefit of combined antiplatelet therapy in the prevention of thrombotic events in high-risk patients.[8,9,13]

(c) Clopidogrel + NSAIDs

A double-blind, placebo-controlled study in 30 healthy subjects given **naproxen** 250 mg twice daily, found that the addition of clopidogrel 75 mg daily increased faecal blood loss compared with **naproxen** alone. Six subjects receiving both drugs had bleeding time prolongation factors above 5, which was greater than expected (clopidogrel alone prolongs bleeding by a factor of about 2) and one subject had subcutaneous haemorrhages of moderate intensity after clopidogrel and **naproxen** treatment.[15] A report describes intracerebral haemorrhage in an 86-year-old woman following 3 weeks use of **celecoxib** 200 mg daily and clopidogrel 75 mg daily. The authors comment that there may possibly have been a pharmacokinetic interaction between clopidogrel and **celecoxib** mediated via the cytochrome P450 isoenzyme CYP2C9, although the haemorrhage could have been secondary to other factors such as age or the individual drugs.[16]

Due to the lack of interaction studies with other NSAIDs, it is unclear whether there is an increased risk of gastrointestinal bleeding with all NSAIDs. The maker advises NSAIDs and clopidogrel should be given together with caution.[11,14]

(d) Dipyridamole + Aspirin

A study in 10 healthy subjects found that the combinations of dipyridamole 50 mg three times daily and a single 180-mg dose of aspirin, or dipyridamole 75 mg three times daily with aspirin 120 mg maximally inhibited platelet functions but did not prolong the bleeding time.[17] The maker of dipyridamole states that the addition of dipyridamole to aspirin does not increase the incidence of bleeding events.[18]

(e) Ticlopidine + Aspirin or NSAIDs

Aspirin combined with ticlopidine appears to inhibit platelet aggregation more than either drug alone.[19,20] The UK maker of ticlopidine[21] warns that combined use increases the risk of bleeding because there is an increase in platelet antiaggregant activity and aspirin also damages the gastro-duodenal lining, which can cause bleeding. The same risk exists with NSAIDs, which can do similar damage. The UK maker recommends that if NSAIDs are necessary, close clinical monitoring is advisable.[21]

1. Mallikaarjun S, Forbes WP, Bramer SL. Interaction potential and tolerability of the coadministration of cilostazol and aspirin. *Clin Pharmacokinet* (1999) 37 (Suppl 2), 87–93.
2. Pletal (Cilostazol). Otsuka America Pharmaceutical Inc. US Prescribing information, May 2004.
3. Pletal (Cilostazol). Otsuka Pharmaceuticals (UK) Ltd. UK Summary of product characteristics, October 2002.
4. Yusuf S, Zhao F, Mehta SR, Chrolavicius S, Tognoni G, Fox KK; The Clopidogrel in Unstable Angina to Prevent Recurrent Events (CURE) Trial Investigators. Effects of clopidogrel in addition to aspirin in patients with acute coronary syndromes without ST-segment elevation. *N Engl J Med* (2001) 345, 494–502.
5. Diener H-C, Bogousslavsky J, Brass LM, Cimminiello C, Csiba L, Kaste M, Leys D, Matias-Guiu J, Rupprecht H-J, on behalf of the MATCH investigators. Aspirin and clopidogrel compared with clopidogrel alone after recent ischaemic stroke or transient ischaemic attack in high-risk patients (MATCH): randomised, double-blind, placebo-controlled trial. *Lancet* (2004) 364, 331–7.
6. Payne DA, Hayes PD, Jones CI, Belham P, Naylor AR, Goodall AH. Combined therapy with clopidogrel and aspirin significantly increases the bleeding time through a synergistic antiplatelet action. *J Vasc Surg* (2002) 35, 1204–9.
7. Gille J, Bernotat J, Böhm S, Behrens P, Löhr JF. Spontaneous hemarthrosis of the knee associated with clopidogrel and aspirin treatment. *Z Rheumatol* (2003) 62, 80–1.
8. Moore M, Power M. Perioperative hemorrhage and combined clopidogrel and aspirin therapy. *Anesthesiology* (2004) 101, 792–4.
9. Yende S, Wunderink RG. Effect of clopidogrel on bleeding after coronary artery bypass surgery. *Crit Care Med* (2001) 29, 2271–5.
10. Chapman TWL, Bowley DMG, Lambert AW, Walker AJ, Ashley SA, Wilkins DC. Haemorrhage associated with combined clopidogrel and aspirin therapy. *Eur J Vasc Endovasc Surg* (2001) 22, 478–9.
11. Plavix (Clopidogrel bisulfate). Sanofi-Aventis. UK Summary of product characteristics, January 2005.
12. Bath P. Role of aspirin in MATCH. *Lancet* (2004) 364, 1662.
13. Yusuf S, Mehta S. Treatment of acute coronary syndromes. Reply. *N Engl J Med* (2002) 346, 207–8.
14. Plavix (Clopidogrel bisulfate). Sanofi-Synthelabo. US Prescribing information, November 2004.
15. Van Hecken A, Depré M, Wynants K, Vanbilloen H, Verbruggen A, Arnout J, Vanhove P, Cariou R, De Schepper PJ. Effect of clopidogrel on naproxen-induced gastrointestinal blood loss in healthy volunteers. *Drug Metabol Drug Interact* (1998) 14, 193–205 .
16. Fisher AA, Le Couteur DG. Intracerebral hemorrhage following possible interaction between celecoxib and clopidogrel. *Ann Pharmacother* (2001) 35, 1567–9.
17. Rajah SM, Penny AF, Crow MJ, Pepper MD, Watson DA. The interaction of varying doses of dipyridamole and acetyl salicylic acid on the inhibition of platelet functions and their effect on bleeding time. *Br J Clin Pharmacol* (1979) 8, 483–9.
18. Persantin (Dipyridamole). Boehringer Ingelheim Ltd. UK Summary of product characteristics, July 2004.
19. Splawinska B, Kuzniar J, Malinga K, Mazurek AP, Splawinski J. The efficacy and potency of antiplatelet activity of ticlopidine is increased by aspirin. *Int J Clin Pharmacol Ther* (1996) 34, 352–6.
20. Gryglewski RJ, Uracz W, Swiês J. Unusual effects of aspirin on ticlopidine induced thrombolysis. *Thorax* (2000) 55 (Suppl 2) S17–S19.
21. Ticlid (Ticlopidine). Sanofi Synthelabo. UK Summary of product characteristics, May 2000.

Antiplatelet drugs + Herbal medicines

Ginkgo biloba **has been associated with platelet, bleeding and clotting disorders and there are isolated reports of serious adverse reactions after concurrent use with antiplatelet drugs such as clopidogrel and ticlopidine. An *animal* study suggests that *Kangen-Karyu* may also enhance the antiplatelet and antithrombotic effects of ticlopidine.**

Clinical evidence, mechanism, importance and management

(a) Ginkgo biloba

A search of Health Canada's database of spontaneous adverse reactions for the period January 1999 to June 2003, found 21 reports of suspected adverse reactions associated with ginkgo and most of these involved platelet, bleeding and clotting disorders. One report of a fatal gastrointestinal haemorrhage was associated with **ticlopidine** and ginkgo**,** both taken over 2 years along with other medications. Another report was of a stroke in a patient taking multiple drugs including **clopidogrel**, aspirin and a herbal product containing ginkgo. Caution should be exercised if ginkgo is used with drugs that affect platelet aggregation.[1] See also 'NSAIDs or Aspirin + Ginkgo biloba', p.87.

(b) Kangen-Karyu

Kangen-Karyu is a Chinese traditional herbal medicine used for 'blood stasis.' A study in *animals* suggested that *Kangen-Karyu* may augment the antiplatelet and antithrombotic effects of **ticlopidine** and that the dosage of ticlopidine should be reduced to prevent adverse effects such as thrombotic thrombocytopenic purpura or haemorrhage.[2]

1. Natural health products and adverse reactions. *Can Adverse React News* (2004) 14, 2–3.
2. Makino T, Wakushima H, Okamoto T, Okukubo Y, Deguchi Y, Kano Y. Pharmacokinetic and pharmacological interactions between ticlopidine hydrochloride and *Kangen-Karyu* – Chinese traditional herbal medicine. *Phytother Res* (2003) 17, 1021–4.

Cilostazol + Food

Food increases the bioavailability of cilostazol, which may increase adverse effects.

Clinical evidence, mechanism, importance and management

A randomised, single-dose, crossover study in 15 healthy subjects found that giving cilostazol 100 mg within 10 minutes of a high fat meal caused an increase in the rate and extent of cilostazol absorption. The maximum plasma concentration of cilostazol was increased by about 95% and the AUC increased by 25%, and the half-life decreased from 15.1 to 5.4 hours when compared with the fasted state.[1] The maker recommends that cilostazol should be taken 30 minutes before or 2 hours after food, because the increase in maximum plasma concentrations of cilostazol taken with food, may be associated with an increased incidence of adverse effects.[2,3]

1. Bramer SL, Forbes WP. Relative bioavailability and effects of a high fat meal on single dose cilostazol pharmacokinetics. *Clin Pharmacokinet* (1999) 37 (Suppl 2), 13–23.
2. Pletal (Cilostazol). Otsuka Pharmaceuticals (UK) Ltd. UK Summary of product characteristics, October 2002.
3. Pletal (Cilostazol). Otsuka America Pharmaceutical Inc. US Prescribing information, May 2004.

Cilostazol + Miscellaneous

Erythromycin, diltiazem and ketoconazole, all inhibitors of the cytochrome P450 isoenzyme CYP3A4, increase the plasma levels of cilostazol. Other inhibitors of CYP3A4 (other azole antifungals, cimetidine, protease inhibitors, other macrolide antibacterials, nefazodone, SSRIs) are predicted to interact similarly, but grapefruit juice does not appear to interact significantly. Omeprazole, an inhibitor of CYP2C19, increases the bioavailability of cilostazol and its active metabolite; lansoprazole may act similarly. However, quinidine, an inhibitor of CYP2D6, does not appear to affect the pharmacokinetics of cilostazol. Cilostazol itself may increase the levels of lovastatin and other substrates of CYP3A4 (and possibly CYP2C19). Cilostazol appears not to interact to a clinically relevant extent with tobacco smoke.

Clinical evidence, mechanism, importance and management

(a) Cytochrome P450 isoenzyme CYP2C19 inhibitors

In a crossover study,[1] in 20 healthy subjects, it was found that **omeprazole** 40 mg daily for one week increased the AUC of a single 100-mg dose of cilostazol by a modest 26%. More importantly though, the AUC of 3,4-dehydro-cilostazol (a metabolite with 4 to 7 times the activity of the parent compound) was increased by 69%.[2,3] **Omeprazole** inhibits the cytochrome P450 isoenzyme CYP2C19, which is involved in the metabolism of cilostazol and may possibly also affect the elimination of the active metabolite. For this reason the US makers suggest that the dose of cilostazol should be halved when given with **omeprazole**,[2] while the UK makers suggest that concurrent use should be avoided.[3] Other CYP2C19 inhibitors such as **lansoprazole** may also interact.[3]

(b) Cytochrome P450 isoenzyme CYP3A4 inhibitors

A study in 16 healthy subjects found that **erythromycin** 500 mg three times daily increased the maximum plasma level and the AUC of a single 100-mg oral dose of cilostazol by 47% and 73% respectively. **Erythromycin** inhibits the cytochrome P450 isoenzyme CYP3A4 resulting in reduced metabolism of cilostazol.[4] Some other macrolide antibiotics e.g. **clarithromycin** (but not **azithromycin**) would be expected to have a similar effect.[2]

Diltiazem is also a moderate inhibitor of CYP3A4. The concurrent use of **diltiazem** 180 mg daily and cilostazol caused a 40% rise in the AUC of cilostazol 100 mg twice daily.[2,3]

In a single-dose study, a greater than twofold increase in the AUC of cilostazol was noted when it was given with **ketoconazole** 400 mg.[3] Other potent CYP3A4 inhibitors such as **itraconazole** are expected to interact similarly.[2]

In view of these effects the US makers suggest halving the dose of cilostazol in the presence of CYP3A4 inhibitors such as **erythromycin**, **diltiazem**, **itraconazole** or **ketoconazole**.[2] However, the UK makers state that CYP3A4 inhibitors are contraindicated, and they specifically name **erythromycin**, **diltiazem** or **ketoconazole**, as well as **cimetidine** and **protease inhibitors**.[3] Just why recommendations differ is not clear. Other CYP3A4 inhibitors such as the **azole antifungals** (**fluconazole**, **miconazole**) and **SSRIs** (**fluoxetine**, **fluvoxamine**, **sertraline**) and **nefazodone** may also interact.[2]

(c) Grapefruit juice

Grapefruit juice has been predicted to increase the activity of cilostazol by inhibiting CYP3A4 and the maximum plasma concentration of cilostazol may be increased.[2] However, the UK makers note that a single 100-mg dose of cilostazol given with 240 ml of grapefruit juice did not have a notable effect on the pharmacokinetics of cilostazol.[3] No special precautions appear necessary.

(d) Lovastatin and other substrates of CYP3A4 or CYP2C19

In a study involving 13 healthy subjects, a single 80-mg oral dose of lovastatin was given alone and then during the use of cilostazol 100 mg twice daily for 7 days. The maximum plasma levels of lovastatin and its beta-hydroxy acid metabolite were not significantly altered by cilostazol, but the AUCs of lovastatin and its metabolite were increased by about 60 and 70%, respectively.[5] Moreover, when 12 subjects were given another dose of lovastatin 80 mg with cilostazol 150 mg at the end of this study, both the maximum level and the AUC of beta-hydroxy lovastatin acid were increased by about twofold.[5] Lovastatin is metabolised by the cytochrome P450 isoenzyme CYP3A4 and although cilostazol can inhibit this enzyme, *in vitro* studies indicate that this occurs only at concentrations several times greater than those found therapeutically. The increases in lovastatin levels described here are lower than those seen with potent CYP3A4 inhibitors (e.g. see 'Statins + Azoles', p.831) but the authors of the study still suggest that the dose of lovastatin may need to be reduced when cilostazol is used concurrently. Absorption of cilostazol decreased by about 15% when it was given with lovastatin, but this was not considered to be clinically relevant.[5]

The UK makers advise caution when cilostazol is given with drugs that are substrates of CYP3A4 (and CYP2C19), especially those with a narrow therapeutic index. They specifically mention **cisapride**, **midazolam**, **nifedipine** and **verapamil**.[3] Further study is needed.

(e) Quinidine and other inhibitors of CYP2D6

A crossover study in 22 healthy subjects found that the pharmacokinetics of a single 100-mg dose of cilostazol were unaffected by pretreatment with two 200-mg doses of quinidine sulfate, one taken 25 hours previously and the other taken one hour previously. Quinidine inhibits the activity of the cytochrome P450 isoenzyme CYP2D6, and it appears that this enzyme does not play a significant role in the metabolism of cilostazol or its primary metabolites. Drugs metabolised by the CYP2D6 pathway are not expected to affect the plasma concentrations of cilostazol.[6]

(f) Tobacco smoking

The makers report that population pharmacokinetic analysis suggests that tobacco smoking reduces the exposure to cilostazol by about 20%,[2] but this is unlikely to have much if any clinical relevance.

1. Suri A, Bramer SL. Effect of omeprazole on the metabolism of cilostazol. *Clin Pharmacokinet* (1999) 37, (Suppl 2), 53–9.
2. Pletal (Cilostazol). Otsuka America Pharmaceutical Inc. US Prescribing information, May 2004.
3. Pletal (Cilostazol). Otsuka Pharmaceuticals (UK) Ltd. UK Summary of product characteristics, October 2002.
4. Suri A, Forbes WP, Bramer SL. Effects of CYP3A inhibition on the metabolism of cilostazol. *Clin Pharmacokinet* (1999) 37 (Suppl 2), 61–8.
5. Bramer SL, Brisson J, Corey AE, Mallikaarjun S. Effect of multiple cilostazol doses on single dose lovastatin pharmacokinetics in healthy volunteers. *Clin Pharmacokinet* (1999) 37 (Suppl 2), 69–77.
6. Bramer SL, Suri A. Inhibition of CYP2D6 by quinidine and its effects on the metabolism of cilostazol. *Clin Pharmacokinet* (1999) 37 (Suppl 2), 41–51.

Clopidogrel + Miscellaneous

No adverse interactions appear to occur with clopidogrel and aluminium/magnesium hydroxide antacids, atenolol, cimetidine, digoxin, estrogens, food, insulin, nifedipine, phenobarbital, phenytoin or tolbutamide.

Clinical evidence, mechanism, importance and management

(a) Antacids or food

Two studies, one in 12 healthy subjects (average age 67 years) and the other in 12 healthy subjects (average age 23 years), found that the bioavailability of a single 75-mg dose of clopidogrel remained unchanged when it was taken with food or two 400-mg tablets of *Maalox* (**aluminium/magnesium hydroxide**) taken 1 hour previously.[1] No special precautions would seem to be needed.

(b) Non-interacting drugs

No clinically significant pharmacodynamic interactions were seen when clopidogrel was given with **atenolol**, **nifedipine** or a combination of **atenolol** and **nifedipine**,[2] and the activity of clopidogrel was not altered by the concurrent use of **cimetidine**,[3] **estrogen**[3] or **phenobarbital**.[3] Another study found that clopidogrel does not alter the plasma levels of **digoxin** and that the pharmacodynamics of clopidogrel do not appear to be affected by digoxin.[4] Data from the CAPRIE study and other clinical trials showed that **ACE inhibitors, antidiabetics** (**insulin, tolbutamide** named),[3] **antiepileptic** therapy (**phenytoin** named),[3] **beta-blockers**, **calcium channel blockers**, **coronary/peripheral vasodilators**, **diuretics** and **hormone replacement therapy** have been safely given with clopidogrel.[5]

1. McEwen J, Strauch G, Perles P, Pritchard G, Moreland TE, Necciari J, Dickinson JP. Clopidogrel bioavailability: absence of influence of food or antacids. *Semin Thromb Hemost* (1999) 25 (Suppl 2), 47–50.
2. Forbes CD, Lowe GDO, Maclaren M, Shaw BG, Dickinson JP, Kieffer G. Clopidogrel compatibility with concomitant cardiac co-medications: a study of its interactions with a beta-blocker and a calcium uptake antagonist. *Semin Thromb Hemost* (1999) 25 (Suppl 2), 55–9.
3. Plavix (Clopidogrel bisulfate). Sanofi-Aventis. UK Summary of product characteristics, January 2005.
4. Peeters PAM, Crijns HJMJ, Tamminga WJ, Jonkman JHG, Dickinson JP, Necciari J. Clopidogrel, a novel antiplatelet agent, and digoxin: absence of pharmacodynamic and pharmacokinetic interaction. *Semin Thromb Hemost* (1999) 25 (Suppl 2), 51–4.
5. Morais J, on behalf of the CAPRIE investigators. Use of concomitant medications in the CAPRIE trial: clopidogrel is unlikely to be associated with clinically significant drug interactions. *Eur Heart J* (1998) 19 (Abstract Suppl) 5.

Clopidogrel + Statins

Statins metabolised by the cytochrome P450 isoenzyme CYP3A4 appear to interfere with the antiplatelet action of clopidogrel, but the clinical significance of this is uncertain; lower doses of these statins seem less likely to interact. Clopidogrel may possibly affect the metabolism of some statins.

Clinical evidence, mechanism, importance and management

(a) Clopidogrel metabolism affected

In a study of 44 patients undergoing elective coronary artery stent implantation, an oral loading dose of clopidogrel 300 mg was given followed by 75 mg daily for 28 days; 9 patients also received **pravastatin** 40 mg daily, 19 received **atorvastatin** 10 to 40 mg daily and 16 patients did not receive any statin therapy. **Atorvastatin**, but not **pravastatin**, attenuated the antiplatelet activity of clopidogrel in a dose-dependent manner (platelet aggregation was 34, 58, 74 and 89% in the presence of 0, 10, 20, and 40 mg of **atorvastatin**, respectively);[1] the patients were also receiving aspirin.[2] Similar results were reported in another study, which found **atorvastatin**, but not **pravastatin** or **fluvastatin**, reduced the antiplatelet effects of clopidogrel.[3]

The study[1] above has been criticised[4] and several other studies have not found any clinical evidence of an interaction between clopidogrel and **atorvastatin**.[4-9] A study specifically set up to investigate this interaction also found that statins in general do not affect the ability of clopidogrel to inhibit platelet function.[8] A further study reported that **atorvastatin** 10 mg daily or **pravastatin** 40 mg daily did not affect the antiplatelet potency of clopidogrel on concurrent use for 5 weeks. In addition, clopidogrel did not influence the hypolipidaemic effect of **atorvastatin**.[9]

A retrospective analysis of a double-blind, placebo controlled study involving 2116 patients with symptomatic coronary artery disease found no statistical difference in clinical events (death/myocardial infarction/stroke), after 28 days or 1 year, when clopidogrel was given with a statin. Furthermore, when the patients were subdivided into those receiving statins predominantly metabolised via the cytochrome P450 isoenzyme CYP3A4 (**atorvastatin**, **lovastatin** or **simvastatin**) or statins not predominantly metabolised by CYP3A4 (**pravastatin** or **fluvastatin**), neither group adversely affected the efficacy of clopidogrel,in preventing short- or long-term ischaemic events, relative to placebo.[6] However, further analysis of this study[6] showed that the patients prescribed clopidogrel plus a statin not metabolised by CYP3A4 appeared to have a better outcome than those on a CYP3A4-metabolised statin (including **atorvastatin**) with respect to a major event at both 28 days[10] and 1 year after percutaneous coronary intervention.[11] Another study found that after placement of coronary artery stents, clopidogrel was associated with significantly higher cardiovascular mortality (7.3%) compared with ticlopidine (2.3%), which is not metabolised by CYP3A4, when the majority of the patients also received a statin which may have exaggerated the difference in antiplatelet activity between clopidogrel and ticlopidine.[12] Furthermore, another study designed specifically to investigate the interaction between statins and clopidogrel, found that pre-treatment with lipophilic statins that are substrates of the CYP3A4 isoenzyme (**atorvastatin** 20 to 40 mg daily or **simvastatin** 10 to 20 mg daily) competitively inhibited the metabolic activation of clopidogrel (loading dose 300 mg orally; maintenance dose 75 mg daily). These statins significantly reduced the platelet inhibitory effects of clopidogrel 5 hours after the loading dose (relative reduction approximately 29%) and, to a lesser extent, after 48 hours during the maintenance phase (relative reduction about 16%). In addition, in 3 out of the 47 patients involved in the study (one receiving no statins, one receiving **simvastatin** 10 mg and one receiving **atorvastatin** 20 mg) clopidogrel exerted no inhibitory effect at all after 5 and 48 hours.[13]

(b) Statin metabolism affected

A report describes 2 cases of rhabdomyolysis when clopidogrel was added to treatment with ciclosporin and **lovastatin** or **simvastatin**. It was thought that the addition of clopidogrel might have destabilised the delicate metabolic equilibrium between the statins and ciclosporin precipitating the development of rhabdomyolysis.[14] Consider also 'Statins + Ciclosporin', p.834

Mechanism

Clopidogrel is an inactive prodrug that is metabolised mainly in the liver. The cytochrome P450 isoenzyme CYP3A4 appears to be primarily responsible for the metabolism and activation of clopidogrel, although other isoenzymes are also involved. Several statins, including atorvastatin, are also metabolised by CYP3A4 and it has been suggested that these statins may competitively inhibit the activation of clopidogrel.[1,15] In addition, the expression and/or activity of CYP3A4 vary widely between individuals and this may conceivably lead to individual variation in metabolism.[10] Pravastatin, a hydrophilic drug, is not significantly metabolised by the cytochrome P450 enzyme system.[1]

Clopidogrel may also inhibit the cytochrome P450 enzyme system and so interfere with the metabolism of a variety of drugs including statins and ciclosporin.[14]

Importance and management

Some studies have shown that statins metabolised by CYP3A4 cause a reduction in the antiplatelet activity of clopidogrel, especially during the initial stages of treatment (following the loading dose of clopidogrel), whereas other, mainly retrospective, studies have found no clinical evidence of reduced efficacy. However, the studies are difficult to compare as some have measured platelet function using different techniques and other studies are based on clinical outcome using varying lengths of treatment and end points. Furthermore, some patients do not respond at all to clopidogrel and this seems unrelated to treatment with any statins.[4]

Dose may be an important factor as to whether or not a significant clinical interaction occurs. A high loading dose of clopidogrel (600 mg) appears to be less likely to be affected by statins,[16] but there is increased risk of serious bleeding. Lower doses of statins (e.g. atorvastatin 10 mg daily)[9] also appear to be less likely to interact. It has been suggested that higher doses of atorvastatin, and perhaps simvastatin, should not be prescribed for patients taking clopidogrel, particularly patients recovering from an acute coronary syndrome, stent (particularly a drug-eluting stent) implantation, or brachytherapy; pravastatin or **rosuvastatin** may be preferred in these patients.[11] However, other workers have said, given the marginal interference and high variability, and until there is evidence to change clinical practice, there is no need to discontinue the statin use during clopidogrel treatment or to prefer hydrophilic statins in patients with clopidogrel comedication.[4,17,18]

Even though the statins metabolised by CYP3A4 appear to reduce the antiplatelet effect of clopidogrel, the overall clinical effect is unclear. The beneficial properties of statins may offset any attenuating effects on the antiplatelet action of clopidogrel.[19] Further prospective studies are needed to determine whether a clinically significant interaction exists.

1. Lau WC, Waskell LA, Watkins PB, Neer CJ, Horowitz K, Hopp AS, Tait AR, Carville DGM, Guyer KE, Bates ER. Atorvastatin reduces the ability of clopidogrel to inhibit platelet aggregation. A new drug–drug interaction. *Circulation* (2003) 107, 32–7.
2. Lau WC, Waskell LA, Neer CJ, Horowitz K, Hopp AS, Tait AR, Bates ER, Watkins PB, Carville DGM, Guyer KE. Atorvastatin–clopidogrel interaction. Response. *Circulation* (2003) 107, e223.
3. Günesdogan B, Neubauer H, Mügge A. Is the clopidogrel effect by patients treated with statins diminished? A flow cytometric evaluation of a possible interaction. *Eur Heart J* (2002) 23 (Abstract Suppl) 725.
4. Serebruany VL, Steinhubl SR, Hennekens CH. Are antiplatelet effects of clopidogrel inhibited by atorvastatin? A research question formulated but not yet adequately tested. *Circulation* (2003) 107, 1568–9.
5. Serebruany VL, Malinin AI, Callahan KP, Gurbel PA, Steinhubl SR. Statins do not affect platelet inhibition with clopidogrel during coronary stenting. *Atherosclerosis* (2001) 159, 239–41.
6. Saw J, Steinhubl SR, Berger PB, Kereiakes DJ, Serebruany VL, Brennan D, Topol EJ; for the Clopidogrel for the Reduction of Events During Observation (CREDO) Investigators. Lack of adverse clopidogrel–atorvastatin clinical interaction from secondary analysis of a randomized, placebo-controlled clopidogrel trial. *Circulation* (2003) 108, 921–4.
7. Wienbergen H, Gitt AK, Schiele R, Juenger C, Heer T, Meisenzahl C, Limbourg P, Bossaller C, Senges J, for the MITRA PLUS Study Group. Comparison of clinical benefits of clopidogrel therapy in patients with acute coronary syndromes taking atorvastatin versus other statin therapies. *Am J Cardiol* (2003) 92, 285–8.
8. Wan Y. Lack of interaction between statins and clopidogrel? *Arch Intern Med* (2004) 164, 2051–7.
9. Mitsios JV, Papathanasiou AI, Rodis FI, Elisaf M, Goudevenos JA, Tselepis AD. Atorvastatin does not affect the antiplatelet potency of clopidogrel when it is administered concomitantly for 5 weeks in patients with acute coronary syndromes. *Circulation* (2004) 109, 1335–8.
10. Ford I, Williams D. Does the use of statins compromise the effectiveness of platelet inhibition by clopidogrel? *Platelets* (2004) 15, 201–5.
11. Bates ER, Mukherjee D, Lau WC. Drug–drug interactions involving antiplatelet agents. *Eur Heart J* (2003) 24, 1707–9.
12. Mueller C, Roskamm H, Neumann F-J, Hunziker P, Marsch S, Perruchoud A, Buettner HJ. A randomized comparison of clopidogrel and aspirin versus ticlopidine and aspirin after the placement of coronary artery stents. *J Am Coll Cardiol* (2003) 41, 969–73.
13. Neubauer H, Günesdogan B, Hanefeld C, Spiecker M, Mügge A. Lipophilic statins interfere with the inhibitory effects of clopidogrel on platelet function – a flow cytometry study. *Eur Heart J* (2003) 24, 1744–9.
14. Uber PA, Mehra MR, Park MH, Scott RL. Clopidogrel and rhabdomyolysis after heart transplantation. *J Heart Lung Transplant* (2003) 22, 107–8.
15. Clarke TA, Waskell LA. The metabolism of clopidogrel is catalyzed by human cytochrome P450 3A and is inhibited by atorvastatin. *Drug Metab Dispos* (2003) 31, 53–9.
16. Müller I, Besta F, Schulz C, Li Z, Massberg S, Gawaz M. Effects of statins on platelet inhibition by a high loading dose of clopidogrel. *Circulation* (2003) 108, 2195–7.
17. Neubauer H, Mugge A. Do statins really interfere with clopidogrel-induced platelet function?: Reply. *Circulation* (2003) 108, 448–9.
18. Shechter M. Do statins really interfere with clopidogrel-induced platelet function? *Circulation* (2003) 108, 448.
19. Schafer AI. Genetic and acquired determinants of individual variability of response to antiplatelet drugs. *Circulation* (2003) 108, 910–11.

Dipyridamole + Antacids, H_2-blockers or Proton pump inhibitors

The effective disintegration, dissolution and eventual absorption of dipyridamole in tablet form depends upon having a low pH in the stomach. Drugs that raise the gastric pH significantly are expected to reduce the bioavailability of dipyridamole.

Clinical evidence, mechanism, importance and management

The solubility of dipyridamole depends very much on the pH. It is very soluble at low pH values and almost insoluble at neutral pH.[1] This indicates that dipyridamole needs a low pH in the stomach if solid formulations of the drug are to disintegrate and dissolve adequately. A study in 11 healthy elderly subjects (6 control subjects with a low fasting gastric pH and 5 achlorhydric subjects with fasting gastric pH greater than 5) found that elevated gastric pH reduced the absorption of a single 50-mg oral dose of dipyridamole. In addition, pretreatment with **famotidine** 40 mg increased pH to above 5 for at least 3 hours and also reduced the absorption of dipyridamole. The dipyridamole AUC was reduced by 37% (not statistically significant) and the maximum serum levels significantly were delayed and reduced.[2]

A consequential conclusion is that any drug that raises the stomach pH significantly would be likely to reduce the dissolution and absorption of dipyridamole. It would therefore be reasonable to expect that antacids, H_2-blockers (e.g. **cimetidine**) and proton pump inhibitors (e.g. **omeprazole**), which can raise the gastric pH, would interact to reduce the bioavailability of dipyridamole. Further study is needed to find out whether this is a clinically relevant interaction or not.

1. Boehringer Ingelheim. Data on file (Study 1482B).
2. Russell TL, Berardi RR, Barnett JL, O'Sullivan TL, Wagner JG, Dressman JB. pH-related changes in the absorption of dipyridamole in the elderly. *Pharm Res* (1994) 11 136–43.

Dipyridamole + Beta-blockers

No adverse reactions normally occur in patients taking beta-blockers who undergo dipyridamole–thallium-201 scintigraphy and echocardiography, but rarely bradycardia and asystole can occur.

Clinical evidence

A 71-year-old woman on **nadolol** 120 mg daily and bendroflumethiazide, with a 3-week history of chest pain, was given a 300-mg dose of oral dipyridamole as part of a diagnostic dipyridamole-thallium imaging test for coronary artery disease. She was given thallium-201 intravenously, 50 minutes after the dipyridamole, but 3 minutes later while exercising she complained of chest pain and then had a cardiac arrest. She was given cardiopulmonary resuscitation and a normal cardiac rhythm was obtained after she was given intravenous aminophylline.[1]

Adverse interactions occurred in another 2 patients on beta-blockers during diagnostic dipyridamole-thallium stress testing. One patient, on **atenolol** developed bradycardia then asystole, which was treated with aminophylline and atropine, and the other patient, on **metoprolol**, developed bradycardia, which resolved after she was given aminophylline.[2]

These reports need to be set in a broad context. A very extensive study of high-dose dipyridamole echocardiography (10 451 tests in 9 122 patients) noted significant adverse effects in only 96 patients, with major adverse reactions occurring in just 7 patients. Three of the 7 developed asystole and two of these patients were taking unnamed beta-blockers.[3]

Another study, over the period 1978 to 1985, involving 1096 patients, 30% of whom were taking **propranolol** and who had undergone intravenous dipyridamole-thallium scintigraphy, found a considerable number of minor adverse reactions (experienced by 46.5% of the patients) including chest pain, but major adverse events occurred in 10 (0.26%) of the patients. Four of these patients experienced a myocardial infarction (2 fatal) and 6 experienced acute bronchospasm.[4] Another study in 170 patients stated that 135 patients were taking nitrates, beta-blockers and/or calcium channel blockers, but neither serious bradycardia nor asystole were reported, although 27 (16%) patients received intravenous aminophylline to resolve threatening, uncomfortable or disabling adverse effects.[5]

Mechanism

Not established. One possible explanation is that both drugs have negative chronotropic effects on the heart.

Importance and management

The value and safety of dipyridamole perfusion scintigraphy and echocardiography have been very extensively studied in very large numbers of patients, and reports of bradycardia and asystole, attributed to an interaction between dipyridamole and beta-blockers, are sparse. Large numbers of patients given this test have apparently taken beta-blockers without developing problems.[4,5] It would therefore appear to be a relatively rare interaction (if such it is). Consider also 'Beta-blockers + Thallium scans', p.644.

1. Blumenthal MS, McCauley CS. Cardiac arrest during dipyridamole imaging. *Chest* (1988) 93, 1103–4.
2. Roach PJ, Magee MA, Freedman SB. Asystole and bradycardia during dipyridamole stress testing in patients receiving beta blockers. *Int J Cardiol* (1993) 42, 92–4.
3. Picano E *et al.* on behalf of the Echo-Persantine International Cooperative Study Group. Safety of intravenous high-dose dipyridamole echocardiography. *Am J Cardiol* (1992) 70, 252–8.
4. Ranhosky A, Kempthorne-Rawson J, and the Intravenous Dipyridamole Thallium Imaging Study Group. The safety of intravenous dipyridamole thallium myocardial perfusion imaging. *Circulation* (1990) 81, 1205–9.
5. Zhu YY, Chung WS, Botvinick EH, Dae MW, Lim AD, Ports TA, Danforth JW, Wolfe CL, Goldschlager N, Chatterjee K. Dipyridamole perfusion scintigraphy: the experience with its application in one hundred seventy patients with known or suspected unstable angina. *Am Heart J* (1991) 121, 33–43.

Dipyridamole + Irbesartan

A study in 13 patients with coronary artery disease found that irbesartan 150 mg daily reduced the extent and severity of perfusion defects after dipyridamole-induced stress.[1]

1. Altun GD, Altun A, Yildiz M, Firat MF, Hacimahmutoglu S, Berkarda S. Irbesartan has a masking effect on dipyridamole stress induced myocardial perfusion defects. *Nucl Med Commun* (2004) 25, 195–9.

Dipyridamole + Xanthines

Caffeine (in tea, coffee, cola, etc.) may interfere with dipyridamole–thallium-201 scintigraphy tests. Similarly, theophylline can also reduce some of the effects of dipyridamole.

Clinical evidence, mechanism, importance and management

Caffeine 4 mg/kg intravenously (roughly equivalent to 2 to 3 cups of coffee), before dipyridamole–thallium-201 myocardial scintigraphy, caused a false-negative test result in a patient.[1] A further study in 8 healthy subjects confirmed that **caffeine** inhibits the haemodynamic response to an infusion of dipyridamole.[2] Similarly, maintenance oral **theophylline** therapy markedly reduced the diagnostic accuracy of myocardial imaging using dipyridamole.[3] In addition, intravenous **aminophylline** accelerated the myocardial washout rate of thallium-201 after a dipyridamole infusion.[4]

It appears that xanthine derivatives such as **caffeine** and **theophylline** might antagonise some of the effects of dipyridamole because they act as competitive antagonists of adenosine (an endogenous vasodilator involved in the action of dipyridamole).[1,2] Due to these opposing effects, parenteral **aminophylline** has been used to treat adverse events associated with intravenous dipyridamole,[5,6] and it is recommended that **aminophylline** should be made available before beginning dipyridamole echocardiography.[6,7]

Patients should therefore abstain from **caffeine** (tea, coffee, chocolate, cocoa, cola, caffeine-containing analgesics etc.)[1,2,7] and other xanthine derivatives such as **theophylline**[3] for 24 hours[2,6] before dipyridamole testing, and if during the test the haemodynamic response is low (e.g. no increase in heart rate) the presence of **caffeine** should be suspected.[2]

1. Smits P, Aengevaeren WRM, Corstens FHM, Thien T. Caffeine reduces dipyridamole-induced myocardial ischemia. *J Nucl Med* (1989) 30, 1723–6.
2. Smits P, Straatman C, Pijpers E, Thien T. Dose-dependent inhibition of the hemodynamic response to dipyridamole by caffeine. *Clin Pharmacol Ther* (1991) 50, 529–37.
3. Daley PJ, Mahn TH, Zielonka JS, Krubsack AJ, Akhtar R, Bamrah VS. Effect of maintenance oral theophylline on dipyridamole–thallium-201 myocardial imaging using SPECT and dipyridamole-induced hemodynamic changes. *Am Heart J* (1988) 115, 1185–92.
4. Takeishi Y, Tono-oka I, Kubota I, Ikeda K, Masakane I, Chiba J, Abe S, Tsuiki K, Tomoike H. Intravenous aminophylline affects myocardial washout of thallium-201 after dipyridamole infusion. *Am J Noninvasive Cardiol* (1992) 6, 116–21.
5. Ranhosky A, Kempthorne-Rawson J, and the Intravenous Dipyridamole Thallium Imaging Study Group. The safety of intravenous dipyridamole thallium myocardial perfusion imaging. *Circulation* (1990) 81, 1205–9.
6. Persantin Ampoules (Dipyridamole). Boehringer Ingelheim Ltd. UK Summary of product characteristics, July 2004.
7. Picano E *et al.* on behalf of the Echo-Persantine International Cooperative Study Group. Safety of intravenous high-dose dipyridamole echocardiography. *Am J Cardiol* (1992) 70, 252–8.

Ifetroban + Miscellaneous

No adverse interaction appears to occur between ifetroban and either heparin, *Mylanta*, ranitidine or warfarin.

Clinical evidence, mechanism, importance and management

(a) Antacids, H_2-blockers

A study in 18 healthy subjects to investigate the possible effects of changes in gastric pH on the pharmacokinetics of ifetroban, found that when given a single 250-mg dose of ifetroban while taking either 30 ml *Mylanta* (**aluminium/magnesium hydroxide**, **simeticone**) four times daily for 5 days or **ranitidine** 150 mg twice daily, no important clinical differences were seen.[1] There would appear to be no reason for avoiding concurrent use.

(b) Heparin

Heparin was given to 37 healthy subjects to reach a stable aPTT of 1.5 times the baseline before 250 mg ifetroban was added for about 5 days. The heparin was then stopped but the ifetroban continued for a further 5 days. The pharmacokinetics of the ifetroban were not changed by the heparin nor was the ifetroban-induced increase in the bleeding time altered by the heparin. Some adverse side-effects were seen but these were attributed to the use of the heparin.[2] On the basis of this study there would seem to be no reason for avoiding concurrent use.

(c) Warfarin

Eighteen patients with deep vein thrombosis taking warfarin and with INRs within the range 2 to 3, were additionally given ifetroban (dose not stated) or a placebo for 6 days. It was found that INRs were not significantly altered by the ifetroban, and no important changes in bleeding times occurred.[3] No special precautions would seem to be needed during concurrent use.

1. Beierle FA, Delaney C, Uderman H, Bourgeois ML, Jemal M, Liao WC. The effect of altered gastric acidity induced by Mylanta or ranitidine on ifetroban pharmacokinetics in healthy volunteers. *J Clin Pharmacol* (1996) 36, 854.
2. Liao W, Delaney C, Jemal M, Norton J, Uderman H, Ford N. The pharmacokinetic and pharmacodynamic (PK/PD) interaction of ifetroban, a TXA_2 receptor antagonist, and heparin. *Clin Pharmacol Ther* (1996) 59, 150.
3. Delaney C, Norton J, Briand R, Lajoie V, Beierle F, Campbell A, Whitsett T, VanNguyen P, Anderson D, Liao W. The pharmacodynamic (PD) interaction of ifetroban (IFET), a thromboxane A_2 (TXA_2) antagonist, and warfarin (W) in patients with venous thrombosis. *J Clin Pharmacol* (1996) 36, 854.

Streptokinase + Aspirin

Patients with acute ischaemic stroke treated with streptokinase have an increased risk of early death due to cerebral haemorrhage if they are also given aspirin. However, a positive effect on life expectancy has been observed in patients with suspected myocardial infarction.

Clinical evidence, mechanism, importance and management

A post hoc analysis of 313 patients with acute ischaemic stroke given intravenous streptokinase 1.5 million units found that the addition of oral aspirin 300 mg daily for 10 days increased the risk of early death. The combined regimen significantly increased early fatalities (from day 3 to 10) with 53 deaths occurring out of 156 patients (34%) compared with 30 of 157 (19%) who received streptokinase alone. Early death was mainly due to cerebral causes (42 versus 24) and associated with intracranial haemorrhage (25 versus 11).[1]

If streptokinase is given to acute ischaemic stroke patients, it would seem sensible to avoid giving aspirin until thrombolysis is accomplished.[1] However, in patients with suspected myocardial infarction, a positive effect of aspirin and streptokinase has been observed.[2]

1. Ciccone A, Motto C, Aritzu E, Piana A, Candelise L, on behalf of the MAST-I Collaborative Group. Negative interaction of aspirin and streptokinase in acute ischemic stroke: further analysis of the Multicenter Acute Stroke Trial-Italy. *Cerebrovasc Dis* (2000) 10, 61–4.
2. Streptase (Streptokinase). ZLB Behring UK Ltd. UK Summary of product characteristics, November 2004.

Streptokinase or Anistreplase + Streptokinase

The thrombolytic effects of streptokinase or anistreplase are likely to be reduced or abolished if they are given some time after a dose of streptokinase because of persistently high levels of streptokinase antibodies. There is also an increased risk of hypersensitivity reactions.

Clinical evidence

A study in 25 patients who had been given streptokinase for the treatment of acute myocardial infarction, found that 12 weeks later 24 patients had enough anti-streptokinase antibodies in circulation to neutralise an entire 1.5 million unit dose. After 4 to 8 months, 18 out of 20 still had enough antibodies to neutralise half of a 1.5 million unit dose.[1] Further study has suggested that after streptokinase use, anti-streptokinase antibodies fall within 24 hours, but then increase gradually and are significantly raised by 4 days after treatment. The antibody titres reach a peak (approximately 200 times that of pretreatment levels) after 2 weeks and then subsequently decline, but remain above baseline values for at least one year.[2] Antibody titres may remain high enough to neutralise the effects of streptokinase for several years after a dose;[3,4] high titres persisting for up to 7.5 years have been reported.[5] However, in contrast, another study found that the neutralising antibody titres had returned to control levels by 2 years.[6] Increased titres of streptokinase antibodies have also been seen in patients receiving topical streptokinase for wound care[7] and following streptococcal infections.[8] Apart from the reduced thrombolytic effect, repeated dosing[9] or high pre-treatment anti-streptokinase antibody titres[10] may increase the risk of allergic reactions.

Anistreplase, like its parent drug streptokinase, has been shown to be neutralised by anti-streptokinase antibodies.[11,12]

Mechanism

Streptokinase use causes the production of anti-streptokinase antibodies. These persist in the circulation so that the clot-dissolving effects of another dose of streptokinase given many months later may be ineffective, or less effective, because it becomes bound and neutralised by the antibodies. Many people already have a very low titre of antibodies resulting from previous streptococcal infections, yet this does not appear to influence thrombolysis.[13] Also, the incidence of allergic and anaphylactic reactions to streptokinase seems to be low after the first time it is given (about 3%).[14] However, hypersensitivity reactions are more likely in patients with high anti-streptokinase antibody levels.[10]

Importance and management

An established and clinically important interaction. One author says[15] that clinically, therapy is not repeated within a year as it would not work. Given that it has been suggested that the effects may be very persistent, it would seem prudent, if a second use is needed, to use a thrombolytic with less antigenic effects such as alteplase. The British National Formulary says that streptokinase should not be used again beyond 4 days of the first use of either streptokinase or anistreplase.[16] In addition, the maker recommends avoidance of streptokinase in patients who have had recent streptococcal infections which have produced high anti-streptokinase titres, such as acute rheumatic fever or acute glomerulonephritis.[8]

1. Jalihal S, Morris GK. Antistreptokinase titres after intravenous streptokinase. *Lancet* (1990) 335, 184–5.
2. Lynch M, Littler WA, Pentecost BL, Stockley RA. Immunoglobulin response to intravenous streptokinase in acute myocardial infarction. *Br Heart J* (1991) 66, 139–42.
3. Elliott JM, Cross DB, Cederholm-Williams SA, White HD. Neutralizing antibodies to streptokinase four years after intravenous thrombolytic therapy. *Am J Cardiol* (1993) 71, 640–5.
4. Lee HS, Cross S, Davidson R, Reid T, Jennings K. Raised levels of antistreptokinase antibody and neutralization titres from 4 days to 54 months after administration of streptokinase or anistreplase. *Eur Heart J* (1993) 14, 84–9.
5. Squire IB, Lawley W, Fletcher S, Holme E, Hillis WS, Hewitt C, Woods KL. Humoral and cellular immune responses up to 7.5 years after administration of streptokinase for acute myocardial infarction. *Eur Heart J* (1999) 20, 1245–52.
6. McGrath K, Hogan C, Hunt D, O'Malley C, Green N, Dauer R, Dalli A. Neutralising antibodies after streptokinase treatment for myocardial infarction: a persisting puzzle. *Br Heart J* (1995) 74, 122–3.
7. Green C. Antistreptokinase titres after topical streptokinase. *Lancet* (1993) 341, 1602–3.
8. Streptase (Streptokinase). ZLB Behring UK Ltd. UK Summary of product characteristics, November 2004.
9. White HD, Cross DB, Williams BF, Norris RM. Safety and efficacy of repeat thrombolytic treatment after acute myocardial infarction. *Br Heart J* (1990) 64, 177–81.
10. Lee HS, Yule S, McKenzie A, Cross S, Reid T, Davidson R, Jennings K. Hypersensitivity reactions to streptokinase in patients with high pre-treatment antistreptokinase antibody and neutralisation titres. *Eur Heart J* (1993) 14, 1640–3.
11. Binette MJ, Agnone FA. Failure of APSAC thrombolysis. *Ann Intern Med* (1993) 119, 637.
12. Brugemann J, van der Meer J, Bom VJJ, van der Schaaf W, de Graeff PA, Lie KI. Anti-streptokinase antibodies inhibit fibrinolytic effects of anistreplase in acute myocardial infarction. *Am J Cardiol* (1993) 72, 462–4.
13. Fears R, Hearn J, Standring R, Anderson JL, Marder VJ. Lack of influence of pretreatment antistreptokinase antibody on efficacy in a multicenter patency comparison of intravenous streptokinase and anistreplase in acute myocardial infarction. *Am Heart J* (1992) 124, 305–14.
14. Gruppo Italiano per lo Studio della Streptochinasi nell'Infarto Miocardico (GISSI). Effectiveness of intravenous thrombolytic treatment in acute myocardial infarction. *Lancet* (1986) i, 397–402.
15. Moriarty AJ. Anaphylaxis and streptokinase. *Hosp Update* (1987) 13, 342.
16. British National Formulary. 49th ed. London: The British Medical Association and The Pharmaceutical Press: 2005. p. 129.

Thrombolytics + Contrast media

In patients with acute ischaemic syndromes undergoing angioplasty procedures, the use of low osmolar ionic contrast media appears to reduce the risk of ischaemic complications compared with nonionic agents.

Clinical evidence, mechanism, importance and management

A study was carried out to assess the thrombogenic potential of contrast media in patients with myocardial infarction or unstable angina undergoing percutaneous transluminal coronary angioplasty (PTCA); 106 patients received **ioxaglate meglumine** 39.3% and **ioxaglate sodium** 19.6% solution *(Hexabrix),* an ionic low osmolar contrast medium, and 105 similar patients received **iohexol** 35% *(Omnipaque 350),* a nonionic low osmolar contrast medium. The use of ionic compared with nonionic low-osmolar contrast media was found to reduce the risk of ischaemic complications acutely and at one month after the procedure.[1] Similar results were found in other studies.[2-6]

A study in *dogs* found that after induction of occlusive coronary artery thrombosis and treatment with **alteplase**, aspirin and heparin, the use of a low-osmolar nonionic contrast medium (**iohexol**) or a high-osmolar ionic contrast medium (**amidotrizoate**) was associated with longer reperfusion delays and shorter periods of coronary perfusion. This effect was not, however, seen with a low-osmolar ionic contrast medium (**ioxaglate**).[7] *In vitro* studies found that radiographic contrast agents (**iohexol**, **amidotrizoate**, or **ioxaglate**) impaired fibrinolysis by **alteplase**, **streptokinase** and **urokinase**,[8] but contrast media varied in their effects on coagulation and platelet activation with the ionic agent **ioxaglate** having greater anticoagulant effects than nonionic agents.[9]

It has been suggested that low osmolar ionic contrast media should be used in preference to nonionic agents in patients with acute ischaemic syndromes undergoing angioplasty procedures.[1,2] However, stable patients undergoing elective angioplasty procedures are less likely to have thrombotic complications and also advances in techniques and anticoagulant/antiplatelet treatment may make the differences between ionic and nonionic contrast media less pronounced.[1]

1. Grines CL, Schreiber TL, Savas V, Jones DE, Zidar FJ, Gangadharan V, Brodsky M, Levin R, Safian R, Puchrowicz-Ochocki S, Castellani MD, O'Neill WW. A randomized trial of low osmolar ionic versus nonionic contrast media in patients with myocardial infarction or unstable angina undergoing percutaneous transluminal coronary angioplasty. *J Am Coll Cardiol* (1996) 27, 1381–6.
2. Aguirre FV, Topol EJ, Donohue TJ, Kern MJ, Leimberger JD, Califf RM and EPIC Investigators. Impact of ionic and non-ionic contrast media on post-PTCA ischemic complications: results from the EPIC trial. *J Am Coll Cardiol* (1995) 25 (Suppl 1), 8A.
3. Gasperetti CM, Feldman MD, Burwell LR, Angello DA, Haugh KH, Owen RM, Powers ER. Influence of contrast media on thrombus formation during coronary angioplasty. *J Am Coll Cardiol* (1991) 18, 443–50.
4. Piessens JH, Stammen F, Vrolix MC, Glazier JJ, Benit E, De Geest H, Willems JL. Effects of an ionic versus a nonionic low osmolar contrast agent on the thrombotic complications of coronary angioplasty. *Cathet Cardiovasc Diagn* (1993) 28, 99–105.
5. Lembo NJ, King SB, Roubin GS, Black AJ, Douglas JS. Effects of nonionic versus ionic contrast media on complications of percutaneous transluminal coronary angioplasty. *Am J Cardiol* (1991) 67, 1046–50.
6. Lefevre T, Adjeroud N, Royer T, Glatt B, Morice MC. Influence of contrast media on the results of percutaneous transluminal coronary angioplasty with provisional stenting: a comparative study. *J Invasive Cardiol* (1998) 10, 380–4.
7. Pislaru S, Pislaru C, Szilard M, Arnout J, Van de Werf F. In vivo effects of contrast media on coronary thrombolysis. *J Am Coll Cardiol* (1998) 32, 1102–8.
8. Dehmer GJ, Gresalfi N, Daly D, Oberhardt B, Tate DA. Impairment of fibrinolysis by streptokinase, urokinase and recombinant tissue-type plasminogen activator in the presence of radiographic contrast agents. *J Am Coll Cardiol* (1995) 25, 1069–75.
9. Corot C, Chronos N, Sabattier V. *In vitro* comparison of the effects of contrast media on coagulation and platelet activation. *Blood Coag Fibrinol* (1996) 7, 602–8.

Ticlopidine + Antacids or Food

Food causes a moderate increase in the absorption of ticlopidine, whereas *Maalox* causes a moderate reduction.

Clinical evidence, mechanism, importance and management

The extent of absorption of a single 250-mg dose of ticlopidine was increased by 20% and occurred more rapidly when 12 healthy subjects took ticlopidine after food, when compared with the fasting state. In contrast, 30 ml of *Maalox* [**aluminium/magnesium hydroxides**] reduced the extent of ticlopidine absorption by about 20%.[1] These modest changes are unlikely to be of much clinical importance. It is suggested that ticlopidine is taken with food to minimise gastric intolerance.[1]

1. Shah J, Fratis A, Ellis D, Murakami S, Teitelbaum P. Effect of food and antacid on absorption of orally administered ticlopidine hydrochloride. *J Clin Pharmacol* (1990) 30, 733–6.

Ticlopidine + Miscellaneous

Ticlopidine-induced increases in bleeding times are opposed by methylprednisolone and prednisolone. Ticlopidine decreases the clearance of phenazone (antipyrine). Beta-blockers, calcium channel blockers and diuretics are reported not to interact with ticlopidine.

Clinical evidence, mechanism, importance and management

(a) Corticosteroids

A study involving 14 healthy subjects found that a single intravenous injection of **methylprednisolone** 20 mg or oral **prednisolone** 15 mg twice daily for 7 days decreased the prolongation of bleeding times caused by ticlopidine 250 to 500 mg twice daily for 7 days, without reducing the antiplatelet effects of ticlopidine.[1] The clinical importance of this is uncertain.

(b) Phenazone (Antipyrine)

A study in 10 healthy subjects found that ticlopidine 250 mg twice daily for 3 weeks decreased the clearance of phenazone (a marker of enzyme inhibition or induction). The AUC increased by 14% and the half-life increased by 27%.[2] This is consistent with the way ticlopidine appears to inhibit the metabolism of theophylline (see 'Theophylline + Clopidogrel or Ticlopidine', p.934) but so far no other drugs seem to be affected to a clinically important extent.

(c) Other non-interacting drugs

The makers of ticlopidine report that in clinical studies in which ticlopidine was given with **beta-blockers**, **calcium channel blockers** and **di uretics** [none of the individual drugs named], no clinically significant adverse interactions were reported.[3,4]

1. Thébault J, Blatrix C, Blanchard J, Panak E. A possible method to control prolongations of bleeding time under antiplatelet therapy with ticlopidine. *Thromb Haemost* (1982) 48, 6–8.
2. Knudsen JB, Bastain W, Sefton CM, Allen JG, Dickinson JP. Pharmacokinetics of ticlopidine during chronic oral administration to healthy volunteers and its effects on antipyrine pharmacokinetics. *Xenobiotica* (1992) 22, 579–89.
3. Ticlid (Ticlopidine). Sanofi Synthelabo. UK Summary of product characteristics, May 2000.
4. Ticlid (Ticlopidine hydrochloride). Roche Pharmaceuticals. US Prescribing information, March 2001.

Urokinase + Streptokinase

Of 6 patients given urokinase 1.5 million units infused over 30 minutes for recurrent myocardial infarction, rigors occurred in 4 patients and 2 of these also had bronchospasm; they had all previously received streptokinase.[1]

1. Matsis P, Mann S. Rigors and bronchospasm with urokinase after streptokinase. *Lancet* (1992) 340, 1552.

18

Antipsychotics, anxiolytics and hypnotics

The anxiolytics include the benzodiazepines, cloral hydrate and other agents used to treat psychoneuroses such as anxiety and tension, and are intended to induce calm without causing drowsiness and sleep. Some of the benzodiazepines and related drugs are also used as anticonvulsants and hypnotics. 'Table 18.1', (below) contains a list of the benzodiazepines that are referred to in this publication.

The antipsychotics are represented by chlorpromazine (and other phenothiazines), butyrophenones and thioxanthenes. Their major use is in the treatment of psychoses such as schizophrenia and mania. These are listed in 'Table 18.2', (p.528). Some of the antipsychotics are also used as antiemetics, and for motor tics and hiccup.

Most of the interactions involving antipsychotic, anxiolytic and hypnotic drugs are covered in this section but there are other monographs elsewhere in this publication where the interacting drug is a benzodiazepine or antipsychotic.

Table 18.1 Benzodiazepines and related drugs

Generic names	*Proprietary names*
Benzodiazepines	
Alprazolam	Adax, Alcelam, Alnax, Alplax, Alpralid, Alprastad, Alpratyrol, Alprax, Alprax , Alpraz, Alprazig, Alprocontin, Alpronax, Alprox, Alzam, Anpress, Antanax, Anxirid, Anzion, Apo-Alpraz, Apraz, Azor, Becede, Bestrol, Calmax, Cassadan, Dizolam, Frontal, Frontin, Gerax, Grifoalpram, Helex, Ibizolam, Kalma, Krama, Marzolam, Mialin, Mitranax, Nalion, Neupax, Neurol, Niravam, Novo-Alprazol, Nu-Alpraz, Pacyl, Pazolam, Pharnax, Prazam, Prenadona, Prinox, PTA, Renax, Restyl, Retan, Sanerva, Saturnil, Siampraxol, Tafil, Tensium, Thiprasolan, Tranax, Trankimazin, Tranquinal, Tricalma Retard, Unilan, Valeans, Xanacine, Xanagis, Xanax, Xanor, Xiemed, Xycalm, Zacetin, Zolam, Zopax, Zotran
Bromazepam	Akamon, Anconevron, Angular, Anxyrex, Atemperator, Benedorm, Brazepam, Bromalex, BromaLich, Bromam, Bromatanil, Bromaz, Bromazanil, Bromaze, Bromazep, Bromazepan, Bromidem, Bromoxon, Bropamil, Brozepax, Compendium, Creosedin, Deptran, durazanil, Equisedin, Estomina, Evagelin, Finaten, Gityl, Lectopam, Lenitin, Lexatin, Lexaurin, Lexilium, Lexomil, Lexostad, Lexotan, Lexotanil, Libronil-R, Molival, neo OPT, Nervium, Neurilan, Neurozepam, Normoc, Notorium, Novazepam, Nulastres, Octanyl, Pascalium, Quietiline, Relaxil, Sedatus, Sipcar, Somalium, Totasedan, Tritopan, Ultramidol, Uni Bromazepax
Brotizolam	Bondormin, Dormex, Lendorm, Lendormin, Lindormin, Noctilan, Sintonal
Chlordiazepoxide	Benpine, Cozep, Defobin, Elenium, Equilibrium, Huberplex, Kalmocaps, Klopoxid, Klorpo, Librium, Multum, Oasil, OCM, Omnalio, Paxium, Psicosedin, Radepur, Reliberan, Risolid, Tropium
Clobazam	Castilium, Frisin, Frisium, Grifoclobam, Karidium, Noiafren, Urbanil, Urbanol, Urbanyl
Clonazepam	Acepran, Antelepsin, Clonagin, Clonapam, Clonax, Clonex, Clonogal, Clozanil, Crismol, Diocam, Epitril, Epizam, Iktorivil, Kenoket, Klonopin, Kriadex, Neuryl, Ozepam, Paxam, Ravotril, Rivatril, Rivotril, Solfidin, Valpax
Clorazepate	Anxielax, Calner, Cloramed, Cloraxene, Diposef, Dipot, Flulium, Justum, Manotran, Medipax, Modival, Novo-Clopate, Polizep, Pomadom, Posene, Sanor, Serene, Tencilan, Trancap, Tranclor, Trancon, Transene, Tranxal, Tranxene, Tranxilene, Tranxilium, Uni-Tranxene, Zetran
Clotiazepam	Clozan, Distensan, Rize, Rizen, Tienor, Veratran
Diazepam	Alboral, Aliseum, Aneurol, Ansilive, Ansiolin, Antenex, Anxicalm, Apaurin, Apollonset, Apozepam, Arzepam, Assival, Atarviton, AT-V, Azepam, Benzopin, Betapam, Bialzepam, Calmociteno, Calmpose, Cardiosedantol, Compaz, Complutine, Cuadel, Daiv, Dezepan, Diactal, Dialar, Diano, Diapam, Diapanil, Diapine, Diapo, Diastat, Diatex, Diaz, Diazemuls, Diazep, Diazepan, Dienpax, Dipezona, Dizan, Dizepam, Doval, Ducene, Elcion, Elongal, Faustan, Freudal, Gewacalm, Glutasedan, Gobanal, Hexalid, Kiatrium, Kratium, Lamra, Laxyl, Lembrol, Medipam, Metamidol, Micronoan, Noan, Novazam, Onapan, Ortopsique, Paceum, Pacinax, Pacium, Pax, Paxum, Pazolini, Placidox, Plidan, Prizem, Propam, Psychopax, Rec-DZ, Relanium, Relazepam, Rimapam, Rupediz, Saromet, Seduxen, Sico Relax, Sipam, Somaplus, Stedon, Stesolid, Tandial, Tensium, Tranquirit, Umbrium, Uni Diazepax, Unisedil, Valaxona, Valclair, Valiquid, Valium, Valix, Valocordin-Diazepam, Valpam, Vatran, Vincosedan, Vival, Zepose, Zeprat, Zopam

Continued

Table 18.1 Benzodiazepines and related drugs (continued)

Generic names	*Proprietary names*
Flunitrazepam	Darkene, Fluni, Flunibeta, Flunimerck, Fluninoc, Flunipam, Flunita, Fluscand, Guttanotte, Hipnosedon, Hypnodorm, Ilman, Insom, Ipnopen, Narcozep, Neo Nifalium, Nilium, Parsimonil, Primum, Rohipnol, Rohypnol, Roipnol, Ronal, Sedex, Somnubene, Valsera, Vulbegal
Flurazepam	Dalmadorm, Dalmane, Dormodor, Felison, Flunox, Fluraz, Fordrim, Morfex, Remdue, Staurodorm, Staurodorm Neu, Valdorm
Ketazolam	Anseren, Ansieten, Ansietil, Marcen, Sedatival, Sedotime, Solatran, Unakalm
Loprazolam	Dormonoct, Havlane, Somnovit, Sonin
Lorazepam	Abinol, Amparax, Ansilor, Anta, Anxira, Aplacasse, Aripax, Ativan, Calmese, Cicletan, Control, Donix, Dorm, duralozam, Emotival, Idalprem, Kalmalin, Larpose, LAtiwen, Laubeel, Lonza, Lorabenz, Lora, Lorafen, Loram, Loramed, Lorans, Lorapam, Lorasifar, Lorax, Lorazep, Lorazepan, Lorenin, Loridem, Lorivan, Lorsedal, Max-Pax, Merlit, Mesmerin, Microzepam, Modium, Nervistop L, Nifalin, Novhepar, Novo-Lorazem, Nu-Loraz, Optisedine, Ora, Orfidal, Placinoral, Proneurit, Razepam , Sedatival, Sedazin, Sedicepan, Serenase, Sidenar, Sinestron, Somagerol, Tavor, Temesta, Titus, Tolid, Tranavan, Trankilium, Tranqipam, Trapax, Tratenamin, Vigiten
Lormetazepam	Aldosomnil, Dilamet, Ergocalm, Loramet, Loretam, Minias, Noctamid, Noctamide, Nocton, Pronoctan, Sedaben, Stilaze
Medazepam	Ansilan, Nobrium, Rudotel, Rusedal
Midazolam	Dalam, Dormicum, Dormid, Dormire, Dormium, Dormonid, Drimnorth, Fulsed, Gobbizolam, Hypnovel, Ipnovel, Midacum, Midazol, Midolam, Noctura, Ormir, Rem, Versed, Zolamid, Zolidan
Nitrazepam	Alodorm, Apodorm, Arem, Dima, Dormalon, Dormo-Puren, Eatan N, Eunoctin, Hypnotex, Imeson, Insoma, Insomin, Mogadan, Mogadon, Nitavan, Nitrados, Nitrapan, Nitravet, Nitrazadon, Nitrazepol, Novanox, Numbon, Ormodon, Pacisyn, Paxadorm, Radedorm, Remnos, Somnite, Sonebon
Oxazepam	Adumbran, Alepam, Alopam, Anxiolit, durazepam, Limbial, Medopam, Mirfudorm, Murelax, Noripam, Opamox, Oxabenz, Oxa, Oxahexal, Oxamin, Oxapax, Oxascand, Oxepam, Ox-Pam, Pausafren T, Praxiten, Purata, Serax, Serenal, Serepax, Seresta, Serpax, Sigacalm, Sobril, Tranquo, Uskan, Vaben
Oxazolam	
Temazepam	Euhypnos, Euipnos, Levanxol, Norkotral Tema, Normison, Nortem, Planum, Pronervon T, Remestan, Restoril, Signopam, Somapam, Temaze, temazep, Temtabs, Tenox
Triazolam	Apo-Triazo, Balidon, Halcion, Rilamir, Somese, Songar, Trilam
Other drugs	
Alpidem	
Buspirone	Anchocalm, Ansial, Ansienon, Ansitec, Ansiten, Antipsichos, Anxiolan, Anxiron, Anxut, Bergamol, Bespar, Biron, Boronex, Busansil, Buscalm, Buscalma, Busp, Buspanil, Buspar, Buspirol, Effiplen, Epsilat, Establix, Hiremon, Hobatstress, Itagil, Kalmiren, Komasin, Lanamont, Lebilon, Ledion, Loxapin, Nadrifor, Nervostal, Neurorestol, Norbal, Pasrin, Paxon, Pendium, Sorbon, Spitomin, Stressigal, Svitalark, Tendan, Tensispes, Trafuril, Umolit
Hydroxyzine	Abacus, AH 3 N, Atano, Atarax, Ataraxone, Aterax, Cerax, Dalun, Drazine, Elroquil N, Fasarax, Hadarax, Hidroxina, Histan, Hizin, Honsa, Hyderax, Hydroxin, Iremofar, Masarax, Navicalm, Neurax, Nexit, Otarex, Phymorax, Polizine, Postarax, Prurizin, R-Rax, Serecid, Taraxin, Trandrozine, Ucerax, Unamine, Vistaril
Zaleplon	Hegon, Hipnodem, Noctiplon, Plenidon, Rhem, Somnipax, Sonata, Starnoc, Zalep, Zaso, Zerene
Zolpidem	Adormix, Ambien, Ambiz, Bikalm, Cymerion, Dalparan, Dormilam, Dormosol, Hypnogen, Ivadal, Ivedal, Lioram, Mondeal, Myslee, Nimadorm, Niotal, Nitrest, Nottem, Nytamel, Sanval, Somit, Somnil, Somnipron, Somno, Sove, Stella, Stilnoct, Stilnox, Sucedal, Sumenan, Zleep, Zodorm, Zodormdura, Zoldem, Zolnod, Zolpihexal, Zolpi-Lich, Zolpinox, Zonoct
Zopiclone	Alchera, Alpaz, Amvey, Datolan, espa-dorm, Eurovan, Foltran, Imoclone, Imovane, Imozop, Insomnium, Limovan, Losopil, Nenia, Neurolil, Nocturno, Nuctane, Optidorm, Relaxon, Rhovane, Siaten, Somnal, Somnol, Somnosan, Ximovan, Z-Dorm, Zedax, Zetix, Zileze, Zimoclone, Zimovane, Zodurat, Zolief, Zometic, Zomni, Zop, Zopicalm Zopicalma, Zopiclodura, Zopicon, Zopimed, Zopinox, Zopi-Puren, Zopitan, Zopivane, Zorclone

Table 18.2 Antipsychotics

Generic names	*Proprietary names*
Phenothiazines	
Butaperazine	
Chlorpromazine	Ampliactil, Amplictil, Chlorazin, Chlormazine , Chlorpromasit, Chlorpromed, Clonazine, Clorpromaz, Conrax, Duncan, Hibernal, Klorproman, Largactil, Largatrex, Longactil, Matcine, Plegomazin, Propaphenin, Prozin, Prozine, Solidon, Taroctyl, Thorazine, Zuledine
Fluphenazine	Anatensol, Cenilene, Dapotum, Deca, Fludecate, Flufenan, Lyogen, Lyorodin, Modecate, Moditen, Moditen Depo, Moditen Depot, Omca, Pacinol, Pharnazine , Phenazin, Potensone, Prolixin, Siqualone
Levomepromazine	Apo-Methoprazine, Levium, Levocina, Levozin, Levozine, Methozane, Neozine, Neurocil, Nozinan, Prazine, Ronexine, Sinogan, Tisercin, Togrel
Mesoridazine	
Pericyazine	Nemactil, Neulactil, Neuleptil
Perphenazine	Conazine, Decentan, Fentazin, Leptopsique, Peratsin, Pernamed, Pernazine, Perphenan, Porazine, Trilafon, Trilifan
Prochlorperazine	Antinaus, Apo-Prochlorazine, Buccastem, Bukatel, Compazine, Compro, Dhaperazine, Emidoxyn, Mitil, Nautisol, Nu-Prochlor, Prochlor, Proclozine, Proziere, Scripto-Metic, Stemetil, Stemzine, Vometil
Promazine	Prazine, Protactyl, Prozine, Sinophenin, Sparine, Talofen
Thioridazine	Aldazine, Melleretten, Melleril, Orsanil, Ridazin, Ridazine, Rideril, Simultan, Thiomed, Thioril, Thiosia, Thiozine, Tinsenol
Trifluoperazine	Eskazine, Flupazine, Modalina, Psyrazine, Stelazine, Stelazine, Stelium, Terflurazine, Triflumed, Trinicalm, Triozine, Triplex
Butyrophenones	
Benperidol	Benquil, Frenactil, Glianimon
Droperidol	Dehidrobenzperidol, Dehydrobenzperidol, Dridol, Droleptan, Droperdal, Droperol, Inapsine, Paxical, Sintodian
Haloperidol	Aloperidin, Alternus, Avant, Dozic, Haldol, Halo, Halomed, Haloper, Haloperil, Halopidol, Halopol, Halozen, Haricon, Haridol, H-Tab, Loperidol, Neupram, Novo-Peridol, Pericate, Perida, Peridor, Polyhadon, Schizopol, Serenace, Serenase, Serenelfi, Sevium, Sigaperidol, Tensidol, Uni Haloper, Zetoridal
Thioxanthenes	
Chlorprothixene	Truxal, Truxaletten
Flupentixol	Depixol, Fluanxol
Tiotixene	Navane, Thixit
Zuclopenthixol	Ciatyl-Z, Cisordinol, Clopixol, Colpixol
Other drugs	
Clozapine	Cloment, Clopine, Clopsine, Clozaril, Denzapine, Elcrit, Fazalco, Froidir, Lanolept, Lapenax, Leponex, Lozapin, Lozapine, Sequax, Sizopin, Zaponex, Zolapin
Loxapine	Desconex, Loxapac, Loxitane
Molindone	Moban
Olanzapine	Joyzol, Midax, Olexar, Ozapin, Psycholanz, Zyprexa
Quetiapine	Alzen, Norsic, Quel, Quetidin, Seroquel, Seroquin, Socalm
Pimozide	Orap, Pirium, Pizide
Risperidone	Belivon, Dagotil, Dropicine, Goval, Radigen, Risnia, Rispen, Risperdal, Risperin, Sequinan, Sizorisp, Spiron, Viverdal, Zargus
Ritanserin	
Sertindole	Serdolect
Sulpiride	Aiglonyl, Aplacid, Arminol, Betamaks, Calmoflorine, Championyl, Darleton, Depral, Digton, Dobren, Dogmatil, Dogmatyl, Dolmatil, Eclorion, Eglonyl, Ekilid, Equilid, Espiride, Guastil, Lebopride, Lisopride, Meresa, Modal, neogama, Nivelan, Noneston, Nufarol, Nylipark, Pontiride, Prosulpin, Psicocen, Restful, Rimastine, Sanblex, Stamoneyrol, Sulp, Sulpilan, Sulpirol, Sulpitil, Sulpivert, Sulpor, Suprium, Synedil, Tepavil, Valirem, Vertigo-Meresa, vertigo-neogama, Vipral
Ziprasidone	Geodon, Zeldox, Zeldox, Zipsydon
Zotepine	Lodopin, Nipolept, Zoleptil

Antipsychotics + Antacids or Sucralfate

Antacids containing aluminium/magnesium hydroxide or magnesium trisilicate can reduce the serum levels of chlorpromazine, which would be expected to reduce the therapeutic response. Sucralfate and an aluminium/magnesium hydroxide antacid can reduce the absorption of sulpiride. *In vitro* studies suggest that this interaction may possibly also occur with other antacids and phenothiazines. There seem to be no clinical studies or reports confirming the anecdotal evidence of a possible reduction in the effects of haloperidol by antacids.

Clinical evidence

(a) Haloperidol

In 1982 a questioner in a letter asked whether haloperidol interacts with antacids because he had a patient doing well on haloperidol who had begun to deteriorate when *Amphojel* (**aluminium hydroxide**) was added. In a written answer it was stated[1] that there are no reports of this interaction but several clinicians had said that based on clinical impressions oral haloperidol and antacids should not be given together.

(b) Phenothiazines

A study in 10 patients taking **chlorpromazine** 600 to 1200 mg daily showed that 30 ml of *Aludrox* (**aluminium/magnesium hydroxide gel**) reduced their urinary excretion of **chlorpromazine** reduced by 10 to 45%.[2]

A study was prompted by the observation of one psychiatric patient, controlled on **chlorpromazine** who relapsed within 3 days of starting to take an unnamed antacid. When 30 ml of *Gelusil* (**aluminium hydroxide** with **magnesium trisilicate**) was given with **chlorpromazine** suspension to 6 patients, the serum **chlorpromazine** levels measured 2 hours later were reduced by about 20% (from 168 to 132 nanograms/ml).[3] *In vitro* studies have also found that other phenothiazines (**trifluoperazine**, **fluphenazine**, **perphenazine**, **thioridazine**) are adsorbed to a considerable extent onto a number of antacids (**magnesium trisilicate**, **bismuth subnitrate**, **aluminium hydroxide** with **magnesium carbonate**) but there do not appear to be any clinical studies of the possible effects of these interactions.[4]

(c) Sulpiride

A study in 6 healthy subjects found that the bioavailability of a single 100-mg dose of sulpiride was reduced by 40% by **sucralfate** 1 g and by 32% by 30 ml of *Simeco* (**aluminium/magnesium hydroxide** and **simeticone**). When either the **sucralfate** or the antacid were taken 2 hours before sulpiride the reduction in bioavailability was only about 25%, and no change in bioavailability was seen in one subject when the **sucralfate** was given 2 hours after the sulpiride.[5]

Mechanism

Chlorpromazine and other phenothiazines become adsorbed onto these antacids,[3,6] which would seem to account for the reduced bioavailability. It is possible that adsorption also occurs with sulpiride, but this has not been proven.

Importance and management

Clinical information seems to be limited to the reports cited. Reductions of up to 45% in serum antipsychotic levels would be expected to be clinically important, but so far only one case seems to have been reported.[3] Separating the doses as much as possible (1 to 2 hours) to avoid admixture in the gut should minimise any effects. This may also prove of use in the interactions with haloperidol and sulpiride (although note; the haloperidol interaction is not confirmed). In the case of chlorpromazine an alternative would be to use calcium carbonate-glycine or magnesium hydroxide gel, which seem to affect its gastrointestinal absorption to a lesser extent.[6] Other phenothiazines and antacids are known to interact *in vitro*,[4] but the clinical importance of these interactions awaits further study.

1. Goldstein BJ. Interaction of antacids with psychotropics. *Hosp Community Psychiatry* (1982) 33, 96.
2. Forrest FM, Forrest IS, Serra MT. Modification of chlorpromazine metabolism by some other drugs frequently administered to psychiatric patients. *Biol Psychiatry* (1970) 2, 53–8.
3. Fann WE, Davis JM, Janowsky DS, Sekerke HJ, Schmidt DM. Chlorpromazine: effects of antacids on its gastrointestinal absorption. *J Clin Pharmacol* (1973) 13, 388–90.
4. Moustafa MA, Babhair SA, Kouta HI. Decreased bioavailability of some antipsychotic phenothiazines due to interactions with adsorbent antacid and antidiarrhoeal mixtures. *Int J Pharmaceutics* (1987) 36, 185–9.
5. Gouda MW, Hikal AH, Babhair SA, ElHofy SA, Mahrous GM. Effect of sucralfate and antacids on the bioavailability of sulpiride in humans. *Int J Pharmaceutics* (1984) 22, 257–63.
6. Pinell OC, Fenimore DC, Davis CM, Moreira O, Fann WE. Drug-drug interaction of chlorpromazine and antacid. *Clin Pharmacol Ther* (1978) 23, 125.

Antipsychotics + Anticholinergics

Antipsychotics and anticholinergics are very often given together advantageously and uneventfully, but occasionally serious and even life-threatening interactions occur. These include heatstroke in hot and humid conditions, severe constipation and adynamic ileus, and atropine-like psychoses. Anticholinergics used to counteract the extrapyramidal adverse effects of antipsychotics may also reduce or abolish their therapeutic effects. Consider also 'Phenothiazines + Tricyclic antidepressants', p.570, and 'Anticholinergics + Anticholinergics', p.501.

Clinical evidence

The use of antipsychotics with anticholinergics can result in a generalised, low grade, but not serious additive increase in the anticholinergic effects of these drugs (blurred vision, dry mouth, constipation, difficulty in urination, see 'Anticholinergics + Anticholinergics', p.501). However, sometimes serious intensification takes place. For the sake of clarity these have been subdivided here into (a) heat stroke, (b) constipation and adynamic ileus, (c) atropine-like psychoses, (d) antagonism of antipsychotic effects and (e) miscellaneous effects.

(a) Heat stroke in hot and humid conditions

Three patients were admitted to hospital in Philadelphia for drug-induced hyperpyrexia during a hot and humid period. In each case their skin and mucous membranes were dry and they were tachycardic (120 bpm). There was no evidence of infection.[1]

Drug combinations implicated in reports of heat stroke, some of them fatal, include:[1-4]

- **chlorpromazine** and **benzatropine**
- **chlorpromazine** and **trifluoperazine**
- **chlorpromazine**, **amitriptyline** and **benzatropine**
- **chlorpromazine**, **chlorprothixene** and **benzatropine**
- **chlorpromazine**, **fluphenazine**, **trihexyphenidyl** and **benzatropine**
- **chlorpromazine**, **trifluoperazine** and **benzatropine**
- **haloperidol** and **benzatropine**
- **promazine** and **benzatropine**.

The danger of heat-stroke in patients on **atropine** or **atropine-like compounds** was recognised in the 1920s, and the warning has been repeated many times.[5,6]

(b) Constipation and adynamic ileus

Paralytic ileus with faecal impaction (fatal in 5 cases) has been reported in a number of patients treated with:

- **chlorpromazine** and **amitriptyline**,[7] **imipramine**,[8] **nortriptyline**,[9] or **trihexyphenidyl**[8]
- **levomepromazine** and **imipramine** with **benzatropine**[8]
- **levomepromazine** and **trihexyphenidyl**[8]
- **thioridazine** and **imipramine** with **trihexyphenidyl**[8]
- **trifluoperazine** and **benzatropine**[10] or **trihexyphenidyl**[8]
- **trifluoperazine** and **benzatropine** with **methylphenidate**.[11]

Severe constipation also occurred in a woman given **thioridazine**, **biperiden** and **doxepin**.[12]

(c) Atropine-like psychoses

In a double-blind study 3 patients given a **phenothiazine** and **benzatropine** for the parkinsonian adverse effects, developed an intermittent toxic confusional state (marked disturbance of short-term memory, impaired attention, disorientation, anxiety, visual and auditory hallucinations) with peripheral anticholinergic signs.[13] Similar reactions occurred in 3 elderly patients given **imipramine** or **desipramine**, with **trihexyphenidyl**,[14] and in another man given **chlorpromazine**, **benzatropine** and **doxepin**.[12]

(d) Antagonism of the antipsychotic effects

A study in psychiatric patients given **chlorpromazine** 300 to 800 mg daily found that when **trihexyphenidyl** 6 to 10 mg daily was added, the plasma **chlorpromazine** concentrations fell from a range of 100 to 300 nanograms/ml to less than 30 nanograms/ml. When the **trihexyphenidyl** was withdrawn the plasma **chlorpromazine** levels rose again and clinical improvement was seen.[15,16]

Other studies confirm that **trihexyphenidyl**[17,18] and **orphenadrine**[19] reduce the plasma levels and effects of **chlorpromazine**. In contrast to these reports, another found that **trihexyphenidyl** increased **chlorpromazine** levels by 41% in 20 young schizophrenics, but no clinical change was seen. The levels dropped again over the first 4 weeks of treatment.[20] Some of the beneficial actions of **haloperidol** on social avoidance behaviour are lost during concurrent treatment with **benzatropine**, but cognitive integrative function is unaffected.[21]

(e) Miscellaneous effects

A study in psychotic patients found that the addition of **biperiden** 2 mg three times daily or **orphenadrine** 50 mg three times daily for 3 weeks had no effect on the steady-state levels of **perphenazine** 24 to 48 mg daily.[22]

An isolated report describes the development of a hypoglycaemic coma in a non-diabetic patient given **chlorpromazine** and **orphenadrine**.[23]

Mechanism

Anticholinergic drugs inhibit the parasympathetic nervous system, which innervates the sweat glands, so that when the ambient temperature rises the major body heat-losing mechanism can be partially or wholly lost.[24] Phenothiazines, thioxanthenes and butyrophenones may also have some anticholinergic effects, but additionally they impair to a varying extent the hypothalamic thermoregulatory mechanisms that control the body's ability to keep a constant temperature when exposed to heat or cold. Thus, when the ambient temperature rises, the body temperature also rises. The tricyclics can similarly disrupt temperature control. Therefore in very hot and humid conditions, when the need to reduce the temperature is great, the additive effects of these drugs can make patients unable to control their temperature,[4] which can be fatal.

Anticholinergic drugs also reduce peristalsis, which in the extreme can result in total gut stasis. Additive effects can occur if two or more anticholinergic drugs are taken.

The toxic psychoses described resemble the CNS effects of atropine or belladonna poisoning and appear to result from the additive effects of the drugs used.

The mechanism for antipsychotic antagonism is not understood. *Animal* studies suggest that the site of interaction is in the gut.[16]

Importance and management

Established and well-documented interactions. While these drugs have been widely used together with apparent advantage and without problems, prescribers should be aware that an unspectacular low-grade anticholinergic toxicity can easily go undetected, particularly in the elderly because the symptoms can be so similar to the general complaints of this group. Also be aware of the serious problems that can sometimes develop, particularly if high doses are used.

- Warn patients to minimise outdoor exposure and/or exercise in hot and humid climates, particularly if they are taking high doses of antipsychotic/anticholinergic drugs.
- Be alert for severe constipation and for the development of complete gut stasis, which can be fatal.
- Be aware that the symptoms of central anticholinergic psychosis can be confused with the basic psychotic symptoms of the patient. Withdrawal of one or more of the drugs, or a dosage reduction and/or appropriate symptomatic treatment can be used to control these interactions.
- Ensure that the concurrent use of anticholinergics to control the extrapyramidal adverse effects of neuroleptics is necessary[25,26] and be aware that the therapeutic effects may possibly be reduced as a result.

Note that tricyclic antidepressants have anticholinergic adverse effects and may therefore interact similarly. The tricyclics also have other interactions with antipsychotics, see 'Phenothiazines + Tricyclic antidepressants', p.570. Some antipsychotics and anticholinergics prolong the QT interval. For interactions resulting from additive effects on the QT interval see 'Drugs that prolong the QT interval + Other drugs that prolong the QT interval', p.170.

1. Westlake RJ, Rastegar A. Hyperpyrexia from drug combinations. *JAMA* (1973) 225, 1250.
2. Zelman S, Guillan R. Heat stroke in phenothiazine-treated patients: a report of three fatalities. *Am J Psychiatry* (1970) 126, 1787–90.
3. Sarnquist F, Larson CP. Drug-induced heat stroke. *Anesthesiology* (1973) 39, 348–50.
4. Reimer DR, Mohan J, Nagaswami S. Heat dyscontrol syndrome in patients receiving antipsychotic, antidepressant and antiparkinson drug therapy. *J Fla Med Assoc* (1974) 61, 573–4.
5. Willcox WH. The nature, prevention, and treatment of heat hyperpyrexia: the clinical aspect. *BMJ* (1920) 1, 392–7.
6. Litman RE. Heat sensitivity due to autonomic drugs. *JAMA* (1952) 149, 635–6.
7. Burkitt EA, Sutcliffe CK. Paralytic ileus after amitriptyline ("Tryptizol"). *BMJ* (1961) 2, 1648–9.
8. Warnes H, Lehmann HE, Ban TA. Adynamic ileus during psychoactive medication: a report of three fatal and five severe cases. *Can Med Assoc J* (1967) 96, 1112–13.
9. Milner G, Hills NF. Adynamic ileus and nortriptyline. *BMJ* (1966) 1, 841–2.
10. Giordano J, Huang A, Canter JW. Fatal paralytic ileus complicating phenothiazine therapy. *South Med J* (1975) 68, 351–3.
11. Spiro RK, Kysilewskyj RM. Iatrogenic ileus secondary to medication. *J Med Soc New Jers* (1973) 70, 565–7.
12. Ayd FJ. Doxepin with other drugs. *South Med J* (1973) 66, 465–71.
13. Davis JM. Psychopharmacology in the aged. Use of psychotropic drugs in geriatric patients. *J Geriatr Psychiatry* (1974) 7, 145.
14. Rogers SC. Imipramine and benzhexol. *BMJ* (1967) 1, 500.
15. Rivera-Calimlim L, Castañeda L, Lasagna L. Effect of mode of management on plasma chlorpromazine in psychiatric patients. *Clin Pharmacol Ther* (1973) 14, 978–86.
16. Rivera-Calimlim L, Castañeda L, Lasagna L. Chlorpromazine and trihexyphenidyl interaction in psychiatric patients. *Pharmacologist* (1973) 15, 212.
17. Chan TL, Sakalis G, Gershon S. Some aspects of chlorpromazine metabolism in humans. *Clin Pharmacol Ther* (1973) 14, 133.
18. Rivera-Calimlim L, Nasrallah H, Strauss J, Lasagna L. Clinical response and plasma levels: effect of dose, dosage schedules, and drug interactions on plasma chlorpromazine levels. *Am J Psychiatry* (1976) 133, 646–52.
19. Loga S, Curry S, Lader M. Interactions of orphenadrine and phenobarbitone with chlorpromazine: plasma concentrations and effects in man. *Br J Clin Pharmacol* (1975) 2, 197–208.
20. Rockland L, Cooper T, Schwartz F, Weber D, Sullivan T. Effects of trihexyphenidyl on plasma chlorpromazine in young schizophrenics. *Can J Psychiatry* (1990) 35, 604–7.
21. Singh MM, Smith JM. Reversal of some therapeutic effects of an antipsychotic agent by an antiparkinsonism drug. *J Nerv Ment Dis* (1973) 157, 50–8.
22. Hansen LB, Elley J, Christensen TR, Larsen N-E, Naestoft J, Hvidberg EF. Plasma levels of perphenazine and its major metabolites during simultaneous treatment with anticholinergic drugs. *Br J Clin Pharmacol* (1979) 7, 75–80.
23. Buckle RM, Guillebaud J. Hypoglycaemic coma occurring during treatment with chlorpromazine and orphenadrine. *BMJ* (1967) 4, 599–600.
24. Kollias J, Bullard RW. The influence of chlorpromazine on physical and chemical mechanisms of temperature regulation in the rat. *J Pharmacol Exp Ther* (1964) 145, 373–81.
25. Prien RF. Unpublished surveys from the NIMH Collaborative Project on Drug Therapy in Chronic Schizophrenia and the VA Collaborative Project on Interim Drug Therapy in Chronic Schizophrenia. *Quoted in: Int Drug Ther Newslett* (1974) 9, 29–32.
26. Klett CJ, Caffey EM. Evaluating the long-term need for antiparkinson drugs by chronic schizophrenics. *Arch Gen Psychiatry* (1972) 26, 374–9.

Antipsychotics + Anticonvulsants

Haloperidol plasma levels are roughly halved by carbamazepine, phenobarbital and phenytoin. Bromperidol, fluphenazine and tiotixene levels are also reduced by carbamazepine. The plasma levels of chlorpromazine and haloperidol do not appear to be affected by oxcarbazepine. Neurotoxicity has been seen with haloperidol and carbamazepine and haloperidol can raise serum carbamazepine levels. Valproate or valproic acid appear not to interact.

Clinical evidence

(a) Carbamazepine

For mention of carbamazepine toxicity and other adverse reactions following the concurrent use of antipsychotics see 'Carbamazepine + Antipsychotics', p.340.

(i) Bromperidol. When 13 schizophrenic patients on bromperidol 12 or 24 mg daily were given carbamazepine 200 mg twice daily for 4 weeks, the plasma levels of bromperidol and reduced bromperidol (a metabolite) were decreased by 37% and 23% respectively. Despite this fall in levels, the Clinical Global Impression scores (a measure of severity of illness) fell slightly.[1]

(ii) Chlorpromazine. **Oxcarbazepine** was substituted for carbamazepine in 4 difficult to treat schizophrenic patients. All patients were also taking chlorpromazine, and in 3 cases other antipsychotic medication (lithium, zuclopenthixol or clozapine). After 3 weeks of taking the **oxcarbazepine** all the 4 patients had rises in their chlorpromazine levels, of 28%, 63%, 76% and 90%. In one case this rise was associated with increased extrapyramidal adverse effects.[2]

(iii) Fluphenazine. A patient on fluphenazine decanoate 37.5 mg weekly had a rise in serum levels from 0.6 to 1.17 nanograms/ml 6 weeks after stopping carbamazepine 800 mg daily. A moderate improvement in his schizophrenic condition occurred.[3]

(iv) Haloperidol. A study in 9 schizophrenics on haloperidol (average dose 30 mg daily) found a 55% reduction in plasma haloperidol levels (a mean fall from 45.5 to 21.2 nanograms/ml) when they were given carbamazepine for 5 weeks [precise dose not stated]. They also took trihexyphenidyl 10 mg daily and oxazepam 30 mg at night as necessary. Carbamazepine serum levels and the control of the disease remained unchanged.[4]

Other studies have similarly found 40 to 60% falls in plasma haloperidol levels in patients taking carbamazepine,[5-7] with the occasional patient having undetectable levels.[6,8] Decreases in plasma haloperidol levels of unspecified amounts have also been described.[9-12] A few patients have had clinical worsening or increased adverse effects.[6-8] Three patients had two to fivefold increases in plasma haloperidol levels and clinical improvement when carbamazepine 1200 to 1400 mg daily was stopped, but extrapyramidal adverse effects developed within 1 to 30 days.[13] Three cases of neurotoxicity (drowsiness, slurred speech, confusion) have also been described in patients on haloperidol and carbamazepine.[9,14,15]

A case report describes 3 schizophrenic patients taking haloperidol who were changed from carbamazepine to **oxcarbazepine**. After 2 weeks their plasma haloperidol levels had dramatically risen (from 6 to 18 nanomol/l, from 6 to 14 nanomol/l and from 17 to 27 nanomol/l). This was accompanied by severe extrapyramidal adverse effects, which necessitated dose reductions in 2 patients.[2]

A study in Japanese schizophrenic patients found that carbamazepine reduced the serum haloperidol levels by an unstated amount, while at the same time the serum carbamazepine levels were raised by about 30% despite a 25% dose reduction.[10] An associated study by the same group of workers found that concurrent use increased the incidence of QTc lengthening.[16]

(v) Tiotixene. A retrospective study in 42 patients found that the mean clearance of tiotixene in those taking enzyme-inducing drugs (carbamazepine, phenytoin, primidone) was threefold greater than in the control group (92.5 compared with 32.8 l/minute). Of the group taking enzyme inducers, 5 patients had non-detectable serum tiotixene levels, and not surprisingly showed no clinical response.[17]

(b) Phenobarbital and/or Phenytoin

A study in epileptic patients, 2 on phenobarbital, 3 on phenytoin, and 5 on both drugs, found that after taking haloperidol 10 mg three times daily for 6 weeks their serum haloperidol levels were about half of those in a control group who were not taking anticonvulsants (19.4 compared to 36.6 nanograms/ml). Anticonvulsant levels remained unchanged.[18] A patient had a marked rise in serum haloperidol levels and clinical improvement when phenytoin 300 mg daily was stopped.[13] A retrospective study found that phenobarbital reduced the haloperidol concentration/dose ratio, suggesting that phenobarbital may affect the metabolism of haloperidol.[12] See also (v) Tiotixene above.

(c) Valproic acid or valproate

A study in 6 patients given haloperidol 6 to 10 mg daily found no significant interaction with valproic acid.[19] Similarly, haloperidol was not found to interact with valproate in another study.[20]

Mechanism

Carbamazepine, phenobarbital and phenytoin are recognised enzyme-inducing agents, therefore it seems highly likely that the reduced plasma bromperidol, chlorpromazine and haloperidol levels occur because their metabolism by the liver is markedly increased by these anticonvulsants. Oxcarbazepine does not appear to interact, probably because it is not an enzyme inducer.

Importance and management

The interactions of haloperidol with carbamazepine, phenytoin and phenobarbital are moderately well documented and appear to be clinically important, but only a few patients have been reported to show clinical worsening. Although there are advantages in adding carbamazepine to haloperidol in treating some patients[21] be alert for the need to increase the haloperidol dosage if any of these anticonvulsants is also given. The authors of one study with phenobarbital and phenytoin suggest a two to threefold increase in the haloperidol dosage may be needed.[18] Another study, in which intramuscular haloperidol was used, recommended shortening the interval between injections rather than raising the dosage, but it was not stated by how much.[22] Remember too that if the anticonvulsants are withdrawn it may be necessary to reduce the haloperidol dosage. Also be alert for the development of dystonic reactions and for a rise in serum carbamazepine levels. Similar precautions seem necessary with tiotixene, and may be needed with bromperidol and chlorpromazine, but this needs confirmation. Limited evidence suggest that no special precautions are necessary with oxcarbazepine, or if sodium valproate is used with haloperidol.

1. Otani K, Ishida M, Yasui N, Kondo T, Mihara K, Suzuki A, Furukori H, Kaneko S, Inoue Y. Interaction between carbamazepine and bromperidol. *Eur J Clin Pharmacol* (1997) 53, 219–22.
2. Raitasuo V, Lehtovaara R, Huttunen MO. Effect of switching carbamazepine to oxcarbazepine on the plasma levels of neuroleptics. A case report. *Psychopharmacology (Berl)* (1994) 116, 115–16.
3. Jann MW, Fidone GS, Hernandez JM, Amrung S, Davis CM. Clinical implications of increased antipsychotic plasma concentrations upon anticonvulsant cessation. *Psychiatry Res* (1989) 28, 153–9.
4. Kidron R, Averbuch I, Klein E, Belmaker RH. Carbamazepine-induced reduction of blood levels of haloperidol in chronic schizophrenia. *Biol Psychiatry* (1985) 20, 219–22.
5. Jann MW, Ereshefsky L, Saklad SR, Seidel DR, Davis CM, Burch NR, Bowden CL. Effects of carbamazepine on plasma haloperidol levels. *J Clin Psychopharmacol* (1985) 5, 106–9.
6. Arana GW, Goff DC, Friedman H, Ornsteen M, Greenblatt DJ, Black B, Shader RI. Does carbamazepine-induced reduction of plasma haloperidol levels worsen psychotic symptoms? *Am J Psychiatry* (1986) 143, 650–1.
7. Kahn EM, Schulz SC, Perel JM, Alexander JE. Change in haloperidol level due to carbamazepine—a complicating factor in combined medication for schizophrenia. *J Clin Psychopharmacol* (1990) 10, 54–7.
8. Fast DK, Jones BD, Kusalic M, Erickson M. Effect of carbamazepine on neuroleptic plasma levels and efficacy. *Am J Psychiatry* (1986) 143, 117–18
9. Brayley J, Yellowlees P. An interaction between haloperidol and carbamazepine in a patient with cerebral palsy. *Aust N Z J Psychiatry* (1987) 21, 605–7.
10. Iwahashi K, Miyatake R, Suwaki H, Hosokawa K, Ichikawa Y. The drug–drug interaction effects of haloperidol on plasma carbamazepine levels. *Clin Neuropharmacol* (1995) 18, 233–6.
11. Jann MW, Chang W-H, Lane H-Y. Differences in haloperidol epidemiologic pharmacokinetic studies. *J Clin Psychopharmacol* (2001) 21, 628–30.
12. Hirokane G, Someya T, Takahashi S, Morita S, Shimoda K. Interindividual variation of plasma haloperidol concentrations and the impact of concomitant medications: the analysis of therapeutic drug monitoring data. *Ther Drug Monit* (1999) 21, 82–6.
13. Jann MW, Fidone GS, Hernandez JM, Amrung S, Davis CM. Clinical implications of increased antipsychotic plasma concentrations upon anticonvulsant cessation. *Psychiatry Res* (1989) 28, 153–9.
14. Kanter GL, Yerevanian BI, Ciccone JR. Case report of a possible interaction between neuroleptics and carbamazepine. *Am J Psychiatry* (1984) 141, 1101–2.
15. Yerevanian BI, Hodgman CH. A haloperidol-carbamazepine interaction in a patient with rapid-cycling bipolar disorder. *Am J Psychiatry* (1985) 142, 785–6.
16. Iwahashi K, Nakamura K, Miyatake R, Suwaki H, Hosokawa K. Cardiac effects of haloperidol and carbamazepine treatment. *Am J Psychiatry* (1996) 153, 135.
17. Ereshefsky L, Saklad SR, Watanabe MD, Davis CM, Jann MW. Thiothixene pharmacokinetic interactions: a study of hepatic enzyme inducers, clearance inhibitors, and demographic variables. *J Clin Psychopharmacol* (1991) 11, 296–301.
18. Linnoila M, Viukari M, Vaisanen K, Auvinen J. Effect of anticonvulsants on plasma haloperidol and thioridazine levels. *Am J Psychiatry* (1980) 137, 819–21.
19. Ishizaki T, Chiba K, Saito M, Kobayashi K, Iizuka R. The effects of neuroleptics (haloperidol and chlorpromazine) on the pharmacokinetics of valproic acid in schizophrenic patients. *J Clin Psychopharmacol* (1984) 4, 254–61.
20. Normann C, Klose P, Hesslinger B, Langosch JM, Berger M, Walden J. Haloperidol plasma levels and psychopathology in schizophrenic patients with antiepileptic co-medication: a clinical trial. *Pharmacopsychiatry* (1997) 30, 204.
21. Klein E, Bental E, Lerer B, Belmaker RH. Carbamazepine and haloperidol *v* placebo and haloperidol in excited psychoses: a controlled study. *Arch Gen Psychiatry* (1984) 41, 165–70.
22. Pupeschi G, Agenet C, Levron J-C, Barges-Bertocchio M-H. Do enzyme inducers modify haloperidol decanoate rate of release? *Prog Neuropsychopharmacol Biol Psychiatry* (1994) 18, 1323–32.

Antipsychotics + Bromocriptine

Concurrent use can be successful, but one report describes the reemergence of schizophrenic symptoms in a patient when bromocriptine was added to treatment with molindone and imipramine.

Clinical evidence, mechanism, importance and management

Single 2-mg doses of bromocriptine have been found to improve the psychopathology of chronic schizophrenia in patients on antipsychotics[1] and a case report describes a reduction in psychopathology when bromocriptine 2.5 mg daily was given with **haloperidol**.[2]

However, a woman with schizoaffective schizophrenia, stabilised on **molindone** 100 mg and imipramine 200 mg daily, relapsed within 5 days of starting treatment with bromocriptine 2.5 mg three times daily for amenorrhoea and galactorrhoea.[3] Within 3 days of stopping the bromocriptine the symptoms of relapse (agitation, delusions, and auditory hallucinations) vanished. The reason suggested by the authors of the report is that the bromocriptine (a dopamine agonist) opposed the actions of the antipsychotic medication (dopamine antagonists) thereby allowing the schizophrenia to re-emerge. Limited evidence suggests that levodopa also may antagonise the effects of antipsychotics, see 'Levodopa + Antipsychotics', p.506, which adds weight to this theory.

1. Cutler NR, Jeste DV, Kaufmann CA, Karoum F, Schran HF, Wyatt RJ. Low dose bromocriptine: a study of acute effects in chronic medicated schizophrenics. *Prog Neuropsychopharmacol Biol Psychiatry* (1984) 8, 277–83.
2. Gattaz WF, Köllisch M. Bromocriptine in the treatment of neuroleptic-resistant schizophrenia. *Biol Psychiatry* (1986) 21, 519–21.
3. Frye PE, Pariser SF, Kim MH, O'Shaughnessy RW. Bromocriptine associated with symptom exacerbation during neuroleptic treatment of schizoaffective schizophrenia. *J Clin Psychiatry* (1982) 43, 252–3.

Antipsychotics + Coffee or Tea

Tea and coffee can cause some drugs to precipitate out of solution, but so far there is no clinical evidence to show that this normally affects the bioavailability of the drugs nor that it has a detrimental effect on treatment.

Clinical evidence, mechanism, importance and management

A single report described 2 patients whose schizophrenia was said to have been exacerbated by an increased consumption of tea and coffee.[1] Subsequent *in vitro* studies[2-6] showed that a number of drugs (**chlorpromazine**, **promethazine**, **fluphenazine**, **orphenadrine**, **promazine**, **prochlorperazine**, **trifluoperazine**, **thioridazine**, **loxapine**, **haloperidol**, **droperidol**) form a precipitate with tea or coffee due to the formation of a drug-tannin complex, which was thought might possibly lower the absorption of these drugs in the gut. Studies with *rats* also showed that tea abolished the cataleptic effects of **chlorpromazine**, which did not appear to be related to the presence of caffeine.[7] However, the drug-tannin complex gives up the drug into solution if it becomes acidified, as in the stomach.[6] Moreover, a clinical study of this interaction showed that the plasma levels of **chlorpromazine**, **fluphenazine**, **trifluoperazine** and **haloperidol** in a group of 16 mentally retarded patients were unaffected by the consumption of tea or coffee.[8] Their behaviour also remained unchanged.[8] So there appears to be little or no direct evidence that this physicochemical interaction is normally of any clinical importance.

1. Mikkelsen EJ. Caffeine and schizophrenia. *J Clin Psychiatry* (1978) 39, 732–5.
2. Kulhanek F, Linde OK, Meisenberg G. Precipitation of antipsychotic drugs in interaction with coffee or tea. *Lancet* (1979) ii, 1130.
3. Hirsch SR. Precipitation of antipsychotic drugs in interaction with tea or coffee. *Lancet* (1979) ii, 1130–1.
4. Lasswell WL, Wilkins JM, Weber SS. In vitro interaction of selected drugs with coffee, tea, and gallotannic acid. *Drug Nutr Interact* (1984) 2, 235–41.
5. Lasswell WL, Weber SS, Wilkins JM. *In vitro* interaction of neuroleptics and tricyclic antidepressants with coffee, tea, and gallotannic acid. *J Pharm Sci* (1984) 73, 1056–8.
6. Curry ML, Curry SH, Marroum PJ. Interaction of phenothiazine and related drugs and caffeinated beverages. *DICP Ann Pharmacother* (1991) 25, 437–8.
7. Cheeseman HJ, Neal MJ. Interaction of chlorpromazine with tea and coffee. *Br J Clin Pharmacol* (1981) 12, 165–9.
8. Bowen S, Taylor KM, Gibb IAM. Effect of coffee and tea on blood levels and efficacy of antipsychotic drugs. *Lancet* (1981) i, 1217–18.

Antipsychotics + Lithium

Chlorpromazine levels can be reduced to subtherapeutic concentrations by lithium. The development of severe extrapyramidal adverse effects or severe neurotoxicity has been seen in one or more patients given lithium with amoxapine, chlorpromazine, chlorprothixene, clopenthixol, flupentixol, fluphenazine, haloperidol, levomepromazine, loxapine, mesoridazine, molindone, perphenazine, prochlorperazine, risperidone, sulpiride, thioridazine, tiotixene, trifluoperazine or zuclopenthixol. Sleep-walking has been described in some patients taking chlorpromazine-like drugs and lithium.

Clinical evidence

(a) Chlorpromazine

In a double-blind study in psychiatric patients it was found that chlorpromazine 400 to 800 mg daily, a dose that normally produced plasma levels of 100 to 300 nanograms/ml, only produced levels of 0 to 70 nanograms/ml when lithium carbonate was also given.[1]

Other studies confirm that normal therapeutic levels of lithium carbonate reduce plasma chlorpromazine levels.[2,3] The peak serum levels and AUC of chlorpromazine were reduced by 40% and 26% respectively, in healthy subjects given lithium carbonate.[2]

A paranoid schizophrenic maintained on chlorpromazine 200 to 600 mg daily for 5 years with no extrapyramidal symptoms developed stiffness of his face, arms and legs, and parkinsonian tremor of both hands within a day of starting to take lithium 900 mg daily. His lithium blood level after 3 days was 0.5 mmol/l. He was later maintained on lithium 1800 mg daily (blood level 1.17 mmol/l), chlorpromazine 200 mg daily and benzatropine 2 mg daily, which improved his condition, but he still complained of stiffness and had a persistent hand tremor.[4]

A number of other reports describe the emergence of severe extrapyramidal adverse effects when chlorpromazine was given with lithium.[5-7] Ventricular fibrillation, thought to be caused by chlorpromazine toxicity, occurred in a patient taking lithium when both drugs were suddenly withdrawn.[8] Severe neurotoxicity has also been seen in a handful of other patients on lithium and chlorpromazine.[9]

(b) Haloperidol

A large-scale retrospective study of the literature over the period 1966 to 1996 using the Medline database identified 41 cases of neurotoxic adverse effects in 41 patients with low therapeutic concentrations of lithium. Of these patients, 10 were taking haloperidol.[9]

Another retrospective study using both Medline and the FDA Spontaneous Reporting System over the period 1969 to 1994 identified 237 cases of severe neurotoxicity involving lithium, of which 59 also involved the concurrent use of haloperidol.[10,11]

Other reports describe encephalopathic syndromes (lethargy, fever, tremulousness, confusion, extrapyramidal and cerebellar dysfunction),[12] neuromuscular symptoms, impaired consciousness and hyperthermia,[13] delirium, severe extrapyramidal symptoms and organic brain damage[14-24]

A small rise in serum lithium levels occurs in the presence of haloperidol, but it is almost certainly of little or no clinical significance.[25]

In contrast to the reports cited above, there are others describing successful and uneventful use.[12,26-29] A retrospective search of Danish hospital records found that 425 patients had been treated with both drugs and none of them had developed serious adverse reactions.[30]

(c) Other antipsychotics

A large-scale retrospective study of the literature over the 1966 to 1996 period using the Medline database identified 41 cases of neurotoxic adverse effects in 41 patients on low therapeutic concentrations of lithium. Of these patients, 51.2% were also taking at least one antipsychotic drug.[9] Another retrospective study using both Medline and the FDA Spontaneous Reporting System over the period 1969 to 1994 identified 237 cases of severe neurotoxicity involving lithium, with 188 involving lithium plus antipsychotics.[10,11] The sudden emergence of extrapyramidal or other adverse effects has also been described in other studies. The antipsychotics implicated in this interaction with lithium are **amoxapine**,[10,11] **bromperidol**,[10,11] **chlorprothixene**,[10,11] **clopenthixol**,[9] **clozapine**,[9-11] **flupentixol**,[14,31] **fluphenazine**,[9-11,14,32] **haloperidol**,[9,14] **levomepromazine**,[9-11] **loxapine**,[10,11,33,34] **mesoridazine**,[10,11] **molindone**,[10,11] **perphenazine**,[10,11] **prochlorperazine**,[10,11] **sulpiride**,[35] **thioridazine**,[9-11,36] **tiotixene**[9-11,15] **trifluoperazine**,[10,11] or **zuclopenthixol**.[9] Examples of some cases are cited in a little more detail below.

A study of 10 patients on **fluphenazine**, **haloperidol** or **thiothixene** found that the addition of lithium worsened their extrapyramidal symptoms.[37] Neurotoxicity (tremor, rigidity, ataxia, tiredness, vomiting, confusion) attributed to an interaction between lithium and **fluphenazine** has been described in another patient. He previously took **haloperidol** and later took **chlorpromazine** with lithium, without problem.[38] Irreversible brain damage has been reported in a patient taking **fluphenazine decanoate** and lithium.[39] Severe neurotoxic complications (seizures, encephalopathy, delirium, abnormal EEGs) developed in 4 patients taking **thioridazine** 400 mg daily or more and lithium. Serum lithium levels remained below 1 mmol/l. Lithium and other phenothiazines had been used in 3 of them for extended periods without problems, and the fourth was subsequently successfully treated with lithium and **fluphenazine**.[40] In one study the concurrent use of lithium, and **chlorpromazine**, **perphenazine**, or **thioridazine** was associated with sleep-walking episodes in 9% of patients.[41] Somnolence, confusion, delirium, creatinine phosphokinase elevation and fever occurred in a man on lithium when given **risperidone**.[42]

Mechanism

Not understood. One suggestion to account for the reduced serum levels of chlorpromazine, which is based on *animal* studies,[43,44] is that chlorpromazine can be metabolised in the gut. Therefore, if lithium delays gastric emptying, more chlorpromazine will be metabolised before it reaches the circulation. Just why severe neurotoxicity and other adverse effects sometimes develop in patients on lithium and antipsychotics is not understood. It is the subject of considerable discussion and debate.[9-11,45,46]

Importance and management

Information about the reduction in chlorpromazine levels caused by lithium is limited, but it would seem to be an established interaction of clinical importance. Serum chlorpromazine levels below 30 nanograms/ml have been shown to be ineffective, whereas clinical improvement is associated with levels within the 150 to 300 nanogram/ml range or more.[47] Thus a fall in levels to below 70 nanograms/ml described in one study would be expected to result in a reduced therapeutic response. Monitor the effects and increase the chlorpromazine dosage if necessary.

The development of severe neurotoxic or severe extrapyramidal adverse effects with combinations of antipsychotics and lithium appears to be uncommon and unexplained but be alert for any evidence of toxicity if lithium is given with any of these drugs. One recommendation is that the onset of neurological manifestations, such as excessive drowsiness or movement disorders, warrants electroencephalography without delay and withdrawal of the drugs, especially as irreversible effects have been seen. A review[48] suggests that the concurrent use of haloperidol seems to be safe if lithium levels are below 1 mmol/l. It is not known whether this also applies to other antipsychotics.

At the moment there seems to be no way of identifying the apparently small number of patients who are particularly at risk, but possible likely factors include a previous history of extrapyramidal reactions with antipsychotics and the use of large doses of antipsychotic.

1. Kerzner B, Rivera-Calimlim L. Lithium and chlorpromazine (CPZ) interaction. *Clin Pharmacol Ther* (1976) 19, 109.
2. Rivera-Calimlim L, Kerzner B, Karch FE. Effect of lithium on plasma chlorpromazine levels. *Clin Pharmacol Ther* (1978) 23, 451–5.
3. Rivera-Calimlim L, Nasrallah H, Strauss J, Lasagna L. Clinical response and plasma levels: effect of dose, dosage schedules, and drug interactions on plasma chlorpromazine levels. *Am J Psychiatry* (1976) 133, 646–52.
4. Addonizio G. Rapid induction of extrapyramidal side effects with combined use of lithium and neuroleptics. *J Clin Psychopharmacol* (1985) 5, 296–8.
5. McGennis AJ. Hazards of lithium and neuroleptics in schizo-affective disorder. *Br J Psychiatry* (1983) 142, 99–100.
6. Yassa R. A case of lithium-chlorpromazine interaction. *J Clin Psychiatry* (1986) 47, 90–1.
7. Habib M, Khalil R, Le Pensec-Bertrand D, Ali-Cherif A, Bongrand MC, Crevat A. Syndrome neurologique persistant après traitement par les sels de lithium: toxicité de l'association lithium-neuroleptiques? *Rev Neurol (Paris)* (1986) 142, 1, 61–4.
8. Stevenson RN, Blanshard C, Patterson DLH. Ventricular fibrillation due to lithium withdrawal – an interaction with chlorpromazine? *Postgrad Med J* (1989) 65, 936–8.
9. Emilien G, Maloteaux JM. Lithium neurotoxicity at low therapeutic doses: hypotheses for causes and mechanism of action following a retrospective analysis of published case reports. *Acta Neurol Belg* (1996) 96, 281–93.
10. Goldman SA. Lithium and neuroleptics in combination: is there enhancement of neurotoxicity leading to permanent sequelae? *J Clin Pharmacol* (1996) 36, 951–62.
11. Goldman SA. FDA MedWatch Report: lithium and neuroleptics in combination: the spectrum of neurotoxicity. *Psychopharmacol Bull* (1996) 32, 299–309.
12. Cohen WJ, Cohen NH. Lithium carbonate, haloperidol, and irreversible brain damage. *JAMA* (1974) 230, 1283–7.
13. Thornton WE, Pray BJ. Lithium intoxication: a report of two cases. *Can Psychiatr Assoc J* (1975) 20, 281–2.
14. Kamlana SH, Kerry RJ, Khan IA. Lithium: some drug interactions. *Practitioner* (1980) 224, 1291–2.
15. Fetzer J, Kader G, Danahy S. Lithium encephalopathy: a clinical, psychiatric, and EEG evaluation. *Am J Psychiatry* (1981) 138, 1622–3.
16. Marhold J, Zimanová J, Lachman M, Král J, Vojtěchovský M. To the incompatibility of haloperidol with lithium salts. *Act Nerv Super (Praha)* (1974) 16, 199–200.
17. Wilson WH. Addition of lithium to haloperidol in non-affective antipsychotic non-responsive schizophrenia: a double blind, placebo controlled, parallel design clinical trial. *Psychopharmacology (Berl)* (1993) 111, 359–66.
18. Loudon JB, Waring H. Toxic reactions to lithium and haloperidol. *Lancet* (1976) ii, 1088.
19. Juhl RP, Tsuang MT, Perry PJ. Concomitant administration of haloperidol and lithium carbonate in acute mania. *Dis Nerv Syst* (1977) 38, 675.
20. Spring G, Frankel M. New data on lithium and haloperidol incompatibility. *Am J Psychiatry* (1981) 138, 818–21.
21. Menes C, Burra P, Hoaken PCS. Untoward effects following combined neuroleptic-lithium therapy. *Can J Psychiatry* (1980) 25, 573–6.
22. Keitner GI, Rahman S. Reversible neurotoxicity with combined lithium-haloperidol administration. *J Clin Psychopharmacol* (1984) 4, 104–5.
23. Thomas CJ. Brain damage with lithium/haloperidol. *Br J Psychiatry* (1979) 134, 552.
24. Thomas C, Tatham A, Jakubowski S. Lithium/haloperidol combinations and brain damage. *Lancet* (1982) i, 626.
25. Schaffer CB, Batra K, Garvey MJ, Mungas DM, Schaffer LC. The effect of haloperidol on serum levels of lithium in adult manic patients. *Biol Psychiatry* (1984) 19, 1495–9.
26. Garfinkel PE, Stancer HC, Persad E. A comparison of haloperidol, lithium carbonate and their combination in the treatment of mania. *J Affect Disord* (1980) 2, 279–88.
27. Baptista T. Lithium-neuroleptic combination and irreversible brain damage. *Acta Psychiatr Scand* (1986) 73, 111.
28. Goldney RD, Spence ND. Safety of the combination of lithium and neuroleptic drugs. *Am J Psychiatry* (1986) 143, 882–4.
29. Biederman J, Lerner Y, Belmaker H. Combination of lithium and haloperidol in schizo-affective disorder. A controlled study. *Arch Gen Psychiatry* (1979) 36, 327–33.
30. Baastrup PC, Hollnagel P, Sørensen R, Schou M. Adverse reactions in treatment with lithium carbonate and haloperidol. *JAMA* (1976) 236, 2645–6.
31. West A. Adverse effects of lithium treatment. *BMJ* (1977) 2, 642.
32. Sachdev PS. Lithium potentiation of neuroleptic-related extrapyramidal side effects. *Am J Psychiatry* (1986) 143, 942.
33. de la Gandara J, Dominguez RA. Lithium and loxapine: a potential interaction. *J Clin Psychiatry* (1988) 49, 126.
34. Fuller MA, Sajatovic M. Neurotoxicity resulting from a combination of lithium and loxapine. *J Clin Psychiatry* (1989) 50, 187.
35. Dinan TG, O'Keane V. Acute extrapyramidal reactions following lithium and sulpiride co-administration: two case reports. *Hum Psychopharmacol* (1991) 6, 67–9.
36. Bailine SH, Doft M. Neurotoxicity induced by combined lithium–thioridazine treatment. *Biol Psychiatry* (1986) 21, 834–7.
37. Addonizio G, Roth SD, Stokes PE, Stoll PM. Increased extrapyramidal symptoms with addition of lithium to neuroleptics. *J Nerv Ment Dis* (1988) 176, 682–5.
38. Alevizos B. Toxic reactions to lithium and neuroleptics. *Br J Psychiatry* (1979) 135, 482.
39. Singh SV. Lithium carbonate/fluphenazine decanoate producing irreversible brain damage. *Lancet* (1982) ii, 278.
40. Spring GK. Neurotoxicity with combined use of lithium and thioridazine. *J Clin Psychiatry* (1979) 40, 135–8.
41. Charney DS, Kales A, Soldatos CR, Nelson JC. Somnambulistic-like episodes secondary to combined lithium-neuroleptic treatment. *Br J Psychiatry* (1979) 135, 418–24.
42. Swanson CL, Price WA, McEvoy JP. Effects of concomitant risperidone and lithium treatment. *Am J Psychiatry* (1995) 152, 1096.
43. Sundaresan PR, Rivera-Calimlim L. Distribution of chlorpromazine in the gastrointestinal tract of the rat and its effects on absorptive function. *J Pharmacol Exp Ther* (1975) 194, 593–602.
44. Curry SH, D'Mello A, Mould GP. Destruction of chlorpromazine during absorption in the rat *in vivo* and *in vitro*. *Br J Pharmacol* (1971) 42, 403–11.
45. Geisler A, Klysner R. Combined effect of lithium and flupenthixol on striatal adenylate cyclase. *Lancet* (1977) i, 430–1.
46. von Knorring L. Possible mechanisms for the presumed interaction between lithium and neuroleptics. *Hum Psychopharmacol* (1990) 5, 287–92.
47. Rivera-Calimlim L, Castañeda L, Lasagna L. Significance of plasma levels of chlorpromazine. *Clin Pharmacol Ther* (1973) 14, 144.
48. Batchelor DH, Lowe MR. Reported neurotoxicity with the lithium/haloperidol combination and other neuroleptics—a literature review. *Hum Psychopharmacol* (1990) 5, 275–80.

Antipsychotics + SSRIs

On the whole no significant adverse interactions appear to occur between the antipsychotics and the SSRIs. However, a number of case reports describe extrapyramidal adverse effects following the use of fluoxetine or paroxetine with an antipsychotic, and galactorrhoea and amenorrhoea developed in one patient given loxapine and fluvoxamine. Fluoxetine and fluvoxamine appear to raise haloperidol levels, which may increase adverse effects.

Clinical evidence, mechanism, importance and management

(a) Chlorpromazine

A study in schizophrenic patients found that over a 12-week period the serum levels of chlorpromazine were not significantly altered by **citalopram** 40 mg daily.[1]

(b) Cyamemazine

A study in patients taking cyamemazine found that **fluvoxamine** 150 mg daily had no effect on its serum levels, but the authors of the report also say that no firm conclusions should be drawn from this finding because the number of patients was too small.[2]

(c) Flupentixol

Parkinson-like symptoms developed in a patient on amitriptyline and flupenthixol when **fluoxetine** was given.[3]

(d) Fluphenazine

A severe dystonic reaction (painful jaw tightness and throat 'closing up') occurred in a man on **fluoxetine** 40 mg daily when he took fluphenazine 2.5 mg on two consecutive nights.[4]

(e) Haloperidol

(i) Citalopram. A study in schizophrenic patients found that over a 12-week period the serum levels of haloperidol were not significantly altered by citalopram 40 mg daily.[1]

(ii) Fluoxetine. A woman taking haloperidol 2 to 5 mg daily for 2 years with only occasional mild extrapyramidal symptoms began to experience severe extrapyramidal symptoms (tongue stiffness, parkinsonism, akathisia) shortly after starting to take fluoxetine 40 mg twice daily and was virtually incapacitated for 3 days. Both drugs were stopped and she recovered over a period of a week.[5] Three other patients developed movement disorders after receiving both drugs,[6-8]
In one case severe anticholinergic adverse effects also occurred.[7]
A report describes 8 patients who had a 20% rise in plasma haloperidol levels when fluoxetine 20 mg daily was added. Although no overall increase in extrapyramidal effects was seen, one patient developed tremor, and another developed akathisia.[9] Similarly 15 patients showed an in-

crease of nearly 30% in haloperidol plasma levels after fluoxetine was given, and 5 of 17 patients had aggravated parkinsonian symptoms.[10] Another report describes a more than 100% rise in plasma haloperidol levels accompanied by clinical improvement in 7 patients given fluoxetine 20 to 40 mg with haloperidol.[11]

(iii) Fluvoxamine. A study in 12 schizophrenic patients found that haloperidol levels were increased by 20%, 39%, and 60% by fluvoxamine 25, 75 and 150 mg daily respectively, which suggested the extent of the interaction was related to the dose of fluvoxamine.[12] A study in 3 schizophrenic patients found that the addition of fluvoxamine caused their serum haloperidol levels to rise, and when the fluvoxamine was stopped the levels fell. This was not a formal pharmacokinetic study, but while taking fluvoxamine 150 to 200 mg daily the haloperidol serum levels of one patient rose from 17 to 38 nanograms/ml. The fluvoxamine was then stopped and 54 days later his serum haloperidol levels had fallen to 9 nanograms/ml. This patient became lethargic and showed worsening of all of the clinical and cognitive functions assessed while taking these drugs.[13] It should be noted that all three patients were also taking benzatropine (see 'SSRIs + Benzatropine', p.980). Another limited study also observed that fluvoxamine causes a rise in the serum levels of haloperidol.[2]

(iv) Paroxetine. In one study the sedative effects and impairment of psychomotor performance caused by haloperidol 3 mg were not increased by paroxetine 30 mg.[14]

(v) Sertraline. In a double-blind, randomised, placebo-controlled study, 21 healthy subjects were given a single 2-mg dose of haloperidol on days 2 to 25. On days 9 to 25 the subjects also received either placebo or sertraline, increased over 7 days to 200 mg daily. All subjects took psychomotor tests on days 1, 2 and 25 to assess the effect of haloperidol. Their cognitive function was impaired for 6 to 8 hours after taking the haloperidol, but this effect had disappeared after 23 hours. Overall, sertraline did not appear to worsen the cognitive impairment caused by haloperidol.[15] Another study found similar pharmacodynamic results, and also found that the pharmacokinetics of haloperidol are unaffected by sertraline.[16]

(f) Levomepromazine

A study in patients taking levomepromazine found that **fluvoxamine** 150 mg daily did not effect its serum levels, but the authors of the report also say that no firm conclusions should be drawn from this finding because the number of patients was too small.[2]

A study in three groups of 8 healthy subjects taking **citalopram** 40 mg daily for 10 days found that a single 50-mg oral dose of levomepromazine increased the initial steady-state levels of the primary metabolite of **citalopram** (desmethylcitalopram) by 10 to 20%, which was not considered to be clinically significant.[17]

A study in schizophrenic patients found that over a 12-week period the serum levels of levomepromazine were not significantly altered by **citalopram** 40 mg daily.[1]

(g) Loxapine

A 38-year-old woman developed amenorrhoea, followed shortly by galactorrhoea, about 6 weeks after starting to take fluvoxamine and loxapine. The galactorrhoea resolved within 3 weeks of stopping the **fluvoxamine**, and menstruation occurred a week later. Her prolactin levels were found to be 80 micrograms/l (normal 4 to 30 micrograms/l).[18]

(h) Molindone

An elderly woman on molindone 10 mg twice daily developed severe and disabling extrapyramidal symptoms (severe bradykinesia, tremor, inability to feed herself, delirium) within about 2 weeks of starting **paroxetine** 10 mg daily. The symptoms resolved when molindone was stopped, and no problems occurred when **fluoxetine** alone was started.[19]

(i) Pericyazine

A New Zealand study describes a patient who developed extrapyramidal symptoms when given pericyazine and **fluoxetine**.[6]

(j) Perphenazine

(i) Citalopram. A study in schizophrenic patients found that over a 12-week period the serum levels of perphenazine were not significantly altered by citalopram 40 mg daily.[1]

(ii) Fluoxetine. The combination of perphenazine and fluoxetine was found to be effective in the treatment of psychotic depression in 30 patients, and the adverse effects (which included dry mouth, blurred vision, constipation, tremor or rigidity, orthostasis and hypotension) were thought to be easier to tolerate than an antipsychotic with a tricyclic antidepressant.[20] However, one woman developed marked extrapyramidal symptoms within 2 weeks of starting perphenazine 4 mg twice daily and fluoxetine 20 mg daily.[21]

(iii) Paroxetine. The effects of a single 100-microgram/kg oral dose of perphenazine on the performance of psychomotor tests were assessed after 4, 6, 8 and 10 hours in 5 subjects. The tests were then repeated after the subjects also took paroxetine 20 mg daily for 10 days. The scores for these tests were worsened by the perphenazine when compared with a placebo and further worsened by the presence of the paroxetine. In addition to oversedation and impairment of the performance of psychomotor tests and memory, 2 of the subjects developed akathisia 10 hours after taking both drugs. The AUC of the perphenazine was increased sevenfold and the maximum plasma levels sixfold.[22]

(k) Pimozide

A patient taking **fluoxetine** and pimozide had a worsening of extrapyramidal symptoms, and another developed marked sinus bradycardia of 35 to 44 bpm with somnolence.[23] This case was the subject of later discussion on the mechanism of the interaction.[24,25] One patient also developed extrapyramidal symptoms,[6] while another became stuporous when given both drugs.[26]

A boy of about 10 years, with various disorders (motor tics, enuresis, attention deficit hyperactivity disorder, Tourettes's disorder, impulsivity, albinism) was treated for a year with pimozide 2 mg twice, and later three times daily.[27] Within 3 days of starting **paroxetine** 10 mg in the morning, he began to complain of his eyes hurting and his mother noted that about 4 hours after taking the **paroxetine** his eyes were rolled back in his head but the problem had resolved by the evening. This oculogyric crisis occurred on a further occasion, and so the **paroxetine** was stopped. There was no other evidence of either extrapyramidal or hyperserotonergic reactions. This case needs to be viewed in its particular context (oculogyric crises are associated with albinism) so that it may not be of general importance.

(l) Sulpiride

Parkinson-like symptoms developed in a patient taking sulpiride and maprotiline when **fluoxetine** was also given.[28]

(m) Thioridazine

A study in schizophrenic patients found that over a 12-week period the serum levels of thioridazine were not significantly altered by **citalopram** 40 mg daily.[1]

(n) Tiotixene

A study in 10 healthy subjects found that **paroxetine** 20 mg daily for 3 days did not significantly affect the pharmacokinetics of a single 20-mg dose of tiotixene.[29]

(o) Trifluoperazine

A New Zealand study describes a patient who developed extrapyramidal symptoms when given trifluoperazine and **fluoxetine**.[6]

(p) Zuclopenthixol

A study in schizophrenic patients found that over a 12-week period the serum levels of zuclopenthixol were not significantly altered by **citalopram** 40 mg daily.[1]

Mechanism

Movement disorders and raised antipsychotic serum levels seem most common with fluoxetine and paroxetine, possibly because they inhibit the metabolism of some antipsychotics by the cytochrome P450 isoenzyme CYP2D6.[22] However, the movement disorders may just be a result of the additive adverse effects of antipsychotics and SSRIs. Fluoxetine alone has been shown to occasionally cause movement disorders.[6,30]

Galactorrhoea is a known adverse effect of loxapine, but just why fluvoxamine apparently increased this effect is not understood.[18]

Importance and management

On the whole significant interactions between the antipsychotics and SSRIs appear rare. The combination can be useful and so the isolated cases of extrapyramidal adverse effects should not prevent concurrent use. However, if extrapyramidal effects become troublesome bear this interaction in mind as a possible cause. The significance of the rise in haloperidol levels caused by fluoxetine and fluvoxamine is unclear, be aware that haloperidol adverse effects may be increased in some patients and consider reducing the haloperidol dose if problems occur. The rise in perphenazine levels caused by paroxetine seems to result in a greater number of more serious adverse effects and so consideration should be given to reducing the dose of perphenazine if paroxetine is started. Citalopram may be a suitable alternative as it does not appear to affect perphenazine levels.

1. Syvälahti EKG, Taiminen T, Saarijärvi S, Lehto H, Niemi H, Ahola V, Dahl M-L, Salokangas RKR. Citalopram causes no significant alterations in plasma neuroleptic levels in schizophrenic patients. *J Int Med Res* (1997) 25, 24–32.
2. Vandel S, Bertschy G, Baumann P, Bouquet S, Bonin B, Francois T, Sechter D, Bizouard P. Fluvoxamine and fluoxetine: Interaction studies with amitriptyline, clomipramine and neuroleptics in phenotyped patients. *Pharmacol Res* (1995) 31, 347–53.
3. Touw DJ, Gernaat HBPE, van der Woude J. Parkinsonisme na toevoeging van fluoxetine aan behandeling met neuroleptica of carbamazepine. *Ned Tijdschr Geneeskd* (1992) 136, 332–4.
4. Ketai R. Interaction between fluoxetine and neuroleptics. *Am J Psychiatry* (1993) 150, 836–7.
5. Tate JL. Extrapyramidal symptoms in a patient taking haloperidol and fluoxetine. *Am J Psychiatry* (1989) 146, 399–400.
6. Coulter DM, Pillans PI. Fluoxetine and extrapyramidal side effects. *Am J Psychiatry* (1995) 152, 122–5.
7. Benazzi F. Urinary retention with fluoxetine–haloperidol combination in a young patient. *Can J Psychiatry* (1996) 41, 606–7.
8. D'Souza DC, Bennett A, Abi-Dargham A, Krystal JH. Precipitation of a psychoneuromotor syndrome by fluoxetine in a haloperidol-treated schizophrenic patient. *J Clin Psychopharmacol* (1994) 14, 361–3.
9. Goff DC, Midha KK, Brotman AW, Waites M, Baldessarini RJ. Elevation of plasma concentrations of haloperidol after the addition of fluoxetine. *Am J Psychiatry* (1991) 148, 790–2.
10. Shim J-C, Kelly DL, Kim Y-H, Yoon Y-R, Park J-H, Shin J-G, Conley RR. Fluoxetine augmentation of haloperidol in chronic schizophrenia. *J Clin Psychopharmacol* (2003) 23, 520–2.
11. Viala A, Aymard N, Leyris A, Caroli F. Corrélations pharmacocliniques lors de l'administration de fluoxétine chez des patients schizophrènes déprimés traités par halopéridol décanoate. *Therapie* (1996) 51, 19–25.
12. Yasui-Furukori N, Kondo T, Mihara K, Inoue Y, Kaneko S. Fluvoxamine dose-dependent interaction with haloperidol and the effects on negative symptoms in schizophrenia. *Psychopharmacology (Berl)* (2004) 171, 223–7.
13. Daniel DG, Randolph C, Jaskiw G, Handel S, Williams T, Abi-Dargham A, Shoaf S, Egan M, Elkashef A, Liboff S, Linnoila M. Coadministration of fluvoxamine increases serum concentrations of haloperidol. *J Clin Psychopharmacol* (1994) 14, 340–3.
14. Cooper SM, Jackson D, Loudon JM, McClelland GR, Raptopoulos P. The psychomotor effects of paroxetine alone and in combination with haloperidol, amylobarbitone, oxazepam, or alcohol. *Acta Psychiatr Scand* (1989) 80 (Suppl 350), 53–5.
15. Williams SA, Wesnes K, Oliver SD, Rapeport WG. Absence of effect of sertraline on time-based sensitization of cognitive impairment with haloperidol. *J Clin Psychiatry* (1996) 57 (Suppl 1), 7–11.
16. Lee MS, Kim YK, Lee SK, Suh KY. A double-blind study of adjunctive sertraline in haloperidol-stabilized patients with chronic schizophrenia. *J Clin Psychopharmacol* (1998) 18, 399–403.
17. Gram LF, Hansen MG, Sindrup SH, Brøsen K, Poulsen JH, Aaes-Jørgensen T, Overø KF. Citalopram: interaction studies with levomepromazine, imipramine and lithium. *Ther Drug Monit* (1993) 15, 18–24.
18. Jeffries J, Bezchlibnyk-Butler K, Remington G. Amenorrhea and galactorrhea associated with fluvoxamine in a loxapine-treated patient. *J Clin Psychopharmacol* (1992) 12, 296–7.
19. Malek-Ahmadi P, Allen SA. Paroxetine-molindone interaction. *J Clin Psychiatry* (1995) 56, 82–3.
20. Rothchild AJ, Samson JA, Bessette MP, Carter-Campbell JT. Efficacy of fluoxetine and perphenazine in the treatment of psychotic depression. *J Clin Psychiatry* (1993) 54, 338–42.
21. Lock JD, Gwirtsman HE, Targ EF. Possible adverse drug interactions between fluoxetine and other psychotropics. *J Clin Psychopharmacol* (1990) 10, 383–4.
22. Özdemir V, Naranjo CA, Herrmann N, Reed K, Sellers EM, Kalow W. Paroxetine potentiates the central nervous system side effects of perphenazine: contribution of cytochrome P4502D6 inhibition in vivo. *Clin Pharmacol Ther* (1997) 62, 334–47.
23. Ahmed I, Dagincourt PG, Miller LG, Shader RI. Possible interaction between fluoxetine and pimozide causing sinus bradycardia. *Can J Psychiatry* (1993) 38, 62–3.
24. Friedman EH. Re: bradycardia and somnolence after adding fluoxetine to pimozide regimen. *Can J Psychiatry* (1994) 39, 634.
25. Ahmed I. Re: bradycardia and somnolence after adding fluoxetine to pimozide regimen. *Can J Psychiatry* (1994) 39, 634.
26. Hansen-Grant S, Silk KR, Guthrie S. Fluoxetine-pimozide interaction. *Am J Psychiatry* (1993) 150, 1751–2.
27. Horrigan JP, Barnhill LJ. Paroxetine–pimozide drug interaction. *J Am Acad Child Adolesc Psychiatry* (1994) 33, 1060–1.
28. Touw DJ, Gernaat HBPE, van der Woude J. Parkinsonisme na toevoeging van fluoxetine aan behandeling met neuroleptica of carbamazepine. *Ned Tijdschr Geneeskd* (1992) 136, 332–3.
29. Guthrie SK, Hariharan M, Kumar AA, Bader G, Tandon R. The effect of paroxetine on thiothixene pharmacokinetics. *J Clin Pharm Ther* (1997) 22, 221–6.
30. Bouchard RH, Pourcher E, Vincent P. Fluoxetine and extrapyramidal side effects. *Am J Psychiatry* (1989) 146, 1352–3.

Antipsychotics + Tobacco or Cannabis smoking

Smokers of tobacco or cannabis may possibly need larger doses of chlorpromazine, fluphenazine, haloperidol or tiotixene than non-smokers.

Clinical evidence

(a) Chlorpromazine

A comparative study found that the frequency of drowsiness in 403 patients taking chlorpromazine was 16% in non-smokers, 11% in light smokers, and 3% in heavy smokers (more than 20 cigarettes daily).[1] Another report describes a patient on chlorpromazine who experienced increased sedation and dizziness and higher plasma chlorpromazine levels when he gave up smoking.[2] A study in 31 patients found that the clearance of chlorpromazine was increased 38% by tobacco smoking, 50% by cannabis smoking, and 107% when both tobacco and cannabis were smoked.[3]

(b) Fluphenazine

In a retrospective study in 40 psychiatric inpatients it was found that the plasma fluphenazine levels of non-smokers were more than double those of smokers (1.83 compared with 0.89 nanograms/ml) when given fluphenazine hydrochloride by mouth. The clearance of both oral and intramuscular fluphenazine was 1.67- and 2.33-fold greater respectively in the smokers than in the non-smokers.[4] No behavioural differences were seen.[4]

(c) Haloperidol

Steady-state haloperidol levels were found to be lower in a group of 23 cigarette smokers than in another group of 27 non-smokers (16.83 compared with 28.8 nanograms/ml) and the clearance was increased by 44%.[5] Other studies have broadly confirmed these findings.[6,7]

(d) Tiotixene

Tobacco smoking increased the clearance of tiotixene in patients taking enzyme inhibitors or no other drugs, but not in patients taking enzyme inducers. Those who smoked were found to need on average 45% more tiotixene than the non-smokers on no other interacting drugs.[8]

Mechanism

Not established. The probable reason is that some of the components of tobacco smoke act as enzyme-inducing agents, which increase the rate at which the liver metabolises these antipsychotics, thereby reducing their serum levels and clinical effects.

Importance and management

Established interactions but of uncertain clinical importance. Be alert for the need to use increased dosages of these antipsychotics in patients who smoke, and reduced dosages if smoking is stopped.

1. Swett C. Drowsiness due to chlorpromazine in relation to cigarette smoking: a report from the Boston Collaborative Drug Surveillance Program. *Arch Gen Psychiatry* (1974) 31, 211–13.
2. Stimmel GL, Falloon IRH. Chlorpromazine plasma levels, adverse effects, and tobacco smoking: case report. *J Clin Psychiatry* (1983) 44, 420–2.
3. Chetty M, Miller R, Moodley SV. Smoking and body weight influence the clearance of chlorpromazine. *Eur J Clin Pharmacol* (1994) 46, 523–6.
4. Ereshefsky L, Jann MW, Saklad SR, Davis CM, Richards AL, Burch NR. Effects of smoking on fluphenazine clearance in psychiatric inpatients. *Biol Psychiatry* (1985) 20, 329–32.
5. Jann MW, Saklad SR, Ereshefsky L, Richards AL, Harrington CA, Davis CM. Effects of smoking on haloperidol and reduced haloperidol plasma concentrations and haloperidol clearance. *Psychopharmacology (Berl)* (1986) 90, 468–70.
6. Perry PJ, Miller DD, Arndt SV, Smith DA, Holman TL. Haloperidol dosing requirements: the contribution of smoking and nonlinear pharmacokinetics. *J Clin Psychopharmacol* (1993) 13, 46–51.
7. Pan L, Vander Stichele R, Rosseel MT, Berlo JA, De Schepper N, Belpaire FM. Effects of smoking, CYP2D6 genotype, and concomitant drug intake on the steady state plasma concentrations of haloperidol and reduced haloperidol in schizophrenic inpatients. *Ther Drug Monit* (1999) 21, 489–97.
8. Ereshefsky L, Saklad SR, Watanabe MD, Davis CM, Jann MW. Thiothixene pharmacokinetic interactions: a study of hepatic enzyme inducers, clearance inhibitors, and demographic variables. *J Clin Psychopharmacol* (1991) 11, 296–301.

Barbiturates + Miscellaneous

Miconazole increases serum pentobarbital levels while the sedative effects of codeine and secobarbital appear to be additive. The hypnotic effects of pentobarbital are reduced or abolished by the concurrent use of caffeine. Caffeine-containing drinks or analgesics should be avoided at bedtime if satisfactory hypnosis is to be achieved.

Clinical evidence, mechanism, importance and management

(a) Caffeine

In a placebo-controlled study caffeine 250 mg and **pentobarbital** 100 mg were given together and alone to 34 patients. It was found that the hypnotic effects of the **pentobarbital** given with caffeine were reduced, and indistinguishable from those of the placebo.[1] Caffeine stimulates the cerebral cortex and impairs sleep, whereas pentobarbital depresses the cortex and promotes sleep. These mutually opposing actions would seem to explain this interaction. This seems to be only direct study of this interaction, but it is well supported by common experience and the numerous studies of the properties of each of these compounds. Patients given barbiturate hypnotics should avoid caffeine-containing drinks (tea, coffee,

Coca-Cola, etc.) or analgesics at or near bedtime if the hypnotic is to be effective. The same is probably true for other non-barbiturate hypnotics, but this needs confirmation.

(b) Codeine

A study found that codeine 60 mg increased the hypnotic actions of **secobarbital** 100 mg resulting in synergism in the sedative effects.[2]

(c) Miconazole

High-dose intravenous **pentobarbital** was given to 5 patients in intensive care to decrease intracranial pressure. When miconazole was added to treatment, all patients had marked rises in plasma **pentobarbital** levels, and a 50 to 90% reduction in total plasma clearance. This is thought to occur because miconazole inhibits the liver enzymes concerned with the metabolism of the barbiturate, thereby reducing its clearance from the body.[3] It would be prudent to monitor the effects of concurrent use to ensure that plasma barbiturate levels do not rise too high. There seems to be no information about other barbiturates.

1. Forrest WH, Bellville JW, Brown BW. The interaction of caffeine with pentobarbital as a nighttime hypnotic. *Anesthesiology* (1972) 36, 37–41.
2. Bellville JW, Forrest WH, Shroff P, Brown BW. The hypnotic effects of codeine and secobarbital and their interaction in man. *Clin Pharmacol Ther* (1971) 12, 607–12.
3. Heinemeyer G, Roots I, Schulz H, Dennhardt R. Hemmung der Pentobarbital-Elimination durch Miconazol bei Intesivtherapie des erhöhten intracraniellen Druckes. *Intensivmed* (1985) 22, 164–7.

Benzodiazepines + Acetazolamide

Although acetazolamide can be used to treat acute mountain sickness at very high altitudes, a case report suggests that it may potentiate the respiratory depressant effects of benzodiazepines such as triazolam.

Clinical evidence, mechanism, importance and management

Acetazolamide is sometimes used by climbers at very high altitudes as a prophylactic against acute mountain sickness. Benzodiazepines are used in this situation to treat insomnia, which is common at high altitude. Benzodiazepines are believed to depress breathing because they reduce the normal respiratory response to hypoxia. This was demonstrated by a Japanese climber in the Himalayas who took acetazolamide 500 mg daily and triazolam 500 micrograms, and then needed to be reminded to hyperventilate in order to relieve his hypoxia while returning from a climb. The acetazolamide did not prevent and may possibly have increased the central ventilatory depression of the triazolam, possibly by increasing its delivery to the brain. The authors of the report advise against taking these two drugs together at high altitudes,[1] thus confirming a previous warning about the risks of taking benzodiazepines at high altitude.[2]

1. Masuyama S, Hirata K, Saito A. 'Ondine's curse': side effect of acetazolamide? *Am J Med* (1989) 86, 637.
2. Sutton JR, Powles ACP, Gray GW, Houston CS. Insomnia, sedation, and high altitude cerebral oedema. *Lancet* (1979) i, 165.

Benzodiazepines + Alosetron

Alosetron 1 mg twice daily for 2 days had no significant effect on the pharmacokinetics of a single 1-mg dose of alprazolam in 12 healthy subjects. No increase in adverse effects was noted with the combination.[1] No special precautions therefore seem necessary on concurrent use.

1. D'Souza DL, Levasseur LM, Nezamis J, Robbins DK, Simms L, Koch KM. Effect of alosetron on the pharmacokinetics of alprazolam. *J Clin Pharmacol* (2001) 41, 452–4.

Benzodiazepines + Amiodarone

An isolated report describes clonazepam toxicity attributed to the concurrent use of amiodarone.

Clinical evidence, mechanism, importance and management

A 78-year-old man with congestive heart failure and coronary artery disease was treated with furosemide, potassium and calcium supplements, a multivitamin preparation, and amiodarone 200 mg daily for sustained ventricular tachycardia. Two months after **clonazepam** 500 micrograms at night was added to treat restless leg syndrome he developed slurred speech, confusion, difficulty in walking, dry mouth and urinary incontinence. This was interpreted as **clonazepam** toxicity. The problems cleared when the **clonazepam** was stopped. The authors of the report suggest that the amiodarone may have inhibited the oxidative metabolism of the **clonazepam** by the liver, thereby allowing it to accumulate. They also point out that this patient may have been more sensitive to these effects because of a degree of hypothyroidism caused by the amiodarone. Hypothyroidism is known to decrease the metabolism of drugs which undergo oxidative metabolism by the liver.[1]

This is an unconfirmed and isolated case and of doubtful general importance. Bear this interaction in mind in the case of an unexpected response to treatment with clonazepam.

1. Witt DM, Ellsworth AJ, Leversee JH. Amiodarone–clonazepam interaction. *Ann Pharmacother* (1993) 27, 1463–4.

Benzodiazepines and related drugs + Antacids

Although antacids can moderately change the rate of absorption of chlordiazepoxide, clorazepate and diazepam, no adverse interaction of clinical importance has been reported.

Clinical evidence

In a three-period study 10 healthy subjects were given **clorazepate** 7.5 mg at night with either water, ***Maalox*** 30 ml, or ***Maalox*** 30 ml three times daily before meals. The mean steady-state serum levels of the active metabolite of clorazepate, desmethyldiazepam, were not affected by ***Maalox***, although they varied widely between individuals.[1] This is in line with another report,[2] but contrasts with a single-dose study, in which the peak plasma concentration of desmethyldiazepam was delayed and reduced by about one-third by the use of ***Maalox***. The 48-hour AUC was reduced by about 10%.[3]

The absorption of a single dose of **chlordiazepoxide** was delayed by ***Maalox***, though the total amount of drug absorbed was not significantly affected.[4] Similar results have been found with **diazepam** and aluminium hydroxide-containing antacids.[5] Another study found that 40 ml of **aluminium hydroxide gel BP** and 30 ml of **sodium citrate** (0.3 mmol/l) marginally hastened the sedative effect of **diazepam** 10 mg when used as an oral premedication before minor surgery. **Magnesium trisilicate mixture BPC** 30 ml tended to delay sedation.[6]

Mechanism

The delay in the absorption of chlordiazepoxide and diazepam is attributed to the effect of the antacid on gastric emptying. Clorazepate on the other hand is a prodrug, which needs acid conditions in the stomach for conversion by hydrolysis and decarboxylation to its active form. Antacids are presumed to inhibit this conversion by raising the pH of the stomach contents.[7]

Importance and management

Most of the reports describe single-dose studies, but what is known suggests that no adverse interaction of any clinical importance is likely during treatment with chlordiazepoxide, diazepam or clorazepate. Whether the delay in absorption has an undesirable effect in those who only take benzodiazepines during acute episodes of anxiety, and who need rapid relief is uncertain. Information about other benzodiazepines is lacking. However, no special precautions would seem to be necessary.

1. Shader RI, Ciraulo DA, Greenblatt DJ, Harmatz JS. Steady-state plasma desmethyldiazepam during long-term clorazepate use: effect of antacids. *Clin Pharmacol Ther* (1982) 31, 180–3.
2. Chun AHC, Carrigan PJ, Hoffman DJ, Kershner RP, Stuart JD. Effect of antacids on absorption of clorazepate. *Clin Pharmacol Ther* (1977) 22, 329–35.
3. Shader RI, Georgotas A, Greenblatt DJ, Harmatz JS, Allen MD. Impaired absorption of desmethyldiazepam from clorazepate by magnesium aluminum hydroxide. *Clin Pharmacol Ther* (1978) 24, 308–15.
4. Greenblatt DJ, Shader RI, Harmatz JS, Franke K, Koch-Weser J. Influence of magnesium and aluminum hydroxide mixture on chlordiazepoxide absorption. *Clin Pharmacol Ther* (1976) 19, 234–9.
5. Greenblatt DJ, Allen MD, MacLaughlin DS, Harmatz JS, Shader RI. Diazepam absorption: effect of antacids and food. *Clin Pharmacol Ther* (1978) 24, 600–9.

6. Nair SG, Gamble JAS, Dundee JW, Howard PJ. The influence of three antacids on the absorption and clinical action of oral diazepam. *Br J Anaesth* (1976) 48, 1175–80.
7. Abruzzo CW, Macasieb T, Weinfeld R, Rider JA, Kaplan SA. Changes in the oral absorption characteristics in man of dipotassium clorazepate at normal and elevated gastric *p*H. *J Pharmacokinet Biopharm* (1977) 5, 377–90.

Benzodiazepines + Anticholinesterases; Centrally acting

Diazepam does not appear to affect the pharmacokinetics of tacrine or rivastigmine.

Clinical evidence, mechanism, importance and management

In a small study a single 2-mg dose of diazepam did not affect the pharmacokinetics of **tacrine** 20 mg every 6 hours when compared with subjects not taking diazepam.[1] Similarly the makers of **rivastigmine** say that no pharmacokinetic interaction has been seen with diazepam in healthy subjects.[2,3] No special precautions would seem necessary if diazepam is given with **tacrine** or **rivastigmine**.

1. deVries TM, Siedlik P, Smithers JA, Brown RR, Reece PA, Posvar EL, Sedman AJ, Koup JR, Forgue ST. Effect of multiple-dose tacrine administration on single-dose pharmacokinetics of digoxin, diazepam, and theophylline. *Pharm Res* (1993) 10 (10 Suppl), S-333.
2. Exelon (Rivastigmine). Novartis Pharmaceuticals UK Ltd. UK Summary of product characteristics, June 2003.
3. Elexon (Rivastigmine). Novartis. US Prescribing information, October 2004.

Benzodiazepines + Anticonvulsants; Carbamazepine

The use of benzodiazepines with carbamazepine is common, although some evidence suggests that the effects of the benzodiazepines are sometimes reduced, and in the case of midazolam almost abolished. Single-dose studies have shown that the sedative effects of zopiclone and carbamazepine are additive, however it has been predicted that when taken long-term carbamazepine will reduce the effects of zopiclone.

Clinical evidence and mechanism

(a) Alprazolam

A patient with atypical bipolar disorder and panic attacks, given alprazolam 7.5 mg daily, had a reduction of more than 50% in plasma alprazolam levels, from 43 to 19.3 nanograms/ml, when given carbamazepine. This was accompanied by a deterioration in his clinical condition, which was controlled with haloperidol.[1]

(b) Clobazam

Carbamazepine reduces the plasma levels of clobazam and increases the levels of norclobazam (the principal metabolite).[2] Similarly, a reduction in steady-state clobazam levels with a rise in norclobazam levels is described in another study in 6 healthy subjects taking carbamazepine.[3] A 66-year-old man on carbamazepine and topiramate experienced fatigue, ataxia, impairment of gait and clumsiness while taking clobazam 10 mg daily. His symptoms resolved when the clobazam was stopped. When he was later given carbamazepine, topiramate, and clobazam 20 mg daily his carbamazepine level rose from 36.8 to 41.9 micromol/l. The carbamazepine level returned to 35.5 micromol/l 5 days after the clobazam was stopped.[4]

(c) Clonazepam

Clonazepam, in slowly increasing doses up to a maximum of 4 to 6 mg/day given over a 6-week period, had no effect carbamazepine serum levels. Some patients were also taking phenobarbital.[5] A study in 7 healthy subjects found that carbamazepine 200 mg daily given over a 3-week period reduced the plasma levels of clonazepam 1 mg daily from a range of 4 to 7 nanograms/ml down to 2.5 to 4 nanograms/ml, and reduced the half-life by about a third.[6] A retrospective analysis of the this interaction in 183 patients found that clonazepam clearance was increased by 22% and carbamazepine clearance was decreased by 20.5% by concurrent use.[7]

(d) Diazepam

A study found that the plasma clearance of a single 10-mg intravenous dose of diazepam was threefold greater, and the half-life shorter in a group of 9 epileptics when compared to 6 healthy subjects. Seven of the epileptics were taking carbamazepine.[8]

(e) Midazolam

The pharmacokinetics and pharmacodynamics of a single 15-mg oral dose of midazolam was studied in 6 epileptic patients taking either carbamazepine, phenytoin or both drugs together, and in 7 control subjects not taking either anticonvulsant. The AUC of midazolam in the epileptics was reduced to 5.7%, and the peak serum levels to 7.4% of the value in the control subjects. The pharmacodynamic effects of the midazolam (subjective drowsiness, body sway with eyes closed and open, as well as more formal tests) were also reduced. Most of the epileptics did not notice any effects from taking midazolam, while the control subjects were clearly sedated for 2 to 4 hours and also experienced amnesia after taking the midazolam.[9]

(f) Zopiclone

A double-blind crossover trial in 12 healthy subjects given a single 7.5-mg dose of zopiclone and carbamazepine 600 mg found only minor changes in the plasma levels of both drugs. Zopiclone levels were higher and carbamazepine levels slightly lower. Psychomotor tests confirmed that both drugs had sedative effects, which were additive, and in a simulated driving test it was found that co-ordination was impaired and reaction times prolonged.[10] However, there do not appear to be any multiple-dose studies. The prediction is that because carbamazepine is a strong inducer of the cytochrome P450 isoenzyme CYP3A4 (by which zopiclone is metabolised) the effect of chronic carbamazepine treatment would be a reduction in zopiclone serum levels and hypnotic effects.[11]

Importance and management

The midazolam and possibly alprazolam interactions with carbamazepine appear to be of greatest clinical significance. Much larger doses of midazolam are likely to be needed in the presence of carbamazepine. An alternative sedative may be needed. **Triazolam** is predicted to interact like midazolam.[9]

Since norclobazam retains some of the activity of clobazam the effects of carbamazepine probably have little clinical significance, and the case of carbamazepine toxicity appears to be isolated and is therefore probably of limited importance.

The pharmacokinetic changes seen with clonazepam seem likely to be too small to be clinically significant, but this needs confirmation.

The evidence for an interaction between zopiclone and carbamazepine is slim, and the effects of long-term use unclear. However, it would seem prudent to be alert for the need to increase the zopiclone dosage in patients taking carbamazepine. More study of this potential interaction is needed.

1. Arana GW, Epstein S, Molloy M, Greenblatt DJ. Carbamazepine-induced reduction of plasma alprazolam concentrations: a clinical case report. *J Clin Psychiatry* (1988) 49, 448–9.
2. Bun H, Monjanel-Mouterde S, Noel F, Durand A, Cano J-P. Effects of age and antiepileptic drugs on plasma levels and kinetics of clobazam and N-desmethylclobazam. *Pharmacol Toxicol* (1990) 67, 136–40.
3. Levy RH, Lane EA, Guyot M, Brachet-Liermain A, Cenraud B, Loiseau P. Analysis of parent drug-metabolite relationship in the presence of an inducer: application to the carbamazepine-clobazam interaction in normal man. *Drug Metab Dispos* (1983) 11, 286–92.
4. Genton P, Nguyen VH, Mesdjian E. Carbamazepine intoxication with negative myoclonus after the addition of clobazam. *Epilepsia* (1998) 39, 1115–1118.
5. Johannessen SI, Strandjord RE, Munthe-Kaas AW. Lack of effect of clonazepam on serum levels of diphenylhydantoin, phenobarbital and carbamazepine. *Acta Neurol Scand* (1977) 55, 506–12.
6. Lai AA, Levy RH, Cutler RE. Time-course of interaction between carbamazepine and clonazepam in normal man. *Clin Pharmacol Ther* (1978) 24, 316–23.
7. Yukawa E, Nonaka T, Yukawa M, Ohdo S, Higuchi S, Kuroda T, Goto Y. Pharmacoepidemiologic investigation of a clonazepam-carbamazepine interaction by mixed effect modeling using routine clinical pharmacokinetic data in Japanese patients. *J Clin Psychopharmacol* (2001) 21, 588–93.
8. Dhillon S, Richens A. Pharmacokinetics of diazepam in epileptic patients and normal volunteers following intravenous administration. *Br J Clin Pharmacol* (1981) 12, 841–4.
9. Backman JT, Olkkola KT, Ojala M, Laaksovirta H, Neuvonen PJ. Concentrations and effects of oral midazolam are greatly reduced in patients treated with carbamazepine or phenytoin. *Epilepsia* (1996) 37, 253–7.
10. Kuitunen T, Mattila MJ, Seppälä T, Aranko K, Mattila ME. Actions of zopiclone and carbamazepine, alone and in combination, on human skilled performance in laboratory and clinical tests. *Br J Clin Pharmacol* (1990) 30, 453–61.
11. Villikka K, Kivistö KT, Lamberg TS, Kantola T, Neuvonen PJ. Concentrations and effects of zopiclone are greatly reduced by rifampicin. *Br J Clin Pharmacol* (1997) 43, 471–4.

Benzodiazepines and related drugs + Anticonvulsants; Miscellaneous

The use of benzodiazepines with anticonvulsants is common and possibly accompanied by some changes in serum levels, which are

normally of limited clinical importance. However, isolated interactions have been reported between chlordiazepoxide or clobazam and phenobarbital; clonazepam and lamotrigine or primidone; and clorazepate and primidone.

Clinical evidence

(a) Chlordiazepoxide

A single case report describes a man given **phenobarbital** and chlordiazepoxide who became drowsy, unsteady, and developed slurred speech, nystagmus, poor memory and hallucinations, all of which disappeared once the **phenobarbital** was withdrawn and the chlordiazepoxide dose reduced from 80 to 60 mg daily, which was well-tolerated.[1]

(b) Clobazam

Phenobarbital slightly reduces the levels of both clobazam and its active metabolite, norclobazam.[2]

A retrospective study compared norclobazam level/dose ratios in patients taking clobazam and enzyme-inducing antiepileptic treatment, without **felbamate** (group B, 28 patients) or with **felbamate** (group C, 16 patients). When compared with 22 patients (group A) receiving clobazam alone or with non-enzyme-inducing antiepileptics the norclobazam level/dose ratio of group B was increased twofold and the group C was increased fivefold.[3]

(c) Clonazepam

Clonazepam, in slowly increasing doses up to a maximum of 4 to 6 mg daily, given over a 6-week period to patients on **phenobarbital** with or without carbamazepine, had no effect on **phenobarbital** levels.[4] A study found that **phenobarbital** caused some small changes in the pharmacokinetics of a single dose of clonazepam but only the small increase in clearance was statistically significant.[5]

The plasma clonazepam levels fell by about 38% in 4 of 8 patients when they were given **lamotrigine**.[6]

An analysis of serum levels of anticonvulsants in children found that those taking clonazepam had markedly higher concentrations of **primidone**, and toxicity was seen.[7]

No significant changes in the pharmacokinetics of clonazepam 1 mg every 12 hours occurred in 18 healthy subjects when they were given **felbamate** 1200 mg every 12 hours for 10 days.[8] No serious adverse reactions were seen.

(d) Clorazepate

A report suggested that the concurrent use of **primidone** and clorazepate may have been responsible for the development of irritability, aggression and depression in 6 of 8 patients.[9]

(e) Diazepam

Phenobarbital 100 mg daily for 8 days had no effect on the metabolism of diazepam in a group of healthy subjects.[10] Some modest additive CNS depression may possibly be expected, but the authors of this report make no comment about this.

(f) Triazolam

Studies in healthy subjects have excluded any pharmacodynamic interaction between **tiagabine** and triazolam.[11]

Mechanism

Uncertain. Changes in the drug metabolism in some cases or simple additive effects in others seem likely. It has been suggested that felbamate inhibits the clearance of norclobazam.[3]

Importance and management

None of the interactions between the benzodiazepines and anticonvulsants described here appear to be of major clinical importance, with the possible exception of the clobazam/felbamate interaction. Bear in mind the possibility of additive sedative or other adverse effects in patients given both drugs. This may also be possible in some rare cases with chlordiazepoxide or clobazam with phenobarbital; clonazepam with lamotrigine or primidone; and clorazepate with primidone.

1. Kane FJ, McCurdy RL. An unusual reaction to combined Librium-barbiturate therapy. *Am J Psychiatry* (1964) 120, 816.
2. Bun H, Monjanel-Mouterde S, Noel F, Durand A, Cano J-P. Effects of age and antiepileptic drugs on plasma levels and kinetics of clobazam and N-desmethylclobazam. *Pharmacol Toxicol* (1990) 67, 136–40.
3. Contin M, Riva R, Albani F, Baruzzi A. Effect of felbamate on clobazam and its metabolite kinetics in patients with epilepsy. *Ther Drug Monit* (1999) 21, 604–8.
4. Johannessen SI, Strandjord RE, Munthe-Kaas AW. Lack of effect of clonazepam on serum levels of diphenylhydantoin, phenobarbital and carbamazepine. *Acta Neurol Scand* (1977) 55, 506–12.
5. Khoo K-C, Mendels J, Rothbart M, Garland WA, Colburn WA, Min BH, Lucek R, Carbone JJ, Boxen baum HG, Kaplan SA. Influence of phenytoin and phenobarbital on the disposition of a single oral dose of clonazepam. *Clin Pharmacol Ther* (1980) 28, 368–75.
6. Eriksson A-S, Hoppu K, Nergårdh A, Boreus L. Pharmacokinetic interactions between lamotrigine and other antiepileptic drugs in children with intractable epilepsy. *Epilepsia* (1996) 37, 769–73.
7. Windorfer A, Sauer W. Drug interactions during anticonvulsant therapy in childhood: diphenylhydantoin, primidone, phenobarbitone, clonazepam, nitrazepam, carbamazepin and dipropylacetate. *Neuropadiatrie* (1977) 8, 29–41.
8. Colucci R, Glue P, Banfield C, Reidenberg P, Meehan J, Radwanski E, Korduba C, Lin C, Dogterom P, Ebels T, Hendricks G, Jonkman JHG, Affrime M. Effect of felbamate on the pharmacokinetics of clonazepam. *Am J Ther* (1996) 3, 294–7.
9. Feldman RG. Chlorazepate in temporal lobe epilepsy. *JAMA* (1976) 236, 2603.
10. Brockmeyer N, Dylewicz P, Habicht H, Ohnhaus EE. The metabolism of diazepam following different enzyme inducing agents. *Br J Clin Pharmacol* (1985) 19. 544P.
11. Richens A, Marshall RW, Dirach J, Jansen JA, Snel S, Pedersen PC. Absence of interaction between tiagabine, a new antiepileptic drug, and the benzodiazepine triazolam. *Drug Metabol Drug Interact* (1998) 14, 159–77.

Benzodiazepines + Anticonvulsants; Phenytoin

Reports are inconsistent: benzodiazepines can cause serum phenytoin levels to rise (toxicity has been seen), fall, or remain unaltered. In addition phenytoin may cause clonazepam, diazepam, midazolam and oxazepam serum levels to fall.

Clinical evidence

(a) Phenytoin levels increased

The observation that toxicity developed in patients on phenytoin when they were given **chlordiazepoxide** or **diazepam** prompted a more detailed study. The serum phenytoin levels of 25 patients taking phenytoin 300 or 400 mg daily and **chlordiazepoxide** or **diazepam** were 80 to 90% higher than those of 99 subjects taking phenytoin without a benzodiazepine.[1]

Further reports attribute increased phenytoin serum levels and phenytoin toxicity to **diazepam**,[2-4] **clobazam**,[5] **clonazepam**,[6-9] and **chlordiazepoxide**.[10]

(b) Phenytoin levels decreased

The serum phenytoin levels of 12 patients fell by about 30% over a 2-month period while they were taking **clonazepam** 1.5 to 12 mg daily. When data from another 12 patients were combined, the mean fall was only 18%.[11] Other studies describe similar findings with **clonazepam**[7,12] and **diazepam**.[13,14]

(c) Phenytoin levels unchanged

In one study **alprazolam** did not affect the serum phenytoin levels of a group of healthy subjects.[15] **Clonazepam** did not alter serum phenytoin levels in one study,[16] and another concluded it produced no predictable change in phenytoin levels.[7]

(d) Benzodiazepine levels reduced

A study in 5 patients given phenytoin 250 to 400 mg daily found that serum **clonazepam** levels were reduced by more than 50%,[17] and another study found that phenytoin decreased the clearance of **clonazepam** by about 50%.[18] In a further study phenytoin reduced the plasma levels of **clobazam** and increased the levels of norclobazam (the principal metabolite).[19]

Diazepam[20] and **oxazepam**[21] may be similarly affected in epileptic patients given phenytoin.

The pharmacokinetics and pharmacodynamics of a single 15-mg oral dose of **midazolam** was studied in 6 epileptic patients taking either carbamazepine, phenytoin or both drugs together, and in 7 control subjects not taking either of these anticonvulsants. The AUC of **midazolam** in the epileptics was reduced to 5.7%, and the peak serum levels to 7.4% of their value in the control subjects. The pharmacodynamic effects (subjective drowsiness, body sway with eyes closed and open, as well as more formal tests) were also reduced. Most of the epileptics did not notice any effects of the **midazolam**, while the control subjects were clearly sedated for 2 to 4 hours after taking the **midazolam** and also experienced amnesia.[22]

Mechanism

The inconsistency of these reports is not understood. Benzodiazepine-induced changes in the metabolism of phenytoin[2,4,10,14] as well as alterations in the apparent volume of distribution have been suggested as possible mechanisms. Enzyme induction by phenytoin may possibly account for the fall in serum benzodiazepine levels.

Importance and management

A confusing picture. Concurrent use certainly need not be avoided (it has proved to be valuable in many cases) but monitor the outcome of concurrent use and consider monitoring serum phenytoin levels so that undesirable changes can be detected. Only diazepam, chlordiazepoxide and clonazepam have been implicated, but it seems possible that other benzodiazepines could also interact.

1. Vajda FJE, Prineas RJ, Lovell RRH. Interaction between phenytoin and the benzodiazepines. *Lancet* (1971) i, 346.
2. Rogers HJ, Haslam RA, Longstreth J, Lietman PS. Phenytoin intoxication during concurrent diazepam therapy. *J Neurol Neurosurg Psychiatry* (1977) 40, 890–5.
3. Kariks J, Perry SW, Wood D. Serum folic acid and phenytoin levels in permanently hospitalized patients receiving anticonvulsant therapy. *Med J Aust* (1971) 2, 368–71.
4. Murphy A, Wilbur K. Phenytion–diazepam interaction. *Ann Pharmacother* (2003) 37, 659–63.
5. Zifkin B, Sherwin A, Andermann F. Phenytoin toxicity due to interaction with clobazam. *Neurology* (1991) 41, 313–14.
6. Eeg-Olofsson O. Experiences with Rivotril in treatment of epilepsy — particularly minor motor epilepsy — in mentally retarded children. *Acta Neurol Scand* (1973) 49 (Suppl 53), 29–31.
7. Huang CY, McLeod JG, Sampson D, Hensley WJ. Clonazepam in the treatment of epilepsy. *Med J Aust* (1974) 2, 5–8.
8. Janz D, Schneider H. Bericht über Wodadiboff II (Workshop on the determination of antiepileptic drugs in body fluids). In 'Antiepileptische Langzeitmedikation'. *Bibl Psychiatr* (1975) 151, 55–7.
9. Windorfer A, Sauer W. Drug interactions during anticonvulsant therapy in childhood: diphenylhydantoin, primidone, phenobarbitone, clonazepam, nitrazepam, carbamazepin and dipropylacetate. *Neuropadiatrie* (1977) 8, 29–41.
10. Kutt H, McDowell F. Management of epilepsy with diphenylhydantoin sodium. *JAMA* (1968) 203, 969–72.
11. Edwards VE, Eadie MJ. Clonazepam — a clinical study of its effectiveness as an anticonvulsant. *Proc Aust Assoc Neurol* (1973) 10, 61–6.
12. Saavedra IN, Aguilera LI, Faure E, Galdames DG. Case report. Phenytoin/clonazepam interaction. *Ther Drug Monit* (1985) 7, 481–4.
13. Siris JH, Pippenger CE, Werner WL, Masland RL. Anticonvulsant drug-serum levels in psychiatric patients with seizure disorders. *N Y State J Med* (1974) 74, 1554–6.
14. Houghton GW, Richens A. The effect of benzodiazepines and pheneturide on phenytoin metabolism in man. *Br J Clin Pharmacol* (1974) 1, P344–P345.
15. Patrias JM, DiPiro JT, Cheung RPF, Townsend RJ. Effect of alprazolam on phenytoin pharmacokinetics. *Drug Intell Clin Pharm* (1987) 21, 2A.
16. Johannessen SI, Strandjord RE, Munthe-Kaas AW. Lack of effect of clonazepam on serum levels of diphenylhydantoin, phenobarbital and carbamazepine. *Acta Neurol Scand* (1977) 55, 506–12.
17. Sjö O, Hvidberg EF, Naestoft J, Lund M. Pharmacokinetics and side-effects of clonazepam and its 7-amino metabolite in man. *Eur J Clin Pharmacol* (1975) 8, 249–54.
18. Khoo K-C, Mendels J, Rothbart M, Garland WA, Colburn WA, Min BH, Lucek R, Carbone JJ, Boxen baum HG, Kaplan SA. Influence of phenytoin and phenobarbital on the disposition of a single oral dose of clonazepam. *Clin Pharmacol Ther* (1980) 28, 368–75.
19. Bun H, Monjanel-Mouterde S, Noel F, Durand A, Cano J-P. Effects of age and antiepileptic drugs on plasma levels and kinetics of clobazam and N-desmethylclobazam. *Pharmacol Toxicol* (1990) 67, 136–40.
20. Hepner GW, Vesell ES, Lipton A, Harvey HA, Wilkinson GR, Schenker S. Disposition of aminopyrine, antipyrine, diazepam, and indocyanine green in patients with liver disease or on anticonvulsant therapy: diazepam breath test and correlations in drug elimination. *J Lab Clin Med* (1977) 90, 440–56.
21. Scott AK, Khir ASM, Steele WH, Hawksworth GM, Petrie JC. Oxazepam pharmacokinetics in patients with epilepsy treated long-term with phenytoin alone or in combination with phenobarbitone. *Br J Clin Pharmacol* (1983) 16, 441–4.
22. Backman JT, Olkkola KT, Ojala M, Laaksovirta H, Neuvonen PJ. Concentrations and effects of oral midazolam are greatly reduced in patients treated with carbamazepine or phenytoin. *Epilepsia* (1996) 37, 253–7.

Benzodiazepines + Anticonvulsants; Valproate

Valproate appears to increase the serum levels of diazepam, lorazepam, while clobazam appears to raise valproate levels. Increased adverse effects have been seen when clonazepam is used with valproate and an isolated case describes sleepwalking in a patient taking valproate and zolpidem.

Clinical evidence

(a) Clobazam

In one study sodium valproate was reported to have no marked effect on clobazam,[1] but a study in children found that clobazam caused an 11% increase in the serum levels of sodium valproate, despite a reduction of at least 10% in valproate dosage.[2]

(b) Clonazepam

The addition of clonazepam to sodium valproate increased the unwanted effects (drowsiness, absence status) in 9 out of 12 paediatric and adolescent patients.[3]

(c) Diazepam

Sodium valproate increased the serum levels of free diazepam twofold in 6 healthy subjects.[4]

(d) Lorazepam

Lorazepam 1 mg every 12 hours for 3 days had no effect on the pharmacokinetics of valproate semisodium 500 mg every 12 hours in healthy subjects. However, valproate semisodium increased the AUC and maximum serum levels of lorazepam by 20 and 8% respectively. Sedation scores were not affected by concurrent treatment, suggesting that the interaction is not clinically significant.[5]

A 40% decrease in the clearance of a 2-mg intravenous bolus dose of lorazepam was seen in 6 out of 8 healthy subjects while they were taking sodium valproate 250 mg twice daily.[6]

A woman on valproate, phenytoin, and carbamazepine went into a coma after she received a total of 6 mg of intravenous lorazepam. She promptly recovered on stopping the valproate.[7]

(e) Zolpidem

A report describes sleepwalking in a patient when sodium valproate 250 mg twice daily was added to treatment with zolpidem 5 mg at night and citalopram 30 mg daily. The patient stopped the valproate and the sleepwalking episodes resolved. Later, the valproate was restarted causing the sleepwalking to recur. This time the symptoms resolved when the zolpidem was stopped.[8]

Mechanism

It seems that sodium valproate reduces the glucuronidation of lorazepam,[5,6] and therefore benzodiazepines that are similarly metabolised are also likely to be affected.

Importance and management

It has been suggested that the combination of clonazepam and sodium valproate should be avoided.[3] However, a very brief letter points out that neither drug affects the serum concentrations of the other and that clonazepam and valproic acid can be given together in patients with absence seizures since some patients have an excellent response to the combination.[9]

It has been recommended that if clobazam is added to sodium valproate it would be prudent to monitor for any increases in valproate serum levels.[2]

Enhanced sedation has been briefly described during the concurrent use of sodium valproate and other unnamed benzodiazepines.[10]

1. Bun H, Monjanel-Mouterde S, Noel F, Durand A, Cano J-P. Effects of age and antiepileptic drugs on plasma levels and kinetics of clobazam and N-desmethylclobazam. *Pharmacol Toxicol* (1990) 67, 136–40.
2. Theis JGW, Koren G, Daneman R, Sherwin AL, Menzano E, Cortez M, Hwang P. Interactions of clobazam with conventional antiepileptics in children. *J Child Neurol* (1997) 12, 208–13.
3. Jeavons PM, Clark JE, Maheshwari MC. Treatment of generalized epilepsies of childhood and adolescence with sodium valproate ('Epilim'). *Dev Med Child Neurol* (1977) 19, 9–25.
4. Dhillon S, Richens A. Valproic acid and diazepam interaction *in vivo*. *Br J Clin Pharmacol* (1982) 13, 553–60.
5. Samara EE, Granneman RG, Witt GF, Cavanaugh JH. Effect of valproate on the pharmacokinetics and pharmacodynamics of lorazepam. *J Clin Pharmacol* (1997) 37, 442–50.
6. Anderson GD, Gidal BE, Kantor ED, Wilensky AJ. Lorazepam-valproate interaction: studies in normal subjects and isolated perfused rat liver. *Epilepsia* (1994) 35, 221–5.
7. Lee S-A, Lee JK, Heo K. Coma probably induced by lorazepam–valproate interaction. *Seizure* (2002) 11, 124–5.
8. Sattar SP, Ramaswamy S, Bhatia SC, Petty F. Somnambulism due to probable interaction of valproic acid and zolpidem. *Ann Pharmacother* (2003) 37, 1429–33.
9. Browne TR. Interaction between clonazepam and sodium valproate. *N Engl J Med* (1979) 300, 679.
10. Völzke E, Doose H. Dipropylacetate (Dépakine®, Ergenyl®) in the treatment of epilepsy. *Epilepsia* (1973) 14, 185–93

Benzodiazepines + Antipsychotics

Marked respiratory depression has been reported in three patients when they were given lorazepam with loxapine, and neuroleptic malignant syndrome has been reported in another three patients on benzodiazepines and antipsychotics. Additive sedative effects appear to occur with zaleplon, zolpidem or zopiclone and some antipsychotics.

Clinical evidence, mechanism, importance and management

(a) Lorazepam

A woman with a manic bipolar affective disorder was admitted to hospital and given lorazepam 2 mg with **loxapine** 25 mg. After 2 hours she was found to be lethargic with sonorous respirations, occasional episodes of apnoea and an irregular respiration as low as 4 breaths per minute. She was given oxygen and recovered spontaneously within 12 hours. She had experienced no previous problems with lorazepam, and had none when it was later given while she was taking perphenazine.[1] Two other cases have been reported where patients given intramuscular lorazepam 1 to 2 mg and oral **loxapine** 50 mg developed prolonged stupor, a significantly lowered respiration rate (8 breaths per minute), and in one case hypotension. Both showed signs of recovery within 3 to 5 hours. Both had taken each of these drugs alone without problems.[2]

(b) Other benzodiazepines

Three cases of neuroleptic malignant syndrome have been reported following the use of **diazepam** with **risperidone**, **clorazepate** with **zuclopenthixol** and **tiapride** with **clonazepam**. In 2 cases this followed the abrupt withdrawal of long-term benzodiazepines. All 3 patients recovered, one without any treatment.[3] These reports are isolated and unexplained. There is no clear reason for avoiding concurrent use, but it should be well monitored.

(c) Zaleplon

A single 50-mg dose of **thioridazine**[4] had no effect on the pharmacokinetics of zaleplon 20 mg, and the psychomotor tests showed only short term additive effects lasting 1 to 4 hours. These short-term CNS additive effects are small and unlikely to be clinically relevant, and so there would seem to be no reason for avoiding concurrent use.

(d) Zolpidem

Single-dose studies found that the pharmacokinetics of 20-mg doses of zolpidem were unaffected by 50 mg of **chlorpromazine**[5,6] or 2 mg of **haloperidol**.[5] The pharmacokinetics of both of these antipsychotics were unaffected by zolpidem, except that in one study the elimination half-life of **chlorpromazine** was increased from about 5 to 8 hours.[6] **Chlorpromazine** increased the sedative effects of zolpidem (as indicated by impaired performances of manual dexterity and Stroop's tests).[5,6] It seems likely that additive sedation will be seen with other sedative drugs.

(e) Zopiclone

No pharmacokinetic interaction was found when 12 healthy subjects were given a single 7.5-mg oral dose of zopiclone with **chlorpromazine** 50 mg. However, the overall performance in a number of psychomotor tests (including digit symbol substitution and simulated driving) was definitely impaired more by the combination of the drugs than by **chlorpromazine** alone. Zopiclone with **chlorpromazine** impaired memory and learning, and caused a marked impairment of the performance of the tests.[7] In practical terms this means that patients given **chlorpromazine** with either of these drugs should be warned that they will almost certainly feel drowsy and be less able to drive or handle potentially hazardous machinery safely.

1. Cohen S, Khan A. Respiratory distress with the use of lorazepam in mania. *J Clin Psychopharmacol* (1987) 7, 199–200.
2. Battaglia J, Thornton L, Young C. Loxapine-lorazepam-induced hypotension and stupor. *J Clin Psychopharmacol* (1989) 9, 227–8.
3. Bobolakis I. Neuroleptic malignant syndrome after antipsychotic drug administration during benzodiazepine withdrawal. *J Clin Psychopharmacol* (2000) 20, 281–3.
4. Hetta J, Broman J-E, Darwish M, Troy SM. Psychomotor effects of zaleplon and thioridazine coadministration. *Eur J Clin Pharmacol* (2000) 56, 211–17.
5. Sauvanet JP, Langer SZ Morselli PL, eds. Imidazopyridines in Sleep Disorders. New York: Raven Press; 1988 p. 165–73.
6. Desager JP, Hulhoven R, Harvengt C, Hermann P, Guillet P, Thiercelin JF. Possible interactions between zolpidem, a new sleep inducer and chlorpromazine, a phenothiazine neuroleptic. *Psychopharmacology (Berl)* (1988) 96, 63–6.
7. Mattila MJ, Vanakoski J, Matilla-Evenden ME, Karonen S-L. Suriclone enhances the actions of chlorpromazine on human psychomotor performance but not on memory or plasma prolactin in healthy subjects. *Eur J Clin Pharmacol* (1994) 46, 215–20.

Benzodiazepines + Aprepitant

Standard clinical doses of aprepitant inhibit the metabolism of midazolam.

Clinical evidence

In a randomised study 16 healthy subjects took either aprepitant 125 mg on day 1 followed by 80 mg daily for 4 days, or 40 mg on day 1 followed by 25 mg daily for 4 days, with a single 2-mg dose of midazolam on days 1 and 5. The aprepitant 40/25 mg dosing schedule had no significant effect on the pharmacokinetics of midazolam. However, the aprepitant 125/80 mg dosing schedule increased the AUC of midazolam by 126% and 229% on days 1 and 5 respectively, and increased the maximum plasma levels of midazolam by 46% and 94% on days 1 and 5 respectively.[1]

Mechanism

Aprepitant inhibits the cytochrome P450 isoenzyme CYP3A4 by which midazolam is metabolised, resulting in increased midazolam levels.

Importance and management

Based on the way midazolam interacts with similarly potent inhibitors of CYP3A4, aprepitant may be expected to increased the drowsiness and length of sedation and amnesia in patients given midazolam. Consider reducing the midazolam dose in patients given aprepitant and monitor the outcome of concurrent use carefully.

1. Majumdar AK, McCrea JB, Panebianco DL, Hesney M, Dru J, Constanzer M, Goldberg MR, Murphy G, Gottesdiener KM, Lines CR, Petty KJ, Blum RA. Effects of aprepitant on cytochrome P450 3A4 activity using midazolam as a probe. *Clin Pharmacol Ther* (2003) 74, 150–6.

Benzodiazepines and related drugs + Atropine or Hyoscine

Atropine and hyoscine do not affect the absorption or the sedative effects of diazepam but atropine may slow the absorption of zopiclone.

Clinical evidence, mechanism, importance and management

(a) Diazepam

A study in 8 healthy subjects given single 10-mg oral doses of diazepam showed that serum diazepam levels were not significantly changed by the concurrent use of atropine 1 mg or hyoscine hydrobromide 1 mg, nor were the sedative effects of the diazepam altered.[1]

(b) Zopiclone

The absorption of a single 7.5-mg dose of zopiclone was reduced by atropine 600 micrograms given intravenously to 12 healthy subjects. Mean plasma zopiclone levels at 1 hour were reduced from 22.7 to 6.5 nanograms/ml and at 2 hours reduced from 49.3 to 31.9 nanograms/ml by atropine. This was presumably due to altered gut motility.[2] The clinical importance of these findings is not known.

1. Gregoretti SM, Uges DRA. Influence of oral atropine or hyoscine on the absorption of oral diazepam. *Br J Anaesth* (1982) 54, 1231–4.
2. Elliott P, Chestnutt WN, Elwood RJ, Dundee JW. Effect of atropine and metoclopramide on the plasma concentrations of orally administered zopiclone. *Br J Anaesth* (1983) 55, 1159P–1160P.

Benzodiazepines and related drugs + Azoles

Fluconazole, itraconazole and ketoconazole very markedly increase the serum levels of oral midazolam and triazolam, thereby increasing and prolonging their sedative and amnesic effects. Similar but smaller effects are seen with alprazolam and itraconazole or ketoconazole, brotizolam with itraconazole, and zolpidem with ketoconazole. Even less effect is seen with etizolam or zopiclone and itraconazole. No important interaction occurs between bromazepam and fluconazole, estazolam and itraconazole, temazepam and itraconazole, zolpidem and fluconazole and probably chlordiazepoxide and ketoconazole.

Clinical evidence

(a) Alprazolam

(i) Itraconazole. A single 800-microgram dose of alprazolam was given to 10 healthy subjects before and after a 6-day course of itraconazole 200 mg daily. The itraconazole increased the AUC and the half-life of alprazolam nearly threefold, and psychomotor function was impaired.[1]

(ii) Ketoconazole. A study in healthy subjects found that ketoconazole 200 mg twice daily decreased the clearance of alprazolam 1 mg by about two-thirds, and prolonged its half-life fourfold, but the maximum serum levels remained unchanged.[2]

(b) Bromazepam

Fluconazole 100 mg daily for 4 days had no effect on the pharmacokinetics or pharmacodynamics of bromazepam in 12 healthy subjects.[3]

(c) Brotizolam

A double blind, placebo-controlled study in 10 healthy subjects found that **itraconazole** 200 mg daily for 4 days increased the 0 to 24-hour AUC, and maximum plasma levels of a single 500-microgram dose of brotizolam given on day 4 by about 2.5-fold and 25% respectively. The elimination half life of brotizolam was also increased, from 4.51 to 23.27 hours, and sedation was increased.[4]

(d) Chlordiazepoxide

After taking **ketoconazole** 400 mg daily for 5 days the clearance of chlordiazepoxide 600 micrograms/kg was decreased by 38% in 12 healthy subjects.[5]

(e) Estazolam

A placebo-controlled study[6] found that **itraconazole** 100 mg daily for 7 days did not affect the pharmacokinetics or pharmacodynamic effects of a single 4-mg dose of estazolam given to 10 healthy subjects on day 4.

(f) Etizolam

A double blind, placebo-controlled study in healthy subjects found that **itraconazole** 100 mg twice daily for 7 days increased the AUC of a single 1-mg dose of etizolam given on day 6 by about 50%. The elimination half life of etizolam was also increased, from 12 to 17.3 hours.[7]

(g) Midazolam

(i) Fluconazole. A study in 12 healthy subjects found that fluconazole 200 mg daily for 5 days reduced the clearance of a single 7.5-mg oral dose of midazolam by 51%, and increased the AUC midazolam 3.5-fold. It was found that the subjects could hardly be wakened during the first hour after taking the midazolam.[8] Another study found that a single 150-mg dose of fluconazole increased the serum levels of a single 10-mg dose of midazolam by about 30%.[9] Yet another study found that the route of administration of the fluconazole (i.e. whether oral or intravenous) made little or no difference to the pharmacodynamic effects of midazolam.[10] Fluconazole caused a fourfold increase in plasma midazolam levels in intensive care unit patients, stabilised on midazolam infusions. The interaction was most marked in patients with renal failure.[11] These reports contrast with another, which found that fluconazole 150 mg only slightly increased the effects of a single 10-mg dose of midazolam.[12]

(ii) Itraconazole. When 9 healthy subjects were given oral midazolam 7.5 mg, before and after taking itraconazole 200 mg daily for 4 days, the itraconazole was found to have increased the midazolam AUC about tenfold, increased the peak plasma levels about threefold, and prolonged the half-life from 2.8 to 7.9 hours. The subjects could hardly be wakened during the first hour after taking the midazolam and most of them experienced amnesia lasting several hours.[13] A later study found that itraconazole 100 mg daily for 4 days increased the midazolam AUC sixfold and the peak plasma levels 2.5-fold.[14] A further study confirmed the marked effect of both itraconazole on oral midazolam, but found that the effects of bolus doses of intravenous midazolam were not increased to a clinically significant extent, although their results suggested that long-term high doses infusions of midazolam need to be titrated according to effect to avoid overdosage.[8]

(iii) Ketoconazole. When 9 healthy subjects were given oral midazolam 7.5 mg before and after taking ketoconazole 400 mg daily for 4 days, the ketoconazole was found to have increased the midazolam AUC from 3.9 to 62 micrograms.ml^{-1}.min, increased the peak plasma levels about fourfold, and prolonged the half-life from 2.8 to 8.7 hours. The subjects could hardly be wakened during the first hour after taking the midazolam and most of them experienced amnesia lasting several hours.[13] Ketoconazole has been shown to reduce the metabolism of midazolam and greatly prolong its effects in another study.[15]

(h) Temazepam

Itraconazole 200 mg daily was given to 10 healthy subjects for 4 days, with a single 20-mg dose of temazepam on day 4. A very small increase in the temazepam AUC was seen, but the psychomotor tests carried out were unchanged.[16]

(i) Triazolam

(i) Fluconazole. Eight healthy subjects were given fluconazole or a placebo daily for 4 days. On day 4 they were also given a single 250-microgram oral dose of triazolam. The triazolam AUCs were increased 1.6-, 2.1- and 4.4-fold by 50, 100 and 200 mg fluconazole respectively, and the maximum plasma triazolam levels were more than doubled by the 200-mg fluconazole dose. The 100- and 200-mg fluconazole doses both produced significant changes in the psychomotor tests of triazolam, but the 50-mg dose did not.[17]

(ii) Itraconazole. The AUC of a single 250-microgram dose of triazolam was increased from 5.9 to 160 nanograms.ml^{-1}.h after 9 healthy subjects were given itraconazole 200 mg daily for 4 days. Peak plasma levels were increased threefold. Marked changes in psychomotor and other responses were seen. The subjects had amnesia and were still very tired and confused as long as 17 hours after taking the triazolam.[18] Another study found that the interaction persists for several days after taking the itraconazole.[19]

(iii) Ketoconazole. A study in healthy subjects [number not stated] found that when they were given triazolam 125 micrograms, preceded by ketoconazole 200 mg taken 17 and 1 hour before, the triazolam half-life was prolonged (from 4 to almost 18 hours in one subject) and the clearance was increased ninefold. Pharmacodynamic testing found an increase in the impairment of a digit-symbol substitution test, and increased effects on EEG beta activity.[20] The AUC of a single 250-microgram dose of triazolam was increased from 5.9 to 132 nanograms.ml^{-1}.hour by ketoconazole 400 mg daily for 4 days. Peak plasma levels were increased threefold. Marked changes in psychomotor and other responses were seen. The subjects had amnesia and were still very tired and confused as long as 17 hours after taking the triazolam.[18] Another study similarly found that ketoconazole inhibited the metabolism of triazolam leading to an increase in its sedative effects.[21]

(j) Zolpidem

(i) Fluconazole. In a placebo-controlled study in healthy subjects[22] itraconazole 100 mg twice daily for 2 days had no significant effect on the pharmacokinetics of a single 5-mg dose of zolpidem given with the third dose of fluconazole.

(ii) Itraconazole. Itraconazole 200 mg daily or a placebo was given to 10 healthy subjects for 4 days. On day 4 they were also given a single 10-mg oral dose of zolpidem. The mean peak serum levels of the zolpidem were increased by 12.5% and the AUC was increased by 35%, but the performance of a number of psychomotor tests (digit symbol substitution, critical flicker fusion, subjective drowsiness, postural sway) remained unaltered.[23] Another study similarly found that itraconazole did not interact significantly with zolpidem.[22]

(iii) Ketoconazole. A study in 12 healthy subjects found that following three 200-mg doses of ketoconazole given every 12 hours, the AUC of zolpidem 5 mg was increased 1.7-fold and the subjects were more sedated, as shown by the digit symbol substitution test.[22]

(k) Zopiclone

Itraconazole 200 mg daily or a placebo was given to 10 healthy young subjects for 4 days. On day 4 they were also given a single 7.5-mg oral dose of zopiclone. The **itraconazole** increased the maximum plasma levels of the zopiclone by 29% (from 49 to 63 nanograms/ml), increased its AUC by 73% and prolonged its half-life from 5 to 7 hours. But despite these increases, there were no statistical or clinical differences between the performance of the psychomotor tests carried out during the placebo and **itraconazole** phases of the study.[24]

Mechanism

Itraconazole, ketoconazole, and to a lesser extent fluconazole are potent inhibitors of the cytochrome P450 isoenzyme CYP3A4. The benzodiazepines, zopiclone and zolpidem are, to varying degrees, metabolised by CYP3A4, with the extent of the interaction related to how significant CYP3A4 is in their metabolism. So, for example midazolam, which is predominantly metabolised by CYP3A4 is greatly affected, whereas CYP3A4 is only a minor metabolic route in the metabolism of diazepam, so it is only slightly affected. Other isoenzymes are also involved in the metabolism of zopiclone and zolpidem so they are only moderately affected. The azoles inhibit CYP3A4 in the liver (hence intravenous benzodiazepines can be affected) but studies have also suggested that ketoconazole inhibits the CYP3A4-mediated metabolism of midazolam[15] and triazolam[21] in the gut wall, which explains why oral benzodiazepines are most affected.

Ketoconazole appears to inhibit the oxidation of chlordiazepoxide by the liver.[5]

Importance and management

The interactions between midazolam or triazolam and itraconazole or ketoconazole are established and clinically important. In very broad terms the dosage of midazolam would need to be reduced by about 75% or more in the presence of these antifungals to avoid excessive sedation, and even then the effects would still be expected to be prolonged. Unless appropriate precautions are taken (very reduced dosages) these interactions can be dangerous. Patients taking itraconazole or ketoconazole are unlikely to be able to drive (for example) for at least 6 hours after receiving midazolam. Patients should also be warned about the likelihood of increased sedation. There is some evidence that bolus doses of intravenous midazolam given in the presence of itraconazole or fluconazole are not increased to a clinically significant degree, and normal doses can be used.[14] However, where high doses of intravenous midazolam are used long term (e.g. during intensive care treatment) it has been suggested that the dosage will need to be titrated to avoid long-lasting hypnotic effects.[8] These precautions are equally applicable to triazolam with itraconazole or ketoconazole and midazolam with ketoconazole. Fluconazole interacts less significantly but even so, the midazolam or triazolam dosage probably needs to be reduced, possibly by as much as half.

The effects of alprazolam and brotizolam are increased and prolonged by ketoconazole and itraconazole, but the extent of this is less than that seen with midazolam or triazolam. However, some dosage reductions may still be necessary.

The effects of itraconazole on temazepam or zopiclone and ketoconazole on zolpidem are small and seem unlikely to be clinically significant in most patients. Nevertheless be aware that there is some possibility of an interaction.

1. Yasui N, Kondo T, Otani K, Furukori H, Kaneko S, Ohkubo T, Nagasaki T, Sugawara K. Effect of itraconazole on the single oral dose pharmacokinetics and pharmacodynamics of alprazolam. *Psychopharmacology (Berl)* (1998) 139, 269–73.
2. Greenblatt DJ, Wright CE, von Moltke LL, Harmatz JS, Ehrenberg BL, Harrel LM, Corbett K, Counihan M, Tobias S, Shader RI. Ketoconazole inhibition of triazolam and alprazolam clearance: differential kinetic and dynamic consequences. *Clin Pharmacol Ther* (1998) 64, 237–47.
3. Ohtani Y, Kotegawa T, Tsutsumi K, Morimoto T, Hirose Y, Nakano S. Effect of fluconazole on the pharmacokinetics and pharmacodynamics of oral and rectal bromazepam: an application of electroencephalography as the pharmacodynamic method. *J Clin Pharmacol* (2002) 42, 183–91.
4. Osanai T, Ohkubo T, Yasui N, Kondo T, Kaneko S. Effect of itraconazole on the pharmacokinetics and pharmacodynamics of a single dose of brotizolam. *Br J Clin Pharmacol* (2004) 58, 476–81.
5. Brown MW, Maldonado AL, Meredith CG, Speeg KV. Effect of ketoconazole on hepatic oxidative drug metabolism. *Clin Pharmacol Ther* (1985) 37, 290–7.
6. Otsuji Y, Okuyama N, Aoshima T, Fukasawa T, Kato K, Gerstenberg G, Miura M, Ohkubo T, Sugawara K, Otani K. No effect of itraconazole on the single oral dose pharmacokinetics and pharmacodynamics of estazolam. *Ther Drug Monit* (2002) 24, 375–8.
7. Araki K, Yasui-Furukori N, Fukasawa T, Aoshima T, Suzuki A, Inoue Y, Tateishi T, Otani K. Inhibition of the metabolism of etizolam by itraconazole in humans: evidence for the involvement of CYP3A4 in etizolam metabolism. *Eur J Clin Pharmacol* (2004) 60, 427–30.
8. Olkkola KT, Ahonen J, Neuvonen PJ. The effect of the systemic antimycotics, itraconazole and fluconazole, on the pharmacokinetics and pharmacodynamics of intravenous and oral midazolam. *Anesth Analg* (1996) 82, 511–16.
9. Mattila MJ, Vainio P, Vanakoski J. Fluconazole moderately increases midazolam effects on performance. *Br J Clin Pharmacol* (1995) 39, 567P.
10. Ahonen J, Olkkola KT, Neuvonen PJ. Effect of route of administration of fluconazole on the interaction between fluconazole and midazolam. *Eur J Clin Pharmacol* (1997) 51, 415–19.
11. Ahonen J, Olkkola KT, Takala A, Neuvonen PJ. Interaction between fluconazole and midazolam in intensive care patients. *Acta Anaesthesiol Scand* (1999) 43, 509–14.
12. Vanakoski J, Mattila MJ, Vainio P, Idänpään-Heikkilä JJ, Törnwall M. 150 mg fluconazole does not substantially increase the effects of 10 mg midazolam or the plasma midazolam concentrations in healthy subjects. *Int J Clin Pharmacol Ther* (1995) 33, 518–23.
13. Olkkola KT, Backman JT, Neuvonen PJ. Midazolam should be avoided in patients receiving systemic antimycotics ketoconazole or itraconazole. *Clin Pharmacol Ther* (1994) 55, 481–5.
14. Ahonen J, Olkkola KT, Neuvonen PJ. Effect of itraconazole and terbinafine on the pharmacokinetics and pharmacodynamics of midazolam in healthy volunteers. *Br J Clin Pharmacol* (1995) 40, 270–2.
15. Lam YWF, Alfaro CL, Ereshefsky L, Miller M. Pharmacokinetic and pharmacodynamic interactions of oral midazolam with ketoconazole, fluoxetine, fluvoxamine, and nefazodone. *J Clin Pharmacol* (2003) 43, 1274–82.
16. Ahonen J, Olkkola KT, Neuvonen PJ. Lack of effect of antimycotic itraconazole on the pharmacokinetics or pharmacodynamics of temazepam. *Ther Drug Monit* (1996) 18, 124–7.
17. Varhe A, Olkkola KT, Neuvonen PJ. Effect of fluconazole dose on the extent of fluconazole-triazolam interaction. *Br J Clin Pharmacol* (1996) 42, 465–70.
18. Varhe A, Olkkola KT, Neuvonen PJ. Oral triazolam is potentially hazardous to patients receiving systemic antimycotics ketoconazole or itraconazole. *Clin Pharmacol Ther* (1994) 56, 601–7.
19. Neuvonen PJ, Varhe A, Olkkola KT. The effect of ingestion time interval on the interaction between itraconazole and triazolam. *Clin Pharmacol Ther* (1996) 60, 326–31.
20. Greenblatt DJ, von Moltke LL, Harmatz JS, Harrel LM, Tobias S, Shader RI, Wright CE. Interaction of triazolam and ketoconazole. *Lancet* (1995) 345, 191.
21. von Moltke LL, Greenblatt DJ, Harmatz JS, Duan SX, Harrel LM, Cotreau-Bibbo MM, Pritchard GA, Wright CE, Shader RI. Triazolam biotransformation by human liver microsomes *in vitro*: effects of metabolic inhibitors and clinical confirmation of a predicted interaction with ketoconazole. *J Pharmacol Exp Ther* (1996) 276, 370–9.
22. Greenblatt DJ, von Moltke LL, Harmatz JS, Mertzanis P, Graf JA, Durol ALB, Counihan M, Roth-Schechter B, Shader RI. Kinetic and dynamic interaction study of zolpidem with ketoconazole, itraconazole, and fluconazole. *Clin Pharmacol Ther* (1998) 64, 661–71.
23. Luurila H, Kivistö KT, Neuvonen PJ. Effect of itraconazole on the pharmacokinetics and pharmacodynamics of zolpidem. *Eur J Clin Pharmacol* (1998) 54, 163–6.
24. Jalava K-M, Olkkola KT, Neuvonen PJ. Effect of itraconazole on the pharmacokinetics and pharmacodynamics of zopiclone. *Eur J Clin Pharmacol* (1996) 51, 331–4.

Benzodiazepines and related drugs + Beta-blockers

Only small and clinically unimportant pharmacokinetic interactions occur between most benzodiazepines and beta-blockers, but there is some evidence that patients on diazepam may possibly be more accident-prone while taking metoprolol, and an isolated report describes marked bradycardia in an elderly woman on propranolol when she started to take clomethiazole.

Clinical evidence, mechanism, importance and management

No significant pharmacokinetic interaction occurs between **alprazolam** and **propranolol**;[1] between **clorazepate** and **propranolol**;[2] between **diazepam** and **atenolol**[3] or **propranolol**;[3] between **lorazepam** and **metoprolol**[4] or **propranolol**;[1] or between **oxazepam** and **labetalol**[5] or **propranolol**.[5]

However, moderate changes, which seem unlikely to be clinically significant were found between **diazepam** and **propranolol** (diazepam clearance reduced by 17%)[1] or **metoprolol** (diazepam clearance reduced by 18%,[6] AUC increased by 25%[3]); and between **bromazepam** and **metoprolol** (**bromazepam** AUC increased by 35%)[4] or **propranolol** (**bromazepam** half-life increased by 22%).[7]

Studies of psychomotor performance have shown that simple reaction times with **oxazepam** combined with either **propranolol** or **labetalol** are increased,[5] and those taking **diazepam** and **metoprolol** have a reduced kinetic visual acuity,[3,8] which is related to driving ability.[9] Moreover, choice reaction times at 2 hours were also found to be lengthened when taking **diazepam** and **metoprolol**, **propranolol** or **atenolol** but at 8 hours they only persisted with **diazepam** and **metoprolol**.[8]

An 84-year-old woman taking **propranolol** 40 mg twice daily for hypertension underwent skin grafting. Her pulse was stable (54 to 64 bpm) until the thirteenth day after the operation when she took two oral doses of **clomethiazole** 192 mg, 9 hours apart. Three hours after taking the second dose her heart rate fell to 43 bpm with a PR interval of 0.24 seconds, and by 5 hours after the dose her pulse rate was down to 36 bpm. Her pulse had risen to 70 bpm twelve hours after stopping both drugs, and had restabilised 2 days later at about 60 bpm with a PR interval of 0.2 seconds. At this time the **propranolol** was restarted, with haloperidol.[10]

Information about interactions between the benzodiazepines and beta-blockers is very limited indeed. The current evidence does not seem to justify any additional caution, but bear this interaction in mind in the case of an unexpected response to treatment. The interaction between **propranolol** and **clomethiazole** appears to be an isolated case and therefore probably of limited clinical significance.

1. Ochs HR, Greenblatt DJ, Verburg-Ochs B. Propranolol interactions with diazepam, lorazepam, and alprazolam. *Clin Pharmacol Ther* (1984) 36, 451–5.
2. Ochs HR, Greenblatt DJ, Locniskar A, Weinbrenner J. Influence of propranolol coadministration or cigarette smoking on the kinetics of desmethyldiazepam following intravenous clorazepate. *Klin Wochenschr* (1986) 64, 1217–21.
3. Hawksworth G, Betts T, Crowe A, Knight R, Nyemitei-Addo I, Parry K, Petrie JC, Raffle A, Parsons A. Diazepam/β-adrenoceptor antagonist interactions. *Br J Clin Pharmacol* (1984) 17, 69S–76S.
4. Scott AK, Cameron GA, Hawksworth GM. Interaction of metoprolol with lorazepam and bromazepam. *Eur J Clin Pharmacol* (1991) 40, 405–9.
5. Sonne J, Døssing M, Loft S, Olesen KL, Vollmer-Larsen A, Victor MA, Hamberg O, Thyssen H. Single dose pharmacokinetics and pharmacodynamics of oral oxazepam during concomitant administration of propranolol and labetalol. *Br J Clin Pharmacol* (1990) 29, 33–7.
6. Klotz U, Reimann IW. Pharmacokinetic and pharmacodynamic interaction study of diazepam and metoprolol. *Eur J Clin Pharmacol* (1984) 26, 223–6.
7. Ochs HR, Greenblatt DJ, Friedman H, Burstein ES, Locniskar A, Harmatz JS, Shader RI. Bromazepam pharmacokinetics: influence of age, gender, oral contraceptives, cimetidine, and propranolol. *Clin Pharmacol Ther* (1987) 41, 562–70.
8. Betts TA, Crowe A, Knight R, Raffle A, Parsons A, Blake A, Hawksworth G, Petrie JC. Is there a clinically relevant interaction between diazepam and lipophilic β-blocking drugs? *Drugs* (1983) 25 (Suppl 2), 279–80.

9. Betts TA, Knight R, Crowe A, Blake A, Harvey P, Mortiboy D. Effect of β-blockers on psychomotor performance in normal volunteers. *Eur J Clin Pharmacol* (1985) 28 (Suppl), 39–49.
10. Adverse Drug Reactions Advisory Committee. Chlormethiazole/propranolol interaction? *Med J Aust* (1979) 2, 553.

Benzodiazepines + Buspirone

No adverse interaction appears to occur if buspirone and alprazolam are given together. When buspirone is used with diazepam the adverse effects appear to be mild and short-lived.

Clinical evidence, mechanism, importance and management

Alprazolam 1 mg every 8 hours, given to 12 healthy subjects with buspirone 10 mg every 8 hours caused a 7% and 8% increase in the maximum plasma levels and AUC of **alprazolam** respectively. The maximum plasma levels of buspirone were not altered, but the AUC of buspirone was increased by 29%. However, these changes were within the normal pharmacokinetic variability of these drugs. No unexpected adverse effects were seen.[1]

Buspirone 15 mg every 8 hours had no effect on plasma levels of **diazepam** 5 mg daily given to 12 healthy subjects for 10 days, but the levels of the metabolite nordiazepam were raised by about 20%. All subjects experienced some mild adverse effects (headache, nausea, dizziness, and in two cases muscle twitching). These symptoms subsided after a few days.[2]

There would seem to be no reason for avoiding the concurrent use of benzodiazepines and buspirone.

1. Buch AB, Van Harken DR, Seidehamel RJ, Barbhaiya RH. A study of pharmacokinetic interaction between buspirone and alprazolam at steady state. *J Clin Pharmacol* (1993) 33, 1104–9.
2. Gammans RE, Mayol RF, Labudde JA. Metabolism and disposition of buspirone. *Am J Med* (1986) 80 (Suppl 3B), 41–51.

Benzodiazepines + Calcium channel blockers

The serum levels and effects of midazolam are markedly increased by diltiazem or verapamil. This also occurs with triazolam and diltiazem, and is predicted to occur with triazolam and verapamil. There appear to be no significant interactions between diazepam and diltiazem, felodipine or nimodipine; between midazolam and nitrendipine; between temazepam and diltiazem; or between triazolam and isradipine.

Clinical evidence

(a) Diazepam

(i) Diltiazem. When single doses of diazepam 5 mg and diltiazem 60 mg were given to 6 subjects it was found that the plasma levels of each drug were not significantly altered by the presence of the other drug.[1] In another study, poor and extensive metabolisers of the cytochrome P450 isoenzyme CYP2C19 (see 'Genetic factors', (p.4)) were given diltiazem 200 mg daily for 3 days before and 7 days after a single 2-mg dose of diazepam. It was found that there were no differences in the interaction between the phenotypes, and both groups showed an increase in the AUC and half-life of diazepam. However, the clinical effects of the pharmacokinetic changes were not assessed.[2]

(ii) Felodipine. The pharmacokinetics of a 10-mg intravenous dose of diazepam were unchanged in 12 healthy subjects after they took felodipine 10 mg daily for 12 days but the AUC and peak serum levels of the diazepam metabolite, desmethyldiazepam were raised by 14 and 16% respectively.[3]

(iii) Nimodipine. The serum levels of diazepam 10 mg daily and nimodipine 30 mg three times daily were unaffected by concurrent use in 24 healthy, elderly subjects, and no clinically relevant changes in haemodynamics, ECG recordings, clinical chemistry or haematology occurred.[4]

(b) Midazolam

(i) Diltiazem. After taking diltiazem 60 mg three times daily for 2 days, 9 healthy female subjects were given midazolam 15 mg orally. The AUC of midazolam was increased fourfold, the maximum serum levels doubled, and the half-life increased by 49%. It was almost impossible for the subjects to stay awake for 90 minutes after taking the midazolam. They suffered several hours of amnesia and there was a marked decrease in the performance of pharmacodynamic tests (digit symbol substitution, Maddox wing test).[5] Diltiazem 60 mg, given to 15 patients 2 hours before induction of anaesthesia with midazolam and alfentanil, increased the AUC and half-life of midazolam by 15 and 43% respectively. Tracheal extubation was performed on average 2.5 hours later than in another group given a placebo instead of diltiazem.[6]

(ii) Lercanidipine. Midazolam appears to increase the absorption of lercanidipine by 40%. The clinical relevance of this interaction is as yet unclear.[7]

(iii) Nitrendipine. A study in 9 healthy subjects found that the pharmacokinetics and pharmacodynamics of midazolam were unaffected by a single 20-mg dose of nitrendipine.[8]

(iv) Verapamil. After taking verapamil 80 mg three times daily for 2 days, 9 healthy female subjects were given midazolam 15 mg orally. The AUC of the midazolam was increased threefold, the maximum serum levels were doubled, and the half-life increased by 41%. It was almost impossible for the subjects to stay awake for 90 minutes after taking the midazolam. They suffered several hours of amnesia and there was a marked decrease in the performance of pharmacodynamic tests (digit symbol substitution, Maddox wing test).[5]

(c) Temazepam

Diltiazem 40 mg had no little or no effect on the hypnotic effects of temazepam in 16 healthy insomniacs.[9]

(d) Triazolam

(i) Diltiazem. A study in 7 healthy subjects found that diltiazem 60 mg three times daily for 3 days increased the AUC of a single 250-microgram dose of triazolam 2.3-fold and almost doubled its peak serum levels. Pharmacodynamic tests showed an increase in the sedative effects of triazolam.[10] Yet another study in 10 healthy subjects found that diltiazem 60 mg three times daily for 2 days increased the AUC of a single 250-microgram dose of triazolam 3.4-fold, and approximately doubled its maximum plasma level and half-life. The pharmacodynamic changes were briefly described as profound and prolonged.[11] In contrast diltiazem 40 mg was found to have little or no effect on the hypnotic effects of triazolam in 16 healthy insomniacs in another study.[9]

(ii) Isradipine

Isradipine 5 mg daily reduced the AUC of a single 250-microgram dose of triazolam by 20% in 9 healthy subjects, but no difference in the pharmacodynamic effects of triazolam were seen.[12]

Mechanism

The evidence suggests that diltiazem and verapamil inhibit the metabolism of midazolam and triazolam by the cytochrome P450 isoenzyme CYP3A4, leading to increased serum levels and increased effects.

Importance and management

The interactions between midazolam and diltiazem, midazolam and verapamil, and triazolam and diltiazem are established and clinically important. The authors of one report say that patients on either of these calcium channel blockers are probably incapable of doing skilled tasks (e.g. car driving) for up to 6 hours after taking midazolam 15 mg, and possibly even after 8 to 10 hours. They suggest that the usual dose of midazolam should be reduced at least 50% to avoid unnecessary deep sleep and prolonged hypnosis, and they also point out that since the half-life of the midazolam is prolonged, the effects will persist regardless of the dose.[5] The same seems likely to be true for triazolam and diltiazem, and the interaction is also predicted to occur with triazolam and verapamil.[11] No special precautions appear to be necessary with diazepam and diltiazem, diazepam and felodipine, diazepam and nimodipine, midazolam and nitrendipine, triazolam and isradipine, or temazepam and diltiazem.

1. Etoh A, Kohno K. Studies on the drug interaction of diltiazem. IV. Relationship between first pass metabolism of various drugs and the absorption enhancing effect of diltiazem. *Yakugaku Zasshi* (1983) 103, 581–8.
2. Kosuge K, Jun Y, Watanabe H, Kimura M, Nishimoto M, Ishizaki T, Ohashi K. Effects of CYP3A4 inhibition by diltiazem on pharmacokinetics and dynamics of diazepam in relation to CYP2C19 genotype status. *Drug Metab Dispos* (2001) 29, 1284–9.
3. Meyer BH, Müller FO, Hundt HKL, Luus HG, de la Rey N, Röthig H-J. The effects of felodipine on the pharmacokinetics of diazepam. *Int J Clin Pharmacol Ther Toxicol* (1992) 30, 117–21.
4. Heine PR, Weyer G, Breuel H-P, Mück W, Schmage N, Kuhlmann J. Lack of interaction between diazepam and nimodipine during chronic oral administration to healthy elderly subjects. *Br J Clin Pharmacol* (1994) 38, 39–43.

5. Backman JT, Olkkola KT, Aranko K, Himberg J-J, Neuvonen PJ. Dose of midazolam should be reduced during diltiazem and verapamil treatments. *Br J Clin Pharmacol* (1994) 37, 221–5.
6. Ahonen J, Olkkola KT, Salmenperä M, Hynynen M, Neuvonen PJ. Effect of diltiazem on midazolam and alfentanil disposition in patients undergoing coronary artery bypass grafting. *Anesthesiology* (1996) 85, 1246–52.
7. Zanidip (Lercanidipine hydrochloride). Napp Pharmaceuticals Ltd. UK Summary of product characteristics, January 2004.
8. Handel J, Ziegler G, Gemeinhardt A, Stuber H, Fischer C, Klotz U. Lack of effect of nitrendipine on the pharmacokinetics and pharmacodynamics of midazolam during steady state. *Br J Clin Pharmacol* (1988) 25, 243–50.
9. Scharf MB, Sachais BA, Mayleben DW, Jennings SW. The effects of a calcium channel blocker on the effects of temazepam and triazolam. *Curr Ther Res* (1990) 48, 516–23.
10. Kosuge K, Nishimoto M, Kimura M, Umemura K, Nakashima M, Ohashi K. Enhanced effect of triazolam with diltiazem. *Br J Clin Pharmacol* (1997) 43, 367–72.
11. Varhe A, Olkkola KT, Neuvonen PJ. Diltiazem enhances the effects of triazolam by inhibiting its metabolism. *Clin Pharmacol Ther* (1996) 59, 369–75.
12. Backman JT, Wang J-S, Wen X, Kivistö KT, Neuvonen PJ. Mibefradil but not isradipine substantially elevates the plasma concentrations of the CYP3A4 substrate triazolam. *Clin Pharmacol Ther* (1999) 66, 401–7.

Benzodiazepines + Colestyramine and Neomycin

The clearance of lorazepam is increased by colestyramine plus neomycin.

Clinical evidence, mechanism, importance and management

A study in 7 healthy subjects found that neomycin 1 g every 6 hours plus colestyramine 4 g every 4 hours reduced the half-life of oral **lorazepam** from 15.8 to 11.7 hours, and increased the clearance of free **lorazepam** by 34%.[1] The reasons for these changes are not clear but parallel studies using intravenous **lorazepam**[1] suggested that neomycin and colestyramine may interfere with the possible enterohepatic circulation of **lorazepam**.

The clinical importance of this interaction is uncertain but probably small. Other benzodiazepines do not appear to have been studied.

1. Herman RJ, Duc Van Pham J, Szakacs CBN. Disposition of lorazepam in human beings: enterohepatic recirculation and first-pass effect. *Clin Pharmacol Ther* (1989) 46, 18–25.

Benzodiazepines + Disulfiram

An isolated report describes temazepam toxicity due to disulfiram. The serum levels of chlordiazepoxide and diazepam are increased by the use of disulfiram and some patients may possibly experience increased drowsiness. Alprazolam, oxazepam and lorazepam are either not affected, or only minimally affected, by disulfiram.

Clinical evidence

A man taking disulfiram 200 mg daily developed confusion, drowsiness, slurred speech and an unsteady gait within a few days of starting to take **temazepam** 20 mg at night. This was interpreted as **temazepam** toxicity. The symptoms disappeared when both drugs were stopped.[1]

After taking disulfiram 500 mg daily for 14 to 16 days, the plasma clearance of single doses of **chlordiazepoxide** and **diazepam** were reduced by 54 and 41% respectively, and the half-lives were increased by 84 and 37% respectively. The plasma levels of **chlordiazepoxide** were approximately doubled. **Oxazepam** was also given following disulfiram treatment but changes in **oxazepam** pharmacokinetics were minimal. The alcoholic subjects (without hepatic cirrhosis) and the healthy subjects interacted similarly.[2]

Other studies show that the pharmacokinetics of **lorazepam** and **alprazolam** are unaffected by disulfiram.[3,4]

Mechanism

Disulfiram inhibits the initial metabolism (*N*-demethylation and oxidation) of both chlordiazepoxide and diazepam by the liver so that an alternative but slower metabolic pathway is used. This results in the accumulation of these benzodiazepines in the body. In contrast, the metabolism (glucuronidation) of oxazepam and lorazepam is minimally affected by disulfiram so that their clearance from the body remains largely unaffected.[2,3]

Importance and management

There seems to be only one report (with temazepam) of a clinically significant interaction between disulfiram and the benzodiazepines, and this report is unconfirmed, as the patient did not take temazepam alone. The other reports only describe potential interactions that have been identified by single-dose studies. These do not necessarily reliably predict what will happen in practice. However, it seems possible that some patients will experience increased drowsiness, possibly because of this interaction, and because drowsiness is a very common adverse effect of disulfiram. Reduce the dosage of the benzodiazepine if necessary. Other benzodiazepines that are metabolised similarly may possibly interact in the same way (e.g. bromazepam, clonazepam, clorazepate, prazepam, ketazolam, clobazam, flurazepam, nitrazepam, medazepam, triazolam) but this needs confirmation. Alprazolam, oxazepam and lorazepam appear to be non-interacting alternatives.

1. Hardman M, Biniwale A, Clarke CE. Temazepam toxicity precipitated by disulfiram. *Lancet* (1994) 344, 1231–2.
2. MacLeod SM, Sellers EM, Giles HG, Billings BJ, Martin PR, Greenblatt DJ, Marshman JA. Interaction of disulfiram with benzodiazepines. *Clin Pharmacol Ther* (1978) 24, 583–9.
3. Sellers EM, Giles HG, Greenblatt DJ, Naranjo CA. Differential effects on benzodiazepine disposition by disulfiram and ethanol. *Arzneimittelforschung* (1980) 30, 882–6.
4. Diquet B, Gujadhur L, Lamiable D, Warot D, Hayoun H, Choisy H. Lack of interaction between disulfiram and alprazolam in alcoholic patients. *Eur J Clin Pharmacol* (1990) 38, 157–60.

Benzodiazepines and related drugs + Ethambutol

Ethambutol appears not to interact with diazepam.

Clinical evidence, mechanism, importance and management

A study in 6 patients, newly diagnosed as having tuberculosis and treated with ethambutol 25 mg/kg, found that although some of the pharmacokinetic parameters of **diazepam** were different to those obtained in healthy control subjects not receiving ethambutol, the changes were not significant.[1] There seems to be nothing in the literature to suggest that ethambutol interacts with other benzodiazepines.

1. Ochs HR, Greenblatt DJ, Roberts G-M, Dengler HJ. Diazepam interaction with antituberculosis drugs. *Clin Pharmacol Ther* (1981) 29, 671–8.

Benzodiazepines + Food

Food can delay and reduce the hypnotic effects of flunitrazepam and loprazolam.

Clinical evidence, mechanism, importance and management

A study in 2 groups of 8 subjects found that when they took single 2-mg doses of **flunitrazepam** or **loprazolam** 2 hours after an evening dinner (spaghetti, meat, salad, an apple and wine) and 1 hour before going to bed, the peak plasma levels of flunitrazepam and loprazolam were reduced by 63% and 41% respectively. The time to reach these levels were delayed by 2.5 and 3.6 hours respectively, and the absorption half-lives of the drugs were considerably prolonged.[1] It seems probable therefore that the onset of sleep with these benzodiazepines may be delayed by food.

1. Bareggi SR, Pirola R, Truci G, Leva S, Smirna S. Effect of after-dinner administration on the pharmacokinetics of oral flunitrazepam and loprazolam. *J Clin Pharmacol* (1988) 28, 371–5.

Benzodiazepines + Grapefruit juice

Grapefruit juice can increase the bioavailability of oral diazepam, midazolam and triazolam but there is evidence that this may be of little practical importance.

Clinical evidence

Grapefruit juice 200 ml was given to 8 healthy subjects followed 60 minutes later by 5 mg of **intravenous midazolam** or 15 minutes later by 15 mg of **oral midazolam**. The pharmacokinetics of the **intravenous midazolam** remained unchanged, but the AUC of the **oral midazolam** was increased by 52%, and its maximum plasma levels rose by 56%.

These changes were also reflected in the psychometric measurements made.[1]

A single oral 250-microgram dose of **triazolam** was given to 10 healthy subjects with either 250 ml grapefruit juice or water. The mean AUC of the **triazolam** was increased 1.5-fold by the grapefruit juice, the peak plasma levels were increased 1.3-fold, and the time when the plasma levels peaked was prolonged from 1.5 to 2.5 hours. A slight decrease in psychomotor performance occurred (more drowsiness and tiredness).[2] Another study of the interaction between **triazolam** and grapefruit juice found that the effects of the grapefruit juice were much more pronounced when multiple doses of grapefruit juice were given. The **triazolam** AUC and half-life was increased by about 50% and 6% when single doses of grapefruit juice were given, and by about 150% and 50% by multiple doses. The effect of grapefruit juice on psychomotor tests was also greater after multiple dosing.[3]

A large scale placebo-controlled study in a total of 120 healthy young medical students used psychomotor tests to measure the effect of benzodiazepines with and without grapefruit juice. Subjects were given **midazolam** 10 mg or **triazolam** 250 micrograms with 300 ml of grapefruit juice. Only a minor increase in the benzodiazepine effects occurred with grapefruit juice, and these effects were of little or no practical importance.[4]

A study in 8 healthy subjects found that 250 ml of grapefruit juice increased the AUC and maximum plasma levels of a single 5-mg oral dose of **diazepam** 3.2-fold and 1.5-fold respectively.[5]

Mechanism

The evidence suggests that grapefruit juice inhibits the metabolism of these benzodiazepines by the cytochrome P450 isoenzyme CYP3A4, so that more is left to enter the circulation.[1] See also 'Grapefruit juice', (p.11).

Importance and management

Established interactions. These increases in bioavailability might be expected to increase the extent of the sedation and amnesia due to these benzodiazepines but in young healthy adults (with midazolam and triazolam at least) this is apparently of little importance. The clinical effects of the interaction with diazepam appear not to have been investigated. What is not clear is whether other factors such as old age or liver cirrhosis might increase the effects. Information about other benzodiazepines appears, as yet, to be lacking.

1. Kupferschmidt HHT, Ha HR, Ziegler WH, Meier PJ, Krähenbühl S. Interaction between grapefruit juice and midazolam in humans. *Clin Pharmacol Ther* (1995) 58, 20–8.
2. Hukkinen SK, Varhe A, Olkkola KT, Neuvonen PJ. Plasma concentrations of triazolam are increased by concomitant ingestion of grapefruit juice. *Clin Pharmacol Ther* (1995) 58, 127–31.
3. Lilja JJ, Kivistö KT, Backman JT, Neuvonen PJ. Effect of grapefruit juice dose on grapefruit juice–triazolam interaction: repeated consumption prolongs triazolam half-life. *Eur J Clin Pharmacol* (2000) 56, 411–15.
4. Vanakoski J, Mattila MJ, Seppälä T. Grapefruit juice does not enhance the effects of midazolam and triazolam in man. *Eur J Clin Pharmacol* (1996) 50, 501–8.
5. Özdemir M, Aktan Y, Boydağ BS, Cingi MI, Musmul A. Interaction between grapefruit juice and diazepam in humans. *Eur J Drug Metab Pharmacokinet* (1998) 23, 55–9.

Benzodiazepines and related drugs + H_2-blockers

The serum levels of adinazolam, alprazolam, chlordiazepoxide, clobazam, clorazepate, diazepam, flurazepam, nitrazepam, triazolam, zaleplon, zolpidem (and probably halazepam and prazepam) are raised by cimetidine, but normally this appears to be of little or no clinical importance and only the occasional patient may experience an increase in the effects (sedation). Clotiazepam, lorazepam, lormetazepam, oxazepam and temazepam are not normally affected by cimetidine. Famotidine, nizatidine and ranitidine do not interact with most benzodiazepines, except possibly triazolam. The picture with midazolam is somewhat confused and increased sedation appears to occur with clomethiazole and cimetidine.

Clinical evidence

(a) Cimetidine

A combined serum level rise of 75% in **diazepam** and its active metabolite, desmethyldiazepam, was found in 10 patients who took cimetidine 300 mg four times daily for 2 weeks, but reaction times and other motor and intellectual tests remained unaffected.[1] Other reports describe a rise in the plasma levels and/or AUC of **diazepam** (associated with increased sedation in one report[2]) due to cimetidine,[3-9] and generalised incoordination has also been described in one individual.[10]

Cimetidine also raises the serum levels of **adinazolam**,[11] **alprazolam**,[12,13] **chlordiazepoxide**,[14] **clobazam**,[15] **clorazepate**,[16] **flurazepam**,[17] **nitrazepam**,[18] and **triazolam**,[12,13,19,20] reduces the clearance of **bromazepam**,[21] increases plasma levels of **zaleplon**[22] and slightly increases sleep duration with **zolpidem**.[23] Cimetidine reduces the clearance of **clomethiazole** and increases sleep duration from a range of 30 to 60 minutes up to at least 2 hours.[24]

Liver cirrhosis increases the effects of cimetidine on the loss of **chlordiazepoxide**.[25] Confusion has been reported in a 50-year-old man taking **clorazepate** when he was given cimetidine,[26] and increased sedation has been seen in some patients taking **adinazolam** and cimetidine.[11] Prolonged hypnosis in an elderly woman[27] and CNS toxicity (including lethargy and hallucinations)[28] in a 49-year-old woman have been attributed to an interaction between **triazolam** and cimetidine but this remains unconfirmed.

In contrast cimetidine does not normally interact with **clobazam**,[29] **clotiazepam**,[30] **lorazepam**,[17,31] **lormetazepam**,[32] **oxazepam**[17,31,33] or **temazepam**,[34,35] although prolonged post-operative sedation was seen in one patient given **oxazepam** and cimetidine.[36]

There is some controversy about whether or not **midazolam** is affected by cimetidine. An increase in sedation,[37,38] an increase in midazolam levels[38-40] and no pharmacokinetic interaction[41] have been reported with the combination.

(b) Famotidine

Famotidine does not interact with **bromazepam**,[42] **clorazepate**,[42] **chlordiazepoxide**,[42] **diazepam**[9,43,44] or **triazolam**.[42]

(c) Nizatidine

Nizatidine does not interact significantly with **diazepam**.[45-47]

(d) Ranitidine

Ranitidine does not interact significantly with **adinazolam**,[48] **clomethiazole**,[49] **diazepam**,[45,50,51] **lorazepam**,[51] or **temazepam**,[35,52] but it can modestly increase the bioavailability (by about 10 to 30%) of oral **triazolam**.[53,54] There is some controversy about whether or not **midazolam** is affected by ranitidine. Increases in sedation have been reported on a number of occasions,[37,39,52,55] but a lack of effect has also been documented.[40,41]

(e) Roxatidine

Roxatidine does not interact with **diazepam** or its active metabolite, desmethyldiazepam.[56]

Mechanism

Cimetidine inhibits the liver enzymes concerned with the metabolism of diazepam, alprazolam, chlordiazepoxide, clomethiazole, clorazepate, flurazepam, nitrazepam, triazolam and zaleplon. As a result their clearance from the body is reduced and their serum levels rise.

Lorazepam, oxazepam and temazepam are metabolised by a different metabolic pathway involving glucuronidation, which is not affected by cimetidine and so they do not usually interact.

Ranitidine, famotidine and nizatidine appear not to inhibit liver microsomal enzymes. There is some evidence that ranitidine increases the absorption of triazolam, and possibly other benzodiazepines, due to changes in gastric pH,[54] although it has been suggested that this effect is negligible.[20] Cimetidine has been said to similarly affect absorption.[3]

Importance and management

The interactions between the benzodiazepines and cimetidine are well documented (not all the references are listed here) but normally they appear to be of little clinical importance, although a few patients may be adversely affected (increased effects, drowsiness, etc.) and possibly this may be more common with clomethiazole. If symptoms occur in any patient on a benzodiazepine and cimetidine reduce the benzodiazepine dose, or alternatively use a non-interacting drug such as lorazepam, lormetazepam, oxazepam or temazepam. Ranitidine does not interact with diazepam or temazepam, and neither nizatidine, ranitidine nor famotidine would be expected to interact with other benzodiazepines that are metabolised similarly (see 'Mechanism' above), although the effects of oral triazolam are possibly very slightly increased. The situation with midazolam is unclear and so it would seem wise to be cautious when using any H_2-blocker with this drug.

1. Greenblatt DJ, Abernethy DR, Morse DS, Harmatz JS and Shader RI. Clinical importance of the interaction of diazepam and cimetidine. *Anesth Analg* (1986) 65, 176–80.
2. Klotz U, Reimann I. Delayed clearance of diazepam due to cimetidine. *N Engl J Med* (1980) 302, 1012–13.
3. McGowan WAW, Dundee JW. The effect of intravenous cimetidine on the absorption of orally administered diazepam and lorazepam. *Br J Clin Pharmacol* (1982) 14, 207–11.
4. Klotz U, Reimann I. Elevation of steady-state diazepam levels by cimetidine. *Clin Pharmacol Ther* (1981) 30, 513–17.
5. Gough PA, Curry SH, Araujo OE, Robinson JD, Dallman JJ. Influence of cimetidine on oral diazepam elimination with measurement of subsequent cognitive change. *Br J Clin Pharmacol* (1982) 14, 739–42.
6. Klotz U, Antilla V-J. Drug interactions with cimetidine: pharmacokinetic studies to evaluate its mechanism. *Naunyn Schmiedebergs Arch Pharmacol* (1980) 311, R77.
7. Bressler R, Carter D, Winters L. Enprostil, in contrast to cimetidine, does not affect diazepam pharmacokinetics. *Adv Therapy* (1988) 5, 306–12.
8. Lima DR, Santos RM, Werneck E, Andrade GN. Effect of orally administered misoprostol and cimetidine on the steady state pharmacokinetics of diazepam and nordiazepam in human volunteers. *Eur J Drug Metab Pharmacokinet* (1991) 16, 161–70.
9. Lockniskar A, Greenblatt DJ, Harmatz JS, Zinny MA, Shader RI. Interaction of diazepam with famotidine and cimetidine, two H_2-receptor antagonists. *J Clin Pharmacol* (1986) 26, 299–303.
10. Anon. Court warns on interaction of drugs. *Doctor* (1979) 9, 1.
11. Hulhoven R, Desager JP, Cox S, Harvengt C. Influence of repeated administration of cimetidine on the pharmacokinetics and pharmacodynamics of adinazolam in healthy subjects. *Eur J Clin Pharmacol* (1988) 35, 59–64.
12. Pourbaix S, Desager JP, Hulhoven R, Smith RB, Harvengt C. Pharmacokinetic consequences of long term coadministration of cimetidine and triazolobenzodiazepines, alprazolam and triazolam, in healthy subjects. *Int J Clin Pharmacol Ther Toxicol* (1985) 23, 447–51.
13. Abernethy DR, Greenblatt DJ, Divoll M, Moschitto LJ, Harmatz JS, Shader RI. Interaction of cimetidine with the triazolobenzodiazepines alprazolam and triazolam. *Psychopharmacology (Berl)* (1983) 80, 275–8.
14. Desmond PV, Patwardhan RV, Schenker S, Speeg KV. Cimetidine impairs elimination of chlordiazepoxide (Librium) in man. *Ann Intern Med* (1980) 93, 266–8.
15. Pullar T, Edwards D, Haigh JRM, Peaker S, Feeley MP. The effect of cimetidine on the single dose pharmacokinetics of oral clobazam and *N*-desmethylclobazam. *Br J Clin Pharmacol* (1987) 23, 317–21.
16. Divoll M, Abernethy DR, Greenblatt DJ. Cimetidine impairs drug oxidizing capacity in the elderly. *Clin Pharmacol Ther* (1982) 31, 218.
17. Greenblatt DJ, Abernethy DR, Koepke HH, Shader RI. Interaction of cimetidine with oxazepam, lorazepam, and flurazepam. *J Clin Pharmacol* (1984) 24, 187–93.
18. Ochs HR, Greenblatt DJ, Gugler R, Müntefering G, Locniskar A, Abernethy DR. Cimetidine impairs nitrazepam clearance. *Clin Pharmacol Ther* (1983) 34, 227–30.
19. Friedman H, Greenblatt DJ, Burstein ES, Scavone JM, Harmatz JS, Shader RI. Triazolam kinetics: interaction with cimetidine, propranolol, and the combination. *J Clin Pharmacol* (1988) 28, 228–33.
20. Cox SR, Kroboth PD, Anderson PH, Smith RB. Mechanism for the interaction between triazolam and cimetidine. *Biopharm Drug Dispos* (1986) 7, 567–75.
21. Ochs HR, Greenblatt DJ, Friedman H, Burstein ES, Locniskar A, Harmatz JS, Shader RI. Bromazepam pharmacokinetics: influence of age, gender, oral contraceptives, cimetidine and propranolol. *Clin Pharmacol Ther* (1987) 41, 562–70.
22. Darwish M. Analysis of potential drug interactions with zaleplon. *J Am Geriatr Soc* (1999) 47, S62.
23. Hulhoven R, Desager JP, Harvengt C, Herman P, Guillet P, Thiercelin JF. Lack of interaction between zolpidem and H_2 antagonists, cimetidine and ranitidine. *Int J Clin Pharmacol Res* (1988) 8, 471–6.
24. Shaw G, Bury RW, Mashford ML, Breen KJ, Desmond PV. Cimetidine impairs the elimination of chlormethiazole. *Eur J Clin Pharmacol* (1981) 21, 83–5.
25. Nelson DC, Schenker S, Hoyumpa AM, Speeg KV, Avant GR. The effects of cimetidine on chlordiazepoxide elimination in cirrhosis. *Clin Res* (1981) 29, 824A.
26. Bouden A, El Hechmi Z, Douki S. Cimetidine-benzodiazepine association confusiogene: a propros d'une observation. *Tunis Med* (1990) 68, 63–4.
27. Parker WA, MacLachlan RA. Prolonged hypnotic response to triazolam-cimetidine combination in an elderly patient. *Drug Intell Clin Pharm* (1984) 18, 980–1.
28. Britton ML, Waller ES. Central nervous system toxicity associated with concurrent use of triazolam and cimetidine. *Drug Intell Clin Pharm* (1985) 19, 666–8.
29. Grigoleit H-G, Hajdú P, Hundt HKL, Koeppen D, Malerczyk V, Meyer BH, Müller FO, Witte PU. Pharmacokinetic aspects of the interaction between clobazam and cimetidine. *Eur J Clin Pharmacol* (1983) 25, 139–42.
30. Ochs HR, Greenblatt DJ, Verburg-Ochs B, Harmatz JS, Grehl H. Disposition of clotiazepam: influence of age, sex, oral contraceptives, cimetidine, isoniazid and ethanol. *Eur J Clin Pharmacol* (1984) 26, 55–9.
31. Patwardhan RV, Yarborough GW, Desmond PV, Johnson RF, Schenker S, Speeg KV. Cimetidine spares the glucuronidation of lorazepam and oxazepam. *Gastroenterology* (1980) 79, 912–16.
32. Doenicke A, Dorow R, Täuber U. Die Pharmakokinetik von Lormetazepam nach Cimetidin. *Anaesthesist* (1991) 40, 675–9.
33. Klotz U, Reimann I. Influence of cimetidine on the pharmacokinetics of desmethyldiazepam and oxazepam. *Eur J Clin Pharmacol* (1980) 18, 517–20.
34. Greenblatt DJ, Abernethy DR, Divoll M, Locniskar A, Harmatz JS, Shader RI. Noninteraction of temazepam and cimetidine. *J Pharm Sci* (1984) 73, 399–401.
35. Elliott P, Dundee JW, Collier PS, McClean E. The influence of two H_2-receptor antagonists, cimetidine and ranitidine, on the systemic availability of temazepam. *Br J Anaesth* (1984) 56, 800P–801P.
36. Lam AM, Parkin JA. Cimetidine and prolonged post-operative somnolence. *Can Anaesth Soc J* (1981) 28, 450–2.
37. Sanders LD, Whitehead C, Gildersleve CD, Rosen M, Robinson JO. Interaction of H_2-receptor antagonists and benzodiazepine sedation. *Anaesthesia* (1993) 48, 286–92.
38. Salonen M, Aantaa E, Aaltonen L, Kanto J. Importance of the interaction of midazolam and cimetidine. *Acta Pharmacol Toxicol (Copenh)* (1986) 58, 91–5.
39. Fee JPH, Collier PS, Howard PJ, Dundee JW. Cimetidine and ranitidine increase midazolam bioavailability. *Clin Pharmacol Ther* (1987) 41, 80–4.
40. Klotz U, Arvela P, Rosenkranz B. Effect of single doses of cimetidine and ranitidine on the steady-state plasma levels of midazolam. *Clin Pharmacol Ther* (1985) 38, 652–5.
41. Greenblatt DJ, Locniskar A, Scavone JM, Blyden GT, Ochs HR, Harmatz JS, Shader RI. Absence of interaction of cimetidine and ranitidine with intravenous and oral midazolam. *Anesth Analg* (1986) 65, 176–80.
42. Chichmanian RM, Mignot G, Spreux A, Jean-Girard C, Hofliger P. Tolérance de la famotidine. Étude due réseau médecins sentinelles en pharmacovigilance. *Therapie* (1992) 47, 239–43.
43. Locniskar A, Greenblatt DJ, Harmatz JS, Zinny MA. Influence of famotidine and cimetidine on the pharmacokinetic properties of intravenous diazepam. *J Clin Pharmacol* (1985) 25, 459–60.
44. Klotz U, Arvela P, Rosenkranz B. Famotidine, a new H_2-receptor antagonist, does not affect hepatic elimination of diazepam or tubular secretion of procainamide. *Eur J Clin Pharmacol* (1985) 28, 671–5.
45. Klotz U, Gottlieb W, Keohane PP, Dammann HG. Nocturnal doses of ranitidine and nizatidine do not affect the disposition of diazepam. *J Clin Pharmacol* (1987) 27, 210–12.
46. Klotz U, Dammann HG, Gottlieb WR, Walter TA, Keohane P. Nizatidine (300 mg nocte) does not interfere with diazepam pharmacokinetics in man. *Br J Clin Pharmacol* (1987) 23, 105–6.
47. Klotz U. Lack of effect of nizatidine on drug metabolism. *Scand J Gastroenterol* (1987) 22 (Suppl 136), 18–23.
48. Suttle AB, Songer SS, Dukes GE, Hak LJ, Koruda M, Fleishaker JC, Brouwer KLR. Ranitidine does not alter adinazolam pharmacokinetics or pharmacodynamics. *Clin Pharmacol Ther* (1991) 49, 178.
49. Mashford ML, Harman PJ, Morphett BJ, Breen KJ, Desmond PV. Ranitidine does not affect chlormethiazole or indocyanine green disposition. *Clin Pharmacol Ther* (1983) 34, 231–3.
50. Klotz U, Reimann IW, Ohnhaus EE. Effect of ranitidine on the steady state pharmacokinetics of diazepam. *Eur J Clin Pharmacol* (1983) 24, 357–60.
51. Abernethy DR, Greenblatt DJ, Eshelman FN, Shader RI. Ranitidine does not impair oxidative or conjugative metabolism: noninteraction with antipyrine, diazepam, and lorazepam. *Clin Pharmacol Ther* (1984) 35, 188–92.
52. Wilson CM, Robinson FP, Thompson EM, Dundee JW, Elliott P. Effect of pre-treatment with ranitidine on the hypnotic action of single doses of midazolam, temazepam and zopiclone. *Br J Anaesth* (1986) 58, 483–6.
53. Vanderveen RP, Jirak JL, Peters GR, Cox SR, Bombardt PA. Effect of ranitidine on the disposition of orally and intravenously administered triazolam. *Clin Pharm* (1991) 10, 539–43.
54. O'Connor-Semmes RL, Kersey K, Williams DH, Lam R, Koch KM. Effect of ranitidine on the pharmacokinetics of triazolam and á-hydroxytriazolam in both young (19-60 years) and older (61-78 years) people. *Clin Pharmacol Ther* (2001) 70, 126–31.
55. Elwood RJ, Hildebrand PJ, Dundee JW, Collier PS. Ranitidine influences the uptake of oral midazolam. *Br J Clin Pharmacol* (1983) 15, 743–5.
56. Labs RA. Interaction of roxatidine acetate with antacids, food and other drugs. *Drugs* (1988) 35 (Suppl 3), 82–9.

Benzodiazepines + 5-HT_3 receptor antagonists

Lorazepam does not appear to interact with granisetron, and temazepam does not appear to interact with ondansetron.

Clinical evidence, mechanism, importance and management

Lorazepam 2.5 mg, given to 12 healthy subjects, clearly affected the performance of a number of psychometric tests. Statistically significant increases occurred in drowsiness, feebleness, muzziness, clumsiness, lethargy, mental slowness, relaxation, dreaminess, incompetence, sadness and withdrawal. However, there was very little evidence that **granisetron** 160 micrograms/kg alone had any effect on the performance of these tests except that clumsiness and inattentiveness were increased, nor was there evidence that **granisetron** added to the effects of **lorazepam** when both drugs were taken concurrently.[1]

In a double-blind, placebo-controlled, crossover study in 24 healthy subjects **ondansetron** 8 mg did not affect the pharmacokinetics of **temazepam** 20 mg. The psychomotor performances of the subjects (subjective and objective sedation, memory and other measurements) were not influenced by the presence of the **ondansetron**.[2]

No additional special precautions would seem to be necessary on concurrent use of either of these pairs of drugs.

1. Leigh TJ, Link CGG, Fell GL. Effects of granisetron and lorazepam, alone and in combination, on psychometric performance. *Br J Clin Pharmacol* (1991) 31, 333–6.
2. Preston GC, Keene ON, Palmer JL. The effect of ondansetron on the pharmacokinetics and pharmacodynamics of temazepam. *Anaesthesia* (1996) 51, 827–30.

Benzodiazepines + Influenza vaccine

The pharmacokinetics of alprazolam, chlordiazepoxide and lorazepam are not affected by influenza vaccine.

Clinical evidence, mechanism, importance and management

The pharmacokinetics of single doses of oral **alprazolam** 1 mg, or intravenous **lorazepam** 2 mg remained unaffected in healthy subjects when given 7 and 21 days after 0.5 ml of intramuscular trivalent influenza vaccine.[1] Similarly, in another study, neither **lorazepam** nor **chlordiazepoxide** metabolism was altered when they were given 1 and 7 days after trivalent influenza virus vaccine.[2] There would seem to be no reason for avoiding the concurrent use of these drugs.

1. Scavone JM, Blyden GT, Greenblatt DJ. Lack of effect of influenza vaccine on the pharmacokinetics of antipyrine, alprazolam, paracetamol (acetaminophen) and lorazepam. *Clin Pharmacokinet* (1989) 16, 180–5.
2. Meredith CG, Christian CD, Johnson RF, Troxell R, Davis GL, Schenker S. Effects of influenza virus vaccine on hepatic drug metabolism. *Clin Pharmacol Ther* (1985) 37, 396–401.

Benzodiazepines + Isoniazid

Isoniazid reduces the clearance of both diazepam and triazolam. Some increase in their effects would be expected. No interaction occurs with oxazepam or clotiazepam.

Clinical evidence

(a) Interacting benzodiazepines

A study in 9 healthy subjects found that isoniazid 90 mg twice daily for 3 days increased the half-life of a single dose of **diazepam** from about 34 to 45 hours, and reduced the total clearance by 26%.[1] A study in 6 healthy subjects found that isoniazid 90 mg twice daily for 3 days, increased the half-life of a single dose of **triazolam** from 2.5 to 3.3 hours, increased the AUC by 46% and reduced the clearance by 43%.[2]

(b) Non-interacting benzodiazepines

A study in 9 healthy subjects found that isoniazid 90 mg twice daily for 3 days had no effect on the pharmacokinetics of a single 30-mg oral dose of **oxazepam**.[2] Similarly the pharmacokinetics of **clotiazepam** were not altered in another study of the effects of isoniazid.[3]

Mechanism

What is known suggests that the isoniazid acts as an enzyme inhibitor, decreasing the metabolism and loss of diazepam and triazolam from the body, thereby increasing and prolonging their effects.

Importance and management

Information is limited but the interactions appear to be established. Their clinical importance is uncertain but be alert for the need to decrease the dosages of diazepam and triazolam if isoniazid is started. There seems to be no direct information about other benzodiazepines, but those undergoing high first-pass extraction and/or liver microsomal metabolism may interact similarly. Oxazepam and clotiazepam appear not to interact.

1. Ochs HR, Greenblatt DJ, Roberts G-M, Dengler HJ. Diazepam interaction with antituberculosis drugs. *Clin Pharmacol Ther* (1981) 29, 671–8.
2. Ochs HR, Greenblatt DJ, Knüchel M. Differential effect of isoniazid on triazolam oxidation and oxazepam conjugation. *Br J Clin Pharmacol* (1983) 16, 743–6.
3. Ochs HR, Greenblatt DJ, Verburg-Ochs B, Harmatz JS, Grehl H. Disposition of clotiazepam: influence of age, sex, oral contraceptives, cimetidine, isoniazid and ethanol. *Eur J Clin Pharmacol* (1984) 26, 55–9.

Benzodiazepines + Kava

A man on alprazolam became semicomatose a few days after starting to take kava.

Clinical evidence, mechanism, importance and management

A 54-year-old man taking **alprazolam**, cimetidine and terazosin was hospitalised in a lethargic and disorientated state 3 days after starting to take kava, which he had bought from a local health food store. He denied having overdosed with any of these drugs. The patient became alert again after several hours.[1] The reason for what happened is not known, but the suggested explanation is that the kava α-pyrones might have had additive sedative effects with those of the **alprazolam**.[1,2] This is an isolated case and its general importance is not known.

1. Almeida JC, Grimsley EW. Coma from the health food store: interaction between kava and alprazolam. *Ann Intern Med* (1996) 125, 940–1.
2. Jussofie A, Schmiz A, Hiemke C. Kavapyrone enriched extract from *Piper methysticum* as modulator of GABA binding site in different regions of rat brain. *Psychopharmacology (Berl)* (1994) 116, 469–74.

Benzodiazepines and related drugs + Macrolides

The serum levels and effects of midazolam and triazolam are markedly increased and prolonged by erythromycin. The same interaction has been seen between triazolam and clarithromycin, troleandomycin or josamycin, and between midazolam and clarithromycin. Plasma levels of zopiclone are markedly increased by erythromycin. Roxithromycin has a weak effect on midazolam and triazolam, and erythromycin has a weak effect on diazepam, flunitrazepam, nitrazepam, temazepam and zaleplon, while azithromycin does not interact with midazolam. Erythromycin possibly increases the effects of alprazolam.

Clinical evidence

(a) Alprazolam

In a double-blind randomised study 12 healthy subjects were given **erythromycin** 400 mg three times daily for 10 days with a single 800-microgram dose of alprazolam on day 8. The alprazolam 48-hour AUC was increased by 61% and the half-life increased from 16 to 40.3 hours. However, no increase in sedation was seen.[1]

(b) Diazepam

In a double-blind crossover study, 6 healthy subjects were given a single 5-mg oral dose of diazepam after taking **erythromycin** 500 mg three times daily for a week. The diazepam AUC was increased by 15%, but its pharmacodynamic were unchanged.[2]

(c) Flunitrazepam

In a double-blind crossover study, 5 healthy subjects were given a single 1-mg oral dose of flunitrazepam after taking **erythromycin** 500 mg three times daily for a week. The flunitrazepam AUC was increased by 25% but its pharmacodynamic effects were unchanged.[2]

(d) Midazolam

(i) Azithromycin. A study in 64 healthy medical students found that azithromycin 750 mg had no effect on the metabolism of a 10- or 15-mg dose of midazolam, and did not alter the performance of a number of psychomotor tests.[3] A study in 10 healthy subjects given **azithromycin** 250 mg daily found that some small changes in pharmacokinetics of midazolam 15 mg (a possible small delay in its onset of action), but its pharmacodynamic effects were unaltered.[4] Other studies confirm that azithromycin does not interact with midazolam.[5,6]

(ii) Clarithromycin. Oral 4 mg and intravenous 50 microgram/kg doses of midazolam were given simultaneously to 16 healthy subjects, before and after they took clarithromycin 500 mg twice daily for 7 days. It was found that clarithromycin reduced the systemic clearance of midazolam by about 64%, which resulted in a doubling of the midazolam-induced sleeping time.[7] Similar results were found in another study.[6]

(iii) Erythromycin. A study in 12 healthy subjects found that erythromycin 500 mg three times daily for 6 days almost tripled the peak plasma levels of a single 15-mg dose of midazolam, more than doubled its half-life and increased the AUC by more than fourfold. The subjects could hardly be wakened during the first hour after being given the midazolam, and most experienced amnesia lasting several hours.[8]

The serum levels of a 500-microgram/kg oral dose of midazolam, given to an 8-year-old boy as pre-medication before surgery, were approximately doubled when he was given intravenous erythromycin. He developed nausea and tachycardia, and after 40 minutes (by which point he had received 200 mg of erythromycin) he lost consciousness.[9] A patient in a coronary care unit given 300 mg of intravenous midazolam over 14 hours slept for about 6 days (apart from brief wakening when given flumazenil). The midazolam half-life was increased by about tenfold. This was attributed to an interaction due to the combined effects of erythromycin 4 g daily and amiodarone 1.7 g over 3 days.[10,11] An interaction between midazolam and erythromycin was suspected in another report, but it was obscured by the state of the patient and the use of other drugs.[12] A study in healthy subjects found that even a single 750-mg dose of erythromycin increased the sedative effects of a single 10-mg dose of midazolam.[13] Two other studies found that erythromycin increased the serum levels of midazolam two to threefold, and markedly worsened the performance of a number of psychomotor tests.[3,5]

(iv) Roxithromycin

Roxithromycin 300 mg daily for 6 days increased the AUC of a single 15-mg dose of midazolam by about 47% in 10 healthy subjects, and lengthened the half-life from 1.7 to 2.2 hours. Only minor psychomotor changes were seen.[14] A modest increase in the effects of midazolam were seen in another study in subjects given roxithromycin 300 mg, but the effects were very much weaker than those seen with erythromycin.[13]

(e) Nitrazepam

When 10 healthy subjects were given **erythromycin** 500 mg three times daily for 4 days, the AUC of a single 5-mg dose of nitrazepam was increased by 25%, the peak plasma levels were increased by 30% and the concentration peak time was reduced by over 50%. However, hardly any changes were seen in psychomotor tests undertaken.[15]

(f) Temazepam

A double-blind, randomised, crossover study in 10 healthy subjects found that **erythromycin** 500 mg three times daily for 6 days had no significant effect on the pharmacokinetics or psychomotor effects of a single 20-mg dose of temazepam.[16]

(g) Triazolam

(i) Azithromycin. A clinical study in 12 healthy subjects found that azithromycin did not affect the pharmacokinetics of a single 125-microgram dose of triazolam.[17] These results were supported by an *in vitro* study, which confirmed that azithromycin was only a weak inhibitor of triazolam metabolism.[17]

(ii) Clarithromycin. An *in vitro* study found clarithromycin to be a relatively potent inhibitor of triazolam metabolism. These results were confirmed in practice with 12 healthy subjects, who were given both drugs. The oral clearance of triazolam was reduced by 77% by clarithromycin when compared with placebo.[17]

(iii) Erythromycin. A study in 16 healthy subjects found that erythromycin 333 mg three times daily for 3 days, reduced the clearance of a single 500-microgram dose of triazolam by about 50%, doubled the AUC, and increased the maximum plasma levels by about one-third (from 2.8 to 4.1 nanograms/ml).[18] Other reports confirm the marked decrease in clearance and an increase in peak levels.[17,19] Repeated visual hallucinations and abnormal body sensations occurred in one patient with acute pneumonia and chronic renal failure on erythromycin 600 mg daily after each dose of triazolam and **nitrazepam**. These symptoms had not occurred before the addition of erythromycin.[20]

(iv) Josamycin. Josamycin has been reported to increase triazolam levels causing an increase in its effects.[21]

(v) Roxithromycin. A study found that roxithromycin 300 mg had only a slight effect on the effects of triazolam.[13]

(vi) Troleandomycin. **Troleandomycin** 2 g daily given to 7 healthy subjects for 7 days increased the peak **triazolam** levels by 107%, the AUC by 275% and the half-life from 1.81 to 6.48 hours. Apparent oral clearance was reduced by 74%. Marked psychomotor impairment and amnesia was seen.[22] **Troleandomycin** has been reported to interact similarly in a patient on **triazolam**, causing an increase in its effects.[21] An *in vitro* study has shown **troleandomycin** to be a potent inhibitor of **triazolam** metabolism.[17]

(h) Zaleplon

The makers say that a single 800-mg dose of **erythromycin** dose increased the plasma levels of zaleplon by 34%.[23]

(i) Zopiclone

Zopiclone 7.5 mg was given to 10 healthy subjects before and after taking **erythromycin** 500 mg three times daily for 6 days. The **erythromycin** increased the plasma concentration of the zopiclone fivefold at 30 minutes and twofold at one hour. Peak plasma levels rose by about 40% and occurred at 1 hour instead of 2 hours. The 1-hour and 2-hour AUCs were increased threefold and twofold respectively, while the total AUC was increased by nearly 80%.[24] These pharmacokinetic changes were reflected in some small changes in a number of psychomotor tests.[24]

Mechanism

Some of the macrolide antibacterials (notable erythromycin and troleandomycin) are potent inhibitors of the cytochrome P450 isoenzyme CYP3A4. The benzodiazepines, zaleplon and zopiclone are, to varying degrees, metabolised by CYP3A4. Those, such as midazolam, that are predominantly metabolised by CYP3A4 are affected more than those such as diazepam, where CYP3A4 plays only a minor part in metabolism. Therefore the macrolides can reduce the loss of some of the benzodiazepines, raising their serum levels and increasing and prolonging their effects.

Importance and management

The interactions of midazolam with erythromycin and triazolam with clarithromycin, erythromycin or troleandomycin appear to be established, and of clinical importance. The dosages of the midazolam and triazolam should be reduced 50 to 75% when these antibacterials are used if excessive effects (marked drowsiness, memory loss) are to be avoided. Remember too that the hypnotic effects are also prolonged so that patients should be warned about hangover effects next morning if they intend to drive. Much less is known about the use of midazolam with clarithromycin and alprazolam with erythromycin but similar precautions may be necessary. The makers of zaleplon say that patients should be advised that increased sedation is possible with erythromycin.

Azithromycin does not interact with midazolam or triazolam, and the effects of roxithromycin on midazolam and triazolam, and of erythromycin on diazepam, flunitrazepam, nitrazepam, temazepam and zopiclone appear to be small and unimportant, or the effects negligible, so that no special precautions seem to be necessary.

1. Yasui N, Otani K, Kaneko S, Ohkubo T, Osanai T, Sugawara K, Chiba K, Ishizaki T. A kinetic and dynamic study of oral alprazolam with and without erythromycin in humans: in vivo evidence for the involvement of CYP3A4 in alprazolam metabolism. *Clin Pharmacol Ther* (1996) 59, 514–19.
2. Luurila H, Olkkola KT, Neuvonen PJ. An interaction between erythromycin and the benzodiazepines diazepam and flunitrazepam. *Therapie* (1995) 50 (Suppl), 484.
3. Mattila MJ, Vanakoski J, Idänpään-Heikkilä JJ. Azithromycin does not alter the effects of oral midazolam on human performance. *Eur J Clin Pharmacol* (1994) 47, 49–52.
4. Backman JT, Olkkola KT, Neuvonen PJ. Azithromycin does not increase plasma concentrations of oral midazolam. *Int J Clin Pharmacol Ther* (1995) 33, 356–9.
5. Zimmermann T, Yeates RA, Laufen H, Scharpf F, Leitold M, Wildfeuer A. Influence of the antibiotics erythromycin and azithromycin on the pharmacokinetics and pharmacodynamics of midazolam. *Arzneimittelforschung* (1996) 46, 213–17.
6. Yeates RA, Laufen H, Zimmermann T. Interaction between midazolam and clarithromycin: comparison with azithromycin. *Int J Clin Pharmacol Ther* (1996) 34, 400–5.
7. Gorski JC, Jones DR, Haehner-Daniels BD, Hamman MA, O'Mara EM, Hall SD. The contribution of intestinal and hepatic CYP3A to the interaction between midazolam and clarithromycin. *Clin Pharmacol Ther* (1998) 64, 133–43.
8. Olkkola KT, Aranko K, Luurila H, Hiller A, Saarnivaara L, Himberg J-J, Neuvonen PJ. A potentially hazardous interaction between erythromycin and midazolam. *Clin Pharmacol Ther* (1993) 53, 298–305.
9. Hiller A, Olkkola KT, Isohanni P, Saarnivaara L. Unconsciousness associated with midazolam and erythromycin. *Br J Anaesth* (1990) 65, 826–8.
10. Gascon M-P, Dayer P, Waldvogel F. Les interactions médicamenteuses du midazolam. *Schweiz Med Wochenschr* (1989) 119, 1834–6.
11. Gascon M-P, Dayer P. In vitro forecasting of drugs which may interfere with the biotransformation of midazolam. *Eur J Clin Pharmacol* (1991) 41, 573–8.
12. Byatt CM, Lewis LD, Dawling S, Cochrane GM. Accumulation of midazolam after repeated dosage in patients receiving mechanical ventilation in an intensive care unit. *BMJ* (1984) 289, 799–800.
13. Mattila MJ, Idänpään-Heikkilä JJ, Törnwall M, Vanakoski J. Oral single doses of erythromycin and roxithromycin may increase the effects of midazolam on human performance. *Pharmacol Toxicol* (1993) 73, 180–5.
14. Backman JT, Aranko K, Himberg J-J, Olkkola KT. A pharmacokinetic interaction between roxithromycin and midazolam. *Eur J Clin Pharmacol* (1994) 46, 551–5.
15. Luurila H, Olkkola KT, Neuvonen PJ. Interaction between erythromycin and nitrazepam in healthy volunteers. *Pharmacol Toxicol* (1995) 76, 255–8.
16. Luurila H, Olkkola KT, Neuvonen PJ. Lack of interaction of erythromycin and temazepam. *Ther Drug Monit* (1994) 16, 548–51.
17. Greenblatt DJ, von Moltke LL, Harmatz JS, Counihan M, Graf JA, Durol ALB, Mertzanis P, Duan SX, Wright CE, Shader RI. Inhibition of triazolam clearance by macrolide antimicrobial agents: in vitro correlates and dynamic consequences. *Clin Pharmacol Ther* (1998) 64, 278–85.
18. Phillips JP, Antal EJ, Smith RB. A pharmacokinetic drug interaction between erythromycin and triazolam. *J Clin Psychopharmacol* (1986) 6, 297–9.
19. Hugues FC, Le Jeunne C, Munera Y. Conséquences en thérapeutique de l'inhibition microsomiale hépatique par les macrolides. *Sem Hop Paris* (1987) 63, 2280–3.
20. Tokinaga N, Kondo T, Kaneko S, Otani K, Mihara K, Morita S. Hallucinations after a therapeutic dose of benzodiazepine hypnotics with co-administration of erythromycin. *Psychiatry Clin Neurosci* (1996) 50, 337–9.
21. Carry PV, Ducluzeau R, Jourdan C, Bourrat C, Vigneou C, Descotes J. De nouvelles interactions avec les macrolides? *Lyon Med* (1982) 248, 189–90.
22. Warot D, Bergougnan L, Lamiable D, Berlin I, Bensimon G, Danjou P, Puech AJ. Troleandomycin-triazolam interaction in healthy volunteers: pharmacokinetic and psychometric evaluation. *Eur J Clin Pharmacol* (1987) 32, 389–93.
23. Sonata (Zaleplon). Wyeth Pharmaceuticals. UK Summary of product characteristics, September 2003.
24. Aranko K, Luurila H, Backman JT, Neuvonen PJ, Olkkola KT. The effect of erythromycin on the pharmacokinetics and pharmacodynamics of zopiclone. *Br J Clin Pharmacol* (1994) 38, 363–7.

Benzodiazepines and related drugs + Metoclopramide

Intravenous but not oral metoclopramide increases the rate of absorption of diazepam and raises its maximum plasma levels. Metoclopramide hastens the absorption of zopiclone.

Clinical evidence, mechanism, importance and management

Metoclopramide given intravenously increased the peak plasma levels of **diazepam** by 38% and increased the rate of absorption (peak levels by 30 minutes instead of 60 minutes),[1] but oral metoclopramide 10 mg did not increase the rate of absorption of oral **diazepam** 0.2 mg/kg in 6 healthy subjects.[2] The reason is not understood. The clinical importance of this interaction is not known, but it is probably small.

The absorption of a single 7.5-mg dose of oral zopiclone was hastened by metoclopramide 10 mg given intravenously to 12 healthy subjects. This was presumably because these drugs alter gut motility. Mean plasma zopiclone levels at 1 hour were 22.7 and 44.4 nanograms/ml and at 2 hours they were 49.3 and 59.6 nanograms/ml, when zopiclone was given alone or with metoclopramide respectively.[3] The clinical importance of these findings is not known.

1. Gamble JAS, Gaston JH, Nair SG, Dundee JW. Some pharmacological factors influencing the absorption of diazepam following oral administration. *Br J Anaesth* (1976) 48, 1181–5.
2. Chapman MH, Woolner DF, Begg EJ, Atkinson HC, Sharman JR. Co-administered oral metoclopramide does not enhance the rate of absorption of oral diazepam. *Anaesth Intensive Care* (1988) 16, 202–5.
3. Elliott P, Chestnutt WN, Elwood RJ, Dundee JW. Effect of atropine and metoclopramide on the plasma concentrations of orally administered zopiclone. *Br J Anaesth* (1983) 55, 1159P–1160P.

Benzodiazepines + Metronidazole

Metronidazole does not interact with alprazolam, diazepam, lorazepam or midazolam.

Clinical evidence, mechanism, importance and management

One study in healthy subjects found that metronidazole 750 mg [for an unstated time] had no effect on the pharmacokinetics of **lorazepam** or **alprazolam**.[1] Another study found that metronidazole 400 mg twice daily for 5 days had no effect on the pharmacokinetics of a single 100-microgram/kg intravenous dose of **diazepam**.[2] *In vivo* and *in vitro* studies have shown that metronidazole has no effect on the pharmacokinetics or pharmacodynamics of **midazolam**.[3] Interactions with other benzodiazepines seem unlikely.

1. Blyden GT, Greenblatt DJ, Scavone JM. Metronidazole impairs clearance of phenytoin but not of alprazolam or lorazepam. *Clin Pharmacol Ther* (1986) 39, 181.
2. Jensen JC, Gugler R. Interaction between metronidazole and drugs eliminated by oxidative metabolism. *Clin Pharmacol Ther* (1985) 37, 407–10.
3. Wang J-S, Backman JT, Kivistö KT, Neuvonen PJ. Effects of metronidazole on midazolam metabolism in vitro and in vivo. *Eur J Clin Pharmacol* (2000) 56, 555–9.

Benzodiazepines + Misoprostol

A study in 12 subjects found that misoprostol 200 micrograms four times daily for 7 days had no effect on the steady-state plasma levels of diazepam 10 mg daily or on the plasma levels of the metabolite nordiazepam.[1] No special precautions would therefore seem to be necessary if misoprostol is given with diazepam.

1. Lima DR, Santos RM, Werneck E, Andrade GN. Effect of orally administered misoprostol and cimetidine on the steady state pharmacokinetics of diazepam and nordiazepam in human volunteers. *Eur J Drug Metab Pharmacokinet* (1991) 16, 161–70.

Benzodiazepines + Nefazodone

Nefazodone increases the plasma levels and effects of alprazolam, midazolam, triazolam and zopiclone, but not lorazepam. Dosage reductions may be needed.

Clinical evidence

(a) Alprazolam

A placebo-controlled study in 12 healthy subjects found that nefazodone 200 mg twice daily caused an almost twofold increase in the plasma levels of alprazolam 1 mg twice daily, taken for 7 days.[1] Another study found that impairment of psychomotor performance and increased sedation occurred when nefazodone was given with alprazolam.[2] A case report describes benzodiazepine withdrawal symptoms in a woman on alprazolam after nefazodone was withdrawn following several years of concurrent use. She needed an alprazolam dosage increase from 500 micrograms to 4 mg daily to control her symptoms.[3]

(b) Lorazepam

A placebo-controlled study in healthy subjects given nefazodone 200 mg twice daily found that no changes in the pharmacokinetics of lorazepam 2 mg twice daily.[1] Another study showed that no impairment of psychomotor performance or increased sedation occurred when nefazodone was given with lorazepam.[2]

(c) Midazolam

A study in 10 healthy subjects found that both the AUC and the maximum plasma level of a single 10-mg dose of midazolam were increased about fivefold and twofold respectively, when they took nefazodone 200 mg twice daily.[4]

(d) Triazolam

A study in 12 healthy subjects found that the maximum plasma levels, the half-life and the AUC of a single 250-microgram dose of triazolam were increased 1.7-fold, 4.6-fold and 4-fold respectively, by nefazodone 200 mg twice daily.[5] Another study showed that impairment of psychomotor performance and increased sedation occurred when nefazodone was given with triazolam.[2]

(e) Zopiclone

An 86-year-old woman taking diltiazem, irbesartan, lorazepam, and pravastatin was started on nefazodone 50 mg twice daily, increasing to 500 mg daily in divided doses, for the treatment of a major depressive episode. Because of associated insomnia zopiclone was added, starting at 15 mg each night, but reduced after 5 days to 7.5 mg, because of morning drowsiness. Plasma levels of (*S*)-zopiclone and (*R*)-zopiclone were 107 and 20.6 nanograms/ml at this time. After several months, nefazodone was replaced by venlafaxine. The (*S*)-zopiclone and (*R*)-zopiclone levels were again measured and found to be only 16.9 and 1.45 nanograms/ml.[6]

Mechanism

Nefazodone appears to inhibit the oxidative metabolism of alprazolam, midazolam, triazolam and zopiclone by the cytochrome P450 isoenzyme CYP3A4 so that they accumulate in the body. Lorazepam is unaffected because it is primarily excreted as a conjugate.

Importance and management

The interactions of nefazodone with alprazolam, midazolam, triazolam and zopiclone are established and clinically important. The practical consequences are that the effects of alprazolam, midazolam and triazolam are expected to be increased but the extent is uncertain. Be alert for any evidence of any psychomotor impairment, drowsiness etc. and reduce the benzodiazepine dosage if necessary. More study is needed. Lorazepam does not interact with nefazodone. As yet there seems to be no direct information about other benzodiazepines.

1. Greene DS, Salazar DE, Dockens RC, Kroboth P, Barbhaiya RH. Coadministration of nefazodone and benzodiazepines: III. A pharmacokinetic interaction study with alprazolam. *J Clin Psychopharmacol* (1995) 15, 399–408.
2. Kroboth P, Folan M, Lush R, Chaikin PC, Barbhaiya RH, Salazar DE. Coadministration of nefazodone and benzodiazepines II: pharmacodynamic assessment. *Clin Pharmacol Ther* (1994) 55, 142.
3. Ninan T. Pharmacokinetically induced benzodiazepine withdrawal. *Psychopharmacol Bull* (2001) 35, 94–100.
4. Lam YWF, Alfaro CL, Ereshefsky L, Miller M. Pharmacokinetic and pharmacodynamic interactions of oral midazolam with ketoconazole, fluoxetine, fluvoxamine, and nefazodone. *J Clin Pharmacol* (2003) 43, 1274–82.
5. Barbhaiya RH, Shukla UA, Kroboth PD, Greene DS. Coadministration of nefazodone and benzodiazepines: II. A pharmacokinetic interaction study with triazolam. *J Clin Psychopharmacol* (1995) 15, 320–6.
6. Alderman CP, Gebauer MG, Gilbert AL, Condon JT. Possible interaction of zopiclone and nefazodone. *Ann Pharmacother* (2001) 35, 1378–80.

Benzodiazepines and related drugs + NSAIDs

Diclofenac reduces the dose of midazolam needed to produce sedation and hypnosis. Diazepam has a small effect on the pharmacokinetics of diclofenac, ibuprofen and naproxen, but diazepam and indometacin appear not to interact adversely although feelings of dizziness may be increased. Zaleplon and ibuprofen appear not to interact. Diazepam may also affect the pharmacokinetics of diclofenac.

Clinical evidence, mechanism, importance and management

(a) Diazepam

Diazepam 10 to 15 mg impaired the performance of a number of psychomotor tests (digit symbol substitution, letter cancellation, tracking and flicker fusion) in 119 healthy medical students. It also caused subjective drowsiness, mental slowness and clumsiness. When **indometacin** 50 or 100 mg was given the effects were little different from diazepam alone, except that the feeling of dizziness (common to both drugs) was increased and caused subjective clumsiness.[1] A study in 8 healthy subjects investigating the effects of diazepam on **ibuprofen** pharmacokinetics found that the **ibuprofen** half-life was increased from 2.39 to 3.59 hours and the clearance was reduced by about one-third when diazepam and **ibuprofen** were given at 10 pm, but no effect was seen with morning dosing.[2] The clinical importance of this is uncertain.

A double-blind crossover study failed to find any clinically important changes in mood or attention in healthy subjects given **naproxen** and diazepam.[3] A single-dose study in 10 healthy subjects found that peak serum concentrations of **naproxen** 500 mg were reduced by 23%, the time to peak concentration was increased (1.36 to 2 hours) and the absorption rate constant was decreased (4.07 to 2.42 h^{-1}) by diazepam 10 mg. Other pharmacokinetic parameters were not affected.[4] No special precautions appear to be necessary.

In another study in 8 healthy subjects diazepam increased the peak serum levels of **diclofenac** by 68 and 112% and increased the AUC by 60% while the clearance was reduced by 36%.[5] The effects of diazepam on **diclofenac** appeared to depend on time of administration and may reflect time-dependent effects of diazepam on gastrointestinal function. More study is needed.

(b) Midazolam

A clinical study found that **diclofenac** 75 mg given intravenously to 10 patients reduced the dose of intravenous midazolam needed to produce sedation and hypnosis by 35%, when compared to 10 control subjects not given **diclofenac**.[6] The clinical importance of this is uncertain.

For the interactions of parecoxib or valdecoxib with midazolam see 'NSAIDs; Parecoxib or Valdecoxib + Miscellaneous', p.101.

(c) Zaleplon

A randomised, single-dose, three-period crossover study in 17 healthy subjects found that **ibuprofen** 600 mg had no effect on the pharmacokinetics of zaleplon 10 mg.[7]

1. Nuotto E, Saarialho-Kere U. Actions and interactions of indomethacin and diazepam on performance in healthy volunteers. *Pharmacol Toxicol* (1988) 62, 293–7.
2. Bapuji AT, Rambhau D, Srinivasu P, Rao BR, Apte SS. Time dependent influence of diazepam on the pharmacokinetics of ibuprofen in man. *Drug Metabol Drug Interact* (1999) 15, 71–81.
3. Stitt FW, Latour R, Frane JW. A clinical study of naproxen-diazepam drug interaction on tests of mood and attention. *Curr Ther Res* (1977) 21, 149–56.
4. Rao BR, Rambhau D. Influence of diazepam on the pharmacokinetic properties of orally administered naproxen. *Drug Invest* (1992) 4, 416–21.
5. Mahender VN, Rambhau D, Rao BR, Rao VVS, Venkateshwarlu G. Time-dependent influence of diazepam on the pharmacokinetics of orally administered diclofenac sodium in human subjects. *Clin Drug Invest* (1995) 10, 296–301.
6. Carrero E, Castillo J, Bogdanovich A, Nalda MA. El diclofenac reduce las dosis sedante e hipnótica de midazolam. *Rev Esp Anestesiol Reanim* (1991) 38, 127.
7. Garcia PS, Carcas A, Zapater P, Rosendo J, Paty I, Leister CA, Troy SM. Absence of an interaction between ibuprofen and zaleplon. *Am J Health-Syst Pharm* (2000) 57, 1137–41.

Benzodiazepines and related drugs + Oral contraceptives

Oral contraceptives can increase the effects of alprazolam, chlordiazepoxide, diazepam, nitrazepam and triazolam, and reduce the effects of oxazepam, lorazepam and temazepam, but whether in practice there is a need for dosage adjustments has not been determined. Chlordiazepoxide, diazepam, nitrazepam and meprobamate can possibly increase the incidence of break-through bleeding.

Clinical evidence

(a) Effects on benzodiazepines

A controlled study found that the mean half-life of intravenous **chlordiazepoxide** 600 micrograms/kg was virtually double (11.6 hours compared with 20.6 hours) and the total clearance was almost two-thirds lower in 6 women on oral contraceptives when compared to 6 women not taking oral contraceptives.[1]

Similar but less marked effects were found in other studies in women taking oral contraceptives given **chlordiazepoxide**,[2] **diazepam**,[3,4] **alprazolam**[5] and to an even lesser extent with **triazolam**[5] and **nitrazepam**.[6] No clinically significant pharmacokinetic changes were seen with **bromazepam**,[7] **clotiazepam**,[8] **midazolam** (given orally[9] intramuscularly[10] or intravenously[9]) or **zolpidem**.[11]

A controlled study, comparing 7 women taking an oral contraceptive with 8 women not taking oral contraceptives found that the mean half-life of intravenous **lorazepam** 2 mg was over 50% shorter in the oral contraceptive group (6 hours compared to 14 hours) and the total clearance was over threefold greater.[1]

A smaller increase in the elimination rate was seen in other controlled studies in women taking oral contraceptives and **lorazepam**,[5,12] or **temazepam**,[5] and in two other studies small decreases in the half-life of **oxazepam** were observed.[1,12]

(b) Effects on contraceptives

A study in 72 patients taking combined oral contraceptives (*Rigevidon*, *Anteovin*) found that break-through bleeding occurred in 36.1% of patients while taking **chlordiazepoxide** 10 to 20 mg daily, **diazepam** 5 to 15 mg daily, **nitrazepam** 5 to 10 mg daily or **meprobamate** 200 to 600 mg daily, but no pregnancies occurred. Only three cases of bleeding occurred with **diazepam** or **nitrazepam**.[13] The average values for break-through bleeding with these two oral contraceptives were 9.1% for *Rigevidon* and 3.3% for *Anteovin* in the absence of other drugs. It was possible to establish a causal relationship between the bleeding and the use of the hypnotic in 77% of the cases either by stopping the drug or by changing it for another.[13]

Mechanism

Oral contraceptives affect the metabolism of the benzodiazepines by the liver in different ways: oxidative metabolism is reduced (alprazolam, chlordiazepoxide, diazepam, etc.), whereas metabolism by glucuronide conjugation is increased (lorazepam, oxazepam, temazepam, etc.). Just why these hypnotics should cause break-through bleeding is not understood.

Importance and management

Established interactions but of uncertain clinical importance. Long-term use of benzodiazepines that are highly oxidised (alprazolam, chlordiazepoxide, diazepam, nitrazepam, etc.) in women taking oral contraceptives should be monitored to ensure that the dosage is not too high. Those taking glucuronidated benzodiazepines (lorazepam, oxazepam, temazepam, etc.) may possibly need a dosage increase but this is not proven. Bromazepam, clotiazepam, midazolam and zolpidem appear not to interact. No firm conclusions could be drawn from the results of one study, which set out to evaluate the importance of this interaction.[14]

The increased incidence of break-through bleeding (more than one-third) due to these hypnotics, is an unpleasant reaction and it suggests that the contraceptive is possibly unreliable, but no outright contraceptive failures were actually reported.[13] Limited evidence from the study suggests that changing the hypnotic or the contraceptive might avoid breakthrough bleeding. Note that the UK Family Planning Association[15] do not consider that additional contraceptive precautions are necessary with clonazepam or clobazam and it seems unlikely that they will be necessary with any benzodiazepine.

1. Patwardhan RV, Mitchell MC, Johnson RF, Schenker S. Differential effects of oral contraceptive steroids on the metabolism of benzodiazepines. *Hepatology* (1983) 3, 248–53.
2. Roberts RK, Desmond PV, Wilkinson GR, Schenker S. Disposition of chlordiazepoxide: sex differences and effects of oral contraceptives. *Clin Pharmacol Ther* (1979) 25, 826–31.
3. Giles HG, Sellers EM, Naranjo CA, Frecker RC, Greenblatt DJ. Disposition of intravenous diazepam in young men and women. *Eur J Clin Pharmacol* (1981) 20, 207–13.

4. Abernethy DR, Greenblatt DJ, Divoll M, Arendt R, Ochs HR, Shader RI. Impairment of diazepam metabolism by low-dose estrogen-containing oral-contraceptive steroids. *N Engl J Med* (1982) 306, 791–2.
5. Stoehr GP, Kroboth PD, Juhl RP, Wender DB, Phillips P, Smith RB. Effect of oral contraceptives on triazolam, temazepam, alprazolam, and lorazepam kinetics. *Clin Pharmacol Ther* (1984) 36, 683–90.
6. Jochemsen R, Van der Graff M, Boejinga JK, Breimer DD. Influence of sex, menstrual cycle and oral contraception on the disposition of nitrazepam. *Br J Clin Pharmacol* (1982) 13, 319–24.
7. Ochs HR, Greenblatt DJ, Friedman H, Burstein ES, Locniskar A, Harmatz JS, Shader RI. Bromazepam pharmacokinetics: influence of age, gender, oral contraceptives, cimetidine, and propranolol. *Clin Pharmacol Ther* (1987) 41, 562–70.
8. Ochs HR, Greenblatt DJ, Verburg-Ochs B, Harmatz JS, Grehl H. Disposition of clotiazepam: influence of age, sex, oral contraceptives, cimetidine, isoniazid and ethanol. *Eur J Clin Pharmacol* (1984) 26, 55–9.
9. Belle DJ, Callaghan JT, Gorski JC, Maya JF, Mousa O, Wrighton SA, Hall SD. The effects of an oral contraceptive containing ethinyloestradiol and norgestrel on CYP3A activity. *Br J Clin Pharmacol* (2002) 53, 67–74.
10. Holazo AA, Winkler MB, Patel IH. Effects of age, gender and oral contraceptives on intramuscular midazolam pharmacokinetics. *J Clin Pharmacol* (1988) 28, 1040–5.
11. Olubodun JO, Ochs HR, Trüten V, Klein A, von Moltke LL, Harmatz JS, Shader RI, Greenblatt DJ. Zolpidem pharmacokinetic properties in young females: influence of smoking and oral contraceptive use. *J Clin Pharmacol* (2002) 42, 1142–6.
12. Abernethy DR, Greenblatt DJ, Ochs HR, Weyers D, Divoll M, Harmatz JS, Shader RI. Lorazepam and oxazepam kinetics in women on low-dose oral contraceptives. *Clin Pharmacol Ther* (1983) 33, 628–32.
13. Somos P. Interaction between certain psychopharmaca and low-dose oral contraceptives. *Ther Hung* (1990) 38, 37–40.
14. Kroboth PD, Smith RB, Stoehr GP, Juhl RP. Pharmacodynamic evaluation of the benzodiazepine–oral contraceptive interaction. *Clin Pharmacol Ther* (1985) 38, 525–32.
15. Belfield T, ed. FPA Contraceptive Handbook: a guide for family planning and other health professionals. 3rd ed. London: Family Planning Association, 1999.

Benzodiazepines + Paracetamol (Acetaminophen)

Paracetamol reduces the excretion of diazepam but plasma levels are little affected.

Clinical evidence, mechanism, importance and management

The 96-hour urinary excretion of a single 10-mg oral dose of **diazepam** and its metabolite, desmethyldiazepam, were reduced from 44 to 12% and from 27% to 8% respectively in 2 female subjects, and from 11 to 4.5% respectively in a male subject by a single 500-mg dose of paracetamol. The reasons are not understood. Plasma levels of **diazepam** and its metabolite were not significantly affected.[1] There would seem to be no reason for avoiding concurrent use. There seems to be no information about other benzodiazepines.

1. Mulley BA, Potter BI, Rye RM, Takeshita K. Interactions between diazepam and paracetamol. *J Clin Pharm* (1978) 3, 25–35.

Benzodiazepines + Probenecid

Probenecid reduces the clearance of adinazolam, lorazepam and nitrazepam. Increased therapeutic and toxic effects (sedation) may be expected. Probenecid does not appear to interact with temazepam.

Clinical evidence

(a) Adinazolam

In a single-dose study, probenecid 2 g increased the psychomotor effects of sustained-release adinazolam 60 mg in 16 healthy subjects. The tests used were symbol-digit substitution, digit span forwards and continuous performance tasks.[1] The peak serum levels of adinazolam and its active metabolite, *N*-desmethyladinazolam, were increased by 37% and 49% respectively, and the clearances were reduced by 16% and 53% respectively. Both drugs have uricosuric actions, but when used together the effects appear not to be additive.[1]

(b) Lorazepam

Probenecid 500 mg every 6 hours approximately halved the clearance of a single 2-mg intravenous dose of lorazepam in 9 healthy subjects. The elimination half-life was more than doubled, from 14.3 to 33 hours.[2]

(c) Nitrazepam

Probenecid 500 mg daily for 7 days reduced the clearance of nitrazepam by 25% in healthy subjects.[3]

(d) Temazepam

Probenecid 500 mg daily for 7 days but did not significantly affect the clearance of temazepam in healthy subjects.[3]

Mechanism

Probenecid inhibits the renal tubular clearance of many drugs and their metabolites, including some of the benzodiazepines. It also inhibits the metabolism (glucuronidation) of nitrazepam and lorazepam by the liver.[2,3] The overall result is that the benzodiazepines accumulate and their effects are increased. Temazepam, which also undergoes glucuronidation, was not affected, possibly as increased sulfation compensated.[3]

Importance and management

Established interactions but of uncertain clinical importance. Be alert for increases in the effects (sedation, antegrade amnesia) of adinazolam, lorazepam and possibly nitrazepam. Reduce the dosage as necessary. There seems to be no direct information about other benzodiazepines, but those that are metabolised like lorazepam and nitrazepam (e.g. oxazepam) may also interact.

1. Golden PL, Warner PE, Fleishaker JC, Jewell RC, Millikin S, Lyon J, Brouwer KLR. Effects of probenecid on the pharmacokinetics and pharmacodynamics of adinazolam in humans. *Clin Pharmacol Ther* (1994) 56, 133–41.
2. Abernethy DR, Greenblatt DJ, Ameer B, Shader RI. Probenecid impairment of acetaminophen and lorazepam clearance: direct inhibition of ether glucuronide formation. *J Pharmacol Exp Ther* (1985) 234, 345–9.
3. Brockmeyer NH, Mertins L, Klimek K, Goos M, Ohnhaus EE. Comparative effects of rifampin and/or probenecid on the pharmacokinetics of temazepam and nitrazepam. *Int J Clin Pharmacol Ther Toxicol* (1990) 28, 387–93.

Benzodiazepines + Protease inhibitors

A study and a case report show that saquinavir markedly decreases midazolam metabolism, resulting in a significant increase in sedation. Ritonavir similarly affects triazolam and, to a lesser extent, alprazolam.

Clinical evidence, mechanism, importance and management

(a) Ritonavir

In a double-blind crossover study in 6 healthy subjects ritonavir 200 mg for 4 doses reduced the clearance of **triazolam** 125 micrograms to less than 4% of control values and increased the half-life from 3 to 41 hours, which resulted in increased and prolonged sedation.[1] A very brief case report also describes prolonged sedation in a patients given ritonavir and **triazolam**.[2]

A double-blind crossover study in 10 healthy subjects found that ritonavir 200 mg for 4 doses decreased the clearance of a single 1-mg dose of **alprazolam** by 59%. The half-life of **alprazolam** was increased from 13.3 to 29.6 hours and the subjects experienced increased and prolonged sedation.[3]

(b) Saquinavir

A double-blind randomised study in 12 healthy subjects found that saquinavir (soft-gel formulation) 1200 mg three times daily increased the bioavailability of oral **midazolam** from 41 to 90% and increased the AUC fivefold. Psychomotor tests showed impaired skills and greater sedation in the presence of saquinavir.[4] When intravenous **midazolam** was given, the sedative effects were only marginally altered.[4] However, a 32-year-old with advanced HIV, on zidovudine, lamivudine, co-trimoxazole and saquinavir 600 mg three times daily, did not wake spontaneously from a 5 mg intravenous dose of midazolam. He was given 300 micrograms of intravenous flumazenil to revert the prolonged sedation, but he was not free from sedation until 5 hours later. On a previous occasion, in the absence of saquinavir, he woke spontaneously 2 hours after the dose of midazolam.[5]

Mechanism

Alprazolam, midazolam and triazolam are metabolised by the cytochrome P450 isoenzyme CYP3A4, which is inhibited, to varying degrees, by the protease inhibitors. Benzodiazepine levels and effects are therefore increased by saquinavir and ritonavir.

Importance and management

This interaction is of general importance, so be alert for the need to reduce the midazolam dosage in the presence of saquinavir. The authors of the study[4] suggest that continuous intravenous midazolam doses should be reduced by 50%, but do not consider dose adjustments to single intravenous doses necessary.[4] The same precautions would seem appropriate with triazolam. However, the maker of saquinavir contraindicates concurrent use with midazolam and triazolam.[6,7]

The UK maker of ritonavir contraindicates its use with **clorazepate, diazepam, estazolam, flurazepam**, midazolam and triazolam as they are highly metabolised and therefore may cause extreme sedation and respiratory depression in the presence of ritonavir.[8] The US maker of ritonavir contraindicates its use with triazolam and midazolam.[9] This interaction is likely to occur with all protease inhibitors and highly metabolised benzodiazepines.

1. Greenblatt DJ, von Moltke LL, Harmatz JS, Durol AL, Daily JP, Graf JA, Mertzanis P, Hoffman JL, Shader RI. Differential impairment of triazolam and zolpidem clearance by ritonavir. *J Acquir Immune Defic Syndr* (2000) 24, 129–36.
2. Shader RI, Greenblatt DJ. Protease inhibitors and drug interaction—an alert. *J Clin Psychopharmacol* (1996) 16, 343–4.
3. Greenblatt DJ, von Moltke LL, Harmatz JS, Durol ALB, Daily JP, Graf JA, Mertzanis P, Hoffman JL, Shader RI. Alprazolam-ritonavir interaction: implications for product labeling. *Clin Pharmacol Ther* (2000) 67, 335–41.
4. Palkama VJ, Ahonen J, Neuvonen PJ, Olkkola KT. Effect of saquinavir on the pharmacokinetics and pharmacodynamics of oral and intravenous midazolam. *Clin Pharmacol Ther* (1999) 66, 33–9.
5. Merry C, Mulcahy F, Barry M, Gibbons S, Back D. Saquinavir interaction with midazolam: pharmacokinetic considerations when prescribing protease inhibitors for patients with HIV disease. *AIDS* (1997) 11, 268–9.
6. Invirase (Saquinavir mesilate). Roche Products Ltd. UK Summary of product characteristics, June 2005.
7. Invirase (Saquinavir). Roche Laboratories Inc. US prescribing information, December 2004.
8. Norvir (Ritonavir). Abbott Laboratories Ltd. UK Summary of product characteristics, January 2005.
9. Norvir (Ritonavir). Abbott Laboratories. US Prescribing information, April 2005.

Benzodiazepines + Proton pump inhibitors

Gait disturbances (attributed to benzodiazepine toxicity) occurred in two patients given triazolam and lorazepam or flurazepam with omeprazole, and another patient on diazepam and omeprazole became wobbly and sedated. Lansoprazole, pantoprazole, or rabeprazole appear not to interact to a clinically relevant extent with diazepam. Diazepam serum levels are increased by esomeprazole but the clinical relevance of this is unknown.

Clinical evidence

(a) Esomeprazole

Esomeprazole inhibits the cytochrome P450 isoenzyme CYP2C19 so the plasma levels of drugs that are metabolised by this isoenzyme might be expected to be increased by concurrent use. This is true for **diazepam**, which showed a 45% decrease in clearance when given with esomeprazole 40 mg.[1]

(b) Lansoprazole

Lansoprazole daily for 10 days was found to have no effect on the pharmacokinetics of a single 100-microgram/kg intravenous dose of **diazepam**.[2]

(c) Omeprazole

Two elderly patients, both smokers, taking **triazolam** and **lorazepam** or **flurazepam**, developed gait disturbances when given omeprazole 20 mg daily. They rapidly recovered when either the benzodiazepines or the omeprazole were stopped.[3] A brief report describes a patient on omeprazole who became wobbly and sedated by small [unspecified] doses of **diazepam**,[4] and another report describes a patient who developed toxic levels of desmethyldiazepam and remained unconscious for 13 days after receiving a high dose of **clorazepate** (1500 mg over about 29 hours) and omeprazole 80 mg daily.[5]

One study found that omeprazole 40 mg daily for a week reduced the clearance of a single 100-microgram/kg intravenous dose of **diazepam** by 54% in 8 healthy subjects,[6] while another study found that omeprazole 20 mg reduced **diazepam** clearance by 27%.[7]

A further study found that omeprazole 40 mg reduced the oral clearance of **diazepam** by 42% in white American subjects but only by 21% in Chinese subjects.[8] Metaboliser status (see 'Genetic factors', (p.4)) was also found to be important in another study of this interaction: only extensive metabolisers of CYP2C19 showed a significant decrease in diazepam clearance when given omeprazole,[9]

(d) Pantoprazole

In a placebo-controlled study in 12 healthy subjects, intravenous pantoprazole 240 mg for 7 days did not change the half-life, clearance and AUC of a 100-microgram/kg intravenous bolus dose of **diazepam**.[10]

(e) Rabeprazole

Rabeprazole 20 mg daily or placebo was given to 15 patients (in 3 groups) for 23 days with a single 100-microgram/kg dose of **diazepam** on day 8. Each group contained at least two poor metabolisers and three extensive metabolisers of the cytochrome P450 isoenzyme CYP2C19 (see 'Genetic factors', (p.4)). No significant changes in the pharmacokinetics of the **diazepam** were seen.[11] Another study similarly found that rabeprazole does not affect the pharmacokinetics of **diazepam** in both poor and extensive metabolisers of CYP2C19.[9]

Mechanism

In vitro studies with human liver microsomes suggest that omeprazole inhibits diazepam metabolism because it inhibits the cytochrome P450 isoenzymes CYP3A, and CYP2C19.[12] Studies in humans suggest that CYP2C19 may be the most important isoenzyme in this interaction.[8] The reaction with lorazepam (and other glucuronidated benzodiazepines) may possibly not be an interaction (so it is suggested) but an adverse effect of giving sedating medications to markedly anaemic patients.[4]

Importance and management

Information is limited, but what is currently known suggests that patients given omeprazole and possibly esomeprazole and diazepam may experience increased benzodiazepine effects (sedation, unstable gait etc). If this occurs the benzodiazepine dosage should be reduced. Lansoprazole, pantoprazole and rabeprazole do not appear to interact with diazepam.

Further *in vitro* study suggests that omeprazole may possibly interact similarly with **midazolam**,[13] although this needs confirmation. There seems to be no information regarding other benzodiazepines.

1. Nexium (Esomeprazole). AstraZeneca UK Ltd. UK Summary of product characteristics, October 2004.
2. Lefebvre RA, Flouvat B, Karolac-Tamisier S, Moerman E, Van Ganse E. Influence of lansoprazole treatment on diazepam plasma concentrations. *Clin Pharmacol Ther* (1992) 52, 458–63.
3. Martí-Massó JF, López de Munain A, López de Dicastillo G. Ataxia following gastric bleeding due to omeprazole–benzodiazepine interaction. *Ann Pharmacother* (1992) 26, 429–30.
4. Shader RI. Question the experts. *J Clin Psychopharmacol* (1993) 13, 459.
5. Konrad A. Protracted episode of reduced consciousness following co-medication with omeprazole and clorazepate. *Clin Drug Invest* (2000) 19, 307–11.
6. Gugler R, Jensen JC. Omeprazole inhibits elimination of diazepam. *Lancet* (1984) i, 969.
7. Andersson T, Andrén K, Cederberg C, Edvardsson G, Heggelund A, Lundborg P. Effect of omeprazole and cimetidine on plasma diazepam levels. *Eur J Clin Pharmacol* (1990) 39, 51–4.
8. Caraco Y, Tateishi T, Wood AJ. Interethnic difference in omeprazole's inhibition of diazepam metabolism. *Clin Pharmacol Ther* (1995) 58, 62–72.
9. Ishizaki T, Chiba K, Manabe K, Koyama E, Hayashi M, Yasuda S, Horai Y, Tomono Y, Yamato C, Toyoki T. Comparison of the interaction potential of a new proton pump inhibitor, E3810, versus omeprazole with diazepam in extensive and poor metabolizers of *S*-mephenytoin 4'-hydroxylation. *Clin Pharmacol Ther* (1995) 58, 155–64.
10. Gugler R, Hartmann M, Rudi J, Brod I, Huber R, Steinijans VW, Bliesath H, Wurst W, Klotz U. Lack of pharmacokinetic interaction of pantoprazole and diazepam in man. *Br J Clin Pharmacol* (1996) 42, 249–52.
11. Merritt GJ, Humphries TJ, Spera AC, Hale JA, Laurent AL. Effect of rabeprazole sodium on the pharmacokinetics of diazepam in healthy male volunteers. *Pharm Res* (1997) 14 (Suppl 11), S-566.
12. Zomorodi K, Houston JB. Diazepam–omeprazole inhibition interaction: an *in vitro* investigation using human liver microsomes. *Br J Clin Pharmacol* (1996) 42, 157–62.
13. Li G, Klotz U. Inhibitory effect of omeprazole on the metabolism of midazolam in vitro. *Arzneimittelforschung* (1990) 40, 1105–7.

Benzodiazepines + Quinolones

Ciprofloxacin causes a marked reduction in the clearance of diazepam, but this does not appear to be clinically important in most individuals. Ciprofloxacin appears not to interact with temazepam and gatifloxacin appears not to interact with midazolam.

Clinical evidence, mechanism, importance and management

(a) Ciprofloxacin

Ciprofloxacin 500 mg twice daily for 3 days was found to have no effect on the pharmacokinetics of **diazepam** in a study in 10 healthy subjects.[1] However, a later study in 12 healthy subjects found that ciprofloxacin 500 mg twice daily for 5 days increased the AUC of a single 5-mg intravenous dose of **diazepam** by 50%, reduced its clearance by 37% and doubled its half-life. These changes caused no significant alteration in the performance of a number of psychometric tests. It was suggested that ciprofloxacin inhibited the cytochrome P450-mediated metabolism of diazepam.[2] Another study by the same group found that ciprofloxacin does not interact with **temazepam**.[3]

It seems unlikely that any marked increases in **diazepam** effects (drowsiness etc.) will occur in most patients, but it may possibly be significant in those who have reduced renal or hepatic clearance (e.g. the elderly).[2] This needs confirmation.

(b) Gatifloxacin

Gatifloxacin 400 mg daily for 5 days had no effect on the pharmacokinetics of **midazolam** in 14 healthy subjects. The pharmacokinetics of gatifloxacin were also unaffected by concurrent use.[4]

1. Wijnands WJA, Trooster JFG, Teunissen PC, Cats HA, Vree TB. Ciprofloxacin does not impair the elimination of diazepam in humans. *Drug Metab Dispos* (1990) 18, 954–7.
2. Kamali F, Thomas SHL, Edwards C. The influence of steady-state ciprofloxacin on the pharmacokinetics and pharmacodynamics of a single dose of diazepam in healthy volunteers. *Eur J Clin Pharmacol* (1993) 44, 365–7.
3. Kamali F, Nicholson E, Edwards C. Ciprofloxacin does not influence temazepam pharmacokinetics. *Br J Clin Pharmacol* (1994) 37, 118P.
4. Grasela DM, LaCreta FP, Kollia GD, Randall DM, Uderman HD. Open-label, nonrandomized study of the effects of gatifloxacin on the pharmacokinetics of midazolam in healthy male volunteers. *Pharmacotherapy* (2000) 20, 330–5.

Benzodiazepines and related drugs + Rifampicin (Rifampin)

Rifampicin causes a very marked increase in the loss from the body of diazepam, midazolam, nitrazepam, triazolam, zaleplon, zolpidem and zopiclone but not temazepam. Benzodiazepines that are metabolised similarly are expected to interact in the same way.

Clinical evidence

(a) Diazepam

The mean half-life of diazepam was reduced from 58 to 14 hours and the clearance was increased fourfold in 7 patients with tuberculosis treated with daily doses of isoniazid 500 mg to 2.2 g, rifampicin 450 to 600 mg and ethambutol 25 mg/kg when compared to healthy control subjects.[1] Rifampicin 600 or 1200 mg daily for 7 days increased the clearance of diazepam in 21 healthy subjects by about threefold.[2]

(b) Midazolam

A pharmacokinetic study in 10 healthy subjects found that rifampicin 600 mg daily for 5 days reduced the AUC of a single 15-mg oral dose of midazolam by 96%, and shortened the half-life by almost two-thirds. The psychomotor effects of the midazolam (as measured by the digit symbol substitution test, Maddox wing test, postural sway and drowsiness) were almost totally lost.[3]

(c) Nitrazepam

A study in healthy subjects found that the total body clearance of nitrazepam in was increased by 83% by rifampicin 600 mg daily for 7 days.[4]

(d) Temazepam

A study found that the pharmacokinetics of temazepam were unchanged by rifampicin.[4]

(e) Triazolam

Triazolam 500 micrograms orally was given to 10 healthy subjects before and after rifampicin 600 mg or a placebo daily for 5 days. The rifampicin reduced the triazolam AUC by 95% and decreased the maximum plasma triazolam levels by 88% when compared with the placebo group. The elimination half-life fell from 2.8 to 1.3 hours. Pharmacodynamic tests (drowsiness, sway, Maddox wing, etc.) showed that the rifampicin abolished the effects of triazolam.[5]

(f) Zaleplon

A non-randomised, multidose, two-period, crossover study in healthy subjects found that rifampicin 600 mg daily for 14 days increased the clearance of a 10-mg dose of zaleplon 5.4-fold, decreasing its maximum serum levels and AUC by 80%.[6]

(g) Zolpidem

In a randomised, placebo-controlled, crossover study, 8 healthy subjects were given rifampicin 600 mg or a placebo daily for 5 days and then on day 6 they were given a single 20-mg oral dose of zolpidem. It was found that the rifampicin reduced the zolpidem AUC by 73%, reduced the maximum plasma concentration by about 60% and reduced its half-life from 2.5 to 1.6 hours. A significant reduction in the effects of zolpidem were also seen, as measured by a number of psychomotor tests (digital symbol substitution, critical flicker fusion, subjective drowsiness, etc.).[7]

(h) Zopiclone

In a two-phase study 8 healthy subjects were given rifampicin 600 mg or a placebo daily for 5 days, with a single 10-mg oral dose of zopiclone on day 6. The rifampicin reduced the zopiclone AUC by 82%, decreased the peak serum levels by 71% and reduced its half-life from 3.8 to 2.3 hours. A significant reduction in the effects of zopiclone was also seen, as measured by the performance of psychomotor tests.[8]

Mechanism

Rifampicin is a potent liver enzyme inducing agent, which increases the metabolism of several benzodiazepines, zaleplon, zolpidem and zopiclone, thereby hastening their loss from the body. The metabolism of midazolam by the cytochrome P450 isoenzyme CYP3A4 in both liver and gut is affected.[3] The enzyme inducing effects of the rifampicin seem to predominate if isoniazid (an enzyme inhibitor) is also present. Temazepam undergoes glucuronidation and is therefore unaffected by rifampicin.

Importance and management

The documentation of these interactions is limited but what has been reported is consistent with the way rifampicin interacts with many other drugs. The clinical importance of some of these interactions between the benzodiazepines and rifampicin has not yet been assessed but what is known suggests that you may need to increase the dosage of diazepam and nitrazepam if rifampicin is given. Be alert for a reduction in the effects of other similarly metabolised benzodiazepines (e.g. chlordiazepoxide, flurazepam). Alprazolam is predicted to interact because CYP3A is involved with its metabolism.[9] The effect of rifampicin on oral midazolam, triazolam, zaleplon, zolpidem and zopiclone is so very large that they are likely to become ineffective and an alternative should be used instead.

Those benzodiazepines that, like temazepam, undergo glucuronidation (e.g. lorazepam, oxazepam) are not expected to be affected by rifampicin and may be useful alternatives.

1. Ochs HR, Greenblatt DJ, Roberts G-M, Dengler HJ. Diazepam interaction with antituberculosis drugs. *Clin Pharmacol Ther* (1981) 29, 671–8.
2. Ohnhaus EE, Brockmeyer N, Dylewicz P, Habicht H. The effect of antipyrine and rifampin on the metabolism of diazepam. *Clin Pharmacol Ther* (1987) 42, 148–56.
3. Backman JT, Olkkola KT, Neuvonen PJ. Rifampin drastically reduces plasma concentrations and effects of oral midazolam. *Clin Pharmacol Ther* (1996) 59, 7–13.
4. Brockmeyer NH, Mertins L, Klimek K, Goos M, Ohnhaus EE. Comparative effects of rifampin and/or probenecid on the pharmacokinetics of temazepam and nitrazepam. *Int J Clin Pharmacol Ther Toxicol* (1990) 28, 387–93.
5. Villikka K, Kivostö KT, Backman JT, Olkkola KT, Neuvonen PJ. Triazolam is ineffective in patients taking rifampin. *Clin Pharmacol Ther* (1997) 61, 8–14.
6. Darwish M. Overview of drug interaction studies with zaleplon. Poster presented at 13th Annual Meeting of Associated Professional Sleep Studies (APSS), Orlando, Florida, June 23rd, 1999.
7. Villikka K, Kivistö KT, Luurila H, Neuvonen PJ. Rifampicin reduces plasma concentrations and effects of zolpidem. *Clin Pharmacol Ther* (1997) 62, 629–34.
8. Villikka K, Kivistö KT, Lamberg TS, Kantola T, Neuvonen PJ. Concentrations and effects of zopiclone are greatly reduced by rifampicin. *Br J Clin Pharmacol* (1997) 43, 471–4.
9. Greenblatt DJ, von Moltke LL, Harmatz JS, Ciraulo DA, Shader RI. Alprazolam pharmacokinetics, metabolism, and plasma levels: clinical implications. *J Clin Psychiatry* (1993) 54, 10 (Suppl), 4–11.

Benzodiazepines + St John's wort (*Hypericum perforatum*)

St John's wort decreases the metabolism of quazepam, although this did not increase the effects of quazepam in one study. Alprazolam appears not to interact, although this needs confirmation.

Clinical evidence, mechanism, importance and management

(a) Alprazolam

Alprazolam 1 or 2 mg was given to 7 healthy subjects on the third day of a 3-day treatment period with St John's wort (*Solaray*; hypericin content standardised at 0.3%) 300 mg three times daily. The pharmacokinetics of alprazolam were unchanged by the St John's wort, but the authors note that 3 days may have been an insufficient time for St John's wort to fully induce cytochrome P450 isoenzymes.[1]

(b) Quazepam

In a placebo-controlled crossover study 13 healthy subjects were given St John's wort (*TruNature*; hypericin content standardised at 0.3%) 300 mg three times daily for 14 days, with a single 15-mg dose of quazepam on day 14. Although St John's wort did not affect the pharmacodynamic effects of quazepam it did decrease the quazepam AUC by 26% and the maximum plasma levels by 29%.This was attributed to the effects of St John's wort on the cytochrome P450 isoenzyme CYP3A4, by which quazepam is metabolised.[2] See also 'Drug-herb interactions', (p.10).

1. Markowitz JS, DeVane CL, Boulton DW, Carson SW, Nahas Z, Risch SC. Effect of St John's wort (*Hypericum perforatum*) on cytochrome P-450 2D6 and 3A4 activity in healthy volunteers. *Life Sci* (2000) 66, 133–9.
2. Kawaguchi A, Ohmori M, Tsuruoka S, Harada K, Miyamori I, Yano R, Nakamura T, Masada M, Fujimura A. Drug interaction between St John's wort and quazepam. *Br J Clin Pharmacol* (2004) 58, 403–10.

Benzodiazepines + Sucrose polyesters

Sucrose polyesters (e.g. *Olestra*) do not appear to interact with diazepam.

Clinical evidence, mechanism, importance and management

A single dose of **diazepam** was given to 8 healthy subjects with 18 g of sucrose polyester. Apart from causing a small delay in time to peak concentration, the sucrose polyester had no effect on the pharmacokinetics of **diazepam**.[1] Sucrose polyesters, are non-absorbable, non-calorific fat replacements. It has been concluded that sucrose polyesters are unlikely to reduce the absorption of oral drugs in general.[2]

1. Roberts RJ, Leff RD. Influence of absorbable and nonabsorbable lipids and lipidlike substances on drug availability. *Clin Pharmacol Ther* (1989) 45, 299–304.
2. Goldman P. Olestra: assessing its potential to interact with drugs in the gastrointestinal tract. *Clin Pharmacol Ther* (1997) 61, 613–18.

Benzodiazepines and related drugs + Tobacco smoking

Smokers may possibly need larger doses of some benzodiazepines and zolpidem than non-smokers.

Clinical evidence, mechanism, importance and management

Some studies have suggested that smoking does not affect the pharmacokinetics of **diazepam**[1,2] **chlordiazepoxide**,[3] **clorazepate**,[4] **lorazepam**,[2] **midazolam**,[2] or **triazolam**,[5] but others have found that the clearance of **alprazolam**,[6] **clorazepate**,[7] **diazepam**,[8] **lorazepam**[9] and **oxazepam**[10,11] from the body is increased by smoking, but not all the changes are significant.[8] The Boston Collaborative Drug Surveillance Program reported a decreased frequency of drowsiness in those taking **diazepam** or **chlordiazepoxide** who smoked,[12] which confirmed the findings of a previous study.[13] It has also been noted that two heavy smokers had a very high clearance and did not experience any sedative effects following the use of **zolpidem**.[14]

The probable reason for the reduction in sedative effects with these drugs is that some of the components of tobacco smoke are enzyme-inducing agents, which increase the rate at which the liver metabolises these benzodiazepines thereby reducing their effects. The inference to be drawn is that smokers may possibly need larger doses than non-smokers to achieve the same therapeutic effects, and smoking also possibly reduces the drowsiness that the benzodiazepines and **zolpidem** can cause. However, one study suggested that caffeine intake,[13] and others suggest age, may affect the response to benzodiazepines, so the picture is not altogether clear. Whether any of these interactions has much clinical relevance awaits assessment.

1. Klotz U, Avant GR, Hoyumpa A, Schenker S, Wilkinson GR. The effects of age and liver disease on the disposition and elimination of diazepam in adult man. *J Clin Invest* (1975) 55, 347–59.
2. Ochs HR, Greenblatt DJ, Knüchel M. Kinetics of diazepam, midazolam, and lorazepam in cigarette smokers. *Chest* (1985) 87, 223–6.
3. Desmond PV, Roberts RK, Wilkinson GR, Schenker S. No effect of smoking on metabolism of chlordiazepoxide. *N Engl J Med* (1979) 300, 199–200.
4. Ochs HR, Greenblatt DJ, Locniskar A, Weinbrenner J. Influence of propranolol coadministration or cigarette smoking on the kinetics of desmethyldiazepam following intravenous clorazepate. *Klin Wochenschr* (1986) 64, 1217–21.
5. Ochs HR, Greenblatt DJ, Burstein ES. Lack of influence of cigarette smoking on triazolam pharmacokinetics. *Br J Clin Pharmacol* (1987) 23, 759–63.
6. Smith RB, Gwilt PR, Wright CE. Single- and multiple-dose pharmacokinetics of oral alprazolam in healthy smoking and nonsmoking men. *Clin Pharm* (1983) 2, 139–43.
7. Norman TR, Fulton A, Burrows GD, Maguire KP. Pharmacokinetics of N-desmethyldiazepam after a single oral dose of clorazepate: the effect of smoking. *Eur J Clin Pharmacol* (1981) 21, 229–33.
8. Greenblatt DJ, Allen MD, Harmatz JS, Shader RI. Diazepam disposition determinants. *Clin Pharmacol Ther* (1980) 27, 301–12.
9. Greenblatt DJ, Allen MD, Locniskar A, Harmatz JS, Shader RI. Lorazepam kinetics in the elderly. *Clin Pharmacol Ther* (1979) 26, 103–13.
10. Greenblatt DJ, Divoll M, Harmatz JS, Shader RI. Oxazepam kinetics: effects of age and sex. *J Pharmacol Exp Ther* (1980) 215, 86–91.
11. Ochs HR, Greenblatt DJ, Otten H. Disposition of oxazepam in relation to age, sex, and cigarette smoking. *Klin Wochenschr* (1981) 59, 899–903.
12. Boston Collaborative Drug Surveillance Program. Clinical depression of the central nervous system due to diazepam and chlordiazepoxide in relation to cigarette smoking and age. *N Engl J Med* (1973) 288, 277–80.
13. Downing RW, Rickels K. Coffee consumption, cigarette smoking and reporting of drowsiness in anxious patients treated with benzodiazepines or placebo. *Acta Psychiatr Scand* (1981) 64, 398–408.
14. Sauvanet JP, Langer SZ, Morselli PL, eds. Imidazopyridines in Sleep Disorders. New York: Raven Press; 1988 p. 165–73.

Benzodiazepines + Vinpocetine

Vinpocetine does not appear to interact adversely with oxazepam.

Clinical evidence, mechanism, importance and management

No changes in the steady-state plasma levels of **oxazepam** 10 mg three times daily were seen in 16 healthy subjects who took vinpocetine 10 mg three times daily, for 7 days.[1] There would therefore seem to be no reason for taking special precautions if these two drugs are given together.

1. Storm G, Oosterhuis, Sollie FAE, Visscher HW, Sommer W, Beitinger H, Jonkman JHG. Lack of pharmacokinetic interaction between vinpocetine and oxazepam. *Br J Clin Pharmacol* (1994) 38, 143–6.

Benzodiazepines and related drugs + Xanthines

Theophylline reduces the serum levels of alprazolam. Caffeine, and to a lesser extent theophylline, may reduce the sedative (and possibly also the anxiolytic) effects of diazepam and clonazepam. Caffeine also opposes the effects of triazolam and zopiclone. Aminophylline antagonises the anaesthesia induced by benzodiazepines.

Clinical evidence

Caffeine, and to a lesser extent **theophylline**, counteract the drowsiness and mental slowness induced by single 10- to 20-mg doses of **diazepam**.[1-4] There is also evidence that **caffeine**, and **clonazepam**[5] or **triazolam**[6] have mutually opposing effects and that **caffeine** may interact similarly with **zopiclone**.[6]

No pharmacokinetic interaction occurred between **zolpidem** and **caffeine** (given as one cup of **coffee** containing **caffeine** 300 mg), and the hypnotic effects of the **zolpidem** were unchanged.[7]

In a comparative study, two groups of patients (one group of 6 patients with chronic obstructive pulmonary disease (COPD) taking **theophylline** and another group of 7 patients with chronic heart failure or atherosclerotic disease (one also with COPD) not taking theophylline) were given **alprazolam** 500 micrograms twice daily for 7 days. On day 7, those taking the **theophylline** were found to have trough serum **alprazolam** levels of 13.25 nanograms/ml, while in the other group the levels were 43.92 nanograms/ml.[8]

A patient who was unrousable and unresponsive following **diazepam** 60 mg given over 10 minutes and nitrous oxide/oxygen anaesthesia, rapidly returned to consciousness when given **aminophylline** 56 mg intravenously.[9] Other reports confirm this antagonism of **diazepam**, even by low doses of **aminophylline** (60 mg to 4.5 mg/kg intravenously).[10-12] **Flunitrazepam**,[13] **lorazepam**,[14] and **midazolam**[15] are also affected. There is some controversy about whether or not **theophylline** antagonises the effects of **midazolam**.[16,17]

Mechanism

Uncertain. One suggestion is that the xanthines can block adenosine receptors.[10] Another is that the xanthines induce the metabolism of the benzodiazepines by the liver so that they are cleared from the body more rapidly.[18]

Importance and management

The documentation is somewhat sparse and there is a need for more study over the range of benzodiazepines, but the overall picture is that these interactions are established. The extent to which these xanthines actually reduce the anxiolytic effects of the benzodiazepines remains uncertain (it needs assessment) but be alert for reduced benzodiazepine effects if both are used. Caffeine in tea or coffee appears to reduce the sedative effects of triazolam and zopiclone. This would appear to be a disadvantage at night, but may possibly be useful the next morning.

1. Mattila MJ, Nuotto E. Caffeine and theophylline counteract diazepam effects in man. *Med Biol* (1983) 61, 337–43.
2. Mattila MJ, Palva E, Savolainen K. Caffeine antagonizes diazepam effects in man. *Med Biol* (1982) 60, 121–3.
3. Henauer SA, Hollister LE, Gillespie HK, Moore F. Theophylline antagonizes diazepam-induced psychomotor impairment. *Eur J Clin Pharmacol* (1983) 25, 743–7.
4. Meyer BH, Weis OF, Müller FO. Antagonism of diazepam by aminophylline in healthy volunteers. *Anesth Analg* (1984) 63, 900–2.
5. Koella WP, Rüther E, Schulz H, eds. Sleep '84. New York: Gustav Fischer Verlag; 1985 p. 314–15.
6. Mattila ME, Mattila MJ, Nuotto E. Caffeine moderately antagonizes the effects of triazolam and zopiclone on the psychomotor performance of healthy subjects. *Pharmacol Toxicol* (1992) 70, 286–9.
7. Salvà P, Costa J. Clinical pharmacokinetics and pharmacodynamics of zolpidem: therapeutic implications. *Clin Pharmacokinet* (1995) 29, 142–53.
8. Tuncok Y, Akpinar O, Guven H, Akkoclu A. The effects of theophylline on serum alprazolam levels. *Int J Clin Pharmacol Ther* (1994) 32, 642–5.
9. Stirt JA. Aminophylline is a diazepam antagonist. *Anesth Analg* (1981) 60, 767–8.
10. Niemand D, Martinell S, Arvidsson S, Svedmyr N, Ekström-Jodal B. Aminophylline inhibition of diazepam sedation: is adenosine blockade of GABA-receptors the mechanism? *Lancet* (1984) i, 463–4.
11. Arvidsson SB, Ekström-Jodal B, Martinell SAG, Niemand D. Aminophylline antagonises diazepam sedation. *Lancet* (1982) 2, 1467.
12. Kleindienst G, Usinger P. Diazepam sedation is not antagonised completely by aminophylline. *Lancet* (1984) 1, 113.
13. Gürel A, Elevli M, Hamulu A. Aminophylline reversal of flunitrazepam sedation. *Anesth Analg* (1987) 66, 333–6.
14. Wangler MA, Kilpatrick DS. Aminophylline is an antagonist of lorazepam. *Anesth Analg* (1985) 64, 834–6.
15. Gallen JS. Aminophylline reversal of midazolam sedation. *Anesth Analg* (1989) 69, 268.
16. Kanto J, Aaltonen L, Himberg J-J, Hovi-Viander M. Midazolam as an intravenous induction agent in the elderly: a clinical and pharmacokinetic study. *Anesth Analg* (1986) 65, 15–20.
17. Sleigh JW. Failure of aminophylline to antagonize midazolam sedation. *Anesth Analg* (1986) 65, 540.
18. Ghoneim MM, Hinrichs JV, Chiang C-K, Loke WH. Pharmacokinetic and pharmacodynamic interactions between caffeine and diazepam. *J Clin Psychopharmacol* (1986) 6, 75–80.

Buspirone + Azoles

The plasma levels of buspirone are markedly increased by itraconazole. Ketoconazole is predicted to interact similarly.

Clinical evidence

In a placebo-controlled study, 8 healthy subjects were given buspirone 10 mg, before and after taking **itraconazole** 100 mg twice daily for 4 days. It was found that the buspirone maximum plasma levels and its AUC were increased 13-fold and 19-fold by the **itraconazole**. These increased buspirone concentrations caused a moderate impairment of psychomotor performance (digital symbol substitution, body sway, drowsiness, etc.) and an increase in adverse effects.[1]

Mechanism

Itraconazole is a potent inhibitor of the cytochrome P450 isoenzyme CYP3A4 by which buspirone is metabolised. Itraconazole therefore increases buspirone levels and effects.

Importance and management

Direct information appears to be limited to this study but the interaction would seem to be established. The dosage of buspirone should be greatly reduced if itraconazole is given concurrently. The makers recommend 2.5 mg daily[2] or twice daily.[3] **Ketoconazole** is predicted to interact similarly because it is also a potent CYP3A4 inhibitor.[1]

1. Kivistö KT, Lamberg TS, Kantola T, Neuvonen PJ. Plasma buspirone concentrations are greatly increased by erythromycin and itraconazole. *Clin Pharmacol Ther* (1997) 62, 348–54.
2. Buspar (Buspirone hydrochloride). Bristol-Myers Squibb Company. US Prescribing information, November 2003.
3. Buspar (Buspirone hydrochloride). Bristol-Myers Pharmaceuticals. UK Summary of product characteristics, July 2005.

Buspirone + Calcium channel blockers

Diltiazem and verapamil can markedly raise the plasma levels of buspirone, increasing the likelihood of adverse effects.

Clinical evidence, mechanism, importance and management

In a randomised crossover study in 9 healthy subjects, the AUC of a single 10-mg dose of buspirone was increased 5.5-fold and the maximum plasma levels 4.1-fold by **diltiazem** 60 mg three times daily for 5 doses.

When **verapamil** 80 mg three times daily was similarly given with buspirone, the buspirone AUC and maximum plasma levels were increased 3.4-fold.

The increased buspirone levels are thought to occur because both **diltiazem** and **verapamil** inhibit the cytochrome P450 isoenzyme CYP3A4, which is concerned with the metabolism of the buspirone.[1]

The practical consequences of this interaction are that the effects of buspirone are likely to be increased by **diltiazem** and **verapamil**. Concurrent use need not be avoided but be alert for the need to reduce the buspirone dosage. The US makers suggest adjusting according to response[2], while the UK makers suggest starting with buspirone 2.5 mg twice daily.[3] Information about other calcium channel blockers appears to be lacking, but, with the possible exception of nifedipine, they do not commonly appear to interact by inhibiting CYP3A4.

1. Lamberg TS, Kivistö KT, Neuvonen PJ. Effects of verapamil and diltiazem on the pharmacokinetics and pharmacodynamics of buspirone. *Clin Pharmacol Ther* (1998) 63, 640–5.
2. Buspar (Buspirone hydrochloride). Bristol-Myers Squibb Company. US Prescribing information, November 2003.
3. Buspar (Buspirone hydrochloride). Bristol-Myers Pharmaceuticals. UK Summary of product characteristics, July 2005.

Buspirone + Herbal medicines

Two patients on buspirone developed marked CNS effects after starting to take herbal medicines including St John's wort and ginkgo biloba.

Clinical evidence, mechanism, importance and management

A 27-year-old woman who had been taking buspirone 30 mg daily for over a month started to take **St John's wort** (*Hypercum 2000 Plus*, Herb Valley, Australia) three tablets daily. After 2 months she complained of nervousness, aggression, hyperactivity, insomnia, confusion and disorientation, which was attributed to the serotonin syndrome. The **St John's wort** was stopped, the buspirone was increased to 50 mg daily and her symptoms resolved over a week.[1] A 42-year-old woman who was taking fluoxetine 20 mg twice daily and buspirone 15 mg twice daily started to develop symptoms of anxiety, with episodes of over-sleeping and memory deficits. It was discovered that she had been self-medicating with **St John's wort**, **ginkgo biloba** and melatonin. She was asked to stop the non-prescribed medication and her symptoms resolved.[2]

The exact mechanism of these interactions are not clear, but it seems most likely they were due to the additive effects of the buspirone or fluoxetine and the herbal medicines, either through their effects on elevating mood or through excess effects on serotonin. See also 'SSRIs + St John's wort (*Hypericum perforatum*)', p.987. The clinical significance of these cases is unclear, but they highlight the importance of considering adverse effects from herbal medicines when they are used with conventional medicines.

1. Dannawi M. Possible serotonin syndrome after combination of buspirone and St John's wort. *J Psychopharmacol* (2002) 16, 401.
2. Spinella M, Eaton LA. Hypomania induced by herbal and pharmaceutical psychotropic medicines following mild traumatic brain injury. *Brain Inj* (2002) 16, 359–67.

Buspirone + Macrolides

The plasma levels of buspirone are markedly increased by erythromycin.

Clinical evidence

In a placebo-controlled study buspirone 10 mg was given to 8 healthy subjects before and after they took **erythromycin** 500 mg three times daily for 4 days. It was found that the buspirone maximum plasma levels and its AUC were increased 5-fold and 6-fold respectively, by the **erythromycin**. These increased buspirone concentrations caused a moderate impairment of psychomotor performance (digital symbol substitution, body sway, drowsiness, etc.) and an increase in adverse effects.[1]

Mechanism

Erythromycin is a potent inhibitor of the cytochrome P450 isoenzyme CYP3A4 by which buspirone is metabolised. Erythromycin therefore increases buspirone levels and hence its effects.

Importance and management

Direct information appears to be limited to this study but the interactions would seem to be established. The dosage of buspirone should be reduced if erythromycin is given concurrently. The makers suggest using buspirone 2.5 mg twice daily,[2,3] adjusted according to response.[3]

Other macrolides (such as **troleandomycin**) are also inhibitors of CYP3A4 and may therefore interact similarly.

1. Kivistö KT, Lamberg TS, Kantola T, Neuvonen PJ. Plasma buspirone concentrations are greatly increased by erythromycin and itraconazole. *Clin Pharmacol Ther* (1997) 62, 348–54.
2. Buspar (Buspirone hydrochloride). Bristol-Myers Pharmaceuticals. UK Summary of product characteristics, July 2005.
3. Buspar (Buspirone hydrochloride). Bristol-Myers Squibb Company. US Prescribing information, November 2003.

Buspirone + Miscellaneous

Buspirone and amitriptyline, cimetidine or terfenadine appear not to interact. An isolated report describes mania in an alcoholic patient on buspirone when given disulfiram. Nefazodone greatly increases buspirone levels.

Clinical evidence, mechanism, importance and management

(a) Amitriptyline

Buspirone 15 mg every 8 hours given with amitriptyline 25 mg every 8 hours for 10 days had no significant effect on the steady-state serum levels of amitriptyline or its metabolite nortriptyline in healthy subjects. No evidence of a pharmacodynamic interaction was seen.[1] There would seem to be no reason for avoiding concurrent use.

(b) Cimetidine

In 10 healthy subjects cimetidine 1 g daily for 7 days had no effect on plasma levels of buspirone 15 mg three times daily. Some small pharmacokinetic changes were seen, but the performance of three psychomotor function tests remained unaltered.[2] There would seem to be no reason for avoiding concurrent use.

(c) Disulfiram

An isolated report describes mania in an alcoholic patient on buspirone 20 mg daily, possibly due to an interaction with disulfiram 400 mg daily[3], but buspirone on its own has also apparently caused mania.[4,5] The reasons are not understood, but until more is known caution should be taken if both drugs are used in combination.

(d) Nefazodone

Nefazodone 250 mg twice daily caused 20-fold increases in the maximum plasma levels and 50-fold increases in the AUC of buspirone 2.5 or 5 mg twice daily. Buspirone 5 mg twice daily raised the nefazodone AUC by 23%, which is unlikely to be clinically significant. The makers recommend that buspirone 2.5 mg daily is used in the presence of nefazodone.[6]

(e) Terfenadine

A single 10-mg dose of buspirone was given to 10 healthy subjects after they had taken terfenadine 120 mg daily for 3 days. There were no significant effects on the pharmacokinetics or pharmacodynamics of buspirone.[7]

1. Gammans RE, Mayol RF, Labudde JA. Metabolism and disposition of buspirone. *Am J Med* (1986) 80 (Suppl 3B), 41–51.
2. Gammans RE, Pfeffer M, Westrick ML, Faulkner HC, Rehm KD, Goodson PJ. Lack of interaction between cimetidine and buspirone. *Pharmacotherapy* (1987) 7, 72–9.
3. McIvor RJ, Sinanan K. Buspirone-induced mania. *Br J Psychiatry* (1991) 158, 136–7.
4. Price WA, Bielefeld M. Buspirone-induced mania. *J Clin Psychopharmacol* (1989) 9, 150–1.
5. McDaniel JS, Ninan PT, Magnuson JV. Possible induction of mania by buspirone. *Am J Psychiatry* (1990) 147, 125–6.
6. Serzone (Nefazodone). Bristol-Myers Squibb Company. US Prescribing information, April 2004.
7. Lamberg TS, Kivistö KT, Neuvonen PJ. Lack of effect of terfenadine on the pharmacokinetics of the CYP3A4 substrate buspirone. *Pharmacol Toxicol* (1999) 84, 165–9.

Buspirone + Rifampicin (Rifampin)

Rifampicin can cause a marked reduction in the plasma levels and effects of buspirone.

Clinical evidence

In a randomised, two-phase crossover study, buspirone 30 mg daily was given to 10 healthy subjects, before and after they took rifampicin 600 mg daily for 5 days. It was found that the rifampicin reduced the total AUC of the buspirone by almost 90% and reduced the peak plasma levels by 87%. The pharmacodynamic effects of the buspirone were reduced accordingly (as measured by digit symbol substitution, critical flicker fusion, body sway and visual analogue scales for subjective drowsiness).[1]

Mechanism

Not fully established but it is almost certain that the rifampicin induces the cytochrome P450 isoenzyme CYP3A4 in the gut and liver, which metabolises buspirone. Therefore the metabolism and clearance of the buspirone are increased.

Importance and management

Direct information appears to be limited to this study but it is consistent with the way rifampicin interacts with many other drugs. This interaction would appear to be clinically important. If both drugs are used be alert for the need to use an increased buspirone dosage.

1. Lambert TS, Kivistö KT, Neuvonen PJ. Concentrations and effects of buspirone are considerably reduced by rifampicin. *Br J Clin Pharmacol* (1998) 45, 381–5.

Buspirone + SSRIs

An isolated report describes the development of the serotonin syndrome with buspirone and citalopram. The combination of buspirone and fluoxetine can be effective, but seizures and worsening of symptoms have been reported. Fluvoxamine may possibly reduce the effects of buspirone.

Clinical evidence, mechanism, importance and management

(a) Citalopram

An isolated report describes the development of the serotonin syndrome and hyponatraemia, thought to be caused by an interaction between citalopram and buspirone.[1] The general importance of this interaction is unknown.

(b) Fluoxetine

A 35-year-old man with a long history of depression, anxiety and panic was started on buspirone 60 mg daily. His anxiety abated, but worsening depression prompted additional treatment with trazodone 200 mg daily for 3 weeks, which had little effect, so fluoxetine 20 mg daily was added. Within 48 hours his usual symptoms of anxiety had returned and persisted even when the dose of buspirone was raised to 80 mg daily. Stopping the buspirone did not increase his anxiety.[2] Another patient with obsessive-compulsive disorder on fluoxetine experienced a marked worsening of his symptoms when buspirone 5 mg twice daily was added.[3] A patient had a grand mal seizure 3 weeks after buspirone 30 mg daily was added to fluoxetine 80 mg daily. The drugs were stopped and an EEG showed no signs of epilepsy, so the seizure was attributed to a drug interaction.[4] Other reports describe the effective concurrent use of fluoxetine and buspirone in patients with treatment-resistant depression[5] and with obsessive-compulsive disorder.[6,7]

The reasons for these adverse reactions are not understood, but there would seem to be little reason for avoiding concurrent use, however bear these interaction in mind when both drugs are used.

(c) Fluvoxamine

A double-blind study in 9 healthy subjects found that after taking fluvoxamine (mean dose 127 mg daily, range 100 to 150 mg daily) for 3 weeks, the plasma levels of a single 30-mg dose of buspirone were increased almost threefold. Even so, the psychological responses to the buspirone were reduced.[8] However, a study in 10 healthy subjects given a single 10-mg dose of buspirone after taking fluvoxamine 100 mg daily for 5 days, found that although the pharmacokinetics of buspirone were altered (AUC increased 2.4-fold) the pharmacodynamic tests remained unchanged.[9]

It has been suggested that fluvoxamine inhibits the liver enzymes concerned with the metabolism of buspirone. Concurrent use need not be avoided but it would be wise to remain alert to the possibility of reduced buspirone effects until more is known.

1. Spigset O, Adielsson G. Combined serotonin syndrome and hyponatraemia caused by a citalopram–buspirone interaction. *Int Clin Psychopharmacol* (1997) 12, 61–3.
2. Bodkin JA, Teicher MH. Fluoxetine may antagonize the anxiolytic action of buspirone. *J Clin Psychopharmacol* (1989) 9, 150.
3. Tanquary J, Masand P. Paradoxical reaction to buspirone augmentation of fluoxetine. *J Clin Psychopharmacol* (1990) 10, 377.
4. Grady TA, Pigott TA, L'Heureux F, Murphy DL. Seizure associated with fluoxetine and adjuvant buspirone therapy. *J Clin Psychopharmacol* (1992) 12, 70–1.
5. Bakish D. Fluoxetine potentiation by buspirone: three case histories. *Can J Psychiatry* (1991) 36, 749–50.
6. Markovitz PJ, Stagno SJ, Calabrese JR. Buspirone augmentation of fluoxetine in obsessive-compulsive disorder. *Am J Psychiatry* (1990) 147, 798–800.
7. Jenike MA, Baer L, Buttolph L. Buspirone augmentation of fluoxetine in patients with obsessive compulsive disorder. *J Clin Psychiatry* (1991) 52, 13–14.
8. Anderson IM, Deakin JFW, Miller HEJ. The effect of chronic fluvoxamine on hormonal and psychological responses to buspirone in normal volunteers. *Psychopharmacology (Berl)* (1996) 128, 74–82.
9. Lamberg TS, Kivistö KT, Laitila J, Mårtensson K, Neuvonen PJ. The effect of fluvoxamine on the pharmacokinetics and pharmacodynamics of buspirone. *Eur J Clin Pharmacol* (1998) 54, 761–6.

Chlorpromazine + Cimetidine

One study found that chlorpromazine serum levels are reduced by cimetidine, while another study suggested that they can be increased.

Clinical evidence, mechanism, importance and management

A study in 8 patients on chlorpromazine 75 to 450 mg daily found that cimetidine 1 g daily in divided doses for a week decreased their steady-state serum chlorpromazine levels by a third, from 37 to 24 micrograms/ml. A two-thirds fall was noted in one patient.[1] The reasons are not understood but a decrease in absorption from the gut has been suggested.[1]

In contrast another report describes 2 schizophrenic patients on chlorpromazine 100 mg four times daily who became excessively sedated when given cimetidine 400 mg twice daily. The sedation disappeared when the chlorpromazine dosage was halved. When the cimetidine was later withdrawn it was found necessary to give the original chlorpromazine dosage.[2] Chlorpromazine serum levels were not measured. There is no simple explanation for these discordant reports, but they emphasise the need to monitor the concurrent use of chlorpromazine and cimetidine. More study is needed. There seems to be no information about other phenothiazines.

1. Howes CA, Pullar T, Sourindhrin I, Mistra PC, Capel H, Lawson DH, Tilstone WJ. Reduced steady-state plasma concentrations of chlorpromazine and indomethacin in patients receiving cimetidine. *Eur J Clin Pharmacol* (1983) 24, 99–102.
2. Byrne A, O'Shea B. Adverse interaction between cimetidine and chlorpromazine in two cases of chronic schizophrenia. *Br J Psychiatry* (1989) 155, 413–15.

Chlorpromazine + Tetrabenazine

An isolated report describes severe Parkinson-like symptoms in a woman with Huntington's chorea when she was given tetrabenazine and chlorpromazine.

Clinical evidence, mechanism, importance and management

A woman with Huntington's chorea, successfully treated with tetrabenazine 100 mg daily for 9 years, became motionless, rigid, mute and only able to respond by blinking her eyes within a day of being given two intramuscular injections of chlorpromazine 25 mg. This was diagnosed as severe drug-induced parkinsonism, which rapidly responded to the withdrawal of both drugs and treatment with benzatropine mesilate given intramuscularly and orally. She had previously tolerated chlorpromazine well.[1] The reason for this reaction is not understood, and as tetrabenazine is used to treat movement disorders its clinical significance is unclear.

1. Moss JH, Stewart DE. Iatrogenic parkinsonism in Huntington's chorea. *Can J Psychiatry* (1986) 31, 865–6.

Clomethiazole + Diazoxide

Clomethiazole and diazoxide given to pregnant women in labour can cause marked respiratory depression in their infants for up to 36 hours after birth.

Clinical evidence

An infusion of 0.8% clomethiazole in a dose of 4 to 24 g was given during labour to 21 pregnant women of 28 to 40 weeks gestation for eclampsia or pre-eclamptic toxaemia. Diazoxide 75 to 150 mg was also given intravenously to 14 of the women for hypertension. All of their babies were born alive but 13 of the 21 suffered hypotonia, hypoventilation or apnoea for 24 to 36 hours after birth. All of the neonates affected, apart from one, came from the group of mothers who had been given diazoxide Three of them died of respiratory distress syndrome, one was only 28 weeks' gestation.[1]

Mechanism

Clomethiazole has some respiratory depressant effects, and is contraindicated in patients with respiratory deficiency, but it is not clear why, having passed across the placenta into the foetus, its effects should apparently be so markedly increased by diazoxide.

Importance and management

Although use of this drug combination in eclampsia is historical, the interaction is included on account of its severity. The author of the report says that the respiratory depression was managed successfully with intermittent positive pressure ventilation, provided that respiratory distress syndrome was not also present.[1]

1. Johnson RA. Adverse neonatal reaction to maternal administration of intravenous chlormethiazole and diazoxide. *BMJ* (1976) 1, 943.

Clomethiazole + Furosemide

Ten female patients aged 66 to 90 were given clomethiazole edisilate 500 mg as syrup each evening as a sedative, and 250 mg each morning with furosemide 20 to 80 mg. No significant changes in the serum levels or effects of clomethiazole or furosemide were detected, and no other significant adverse reactions were seen.[1]

1. Reid J, Judge TG. Chlormethiazole night sedation in elderly subjects receiving other medications. *Practitioner* (1980) 224, 751–3.

Clozapine + Anticholinergics

The anticholinergic effects of clozapine are additive with those of other anticholinergic drugs, which has led to urinary retention and delirium.

Clinical evidence, mechanism, importance and management

The makers of clozapine warn that the anticholinergic effects of some drugs may be additive with those of clozapine, which may lead to adverse effects such as dry mouth and constipation.[1,2] Confirmation of the clinical relevance of this proposed interaction was seen in a patient who developed severe urinary retention while taking clozapine and **meclozine**.[3]

A man with a schizoaffective disorder on **nortriptyline**, **perphenazine** and propranolol was additionally given clozapine 150 mg daily. Some improvement was seen after 8 days, and over the next week the propranolol was gradually discontinued while the clozapine dosage was raised to 225 mg daily. The patient then began to complain of extreme fatigue and slurred speech, and by day 17 was delirious and confused. His serum **nortriptyline** levels were found to have doubled (from 93 to 185 nanograms/ml) from the time the clozapine was started. He recovered within 5 days of stopping all of the drugs, after which the clozapine was restarted.[4] The authors of the report interpreted the symptoms as an anticholinergic delirium arising from the additive anticholinergic effects of the clozapine, **nortriptyline** and **perphenazine**, made worse by the increased levels of **nortriptyline**.[4] Just why the **nortriptyline** levels rose is not clear, but one possible explanation is that the **nortriptyline** and clozapine compete for the same liver enzymes concerned with their metabolism, resulting in a reduction in the clearance of the **nortriptyline**. 'Table 16.1', (p.500) and 'Table 16.2', (p.502) give lists of drugs that have anticholinergic activity.

Consider also 'Antipsychotics + Anticholinergics', p.529.

1. Clozaril (Clozapine). Novartis Pharmaceuticals UK Ltd. UK Summary of product characteristics, September 2004.
2. Clozaril (Clozapine). Novartis Pharmaceuticals Corporation. US Prescribing information, November 2004.
3. Cohen MAA, Alfonso CA, Mosquera M. Development of urinary retention during treatment with clozapine and meclizine. *Am J Psychiatry* (1994) 151, 619–20.
4. Smith T, Riskin J. Effect of clozapine on plasma nortriptyline concentration. *Pharmacopsychiatry* (1994) 27, 41–2.

Clozapine + Anticonvulsants

Clozapine serum levels are approximately halved by carbamazepine and possibly by phenytoin. An isolated case of fatal pancytopenia has been seen in one patient taking clozapine and carbamazepine, and neuroleptic malignant syndrome occurred in another. Sodium valproate can apparently lower serum clozapine levels, and an isolated case report suggests that lamotrigine may raise them.

Clinical evidence

(a) Carbamazepine

A study by a therapeutic drug monitoring service for clozapine found that the concentration/dose ratio of 17 patients taking carbamazepine was 50% of that found in 124 other patients taking clozapine alone.[1] A 47% decrease in the serum levels of clozapine were seen in another 12 patients when they were given carbamazepine. **Oxcarbazepine** did not interact.[2] The plasma clozapine levels of 2 patients who had been taking clozapine 600 or 800 mg daily and carbamazepine 600 or 800 mg daily for several months were increased from 1.4 to 2.4 and from 1.5 to 3 micromol/l respectively within 2 weeks of stopping the carbamazepine.[3]

A man with mania on carbamazepine 1200 mg daily and lithium developed muscle rigidity, mild hyperpyrexia, tachycardia, sweating and somnolence (diagnosed as neuroleptic malignant syndrome) 3 days after his lithium was stopped and clozapine 25 mg daily started. The symptoms immediately improved when the clozapine was stopped.[4]

A patient on carbamazepine, lithium, benzatropine and clonazepam developed fatal pancytopenia about 10 weeks after starting clozapine 400 mg daily.[5] A retrospective study of the records of other patients given clozapine and carbamazepine found a significant increase in granulopenia.[6] A previous report had failed to find this due to a statistical error.[7]

A case report describes 2 schizophrenic patients taking clozapine who were changed from carbamazepine to **oxcarbazepine**. After 3 weeks their plasma clozapine levels had risen from 1.4 to 1.7 micromol/l and from 1.5 to 2.5 micromolmol/l respectively.[8]

(b) Lamotrigine

A 35-year-old man, who had been taking clozapine for 3 years, became dizzy and sedated about a month after starting to take lamotrigine. His plasma clozapine levels were found to have increased to 1020 micrograms/l. When the lamotrigine was stopped his levels fell to 450 micrograms/l.[9]

(c) Phenytoin

Two patients developed reduced clozapine levels (falls of 65 to 85%) and worsening psychoses when phenytoin was added to their treatment.[10] Another patient developed neutropenia, which was attributed to concurrent use of phenytoin and clozapine. When the phenytoin was stopped clozapine levels rose from 114 to 137 nanograms/ml, suggesting a pharmacokinetic interaction,[11] rather than just additive adverse effects.

(d) Valproate

A controlled study in 11 psychotic patients found that when sodium valproate (at an average dose of 1060 mg daily) was added to clozapine, the steady-state serum clozapine levels were increased by 39% and the levels of the demethylated metabolite increased by 23%. However, correction of these levels for dose and weight reduced the total clozapine metabolite values to only 6% above those of the controls. No increase in clozapine adverse effects was seen.[12] Another study found that sodium valproate and clozapine had no significant effect on the pharmacokinetics of each other.[13] In contrast, a study in 4 schizophrenics stabilised on clozapine 550 to 650 mg daily found that when semisodium valproate 750 to 1000 mg daily was added, the serum clozapine levels began to fall, and by 3 weeks had dropped by an average of 41%. No deterioration in clinical condition occurred.[14] A 15% decrease in clozapine levels was seen in another study in 7 patients given clozapine and sodium valproate.[15] An isolated report describes sedation, confusion, slurred speech and impaired functioning on two occasions when semisodium valproate was added to clozapine treatment in a 37-year-old man.[16]

Mechanism

Not established, but it seems likely that both carbamazepine and phenytoin (recognised potent enzyme inducers) increase the metabolism of the clozapine by the liver, thereby reducing its effects. It has been suggested that this is because carbamazepine and phenytoin induce the activity of the cytochrome P450 isoenzyme CYP1A2.[1,11] Carbamazepine may also have an effect via CYP3A4. The case of pancytopenia may possibly have been due to the additive bone marrow depressant effects of the clozapine and carbamazepine.

Importance and management

The interaction between clozapine and carbamazepine is much more firmly established than that between clozapine and phenytoin, but both appear to be clinically important. Monitor symptoms and be alert for the need to increase the clozapine dosage if either carbamazepine or phenytoin is given concurrently, and reduce the dosage if either is withdrawn. However, because of the substantial risk of bone marrow suppression the makers of clozapine advise that carbamazepine should not be given concurrently.[17,18]

As yet there only appears to be one case report with lamotrigine, so the situation is unclear. There appears to be no pharmacokinetic mechanism for this interaction, so it awaits confirmation.

The situation with sodium valproate is not entirely clear. There are cases of successful concurrent use,[16] but in the light of the reports cited here it would clearly be prudent to monitor concurrent use closely.

1. Jerling M, Lindström L, Bondesson U, Bertilsson L. Fluvoxamine inhibition and carbamazepine induction of the metabolism of clozapine: evidence from a therapeutic drug monitoring service. *Ther Drug Monit* (1994) 16, 368–74.
2. Tiihonen J, Vartiainen H, Hakola P. The carbamazepine-induced changes in plasma levels of neuroleptics. *Pharmacopsychiatry* (1995) 28, 26–8.
3. Raitasuo V, Lehtovaara R, Huttunen MO. Carbamazepine and plasma levels of clozapine. *Am J Psychiatry* (1993) 150, 169.
4. Müller T, Becker T, Fritze J. Neuroleptic malignant syndrome after clozapine plus carbamazepine. *Lancet* (1988) 2, 1500.
5. Gerson SL, Lieberman JA, Friedenberg WR, Lee D, Marx JJ, Meltzer H. Polypharmacy in fatal clozapine-associated agranulocytosis. *Lancet* (1991) 338, 262–3.
6. Langbehm DR, Alexander B. Increased risk of side-effects in psychiatric patients treated with clozapine and carbamazepine: a reanalysis. *Pharmacopsychiatry* (2000) 33,196.
7. Junghan U, Albers M, Woggon B. Increased risk of hematological side-effects in psychiatric patients treated with clozapine and carbamazepine? *Pharmacopsychiatry* (1993) 26, 262.
8. Raitasuo V, Lehtovaara R, Huttunen MO. Effect of switching carbamazepine to oxcarbazepine on the plasma levels of neuroleptics: a case report. *Psychopharmacology (Berl)* (1994) 116, 115–16.
9. Kossen M, Selten JP, Kahn RS. Elevated clozapine plasma level with lamotrigine. *Am J Psychiatry* (2001) 158, 1930.
10. Miller DD. Effect of phenytoin on plasma clozapine concentrations in two patients. *J Clin Psychiatry* (1991) 52, 23–5.
11. Shad MU. A complex interaction between clozapine and phenytoin. *J Pharm Technol* (2004) 20, 280–2.
12. Centorrino F, Baldessarini RJ, Kando J, Frankenburg FR, Volpicelli SA, Puopolo PR, Flood JG. Serum concentrations of clozapine and its major metabolites: effects of cotreatment with fluoxetine or valproate. *Am J Psychiatry* (1994) 151, 123–5.

13. Facciolà G, Avenoso A, Scordo MG, Madia AG, Ventimiglia A, Perucca E, Spina E. Small effects of valproic acid on the plasma concentrations of clozapine and its major metabolites in patients with schizophrenic or affective disorders. *Ther Drug Monit* (1999) 21, 341–5.
14. Finley P, Warner D. Potential impact of valproic acid therapy on clozapine disposition. *Biol Psychiatry* (1994) 36, 487–8.
15. Longo LP, Salzman C. Valproic acid effects on serum concentrations of clozapine and norclozapine. *Am J Psychiatry* (1995) 152, 650.
16. Costello LE, Suppes T. A clinically significant interaction between clozapine and valproate. *J Clin Psychopharmacol* (1995) 15, 139–141.
17. Clozaril (Clozapine). Novartis Pharmaceuticals UK Ltd. UK Summary of product characteristics, September 2004.
18. Clozaril (Clozapine). Novartis Pharmaceuticals Corporation. US Prescribing information, November 2004.

Clozapine + Antihypertensives

There are isolated cases of apparent interactions between clozapine, and enalapril, lisinopril or propranolol, Additive hypotensive effects are possible with clozapine and any antihypertensive agent.

Clinical evidence, mechanism, importance and management

A patient taking **enalapril** 5 mg twice daily fainted within an hour of being given an initial 25-mg dose of clozapine. Later he was stabilised without problems on **enalapril** 2.5 mg twice daily and clozapine, initially 12.5 mg daily, later rising to 800 mg daily. Another patient taking **enalapril** 5 mg daily fainted within 5 hours of being given clozapine 25 mg. He needed resuscitation, but was later stabilised on clozapine in doses up to 600 mg daily.[1] The clozapine blood levels of a 39-year-old man rose from 490 to 966 nanograms/ml after the addition of **lisinopril** 5 mg daily. When the **lisinopril** dose was increased to 10 mg daily, the levels further rose to 1092 nanograms/ml. The dose of clozapine was reduced, and **lisinopril** replaced by diltiazem, after which his levels began to return to normal.[2]

Coma developed in a woman taking **propranolol** 40 mg daily 1.5 to 2 hours after she was given a single 150-mg dose of clozapine. She had stopped taking fluphenazine 24 hours earlier. The patient recovered, and was subsequently slowly titrated up to a daily clozapine dose of 100 mg in addition to the **propranolol**, without any problems. Although the authors state that an interaction between **propranolol** and clozapine was the likely cause of the coma, the effects of fluphenazine cannot be wholly ruled out.[3]

Clozapine has alpha-blocking effects and therefore may cause orthostatic hypotension. The makers note that this is more likely in the presence of other antipsychotics or benzodiazepines and during initial titration with rapid dose increases. Because of the potential for additive effects they recommend caution when giving clozapine to patients on any hypotensive drug.[4,5]

1. Aronowitz JS, Chakos MH, Safferman AZ, Lieberman JA. Syncope associated with the combination of clozapine and enalapril. *J Clin Psychopharmacol* (1994) 14, 429–30.
2. Abraham G, Grunberg B, Gratz S. Possible interaction of clozapine and lisinopril. *Am J Psychiatry* (2001) 158, 969.
3. Vetter PH, Proppe DG. Clozapine induced coma. *J Nerv Ment Dis* (1992) 180, 58–9.
4. Clozaril (Clozapine). Novartis Pharmaceuticals UK Ltd. UK Summary of product characteristics, September 2004.
5. Clozaril (Clozapine). Novartis Pharmaceuticals Corporation. US Prescribing information, November 2004.

Clozapine + Azoles

Itraconazole and ketoconazole do not interact with clozapine.

Clinical evidence, mechanism, importance and management

A double-blind study in 7 schizophrenic patients on clozapine found that when **itraconazole** 200 mg daily was given for a week, no changes in clozapine or desmethylclozapine serum levels were seen.[1]

A single 50-mg dose of clozapine was given to 5 schizophrenic patients before and after a 7-day course of **ketoconazole** 400 mg daily. The **ketoconazole** had no significant effect on the pharmacokinetics of the clozapine.[2]

The conclusion is that the cytochrome P450 isoenzyme CYP3A4 is of only minor importance in clozapine metabolism, and that because no interaction takes place between clozapine and **itraconazole** or clozapine and **ketoconazole**, both it and other inhibitors of CYP3A4 can be used with clozapine.[1,2] However, note that raised clozapine levels have been attributed to treatment with erythromycin, see 'Clozapine + Erythromycin', p.560.

1. Raaska K, Neuvonen PJ. Serum concentrations of clozapine and *N*-desmethylclozapine are unaffected by the potent CYP3A4 inhibitor itraconazole. *Eur J Clin Pharmacol* (1998) 54, 167–70.
2. Lane H-Y, Chiu C-C, Kazmi Y, Desai H, Lam YWF, Jann MW, Chang W-H. Lack of CYP3A4 inhibition by grapefruit juice and ketoconazole upon clozapine administration *in vivo*. *Drug Metabol Drug Interact* (2001) 18, 263–78.

Clozapine + Benzodiazepines

A handful of reports describe severe hypotension, respiratory depression, unconsciousness and potentially fatal respiratory arrest in patients on benzodiazepines and clozapine. Dizziness and sedation are also increased.

Clinical evidence

A schizophrenic patient failed to respond to fluphenazine, **diazepam**, **clobazam** and **lormetazepam** after a trial over several weeks. The fluphenazine was stopped and clozapine started at a dose of 25 mg at noon and 100 mg at night. Toxic delirium and severe hypersalivation developed 3 hours later. The patient collapsed (systolic pressure 50 mmHg, diastolic unrecordable) and stopped breathing. Resuscitation was started, and the patient remained unconscious for 30 minutes. After a few drug-free days he was successfully re-started on clozapine 12.5 mg, which was very slowly titrated upwards, and a low benzodiazepine dosage.[1]

Another patient on clozapine died suddenly and unexpectedly during the night, apparently due to respiratory arrest, after being given three 2-mg intravenous doses of **lorazepam** the previous day.[2]

There are at least 6 other cases of severe hypotension, respiratory depression or loss of consciousness in patients on clozapine and **flurazepam**, **lorazepam** or **diazepam**,[1,3-5] as well as two cases of marked sedation, hypersalivation and ataxia in patients on **lorazepam** and clozapine.[6] Two of these reports[1,3] are from the same group of workers and it is not clear whether they are about the same or different patients.

Mechanism

Not understood. Clozapine on its own very occasionally causes respiratory arrest and hypotension.

Importance and management

The authors of the first of these reports[1] say that the relative risk of the cardiovascular/respiratory reaction is only 2.1%. Another report[2] says that the death cited above is the only life-threatening event among 162 patients given clozapine and benzodiazepines between 1986 and 1991 so that the incidence of serious problems is quite low. Even so, concurrent use should be very well monitored because of the severity of the reaction, even if it is rare.

1. Grohmann R, Rüther E, Sassim N, Schmidt LG. Adverse effects of clozapine. *Psychopharmacology (Berl)* (1989) 99, S101–S104.
2. Klimke A, Klieser E. Sudden death after intravenous application of lorazepam in a patient treated with clozapine. *Am J Psychiatry* (1994) 151, 780.
3. Sassim N, Grohmann R. Adverse drug reactions with clozapine and simultaneous application of benzodiazepines. *Pharmacopsychiatry* (1988) 21, 306–7.
4. Friedman LJ, Tabb SE, Worthington JJ, Sanchez CJ, Sved M. Clozapine – a novel antipsychotic agent. *N Engl J Med* (1991) 325, 518–9.
5. Tupala E, Niskanen L, Tiihonen J. Transient syncope and ECG changes associated with the concurrent administration of clozapine and diazepam. *J Clin Psychiatry* (1999) 60, 619–20.
6. Cobb CD, Anderson CB, Seidel DR. Possible interaction between clozapine and lorazepam. *Am J Psychiatry* (1991) 148, 1606–7.

Clozapine + Bone marrow suppressants

The makers caution the use of clozapine with other drugs that can cause bone marrow suppression. Low white cells counts have been seen in patients on clozapine and chloroquine, co-trimoxazole, methazolamide, nitrofurantoin, olanzapine or thiamazole.

Clinical evidence, mechanism, importance and management

Because clozapine can cause blood dyscrasias and potentially fatal agranulocytosis, the makers say that it should not be given with other drugs that have a well-known potential to cause agranulocytosis.[1,2] The UK maker lists **carbamazepine** (see also 'Clozapine + Anticonvulsants', p.558), **chloramphenicol**, **cytotoxics**, **pyrazolone analgesics** (e.g. **phenylbutazone**), **penicillamine**, **sulphonamides** (e.g.**co-trimoxazole**) and, because they cannot be stopped if an adverse reaction occurs, they advise against the use of **depot antipsychotics**.[1] There are several cases that confirm the clinical significance of these predicted interactions.

A woman was treated with **thiamazole** for Graves' disease and at times with various different antipsychotics including haloperidol, flupentixol, zuclopenthixol and perphenazine for schizophrenia. Because of the severe extrapyramidal reactions and failure to control the schizophrenia, clozapine, increased over 5 days to 250 mg daily was started instead. Within 5 days her white cell count had fallen to 2200/mm^3, which rose to 4000/mm^3, a month after both drugs were stopped. Later, after the **thiamazole** was stopped she was successfully treated with the same dose of clozapine.[3]

A patient who had been taking clozapine 500 mg daily for 8 months developed granulocytopenia within 8 days of starting **nitrofurantoin** 200 mg daily.[4]

An 86-year old woman developed neutropenia 2 weeks after **methazolamide** for glaucoma was added to clozapine. Both drugs were stopped and her white cell count recovered. She later started clozapine without problem and so the toxic effect was attributed to the combined use of two drugs.[5]

Neutropenia developed 4 days after **co-trimoxazole** was started in a 47-year-old woman who had been stabilised on clozapine for 5 years. **Co-trimoxazole** was stopped and the white cell counts returned to normal over the next 2 weeks.[6]

Three patients have been described who showed a delay in recovery from clozapine-induced agranulocytosis when given **olanzapine**, and it has been suggested that **olanzapine** should therefore be avoided until the patient's haematological status has normalised.[7]

However, in contrast, a patient on clozapine 25 mg daily had no significant changes in his white cell count after taking **chloroquine** for malaria prophylaxis, over the course of a month.[8]

1. Clozaril (Clozapine). Novartis Pharmaceuticals UK Ltd. UK Summary of product characteristics, September 2004.
2. Clozaril (Clozapine). Novartis Pharmaceuticals Corporation. US Prescribing information, November 2004.
3. Rocco PL. Concurrent treatment with clozapine and methimazole inducing granulocytopenia: a case report. *Hum Psychopharmacol* (1993) 8, 445–6.
4. Juul Povlsen U, Noring U, Fog R, Gerlach J. Tolerability and therapeutic effect of clozapine. *Acta Psychiatr Scand* (1985) 71, 176–85.
5. Burke WJ, Ranno AE. Neutropenia with clozapine and methazolamide. *J Clin Psychopharmacol* (1994) 14, 357–8.
6. Henderson DC, Borba CP. Trimethoprim-sulfamethoxazole and clozapine. *Psychiatr Serv* (2001) 52, 111–12.
7. Flynn SW, Altman S, MacEwan GW, Black LL, Greenidge LL, Honer WG. Prolongation of clozapine-induced granulocytopenia associated with olanzapine. *J Clin Psychopharmacol* (1997) 17, 494–5.
8. König P, Künz A. Compatibility of clozapine and chloroquine. *Lancet* (1991) 338, 948.

Clozapine + Caffeine

Caffeine increases serum clozapine levels, which may increase the incidence of clozapine adverse effects.

Clinical evidence

In a double-blind crossover study 6 coffee-drinking patients on clozapine were given decaffeinated or caffeine-containing instant coffee for 7 days. The plasma levels of clozapine were 26% higher while the patients were taking caffeine.[1] A study in 12 healthy subjects[2] found that caffeine 400 to 1000 mg daily, raised the AUC and decreased the clearance of a single 12.5-mg dose of clozapine by 19% and 14% respectively. A previous study in 7 patients had found that clozapine levels decreased by 47% when the subjects avoided caffeine for 5 days, and increased again when caffeine consumption was resumed.[3]

A 66-year-old woman on clozapine 300 mg daily developed supraventricular tachycardia (180 bpm) when she was given 500 mg of intravenous caffeine sodium benzoate to increase seizure length during an ECT session. Verapamil was needed to revert the arrhythmia. Before taking clozapine she had received caffeine sodium benzoate in doses of up to 1 g during ECT sessions without problems.[4] Another patient on clozapine for schizophrenia had an exacerbation of his psychotic symptoms, which was attributed to caffeinated coffee (5 to 10 cups daily). The problem resolved when the patient stopped drinking caffeine. He had previously not had any problems with caffeine while taking haloperidol 30 mg and procyclidine 30 mg daily.[5] A 31-year-old woman on clozapine 550 mg daily developed increased daytime sleepiness, sialorrhoea and withdrawn behaviour after taking about 1200 mg of caffeine daily (as drinks and tablets). Her plasma clozapine levels fell from 1500 to 630 nanograms/ml when her caffeine intake was stopped.[6]

Mechanism

Caffeine inhibits the cytochrome P450 isoenzyme CYP1A2, which is one of the major isoenzymes involved in the metabolism of caffeine. Consequently clozapine serum levels and effects increase.[2,3,7]

Importance and management

This would appear to be an established and clinically important interaction, but unlikely to be a problem if clozapine serum levels are established and well monitored, and caffeine intake remains fairly stable and moderate. Possible exceptions are if large doses of caffeine are given during ECT treatment or if for some other reason the caffeine intake suddenly increases or decreases markedly.

1. Raaska K, Raitasuo V, Laitila J, Neuvonen PJ. Effect of caffeine-containing versus decaffeinated coffee on serum clozapine concentrations in hospitalised patients. *Basic Clin Pharmacol Toxicol* (2004) 94, 13–18.
2. Hägg S, Spigset O, Mjörndal T, Dahlqvist R. Effect of caffeine on clozapine pharmacokinetics in healthy volunteers. *Br J Clin Pharmacol* (2000) 49, 59–63.
3. Carrillo JA, Herraiz AG, Ramos SI, Benitez J. Effects of caffeine withdrawal from the diet on the metabolism of clozapine in schizophrenic patients. *J Clin Psychopharmacol* (1998) 18, 311–16.
4. Beale MD, Pritchett JT, Kellner CH. Supraventricular tachycardia in a patient receiving ECT, clozapine, and caffeine. *Convuls Ther* (1994) 10, 228–31.
5. Vainer JL, Chouinard G. Interaction between caffeine and clozapine. *J Clin Psychopharmacol* (1994) 14, 284–5.
6. Odom-White A, de Leon J. Clozapine levels and caffeine. *J Clin Psychiatry* (1996) 57, 175–6.
7. Carrillo JA, Jerling M, Bertilsson L. Comments to "Interaction between caffeine and clozapine". *J Clin Psychopharmacol* (1995) 15, 376–7.

Clozapine + Ciprofloxacin

An isolated report describes the development of agitation in an elderly man on clozapine, tentatively attributed to elevated serum levels caused by an interaction with ciprofloxacin. A study supports this observation.

Clinical evidence, mechanism, importance and management

An elderly man with multi-infarct dementia and behavioural disturbances' taking clozapine, glibenclamide (glyburide), trazodone and melatonin, was hospitalised for agitation on the last day of a 10-day course of ciprofloxacin 500 mg twice daily. When the ciprofloxacin course was completed, his plasma clozapine serum levels fell from 90 nanograms/ml to undetectable concentrations (lower limit of detection being 50 nanograms/ml).[1]

Ciprofloxacin 250 mg twice daily for 7 days was given to 7 schizophrenic patients, stabilised on clozapine. The mean serum clozapine and *N*-desmethylclozapine concentrations were increased by 29 and 31% respectively, but no additional adverse effects were reported. Interindividual variation in serum levels was high, so it seems likely that some patients may demonstrate a clinically significant interaction.[2] It seems likely that this reaction occurs because ciprofloxacin inhibits the cytochrome P450 isoenzyme CYP1A2, the major isoenzyme involved in the metabolism of clozapine, resulting in elevated clozapine levels. Monitor the outcome carefully if ciprofloxacin is added to clozapine treatment. There seem as yet to be no other reports of a in interaction between clozapine and other quinolones.

1. Markowitz JS, Gill HS, Devane CL, Mintzer JE. Fluoroquinolone inhibition of clozapine metabolism. *Am J Psychiatry* (1997) 153, 881.
2. Raaska K, Neuvonen PJ. Ciprofloxacin increases serum clozapine and *N*-desmethylclozapine: a study in patients with schizophrenia. *Eur J Clin Pharmacol* (2000) 56, 585–9.

Clozapine + Erythromycin

A study in healthy subjects found no evidence of an interaction between clozapine and erythromycin, but three case reports describe clozapine toxicity (seizures in one patient, drowsiness, incoordination and incontinence in another and neutropenia in the third) when the patients were given erythromycin.

Clinical evidence

A randomised crossover study in 12 healthy subjects found erythromycin 500 mg three times daily did not affect the pharmacokinetics of a single 12.5-mg dose of clozapine.[1]

In contrast, a schizophrenic man, stable on clozapine 800 mg daily was additionally started on erythromycin 250 mg four times daily for a fever and sore throat caused by pharyngitis. After a week he had a single tonic-clonic seizure and his serum clozapine levels were found to be 1.3 mg/ml. Both drugs were stopped, and the clozapine restarted 2 days later, initially at only 400 mg daily, but after several weeks had increased to 800 mg daily, giving serum clozapine levels of 700 micrograms/ml.[2] Another schizophrenic on clozapine 600 mg daily became drowsy, with slurred speech, incontinence, difficulty in walking and incoordination within 2 to 3 days of starting to take erythromycin 333 mg three times daily. His serum clozapine level was found to be 1.15 mg/l and he had leucocytosis. He recovered when both drugs were stopped. When he was later restarted on the same clozapine dosage, but without the erythromycin, his steady-state trough clozapine serum level was 385 micrograms/l.[3] Another case also describes a reduced white cell count when erythromycin was added to established clozapine therapy, but no clozapine levels were available.[4]

Mechanism

Uncertain. One suggestion is that erythromycin might have inhibited the cytochrome P450 isoenzyme CYP3A4, which has a minor role in the metabolism of clozapine, leading to a reduced clearance, which resulted in increased serum clozapine levels and toxicity.[2,3]

Importance and management

Information appears to be limited to this study and the three case reports. As clozapine is metabolised mainly by the cytochrome P450 isoenzyme CYP1A2 a significant interaction seems unlikely, although the case reports do suggest that rarely some patients may be affected. Also note that clozapine has not been found to interact with other potent inhibitors of CYP3A4, see 'Clozapine + Azoles', p.559. Bear this interaction in mind in the case of an unexpected response to treatment.

1. Hägg S, Spigset O, Mjörndal T, Granberg K, Persbo-Lundqvist G, Dahlqvist R. Absence of interaction between erythromycin and a single dose of clozapine. *Eur J Clin Pharmacol* (1999) 55, 221–6.
2. Funderburg LG, Vertrees JE, True JE, Miller AL. Seizure following addition of erythromycin to clozapine treatment. *Am J Psychiatry* (1994) 151, 1840–1.
3. Cohen LG, Chesley S, Eugenio L, Flood JG, Fisch J, Goff DC. Erythromycin-induced clozapine toxic reaction. *Arch Intern Med* (1996) 156, 675–7.
4. Usiskin SI, Nicolson R, Lenane M, Rapoport JL. Retreatment with clozapine after erythromycin-induced neutropenia. *Am J Psychiatry* (2000) 157, 1021.

Clozapine + H_2-blockers

A single case report describes increased serum clozapine levels and toxicity due to cimetidine, but not ranitidine.

Clinical evidence, mechanism, importance and management

A man with chronic paranoid schizophrenia was treated with atenolol and clozapine 900 mg daily. When **cimetidine** 400 mg twice daily was added for gastritis, his serum clozapine levels rose by almost 60% (from a range of 992 to 1081 nanograms/ml to a range of 1559 to 1701 nanograms/ml) but without any problems. Within 3 days of raising the dosage of **cimetidine** to 400 mg three times daily he developed evidence of clozapine toxicity (marked diaphoresis, dizziness, vomiting, weakness, orthostatic hypotension), all of which resolved over 5 days when the clozapine dosage was lowered to 200 mg daily and the **cimetidine** stopped. The serum clozapine levels during this period were not reported. When **cimetidine** was replaced by **ranitidine** 150 mg twice daily his clozapine serum levels were not affected.[1]

The suggested reason for this interaction is that the **cimetidine** (a potent non-specific enzyme inhibitor) reduces the liver metabolism of the clozapine so that it accumulates, causing toxicity. **Ranitidine** does not cause enzyme inhibition and therefore does not interact.

Information appears to be limited to this report but it is consistent with the way **cimetidine** interacts with many other drugs. **Ranitidine**, or possibly other H_2-blockers such as **famotidine** or **nizatidine**, which do not inhibit liver enzymes, would seem to be preferable and safer alternatives. This needs confirmation. More study is needed.

1. Szymanski S, Lieberman JA, Picou D, Masiar S, Cooper T. A case report of cimetidine-induced clozapine toxicity. *J Clin Psychiatry* (1991) 52, 21–2.

Clozapine + Lithium

A few patients given lithium carbonate and clozapine have experienced adverse reactions including myoclonus, neuroleptic malignant syndrome, seizures, delirium and psychoses.

Clinical evidence

A schizophrenic man, poorly controlled on clozapine 750 mg daily for 6 weeks, was given lithium, initially 900 mg and then subsequently 1200 mg daily. His serum lithium level was 0.86 mmol/l. Within a week he began to experience paroxysmal jerky movements of his upper and lower extremities lasting about 30 minutes. This myoclonus resolved when both drugs were stopped, and did not recur when clozapine was restarted alone.[1] Another patient developed neuroleptic malignant syndrome (stiffness, rigidity, tachycardia, diaphoresis, hypertension) 3 to 4 weeks after clozapine was added to his lithium treatment. The symptoms disappeared within 2 to 3 days of stopping the clozapine.[2] An elderly man also developed neuroleptic malignant syndrome 3 days after starting to take clozapine 25 mg daily. He was also taking carbamazepine, and had stopped taking lithium 3 days earlier.[3]

Four out of 10 patients on lithium carbonate (mean dose of 1400 mg daily) and clozapine (mean maximum dose 900 mg daily) developed reversible neurological symptoms including involuntary jerking of the limbs and tongue, facial spasm, tremor, confusion, generalised weakness, stumbling gait, leaning and falling to the right. One of them also became delirious. Serum lithium levels remained unchanged, and the problems resolved when the lithium was stopped. Three of the four had a recurrence of the symptoms when rechallenged with the drug combination.[4] A man on clozapine and lithium carbonate developed psychosis with delusions and visual hallucinations over a 5-day period when clozapine was tapered off and stopped. This was accompanied by a doubling in his serum lithium levels. He recovered completely when the drugs were stopped.[5] Two patients on clozapine developed seizures: one developed a tonic-clonic seizure within 4 days of adding lithium carbonate 900 mg to clozapine 600 mg daily, and the other a grand mal seizure within 6 days of adding lithium carbonate 900 mg to clozapine 900 mg daily.[6]

Mechanism

Not understood.

Importance and management

Some patients develop a toxic reaction when given both drugs, and others do not, for reasons that are not understood. Concurrent use should therefore be extremely well monitored. One group of workers suggest that lithium levels of no more than 0.5 mmol/l may give therapeutic benefits while minimising adverse effects.[4]

1. Lemus CZ, Lieberman JA, Johns CA. Myoclonus during treatment with clozapine and lithium: the role of serotonin. *Hillside J Clin Psychiatry* (1989) 11, 127–30.
2. Pope HG, Cole JO, Choras PT, Fulwiler CE. Apparent neuroleptic malignant syndrome with clozapine and lithium. *J Nerv Ment Dis* (1986) 174, 493–5.
3. Müller T, Becker T, Fritze J. Neuroleptic malignant syndrome after clozapine plus carbamazepine. *Lancet* (1988) ii, 1500.
4. Blake LM, Marks RC, Luchins DJ. Reversible neurologic symptoms with clozapine and lithium. *J Clin Psychopharmacol* (1992) 12, 297–9.
5. Hellwig B, Hesslinger B, Walder J. Tapering off clozapine in a clozapine-lithium co-medication may cause an acute organic psychosis. A case report. *Pharmacopsychiatry* (1995) 28, 187.
6. Garcia G, Crismon ML, Dorson PG. Seizures in two patients after the addition of lithium to a clozapine regimen. *J Clin Psychopharmacol* (1994) 14, 426–7.

Clozapine + Miscellaneous

There are isolated cases of apparent interactions between clozapine, and ampicillin, buspirone, caffeine, haloperidol, loperamide, modafinil, nicotinic acid, tryptophan, tobacco smoking or vitamin C. Influenza vaccine does not appear to interact.

Clinical evidence, mechanism, importance and management

(a) Ampicillin

An isolated report describes a 17-year-old on clozapine (12.5 mg increased to 50 mg three times daily) who was additionally given ampicillin 500 mg four times daily, starting on day 15 of clozapine treatment. On the next day the patient became easily distracted, very drowsy and salivated excessively. These adverse reactions stopped when the ampicillin was replaced by doxycycline.[1]

(b) Buspirone

A man who had been taking clozapine for a year developed acute and potentially lethal gastrointestinal bleeding and marked hyperglycaemia about 5 weeks after starting buspirone, and a week after the buspirone dosage was raised to 20 mg daily. No gut pathology (e.g. ulceration) was detected and there were no problems when he was subsequently given clozapine alone, so the reaction was attributed to the drug combination.[2]

(c) Grapefruit juice

Grapefruit juice did not affect the metabolism of clozapine in two studies in a total of 36 schizophrenic patients.[3,4]

(d) Haloperidol

A 68-year-old man on clozapine 600 mg daily and venlafaxine, lorazepam, aspirin, vitamin E and multivitamins was started on haloperidol 4 mg daily to control persistent paranoid delusions and hallucinations. After 27 days he was found collapsed and was lethargic, tachycardic, feverish and delirious. Because neuroleptic malignant syndrome was suspected the antipsychotics were withheld, and the patient recovered over the following 7 days. Clozapine was later re-started without a recurrence of symptoms.[5]

(e) Influenza vaccine

In an open-label study in 14 patients the metabolism of clozapine was not altered following a single intramuscular dose of influenza vaccine (*Influvac* 2001 to 2002 formula, Solvay).[6]

(f) Loperamide

A patient on clozapine 500 mg daily died after taking loperamide 6 mg daily during an episode of food poisoning. The authors of the report attribute the death to toxic megacolon brought on by the additive effects of clozapine and loperamide on gut transit.[7] Toxic megacolon can sometimes occur with loperamide alone, especially in the presence of an infection. Also, the makers of clozapine say that care is necessary in patients given clozapine with drugs known to cause constipation (see also 'Clozapine + Anticholinergics', p.557) because on rare occasions clozapine alone has been shown to cause significant impairment of intestinal function (such as paralytic ileus).[8,9]

(g) Modafinil

A 42-year-old man taking clozapine 450 mg daily was given modafinil, titrated up to 300 mg daily, to combat sedation. After about a month of concurrent use he developed dizziness and an unsteady gait and his clozapine level was found to be 1400 nanograms/ml. While taking clozapine 400 mg daily his level was 761 nanograms/ml, and because the 50 mg increase was not thought large enough to almost double his clozapine level an interaction with modafinil was suspected.[10]

(h) Nefazodone

A 40-year-old man who had been successfully treated with risperidone and clozapine 425 to 475 mg daily was started on nefazodone 200 mg daily increasing to 300 mg daily, for the treatment of persistent depression. After a week on the higher dose he became dizzy and hypotensive and it was noted that his clozapine level had risen from 133 to 233 nanograms/ml. This was thought to be due to an inhibitory effect of nefazodone on the cytochrome P450 isoenzyme CYP3A4,[11] although note that potent inhibitors of CYP3A4 (such as 'erythromycin', (p.560) or the 'azoles', (p.559)) rarely appear to increase clozapine levels.

(i) Nicotinic acid/Tryptophan/Vitamin C

A man with schizophrenia taking tryptophan, lorazepam, vitamin C, benzatropine and nicotinic acid, developed a severe urticarial rash covering his face, neck and trunk 3 days after starting clozapine 150 mg daily. All of the drugs except lorazepam were stopped, and the rash subsided. It did not recur when clozapine was restarted, even at a dose of 600 mg daily, nor when small doses of benzatropine and fluphenazine were briefly added. The authors draw the inference that tryptophan, vitamin C and nicotinic acid may have been responsible for this alleged interaction.[12]

(j) Reboxetine

A small study in 7 patients found that reboxetine 8 mg daily had no effect on the metabolism of clozapine or its major metabolite.[13]

(k) Tobacco smoke

Tobacco smoking might be expected to lower serum clozapine levels because the smoke contains aromatic hydrocarbons that are potent inducers, of the cytochrome P450 isoenzyme CYP1A2 but studies of this likely interaction have been equivocal. One group of workers found no differences in clozapine levels with smoking,[14] while another group found that smokers had lower clozapine levels.[15] In addition, a case report describes clozapine-induced seizures in a man when he gave up smoking, although no levels were available so the authors point out it is difficult to be sure that smoking cessation was the cause.[16] A retrospective study found that the clozapine clearance was 86% higher in 9 smokers than in 3 non-smokers, although it should be noted that this study was not specifically looking at the effects of smoking.[17]

1. Csík V, Molnár J. Possible adverse interaction between clozapine and ampicillin in an adolescent with schizophrenia. *J Child Adolesc Psychopharmacol* (1994) 4, 123–8.
2. Good MI. Lethal interaction of clozapine and buspirone? *Am J Psychiatry* (1997) 154, 1472–3.
3. Lane H-Y, Chiu C-C, Kazmi Y, Desai H, Lam YWF, Jan MW, Chang W-H. Lack of CYP3A4 inhibition by grapefruit juice and ketoconazole upon clozapine administration *in vivo*. *Drug Metabol Drug Interact* (2001) 18, 263–78.
4. Lane H-Y, Jann MW, Chang Y-C, Chiu C-C, Huang M-C, Lee S-H, Chang W-H. Repeated ingestion of grapefruit juice does not alter clozapine's steady-state plasma levels, effectiveness, and tolerability. *J Clin Psychiatry* (2001) 62, 812–17.
5. Garcia G, Ghani S, Poveda RA, Dansky BL. Neuroleptic malignant syndrome with antidepressant/antipsychotic drug combination. *Ann Pharmacother* (2001) 35, 784–5.
6. Raaska K, Raitasuo V, Neuvonen PJ. Effect of influenza vaccination on serum clozapine and its main metabolite concentrations in patients with schizophrenia. *Eur J Clin Pharmacol* (2001) 57, 705–8.
7. Eronen M, Putkonen H, Hallikainen T, Vartiainen H. Lethal gastroenteritis associated with clozapine and loperamide. *Am J Psychiatry* (2003) 160, 2242–3.
8. Clozaril (Clozapine). Novartis Pharmaceuticals UK Ltd. UK Summary of product characteristics, September 2004.
9. Clozaril (Clozapine). Novartis Pharmaceuticals Corporation. US Prescribing information, November 2004.
10. Dequardo JR. Modafinil-associated clozapine toxicity. *Am J Psychiatry* (2002) 159, 1243–4.
11. Khan AY, Preskorn SH. Increase in plasma levels of clozapine and norclozapine after administration of nefazodone. *J Clin Psychiatry* (2001) 62, 375–6.
12. Goumeniouk AD, Ancill RJ, MacEwan GW, Koczapski AB. A case of drug-drug interaction involving clozapine. *Can J Psychiatry* (1991) 36, 234–5.
13. Spina E, Avenoso A, Scordo MG, Ancione M, Madia A, Levita A. No effect of reboxetine on plasma concentrations of clozapine, risperidone, and their active metabolites. *Ther Drug Monit* (2001) 23, 675–8.
14. Hasegawa M, Gutierrez-Esteinou R, Way L, Meltzer HY. Relationship between clinical efficacy and clozapine concentrations in plasma in schizophrenia: effect of smoking. *J Clin Psychopharmacol* (1993) 13, 383–90.
15. Haring C, Meise U, Humpel C, Fleischhacker WW, Hinterhuber H. Dose-related plasma effects of clozapine: influence of smoking behaviour, sex and age. *Psychopharmacology (Berl)* (1989) 99, S38–S40.
16. McCarthy RH. Seizures following smoking cessation in a clozapine responder. *Pharmacopsychiatry* (1994) 27, 210–11.
17. Mookhoek EJ, Loonen AJM. Retrospective evaluation of the effect of omeprazole on clozapine metabolism. *Pharm World Sci* (2004) 26, 180–2.

Clozapine + Proton pump inhibitors

Omeprazole appears to reduce the serum levels of clozapine.

Clinical evidence, mechanism, importance and management

A retrospective study identified 13 patients taking clozapine and **omeprazole** who were subsequently changed to a combination of clozapine and **pantoprazole**. After **pantoprazole** was substituted for **omeprazole** the mean clozapine serum level rose from 445 to 579 nanograms/ml in 3 non-smokers, but fell from 364 to 323 nanograms/ml in 10 smokers. Both **omeprazole** and smoking are known to induce the cytochrome P450 isoenzyme CYP1A2, which is the major isoenzyme involved in the metabolism of clozapine. The authors suggest that when **omeprazole** was stopped in the non-smokers there was no CYP1A2 inhibition, hence clozapine levels rose, whereas CYP1A2 inhibition continued in the smokers, so their levels were only slightly affected.[1]

A case report describes two patients (both smokers) whose clozapine levels fell from 762 to 443 nanograms/ml and from 369 to 204 nanograms/ml respectively, after **omeprazole** was started. However, no changes in clinical condition were noted.[2]

Although other proton pump inhibitors do not appear to have been studied both **esomeprazole** and **lansoprazole** also inhibit CYP1A2 and so may possibly interact similarly. **Rabeprazole** and **pantoprazole** are not known to inhibit CYP1A2 so an interaction seems unlikely, although this needs confirmation.

1. Mookhoek EJ, Loonen AJM. Retrospective evaluation of the effect of omeprazole on clozapine metabolism. *Pharm World Sci* (2004) 26, 180–2.
2. Frick A, Kopitz J, Bergemann N. Omeprazole reduces clozapine plasma concentrations. *Pharmacopsychiatry* (2003) 36, 121–3.

Clozapine + Rifampicin (Rifampin)

An isolated report describes a marked fall in the serum levels of a patient on clozapine when he was treated with rifampicin.

Clinical evidence, mechanism, importance and management

A schizophrenic patient on clozapine developed tuberculosis and was started on rifampicin, isoniazid and pyrazinamide. Within 2 to 3 weeks his trough serum clozapine levels had fallen dramatically from about 250 to 40 nanograms/ml but rose again rapidly when the rifampicin was replaced by ciprofloxacin. It was suggested that rifampicin (a potent non-specific enzyme inducing agent) increased the metabolism of clozapine, probably by the cytochrome P450 isoenzymes CYP1A2 and CYP3A, thereby increasing the loss of the clozapine from the body.[1]

This appears to be an isolated case but it is consistent with the way rifampicin interacts with other drugs. Clozapine serum levels should be well monitored if rifampicin is added, being alert for the need to increase its dosage. An alternative (as in this case) is to use another antibacterial. However, note that there are reports of an interaction between 'clozapine and ciprofloxacin', (p.560).

1. Joos AAB, Frank UG, Kaschka WP. Pharmacokinetic interaction of clozapine and rifampicin in a forensic patient with an atypical mycobacterial infection. *J Clin Psychopharmacol* (1998) 18, 83–5.

Clozapine + Risperidone

The concurrent use of clozapine and risperidone can be effective and well tolerated but two isolated reports describe a rise in serum clozapine levels when risperidone was added and another describes the development of atrial ectopics. Dystonia has been seen when clozapine was replaced by risperidone.

Clinical evidence

A man with a schizoaffective disorder taking clozapine was also started on risperidone, firstly 0.5 mg twice daily, and then after a week 1 mg twice daily. Clinical improvement was seen and it was found that after 2 weeks his serum clozapine levels had risen by 74% from 344 to 598 nanograms/ml, without any adverse effects.[1] The serum clozapine levels of another patient more than doubled when risperidone was given. No signs of clozapine toxicity were seen, but mild oculogyric crises were reported.[2] A schizophrenic on clozapine and trihexyphenidyl who developed tachycardia of 120 bpm, which was controlled with propranolol, developed atrial ectopics when risperidone 1.5 mg daily was added. The ectopics stopped when the risperidone was withdrawn and started again when it was re-introduced. Clozapine plasma levels were normal throughout the duration of risperidone treatment.[3] Four patients have been described who developed dystonia after they were transferred from clozapine to risperidone.[4] A single case of agranulocytosis has been seen 6 weeks after risperidone was added to stable clozapine treatment. The patient needed 3 doses of GCSF before the white cell count returned to normal.[5] Another case report describes neuroleptic malignant syndrome in a 20-year-old man within 2 days of clozapine being added to risperidone treatment. The drugs were stopped and he recovered over the following 10 days. He subsequently received clozapine alone without problem.[6]

Contrasting with these reports is a study in 12 schizophrenic patients, which found that the addition of risperidone to clozapine was both effective and well tolerated, although 4 patients complained of mild akathisia. Serum clozapine levels were not significantly changed.[7] A retrospective study in 18 patients also found that risperidone did not alter clozapine serum levels.[8]

Mechanism, importance and management

The suggested reason for the raised clozapine levels is that both drugs compete for metabolism by the cytochrome P450 isoenzyme CYP2D6 resulting in a reduction in the metabolism of the clozapine.[1,2] The dystonias are attributed to cholinergic rebound and ongoing dopamine blockade caused by a rapid switch of medication. The recommendation is that withdrawal should be tapered and possibly that an anticholinergic agent should be given.[4] The raised clozapine levels seem to be isolated cases and therefore of doubtful general significance.

1. Tyson SC, Devane LC, Risch SC. Pharmacokinetic interaction between risperidone and clozapine. *Am J Psychiatry* (1995) 152, 1401–2.
2. Koreen AR, Lieberman JA, Kronig M, Cooper TB. Cross-tapering clozapine and risperidone. *Am J Psychiatry* (1995) 152, 1690.
3. Chong SA, Tan CH, Lee HS. Atrial ectopics with clozapine-risperidone combination. *J Clin Psychopharmacol* (1997) 17, 130–1.
4. Simpson GM, Meyer JM. Dystonia while changing from clozapine to risperidone. *J Clin Psychopharmacol* (1996) 16, 260–1.
5. Godleski LS, Sernyak MJ. Agranulocytosis after addition of risperidone to clozapine treatment. *Am J Psychiatry* (1996) 153, 735–6.
6. Kontaxakis VP, Havaki-Kontaxaki BJ, Stamouli SS, Christodoulou GN. Toxic interaction between risperidone and clozapine: a case report. *Prog Neuropsychopharmacol Biol Psychiatry* (2002) 26, 407–9.
7. Henderson DC, Goff DC. Risperidone as an adjunct to clozapine therapy in chronic schizophrenics. *J Clin Psychiatry* (1996) 57, 395–7.
8. Raaska K, Raitasuo V, Neuvonen PJ. Therapeutic drug monitoring data: risperidone does not increase serum clozapine concentration. *Eur J Clin Pharmacol* (2002) 58, 587–91.

Clozapine + SSRIs

Fluoxetine, paroxetine, sertraline and possibly citalopram can raise serum clozapine levels. Particularly large increases can occur with fluvoxamine. Clozapine toxicity has been seen in some patients.

Clinical evidence

(a) Citalopram

Preliminary studies in 5 patients found that their mean plasma clozapine levels were unchanged by citalopram.[1] Another study in 8 patients found similar results.[2] However, a patient who was stable on clozapine developed sedation, hypersalivation and confusion shortly after he started to take citalopram 40 mg daily. When total clozapine serum levels were measured they were found to be 1097 nanograms/ml. The citalopram dose was reduced to 20 mg daily, the symptoms resolved over the following 2 weeks, and the total clozapine level dropped to 792 nanograms/ml.[3]

(b) Fluoxetine

Several studies and case reports have found increased clozapine levels of 30 to 75%, and increased levels of the metabolite norclozapine of 34 to 52% after fluoxetine was added to established clozapine treatment.[4-6] In one case the levels of clozapine and norclozapine were raised over fivefold, accompanied by hypertension. Clozapine levels became subtherapeutic 2 weeks after fluoxetine was withdrawn, necessitating an increase in dosage.[7]

A patient who had been taking clozapine 500 mg and lorazepam 3 mg daily, developed myoclonic jerks of his whole body 79 days after fluoxetine 20 mg was added. These decreased over the next 2 days when the fluoxetine and lorazepam were stopped.[8]

In contrast, there are reports of successful use,[9] and no pharmacokinetic changes[10] when clozapine and fluoxetine were used together.

(c) Fluvoxamine

Up to tenfold elevations in plasma clozapine levels have been seen in several studies and case reports when clozapine was given with fluvoxamine.[11-20] These elevations occurred as early as 20 days after combined treatment was started,[16] but were often not associated with any significant adverse effects, even after treatment had continued for a year in one patient.[14] Another study, which compared 12 patients on clozapine with 11 patients on clozapine and fluvoxamine, found that in the combined treatment group, clozapine doses were about half those used when clozapine was given alone. A trend towards decreased granulocyte levels was also seen in the clozapine/fluvoxamine group, but not when clozapine was used alone.[21]

Another patient had extremely high plasma clozapine levels of up to 4160 micrograms/l as a result of taking fluvoxamine.[22]

Other cases have also demonstrated worsening psychosis[23] or extrapyramidal adverse effects[24] (including, rigidity, tremors and akathisia) and sedation within days of giving fluvoxamine with clozapine.

(d) Paroxetine

The serum levels of clozapine and norclozapine rose by 57% and 50% in 16 schizophrenics after taking an average of 31.2 mg of paroxetine daily. One patient on clozapine 300 mg daily developed reversible cerebral intoxication when given paroxetine 40 mg daily.[5] Another patient with a delusional disorder developed an anticholinergic syndrome with doubled serum clozapine levels within about 3 weeks of the addition of paroxetine.[25] In contrast, a study in 14 patients on clozapine 2.5 to 3 mg/kg daily found that the addition of paroxetine 20 mg daily had no effect on the serum levels of clozapine.[19]

(e) Sertraline

The serum levels of clozapine and norclozapine increased by 30% and 52% in 10 schizophrenics when they started to take an average of 92.5 mg of sertraline daily.[5] Another patient on clozapine 600 mg daily had a fall in total clozapine serum levels of 40% within a month of stopping sertraline 300 mg daily.[26]

The serum clozapine levels of a schizophrenic patient doubled within a month of adding sertraline 50 mg daily and her psychosis worsened. When the sertraline was stopped she improved and her serum clozapine levels fell once again.[23]

A case report describes sudden cardiac death in a 26-year-old man, which the authors attributed to an interaction between clozapine and sertraline.[27] However, this interaction has been questioned as it is said that the patient had other risk factors that were more likely to have caused the fatality.[28]

Mechanism

The SSRIs (including **escitalopram**) are known to inhibit the cytochrome P450 isoenzyme CYP2D6 to a varying extent. Fluvoxamine is also a potent inhibitor of CYP1A2. Both of these isoenzymes are involved in the metabolism of clozapine, the most significant being CYP1A2, so their inhibition causes clozapine levels to rise.

The levels of clozapine and norclozapine rise together, on the basis of which it has been suggested that the metabolic step inhibited is after the *N*-dealkylation step.[5]

Importance and management

These interactions are established. Concurrent use need not be avoided, but it would be prudent to monitor the outcome closely because of the rises in serum clozapine and norclozapine levels that can occur, and because of the rare potential for deterioration in clinical status. Adjust the clozapine dosage as necessary. The authors of one study suggest particularly close monitoring if the daily clozapine dosage exceeds 300 mg or 3.5 mg/kg.[5] The interaction is greatest with fluvoxamine, so other SSRIs may be a more prudent choice.

1. Taylor D, Ellison Z, Ementon Shaw L, Wickham H, Murray R. Co-administration of citalopram and clozapine: effect on plasma clozapine levels. *Int Clin Psychopharmacol* (1998) 13, 19–21.
2. Avenoso A, Facciolà G, Scordo MG, Gitto C, Ferrante GD, Madia AG, Spina E. No effect of citalopram on plasma levels of clozapine, risperidone and their active metabolites in patients with chronic schizophrenia. *Clin Drug Invest* (1998) 16, 393–8.
3. Borba CP, Henderson DC. Citalopram and clozapine: potential drug interaction. *J Clin Psychiatry* (2000) 61, 301–2.
4. Centorrino F, Baldessarini RJ, Kando J, Frankenburg FR, Volpicelli SA, Puopolo PR, Flood JG. Serum concentrations of clozapine and its major metabolites: effects of cotreatment with fluoxetine or valproate. *Am J Psychiatry* (1994) 151, 123–5.
5. Centorrino F, Baldessarini RJ, Frankenburg FR, Kando J, Volpicelli SA, Flood JG. Serum levels of clozapine and norclozapine in patients treated with selective serotonin reuptake inhibitors. *Am J Psychiatry* (1996) 153, 820–2.
6. Spina E, Avenoso A, Facciolà G, Fabrazzo M, Monteleone P, Maj M, Perucca E, Caputi AP. Effect of fluoxetine on the plasma concentrations of clozapine and its major metabolites in patients with schizophrenia. *Int Clin Psychopharmacol* (1998) 13, 141–5.
7. Sloan D, O'Boyle J. Hypertension and increased serum clozapine associated with clozapine and fluoxetine in combination. *Ir J Psychol Med* (1977) 14, 149–51.
8. Kingsbury SJ, Puckett KM. Effects of fluoxetine on serum clozapine levels. *Am J Psychiatry* (1995) 152, 473–4.
9. Cassady SL, Thaker GK. Addition of fluoxetine to clozapine. *Am J Psychiatry* (1992) 149, 1274.
10. Eggert AE, Crismon ML, Dorson PG. Lack of effect of fluoxetine on plasma clozapine concentrations. *J Clin Psychiatry* (1994) 55, 454–5.
11. Hiemke C, Weigmann H, Müller H, Dahmen N, Wetzel H, Fuchs E. Elevated clozapine plasma levels after addition of fluvoxamine. *Abstr Soc Neurosci* (1993) 19, 382.
12. Weigmann H, Müller H, Dahmen N, Wetzel H, Hiemke C. Interactions of fluvoxamine with the metabolism of clozapine. *Pharmacopsychiatry* (1993) 26, 209.
13. Jerling M, Lindström L, Bondesson U, Bertilsson L. Fluvoxamine inhibition and carbamazepine induction of the metabolism of clozapine: evidence from a therapeutic drug monitoring service. *Ther Drug Monit* (1994) 16, 368–74.
14. Dumortier G, Lochu A, Colen de Melo P, Ghribi O, Roche Rabreau D, Degrassat K, Desce JM. Elevated clozapine plasma concentrations after fluvoxamine initiation. *Am J Psychiatry* (1996) 153, 738–9.
15. Olesen OV, Starup G, Linnet K. Alvorlig lægmiddelinteraktion mellem clozapin – Leponex og fluvoxamin – Fevarin. *Ugeskr Laeger* (1996) 158, 6931–2.
16. Dequardo JR, Roberts M. Elevated clozapine levels after fluvoxamine initiation. *Am J Psychiatry* (1996) 153, 840–1.
17. Koponen HJ, Leinonen E, Lepola U. Fluvoxamine increases the clozapine serum levels significantly. *Eur Neuropsychopharmacol* (1996) 6, 69–71.
18. Hiemke C, Weigmann H, Härtter S, Dahmen N, Wetzel H, Müller H. Elevated levels of clozapine in serum after addition of fluvoxamine. *J Clin Psychopharmacol* (1994) 14, 279–81.
19. Wetzel H, Anghelescu I, Szegedi A, Wiesner J, Weigmann H, Hörtter S, Hiemke C. Pharmacokinetic interactions of clozapine with selective serotonin reuptake inhibitors: differential effects of fluvoxamine and paroxetine in a prospective study. *J Clin Psychopharmacol* (1998) 18, 2–9.
20. Wang C-Y, Zhang Z-J, Li W-B, Zhai Y-M, Cai Z-J, Weng Y-Z, Zhu R-H, Zhao J-P, Zhou H-H. The differential effects of steady-state fluvoxamine on the pharmacokinetics of olanzapine and clozapine in healthy volunteers. *J Clin Pharmacol* (2004) 44, 785–92.
21. Hinze-Selch D, Deuschle M, Weber B, Heuser I, Pollmächer T. Effect of coadministration of clozapine and fluvoxamine versus clozapine monotherapy on blood cell counts, plasma levels of cytokines and body weight. *Psychopharmacology (Berl)* (2000) 149, 163–9.
22. Heeringa M, Beurskens R, Schouten W, Verduijn MM. Elevated plasma levels of clozapine after concomitant use of fluvoxamine. *Pharm World Sci* (1999) 21, 243–4
23. Chong SA, Tan CH, Lee HS. Worsening of psychosis with clozapine and selective serotonin reuptake inhibitor combination: two case reports. *J Clin Psychopharmacol* (1997) 17, 68–9.
24. Kuo F-J, Lane H-Y, Chang W-H. Extrapyramidal symptoms after addition of fluvoxamine to clozapine. *J Clin Psychopharmacol* (1998) 18, 483–4.
25. Joos AAB, König F, Frank UG, Kaschka WP, Mörike KE, Ewald R. Dose-dependent pharmacokinetic interaction of clozapine and paroxetine in an extensive metabolizer. *Pharmacopsychiatry* (1997) 30, 266–70.
26. Pinniniti NR, De Leon J. Interaction of sertraline with clozapine. *J Clin Psychopharmacol* (1997) 17, 119.
27. Hoehns JD, Fouts MM, Kelly MW, Tu KB. Sudden cardiac death with clozapine and sertraline combination. *Ann Pharmacother* (2001) 35, 862–6.
28. Gillespie JA. Comment: sudden cardiac death with clozapine and sertraline combination. *Ann Pharmacother* (2001) 35, 1671.

Droperidol + MAOIs

An isolated report describes hypotension in a patient given droperidol shortly after the withdrawal of phenelzine.

Clinical evidence, mechanism, importance and management

Four days after the withdrawal of **phenelzine** and perphenazine, a patient was given operative premedication of droperidol 20 mg and hyoscine 400 micrograms, orally. About 2 hours later he was observed to be pale, sweating profusely and slightly cyanosed, with a blood pressure of 75/60 mmHg and a pulse rate of 60 bpm. He was not excitable, and no changes in respiration were seen. The blood pressure gradually rose to 115/80 mmHg over the next 45 minutes, but did not return to his normal level of 160/100 mmHg for 36 hours. The same premedication was given 11 days later without any adverse effects.[1] The response was attributed to the residual effects of **phenelzine** treatment. Its general significance is unclear.

1. Penlington GN. Droperidol and monoamine-oxidase inhibitors. *BMJ* (1966) 1, 483–4.

Fluphenazine + Ascorbic acid (Vitamin C)

A single case report describes a fall in serum fluphenazine levels and deterioration in a patient when given ascorbic acid (vitamin C).

Clinical evidence, mechanism, importance and management

A man with a history of manic behaviour, taking fluphenazine 15 mg daily, had a 25% fall in his plasma fluphenazine levels, from 0.93 to 0.705 nanograms/ml, over a 13-day period accompanied by a deterioration in behaviour while taking ascorbic acid 500 mg twice daily.[1] The reason is not understood. There seem to be no other reports of this interaction with fluphenazine or any other phenothiazine so that this interaction would appear not to be of general importance.

1. Dysken MW, Cumming RJ, Channon RA, Davis JM. Drug interaction between ascorbic acid and fluphenazine. *JAMA* (1979) 241, 2008.

Fluphenazine + Spiramycin

Acute dystonia occurred in a man on fluphenazine, which was attributed to an interaction with spiramycin.

Clinical evidence, mechanism, importance and management

A man with schizoaffective disorder taking lorazepam, orphenadrine, fluvoxamine and fluphenazine decanoate 12.5 mg every 2 weeks, developed acute and painful dystonia of the trunk, neck, right arm and leg about a week after his last fluphenazine injection and on the fourth day of taking spiramycin 6 million units daily for gingivitis. The problem resolved when he was given biperiden.[1] The reasons for this adverse reaction are not understood, nor is it entirely clear whether this was an interaction between fluphenazine and spiramycin, although the author suggested that a causal link existed. This seems to be the only report of an alleged interaction between fluphenazine and a macrolide antibacterial and it is therefore of little or no general importance.

1. Benazzi F. Spiramycin-associated acute dystonia during neuroleptic treatment. *Can J Psychiatry* (1997) 42, 665–6.

Glutethimide + Tobacco smoking

A study in 7 subjects found that glutethimide worsened psychomotor performance in smokers more than in non-smokers, possibly due to an increase in its absorption.[1] However there would seem to be no need for particular caution if smokers take glutethimide.

1. Crow JW, Lain P, Bochner F, Shoeman DW, Azarnoff DL. Glutethimide and 4-OH glutethimide: pharmacokinetics and effect on performance in man. *Clin Pharmacol Ther* (1978) 22, 458–64.

Haloperidol + Antituberculars

The serum levels of haloperidol can be reduced by rifampicin (rifampin), and possibly raised by isoniazid.

Clinical evidence

A study in schizophrenic patients on haloperidol, 7 of whom were also on a range of antitubercular drugs (**ethambutol**, **isoniazid**, **rifampicin**), and 18 of whom were on **isoniazid** only, showed that those on multiple drugs, which included **rifampicin** had significantly reduced haloperidol serum levels. The half-life of haloperidol in 2 patients on **rifampicin** was 4.9 hours compared with 9.4 hours in 3 other patients not taking **rifampicin**.[1] Three of the patients on **isoniazid** (without rifampicin or ethambutol) had increased serum haloperidol levels.[1]

The trough serum haloperidol levels of 15 schizophrenics fell to 37.4% of the expected level after they took **rifampicin** 600 mg daily for 7 days.[2] After 28 days the serum level had dropped further to 30% of the expected level. In another group of 5 patients stabilised on haloperidol and **rifampicin**, the serum haloperidol levels rose to 229% of the previous level 7 days after stopping **rifampicin**, and to 329% after 28 days.[2] The clinical effects of the haloperidol appeared to be reduced by the **rifampicin**.[2]

Mechanism

The likeliest explanation is that the rifampicin, a recognised enzyme inducing agent, increases the metabolism and loss of the haloperidol from the body.

Importance and management

The interaction between haloperidol and rifampicin would appear to be established and clinically important. Be alert for any evidence of reduced haloperidol effects if rifampicin alone is used, and possibly increased effects if isoniazid alone is used. Adjust the haloperidol dosage if necessary.

1. Takeda M, Nishinuma K, Yamashita S, Matsubayashi T, Tanino S, Nishimura T. Serum haloperidol levels of schizophrenics receiving treatment for tuberculosis. *Clin Neuropharmacol* (1986) 9, 386–97.
2. Kim Y-H, Cha I-J, Shim J-C, Shin J-G, Yoon Y-R, Kim Y-K, Kim J-I, Park G-H, Jang I-J, Woo J-I, Shin S-G. Effect of rifampin on the plasma concentration and the clinical effect of haloperidol concomitantly administered to schizophrenic patients. *J Clin Psychopharmacol* (1996) 16, 247–52.

Haloperidol + Buspirone

Two studies found that buspirone can cause a rise in plasma haloperidol levels, while another found no interaction occurred.

Clinical evidence, mechanism, importance and management

A pharmacokinetic study in 27 schizophrenic patients taking haloperidol 10 to 40 mg daily found that buspirone 5 mg three times daily for 2 weeks, followed by 10 mg three times daily for 4 weeks, did not significantly affect the steady-state plasma haloperidol levels.[1]

These findings contrast with those of a 6-week study, in which 6 out of 7 schizophrenics had 15 to 122% rises in plasma haloperidol levels when they were given buspirone.[2] The authors also mention a single-dose study in healthy subjects, which found a 30% rise in haloperidol levels when subjects were given buspirone.[2]

It is not known why these findings differ, but since no adverse reactions have been reported, there would seem to be no reason for avoiding concurrent use. However, be aware that some patients seem to experience large rises in haloperidol levels, so consider this interaction if the effects of haloperidol seem excessive.

1. Huang HF, Jann MW, Wei F-C, Chang T-P, Chen J-S, Juang D-J, Lin S-K, Lam YFW, Chien C-P, Chang W-H. Lack of pharmacokinetic interaction between buspirone and haloperidol in patients with schizophrenia. *J Clin Pharmacol* (1996) 36, 963–9.
2. Goff DC, Midha KK, Brotman AW, McCormick S, Waites M, Amico ET. An open trial of buspirone added to neuroleptics in schizophrenic patients. *J Clin Psychopharmacol* (1991) 11, 193–7.

Haloperidol + Dexamfetamine

Acute dystonia occurred in two healthy subjects when they were given haloperidol with dexamfetamine.

Clinical evidence, mechanism, importance and management

Two healthy young women were given haloperidol 5 mg and dexamfetamine 5 mg as part of a neuropharmacological study. After 29 hours one of them developed stiffness of neck and limbs, parkinsonian facies, her tongue protruded and she had oropharyngeal spasm. After 34 hours the other woman developed an oculogyric crisis and acute dystonia of the neck with her back slightly arched. Both recovered rapidly after being given 10 mg of intramuscular procyclidine.[1]

The reasons for this interaction are not fully understood, but the authors of the study suggest that the acute dystonia was due to a potentiation of dopamine release. The clinical significance of this interaction is unclear.

1. Capstick C, Checkley S, Gray J, Dawe S. Dystonia induced by amphetamine and haloperidol. *Br J Psychiatry* (1994) 165, 276.

Haloperidol + Granisetron

Granisetron appears not to increase the adverse effects of haloperidol.

Clinical evidence, mechanism, importance and management

A study in 12 healthy subjects found that while haloperidol 3 mg alone caused some impaired psychometric performance (increased drowsiness, muzziness, lethargy, mental slowness, etc.), the addition of granisetron 160 micrograms/kg did not seem to make performance significantly worse.[1] If both drugs are used, no additional precautions would seem necessary.

1. Leigh TJ, Link CGG, Fell GL. Effects of granisetron and haloperidol, alone and in combination, on psychometric performance and the EEG. *Br J Clin Pharmacol* (1992) 34, 65–70.

Haloperidol + Imipenem

Marked but transient hypotension was seen in 3 patients on intravenous imipenem when they were given low dose intravenous haloperidol.

Clinical evidence, mechanism, importance and management

Three patients in intensive care who were being treated with intravenous imipenem 500 mg (with cilastatin) every 6 hours for 2, 3 and 7 days respectively, developed a rapid and short-lived episode of hypotension when given a 2.5-mg dose of intravenous haloperidol. For example, the blood pressure of one of the patients fell from 117/75 mmHg to 91/49 mmHg. After 30 minutes her blood pressure had risen to 100/57 mmHg. No treatment for hypotension was given to any of the patients and the reaction was brief and self-limiting. Two of them were also taking famotidine and erythromycin. No acute ECG changes were seen.[1]

The reason for this fall in blood pressure is not understood, but the authors attribute what happened to the concurrent use of haloperidol and imipenem, although they point out that intravenous haloperidol alone can cause orthostatic hypotension. One suggestion is that competitive protein binding displacement might have increased the levels of free haloperidol.[1]

The authors advise that if haloperidol is used low doses should be given and the outcome well monitored. They say that no pressor agent was needed in these cases, but they suggest the possible use of metaraminol, phenylephrine or noradrenaline (norepinephrine) rather than dopamine, the vasopressor effects of which might be blocked or reversed by haloperidol.[1] This interaction seems not to have been reported to occur with oral haloperidol.

1. Franco-Bronson K, Gajwani P. Hypotension associated with intravenous haloperidol and imipenem. *J Clin Psychopharmacol* (1999) 19, 480–1.

Haloperidol + Indometacin

Profound drowsiness and confusion have been described in patients given haloperidol and indometacin.

Clinical evidence, mechanism, importance and management

A double-blind crossover study in 20 patients to find out the possible advantages of combining haloperidol 5 mg daily with indometacin 25 mg three times daily was eventually abandoned because 13 patients (11 on haloperidol and 2 on placebo) failed to complete the trial. Profound drowsiness or tiredness caused 6 of the haloperidol-treated patients to be withdrawn from the trial. The authors of the paper said[1] that the combined treatment produced drowsiness and confusion that was greater than anything expected with haloperidol alone, and sufficiently severe to affect independent functioning in some cases.

Evidence of this interaction appears to be very limited. If concurrent use is thought appropriate, warn patients about this potentially severe effect. It might be wiser to avoid concurrent use because many patients requiring this type of treatment may not be hospitalised and under the day-to-day scrutiny of the prescriber.

1. Bird HA, Le Gallez P, Wright V. Drowsiness due to haloperidol/indomethacin in combination. *Lancet* (1983) i, 830–1.

Haloperidol + Quinidine

Blood levels of haloperidol can be markedly increased if quinidine is added.

Clinical evidence, mechanism, importance and management

An experimental study in 13 healthy subjects found that 1 hour after taking quinidine bisulfate 250 mg, the maximum plasma levels and the AUC of a single 5-mg dose of haloperidol were approximately doubled. The reasons are not understood.[1] The clinical importance of this has not been assessed, but it seems likely that the effects and adverse effects of haloperidol will be increased if quinidine is added. Be alert for this interaction if both drugs are given.

See also 'Drugs that prolong the QT interval + Other drugs that prolong the QT interval', p.170.

1. Young D, Midha KK, Fossler MJ, Hawes EM, Hubbard JW, McKay G, Korchinski ED. Effect of quinidine on the interconversion kinetics between haloperidol and reduced haloperidol in humans: implications for the involvement of cytochrome P450IID6. *Eur J Clin Pharmacol* (1993) 44, 433–8.

Haloperidol + Venlafaxine

Venlafaxine can increase the serum levels of haloperidol. This is consistent with an isolated report of a man who developed urinary retention when venlafaxine was added to a previously well tolerated regimen of haloperidol and alprazolam.

Clinical evidence, mechanism, importance and management

A study in 24 healthy subjects found that steady-state venlafaxine 75 mg every 12 hours reduced the renal clearance of a single 2-mg dose of haloperidol by 42%, resulting in a 70% rise in the AUC and an 88% rise in the maximum serum levels.[1-3] This rise in haloperidol levels would seem to be consistent with an isolated report of a 75-year-old man taking haloperidol 1 mg and alprazolam 500 micrograms daily, who suddenly developed urinary retention when the venlafaxine 37.5 mg daily was added. Urinary retention resolved spontaneously when all the drugs were stopped.[4]

It was suggested that venlafaxine inhibits the cytochrome P450 isoenzyme CYP2D6, which is concerned with the metabolism of haloperidol. As a result the serum levels of the haloperidol rise, thereby increasing its anticholinergic effects.[4]

The evidence is very limited but be aware that increased haloperidol adverse effects may occur if venlafaxine is also given. It may be necessary to reduce the haloperidol dosage.

1. Efexor XL (Venlafaxine hydrochloride). Wyeth Pharmaceuticals. UK Summary of product characteristics, December 2004.
2. Wyeth, Personal communication, April 2001.
3. Effexor XR (Venlafaxine). Wyeth Pharmaceuticals Inc. US Prescribing information, January 2005.
4. Benazzi F. Urinary retention with venlafaxine-haloperidol combination. *Pharmacopsychiatry* (1997) 30, 27.

Olanzapine + Anticonvulsants

Carbamazepine lowers olanzapine levels, and the combination of olanzapine and valproate appears to increase the risk of hepatic injury in children.

Clinical evidence, mechanism, importance and management

(a) Carbamazepine

Multiple-dose studies in healthy subjects have shown that carbamazepine increases the metabolism of olanzapine (by induction of the cytochrome P450 isoenzyme CYP1A2). The clearance of olanzapine was increased 44% and its terminal elimination half-life was reduced 20%, but these changes were not considered significant enough to necessitate dosage adjustments of either drug.[1] Another study found that 5 patients taking olanzapine and carbamazepine had a concentration/dose ratio 36% lower than 22 patients taking olanzapine alone.[2] A later study by the same authors found similar results, and also found that this increased olanzapine metabolism was probably due to an increase in glucuronidation, which was induced by the carbamazepine.[3]

A retrospective study identified 10 patients taking olanzapine and carbamazepine. The patients on carbamazepine were taking olanzapine doses that were double those of subjects on olanzapine alone. When corrected for dose it was found that the concentration dose ratio of olanzapine was 71% lower in those also taking carbamazepine.[4] It would seem prudent to closely monitor the outcome of concurrent use and adjust the olanzapine dose as necessary.

(b) Valproate

A retrospective study identified 52 children (under 18-years-old) who were treated with olanzapine alone (17), semisodium valproate alone (23) or both drugs together (12). At least one peak liver enzyme level (ALT, AST or lactate dehydrogenase) was found to be above the normal range in 59% of those on olanzapine alone, 26% of those on valproate alone, and 100% of patients on the combination. Liver enzymes were persistently elevated in 42% of the patients on combination treatment, and 2 of these patients had levels that were three times the upper limit of normal. Treatment was discontinued due to pancreatitis in one and steatohepatitis in the other. The authors recommend measuring liver enzymes every 3 to 4 months for the first year of treatment, thereafter monitoring every 6 months if no adverse effects are detected.[5]

1. Zyprexa (Olanzapine). Eli Lilly. Clinical and Laboratory Experience A Comprehensive Monograph, August 1996.
2. Olesen OV, Linnet K. Olanzapine serum concentrations in psychiatric patients given standard doses: the influence of comedication. *Ther Drug Monit* (1999) 21, 87–90.
3. Linnet K, Olesen OV. Free and glucuronidated olanzapine serum concentrations in psychiatric patients: influence of carbamazepine comedication. *Ther Drug Monit* (2002) 24, 512–17.
4. Skogh E, Reis M, Dahl M-L, Lundmark J, Bengtsson F. Therapeutic drug monitoring data on olanzapine and its N-demethyl metabolite in the naturalistic clinical setting. *Ther Drug Monit* (2002) 24, 518–26.
5. Gonzalez-Heydrich J, Raches D, Wilens TE, Leichtner A, Mezzacappa E. Retrospective study of hepatic enzyme elevations in children treated with olanzapine, divalproex, and their combination. *J Am Acad Child Adolesc Psychiatry* (2003) 12, 1227–33.

Olanzapine + Miscellaneous

Activated charcoal causes a fall in fluvoxamine levels and venlafaxine moderately raises olanzapine levels. Additive dopaminergic effects have been seen in one patient on olanzapine and haloperidol. Olanzapine appears not to interact to a clinically relevant extent with aluminium/magnesium hydroxide antacids, cimetidine or diazepam. However, excessive sedation may occur with parenteral benzodiazepines and intramuscular olanzapine.

Clinical evidence, mechanism, importance and management

(a) Antacids

The makers of olanzapine say that single doses of an **aluminium/magnesium-containing antacid** had no effect on the pharmacokinetics of olanzapine.[1] No special precautions would seem to be needed during concurrent use.

(b) Benzodiazepines

In vivo studies have found that no pharmacokinetic interaction occurs between olanzapine and **diazepam**.[1] This confirms *in vitro* studies using human liver microsomes,[1] which demonstrated that olanzapine did not inhibit the cytochrome P450 isoenzymes CYP3A4 or CYP2C19, which are concerned with the metabolism of **diazepam**. It was noted that mild increases in heart rate, sedation and dry mouth were seen in patients taking both drugs, but no dosage adjustments were thought to be necessary.[2] There would therefore appear to be no reason for avoiding concurrent use.

Intramuscular **lorazepam** 2 mg, given 1 hour after intramuscular olanzapine 5 mg increased the drowsiness seen with either drug alone.[3,4] Intramuscular olanzapine has been associated with hypotension, bradycardia, respiratory depression, and rarely death, particularly in patients who have also received benzodiazepines. The makers therefore say that concurrent use is not recommended. If both drugs are needed, parenteral benzodiazepines should not be given for 1 hour after intramuscular olanzapine. If a parenteral benzodiazepine has already been given, intramuscular olanzapine should only be given with careful consideration and monitoring of sedation and respiration.[4]

(c) Charcoal, activated

The makers report that activated charcoal reduces the bioavailability of oral olanzapine by 50 to 60%,[1,3] and recommend that administration be separated by 2 hours.[1]

(d) Cimetidine

The makers say that cimetidine has no effect on the bioavailability of olanzapine.[3] No special precautions would seem to be needed during concurrent use.

(e) Haloperidol

A 67-year-old man with a long history of bipolar disorder was taking haloperidol 10 mg daily, with valproate and benzatropine. Because he had previously had parkinsonian symptoms, olanzapine was started, to be increased as the haloperidol was decreased. On day 6 his parkinsonian symptoms became particularly marked. The haloperidol was stopped and 2 days later the symptoms had resolved. It is thought that either the small amount of dopaminergic activity of olanzapine combined with that of the haloperidol brought on these symptoms, or that olanzapine affected the metabolism of haloperidol, caused increased levels and therefore greater dopaminergic activity.[5] The significance of this interaction is not clear, but it would be wise to be aware of this interaction if both drugs are used.

(f) Venlafaxine

A retrospective study found that venlafaxine caused a 27% increase in olanzapine plasma levels. The clinical significance of this finding is unclear.[6]

1. Zyprexa (Olanzapine). Eli Lilly and Company Ltd. UK Summary of product characteristics, February 2005.
2. Zyprexa (Olanzapine). Eli Lilly. Clinical and Laboratory Experience A Comprehensive Monograph. August 1996.
3. Zyprexa (Olanzapine). Eli Lilly and Company. US Prescribing information, September 2004.
4. Zyprexa powder for solution for injection (Olanzapine). Eli Lilly and Company Ltd. UK Summary of product characteristics, February 2005.
5. Gomberg RF. Interaction between olanzapine and haloperidol. *J Clin Psychopharmacol* (1999) 19, 272–3.
6. Gex-Fabry M, Balant-Gorgia AE, Balant LP. Therapeutic drug monitoring of olanzapine: the combined effect of age, gender, smoking, and comedication. *Ther Drug Monit* (2003) 25, 46–53.

Olanzapine + Ritonavir

Ritonavir almost halves olanzapine levels.

Clinical evidence, mechanism, importance and management

A single 10-mg dose of olanzapine was given to 14 healthy, non-smoking subjects after they had taken ritonavir for 11 days (initially 300 mg twice daily, escalating to 500 mg twice daily). Ritonavir decreased the AUC and maximum plasma levels of olanzapine by 53% and 40% respectively, and reduced the half-life from 32 to 16 hours.[1]

The authors suggest that ritonavir increased the metabolism of olanzapine by inducing the cytochrome P450 isoenzyme CYP1A2, which is the main metabolic route of olanzapine. They also suggest that increased glucuronidation, mediated by glucuronyl transferases induced by ritonavir, may have contributed.

It seems likely that increased olanzapine doses may be needed in the presence of ritonavir. If concurrent use is necessary monitor for olanzapine efficacy and increase the dose if necessary.

1. Penzak SR, Hon YY, Lawhorn WD, Shirley KL, Spratlin V, Jann MW. Influence of ritonavir on olanzapine pharmacokinetics in healthy volunteers. *J Clin Psychopharmacol* (2002) 22, 366–70.

Olanzapine + SSRIs

Fluvoxamine causes a rise in serum olanzapine levels, which is associated with increased adverse effects. Fluoxetine, paroxetine and sertraline appear to moderately raise olanzapine levels while citalopram appears to have no effect. A case of retarded ejaculation has been seen in one patient on olanzapine and paroxetine.

Clinical evidence, mechanism, importance and management

(a) Fluvoxamine

In a placebo-controlled study, fluvoxamine 50 to 100 mg daily was given to 10 male smokers daily for 11 days, with olanzapine 2.5 to 7.5 mg daily on days 4 to 11. During the initial 4 days of concurrent use somnolence was increased by 19 to 115% when compared to the group on olanzapine and placebo but the subjects accommodated to this over the next 4 days. Fluvoxamine increased the olanzapine maximum plasma levels and AUC by 84 and 119% respectively and the olanzapine clearance fell by 50%.[1] A retrospective study found that in patients taking fluvoxamine and olanzapine the concentration/dose ratio was 2.3-fold higher than those on olanzapine alone.[2] In another study 10 schizophrenic patients were given fluvoxamine 50 mg daily from days 1 to 14 followed by fluvoxamine 100 mg daily from days 15 to 28. A single 10-mg dose of olanzapine was given on day 10 and again on day 24. The maximum plasma levels of olanzapine were raised by 12% and 64% and the clearance was reduced by about 25% and 35%, by 50 and 100 mg of fluvoxamine respectively. Increased sedation was also seen, which was more frequent with fluvoxamine 100 mg daily.[3] Other studies have found 50 to 81% increases in olanzapine levels with fluvoxamine 100 mg daily, which took up to 8 weeks to occur. There was a marked variation between individuals in the extent of the interaction.[4-6]

The olanzapine plasma levels of a 21-year-old woman were 6 times the recommended upper limit while she was taking fluvoxamine. During this time she developed rigidity and tremor. After the olanzapine dose was reduced from 15 mg to 5 mg daily the levels were still almost double the recommended level.[7]

(b) Other SSRIs

The makers say that **fluoxetine** 60 mg daily for 8 days caused an increase of 16% in olanzapine maximum serum levels and a 16% decrease in clearance. These differences were considered to be too small to necessitate dosage adjustments.[8] Similar results were found in a published study.[9]

A patient taking fluvoxamine had olanzapine levels double the upper recommended limit while taking fluvoxamine. When **paroxetine** was substituted for fluvoxamine the olanzapine levels became almost normal.[7] Another patient taking **paroxetine** developed retarded ejaculation 2 months after he started to take olanzapine 15 mg daily. This adverse effect resolved when the olanzapine was given in divided doses.[10]

A retrospective study found that **sertraline** had no effect on the concentration/dose ratio of olanzapine, suggesting that it does not interact.[2]

Another study found that **paroxetine**, **fluoxetine** and **sertraline** increased olanzapine levels by about 32%, but **citalopram** had no effect.[6]

Mechanism

Fluvoxamine inhibits the cytochrome P450 isoenzyme CYP1A2, which is involved in the metabolism of olanzapine,[1] resulting in increased olanzapine levels and adverse effects. All SSRIs affect CYP2D6 (to differing extents). This isoenzyme is also involved in olanzapine metabolism, although to a lesser extent than CYP1A2. Therefore SSRIs other than fluvoxamine have only a small effect on olanzapine levels.

Importance and management

The makers of olanzapine suggest that lower olanzapine doses may be needed if fluvoxamine is given.[8,11] Monitor for fluvoxamine adverse effects. Other SSRIs appear not to interact significantly, although the case report with paroxetine suggests that additive adverse effects are a possibility.

1. Mäenpää J, Wrighton S, Bergstrom R, Cerimele B, Tatum D, Hatcher B, Callaghan JT. Pharmacokinetic (PK) and pharmacodynamic (PD) interactions between fluvoxamine and olanzapine. *Clin Pharmacol Ther* (1997) 61, 225.
2. Weigmann H, Gerek S, Zeisig A, Müller M, Härtter S, Heimke C. Fluvoxamine but not sertraline inhibits the metabolism of olanzapine: evidence from a therapeutic drug monitoring service. *Ther Drug Monit* (2001) 23, 410–13.
3. Chiu C-C, Lane H-Y, Huang M-C, Liu H-C, Jann MW, Hon Y-Y, Chang W-H, Lu M-L. Dose-dependent alterations in the pharmacokinetics of olanzapine during coadministration of fluvoxamine in patients with schizophrenia. *J Clin Pharmacol* (2004) 44, 1385–90.
4. Wang C-Y, Zhang Z-J, Li W-B, Zhai Y-M, Cai Z-J, Weng Y-Z, Zhu R-H, Zhao J-P, Zhou H-H. The differential effects of steady-state fluvoxamine on the pharmacokinetics of olanzapine and clozapine in healthy volunteers. *J Clin Pharmacol* (2004) 44, 785–92.
5. Hiemke C, Peled A, Jabarin M, Hadjez J, Weigmann H, Härtter S, Ilan M, Ritsner M, Silver H. Fluvoxamine augmentation of olanzapine in chronic schizophrenia: pharmacokinetic interactions and clinical effects. *J Clin Psychopharmacol* (2002) 22, 502–6.
6. Gex-Fabry M, Balant-Gorgia AE, Balant LP. Therapeutic drug monitoring of olanzapine: the combined effect of age, gender, smoking, and comedication. *Ther Drug Monit* (2003) 25, 46–53.
7. de Jong J, Hoogenboom B, van Troostwijk LD, de Haan L. Interaction of olanzapine with fluvoxamine. *Psychopharmacology (Berl)* (2001) 155, 219–20.
8. Zyprexa (Olanzapine). Eli Lilly and Company. US Prescribing information, September 2004.
9. Gossen D, de Suray J-M, Vandenhende F, Onkelinx C, Gangji D. Influence of fluoxetine on olanzapine pharmacokinetics. *AAPS PharmSci* (2002) 4, E11.
10. Bizouard P, Vandel S, Kantelip JP. Olanzapine-induced retarded ejaculation: role of paroxetine comedication? A case report. *Therapie* (2001) 56, 441–7.
11. Zyprexa (Olanzapine). Eli Lilly and Company Ltd. UK Summary of product characteristics, February 2005.

Olanzapine + Tobacco smoking

Smoking increases the clearance of olanzapine.

Clinical evidence, mechanism, importance and management

Retrospective study has found that cigarette smoking reduced olanzapine concentrations by 12%[1] and that smokers needed higher doses of olanzapine than non-smokers (10 mg compared to 12.5 mg) yet had lower olanzapine levels (60 nanomol/l compared to 92 nanomol/l).[2]

A study in 17 psychiatric patients found that the olanzapine concentration dose ratio was directly related to CYP1A2 activity, which was sixfold higher in smokers than non-smokers. When corrected for dose, the non-smokers had olanzapine levels of 7.9 nanograms/ml compared with 1.56 nanograms/ml in smokers.[3]

The makers of olanzapine say that smokers show a 40% greater clearance than non-smokers.[4] The consequences are that the effects of olanzapine will be reduced to some extent by smoking. However, the makers say that dosage adjustments are not routinely recommended in smokers.[4,5]

1. Gex-Fabry M, Balant-Gorgia AE, Balant LP. Therapeutic drug monitoring of olanzapine: the combined effect of age, gender, smoking, and comedication. *Ther Drug Monit* (2003) 25, 46–53.
2. Skogh E, Reis M, Dahl M-L, Lundmark J, Bengtsson F. Therapeutic drug monitoring data on olanzapine and its N-demethyl metabolite in the naturalistic clinical setting. *Ther Drug Monit* (2002) 24, 518–26.
3. Carillo JA, Herráiz AG, Ramos SI, Gervasini G, Vizcaíno S, Benítez J. Role of the smoking-induced cytochrome P450 (CYP)1A2 and polymorphic CYP2D6 in steady-state concentration of olanzapine. *J Clin Psychopharmacol* (2003) 23, 119–27.
4. Zyprexa (Olanzapine). Eli Lilly and Company. US Prescribing information, September 2004.
5. Zyprexa (Olanzapine). Eli Lilly and Company Ltd. UK Summary of product characteristics, February 2005.

Olanzapine + Tricyclic antidepressants

No pharmacokinetic interaction occurs between imipramine and olanzapine, but the additive effects of clomipramine and olanzapine was thought to cause a seizure in one patient.

Clinical evidence, mechanism, importance and management

A randomised, open-label three-way crossover study in 9 healthy men given single doses of olanzapine 5 mg and **imipramine** 75 mg found no clinically relevant pharmacokinetic or pharmacodynamic interactions between the two drugs.[1] This would seem to confirm *in vitro* studies using human liver microsomes,[2] which demonstrated that olanzapine causes minimal inhibition of the cytochrome P450 isoenzyme CYP2D6, an enzyme involved in the metabolism of the tricyclic antidepressants. However, one case report describes seizures, thought to be caused by the additive effects of olanzapine and **clomipramine**. Neither drug alone had produced this reaction in the patient.[3] No special precautions would seem to be necessary if both drugs are used concurrently, but be aware that they both have the potential to lower the seizure threshold and that the effect may be additive.

1. Callaghan JT, Cerimele BJ, Kassahun KJ, Nyhart EH, Hoyes-Beehler PJ, Kondraske GV. Olanzapine: interaction study with imipramine. *J Clin Pharmacol* (1997) 37, 971–8.
2. Zyprexa (Olanzapine). Eli Lilly and Company Ltd. UK Summary of product characteristics, February 2005.
3. Deshauer D, Albuquerque J, Alda M, Grof P. Seizures caused by possible interaction between olanzapine and clomipramine. *J Clin Psychopharmacol* (2000) 20, 283–4.

Perphenazine + Disulfiram

A single case report describes a man on perphenazine whose psychotic symptoms re-emerged when he began to take disulfiram.

Clinical evidence, mechanism, importance and management

A man stabilised on perphenazine 8 mg twice daily developed marked psychosis soon after starting to take disulfiram 100 mg daily.[1] His serum perphenazine levels had fallen from a range of 2 to 3 nanomol/l to less than 1 nanomol/l. Doubling the dosage of perphenazine had little effect, and no substantial clinical improvement or rise in serum levels occurred until he was given intramuscular perphenazine enantate 50 mg weekly, at which point the levels rose to about 4 nanomol/l. The results of clinical biochemical tests suggested that the disulfiram was acting as an enzyme-inducing agent, so that the perphenazine was being metabolised and cleared from the body more rapidly. Disulfiram normally acts as an enzyme inhibitor. Too little is known to assess the general importance of this interaction, and there seems to be no information about an interaction with other phenothiazines.

1. Hansen LB, Larsen N-E. Metabolic interaction between perphenazine and disulfiram. *Lancet* (1982) ii, 1472.

Phenothiazines + Antimalarials

Chloroquine, amodiaquine and *Fansidar* (sulfadoxine/pyrimethamine) can markedly increase serum chlorpromazine levels.

Clinical evidence

A total of 15 schizophrenic patients (in three groups of five) given **chlorpromazine** 400 or 500 mg daily for at least 2 weeks were given single doses of either **chloroquine sulphate** 400 mg, **amodiaquine hydrochloride** 600 mg or three tablets of *Fansidar* (**pyrimethamine** 25 mg with **sulfadoxine** 500 mg) an hour before the **chlorpromazine**. Serum **chlorpromazine** levels 3 hours later were found to be raised about threefold by the **chloroquine** and **amodiaquine**, and almost fourfold by the *Fansidar*. The plasma levels of 7-hydroxychlorpromazine, one of the major metabolites of **chlorpromazine**, were also elevated, but not those of the other metabolite, chlorpromazine sulphoxide. The serum **chlorpromazine** levels of the patients given **chloroquine** or *Fansidar* were, to some extent, still elevated 4 days later. There was subjective evidence that the patients were more heavily sedated when given the antimalarials.[1]

Mechanism

Not understood. Both chloroquine and *Fansidar* have relatively long half-lives compared with amodiaquine, which may explain the persistence of their effects.

Importance and management

Direct information about this interaction seems to be limited to this study. Its clinical importance is uncertain but it seems possible that these antimalarials could cause chlorpromazine toxicity. Monitor the effects of concurrent use closely and anticipate the need to reduce the chlorpromazine dosage. More study is needed. See also 'Drugs that prolong the QT interval + Other drugs that prolong the QT interval', p.170.

1. Makanjuola ROA, Dixon PAF, Oforah E. Effects of antimalarial agents on plasma levels of chlorpromazine and its metabolites in schizophrenic patients. *Trop Geogr Med* (1988) 40, 31–3.

Phenothiazines + Barbiturates

The levels of chlorpromazine and possibly thioridazine are decreased by phenobarbital. Phenothiazines also appear to reduce barbiturate levels. However, the clinical importance of these reductions is uncertain. Pentobarbital, promethazine and hyoscine in combination are said to increase the incidence of operative agitation.

Clinical evidence

(a) Phenothiazine levels reduced

A study in 12 schizophrenics on **chlorpromazine** 100 mg three times daily found that **phenobarbital** 50 mg three times daily reduced plasma **chlorpromazine** levels by 25 to 30%, which was accompanied by changes in certain physiological measurements, which clearly reflected a reduced response. The conclusion was made that there was no advantage to be gained by concurrent use.[1]

In another study in 7 patients, the plasma levels of **thioridazine** were reduced by **phenobarbital**, but the clinical effects of this were uncertain.[2] However, another study found that **phenobarbital** caused no changes in serum **thioridazine** levels, but the levels of its active metabolite (mesoridazine) were reduced.[3]

(b) Phenobarbital levels reduced

A study in epileptic patients found that their serum phenobarbital levels fell by 29% when they were treated with phenothiazines, which included **chlorpromazine**, **thioridazine** or **mesoridazine**, and increased when the phenothiazine was withdrawn.[4]

This study confirms another, in which **thioridazine** 100 to 200 mg daily was found to reduce serum phenobarbital levels by about 25%.[5] There is also some limited evidence that the concurrent use of pentobarbital, **promethazine** and hyoscine increases the incidence of pre-operative, operative and postoperative agitation, and it has been suggested that this triple combination should be avoided.[6]

Mechanism

Uncertain. The barbiturates are potent liver enzyme inducing agents, and so it is presumed that they increase the metabolism of the phenothiazines by the liver.

Importance and management

These interactions appear to be established, but the documentation is limited. Their importance is uncertain, but be alert for evidence of reductions in response during concurrent use of phenothiazines and barbiturates, and to increased responses if one of the drugs is withdrawn. So far only chlorpromazine, thioridazine, mesoridazine and phenobarbital are implicated, but it seems possible that other phenothiazines and barbiturates will behave similarly.

1. Loga S, Curry S, Lader M. Interactions of orphenadrine and phenobarbitone with chlorpromazine: plasma concentrations and effects in man. *Br J Clin Pharmacol* (1975) 2, 197–208.
2. Ellenor GL, Musa MN, Beuthin FC. Phenobarbital-thioridazine interaction in man. *Res Commun Chem Pathol Pharmacol* (1978) 21, 185–8.
3. Linnoila M, Viukari M, Vaisanen K, Auvinen J. Effect of anticonvulsants on plasma haloperidol and thioridazine levels. *Am J Psychiatry* (1980) 137, 819–21.
4. Haidukewych D, Rodin EA. Effect of phenothiazines on serum antiepileptic drug concentrations in psychiatric patients with seizure disorder. *Ther Drug Monit* (1985) 7, 401–4.
5. Gay PE, Madsen JA. Interaction between phenobarbital and thioridazine. *Neurology* (1983) 33, 1631–2.
6. Macris SG, Levy L. Preanesthetic medication: untoward effects of certain drug combinations. *Anesthesiology* (1965) 26, 256.

Phenothiazines + HRT or Oral contraceptives

Oestrogens can increase the plasma levels of butaperazine. A single report describes a marked rise in serum chlorpromazine levels in a woman on a combined oral contraceptive.

Clinical evidence, mechanism, importance and management

When a severe dystonic reaction to a single dose of **prochlorperazine** was seen in a pregnant woman (presumed to be due to increased plasma **butaperazine** levels resulting from the high oestrogen levels), a further study was undertaken in 4 postmenopausal schizophrenic women. **Conjugated oestrogens** (*Premarin*) 1.25 mg daily increased the plasma **butaperazine** levels by 48% (from 231 to 343 nanograms/ml) and increased the AUC by 92%.[1]

A case report describes a woman who had been taking **chlorpromazine** 100 mg three times daily for one week without problems when a combined oral contraceptive (**ethinylestradiol/norgestrel**) was started. Four days later she developed severe dyskinesias and tremor, and her **chlorpromazine** levels were found to have increased by about sixfold.[2] This case was briefly mentioned in an earlier report by the same authors.[3]

The reasons are not understood but increased absorption or reduced liver metabolism of the phenothiazines are suggested.[1,2] The general clinical importance of these findings is not known, and documentation is very limited. There seem to be no other reports of adverse reactions, and the available data are insufficient to justify any general precautions. Further study is needed.

1. El-Yousef MK, Manier DH. Estrogen effects on phenothiazine derivative blood levels. *JAMA* (1974) 228, 827–8.
2. Chetty M, Miller R. Oral contraceptives increase the plasma concentrations of chlorpromazine. *Ther Drug Monit* (2001) 23, 556–8.
3. Chetty M, Miller R, Moodley SV. Smoking and body weight influence the clearance of chlorpromazine. *Eur J Clin Pharmacol* (1994) 46, 523–6.

Phenothiazines + Trazodone

Undesirable hypotension occurred in two patients on chlorpromazine or trifluoperazine given trazodone. Thioridazine causes a moderate rise in trazodone plasma levels.

Clinical evidence, mechanism, importance and management

A depressed patient on **chlorpromazine** began to complain of dizziness and unstable gait within 2 weeks of starting to take trazodone 100 mg one to three times daily. His blood pressure had fallen to between 92/58 and 126/72 mmHg. Within 2 days of stopping the trazodone his blood pressure had restabilised.[1]

A patient on **trifluoperazine** was given trazodone 100 mg daily and within 2 days she complained of dizziness and was found to have a blood pressure of 86/52 mmHg. Within a day of stopping the trazodone her blood pressure was back to 100/65 mmHg.[1]

It would seem that the hypotensive adverse effects of the two drugs can be additive. Patients given phenothiazines and trazodone should be monitored for signs of excessive hypotension.

A study, undertaken to confirm the involvement of the cytochrome P450 isoenzyme CYP2D6 in the metabolism of trazodone, found that when 11 depressed patients were given trazodone 150 to 300 mg at bedtime for 18 weeks, and then additionally **thioridazine** 20 mg twice daily for a week, the plasma levels of the trazodone and its active metabolite (*m*-chlorophenylpiperazine) rose by 36% and 54% respectively.[2] No adverse reactions were described and there would seem to be no reason for avoiding concurrent use.

1. Asayesh K. Combination of trazodone and phenothiazines: a possible additive hypotensive effect. *Can J Psychiatry* (1986) 31, 857–8.
2. Yasui N, Otani K, Kaneko S, Ohkubo T, Osanai T, Ishida M, Mihara K, Kondo T, Sugawara K, Fukushima Y. Inhibition of trazodone metabolism by thioridazine in humans. *Ther Drug Monit* (1995) 17, 333–5.

Phenothiazines + Tricyclic antidepressants

Concurrent treatment with tricyclic antidepressants and phenothiazines is common, but the tricyclic levels are increased by many of the phenothiazines, and the levels of some phenothiazines are also increased by the tricyclics. It has been suggested that concurrent use might contribute to an increased incidence of tardive dyskinesia. Nevertheless, fixed-dose combined preparations are available. Tricyclics have also been shown to reverse the therapeutic effects of chlorpromazine.

Clinical evidence

(a) Effect of phenothiazines on tricyclic antidepressants

An extended study of 4 patients given intramuscular **fluphenazine decanoate** 12.5 mg weekly, with benzatropine 2 mg three times daily and **imipramine** 300 mg daily, found that the mean combined plasma concentrations of **imipramine** and its metabolite, desipramine, were 850 nanograms/ml. This appeared high when compared with 60 other patients who were taking **imipramine** 225 mg daily and had levels of 180 nanograms/ml.[1]

A comparative study of 99 patients taking **amitriptyline** or **nortriptyline** alone, and 60 other patients additionally taking an average of **perphenazine** 10 mg daily, found that although the tricyclic antidepressant dosage levels were the same, the plasma tricyclic antidepressant levels of the **perphenazine** group were up to 70% higher.[2]

Other studies have described increased tricyclic antidepressant levels with phenothiazines. There is currently evidence for this interaction between:

- **imipramine**,[3-5] and **chlorpromazine**
- **nortriptyline**,[6] and **levomepromazine**
- **amitriptyline**,[7] **imipramine**,[5,8] **desipramine**[9] or **nortriptyline**[6,10,11] and **perphenazine**
- **desipramine**,[12] **imipramine**[13] or **nortriptyline**,[6] and **thioridazine**

However, other studies have found no interaction between:

- **amitriptyline**[6,10,14] or **nortriptyline**[15] and **perphenazine**
- **amitriptyline**[6] and **thioridazine**
- **amitriptyline**[6] and **levomepromazine**
- **amitriptyline**,[10] or **nortriptyline**[10] and **zuclopenthixol**.

It should be noted that in the case of **amitriptyline**, although the levels were not affected, levels of nortriptyline, its metabolite, were raised.[6]

(b) Effect of tricyclic antidepressant on phenothiazines

In a controlled study in 8 schizophrenic patients taking **butaperazine** 20 mg daily, 6 of them on **desipramine** 150 mg or more daily had a rise in serum **butaperazine** levels of between 50 and 300%. The other 2 patients, taking **desipramine** 100 mg or less, showed no changes.[16] Other studies have found a rise in phenothiazine levels when tricyclic antidepressants are added. So far, interactions with **chlorpromazine** and **amitriptyline**,[17] **imipramine**[17] or **nortriptyline**[18] have been documented.

One study in 7 chronic schizophrenics also reported that giving **nortriptyline** 50 mg three times daily to patients taking **chlorpromazine** 100 mg three times daily resulted in profound worsening of the clinical state, with marked increases in agitation and tension, despite the fact the **chlorpromazine** levels were actually raised. The **nortriptyline** was withdrawn.[18] A temporary reversion to a disruptive behaviour pattern has been seen in other patients on **chlorpromazine** when given **amitriptyline**.[19]

Mechanism

The rise in the serum levels of both drugs is thought to be due to a mutual inhibition of the liver enzymes concerned with the metabolism of both drugs, which results in their accumulation.[3,4,8,16,18]

Importance and management

Established interactions, but the advantages and disadvantages of concurrent use are still the subject of debate. These two groups of drugs are widely used together in the treatment of schizophrenic patients who show depression, and for mixed anxiety and depression. A number of fixed-dose combinations have been marketed, e.g. *Triptafen*, *Etrafon*, *Triaval* (amitriptyline and perphenazine), *Motival*, *Motipress* (nortriptyline and fluphenazine). However, the safety of using both drugs together has been questioned.

One of the problems of phenothiazine treatment is the development of tardive dyskinesias, and some evidence suggests that the higher the dosage, the greater the incidence.[20] The symptoms can be transiently masked by increasing the dosage,[21] thus the presence of a tricyclic antidepressant might not only be a factor causing tardive dyskinesia to develop, but might also mask the condition, or so it has been suggested.[16,22] It has been recommended that the addition of full antidepressant doses of nortriptyline to average antipsychotic doses of chlorpromazine should be avoided because the therapeutic actions of the chlorpromazine may be reversed.[18] See also 'Antipsychotics + Anticholinergics', p.529.

Attention has also been drawn to excessive weight gain associated with several months use of amitriptyline with thioridazine for the treatment of chronic pain,[23] but note that excessive weight gain is a recognised adverse effect of the antipsychotics alone. The tricyclic antidepressants and many antipsychotics increase the QT interval, see 'Drugs that prolong the QT interval + Other drugs that prolong the QT interval', p.170 for further information.

1. Siris SG, Cooper TB, Rifkin AE, Brenner R, Lieberman JA. Plasma imipramine concentrations in patients receiving concomitant fluphenazine decanoate. *Am J Psychiatry* (1982) 139, 104–6.
2. Linnoila M, George L, Guthrie S. Interaction between antidepressants and perphenazine in psychiatric patients. *Am J Psychiatry* (1982) 139, 1329–31.
3. Gram LF, Overø KF. Drug interaction: inhibitory effect of neuroleptics on metabolism of tricyclic antidepressants in man. *BMJ* (1972) 1, 463–5.
4. Crammer JL, Rolfe B. Interaction of imipramine and chlorpromazine in man. *Psychopharmacologia* (1972) 26 (Suppl), 81.
5. Gram LF. Lægemiddelinteraktion: hæmmende virkning af neurolepltica på tricycliske antidepressivas metabolisering. *Nord Psykiatr Tidsskr* (1971) 25, 357–60.
6. Jerling M, Bertilsson L, Sjöqvist F. The use of therapeutic drug monitoring data to document kinetic drug interactions: an example with amitriptyline and nortriptyline. *Ther Drug Monit* (1994) 16, 1–12.
7. Perel JM, Stiller RL, Feldman BL, Lin FC, Narayanan S. Therapeutic drug monitoring (TDM) of the amitriptyline (AT)/perphenazine (PER) interaction in depressed patients. *Clin Chem* (1985) 31, 939–40.
8. Gram LF, Overø KF, Kirk L. Influence of neuroleptics and benzodiazepines on metabolism of tricyclic antidepressants in man. *Am J Psychiatry* (1974) 131, 863–6.
9. Nelson JC, Jatlow PI. Neuroleptic effect on desipramine steady-state plasma concentrations. *Am J Psychiatry* (1980) 137, 1232–4.
10. Linnet K. Comparison of the kinetic interactions of the neuroleptics perphenazine and zuclopenthixol with tricyclic antidepressives. *Ther Drug Monit* (1995) 17, 308–11.
11. Mulsant BH, Foglia JP, Sweet RA, Rosen J, Lo KH, Pollock BG. The effects of perphenazine on the concentration of nortriptyline and its hydroxymetabolites in older patients. *J Clin Psychopharmacol* (1997) 17, 318–21.
12. Hirschowitz J, Bennett JA, Zemlan FP, Garver DL. Thioridazine effect on desipramine plasma levels. *J Clin Psychopharmacol* (1983) 3, 376–9.
13. Maynard GL, Soni P. Thioridazine interferences with imipramine metabolism and measurement. *Ther Drug Monit* (1996) 18, 729–31.
14. Cooper SF, Dugal R, Elie R, Albert J-M. Metabolic interaction between amitriptyline and perphenazine in psychiatric patients. *Prog Neuropsychopharmacol* (1979) 3, 369–76.
15. Kragh-Sørensen P, Borgå O, Garle M, Bolvig Hansen L, Hansen CE, Hvidberg EF, Larsen N-E, Sjöqvist F. Effect of simultaneous treatment with low doses of perphenazine on plasma and urine concentrations of nortriptyline and 10-hydroxynortriptyline. *Eur J Clin Pharmacol* (1977) 11, 479–83.
16. El-Yousef MK, Manier DH. Tricyclic antidepressants and phenothiazines. *JAMA* (1974) 229, 1419.
17. Rasheed A, Javed MA, Nazir S, Khawaja O. Interaction of chlorpromazine with tricyclic antidepressants in schizophrenic patients. *J Pakistan Med Assoc* (1994) 44, 233–4.
18. Loga S, Curry S, Lader M. Interaction of chlorpromazine and nortriptyline in patients with schizophrenia. *Clin Pharmacokinet* (1981) 6, 454–62.
19. O'Connor JW. Personal communication, February 1983.
20. Crane GE. Persistent dyskinesia. *Br J Psychiatry* (1973), 122, 395–405.
21. Crane GE. Tardive dyskinesia in patients treated with major neuroleptics: a review of the literature. *Am J Psychiatry* (1968) 124 (Suppl), 40–8.
22. Ayd FJ. Pharmacokinetic interaction between tricyclic antidepressants and phenothiazine neuroleptics. *Int Drug Ther Newslett* (1974) 9, 31–2.
23. Pfister AK. Weight gain from combined phenothiazine and tricyclic therapy. *JAMA* (1978) 239, 1959.

Pimozide + Drugs that prolong the QT interval

Pimozide should not be given with other drugs that can prolong the QT interval because of the risk of potentially fatal cardiac arrhythmias.

Clinical evidence, mechanism, importance and management

Between 1971 and 1995 the UK Committee on Safety of Medicines (CSM) received a total of 40 reports (16 fatal) of serious cardiac arrhythmias in patients taking pimozide. Pimozide is contraindicated in patients with a prolonged QT interval or with a history of cardiac arrhythmias. Patients on pimozide should have an annual ECG, and if the QT interval is prolonged the treatment should be reviewed and either withdrawn or the dosage reduced under close supervision. The CSM advises the avoidance of pimozide with the following drugs and groups of drugs that can also prolong the QT interval: other **antipsychotics** (including depot preparations), **tricyclic antidepressants**, and other drugs known to prolong the QT interval such as **antimalarials**, **antiarrhythmic agents**, **astemizole**, **terfenadine**, or drugs that can cause electrolyte disturbances, especially **diuretics**.[1] See also 'Drugs that prolong the QT interval + Other drugs that prolong the QT interval', p.170.

1. Committee on Safety of Medicines. Cardiac arrhythmias with pimozide (Orap). *Current Problems* (1995) 21, 2.

Pimozide + Macrolides

Clarithromycin can increase the serum levels of pimozide, which is believed to increase its serious cardiotoxicity. The makers predict that other macrolides will interact similarly.

Clinical evidence, mechanism, importance and management

The sudden death of a patient taking pimozide and **clarithromycin** prompted a study of a possible interaction between the two drugs. Using human liver microsomes it was found that pimozide is partly metabolised by the cytochrome P450 isoenzyme CYP3A, and that 2 micromol of **clarithromycin** inhibits this enzyme by at least 80%.[1] The practical consequences of this were seen in a later study in 12 healthy subjects, which found that **clarithromycin** 500 mg twice daily for 5 days more than doubled the AUC of a single 6-mg oral dose of pimozide and raised its maximum serum levels by almost 50%. The QT_c interval was prolonged from 19 to 28 milliseconds.[2] The results were the same in both poor and extensive CYP2D6 metabolisers (see 'Genetic factors', (p.4)). The authors of this study concluded that **clarithromycin** can therefore increase the cardiotoxicity of pimozide during chronic use, irrespective of the CYP2D6 status of the patient.[2] Pimozide alone has been associated with ventricular arrhythmias, prolongation of the QT interval, T-wave changes and sudden and unexpected death, even in the young with no previous evidence of cardiac disease.[3] Due to the severity of this interaction and because the macrolides are inhibitors of CYP3A4 the UK makers contraindicate their use with pimozide,[4] whereas the US makers contraindicate pimozide with **azithromycin**, **clarithromycin**, **dirithromycin**, **erythromycin** and **troleandomycin**.[5]

1. Flockhart DA, Richard E, Woosely RL, Pearle PL, Drici M-D. A metabolic interaction between clarithromycin and pimozide may result in cardiac toxicity. *Clin Pharmacol Ther* (1996) 59, 189.
2. Desta Z, Kerbusch T, Flockhart DA. Effect of clarithromycin on the pharmacokinetics and pharmacodynamics of pimozide in healthy poor and extensive metabolizers of cytochrome P450 2D6 (CYP2D6). *Clin Pharmacol Ther* (1999) 65, 10–20.
3. Committee on Safety of Medicines. Cardiotoxic effects of pimozide. *Current Problems* (1990) 29.
4. Orap (Pimozide). Janssen-Cilag Ltd. UK Summary of product characteristics, April 2002.
5. Orap (Pimozide). Gate Pharmaceuticals. US Prescribing information, June 2004.

Prochlorperazine + Metoclopramide

A single case report describes tongue swelling and respiratory obstruction in a patient given prochlorperazine followed by metoclopramide.

Clinical evidence, mechanism, importance and management

A 19-year-old woman experienced progressive swelling of the tongue, partial upper-airways obstruction and a sensation of choking over a period of 12 hours following intramuscular doses of metoclopramide to a total of 30 mg. She had received a 12.5-mg intramuscular dose of prochlorperazine for nausea 24 hours earlier. On examination her tongue was strikingly blue, but within 15 minutes of receiving benzatropine 2 mg it returned to its normal size and colour. The respiratory distress also disappeared.[1] The reason for the reaction, suggested by the authors of the report, is that the dystonic adverse effects of both drugs were additive.[1] However, it should be noted that oedema of the tongue has also been described with metoclopramide alone.[2] Young patients, especially women, are particularly susceptible to the adverse effects of metoclopramide, and this patient received the standard total daily dose over just 12 hours, so an interaction is by no means established.

1. Alroe C, Bowen P. Metoclopramide and prochlorperazine: "the blue-tongue sign". *Med J Aust* (1989) 150, 724–5.
2. Robinson OPW. Metoclopramide—side effects and safety. *Postgrad Med J* (1973) 49 (Suppl July), 77–80.

Promazine + Attapulgite-pectin

An attapulgite-pectin antidiarrhoeal preparation caused a small reduction in the absorption of promazine in one subject.

Clinical evidence, mechanism, importance and management

A study in one healthy subject found that attapulgite-pectin reduced the absorption of a single 50-mg dose of promazine by about 25%, possibly due to adsorption of the phenothiazine onto the attapulgite.[1] The clinical importance of this interaction and whether other phenothiazines behave similarly appears not to have been studied. If a problem does occur, separating administration as much as possible (2 hours or more) to avoid admixture in the gut has been shown to minimise the effects of this type of interaction with other drugs.

1. Sorby DL, Liu G. Effects of adsorbents on drug absorption II. Effect of an antidiarrhea mixture on promazine absorption. *J Pharm Sci* (1966) 55, 504–10.

Quetiapine + Antipsychotics

Quetiapine does not appear to interact with haloperidol or risperidone. Thioridazine moderately increases quetiapine levels and a case report describes a seizure in a patient taking olanzapine and quetiapine.

Clinical evidence, mechanism, importance and management

In patients with schizophrenia or bipolar disorder given quetiapine 300 mg twice daily, **thioridazine** 200 mg twice daily reduced the steady-state quetiapine AUC, and its maximum and minimum plasma levels by about 41%, 48% and 33% respectively. It was suggested that this was due increase metabolism of quetiapine, although the mechanism for this effect was unclear.[1] These reductions are only moderate and their importance is not known, but until more information is available it would seem prudent to monitor concurrent use, being alert for the need to raise the quetiapine dosage.

Haloperidol 7.5 mg twice daily and **risperidone** 3 mg twice daily for 9 days had no significant effect on the pharmacokinetics of quetiapine 300 mg twice daily in the same study.[1] However, there is a case report describing considerable QT prolongation in a patient who took quetiapine 2 g whilst on **risperidone**. The authors consider this significant as the overdose was small, and because no QT prolongation was seen in toxicity studies of quetiapine when doses as large as 9.6 g were used,[2] although there is a single case of prolonged QTc interval associated with an overdose of 9.6 g.[3] No special precautions would therefore appear to be routinely necessary if either of these drugs and quetiapine are used concurrently.

A case report describes a seizure lasting 30 to 60 seconds in a 27-year-old woman one day after quetiapine 100 mg daily was added to treatment with **olanzapine** 15 mg daily and sertraline 100 mg daily. The seizure was attributed to an interaction between quetiapine and **olanzapine**, although it seems possible that the sertraline also may have contributed.[4]

Concurrent use need not be avoided, but this case highlights the importance of considering seizure potential when prescribing multiple antipsychotic medications.

1. Potkin SG, Thyrum PT, Alva G, Bera R, Yeh C, Arvanitis LA. The safety and pharmacokinetics of quetiapine when coadministered with haloperidol, risperidone, or thioridazine. *J Clin Psychopharmacol* (2002) 22, 121–30.
2. Beelen AP, Yeo K-TJ, Lewis LD. Asymptomatic QTc prolongation associated with quetiapine fumarate overdose in a patient being treated with risperidone. *Hum Exp Toxicol* (2001) 20, 215–19.
3. Gajwani P, Pozuelo L, Tesar GE. QT interval prolongation associated with quetiapine (Seroquel) overdose. *Psychosomatics* (2000) 41, 63–5.
4. Hedges DW, Jeppson KG. New-onset seizure associated with quetiapine and olanzapine. *Ann Pharmacother* (2002) 36, 437–9.

Quetiapine + Miscellaneous

The plasma levels of quetiapine are reduced by phenytoin and predicted to be reduced by carbamazepine, barbiturates and rifampicin. Cautionary predictive warnings have been also issued by the makers about interactions with macrolides and azoles, but no interaction occurs with cimetidine, fluoxetine, imipramine or lorazepam.

Clinical evidence, mechanism, importance and management

(a) Antidepressants

Fluoxetine 60 mg daily or **imipramine** 75 mg twice daily for 5 days had no clinically significant effect on the steady-state plasma levels of quetiapine 300 mg twice daily.[1] No special precautions would therefore appear to be necessary if either of these drugs and quetiapine are used concurrently.

(b) Cimetidine

Quetiapine 150 mg three times daily was given to 7 psychotic men with cimetidine 400 mg three times daily for 4 days. There were some slight alterations in the pharmacokinetics of the quetiapine, but these were within the intraindividual changes seen and so were not considered significant.[2] There would therefore appear to be no reason for avoiding concurrent use.

(c) Enzyme inducers

When 17 psychotic patients on quetiapine 250 mg three times daily were given **phenytoin** 100 mg three times daily for 10 days, the oral clearance of quetiapine was increased fivefold.[3] This increased clearance appears to occur because **phenytoin** is a specific inducer of the cytochrome P450 isoenzyme CYP3A4, which is also concerned with the metabolism of quetiapine (confirmed by *in vitro* studies). The makers of quetiapine[4] report that **carbamazepine** reduces the quetiapine AUC by 87%. They suggest that dosage adjustments [increases] may be necessary if quetiapine is given with **carbamazepine**, **phenytoin** or other enzyme inducers (such as **barbiturates** or **rifampicin**). This is a reasonable prediction but no direct clinical evidence is yet available. However, be alert for the need to use an increased quetiapine dosage in patients treated with any of these drugs.

See 'Carbamazepine + Antipsychotics', p.340 for comment on the effect of quetiapine on carbamazepine.

(d) Enzyme inhibitors

There appear to be no reported studies investigating the possible interaction between quetiapine and drugs that are specific inhibitors of the cytochrome P450 isoenzyme CYP3A4 (by which quetiapine is primarily metabolised). On theoretical grounds CYP3A4 inhibitors might be expected to raise serum quetiapine levels, thereby increasing its adverse effects. The UK makers[4] particularly mention caution with **macrolides** and **azole antifungals**, and suggest that lower quetiapine doses should be considered. The US makers say that **ketoconazole** 200 mg daily for 4 days reduced the clearance of quetiapine by 84% and caused a fourfold increase in plasma levels. They additionally advise caution with **itraconazole** and **fluconazole** and **erythromycin**.[5]

(e) Lorazepam

The pharmacokinetics and pharmacodynamic effects of a single 2-mg dose of lorazepam were studied in 10 psychotic men taking quetiapine 250 mg three times daily. It was found that the maximum serum lorazepam levels were not significantly changed by quetiapine, and the alterations in the performance of a number of psychometric tests were small and considered not to be clinically relevant.[6]

1. Potkin SG, Thyrum PT, Alva G, Carreon D, Yeh C, Kalali A, Arvanitis LA. Effect of fluoxetine and imipramine on the pharmacokinetics and tolerability of the antipsychotic quetiapine. *J Clin Psychopharmacol* (2002) 22, 174–82.
2. Strakowski SM, Keck PE, Wong YWJ, Thyrum PT, Yeh C. The effect of multiple doses of cimetidine on the steady-state pharmacokinetics of quetiapine in men with selected psychotic disorders. *J Clin Psychopharmacol* (2002) 22, 201–5.
3. Wong YWJ, Yeh C, Thyrum PT. The effects of concomitant phenytoin administration on the steady-state pharmacokinetics of quetiapine. *J Clin Psychopharmacol* (2001) 21, 89–93.
4. Seroquel (Quetiapine). AstraZeneca UK Ltd. UK Summary of product characteristics, June 2005.
5. Seroquel (Quetiapine). AstraZeneca. US Prescribing information, July 2004.
6. Potkin SG. The pharmacokinetics and pharmacodynamics of lorazepam given before and during treatment with ICI 204,636 (Seroquel) in men with selected psychotic disorders. (5077IL/0027). Zeneca Pharma. Data on file (Study 27).

Risperidone + Amitriptyline

No pharmacokinetic interaction normally occurs between risperidone and amitriptyline, but extrapyramidal reactions have been reported in one patient.

Clinical evidence, mechanism, importance and management

A study in 12 schizophrenic patients found that amitriptyline 50 to 100 mg daily had no effect on the serum levels of risperidone 3 mg twice daily.[1] However, a 26-year old man on amitriptyline 25 mg daily developed extrapyramidal reactions after his dosage of risperidone was increased from 2 to 4 mg daily.[2] On another occasion extrapyramidal adverse effects developed after risperidone 2 mg daily was added to treatment with amitriptyline 25 mg and fluoxetine 20 mg daily.[2] Both pharmacokinetic and pharmacodynamic reasons for this reaction have been suggested.[3] The cases illustrate that there is the potential for an adverse interaction between these drugs , which should be borne in mind when prescribing both drugs.

1. Sommers DK, Snyman JR, van Wyk M, Blom MW, Huang ML, Levron JC. Lack of effect of amitriptyline on risperidone pharmacokinetics in schizophrenic patients. *Int Clin Psychopharmacol* (1997) 12, 141–5.
2. Brown ES. Extrapyramidal side effects with low-dose risperidone. *Can J Psychiatry* (1997) 42, 325–6.
3. Caley CF. Extrapyramidal reactions from concurrent SSRI and atypical antipsychotic use. *Can J Psychiatry* (1998) 43, 307–8.

Risperidone + Anticholinesterases; Centrally acting

No pharmacokinetic interaction appears to occur between risperidone and donepezil or galantamine, but extrapyramidal symptoms occurred in one patient given donepezil and risperidone.

Clinical evidence, mechanism importance and management

(a) Donepezil

In a randomised crossover study 24 healthy subjects were given risperidone 500 micrograms twice daily with donepezil 5 mg daily. Although donepezil caused slight changes in the levels of risperidone and 9-hydroxyrisperidone they did not exceed the limits for bioequivalence. Concurrent use did not increase adverse effects.[1] In one study 16 schizophrenic patients on risperidone were given donepezil 5 mg daily for 7 days without any alteration in their risperidone and 9-hydroxyrisperidone levels. The pharmacokinetics of donepezil were similar in the risperidone-treated patients and healthy controls taking donepezil alone.[2]

However, a case report describes the emergence of parkinsonian symptoms in an 80-year-old woman after she was given donepezil 5 mg daily and, after 12 days, risperidone 1 mg daily. Risperidone was discontinued and she recovered without treatment.[3]

(b) Galantamine

In a randomised, crossover study 16 patients over 60-years-old were given a 14-day dose escalation of galantamine after which they were given galantamine 12 mg twice daily for 13 doses with risperidone 500 micrograms twice daily for 13 doses. Although galantamine caused slight changes in the levels of risperidone and 9-hydroxyrisperidone, their combined level (the active moiety) was unchanged. The combination was well-tolerated so no additional precautions would seem to be necessary on concurrent use.[4]

1. Zhao Q, Xie C, Pesco-Koplowitz L, Jia X, Parier J-L. Pharmacokinetic and safety assessments of concurrent administration of risperidone and donepezil. *J Clin Pharmacol* (2003) 43, 180–6.
2. Reyes JF, Preskorn SH, Khan A, Kumar D, Cullen EI, Perdomo CA, Pratt RD. Concurrent administration of donepezil HCl and risperidone in patients with schizophrenia: assessment of pharmacokinetic changes and safety following multiple oral doses. *Br J Clin Pharmacol* (2004) 58, 50–7.
3. Liu H-C, Lin S-K, Sung S-M. Extrapyramidal side-effect due to drug combination of risperidone and donepezil. *Psychiatry Clin Neurosci* (2002) 54, 479.
4. Huang F, Lasseter KC, Janssens L, Verhaeghe T, Lau H, Zhao Q. Pharmacokinetic and safety assessments of galantamine and risperidone after the two drugs are administered alone and together. *J Clin Pharmacol* (2002) 42, 1341–51.

Risperidone + Anticonvulsants

Carbamazepine can greatly reduce risperidone plasma levels. There are case reports of adverse effects with risperidone and sodium valproate, but they do not seem to be of general importance.

Clinical evidence, mechanism, importance and management

(a) Carbamazepine

A 22-year-old man taking risperidone 4 mg daily and carbamazepine 600 mg daily for schizophrenia had lower than expected risperidone levels, so his dose was doubled and the carbamazepine tailed off. Ten days after carbamazepine had been discontinued it was noted that his plasma 9-hydroxyrisperidone level was 49 micrograms/l; it had only been 19 micrograms/l when he was taking carbamazepine.[1] There are 4 other cases of this interaction between risperidone and carbamazepine.[2-4] In one case, the addition of carbamazepine to established risperidone treatment resulted in a fall in the risperidone and 9-hydroxyrisperidone levels of about 75% and 65% respectively, accompanied by the return of the patients psychotic symptoms.[4] In 2 other cases, a 20-year-old and an 81-year-old man developed parkinsonian symptoms when carbamazepine was stopped. The symptoms resolved when the doses of risperidone were reduced by about two-thirds.[2]

These cases are supported by a study in 5 patients on carbamazepine and risperidone for schizophrenia or bipolar disorders. The dose-normalised plasma level of risperidone and its active metabolite, 9-hydroxyrisperidone were 1.4 and 6.2 nanomol/l.mg with carbamazepine, compared to 4.4 and 17.3 nanomol/l.mg without carbamazepine.[5] Another study in 11 patients who had been taking risperidone for 2 to 68 weeks found that carbamazepine 200 mg twice daily for a week approximately halved the plasma levels of risperidone and its active moiety (risperidone plus 9-hydroxyrisperidone).[6]

Carbamazepine is a known potent enzyme inducer, which appears to increase the metabolism of risperidone by the cytochrome P450 isoenzyme CYP2D6 (although other isoenzymes may play a part). The extent of the interaction appears to be related to CYP2D6 genotype (see 'Genetic factors', (p.4)).

It would now seem important to monitor the levels of risperidone and 9-hydroxyrisperidone in patients given carbamazepine, being alert for the need to raise the risperidone dosage, possibly by as much as two-thirds.

For mention that risperidone may moderately increase carbamazepine levels see 'Carbamazepine + Antipsychotics', p.340.

(b) Sodium valproate

A study comparing 10 patients on sodium valproate and risperidone with 23 patients on risperidone alone found no significant difference between the two groups, suggesting that sodium valproate and risperidone can be safely used together.[5] However, the valproate levels of a 10-year-old boy increased from 143 to 191 mg/l 5 days after he started to take risperidone (initially 2 mg daily, then later 3 mg daily). This was attributed to an interaction, the exact mechanism of which is unclear.[7] Another case report describes the development of generalised acute oedema in a schizophrenic patient when risperidone (titrated to 10 mg daily) was added to established sodium valproate treatment. The oedema was unresponsive to diuretics, but resolved when the risperidone dose was reduced to 2 mg. When the risperidone dose was later increased to 8 mg the oedema reappeared, so the risperidone was withdrawn.[8] No special precautions seem necessary on concurrent use, but it is worth bearing this case in mind when these two drugs are used together.

1. de Leon J, Bork J. Risperidone and cytochrome P450 3A. *J Clin Psychiatry* (1997) 58, 450.
2. Takahashi H, Yoshida K, Higuchi H, Shimizu T. Development of parkinsonian symptoms after discontinuation of carbamazepine in patients concurrently treated with risperidone: two case reports. *Clin Neuropharmacol* (2001) 24, 358–60.
3. Alfaro CL, Nicolson R, Lenane M, Rapoport JL. Carbamazepine and/or fluvoxamine drug interaction with risperidone in a patient on multiple psychotropic medications. *Ann Pharmacother* (2000) 34, 122–3.
4. Spina E, Scordo MG, Avenoso A, Perucca E. Adverse drug interaction between risperidone and carbamazepine in a patient with chronic schizophrenia and deficient CYP2D6 activity. *J Clin Psychopharmacol* (2001) 21, 108–9.
5. Spina E, Avenoso A, Facciolà G, Salemi M, Scordo MG, Giacobello T, Madia AG, Perucca E. Plasma concentrations of risperidone and 9-hydroxyrisperidone: effect of comedication with carbamazepine or valproate. *Ther Drug Monit* (2000) 22, 481–5.
6. Ono S, Mihara K, Suzuki A, Kondo T, Yasui-Furukori N, Furukori H, de Vries R, Kaneko S. Significant pharmacokinetic interaction between risperidone and carbamazepine: its relationship with CYP2D6 genotypes. *Psychopharmacology (Berl)* (2002) 162, 50–54.
7. van Wattum PJ. Valproic acid and risperidone. *J Am Acad Child Adolesc Psychiatry* (2001) 40, 866–7.
8. Sanders RD, Lehrer DS. Edema associated with addition of risperidone to valproate treatment. *J Clin Psychiatry* (1998) 59, 689–90.

Risperidone + Protease inhibitors

The neuroleptic malignant syndrome occurred in one patient and extrapyramidal adverse effects in another given risperidone with indinavir and ritonavir.

Clinical evidence, mechanism importance and management

A 35-year-old man with AIDS was diagnosed with a Tourette's-like disorder and started on risperidone 1 mg twice daily. After 2 weeks the risperidone was increased to 2 mg twice daily and he was started on **indinavir** 800 mg twice daily with **ritonavir** 200 mg twice daily. He discontinued the antiretrovirals after 5 days due to nausea, but started them again 1 month later when the tic disorder had improved. After 1 week he became short of breath and fatigued with worsening tremor and other extrapyramidal adverse effects. The antiretrovirals were stopped and the risperidone dose increased to 3 mg twice daily. Over the next 3 days his symptoms worsened and began to interfere with daily living. Risperidone was discontinued and clonazepam started, and his symptoms resolved.[1] Another patient developed neuroleptic malignant syndrome 3 days after starting to take risperidone with **indinavir** and **ritonavir**. This patient also recovered when the risperidone was stopped.[2]

Indinavir inhibits the cytochrome P450 isoenzyme CYP3A4 and **ritonavir** inhibits CYP2D6 and CYP3A4, which are the main enzymes involved in the metabolism of risperidone. The extrapyramidal symptoms and the neuroleptic malignant syndrome in the two patients may have been due to increased levels of risperidone caused by inhibition of its metabolism by **indinavir** and **ritonavir**.[1]

These appear to be the only reports of an interaction between risperidone and protease inhibitors, and their general significance is unclear. Until more is known it would be prudent to monitor patients on risperidone who are given these protease inhibitors for risperidone adverse effects.

1. Kelly DV, Béïque LC, Bowmer MI. Extrapyramidal symptoms with ritonavir/indinavir plus risperidone. *Ann Pharmacother* (2002) 36, 827–30.
2. Lee SI, Klesmer J, Hirsch BE. Neuroleptic malignant syndrome associated with the use of risperidone, ritonavir and indinavir: a case report. *Psychosomatics* (2000) 41, 453–4.

Risperidone + Reboxetine

No clinically relevant pharmacokinetic interaction appears to occur between risperidone and reboxetine.

Clinical evidence, mechanism, importance and management

Reboxetine 8 mg daily was given to 7 schizophrenic patients stabilised on risperidone 8 mg daily for a period of 3 weeks. Reboxetine had no significant effects on the pharmacokinetics of either risperidone or its active metabolite 9-hydroxyrisperidone, suggesting that no additional precautions are necessary if reboxetine and risperidone are used together.[1]

1. Spina E, Avenoso A, Scordo MG, Ancione M, Madia A, Levita A. No effect of reboxetine on plasma concentrations of clozapine, risperidone, and their active metabolites. *Ther Drug Monit* (2001) 23, 675–8.

Risperidone + SSRIs

Fluvoxamine, fluoxetine and paroxetine appear to raise risperidone levels. The combination of SSRIs and risperidone is generally useful, but has resulted in a number of adverse effects including priapism, extrapyramidal effects and the serotonin syndrome.

Clinical evidence

(a) Citalopram

A study in 7 patients found that citalopram had no effect on the plasma levels of risperidone or its active metabolite 9-hydroxyrisperidone.[1] A 29-year-old man with idiopathic priapism, about one 4-hour erection every 1 to 2 months, which typically woke him up, began to experience much longer bouts lasting 6 to 8 hours when he was given risperidone 4 mg daily. Within about 4 weeks of adding citalopram 40 mg daily to a slightly reduced risperidone dose (3 mg daily), he began to have almost daily erections lasting 12 hours. Three days after his dosages were changed to risperidone 3 mg twice daily plus citalopram 20 mg daily he had an episode of such persistent priapism that emergency detumescence was needed. When both drugs were stopped he improved markedly and then only had occasional 4-hour erections as before.[2]

(b) Fluoxetine

A pharmacokinetic study in 10 psychotic patients found that fluoxetine 20 mg daily raised the levels of risperidone 2 or 3 mg twice daily from 12 to 19 nanograms/ml after 3 weeks and to 56 nanograms/ml after 4 weeks. All patients experienced a rise in risperidone levels, but this varied from two to tenfold. One patient withdrew from the study because of severe akathisia and another two patients needed treatment with biperiden to control parkinsonian adverse effects.[3] Similar finding were found in another study.[4]

A 30-year-old woman taking valproate, clonazepam, and risperidone 3 mg daily for schizophrenia was also given fluoxetine 5 mg daily for a depressive disorder. The depression improved, but she noticed painful bilateral breast enlargement, which resolved when risperidone was stopped. Similar symptoms were noted when the risperidone was later restarted.[5]

An 18-year old developed extrapyramidal adverse effects, and later persistent dyskinetic tongue movements when given fluoxetine and risperidone,[6] and a 46-year-old man on risperidone 2 mg daily developed urinary retention, extrapyramidal adverse effects, sedation and constipation, which developed over 10 days after fluoxetine 20 mg daily was started.[7]

(c) Fluvoxamine

A 24-year-old woman taking risperidone 3 mg twice daily developed fever, limb rigidity, confusion 3 days after starting fluvoxamine 50 mg daily. She required ventilation after her condition worsened and was eventually diagnosed as having either the serotonin syndrome or neuroleptic malignant syndrome. Both drugs were stopped and her condition resolved. She was later successfully treated with fluvoxamine 100 mg twice daily.[8]

(d) Paroxetine

Paroxetine 20 mg daily was given to 10 patients stabilised on risperidone 2 to 4 mg twice daily. After 4 weeks treatment paroxetine had increased the levels of risperidone and its active metabolite, 9-hydroxyrisperidone, by 45%. Although the combination was generally well-tolerated one patient developed parkinsonian adverse effects.[9]

A case report describes two elderly patients taking paroxetine who developed the serotonin syndrome within a couple of days of a risperidone dose increase. One patient had recently been changed from venlafaxine to paroxetine, which may have contributed to the reaction[10] (see 'Venlafaxine + SSRIs', p.1008).

Mechanism

Fluoxetine and paroxetine inhibit the cytochrome P450 isoenzyme CYP2D6 by which risperidone is metabolised, hence risperidone levels rise. This can lead to extrapyramidal adverse effects and, it has been suggested, the increased prolactin levels and gynaecomastia seen in one patient.[5]

Many of the other reactions (sedation, urinary retention, priapism) appear to be a result of additive adverse effects of the SSRIs and risperidone. The serotonin syndrome can result when two drugs with serotonin effects are given together, see 'Additive or synergistic interactions', (p.9).

Importance and management

The elevated risperidone levels seen with fluoxetine and paroxetine appear to be well-documented and clinically significant. The makers of risperidone[11,12] say that when adding either of these SSRIs the risperidone dose should be re-evaluated (presumably decreased). A one-third reduction in the risperidone dose has been suggested with fluoxetine.[4] The case reports of the serotonin syndrome appear to be rare, but they should be borne in mind when prescribing SSRIs and risperidone.

1. Avenoso A, Facciolà G, Scordo MG, Gitto C, Ferrante GD, Madia AG, Spina E. No effect of citalopram on plasma levels of clozapine, risperidone and their active metabolites in patients with chronic schizophrenia. *Clin Drug Invest* (1998) 16, 393–8.
2. Freudenreich O. Exacerbation of idiopathic priapism with risperidone-citalopram combination. *J Clin Psychiatry* (2002) 63, 249–50.
3. Spina E, Avenoso A, Scordo MG, Ancione M, Madia A, Gatti G, Perucca E. Inhibition of risperidone metabolism by fluoxetine in patients with schizophrenia: a clinically relevant pharmacokinetic interaction. *J Clin Psychopharmacol* (2002) 22, 419–23.
4. Bondolfi G, Eap CB, Bertschy G, Zullino D, Vermeulen A, Baumann P. The effect of fluoxetine on the pharmacokinetics and safety of risperidone in psychotic patients. *Pharmacopsychiatry* (2002) 35, 50–56.
5. Benazzi F. Gynecomastia with risperidone-fluoxetine combination. *Pharmacopsychiatry* (1999) 32, 41.
6. Daniel DG, Egan M, Hyde T. Probable neuroleptic induced tardive dyskinesia in association with combined SSRI and risperidone treatment. *Schizophr Res* (1996) 18, 149.
7. Bozikas V, Petrikis P, Karavatos A. Urinary retention caused after fluoxetine-risperidone combination. *J Psychopharmacol* (2001) 15, 142–3.
8. Reeves RR, Mack JE, Bedingfield JJ. Neurotoxic syndrome associated with risperidone and fluvoxamine. *Ann Pharmacother* (2002) 36, 440–3.
9. Spina E, Avenoso A, Facciolà G, Scordo MG, Ancione M, Madia AG. Plasma concentrations of risperidone and 9-hydroxyrisperidone during combined treatment with paroxetine. *Ther Drug Monit* (2001) 23, 223–7.
10. Karki SD, Masood G-R. Combination risperidone and SSRI-induced serotonin syndrome. *Ann Pharmacother* (2003) 37, 388–91.
11. Risperdal (Risperidone). Janssen-Cilag Ltd. UK Summary of product characteristics, March 2005.
12. Risperdal (Risperidone). Janssen Pharmaceutica Products. US Prescribing information, February 2005.

Risperidone + Venlafaxine

No clinically relevant pharmacokinetic interaction appears to occur between risperidone and venlafaxine.

Clinical evidence, mechanism, importance and management

Steady-state venlafaxine 75 mg every 12-hours was found to increase the AUC of a single 1-mg oral dose of risperidone by about 32%, but the pharmacokinetic profile of the risperidone plus its active metabolite (9-hydroxyrisperidone) was not significantly changed, nor were any adverse events seen.[1] There would seem to be no reason for avoiding concurrent use.

1. Amchin J, Zarycranski W, Taylor KP, Albano D, Klockowski PM. Effect of venlafaxine on the pharmacokinetics of risperidone. *J Clin Pharmacol* (1999) 39, 297–309.

Ritanserin + Miscellaneous

Ritanserin does not interact with alcohol, cimetidine or ranitidine.

Clinical evidence, mechanism, importance and management

A study in 20 healthy subjects given ritanserin 10 mg with and without **alcohol** 0.5 g/kg found no pharmacokinetic or pharmacodynamic interactions between these drugs.[1] **Cimetidine** 800 mg daily or **ranitidine** 300 mg daily given to 9 healthy subjects for 11 days caused only small changes in the pharmacokinetics of a single 10-mg dose of ritanserin given on day 3. These changes were attributed to altered absorption,[2] but were of little or no clinical significance.

1. Estevez F, Parrillo S, Giusti M, Monti JM. Single-dose ritanserin and alcohol in healthy volunteers: a placebo-controlled trial. *Alcohol* (1995) 12, 541–5.
2. Trenk D, Seiler K-U, Buschmann M, Szathmary S, Benn H-P, Jähnchen E. Effect of concomitantly administered cimetidine or ranitidine on the pharmacokinetics of the 5-HT_2-receptor antagonist ritanserin. *J Clin Pharmacol* (1993) 33, 330–4.

Sertindole + Miscellaneous

The makers of sertindole contraindicate the concurrent use of cimetidine, diltiazem, erythromycin, itraconazole, ketoconazole, terfenadine and verapamil because of an increased risk of cardiac arrhythmias. Carbamazepine and phenytoin reduce plasma sertindole levels whereas fluoxetine and paroxetine increase them. No clinically relevant interactions occur with alprazolam, antacids, food or tobacco smoking.

Clinical evidence, mechanism, importance and management

(a) Antacids, Food

A **standardised breakfast** or ***Maalox*** 45 ml had no significant effect on the AUC of a single 4-mg dose of sertindole in 16 healthy subjects, and only minor and unimportant changes occurred in maximum serum levels and in the time to achieve them.[1,2] No special precautions are needed if sertindole is given with **food** or ***Maalox***.

(b) Anticonvulsants

The metabolism of sertindole is markedly increased by enzyme inducers such as **phenytoin** and **carbamazepine** and plasma sertindole levels may be reduced 2 to 3-fold. The makers therefore say that the daily dosage of sertindole may need to be increased towards the upper end of the maximum dosage range to accommodate this interaction.[3,4]

(c) Antifungals

No formal studies have been carried out on the use of sertindole with either **itraconazole** or **ketoconazole**, but because both of these antifungals are potent inhibitors of CYP3A it is expected that a marked rise in serum sertindole levels may occur. The makers therefore say that concurrent use is contraindicated[3] because elevated serum levels are associated with a prolongation of the QTc interval and an increased risk of cardiac arrhythmias.

(d) Benzodiazepines

A pharmacokinetic study in 14 healthy subjects found only minor changes in pharmacokinetics of a single 1-mg dose of **alprazolam** due to the presence of sertindole 12 mg daily. The changes were considered to be clinically unimportant.[5]

(e) Calcium channel blockers

Studies in patients found that **diltiazem**, **nifedipine** or **verapamil** resulted in a 20% reduction in the sertindole clearance, attributed to inhibition of CYP3A metabolism.[4] The makers contraindicate concurrent use (**diltiazem** and **verapamil** are specifically named) as raised sertindole levels may prolong the QT interval.[3]

(f) Cimetidine

Because cimetidine is a potent inhibitor of the cytochrome P450 isoenzyme CYP3A it is expected that sertindole levels may be increased. The makers therefore contraindicate concurrent use,[3] see (g) below.

(g) Drugs affecting the QTc interval

Sertindole increases the QTc interval in a small proportion of patients. The makers found in clinical trials that 24 out of a total of 1446 patients (1.66%) showed increases ranging from 500 to 581 milliseconds. The mean increase was 21 milliseconds.[6] The importance of these increases is that they may lead to the development of potentially life-threatening ventricular arrhythmias (torsade de pointes) and the makers therefore recommend that ECGs should be taken before and during treatment, and that if the QT_c interval exceeds 520 milliseconds the sertindole should be stopped. In the context of adverse interactions there is the potential risk that other drugs that also increase the QTc interval may have an additive effect. See 'Drugs that prolong the QT interval + Other drugs that prolong the QT interval', p.170.

(h) Erythromycin

A single 4-mg dose of sertindole was given to 10 healthy subjects before and after a course of erythromycin 250 mg every 6 hours for 10 days. The mean maximum serum levels were increased by 15%, probably because erythromycin inhibits the cytochrome P450 isoenzyme CYP3A4, but this was not considered to be clinically significant. The incidence of adverse events also rose (diarrhoea, abdominal pain, dizziness) but no ECG changes were seen.[7,8] Nevertheless the makers contraindicate erythromycin because raised sertindole levels may prolong the QT interval.[3] Also note that intravenous erythromycin is itself associated with prolongation of the QT interval.

(i) SSRIs

Fluoxetine and **paroxetine** are inhibitors of the cytochrome P450 isoenzyme CYP2D6. Concurrent use results in a 2- to 3-fold increase in sertindole plasma levels. The makers advise that low maintenance doses of sertindole may be needed and recommend close ECG monitoring when doses are adjusted[3] An isolated case report describes a man with paranoid psychosis and unipolar depression whose condition unexpectedly seriously worsened when **paroxetine** was stopped while continuing to take sertindole.[9]

(j) Terfenadine

A single 120-mg dose of terfenadine was given to 14 healthy subjects who had taken sertindole 20 mg daily for 5 days. The pharmacokinetics of neither drug was significantly changed, nor that of the metabolite of terfenadine (carboxyterfenadine), although it was concluded that sertindole may be a modest inhibitor of the first pass metabolism of terfenadine.[10,11] However, it was found that the combination caused an additive increase of 49 milliseconds in the QTc interval and therefore these two drugs are contraindicated by the maker.[3]

(k) Tobacco smoking

The clearance of sertindole is increased by tobacco smoking (probably because of the induction of the cytochrome P450 isoenzyme CYP3A) but no sertraline dosage alteration is thought necessary.[4]

1. Granneman GR, Wozniak P, Ereshefsky L, Silber C, Mack R. Effect of food and antacid on the bioavailability of sertindole (M94–164). Poster presentation at the American College of Neuropsychopharmacology Annual Meeting, San Juan, Puerto Rico, December 1996.
2. Wong S, Linnen P, Mack R, Granneman GR. Effects of food, antacid, and dosage form on the pharmacokinetics and relative bioavailability of sertindole in healthy volunteers. *Biopharm Drug Dispos* (1997) 18, 533–41.
3. Serdolect (Sertindole). Lundbeck Ltd. UK Summary of product characteristics, June 2003.
4. Granneman GR, Wozniak P, Ereshefsky L, Silber C, Mack R. Population pharmacokinetics of sertindole during long-term treatment of patients with schizophrenia. Poster presentation at the American College of Neuropsychopharmacology Annual Meeting, San Juan, Puerto Rico, December 1996.
5. Wong SL, Locke C, Staser J, Granneman GR. Lack of multiple dosing effect of sertindole on the pharmacokinetics of alprazolam in healthy volunteers. *Psychopharmacology (Berl)* (1998) 135, 236–41.
6. Lundbeck Ltd, Personal communications, July and August 1997.
7. Granneman GR, Wozniak P, Ereshefsky L, Silber C, Mack R. Effect of erythromycin on the pharmacokinetics of sertindole (M94–145). Poster presentation at the American College of Neuropsychopharmacology Annual Meeting, San Juan, Puerto Rico, December 1996.
8. Wong SL, Cao G, Mack RJ, Granneman GR. The effect of erythromycin on the CYP3A component of sertindole clearance in healthy volunteers. *J Clin Pharmacol* (1997) 37, 1056–61.
9. Walker-Kinnear M, McnNaughton S. Paroxetine discontinuation syndrome in association with sertindole therapy. *Br J Psychiatry* (1997) 170, 389.
10. Granneman GR, Wozniak P, Ereshefsky L, Silber C, Mack R. Effect of sertindole on the pharmacokinetics of terfenadine (M94–146). Poster presentation at the American College of Neuropsychopharmacology Annual Meeting, San Juan, Puerto Rico, December 1996.
11. Wong SL, Cao G, Mack R, Granneman GR. Lack of CYP3A inhibition effects of sertindole on terfenadine in healthy volunteers. *Int J Clin Pharmacol Ther* (1998) 36, 146–51.

Thioridazine + Naltrexone

Extreme lethargy occurred in two patients on thioridazine when they were given naltrexone.

Clinical evidence, mechanism, importance and management

Two schizophrenic patients stabilised on thioridazine 50 to 200 mg three times daily for at least one year took part in a pilot project to assess the efficacy of naltrexone for the treatment of tardive dyskinesia. Both tolerated the first challenge dose of intravenous naltrexone 800 micrograms without problems but experienced extreme lethargy and slept almost continuously after the second naltrexone dose of 50 to 100 mg orally. The severe lethargy resolved within 12 hours of stopping the naltrexone.[1] The reasons for this reaction are not understood. Information seems to be limited to this report and the general importance of this interaction is unknown. There seems to be nothing documented about other phenothiazines.

1. Maany I, O'Brien CP, Woody G. Interaction between thioridazine and naltrexone. *Am J Psychiatry* (1987) 144, 966.

Thioridazine + Phenylpropanolamine

A single case report describes fatal ventricular fibrillation attributed to the use of thioridazine with phenylpropanolamine.

Clinical evidence, mechanism, importance and management

A 27-year-old schizophrenic woman who was taking thioridazine 100 mg daily and procyclidine 2.5 mg twice daily was found dead in bed 2 hours after taking a single capsule of *Contac C* (phenylpropanolamine 50 mg with chlorphenamine 4 mg). The principal cause of death was attributed to ventricular fibrillation.[1] Just why this happened is not understood but it is suggested that it may have been due to the combined effects of the thioridazine (known to be cardiotoxic and to cause T-wave abnormalities) and the phenylpropanolamine (possibly able to cause ventricular arrhythmias).

The general importance of this alleged interaction is uncertain but the authors of the report suggest that ephedrine-like agents such as phenylpropanolamine should not be given to patients on thioridazine or **mesoridazine**.

1. Chouinard G, Ghadirian AM, Jones BD. Death attributed to ventricular arrhythmia induced by thioridazine in combination with a single Contac C capsule. *Can Med Assoc J* (1978) 119, 729–31.

Tiotixene + Enzyme inhibitors

A group of patients taking enzyme inhibitors (cimetidine, doxepin, isoniazid, nortriptyline, propranolol) had a tiotixene clearance of 9.51 l/minute, which was 71% less than patients on tiotixene alone.[1] It seems possible that the tiotixene dose will need to be reduced in those taking these drugs but this needs confirmation. Monitor concurrent use for tiotixene adverse effects and adjust the dose accordingly.

1. Ereshefsky L, Saklad SR, Watanabe MD, Davis CM, Jann MW. Thiothixene pharmacokinetic interactions: a study of hepatic enzyme inducers, clearance inhibitors, and demographic variables. *J Clin Psychopharmacol* (1991) 11, 296–301.

Ziprasidone + Carbamazepine

Ziprasidone appears not interact to a clinically relevant extent with low doses of carbamazepine.

Clinical evidence, mechanism importance and management

In a randomised, parallel study, healthy subjects were given ziprasidone 20 mg twice daily with either placebo (10 subjects), or carbamazepine 200 mg twice daily for 2.5 days (9 subjects). It was found that the 12-hour AUC and maximum serum levels of the ziprasidone were reduced by 36% and 27% respectively in the carbamazepine group. It was concluded that while induction of the cytochrome P450 isoenzyme CYP3A4 by carbamazepine is responsible for this modest reduction in the steady-state levels of ziprasidone, the extent is not clinically relevant.[1] No special precautions would seem to be needed with this dosage of carbamazepine,[1] but there is the possibility that higher doses may interact to a greater extent.

1. Miceli JJ, Anziano RJ, Robarge L, Hansen RA. Laurent A. The effect of carbamazepine on the steady-state pharmacokinetics of ziprasidone in healthy volunteers. *Br J Clin Pharmacol* (2000) 49 (Suppl 1), 65S–70S.

Ziprasidone + Ketoconazole

Ziprasidone does not appear to interact with ketoconazole to a clinically relevant extent.

Clinical evidence, mechanism importance and management

In a randomised, placebo-controlled, crossover study, 14 healthy subjects were given a 40-mg dose of ziprasidone before and after taking ketoconazole 400 mg daily for 6 days. It was found that ketoconazole increased the AUC and maximum serum levels of ziprasidone by 33% and 34% respectively.

The modest rise in levels probably occurs because ketoconazole inhibits the cytochrome P450 isoenzyme CYP3A4 by which ziprasidone is metabolised. However, it was concluded that the increase is not clinically relevant.[1] No special precautions would therefore seem to be needed on concurrent use.

1. Miceli JJ, Smith M, Robarge L, Morse T, Laurent A. The effects of ketoconazole on ziprasidone pharmacokinetics – a placebo-controlled crossover study in healthy volunteers. *Br J Clin Pharmacol* (2000) 49 (Suppl 1), 71S–76S.

Ziprasidone + Miscellaneous

The makers warn of the possible risks of giving ziprasidone with drugs that prolong the QT interval, and of the possible antagonism which may occur with levodopa and other dopamine agonists. Ziprasidone appears not interact to a clinically relevant extent with an aluminium/magnesium hydroxide antacid, benzatropine, cimetidine, lorazepam, propranolol or tobacco smoking.

Clinical evidence, mechanism importance and management

(a) Antacids or Cimetidine

Single 40-mg oral doses of ziprasidone were given to 10 healthy subjects either alone, with cimetidine 800 mg daily for 2 days, or with three 30-ml doses of *Maalox* (**aluminium/magnesium hydroxide**). The only change in the pharmacokinetics of ziprasidone was a 6% increase in the AUC with cimetidine. It was concluded that no special precautions are needed if either of these drugs and ziprasidone are given concurrently, and that any inhibition of cytochrome P450 isoenzyme CYP3A4 is irrelevant because alternative metabolic pathways are available. The results of the study with cimetidine also suggest that other non-specific inhibitors of cytochrome P450 are unlikely to alter the ziprasidone pharmacokinetics.[1]

(b) Drugs that prolong the QT interval

Trials in healthy subjects found that ziprasidone 160 mg increased the QTc interval by about 10 milliseconds. While only a relatively moderate increase in the QT interval actually occurs with ziprasidone, because of the possibility of additive effects with some other drugs (and the attendant risk of torsade de pointes), to be on the safe side the makers of ziprasidone contraindicate its use with other drugs that can prolong the QT interval.[2] A list of QT-prolonging drugs is to be found in 'Table 7.3', (p.169).

(c) Effects on the cytochrome P450 isoenzymes

In vitro studies using human liver microsomal enzymes have shown that ziprasidone has little inhibitory effects on the cytochrome P450 isoenzymes CYP1A2, CYP2C9, CYP2C19, CYP2D6 and CYP3A4,[3] and a study in healthy subjects confirmed that *in vivo* ziprasidone does not inhibit CYP2D6 (using dextromethorphan as a model drug).[4] It is therefore unlikely that ziprasidone will interact with drugs whose metabolism is primarily carried out by these isoenzymes.

(d) Levodopa and dopamine agonists

The mechanism by which ziprasidone acts to control schizophrenia is not understood, but it is known to be an antagonist of dopamine type 2 (D_2) receptors and therefore it may possibly oppose the effects of levodopa and other dopamine agonists. There seem to be no clinical reports of problems during concurrent use, but good monitoring would be advisable if ziprasidone is given with any dopamine agonist.

(e) Miscellaneous drugs

The makers say that population pharmacokinetic analysis of schizophrenic patients who were enrolled in clinical trials showed that no significant pharmacokinetic interactions occurred with **benzatropine**, **lorazepam** or **propranolol**.[2] The makers also point out that since ziprasidone is not metabolised by the cytochrome P450 isoenzyme CYP1A2, smoking should not affect its pharmacokinetics. This is borne out by studies in patients, which did not reveal any differences in the pharmacokinetics of ziprasidone between **tobacco smokers** and non-smokers.[2]

1. Wilner KD, Hansen RA, Folger CJ, Geoffroy P. The pharmacokinetics of ziprasidone in healthy volunteers treated with cimetidine or antacid. *Br J Clin Pharmacol* (2000) 49 (Suppl 1), 57S–60S.
2. Geodon (Ziprasidone). Pfizer Inc. US prescribing information, May 2005.

3. Prakash C, Kamel A, Cui D, Whalen RD, Miceli JJ, Tweedie D. Identification of the major human liver cytochrome P450 isoform(s) responsible for the formation of the primary metabolites of ziprasidone and prediction of possible drug interactions. *Br J Clin Pharmacol* (2000) 49 (Suppl 1), 35S–42S.
4. Wilner KD, DeMattos SB, Anziano RJ, Apseloff G, Gerber N. Lack of CYP 2D6 inhibition by ziprasidone in healthy volunteers. *Biol Psychiatry* (1997) 42, 42S.

Zotepine + Miscellaneous

There appears to be little or no information about adverse interactions between zotepine and other drugs, but the makers warn about the concurrent use of antihypertensives, anaesthetics, antipsychotics, and drugs that prolong the QTc interval.

Clinical evidence, mechanism, importance and management

(a) Antihypertensives

Zotepine has alpha-adrenergic blocking properties, which may cause orthostatic hypotension, especially when treatment is first started or if the dosage is increased. The makers advise caution when it is given with hypotensive agents, including some **anaesthetic agents**, the implication being that any orthostatic hypotension may possibly be worsened. If patients feel faint and dizzy when they stand up, they should be advised to get up more slowly, and if necessary, a smaller dosage should be used.[1]

(b) Antipsychotics

The makers point out that as with some other antipsychotics, zotepine has clear pro-convulsive effects, which may be additive with other antipsychotics, particularly if high doses of either or both drugs are used. They therefore recommend that zotepine doses above 300 mg daily or the concurrent use of high doses of other antipsychotics should be avoided.[1]

(c) Desipramine

No pharmacokinetic interaction was seen when zotepine was given with desipramine, indicating that the cytochrome P450 isoenzyme CYP2D6 is not involved in the metabolism of zotepine.[1]

(d) Diazepam, Fluoxetine

In a clinical interaction study, fluoxetine and diazepam increased the plasma concentrations of zotepine and norzotepine. The makers advise caution if these drugs are given concurrently.[1]

(e) QTc prolonging drugs

The makers of zotepine advise caution when treating patients taking drugs known to prolong the QTc interval (or those with coronary heart disease or at risk of hypokalaemia) because zotepine also shows a dose-related QTc interval prolongation,[1] the implication being that the effects may be additive. See also 'Drugs that prolong the QT interval + Other drugs that prolong the QT interval', p.170.

1. Zoleptil (Zotepine). Orion Pharma UK Ltd. UK Summary of product characteristics, April 2002.

19

Antivirals

This section is concerned with the drugs used to treat viral infections. These drugs may be grouped by the viral infections they are used to treat, and also by drug class (see 'Table 19.1', (p.579)). Where antivirals affect other drugs the interactions are generally covered elsewhere.

Antivirals active against herpes

(a) Nucleoside analogues

The nucleoside analogues are principally eliminated unchanged by the kidneys by a process of active tubular secretion as well as glomerular filtration. The few interactions with these drugs mainly involve altered renal clearance (e.g. probenecid), but since they have a wide therapeutic range, even these interactions are of debatable clinical relevance. Cytochrome P450 mediated interactions are not important for this group of drugs.

Antiretrovirals active against HIV

Treatment of HIV infection commonly requires a combination of 3 to 4 antiretrovirals, termed highly active antiretroviral therapy (HAART). In addition, patients often receive a large number of other drugs for comorbid conditions. This markedly increases the risk of drug interactions and complicates their assessment.

(a) Fusion inhibitors

The fusion inhibitor, enfuvirtide, is a peptide. It does not cause cytochrome P450-mediated drug interactions, and is not affected by potent enzyme inducers (rifampicin) or inhibitors (ritonavir).

(b) Non-nucleoside reverse transcriptase inhibitors (NNRTIs)

The NNRTIs are extensively metabolised by the cytochrome P450 system, particularly isoenzyme CYP3A4. They are also inducers (nevirapine, efavirenz) or inhibitors (delavirdine) of CYP3A4. NNRTIs would therefore be expected to interact with each other, and with protease inhibitors, but not with NRTIs. They also have the potential to interact with other drugs metabolised by CYP3A4, and are affected by CYP3A4 inhibitors and inducers. Delavirdine and efavirenz may also inhibit some other P450 isoenzymes. For a summary, see 'Table 19.2', (p.580).

(c) Nucleoside reverse transcriptase inhibitors (NRTIs)

NRTIs are prodrugs, which need to be activated by phosphorylation within cells to a triphosphate anabolite. Drugs may therefore interact with NRTIs by increasing or decreasing intracellular activation. NRTIs may also interact with each other by this mechanism. This interaction mechanism is studied *in vitro*, and clinical data are often not available, or the clinical relevance is unclear. Nevertheless, it is generally recommended that drugs inhibiting the intracellular activation of NRTIs are not used concurrently (e.g. 'doxorubicin and stavudine', (p.605), or 'zidovudine and stavudine', (p.599)). 'Hydroxycarbamide', (p.598) may increase the intracellular activation of NRTIs.

NRTIs are water soluble, and are mainly eliminated by the kidneys (lamivudine, zalcitabine, didanosine and stavudine) or undergo hepatic glucuronidation (zidovudine, abacavir). The few important interactions with these drugs primarily involve altered renal clearance. For zidovudine (and possibly abacavir) some interactions occur via altered glucuronidation, but the clinical relevance of these are less clear (e.g. 'rifampicin', (p.592)). Cytochrome P450-mediated interactions are not important for this class of drugs.

Some of the didanosine preparations (e.g. chewable tablets) are formulated with antacid buffers that are intended to facilitate didanosine absorption by minimising acid-induced hydrolysis in the stomach. These preparations can therefore alter the absorption of other drugs that are affected by antacids (e.g. azole antifungals, quinolone antibacterials, tetracyclines). This interaction may be minimised by separating administration by at least 2 hours. Alternatively, the newer enteric-coated preparation of didanosine (gastro-resistant capsules) may be used.

(d) Protease Inhibitors

These are extensively metabolised by the cytochrome P450 system, particularly isoenzyme CYP3A4. All of them inhibit CYP3A4, with ritonavir being the most potent inhibitor, followed by indinavir, nelfinavir, amprenavir, and saquinavir. The protease inhibitors therefore have the potential to interact with other drugs metabolised by CYP3A4, and are also affected by CYP3A4 inhibitors and inducers. Ritonavir and nelfinavir also affect some other cytochrome P450 isoenzymes, as summarised in 'Table 19.2', (p.580). In addition, protease inhibitors are substrates as well as inhibitors of P-glycoprotein. Protease inhibitors therefore have the potential to interact with each other, and with NNRTIs, but are not likely to interact with NRTIs.

The plasma level of protease inhibitors is thought to be critical in maintaining efficacy and minimising the potential for development of viral resistance. Therefore even modest reductions in levels are potentially clinically important.

General references

1. Barry M, Mulcahy F, Merry C, Gibbons S, Back D. Pharmacokinetics and potential interactions amongst antiretroviral agents used to treat patients with HIV infection. *Clin Pharmacokinet* (1999) 36, 289–304.
2. de Maat MMR, Ekhart GC, Huitema ADR, Koks CHW, Mulder JW, Beijnen JH. Drug interactions between antiretroviral drugs and comedicated agents. *Clin Pharmacokinet* (2003) 42, 223–82.

Table 19.1 Antivirals

Generic names	*Proprietary names*
Antivirals for hepatitis viruses	
Nucleotide analogues	
Adefovir	Adsera, Hepsera
Miscellaneous	
Interferon alfa	Alfaferone, Alfater, Beferon, Biaferone, Blauferon, Cilferon-A, Egiferon, Finnferon-Alpha, Inmutag, Interferon Alfanative, Intermax-Alpha, Isiferone, Multiferon, OIF, Sumiferon
Peginterferon alfa	
Ribavirin	Copegus, Desiken, Rebetol, Ribav, Ribavin, Ribaviron C, Vilona, Viramid, Virazide, Virazole
Antivirals for herpes viruses	
Guanine nucleoside analogues	
Aciclovir	Abduce, Acerpes, Acic, Aciclin, Aciclo, Aciclobene, Aciclobeta, Aciclodan, Aciclomed, Aciclosina, Aciclostad, Aciclotyrol, Aciclovivax, Acic-Ophtal, Acicvir, Acifur, Acihexal, Acilax, Acitop, Aciveral, Acivir, Aclovir, Aclovirax, Activir, ACV, ACY, Acyclostad, Acyclo-V, Acyclox, Acyrax, Acyvir, Alovir, Amodivyr, Anclomax, Anti, Antivirax, Aviral, Avirase, Avirex-T, Avirox, Avix, Avorax, Avyclor, Avyplus, Avysal, Bearax, Bel Labial, Biozirox, Cargosil, Cevinolon, Ciclavix, Ciclocris, Cicloferon, Cicloviral, Citivir, Clearsore, Clinovir, Clovin, Clovir, Clovira, Clovirax, Colsor, Cusiviral, Cyclivex, Cyclomed, Cyclorax, Cyclovax, Cyclovir, Cycloviran, Declovir, Divicil, Dravyr, Dynexan Herpescreme, Efriviral, Entir, Epsin, Erpaclovir, Erpizon, Esavir, Etasisen, Eurovir, Exaliver, Exavir, Exviral, Ezopen, Farocid, Faulviral, Fibral, Fuviron, Geavir, Hagevir, Heclivir, Helposol, Helvevir, Hepirax, Hermixsofex, Hermocil, Herpavir, Herpenon, Herpesil, Herpesin, Herpesnil, Herpetad, Herpex, Herpilem, Herpolips, Herpomed, Herpotern, Herzkur, Iliaclor, Immunovir, Ipaviran, Ipsovir, Isavir, Juviral, Kendix, Laciken, Lermex, Lisovyr, Lovir, Lovire, Lovrak, Maclov, Mapox, Marvir, Maynar, Medovir, Milavir, Neclovir, Neldim, Neviran, Norum, Nycovir, Ocurax, Oftavir, Opthavir, Orivir, Poviral, Provirsan, Pulibex, Ranvir, Rexan, Riduvir, Sanavir, Sifiviral, Simplex-Fieberblasen, Soothelip, Soviclor, Stadovir, Supra-Vir, Supraviran, Synclovir, Telviran, Uni Vir, Uniplex, Vacrax, Vermis, Verpir, Vidaclovir, Vilerm, Viraban, Viralief, Virasorb, Virax, Viraxy, Virest, Virherpes, Virless, Virmen, Viro, Viroclear, Virogon, Virokill, Virolan, Virolex, ViroMed, Vironida, Virovir, Virucalm, Virucid, Viruderm, Virupos, Viruseen, Virusteril, Virzin, Vivax , Vivir, Voraclor, Vyrohexal, Wariviron, Xiclovir, Xorox, Zeramil, Zetavir, Zevin, Zidovimm, Ziverone, Zocovin, Zolaten, Zoliparin, Zoral, Zorax, Zoraxin, Zov800, Zovir, Zovirax, Zoylex, Zyclir
Famciclovir	Ancivin, Famtrex, Famvir, Fanclomax, Oravir, Penvir, Zosvir
Ganciclovir	Ciganclor, Citovirax, Cymevan, Cymeven, Cymevene, Cytovene, Ganvirax, Gasmilen, Grinevel, Virgan, Vitrasert
Penciclovir	Denavir, Famvir, Vectavir
Valaciclovir	Pervioral, Rapivir, Talavir, Vadiral, Valavir, Valcivir, Valherpes, Valtrex, Viranet, Virmax, Virval, Zelitrex
Valganciclovir	Darilin, Rovalcyte, Valcyte
Other nucleoside analogues	
Idoxuridine	Herpesine, Herpid, Herplex, Herplex-D, Idina, Iducher, Idulea, Idustatin, Oftan IDU, Ridinox, Stoxil, Virasolve, Virexen, Virunguent, Zostrum
Trifluridine	Adrocil, TFT, TFT Ophtiole, Thilol, Triflumann, Triherpine, Viridin, Viromidin, Virophta, Viroptic
Vidarabine	Arasena-A, Tekarin, Virerpin
Nucleotide analogues	
Cidofovir	Vistide
Fomivirsen	Vitravene
Miscellaneous	
Foscarnet sodium	Foscavir, Triapten
Inosine pranobex	delimmun, Imunovir, Isoprinosin, Isoprinosine, Isovir, Pranosine, Virustop, Viruxan
Antivirals for HIV infection (antiretrovirals)	
HIV infusion inhibitors	
Enfuvirtide	Fuzeon
Non-nucleoside reverse transcriptase inhibitors (NNRTIs)	
Delavirdine	Rescriptor
Efavirenz	Efavir, Filginase, Stocrin, Sustiva
Nevirapine	Filide, Nerapin, Nevimune, Nevipan, Neviralea, Protease, Ritvir, Viramune
Nucleoside reverse transcriptase inhibitors (NRTIs)	
Abacavir	Abamune, Ziagen, Ziagenavir
Didanosine	Aso DDI, Bandotan, Dibistic, Dinex, Megavir, Ronvir, Videx
Emtricitabine	Emtriva

Continued

Table 19.1 Antivirals *(continued)*

Generic names	*Proprietary names*
Lamivudine	3TC, 3TC/Epivir, Birvac, Epivir, Ganvirel, Heptovir, Hivirux, Imunoxa, Kess, Ladiwin, Lamidac, Lamilea, Lamirex, Lamivir, Oralmuv, Ultraviral, Vuclodir, Vudirax, Zeffix
Stavudine	Birac, Lion, Revixil, Stamar, Stavir, Stelea, STV, Tonavir, Virostav, Zerit, Zeritavir
Zalcitabine	Hivid, Inxibir
Zidovudine	Azetavir, Azoazol, Azotine, Crisazet, Enper, Exovir, Iduvo, Pranadox, Produvir, Retrovir, Revirax, T.O.Vir, T-ZA, Virozid, Zetrotax, Zidorex, Zidovir, Zidovusan, Zydowin
Nucleotide reverse transcriptase inhibitors	
Tenofovir	Viread
Protease inhibitors	
Amprenavir	Agenerase
Atazanavir	Reyataz
Fosamprenavir	Lexiva, Telzir
Indinavir	Avural, Crixivan, Elvenavir, Forli, Indilea, Indinax, Indivan, Inhibisam
Lopinavir	
Nelfinavir	Filosfil, Nalvir, Nelfilea, Nelvir, Viracept
Ritonavir	Norvir, Ritomune
Saquinavir	Fortovase, Invirase
Antivirals for influenza	
Amantadine	Adekin, Aman, Amant, Amanta, Amantagamma, Amantan, Amantrel, Amixx, A-Parkin, Atarin, Endantadine, Hofcomant, Infex, Lysovir, Mantadan, Mantadix, Mantidan, Paritrel, Parkadina, PK-Merz, Prayanol, Profil, Symmetrel, tregor, Viregyt, Viregyt-K, Virosol, Virucid
Oseltamivir	Tamiflu
Rimantadine	Flumadine, Germic, Oclovir
Zanamivir	Relenza

Table 19.2 Summary of the effect of the protease inhibitors and NNRTIs on cytochrome P450 isoenzymes

Antiviral	*Substrate*	*Inhibits*	*Induces*
Protease inhibitors			
Amprenavir or Fosamprenavir	CYP3A4	CYP3A4	
Atazanavir	CYP3A4	CYP3A4	
Indinavir	CYP3A4	CYP3A4	
Lopinavir	CYP3A4	CYP3A4, CYP2D6	
Nelfinavir	CYP3A4, CYP2C19, CYP2C9, CYP2D6	CYP3A4	
Ritonavir	CYP3A4, CYP2D6	CYP3A4, CYP2D6	CYP3A4
Saquinavir	CYP3A4	CYP3A4	
NNRTIs (Non-nucleoside reverse transcriptase inhibitors)			
Delavirdine	CYP3A4, CYP2D6	CYP3A4, CYP2C9, CYP2D6, CYP2C19	
Efavirenz	CYP3A4, CYP2B6	CYP3A4, CYP2C9, CYP2C19	CYP3A4
Nevirapine	CYP3A4		CYP3A4

Aciclovir and related drugs + Cimetidine

Single-dose studies have found that cimetidine increases the AUC of aciclovir and valaciclovir, but this is thought unlikely to be clinically important. No clinically important interaction appears to occur if famciclovir is given with cimetidine.

Clinical evidence

(a) Aciclovir or Valaciclovir

Twelve healthy subjects were given a 1-g dose of valaciclovir alone or with cimetidine 800 mg, taken 10 hours and 1 hour before. The 0 to 3-hour AUC for the prodrug valaciclovir was increased 73% by cimetidine, and the 0 to 24-hour AUC for the active metabolite aciclovir was increased by 27%. The renal clearance of aciclovir was reduced by 22%, although the total urinary recovery of aciclovir was unchanged.[1]

(b) Famciclovir

Cimetidine 400 mg was given twice daily for 8 days to 12 healthy subjects with a single 500-mg dose of the famciclovir, a prodrug for penciclovir, on the last day. The AUC of penciclovir was increased by about 18% by cimetidine, but there was no change in renal clearance.[2,3]

Mechanism

The increase in aciclovir AUC with cimetidine is attributable to a reduction in its renal excretion, probably due to competition for secretion by the kidney tubules.[1] The effects on aciclovir of combining the renal tubular secretion competitor 'probenecid', (below) and cimetidine were greater than either drug alone.[1] Cimetidine does not significantly alter the pharmacokinetics of famciclovir/penciclovir.[3]

Importance and management

These interactions are established but, because aciclovir has such a wide therapeutic index,[4] the authors of the study suggest that its interaction with cimetidine is probably clinically unimportant.[1] It seems likely that no changes in the usual dosages of aciclovir or valaciclovir will be needed in patients also taking cimetidine. However, the UK maker states that caution is required with high doses of valaciclovir, and that alternatives to cimetidine could be considered in this situation.[4] No special precautions would seem necessary if cimetidine is used with famciclovir.

1. De Bony F, Tod M, Bidault R, On NT, Posner J, Rolan P. Multiple interactions of cimetidine and probenecid with valaciclovir and its metabolite acyclovir. *Antimicrob Agents Chemother* (2002) 46, 458–63.
2. Pratt SK, Fowles SE, Pierce DM, Prince WT. An investigation of the potential interaction between cimetidine and famciclovir in non-patient volunteers. *Br J Clin Pharmacol* (1991) 32, 656P–657P.
3. Daniels S, Schentag JJ. Drug interaction studies and safety of famciclovir in healthy volunteers: a review. *Antiviral Chem Chemother* (1993) 4 (Suppl 1), 57–64.
4. Valtrex (Valaciclovir). GlaxoSmithKline UK. UK Summary of product characteristics, November 2004.

Aciclovir and related drugs + Mycophenolate

Aciclovir or ganciclovir and mycophenolate mofetil appear not to interact pharmacokinetically to a clinically relevant extent, but the makers recommend care, especially in renal impairment.

Clinical evidence, mechanism, importance and management

(a) Aciclovir

Healthy subjects were given single doses of oral aciclovir 800 mg or mycophenolate mofetil 1 g or both drugs together in a three-period crossover study. The AUC and renal clearances of both drugs were not significantly altered by concurrent use, although the AUC of the glucuronide metabolite of mycophenolate was higher. It was concluded that any changes were unlikely to be clinically significant.[1] However, UK the maker of aciclovir states that *increases* in the AUCs of aciclovir have been shown when the drugs are given together.[2] Similarly, the makers of mycophenolate states that, in renal impairment there may be competition for tubular secretion and that further increases in concentrations of both aciclovir and mycophenolate may occur.[3,4]

Note that some data suggests that mycophenolate potentiates the antiherpes virus activity of aciclovir, which may be clinically useful.[5]

(b) Ganciclovir or Valganciclovir

A three-way crossover study in 12 transplant patients found no pharmacokinetic interaction between a single 1.5-g oral dose of mycophenolate mofetil and intravenous ganciclovir 5 mg/kg, but renal clearance of ganciclovir was slightly reduced, by 12%.[6] However, the makers note that it is anticipated that the concurrent use of these two drugs will result in increases in ganciclovir levels, and levels of the inactive metabolite of mycophenolate, due to competition for renal tubular secretion. They suggest careful monitoring in patients with renal impairment given both drugs.[3,4,7] These cautions are also applied to the ganciclovir prodrug valganciclovir.[8,9]

Five cases of neutrophil dysplasia in transplant patients appeared to be related to the combination of ganciclovir and mycophenolate, rather than mycophenolate alone.[10] This emphasises the need for caution with concurrent use.

Note that some data suggests that mycophenolate potentiates the antiherpes virus activity of ganciclovir, which may be clinically useful.[5]

1. Shah J, Juan D, Bullingham R, Wong B, Wong R, Fu C. A single dose drug interaction study of mycophenolate mofetil and acyclovir in normal subjects. *J Clin Pharmacol* (1994) 34, 1029.
2. Zovirax IV (Aciclovir). GlaxoSmithKline UK. UK Summary of product characteristics, December 2004.
3. CellCept (Mycophenolate mofetil). Roche Products Ltd. UK Summary of product characteristics, April 2005.
4. CellCept (Mycophenolate mofetil). Roche Pharmaceuticals. US Prescribing information, October 2004.
5. Neyts J, Andrei G, De Clercq E. The novel immunosuppressive agent mycophenolate mofetil markedly potentiates the antiherpesvirus activities of acyclovir, ganciclovir, and penciclovir in vitro and in vivo. *Antimicrob Agents Chemother* (1998) 42, 216–22.
6. Wolfe EJ, Mathur V, Tomlanovich S, Jung D, Wong R, Griffy K, Aweeka FT. Pharmacokinetics of mycophenolate mofetil and intravenous ganciclovir alone and in combination in renal transplant recipients. *Pharmacotherapy* (1997) 17, 591–8.
7. Cymevene IV (Ganciclovir sodium). Roche Products Ltd. UK Summary of product characteristics, April 2004.
8. Valcyte (Valganciclovir hydrochloride). Roche Products Ltd. UK Summary of product characteristics, June 2003.
9. Valcyte (Valganciclovir hydrochloride). Roche Pharmaceuticals. US Prescribing information, September 2003.
10. Kennedy GA, Kay TD, Johnson DW, Hawley CM, Campbell SB, Isbel NM, Marlton P, Cobcroft R, Gill D, Cull G. Neutrophil dysplasia characterised by a pseudo-Pelger–Huet anomaly occurring with the use of mycophenolate mofetil and ganciclovir following renal transplantation: a report of five cases. *Pathology* (2002) 34, 263–6.

Aciclovir and related drugs + Probenecid

Probenecid reduces the renal excretion and increases the plasma levels of aciclovir, valaciclovir and ganciclovir. Famciclovir and valganciclovir are predicted to interact similarly.

Clinical evidence

(a) Aciclovir or Valaciclovir

Twelve healthy subjects were given 1 g of valaciclovir alone or with probenecid 1 g taken 2 hours earlier. The 0 to 3-hour AUC for the prodrug valaciclovir was increased by 22% by probenecid, and the 0 to 24-hour AUC for the active metabolite aciclovir was increased by 48% by probenecid. The renal clearance of aciclovir was reduced by 33%, although the total urinary recovery of aciclovir was unchanged.[1] An earlier study had found that oral probenecid 1 g caused a similar increase in the AUC of intravenous aciclovir.[2]

(b) Ganciclovir

A pharmacokinetic study[3] in HIV+ patients found that probenecid 500 mg every 6 hours increased the AUC of oral ganciclovir 1 g every 8 hours by 53.1%, and the renal clearance was reduced 12.3%.

Mechanism

The increases in aciclovir and ganciclovir AUCs are attributable to a reduction in their renal excretion by probenecid, probably due to competition for secretion by the kidney tubules.[1,3] The effects on aciclovir of combining probenecid and 'cimetidine', (above) were greater than either drug alone.[1]

Importance and management

These interactions are established, but because aciclovir has such a wide therapeutic index,[4] the authors of the study suggest that its interaction with cimetidine is probably clinically unimportant.[1] It seems likely that no changes in the usual dosages of aciclovir or valaciclovir will be needed in patients also taking probenecid. However, the UK maker states that caution is required with high doses of valaciclovir, and that alternatives to probenecid could be considered in this situation.[4] The US maker suggests that the dosage of probenecid may need to be altered.[5] Similarly, it may be prudent to be alert for increased ganciclovir effects and toxicity if probenecid is used concurrently. **Valganciclovir** is a prodrug of ganciclovir, and the makers recommend that patients taking valganciclovir with probenecid should be closely monitored for ganciclovir toxicity.[6,7] The makers of **famciclovir** suggest that a similar interaction might also occur with probenecid and famciclovir, resulting in an increase in the plasma levels of penciclovir (the active metabolite of famciclovir).[8,9]

1. De Bony F, Tod M, Bidault R, On NT, Posner J, Rolan P. Multiple interactions of cimetidine and probenecid with valaciclovir and its metabolite acyclovir. *Antimicrob Agents Chemother* (2002) 46, 458–63.
2. Laskin OL, de Miranda P, King DH, Page DA, Longstreth JA, Rocco L, Lietman PS. Effects of probenecid on the pharmacokinetics and elimination of acyclovir in humans. *Antimicrob Agents Chemother* (1982) 21, 804–7.
3. Gaines K, Wong R, Jung D, Cimoch P, Lavelle J, Pollard R. Pharmacokinetic interactions with oral ganciclovir: zidovudine, didanosine, probenecid. *Abstract book of the 10th Int Conf AIDS 1994 August 7–12, Yokohama (Japan)* (1994) 1,7.
4. Valtrex (Valaciclovir). GlaxoSmithKline UK. UK Summary of product characteristics, November 2004.
5. Valtrex (Valacyclovir hydrochloride). GlaxoSmithKline. US Prescribing information, November 2004.
6. Valcyte (Valganciclovir hydrochloride). Roche Products Ltd. UK Summary of product characteristics, June 2003.
7. Valcyte (Valganciclovir hydrochloride). Roche Pharmaceuticals. US Prescribing information, September 2003.
8. Famvir (Famciclovir). Novartis Pharmaceuticals UK Ltd. UK Summary of product characteristics, December 2004.
9. Famvir (Famciclovir). Novartis Pharmaceuticals Corp. US Prescribing information, February 2002.

Adefovir + Miscellaneous

There is no pharmacokinetic interaction between adefovir and co-trimoxazole, lamivudine, paracetamol or tenofovir. Ibuprofen modestly raises adefovir levels, but this is not clinically important. Adefovir modestly raises didanosine levels, and saquinavir modestly raises adefovir levels, but neither change is clinically important. Adefovir does not interact with zidovudine, delavirdine, efavirenz, nevirapine, indinavir or nelfinavir.

Clinical evidence, mechanism, importance and management

(a) Antiretrovirals

At doses 6 to 12 times higher than the 10-mg dose of adefovir recommended for hepatitis B infection, there was no interaction with the NRTIs **lamivudine** or **zidovudine**, the NNRTIs **delavirdine**, **efavirenz** or **nevirapine**, or the protease inhibitors **indinavir** or **nelfinavir**.[1] Concurrent use of adefovir 60 mg with **saquinavir** soft capsules increased the adefovir AUC by 20%, which is not clinically relevant.[1] Concurrent use of adefovir 60 mg with **didanosine** buffered tablets increased the **didanosine** AUC by 29%, which is not clinically relevant.[1]

(b) Drugs undergoing, or affecting, tubular secretion

Adefovir is excreted by the kidneys, by a combination of glomerular filtration and active secretion via the renal transporter, human Organic Anion Transporter 1 (hOAT1). The potential for pharmacokinetic interactions with **co-trimoxazole**, **ibuprofen**, **lamivudine**, **paracetamol** and **tenofovir** (other drugs that also undergo, or may affect tubular secretion) has been investigated.[1,2]

(i) Co-trimoxazole. The makers note that there was no pharmacokinetic interaction between adefovir 10 mg and **trimethoprim/sulfamethoxazole**.[1,2]

(ii) Ibuprofen. The concurrent use of adefovir 10 mg and ibuprofen 800 mg three times daily modestly increased the AUC and maximum level of adefovir by 23% and 33%, respectively. These changes were considered to be due to higher bioavailability rather than a reduction in renal clearance, and are not considered clinically relevant. Adefovir did not alter ibuprofen pharmacokinetics.[1,2]

(iii) Lamivudine. The makers note that there was no pharmacokinetic interaction between adefovir 10 mg and lamivudine 100 mg.[1,2]

(iv) Paracetamol. The makers note that there was no pharmacokinetic interaction between adefovir 10 mg and paracetamol.[1,2]

(v) Tenofovir. There was no pharmacokinetic interaction between adefovir 10 mg and tenofovir in a single-dose study in healthy subjects. However, the makers still advise close monitoring during concurrent use, since the clinical safety, including renal effects, has not yet been assessed.[1,2]

1. Hepsera (Adefovir dipivoxil). Gilead Sciences International Ltd. UK Summary of product characteristics, May 2004.
2. Hepsera (Adefovir dipivoxil). Gilead Sciences, Inc. US Prescribing information, August 2004.

Cidofovir + Probenecid

Probenecid reduces the nephrotoxicity of cidofovir, and it is recommended it should always be used concurrently.[1,2] Therefore, when using cidofovir/probenecid the interactions of probenecid should be considered. Of particular note, zidovudine should be temporarily discontinued or the dosage halved when cidofovir/probenecid is used[1,2] (see also 'NRTIs + Probenecid', p.601).

1. Vistide (Cidofovir). Pharmacia Ltd. UK Summary of product characteristics, September 2004.
2. Vistide (Cidofovir). Gilead Sciences, Inc. US Prescribing information, September 2000.

Enfuvirtide + Cytochrome P450 isoenzyme substrates

Enfuvirtide had no effect on the metabolism of dapsone or debrisoquine, and had little effect on the metabolism of caffeine, chlorzoxazone, and mephenytoin. Thus, it is not anticipated that enfuvirtide would cause clinically important drug interactions with drugs metabolised by the cytochrome P450 isoenzymes.

Clinical evidence, mechanism, importance and management

A single oral dose of five drugs (**caffeine** 100 mg, **chlorzoxazone** 250 mg, **dapsone** 100 mg, **debrisoquine** 10 mg and **mephenytoin** 100 mg) was given to 12 subjects with HIV infection, once before, and once after receiving subcutaneous enfuvirtide 90 mg twice daily for 6 days. Enfuvirtide had no effect on the urinary **dapsone** recovery ratio (a measure of the activity of the cytochrome P450 isoenzyme CYP3A4), plasma monoacetyldapsone-to-**dapsone** ratio (a measure of *N*-acetyltransferase (NAT) activity) or urinary **debrisoquine** recovery ratio (a measure of CYP2D6 activity). Enfuvirtide had little effect (less than ±30%) on the plasma paraxanthine-to-**caffeine** ratio (a measure of CYP1A2 activity), the plasma 6-hydroxychlorzoxazone-to-**chlorzoxazone** ratio (CYP2E1) and urinary recovery of 4-hydroxy**mephenytoin** (CYP2C19). Subjects in this study were taking up to 3 NRTIs in stable doses, and were not taking any NNRTIs or protease inhibitors.[1]

This type of study is being increasingly used to assess the potential for new drugs to cause clinically important cytochrome P450-mediated drug interactions. The results indicate that enfuvirtide is unlikely to cause clinically important changes in the pharmacokinetics of drugs metabolised by CYP3A4, NAT and CYP2D6. They also give some reassurance that drugs metabolised by CYP1A2, CYP2E1 and CYP2C19 are unlikely to be affected, although the modest changes seen introduce some caution. No substrate for CYP2C9 was included in this study, but enfuvirtide does not affect CYP2C9 *in vitro*.[1]

1. Zhang X, Lalezari JP, Badley AD, Dorr A, Kolis SJ, Kinchelow T, Patel IH. Assessment of drug-drug interaction potential of enfuvirtide in human immunodeficiency virus type 1–infected patients. *Clin Pharmacol Ther* (2004) 75, 558–68.

Enfuvirtide + Protease inhibitors

Ritonavir caused a minor increase in enfuvirtide exposure, which is not clinically relevant. Saquinavir/ritonavir had little effect on enfuvirtide.

Clinical evidence, mechanism, importance and management

Subcutaneous enfuvirtide 90 mg twice daily was given for 7 days to 24 subjects with HIV infection, with either **ritonavir** 200 mg twice daily or **saquinavir/ritonavir** 1000 mg/100 mg twice daily given for the last 4 days. **Ritonavir** caused a minor 24% rise in the enfuvirtide AUC, and **saquinavir/ritonavir** caused a 14% increase. Such small increases in

Clinical evidence, mechanism, importance and management

Patients with cryoglobulinaemia were treated with 3 million units of recombinant **interferon alfa-2a** (35 patients) or natural **interferon beta** (3 patients), usually given daily for 3 months then on alternate days for periods of 6 to 17 months. Severe toxicity developed in 3 patients, who were the only ones amongst the group to also be treated with ACE inhibitors. Granulocytopenia developed in 2 patients within a few days of starting **enalapril** 10 mg daily or **captopril** 50 mg daily, and subsided 1 to 2 weeks after both drugs were stopped. Another patient, already on **enalapril** 5 mg daily, developed severe granulocytopenia when interferon was started, and again when re-challenged with both drugs. None of the other 35 patients on interferon alone developed any significant haematological problems. The reasons for this severe reaction are not understood but the authors of the report suggest that it may be an autoimmune response.[1]

A follow-up letter commenting on this report described 2 further patients with hepatitis C infection, cryoglobulinaemia and glomerulonephritis, who were treated for several weeks with **captopril** 75 mg or **enalapril** 20 mg daily, and who had granulocytopenia within 9 days of being given 3 million units of recombinant **interferon alfa-2a** daily or on alternate days. However, this resolved without any change in treatment. Another patient with multiple myeloma given **interferon alfa-2a** 3 million units 3 times weekly and long-term **benazepril** 10 mg daily had a normal granulocyte count after 3 months.[2]

Whatever the explanation for the findings, the extent of this severe and potentially life-threatening response certainly suggests that if the decision is made to give ACE inhibitors and interferons concurrently, the outcome should be very closely monitored.

1. Casato M, Pucillo LP, Leoni M, di Lullo L, Gabrielli A, Sansonno D, Dammacco F, Danieli G, Bonomo L. Granulocytopenia after combined therapy with interferon and angiotensin-converting enzyme inhibitors: evidence for a synergistic hematologic toxicity. *Am J Med* (1995) 99, 386–91.
2. Jacquot C, Caudwell V, Belenfant X. Granulocytopenia after combined therapy with interferon and angiotensin-converting enzyme inhibitors: evidence for a synergistic hematologic toxicity. *Am J Med* (1996) 101, 235–6.

Interferons + Analgesics or Corticosteroids

Prednisone and paracetamol have disparate effects on some measures of the antiviral activity of interferon, but the clinical relevance of these is unclear. Isolated cases of acute hepatitis have been seen when interferon is given with paracetamol.

Clinical evidence, mechanism, importance and management

A single intramuscular dose of recombinant human **interferon alfa-2a** 18 million units was given to 8 healthy subjects alone, or after one day of either **aspirin** 650 mg every 4 hours, **paracetamol** 650 mg every 4 hours or **prednisone** 40 mg daily, for a total of 8 days. None of these additional drugs reduced the interferon adverse effects of fever, chills, headache or myalgia. Neither **paracetamol** nor **aspirin** affected measures of interferon antiviral activity, but **prednisone** appeared to reduce one of the two measures of interferon activity.[1] In a later similar study by the same research group, the effect of the same drugs and doses (started 3 days before the interferon) was evaluated with a lower dose of **interferon alfa-2a** (3 million units). When data for **aspirin**, **paracetamol** or **prednisone** was combined the subjects had a 47% reduction in symptom score compared with controls not taking any of these three drugs. The **prednisone** group also had fewer hours of fever. In this study, neither **prednisone** nor **aspirin** consistently altered measures of the antiviral activity of interferon, but **paracetamol** appeared to enhance them.[2] Taken together, the results of these two studies suggest that these drugs may reduce the flu-like adverse effects of interferon, perhaps more so at lower doses of interferon. The clinical relevance of the measures of antiviral activity of interferon is uncertain, so the disparate effects found with **paracetamol** and **prednisone** are unclear.

The authors of a report describing an unusual acute form of hepatitis, occurring in 3 patients on **interferon alfa-2a**, vinblastine and **paracetamol**, suggested that this might have been due to a drug interaction.[3] Another 2 similar cases have been reported with **interferon alfa-2b** and **paracetamol**, but no liver toxicity occurred when one of these patients was given **indometacin** with interferon instead.[4] The general relevance of these isolated reports is unclear.

1. Witter FR, Woods AS, Griffin MD, Smith CR, Nadler P, Lietman PS. Effects of prednisone, aspirin and acetaminophen on an *in vivo* biologic response to interferon in humans. *Clin Pharmacol Ther* (1988) 44, 239–43.
2. Hendrix CW, Petty BG, Woods A, Kuwahara SK, Witter FR, Soo W, Griffin DE, Lietman PS. Modulation of α-interferon's antiviral and clinical effects by aspirin, acetaminophen, and prednisone in healthy volunteers. *Antiviral Res* (1995) 28, 121–31.
3. Kellokumpu-Lehtinen P, Iisalo E, Nordman E. Hepatotoxicity of paracetamol in combination with interferon and vinblastine. *Lancet* (1989) 1, 1143.
4. Fabris P, Dalla Palma M, de Lalla F. Idiosyncratic acute hepatitis caused by paracetamol in two patients with melanoma treated with high-dose interferon-α. *Ann Intern Med* (2001) 134, 345.

Interferons + Ribavirin

There appears to be no pharmacokinetic interaction between interferon alfa or peginterferon alfa and ribavirin. The combination has improved efficacy against hepatitis C.

Clinical evidence, mechanism, importance and management

There was no evidence of any changes in pharmacokinetic parameters when ribavirin and **interferon alfa-2b** were given together, and trends suggested that there were reduced titres of hepatitis C in a study in patients with chronic hepatitis C.[1] Another study using the pegylated form of interferon alfa-2b (**peginterferon alfa-2b**) also found no pharmacokinetic interactions with ribavirin.[2] Similarly, the makers note that there was no pharmacokinetic interaction between **peginterferon alfa-2a** and ribavirin.[3] The combination of **interferon alfa** and ribavirin has enhanced efficacy against hepatitis C.[4,5]

1. Khakoo S, Glue P, Grellier L, Wells B, Bell A, Dash C, Murray-Lyon I, Lypnyj D, Flannery B, Walters K, Dusheiko GM. Ribavirin and interferon alfa-2b in chronic hepatitis C: assessment of possible pharmacokinetic and pharmacodynamic interactions. *Br J Clin Pharmacol* (1998) 46, 563–70.
2. Glue P, Rouzier-Panis R, Raffanel C, Sabo R, Gupta SK, Salfi M, Jacobs S, Clement RP. A dose-ranging study of pegylated interferon alfa-2b and ribavirin in chronic hepatitis C. The Hepatitis C Intervention Therapy Group. *Hepatology* (2000) 32, 647–53.
3. Pegasys (Peginterferon alfa-2a). Roche Products Ltd. UK Summary of product characteristics, February 2005.
4. Schalm SW, Hansen BE, Chemello L, Bellobuono A, Brouwer JT, Weiland O, Cavalletto L, Schvarcz R, Ideo G, Alberti A. Ribavirin enhances the efficacy but not the adverse effects of interferon in chronic hepatitis C. Meta-analysis of individual patient data from European centers. *J Hepatol* (1997) 26, 961–6.
5. Kjaergard LL, Krogsgaard K, Gluud C. Interferon alfa with or without ribavirin for chronic hepatitis C: systematic review of randomised trials. *BMJ* (2001) 323, 1151–5.

NNRTIs + Antacids, H_2-blockers or Proton pump inhibitors

Antacids roughly halve the AUC of delavirdine, and H_2-blockers or proton pump inhibitors would be expected to interact similarly. Aluminium/magnesium antacids do not interact to a clinically relevant extent with efavirenz or nevirapine, and famotidine does not alter the absorption of efavirenz.

Clinical evidence, mechanism, importance and management

(a) Delavirdine

Delavirdine is poorly soluble at pHs greater than 3, so the effect of giving delavirdine 300 mg 10 minutes after an antacid [type and dose not stated] was studied in 12 healthy subjects. The AUC and maximum serum levels of delavirdine were reduced by 48% and 57% respectively, suggesting that delavirdine should not be given with antacids.[1] The maker recommends separating administration by at least one hour.[2] Although it has not been studied, it is predicted that other drugs that reduce gastric acidity, such as H_2-blockers and proton pump inhibitors, will also reduce the absorption of delavirdine, and their long-term use with delavirdine is not recommended.[2]

(b) Efavirenz

The maker notes that neither **aluminium/magnesium hydroxide** antacids nor **famotidine** had any effect on the absorption of efavirenz.[3] No special precautions are expected to be necessary with drugs that reduce gastric acidity.

(c) Nevirapine

In a study in 24 healthy subjects it was found that 30 ml of *Maalox* (**aluminium/magnesium hydroxide**) caused some moderate changes in the pharmacokinetics of nevirapine 200 mg, but none of them was considered to be clinically relevant.[4] No special precautions would seem to be necessary.

1. Cox SR, Della-Coletta AA, Turner SW, Freimuth WW. Single-dose pharmacokinetic (PK) studies with delavirdine (DLV) mesylate: dose proportionality and effects of food and antacid. *Intersci Conf Antimicrob Agents Chemother* (1994) 34, 82.
2. Rescriptor (Delavirdine). Pharmacia & Upjohn Company. US Prescribing information, November 2003.
3. Sustiva (Efavirenz). Bristol-Myers Squibb Pharmaceuticals Ltd. UK Summary of product characteristics, March 2005.
4. Lamson M, Cort S, Macy H, Love J, Korpalski D, Pav J, Keirns J. Effects of food or antacid on the bioavailability of nevirapine 200 mg tablets. 11th International Conference on AIDS, Vancouver, 1996. Abstract Tu.B.2323.

NNRTIs + Azoles

Nevirapine reduces the AUC of ketoconazole by about two-thirds, and the makers advise avoidance of the combination. Fluconazole increases nevirapine exposure, and the combination should be used with caution. Fluconazole causes a modest rise in efavirenz steady-state levels. Delavirdine does not appear to interact with fluconazole, but its plasma levels may be raised by ketoconazole.

Clinical evidence, mechanism, importance and management

(a) Delavirdine

Delavirdine mesilate 300 mg three times daily was given to 13 HIV+ subjects for 30 days. **Fluconazole** 400 mg daily was given to 8 of them on days 16 to 30. No differences in the pharmacokinetics of either drug were noted between the two groups.[1] On the basis of these results, it would appear that no dosage adjustments are needed if these drugs are used together.

The maker notes that the minimum level of delavirdine was 50% higher than population pharmacokinetic data in 26 patients on **ketoconazole**.[2]

The makers of **voriconazole** suggest that patients given delavirdine should be carefully monitored for evidence of drug toxicity and/or loss of efficacy during concurrent use. This is because *in vitro* study suggests that delavirdine may inhibit the metabolism of **voriconazole**. The makers also predict that **voriconazole** may inhibit the metabolism of NNRTIs.[3,4]

(b) Efavirenz

Fluconazole 400 mg daily for one day, then 200 mg daily for 6 days was given to 20 healthy subjects with efavirenz 400 mg daily. The pharmacokinetics of **fluconazole** were not affected, and although the AUC of efavirenz was raised by 15%, no clinically significant effects are anticipated.[5]

A study in healthy subjects found that efavirenz 400 mg daily decreased the steady state maximum serum levels and the AUC of **voriconazole** 200 mg twice daily for 8 days by 61 and 77% respectively. This is almost certainly because the metabolism of the **voriconazole** by the cytochrome P450 isoenzyme CYP3A4 is induced by efavirenz. At the same time the steady state maximum serum levels and the AUC of efavirenz are increased by 38 and 44% respectively, because its metabolism is reduced by the **voriconazole**. On the basis of these studies the makers of **voriconazole** contraindicate the concurrent use of efavirenz.[3,4]

(c) Nevirapine

The makers of nevirapine quote a study in which nevirapine 200 mg twice daily was given with **ketoconazole** 400 mg daily. The **ketoconazole** AUC was reduced by 63% and its maximum plasma levels were reduced by 40%. In addition, the nevirapine plasma levels were raised by 15 to 28% compared with historical control data.[6]

In another study, the concurrent use of **fluconazole** and nevirapine increased the exposure to nevirapine by about 100% compared with historical control data, although nevirapine did not have any clinically relevant effect on **fluconazole**.[6] The maker suggests that **ketoconazole** and nevirapine should not be used together, and that patients should be closely monitored if **fluconazole** and nevirapine are used concurrently.[6]

The makers of **voriconazole** suggest that patients given delavirdine should be carefully monitored for evidence of drug toxicity and/or loss of efficacy during concurrent use. They predict that the metabolism of **voriconazole** may also be induced by nevirapine, while **voriconazole** may inhibit the metabolism of NNRTIs.[3,4]

1. Borin MT, Cox SR, Herman BD, Carel BJ, Anderson RD, Freimuth WW. Effect of fluconazole on the steady-state pharmacokinetics of delavirdine in human immunodeficiency virus-positive patients. *Antimicrob Agents Chemother* (1997) 41, 1892–7.
2. Rescriptor (Delavirdine). Pharmacia & Upjohn Company. US prescribing information, June 2001.
3. VFEND (Voriconazole). Pfizer Ltd. UK Summary of product characteristics, March 2005.
4. VFEND (Voriconazole). Pfizer Ltd. US Prescribing information, March 2005.
5. Benedek IH, Fiske WD, White SJ, Kornhauser DM. Plasma levels of fluconazole (FL) are not altered by coadministration of DMP 266 in healthy volunteers. *Intersci Conf Antimicrob Agents Chemother* (1997) 37, 1.
6. Viramune (Nevirapine). Boehringer Ingelheim Ltd. UK Summary of product characteristics, April 2005.

NNRTIs + Fluoxetine

A case of serotonin syndrome in a women on fluoxetine coincided with starting a new antiretroviral regimen including efavirenz. Symptoms resolved on halving the fluoxetine dose. It was suggested that efavirenz inhibited the metabolism of fluoxetine.[1] Until further information is available, caution may be warranted.

1. DeSilva KE, Le Flore DB, Marston BJ, Rimland D. Serotonin syndrome in HIV-infected individuals receiving antiretroviral therapy and fluoxetine. *AIDS* (2001) 15, 1281–5.

NNRTIs + Food

Food has no clinically relevant effect on the levels of delavirdine, efavirenz or nevirapine. See also 'NNRTIs; Delavirdine + Acids', p.591.

Clinical evidence, mechanism, importance and management

(a) Delavirdine

A randomised crossover study in 13 HIV+ patients on delavirdine 400 mg daily found that there were no changes in the steady-state serum levels of delavirdine whether taken with or without food for 2 weeks.[1] This differed from a previous single-dose study, which had found a 26% fall in the AUC of delavirdine given with food.[2] There would appear to be no need to avoid taking delavirdine with food. For mention that orange juice increased the absorption of delavirdine in patients with gastric hypoacidity, see 'NNRTIs; Delavirdine + Acids', p.591.

(b) Efavirenz

The maker of efavirenz notes that taking a 600-mg dose with a **high-fat meal** increased the AUC by 28% when compared with fasting conditions, and increased the maximum concentration by 79%. This is not considered clinically relevant, and efavirenz may be taken with or without food.[3]

(c) Nevirapine

In a study in 24 healthy subjects it was found that a **high-fat breakfast** caused some moderate changes in the pharmacokinetics of oral nevirapine 200 mg, but the AUC was not affected and none of the changes were considered to be clinically relevant.[4] No special precautions would seem to be necessary.

1. Morse GD, Fischl MA, Cox SR, Thompson L, Della-Coletta AA, Freimuth WW. Effect of food on the steady-state (SS) pharmacokinetics of delavirdine mesylate (DLV) in HIV+ patients. *Intersci Conf Antimicrob Agents Chemother* (1995) 35, 210.
2. Cox SR, Della-Coletta AA, Turner SW, Freimuth WW. Single-dose pharmacokinetic (PK) studies with delavirdine (DLV) mesylate: dose proportionality and effects of food and antacid. *Intersci Conf Antimicrob Agents Chemother* (1994) 34, 82.
3. Sustiva (Efavirenz). Bristol-Myers Squibb Pharmaceuticals Ltd. UK Summary of product characteristics, March 2005.
4. Lamson MJ, Cort S, Sabo JP, MacGregor TR, Keirns JJ, Effects of food or antacid on the bioavailability of nevirapine 200 mg in 24 healthy volunteers. *Pharm Res* (1995) 12 (9 Suppl), S-101.

NNRTIs + Macrolides

Delavirdine may increase the levels of clarithromycin, whereas efavirenz and nevirapine may reduce them and increase the levels of clarithromycin's active metabolite. Clarithromycin does not appear to affect the pharmacokinetics of delavirdine, efavirenz or nevirapine to a clinically relevant extent. There is no pharmacokinetic interaction between azithromycin and efavirenz. A case of a neuropsychiatric reaction has been attributed to the use of clarithromycin in a man on nevirapine.

Clinical evidence

(a) Delavirdine

Clarithromycin 500 mg twice daily for 15 days did not cause a clinically significant change in the pharmacokinetics of delavirdine 300 mg three times daily in 7 HIV+ patients when compared with 4 other HIV+ patients taking only delavirdine. The combination was well tolerated and no serious events occurred.[1] However, the maker notes that the AUC of **clarithromycin** was increased by 100% by delavirdine.[2]

(b) Efavirenz

The maker notes that the concurrent use of **clarithromycin** 500 mg twice daily and efavirenz 400 mg daily for 7 days reduced the AUC of **clarithromycin** by 39% and increased the AUC of its active hydroxy metabolite by 34%. Moreover, 46% of subjects receiving the combination developed a rash.[3]

The maker also notes that there was no clinically significant pharmacokinetic interaction when a single dose of **azithromycin** was given to healthy subjects on efavirenz.[3]

(c) Nevirapine

The maker notes that the AUC of nevirapine was increased by 26% by **clarithromycin**, but this was not statistically significant. The AUC of **clarithromycin** was reduced by 30% and the AUC of its active hydroxy metabolite was increased by 58%.[4] A man developed hyperactivity (poor concentration, anxiety, suicidal and homicidal ideation) when on **clarithromycin** and antiretroviral therapy including nevirapine. This was thought to be due to accumulation of the hydroxy metabolite of **clarithromycin**.[5]

Mechanism

The cytochrome P450 isoenzyme CYP3A4 is inhibited by clarithromycin. Delavirdine is also reported to inhibit CYP3A4, whereas efavirenz and nevirapine induce CYP3A4. The NNRTIs are also substrates of this isoenzyme. Therefore alterations in the metabolism of these drugs by CYP3A4 results in the altered levels seen.

Importance and management

Not established. It appears that these macrolides have minimal effects on the pharmacokinetics of the NNRTIs. However, delavirdine may increase levels of clarithromycin. The makers of delavirdine recommend that when the drugs are used concurrently the dose of clarithromycin should be reduced only in patients with renal impairment.[2] In contrast, efavirenz and nevirapine may increase the levels of the active hydroxy metabolite of clarithromycin. The maker of nevirapine suggests that no dose adjustment of clarithromycin is needed.[4] However, the maker of efavirenz says that the clinical significance of these changes is not known, but they suggest alternatives to clarithromycin should be considered.[3] Further study and experience of the combinations is needed. Until then, caution is warranted.

1. Cox SR, Borin MT, Driver MR, Levy B, Freimuth WW. Effect of clarithromycin on the steady-state pharmacokinetics of delavirdine in HIV-1 patients. American Society for Microbiology, 2nd National Conference on Human Retroviruses, 1995. Abstract 487.
2. Rescriptor (Delavirdine). Pharmacia & Upjohn Company. US prescribing information, June 2001.
3. Sustiva (Efavirenz). Bristol-Myers Squibb Pharmaceuticals Ltd. UK Summary of product characteristics, March 2005.
4. Viramune (Nevirapine). Boehringer Ingelheim Ltd. UK Summary of product characteristics, April 2005.
5. Prime K, French P. Neuropsychiatric reaction induced by clarithromycin in a patient on highly active antiretroviral therapy (HAART). *Sex Transm Infect* (2001) 77, 297–8.

NNRTIs + NNRTIs

Nevirapine modestly reduces the levels of efavirenz, whereas efavirenz has no effect on nevirapine levels.

Clinical evidence, mechanism, importance and management

The steady-state pharmacokinetics of **nevirapine** were not altered by **efavirenz** in one study in 14 patients. However, the AUC of **efavirenz** was reduced by 22% and the minimum plasma concentration by 36%.[1] The maker of **nevirapine** suggests that a dose increase of **efavirenz** to 800 mg once daily may be warranted when used concurrently.[1]

1. Viramune (Nevirapine). Boehringer Ingelheim Ltd. UK Summary of product characteristics, April 2005.

NNRTIs + NRTIs

Delavirdine absorption is reduced by the buffered preparation of didanosine and therefore doses should be given at least an hour apart. This interaction would not be expected with the enteric-coated preparation of didanosine. Delavirdine does not affect the pharmacokinetics of zidovudine. There is no pharmacokinetic interaction between efavirenz and zidovudine with lamivudine. There is no clinically relevant pharmacokinetic interaction between nevirapine and didanosine, lamivudine, stavudine, zalcitabine or zidovudine.

Clinical evidence, mechanism, importance and management

(a) Delavirdine

A study in 34 HIV+ patients stabilised on **zidovudine** 200 mg three times daily found that delavirdine mesilate 400 to 1200 mg daily for 9 days had no clinically significant effect on the pharmacokinetics of **zidovudine**.[1]

In a steady-state study, 9 HIV+ patients stabilised on **didanosine** 200 mg twice times daily were also given delavirdine mesilate 400 mg three times daily for 14 days. **Didanosine** caused a 37% reduction in the maximum delavirdine serum levels, but when the drugs were given 1 hour apart no significant effect occurred.[2] A single-dose study in 12 HIV+ patients found similar results.[3] The buffered preparation of **didanosine** contains antacids to increase its absorption, and antacids decrease the absorption of delavirdine (see 'NNRTIs + Antacids, H_2-blockers or Proton pump inhibitors', p.585). The authors of one report suggest that separating the doses by about one hour is preferable.[2] The enteric-coated preparation of **didanosine**, which does not contain antacids, would not be expected to reduce the absorption of delavirdine.

(b) Efavirenz

The maker notes that there were no clinically significant pharmacokinetic interactions between efavirenz and the combination of **zidovudine** and **lamivudine** in patients with HIV.[4]

(c) Nevirapine

The pharmacokinetics of **didanosine** and **zidovudine** with or without nevirapine were assessed in 175 HIV+ subjects. The bioavailability of **didanosine** was not affected, but the bioavailability of **zidovudine** was decreased by about one-third by nevirapine.[5] In a steady-state study in 24 HIV+ patients, nevirapine 200 mg every 12 hours was added to regimens of **didanosine** or **didanosine** with **zidovudine** or **zidovudine** with **zalcitabine** for a 4-week period. No significant changes in the pharmacokinetics of **didanosine** or **zalcitabine** were seen. However, in the **didanosine/zidovudine** group the peak **zidovudine** plasma levels and AUC were reduced by 27% and 32% respectively. The **zidovudine** pharmacokinetics in the **zidovudine/zalcitabine** group were not affected.[6] The reasons for these changes are not clear, but the clinical consequences are thought to be small, and the safety data indicate that the concurrent use of these drugs is safe and well tolerated. The makers say that no dosage adjustments are needed if **didanosine**, **zalcitabine** or **zidovudine** is taken with nevirapine.[7]

The makers also state that nevirapine had no effect on the AUC of **stavudine** in a study in 25 patients, and that nevirapine appears to have no effect on **lamivudine** clearance, based on a population pharmacokinetic study.[7]

1. Morse GD, Cox SR, DeRemer MF, Batts DH, Freimuth WW. Zidovudine (ZDV) pharmacokinetics (PK) during an escalating, multiple-dose study of delavirdine (DLV) mesylate. *Intersci Conf Antimicrob Agents Chemother* (1994) 34, 132.
2. Cox SR, Cohn SE, Greisberger C, Reichman RC, Della-Coletta AA, Freimuth WW, Morse GD. Evaluation of the steady-state (SS) pharmacokinetic interaction between didanosine (ddI) and delavirdine mesylate (DLV) in HIV+ patients. *Intersci Conf Antimicrob Agents Chemother* (1995) 35, 210.
3. Morse GD, Fischl MA, Shelton MJ, Cox SR, Driver M, DeRemer M, Freimuth WW. Single-dose pharmacokinetics of delavirdine mesylate and didanosine in patients with human immunodeficiency virus infection. *Antimicrob Agents Chemother* (1997) 41, 169–74.
4. Sustiva (Efavirenz). Bristol-Myers Squibb Pharmaceuticals Ltd. UK Summary of product characteristics, March 2005.
5. Zhou XJ, Sheiner LB, D'Aquila RT, Hughes MD, Hirsch MS, Fischl MA, Johnson VA, Myers M, Sommadossi JP and the NIAID ACTG241 Investigators. Population pharmacokinetics of nevirapine, zidovudine and didanosine after combination therapy in HIV-infected patients. *Clin Pharmacol Ther* (1998) 63,182.
6. MacGregor TR, Lamson MJ, Cort S, Pav JW, Saag MS, Elvin AT, Sommadossi J-P, Myers M, Keirns JJ. Steady state pharmacokinetics of nevirapine, didanosine, zalcitabine, and zidovudine combination therapy in HIV-1 positive patients. *Pharm Res* (1995) 12 (9 Suppl), S-101.
7. Viramune (Nevirapine). Boehringer Ingelheim Ltd. UK Summary of product characteristics, April 2005.

NNRTIs + Protease inhibitors

In general, efavirenz and nevirapine decrease the levels of protease inhibitors, whereas delavirdine has the opposite effect. Ritonavir is used to elevate levels of other protease inhibitors, and has been tried for this purpose when efavirenz or nevirapine are required. Amprenavir and nelfinavir decrease the levels of delavirdine. The protease inhibitors do not appear to affect the levels of efavirenz or nevirapine.

Clinical evidence, mechanism, importance and management

(a) Delavirdine

For a summary of the studies of the pharmacokinetic interactions of delavirdine and various protease inhibitors, see 'Table 19.3', (below). In general, these studies show that delavirdine can markedly increase protease inhibitor exposure. In addition, **amprenavir** and **nelfinavir** have been shown to approximately halve the AUC of delavirdine.

Delavirdine and the protease inhibitors are known to be both inhibitors of, and metabolised by, the cytochrome P450 isoenzyme CYP3A4, see 'Table 19.2', (p.580).

It has been suggested that delavirdine could be used clinically to boost the exposure to protease inhibitors, and this has been tried in at least one study.[1] However, this combination is complicated by the reduction in delavirdine levels with some protease inhibitors, and the combination may not be appropriate if the antiviral effect of delavirdine is required.[2] Moreover, if the combination is used, patients should be closely monitored for toxicity since in one study of **nelfinavir** and delavirdine, 4 out of 24 subjects had to stop both drugs before completing the study because of neutropenia, which resolved over several days.[3] Further study is needed to determine the appropriate dosage regimens for concurrent use.

(b) Efavirenz

For a summary of the studies of the pharmacokinetic interactions of efavirenz and various protease inhibitors, see 'Table 19.3', (below). None of the protease inhibitors affected efavirenz levels. Efavirenz is an inducer of the cytochrome P450 isoenzyme CYP3A4, and so would be expected to reduce the levels of the protease inhibitors.

Two reports in patients with HIV have shown that using efavirenz with **amprenavir** results in sub-therapeutic **amprenavir** levels, and that the addition of low-dose **ritonavir** reverses this effect[4,5] (see also 'Protease inhibitors + Protease inhibitors', p.614). Authors of another study have suggested that if **amprenavir** is to be used with efavirenz, the dose of **amprenavir** should be increased to 1200 mg three times daily to ensure the minimum serum levels remain high enough for sufficient antiretroviral activity.[6]

Table 19.3 Summary of the pharmacokinetic interactions of NNRTIs and protease inhibitors

Drug combination	*No. of healthy subjects (unless specified)*	*Change in AUC (unless specified)*		*Refs*
		NNRTI	*Protease inhibitor*	
Delavirdine studies (usually 400 mg three times daily or 600 mg twice daily)				
Amprenavir	6 HIV+ children		3-fold increase in Cmax[a] 5 to 10-fold increase in Cmin[a]	1
Amprenavir 1200 mg Amprenavir 1200 mg twice daily alone then 600 mg twice daily in combination	12 11	21% increase 47% decrease	4-fold increase 32% increase vs twice the dose given alone	2
Amprenavir 600 mg twice daily	18	61% decrease	130% increase	3
Indinavir 800 mg alone then 600 mg in combination	14	No change	44% increase vs higher dose given alone	4, 5
Nelfinavir 750 mg three times daily	24	42% decrease	92% increase	6
Ritonavir 300 mg twice daily	Not stated	No change in steady state level	No change in steady state level	4
Ritonavir 600 mg twice daily	12 HIV+	No change[a]	64% increase 81% increase in Cmin	7
Ritonavir 100 mg twice daily	19	No change	80% increase	8
Saquinavir 600 mg three times daily		No change in steady state level	5-fold increase in steady state level	4
Efavirenz studies (600 mg once daily)				
Amprenavir	2 HIV+ children		Undetectable levels in less than 4 hours[b]	1
Amprenavir 1200 mg twice daily	7 HIV+		About an 80% decrease in trough levels[b]	9
Amprenavir 1200 mg twice daily	11 HIV+	No change[a]	24% decrease 43% decrease in Cmin	10
Indinavir 800 mg three times daily alone then 1000 mg three times daily in combination			33% to 46% decrease vs lower dose given alone	11
Indinavir 800 mg with Ritonavir 100 mg twice daily	14	No change[a]	25% decrease (indinavir) 36% decrease (ritonavir)	12
Nelfinavir 750 mg three times daily		No change	20% increase	13
Saquinavir 1200 mg three times daily			62% decrease	11
Ritonavir 400 mg twice daily with Saquinavir 400 mg twice daily	12	No change[a]	No change in Cmin (ritonavir) 10% decrease in Cmin (saquinavir)	14
Nevirapine studies (200 mg once daily increased to twice daily)				
Indinavir 800 mg three times daily	19 HIV+	No change[a]	28% decrease 48% decrease in Cmin	15

Continued

Table 19.3 Summary of the pharmacokinetic interactions of NNRTIs and protease inhibitors *(continued)*

Drug combination	*No. of healthy subjects (unless specified)*	*Change in AUC (unless specified)*		*Refs*
		NNRTI	*Protease inhibitor*	
Indinavir 800 mg three times daily alone or 1000 mg three times daily in combination	124 HIV+	No change	27% decrease in Cmin vs therapy alone at lower dose	16
Lopinavir/ritonavir 300/75 mg/m^2 twice daily	27 HIV+ children		22% decrease, 55% decrease in Cmin (lopinavir)	17
Nelfinavir 750 mg three times daily	7 HIV+	No change[a]	50% decrease	18
Nelfinavir 750 mg three times daily	12 HIV+	No change[a]	No change	19, 20
Nelfinavir 750 mg three times daily	13 HIV+		No change	21
Ritonavir 600 mg twice daily	25 HIV+	No change	No change	22
Saquinavir 600 mg three times daily	21 HIV+	No change	27% decrease	23
Saquinavir/ritonavir	20 HIV+	No change[a]	No change	22

[a] Versus historical control data

[b] Therapeutic levels subsequently acheived by the addition of low-dose ritonavir

1. Wintergerst U, Engelhorn C, Kurowski M, Hoffmann F, Notheis G, Belohradsky BH. Pharmacokinetic interaction of amprenavir in combination with efavirenz or delavirdine in HIV-infected children. *AIDS* (2000) 14, 1866–8.
2. Tran JQ, Petersen C, Garrett M, Hee B, Kerr BM. Pharmacokinetic interaction between amprenavir and delavirdine: evidence of induced clearance by amprenavir. *Clin Pharmacol Ther* (2002) 72, 615–26.
3. Justesen US, Klitgaard NA, Brosen K, Pedersen C. Pharmacokinetic interaction between amprenavir and delavirdine after multiple-dose administration in healthy volunteers. *Br J Clin Pharmacol* (2003) 55, 100–6.
4. Cox SR, Ferry JJ, Batts DH, Carlson GF, Schneck DW, Herman BD, Della-Coletta AA, Chambers JH, Carel BJ, Stewart F, Buss N, Brown A. Delavirdine (D) and marketed protease inhibitors (PIs): pharmacokinetic (PK) interaction studies in healthy volunteers. 4th Conference on Retroviruses and Opportunistic Infections, Washington, 1997. Abstract 372.
5. Ferry JJ, Herman BD, Carel BJ, Carlson GF, Batts DH. Pharmacokinetic drug-drug interaction study of delavirdine and indinavir in healthy volunteers. *J Acquir Immune Defic Syndr Hum Retrovirol* (1998) 18, 252–9.
6. Cox SR, Schneck DW, Herman BD, Carel BJ, Gullotti BR, Kerr BM, Freimuth WW. Delavirdine (DLV) and nelfinavir (NFV): A pharmacokinetic (PK) drug-drug interaction study in healthy adult volunteers. 5th Conference on Retroviruses and Opportunistic Infections, Chicago, 1998. Abstract 345.
7. Shelton MJ, Hewitt RG, Adams J, Della-Coletta A, Cox S, Morse GD. Pharmacokinetics of ritonavir and delavirdine in human immunodeficiency virus-infected patients. *Antimicrob Agents Chemother* (2003) 47, 1694–9.
8. Tran JQ, Petersen C, Garrett M, Smith M, Hee B, Lillibridge J, Kerr B. Delavirdine significantly increases exposure of low dose ritonavir in healthy volunteers. *Intersci Conf Antimicrob Agents Chemother* (2001) 41, 15.
9. Duval X, Le Moing V, Longuet P, Leport C, Vildé J-L, Lamotte C, Peytavin G, Farinotti R. Efavirenz-induced decrease in plasma amprenavir levels in human immunodeficiency virus-infected patients and correction by ritonavir. *Antimicrob Agents Chemother* (2000) 44, 2593.
10. Falloon J, Piscitelli S, Vogel S, Sadler B, Mitsuya H, Kavlick MF, Yoshimura K, Rogers M, LaFon S, Manion DJ, Lane HC, Masur H. Combination therapy with amprenavir, abacavir, and efavirenz in human immunodeficiency virus (HIV)-infected patients failing a protease-inhibitor regimen: pharmacokinetic drug interactions and antiviral activity. *Clin Infect Dis* (2000) 30, 313–18.
11. Sustiva (Efavirenz). Bristol-Myers Squibb Pharmaceuticals Ltd. UK Summary of product characteristics, March 2005.
12. Aarnoutse RE, Grintjes KJT, Telgt DSC, Stek M, Hugen PWH, Reiss P, Koopmans PP, Hekster YA, Burger DM. The influence of efavirenz on the pharmacokinetics of a twice-daily combination of indinavir and low-dose ritonavir in healthy volunteers. *Clin Pharmacol Ther* (2002) 71, 57–67.
13. Fiske WD, Benedek IH, White SJ, Pepperess KA, Joseph JL, Kornhauser DM. Pharmacokinetic interaction between efavirenz (EFV) and nelfinavir mesylate (NFV) in healthy volunteers. 5th Conference on Retroviruses and Opportunistic Infections, Chicago, 1998. Abstract 349.
14. Piliero PJ, Preston SL, Japour A, Stevens RC, Morvillo C, Drusano GL. Pharmacokinetics of the combination of ritonavir plus saquinavir, with and without efavirenz, in healthy volunteers. *Intersci Conf Antimicrob Agents Chemother* (2001) 41, 15.
15. Murphy RL, Sommadossi J-P, Lamson M, Hall DB, Myers M, Dusek A. Antiviral effect and pharmacokinetic interaction between nevirapine and indinavir in persons infected with human immunodeficiency virus type 1. *J Infect Dis* (1999) 179, 1116–23.
16. Launay O, Peytavin G, Flandre P, Gerard L, Levy C, Joly V, Aboulker JP, Yeni P. Pharmacokinetic (PK) interaction between nevirapine (NVP) and indinavir (IDV) in ANRS 081 trial. *Intersci Conf Antimicrob Agents Chemother* (2000) 40, 331.
17. Hsu A, Bertz R, Renz C, Lam W, Rode R, Deetz C, Schweitzer SM, Berstein B, Brun S, Granneman GR, Sun E. Assessment of the pharmacokinetic interaction between lopinavir/ritonavir (ABT-378/r) and nevirapine (NVP) in HIV-infected pediatric subjects. *AIDS* (2000) 14 (Suppl. 4), S100.
18. Merry C, Barry MG, Mulcahy F, Ryan M, Tjia JF, Halifax KL, Breckenridge AM, Back DJ. The pharmacokinetics of combination therapy with nelfinavir plus nevirapine. *AIDS* (1998) 12, 1163–7.
19. Skowron G, Leoung G, Dusek A, Anderson R, Grosso R, Lamson M, Beebe S. Stavudine (d4T), nelfinavir (NFV) and nevirapine (NVP): Preliminary safety, activity and pharmacokinetic (PK) interactions. 5th Conference on Retroviruses and Opportunistic Infections, Chicago, 1998. Abstract 350.
20. Skowron G, Leoung G, Kerr B, Dusek A, Anderson R, Beebe S, Grosso R. Lack of pharmacokinetic interaction between nelfinavir and nevirapine. AIDS (1998) 12, 1243–4.
21. Vilaro J, Mascaro J, Colomer J, Cucurull J, Garcia D, Yanez A. The pharmacokinetics of combination therapy with nelfinavir (NFV) plus nevirapine (NVP) in HIV positive patients. *Intersci Conf Antimicrob Agents Chemother* (2001) 41, 16.
22. Viramune (Nevirapine). Boehringer Ingelheim LTD. UK Summary of product characteristics, April 2005.
23. Sahai J, Cameron W, Salgo M, Stewart F, Myers M, Lamson M, Gagnier P. Drug interaction study between saquinavir (SQV) and nevirapine (NVP). 4th Conference on Retroviruses and Opportunistic Infections, Washington, 1997. Abstract 613.

Similarly, the doses of **atazanavir**,[7] **indinavir**[8] or **indinavir** with **ritonavir**[9] may need to be increased when efavirenz is used. The maker of **atazanavir** recommends that the dose should be increased from 300 mg to 400 mg when used with efavirenz 600 mg daily.[7] The maker of efavirenz suggests that **indinavir** 1 g every 8 hours should be used.[8] The maker also notes that efavirenz markedly reduced **saquinavir** concentrations, and advises that **saquinavir** should not be used as the sole protease inhibitor with efavirenz.[8] Another study showed that **ritonavir** with **saquinavir** were little affected by efavirenz.[10] However, the maker notes that increased adverse effects including elevated transaminase levels occurred with the combination of efavirenz and **ritonavir**, and consequently recommends monitoring of liver enzyme levels with this combination.[8] **Nelfinavir** levels were modestly increased by 20% by efavirenz in one study, but no dose modification was considered necessary.[11]

If efavirenz is used with protease inhibitors, therapy should be closely monitored.

(c) Nevirapine

For a summary of the studies of the pharmacokinetic interactions of nevirapine and various protease inhibitors, see 'Table 19.3', (p.588). The protease inhibitors do not appear to affect the levels of nevirapine. Nevirapine is an inducer of the cytochrome P450 isoenzyme CYP3A4, and so would be expected to reduce the levels of some of the protease inhibitors (see 'Table 19.2', (p.580)).

Nevirapine decreases exposure to **indinavir**. The authors of one study concluded that no change to the **indinavir** dosage would be required, unless other parameters (e.g. the viral load) suggested it was necessary.[12] However, other researchers suggested that the **indinavir** dose may need to be increased from 800 mg to 1 g three times daily in the presence of nevirapine.[13]

Two studies have shown that nevirapine had no effect on **nelfinavir** levels,[14,15] whereas another study reported a 50% decrease in the **nelfinavir** AUC.[16] This latter finding may be due to sampling before **nelfinavir** had reached steady state, particularly as it undergoes autoinduction of metabolism.[17] It is likely that no dosage changes in **nelfinavir** are required, although some recommend an increase as a precaution.[18]

Nevirapine modestly reduced the levels of **lopinavir** in children.[19] The maker of nevirapine suggests that a dose increase of **lopinavir/ritonavir** may be considered where reduced susceptibility is suspected.[20]

Nevirapine modestly reduced the levels of **saquinavir**.[21] The importance of this is uncertain, but the makers of nevirapine point out that this may possibly be significant because the serum levels of **saquinavir** achieved with hard gelatin capsules are already marginal.[20] Nevirapine had no clinically significant pharmacokinetic effect on the combination of **saquinavir** with **ritonavir**[20] or on **ritonavir** alone,[20] and no dosage adjustments are required.

If nevirapine is used with protease inhibitors, therapy should be closely monitored.

1. Harris M, Alexander C, O'Shaughnessy M, Montaner JSG. Delavirdine increases drug exposure of ritonavir-boosted protease inhibitors. *AIDS* (2002) 16, 798–9.
2. Justesen US, Klitgaard NA, Brosen K, Pedersen C. Pharmacokinetic interaction between amprenavir and delavirdine after multiple-dose administration in healthy volunteers. *Br J Clin Pharmacol* (2003) 55, 100–6.
3. Cox SR, Schneck DW, Herman BD, Carel BJ, Gullotti BR, Kerr BM, Freimuth WW. Delavirdine (DLV) and nelfinavir (NFV): A pharmacokinetic (PK) drug-drug interaction study in healthy adult volunteers. 5th Conference on Retroviruses and Opportunistic Infections, Chicago, 1998. Abstract 345.
4. Wintergerst U, Engelhorn C, Kurowski M, Hoffmann F, Notheis G, Belohradsky BH. Pharmacokinetic interaction of amprenavir in combination with efavirenz or delavirdine in HIV-infected children. *AIDS* (2000) 14, 1866–8.
5. Duval X, Le Moing V, Longuet P, Leport C, Vildé J-L, Lamotte C, Peytavin G, Farinotti R. Efavirenz-induced decrease in plasma amprenavir levels in human immunodeficiency virus-infected patients and correction by ritonavir. *Antimicrob Agents Chemother* (2000) 44, 2593.
6. Falloon J, Piscitelli S, Vogel S, Sadler B, Mitsuya H, Kavlick MF, Yoshimura K, Rogers M, LaFon S, Manion DJ, Lane HC, Masur H. Combination therapy with amprenavir, abacavir, and efavirenz in human immunodeficiency virus (HIV)-infected patients failing a protease-inhibitor regimen: pharmacokinetic drug interactions and antiviral activity. *Clin Infect Dis* (2000) 30, 313–18.
7. Reyataz Hard Capsules (Atazanavir). Bristol-Myers Squibb Pharmaceuticals Ltd. UK Summary of product characteristics, February 2005.
8. Sustiva (Efavirenz). Bristol-Myers Squibb Pharmaceuticals Ltd. UK Summary of product characteristics, March 2005.
9. Aarnoutse RE, Grintjes KJT, Telgt DSC, Stek M, Hugen PWH, Reiss P, Koopmans PP, Hekster YA, Burger DM. The influence of efavirenz on the pharmacokinetics of a twice-daily combination of indinavir and low-dose ritonavir in healthy volunteers. *Clin Pharmacol Ther* (2002) 71, 57–67.
10. Piliero PJ, Preston SL, Japour A, Stevens RC, Morvillo C, Drusano GL. Pharmacokinetics of the combination of ritonavir plus saquinavir, with and without efavirenz, in healthy volunteers. *Intersci Conf Antimicrob Agents Chemother* (2001) 41, 15.
11. Fiske WD, Benedek IH, White SJ, Pepperess KA, Joseph JL, Kornhauser DM. Pharmacokinetic interaction between efavirenz (EFV) and nelfinavir mesylate (NFV) in healthy volunteers. 5th Conference on Retroviruses and Opportunistic Infections, Chicago, 1998. Abstract 349.
12. Murphy RL, Sommadossi J-P, Lamson M, Hall DB, Myers M, Dusek A. Antiviral effect and pharmacokinetic interaction between nevirapine and indinavir in persons infected with human immunodeficiency virus type 1. *J Infect Dis* (1999) 179, 1116–23.
13. Launay O, Peytavin G, Flandre P, Gerard L, Levy C, Joly V, Aboulker JP, Yeni P. Pharmacokinetic (PK) interaction between nevirapine (NVP) and indinavir (IDV) in ANRS 081 trial. *Intersci Conf Antimicrob Agents Chemother* (2000) 40, 331.
14. Skowron G, Leoung G, Dusek A, Anderson R, Grosso R, Lamson M, Beebe S. Stavudine (d4T), nelfinavir (NFV) and nevirapine (NVP): Preliminary safety, activity and pharmacokinetic (PK) interactions. 5th Conference on Retroviruses and Opportunistic Infections, Chicago, 1998. Abstract 350.
15. Vilaro J, Mascaro J, Colomer J, Cucurull J, Garcia D, Yanez A. The pharmacokinetics of combination therapy with nelfinavir (NFV) plus nevirapine (NVP) in HIV positive patients. *Intersci Conf Antimicrob Agents Chemother* (2001) 41, 16.
16. Merry C, Barry MG, Mulcahy F, Ryan M, Tjia JF, Halifax KL, Breckenridge AM, Back DJ. The pharmacokinetics of combination therapy with nelfinavir plus nevirapine. *AIDS* (1998) 12, 1163–7.
17. Skowron G, Leoung G, Kerr B, Dusek A, Anderson R, Beebe S, Grosso R. Lack of pharmacokinetic interaction between nelfinavir and nevirapine. *AIDS* (1998) 12, 1243–4.
18. Mulcahy F, Barry M, Merry C, Back D. Nelfinavir and nevirapine interaction? *AIDS* (1998) 12, 2361.
19. Hsu A, Bertz R, Renz C, Lam W, Rode R, Deetz C, Schweitzer SM, Berstein B, Brun S, Granneman GR, Sun E. Assessment of the pharmacokinetic interaction between lopinavir/ritonavir (ABT-378/r) and nevirapine (NVP) in HIV-infected pediatric subjects. *AIDS* (2000) 14 (Suppl. 4), S100.
20. Viramune (Nevirapine). Boehringer Ingelheim Ltd. UK Summary of product characteristics, April 2005.
21. Sahai J, Cameron W, Salgo M, Stewart F, Myers M, Lamson M, Gagnier P. Drug interaction study between saquinavir (SQV) and nevirapine (NVP). 4th Conference on Retroviruses and Opportunistic Infections, Washington, 1997. Abstract 613.

NNRTIs + Rifamycins

Rifabutin and rifampicin (rifampin) cause a very marked fall in delavirdine serum levels. Rifabutin does not affect efavirenz or nevirapine levels, whereas rifampicin causes a moderate fall in efavirenz and nevirapine levels. Delavirdine may increase rifabutin levels. Efavirenz may decrease rifabutin levels. Nevirapine does not appear to affect rifabutin or rifampicin levels.

Clinical evidence, mechanism, importance and management

(a) Delavirdine

A controlled study in 7 HIV+ patients on delavirdine mesilate 400 mg three times daily for 30 days found that the addition of **rifabutin** 300 mg daily from days 16 to 30 caused a fivefold increase in the delavirdine clearance, and an 84% fall in the steady-state plasma levels.[1] This was presumably due to the enzyme inducing effects of the **rifabutin**. A similar study using **rifampicin** in place of **rifabutin** found that **rifampicin** caused a 27-fold increase in clearance of delavirdine, and the steady-state plasma levels became almost undetectable.[2]

In another study,[3] where the dose of delavirdine was titrated to achieve a trough level of at least 5 micromol/l, the AUC of **rifabutin** was found to increase by 242%.

It has been recommended that the combination of delavirdine and **rifampicin** should be considered as contraindicated because the effects of the interaction are so large.[2] The US Centers for Disease Control and Prevention recommends that neither **rifabutin** nor **rifampicin** should be used with delavirdine.[4]

(b) Efavirenz

The concurrent use of efavirenz 600 mg once daily and **rifabutin** 300 mg once daily for 2 weeks resulted in a modest decrease in **rifabutin** levels, but no change in efavirenz levels in a study in 24 healthy subjects.[5] The US Centers for Disease Control and Prevention state that the combination is probably clinically useful, and they suggest increasing the dose of **rifabutin** to 450 mg or 600 mg daily, or 600 mg two to three times weekly.[4] However, in one analysis, 8 of 35 patients (23%) on efavirenz given **rifabutin** 450 mg once daily were found to have subtherapeutic **rifabutin** levels, and they were switched to isoniazid therapy.[6] Concurrent use should therefore be closely monitored.

The concurrent use of HAART including efavirenz 600 mg once daily with antitubercular therapy including **rifampicin** 480 to 720 mg daily decreased the efavirenz AUC by 22% and the trough concentration by 25% (although large interpatient variability was observed) in patients with HIV and tuberculosis. Overall the pharmacokinetics of efavirenz 800 mg daily with **rifampicin** were similar to those of efavirenz 600 mg daily without **rifampicin**. The pharmacokinetics of **rifampicin** were not substantially altered by efavirenz.[7] Similar findings were reported in a study in healthy subjects.[8] The authors of the first study suggest that it may be advisable to increase the efavirenz dose to 800 mg daily when used with **rifampicin**,[7] and the UK maker also recommends this.[9]

(c) Nevirapine

Results of a clinical study from the makers of nevirapine showed that the pharmacokinetics of nevirapine were only minimally affected by **rifabutin** in 19 patients, when compared with historical data.[10] The UK maker notes that concurrent use of **rifabutin** with nevirapine caused clinically insignificant changes in **rifabutin** and nevirapine pharmacokinetics. The only statistically significant changes were a 9% increase in nevirapine clearance and a 20% increase in maximum steady-state **rifabutin** levels.[11]

The maker states that the AUC of nevirapine was reduced by 58% by **rifampicin** in 14 subjects, when compared with historical data.[11] There was no change in steady-state **rifampicin** pharmacokinetics.[11] A study in HIV+ patients with tuberculosis found that the **rifampicin** caused a 31% decrease in nevirapine AUC and a non-significant 21% decrease in trough concentration.[12]

Based on the available pharmacokinetic data, the maker suggests that the concurrent use of **rifampicin** with nevirapine is not recommended, and that **rifabutin** may be considered instead, with close monitoring of adverse effects.[11] The US Centers for Disease Control and Prevention state that the combination of nevirapine and **rifabutin** can be used, while the combination of nevirapine and **rifampicin** should only be used if clearly indicated and with careful monitoring, because of insufficient data on whether dose adjustments are necessary.[4] However, it has been suggested that there is probably no need to increase the nevirapine dose, since the trough levels were still sufficiently above the level needed for antiviral activity.[12] Moreover, subsequent observational data supported the continued efficacy of nevirapine when it was used with **rifampicin**.[13] Similarly, others have reported the successful use of nevirapine with twice weekly **rifampicin** with little effect on trough nevirapine levels.[14] Further study is needed.

1. Borin MT, Chambers JH, Carel BJ, Freimuth WW, Aksentijevich S, Piergies AA. Pharmacokinetic study of the interaction between rifabutin and delavirdine mesylate in HIV-1 infected patients. *Antiviral Res* (1997) 35, 53–63.
2. Borin MT, Chambers JH, Carel BJ, Gagnon S, Freimuth WW. Pharmacokinetic study of the interaction between rifampin and delavirdine mesylate. *Clin Pharmacol Ther* (1997) 61, 544–53.
3. Cox SR, Herman BD, Batts DH, et al. Delavirdine and rifabutin: pharmacokinetic evaluation in HIV-1 patients with concentration-targeting of delavirdine [abstract no. 344]. 5th Conference on Retroviruses and Opportunistic Infections, Chicago, 1998.
4. Centers for Disease Control and Prevention. Updated guidelines for the use of rifamycins for the treatment of tuberculosis among HIV-infected patients taking protease inhibitors or non-nucleoside reverse transcriptase inhibitors. *MMWR* (2004) 53, 37.
5. Benedek IH, Fiske WD, White SJ, Stevenson D, Joseph JL, Kornhauser DM. Pharmacokinetic interaction between multiple doses of efavirenz and rifabutin in healthy volunteers [abstract no. 461]. *Clin Infect Dis* (1998) 27, 1008.
6. Spradling P, Drociuk D, McLaughlin S, Lee LM, Peloquin CA, Gallicano K, Pozsik C, Onorato I, Castro KG, Ridzon R. Drug-drug interactions in inmates treated for human immunodeficiency virus and *Mycobacterium tuberculosis* infection or disease: an institutional tuberculosis outbreak. *Clin Infect Dis* (2002) 35, 1106–12.
7. López-Cortés LF, Ruiz-Valderas R, Viciana P, Alarcón-González A, Gómez-Mateos J, León-Jimenez E, Sarasa-Nacenta M, López-Pua Y, Pachón J. Pharmacokinetic interactions between efavirenz and rifampicin in HIV-infected patients with tuberculosis. *Clin Pharmacokinet* (2002) 41, 681–90.
8. Benedek I, Joshi A, Fiske WD, et al. Pharmacokinetic interaction between efavirenz and rifampin in healthy volunteers. *12th World AIDS Conference;* (1998) June 28-Jul 3; Geneva, 829.
9. Sustiva (Efavirenz). Bristol-Myers Squibb Pharmaceuticals Ltd. UK Summary of product characteristics, March 2005.
10. Maldonado S, Lamson M, Gigliotti M, Pav JW, Robinson P. Pharmacokinetic interaction between nevirapine and rifabutin. *Intersci Conf Antimicrob Agents Chemother* (1999) 39, 21.
11. Viramune (Nevirapine). Boehringer Ingelheim Ltd. UK Summary of product characteristics, April 2005.
12. Ribera E, Pou L, Lopez RM, Crespo M, Falco V, Ocaña I, Ruiz I, Pahissa A. Pharmacokinetic interaction between nevirapine and rifampicin in HIV-infected patients with tuberculosis. *J Acquir Immune Defic Syndr* (2001) 28, 450–3.
13. Oliva J, Moreno S, Sanz J, Ribera E, Pérez Molina JAÒ, Rubio R, Casas E, Mariño A. Coadministration of rifampin and nevirapine in HIV-infected patients with tuberculosis. *AIDS* (2003) 17, 637–8.
14. Dean GL, Back DJ, de Ruiter A. Effect of tuberculosis therapy on nevirapine trough plasma concentrations. *AIDS* (1999) 13, 2489–90.

NNRTIs + St John's wort *(Hypericum perforatum)*

There is evidence that St John's wort may decrease blood levels of nevirapine, and this would also be expected for delavirdine and efavirenz.

Clinical evidence, mechanism, importance and management

Routine clinic plasma levels of **nevirapine** were noted to be lower in 5 men who were also taking St John's wort. Based on a pharmacokinetic modelling analysis, it was estimated that St John's wort increased the oral clearance of **nevirapine** by about 35%.[1] This finding supports predictions based on the known metabolism of non-nucleoside reverse transcriptase inhibitors involving the cytochrome P450 isoenzyme CYP3A4 (see 'Table 19.2', (p.580)). It confirms advice issued by the UK Committee on Safety of Medicines,[2] that St John's wort may decrease blood levels of the non-nucleoside reverse transcriptase inhibitors with possible loss of HIV suppression, so combined use should be avoided.

1. de Maat MMR, Hoetelmans RMW, Mathôt RAA, van Gorp ECM, Meenhorst PL, Mulder JW, Beijnen JH. Drug interaction between St John's wort and nevirapine. *AIDS* (2001) 15, 420–1.
2. Committee on Safety of Medicines. Message from Professor A Breckenridge (Chairman of CSM) and Fact Sheet for Health Care Professionals, 29th February 2000.

NNRTIs + Tenofovir

The maker briefly notes that there was no pharmacokinetic interaction between tenofovir and efavirenz.[1,2] Some clinical data have shown a high rate of treatment failure with a once daily combination of tenofovir 300 mg, enteric-coated didanosine 250 mg and either efavirenz 600 mg once daily or nevirapine 400 mg once daily.[3] These combinations should be used with caution.[3]

1. Viread (Tenofovir disoproxil fumarate). Gilead Sciences International Ltd. UK Summary of product characteristics, March 2005.
2. Viread (Tenofovir disoproxil). Gilead Sciences Inc. US prescribing information, May 2005.
3. Hodder SL. Re: Important new clinical data. Potential early virologic failure associated with the combination antiretroviral regimen of tenofovir disoproxil fumarate, didanosine, and either efavirenz or nevirapine in HIV treatment-naïve patients with high baseline viral loads. Bristol-Myers Squibb Company, November 2004. Available at: http://www.fda.gov/aashi/aids/listserv/bms.pdf (accessed 04/07/05).

NNRTIs; Delavirdine + Acids

In patients with poor gastric acid production, orange juice and glutamic acid increase the absorption of delavirdine.

Clinical evidence, mechanism, importance and management

When **glutamic acid** 1.36 g three times daily was given with delavirdine 400 mg three times daily to 8 HIV+ subjects with gastric hypoacidity, the AUC of delavirdine was increased by 50%.[1] Similarly, **orange juice** increased delavirdine absorption by 50% to 70% in subjects with gastric hypoacidity, but had less effect (0 to 30%) in those with normal gastric acidity. However, despite the use of **orange juice,** the AUC of delavirdine was still about 50% lower in patients with gastric hypoacidity than those without.[2]

Delavirdine is a weak base that is poorly soluble at neutral pH (note that antacids reduce its absorption, see 'NNRTIs + Antacids, H_2-blockers or Proton pump inhibitors', p.585). Therefore, in subjects with gastric hypoacidity, absorption of delavirdine is reduced, and substances that lower gastric pH increase its absorption. However, the clinical value of using **glutamic acid** or acidic beverages with delavirdine is unknown.

1. Morse GD, Adams JM, Shelton MJ, Hewitt RG, Cox SR, Chambers JH. Gastric acidification increases delavirdine mesylate (DLV) exposure in HIV+ subjects with gastric hypoacidity (GH). *Clin Pharmacol Ther* (1996) 59, 141.
2. Shelton MJ, Hewitt RG, Adams JM, Cox SR, Chambers JH, Morse GD. Delavirdine malabsorption in HIV-infected subjects with spontaneous gastric hypoacidity. *J Clin Pharmacol* (2003) 43, 171–9.

NRTIs + Aciclovir or Famciclovir

The concurrent use of zidovudine and aciclovir normally appears to be uneventful, but an isolated report describes overwhelming fatigue in one patient given zidovudine and intravenous aciclovir. Famciclovir did not alter the pharmacokinetics of zidovudine or emtricitabine.

Clinical evidence, mechanism, importance and management

(a) Aciclovir

A study in 20 HIV+ men found no pharmacokinetic interaction between **zidovudine** 100 mg and aciclovir 400 or 800 mg, both given every 4 hours, 5 times a day, and the combination was well tolerated over a 6-month period.[1] When 41 HIV+ patients on **zidovudine** were given aciclovir, no changes in the pharmacokinetics of the **zidovudine** occurred and the adverse effects were unchanged.[2] In a group of AIDS patients on

zidovudine, some of whom were also given aciclovir, no obvious problems developed that could be attributed to the use of the aciclovir.[3] In contrast, a man with herpes who had been treated with intravenous aciclovir 250 mg every 8 hours for 3 days, developed overwhelming fatigue and lethargy within about an hour of starting oral **zidovudine** 200 mg every 4 hours. This lessened slightly on changing from intravenous to oral aciclovir, which was continued for 3 days, and symptoms resolved when the aciclovir was withdrawn. The symptoms developed again when intravenous aciclovir was given as a test.[4] This isolated case of fatigue is not understood, and no other cases appear to have been reported. There would seem to be no reason for avoiding concurrent use.

(b) Famciclovir

Only minimal changes in **zidovudine** pharmacokinetics were seen when 12 HIV+ patients stabilised on **zidovudine** 400 mg to 1 g daily were given a single 500-mg dose of famciclovir.[5]

In a study in 12 healthy subjects there was no important pharmacokinetic interaction between single doses of **emtricitabine** 200 mg and famciclovir 500 mg.[6]

1. Hollander H, Lifson AR, Maha M, Blum R, Rutherfod GW, Nusinoff-Lehrman S. Phase I study of low-dose zidovudine and acyclovir in asymptomatic human immunodeficiency virus seropositive individuals. *Am J Med* (1989) 87, 628–32.
2. Tartaglione TA, Collier AC, Opheim K, Gianola FG, Benedetti J, Corey L. Pharmacokinetic evaluations of low- and high-dose zidovudine plus high-dose acyclovir in patients with symptomatic human immunodeficiency virus infection. *Antimicrob Agents Chemother* (1991) 35, 2225–31.
3. Richman DD, Fischl MA, Grieco MH, Gottlieb MS, Volberding PA, Laskin OL, Leedom JM, Groopman JE, Mildvan D, Hirsch MS, Jackson GG, Durack DT, Nusinoff-Lehrman S and the AZT Collaborative Working Group. The toxicity of azidothymidine (AZT) in the treatment of patients with AIDS and AIDS-related complex. A double-blind, placebo-controlled trial. *N Engl J Med* (1987) 317, 192–7.
4. Bach MC. Possible drug interaction during therapy with azidothymidine and acyclovir for AIDS. *N Engl J Med* (1987) 316, 547.
5. Rousseau F, Scott S, Pratt S, Fowles S, Sparrow P, Lascoux C, Lehner V, Sereni D. Safe coadministration of famciclovir and zidovudine. *Intersci Conf Antimicrob Agents Chemother* (1994) 34, 83.
6. Wang LH, Blum MR, Hui J, Hulett L, Chittick GE, Rousseau F. Lack of significant pharmacokinetic interactions between emtricitabine and other nucleoside antivirals in healthy volunteers. *Intersci Conf Antimicrob Agents Chemother* (2001) 41, 18.

NRTIs + Antacids

Aluminium/magnesium hydroxide caused a 25% reduction in the bioavailability of zalcitabine. Antacids would not be expected to have any additional effect on buffered didanosine preparations.

Clinical evidence, mechanism, importance and management

(a) Didanosine

Didanosine is acid labile. To increase its absorption, some didanosine preparations (e.g. buffered tablets) have been formulated with antacids.[1] Additional concurrent antacids would not be expected to have any further clinically relevant effect. No special precautions are needed.

(b) Zalcitabine

A study in 12 HIV+ patients given a single 1.5-mg dose of zalcitabine found that 30 ml of *Maalox* [**aluminium/magnesium hydroxide**] caused a 25% reduction in the bioavailability of the zalcitabine.[2] The changes are moderate and of uncertain clinical importance, but this still awaits formal assessment. The maker recommends not taking zalcitabine at the same time as **aluminium/magnesium**-containing antacids.[3,4]

1. Videx Tablets (Didanosine). Bristol-Myers Squibb Pharmaceuticals Ltd. UK Summary of product characteristics, March 2005.
2. Massarella JW, Holazo AA, Koss-Twardy S, Min B, Smith B, Nazareno LA. The effects of cimetidine and Maalox® on the pharmacokinetics of zalcitabine in HIV-positive patients. *Pharm Res* (1994) 11 (10 Suppl), S-415.
3. Hivid (Zalcitabine). Roche Products Ltd. UK Summary of product characteristics, November 2004.
4. Hivid (Zalcitabine). Roche Pharmaceuticals. US Prescribing information, September 2002.

NRTIs + Anticonvulsants

Valproate increases the bioavailability of zidovudine. Phenytoin and phenobarbital are predicted to slightly decrease abacavir levels. See also 'Phenytoin + Zidovudine', p.377.

Clinical evidence

(a) Abacavir

The UK makers of abacavir say that potent enzyme inducers such as **phenobarbital** and **phenytoin** may slightly decrease abacavir concentrations.[1] As yet, there appears to be no other information on this.

(b) Zidovudine

The AUC and mean plasma levels of zidovudine 100 mg every 8 hours was increased by 80% in 6 HIV+ subjects when they were given **valproic acid** 250 or 500 mg every 8 hours for 4 days. No adverse reactions, changes in hepatic or renal function, or alterations in the blood picture were reported.[2] A case report describes an AIDS patient on zidovudine 100 mg five times daily who had a two- to threefold increase in trough and peak serum zidovudine levels, and a 74% increase in the CSF zidovudine levels while taking **valproic acid** 500 mg three times daily.[3] For the possible effect of zidovudine on phenytoin levels, see 'Phenytoin + Zidovudine', p.377.

Mechanism

The evidence indicates that the metabolism (glucuronidation) of zidovudine is inhibited by valproate so that its bioavailability is increased.[2,3] The glucuronidation of abacavir is predicted to be increased by drugs that can induce UDP-glucuronyltransferase, such as phenobarbital and phenytoin.[1]

Importance and management

Information seems to be limited to the papers cited, but an interaction between zidovudine and valproate would appear to be established. It would therefore seem prudent to monitor for any evidence of increased zidovudine effects and possible toxicity if valproate is added. The other antiretroviral NRTIs do not undergo significant glucuronidation (see 'Antivirals', (p.578)), and would therefore not be expected to interact with sodium valproate.

1. Ziagen (Abacavir sulfate). GlaxoSmithKline UK. UK Summary of product characteristics, December 2004.
2. Lertora JJL, Rege AB, Greenspan DL, Akula S, George WJ, Hyslop NE, Agrawal KC. Pharmacokinetic interaction between zidovudine and valproic acid in patients infected with human immunodeficiency virus. *Clin Pharmacol Ther* (1994) 56, 272–8.
3. Akula SK, Rege AB, Dreisbach AW, Dejace PMJT, Lertora JJL. Valproic acid increases cerebrospinal fluid zidovudine levels in a patient with AIDS. *Am J Med Sci* (1997) 313, 244–6.

NRTIs + Antituberculars

Didanosine, stavudine and zalcitabine are not expected to interact with rifabutin, but rifabutin may modestly increase the clearance of zidovudine. An isolated case describes undetectable rifabutin levels in a patient on antiretrovirals including buffered didanosine. Rifampicin (rifampin) appears to modestly increase the clearance of zidovudine, and is predicted to interact similarly with abacavir. However, no dose adjustments are recommended for combinations of these NRTIs and rifamycins.

The clearance of isoniazid is increased by zalcitabine, and there is a theoretical increased risk of peripheral neuropathy. Isoniazid, pyrazinamide and ethambutol appear not to interact with zidovudine.

Clinical evidence, mechanism, importance and management

(a) Abacavir

The UK maker of abacavir[1] says that potent enzyme inducers such as **rifampicin (rifampin)** may slightly decrease abacavir plasma concentrations due to their ability to induce UDP-glucuronyltransferases (see also Zidovudine, below). As yet, there appears to be no other information on this.

(b) Didanosine

Rifabutin 300 to 600 mg daily for 12 days did not significantly affect the pharmacokinetics of **didanosine** [buffered preparation] 167 to 250 mg twice daily in 12 patients with AIDS.[2] Similarly, in this study the steady-state pharmacokinetics of **rifabutin** were not affected by didanosine (buffered sachet preparation).[3] This study suggests that the buffer used in the didanosine preparation had no effect on **rifabutin** absorption.[3] However, a case has been reported of a patient on lopinavir/ritonavir, efavirenz, lamivudine and didanosine (buffered preparation) who had impaired

rifabutin absorption. When **rifabutin** was taken 30 minutes after didanosine, **rifabutin** levels were undetectable, but when **rifabutin** was taken 3 hours after didanosine, **rifabutin** levels were apparent.[4]

The controlled study[3] suggests that no special precautions are necessary if both drugs are given. However, the case report[4] introduces an element of caution, especially if other drugs that may affect **rifabutin** pharmacokinetics are used. It remains to be seen if this stays as an isolated case. If indeed **rifabutin** absorption is affected by antacids (there appear to be no clinical data on this), then giving the drugs at least 2 hours apart, or using the enteric-coated didanosine preparation should avoid the interaction.[4]

(c) Stavudine

A study in 10 HIV+ subjects found that the addition of **rifabutin** 300 mg daily to stavudine 30 or 40 mg twice daily caused no significant effects on the pharmacokinetics of the stavudine and the incidence of adverse effects did not increase.[5] No special precautions would seem necessary if both drugs are given.

(d) Zalcitabine

A study in 12 HIV+ patients found that when zalcitabine 1.5 mg three times daily was given with **isoniazid** 300 mg daily the pharmacokinetics of the zalcitabine remained unchanged but the clearance of the **isoniazid** was about doubled.[6] The UK maker of zalcitabine[7] recommends caution with the combination because of the possibility of an increased risk of peripheral neuropathy (see also 'NRTIs + Drugs causing peripheral neuropathy', p.595); the US maker recommends that the combination should be avoided where possible.[8] Monitor concurrent use well.

The UK maker of **rifabutin** says that no significant interactions may be expected between **rifabutin** and zalcitabine.[9]

(e) Zidovudine

The pharmacokinetics of **rifabutin** are not affected by the concurrent use of zidovudine in AIDS patients.[10,11] **Rifabutin** does not affect the pharmacokinetics of zidovudine in HIV+ patients,[12] although one review of concurrent treatment found a trend towards increased clearance of zidovudine by **rifabutin**.[13] No increase in adverse effects appears to occur with the combination of **rifabutin** and zidovudine.[11] In a retrospective study of healthy subjects and HIV+ individuals, the clearance of zidovudine was increased by 132% by **rifampicin (rifampin)** and by 50% by **rifabutin**, suggesting that the enzyme-inducing effects of **rifabutin** are very much less than those of **rifampicin**, so less significant interactions would be expected.[14]

A comparative study in HIV+ patients given zidovudine and antitubercular treatment (**isoniazid**, **rifampicin**, **pyrazinamide**, **ethambutol** initially, then **isoniazid** and **rifampicin**) for 8 months found no evidence of an adverse interaction. However, marked anaemia occurred in those subjects given both groups of drugs, but it was not necessary to permanently stop zidovudine in any patient. The authors advise careful monitoring for haematological toxicity.[15] Another study in 4 HIV+ patients found that **rifampicin** lowered the AUC and increased the clearance of zidovudine in all patients, probably due to the enzyme-inducing activity of the **rifampicin**, which increases the glucuronidation of zidovudine. When the **rifampicin** was stopped in one patient, his zidovudine AUC doubled.[16] A later study of the same interaction in 8 HIV+ men found that **rifampicin** significantly induced the glucuronidation of zidovudine and suggested that the effect wore off 14 days after stopping the **rifampicin**. The authors of this study suggest that dosage alterations may not be necessary with concurrent use.[17]

1. Ziagen (Abacavir sulfate). GlaxoSmithKline UK. UK Summary of product characteristics, December 2004.
2. Sahai J, Foss N, Li R, Narang PK, Cameron DW. Rifabutin and didanosine interaction in AIDS patients. *Clin Pharmacol Ther* (1993) 53, 197.
3. Li RC, Narang PK, Sahai J, Cameron W, Bianchine JR. Rifabutin absorption in the gut unaltered by concomitant administration of didanosine in AIDS patients. *Antimicrob Agents Chemother* (1997) 41, 1566–70.
4. Marzolini C, Chave J-P, Telenti A, Brenas-Chinchon L, Biollaz J. Impaired absorption of rifabutin by concomitant administration of didanosine. *AIDS* (2001) 15, 2203–4.
5. Piscitelli SC, Kelly G, Walker RE, Kovacs J, Falloon J, Davey RT, Raje S, Masur H, Polis MA. A multiple drug interaction study of stavudine with agents for opportunistic infections in human immunodeficiency virus-infected patients. *Antimicrob Agents Chemother* (1999) 43, 647–50.
6. Lee BL, Täuber MG, Chambers HF, Gambertoglio J, Delahunty T. The effect of zalcitabine on the pharmacokinetics of isoniazid in HIV-infected patients. *Intersci Conf Antimicrob Agents Chemother* (1994) 34, 3.
7. Hivid (Zalcitabine). Roche Products Ltd. UK Summary of product characteristics, November 2004.
8. Hivid (Zalcitabine). Roche Pharmaceuticals. US Prescribing information, September 2002.
9. Mycobutin (Rifabutin). Pharmacia Ltd. UK Summary of product characteristics, January 2003.
10. Narang PK, Nightingale S, Lewis RC, Colborn D, Wynne B, Li R. Concomitant zidovudine (ZDV) dosing does not affect rifabutin (RIF) disposition in AIDS patients. 9th International Conference AIDS & 4th STD World Congress, Berlin, June 6–11, 1993. Abstract PO-B31-2216.
11. Li RC, Nightingale S, Lewis RC, Colburn DC, Narang PK. Lack of effect of concomitant zidovudine on rifabutin kinetics in patients with AIDS-related complex. *Antimicrob Agents Chemother* (1996) 40, 1397–1402.
12. Gallicano K, Sahai J, Swick L, Seguin I, Pakuts A, Cameron DW. Effect of rifabutin on the pharmacokinetics of zidovudine in patients infected with human immunodeficiency virus. *Clin Infect Dis* (1995) 21, 1008–11.
13. Narang PK, Sale M. Population based assessment of rifabutin (R) effect on zidovudine (ZDV) disposition in AIDS patients. *Clin Pharmacol Ther* (1993) 53, 219.
14. Narang PK, Gupta S, Li RC, Strolin-Benedetti M, Della Bruna C, Bianchine JR. Assessing dosing implications of enzyme inducing potential: rifabutin (RIF) vs. rifampin (RFM). *Intersci Conf Antimicrob Agents Chemother* (1993) 33, 228.
15. Antoniskis D, Easley AC, Espina BM, Davidson PT, Barnes PF. Combined toxicity of zidovudine and antituberculosis chemotherapy. *Am Rev Respir Dis* (1992) 145, 430–4.
16. Burger DM, Meenhorst PL, Koks CHW, Beijnen JH. Pharmacokinetic interaction between rifampin and zidovudine. *Antimicrob Agents Chemother* (1993) 37, 1426–31.
17. Gallicano KD, Sahai J, Shukla VK, Seguin I, Pakuts A, Kwok D, Foster BC, Cameron DW. Induction of zidovudine glucuronidation and amination pathways by rifampicin in HIV-infected patients. *Br J Clin Pharmacol* (1999) 48, 168–79.

NRTIs + Azoles

Fluconazole has no significant effect on the pharmacokinetics of didanosine or stavudine, but it may cause an increase in serum zidovudine levels although the clinical importance of this is uncertain. Fluconazole serum levels remain unchanged. Itraconazole appears not to affect the pharmacokinetics of zidovudine. Serum levels of itraconazole are markedly reduced by buffered didanosine, but the interaction can be avoided if itraconazole is taken at least 2 hours before didanosine. Similarly, buffered didanosine does not interact with ketoconazole given at least 2 hours earlier. Enteric-coated didanosine has no clinically relevant effect on the pharmacokinetics of fluconazole, itraconazole or ketoconazole. The frequency of haematological toxicity with zidovudine was not increased by ketoconazole.

Clinical evidence

(a) Didanosine

(i) Buffered preparation. A 35-year-old patient with AIDS was given **itraconazole** capsules 200 mg twice daily following an episode of cryptococcal meningitis. When he relapsed it was noted that he had been taking the **itraconazole** at the same time as his buffered didanosine. Subsequent study in this patient indicated a marked delay in **itraconazole** absorption when it was taken with didanosine. Two hours after the dose, plasma **itraconazole** concentrations of 1.6 micrograms/ml were observed without didanosine, but were undetectable with didanosine. A peak **itraconazole** level of 1.4 micrograms/ml was observed when it was given 8 hours after a dose of didanosine.[1] A mean peak serum **itraconazole** level of 0.9 micrograms/ml was seen in 6 healthy subjects 3 hours after a single 200-mg oral dose of **itraconazole**, but the levels were undetectable when [buffered] didanosine 300 mg was given with the **itraconazole**.[2] A later study in 12 HIV+ patients found that the AUC of **itraconazole** after a single 200-mg dose was not significantly different when buffered didanosine 200 mg was given 4 hours before or 2 hours after **itraconazole**.[3]

A group of 12 HIV+ subjects taking buffered didanosine 100 to 250 mg twice daily were also given **fluconazole** for 7 days (two 200-mg doses on the first day, followed by 200 mg daily). The pharmacokinetics of the didanosine remained unchanged in the presence of the **fluconazole**, and concurrent use was well tolerated. **Fluconazole** pharmacokinetics were not assessed.[4]

Twelve HIV+ patients were given buffered didanosine 375 mg twice daily either alone or 2 hours after **ketoconazole** 200 mg daily, for 4 days. Didanosine maximum plasma levels were slightly reduced by 12% and no significant changes in the pharmacokinetics of the **ketoconazole** were seen when dosing was separated in this way.[5]

(ii) Enteric-coated preparation. Enteric-coated didanosine 400 mg had no significant effect on the pharmacokinetics of **fluconazole** 200 mg in 1 healthy subjects, and no clinically relevant effect on the pharmacokine of **itraconazole** 200 mg in 25 healthy subjects.[6] Similarly, enteric-c didanosine 400 mg had no clinically relevant effect on the pharmac ics of **ketoconazole** 200 mg in 24 healthy subjects. Three of th had increased concentrations of **ketoconazole** with didanosin values for **ketoconazole** alone appeared unusually low. Whe were excluded, no effect on AUC was seen in the remaining

(b) Stavudine

A study in 10 HIV+ subjects on stavudine 40 mg twice daily, found that the addition of **fluconazole** 200 mg daily for one week had no significant effect on the pharmacokinetics of the stavudine.[8]

(c) Zidovudine

On two occasions, 12 HIV+ men were given 200 mg of zidovudine every 8 hours with and without **fluconazole** 400 mg daily for 7 days. While taking **fluconazole** the AUC of the zidovudine increased by 74%, the maximum serum levels increased by 84%, the terminal half-life was increased by 128% and the clearance was reduced by 43%.[9] In contrast, another study in 10 HIV+ patients found only a very small change in the pharmacokinetics of a single 500-mg dose of zidovudine given before and after 7 days treatment with **fluconazole** (e.g. a 7% increase in zidovudine AUC). In another 10 patients, zidovudine had no effect on the pharmacokinetics of a single dose of **fluconazole**.[10]

Itraconazole 200 mg daily for 2 weeks was reported to have no effect on the pharmacokinetics of zidovudine in 7 patients, but the serum levels in 2 patients were higher.[11]

A study of zidovudine use in 282 AIDS patients found that haematological abnormalities (anaemia, leucopenia, neutropenia) were very common, but the concurrent use of **ketoconazole** in some of these patients did not increase the haematological toxicity.[12]

Mechanism

Itraconazole capsules and ketoconazole depend on stomach acidity for absorption. A raised gastric pH due to the antacids in the buffered didanosine formulation appears to reduce itraconazole absorption (see also, 'Azoles + Antacids, H_2-blockers or Sucralfate', p.135). The didanosine itself appears to have no part to play in this interaction. The enteric-coated preparation of didanosine does not contain any antacids.

In vitro data suggest that the altered zidovudine pharmacokinetics may, in part, be due to fluconazole inhibiting zidovudine glucuronidation.[13]

Importance and management

The most significant interaction occurs between the buffered preparation of didanosine and itraconazole. Patients should avoid taking both drugs at the same time, but giving the itraconazole at least 2 hours before the didanosine appears to solve any problem. Any possible interaction with ketoconazole can similarly be avoided by giving ketoconazole at least 2 hours before didanosine. Alternatively, the interaction may be avoided by using the newer enteric-coated preparation of didanosine.

There is no pharmacokinetic interaction between stavudine and fluconazole. No interaction would be expected with other similar NRTIs such as **lamivudine** and **zalcitabine** (see 'Antivirals', (p.578)).

There is evidence of a minor interaction between zidovudine and fluconazole, but this is unlikely to be clinically significant.

1. Moreno F, Hardin TC, Rinaldi MG, Graybill JR. Itraconazole-didanosine excipient interaction. *JAMA* (1993) 269, 1508.
2. May DB, Drew RH, Yedinak KC, Bartlett JA. Effect of simultaneous didanosine administration on itraconazole absorption in healthy volunteers. *Pharmacotherapy* (1994) 14, 509–13.
3. Hardin TC, Sharkey-Mathis PK, Rinaldi MG, Graybill JR. Evaluation of the pharmacokinetic interaction between itraconazole and didanosine in HIV-infected subjects. *Intersci Conf Antimicrob Agents Chemother* (1995) 35, 6.
4. Bruzzese VL, Gillum JG, Israel DS, Johnson GL, Kaplowitz LG, Polk RE. Effect of fluconazole on pharmacokinetics of 2′,3′-dideoxyinosine in persons seropositive for human immunodeficiency virus. *Antimicrob Agents Chemother* (1995) 39, 1050–53.
5. Knupp CA, Brater DC, Relue J, Barbhaiya RH. Pharmacokinetics of didanosine and ketoconazole after coadministration to patients seropositive for the human immunodeficiency virus. *J Clin Pharmacol* (1993) 33, 912–17.
6. Damle B, Hess H, Kaul S, Knupp C. Absence of clinically relevant drug interactions following simultaneous administration of didanosine-encapsulated, enteric-coated bead formulation with either itraconazole or fluconazole. *Biopharm Drug Dispos* (2002) 23, 59–66.
7. Damle BD, Mummaneni V, Kaul S, Knupp C. Lack of effect of simultaneously administered didanosine encapsulated enteric bead formulation (Videx EC) on oral absorption of indinavir, ketoconazole, or ciprofloxacin. *Antimicrob Agents Chemother* (2002) 46, 385–91.
8. Piscitelli SC, Kelly G, Walker RE, Kovacs J, Falloon J, Davey RT, Raje S, Masur H, Polis MA. A multiple drug interaction study of stavudine with agents for opportunistic infections in human immunodeficiency virus-infected patients. *Antimicrob Agents Chemother* (1999) 43, 647–50.
9. Sahai J, Gallicano K, Pakuts A, Cameron DW. Effect of fluconazole on zidovudine pharmacokinetics in patients infected with human deficiency virus. *J Infect Dis* (1994) 169, 1103–7.
10. Brockmeyer NH, Tillmann I, Mertins L, Barthel B, Goos M. Pharmacokinetic interaction of fluconazole and zidovudine in HIV-positive patients. *Eur J Med Res* (1997) 2, 377–83.
11. Henrivaux P, Fairon Y, Fillet G. Pharmacokinetics of AZT among HIV infected patients treated by itraconazole. 5th Int Conf AIDS, Montreal. 1989, Abstract M.B.P.340.
12. Richman DD, Fischl MA, Grieco MH, Gottlieb MS, Volberding PA, Laskin OL, Leedom JM, Groopman JE, Mildvan D, Hirsch MS, Jackson GG, Durack DT, Nusinoff-Lehrman S and the AZT Collaborative Working Group. The toxicity of azidothymidine (AZT) in the treatment of patients with AIDS and AIDS-related complex. A double-blind, placebo-controlled trial. *N Engl J Med* (1987) 317, 192–7.

Asgari M, Back DJ. Effect of azoles on the glucuronidation of zidovudine by human liver UDP-glucuronyltransferase. *J Infect Dis* (1995) 172, 1634–5.

NRTIs + Cytokines

Interferon alfa does not alter the pharmacokinetics of didanosine or lamivudine to a clinically relevant extent. Interferon alfa and, particularly, interferon beta can cause an increase in the serum levels of zidovudine. Interleukin-2 appears not to interact significantly with zidovudine.

Clinical evidence

(a) Interferon

AIDS patients who had been taking **zidovudine** 200 mg every 4 hours for 8 weeks were also given subcutaneous **recombinant beta interferon** 45 million units daily. After 3 and 15 days the **zidovudine** metabolism was reduced by 75% and 97% respectively. By day 15 the **zidovudine** half-life was increased about twofold.[1] Another study in 6 children aged 3 months to 17 years found that after 5 weeks of concurrent use the AUC of **zidovudine** was increased by 36% by **interferon alfa**, the maximum serum levels were raised by 69% and the clearance was reduced by 20%.[2]

Interferon alfa 1 to 15 million units daily was given to 26 HIV+ patients taking **didanosine** sachets 100 to 375 mg twice daily. The interferon appeared to have no clinically significant effects on the pharmacokinetics of the **didanosine**.[3] Similarly, a single subcutaneous injection of **interferon alfa** 10 million units had no clinically significant effects on the pharmacokinetics of **lamivudine** 100 mg daily for 7 days in 19 healthy subjects (the **lamivudine** AUC was decreased by about 10%). **Lamivudine** did not appear to alter the pharmacokinetics of **interferon alfa**.[4]

(b) Interleukin-2

A study found that a 4-week course of interleukin-2 (0.25 million units/m^2 daily) by continuous infusion had no clinically significant effect on the pharmacokinetics of a 100-mg intravenous dose of **zidovudine**.[5] Another study in 8 HIV+ males given oral **zidovudine** 200 mg every 4 hours found similar results.[3] No special precautions would seem necessary.

Mechanism

Beta interferon appears to inhibit the metabolism (glucuronidation) of the zidovudine by the liver.

Importance and management

Information seems to be limited to these reports. The results of the first report suggest that the zidovudine dosage may need to be reduced if beta interferon is added in order to avoid increased zidovudine toxicity. A dosage reduction of two-thirds, or even more, would seem to be needed. More study is needed to confirm these observations. Interferon alfa appears to interact to a lesser extent. The makers warn that the risk of haematological toxicity may be increased if zidovudine and interferon are used together,[6,7] and the UK makers recommend extra care.[6] Interferon alfa does not appear to interact pharmacokinetically with didanosine or lamivudine.

1. Nokta M, Loh JP, Douidar SM, Ahmed AE, Pollard RB. Metabolic interaction of recombinant interferon-β and zidovudine in AIDS patients. *J Interferon Res* (1991) 11, 159–64.
2. Diaz C, Yogev R, Rodriguez J, Rege A, George W, Lertora J. ACTG-153: Zidovudine pharmacokinetics when used in combination with interferon alpha. *Intersci Conf Antimicrob Agents Chemother* (1994) 34, 79.
3. Piscitelli SC, Amantea MA, Vogel S, Bechtel C, Metcalf JA, Kovacs JA. Effects of cytokines on antiviral pharmacokinetics: an alternative approach to assessment of drug interactions using bioequivalence guidelines. *Antimicrob Agents Chemother* (1996) 40, 161–5.
4. Johnson MA, Jenkins JM, Bye C. A study of the pharmacokinetic interaction between lamivudine and alpha interferon. *Eur J Clin Pharmacol* (2000) 56, 289–92.
5. Skinner MH, Pauloin D, Schwartz D, Merigan TC, Blaschke TF. IL-2 does not alter zidovudine kinetics. *Clin Pharmacol Ther* (1989) 45, 128.
6. Retrovir (Zidovudine). GlaxoSmithKline UK. UK Summary of product characteristics, September 2004.
7. Retrovir (Zidovudine). GlaxoSmithKline. US Prescribing information, April 2003.

NRTIs + Dapsone

Buffered didanosine does not alter the pharmacokinetics of dapsone, but there is some circumstantial evidence to suggest that it may reduce the prophylactic effects of dapsone in preventing *Pneumocystis carinii* pneumonia. Dapsone has no effect on the pharmacokinetics of zalcitabine, whereas zalcitabine causes a small rise in the serum levels of dapsone, and there is a theoretical increased risk of peripheral neuropathy with the combination.

Dapsone appears not to affect the pharmacokinetics of zidovudine, although concurrent use may be associated with increased blood dyscrasias.

Clinical evidence, mechanism, importance and management

(a) Didanosine

An early report of the use of buffered didanosine described the development of *Pneumocystis carinii* pneumonia (PCP) in 11 out of 28 HIV+ patients taking dapsone prophylaxis compared with only 1 of 12 taking aerosolised pentamidine and none of 17 taking co-trimoxazole. Of the 11 patients where prophylaxis failed, 4 died from respiratory failure.[1] The authors suggested that the most likely explanation of the high failure rate of dapsone with didanosine, was reduced dapsone absorption due to the citrate-phosphate buffer in the didanosine formulation.[1] This has led to some recommending that the drugs be taken at least 2 hours apart.

However, in a controlled study in 6 HIV+ subjects, dapsone pharmacokinetics were not altered by taking a dose of buffered didanosine within 5 minutes.[2] Similarly, dapsone pharmacokinetics were not altered by the aluminium/magnesium antacids and other excipients of the didanosine tablets in 6 healthy subjects.[2] Another study in healthy subjects also failed to confirm that a marked rise in gastric pH affects the absorption of dapsone, see 'Dapsone + Antacids', p.208. Furthermore, low dapsone levels have been found in patients on a weekly dapsone regimen who took dapsone at least 2 hours before or 6 hours after didanosine, and in patients on zidovudine or no antiretrovirals (although this study did not look at whether dapsone levels were correlated with efficacy).[3] In a retrospective analysis, other authors found no evidence to confirm a correlation between failure of PCP prophylaxis with dapsone and use of drugs that increase gastric pH (didanosine, H_2-blockers, antacids).[4]

It has therefore been adequately demonstrated that the buffered preparation of didanosine and antacids do not affect dapsone absorption. The explanation for the apparent failure of PCP prophylaxis in the original report[1] is unresolved. Despite the use of both didanosine and dapsone in the management of HIV and opportunistic infections there do not appear to be any further reports of problems with the combination.

(b) Zalcitabine

A pharmacokinetic study in 12 HIV+ patients who were given zalcitabine 1.5 mg three times daily and dapsone 100 mg daily, alone or together, found that dapsone did not significantly affect the kinetics of the zalcitabine. However, zalcitabine decreased the clearance of dapsone by 21%, increased its maximum serum levels by 19% and increased its half-life by 34%.[5] These changes are relatively small and seem unlikely to have much clinical relevance, but until this is confirmed it would seem prudent to monitor the concurrent use of these two drugs. The UK maker[6] recommends caution with the combination because of the possibility of an increased risk of peripheral neuropathy (see also 'NRTIs + Drugs causing peripheral neuropathy', below); the US maker advises avoiding the combination where possible.[7]

(c) Zidovudine

Dapsone 100 mg daily had no effect on the pharmacokinetics of a single 200-mg dose of zidovudine in 8 HIV+ subjects.[8] In a further study, which considered the safety of dapsone in combination with zidovudine, dapsone was shown to increase the risk of blood dyscrasias that occur with zidovudine treatment.[9] Therefore it would seem that dapsone and zidovudine can be given concurrently, but monitoring for an increase in adverse events would seem advisable.

1. Metroka CE, McMechan MF, Andrada R, Laubenstein LJ, Jacobus DP. Failure of prophylaxis with dapsone in patients taking dideoxyinosine. *N Engl J Med* (1992) 325, 737.
2. Sahai J, Garber G, Gallicano K, Oliveras L, Cameron DW. Effects of the antacids in didanosine tablets on dapsone pharmacokinetics. *Ann Intern Med* (1995) 123, 584–7.
3. Opravil M, Joos B, Lüthy R. Levels of dapsone and pyrimethamine in serum during once-weekly dosing for prophylaxis of *Pneumocystis carinii* pneumonia and toxoplasmic encephalitis. *Antimicrob Agents Chemother* (1994) 38, 1197–9.
4. Huengsberg M, Castelino S, Sherrard J, O'Farrell N, Bingham J. Does drug interaction cause failure of PCP prophylaxis with dapsone? *Lancet* (1993) 341, 48.
5. Lee BL, Tauber MG, Chambers HF, Gambertoglio J, Delahunty T. Zalcitabine (DDC) and dapsone (DAP) pharmacokinetic (PK) interaction in HIV-infected patients. *Clin Pharmacol Ther* (1995) 57, 186.
6. Hivid (Zalcitabine). Roche Products Ltd. UK Summary of product characteristics, November 2004.
7. Hivid (Zalcitabine). Roche Pharmaceuticals. US Prescribing information, September 2002.
8. Lee BL, Safrin S, Makrides V, Gambertoglio JG. Zidovudine, trimethoprim, and dapsone pharmacokinetic interactions in patients with human immunodeficiency virus infection. *Antimicrob Agents Chemother* (1996) 40, 1231–6.
9. Pinching AJ, Helbert M, Peddle B, Robinson D, Janes K, Gor D, Jeffries DJ, Stoneham C, Mitchell D, Kocsis AE, Mann J, Forster SM, Harris JRW. Clinical experience with zidovudine for patients with acquired immune deficiency syndrome and acquired immune deficiency syndrome-related complex. *J Infect* (1989) 18 (Suppl 1), 33–40.

NRTIs + Drugs causing pancreatitis

Additive pancreatic toxicity has been described with zalcitabine and intravenous pentamidine, and is expected with didanosine or stavudine and other drugs that can cause pancreatitis. An isolated case describes pancreatitis with lamivudine and azathioprine.

Clinical evidence

(a) Lamivudine

A single case report describes a 51-year-old woman with a kidney transplant who developed pancreatitis after starting lamivudine. **Azathioprine** had been discontinued only 3 days before and it is possible (although the evidence is weak) that the residual serum **azathioprine** had interacted with lamivudine to cause the pancreatitis.[1]

(b) Zalcitabine

Fatal fulminant pancreatitis occurred in a patient given zalcitabine and intravenous **pentamidine**.[2]

Mechanism

Possible additive toxicity.

Importance and management

Of the NRTIs, didanosine, stavudine and zalcitabine have been associated with fatal pancreatitis.[2-6] The makers of zalcitabine recommend that if therapy with a drug that has the potential to cause pancreatitis is required, treatment with zalcitabine should be interrupted.[2,5] They specifically apply this to the use of pentamidine to treat pneumocystis carinii pneumonia.[2,5] The makers of didanosine have a similar recommendation and state that if concurrent therapy is unavoidable, there should be close observation.[3,6] Similarly, other authors recommend temporarily discontinuing didanosine in patients needing systemic pentamidine or **sulfonamide**-containing regimens.[7] The UK maker of stavudine recommends that patients receiving concurrent treatment with drugs known to cause pancreatitis should be carefully observed.[4] Note that **hydroxycarbamide** may increase the risk of pancreatitis with didanosine and stavudine, see 'NRTIs + Hydroxycarbamide', p.598. The UK maker states that lamivudine is rarely associated with pancreatitis,[8] and no firm conclusions can be drawn from the case discussed above.

1. Van Vlierberghe H, Elewaut A. Development of a necrotising pancreatitis after starting lamivudine in a kidney transplant patient with fibrosing cholestatic hepatitis: A possible role of the interaction lamivudine and azathioprine. *Gastroenterology* (1997) 112 (4 Suppl), A1407.
2. Hivid (Zalcitabine). Roche Products Ltd. UK Summary of product characteristics, November 2004.
3. Videx Tablets (Didanosine). Bristol-Myers Squibb Pharmaceuticals Ltd. UK Summary of product characteristics, March 2005.
4. Zerit (Stavudine). Bristol-Myers Squibb Pharmaceuticals Ltd. UK Summary of product characteristics, January 2005.
5. Hivid (Zalcitabine). Roche Pharmaceuticals. US Prescribing information, September 2002.
6. Videx EC (Didanosine). Bristol-Myers Squibb Company. US Prescribing information, January 2004.
7. Yarchoan R, Mitsuya H, Pluda JM, Marczyk KS, Thomas RV, Hartman NR, Brouwers P, Perno C-F, Allain J-P, Johns DG, Broder S. The National Cancer Institute phase I study of 2',3'-dideoxyinosine administration in adults with AIDS or AIDS-related complex: analysis of activity and toxicity profiles. *Rev Infect Dis* (1990) 12 (Suppl 5), S522–S533.
8. Epivir (Lamivudine). GlaxoSmithKline UK. UK Summary of product characteristics, December 2004.

NRTIs + Drugs causing peripheral neuropathy

Of the NRTIs, didanosine and, particularly, zalcitabine can cause peripheral neuropathy. The makers recommend caution with the concurrent use of these NRTIs with other drugs known to cause peripheral neuropathy. Stavudine may also cause peripheral neuropathy.

Clinical evidence, mechanism, importance and management

Zalcitabine may cause a severe irreversible peripheral neuropathy.[1] B cause of the possible increased risk of developing peripheral neurop the makers recommend that **zalcitabine** should be used with caution tients on other drugs that have the potential to cause peripheral r thy. If peripheral neuropathy occurs, **zalcitabine** should be stopped. The makers list drugs that have been associated wit neuropathy; **'antiretroviral nucleoside analogues'**, (p.599), **chloramphenicol**, **cisplatin**, **'dapsone'**, (p.594), **disulfiram**, **ethionamide**, **glutethimide**, **gold**, **hydralazine**, **iodoquinol**, **'isoniazid'**, (p.592), **metronidazole**, **nitrofurantoin**, **phenytoin**, **ribavirin**, and **vincristine**.[1,2]

They also state that concurrent use of **amphotericin**, **'foscarnet'**, (p.583) or the **aminoglycosides** should be well monitored because these drugs may possibly decrease the renal clearance of the **zalcitabine**, thereby increasing its plasma levels and the risk of developing peripheral neuropathy or other adverse effects.[1,2] These predicted interactions still await formal assessment.

The maker of **didanosine** states that the risk of peripheral neuropathy may be increased in patients on drugs known to cause this effect. They recommend careful monitoring of concurrent use.[3] **Hydroxycarbamide** may increase the risk of peripheral neuropathy with **didanosine**, see 'NRTIs + Hydroxycarbamide', p.598.

Stavudine may also cause dose-limiting peripheral neuropathy,[4] which would be expected to be additive with other drugs that cause peripheral neuropathy.

1. Hivid (Zalcitabine). Roche Products Ltd. UK Summary of product characteristics, November 2004.
2. Hivid (Zalcitabine). Roche Pharmaceuticals. US Prescribing information, September 2002.
3. Videx Tablets (Didanosine). Bristol-Myers Squibb Pharmaceuticals Ltd. UK Summary of product characteristics, March 2005.
4. Zerit (Stavudine). Bristol-Myers Squibb Pharmaceuticals Ltd. UK Summary of product characteristics, January 2005.

NRTIs + Food

Food can reduce the extent of absorption of didanosine, possibly causing a loss in efficacy. Food affects the rate, but not the extent, of absorption of abacavir, lamivudine, and stavudine. The extent of absorption of zalcitabine is reduced slightly by food. Food may also modestly reduce the extent of absorption of zidovudine.

Clinical evidence, mechanism, importance and management

(a) Abacavir

The maker of abacavir notes that food delayed its rate, but not extent, of absorption. Therefore, abacavir can be taken with or without food.[1,2]

(b) Didanosine

(i) Buffered preparations. Didanosine (as two 150-mg chewable tablets) was given to 10 HIV+ subjects 30 minutes before breakfast, 1 hour before breakfast, 1 hour after breakfast, and 2 hours after breakfast. When the dose was given before breakfast the results were very similar to those obtained with subjects in the fasting state. When given after a breakfast, the didanosine AUC and maximum plasma concentration were both decreased by about 50%.[3] Similar results were found in another study.[4] A further study[5] using sachets containing didanosine, sucrose and citrate-phosphate buffer, similarly found that food reduced the bioavailability by 41% (from 29 to 17%). The reason would appear to be that food delays gastric emptying so that the didanosine is exposed to prolonged contact with gastric acid, which causes decomposition (see 'Antivirals', (p.578)), with a resultant fall in bioavailability.[6] To achieve maximum bioavailability the didanosine buffered preparations should be taken on an empty stomach at least 30 minutes before food.

(ii) Enteric-coated preparation. Giving didanosine gastro-resistant capsules with a high-fat meal or a light meal reduced the AUC by 19% and 27%, respectively, compared with the fasting state. A similar 24% decrease in AUC was also seen when taken 1 hour before a light meal. However, the effect on AUC was negligible when taken 1.5 to 3 hours prior to a light meal.[7] Sprinkling the capsule contents on yoghurt or apple sauce also decreased the AUC by 20% or 18%, respectively.[7] Despite these modest changes in AUC, the UK maker recommends that didanosine gastro-resistant capsules are taken intact with at least 100 ml of water on an empty stomach at least 2 hours before or 2 hours after a meal.[7]

(c) Lamivudine

The maker notes that food delayed rate, but not extent, of absorption of lamivudine. Therefore, lamivudine can be taken with or without food.[8,9]

(d) Stavudine

The UK maker of stavudine notes that a standardised high-fat meal re-uced, and delayed the time to reach, the maximum plasma concentration (specific details not given), but did not alter the extent of systemic exposure compared with the fasting state. Nevertheless, they recommend that, for optimal absorption, stavudine should be taken on an empty stomach at least 1 hour prior to meals. However, if this is not possible, they suggest administration with a light meal; in addition the contents of the capsule may be mixed with food.[10] The US maker states that stavudine can be taken with food or on an empty stomach.[11]

(e) Zalcitabine

The makers of zalcitabine[12,13] note that food decreased the maximum plasma concentration by 39% and prolonged the time to achieve maximum concentrations from 0.8 to 1.6 hours compared with the fasting state. The extent of absorption was decreased by 14%. The UK maker states that zalcitabine can be taken with or without food.[12]

(f) Zidovudine

Zidovudine was given to 13 AIDS patients either with breakfast or when fasting. The maximum plasma level of zidovudine was 2.8-times greater in the fasted patients, and the AUC was reduced by 22% when zidovudine was given with food.[14] Zidovudine rate and extent of absorption was reduced in another study by a standard breakfast (14% decrease in AUC with a 200-mg dose and 33% with a 100-mg dose).[15] In a study[16] of 8 patients a high-fat meal reduced the maximum zidovudine serum levels by about 50%. In all these cases inter-individual variation in zidovudine absorption was high.[14-16] However, when a sustained-release formulation of zidovudine was used, the absorption was delayed, but the AUC was increased by 28% by a high-fat meal.[17] In contrast zidovudine AUC was not affected by 25 g of a **protein supplement**.[18]

Inter-individual variation appears high and the practical consequences of the changes caused are uncertain. Some have suggested zidovudine should be taken on an empty stomach;[15,16] the US maker states that zidovudine can be taken with or without food,[19] but the UK maker gives no specific recommendations regarding administration in relation to food.[20]

1. Ziagen (Abacavir sulfate). GlaxoSmithKline UK. UK Summary of product characteristics, December 2004.
2. Ziagen (Abacavir sulfate). GlaxoSmithKline. US Prescribing information, July 2002.
3. Knupp CA, Milbrath R, Barbhaiya RH. Effect of time of food administration on the bioavailability of didanosine from a chewable tablet formulation. *J Clin Pharmacol* (1993) 33, 568–73.
4. Shyu WC, Knupp CA, Pittman KA, Dunkle L, Barbhaiya RH. Food-induced reduction in bioavailability of didanosine. *Clin Pharmacol Ther* (1991) 50, 503–7.
5. Hartman NR, Yarchoan R, Pluda JM, Thomas RV, Wyvill KM, Flora KP, Broder S, Johns DG. Pharmacokinetics of 2′,3′-dideoxyinosine in patients with severe human immunodeficiency infection. II. The effects of different oral formulations and the presence of other medications. *Clin Pharmacol Ther* (1991) 50, 278–85.
6. Videx Tablets (Didanosine). Bristol-Myers Squibb Pharmaceuticals Ltd. UK Summary of product characteristics, March 2005.
7. Videx EC (Didanosine). Bristol-Myers Squibb Pharmaceuticals Ltd. UK Summary of product characteristics, March 2005.
8. Epivir (Lamivudine). GlaxoSmithKline UK. UK Summary of product characteristics, December 2004.
9. Epivir (Lamivudine). GlaxoSmithKline. US Prescribing information, December 2004.
10. Zerit (Stavudine). Bristol-Myers Squibb Pharmaceuticals Ltd. UK Summary of product characteristics, January 2005.
11. Zerit (Stavudine). Bristol-Myers Squibb Company. US Prescribing information, June 2004.
12. Hivid (Zalcitabine). Roche Products Ltd. UK Summary of product characteristics, November 2004.
13. Hivid (Zalcitabine). Roche Pharmaceuticals. US Prescribing information, September 2002.
14. Lotterer E, Ruhnke M, Trautmann M, Beyer R, Bauer FE. Decreased and variable systemic availability of zidovudine in patients with AIDS if administered with a meal. *Eur J Clin Pharmacol* (1991) 40, 305–8.
15. Ruhnke M, Bauer FE, Seifert M, Trautmann M, Hille H, Koeppe P. Effects of standard breakfast on pharmacokinetics of oral zidovudine in patients with AIDS. *Antimicrob Agents Chemother* (1993) 37, 2153–8.
16. Unadkat JD, Collier AC, Crosby SS, Cummings D, Opheim KE, Corey L. Pharmacokinetics of oral zidovudine (azidothymidine) in patients with AIDS when administered with and without a high-fat meal. *AIDS* (1990) 4, 229–32.
17. Hollister AS, Frazer HA. The effects of a high fat meal on the serum pharmacokinetics of sustained-release zidovudine. *Clin Pharmacol Ther* (1994) 55, 193.
18. Sahai J, Gallicano K, Garber G, McGilveray I, Hawley-Foss N, Turgeon N, Cameron DW. The effect of a protein meal on zidovudine pharmacokinetics in HIV-infected patients. *Br J Clin Pharmacol* (1992) 33, 657–60.
19. Retrovir (Zidovudine). GlaxoSmithKline. US Prescribing information, April 2003.
20. Retrovir (Zidovudine). GlaxoSmithKline UK. UK Summary of product characteristics, September 2004.

NRTIs + Ganciclovir

Concurrent use of zidovudine and ganciclovir produces a very marked increase in haematological toxicity, without any apparent increase in efficacy. Didanosine serum levels are raised by ganciclovir, but there is some evidence suggesting reduced efficacy of ganciclovir prophylaxis. Ganciclovir does not appear to interact with stavudine, and there is no clinically important pharmacoki-

netic interaction between ganciclovir and zalcitabine. Until further information is available, the makers of lamivudine advise the avoidance of intravenous ganciclovir.

Clinical evidence

(a) Didanosine

Buffered didanosine 200 mg twice daily was given to 12 HIV+ patients with oral ganciclovir 1 g three times daily. When the didanosine was given 2 hours before ganciclovir, the maximum serum levels and AUC of didanosine were raised by about 47% and 83%, respectively, and those of ganciclovir were decreased by about 26% and 22%, respectively. When the didanosine was given simultaneously with ganciclovir, the maximum serum levels and AUC of didanosine were similarly raised by about 53% and 77%, but those of ganciclovir were unchanged. The renal clearance of didanosine was not significantly changed by ganciclovir.[1] Similar increases in didanosine levels with ganciclovir given intravenously[2] and high-dose oral ganciclovir 2 g every 8 hours have also been reported.[3] However, in contrast, an earlier study found that the pharmacokinetics of didanosine (sachet preparation) were not altered by intravenous ganciclovir.[4]

Rates of dose-limiting intolerance to the combination of didanosine and ganciclovir were reported to be similar to those seen with didanosine alone in one small study (15 of 32 patients tolerated usual doses of didanosine with the ganciclovir).[5] Analysis of the results of a large randomised study unexpectedly suggested that there was an increased risk of cytomegalovirus disease in those patients taking ganciclovir and didanosine when compared with those not on didanosine.[6]

(b) Lamivudine

The UK maker of lamivudine says that concurrent use with intravenous ganciclovir is not recommended until further information becomes available,[7] although they give no rationale for this advice. They do not mention oral ganciclovir.[7]

(c) Stavudine

In a study of 11 HIV+ patients, oral ganciclovir 1 g three times daily had no significant effect on the pharmacokinetics of stavudine 40 mg twice daily, nor were the ganciclovir pharmacokinetics affected by the stavudine.[8] There were no serious or severe adverse events attributed to the combination.

(d) Zalcitabine

In a study in 10 HIV+ patients zalcitabine 750 micrograms every 8 hours increased the AUC of oral ganciclovir 1 g three times daily by 22%. There was no change in zalcitabine pharmacokinetics. There were no serious or severe adverse events attributed to the combination.[8]

(e) Zidovudine

The efficacy of zidovudine 100 or 200 mg every 4 hours, given alone or combined with intravenous ganciclovir 5 mg/kg twice daily for 14 days, then once daily for 5 days of each week, was assessed in 40 patients for the treatment of cytomegalovirus (CMV). Severe haematological toxicity occurred in all of the first 10 patients given zidovudine 1.2 g daily and ganciclovir. Consequently the dose of zidovudine was reduced to 600 mg daily. Overall 82% of the 40 patients enrolled experienced profound and rapid toxicity (anaemia, neutropenia, leucopenia, gastrointestinal disturbances). Zidovudine dosage reductions to 300 mg daily were needed in many patients. No change in the pharmacokinetics of zidovudine or ganciclovir was noted.[9]

Another study in 6 AIDS patients with CMV retinitis given zidovudine and ganciclovir found increased bone marrow toxicity but no improved efficacy over ganciclovir alone.[10] Increased toxicity (myelotoxicity and pancytopenia) following the use of both drugs has also been reported elsewhere.[11,12]

In contrast to the first study,[9] a specific study on the pharmacokinetics of zidovudine and ganciclovir in HIV+ subjects reported that oral ganciclovir increased the maximum levels of zidovudine by 38% and the AUC by 15%, without altering renal clearance. Zidovudine did not alter ganciclovir pharmacokinetics.[1]

Mechanism

The reason for the increased levels of didanosine and zidovudine when given with ganciclovir is unknown. It does not appear to be due to competition for active secretion by the kidney tubules.[1]

The toxicity of the zidovudine/ganciclovir combination may be simply additive,[9] but *in vitro* studies with three human cell lines found synergistic cytotoxicity when both drugs were used.[13]

There is some *in vitro* evidence that ganciclovir antagonises the anti-HIV activity of zidovudine and didanosine.[14]

Importance and management

The interactions between ganciclovir and didanosine or zidovudine would appear to be established, but the clinical importance is uncertain. Zidovudine seems to be associated with greater toxicity than didanosine. However, there is also some evidence suggesting reduced efficacy of ganciclovir in the presence of didanosine, and this requires further study. Close and careful monitoring is required if either combination is used. The UK maker of ganciclovir suggests that zidovudine should not be given during ganciclovir induction treatment, and patients should be closely monitored for neutropenia when maintenance ganciclovir is used with zidovudine.[15]

Ganciclovir does not appear to alter the pharmacokinetics of stavudine or zalcitabine. Zalcitabine increased ganciclovir levels to a minor extent, although this is probably not clinically important.

1. Cimoch PJ, Lavelle J, Pollard R, Griffy KG, Wong R, Tarnowski TL, Casserella S, Jung D. Pharmacokinetics of oral ganciclovir alone and in combination with zidovudine, didanosine, and probenecid in HIV-infected subjects. *J Acquir Immune Defic Syndr Hum Retrovirol* (1998) 17, 227–34.
2. Frascino RJ, Anderson RD, Griffy KG, Jung D, Yu S. Two multiple dose crossover studies of IV ganciclovir (GCV) and didanosine (ddI) in HIV infected persons. *Intersci Conf Antimicrob Agents Chemother* (1995) 35, 6.
3. Jung D, Griffy K, Dorr A, Raschke R, Tarnowski TL, Hulse J, Kates RE. Effect of high-dose oral ganciclovir on didanosine disposition in human immunodeficiency virus (HIV)-positive patients. *J Clin Pharmacol* (1998) 38, 1057–62.
4. Hartman NR, Yarchoan R, Pluda JM, Thomas RV, Wyvill KM, Flora KP, Broder S, Johns DG. Pharmacokinetics of 2′,3′-dideoxyinosine in patients with severe human immunodeficiency infection. II. The effects of different oral formulations and the presence of other medications. *Clin Pharmacol Ther* (1991) 50, 278–85.
5. Jacobson MA, Owen W, Campbell J, Brosgart C, Abrams DI. Tolerability of combined ganciclovir and didanosine for the treatment of cytomegalovirus disease associated with AIDS. *Clin Infect Dis* (1993) 16 (Suppl 1), S69–S73.
6. Brosgart CL, Louis TA, Hillman DW, Craig CP, Alston B, Fisher E, Abrams DI, Luskin-Hawk RL, Sampson JH, Ward DJ, Thompson MA, Torres RA. A randomized, placebo-controlled trial of the safety and efficacy of oral ganciclovir for prophylaxis of cytomegalovirus disease in HIV-infected individuals. *AIDS* (1998) 12, 269–77.
7. Epivir (Lamivudine). GlaxoSmithKline UK. UK Summary of product characteristics, December 2004.
8. Jung D, AbdelHameed MH, Teitelbaum P, Dorr A, Griffy K. The pharmacokinetics and safety profile of oral ganciclovir combined with zalcitabine or stavudine in asymptomatic HIV- and CMV-seropositive patients. *J Clin Pharmacol* (1999) 39, 505–12.
9. Hochster H, Dieterich D, Bozzette S, Reichman RC, Connor JD, Liebes L, Sonke RL, Spector SA, Valentine F, Pettinelli C, Richman DD. Toxicity of combined ganciclovir and zidovudine for cytomegalovirus disease associated with AIDS. An AIDS clinical trials group study. *Ann Intern Med* (1990) 113, 111–17.
10. Millar AB, Miller RF, Patou G, Mindel A, Marsh R, Semple SJG. Treatment of cytomegalovirus retinitis with zidovudine and ganciclovir in patients with AIDS: outcome and toxicity. *Genitourin Med* (1990) 66, 156–8.
11. Jacobson MA, de Miranda P, Gordon SM, Blum MR, Volberding P, Mills J. Prolonged pancytopenia due to combined ganciclovir and zidovudine therapy. *J Infect Dis* (1988) 158, 489–90.
12. Pinching AJ, Helbert M, Peddle B, Robinson D, Janes K, Gor D, Jeffries DJ, Stoneham C, Mitchell D, Kocsis AE, Mann J, Forster SM, Harris JRW. *J Infect* (1989) 18 (Suppl 1), 33–40.
13. Prichard MN, Prichard LE, Baguley WA, Nassiri MR, Shipman C. Three-dimensional analysis of the synergistic cytotoxicity of ganciclovir and zidovudine. *Antimicrob Agents Chemother* (1991) 35, 1060–5.
14. Medina DJ, Hsiung GD, Mellors JW. Ganciclovir antagonizes the anti-human immunodeficiency virus type 1 activity of zidovudine and didanosine in vitro. *Antimicrob Agents Chemother* (1992) 36, 1127–30.
15. Cymevene IV (Ganciclovir sodium). Roche Products Ltd. UK Summary of product characteristics, April 2004.

NRTIs + H_2-blockers

The concurrent use of didanosine and ranitidine results in a minor increase in the serum levels of didanosine, and a minor decrease in the serum levels of ranitidine. Both changes seem to be clinically unimportant. Cimetidine raises serum zalcitabine levels, but this is of uncertain importance. Cimetidine, but not ranitidine, reduces the renal secretion of zidovudine, but neither has a significant effect on zidovudine serum levels. Cimetidine and ranitidine do not interact with lamivudine.

Clinical evidence, mechanism, importance and management

(a) Didanosine

Didanosine 375 mg (buffered sachet preparation) was given to 12 HIV+ subjects either alone, or 2 hours after a single 150-mg dose of **ranitidine**. The didanosine AUC was increased by 14% by the **ranitidine**.[1] The reason is not known but the **ranitidine** possibly enhanced the effects of citrate-phosphate buffer with which the didanosine sachet was form

The **ranitidine** AUC was reduced by 16% for reasons that are not understood, but it is possible that antacids (such as the citrate-phosphate buffer) reduce the absorption of **ranitidine**[1] (see 'H$_2$-blockers + Antacids', p.734).

These bioavailability changes appear to be too small to matter clinically, and no particular precautions would seem necessary if the drugs are taken in this way. It is not known whether other H$_2$-blockers behave similarly.

(b) Lamivudine

Lamivudine is cleared predominantly from the body by the kidneys using the organic cationic transport system, but the maker notes that **cimetidine** and **ranitidine**, which partly use this mechanism, do not interact with lamivudine.[2]

(c) Zalcitabine

A study in 12 HIV+ patients given a single 1.5-mg dose of zalcitabine found that **cimetidine** 800 mg caused a 24% reduction in the renal clearance of zalcitabine, assumed to be due to a reduction in renal tubular secretion, and a 36% increase in the AUC.[3]

These changes are relatively moderate and of uncertain clinical importance, but this still awaits formal assessment. Monitor concurrent use for possible toxicity.

(d) Zidovudine

Zidovudine 600 mg daily was given to 5 HIV+ men and one man with AIDS in a randomised crossover study. The zidovudine was given either alone, with **cimetidine** 300 mg four times daily, or with **ranitidine** 150 mg twice daily, each for 7 days. **Cimetidine** reduced the renal elimination of the zidovudine by 56%, but had no effect on the AUC of zidovudine. It was suggested that the reduction in clearance was due to inhibition of tubular secretion. **Ranitidine** had no effect on zidovudine pharmacokinetics. No clinical toxicity occurred and the immunological parameters measured (CD4 and CD8 cells) were not significantly altered. The authors concluded that no change in the dosage of zidovudine is needed if either of these H$_2$-blockers is given concurrently.[4] Information about other H$_2$-blockers seems to be lacking.

1. Knupp CA, Graziano FM, Dixon RM, Barbhaiya RH. Pharmacokinetic-interaction study of didanosine and ranitidine in patients seropositive for human immunodeficiency virus. *Antimicrob Agents Chemother* (1992) 36, 2075–9.
2. Epivir (Lamivudine). GlaxoSmithKline UK. UK Summary of product characteristics, December 2004.
3. Massarella JW, Holazo AA, Koss-Twardy S, Min B, Smith B, Nazareno LA. The effects of cimetidine and Maalox® on the pharmacokinetics of zalcitabine in HIV-positive patients. *Pharm Res* (1994) 11 (10 Suppl), S-415.
4. Fletcher CV, Henry WK, Noormohamed SE, Rhame FS, Balfour HH. The effect of cimetidine and ranitidine administration with zidovudine. *Pharmacotherapy* (1995) 15, 701–8.

NRTIs + Hydroxycarbamide

Hydroxycarbamide appears to increase the antiviral activity of NRTIs, particularly didanosine. However, the combination of hydroxycarbamide and didanosine may carry a higher risk of adverse effects including neuropathy and pancreatitis, especially if stavudine is also given.

Clinical evidence, mechanism, importance and management

Data from *in vitro* studies have shown that hydroxycarbamide increases the antiviral activity of NRTIs, particularly **didanosine**, possibly by increasing their intracellular activation (phosphorylation).[1,2] The combination is therefore under clinical investigation. Some randomised trials[3,4] have shown that the addition of hydroxycarbamide to reverse transcriptase inhibitors improves virologic response, whereas others have not demonstrated this.[5]

Of concern is that a number of studies have shown increased toxicity. One study reported that the relative risk of neuropathy with **didanosine** plus hydroxycarbamide was 2.35 compared with **didanosine** alone, and increased to 7.8 when **stavudine** was also added.[6] Another study reported an increased incidence of neuropathy, and an increased incidence of fatigue and nausea and vomiting.[7] The risk of pancreatitis may also be increased. In one study, 3 patients randomised to indinavir, **didanosine**, **stavudine** and hydroxycarbamide developed pancreatitis and died, compared with no deaths in those receiving the same antivirals without hydroxycarbamide.[8] Another non-fatal case of pancreatitis has been reported when hydroxycarbamide was added to **stavudine**, **didanosine** and nevirapine therapy.[9] The maker has issued a warning about the risks of pancreatitis with **didanosine**, particularly in combination with hydroxycarbamide and **stavudine**.[10]

Further studies are needed to define the role of hydroxycarbamide in combination with NRTIs in HIV infection.

1. Palmer S, Cox S. Increased activation of the combination of 3'-azido-3'-deoxythymidine and 2'-deoxy-3'-thiacytidine in the presence of hydroxyurea. *Antimicrob Agents Chemother* (1997) 41, 460–4.
2. Rana KZ, Simmons KA, Dudley MN. Hydroxyurea reduces the 50% inhibitory concentration of didanosine in HIV-infected cells. *AIDS* (1999) 13, 2186–88.
3. Lafeuillade A, Hittinger G, Chadapaud S, Maillefet S, Rieu A, Poggi C. The HYDILE trial: efficacy and tolerance of a quadruple combination of reverse transcriptase inhibitors versus the same regimen plus hydroxyurea or hydroxyurea and interleukin-2 in HIV-infected patients failing protease inhibitor–based combinations. *HIV Clin Trials* (2002) 3, 263–71.
4. Rodriguez CG, Vila J, Capurro AF, Maidana MM, Boffo Lissin LD. Combination therapy with hydroxyurea versus without hydroxyurea as first line treatment options for antiretroviral-naive patients. *HIV Clin Trials* (2000) 1, 1–8.
5. Zala C, Salomon H, Ochoa C, Kijak G, Federico A, Perez H, Montaner JSG, Cahn P. Higher rate of toxicity with no increased efficacy when hydroxyurea is added to a regimen of stavudine plus didanosine and nevirapine in primary HIV infection. *J Acquir Immune Defic Syndr* (2002) 29, 368–73.
6. Moore RD, Wong W-ME, Keruly JC, McArthur JC. Incidence of neuropathy in HIV-infected patients on monotherapy versus those on combination therapy with didanosine, stavudine and hydroxyurea. *AIDS* (2000) 14, 273–8.
7. Rutschmann OT, Vernazza PL, Bucher HC, Opravil M, Ledergerber B, Telenti A, Malinverni R, Bernasconi E, Fagard C, Leduc D, Perrin L, Hirschel B. Long-term hydroxyurea in combination with didanosine and stavudine for the treatment of HIV-1 infection. *AIDS* (2000) 14, 2145–51.
8. Havlir DV, Gilbert PB, Bennett K, Collier AC, Hirsch MS, Tebas P, Adams EM, Wheat LJ, Goodwin D, Schnittman S, Holohan MK, Richman DD; ACTG 5025 Study Team. Effects of treatment intensification with hydroxyurea in HIV-infected patients with virologic suppression. *AIDS* (2001) 1379–88.
9. Longhurst HJ, Pinching AJ. Pancreatitis associated with hydroxyurea in combination with didanosine. *BMJ* (2001) 322, 81.
10. ddI, d4T, hydroxyurea: new pancreatitis warning. *AIDS Treat News* (1999) Nov 19; (no. 331): 1–3.

NRTIs + Macrolides

Clarithromycin causes some reduction in the bioavailability of zidovudine, but this is minimised if the two drugs are given not less than 2 hours apart. Clarithromycin does not appear to interact with didanosine, stavudine or zalcitabine, and azithromycin does not interact with didanosine or zidovudine.

Clinical evidence

(a) Didanosine

Azithromycin 1.2 g daily for 14 days was given to 12 HIV+ subjects with didanosine 200 mg twice daily without any significant change in the pharmacokinetics of either drug.[1]

Clarithromycin 1 g twice daily for 7 days was given to 4 HIV+ patients and 8 AIDS patients already taking oral didanosine. For the group as a whole the pharmacokinetics of the didanosine remained unchanged, but there were large differences in the AUC between subjects that could have hidden an interaction.[2]

(b) Stavudine

A study in 10 HIV+ subjects found that the addition of **clarithromycin** 500 mg twice daily to stavudine 30 or 40 mg twice daily caused no significant effects on the pharmacokinetics of the stavudine and the incidence of adverse effects did not increase.[3] No special precautions would seem necessary if both drugs are given.

(c) Zalcitabine

A 7-day course of **clarithromycin** 500 mg twice daily was given to 12 HIV+ subjects already taking zalcitabine. The addition of **clarithromycin** caused no change to the pharmacokinetics of zalcitabine.[4]

(d) Zidovudine

Azithromycin 600 mg to 1.2 g daily for 14 days was given to 12 HIV+ subjects with zidovudine 100 mg five times daily without any significant change in zidovudine pharmacokinetics.[1] Similarly, **azithromycin** 1 g given weekly to 9 HIV+ subjects caused no change in the pharmacokinetics of zidovudine 10 mg/kg daily. The **azithromycin** pharmacokinetics also remained unchanged.[5]

Zidovudine 100 mg every 4 hours 5 times a day and oral **clarithromycin** 500 mg, 1 g or 2 g every 12 hours, both together and alone, were given to 15 HIV+ patients. The pharmacokinetics of the **clarithromycin** were not substantially changed but the zidovudine levels and AUCs were reduced by 23 to 58% and 12 to 36% respectively. However, these effects were not seen in all patients.[6,7] Another study similarly found that **clarithromycin** caused a moderate reduction in the AUC of oral zidovudine (by up to 27%). No changes were seen when the zidovudine was given 4 or more hours after the **clarithromycin**.[8] Zidovudine and **clarithromycin** were given to 16 AIDS patients 2 hours apart for 4 days. The maximum plasma levels of the zidovudine rose by about 50%, but the minimum levels and the AUC over 8 hours did not change.[9]

Mechanism

Not understood but possibly due to some changes in absorption.

Importance and management

The overall picture is slightly confusing, but it seems that some reductions in zidovudine levels are likely if clarithromycin is taken at the same time, but no important changes seem to occur if the administration of the drugs is separated. The authors of one study recommend that the clarithromycin is given at least 2 hours before or after the zidovudine.[7] The authors of the report on didanosine conclude that clarithromycin may safely be given with didanosine,[2] and it also seems likely that didanosine and azithromycin, zidovudine and azithromycin, stavudine and clarithromycin, or zalcitabine and clarithromycin can be used safely together. More study is needed to confirm this.

1. Amsden G, Flaherty J, Luke D. Lack of an effect of azithromycin on the disposition of zidovudine and dideoxyinosine in HIV-infected patients. *J Clin Pharmacol* (2001) 41, 210–16.
2. Gillum JG, Bruzzese VL, Israel DS, Kaplowitz LG, Polk RE. Effect of clarithromycin on the pharmacokinetics of 2′,3′-dideoxyinosine in patients who are seropositive for human immunodeficiency virus. *Clin Infect Dis* (1996) 22, 716–18.
3. Piscitelli SC, Kelly G, Walker RE, Kovacs J, Falloon J, Davey RT, Raje S, Masur H, Polis MA. A multiple drug interaction study of stavudine with agents for opportunistic infections in human immunodeficiency virus-infected patients. *Antimicrob Agents Chemother* (1999) 43, 647–50.
4. Pastore A, van Cleef G, Fisher EJ, Gillum JG, LeBel M, Polk RE. Dideoxycytidine (ddC) pharmacokinetics and interaction with clarithromycin in patients seropositive for HIV. 4th Conference on Retroviruses and Opportunistic Infections, Washington DC, January 22nd-26th 1997. Abstract 613.
5. Chave J-P, Munafo A, Chatton J-Y, Dayer P, Glauser MP, Biollaz J. Once-a-week azithromycin in AIDS patients: tolerability, kinetics, and effects on zidovudine disposition. *Antimicrob Agents Chemother* (1992) 36, 1013–18.
6. Gustavson LE, Chu S-Y, Mackenthun A, Gupta SD, Craft JC. Drug interaction between clarithromycin and oral zidovudine in HIV-1 infected patients. *Clin Pharmacol Ther* (1993) 53, 163.
7. Polis MA, Piscitelli SC, Vogel S, Witebsky FG, Conville PS, Petty B, Kovacs JA, Davey RT, Walker RE, Falloon J, Metcalf JA, Craft C, Lane HC, Masur H. Clarithromycin lowers plasma zidovudine levels in persons with human immunodeficiency virus infection. *Antimicrob Agents Chemother* (1997) 41, 1709–14.
8. Petty B, Polis M, Haneiwich S, Dellerson M, Craft JC, Chaisson R. Pharmacokinetic assessment of clarithromycin plus zidovudine in HIV patients. Interdsci Conf Antimicrob Ag Chemother, Anaheim, Calif, Oct 11–14, 1992, 32, 114.
9. Vance E, Watson-Bitar M, Gustavson L, Kazanjian P. Pharmacokinetics of clarithromycin and zidovudine in patients with AIDS. *Antimicrob Agents Chemother* (1995) 39, 1355–60.

NRTIs + NRTIs

***In vitro*, zidovudine decreases the intracellular activation of stavudine, and antagonism has been demonstrated clinically. Lamivudine decreases the *in vitro* activation of zalcitabine. It is recommended that concurrent use of stavudine with zidovudine, and lamivudine with zalcitabine should be avoided. There are some reports of additive toxicity with didanosine/stavudine (pancreatitis and neuropathy), didanosine/zalcitabine (neuropathy), and lamivudine/zidovudine (blood dyscrasias), so treatment should be carefully monitored. Additive risk for neuropathy and pancreatitis would also be predicted for stavudine/zalcitabine. In general the other NRTIs are well tolerated in combination, with minimal pharmacokinetic changes occurring.**

Clinical evidence, mechanism, importance and management

(a) Abacavir + Lamivudine

A single dose of lamivudine 150 mg was given with abacavir 600 mg to 13 HIV+ subjects. The pharmacokinetics of abacavir were not significantly affected but the lamivudine maximum plasma levels and AUC were decreased by 35 and 15%. These changes were considered to be consistent with a change in absorption. The extent of the change is not thought to be clinically significant and so no dose alteration would seem necessary on concurrent use.[1]

(b) Abacavir + Zidovudine

A single dose of zidovudine 300 mg was given with abacavir 600 mg to 13 HIV+ subjects. The pharmacokinetics of abacavir were not significantly affected. The zidovudine maximum plasma level decreased by 20%, but the AUC was unchanged. This change is not thought to be clinically significant and so no dose alteration would seem necessary on concurrent use.[1] These results were confirmed in a steady-state study in which 79 HIV+ subjects received 8 weeks treatment with abacavir 600 to 1800 mg daily, in divided doses and zidovudine 600 mg daily, in divided doses.[2]

(c) Didanosine + Lamivudine

Lamivudine is cleared predominantly from the body by the kidneys using the organic cationic transport system. Didanosine is not cleared by this mechanism and so is unlikely to interact pharmacokinetically with lamivudine.[3] Didanosine does not affect the intracellular activation of lamivudine *in vitro*.[4]

(d) Didanosine + Stavudine

Didanosine does not interfere with the intracellular activation of stavudine *in vitro*.[5] Didanosine 100 mg twice daily was given to 10 HIV+ subjects with stavudine 40 mg twice daily for 9 doses. The didanosine pharmacokinetics were unchanged by concurrent use. The half-life of the stavudine increased from 1.56 to 1.96 hours, but the AUC was unchanged and adverse effects were minimal. The authors of the report concluded that no clinically significant pharmacokinetic interaction, and no change in acute safety and tolerance, are likely if both drugs are given concurrently.[6] However, both didanosine and stavudine can cause peripheral neuropathy and pancreatitis, and there is some evidence that this risk may be additive. In one early study, combination treatment with stavudine and didanosine was given to 13 HIV+ subjects for 8 weeks. Neuropathy occurred in 3 patients, with only 2 restarting treatment.[7] In another study, the relative risk of neuropathy was 1.39 for stavudine alone relative to didanosine alone, and 3.5 for combined use of both drugs.[8] In 1999, the maker of didanosine issued a stronger warning about the risk of pancreatitis with didanosine, and noted this risk was higher in patients also taking stavudine,[9] see also 'NRTIs + Hydroxycarbamide', p.598. Combined use should be carefully monitored. See also 'NRTIs + Drugs causing peripheral neuropathy', p.595, and 'NRTIs + Drugs causing pancreatitis', p.595.

(e) Didanosine + Zalcitabine

In vitro, didanosine had no significant effect on the intracellular activation of zalcitabine.[10] A 29-year-old man with persistent mild neuropathy due to zalcitabine developed severe neuropathy when given didanosine 3 weeks after discontinuing zalcitabine. As the didanosine neuropathy developed so rapidly it was suggested that it was caused by additive toxicity with zalcitabine.[11] Note also that both drugs are associated with pancreatitis. The makers advise caution and careful monitoring if drugs that share these serious side effects are used concurrently. See also 'NRTIs + Drugs causing peripheral neuropathy', p.595, and 'NRTIs + Drugs causing pancreatitis', p.595.

(f) Didanosine + Zidovudine

A study in 8 HIV+ patients found that when given zidovudine 250 mg and didanosine 250 mg (buffered sachet formulation) together, the pharmacokinetics of the didanosine were unaltered but the zidovudine AUC was raised by 35%, possibly due to altered absorption.[12] Conversely, in another study zidovudine plasma levels were lower in 4 out of 5 HIV+ patients when given didanosine (chewable tablets) and there was an average 14% reduction in the zidovudine AUC. The zidovudine clearance was increased by 29% but the didanosine pharmacokinetics were unchanged.[13] A study in over 50 subjects ranging in age from 3 months to 21 years found that when compared with day 3 (start of concurrent use), no significant changes in AUCs occurred after 4 or 12 weeks of concurrent zidovudine 60 to 180 mg/m^2 every 6 hours and didanosine 60 to 180 mg/m^2 every 12 hours (given 2 minutes after an antacid).[14] Several other studies have not found a pharmacokinetic interaction or evidence of increased toxicity when didanosine and zidovudine are used concurrently.[15-18]

The reports are slightly contradictory, but the weight of evidence seems to be that no clinically relevant interaction occurs.

(g) Emtricitabine + Stavudine

There was no important pharmacokinetic interaction between single doses of emtricitabine 200 mg and stavudine 40 mg in 6 healthy subjects.[19]

(h) Emtricitabine + Zidovudine

The AUC and maximum level of zidovudine 300 mg were increased by 26% and 66%, respectively, by emtricitabine 200 mg in a single-dose study in 6 healthy subjects. The pharmacokinetics of emtricitabine were not altered.[19] The authors suggest that these increases in zidovudine lev are unlikely to be clinically relevant based on experience of using th drugs together for 48 weeks in a phase III clinical trial.[19] Further experience is needed.

(i) Lamivudine + Stavudine

Nucleoside reverse transcriptase inhibitors such as lamivudine need to be activated by phosphorylation within cells to a triphosphate anabolite. Since stavudine does not affect this phosphorylation *in vitro*[4] it is predicted that no interaction is likely to occur by this mechanism. The maker briefly states that no clinically relevant pharmacokinetic interaction has been noted between stavudine and lamivudine.[20,21]

(j) Lamivudine + Zalcitabine

Lamivudine is cleared predominantly from the body by the kidneys using the organic cationic transport system. Zalcitabine is not cleared by this mechanism and so is unlikely to interact pharmacokinetically with lamivudine.[3] However, the makers say that lamivudine is not recommended to be used with zalcitabine, since lamivudine may inhibit the intracellular activation of zalcitabine.[3,10,22,23]

(k) Lamivudine + Zidovudine

Lamivudine 300 mg twice daily was given to 12 HIV+ patients for 2 days, and then on day 3 they were given lamivudine 300 mg plus zidovudine 200 mg. No major changes in the pharmacokinetics of the zidovudine occurred and it was concluded that dosage adjustments are not needed if these two drugs are given concurrently.[24] Another study showed the same results,[1] and an extensive study in over 200 patients has shown that combined use can be safe and effective.[25]

However there are case reports of blood dyscrasias occurring with concurrent use. Zidovudine 500 to 600 mg daily was given with lamivudine 300 mg daily to 8 HIV+ men. Zidovudine or lamivudine alone had previously been given to 6 of these 8 without problem. However, when the drugs were combined, blood dyscrasias occurred in all patients within 7 weeks. Anaemia, with a 50% fall in haemoglobin occurred in 7 patients, while the other patient developed leucopenia and thrombocytopenia. The drug combination was stopped, blood transfusions were given, and all patients improved or recovered over 5 weeks. Zidovudine or lamivudine alone was later started in 5 patients without further haematological problems.[26] Similar precipitous falls in haemoglobin occurred in another 2 patients when lamivudine 300 mg daily was added to their long-term zidovudine treatment. Again both recovered when the drugs were stopped and blood was given.[27] Anaemia is a common adverse effect of zidovudine, but these patients had no problems until the lamivudine was added. The available evidence indicates that concurrent use can be safe and effective, with the adverse interactions cited here being uncommon. It has been suggested that a complete baseline blood count should be done when combined treatment is started, and then every month for the first 3 months of treatment.[27]

(l) Stavudine + Zalcitabine

In vitro, stavudine had no significant effect on the intracellular activation of zalcitabine.[10] Both stavudine and zalcitabine have the potential to cause peripheral neuropathy and pancreatitis. Combined use of drugs causing these serious side effects should be closely monitored (see also 'NRTIs + Drugs causing peripheral neuropathy', p.595, and 'NRTIs + Drugs causing pancreatitis', p.595).

(m) Stavudine + Zidovudine

Nucleoside reverse transcriptase inhibitors such as stavudine need to be phosphorylated within cells to a triphosphate anabolite before they become effective. *In vitro* studies using mononucleated blood cells found that zidovudine significantly inhibited this phosphorylation.[5] Antagonism between zidovudine and stavudine has also been seen *in vivo* in a clinical trial.[28] The makers currently do not recommend the combination.[20,21]

(n) Zalcitabine + Zidovudine

In vitro, zalcitabine had no significant effect on the intracellular activation of zidovudine.[10] In a study in 56 advanced HIV+ patients taking zidovudine 50 to 200 mg every 8 hours and zalcitabine 5 to 10 micrograms/kg every 8 hours, neither drug affected the pharmacokinetics of the other nor was toxicity increased.[29] No special precautions would appear to be necessary.

1. Wang LH, Chittick GE, McDowell JA. Single-dose pharmacokinetics and safety of abacavir (1592U89), zidovudine, and lamivudine administered alone and in combination in adults with human immunodeficiency virus infection. *Antimicrob Agents Chemother* (1999) 43, 1708–15.
2. McDowell JA, Lou Y, Symonds WS, Stein DS. Multiple-dose pharmacokinetics and pharmacodynamics of abacavir alone and in combination with zidovudine in human immunodeficiency virus-infected adults. *Antimicrob Agents Chemother* (2000) 44, 2061–7.
3. Epivir (Lamivudine). GlaxoSmithKline UK. UK Summary of product characteristics, December 2004.
4. Kewn S, Veal GJ, Hoggard PG, Barry MG, Back DJ. Lamivudine (3TC). Phosphorylation and drug interactions *in vitro*. *Biochem Pharmacol* (1997) 54, 589–95.
5. Hoggard PG, Kewn S, Barry MG, Khoo SH, Back DJ. Effects of drugs on 2',3'-dideoxy-2',3'-didehydrothymidine phosphorylation in vitro. *Antimicrob Agents Chemother* (1997) 41, 1231–6.
6. Seifert RD, Stewart MB, Sramek JJ, Conrad J, Kaul S, Cutler NR. Pharmacokinetics of co-administered didanosine and stavudine in HIV-seropositive male patients. *Br J Clin Pharmacol* (1994) 38, 405–10.
7. Kalathoor S, Sinclair J, Andron L, Sension MG, High K. Combination therapy with stavudine and didanosine. 4th Conference on Retroviruses and Opportunistic Infections, Washington DC, Jan 22-26 1997. Abstract 552.
8. Moore RD, Wong W-ME, Keruly JC, McArthur JC. Incidence of neuropathy in HIV-infected patients on monotherapy versus those on combination therapy with didanosine, stavudine, and hydroxyurea. *AIDS* (2000) 14, 273–8.
9. ddI, d4T, hydroxyurea: new pancreatitis warning. *AIDS Treat News* (1999) Nov 19 (No. 331), 1–3.
10. Hivid (Zalcitabine). Roche Products Ltd. UK Summary of product characteristics, November 2004.
11. LeLacheur SF, Simon GL. Exacerbation of dideoxycytidine-induced neuropathy with dideoxyinosine. *J Acquir Immune Defic Syndr* (1991) 4, 538–9.
12. Barry M, Howe JL, Ormesher S, Back DJ, Breckenridge AM, Bergin C, Mulcahy F, Beeching N, Nye F. Pharmacokinetics of zidovudine and dideoxyinosine alone and in combination in patients with acquired immunodeficiency syndrome. *Br J Clin Pharmacol* (1994) 37, 421–6.
13. Burger DM, Meenhorst PL, Kroon FP, Mulder JW, Koks CHW, Bult A, Beijnen JH. Pharmacokinetic interaction study of zidovudine and didanosine. *J Drug Dev* (1994) 6, 187–94.
14. Mueller BU, Pizzo PA, Farley M, Husson RN, Goldsmith J, Kovacs A, Woods L, Ono J, Church JA, Brouwers P, Jarosinski P, Venzon D, Balis FM. Pharmacokinetic evaluation of the combination of zidovudine and didanosine in children with human immunodeficiency virus infection. *J Pediatr* (1994) 125, 142–6.
15. Collier AC, Coombs RW, Fischl MA, Skolnik PR, Northfelt D, Boutin P, Hooper CJ, Kaplan LD, Volberding PA, Davis LG, Henrard DR, Weller S, Corey L. Combination therapy with zidovudine and didanosine compared with zidovudine alone in HIV-1 infection. *Ann Intern Med* (1993) 119, 786–93.
16. Sahai J, Gallicano K, Seguin I, Garber G, Cameron W. Interaction between zidovudine (ZDV) and didanosine (ddI). *Intersci Conf Antimicrob Agents Chemother* (1994) 34, 82.
17. Sahai J, Gallicano K, Garber G, Pakuts A, Cameron W. Pharmacokinetics of simultaneously administered zidovudine and didanosine in HIV-seropositive male patients. *J Acquir Immune Defic Syndr Hum Retrovirol* (1995) 10, 54–60.
18. Gibb D, Barry M, Ormesher S, Nokes L, Seefried M, Giaquinto C, Back D. Pharmacokinetics of zidovudine and dideoxyinosine alone and combination in children with HIV infection. *Br J Clin Pharmacol* (1995) 39, 527–30.
19. Wang LH, Blum MR, Hui J, Hulett L, Chittick GE, Rousseau F. Lack of significant pharmacokinetic interactions between emtricitabine and other nucleoside antivirals in healthy volunteers. *Intersci Conf Antimicrob Agents Chemother* (2001) 41, 18.
20. Zerit (Stavudine). Bristol-Myers Squibb Pharmaceuticals Ltd. UK Summary of product characteristics, January 2005.
21. Zerit (Stavudine). Bristol-Myers Squibb Company. US Prescribing information, June 2004.
22. Hivid (Zalcitabine). Roche Pharmaceuticals. US Prescribing information, September 2002.
23. Epivir (Lamivudine). GlaxoSmithKline. US Prescribing information, December 2004.
24. Rana KZ, Horton CM, Yuen GJ, Pivarnik PE, Mikolich DM, Fisher AE, Mydlow PK, Dudley MN. Effect of lamivudine on zidovudine pharmacokinetics in asymptomatic HIV-infected individuals. *Intersci Conf Antimicrob Agents Chemother* (1994) 34, 83.
25. Staszewski S, Loveday C, Picazo JJ, Dellamonica P, Skinhøj P, Johnson MA, Danner SA, Harrigan PR, Hill AM, Verity L, McDade H; for the Lamivudine European HIV Working Group. Safety and efficacy of lamivudine-zidovudine combination therapy in zidovudine-experienced patients. A randomized controlled comparison with zidovudine monotherapy. *JAMA* (1996) 276, 111–17.
26. Tseng A, Fletcher D, Gold W, Conly J, Keystone D, Walmsley S. Precipitous declines in hemoglobin with combination AZT/3TC. 4th Conference on Retroviruses and Opportunistic Infections, Washington, Jan 22-26, 1997. Abstract 559.
27. Hester EK, Peacock JE. Profound and unanticipated anemia with lamivudine-zidovudine combination therapy in zidovudine-experienced patients with HIV infection. *AIDS* (1998) 12, 439–51.
28. Havlir DV, Tierney C, Friedland GH, Pollard RB, Smeaton L, Sommadossi JP, Fox L, Kessler H, Fife KH, Richman DD. In vivo antagonism with zidovudine plus stavudine combination therapy. *J Infect Dis* (2000) 182, 321–5.
29. Meng T-C, Fischl MA, Boota AM, Spector SA. Bennett D, Bassiakos Y, Lai S, Wright B, Richman DD. Combination therapy with zidovudine and dideoxycytidine in patients with advanced human immunodeficiency virus infection. *Ann Intern Med* (1992) 116, 13–20.

NRTIs + Paracetamol (Acetaminophen)

Limited and unconfirmed evidence suggests that paracetamol possibly increases the bone marrow suppressant effects of zidovudine. Single case reports describe severe liver toxicity when patients were given paracetamol with either zidovudine or didanosine.

Clinical evidence

(a) Didanosine

Increasing abdominal pain occurred in a 47-year-old HIV+ man one month after starting didanosine (his other medications included nevirapine, hydroxycarbamide, aciclovir and lorazepam). He had been treating the pain with paracetamol, and had taken 4 g over 3 days. Severe hepatitis and pancreatitis was diagnosed, which slowly resolved over the following 3 weeks.[1]

(b) Zidovudine

An early study of zidovudine use in 282 AIDS patients found that haematological abnormalities (anaemia, leucopenia, neutropenia) were very common and 21% needed multiple red cell transfusions. Some of the patients also received paracetamol, which increased the haematological toxicity (neutropenia) by an unstated amount.[2]

Short-term clinical studies using paracetamol 650 mg up to every 4 hours found that it had no clinically significant effects on the pharmacokinetics of zidovudine,[3-6] although in one case clearance was slightly increased.[7] An 8-month study in a single patient suggested that long-term concurrent use did not affect the pharmacokinetics of either drug. However, in this individual very rapid absorption and a high peak serum level of zidovudine were seen, so for safety the zidovudine dosage was reduced from 200 mg every 4 hours to 100 mg every 6 hours.[8]

A patient on zidovudine and co-trimoxazole took 3.3 g of paracetamol over 36 hours. Within 2 days he developed severe hepatotoxicity, and as other causes were excluded the reaction was attributed to paracetamol. The authors suggested that zidovudine may have augmented the paracetamol toxicity.[9] However, in a single-dose study, reduced paracetamol glucuronidation and increased formation of hepatotoxic metabolites was seen in patients with advanced HIV infection compared with healthy HIV+ subjects and those without HIV, and this effect was independent of zidovudine therapy.[10] In contrast, in another study, disease state (AIDS versus healthy HIV+ subjects) was not found to alter paracetamol metabolism, and zidovudine was found to *increase* paracetamol glucuronidation in some patients.[11]

Mechanism

Not understood. Paracetamol does not increase the serum levels of zidovudine,[3-5,7] which might have provided an explanation for the apparent increased toxicity. One *in vitro* study found that paracetamol does not affect the glucuronidation of zidovudine,[12] whereas another found that paracetamol did inhibit its metabolism to the glucuronide.[13] The effect of zidovudine on paracetamol metabolism is also unclear.

Didanosine may cause pancreatitis or hepatic disease, and zidovudine may also rarely cause hepatic disease. It has been suggested that the hepatotoxicity of didanosine and paracetamol are augmented when they are given together.[1]

Importance and management

The authors suggest extreme caution when potentially hepatotoxic drugs such as paracetamol are used with didanosine.[1] Note that paracetamol is a widely used non-prescription analgesic, and this appears to be the first report of potential combined toxicity with didanosine. Further study is needed to assess any association of combined use of these drugs with hepatotoxicity.

The short-term use of zidovudine and paracetamol does not appear to alter the pharmacokinetics of either drug. Whether paracetamol can increase the haematological toxicity of zidovudine and whether the drugs have combined hepatotoxicity is unclear from the available data. More study is needed.

1. Lederman JC, Nawaz H. Toxic interaction of didanosine and acetaminophen leading to severe hepatitis and pancreatitis: a case report and review of the literature. *Am J Gastroenterol* (2001) 96, 3474–5.
2. Richman DD, Fischl MA, Grieco MH, Gottlieb MS, Volberding PA, Laskin OL, Leedom JM, Groopman JE, Mildvan D, Hirsch MS, Jackson GG, Durack DT, Nusinoff-Lehrman S and the AZT Collaborative Working Group. The toxicity of azidothymidine (AZT) in the treatment of patients with AIDS and AIDS-related complex. A double-blind, placebo-controlled trial. *N Engl J Med* (1987) 317, 192–7.
3. Steffe EM, King JH, Inciardi JF, Flynn NF, Goldstein E, Tonjes TS, Benet LZ. The effect of acetaminophen on zidovudine metabolism in HIV-infected patients. *J Acquir Immune Defic Syndr* (1990) 3, 691–4.
4. Ptachcinski J, Pazin G, Ho M. The effect of acetaminophen on the pharmacokinetics of zidovudine. *Pharmacotherapy* (1989) 9, 190.
5. Pazin GJ, Ptachcinski RJ, Sheehan M, Ho M. Interactive pharmacokinetics of zidovudine and acetaminophen. 5th International Conference on AIDS, Montreal, 1989. Abstract M.B.P.338.
6. Burger DM, Meenhorst PL, Underberg WJM, van der Heijde JF, Koks CHW, Beijnen JH. Short-term, combined use of paracetamol and zidovudine does not alter the pharmacokinetics of either drug. *Neth J Med* (1994) 44, 161–5.
7. Sattler FR, Ko R, Antoniskis D, Shields M, Cohen J, Nicoloff J, Leedom J, Koda R. Acetaminophen does not impair clearance of zidovudine. *Ann Intern Med* (1991) 114, 937–40.
8. Burger DM, Meenhorst PL, Koks CHW, Beijnen JH. Pharmacokinetics of zidovudine and acetaminophen in a patient on chronic acetaminophen therapy. *Ann Pharmacother* (1994) 28, 327–30.
9. Shriner K, Goetz MB. Severe hepatotoxicity in a patient receiving both acetaminophen and zidovudine. *Am J Med* (1992) 93, 94–6.
10. Esteban A, Pérez-Mateo M, Boix V, González M, Portilla J, Mora A. Abnormalities in the metabolism of acetaminophen in patients infected with the human immunodeficiency virus (HIV). *Methods Find Exp Clin Pharmacol* (1997) 19, 129–32.
11. O'Neil WM, Pezzullo JC, Di Girolamo A, Tsoukas CM, Wainer IW. Glucuronidation and sulphation of paracetamol in HIV-positive patients and patients with AIDS. *Br J Clin Pharmacol* (1999) 48, 811–18.
12. Kamali F, Rawlins MD. Influence of probenecid and paracetamol (acetaminophen) on zidovudine glucuronidation in human liver *in vitro*. *Biopharm Drug Dispos* (1992) 13, 403–9.
13. Schumann L, Unadkat JD. Does acetaminophen potentiate the hematotoxicity of zidovudine (ZDV or AZT) by inhibition of its metabolism to the glucuronide? *Pharm Res* (1988) 5 (Suppl), S-177.

NRTIs + Probenecid

Probenecid reduces the loss of zalcitabine and zidovudine, increasing their serum levels. The zalcitabine/probenecid combination is well tolerated, but the incidence of adverse effects is reported to be very much increased with the probenecid and zidovudine combination. Patients should be monitored for any signs of toxicity.

Clinical evidence

(a) Zalcitabine

In a single-dose study, 12 HIV+ or AIDS patients were given zalcitabine 1.5 mg alone or with probenecid 500 mg, given 8 and 2 hours before then 4 hours after. The renal clearance of the zalcitabine was decreased 42% by probenecid, the half-life increased 47% and AUC increased 54%.[1]

(b) Zidovudine

The concurrent use of zidovudine and probenecid 500 mg every 8 hours for 3 days increased the zidovudine AUC in 12 patients with AIDS or AIDS-related complex by an average of 80% (range 14 to 192%).[2]

Other studies in patients[3-5] and healthy subjects[6] found that probenecid roughly doubled the AUC of zidovudine when given in a variety of dosing schedules.[3,4] However, the effects on zidovudine pharmacokinetics were minimal if the two drugs were given 6 hours apart.[5] Another report describes a very high incidence of rashes in 6 out of 8 HIV+ men given zidovudine with probenecid 500 mg every 6 hours. The rash and other symptoms (such as malaise, fever and myalgia) were sufficiently severe for the probenecid to be withdrawn in 4 of them.[7] A later study found that when using only 250 mg of probenecid every 8 hours the zidovudine AUC was increased 70% but the adverse effects still occurred, although the incidence was possibly somewhat lower.[8]

Mechanism

Experimental clinical evidence indicates that probenecid reduces the metabolism (glucuronidation) of the zidovudine by the liver enzymes, thereby reducing its loss from the body.[2,4,6,9,10] The interaction with zalcitabine is presumably due to inhibition of zalcitabine secretion in the renal tubules.[1]

Importance and management

The concurrent use of zidovudine and probenecid should be well monitored to ensure that zidovudine levels do not rise excessively. Reduce the zidovudine dosage as necessary. However, the apparent increase in adverse effects during concurrent use[7] should be borne in mind.

The concurrent use of zalcitabine and probenecid was well tolerated, and because the zalcitabine half-life is short compared to its dosing schedule significant accumulation would not be expected.

It would seem prudent to monitor for any signs of toxicity if either drug combination is used long-term. The safety of combined use needs further assessment.

1. Massarella JW, Nazareno LA, Passe S, Min B. The effect of probenecid on the pharmacokinetics of zalcitabine in HIV-positive patients. *Pharm Res* (1996) 13, 449–52.
2. Kornhauser DM, Petty BG, Hendrix CW, Woods AS, Nerhood LJ, Bartlett JG, Lietman PS. Probenecid and zidovudine metabolism. *Lancet* (1989) 2, 473–5.
3. Hedaya MA, Elmquist WF, Sawchuk RJ. Probenecid inhibits the metabolic and renal clearances of zidovudine (AZT) in human volunteers. *Pharm Res* (1990) 7, 411–17.
4. de Miranda P, Good SS, Yarchoan R, Thomas RV, Blum MR, Myers CE, Broder S. Alteration of zidovudine pharmacokinetics by probenecid in patients with AIDS or AIDS-related complex. *Clin Pharmacol Ther* (1989) 46, 494–500.
5. McDermott J, Kennedy J, Ellis-Pegler RB, Thomas MG. Pharmacokinetics of zidovudine plus probenecid. *J Infect Dis* (1992) 166, 687–8.
6. Campion JJ, Bawdon RE, Baskin LB, Barton CI. Effect of probenecid on the pharmacokinetics of zidovudine and zidovudine glucuronide. *Pharmacotherapy* (1990) 10, 235.
7. Petty BG, Kornhauser DM, Lietman PS. Zidovudine with probenecid: a warning. *Lancet* (1990) 1, 1044–5.
8. Petty BG, Barditch-Crovo PA, Nerhood L, Kornhauser DM, Kuwahara S, Lietman PS. Unexpected clinical toxicity of probenecid (P) with zidovudine (Z) in patients with HIV infection. *Intersci Conf Antimicrob Agents Chemother* (1991) 31, 323.

9. Sim SM, Back DJ, Breckenridge AM. The effect of various drugs on the glucuronidation of zidovudine (azidothymidine; AZT) by human liver microsomes. *Br J Clin Pharmacol* (1991) 32, 17–21.
10. Kamali F, Rawlins MD. Influence of probenecid and paracetamol (acetaminophen) on zidovudine glucuronidation in human liver *in vitro*. *Biopharm Drug Dispos* (1992) 13, 403–9.

NRTIs + Protease inhibitors

Buffered didanosine decreases the AUC of indinavir, and the drugs should be given one hour apart. Buffered didanosine is predicted to interact similarly with atazanavir, and possibly amprenavir. [Note that many other protease inhibitors should be given separately from didanosine, because of the need to administer them with 'food', (p.611), and didanosine preparations without]. The changes in pharmacokinetics seen when giving other combinations of protease inhibitors with NRTIs do not appear to be clinically significant. Protease inhibitors do not affect the intracellular activation of NRTIs.

Clinical evidence, mechanism, importance and management

The protease inhibitors **indinavir**, **ritonavir**, and **saquinavir** had no effect on intracellular activation of various NRTIs (**didanosine**, **lamivudine**, **stavudine**, **zalcitabine** and **zidovudine**).[1] No interaction would be expected by this mechanism. Other potential interactions are discussed below.

(a) Abacavir

A phase I study in HIV+ patients given **amprenavir** 900 mg twice daily with abacavir 300 mg twice daily for 3 weeks found that neither drug had any clinically significant effect on the pharmacokinetics of the other.[2] The maker of **amprenavir** notes that its AUC and minimum and maximum levels were increased by 29%, 27%, and 47%, respectively by abacavir, but no dosage adjustments are recommended.[3,4]

The maker of a preparation containing **lopinavir/ritonavir** notes that it induces glucuronidation and therefore has the potential to reduce abacavir plasma levels. However this, and its clinical relevance, have yet to be studied.[5,6]

(b) Didanosine

The concurrent use of [buffered] didanosine and **indinavir** reduced the AUC of **indinavir** by 80%, but when given one hour before didanosine the pharmacokinetics of **indinavir** were not significantly affected.[7] Similarly, another study found that the pharmacokinetics of **indinavir** 800 mg were unchanged when the dose was given one hour after buffered didanosine 400 mg.[8] An enteric-coated preparation of didanosine had no effect on the pharmacokinetics of **indinavir** in a single-dose study in 23 healthy subjects.[9] **Indinavir** may require a normal acidic gastric pH for optimal absorption, whereas some didanosine preparations are formulated with buffering agents to raise gastric pH. Any increase in pH would therefore be expected to reduce **indinavir** absorption.[10] The makers of **indinavir** recommend that **indinavir** and didanosine should be given at least one hour apart.[10,11]

Based on the data for other protease inhibitors, the makers of **amprenavir** suggest that it should be given at least one hour apart from didanosine.[3,4] Similarly, the maker of **atazanavir** predicts that buffered drugs may decrease atazanavir plasma levels, and administration should be separated.[12,13] These recommendations would not apply to the enteric-coated preparation of didanosine.[9] Note that both 'didanosine', (p.596) and '**indinavir**', (p.611), are preferably taken on an empty stomach, whereas '**amprenavir**', (p.611), can be given with or without food, and '**atazanavir**', (p.611), should be taken with food.

The pharmacokinetics of **nelfinavir** were not significantly altered after concurrent use with didanosine.[14] Note that '**nelfinavir**', (p.611), should preferably be taken with food, and all 'didanosine preparations', (p.596) without.

Buffered didanosine 200 mg twice daily was given with **ritonavir** 600 mg twice daily to 13 HIV+ subjects. Administration of the two drugs was separated by 2.5 hours, and treatment was given for 4 days. [Note that treatment was staggered in this way since '**ritonavir**, (p.611), should be given with food, and 'didanosine', (p.596) without]. There was little or no change in the pharmacokinetics of **ritonavir**, and the maximum serum levels and AUC of didanosine were reduced by 16 and 13% respectively, which was not considered to be clinically significant. It was suggested that these changes may have been due to altered absorption in the presence of **ritonavir**.[15]

Note also that '**saquinavir**', (p.611), should preferably be taken with food, and all 'didanosine preparations', (p.596) without.

(c) Lamivudine

Lamivudine metabolism does not involve the cytochrome P450 isoenzyme CYP3A4. Therefore it is unlikely that it will interact with drugs, such as the protease inhibitors, which are metabolised by this system.[16] The maker of **amprenavir** notes that there was no pharmacokinetic interaction with lamivudine.[3,4] The maker of **lopinavir/ritonavir** notes that lamivudine did not alter the pharmacokinetics of **lopinavir**.[5,6]

(d) Stavudine

The AUC of stavudine was increased by 25% when stavudine 40 mg twice daily was given with **indinavir** 800 mg every 8 hours for a week, which was not considered to be clinically significant. The serum levels of **indinavir** were unchanged.[17]

The maker of **lopinavir/ritonavir** notes that stavudine did not alter the pharmacokinetics of **lopinavir**.[5,6]

In an early pilot study, combined **nelfinavir** and stavudine was well tolerated, and the adverse effects were similar to those seen when stavudine was given alone, although the incidence of diarrhoea did increase.[18] The maker of **nelfinavir** notes that clinically significant interactions have not been observed with stavudine.[19,20]

(e) Zalcitabine

The maker of zalcitabine notes that there is no pharmacokinetic interaction with **saquinavir**.[21,22] They state that pharmacokinetic interactions with protease inhibitors would not be expected, since zalcitabine is mainly excreted unchanged in the urine.[21]

(f) Zidovudine

The AUC and maximum levels of zidovudine were increased by 31% and 40%, respectively, when given with **amprenavir**. The pharmacokinetics of **amprenavir** were unchanged. The UK maker of **amprenavir** states that no dose adjustment of either drug is necessary when **amprenavir** and zidovudine are used together.[3]

The maker of **lopinavir/ritonavir** notes that it induces glucuronidation and therefore has the potential to reduce zidovudine levels. However this, and its clinical relevance, have yet to be studied.[5,6]

A study found that the AUC of zidovudine was increased by 17% and that of **indinavir** by 13% when zidovudine 200 mg every 8 hours and **indinavir** 1 g every 8 hours were given together for a week.[17] These changes are not clinically relevant.

A crossover study in 18 HIV+ subjects found that the pharmacokinetics of **ritonavir** 300 mg every 6 hours were unchanged when given with zidovudine 200 mg every 8 hours. However, the maximum plasma levels and AUC of the zidovudine were both reduced by about 25%. The lack of change in the other pharmacokinetic parameters suggested that these changes were not due to altered metabolism.[23]

The UK maker of **saquinavir** notes that there was no pharmacokinetic interaction with zidovudine.[24]

1. Hoggard PG, Manion V, Barry MG, Back DJ. Effect of protease inhibitors on nucleoside analogue phosphorylation *in vitro*. *Br J Clin Pharmacol* (1998) 45, 164–7.
2. McDowell J, Sadler BM, Millard J, Nunnally P, Mustafa N. Evaluation of potential pharmacokinetic (PK) drug interaction between 141W94 and 1592U89 in HIV+ patients. *Intersci Conf Antimicrob Agents Chemother* (1997) 37, 13.
3. Agenerase (Amprenavir). GlaxoSmithKline UK. UK Summary of product characteristics, December 2004.
4. Agenerase (Amprenavir). GlaxoSmithKline. US Prescribing information, May 2005.
5. Kaletra (Lopinavir/ritonavir). Abbott Laboratories Ltd. UK Summary of product characteristics, January 2005.
6. Kaletra (Lopinavir/ritonavir). Abbott Laboratories. US Prescribing information, April 2005.
7. Mummaneni V, Kaul S, Knupp CA. Single oral dose pharmacokinetic interaction study of didanosine and indinavir sulfate in healthy subjects (abstract 34). *J Clin Pharmacol* (1997) 37, 865.
8. Shelton MJ, Mei H, Hewitt RG, Defrancesco R. If taken 1 hour before indinavir (IDV), didanosine does not affect IDV exposure, despite persistent buffering effects. *Antimicrob Agents Chemother* (2001) 45, 298–300.
9. Damle BD, Mummaneni V, Kaul S, Knupp C. Lack of effect of simultaneously administered didanosine encapsulated enteric bead formulation (Videx EC) on oral absorption of indinavir, ketoconazole, or ciprofloxacin. *Antimicrob Agents Chemother* (2002) 46, 385–91.
10. Crixivan (Indinavir sulfate). Merck Sharp & Dohme Ltd. UK Summary of product characteristics, January 2005.
11. Crixivan (Indinavir sulfate). Merck & Co., Inc. US Prescribing information, May 2004.
12. Reyataz Hard Capsules (Atazanavir). Bristol-Myers Squibb Pharmaceuticals Ltd. UK Summary of product characteristics, February 2005.
13. Reyataz (Atazanavir sulfate). Bristol-Myers Squibb Company. US Prescribing information, June 2005.
14. Pedneault L, Elion R, Adler M, Anderson R, Kelleher T, Knupp C, Kaul S, Kerr B, Cross A, Dunkle L. Stavudine (d4T), didanosine (ddI), and nelfinavir combination therapy in HIV-infected subjects: antiviral effect and safety in an ongoing pilot study. 4th Conference on Retroviruses and Opportunistic Infections, Washington, 1997. Abstract 241.

15. Cato A, Qian J, Hsu A, Vomvouras S, Piergies AA, Leonard J, Granneman R. Pharmacokinetic interaction between ritonavir and didanosine when administered concurrently to HIV-infected patients. *J Acquir Immune Defic Syndr Hum Retrovirol* (1998) 18, 466–72.
16. Epivir (Lamivudine). GlaxoSmithKline UK. UK Summary of product characteristics, December 2004.
17. The Indinavir (MK 639) Pharmacokinetic Study Group. Indinavir (MK 639) drug interaction studies. 11th International Conference on AIDS, Vancouver, 1996. Abstract Mo.B.174.
18. Gathe J, Burkhardt B, Hawley P, Conant M, Peterkin J, Chapman S. A randomized phase II study of Viracept™, a novel HIV protease inhibitor, used in combination with stavudine (D4T) vs. stavudine (D4T) alone. 11th International Conference on AIDS, Vancouver, 1996. Abstract Mo.B.413.
19. Viracept (Nelfinavir mesilate). Roche Products Ltd. UK Summary of product characteristics, June 2005.
20. Viracept (Nelfinavir mesilate). Agouron Pharmaceuticals, Inc. US Prescribing information, September 2004.
21. Hivid (Zalcitabine). Roche Products Ltd. UK Summary of product characteristics, November 2004.
22. Hivid (Zalcitabine). Roche Pharmaceuticals. US Prescribing information, September 2002.
23. Cato A, Qian J, Hsu A, Levy B, Leonard J, Granneman R. Multidose pharmacokinetics of ritonavir and zidovudine in human immunodeficiency virus-infected patients. *Antimicrob Agents Chemother* (1998) 42, 1788–93.
24. Invirase (Saquinavir mesilate). Roche Products Ltd. UK Summary of product characteristics, June 2005.

NRTIs + Ribavirin

In vitro **studies suggest that ribavirin may reduce the anti-HIV activity of lamivudine, stavudine, zalcitabine and zidovudine. However, there are some clinical data to suggest that these antiretrovirals are still active when ribavirin is used. Ribavirin does not appear to affect the pharmacokinetics of didanosine, but** ***in vitro*** **evidence suggests it may increase the activity of didanosine, and a fatal case of lactic acidosis with pancreatitis has been reported.**

Clinical evidence, mechanism, importance and management

(a) Didanosine

In vitro, ribavirin increases the intracellular activation of didanosine, and the makers note that this could result in increased adverse effects.[1-3] At least one case of fatal lactic acidosis and pancreatitis has been reported with the combination of ribavirin and didanosine therapy.[4] However, no increase in adverse effects was seen in one study in which ribavirin 600 mg daily was given to 16 HIV+ patients who had already been taking didanosine 125 to 200 mg twice daily for 4 weeks. Ribavirin was given 6 hours after the morning dose of didanosine. Over the 8 or 20 weeks of the study, no pharmacokinetic interaction was seen and the combination was well tolerated.[5] In another study, ribavirin 6 or 10 mg/kg daily was given with didanosine 120 mg/m^2 every 12 hours to 11 HIV+ children (aged 3 months to 12 years) for 24 weeks. No significant changes were found in the pharmacokinetics of didanosine.[6] The combination of didanosine and ribavirin should be used with caution, with consideration given to monitoring of serum lactate and amylase or lipase levels.[4]

(b) Lamivudine, Stavudine, Zalcitabine, and Zidovudine

In vitro, ribavirin reduced the intracellular activation and antiretroviral activity of lamivudine,[7] stavudine,[2,8] zalcitabine,[9] and zidovudine.[2,10,11] The maker of zidovudine specifically recommends avoiding concurrent use of ribavirin.[10,12] However, there was no decrease in antiviral activity of stavudine (as assessed by plasma HIV RNA levels) after 3 months of combined treatment with ribavirin and interferon for hepatitis C infection in patients with HIV (although there was a trend towards decreased concentrations of intracellular stavudine triphosphate).[13] Similarly, in another study in 21 patients (8 treated with zidovudine and 13 treated with stavudine) there was no significant variation in HIV viral load or CD4 cell counts after 3 or 6 months of ribavirin therapy compared with baseline values (although 3 subjects did have an increase in HIV viral load, leading to discontinuation of ribavirin in one).[14] These studies suggest that ribavirin can be used for the treatment of hepatitis C in patients with HIV infection without significantly reducing the antiretroviral activity of stavudine or zidovudine in most patients. The UK maker of ribavirin recommends that plasma HIV RNA levels are closely monitored in patients treated with ribavirin and stavudine or zidovudine to ensure continued efficacy,[2] and this seems wise.

1. Videx EC (Didanosine). Bristol-Myers Squibb Pharmaceuticals Ltd. UK Summary of product characteristics, March 2005.
2. Copegus (Ribavirin). Roche Products Ltd. UK Summary of product characteristics, May 2003.
3. Videc EC (Didanosine). Bristol-Myers Squibb Company. US Prescribing information, January 2004.
4. Butt AA. Fatal lactic acidosis and pancreatitis associated with ribavirin and didanosine therapy. *AIDS Read* (2003) 13, 344–8.
5. Japour AJ, Lertora JJ, Meehan PM, Erice A, Connor JD, Griffith BP, Clax PA, Holden-Wiltse J, Hussey S, Walesky M, Cooney E, Pollard R, Timpone J, McLaren C, Johanneson N, Wood K, Booth DK, Bassiakos Y, Crumpacker CS, for the AIDS Clinical Trials Group 231 Protocol Team. A phase-1 study of the safety, pharmacokinetics, and antiviral activity of combination didanosine and ribavirin in patients with HIV-1 disease. *J Acquir Immune Defic Syndr Hum Retrovirol* (1996) 13, 235–46.
6. Lertora JJL, Harrison M, Dreisbach AW, Van Dyke R. Lack of pharmacokinetic interaction between DDI and ribavirin in HIV infected children. *J Investig Med* (1999) 47, 106A.
7. Huh A, Nam J, Chang K, Yeom J, Song Y, Kim S, Lee J, Kim J. Antagonistic effect of ribavirin on lamivudine against HIV-1 infection (abstract I-1939). *Intersci Conf Antimicrob Agents Chemother* (2001) 41, 348.
8. Hoggard PG, Kewn S, Barry MG, Khoo SH, Back DJ. Effects of drugs on 2',3'-dideoxy-2',3'-didehydrothymidine phosphorylation in vitro. *Antimicrob Agents Chemother* (1997) 41, 1231–6.
9. Hivid (Zalcitabine). Roche Products Ltd. UK Summary of product characteristics, November 2004.
10. Retrovir (Zidovudine). GlaxoSmithKline UK. UK Summary of product characteristics, September 2004.
11. Vogt MW, Hartshorn KL, Furman PA, Chou TC, Fyfe JA, Coleman LA, Crumpacker C, Schooley RT, Hirsch MS. Ribavirin antagonizes the effect of azidothymidine on HIV replication. *Science* (1987) 235, 1376–9.
12. Retrovir (Zidovudine). GlaxoSmithKline. US Prescribing information, April 2003.
13. Salmon-Céron D, Lassalle R, Pruvost A, Benech H, Bouvier-Alias M, Payan C, Goujard C, Bonnet E, Zoulim F, Morlat P, Sogni P, Pérusat S, Tréluyer J-M, Chêne G, and the CORIST-ANRS HC1 Study Group. Interferon-ribavirin in association with stavudine has no impact on plasma human immunodeficiency virus (HIV) type 1 level in patients coinfected with HIV and hepatitis C virus: a CORIST-ANRS HC1 trial. *Clin Infect Dis* (2003) 36, 1295–1304.
14. Zylberberg H, Benhamou Y, Lagneaux JL, Landau A, Chaix M-L, Fontaine H, Bochet M, Poynard T, Katlama C, Pialoux G, Bréchot C, Pol S. Safety and efficacy of interferon-ribavirin combination therapy in HCV-HIV coinfected subjects: an early report. *Gut* (2000) 47, 694–7.

NRTIs + Tenofovir

Tenofovir increases the levels of didanosine, and cases of pancreatitis have been reported for the combination. There is no pharmacokinetic interaction between tenofovir and abacavir, emtricitabine, lamivudine or stavudine. However, the triple therapy combinations of tenofovir and lamivudine with either abacavir or didanosine were unexpectedly associated with a high level of treatment failure, and should be avoided.

Clinical evidence, mechanism, importance and management

(a) Abacavir

There was no clinically relevant pharmacokinetic interaction between tenofovir and abacavir in 8 healthy subjects.[1,2] However, the combination of tenofovir with lamivudine and abacavir was unexpectedly associated with a high rate of treatment failure (early virological non-response) in clinical trials.[3] Consequently, the maker and others recommend that this triple therapy should not be used alone, and if these three drugs are used with other antiretrovirals, virological response should be closely monitored.[3]

(b) Didanosine

The AUC of buffered didanosine was increased by 44% when it was given 1 hour before tenofovir.[4,5] Similarly the AUC of enteric-coated didanosine was increased by 48% and 60% when didanosine was given 2 hours before and with tenofovir, respectively.[1] The pharmacokinetics of tenofovir were unchanged.[5,6] Another study found that the AUC of enteric-coated didanosine 250 mg when given with tenofovir (simultaneously or 2 hours apart, fasted or with food) was about equivalent to that seen with didanosine 400 mg alone.[1] It is appears that these studies have so far been presented only as conference abstracts, and have been discussed in a review.[7]

The main concern with raised didanosine levels is the increased risk of adverse effects, particularly pancreatitis and peripheral neuropathy. One retrospective analysis found that 5 of 185 patients receiving didanosine with tenofovir developed pancreatitis compared with one of 182 on didanosine without tenofovir and none of 208 on tenofovir without didanosine, suggesting an increased risk of pancreatitis with the combination. All 6 cases of pancreatitis were in women without renal impairment, who weighed less than 60 kg. Five had received a reduced dose of didanosine (250 mg) and one had received 400 mg. Pancreatitis developed after 12 to 24 weeks.[8] However, another analysis failed to find an enhanced risk of toxicity with the combination of didanosine and tenofovir at full dose during the first 6 months of therapy.[9] Other cases of pancreatitis[10,11] or lactic acidosis and renal failure[12,13] have been reported.

Furthermore, a once daily combination of tenofovir 300 mg, enteric-coated didanosine 250 mg and lamivudine 300 mg was unexpectedly associated with a high rate of treatment failure (early virological non-response) in a clinical trial in treatment-naïve patients.[14] Consequently, the European Agency for the Evaluation of Medicinal products recommended that this triple therapy should not be used alone, particularly as a once-daily regimen.[14] Similarly, other results have shown a high rate of treatment failure with a once daily combination of tenofovir 300 mg, enteric-coated didanosine 250 mg and either efavirenz or nevirapine.[15]

The pharmacokinetic interaction is established, and raised didanosine levels would be expected when given with tenofovir. The US maker recommends that the dose of didanosine be reduced to 250 mg once daily when given with tenofovir in patients weighing more than 60 kg.[1] However, there is no recommendation as to an appropriate dose in patients weighing less than 60 kg. It may be appropriate to reduce the dose further in these patients. Whenever the combination is used, patients should be carefully monitored for didanosine-related adverse effects (e.g. pancreatitis, peripheral neuropathy) and for antiviral efficacy.

(c) Emtricitabine

The maker briefly notes that there was no pharmacokinetic interaction between tenofovir and emtricitabine.[1]

(d) Lamivudine

The maker briefly notes that there was no pharmacokinetic interaction between tenofovir and lamivudine.[5]

However, for studies showing a high rate of virological failure with the combination of tenofovir, lamivudine and one other NRTI, see (a) abacavir, above and (b) didanosine, above.

(e) Stavudine

There is information that tenofovir 300 mg does not alter levels of stavudine 100 mg.[6]

1. Viread (Tenofovir disoproxil). Gilead Sciences, Inc. US Prescribing information, May 2005.
2. Kearney BP, Isaacson E, Sayre J, Ebrahimi R, Cheng AK. The pharmacokinetics of abacavir, a purine nucleoside analog, are not affected by tenofovir DF. *Intersci Conf Antimicrob Agents Chemother* (2003) 43, 36.
3. Manion DJ. Important drug warning. Re: early virologic non-response in patients with HIV infection treated with lamivudine, abacavir and tenofovir. GlaxoSmithKline, July 2003. Available at http://www.fda.gov/medwatch/SAFETY/2003/ziagen_deardoc_07-25-03.pdf (accessed 15/07/05).
4. Videx EC (Didanosine). Bristol-Myers Squibb Pharmaceuticals Ltd. UK Summary of product characteristics, March 2005.
5. Viread (Tenofovir disoproxil fumarate). Gilead Sciences International Ltd. UK Summary of product characteristics, March 2005.
6. Anon. E. Tenofovir drug interactions: ddI and d4T. *Treatmentupdate* (2003) 15 (Part 2), 7.
7. Pecora Fulco P, Kirian MA. Effect of tenofovir on didanosine absorption in patients with HIV. *Ann Pharmacother* (2003) 37, 1325–8.
8. Martínez E, Milinkovic A, de Lazzari E, Ravasi G, Blanco JL, Larrousse M, Mallolas J, García F, Miró JM, Gatell JM. Pancreatic toxic effects associated with co-administration of didanosine and tenofovir in HIV-infected adults. *Lancet* (2004) 364, 65–7.
9. Barrios A, Maida I, Perez-Saleme L, Negredo E, Clotet B, Vilaro J, Domingo P, Estrada V, Santos J, Asensi V, Labarga P, Terron J, Vergara A, Garcia-Benayas T, Martin-Carbonero L, Barreiro P, Gonzalez-Lahoz J, Soriano V. Safety and efficacy of combinations based on didanosine 400 mg od plus tenofovir 300 mg od. *Intersci Conf Antimicrob Agents Chemother* (2003) 43, 314.
10. Blanchard JN, Wohlfeiler M, Canas A, King K, Lonergan JT. Pancreatitis with didanosine and tenofovir disoproxil fumarate. *Clin Infect Dis* (2003) 37, e57–e62. Erratum. *Ibid.* 995.
11. Kirian MA, Higginson RT, Pecora Fulco P. Acute onset of pancreatitis with concomitant use of tenofovir and didanosine. *Ann Pharmacother* (2004) 38, 1660–3.
12. Murphy MD, O'Hearn M, Chou S. Fatal lactic acidosis and acute renal failure after addition of tenofovir to an antiretroviral regimen containing didanosine. *Clin Infect Dis* (2003) 36, 1082–5.
13. Guo Y, Fung HB. Fatal lactic acidosis associated with coadministration of didanosine and tenofovir disoproxil fumarate. *Pharmacotherapy* (2004) 24, 1089–94.
14. EMEA Public Statement. High rate of virologic failure in patients with HIV infection treated with a once-daily triple nucleosides/nucleotide reverse transcriptase inhibitors combination containing didanosine, lamivudine and tenofovir. London, 22 October 2003. Available at: http://www.emea.eu.int/pdfs/human/press/pus/509403en.pdf (accessed 14/07/05).
15. Hodder SL. Re: Important new clinical data. Potential early virologic failure associated with the combination antiretroviral regimen of tenofovir disoproxil fumarate, didanosine, and either efavirenz or nevirapine in HIV treatment-naïve patients with high baseline viral loads. Bristol-Myers Squibb Company, November 2004. Available at http://www.fda.gov/oashi/aids/listserv/bms.pdf (accessed 14/07/05).

NRTIs + Trimethoprim ± Sulfamethoxazole

Co-trimoxazole reduces the loss of lamivudine, zalcitabine and zidovudine in the urine, and trimethoprim alone interacts with zalcitabine and zidovudine in the same way. However, the extent of the interaction does not usually appear to be clinically significant. No clinically significant adverse pharmacokinetic interaction occurs if didanosine is given with sulfamethoxazole or trimethoprim either separately or together.

Clinical evidence

(a) Didanosine

A study in 10 HIV+ subjects investigated the pharmacokinetics of didanosine 200 mg, trimethoprim 200 mg and sulfamethoxazole 1 g in combination. Most pharmacokinetic parameters were unchanged. However, didanosine clearance was reduced by 35%, trimethoprim clearance was decreased by 32% and sulfamethoxazole clearance was increased by 39%, when all 3 agents were given together. When only 2 of the 3 drugs were given, trimethoprim caused a 27% decrease in the clearance of didanosine, and didanosine caused an 82% increase in the clearance of sulfamethoxazole.[1] Despite these alterations in clearance, the maximum serum concentration, AUC and half-life of each of the three drugs were minimally affected when they were given together.[1]

(b) Lamivudine

In a study of 14 HIV+ patients taking co-trimoxazole 960 mg daily for 5 days, it was found that the AUC of a single 300-mg dose of lamivudine given on day 4 was increased by 43% and the renal clearance was decreased by 35%. The pharmacokinetics of the trimethoprim and the sulfamethoxazole were unaffected.[2]

(c) Stavudine

The UK maker notes that an interaction with trimethoprim is possible, since both drugs are actively secreted by the renal tubules.[3]

(d) Zalcitabine

In a steady-state study, 8 HIV+ patients received zalcitabine 1.5 mg three times daily with and without trimethoprim 200 mg twice daily. The trimethoprim increased the AUC and decreased the clearance of the zalcitabine by about 35%.[4]

(e) Zidovudine

A study in 9 HIV+ patients given zidovudine 3 mg/kg by infusion over 1 hour found that neither trimethoprim 150 mg nor co-trimoxazole 960 mg affected the metabolic clearance of the zidovudine. However, the renal clearances of zidovudine were reduced by 48 and 58% respectively, and the renal clearances of its glucuronide were reduced by 20 and 27% respectively.[5] Another study also found that co-trimoxazole did not alter zidovudine pharmacokinetics.[6] Another 5 HIV+ patients had a 30% increase in the AUC of zidovudine when they were given trimethoprim [dosages not stated].[7] Zidovudine renal clearance was reduced by 58% in 8 HIV+ subjects when they were also given trimethoprim 200 mg, but the 6-hour AUC of the zidovudine glucuronide/zidovudine ratio was unchanged, suggesting that the metabolism was unaffected.[8]

Increases in the half-lives of trimethoprim, sulfamethoxazole and *N*-acetyl sulfamethoxazole of 72, 39 and 115% respectively were seen when co-trimoxazole was given to 4 patients with AIDS taking zidovudine 250 mg every 8 hours for 8 days.[9]

A study of zidovudine use in 282 AIDS patients found that haematological abnormalities (anaemia, leucopenia, neutropenia) were common. However, the frequency was not increased in the patients [number unknown] also taking co-trimoxazole.[10]

Mechanism

A likely reason is that the trimethoprim inhibits the secretion of both zidovudine and its glucuronide by the kidney tubules. It is not known why the half-life of co-trimoxazole is increased. The other NRTIs that interact are likely to do so by the same mechanism.

Importance and management

Established interactions. With the NRTIs that are actively excreted via the kidneys (e.g. lamivudine, stavudine, and zalcitabine), it is unlikely that dosage alterations are necessary unless the patient has renal impairment. However, when concurrent therapy is needed, patients should be closely monitored for signs of toxicity. Moreover, the UK makers of lamivudine recommend that the use of lamivudine with high-dose co-trimoxazole for the treatment of *Pneumocystis carinii* pneumonia and toxoplasmosis should be avoided.[11] Since renal clearance represents only 20 to 30% of the total clearance of zidovudine, the authors of two of these reports[5,8] suggest that this interaction is unlikely to be clinically important for zidovudine unless the glucuronidation by the liver is impaired by liver disease or other drugs. Didanosine also does not appear to interact to a clinically relevant extent.

Nevertheless concurrent use should be well monitored, especially because co-trimoxazole alone has been associated with a high incidence of adverse effects in patients with AIDS.[12]

1. Srinivas NR, Knupp CA, Batteiger B, Smith RA, Barbhaiya RH. A pharmacokinetic interaction study of didanosine coadministered with trimethoprim and/or sulphamethoxazole in HIV seropositive asymptomatic male patients. *Br J Clin Pharmacol* (1996) 41, 207–15.
2. Moore KHP, Yuen GJ, Raasch RH, Eron JJ, Martin D, Mydlow PK, Hussey EK. Pharmacokinetics of lamivudine administered alone and with trimethoprim-sulfamethoxazole. *Clin Pharmacol Ther* (1996) 59, 550–8.
3. Zerit (Stavudine). Bristol-Myers Squibb Pharmaceuticals Ltd. UK Summary of product characteristics, January 2005.
4. Lee BL, Täuber MG, Chambers HF, Gambertoglio J, Delahunty T. The effect of trimethoprim (TMP) on the pharmacokinetics (PK) of zalcitabine (ddC) in HIV-infected patients. *Intersci Conf Antimicrob Agents Chemother* (1995) 35, 6.
5. Chatton JY, Munafo A, Chave JP, Steinhäuslin F, Roch-Ramel F, Glauser MP, Biollaz J. Trimethoprim, alone or in combination with sulphamethoxazole, decreases the renal excretion of zidovudine and its glucuronide. *Br J Clin Pharmacol* (1992) 34, 551–4.
6. Cañas E, Pachon J, Garcia-Pesquera F, Castillo JR, Viciana P, Cisneros JM, Jimenez-Mejias M. Absence of effect of trimethoprim-sulfamethoxazole on pharmacokinetics of zidovudine in patients infected with human immunodeficiency virus. *Antimicrob Agents Chemother* (1996) 40, 230–33.
7. Lee BL, Safrin S, Makrides V, Benowitz NL, Gambertoglio JG, Mills J. Trimethoprim decreases the renal clearance of zidovudine. *Clin Pharmacol Ther* (1992) 51,183.
8. Lee BL, Safrin S, Makrides V, Gambertoglio JG. Zidovudine, trimethoprim, and dapsone pharmacokinetic interactions in patients with human immunodeficiency virus infection. *Antimicrob Agents Chemother* (1996) 40, 1231–6.
9. Berson A, Happy K, Rousseau F, Grateau G, Farinotti R, Séréni D. Effect of zidovudine (AZT) on cotrimoxazole (TMP-SMX) kinetics: preliminary results. 9th International Conference on AIDS & 5th STD World Congress, Berlin, June 6-11 1993. Abstract PO-B30-2193.
10. Richman DD, Fischl MA, Grieco MH, Gottlieb MS, Volberding PA, Laskin OL, Leedom JM, Groopman JE, Mildvan D, Hirsch MS, Jackson GG, Durack DT, Nusinoff-Lehrman S and the AZT Collaborative Working Group. The toxicity of azidothymidine (AZT) in the treatment of patients with AIDS and AIDS-related complex. A double-blind, placebo-controlled trial. *N Engl J Med* (1987) 317, 192–7.
11. Epivir (Lamivudine). GlaxoSmithKline UK. UK Summary of product characteristics, December 2004.
12. Medina I, Mills J, Leoung G, Hopewell PC, Lee B, Modin G, Benowitz N, Wofsy CB. Oral therapy for *Pneumocystis carinii* pneumonia in the acquired immunodeficiency syndrome: a controlled trial of trimethoprim-sulfamethoxazole versus trimethoprim-dapsone. *N Engl J Med* (1990) 323, 776–82.

NRTIs; Didanosine + Allopurinol

Allopurinol raises didanosine levels, possibly advantageously.

Clinical evidence, mechanism, importance and management

Buffered didanosine 400 mg was given to 14 healthy subjects with and without allopurinol 300 mg daily for 7 days. The allopurinol significantly increased didanosine absorption, shown by a twofold increase in the AUC and a 69% rise in the maximum serum concentration.[1] Similar findings were seen in patients with HIV infection.[2] Moreover, the addition of allopurinol 300 mg daily allowed the dosage of didanosine to be halved from 400 mg to 200 mg daily in 4 patients on buffered didanosine, hydroxycarbamide and chloroquine. Didanosine plasma levels and antiviral efficacy were unchanged.[3] The maker notes that allopurinol may increase the exposure to didanosine via its inhibitory effects on xanthine oxidase, an enzyme involved in didanosine metabolism.[4] This interaction has been studied for its therapeutic benefit.[3] However, if the dose of didanosine is not reduced, there is the potential for an increase in didanosine adverse effects.

The UK maker recommends close monitoring for adverse effects but the US maker does not recommend use together.[4,5]

1. Liang D, Breaux K, Nornoo A Phadungpojna S, Rodriguez-Barradas M, Bates TR. Pharmacokinetic interaction between didanosine (ddI) and allopurinol in healthy volunteers. *Intersci Conf Antimicrob Agents Chemother* (1999) 39, 25.
2. Liang D, Breaux K, Rodriguez-Barradas M, Bates TR. Allopurinol increases didanosine absorption in HIV-infected patients. *Intersci Conf Antimicrob Agents Chemother* (2001) 41, 16.
3. Boelaert JR, Dom GM, Huitema ADR, Beijnen JH, Lange JMA. The boosting of didanosine by allopurinol permits a halving of the didanosine dosage. *AIDS* (2002) 16, 2221–3.
4. Videx EC (Didanosine). Bristol-Myers Squibb Pharmaceuticals Ltd. UK Summary of product characteristics, March 2005.
5. Videx EC (Didanosine). Bristol-Myers Squibb Company. US Prescribing information, January 2004.

NRTIs; Didanosine + Loperamide or Metoclopramide

Loperamide and metoclopramide do not appear to interact with didanosine.

Clinical evidence, mechanism, importance and management

The pharmacokinetics of oral buffered didanosine 300 mg were not altered to a clinically relevant extent by 4 mg of loperamide given 19, 13, 7 and 1 hour before the didanosine in 6 men and 6 women who were HIV+. The rate of didanosine absorption was slightly decreased but the extent of absorption was unchanged. Similarly, the pharmacokinetics of oral buffered didanosine 300 mg were found to be unaffected by 10 mg of intravenous metoclopramide.[1] It appears that neither delaying nor accelerating gastrointestinal transit time appreciably alters the pharmacokinetics of didanosine, which is acid labile. On the basis of this study the authors conclude that neither the dose nor the frequency of didanosine administration need be altered if either loperamide or metoclopramide is given concurrently.[1]

1. Knupp CA, Milbrath RL, Barbhaiya RH. Effect of metoclopramide and loperamide on the pharmacokinetics of didanosine in HIV seropositive asymptomatic male and female patients. *Eur J Clin Pharmacol* (1993) 45, 409–13.

NRTIs; Stavudine + Doxorubicin

***In vitro* evidence suggests that doxorubicin may inhibit the activation of stavudine.**

Clinical evidence, mechanism, importance and management

Nucleoside reverse transcriptase inhibitors such as stavudine need to be phosphorylated within cells before they become effective. *In vitro* studies using mononucleated blood cells found that doxorubicin may interfere with stavudine phosphorylation at clinically relevant concentrations.[1] The clinical importance of this interaction awaits assessment.

1. Hoggard PG, Kewn S, Barry MG, Khoo SH, Back DJ. Effects of drugs on 2',3'-dideoxy-2',3'-didehydrothymidine phosphorylation in vitro. *Antimicrob Agents Chemother* (1997) 41, 1231–6.

NRTIs; Zidovudine + Benzodiazepines

Oxazepam causes a modest increase in the bioavailability of zidovudine, and the combination can increase the incidence of headaches. Lorazepam possibly behaves similarly.

Clinical evidence, mechanism, importance and management

A pharmacokinetic study in 6 HIV patients found that **oxazepam** did not significantly affect the bioavailability of zidovudine. All of them were sleepy and fatigued while taking **oxazepam** (as expected), but 5 of the 6 complained of headaches while taking both drugs, compared with only 1 of 6 while taking zidovudine only and none while taking **oxazepam** only. The authors of the report suggest that if headaches occur during concurrent use, the benzodiazepine should be stopped.[1] A previous *in vitro* study using human liver microsomes confirmed that **oxazepam** inhibits the metabolism of zidovudine to its glucuronide, and **lorazepam** behaves in the same way.[2] The same precautions suggested for **oxazepam** would therefore also appear to apply to **lorazepam**.

1. Mole L, Israelski D, Bubp J, O'Hanley P, Merigan T, Blaschke T. Pharmacokinetics of zidovudine alone and in combination with oxazepam in the HIV infected patient. *J Acquir Immune Defic Syndr* (1993) 6, 56–60.
2. Unadkat JD, Chien J. Lorazepam and oxazepam inhibit the metabolism of zidovudine (ZDV or azidothymidine) in an *in vitro* human liver microsomal system. *Pharm Res* (1988) 5 (Suppl), S177.

NRTIs; Zidovudine + Drugs inhibiting glucuronidation

Moderate pharmacokinetic changes not requiring dose adjustments have been seen between zidovudine and atovaquone. Dipyridamole, indometacin and naproxen did not alter zidovudine pharmacokinetics. *In vitro* evidence suggests that zidovudine may interact with chloramphenicol and ethinylestradiol.

Clinical evidence and mechanism

(a) Aspirin or NSAIDs

A study of zidovudine use in 282 AIDS patients found that haematological abnormalities were not increased by aspirin in 47 patients.[1] An *in vitro* study using human liver microsomes found that **indometacin** and

naproxen inhibited the glucuronidation of zidovudine by 50% or more, and aspirin also had some inhibitory effect.[2] This suggested that these drugs might possibly increase the effects and the toxicity of zidovudine. However, other clinical studies found no changes in the pharmacokinetics of a single dose of zidovudine given with **indometacin** 25 mg twice daily for 3 days[3] or **naproxen** 500 mg to 1 g daily for 3 or 4 days.[3,4]

(b) Atovaquone

A study in 14 HIV+ patients given atovaquone 750 mg every 12 hours and zidovudine 200 mg every 8 hours found that under steady-state conditions the zidovudine had no effect on the pharmacokinetics of atovaquone.[5] This confirmed the findings of a previous study.[6] However, the AUC of the zidovudine was increased by 31%, and its clearance was reduced by 25% by concurrent use of atovaquone. The reason appears to be that the atovaquone inhibits the metabolism (glucuronidation) of the zidovudine.[5]

(c) Chloramphenicol

An *in vitro* study using human liver microsomes found that chloramphenicol inhibited the glucuronidation of zidovudine by 50% or more, suggesting that the effects and toxicity of zidovudine may be increased.[2] The effect of concurrent use in patients awaits assessment.

(d) Dipyridamole

A study in 11 asymptomatic HIV+ patients found that dipyridamole 75 to 100 mg every 4 hours for 5 days caused no significant changes in the pharmacokinetics of zidovudine 500 mg daily, but the dipyridamole adverse effects (headaches, nausea) when taking the higher dose were found to be intolerable.[7]

(e) Ethinylestradiol

An *in vitro* study using human liver microsomes found that ethinylestradiol inhibited the glucuronidation of zidovudine by 50% or more, suggesting that the effects and toxicity of zidovudine may be increased.[2] The effect of concurrent use in patients awaits assessment.

Importance and management

Many drugs that inhibit the glucuronidation of zidovudine appear to have only a modest effect on zidovudine levels, which are unlikely to be clinically important in most patients. However, the authors of the report with atovaquone suggest that increases could possibly be important in patients also taking other drugs causing bone marrow toxicity (such as ganciclovir, amphotericin B, flucytosine). If bone marrow toxicity is seen, it is suggested that the zidovudine dosage may need to be reduced by a third.[5]

1. Richman DD, Fischl MA, Grieco MH, Gottlieb MS, Volberding PA, Laskin OL, Leedom JM, Groopman JE, Mildvan D, Hirsch MS, Jackson GG, Durack DT, Nusinoff-Lehrman S and the AZT Collaborative Working Group. The toxicity of azidothymidine (AZT) in the treatment of patients with AIDS and AIDS-related complex. A double-blind, placebo-controlled trial. *N Engl J Med* (1987) 317, 192–7.
2. Sim SM, Back DJ, Breckenridge AM. The effect of various drugs on the glucuronidation of zidovudine (azidothymidine; AZT) by human liver microsomes. *Br J Clin Pharmacol* (1991) 32, 17–21.
3. Barry M, Howe J, Back D, Breckenridge A, Brettle R, Mitchell R, Beeching N, Nye F. Effect of non-steroidal anti-inflammatory drugs on zidovudine pharmacokinetics. *Br J Clin Pharmacol* (1992) 34, 446P.
4. Sahai J, Gallicano K, Garber G, Pakuts A, Hawley-Foss N, Huang L, McGilveray I, Cameron DW. Evaluation of the in vivo effect of naproxen on zidovudine pharmacokinetics in patients infected with human immunodeficiency virus. *Clin Pharmacol Ther* (1992) 52, 464–70.
5. Lee BL, Täuber MG, Sadler B, Goldstein D, Chambers HF. Atovaquone inhibits the glucuronidation and increases the plasma concentrations of zidovudine. *Clin Pharmacol Ther* (1996) 59, 14–21.
6. Sadler BM, Blum MR. Relationship between steady-state plasma concentrations of atovaquone (C_{ss}) and the use of various concomitant medications in AIDS patients with *Pneumocystis carinii* pneumonia. 9th International Conference AIDS & 4th STD World Congress, Berlin, June 6–11 1993. Abstract PO-B31-2213.
7. Hendrix CW, Flexner C, Szebeni J, Kuwahara S, Pennypacker S, Weinstein JN, Lietman PS. Effect of dipyridamole on zidovudine pharmacokinetics and short-term tolerance in asymptomatic human immunodeficiency virus-infected subjects. *Antimicrob Agents Chemother* (1994) 38, 1036–40.

NRTIs; Zidovudine + Lithium

Lithium can apparently oppose the neutropenic effects of zidovudine.

Clinical evidence, mechanism, importance and management

A study in 5 patients with AIDS found that serum lithium carbonate levels of 0.6 to 1.2 mmol/l increased their neutrophil counts sufficiently to allow the re-introduction of zidovudine previously withdrawn due to neutropenia. Withdrawal of the lithium resulted in a rapid fall in neutrophil levels in two patients.[1] The reasons for this effect on neutrophil production are not understood.

This report suggests that no adverse reaction occurs in patients taking zidovudine and lithium, and that there may be some advantages.

1. Roberts DE, Berman SM, Nakasato S, Wyle FA, Wishnow RM, Segal GP. Effect of lithium carbonate on zidovudine-associated neutropenia in the acquired immunodeficiency syndrome. *Am J Med* (1988) 85, 428–31.

NRTIs; Zidovudine + Megestrol

There is no pharmacokinetic interaction between megestrol acetate and zidovudine.

Clinical evidence, mechanism, importance and management

Megestrol acetate 800 mg once daily for 13 days had no effect on the steady-state pharmacokinetics of zidovudine or its glucuronide metabolite in 12 asymptomatic HIV+ subjects.[1] Megestrol does not appear to affect the metabolism of zidovudine. No dose adjustments appear necessary.

1. Van Harken DR, Pei JC, Wagner J, Pike IM. Pharmacokinetic interaction of megestrol acetate with zidovudine in human immunodeficiency virus-infected patients. *Antimicrob Agents Chemother* (1997) 41, 2480–3.

NRTIs; Zidovudine + Myelosuppressive drugs

There have been reports of serious myelotoxicity with vancomycin/zidovudine and antineoplastics/zidovudine. Moderate pharmacokinetic changes not requiring dose adjustments *per se* have been seen between zidovudine and chemotherapy regimens used for Kaposi's sarcoma, Hodgkin's disease, and Non-Hodgkin's lymphoma.

Clinical evidence and mechanism

(a) Antineoplastics

In one preliminary report, the addition of **vinblastine** to zidovudine resulted in severe bone marrow depression.[1] Similarly, 9 of 21 patients could not tolerate zidovudine while receiving a chemotherapy regimen (**cyclophosphamide**, **doxorubicin**, **teniposide**, **prednisone**, **vincristine** and **bleomycin**) because of haematological toxicity.[2]

The pharmacokinetic interaction of chemotherapy with zidovudine was assessed in HIV+ patients being treated for Kaposi's sarcoma, non-Hodgkin's lymphoma or Hodgkin's disease. The antineoplastics used were **bleomycin**, **cyclophosphamide**, **doxorubicin**, **epirubicin**, **etoposide**, **vinblastine**, **vincristine**, **vindesine** and **vinorelbine**. The zidovudine metabolism was unchanged, but a 43% decrease was noted in the maximum plasma levels of zidovudine and the time to peak level was prolonged by 51%, which was independent of the chemotherapy given.[3] The authors concluded that dose changes of zidovudine were not needed with the antineoplastics used, based on these pharmacokinetic changes alone, since the zidovudine AUC remained unchanged and maximum plasma levels have not been shown to clearly correlate with virustatic activity.[3] Thus it appears that any interaction is likely to be attributable to additive myelosuppressive effects.

(b) Vancomycin

A report describes marked neutropenia in 4 HIV+ patients on zidovudine when given vancomycin (which can also, rarely, have neutropenic effects).[4]

Importance and management

On theoretical grounds any drug causing bone marrow suppression might be additive with the effects of zidovudine. The UK maker recommends that extra care be taken in monitoring haematological parameters if concurrent treatment with any myelosuppressive drug and zidovudine is required.[5] They specifically mention systemic **pentamidine**, '**dapsone**', (p.594), **pyrimethamine**, '**co-trimoxazole**', (p.604), **amphotericin**, **flucytosine**, '**ganciclovir**', (p.596), '**interferon**', (p.594), **vinblastine**, and **doxorubicin**.[5] However, they also state that limited clinical data do not indicate a significantly increased risk of adverse reactions to zidovudine when used with prophylactic **co-trimoxazole,** aerosolised **pentamidine,** and **pyrimethamine**.[5]

1. Charakhanian S, De Sabb R, Vaseghi M, Cardon B, Rozenbaum W. Evaluation of the association of zidovudine and vinblastine in treatment of AIDS-related Kaposi's sarcoma. 5th International Conference on AIDS, Montreal, 1989. Abstract MBP368.
2. Tirelli U, Errante D, Oksenhendler E, Spina M, Vaccher E, Serraino D, Gastaldi R, Repetto L, Rizzardini G, Carbone A, et al. French-Italian Cooperative Study Group. Prospective study with combined low-dose chemotherapy and zidovudine in 37 patients with poor-prognosis AIDS-related non-Hodgkin's lymphoma. *Ann Oncol* (1992) 3, 843–7.
3. Toffoli G, Errante D, Corona G, Vaccher E, Bertola A, Robieux I, Aita P, Sorio R, Tirelli U, Boiocchi M. Interactions of antineoplastic chemotherapy with zidovudine pharmacokinetics in patients with HIV-related neoplasms. *Chemotherapy* (1999) 45, 418–28.
4. Kitchen LW, Clark RA, Hanna BJ, Pollock B, Valainis GT. Vancomycin and neutropenia in AZT-treated AIDS patients with staphylococcal infections. *J Acquir Immune Defic Syndr* (1990) 3, 925–6.
5. Retrovir (Zidovudine). GlaxoSmithKline UK. UK Summary of product characteristics, September 2004.

Oseltamivir or Zanamivir + Miscellaneous

Antacids and aspirin do not affect the pharmacokinetics of oseltamivir. Aspirin and a variety of other drugs used for influenza management do not affect the antiviral activity of zanamivir *in vitro*.

Clinical evidence, mechanism, importance and management

(a) Antacids

In a single-dose study, the pharmacokinetics of 150 mg of oseltamivir and its active carboxylate metabolite were not affected by antacids. The antacids used were a suspension of **aluminium/magnesium hydroxide** *(Maalox)* and tablets of **calcium carbonate** *(Titralac)*.[1]

(b) Aspirin and other drugs used for influenza management

There was no pharmacokinetic interaction between aspirin and oseltamivir in a study where 12 healthy subjects were given a single 900-mg dose of aspirin before, during and/or after oseltamivir 75 mg twice daily for 9 doses.[2] A possible interaction was postulated since both drugs are hydrolysed by esterases and secreted by anionic tubular secretion.[2]

The *in vitro* antiviral potency of zanamivir was not affected by aspirin, **paracetamol**, **ibuprofen**, **phenylephrine**, **oxymetazoline**, **promethazine**, or **co-amoxiclav**.[3]

1. Snell P, Oo C, Dorr A, Barrett J. Lack of pharmacokinetic interaction between the oral anti-influenza neuraminidase inhibitor prodrug oseltamivir and antacids. *Br J Clin Pharmacol* (2002) 54, 372–7.
2. Oo C, Barrett J, Dorr A, Liu B, Ward P. Lack of pharmacokinetic interaction between the oral anti-influenza prodrug oseltamivir and aspirin. *Antimicrob Agents Chemother* (2002) 46, 1993–5.
3. Daniel MJ, Barnett JM, Pearson BA. The low potential for drug interactions with zanamivir. *Clin Pharmacokinet* (1999) 36 (Suppl 1), 41–50.

Protease inhibitors + Antacids, H_2-blockers or Proton pump inhibitors

Omeprazole has been shown to decrease indinavir levels. Omeprazole markedly reduced plasma levels of atazanavir. Other drugs that increase gastric pH are also predicted to reduce plasma levels of atazanavir, and possibly also amprenavir.

Clinical evidence

(a) Atazanavir

The AUC of atazanavir was reduced by 76% and the trough plasma level by 78% when atazanavir/ritonavir 300 mg/100 mg was given with **omeprazole** 40 mg. Increasing the dose of atazanavir/ritonavir to 400 mg/100 mg did not negate the effects of this interaction.[1]

(b) Indinavir

A study in 8 healthy subjects given **omeprazole** 40 mg daily with a single 800-mg dose of indinavir found that although not all subjects had significant pharmacokinetic changes, half of them showed a clinically significant decrease in the plasma levels of indinavir.[2] A review by the same authors, of 9 patients taking **omeprazole** with indinavir found that 4 had plasma levels of indinavir lower than expected. In two patients, increasing the indinavir dose from 800 mg to 1 g three times daily resulted in acceptable plasma levels.[3] In a later randomised controlled trial, **omeprazole** 40 mg once daily for 7 days reduced the AUC of indinavir 800 mg by 47% in 14 subjects. However, the addition of **ritonavir** 200 mg to the indinavir negated the effect of the **omeprazole**.[4]

Mechanism

The UK maker of indinavir states that a normal (acidic) gastric pH may be necessary for optimum absorption of indinavir.[5] Any drug that increases the gastric pH could therefore potentially reduce absorption. Note that 'buffered didanosine tablets', (p.602) have also been shown to reduce indinavir levels. Altered gastric pH may also account for the interaction between omeprazole and atazanavir.[1]

Importance and management

The interaction between omeprazole and indinavir would appear to be established. Omeprazole should probably not be used with indinavir unless ritonavir is used to boost the indinavir levels.[4] This would likely apply to other proton pump inhibitors used with indinavir as well.

The interaction of omeprazole with atazanavir/ritonavir is also established. Based on the available data, the European Agency for the Evaluation of Medicinal Products state that atazanavir or atazanavir/ritonavir should not be given with omeprazole or other proton pump inhibitors.[1] Similarly, until more is known, caution is required with other drugs that increase the gastric pH (such as **antacids**, drug formulations containing buffers and **H_2-blockers**).[6] The makers of atazanavir recommend it should be given 2 hours before or 1 hour after buffered medicinal products.[6,7] This would include didanosine buffered tablets (see 'NRTIs + Protease inhibitors', p.602).

Based on the limited data with other protease inhibitors, the maker of **amprenavir** also recommends it should not be given within 1 hour of antacids.[8,9]

1. EMEA public statement. Important new pharmacokinetic data demonstrating that REYATAZ (atazanavir sulfate) combined with NORVIR (ritonavir) and omeprazole should not be co-administered. London, 21 December 2004. Available at http://www.emea.eu.int/pdfs/human/press/pus/20264904en.pdf (accessed 14/07/05).
2. Hugen PWH, Burger DM, ter Hofstede HJM, Koopmans PP. Concomitant use of indinavir and omeprazole; risk of antiretroviral subtherapy. *AIDS* (1998) 12 (Suppl 4), S29.
3. Burger DM, Hugen PWH, Kroon FP, Groeneveld P, Brinkman K, Foudraine NA, Sprenger H, Koopmans PP, Hekster YA. *AIDS* (1998) 12, 2080–2.
4. Rublein JC, Donovan BJ, Hollowell SB, Min SS, Theodore D, Raasch RH, Kashuba ADM. Effect of omeprazole on the plasma concentrations of indinavir in HIV-negative subjects. *Intersci Conf Antimicrob Agents Chemother* (2003) 43, 35.
5. Crixivan (Indinavir sulfate). Merck Sharp & Dohme Ltd. UK Summary of product characteristics, January 2005.
6. Reyataz (Atazanavir sulfate). Bristol-Myers Squibb Pharmaceuticals Ltd. UK Summary of product characteristics, February 2005.
7. Reyataz (Atazanavir sulfate). Bristol-Myers Squibb Company. US Prescribing information, June 2005.
8. Agenerase (Amprenavir). GlaxoSmithKline UK. UK Summary of product characteristics, December 2004.
9. Agenerase (Amprenavir). GlaxoSmithKline. US Prescribing information, May 2005.

Protease inhibitors + Anticonvulsants; Barbiturates

It is likely that phenobarbital and other barbiturates will increase the metabolism of the protease inhibitors, thereby reducing their levels and possibly resulting in antiretroviral therapy failure. However, one case suggested that this may not have occurred with primidone and ritonavir/saquinavir, although this should be viewed with caution.

Clinical evidence, mechanism, importance and management

The makers of **indinavir**,[1,2] **lopinavir**,[3,4] **nelfinavir**[5,6] and **saquinavir**[7,8] all predict that their levels may be reduced by **phenobarbital**, due to induction of the cytochrome P450 isoenzyme CYP3A4. There do not appear to be any controlled studies to demonstrate the extent of the pharmacokinetic interaction with different protease inhibitors. Data from one case report of carbamazepine toxicity with '**ritonavir/saquinavir**', (p.608), provide indirect evidence to suggest the interaction with **primidone** is not clinically important. In this report, a patient on an antiretroviral regimen including **ritonavir** and **saquinavir** had his anticonvulsant therapy changed from carbamazepine to **primidone** 500 mg daily. The authors noted that during follow-up (duration not stated), viral load was still undetectable and seizures remained under control.[9] **Primidone** is metabolised to **phenobarbital**, and might have been expected to cause antiretroviral therapy failure. The combination of protease inhibitors and barbiturates should be used with caution.

1. Crixivan (Indinavir sulfate). Merck Sharp & Dohme Ltd. UK Summary of product characteristics, January 2005.
2. Crixivan (Indinavir sulfate). Merck & Co., Inc. US Prescribing information, May 2004.

3. Kaletra Soft Capsules (Lopinavir/ritonavir). Abbott Laboratories Ltd. UK Summary of product characteristics, January 2005.
4. Kaletra (Lopinavir/ritonavir). Abbott Laboratories. US Prescribing information, April 2005.
5. Viracept (Nelfinavir mesilate). Roche Products Ltd. UK Summary of product characteristics, June 2005.
6. Viracept (Nelfinavir mesilate). Agouron Pharmaceuticals, Inc. US Prescribing information, September 2004.
7. Fortovase (Saquinavir). Roche Products Ltd. UK Summary of product characteristics, January 2005.
8. Invirase (Saquinavir mesilate). Roche Pharmaceuticals. US Prescribing information, December 2004.
9. Berbel Garcia A, Latorre Ibarra A, Porta Etessam J, Martinez Salio A, Perez Martinez DA, Saiz Diaz R, Toledo Heras M. Protease inhibitor-induced carbamazepine toxicity. *Clin Neuropharmacol* (2000) 23, 216–18.

Protease inhibitors + Anticonvulsants; Carbamazepine

Case reports suggest that ritonavir markedly increases carbamazepine levels and toxicity. Carbamazepine reduces indinavir levels and efficacy, and would also be expected to decrease levels of other protease inhibitors. Carbamazepine should be used with caution in combination with protease inhibitors, if at all, because of the risks of antiviral treatment failure.

Clinical evidence

(a) Indinavir

A report describes the case of a 48-year-old man whose antiretroviral therapy (indinavir 800 mg every 8 hours, lamivudine 150 mg twice daily and zidovudine 200 mg three times daily) became ineffective after a 10-week course of carbamazepine for postherpetic neuralgia. Over this time indinavir levels were up to 16 times lower than those measured in the absence of carbamazepine.[1] In two further cases, patients treated with carbamazepine had partial failure of indinavir-containing regimens, which prompted a change in their therapy to include ritonavir rather than indinavir.[2,3]

In 3 of the case reports described below, in which ritonavir increased carbamazepine levels,[2-4] patients had previously received indinavir (800 mg three times daily[2,4]), carbamazepine (600 mg daily[2,3] or 400 mg three times daily[4]) without experiencing carbamazepine toxicity (therapeutic carbamazepine levels were reported in 2 of the cases[2,3]). This suggests that indinavir does not increase carbamazepine levels. However, in the case described above,[1] carbamazepine levels reached the therapeutic range for epilepsy even though the dosage of carbamazepine was only 200 mg daily, suggesting indinavir may increase carbamazepine levels.

(b) Ritonavir

An epileptic 20-year-old HIV+ man who had his seizures controlled with carbamazepine 350 mg twice daily and zonisamide 140 mg twice daily was admitted to hospital for review of his antiretrovirals. He was started on ritonavir 200 mg three times daily, but after the first dose of ritonavir his serum carbamazepine levels rose from 9.5 to 17.8 micrograms/ml. This was accompanied by intractable vomiting and vertigo, so after 2 days the ritonavir was stopped. Symptoms resolved over the next few days. Subsequently ritonavir 200 mg daily was started, with the same effect, so the dose of carbamazepine was reduced to one third, which resulted in carbamazepine levels of 6.2 micrograms/ml. Levels of ritonavir were not measured.[5] Three other cases also document two- to threefold rises in carbamazepine levels with associated toxicity caused by the addition of ritonavir.[2-4] In one case a carbamazepine dose reduction from 600 to 100 mg daily was needed to keep the levels within the therapeutic range before ritonavir was discontinued.[3]

Mechanism

Ritonavir is a potent inhibitor of the cytochrome P450 isoenzyme CYP3A4 and consequently markedly increases carbamazepine levels. Other protease inhibitors would be expected to interact similarly, although to a lesser degree (see also 'Antivirals', (p.578)). Moreover, carbamazepine is an inducer of CYP3A4 and therefore increases the metabolism of the protease inhibitor causing levels to become subtherapeutic.

Importance and management

Although the evidence is limited, these interactions seem to be established. It would therefore appear that the combination of carbamazepine and protease inhibitors should be avoided where possible (mainly because of the risk of antiviral treatment failure). If both must be used then extremely close monitoring of both protease inhibitor levels/efficacy and carbamazepine levels/toxicity is warranted. The authors of one report suggest that amitriptyline or gabapentin would be possible alternatives for carbamazepine used for pain, or valproic acid or lamotrigine for carbamazepine used for seizures.[1]

1. Hugen PWH, Burger DM, Brinkman K, ter Hofstede HJM, Schuurman R, Koopmans PP, Hekster YA. Carbamazepine-indinavir interaction causes antiretroviral therapy failure. *Ann Pharmacother* (2000) 34, 465–70.
2. Berbel Garcia A, Latorre Ibarra A, Porta Etessam J, Martinez Salio A, Perez Martinez DA, Saiz Diaz R, Toledo Heras M. Protease inhibitor-induced carbamazepine toxicity. *Clin Neuropharmacol* (2000) 23, 216–18.
3. Burman W, Orr L. Carbamazepine toxicity after starting combination antiretroviral therapy including ritonavir and efavirenz. *AIDS* (2000) 14, 2793–4.
4. Mateu-de Antonio J, Grau S, Gimeno-Bayón J-L, Carmona A. Ritonavir-induced carbamazepine toxicity. *Ann Pharmacother* (2001) 35, 125–6.
5. Kato Y, Fujii T, Mizoguchi N, Takata N, Ueda K, Feldman MD, Kayser SR. Potential interaction between ritonavir and carbamazepine. *Pharmacotherapy* (2000) 20, 851–4.

Protease inhibitors + Anticonvulsants; Phenytoin

Ritonavir appears to increase phenytoin levels, whereas nelfinavir and lopinavir/ritonavir modestly reduced phenytoin levels. Phenytoin decreases lopinavir levels, and possibly also indinavir levels, but did not alter nelfinavir levels. Phenytoin should be used with caution in combination with protease inhibitors with close monitoring of antiviral efficacy and phenytoin levels.

Clinical evidence

(a) Indinavir

A 39-year-old HIV+ man, on phenytoin 300 mg daily, was started on indinavir 800 mg three times daily. When the phenytoin dose was reduced to 200 mg daily, the viral load dropped by almost half and his CD4+ count doubled.[1]

(b) Lopinavir/ritonavir

Combined use of phenytoin 300 mg once daily and lopinavir/ritonavir 400 mg/100 mg twice daily resulted in a 30% decrease in the AUC of lopinavir and a 23% decrease in the AUC of phenytoin in studies in healthy subjects.[2]

(c) Nelfinavir

An HIV+ man taking phenytoin and phenobarbital for epilepsy had been on nelfinavir 750 mg three times daily and stavudine 30 mg twice daily for nearly 3 months when he had a tonic-clonic seizure. After starting nelfinavir and stavudine, serum phenytoin levels were found to have dropped from around 10 mg/l to around 5 mg/l.[3] Similarly, nelfinavir 1.25 g twice daily for 7 days decreased the AUC of phenytoin by about 30% and the maximum serum level by 21%, in healthy subjects, whereas the nelfinavir levels were not altered.[4]

(d) Ritonavir

A case report describes the intentional use of ritonavir 600 mg twice daily in a 14-year-old boy who had been having seizures for 28 days, despite the use of several anticonvulsants. Phenytoin at 20 mg/kg daily had originally failed to produce satisfactory plasma levels, although it did reduce the rate of seizures. After starting the ritonavir his seizures were controlled and the phenytoin level became therapeutic. Seizures started again after the ritonavir was stopped.[5]

Mechanism

Phenytoin is an inducer of the cytochrome P450 isoenzyme CYP3A4, and would be expected to increase the metabolism of the protease inhibitors, although nelfinavir levels were not altered. Phenytoin is principally metabolised by CYP2C9 and CYP2C19, and would therefore, not be expected to be substantially affected by most protease inhibitors. However, both increases and modest decreases in phenytoin levels have been seen.

Importance and management

Although information is limited, some of these interactions are expected. Phenytoin may decrease plasma levels of indinavir and lopinavir, and the makers of **saquinavir**[6,7] also predict that its levels will be reduced by phenytoin. Phenytoin appears not to alter nelfinavir levels.

In addition, protease inhibitors appear to alter phenytoin levels. Therefore an alternative anticonvulsant, such as sodium valproate, which does not affect cytochrome P450 isoenzymes, may be more appropriate in patients on protease inhibitors. However, if there is no option but to use phenytoin, close monitoring of antiviral efficacy and phenytoin levels is essential.

1. Campagna KD, Torbert A, Bedsole GD, Ravis WR. Possible induction of indinavir metabolism by phenytoin. *Pharmacotherapy* (1997) 17, 182.
2. Lim ML, Min SS, Eron JJ, Bertz RJ, Robinson M, Gaedigk A, Kashuba ADM. Coadministration of lopinavir/ritonavir and phenytoin results in two-way drug interaction through cytochrome P-450 induction. *J Acquir Immune Defic Syndr* (2004) 36, 1034–40.
3. Honda M, Yasuoka A, Aoki M, Oka S. A generalized seizure following initiation of nelfinavir in a patient with human immunodeficiency virus type 1 infection, suspected due to interaction between nelfinavir and phenytoin. *Intern Med* (1999) 38, 302–3.
4. Shelton MJ, Cloen D, Becker M, Hsyu PH, Wilton JH, Hewitt RG. Evaluation of the pharmacokinetic interaction between phenytoin and nelfinavir in healthy volunteers at steady state. *40th Intersci Conf Antimicrob Agents Chemother* (2000) Sep 17-20; Toronto. Abstract 426.
5. Broderick A, Webb DW, McMenamin J, Butler K. A novel use of ritonavir. *AIDS* (1998) 12 (Suppl 4), S29.
6. Fortovase (Saquinavir). Roche Products Ltd. UK Summary of product characteristics, January 2005.
7. Invirase (Saquinavir mesilate). Roche Pharmaceuticals. US Prescribing information, December 2004.

Protease inhibitors + Antidepressants

Fluoxetine modestly raises the levels of ritonavir, and ritonavir is predicted to raise levels of fluoxetine, paroxetine and sertraline. A few cases of the serotonin syndrome have been attributed to the use of fluoxetine and ritonavir. Ritonavir raises desipramine levels and is predicted to also raise the levels of other tricyclic antidepressants. A lower starting dose of desipramine is suggested and monitoring is advisable. In a single-dose study, venlafaxine lowered indinavir levels, which may affect treatment efficacy.

Clinical evidence, mechanism, importance and management

(a) SSRIs and Trazodone

Ritonavir 600 mg was given to 16 healthy subjects before and after 8 days of treatment with **fluoxetine** 30 mg twice daily. The maximum plasma levels of **ritonavir** were unaffected, but the AUC rose by 19%. These changes were not considered large enough to warrant changing the dose of **ritonavir**.[1] The study was criticised for not achieving steady state before assessing the pharmacokinetics and thus possibly underestimating the interaction.[2] However, the authors point out that **fluoxetine** levels were equivalent to those seen at steady state, and multiple dosing of **ritonavir** is likely to induce its own metabolism, so if anything, the interaction would be lessened at steady state.[3]

The makers of **ritonavir** predict that the levels of SSRIs (**fluoxetine**, **paroxetine**, **sertraline**) may also be elevated [not investigated in the study quoted] due to the inhibitory effect of **ritonavir** on various cytochrome P450 isoenzymes.[4,5] They suggest careful monitoring of adverse effects when these drugs are used with **ritonavir**;[4] dose reduction of the SSRI may be required.[5] Two cases of serotonin syndrome were attributed to adding **ritonavir** to established **fluoxetine** therapy. In one patient this was managed by halving the **fluoxetine** dose, and in the other **ritonavir** was withdrawn. Another case occurred in a patient on **fluoxetine** and **trazodone** when **ritonavir** was added, and this resolved on discontinuing the **trazodone** and halving the **ritonavir** dose.[6]

(b) Tricyclic antidepressants

A single 100-mg dose of **desipramine** was given to 14 healthy subjects before and after 10 days of **ritonavir** 500 mg twice daily. The AUC and half-life of **desipramine** increased nearly 2.5-fold and 2-fold respectively. The maximum plasma levels were also increased by 22.1%. These changes are considered to be clinically significant, so the authors suggest that a lower initial dose of **desipramine** should be used if it is to be started in patients on **ritonavir**, and careful monitoring should be carried out in the first few weeks of treatment.[7] These effects are likely to be due to the inhibitory effects of **ritonavir** on the cytochrome P450 isoenzyme CYP2D6.[8] Because of this, the makers of **ritonavir** also predict that the levels of other tricyclic antidepressants (e.g. **amitriptyline**, **imipramine**, **nortriptyline**) will also be raised, and they suggest careful monitoring of adverse effects if these drugs are used with **ritonavir**;[4] dose reduction of the tricyclic may be required.[5] *In vitro* data show that other protease inhibitors also inhibit **desipramine** hydroxylation (in order of potency; **indinavir**, **saquinavir**, and **nelfinavir**), but less so than **ritonavir**.[8]

(c) Venlafaxine

In a study, 9 healthy subjects were given a single dose of **indinavir** before and after 10 days of venlafaxine 150 mg daily in divided doses. **Indinavir** did not affect the venlafaxine, but venlafaxine reduced the AUC and maximum plasma levels of **indinavir** by 28 and 36% respectively. This is possibly enough to reduce the efficacy of **indinavir**.[9] Quite why this happens is not clear. More study is needed to establish the effects of multiple doses.

1. Ouellet D, Hsu A, Qian J, Lamm JE, Cavanaugh JH, Leonard JM, Granneman GR. Effect of fluoxetine on the pharmacokinetics of ritonavir. *Antimicrob Agents Chemother* (1998) 42, 3107–12.
2. Bellibas SE. Ritonavir-fluoxetine interaction. *Antimicrob Agents Chemother* (1999) 43, 1815.
3. Ouellet D, Hsu A. Ritonavir-fluoxetine interaction. *Antimicrob Agents Chemother* (1999) 43, 1815.
4. Norvir (Ritonavir). Abbott Laboratories Ltd. UK Summary of product characteristics, January 2005.
5. Norvir (Ritonavir). Abbott Laboratories. US Prescribing information, April 2005.
6. DeSilva KE, Le Flore DB, Marston BJ, Rimland D. Serotonin syndrome in HIV-infected individuals receiving antiretroviral therapy and fluoxetine. *AIDS* (2001) 15, 1281–5.
7. Bertz RI, Cao G, Cavanaugh JH, Hsu A, Granneman GR, Leonard JM. Effect of ritonavir on the pharmacokinetics of desipramine. 11th International Conference on AIDS, Vancouver, 1996. Abstract Mo.B.1201.
8. Von Moltke LL, Greenblatt DJ, Duan SX, Daily JP, Harmatz JS, Shader RI. Inhibition of desipramine hydroxylation (cytochrome P450-2D6) in vitro by quinidine and by viral protease inhibitors: relation to drug interactions in vivo. *J Pharm Sci* (1998) 87, 1184–9.
9. Levin GM, Nelson LA, DeVane CL, Preston SL, Eisele G, Carson SW. A pharmacokinetic drug-drug interaction study of venlafaxine and indinavir. *Psychopharmacol Bull* (2001) 35, 62–71.

Protease inhibitors + Azoles

Ketoconazole raises the AUCs of the protease inhibitors, but on the information available so far this rarely seems to warrant a dose adjustment. Ritonavir markedly raises ketoconazole levels; therefore limiting the dose of ketoconazole is recommended when ritonavir is used alone or in combination with other protease inhibitors. Amprenavir modestly raises ketoconazole levels and saquinavir alone has no effect.

Itraconazole appears to markedly raise the levels of saquinavir, and may also raise the levels of other protease inhibitors. Ritonavir, indinavir and amprenavir may increase itraconazole levels. Fluconazole appears not to interact with ritonavir or indinavir, but may raise nelfinavir and saquinavir levels to a modest extent.

Clinical evidence

(a) Fluconazole

Fluconazole 400 mg on day one, followed by 200 mg daily for 4 days did not affect any of the pharmacokinetic parameters of **ritonavir** 200 mg every 6 hours by more than 15%, when given to 8 healthy subjects.[1] Similarly, fluconazole had no effect on the pharmacokinetics of **ritonavir** in 3 HIV+ subjects.[2] The pharmacokinetics of both **indinavir** 1 g every 8 hours and fluconazole 400 mg daily were not significantly affected by concurrent use in 11 HIV+ patients.[3] Another study also found no significant interaction between **indinavir** and fluconazole.[4] A population pharmacokinetic analysis estimated that fluconazole decreased **nelfinavir** clearance by 26 to 30%, but this was not considered clinically significant.[5] However, fluconazole 400 mg on day 2, followed by 200 mg daily for 6 days increased the median AUC of **saquinavir** by 50%, and the maximum level by 56% in 5 HIV+ subjects.[2]

(b) Itraconazole

Shortly after itraconazole was added to their treatment, 2 patients on **indinavir** and another on **saquinavir/ritonavir** were noted to have reactions similar to those seen with protease inhibitors alone (eczematous eruptions, raised serum transaminases). This was attributed to raised levels of both medications, arising from concurrent use. A very prolonged itraconazole half-life was measured in the patient on **saquinavir/ritonavir**.[6] In another study, itraconazole caused a median fivefold increase in the AUC of **saquinavir**, and it was considered that itraconazole may be an alternative to **ritonavir** for boosting **saquinavir** levels.[7] The UK makers of **indinavir** say that giving **indinavir** 600 mg every 8 hours with itraconazole 200 mg twice daily produces an AUC similar to that achieved when **indinavir** 800 mg every 8 hours is given alone.[8] The maker of **amprenavir** notes that it is possible that plasma levels of itraconazole may be raised by concurrent use.[9] The maker of itraconazole[10,11] says that **ritonavir** and **indinavir** may increase the bioavailability of itraconazole, since they are potent inhibitors of CYP3A4.

(c) Ketoconazole

In one early clinical study, patients who received the combination of ketoconazole and **saquinavir** had a greater drop in viral load after 3 months than those receiving no ketoconazole.[12] However, in one pharmacokinetic study, ketoconazole 200 mg for 7 days then 400 mg daily for 7 days had no consistent effect on **saquinavir** peak and trough plasma levels in 7 HIV+ patients, although inter-individual variability was great. **Saquinavir** [as hard gelatin capsules[13]] was given at the low dose of 600 mg three times daily.[14] Conversely, when **saquinavir** (soft gel capsule formulation) 1.2 g three times daily was given to 12 healthy subjects with ketoconazole 400 mg daily for 7 days, the **saquinavir** AUC and maximum plasma levels were raised by 190% and 171%, respectively.[13] A similar study in 22 HIV+ patients, using ketoconazole 200 mg daily, found that the **saquinavir** AUC and maximum plasma levels were raised by 69% and 36% respectively.[13]

Pharmacokinetic changes have also been seen with concurrent use of ketoconazole with **amprenavir**[15] (AUC increased by 32%), **indinavir**[16] (AUC raised by 62%) or **nelfinavir**[17] (AUC raised by 35%). In 12 HIV+ patients, ketoconazole 200 or 400 mg increased the AUC of **saquinavir** and **ritonavir** in combination (both 400 mg twice daily) by 37% and 29% respectively. The distribution of **ritonavir** was also affected, with disproportionate rises seen in CSF concentrations. All these changes appeared to be unrelated to the dose of ketoconazole used.[18] Conversely, the pharmacokinetics of **atazanavir** 400 mg daily were not affected after 7 days of concurrent treatment with ketoconazole 200 mg daily.[19] A single 200-mg dose of ketoconazole had no effect on the pharmacokinetics of **lopinavir**.[20]

The pharmacokinetics of ketoconazole are also affected by some protease inhibitors. In a single-dose study **amprenavir** 1.2 g caused a 44% rise in the AUC of ketoconazole 400 mg.[15] **Ritonavir** increased the AUC of ketoconazole 3.4-fold and the maximum plasma level 1.6-fold.[21] In another study, the AUC of a single 200-mg dose of ketoconazole was increased threefold in patients on **lopinavir/ritonavir** 400/100 mg twice daily.[20] The peak plasma level of ketoconazole 400 mg daily when given with **saquinavir/ritonavir** was similar to that usually seen with ketoconazole 800 mg alone.[18] Moreover, in this study, dose escalation to higher doses of ketoconazole was discontinued after the first patient given ketoconazole 600 mg daily stopped treatment early because of adverse gastrointestinal effects.[18] However, **saquinavir** alone did not affect ketoconazole pharmacokinetics.[13]

(d) Voriconazole

In a study in 18 healthy subjects, the pharmacokinetics of both **indinavir** 800 mg three times daily and voriconazole 200 mg twice daily were unaffected by at least a week of concurrent use.[22] However, *in vitro* studies suggest that the metabolism of HIV-protease inhibitors may be inhibited by voriconazole, and the metabolism of voriconazole may be inhibited by HIV-protease inhibitors. The makers therefore suggest that patients be carefully monitored for evidence of drug toxicity and/or loss of efficacy during concurrent use of other HIV-protease inhibitors (**amprenavir**, **nelfinavir** and **saquinavir** are specifically mentioned).[23]

In healthy subjects **ritonavir** 400 mg twice daily for 9 days decreased the steady state maximum levels and AUC of oral voriconazole (400 mg twice daily for 1 day, then 200 mg twice daily for 8 days) by 66% and 82% respectively.[24] The pharmacokinetics of the **ritonavir** remained unchanged.[24]

Mechanism

Ketoconazole and itraconazole are known to inhibit the cytochrome P450 isoenzyme CYP3A4, and the protease inhibitors also inhibit and share this pathway of metabolism.[4,13,15,18] Thus enzyme inhibition, and competition for metabolism results in raised serum levels of both drugs. Ketoconazole may also inhibit P-glycoprotein transport of saquinavir and ritonavir, causing a decrease in their clearance, and raising serum levels.[13,18] Inhibition of P-glycoprotein may reduce efflux of protease inhibitors from the CSF, so increasing CSF levels.[18] Fluconazole is not such a potent enzyme inhibitor and is therefore not expected to interact.[1,3]

Importance and management

The magnitude of the changes in protease inhibitor pharmacokinetics seen with ketoconazole are unlikely to warrant dose changes of the protease inhibitors or cause significant increase in their adverse effects. No dose adjustments are considered necessary by some makers of amprenavir,[9] indinavir,[8] nelfinavir,[25,26] or saquinavir (when the drugs are used concurrently for a limited time).[27,28] However, the US maker of indinavir recommends that the dose of indinavir be reduced to 600 mg every 8 hours when used with ketoconazole.[29] Whether ketoconazole's ability to boost CSF exposure to protease inhibitors has a role in improving therapeutic efficacy in the CNS remains to be seen.[18]

The data on the effect of protease inhibitors on ketoconazole are more limited. Amprenavir caused a modest increase in ketoconazole levels, and the UK makers of amprenavir suggest that no ketoconazole dose adjustment is necessary,[9] although the US makers recommend increased monitoring for adverse effects and state that a dose reduction may be needed in patients receiving more than 400 mg daily.[30] Saquinavir alone did not affect ketoconazole levels. However, a marked effect was seen for ritonavir alone and when combined with lopinavir or saquinavir. This may increase the adverse effects of ketoconazole. The makers of a combination product containing lopinavir/ritonavir say that doses greater than 200 mg a day of ketoconazole are not recommended.[31,32] The makers of ritonavir say that doses of ketoconazole 200 mg a day or greater should not be used with ritonavir without assessing the risk and benefits.[21,33] Similarly, the UK maker of ketoconazole says that a dose reduction of ketoconazole should be considered when given with ritonavir.[34]

The information with itraconazole is more limited. On the basis of the available data, it is possible that itraconazole has greater effects than ketoconazole on protease inhibitor levels. The US makers of amprenavir recommend increased monitoring for adverse effects and state that the dose of itraconazole may need to be reduced if it is greater than 400 mg daily.[30] The makers of indinavir advise modestly reducing the indinavir dose to 600 mg every 8 hours if it is to be given with itraconazole.[8,29] The UK maker of saquinavir recommends monitoring for saquinavir toxicity if itraconazole is used.[27] Some protease inhibitors, especially ritonavir and possibly indinavir, may increase itraconazole levels. The maker of a combination product containing lopinavir/ritonavir says that doses greater than 200 mg a day of itraconazole are not recommended.[31,32]

The small to modest changes in protease inhibitor pharmacokinetics seen with fluconazole are unlikely to be of clinical significance. Some authors suggest using an alternative azole in place of ketoconazole where possible.[13] Fluconazole would seem an appropriate choice.

The makers of voriconazole say that the concurrent use of ritonavir (at doses of 400 mg and above twice daily) is contraindicated,[23,24] presumably because the efficacy of the voriconazole is expected to be markedly reduced.

1. Cato A, Cao G, Hsu A, Cavanaugh J, Leonard J, Granneman R. Evaluation of the effect of fluconazole on the pharmacokinetics of ritonavir. *Drug Metab Dispos* (1997) 25, 1104–1106.
2. Koks CHW, Crommentuyn KML, Hoetelmans RMW, Burger DM, Koopmans PP, Mathôt RAA, Mulder JW, Meenhorst PL, Beijnen JH. The effect of fluconazole on ritonavir and saquinavir pharmacokinetics in HIV-1-infected individuals. *Br J Clin Pharmacol* (2001) 51, 631–5.
3. De Wit S, Debier M, De Smet M, McCrea J, Stone J, Carides A, Matthews C, Deutsch P, Clumeck N. Effect of fluconazole on indinavir pharmacokinetics in human immunodeficiency virus-infected patients. *Antimicrob Agents Chemother* (1998) 42, 223–7.
4. The indinavir (MK 639) pharmacokinetic study group. Indinavir (MK 639) drug interaction studies. 11th International Conference on AIDS, Vancouver, 1996. Abstract Mo.B.174.
5. Jackson KA, Rosenbaum SE, Kerr BM, Pithavala YK, Yuen G, Dudley MN. A population pharmacokinetic analysis of nelfinavir mesylate in human immunodeficiency virus-infected patients enrolled in a phase III clinical trial. *Antimicrob Agents Chemother* (2000) 44, 1832–7.
6. MacKenzie-Wood AR, Whitfeld MJ, Ray JE. Itraconazole and HIV protease inhibitors: an important interaction. *Med J Aust* (1999) 170, 46–7.
7. Koks CHW, Van Heeswijk RPG, Veldkamp AI, Meenhorst PL, Mulder J-W, van der Meer JTM, Beijnen JH, Hoetelmans RMW. Itraconazole as an alternative for ritonavir liquid formulation when combined with saquinavir. *AIDS* (2000) 14, 89–90.
8. Crixivan (Indinavir sulfate). Merck Sharp & Dohme Ltd. UK Summary of product characteristics, January 2005.
9. Agenerase (Amprenavir). GlaxoSmithKline UK. UK Summary of product characteristics, December 2004.
10. Sporanox (Itraconazole). Janssen-Cilag Ltd. UK Summary of product characteristics, November 2002.
11. Sporanox (Itraconazole). Janssen Pharmaceutica Products L.P. US Prescribing information, January 2004.
12. Jordan WC. The effectiveness of combined saquinavir and ketoconazole treatment in reducing HIV viral load. *J Natl Med Assoc* (1998) 90, 622–4.
13. Grub S, Bryson H, Goggin T, Lüdin E, Jorga K. The interaction of saquinavir (soft gelatin capsule) with ketoconazole, erythromycin and rifampicin: comparison of the effect in healthy volunteers and in HIV-infected patients. *Eur J Clin Pharmacol* (2001) 57, 115–21.
14. Collazos J, Martínez E, Mayo J, Blanco M-S. Effect of ketoconazole on plasma concentrations of saquinavir. *J Antimicrob Chemother* (2000) 46, 151–2.
15. Polk RE, Crouch MA, Israel DS, Pastor A, Sadler BM, Chittick GE, Symonds WT, Gouldin W, Lou Y. Pharmacokinetic interaction between ketoconazole and amprenavir after single doses in healthy men. *Pharmacotherapy* (1999) 19, 1378–84.
16. McCrea J, Woolf E, Sterrett A, Matthews C, Deutsch P, Yeh KC, Waldman S, Bjornsson T. Effects of ketoconazole and other P450 inhibitors on the pharmacokinetics of indinavir. *Pharm Res* (1996) 13 (Suppl 9), S465.
17. Kerr B, Lee C, Yuen G, Anderson R, Daniels R, Grettenberger H, Liang B-H, Quart B, Sandoval T, Shetty B, Wu E, Zhang K. Overview of *in-vitro* and *in-vivo* drug interaction studies of nelfinavir mesylate (NFV), a new HIV-1 protease inhibitor. 4th Conference on Retroviruses and Opportunistic Infections, Washington DC, 1997. Session 39, Slide 373.

18. Khaliq Y, Gallicano K, Venance S, Kravcik S, Cameron DW. Effect of ketoconazole on ritonavir and saquinavir concentrations in plasma and cerebrospinal fluid from patients infected with human immunodeficiency virus. *Clin Pharmacol Ther* (2000) 68, 637–46.
19. O'Mara EM, Randall D, Mummaneni V, Uderman H, Knox L, Schuster A, Geraldes M, Raymond R. Steady-state pharmacokinetic interaction study between BMS-232632 and ketoconazole in healthy subjects. *Intersci Conf Antimicrob Agents Chemother* (2000) 40, 335.
20. Bertz R, Hsu A, Lam W, Williams L, Renz C, Karol M, Dutta S, Carr R, Zhang Y, Wang Q, Schweitzer S, Foit C, Andre A, Bernstein B, Granneman GR, Sun E. Pharmacokinetic interactions between lopinavir/ritonavir (ABT-378r) and other non-HIV drugs (abstract P291). *AIDS* (2000) 14 (Suppl 4), S100.
21. Norvir (Ritonavir). Abbott Laboratories Ltd. UK Summary of product characteristics, January 2005.
22. Purkins L, Wood N, Kleinermans D, Love ER. No clinically significant pharmacokinetic interactions between voriconazole and indinavir in healthy volunteers. *Br J Clin Pharmacol* (2003) 56 (Suppl 1), 62–8.
23. VFEND (Voriconazole). Pfizer Ltd. UK Summary of product characteristics, March 2005.
24. VFEND (Voriconazole). Pfizer Ltd. US Prescribing information, March 2005.
25. Viracept (Nelfinavir mesilate). Roche Products Ltd. UK Summary of product characteristics, June 2005.
26. Viracept (Nelfinavir mesilate). Agouron Pharmaceuticals, Inc. US Prescribing information, September 2004.
27. Fortovase (Saquinavir). Roche Products Ltd. UK Summary of product characteristics, January 2005.
28. Fortavase (Saquinavir). Roche Pharmaceuticals. US Prescribing information, December 2003.
29. Crixivan (Indinavir sulfate). Merck & Co., Inc. US Prescribing information, May 2004.
30. Agenerase (Amprenavir). GlaxoSmithKline. US Prescribing information, May 2005.
31. Kaletra Soft Capsules (Lopinavir/ritonavir). Abbott Laboratories Ltd. UK Summary of product characteristics, January 2005.
32. Kaletra (Lopinavir/ritonavir). Abbott Laboratories. US Prescribing information, April 2005.
33. Norvir (Ritonavir). Abbott Laboratories. US Prescribing information, April 2005.
34. Nizoral (Ketoconazole). Janssen-Cilag Ltd. UK Summary of product characteristics, May 2001.

Protease inhibitors + Co-trimoxazole

Minor pharmacokinetic changes have been seen when co-trimoxazole is given with the protease inhibitors, but these changes are not considered to be clinically significant.

Clinical evidence, mechanism, importance and management

A study in 12 healthy subjects given **indinavir** 400 mg every 6 hours with co-trimoxazole 960 mg every 12 hours found that there was no change in the AUC of **indinavir**, but a 17% decrease in **indinavir** trough levels. In addition, there was an 18% increase in the AUC of **trimethoprim**, and a 5% increase in the AUC of **sulfamethoxazole**. None of these changes were considered to be clinically important.[1]

Ritonavir 500 mg twice daily caused a 20% increase in the AUC of **trimethoprim** and a 20% decrease in the AUC of **sulfamethoxazole** when a single 960-mg dose of co-trimoxazole was given to 15 healthy subjects. These changes were considered too small to be of clinical relevance.[2,3] The pharmacokinetics of **ritonavir** were not assessed.

The combination of **saquinavir** 600 mg three times daily and co-trimoxazole 960 mg three times weekly caused no changes in the pharmacokinetics of **saquinavir**.[4] The makers of a combination product containing **lopinavir** state that they do not anticipate any interaction between **lopinavir** and co-trimoxazole.[5,6]

There would seem to be no reason for avoiding the use of co-trimoxazole with any of the protease inhibitors.

1. Sturgill MG, Seibold JR, Boruchoff SE, Yeh KC, Haddix H, Deutsch P. Trimethoprim/sulfamethoxazole does not affect the steady-state disposition of indinavir. *J Clin Pharmacol* (1999) 39, 1077–84.
2. Bertz RJ, Cao G, Cavanaugh JH, Hsu A, Granneman GR, Leonard JM. Effect of ritonavir on the pharmacokinetics of trimethoprim/sulfamethoxazole. 11th International Conference on AIDS, Vancouver, 1996. Abstract Mo.B.1197.
3. Norvir (Ritonavir). Abbott Laboratories Ltd. UK Summary of product characteristics, January 2005.
4. Maserati R, Villani P, Cocchi L, Regazzi MB. Co-trimoxazole administered for *Pneumocystis carinii* pneumonia prophylaxis does not interfere with saquinavir pharmacokinetics. *AIDS* (1998) 12, 815–6.
5. Kaletra Soft Capsules (Lopinavir/ritonavir). Abbott Laboratories Ltd. UK Summary of product characteristics, January 2005.
6. Kaletra (Lopinavir/ritonavir). Abbott Laboratories. US Prescribing information, April 2005.

Protease inhibitors + Food

Food increases the bioavailability of atazanavir, lopinavir, nelfinavir and saquinavir, but decreases that of indinavir. Food only minimally affects the bioavailability of amprenavir and ritonavir. Mixing ritonavir with enteral feeds does not affect the pharmacokinetics of ritonavir, when this is given after a light meal.

Clinical evidence, mechanism, importance and management

(a) Absorption decreased

(i) Indinavir. A single 600-mg dose of indinavir was given to 7 HIV+ subjects immediately after various types of meal. The **protein**, **carbohydrate**, **fat** and **high-viscosity meals** reduced the AUC of indinavir by 68%, 45%, 34% and 30% respectively. The fat meal was associated with the largest inter-subject variation in bioavailability. The effect of the protein meal was attributed to the fact that it raised gastric pH and therefore impaired the absorption of indinavir (a weak base). The impairment of indinavir absorption caused by the other meals, which did not alter gastric pH, may have been due to delayed gastric emptying.[1] A similar study comparing a full breakfast with light breakfasts (toast or cereal) on indinavir absorption found that the full breakfast reduced the absorption of indinavir by 78% and the maximum serum levels by 86%, whilst the light breakfasts had no significant effect.[2] The makers advise that indinavir is given 1 hour before or 2 hours after meals, or with light meals only.[3,4]

(b) Absorption increased

(i) Atazanavir. The makers of atazanavir note that administration with a light or high-fat meal decreased the wide variation in plasma levels. They recommend that atazanavir should be taken with food to enhance bioavailability and minimise variability.[5,6]

(ii) Lopinavir. A moderate-fat meal increased the AUC and maximum level of lopinavir capsules by 48% and 23%, respectively, and a high-fat meal by 96% and 43% respectively. The corresponding increases for lopinavir solution were 80% and 54% for the moderate-fat meal, and 130% and 56% for the high-fat meal.[7] The makers of a combination product of lopinavir/ritonavir say that it should be taken with food.[7,8]

(iii) Nelfinavir. When nelfinavir 400 or 800 mg was given to 12 healthy subjects in the fasted state, the AUC was only 27% to 50% of that observed when nelfinavir was given with a meal.[9] Nelfinavir should preferably be taken with food.[10,11]

(iv) Saquinavir. The AUC of saquinavir (soft capsules) was increased 6.7-fold (570%) when given after a heavy breakfast compared with the fasting state, and increased by 46% when given after a heavy breakfast compared with a light meal.[12] The effect of food persists for up to 2 hours, so saquinavir (soft capsules) should be taken up to 2 hours after a, preferably substantial, meal.[12] When used in combination with ritonavir, the AUC of saquinavir (soft capsules) was increased only 24% when taken after a high-fat compared with a normal breakfast. Therefore, when used with ritonavir, the UK maker recommends that saquinavir (soft capsules) should be taken within 2 hours after either a moderate or substantial meal;[12,13] the US maker states that a light meal is sufficient in the presence of ritonavir.[13] Similarly, the AUC of saquinavir (hard capsules) was increased 6.7-fold, and the maximum plasma level 11.8-fold, when given after a heavy breakfast compared with the fasted state.[14] Saquinavir (hard capsules) should be taken up to 2 hours after a meal.[14,15]

(c) Absorption minimally affected

(i) Amprenavir. Food resulted in a 25% reduction in the AUC of amprenavir, but no change in the steady-state trough level. Consequently, the makers say it can be given with or without food,[16] but the US maker says not with a high-fat meal.[17]

(ii) Ritonavir. The US maker notes that the extent of absorption of ritonavir capsules was 13% higher when given with a meal compared with the fasting state, whereas that of the oral solution was decreased 7%.[18] Although these changes are modest the makers state that ritonavir capsules and solution are preferably taken with food.[18-20] There is also some evidence that mixing ritonavir with **enteral feeds** does not affect ritonavir pharmacokinetics. A 600-mg dose of **ritonavir** oral solution was mixed with 240 ml of **enteral feeds** (either *Advera* or *Ensure*), **chocolate milk** or water within 1 hour prior to dosing. When given within 15 minutes after a low-fat meal, the pharmacokinetics of ritonavir in either of the **enteral feeds** or the **milk** were almost identical to those when ritonavir was given in water.[21]

1. Carver PL, Fleisher D, Zhou SY, Kaul D, Kazanjian P, Li C. Meal composition effects on the oral bioavailability of indinavir in HIV-infected patients. *Pharm Res* (1999) 16, 718–24.
2. Stone JA, Ju WD, Steritt A, Woolf EJ, Yeh KC, Deutsch P, Waldman S, Bjornsson TD. Effect of food on the pharmacokinetics of indinavir in man. *Pharm Res* (1996) 13 (Suppl 9), S414.
3. Crixivan (Indinavir sulfate). Merck Sharp & Dohme Ltd. UK Summary of product characteristics, January 2005.
4. Crixivan (Indinavir sulfate). Merck & Co., Inc. US Prescribing information, May 2004.
5. Reyataz Hard Capsules (Atazanavir). Bristol-Myers Squibb Pharmaceuticals Ltd. UK Summary of product characteristics, February 2005.
6. Reyataz (Atazanavir sulfate). Bristol-Myers Squibb Company. US Prescribing information, June 2005.

7. Kaletra (Lopinavir/ritonavir). Abbott Laboratories Ltd. UK Summary of product characteristics, January 2005.
8. Kaletra (Lopinavir/ritonavir). Abbott Laboratories. US Prescribing information, April 2005.
9. Quart BD, Chapman SK, Peterkin J, Webber S, Oliver S. Phase I safety, tolerance, pharmacokinetics and food effect studies of AG1343--a novel HIV protease inhibitor. The American Society for Microbiology in collaboration with NIH and CDC. 2nd National Conference Human Retroviruses and Related Infections, Washington DC, 1995. Abstract LB3.
10. Viracept (Nelfinavir mesilate). Roche Products Ltd. UK Summary of product characteristics, June 2005.
11. Viracept (Nelfinavir mesilate). Agouron Pharmaceuticals, Inc. US Prescribing information, September 2004.
12. Fortovase (Saquinavir). Roche Products Ltd. UK Summary of product characteristics, January 2005.
13. Fortovase (Saquinavir). Roche Pharmaceuticals. US Prescribing information, December 2003.
14. Invirase (Saquinavir mesilate). Roche Products Ltd. UK Summary of product characteristics, June 2005.
15. Invirase (Saquinavir mesilate). Roche Pharmaceuticals. US Prescribing information, December 2004.
16. Agenerase (Amprenavir). GlaxoSmithKline UK. UK Summary of product characteristics, December 2004.
17. Agenerase (Amprenavir). GlaxoSmithKline. US Prescribing information, May 2005.
18. Norvir Soft Capsules (Ritonavir). Abbott Laboratories. US prescribing information, April 2005.
19. Norvir Oral Solution (Ritonavir). Abbott Laboratories Ltd. UK Summary of product characteristics, January 2005.
20. Norvir Soft Capsules (Ritonavir). Abbott Laboratories Ltd. UK Summary of product characteristics, January 2005.
21. Bertz R, Shi H, Cavanaugh J, Hsu A. Effect of three vehicles, Advera®, Ensure® and chocolate milk, on the bioavailability of an oral liquid formulation of Norvir (Ritonavir). *Intersci Conf Antimicrob Agents Chemother* (1996) 36, 5.

Protease inhibitors + Garlic

A garlic supplement reduced the plasma levels of saquinavir by 50%. Therefore, garlic supplements should probably be avoided in those on saquinavir as the sole protease inhibitor. Another garlic supplement did not have an important effect on the plasma levels of a single dose of ritonavir.

Clinical evidence

Garlic reduced the AUC and maximum and minimum plasma concentrations of **saquinavir** by about 50% in a study in 9 healthy subjects. The garlic was taken in the form of a dietary supplement (*GarliPure, Maximum Allicin Formula* caplets) twice daily for 20 days. **Saquinavir** 1.2 g three times daily was given for 4-day periods before, during, and after the garlic supplement. Fourteen days after the garlic supplement the **saquinavir** pharmacokinetics had still not returned to baseline values. Of the 9 subjects, 6 had a substantial drop in **saquinavir** AUC while taking garlic, then a rise when garlic was stopped. The remaining 3 had no change in **saquinavir** AUC while taking garlic, then a drop when garlic was stopped.[1]

Gastrointestinal toxicity was noted in 2 patients taking garlic or garlic supplements when they started **ritonavir**-containing regimens.[2] However, 4 days use of garlic extract 10 mg (equivalent to 1 g of fresh garlic) twice daily did not significantly affect the pharmacokinetics of a single 400-mg dose of **ritonavir** in a study in 10 healthy subjects. There was a nonsignificant 17% decrease in **ritonavir** AUC. The garlic was given in the form of capsules (*Natural Source Odourless Garlic Life Brand*).[3]

Mechanism

The mechanism of this interaction is uncertain, but it is thought that garlic reduced the bioavailability of saquinavir by increasing its metabolism in the intestine.[1] Why there was a disparity in the effect of garlic on saquinavir between patients is unclear.

Importance and management

Although information is limited, a reduction in saquinavir plasma levels of this magnitude could diminish its antiviral efficacy. All garlic supplements should probably be avoided in those on saquinavir as the sole protease inhibitor. While the pharmacokinetic effect on single-dose ritonavir was not clinically important, this requires confirmation in a multiple-dose study.

1. Piscitelli SC, Burstein AH, Welden N, Gallicano KD, Falloon J. The effect of garlic supplements on the pharmacokinetics of saquinavir. *Clin Infect Dis* (2002) 34, 234–8.
2. Laroche M, Choudhri S, Gallicano K, Foster B. Severe gastrointestinal toxicity with concomitant ingestion of ritonavir and garlic. *Can J Infect Dis* (1998) 9 (Suppl A), 76A.
3. Gallicano K, Foster B, Choudhri S. Effect of short-term administration of garlic supplements on single-dose ritonavir pharmacokinetics in healthy volunteers. *Br J Clin Pharmacol* (2003) 55, 199–202.

Protease inhibitors + Grapefruit or Seville orange juice

Grapefruit juice does not have any clinically significant effects on the pharmacokinetics of either indinavir or saquinavir. Seville orange juice did not alter indinavir pharmacokinetics.

Clinical evidence, mechanism, importance and management

(a) Indinavir

Grapefruit juice (8 oz, about 200 ml) reduced the AUC of indinavir 400 mg by 27% in a single-dose study in 10 healthy subjects, although this was not considered clinically significant.[1] Conversely, neither grapefruit juice (8 oz) nor Seville orange juice (8 oz) had any effect on the pharmacokinetics of indinavir in another study in 13 healthy subjects. In this study indinavir 800 mg was given every 8 hours for 4 doses with water, with grapefruit juice or Seville orange juice given with the last 2 doses.[2] Similarly, grapefruit juice (6 oz double strength) had no effect on the steady-state pharmacokinetics of indinavir in 15 HIV+ subjects (a non-significant 4.8% increase in AUC was seen).[3]

(b) Saquinavir

In a study of the effects of concurrent use of grapefruit juice 400 ml and saquinavir (*Invirase;* hard capsules) 600 mg, the grapefruit juice was found to increase the AUC of saquinavir by 50%, possibly by affecting the cytochrome P450 isoenzyme CYP3A4 in the intestines.[4] This modest increase is unlikely to be clinically relevant with normal amounts of grapefruit juice, and the UK makers of saquinavir advise that no dosage adjustment is necessary.[5,6] Various components of grapefruit juice have been shown to inhibit the metabolism of saquinavir *in vitro.*[7]

1. McCrea J, Woolf E, Sterrett A, Matthews C, Deutsch P, Yeh KC, Waldman S, Bjornsson T. Effects of ketoconazole and other P-450 inhibitors on the pharmacokinetics of indinavir. *Pharm Res* (1996) 13 (Suppl 9), S485.
2. Penzak SR, Acosta EP, Turner M, Edwards DJ, Hon YY, Desai HD, Jann MW. Effect of Seville orange juice and grapefruit juice on indinavir pharmacokinetics. *J Clin Pharmacol* (2002) 42, 1165–70.
3. Wynn H, Shelton MJ, Bartos L, Difrancesco R, Hewitt RG. Grapefruit juice (GJ) increases gastric pH, but does not affect indinavir (IDV) exposure, in HIV patients. *Intersci Conf Antimicrob Agents Chemother* (1999) 39, 25.
4. Kupferschmidt HHT, Fattinger KE, Ha HR, Follath F, Krähenbühl S. Grapefruit juice enhances the bioavailability of the HIV protease inhibitor saquinavir in man. *Br J Clin Pharmacol* (1998) 45, 355–9.
5. Fortovase (Saquinavir). Roche Products Ltd. UK Summary of product characteristics, January 2005.
6. Invirase (Saquinavir mesilate). Roche Products Ltd. UK Summary of product characteristics, June 2005.
7. Eagling VA, Profit L, Back DJ. Inhibition of the CYP3A4-mediated metabolism and P-glycoprotein-mediated transport of the HIV-1 protease inhibitor saquinavir by grapefruit juice components. *Br J Clin Pharmacol* (1999) 48, 543–52.

Protease inhibitors + Macrolides

Nelfinavir significantly elevates the serum levels of azithromycin, but the clinical significance of this is uncertain. Single doses of azithromycin have no effect on the levels of indinavir and nelfinavir. Ritonavir increases clarithromycin levels, and dosage adjustments may be needed in those with renal impairment. Atazanavir also increases clarithromycin levels. Indinavir and saquinavir may modestly increase clarithromycin levels, but not to a clinically important extent, and amprenavir did not alter clarithromycin pharmacokinetics. Clarithromycin has no important effect on the pharmacokinetics of amprenavir, atazanavir, indinavir or ritonavir. Although both clarithromycin and erythromycin markedly raise saquinavir levels, this is not considered clinically important for short courses of these antibacterials.

Clinical evidence

(a) Azithromycin

(i) Indinavir. A single 1.2 g dose of azithromycin had no effect on the pharmacokinetics of indinavir in healthy subjects who had taken indinavir 800 mg three times daily for 5 days.[1]

(ii) Nelfinavir. A single 1.2 g dose of azithromycin was given to 12 healthy subjects who had taken nelfinavir 750 mg every 8 hours for 8 days. The pharmacokinetics of nelfinavir were minimally affected, but the AUC and maximum serum levels of azithromycin were about doubled.[2]

(b) Clarithromycin

(i) Amprenavir. In a study in 12 healthy adults, amprenavir 1.2 g twice daily was given with clarithromycin 500 mg twice daily, for 4 days. The AUC and maximum serum levels of amprenavir were increased by 18% and 15% respectively, whereas the pharmacokinetics of clarithromycin were not significantly altered. None of the changes were considered to be clinically significant.[3]

(ii) Atazanavir. The concurrent use of atazanavir 400 mg once daily and clarithromycin 500 mg twice daily for 4 days increased the AUC of clarithromycin by 94%, and reduced the AUC of the active metabolite 14-hydroxyclarithromycin by 70%. In addition, there was a minor 28% increase in the AUC of atazanavir.[4]

(iii) Indinavir. A study found no clinically important alterations in the pharmacokinetics of indinavir in 11 healthy subjects (the only significant change was a 52% increase in the trough level) when clarithromycin 500 mg every 12 hours was given with indinavir 800 mg every 8 hours. The AUC of clarithromycin was increased by about 50%, and that of 14-hydroxyclarithromycin reduced by about 50%, but neither of these changes were considered clinically important because of the wide safety margin of clarithromycin.[5]

(iv) Ritonavir. A study of ritonavir 200 mg every 8 hours given with clarithromycin 500 mg every 12 hours found that there were only minimal changes in ritonavir pharmacokinetics (12.5% increase in AUC and 15.3% increase in maximum plasma level). However, the AUC of clarithromycin increased by 77% with an almost total inhibition of formation of 14-hydroxyclarithromycin (99.7% decrease in AUC).[6]

(v) Saquinavir. The concurrent use of saquinavir *(Fortovase)* 1.2 g three times daily and clarithromycin 500 mg twice daily resulted in 177% and 187% increases in the AUC and maximum serum levels of saquinavir, respectively. Clarithromycin AUC and maximum serum levels were about 40% higher than when given alone.[7]

(c) Erythromycin

The concurrent use of saquinavir *(Fortovase)* 1.2 g three times daily and erythromycin 250 mg four times daily doubled the AUC and maximum serum levels of saquinavir in HIV-infected subjects.[8]

Mechanism

Ritonavir is a potent inhibitor of the cytochrome P450 isoenzyme CYP3A4 and consequently markedly inhibits the 14-hydroxylation of clarithromycin. Other protease inhibitors would be expected to interact similarly, although to a lesser degree (see also 'Antivirals', (p.578)). Clarithromycin is a weak inhibitor of CYP3A4, and generally has only a small effect on the protease inhibitors, except for saquinavir. The effect of clarithromycin on saquinavir, and nelfinavir on azithromycin may involve inhibition of P-glycoprotein.[2,3]

Importance and management

The interaction of amprenavir or indinavir with clarithromycin does not appear to be clinically significant. Similarly, although large increases in saquinavir levels have been seen, the makers say that for short courses no dosage adjustment is needed.[7] However, with ritonavir, clarithromycin becomes more dependent on renal clearance and so the authors concluded that the interaction may be significant in patients with renal failure.[6] The makers of ritonavir and clarithromycin suggest that no dosage reductions should be needed in those with normal renal function, but they recommend a 50% reduction in clarithromycin dose for those with a creatinine clearance of 30 to 60 ml/minute and a 75% reduction for clearances of less than 30 ml/minute.[9-12] Some advise avoidance of clarithromycin dosages exceeding 1 g daily.[9,10] Although there are no formal studies, a similar interaction is predicted with **lopinavir/ritonavir**, and the makers of this combination product state that a dose reduction of clarithromycin should be considered in those with renal or hepatic impairment.[13,14] Atazanavir also reduces the conversion of clarithromycin to its active metabolite, and is often given with ritonavir. However, the maker cautions that reducing the dose of clarithromycin to avoid high levels of the parent drug may result in subtherapeutic levels of the active metabolite. The US maker says that, other than for *Mycobacterium avium* complex infections, an alternative to clarithromycin should be considered.[15] If the combination is used they suggest a 50% dose reduction for the clarithromycin. The UK maker gives no recommendations about dose reductions of clarithromycin, and just recommend caution if the combination is required.[16]

The increase in azithromycin levels with nelfinavir is likely to be of clinical significance,[2] and although the outcome is presumed to be positive, this has yet to be assessed in practice. If concurrent use is necessary, monitor the outcome carefully. Single doses of azithromycin did not affect the pharmacokinetics of nelfinavir or indinavir. The makers of a combination product of lopinavir/ritonavir do not expect a clinically significant interaction with azithromycin.[13,14]

Despite the increases in saquinavir levels, the UK maker says that no dose adjustment is needed when saquinavir is given with erythromycin.[7] The UK maker of nelfinavir suggests that an interaction with erythromycin is unlikely, although this cannot be excluded.[17] The UK maker of ritonavir suggests that because erythromycin levels may rise, due to inhibition of its metabolism by ritonavir, care should be taken if both drugs are prescribed concurrently.[9] A similar warning has been issued by the UK maker of amprenavir about erythromycin.[18]

1. Foulds G, LaBoy-Goral L, Wei GCG, Apseloff G. The effect of azithromycin on the pharmacokinetics of indinavir. *J Clin Pharmacol* (1999) 39, 842–6.
2. Amsden GW, Nafziger AN, Foulds G, Cabelus LJ. A study of the pharmacokinetics of azithromycin and nelfinavir when coadministered in healthy volunteers. *J Clin Pharmacol* (2000) 40, 1522–7.
3. Brophy DF, Israel DS, Pastor A, Gillotin C, Chittick GE, Symonds WT, Lou Y, Sadler BM, Polk RE. Pharmacokinetic interaction between amprenavir and clarithromycin in healthy male volunteers. *Antimicrob Agents Chemother* (2000) 44, 978–84.
4. Mummaneni V, Randall D, Chabuel D, Geraldes M, O'Mara E. Steady-state pharmacokinetic interaction study of atazanavir with clarithromycin in healthy subjects. *Intersci Conf Antimicrob Agents Chemother* (2002) 42, 275.
5. Boruchoff SE, Sturgill MG, Grasing KW, Seibold JR, McCrea J, Winchell GA, Kusma SE, Deutsch PJ. The steady-state disposition of indinavir is not altered by the concomitant administration of clarithromycin. *Clin Pharmacol Ther* (2000) 67, 351–9.
6. Ouellet D, Hsu A, Granneman GR, Carlson G, Cavanaugh J, Guenther H, Leonard JM. Pharmacokinetic interaction between ritonavir and clarithromycin. *Clin Pharmacol Ther* (1998) 64, 355–62.
7. Fortovase (Saquinavir). Roche Products Ltd. UK Summary of product characteristics, January 2005.
8. Grub S, Bryson H, Goggin T, Lüdin E, Jorga K. The interaction of saquinavir (soft gelatin capsule) with ketoconazole, erythromycin and rifampicin: comparison of the effect in healthy volunteers and in HIV-infected patients. *Eur J Clin Pharmacol* (2001) 57, 115–21.
9. Norvir (Ritonavir). Abbott Laboratories Ltd. UK Summary of product characteristics, January 2005.
10. Klaricid (Clarithromycin). Abbott Laboratories Ltd. UK Summary of product characteristics, October 2002.
11. Norvir (Ritonavir). Abbott Laboratories. US Prescribing information, April 2005.
12. Biaxin (Clarithromycin). Abbott Laboratories. US Prescribing information, January 2005.
13. Kaletra Soft Capsules (Lopinavir/ritonavir). Abbott Laboratories Ltd. UK Summary of product characteristics, January 2005.
14. Kaletra (Lopinavir/ritonavir). Abbott Laboratories. US Prescribing information, April 2005.
15. Reyataz (Atazanavir sulfate). Bristol-Myers Squibb Company. US Prescribing information, June 2005.
16. Reyataz Hard Capsules (Atazanavir). Bristol-Myers Squibb Pharmaceuticals Ltd. UK Summary of product characteristics, February 2005.
17. Viracept (Nelfinavir mesilate). Roche Products Ltd. UK Summary of product characteristics, June 2005.
18. Agenerase (Amprenavir). GlaxoSmithKline UK. UK Summary of product characteristics, December 2004.

Protease inhibitors + Mefloquine

Limited data suggest there is no pharmacokinetic interaction between mefloquine and indinavir or nelfinavir. Ritonavir does not alter mefloquine pharmacokinetics, but there is some evidence that mefloquine may decrease ritonavir levels.

Clinical evidence

Two HIV+ patients using HAART, one on **indinavir** 800 mg three times daily, the other on **nelfinavir** 1.25 g twice daily were given mefloquine 250 mg weekly, before a trip to Africa. Mefloquine achieved therapeutic levels, and its half-life was similar to that found in healthy subjects. In addition, no consistent changes in the plasma levels of the protease inhibitors were found.[1]

Ritonavir 200 mg twice daily for one week had no significant effect on the pharmacokinetics of mefloquine in 12 healthy subjects.[2] Conversely, mefloquine (250 mg once daily for 3 days, then 250 mg weekly) significantly reduced the steady-state AUC, and maximum and minimum plasma levels of **ritonavir** 200 mg twice daily, by 31%, 36%, and 43% respectively, but had no effect on the single-dose **ritonavir** pharmacokinetics.[2]

Mechanism

Despite being inhibitors of the cytochrome P450 isoenzyme CYP3A4, the protease inhibitors do not appear to alter mefloquine pharmacokinetics.[1,2] It was suggested that the decrease in ritonavir levels was due to decreased absorption, perhaps due to mefloquine-induced inhibition of bile acid production or induction of P-glycoprotein.[2]

Importance and management

The limited evidence suggests that protease inhibitors do not affect mefloquine pharmacokinetics. The data on the effect of mefloquine on ritonavir are less clear. Until further evidence is available, it may be prudent to closely monitor ritonavir levels/efficacy if mefloquine is required.

1. Schippers EF, Hugen PWH, den Hartigh J, Burger DM, Hoetelmans RMW, Visser LG, Kroon FP. No drug-drug interaction between nelfinavir or indinavir and mefloquine in HIV-1 infected patients. *AIDS* (2000) 14, 2794–5.
2. Khaliq Y, Gallicano K, Tisdale C, Carignan G, Cooper C, McCarthy A. Pharmacokinetic interaction between mefloquine and ritonavir in healthy volunteers. *Br J Clin Pharmacol* (2001) 51, 591–600.

Protease inhibitors + Miscellaneous

Indinavir levels are raised by interleukin-2, but not affected by influenza vaccine or quinidine. Lopinavir/ritonavir and atazanavir/ritonavir are predicted to increase quinidine levels. Nelfinavir does not appear to interact with pancreatic enzyme supplements. In one case report, the combination of ritonavir/saquinavir and fusidic acid raised plasma levels of all three drugs.

Clinical evidence, mechanism, importance and management

(a) Fusidic acid

A 32-year-old HIV+ man was admitted with suspected fusidic acid toxicity after taking fusidic acid 500 mg three times daily for one week, with his usual treatment of **ritonavir** 400 mg twice daily, **saquinavir** 400 mg twice daily and stavudine 40 mg twice daily. His plasma fusidic acid level was found to be twice the expected level, and his **ritonavir** and **saquinavir** levels were also elevated. He improved spontaneously, but 4 days later he returned with jaundice, nausea and vomiting. All medications were stopped, but after 6 days his fusidic acid level was still 1.3 times that expected, his **saquinavir** level was 16.3 micrograms/ml (expected range 1 to 4 micrograms/ml) and his **ritonavir** level was 43.4 micrograms/ml (expected range 4 to 12 micrograms/ml). He was later able to restart his antivirals without problem. It is possible that there was mutual inhibition of drug metabolism. The authors recommend avoiding this drug combination.[1] Further study is needed.

(b) Influenza vaccine

Influenza whole virus vaccine was given to 9 patients on **indinavir** containing HAART. No significant changes were found in **indinavir** pharmacokinetics.[2]

(c) Interleukins

In a pharmacokinetic study in 9 HIV+ patients, the subjects were kept on their usual antiretrovirals and additionally given a 4-week course of **indinavir** 800 mg three times daily followed by infusions of interleukin-2 of 3 to 12 million units daily for 5 days. The AUC of **indinavir** increased in 8 of the 9 subjects (average increase 88%). During this time interleukin-6 was also elevated, so it was thought that the increased **indinavir** concentrations were due to the inhibitory effects of interleukin-6 on the cytochrome P450 isoenzyme CYP3A4. Increased **indinavir** trough levels were also seen in a further 8 patients not participating in the pharmacokinetic study.[3]

(d) Pancreatic enzymes

Combined use of pancreatic enzymes (pancrelipase 20,000 USP units, amylase 65,000 USP units and protease 65,000 USP units) and **nelfinavir** 1.25 g twice daily for 14 days resulted in no significant changes in the pharmacokinetics of **nelfinavir** in 9 HIV+ subjects.[4]

(e) Quinidine

Quinidine sulphate 200 mg was given to 10 healthy subjects, followed 1 hour later by a single 400-mg dose of **indinavir**. Quinidine had no clinically significant effects on the pharmacokinetics of **indinavir**.[5] **Lopinavir/ritonavir** is predicted to increase quinidine levels, and the combination should be closely monitored.[6,7] **Atazanavir/ritonavir** is predicted to increase quinidine levels, and the UK maker contraindicates the combination[8] while the US maker recommends monitoring quinidine concentrations.[9]

1. Khaliq Y, Gallicano K, Leger R, Foster B, Badley A. A drug interaction between fusidic acid and a combination of ritonavir and saquinavir. *Br J Clin Pharmacol* (2000) 50, 82–3.
2. Maserati R, Villani P, Barasolo G, Mongiovetti M, Regazzi MB. Influenza immunization and indinavir pharmacokinetics. *Scand J Infect Dis* (2000) 32, 449–50.
3. Piscitelli SC, Vogel S, Figg WD, Raje S, Forrest A, Metcalf JA, Baseler M, Falloon J. Alteration in indinavir clearance during interleukin-2 infusions in patients infected with the human immunodeficiency virus. *Pharmacotherapy* (1998) 18, 1212–16.
4. Price J, Shalit P, Carlsen J, Becker MI, Frye J, Hsyu P. Pharmacokinetic interaction between Ultrase® MT-20 and nelfinavir in HIV-infected individuals. *Intersci Conf Antimicrob Agents Chemother* (1999) 39, 20.
5. McCrea J, Woolf E, Sterrett A, Matthews C, Deutsch P, Yeh KC, Waldman S, Bjornsson T. Effects of ketoconazole and other P-450 inhibitors on the pharmacokinetics of indinavir. *Pharm Res* (1996) 13 (9 Suppl), S485.
6. Kaletra (Lopinavir/ritonavir). Abbott Laboratories Ltd. UK Summary of product characteristics, January 2005.
7. Kaletra (Lopinavir/ritonavir). Abbott Laboratories. US Prescribing information, April 2005.
8. Reyataz (Atazanavir sulfate). Bristol-Myers Squibb Pharmaceuticals Ltd. UK Summary of product characteristics, February 2005.
9. Reyataz (Atazanavir sulfate). Bristol-Myers Squibb Company. US Prescribing information, June 2005.

Protease inhibitors + Protease inhibitors

Various combinations of protease inhibitors have been tried, or are used, to boost the levels and consequently the efficacy of one of the protease inhibitors. Ritonavir is the most potent at boosting levels of the other protease inhibitors, and is currently used in combination with lopinavir and saquinavir in particular, and also atazanavir. There is no important pharmacokinetic interaction between amprenavir/indinavir, amprenavir/nelfinavir, and amprenavir/saquinavir, and probably also indinavir/nelfinavir. Amprenavir and lopinavir may act to lower the concentrations of each other.

Clinical evidence

(a) Amprenavir + Indinavir

The steady-state AUC of amprenavir was 33% higher when amprenavir 750 or 800 mg three times daily was given with indinavir 800 mg three times daily. In this study, the AUC of indinavir was 38% lower than historical control data.[1] Similarly, amprenavir intrinsic clearance was reduced by 54% by indinavir in a model-based pharmacokinetic analysis of data from a clinical trial.[2] This agrees with *in vitro* data.[3] It was suggested[1] that the effect of amprenavir on indinavir was due to the lipid-like formulation of amprenavir reducing the absorption of indinavir (analogous to 'food', (p.611)). The changes in amprenavir levels were not considered to be clinically relevant.[1] The UK makers say that no dose adjustment of either drug is needed when they are given together.[4]

(b) Amprenavir + Lopinavir/ritonavir

Preliminary data suggest that the combination of amprenavir 600 mg twice daily with lopinavir/ritonavir 400/100 mg twice daily resulted in amprenavir trough plasma levels that were lower than with the combination of amprenavir/ritonavir at the same doses. Similarly the lopinavir levels were lower than those without amprenavir.[5] Others have reported similar findings.[6] Therefore, amprenavir and lopinavir may act to lower the concentrations of each other.

(c) Amprenavir + Nelfinavir

The trough concentration of amprenavir was increased by 189% when amprenavir 750 or 800 mg three times daily was given with nelfinavir 750 mg three times daily, but the AUC and maximum level were not significantly altered. In this study, the pharmacokinetics of nelfinavir were not altered when compared with historical control data.[1] Amprenavir intrinsic clearance was reduced by about 40% by nelfinavir in a model-based pharmacokinetic analysis of data from a clinical trial,[2] which agrees with *in vitro* data.[3] The increase in amprenavir trough concentration could result in improved antiviral efficacy, but further study is needed.[1] The UK makers say that no dose adjustment of either drug is needed when they are given together.[4,7]

(d) Amprenavir + Ritonavir

The AUC, minimum and maximum levels of amprenavir were increased by 131%, 484% and 33% when amprenavir 1.2 g twice daily was given with ritonavir 200 mg twice daily.[4] This agrees with *in vitro* data.[3] The maker recommends that doses of both protease inhibitors be reduced when they are used together.[4,8] Based on modelling of pharmacokinetic data, a dose of amprenavir 600 mg with ritonavir 100 mg, both twice daily, has been suggested.[9] This combination has shown good clinical efficacy in at least one study,[10] and resulted in satisfactory amprenavir levels when efavirenz was also used[11] (see also 'NNRTIs + Protease inhibitors', p.588).

(e) Amprenavir + Saquinavir

The steady-state AUC of amprenavir was reduced by 32% when amprenavir 750 or 800 mg three times daily was given with saquinavir (soft gel capsule) 800 mg three times daily, and the maximum plasma level was reduced by 37%. In this study, the pharmacokinetics of saquinavir were not changed when compared with historical control data.[1] Conversely, amprenavir intrinsic clearance was not altered by saquinavir in a model-based pharmacokinetic analysis of data from a clinical trial,[2] which agrees with *in vitro* data.[3] It was suggested that, since amprenavir was given with food in the first study, and 'food', (p.611) modestly reduces amprenavir levels, this may have accounted for the reduced amprenavir levels.[1] The UK makers say that no dose adjustment of either drug is needed when they are given together.[4]

(f) Atazanavir + Ritonavir

The addition of ritonavir 100 mg to atazanavir 300 mg increased the AUC of atazanavir about twofold, and the trough plasma level sevenfold, in healthy subjects. The effect on the trough level was less marked in patients (about a threefold increase).[12] The maker of atazanavir recommends that it is given with ritonavir when used in patients who have already received antiretroviral treatment.[12,13]

(g) Indinavir + Lopinavir/ritonavir

The pharmacokinetics of a single 600-mg dose of indinavir after 10 days of lopinavir/ritonavir 400/100 mg twice daily in healthy subjects were compared with historical data in HIV-infected patients. Based on this comparison, it was suggested that lopinavir/ritonavir 400/100 mg twice daily given with indinavir 600 mg twice daily may produce a similar indinavir AUC and a higher trough concentration to indinavir 800 mg three times daily alone.[14,15]

(h) Indinavir + Nelfinavir

The combination of indinavir 1.2 g every 12 hours with nelfinavir 1.25 g every 12 hours produced plasma levels that were equivalent to the standard dose of indinavir 800 mg every 8 hours in HIV+ subjects. This suggests that nelfinavir only modestly inhibits indinavir metabolism. In this multiple-dose study, indinavir did not affect the pharmacokinetics of nelfinavir.[16] In contrast, a 750-mg single dose of nelfinavir, given after indinavir 800 mg every 8 hours for 7 days resulted in an 83% increase in nelfinavir AUC and a 22% increase in elimination half-life.[7]

(i) Indinavir + Ritonavir

The effects of a range of doses of ritonavir (200, 300, or 400 mg every 12 hours) on indinavir pharmacokinetics were assessed in 39 healthy subjects. The AUC of indinavir 400 or 600 mg was increased two- to fivefold by the ritonavir. It is suggested that the combination of indinavir 400 mg every 12 hours with ritonavir 400 mg every 12 hours will result in an AUC of indinavir roughly equivalent to that of indinavir 800 mg every 8 hours, without any effect on the pharmacokinetics of ritonavir.[17] In another similar study, when compared with historical data for indinavir 800 mg every 8 hours, the AUC of indinavir was at least 1.4, 2.3, and 3.3 times higher when given indinavir/ritonavir in twice daily doses of 400/400 mg, 800/100 mg, and 800/200 mg, respectively. The regimens also produced markedly higher trough indinavir levels. The 800/100 mg regimen was the best tolerated. Thus the optimum combination was suggested to be indinavir 800 mg twice daily with ritonavir 100 mg or 200 mg twice daily.[18] The same indinavir/ritonavir 800/100 mg twice daily regimen was similarly suggested by the authors of another study.[19] The maker of indinavir notes that caution is needed when indinavir is used at a dose of 800 mg twice daily with ritonavir, because of the possibility of an increased risk of nephrolithiasis. They strongly recommend appropriate hydration.[20]

(j) Indinavir + Saquinavir

In a single-dose study, the concurrent use of indinavir and saquinavir 600 mg (hard capsule) or 800 mg or 1200 mg (soft capsule) increased the AUC of saquinavir by 500%, 620% and 360%, respectively.[20] This is supported by *in vitro* data.[21] However, in another *in vitro* study of antiviral activity, the combination of saquinavir and indinavir was antagonistic.[22] Further study is needed.

(k) Lopinavir/ritonavir + Ritonavir

Ritonavir is used to increase the plasma levels of lopinavir. The marketed dose combination is lopinavir/ritonavir 400/100 mg twice daily.[14] When an additional 100 mg of ritonavir twice daily was added to the marketed combination, the AUC of lopinavir increased by 33% and the trough concentration by 64%.[14]

(l) Lopinavir/ritonavir + Saquinavir

The pharmacokinetics of a single 800-mg dose of saquinavir (soft capsule), after 10 days of lopinavir/ritonavir 400/100 mg twice daily in healthy subjects, were compared with historical data in HIV-infected patients. Based on this comparison, it was suggested that lopinavir/ritonavir 400/100 mg twice daily given with saquinavir 800 mg twice daily may produce a similar saquinavir AUC and a higher saquinavir trough concentration to those of saquinavir 1.2 g given three times daily alone.[14,15]

(m) Nelfinavir + Ritonavir

Single-dose data indicate that ritonavir increases the AUC of nelfinavir by 1.8 to 2.5-fold, whereas the AUC of ritonavir is unchanged.[23] In a multiple-dose study in healthy subjects, ritonavir 100 or 200 mg twice daily increased the steady-state AUC of nelfinavir 1.25 g twice daily by 20 and 39%, after morning and evening doses respectively. The AUC of the nelfinavir metabolite (M8) was increased by 74% and 86% respectively. There was no difference in the effect of the two doses of ritonavir on nelfinavir AUC.[24]

(n) Nelfinavir + Saquinavir

A single 1.2 g dose of saquinavir (soft gel capsules), given after 3 days of nelfinavir 750 mg every 8 hours had no effect on the pharmacokinetics of nelfinavir, but the nelfinavir caused a fourfold increase in the AUC of saquinavir.[25] Similar two- to twelvefold increases have been found in other studies in HIV+ subjects.[26-29] A study in which 157 patients received 12 weeks of combined saquinavir/nelfinavir treatment [doses unstated] found that the combination was well tolerated.[30] It appears that nelfinavir inhibits the hepatic clearance of saquinavir.[31]

(o) Ritonavir + Saquinavir

A study in 6 patients with advanced HIV disease found that while taking saquinavir 600 mg three times daily the addition of ritonavir 300 mg twice daily increased the maximum saquinavir plasma levels 33-fold, and increased the AUC 58-fold at steady state.[32] A pilot study in HIV+ patients given both drugs together (saquinavir 800 mg daily, ritonavir 400 to 600 mg daily) found that the ritonavir serum levels were unaffected. However, the saquinavir levels were substantially higher than those achieved with saquinavir alone in daily doses of 3.6 to 7.2 g.[33] A study of a range of ritonavir and saquinavir *(Invirase)* doses (200 to 600 mg) in 57 healthy subjects found that saquinavir did not affect ritonavir pharmacokinetics, but ritonavir increased the AUC of saquinavir 50 to 132-fold. The authors suggested that giving both drugs in the dosage 400 mg every 12 hours might be optimal.[34] Subsequent study has revealed that the effect of ritonavir on saquinavir is not related to the ritonavir dose in the range of 100 to 400 mg twice daily,[35-37] and that the use of a combination with a higher dose of saquinavir and a lower dose of ritonavir may be preferable, as the lower doses of ritonavir are associated with fewer adverse effects.[37] A dose of saquinavir 1 g twice daily with ritonavir 100 mg twice daily is currently suggested by the maker of saquinavir.[38-41]

Mechanism

Protease inhibitors are inhibitors and substrates of the cytochrome P450 isoenzyme CYP3A4, with ritonavir being the most potent inhibitor and saquinavir the least (see 'Antivirals', (p.578)). They probably interact by competitively inhibiting each other's gut (preabsorption) and hepatic (postabsorption) metabolism, so resulting in increased absorption and decreased elimination.[31,34] A mechanism involving inhibition of P-glycoprotein may also be involved.[31]

Importance and management

Ritonavir inhibits the metabolism of amprenavir, atazanavir, indinavir, lopinavir, nelfinavir, and especially saquinavir. Ritonavir is therefore used in combination with other protease inhibitors to boost their levels, and allow a reduction in the protease inhibitor dose and the frequency of dosing, or to allow combination with antiretrovirals that induce CYP3A4 (e.g. nevirapine, see 'NNRTIs + Protease inhibitors', p.588). The combinations of lopinavir/ritonavir and saquinavir/ritonavir are currently the most established. Atazanavir is also used with ritonavir. There appears to be no clinically important pharmacokinetic interactions between amprenavir/indinavir, amprenavir/nelfinavir, amprenavir/saquinavir and, probably also indinavir/nelfinavir. Preliminary data suggest amprenavir and lopinavir may interact to reduce the levels of each other. The pharmacokinetic interactions and dose recommendations of the protease inhibitor combinations are summarised in 'Table 19.4', (below). When considering appropriate protease inhibitor combinations, in addition to pharmacokinetic interactions, cross resistance patterns and adverse effects should also be considered.[42]

1. Sadler BM, Gillotin C, Lou Y, Eron JJ, Lang W, Haubrich R, Stein DS. Pharmacokinetic study of human immunodeficiency virus protease inhibitors used in combination with amprenavir. *Antimicrob Agents Chemother* (2001) 45, 3663–8.
2. Pfister M, Labbé L, Lu J-F, Hammer SM, Mellors J, Bennett KK, Rosenkranz S, Sheiner LB, and the AIDS Clinical Trial Group Protocol 398 Investigators. Effect of coadministration of nelfinavir, indinavir, and saquinavir on the pharmacokinetics of amprenavir. *Clin Pharmacol Ther* (2002) 72, 133–41.
3. Decker CJ, Laitinen LM, Bridson GW, Raybuck SA, Tung RD, Chaturvedi PR. Metabolism of amprenavir in liver microsomes: role of CYP3A4 inhibition for drug interactions. *J Pharm Sci* (1998) 87, 803–7.
4. Agenerase (Amprenavir). GlaxoSmithKline UK. UK Summary of product characteristics, December 2004.
5. Mauss S, Schmutz G, Kuschak D. Unfavourable interaction of amprenavir and lopinavir in combination with ritonavir? *AIDS* (2002) 16, 296–7.
6. Khanlou H, Graham E, Brill M, Farthing C. Drug interaction between amprenavir and lopinavir/ritonavir in salvage therapy. *AIDS* (2002) 16, 797–8.
7. Viracept (Nelfinavir mesilate). Roche Products Ltd. UK Summary of product characteristics, June 2005.
8. Agenerase (Amprenavir). GlaxoSmithKline. US Prescribing information, May 2005.
9. Sale M, Sadler BM, Stein DS. Pharmacokinetic modeling and simulations of interaction of amprenavir and ritonavir. *Antimicrob Agents Chemother* (2002) 46, 746–54.
10. Duval X, Lamotte C, Race E, Descamps D, Damond F, Clavel F, Leport C, Peytavin G, Vilde J-L. Amprenavir inhibitory quotient and virological response in human immunodeficiency virus-infected patients on an amprenavir-containing salvage regimen without or with ritonavir. *Antimicrob Agents Chemother* (2002) 46, 570–4.
11. Goujard C, Vincent I, Meynard J-L, Choudet N, Bollens D, Rousseau C, Demarles D, Gillotin C, Bidault R, Taburet A-M. Steady-state pharmacokinetics of amprenavir coadministered with ritonavir in human immunodeficiency virus type 1-infected patients. *Antimicrob Agents Chemother* (2003) 47, 118–23.
12. Reyataz Hard Capsules (Atazanavir). Bristol-Myers Squibb Pharmaceuticals Ltd. UK Summary of product characteristics, February 2005.
13. Reyataz (Atazanavir sulfate). Bristol-Myers Squibb Company. US Prescribing information, June 2005.
14. Kaletra (Lopinavir/ritonavir). Abbott Laboratories Ltd. UK Summary of product characteristics, January 2005.
15. Abbott Laboratories Ltd. Personal communication, August 2001.
16. Riddler SA, Havlir D, Squires KE, Kerr B, Lewis RH, Yeh K, Hawe Wynne L, Zhong L, Peng Y, Deutsch P, Saah A. Coadministration of indinavir and nelfinavir in human immunodeficiency virus type 1-infected adults: safety, pharmacokinetics, and antiretroviral activity. *Antimicrob Agents Chemother* (2002) 46, 3877–82.
17. Hsu A, Granneman GR, Cao G, Carothers L, Japour A, El-Shourbagy T, Dennis S, Berg J, Erdman K, Leonard JM, Sun E. Pharmacokinetic interaction between ritonavir and indinavir in healthy volunteers. *Antimicrob Agents Chemother* (1998) 42, 2784–91.
18. Saah AJ, Winchell GA, Nessly ML, Seniuk MA, Rhodes RR, Deutsch PJ. Pharmacokinetic profile and tolerability of indinavir-ritonavir combinations in healthy volunteers. *Antimicrob Agents Chemother* (2001) 45, 2710–15.
19. van Heeswijk RP, Veldkamp AI, Hoetelmans RM, Mulder JW, Schreij G, Hsu A, Lange JM, Beijnen JH, Meenhorst PL. The steady-state plasma pharmacokinetics of indinavir alone and in combination with a low dose of ritonavir in twice daily dosing regimens in HIV-1-infected individuals. *AIDS* (1999) 13, F95–9.
20. Crixivan (Indinavir sulfate). Merck Sharp & Dohme Ltd. UK Summary of product characteristics, January 2005.
21. Fitzsimmons ME, Collins JM. Selective biotransformation of the human immunodeficiency virus protease inhibitor saquinavir by human small-intestinal cytochrome P4503A4: Potential contribution to high first-pass metabolism. *Drug Metab Dispos* (1997) 25, 256–66.
22. Merrill DP, Manion DJ, Chou T-C, Hirsch MS. Antagonism between human immunodeficiency virus type 1 protease inhibitors indinavir and saquinavir in vitro. *J Infect Dis* (1997) 176, 265–8.
23. Washington CB, Flexner C, Sheiner LB, Rosenkranz SL, Segal Y, Aberg JA, Blaschke TF, AIDS Clinical Trials Group Protocol (ACTG 378) study team. *Clin Pharmacol Ther* (2003) 73, 406–16.
24. Kurowski M, Kaeser B, Sawyer A, Popescu M, Mrozikiewicz A. Low-dose ritonavir moderately enhances nelfinavir exposure. *Clin Pharmacol Ther* (2002) 72, 123–32.
25. Kerr B, Yuep G, Daniels R, Quart B, Kravcik S, Sahai J, Anderson R. Strategic approach to nelfinavir mesylate (NFV) drug interactions involving CYP3A metabolism. 6th European Conference on Clinical Aspects and Treatment of HIV-infection, Hamburg, Germany, 1997. Abstract.
26. Merry C, Ryan M, Mulchay F, Halifax K, Barry M, Back D. The effect of nelfinavir on plasma saquinavir levels. 6th European Conference on Clinical Aspects and Treatment of HIV-infection, Hamburg, Germany, 1997. Abstract 455.
27. Merry C, Barry MG, Mulcahy FM, Back DJ. Saquinavir pharmacokinetics alone and in combination with nelfinavir in HIV infected patients. 5th Conference on Retroviruses and Opportunistic Infections, Chicago, 1998. Abstract 352.
28. Gallicano K, Sahai J, Kravcik S, Seguin I, Bristow N, Cameron DW. Nelfinavir (NFV) increases plasma exposure of saquinavir in hard gel capsule (SQV-HGC) in HIV+ patients. 5th Conference on Retroviruses and Opportunistic Infections, Chicago, 1998. Abstract 353.
29. Hoetelmans RMW, Reijers MHE, Wit FW, ten Kate RW, Weige HM, Frissen PHJ, Bruisten SM, Beijnen JH, Lange JMA. Saquinavir (SQV) pharmacokinetics in combination with nelfinavir (NFV) in the ADAM study. 6th European Conference on Clinical Aspects and Treatment of HIV-infection, Hamburg, Germany, 1997. Abstract 255.
30. Posniak A and the SPICE study team. Study of protease inhibitors in combination in Europe (SPICE). 6th European Conference on Clinical Aspects and Treatment of HIV-infection, Hamburg, Germany, 1997. Abstract 209.
31. Lu J-F, Blaschke TF, Flexner C, Rosenkranz SL, Sheiner LB, and AIDS Clinical Trials Group protocol 378 investigators. Model-based analysis of the pharmacokinetic interactions between ritonavir, nelfinavir, and saquinavir after simultaneous and staggered oral administration. *Drug Metab Dispos* (2002) 30, 1455–61.

Table 19.4 Summary of the pharmacokinetic interactions and makers' dosage recommendations (unless stated otherwise) for combined use of protease inhibitors

Interacting protease inhibitor	*Affected protease inhibitor with recommended dose adjustment*					
	Amprenavir	*Indinavir*	*Lopinavir/ritonavir*	*Nelfinavir*	*Ritonavir*	*Saquinavir*
Amprenavir		Minor AUC decrease No dose change	Lopinavir minimum levels decreased	Pharmacokinetics unaltered No dose change	Pharmacokinetics unaltered 100 mg twice daily	Pharmacokinetics unaltered No dose change
Indinavir	Minor AUC decrease No dose change		(No dose change)[a]	Pharmacokinetics unaltered[b]	No important pharmacokinetic changes 100 or 200 mg twice daily[c]	AUC increased
Lopinavir/ritonavir	Minimum levels decreased	AUC increased (600 mg twice daily)[a]				AUC increased (800 mg twice daily)[a]
Nelfinavir	Minimum levels increased No dose change	Minor AUC increase[b]			Pharmacokinetics unaltered	AUC increased
Ritonavir	AUC increased 600 mg twice daily	AUC increased (800 mg twice daily)[d]	Minor AUC increase	Modest AUC increase[b]		AUC markedly increased 1000 mg twice daily
Saquinavir	Pharmacokinetics unaltered No dose change		(No dose change)[a]	Pharmacokinetics unaltered	Pharmacokinetics unaltered 100 mg twice daily[e]	

[a] Dose is a suggestion only, based on limited pharmacokinetic evidence.
[b] Multiple-dose study (single-dose study showed greater effect).
[c] As suggested by Saah AJ, Winchell GA, Nessly ML, Seniuk MA, Rhodes RR, Deutsch PJ. Pharmacokinetic profile and tolerability of indinavir-ritonavir combinations in healthy volunteers. *Antimicrob Agents Chemother* (2001) 45, 2710–15.
[d] Appropriate hydration needed because of the possibility of an increased risk of nephrolithiasis.
[e] As a pharmacokinetic booster.

32. Merry C, Barry MG, Mulcahy F, Ryan M, Heavey J, Tjia JF, Gibbons SE, Breckenridge AM, Back DJ. Saquinavir pharmacokinetics alone and in combination with ritonavir in HIV-infected patients. *AIDS* (1997) 11, F29–F33.
33. Cameron DW, Hsu A, Granneman GR, Sun E, McMahon D, Farthing C, Poretz D, Markowitz M, Cohen C, Follansbee S, Mellors J, Ho D, Xu Y, Rode R, Salgo M, Leonard J. Pharmacokinetics of ritonavir-saquinavir combination therapy. *AIDS* (1996) 10 (Suppl 2), S16.
34. Hsu A, Granneman GR, Cao G, Carothers L, El-Shourbagy T, Baroldi P, Erdman K, Brown F, Sun E, Leonard JM. Pharmacokinetic interactions between two human immunodeficiency virus protease inhibitors, ritonavir and saquinavir. *Clin Pharmacol Ther* (1998) 63, 453–64.
35. Kilby JM, Hill A, Buss N. The effect of ritonavir on saquinavir plasma concentration is independent of ritonavir dosage: combined analysis of pharmacokinetic data from 97 subjects. *HIV Med* (2002) 3, 97–104.
36. Kurowski M, Arslan A, Moecklinghoff C, Sawyer W, Hill A. Effects of ritonavir on saquinavir plasma concentration: analysis of 271 patients in routine clinical practice (P261A). *AIDS* (2000) 14 (Suppl 4), 591.
37. Buss N, Snell P, Bock J, Hsu A, Jorga K. Saquinavir and ritonavir pharmacokinetics following combined ritonavir and saquinavir (soft gelatin capsules) administration. *Br J Clin Pharmacol* (2001) 52, 255–64.
38. Fortovase (Saquinavir). Roche Products Ltd. UK Summary of product characteristics, January 2005.
39. Invirase (Saquinavir mesilate). Roche Products Ltd. UK Summary of product characteristics, June 2005.
40. Fortovase (Saquinavir). Roche Pharmaceuticals. US Prescribing information, December 2003.
41. Invirase (Saquinavir mesilate). Roche Pharmaceuticals. US Prescribing information, December 2004.
42. Norvir (Ritonavir). Abbott Laboratories Ltd. UK Summary of product characteristics, January 2005.

Protease inhibitors + Rifamycins

Rifabutin bioavailability is increased by amprenavir, atazanavir, indinavir, nelfinavir and, especially, ritonavir, with an increased risk of toxicity. Rifabutin decreases the bioavailability of indinavir, nelfinavir and, particularly, saquinavir (with an increased risk of therapeutic failure) but has no effect on amprenavir and atazanavir. The combination of rifabutin with protease inhibitors may be used, but dosage adjustments of rifabutin or both drugs are often necessary, see 'Table 19.5', (below).

Rifampicin (rifampin) bioavailability is increased by indinavir, but amprenavir has no effect. Rifampicin markedly reduces the bioavailability of amprenavir, indinavir, lopinavir, nelfinavir and saquinavir. Consequently, the use of many of the protease inhibitors with rifampicin is contraindicated, although dual protease inhibitor therapy e.g. with ritonavir and saquinavir may make concurrent use possible.

Table 19.5 Summary of the recommendations for the use of protease inhibitors with rifamycins

Protease inhibitor	*Rifabutin*	*Rifampicin*	*Refs*
Protease inhibitors			
Amprenavir	Rifabutin dose at least halved Amprenavir dose unchanged	Not recommended (amprenavir levels markedly reduced)	1
Indinavir	Rifabutin dose reduced by 50% Indinavir dose increased (1 to 1.2 g every 8 hours)	Not recommended (indinavir levels markedly reduced, rifampicin levels raised)	2, 3, 4
Nelfinavir	Rifabutin dose at least halved Nelfinavir dose unchanged or increased to 1 g tid	Not recommended (nelfinavir levels markedly reduced)	5, 6
Ritonavir alone	Rifabutin dose should be substantially reduced (by at least 75%)†	May be used at usual doses, although limited data (ritonavir levels reduced)	6
Saquinavir alone	Not recommended (saquinavir levels reduced)	Not recommended (saquinavir levels markedly reduced)	7
Ritonavir boosted protease inhibitors			
Atazanavir/ritonavir	Rifabutin dose reduced by up to 75% (150 mg every other day or three times per week) Atazanavir/ritonavir dose unchanged	Not recommended (atazanavir levels predicted to be markedly reduced)	8
Lopinavir/ritonavir	Rifabutin dose reduced by at least 75% Lopinavir/ritonavir dose unchanged	Not recommended (lopinavir levels markedly reduced)	9, 10
Saquinavir/ritonavir	Rifabutin dose at least halved	Rifampicin dose unchanged	6

† Formerly considered contraindicated (rifabutin levels markedly increased with risk of toxicity)

1. Hsu A, Granneman GR, Cao G, Carothers L, Japour A, El-Shourbagy T, Dennis S, Berg J, Erdman K, Leonard JM, Sun E. Pharmacokinetic interaction between ritonavir and indinavir in healthy volunteers. *Antimicrob Agents Chemother* (1998) 42, 2784–91.
2. Fitzsimmons ME, Collins JM. Selective biotransformation of the human immunodeficiency virus protease inhibitor saquinavir by human small-intestinal cytochrome P4503A4: Potential contribution to high first-pass metabolism. *Drug Metab Dispos* (1997) 25, 256–66.
3. Riddler SA, Havlir D, Squires KE, Kerr B, Lewis RH, Yeh K, Hawe Wynne L, Zhong L, Peng Y, Deutsch P, Saah A. Coadministration of indinavir and nelfinavir in human immunodeficiency virus type 1-infected adults: safety, pharmacokinetics, and antiretroviral activity. *Antimicrob Agents Chemother* (2002) 46, 3877–82.
4. Kerr B, Yuep G, Daniels R, Quart B, Kravcik S, Sahai J, Anderson R. Strategic approach to nelfinavir mesylate (NFV) drug interactions involving CYP3A metabolism. 6th European Conference on Clinical Aspects and Treatment of HIV-infection, Hamburg, Germany, 1997. Abstract.
5. Hoetelmans RMW, Reijers MHE, Wit FW, ten Kate RW, Weige HM, Frissen PHJ, Bruisten SM, Beijnen JH, Lange JMA. Saquinavir (SQV) pharmacokinetics in combination with nelfinavir (NFV) in the ADAM study. 6th European Conference on Clinical Aspects and Treatment of HIV-infection, Hamburg, Germany, 1997. Abstract 255.
6. Merry C, Barry MG, Mulcahy F, Ryan M, Heavey J, Tjia JF, Gibbons SE, Breckenridge AM, Back DJ. Saquinavir pharmacokinetics alone and in combination with ritonavir in HIV-infected patients. *AIDS* (1997) 11, F29–F33.
7. Pfister M, Labbé L, Lu J-F, Hammer SM, Mellors J, Bennett KK, Rosenkranz S, Sheiner LB, and the AIDS Clinical Trial Group Protocol 398 Investigators. Effect of coadministration of nelfinavir, indinavir, and saquinavir on the pharmacokinetics of amprenavir. *Clin Pharmacol Ther* (2002) 72, 133–41.
8. Crixivan (Indinavir sulfate). Merck Sharp & Dohme Ltd. UK Summary of product characteristics, January 2005.
9. Saah AJ, Winchell GA, Nessly ML, Seniuk MA, Rhodes RR, Deutsch PJ. Pharmacokinetic profile and tolerability of indinavir-ritonavir combinations in healthy volunteers. *Antimicrob Agents Chemother* (2001) 45, 2710–15.
10. van Heeswijk RP, Veldkamp AI, Hoetelmans RM, Mulder JW, Schreij G, Hsu A, Lange JM, Beijnen JH, Meenhorst PL. The steady-state plasma pharmacokinetics of indinavir alone and in combination with a low dose of ritonavir in twice daily dosing regimens in HIV-1-infected individuals. *AIDS* (1999) 13, F95–9.

Clinical evidence

(a) Amprenavir

Amprenavir 1200 mg twice daily was given with **rifabutin** 300 mg daily or **rifampicin** (**rifampin**) 600 mg daily, to two groups of 11 healthy subjects for 10 and 4 days respectively. Amprenavir caused an almost threefold increase in the AUC of **rifabutin**, but the **rifabutin** did not significantly affect the pharmacokinetics of amprenavir. The combination was poorly tolerated, with 5 of 11 subjects stopping treatment between days one and 9 due to adverse events.[1] In the **rifampicin** group, the effects were reversed; amprenavir did not affect the pharmacokinetics of **rifampicin**, but **rifampicin** caused the amprenavir AUC to drop by 82%. The maximum plasma levels were also significantly affected, dropping by 70% from 9.2 to 2.78 micrograms/ml when **rifampicin** was added.[1]

(b) Atazanavir

The maker notes that atazanavir 400 mg daily given with **rifabutin** 150 mg once daily for 14 days did not have any important effect on the AUC of atazanavir. However, the AUC for **rifabutin** 150 mg was 2.3-fold higher than historical data for a standard 300-mg dose.[2]

(c) Indinavir

A study in 11 AIDS patients given indinavir 800 mg every 8 hours and **rifampicin** 600 mg daily for 14 days found that the AUC of **rifampicin** was increased by 73% by indinavir.[3] In a similar study looking at the effects of the **rifampicin** on indinavir, the indinavir AUC and maximum serum levels were decreased by 92 and 86% respectively.[4]

When **rifabutin** 300 mg was given with **indinavir** 800 mg every 8 hours to 10 healthy subjects for 10 days, the indinavir maximum serum levels and AUC were reduced by about a third, whereas the **rifabutin** maximum serum levels and AUC were increased two- to threefold.[5,6] In another study, the pharmacokinetics of the combined use of an increased dose of indinavir (1 g every 8 hours) and a 50% reduction in **rifabutin** dose (150 mg daily) was investigated in healthy and HIV+ subjects. The indinavir AUC was the same with this increased dose as with indinavir 800 mg every 8 hours alone. However, despite the halving of **rifabutin** dose, the AUC was still up to 70% higher than with the 300-mg dose alone.[7] When the combination was used in practice, there were no treatment failures in 25 patients being treated with **rifabutin** while on HAART (containing indinavir and/or nelfinavir). The **rifabutin** was given as 300 mg twice weekly and the indinavir dose was increased from 800 to 1200 mg every 8 hours to achieve satisfactory levels.[8]

(d) Nelfinavir

Rifampicin 600 mg daily for 7 days decreased the AUC of **nelfinavir** 750 mg every 8 hours for 6 days by 82%.[9]

In an associated study in which **rifabutin** 300 mg daily for 8 days was given with nelfinavir 750 mg every 8 hours for 7 to 8 days, the nelfinavir AUC was reduced by 32% and the **rifabutin** AUC was increased by 207%.[9] When nelfinavir 750 mg every 8 hours was given with half the dose of **rifabutin** (150 mg daily), the nelfinavir AUC was reduced by a similar amount (23%), whereas the **rifabutin** AUC was increased by a lower amount (83%).[10]

(e) Ritonavir

In a study where ritonavir 500 mg twice daily was given with **rifabutin** 150 mg daily to 5 healthy subjects for 8 days, the maximum serum level of **rifabutin** was increased threefold and the AUC was increased fourfold (and the AUC of its active metabolite, 25-*O*-desacetylrifabutin, 35-fold). Seven subjects had to be withdrawn due to adverse events, primarily leucopenia.[11] Retrospective analysis of regimens containing ritonavir found that concurrent use of **rifabutin** was associated with a higher incidence of **rifabutin**-related adverse effects including arthralgia, joint stiffness, uveitis and leucopenia.[12]

When ritonavir 500 mg every 12 hours was given concurrently with **rifampicin** 300 or 600 mg daily for 10 days, the AUC of ritonavir was 35% lower and the maximum level 25% lower than in subjects receiving ritonavir alone.[13]

(f) Ritonavir combined with other protease inhibitors

(i) Lopinavir. Lopinavir/ritonavir 400/100 mg twice daily increased the AUC of **rifabutin** 150 or 300 mg daily threefold when both drugs were given to healthy subjects for 10 days. The AUC of lopinavir was increased by 17%.[14] **Rifampicin** 600 mg daily decreased the AUC of lopinavir (given as lopinavir/ritonavir 400/100 mg twice daily) by 75% when given together to healthy subjects for 10 days.[14]

(ii) Nelfinavir. A 7-month-old infant with HIV and tuberculosis was started on **rifampicin**-based antituberculosis therapy and HAART therapy containing nelfinavir. Nelfinavir plasma levels were found to be very low, so ritonavir was added. This improved nelfinavir levels, and also greatly increased those of the principal active metabolite of nelfinavir. The regimen was well tolerated and had good clinical response.[15]

(iii) Saquinavir. It was suggested that the combination of ritonavir and saquinavir (both 400 mg twice daily) could cancel out the effects of **rifampicin** on saquinavir, so therapeutic levels of all three drugs could be achieved. This assumption was confirmed in 2 HIV+ subjects.[16] Similarly, combined use of ritonavir and saquinavir (hard capsules), both 400 mg twice daily, with intermittent **rifabutin** dosing (300 mg weekly or 150 mg every 3 days) for 8 weeks was reported to be safe and manageable. **Rifabutin** did not significantly alter the protease inhibitor levels, and the **rifabutin** pharmacokinetics were similar to those usually seen with **rifabutin** 300 mg daily alone.[17] However, in one analysis, the use of **rifabutin** 150 mg twice weekly with low-dose ritonavir and a second protease inhibitor was associated with low rifabutin levels, leading to the suggestion that higher doses of **rifabutin** may be necessary with low-dose ritonavir containing HAART.[18]

(g) Saquinavir

The AUC of saquinavir 600 mg three times daily was reduced by about 40% by **rifabutin** 300 mg daily, in 12 HIV+ subjects.[19] Similarly, the AUC of saquinavir (soft capsules) 1.2 g three times daily was decreased by 47% by **rifabutin** 300 mg once daily in 14 HIV+ patients. In addition, the **rifabutin** AUC was increased by 44%.[20] **Rifampicin** 600 mg once daily decreased the AUC of saquinavir (soft capsules) 1.2 g three times daily by 70%.[21]

Mechanism

Rifampicin is a potent inducer of the cytochrome P450 isoenzyme CYP3A4, by which the protease inhibitors are at least partially metabolised, and therefore markedly reduces protease inhibitor levels. Rifabutin is a moderate inducer of CYP3A4. The protease inhibitors are inhibitors of CYP3A4, with ritonavir being the most potent, and can therefore increase the levels of the rifamycins.

Importance and management

Established interactions of clinical importance. The protease inhibitors increase the levels of rifabutin, with a consequent increase in adverse effects unless the rifabutin dose is reduced. Ritonavir is the most potent protease inhibitor in this regard, and the combination has been considered contraindicated. However, the Centers for Disease Control and Prevention[22] now say that it may be used if the dose of rifabutin is markedly reduced. In addition, rifabutin decreases the levels of some protease inhibitors, particularly saquinavir, increasing the risk of treatment failure. Rifabutin should not be used when saquinavir is the sole protease inhibitor. However, there is some evidence that rifabutin can be used with ritonavir-boosted saquinavir. 'Table 19.5', (p.617) summarises the clinical recommendations for the concurrent use of protease inhibitors and rifabutin. Therapy should be well monitored.

Rifampicin markedly reduces the levels of many of the protease inhibitors, and the combinations are generally not recommended, because of the risk of reduced antiviral efficacy and emergence of resistant viral strains. However, there are limited data that ritonavir as sole protease inhibitor, or ritonavir used as a pharmacokinetic enhancer with other protease inhibitors such as saquinavir, can be used with rifampicin.[22] Thus, for the treatment of active tuberculosis in patients with HIV, rifampicin-based regimens (preferred treatment) can possibly be used with antiretroviral regimens including ritonavir.[22]

1. Polk RE, Brophy DF, Israel DS, Patron R, Sadler BM, Chittick GE, Symonds WT, Lou Y, Kristoff D, Stein DS. Pharmacokinetic interaction between amprenavir and rifabutin or rifampin in healthy males. *Antimicrob Agents Chemother* (2001) 45, 502–508.
2. Reyataz Hard Capsules (Atazanavir). Bristol-Myers Squibb Pharmaceuticals Ltd. UK Summary of product characteristics, February 2005.

3. Jaruratanasirikul S, Sriwiriyajan S. Pharmacokinetics of rifampicin administered alone and with indinavir. *J Antimicrob Chemother* (1999) 44 (Suppl A), 58.
4. McCrea J, Wyss D, Stone J, Carides A, Kusma S, Kleinbloesem C, Al-Hamdan Y, Yeh K, Deutsch P. Pharmacokinetic interaction between indinavir and rifampin. *Clin Pharmacol Ther* (1997) 61, 152.
5. Winchell GA, McCrea JB, Carides A, Kusma SE, Chiou R, Deutsch P, Yeh KC, Waldman S, Bjornsson TD. Pharmacokinetic interaction between indinavir and rifabutin. *Clin Pharmacol Ther* (1997) 61, 153.
6. The indinavir (MK 639) pharmacokinetic study group. Indinavir (MK 639) drug interaction studies. 11th International Conference on AIDS, Vancouver, 1996. Abstract Mo.B.174.
7. Hamzeh FM, Benson C, Gerber J, Currier J, McCrea J, Deutsch P, Ruan P, Wu H, Lee J, Flexner C, for the AIDS Clinical Trials Group 365 Study Team. Steady-state pharmacokinetic interaction of modified-dose indinavir and rifabutin. *Clin Pharmacol Ther* (2003) 73, 159–69.
8. Narita M, Stambaugh JJ, Hollender ES, Jones D, Pitchenik AE, Ashkin D. Use of rifabutin with protease inhibitors for human immunodeficiency virus-infected patients with tuberculosis. *Clin Infect Dis* (2000) 30, 779–83. Erratum. *ibid,* 992.
9. Kerr B, Yuep G, Daniels R, Quart B, Kravcik S, Sahai J, Anderson R. Strategic approach to nelfinavir mesylate (NFV) drug interactions involving CYP3A metabolism. 6th European Conference on Clinical Aspects and Treatment of HIV-infection, Hamburg, 1997, 256.
10. Viracept (Nelfinavir mesilate). Roche Products Ltd. UK Summary of product characteristics, June 2005.
11. Cato A, Cavanaugh J, Shi H, Hsu A, Leonard J, Granneman R. The effect of multiple doses of ritonavir on the pharmacokinetics of rifabutin. *Clin Pharmacol Ther* (1998) 63, 414–21.
12. Sun E, Heath-Chiozzi M, Cameron DW, Hsu A, Granneman RG, Maurath CJ, Leonard JM. Concurrent ritonavir and rifabutin increases risk of rifabutin-associated adverse events (Mo.B.171). *11th International Conference on AIDS, Vancouver,* (1996), 18.
13. Norvir (Ritonavir). Abbott Laboratories. US prescribing information, April 2005.
14. Bertz R, Hsu A, Lam W, Williams L, Renz C, Karol M, Dutta S, Carr R, Zhang Y, Wang Q, Schweitzer S, Foit C, Andre A, Bernstein B, Granneman GR, Sun E. Pharmacokinetic interactions between lopinavir/ritonavir (ABT-378r) and other non-HIV drugs (abstract P291). *AIDS* (2000) 14 (Suppl 4), S100.
15. Bergshoeff AS, Wolfs TFW, Geelen SPM, Burger DM. Ritonavir-enhanced pharmacokinetics of nelfinavir/M8 during rifampin use. *Ann Pharmacother* (2003) 37, 521–5.
16. Veldkamp AI, Hoetelmans RMW, Beijnen JH, Mulder JW, Meenhorst PL. Ritonavir enables combined therapy with rifampicin and saquinavir. *Clin Infect Dis* (1999) 29, 1586.
17. Gallicano K, Khaliq Y, Carignan G, Tseng A, Walmsley S, Cameron DW. A pharmacokinetic study of intermittent rifabutin dosing with a combination of ritonavir and saquinavir in patients infected with human immunodeficiency virus. *Clin Pharmacol Ther* (2001) 70, 149–58.
18. Spradling P, Drociuk D, McLaughlin S, Lee LM, Peloquin CA, Gallicano K, Pozsik C, Onorato I, Castro KG, Ridzon R. Drug-drug interactions in inmates treated for human immunodeficiency virus and *Mycobacterium tuberculosis* infection or disease: an institutional tuberculosis outbreak. *Clin Infect Dis* (2002) 35, 1106–12.
19. Sahai J, Stewart F, Swick L, Gallicano K, Garber G, Seguin I, Tucker A, Bristow N, Cameron W. Rifabutin (RBT) reduces saquinavir (SAQ) plasma levels in HIV-infected patients. *Intersci Conf Antimicrob Agents Chemother* (1996) 36, 6.
20. Moyle GJ, Buss NE, Goggin T, Snell P, Higgs C, Hawkins DA. Interaction between saquinavir soft-gel and rifabutin in patients infected with HIV. *Br J Clin Pharmacol* (2002) 54, 178–82.
21. Fortovase (Saquinavir). Roche Products Ltd. UK Summary of product characteristics, January 2005.
22. Centers for Disease Control and Prevention. Updated guidelines for the use of rifamycins for the treatment of tuberculosis among HIV-infected patients taking protease inhibitors or non-nucleoside reverse transcriptase inhibitors. *MMWR* (2004) 53, 37.

Protease inhibitors + St John's wort (*Hypericum perforatum*)

St John's wort causes a marked reduction in the serum levels of indinavir, which may result in HIV treatment failure. Other protease inhibitors (amprenavir, atazanavir, lopinavir, nelfinavir, ritonavir, saquinavir) are predicted to interact similarly.

Clinical evidence

In a single-drug pharmacokinetic study 8 healthy subjects were given three 800-mg oral doses of **indinavir** on day 1 of to achieve steady-state serum levels, and then an 800-mg dose on day 2. For the next 14 days they were given St John's wort extract 300 mg three times daily. Starting on day 16, the indinavir dosing was repeated. It was found that the St John's wort reduced the mean AUC of **indinavir** by 57% and decreased the 8-hour **indinavir** trough serum level by 81%.[1]

Mechanism

Not fully understood, but it seems highly likely that the St John's wort induces the activity of the cytochrome P450 isoenzyme CYP3A4, thereby increasing the metabolism and loss of the indinavir from the body.

Importance and management

Direct information seems to be limited to this study, but the interaction would appear to be established. Such a large reduction in the serum levels of indinavir is likely to result in treatment failures and therefore St John's wort should be avoided. There seems to be no direct information about other protease inhibitors but since they are also metabolised by CYP3A4 it is reasonable to expect that they will be similarly affected by St John's wort. The advice of the UK Committee on Safety of Medicines is that patients on protease inhibitors should avoid St John's wort and that anyone already taking both should stop the St John's wort and have their HIV RNA viral load measured.[2] The makers give similar advice,[3,4] and also note that protease inhibitor levels may increase on stopping St John's wort, and the dose may need adjusting.[3] They note the inducing effect may persist for up to 2 weeks after stopping treatment with St John's wort.[3]

1. Piscitelli SC, Burstein AH, Chaitt D, Alfaro RM, Falloon J. Indinavir concentrations and St John's wort. *Lancet* (2000) 355, 547–8.
2. Committee on Safety of Medicines. Message from Professor A Breckenridge (Chairman of CSM) and Fact Sheet for Health Care Professionals, 29th February 2000.
3. Crixivan (Indinavir sulfate). Merck Sharp & Dohme Ltd. UK Summary of product characteristics, January 2005.
4. Crixivan (Indinavir sulfate). Merck & Co., Inc. US Prescribing information, May 2004.

Protease inhibitors + Tenofovir

Lopinavir/ritonavir modestly increased the levels of tenofovir. Tenofovir modestly decreased atazanavir levels, and this was less when ritonavir was also given. Indinavir did not interact pharmacokinetically with tenofovir.

Clinical evidence, mechanism, importance and management

(a) Atazanavir and atazanavir/ritonavir

The AUC of atazanavir was decreased by 25%, and the trough level by 40% when atazanavir was given with tenofovir.[1,2] When ritonavir 100 mg once daily was added to atazanavir 300 mg once daily, tenofovir 300 mg once daily reduced the AUC of atazanavir by a similar amount (25%), but had less effect on the trough level (23% reduction).[3] The US maker notes that unboosted atazanavir should be used with caution with tenofovir because of the potential for reduced efficacy and development of resistance.[4,5] Atazanavir/ritonavir (boosted atazanavir) and tenofovir have been used successfully in a clinical study.[1,2]

(b) Indinavir

The maker briefly notes that there was no pharmacokinetic interaction between tenofovir and indinavir 800 mg three times daily.[1,6]

(c) Lopinavir/ritonavir

The concurrent use of lopinavir/ritonavir 400 mg/100 mg twice daily and tenofovir resulted in a 30% increase in the AUC and a 50% increase in the trough level of tenofovir, but no change in the pharmacokinetics of lopinavir/ritonavir.[1,6] The clinical relevance of these modest changes has not been assessed, but is unlikely to be important.

1. Viread (Tenofovir disoproxil fumarate). Gilead Sciences International Ltd. UK Summary of product characteristics, March 2005.
2. Reyataz Hard Capsules (Atazanavir). Bristol-Myers Squibb Pharmaceuticals Ltd. UK Summary of product characteristics, February 2005.
3. Taburet A-M, Piketty C, Chazallon C, Vincent I, Gérard L, Calvez V, Clavel F, Aboulker J-P, Girard P-M, and the ANRS Protocol 107 Puzzle 2 Investigators. Interactions between atazanavir-ritonavir and tenofovir in heavily pretreated human immunodeficiency virus-infected patients. *Antimicrob Agents Chemother* (2004) 48, 2091–6.
4. Hodder S, Bristol-Myers Squibb Company, Klein R, Struble K, FDA. Letter to health care providers. Re: Important new pharmacokinetic data for REYATAZ™ (atazanavir sulfate) in combination with Viread® (tenofovir disoproxil fumarate). August 8, 2003. Available at http://www.fda.gov/oashi/aids/listserve/listserve2003.html (accessed 18/07/05).
5. Reyataz (Atazanavir sulfate). Bristol-Myers Squibb Company. US Prescribing information, June 2005.
6. Viread (Tenofovir disoproxil fumarate). Gilead Sciences Inc. US prescribing information, May 2005.

Protease inhibitors; Fosamprenavir + Miscellaneous

Fosamprenavir is a prodrug of amprenavir, and is rapidly and almost completely hydrolysed to amprenavir and inorganic phosphate primarily in the lining of the gut.[1,2] The interactions of fosamprenavir are therefore primarily those of amprenavir.

1. Telzir Tablets (Fosamprenavir calcium). GlaxoSmithKline UK. UK Summary of product characteristics, December 2004.
2. Lexiva (Fosamprenavir calcium). GlaxoSmithKline. US Prescribing information, June 2005.

Protease inhibitors; Indinavir + Milk thistle

One study found that milk thistle lowered the trough level of indinavir by 25%, but this may have been a time-dependent effect rather than a drug interaction. Nevertheless, this modest effect may not be clinically important.

Clinical evidence, mechanism, importance and management

Milk thistle (*Silybum marianum*) 175 mg three times daily (*Thisilyn; Nature's Way,* standardised for silymarin content) for 3 weeks caused a 9% reduction in indinavir AUC and a 25% reduction in trough plasma level, but only the value for the trough level reached statistical significance.[1] The authors suggested that the effect on the trough level could represent a time-dependent effect of indinavir pharmacokinetics, since the plasma levels without milk thistle were found to be similarly lower after a washout phase. Based on *animal* data, the authors had expected milk thistle to increase indinavir levels by inhibiting metabolism. They did not consider their findings to be clinically important in terms of dosing of indinavir or, by extrapolation, other protease inhibitors.[1] However, although others agreed with this conclusion when ritonavir-boosted protease inhibitor therapy is used, they state that the effect of milk thistle on unboosted protease inhibitors is unclear.[2] Further study is needed.

1. Piscitelli SC, Formentini E, Burstein AH, Alfaro R, Jagannatha S, Falloon J. Effect of milk thistle on the pharmacokinetics of indinavir in healthy volunteers. *Pharmacotherapy* (2002) 22, 551–6.
2. Anon. Milk thistle and indinavir. *Treatmentupdate* (2002) 14, 4–5.

Protease inhibitors; Nelfinavir + Calcium

Calcium supplements did not affect the plasma levels of nelfinavir.

Clinical evidence, mechanism, importance and management

Calcium supplements had no effect on plasma levels of nelfinavir or its M8 metabolite in 15 patients receiving nelfinavir 1.25 g twice daily as part of a HAART regimen. Calcium was given as calcium carbonate 1350 mg twice daily to 9 patients, and calcium gluconate/calcium carbonate 2950/300 mg twice daily to 6 patients, both for 14 days. Plasma levels of nelfinavir were measured before a dose and 3 hours after a dose.[1] Similar results were reported in another study.[2] No nelfinavir dosage adjustments appear necessary if calcium supplements are given.

1. Jensen-Fangel S, Justesen US, Black FT, Pedersen C, Obel N. The use of calcium carbonate in nelfinavir-associated diarrhoea in HIV-1-infected patients. *HIV Med* (2003) 4, 48–52.
2. Kopp Hutzler B, Perez-Rodriguez E, Norton S, Hsyu PH. Pharmacokinetics (PK) interactions between nelfinavir (NFV) and calcium supplements (P277). *AIDS* (2000) 14 (Suppl 4), S96.

Ribavirin + Antacids

The UK makers of ribavirin note that there was a minor 14% decrease in the AUC of ribavirin when it was given with an antacid containing aluminium, magnesium, and simeticone, but this is not considered clinically relevant.[1,2] No special precautions are needed.

1. Copegus (Ribavirin). Roche Products Ltd. UK Summary of product characteristics, May 2003.
2. Rebetol (Ribavirin). Schering-Plough Ltd. UK Summary of product characteristics, June 2005.

Rimantadine + Cimetidine

Cimetidine causes a small but probably clinically unimportant rise in the plasma levels of rimantadine.

Clinical evidence, mechanism, importance and management

After taking cimetidine 300 mg four times daily for 6 days, the AUC of a single 100-mg dose of rimantadine was increased by 20% and the apparent total clearance reduced by 18% in 23 healthy subjects. The authors of the study suggest that these changes are likely to have little, if any, clinical consequences.[1] However, this needs confirmation in patients.

1. Holazo AA, Choma N, Brown SY, Lee LF, Wills RJ. Effect of cimetidine on the disposition of rimantadine in healthy subjects. *Antimicrob Agents Chemother* (1989) 33, 820–3.

Tenofovir + Miscellaneous

Tenofovir absorption is increased by food. Caution is recommended with drugs causing renal toxicity. Tenofovir did not alter the pharmacokinetics of a combined oral contraceptive, methadone, or ribavirin.

Clinical evidence, mechanism, importance and management

(a) Cidofovir

Tenofovir is actively secreted by human organic anion transporter 1 (hOAT1) in the kidneys. Therefore, the makers suggest that if it is given with other drugs that are also secreted by this renal transporter, such as cidofovir, increased levels of tenofovir or the other drug could result. They specifically recommend that tenofovir and cidofovir are not given together, unless clearly necessary, when renal function should be monitored weekly.[1]

(b) Contraceptives

The maker notes that tenofovir did not alter the pharmacokinetics of a combined oral contraceptive (**ethinylestradiol/norgestimate**) in 20 subjects.[2]

(c) Food

Administration of tenofovir with a high-fat meal increased the AUC by about 40%, and the maximum level by about 14% compared with the fasted state. The maker recommends that tenofovir be taken with food.[1]

(d) Methadone

The maker notes that tenofovir did not alter the pharmacokinetics of methadone in 13 subjects on stable methadone maintenance doses, and that no symptoms of opiate toxicity or opiate withdrawal were detected.[2]

(e) Other nephrotoxic drugs

Tenofovir has the potential to cause nephrotoxicity, and the maker recommends monthly monitoring of renal function. Although the concurrent administration of other nephrotoxic drugs has not been studied, the makers suggest that renal function should be monitored more frequently (weekly) if concurrent use is unavoidable. They specifically name **aminoglycosides**, **amphotericin B**, **foscarnet**, **ganciclovir**, **interleukin-2**, **pentamidine** and **vancomycin**.[1]

(f) Ribavirin

The maker notes that tenofovir did not alter the pharmacokinetics of ribavirin 600 mg in 22 subjects.[2]

1. Viread (Tenofovir disoproxil fumarate). Gilead Sciences International Ltd. UK Summary of product characteristics, March 2005.
2. Viread (Tenofovir disoproxil fumarate). Gilead Sciences, Inc. US prescribing information, May 2005.

Valaciclovir + Antacids

Valaciclovir does not interact with an aluminium/magnesium hydroxide antacid.

Clinical evidence, mechanism, importance and management

On three separate occasions, 18 healthy subjects were given a single 1-g oral dose of valaciclovir either alone, 65 minutes before, or 30 minutes after taking 30 ml of *Maalox* (**aluminium/magnesium hydroxide**). The pharmacokinetics of aciclovir (which is produced from valaciclovir in the body) remained unchanged. It was concluded that no special precautions are needed if these drugs are taken together, and the authors of the report also suggest that it is unlikely that other antacids will interact.[1]

1. de Bony F, Bidault R, Peck R, Posner J. Lack of interaction between valaciclovir, the L-valyl ester of acyclovir, and Maalox antacid. *J Antimicrob Chemother* (1996) 37, 383–7.

Valaciclovir + Hydrochlorothiazide

Hydrochlorothiazide does not interact adversely with valaciclovir.

Clinical evidence, mechanism, importance and management

A study in a group of elderly subjects (65 to 83 years old) given valaciclovir 500 mg or 1 g three times daily for 8 days found that its safety profile was unchanged in the presence of hydrochlorothiazide, and was similar to that in young healthy subjects.[1] The pharmacokinetics of the active metabolite aciclovir following valaciclovir were not significantly different.[1] There would seem to be no reason for avoiding concurrent use.

1. Wang LH, Schultz M, Weller S, Smiley ML, Blum MR. Pharmacokinetics and safety of multiple-dose valaciclovir in geriatric volunteers with and without concomitant diuretic therapy. *Antimicrob Agents Chemother* (1996) 40, 80–5.

Vidarabine + Allopurinol

There is evidence that if allopurinol and vidarabine (adenine arabinoside) are given together the toxicity of vidarabine may be increased.

Clinical evidence

Two patients with chronic lymphocytic leukaemia treated with allopurinol 300 mg daily developed severe neurotoxicity (coarse rhythmic tremors of the extremities and facial muscles, and impaired mentation) 4 days after vidarabine was added for the treatment of viral infections.[1] A retrospective search to find other patients who had taken both drugs for 4 days revealed a total of 17 patients, 5 of whom had experienced adverse reactions including tremors, nausea, pain, itching and anaemia.[1] Another possible case of neurological toxicity has also been reported.[2]

Mechanism

Uncertain. One suggestion is that the allopurinol causes hypoxanthine arabinoside, the major metabolite of vidarabine, to accumulate by inhibiting xanthine oxidase. A study with *rat* liver cytosol found that allopurinol greatly increased the half-life of this metabolite.[3]

Importance and management

Information seems to be limited to these reports, and so the general clinical importance of this possible interaction is uncertain, but it would be prudent to exercise particular care if these drugs are used together.

1. Friedman HM, Grasela T. Adenine arabinoside and allopurinol – possible adverse drug interaction. *N Engl J Med* (1981) 304, 423.
2. Collignon PJ, Sorrell TC. Neurological toxicity associated with vidarabine (adenine arabinoside) therapy. *Aust N Z J Med* (1983) 13, 627–9.
3. Drach JC, Rentea RG, Cowen ME. The metabolic degradation of 9-β-D-arabinofuranosyladenine (ara-A) *in vitro*. *Fedn Proc* (1973) 32, 777.

20

Beta-blockers

The adrenoceptors of the sympathetic nervous system are of two main types, namely alpha and beta. The beta-adrenoceptor blocking drugs (better known as the beta-blockers) block the beta-receptors and this property is therapeutically exploited to reduce, for example, the normal sympathetic stimulation of the heart. The activity of the heart in response to stress and exercise is reduced, its consumption of oxygen is diminished, and in this way the angina of effort can be treated. Beta-blockers given orally can also be used in the management of cardiac arrhythmias, hypertension, myocardial infarction, and heart failure. They may also be used for some symptoms of anxiety and for migraine prophylaxis. Some beta-blockers are used in the form of eye-drops for glaucoma and ocular hypertension.

Not all beta-receptors are identical but can be further subdivided into two groups, beta-1 and beta-2. The former are found in the heart and the latter in the bronchi. Since one of the unwanted adverse effects of generalised beta-blockade can be the loss of the normal noradrenaline-stimulated bronchodilation (leading to bronchospasm), cardioselective beta-1 blocking drugs (e.g. atenolol, metoprolol) were developed, which have less effect on beta-2 receptors. However, it should be emphasised that the selectivity is not absolute because bronchospasm can still occur with these drugs, particularly at high doses. 'Table 20.1', (p.623) lists the cardioselective beta-blockers, and 'Table 20.2', (p.623) the non-selective beta-blockers. Some beta-blockers also have alpha-1 blocking activity, which causes vasodilatation, and these are listed in 'Table 20.3', (p.624). Some beta-blockers, such as celiprolol and nebivolol, also have vasodilator activity but produce this by mechanisms other than blocking alpha-1 receptors. Other beta-blockers also possess intrinsic sympathomimetic activity in that they can activate beta-receptors and are therefore partial agonists; these are listed in 'Table 20.4', (p.624). Sotalol has additional class III antiarrhythmic activity.

Beta-blockers may be involved in pharmacodynamic interactions with other drugs that are based on enhancement or antagonism of pharmacological effects. Beta-blockers may be lipophilic drugs (such as metoprolol) or hydrophilic (such as atenolol). The lipophilic beta-blockers are more likely to be involved in pharmacokinetic interactions than the hydrophilic drugs. Many of the lipophilic beta-blockers are principally metabolised by the cytochrome P450 isoenzyme CYP2D6, and drugs that are inhibitors or inducers of this isoenzyme (see 'Table 1.3', (p.6)) increase or decrease their levels. Propranolol is also metabolised by CYP1A2 (see 'Beta-blockers + SSRIs', p.641).

This section is generally concerned with those drugs that affect the activity of the beta-blockers. Where the beta-blockers are the affecting drug, the interaction is dealt with elsewhere.

Table 20.1 Cardioselective beta-blockers (beta-1 receptor selectivity)

Generic Names	*Proprietary names*
Acebutolol	ACB, Acecor, Beloc, Diasectral, Espesil, Grifobutol, Monitan, Prent, Rhotral, Sali-Prent, Secadrex, Sectral, Sectrazide, Tredalat
Atenolol	Ablock, Adco-Loten, Adoll, Amlopres AT, Amlosafe-AT, Amlostat-AT, Amolin, Ancoren, Angipress, Anselol, Antipressan, Apo-Atenol, Apress, Arcablock, Ate, Ate Lich, Atebeta, Ateblocor, Atecard, Atecor, Atedon, Atedurex, Atehexal, Atel, Aten, Atenblock, Atendol, Ateneo, Atenet, Atenetic, Ateni, AteNif beta, Atenigron, Atenil, Atenix, AtenixCo, Ateno, ateno-basan, Atenobene, Atenoblock, Atenoblok, Atenodan, Atenogamma, Atenogen, Atenol, Atenomel, Atenopress, Atenor, Atenoric Atenotyrol, Atermin, Atinorm, Azectol, Beta, Beta Nicardia, Beta-Adalat, Beta-Adalate, Betacar, Betasyn, Betatop, Blocotenol, Blokium, Blotex, Bresben, Cardaxen, Cardif Beta, Cardules Plus, Carmian, Catenol, Chlotenol, Clortanol, Coratol, Corotenol, Co-tenidone, Cotenolol-Neo, Cotesifar, CP-Atenol, Cuxanorm, Depten, Diu-Atenolol, Diube, Duratenol, Eupres, Evitocor, Fealin, Felobits, Galol, Grifotenol, Hemon, Hexa-Blok, Hipres, Huma-Atenol, Hypernol, Igroseles, Jenatenol, Juvental, Kalten, Labotensil, Lerez-AT, Lonol, Loten, Lo-Ten, Martenol, Mesonex, Mezarid, Mixer, Myocord, Neatenol, Neocardon, Neotenol, Nif-Atenil, Nifatenol, Nifelat, Nifetex, Nifetolol, Nif-Ten, Nolol, Normalol, Normaten, Normiten, Normopresil, Normopress, Nortelol, Noten, Novo-Atenol, Nu-Atenol, Obosan, Oraday, Plenacor, Polinorm, Prenolol, Prenomod, Prenoretic, Prenormine, Presolar, Prinorm, Ranlol, Seles Beta, Selobloc, Sigabloc, Silder, Synarome, Tanser, Target, Telvodin, Ten-Bloka, Tenchlor, Teneretic, Tenidon, Tenif, Teno, Tenoblock, Tenochek, Tenoclor, Tenocor, Tenofed, Tenol, Tenolol, Tenolone, Tenomax, Tenoprin, Tenordate, Tenoret, Tenoretic, Tenoric, Tenormin, Tenormine, Tensig, Tensotin, Ternolol, Tessifol, Totaretic, Tradiver, Trantalol, Tredol, TRI-Normin, Typofen, Umoder, Uniloc, Urosin, Vascoten, Velorin, Venapulse, Vericordin
Betaxolol	Armament, Bemaz, Beof, Beofta, Bertocil, Betac, Betasel, Betoptic, Betoptic S, Betoptima, Betoquin, Davixolol, Eifel, Kerlon, Kerlone, Kerlong, Lokren, Optipres, Pertaxol, Tonobexol
Bevantolol	
Bisoprolol	Biconcor, Bicor, Bilol, Bipranix, Biso, Biso Lich, BisoAPS, Bisobeta, Bisobloc, Bisoblock, Bisocor, Bisogamma, Bisogen, Bisohexal, Bisolol, Bisomerck, Bisopine, Bisoplus, Bisopral, Biso-Puren, Bisostad, Bisotyrol, Cardensiel, Cardicor, Cardiloc, Cardiocor, Co-Bisoprolol, Concor, Concor Cor, Congescor, Corbis, Coviogal, Darbalan, Detensiel, Emcolol, Emconcor, Emcor, Emcoretic, Euradal, Fondril, Godal, Isoten, Jutabis, Lodoz, Maintate, Maxsoten, Monocor, Nanalan, Orloc, Pactens, Pluscor, Rivacor, Sequacor, Soloc, Soprol, Vivacor, Wytens, Zebeta, Ziac, Ziak
Celiprolol	Cardem, Celectol, Celipro, Celiprogamma, Celol, Cordiax, Dilanorm, Selectol, Selecturon, Tenoloc
Esmolol	Brevibloc, Dublon, Miniblock
Levobetaxolol	Betaxon
Metoprolol	Beatrolol, Belnif, Beloc, Beloc-Zok, Beloken, Betaloc, Bioprol, Cardeloc, Cardoxone, Co-Betaloc, Corvitol, CP-Metolol, Denex, Diubeloc, Dura-Zok, Egilok, Emzok, Huma-Metoprol, Igroton-Lopresor, Jeprolol, Jutabloc, Lanoc, Logimat, Logimax, Logroton, Lopresor, Lopressor, Melol, Meprolol, Mepronet, Metblock, Meto, Metobeta, Metoblock, Metocar, Metocard, Metocor, Metodoc, Metodura, Metohexal, Meto-Isis, Metok, Metolar, Metolol, MetoMed, Metomerck, Metop, Metopal, Metopresol, Metopress, Metoprogamma, Metoprolin, Metostad, Meto-Tablinen, Meto-thiazid, Metotyrol, Metozoc, Minax, Mobloc, Neobloc, Novo-Metoprol, Nu-Metop, Prelis, Proken M, Prolaken, Promiced, Prontol, Revelol, Ritmetol, Ritmolol, Sefloc, Selectadril, Selocomp ZOC, Selokeen, Seloken, Selokomb, Selopral, Selopres, Selopresin, Selopress, Selozide, Selozok, Selo-Zok, Serdol, Sermetrol, Sigaprolol, Slow-Lopresor, Spesicor, Toprol, Treloc, Triloc, Vasocardin, Zok-Zid
Nebivolol	Lobivon, Nebilet, Nebiloc , Nebilox, Nebolet, Nobiten, Nodon, Silostar, Temerit
Practolol	
Talinolol	Cordanum

Table 20.2 Non-selective beta-blockers (block beta-1 and beta-2 receptors)

Generic names	*Proprietary names*
Alprenolol	
Befunolol	Bentos, Betaclar, Glauconex, Thilonium
Bopindolol	Sandonorm, Sandoretic
Bupranolol	Betadrenol, Betamed
Carazolol	Conducton
Carteolol	Arteolol, Arteopilo, Arteoptic, Carpilo, Carteabak, Carteodose, Carteol, Carteopil, Cartrol, Elebloc, Endak, Fortinol, Glauteolol, Mikelan, Napolit, Poenglaucol, Singlauc, Teoptic, Zymoptic
Carvedilol	Acridilole, Betaplex, Biocard, Blocar, Cardilol, Cardiol, Cardivas, Carloc, Carvedexxon, Carvetone, Carvil, Carvipress, Co-Dilatrend, Coreg, Coritensil, Coropres, Dilaplus, Dilatrend, Dilbloc, Dimitone, Divelol, Dualten, Eucardic, Hybridil, Kredex, Lodipres, Querto, Talliton
Indenolol	Securpres
Labetalol	Albetol, Coreton, Hybloc, Ipolab, Normodyne, Presolol, Trandate, Trandiur
Levobunolol	Ak-Beta, Betagan, Betagen, Levunolol, Ophtho-Bunolol, Probeta, Vistagan
Mepindolol	Corindocomb, Corindolan
Metipranolol	Betacarpin, Betamann, Betanol, Beta-Ophtiole, Normoglaucon, OptiPranolol, Ripix, Trimecryton, Trimepranol, Tri-Torrat, Turoptin
Nadolol	Anabet, Apo-Nadol, Corgard, Corgaretic, Corzide, Solgol, Sotaziden N

Continued

Table 20.2 Non-selective beta-blockers (block beta-1 and beta-2 receptors) *(continued)*

Generic names	*Proprietary names*
Oxprenolol	Captol, Corbeton, Impresso, Slow-Trasicor, Slow-Trasitensine, Trasicor, Trasidrex, Trasitensin, Trasitensine, Trepress
Penbutolol	Betapressin, Betarelix, Betasemid, Levatol
Pindolol	Apo-Pindol, Barbloc, Durapindol, Glauco-Stulln, Hexapindol, Novo-Pindol, Nu-Pindol, Pinden, Pindocor, Pindol, Pinloc, Viskaldix, Viskazide, Viskeen, Visken, Viskene, Viskenit
Propranolol	Acifol, Angilol, Antitensin, Atensin, Avlocardyl, Bedranol, Beptazine, Betabloc, Betadipresan, Betalol, Betapress, Beta-Prograne, Betaspan, Beta-Tablinen, Beta-Turfa, Cardenol, Cardiblok, Cardilol, Cardinol, Ciplar, Corbeta, Corbetazine, Coriodal, Corpendol, Deralin, Dociretic, Dociton, Efektolol, Elbrol, Emforal, Half Beta-Prograne, Half Inderal, Hemipralon, Huma-Pronol, Inderal, Inderalici, Inderetic, Inderide, InnoPran, Inpanol, Neo Propranol, Normpress, Obsidan, Obsilazin N, Palon, Perlol, Pertenso N, Pirimetan, Pradinolol, Pralol, Pranolol, Prodorol, Prolol, Propacor, Propal, Propalem, Propalong, Propayerst, Prophylux, Propra, Proprahexal, Propral, Propranur, Propra-ratiopharm, Pur-Bloka, Ranoprin, Rebaten, Sanpronol, Slo-Pro, Slow Deralin, Sumial, Syntonol, Syprol, Tenadren, Triamteren, Uni Propralol, Zopax Plus
Sotalol	Beta-Cardone, Betapace, Cardol, CorSotalol, Darob, Dutacor, Favorex, Gilucor, Hipecor, Jutalex, Rentibloc, Rytmobeta, Solavert, Sota, Sota Lich, Sotab, Sotabeta, Sotacor, Sotagamma, Sotahexal, Sotalex, Sotalin, Sotalodoc, Sotamed, Sotanorm, Sotaper, Sotapor, Sota-Puren, Sota-saar, Sotastad, Sotazide, Sotoger, Ventricor
Tertatolol	Artex, Artexal
Timolol	Apo-Timol, Apo-Timop, Aquanil, Arutimol, Betim, Betimol, Blocadren, Blocanol, Chibro-Timoptol, Combigan, Cosopt, Cusimolol, Digaol, Dispatim, Dorsof T, Dorzoflax, Dropiltim, Droptimol, Equiton, Flumetol, Fotil, Gaoptol, Glafemak, Glatim, Glaucocin, Glauco-Oph, Glaucosan, Glaucotensil, Glausolets, Glautimol, Glucomol, Glucotim, Horex, Hypermol, Isatol, Klonalol, Latof-T, Lithimole, Loptomit, Moducren, Moducrin, Noval, Novo-Timol, Nyogel, Nyolol, Octil, Ocupres, Ocutim, Ofal, Oftamolol, Oftan, Oftensin, Oftimolo, Ophtilan, Ophtim, Optimol, Pilobloc, Pilobloq, Pilotim, Plostim, Poentimol, Prestim, Proflax, Protevis, Servatrin, Shemol, Temserin, Tenopt, Tesol, Thilotim, Tiloptic, Timabak, Timacar, Timacor, Timax, Timed, Timicon, Timisol, Timocomod, Timo-COMOD, Timodose, Timodrop, TimoEDO, Timoftal, Timoftol, Timogal, Timogel, Timoglau, Timohexal, Timolabak, Timolen, Timoler, Timolide, Timolo, Timolux, Timomann, Timo-Optal, Timop, Tim-Ophtal, Timoptic, Timoptol, Timosan, Timosil, Timosine, Timosoft, Timo-Stulln, Timozzard, Timpilo, Timsopt, Tiof, T+P, TP-Ophtal, V-Optic, Waucosin, Xalacom, Xalcom, Yesan, Yvano

Table 20.3 Drugs with both alpha and beta-blocking activity

Generic names	*Proprietary names*
Carvedilol	Acridilole, Betaplex, Biocard, Blocar, Cardilol, Cardiol, Cardivas, Carloc, Carvedexxon, Carvetone, Carvil, Carvipress, Co-Dilatrend, Coreg, Coritensil, Coropres, Dilaplus, Dilatrend, Dilbloc, Dimitone, Divelol, Dualten, Eucardic, Hybridil, Kredex, Lodipres, Querto, Talliton
Labetalol	Albetol, Coreton, Hybloc, Ipolab, Normodyne, Presolol, Trandate, Trandiur

Table 20.4 Drugs with intrinsic sympathomimetic activity (partial agonists)

Generic names	*Proprietary names*
Acebutolol	ACB, Acecor, Beloc, Diasectral, Espesil, Grifobutol, Monitan, Prent, Rhotral, Sali-Prent, Secadrex, Sectral, Sectrazide, Tredalat
Alprenolol	
Carteolol	Arteolol, Arteopilo, Arteoptic, Carpilo, Carteabak, Carteodose, Carteol, Cartrol, Elebloc, Endak, Fortinol, Glauteolol, Mikelan, Napolit, Poenglaucol, Singlauc, Teoptic, Zymoptic
Celiprolol	Cardem, Celectol, Celipro, Celiprogamma, Celol, Cordiax, Dilanorm, Selectol, Selecturon, Tenoloc
Mepindolol	Corindocomb, Corindolan
Oxprenolol	Captol, Corbeton, Impresso, Slow-Trasicor, Slow-Trasitensine, Trasicor, Trasidrex, Trasitensin, Trasitensine, Trepress
Pindolol	Apo-Pindol, Barbloc, Durapindol, Glauco-Stulln, Hexapindol, Novo-Pindol, Nu-Pindol, Pinden, Pindocor, Pindol, Pinloc, Viskaldix, Viskazide, Viskeen, Visken, Viskene, Viskenit

Beta-blockers + Acetylcholine

An isolated case describes bronchospasm in a patient on metoprolol given intra-ocular acetylcholine.

Clinical evidence, mechanism, importance and management

An elderly patient with a history of hypertension, obstructive pulmonary disease and stable angina, taking several drugs including **metoprolol**, experienced severe bronchospasm and pulmonary oedema immediately following the intra-ocular injection of **acetylcholine chloride** during cataract surgery. Her blood pressure rapidly increased, and she had tachycardia. She had also received phenylephrine eye drops before surgery. The patient may have been more sensitive to the pulmonary effects of acetylcholine, such as bronchospasm, because of pre-existing disease and metoprolol therapy. Phenylephrine may also have been involved,[1] (see also 'Beta-blockers + Sympathomimetics; Directly-acting', p.643. The general clinical relevance of this single case is uncertain.

1. Rasch D, Holt J, Wilson M, Smith RB. Bronchospasm following intraocular injection of acetylcholine in a patient taking metoprolol. *Anesthesiology* (1983) 59, 583–5.

Beta-blockers + Allopurinol

Allopurinol 300 mg daily for 6 days did not affect the steady-state pharmacokinetics of atenolol 100 mg daily in 6 healthy subjects.[1] No special precautions would appear to be necessary on concurrent use.

1. Schäfer-Korting M, Kirch W, Axthelm T, Köhler H, Mutschler E. Atenolol interaction with aspirin, allopurinol, and ampicillin. *Clin Pharmacol Ther* (1983) 33, 283–8.

Beta-blockers + 5-Alpha-reductase inhibitors

Finasteride 5 mg daily for 10 days caused no change in the pharmacokinetics or pharmacodynamics of a single 80-mg dose of propranolol in healthy subjects,[1] and the makers say that finasteride was used with beta-blockers in clinical trials without any evidence of an interaction.[2,3] Similarly, 'dutasteride', (p.1020) does not appear to interact with beta-blockers.

1. Gregoire S, Williams R, Gormely G, Lin E. Effect of finasteride (Mk-906), a new potent 5 alpha reductase inhibitor on the disposition of D and L-propranolol. *J Clin Pharmacol* (1990) 30, 847.
2. Proscar (Finasteride). Merck Sharp & Dohme Ltd. UK Summary of product characteristics, December 2003.
3. Proscar (Finasteride). Merck and Co. Inc. US Prescribing information, April 2004.

Beta-blockers + Antacids or Antidiarrhoeals

Although some antacids and antidiarrhoeals may cause a modest reduction in the absorption of atenolol, propranolol, sotalol and other beta-blockers, and possibly a slight increase in the absorption of metoprolol, the clinical importance of these interactions is probably minimal.

Clinical evidence

(a) Atenolol

Aluminium hydroxide 5.6 g given to 6 healthy subjects caused an insignificant 20% fall in the plasma levels of a single 100-mg dose of atenolol, and had no effect on the reduction in exercise heart rate. **Aluminium hydroxide** had no significant effect on atenolol pharmacokinetics when both drugs were given together for 6 days.[1] Conversely, a single 500-mg dose of **calcium** (as the lactate, gluconate and carbonate) caused a 51% reduction in the peak plasma level, a 32% reduction in AUC, and an increase in elimination half-life from 6.2 to 11 hours after a single 100-mg dose of atenolol in 6 healthy subjects. The effect of atenolol on heart rate was decreased by 12%. However, these changes were no longer significant after 6 days of concurrent use, except for a 21% reduction in peak plasma atenolol levels. In a further 6 hypertensive subjects, neither **calcium** 500 mg daily nor **aluminium hydroxide** 5.6 g daily had any influence on the blood pressure lowering effect of atenolol 100 mg daily for 4 weeks.[1]

Another study found that 30 ml of *Novalucol forte* (an **aluminium/magnesium-containing antacid**) reduced the peak plasma level and AUC of a single 100-mg dose of atenolol by 37 and 33% respectively in 6 healthy subjects.[2]

(b) Indenolol

A study in *rats* found that when indenolol was given with either *Simeco* (**aluminium/magnesium hydroxide** with **simeticone**) or *Kaopectate* (**kaolin-pectin**), the 6-hour AUCs were reduced by 15 and 30% respectively.[3]

(c) Metoprolol

In 6 healthy subjects, 30 ml of *Novalucol forte* (an **aluminium/magnesium-containing antacid**) increased the peak plasma level and AUC of a single 100-mg dose of metoprolol by 25 and 11%, respectively.[2]

(d) Propranolol

Aluminium hydroxide gel 30 ml affected neither the plasma concentrations nor the reduction in exercise heart rate in 6 healthy subjects after a single 40-mg dose of propranolol.[4] In contrast, a study in 5 healthy subjects found that 30 ml of an **aluminium hydroxide gel** given with a single 80-mg dose of propranolol reduced the plasma propranolol levels and the AUC by almost 60%.[5] *In vitro* and *animal* data suggest that **bismuth subsalicylate**, **kaolin-pectin** and **magnesium trisilicate** can also reduce the absorption of propranolol.[6,7]

(e) Sotalol

A study in 5 healthy subjects found that single-doses of **aluminium hydroxide** suspension (*Neutragel*) or **calcium carbonate** suspension given after an overnight fast had negligible effects on the pharmacokinetics of a single 160-mg dose of sotalol, whereas a single-dose of **magnesium hydroxide** slightly reduced the AUC of sotalol by 16%.[8] A further study in 6 healthy subjects found that when 20 ml of *Maalox* (**aluminium/magnesium hydroxide**) was given at the same time as 160 mg of sotalol, the maximum plasma level of the sotalol was reduced by 26% and its AUC was reduced by 21%. Changes in heart rates reflected these pharmacokinetic changes.[9] When the *Maalox* was given 2 hours after the sotalol no interaction occurred.[9]

Mechanism

Uncertain. The reduction in absorption could possibly be related to a delay in gastric emptying caused by the antacid, delayed dissolution due to an increase in gastric pH, or to the formation of a complex of the two drugs in the gut, which reduces absorption. However, one *in vitro* study indicated that sotalol was only subject to minor absorption or complexation interactions.[9] Another study found that 35 to 40% of sotalol was bound by magnesium hydroxide, but this may be reversible under physiological conditions and therefore unlikely to be relevant during long-term clinical use.[8]

Importance and management

The documentation is limited, in some instances somewhat contradictory, and largely confined to single-dose or *animal* studies, which may not be clinically relevant. Some changes in absorption may possibly occur but no study seems to have shown that there is a significant effect on the therapeutic effectiveness of the beta-blockers. The one study using atenolol in patients found that the pharmacokinetic changes seen with single-doses of aluminium or calcium containing antacids were not clinically significant.[1] However, be alert for any changes during concurrent use. Separating the dosages by 2 hours was shown to avoid the interaction in one study,[9] and would seem a simple way of avoiding problems should they occur.

1. Kirch W, Schäfer-Korting M, Axthelm T, Köhler H, Mutschler E. Interaction of atenolol with furosemide and calcium and aluminium salts. *Clin Pharmacol Ther* (1981) 30, 429–35.
2. Regårdh CG, Lundborg P, Persson BA. The effect of antacid, metoclopramide and propantheline on the bioavailability of metoprolol and atenolol. *Biopharm Drug Dispos* (1981) 2, 79–87.
3. Tariq M, Babhair SA. Effect of antacid and antidiarrhoeal drugs on the bioavailability of indenolol. *IRCS Med Sci* (1984) 12, 87–8.
4. Hong CY, Hu SC, Lin SJ, Chiang BN. Lack of influence of aluminium hydroxide on the bioavailability and beta-adrenoceptor blocking activity of propranolol. *Int J Clin Pharmacol Ther Toxicol* (1985) 23, 244–46.
5. Dobbs JH, Skoutakis VA, Acchardio SR, Dobbs BR. Effects of aluminium hydroxide on the absorption of propranolol. *Curr Ther Res* (1977) 21, 887–92.
6. Moustafa MA, Gouda MW, Tariq M. Decreased bioavailability of propranolol due to interactions with adsorbent antacids and antidiarrhoeal mixtures. *Int J Pharmaceutics* (1986) 30, 225–8.

7. McElnay JC, D'Arcy PF, Leonard JK. The effect of activated dimethicone, other antacid constituents, and kaolin on the absorption of propranolol. *Experientia* (1982) 38, 605–7.
8. Kahela P, Anttila M, Sundqvist H. Antacids and sotalol absorption. *Acta Pharmacol Toxicol (Copenh)* (1981) 49, 181–3.
9. Läer S, Neumann J, Scholz H. Interaction between sotalol and an antacid preparation. *Br J Clin Pharmacol* (1997) 43, 269–72.

Beta-blockers + Anticholinesterases

A small number of reports describe marked bradycardia and hypotension during the recovery period from anaesthesia and neuromuscular blockade, in patients on beta-blockers given anticholinesterase drugs, but normally no adverse reaction seems to occur. (See also 'Anaesthetics, general + Beta-blockers', p.885). Myasthenic symptoms and myasthenia gravis have occurred with oral and topical beta-blockers, and so beta-blockers could oppose the efficacy of anticholinesterases in treating myasthenia gravis.

Clinical evidence

(a) Bradycardia

A patient on **nadolol** 40 mg daily, recovering from surgery during which suxamethonium (succinylcholine) had been used for tracheal intubation and pancuronium for general muscular relaxation, developed prolonged bradycardia of 32 to 36 bpm and hypotension (systolic pressure 60 to 70 torr) when **neostigmine** and atropine were given to reverse the neuromuscular blockade. Isoprenaline and phenylephrine infusions were required to maintain a systolic blood pressure of 90 torr, and were gradually reduced over 3 days. **Propranolol** was substituted for **nadolol**, and about 10 weeks later she underwent general anaesthesia again (this time without a neuromuscular blocker/**neostigmine**) and she recovered uneventfully.[1] A patient on **propranolol** 20 mg twice daily, recovering from surgery during which alcuronium had been used, received glycopyrronium and **neostigmine** without any change in heart rate. However, one hour later he developed severe bradycardia (a fall from 65 to 40 bpm) and hypotension (systolic blood pressure 70 mmHg) when given intravenous **physostigmine** 2 mg over 5 minutes, for extreme drowsiness attributed to the premedication. This responded to glycopyrronium.[2] Prolonged bradycardia and hypotension, requiring isoprenaline then adrenaline (epinephrine), were seen in an elderly woman on **atenolol** 50 mg daily and nitrates when she was given **neostigmine** and atropine for the reversal of muscle relaxation at the end of general anaesthesia.[3] Another report similarly describes bradycardia in a patient on **propranolol** when intravenous **neostigmine** was used to reverse pancuronium-induced blockade. This responded to atropine.[4]

However, a study in 8 hypertensive patients taking long-term **atenolol** or **propranolol** found no significant changes in heart rate and no serious adverse reactions when they were given low-dose oral **pyridostigmine** 30 mg three times daily for 2 days.[5]

(b) Anticholinesterase effects

Three patients developed myasthenic symptoms when treated with **beta-blockers** (two on **propranolol** and one on **oxprenolol**). Two of them were effectively treated with **pyridostigmine**.[6] Another patient developed fulminant myasthenia gravis within 2 weeks of starting treatment with **acebutolol**.[7] Similarly, in a patient with myasthenia gravis, the use of **timolol** eye drops was associated with deterioration of muscle strength,[8] and in another, serious deterioration in myasthenia.[9]

However, in a study in 10 myasthenic patients with mild to moderate symptoms, intravenous **propranolol** 100 micrograms/kg did not result in worsening of neuromuscular transmission (assessed by muscle function tests and repetitive nerve stimulation). Moreover, 8 of those with mild symptoms reduced their **pyridostigmine** dose during the study to allow the effects of the additional drug to be more readily seen.[10]

Mechanism

It would appear that the bradycardic effects of the beta-blockers and the acetylcholine-like effects of these anticholinesterase drugs can be additive. These were inadequately controlled by the use of atropine in some of the instances cited. The myasthenic symptoms may be due beta-blockers exerting a depressant effect on the neuromuscular junction.[7,8]

Importance and management

The information available indicates that marked adverse reactions after surgery are uncommon, but concurrent use should be well monitored to ensure that the occasional problem is dealt with promptly. Be alert when using any intravenous anticholinesterase in a patient on beta-blockers.

Limited information suggests beta-blockers given orally or topically could oppose the efficacy of anticholinesterases in the treatment of myasthenia gravis. However, one study suggests that, in cardiovascular emergencies, propranolol may be given to patients with myasthenia gravis, provided that resuscitation equipment and specific antidotes are available.[10] Strictly speaking this is a drug-disease rather than a drug-drug interaction.

1. Seidl DC, Martin DE. Prolonged bradycardia after neostigmine administration in a patient taking nadolol. *Anesth Analg* (1984) 63, 365–7.
2. Baraka A, Dajani A. Severe bradycardia following physostigmine in the presence of beta-adrenergic blockade. *Middle East J Anesthesiol* (1984) 7, 291–3.
3. Eldor J, Hoffman B, Davidson JT. Prolonged bradycardia and hypotension after neostigmine administration in a patient receiving atenolol. *Anaesthesia* (1987) 42, 1294–7.
4. Sprague DH. Severe bradycardia after neostigmine in a patient taking propranolol to control paroxysmal atrial tachycardia. *Anesthesiology* (1975) 42, 208–10.
5. Arad M, Roth A, Zelinger J, Zivner Z, Rabinowitz B, Atsmon J. Safety of pyridostigmine in hypertensive patients receiving beta blockers. *Am J Cardiol* (1992) 69, 518–22.
6. Herishanu Y, Rosenberg P. Beta-blockers and myasthenia gravis. *Ann Intern Med* (1975) 83, 834–5.
7. Confavreux C, Charles N, Aimard G. Fulminant myasthenia gravis soon after initiation of acebutolol therapy. *Eur Neurol* (1990) 30, 279–81.
8. Verkijk A. Worsening of myasthenia gravis with timolol maleate eyedrops. *Ann Neurol* (1985) 17, 211–12.
9. Shaivitz SA. Timolol and myasthenia gravis. *JAMA* (1979) 242, 1611–12.
10. Jonkers I, Swerup C, Pirskanen R, Bjelak S, Matell G. Acute effects of intravenous injection of beta-adrenoreceptor- and calcium channel antagonists and agonists in myasthenia gravis. *Muscle Nerve* (1996) 19, 959–65.

Beta-blockers + Aspirin or NSAIDs

Indometacin reduces the antihypertensive effects of the beta-blockers. Piroxicam usually interacts similarly, while sulindac usually does not. Limited information suggests that normally diclofenac, imidazole salicylate, oxaprozin and tenoxicam do not interact. Ibuprofen and naproxen have reduced the effect of beta-blockers in some studies but not others. Isolated cases of hypertension have been reported with naproxen and ibuprofen. Multiple-dose aspirin, both in high and low dose, did not reduce the efficacy of antihypertensives in three studies, but one single-dose study showed antagonism of the effect of beta-blockers. Another study suggested aspirin may attenuate the benefit of carvedilol in heart failure. Indometacin has also been reported to cause a marked hypertensive response in two women with pre-eclampsia treated with pindolol and propranolol. Celecoxib, but not rofecoxib, inhibits the metabolism of metoprolol.

Clinical evidence

(a) Aspirin and other salicylates

A study in patients on various antihypertensives [not specified] found that aspirin, in both low dose (650 mg daily) and high doses (3.9 g daily), did not cause clinically significant increases in blood pressure.[1] Similarly, a study in 11 patients taking a number of antihypertensives (which included a few patients on **propranolol** and **pindolol**) found that aspirin 650 mg three times daily for 7 days did not affect the control of blood pressure.[2] In contrast, another study found that 5 g of aspirin given over 24 hours prevented the antihypertensive effects of a single 1-mg intravenous dose of **pindolol**, and a single 1- to 1.5-g dose of aspirin reduced the antihypertensive effect of a single 5-mg intravenous dose of **propranolol**.[3] Aspirin was reported not to affect the control of hypertension by **metipranolol**.[4] A retrospective study of patients with heart failure treated with **carvedilol** found that aspirin did not significantly affect systolic blood pressure or heart rate but did observe that left ventricular ejection fraction improved less in those patients taking aspirin in addition to **carvedilol**.[5]

A single-dose study in 6 healthy subjects found that aspirin 500 mg did not affect the pharmacokinetics of **atenolol**.[6] Another study in 6 healthy subjects found that aspirin did not affect the pharmacokinetics of **metoprolol**, but the maximum plasma levels of aspirin were increased by **metoprolol** although this was not considered to be clinically relevant.[7]

Sodium salicylate did not affect either the pharmacokinetics of **alprenolol** or its effects on heart rate and blood pressure during exercise in a single-dose study in healthy subjects.[8] **Imidazole salicylate** did not affect the blood pressure control of patients treated with **atenolol**.[9]

(b) Celecoxib or Rofecoxib

In an open, randomised crossover study in 12 healthy subjects, celecoxib 200 mg twice daily for 7 days increased the AUC of a single 50-mg dose of **metoprolol** by 64%. In contrast, rofecoxib 25 mg daily for 7 days did not significantly affect the pharmacokinetics of **metoprolol**.

(c) Diclofenac

A study in 16 patients taking **atenolol**, **metoprolol**, **propranolol** or **pindolol** and/or a diuretic found that diclofenac 50 mg three times daily had no effect on the control of blood pressure.[10]

(d) Flurbiprofen

A study in 10 patients with hypertension found that flurbiprofen 100 mg daily for 7 days did not affect the pharmacokinetics of single-doses of either **propranolol** 80 mg or **atenolol** 100 mg. However, the hypotensive effects of **propranolol** but not **atenolol** were reduced by the flurbiprofen.[11]

(e) Ibuprofen

In a randomised study, ibuprofen 400 mg every 8 hours caused significant increases in blood pressure (mean increases of about 5 to 7 mmHg) in 6 hypertensive patients treated with thiazides and beta-blockers.[12] The antihypertensive effect of **pindolol** was antagonised by ibuprofen in one patient.[13] However, ibuprofen 400 mg four times daily had no effect on the control of blood pressure in patients on **propranolol** in one randomised controlled study.[14]

(f) Indometacin

A study found that when indometacin 25 mg three times daily was given to hypertensive patients on thiazides with or without beta-blockers, their blood pressure increased by 8 to 10 mmHg.[1] The diastolic blood pressures of 7 hypertensive patients treated with **pindolol** 15 mg daily or **propranolol** 80 to 160 mg daily rose from 82 to 96 mmHg when they were given indometacin 100 mg daily over a 10-day period. Changes in systolic pressures were not statistically significant.[15]

In another study, indometacin 50 mg twice daily raised the systolic/diastolic blood pressures of patients on **propranolol** 60 to 320 mg daily by 14/5 mmHg when lying and 16/9 mmHg when standing.[16] This interaction has also been seen in other studies in patients on **metipranolol**,[4] **propranolol**,[2,17] **oxprenolol**,[18,19] **atenolol**,[9,20,21] and **labetalol**.[22] Two women with pre-eclampsia treated with **propranolol** or **pindolol** became markedly hypertensive (rises in blood pressure from 135/85 to 240/140 mmHg, and from 130/70 to 230/130 mmHg, respectively) within 4 to 5 days of being given indometacin to inhibit premature contractions.[23]

(g) Naproxen

A study in hypertensive patients treated with **timolol** and hydrochlorothiazide with amiloride found that naproxen 250 mg twice daily caused a significant 4 mmHg rise in diastolic blood pressure, but did not significantly increase systolic blood pressure.[24] Similarly, in another study, naproxen 500 mg twice daily caused an average 4 mmHg rise in systolic blood pressure in patients on **atenolol**, but did not significantly increase diastolic blood pressure.[25] In contrast, another study found that naproxen caused no changes in hypertension controlled with **propranolol**,[26] and a study in patients with on antihypertensives [drugs not specified] found that naproxen did not cause clinically significant increases in blood pressure.[1] A case report describes one patient on **propranolol** who had a marked rise in blood pressure when given naproxen.[27]

(h) Oxaprozin

A study in 32 hypertensive arthritic patients found that oxaprozin 1.2 g daily for 4 weeks did not affect the antihypertensive effects of **metoprolol** 100 mg twice daily, although at 2 weeks there was a significant increase in systolic blood pressure.[28]

(i) Piroxicam

A double-blind study found that about one-quarter of the patients given piroxicam 20 mg daily and **propranolol** 80 to 160 mg daily developed diastolic pressure rises of 10 mmHg or more when lying or standing.[29,30] Increases in both systolic and diastolic pressures (8.1/5.2 mmHg lying and 8.5/8.9 mmHg standing) were seen in another study in 3 patients.[31] In contrast, patients taking **propranolol** and piroxicam 20 mg daily showed systolic/diastolic blood pressure rises of 5.8/2.4 mmHg when lying and 3.5/0.5 mmHg when standing after 2 weeks, but these increases were not statistically significant.[32] Blood pressure showed a trend towards higher levels in another study in 20 patients given **timolol** and piroxicam 20 mg daily.[24]

A study in 6 healthy subjects given **atenolol** 100 mg daily and piroxicam 20 mg daily for 7 days found no pharmacokinetic interaction. An associated study in another 6 healthy subjects given **metoprolol** 100 mg twice daily and piroxicam 20 mg daily for 7 days found that **metoprolol** levels were increased by piroxicam, but not to a statistically significant extent.[33]

(j) Sulindac

Sulindac 200 mg twice daily had little or no effect on the control of hypertension in patients taking hydrochlorothiazide with amiloride and **atenolol**, **metoprolol**, **propranolol** or **pindolol**.[10] In another study, diastolic blood pressure was slightly and significantly lower when sulindac was given with **timolol**.[24] No statistically significant rises in blood pressure occurred in other studies in patients on **propranolol**[26,29-31] or **atenolol**[21,25] or unspecified antihypertensives[1] given sulindac 200 mg twice daily. In contrast, another study claimed that patients given **propranolol** and sulindac 200 mg twice daily had systolic/diastolic blood pressure rises of 10.3/4.8 mmHg when standing and 2.4/7.1 mmHg when lying after 2 weeks, but only the increase in standing systolic blood pressure statistically significant.[32] Similarly, a crossover study in 26 hypertensive patients on **labetalol** found that sulindac 200 mg twice daily for 7 days raised the mean systolic blood pressure by 6 mmHg when sitting, and by 9 to 14 mmHg when standing, which was considered potentially clinically significant. Diastolic pressures were not affected.[22]

(k) Tenoxicam

The control of hypertension in 16 patients on **atenolol** was found not to be affected by tenoxicam 40 mg daily.[34]

Mechanism

Indometacin alone can raise blood pressure (13 hypertensive patients given indometacin 150 mg daily for 3 days had a mean systolic blood pressure rise from 118 to 131 mmHg).[35] One suggested reason is that indometacin inhibits the synthesis and release of two prostaglandins (PGA and PGE), which have a potent dilating effect on peripheral arterioles throughout the body. In their absence the blood pressure rises. Thus the hypotensive actions of the beta-blockers are opposed by the hypertensive actions of indometacin. This mechanism has been questioned and it is possible that other physiological and pharmacological mechanisms have a part to play.[1,36,37] One study found that although indometacin caused increases in blood pressure in treated hypertensive patients, other inhibitors of prostaglandin synthesis (aspirin, naproxen and sulindac) did not.[1] Further, all four drugs caused similar reductions in plasma renin activity and aldosterone concentration, which suggests that the effect of indometacin on blood pressure may not be dependent on such changes.[1]

Celecoxib, but not rofecoxib, inhibits the metabolism of metoprolol by the cytochrome P450 isoenzyme CYP2D6.[38]

Importance and management

Some of the interactions between beta-blockers and NSAIDs have been well studied and are of clinical importance, but others are not. The concurrent use of beta-blockers and indometacin need not be avoided (except perhaps in patients with eclampsia or pre-eclampsia) but anticipate the need to increase the dosage of the beta-blocker. Alternatively, exchange the indometacin for a non-interacting NSAID. Piroxicam may interact like indometacin while normally sulindac only interacts minimally or not at all. Limited data suggest that diclofenac, imidazole salicylate, oxaprozin and tenoxicam interact minimally. Some studies have shown ibuprofen and naproxen to interact, but others have not. Because the occasional patient may show a marked interaction even with these NSAIDs, it would be prudent to monitor the effects when any NSAID is given. Direct information about other NSAIDs seems not to be available. Many of the antihypertensive agents appear to be affected by this interaction so that exchanging one for another may not avoid the problem.

A few multiple-dose studies have not found aspirin to alter the antihypertensive effect of beta-blockers, even in high doses, but one single-dose study reported an interaction. Another study suggested that aspirin might attenuate the benefit of carvedilol in heart failure.

Although celecoxib increased levels of metoprolol, increases in plasma metoprolol levels of this size are unlikely to be clinically relevant.

1. Chalmers JP, West MJ, Wing LMH, Bune AJC, Graham JR. Effects of indomethacin, sulindac, naproxen, aspirin, and paracetamol in treated hypertensive patients. *Clin Exp Hypertens A* (1984) 6, 1077–93.
2. Mills EH, Whitworth JA, Andrews J, Kincaid-Smith P. Non-steroidal anti-inflammatory drugs and blood pressure. *Aust N Z J Med* (1982) 12, 478–82.
3. Sziegoleit W, Rausch J, Polák G, György M, Dekov E, Békés M. Influence of acetylsalicylic acid on acute circulatory effects of the beta-blocking agents pindolol and propranolol in humans. *Int J Clin Pharmacol Ther Toxicol* (1982) 20, 423–30.
4. Macek K, Jurin I. Effects of indomethacine and aspirin on the antihypertensive action of metipranolol — a clinical study. *Eur J Pharmacol* (1990) 183, 839–40.
5. Lindenfeld J, Robertson AD, Lowes BD, Brisow MR. Aspirin impairs reverse myocardial remodelling in patients with heart failure treated with beta-blockers. *J Am Coll Cardiol* (2001) 38, 1950–6.
6. Schäfer-Korting M, Kirch W, Axthelm T, Köhler H, Mutschler E. Atenolol interaction with aspirin, allopurinol, and ampicillin. *Clin Pharmacol Ther* (1983) 33, 283–8.
7. Spahn H, Langguth P, Kirch W, Mutschler E, Ohnhaus EE. Pharmacokinetics of salicylates administered with metoprolol. *Arzneimittelforschung* (1986) 36, 1697–9.
8. Johnsson G, Regårdh CG, Sölvell L. Lack of biological interaction of alprenolol and salicylate in man. *Eur J Clin Pharmacol* (1973) 6, 9–14.
9. Abdel-Haq B, Magagna A, Favilla S, Salvetti A. The interference of indomethacin and of imidazole salicylate on blood pressure control of essential hypertensive patients treated with atenolol. *Int J Clin Pharmacol Ther Toxicol* (1987) 25, 598–600.
10. Stokes GS, Brooks PM, Johnston HJ, Monaghan JC, Okoro EO, Kelly D. The effects of sulindac and diclofenac in essential hypertension controlled by treatment with a beta blocker and/or diuretic. *Clin Exp Hypertens A* (1991) A13, 1169–78.
11. Webster J, Petrie JC, McLean I, Hawksworth GM. Flurbiprofen interaction with single doses of atenolol and propranolol. *Br J Clin Pharmacol* (1984) 18, 861–6.
12. Radack KL, Deck CC, Bloomfield SS. Ibuprofen interferes with the efficacy of antihypertensive drugs. A Randomized, double-blind, placebo-controlled trial of ibuprofen compared with acetaminophen. *Ann Intern Med* (1987) 107, 628–35.
13. Reid ALA. Antihypertensive effect of thiazides. *Med J Aust* (1981) 2, 109–10.
14. Davies JG, Rawlins DC, Busson M. Effect of ibuprofen on blood pressure control by propranolol and bendrofluazide. *J Int Med Res* (1988) 16, 173–81.
15. Durão V, Prata MM, Gonçalves LMP. Modification of antihypertensive effects of β-adrenoceptor blocking agents by inhibition of endogenous prostaglandin synthesis. *Lancet* (1977) ii, 1005–7.
16. Watkins J, Abbott EC, Hensby CN, Webster J, Dollery CT. Attenuation of hypotensive effects of propranolol and thiazide diuretics by indomethacin. *BMJ* (1980) 281, 702–5.
17. Lopez-Ovejero JA, Weber MA, Drayer JIM, Sealey JE, Laragh JH. Effects of indomethacin alone and during diuretic or beta-adrenoceptor blockade therapy on blood pressure and the renin system in essential hypertension. *Clin Sci Mol Med* (1978) 55, 203S–205S.
18. Salvetti A, Arzilli F, Pedrinelli R, Beggi P, Motolese M. Interaction between oxprenolol and indomethacin on blood pressure in essential hypertensive patients. *Eur J Clin Pharmacol* (1982) 22, 197–201.
19. Sörgel F, Hemmerlein M, Lang E. Wirkung von Pirprofen und Indometacin auf die Effekte von Oxprenolol und Furosemid. *Arzneimittelforschung* (1984) 34, 1330–2.
20. Ylitalo P, Pitkäjärvi T, Pyykönen M-L, Nurmi A-K, Seppälä E, Vapaatalo H. Inhibition of prostaglandin synthesis by indomethacin interacts with the antihypertensive effect of atenolol. *Clin Pharmacol Ther* (1985) 38, 443–9.
21. Salvetti A, Pedrinelli R, Alberici A, Magagna A and Abdel-Haq B. The influence of indomethacin and sulindac on some pharmacological actions of atenolol in hypertensive patients. *Br J Clin Pharmacol* (1984) 17, 108S–111S.
22. Abate MA, Neeley JL, Layne RD, D'Alessandri R. Interaction of indomethacin and sulindac with labetalol. *Br J Clin Pharmacol* (1991) 31, 363–6.
23. Schoenfeld A, Freedman S, Hod M, Ovadia Y. Antagonism of antihypertensive drug therapy in pregnancy by indomethacin? *Am J Obstet Gynecol* (1989) 161, 1204–5.
24. Wong DG, Spence JD, Lamki L, Freeman D, McDonald JWD. Effect of non-steroidal anti-inflammatory drugs on control of hypertension by beta-blockers and diuretics. *Lancet* (1986) i, 997–1001.
25. Abate MA, Layne RD, Neeley JL, D'Alessandri R. Effect of naproxen and sulindac on blood pressure response to atenolol. *DICP Ann Pharmacother* (1990) 24, 810–3.
26. Schuna AA, Vejraska BD, Hiatt JG, Kochar M, Day R, Goodfriend TL. Lack of interaction between sulindac or naproxen and propranolol in hypertensive patients. *J Clin Pharmacol* (1989) 29, 524–8.
27. Anon. Adverse Drug Reactions Advisory Committee. Seven case studies. *Med J Aust* (1982) 2, 190–1.
28. Halabi A, Linde M, Zeidler H, König J, Kirch W. Double-blind study on the interaction of oxaprozin with metoprolol in hypertensives. *Cardiovasc Drugs Ther* (1989) 3, 441–3.
29. Ebel DL, Rhymer AR, Stahl E. Effect of sulindac, piroxicam and placebo on the hypotensive effect of propranolol in patients with mild to moderate essential hypertension. *Adv Therapy* (1985) 2, 131–42.
30. Ebel DL, Rhymer AR, Stahl E, Tipping R. Effect of Clinoril (sulindac, MSD), piroxicam and placebo on the hypotensive effect of propranolol in patients with mild to moderate essential hypertension. *Scand J Rheumatol* (1986) (Suppl), 62, 41–49.
31. Pugliese F, Simonetti BM, Cinotti GA, Ciabattoni G, Catella F, Vastano S, Ghidini Ottonelli A, Pierucci A. Differential interaction of piroxicam and sulindac with the anti-hypertensive effect of propranolol. *Eur J Clin Invest* (1984) 14, 54.
32. Baez MA, Alvarez CR, Weidler DJ. Effects of the non-steroidal anti-inflammatory drugs, piroxicam or sulindac, on the antihypertensive actions of propranolol and verapamil. *J Hypertens* (1987) 5 (Suppl): S563–S566.
33. Spahn H, Langguth P, Krauss D, Kirch W, Mutschler E. Pharmacokinetics of atenolol and metoprolol administered together with piroxicam. *Arch Pharm (Wienham)* (1987) 320, 103–7.
34. Hartmann D, Stief G, Lingenfelder M, Güzelhan C, Horsch AK. Study on the possible interaction between tenoxicam and atenolol in hypertensive patients. *Arzneimittelforschung* (1995) 45, 494–8.
35. Barrientos A, Alcazar V, Ruilope L, Jarillo D, Rodicio JL. Indomethacin and beta-blockers in hypertension. *Lancet* (1978) i, 277.
36. Frölich JC, Whorten AR, Walker L, Smigel M, Oates JA, France R, Hollifield JW, Data JL, Gerber JG, Nies AS, Williams W, Robertson GL. Renal prostaglandins: regional differences in synthesis and role in renin release and ADH action. 7th Int Congr Nephrol, Montreal, 1978. 107–114.
37. Walker LA, Frölich JC. Renal prostaglandins and leukotrienes. *Rev Physiol Biochem Pharmacol* (1987) 107, 1–72.
38. Werner U, Werner D, Rau T, Fromm MF, Hinz B, Brune K. Celecoxib inhibits metabolism of cytochrome P450 2D6 substrate metoprolol in humans. *Clin Pharmacol Ther* (2003) 74, 130–7.

Beta-blockers + Barbiturates

The plasma levels and the effects of beta-blockers that are mainly removed from the body by liver metabolism (e.g. alprenolol, metoprolol, timolol) are reduced by the barbiturates. Alprenolol concentrations are halved, but the others are possibly not affected as much. Beta-blockers that are mainly lost unchanged in the urine (e.g. atenolol, sotalol, nadolol) would not be expected to be affected by the barbiturates.

Clinical evidence

Pentobarbital 100 mg daily for 10 days at bedtime reduced the plasma levels of **alprenolol** 400 mg twice daily by 59% in 6 hypertensive patients. On day 11, the mean pulse rate at rest had risen from 70 to 74 bpm and blood pressure had risen from 134/89 to 145/97 mmHg. The changes were seen within 4 to 5 days of starting the barbiturate, and decreased within 8 to 9 days of stopping it.[1] These results confirm previous studies by the same research group using **pentobarbital** 100 mg daily in healthy subjects.[2,3] In one of these studies, **pentobarbital** was found to cause a 38% reduction in plasma **alprenolol** levels 90 minutes after a single 200-mg dose of **alprenolol**, and a 43% reduction in AUC, with no change in elimination half-life. There was also a 20% reduction in the effects of the beta-blocker on heart rate during exercise.[3] In the other study, the AUC of oral **alprenolol** was reduced by about 80%, but that of intravenous **alprenolol** was unaffected.[2]

Another study has shown that **pentobarbital** 100 mg daily for 10 days reduced the AUC of **metoprolol** 100 mg by 32% (range 2 to 46%) in 8 healthy subjects.[4] **Phenobarbital** 100 mg daily for 7 days reduced the AUC of **timolol** by 24% in 12 healthy subjects, but this was not statistically significant.[5]

Mechanism

Barbiturates are potent liver enzyme inducing agents that can increase the metabolism and clearance of other drugs from the body. Beta-blockers that are removed from the body principally by liver metabolism (e.g. alprenolol, metoprolol, timolol) can therefore possibly be cleared more quickly in the presence of a barbiturate.

Importance and management

The interaction between alprenolol and pentobarbital is well documented and likely to be of modest clinical importance when the beta-blocker is being used to treat hypertension, and possibly angina. Monitor the effects of alprenolol and increase the dose as necessary. Other barbiturates would be expected to interact similarly.

A reduced response is possible with any of the beta-blockers that are extensively metabolised (e.g. alprenolol, propranolol, metoprolol, timolol), but the effects on the AUCs of metoprolol and timolol appear to be less than with alprenolol. Detailed information about the clinical importance of this interaction with propranolol and other beta-blockers is lacking, but is likely to be minor. Any possible interaction can almost certainly be avoided by using one of the beta-blockers that are primarily lost unchanged in the urine (e.g. atenolol, nadolol).

1. Seideman P, Borg K-O, Haglund K, von Bahr C. Decreased plasma concentrations and clinical effects of alprenolol during combined treatment with pentobarbitone in hypertension. *Br J Clin Pharmacol* (1987) 23, 267–71.
2. Alvan G, Piafsky K, Lind M, von Bahr C. Effect of pentobarbital on the disposition of alprenolol. *Clin Pharmacol Ther* (1977) 22, 316–21.
3. Collste P, Seideman P, Borg K-O, Haglund K, von Bahr C. Influence of pentobarbital on effects and plasma levels of alprenolol and 4-hydroxy-alprenolol. *Clin Pharmacol Ther* (1979) 25, 423–7.
4. Haglund K, Seideman P, Collste P, Borg K-O, von Bahr C. Influence of pentobarbital on metoprolol plasma levels. *Clin Pharmacol Ther* (1979) 26, 326–9.
5. Mäntylä R, Männistö P, Nykänen S, Koponen A, Lamminsivu U. Pharmacokinetic interactions of timolol with vasodilating drugs, food and phenobarbitone in healthy human volunteers. *Eur J Clin Pharmacol* (1983) 24, 227–30.

Beta-blockers + Bile-acid binding resins

Although both colestyramine and colestipol can reduce the absorption of propranolol to some extent, this does not seem to reduce its effects. Colesevelam did not affect the absorption of metoprolol.

Clinical evidence

(a) Colesevelam

A single-dose study in 33 healthy subjects found that colesevelam 4.5 g did not alter the plasma levels of sustained-release **metoprolol** 100 mg to a clinically significant extent.[1]

(b) Colestipol

When single 120-mg doses of **propranolol** and 10-g doses of colestipol were taken together by 6 healthy subjects, the peak plasma **propranolol** levels were raised by 30%. However, if an additional 10 g dose of colestipol was taken 12 hours before the **propranolol** the peak plasma levels were decreased by 36%, and the AUC was reduced by about 30%. No changes in blood pressure or pulse rates were seen.[2]

(c) Colestyramine

When single 120-mg doses of **propranolol** and 8-g doses of colestyramine were taken together by 6 healthy subjects, the peak **propranolol** plasma levels were reduced by almost 25% and the AUC was reduced 13%. An additional dose of colestyramine 12 hours before the **propranolol** reduced the AUC by 43%. However, no changes in blood pressure or pulse rate were seen.[2] Preliminary results of another study found no significant changes in blood levels of **propranolol** occurred in 5 patients with type II hyperlipidaemia on **propranolol** 40 mg four times daily after they were given a single unstated dose of colestyramine.[3]

Mechanism

Uncertain. It seems probable that both the colestyramine and colestipol can bind to the propranolol in the gut, thereby reducing its absorption.

Importance and management

Information is limited. Even though both colestyramine and colestipol can apparently reduce the absorption of single-dose propranolol, no changes in its effects were reported,[2] suggesting that the interaction is of minimal clinical importance. There is no obvious reason for avoiding concurrent use. There seems to be no information about other beta-blockers. Colesevelam did not affect the absorption of metoprolol.

1. Donovan JM, Stypinski D, Stiles MR, Olson TA, Burke SK. Drug interactions with colesevelam hydrochloride, a novel, potent lipid-lowering agent. *Cardiovasc Drugs Ther* (2000) 14, 681–90.
2. Hibbard DM, Peters JR, Hunninghake DB. Effects of cholestyramine and colestipol on the plasma concentrations of propranolol. *Br J Clin Pharmacol* (1984) 18, 337–42.
3. Schwartz DE, Schaeffer E, Brewer HB, Franciosa JA. Bioavailability of propranolol following administration of cholestyramine. *Clin Pharmacol Ther* (1982) 31, 268.

Beta-blockers + Calcium channel blockers; Dihydropyridines

The use of beta-blockers with felodipine, isradipine, lacidipine, nicardipine, nimodipine and nisoldipine normally appears to be useful and safe. However, severe hypotension and heart failure have occurred rarely with nifedipine and nisoldipine. Changes in the pharmacokinetics of the beta-blockers and calcium channel blockers may also occur, but these changes do not appear to be clinically important.

Clinical evidence

(a) Felodipine

A double-blind crossover study in 8 healthy subjects found that over a 5-day period, **metoprolol** 100 mg twice daily did not affect the pharmacokinetics of felodipine 10 mg twice daily. On the other hand, the bioavailability and peak plasma levels of **metoprolol** were increased by 31% and 38% respectively.[1] Another study in 10 healthy subjects given felodipine 10 mg with either **metoprolol** 100 mg, **pindolol** 5 mg, **propranolol** 80 mg or **timolol** 10 mg found no changes in heart rate, PR interval or blood pressure that might be considered to be harmful to patients with hypertension or angina. However, 7 of the 10 subjects reported some increase in adverse reactions.[2]

(b) Isradipine

A preliminary report of a study in 24 healthy subjects found that **propranolol** 40 mg twice daily given with isradipine 5 mg twice daily caused some modest changes in the pharmacokinetics of both drugs (peak **propranolol** plasma levels increased by 17%, peak isradipine plasma levels reduced by 18%), but the AUCs were not significantly altered.[3] However, an earlier preliminary report by the same research group in 17 subjects found an increase in the **propranolol** AUC of 28%, a reduction in the isradipine AUC of 22% and a 59% increase in the peak **propranolol** levels.[4]

(c) Lacidipine

Twelve patients with mild to moderate hypertension not satisfactorily controlled by **atenolol** alone were given lacidipine 4 mg once daily with or without **atenolol** 100 mg daily for 14 days. There was no evidence of a significant change in drug levels, but there was a significant additive reduction in blood pressure during concurrent use compared to the reductions observed with either drug alone.[5]

Single-dose studies in 24 healthy subjects found that **propranolol** 160 mg reduced the peak plasma levels and AUC of lacidipine 4 mg by 38 and 42% respectively, while the peak plasma levels and AUC of the **propranolol** were increased by 35 and 26% respectively. There was a modest additive reduction of 4 to 6 mmHg in blood pressure, and the combination reduced heart rate, but not to an extent greater than **propranolol** alone. No significant adverse effects were seen.[6] However, a further preliminary report of a study by the same authors, in which 12 hypertensive patients were given **propranolol** 160 mg twice daily and lacidipine 4 mg daily for 2 weeks, found a non-significant 30% increase in systemic availability of lacidipine, and no change in **propranolol** pharmacokinetics. In addition, no clinically significant alterations in ECG recordings, blood pressure, or pulse rate were seen.[7]

(d) Lercanidipine

The maker notes that when lercanidipine was given with **metoprolol**, the bioavailability of lercanidipine was reduced by 50% while the bioavailability of **metoprolol** was not changed. They suggest that some adjustment of the lercanidipine dose may be needed.[8]

(e) Nicardipine

Nicardipine 30 mg did not affect the pharmacokinetics or pharmacodynamics of **atenolol** 100 mg in a single-dose study in healthy subjects.[9]

In another study, 14 healthy subjects were given nicardipine 50 mg every 12 hours and **metoprolol** 100 mg every 12 hours, alone or together, for 11 doses. **Metoprolol** plasma levels were raised by 28% by the nicardipine in the 7 subjects who were extensive metabolisers, but had no significant effect in the poor metabolisers. The extent of the beta-blockade was unchanged in all of them.[10]

Preliminary analysis of another study in healthy subjects found that the pharmacokinetics of both **propranolol** 80 mg twice daily and nicardipine 30 mg three times daily were unaffected when they were given together for 6 days.[11] However, this contrasts with two single-dose studies, which found that nicardipine 30 mg increased the AUC and peak plasma levels of a single 80-mg dose of **propranolol** by 47% and 80%, respectively,[12] and in the other study raised the AUC and peak plasma levels of an 80-mg dose of sustained-release **propranolol** to a lesser extent (17% and 22%, respectively).[13] A related single-dose study found that in elderly healthy subjects nicardipine 30 mg increased the maximum plasma levels and AUC of **propranolol** 40 mg by 99.6% and 80.8% respectively. Nicardipine caused a further decrease in blood pressure, and attenuated the reduction in heart rate seen with **propranolol** alone.[14]

A study in 8 healthy subjects found that the increase in heart rate during exercise associated with a single 40-mg dose of nicardipine was reduced by one drop of **timolol** 0.5% to each eye. Systolic blood pressure was also reduced during concurrent use, but nicardipine did not cause any further reduction in the intraocular pressure reduction produced by **timolol**.[15]

(f) Nifedipine

Nifedipine 10 mg three times daily did not alter the pharmacokinetics of **atenolol** 100 mg once daily,[16,17] **metoprolol** 100 mg twice daily[16,17] or **propranolol** 80 mg twice daily.[16] However, another study found that nifedipine 10 mg three times daily caused an increase in the peak plasma concentration and AUC of **propranolol** 80 mg twice daily of 56% and 23%, respectively.[18] There was no effect on **betaxolol**,[18] and in a single-dose study, there was no pharmacokinetic interaction between nifedipine and **atenolol**.[19] Another study found that the absorption of a single-dose of **propranolol** appeared to be faster leading to higher initial concentrations when it was given after nifedipine.[20] Regardless of the pharmacokinetic changes, none of these studies in healthy subjects found any adverse haemodynamic effects from the combination of nifedipine and these beta-blockers.[16,18,19] Similarly, in studies in patients with normal left ventricular function there was no evidence of adverse haemodynamic effects when nifedipine (single-dose sublingual[21,22] or intravenously,[23] or daily dose orally[23]) was given with **atenolol**,[23] **celiprolol**[22] or **propranolol**.[21,24] However, there are a few earlier isolated case reports of hypotension and heart failure with the combination.

Two patients with angina being treated with **alprenolol** or **propranolol** developed heart failure when they were given nifedipine 10 mg three times daily. The signs of heart failure disappeared when the nifedipine was withdrawn.[25] One out of 15 patients with hypertension and exertional angina progressively developed hypotension (90/60 mmHg) when given nifedipine 10 mg twice daily in addition to treatment with **atenolol** 50 mg daily and a diuretic for 1 month.[26] Severe and prolonged hypotension (blood pressure initially not recordable, then 60 mmHg systolic) developed in a patient with angina treated with **propranolol** 160 mg four times daily 18 days after nifedipine 10 mg three times daily was substituted for 'isosorbide', and this may have been a factor that led to fatal myocardial infarction.[27] Heart failure is also described in another patient with angina on **atenolol** and various other drugs when nifedipine 20 mg three times daily was given.[28]

A patient developed hypotension and severe bradycardia on two occasions after being given her usual antihypertensive medication of **labetalol** and extended-release nifedipine crushed and via a nasogastric tube. Crushing the nifedipine tablet altered its release characteristics so that the total dose was released quickly causing profound hypotension. The **labetalol** produced additional hypotensive effects and prevented a compensatory increase in heart rate.[29]

(g) Nimodipine

In a preliminary report of a study in 12 healthy subjects, nimodipine 30 mg three times daily for 4 days had no significant effect on the changes in heart rate, blood pressure or cardiac output seen with either **propranolol** 40 mg or **atenolol** 25 mg three times daily, or on the pharmacokinetics of the beta-blockers.[30]

(h) Nisoldipine

A single 20-mg dose of nisoldipine increased the steady-state AUC and peak plasma concentrations of **propranolol** 160 mg daily by 35% and 55% respectively. After combined treatment for 7 days, the AUC of **propranolol** was increased by 60% and the peak plasma concentration was increased by 55%. The combination enhanced blood pressure reduction to a small extent, but nisoldipine did not significantly reduce the effect of **propranolol** on heart rate.[31] Similarly, another study found that a single 20-mg dose of nisoldipine increased the AUC and peak plasma concentrations of a single 40-mg dose of **propranolol** by 43% and 68% respectively, and that the AUC and peak plasma concentrations of nisoldipine increased 30% and 57%. In this study, nisoldipine was reported to enhance beta-blockade.[32] However, the same research group later found that the steady-state pharmacokinetics of **propranolol** 80 mg twice daily and nisoldipine 10 mg twice daily were not affected by concurrent use for 7 days, but nisoldipine attenuated the decrease in forearm blood flow seen with propranolol.[33] The maker of nisoldipine notes that severe hypotension can occur when it is given at the same time as beta-blockers, and that, in isolated cases, signs of heart failure can also occur.[34]

Mechanism

Not understood. Where pharmacokinetic changes are seen, a possible reason is that the metabolism of the beta-blockers is altered by changes in blood flow through the liver. The pharmacodynamic changes with nifedipine may be explained by the fact that nifedipine reduces the contractility of the heart muscle. This is counteracted by a sympathetic reflex increase in heart rate due to nifedipine-induced peripheral vasodilation, so that the ventricular output stays the same or is even improved. The presence of a beta-blocker may oppose this to some extent by slowing the heart rate, which allows the negative inotropic effects of nifedipine to go unchecked.

Importance and management

The concurrent use of beta-blockers and the dihydropyridine calcium channel blockers is common, and normally valuable. However, isolated cases of severe hypotension and heart failure have been seen in a few patients on beta-blockers given nifedipine or nisoldipine. It has been suggested that those likely to be most at risk are patients with impaired left ventricular function[35] (which is a caution for the use of nifedipine anyway) and/or those taking beta-blockers in high dosage. Bear this in mind. It should also be noted that the topical use of beta-blockers such as timolol (as eye drops) may reduce heart rate and blood pressure. Changes in the pharmacokinetics of the beta-blockers and calcium channel blockers may also occur, but these do not appear to be clinically important. It may also be worth noting that all but one of the cases with nifedipine occurred with 'short-acting' formulations, which are now considered unsuitable for long-term management of angina or hypertension since they are associated with larger variations in blood pressure and heart rate. The remaining case was associated with the incorrect use of an extended-release nifedipine preparation.

1. Smith SR, Wilkins MR, Jack DB, Kendall MJ, Laugher S. Pharmacokinetic interactions between felodipine and metoprolol. *Eur J Clin Pharmacol* (1987) 31, 575–8.
2. Carruthers SG, Bailey DG. Tolerance and cardiovascular effects of single dose felodipine/β-blocker combinations in healthy subjects. *J Cardiovasc Pharmacol* (1987) 10 (Suppl 1), S169–S176.
3. Schran HF, Shepherd AM, Choc MM, Gonasun LM, Brodie CL. The effect of concomitant administration of isradipine and propranolol on their steady-state bioavailability. *Pharmacologist* (1989) 31, 153.
4. Shepherd AMM, Brodie CL, Carrillo DW, Kwan CM. Pharmacokinetic interaction between isradipine and propranolol. *Clin Pharmacol Ther* (1988) 43,194.
5. Lyons D, Fowler G, Webster J, Hall ST, Petrie JC. An assessment of lacidipine and atenolol in mild to moderate hypertension. *Br J Clin Pharmacol* (1994) 37, 45–51.
6. Hall ST, Harding SM, Hassani H, Keene ON, Pellegatti M. The pharmacokinetic and pharmacodynamic interaction between lacidipine and propranolol in healthy volunteers. *J Cardiovasc Pharmacol* (1991) 18, (Suppl 11), S13–S17.
7. Hall ST, Saul P, Keene ON, Hassani H. Pharmacodynamic and pharmacokinetic interaction between lacidipine and propranolol. *Pharm Res* (1992) 9 (10 Suppl), S88.
8. Zanidip (Lercanidipine hydrochloride). Napp Pharmaceuticals Ltd. UK Summary of product characteristics, January 2004.
9. Vercruysse I, Schoors DF, Musch G, Massart DL, Dupont AG. Nicardipine does not influence the pharmacokinetics and pharmacodynamics of atenolol. *Br J Clin Pharmacol* (1990) 30, 499–500.
10. Laurent-Kenesi M-A, Funck-Brentano C, Poirier J-M, Decolin D, Jaillon P. Influence of CYP2D6-dependent metabolism on the steady-state pharmacokinetics and pharmacodynamics of metoprolol and nicardipine, alone and in combination. *Br J Clin Pharmacol* (1993) 36, 531–8.
11. Macdonald FC, Dow RJ, Wilson RAG, Yee KF, Finlayson J. A study to determine potential interactions between nicardipine and propranolol in healthy volunteers. *Br J Clin Pharmacol* (1987), 23, 626P.
12. Schoors DF, Vercruysse I, Musch G, Massart DL, Dupont AG. Influence of nicardipine on the pharmacokinetics and pharmacodynamics of propranolol in healthy volunteers. *Br J Clin Pharmacol* (1990) 29, 497–501.
13. Vercruysse I, Massart DL, Dupont AG. Increase in plasma propranolol caused by nicardipine is dependent on the delivery rate of propranolol. *Eur J Clin Pharmacol* (1995) 49, 121–5.
14. Hartmann C, Vercruysse I, Metz T, Massart DL, Dupont AG. Influence of nicardipine on the pharmacokinetics of propranolol in the elderly. *Br J Clin Pharmacol* (1995) 39, 540P.
15. Yatsuka YI, Tsutsumi K, Kotegawa T, Nakamura K, Nakano S, Nakatsuka K. Interaction between timolol eyedrops and oral nicardipine or oral diltiazem in healthy Japanese subjects. *Eur J Clin Pharmacol* (1998) 54, 149–54.
16. Gangji D, Juvent M, Niset G, Wathieu M, Degreve M, Bellens R, Poortmans J, Degre S, Fitzsimons TJ, Herchuelz A. Study of the influence of nifedipine on the pharmacokinetics and pharmacodynamics of propranolol, metoprolol and atenolol. *Br J Clin Pharmacol* (1984) 17, 29S–35S.
17. Kendall MJ, Jack DB, Laugher SJ, Lobo J, Smith RS. Lack of a pharmacokinetic interaction between nifedipine and the β-adrenoceptor blockers metoprolol and atenolol. *Br J Clin Pharmacol* (1984) 18, 331–5.
18. Vinceneux Ph, Canal M, Domart Y, Roux A, Cascio B, Orofiamma B, Larribaud J, Flouvat B, Carbon C. Pharmacokinetic and pharmacodynamic interactions between nifedipine and propranolol or betaxolol. *Int J Clin Pharmacol Ther Toxicol* (1986) 24, 153–8.
19. Rosenkranz B, Ledermann H, Frölich JC. Interaction between nifedipine and atenolol: pharmacokinetics and pharmacodynamics in normotensive volunteers. *J Cardiovasc Pharmacol* (1986) 8, 943–9.
20. Bauer LA, Murray K, Horn JR, Opheim K, Olsen J. Influence of nifedipine therapy on indocyanine green and oral propranolol pharmacokinetics. *Eur J Clin Pharmacol* (1989) 37, 257–60.
21. Elkayam U, Roth A, Weber L, Kulick D, Kawanishi D, McKay C, Rahimtoola SH. Effects of nifedipine on hemodynamics and cardiac function in patients with normal left ventricular ejection fraction already treated with propranolol. *Am J Cardiol* (1986) 58, 536–40.
22. Silke B, Verma SP, Guy S. Hemodynamic interactions of a new beta blocker, celiprolol, with nifedipine in angina pectoris. *Cardiovasc Drugs Ther* (1991) 5, 681–8.
23. Rowland E, Razis P, Sugrue D, Krikler DM. Acute and chronic haemodynamic and electrophysiological effects of nifedipine in patients receiving atenolol. *Br Heart J* (1983) 50, 383–9.
24. Vetrovec GW, Parker VE. Nifedipine, beta blocker interaction: effect on left ventricular function. *Clin Res* (1984) 32, 833A.
25. Anastassiades CJ. Nifedipine and beta-blocker drugs. *BMJ* (1980) 281, 1251–2.
26. Opie LH, White DA. Adverse interaction between nifedipine and β-blockade. *BMJ* (1980) 281, 1462.
27. Staffurth JS, Emery P. Adverse interaction between nifedipine and beta-blockade. *BMJ* (1981) 282, 225.
28. Robson RH, Vishwanath MC. Nifedipine and beta-blockade as a cause of cardiac failure. *BMJ* (1982) 284, 104.
29. Schier JG, Howland MA, Hoffman RS, Nelson LS. Fatality from administration of labetalol and crushed extended-release nifedipine. *Ann Pharmacother* (2003) 37, 1420–3.
30. Horstmann R, Weber H, Wingender W, Rämsch K-D, Kuhlmann J. Does nimodipine interact with beta adrenergic blocking agents? *Eur J Clin Pharmacol* (1989) 36, A258.
31. Elliott HL, Meredith PA, McNally C, Reid JL. The interactions between nisoldipine and two β-adrenoceptor antagonists—atenolol and propranolol. *Br J Clin Pharmacol* (1991) 32, 379–85.
32. Levine MAH, Ogilvie RI, Leenen FHH. Pharmacokinetic and pharmacodynamic interactions between nisoldipine and propranolol. *Clin Pharmacol Ther* (1988) 43, 39–48.
33. Shaw-Stiffel TA, Walker SE, Ogilvie RI, Leenen FH. Pharmacokinetic and pharmacodynamic interactions during multiple-dose administration of nisoldipine and propranolol. *Clin Pharmacol Ther* (1994) 55, 661–9.
34. Syscor MR (Nisoldipine). Forest Laboratories UK Ltd. UK Summary of product characteristics, August 1998.
35. Brooks N, Cattell M, Pigeon J, Balcon R. Unpredictable response to nifedipine in severe cardiac failure. *BMJ* (1980) 281, 1324.

Beta-blockers + Calcium channel blockers; Diltiazem

The cardiac depressant effects of diltiazem and beta-blockers are additive, and although concurrent use can be beneficial, close monitoring is recommended. A number of patients, (usually those with pre-existing ventricular failure or conduction abnormalities) have developed serious and potentially life-threatening bradycardia. Diltiazem increases the serum levels of propranolol and metoprolol, but not those of atenolol, but these changes are probably not clinically important.

Clinical evidence

(a) Cardiac depressant effects

Ten patients were admitted to an intensive coronary care unit during one year with severe bradycardia (heart rates of 24 to 44 bpm) while receiving diltiazem 90 to 360 mg daily and **propranolol** 30 to 120 mg daily, **atenolol** 50 to 100 mg daily, or **pindolol** 90 mg daily. All were relatively elderly and presented with lethargy, dizziness, syncope, chest pain, and in one case pulmonary oedema. The ECG abnormalities were localised in the sinus node, the primary rhythm disorders being junctional escape rhythms, sinus bradycardia and sinus pause. These resolved within 24 hours of withdrawing the drugs, although a temporary pacemaker was needed in 4 patients.[1]

Symptomatic and severe bradyarrhythmias of this kind have been described in case reports in 16 other patients taking diltiazem with **atenolol**,[2] **carteolol**,[3] **metoprolol**,[2,4,5] **nadolol**,[6] **pindolol**,[7] **propranolol**,[2,4,6,8] or **sotalol**.[3,7] AV block with unusual ECG changes (T-wave inversion and ST-segment depression) was found in a 16-year-old girl following an overdose of diltiazem and **propranolol**.[9] In a later prospective study of hospital admissions due to cardiovascular adverse drug reactions, bradycardia, hypotension, syncope and worsening heart failure were noted in 21 patients taking beta-blockers with diltiazem. The beta-blockers involved were **propranolol** (13 patients), **atenolol** (5), **metoprolol** (2) and **oxprenolol** (1).[10] Similarly severe sinus bradycardia occurred in 8 of 59 patients in three early clinical studies of the combination of diltiazem and **propranolol**.[11-13] One patient developed congestive heart failure on the combination.[13] Four other similar clinical trials did not report any adverse effects.[14-17] In a single-dose study, one drop of **timolol** 0.5% eye drops did not cause an additional reduction in heart rate when given to healthy subjects with diltiazem 60 mg.[18]

(b) Pharmacokinetics

In healthy subjects, diltiazem increased the AUC of **propranolol** and **metoprolol** by 48 and 33% respectively, and increased the maximum serum concentrations by 45 and 71%, but **atenolol** was not significantly affected.[19] Another study found that diltiazem caused a 24 to 27% reduction in **propranolol** clearance.[20]

Mechanism

The bradycardic effects of the beta-blockers can be additive with the delay in conduction through the atrioventricular node caused by diltiazem.[7] This advantageously increases the antianginal effects in most patients, but in a few these effects may exacerbate existing cardiac abnormalities. Diltiazem apparently also inhibits the metabolism of propranolol and metoprolol, but not atenolol.[19]

Importance and management

Concurrent use is unquestionably valuable and uneventful in many patients, but severe adverse effects can develop. This is well established. A not dissimilar adverse interaction can occur with 'verapamil', (below). On the basis of 6 reports, the incidence of symptomatic bradyarrhythmia was estimated to be about 10 to 15%.[1] It can occur with different beta-blockers, even with very low doses, and any time from within a few hours of starting treatment to 2 years of concurrent use.[1] The main risk factors seem to be ventricular dysfunction, or sinoatrial or AV nodal conduction abnormalities.[1] Note that these are usually contraindications to the use of diltiazem. Patients with normal ventricular function and no evidence of conduction abnormalities are usually not at risk. Concurrent use should be well monitored for evidence of adverse effects. Changes in the pharmacokinetics of the beta-blockers may also occur, but these changes are probably not clinically important.

1. Sagie A, Strasberg B, Kusnieck J, Sclarovsky S. Symptomatic bradycardia induced by the combination of oral diltiazem and beta blockers. *Clin Cardiol* (1991) 14, 314–16.
2. Yust I, Hoffman M, Aronson RJ. Life-threatening bradycardic reactions due to beta blocker-diltiazem interactions. *Isr J Med Sci* (1992) 28, 292–4.
3. Lamaison D, Vacher D, Berenfeld A, Schandrin C, Lavarenne V. Association de diltiazem à libération prolongée et d'un bêta-bloquant dans l'hypertension artérielle. Deux cas de choc cardiogénique avec bradycardie extrême. *Therapie* (1990) 45, 411–13.
4. Lan Cheong Wah LSH, Robinet G, Guiavarc'h M, Garo B, Boles JM. États de choc au cours de l'association diltiazem-β-bloquant. *Rev Med Interne* (1992) 13, 80.
5. Kjeldsen SE, Syvertsen J-O, Hedner T. Cardiac conduction with diltiazem and beta-blockade combined. A review and report on cases. *Blood Pressure* (1996) 5, 260–3.
6. Hossack KF. Conduction abnormalities due to diltiazem. *N Engl J Med* (1982) 307, 953–4.
7. Hassell AB, Creamer JE. Profound bradycardia after the addition of diltiazem to a beta-blocker. *BMJ* (1989) 298, 675.
8. Ishikawa T, Imamura T, Koiwaya Y, Tanaka K. Atrioventricular dissociation and sinus arrest induced by oral diltiazem. *N Engl J Med* (1983) 309, 1124–5.
9. Satar S, Acikalin A, Akpinar O. Unusual electrocardiographic changes with propranolol and diltiazem overdosage: a case report. *Am J Ther* (2003) 10, 299–302.
10. Edoute Y, Nagachandran P, Svirski B, Ben-Ami H. Cardiovascular adverse drug reaction associated with combined β-adrenergic and calcium entry-blocking agents. *J Cardiovasc Pharmacol* (2000) 35, 556–9.
11. O'Hara MJ, Khurmi NS, Bowles MJ, Raftery BB. Diltiazem and propranolol combination for the treatment of chronic stable angina pectoris. *Clin Cardiol* (1987) 10, 115–23.
12. Hung J, Lamb IH, Connolly SJ, Jutzy KR, Goris ML, Schroeder JS. The effect of diltiazem and propranolol, alone and in combination, on exercise performance and left ventricular function in patients with stable effort angina: a double-blind, randomized, and placebo-controlled study. *Circulation* (1983) 68, 560–7.
13. Strauss WE, Parisi AF. Superiority of combined diltiazem and propranolol therapy for angina pectoris. *Circulation* (1985) 71, 951–7.
14. Tilmant PY, Lablanche JM, Thieuleux FA, Dupuis BA, Bertrand ME. Detrimental effect of propranolol in patients with coronary arterial spasm countered by combination with diltiazem. *Am J Cardiol* (1983) 52, 230–33.
15. Rocha P, Baron B, Delestrain A, Pathe M, Cazor J-L, Kahn J-C. Hemodynamic effects of intravenous diltiazem in patients treated chronically with propranolol. *Am Heart J* (1986) 111, 62–8.
16. Humen DP, O'Brien P, Purves P, Johnson D, Kostuk WJ. Effort angina with adequate beta-receptor blockade: comparison with diltiazem alone and in combination. *J Am Coll Cardiol* (1986) 7, 329–35.
17. Kenny J, Daly K, Bergman G, Kerkez S, Jewitt DE. Beneficial effects of diltiazem combined with beta blockade in angina pectoris. *Eur Heart J* (1985) 6, 418–23.
18. Yatsuka YI, Tsutsumi K, Kotegawa T, Nakamura K, Nakano S, Nakatsuka K. Interaction between timolol eyedrops and oral nicardipine or oral diltiazem in healthy Japanese subjects. *Eur J Clin Pharmacol* (1998) 54, 149–54.
19. Tateishi T, Nakashima H, Shitou T, Kumagai Y, Ohashi K, Hosada S, Ebihara A. Effect of diltiazem on the pharmacokinetics of propranolol, metoprolol and atenolol. *Eur J Clin Pharmacol* (1989) 36, 67–70.
20. Hunt BA, Bottorff MB, Herring VL, Self TH, Lalonde RL. Effects of calcium channel blockers on the pharmacokinetics of propranolol stereoisomers. *Clin Pharmacol Ther* (1990) 47, 584–91.

Beta-blockers + Calcium channel blockers; Verapamil

The cardiac depressant effects of verapamil and beta-blockers are additive, and although concurrent use can be beneficial, serious cardiodepression (bradycardia, asystole, sinus arrest) sometimes occurs. It has been suggested that the combination should only be given to those who can initially be closely supervised. An adverse interaction can occur even with beta-blockers given as eye drops.

Clinical evidence

(a) Adverse interactions

(i) Intravenous administration. Ventricular asystole developed when intravenous verapamil was given after the unsuccessful use of intravenous **practolol**, to treat supraventricular tachycardia in a 70-year-old man and a 6-month-old baby.[1] In a later study, the combination of intravenous verapamil and intravenous **practolol** produced a marked reduction in cardiac contractility, which was more evident when **practolol** was given first.[2]

(ii) Oral administration. In one series, 34 out of 42 patients on beta-blockers (daily dose: **atenolol** 100 mg (34 patients), **atenolol** 50 mg (2), **propranolol** 160 mg (4), **pindolol** 20 mg (1), or **metoprolol** 100 mg (1)) and verapamil 360 mg daily experienced a reduction in anginal episodes over a mean period of 6.5 months while taking both drugs. However, 12 patients needed a reduced dosage or withdrawal of one or both drugs. One had non-specific symptoms (drugs withdrawn), 2 had bradyarrhythmias (drugs withdrawn) and 6 experienced dyspnoea (3 withdrawals and 3 dosage reductions) presumed to be secondary to left ventricular failure. Other complications were tiredness (2 patients) and postural hypotension (1 patient), which were dealt with by reducing the dosage.[3] In another study in 15 patients with angina given **atenolol** and verapamil, 4 experienced profound lethargy, one had left ventricular failure and 4 had brady-

arrhythmias.[4]

Other case reports and studies describe heart failure,[5,6] dyspnoea,[5,7,8] sinus arrest,[9,10] heart block,[9,11-13] hypotension,[5,6,8,10,13-16] and bradycardia[4,5,8,10,11,14-18] in patients on verapamil and **alprenolol**,[9] **atenolol**,[6,9,10,12] **metoprolol**,[5,11,13,15] **propranolol**[7,8,14,16-18] or **pindolol**.[5] In two further cases, bradycardia occurred in patients on verapamil using **timolol** eye drops.[19,20] A further report describes bradycardia in a patient who was given **timolol** eye drops whilst taking verapamil and 'flecainide', (p.634). A number of reports noted that patients experiencing this interaction had reasonable left ventricular function.[5,10,12,19] Heart block and hypotension or cardiogenic shock has also been reported after verapamil was given with **atenolol**[21] or **propranolol** in overdose.[22]

(b) Pharmacokinetic interactions

Verapamil raised the **metoprolol** AUC in 10 patients by 33% and the peak plasma levels by 41%. The minimum pulse rate and systolic blood pressure (1 to 3 hours post-dose) were also lower than with **metoprolol** alone.[15] Similarly, in a single-dose study in 9 healthy subjects, the AUC and maximum plasma level of **metoprolol** increased by 35% and 64% respectively, and the AUC and half-life of verapamil increased by 57% and 29% respectively, on concurrent use.[23]

The pharmacokinetics of **atenolol** were not altered by verapamil in one study in a single patient.[24] In a study in 15 patients the plasma levels of verapamil and **atenolol** varied greatly during individual and concurrent use but mean concentrations were not significantly changed.[4] Although the mean AUC was not significantly increased in another study in 10 patients, individual patients had **atenolol** AUC increases of up to 112%.[25]

In healthy subjects, verapamil reduced the clearance of **propranolol** by 26 to 32% and increased its AUC by 46 to 58% after 6 days of concurrent use.[26] Similarly, in 5 patients verapamil increased the peak plasma levels of **propranolol** by 94%, and its AUC by 66%.[18] **Propranolol** did not affect the pharmacokinetics of verapamil.[18] However, in another study in healthy subjects no pharmacokinetic interaction was noted between **propranolol** and verapamil after concurrent use for 6 days.[27]

In a single-dose study, *(R)*-verapamil reduced the AUC of **talinolol** by 24% in 9 healthy subjects.[28]

Mechanism

Both beta-blockers and verapamil have negative inotropic (cardiac depressant) effects on the heart, which can be additive.[27] Given together they can cause marked bradycardia and may even depress the contraction of the ventricle completely. Verapamil can also raise the serum levels of beta-blockers that are extensively metabolised in the liver (e.g. metoprolol, propranolol), possibly by inhibiting their metabolism.[29] It is thought that verapamil affects talinolol bioavailability by modulating intestinal P-glycoprotein.[28,30]

Importance and management

Well documented and well established interactions. Although concurrent use can be uneventful and successful, the reports cited here amply demonstrate that it may not always be safe. The difficulty is identifying the patients most at risk. In the UK, the British National Formulary says that oral concurrent use should only be considered if myocardial function is well preserved, and that verapamil should not be injected in patients recently given beta-blockers because of the risk of hypotension and asystole. The British National Formulary also notes that, although 30 minutes has been suggested as a sufficient interval before giving a beta blocker when verapamil injection has been given first, the safety of this has not been established.[31]

It has been advised that the initiation of treatment should be restricted to hospital practice, where the dose of each drug can be carefully titrated and the patient closely supervised, particularly during the first few days when adverse effects are most likely to develop.[3,4,18] Some have suggested that beta-blockers that are extensively metabolised (e.g. metoprolol, propranolol) may possibly carry some additional risk because verapamil raises their serum levels.[24] However, others contend that, since the interaction occurs with atenolol, the pharmacodynamic effects are more important than any pharmacokinetic changes.[4,10,18] Note that changes of this size, or even more, in the AUC of beta-blockers have proved not to be clinically important with other enzyme inhibiting drugs.

1. Boothby CB, Garrard CS, Pickering D. Verapamil in cardiac arrhythmias. *BMJ* (1972) 2, 349.
2. Seabra-Gomes R, Rickards A, Sutton R. Hemodynamic effects of verapamil and practolol in man. *Eur J Cardiol* (1976) 4, 79–85.
3. McGourty JC, Silas JH, Solomon SA. Tolerability of combined treatment with verapamil and beta-blockers in angina resistant to monotherapy. *Postgrad Med J* (1985) 61, 229–32.
4. Findlay IN, MacLeod K, Gillen G, Elliott AT, Aitchison T, Dargie HJ. A double blind placebo controlled comparison of verapamil, atenolol, and their combination in patients with chronic stable angina pectoris. *Br Heart J* (1987) 57, 336–43.
5. Wayne VS, Harper RW, Laufer E, Federman J, Anderson ST, Pitt A. Adverse interaction between beta-adrenergic blocking drugs and verapamil-report of three cases. *Aust N Z J Med* (1982) 12, 285–9.
6. Sakurai H, Kei M, Matsubara K, Yokouchi K, Hattori K, Ichihashi R, Hirakawa Y, Tsukamoto H, Saburi Y. Cardiogenic shock triggered by verapamil and atenolol—a case report of therapeutic experience with intravenous calcium. *Jpn Circ J* (2000) 64, 893–6.
7. Balasubramian V, Bowles M, Davies AB, Raferty EB. Combined treatment with verapamil and propranolol in chronic stable angina. *Br Heart J* (1981) 45, 349–50.
8. Leon MB, Rosing DR, Bonow RO, Lipson LC, Epstein SE. Clinical efficacy of verapamil alone and combined with propranolol in treating patients with chronic stable angina pectoris. *Am J Cardiol* (1981) 48, 131–9.
9. McQueen EG. New Zealand Committee on Adverse Reactions: 14th Annual Report 1979. *N Z Med J* (1980) 91, 226–9.
10. Misra M, Thakur R, Bhandari K. Sinus arrest caused by atenolol-verapamil combination. *Clin Cardiol* (1987) 10, 365–7.
11. Eisenberg JNH, Oakley GDG. Probable adverse interaction between oral metoprolol and verapamil. *Postgrad Med J* (1984) 60, 705–6.
12. Hutchison SJ, Lorimer AR, Lakhdar A, McAlpine SG. β-blockers and verapamil: a cautionary tale. *BMJ* (1984) 289, 659–60.
13. Lee DW, Cohan B. Refractory cardiogenic shock and complete heart block after verapamil SR and metoprolol treatment. *Angiology* (1995) 46, 517–19.
14. Ljungström A, Åberg H. Interaktion mellan betareceptorblockerare och verapamil. *Lakartidningen* (1973) 70, 3548.
15. Keech AC, Harper RW, Harrison PM, Pitt A, McLean AJ. Pharmacokinetic interaction between oral metoprolol and verapamil for angina pectoris. *Am J Cardiol* (1986) 58, 551–2.
16. Zatuchni J. Bradycardia and hypotension after propranolol HCl and verapamil. *Heart Lung* (1985) 14, 94–5.
17. Rumboldt Z, Baković Z, Bagatin J. Opasna kardiodepresivna interakcija izmedu verapamila i propranolola. *Lijec Vjesn* (1979) 101, 430–2.
18. McCourty JC, Silas JH, Tucker GT, Lennard MS. The effect of combined therapy on the pharmacokinetics and pharmacodynamics of verapamil and propranolol in patients with angina pectoris. *Br J Clin Pharmacol* (1988) 25, 349–57.
19. Sinclair NI, Benzie JL. Timolol eye drops and verapamil — a dangerous combination. *Med J Aust* (1983) 1, 548.
20. Pringle SD, MacEwen CJ. Severe bradycardia due to interaction of timolol eye drops and verapamil. *BMJ* (1987) 294, 155–6.
21. Frierson J, Bailly D, Shultz T, Sund S, Dimas A. Refractory cardiogenic shock and complete heart block after unsuspected verapamil-SR and atenolol overdose. *Clin Cardiol* (1991) 14, 933–5.
22. Waxman AB, White KP, Trawick DR. Electromechanical dissociation following verapamil and propranolol ingestion: a physiologic profile. *Cardiology* (1997) 88, 478–81.
23. Bauer LA, Horn JR, Maxon MS, Easterling TR, Shen DD, Strandness DE. Effect of metoprolol and verapamil administered separately and concurrently after single doses on liver blood flow and drug disposition. *J Clin Pharmacol* (2000) 40, 533–43.
24. McLean AJ, Knight R, Harrison PM, Harper RW. Clearance-based oral drug interaction between verapamil and metoprolol and comparison with atenolol. *Am J Cardiol* (1985) 55, 1628–9.
25. Keech AC, Harper RW, Harrison PM, Pitt A, McLean AJ. Extent and pharmacokinetic mechanisms of oral atenolol-verapamil interaction in man. *Eur J Clin Pharmacol* (1988) 35, 363–6.
26. Hunt BA, Bottorff MB, Herring VL, Self TH, Lalonde RL. Effects of calcium channel blockers on the pharmacokinetics of propranolol stereoisomers. *Clin Pharmacol Ther* (1990) 47, 584–91.
27. Murdoch DL, Thomson GD, Thompson GG, Murray GD, Brodie MJ, McInnes GT. Evaluation of potential pharmacodynamic interactions between verapamil and propranolol in normal subjects. *Br J Clin Pharmacol* (1991) 31, 323–32.
28. Schwarz U, Krappweis J, Berndt A, Gramatté T. Unexpected verapamil on oral bioavailability of the β-blocker talinolol in humans. *Naunyn Schmiedebergs Arch Pharmacol* (1998) 357, (4 Suppl), R167.
29. Kim M, Shen DD, Eddy AC, Nelson WL. Inhibition of the enantioselective oxidative metabolism of metoprolol by verapamil in human liver microsomes. *Drug Metab Dispos* (1993) 21, 309–17.
30. Gramatté T, Oertel R. Intestinal secretion of intravenous talinolol is inhibited by luminal *R*-verapamil. *Clin Pharmacol Ther* (1999) 66, 239–45.
31. British National Formulary. 49th ed. London: The British Medical Association and Royal Pharmaceutical Society of Great Britain; 2005. p. 114.

Beta-blockers + Dextromoramide

An isolated report describes two patients who developed marked bradycardia and severe hypotension when given propranolol and dextromoramide following the induction of anaesthesia.

Clinical evidence, mechanism, importance and management

Two women about to undergo partial thyroidectomy were given **propranolol** 30 mg and dextromoramide 1.25 or 4 mg by injection during the pre-operative period, following the induction of anaesthesia with a barbiturate. Each woman developed marked bradycardia and severe hypotension, which responded rapidly to intravenous atropine.[1] The reasons for this response are not understood.

1. Cabanne F, Wilkening M, Caillard B, Foissac JC, Aupecle P. Interférences médicamenteuses induites par l'association propranolol-dextromoramide. *Anesth Analg Reanim* (1973) 30, 369–75.

Beta-blockers + Dextropropoxyphene (Propoxyphene)

A single-dose study has shown that the bioavailability of metoprolol is markedly increased by dextropropoxyphene. The bioavailability of propranolol is also increased, but to a lesser extent. However, there seem to be no reports of adverse reactions.

Clinical evidence, mechanism, importance and management

Preliminary results of a study suggest that after taking dextropropoxyphene for a day [dose not stated] the bioavailability of a single 100-mg oral dose of **metoprolol** was increased by almost 260% and the total body clearance was reduced by 18% in healthy subjects. The bioavailability of a single 40-mg oral dose of **propranolol** was increased by about 70%.[1] The probable reason is that the dextropropoxyphene inhibits the metabolism of these beta-blockers by the liver, so that they are cleared from the body more slowly.

Be alert for evidence of an increased response to **metoprolol** or **propranolol** if dextropropoxyphene is added, but so far there seems to be no evidence that concurrent use causes problems. No interaction would be expected with those beta-blockers that are largely excreted unchanged in the urine (e.g. **nadolol**, **sotalol**, **atenolol**)

1. Lundborg P, Regård CG. The effect of propoxyphene pretreatment on the disposition of metoprolol and propranolol. *Clin Pharmacol Ther* (1981) 29, 263–4.

Beta-blockers + Diphenhydramine

Diphenhydramine inhibits the metabolism of metoprolol, but this is probably not clinically important.

Clinical evidence

In a placebo-controlled study, a single 100-mg dose of **metoprolol** was given to 16 healthy subjects on day 3 of a 5-day course of diphenhydramine 50 mg three times daily. Diphenhydramine decreased the clearance of **metoprolol** by 46% and increased its AUC by 61% in the 10 subjects who were extensive metabolisers, but had no significant effect in the 6 poor metabolisers. However, the **metoprolol** AUC in the extensive metabolisers on diphenhydramine was still only about one-third of that in the poor metabolisers on placebo. The effect of **metoprolol** on heart rate and systolic blood pressure during exercise was also increased by diphenhydramine in extensive metabolisers. However, as before, it was not as great as the effect of **metoprolol** alone in poor metabolisers.[1]

Mechanism

Diphenhydramine inhibits the cytochrome P450 isoenzyme CYP2D6, which is responsible, in part, for the metabolism of metoprolol and some other beta-blockers (e.g. **propranolol**, **timolol**). CYP2D6 shows polymorphism, with some individuals lacking CYP2D6 activity (poor metabolisers), in whom diphenhydramine would have no effect. See 'Genetic factors', (p.4) for more on polymorphism.

Importance and management

Information appears to be limited to this study. Increases in plasma metoprolol levels of this size are unlikely to be clinically relevant. Indeed, despite the likely widespread use of 'extensively-metabolised' beta-blockers and diphenhydramine, no problems seem to have been reported.

1. Hamelin BA, Bouayad A, Méthot J, Jobin J, Desgagnés P, Poirier P, Allaire J, Dumesnil J, Turgeon J. Significant interaction between the nonprescription antihistamine diphenhydramine and the CYP2D6 substrate metoprolol in healthy men with high or low CYP2D6 activity. *Clin Pharmacol Ther* (2000) 67, 466–77.

Beta-blockers + Ergot derivatives

The use of beta-blockers with ergot derivatives in the management of migraine is not uncommon, but three cases of severe peripheral vasoconstriction and one of hypertension have been described.

Clinical evidence

A man with recurrent migraine headaches, reasonably well-controlled over a 6-year period with 2 daily suppositories of *Cafergot* (containing **ergotamine tartrate**) developed progressively painful and purple feet a short while after starting to take **propranolol** 30 mg daily. When he eventually resumed taking the *Cafergot* alone there was no further evidence of peripheral vasoconstriction.[1]

A similar situation occurred in a woman taking **oxprenolol** and **ergotamine tartrate** [dosages unknown] for some considerable time, as well as a number of other drugs. Arteriography showed severe spasm in a number of arteries, which responded eventually to an intra-arterial infusion of glyceryl trinitrate and heparin.[2] Severe pain in the legs and feet occurred in another man after taking **methysergide** 3 mg and **propranolol** 120 mg daily for 2 weeks. This failed to respond to various therapies, and in 6 days it was necessary to amputate both his legs below the knee because of gangrene.[2] A woman on **propranolol** for migraine prophylaxis became hypertensive (BP 180/120 mmHg) with a crushing substernal pain immediately after being given oxygen, prochlorperazine 5 mg and intravenous **dihydroergotamine** 750 micrograms for treating an acute migraine headache. She recovered uneventfully. She was later found to be hyperthyroid.[3]

Paradoxical exacerbation of migraine in a patient given **propranolol** 60 mg daily for angina has also been described. When taking **propranolol**, the headaches also became refractory to **ergotamine**. The migraine attacks ceased when the **propranolol** was withdrawn.[4]

These reports contrast with another stating that the use of **propranolol** with **ergotamine** was both effective and uneventful in 50 patients.[5]

Mechanism

Uncertain. One suggestion is that additive vasoconstriction occurs.[1,2] Ergot derivatives cause vasoconstriction, and the beta-blockers do the same by blocking the normal (beta-2-stimulated) sympathetic vasodilatation. The beta-blockers also reduce blood flow by reducing cardiac output.

Importance and management

Concurrent use is usually safe and effective, and there are only five reports of adverse interactions. It was suggested that at least one of these could have been due to the ergotamine alone (i.e. ergotism).[5] However, it would clearly be prudent to be extra alert for any signs of an adverse response, particularly those suggestive of reduced peripheral circulation (coldness, numbness or tingling of the hands and feet).

1. Baumrucker JF. Drug interaction — propranolol and cafergot. *N Engl J Med* (1973) 288, 916–17.
2. Venter CP, Joubert PH, Buys AC. Severe peripheral ischaemia during concomitant use of beta blockers and ergot alkaloids. *BMJ* (1984) 289, 288–9.
3. Gandy W. Dihydroergotamine interaction with propranolol. *Ann Emerg Med* (1990) 19, 221.
4. Blank NK, Rieder MJ. Paradoxical response to propranolol in migraine. *Lancet* (1973) ii, 1336.
5. Diamond S. Propranolol and ergotamine tartrate (cont.). *N Engl J Med* (1973) 289, 159.

Beta-blockers + Erythromycin

The serum levels of talinolol and possibly nadolol are increased by erythromycin, but the clinical importance of this is uncertain. The combined use of sotalol and intravenous erythromycin should generally be avoided because of the possible additive effects on QT interval prolongation.

Clinical evidence, mechanism, importance and management

A single-dose study in 8 healthy subjects found that the AUC and serum levels of **talinolol** 50 mg were increased by 51% and 26% respectively, by erythromycin 2 g. It was suggested that the increased bioavailability of **talinolol** was due to increased intestinal absorption caused by the inhibition of P-glycoprotein by erythromycin.[1] Another study, in which 7 healthy subjects were given a single 80-mg dose of **nadolol** after erythromycin 500 mg plus neomycin 500 mg every 6 hours for 2 days, suggested an increase in the rate of beta-blocker absorption (reduced time to maximum plasma level, but no effect on AUC). A decrease in the elimination half-life was also seen.[2] More study is needed to determine the clinical significance of these findings, and to establish whether or not other beta-blockers are significantly affected.

Sotalol prolongs the QT interval and should generally not be given with other drugs that do the same, such as intravenous erythromycin, because of the increased risk of torsade de pointes arrhythmia (see also 'Drugs that prolong the QT interval + Other drugs that prolong the QT interval', p.170).

1. Schwarz UI, Gramatté T, Krappweis J, Oertel R, Kirch W. P-glycoprotein inhibitor erythromycin increases oral bioavailability of talinolol in humans. *Int J Clin Pharmacol Ther* (2000) 38, 161–7.
2. du Souich P, Caillé G, Larochelle P. Enhancement of nadolol elimination by activated charcoal and antibiotics. *Clin Pharmacol Ther* (1983) 33, 585–90.

Beta-blockers + Flecainide

The combined use of flecainide and beta-blockers may have additive cardiac depressant effects. An isolated case of bradycardia and fatal AV block has been reported during the use of flecainide with sotalol, and bradycardia has been reported in a patient on flecainide given timolol eye drops.

Clinical evidence, mechanism, importance and management

A study on cardiac function and drug clearance in 10 healthy subjects found that when **propranolol** 80 mg three times daily was given with flecainide 200 mg twice daily for 4 days the AUCs of both drugs were increased by 20 to 30%, and they had some additive negative inotropic effects.[1] There is a report of a patient on flecainide 100 mg twice daily who developed bradycardia and fatal atrioventricular conduction block 3 hours after the second dose of **sotalol** 40 mg.[2] Another report describes a patient with chronic atrial fibrillation that had been stable for 5 years during treatment with flecainide and verapamil. Within 3 days of starting **timolol** 0.1% eye drops twice daily, she developed bradycardia with a heart rate of 35 to 40 bpm. The eye drops were stopped and 16 hours after the last dose, her heart rate had increased to 90 to 100 bpm.[3] Careful monitoring has therefore been recommended if beta-blockers are added to therapy with other antiarrhythmic agents. Serious cardiac depression has been seen following the use of flecainide with other drugs that have negative inotropic effects such as 'verapamil', (p.172).

1. Holtzman JL, Kvam DC, Berry DA, Mottonen L, Borrell G, Harrison LI, Conard GJ. The pharmacodynamic and pharmacokinetic interaction of flecainide acetate with propranolol: effects on cardiac function and drug clearance. *Eur J Clin Pharmacol* (1987) 33, 97–9.
2. Warren R, Vohra J, Hunt D, Hamer A. Serious interactions of sotalol with amiodarone and flecainide. *Med J Aust* (1990) 152, 277.
3. Minish T, Herd A. Symptomatic bradycardia secondary to interaction between timolol maleate, verapamil, and flecainide: a case report. *J Emerg Med* (2002) 22, 247–9.

Beta-blockers + Food or Drinks

Food can increase, decrease or not affect the bioavailability of beta-blockers, but none of the changes has been shown to be of clinical importance. The hypotensive effect of propranolol may be enhanced by fish oil. The bioavailability of celiprolol is markedly reduced by both grapefruit juice and orange juice, and that of talinolol is reduced by grapefruit juice.

Clinical evidence, mechanism, importance and management

(a) Grapefruit juice or orange juice

(i) Celiprolol. In a study 12 healthy subjects were given grapefruit juice 200 ml three times daily for 2 days and celiprolol 100 mg with the second of four 200 ml volumes of grapefruit juice on day 3 followed by 2 further 200 ml volumes of grapefruit juice on day 4. The AUC and peak plasma levels of celiprolol were reduced by about 87% and 95% of placebo phase values respectively. The half-life of celiprolol was slightly prolonged. However, no difference was demonstrated in blood pressure or heart rate.[1] In a similar study in 10 healthy subjects, 200 ml of 'normal-strength' orange juice 2 to 4 times daily for 4 days was found to reduce the AUC and peak plasma levels of a single 100-mg dose of celiprolol given on day 3 by 83% and 89% respectively. The half-life of celiprolol was prolonged from 4.6 to 10.8 hours and the renal excretion of celiprolol was reduced by 77%. However, no difference was demonstrated in blood pressure or heart rate.[2]
The mechanism is not known, but suggestions include an effect on intraduodenal pH and lipid solubility of celiprolol, or the formation of a complex between celiprolol and an ingredient of grapefruit or orange juice that interfered with celiprolol absorption. Alternatively, inhibition of uptake transporter proteins in the intestine may have reduced absorption.[1,2] Although the clinical relevance has not been assessed, the marked reduction in celiprolol bioavailability in the presence of grapefruit or orange juice suggests this interaction may be of clinical significance in some patients.[1,2] Caution is warranted.

(ii) Talinolol. Grapefruit juice 300 ml decreased the AUC of a single dose of talinolol 50 mg by 44%, and increased the maximum level by 42%, and increased the oral clearance by 62%. Similar results were seen after repeated administration of grapefruit juice over 6 days. However, the haemodynamic effects of talinolol were not altered by grapefruit juice.[3] Because P-glycoprotein levels did not appear to be affected by grapefruit juice, it was suggested that constituents in the juice might inhibit an uptake process other than P-glycoprotein. [Note that, in contrast, a study in *animals* found that the bioavailability of talinolol was increased by grapefruit juice.[4]] The decreases in talinolol levels are unlikely to be clinically relevant.

(b) Fish oil

In a study 36 patients with mild hypertension were given either **propranolol** 80 mg daily or fish oil 9 g daily (as capsules and equivalent to **eicosapentanoic acid** 1.8 g and **docosahexaenoic acid** 1.1 g daily) for 36 weeks followed by 4 weeks of placebo. A further group of 16 patients were given **propranolol** 80 mg daily for 12 weeks**, propranolol** plus fish oil 9 g daily for 12 weeks, **propranolol** plus fish oil placebo for 12 weeks and finally propranolol placebo for 4 weeks. Fish oil alone decreased blood pressure to a similar extent to **propranolol**, and decreases in blood pressure with the combination were greater than with either **propranolol** or fish oil alone.[5]

The mechanism is uncertain, but fish oil might be expected to enhance the hypotensive effect of beta-blockers.

(c) Food

Food increased the AUC of **propranolol** by 50 to 80%,[6-8] **metoprolol** by about 40%[6] and of **labetalol** by about 40%[9] probably by changing the extent of their metabolism during their first pass through the liver.[7-9] Food did not affect the extent of absorption of a sustained-release formulation of **propranolol**.[7] Food had very little effect on the absorption of **oxprenolol**[10,11] or **pindolol**,[12] whereas the AUC of **atenolol** was reduced by about 20%.[13] A later study suggested **atenolol** (and possibly other hydrophilic beta-blockers) become tightly associated with bile acid micelles, preventing their absorption.[14] None of these changes has been shown to be of clinical importance, nor is it clear whether it matters if patients take these drugs in a regular pattern in relation to meals. Beta-blocker serum concentrations vary widely between patients (a 20-fold difference in propranolol AUC has been noted between individuals),[6] and individualising the dose is therefore the major issue.

1. Lilja JJ, Backman JT, Laitila J, Luurila H, Neuvonen PJ. Itraconazole increases but grapefruit juice greatly decreases plasma concentrations of celiprolol. *Clin Pharmacol Ther* (2003) 73, 192–8.
2. Lilja JJ, Juntti-Patinen L, Neuvonen PJ. Orange juice substantially reduces the bioavailability of the β-adrenergic-blocking agent celiprolol. *Clin Pharmacol Ther* (2004) 75, 184–90.
3. Schwarz UI, Seemann D, Oertel R, Miehlke S, Kuhlisch E, Fromm MF, Kim RB, Bailey DG, Kirch W. Grapefruit juice ingestion significantly reduces talinolol bioavailability. *Clin Pharmacol Ther* (2005) 77, 291–301.
4. Spahn-Langguth H. Langguth P. Grapefruit juice enhances intestinal absorption of the P-glycoprotein substrate talinolol. *Eur J Pharm Sci* (2001) 12, 361–7.
5. Singer P, Melzer S, Goschel M, Augustin S. Fish oil amplifies the effect of propranolol in mild essential hypertension. *Hypertension* (1990) 16, 682–91.
6. Melander A, Danielson K, Scherstén B, Wåhlin E. Enhancement of the bioavailability of propranolol and metoprolol by food. *Clin Pharmacol Ther* (1977) 22, 108–12.
7. Liedholm H, Melander A. Concomitant food intake can increase the bioavailability of propranolol by transient inhibition of its presystemic primary conjugation. *Clin Pharmacol Ther* (1986) 40, 29–36.
8. McLean AJ, Isbister C, Bobik A, Dudley F. Reduction of first-pass hepatic clearance of propranolol by food. *Clin Pharmacol Ther* (1981) 30, 31–4.
9. Daneshmend TK, Roberts CJC. The influence of food on the oral and intravenous pharmacokinetics of a high clearance drug: a study with labetalol. *Br J Clin Pharmacol* (1982) 14, 73–8.
10. Dawes CP, Kendall MJ, Welling PG. Bioavailability of conventional and slow-release oxprenolol in fasted and nonfasted individuals. *Br J Clin Pharmacol* (1979) 7, 299–302.
11. John VA, Smith SE. Influence of food intake on plasma oxprenolol concentrations following oral administration of conventional and Oros preparations. *Br J Clin Pharmacol* (1985) 19, 191S–195S.
12. Kiger JL, Lavene D, Guillaume MF, Guerret M, Longchampt J. The effect of food and clopamide on the absorption of pindolol in man. *Int J Clin Pharmacol Biopharm* (1976) 13, 228–32.
13. Melander A, Stenberg P, Liedholm H, Scherstén B, Wåhlin-Boll E. Food-induced reduction in bioavailability of atenolol. *Eur J Clin Pharmacol* (1979) 16, 327–30.
14. Barnwell SG, Laudanski T, Dwyer M, Story MJ, Guard P, Cole S, Attwood D. Reduced bioavailability of atenolol in man: the role of bile acids. *Int J Pharmaceutics* (1993) 89, 245–50.

Beta-blockers + Haloperidol

An isolated case report describes severe hypotension and cardiopulmonary arrest in a woman shortly after she was given haloperidol and propranolol. Plasma levels of haloperidol in three patients were not significantly changed by propranolol. The concurrent use of sotalol and haloperidol should generally be avoided because of the possible increased risk of QT prolongation.

Clinical evidence, importance and management

A middle-aged woman with schizophrenia and hypertension experienced three episodes of severe hypotension within 30 to 120 minutes of being given **propranolol** 40 to 80 mg and haloperidol 10 mg.[1] On two of the occasions she had a cardiopulmonary arrest. She fainted each time, became cyanotic, had no palpable pulses and had severe hypotension, but rapidly responded to cardiopulmonary resuscitation. She suffered no adverse consequences.[1]

A study found that the steady-state plasma levels of haloperidol 6 to 15 mg daily were not significantly changed in 3 patients by incremental doses of long-acting **propranolol** up to 480 mg daily.[2]

The reasons for the severe hypotension in one case are not understood. Haloperidol alone can cause hypotension, as can **propranolol**.

This seems to be the only case of this interaction on record. Bearing in mind the widespread use of **propranolol**, other beta-blockers and haloperidol, this interaction is obviously rare. There would seem to be little reason for avoiding concurrent use.

Note that both haloperidol and **sotalol** can prolong the QT interval and should therefore not generally be used together, see 'Drugs that prolong the QT interval + Other drugs that prolong the QT interval', p.170.

1. Alexander HE, McCarty K, Giffen MB. Hypotension and cardiopulmonary arrest associated with concurrent haloperidol and propranolol therapy. *JAMA* (1984) 252, 87–8.
2. Greendyke RM, Kanter DR. Plasma propranolol levels and their effect on plasma thioridazine and haloperidol concentrations. *J Clin Psychopharmacol* (1987) 7, 178–82

Beta-blockers + H_2-blockers; Cimetidine

The blood levels of some extensively metabolised beta-blockers (e.g. metoprolol, propranolol) can be doubled by cimetidine, but normally this appears to be clinically unimportant. No important interaction normally seems to occur with other beta-blockers. An isolated report describes profound bradycardia in a patient given atenolol and cimetidine. Marked hypotension occurred in two patients on labetalol and cimetidine, and an irregular heart beat in yet another taking metoprolol and cimetidine.

Clinical evidence

(A) Beta-blockers showing raised levels

(a) Atenolol

A brief mention of a patient taking a beta-blocker for angina who developed profound sinus bradycardia (36 bpm) and hypotension when additionally treated with cimetidine was made in a report.[1] The beta-blocker was not specified, but it was identified as atenolol elsewhere in a letter.[2] However, see also (B) below.

(b) Bisoprolol

A study in 6 healthy subjects found that the maximum plasma level, AUC and clearance of bisoprolol were not significantly affected by cimetidine[3,4] although an analysis of the results by other authors suggested that cimetidine may cause a significant reduction in the renal clearance of bisoprolol.[5]

(c) Labetalol

The AUC and bioavailability of a single 200-mg oral dose of labetalol was increased by 66% and 56% respectively, in 6 healthy subjects who took cimetidine 400 mg four times daily for 4 days.[6] One subject developed postural hypotension (70/40 mmHg), felt light-headed and almost fainted on standing.[6] Conversely, the AUC of intravenous labetalol was unaffected by cimetidine.[6]

(d) Metoprolol

A study in 6 healthy subjects given metoprolol 100 mg twice daily for a week found that the cimetidine 1 g daily in divided doses increased the peak plasma levels of metoprolol by 70% and the AUC by 61%, but this did not increase the effect of metoprolol on the heart rate during exercise.[7-9] Metoprolol did not affect cimetidine pharmacokinetics.[9]

Three other studies confirmed that cimetidine increased metoprolol serum levels after single or multiple doses, and that this did not increase the effect of metoprolol on the heart rate during exercise.[10-13] However, two other studies found cimetidine did not affect serum levels of a single 100-mg metoprolol dose.[14,15] An isolated case describes one patient who complained of a "very irregular heart beat" while taking both drugs, which was much less marked when he took the two drugs separated by as much time as possible.[16]

(e) Nebivolol

Cimetidine 400 mg twice daily increased the AUC and peak plasma levels of a single 5-mg dose of nebivolol by 48% and 23% respectively, but did not alter the effect of nebivolol on blood pressure or heart rate.[17]

(f) Pindolol

Cimetidine 1 g daily in divided doses increased the AUC and peak plasma levels of pindolol 10 mg twice daily by 30% and 33% respectively, although these changes were not statistically significant.[18] In another study, cimetidine 400 mg twice daily increased the AUC of the pindolol by about 40% and decreased the renal clearance by about 35%.[19]

(g) Propranolol

Cimetidine 300 mg four times daily for a week was given to 12 healthy subjects with propranolol 80 mg every 12 hours from day 3 onwards. The mean steady-state blood levels of propranolol were raised by 47%, the AUC by 47% and the half-life was prolonged by 17%, but cimetidine did not alter the effect of propranolol on heart rate.[20] A number of other single-dose and steady-state studies confirmed that cimetidine caused rises of 35 to 136% in the blood levels and AUC of propranolol,[7-9,21-28] but that this did not increase the effect of the beta-blocker on blood pressure,[22,24,25] or on heart rate at either at rest or during exercise.[7,22-25] In contrast, one study did show a further reduction in heart rate when cimetidine was given with propranolol.[29] A letter describes one patient given cimetidine 1 g daily for 6 weeks who had an increase in serum propranolol level of about threefold and an AUC increase of 340% when a single 80-mg dose of propranolol was given.[1] In one study, the increase in steady-state propranolol AUC tended to be higher when cimetidine was given simultaneously with propranolol than when they were given separated by 10 hours (41% versus 26%), but the difference was not significant.[30]

In one study propranolol did not affect cimetidine pharmacokinetics.[9]

(B) Beta-blockers not affected

Three well controlled studies in healthy subjects and patients found that cimetidine did not significantly alter blood levels of **atenolol**, nor did it alter the affect of **atenolol** on heart rate.[7-9,14,15,18] **Atenolol** did not affect cimetidine pharmacokinetics.[9]

Similarly, the blood levels and pharmacokinetics of **betaxolol**,[26] **carvedilol**,[31] **nadolol**,[24] and **penbutolol**[18,32] were unaffected by cimetidine, and the effects of the beta-blockers on heart rate and blood pressure were not changed.[24,32] A study *in animals* found that the pharmacokinetics of **acebutolol** were not affected by cimetidine, which suggests that a clinical interaction is unlikely.[33]

A double-blind study in 12 healthy subjects found that cimetidine 400 mg twice daily for 3 days did not modify the effect of a single drop of 0.5% **timolol** put into each eye on heart rate or intraocular pressure to a statistically significant or clinically relevant extent.[34]

Mechanism

The blood levels of beta-blockers extensively metabolised in the liver by the cytochrome P450 isoenzyme CYP2D6 (e.g. propranolol, metoprolol and nebivolol) are increased because cimetidine reduces their metabolism by inhibiting the activity of the liver enzymes. It is unclear why cimetidine affects labetalol, a beta-blocker that is extensively metabolised, but not by CYP2D6.[6] Other extensively metabolised beta-blockers not affected by cimetidine include betaxolol, carvedilol, and penbutolol. Pindolol is partly excreted by an active renal tubular secretion mechanism, and cimetidine increases pindolol blood levels by inhibiting this mechanism.[19] Cimetidine may reduce renal clearance of bisoprolol by a similar mechanism.[4] Those beta-blockers that are largely excreted unchanged in the urine (e.g. atenolol, nadolol) are not affected by cimetidine.[15,24]

Importance and management

Well studied and established interactions but, despite the considerable rises in blood levels that can occur with some beta-blockers, the effects normally appear to be clinically unimportant. Concurrent use is common, but only one isolated case of profound bradycardia involving atenolol appears to have been reported (see case cited above). Marked hypotension also seems to be rare. Combined use need not be avoided, however it has been suggested that patients with impaired liver function who are given beta-blockers that are extensively metabolised in the liver (e.g. metoprolol, propranolol) might possibly develop grossly elevated blood levels, which could cause adverse effects. This needs confirmation.

1. Donovan MA, Heagerty AM, Patel L, Castleden M, Pohl JEF. Cimetidine and bioavailability of propranolol. *Lancet* (1981) i, 164.
2. Rowley-Jones D, Flind AC. Drug interactions with cimetidine. *Pharm J* (1981) 283, 659.
3. Kirch W, Rose I, Klingmann I, Pabst J, Ohnhaus EE. Interaction of bisoprolol with cimetidine and rifampicin. *Eur J Clin Pharmacol* (1986) 31, 59–62.
4. Kirch W, Ohnhaus EE, Pabst J. Reply. *Eur J Clin Pharmacol* (1987) 33, 110.
5. Somogyi A, Muirhead M. Interaction of cimetidine with bisoprolol. *Eur J Clin Pharmacol* (1987) 33, 109–110.
6. Daneshmend TK, Roberts CJC. The effects of enzyme induction and enzyme inhibition on labetalol pharmacokinetics. *Br J Clin Pharmacol* (1984) 18, 393–400.
7. Kirch W, Spahn H, Köhler H, Mutschler E. Accumulation and adverse effects of metoprolol and propranolol after concurrent administration of cimetidine. *Arch Toxicol* (1983) (Suppl 6), 379–83.
8. Kirch W, Spahn H, Köhler H, Mutschler E. Interaction of metoprolol, propranolol and atenolol with cimetidine. *Clin Sci* (1982) 63, 451S–453S.
9. Kirch W, Spahn H, Köhler H, Mutschler E. Influence of β-receptor antagonists on the pharmacokinetics of cimetidine. *Drugs* (1983) 25 (Suppl 2), 127–30.
10. Kendall MJ, Laugher SJ, Wilkins MR. Ranitidine, cimetidine and metoprolol: a pharmacokinetic interaction study. *Gastroenterology* (1986) 90, 1490.
11. Kirch W, Rämsch K, Janisch HD, Ohnhaus EE. The influence of two histamine H_2-receptor antagonists, cimetidine and ranitidine, on plasma levels and clinical effect of nifedipine and metoprolol. *Arch Toxicol* (1984) (Suppl 7), 256–9.
12. Chellingsworth MC, Laugher S, Akhlaghi S, Jack DB, Kendall MJ. The effects of ranitidine and cimetidine on the pharmacokinetics and pharmacodynamics of metoprolol. *Aliment Pharmacol Ther* (1988) 2, 521–7.
13. Toon S, Davidson EM, Garstang FM, Batra H, Bowes RJ, Rowland M. The racemic metoprolol H_2-antagonist interaction. *Clin Pharmacol Ther* (1988) 43, 283–9.
14. Houtzagers JJR, Streurman O, Regårdh CG. The effect of pretreatment with cimetidine on the bioavailability and disposition of atenolol and metoprolol. *Br J Clin Pharmacol* (1982) 14, 67–72.
15. Ellis ME, Hussain M, Webb AK, Barker NP, Fitzsimons TJ. The effect of cimetidine on the relative cardioselectivity of atenolol and metoprolol in asthmatic patients. *Br J Clin Pharmacol* (1984) 17, 59S–64S.
16. Anon. Adverse Drug Reactions Advisory Committee. Seven case studies. *Med J Aust* (1982) 2, 190–1.
17. Kamali F, Howes A, Thomas SHL, Ford GA, Snoeck E. A pharmacokinetic and pharmacodynamic interaction study between nebivolol and the H_2-receptor antagonists cimetidine and ranitidine. *Br J Clin Pharmacol* (1997) 43, 201–4.
18. Mutschler E, Spahn H, Kirch W. The interaction between H2-receptor antagonists and β-adrenoceptor blockers. *Br J Clin Pharmacol* (1984) 17, 51S–57S.
19. Somogyi AA, Bochner F, Sallustio BC. Stereoselective inhibition of pindolol renal clearance by cimetidine in humans. *Clin Pharmacol Ther* (1992) 51, 379–87.
20. Donn KH, Powell JR, Rogers JF, Eshelman FN. The influence of H2-receptor antagonists on steady-state concentrations of propranolol and 4-hydroxypropranolol. *J Clin Pharmacol* (1984) 24, 500–8.
21. Kirch W, Köhler H, Spahn H, Mutschler E. Interaction of cimetidine with metoprolol, propranolol or atenolol. *Lancet* (1981) ii, 531–2.
22. Reimann IW, Klotz U, Frölich JC. Effects of cimetidine and ranitidine on steady-state propranolol kinetics and dynamics. *Clin Pharmacol Ther* (1982) 32, 749–57.
23. Reimann IW, Klotz U, Siems B, Frölich JC. Cimetidine increases steady-state plasma levels of propranolol. *Br J Clin Pharmacol* (1981) 12, 785–90.
24. Duchin KL, Stern MA, Willard DA, McKinstry DN. Comparison of kinetic interactions of nadolol and propranolol with cimetidine. *Am Heart J* (1984) 108, 1084–6.
25. Markiewicz A, Hartleb M, Lelek A, Boldys H, Nowak A. The effect of treatment with cimetidine and ranitidine on bioavailability of, and circulatory response to, propranolol. *Zbl Pharm* (1984) 123, 516–18.
26. Rey E, Jammet P, d'Athis P, de Lauture D, Christoforov B, Weber S, Olive G. Effect of cimetidine on the pharmacokinetics of the new beta-blocker betaxolol. *Arzneimittelforschung* (1987) 37, 953–6.
27. Heagerty AM, Donovan MA, Castleden CM, Pohl JF, Patel L, Hedges A. Influence of cimetidine on pharmacokinetics of propranolol. *BMJ* (1981) 282, 1917–19.
28. Heagerty AM, Donovan MA, Casteleden CM, Pohl JEF, Patel L. The influence of histamine (H_2) antagonists on propranolol pharmacokinetics. *Int J Clin Pharmacol Res* (1982) 2, 203–5.
29. Feely J, Wilkinson GR, Wood AJJ. Reduction in liver blood flow and propranolol metabolism by cimetidine. *N Engl J Med* (1981) 304, 692–5.
30. Asgharnejad M, Powell JR, Donn KH, Danis M. The effect of cimetidine dose timing on oral propranolol kinetics in adults. *J Clin Pharmacol* (1988) 28, 339–43.
31. Data on file, database on carvedilol, SmithKline Beecham, quoted by Ruffolo RR, Boyle DA, Venuti RP, Lukas MA. Carvedilol (Kredex®): a novel multiple action cardiovascular agent. *Drugs Today* (1991) 27, 465–92.
32. Spahn H, Kirch W, Hajdu P, Mutschler E, Ohnhaus EE. Penbutolol pharmacokinetics: the influence of concomitant administration of cimetidine. *Eur J Clin Pharmacol* (1986) 29, 555–60.
33. Mostafavi SA, Foster RT. Influence of cimetidine co-administration on the pharmacokinetics of acebutolol enantiomers and its metabolite diacetolol in a rat model: the effect of gastric pH on double-peak phenomena. *Int J Pharm* (2003) 255, 81–6.
34. Ishii Y, Nakamura K, Tsutsumi K, Kotegawa, Nakano S, Natasuka K. Drug interaction between cimetidine and timolol ophthalmic solution: effect on heart rate and intraocular pressure in healthy Japanese volunteers. *J Clin Pharmacol* (2000) 40, 193–9.

Beta-blockers + H_2-blockers; Famotidine

Famotidine does not interact with beta-blockers.

Clinical evidence, mechanism, importance and management

A survey of 15 patients taking beta-blockers (**acebutolol**, **atenolol**, **betaxolol**, **nadolol**, **pindolol**, **propranolol** or **sotalol**) for 6 to 8 weeks found no evidence of changes in antihypertensive effects or bradycardia while they were taking famotidine 40 mg daily.[1] No interaction would be expected, and no special precautions would seem necessary if famotidine is taken with these or any other beta-blocker.

1. Chichmanian RM, Mignot G, Spreux A, Jean-Girard C, Hofliger P. Tolérance de la famotidine. Étude due réseau médecins sentinelles en pharmacovigilance. *Therapie* (1992) 47, 239–43.

Beta-blockers + H_2-blockers; Nizatidine

The bradycardic effects of atenolol are increased by nizatidine.

Clinical evidence, mechanism, importance and management

After taking **atenolol** 100 mg daily for 7 days the mean resting heart rate of 12 healthy subjects fell from 63.7 to 53.1 bpm 3 hours after dosing. A further fall of 6 bpm occurred when they were additionally given nizatidine 300 mg daily for 7 days. Nizatidine alone caused a fall in heart rate of about 8 bpm.[1] Thus the effects of nizatidine and **atenolol** on heart rate appear to be additive. It seems likely that nizatidine would have the same effects in the presence of other beta-blockers. The clinical significance of these effects is uncertain, but it might be important in elderly patients.[1] More study is needed.

1. Halabi A, Kirch W. Negative chronotropic effects of nizatidine. *Gut* (1991) 32, 630–4.

Beta-blockers + H_2-blockers; Ranitidine

Ranitidine does not alter the steady-state plasma levels of atenolol, nebivolol, propranolol or tertatolol and their therapeutic effects remain unchanged. Some studies have shown moderate rises in metoprolol levels, but these are not clinically important.

Clinical evidence

The plasma levels of **metoprolol** 100 mg twice daily were unaffected by ranitidine 300 mg daily for 7 days in 12 healthy subjects.[1] Two other studies have confirmed that ranitidine did not significantly affect the plasma levels of **metoprolol**.[2-5] However, these studies found increases of up to 38% in the AUC of single intravenous or oral doses of **metoprolol**,[2-5] and another study found that ranitidine increased the AUC and plasma concentrations of **metoprolol** 100 mg twice daily, by 55 and 34%, respectively.[6-8] All of these studies found that ranitidine did not alter the effect of **metoprolol** on heart rate during exercise.[1,2,5,6]

Ranitidine 300 mg daily for 6 days did not affect the steady-state plasma levels of **propranolol** 160 mg daily nor did it alter the effect of **propranolol** on heart rate or blood pressure in 5 healthy subjects.[9] Similarly no changes in plasma **propranolol** levels were seen in other multiple-dose[10] or single-dose studies.[11-14]

Similarly, in other studies, ranitidine 150 mg twice daily did not significantly alter the pharmacokinetic or pharmacodynamic effects of a single 5-mg dose of nebivolol,[15] a single 5-mg dose of **tertatolol**,[16] or **atenolol** 100 mg daily for 7 days.[6,8]

Mechanism

The rises in metoprolol serum levels caused by ranitidine in the two single-dose metoprolol studies are not understood, nor is it clear why one of four studies found an increase after multiple doses.

Importance and management

The possible effects of ranitidine on the plasma levels and effects of propranolol and metoprolol have been well studied. Although some studies have shown moderate rises in metoprolol levels, particularly after single-doses, these increases are of a magnitude that is unlikely to be clinically important. Less is known about atenolol, nebivolol and tertatolol, although no clinically relevant interactions have been seen. There is nothing to suggest that the concurrent use of ranitidine and any beta-blocker should be avoided, nor that there is any need to take particular precautions.

1. Toon S, Davidson EM, Garstang FM, Batra H, Bowers RJ, Rowland M. The racemic metoprolol H_2-antagonist interaction. *Clin Pharmacol Ther* (1988) 43, 283–9.
2. Kelly JG, Salem SAM, Kinney CD, Shanks RG, McDevitt DG. Effects of ranitidine on the disposition of metoprolol. *Br J Clin Pharmacol* (1985) 19, 219–24.
3. Kelly JG, Shanks RG, McDevitt DG. Influence of ranitidine on plasma metoprolol concentrations. *BMJ* (1983) 287, 1218–19.
4. Kendall MJ, Laugher SJ, Wilkins MR. Ranitidine, cimetidine and metoprolol-a pharmacokinetic interaction study. *Gastroenterology* (1986) 90, 1490.
5. Chellingsworth MC, Laugher S, Akhlaghi S, Jack DB, Kendall MJ. The effects of ranitidine and cimetidine on the pharmacokinetics and pharmacodynamics of metoprolol. *Aliment Pharmacol Ther* (1988) 2, 521–7.
6. Spahn H, Mutschler E, Kirch W, Ohnhaus EE, Janisch HD. Influence of ranitidine on plasma metoprolol and atenolol concentrations. *BMJ* (1983) 286, 1546–7.
7. Kirch W, Rämsch K, Janisch HD, Ohnhaus EE. The influence of two histamine H_2-receptor antagonists, cimetidine and ranitidine, on the plasma levels and clinical effect of nifedipine and metoprolol. *Arch Toxicol* (1984) 7 (Suppl), 256–9.
8. Mutschler E, Spahn H, Kirch W. The interaction between H_2-receptor antagonists and beta-adrenoceptor blockers. *Br J Clin Pharmacol* (1984) 17, 51S–57S.
9. Reimann IW, Klotz U, Frölich JC. Effects of cimetidine and ranitidine on steady-state propranolol kinetics and dynamics. *Clin Pharmacol Ther* (1982) 32, 749–57.
10. Donn KH, Powell JR, Rogers JF, Eshelman FN. The influence of H_2-receptor antagonists on steady-state concentrations of propranolol and 4-hydroxypropranolol. *J Clin Pharmacol* (1984) 24, 500–8.
11. Markiewicz A, Hartleb M, Lelek H, Boldys H, Nowak A. The effect of treatment with cimetidine and ranitidine on bioavailability of, and circulatory response to, propranolol. *Zbl Pharm* (1984) 123, 516–18.
12. Heagerty AM, Castleden CM, Patel L. Failure of ranitidine to interact with propranolol. *BMJ* (1982) 284, 1304.
13. Heagerty AM, Donovan MA, Casteleden CM, Pohl JEF, Patel L. The influence of histamine (H_2) antagonists on propranolol pharmacokinetics. *Int J Clin Pharmacol Res* (1982) 2, 203–5.
14. Patel L, Weerasuriya K. Effect of cimetidine and ranitidine on propranolol clearance. *Br J Clin Pharmacol* (1983) 15, 152P.
15. Kamali F, Howes A, Thomas SHL, Ford GA, Snoeck E. A pharmacokinetic and pharmacodynamic interaction study between nebivolol and the H_2-receptor antagonists cimetidine and ranitidine. *Br J Clin Pharmacol* (1997) 43, 201–4.
16. Kirch W, Milferstädt S, Halabi A, Rocher I, Efthymiopoulos C, Jung L. Interaction of tertatolol with rifampicin and ranitidine pharmacokinetics and antihypertensive activity. *Cardiovasc Drugs Ther* (1990) 4, 487–92.

Beta-blockers + Hydralazine

Plasma levels of propranolol and other extensively metabolised beta-blockers (metoprolol, oxprenolol) are increased by hydralazine, but no increase in adverse effects seems to have been reported.

Clinical evidence

(a) Effect of hydralazine on beta-blockers

Single 25- and 50-mg doses of hydralazine increased the AUC of a single 40-mg dose of **propranolol** in 5 healthy subjects by 60% and 110%, and raised the peak plasma concentrations by 144 and 240% respectively.[1] Similarly, in another single-dose study, hydralazine increased the AUC of **propranolol** by 62 to 77%.[2] However, a further single-dose study using sustained-release **propranolol** found that hydralazine had no effect on **propranolol** pharmacokinetics.[3]

In other studies hydralazine increased the AUC of sustained-release **oxprenolol** by 41% at steady-state,[4] and of **metoprolol** by 30% after a single-dose[5] and by 38% at steady-state.[6] In contrast, single-dose studies found that hydralazine did not affect the AUC of **acebutolol** or **nadolol**.[5]

(b) Effect of beta-blockers on hydralazine

Oxprenolol was found not to have a significant effect on the pharmacokinetics of hydralazine.[4]

Mechanism

Uncertain. Hydralazine appears to increase the bioavailability only of those beta-blockers that undergo high hepatic extraction (e.g. propranolol, metoprolol) and not those that are largely excreted unchanged in the urine (e.g. atenolol, nadolol). Hepatic extraction is discussed in more detail under 'Changes in first-pass metabolism', (p.4). It has been suggested that hydralazine may alter hepatic blood flow or inhibit hepatic enzymes,[1,5,6] although other mechanisms may also be involved.[3,7,8]

Importance and management

Moderately well documented and established interactions, but the increased beta-blocker serum levels appear to cause no adverse clinical effect. Concurrent use is usually valuable in the treatment of hypertension. No particular precautions seem to be necessary, but the outcome should be monitored.

1. Schneck DW, Vary JE. Mechanism by which hydralazine increases propranolol bioavailability. *Clin Pharmacol Ther* (1984) 35, 447–53.
2. McLean AJ, Skews H, Bobik A, Dudley FJ. Interaction between oral propranolol and hydralazine. *Clin Pharmacol Ther* (1980) 27, 726–32.
3. Byrne AJ, McNeil JJ, Harrison PM, Louis W, Tonkin AM, McLean AJ. Stable oral availability of sustained release propranolol when co-administered with hydralazine or food: evidence implicating substrate delivery rate as a determinant of presystematic drug interactions. *Br J Clin Pharmacol* (1984) 17, 45S–50S.
4. Hawksworth GM, Dart AM, Chiang K, Parry K, Petrie JC. Effect of oxprenolol on the pharmacokinetics and pharmacodynamics of hydralazine. *Drugs* (1983) 25 (Suppl 2), 136–40.
5. Jack DB, Kendall MJ, Dean S, Laugher SJ, Zaman R, Tenneson ME. The effect of hydralazine on the pharmacokinetics of three different beta adrenoceptor antagonists: metoprolol, nadolol, and acebutolol. *Biopharm Drug Dispos* (1982) 3, 47–54.
6. Lindeberg S, Holm B, Lundborg P, Regårdh CG, Sandström B. The effect of hydralazine on steady-state plasma concentrations of metoprolol in pregnant hypertensive women. *Eur J Clin Pharmacol* (1988) 35, 131–5.
7. Svensson CK, Cumella JC, Tronolone M, Middleton E, Lalka D. Effects of hydralazine, nitroglycerin, and food on estimated hepatic blood flow. *Clin Pharmacol Ther* (1985) 37, 464–8.
8. Svensson CK, Knowlton PW, Ware JA. Effect of hydralazine on the elimination of antipyrine in the rat. *Pharm Res* (1987) 4, 515–18.

Beta-blockers + Hydroxychloroquine

Hydroxychloroquine may increase the blood levels of metoprolol, but this is probably not clinically important.

Clinical evidence, mechanism, importance and management

Hydroxychloroquine 400 mg daily for 8 days increased the AUC and peak plasma levels of a single 100-mg dose of **metoprolol** by 65% and 72% respectively,[1] in 7 healthy subjects who were extensive metabolisers, see 'Genetic factors', (p.4). Hydroxychloroquine may inhibit the metabolism of **metoprolol** by the cytochrome P450 isoenzyme CYP2D6. The clinical significance of this interaction is unknown, but changes of this size in the AUC of beta-blockers caused by other enzyme inhibiting drugs have proved not to be clinically important. Other beta-blockers that are extensively metabolised (e.g. **propranolol**) may behave similarly. More study is needed.

1. Somer M, Kallio J, Pesonen U, Pyykkö K, Huupponen R, Scheinin M. Influence of hydroxychloroquine on the bioavailability of oral metoprolol. *Br J Clin Pharmacol* (2000) 49, 549–54.

Beta-blockers + Metoclopramide

A patient with scleroderma suffered a fatal cardiac arrest after receiving postoperative intravenous labetalol and intravenous metoclopramide. Metoclopramide increased the rate of absorption of a conventional formulation of propranolol, but did not affect a sustained-release preparation.

Clinical evidence, mechanism, importance and management

(a) Labetalol

A 38-year-old patient with scleroderma, hypertension (treated with lisinopril) and gangrene of her left index finger underwent minor hand surgery. While in postoperative care her blood pressure rose to 153/120 mmHg and she was given intravenous labetalol 10 mg. About 15 minutes later she experienced nausea and vomiting, which was treated with intravenous metoclopramide 10 mg. About 5 minutes later her heart rate decreased to 38 bpm and she became unresponsive with no palpable pulse: an ECG showed junctional bradycardia. She was initially resuscitated but died about 13 hours later after a further episode of bradycardia, despite full supportive treatment. It was noted that the bradycardia did not respond well to atropine, and there was persistent hypotension, despite escalating vasopressor use. Scleroderma and lisinopril may have contributed to the failure to resuscitate the patient. However, bradycardia or heart block and hypotension may occur with intravenous metoclopramide. In this patient the use of labetalol may have exacerbated the effects of metoclopramide by causing reductions in ventricular contractility due to its beta-adrenergic effects and limiting vasoconstrictive compensatory mechanisms due to alpha-adrenergic effects.[1]

(b) Propranolol

Oral metoclopramide syrup 20 mg, given 30 minutes before sustained-release propranolol 160 mg had no effect on the pharmacokinetics of propranolol in 12 healthy subjects.[2] In contrast, an earlier brief report found that the rate of absorption of a conventional formulation of propranolol 80 mg was increased by intravenous metoclopramide 10 mg in 4 healthy subjects. In the first 2 hours after dosing, propranolol levels were increased by 1.3 to 2.5-fold.[3] However, these changes are unlikely to be clinically relevant.

1. Tung A, Sweitzer B, Cutter T. Cardiac arrest after labetalol and metoclopramide administration in a patient with scleroderma. *Anesth Analg* (2002) 95, 1667–8.
2. Charles BG, Renshaw PJ, Kay JJ, Ravenscroft PJ. Effect of metoclopramide on the bioavailability of long-acting propranolol. *Br J Clin Pharmacol* (1981) 517–18.
3. George CF, Castleden M. Propranolol absorption. *BMJ* (1977) 1, 47.

Beta-blockers + Morphine

Morphine may moderately raise the serum levels of esmolol, but this is unlikely to be clinically important. The fatal doses of morphine and propranolol are markedly reduced in *animals* when given together, but the clinical relevance of this in man is uncertain.

Clinical evidence, mechanism, importance and management

After being given a 3-mg injection of morphine sulphate the steady-state levels of a 300 microgram/kg per minute infusion of **esmolol**, given over 4 hours to 10 healthy men were generally higher, but were only statistically significantly higher (by 46%) in 2 of the subjects, and were considered to be of no clinical importance. The pharmacokinetics of morphine were unchanged.[1]

Studies in *animals* have shown that the median fatal dose of **propranolol** was reduced two to sevenfold by morphine in *mice*[2] and the median lethal dose of morphine was reduced fifteen to sixteenfold in *rats*[3] by **propranolol**. The same interaction has also been seen in *dogs*.[3] There do not appear to be any published reports of synergistic toxicity involving morphine and **propranolol**, so the clinical relevance of this is uncertain.

1. Lowenthal DT, Porter RS, Saris SD, Bies CM, Slegowski MB, Staudacher A. Clinical pharmacology, pharmacodynamics and interactions with esmolol. *Am J Cardiol* (1985) 56, 14–18F.
2. Murmann W, Almirante L, Saccani-Guelfi M. Effects of hexobarbitone, ether, morphine, and urethane upon the acute toxicity of propranolol and D-(-)-INPEA. *J Pharm Pharmacol* (1966) 18, 692–4.
3. Davis WM, Hatoum NS. Possible toxic interaction of propranolol and narcotic analgesics. *Drug Intell Clin Pharm* (1981) 15, 290–1.

Beta-blockers + Oral contraceptives

The blood levels of metoprolol are increased in women taking oral contraceptives, but the clinical importance is probably very small. Acebutolol, oxprenolol and propranolol are minimally affected.

Clinical evidence

The peak plasma levels and the AUC of a single 100-mg dose of **metoprolol** were 36 and 70% higher respectively in 12 women on low-dose combined oral contraceptives when compared with a similar group not taking contraceptives, with no effect on the elimination half-life.[1] In a further study by the same research group, the AUC of **metoprolol** was 71% higher, the AUC of **oxprenolol** was 26% higher, the AUC of **propranolol** was 42% higher and the AUC of acebutolol was marginally lower in women on combined oral contraceptives compared to those not on contraceptives, but only the **metoprolol** difference was statistically significant.[2] In another study, the total clearance of a single 80-mg dose of **propranolol** was increased (although not significantly) in 8 women given **ethinylestradiol** 50 micrograms daily alone, and an even smaller increase was seen while taking a combined oral contraceptive containing **ethinylestradiol** and **norethisterone**.[3]

Mechanism

The reason for the changes appears to be that ethinylestradiol alters the metabolism of these beta-blockers. In the case of propranolol its conjugation and oxidation are increased by the ethinylestradiol.[3]

Importance and management

The changes seen with propranolol, oxprenolol and acebutolol are almost certainly too small to matter, but with metoprolol the changes are somewhat larger. Even so, changes of this size caused by the interactions of other drugs with beta-blockers are not usually clinically relevant. No special precautions therefore seem necessary if any of these beta-blockers are given to women taking combined oral contraceptives containing ethinylestradiol, or those taking ethinylestradiol alone. However, be aware that some of the indications for beta-blockers are cautions for, or preclude the use of, combined oral contraceptives.

1. Kendall MJ, Quarterman CP, Jack DB, Beeley L. Metoprolol pharmacokinetics and the oral contraceptive pill. *Br J Clin Pharmacol* (1982) 14, 120–2.
2. Kendall MJ, Jack DB, Quarterman CP, Smith SR, Zaman R. β-adrenoceptor blocker pharmacokinetics and the oral contraceptive pill. *Br J Clin Pharmacol* (1984) 17, 87S–89S.
3. Walle T, Fagan TC, Walle UK, Topmiller MJ. Stimulatory as well as inhibitory effects of ethinyloestradiol on the metabolic clearances of propranolol in young women. *Br J Clin Pharmacol* (1996) 41, 305–9.

Beta-blockers + Phenothiazines

The concurrent use of chlorpromazine and propranolol, or thioridazine and pindolol, can result in a marked rise in the plasma levels of both drugs. Propranolol also markedly increases plasma thioridazine levels. There are isolated reports of possible adverse interactions. Concurrent use of sotalol and phenothiazines that prolong the QT interval should generally be avoided.

Clinical evidence

(a) Plasma beta-blocker levels

The mean steady-state levels of **propranolol** 80 mg every 8 hours of 4 normal subjects and one hypertensive patient were raised by 70% (from 41.5 to 70.2 nanograms/ml) when they were given **chlorpromazine** 50 mg every 8 hours.[1] The increase was considerable in some subjects but barely detectable in others. A sixth subject on **propranolol** promptly fainted when getting out of bed after the first dose of **chlorpromazine**. He was found to have a pulse rate of 35 to 40 bpm and a blood pressure of 70/0 mmHg. He rapidly recovered, achieving a pulse rate of 85 and blood pressure of 120/70 when given atropine 3 mg. However, it is unclear whether the adverse effect was due to **chlorpromazine** alone, or to an interaction with **propranolol**.[1]

A brief mention of an episode of minor hypotension with **chlorpromazine** that appeared to have been exacerbated by **sotalol** has been noted in a diabetic girl.[2] Serum **pindolol** levels were 2.5-fold higher in 7 patients treated with **thioridazine** than in 17 patients treated with haloperidol, phenytoin, and/or phenobarbital.[3]

(b) Plasma phenothiazine levels

Propranolol (mean daily dose 8.1 mg/kg) increased the serum **chlorpromazine** levels of 7 schizophrenics by about 100 to 500%, and raised the plasma levels of the active metabolites of **chlorpromazine** by about 50 to 100%.[4] The same or similar work by the same authors is described elsewhere.[5] One of the patients was withdrawn from the study because he suffered a cardiovascular collapse while taking both drugs.[5] It has been suggested that the value of **propranolol** in the treatment of schizophrenia probably results from the rise in serum **chlorpromazine** levels.[5]

A schizophrenic patient taking **chlorpromazine** and **tiotixene** experienced delirium, grand mal seizures and skin photosensitivity, attributed to a rise in the serum levels of the antipsychotic drugs caused by **propranolol** in increasing doses up to a total of 1200 mg daily.[6]

Two patients stabilised on **thioridazine** 600 or 800 mg daily had three and fivefold rises in plasma levels, respectively when given **propranolol** in increasing doses up to a total of 800 mg daily over 26 to 40 days. No **thioridazine** toxicity was seen although plasma levels had risen into the toxic range.[7] Similarly, in another study **thioridazine** levels rose by about 55 to 370% in 5 patients taking **propranolol** 320 to 520 mg daily.[8] **Pindolol** 40 mg daily also increased serum **thioridazine** levels by about 50% in 8 patients.[3]

Mechanism

Pharmacokinetic evidence[1] and *animal* studies[9] suggest that propranolol and chlorpromazine mutually inhibit the liver metabolism of the other drug so that both accumulate within the body. The mechanism of the interaction between propranolol and thioridazine is probably similar. Both beta-blockers and phenothiazines can cause hypotension, and these effects could be additive.

Importance and management

The interaction between propranolol and chlorpromazine appears to be established although information is limited. Concurrent use should be well monitored and the dosages reduced if necessary. The same precautions apply with propranolol and thioridazine.[7] There seems to be no information about any other interaction between beta-blockers and phenothiazines, but if the mechanism of interaction suggested above is true, it seems possible that other beta-blockers that are mainly cleared from the body by liver metabolism (e.g. alprenolol, metoprolol) might interact similarly with chlorpromazine, whereas those mainly cleared unchanged in the urine (e.g. atenolol, nadolol) are less likely to interact, although additive hypotensive effects would still be expected.

Note that **sotalol** and some phenothiazines (including chlorpromazine and thioridazine prolong the QT interval (see 'Table 7.3', (p.169) for a full list). Combined use should therefore generally be avoided, because of the increased risk of torsade de pointes. See also 'Drugs that prolong the QT interval + Other drugs that prolong the QT interval', p.170.

1. Vestal RE, Kornhauser DM, Hollifield JW, Shand DG. Inhibition of propranolol metabolism by chlorpromazine. *Clin Pharmacol Ther* (1979) 25, 19–24.
2. Baker L, Barcai A, Kaye R, Haque N. Beta adrenergic blockade and juvenile diabetes: acute studies and long-term therapeutic trial. *J Pediatr* (1969) 75, 19–29.
3. Greendyke RM, Gulya A. Effect of pindolol administration on serum levels of thioridazine, haloperidol, phenytoin, and phenobarbital. *J Clin Psychiatry* (1988) 49, 105–7.
4. Peet M, Middlemiss DN, Yates RA. Pharmacokinetic interaction between propranolol and chlorpromazine in schizophrenic patients. *Lancet* (1980) ii, 978.
5. Peet M, Middlemiss DN, Yates RA. Propranolol in schizophrenia II. Clinical and biochemical aspects of combining propranolol with chlorpromazine. *Br J Psychiatry* (1981) 138, 112–17.
6. Miller FA, Rampling D. Adverse effects of combined propranolol and chlorpromazine therapy. *Am J Psychiatry* (1982) 139, 1198–9.
7. Silver JM, Yudofsky SC, Kogan M, Katz BL. Elevation of thioridazine plasma levels by propranolol. *Am J Psychiatry* (1986) 143, 1290–2.
8. Greendyke RM, Kanter DR. Plasma propranolol levels and their effect on plasma thioridazine and haloperidol concentrations. *J Clin Psychopharmacol* (1987) 7, 178–82.
9. Shand DG, Oates JA. Metabolism of propranolol by rat liver microsomes and its inhibition by phenothiazine and tricyclic antidepressant drugs. *Biochem Pharmacol* (1971) 20, 1720–3.

Beta-blockers + Phenylpropanolamine

A small rise in blood pressure may occur in patients on beta-blockers who take single-doses of phenylpropanolamine. A marked rise in blood pressure has been seen in one patient on oxprenolol and methyldopa when given phenylpropanolamine. Propranolol attenuates the blood pressure rise seen with phenylpropanolamine.

Clinical evidence, mechanism, importance and management

(a) Effect on beta-blockers

A study in 7 hypertensive patients stable on beta-blockers (5 on **atenolol**, and the other 2 on **metoprolol** or **propranolol**) found that single 25-mg doses of rapid-release phenylpropanolamine (*Super Odrinex*) increased the mean peak systolic/diastolic blood pressures by about 8/5 mmHg over a 6-hour period.[1] Another study in 13 patients on various antihypertensives including 5 on unnamed beta-blockers found that a single-dose of *Dimetapp Extentabs* (phenylpropanolamine 75 mg with brompheniramine 12 mg) caused systolic/diastolic blood pressure rises of 1.7/0.9 mmHg over a 4-hour period, which was not statistically or clinically significant.[2] These rises in blood pressure after single-doses are small and relatively short-lived, and probably of little clinical importance. However, cold remedies are frequently taken up to every 4 hours over a number of days, and the effect of these doses on control of hypertension does not appear to have been assessed. Note that a marked rise in blood pressure was seen in one patient on methyldopa and **oxprenolol** when given phenylpropanolamine, see 'Methyldopa + Sympathomimetics; Indirectly-acting', p.675.

(b) Effect on phenylpropanolamine

In a placebo-controlled study in 6 healthy subjects, **propranolol** given either orally as a pretreatment or intravenously after phenylpropanolamine was found to antagonise the rise in blood pressure induced by the phenylpropanolamine. Oral phenylpropanolamine 75 mg alone increased blood pressure from 116/63 to 148/83 mmHg; pretreatment with oral **propranolol** 80 mg every 6 hours reduced the baseline blood pressure to 107/62 mmHg and antagonised the increase with phenylpropanolamine to 119/72 mmHg. Intravenous **propranolol** 0.3 mg/kg given after the phenylpropanolamine decreased blood pressure from 144/87 to 121/84 mmHg.[3]

1. O'Connell MB, Gross CR. The effect of single-dose phenylpropanolamine on blood pressure in patients with hypertension controlled by β blockers. *Pharmacotherapy* (1990) 10, 85–91.
2. Petrulis AS, Imperiale TF, Speroff T. The acute effect of phenylpropanolamine and brompheniramine on blood pressure in controlled hypertension. *J Gen Intern Med* (1991) 6, 503–6.
3. Pentel PR, Asinger RW, Benowitz, NL. Propranolol antagonism of phenylpropanolamine-induced hypertension. *Clin Pharmacol Ther* (1985) 37, 488–94.

Beta-blockers + Propafenone

Plasma metoprolol and propranolol levels can be markedly raised (two to fivefold) by propafenone. Toxicity may develop.

Clinical evidence

Four patients with ventricular arrhythmias given **metoprolol** 150 to 200 mg daily had a two to fivefold rise in steady-state **metoprolol** serum levels when they were given propafenone 150 mg three times daily. In 4 other patients treated with **metoprolol** 50 mg three times daily and propafenone 150 mg three times daily, it was found that stopping **metoprolol** did not affect propafenone plasma levels. One of them developed distressing nightmares, and another had acute left ventricular failure with pulmonary oedema and haemoptysis, which disappeared when the **metoprolol** dosage was reduced or stopped. Single-dose studies in healthy subjects found a twofold decrease in the clearance of **metoprolol** and a further 20% reduction in exercise-induced tachycardia at 90 minutes when propafenone was given.[1]

A patient developed neurotoxicity (including vivid nightmares, fatigue, headache) when given **metoprolol** 100 mg daily in divided doses, which worsened while it was being withdrawn and replaced by propafenone 300 mg daily. The symptoms disappeared when both drugs were withdrawn.[2]

Propafenone 225 mg every 8 hours more than doubled the steady-state levels of **propranolol** 50 mg every 8 hours in 12 healthy subjects. The beta-blocking effects were only modestly increased. The propafenone pharmacokinetics remained unchanged.[3]

Mechanism

It is suggested that the propafenone reduces the metabolism of the metoprolol and propranolol by the liver, thereby reducing their clearance and raising serum levels.[1,3]

Importance and management

Information is limited but the interaction would seem to be established. Concurrent use need not be avoided but anticipate the need to reduce the dosage of metoprolol and propranolol. Monitor closely because some patients may experience adverse effects. If the suggested mechanism of interaction is correct it is possible that other beta-blockers that undergo liver metabolism will interact similarly but not those largely excreted unchanged in the urine (e.g. atenolol, nadolol). This needs confirmation.

1. Wagner F, Kalusche D, Trenk D, Jähnchen E, Roskamm H. Drug interaction between propafenone and metoprolol. *Br J Clin Pharmacol* (1987) 24, 213–20.
2. Ahmad S. Metoprolol-induced delirium perpetuated by propafenone. *Am Fam Physician* (1991) 44, 1142–3.
3. Kowey PR, Kirsten EB, Fu C-HJ, Mason WD. Interaction between propranolol and propafenone in healthy volunteers. *J Clin Pharmacol* (1989) 29, 512–17.

Beta-blockers + Proton pump inhibitors

Omeprazole does not interact with metoprolol or propranolol, and lansoprazole does not interact with propranolol.

Clinical evidence, mechanism, importance and management

Omeprazole 20 mg daily for 8 days had no effect on the steady-state plasma levels of **propranolol** 80 mg twice daily, and no effect on resting and exercised heart rates or blood pressure in 8 healthy subjects.[1] Another study found that **omeprazole** 40 mg daily for 8 days had no effect on the steady-state plasma levels of **metoprolol** 100 mg daily.[2]

A double-blind crossover study in 18 healthy subjects found that **lanso-**

prazole 60 mg daily for 7 days did not significantly affect the pharmacokinetics of a single 80-mg dose of **propranolol**.[3]

No special precautions would seem necessary if these proton pump inhibitors are used with **propranolol** or **metoprolol**.

1. Henry D, Brent P, Whyte I, Mihaly G, Devenish-Meares S. Propranolol steady-state pharmacokinetics are unaltered by omeprazole. *Eur J Clin Pharmacol* (1987) 33, 369–73.
2. Andersson T, Lundborg P, Regårdh CG. Lack of effect of omeprazole treatment on steady-state plasma levels of metoprolol. *Eur J Clin Pharmacol* (1991) 40, 61–5.
3. Karol MD, Locke CS, Cavanaugh JH. Lack of interaction between lansoprazole and propranolol, a pharmacokinetic and safety assessment. *J Clin Pharmacol* (2000) 40, 301–8.

Beta-blockers + Quinidine

An isolated report describes a patient on quinidine who developed marked bradycardia when using timolol eye drops. Others describe orthostatic hypotension with quinidine and atenolol or propranolol. Both sotalol and quinidine can prolong the QT interval, which may therefore increase the risk of torsade de pointes arrhythmia if they are used together. Quinidine can raise plasma metoprolol, propranolol, and timolol levels, but the clinical relevance of this is uncertain.

Clinical evidence

(a) Atenolol

Orthostatic hypotension occurred in a 56-year-old woman on isosorbide dinitrate, diltiazem and quinidine sulfate 300 mg four times daily, 3 days after starting atenolol 50 mg daily. This resolved within 2 days of stopping atenolol. Before starting the quinidine, she had previously been treated with atenolol and the other drugs without problems.[1]

(b) Metoprolol

A metabolic study found that a single 50-mg dose quinidine caused marked inhibition of the metabolism of a single 100-mg dose of metoprolol in 5 healthy subjects who were extensive metabolisers, making them effectively into poor metabolisers. The plasma levels of metoprolol were approximately tripled. Quinidine had no effect on metoprolol pharmacokinetics in 5 poor metabolisers.[2] Similar findings were reported in another study when quinidine 50 mg daily was given with metoprolol 100 mg twice daily for 7 days. However, the effect on heart-rate reduction was small given the increase in serum metoprolol concentrations.[3]

(c) Propranolol

A single-dose pharmacokinetic study showed that quinidine 200 mg given with propranolol 20 mg doubled the AUC and the peak plasma levels of propranolol. Maximum heart rates during exercise were suppressed by a further 45%.[4] A similar study by the same research group found that propranolol AUCs were approximately tripled.[5] A further study found that quinidine doubled the AUC of propranolol and halved its clearance resulting in increased beta-blockade.[6] After a single 200-mg dose of quinidine the peak plasma quinidine levels were over 50% higher and its clearance almost 40% lower in 7 patients taking propranolol 40 to 400 mg daily when compared with 8 control patients, but the quinidine elimination half-life did not differ.[7] However, this interaction was not found in two other studies.[8,9]

A man on propranolol 40 mg four times daily developed orthostatic hypotension with symptoms of dizziness and faintness on standing when he was additionally treated with quinidine 200 mg four times daily. This resolved when quinidine was withdrawn.[10] The same authors subsequently briefly reported another two cases of orthostatic hypotension with quinidine and unnamed beta-blockers.[11]

(d) Sotalol

Although one study reports the safe concurrent use of sotalol and quinidine,[12] both drugs can prolong the QT interval, which may increase the risk of torsade de pointes arrhythmia if they are used together.

(e) Timolol

An elderly man taking quinidine sulfate 500 mg three times daily for atrial premature beats was hospitalised with dizziness 12 weeks after starting to use 0.5% timolol eye drops for open-angle glaucoma. He was found to have a sinus bradycardia of 36 bpm. The symptoms abated when the drugs were withdrawn and normal sinus rhythm returned after 24 hours. The same symptoms developed within 30 hours of re-starting both drugs, but disappeared when the quinidine was withdrawn.[13] In a later study in healthy subjects, a single 50-mg oral dose of quinidine was given 30 minutes before 2 drops of 0.5% timolol ophthalmic solution, put into each *nostril*. In 13 extensive metabolisers, quinidine caused a further decrease in heart rate and increase in plasma timolol concentrations compared with timolol alone. Giving quinidine with timolol in these extensive metabolisers gave results similar to timolol alone in 5 poor metabolisers,[14] In another study, quinidine augmented the plasma levels and cardiac effects of intravenous timolol.[15]

Mechanism

Quinidine appears to increase metoprolol, propranolol and timolol plasma levels by inhibiting the cytochrome P450 isoenzyme CYP2D6, thereby reducing their clearance.[2,6,14] As CYP2D6 shows polymorphism, these interactions would be most apparent in patients with high CYP2D6 activity (extensive metabolisers), making them effectively into poor metabolisers. See 'Genetic factors', (p.4) for further information on polymorphism.

Importance and management

The pharmacokinetic interaction would seem to be established, but of uncertain clinical importance. Only one isolated case of possible excessive beta-blockade has been reported (with quinidine and timolol eye drops). Concurrent use need not be avoided (and may be beneficial in the treatment of atrial fibrillation). The general relevance of the isolated reports of orthostatic hypotension with atenolol or propranolol and beta-blockers is uncertain.

The general consensus is that the combination of two drugs that prolong the QT interval such as quinidine and sotalol should usually be avoided, or only used with great caution. See also 'Drugs that prolong the QT interval + Other drugs that prolong the QT interval', p.170.

1. Manolis AS, Estes NA. Orthostatic hypotension due to quinidine and atenolol. *Am J Med* (1987) 82, 1083–4.
2. Leemann T, Dayer P, Meyer UA. Single-dose quinidine treatment inhibits metoprolol oxidation in extensive metabolizers. *Eur J Clin Pharmacol* (1986) 29, 739–41.
3. Schlanz KD, Yingling KW, Verme CN, Lalonde RL, Harrison DC, Bottorff MB. Loss of stereoselective metoprolol metabolism following quinidine inhibition of P450IID6. *Pharmacotherapy* (1991) 11, 272.
4. Sakurai T, Kawai C, Yasuhara M, Okumura K, Hori R. Increased plasma concentration of propranolol by a pharmacokinetic interaction with quinidine. *Jpn Circ J* (1983) 47, 872–3.
5. Yasuhara M, Yatsuzuka A, Yamada K, Okumura K, Hori R, Sakurai T, Kawai C. Alteration of propranolol pharmacokinetics and pharmacodynamics by quinidine in man. *J Pharmacobiodyn* (1990) 13, 681–7.
6. Zhou H-H, Anthony LB, Roden DM, Wood AJJ. Quinidine reduces clearance of (+)-propranolol more than (–)-propranolol through marked reduction in 4-hydroxylation. *Clin Pharmacol Ther* (1990) 47, 686–93.
7. Kessler KM, Humphries WC, Black M, Spann JF. Quinidine pharmacokinetics in patients with cirrhosis or receiving propranolol. *Am Heart J* (1978) 96, 627–35.
8. Kates RE, Blanford MF. Disposition kinetics of oral quinidine when administered concurrently with propranolol. *J Clin Pharmacol* (1979) 19, 378–83.
9. Fenster P, Perrier D, Mayersohn M, Marcus FI. Kinetic evaluation of the propranolol-quinidine combination. *Clin Pharmacol Ther* (1980) 27, 450–3.
10. Loon NR, Wilcox CS, Folger W. Orthostatic hypotension due to quinidine and propranolol. *Am J Med* (1986) 81, 1101–4.
11. Loon NR, Wilcox CS. Orthostatic hypotension due to quinidine and propranolol. The reply. *Am J Med* (1987) 82, 1276–7.
12. Dorian P, Newman D, Berman N, Hardy J, Mitchell J. Sotalol and type IA drugs in combination prevent recurrence of sustained ventricular tachycardia. *J Am Coll Cardiol* (1993) 22, 106–13.
13. Dinai Y, Sharir M, Naveh N, Halkin H. Bradycardia induced by interaction between quinidine and ophthalmic timolol. *Ann Intern Med* (1985) 103, 890–1.
14. Edeki TI, He H, Wood AJJ. Pharmacogenetic explanation for excessive β-blockade following timolol eye drops. *JAMA* (1995) 274, 1611–13.
15. Kaila T, Huupponen R, Karhuvaara S, Havula P, Scheinin M, Iisalo E, Salminen L. Beta-blocking effects of timolol at low plasma concentrations. *Clin Pharmacol Ther* (1991) 49, 53–8.

Beta-blockers + Quinolones

Ciprofloxacin reduces the loss of metoprolol from the body, but this is probably clinically unimportant. The concurrent use of sotalol and quinolones that prolong the QT interval should generally be avoided.

Clinical evidence, mechanism, importance and management

(a) Ciprofloxacin

Preliminary evidence suggests pretreatment with five doses of ciprofloxacin 500 mg given every 12 hours increased the AUC of ***(+)*-metoprolol** in 7 healthy subjects given a single 100-mg dose of **metoprolol** by 54% and reduced its clearance by 38.5%. The AUC of ***(–)*-metoprolol** was increased by 29% and its clearance reduced by 12%.[1] This interaction would appear to occur because ciprofloxacin inhibits the activity of the cytochrome P450 isoenzymes concerned with the metabolism and clearance of **metoprolol**, although this is questionable as **metoprolol** is metabolised, predominantly, by CYP2D6 while ciprofloxacin inhibits CYP1A2. Changes of this size, or even more, in the AUC of beta-blockers have proved not to be clinically important with other enzyme inhibiting drugs, and it seems probable that this will be the case with ciprofloxacin, but this needs confirmation.

(b) Quinolones that prolong the QT interval

Two cases of torsade de pointes were noted in patients taking a fluoroquinolone with **sotalol** in an analysis of cases of torsade de pointes associated with fluoroquinolones on the FDA Adverse Events Reporting System database (there were 37 cases identified, and 19 occurred in patients also taking other drugs known to prolong the QT interval).[2] **Sotalol** has class III antiarrhythmic effects and prolongs the QT interval, and this could be additive with the effects of quinolones that prolong the QT interval (e.g. **gatifloxacin**, **moxifloxacin**, **sparfloxacin**, see 'Table 7.3', (p.169)).The concurrent use of **sotalol** and these quinolones should generally be avoided (see 'Drugs that prolong the QT interval + Other drugs that prolong the QT interval', p.170).

1. Waite NM, Rutledge DR, Warbasse LH, Edwards DJ. Disposition of the (+) and (−) isomers of metoprolol following ciprofloxacin treatment. *Pharmacotherapy* (1990) 10, 236.
2. Frothingham R. Rates of torsades de pointes associated with ciprofloxacin, ofloxacin, levofloxacin, gatifloxacin, and moxifloxacin. *Pharmacotherapy* (2001) 21, 1468–72.

Beta-blockers + Rifamycins

Rifampicin increases the loss of bisoprolol, carvedilol, celiprolol, metoprolol, propranolol, tertatolol and talinolol from the body, and reduces their serum levels. The extent to which this reduces the effects of these beta-blockers is uncertain, but it is probably small. A patient on atenolol experienced a reduction in exercise tolerance when given rifampicin, but not when given rifabutin.

Clinical evidence

Rifampicin (**rifampin**) 600 mg daily for 3 weeks increased the oral clearance of **propranolol** in 6 healthy subjects by almost threefold. Increasing the **rifampicin** dosage to 900 or 1200 mg daily did not further increase the clearance. Four weeks after withdrawing the **rifampicin** the blood levels of **propranolol** had returned to normal.[1] In a similar study the oral clearance of **propranolol** was increased by about fourfold by **rifampicin** 600 mg daily for 3 weeks in both poor and extensive metabolisers of **propranolol**.[2]

The AUC of **bisoprolol** 10 mg daily was reduced by 34% in healthy subjects given **rifampicin** 600 mg daily.[3] **Rifampicin** 600 mg daily for 12 days caused a 60% decrease in the maximum serum levels and the AUC of **carvedilol**.[4] In other studies in healthy subjects, **rifampicin** 600 mg daily reduced the AUC of single doses of **celiprolol** 200 mg by 55%[5] and of **metoprolol** 100 mg by 33%.[6] **Rifampicin** 600 mg daily for a week increased the clearance of **tertatolol** almost threefold and reduced the half-life from 9 to 3.4 hours. A slight reduction in the effects of **tertatolol** on blood pressure was seen and heart rates were raised from 68 to 74 bpm.[7] **Rifampicin** 600 mg daily decreased the AUC of a single-dose of **talinolol** 30 mg intravenously or 100 mg orally by 21 and 35%, respectively, in 8 healthy subjects.[8]

A case report describes a man on **atenolol** for angina whose exercise threshold before developing angina symptoms appreciably worsened when he was given **rifampicin**. **Rifampicin** was stopped, and after a week **rifabutin** was started. **Rifabutin** did not cause any change in his baseline exercise tolerance.[9]

Mechanism

Rifampicin is a potent liver enzyme inducing agent that increases the metabolism and loss of extensively metabolised beta-blockers such as propranolol and metoprolol. However, rifampicin may interact by mechanisms other than enzyme induction. Rifampicin also increases duodenal P-glycoprotein expression, so increased clearance of talinolol (which is not metabolised) may be due to induction of P-glycoprotein excretion.[8] The case of possible reduced effect of atenolol with rifampicin is not explained, since atenolol is principally excreted unchanged by the kidneys.

Importance and management

These interactions are established. Their clinical importance is uncertain but probably small.[7] Nevertheless, concurrent use should be monitored. Increase the dosage of the beta-blocker if there is any evidence that the therapeutic response is inadequate. Beta-blockers that undergo extensive liver metabolism would be expected to be affected by the enzyme-inducing effects of rifampicin (e.g. propranolol, metoprolol, alprenolol). Those beta-blockers mainly lost unchanged in the urine (atenolol, nadolol) would not be expected to be affected, but it appears that a reaction may occur with non-metabolised drugs, such as talinolol, that are substrates for P-glycoprotein. However, note there is one case of a possible reduced effect of atenolol with rifampicin. More study is required.

1. Herman RJ, Nakamura K, Wilkinson GR, Wood AJJ. Induction of propranolol metabolism by rifampicin. *Br J Clin Pharmacol* (1983) 16, 565–9.
2. Shaheen O, Biollaz J, Koshakji RP, Wilkinson GR, Wood AJJ. Influence of debrisoquin phenotype on the inducibility of propranolol metabolism. *Clin Pharmacol Ther* (1989) 45, 439–43.
3. Kirch W, Rose I, Klingmann I, Pabst J, Ohnhaus EE. Interaction of bisoprolol with cimetidine and rifampicin. *Eur J Clin Pharmacol* (1986) 31, 59–62.
4. Data on file, database on carvedilol, SmithKline Beecham, quoted by Ruffolo RR, Boyle DA, Venuti RP, Lukas MA. Carvedilol (Kredex®): a novel multiple action cardiovascular agent. *Drugs Today* (1991) 27, 465–92.
5. Lilja JJ, Niemi M, Neuvonen PJ. Rifampicin reduces plasma concentrations of celiprolol. *Eur J Clin Pharmacol* (2004) 59, 819–24.
6. Bennett PN, John VA, Whitmarsh VB. Effect of rifampicin on metoprolol and antipyrine kinetics. *Br J Clin Pharmacol* (1982) 13, 387–91.
7. Kirch W, Milferstädt S, Halabi A, Rocher I, Efthymiopoulos C, Jung L. Interaction of tertatolol with rifampicin and ranitidine pharmacokinetics and antihypertensive activity. *Cardiovasc Drugs Ther* (1990) 4, 487–92.
8. Westphal K, Weinbrenner A, Zschiesche M, Franke G, Knoke M, Oertel R, Fritz P, von Richter O, Warzok R, Hachenberg T, Kauffmann H-M, Schrenk D, Terhaag B, Kroemer HK, Siegmund W. Induction of P-glycoprotein by rifampin increases intestinal secretion of talinolol in human beings: a new type of drug/drug interaction. *Clin Pharmacol Ther* (2000) 68, 345–55.
9. Goldberg SV, Hanson D, Peloquin CA. Rifamycin treatment of tuberculosis in a patient receiving atenolol: less interaction with rifabutin than with rifampin. *Clin Infect Dis* (2003), 37, 607–8.

Beta-blockers + SSRIs

Fluoxetine can increase serum pindolol and carvedilol levels, but the clinical effects of this are minimal. Two isolated reports describe lethargy and bradycardia in men on metoprolol or propranolol shortly after starting to take fluoxetine. Sotalol was found not to interact with fluoxetine in one of them. Fluvoxamine may increase levels of propranolol, but not of atenolol, and there is an isolated case of lethargy and bradycardia in a man on propranolol within days of starting fluvoxamine. Paroxetine may increase levels of metoprolol resulting in increased beta-blocking effects. Sertraline does not interact with atenolol, and there are no reports of interactions between citalopram and beta-blockers, although citalopram and escitalopram may raise metoprolol levels.

Clinical evidence

(a) Citalopram

The UK makers of citalopram say that no pharmacodynamic interactions have been noted in clinical studies in which citalopram was given with beta-blockers.[1] However the US makers say that although the concurrent use of **metoprolol** and citalopram had no clinically significant effect on heart rate and blood pressure the plasma levels of **metoprolol** were increased twofold, which may decrease its cardioselectivity.[2]

(b) Escitalopram

Escitalopram 20 mg daily increased the AUC and maximum serum levels of a single 100-mg dose of **metoprolol** by 82% and 50% respectively. However, no clinically significant effect on heart rate or blood pressure was seen.[3]

(c) Fluoxetine

Metoprolol 100 mg daily improved the angina of a man who had undergone a coronary artery bypass 4 years earlier. A month later he was given fluoxetine 20 mg daily for depression. Within 2 days he complained of profound lethargy, and his resting heart rate was found to have fallen from 64 to 36 bpm. The fluoxetine was withdrawn, and within 5 days his heart rate returned to 64 bpm. The **metoprolol** was replaced by **sotalol** 80 mg twice daily and fluoxetine reintroduced without problems.[4]

A patient on **propranolol** 40 mg twice daily developed bradycardia of 30 bpm, heart block and syncope 2 weeks after starting fluoxetine 20 mg daily. This patient possibly also had some pre-existing conduction disease contributing to the effect.[5]

When 9 healthy subjects were given **pindolol** 5 mg every 6 hours with fluoxetine 20 mg daily for 3 days and then 60 mg daily for another 7 days, the **pindolol** AUC rose by about 75% and its clearance fell by about 45% when compared with a single 5-mg dose of **pindolol**. Only mild to moderate alterations in pulse rate and blood pressure were seen.[6] Some studies including a high proportion of patients with first-episode depression have suggested that the antidepressant response of fluoxetine is accelerated by **pindolol**[7] while other studies in patients with predominantly chronic or recurrent depression did not find an enhanced response.[8] A double-blind crossover study in 10 patients with heart failure, maintained on **carvedilol** 25 to 50 mg twice daily, found that the addition of fluoxetine 20 mg daily for 28 days increased the AUC of ***(R)*-carvedilol** by 77%, and decreased the clearance of both enantiomers by 44 to 56%. However, these pharmacokinetic changes were of little clinical significance, since there were no changes in blood pressure, heart rate, and heart rate variability.[9]

(d) Fluvoxamine

A 79-year-old man who had taken **propranolol** for prophylaxis of migraine for several years developed fatigue and lightheadedness within a few days of starting fluvoxamine. He was admitted to hospital with syncope and bradycardia of 38 bpm but recovered after both drugs were discontinued.[10] Fluvoxamine 100 mg daily raised the plasma levels of **propranolol** 160 mg daily fivefold in healthy subjects, but the bradycardic effects were only slightly increased, by 3 bpm. The diastolic pressure following exercise was only slightly reduced but the general hypotensive effects remained unaltered.[11] When **atenolol** 100 mg daily was given, no changes in its plasma levels were seen, but the heart-slowing effects were slightly increased and the hypotensive effects slightly decreased by fluvoxamine.[11]

(e) Paroxetine

A study in 8 healthy subjects found that paroxetine 20 mg daily for 6 days increased the AUCs of ***(R)*-** and ***(S)*-metoprolol** by eightfold and fivefold respectively after a single 100-mg dose of **metoprolol**. The maximum plasma concentration and elimination half-life were increased about twofold. The beta-blocking effects of **metoprolol** were more sustained after paroxetine and the reduction in exercise systolic pressure by **metoprolol** was more pronounced after paroxetine treatment than when taken alone.[12]

(f) Sertraline

No changes in the beta-blocking effects of **atenolol** were found in a single-dose study in 10 healthy subjects given sertraline 100 mg five hours before **atenolol** 50 mg.[13,14]

Mechanism

Fluoxetine and paroxetine inhibit the cytochrome P450 isoenzyme CYP2D6 thus inhibiting the metabolism of some beta-blockers (e.g. propranolol, metoprolol, carvedilol) so that they accumulate, the result being that their effects, such as bradycardia, may be increased.[4] Citalopram and escitalopram may also inhibit CYP2D6. *In vitro* studies with human liver microsomes found that fluoxetine and paroxetine are potent inhibitors of metoprolol metabolism and fluvoxamine, sertraline and citalopram less potent.[15] However, fluvoxamine also potently inhibits the metabolism of propranolol by CYP1A2.[10,16] Beta-blockers that are not extensively metabolised, such as atenolol and sotalol, would not be expected to be affected. Bradycardia occurs rarely with fluoxetine alone.

Pindolol may augment the antidepressant effect of fluoxetine by its antagonistic effects at 5-HT_{1A} receptors.[7,8,17]

Importance and management

Pharmacokinetic interactions have been found between fluoxetine, fluvoxamine or paroxetine and some beta-blockers, but despite marked pharmacokinetic changes, the clinical effects are not generally significant. However, be aware that there are a few isolated reports of severe bradycardia with beta-blockers and fluoxetine or fluvoxamine. If problems arise, the interaction can apparently be avoided by giving a water-soluble beta-blocker (such as atenolol), which is not extensively metabolised. Alternatively, sertraline and citalopram seem to be less likely than the other SSRIs to interact with extensively-metabolised beta-blockers.[15] However, because metoprolol is considered to have a narrow therapeutic index in the treatment of heart failure, the UK makers of escitalopram say that caution and possible dosage adjustments are warranted on concurrent use.[18] The clinical significance of this potential interaction is not established. Remember that fluoxetine and particularly its metabolite have long half-lives so that this interaction may possibly still occur for some days after the fluoxetine has been stopped.

The combination of pindolol with fluoxetine may be advantageous in the treatment of depression in some patients.[7,8]

1. Cipramil (Citalopram). Lundbeck Ltd. UK Summary of product characteristics, April 2003.
2. Celexa (Citalopram). Forest Pharmaceuticals Inc. US Prescribing information, February 2005.
3. Lexapro (Escitalopram). Forest Pharmaceuticals Inc. US Prescribing information, February 2005.
4. Walley T, Pirmohamed M, Proudlove C, Maxwell D. Interaction of metoprolol and fluoxetine. *Lancet* (1993) 341, 967–8.
5. Drake WM, Gordon GD. Heart block in a patient on propranolol and fluoxetine. *Lancet* (1994) 343, 425–6.
6. Goldberg MJ, Bergstrom RF, Cerimele BJ, Thomassom HR, Hatcher BL, Simcox EA. Fluoxetine effects on pindolol pharmacokinetics. *Clin Pharmacol Ther* (1997) 61, 178.
7. Pérez V, Gilaberte I, Faries D, Alvarez E, Artigas F. Randomised, double-blind, placebo-controlled trial of pindolol in combination with fluoxetine antidepressant treatment. *Lancet* (1997) 349, 1594–7.
8. Berman RM, Anand A, Cappiello A, Miller HL, Hu XS, Oren DA, Charney DS. The use of pindolol with fluoxetine in the treatment of major depression: final results from a double-blind, placebo-controlled trial. *Biol Psychiatry* (1999) 45, 1170–7.
9. Graff DW, Williamson KM, Pieper JA, Carson SW, Adams KF, Cascio WE, Patterson JH. Effect of fluoxetine on carvedilol pharmacokinetics, CYP2D6 activity, and autonomic balance in heart failure patients. *J Clin Pharmacol* (2001) 41, 97–106.
10. Morocco AP, Hendrickson RG. Propranolol-induced symptomatic bradycardia after initiation of fluvoxamine therapy. *J Toxicol Clin Toxicol* (2001) 39, 490–1.
11. Data on file (Duphar), quoted by Benfield P, Ward A. Fluvoxamine, a review of its pharmacodynamic and pharmacokinetic properties and therapeutic efficacy in depressive illness. *Drugs* (1986) 32, 313–34.
12. Hemeryck A, Lefebvre RA, De Vriendt C, Belpaire FM. Paroxetine affects metoprolol pharmacokinetics and pharmacodynamics in healthy volunteers. *Clin Pharmacol Ther* (2000) 67, 283–9.
13. Warrington SJ. Clinical implications of the pharmacology of sertraline. *Int Clin Psychopharmacol* (1991) 6 (Suppl 2), 11–21.
14. Ziegler MG, Wilner KD, Sertraline does not alter the β-adrenergic blocking activity of atenolol in healthy male volunteers. *J Clin Psychiatry* (1996) 57, (Suppl 1), 12–15.
15. Belpaire FM, Wijnant P, Temmerman A, Rasmussen BB, Brøsen K. The oxidative metabolism of metoprolol in human liver microsomes: inhibition by the selective serotonin reuptake inhibitors. *Eur J Clin Pharmacol* (1998) 54, 261–4.
16. Brøsen K, Skelbo E, Rasmussen BB, Poulsen HE, Loft S. Fluvoxamine is a potent inhibitor of cytochrome P4501A2. *Biochem Pharmacol* (1993) 45, 1211–14.
17. Dawson LA, Nguyen HQ, Smith DI, Schechter LE. Effects of chronic fluoxetine treatment in the presence and absence of (+/-)pindolol: a microdialysis study. *Br J Pharmacol* (2000) 130, 797–804.
18. Cipralex (Escitalopram). Lundbeck Ltd. UK Summary of product characteristics, March 2004.

Beta-blockers + Sucrose polyesters

There is evidence that sucrose polyesters (e.g. *Olestra*) do not interact with propranolol.

Clinical evidence, mechanism, importance and management

Eight healthy subjects were given sucrose polyester 18 g and a single unstated dose of **propranolol**. Sucrose polyester had no effect on the pharmacokinetics of **propranolol**.[1] Sucrose polyesters, are non-absorbable, non-calorific fat replacements. It has been concluded that sucrose polyesters are unlikely to reduce the absorption of oral drugs in general.[2]

1. Roberts RJ, Leff RD. Influence of absorbable and nonabsorbable lipids and lipidlike substances on drug bioavailability. *Clin Pharmacol Ther* (1989) 45, 299–304.
2. Goldman P. Olestra: assessing its potential to interact with drugs in the gastrointestinal tract. *Clin Pharmacol Ther* (1997) 61, 613–18.

Beta-blockers + Sulfinpyrazone

The antihypertensive effects of oxprenolol can be reduced or abolished by sulfinpyrazone. The pharmacokinetics of metoprolol are not affected by sulfinpyrazone.

Clinical evidence

Oxprenolol 80 mg twice daily was given to 10 hypertensive subjects for 15 days, which reduced their mean supine blood pressure from 161/101 to 149/96 mmHg, and their heart rate from 72 to 66 bpm. When they were additionally given sulfinpyrazone 400 mg twice daily for 15 days, their mean blood pressure climbed again to about its former level. The reduction in mean heart rate remained unaffected. Sulfinpyrazone halved the reduction in cardiac workload seen with **oxprenolol** alone.[1]

A study in 9 healthy subjects found that sulfinpyrazone 400 mg twice daily did not affect the pharmacokinetics of **metoprolol** 100 mg twice daily. No adverse effects were noted in healthy subjects during concurrent use.[2]

Mechanism

Not understood. One idea is that the sulfinpyrazone inhibits the production of vasodilatory (antihypertensive) prostaglandins by the kidney. This would oppose the actions of the oxprenolol.

Importance and management

Information seems to be limited. If sulfinpyrazone is given to patients taking oxprenolol for hypertension, the effects should be monitored. It seems likely that this interaction could be accommodated by raising the dosage of the oxprenolol but this needs confirmation. The effect of this interaction on cardiac workload appears to be less important, but it would still be prudent to monitor concurrent use if oxprenolol is used for angina. Sulfinpyrazone did not alter the pharmacokinetics of metoprolol.

1. Ferrara LA, Mancini M, Marotta T, Pasanisi F, Fasano ML. Interference by sulphinpyrazone with the antihypertensive effects of oxprenolol. *Eur J Clin Pharmacol* (1986) 29, 717–19.
2. Cortellaro M, Boschetti C, Antoniazzi V, Polli EE, de Gaetano G, De Blasi A, Gerna M, Pezzi L, Garattini S. A pharmacokinetic and platelet function study of the combined administration of metoprolol and sulfinpyrazone to healthy volunteers. *Thromb Res* (1984) 34, 65–74.

Beta-blockers + Sympathomimetics; Directly-acting

Effects on blood pressure and heart rate: The hypertensive effects of adrenaline (epinephrine) can be markedly increased in patients taking non-selective beta-blockers such as propranolol. A severe and potentially life-threatening hypertensive reaction and/or marked bradycardia can develop. Cardioselective beta-blockers such as atenolol and metoprolol interact minimally. An isolated report describes a fatal hypertensive reaction with propranolol and phenylephrine, but concurrent use normally seems to be uneventful. Paradoxically, marked hypotension occurred in one patient given low-dose carvedilol and dobutamine.
Anaphylaxis: Some evidence suggests anaphylactic shock in patients on beta-blockers may be resistant to treatment with adrenaline (epinephrine).

Clinical evidence

A. Effects on blood pressure and heart rate

(a) Adrenaline (Epinephrine)

An early study in 10 healthy subjects found that intravenous adrenaline (epinephrine) 5 micrograms/minute alone increased heart rates and caused minimal changes in blood pressure. However, after pretreatment with intravenous **propranolol** 10 mg, the same dose of adrenaline caused a fall in heart rate of 12 bpm and an increase in arterial pressure of 20/10 mmHg.[1] One case report describes 6 patients on **propranolol** 20 to 80 mg daily, undergoing plastic surgery, who experienced marked hypertensive reactions (blood pressures in the range of 190/110 to 260/150 mmHg) and bradycardia when their eyelids and/or faces were infiltrated with 8 to 40 ml of local anaesthetic solutions of lidocaine containing 1:100 000 or 1:200 000 (10 or 5 micrograms/ml) of adrenaline. Cardiac arrest occurred in one patient.[2]

Similar marked increases in blood pressure, associated with marked bradycardia, sometimes severe, have been described in other studies and case reports involving **propranolol**.[3-11] In contrast, only a small blood pressure rise was seen in a comparative study with **metoprolol**.[4] This was confirmed in another study in which patients given identical infusions of adrenaline developed a hypertensive/bradycardic reaction while taking **propranolol** but not while taking **metoprolol**.[5] After pretreatment with a single 5-mg dose of **pindolol**, only small reductions in blood pressure (4 mmHg) and heart rate (about 5 bpm) were seen with the intra-oral injection of 3.6 ml of 2% lidocaine containing 1:80 000 adrenaline (45 micrograms adrenaline) in healthy subjects.[12] In 24 healthy subjects given either **nadolol**, **atenolol** or placebo for 1 week followed by an infusion of adrenaline, mean arterial pressure and calf vascular resistance rose markedly in the **nadolol**-treated group but not the **atenolol** group. Marked bradycardia also occurred in those given **nadolol** and adrenaline.[13]

In 6 healthy subjects, giving adrenaline after intravenous **labetalol** 1 mg/kg resulted in a 13 to 21 mmHg increase in mean arterial pressure and a 23 to 29 bpm reduction in heart rate compared with adrenaline alone.[14]

(b) Corbadrine

A transient hypertensive reaction has been seen in a patient on **propranolol** when given injections of 2% mepivacaine with 1:20 000 corbadrine for dental anaesthesia.[15]

(c) Dobutamine

A 54-year-old man with severe heart failure was given **carvedilol** 3.125 to 6.25 mg twice daily. His symptoms worsened and he was admitted for treatment with intravenous dobutamine; the **carvedilol** was discontinued and other medications apart from furosemide were withheld short-term. Dobutamine was started at 1 microgram/kg per minute intravenously and gradually increased to 5 micrograms/kg per minute. However, with each 1 microgram/kg increment the systolic blood pressure dropped to about 70 mmHg for 5 to 10 minutes and then quickly returned to the baseline level of 80 to 84 mmHg. When the patient received dobutamine 5 micrograms/kg per minute, his systolic blood pressure dropped to 56 mmHg and the dobutamine was discontinued. The blood pressure returned to normal over the next 30 minutes. Two months later when the patient was no longer taking **carvedilol** he was again treated with intravenous dobutamine and his systolic blood pressure increased.[16]

(d) Phenylephrine

A woman on **propranolol** 40 mg four times daily for hypertension was given one drop of a 10% phenylephrine hydrochloride solution in each eye during an ophthalmic examination. About 45 minutes later she complained of a sudden and sharp bi-temporal pain and shortly afterwards became unconscious. She later died of an intracerebral haemorrhage due to the rupture of a berry aneurysm. She had received a similar dose of phenylephrine on a previous occasion in the absence of **propranolol** without any problems.[17]

However, no change in blood pressure was seen in a study in both normotensive subjects and patients taking **metoprolol** who were given 0.5 to 4-mg doses of phenylephrine intranasally every hour to a total of 7.5 to 15 mg (4 to 30 times the usual dose).[18] Similarly, in a placebo-controlled study in 12 hypertensive patients, neither **propranolol** nor **metoprolol** significantly altered the dose of intravenous phenylephrine required to cause a 25 mmHg increase in systolic blood pressure.[19]

B. Anaphylaxis: resistance to treatment

A patient on **propranolol** who suffered an anaphylactic reaction after receiving an allergy injection for desensitisation failed to respond to adrenaline (epinephrine) and required intubation.[20] Resistance to adrenaline treatment for anaphylaxis occurred in another patient using **timolol** eye drops.[21] It has also been proposed that the incidence and severity of anaphylactic reactions may be increased in those on beta-blockers,[22-24] one idea being that the adrenoceptors concerned with suppressing the release of the mediators of anaphylaxis may be blocked by either beta$_1$- or beta$_2$-antagonists.[22] However, one study failed to find any evidence to support an increased incidence of systemic reactions in patients taking beta-blockers receiving allergen immunotherapy.[25] See also 'Beta-blockers + X-ray contrast media', p.645, for other anaphylactic reactions potentially exacerbated by beta-blockers.

A beta-agonist bronchodilator (e.g. isoprenaline, salbutamol) may be effective in patients on beta-blockers with anaphylaxis resistant to adrenaline,[22] and glucagon was effective in treating a severe anaphylactoid reaction in one patient on a beta-blocker.[24] Reports of severe hypertension, sometimes with bradycardia following the use of adrenaline to treat allergic reactions, including presumed anaphylaxis, in patients on **propranolol**,[6-8] are described under A. above.

Mechanism

Adrenaline (epinephrine) stimulates alpha- and beta-receptors of the cardiovascular system, the former results in vasoconstriction (mainly alpha-1) and the latter in both vasodilatation (mainly beta-2) and stimulation of the heart (mainly beta-1). The net result is usually a modest increase in heart rate and a small rise in blood pressure. However, if the beta-receptors are blocked by a non-selective beta-blocker such as propranolol or nadolol (see 'Table 20.2', (p.623) for a list), the unopposed alpha vasoconstriction causes a marked rise in blood pressure, followed by reflex bradycardia. Cardioselective beta-blockers such as atenolol and metoprolol (see 'Table 20.1', (p.623) for a list), which are more selective for beta-1 receptors, do not prevent the vasodilator action of adrenaline at beta-2 receptors to the same extent, and therefore the effect of any interaction is relatively small. Consequently, adrenaline has been used to assess the degree of beta-blockade after propranolol and other beta-blockers.[13,26] Phenylephrine is largely an alpha-stimulator, therefore beta-blockers should have a minimal effect on its action.

Dobutamine is a beta-1, beta-2 and alpha-1 adrenergic agonist and carvedilol is a non-selective beta-blocker, but at low doses it is primarily a selective beta-1 adrenergic antagonist and it is also an alpha-1 antagonist. It was proposed that the drop in blood pressure was caused by vasodilation due to vascular beta-2 receptor activation, which was not blocked by low doses of carvedilol.[16]

Importance and management

The interaction between propranolol and adrenaline (epinephrine) is established. It may be serious and potentially life-threatening, depending on the dosage of adrenaline used. Marked and serious blood pressure rises and severe bradycardia have occurred in patients given 300 micrograms of adrenaline (0.3 ml of 1:1000) subcutaneously[6-8] or 40 to 400 micrograms by infiltration of the skin and eyelids during plastic surgery.[2] Adrenaline 15 micrograms given intravenously can cause an almost 40% fall in heart rate.[9] Patients on non-selective beta-blockers such as propranolol (see 'Table 20.2', (p.623) for a list) should only be given adrenaline in very reduced dosages because of the marked bradycardia and hypertension that can occur. A less marked effect is likely with the cardioselective beta-blockers such as atenolol and metoprolol (see 'Table 20.1', (p.623) for a list).[4] Local anaesthetics used in dental surgery usually contain very low concentrations of adrenaline (e.g. 5 to 20 micrograms/ml, i.e. 1:200 000 to 1:50 000) and only small volumes are usually given, so that an undesirable interaction is unlikely.

No interaction between phenylephrine and the beta-blockers would be expected, and apart from the single unexplained case cited above,[17] the literature appears to be silent. Concurrent use normally appears to be clinically unimportant,[18,19] particularly bearing in mind the widespread use of beta-blockers and the ready availability of phenylephrine in the form of non-prescription cough-and-cold remedies and nasal decongestants.

Acute hypertensive episodes have been controlled with chlorpromazine or phentolamine (both of which are alpha-blockers). Hydralazine,[2,10] nifedipine[7] and aminophylline[10] have also been used. Reflex bradycardia may be managed with atropine and the pre-emptive use of glycopyrrolate has also been suggested.[10]

The paradoxical case of hypotension with dobutamine and carvedilol suggests that this combination should be monitored carefully.[16]

1. Harris WS, Schoenfeld CD, Brooks RH, Weissler AM. Effect of beta adrenergic blockade on the hemodynamic responses to epinephrine in man. *Am J Cardiol* (1966) 17, 484–92.
2. Foster CA, Aston SJ. Propranolol-epinephrine interaction: a potential disaster. *Plast Reconstr Surg* (1983) 72, 74–8.
3. Kram J, Bourne HR, Melmon KL, Maibach H. Propranolol. *Ann Intern Med* (1974) 80, 282–3.
4. van Herwaarden CLA, Binkhorst RA, Fennis JFM, van'T Laar A. Effects of adrenaline during treatment with propranolol and metoprolol. *BMJ* (1977) 2, 1029.
5. Houben H, Thien T, Laor VA. Effect of low-dose epinephrine infusion on hemodynamics after selective and non-selective beta-blockade in hypertension. *Clin Pharmacol Ther* (1982) 31, 685.
6. Hansbrough JF, Near A. Propranolol-epinephrine antagonism with hypertension and stroke. *Ann Intern Med* (1980) 92, 717.
7. Whelan TV. Propranolol, epinephrine and accelerated hypertension during hemodialysis. *Ann Intern Med* (1987) 106, 327.
8. Gandy W. Severe epinephrine-propranolol interaction. *Ann Emerg Med* (1989) 18, 98–9.
9. Mackie K, Lam A. Epinephrine-containing test dose during beta-blockade. *J Clin Monit* (1991) 7, 213–6.
10. Centeno RF, Yu YL. The propranolol-epinephrine interaction revisited: a serious and potentially catastrophic adverse drug interaction in facial plastic surgery. *Plast Reconstr Surg* (2003) 111, 944–5.
11. Lampman RM, Santinga JT, Bassett DR, Savage PJ. Cardiac arrhythmias during epinephrine-propranolol infusions for measurement on in vivo insulin resistance. *Diabetes* (1981) 30, 618–20.
12. Sugimura M, Hirota Y, Shibutani T, Niwa H, Hori T, Kim Y, Matsuura H. An echocardiographic study of interactions between pindolol and epinephrine contained in a local anesthetic solution. *Anesth Prog* (1995) 42, 29–35.
13. Hiatt WR, Wolfel EE, Stoll S, Nies AS, Zerbe GO, Brammell HL, Horwitz LD. Beta-2 Adrenergic blockade evaluated with epinephrine after placebo, atenolol, and nadolol. *Clin Pharmacol Ther* (1985) 37, 2–6.
14. Richards DA, Prichard BNC, Hernández R. Circulatory effects of noradrenaline and adrenaline before and after labetalol. *Br J Clin Pharmacol* (1979) 7, 371–8.
15. Mito RS, Yagiela JA. Hypertensive response to levonordefrin in a patient receiving propranolol: report of a case. *J Am Dent Assoc* (1988) 116, 55–7.
16. Lindenfield J, Lowes BD, Bristow MR. Hypotension with dobutamine: β-adrenergic antagonist selectivity at low doses of carvedilol. *Ann Pharmacother* (1999) 33, 1266–9.
17. Cass E, Kadar D, Stein HA. Hazards of phenylephrine topical medication in persons taking propranolol. *Can Med Assoc J* (1979) 120, 1261–2.
18. Myers MG, Iazzetta JJ. Intranasally administered phenylephrine and blood pressure. *Can Med Assoc J* (1982) 127, 365–8.
19. Myers MG. Beta adrenoceptor antagonism and pressor response to phenylephrine. *Clin Pharmacol Ther* (1984) 36, 57–63.
20. Newman BR, Schultz LK. Epinephrine-resistant anaphylaxis in a patient taking propranolol hydrochloride. *Ann Allergy* (1981) 47, 35–7.
21. Moneret-Vautrin DA, Kanny G, Faller JP, Levan D, Kohler C.Choc anaphylactique grave avec arrêt cardiaque au café et à la gomme arabique, potentialisé par un collyre bêta-bloquant. *Rev Med Interne* (1993) 14, 107–11.
22. Toogood JH. Beta-blocker therapy and the risk of anaphylaxis. *Can Med Assoc J* (1987) 136, 929–33.
23. Berkelman RL, Finton RJ, Elsea WR. Beta-adrenergic antagonists and fatal anaphylactic reactions to oral penicillin. *Ann Intern Med* (1986) 104, 134.
24. Lang DM. Anaphylactoid and anaphylactic reactions. Hazards of beta-blockers. *Drug Safety* (1995) 12, 299–304.
25. Hepner MJ, Ownby DR, Anderson JA, Rowe MS, Sears-Ewald D, Brown EB. Risk of systemic reactions in patients taking beta-blocker drugs receiving allergen immunotherapy injections. *J Allergy Clin Immunol* (1990) 86, 407–11.
26. Varma DR, Sharma KK, Arora RC. Response to adrenaline and propranolol in hyperthyroidism. *Lancet* (1976), i, 260.

Beta-blockers + Thallium scans

Beta-blockers may reduce the sensitivity of stress thallium scans used for the diagnosis of coronary heart disease.

Clinical evidence, mechanism, importance and management

A retrospective comparison of patients given **201-thallous chloride** during exercise for the diagnosis of coronary heart disease showed that there was a marked reduction in the sensitivity to stress thallium scans in those on beta-blockers when compared with other patients not taking beta-blockers.[1,2] Similar results have been reported in other studies.[3-5] **Propranolol** may decrease blood flow to non-ischaemic heart muscle, or prevent ischaemia during exercise, which may lead to a reduction in the sensitivity of thallium scans and reducing diagnostic accuracy.[5] The suggestion was made that consideration should be given to discontinuing beta-blockers before evaluating these patients.[1,2,4,5] Strictly speaking this is not a drug-drug interaction. Beta-blockers do not appear to affect dipyridamole stress-testing, see 'Dipyridamole + Beta-blockers', p.523.

1. Henkin RE, Chang W, Provus R. The effect of beta-blockers on thallium scans. *J Nucl Med* (1982) 23, P63.
2. Martin GJ, Henkin RE, Scanlon PJ. Beta blockers and the sensitivity of the thallium treadmill test. *Chest* (1987) 92, 486–7.
3. Pohost GM, Alpert NM, Ingwall JS, Strauss HW. Thallium redistribution: mechanisms and clinical utility. *Semin Nucl Med* (1980) 10, 70–92.
4. Hockings B, Saltissi S, Croft DN, Webb-Peploe MM. Effect of beta adrenergic blockade on thallium-201 myocardial perfusion imaging. *Br Heart J* (1983) 49, 83–9.
5. Osbakken MD, Okada RD, Boucher CA, Strauss HW, Pohost GM. Comparison of exercise perfusion and ventricular function imaging: an analysis of factors affecting the diagnostic accuracy of each technique. *J Am Coll Cardiol* (1984) 3, 272–83.

Beta-blockers + Tobacco smoking ± Coffee and Tea

Beta-blockers reduce heart rate and blood pressure. These therapeutically useful effects are exploited in the treatment of angina and hypertension, but are reduced to some extent if patients smoke. Some increase in the dosage of the beta-blocker may be necessary. Drinking tea or coffee may have a similar but smaller effect.

Clinical evidence

(a) Tobacco smoking

A double-blind study in 10 smokers with angina pectoris, taking daily doses of either **propranolol** 240 mg, **atenolol** 100 mg or a placebo, found that smoking reduced their plasma **propranolol** levels by 25% when compared with a non-smoking phase. Plasma **atenolol** levels were not significantly altered. Both of the beta-blockers reduced heart rate at rest and during exercise, but the reductions were less when subjects smoked (effects attenuated by 8 to 14%).[1]

Other studies found that serum **propranolol** levels in smokers were about half those in non-smokers.[2,3] Smoking caused an increase in blood pressure and heart rate in patients with angina and these effects were still evident, to a reduced extent, during **propranolol** treatment. In addition smoking abolished the beneficial effects of **propranolol** on ST-segment depression.[4]

(b) Caffeine

Two 150-ml cups of coffee (made from 24 g of coffee) increased the blood pressures of 12 healthy subjects taking **propranolol** 240 mg, **metoprolol** 300 mg or a placebo. Mean systolic/diastolic blood pressure rises were 7%/22% with **propranolol**, 7%/19% with **metoprolol** and 4%/16% mmHg with placebo. The beta-blockers and placebo were given in divided doses over 15 hours before the test.[5]

(c) Tobacco smoking and caffeine

Eight patients with mild hypertension taking **propranolol** 80 mg twice daily, **oxprenolol** 80 mg twice daily or **atenolol** 100 mg daily over a 6-week period had their blood pressure monitored after smoking 2 tipped cigarettes and drinking coffee, containing 200 mg of caffeine. Their mean systolic/diastolic blood pressure rises over the following 2 hours were 8.5/8 mmHg in those on **propranolol**, 12.1/9.1 mmHg in those on **oxprenolol** and 5.2/4.4 mmHg in those on **atenolol**.[6]

Mechanism

Smoking tobacco increases heart rate, blood pressure and the severity of myocardial ischaemia, probably as a direct effect of the nicotine and due to the reduced oxygen-carrying capacity of the blood.[1,4] These actions oppose and may even totally abolish the beneficial actions of the beta-blockers. In addition, smoking stimulates the liver enzymes concerned with the metabolism of some beta-blockers (e.g. propranolol, metoprolol) so that their serum levels are reduced.

Caffeine causes the release of catecholamines into the blood, such as adrenaline, which could account for the increases in heart rate and blood pressure that are seen.[6] The blood pressure rise may be exaggerated in the presence of non-cardioselective beta-blockers, which block vasodilatation leaving the alpha (vasoconstrictor) effects of adrenaline unopposed. This too opposes the actions of the beta-blockers.

Importance and management

Established interactions. Smoking tobacco and (to a very much lesser extent) drinking tea or coffee oppose the effects of the beta-blockers in the treatment of angina or hypertension. Patients should be encouraged to stop smoking because, quite apart from its other toxic effects, it aggravates myocardial ischaemia, increases heart rate and can impair blood pressure control. If patients continue to smoke, it may be necessary to raise the dosages of the beta-blockers. The effects of the caffeine in tea, coffee, cola drinks, etc. are quite small and there seems to be no strong reason to forbid them, but the excessive consumption of large amounts may not be a good idea, particularly in those who also smoke.

1. Fox K, Deanfield J, Krikler S, Ribeiro P, Wright C. The interaction of cigarette smoking and β-adrenoceptor blockade. *Br J Clin Pharmacol* (1984) 17, 92S–93S.
2. Vestal RE, Wood AJJ, Branch RA, Shand DG, Wilkinson GR. Effects of age and cigarette smoking on propranolol disposition. *Clin Pharmacol Ther* (1979) 26, 8–15.
3. Gardner SK, Cady WJ, Ong YS. Effect of smoking on the elimination of propranolol hydrochloride. *Int J Clin Pharmacol Ther Toxicol* (1980) 18, 421–4.
4. Fox K, Jonathan A, Williams H, Selwyn A. Interaction between cigarettes and propranolol in treatment of angina pectoris. *BMJ* (1980) 281, 191–3.
5. Smits P, Hoffmann H, Thien T, Houben H, van't Laar A. Hemodynamic and humoral effects of coffee after β_1-selective and nonselective β-blockade. *Clin Pharmacol Ther* (1983) 34, 153–8.
6. Freestone S and Ramsey LE. Effect of β-blockade on the pressor response to coffee plus smoking in patients with mild hypertension. *Drugs* (1983) 25 (Suppl 2), 141–5.

Beta-blockers + Vitamin C (Ascorbic acid)

Vitamin C reduces the bioavailability of propranolol but the extent is too small to matter.

Clinical evidence, mechanism, importance and management

A study in 5 healthy subjects given a single 80-mg dose of **propranolol** found that a single 2-g dose of vitamin C reduced the maximum plasma levels of **propranolol** by 28%, reduced the AUC by 37% and reduced its recovery in the urine by 66%. The fall in heart rate was also slightly reduced. The reason for this interaction appears to be that vitamin C reduces both the absorption and the metabolic conjugation of **propranolol**.[1] However, none of the changes seen would appear to be of clinical relevance.

1. Gonzalez JP, Valdivieso A, Calvo R, Rodríguez-Sasiaín JM, Jimenez R, Aguirre C, du Souich P. Influence of vitamin C on the absorption and first pass metabolism of propranolol. *Eur J Clin Pharmacol* (1995) 48, 295–7.

Beta-blockers + X-ray contrast media

There is some evidence that use of beta-blockers is a risk factor for anaphylactoid reactions to X-ray contrast media. Severe hypotension has been seen in two patients on beta-blockers given sodium meglumine amidotrizoate as a contrast agent and in a further patient on atenolol given iohexol.

Clinical evidence

A case-control study of anaphylactoid reactions to X-ray contrast media found that the risk of bronchospasm during intravenous contrast media procedures was associated with beta-blocker use and also with asthma, while the risk of major and life-threatening anaphylactoid reactions were associated with cardiovascular disorders. Use of beta-blockers also increased the risk of hospitalisation in those patients who had a severe anaphylactoid reaction.[1]

Two patients, one taking **nadolol** and the other **propranolol**, developed severe hypotensive reactions when given **sodium meglumine amidotrizoate** as a contrast agent for X-ray urography. Both patients developed slowly progressive erythema on the face and arms followed by tachycardia and a weak pulse. Each was successfully treated with subcutaneous adrenaline (epinephrine) and hydrocortisone.[2]

Another patient who had developed a transient rash during cardiac catheterisation 6 years earlier and who was subsequently treated with **atenolol** developed generalised urticaria and severe hypotension immediately after an injection of **iohexol** for coronary angiography. The hypotension was refractory to aggressive standard treatment with adrenaline, atropine and dopamine and the patient remained in shock (BP 60/34 mmHg). Noradrenaline (norepinephrine) infusion produced a modest improvement (BP 80/40 mmHg), but significant improvement in blood pressure occurred only after intravenous injections of glucagon 1 mg.[3]

See also, Anaphylaxis under 'Beta-blockers + Sympathomimetics; Directly-acting', p.643.

Mechanism

Iodinated contrast media are associated with hypersensitivity reactions due to the release of histamine. It is suggested that beta-blockers compromise the ability of the body to cope with the effects of histamine release.[2]

Importance and management

Limited documentation. Withdrawal of the beta-blocker 2 to 3 days before use of contrast media has been suggested,[2] but because of the potential for beta-blocker withdrawal syndromes this must be considered on an individual risk/benefit basis.[1] Pretreatment with a diphenhydramine and a corticosteroid such as prednisone may reduce the risk of reactions.[3] Use of low osmolality contrast media may reduce the risk of adverse reactions including anaphylaxis.[1,4] However, even mild reactions to contrast media may sensitise the patient and a serious anaphylactoid reaction may occur on further exposure despite pretreatment and the use of low osmolality contrast media.[3]

When anaphylactic reactions do occur in patients on beta-blockers, it may be preferable to use a beta-agonist bronchodilator such as isoprenaline rather than adrenaline (epinephrine).[2] Glucagon, which has inotropic and chronotropic actions that are only minimally antagonised by beta-blockers, may also be effective in reversing anaphylactoid shock in patients taking beta-blockers.[3]

1. Lang DM, Alpern MB, Visintainer PF, Smith ST. Elevated risk of anaphylactoid reaction from radiographic contrast media is associated with both β-blocker exposure and cardiovascular disorders. *Arch Intern Med* (1993) 153, 2033–40.
2. Hamilton G. Severe adverse reactions to urography in patients taking beta-adrenergic blocking agents. *Can Med Assoc J* (1985) 133, 122.
3. Javeed N, Javeed H, Javeed S, Moussa G, Wong P, Rezai F. Refractory anaphylactoid shock potentiated by beta-blockers. *Cathet Cardiovasc Diagn* (1996) 39, 383–4.
4. Greenberger PA, Patterson R. The prevention of immediate generalized reactions to radiocontrast media in high-risk patients. *J Allergy Clin Immunol* (1991) 87, 867–72.

Beta-blockers; Atenolol + Ampicillin

Plasma atenolol levels are halved by 1-g doses of ampicillin. The clinical importance of this is uncertain, but probably small. No important interaction occurs with ampicillin 250 mg every 6 hours.

Clinical evidence

A single 1-g dose of ampicillin reduced the AUC of a single 100-mg dose of atenolol by 40%, and decreased its bioavailability from 60 to 36% in 6 healthy subjects. Similarly, when atenolol 100 mg was given with ampicillin 1 g daily for 6 days, the mean steady-state plasma atenolol level was reduced by 52% (from 199 to 95 nanograms/ml), and the AUC was reduced by 52%. The blood pressure lowering effect of atenolol at rest was not affected, but after exercise a small rise in systolic pressure of up to 17 mmHg occurred, whereas diastolic pressure was unchanged. The effects of atenolol on reducing heart rate during exercise were diminished from 24% to 11% at 12 hours.[1]

Another study showed that when a single 50-mg oral dose of atenolol was given with a single 1-g oral dose of ampicillin the AUC of atenolol was reduced by 51.5%, whereas when ampicillin 250 mg four times daily was given for 24 hours, the AUC was only reduced by 18.2%.[2]

Mechanism

Uncertain. Ampicillin apparently affects the absorption of the atenolol.

Importance and management

Information is limited, but the interaction appears to be established. The clinical importance awaits full evaluation but the modest effects on blood pressure and heart rate[1] suggest that it is of limited importance. Information about other beta-blockers and penicillins is lacking.

1. Schäfer-Korting M, Kirch W, Axthelm T, Köhler H, Mutschler E. Atenolol interaction with aspirin, allopurinol, and ampicillin. *Clin Pharmacol Ther* (1983) 33, 283–8.
2. McLean AJ, Tonkin A, McCarthy P, Harrison P. Dose-dependence of atenolol-ampicillin interaction. *Br J Clin Pharmacol* (1984) 18, 969–71.

Beta-blockers; Celiprolol + Itraconazole

Itraconazole markedly increased the bioavailability of celiprolol, although this is not predicted to be clinically relevant.

Clinical evidence, mechanism, importance and management

In a study in 12 healthy subjects itraconazole 200 mg twice daily for 5 doses increased the AUC of a single 100-mg dose of celiprolol by 80%, without increasing the half-life. However, itraconazole did not increase the effect of celiprolol on heart rate or blood pressure.[1]

It was suggested that itraconazole probably increases the absorption of celiprolol by inhibiting P-glycoprotein in the intestinal wall.[1]

Although the increase in plasma levels was marked, it was suggested it is unlikely to be clinically relevant because celiprolol has a wide therapeutic range.[1]

1. Lilja JJ, Backman JT, Laitila J, Luurila H, Neuvonen PJ. Itraconazole increases but grapefruit juice greatly decreases plasma concentrations of celiprolol. *Clin Pharmacol Ther* (2003) 73, 192–8.

Beta-blockers; Propranolol + Misoprostol

Misoprostol does not significantly alter propranolol pharmacokinetics.

Clinical evidence, mechanism, importance and management

Misoprostol 400 micrograms twice daily raised the AUC of propranolol 80 mg twice daily by about 20 to 40% in 12 healthy subjects, and this remained raised 7 days after misoprostol was discontinued.[1] However, as these findings were unexpected, the authors conducted a randomised, crossover, placebo-controlled study and ensured propranolol was at steady state before assessing the effect of misoprostol. No significant effects on the pharmacokinetics of propranolol were found.[2] No special precautions would therefore seem necessary during concurrent use.

1. Bennett PN, Fenn GC, Notarianni LJ. Potential drug interactions with misoprostol: effects on the pharmacokinetics of antipyrine and propranolol. *Postgrad Med J* (1988) 64 (Suppl 1), 21–4.
2. Bennett PN, Fenn GC, Notarianni LJ, Lee CE. Misoprostol does not alter the pharmacokinetics of propranolol. *Postgrad Med J* (1991) 67, 455–7.

Beta-blockers; Sotalol + Potassium-depleting drugs

The use of potassium-depleting diuretics can precipitate the development of potentially life-threatening torsade de pointes arrhythmia in patients taking sotalol unless potassium levels are maintained. This would also be expected with other potassium-depleting drugs such as corticosteroids, some laxatives, and intravenous amphotericin.

Clinical evidence

A 4-year study in cardiac clinics in South Africa identified 13 patients who developed syncope and a prolonged QT interval while taking sotalol 80 to 480 mg daily. Eleven patients were being treated for hypertension, one for ventricular asystoles, and one for both. Polymorphous ventricular tachycardia was seen in 12 of the patients, and torsade de pointes were seen in 10 of these 12. Arrhythmias occurred within 72 hours of starting sotalol in 6 patients, and at varying intervals from 10 days to 3 years in the other 6 patients. Twelve patients were taking a combined preparation (*Sotazide*) containing sotalol 160 mg and **hydrochlorothiazide** 25 mg. Definite hypokalaemia (defined by the study as serum potassium of less than 3.5 mmol/l) was detected in 8 of the 13 patients. Four of the patients were also taking other drugs known to prolong the QT interval, namely disopyramide and tricyclic antidepressants. The problems resolved in all of the cases within 12 hours of stopping the sotalol and giving potassium supplements when indicated.[1]

Mechanism

Potassium-depleting drugs may cause hypokalaemia, which increases the potential for torsade de pointes arrhythmia with sotalol.

Importance and management

This interaction is established, clinically important and potentially life threatening. Prolongation of the QT interval and the development of torsade de pointes in patients on sotalol, particularly with high doses, is a recognised adverse effect, but it can occur even with small doses of sotalol if potassium depletion is allowed to develop. It is clearly very important therefore to ensure that potassium levels are maintained if potassium-depleting drugs are given with sotalol. A list of potassium-depleting diuretics is given in 'Table 24.1', (p.717). Other drugs that may cause potassium depletion include **corticosteroids**, some **laxatives**, and intravenous **amphotericin**.

1. McKibbin JK, Pocock WA, Barlow JB, Scott Millar RN, Obel IWP. Sotalol, hypokalaemia, syncope, and torsade de pointes. *Br Heart J* (1984) 51, 157–62.

Beta-blockers; Sotalol + Terfenadine

Episodes of torsade de pointes arrhythmia developed in a woman taking sotalol when terfenadine was added.

Clinical evidence, mechanism, importance and management

A 71-year-old woman with a history of atrial fibrillation was successfully treated with sotalol 80 mg twice daily. She started to take 60 mg terfenadine twice daily, and 8 days later she developed repeated self-limiting episodes of torsade de pointes arrhythmia. On one occasion she required resuscitation. Both drugs were stopped and no further episodes of arrhythmia occurred 72 hours after temporary pacing was discontinued.[1] It seems likely that what happened resulted from the additive effects of both drugs on the QT interval, which can lead to the development of torsade de pointes. This case confirms a previous mention of the possibility of this interaction.[2]

Although this seems to be the first report of this interaction, it is consistent with the known pharmacology of both drugs. Torsade de pointes is potentially life threatening so the concurrent use of these two drugs should generally be avoided. See also 'Drugs that prolong the QT interval + Other drugs that prolong the QT interval', p.170.

1. Feroze H, Suri R, Silverman DI. Torsades de pointes from terfenadine and sotalol given in combination. *Pacing Clin Electrophysiol* (1996) 19, 1519–21.
2. Woosley RL, Chen Y, Freiman JP, Gillis RA. Mechanism of the cardiotoxic actions of terfenadine. *JAMA* (1993) 269, 1532–6.

Beta-blockers; Talinolol + Sulfasalazine

Sulfasalazine markedly reduces the absorption of talinolol.

Clinical evidence

The AUC of talinolol 50 mg was reduced to by 91% (from 958 to 84 nanograms/ml per hour) in 8 healthy subjects given sulfasalazine 4 g. The maximum serum levels were also markedly reduced, from 112 to 23 nanograms/ml in 3 subjects, and to undetectable levels in the other 5 subjects.[1]

Mechanism

Not known. It is suggested that the talinolol is adsorbed onto the sulfasalazine, thereby preventing its absorption.[1]

Importance and management

Information is limited to this study, but it would appear to be an established and probably clinically important interaction. The efficacy of the talinolol would be expected to be markedly reduced, but this does not appear to have been studied. If the mechanism suggested by the authors is true, their advice to separate the dosages by 2 to 3 hours should minimise this interaction.[1] More study is needed to confirm how effective this action is, and whether other beta-blockers behave similarly.

1. Terhaag B, Palm U, Sahre H, Richter K, Oertel R. Interaction of talinolol and sulfasalazine in the human gastrointestinal tract. *Eur J Clin Pharmacol* (1992) 42, 461–2.

21

Calcium channel blockers

This section is primarily concerned with those interactions where the activity of the calcium channel blockers (sometimes called calcium antagonists) is changed by the presence of another drug. 'Table 21.1', (p.649) lists the calcium channel blockers with interactions described in this publication. However, not all of their interactions are necessarily dealt with in this section because, where the calcium channel blocker is the affecting agent, the relevant monograph may be categorised under the heading of the drug affected.

The calcium channel blockers have an increasingly wide application and are used for paroxysmal supraventricular tachycardia, angina, arrhythmias, hypertension, congestive heart failure, pulmonary disorders, gastrointestinal disorders and migraine headaches.

Table 21.1 Calcium channel blockers

Generic names	*Proprietary names*
Amlodipine	Agen, Akridipin, Amdipin, Amloc, Amlodac, Amlodin, Amlodine, Amlopine, Amloprax, Amlopres, Amlor, Amlosafe, Amlostad, Amlostat, Amlostin, Amlotabs, Amlotens, Amlotrust, Amlovasc, Amvaz, Amze, Anexa, Angiofilina, Anlodibal, Antacal, Astudal, Ateriosan, Avirin, Calchek, Calpres, Cardilopin, Cardionox, Cardiorex, Cordarex, Cordipina, Coroval, Ilduc, Istin, Lama, Lodipen, Mibral, Mitokor, Monopina, Myodura, Nemodine, Nicord, Normodipine, Norvas, Norvasc, Orcal, Pelmec, Presdeten, Presilam, Pressat, Prilpressin, Roxflan, S-Amlip, Sinop, Tensaliv, Tensodin, Terloc, Tervalon, Zorem, Zundic
Barnidipine	Cyress, Dilacor, Hypoca, Libradin, Vasexten
Bepridil	Unicordium
Diltiazem	Acalix, Acasmul, Adizem, Alandiem, Aldizem, Alfener, Altiazem, Angiodrox, Angiolong, Angiotrofin, Angiozem, Angitil, Angizem, Apo-Diltiaz, Balcor, Beatizem, Bi-Tildiem, Blocalcin, Cal-Antagon, Calcicard, Cardil, Cardiser, Cardium, Cardizem, Carreldon, Cartia, Cascor, Clobendian, Coramil, Coras, Corazem, Coridil, Corolater, Cronodine, Deltazen, Denazox, Diacardin, Diacor, Diacordin, Dilaclan, Dilacor, Diladel, Dilatam, Dilcard, Dilcardia, Dilcontin, Dilcor, Dilem, Dilfar, Dilgard, Diliter, Dilizem, Dilmin, Diloc, Dilongo, Dilpral, Dilrene, Dilsal, Dil-Sanorania, Dilta, Diltabeta, Diltahexal, Diltam, Diltan, Diltaretard, Diltec, Diltelan, Diltem, Diltenk, Dilti, Diltia, Diltiacor, Diltiagamma, Diltiangina, Diltiastad, Diltiem, Diltipress, Diltiuc, Diltiwas, Dilt-XR, Dilzanol, Dilzanton, Dilzem, Dilzene, Dilzen-G, Dinisor, Dipen, Disogram, Ditizem, Doclis, DTM, Elvesil, Entrydil, Ergoclavin, Escozem, Etizem, Etyzem, Grifodilzem, Hart, Herbesser, Incoril, Iski, Kaizem, Kaltiazem, Lacerol, Levodex, Longazem, Masdil, Mavitalon, Mono-Tildiem, Mycarzem, Myonil, Novo-Diltazem, Nu-Diltiaz, Optil, Progor, Ritmocit, Rubiten, Slozem, Surazem, Taztia, Ternel, Tiadil, Tiakem, Tiazac, Tilazem, Tildiem, Tilker, Trumsal, Uni Masdil, Vasocardol, Viazem, Wontizem, Zem, Zemtard, Zildem, Zilden
Felodipine	Cardioplen, Felim, Felo, Felobeta, Felocor, Feloday, Felodil, Felodin, Felodip, Felodur, Felogamma, Felogard, Felo-Puren, Felotens, Fensel, Flodil, Hydac, Keloc, Modip, Munobal, Neofel, Penedil, Perfudal, Plendil, Plendur, Presid, Preslow, Prevex, Renedil, Splendil, Vascalpha
Gallopamil	Algocor, Gallobeta, Procorum
Isradipine	Clivoten, Dilatol, Dynacirc, Esradin, Icaz, Lomir, Prescal, Vascal
Lacidipine	Aponil, Balnox, Caldine, Lacimen, Lacipil, Lacirex, Lacitens, Ladip, Midotens, Midotens, Motens, Sinopil, Tens, Viapres
Lercanidipine	Cardiovasc, Carmen, Corifeo, Lercadip, Lercan, Lercaton, Lerdip, Lerez, Lerzam, Vasodip, Zanedip, Zanicor, Zanidip
Manidipine	Artedil, Calslot, Iperten, Madiplot, Manivasc, Vascoman
Nicardipine	Antagonil, Bionicard, Cardene, Cardepine, Cardibloc, Cardioten, Cardip, Dagan, Flusemide, Karden, Lecibral, Lincil, Lisanirc, Loxen, Lucenfal, Nerdipina, Nerdipine, Neucor, Nicant, Nicapress, Nicardal, Nicarpin, Nicaven, Nimicor, Niven, Perdipina, Perdipine, Rydene, Vasodin, Vasonase
Nifedipine	Adalat, Adalate, Adefin, Adipine, Afeditab, Angiopine, Antiblut, Apo-Nifed, Aprical, Atenses, Buconif, Calchan, Calcigard, Carbloc, Cardalin, Cardicon, Cardifen, Cardilat, Cardilate MR, Cardiopine, Cardipin, Cardules, Chronadalate, Cipalat, Citilat, Coracten, Coral, Cordafen, Cordaflex, Cordicant, Cordilat, Cordipin, Cordipin, Corinfar, Corogal, Coronovo, Corotrend, Depicor, Depin, Dilaflux, Dilcor, duranifin, Ecodipine, Edip, Euxat, Fedip, Fenamon, Fenidina, Flecor-N, Fortipine, Fusepina, Glopir, Hexadilat, Hypan, Hypolar Retard, Jedipin, Jutadilat, Loncord, Macorel, Majolat, Medipina, Megalat, Myogard, Nadipinia, Nefelid, Nelapine, Neo Fedipina, Nifadil, Nifal, Nifangin, Nifdemin, Nife, nife-basan, Nifebene, Nifecard, Nifecard XL, Nifeclair, Nifecodan, Nifecor, Nifed, Nifed Sol, Nifedalat, Nifedate, Nifedax, Nifedel, Nifediac, Nifedical, Nifedicor, Nifedicron, Nifedin, Nifedine, Nifedipat, Nifedipres, Nifedipress, Nifehexal, Nifelat, Nifelat, Nifesal, Nifezzard, Nifical, Nifiran, Nifopress, Nipin, Nipress, Normopres, Novo-Nifedin, Nu-Nifed, Nyefax, Nypine, Osmo-Adalat, Ospocard, Oxcord, Pabalat, Pertensal, Pidilat, Pressolat, Procardia, Prudencial, Slofedipine, Sponif, Sulotil, Supracordin, Tensipine, Vascard, Vasofed, Vidalat, Viscard, Waridipin, Zenusin
Nilvadipine	Escor, Nivadil, Peroma, Tensan
Nimodipine	AC Vascular, Acival, Admon, Ampina, Aniduv, Aurodipine, Befimat, Brainal, Brainox, Calnit, Cebrofort, Cletonol, Curban, Dilceren, Eugerial, Figozant, Finacilen, Genovox, Grifonimod, Kenesil, Kenzolol, Macobal, Modina, Modus, Myodipine, Naborel, Nelbinex, Neurogeron, Nimodil, Nimodilat, Nimotop, Nimotop, Nimovas, Nivas, Noodipina, Nortolan, Norton, Oxigen, Periplum, Regental, Remontal, Rosital, Sobrepina, Stigmicarpin, Tenocard, Thrioniren, Trinalion, Vasodipina, Vasoflex, Vasotop, Vastripine, Ziremex
Nisoldipine	Baymycard, Cornel, Nisodipen, Nivas, Sular, Syscor
Nitrendipine	Aroselin, Baylotensin, Bayotensin, Baypresol, Baypress, Caltren, Cardiazem, Crivion, Deiten, Ditrenil, Farnitran, Gericin, G-Press, Grifonitren, Hiperdipina, Hipertenol, Jutapress, Lanocardique, Leonitren, Lisba, Lostradyl, Lusopress, Midonat, Miniten, Nelconil, Nidrel, Nifecard, Niprina, Nirapel, Nitre, Nitregamma, Nitren, Nitren Lich, Nitrencord, Nitrendicor, Nitrendidoc, Nitrendil, Nitrendimerck, Nitrensal, Nitrepress, Nitre-Puren, Pallohyman, Potional, Presabet, Pressodipin, Spidox, Sub Tensin, Tensofar, Tensogradal, Tepanil, Tocrat, Ufocard, Unipres, Vastensium
Prenylamine	
Tiapamil	
Verapamil	Akilen, Anpec, Apoacor, Apo-Verap, Brovicarpine, Calan, Calaptin, Calcicard, Cardinorm, Cardiolen, Caveril, Chinopamil, Chronovera, Cintsu, Civicor, Cordilat, Cordilox, Covera, Cronovera, Dilacard, Dilacoran, durasoptin, Elanver, Falicard, Flamon, Geangin, Half Securon, Hexasoptin, Ikacor, Ikapress, Isopamil, Isoptin, Isoptina, Isoptine, Isoptino, Lekoptin, Lodixal, Manidon, Neo Verpamil, Novo-Veramil, Nu-Verap, Presocor, Quasar, Ravamil, Securon, Univer, Vasomil, Vera, Verabeta, Veracaps, Veracor, Veragamma, Verahexal, Verakard, Veral, Vera-Lich, Veraloc, Veramex, Veramil, Veranorm, Verap, Verapabene, Verapal, Verapam, Verapin, Verapress, Veraptin, Verasal, Verastad, Veraval, Verelan, Verisop, Vermin, Vermine, Verogalid, Veroptinstada, Verpamil, Vertab, Zolvera

Calcium channel blockers + Antihistamines

An isolated report describes increased adverse effects in two patients when terfenadine was added to nifedipine or verapamil therapy.
No pharmacokinetic or pharmacodynamic interaction appears to occur between diltiazem and mizolastine. Nifedipine may increase levels of mizolastine.

Clinical evidence, mechanism, importance and management

A double-blind crossover study in 12 healthy subjects on **diltiazem** 60 mg three times daily found that the concurrent use of **mizolastine** 10 mg daily had no effect on ECGs or blood pressures. No significant increases in adverse effects were seen and the pharmacokinetics of the **diltiazem** remained unchanged.[1] There would seem to be no reason for avoiding concurrent use.

The makers[2,3] of both **nifedipine** and **mizolastine** suggest that concurrent use may raise **mizolastine** levels by inhibition of the cytochrome P450 isoenzyme CYP3A4 and caution is advised if they are used concurrently,[1] presumably because mizolastine has a weak potential to prolong the QT interval.

An isolated report describes severe angina in a patient stabilised on **nifedipine** 10 mg three times daily when she took **terfenadine** 60 mg for seasonal allergy. A second patient on **verapamil** 80 mg three times daily also experienced adverse effects (including severe headache and confusion) when a single 60-mg dose of **terfenadine** was taken.[4] Calcium channel blockers are metabolised by the cytochrome P450 isoenzyme CYP3A4, but there appear to be no other reports of interactions with either **terfenadine** or **astemizole** (substrates of CYP3A4). Nevertheless, the makers of **lercanidipine** advise caution during concurrent use.[5]

1. Miget N, Herrmann WM, Bergougnan L, Dubruc C, Weber F, Rosenzweig P. Lack of interaction between mizolastine and diltiazem in healthy volunteers. *Methods Find Exp Clin Pharmacol* (1996) 18 (Suppl B), 204.
2. Coracten SR (Nifedipine). Celltech Pharmaceuticals Ltd. UK Summary of product characteristics, July 2003.
3. Mizollen (Mizolastine). Schwarz Pharma Ltd. UK Summary of product characteristics, October 2003.
4. Falkenberg HM. Possible interaction report. *Can Pharm J* (1988) 121, 294.
5. Zanidip (Lercanidipine hydrochloride). Napp Pharmaceuticals Ltd. UK Summary of product characteristics, January 2004.

Calcium channel blockers + Antineoplastics

The absorption of verapamil can be modestly reduced by antineoplastic regimens containing cyclophosphamide, vincristine, and procarbazine, or vindesine, doxorubicin, cisplatin.

Clinical evidence, mechanism, importance and management

A study in 9 patients with a variety of malignant diseases found that treatment with antineoplastics reduced the absorption of a single 160-mg oral dose of **verapamil**. The **verapamil** AUC in 8 patients was reduced by 40% (range 7 to 58%), and one patient conversely had a 26% increase. Five patients received a modified **COPP** regimen (**cyclophosphamide, vincristine, procarbazine**, prednisone) and four received **VAC** (**vindesine, doxorubicin, cisplatin**).[1] It is believed that these antineoplastics damage the lining of the upper part of the small intestine, which impairs the absorption of **verapamil**. The clinical relevance of this reduction does not appear to have been studied. Note that **verapamil** may affect levels of 'anthracyclines', (p.449), 'etoposide', (p.466), and 'docetaxel', (p.490). In addition, **nifedipine** may affect the levels of 'vincristine', (p.498).

1. Kuhlmann J, Woodcock B, Wilke J, Rietbrock N. Verapamil plasma concentrations during treatment with cytostatic drugs. *J Cardiovasc Pharmacol* (1985) 7, 1003–6.

Calcium channel blockers + Antivirals

Symptomatic orthostasis occurred in a patient treated with nelfinavir or ritonavir/indinavir and nifedipine. Another patient had similar symptoms when nelfinavir was added to felodipine therapy. Nimodipine may increase the bioavailability of zidovudine. Atazanavir increases diltiazem bioavailability and is predicted to have the same effect on verapamil. Similarly, raised calcium channel blocker levels are predicted when lercanidipine is given with ritonavir and when nimodipine is given with the protease inhibitors.

Clinical evidence, mechanism, importance and management

(a) Diltiazem

A study in healthy subjects found that **atazanavir** 400 mg once daily with diltiazem 180 mg once daily resulted in a two- to threefold increase in the bioavailability of diltiazem and its metabolite desacetyl-diltiazem. The pharmacokinetics of **atazanavir** were not affected by diltiazem. There was an increase in the maximum PR interval with combined use compared to that found with **atazanavir** alone.[1,2] The makers recommend that if diltiazem is given with **atazanavir/ritonavir** the initial dose of diltiazem should be reduced by 50% with subsequent dose titration and ECG monitoring.[1,2]

(b) Felodipine

A woman receiving metoprolol 50 mg daily and felodipine 5 mg daily for hypertension developed bilateral leg oedema, orthostatic hypotension, and other symptoms including dizziness and fatigue, 3 days after starting HAART following a needle-stick injury. The antiretroviral therapy included zidovudine, lamivudine, and **nelfinavir** 2 g daily. Antihypertensive treatment was stopped and the adverse effects abated within 3 days. The patient was then successfully switched to a diuretic-based regimen without recurrence of oedema. It was thought that the **nelfinavir** (an inhibitor of the cytochrome P450 isoenzyme CYP3A4) reduced the metabolism of the felodipine leading to higher concentrations and the adverse effects. Several other protease inhibitors are also potent inhibitors of CYP3A4 and may also interact with felodipine.[3]

(c) Lercanidipine

The maker of lercanidipine warns that as it is metabolised by the cytochrome P450 isoenzyme CYP3A4, concurrent use of **ritonavir**, a potent inhibitor of CYP3A4, should be avoided.[4]

(d) Nifedipine

A 51-year-old HIV+ man with coronary artery disease, hypertension and osteoarthritis, and taking atenolol, was started on extended-release nifedipine 60 mg daily. When his blood pressure control improved he was started on zidovudine 300 mg, lamivudine 150 mg, and **nelfinavir** 1.25 g all twice daily. Within 3 days of starting the antiretroviral therapy he experienced dizziness, weakness and hypotension and developed complete heart block with a junctional escape rhythm. His ECG returned to normal within 24 hours of stopping the antiretroviral therapy, but he developed orthostatic symptoms within 2 days of restarting **nelfinavir**. He later tolerated a regimen consisting of stavudine, didanosine and efavirenz without any episodes of dizziness, hypotension or bradycardia. However, when he was given zidovudine, abacavir, **ritonavir**, and **indinavir**, he experienced hypotension, decreased heart rate, weakness and fatigue. His symptoms were controlled by modifying his antihypertensive therapy, including discontinuation of atenolol and reduction of the dose of nifedipine to 30 mg daily.[5]

The hypotensive effects observed in this patient were probably due to the inhibition of cytochrome P450 isoenzyme CYP3A4-mediated metabolism of nifedipine by **nelfinavir**, **ritonavir**, and **indinavir**.[5] The UK makers of nifedipine warn of the theoretical possibility that these and other protease inhibitors, including **amprenavir** and **saquinavir**, may inhibit the metabolism of nifedipine. They recommend that blood pressure monitoring is required and a reduction in nifedipine dose may be necessary.[6]

(e) Nimodipine

Studies in *animals* have shown that the AUC of **zidovudine** is increased and its volume of distribution and clearance rate decreased when it is given with nimodipine. The clinical relevance of the interaction is not known, but as the adverse effects of **zidovudine** are dose related, the possibility of this interaction should be borne in mind in patients treated with both drugs.[7]

The UK maker of nimodipine warns that concurrent administration with potent CYP3A4 inhibitors including protease inhibitors (e.g. **indinavir, nelfinavir, ritonavir, saquinavir**) may lead to substantially increased plasma concentrations of nimodipine and should be avoided; if concurrent administration is unavoidable then the patient's blood pressure should be carefully monitored.[7]

(f) Verapamil

The makers of **atazanavir/ritonavir** say that it may raise verapamil levels and therefore caution is advised if they are given concurrently.[1]

1. Reyataz (Atazanavir sulfate). Bristol-Myers Squibb Pharmaceuticals Ltd. UK Summary of product characteristics, February 2005.
2. Reyataz (Atazanavir sulfate). Bristol-Myers Squibb Company. US Prescribing information, June 2005.
3. Izzedine H, Launay-Vacher V, Deray G, Hulot J-S. Nelfinavir and felodipine: A cytochrome P450 3A4-mediated drug interaction. *Clin Pharmacol Ther* (2004) 75, 362–3.
4. Zanidip (Lercanidipine hydrochloride). Napp Pharmaceuticals Ltd. UK Summary of product characteristics, January 2004.
5. Rossi DR, Rathbun RC, Slater LN. Symptomatic orthostasis with extended-release nifedipine and protease inhibitors. *Pharmacotherapy* (2002) 22, 1312–16.
6. Adalat Retard (Nifedipine). Bayer plc. UK Summary of product characteristics, April 2005.
7. Nimotop (Nimodipine). Bayer plc. UK Summary of product characteristics, June 2002.

Calcium channel blockers + Aprepitant

When given together, markedly increased levels of both aprepitant and diltiazem are seen.

Clinical evidence, mechanism, importance and management

The US maker notes that aprepitant 230 mg daily with **diltiazem** 120 mg three times daily for 5 days increased the AUC of aprepitant twofold and increased the **diltiazem** AUC 1.7-fold in patients with hypertension. Nevertheless, aprepitant did not alter the effects of **diltiazem** on heart rate or blood pressure.[1]

Both aprepitant and **diltiazem** are substrates and inhibitors of the cytochrome P450 isoenzyme CYP3A4, therefore they inhibit each others metabolism.

The clinical relevance of this interaction is uncertain, but the makers recommend caution with **diltiazem** and other moderate inhibitors of CYP3A4.[1]

1. Emend (Aprepitant). Merck & Co., Inc. US Prescribing information, March 2005.

Calcium channel blockers + Azoles

Itraconazole can markedly raise the serum levels of felodipine, which increases its adverse effects, in particular ankle and leg swelling. A few case reports suggest that isradipine and nifedipine can interact similarly with itraconazole, and that fluconazole can also interact with nifedipine. Ketoconazole can markedly raise the plasma levels of lercanidipine and nisoldipine.

Clinical evidence

(a) Felodipine

When **itraconazole** 200 mg daily or a placebo was given to 9 healthy subjects for 4 days followed by a single 5-mg dose of felodipine, it was found that the felodipine AUC was increased sixfold and the maximum plasma levels were increased eightfold. The effects of the felodipine on blood pressure and heart rate were also increased.[1]

A 52-year-old woman taking felodipine 10 mg daily for hypertension for a year, without problems, developed ankle and leg swelling within 7 days of starting **itraconazole** 100 mg daily for tinea pedis. The oedema disappeared within 2 to 4 days of stopping the **itraconazole**.[2] Virtually the same reaction occurred in another woman taking both drugs. Later tests found that her 0 to 6-hour AUC of a single 5-mg dose of felodipine was increased at least fourfold (possibly up to tenfold) while taking **itraconazole** and ankle swelling was noted.[2]

(b) Isradipine

Ankle swelling was noted in one patient on isradipine 5 mg daily when **itraconazole** 200 mg twice daily was also taken.[2]

(c) Lercanidipine

An interaction study found that **ketoconazole** increased the lercanidipine AUC and peak plasma levels 15-fold and 8-fold respectively.[3]

(d) Nifedipine

A report describes massive pitting oedema in the legs and ankles of a patient taking nifedipine when **itraconazole** 100 mg twice daily was also taken.[4] Another patient similarly had ankle oedema and markedly raised serum nifedipine levels (trough levels raised almost fivefold) when **itraconazole** was also taken.[5] A patient with malignant phaeochromocytoma whose persistent hypertension was controlled with nifedipine had a rise in blood pressure when **fluconazole** 200 mg daily was stopped. His blood pressure fell again when the **fluconazole** was restarted. A later study found that his maximum nifedipine plasma levels and 0 to 5-hour AUC were raised about threefold by **fluconazole**.[6]

(e) Nisoldipine

A study in 7 healthy subjects found that **ketoconazole** 200 mg daily for 5 days increased the AUC and peak plasma levels of a single 5-mg dose of nisoldipine by 24-fold and 11-fold respectively. The levels of nisoldipine metabolite were similarly increased.[7]

Mechanism

Ankle swelling due to precapillary vasodilatation is a not an uncommon adverse effect of the dihydropyridine calcium channel blockers, which appears to be dose-related. Calcium channel blockers are metabolised in the gut wall and liver by the cytochrome P450 CYP3A subfamily of isoenzymes, which are inhibited by itraconazole, ketoconazole and to an extent fluconazole, so that in the presence of these antifungals the levels of the calcium channel blockers are raised and the adverse effects increased.

Importance and management

The interaction between felodipine and itraconazole would appear to be established and clinically important. It also seems that isradipine, lercanidipine, nifedipine and nisoldipine can interact similarly with fluconazole, itraconazole or ketoconazole and it is possible that other calcium channel blockers including **diltiazem** and **nimodipine** may behave in the same way. If itraconazole, ketoconazole, or fluconazole is given to a patient on established treatment with any calcium channel blocker be alert for the need to lower the dosage. The makers of lercanidipine[3] contraindicates itraconazole and ketoconazole, and the UK maker of nisoldipine[8] additionally contraindicates fluconazole.

1. Jalava K-M, Olkkola KT, Neuvonen PJ. Itraconazole greatly increases plasma concentrations and effects of felodipine. *Clin Pharmacol Ther* (1997) 61, 410–15.
2. Neuvonen PJ, Suhonen R. Itraconazole interacts with felodipine. *J Am Acad Dermatol* (1995) 33, 134–5.
3. Zanidip (Lercanidipine hydrochloride). Napp Pharmaceuticals Ltd. UK Summary of product characteristics, January 2004.
4. Rosen T. Debilitating edema associated with itraconazole therapy. *Arch Dermatol* (1994) 130, 260–1.
5. Tailor SAN, Gupta AK, Walker SE, Shear NH. Peripheral edema due to nifedipine-itraconazole interaction: a case report. *Arch Dermatol* (1996) 132, 350–2.
6. Kremens B, Brendel E, Bald M, Czyborra P, Michel MC. Loss of blood pressure control on withdrawal of fluconazole during nifedipine therapy. *Br J Clin Pharmacol* (1999) 47, 707–8.
7. Heinig R, Adelmann HG, Ahr G. The effect of ketoconazole on the pharmacokinetics, pharmacodynamics and safety of nisoldipine. *Eur J Clin Pharmacol* (1999) 55, 57–60.
8. Syscor MR (Nisoldipine). Forest Laboratories UK Ltd. UK Summary of product characteristics, August 1998.

Calcium channel blockers + Bile acids

Chenodeoxycholic acid and ursodeoxycholic acid reduce the bioavailability of nitrendipine.

Clinical evidence, mechanism, importance and management

A single-dose study in 6 healthy subjects given **nitrendipine** 10 mg with or without either **chenodeoxycholic acid** 200 mg or 600 mg, or **ursodeoxycholic acid** 50 mg, found that **ursodeoxycholic acid** reduced the peak plasma level and AUC of **nitrendipine** by 54% and 75% respectively. **Chenodeoxycholic acid** 200 mg decreased the AUC and peak plasma level of **nitrendipine** by about 20% but the 600-mg dose reduced the peak plasma level and AUC of **nitrendipine** by 54% and 68% respectively. The reduction in bioavailability of **nitrendipine** was possibly due to the effects of the bile acids on tablet disintegration or more probably on drug solubilisation. The clinical importance of the interaction is not known.[1]

1. Sasaki M, Maeda A, Sakamoto K-I, Fujimura A. Effect of bile acids on absorption of nitrendipine in healthy subjects. *Br J Clin Pharmacol* (2001) 52, 699–701.

Calcium channel blockers + Bile-acid binding resins

Colesevelam reduces the bioavailability of verapamil and colestipol reduces the bioavailability of diltiazem.

Clinical evidence, mechanism, importance and management

(a) Colesevelam

A study in 31 healthy subjects found that a single 4.5-g dose of colesevelam reduced the peak plasma levels and AUC of a single 240-mg dose of **verapamil** by about 33% and about 15% respectively. These changes were not considered to be clinically significant.[1]

(b) Colestipol

A study in 12 healthy subjects found that colestipol reduced the AUC and peak plasma levels of a single 120-mg dose of sustained-release **diltiazem** by 22% and 36% respectively and those of a single 120-mg dose of immediate-release **diltiazem** by 27% and 33% respectively. In a further study sustained-release **diltiazem** 120 mg was given either without colestipol, or 1 hour before or 4 hours after multiple doses of colestipol. The AUC of **diltiazem** was decreased by 17% when it was taken 1 hour before colestipol and by 22% when taken 4 hours after colestipol. This suggests that the effects of colestipol on **diltiazem** bioavailability are not reduced by separating their administration. However, it is not known whether the interaction will result in reduced **diltiazem** efficacy, but caution is advised if these drugs are used concurrently.[2]

1. Donovan JM, Stypinski D, Stiles MR, Olson TA, Burke SK. Drug interactions with colesevelam hydrochloride, a novel, potent lipid-lowering agent. *Cardiovasc Drugs Ther* (2000) 14, 681–90.
2. Turner SW, Jungbluth GL, Knuth DW. Effect of concomitant colestipol hydrochloride administration on the bioavailability of diltiazem from immediate- and sustained-release formulations. *Biopharm Drug Dispos* (2002) 23, 369–77.

Calcium channel blockers + Calcium channel blockers

Plasma levels of both nifedipine and diltiazem are increased by concurrent use and blood pressure is reduced accordingly. This has been claimed to be an advantageous interaction but caution is advised. There are isolated reports of intestinal occlusion attributed to the concurrent nifedipine and diltiazem. If nimodipine is used with another calcium channel blocker, monitoring, with possible dose reduction or discontinuation of the other calcium channel blocker is recommended.

Clinical evidence

Pretreatment of 6 healthy subjects with **diltiazem** 30 or 90 mg three times daily for 3 days was found to increase the AUC of a single 20-mg dose of **nifedipine** two- and threefold respectively.[1] Similar and related results are reported elsewhere.[2] In another study it was found that **nifedipine** 10 mg three times daily for 3 days increased the maximum plasma levels of a single 60-mg dose of **diltiazem** by 54% and increased its AUC by 49%.[3]

A patient on **nifedipine** 20 mg twice daily developed abdominal distension and vomiting 2 days after also being given **diltiazem** 100 mg twice daily. Both calcium channel blockers were stopped and abdominal X-ray suggested paralytic ileus, which resolved but then recurred when the drugs were restarted. The excessive relaxation of the intestine was attributed to elevated **nifedipine** plasma levels, which were said to be caused by **diltiazem.**[4] Another report attributes complete or partial intestinal occlusion in a patient on **diltiazem** on three occasions, each time when **nifedipine** was added.[5]

Mechanism

A reduction in the metabolism of both the nifedipine and diltiazem in the liver seems to be the explanation.[3] An increased relaxant effect on smooth muscle is suggested for the cases of intestinal occlusion.[5]

Importance and management

Established interactions but of uncertain clinical importance. The authors of these reports suggest that the effects of the concurrent use of diltiazem and nifedipine are usually beneficial rather than adverse, and that the dosage of the nifedipine can be reduced. Although fewer adverse effects and better compliance have been predicted,[1] the makers of nifedipine[6] advise caution when it is used with diltiazem because of possible increases in nifedipine levels. Information about the use of combinations of other calcium channel blockers appears to be lacking. However, the UK makers of **nimodipine**[7] advise that if it is used with other antihypertensive drugs, including other calcium channel blockers such as nifedipine, diltiazem, or verapamil, blood pressure monitoring and careful dose titration of nimodipine should be carried out with possible reduction or discontinuation of the other calcium channel blocker.

1. Tateishi T, Ohashi K, Sudo T, Sakamoto K, Toyosaki N, Hosoda S, Toyo-oka T, Kumagai Y, Sugimoto K, Fujimura A, Ebihara A. Dose dependent effect of diltiazem on the pharmacokinetics of nifedipine. *J Clin Pharmacol* (1989) 29, 994–7.
2. Ohashi K, Tateishi T, Sudo T, Sakamoto K, Toyosaki N, Hosoda S, Toyo-oka T, Sugimoto K, Kumagai Y, Ebihara A. Effects of diltiazem on the pharmacokinetics of nifedipine. *J Cardiovasc Pharmacol* (1990) 15, 96–101.
3. Tateishi T, Ohashi K, Sudo T, Sakamoto K, Fujimura A, Ebihara A. The effect of nifedipine on the pharmacokinetics and dynamics of diltiazem: the preliminary study in normal volunteers. *J Clin Pharmacol* (1993) 33, 738–40.
4. Harada T, Ohtaki E, Sumiyoshi T, Hosoda S. Paralytic ileus induced by the combined use of nifedipine and diltiazem in the treatment of vasospastic angina. *Cardiology* (2002) 97, 113–14.
5. Lamaison D, Abrieu V, Fialip J, Dumas R, Andronikoff M, Lavarenne J. Occlusion intestinale aiguë et antagonistes calciques. *Therapie* (1989) 44, 201–2.
6. Adalat Retard (Nifedipine). Bayer plc. UK Summary of product characteristics, April 2005.
7. Nimotop (Nimodipine). Bayer plc. UK Summary of product characteristics, June 2002.

Calcium channel blockers + Calcium compounds

The concurrent use of verapamil and intravenous calcium compounds can be therapeutically useful, but an isolated report describes antagonism of the antiarrhythmic effects of verapamil due to the use of oral calcium and calciferol.

Clinical evidence, mechanism, importance and management

Verapamil is effective in treating atrial fibrillation and supraventricular arrhythmias, and if preceded by an intravenous infusion of calcium gluconate or chloride, its hypotensive and possible negative inotropic effects are reduced or prevented without compromising its antiarrhythmic effects.[1-5] Concurrent use is therefore normally valuable,[6] but an isolated report describes an adverse response:

An elderly woman with atrial fibrillation, successfully treated for over a year with **verapamil**, developed atrial fibrillation within a week of starting to take an oral calcium compound 1.2 g with calciferol (vitamin D) 3000 units daily for diffuse osteoporosis. Her serum calcium levels had risen from 2.45 to 2.7 mmol/l. Normal sinus rhythm was restored by giving 500 ml of saline and repeated doses of furosemide 20 mg and **verapamil** 5 mg by intravenous injection.[7]

Verapamil acts by inhibiting the passage of calcium ions into cardiac muscle cells and it would appear that in this case the increased concentration of calcium ions outside the cells opposed the effects of the **verapamil**.

The general importance of this isolated case is uncertain, but it would clearly be prudent to monitor concurrent use for any signs of reduced **verapamil** effects.

1. Roguin N, Shapir Y, Blazer S, Zeltzer M, Berant M. The use of calcium gluconate prior to verapamil in infants with paroxysmal supraventricular tachycardia. *Clin Cardiol* (1984) 7, 613–16.
2. Salerno DM, Anderson B, Sharkey PJ, Iber C. Intravenous verapamil for treatment of multifocal atrial tachycardia with and without calcium pretreatment. *Ann Intern Med* (1987) 107, 623–8.
3. Haft JI, Habbab MA. Treatment of atrial arrhythmias: effectiveness of verapamil when preceded by calcium infusion. *Arch Intern Med* (1986) 146, 1085–9.
4. Schoen MD, Parker RB, Hoon TJ, Hariman RJ, Bauman JL, Beckman KJ. Evaluation of the pharmacokinetics and electrocardiographic effects of intravenous verapamil with intravenous calcium chloride pretreatment in normal subjects. *Am J Cardiol* (1991) 67, 300–4.
5. Weiss AT, Lewis BS, Halon DA, Hasin Y, Gotsman MS. The use of calcium with verapamil in the management of supraventricular tachyarrhythmias. *Int J Cardiol* (1983) 4, 275–80.
6. Moser LR, Smythe MA, Tisdale JE. The use of calcium salts in the prevention and management of verapamil-induced hypotension. *Ann Pharmacother* (2000) 34, 622–9.
7. Bar-Or D, Yoel G. Calcium and calciferol antagonise effect of verapamil in atrial fibrillation. *BMJ* (1981) 282, 1585–6.

Calcium channel blockers + Ceftriaxone and Clindamycin

An isolated report describes the development of complete heart block in a man on long-term verapamil, attributed to the use of intravenous ceftriaxone and clindamycin. The validity of this interaction has been questioned.

Clinical evidence, mechanism, importance and management

A 59-year-old man who had been on **SR verapamil** 240 mg twice daily for 2 years and phenytoin 300 mg daily for several years, developed complete heart block an hour after being given intravenous ceftriaxone 1 g and clindamycin 900 mg for bilateral pneumonia. He needed cardiopulmonary resuscitation and the insertion of a temporary pacemaker, but spontaneously recovered normal sinus rhythm after 16 hours. He made a full recovery. The reasons for this serious reaction are not known, but the authors of the report postulate that these two antibacterials precipitated acute **verapamil** toxicity, possibly by displacing it from its plasma protein binding sites. Although both antibacterials are highly protein-bound (93% or more),[1] they are acidic and do not bind to the same sites as the **verapamil** (a base), so that this mechanism of interaction seems very unlikely. This seems to be the first and only report of this reaction, and the suggestion by the authors that it was due to a drug interaction has been seriously questioned.[2] There seems to be no evidence that either of these antibacterials normally interact with **verapamil** if given orally.

1. Kishore K, Raina A, Misra V, Jonas E. Acute verapamil toxicity in a patient with chronic toxicity: possible interaction with ceftriaxone and clindamycin. *Ann Pharmacother* (1993) 27, 877–80.
2. Horn JR, Hansten PD. Comment: pitfalls in reporting drug interactions. *Ann Pharmacother* (1993) 27, 1545–6.

Calcium channel blockers + Clonidine

Two hypertensive patients taking verapamil developed complete heart block when clonidine was added. No adverse interaction appears to occur between nifedipine and clonidine.

Clinical evidence

A 54-year-old woman with refractory hypertension (240/140 mmHg) and hyperaldosteronism had a reduction in her blood pressure, to 180/100 mmHg, after 10 days of treatment with **verapamil** 160 mg three times daily and spironolactone 100 mg daily. She was additionally given clonidine 150 micrograms twice daily, and after the second dose she became confused and her blood pressure was found to have fallen to 90/70 mmHg, with a heart rate of 50 bpm. She had developed complete AV block, which resolved when all therapy was stopped. A 65-year-old woman, with persistent hypertension did not have a satisfactory reduction in blood pressure with extended-release **verapamil** 240 mg daily (blood pressure 165/100 mmHg). Clonidine 150 micrograms twice daily was then added, and the next day a routine ECG showed that she had a nodal rhythm of 80 bpm, which developed into complete AV block. Her blood pressure had fallen to 130/80 mmHg.[1]

Clonidine 250 micrograms daily for 2 weeks increased the hypotensive effects of **nifedipine** 20 mg twice daily by about 5 mmHg (mean blood pressure) in 12 patients.[2]

Mechanism

Not fully understood. Verapamil very occasionally causes AV node disturbances, but both of these patients had normal sinus rhythm before the clonidine was added. Clonidine alone has been associated with AV node dysfunction in hypertensive patients. It would seem therefore that these effects were additive in these two patients.[1]

Importance and management

Information about the interaction between verapamil and clonidine seems to be limited to this report.[1] Its authors say that a review of the literature from 1966 to 1992 revealed no reports of any adverse interactions between these drugs. Nonetheless, they suggest that it would now be prudent to give these two drugs together with caution and good monitoring in any patient, even in those without sinus or AV node dysfunction. There seems to be no particular need for additional caution when nifedipine is given with clonidine.

1. Jaffe R, Livshits T, Bursztyn M. Adverse interaction between clonidine and verapamil. *Ann Pharmacother* (1994) 28, 881–3.
2. Salvetti A, Pedrinelli R, Magagna A, Stornello M, Scapellato L. Calcium antagonists: interactions in hypertension. *Am J Nephrol* (1986) 6 (Suppl 1), 95–9.

Calcium channel blockers + Co-trimoxazole

Co-trimoxazole normally appears not to interact with nifedipine, but adverse effects (leg cramps, facial flushing) have been reported in one patient.

Clinical evidence, mechanism, importance and management

The observation of a patient on **nifedipine** who developed leg cramps and facial flushing (possibly as a result of raised plasma **nifedipine** levels) when given co-trimoxazole, prompted further study of this possible interaction in 9 healthy subjects. After taking co-trimoxazole 960 mg twice daily for 3 days the pharmacokinetics and hypotensive effects of single 20-mg doses of **nifedipine** were found to be unchanged.[1] No special precautions would therefore normally seem to be necessary on concurrent use.

1. Edwards C, Monkman S, Cholerton S, Rawlins MD, Idle JR, Ferner RE. Lack of effect of co-trimoxazole on the pharmacokinetics and pharmacodynamics of nifedipine. *Br J Clin Pharmacol* (1990) 30, 889–91.

Calcium channel blockers + Dantrolene

An isolated report describes acute hyperkalaemia and cardiovascular collapse when dantrolene was given in the presence of verapamil, but not nifedipine.

Clinical evidence, mechanism, importance and management

A 60-year-old man with coronary artery disease taking **verapamil** 80 mg three times daily, with a history of malignant hyperthermia and undergoing surgery, had marked myocardial depression and hyperkalaemia of 7.1 mmol/l within about 2.5 hours of being given **dantrolene** 220 mg intravenously.[1] Six months later similar preoperative and intraoperative procedures were undertaken uneventfully when the **verapamil** was replaced by **nifedipine** 10 mg three times daily. Hyperkalaemia and cardiovascular collapse have been seen in *pigs* and *dogs* given **dantrolene** and **verapamil** or **diltiazem**, but not with **nifedipine** or **amlodipine**.[2-6]

These observations would seem to link with a report of 3 patients taking **verapamil**, who developed hypotension and sinus bradycardia, all of whom were noted to be hyperkalaemic. In two cases their severe left ventricular dysfunction reversed when they were given intravenous calcium.[7] Studies in *dogs* confirmed that hyperkalaemia reduced myocardial contractility in the presence of **verapamil**, and this was reversed by calcium.[7]

The overall picture is that hyperkalaemia can apparently increase the myocardial depression caused by **verapamil**, and it seems possible that drugs other than **dantrolene**, which can raise blood potassium levels, may be among the factors that may predispose patients to severe left ventricular dysfunction. As a result of the potentially fatal ventricular arrhythmias observed in *animals* some makers contraindicate the use of either **diltiazem**[8,9] or **verapamil**[10] with **dantrolene**. More study is needed.

1. Rubin AS, Zablocki AD. Hyperkalemia, verapamil, and dantrolene. *Anesthesiology* (1987) 66, 246–9.
2. Lynch C, Durbin CG, Fisher NA, Veselis RA, Althaus JS. Effects of dantrolene and verapamil on atrioventricular conduction and cardiovascular performance in dogs. *Anesth Analg* (1986) 65, 252–8.
3. San Juan AC, Port JD, Wong KC. Hyperkalemia after dantrolene administration in dogs. *Anesth Analg* (1986) 65, S131.
4. Saltzman LS, Kates RA, Corke BC, Norfleet EA, Heath KR. Hyperkalemia and cardiovascular collapse after verapamil and dantrolene administration in swine. *Anesth Analg* (1984) 63, 473–8.
5. Saltzman LS, Kates RA, Norfleet EA, Corke BC, Heath KS. Hemodynamic interactions of diltiazem-dantrolene and nifedipine and nifedipine-dantrolene. *Anesthesiology* (1984) 61, A11.
6. Freysz M, Timour Q, Bernaud C, Bertrix L, Faucon G. Cardiac implications of amlodipine-dantrolene combinations. *Can J Anaesth* (1996) 43, 50–5.
7. Jolly SR, Keaton N, Movahed A, Rose GC, Reeves WC. Effect of hyperkalemia on experimental myocardial depression by verapamil. *Am Heart J* (1991) 121, 517–23.
8. Dilzem SR (Diltiazem hydrochloride). Zeneus Pharma Ltd. UK Summary of product characteristics, November 2003.

9. Tildiem Retard (Diltiazem hydrochloride). Sanofi-Aventis. UK Summary of product characteristics, April 2004.
10. Univer (Verapamil hydrochloride). Zeneus Pharma Ltd. UK Summary of product characteristics, August 2003.

Calcium channel blockers + Diuretics

Diuretics may not affect the pharmacokinetics of calcium channel blockers. Combinations of these drugs are used clinically for their additive antihypertensive effects but care is required to avoid hypotension.

Clinical evidence, mechanism, importance and management

A study in 21 healthy subjects given **diltiazem** 60 mg 4 times daily (for 21 doses) and **hydrochlorothiazide** 25 mg twice daily (for 11 doses) either alone or in combination found that at steady-state there was no clinically significant pharmacokinetic interaction between the two drugs.[1] However, the makers[2] say that patients on **diltiazem** and also receiving diuretics should be strictly monitored. The pharmacokinetics of **isradipine** and **hydrochlorothiazide** are not affected by concurrent administration,[3] and the pharmacokinetics of **nifedipine** are not affected by either **hydrochlorothiazide** or **triamterene**.[4] **Spironolactone** 50 mg was found not to affect the pharmacokinetics of **felodipine** or its clinical effects.[5]

The makers say that **amlodipine** has been safely administered with **thiazide diuretics** and no dosage adjustment of **amlodipine** is required.[6] Additive antihypertensive effects are expected when diuretics such as **hydrochlorothiazide** are used in combination with calcium channel blockers, including **felodipine**,[7,8] **lacidipine**,[9] **lercanidipine**,[10] **nicardipine**,[11] **nifedipine**,[12] and such combinations are used clinically, but care is required to avoid hypotension.[7,11]

1. Weir SJ, Dimmitt DC, Lanman RC, Morrill MB, Geising DH. Steady-state pharmacokinetics of diltiazem and hydrochlorothiazide administered alone and in combination. *Biopharm Drug Dispos* (1998) 19, 365–71.
2. Dilzem SR (Diltiazem hydrochloride). Zeneus Pharma Ltd. UK Summary of product characteristics, November 2003.
3. Prescal (Isradipine). Novartis Pharmaceuticals UK Ltd. UK Summary of product characteristics, February 2002.
4. Adalat Retard (Nifedipine). Bayer plc. UK Summary of product characteristics, April 2005.
5. Janzon K, Edgar B, Lundborg P, Regardh CG. The influence of cimetidine and spironolactone on the pharmacokinetics and haemodynamic effects of felodipine in healthy subjects. *Acta Pharmacol Toxicol (Copenh)* (1986) 59 (Suppl 4), 98.
6. Istin (Amlodipine besilate). Pfizer Ltd. UK Summary of product characteristics, April 2005.
7. Plendil (Felodipine). AstraZeneca UK Ltd. UK Summary of product characteristics, September 2003.
8. Vascalpha (Felodipine). Alpharma Ltd. UK Summary of product characteristics, August 2003.
9. Motens (Lacidipine). Boehringer Ingelheim Ltd. UK Summary of product characteristics, July 2003.
10. Zanidip (Lercanidipine hydrochloride). Napp Pharmaceuticals Ltd. UK Summary of product characteristics, January 2004.
11. Cardene (Nicardipine hydrochloride). Yamanouchi Pharma Ltd. UK Summary of product characteristics, April 2004.
12. Coracten SR (Nifedipine). Celltech Pharmaceuticals Ltd. UK Summary of product characteristics, July 2003.

Calcium channel blockers + Fluoxetine

Two patients on verapamil and two on nifedipine developed increased adverse effects (oedema, headaches, nausea, flushing, orthostatic hypotension) due to the concurrent use of fluoxetine. Fluoxetine appears to increase nimodipine levels and fluoxetine levels may be decreased by nimodipine. There does not appear to be a pharmacokinetic interaction between lercanidipine and fluoxetine.

Clinical evidence

(a) Lercanidipine

A study in elderly subjects found that fluoxetine had no clinically relevant effects on the pharmacokinetics of lercanidipine.[1]

(b) Nifedipine

A patient on nifedipine 60 mg daily developed nausea and flushing after also starting to take fluoxetine 20 mg every other day. The adverse effects gradually disappeared over the next 2 to 3 weeks when the nifedipine dosage was halved.[2] An 80-year-old woman on nifedipine developed tachycardia, hypotension and profound weakness 10 days after starting fluoxetine 20 mg daily. On admission to hospital 8 days later she was unable to stand, her standing blood pressure was 90/50 mmHg and her heart rate was 120 bpm. She fully recovered within a week of stopping the fluoxetine.[3]

(c) Nimodipine

In elderly patients nimodipine 30 mg twice daily given with fluoxetine 20 mg daily resulted in an increase in plasma levels of nimodipine, a reduction in plasma levels of fluoxetine, and a trend towards increased levels of the metabolite norfluoxetine.[4]

(d) Verapamil

A woman on verapamil 240 mg daily developed oedema of the feet and ankles, and neck vein distention within 6 weeks of starting fluoxetine 20 mg every other day. The oedema resolved within 2 to 3 weeks of reducing the verapamil dosage to 120 mg daily.[2] Another patient taking verapamil 240 mg daily for the prophylaxis of migraine developed morning headaches (believed by the patient not to be migraine) about one week after increasing his fluoxetine dosage from 20 to 40 mg daily. The headaches stopped when the verapamil dosage was reduced and then stopped.[2]

Mechanism

The calcium channel blockers are metabolised by the cytochrome P450 isoenzyme CYP3A4, which can be inhibited by fluoxetine, which results in a marked reduction in the metabolism and clearance of the calcium channel blockers. The reactions reported appear to be the exaggeration of the adverse effects of these calcium channel blockers, possibly due to an increase in their levels.

Importance and management

Although information on nifedipine and verapamil appears to be limited to these reports,[2,3] it would seem reasonable to monitor their concurrent use with fluoxetine, being alert for the need to reduce the drug dosages. The clinical significance of the interaction between nimodipine and fluoxetine is not known.[4] More study is needed. Information about other calcium channel blockers with fluoxetine appears to be lacking.

1. Zanidip (Lercanidipine hydrochloride). Napp Pharmaceuticals Ltd. UK Summary of product characteristics, January 2004.
2. Sternbach H. Fluoxetine-associated potentiation of calcium-channel blockers. *J Clin Psychopharmacol* (1991) 11, 390–1.
3. Azaz-Livshits TLT, Danenberg HD. Tachycardia, orthostatic hypotension and profound weakness due to concomitant use of fluoxetine and nifedipine. *Pharmacopsychiatry* (1997) 30, 274–5.
4. Nimotop (Nimodipine). Bayer plc. UK Summary of product characteristics, June 2002.

Calcium channel blockers + Food

The bioavailability of manidipine may be increased by food and the plasma levels of other lipophilic calcium channel blockers may also be affected. Food appears not to have an important effect on the absorption of bepridil, nifedipine or verapamil in standard or sustained-release formulations although the release characteristics of one modified-release preparation of nifedipine were affected.

Clinical evidence

(a) Bepridil

The absorption of two 200-mg capsules of bepridil in 15 healthy subjects was delayed by food (time to peak plasma level prolonged from 2.6 to 3.8 hours) but the amount absorbed was unchanged.[1] It seems likely that steady-state levels will be unaffected by food.

(b) Manidipine

The bioavailability of single 20-mg doses of manidipine was increased by 42% when given to 12 healthy subjects after a standard breakfast rather than in the fasting state. Peak plasma levels were increased by about 25% (not significant) by food, and the rate of absorption was unaffected.[2]

(c) Nifedipine

Some single-dose studies suggested that food might delay[3] the absorption of nifedipine and reduce its peak levels,[4,5] but a multiple dose study found that food did not have an important effect on the steady-state levels of nifedipine in a 'biphasic' formulation.[6] A further single-dose study in healthy subjects found that the bioavailability of two modified-release preparations of nifedipine (*Adalat OROS* or *Nifedicron*) were not significantly different when they were given in the fasting state, although the maximum plasma levels were 31 and 53 micrograms/litre respectively. The bioavailability and maximum plasma level (38 micrograms/litre) of *Adalat OROS* were similar after a high-fat breakfast to those in the fasting state. However, the maximum plasma level of *Nifedicron* increased to 128 micrograms/litre after a high-fat breakfast. Although the bioavailability of *Nifedicron* was only modestly increased by food, the increase in plasma levels indicates a loss of modified-release characteristics and suggests that the effect of food on nifedipine may depend on the product formulation.[7]

(d) Verapamil

The absorption of verapamil from a multiparticulate sustained release preparation were not affected when it was given with food.[8]

Mechanism

The increase in bioavailability of manidipine in the presence of food may be because it is lipophilic and solubilised by food and bile secretions. Similar effects have been observed for other lipophilic dihydropyridine calcium channel blockers such as **benidipine**, **felodipine** and **nisoldipine**.[2]

Importance and management

Food increases the extent of absorption of manidipine and so it has been recommended that manidipine should be given with food.[2] Because of the increase in peak plasma concentrations, the makers of **lercanidipine**[9] and nisoldipine[10] recommend they are given (at least 15 minutes[9]) before meals.

1. Easterling DE, Stellar SM, Nayak RK, Desiraju RK. The effect of food on the bioavailability of bepridil. *J Clin Pharmacol* (1984) 24, 416–17.
2. Rosillon D, Stockis A, Poli G, Acerbi D, Lins R, Jeanbaptiste B. Food effect on the oral bioavailability of manidipine: single dose, randomized, crossover study in healthy male subjects. *Eur J Drug Metab Pharmacokinet* (1998) 23, 197–202.
3. Ochs HR, Rämsch K-D, Verburg-Ochs B, Greenblatt DJ, Gerloff J. Nifedipine: kinetics and dynamics after single oral doses. *Klin Wochenschr* (1984) 62, 427–9.
4. Reitberg DP, Love SJ, Quercia GT, Zinny MA. Effect of food on nifedipine pharmacokinetics. *Clin Pharmacol Ther* (1987) 42, 72–5.
5. Challenor VF, Waller DG, Gruchy BS, Renwick AG, George CF. Food and nifedipine pharmacokinetics. *Br J Clin Pharmacol* (1987) 23, 248–9.
6. Rimoy GH, Idle JR, Bhaskar NK, Rubin PC. The influence of food on the pharmacokinetics of 'biphasic' nifedipine at steady state in normal subjects. *Br J Clin Pharmacol* (1989) 28, 612–15.
7. Schug BS, Brendel E, Wonnemann M, Wolf D, Wargenau M, Dingler A, Blume HH. Dosage form-related food interaction observed in a marketed once-daily nifedipine formulation after a high-fat American breakfast. *Eur J Clin Pharmacol* (2002) 58, 119–25.
8. Devane JG, Kelly JG. Effect of food on the bioavailability of a multiparticulate sustained-release verapamil formulation. *Adv Therapy* (1991) 8, 48–53.
9. Zanidip (Lercanidipine hydrochloride). Napp Pharmaceuticals Ltd. UK Summary of product characteristics, January 2004.
10. Syscor MR (Nisoldipine). Forest Laboratories UK Ltd. UK Summary of product characteristics, August 1998.

Calcium channel blockers + Grapefruit juice

Grapefruit juice very markedly increases the bioavailability of felodipine and nisoldipine and alters their haemodynamic effects. The bioavailability of nicardipine, nifedipine, nimodipine or nitrendipine is increased without significantly altering haemodynamic effects, whereas the bioavailability of amlodipine, diltiazem and verapamil is only minimally affected.

Clinical evidence

Drinking 200 to 250 ml of grapefruit juice can increase the bioavailability of **felodipine** two to threefold in healthy subjects and patients with hypertension.[1-11] Its effects are proportionately increased. One study found that diastolic pressures were reduced by 20% (11% with water) and heart rates increased by 22% (9% with water) when blood **felodipine** levels were at their highest after a drink of grapefruit juice.[1] Adverse effects such as headaches, facial flushing and lightheadedness were also increased.[1] The interaction develops after taking the first glass of grapefruit juice and persists for about 24 hours.[7,12]

The bioavailabilities of **nicardipine**,[13] **nifedipine**,[1,14-17] **nimodipine**[18,19] and **nitrendipine**[20] have also been found to be increased, even about doubled in some instances, but usually only minor changes in haemodynamic effects (blood pressure and heart rate) were reported in healthy subjects.[17,19-21] However, the effect may be more pronounced in some hypertensive patients.[17]

A study in 10 hypertensive patients found that a single drink of grapefruit juice had no significant effects on the pharmacokinetics of **verapamil**.[22] However, studies in healthy subjects[23,24] found that grapefruit juice given 2 to 4 times daily for 3 to 5 days increased the AUC of **verapamil** by about 40%. Pharmacodynamic parameters (blood pressure heart rate and PR interval) were not significantly altered by grapefruit juice in one study,[23] but prolongation of PR intervals occurred in the other[24] and were of borderline significance, with increases to above 350 milliseconds in 2 subjects (maximal PR intervals of 200 to 260 milliseconds were usually observed).

One study in 8 healthy subjects found that when **nisoldipine** was given with grapefruit juice it produced significantly larger decreases in blood pressure for 8 hours compared to **nisoldipine** alone. The effect of grapefruit juice decreased with time but lasted for at least 3 days.[25] However, in a further study in healthy subjects, grapefruit juice increased the maximum nisoldipine plasma levels fivefold, but only minor effects on blood pressure and heart rate were found.[21]

Other studies found that the bioavailability of **amlodipine** was at most only slightly increased by grapefruit juice.[26-28] Similarly, in one study grapefruit juice had no significant effect on the bioavailability of **diltiazem**,[29] and in another it increased the AUC of **diltiazem** by about 20% but differences in blood pressure and heart rate were not significant.[30]

Some studies have found that grapefruit pulp, segments, or extract may increase the AUCs of **nifedipine**, **nisoldipine** and **felodipine** by 1.3-fold, 1.3-fold and threefold respectively.[31,32]

Mechanism

Uncertain. It has been suggested that the increases in bioavailability are due to components of the fruit juice including flavonoids such as naringin,[1,5,21] (but not quercetin[14]), sesquiterpenoids,[33] or furanocoumarins including bergamottin (also found in Seville oranges and lime juice) and 6',7'-dihydroxybergamottin.[9,25,34,35] These components inhibit the activity of the cytochrome P450 isoenzymes CYP3A subfamily in the intestinal wall so that the metabolism of these calcium channel blockers is reduced, thereby reducing their loss from the body and increasing their effects. Grapefruit juice has little effect on hepatic CYP3A4 and this is borne out by the fact that it interacts with oral but not intravenous preparations. See also 'Grapefruit juice', (p.11).

It has been suggested that the sensitivity of the interaction with grapefruit juice may be related to the oral bioavailability of the calcium channel blocker.[30] Thus, amlodipine and diltiazem with high bioavailability are least affected, nifedipine is intermediate, and felodipine,[30] which has a lower bioavailability, is most sensitive to the activity of grapefruit juice. The exception is verapamil, which has low bioavailability and appears to be only slightly affected by grapefruit juice, but this is possibly because cytochrome P450 isoenzymes other than CYP3A4 are involved in its metabolism.[30]

Furanocoumarins and possibly other components of grapefruit juice may also increase the levels of calcium channel blockers by inhibition of intestinal P-glycoprotein efflux transport.[9,25,30]

Importance and management

These are established interactions and the makers of felodipine[36,37] say that it should not be taken with grapefruit juice. It has been suggested that **whole grapefruit** or products made from **grapefruit peel** such as marmalade should also be avoided in patients on felodipine.[32] The makers of **lercanidipine**,[38] nifedipine,[39,40] nimodipine[41] nisoldipine[42] and verapamil[43,44] also contraindicate grapefruit juice, although this interaction is normally of little clinical relevance with most calcium channel blockers in the majority of patients. Generally speaking the concurrent use of grapefruit juice and most calcium channel blockers other than felodipine, and possibly nisoldipine, need not be avoided. However, it would be worth checking the diet of any patient who complains of increased adverse effects with any of the calcium channel blockers that are known to interact with grapefruit juice. Any problems can be solved either by reducing the dosage of the calcium channel blocker, swapping it for another (diltiazem appears not to interact), or by stopping the grapefruit juice.

1. Bailey DG, Spence JD, Munoz C, Arnold JMO. Interaction of citrus juices with felodipine and nifedipine. *Lancet* (1991) 337, 268–9.
2. Edgar B, Bailey DG, Bergstrand R, Johnsson G, Lurje L. Formulation dependent interaction between felodipine and grapefruit juice. *Clin Pharmacol Ther* (1990) 47, 181.

3. Bailey DG, Spence JD, Edgar B, Bayliff CD, Arnold JMO. Ethanol enhances the hemodynamic effects of felodipine. *Clin Invest Med* (1989) 12, 357–62.
4. Edgar B, Bailey D, Bergstrand R, Johnsson G, Regårdh CG. Acute effects of drinking grapefruit juice on the pharmacokinetics and dynamics on felodipine – and its potential clinical relevance. *Eur J Clin Pharmacol* (1992) 42, 313–17.
5. Bailey DG, Arnold JMO, Munoz C, Spence JD. Grapefruit juice–felodipine interaction: mechanism, predictability, and effect of naringin. *Clin Pharmacol Ther* (1993) 53, 637–42.
6. Bailey DG, Bend JR, Arnold JMO, Tran LT, Spence JD. Erythromycin-felodipine interaction: magnitude, mechanism, and comparison with grapefruit juice. *Clin Pharmacol Ther* (1996) 60, 25–33.
7. Lundahl JUE, Regårdh CG, Edgar B, Johnsson G. The interaction effect of grapefruit juice is maximal after the first glass. *Eur J Clin Pharmacol* (1998) 54, 75–81.
8. Lundahl J, Regårdh CG, Edgar B, Johnsson G. Effects of grapefruit juice ingestion – pharmacokinetics and haemodynamics of intravenously and orally administered felodipine in healthy men. *Eur J Clin Pharmacol* (1997) 52, 139–45.
9. Malhotra S, Bailey DG, Paine MF, Watkins PB. Seville orange juice-felodipine interaction: comparison with dilute grapefruit juice and involvement of furocoumarins. *Clin Pharmacol Ther* (2001) 69, 14–23.
10. Dresser GK, Bailey DG, Carruthers SG. Grapefruit juice—felodipine interaction in the elderly. *Clin Pharmacol Ther* (2000) 68, 28–34.
11. Bailey DG, Arnold JMO, Bend JR, Tran LT, Spence JD. Grapefruit juice-felodipine interaction: reproducibility and characterization with the extended release drug formulation. *Br J Clin Pharmacol* (1995) 40, 135–40.
12. Lundahl J, Regårdh CG, Edgar B, Johnsson G. Relationship between time of intake of grapefruit juice and its effect on pharmacokinetics and pharmacodynamics of felodipine in healthy subjects. *Eur J Clin Pharmacol* (1995) 49, 61–7.
13. Uno T, Ohkubo T, Sugawara K, Higashiyama A, Motomura S, Ishizaki T. Effect of grapefruit juice on the stereoselective disposition of nicardipine in humans: evidence for dominant presystemic elimination at the gut site. *Eur J Clin Pharmacol* (2002) 56, 643–9.
14. Rashid J, McKinstry C, Renwick AG, Dirnhuber M, Waller DG, George CF. Quercetin, an *in vitro* inhibitor of CYP3A, does not contribute to the interaction between nifedipine and grapefruit juice. *Br J Clin Pharmacol* (1993) 36, 460–3.
15. Sigusch H, Hippius M, Henschel L, Kaufmann K, Hoffmann A. Influence of grapefruit juice on the pharmacokinetics of a slow release nifedipine formulation. *Pharmazie* (1994) 49, 522–4.
16. Rashid TJ, Martin U, Clarke H, Waller DG, Renwick AG, George CF. Factors affecting the absolute bioavailability of nifedipine. *Br J Clin Pharmacol* (1995) 40, 51–8.
17. Pisařík P. Blood pressure-lowering effect of adding grapefruit juice to nifedipine and terazosin in a patient with severe renovascular hypertension. *Arch Fam Med* (1996) 5, 413–6.
18. Fuhr U, Maier A, Blume H, Mück W, Unger S, Staib AH. Grapefruit juice increases oral nimodipine bioavailability. *Eur J Clin Pharmacol* (1994) 47, A100.
19. Fuhr U, Maier-Brüggemann A, Blume H, Mück W, Unger S, Kuhlmann J, Huschka C, Zaigler M, Rietbrock S, Staib AH. Grapefruit juice increases oral nimodipine bioavailability. *Int J Clin Pharmacol Ther* (1998) 36, 126–32.
20. Soons PA, Vogels BAPM, Roosemalen MCM, Schoemaker HC, Uchida E, Edgar B, Lundahl J, Cohen AF, Breimer DD. Grapefruit juice and cimetidine inhibit stereoselective metabolism of nitrendipine in humans. *Clin Pharmacol Ther* (1991) 50, 394–403.
21. Bailey DG, Arnold JMO, Strong HA, Munoz C, Spence JD. Effect of grapefruit juice and naringin on nisoldipine pharmacokinetics. *Clin Pharmacol Ther* (1993) 54, 589–94.
22. Zaidenstein R, Dishi V, Gips M, Soback S, Cohen N, Weissgarten J, Blatt A, Golik A. The effect of grapefruit juice on the pharmacokinetics of orally administered verapamil. *Eur J Clin Pharmacol* (1998) 54, 337–40.
23. Ho P-C, Ghose K, Saville D, Wanwimolruk S. Effect of grapefruit juice on pharmacokinetics and pharmacodynamics of verapamil enantiomers in healthy volunteers. *Eur J Clin Pharmacol* (2000) 56, 693–8.
24. Fuhr U, Müller-Peltzer H, Kern R, Lopez-Rojas P, Jünemann M, Harder S, Staib AH. Effects of grapefruit juice and smoking on verapamil concentrations in steady state. *Eur J Clin Pharmacol* (2002) 58, 45–53.
25. Takanaga H, Ohnishi A, Murakami H, Matsuo H, Higuchi S, Urae A, Irie S, Furuie H, Matsukuma K, Kimura M, Kawano K, Orii Y, Tanaka T, Sawada Y. Relationship between time after intake of grapefruit juice and the effect on pharmacokinetics and pharmacodynamics of nisoldipine in healthy subjects. *Clin Pharmacol Ther* (2000) 67, 201–14.
26. Josefsson M, Zackrisson A-L, Ahlner J. Effect of grapefruit juice on the pharmacokinetics of amlodipine in healthy volunteers. *Eur J Clin Pharmacol* (1996) 51, 189–93.
27. Vincent J, Harris SI, Foulds G, Dogolo LC, Willavize S, Friedman HL. Lack of effect of grapefruit juice on the pharmacokinetics and pharmacodynamics of amlodipine. *Br J Clin Pharmacol* (2000) 50, 455–63.
28. Josefsson M, Ahlner J. Amlodipine and grapefruit juice. *Br J Clin Pharmacol* (2002) 53, 405.
29. Sigusch H, Henschel L, Kraul H, Merkel U, Hoffman A. Lack of effect of grapefruit juice on diltiazem bioavailability in normal subjects. *Pharmazie* (1994) 49, 675–9.
30. Christensen H, Åsberg A, Holmboe A-B. Berg KJ. Coadministration of grapefruit juice increases systemic exposure of diltiazem in healthy volunteers. *Eur J Clin Pharmacol* (2002) 58, 515–20.
31. Ohtani M, Kawabata S, Kariya S, Uchino K, Itou K, Kotaki H, Kasuyama K, Morikawa A, Seo I, Nishida N. Effect of grapefruit pulp on the pharmacokinetics of the dihydropyridine calcium antagonists nifedipine and nisoldipine. *Yakugaku Zasshi* (2002) 122, 323–9.
32. Bailey DG, Dresser GK, Kreeft JH, Munoz C, Freeman DJ, Bend JR. Grapefruit-felodipine interaction: effect of unprocessed fruit and probable active ingredients. *Clin Pharmacol Ther* (2000) 68, 468–77.
33. Chayen R, Rosenthal T. Interaction of citrus juices with felodipine and nifedipine. *Lancet* (1991) 337, 854.
34. Bailey DG, Dresser GK, Bend JR. Bergamottin, lime juice, and red wine as inhibitors of cytochrome P450 3A4 activity: comparison with grapefruit juice. *Clin Pharmacol Ther* (2003) 73, 529–37.
35. Goosen TC, Cillié D, Bailey DG, Yu C, He K, Hollenberg PF, Woster PM, Cohen L, Williams JA, Rheeders M, Dijkstra HP. Bergamottin contribution to the grapefruit juice—felodipine interaction and disposition in humans. *Clin Pharmacol Ther* (2004) 76, 607–17.
36. Plendil (Felodipine). AstraZeneca UK Ltd. UK Summary of product characteristics, September 2003.
37. Vascalpha (Felodipine). Alpharma Ltd. UK Summary of product characteristics, August 2003.
38. Zanidip (Lercanidipine hydrochloride). Napp Pharmaceuticals Ltd. UK Summary of product characteristics, January 2004.
39. Adalat Retard (Nifedipine). Bayer plc. UK Summary of product characteristics, April 2005.
40. Coracten SR (Nifedipine). Celltech Pharmaceuticals Ltd. UK Summary of product characteristics, July 2003.
41. Nimotop (Nimodipine). Bayer plc. UK Summary of product characteristics, June 2002.
42. Syscor MR (Nisoldipine). Forest Laboratories UK Ltd. UK Summary of product characteristics, August 1998.
43. Securon (Verapamil hydrochloride). Abbott Laboratories Ltd. UK Summary of product characteristics, August 2003.
44. Univer (Verapamil hydrochloride). Zeneus Pharma Ltd. UK Summary of product characteristics, August 2003.

Calcium channel blockers + H_2-blockers

The plasma levels of diltiazem, isradipine and nifedipine are increased by cimetidine and it may possibly be necessary to reduce the dosages. High doses of cimetidine may increase the bioavailability of lercanidipine. Although studies suggest no important interactions occur between nicardipine or nisoldipine and cimetidine, the makers advise caution. Plasma felodipine, lacidipine, nimodipine, and nitrendipine levels are also increased but this seems to be clinically unimportant. Amlodipine and cimetidine do not interact. It is uncertain whether cimetidine interacts significantly with verapamil. Ranitidine appears to interact only minimally with calcium channel blockers but famotidine may possibly reduce their cardiac effects undesirably.

Clinical evidence

(a) Amlodipine

A crossover study in 12 healthy subjects found that **cimetidine** 400 mg twice daily for 14 days had no effect on the pharmacokinetics of amlodipine 10 mg.[1]

(b) Diltiazem

Cimetidine 300 mg before meals and at bedtime for a week increased the AUC of a single 60-mg oral dose of diltiazem by 50% in 6 healthy subjects and increased peak plasma levels by 57% (from 46.4 to 73.1 nanograms/ml). **Ranitidine** 150 mg twice daily for a week increased the AUC of diltiazem by 15% but this was not statistically significant.[2] Increases in the serum levels and AUC of diltiazem of 40% and 25 to 50% respectively were seen in another study using **cimetidine**.[3]

(c) Felodipine

Cimetidine 1 g daily increased the AUC of felodipine 10 mg by 56%, and raised the peak serum level by 54% in 12 subjects. There was a short lasting effect on their heart rates but the clinical effects were minimal.[4]

(d) Isradipine

The maker of isradipine[5] notes that **cimetidine** increases the bioavailability of isradipine by about 50%.

(e) Lacidipine

A single 800-mg dose of **cimetidine** increased the maximum plasma level of a single 4-mg dose of lacidipine by 59% and increased the AUC by 74% in one study in healthy subjects. Pulse rates and blood pressures were unaffected.[6]

(f) Lercanidipine

Cimetidine 800 mg daily causes no significant alteration in plasma levels of lercanidipine but the maker says that the bioavailability of lercanidipine and its hypotensive effects may be increased by higher doses of **cimetidine**.[7]

(g) Nicardipine

No adverse interaction was seen in 22 patients given calcium channel blockers including **nicardipine** with oral **famotidine** for 6 to 8 weeks.[8] No changes in the pharmacokinetics or pharmacodynamics of a 12-hour intravenous infusion of **nicardipine** 24 mg were seen in 12 healthy subjects given intravenous **cimetidine** 300 mg every 6 hours for 48 hours.[9]

(h) Nifedipine

Cimetidine 1 g daily for a week increased the AUC of nifedipine 40 mg daily by about 60% and increased the maximum plasma levels by about 90%, from 46.1 to 87.7 nanograms/ml. **Ranitidine** 150 mg twice daily for a week caused an insignificant rise of about 25% in maximum nifedipine plasma levels and AUC.[10] Seven hypertensive patients had a fall in mean blood pressure from 127 to 109 mmHg after taking nifedipine 40 mg daily for 4 weeks, and a further fall to 95 mmHg after they also took **cimetidine** 1 g daily for 3 weeks. When they took **ranitidine** 300 mg instead of cimetidine, there was an insignificant fall in blood pressure.[10,11]

Other studies clearly confirm that **cimetidine** causes a very significant rise in plasma nifedipine levels and an increase in its effects, whereas **ranitidine** interacts only minimally.[12-18]

A study found no pharmacokinetic interaction between nifedipine and **famotidine**, but the famotidine reversed the effects of nifedipine on systolic time intervals and significantly reduced the stroke volume and cardiac output.[19,20] No adverse interaction was seen in 22 patients given calcium channel blockers including nifedipine with **famotidine** for 6 to 8 weeks.[8]

(i) Nimodipine

Seven days of treatment with **cimetidine** 1 g daily increased the bioavailability of **nimodipine** 30 mg three times daily in 8 healthy subjects by 75%, but the haemodynamic effects were unchanged. **Ranitidine** did not interact.[21]

(j) Nisoldipine

A study in 8 healthy subjects found that taking **cimetidine** 1 g in divided doses on the day before the study and then three 200 mg doses every 4 hours on the study day, increased the bioavailability of a single 10-mg dose of nisoldipine by about 50%, but the haemodynamic effects of the nisoldipine were unaltered.[22] **Ranitidine** does not interact with nisoldipine.[23]

(k) Nitrendipine

Cimetidine 800 mg given before and 400 mg in divided doses, given after a single 20-mg dose of nitrendipine was found to increase its bioavailability by 154% but the haemodynamic effects were unchanged.[24] Another study found that **ranitidine** increased the AUC of oral nitrendipine 20 mg daily for 1 week by about 50% and decreased its clearance, but there were no changes in the haemodynamic measurements (systolic time intervals, impedance cardiography).[25,26] A further study found that ranitidine increases the AUC of nitrendipine by 89%, but this does not appear to be clinically significant.[27]

(l) Verapamil

A study in 8 healthy subjects found that **cimetidine** 300 mg every 6 hours for 8 days did not affect the pharmacokinetics of a single 10-mg intravenous dose of verapamil, but the bioavailability of a 120-mg oral dose of verapamil was increased from 26 to 49%. A small insignificant change in clearance occurred but no change in AUC. The changes in the PR interval caused by the verapamil were unaltered in the presence of **cimetidine**.[28]

Another study found that **cimetidine** 300 mg four times daily for 5 days reduced the clearance of a single intravenous dose of verapamil by 21% and increased its elimination half-life by 50%.[29] **Cimetidine** 400 mg twice daily for a week increased the bioavailability of verapamil from 35 to 42% and its clearance fell from 45.9 to 33.2 ml/minute per kg in another study.[30] A further study found a small increase in the bioavailability of both enantiomers of verapamil.[31] In contrast, other studies have found that the pharmacokinetics of verapamil were unaffected by **cimetidine**.[32,33]

Mechanism

It is believed that cimetidine increases nifedipine levels by inhibiting its oxidative metabolism by the liver. Like ranitidine it may also increase the bioavailability of nifedipine by lowering gastric acidity.[14] The mechanisms of the other interactions are probably similar.

Importance and management

The interactions of cimetidine with diltiazem and nifedipine are established. Concurrent use need not be avoided but the increase in the calcium channel blocker effects should be taken into account. It has been suggested that the dosage of diltiazem should be reduced by 30 to 50%[34,35] and that of nifedipine by 40 to 50%.[34,35] Monitoring is advised if isradipine is given with cimetidine and a reduction in isradipine dose may be required.[5]

The evidence available suggests that although cimetidine increases the serum levels of felodipine, lacidipine, nimodipine, nisoldipine and nitrendipine, the haemodynamic changes are unimportant. However, this needs confirmation. Furthermore, the maker of nisoldipine warns that the antihypertensive effect may be potentiated by cimetidine.[23] Similarly, high doses of cimetidine may increase the hypotensive effects of lercanidipine and caution is advised.[7] Although some studies indicate no interaction between nicardipine and cimetidine, the maker notes that cimetidine increases nicardipine plasma levels and monitoring is recommended.[36] The interaction between verapamil and cimetidine is not well established, but monitor the effects until more is known. It has been suggested that the verapamil dose may need to be reduced by 50%.[35] Amlodipine and cimetidine do not interact.

Ranitidine does not interact significantly with diltiazem, nimodipine, nisoldipine or nifedipine and is possibly a non-interacting alternative for cimetidine with other calcium channel blockers.

Famotidine does not have a pharmacokinetic interaction with nifedipine, but its negative inotropic effects may possibly be undesirable in the elderly or those with heart failure,[19,20] and therefore some care may be needed.

1. Quoted as unpublished data, Pfizer Central Research by Abernethy DR. Amlodipine: pharmacokinetic profile of a low-clearance calcium antagonist. *J Cardiovasc Pharmacol* (1991) 17 (Suppl 1), S4–S7.
2. Winship LC, McKenney JM, Wright JT, Wood JH, Goodman RP. The effect of ranitidine and cimetidine on single-dose diltiazem pharmacokinetics. *Pharmacotherapy* (1985) 5, 16–19.
3. Mazhar M, Popat KD, Sanders C. Effect of cimetidine on diltiazem blood levels. *Clin Res* (1984) 32, 741A.
4. Janzon K, Edgar B, Lundborg P, Regårdh CG. The influence of cimetidine and spironolactone on the pharmacokinetics and haemodynamic effects of felodipine in healthy subjects. *Acta Pharmacol Toxicol (Copenh)* (1986) 59 (Suppl 4), 98.
5. Prescal (Isradipine). Novartis Pharmaceuticals UK Ltd. UK Summary of product characteristics, February 2002.
6. Dewland PM. A study to assess the effect of food and a single 800 mg oral dose of cimetidine on the pharmacokinetics of a single 4 mg oral dose of calcium-channel inhibitor, GR43659X (lacidipine). Boehringer Ingelheim report GMH/88/030.
7. Zanidip (Lercanidipine hydrochloride). Napp Pharmaceuticals Ltd. UK Summary of product characteristics, January 2004.
8. Chichmanian RM, Mignot G, Spreux A, Jean-Girard C, Hofliger P. Tolérance de la famotidine. Étude du réseau médecins sentinelles en pharmacovigilance. *Therapie* (1992) 47, 239–43.
9. Lai C-M, McEntegart CM, Maher KE, Bell VA, Turlapaty P, Quon CY. The effects of iv cimetidine on the pharmacokinetics (PK) and pharmacodynamics (PD) of iv nicardipine in man. *Pharm Res* (1994) 11 (Suppl 10), S386.
10. Kirch W, Janisch HD, Heidemann H, Rämsch K, Ohnhaus EE. Einfluss von Cimetidin und Ranitidin auf Pharmakokinetik und antihypertensiven Effekt von Nifedipin. *Dtsch Med Wochenschr* (1983) 108, 1757–61.
11. Kirch W, Rämsch K, Janisch HD, Ohnhaus EE. The influence of two histamine H_2-receptor antagonists, cimetidine and ranitidine, on the plasma levels and clinical effect of nifedipine and metoprolol. *Arch Toxicol* (1984) (Suppl 7), 256–9.
12. Kirch W, Hoensch H, Ohnhaus EE, Janisch HD. Ranitidin-Nifedipin-Interaktion. *Dtsch Med Wochenschr* (1984) 109, 1223.
13. Smith SR, Kendall MJ, Lobo J, Beerahee A, Jack DB, Wilkins MR. Ranitidine and cimetidine: drug interactions with single dose and steady-state nifedipine administration. *Br J Clin Pharmacol* (1987) 23, 311–15.
14. Adams LJ, Antonow DR, McClain CJ, McAllister R. Effect of ranitidine on bioavailability of nifedipine. *Gastroenterology* (1986) 90, 1320.
15. Kirch W, Ohnhaus EE, Hoensch H, Janisch HD. Ranitidine increases bioavailability of nifedipine. *Clin Pharmacol Ther* (1985) 37, 204.
16. Schwartz JB, Upton RA, Lin ET, Williams RL, Benet LZ. Effect of cimetidine or ranitidine administration on nifedipine pharmacokinetics and pharmacodynamics. *Clin Pharmacol Ther* (1988) 43, 673–80.
17. Renwick AG, Le Vie J, Challenor VF, Waller DG, Gruchy B, George CF. Factors affecting the pharmacokinetics of nifedipine. *Eur J Clin Pharmacol* (1987) 32, 351–5.
18. Khan A, Langley SJ, Mullins FGP, Dixon JS, Toon S. The pharmacokinetics and pharmacodynamics of nifedipine at steady state during concomitant administration of cimetidine or high dose ranitidine. *Br J Clin Pharmacol* (1991) 32, 519–22.
19. Kirch W, Halabi A, Linde M, Ohnhaus EE. Negativ-inotrope Wirkung von Famotidin. *Schweiz Med Wochenschr* (1988) 118, 1912–14.
20. Kirch W, Halabi A, Linde M, Santos SR, Ohnhaus EE. Negative effects of famotidine on cardiac performance assessed by noninvasive hemodynamic measurements. *Gastroenterology* (1989) 96, 1388–92.
21. Mück W, Wingender W, Seiberling M, Woelke E, Rämsch K-D, Kuhlmann J. Influence of the H2-receptor antagonists cimetidine and ranitidine on the pharmacokinetics of nimodipine in healthy volunteers. *Eur J Clin Pharmacol* (1992) 42, 325–8.
22. Van Harten J, van Brummelen P, Lodewijks MThM, Danhof M, Breimer DD. Pharmacokinetics and hemodynamic effects of nisoldipine and its interaction with cimetidine. *Clin Pharmacol Ther* (1988) 43, 332–41.
23. Syscor MR (Nisoldipine). Forest Laboratories UK Ltd. UK Summary of product characteristics, August 1998.
24. Soons PA, Vogels BAPM, Roosemalen MCM, Schoemaker HC, Uchida E, Edgar B, Lundahl J, Cohen AF, Breimer DD. Grapefruit juice and cimetidine inhibit stereoselective metabolism of nitrendipine in humans. *Clin Pharmacol Ther* (1991) 50, 394–403.
25. Kirch W, Nahoui R, Ohnhaus EE. Ranitidine/nitrendipine interaction. *Clin Pharmacol Ther* (1988) 43, 149.
26. Halabi A, Nahoui R, Kirch W. Influence of ranitidine on kinetics of nitrendipine and on noninvasive hemodynamic parameters. *Ther Drug Monit* (1990) 12, 303–4.
27. Santos SR, Storpirtis S, Moreira-Filho L, Donzella H, Kirch W. Ranitidine increases the bioavailability of nitrendipine in patients with arterial hypertension. *Braz J Med Biol Res* (1992) 25, 337–47.
28. Smith MS, Benyunes MC, Bjornsson TD, Shand DG, Pritchett ELC. Influence of cimetidine on verapamil kinetics and dynamics. *Clin Pharmacol Ther* (1984) 36, 551–4.
29. Loi C-M, Rollins DE, Dukes GE, Peat MA. Effect of cimetidine on verapamil disposition. *Clin Pharmacol Ther* (1985) 37, 654–7.
30. Mikus G, Stuber H. Influence of cimetidine treatment on the physiological disposition of verapamil. *Naunyn Schmiedebergs Arch Pharmacol* (1987) 335 (Suppl), R106.
31. Mikus G, Eichelbaum M, Fischer C, Gumulka S, Klotz U, Kroemer HK. Interaction of verapamil and cimetidine: stereochemical aspects of drug metabolism, drug disposition and drug action. *J Pharmacol Exp Ther* (1990) 253, 1042–8.
32. Abernethy DR, Schwartz JB, Todd EL. Lack of interaction between verapamil and cimetidine. *Clin Pharmacol Ther* (1985) 38, 342–9.
33. Wing LMH, Miners JO, Lillywhite KJ. Verapamil disposition—effects of sulphinpyrazone and cimetidine. *Br J Clin Pharmacol* (1985) 19, 385–91.
34. Piepho RW, Culbertson VL, Rhodes RS. Drug interactions with the calcium-entry blockers. *Circulation* (1987) 75 (Suppl V), V181–V194.
35. Piepho RW. Individualization of calcium entry–blocker dosage for systemic hypertension. *Am J Cardiol* (1985) 56, 105H–111H.
36. Cardene SR (Nicardipine hydrochloride). Yamanouchi Pharma Ltd. UK Summary of product characteristics, April 2004.

Calcium channel blockers + Macrolides

Erythromycin markedly increases the bioavailability of felodipine. Isolated reports describe increased felodipine or verapamil effects and toxicity in patients when given erythromycin or

clarithromycin. A prolonged QT interval in one patient may have been due to increased levels of erythromycin in the presence of verapamil.

Clinical evidence

(a) Felodipine

Twelve healthy subjects were given felodipine 10 mg before and after taking **erythromycin** 250 mg four times daily for a day.[1] The felodipine AUC was increased almost threefold by the **erythromycin**, the maximum plasma levels were more than doubled and the half-life prolonged from 6.9 to 11.1 hours.[1]

A hypertensive woman on felodipine 10 mg daily developed tachycardia, flushing and massive ankle oedema within 2 to 3 days of starting to take **erythromycin** 250 mg twice daily. Her blood pressure had fallen from 120/90 to 110/70 mmHg. She fully recovered within a few days stopping the **erythromycin**.[2]

(b) Verapamil

A 53-year-old woman on haemodialysis 3 times a week, and a range of medicines including digoxin, was given **clarithromycin** 250 mg and verapamil 120 mg both twice daily because of an acute exacerbation of chronic obstructive pulmonary disease and a recurrence of atrial fibrillation. After 24 hours she experienced dizziness and episodes of fainting and her supine blood pressure a day later was 89/39 mmHg and her pulse rate 50 bpm. Verapamil was stopped and she recovered within 2 days after which verapamil was re-started at a dose of 40 mg before each dialysis session.[3] Another report[4] describes a 77-year-old woman with hypertension, taking propranolol and verapamil, who developed marked bradycardia (37 to 50 bpm), within 4 days of starting a course of **clarithromycin** 500 mg twice daily. The problem was solved by temporarily reducing the dose of the verapamil from 80 mg to 40 mg twice daily and the propranolol to a half until the **clarithromycin** course was over. Essentially the same thing happened 2 years later while taking the same drugs when **erythromycin** 333 mg three times daily was added.

A 79-year-old woman on verapamil 240 mg twice daily and ramipril was admitted to hospital with extreme fatigue and dizziness one week after starting a course of **erythromycin** 2 g daily for a respiratory-tract disorder. Her blood pressure was 80/60 mmHg and her respiratory rate was 18 breaths per minute. ECG showed complete AV block, escape rhythm of 50 bpm, pattern of left bundle-branch block and QTc interval prolongation (583 milliseconds compared with 436 milliseconds 20 days before admission). Verapamil and **erythromycin** were stopped and intravenous fluids, dopamine and calcium were given. Her blood pressure increased to 110/70 mmHg and after 4 days the QTc interval prolongation had resolved and her heart rate was 76 bpm.[5]

Mechanism

Calcium channel blockers are metabolised in the gut wall and liver by the cytochrome P450 CYP3A subfamily of isoenzymes, which are inhibited by erythromycin and clarithromycin, so that in their presence a normal oral dose becomes in effect an overdose with its attendant adverse effects.[1,2,4]

Verapamil, erythromycin[5] and possibly clarithromycin are also P-glycoprotein inhibitors, which may contribute to the pharmacokinetic interaction by reducing the elimination of the calcium channel blocker,[3] or by increasing macrolide absorption.[5]

Importance and management

Information seems to be limited but the interaction would appear to be established and clinically important. Anticipate the need to reduce the felodipine or verapamil dosage if erythromycin or clarithromycin is added. One report suggests that the cardiac toxicity of erythromycin may be increased by verapamil.[5] There seem to be no reports of interactions between any of the other calcium channel blockers and macrolide. However, because of the theoretical possibility of an interaction, many of the makers of calcium channel blockers including warn of the possibility of increased plasma levels and the need to either avoid use with macrolides such as erythromycin, or **troleandomycin**, or to monitor and reduce doses where necessary.

1. Bailey DG, Bend JR, Arnold JMO, Tran LT, Spence JD. Erythromycin-felodipine interaction: magnitude, mechanism, and comparison with grapefruit juice. *Clin Pharmacol Ther* (1996) 60, 25–33.
2. Liedholm H, Nordin G. Erythromycin–felodipine interaction. *DICP Ann Pharmacother* (1991) 25, 1007–8.
3. Kaeser YA, Brunner F, Drewe J, Haefeli WE. Severe hypotension and bradycardia associated with verapamil and clarithromycin. *Am J Health-Syst Pharm* (1998) 55, 2417–18.
4. Steenbergen JA, Stauffer VL. Potential macrolide interaction with verapamil. *Ann Pharmacother* (1998) 32, 387–8.
5. Goldschmidt N, Azaz-Livshits T, Gotsman I, Nir-Paz R, Ben-Yehuda A, Muszkat M. Compound cardiac toxicity of oral erythromycin and verapamil. *Ann Pharmacother* (2001) 35, 1396–9.

Calcium channel blockers + Magnesium compounds

Two pregnant women developed bilateral hand contractures after receiving magnesium sulfate either alone or with nifedipine. Two other pregnant women developed muscular weakness and then paralysis when they were given both nifedipine and intravenous magnesium sulfate.

Clinical evidence

A report describes symptomatic hypocalcaemia (serum calcium levels 5.4 mg/dl) in a woman at 33 weeks' gestation after she received magnesium sulfate plus **nifedipine**.[1] However, this report also describes this effect in a patient taking magnesium sulfate alone. Both women experienced bilateral hand contractures and were successfully treated with calcium gluconate.[1]

A pregnant woman at 32 weeks' gestation was effectively treated for premature uterine contractions with **nifedipine**, 60 mg orally over 3 hours, and later 20 mg every 8 hours. When contractions began again 12 hours later she was given magnesium sulfate 500 mg intravenously. She developed jerky movements of the extremities, complained of difficulty in swallowing, paradoxical respirations and an inability to lift her head from the pillow. The magnesium was stopped and the muscle weakness disappeared over the next 25 minutes.[2]

A woman at 28 weeks' gestation with mild pre-eclampsia was started on an infusion of magnesium sulfate 2 g/hour. Her plasma magnesium levels were found to be 2.75 mmol/l. No untoward reactions developed when she took a 20-mg dose of **nifedipine**, but 30 minutes after taking a second dose [by implication 3 to 4 hours later] she complained of flushing and sweating and had difficulty in lifting her head and limbs. Shortly afterwards almost complete muscular paralysis developed. The magnesium sulfate was stopped and a dramatic improvement followed within 15 minutes of an intravenous injection of calcium gluconate 1 g.[3]

Mechanism

The probable reason for neuromuscular effects is that both drugs can seriously reduce the amount of calcium ions needed for normal muscular contraction. Nifedipine (a calcium channel blocker) inhibits the inflow of extracellular calcium across cell membranes. Magnesium probably acts in the same way, and also reduces intracellular calcium by activating adenyl cyclase and increasing cAMP. In addition magnesium stimulates calcium-dependent ATPase which promotes calcium uptake by the sarcoplasmic reticulum. The result is muscular paralysis, which is reversed by giving large amounts of calcium. Magnesium sulfate is also known to have neuromuscular blocking activity.

Importance and management

Direct information on the neuromuscular effects of the combination of nifedipine and magnesium seems to be limited, but the interaction appears to be established. Magnesium sulfate alone may cause hypocalcaemia and nifedipine is said to increase this effect.[1] The makers of nifedipine advise particular caution when it is used in combination with intravenous magnesium sulfate in pregnant women,[4] but do not state why. The same interaction would be expected to occur with other calcium channel blockers.

1. Koontz SL, Friedman SA, Schwartz ML. Symptomatic hypocalcemia after tocolytic therapy with magnesium sulfate and nifedipine. *Am J Obstet Gynecol* (2004) 190, 1773–6.
2. Snyder SW, Cardwell MS. Neuromuscular blockade with magnesium sulfate and nifedipine. *Am J Obstet Gynecol* (1989) 161, 35–6.
3. Ben-Ami M, Giladi Y, Shalev E. The combination of magnesium sulphate and nifedipine: a cause of neuromuscular blockade. *Br J Obstet Gynaecol* (1994) 101, 262–3.
4. Adalat Retard (Nifedipine). Bayer plc. UK Summary of product characteristics, April 2005.

Calcium channel blockers + Nitrates

Enhanced hypotensive effects may occur when calcium channel blockers are given with nitrates. The makers of amlodipine say that long-acting nitrates and sublingual glyceryl trinitrate have been given safely with amlodipine.[1] Increased hypotensive effects and faintness due to additive vasodilating effects have been noted when diltiazem has been given with nitrate derivatives. In patients treated with calcium channel blockers, the dosage of concurrent nitrate derivatives should be increased gradually.[2]

1. Istin (Amlodipine besilate). Pfizer Ltd. UK Summary of product characteristics, April 2005.
2. Tildiem Retard (Diltiazem hydrochloride). Sanofi-Aventis. UK Summary of product characteristics, April 2004.

Calcium channel blockers + NSAIDs

Two reports describe abnormal bruising and prolonged bleeding times in two patients and one healthy subject on verapamil also taking aspirin. There are conflicting reports as to whether or not gastrointestinal bleeding is increased by giving NSAIDs with calcium channel blockers.
Diclofenac reduces verapamil serum levels and raises those of isradipine but these changes are probably unimportant.
Most NSAIDs can increase blood pressure in hypertensive patients. Ibuprofen causes a small reduction in the antihypertensive effects of amlodipine. Indometacin appears not to reduce the hypotensive effects of amlodipine, felodipine, nicardipine, nimodipine or verapamil but it possibly interacts with nifedipine. Diclofenac and sulindac appear not to interact with nifedipine, nor ibuprofen, naproxen, piroxicam or sulindac with verapamil, nor naproxen with nicardipine. Low-dose aspirin does not alter the antihypertensive effect of felodipine.

Clinical evidence

(a) Aspirin

(i) Felodipine. In the Hypertension Optimal Treatment (HOT) study, 18 790 treated hypertensive patients, about 82% of whom received a calcium channel blocker, usually felodipine alone or in combination, were also given either aspirin 75 mg daily or placebo for an average of 3.8 years. It was found that long-term low-dose aspirin does not interfere with the blood pressure-lowering effects of the antihypertensive drugs studied.[1]

(ii) Verapamil. Abnormal bruising and prolonged bleeding times occurred in a woman on verapamil 80 mg three times daily when she took aspirin 650 mg several times a week for headaches. The bruising ceased when the verapamil was stopped. Her normal bleeding time of 1 minute rose to 4.5 minutes while she was taking verapamil, and to 9 minutes while she was taking verapamil and aspirin. A healthy subject taking the same dose of verapamil and aspirin observed the appearance of new petechiae and her bleeding time rose from a normal 4.5 minutes to more than 15 minutes in the presence of both drugs.[2] An 85-year-old man taking enteric-coated aspirin 325 mg daily developed widespread and serious ecchymoses of his arms and legs and a retroperitoneal bleed about 3 weeks after starting verapamil 240 mg daily.[3]

(b) Diclofenac

Hypertensive subjects on slow-release **verapamil** 240 mg daily had a 26% reduction in the AUC of verapamil when they took diclofenac 75 mg twice daily.[4] The AUC of **isradipine** 5 mg twice daily for a week was unaffected in 18 healthy subjects by a single 50-mg dose of diclofenac but the maximum serum levels were raised by about 20%. Platelet aggregation was unaffected and the pharmacokinetics of the diclofenac were unchanged.[5]

A study in elderly women with hypertension found that diclofenac sodium 25 mg three times daily for one week had no effect on the control of their blood pressure with **nifedipine**.[6]

(c) Ibuprofen

Fifty-three hypertensive patients had no changes in their blood pressure control with **verapamil** 240 or 480 mg daily when they also took ibuprofen 400 mg three times daily for 3 weeks.[7] No special precautions seem necessary. However, another study in 12 patients with mild or moderate essential hypertension controlled with **amlodipine** 10 mg daily, found that ibuprofen 400 mg three times daily for 3 days increased the mean blood pressure by 7.8/3.9 mmHg.[8]

(d) Indometacin

Indometacin 100 mg daily for a week did not significantly affect the hypotensive effects of **nifedipine** 20 mg twice daily in 10 patients with mild to moderate essential hypertension.[9]

Four other studies, two in healthy subjects[10,11] and two in patients with hypertension[12,13] also found that indometacin did not alter the blood pressure-lowering effects of **amlodipine**,[12] **felodipine**,[10,12] **nicardipine**[11] or **verapamil**.[13]

The haemodynamic effects of **nimodipine** 30 mg three times daily were not affected to a clinically relevant extent by indometacin 25 mg twice daily in 24 healthy elderly subjects, although the AUC of **nimodipine** and its maximum plasma levels were slightly increased.[14]

In contrast, in another study indometacin 100 mg in divided doses over 24 hours was found to raise the mean arterial pressure in 5 out of 8 hypertensive patients on **nifedipine** 15 to 40 mg daily by 17 to 20 mmHg.[15]

(e) Naproxen

Naproxen 375 mg twice daily had no effect on the pharmacokinetics of **verapamil** in hypertensive subjects.[4] Fifty-five hypertensive patients had no changes in their blood pressure control with **verapamil** 240 to 480 mg daily when they were given naproxen 250 mg twice daily for 3 weeks.[7]

A placebo-controlled study in 100 patients on **nicardipine** 30 mg three times daily found that naproxen 375 mg twice daily caused no clinically relevant changes in the control of their blood pressure.[16]

(f) Piroxicam

A study in hypertensive patients given up to 440 mg of **verapamil** daily found that piroxicam 20 mg once daily for 4 weeks did not significantly alter the antihypertensive effects of **verapamil**.[17]

(g) Sulindac

A study in elderly women with hypertension found that sulindac 100 mg three times daily for one week had no effect on the control of their blood pressure with **nifedipine**.[6]

A study in hypertensive patients given up to 440 mg of **verapamil** daily found that sulindac 200 mg twice daily for 4 weeks did not significantly alter the antihypertensive effects of **verapamil**.[17]

Mechanism, importance and management

Antiplatelet effects

The prolonged bleeding times noted with verapamil[2] are probably a result of inhibition of platelet aggregation, because calcium channel blockers interfere with the movement of calcium ions through cell membranes, which can affect platelet function. This appears to be additive with the effects of other antiplatelet drugs. A prospective cohort study[18] in 1636 elderly hypertensive patients and a case-control study[19] found that calcium channel blockers were associated with an increased risk of gastrointestinal bleeding compared with beta-blockers; in one of the studies, verapamil had the highest rate of bleeding, followed by diltiazem and nifedipine.[18] It was suggested that vasodilation produced by calcium channel blockers in conjunction with inhibition of platelet aggregation may increase the risk of bleeding, or at least prevent the normal vasoconstrictive response to bleeding,[18] although a protective effect of beta-blockers rather than an adverse effect of calcium channel blockers may also be the reason.[20] Two studies indicated that gastrointestinal bleeding was not increased by calcium channel blockers.[20,21] A post-hoc analysis of the Syst-Eur data found that there was no interaction between chronic NSAID intake and antihypertensive therapy based on **nitrendipine** in terms of incidence of gastrointestinal bleeding. Further, the results suggested that chronic NSAID therapy tended to be associated with a lower incidence of bleeding in patients on nitrendipine-based therapy than those on placebo.[22] Therefore clinically significant interactions between NSAIDs and calcium channel blockers that result in bleeding appear rare.

Effects on blood pressure

NSAIDs may increase blood pressure in hypertensive patients. The effect occurs with both COX-1 and COX-2 inhibitors but most studies have involved non-specific COX inhibitors.[23] A meta-analysis of 50 trials in 771 patients or healthy subjects found that NSAIDs elevated mean supine blood pressure by 5 mmHg. Piroxicam, indometacin and ibuprofen produced the greatest increases (statistically significant for piroxicam). Aspirin and sulindac produced the smallest increases in blood pressure and the effects of tiaprofenic acid, diclofenac, naproxen and flurbiprofen were intermediate. Further, the increases were more marked in hypertensive patients than in normotensive subjects (both given antihypertensives).[24] Low-dose aspirin appears not to affect the blood pressure-lowering effects of antihypertensive drugs including calcium channel blockers.[1]

The effects on blood pressure may be due to inhibition of vasodilator and natriuretic prostaglandins in the kidney and/or a decrease in vascular or endothelial prostaglandin synthesis resulting in salt retention and vasoconstriction.[23]

Although the risks of NSAIDs with calcium channel blockers may be less than those with other antihypertensive drugs, until more information is available, caution has been recommended. It has been suggested that the use of NSAIDs (with the possible exception of low-dose aspirin) should be kept to a minimum in patients with hypertension. The effects may be greater in the elderly and in those with blood pressures that are relatively high, as well as in those with high salt intake.[23,25]

1. Zanchetti A, Hansson L, Leonetti G, Rahn K-H, Ruilope L, Warnold I, Wedel H. Low-dose aspirin does not interfere with the blood pressure-lowering effects of antihypertensive therapy. *J Hypertens* (2002) 20, 1015–22.
2. Ring ME, Martin GV, Fenster PE. Clinically significant antiplatelet effects of calcium-channel blockers. *J Clin Pharmacol* (1986) 26, 719–20.
3. Verzino E, Kaplan B, Ashley JV, Burdette M. Verapamil–aspirin interaction. *Ann Pharmacother* (1994) 28, 536–7.
4. Peterson C, Basch C, Cohen A. Differential effects of naproxen and diclofenac on verapamil pharmacokinetics. *Clin Pharmacol Ther* (1990) 49, 129.
5. Sommers De K, Kovarik JM, Meyer EC, van Wyk M, Snyman JR, Blom M, Ott S, Grass P, Kutz K. Effects of diclofenac on isradipine pharmacokinetics and platelet aggregation in volunteers. *Eur J Clin Pharmacol* (1993) 44, 391–3.
6. Takeuchi K, Abe K, Yasujima M, Sato M, Tanno M, Sato K, Yoshinaga K. No adverse effect of non-steroidal anti-inflammatory drugs, sulindac and diclofenac sodium, on blood pressure control with a calcium antagonist, nifedipine, in elderly hypertensive patients. *Tohoku J Exp Med* (1991) 165, 201–8.
7. Houston MC, Weir M, Gray J, Ginsberg D, Szeto C, Kaihlenen PM, Sugimoto D, Runde M, Lefkowitz M. The effects of nonsteroidal anti-inflammatory drugs on blood pressures of patients with hypertension controlled by verapamil. *Arch Intern Med* (1995) 155, 1049–54.
8. Minuz P, Pancera P, Ribul M, Priante F, Degan M, Campedelli A, Arosio E, Lechi A. Amlodipine and haemodynamic effects of cyclo-oxygenase inhibition. *Br J Clin Pharmacol* (1995) 39, 45–50.
9. Salvetti A, Pedrinelli R, Magagna A, Stornello M, Scapellato L. Calcium antagonists: interactions in hypertension. *Am J Nephrol* (1986) 6 (Suppl 1), 95–99.
10. Hardy BG, Bartle WR, Myers M, Bailey DG, Edgar B. Effect of indomethacin on the pharmacokinetics and pharmacodynamics of felodipine. *Br J Clin Pharmacol* (1988) 26, 557–62.
11. Debbas NMG, Raoof NT, Al Qassab HK, Jackson SHD, Turner P. Does indomethacin antagonise the effects of nicardipine? *Acta Pharmacol Toxicol (Copenh)* (1986) 59 (Suppl V), 181.
12. Morgan T, Anderson A. The effect of nonsteroidal anti-inflammatory drugs on blood pressure in patients treated with different antihypertensive drugs. *J Clin Hypertens* (2003) 5, 53–7.
13. Perreault MM, Foster RT, Lebel M, Du Souich P, Larochelle P, Cusson JR. Pharmacodynamic effects of indomethacin in essential hypertensive patients treated with verapamil. *Clin Invest Med* (1993) 16 (Suppl 4), B17.
14. Mück W, Heine PR, Schmage N, Niklaus H, Horkulak J, Breuel H-P. Steady-state pharmacokinetics of nimodipine during chronic administration of indometacin in elderly healthy volunteers. *Arzneimittelforschung* (1995) 45, 460–2.
15. Thatte UM, Shah SJ, Dalvi SS, Suraokar S, Temulkar P, Anklesaria P, Kshirsager NA. Acute drug interaction between indomethacin and nifedipine in hypertensive patients. *J Assoc Physicians India* (1988) 36, 695–8.
16. Klassen DK, Jane LH, Young DY, Peterson CA. Assessment of blood pressure during naproxen therapy in hypertensive patients treated with nicardipine. *Am J Hypertens* (1995) 8, 146–53.
17. Baez MA, Alvarez CR, Weidler DJ. Effects of the non-steroidal anti-inflammatory drugs, piroxicam or sulindac, on the antihypertensive actions of propranolol and verapamil. *J Hypertens* (1987) 5 (Suppl 5) S563–S566.
18. Pahor M, Guralnik JM, Furberg CD, Carbonin P, Havlik RJ. Risk of gastrointestinal haemorrhage with calcium antagonists in hypertensive persons over 67 years old. *Lancet* (1996) 347, 1061–5.
19. Kaplan RC, Heckbert SR, Koepsell TD, Rosendaal FR, Psaty BM. Use of calcium channel blockers and risk of hospitalized gastrointestinal tract bleeding. *Arch Intern Med* (2000) 160, 1849–55.
20. Suissa S, Bourgault C, Barkun A, Sheehy O, Ernst P. Antihypertensive drugs and the risk of gastrointestinal bleeding. *Am J Med* (1998) 105, 230–5.
21. Kelly JP, Laszlo A, Kaufman DW, Sundstrom A, Shapiro S. Major upper gastrointestinal bleeding and the use of calcium channel blockers. *Lancet* (1999) 353, 559.
22. Celis H, Thijs L, Staessen JA, Birkenhäger WH, Bulpitt CJ, de Leeuw PW, Leonetti G, Nachev C, Tuomilehto J, Fagard RH for the Syst-Eur investigators. Interaction between nonsteroidal anti-inflammatory drug intake and calcium-channel blocker-based antihypertensive treatment in the Syst-Eur trial. *J Hum Hypertens* (2001) 15, 613–18.
23. Beilin LJ. Non-steroidal anti-inflammatory drugs and antihypertensive drug therapy. *J Hypertens* (2002) 20, 849–50.
24. Johnson AG, Nguyen TV, Day RO. Do nonsteroidal anti-inflammatory drugs affect blood pressure? A meta-analysis. *Ann Intern Med* (1994) 121, 289–300.
25. Johnson AG. NSAIDs and blood pressure. Clinical importance for older patients. *Drugs Aging* (1998) 12, 17–27.

Calcium channel blockers + Proton pump inhibitors

The clearance of both nifedipine and omeprazole is modestly reduced by concurrent use, but these changes seem unlikely to be of clinical importance. Pantoprazole does not affect the pharmacokinetics of nifedipine.

Clinical evidence, mechanism, importance and management

(a) Omeprazole

After taking omeprazole 20 mg daily for 7 days the clearance of **nifedipine** was reduced 21% in 10 healthy subjects. The same subjects had a 14% reduction in the clearance of a 40-mg intravenous dose of omeprazole after 5 days of treatment with **nifedipine** 10 mg three times daily.[1] In a related study the same group of workers found that omeprazole 20 mg daily for 8 days increased the AUC of **nifedipine** by 26%, but no changes in blood pressures or heart rates were seen.[2] None of these changes is large and they seem not to be of clinical importance.

(b) Pantoprazole

In an open, randomised, crossover study 24 healthy subjects were given pantoprazole 40 mg daily for 10 days, with sustained-release **nifedipine** 20 mg twice daily from day 6 to 10. The pharmacokinetics of the **nifedipine** were unchanged by the pantoprazole.[3] No special precautions would seem to be necessary if pantoprazole and **nifedipine** are given concurrently.

1. Danhof M, Soons PA, van den Berg G, Van Brummelen P, Jansen JBMJ. Interactions between nifedipine and omeprazole. *Eur J Clin Pharmacol* (1989) 36 (Suppl), A258.
2. Soons PA, van den Berg G, Danhof M, van Brummelen P, Jansen JBMJ, Lamers CBHW, Breimer DD. Influence of single- and multiple-dose omeprazole treatment on nifedipine pharmacokinetics and effects in healthy subjects. *Eur J Clin Pharmacol* (1992) 42, 319–24.
3. Bliesath H, Huber R, Steinijans VW, Koch HJ, Kunz K, Wurst W. Pantoprazole does not interact with nifedipine in man under steady-state conditions. *Int J Clin Pharmacol Ther* (1996) 34, 51–5.

Calcium channel blockers + Quinupristin/Dalfopristin

Quinupristin/dalfopristin may inhibit the metabolism of nifedipine.

Clinical evidence, mechanism, importance and management

The makers say that the plasma levels of nifedipine may be increased if it is given with quinupristin/dalfopristin, and nifedipine dosage reductions may be necessary.[1,2] This is probably because quinupristin/dalfopristin inhibits the cytochrome P450 isoenzyme CYP3A4-mediated metabolism of nifedipine.[3] The makers advise blood pressure monitoring and, if necessary, a reduction of nifedipine dosage during concurrent use.[2] It is predicted that other calcium channel blockers (e.g. verapamil, diltiazem) will also have their levels raised by quinupristin/dalfopristin.[3]

1. Coracten SR (Nifedipine). Celltech Pharmaceuticals Ltd. UK Summary of product characteristics, July 2003.
2. Adalat Retard (Nifedipine). Bayer plc. UK Summary of product characteristics, April 2005.
3. Rubinstein E, Prokocimer P, Talbot GH. Safety and tolerability of quinupristin/dalfopristin: administration guidelines. *J Antimicrob Chemother* (1999) 44 (Suppl A) 37–46.

Calcium channel blockers + Rifampicin (Rifampin)

The plasma levels of diltiazem, nifedipine, nilvadipine, verapamil and possibly those of barnidipine, isradipine, lercanidipine, manidipine, nicardipine, nimodipine, and nisoldipine are markedly reduced by rifampicin. They may become therapeutically ineffective unless their dosages are raised.

Clinical evidence

(a) Barnidipine, Manidipine

A brief report states that elderly patients with hypertension, well-controlled on calcium channel blockers including barnidipine or manidipine had blood pressure rises when rifampicin was added. Increased dosages or additional antihypertensives were needed to control the blood pressures, and reduced doses when the rifampicin was withdrawn.[1]

(b) Diltiazem

A study in 12 subjects found that the peak serum level following a single 120-mg oral dose of diltiazem alone was 186 nanograms/ml, but after taking rifampicin 600 mg daily for 8 days maximum serum diltiazem levels were less than 8 nanograms/ml.[2]

(c) Nifedipine

A hypertensive woman well controlled on nifedipine 40 mg twice daily, had a blood pressure rise from under 160/90 mmHg to 200/110 mmHg within 2 weeks of starting to take antitubercular treatment, which included rifampicin 450 mg daily. When the rifampicin was stopped and then restarted, the blood pressure fell and then rose again. The peak nifedipine plasma levels and the AUC fell by about 60% in the presence of rifampicin.[3] Another patient had reduced nifedipine levels (peak plasma levels and AUCs roughly halved) and an increase in anginal attacks when given rifampicin,[4] and yet another patient taking nifedipine had a loss of blood pressure control when given rifampicin.[5]

Six healthy subjects were given nifedipine 20 micrograms/kg intravenously and nifedipine 20 mg orally on separate days before and after taking rifampicin 600 mg daily for 7 days. The pharmacokinetics of the intravenous nifedipine were not significantly changed by the rifampicin, but the oral clearance increased from 1.5 to 20.9 litres/minute and the bioavailability fell from 41.2 to 5.3%.[6] A pharmacokinetic study in 6 healthy subjects found that when a single 10-mg oral dose of nifedipine was taken 8 hours after a single 1.2-g dose of rifampicin its bioavailability was reduced to 36%, its half-life was more than halved and its clearance increased threefold.[7]

(d) Nilvadipine

A study in 5 healthy normotensive subjects found that rifampicin 450 mg daily for 6 days reduced the peak plasma level and AUC of a single 4-mg dose of nilvadipine by about 20-fold and 30-fold respectively. The hypotensive effect and reflex tachycardia associated with nilvadipine alone in these subjects was also abolished by rifampicin.[8]

(e) Nisoldipine

There is some evidence that nisoldipine is ineffective in reducing blood pressure in the presence of rifampicin.[1,3]

(f) Verapamil

The observation that a patient whose hypertension was not reduced by verapamil while on antitubercular drugs, prompted a study in 4 other patients.[9] No verapamil could be detected in the plasma of 3 patients who took a single 40-mg dose of verapamil with rifampicin 450 to 600 mg daily, isoniazid 5 mg/kg daily, and ethambutol 15 mg/kg daily of verapamil. A maximum verapamil level of 20 nanograms/ml was found in the fourth patient. Six other subjects not taking antitubercular drugs had a maximum verapamil plasma concentration of 35 nanograms/ml.[9] Similar results have been reported by the same authors in another study.[10]

Supraventricular tachycardia was inadequately controlled in a patient taking rifampicin 600 mg daily and isoniazid 300 mg daily, despite a verapamil dose of 480 mg every 6 hours.[11] Substitution of the rifampicin by ethambutol resulted in a fourfold rise in serum verapamil levels.[11] A later study in 6 healthy subjects found that after taking rifampicin 600 mg daily for 2 weeks the oral bioavailability of verapamil was reduced from 26 to 2%, and the effects of verapamil on the ECG were abolished.[12] Yet another study in elderly patients similarly found that rifampicin 600 mg daily markedly increased the clearance of verapamil 120 mg twice daily. The effects of verapamil on AV conduction were almost abolished.[13]

Mechanism

Rifampicin reduces the effectiveness of nifedipine and verapamil to a greater extent after oral than after intravenous use. The evidence suggests that the rifampicin (known to be a potent enzyme inducing agent) increases the cytochrome P450 isoenzyme CYP3A4-mediated metabolism of calcium channel blockers in the gastrointestinal wall,[6,13,14] thereby increasing their clearance from the body.

Importance and management

The interactions between diltiazem, nifedipine, or verapamil and rifampicin are established and of clinical importance. There is some evidence that barnidipine, manidipine, nilvadipine, and nisoldipine interact with rifampicin and the makers of a number of other calcium channel blockers warn of similar interactions. Monitor the effects closely if rifampicin is given with any calcium channel blocker, being alert for the need to make a marked increase in their dosage. However, note that the makers of nifedipine,[15] **nimodipine**[16] and nisoldipine[17] contraindicate their use with rifampicin.

1. Yoshimoto H, Takahashi M, Saima S. Influence of rifampicin on antihypertensive effects of dihydropiridine calcium-channel blockers in four elderly patients. *Nippon Ronen Igakkai Zasshi* (1996) 33, 692–6.
2. Drda KD, Bastian TL, Self TH, Lawson J, Lanman RC, Burlew BS, Lalonde RL. Effects of debrisoquine hydroxylation phenotype and enzyme induction with rifampin on diltiazem pharmacokinetics and pharmacodynamics. *Pharmacotherapy* (1991) 11, 278.
3. Tada Y, Tsuda Y, Otsuka T, Nagasawa K, Kimura H, Kusaba T, Sakata T. Case report: nifedipine-rifampicin interaction attenuates the effect on blood pressure in a patient with essential hypertension. *Am J Med Sci* (1992) 303, 25–7.
4. Tsuchihashi K, Fukami K, Kishimoto H, Sumiyoshi T, Haze K, Saito M, Hiramori K. A case of variant angina exacerbated by administration of rifampicin. *Heart Vessels* (1987) 3, 214–17.
5. Takasugi T. A case of hypertension suggesting nifedipine and rifampicin drug interaction. *Igaku To Yakugaku* (1989) 22, 132–5.
6. Holtbecker N, Fromm MF, Kroemer HK, Ohnhaus EE, Heidemann H. The nifedipine-rifampin interaction: Evidence for induction of gut wall metabolism. *Drug Metab Dispos* (1996) 24, 1121–3.
7. Ndanusa BU, Mustapha A, Abdu-Aguye I. The effect of single dose of rifampicin on the pharmacokinetics of oral nifedipine. *J Pharm Biomed Anal* (1997) 15, 1571–5.
8. Saima S, Furuie K, Yoshimoto H, Fukuda J, Hayashi T, Echizen H. The effects of rifampicin on the pharmacokinetics and pharmacodynamics of orally administered nilvadipine to healthy subjects. *Br J Clin Pharmacol* (2002) 53, 203–6.
9. Rahn KH, Mooy J, Böhm R, vd Vet, A. Reduction of bioavailability of verapamil by rifampin. *N Engl J Med* (1985) 312, 920–1.
10. Mooy J, Böhm R, van Baak M, van Kemenade J, vd Vet A, Rahn KH. The influence of antituberculosis drugs on the plasma level of verapamil. *Eur J Clin Pharmacol* (1987) 32, 107–9.
11. Barbarash RA. Verapamil-rifampin interaction. *Drug Intell Clin Pharm* (1985) 19, 559–60.
12. Barbarash RA, Bauman JL, Fischer JH, Kondos GT, Batenhorst RL. Near-total reduction in verapamil bioavailability by rifampin: electrocardiographic correlates. *Chest* (1988) 94, 954–9.
13. Fromm MF, Dilger K, Busse D, Kroemer HK, Eichelbaum M, Klotz U. Gut wall metabolism of verapamil in older people: effects of rifampicin-mediated enzyme induction. *Br J Clin Pharmacol* (1998) 45, 247–55.
14. Fromm MF, Busse D, Kroemer HK, Eichelbaum M. Differential induction of prehepatic and hepatic metabolism of verapamil by rifampin. *Hepatology* (1996) 24, 796–801.
15. Adalat Retard (Nifedipine). Bayer plc. UK Summary of product characteristics, April 2005.
16. Nimotop (Nimodipine). Bayer plc. UK Summary of product characteristics, June 2002.
17. Syscor MR (Nisoldipine). Forest Laboratories UK Ltd. UK Summary of product characteristics, August 1998.

Calcium channel blockers + St John's wort (*Hypericum perforatum*)

St John's wort significantly reduces the bioavailability of verapamil.

Clinical evidence, mechanism, importance and management

In a study, racemic **verapamil** 24 mg was given as a jejunal perfusion over 100 minutes to 8 healthy subjects both before and after treatment with St John's wort tablets 300 mg three times daily for 14 days. St John's wort did not affect jejunal permeability or the absorption of either ***R*- or *S*-verapamil**. The AUCs of ***R*- and *S*-verapamil** were decreased by 78% and 80% respectively and the peak plasma levels by 76% and 78% respectively. The terminal half-life was not changed significantly. The AUC for ***R*-verapamil** was sixfold higher than that of ***S*-verapamil** and St John's wort did not change this ratio.[1]

It appears that St John's wort decreased the bioavailability of both ***R*- and *S*-verapamil** by inducing their metabolism by the cytochrome P450 isoenzyme CYP3A4 in the gut. An effect on P-glycoprotein-mediated transport is not likely, as intestinal permeability was not significantly altered.[1] The clinical importance of this interaction is not known but it may be prudent to avoid concurrent use. There appears to be no information about other calcium channel blockers, but as they are also affected by other CYP3A4 enzyme inducers, it would seem prudent to monitor concurrent use carefully. More study is required.

1. Tannergren C, Engman H, Knutson L, Hedeland M, Bondesson U, Lennernäs H. St John's wort decreases the bioavailability of *R*- and *S*-verapamil through induction of first-pass metabolism. *Clin Pharmacol Ther* (2004) 75, 298–309.

Calcium channel blockers + Sulfinpyrazone

The clearance of verapamil is markedly increased by sulfinpyrazone.

Clinical evidence, mechanism, importance and management

A study in 8 healthy subjects found that sulfinpyrazone 800 mg daily for a week, increased the clearance of a single oral dose of **verapamil** by about threefold, possibly due to an increase in its liver metabolism.[1] The clinical importance of this is uncertain, but be alert for reduced **verapamil** effects. It seems probable that the dosage may need to be increased.

1. Wing LMH, Miners JO, Lillywhite KJ. Verapamil disposition—effects of sulphinpyrazone and cimetidine. *Br J Clin Pharmacol* (1985) 19, 385–91.

Calcium channel blockers + Vancomycin

An isolated case report suggests that the hypotensive effects of the rapid infusion of vancomycin may occur more readily in those who are already vasodilated with nifedipine, but it seems likely that the effects seen were due to the rapid infusion alone.

Clinical evidence, mechanism, importance and management

A man with severe systemic sclerosis was hospitalised for Raynaud's phenomenon and dental extraction. After being started on **nifedipine** 40 mg daily, he was given intravenous vancomycin 1 g in 200 ml of dextrose 5% over 30 minutes. After 20 minutes he experienced a severe headache and was found to have a marked macular erythema on the upper trunk, head, neck and arms. His blood pressure fell to 100/60 mmHg and his pulse rate was 90 bpm. He recovered spontaneously.[1] The authors of the report acknowledge the possibility of 'red-man syndrome' caused by the vancomycin, and suggest that it may occur more readily in those already vasodilated with nifedipine. However, given that this is an isolated report, and the vancomycin was given over 3 times faster than the recommended rate, it seems likely that this is purely an adverse effect of vancomycin.

1. Daly BM, Sharkey I. Nifedipine and vancomycin-associated red man syndrome. *Drug Intell Clin Pharm* (1986) 20, 986.

Calcium channel blockers + X-ray contrast media

The hypotensive effects of an intravenous bolus of an ionic X-ray contrast medium can be increased by the presence of calcium channel blockers. No interaction or only a small interaction appears to occur with non-ionic contrast media.

Clinical evidence, mechanism, importance and management

It is well recognised that ionic X-ray contrast media used for ventriculography reduce the systemic blood pressure due to peripheral vasodilation. They also have a direct depressant effect on the heart muscle. A comparative study of the haemodynamic response of 65 patients found that the hypotensive effect of a bolus dose of an ionic agent (0.5 ml/kg of **meglumine amidotrizoate** and **sodium amidotrizoate** with edetate sodium or disodium) was increased by the concurrent use of **nifedipine** or **diltiazem.** Haemodynamic effects occurred earlier (3.1 seconds instead of 12.9 seconds), were more profound (a fall in systolic pressure of 48.4 instead of 36.9 mmHg) and more prolonged (62 seconds instead of 36 seconds).[1] A similar interaction was seen in *dogs* given **verapamil.**[2] No interaction or only a minimal interaction was seen in the patients and *dogs* when non-ionic contrast media (**iopamidol** or **iohexol**) were used instead.[1,2]

1. Morris DL, Wisneski JA, Gertz EW, Wexman M, Axelrod R, Langberg JJ. Potentiation by nifedipine and diltiazem of the hypotensive response after contrast angiography. *J Am Coll Cardiol* (1985) 6, 785–91.
2. Higgins CB, Kuber M, Slutsky RA. Interaction between verapamil and contrast media in coronary arteriography: comparison of standard ionic and new nonionic media. *Circulation* (1983) 68, 628–35.

22

Cardiovascular drugs, miscellaneous

The drugs dealt with in this section include the centrally acting drugs (clonidine, methyldopa), adrenergic neurone blockers (guanethidine), some vasodilator antihypertensives (hydralazine, diazoxide), nitrates (glyceryl trinitrate), potassium channel activators (nicorandil), peripheral vasodilators (pentoxifylline), calcium sensitisers (levosimendan) and endothelin antagonists (bosentan). 'Table 22.1', (p.664) lists the drugs dealt with here and their proprietary names. Where these drugs are the affecting agent rather than the drug affected, the interactions are described elsewhere.

Table 22.1 *Antihypertensive drugs*

Generic names	*Proprietary names*
Adrenergic neurone blockers	
Guanethidine	Ismelin
Calcium sensitiser	
Levosimendan	
Centrally-acting agents	
Clonidine	Adesipress-TTS, Arkamin, Aruclonin, Atensina, Catapres, Catapresan, Catapressan, Clonesina, Clonid-Ophtal, Clonidural, Clonistada, Clonnirit, Dispaclonidin, Dixarit, Duraclon, Edolglau, Epiclodina, Haemiton, Hypodine , Isoglaucon, Menograine, Mirfat, Neo Clodil, Normopresan, Paracefan
Guanfacine	Estulic, Tenex
Guanabenz	Lisapres, Wytensin
Methyldopa	Aldomet, Aldometil, Aldomin, Aldotensin, Aloset, Alphadopa, Amender, Biotenzol, Cardiodopa, Dopagrand, Dopagyt, Dopamed, Dopamet, Dopametil, Dopasian, Dopatral, Dopegyt, Ductomet, Etildopanan, Hydopa, Hy-Po-Tone, Isomet, Kindomet, Medopa, Medopren, Mefpa, Meldopa, Metilcord, Metpata , Normopress, Nu-Medopa, Presinol, Prodopa, Siamdopa, Tensioval, Toparal
Moxonidine	Cynt, Fisiotens, Gilutens, Moxamar, Moxaviv, Moxocard, moxodura, Moxoham, Moxon, Moxonur, Moxotel, Moxovasc, Normatens, Normoxin, Physiotens, Ratiomox
Directly-acting vasodilators	
Diazoxide	Eudemine, Hyperstat, Proglicem, Proglycem, Sefulken, Tensuril
Hydralazine	Alphapress, Apresolin, Apresolina, Apresoline, Bionobal, Cesoline, Hidral, Hydrapres, Hyperphen, Nepresol, Novo-Hylazin, Nu-Hydral
Minoxidil	Alopexy, Alostil, Aloxidil, Apo-Gain, Axelan, Biocrinal, Carexidil, Crinalsofex, Dermolantyl, Dinaxil Capilar, Ebersedin, Epokelan, Folcress, Growell, Hairgaine, Hairgrow, Hair-Treat, Headway, Lacovin, Locemix, Loniten, Lonnoten, Lonolox, Lonoten, Lotorin, Macbirs Minoxidil, Manoxidil , Minocalve, Minovital, Minox, Minoxi, Minoximen, Minoxitrim, Modil, Monoxidil, Neocapil, Neo-Pruristam, Neoxidil, Noxidil, Nuhair, Oxofenil, Recrea, Regaine, Regro, Regrowth, Revexan, Rogaine, Stemeral, Toneon, Tricolocion, Tricoplus, Tricovivax, Tricoxane, Tricoxidil, Ylox
Sodium nitroprusside	Doketrol, Hypoten, Nipride, Niprusodio, Nipruss, Nitan, Nitopro, Nitriate, Nitropresabbott, Nitropress, Nitroprus, Nitroprussiat, SNP, Sonide
Tolazoline	Divascol
Endothelin antagonists	
Bosentan	Tracleer
Nitrates	
Glyceryl trinitrate (Nitroglycerin)	Adesitrin, Amitacon, Anginine, Angiolingual, Angised, Anglix, Aquo-Trinitrosan, Buccard, Cardinit, Cardiplast, Corangin Nitrokapseln, Cordipatch, Cordiplast, Coro-Nitro, Dauxona, Deponit, Dermatrans, Diafusor, Discotrine, Enetege, Epinitril, Gen-Nitro, Gepan, Glytrin, GTO Oil, Keritrina, Lanesta, Lenitral, Lycinate, Maycor Nitrospray, Millisrol, Minitran, Minitran, MinitranS, Myonit, Myovin, Natispray, Niglinar, Nirmin, Nitradisc, Nitraket, Nitrangin, Nitrek, Nit-Ret, Nitriderm TTS, Nitrilex, Nitro, Nitro Mack, Nitro Pohl, Nitro Solvay, Nitro-Bid, Nitrocine, Nitrocontin, Nitrocor, Nitro-Derm, Nitroderm TTS, Nitrodisc, Nitro-Dur, Nitro-Dyl, Nitrogard, Nitrogesic, Nitrogray, Nitroject, Nitrokor, Nitrol, Nitrolingual, Nitromex, Nitromin, Nitromint, Nitronal, Nitrong, Nitroplast, NitroQuick, Nitroretard-Faran, Nitrospray, Nitrostat, Nitrosylon, NitroTab, Nitro-Time, Nitroven, Nysconitrine, Pancoran, Percutol, Perganit, Perlinganit, Plastranit, Rectogesic, Rho-Nitro, Sodemethin, Solinitrina, Supranitrin, Suscard, Sustac, Top-Nitro, Transdermal-NTG, Transderm-Nitro, Transiderm-Nitro, Tridil, Trinipatch, Triniplas, Trinispray, Trinitrina, Trinitrine, Trinitrine Simple Laleuf, Trinitrosan, Trintek, Venitrin, Vernies, Willlong
Peripheral vasodilators	
Pentoxifylline	Agapurin, Artal, Chemopent, Chinotal, Claudicat, Dinostral, Dospan Pento, Durapental, Elastab, Elorgan, Fixoten, Flexital, Haemodyn, Hatial, Hemovas, Ikatral Periferico, Kentadin, Kinetal, Neotren, Oxopurin, Penlol, Pentilin, Pento, Pentoflux, Pentohexal, Pentolab, Pentomer, Pentong, Pento-Puren, Pentox, Pentoxi, Pentoximed, Pentoxin, Peridane, Previscan, Ralofekt, Rentylin, Retimax, Sufisal, Tarontal, Torental, Trenlin, Trental, Vascer, Vasofyl, Vasonit
Potassium channel activators	
Nicorandil	Adancor, Angicor, Corflo, Dancor, Ikorel, Nikoril, Sigmart, Zynicor
Rauwolfia alkaloids	
Reserpine	Serfinato
Serotonin blockers	
Ketanserin	Ketensin, Serefrex, Serepress, Sufrexal
Miscellaneous	
Perhexiline	Pexsig
Tirilazad	Freedox

Antihypertensives + Phenothiazines

The hypotensive adverse effects of chlorpromazine and other phenothiazines may be additive with the effects of antihypertensives. Patients may feel faint and dizzy if they stand up quickly. Guanethidine-like drugs are the probable exception because their effects may be opposed by the phenothiazines (see 'Guanethidine + Antipsychotics', p.670). An isolated report describes paradoxical hypertension in a patient given methyldopa and trifluoperazine.

Clinical evidence

(a) Clonidine

In one report, a patient experienced dizziness and hypotension (systolic blood pressure 76 mmHg) about an hour after being given **chlorpromazine** 100 mg, clonidine 100 micrograms and **furosemide** 40 mg. Another patient also experienced hypotension 2 hours after being given clonidine 100 micrograms and a 1-mg intramuscular dose of **haloperidol** (a butyrophenone with general properties similar to phenothiazines).[1]

There is also an isolated and unexplained case of a psychotic patient on **fluphenazine decanoate** who began to exhibit delirium, agitation disorientation, short-term memory loss, confusion and clouded consciousness within 10 days of starting to take clonidine 200 micrograms daily. These symptoms disappeared when the clonidine was stopped and returned when it was re-started. He had previously been successfully treated with **haloperidol** and clonidine.[2]

(b) Methyldopa

In one study, 8 normotensive patients given methyldopa 500 mg to 1 g daily with **chlorpromazine** 200 to 400 mg daily for schizophrenia experienced orthostatic dizziness and had reductions in their standing systolic blood pressure.[3] In contrast, an isolated report describes a paradoxical rise in blood pressure in a patient with systemic lupus erythematosus and renal failure when treated with methyldopa and **trifluoperazine**. When the **trifluoperazine** was stopped, the blood pressure fell.[4]

(c) Nifedipine

A patient on **chlorpromazine** given nifedipine [dosage not stated] for 2 days before surgery developed marked hypotension during surgery, which was eventually controlled with noradrenaline (norepinephrine).[5]

Mechanism

Simple addition of the hypotensive effects of both drugs seems to be the explanation for the increased hypotension and orthostasis. However, note that in contrast to the case report above, *animal* studies have shown that chlorpromazine reduces the antihypertensive effect of clonidine.[6] The suggested explanation for the hypertensive interaction with methyldopa and trifluoperazine is that the phenothiazine blocked the reuptake of the 'false transmitter' (alpha-methyl noradrenaline) that is produced during therapy with methyldopa.[4]

Importance and management

The increased hypotension and orthostasis that can occur if chlorpromazine or other phenothiazines are used with antihypertensive drugs is established. Note that, of the phenothiazines, **levomepromazine** is particularly associated with postural hypotension. Monitor the reaction, particularly during the first period of treatment and warn patients that if they feel faint and dizzy they should lie down, and that they should remain lying down until symptoms abate completely. Dosage adjustment may be necessary. See also 'Beta-blockers + Phenothiazines', p.638 and 'ACE inhibitors + Antipsychotics', p.15.

Guanethidine-like drugs behave differently because their antihypertensive actions can be opposed to some extent by the phenothiazines (see 'Guanethidine + Antipsychotics', p.670). Similarly, the makers of clonidine note that a reduced antihypertensive effect may occur with antipsychotics with alpha-blocking properties (e.g. chlorpromazine), as well as mentioning the risk of orthostatic hypotension.[7] Consider also 'Clonidine + Tricyclic and related antidepressants', p.667. Although antagonism of the antihypertensive effect of clonidine has been seen in *animals* given chlorpromazine, there appear to be no clinical reports.

1. Fruncillo RJ, Gibbons WJ, Vlasses PH, Ferguson RK. Severe hypotension associated with concurrent clonidine and antipsychotic medication. *Am J Psychiatry* (1985) 142, 274.
2. Allen RM, Flemenbaum A. Delirium associated with combined fluphenazine-clonidine therapy. *J Clin Psychiatry* (1979) 40, 236–7.
3. Chouinard G, Pinard G, Prenoveau Y, Tetreault L. Alpha methyldopa-chlorpromazine interaction in schizophrenic patients. *Curr Ther Res* (1973) 15, 60–72.
4. Westhervelt FB, Atuk NO. Methyldopa-induced hypertension. *JAMA* (1974) 227, 557.
5. Stuart-Taylor ME, Crosse MM. A plea for noradrenaline. *Anaesthesia* (1989) 44, 916–7.
6. van Zwieten PA. The interaction between clonidine and various neuroleptic agents and some benzodiazepine tranquillizers. *J Pharm Pharmacol* (1977) 29, 229–34.
7. Catapres Tablets (Clonidine hydrochloride). Boehringer Ingelheim Ltd. UK Summary of product characteristics, November 2003.

Antihypertensives + Phenylpropanolamine

A single dose of a sustained-release preparation of phenylpropanolamine and brompheniramine was found to cause a minor and clinically insignificant rise in the blood pressures of patients on various antihypertensives.

Clinical evidence, mechanism, importance and management

A randomised double-blind crossover study in 13 patients with hypertension controlled with **unnamed diuretics** (7), **ACE inhibitors** (6), **beta-blockers** (5), **calcium channel blockers** (1) and a **centrally acting alpha-agonist** (1) found that a single dose of *Dimetapp Extentabs* (phenylpropanolamine 75 mg with brompheniramine 12 mg) caused only a minor systolic/diastolic blood pressure rise of 1.7/0.9 mmHg over 4 hours.[1] This sustained release preparation in this dosage has therefore no clinically important effect on the blood pressure, but (as the authors point out) these results do not necessarily apply to different doses and immediate-release preparations. A marked rise in blood pressure was seen in one patient on **methyldopa** and **oxprenolol** when given phenylpropanolamine, see 'Methyldopa + Sympathomimetics; Indirectly-acting', p.675. Consider also 'Beta-blockers + Phenylpropanolamine', p.639.

1. Petrulis AS, Imperiale TF, Speroff T. The acute effect of phenylpropanolamine and brompheniramine on blood pressure in controlled hypertension. *J Gen Intern Med* (1991) 6, 503–6.

Bosentan + Azoles

Ketoconazole increased bosentan levels twofold, but the clinical significance of this is unclear. However, fluconazole is predicted to have a greater effect. As elevated bosentan levels are associated with an increased risk of liver toxicity the makers do not recommend the concurrent use of azoles.

Clinical evidence, mechanism, importance and management

In a randomised crossover study, 10 healthy subjects were given bosentan 62.5 mg twice daily for 11 doses, either alone or with **ketoconazole** 200 mg daily each morning. The maximum plasma level of bosentan was increased 2.1-fold, and the AUC was increased 2.3-fold (range 1.4- to 4-fold) when given with **ketoconazole**. This interaction was attributed to **ketoconazole** inhibiting the cytochrome P450 isoenzyme CYP3A4, which mediates the metabolism of bosentan.[1]

Other potent CYP3A4 inhibitors (e.g. **itraconazole**) are expected to interact similarly to **ketoconazole**.[2] However, because **fluconazole** also inhibits CYP2C9, another enzyme involved in the metabolism of bosentan, and to some extent CYP3A4, it is anticipated that it could cause large increases in bosentan levels.

The clinical significance of raised bosentan levels is unclear. Bosentan has been tolerated in single-doses of up to 2400 mg in healthy subjects, although elevations in liver transaminases have been seen during long-term high-dose treatment.[1] Even so, the makers do not recommend the combination of **fluconazole** with bosentan because of the risk of liver toxicity.[2] Similarly using **ketoconazole** or **itraconazole** in combination with **voriconazole** (an inhibitor of CYP2C9) and bosentan is also not recommended.[2]

Until more is known, it may be prudent to carefully monitor liver function when the combination is used. The makers suggest that no dosage adjustment is likely to be required when **ketoconazole** is used with bosentan.[2]

1. van Giersbergen PLM, Halabi A, Dingemanse J. Single- and multiple-dose pharmacokinetics of bosentan and its interaction with ketoconazole. *Br J Clin Pharmacol* (2002) 53, 589–95.
2. Tracleer (Bosentan monohydrate). Actelion Pharmaceuticals UK. UK Summary of product characteristics, September 2004.

Bosentan + Food

In a study in 16 healthy subjects the pharmacokinetics of bosentan were not significantly changed by the presence of food. Bosentan may therefore be given without regard to meal times.[1]

1. Dingemanse J, Bodin F, Weidekamm E, Kutz K, van Giersbergen P. Influence of food intake and formulation on the pharmacokinetics and metabolism of bosentan, a dual enothelin receptor antagonist. *J Clin Pharmacol* (2002) 42, 283–9.

Clonidine + Beta-blockers

The use of clonidine with beta-blockers can be therapeutically valuable, but a sharp and serious rise in blood pressure ('rebound hypertension') can follow the sudden withdrawal of clonidine, which may be worsened by the presence of a beta-blocker. Isolated cases of marked bradycardia and hypotension have been seen in patients given clonidine with esmolol. There are also two reports describing paradoxical hypertension with the combination of clonidine and beta-blockers.

Clinical evidence

(a) Exacerbation of the clonidine-withdrawal hypertensive rebound

A woman with a blood pressure of 180/140 mmHg was treated with clonidine and **timolol**. When the clonidine was stopped in error, she developed a violent throbbing headache and became progressively confused, ataxic and semicomatose, and had a grand mal convulsion. Her blood pressure was found to have risen to over 300/185 mmHg.[1]

A number of other reports describe similar cases of hypertensive rebound (a sudden and serious rise in blood pressure) within 24 and 72 hours of stopping the clonidine, apparently worsened by the presence of **propranolol**.[2-6] The symptoms resemble those of phaeochromocytoma, and include tremor, apprehension, flushing, nausea, vomiting, severe headache and a serious rise in blood pressure. One patient died from a cerebellar haemorrhage.[5]

(b) Bradycardia and hypotension

A man anaesthetised with thiopental and diamorphine, with oxygen, nitrous oxide, enflurane and atracurium was given clonidine 50 micrograms to control hypertension. After 15 minutes he became tachycardic with heart rates of up to 170 bpm. **Esmolol** 75 mg was given by slow infusion, whereupon his heart rate fell to 20 bpm. He responded to atropine 1.2 mg, adrenaline (epinephrine) 1 mg and calcium chloride 10 ml with a stable heart rate of 110 bpm.[7] Of 32 patients receiving **esmolol** during surgery in a clinical trial, one patient developed marked hypotension and bradycardia, which responded to ephedrine 10 mg. It was noted that this patient had been receiving clonidine.[8]

(c) Antagonism of the hypotensive effects

The combination of **sotalol** 160 mg daily and clonidine 450 micrograms daily caused a marked rise in blood pressure in 6 of 10 patients compared with either clonidine alone (3 patients) or **sotalol** alone (3 patients). Two of the 10 had blood pressures that were lower than with either drug alone, and the remaining 2 patients had no appreciable change in blood pressure.[9] Two cases of hypertension involving clonidine with **propranolol** have also been described.[10]

(d) Peripheral vascular disorders

The maker of clonidine notes that the concurrent use of a beta-blocker may possibly potentiate peripheral vascular disorders.[11] This is based on the known pharmacology of the drugs,[12] and no specific cases appear to have been reported.

Mechanism

The normal additive hypotensive effects of these drugs result from the two acting in concert at different but complementary sites in the cardiovascular system. Just why antagonism sometimes occurs is unexplained. The hypertensive rebound following clonidine withdrawal is thought to be due to an increase in the levels of circulating catecholamines. With the beta (vasodilator) effects blocked by a beta-blocker, the alpha (vasoconstrictor) effects of the catecholamines are unopposed and the hypertension is further exaggerated.

Importance and management

It is well-known that beta-blockers seriously worsen the rebound hypertension following clonidine withdrawal. Control this adverse effect by stopping the beta-blocker several days before starting a gradual withdrawal of clonidine.[13] A successful alternative is to replace the clonidine and the beta-blocker with labetalol,[14] which is both an alpha- and a beta-blocker: the blood catecholamine levels still rise markedly (20-fold) and the patient may experience tremor, nausea, apprehension and palpitations, but no serious blood pressure rise or headaches occur.[14] The dosage of labetalol will need to be titrated to the patient, with regular checks on the blood pressure over 2 to 3 days. If a hypertensive episode develops, control it with an alpha-blocking agent such as phentolamine.[2] Diazoxide is also effective.[1,5] Re-introduction of oral or intravenous clonidine should also stabilise the situation. It is clearly important to emphasise to patients taking clonidine and beta-blockers that they must keep taking their drugs.

Clonidine and atenolol[15,16] (a cardio-selective beta-blocker) have additive hypotensive effects and smaller doses of clonidine can be given, which decreases its troublesome adverse effects (sedation and dry mouth). In contrast, with propranolol[15] or nadolol[16] (nonselective beta-blockers) the blood pressure reductions were the same as with either drug alone. The weight of evidence suggests that paradoxical hypertension is rare.[9,10]

1. Bailey RR, Neale TJ. Rapid clonidine withdrawal with blood pressure overshoot exaggerated by beta-blockade. *BMJ* (1976) i, 942–3.
2. Bruce DL, Croley TF, Less JS. Preoperative clonidine withdrawal syndrome. *Anesthesiology* (1979) 51, 90–2.
3. Cairns SA, Marshall AJ. Clonidine withdrawal. *Lancet* (1976) i, 368.
4. Strauss FG, Franklin SS, Lewin AJ, Maxwell MH. Withdrawal of antihypertensive therapy. Hypertensive crisis in renovascular hypertension. *JAMA* (1977) 238, 1734–6.
5. Vernon C, Sakula A. Fatal rebound hypertension after abrupt withdrawal of clonidine and propranolol. *Br J Clin Pract* (1979) 33, 112,121.
6. Reid JL, Wing LMH, Dargie HJ, Hamilton CA, Davies DS, Dollery CT. Clonidine withdrawal in hypertension. Changes in blood pressure and plasma and urinary noradrenaline. *Lancet* (1977) i, 1171–4.
7. Perks D, Fisher GC. Esmolol and clonidine — a possible interaction. *Anaesthesia* (1992) 47, 533–4.
8. Kanitz DD, Ebert TJ, Kampine JP. Intraoperative use of bolus doses of esmolol to treat tachycardia. *J Clin Anesth* (1990) 2, 238–42.
9. Saarimaa H. Combination of clonidine and sotalol in hypertension. *BMJ* (1976) i, 810.
10. Warren SE, Ebert E, Swerdlin A-H, Steinberg SM, Stone R. Clonidine and propranolol paradoxical hypertension. *Arch Intern Med* (1979) 139, 253.
11. Catapres (Clonidine hydrochloride). Boehringer Ingelheim Ltd. UK Summary of product characteristics, November 2003.
12. Boehringer Ingelheim. Personal communication, 29 March 2005.
13. Harris AL. Clonidine withdrawal and blockade. *Lancet* (1976) i, 596.
14. Rosenthal T, Rabinowitz B, Boichis H, Elazar E, Brauner A, Neufeld HN. Use of labetalol in hypertensive patients during discontinuation of clonidine therapy. *Eur J Clin Pharmacol* (1981) 20, 237–40.
15. Lilja M, Jounela AJ, Juustila H, Mattila MJ. Interaction of clonidine and β-blockers. *Acta Med Scand* (1980) 207, 173–6.
16. Fogari R, Corradi L. Interaction of clonidine and beta blocking agents in the treatment of essential hypertension. In 'Low dose oral and transdermal therapy of hypertension' (Proceedings of Conference 1984), edited by Weber MA, Drayer JIM, Kolloch R. Springer-Verlag, 1985, pp. 118–21.

Clonidine + Bupropion

Bupropion 100 mg three times daily for 9 days did not reduce the hypotensive effect of a single 300-microgram oral dose of clonidine in 8 healthy subjects.[1]

1. Cubeddu LX, Cloutier G, Gross K, Grippo R, Tanner L, Lerea L, Shakarjian M, Knowlton G, Harden TK, Arendshorst W and Rogers JF. Bupropion does not antagonize cardiovascular actions of clonidine in normal subjects and spontaneously hypertensive rats. *Clin Pharmacol Ther* (1984) 35, 576–84.

Clonidine and related drugs + CNS depressants

Increased sedation may occur if alcohol or other CNS depressants are taken with clonidine, guanfacine or guanabenz.

Clinical evidence, mechanism, importance and management

Sedation is a common adverse effect of clonidine and other central alpha-adrenoceptor agonists such as **guanfacine** and **guanabenz**, particularly during the initial stages of therapy.[1-3] Patients starting on these drugs should be warned that their tolerance to **alcohol** and other CNS depressant drugs may be diminished. Patients who are affected should not drive or operate machinery. See also 'Moxonidine + Miscellaneous', p.676.

1. Catapres (Clonidine hydrochloride). Boehringer Ingelheim Ltd. UK Summary of product characteristics, November 2003.
2. Tenex (Guanfacine hydrochloride). ESP Pharma Inc. US Prescribing information [undated – accessed 27/07/05].
3. Catapres tablets (Clonidine hydrochloride). Boehringer Ingelheim Pharmaceuticals Inc. US Prescribing information, April 1998.

Clonidine + Oral contraceptives

The sedative effects of intravenous clonidine have been increased by a combined oral contraceptive.

Clinical evidence, mechanism, importance and management

A study[1] in a group of 10 women found that the sedative effects of a single 1.3-microgram/kg dose of intravenous clonidine were increased by a combined oral contraceptive (**ethinylestradiol/levonorgestrel** 30 micrograms/150 or 250 micrograms). The clinical importance of this is uncertain.

1. Chalmers JS, Fulli-Lemaire I, Cowen PJ. Effects of the contraceptive pill on sedative responses to clonidine and apomorphine in normal women. *Psychol Med* (1985) 15, 363–7.

Clonidine + Prazosin

There is evidence that prazosin can reduce the antihypertensive effects of clonidine, whereas some other evidence suggests that this does not occur.

Clinical evidence, mechanism, importance and management

The hypotensive effect of a 150-microgram intravenous dose of clonidine was reduced by 47% in 18 patients with essential hypertension after 4 days' treatment with prazosin (mean dose 11 mg three times daily).[1] A later crossover study by the same research group in 17 patients with essential hypertension (mean blood pressures 170/103 mmHg) found that clonidine 300 micrograms daily for 4 days reduced blood pressures by 38/18 mmHg and prazosin 6 mg daily for 3 days reduced blood pressures by 10/4 mmHg. However, when prazosin and clonidine were given together the blood pressures were only reduced to a similar extent as prazosin alone (12/6 mmHg).[2] Similarly, some earlier studies had suggested that the combination of clonidine and prazosin produced only a modest,[3] or no additive antihypertensive effect.[4] Conversely, other studies using the combination have not reported a reduced antihypertensive effect.[5,6] In the presence of prazosin the rebound hypertension following clonidine withdrawal was said to be moderate (a rise from 145/85 to 169/104 mmHg).[6]

Clonidine is an $alpha_2$ agonist, whereas prazosin is an $alpha_1$-blocker. Consequently, it has been postulated that the drugs may be partially antagonistic when given together, and the authors of the first study cite a number of *animal* studies to support this.[1] Although not conclusive, it seems possible that concurrent use may not always be favourable. Monitor the effects.

1. Kapocsi J, Farsang C, Vizi ES. Prazosin partly blocks clonidine-induced hypotension in patients with essential hypertension. *Eur J Clin Pharmacol* (1987) 32, 331–4.
2. Farsang C, Varga K, Kapocsi J. Prazosin-clonidine and prazosin-guanfacine interactions in hypertension. *Pharmacol Res Commun* (1988) 20 (Suppl 1), 85–6.
3. Kuokkanen K, Mattila MJ. Antihypertensive effects of prazosin in combination with methyldopa, clonidine or propranolol. *Ann Clin Res* (1979) 11, 18–24.
4. Hubbel FA, Weber MA, Drayer JIM, Rose DE. Combined central and peripheral sympathetic blockade: absence of additive antihypertensive effects. *Am J Med Sci* (1983) 285: 18–26.
5. Stokes GS, Gain JM, Mahoney JE, Raaftos J, Steward JH. Long term use of prazosin in combination or alone for treating hypertension. *Med J Aust* (1977) 2 (Suppl), 13–16.
6. Andréjak M, Fievet P, Makdassi R, Comoy E, de Fremont JF, Coevoet B, Fournier A. Lack of antagonism in the antihypertensive effects of clonidine and prazosin in man. *Clin Sci* (1981) 61, 453s–455s.

Clonidine + Rifampicin (Rifampin)

Rifampicin does not interact with clonidine.

Clinical evidence, mechanism, importance and management

Rifampicin 600 mg twice daily for 7 days had no effect on the elimination kinetics of clonidine nor on the pulse rates or blood pressures of 6 subjects taking clonidine 200 micrograms twice daily.[1] No special precautions would seem necessary on concurrent use.

1. Affrime MB, Lowenthal DT, Rufo M. Failure of rifampin to induce the metabolism of clonidine in normal volunteers. *Drug Intell Clin Pharm* (1981) 15, 964–6.

Clonidine + Tricyclic and related antidepressants

The tricyclic antidepressants, clomipramine, desipramine and imipramine reduce or abolish the antihypertensive effects of clonidine. Other tricyclics are expected to behave similarly. A hypertensive crisis developed in a woman on clonidine given imipramine, and severe pain occurred in a man on amitriptyline and diamorphine given intrathecal clonidine. Conversely, the tetracyclics, maprotiline and mianserin do not appear to alter the antihypertensive effects of clonidine. An isolated case report describes a hypertensive crisis in a patient on mirtazapine and clonidine. Hypotension occurred in a boy on clonidine and trazodone.

Clinical evidence

(a) Tetracyclic and related antidepressants

Maprotiline 100 mg in 4 divided doses over 22 hours did not alter the effect of a single dose of clonidine on blood pressure or heart rate in 8 healthy subjects.[1] **Mianserin** 20 mg three times daily for 2 weeks had no effect on the control of blood pressure in 5 patients receiving clonidine.[2,3] Similarly, **mianserin** pretreatment did not significantly alter the hypotensive action of a single dose of clonidine in healthy subjects.[2,4] In contrast, an isolated report describes hypertensive urgency in a man with end-stage renal disease on clonidine, metoprolol and losartan when **mirtazapine** (a **mianserin** analogue) was added for depression.[5]

(b) Trazodone

A 12-year-old boy on clonidine 100 micrograms three times daily and dexamfetamine 15 mg twice daily was started on trazodone 50 mg at bedtime. After a few weeks his trazodone dosage was increased to 100 mg at bedtime. Within 45 minutes of taking his first increased dose he had a hypotensive episode with bradycardia and sedation. The trazodone dose was reduced back to 50 mg, but the drug was discontinued 2 weeks later because of low blood pressure.[6]

(c) Tricyclic antidepressants

Desipramine 75 mg daily for 2 weeks caused the lying and standing blood pressures of 4 out of 5 hypertensive patients on clonidine 600 to 1800 micrograms daily (with chlortalidone or hydrochlorothiazide) to rise by 22/15 mmHg and 12/10 mmHg respectively.[7]

This interaction has been seen in other patients taking **clomipramine**, **desipramine** and **imipramine**.[8-11] In one study, the antihypertensive effects of a single intravenous dose of clonidine were reduced by about 50% in 6 patients given **desipramine** for 3 weeks.[12] Similarly the blood pressure lowering effect of a single 300-microgram dose of clonidine was reduced by 40 to 50% in 8 healthy subjects when it was given on day 9 of treatment with **imipramine** 25 mg three times daily.[13] An elderly woman on clonidine 200 micrograms daily developed severe frontal headache, dizziness, chest and neck pain and tachycardia of 120 bpm with hypertension (230/124–130 mmHg) on the second day of taking **imipramine** 50 mg for incontinence.[14]

Rebound hypertension and tachycardia seen on the withdrawal of clonidine, may have been made worse by the presence of **amitriptyline** in a 73-year-old woman.[15]

A man with severe pain, well controlled with **amitriptyline**, sodium valproate and intrathecal boluses of diamorphine, experienced severe pain within 5 minutes of an intrathecal test dose of clonidine 75 micrograms.[16]

Mechanism

Not understood. One idea is that the tricyclics desensitise or block central alpha$_2$-receptors.[17] This would explain the interaction with mirtazapine (a mianserin analogue), which also has alpha-blocking properties.[5] However, mianserin (also an alpha-blocker) did not interact.[2] Another idea is that tricyclics block noradrenaline uptake. However, maprotiline, which also blocks noradrenaline uptake, did not interact.[1] Trazodone, which also has alpha-blocking properties was predicted to inhibit the effect of clonidine based on a study in *animals* where it antagonised the hypotensive effect of clonidine when given centrally (note this effect was not seen when it was administered intravenously).[18] The case of hypotension described could be explained by the hypotensive effect of trazodone alone, but may have been compounded by the hypotensive effect of clonidine.

Importance and management

The interaction between clonidine and the tricyclics is established and clinically important. The incidence is uncertain but it is not seen in all patients.[7] Avoid concurrent use unless the effects can be monitored. Increasing the dosage of clonidine may possibly be effective. The clonidine dosage was apparently successfully titrated in 10 out of 11 hypertensive patients already on amitriptyline or imipramine.[19] Only clomipramine, desipramine and imipramine have been implicated so far, but other tricyclics would be expected to behave similarly (amitriptyline, **nortriptyline** and **protriptyline** have been shown to interact in *animals*[20]). The tetracyclic antidepressants maprotiline and mianserin do not generally appear to interact with clonidine. The isolated case of hypotension with trazodone is of unknown general importance.

1. Gundert-Remy U, Amann E, Hildebrandt R, Weber E. Lack of interaction between the tetracyclic antidepressant maprotiline and the centrally acting antihypertensive drug clonidine. *Eur J Clin Pharmacol* (1983) 25, 595–9.
2. Elliott HL, Whiting B, Reid JL. Assessment of the interaction between mianserin and centrally-acting antihypertensive drugs. *Br J Clin Pharmacol* (1983) 15, 323S–328S.
3. Elliott HL, McLean K, Sumner DJ, Reid JL. Absence of an effect of mianserin on the actions of clonidine or methyldopa in hypertensive patients. *Eur J Clin Pharmacol* (1983) 24, 15–19.
4. Elliott HL, McLean K, Sumner DJ, Reid JL. Pharmacodynamic studies on mianserin and its interaction with clonidine. *Eur J Clin Pharmacol* (1981) 21, 97–102.
5. Abo-Zena RA, Bobek MB, Dweik RA. Hypertensive urgency induced by an interaction of mirtazapine and clonidine. *Pharmacotherapy* (2000) 20, 476–8.
6. Bhatara VS, Kallepalli BR, Misra LK, Awadallah S. A possible clonidine-trazodone-dextroamphetamine interaction in a 12-year-old boy. *J Child Adolesc Psychopharmacol* (1996) 6, 203–9.
7. Briant RH, Reid JL, Dollery CT. Interaction between clonidine and desipramine in man. *BMJ* (1973) i, 522–3.
8. Coffler DE. Antipsychotic drug interaction. *Drug Intell Clin Pharm* (1976) 10, 114–15.
9. Andrejak M, Fournier A, Hardin J-M, Coevoet B, Lambrey G, De Fremont J-F, Quichaud J. Suppression de l'effet antihypertenseur de la clonidine par la prise simultaneé d'un antidépresseur tricyclique. *Nouv Presse Med* (1977) 6, 2603.
10. Lacomblez L, Warot D, Bouche P, Derouesné C. Suppression de l'effet antihypertenseur de la clonidine par la clomipramine. *Rev Med Interne* (1988) 9, 291–3.
11. Manchon ND, Bercoff E, Lemarchand P, Chassagne P, Senant J, Bourreille J. Fréquence et gravité des interactions médicamenteuses dan une population âgée: étude prospective concernant 63 malades. *Rev Med Interne* (1989) 10, 521–5.
12. Checkley SA, Slade AP, Shur E, Dawling S. A pilot study of the mechanism of action of desipramine. *Br J Psychiatry* (1981) 138, 248–51.
13. Cubeddu LX, Cloutier G, Gross K, Grippo PA-CR, Tanner L, Lerea L, Shakarjian M, Knowlton G, Harden TK, Arendshorst W, Rogers JF. Bupropion does not antagonize cardiovascular actions of clonidine in normal subjects and spontaneously hypertensive rats. *Clin Pharmacol Ther* (1984) 35, 576–84.
14. Hui KK. Hypertensive crisis induced by interaction of clonidine with imipramine. *J Am Geriatr Soc* (1983) 31, 164–5.
15. Stiff JL, Harris DB. Clonidine withdrawal complicated by amitriptyline therapy. *Anesthesiology* (1983) 59, 73–4.
16. Hardy PAJ, Wells JCD. Pain after spinal intrathecal clonidine. An adverse interaction with tricyclic antidepressants? *Anaesthesia* (1988) 43, 1026–7.
17. van Spanning HW, van Zwieten PA. The interference of tricyclic antidepressants with the central hypotensive effect of clonidine. *Eur J Pharmacol* (1973) 24, 402–4.
18. van Zwieten PA. Inhibition of the central hypotensive effect of clonidine by trazodone, a novel antidepressant. *Pharmacology* (1977) 15, 331–6.
19. Raftos J, Bauer GE, Lewis RG, Stokes GS, Mitchell AS, Young AA, Maclachlan I. Clonidine in the treatment of severe hypertension. *Med J Aust* (1973) 1, 786–93.
20. van Zwieten PA. Interaction between centrally active hypotensive drugs and tricyclic antidepressants. *Arch Int Pharmacodyn Ther* (1975) 214, 12–30.

Diazoxide + Hydralazine

Severe hypotension, in some cases fatal, has followed the administration of high doses of intravenous diazoxide before or after hydralazine.

Clinical evidence

A previously normotensive 25-year-old woman had a blood pressure of 250/150 mmHg during the 34th week of pregnancy, which failed to respond to intravenous magnesium sulfate 4 g. Her blood pressure fell transiently to 170/120 mmHg when she was given hydralazine 15 mg intravenously. One hour later intravenous diazoxide 5 mg/kg resulted in a blood pressure fall to 60/0 mmHg. Despite large doses of noradrenaline (norepinephrine), the hypotension persisted and the woman died.[1]

Other cases of severe hypotension in patients given high doses of intravenous diazoxide and intravenous or oral hydralazine are described in this[1] and other studies and reports.[2-4] In some instances the patients had also received other antihypertensive agents such as methyldopa[1] or reserpine.[1,4] At least three of the cases had a fatal outcome.[4]

Mechanism

Not fully understood. The hypotensive effects (vasodilatory) of the two drugs are additive, and it would seem that in some instances the normal compensatory responses of the cardiovascular system to maintain an adequate blood pressure reach their limit. This can occur with intravenous diazoxide alone.[2]

Importance and management

Concurrent use of intravenous diazoxide and hydralazine should be undertaken extremely cautiously with thorough monitoring. Note that the doses of diazoxide used in the above reports were frequently higher than those currently recommended for hypertensive crises.[5] In addition, there are now many more options available for the treatment of very severe hypertension, and the British National Formulary considers intravenous diazoxide to be one of the less suitable choices.[5] Moreover, diazoxide was frequently associated with clinically important hypotension when used in pregnancy, and is not considered a good choice in this situation.[6]

1. Henrich WL, Cronin R, Miller PD, Anderson RJ. Hypotensive sequelae of diazoxide and hydralazine therapy. *JAMA* (1977) 237, 264–5.
2. Kumar GK, Dastoor FC, Robayo JR, Razzaque MA. Side effects of diazoxide. *JAMA* (1976) 235, 275–6.
3. Tansey WA, Williams EG, Landesman RH and Schwarz MJ. Diazoxide. *JAMA* (1973) 225, 749.
4. Davey M, Moodley J, Soutter P. Adverse effects of a combination of diazoxide and hydrallazine therapy. *S Afr Med J* (1981) 59, 496–7.
5. British National Formulary. 49th ed. London: The British Medical Association and The Pharmaceutical Press; 2005. p. 93.
6. Duley L, Henderson-Smart DJ. Drugs for treatment of very high blood pressure during pregnancy. *Cochrane Database Syst Rev* (2002) 4, CD001449.

Diazoxide + Other drugs with hyperglycaemic activity

The risk of hyperglycaemia is increased if diazoxide is given with other drugs with hyperglycaemic activity (e.g. the thiazides, chlorpromazine, corticosteroids, combined oral contraceptives).

Clinical evidence, mechanism, importance and management

An isolated report[1] describes a child on long-term treatment for hypoglycaemia with diazoxide 8 mg/kg daily in divided doses and **bendroflumethiazide** 1.25 mg daily, who developed a diabetic precoma and severe hyperglycaemia after taking a single 30-mg dose of **chlorpromazine**. The reason is not understood but one idea is that all three drugs had additive hyperglycaemic effects. Enhanced hyperglycaemia has been seen in other patients given diazoxide and **trichlormethiazide**.[2] Caution is clearly needed to ensure that the hyperglycaemic effects do not become excessive. The makers of diazoxide also mention that the risk of hyperglycaemia may be increased by **corticosteroids** or oestrogen-progestogen combinations (e.g. **combined oral contraceptives**).[3]

1. Aynsley-Green A, Illig R. Enhancement by chlorpromazine of hyperglycaemic action of diazoxide. *Lancet* (1975) ii, 658–9.
2. Seltzer HS, Allen EW. Hyperglycemia and inhibition of insulin secretion during administration of diazoxide and trichlormethiazide in man. *Diabetes* (1969) 18, 19–28.
3. Eudemine Tablets (Diazoxide). Celltech Pharmaceuticals Ltd. UK Summary of product characteristics, August 2002.

Glyceryl trinitrate (Nitroglycerin) + Anticholinergics

Drugs with anticholinergic effects, such as the tricyclic antidepressants and disopyramide, depress salivation and many patients complain of having a dry mouth. In theory sublingual

glyceryl trinitrate tablets will dissolve less readily under the tongue in these patients, thereby reducing their absorption and effects. However, no formal studies seem to have been done to confirm that this actually happens. 'Table 16.1', (p.500), and 'Table 16.2', (p.502) list drugs that have anticholinergic effects. A possible alternative is to use a glyceryl trinitrate spray in patients who suffer from dry mouth.

Glyceryl trinitrate (Nitroglycerin) + Aspirin

Some limited evidence suggests that analgesic doses of aspirin can increase the serum levels of glyceryl trinitrate given sublingually, possibly resulting in an increase in its adverse effects such as hypotension and headache. Paradoxically, long-term aspirin use appears to reduce the effects of intravenous glyceryl trinitrate used for vasodilatation in patients following coronary artery bypass surgery.

Clinical evidence

(a) Glyceryl trinitrate (sublingual) effects increased

When aspirin 1 g was given to 7 healthy subjects followed one hour later by 800 micrograms of glyceryl trinitrate sublingual spray, the mean plasma glyceryl trinitrate levels 30 minutes after administration were increased by 54% (from 0.24 to 0.37 nanograms/ml). The haemodynamic effects of the glyceryl trinitrate (including heart rate and reduced diastolic blood pressure) were enhanced. Some changes were seen when aspirin 500 mg was given every 2 days (described as an anti-aggregant dose) but the effects were not statistically significant.[1]

(b) Glyceryl trinitrate (intravenous) effects reduced

A study in patients following coronary artery bypass surgery found that those who had been taking aspirin 150 or 300 mg daily (33 patients) for at least 3 months, needed more glyceryl trinitrate to control blood pressure during the recovery period than those who had not taken aspirin (33 patients). To achieve the blood pressure criteria required, the aspirin-group needed an 8.2 microgram/minute infusion of glyceryl trinitrate. The dose remained relatively high at 3.3 microgram/minute even after 8 hours, whereas the non-aspirin group only needed 5.5 micrograms/minute, which was reduced to 1.9 micrograms/minute after 8 hours.[2]

Mechanism

Not understood. Prostaglandin-synthetase inhibitors such as aspirin can suppress the vasodilator effects of glyceryl trinitrate, to some extent, by blocking prostaglandin release. However, it seems that a much greater pharmacodynamic interaction also occurs, in which aspirin reduces the flow of blood through the liver so that the metabolism of the glyceryl trinitrate is reduced, thus increasing its effects.

Importance and management

A confusing and unexplained situation. It seems possible that patients taking sublingual glyceryl trinitrate may experience an exaggeration of its adverse effects such as hypotension and headaches if they are taking analgesic doses of aspirin. Also be aware that long-term aspirin use may reduce the vasodilatory effects of intravenous glyceryl trinitrate. The antiplatelet effects of aspirin and glyceryl trinitrate appear to be additive.[3]

1. Weber S, Rey E, Pipeau C, Lutfalla G, Richard M-O, Daoud-El-Assaf H, Olive G, Degeorges M. Influence of aspirin on the hemodynamic effects of sublingual nitroglycerin. *J Cardiovasc Pharmacol* (1983) 5, 874–7.
2. Key BJ, Keen M, Wilkes MP. Reduced responsiveness to nitro-vasodilators following prolonged low dose aspirin administration in man. *Br J Clin Pharmacol* (1992) 34, 453P–454P.
3. Karlberg K-E, Ahlner J, Henriksson P, Torfgård K, Sylvén C. Effects of nitroglycerin on platelet aggregation beyond the effects of acetylsalicylic acid in healthy subjects. *Am J Cardiol* (1993) 71, 361–4.

Glyceryl trinitrate (Nitroglycerin) + Nifedipine

The effect of sublingual glyceryl trinitrate was not altered by pretreatment with nifedipine in two studies. Nifedipine and intravenous glyceryl trinitrate had additive vasodilator effects in one study, but the preliminary results of another study found that patients undergoing coronary artery bypass surgery on nifedipine 20 mg twice daily required more intravenous glyceryl trinitrate than those on nifedipine 10 mg twice daily or those not on nifedipine.

Clinical evidence, mechanism, importance and management

(a) Sublingual glyceryl trinitrate

In 9 patients with stable chronic angina, there was no significant haemodynamic interaction between sublingual glyceryl trinitrate and a single-dose of nifedipine, or nifedipine three times daily for 5 days.[1] In another study in healthy subjects, the venodilatory effect of sublingual glyceryl trinitrate was not altered by pretreatment with nifedipine 10 mg.[2] No special precautions are required during concurrent use.

(b) Intravenous glyceryl trinitrate

In 7 patients with severe congestive heart failure, a single-dose of oral nifedipine increased stroke volume, with a peak effect at 30 minutes. The addition of an intravenous dose of glyceryl trinitrate at 2 hours further increased stroke volume and increased cardiac index.[3] Therefore the addition of nitroglycerin enhanced the vasodilator action of nifedipine. Conversely, in the preliminary findings of a comparative study of 3 groups of patients undergoing coronary bypass graft surgery, those on nifedipine 20 mg twice daily needed about 40% higher initial doses of intravenous glyceryl trinitrate (to reduce cardiac workload, maintain graft patency and control blood pressure) than two other groups, one of them taking nifedipine 10 mg twice daily for hypertension, and the other a control group of normotensive patients. Moreover, these higher doses had little effect on the initial mean systolic blood pressure of half of the group taking nifedipine 20 mg twice daily, and they needed an additional infusion of nitroprusside.[4] It was suggested that since glyceryl trinitrate is converted to nitric oxide to elicit its vasodilator effect, it is possible that the nifedipine inhibits the enzymic production of the nitrous oxide. This appears to be the only study to suggest a negative interaction, and the clinical relevance of its findings are unclear. Note that this study was non-randomised, and there may have been other important differences between the patients in each group.

1. Boje KM, Fung H-L, Yoshitomi K, Parker JO. Haemodynamic effects of combined oral nifedipine and sublingual nitroglycerin in patients with chronic stable angina. *Eur J Clin Pharmacol* (1987) 33, 349–54.
2. Gascho JA, Apollo WP. Effects of nifedipine on the venodilatory response to nitroglycerin. *Am J Cardiol* (1990) 65, 99–102.
3. Kubo SH, Fox SC, Prida XE, Cody RJ. Combined hemodynamic effects of nifedipine and nitroglycerin in congestive heart failure. *Am Heart J* (1985) 110, 1032–4.
4. Key BJ, Wilkes MP, Keen M. Reduced responsiveness to glyceryl trinitrate following antihypertensive treatment with nifedipine in man. *Br J Clin Pharmacol* (1993) 36, 499P.

Guanethidine + Amfetamines and related drugs

The antihypertensive effects of guanethidine can be reduced or abolished by drugs including dexamfetamine, ephedrine, metamfetamine and methylphenidate. The blood pressure may even rise higher than before treatment with the antihypertensive.

Clinical evidence

When 16 hypertensive patients on guanethidine 25 to 35 mg daily were given single-doses of **dexamfetamine** 10 mg orally, **ephedrine** 90 mg orally, **metamfetamine** 30 mg intramuscularly or **methylphenidate** 20 mg orally, the hypotensive effects of the guanethidine were completely abolished, and in some instances the blood pressures rose higher than before treatment with the guanethidine.[1]

Another report describes the same interaction between guanethidine and **dexamfetamine**.[2]

Mechanism

These drugs are all indirectly acting sympathomimetic amines, which not only prevent guanethidine-like drugs from entering the adrenergic neurones of the sympathetic nervous system, but also displace the antihypertensive drug already there.[3] As a result the blood pressure lowering effects are lost. In addition these amines release noradrenaline from the neurones, which raises the blood pressure. Thus the antihypertensive effects are not only opposed, but the pressure may even be raised higher than before treatment.[3-8]

Importance and management

Well documented, well established and clinically important interactions. Other drugs, such as **phenylpropanolamine**, which is also an indirectly-acting sympathomimetic are likely to interact similarly. Patients taking guanethidine should avoid indirectly-acting sympathomimetics, see 'Table 33.1', (p.960) for a list. Warn them against the temptation to use proprietary non-prescription nasal decongestants containing any of these amines to relieve the nasal stuffiness commonly associated with the use of guanethidine and related drugs. The same precautions apply to the sympathomimetics used as appetite suppressants. However, one brief report stated that **diethylpropion** has been used with guanethidine without any adverse events.[9] Note that guanethidine increases the hypertensive effects of 'directly-acting sympathomimetics', (p.969).

1. Gulati OD, Dave BT, Gokhale SD, Shah KM. Antagonism of adrenergic neurone blockade in hypertensive subjects. *Clin Pharmacol Ther* (1966) 7, 510–4.
2. Ober KF, Wang RIH. Drug interactions with guanethidine. *Clin Pharmacol Ther* (1973) 14, 190–5.
3. Flegin OT, Morgan DH, Oates JA, Shand DG. The mechanism of the reversal of the effect of guanethidine by amphetamines in cat and man. *Br J Pharmacol* (1970) 39, 253P–254P.
4. Day MD, Rand MJ. Antagonism of guanethidine and bretylium by various agents. *Lancet* (1962) 2, 1282–3.
5. Day MD, Rand MJ. Evidence for a competitive antagonism of guanethidine by dexamphetamine. *Br J Pharmacol* (1963) 20, 17–28.
6. Day MD. Effect of sympathomimetic amines on the blocking action of guanethidine, bretylium and xylocholine. *Br J Pharmacol* (1962) 18, 421–39.
7. Starke K. Interactions of guanethidine and indirectly-acting sympathomimetic amines. *Arch Int Pharmacodyn Ther* (1972) 195, 309–14.
8. Boura ALA, Green AF. Comparison of bretylium and guanethidine: tolerance and effects on adrenergic nerve function and responses to sympathomimetic amines. *Br J Pharmacol* (1962) 19, 13–41.
9. Seedat YK, Reddy J. Diethylpropion hydrochloride (Tenuate Dospan) in the treatment of obese hypertensive patients. *S Afr Med J* (1974) 48, 569.

Guanethidine + Antipsychotics

Large doses of chlorpromazine may reduce or even abolish the antihypertensive effects of guanethidine, although in some patients the inherent hypotensive effects of the chlorpromazine may possibly predominate. Molindone is reported not to interact with guanethidine, and a single-dose of prochlorperazine did not interact.

Clinical evidence

Two severely hypertensive patients, stable on guanethidine 80 mg daily, were given **chlorpromazine** 200 to 300 mg daily. The diastolic blood pressure of one rose over 10 days from 94 to 112 mmHg and continued to rise to 116 mmHg even when the **chlorpromazine** was withdrawn. The diastolic pressure of the other rose from 105 to 127 mmHg, and then to 150 mmHg even after the **chlorpromazine** had been withdrawn.[1]

Other reports similarly describe marked rises in blood pressure in patients on guanethidine given **chlorpromazine** 100 to 400 mg daily.[2-4]

However, a single dose of **prochlorperazine** 25 mg did not significantly antagonise the effect of guanethidine 15 to 20 mg daily in 5 patients.[5] In another study in 7 patients on guanethidine 50 to 95 mg daily, the addition of **molindone** 30 to 120 mg daily had no effect on blood pressure.[6]

Mechanism

Chlorpromazine prevents the entry of guanethidine into the adrenergic neurones of the sympathetic nervous system resulting in a loss of its blood pressure lowering effects. This is essentially the same mechanism of interaction as that seen with the 'tricyclic antidepressants', (p.671).

Importance and management

Direct information is limited but the interaction is established and can be clinically important. It may take several days to develop. Not all patients may react to the same extent.[2,7] Monitor concurrent use and raise the guanethidine dosage if necessary. It is uncertain how much chlorpromazine is needed before a significant effect occurs, but the smallest dose of chlorpromazine used in the studies was 100 mg with 90 mg guanethidine, which raised the blood pressure by 40/23 mmHg.[2] The inherent hypotensive effects of the chlorpromazine may possibly reduce the effects of this interaction. Other phenothiazines might be expected to interact similarly. The effects should be monitored. However, molindone is reported not to interact, and a single-dose of prochlorperazine did not interact.

See also 'Guanethidine + Antipsychotics; Haloperidol or Tiotixene', below.

1. Fann WE, Janowsky DS, Davis JM, Oates JA. Chlorpromazine reversal of the antihypertensive action of guanethidine. *Lancet* (1971) ii, 436–7.
2. Janowsky DS, El-Yousef MK, Davis JM, Fann WE, Oates JA. Guanethidine antagonism by antipsychotic drugs. *J Tenn Med Assoc* (1972) 65, 620–2.
3. Janowsky DS, El-Yousef MK, Davis JM, Fann WE. Antagonism of guanethidine by chlorpromazine. *Am J Psychiatry* (1973) 130, 808–12.
4. Davis JM. Psychopharmacology in the aged. Use of psychotropic drugs in geriatric patients. *J Geriatr Psychiatry* (1974) 7, 145–59.
5. Ober KF, Wang RIH. Drug interactions with guanethidine. *Clin Pharmacol Ther* (1973) 14, 190–5.
6. Simpson LL. Combined use of molindone and guanethidine in patients with schizophrenia and hypertension. *Am J Psychiatry* (1979) 136, 1410–14.
7. Tuck D, Hamberger B and Sjoqvist F. Drug interactions: effect of chlorpromazine on the uptake of monoamines into adrenergic neurones in man. *Lancet* (1972) ii, 492.

Guanethidine + Antipsychotics; Haloperidol or Tiotixene

The antihypertensive effects of guanethidine can be reduced by haloperidol or thiothixene.

Clinical evidence

Three hypertensive patients taking guanethidine 60 to 150 mg daily had rises in their blood pressure when haloperidol 6 to 9 mg daily was added. Blood pressure rose from 132/95 to 149/99 mmHg in the first patient; from 125/84 to 148/100 mmHg in the second patient; and from 138/91 to 154/100 mmHg in the third patient. Tiotixene 60 mg daily was later given to one of the patients and the blood pressure rose from 126/87 to 156/110 mmHg.[1] These results have been reported elsewhere.[2,3]

Mechanism

Haloperidol and thiothixene prevent the entry of guanethidine into the adrenergic neurones of the sympathetic nervous system, so that its blood pressure lowering effects are reduced or lost. This is essentially the same mechanism of interaction as that seen with the 'tricyclic antidepressants', (p.671), and 'chlorpromazine', (above).

Importance and management

Information seems to be limited to this report, but it is supported by the well-documented pharmacology of these drugs. It appears to be clinically important. If haloperidol or thiothixene are given to patients on guanethidine, monitor their blood pressures and raise the guanethidine dosage as necessary.[3] There is no direct evidence of an interaction between guanethidine and other butyrophenones or thioxanthenes but it would be prudent to adopt the same precautions.

1. Janowsky DS, El-Yousef MK, Davis JM, Fann WE, Oates JA. Guanethidine antagonism by antipsychotic drugs. *J Tenn Med Assoc* (1972) 65, 620–2.
2. Davis JM. Psychopharmacology in the aged. Use of psychotropic drugs in geriatric patients. *J Geriatr Psychiatry* (1974) 7, 145–59.
3. Janowsky DS, El-Yousef MK, Davis JM, Fann WE. Antagonism of guanethidine by chlorpromazine. *Am J Psychiatry* (1973) 130, 808–12.

Guanethidine + Levodopa

When two patients on guanethidine were given levodopa it was possible to reduce the guanethidine dosage in one and stop adjunctive diuretic therapy in the other.

Clinical evidence, mechanism, importance and management

A brief report describes a patient on guanethidine and a diuretic who, when given levodopa [dose not stated], required a reduction in his daily dose of guanethidine, from 60 to 20 mg. Another patient similarly treated was able to discontinue the diuretic.[1] The suggested reason is that the hypotensive adverse effects of the levodopa are additive with the effects of the guanethidine. Direct information seems to be limited to this report but it would be wise to confirm that excessive hypotension does not develop if levodopa is added to treatment with guanethidine.

1. Hunter KR, Stern GM, Laurence DR. Use of levodopa with other drugs. *Lancet* (1970) ii, 1283–5.

Guanethidine + MAOIs

The antihypertensive effects of guanethidine can be reduced by nialamide, and probably therefore other similar MAOIs.

Clinical evidence, mechanism, importance and management

Four out of 5 hypertensive patients on guanethidine 25 to 35 mg daily had a rise in blood pressure from 140/85 to 165/100 mmHg six hours after being given a single 50-mg dose of **nialamide**.[1] The reason is not understood but one idea is that MAOIs possibly oppose the guanethidine-induced loss of noradrenaline from sympathetic neurones. In *animal* studies, effective antagonism of guanethidine was shown by those MAOIs that also possess sympathomimetic effects (**phenelzine** and **tranylcypromine**), but not by **iproniazid** or **nialamide**,[2] and the antagonism was weaker than that seen with some other sympathomimetics.[3]

Direct clinical information seems to be limited to the single dose study,[1] but it would be prudent to monitor the effects if any MAOI is given to patients taking any guanethidine-like drug. The makers of guanethidine actually contraindicate the use of MAOIs because of the possibility of the release of large quantities of catecholamines and the risk of hypertensive crisis. They recommend that at least 14 days should elapse between stopping an MAOI and starting guanethidine.[4]

1. Gulati OD, Dave BT, Gokhale SD, Shah KM. Antagonism of adrenergic neuron blockade in hypertensive subjects. *Clin Pharmacol Ther* (1966) 7, 510–4.
2. Day MD. Effect of sympathomimetic amines on the blocking action of guanethidine, bretylium and xylocholine. *Br J Pharmacol* (1962) 18, 421–39.
3. Day MD, Rand MJ. Antagonism of guanethidine and bretylium by various agents. *Lancet* (1962) 2, 1282–3.
4. Ismelin ampoules (Guanethidine monosulfate). Sovereign Medical. UK Summary of product characteristics, November 2001.

Guanethidine + NSAIDs

Phenylbutazone and kebuzone reduce the antihypertensive effects of guanethidine.

Clinical evidence, mechanism, importance and management

A mean systolic blood pressure rise of 20 mmHg (from 169 to 189 mmHg) was seen when 20 patients on guanethidine 75 mg daily were given **phenylbutazone** or **kebuzone** 750 mg daily.[1] This rise represents about a 35% reduction in the antihypertensive effect of guanethidine. The mechanism of this interaction is uncertain but it is probably due to salt and water retention caused by these pyrazolone compounds. Direct evidence seems to be limited to this report, but it is in line with what is known about these NSAIDs. Patients taking guanethidine should be monitored if **phenylbutazone**, **kebuzone** or **oxyphenbutazone** are given concurrently. There does not appear to be any information on guanethidine and other NSAIDs, but **indometacin** in particular is well known to reduce the efficacy of other classes of antihypertensives, see for example 'ACE inhibitors + NSAIDs', p.27.

1. Polak F. Die hemmende Wirkung von Phenylbutazon auf die durch einige Antihypertonika hervorgerufene Blutdrucksenkung bei Hypertonikern. *Z Gesamte Inn Med* (1967) 22, 375–6.

Guanethidine + Tricyclic or Tetracyclic antidepressants

The antihypertensive effects of guanethidine are reduced or abolished by amitriptyline, desipramine, imipramine, nortriptyline and protriptyline. Doxepin in doses of 300 mg or more daily interacts similarly, but in smaller doses appears not to do so, although one case is reported with doxepin 100 mg daily. A few case reports suggest that maprotiline and mianserin do not interact.

Clinical evidence

(a) Tricyclic antidepressants

Five hypertensive patients, controlled on guanethidine sulfate 50 to 150 mg daily, showed a mean arterial blood pressure rise of 27 mmHg when given **desipramine** 50 or 75 mg or **protriptyline** 20 mg daily for 1 to 9 days. The full antihypertensive effects of the guanethidine were not re-established until 5 days after the antidepressants were withdrawn.[1]

The same interaction has been described in other reports between guanethidine and **desipramine**,[2,3] **imipramine**,[4] **amitriptyline**,[5-7] **protriptyline**[3] and **nortriptyline**.[8] The interaction may take several days to develop fully and can last an average of 5 days after discontinuation of the tricyclic.[2] Some studies, and clinical experience have shown that **doxepin** does not begin to interact until doses of about 200 to 250 mg daily are used, then at 300 mg or more daily it interacts to the same extent as other tricyclics.[9-13] However, in one case excessive hypertension occurred in a man on guanethidine given 100 mg of **doxepin** daily.[14]

(b) Tetracyclic antidepressants

Maprotiline 25 mg three times daily caused no appreciable change in blood pressure in two patients on guanethidine.[7] Similarly, in a study in two patients, **mianserin** 20 mg three times daily for 2 days did not alter the antihypertensive efficacy of guanethidine.[15]

Mechanism

The guanethidine-like drugs exert their hypotensive actions firstly by entering the adrenergic nerve endings associated with blood vessels using the noradrenaline uptake mechanism. The tricyclics successfully compete for the same mechanism so that the antihypertensives fail to reach their site of action, and as a result, the blood pressure rises once again.[16] The differences in the rate of development, duration and extent of the interactions reflect the pharmacokinetic differences between the various tricyclics, as well as individual differences between patients.

Importance and management

A very well documented and well established interaction of clinical importance. Not every combination of guanethidine and tricyclic antidepressant has been studied but all are expected to interact similarly. Concurrent use should be avoided unless the effects are very closely monitored and the interaction balanced by raising the dosage of the antihypertensive. Note that the use of guanethidine and related adrenergic neurone blockers has largely been superseded by other antihypertensive drug classes.

1. Mitchell JR, Arias L, Oates JA. Antagonism of the antihypertensive actions of guanethidine sulfate by desipramine hydrochloride. *JAMA* (1967) 202, 973–6.
2. Oates JA, Mitchell JR, Feagin OT, Kaufmann JS, Shand DG. Distribution of guanidinium antihypertensives-mechanism of their selective action. *Ann N Y Acad Sci* (1971) 179, 302–9.
3. Mitchell JR, Cavanaugh JH, Arias L, Oates JA. Guanethidine and related agents. III. Antagonism by drugs which inhibit the norepinephrine pump in man. *J Clin Invest* (1970) 49, 1596–1604.
4. Leishman AWD, Matthews HL, Smith AJ. Antagonism of guanethidine by imipramine. *Lancet* (1963) i, 112.
5. Meyer JF, McAllister CK, Goldberg LI. Insidious and prolonged antagonism of guanethidine by amitriptyline. *JAMA* (1970) 213, 1487–8.
6. Ober KF, Wang RIH. Drug interactions with guanethidine. *Clin Pharmacol Ther* (1973) 14, 190–5.
7. Smith AJ, Bant WP. Interactions between post-ganglionic sympathetic blocking drugs and anti-depressants. *J Int Med Res* (1975) 3 (Suppl 2), 55–60.
8. McQueen EG. New Zealand Committee on Adverse Reactions: Ninth Annual Report 1974. *N Z Med J* (1974) 80, 305–11.
9. Oates JA, Fann WE, Cavanaugh JH. Effect of doxepin on the norepinephrine pump. A preliminary report. *Psychosomatics* (1969) 10 (Suppl), 12–13.
10. Fann WE, Cavanaugh JH, Kaufmann JS, Griffith JD, Davis JM, Janowsky DS, Oates JA. Doxepin: effects on transport of biogenic amines in man. *Psychopharmacologia* (1971) 22, 111–25.
11. Gerson IM, Friedman R, Unterberger H. Non-antagonism of anti-adrenergic agents by dibenzoxepine (preliminary report). *Dis Nerv Syst* (1970) 31, 780–2.
12. Ayd FJ. Long-term administration of doxepin (Sinequan). *Dis Nerv Syst* (1971) 32, 617–22.
13. Ayd FJ. Doxepin with other drugs. *South Med J* (1973) 66, 465–71.
14. Poe TE, Edwards JL, Taylor RB. Hypertensive crisis possibly due to drug interaction. *Postgrad Med* (1979) 66, 235–7.
15. Burgess CD, Turner P, Wadsworth J. Cardiovascular responses to mianserin hydrochloride: a comparison with tricyclic antidepressant drugs. *Br J Clin Pharmacol* (1978) 5, 21S–28S.
16. Cairncross KD. On the peripheral pharmacology of amitriptyline. *Arch Int Pharmacodyn Ther* (1965) 154, 438–48.

Guanfacine + Phenobarbital or Phenytoin

In two patients, concurrent use of phenobarbital or phenytoin increased the metabolism of guanfacine.

Clinical evidence, mechanism, importance and management

When phenobarbital 10 mg daily was given to a hypertensive patient with chronic renal failure on guanfacine 4 mg daily, reduced effectiveness of the antihypertensive was noted and the dose was progressively raised over about 18 months to 12 mg daily. Phenobarbital was eventually stopped. Single measurements of the kinetics of guanfacine while the patient was on phenobarbital and 2 months after cessation of phenobarbital showed that the half-life of guanfacine increased fourfold on stopping the phenobarbital.[1] The maker also reports a similar case with phenytoin and guanfacine.[2] Phenobarbital and phenytoin probably induce the metabolism of guanfacine. Patients on these drugs are likely to need more frequent doses of guanfacine.

1. Kiechel JR, Lavene D, Guerret M, Comoy E, Godin M, Fillastre JP. Pharmacokinetic aspects of guanfacine withdrawal syndrome in a hypertensive patient with chronic renal failure. *Eur J Clin Pharmacol* (1983) 25, 463–6.
2. Tenex (Guanfacine hydrochloride). ESP Pharma Inc. US Prescribing information [undated – accessed 27/07/05].

Guanfacine + Tricyclic antidepressants

A single report describes a reduced antihypertensive response to guanfacine in a patient given amitriptyline and later imipramine. The sedative effects of guanfacine and tricyclics are predicted to be additive.

Clinical evidence

A 38-year-old woman with hypertension, stable on guanfacine 2 mg daily, had a rise in her blood pressure from 138/89 mmHg to 150/100 mmHg after taking amitriptyline 75 mg daily for 7 to 14 days. The pressure fell again when the amitriptyline was stopped. A month later her blood pressure rose to 142/98 mmHg after she took imipramine 50 mg daily for two days, and fell again when it was stopped.[1]

Mechanism

Uncertain. A possible reason is that, like clonidine (another alpha-2 agonist), the uptake of guanfacine into neurones within the brain is blocked by tricyclic antidepressants, thereby reducing its effects.

Importance and management

Direct information is limited to this report, but it is supported by *animal* studies[2] and consistent with the way another alpha-2 agonist interacts with tricyclic antidepressants (see 'Clonidine + Tricyclic and related antidepressants', p.667). Be alert for this interaction in any patient given guanfacine and any tricyclic antidepressant. **Guanabenz** is another alpha-2 agonist that might interact similarly, but as yet there is no direct clinical evidence that it does so. Note that the sedative effects of guanfacine or **guanabenz** and tricyclics would be predicted to be additive.

1. Buckley M, Feeley J. Antagonism of antihypertensive effect of guanfacine by tricyclic antidepressants. *Lancet* (1991) 337, 1173–4.
2. Ohkubo K, Suzuki K, Oguma T, Otorii T. Central hypotensive effects of guanfacine in anaesthetised rabbits. *Nippon Yakurigaku Zasshi* (1982) 79, 263–74.

Hydralazine + Adrenaline (Epinephrine)

The makers note that patients on hydralazine who develop hypotension while undergoing surgery should *not* be treated with adrenaline (epinephrine).[1] This is because hydralazine frequently causes tachycardia[2] and adrenaline would enhance this.[1]

1. Apresoline (Hydralazine hydrochloride). Sovereign Medical. UK Summary of product characteristics, April 2003.
2. Lin M-S, McNay JL, Shepherd AMM, Musgrave GE, Keeton TK. Increased plasma norepinephrine accompanies persistent tachycardia after hydralazine. *Hypertension* (1983) 5, 257–63.

Hydralazine + Food

The effect of food on hydralazine absorption is uncertain: food increased the AUC of hydralazine in two studies, had no effect in one study, and decreased it in three others. A bolus dose of enteral feed decreased the AUC of hydralazine, but an enteral feed infusion had no effect.

Clinical evidence, mechanism, importance and management

Food *enhanced* the bioavailability of single 50-mg doses of hydralazine in healthy subjects by two to threefold in one study.[1] Similar findings were reported by the same research group with conventional hydralazine tablets, but not slow-release tablets.[2] In contrast, others found that food had no effect on the AUC of hydralazine in healthy subjects.[3] Furthermore, other studies have found that food decreases the AUC of hydralazine by 46% when it is given as oral solution,[4] by 44% after conventional tablets,[5] and by 29% (not significant) after a slow-release preparation.[5] A reduction in antihypertensive effect was noted in the first of these studies,[4] but no significant alteration in antihypertensive effect was seen in the second.[5] Similarly, another study reported a 55% decrease in the AUC of hydralazine when it was given with a meal, and 62% with a bolus dose of **enteral feed**, but no significant change when it was given during an **enteral feed infusion**.[6]

The widely different findings of these studies may be related to the problems in analysing hydralazine and its metabolites, all of which are unstable. All these studies were single-dose, and no studies have adequately assessed the possible clinical importance of any pharmacokinetic changes in long-term clinical use. Note that the bioavailability of hydralazine varies widely between individuals dependent on their acetylator status. No recommendations can be made as to whether or not hydralazine should be taken at a set time in relation to meals.

1. Melander A, Danielson K, Hanson A, Rudell B, Schersten B, Thulin T, Wåhlin E. Enhancement of hydralazine bioavailability by food. *Clin Pharmacol Ther* (1977) 22, 104–7.
2. Liedholm H, Wåhlin-Boll E, Hanson A, Melander A. Influence of food on the bioavailability of 'real' and 'apparent' hydralazine from conventional and slow-release preparations. *Drug Nutr Interact* (1982) 1, 293–302.
3. Walden RJ, Hernadez R, Witts D, Graham BR, Prichard BN. Effect of food on the absorption of hydralazine in man. *Eur J Clin Pharmacol* (1981) 20, 53–8.
4. Shepherd AM, Irvine NA, Ludden TM. Effect of food on blood hydralazine levels and response in hypertension. *Clin Pharmacol Ther* (1984) 36, 14–18.
5. Jackson SHD, Shepherd AMM, Ludden TM, Jamieson MJ, Woodworth J, Rogers D, Ludden LK, Muir KT. Effect of food on oral bioavailability of apresoline and controlled release hydralazine in hypertensive patients. *J Cardiovasc Pharmacol* (1990) 16, 624–8.
6. Semple HA, Koo W, Tam YK, Ngo LY, Coutts RT. Interactions between hydralazine and oral nutrients in humans. *Ther Drug Monit* (1991) 13, 304–8.

Hydralazine + NSAIDs

Indometacin abolished the hypotensive effects of intravenous hydralazine in one study, but did not affect it in another. Intravenous diclofenac reduced the effects of intravenous dihydralazine.

Clinical evidence, mechanism, importance and management

In healthy subjects, **indometacin** 50 mg every 6 hours for 4 doses abolished the hypotensive response to intravenous hydralazine 150 micrograms/kg, and the subjects only responded when given another dose of hydralazine 30 minutes later.[1] In contrast, another study in healthy subjects[2] found that **indometacin** 25 mg four times daily for 2.5 days did not affect the hypotensive response to a single 200-microgram/kg intravenous dose of hydralazine. Thus it is not clear if **indometacin** interacts with hydralazine given intravenously, and equally uncertain if an interaction occurs when hydralazine is given orally. On the other hand, a single-dose study in 4 hypertensive subjects found that the actions of intravenous **dihydralazine** (effects on blood pressure, urinary excretion, heart rate and sodium clearance) were reduced by intravenous **diclofenac**.[3] NSAIDs can cause increases in blood pressure due to their effects on sodium and water retention. Various NSAIDs have been reported to reduce the efficacy of other antihypertensive drug classes, for example see 'ACE inhibitors + NSAIDs', p.27. It would be prudent to monitor concurrent use of hydralazine and NSAIDs.

1. Cinquegrani MP, Liang C-S. Indomethacin attenuates the hypotensive action of hydralazine. *Clin Pharmacol Ther* (1986) 39, 564–70.
2. Jackson SHD, Pickles H. Indomethacin does not attenuate the effects of hydralazine in normal subjects. *Eur J Clin Pharmacol* (1983) 25, 303–5.
3. Reimann IW, Ratge D, Wisser H, Fröhlich JC. Are prostaglandins involved in the antihypertensive effect of dihydralazine? *Clin Sci* (1981) 61, 319S–321S.

Ketanserin + Beta-blockers

There is no pharmacokinetic interaction between ketanserin and propranolol, but additive hypotensive effects may occur. Very marked acute hypotension has been seen in two patients on atenolol when they were first given ketanserin.

Clinical evidence, mechanism, importance and management

A study in 6 patients and 2 healthy subjects given ketanserin 40 mg twice daily for 3 weeks found that **propranolol** 80 mg twice daily for 6 days did not significantly alter the steady-state plasma levels of ketanserin.[1] Another study in healthy subjects, using single doses of both drugs, found that neither drug affected the pharmacokinetics of the other.[2] In a third study, **propranolol** 80 mg twice daily had no effect on the pharmacokinetics of a single 10-mg intravenous dose of ketanserin. However, ketanserin 40 mg twice daily modestly decreased the clearance of a single 160-mg dose of **propranolol** by 29% and increased the maximum serum level by 38%, although neither of these changes were statistically significant and are also unlikely to be clinically relevant.[3] The hypotensive effects of ketanserin were slightly increased by **propranolol** in the first study,[1] and additive hypotensive effects were seen in another study in patients with essential hypertension.[4]

Acute hypotension is reported to have occurred in two patients taking **atenolol** within an hour of taking a 40-mg oral dose of ketanserin. One of them briefly lost consciousness.[5]

Concurrent use of ketanserin and beta-blockers can be valuable and uneventful, but a few patients may experience marked hypotensive effects when first given ketanserin. Patients should be warned.

1. Trenk D, Lühr A, Radkow N, Jähnchen E. Lack of effect of propranolol on the steady-state plasma levels of ketanserin. *Arzneimittelforschung* (1985) 35, 1286–8.
2. Williams FM, Leeser JE, Rawlins MD. Pharmacodynamics and pharmacokinetics of single doses of ketanserin and propranolol alone and in combination in healthy volunteers. *Br J Clin Pharmacol* (1986) 22, 301–8.
3. Ochs HR, Greenblatt DJ, Höller M, Labedzky L. The interactions of propranolol and ketanserin. *Clin Pharmacol Ther* (1987) 41, 55–60.
4. Hedner T, Persson B. Antihypertensive properties of ketanserin in combination with β-adrenergic blocking agents. *J Cardiovasc Pharmacol* (1985) 7 (Suppl 7), S161–S163.
5. Waller PC, Cameron HA, Ramsey LE. Profound hypotension after the first dose of ketanserin. *Postgrad Med J* (1987) 63, 305–7.

Ketanserin + Diuretics

Sudden deaths, probably from cardiac arrhythmias, were markedly increased in patients taking potassium-depleting diuretics and high doses of ketanserin. No interaction occurred with low doses of ketanserin in those with normal potassium levels. Potassium-sparing diuretics do not interact in this way.

Clinical evidence

A large multi-national study[1] involving 3899 patients found that a harmful and potentially fatal interaction could occur in those given ketanserin 40 mg three times daily and **potassium-depleting diuretics**. Of 249 patients taking both drugs, 35 died (16 suddenly) compared with only 15 (5 suddenly) of 260 patients taking a placebo and **potassium-depleting diuretics**. No significant increase in the number of deaths occurred in those on ketanserin and **potassium-sparing diuretics**.

It was found that the corrected QT interval was prolonged as follows: ketanserin alone 18 milliseconds, ketanserin with **potassium-sparing diuretics** 24 milliseconds, ketanserin with **potassium-depleting diuretics** 30 milliseconds. Preliminary results of a later study in 33 patients using a smaller dose of ketanserin (20 mg twice daily) with **potassium-depleting diuretics** (**furosemide**, **thiazides**) found no evidence of a prolonged the QT_c interval in patients with normal potassium levels.[2] The pharmacokinetics of a single 20-mg dose of ketanserin were not altered by single 25-mg doses of **hydrochlorothiazide**.[3]

Mechanism

Potassium-depleting diuretics may cause hypokalaemia, which increases the risk of QT-prolongation and torsade de pointes arrhythmia, which can result in sudden death. Ketanserin also prolongs the QT interval in a dose-related way, and its effects would be expected to be additive with that of diuretic-induced hypokalaemia. See also 'Drugs that prolong the QT interval + Other drugs that prolong the QT interval', p.170.

Importance and management

The use of potassium-depleting diuretics (see 'Table 24.1', (p.717)) with ketanserin 40 mg three times daily should be avoided. Lower doses of ketanserin (20 mg twice daily) have less effect on the QT interval, and can probably be used cautiously with potassium-depleting diuretics as long as serum potassium levels are maintained. Potassium-sparing diuretics do not interact.

1. Prevention of Atherosclerotic Complications with Ketanserin Trial Group. Prevention of atherosclerotic complications: controlled trial of ketanserin. *BMJ* (1989) 298, 424–30.
2. Van Gool R, Symoens J. Ketanserin in combination with diuretics: effect on QTc-interval. *Eur Heart J* (1990) 11 (Suppl), 57.
3. Botha JH, McFadyen ML, Leary WPP, Janssens M. No effect of single-dose hydrochlorothiazide on the pharmacokinetics of single-dose ketanserin. *Curr Ther Res* (1991) 49, 225–30.

Ketanserin + Miscellaneous

Ketanserin should not be given with certain antiarrhythmics, naftidrofuryl or tricyclic antidepressants because of the risk of potentially fatal cardiac arrhythmias. Similarly, caution is also required with potassium-depleting drugs. Drowsiness and dizziness are common adverse effects, which may possibly be additive with the effects of other CNS depressants.

Clinical evidence, mechanism, importance and management

Ketanserin has weak class III antiarrhythmic activity and can prolong the QT_c interval. For safety reasons it has therefore been advised that it should be avoided in patients with existing QT_c prolongation, atrioventricular or sinoauricular block of higher degree, or severe bradycardia of less than 50 bpm.[1] For the same reason the concurrent use of drugs that affect repolarisation (**class Ia**, **Ic** and **III arrhythmics**) or those that cause conduction disturbances (**naftidrofuryl**, **tricyclic antidepressants**) should be avoided.[1] See also 'Drugs that prolong the QT interval + Other drugs that prolong the QT interval', p.170. Because hypokalaemia can also prolong the QT interval, it is important that potassium levels are maintained when ketanserin is used with **potassium-depleting drugs** such as the thiazide or loop '**diuretics**', (p.673).

Dizziness and drowsiness are common adverse effects of ketanserin and therefore it seems likely that these will be additive with other **CNS depressants** and **alcohol**, which may possibly make driving more hazardous, but this needs confirmation.

1. Distler A. Clinical aspects during therapy with the serotonin antagonist ketanserin. *Clin Physiol Biochem* (1990) 8 (Suppl 3), 64–80.

Ketanserin + Nifedipine

Two patients experienced an increase in cardiac arrhythmias when given ketanserin and nifedipine.

Clinical evidence, mechanism, importance and management

A study in 20 subjects aged 60 years or more, with normal or slightly raised blood pressures, found that the concurrent use of ketanserin and nifedipine for a week did not, on average, affect their blood pressures, heart rates, or the QT intervals, but 2 of the subjects monitored over 24 hours showed a marked increase in the frequency of ectopic beats, couplets and ventricular tachycardia.[1] The reasons are not understood. The authors of this study say that their findings do not exclude the possibility that the combined use of these two drugs might therefore increase arrhythmia in some elderly patients.[1] Concurrent use should be monitored.

1. Alberio L, Beretta-Piccoli C, Tanzi F, Koch P, Zehender M. Kardiale Interaktionen zwischen Ketanserin und dem Calcium-Antagonisten Nifedipin. *Schweiz Med Wochenschr* (1992) 122, 1723–7.

Levosimendan + Miscellaneous

Orthostatic hypotension occurred when levosimendan was given with isosorbide mononitrate. The haemodynamic effects of levosimendan were not significantly altered by captopril, carvedilol or felodipine. Levosimendan does not alter the effects of warfarin on blood coagulation. Itraconazole does not alter the pharmacokinetics of levosimendan. Levosimendan appears not to interact adversely with alcohol.

Clinical evidence, mechanism, importance and management

(a) Alcohol

A double-blind, randomised, crossover study in 12 healthy subjects given oral alcohol 0.8 g/kg with intravenous levosimendan 1 mg found no clinically significant pharmacokinetic or pharmacodynamic interactions.[1]

(b) Captopril

Captopril in doses of up to 50 mg twice daily did not change the haemodynamic effects of a single 1- or 2-mg intravenous dose of levosimendan in 24 patients with heart failure. No additional decrease in blood pressure was observed.[2] No special precautions appear to be required if levosimendan is given to patients on captopril.

(c) Carvedilol

Carvedilol 25 mg twice daily for 7 to 9 days did not alter the effects of a single 2-mg intravenous dose of levosimendan on cardiac contractility in 12 healthy subjects. In addition, the heart rate and diastolic blood pressure responses were not altered, but the systolic blood pressure response was blunted.[3] Levosimendan may be used in patients on carvedilol.

(d) Felodipine

A study of the use of oral levosimendan 500 micrograms four times daily and felodipine 5 mg once daily in 24 men with coronary heart disease found that concurrent use was well tolerated. The felodipine did not antagonise the positive inotropic effects of the levosimendan and had no effect on exercise capacity. Both drugs increased the heart rate during exercise, and there was a slight additional effect with the combination (5 to 8 bpm for levosimendan alone versus 6 to 10 bpm for the combination).[4] There would appear to be no reason for avoiding concurrent use.

(e) Itraconazole

A study in 12 healthy subjects found that the pharmacokinetics of a single 2-mg oral dose of levosimendan were unchanged by itraconazole 200 mg daily for 5 days, and heart rates PQ, QTc and QRS intervals were unaltered. It was concluded that because itraconazole, a potent inhibitor of the cytochrome P450 isoenzyme CYP3A4, does not interact significantly with levosimendan, interactions with other CYP3A4 inhibitors are unlikely.[5]

(f) Isosorbide mononitrate

The combined use of an infusion of levosimendan (12 micrograms/kg over 10 minutes, then 0.2 micrograms/kg/minute for 110 minutes) and a single 20-mg oral dose of isosorbide mononitrate had no additional effects on haemodynamic parameters (heart rate, blood pressure, leg blood flow, cardiac output) in 12 healthy subjects at rest. However, during an orthostatic test, the circulatory response of the combination was significantly potentiated, and three subjects were unable to remain standing for the stipulated time.[6] Care is therefore required when levosimendan and isosorbide mononitrate or similar drugs are used concurrently.

(g) Warfarin

In an open, randomised, crossover study, 10 healthy subjects were given a single 25-mg oral dose of warfarin both before and on day 4 of a 9-day course of oral levosimendan 500 micrograms four times daily. No clinically relevant changes in the anticoagulant effects of the warfarin were seen, and levosimendan alone had no effect on blood coagulation. In addition, there was no important pharmacokinetic interaction between warfarin and levosimendan. No interactions would therefore be expected if both drugs are used concurrently.[7]

1. Antila S, Järvinen A, Akkila J, Honkanen T, Karlsson M, Lehtonen L. Studies on psychomotoric effects and pharmacokinetic interactions of the new calcium sensitizing drug levosimendan and ethanol. *Arzneimittelforschung* (1997) 47, 816–20.
2. Antila S, Eha J, Heinpalu M, Lehtonen L, Loogna I, Mesikepp A, Planken U, Sandell E-P. Haemodynamic interactions of a new calcium sensitizing drug levosimendan and captopril. *Eur J Clin Pharmacol* (1996) 49, 451–8.
3. Lehtonen L, Sundberg S. The contractility enhancing effect of the calcium sensitiser levosimendan is not attenuated by carvedilol in healthy subjects. *Eur J Clin Pharmacol* (2002) 58, 449–52.
4. Põder P, Eha J, Antila S, Heinpalu M, Planken Ü, Loogna I, Mesikepp A, Akkila J, Lehtonen L. Pharmacodynamic interactions of levosimendan and felodipine in patients with coronary heart disease. *Cardiovasc Drugs Ther* (2003) 17, 451–8.
5. Antila S, Honkanen T, Lehtonen L, Neuvonen PJ. The CYP3A4 inhibitor itraconazole does not affect the pharmacokinetics of a new calcium-sensitizing drug levosimendan. *Int J Clin Pharmacol Ther* (1998) 36, 446–9.
6. Sundberg S, Lehtonen L. Haemodynamic interactions between the novel calcium sensitiser levosimendan and isosorbide-5-mononitrate in healthy subjects. *Eur J Clin Pharmacol* (2000) 55, 793–9.
7. Antila S, Jarvinen A, Honkanen T, Lehtonen L. Pharmacokinetic and pharmacodynamic interactions between the new calcium sensitiser levosimendan and warfarin. *Eur J Clin Pharmacol* (2000) 56, 705–10.

Methyldopa + Barbiturates

Methyldopa plasma levels are not altered by the use of phenobarbital.

Clinical evidence, mechanism, importance and management

Indirect evidence from one study in hypertensive subjects suggested that phenobarbital could reduce methyldopa levels[1] but later work, which directly measured the plasma levels of methyldopa, did not find any evidence of a pharmacokinetic interaction.[2,3]

1. Káldor A, Juvancz P, Demeczky M, Sebestyen, Palotas J. Enhancement of methyldopa metabolism with barbiturate. *BMJ* (1971) 3, 518–19.
2. Kristensen M, Jørgensen M, Hansen T. Plasma concentration of alfamethyldopa and its main metabolite, methyldopa-O-sulphate, during long term treatment with alfamethyldopa with special reference to possible interaction with other drugs given simultaneously. *Clin Pharmacol Ther* (1973) 14, 139–40.
3. Kristensen M, Jørgensen M, Hansen T. Barbiturates and methyldopa metabolism. *BMJ* (1973) 1, 49.

Methyldopa + Cephalosporins

Two reports describe the development of pustular eruptions in two women taking methyldopa and cefradine or cefazolin. The use of methyldopa may have been coincidental.

Clinical evidence, mechanism, importance and management

A 74-year-old black woman on methyldopa and insulin developed pruritus on her arms and legs within 2 hours of starting to take **cefradine** 250 mg every 6 hours. **Cefradine** was stopped after 7 doses. Over the next 2 days, fever and a widespread pustular eruption developed.[1] Another 65-year-old black woman on methyldopa and furosemide experienced severe pruritus within 8 hours of starting to receive intravenous **cefazolin sodium** 1 g every 12 hours. Over the next 2 days superficial and coalescing pustules appeared on her trunk, arms and legs.[2] The authors of the first report attributed the reaction to **cefradine**.[1] The authors of the second report note that the concurrent use of methyldopa may or may not have been a contributing factor in both reports.[2] There seem to be no other reports of this reaction.

1. Kalb RE, Grossman ME. Pustular eruption following administration of cephradine. *Cutis* (1986) 38, 58–60.
2. Stough D, Guin JD, Baker GF, Haynie L. Pustular eruptions following administration of cefazolin: a possible interaction with methyldopa. *J Am Acad Dermatol* (1987) 16, 1051–2.

Methyldopa + Colestyramine or Colestipol

Colestyramine and colestipol are reported to have no important effect on the absorption of methyldopa.[1]

1. Hunninghake DB, King S. Effect of cholestyramine and colestipol on the absorption of methyldopa and hydrochlorothiazide. *Pharmacologist* (1978) 20, 220.

Methyldopa + Disulfiram

An isolated report describes a patient with hypertension unresponsive to methyldopa in the presence of disulfiram.

Clinical evidence, mechanism, importance and management

The hypertension of an alcoholic patient on disulfiram did not respond to moderate to high doses of intravenous methyldopa, but responded to oral low-dose clonidine. The postulated reason is that disulfiram blocks the activity of dopamine beta-hydroxylase, the enzyme responsible for the conversion of the methyldopa to its active form.[1] The general importance of this alleged interaction is uncertain.

1. McCord RW, LaCorte WS. Hypertension refractory to methyldopa in a disulfiram-treated patient. *Clin Res* (1984) 32, 923A.

Methyldopa + Haloperidol

Two cases of marked mental retardation have been attributed to the use of methyldopa and haloperidol. Another patient became irritable and aggressive. In a small pilot study, the combination of methyldopa and haloperidol lowered blood pressure, and symptomatic hypotension occurred in one patient. The combination also caused marked sedation.

Clinical evidence

Two patients who had been taking methyldopa 1 to 1.5 g daily for hypertension, without problems, developed a dementia syndrome (mental retardation, loss of memory, disorientation, etc.) within 3 days of starting to take haloperidol 6 to 8 mg daily for anxiety. The symptoms totally cleared within 72 hours of stopping the haloperidol.[1] Another patient treated with haloperidol for schizophrenia and methyldopa for hypertension became very irritable and aggressive. When the methyldopa was replaced with hydrochlorothiazide, the patient's behaviour improved dramatically.[2]

In a pilot study of the therapeutic potential of using haloperidol 10 mg daily with methyldopa 500 mg daily for 4 weeks in the treatment of schizophrenia, the supine diastolic blood pressure decreased significantly from 65 to 59.5 mmHg. Six of the 10 patients complained of dizziness, and one patient needed a reduction in the drug doses because of transient hypotension. Somnolence occurred in 8 of the 10 patients.[3]

Mechanism

The hypotensive effects of methyldopa and haloperidol might be expected to be additive. The CNS effects are not understood, although methyldopa can cause sedation, depression and dementia, and haloperidol can cause drowsiness, dizziness and depression.

Importance and management

Concurrent use need not be avoided, but it would be prudent to be on the alert for excessive sedation, excessive reductions in blood pressure or the development of other unexpected adverse effects, particularly in the initial stages of combined therapy.

1. Thornton WE. Dementia induced by methyldopa with haloperidol. *N Engl J Med* (1976) 294, 1222.
2. Nadel I, Wallach M. Drug interaction between haloperidol and methyldopa. *Br J Psychiatry* (1979) 135, 484.
3. Chouinard G, Pinard G, Serrano M, Tetreault L. Potentiation of haloperidol by α-methyldopa in the treatment of schizophrenic patients. *Curr Ther Res* (1973) 15, 473–83.

Methyldopa + Iron compounds

The antihypertensive effects of methyldopa can be reduced by ferrous sulfate. Ferrous gluconate appears to interact similarly.

Clinical evidence

Ferrous sulfate 325 mg three times daily was given to 5 hypertensive patients who had been taking methyldopa 250 mg to 1.5 g daily for more than a year. After 2 weeks the blood pressures of all of them had risen, and the systolic pressures of 3 of them had risen by more than 15 mmHg. Four had diastolic pressure rises, two of them exceeding 10 mmHg.[1] The renal excretion of unmetabolised methyldopa was reduced by 88% and 79% when methyldopa was given with **ferrous sulfate** and **ferrous gluconate** respectively.[1] A further study found that if the **ferrous sulfate** was given 2 hours before, 1 hour before or with the methyldopa, its bioavailability was reduced by 42%, 55% and 83% respectively.[2]

Mechanism

It appears that iron chelates or complexes with the methyldopa in the gut, reducing its absorption by about 50%.[1,3,4] The increase in the metabolic sulfonation of the methyldopa also seems to have a part to play.

Importance and management

Information is limited, but this interaction appears to be established and clinically important. Monitor the effects of concurrent use and increase the methyldopa dosage as necessary. Separating the dosages by up to 2 hours apparently only partially reduces the effects of this interaction. Ferrous gluconate appears to interact like ferrous sulfate, and all iron compounds would be expected to interact similarly.

1. Campbell N, Paddock V, Sundaram R. Alteration of methyldopa absorption, metabolism, and blood pressure control caused by ferrous sulfate and ferrous gluconate. *Clin Pharmacol Ther* (1988) 43, 381–6.
2. Campbell NRC, Hasinoff BB. Iron supplements: a common cause of drug interactions. *Br J Clin Pharmacol* (1991) 31, 251–55.
3. Campbell NRC, Campbell RRA, Hasinoff BB. Ferrous sulfate reduces methyldopa absorption: methyldopa: iron complex formation as a likely mechanism. *Clin Invest Med* (1990) 13, 329–32.
4. Greene RJ, Hall AD, Hider RC. The interaction of orally administered iron with levodopa and methyldopa therapy. *J Pharm Pharmacol* (1990) 42, 502–4.

Methyldopa + Oxazepam

A single case report suggests that blood pressure control in essential hypertension with methyldopa may possibly be made more difficult in the presence of oxazepam.

Clinical evidence, mechanism, importance and management

A 54-year-old woman with insomnia and essential hypertension had unexplained variability in blood pressure while taking methyldopa 750 mg three times daily and a thiazide diuretic. Within a week of stopping oxazepam 60 mg at night, she developed grand mal convulsions and hypertension (190/90 mmHg standing, 240/140 mmHg lying). Her hypertension was then successfully controlled by switching to atenolol and prazosin. The authors of this report suggest that short-acting benzodiazepines such as oxazepam can cause transient hypotension after a dose, but that hypertension may occur on withdrawal. These effects may complicate the management of hypertension.[1] The general importance of this possible interaction is not established, but it seems likely to be limited.

1. Stokes GS. Can short-acting benzodiazepines exacerbate essential hypertension? *Cardiovasc Rev Rep* (1989) 10, 60–1.

Methyldopa + Phenoxybenzamine

An isolated case report describes total urinary incontinence in a patient treated with methyldopa and phenoxybenzamine after bilateral lumbar sympathectomy.

Clinical evidence, mechanism, importance and management

A woman who had previously had bilateral lumbar sympathectomy for Raynaud's disease developed total urinary incontinence when given methyldopa 500 mg to 1.5 g and phenoxybenzamine 12.5 mg daily, but not with either drug alone. This would seem to be the outcome of the additive effects of the sympathectomy and the two drugs on the sympathetic control of the bladder sphincters.[1] Stress incontinence has previously been described with these drugs. The general importance of this interaction is probably small.

1. Fernandez PG, Sahni S, Galway BA, Granter S, McDonald J. Urinary incontinence due to interaction of phenoxybenzamine and α-methyldopa. *Can Med Assoc J* (1981) 124, 174.

Methyldopa + Sympathomimetics; Indirectly-acting

Indirectly-acting sympathomimetics might be expected to cause a blood pressure rise in patients taking methyldopa, and an isolated case report describes such a reaction in a patient who took phenylpropanolamine, but in practice this interaction normally seems to be of little or no general practical importance. The mydriatic effects of ephedrine are reported to be reduced by methyldopa.

Clinical evidence, mechanism, importance and management

In a study in 5 hypertensive subjects taking methyldopa 2 to 3 g daily, the pressor (rise in blood pressure) effects of **tyramine** were doubled.[1] In another study the pressor effect of **tyramine** was 50/16 mmHg compared with 18/10 mmHg before methyldopa treatment.[2]

A man with renal hypertension, whose blood pressure was well controlled with methyldopa 250 mg twice daily and oxprenolol 160 mg three times daily, had a rise in blood pressure from under 140/80 mmHg to 200/150 mmHg within 2 days of starting to take two tablets of *Triogesic* (**phenylpropanolamine** 12.5 mg and paracetamol 500 mg) three times daily. His blood pressure fell when the *Triogesic* was withdrawn.[3]

The reason for this is uncertain. One suggestion is that the methyldopa causes the replacement of noradrenaline at adrenergic nerve endings by methylnoradrenaline, which has weaker pressor (alpha) activity but greater vasodilator (beta) activity. With the vasodilator activity blocked by the oxprenolol, the vasoconstrictor (pressor) activity of the **phenylpropanolamine** would be unopposed and exaggerated. Alternatively it could have been that he was unusually sensitive to the pressor effects of **phenylpropanolamine**.

Despite the information derived from the studies outlined above[1,2] and the single report cited, there seems to be nothing else in the literature to suggest that indirectly-acting sympathomimetics normally cause an adverse reaction with methyldopa. One report briefly mentions that the antihypertensive effects of various drugs including methyldopa were not affected by **diethylpropion**.[4]

In 9 patients with untreated hypertension, the normal mydriatic effects of **ephedrine** were reduced by 54% after they started treatment with methyldopa 500 mg to 1.5 g daily.[5]

1. Pettinger W, Horwitz D, Spector S, Sjoerdsma A. Enhancement by methyldopa of tyramine sensitivity in man. *Nature* (1963) 200, 1107–8.
2. Dollery CT, Harington M, Hodge JV. Haemodynamic studies with methyldopa: effect on cardiac output and response to pressor amines. *Br Heart J* (1963) 25, 670–6.
3. McLaren EH. Severe hypertension produced by interaction of phenylpropanolamine with methyldopa and oxprenolol. *BMJ* (1976) 3, 283–4.
4. Seedat YK, Reddy J. Diethylpropion hydrochloride (Tenuate, Dospan) in the treatment of obese hypertensive patients. *S Afr Med J* (1974) 48, 569.
5. Sneddon JM, Turner P. Ephedrine mydriasis in hypertension and the response to treatment. *Clin Pharmacol Ther* (1969) 10, 64–71.

Methyldopa + Tricyclic and Tetracyclic antidepressants

The antihypertensive effects of methyldopa are not normally adversely affected by desipramine, but an isolated report describes hypertension, tachycardia, tremor and agitation in a man on methyldopa and amitriptyline. The tetracyclic mianserin appears not to interact.

Clinical evidence

A man with hypertension controlled by methyldopa 250 mg three times daily and a thiazide diuretic, experienced tremor, agitation, tachycardia (148 bpm) and hypertension (a rise from under 150/90 mmHg to 170/110 mmHg) within 10 days of starting to take **amitriptyline** 25 mg three times daily. A week after stopping all treatment his pulse rate was 100 bpm and his blood pressure 160/90 mmHg.[1] In contrast, a double-blind crossover study in 5 subjects (one with mild hypertension) found that **desipramine** 25 mg three times daily for 3 days had no significant effect on the hypotensive effects of a single 750-mg dose of methyldopa.[2] Another study including 3 hypertensive patients on methyldopa 2.5 to 3 g daily found that **desipramine** 75 mg daily for 5 to 6 days did not antagonise the action of methyldopa. In fact, the blood pressure fell slightly.[3] **Mianserin** 20 mg three times daily for 2 weeks had no effect on the control of blood pressure in 6 patients receiving methyldopa, although 2 patients developed symptomatic hypotension after the first dose of **mianserin**.[4,5]

Mechanism

Not understood. Antagonism of the antihypertensive actions of methyldopa by tricyclic antidepressants is seen in *animals* and it seems to occur within the brain.[6,7]

Importance and management

Normally no adverse interaction occurs, nevertheless it would seem prudent to monitor the effects of concurrent use if amitriptyline or any other tricyclic antidepressant is given to patients on methyldopa. Note that methyldopa sometimes induces depression, so it is generally considered contraindicated in depressed patients.

1. White AG. Methyldopa and amitriptyline. *Lancet* (1965) ii, 441.
2. Reid JL, Porsius AJ, Zamboulis C, Polak G, Hamilton CA, Dean CR. The effects of desmethylimipramine on the pharmacological actions of alpha methyldopa in man. *Eur J Clin Pharmacol* (1979) 16, 75–80.
3. Mitchell JR, Cavanaugh JH, Arias L, Oates JA. Guanethidine and related agents. III. Antagonism by drugs which inhibit the norepinephrine pump in man. *J Clin Invest* (1970) 49, 1596–1604.
4. Elliott HL, Whiting B, Reid JL. Assessment of the interaction between mianserin and centrally-acting antihypertensive drugs. *Br J Clin Pharmacol* (1983) 15, 323S–328S.
5. Elliott HL, McLean K, Sumner DJ, Reid JL. Absence of an effect of mianserin on the actions of clonidine or methyldopa in hypertensive patients. *Eur J Clin Pharmacol* (1983) 24, 15–19.
6. van Spanning HW, van Zwieten PA. The interaction between alpha-methyl-dopa and tricyclic antidepressants. *Int J Clin Pharmacol Biopharm* (1975) 11, 65–7.
7. van Zwieten PA. Interaction between centrally acting hypotensive drugs and tricyclic antidepressants. *Arch Int Pharmacodyn Ther* (1975) 214, 12–30.

Minoxidil + Glibenclamide (Glyburide)

Glibenclamide 2.5 mg did not alter the hypotensive effects of oral minoxidil. However, there was some evidence that a 5-mg dose of glibenclamide appeared to reduce the hypotensive effect to some extent, but the clinical importance of this is not yet known.

Clinical evidence, mechanism, importance and management

A single-dose study in 9 healthy subjects found that glibenclamide 2.5 mg did not alter the hypotensive effect of oral minoxidil 5 mg. However, in a further 4 subjects a 5-mg dose of glibenclamide appeared to cause some loss in the hypotensive effect of minoxidil, but this was not statistically significant. The suggested reason is that these two drugs have opposing effects on the potassium channels of the smooth muscle of blood vessels.[1] In this study, subjects were pre-treated with propranolol to prevent reflex tachycardia when given minoxidil, which is how minoxidil is used clinically.[1] What is not yet clear is whether any interaction occurs between minoxidil and glibenclamide in the clinical setting.

1. Stein CM, Brown N, Carlson MG, Campbell P, Wood AJJ. Coadministration of glyburide and minoxidil, drugs with opposing effects on potassium channels. *Clin Pharmacol Ther* (1997) 61, 662–8.

Minoxidil + Guanethidine or Sympathomimetics

The maker notes that excessive blood pressure reductions may occur if minoxidil is used in patients on guanethidine, because of the adrenergic blocking effects of guanethidine.[1,2] If excessive hypotension occurs with minoxidil, this should *not* be treated with adrenaline (epinephrine) or noradrenaline (norepinephrine), because this may result in excessive tachycardia.[1]

1. Loniten tablets (Minoxidil). Pharmacia Ltd. UK Summary of product characteristics, April 2001.
2. Loniten tablets (Minoxidil). Pharmacia & Upjohn Co. US Prescribing information, March 2002.

Minoxidil topical + Miscellaneous

There are no reports of topical minoxidil being absorbed and causing interactions with other medicines.[1] However, the makers note that, theoretically at least, topical drugs that alter the stratum corneum barrier such as tretinoin or dithranol could result in increased absorption of minoxidil if applied concurrently. They suggest that one possible effect of minoxidil absorption would be potentiation of orthostatic hypotension caused by vasodilator drugs.[1]

1. Regaine (Minoxidil). Pharmacia Ltd. UK Summary of product characteristics, May 2004.

Moxonidine + Miscellaneous

On theoretical grounds the makers of moxonidine advise withdrawing beta-blockers before withdrawing moxonidine. They

also advise avoiding alcohol and tricyclic antidepressants during the use of moxonidine. Moxonidine alone can cause sedation, and increases the sedative effects of lorazepam, therefore care is needed with other benzodiazepines, hypnotics and sedatives because of possible increased sedation. No clinically significant pharmacokinetic interactions occur with digoxin, glibenclamide (glyburide), hydrochlorothiazide, moclobemide, or quinidine.

Clinical evidence, mechanism, importance and management

(a) Benzodiazepines and other sedatives and hypnotics

The cognitive function of 24 healthy subjects was not impaired by moxonidine 400 micrograms daily, but the presence of moxonidine was found to increase the impairment caused by **lorazepam** 1 mg daily.[1] For this reason the makers warn that the sedative effects of the benzodiazepines may possibly be enhanced by moxonidine.[2] Sedation and dizziness may occur with moxonidine, which the makers suggest may be additive with the effects of sedatives and hypnotics.[2] They also advise the avoidance of **alcohol**.[2]

(b) Beta-blockers

The presence of a beta-blocker can exacerbate the rebound hypertension that follows the withdrawal of clonidine (see 'Clonidine + Beta-blockers', p.666). Moxonidine is reported to have less affinity for central alpha-receptors than clonidine, and no such rebound hypertension has actually been seen when moxonidine is withdrawn. However, for safety's sake the makers advise that any beta-blocker should be stopped first, followed by the moxonidine a few days later.[2,3]

(c) Digoxin

No clinically relevant pharmacokinetic interaction was seen at steady state between moxonidine 200 micrograms twice daily and digoxin 200 micrograms daily in 15 healthy subjects.[4]

(d) Glibenclamide (Glyburide)

Glibenclamide 2.5 mg daily had no effect on the steady-state pharmacokinetics of moxonidine 200 micrograms twice daily in 18 healthy subjects. There was a minor 12% decrease in the AUC of glibenclamide, and a 14% increase in clearance, but these changes are unlikely to be of any clinical relevance.[5]

(e) Hydrochlorothiazide

No clinically relevant pharmacokinetic interaction was seen at steady state between moxonidine 200 micrograms twice daily and hydrochlorothiazide 25 mg twice daily.[6]

(f) Moclobemide

A study in healthy subjects given moxonidine 400 micrograms daily and a single 300-mg dose of moclobemide found no pharmacokinetic interaction. Moxonidine alone or with moclobemide did not significantly affect cognitive function.[1]

(g) Quinidine

In a single-dose study in 6 healthy subjects, quinidine sulfate 400 mg, given one hour before moxonidine 200 micrograms, caused a minor 11% increase in the AUC of moxonidine and decreased its clearance by 10%. These small changes were thought to be due to metabolic inhibition, though are unlikely to be of any clinical relevance.[7]

(h) Tricyclic antidepressants

The makers of moxonidine advise avoiding tricyclic antidepressants, because of the lack of clinical experience of combined use.[2] Presumably, this is because moxonidine is related to clonidine, and tricyclics may antagonise the blood pressure lowering effects of clonidine, see 'Clonidine + Tricyclic and related antidepressants', p.667. Tricyclics can also cause postural hypotension, and can cause sedation, both of which could potentially be additive with those of moxonidine. If the combination is used, it would be prudent to carefully monitor blood pressure and sedation.

1. Wesnes K, Simpson PM, Jansson B, Grahnén A, Wemann H-J, Küppers H. moxonidine and cognitive function: interactions with moclobemide and lorazepam. *Eur J Clin Pharmacol* (1997) 52, 351–8.
2. Moxonidine (Physiotens). Solvay Healthcare. UK Summary of product characteristics, March 2002.
3. Solvay Healthcare. Personal communication, September 1996.
4. Pabst G, Weimann H-J, Weber W. Lack of pharmacokinetic interactions between moxonidine and digoxin. *Clin Pharmacokinet* (1992) 23, 477–81.
5. Müller M, Weimann H-J, Eden G, Weber W, Michaelis K, Dilger C, Achtert G. Steady state investigation of possible pharmacokinetic interactions of moxonidine and glibenclamide. *Eur J Drug Metab Pharmacokinet* (1993) 18, 277–83.
6. Weimann H-J, Rudolph M. Clinical pharmacokinetics of moxonidine. *J Cardiovasc Pharmacol* (1992) 20 (Suppl 4), S37–S41.
7. Wise SD, Chan C, Schaefer HG, He MM, Pouliquen IJ, Mitchell MI. Quinidine does not affect the renal clearance of moxonidine. *Br J Clin Pharmacol* (2002) 54, 251–4.

Nicorandil + Miscellaneous

Neither cimetidine nor rifampicin had any clinically relevant effect on the pharmacokinetics of nicorandil. Nicorandil did not alter the anticoagulant effects of acenocoumarol. In clinical trials, nicorandil was used with a wide range of drugs without any evidence of adverse interactions. Nevertheless, there is the possibility it may potentiate the hypotensive effects of other vasodilators, tricyclic antidepressants and alcohol. It should not be used with phosphodiesterase inhibitors, see 'Sildenafil + Cardiovascular drugs', p.1029.

Clinical evidence, mechanism, importance and management

(a) Acenocoumarol

Nicorandil 10 mg twice daily for 4 days then 20 mg twice daily for 7 days did not alter the INR in 11 patients stable on acenocoumarol.[1]

(b) Cimetidine

Cimetidine 400 mg twice daily for 7 days had no effect on the pharmacokinetics of nicorandil 20 mg twice daily for 7 days, except that the nicorandil AUC showed a minor 10% increase, which is not clinically important.[1]

(c) Miscellaneous drugs

Combined data from clinical studies in 1152 patients using nicorandil found no evidence of increased adverse effects or an increased number of withdrawals in patients taking unnamed **beta-blockers** (210 patients), **calcium channel blockers** (117), **long-acting nitrates** (130), **bepridil** (18), **diltiazem** (91), **verapamil** (9), **amiodarone** (23) or **molsidomine** (30). It has also been reported that unnamed **antihypertensives**, **antidiabetic** or **hypolipidaemic** agents do not appear to interact adversely.[2] No adverse ECG effects have been seen (including QT or ST segment modifications) with nicorandil.[2] However, the makers suggest that nicorandil may possibly potentiate the blood pressure lowering effects of other **vasodilators**, **tricyclic antidepressants** or **alcohol**.[3] For mention that phosphodiesterase inhibitors (e.g. sildenafil, tadalafil, vardenafil) should not be used with nicorandil, see 'Sildenafil + Cardiovascular drugs', p.1029.

(d) Rifampicin

Rifampicin 600 mg daily for 5 days had no effect on the pharmacokinetics of nicorandil 20 mg twice daily for 5 days, accept that the elimination half-life showed a minor 17% decrease, which is not clinically important.[1]

1. Frydman A. Pharmacokinetic profile of nicorandil in humans: an overview. *J Cardiovasc Pharmacol* (1992) 20 (Suppl 3), S34–S44.
2. Witchitz S, Darmon J-Y. Nicorandil safety in the long-term treatment of coronary heart disease. *Cardiovasc Drugs Ther* (1995) 9, 237–43.
3. Ikorel (Nicorandil). Rhone-Poulenc Rorer Ltd. UK Summary of product characteristics, June 2004.

Pentoxifylline + Cimetidine

Cimetidine increases plasma pentoxifylline levels to a moderate extent, and may increase the incidence of adverse effects.

Clinical evidence, mechanism, importance and management

A study in 10 healthy subjects found that the mean steady-state plasma levels of controlled-release pentoxifylline 400 mg every 8 hours were raised by 27.4% when cimetidine 300 mg four times daily for 7 days was added.[1] Adverse effects such as headache, nausea, and vomiting were said to be more common and bothersome while taking the cimetidine.[1]

The reason for this interaction is not known. However, cimetidine is known to inhibit the metabolism of 'theophylline', (p.937), to which pentoxifylline is structurally related.

The findings of this study suggest that this interaction may be clinically relevant. If cimetidine is required in a patient on pentoxifylline, monitor for adverse effects, and decrease the pentoxifylline dose if problems occur.

1. Mauro VF, Mauro LS, Hageman JH. Alteration of pentoxifylline pharmacokinetics by cimetidine. *J Clin Pharmacol* (1988) 28, 649–54.

Pentoxifylline + Ciprofloxacin

Evidence from one study suggests that ciprofloxacin increases the serum levels of pentoxifylline, and may increase the incidence of adverse effects. In some clinical trials ciprofloxacin has been used to boost the levels of pentoxifylline.

Clinical evidence

Because patients taking pentoxifylline and ciprofloxacin often complained of headache, the possibility of a pharmacokinetic interaction was studied in 6 healthy subjects. The study showed that ciprofloxacin 500 mg daily for 3 days increased the peak serum levels of a single 400-mg dose of pentoxifylline by almost 60% (from 114.5 to 179.5 nanograms/ml), and increased the AUC by 15%. All 6 subjects complained of a frontal headache.[1]

Mechanism

The evidence suggests that the ciprofloxacin inhibits the metabolism of the pentoxifylline, a xanthine derivative) by the liver. Compare 'Theophylline + Quinolones', p.951.

Importance and management

Information on this interaction and its clinical relevance is limited. The author of the pharmacokinetic study suggests that, if the drugs need to be used together, the dosage of pentoxifylline should be halved.[1] In the absence of other information, if a short-course of ciprofloxacin is required in a patient on pentoxifylline, this may be a sensible precaution. Alternatively, because the increase in AUC was minor, it may be sufficient to recommend a reduction in pentoxifylline dose only in those who experience adverse effects (e.g. nausea, headache). Note that ciprofloxacin has been used to boost pentoxifylline levels in trials investigating the possible therapeutic value of pentoxifylline's ability to inhibit various cytokines. For example, ciprofloxacin 500 mg twice daily was used with pentoxifylline 800 mg three times daily for up to one year in patients with myelodysplastic syndrome.[2]

1. Cleary JD. Ciprofloxacin (CIPRO) and pentoxifylline (PTF): a clinically significant drug interaction. *Pharmacotherapy* (1992) 12, 259–60.
2. Raza A, Qawi H, Lisak L, Andric T, Dar S, Andrews C, Venugopal P, Gezer S, Gregory S, Loew J, Robin E, Rifkin S, Hsu W-T, Huang R-W. Patients with myelodysplastic syndromes benefit from palliative therapy with amifostine, pentoxifylline, and ciprofloxacin with or without dexamethasone. *Blood* (2000) 95, 1580–87.

Perhexiline + SSRIs

Case reports describe an increase in perhexiline serum levels resulting in toxicity due to citalopram, fluoxetine or paroxetine.

Clinical evidence, mechanism, importance and management

An 86-year-old woman on perhexiline was admitted to hospital because of ataxia, falls, lethargy, nausea and an inability to cope at home. She had started to take **paroxetine** 20 mg daily 5 weeks earlier. Her serum perhexiline levels were 2.02 mg/l compared with the normal range of 0.15 to 0.6 mg/l.[1] Perhexiline toxicity was also seen in two other elderly women following the use of **paroxetine** in one case, and **fluoxetine** in the other. The perhexiline serum levels fell when both drugs were stopped, but in one case the fall was very slow.[2] Another case report describes toxicity and raised perhexiline levels in an elderly man shortly after **citalopram** was added to his therapy.[3]

The reason for the rise in perhexiline levels is not known, but it seems likely that these SSRIs can inhibit its metabolism, probably via the cytochrome P450 isoenzyme CYP2D6. The general importance of these interactions is also not known, but it would now be prudent to monitor the outcome of concurrent use for perhexiline toxicity and consider monitoring perhexiline serum levels where possible. The perhexiline dosage may need to be reduced. More study is needed.

1. Alderman CP. Perhexiline-paroxetine interaction. *Aust J Hosp Pharm* (1998) 28, 254–5.
2. Alderman CP, Hundertmark JD, Soetratma TW. Interaction of serotonin re-uptake inhibitors with perhexiline. *Aust N Z J Psychiatry* (1997) 31, 601–3.
3. Nyfort-Hansen K. Perhexiline toxicity related to citalopram use. *Med J Aust* (2002) 176, 560–61.

Sodium nitroprusside + Miscellaneous

The maker notes that smaller doses of sodium nitroprusside might be required in patients receiving antihypertensive drugs.[1] In any event the required dose varies considerably between patients and so should be titrated to effect.[1] When used for controlled hypotension during anaesthesia, the hypotensive effect of other drugs should be remembered. The maker specifically names the anaesthetic agents.[1]

1. Sodium Nitroprusside. Mayne Pharma plc. UK Summary of product characteristics, August 2000.

Tirilazad mesilate + Miscellaneous

Phenobarbital and phenytoin reduce the serum levels of tirilazad mesilate whereas ketoconazole increases them. No pharmacokinetic interaction appears to occur between cimetidine or nimodipine and tirilazad.

Clinical evidence, mechanism, importance and management

(a) Cimetidine

A study in 16 healthy men found that cimetidine 300 mg every 6 hours for 4 days had no effect on the pharmacokinetics of a single 2-mg/kg dose of tirilazad mesilate given by infusion over 10 minutes on day 2, nor on U-89678, its metabolite.[1] No special precautions would seem necessary if cimetidine is given with tirilazad mesilate.

(b) Ketoconazole

Tirilazad mesilate, 10 mg/kg orally or 2 mg/kg intravenously, was given to 12 healthy men and women, either alone or on day 4 of a 7-day regimen of ketoconazole 200 mg daily. The ketoconazole more than doubled the absolute bioavailability of the oral tirilazad mesilate (from 8.7 to 20.9%), apparently because its metabolism by the cytochrome P450 isoenzyme CYP3A in the gut wall and during the first pass through the liver was inhibited.[2] The clinical importance of this interaction awaits assessment.

(c) Nimodipine

In a single-dose study in 12 healthy men, there was no pharmacokinetic or pharmacodynamic interaction between intravenous tirilazad mesilate 2 mg/kg and oral nimodipine 60 mg.[3] No special precautions would seem necessary if nimodipine is given with tirilazad mesilate

(d) Phenobarbital

The pharmacokinetics of tirilazad mesilate (1.5 mg/kg as 10 minute intravenous infusions 6-hourly for 29 doses) were studied in 15 healthy subjects before and after taking 100 mg phenobarbital daily for 8 days. The phenobarbital increased the clearance of the tirilazad by 25% in the male subjects and 29% in the female, and the AUC of the metabolite of tirilazad (U-89678) was reduced by 51% in the males and 69% in the females. The reason is thought to be that the phenobarbital acts as an enzyme inducing agent, which increases the metabolism of the tirilazad.[4] The clinical importance of these reductions awaits assessment, but be alert for evidence of reduced effects if both drugs are given. It is doubtful if the full enzyme-inducing effects of the phenobarbital would have been reached in this study after only one week, so anticipate a greater effect if it is given for a longer period.

(e) Phenytoin

After taking 200 mg phenytoin every 8 hours for 11 doses followed by 100 mg every 8 hours for 5 doses, the AUC (over 6 hours) of tirilazad mesilate was reduced by 35% in 12 healthy subjects. The AUC of a metabolite with possible activity (U-89678) was reduced by 87%.[5] Another report by the same group of workers[6] found that phenytoin every 8 hours for 7 days (9 doses of 200 mg followed by 13 doses of 100 mg) reduced the clearance of tirilazad by 92% and of U-89678 by 93%. In another report the authors noted that phenytoin increased the metabolism of tirilazad and its metabolite in men and women to similar extents.[7] The clinical importance of these reductions is still to be assessed, but you should be alert for any evidence of reduced tirilazad effects if both drugs are given.

1. Fleishaker JC, Hulst LK, Peters GR. Lack of pharmacokinetic interaction between cimetidine and tirilazad mesylate. *Pharm Res* (1994) 11, 341–4.
2. Fleishaker JC, Pearson PG, Wienkers LC, Pearson LK, Peters GR. Biotransformation of tirilazad in humans: 2. Effect of ketoconazole on tirilazad clearance and oral bioavailability. *J Pharmacol Exp Ther* (1996) 277, 991–8.
3. Fleishaker JC, Hulst LK, Peters GR. Lack of a pharmacokinetic/pharmacodynamic interaction between nimodipine and tirilazad mesylate in healthy volunteers. *J Clin Pharmacol* (1994) 34, 837–41.
4. Fleishaker JC, Pearson LK, Peters GR. Gender does not affect the degree of induction of tirilazad clearance by phenobarbital. *Eur J Clin Pharmacol* (1996) 50, 139–45.
5. Fleishaker JC, Hulst LK, Peters GR. The effect of phenytoin on the pharmacokinetics of tirilazad mesylate in healthy male volunteers. *Clin Pharmacol Ther* (1994) 56, 389–97.
6. Fleishaker JC, Pearson LK, Peters GR. Induction of tirilazad clearance by phenytoin. *Biopharm Drug Dispos* (1998) 19, 91–6.
7. Fleishaker JC, Pearson LK, Peters GR. Effect of gender on the degree of induction of tirilazad clearance by phenytoin. *Clin Pharmacol Ther* (1996) 59, 168.

Tolazoline + H_2-blockers

Cimetidine and ranitidine can reduce or abolish the effects of tolazoline used as a pulmonary vasodilator in children.

Clinical evidence

A newborn infant with persistent foetal circulation was given a continuous infusion of tolazoline to reduce pulmonary hypertension. The oxygenation improved but gastrointestinal bleeding occurred. When **cimetidine** was given, the condition of the child deteriorated with a decrease in oxygen saturation and arterial pO_2 values.[1]

This report is similar to another in which the tolazoline-induced fall in pulmonary arterial pressure in a child was reversed when **cimetidine** was given for acute gastrointestinal haemorrhage.[2] Another study found that intravenous **ranitidine** 3 mg/kg abolished the fall in pulmonary and systemic vascular resistance in 12 children who had been treated with tolazoline 1 to 2 mg/kg as a pulmonary vasodilator.[3]

Mechanism

Tolazoline dilates the pulmonary vascular system by stimulating both H_1- and H_2-receptors. Cimetidine and ranitidine block H_2-receptors so that at least part of the effects of tolazoline are abolished. It has been suggested that this interaction is confined to children.[2]

Importance and management

An established interaction. Cimetidine and ranitidine are not suitable agents for prophylaxis of the gastrointestinal adverse effects of tolazoline in children. Other H_2-blockers would be expected to behave similarly.

1. Roll C, Hanssler L. Interaktion von Tolazolin und Cimetidin bei persistierender fetaler Zirkulation des Neugeborenen. *Monatsschr Kinderheilkd* (1993) 141, 297–9.
2. Jones ODH, Shore DF, Rigby ML. The use of tolazoline hydrochloride as a pulmonary vasodilator in potentially fatal episodes of pulmonary vasoconstriction after cardiac surgery in children. *Circulation* (1981) 64 (Suppl II), 134–9.
3. Bush A, Busst CM, Knight WB, Shinebourne EA. Cardiovascular effects of tolazoline and ranitidine. *Arch Dis Child* (1987) 62, 241–6.

23

Digitalis glycosides

Plant extracts containing cardiac glycosides have been in use for thousands of years. The ancient Egyptians were familiar with squill, as were the Romans who used it as a heart tonic and diuretic. The foxglove was mentioned in the writings of Welsh physicians in the thirteenth century and features in 'An Account of the Foxglove and some of its Medical Uses', published by William Withering in 1785, in which he described its application in the treatment of 'dropsy' or the oedema that results from heart failure.

The most commonly used cardiac glycosides are those obtained from the members of the foxglove family, *Digitalis purpurea* and *Digitalis lanata*. The leaves of these two plants are the source of a number of purified glycosides (digoxin, digitoxin, gitoxin, lanatoside C and others), of gitalin (an amorphous mixture largely composed of digitoxin and digoxin), and of powdered whole leaf digitalis. Occasionally ouabain or strophanthin (also of plant origin) are used for particular situations, while for a number of years the Russians have exploited cardiac glycosides from lily of the valley. Bufalin is a cardioactive compound obtained from toads and is found in a number of Chinese medicines. 'Table 23.1', (below) lists many of the cardiac glycosides that have been used medicinally.

Digitalisation

The cardiac glycosides have two main actions and two main applications. They reduce conductivity within the atrioventricular (AV) node, hence are used for treating supraventricular tachycardias (especially atrial fibrillation), and they have a positive inotropic effect (i.e. increase the force of contraction), hence are used for congestive heart failure, although to a much lesser extent these days.

Because the most commonly used glycosides are derived from digitalis, the achievement of the desired therapeutic serum concentration of any cardiac glycoside is usually referred to as digitalisation. Treatment may be started with a large loading dose so that the therapeutic concentrations are achieved reasonably quickly, but once these have been reached the amount is reduced to a maintenance dose. This has to be done carefully because there is a relatively narrow gap between therapeutic and toxic serum concentrations. Normal therapeutic levels are about one-third of those that are fatal, and serious toxic arrhythmias begin at about two-thirds of the fatal levels. The normal range for digoxin levels is 1.02 to 2.56 nanomol/l. The ranges are often given in nanograms/ml. To convert nanograms/ml to nanomol/l multiply by 1.28.

If a patient is over-digitalised, signs of toxicity will occur, which may include loss of appetite, nausea and vomiting and bradycardia. These symptoms are often used as clinical indicators of toxicity, and a pulse rate of less than 60 bpm is usually considered to be an indication of over-treatment. Other symptoms include visual disturbances, headache, drowsiness and occasionally diarrhoea. Death may result from cardiac arrhythmias. Patients treated for cardiac arrhythmias can therefore demonstrate arrhythmias when they are both under- as well as over-digitalised.

Interactions of the cardiac glycosides

The pharmacological actions of these glycosides are very similar, but their rates and degree of absorption, metabolism and clearance are different and this determines the dosages used. For example, digoxin is mainly renally cleared whereas digitoxin undergoes a degree of metabolism by the liver. It is therefore most important not to extrapolate an interaction seen with one glycoside and apply it uncritically to any other. Because the therapeutic ratio of the cardiac glycosides is low, a quite small change in serum levels may lead to inadequate digitalisation or to toxicity. For this reason interactions that have a relatively modest effect on serum levels may sometimes have serious consequences.

Many interactions between digoxin and other drugs are mediated by P-glycoprotein. Drugs that inhibit the activity of P-glycoprotein in the renal tubules may reduce the elimination of digoxin in the urine and this may result in toxic serum levels. Further, the induction or inhibition of P-glycoprotein in the gut may affect the oral absorption of digoxin. See also 'Drug transporter proteins', (p.8).

Table 23.1 Cardiac glycosides

Generic names	*Proprietary names*
Acetyldigitoxin	
Acetyldigoxin	Corotal, Digostada, Digotab, Digox, Lanatilin, Novodigal, Stillacor
Convallaria	
Cymarin	
Deslanoside	Cedilanide
Digitalin	Augentonikum N
Digitalis leaf	
Prepared digitalis	
Digitoxin	Coramedan, Crystodigin, Digimed, Digimerck, Digitaline, Digitrin, Ditaven
Digoxin	Cardocor, Cardiogoxin, Cardioxin, Cimecard, Digacin, Digocard-G, Digoregen, Digosin, Digoxil, Dilanacin, Eudigox, Grexin, Hemigoxine Nativelle, Lanacordin, Lanacrist, Lanicor, Lanoxicaps, Lanoxin, Lenoxin, Mapluxin, Novodigal, Purgoxin, Sigmaxin, Toloxin
Gitoformate	
Lanatoside C	Develanid
Meproscillarin	
Metildigoxin	Lanirapid, Lanitop
Ouabain (Strophanthin-G)	Strodival
Proscillaridin	Talusin
Strophanthin-K	Kombetin

Digitalis glycosides + ACE inhibitors

No significant interaction has been seen between digoxin and cilazapril, enalapril, imidapril, lisinopril, moexipril, perindopril, quinapril, ramipril, spirapril or trandolapril. Some studies have found that serum digoxin levels rise by about 20% or more if captopril is used, but others have found no significant changes. It has been suggested that any interaction is likely to occur only in those patients who have pre-existing renal impairment. Digitoxin and captopril appear not to interact.

Clinical evidence

(a) Digoxin + Captopril

The serum digoxin levels of 16 patients with severe chronic congestive heart failure rose by 21%, from 1.4 to 1.7 nanomol/l, while taking captopril (average dose 93.7 mg daily). Serum digoxin levels were above the therapeutic range at 2.6 nanomol/l on 3 out of 63 occasions, but no toxicity was seen. All patients had impaired renal function and were being treated with diuretics.[1,2] Another study[3] found an approximate 30% rise in serum digoxin levels in patients with congestive heart failure class II and a further study[4] found an approximate 60% rise in peak serum digoxin levels in patients with congestive heart failure class IV. Conversely, another study in 31 patients with stable congestive heart failure, given captopril 25 mg three times daily, found no significant changes in serum digoxin levels over a 6-month period.[5] Two other studies in healthy subjects[6] and patients with congestive heart failure[7] also found no evidence of an interaction.

(b) Digoxin + Other ACE inhibitors

Cilazapril 5 mg for 14 days did not alter the trough plasma digoxin levels in healthy subjects.[8] **Enalapril** 20 mg daily for 30 days had no significant effect on the pharmacokinetics of digoxin 250 micrograms daily in 7 patients with congestive heart failure.[9] **Imidapril** 10 mg daily had no effect on the serum digoxin levels of 12 healthy subjects, but slight reductions in levels of the active form imidaprilat and in ACE-inhibition of about 15% were seen, which were of uncertain clinical relevance.[10] **Lisinopril** 5 mg daily for 4 weeks had no significant effect on the serum digoxin levels of another 9 patients.[11] This confirms the findings of a single-dose study.[12] **Moexipril** has been reported, by the maker, to have had no important pharmacokinetic interaction with digoxin in healthy subjects.[13] They also have clinical trials that show no evidence of clinically important adverse interactions when **moexipril** was used with digoxin.[14] **Perindopril** 2 to 4 mg daily for a month had no effect on the steady-state serum digoxin levels of 10 patients with mild chronic heart failure.[15] **Quinapril** is also reported not to alter the steady-state levels of digoxin in healthy subjects,[16] and patients with congestive heart failure.[17] **Ramipril** 5 mg daily for 14 days had no effect on the serum digoxin levels of 12 healthy subjects.[18] **Spirapril** 12 to 48 mg daily did not significantly affect the pharmacokinetics nor the steady-state serum levels of digoxin in 15 healthy subjects on digoxin 250 micrograms twice daily.[19] **Trandolapril** has been shown to have no significant pharmacokinetic interaction with digoxin in healthy subjects.[20] The makers also note that in patients with left ventricular dysfunction after myocardial infarction, no clinical interactions have been found between **trandolapril** and digoxin.[21,22]

(c) Digitoxin + Captopril

A study in 12 healthy subjects given digitoxin 70 micrograms daily for up to 58 days found no evidence that the addition of captopril 25 mg daily had a relevant effect on the pharmacokinetics of digitoxin, or its effects on the heart.[23]

Mechanism

Not fully understood. It has been suggested that an interaction is only likely to occur in those who have renal impairment because the glomerular filtration rate of these patients may be maintained by the vasoconstrictor action of angiotensin II on the postglomerular blood vessels, which would be impaired by ACE inhibition. As a result some of the loss of digoxin through the tubules is reduced.[6]

Importance and management

The overall picture is that no clinically important adverse interaction occurs between digoxin and ACE inhibitors in patients with normal renal function, and that serum digoxin monitoring is only needed in those who have a high risk of reversible ACE inhibitor induced renal failure (e.g. patients with congestive heart failure during chronic diuretic treatment, with bilateral renal artery stenosis or unilateral renal artery stenosis in a solitary kidney).[6] However, note these later two conditions are contraindications to the use of ACE inhibitors. The critical factor does not seem to be the particular ACE inhibitor used but the existence of abnormal renal function or conditions that increase the risk of renal impairment. This needs confirmation.

No interaction apparently occurs between digitoxin and captopril in healthy subjects, but this needs confirmation in patients.

1. Cleland JGF, Dargie HJ, Hodsman GP, Robertson JIS, Ball SG. Interaction of digoxin and captopril. *Br J Clin Pharmacol* (1984) 17, 214P.
2. Cleland JGF, Dargie HJ, Pettigrew A, Gillen C, Robertson JIS. The effects of captopril on serum digoxin and urinary urea and digoxin clearances in patients with congestive heart failure. *Am Heart J* (1986) 112, 130–5.
3. Mazurek W, Haczyński J, Interakcja kaptoprilu i digoksyny. *Pol Tyg Lek* (1993) 48, 834–5.
4. Kirimli O, Kalkan S, Guneri S, Tuncok Y, Akdeniz B, Ozdamar M, Guven H. The effects of captopril on serum digoxin levels in patients with severe congestive heart failure. *Int J Clin Pharmacol Ther* (2001) 39, 311–14.
5. Magelli C, Bassein L, Ribani MA, Liberatore S, Ambrosioni E, Magnani B. Lack of effect of captopril on serum digoxin in congestive heart failure. *Eur J Clin Pharmacol* (1989) 36, 99–100.
6. Rossi GP, Semplicini A, Bongiovi S, Mozzato MG, Paleari CD, Pessina AC. Effect of acute captopril administration on digoxin pharmacokinetics in normal subjects. *Curr Ther Res* (1989) 46, 439–44.
7. Miyakawa T, Shionoiri H, Takasaki I, Kobayashi K, Ishii M. The effect of captopril on pharmacokinetics of digoxin in patients with mild congestive heart failure. *J Cardiovasc Pharmacol* (1991) 17, 576–80.
8. Kleinbloesem CH, van Brummelen P, Francis RJ, Wiegand U-W. Clinical pharmacology of cilazapril. *Drugs* (1991) 41 (Suppl 1), 3–10.
9. Douste-Blazy Ph, Blanc M, Montastruc JL, Conte D, Cotonat J, Galinier F. Is there any interaction between digoxin and enalapril? *Br J Clin Pharmacol* (1986) 22, 752–3.
10. Harder S, Thürmann PA. Pharmacokinetic and pharmacodynamic interaction trial after repeated oral doses of imidapril and digoxin in healthy volunteers. *Br J Clin Pharmacol* (1997) 43, 475–80.
11. Vandenburg MJ, Kelly JG, Wiseman HT, Mannering D, Long C, Glover DR. The effect of lisinopril on digoxin pharmacokinetics in patients with congestive heart failure. *Br J Clin Pharmacol* (1988) 21, 656P–657P.
12. Vandenburg MJ, Morris F, Marks C, Kelly JG, Dews IM, Stephens JD. A study of the potential pharmacokinetic interaction of lisinopril and digoxin in normal volunteers. *Xenobiotica* (1988) 18, 1179–84.
13. Perdix (Moexipril). Schwarz Pharma Ltd. UK Summary of product characteristics, May 2005.
14. Perdix (Moexipril). Schwarz Pharma. Product Monograph. Data on file, September 1995.
15. Vandenburg MJ, Stephens JD, Resplandy G, Dews IM, Robinson J, Desche P. Digoxin pharmacokinetics and perindopril in heart failure patients. *J Clin Pharmacol* (1993) 33, 146–9.
16. Ferry JJ, Sedman AJ, Hengy H, Vollmer KO, Dunkey A, Klotz U, Colburn WA. Concomitant multiple dose quinapril administration does not alter steady-state pharmacokinetics of digoxin. *Pharm Res* (1987) 4, S98.
17. Kromer EP, Elsner D, Riegger GAJ. Digoxin, converting-enzyme inhibition (quinapril) and the combination in patients with congestive heart failure functional class II and sinus rhythm. *J Cardiovasc Pharmacol* (1990) 16, 9–14.
18. Doering W, Maass L, Irmisch R and König E. Pharmacokinetic interaction study with ramipril and digoxin in healthy volunteers. *Am J Cardiol* (1987) 59, 60D–64D.
19. Johnson BF, Wilson J, Johnson J, Flemming J. Digoxin pharmacokinetics and spirapril, a new ACE inhibitor. *J Clin Pharmacol* (1991) 31, 527–30.
20. New horizons in antihypertensive therapy. Gopten® Trandolapril. Knoll AG, 1992.
21. Gopten (Trandolapril). Abbott Laboratories Ltd. UK Summary of product characteristics, September 2004.
22. Mavik (Trandolapril). Abbott Laboratories. US Prescribing information, July 2003.
23. de Mey C, Elich D, Schroeter V, Butzer R, Belz GG. Captopril does not interact with the pharmacodynamics and pharmacokinetics of digitoxin in healthy man. *Eur J Clin Pharmacol* (1992) 43, 445–7.

Digitalis glycosides + Acipimox

One study suggests that acipimox does not interact with digoxin.

Clinical evidence, mechanism, importance and management

Acipimox 250 mg three times daily for a week was found to have no significant effect on the plasma **digoxin** levels, clinical condition, ECGs, plasma urea or electrolyte levels of 6 elderly patients.[1] No special precautions during concurrent use would seem necessary.

1. Chijioke PC, Pearson RM, Benedetti S. Lack of acipimox-digoxin interaction in patient volunteers. *Hum Exp Toxicol* (1992) 11, 357–9.

Digitalis glycosides + Allopurinol

Allopurinol does not appear to affect serum digoxin levels.

Clinical evidence, mechanism, importance and management

No significant changes in the serum **digoxin** levels of 5 healthy subjects occurred over a 7-day period while they were taking allopurinol 300 mg daily.[1] No additional precautions would appear to be necessary on concurrent use.

1. Havelund T, Abildtrup N, Birkebaek N, Breddam E, Rosager AM. Allopurinols effekt på koncentrationen af digoksin i serum. *Ugeskr Laeger* (1984) 146, 1209–11.

Digitalis glycosides + Alpha blockers

A rapid and marked rise in serum digoxin levels occurred in one study when prazosin was given. Alfuzosin, doxazosin, tamsulosin and terazosin appear not to interact with digoxin.

Clinical evidence, mechanism, importance and management

(a) Alfuzosin

The makers of alfuzosin report that no pharmacodynamic or pharmacokinetic interaction was observed in healthy subjects given alfuzosin with **digoxin**.[1,2]

(b) Doxazosin

Doxazosin is highly bound to plasma proteins (98%), but the maker notes that *in vitro* data in human plasma indicated that doxazosin did not affect the protein binding of **digoxin**.[3,4] Although there appears to be no clinical evidence of an interaction between **digoxin** and doxazosin, an *in vitro* study found that doxazosin inhibited P-glycoprotein-mediated transcellular transport of **digoxin** suggesting an interaction is possible as digoxin renal transport may be inhibited.[5] More study is needed.

(c) Prazosin

Prazosin 2.5 mg twice daily increased the mean steady-state plasma **digoxin** level by 43% from 0.94 to 1.34 nanograms/ml after one day, and by 60% from 0.94 to 1.51 nanograms/ml after 3 days in 20 patients, although the individual response varied from an increase to a decrease, or no effect. Three days after the prazosin was stopped, by which time it would be totally cleared from the body, the serum **digoxin** levels had fallen to their previous values.[6] The reason for this response is not understood. There do not appear to be any other reports in the literature, and the maker notes that, in clinical experience, prazosin has been given with **digoxin** without any adverse drug interaction.[7,8] However, bear this interaction in mind in the case of an unexpected response to treatment.

(d) Tamsulosin

A placebo-controlled study in 10 healthy subjects found that tamsulosin 800 micrograms daily had no effect on the pharmacokinetics of a single intravenous dose of **digoxin** 500 micrograms. The most frequently reported adverse effect was dizziness and the safety profile was considered acceptable.[9] The makers note that dosage adjustments are not necessary when tamsulosin is given with **digoxin**.[10]

(e) Terazosin

The maker of terazosin states that terazosin has been given without interaction with cardiac glycosides.[11]

1. Xatral (Alfuzosin). Sanofi-Aventis. UK Summary of product characteristics, March 2003.
2. Uroxatral (Alfuzosin). Sanofi-Synthelabo Inc. US Prescribing information, June 2003.
3. Cardura (Doxazosin). Pfizer Ltd. UK Summary of product characteristics, May 2003.
4. Cardura (Doxazosin). Pfizer Inc. US Prescribing information, April 2002.
5. Takara K, Kakumoto M, Tanigawara Y, Funakoshi J, Sakaeda T, Okumura K. Interaction of digoxin with antihypertensive drugs *via* MDR1. *Life Sci* (2002) 70, 1491–1500.
6. Çopur S, Tokgözoğlu L, Oto A, Oram E, Uğurlu Ş. Effects of oral prazosin on total plasma digoxin levels. *Fundam Clin Pharmacol* (1988) 2, 13–17.
7. Hypovase (Prazosin). Pfizer Ltd. UK Summary of product characteristics, December 2004.
8. Minipress (Prazosin). Pfizer Inc. US Prescribing information, September 2000.
9. Miyazawa Y, Starkey LP, Forrest A, Schentag JJ, Kamimura H, Swarz H, Ito Y. Effects of the concomitant administration of tamsulosin (0.8 mg) on the pharmacokinetic and safety profile of intravenous digoxin (Lanoxin®) in normal healthy subjects: a placebo-controlled evaluation. *J Clin Pharm Ther* (2002) 27, 13–19.
10. Flomax (Tamsulosin). Boehringer Ingelheim Pharmaceuticals Inc. US Prescribing information, August 2002.
11. Hytrin (Terazosin). Abbott Laboratories Ltd. UK Summary of product characteristics, October 2000.

Digitalis glycosides + Alpha glucosidase inhibitors

Some but not all studies have found that digoxin plasma levels can be markedly reduced by acarbose. Voglibose does not appear to interact adversely with digoxin.

Clinical evidence, mechanism, importance and management

(a) Acarbose

A woman on **digoxin** 250 micrograms daily, insulin, nifedipine, isosorbide dinitrate, clorazepate and nabumetone had subtherapeutic plasma **digoxin** levels of 0.48 to 0.64 nanograms/ml while taking acarbose, even when her **digoxin** dosage was raised by adding 125 micrograms two days of the week. Later, in the absence of acarbose and with the original **digoxin** dosage, her plasma levels were 1.9 nanograms/ml.[1] Two other patients similarly showed markedly reduced plasma **digoxin** levels while taking acarbose. When the acarbose was stopped, the plasma **digoxin** levels rose from 0.23 to 1.6 nanograms/ml and 0.56 to 1.9 nanograms/ml respectively.[2] Another patient with heart failure and type 2 diabetes treated with **digoxin** and voglibose, was found to have subtherapeutic levels of **digoxin** when his treatment was changed from voglibose to acarbose. The serum levels unexpectedly remained subtherapeutic for at least a month when treatment was switched back to voglibose.[3] A pharmacokinetic study in 7 healthy subjects, using either a 200-mg dose of acarbose or pretreatment with 100-mg doses taken three times daily, similarly found that the serum levels and AUC of a single 500-microgram dose of **digoxin** were reduced. Maximum **digoxin** serum levels were reduced by about 30 to 40% and the AUC was reduced by about 40%.[4]

The reasons for this interaction are not understood but a reduction in the absorption of the **digoxin** from the gut has been suggested.[4]

These reports contrast with other studies that found no significant interaction between single-dose **digoxin** and acarbose at therapeutic doses in healthy subjects.[5,6]

Just why there is an inconsistency between these reports is not understood but it would clearly be prudent to consider monitoring **digoxin** levels if both drugs are used, being alert for any evidence of reduced levels.

(b) Voglibose

A randomised, two-way crossover study in 8 healthy subjects taking **digoxin** 250 micrograms daily after breakfast for 8 days found that voglibose 200 micrograms three times daily had no effect on the pharmacokinetics of the **digoxin**.[7] There would therefore appear to be no reason for avoiding concurrent use. No special precautions are needed.

1. Serrano JS, Jiménez CM, Serrano MI, Balboa B. A possible interaction of potential clinical interest between digoxin and acarbose. *Clin Pharmacol Ther* (1996) 60, 589–92.
2. Ben-Ami H, Krivoy N, Nagachandran P, Roguin A, Edoute Y. An interaction between digoxin and acarbose. *Diabetes Care* (1999) 22, 860–1.
3. Nagai Y, Hayakawa T, Abe T, Nomura G. Are there different effects of acarbose and voglibose on serum levels of digoxin in a diabetic patient with congestive heart failure? *Diabetes Care* (2000) 23, 1703.
4. Miura T, Ueno K, Tanaka K, Sugiura Y, Mizutani M, Takatsu F, Takano Y, Shibakawa M. Impairment of absorption of digoxin by acarbose. *J Clin Pharmacol* (1998) 38, 654-7.
5. Cohen E, Almog S, Staruvin D, Garty M. Do therapeutic doses of acarbose alter the pharmacokinetics of digoxin? Isr Med Assoc J. *(2002) 4, 772–5.* (2002) 4, 772–5.
6. Hillebrand I, Graefe KH, Bischoff H, Frank G, Raemsch KD, Berchtold P. Serum digoxin and propranolol levels during acarbose-treatment. *Diabetologia* (1981) 21, 282–3.
7. Kusumoto M, Ueno K, Fujimura Y, Kameda T, Mashimo K, Takeda K, Tatami R, Shibakawa M. Lack of kinetic interaction between digoxin and voglibose. *Eur J Clin Pharmacol* (1999) 55, 79-80.

Digitalis glycosides + Aminoglutethimide

The clearance of digitoxin is markedly increased by aminoglutethimide and a reduction in its effects would be expected.

Clinical evidence, mechanism, importance and management

The clearance of **digitoxin** was increased by 109% in 5 patients who took aminoglutethimide 250 mg four times a day.[1] The likely reason is that aminoglutethimide increases the metabolism of the **digitoxin** by the liver. This increase in clearance would be expected to be clinically important, but this does not appear to have been assessed. Check that patients do not become under-digitalised during concurrent treatment. No interaction would be expected with **digoxin** because it is largely excreted unchanged in the urine and therefore metabolism by the liver has little part to play in its clearance.

1. Lønning PE, Kvinnsland S and Bakke OM. Effect of aminoglutethimide on antipyrine, theophylline and digitoxin disposition in breast cancer. *Clin Pharmacol Ther* (1984) 36, 796–802.

Digitalis glycosides + Aminoglycosides

Serum levels of digoxin can be reduced by the concurrent use of neomycin and increased by gentamicin.

Clinical evidence

(a) Gentamicin

In a study in 12 patients with congestive heart failure treated with **digoxin** 250 micrograms daily, the addition of gentamicin 80 mg intramuscularly twice daily for 7 days was found to increase serum **digoxin** levels by 129%. In a further 12 patients with congestive heart failure and diabetes, gentamicin increased **digoxin** levels more than twofold to 2.56 nanomol/l. However, no symptoms of **digoxin** toxicity were seen. it should be noted that serum creatinine levels were higher in both groups than those in healthy controls even before receiving gentamicin and were further increased after gentamicin.[1]

(b) Neomycin

Neomycin 1 to 3 g orally was found to reduce and delay the absorption of a single 500-microgram dose of **digoxin** in healthy subjects.[2] The AUC was reduced by 41 to 51%. Absorption was affected even when the neomycin was given 3 to 6 hours before the **digoxin**. In a steady-state study, neomycin 2 g given with **digoxin** 250 to 500 micrograms daily reduced the serum concentration of **digoxin** by 8 to 49% (mean 28.2%).[2]

Mechanism

Higher digoxin levels and serum creatinine levels in diabetic compared with non-diabetic patients may be due to differences in renal function,[1] with concurrent gentamicin causing further renal function impairment and even higher digoxin levels. The reduction in digoxin toxicity is not fully understood but changes in ionic transport may be involved. The inhibition by gentamicin of Na^+/K^+ ATPase, which acts as a specific receptor for digoxin, may also be a factor.[1]

Neomycin can cause a general but reversible malabsorption syndrome, which affects the absorption of several drugs. The extent of this is probably offset in some patients, because the neomycin also reduces the breakdown of digoxin by the bacteria in the gut.[3]

Importance and management

Information is limited, but patients should be monitored for increased digoxin effects if gentamicin is given, especially those with diabetes or any other patient with impaired renal function. Initially, checking pulse rate is probably adequate. There seems to be no information about other parenteral aminoglycosides.

Patients should be monitored for reduced digoxin effects if neomycin is given and suitable dosage adjustments made if necessary. Separating the dosages of the two drugs does not prevent this interaction. Other aminoglycosides that can be given orally such as **kanamycin** and **paromomycin** might possibly interact similarly to neomycin, but this requires confirmation.

1. Alkadi HO, Nooman MA, Raja'a YA. Effect of gentamicin on serum digoxin level in patients with congestive heart failure. *Pharm World Sci* (2004) 26, 107–9.
2. Lindenbaum J, Maulitz RM, Butler VP. Inhibition of digoxin absorption by neomycin. *Gastroenterology* (1976) 71, 399–404.
3. Lindenbaum J, Tse-Eng D, Butler VP, Rund DG. Urinary excretion of reduced metabolites of digoxin. *Am J Med* (1981) 71, 67–74.

Digitalis glycosides + 5-Aminosalicylates

Serum digoxin levels can be reduced by sulfasalazine. The makers of balsalazide suggest that there may be an interaction with digoxin.

Clinical evidence, mechanism, importance and management

The observation that a patient taking **sulfasalazine** 8 g daily had low serum **digoxin** levels, prompted a crossover study in 10 healthy subjects who were given **digoxin** syrup 500 micrograms, both alone, and after 6 days of treatment with **sulfasalazine** 2 to 6 g daily. **Digoxin** absorption was reduced, ranging from 0 to 50% depending on the dosage of **sulfasalazine** used.[1] Serum **digoxin** levels were reduced accordingly.[1] The reasons are not understood. This seems to be the only report of this interaction. Concurrent use need not be avoided, but it would be prudent to check for under-digitalisation, initially by checking symptoms and pulse rate, and then taking digoxin levels if an interaction is suspected. In the one patient examined, separating the dosages appeared not to prevent this interaction.[1]

Although no **digoxin/balsalazide** interaction has been reported, the makers of **balsalazide** cautiously suggest the possibility of an interaction.[2] They recommend that plasma levels of **digoxin** should be monitored in digitalised patients starting **balsalazide**.[3]

1. Juhl RP, Summers RW, Guillory JK, Blaug SM, Cheng FH, Brown DD. Effect of sulfasalazine on digoxin bioavailability. *Clin Pharmacol Ther* (1976) 20, 387–94.
2. Colazide (Balsalazide). Shire Pharmaceuticals Ltd. UK Summary of product characteristics, December 2002.
3. Astra Pharmaceuticals. Personal communication, November and December 1997.

Digitalis glycosides + Aminosalicylic acid

Aminosalicylic acid causes a small reduction in digoxin levels in healthy subjects but the importance of this in patients is uncertain.

Clinical evidence, mechanism, importance and management

In one study the bioavailability of a single 750-microgram dose of **digoxin** (using urinary excretion as a measure) was reduced by 20% in 10 healthy subjects who were given aminosalicylic acid 2 g four times daily for 2 weeks.[1] This seems to be just another aspect of the general malabsorption caused by aminosalicylic acid. The importance of this interaction in patients is not known (it is probably small) but it would be prudent to monitor concurrent use.

1. Brown DD, Juhl RP, Warner SL. Decreased bioavailability of digoxin due to hypocholesterolemic interventions. *Circulation* (1978) 58, 164–72.

Digitalis glycosides + Amiodarone

Digoxin levels can be approximately doubled by amiodarone. Some individuals may show even greater increases. Digitalis toxicity will occur if the dosage of digoxin is not reduced appropriately. The same interaction also appears to occur with digitoxin.

Clinical evidence

(a) Digoxin

The observation that patients on digoxin developed digoxin toxicity when given amiodarone[1] prompted a study of this interaction. Seven patients stabilised on digoxin for 14 days showed a mean rise in plasma digoxin levels of 69%, from 1.17 to 1.98 micrograms/l, when given amiodarone 200 mg three times daily. Two other patients similarly treated also showed this interaction.[1]

Numerous studies in large numbers of patients have confirmed this interaction with reported increases in serum digoxin levels of 75%,[2] 90%,[3] 95%[4] and 104%.[5] The occasional patient may show three- to fourfold increases, whereas others may show little or no change.[3,6] Children seem particularly sensitive, with threefold, and even as much as ninefold rises.[7] Other reports confirm that the digoxin levels are markedly increased or roughly doubled, and toxicity can occur.[6,8-15] In contrast, one group of workers state that they observed no change in serum digoxin levels in 5 patients given amiodarone.[16,17] There is also some evidence that in the treatment of resistant atrial tachyarrhythmias the risk of arrhythmias may be increased by concurrent use,[18] and another study found that combined use had an unfavourable effect on survival in patients with atrial fibrillation and sinus rhythm.[19]

(b) Digitoxin

Two elderly patients (aged 77 and 78) taking digitoxin 100 micrograms daily were additionally given loading doses of amiodarone followed by maintenance doses of 200 to 400 mg daily. Within 2 months in one case, and 4 months in the other, they were hospitalised because of bradycardia, dyspnoea, nausea and malaise. One of them had total AV block (38 bpm). The serum digitoxin levels of both of them were found to be elevated (54 and 45 micrograms/l respectively) well above the normal therapeutic range of 9 to 30 micrograms/l. Serum amiodarone and desethylamiodarone levels were normal. Both patients recovered when the digitoxin was stopped.[20]

Mechanism

Not fully understood. Amiodarone reduces both the renal and non-renal excretion of digoxin.[21] P-glycoprotein is involved in the renal tubular secretion of digoxin. An *in vitro* study found that amiodarone (and possibly desethylamiodarone) inhibit P-glycoprotein-mediated transcellular transport of digoxin. This suggests that any interaction may occur, at least in part, by inhibiting digoxin renal tubular secretion.[22] See also 'Drug transporter proteins', (p.8).

Other possible mechanisms that have been suggested include changes in thyroid function,[23] protein-binding displacement[24,25] or increased absorption.[26]

It is thought that amiodarone can also inhibit the metabolism of digitoxin by the liver, which would explain why its serum levels are increased.[20]

Importance and management

The digoxin/amiodarone interaction is well documented, well established and of considerable clinical importance. It occurs in most patients. It is clearly evident after a few days and develops over the course of 1 to 4 weeks.[4] If no account is taken of this interaction the patient may develop digitalis toxicity. Reduce the digoxin dosage by between one-third to one-half when amiodarone is added,[1,2,11,26] with further adjustment of the dosage after a week or two, and possibly a month or more,[11] depending on digoxin levels. Particular care is needed in children, who may show much larger rises in digoxin levels than adults. Amiodarone is excreted very slowly so that the effects of this interaction will persist for several weeks after its withdrawal.[15] Also note that some authors suggest that concurrent use may possibly worsen the prognosis in some patients.[18,19]

Far less is known about the digitoxin/amiodarone interaction but the limited evidence available suggests that all of the precautions appropriate for digoxin should be used for digitoxin as well. Note that the interaction may possibly take months to develop.

1. Moysey JO, Jaggarao NSV, Grundy EN, Chamberlain DA. Amiodarone increases plasma digoxin concentrations. *BMJ* (1981) 282, 272.
2. Fornaro G, Rossi P, Padrini R, Piovan D, Ferrari M, Fortina A, Tomassini G, Aquili C. Ricerca farmacologico-clinica sull'interazione digitale-amiodarone in pazienti cardiopatici con insufficiencza cardiaca di vario grado. *G Ital Cardiol* (1984) 14, 990–8.
3. Oetgen WJ, Sobol SM, Tri TB, Heydorn WH, Rakita L. Amiodarone-digoxin interaction. Clinical and experimental observations. *Chest* (1984) 86, 75–9.
4. Vitale P, Jacono A, Gonzales y Reyero E, Zeuli L. Effect of amiodarone on serum digoxin levels in patients with atrial fibrillation. *Clin Trials J* (1984) 21, 199–206.
5. Nademanee K, Kannan R, Hendrickson J, Ookhtens M, Kay I, Singh BN. Amiodarone-digoxin interaction: clinical significance, time course of development, potential pharmacokinetic mechanisms and therapeutic implications. *J Am Coll Cardiol* (1984) 4, 111–16.
6. Nager G, Nager F. Interaktion zwischen Amiodaron und Digoxin. *Schweiz Med Wochenschr* (1983) 113, 1727–30.
7. Koren G, Hesslein PS, MacLeod SM. Digoxin toxicity associated with amiodarone therapy in children. *J Pediatr* (1984) 104, 467–70.
8. Nademanee K, Kannan R, Hendrickson JA, Burnam M, Kay I, Singh B. Amiodarone-digoxin interaction during treatment of resistant cardiac arrhythmias. *Am J Cardiol* (1982) 49, 1026.
9. McQueen EG. New Zealand Committee on Adverse Drug Reactions. 17th Annual Report 1982. *N Z Med J* (1983) 96, 95–9.
10. McGovern B, Garan H, Kelly E, Ruskin JN. Adverse reactions during treatment with amiodarone hydrochloride. *BMJ* (1983) 287, 175–80.
11. Marcus FI, Fenster PE. Drug therapy. Digoxin interactions with other cardiac drugs. *J Cardiovasc Med* (1983) 8, 25–8.
12. Strocchi E, Malini PL, Graziani A, Ambrosioni E, Magnani B. L'interazione tra digossina ed amiodarone. *G Ital Cardiol* (1984) 14, 12–15.
13. Robinson KC, Walker S, Johnston A, Mulrow JP, McKenna WJ, Holt DW. The digoxin-amiodarone interaction. *Circulation* (1986) 74, II-225.
14. Johnston A, Walker S, Robinson KC, McKenna WJ and Holt DW. The digoxin-amiodarone interaction. *Br J Clin Pharmacol* (1987) 24, 253P.
15. Robinson K, Johnston A, Walker S, Mulrow JP, McKenna WJ, Holt DW. The digoxin-amiodarone interaction. *Cardiovasc Drugs Ther* (1989) 3, 25–28.
16. Achilli A, Serra N. Amiodarone increases plasma digoxin concentrations. *BMJ* (1981) 282, 1630.
17. Achilli A, Giacci M, Capezzuto A, de Luca F, Guerra R, Serra N. Interazione digossina-chinidina e digossina-amiodarone. *G Ital Cardiol* (1981) 11, 918–25.
18. Bajaj BP, Baig MW, Perrins EJ. Amiodarone-induced torsades de pointes: the possible facilitatory role of digoxin. *Int J Cardiol* (1991) 33, 335–8.
19. Mortara A, Cioffi G, Opasich C, Pozzoli M, Febo O, Riccardi G, Cobelli F, Tavazzi L. Combination of amiodarone plus digoxin in chronic heart failure: an adverse effect on survival independently of the presence of sinus rhythm or atrial fibrillation. *Circulation* (1996) 94 (8 Suppl), I-21.
20. Läer S, Scholz H, Buschmann I, Thoenes M, Meinertz T. Digitoxin intoxication during concomitant use of amiodarone. *Eur J Clin Pharmacol* (1998) 54, 95–6.
21. Fenster PE, White NW, Hanson CD. Pharmacokinetic evaluation of the digoxin-amiodarone interaction. *J Am Coll Cardiol* (1985) 5, 108–12.
22. Kakumoto M, Takara K, Sakaeda T, Tanigawara Y, Kita T, Okumura K. MDR1-mediated interaction of digoxin with antiarrhythmic or antianginal drugs. *Biol Pharm Bull* (2002) 25, 1604–7.
23. Ben-Chetrit E, Ackerman Z, Eliakim M. Case-report: Amiodarone-associated hypothyroidism — a possible cause of digoxin intoxication. *Am J Med Sci* (1985) 289, 114–16.
24. Douste-Blazy Ph, Montastruc JL, Bonnet B, Auriol P, Conte D, Bernadet P. Influence of amiodarone on plasma and urine digoxin concentrations. *Lancet* (1984) i, 905.
25. Mingardi G. Amiodarone and plasma digoxin levels. *Lancet* (1984) i, 1238.
26. Santostasi G, Fantin M, Maragno I, Gaion RM, Basadonna O, Dalla-Volta S. Effects of amiodarone on oral and intravenous digoxin kinetics in healthy subjects. *J Cardiovasc Pharmacol* (1987) 9, 385–90.

Digitalis glycosides + Angiotensin II receptor antagonists

Candesartan, eprosartan, irbesartan, losartan, and valsartan appear not to interact with digoxin but telmisartan may cause a rise in serum digoxin levels.

Clinical evidence

(a) Candesartan

There was no pharmacokinetic interaction between candesartan 16 mg daily and **digoxin** given as a loading dose of 750 micrograms then 250 micrograms daily in 12 healthy subjects.[1]

(b) Eprosartan

A study in 12 healthy men given single 600-microgram doses of **digoxin** found that eprosartan 200 mg 12-hourly for 4 days had no significant effect on the **digoxin** pharmacokinetics.[2]

(c) Irbesartan

A study in 10 healthy subjects taking **digoxin** for 2 weeks showed no changes in the AUC or maximum serum levels of the **digoxin** during the second week while also taking irbesartan 150 mg daily.[3]

(d) Losartan

The pharmacokinetics of **digoxin** were found to be unaltered when 13 healthy subjects were given a single 500-microgram oral or intravenous dose of **digoxin** before and after taking losartan 50 mg daily for a week.[4]

(e) Telmisartan

A study in 12 healthy subjects given a 500-microgram loading dose of **digoxin** followed by 250 micrograms daily found that the maximum serum concentration, the trough serum concentration and AUC were increased by 50, 13 and 22% respectively when telmisartan 120 mg daily was given for 7 days.[5] No clinically relevant changes in vital signs or ECGs were noted.

(f) Valsartan

There was no adverse interaction between a single 160-mg dose of valsartan and **digoxin** 250 micrograms in a study in 12 healthy subjects.[6]

Mechanism

It has been suggested that telmisartan may have caused digoxin to be more rapidly absorbed.[5] An *in vitro* study found that candesartan and losartan do not appear to inhibit P-glycoprotein-mediated transcellular transport. Therefore interactions resulting in reduced digoxin renal excretion are unlikely.[7]

Importance and management

No special precautions seem to be necessary when digoxin is used with candesartan, eprosartan, irbesartan, losartan, or valsartan. However, note that information for eprosartan, losartan, and valsartan is from single-dose studies, although the authors of the eprosartan study consider that a clinically relevant interaction with multiple doses of digoxin is unlikely.[2] The small increase in trough serum digoxin level with telmisartan suggests that the dose of digoxin need not automatically be reduced when telmisartan is started, but consideration should be given to monitoring digoxin levels.

1. Jonkman JH, van Lier JJ, van Heiningen PN, Lins R, Sennewald R, Hogemann A. Pharmacokinetic drug interaction studies with candesartan cilexetil. *J Hum Hypertens* (1997) 11 (Suppl 2), S31–S35.
2. Martin DE, Tompson D, Boike SC, Tenero D, Ilson B, Citerone D, Jorkasky DK. Lack of effect of eprosartan on the single dose pharmacokinetics of orally administered digoxin in healthy male volunteers. *Br J Clin Pharmacol* (1997) 43, 661–4.
3. Marino MR, Vachharajani NN. Drug interactions with irbesartan. *Clin Pharmacokinet* (2001) 40, 605–14.
4. De Smet M, Schoors DF, De Meyer G, Verbesselt R, Goldberg MR, Fitzpatrick V, Somers G. Effect of multiple doses of losartan on the pharmacokinetics of single doses of digoxin in healthy volunteers. *Br J Clin Pharmacol* (1995) 40, 571–5.
5. Stangier J, Su C-APF, Hendricks MGC, van Lier JJ, Sollie FAE, Oosterhuis B, Jonkman JHG. The effect of telmisartan on the steady-state pharmacokinetics of digoxin in healthy male volunteers. *J Clin Pharmacol* (2000) 40, 1373–9.
6. Ciba Laboratories. Data on file, Protocols 07, 36–40, 42, 43, 52.
7. Takara K, Kakumoto M, Tanigawara Y, Funakoshi J, Sakaeda T, Okumura K. Interaction of digoxin with antihypertensive drugs *via* MDR1. *Life Sci* (2002) 70, 1491–1500.

Digitalis glycosides + Antacids

Although some studies suggest that antacids can reduce the bioavailability of digoxin and digitoxin, there is other evidence suggesting that no clinically relevant interactions occur.

Clinical evidence

(a) Digoxin

(i) Evidence of an interaction. A study in 10 healthy subjects given digoxin 750 micrograms with 60 ml of either 4% **aluminium hydroxide gel**, 8% **magnesium hydroxide gel** or **magnesium trisilicate** showed that the cumulative 6-day urinary excretion, expressed as a percentage of the original dose, was: control 40%; **aluminium hydroxide** 31%; **magnesium hydroxide** 27%; **magnesium trisilicate** 29%.[1]
Other studies describe reductions in digoxin absorption of 11% with **aluminium hydroxide**, 15% with **bismuth carbonate** and **light magnesium carbonate**, and 99.5% with **magnesium trisilicate**.[2]
When digoxin was given with 30 ml of an **aluminium/magnesium hydroxide** antacid and mexiletine, the digoxin AUC was approximately halved. As 'mexiletine', (p.704) does not appear to interact with digoxin the interaction was attributed to the antacid.[3]

(ii) Evidence of no interaction. A study in 4 patients chronically treated with digoxin 250 to 500 micrograms daily, showed that concurrent treatment with either 10 ml of **aluminium hydroxide mixture BP** or **magnesium trisilicate mixture BP**, three times daily, did not reduce the bioavailability of the digoxin and none of the patients showed any reduction in the control of their symptoms.[4]
Other bioavailability studies have not found a significant interaction between digoxin capsules and **aluminium/magnesium hydroxide**.[5]

(b) Other cardiac glycosides

In vitro studies with **digitoxin** suggest that it might possibly interact like digoxin and be absorbed by various antacids[6] but **lanatoside C** probably does not interact.[7] Bioavailability studies have not found a significant interaction between **beta-acetyldigoxin** and **aluminium/magnesium hydroxide**.[8]

A study in 10 patients with heart failure showed that their steady-state serum **digitoxin** levels were slightly, but not significantly raised (from 13.6 to 15.1 nanograms/ml) while taking 20 ml of **aluminium/magnesium hydroxide** gel three or four times daily, separated from the **digitoxin** dosage by at least 1 to 2 hours.[9]

Mechanism

Not established. One suggestion is that the digoxin can become adsorbed onto the antacids and therefore unavailable for absorption.[1,6] This is probably also true for digitoxin. However, some results are not consistent with this idea.

Importance and management

The digoxin/antacid and digitoxin/antacid interactions are only moderately well documented, and the evidence is inconsistent. No clearly clinically relevant interactions have been reported. Separating the dosages by 1 to 2 hours to minimise admixture is effective with many other drugs that interact in the gut, and seems to work with digitoxin. However, unless further information becomes available it seems unlikely that separating administration is necessary, although it may be worth bearing in mind if, on rare occasions, a patient experiences an interaction.

1. Brown DD, Juhl RP, Lewis K, Schrott M, Bartels B. Decreased bioavailability of digoxin due to antacids and kaolin-pectin. *N Engl J Med* (1976) 295, 1034–7.
2. McElnay JC, Harron DWG, D'Arcy PF, Eagle MRG. Interaction of digoxin with antacid constituents. *BMJ* (1978) i, 1554.
3. Saris SD, Lowenthal DT, Affrime MB. Steady-state digoxin concentration during oral mexiletine administration. *Curr Ther Res* (1983) 34, 662–66.
4. Cooke J, Smith JA. Absence of interaction of digoxin with antacids under clinical conditions. *BMJ* (1978) 2, 1166.
5. Allen MD, Greenblatt DJ, Harmatz JS, Smith TW. Effect of magnesium-aluminum hydroxide and kaolin-pectin on the absorption of digoxin from tablets and capsules. *J Clin Pharmacol* (1981) 21, 26–30.
6. Khalil SAH. The uptake of digoxin and digitoxin by some antacids. *J Pharm Pharmacol* (1974) 26, 961–7.
7. Aldous S, Thomas R. Absorption and metabolism of lanatoside C. *Clin Pharmacol Ther* (1977) 21, 647–58.
8. Bonelli J, Hruby K, Magometschnigg D, Hitzenberger G, Kaik G. The bioavailability of β-acetyldigoxine alone and combined with aluminium hydroxide and magnesium hydroxide (Alucol®). *Int J Clin Pharmacol* (1977) 15, 337–9.
9. Kuhlmann J. Plasmaspiegel und renale Elimination von Digitoxin bei Langzeittherapie mit Aluminium-Magnesium-Hydroxid-Gel. *Dtsch Med Wochenschr* (1984) 109, 59–61.

Digitalis glycosides + Anticholinesterases; Centrally acting

There is no pharmacokinetic interaction between digoxin and tacrine. The bradycardic effects of anticholinesterases and digoxin may possibly be additive.

Clinical evidence, mechanism, importance and management

A single-dose study in 12 healthy subjects found that the pharmacokinetics of **donepezil** 5 mg and **digoxin** 250 micrograms were not affected by concurrent use and no clinically relevant changes in cardiac conduction parameters occurred.[1]

In one study in healthy subjects given a single 500-microgram dose of **digoxin**, the pharmacokinetics of the **digoxin** were unchanged in those patients also taking **tacrine** 20 mg 6-hourly.[2] Although no special precautions would seem necessary on a pharmacokinetic basis, check to see that the combined bradycardic effects of **digoxin** and **tacrine** do not become excessive.

Similarly, the makers of **galantamine**[3] say that no pharmacokinetic interactions have been seen with **digoxin**, but caution about the possibility of a pharmacodynamic interaction that may result in bradycardia. The makers of **rivastigmine**[4] say that the combination has no pharmacokinetic interaction, nor does it interfere with cardiac conduction. It would however seem prudent to monitor heart rate if any of these combinations are used.

1. Tiseo PJ, Perdomo CA, Friedhoff LT. Concurrent administration of donepezil HCl and digoxin: assessment of pharmacokinetic changes. *Br J Clin Pharmacol* (1998) 46 (Suppl 1), 40–4.
2. deVries TM, Siedlik P, Smithers JA, Brown RR, Reece PA, Posvar EL, Sedman AJ, Koup JR, Forgue ST. Effect of multiple-dose tacrine administration on single-dose pharmacokinetics of digoxin, diazepam, and theophylline. *Pharm Res* (1993) 10 (10 Suppl), S-333.
3. Reminyl (Galantamine hydrobromide). Shire Pharmaceuticals Ltd. UK Summary of product characteristics, November 2004.
4. Exelon (Rivastigmine). Novartis Pharmaceuticals UK Ltd. UK Summary of product characteristics, June 2003.

Digitalis glycosides + Anticonvulsants; Miscellaneous

Carbamazepine does not appear to interact significantly with digoxin, and topiramate causes only a small reduction in digoxin serum levels. Levetiracetam and tiagabine do not appear to interact with digoxin. See also 'Digitalis glycosides + Anticonvulsants; Phenytoin', p.686.

Clinical evidence, mechanism, importance and management

(a) Carbamazepine

Bradycardia seen in 3 patients on **digitalis** and carbamazepine was tentatively attributed to their concurrent use,[1] but as yet this has not been confirmed by other observations.

(b) Levetiracetam

In a double-blind, crossover, placebo-controlled study 11 healthy subjects were given an initial loading dose of **digoxin** 500 micrograms followed by

250 micrograms daily with levetiracetam 1 g twice daily for one week. Levetiracetam did not significantly affect the pharmacokinetics or pharmacodynamics of **digoxin**, and the pharmacokinetics of levetiracetam were not significantly altered by **digoxin**.[2] No additional precautions seem necessary on concurrent use.

(c) Tiagabine

In an open-label, crossover study, 13 healthy subjects were given a loading dose of **digoxin** 500 micrograms twice daily for one day then 250 micrograms daily for 8 days, either alone or with tiagabine 4 mg three times daily for 9 days. It was found that the pharmacokinetics of **digoxin** were not significantly altered by tiagabine.[3]

(d) Topiramate

Topiramate 100 mg twice daily for 9 days caused a small reduction in the serum **digoxin** levels of 12 healthy subjects.[4,5] The maximum serum levels and the AUC were reduced by 15.8% and 12% respectively, and the oral **digoxin** clearance was increased by 13%.[5] The makers suggest good monitoring of **digoxin** if topiramate is added or withdrawn,[5] but changes in the pharmacokinetics of **digoxin** of this magnitude seem unlikely to be clinically relevant in most patients.

See also 'Digitalis glycosides + Anticonvulsants; Phenytoin', p.686.

1. Killian JM, Fromm GH. Carbamazepine in the treatment of neuralgia. Use and side effects. *Arch Neurol* (1968) 19, 129–36.
2. Levy RH, Ragueneau-Majlessi I, Baltes E. Repeated administration of the novel antiepileptic agent levetiracetam does not alter digoxin pharmacokinetics and pharmacodynamics in healthy volunteers. *Epilepsia* (2000) 41 (Suppl 7), 227–8.
3. Snel S, Jansen JA, Pedersen PC, Jonkman JHG, van Heiningen PNM. Tiagabine, a novel antiepileptic agent: lack of pharmacokinetic interaction with digoxin. *Eur J Clin Pharmacol* (1998) 54, 355–7.
4. Liao S, Palmer M. Digoxin and topiramate drug interaction study in male volunteers. *Pharm Res* (1993) 10 (10 Suppl), S405.
5. Topamax (Topiramate). Janssen-Cilag Ltd. UK Summary of product characteristics, August 2004.

Digitalis glycosides + Anticonvulsants; Phenytoin

Phenytoin reduces serum digoxin levels and digitoxin levels. Cases of bradycardia have been seen in digitalised patients given phenytoin. Phenytoin was formerly used for the treatment of digitalis-induced cardiac arrhythmias, but sudden cardiac arrest has been reported.

Clinical evidence

(a) Bradycardia and cardiac arrest

A patient with suspected digitalis-induced cardiac arrhythmias developed bradycardia, then became asystolic and died, following the intravenous injection of phenytoin.[1] The discussion of this case briefly mentions a further 6 fatalities in patients similarly treated.[1] A patient with Down's syndrome and mitral valve insufficiency taking **digoxin** 250 micrograms daily developed bradycardia of 34 bpm and complete heart block when his phenytoin dose was increased from 200 to 300 mg daily.[2]

(b) Reduced serum digoxin levels

A study in 6 healthy subjects given **β-acetyldigoxin** 400 micrograms daily found that the half-life of digoxin was reduced by 30% (from 33.9 to 23.7 hours) and the AUC was reduced by 23% after they took phenytoin 200 mg twice daily for a week. Total digoxin clearance increased by 27% (from 258.6 to 328.3 ml/minute).[3]

(c) Reduced plasma digitoxin levels

The plasma digitoxin levels of a man fell on 3 occasions when he was given phenytoin. On the third occasion while taking digitoxin 200 micrograms daily, the addition of phenytoin 900 mg daily caused a 60% fall (from 25 to 10 nanograms/ml) in digitoxin levels over a 7 to 10 day period.[4]

Mechanism

Phenytoin has a stabilising effect on the myocardial cells so that the toxic threshold of digoxin at which arrhythmias occur is raised. However, the bradycardic effects of the digitalis glycoside are not opposed and the lethal dose is unaltered, so that the cardiac arrest reported would appear to be the result of excessive bradycardia. It seems possible that the fall in plasma digitoxin levels may be due to a phenytoin-induced increase in the metabolism of the digitoxin by the liver.[5]

Importance and management

Phenytoin was formerly used for treating digitalis-induced arrhythmias, but this use now appears to be obsolete. Intravenous phenytoin should not be used in patients with a high degree of heart block or marked bradycardia because of the risk that cardiac arrest may occur. Information about the effects of phenytoin on digitalis glycoside levels seems to be confined to these single reports, but it would now be prudent to check that patients on digoxin or digitoxin who are subsequently given phenytoin do not become under-digitalised.

1. Zoneraich S, Zoneraich O, Siegel J. Sudden death following intravenous sodium diphenylhydantoin. *Am Heart J* (1976) 91, 375–7.
2. Viukari NMA, Aho K. Digoxin-phenytoin interaction. *BMJ* (1970) 2, 51.
3. Rameis H. On the interaction between phenytoin and digoxin. *Eur J Clin Pharmacol* (1985) 29, 49–53.
4. Solomon HM, Reich S, Spirt N, Abrams WB. Interactions between digitoxin and other drugs *in vitro* and *in vivo*. *Ann N Y Acad Sci* (1971) 179, 362–9.
5. Rameis H. The importance of prospective planning of pharmacokinetic trials. Considerations of studies on the phenytoin-digoxin-(P-D) and phenytoin-digitoxin-(P-DT) interaction. *Int J Clin Pharmacol Ther Toxicol* (1992) 30, 528–9.

Digitalis glycosides + Antineoplastics

Treatment with radiation and/or antineoplastic cytotoxics can damage the lining of the intestine so that digoxin is much less readily absorbed when given in tablet form. This appears to be resolved by giving the digoxin in liquid or liquid-in-capsule form, or by substituting digitoxin.

Clinical evidence

A study in 13 patients with various forms of neoplastic disease showed that radiation therapy and/or various high-dose cytotoxic regimens (including **carmustine**, **cyclophosphamide**, **melphalan**, **cytarabine** and **methotrexate**) reduced the absorption of **digoxin** from tablets (*Lanoxin*) by almost 46%, but the reduction was not significant (15%) when the **digoxin** was given as capsules (*Lanoxicaps*).[1]

Other studies confirm that a 50% reduction in serum **digoxin** levels (using **β-acetyldigoxin**) occurred in patients given **cyclophosphamide**, **vincristine**, **procarbazine** and prednisone (COPP); **cyclophosphamide**, **vincristine** and prednisone (COP); **cyclophosphamide**, **vincristine**, **cytarabine** and prednisone (COAP); and **doxorubicin**, **bleomycin** and prednisone (ABP). These effects disappeared about a week after cytotoxic therapy finished.[2] Radiation has a smaller effect.[3] **Digitoxin** absorption does not seem to be affected by antineoplastics.[4]

Mechanism

The reduced absorption is thought to result from damage to the intestinal epithelium caused by the antineoplastic cytotoxics.[5]

Importance and management

The interaction appears to be established. Patients on digoxin and receiving treatment with antineoplastic cytotoxics should be monitored for signs of under-digitalisation. The problem can be overcome by replacing digoxin tablets with digoxin in liquid form or in solution inside a capsule. The effects of the interaction are short-lived so that a downward readjustment may be necessary about a week after treatment is withdrawn. An alternative is to use digitoxin, which does not appear to be affected.

1. Bjornsson TD, Huang AT, Roth P, Jacob DS, Christenson R. Effects of high-dose cancer chemotherapy on the absorption of digoxin in two different formulations. *Clin Pharmacol Ther* (1986) 39, 25–8.
2. Kuhlmann J, Zilly W, Wilke J. Effects of cytostatic drugs on plasma levels and renal excretion of β-acetyldigoxin. *Clin Pharmacol Ther* (1981) 30, 518–27.
3. Sokol GH, Greenblatt DJ, Lloyd BL, Georgotas A, Allen MD, Harmatz JS, Smith TW, Shader RI. Effect of abdominal radiation therapy on drug absorption in humans. *J Clin Pharmacol* (1978) 18, 388–96.
4. Kuhlmann J, Wilke J, Rietbrock N. Cytostatic drugs are without significant effect on digitoxin plasma level and renal excretion. *Clin Pharmacol Ther* (1982) 32, 646–51.
5. Jusko WB, Conti DR, Molson A, Kuritzky P, Giller J, Schultz R. Digoxin absorption from tablets and elixir: the effect of radiation-induced malabsorption. *JAMA* (1974) 230, 1554–5.

Digitalis glycosides + Aprepitant

Aprepitant does not affect the pharmacokinetics of digoxin.

Clinical evidence, mechanism, importance and management

A double-blind, placebo-controlled, randomised, crossover study in 11 healthy subjects found that the pharmacokinetics of **digoxin** 250 micrograms daily was not affected by aprepitant 125 mg given on day 7 and 80 mg given daily on days 8 to 11. *In vitro* evidence indicates that aprepitant is a substrate and weak inhibitor of P-glycoprotein. However, at the doses used for the prevention of chemotherapy-induced nausea and vomiting, it appears unlikely to interact with P-glycoprotein substrates such as **digoxin**.[1]

1. Feuring M, Lee Y, Orlowski LH, Michiels N, De Smet M, Majumdar AK, Petty KJ, Goldberg MR, Murphy MG, Gottesdiener KM, Hesney M, Brackett LE, Wehling M. Lack of effect of aprepitant on digoxin pharmacokinetics in healthy subjects. *J Clin Pharmacol* (2003) 43, 912–17.

Digitalis glycosides + Argatroban

No significant pharmacokinetic interaction occurs between digoxin and argatroban.

Clinical evidence, mechanism, importance and management

A placebo-controlled, crossover study in 12 healthy subjects found that the pharmacokinetics of steady-state **digoxin** 375 micrograms daily were not affected by an infusion of argatroban 2 micrograms/kg per minute for 120 hours. Steady-state argatroban levels were obtained within 3 hours and maintained throughout the infusion. Dosage adjustments should not be necessary during concurrent use.[1]

1. Inglis AML, Sheth SB, Hursting MJ, Tenero DM, Graham AM, DiCicco RA. Investigation of the interaction between argatroban and acetaminophen, lidocaine, or digoxin. *Am J Health-Syst Pharm* (2002) 59, 1258–66.

Digitalis glycosides + Aspirin

Aspirin may cause a moderate rise in serum digoxin levels, but no interaction of clinical relevance seems to occur.

Clinical evidence, mechanism, importance and management

Although aspirin can double the serum concentrations of **digoxin** in *dogs*, a study in 8 healthy subjects found no interaction, even when high doses (975 mg three times daily) were given.[1] However, in another study in 9 healthy subjects given aspirin 1.5 g daily for 10 days increased the serum **digoxin** levels by 31%.[2] Bearing in mind that both drugs have been in use for a very considerable number of years, the lack of reports in the literature describing problems suggests that no clinically important interaction normally occurs.

1. Fenster PE, Comess KA, Hanson CD and Finley PR. Kinetics of digoxin-aspirin combination. *Clin Pharmacol Ther* (1982) 32, 428–30.
2. Isbary J, Doering W, König E.Der Einfluβ von Tiaprofensäure auf die Digoxinkonzentration im Serum (DKS) im Vergleich zu anderen Antirheumatika (AR). *Z Rheumatol* (1982) 41, 164.

Digitalis glycosides + Barbiturates

Blood levels of digitoxin can be halved by the concurrent use of phenobarbital. Its effects may be expected to be reduced accordingly. However, another study found that phenobarbital did not affect digitoxin, digoxin or beta-acetyldigoxin pharmacokinetics.

Clinical evidence

Phenobarbital 60 mg three times daily for 12 weeks, halved the steady-state plasma levels of **digitoxin** 100 micrograms daily.[1] In associated studies the half-life of **digitoxin** decreased from 7.8 to 4.5 days during **phenobarbital** treatment.[1] In another study[2] the rate of conversion of **digitoxin** to digoxin increased from 4% to 27% in one patient who took **phenobarbital** 96 mg daily for 13 days.

In contrast, a study in groups of 10 healthy subjects given either **digitoxin** 400 micrograms, **digoxin** 1000 micrograms or **acetyldigitoxin** 800 micrograms daily did not find any changes in the serum concentrations of any of these glycosides when **phenobarbital** 100 mg was given three times daily for 7 to 9 days.[3]

Mechanism

Phenobarbital and other barbiturates are well-known potent liver enzyme inducing agents which, it would seem, can increase the metabolism and conversion of digitoxin to digoxin.[1,2] The lack of interaction in one study may possibly have been because the barbiturate was taken for a relatively short time.[3]

Importance and management

An established interaction, although its clinical importance is somewhat uncertain because there seem to be few reports of the effects of using digitoxin with phenobarbital, or of problems in practice. Nevertheless, patients taking both drugs should be monitored for expected under-digitalisation and the dosage of digitoxin increased if necessary. It seems likely that digoxin itself will not be affected by the barbiturates because it is largely excreted unchanged in the urine. Other barbiturates would be expected to behave like phenobarbital.

1. Solomon HM, Abrams WB. Interactions between digitoxin and other drugs in man. *Am Heart J* (1972) 83, 277–80.
2. Jelliffe RW, Blankenhorn DH. Effect of phenobarbital on digitoxin metabolism. *Clin Res* (1966) 14, 160.
3. Káldor A, Somogyi G, Debreczeni LA, Gachályi B. Interaction of heart glycosides and phenobarbital. *Int J Clin Pharmacol* (1975) 12, 403–7.

Digitalis glycosides + Benzodiazepines and related drugs

Digoxin toxicity occurred in two elderly patients and rises in serum digoxin levels have been seen in others when they were given alprazolam. A reduction in the urinary clearance of digoxin has been described during the use of diazepam, but no interaction seems to occur with metaclazepam, zaleplon or zolpidem.

Clinical evidence

(a) Alprazolam

An elderly woman on **digoxin**, maprotiline, isosorbide dinitrate, furosemide and potassium chloride showed signs of **digoxin** toxicity during the second week of taking alprazolam 1 mg daily. Her serum **digoxin** levels were later found to have risen almost 300%, from 1.6 to 4.3 nanograms/ml, and her apparent digoxin clearance had fallen from 126.3 to 49.8 l/day.[1] A later study in 12 patients confirmed that **digoxin** levels can be significantly raised by alprazolam, particularly in those over 65-years-old. One elderly man developed clinical **digoxin** toxicity.[2] In contrast, a two-way crossover study in 8 healthy subjects found no changes in the clearance of **digoxin** after they took alprazolam 1.5 mg daily.[3]

(b) Diazepam

The observation that 3 patients developed raised **digoxin** levels while also taking diazepam prompted a further study in 7 healthy subjects.[4] After taking diazepam 5 mg with a single 500-microgram dose of **digoxin**, and another diazepam 5 mg 12 hours later, all of them had a substantial reduction in urinary excretion and 5 of them showed a moderate increase in the **digoxin** half-life. No further details were given.[4]

(c) Metaclazepam

No statistically significant interaction was seen in 9 patients on **β-acetyldigoxin** when they were given metaclazepam.[5]

(d) Zaleplon

Zaleplon 10 mg daily given to 20 healthy subjects for 5 days had no significant effects on the steady-state pharmacokinetics of **digoxin** 375 micrograms daily. There were no significant differences in QTc or PR intervals.[6]

(e) Zolpidem

No significant pharmacokinetic interaction occurs between zolpidem and **digoxin**.[7]

Mechanism

Uncertain. The suggestion is that diazepam may possibly alter the extent of the protein binding of digoxin within the plasma, which may have some influence on the renal tubular excretion,[4] but see comments on protein binding interactions in 'Drug distribution interactions', (p.3). The reason for the digoxin/alprazolam interaction is not understood.

Importance and management

The digoxin/alprazolam interaction is established and clinically important. Monitor the effects of digoxin (e.g. bradycardia) in any patient if alprazolam is added and reduce the digoxin dosage as necessary. What is known suggests that toxicity is more likely in those over 65-years-old. Other benzodiazepines and digoxin have been used for a considerable time but there seem to be no other reports of adverse interactions.

1. Tollefson G, Lesar T, Grothe D, Garvey M. Alprazolam-related digoxin toxicity. *Am J Psychiatry* (1984) 141, 1612–14.
2. Guven H, Tuncok Y, Guneri S, Cavdar C, Fowler J. Age-related digoxin-alprazolam interaction. *Clin Pharmacol Ther* (1993) 54, 42–4.
3. Ochs HR, Greenblatt DJ, Verburg-Ochs B. Effect of alprazolam on digoxin kinetics and creatinine clearance. *Clin Pharmacol Ther* (1985) 38, 595–8.
4. Castillo-Ferrando JR, Garcia M, Carmona J. Digoxin levels and diazepam. *Lancet* (1980) ii, 368.
5. Völker D, Müller R, Günther C, Bode R. Digoxin-Plasmaspiegel während der Behandlung mit Metaclazepam. *Arzneimittelforschung* (1988) 38, 923–5.
6. Sanchez Garcia P, Paty I, Leister CA, Guerra P, Frías J, García Pérez LE, Darwish M. Effect of zaleplon on digoxin pharmacokinetics and pharmacodynamics. *Am J Health-Syst Pharm* (2000) 57, 2267–70.
7. Salvà P, Costa J. Clinical pharmacokinetics and pharmacodynamics of zolpidem: therapeutic implications. *Clin Pharmacokinet* (1995) 29, 142–53.

Digitalis glycosides + Beta-agonist bronchodilators

Oral salbutamol (albuterol) causes a small reduction in serum digoxin levels. Beta-agonists can cause hypokalaemia, which could lead to the development of digitalis toxicity.

Clinical evidence, mechanism, importance and management

A study in 10 healthy subjects who had taken **digoxin** 500 micrograms daily for 10 days[1] found that 3 hours after taking 3 to 4 mg of oral **salbutamol** (albuterol) their serum **digoxin** levels had fallen by 0.3 nanomol/l and their serum potassium levels had fallen by 0.58 millimol/l. A follow-up study suggested that the **digoxin** distribution to skeletal muscle may have been increased.[2]

Note that all beta-agonists can cause a fall in serum potassium, which could possibly affect the response of patients to **digoxin**. The clinical importance of these changes is uncertain but concurrent use should be monitored. Consider taking potassium levels if the effects of **digoxin** seem excessive.

1. Edner M, Jogestrand T. Oral salbutamol decreases serum digoxin concentration. *Eur J Clin Pharmacol* (1990) 38, 195–7.
2. Edner M, Jogestrand T, Dahlqvist R. Effect of salbutamol on digoxin pharmacokinetics. *Eur J Clin Pharmacol* (1992) 42, 197–201.

Digitalis glycosides + Beta-blockers

In general digoxin and beta-blockers appear not to interact, however there is always the risk of additive bradycardia. A few cases of excessive bradycardia have been reported when propranolol was used to control digitalis-induced arrhythmias. Talinolol and carvedilol appear to increase the bioavailability of digoxin. Digoxin dose reductions may be required in children given carvedilol.

Clinical evidence

(a) Pharmacokinetic interactions

In healthy subjects given a single 500-micrograms dose of **digoxin**, **talinolol** 100 mg orally substantially increased the bioavailability of **digoxin**. The 0 to 72-hour AUC and the maximum serum levels of **digoxin** were increased by 23 and 45% respectively.[1] Conversely, intravenous **talinolol** 30 mg had no effect on **digoxin** pharmacokinetics.[1]

A 12-year-old boy with dilated cardiomyopathy treated with **digoxin** 250 micrograms in the morning and 125 micrograms in the evening was subsequently given **carvedilol** 70 micrograms/kg twice daily. Several days later he became anorexic and started vomiting and his **digoxin** serum level was found to have increased from 2 to 3 nanomol/l up to 5.4 nanomol/l. **Digoxin** was stopped and subsequently restarted at half the original dose.[2] In one study, 8 children aged 2 weeks to 8 years were given **digoxin** for ventricular failure secondary to congenital heart disease. When they were also given **carvedilol** 0.06 to 1.06 mg/kg daily the clearance of **digoxin** was approximately halved and 2 children experienced **digoxin** toxicity.[2]

A single-dose study in healthy adults given **carvedilol** 25 mg found that maximum plasma levels of a 500-microgram dose of **digoxin** were increased by 0.97 nanograms/ml (60%) and the AUC was increased by about 20%, but the clinical effects of these changes were considered likely to be small.[3] No significant pharmacokinetic interaction was found in other single-dose studies in adults given **carvedilol** and **digitoxin**,[4] or **carvedilol** and intravenous **digoxin**.[3]

In a multiple-dose study in adult patients with hypertension, **carvedilol** raised the maximum serum levels and AUC of **digoxin** 250 micrograms daily by 32% and 14% respectively after 2 weeks' treatment. Again, these changes were considered unlikely to be clinically significant.[5]

A single dose of intravenous **esmolol** did not affect the pharmacokinetics of multiple-dose **digoxin**, except that a small increase was seen in the 6-hour AUC of **digoxin**.[6] The pharmacokinetics of multiple-dose **digoxin** have been shown to be unaffected by **acebutolol**,[7] **bevantolol** 200 mg daily,[8] **bisoprolol** 10 mg daily,[9] or **sotalol** 80 to 320 mg daily.[10]

(b) Pharmacodynamic interactions

Increased bradycardia is expected to occur with **digoxin**/beta-blocker combinations, but reports of this becoming a problem seem rare. One report notes marked bradycardia of 35 to 50 bpm in a 91-year-old patient on **digoxin** and using **timolol** 0.25% eye drops.[11] Bradycardia persisted on withdrawal of **digoxin**, and improved only after discontinuation of the timolol as well. Two cases, where **propranolol** 10 mg orally was used to treat arrhythmias associated with **digoxin** toxicity, are reported.[12] The first patient (who had heart failure) became bradycardic, asystolic and then died, while the second patient became bradycardic (30 bpm) but recovered after being given atropine. A further fatality was reported when intravenous **propranolol** was used.[13] In a placebo-controlled study of the use of **sotalol** in digitalised patients with chronic atrial fibrillation, 2 of 24 **sotalol** recipients were withdrawn due to bradycardia compared with none of 10 given placebo. However, the combination was still considered valuable.[10]

In healthy subjects, the pharmacodynamics of **digoxin** were unaffected by **bevantolol**,[8] and **esmolol**,[6] with no significant changes in heart rate or blood pressure occurring.

Mechanism

In most cases where the situation has had an adverse outcome the interaction seems to be due to the additive effects on the slowing of the heart.

It has been suggested that the pharmacokinetic interaction with talinolol is due to competition with digoxin for intestinal P-glycoprotein, although this needs confirmation.[1] It would seem possible that this mechanism also accounts for the interaction between digoxin and carvedilol. However, an *in vitro* study found that carvedilol (but not atenolol or metoprolol) inhibits P-glycoprotein-mediated transcellular transport of digoxin,[14] which may mean renal tubular secretion of digoxin is inhibited. It is conceivable that P-glycoprotein inhibition by carvedilol enhances the intestinal absorption of digoxin and also decreases its renal excretion. This may explain why the interaction is possibly more significant in children as they have a higher renal clearance rate of digoxin than adults.[2]

It has also been suggested that the interaction between digoxin and talinolol may be dosage form dependent. More study is needed.

Importance and management

Concurrent use appears, on the whole, beneficial, but the potential for additive bradycardia should be borne in mind. Use of beta-blockers in cases of digoxin toxicity should be undertaken with great care. In addition, it may be prudent to monitor digoxin levels with talinolol, and also with carvedilol in children. It has been suggested that the dose of digoxin should be reduced by at least 25% in children given carvedilol with further adjustments as required.[2]

1. Westphal K, Weinbrenner A, Giessmann T, Stuhr M, Gerd F, Zschiesche M, Oertel R, Terhaag B, Kroemer HK, Siegmund W. Oral bioavailability of digoxin is enhanced by talinolol: Evidence for involvement of P-glycoprotein. *Clin Pharmacol Ther* (2000) 68, 6–12.
2. Ratnapalan S, Griffiths K, Costei AM, Benson L, Koren G. Digoxin-carvedilol interactions in children. *J Pediatr* (2003) 142, 572–4.
3. De Mey C, Brendel E, Enterling D. Carvedilol increases the systemic bioavailability of oral digoxin. *Br J Clin Pharmacol* (1990) 29, 486–90.
4. Harder S, Brei R, Caspary S, Merz PG. Lack of a pharmacokinetic interaction between carvedilol and digitoxin or phenprocoumon. *Eur J Clin Pharmacol* (1993) 44, 583–6.
5. Wermeling DP, Feild CJ, Smith DA, Chandler MHH, Clifton GD, Boyle DA. Effects of long-term oral carvedilol on the steady-state pharmacokinetics of oral digoxin in patients with mild to moderate hypertension. *Pharmacotherapy* (1994) 14, 600–6.
6. Lowenthal DT, Porter RS, Achari R, Turlapaty P, Laddu AR and Matier WL. Esmolol-digoxin drug interaction. *J Clin Pharmacol* (1987) 27, 561–6.
7. Ryan JR. Clinical pharmacology of acebutolol. *Am Heart J* (1985) 109, 1131–6.
8. Quoted as data on file, Parke-Davis, by Frishman WH, Goldberg RJ, Benfield P. Bevantolol. A preliminary review of its pharmacodynamic and pharmacokinetic properties, and therapeutic efficacy in hypertension and angina pectoris. *Drugs* (1988) 35, 1–21.
9. Vechlekar DL, Cheung WK, Pearse S, Greene DS, Dukart G, Unczowsky R, Weiss AI, Silber BM, Faulkner RD. Bisoprolol does not alter the pharmacokinetics of digoxin. *Pharm Res* (1988) 5 (Suppl), S176.
10. Singh S, Saini RK, DiMarco J, Kluger J, Gold R, Chen Y. Efficacy and safety of sotalol in digitalized patients with chronic atrial fibrillation. *Am J Cardiol* (1991) 68, 1227–30.
11. Rynne MV. Timolol toxicity: ophthalmic medication complicating systemic disease. *J Maine Med Assoc* (1980) 71, 82.
12. Watt DAL. Sensitivity to propranolol after digoxin intoxication. *BMJ* (1968) 3, 413–14.
13. Schamroth L. The immediate effects of intravenous propranolol in various cardiac arrhythmias. *Am J Cardiol* (1966) 18, 438.
14. Takara K, Kakumoto M, Tanigawara Y, Funakoshi J, Sakaeda T, Okumura K. Interaction of digoxin with antihypertensive drugs *via* MDR1. *Life Sci* (2002) 70, 1491–1500.

Digitalis glycosides + Beta-lactam antibacterials

No interaction normally occurs between digoxin and amoxicillin, cefazolin, flucloxacillin, phenoxymethylpenicillin or ticarcillin/clavulanic acid. No pharmacokinetic interaction occurs between ampicillin and digitoxin.

Clinical evidence

Ampicillin 500 mg four times daily for 5 days had no significant effect on the pharmacokinetics of a single 1-mg dose of **digitoxin** in 6 healthy subjects.[1] No significant changes in **digoxin** serum concentrations were found in 16 elderly patients given **amoxicillin** (2 patients also took erythromycin and one **flucloxacillin**), and 2 patients who took **flucloxacillin** and **phenoxymethylpenicillin**. However, a few patients complained of some 'toxic' symptoms (nausea, vomiting, anorexia, headache, fatigue, blurred vision, confusion), which the authors of the report attributed to the underlying illness or the antibacterials rather than to an interaction.[2] There was no significant change in digoxin pharmacokinetics in 15 patients given **ticarcillin/clavulanic acid** 1 g/200 mg intramuscularly every 12 hours for one week.[3] There was no reduction in the excretion of **digoxin** metabolites from the gut (see Mechanism) in 3 patients taking **cefazolin,** and a reduction occurred in only 1 of 10 patients taking penicillins (**ampicillin** 6, **oxacillin** 3, **penicillin** 1).[4]

Mechanism

Up to 10% of patients on oral digoxin excrete it in substantial amounts in the faeces and urine as inactive metabolites (digoxin reduction products or DRPs). This metabolism seems to be due to gut flora,[5] in particular *Eubacterium lentum*, which is anaerobic and Gram positive. In the presence of some antibacterials that inhibit this organism, more digoxin is available for absorption, which results in a rise in serum levels (see 'Digitalis glycosides + Macrolides', p.702). At the same time the inactive metabolites derived from the gut disappear.[6] Despite *in vitro* susceptibility of *E. lentum* to a range of antibacterials, including penicillins, there is little information to suggest an interaction between digoxin and penicillins[7] or other beta-lactam antibacterials.[4] One explanation could be that these antibacterials do not achieve sufficient concentrations in the gastrointestinal tract to inhibit *E. lentum.*[7]

Importance and management

The silence of the literature on adverse interactions between digoxin and beta-lactam antibacterials, and the limited evidence given above suggest that interactions are unlikely.

1. Lucena MI, Moreno A, Fernandez MC, Garcia-Morillas M, Andrade R. Digitoxin elimination in healthy subjects taking ampicillin. *Int J Clin Pharmacol Res* (1987) VII, 33–7.
2. Rhodes KM, Brown SN. Do the penicillin antibiotics interact with digoxin? *Eur J Clin Pharmacol* (1994) 46, 479–80.
3. Cazzola M, Matera MG, Santangelo G, Angrisani M, Loffreda A, de Prisco F, Paizis G, Rossi F. Serum digoxin levels after concomitant ticarcillin and clavulanic acid administration. *Ther Drug Monit* (1994) 16, 46–8.
4. Dobkin JF, Saha JR, Butler VP, Lindenbaum J. Effects of antibiotic therapy on digoxin metabolism. *Clin Res* (1982) 30, 517A.
5. Lindenbaum J, Rund DG, Butler VP, Tse-Eng D, Saha JR. Inactivation of digoxin by the gut flora: reversal by antibiotic therapy. *N Engl J Med* (1981) 305, 789–94.
6. Lindenbaum J, Tse-Eng D, Butler VP, Rund DG. Urinary excretion of reduced metabolites of digoxin. *Am J Med* (1981) 71, 67–74.
7. Ten Eick AP, Reed MD. Hidden dangers of coadministration of antibiotics and digoxin in children: focus on azithromycin. *Curr Ther Res* (2000) 61, 148–60.

Digitalis glycosides + Bosentan

Bosentan does not appear to affect the pharmacokinetics of digoxin.

Clinical evidence, mechanism, importance and management

Bosentan 500 mg twice daily for a week did not significantly affect steady-state peak or trough serum **digoxin** levels in 18 healthy subjects given 375 micrograms daily. There was a small reduction of about 12% in the AUC of **digoxin**, although this was not considered to be clinically relevant. There were no changes in ECG recordings and vital signs.[1]

The results suggest that bosentan does not interact with **digoxin**, and that concurrent use need not be avoided. However, the authors note that further studies over the longer term, and in patients with renal impairment may be necessary to confirm this.

1. Weber C, Banken L, Birnboeck H, Nave S, Schulz R. The effect of bosentan on the pharmacokinetics of digoxin in healthy male subjects. *Br J Clin Pharmacol* (1999) 47, 701–6.

Digitalis glycosides + Calcium channel blockers

Concurrent use can be valuable, but bepridil may cause a 34 to 48% rise in serum digoxin levels, which can cause toxicity. Dosage adjustments may be needed. Felodipine, gallopamil, lacidipine, nicardipine and nisoldipine cause small but normally clinically unimportant increases in digoxin levels, while amlodipine, isradipine and nimodipine appear not to interact. The situation with nitrendipine is uncertain but it possibly causes only a small rise in digoxin levels. The interactions of digoxin with diltiazem, nifedipine and verapamil are dealt with elsewhere.

Clinical evidence

(a) Amlodipine

Amlodipine 5 mg daily had no significant effect on the serum levels or renal clearance of **digoxin** 375 micrograms daily given to 21 healthy subjects.[1]

(b) Bepridil

Bepridil 300 mg daily for a week raised the serum levels of **digoxin** 375 micrograms daily in 12 healthy subjects by 34% (from 0.93 to 1.25 nanograms/ml).[2] Five of them had mild to moderate headache, nausea and dizziness for 1 to 3 days shortly after concurrent use started. The bradycardic effects of the two drugs were found to be additive, while the negative inotropic effects of the bepridil and the positive inotropism of the increased serum **digoxin** levels were almost balanced.[2]

In another study in 23 subjects given **digoxin** 250 micrograms and bepridil 300 mg daily for 14 days, peak plasma **digoxin** levels rose by 48% (from 1.49 to 2.2 nanograms/ml) and the AUC rose by 21%.[3]

(c) Felodipine

Felodipine 10 mg twice daily for 8 weeks raised the serum **digoxin** levels in 11 patients by 15%, which was not clinically significant.[4] In another study, 14 patients were given felodipine 10 mg daily for a week. Plain tablets raised the steady-state **digoxin** serum levels by 11%, but extended-release tablets had no significant effect.[5] A third study found that, when taking felodipine, peak plasma **digoxin** levels were transiently raised by about 40% one hour after intake, but that **digoxin** AUCs were not significantly increased.[6]

(d) Gallopamil

Gallopamil 50 mg three times daily for 2 weeks raised the serum levels of **digoxin** 375 micrograms daily by 16% (from 0.58 to 0.67 nanograms/ml) in 12 healthy subjects.[7]

(e) Isradipine

Isradipine (given as 2.5 mg every 12 hours for 2 days, 5 mg every 12 hours for 2 days and then 5 mg three times daily for 10 days) did not interact significantly with a single 1000-microgram intravenous dose of **digoxin** given to 24 healthy subjects.[8] A similar study by the same group found that the same dosage regimen of isradipine given with oral **digoxin** 250 micrograms twice daily caused a small increase in peak-serum **digoxin** levels but no changes in steady-state levels or AUC.[9]

(f) Lacidipine

No significant changes in the **digoxin** AUC or minimum serum levels were found in 12 healthy subjects taking **digoxin** 250 micrograms daily for 7 days when given a single 4-mg oral dose of lacidipine, but the maximum serum levels were increased by 34%. These changes were not considered to be clinically significant.[10]

(g) Lercanidipine

The maximum serum levels of **digoxin** rose by 33% in healthy subjects also given lercanidipine.[11]

(h) Nicardipine

The plasma levels of **digoxin** 130 to 250 micrograms daily, increased by 15% (said not to be statistically significant) in 10 patients given nicardipine 20 mg three times a day for 14 days.[12] Another 20 patients with congestive heart failure also had no significant changes in steady-state serum **digoxin** levels while taking nicardipine 30 mg three times daily for 5 days.[13] Yet another study in 9 patients confirmed the absence of an interaction.[14]

(i) Nimodipine

Nimodipine 30 mg twice daily caused no change in the pharmacokinetics or haemodynamic effects of **β-acetyldigoxin** in 12 healthy subjects.[15]

(j) Nisoldipine

Nisoldipine 20 mg daily increased plasma trough **digoxin** levels of 10 patients with heart failure by about 15%.[16] This study is also reported elsewhere.[17] Nisoldipine 10 mg twice daily caused no changes in the pharmacokinetics or haemodynamic effects of **digoxin** in 8 healthy subjects.[15]

(k) Nitrendipine

A study in 8 healthy subjects, who had been taking **digoxin** 250 micrograms twice daily for 2 weeks, showed that nitrendipine 10 mg daily caused a slight but insignificant rise in plasma **digoxin** levels. Nitrendipine 20 mg daily increased the **digoxin** AUC by 15% and the maximum plasma **digoxin** levels rose from 1.34 to 2.1 nanograms/ml. Clearance fell by 13% (from 315 to 275 ml/minute). One subject dropped out of the study because of dizziness, nausea and vomiting, palpitations, insomnia and nervousness.[18,19]

Another study found that plasma **digoxin** levels were approximately doubled when nitrendipine was given,[20] but other studies in healthy subjects and patients found that nitrendipine 20 mg twice daily caused no changes in the pharmacokinetics or haemodynamic effects of **digoxin**,[15,21] or **β-acetyldigoxin**.[22]

Mechanism

Where an interaction occurs it is probably due to changes in the renal excretion of the digoxin. An *in vitro* study found that several calcium channel blockers including bepridil, nicardipine, and to a lesser extent nisoldipine (as well as barnidipine, benidipine, efonidipine, manidipine, nilvadipine, and verapamil) inhibited P-glycoprotein-mediated transcellular transport of digoxin. This suggests that any interaction may occur, at least in part, by affecting digoxin renal tubular excretion. Nitrendipine (and also diltiazem and nifedipine) only weakly inhibited the transcellular transport of digoxin.[23] Consider also 'Drug transporter proteins', (p.8).

Importance and management

The extent of the information varies from drug to drug, but the concurrent use of digoxin and calcium channel blockers can be therapeutically valuable. Monitor the effects of digoxin (e.g. bradycardia) in patients given digoxin and bepridil or lercanidipine, and consider taking levels if the effects of digoxin seem excessive. Reduce the digoxin dosage as necessary. The other calcium channel blockers listed here either cause only minimal increases in digoxin levels, which are unlikely to be clinically important in most patients, or do not interact at all. The situation with nitrendipine needs clarification. For the interactions of digoxin with other calcium channel blockers see 'diltiazem', (p.690), 'nifedipine', (p.691), and 'verapamil', (p.692).

1. Schwartz JB. Effects of amlodipine on steady-state digoxin concentrations and renal digoxin clearance. *J Cardiovasc Pharmacol* (1988) 12, 1–5.
2. Belz GG, Wistuba S, Matthews JH. Digoxin and bepridil: pharmacokinetic and pharmacodynamic interactions. *Clin Pharmacol Ther* (1986) 39, 65–71.
3. Doose DR, Wallen S, Nayak RK, Minn FL. Pharmacokinetic interaction of bepridil and digoxin at steady-state. *Clin Pharmacol Ther* (1987) 41, 204.
4. Dunselman PHJM, Scaf AHJ, Kuntze CEE, Lie KI, Wesseling H. Digoxin-felodipine interaction in patients with congestive heart failure. *Eur J Clin Pharmacol* (1988) 35, 461–5.
5. Kirch W, Laskowski M, Ohnhaus EE, Åberg J. Effects of felodipine on plasma digoxin levels and haemodynamics in patients with heart failure. *J Intern Med* (1989) 225, 237–39.
6. Rehnqvist N, Billing E, Moberg L, Lundman T, Olsson G. Pharmacokinetics of felodipine and effect on digoxin plasma levels in patients with heart failure. *Drugs* (1987) 34 (Suppl 3), 33–42.
7. Belz GG, Doering W, Munkes R, Matthews J. Interaction between digoxin and calcium antagonists and antiarrhythmic drugs. *Clin Pharmacol Ther* (1983) 33, 410–17.
8. Johnson BF, Wilson J, Marwaha R, Hoch K, Johnson J. The comparative effects of verapamil and a new dihydropyridine calcium channel blocker on digoxin pharmacokinetics. *Clin Pharmacol Ther* (1987) 42, 66–71.
9. Rodin SM, Johnson BF, Wilson J, Ritchie P, Johnson J. Comparative effects of verapamil and isradipine on steady-state digoxin kinetics. *Clin Pharmacol Ther* (1988) 43, 668–72.
10. Hall ST, Harding SM, Anderson DM, Ward C, Stevens LA. The effect of single 4 mg oral dose of calcium antagonist lacidipine on the pharmacokinetics of digoxin. In: Carpi C, Zanchetti A, eds. IVth Int Symp Calcium Antagonists: Pharmacology and Clinical Research. Florence, May 1989: 161.
11. Zanidip (Lercanidipine hydrochloride). Napp Pharmaceuticals Ltd. UK Summary of product characteristics, January 2004.
12. Lessem J, Bellinetto A. Interaction between digoxin and the calcium antagonists nicardipine and tiapamil. *Clin Ther* (1983) 5, 595–602.
13. Debruyne D, Commeau Ph, Grollier G, Huret B, Scanu P, Moulin M. Nicardipine does not significantly affect serum digoxin concentrations at the steady state of patients with congestive heart failure. *Int J Clin Pharmacol Res* (1989) IX, 15–19.
14. Scanu P, Commeau P, Huret B, Gérard JL, Debruyne D, Moore N, Lamy E, Dorey H, Grolier G, Potier JC. Pharmacocinétique et effets pharmacodynamiques de la digoxine dans les myocardiopathies dilatées. Influence de la nicardipine. *Arch Mal Coeur Vaiss* (1987) 80, 1773–83.
15. Ziegler R, Horstmann R, Wingender W, Kuhlmann J. Do dihydropyridines influence pharmacokinetic and hemodynamic parameters of digoxin? *J Clin Pharmacol* (1987) 27, 712.
16. Kirch W, Stenzel J, Dylewicz P, Hutt HJ, Santos SR, Ohnhaus EE. Influence of nisoldipine on haemodynamic effects and plasma levels of digoxin. *Br J Clin Pharmacol* (1986) 22, 155–9.
17. Kirch W, Stenzel J, Santos SR, Ohnhaus EE. Nisoldipine, a new calcium channel antagonist, elevates plasma levels of digoxin. *Arch Toxicol* (1987) (Suppl 11), 310–12.
18. Kirch W, Logemann C, Heidemann H, Santos SR, Ohnhaus EE. Effect of two different doses of nitrendipine on steady-state plasma digoxin levels and systolic time intervals. *Eur J Clin Pharmacol* (1986) 31, 391–5.
19. Kirch W, Logemann C, Heidemann H, Santos SR, Ohnhaus EE. Nitrendipine/digoxin interaction. *J Cardiovasc Pharmacol* (1987) 10 (Suppl 10), S74–S75.
20. Kirch W, Hutt HJ, Heidemann H, Rämsch K, Janisch HD, Ohnhaus EE. Drug interactions with nitrendipine. *J Cardiovasc Pharmacol* (1984) 6 (Suppl 7), S982–S985.
21. Debbas NMG, Johnston A, Jackson SHD, Banim SO, Camm AJ, Turner P. The effect of nitrendipine on predose digoxin serum concentration. *Br J Clin Pharmacol* (1988) 25, 151P.
22. Ziegler R, Wingender W, Boehme K, Raemsch K, Kuhlmann J. Study of pharmacokinetic and pharmacodynamic interaction between nitrendipine and digoxin. *J Cardiovasc Pharmacol* (1987) 9 (Suppl 4), S101–S106.
23. Takara K, Kakumoto M, Tanigawara Y, Funakoshi J, Sakaeda T, Okumura K. Interaction of digoxin with antihypertensive drugs *via* MDR1. *Life Sci* (2002) 70, 1491–1500.

Digitalis glycosides + Calcium channel blockers; Diltiazem

Serum digoxin levels are reported to be unchanged by diltiazem in a number of studies but others describe increases ranging from 20 to 85%. Serum digitoxin levels have also been reported to rise, but only by about 20%.

Clinical evidence

(a) Digoxin

(i) Evidence of no interaction. Diltiazem 30 or 60 mg four times daily had no significant effect on the serum levels of digoxin 250 micrograms daily in 9 patients with cardiac diseases.[1] Two similar studies in 12 patients[2] and 8 healthy subjects,[3] on digoxin given diltiazem 120 to 360 mg daily confirmed the absence of an interaction. Two further studies in healthy subjects,[4,5] found that diltiazem 120 mg daily did not affect the pharmacokinetics of a single 1-mg intravenous dose of digoxin.

(ii) Evidence of an interaction. A study in 17 Japanese patients (some with rheumatic valvular disease) taking either digoxin or **metildigoxin** found that diltiazem 60 mg three times daily for 2 weeks increased their serum digoxin levels measured at 24 hours by 36 and 51% respectively.[6] Another

study in 8 patients with chronic heart failure secondary to ischaemic disease, taking digoxin 250 micrograms daily, found that diltiazem 60 mg three times daily increased the digoxin AUC and mean steady state serum levels by about 50%, its peak serum level by 37% and elimination half-life by 29%. Diltiazem had no significant effects on haemodynamic parameters.[7]

Other studies in Western patients[8,9] and healthy subjects[10-13] have shown rises of 20 to 85% in plasma digoxin levels during diltiazem use. In one case report a 143% increase was seen.[14] The authors of two of these studies noted that the effect was highly individual with some subjects showing no increase and some a large increase.[9,11]

(b) Digitoxin

Five out of 10 patients on digitoxin showed a 6 to 31% (mean 21%) rise in plasma digitoxin levels while taking diltiazem 180 mg daily for 4 to 6 weeks.[15]

Mechanism

Not understood. In those individuals showing an interaction, falls in total digoxin clearance of about 25% have been described.[7,9,10,16,17] Although several calcium channel blockers may inhibit the P-glycoprotein mediated renal clearance of digoxin, the results of an *in vitro* study[18] suggest that this may not occur with diltiazem.

Importance and management

A thoroughly investigated and well documented interaction but there is no clear explanation for the inconsistent results. All patients on digoxin given diltiazem should be well monitored for signs of over-digitalisation (e.g. bradycardia) with digoxin levels measured as necessary. Dosage reductions may be necessary. Those most at risk are patients with digoxin levels near the top end of the range. Similar precautions would appear to be necessary with digitoxin, although the documentation of this interaction is very limited.

1. Elkayam U, Parikh K, Torkan B, Weber L, Cohen JL, Rahimtoola SH. Effect of diltiazem on renal clearance and serum concentration of digoxin in patients with cardiac disease. *Am J Cardiol* (1985) 55, 1393–5.
2. Schrager BR, Pina I, Frangi M, Applewhite S, Sequeira R, Chahine RA. Diltiazem, digoxin interaction? *Circulation* (1983) 68 (Suppl), III-368.
3. Boden WE, More G, Sharma S, Bough EW, Korr KS, Young PM, Shulman RS. No increase in serum digoxin concentrations with high dose diltiazem. *Am J Med* (1986) 81, 425–8.
4. Beltrami TR, May JJ, Bertino JS. Lack of effects of diltiazem on digoxin pharmacokinetics. *J Clin Pharmacol* (1985) 25, 390–392.
5. Jones WN, Kern KB, Rindone JP, Mayersohn M, Bliss M, Goldman S. Digoxin-diltiazem interaction: a pharmacokinetic evaluation. *Eur J Clin Pharmacol* (1986) 31, 351–3.
6. Oyama Y, Fujii S, Kanda K, Akino E, Kawasaki H, Nagata M, Goto K. Digoxin-diltiazem interaction. *Am J Cardiol* (1984) 53, 1480–1.
7. Mahgoub AA, El-Medany AH, Abdulatif AS. A comparison between the effects of diltiazem and isosorbide dinitrate on digoxin pharmacodynamics and kinetics in the treatment of patients with chronic ischemic heart failure. *Saudi Med J* (2002) 23, 725–31.
8. Andrejak M, Hary L, Andrjak M-Th, Lesbre J Ph. Diltiazem increases steady state digoxin serum levels in patients with cardiac disease. *J Clin Pharmacol* (1987) 27, 967–70.
9. Kuhlmann J. Effects of nifedipine and diltiazem on plasma levels and renal excretion of beta-acetyldigoxin. *Clin Pharmacol Ther* (1985) 37, 150–6.
10. Rameis H, Magometschnigg D, Ganzinger U. The diltiazem-digoxin interaction. *Clin Pharmacol Ther* (1984) 36, 183–9.
11. North DS, Mattern AL, Hiser WW. The influence of diltiazem hydrochloride on trough serum digoxin levels. *Drug Intell Clin Pharm* (1986) 20, 500–3.
12. Gallet M, Aupetit JF, Lopez M, Manchon J, Lestaevel M, Lefrancois JJ. Interaction diltiazem-digoxine. Évolution de la digoxinémie et des paramtres électrocardiographiques chez le sujet sain. *Arch Mal Coeur* (1986) 79, 1216–20.
13. Larman RC. A pharmacokinetic evaluation of the digoxin-diltiazem interaction. *J Pharm Sci* (1987) 76, S79.
14. King T, Mallet L. Diltiazem-digoxin interaction in an elderly woman: a case report. *J Geriatr Drug Ther* (1991) 5, 79–83.
15. Kuhlmann J. Effects of verapamil, diltiazem, and nifedipine on plasma levels and renal excretion of digitoxin. *Clin Pharmacol Ther* (1985) 38, 667–73.
16. Yoshida A, Fujita M, Kurosawa N, Nioka M, Shichinohe T, Arakawa M, Fukuda R, Owada E, Ito K. Effects of diltiazem on plasma level and urinary excretion of digoxin in healthy subjects. *Clin Pharmacol Ther* (1984) 35, 681–5.
17. Suematsu F, Yukawa E, Yukawa M, Minemoto M, Ohdo S, Higuchi S, Goto Y. Pharmacoepidemiologic detection of calcium channel blocker-induced change on digoxin clearance using multiple trough screen analysis. *Biopharm Drug Dispos* (2002) 23, 173–81.
18. Takara K, Kakumoto M, Tanigawara Y, Funakoshi J, Sakaeda T, Okumura K. Interaction of digoxin with antihypertensive drugs *via* MDR1. *Life Sci* (2002) 70, 1491–1500.

Digitalis glycosides + Calcium channel blockers; Nifedipine

Serum digoxin levels are normally unchanged or increased only to a small extent by nifedipine. However, one unexplained and conflicting study indicated that a 45% rise could occur. Digitoxin appears not to interact.

Clinical evidence

(a) Digoxin

(i) Serum digoxin levels unchanged. Studies in 25 patients[1-3] and 28 healthy subjects[4-6] showed that serum digoxin levels were not significantly altered by nifedipine 30 to 60 mg daily. Similarly no significant changes in the pharmacokinetics of a single intravenous dose of digoxin were found in 6 patients[7] or 16 healthy subjects[8,9] taking nifedipine 40 to 90 mg daily. No changes in the pharmacokinetics of nifedipine were seen.[8]

(ii) Serum digoxin levels increased. Nifedipine 30 mg increased the plasma levels of digoxin 375 micrograms daily by 45% (from 0.505 to 0.734 nanograms/ml) over 14 days in 12 healthy subjects.[10] A 15% increase was also seen in a study[11] in 7 healthy subjects given 15 to 60 mg nifedipine daily with digoxin 250 micrograms twice daily. These studies have been reported elsewhere.[12,13]

Nifedipine 20 mg twice daily increased the steady-state serum digoxin levels of 9 patients by 15% (from 0.87 to 1.04 nanograms/ml).[14]

(b) Digitoxin

A study in 18 subjects showed that nifedipine 40 to 60 mg daily had no significant effect on their steady-state plasma digitoxin levels over a 6-week period.[15]

Mechanism

Not understood. Changes and lack of changes in both the renal and non-renal excretion of digoxin have been reported. A retrospective analysis of pharmacokinetic data suggests that clearance of digoxin may be reduced by 10% in patients also taking nifedipine.[16] Although several calcium channel blockers may inhibit the P-glycoprotein mediated renal clearance of digoxin, the results of an *in vitro* study[17] suggest that this may not occur with nifedipine.

Importance and management

The digoxin/nifedipine interaction is well documented but the findings are inconsistent. The weight of evidence appears to be that serum digoxin levels are normally unchanged or only very moderately increased by nifedipine. Concurrent use appears normally to be safe and effective.[18] One report suggests that nifedipine has some attenuating effect on the digoxin-induced inotropism.[19] Another points out that under some circumstances (renal insufficiency or pre-existing digoxin overdosage) some risk of an undesirable interaction still exists.[11] If undesirable bradycardia occurs in a patient taking digoxin and nifedipine consider taking digoxin levels, and adjust the dose accordingly. Nifedipine appears not to interact with digitoxin significantly.

1. Schwartz JB, Raizner A, Akers S. The effect of nifedipine on serum digoxin concentrations in patients. *Am Heart J* (1984) 107, 669–73.
2. Kuhlmann J, Marcin S, Frank KH. Effects of nifedipine and diltiazem on the pharmacokinetics of digoxin. *Naunyn Schmiedebergs Arch Pharmacol* (1983) 324 (Suppl), R81.
3. Kuhlmann J. Effects of nifedipine and diltiazem on plasma levels and renal excretion of beta-acetyldigoxin. *Clin Pharmacol Ther* (1985) 37, 150–6.
4. Schwartz JB, Migliore PJ. Nifedipine does not alter digoxin level or clearance. *J Am Coll Cardiol* (1984) 3, 478.
5. Schwartz JB, Migliore PJ. Effect of nifedipine on serum digoxin concentration and renal clearance. *Clin Pharmacol Ther* (1984) 36, 19–24.
6. Pedersen KE, Madsen JL, Klitgaard NA, Kjoer K, Hvidt S. Non-interaction between nifedipine and digoxin. *Dan Med Bull* (1986) 33, 109–10.
7. Garty M, Shamir E, Ilfeld D, Pitlik S, Rosenfeld JB. Non interaction of digoxin and nifedipine in cardiac patients. *J Clin Pharmacol* (1986) 26, 304–5.
8. Koren G, Zylber-Katz E, Granit L, Levy M. Pharmacokinetic studies of nifedipine and digoxin co-administration. *Int J Clin Pharmacol Ther Toxicol* (1986) 24, 39–42.
9. Pedersen KE, Dorph-Pedersen A, Hvidt S, Klitgaard NA, Kjaer K, Nielsen-Kudsk F. Effect of nifedipine on digoxin kinetics in healthy subjects. *Clin Pharmacol Ther* (1982) 32, 562–5.
10. Belz GG, Doering W, Munkes R, Matthews J. Interaction between digoxin and calcium antagonists and antiarrhythmic drugs. *Clin Pharmacol Ther* (1983) 33, 410–17.
11. Kirch W, Hutt HJ, Dylewicz P, Gräf KJ, Ohnhaus EE. Dose-dependence of the nifedipine-digoxin interaction? *Clin Pharmacol Ther* (1986) 39, 35–9.
12. Belz GG, Aust PE, Munkes R. Digoxin plasma concentrations and nifedipine. *Lancet* (1981) i, 844–5.
13. Hutt HJ, Kirch W, Dylewicz P, Ohnhaus EE. Dose-dependence of the nifedipine/digoxin interaction? *Arch Toxicol* (1986) (Suppl 9), 209–12.
14. Kleinbloesem CH, van Brummelen P, Hillers J, Moolenaar AJ, Breimer DD. Interaction between digoxin and nifedipine at steady state in patients with atrial fibrillation. *Ther Drug Monit* (1985) 7, 372–6.
15. Kuhlmann J. Effects of quinidine, verapamil and nifedipine on the pharmacokinetics and pharmacodynamics of digitoxin during steady-state conditions. *Arzneimittelforschung* (1987) 37, 545–8.
16. Suematsu F, Yukawa E, Yukawa M, Minemoto M, Ohdo S, Higuchi S, Goto Y. Pharmacoepidemiologic detection of calcium channel blocker-induced change on digoxin clearance using multiple trough screen analysis. *Biopharm Drug Dispos* (2002) 23, 173–81.
17. Takara K, Kakumoto M, Tanigawara Y, Funakoshi J, Sakaeda T, Okumura K. Interaction of digoxin with antihypertensive drugs *via* MDR1. *Life Sci* (2002) 70, 1491–1500.

18. Cantelli I, Pavesi PC, Parchi C, Naccarella F, Bracchetti D. Acute hemodynamic effects of combined therapy with digoxin and nifedipine in patients with chronic heart failure. *Am Heart J* (1983) 106, 308–15.
19. Hansen PB, Buch J, Rasmussen OØ, Waldorff S, Steiness E. Influence of atenolol and nifedipine on digoxin-induced inotropism in humans. *Br J Clin Pharmacol* (1984) 18, 817–22.

Digitalis glycosides + Calcium channel blockers; Verapamil

Serum digoxin levels are increased by about 40% by verapamil 160 mg daily, and by about 70% by verapamil 240 mg daily. Digoxin toxicity may develop if the dosage is not reduced. Deaths have occurred. A rise of about 35% occurs with digitoxin.

Clinical evidence

(a) Digoxin

After 2 weeks' treatment with verapamil 240 mg daily, in 3 divided doses, the mean serum digoxin levels of 49 patients with chronic atrial fibrillation had risen by 72%. The rise was seen in most patients, and it occurred largely within the first 7 days. A rise of about 40% has been seen with verapamil 160 mg daily.[1,2]

Reports in a total of 21 healthy subjects,[3,4] and 54 patients[5-7] describe rises in serum digoxin levels of 22 to 147% when verapamil 240 to 360 mg daily was added to digoxin. Similar rises are reported elsewhere.[2,8-10]

A rise in digoxin levels of about 50% was seen in chronic haemodialysis patients given verapamil 120 to 240 mg daily.[11] Nine healthy subjects showed a 53% rise in digoxin levels while taking verapamil 240 mg three times daily for two weeks.[3] Toxicity[12] and a fatality[13] occurred in patients whose digoxin levels became markedly increased by verapamil. Both asystole and sinus arrest have been described.[14,15] A single dose study indicated that cirrhosis magnifies the extent of this interaction.[16]

(b) Digitoxin

Eight out of 10 patients showed a mean 35% rise (range 14 to 97%) in plasma digitoxin levels over a 4 to 6 week period while taking verapamil 240 mg daily, in three divided doses. Two patients showed no changes, and no changes in the pharmacokinetics of a single dose of digitoxin were found in 3 other healthy subjects.[17,18]

Mechanism

The rise in serum digoxin levels is due to reductions in renal and especially extra-renal (biliary) clearance; a diminution in the volume of distribution also takes place.[2,7,8,19] It has been suggested that P-glycoprotein may be involved.[20] An *in vitro* study found that verapamil can inhibit the P-glycoprotein-mediated transcellular transport of digoxin,[21] which suggests that any interaction may occur, at least in part, by inhibiting the renal tubular excretion of digoxin. Impaired extra-renal excretion is suggested as the reason for the rise in serum digitoxin levels.[17]

The increased plasma levels of digoxin caused by verapamil are reported to increase both inotropism[22] and toxic effects.[23] Verapamil may enhance the digoxin-induced elevation of intracellular sodium, which may increase the risk of arrhythmias.[23,24]

Importance and management

The interaction between digoxin and verapamil is well documented, well established and it occurs in most patients.[8,25] Serum digoxin levels should be well monitored and downward dosage adjustments made to avoid digoxin toxicity (deaths have occurred[13]). An initial 33 to 50% dosage reduction has been recommended.[26,27] The interaction develops within 2 to 7 days, approaching or reaching a maximum within 14 days or so.[1,6] The magnitude of the rise in serum digoxin is dose-dependent[28] with a significant increase if the verapamil dosage is increased from 160 to 240 mg daily,[1] but with no further significant increase if the dose is raised any higher.[4] The mean rise with verapamil 160 mg daily is about 40%, and with 240 mg or more is about 60 to 80%, but the response is variable. Some patients may show rises of up to 150% while others show only a modest increase. One study found that although the rise in serum digoxin levels was 60% within a week, this had lessened to about 30% five weeks later.[8] Regular monitoring and dosage adjustments would seem to be necessary.

The documentation of the digitoxin and verapamil interaction is limited, but the interaction appears to be established. Downward dosage adjustment may be necessary, particularly in some patients.[17]

1. Klein HO, Lang R, Weiss E, Di Segni E, Libhaber C, Guerrero J, Kaplinsky E. The influence of verapamil on serum digoxin concentration. *Circulation* (1982) 65, 998–1003.
2. Lang R, Klein HO, Weiss E, Libhaber C, Kaplinsky E. Effect of verapamil on digoxin blood level and clearance. *Chest* (1980) 78, 525.
3. Doering W. Effect of coadministration of verapamil and quinidine on serum digoxin concentration. *Eur J Clin Pharmacol* (1983) 25, 517–21.
4. Belz GG, Doering W, Munkes R, Matthews J. Interaction between digoxin and calcium antagonists and antiarrhythmic drugs. *Clin Pharmacol Ther* (1983) 33, 410–17.
5. Klein HO, Lang R, Di Segni E, Kaplinsky E. Verapamil-digoxin interaction. *N Engl J Med* (1980) 303, 160.
6. Merola P, Badin A, Paleari DC, De Petris A, Maragno I. Influenza del verapamile sui livelli plasmatici di digossina nell'uomo. *Cardiologia* (1982) 27, 683–7.
7. Hedman A, Angelin B, Arvidsson A, Beck O, Dahlqvist R, Nilsson B, Olsson M, Schenck-Gustafsson K. Digoxin-verapamil interaction: reduction of biliary but not renal digoxin clearance. *Clin Pharmacol Ther* (1991) 49, 256–62.
8. Pedersen KE, Dorph-Pedersen A, Hvidt S, Klitgaard NA, Pedersen KK. The long-term effect of verapamil on plasma digoxin concentration and renal digoxin clearance in healthy subjects. *Eur J Clin Pharmacol* (1982) 22, 123–7.
9. Klein HO, Lang R, Di Segni E, Sareli P, David D, Kaplinsky E. Oral verapamil versus digoxin in the management of chronic atrial fibrillation. *Chest* (1980) 78, 524.
10. Schwartz JB, Keefe D, Kates RE, Harrison DC. Verapamil and digoxin. Another drug-drug interaction. *Clin Res* (1981) 29, 501A.
11. Rendtorff C, Johannessen AC, Halck S, Klitgaard NA. Verapamil-digoxin interaction in chronic hemodialysis patients. *Scand J Urol Nephrol* (1990) 24, 137–9.
12. Gordon M, Goldenberg LMC. Clinical digoxin toxicity in the aged in association with co-administered verapamil. A report of two cases and a review of the literature. *J Am Geriatr Soc* (1986) 34, 659–62.
13. Zatuchni J. Verapamil-digoxin interaction. *Am Heart J* (1984) 108, 412–3.
14. Kounis NG. Asystole after verapamil and digoxin. *Br J Clin Pract* (1980) 34, 57–8.
15. Kounis NG, Mallioris C. Interactions with cardioactive drugs. *Br J Clin Pract* (1986) 40, 537–8.
16. Maragno I, Gianotti C, Tropeano PF, Rodighiero V, Gaion RM, Paleari C, Prandoni R, Menozzi L. Verapamil-induced changes in digoxin kinetics in cirrhosis. *Eur J Clin Pharmacol* (1987) 32, 309–11.
17. Kuhlmann J, Marcin S. Effects of verapamil on pharmacokinetics and pharmacodynamics of digitoxin in patients. *Am Heart J* (1985) 110, 1245–50.
18. Kuhlmann J. Effects of verapamil, diltiazem, and nifedipine on plasma levels and renal excretion of digitoxin. *Clin Pharmacol Ther* (1985) 38, 667–73.
19. Pedersen KE, Dorph-Pedersen A, Hvidt S, Klitgaard NA, Nielsen-Kudsk F. Digoxin-verapamil interaction. *Clin Pharmacol Ther* (1981) 30, 311–16.
20. Verschraagen M, Koks CHW, Schellens JHM, Beijnen JH. P-glycoprotein system as a determinant of drug interactions: the case of digoxin-verapamil. *Pharmacol Res* (1999) 40, 301–6.
21. Takara K, Kakumoto M, Tanigawara Y, Funakoshi J, Sakaeda T, Okumura K. Interaction of digoxin with antihypertensive drugs *via* MDR1. *Life Sci* (2002) 70, 1491–1500.
22. Pedersen KE, Thayssen P, Klitgaard NA, Christiansen BD, Nielsen-Kudsk F. Influence of verapamil on the inotropism and pharmacokinetics of digoxin. *Eur J Clin Pharmacol* (1983) 25, 199–206.
23. Pedersen KE. The influence of calcium antagonists on plasma digoxin concentration. *Acta Med Scand* (1984) (Suppl 681), 31–6.
24. Pedersen KE, Christiansen BD, Kjaer K, Klitgaard NA, Nielsen-Kudsk F. Verapamil-induced changes in digoxin kinetics and intraerythrocytic sodium concentration. *Clin Pharmacol Ther* (1983) 34, 8–13.
25. Belz GG, Aust PE, Munkes R. Digoxin plasma concentrations and nifedipine. *Lancet* (1981) i, 844–5.
26. Marcus FI. Pharmacokinetic interactions between digoxin and other drugs. *J Am Coll Cardiol* (1985) 5, 82A–90A.
27. Klein HO, Kaplinsky E. Verapamil and digoxin: their respective effects on atrial fibrillation and their interaction. *Am J Cardiol* (1982) 50, 894–902.
28. Schwartz JB, Keefe D, Kates RE, Kirsten E, Harrison DC. Acute and chronic pharmacodynamic interaction of verapamil and digoxin in atrial fibrillation. *Circulation* (1982) 65, 1163–70.

Digitalis glycosides + Calcium compounds

The effects of digitalis glycosides can be increased by rises in blood calcium levels, and the use of intravenous calcium may result in the development of potentially life-threatening digitalis-induced cardiac arrhythmias.

Clinical evidence

Two patients developed cardiac arrhythmias and died after being given **digitalis** intramuscularly and either **calcium chloride** or **calcium gluconate** intravenously. No absolutely certain causative relationship was established.[1]

There is other evidence that increases or decreases in blood **calcium** levels can increase or decrease, respectively, the effects of **digitalis**. A patient with congestive heart failure and atrial fibrillation was resistant to the actions of **digoxin** serum levels of 1.5 to 3 nanograms/ml until his serum **calcium** levels were raised from 6.7 to about 8.5 mg/dl by oral **calcium and vitamin D**.[2] **Disodium edetate**,[3-5] which lowers blood calcium levels, has been used successfully in the treatment of digitalis toxicity, although less toxic agents are generally preferred.

Mechanism

The actions of the cardiac glycosides (even now not fully understood) are closely tied up with movement of calcium ions into heart muscle cells.

Increased concentrations of calcium outside these cells increase the inflow of calcium and this enhances the activity of the glycosides. This can lead to effective over-digitalisation and even potentially life-threatening arrhythmias.

Importance and management

The report cited[1] (published in 1936) seems to be the only direct clinical evidence of a serious adverse interaction, although there is plenty of less direct evidence that an interaction is possible. Intravenous calcium should be avoided in patients on cardiac glycosides. If that is not possible, it has been suggested[6] that it should be given slowly or only in small amounts in order to avoid transient serum calcium levels higher than 15 mEq/l.

1. Bower JO, Mengle HAK. The additive effects of calcium and digitalis. A warning with a report of two deaths. *JAMA* (1936) 106, 1151.
2. Chopra D, Janson P, Sawin CT. Insensitivity to digoxin associated with hypocalcaemia. *N Engl J Med* (1977) 296, 917–8.
3. Jick S and Karsh R. The effect of calcium chelation on cardiac arrhythmias and conduction disturbances. *Am J Cardiol* (1959) 43, 287.
4. Szekely P, Wynne NA. Effects of calcium chelation on digitalis-induced cardiac arrhythmias. *Br Heart J* (1963) 25, 589–94.
5. Rosenbaum JL, Mason D, Seven MJ. The effect of disodium EDTA on digitalis intoxication. *Am J Med Sci* (1960) 240, 111–18.
6. Nola GT, Pope S, Harrison DC. Assessment of the synergistic relationship between serum calcium and digitalis. *Am Heart J* (1970) 79, 499–507.

Digitalis glycosides + Chinese herbal medicines

Bufalin can interfere with the assay of cardiac glycosides. Danshen appears not to interact with digoxin, but it can falsify the results of serum immunoassay methods. Digoxin toxicity in an elderly man was attributed to the use of a herbal laxative containing liquorice.

Clinical evidence, mechanism, importance and management

(a) Bufalin (Chan Su, Kyushin, and Lu-Shen-Wan)

Bufalin, a cardioactive substance of amphibian origin and Chinese medicines such as Chan Su, Lu-Shen-Wan and Kyushin that contain bufalin can interfere with some immunoassay methods of **digitoxin** and **digoxin**, particularly the fluorescence polarisation immunoassay.[1-3] The digoxin-like immunoreactivity of Kyushin was found to be equivalent to varying amounts of **digoxin** because of differences in the cross-reactivity of the antibody used in different immunoassays.[3] A chemiluminescent assay for **digitoxin**[2,4] and **digoxin**[2] did not cross-react with bufalin.

Bufalin and an extract of Chan Su displaced **digitoxin** from protein-binding sites *in vitro*.[4] Whether this would result in elevated free **digitoxin** levels and toxicity *in vivo* is not known. However, this is probably unlikely, since *in vivo* the free drug would be available for metabolism (see 'Drug distribution interactions', (p.3)). Another possibility, given the similarities between bufalin and cardiac glycosides, is that toxicity could result from additive cardiac effects.

(b) Danshen

Danshen appears not to have been reported to affect serum **digoxin** levels, but it can falsify laboratory measurements. A study found that a fluorescent polarization immunoassay method (Abbott Laboratories) for **digoxin** gave falsely high readings in the presence of danshen, whereas a microparticle enzyme immunoassay (Abbott Laboratories) gave falsely low readings. These false readings could be eliminated by monitoring the free (i.e. unbound) **digoxin** concentrations[5] or by choosing assay systems that are unaffected by the presence of danshen (said to be the Roche and Beckman systems).[1]

(c) Liquorice (Kanzo)

An 84-year-old man on **digoxin** 125 micrograms daily and furosemide complained of loss of appetite, fatigue and oedema of the lower extremities 5 days after starting to take a Chinese herbal laxative containing liquorice (kanzo) 400 mg and rhubarb (daio) 1.6 g three times daily. It was suggested that heart failure occurred because of **digoxin** toxicity induced by liquorice-associated electrolyte imbalance which may also have been exacerbated by the age of the patient, the diuretic and his existing cardiovascular disease.[6]

1. Chow L, Johnson M, Wells A, Dasgupta A. Effect of the traditional Chinese medicines Chan Su, Lu-Shen-Wan, Dan Shen, and Asian ginseng on serum digoxin measurement by Tina-quant (Roche) and Synchron LX System (Beckman) digoxin immunoassays. *J Clin Lab Anal* (2003) 17, 22–7.
2. Dasgupta A, Datta P. Rapid detection of cardioactive bufalin toxicity using fluorescence polarization immunoassay for digitoxin. *Ther Drug Monit* (1998) 20, 104–8.
3. Fushimi R, Koh T, Iyama S, Yasuhara M, Tachi J, Kohda K, Amino N, Miyai K. Digoxin-like immunoreactivity in Chinese medicine. *Ther Drug Monit* (1990) 12, 242–5.
4. Datta P, Dasgupta A. Interactions between drugs and Asian medicine: displacement of digitoxin from protein binding site by bufalin, the constituent of Chinese medicines Chan Su and Lu-Shen-Wan. *Ther Drug Monit* (2000) 22, 155–9.
5. Wahed A, Dasgupta A. Positive and negative in vitro interference of Chinese medicine dan shen in serum digoxin measurement. Elimination of interference by monitoring free digoxin concentration. *Am J Clin Pathol* (2001) 116, 403–8.
6. Harada T, Ohtaki E, Misu K, Sumiyoshi T, Hosoda S. Congestive heart failure caused by digitalis toxicity in an elderly man taking a licorice-containing Chinese herbal laxative. *Cardiology* (2002) 98, 218.

Digitalis glycosides + Chloroquine or Hydroxychloroquine

The blood levels of digoxin were found to be increased by over 70% in two elderly patients when they were treated with hydroxychloroquine. A similar increase has been seen with chloroquine in *dogs*.

Clinical evidence, mechanism, importance and management

Two women of 65 and 68 who had been taking **digoxin** 250 micrograms daily for 2 to 3 years for arrhythmias were treated with hydroxychloroquine 250 mg twice daily for rheumatoid arthritis. When the hydroxychloroquine was withdrawn the plasma **digoxin** levels of both women fell by 70 to 75% (from 3 to 0.7 nanomol/l and from 3.1 to 0.9 nanomol/l respectively). Neither showed any evidence of toxicity during concurrent use, and one of them claimed that the regularity of her heart rhythm had been improved.[1] The reason for this apparent interaction is not understood and its general significance is uncertain.

No interaction between digoxin and chloroquine has been described in man, but increases in peak serum **digoxin** levels of about 77% have been seen in *dogs*.[2]

1. Leden I. Digoxin-hydroxychloroquine interaction? *Acta Med Scand* (1982) 211, 411–12.
2. McElnay JC, Sidahmed AM, D'Arcy PF and McQuade RD. Chloroquine-digoxin interaction. *Int J Pharmaceutics* (1985) 26, 267–74.

Digitalis glycosides + Cibenzoline (Cifenline)

Cibenzoline did not affect plasma digoxin levels.

Clinical evidence, mechanism, importance and management

A study in 12 healthy subjects taking **digoxin** 250 to 375 micrograms daily showed that cibenzoline 160 mg twice daily for 7 days had no effect on the pharmacokinetics of the **digoxin**.[1] An *in vitro* study found that cibenzoline only slightly inhibited the P-glycoprotein-mediated transcellular transport of **digoxin** and therefore inhibition of the renal tubular secretion of **digoxin** is unlikely.[2]

1. Khoo K-C, Givens SV, Parsonnet M, Massarella JW. Effect of oral cibenzoline on steady-state digoxin concentrations in healthy volunteers. *J Clin Pharmacol* (1988) 28, 29–35.
2. Kakumoto M, Takara K, Sakaeda T, Tanigawara Y, Kita T, Okumura K. MDR1-mediated interaction of digoxin with antiarrhythmic or antianginal drugs. *Biol Pharm Bull* (2002), 25, 1604–7.

Digitalis glycosides + Cicletanine

Cicletanine appears not to affect plasma digoxin levels.

Clinical evidence, mechanism, importance and management

Single 50-mg and 100-mg doses of cicletanine were found to have no effect on the plasma **digoxin** levels of 6 patients stabilised on **digoxin** 125 to 250 micrograms daily.[1] This absence of an interaction needs further confirmation with multiple dose studies.

1. Clement DL, Teirlynck O, Belpaire F. Lack of effect of cicletanine on plasma digoxin levels. *Int J Clin Pharmacol Res* (1988) 8, 9–11.

Digitalis glycosides + Ciclosporin

Ciclosporin causes marked rises in serum digoxin levels in some patients.

Clinical Evidence

Digoxin toxicity developed in 4 patients when they were given ciclosporin prior to cardiac transplantation. In the two cases described in detail, ciclosporin 10 mg/kg daily was added to **digoxin** 375 micrograms daily. Fourfold rises in **digoxin** levels, from 1.5 to 5.7 nanomol/l and from 2.6 to 10.6 nanomol/l, were seen within 2 to 3 days. This was accompanied by rises in serum creatinine levels from 110 to 120 micromol/l and from 84 to 181 micromol/l respectively, which were considered insufficient to explain the rise in **digoxin** levels. As a consequence of these findings, the same authors conducted a study in 4 patients given ciclosporin and **digoxin**. Two patients developed acute renal failure. In the other 2 patients, the volume of distribution of **digoxin** was decreased by 69 and 72%, while the clearance was reduced by 47 and 58%.[1] In a further 7 patients, **digoxin** pharmacokinetics were assessed prior to cardiac transplantation, then after transplantation during maintenance ciclosporin therapy.[2] The total body clearance of **digoxin** remained unchanged, which appeared to be at odds with the earlier results.[1] It was suggested that haemodynamic improvements brought about by successful cardiac transplantation may have counterbalanced any inhibitory effect ciclosporin had on renal clearance.[2]

Mechanism

Not fully understood. The authors of the studies concluded that ciclosporin has no specific inhibitory effect on the renal elimination of digoxin, but that it causes a non-specific reduction in renal function after acute administration, which reduces digoxin elimination.[2] Conversely, another study in *animals* suggested that ciclosporin can reduce the secretion of digoxin by the kidney tubular cells by inhibiting P-glycoprotein.[3]

Importance and management

Information seems limited to the studies cited. The effects of concurrent use should be monitored very closely, and the digoxin dosage should be adjusted as necessary.

1. Dorian P, Cardella C, Strauss M, David T, East S, Ogilvie R. Cyclosporine nephrotoxicity and cyclosporine-digoxin interaction prior to heart transplantation. *Transplant Proc* (1987) 19, 1825–7.
2. Robieux I, Dorian P, Klein J, Chung D, Zborowska-Sluis D, Ogilvie R, Koren G. The effects of cardiac transplantation and cyclosporine therapy on digoxin pharmacokinetics. *J Clin Pharmacol* (1992) 32, 338–43.
3. Okamura N, Hirai M, Tanigawara Y, Tanaka K, Yasuhura M, Ueda K, Komano T, Hori R. Digoxin-cyclosporin A interaction: modulation of the multidrug transporter P-glycoprotein in the kidney. *J Pharmacol Exp Ther* (1993) 266, 1614–9.

Digitalis glycosides + Colesevelam

The absorption of a single dose of digoxin is not affected by colesevelam.

Clinical evidence, mechanism, importance and management

A single-dose, cross-over study in which 26 healthy subjects were given **digoxin** 250 micrograms with or without **colesevelam** 4.5 g, followed by a standard meal, found that **colesevelam** did not significantly affect the absorption of **digoxin**.[1] Because the bile-acid binding resins 'colestyramine', (p.694) and 'colestipol', (p.694) may interact with digoxin it was suggested that **colesevelam** could also interact, although this appears not to be the case. This finding requires confirmation in long-term studies.

1. Donovan JM, Stypinski D, Stiles MR, Olson TA, Burke SK. Drug interactions with colesevelam hydrochloride, a novel, potent lipid-lowering agent. *Cardiovasc Drugs Ther* (2000) 14, 681–90.

Digitalis glycosides + Colestipol

Colestipol appears not to interfere with the absorption of either digoxin or digitoxin if it is given at least 1.5 hours after the digitalis glycoside.

Clinical evidence

(a) Digitalis levels reduced

Four patients with **digitoxin** toxicity were given colestipol 10 g at once and 5 g every 6 to 8 hours thereafter to reduce their **digitoxin** serum levels. The average **digitoxin** half-life fell to 2.75 days compared with an untreated control patient in whom the **digitoxin** half-life was 9.3 days. In another patient with **digoxin** toxicity similarly treated the **digoxin** half-life was 16 hours compared with 1.8 to 2 days in two other control patients.[1]

(b) Digitalis levels unaffected

Ten patients on long-term treatment with either **digoxin** 125 to 250 micrograms daily or **digitoxin** 100 to 200 micrograms daily were treated with colestipol 15 g daily or a placebo, taken 1.5 hour after the digitalis. Their serum digitalis levels were not significantly altered over a 1-year period by the colestipol.[2]

A comparative study in 11 patients with plasma **digitoxin** levels greater than 40 nanograms/ml found that when the **digitoxin** was stopped and colestipol 5 g four times daily was given before meals, the **digitoxin** half-life (6.3 days) was unaffected when compared with 11 other patients not given colestipol (6.8 days).[3]

Mechanism

Colestipol is an ion-exchange resin which can bind to digitalis glycosides.[1] In cases of toxicity colestipol may possibly reduce serum digitalis levels because under these circumstances the excretion of digitalis in the bile increases and more becomes available for binding in the gut.[2]

Importance and management

This interaction is not well established. Giving either digoxin or digitoxin 1.5 hours before colestipol appears to avoid any possible interaction in the gut.[2] It is usually recommended that other drugs are given 1 hour before or 4 hours after colestipol.

1. Bazzano G, Bazzano GS. Digitalis intoxication. Treatment with a new steroid-binding resin. *JAMA* (1972) 220, 828–30.
2. Bazzano G, Bazzano GS. Effect of digitalis-binding resins on cardiac glycosides plasma levels. *Clin Res* (1972) 20, 24.
3. van Bever RJ, Duchateau AMJA, Pluym BFM, Merkus FWHM. The effect of colestipol on digitoxin plasma levels. *Arzneimittelforschung* (1976) 26, 1891–3.

Digitalis glycosides + Colestyramine

The levels of both digoxin and digitoxin can be reduced by colestyramine, but the clinical importance of this is uncertain. Minimise the possible effects of this interaction by separating administration.

Clinical evidence

(a) Digitalis glycoside levels unaffected

Ten patients on long-term treatment with either **digoxin** 125 to 250 micrograms daily or **digitoxin** 100 to 200 micrograms daily were given colestyramine 12 g daily or a placebo taken 1.5 hour after the digitalis. Their plasma digitalis levels were not significantly altered by the colestyramine over a 1-year period.[1] The half-life of **digitoxin** is reported to have remained unchanged when colestyramine was given.[2]

(b) Digitalis glycoside levels reduced

A study in 12 healthy subjects given **digoxin** 750 micrograms showed that the cumulative 6-day recovery of **digoxin** from the urine was reduced by almost 20% (from 40.5 to 33.1%) when colestyramine 4 g was given.[3] Two patients with congestive heart failure and toxic serum levels of **digoxin** of 3 and 4 nanograms/ml were given colestyramine 4 g every 4 hours for 4 doses. The levels of **digoxin** fell to therapeutic levels within 13 to 24 hours.[4]

Other reports describe a fall in serum **digoxin** levels during the concurrent use of colestyramine[5-7] and an increase in the loss of **digoxin** and its metabolites in the faeces during long-term use.[8] Another study showed that giving **digoxin** as a solution in a capsule reduced the effects of this interaction.[7] Other studies have found that colestyramine reduces the half-life of **digitoxin** by 35 to 40%.[9,10]

Mechanism

Not totally understood. Colestyramine appears to bind with digitoxin in the gut, thereby reducing its bioavailability and interfering with the enterohepatic cycle so that its half-life is shortened. Digoxin may interact similarly.[4]

Importance and management

The overall picture is far from clear. Some interaction seems possible but the extent to which it impairs the treatment of patients on these glycosides is uncertain. Be alert for any evidence of under-digitalisation if digoxin or, more particularly, digitoxin are given with colestyramine. The studies suggest that colestyramine should not be given less than 1.5 to 2 hours after the digitalis to minimise the possibility of an interaction.[1] Note that the standard recommendation is to give other drugs 1 hour before or 4 to 6 hours after colestyramine. An alternative is to use **metildigoxin**, which one study suggests may be minimally affected by colestyramine.[11]

1. Bazzano G, Bazzano GS. Effects of digitalis binding resins on cardiac glycoside plasma levels. *Clin Res* (1972) 20, 24.
2. Pabst J, Leopold G, Schad W, Meub R. Bioavailability of digitoxin during chronic administration and influence of food and cholestyramine on the bioavailability after a single dose. *Naunyn Schmiedebergs Arch Pharmacol* (1979) 307, R70.
3. Brown DD, Juhl RP, Warner SL. Decreased bioavailability of digoxin produced by dietary fiber and cholestyramine. *Am J Cardiol* (1977) 39, 297.
4. Roberge RJ, Sorensen T. Congestive heart failure and toxic digoxin levels: role of cholestyramine. *Vet Hum Toxicol* (2000) 42, 172–3.
5. Smith TW. New approaches to the management of digitalis intoxication, In 'Symposium on Digitalis'. *Gyldendal Norsk Forlag* (1977) 39, 312.
6. Brown DD, Juhl RP, Warner SL. Decreased bioavailability of digoxin due to hypocholesterolemic interventions. *Circulation* (1978) 58, 164–72.
7. Brown DD, Schmid J, Long RA, Hull JH. A steady-state evaluation of the effects of propantheline bromide and cholestyramine on the bioavailability of digoxin when administered as tablets or capsules. *J Clin Pharmacol* (1985) 25, 360–4.
8. Hall WH, Shappell SD, Doherty JE. Effect of cholestyramine on digoxin absorption and excretion in man. *Am J Cardiol* (1977) 39, 213–16.
9. Caldwell JH, Bush CA, Greenberger NJ. Interruption of the enterohepatic circulation of digitoxin by cholestyramine. *J Clin Invest* (1971) 50, 2638–44.
10. Carruthers SG, Dujovne CA. Cholestyramine and spironolactone and their combination in digitoxin elimination. *Clin Pharmacol Ther* (1980) 27, 184–7.
11. Blondheim SH, Alkan WJ, Brunner D. Frontiers of Internal Medicine. Basel: Karger; 1975 p. 409–11.

Digitalis glycosides + Co-trimoxazole or Trimethoprim

Serum digoxin levels can be increased by about 22% by trimethoprim but some individuals may show a much greater rise.

Clinical evidence

(a) Elderly patients

After taking trimethoprim 200 mg twice daily for 14 days the mean serum **digoxin** levels in 9 elderly patients (aged 62 to 92) had risen by an average of 22%, from 1.17 to 1.5 nanomol/l. One patient showed a 75% rise. A 34% increase in mean serum creatinine was also seen. When the trimethoprim was withdrawn, the serum **digoxin** levels returned to their previous value.[1,2]

(b) Young healthy adult subjects

Trimethoprim 200 mg twice daily for 10 days did not affect total body clearance of **digoxin** after a single 1-mg intravenous dose in 6 young healthy subjects (aged 24 to 31). Renal clearance was reduced, but this was compensated for by an increase in extrarenal clearance.[2]

Mechanism

It is suggested that trimethoprim reduces the renal excretion of digoxin.[1,2] The paradoxical finding between the elderly patients and the young healthy subjects may be the age difference, probably as the elderly patients may not be able to accommodate an increase in extrarenal digoxin clearance.

Importance and management

Information seems to be limited to the information cited. Although the serum digoxin rise in the elderly was modest, it would seem prudent to monitor the effects because some individuals can apparently experience a marked rise. Reduce the digoxin dosage if necessary. Trimethoprim is contained in co-trimoxazole but it is not known whether prophylactic doses of co-trimoxazole (160 mg trimethoprim a day, from 960 mg co-trimoxazole) will interact to a clinically significant degree. An interaction would seem likely with high-dose co-trimoxazole regimens and care with any co-trimoxazole regimen is needed in the elderly.

1. Kastrup J, Bartram R, Petersen P, Hansen JM. Trimetoprims indvirkning på serum-digoksin og serum-kreatinin. *Ugeskr Laeger* (1983) 145, 2286–8.
2. Petersen P, Kastrup J, Bartram R, Hansen JM. Digoxin-trimethoprim interaction. *Acta Med Scand* (1985) 217, 423–7.

Digitalis glycosides + Danaparoid

No clinically significant interaction appears to occur between digoxin and danaparoid.

Clinical evidence, mechanism, importance and management

In a study, 6 healthy subjects were given a single bolus dose of danaparoid 3250 anti-Xa units during day 7 of an 8-day course of digoxin 250 micrograms daily. The AUC of digoxin was slightly decreased, although this did not appear to be clinically significant. Digoxin did not alter the effects of danaparoid on clotting tests (including aPTT).[1]

1. de Boer A, Stiekema JCJ, Danhof M, Moolenaar AJ, Breimer DD. Interaction of ORG 10172, a low molecular weight heparinoid, and digoxin in healthy volunteers. *Eur J Clin Pharmacol* (1991) 41, 245–50.

Digitalis glycosides + Dexmedetomidine

An isolated report describes bradycardia in an infant on digoxin when she was given dexmedetomidine.

Clinical evidence, mechanism, importance and management

A 5-week-old infant with an atrioventricular septal defect, treated with **digoxin** 10 micrograms twice daily and furosemide for mild congestive heart failure, developed respiratory failure requiring intubation and mechanical ventilation. She was given dexmedetomidine for sedation and received a loading dose of 0.5 micrograms/kg over 15 minutes, followed by an infusion of 0.44 micrograms/kg per hour. During the loading dose period her heart rate decreased from 133 to 116 bpm. Throughout the next 13 hours the rate continued to decrease to about 90 bpm, with episodes of sinus bradycardia (heart rate around 50 bpm). Within 1 hour of discontinuing dexmedetomidine, the heart rate increased to its baseline value and no further episodes of bradycardia were observed. The reasons for the interaction are not known, but caution is advised if dexmedetomidine is used for sedation in patients on **digoxin**.[1]

1. Berkenbosch JW, Tobias JD. Development of bradycardia during sedation with dexmedetomidine in an infant concurrently receiving digoxin. *Pediatr Crit Care Med* (2003) 4, 203–5.

Digitalis glycosides + Dietary fibre and Laxatives

Bisacodyl reduces serum digoxin levels to a small extent. Large amounts of dietary fibre, guar gum and bulk-forming laxatives containing ispaghula or psyllium appear to have no significant effect on the absorption of digoxin from the gut. Single-dose studies show that macrogol 4000, a laxative polymer, reduces the serum levels of digoxin.

Clinical evidence

(a) Bisacodyl

Bisacodyl reduced the mean serum **digoxin** levels of 11 healthy subjects by about 12%. When the bisacodyl was taken 2 hours before the **digoxin**, serum **digoxin** levels were slightly raised, but not to a statistically significant extent.[1]

(b) Fibre

The serum **digoxin** levels of 12 patients taking 125 to 250 micrograms daily 15 to 30 minutes before breakfast were unchanged over a 10-day period while on a diet supplemented each day with 22 g of dietary fibre. The fibre was given in this way to simulate the conditions that might be encountered clinically (for example to reduce the symptoms of diverticular disease).[2]

Wheat bran 7.5 g twice daily caused a small reduction of 10% in plasma **digoxin** levels of 14 geriatric patients after 2 weeks, but no significant change after 4 weeks.[3] Bran fibre 11 g caused a 6 to 7% reduction in the absorption and the steady-state serum levels of **digoxin** in 16 healthy subjects.[4] The cumulative urinary recovery of single oral doses of **digoxin** in healthy subjects was reduced almost 20% by 5 g of fibre, whereas 0.75 g of fibre had no effect.[5]

(c) Guar gum

Guarem (95% guar gum) 5 g reduced the peak serum levels of a single 500-microgram oral dose of **digoxin** by 21% and the 0 to 6-hour AUC was reduced by 16% in 10 healthy subjects, but the amount excreted in the urine over 24 hours was only minimally reduced.[6] Guar gum 18 g with a test meal did not affect steady-state plasma **digoxin** levels in 11 healthy subjects given **digoxin** 1000 micrograms on day 1, then 750 micrograms on day 2, then 500 micrograms daily for 3 days.[7]

(d) Ispaghula or psyllium

An ispaghula preparation (*Vi-Siblin S*) was found to have no significant effect on serum **digoxin** levels of 16 geriatric patients.[3] The same lack of effect was seen in another study in 15 patients given 3.6 g of a psyllium preparation (*Metamucil*) three times a day.[8]

(e) Macrogol 4000

An open, randomised, two-way crossover study in 18 healthy subjects found that 20 g of macrogol 4000 daily over an 8-day period reduced the maximum serum levels of a single 500-microgram dose of **digoxin** by 40%, and reduced the AUC by 30%. Heart rate and the PR interval were unchanged.[9] More study is needed to assess the effects of this interaction on steady-state **digoxin** levels.

Mechanism

Not established. Digoxin can bind to some extent to fibre within the gut.[10] However, *in vitro* studies (with bran, carrageenan, pectin, sodium pectinate, xylan and carboxymethylcellulose) have shown that most of the binding is reversible.[11]

Importance and management

Information seems to be limited to these reports. The reduction in serum digoxin levels caused by bisacodyl is small, probably of little clinical importance, and apparently preventable by giving the bisacodyl 2 hours before the digoxin. Neither dietary fibre (bran), guar gum nor the two bulk-forming laxatives (*Vi-Siblin* and *Metamucil*) have a clinically important effect on serum digoxin levels. No special precautions would appear to be necessary. The importance of the interaction between digoxin and macrogol 4000 awaits further assessment but on the current evidence it would be prudent to be alert for the need to increase the digoxin dosage.

1. Wang D-J, Chu K-M, Chen J-D. Drug interaction between digoxin and bisacodyl. *J Formos Med Assoc* (1990) 89, 913, 915–9.
2. Woods MN, Ingelfinger JA. Lack of effect of bran on digoxin absorption. *Clin Pharmacol Ther* (1979) 26, 21–3.
3. Nordström M, Melander A, Robertsson E, Steen B. Influence of wheat bran and of a bulk-forming ispaghula cathartic on the bioavailability of digoxin in geriatric in-patients. *Drug Nutr Interact* (1987) 5, 67–9.
4. Johnson BF, Rodin SM, Hoch K, Shekar V. The effect of dietary fiber on the bioavailability of digoxin in capsules. *J Clin Pharmacol* (1987) 27, 487–90.
5. Brown DD, Juhl RP, Warner SL. Decreased bioavailability of digoxin due to hypocholesterolemic interventions. *Circulation* (1978) 58, 164–72.
6. Huupponen R, Seppälä P, Iisalo E. Effect of guar gum, a fibre preparation, on digoxin and penicillin absorption in man. *Eur J Clin Pharmacol* (1984) 26, 279–81.
7. Lembcke B, Häsler K, Kramer P, Caspary WF, Creuzfeldt W. Plasma digoxin concentrations during administration of dietary fibre (guar gum) in man. *Z Gastroenterol* (1982) 20, 164–7.
8. Walan A, Bergdahl B, Skoog M-L. Study of digoxin bioavailability during treatment with a bulk forming laxative (*Metamucil*). *Scand J Gastroenterol* (1977) 12 (Suppl 45), 111.
9. Ragueneau I, Poirier J-M, Radembino N, Sao AB, Funck-Brentano C, Jaillon P. Pharmacokinetic and pharmacodynamic drug interactions between digoxin and macrogol 4000, a laxative polymer, in healthy volunteers. *Br J Clin Pharmacol* (1999) 48, 453–6.
10. Floyd RA. Digoxin interaction with bran and high fiber foods. *Am J Hosp Pharm* (1978) 35, 660.
11. Hamamura J, Burros BC, Clemens RA, Smith CH. Dietary fiber and digoxin. *Fedn Proc* (1985) 44, 759.

Digitalis glycosides + Dihydroergocryptine

Dihydroergocryptine appears not to interact with digoxin.

Clinical evidence, mechanism, importance and management

In a randomised non-blinded crossover study in 12 healthy subjects dihydroergocryptine 20 mg did not affect the pharmacokinetics of a single 500-microgram dose of **digoxin**. No clinically significant changes were seen in the ability of the heart to initiate and conduct impulses, or repolarise. The slight drop in blood pressure during the first 2 to 4 hours after **digoxin** was more pronounced in the presence of dihydroergocryptine, but there was no evidence of impaired orthostatic blood pressure control.[1] No special precautions would seem necessary during concurrent use.

1. Retzow A, Althaus M, de Mey C, Mazur D, Vens-Cappell B. Study on the interaction of the dopamine agonist α-dihydroergocryptine with the pharmacokinetics of digoxin. *Arzneimittelforschung* (2000) 50, 591–6.

Digitalis glycosides + Diprafenone

Diprafenone caused a moderate increase in the peak digoxin levels.

Clinical evidence

Twelve healthy subjects were given **digoxin** 500 micrograms daily with or without diprafenone 300 mg daily for a week. The diprafenone caused a 14% increase in trough serum **digoxin** levels from 1.4 to 1.6 nanograms/ml, a 41% increase in peak steady-state serum levels from 3.9 to 5.5 nanograms/ml and an increase in the AUC of 17%. When the diprafenone was stopped the serum **digoxin** concentrations returned to their former levels.[1]

Mechanism

It is believed that the diprafenone reduces the excretion of digoxin by the kidneys, possibly by inhibition of P-glycoprotein-mediated renal transport.

Importance and management

Information is limited but the interaction appears to be established. The rise in digoxin levels and AUC may possibly be enough to cause problems, therefore it would be prudent to monitor the effects of digoxin in the presence of diprafenone.

1. Koytchev R, Alken R-G, Mayer O. Effect of diprafenone on the pharmacokinetics of digoxin. *Eur J Clin Pharmacol* (1996) 50, 97–100.

Digitalis glycosides + Dipyridamole

Dipyridamole may cause modest increases in the absorption of digoxin.

Clinical evidence, mechanism, importance and management

A study in 12 healthy subjects found that dipyridamole 150 mg twice daily for 5 doses increased the 0 to 4 and 0 to 24 hour AUCs of a single 500-microgram oral dose of **digoxin** by 20% and 13% respectively. This was attributed to an increase in **digoxin** absorption possibly mediated by intestinal P-glycoprotein inhibition.[1] *In vitro* studies[1,2] found that dipyridamole inhibits P-glycoprotein-mediated transport of **digoxin**, but in one study this was only at higher levels than those achieved clinically.[2] The changes in **digoxin** pharmacokinetics in the presence of dipyridamole are probably not clinically significant.

1. Verstuyft C, Strabach S, El Morabet H, Kerb R, Brinkmann U, Dubert L, Jaillon P, Funck-Brentano C, Trugnan G, Becquemont L. Dipyridamole enhances digoxin bioavailability via P-glycoprotein inhibition. *Clin Pharmacol Ther* (2003) 73, 51–60.
2. Kakumoto M, Takara K, Sakaeda T, Tanigawara Y, Kita T, Okumura K. MDR1-mediated interaction of digoxin with antiarrhythmic or antianginal drugs. *Biol Pharm Bull* (2002) 25, 1604–7.

Digitalis glycosides + Disopyramide or Procainamide

Neither disopyramide nor procainamide normally cause a significant change in serum digoxin levels. A single report describes toxicity in a patient on digitoxin and disopyramide.

Clinical evidence, mechanism, importance and management

(a) Disopyramide

A number of studies have clearly shown that disopyramide causes only a very small increase or no increase at all in the serum concentrations of **digoxin**.[1-6] A small but insignificant reduction in heart rate has been seen[7] but the weight of evidence suggests that no adverse interaction occurs if digoxin and disopyramide are used together. However, a very brief report describes toxicity and serious arrhythmia in one patient given **digitoxin** and disopyramide.[8]

(b) Procainamide

A study in patients who had been taking **digoxin** for at least 7 days showed that procainamide did not affect their serum **digoxin** levels.[2] However, it should be noted that the makers of procainamide say that, in digitalis toxicity, procainamide may further depress conduction, which may result in ventricular asystole or fibrillation.[9] Considerable care and good monitoring would therefore seem necessary if both drugs are used.

1. Doering W. Quinidine-digoxin interaction. *N Engl J Med* (1979) 301, 400–4.
2. Leahey EB, Reiffel JA, Giardina E-GV, Bigger JT. The effect of quinidine and other oral antiarrhythmic drugs on serum digoxin: a prospective study. *Ann Intern Med* (1980) 92, 605–8.
3. Manolas EG, Hunt D, Sloman G. Effects of quinidine and disopyramide on serum digoxin concentrations. *Aust N Z J Med* (1980) 10, 426–9.
4. Wellens HJ, Gorgels AP, Braat SJ, Bär FW, Vanagt EJ, Phaf B. Effect of oral disopyramide on serum digoxin levels. A prospective study. *Am Heart J* (1980) 100, 934–5.
5. Risler T, Burk M, Peters U, Grabensee B, Seipel L. On the interaction between digoxin and disopyramide. *Clin Pharmacol Ther* (1983) 34, 176–80.
6. García-Barreto D, Groning E, González-Gómez A, Pérez A, Hernández-Cañero A, Toruncha A. Enhancement of the antiarrhythmic action of disopyramide by digoxin. *J Cardiovasc Pharmacol* (1981) 3, 1236–42.
7. Elliott HL, Kelman AW, Sumner DJ, Bryson SM, Campbell BC, Hillis WS, Whiting B. Pharmacodynamic and pharmacokinetic evaluation of the interaction between digoxin and disopyramide. *Br J Clin Pharmacol* (1982) 14, 141P.
8. Manchon ND, Bercoff E, Lemarchand P, Chassagne P, Senant J, Bourreille J. Fréquence et gravité des interactions médicamenteuses dans une population âgée: étude prospective concernant 63 malades. *Rev Med Interne* (1989) 10, 521–5.
9. Pronestyl (Procainamide).E.R. Squibb & Sons Ltd. ABPI Datasheet Compendium 1999–2000, 1649–51.

Digitalis glycosides + Diuretics; Potassium-depleting

The potassium loss caused by potassium-depleting diuretics (see 'Table 24.1', (p.717)) increases the toxicity of the digitalis glycosides.

Clinical evidence

(a) Evidence suggesting an interaction

A comparative study[1] of the medical records of 418 patients on digitalis over the period 1950 to 1952, and of 679 patients over the period 1964 to 1966, showed that the incidence of digitalis toxicity had more than doubled. Of the earlier group 8.6% developed toxicity (58% on diuretics, mainly of the **organomercurial type**) compared with 17.2% of the latter group (81% taking diuretics, mainly **chlorothiazides**, **furosemide**, **etacrynic acid**, **chlortalidone**). It was concluded that the increased toxicity was related to the increased usage of potassium-depleting diuretics.

A retrospective study of over 400 patients on **digoxin** showed that almost one in five had some toxic reactions attributable to the use of the glycoside. Of these, 16% had demonstrable hypokalaemia (defined as serum potassium less than 3.5 mmol/l). Almost half of the patients who showed toxicity were taking potassium-depleting diuretics, notably **hydrochlorothiazide** or **furosemide**.[2] Similar results were found in other studies[3-9] in a considerable number of patients. There are other reports not listed here. In addition there is also some evidence that **furosemide** may raise serum **digoxin** levels,[10] although two other studies found no evidence that **furosemide** affects the urinary excretion of **digoxin**.[11,12]

(b) Evidence suggesting no interaction

A retrospective study of patients who developed digitalis toxicity showed that the likelihood of its development in those with potassium levels below 3.5 mmol/l was no greater than those with normal potassium levels.[13]

Two other studies in a total of almost 200 patients failed to detect any association between the development of digitalis toxicity and the use of diuretics or changes in potassium levels.[14,15]

Mechanism

Not fully understood. The cardiac glycosides inhibit sodium-potassium ATP-ase, which is concerned with the transport of sodium and potassium ions across the membranes of the myocardial cells. This is associated with an increase in the availability of calcium ions concerned with the contraction of the cells. Potassium loss caused by these diuretics exacerbates the potassium loss from the myocardial cells, thereby increasing the activity and the toxicity of the digitalis. Some loss of magnesium may also have a part to play. The mechanism of this interaction is still being debated.

Importance and management

A direct link between the use of these diuretics and the development of digitalis toxicity is not established beyond doubt, but concurrent use can result in digitalis toxicity. It is therefore important that potassium levels remain within the accepted normal range during digitalis treatment. Potassium levels should be routinely monitored when diuretics are given and it may be prudent to recheck levels if patients develop symptoms of digitalis toxicity.

1. Jørgenson AW, Sørensen OH. Digitalis intoxication. A comparative study on the incidence of digitalis intoxication during the periods 1950–52 and 1964–66. *Acta Med Scand* (1970) 188, 179–83.
2. Shapiro S, Slone D, Lewis GP, Jick H. The epidemiology of digoxin. A study in three Boston Hospitals. *J Chron Dis* (1969) 22, 361–71.
3. Tawakkol AA, Nutter DO, Massumi RA. A prospective study of digitalis toxicity in a large city hospital. *Med Ann Dist Columbia* (1967) 36, 402–9.
4. Soffer A. The changing clinical picture of digitalis intoxication. *Arch Intern Med* (1961) 107, 681–8.
5. Rodensky PL, Wasserman F. Observations on digitalis intoxication. *Arch Intern Med* (1961) 108, 171–88.
6. Steiness E, Olesen KH. Cardiac arrhythmias induced by hypokalaemia and potassium loss during maintenance digoxin therapy. *Br Heart J* (1976) 38, 167–72.
7. Binnion PF. Hypokalaemia and digoxin-induced arrhythmias. *Lancet* (1975) i, 343–4.
8. Poole-Wilson PA, Hall R, Cameron IR. Hypokalaemia, digitalis and arrhythmias. *Lancet* (1975) i, 575–6.
9. Shapiro W, Taubert K. Hypokalaemia and digoxin-induced arrhythmias. *Lancet* (1975) ii, 604–5.
10. Tsutsumi E, Fujiki H, Takeda H, Fukushima H. Effect of furosemide on serum clearance and renal excretion of digoxin. *J Clin Pharmacol* (1979) 19, 200–204.
11. Malcolm AD, Leung FY, Fuchs JCA, Duarte JE. Digoxin kinetics during furosemide administration. *Clin Pharmacol Ther* (1977) 21, 567–574.
12. Brown DD, Dormois JC, Abraham GN, Lewis K, Dixon K. Effect of furosemide on the renal excretion of digoxin. *Clin Pharmacol Ther* (1976) 20, 395–400.
13. Ogilvie RI, Ruedy J. An educational program in digitalis therapy. *JAMA* (1972) 222, 50–55.
14. Smith TW, Haber E. Digoxin intoxication: the relationship of clinical presentation to serum digoxin concentration. *J Clin Invest* (1970) 49, 2377–86.
15. Beller GA, Smith TW, Abelmann WH, Haber E, Hood WB. Digitalis intoxication. A prospective clinical study with serum level correlations. *N Engl J Med* (1971) 284, 989–97.

Digitalis glycosides + Diuretics; Potassium-sparing

Serum digoxin levels may be increased by 25% by spironolactone, but because spironolactone or its metabolite, canrenone, can interfere with some digoxin assay methods, the evaluation of this interaction is difficult. The effects of digitoxin are reported to be both increased and decreased by spironolactone. Amiloride has little effect on digoxin levels in healthy subjects, but it may reduce its inotropic effects. In patients with renal impairment it possibly raises plasma digoxin levels.

Clinical evidence

(a) Digoxin

(i) Amiloride. Amiloride 5 mg twice daily for 8 days almost doubled the renal clearance of digoxin from 1.3 to 2.4 ml/kg per minute in 6 healthy subjects, but reduced the extra-renal clearance from 2.1 to 0.1 ml/kg per minute. The balance of the two effects was to cause a small fall in total clearance and a small rise in plasma digoxin levels.[1] The positive inotropic effects of digoxin were reduced, but whether this is clinically important is uncertain.

In contrast, a later study in 8 healthy subjects found that a single 75-mg (sic) oral dose of amiloride given 3 hours before an infusion of digoxin did not reduce the inotropic effects of digoxin.[2]

(ii) Spironolactone. The plasma digoxin levels of 9 patients were increased by about 20% (from 0.8 to 1 nanograms/ml) when they were given spironolactone 100 mg daily. One patient showed a three to fourfold rise in digoxin levels.[3]

The clearance of a single 750-microgram intravenous dose of digoxin was reduced by about 25% in 4 patients and 4 healthy subjects following 5 days' treatment with spironolactone 100 mg twice daily.[4] A marked fall in serum digoxin was reported in an elderly patient when spironolactone was withdrawn[5] but the accuracy of the assay method used is uncertain (see Importance and management below). One study found that no clinically important reduction in digoxin clearance occurred when *Aldactazide* (spironolactone-hydrochlorothiazide) was given.[6]

(b) Digitoxin

A study in 6 healthy subjects who had been taking digitoxin 100 or 150 micrograms daily for 30 days showed that spironolactone 300 mg daily increased the digitoxin half-life by a third (from 142 to 192 hours).[7]

In contrast, other studies have found that the digitoxin half-life was reduced (from 256 to 205 hours).[8]

Mechanism

Not fully understood. Spironolactone inhibits the excretion of digoxin by the kidney (by 13%) but does not affect its biliary clearance.[9] Spironolactone probably causes a reduction in the volume of distribution of digoxin.

It has been suggested that amiloride may have increased the production of aldosterone, which suppressed the positive inotropic effects of digoxin.[1] Studies in patients with congestive heart failure are needed.

Importance and management

The digoxin/spironolactone interaction appears to be established. What is known suggests that a rise in digoxin levels of up to 25% is likely to occur, although much greater increases can apparently occur in some patients.[3] Monitor concurrent use carefully for signs of over-digitalisation. The reports cited here appear to be reliable, but the total picture of this interaction is confused by a number of other reports (not cited) of doubtful reliability. The problem is that spironolactone or its metabolite, canrenone, can interfere with some assay methods.[10] In one report, radioimmunoassay (RIA) and affinity-column-mediated immunoassay (ACMIA) were particularly affected by spironolactone and its metabolites.[11] Conversely, falsely low digoxin readings with the AxSym MEIA assay method led to digoxin overdose and toxicity in one patient.[12] This means that monitoring is difficult unless the digoxin assay method is known to be reliable. Measurement of free digoxin levels or use of a chemiluminescent assay (CLIA) for digoxin has been reported to mostly eliminate interference from spironolactone, potassium canrenoate and canrenone.[13]

The situation with digitoxin is even more confusing because the reports are contradictory and the outcome uncertain. Concurrent use should be well monitored.

Patients with poor renal function would be expected to show a rise in digoxin levels when given amiloride (due to the increased reliance on renal clearance) but the clinical importance of this awaits confirmation.

1. Waldorff S, Hansen PB, Kjærgård H, Buch J, Egeblad H, Steiness E. Amiloride-induced changes in digoxin dynamics and kinetics: abolition of digoxin-induced inotropism with amiloride. *Clin Pharmacol Ther* (1981) 30, 172–6.
2. Richter JP, Sommers De K, Snyman JR, Millard SM. The acute effects of amiloride and potassium canrenoate on digoxin-induced positive inotropism in healthy volunteers. *Eur J Clin Pharmacol* (1993) 45, 195–6.
3. Steiness E. Renal tubular secretion of digoxin. *Circulation* (1974) 50. 103–7.
4. Waldorff S, Andersen JD, Heebøll-Nielsen N, Nielsen OG, Moltke E, Sørensen U, Steiness E. Spironolactone-induced changes in digoxin kinetics. *Clin Pharmacol Ther* (1978) 24, 162–7.
5. Paladino JA, Davidson KH, McCall BB. Influence of spironolactone on serum digoxin concentration. *JAMA* (1984) 251, 470–1.
6. Finnegan TP, Spence JD, Cape R. Potassium-sparing diuretics: interaction with digoxin in elderly men. *J Am Geriatr Soc* (1984) 32, 129–31.
7. Carruthers SG, Dujovne CA. Cholestyramine and spironolactone and their combination in digitoxin elimination. *Clin Pharmacol Ther* (1980) 27, 184–7.
8. Wirth KE, Frölich JC, Hollifield JW, Falkner FC, Sweetman BS, Oates JA. Metabolism of digitoxin in man and its modification by spironolactone. *Eur J Clin Pharmacol* (1976) 9, 345–54.
9. Hedman A, Angelin B, Arvidsson A, Dahlqvist R. Digoxin-interactions in man: spironolactone reduces renal but not biliary digoxin clearance. *Eur J Clin Pharmacol* (1992) 42, 481–5.
10. Steimer W, Müller C, Eber B. Digoxin assays: frequent, substantial, and potentially dangerous interference by spironolactone, canrenone, and other steroids. *Clin Chem* (2002) 48, 507–16.
11. Pleasants RA, Williams DM, Porter RS, Gadsden RH. Reassessment of cross-reactivity of spironolactone metabolites with four digoxin immunoassays. *Ther Drug Monit* (1989) 11, 200–4.
12. Steimer W, Müller C, Eber B, Emmanuilidis K. Intoxication due to negative canrenone interference in digoxin drug monitoring. *Lancet* (1999) 354, 1176–7.
13. Dasgupta A, Saffer H, Wells A, Datta P. Bidirectional (positive/negative) interference of spironolactone, canrenone, and potassium canrenoate on serum digoxin measurement: elimination of interference by measuring free digoxin or using a chemiluminescent assay for digoxin. *J Clin Lab Anal* (2002) 16, 172–7.

Digitalis glycosides + Dofetilide

Dofetilide does not affect the pharmacokinetics of digoxin.

Clinical evidence, mechanism, importance and management

In a placebo-controlled study in 13 subjects, dofetilide 250 micrograms twice daily for 5 days had no effect on the steady-state pharmacokinetics of **digoxin**, given at a dose of 250 micrograms daily after a loading dose.[1]

1. Kleinermans D, Nichols DJ, Dalrymple I. Effect of dofetilide on the pharmacokinetics of digoxin. *Am J Cardiol* (2001) 87, 248–50.

Digitalis glycosides + Drugs that reduce potassium levels

A number of drugs, including amphotericin B, carbenoxolone and corticosteroids cause potassium loss, which could lead to the development of digitalis toxicity.

Clinical evidence, mechanism, importance and management

Among the well-recognised adverse effects of **amphotericin B** treatment is hypokalaemia, which can be severe. Although there seem to be no reports of adverse interactions, it would be logical to expect that digitalis toxicity could develop in patients given both drugs if the potassium levels fall. Amiloride has been successfully used to counteract the potassium loss caused by **amphotericin B**.[1]

The adverse effects of **carbenoxolone** include an increase in blood pressure (both systolic and diastolic), fluid retention and reduced serum potassium levels. The incidence of these adverse effects is said in some reports to be as high as 50%; others quote lower figures. Hypertension and fluid retention occur early in **carbenoxolone** treatment, whereas the hypokalaemia develops later and may occur in the absence of the other two adverse effects.[2-5] **Carbenoxolone** is therefore unsuitable for patients with congestive heart failure, or those taking digitalis glycosides, unless measures to avoid hypokalaemia are taken.

Systemic corticosteroids can increase the loss of potassium, particularly those that are naturally occurring (**cortisone, deoxycortone, hydrocortisone**) whereas the synthetic derivatives (**betamethasone, dexamethasone, methylprednisolone, prednisolone, prednisone, triamcinolone**) have much less mineralocorticoid activity. There is therefore the possibility of potassium depletion, particularly when used long-term, which may increase the risk of digitalis toxicity. These corticosteroids also cause sodium and water retention, resulting in oedema and hypertension, which can lead to cardiac failure in some individuals.

It is therefore important to monitor the use of **digoxin** and any of these drugs well. Potassium levels should be routinely monitored in any patient on **amphotericin B**, but it is particularly important in those taking **digoxin**. With other drugs where potassium monitoring is not routine one should watch for signs of **digoxin** toxicity (e.g. bradycardia) and consider measuring potassium levels. No problems of this kind would be expected with corticosteroids used topically or by inhalation because the amounts absorbed are likely to be relatively small.

1. Smith SR, Galloway MJ, Reilly JT, Davies JM. Amiloride prevents amphotericin B related hypokalaemia in neutropenic patients. *J Clin Pathol* (1988) 41, 494–7.
2. Geismar P, Mosbech J, Myren J. A double-blind study of the effect of carbenoxolone sodium in the treatment of gastric ulcer. *Scand J Gastroenterol* (1973) 8, 251–6.
3. Turpie AGG, Thomson TJ. Carbenoxolone sodium in the treatment of gastric ulcer with special reference to side-effects. *Gut* (1965) 6, 591–4.
4. Langman MJS, Knapp DR, Wakley EJ. Treatment of chronic gastric ulcer with carbenoxolone and gefarnate: a comparative trial. *BMJ* (1973) 3, 84–6.
5. Davies GJ, Rhodes J, Calcraft BJ. Complications of carbenoxolone therapy. *BMJ* (1974) 3, 400–402.

Digitalis glycosides + Edrophonium

Excessive bradycardia and AV-block may occur in patients on digitalis glycosides given edrophonium.

Clinical evidence, mechanism, importance and management

The rapid intravenous injection of edrophonium 10 mg has been used in the differentiation of cardiac arrhythmias, but in one study, 4 of 10 digitalised patients given edrophonium developed atrial tachycardia with AV block. The effect was transient; recovery of baseline ECGs occurred 15 to 20 minutes after administration.[1] Nevertheless, the authors recommended that edrophonium should not be given to patients with atrial flutter or tachycardia who are taking digitalis glycosides. This recommendation is reinforced by the case of an elderly woman[2] who developed bradycardia, AV block and asystole following concurrent use. She recovered after being given atropine 1 mg.

1. Reddy RCV, Gould L, Gomprecht RF. Use of edrophonium (Tensilon) in the evaluation of cardiac arrhythmias. *Am Heart J* (1971) 82, 742–9.
2. Gould L, Zahir M, Gomprecht RF. Cardiac arrest during edrophonium administration. *Am Heart J* (1971) 81, 437–8.

Digitalis glycosides + Enoximone

Studies in patients on long-term treatment with digitalis glycosides (digoxin or digitoxin) showed that oral enoximone 100 mg three times daily for a week had no significant effect on the plasma levels of either of these glycosides.[1,2] Cardiac function was improved.

1. Glauner T, Hertrich F, Winkelmann B, Dieterich HA, Trenk D, Jähnchen E. Lack of effect of enoximone on steady-state plasma concentrations of digoxin and digitoxin. *Eur Heart J* (1988) 9 (Suppl 1), 151.
2. Trenk D, Hertrich F, Winkelmann B, Glauner T, Dieterich HA, Jähnchen E. Lack of effect of enoximone on the pharmacokinetics of digoxin in patients with congestive heart failure. *J Clin Pharmacol* (1990) 30, 235–40.

Digitalis glycosides + Etanercept

No clinically significant interaction appears to occur between digoxin and etanercept.

Clinical evidence, mechanism, importance and management

A study in 12 healthy subjects given an oral loading dose of **digoxin** 500 micrograms twice daily on day 1 followed by 250 micrograms daily found that subcutaneous etanercept 25 mg twice weekly did not significantly affect the pharmacokinetics of **digoxin**. The maximum serum levels and AUC of etanercept were 4.2% and 12.5% lower respectively, during concurrent use but this was not considered clinically significant. The combination was well tolerated and there were no changes in ECG parameters.[1] No special precautions therefore seem necessary.

1. Zhou H, Parks V, Patat A, Le Coz F, Simcoe D, Korth-Bradley J. Absence of a clinically relevant interaction between etanercept and digoxin. *J Clin Pharmacol* (2004) 44, 1244–51.

Digitalis glycosides + Fenoldopam

Fenoldopam appears to cause a small and clinically unimportant reduction in serum digoxin levels in most patients, but more marked changes may occur in a few individuals.

Clinical evidence, mechanism, importance and management

Ten patients with congestive heart failure on chronic **digoxin** treatment (doses not stated) were additionally given fenoldopam 100 mg three times daily for 9 days. The mean AUC and steady-state **digoxin** levels were reduced by about 20%. In two patients, the steady-state serum levels of **digoxin** fell by 48%, from 1.36 to 0.71 nanograms/ml, and 68%, from 1.93 to 0.61 nanograms/ml respectively, and in a further patient, rose by 45% (from 1.03 to 1.49 nanograms/ml).[1] Most patients appear therefore not to show marked changes in serum **digoxin** levels, but a few individuals may possibly need some dosage adjustment. Monitor the effects of concurrent use.

1. Strocchi E, Tartagni F, Malini PL, Valtancoli G, Ambrosioni E, Pasinelli F, Riva E, Fuccella LM. Interaction study of fenoldopam-digoxin in congestive heart failure. *Eur J Clin Pharmacol* (1989) 37, 395–7.

Digitalis glycosides + Finasteride

Finasteride does not appear to affect the pharmacokinetics of digoxin.

Clinical evidence, mechanism, importance and management

In a double-blind randomised study, 17 healthy subjects were given a single 400-microgram dose of **digoxin** during a course of finasteride 5 mg daily for 10 days. Finasteride had no significant effect on the pharmacokinetics of **digoxin**.[1] No adverse effects are expected on concurrent use.

1. Gregoire S, Williams R, Gormely G, Lin E. Effect of finasteride (MK-906) on the disposition of digoxin. *J Clin Pharmacol* (1990) 30, 847.

Digitalis glycosides + Flecainide

Plasma digoxin levels are unaltered or only modestly increased by the use of flecainide, but this is not likely to be important in most patients.

Clinical evidence

The plasma **digoxin** levels of 10 patients with congestive heart failure remained unaltered when they took flecainide 100 to 200 mg twice daily for 7 days. The same result was seen in 4 patients over a 4-week period.[1]

In contrast, a study in 15 healthy subjects showed that flecainide 200 mg twice daily increased their trough and peak plasma levels of **digoxin** 250 micrograms 24% and 13% respectively.[2] The changes observed in vital signs were not clinically significant. Based on the results of a single-dose study the steady-state **digoxin** levels were predicted to rise by about 15% during the use of flecainide 200 mg twice daily.[3]

Mechanism

Uncertain. It is suggested that any changes may be due to alterations in the volume of distribution.[3]

Importance and management

Documentation is limited but what is known suggests that either no interaction occurs, or any changes are small and unlikely to be clinically relevant in most patients. However, the UK makers of flecainide recommend that digoxin plasma levels should be measured not less than six hours after any digoxin dose, before or after the administration of flecainide.[4] The US makers do not advise any additional monitoring.[5] The authors of one of the reports[2] suggest that patients with high drug levels, atrioventricular nodal dysfunction, or both, should be monitored during concurrent treatment.

1. McQuinn RL, Kvam DC, Parrish SL, Fox TL, Miller AM, Franciosa JA. Digoxin levels in patients with congestive heart failure are not altered by flecainide. *Clin Pharmacol Ther* (1988) 43, 150.
2. Weeks CE, Conard GJ, Kvam DC, Fox JM, Chang SF, Paone RP, Lewis GP. The effect of flecainide acetate, a new antiarrhythmic, on plasma digoxin levels. *J Clin Pharmacol* (1986) 26, 27–31.
3. Tjandramaga TB, Verbesselt R, Van Hecken A, Mullie A, De Schepper PJ. Oral digoxin pharmacokinetics during multiple-dose flecainide treatment. *Arch Int Pharmacodyn Ther* (1982) 260, 302–3.
4. Tambocor (Flecainide). 3M Health Care Ltd. UK Summary of product characteristics, July 2003.
5. Tambocor (Flecainide). 3M Pharmaceuticals. US Prescribing information, June 1998.

Digitalis glycosides + Fondaparinux

No significant interaction appears to occur between digoxin and fondaparinux.

Clinical evidence, mechanism, importance and management

A phase I randomised study in 24 healthy subjects found that the pharmacokinetics of oral **digoxin** 250 micrograms twice daily for one day then 250 micrograms daily for 6 days was unaffected by subcutaneous fondaparinux 10 mg daily. The pharmacokinetics of fondaparinux were not affected by **digoxin**. The combination was well tolerated and no clinically significant changes in vital signs and ECGs were observed.[1] No additional precautions therefore seem necessary on concurrent use.

1. Mant T, Fournié P, Ollier C, Donat F, Necciari J. Absence of interaction of fondaparinux sodium with digoxin in healthy volunteers. *Clin Pharmacokinet* (2002), 41 (Suppl 2), 39–45.

Digitalis glycosides + Ginkgo biloba

A study in 8 healthy subjects found that ginkgo biloba leaf extract 80 mg three times daily had no significant effects on the pharmacokinetics of a single 500-microgram dose of digoxin.[1]

1. Mauro VF, Mauro LS, Kleshinski JF, Khuder SA, Wang Y, Erhardt PW. Impact of Ginkgo biloba on the pharmacokinetics of digoxin. *Am J Ther* (2003) 10, 247–51.

Digitalis glycosides + Ginseng

A man on digoxin developed grossly elevated serum digoxin levels, without symptoms of toxicity, while taking Siberian ginseng. Both Chinese and Siberian ginseng may interfere with some digoxin assays.

Clinical evidence, mechanism, importance and management

A 74-year-old man stabilised on **digoxin** for many years (serum levels normally in the range 0.9 to 2.2 nanograms/ml) was found during a routine check to have levels of 5.2 nanograms/ml but without evidence of toxicity or bradycardia or any other ECG changes.[1] The levels remained high even when the **digoxin** was stopped. Later it turned out he was also taking **Siberian ginseng** capsules. When the ginseng was stopped, the **digoxin** levels returned to the usual range, and **digoxin** therapy was resumed. Later rechallenge with the ginseng caused a rise in his serum **digoxin** levels. No digoxin or digitoxin contamination was found in the capsules, and the authors of the report also rejected the idea that the eleutherosides (chemically related to cardiac glycosides) in ginseng might have been converted *in vivo* into **digoxin**, or that the renal elimination of **digoxin** might have been impaired, since the patient showed no signs of toxicity. One possible explanation is that the ginseng affected the accuracy of the **digoxin** assay so that it gave false results.[1]

Asian or **Chinese ginseng** *(Panax ginseng)* and **Siberian ginseng** *(Eleutherococcus senticosus)* have both been found to interfere with some **digoxin** assays including fluorescence polarisation immunoassay (FPIA) and microparticle enzyme immunoassay (MEIA).[2]

Whether serum digoxin levels are actually affected is uncertain, but the case report acts as a reminder that herbal remedies can sometimes interact. Be aware that ginseng can possibly elevate serum **digoxin** levels or affect the assay of **digoxin**.

1. McRae S. Elevated serum digoxin levels in a patient taking digoxin and Siberian ginseng. *Can Med Assoc J* (1996) 155, 293–5.
2. Dasgupta A, Wu S, Actor J, Olsen M, Wells A, Datta P. Effect of Asian and Siberian ginseng on serum digoxin measurement by five digoxin immunoassays. Significant variation in digoxin-like immunoreactivity among commercial ginsengs. *Am J Clin Pathol* (2003) 119, 298–303.

Digitalis glycosides + Grapefruit juice

Plasma digoxin levels are generally unaltered or only modestly increased by grapefruit juice, but in some individuals significant changes may occur.

Clinical evidence

An open crossover study in 12 healthy subjects found that when they were given either grapefruit juice 220 ml or water, 30 minutes before and 3.5, 7.5, and 11.5 hours after a single 500-microgram dose of **digoxin** taken with 50 ml of grapefruit juice or water respectively, the 0 to 4-hour and 0 to 24-hour **digoxin** AUCs were increased by about 10%. A mean non-significant increase of about 20% in the maximum plasma levels of **digoxin** occurred and renal clearance was unaffected. However, in 2 subjects taking grapefruit juice, the ECGs taken 90 minutes after **digoxin** ingestion revealed an asymptomatic first-degree atrioventricular block. Plasma levels in these subjects had increased by 50% to 2.4 and 2.8 nanograms/ml respectively.[1]

Another study found that grapefruit juice decreased the rate but not the extent of absorption of **digoxin** and had no effect on AUC or renal clearance, but there was significant interindividual variability.[2]

Mechanism

The modest increases in digoxin levels may be due to increased intestinal absorption of digoxin, possibly due to inhibition of P-glycoprotein-mediated digoxin transport by grapefruit juice, although this mechanism has been questioned.[1]

Importance and management

Although grapefruit juice appears to have little effect on digoxin bioavailability, it is possible that in some individuals the interaction could be of clinical significance.[2] Bear this interaction in mind in the case of an unexpected response to digoxin. More study is needed.

1. Becquemont L, Verstuyft C, Kerb R, Brinkmann U, Lebot M, Jaillon P, Funck-Brentano C. Effect of grapefruit juice on digoxin pharmacokinetics in humans. *Clin Pharmacol Ther* (2001) 70, 311–6.
2. Parker RB, Yates CR, Soberman JE, Laizure SC. Effects of grapefruit juice on intestinal P-glycoprotein: evaluation using digoxin in humans. *Pharmacotherapy* (2003) 23, 979–87.

Digitalis glycosides + Guanadrel

Guanadrel did not affect the pharmacokinetics of a single dose of digoxin.

Clinical evidence, mechanism, importance and management

No change in the pharmacokinetics of a single intravenous dose of **digoxin** occurred in 13 healthy subjects after taking guanadrel 10 mg orally every 12 hours for 3 days before and 5 days after the **digoxin** dose. One subject experienced a 10-minute episode of asymptomatic second-degree heart block (Wenckebach) 3 hours after the dose of **digoxin**, the reason for which was not clear.[1] There seem to be no reports of adverse interactions between the digitalis glycosides and any of the guanethidine-like antihypertensive drugs.

1. Wright CE, Andreadis NA. Digoxin pharmacokinetics when administered concurrently with guanadrel sulfate. *Drug Intell Clin Pharm* (1986) 20, 465.

Digitalis glycosides + H_2-blockers

Small changes in serum digoxin levels, both rises and falls, have been seen in patients given cimetidine, but these do not appear to be of clinical importance. Ranitidine appears not to interact with metildigoxin.

Clinical evidence, mechanism, importance and management

While taking **cimetidine** 300 mg every 6 or 12 hours the steady-state serum **digoxin** levels of 11 patients with congestive heart failure fell on average by 25% (from 2 to 1.5 nanograms/ml), but none of them showed any ECG changes or signs that their condition had worsened.[1] Four other patients with stable congestive heart failure showed no significant changes in the pharmacokinetics of **digoxin** 125 to 250 micrograms daily when treated with **cimetidine** 300 mg 6 hourly.[2] Three single dose studies in a total of 19 healthy subjects, and 6 patients with duodenal ulcers[3] found that **cimetidine** 600 to 1200 mg daily had no significant effect on the absorption[4] or the kinetics[3,5] of **digoxin**. Another study found a small increase in **digoxin** levels in healthy subjects, but only a small statistically insignificant rise in the steady-state levels of 11 patients given **cimetidine** 400 mg four times daily.[6] Six patients with chronic congestive heart failure given **metildigoxin** showed no changes in their serum **digoxin** levels when they were given **ranitidine** 150 mg twice daily for a week.[7]

No interaction of clinical importance with either of these H_2-blockers has been established and no special precautions would seem to be necessary.

1. Fraley DS, Britton HL, Schwinghammer TL, Kalla R. Effect of cimetidine on steady-state serum digoxin concentrations. *Clin Pharm* (1983) 2, 163–5.
2. Mouser B, Nykamp D, Murphy JE, Krissman PH. Effect of cimetidine on oral digoxin absorption. *DICP Ann Pharmacother* (1990) 24, 286–8.
3. Garty M, Perry G, Shmueli H, Ilfeld D, Boner G, Pitlik S, Rosenfeld J. Effect of cimetidine on digoxin disposition in peptic ulcer patients. *Eur J Clin Pharmacol* (1986) 30, 489–91.
4. Jordaens L, Hoegaerts J, Belpaire F. Non-interaction of cimetidine with digoxin absorption. *Acta Clin Belg* (1981) 36, 109–10.
5. Ochs HR, Gugler R, Guthoff T, Greenblatt DJ. Effect of cimetidine on digoxin kinetics and creatinine clearance. *Am Heart J* (1984) 107, 170–2.
6. Crome P, Curl B, Holt D, Volans GN, Bennett PN, Cole DS. Digoxin and cimetidine: investigation of the potential for a drug interaction. *Hum Toxicol* (1985) 4, 391–9.
7. Enomoto N, Kurasawa T, Ichikawa M, Shimuzu T, Matsuyama T, Sakai K, Shimamura K, Oda M. Lack of interaction of β-methyldigoxin with ranitidine in patients with chronic congestive heart failure. *Eur J Clin Pharmacol* (1992) 43, 205–6.

Digitalis glycosides + Herbal medicines; Digoxin-like

Although few interactions between herbal remedies and digoxin or digitoxin have been reported, many herbal remedies contain digitalis glycosides, which could in theory have additive effects with digoxin or digitoxin.

Clinical evidence, mechanism, importance and management

A 26-year-old woman developed severe and unexplained chest pain, and was later noted to have a heart rate of 39 bpm and a blood pressure of 59/36 mmHg, but these rose to normal with conservative management. She was found to have a digoxin level of 0.9 nanograms/ml and was diagnosed as having digoxin toxicity, despite not taking any prescribed digoxin. The digoxin was thought to have come from an un-named herbal remedy for stress, which contained **black cohosh root** *(Cimicifuga racemosa)*, **cayenne pepper fruit** *(Capsicum annuum)*, **hops flowers** *(Humulus lupulus)*, **skullcap herb** (*Scutellaria lateriflora*), **valerian root** (*Valeriana officinalis*) and **wood betony herb** *(Pedicularis canadensis)*, all of which contain digoxin-like compounds which are detected by digoxin antibody immunoassays.[1]

In a study, 46 commercially packaged herb teas and 78 teas prepared from herbs were assayed for digoxin-like factors by their cross-reactivity with digoxin antibody, and these values were used to give approximate equivalent daily doses of digoxin. Three packaged teas (***Breathe Easy***, **blackcurrant**, and **jasmine**) and 3 herbs (**pleurisy root**, **chaparral**, **peppermint**) were found to theoretically provide a therapeutic daily dose of digoxin if 5 cups a day were drunk.[2]

It is therefore apparent that if a patient taking digoxin also consumed these herbal remedies or teas they could develop symptoms of digoxin toxicity. However, theoretical interaction with herbal remedies are not always translated into practice. For example, **hawthorn** is used in cardiac disorders and the leaves and berries are reported to contain digoxin-like substances,[2,3] but a study in healthy subjects found no pharmacokinetic or pharmacodynamic interaction between digoxin and an extract of **hawthorn** leaves and flowers (*Crataegus oxyacantha*).[4] Therefore although these predicted interactions should be borne in mind when using digoxin and herbal remedies they cannot be taken as total proof that an interaction will occur.

See also 'Digitalis glycosides + Chinese herbal medicines', p.693 and 'Digitalis glycosides + Ginseng', p.700.

1. Scheinhost ME. Digoxin toxicity in a 26-year-old woman taking a herbal dietary supplement. *J Am Osteopath Assoc* (2001), 101, 444–6.
2. Longerich L, Johnson E, Gault MH. Digoxin-like factors in herbal teas. *Clin Invest Med* (1993) 16, 210–8.
3. Miller LG. Herbal medicines: selected clinical considerations focusing on known or potential drug-herb interactions. *Arch Intern Med* (1998) 158, 2200–11.
4. Tankanow R, Tamer HR, Streetman DS, Smith SG, Welton JL, Annesley T, Aaronson KD, Bleske BE. Interaction study between digoxin and a preparation of hawthorn (*Crataegus oxyacantha*). *J Clin Pharmacol* (2003) 43, 637–42.

Digitalis glycosides + Itraconazole

Itraconazole can cause a marked increase in serum digoxin levels. Toxicity may occur unless the digoxin dosage is suitably reduced. Itraconazole may also oppose the positive inotropic effects of digoxin.

Clinical evidence

In a double-blind placebo-controlled crossover study 10 healthy subjects taking **digoxin** 250 micrograms daily were given either itraconazole 200 mg daily or placebo for 10 days, and then the two were swapped over for a further 10 days. The serum **digoxin** levels were reduced from about 1.7 nanomol/l to about 1 nanomol/l by itraconazole. Steady-state **digoxin** levels were not fully achieved during the 10-day period.[1]

A further study in 3 patients with congestive heart failure taking **digoxin** found ECG changes (premature ventricular contractions, AV block and ST depression) when they were given itraconazole.[2]

A 68-year-old man on **digoxin** 250 micrograms twice daily and ibuprofen developed nausea and fatigue (interpreted later as **digoxin** toxicity) after starting itraconazole 400 mg daily for an infected elbow. The symptoms disappeared when both the itraconazole and ibuprofen were stopped, but returned when the itraconazole was restarted. After 7 days his heart rate had fallen from 60 to 40 bpm and his **digoxin** level had doubled, from 1.6 to 3.2 nanograms/ml. He was later satisfactorily restabilised on a quarter of the **digoxin** dosage while taking the same dose of itraconazole.[3] Several other patients developed **digoxin** toxicity (a sixfold increase in one case) after taking itraconazole for 9 to 13 days.[4-9] Two cases of **digoxin** toxicity have been reported during concurrent itraconazole therapy in renal transplant patients, but other factors may have contributed to the high levels of **digoxin** in these 2 patients.[10]

Mechanism

Itraconazole inhibits the action of P-glycoprotein, which transports digoxin out of kidney tubule cells into the urine,[11-14] and therefore digoxin urinary clearance is reduced and serum levels are increased.[5,15]

Importance and management

An established and clinically important interaction of uncertain incidence but probably affecting most patients. Monitor the effects of digoxin (e.g. bradycardia, nausea, vomiting) if itraconazole is started, anticipating the need to reduce the digoxin dosage. Halving the dose was suggested in one study.[2] Two of the patients cited above were restabilised on a quarter of the digoxin dosage[3,4] and another on about one-third while taking itraconazole.[5] More recent findings suggest that itraconazole may possess significant negative inotropic properties, and the UK Committee on Safety of Medicines suggest that it should be used with caution in patients at risk of heart failure.[16] This suggests that itraconazole would oppose the pharmacological effects of digoxin.

1. Jalava K-M, Partanen J, Neuvonen PJ. Digoxin-itraconazole interaction. *Therapie* (1995) 50 (Suppl), 185.
2. Wagasugi H, Isizuka R, Koreeda N, Yano I, Futami T, Nohara R, Sasayoma S, Inui K. Effect of itraconazole on digoxin clearance in patients with congestive heart failure. *Yakugaku Zasshi* (2000) 120, 807–11.
3. Rex J. Itraconazole-digoxin interaction. *Ann Intern Med* (1992) 116, 525.
4. Kauffman CA, Bagnasco FA. Digoxin toxicity associated with itraconazole therapy. *Clin Infect Dis* (1992) 15, 886–7.
5. Sachs MK, Blanchard LM, Green PJ. Interaction of itraconazole and digoxin. *Clin Infect Dis* (1993) 16, 400–3.
6. Alderman CP, Jersmann HPA. Digoxin-itraconazole interaction. *Med J Aust* (1993) 159, 838–9.
7. McClean KL, Sheehan GJ. Interaction between itraconazole and digoxin. *Clin Infect Dis* (1994) 18, 259–60.
8. Meyboom RH, de Jonge K, Veentjer H, Dekens-Konter JA, de Koning GH. Potentiering van digoxine door itraconazol. *Ned Tijdschr Geneeskd* (1994) 138, 2353–6.
9. Cone LA, Himelman RB, Hirschberg JN, Hutcheson JW. Itraconazole-related amaurosis and vomiting due to digoxin toxicity. *West J Med* (1996) 165, 322.
10. Mathis AS, Friedman GS. Coadministration of digoxin with itraconazole in renal transplant recipients. *Am J Kidney Dis* (2001) 37, 1–8.
11. Ito S, Koren G. Comment: possible mechanism of digoxin-itraconazole interaction. *Ann Pharmacother* (1997) 31, 1091–2.
12. Woodland C, Ito S, Koren G. A model for the prediction of digoxin–drug interactions at the renal tubular cell level. *Ther Drug Monit* (1998) 20, 134–8.
13. Angirasa AK, Koch AZ. P-glycoprotein as the mediator of itraconazole–digoxin interaction. *J Am Podiatr Med Assoc* (2002) 92, 471–2.
14. Jalava K-M, Partanen J, Neuvonen PJ. Itraconazole decreases renal clearance of digoxin. *Ther Drug Monit* (1997) 19, 609–13.
15. Alderman CP, Allcroft PD. Digoxin-itraconazole interaction: possible mechanisms. *Ann Pharmacother* (1997) 31, 438–40.
16. Committee on Safety of Medicines/Medicines Control Agency. Cardiodepressant effects of itraconazole. *Current Problems* (2001) 27, 11.

Digitalis glycosides + Kaolin-pectin

Plasma digoxin levels can be reduced by kaolin-pectin, but the reduction is small and probably of minimal clinical importance.

Clinical evidence

The concurrent use of kaolin-pectin suspension and **digoxin** reduced the peak plasma **digoxin** levels of 7 patients by 36%, while the 0 to 24-hour AUC was reduced by 15%. Conversely, when two doses of kaolin-pectin were taken, the first 2 hours before and the other 2 hours after the **digoxin**, no significant changes were seen.[1]

Single dose studies have found 42 and 62% reductions in the bioavailability of **digoxin** caused by kaolin-pectin.[2,3] Another study showed an interaction with **digoxin** tablets but not with **digoxin** capsules.[4]

Mechanism

Not understood. The digoxin may possibly become adsorbed onto the kaolin so that less is available for absorption. Another possibility is that the kaolin reduces the motility of the gut, which normally increases mixing and brings the digoxin into contact with the absorbing surface.

Importance and management

Steady-state studies reflect the every-day situation much more closely than single dose studies, and the one cited above[1] indicates that the total reduction in digoxin absorption is small (15%). This is unlikely to be of clinical importance. However, if an interaction does occur the effects can seemingly be minimised by separating the dosages by 2 hours.

1. Albert KS, Elliott WJ, Abbott RD, Gilbertson TJ, Data JL. Influence of kaolin-pectin suspension on steady-state plasma digoxin levels. *J Clin Pharmacol* (1981) 21, 449–55.
2. Brown DD, Juhl RP, Lewis K, Schrott M, Bartels B. Decreased bioavailability of digoxin due to antacids and kaolin-pectin. *N Engl J Med* (1976) 295, 1034–7.
3. Albert KS, Ayres JW, Disanto AR, Weidler DJ, Sakmar E, Hallmark MR, Stoll RG, DeSante KA, Wagner JG. Influence of kaolin-pectin suspension on digoxin bioavailability. *J Pharm Sci* (1978) 67, 1582–6.
4. Allen MD, Greenblatt DJ, Harmatz JS, Smith TW. Effect of magnesium aluminum hydroxide and kaolin-pectin on absorption of digoxin from tablets and capsules. *J Clin Pharmacol* (1981) 21, 26–30.

Digitalis glycosides + Ketanserin

Ketanserin is unlikely to affect the serum levels of either digoxin or digitoxin.

Clinical evidence, mechanism, importance and management

Ketanserin 40 mg twice daily did not cause significant changes in the pharmacokinetics of single doses of either **digoxin** 1250 micrograms or **digitoxin** 1000 micrograms in healthy subjects, and it was concluded that ketanserin is unlikely to alter serum concentrations of either glycoside during clinical use.[1]

1. Ochs HR, Verburg-Ochs B, Höller M, Greenblatt DJ. Effect of ketanserin on the kinetics of digoxin and digitoxin. *J Cardiovasc Pharmacol* (1985) 7, 205–7.

Digitalis glycosides + Lanthanum

Lanthanum did not significantly affect the pharmacokinetics of digoxin in a single dose study.

Clinical evidence, mechanism, importance and management

In an open-label crossover study 14 healthy subjects were given lanthanum 1 g for 3 doses on one day, followed by a fourth dose the next day. A single 500-microgram dose of **digoxin** was given 30 minutes after the fourth dose of lanthanum. The **digoxin** half-life was increased during concurrent treatment from 11.4 to 14.8 hours but this was not considered to be clinically significant. Other pharmacokinetic parameters were not significantly affected.[1] Further multiple dose studies are needed to confirm this lack of interaction in patients.

1. Fiddler G. Fosrenol™ (lanthanum carbonate) does not affect the pharmacokinetics of concomitant treatment with digoxin. *J Am Soc Nephrol* (2002) 13, 749A.

Digitalis glycosides + Lithium

No pharmacokinetic interaction occurs between digoxin and lithium but the addition of digoxin to lithium possibly has a detrimental short-term effect on the control of mania. An isolated report describes severe bradycardia in one patient given both drugs.

Clinical evidence, mechanism, importance and management

A study in 6 healthy subjects taking lithium carbonate sufficient to achieve mean steady-state serum levels of 0.76 mmol/l (range 0.4 to 1 mmol/l) showed that the pharmacokinetics of a 750-microgram intravenous dose of **digoxin** were unchanged, and that there were no significant effects on sodium pump activity or electrolyte concentrations.[1] However an experimental 7-day study in patients with manic-depressive psychoses found that there was a greater improvement in those given lithium plus placebo than those given lithium plus **digoxin**. This may be a reflection of changes in Na-K ATP-ase.[2] An isolated report describes tremor, confusion and severe nodal bradycardia in a patient given both drugs. The bradycardia worsened (30 bpm) even after both drugs were stopped.[3] The clinical significance of all of these findings is uncertain. More study is needed.

1. Cooper SJ, Kelly JG, Johnston GD, Copeland S, King DJ, McDevitt DG. Pharmacodynamics and pharmacokinetics of digoxin in the presence of lithium. *Br J Clin Pharmacol* (1984) 18, 21–5.
2. Chambers CA, Smith AHW, Naylor GJ. The effect of digoxin on the response to lithium therapy in mania. *Psychol Med* (1982) 12, 57–60.
3. Winters WD, Ralph DD. Digoxin-lithium drug interaction. *Clin Toxicol* (1977) 10, 487–8.

Digitalis glycosides + Macrolides

Some patients unpredictably show a rapid and marked two to fourfold increase in serum digoxin levels when given azithromycin, clarithromycin, erythromycin or roxithromycin. Increases in serum digoxin levels may also occur with telithromycin. The same interaction has been seen with digitoxin and azithromycin. Digitalis toxicity can occur.

Clinical evidence

A. Digitoxin

A man with congestive heart failure taking digitoxin 70 micrograms daily for 5 days of each week, and enalapril and furosemide, was admitted to hospital with nausea and bradycardia of 26 bpm 4 days after starting a 3-day course of **azithromycin** [dosage not stated]. His serum digitoxin levels were found to be raised from his usual baseline range of 13 to 25 nanomol/l up to 44 nanomol/l. His renal function was normal. Another patient treated with intravenous digitoxin 250 micrograms once daily showed a marked rise from his steady-state digitoxin range of 15 to 20 nmol/l after being given **azithromycin** 500 mg daily for 3 days. The digitoxin was withdrawn one day later but even so the levels climbed to a peak of 41.9 nanomol/l after a further 3 days, and remained in the toxic range for yet another 3 days.[1]

B. Digoxin

(a) Azithromycin

A 31-month-old boy with Down's syndrome and tetralogy of Fallot (a congenital heart defect resulting in reduced blood flow to the lungs) was discharged from hospital after repair of his heart defect. He was on digoxin 60 micrograms twice daily, furosemide, and potassium chloride. Eight days later when readmitted with symptoms of heart failure, intermittent fever and wheezing he was started on azithromycin (10 mg/kg on day 1, then 50 mg/kg daily for 4 days). Three days later his steady-state serum digoxin levels had risen from 1.79 to 2.37 nanograms/ml and he experienced anorexia, nausea, and second degree atrioventricular block. All the symptoms resolved when the digoxin was withdrawn. Digoxin was restarted at 50 micrograms twice daily after the azithromycin course was completed and steady-state digoxin levels of 1.42 nanograms/ml were noted.[2]

The makers of azithromycin say that, as of October 2000, there were 230 cases of the concurrent use of azithromycin and digoxin on their database. Of these, 78 cases had adverse events indicating possible digoxin toxicity. However on review, 21 cases were clearly excluded. Of the remaining cases, only 13 provided digoxin levels, and of these, high serum digoxin concentrations were reported in 6, but generally insufficient data made interpretation difficult.[3] The makers concluded that the possibility that a patient may experience an increase in digoxin concentrations during azithromycin therapy cannot be entirely excluded.

(b) Clarithromycin

A woman on warfarin, heparin, carbamazepine and digoxin was admitted to hospital with syncope, vomiting and an irregular heart rhythm shortly after starting clarithromycin 1 g daily. Her serum digoxin levels were found to be raised. The clarithromycin was decreased, the carbamazepine and digoxin stopped, and she was treated with digoxin-specific antibody fragments *(Digibind)* and intravenous fluids. Her serum digoxin levels fell again and the digitalis toxicity disappeared.[4]

The makers of clarithromycin have a few other cases on their records of raised digoxin levels in patients following treatment with clarithromycin[4] and there are other reports of this interaction in the literature.[5-17] One study found a significant correlation between the dose of clarithromycin and the increase in digoxin serum levels. Doses of clarithromycin ranging from 3 to 9 mg/kg daily produced an increase in digoxin concentrations ranging from about 30 to 100%; at a dose of clarithromycin 400 mg daily, digoxin levels were increased by about 70%.[18]

(c) Erythromycin

An elderly woman with a prosthetic heart valve being treated for left ventricular dysfunction with warfarin, furosemide, hydralazine, isosorbide dinitrate and digoxin, was given erythromycin. She took only four 250-mg doses. Four days later her serum digoxin levels were found to have risen to 2.6 nanograms/ml from a normal steady-state range of 1.4 to 1.7 nanograms/ml, and she showed evidence of digitalis toxicity.[19] Another four similar cases have also been reported.[20-22]

A study in a man who was resistant to digoxin found that erythromycin 1 g daily increased the AUC of digoxin by 300%.[23] A neonate given oral digoxin 5 micrograms/kg daily developed digoxin toxicity two days after erythromycin (10 mg three times daily, then 17 mg three times daily) was given. Digoxin levels rose from 1.8 to 16 nanograms/ml.[24]

(d) Rokitamycin

Rokitamycin did not affect serum digoxin levels in a study in 10 subjects.[25]

(e) Roxithromycin

A 76-year-old woman on digoxin and a number of other drugs (enalapril, isosorbide mononitrate, furosemide, diltiazem, glyceryl trinitrate, slow-release potassium, prednisolone, omeprazole, calcitriol) developed signs of digoxin toxicity (nausea, vomiting, first degree heart block) within 4 days of starting to take roxithromycin 150 mg twice daily. Her serum digoxin levels were found to be raised about fourfold.[26]

(f) Telithromycin

A study in 26 healthy subjects given digoxin 500 micrograms twice daily on the first day followed by 250 micrograms twice daily found that telithromycin 800 mg daily increased the digoxin AUC by 37% and the maximum blood levels by 74%. Trough plasma levels remained within the therapeutic range. No signs of digoxin toxicity were observed on ECGs.[27]

Mechanism

Up to 10% of patients on oral digoxin excrete it in substantial amounts in the faeces and urine as inactive metabolites (digoxin reduction products or DRPs). This metabolism seems to be the responsibility of the gut flora,[20] in particular *Eubacterium lentum*, which is anaerobic and Gram positive.[22,28] In the presence of antibacterials that inhibit this organism, much more digoxin becomes available for absorption, which results in a marked rise in serum levels. At the same time the inactive metabolites derived from the gut disappear.[20,29] However, it is worth noting that most classes of antibacterials do not appear to interact with digoxin despite inhibiting *E. lentum in vitro*.[28] See also 'Digitalis glycosides + Beta-lactam antibacterials', p.689. Further, the increased gastric emptying due to erythromycin may also increase the bioavailability of digoxin[30] or digitoxin.[28]

An alternative explanation for the digoxin/erythromycin and clarithromycin interactions, is that the antibacterials inhibit the intestinal[31,32] or renal[14,18] P-glycoprotein transport of digoxin, which would increase the oral bioavailability and reduce the nonglomerular renal clearance respectively.[33]

None of these suggested mechanisms may be the whole story.

Importance and management

The interactions between digoxin and clarithromycin, and digoxin and erythromycin, appear to be established but unpredictable. Information is limited to a relatively small number of patients, and there is only one report about digoxin/roxithromycin. Although only a small proportion of patients (up to 10%) is likely to be at risk, the 'excreter' category of any particular patient is probably not known (see Mechanism), and it is therefore important to monitor all patients well for signs of increased digoxin effects when any of these macrolide antibacterials is first given, reducing the digoxin dosage as necessary. The interaction between digoxin and clarithromycin may be dependent on clarithromycin dosage.[18] It has been suggested that the elderly may be more susceptible because of a reduction in renal function[8] and the age of the patients in the case reports seem to support this suggestion. Careful monitoring has been recommended in all elderly patients receiving digoxin and clarithromycin, while in those with impaired renal function caution is advised.[34]

The interaction between azithromycin and digoxin also appears to be established, but published information is limited, however the same precautions suggested for clarithromycin and erythromycin would seem to be appropriate. The number of spontaneous case reports submitted to the makers indicates that the potential for this interaction should be studied further.[28] In addition, remember that azithromycin has a long serum half-life (60 hours), which means that it can continue to interact for several days after it has been withdrawn.

1. Thalhammer F, Hollenstein UM, Locker GJ, Janata K, Sunder-Plassmann G, Frass M, Burgmann H. Azithromycin-related toxic effects of digitoxin. *Br J Clin Pharmacol* (1998) 45, 91–2.
2. Ten Eick AP, Sallee D, Preminger T, Weiss A, Reed DM. Possible drug interaction between digoxin and azithromycin in a young child. *Clin Drug Invest* (2000) 20, 61–4.
3. Pfizer Ltd. Personal Communication, February 2001.
4. Abbott Labs, Personal communication 1995.
5. Midoneck SR, Etingin OR. Clarithromycin-related toxic effects of digoxin. *N Engl J Med* (1995) 333, 1505.
6. Taylor JW, Gammenthaler SA, Rape JM. Clarithromycin (Biaxin) induced digoxin toxicity. Presented at the American Society of Healthcare Pharmacists Midyear Clinical Meeting, Miami, December 1994.
7. Ford A, Crocker Smith L, Baltch AL, Smith RP. Clarithromycin-induced digoxin toxicity in a patient with AIDS. *Clin Infect Dis* (1995) 21, 1051–2.
8. Brown BA, Wallace RJ, Griffith DE, Warden R. Clarithromycin-associated digoxin toxicity in the elderly. *Clin Infect Dis* (1997) 24, 92–3.
9. Guillemet C, Alt M, Arpin-Bott MP, Imler M. Clarithromycine-digoxine: une interaction méconnue chez certains patients? *Presse Med* (1997) 26, 512.
10. Nordt S, Williams S, Manoguerra A, Clark R. Clarithromycin-induced digoxin poisoning. *J Toxicol Clin Toxicol* (1997) 35, 501–2.
11. Guerriero SE, Ehrenpreis E, Gallagher KL. Two cases of clarithromycin-induced digoxin toxicity. *Pharmacotherapy* (1997) 17, 1035–7.
12. Laberge P, Martineau P. Clarithromycin-induced digoxin intoxication. *Ann Pharmacother* (1997) 31, 999–1001.
13. Trivedi S, Hyman J, Lichstein E. Clarithromycin and digoxin toxicity. *Ann Intern Med* (1998) 128, 604.
14. Wakasugi H, Yano I, Ito T, Hashida T, Futami T, Nohara R, Sasayama S, Inui K-I. Effect of clarithromycin on renal excretion of digoxin: interaction with P-glycoprotein. *Clin Pharmacol Ther* (1998) 64, 123–8.
15. Nawarskas JJ, McCarthy DM, Spinler SA. Digoxin toxicity secondary to clarithromycin therapy. *Ann Pharmacother* (1997) 31, 864–6.
16. Nordt SP, Williams SR, Manoguerra AS, Clark RF. Clarithromycin induced digoxin toxicity. *J Accid Emerg Med* (1998) 15, 194–5.
17. Juurlink DN, Ito S. Comment: clarithromycin-digoxin interaction. *Ann Pharmacother* (1999) 33, 1375–6.
18. Tanaka H, Matsumoto K, Ueno K, Kodama M, Yoneda K, Katayama Y, Miyatake K. Effect of clarithromycin on steady-state digoxin concentrations. *Ann Pharmacother* (2003) 37, 178–81.
19. Friedman HS, Bonventre MV. Erythromycin-induced digoxin toxicity. *Chest* (1982) 82, 202.
20. Lindenbaum J, Rund DG, Butler VP, Tse-Eng D, Saha JR. Inactivation of digoxin by the gut flora: reversal by antibiotic therapy. *N Engl J Med* (1981) 305, 789–94.
21. Maxwell DL, Gilmour-White SK, Hall MR. Digoxin toxicity due to interaction of digoxin with erythromycin. *BMJ* (1989) 298, 572.
22. Morton MR, Cooper JW. Erythromycin-induced digoxin toxicity. *DICP Ann Pharmacother* (1989) 23, 668–70.
23. Nørregaard-Hansen K, Klitgaard NA, Pedersen KE. The significance of the enterohepatic circulation on the metabolism of digoxin in patients with the ability of intestinal conversion of the drug. *Acta Med Scand* (1986) 220, 89–92.
24. Coudray S, Janoly A, Belkacem-Kahlouli A, Bourhis Y, Bleyzac N, Bourgeois J, Putet G, Aulagner G. L'érythromycine responsable d'une intoxication sévère par la digoxine dans un service de réanimation néonatale. *J Pharm Clin* (2001) 20, 129–31.
25. Ishioka T. Effect of a new macrolide antibiotic 3″-O-propionyl-leucomycin A_5 (Rokitamycin) on serum concentrations of theophylline and digoxin in the elderly. *Acta Ther* (1987) 13, 17–23.
26. Corallo CE, Rogers IR. Roxithromycin-induced digoxin toxicity. *Med J Aust* (1996) 165, 433–4.
27. Montay G, Shi J, Leroy B, Bhargava V. Effects of telithromycin on the pharmacokinetics of digoxin in healthy men. *Intersci Conf Antimicrob Agents Chemother* (2002) 42, 28.
28. Ten Eick AP, Reed MD. Hidden dangers of coadministration of antibiotics and digoxin in children: focus on azithromycin. *Curr Ther Res* (2000) 61, 148–60.
29. Lindenbaum J, Tse-Eng D, Butler VP, Rund DG. Urinary excretion of reduced metabolites of digoxin. *Am J Med* (1981) 71, 67–74.
30. Sutton A, Pilot M-A. Digoxin toxicity and erythromycin. *BMJ* (1989) 298, 1101.
31. Berndt A, Gramatté T, Kirch W. Digoxin-erythromycin interaction: in vitro evidence for competition for intestinal P-glycoprotein. *Eur J Clin Pharmacol* (1996) 50, 538.
32. Tsutsumi K, Kotegawa T, Kuranari M, Otani Y, Morimoto T, Matsuki S, Nakano S. The effect of erythromycin and clarithromycin on the pharmacokinetics of intravenous digoxin in healthy volunteers. *J Clin Pharmacol* (2002) 42, 1159–64.
33. Rengelshausen J, Göggelmann C, Burhenne J, Riedel K-D, Ludwig J, Weiss J, Mikus G, Walter-Sack I, Haefeli WE. Contribution of increased oral bioavailability and reduced nonglomerular renal clearance of digoxin to the digoxin–clarithromycin interaction. *Br J Clin Pharmacol* (2003) 56, 32–8.
34. Zapater P, Reus S, Tello A, Torrús D, Pérez-Mateo M, Horga JF. A prospective study of the clarithromycin–digoxin interaction in elderly patients. *J Antimicrob Chemother* (2002) 50, 601–6.

Digitalis glycosides + Medroxyprogesterone acetate or Megestrol

Medroxyprogesterone acetate or megestrol do not appear to interact to a clinically relevant extent with digitoxin.

Clinical evidence, mechanism, importance and management

Steady-state **digitoxin** levels were monitored in 3 patients before and after 5 weeks treatment with oral medroxyprogesterone acetate 500 mg twice daily or megestrol 160 mg daily. Only small and clinically irrelevant changes in **digitoxin** levels and clearance were seen.[1]

1. Lundgren S, Kvinnsland S, Utaaker E, Bakke O, Ueland PM. Effect of oral high-dose progestins on the disposition of antipyrine, digitoxin, and warfarin in patients with advanced breast cancer. *Cancer Chemother Pharmacol* (1986) 18, 270–5.

Digitalis glycosides + Methyldopa

Methyldopa does not appear to affect serum digoxin levels, but marked bradycardia has been seen in two elderly women given both drugs.

Clinical evidence

Methyldopa 250 mg daily had no effect on the steady-state serum levels of **digoxin** 250 micrograms daily in 8 healthy subjects.[1]

Two elderly women with hypertension and left ventricular failure developed marked bradycardia when they were given **digoxin** and methyldopa 750 mg or 3.75 g daily but not with **digoxin** alone. Average heart rates were 50 and 48 bpm while minimum heart rates were 32 and 38 bpm respectively. They were subsequently discharged on **digoxin** and hydralazine with heart rates within the normal range.[2]

Mechanism

Uncertain. Both digoxin and methyldopa[3] can cause some bradycardia, but these effects seem to have been more than simply the sum of the individual drug effects on the autonomic nervous system.[2]

Importance and management

Information is limited but it would seem that concurrent use need not be avoided, but monitor the effects for any evidence of undesirable bradycardia.

1. May CA, Vlasses PH, Rocci ML, Rotmensch HH, Swanson BN, Tannenbaum RP, Ferguson RK, Abrams WB. Methyldopa does not alter the disposition of digoxin. *J Clin Pharmacol* (1984) 24, 386–9.
2. Davis JC, Reiffel JA, Bigger JT. Sinus node dysfunction caused by methyldopa and digoxin. *JAMA* (1981) 245, 1241–3.
3. Lund-Johansen P. Hemodynamic changes in long term α-methyldopa therapy of essential hypertension. *Acta Med Scand* (1972) 192, 221–6.

Digitalis glycosides + Metoclopramide

The serum levels of digoxin may be reduced by about a third if metoclopramide is given with slowly dissolving forms of digoxin. No interaction is likely with digoxin in liquid form or in fast-dissolving preparations.

Clinical evidence

A study in 11 patients taking slowly dissolving **digoxin** tablets *(Orion)* found that metoclopramide 10 mg three times a day for 10 days reduced the serum **digoxin** levels by 36%, from 0.72 to 0.46 nanograms/ml.[1] The **digoxin** concentrations rose to their former levels when the metoclopramide was withdrawn.

Another study in healthy subjects found metoclopramide 10 mg three times daily caused a 19% reduction in the AUC of **digoxin** and a 27% reduction in peak serum **digoxin** levels (**digoxin** formulation not stated).[2] Yet another study in healthy subjects clearly showed that metoclopramide decreased the absorption of **digoxin** from tablets *(Lanoxin)* but not capsules *(Lanoxicaps)*.[3]

Mechanism

It would seem[4-6] that the metoclopramide increases the motility of the gut to such an extent that full dissolution and absorption of some digoxin formulations is unfinished by the time digoxin is lost in the faeces.

Importance and management

Information is very limited, but the interaction seems to be established. It is not likely to occur with solid form, fast-dissolving digoxin preparations (e.g. liquid-filled capsules) or digoxin in liquid form, but only those preparations which are slowly dissolving (i.e. some tablet formulations). A reduction in digoxin levels of a third could result in under-digitalisation. There seems to be no information about **digitoxin**.

1. Manninen V, Apajalahti A, Melin J, Karesoja M. Altered absorption of digoxin in patients given propantheline and metoclopramide. *Lancet* (1973) i, 398–400.
2. Kirch W, Janisch HD, Santos SR, Duhrsen U, Dylewicz P, Ohnhaus EE. Effect of cisapride and metoclopramide on digoxin bioavailability. *Eur J Drug Metab Pharmacokinet* (1986) 11, 249–50.
3. Johnson BF, Bustrack JA, Urbach DR, Hull JH, Marwaha R. Effect of metoclopramide on digoxin absorption from tablets and capsules. *Clin Pharmacol Ther* (1984) 36, 724–30.
4. Manninen V, Apajalahti A, Simonen H, Reissell P. Effect of propantheline and metoclopramide on the absorption of digoxin. *Lancet* (1973) i, 1118–9.
5. Medin S, Nyberg L. Effect of propantheline and metoclopramide on the absorption of digoxin. *Lancet* (1973) i, 1393.
6. Fraser EJ, Leach RH, Poston JW, Bold AM, Culank LS, Lipede AB. Dissolution-rates and bioavailability of digoxin tablets. *Lancet* (1973) i, 1393.

Digitalis glycosides + Mexiletine

Serum digoxin levels are not significantly altered by mexiletine.

Clinical evidence, mechanism, importance and management

Mexiletine 200 mg 8-hourly for 4 days slightly reduced the serum levels of **digoxin** 250 micrograms daily from 0.32 to 0.27 nanograms/ml in 10 healthy subjects.[1] Two other studies in a total of 17 patients[2,3] confirmed that mexiletine does not significantly affect serum **digoxin** levels.

1. Saris SD, Lowenthal DT, Affrime MB. Steady-state digoxin concentration during oral mexiletine administration. *Curr Ther Res* (1983) 34, 662–66.
2. Leahey EB, Reiffel JA, Giardina E-GV, Bigger T. The effect of quinidine and other oral antiarrhythmic drugs on serum digoxin. *Ann Intern Med* (1980) 92, 605–8.
3. Day T, Hunt D. Interaction between mexiletine and digoxin. *Med J Aust* (1983) 2, 630.

Digitalis glycosides + Mizolastine

Mizolastine can cause a small but clinically irrelevant rise in serum digoxin levels.

Clinical evidence, mechanism, importance and management

A double-blind placebo-controlled crossover study in 12 healthy subjects found that mizolastine 10 mg daily for a week caused a 17% increase in the maximum serum levels of **digoxin** 250 micrograms daily. The **digoxin** AUC and half-life were unchanged and the haemodynamic parameters measured (blood pressure, ECG) were unaltered.[1] No special precautions would seem necessary during concurrent use.

1. Chaufour S, Le Coz F, Denolle T, Dubruc C, Cimarosti I, Deschamps C, Ulliac N, Delhotal-Landes B, Rosenweig P. Lack of effect of mizolastine on the safety and pharmacokinetics of digoxin administered orally in repeated doses to healthy volunteers. *Int J Clin Pharmacol Ther* (1998) 36, 286–91.

Digitalis glycosides + Montelukast

Montelukast 10 mg was given to 11 healthy subjects for 12 days, with a single 500-microgram dose of digoxin on day 7 in a randomised two-period crossover study. It was found that the pharmacokinetic profile of the digoxin was unchanged by the montelukast.[1] No special precautions are needed if both drugs are used concurrently.

1. Depre M, Van Hecken A, Verbesselt R, Wynants K, De Lelepeire I, Freeman A, Holland S, Shahane A, Gertz B, De Schepper PJ. Effect of multiple doses of montelukast, a CysLT1 receptor agonist, on digoxin pharmacokinetics in healthy volunteers. *J Clin Pharmacol* (1999) 39, 941–4.

Digitalis glycosides + Moracizine

Moracizine does not significantly increase serum digoxin levels in patients with normal renal function. However, some adverse conduction effects have been seen.

Clinical evidence

Thirteen patients on **digoxin** 125 to 250 micrograms daily showed a non-significant rise in their serum **digoxin** levels of 10 to 15% when they were given moracizine 10 mg/kg daily in three divided doses for 2 weeks. Nine patients taking **digoxin** and moracizine for 1 to 6 months showed no significant changes in their serum **digoxin** levels.[1]

No changes in the pharmacokinetics of **digoxin** were seen in a single-dose study of intravenous **digoxin** and moracizine in 9 healthy subjects[2] nor in another study in patients on maintenance treatment with **digoxin** over a 13-day period. However, cardiac arrhythmias (AV junctional rhythm and heart block) were seen, which resolved when the moracizine was stopped.[3]

Mechanism

Not established. There does not appear to be a pharmacokinetic interaction between moracizine and digoxin. Concurrent use can cause a significant increase in the PR interval and QRS duration, which can result in AV block.[4]

Importance and management

Although no clinically important changes in serum digoxin levels appear to occur during concurrent use, the occurrence of arrhythmias in a few patients indicates that good monitoring is advisable. It has been pointed out that the additive effects of both drugs on intranodal and intraventricular conduction may be excessive in some patients with heart disease.[4] More study is needed.

1. Kennedy HL, Sprague MK, Redd RM, Wiens RD, Blum RI, Buckingham TA. Serum digoxin concentrations during ethmozine antiarrhythmic therapy. *Am Heart J* (1986) 111, 667–72.
2. MacFarland RT, Moeller VR, Pieniaszek HJ, Whitney CC, Marcus FI. Assessment of the potential pharmacokinetic interaction between digoxin and ethmozine. *J Clin Pharmacol* (1985) 25, 138–43.
3. Antman EM, Arnold JMO, Friedman PL, White H, Bosak M, Smith TW. Drug interactions with cardiac glycosides: evaluation of a possible digoxin-ethmozine pharmacokinetic interaction. *J Cardiovasc Pharmacol* (1987) 9, 622–7.
4. Siddoway LA, Schwartz SL, Barbey JT, Woosley RL. Clinical pharmacokinetics of moricizine. *Am J Cardiol* (1990) 65, 21D–25D.

Digitalis glycosides + Nefazodone

Nefazodone causes a moderate increase in serum digoxin levels but this is of uncertain clinical importance. Digoxin does not appear to affect the pharmacokinetics of nefazodone.

Clinical evidence

Eighteen healthy subjects were given **digoxin** 200 micrograms daily for 8 days, then nefazodone 200 mg twice daily for 8 days, and then both drugs together for 8 days. Nefazodone increased the digoxin AUC by 15%, and increased the peak and trough serum levels of digoxin by 29% and 27% respectively. However, no clinically significant changes in ECG measurements occurred (PR, QRS and QT intervals), nor was the heart rate nor any other vital sign altered. The pharmacokinetics of the nefazodone were unchanged.[1]

Mechanism

Not understood.

Importance and management

This interaction appears to be established, but its clinical importance is uncertain. Because digoxin has a narrow therapeutic index, it would seem prudent to monitor the outcome of concurrent use, being alert for the need to reduce the digoxin dosage. More study is needed.

1. Dockens RC, Greene DS, Barbhaiya RH. Assessment of pharmacokinetic and pharmacodynamic drug interactions between nefazodone and digoxin in healthy male volunteers. *J Clin Pharmacol* (1996) 36, 160–7.

Digitalis glycosides + Neuromuscular blockers

Serious cardiac arrhythmias can develop in patients receiving digitalis glycosides who are given suxamethonium (succinylcholine) or pancuronium.

Clinical evidence

Eight out of 17 digitalised patients (anaesthetised with thiamylal and then maintained with nitrous oxide and oxygen) developed serious ventricular arrhythmias following the intravenous injection of **suxamethonium (succinylcholine)** 40 to 100 mg. Four out of the 8 patients reverted to their previous rhythm when they were given tubocurarine 15 to 30 mg, with one patient returning to a regular nodal rhythm from ventricular tachycardia.[1]

Of the other 9 patients, 3 had immediate and definite ST-T wave changes, and the remaining 6 had no demonstrable changes.[1] There are other reports of this interaction,[2-4] including one that describes sinus tachycardia and atrial flutter in 6 out of 18 patients on **digoxin** after they were given **pancuronium**.[4]

Mechanism

Not understood. One possibility is that the suxamethonium may cause the rapid removal of potassium from the myocardial cells. Another idea is that it affects catecholamine-releasing cholinergic receptors.

Importance and management

Information is limited but the interaction appears to be established. Suxamethonium should be used with great caution in patients taking digitalis glycosides. Similarly, caution would seem appropriate with pancuronium.

1. Dowdy EG, Fabian LW. Ventricular arrhythmias induced by succinylcholine in digitalized patients: A preliminary report. *Anesth Analg* (1963) 42, 501–13.
2. Pérez HR. Cardiac arrhythmia after succinylcholine. *Anesth Analg* (1970) 49, 33–8.
3. Smith RB, Petrusack J. Succinylcholine, digitalis, and hypercalcaemia: a case report. *Anesth Analg* (1972) 51, 202–5.
4. Bartolone RS, Rao TLK. Dysrhythmias following muscle relaxant administration in patients receiving digitalis. *Anesthesiology* (1983) 58, 567–9.

Digitalis glycosides + NSAIDs

Diclofenac and indometacin can cause potentially toxic rises in digitalis glycoside levels, while azapropazone, fenbufen and tiaprofenic acid raise levels to a lesser degree. Two studies found that ibuprofen raised serum digoxin levels, whereas another found no evidence of an interaction. Isoxicam, ketoprofen, lornoxicam, meloxicam, nimesulide, piroxicam, and rofecoxib do not appear to interact significantly with digoxin. In contrast, phenylbutazone appears to lower plasma digitalis glycoside levels. NSAIDs can cause deterioration of renal function, which could result in digoxin toxicity.

Clinical evidence

(a) Azapropazone

Azapropazone 900 mg daily did not significantly alter the AUC of a single 500-microgram intravenous dose of **digitoxin** in 8 arthritic patients, but its mean half-life was increased by about 10%. Two of the patients showed individual half-life increases of almost a third.[1]

(b) Diclofenac

A study in 7 healthy subjects found that diclofenac 100 mg daily for 10 days increased the serum levels of **digoxin** by 29%.[2] Another study in 6 healthy subjects similarly found that diclofenac 50 mg three times daily raised the serum **digoxin** levels by about a third.[3] **Digitoxin** 100 micrograms had no effect on the plasma levels of diclofenac 50 mg twice daily in 8 subjects; **digitoxin** levels were not reported.[4]

(c) Etoricoxib

A study in healthy subjects on **digoxin** found that the addition of etoricoxib 120 mg daily for 10 days did not alter the steady-state AUC of **digoxin** or its renal elimination, but the maximum serum **digoxin** levels were increased by about 33%.[5] This change is unlikely to be clinically relevant in most patients but it might possibly affect a very small number whose **digoxin** levels are already high.

(d) Fenbufen

Fenbufen 900 mg daily was found to cause an insignificant rise in the serum levels of **digoxin**.[6]

(e) Ibuprofen

The serum **digoxin** levels of 12 patients were reported to have risen by about 60% after they were treated with at least 1600 mg of ibuprofen daily for a week. However, after a month the **digoxin** levels had returned to their former amount.[7] These findings may be unreliable because half of the patients were not satisfactorily compliant with treatment. Another study found that ibuprofen 1200 mg daily for 10 days raised the serum **digoxin** levels of 9 healthy subjects by 25%.[2] Yet another study found that ibuprofen 600 mg three times daily for 10 days had no effect on steady-state serum **digoxin** levels of 8 patients.[8]

(f) Indometacin

(i) Neonates. A study in 11 premature neonates (gestational age 25 to 33 weeks) given **digoxin** showed that when they were given indometacin (mean total dose of 320 micrograms/kg over 12 to 24 hours) for the treatment of patent ductus arteriosus, their mean serum **digoxin** levels rose on average by 40%. The **digoxin** was stopped in 5 of them because serum concentrations were potentially toxic.[9] This confirms the observation of digitalis toxicity in 3 similarly treated premature neonates,[10] and of toxic serum **digoxin** concentrations in another neonate.[11] A further report describes very high **digoxin** levels (8.2 nanograms/ml) without symptoms of toxicity in a full-term neonate.[12]

(ii) Adults. Indometacin 50 mg three times daily for 10 days increased steady-state serum **digoxin** levels of 10 patients by about 40% (from 0.73 to 1.02 nmol/l), with a range of 0 to 100%.[8] Indometacin 150 mg daily for 10 days increased the serum **digoxin** levels of 9 healthy subjects by 25%.[2] This contrasts with the results of single-dose studies in 2 groups of 6 healthy adult subjects[13,14] who were given a 4-hour infusion of **digoxin**. Both studies suggested that no interaction occurs.

(g) Isoxicam

Isoxicam 200 mg daily did not affect the steady-state plasma levels of 12 healthy subjects taking **beta-acetyldigoxin**.[15] This confirms the findings of a previous study.[16]

(h) Ketoprofen

Ketoprofen 50 mg four times daily for 4 days had no effect on the serum **digoxin** levels of 12 patients.[17]

(i) Lornoxicam

The concurrent use of lornoxicam 4 mg twice daily for 14 days and **digoxin** 250 micrograms daily in 12 healthy subjects had only a small effect on the pharmacokinetics of each drug. The apparent clearance of the **digoxin** was decreased by 14% while the maximum serum level of the lornoxicam was decreased by 21% and its elimination half-life increased by 36%.[18]

(j) Meloxicam

Meloxicam 15 mg daily for 8 days had no effect on the pharmacokinetics of **digoxin** (given as **beta-acetyldigoxin**) in 12 healthy subjects.[19]

(k) Nimesulide

Nimesulide 100 mg twice daily for 7 days had little effect on the pharmacokinetics of **digoxin** 250 micrograms daily in 9 patients with mild heart failure. No major change in their clinical condition occurred.[20]

(l) Phenylbutazone

Phenylbutazone 200 or 400 mg daily halved the plasma levels of **digitoxin** 100 micrograms daily in 6 patients, on two separate occasions. **Digitoxin** levels returned to their former values within roughly the same period of time after phenylbutazone was withdrawn.[21] A similar response has been described elsewhere in one patient.[22] Six healthy subjects showed an a decrease of about 20% in their serum **digoxin** levels while taking phenylbutazone 200 mg three times daily for 4 days.[3]

(m) Piroxicam

In 10 patients taking **digoxin** for mild cardiac failure, piroxicam 10 or 20 mg daily for 15 days had no effect on the steady-state **digoxin** levels, nor were consistent effects seen on the pharmacokinetics of **digoxin**.[23] Piroxicam 20 mg daily for 10 days was found to have no effect on serum **digoxin** levels of 6 healthy subjects.[2]

(n) Rofecoxib

Rofecoxib 75 mg once daily did not cause significant changes in the plasma pharmacokinetics or renal elimination of single 500-microgram doses of **digoxin** elixir.[24]

(o) Tiaprofenic acid

Tiaprofenic acid 200 mg three times daily for 10 days caused a non-significant 15% rise, from 0.97 to 1.12 nanograms/ml, in the serum **digoxin** levels of 12 healthy subjects.[25]

Mechanism

The reasons for the altered digoxin pharmacokinetics in some of the studies are not clear. However, in the studies in neonates, the elevated digoxin levels were clearly related to indometacin-induced deterioration in renal function.[9,11,12] It should be noted that all NSAIDs have the potential to cause renal impairment.

It is suggested that phenylbutazone lowers digitoxin levels by increasing its rate of metabolism by the liver.[21]

Importance and management

The interaction between digoxin and diclofenac is established but the clinical importance is uncertain. It would be prudent to monitor concurrent use to ensure that the digoxin serum levels remain at acceptable levels. Reduce the digoxin dosage if necessary. The interaction also seems established in neonates, but documentation is limited. It has been suggested that the digoxin dosage should be halved if indometacin is given to premature or full-term infants and the serum digoxin levels and urinary output monitored. Also be alert for moderate increases in serum digoxin levels in adults if indometacin is added. The importance of the interaction with azapropazone, etoricoxib, fenbufen and tiaprofenic acid is not known. In most cases changes to doses are unlikely to be necessary, but remain aware of the potential for interaction. No special precautions would appear to be necessary with isoxicam, ketoprofen, meloxicam, piroxicam, and rofecoxib. More study is needed in most cases, but especially with ibuprofen, where the evidence is conflicting. Monitor the effects of digoxin (e.g. heart rate) if ibuprofen is started or stopped.

The interaction with phenylbutazone appears to be in direct contrast to that with the other NSAIDs, but documentation is limited. The dosage of digoxin and digitoxin may possibly need to be increased to avoid underdigitalisation if phenylbutazone is added to established treatment. You should monitor concurrent use well.

1. Faust-Tinnefeldt G, Gilfrich HJ. Digitoxin-Kinetik unter antirheumatischer Therapie mit Azapropazon. *Arzneimittelforschung* (1977) 27, 2009–11.
2. Isbary J, Doering W, König E. Der Einfluβ von Tiaprofensäure auf die Digoxinkonzentration im Serum (DKS) im Vergleich zu anderen Antirheumatika (AR). *Z Rheumatol* (1982) 41, 164.
3. Rau R, Georgiopoulos G, Neumann P, Gross D. Die Beeinflussung des Digoxinblutspiegels durch Antirheumatika. *Akt Rheum* (1980) 5, 349–58.
4. Schumacher A, Faust-Tinnefeldt G, Geissler HE, Gilfrich HJ, Mutschler E. Untersuchungen potentieller Interaktionen von Diclofenac-Natrium (Voltaren) mit einem Antazidum und mit Digitoxin. *Therapiewoche* (1983) 33, 2619–25.
5. Arcoxia (Etoricoxib). Merck Sharp & Dohme Ltd. UK Summary of product characteristics, May 2005.
6. Dunky A, Eberi R. Anti-inflammatory effects of a new anti-rheumatic drug fenbufen in rheumatoid arthritis. *XIV Int Congr Rheumatology, June 26–July 1* (1977). Abstract No 379.
7. Quattrocchi FP, Robinson JD, Curry RW, Grieco ML, Schulman SG. The effect of ibuprofen on serum digoxin concentrations. *Drug Intell Clin Pharm* (1983) 17, 286–8.
8. Jørgensen HS, Christensen HR, Kampmann JP. Interaction between digoxin and indomethacin or ibuprofen. *Br J Clin Pharmacol* (1991) 31, 108–110.
9. Koren G, Zarfin Y, Perlman M, MacLeod SM. Effects of indomethacin on digoxin pharmacokinetics in preterm infants. *Pediatr Pharmacol* (1984) 4, 25–30.
10. Mayes LC, Boerth RC. Digoxin-indomethacin interaction. *Pediatr Res* (1980) 14, 469.
11. Schimmel MS, Inwood RL, Eidelman AI, Eylath U. Toxic digitalis levels associated with indomethacin therapy in a neonate. *Clin Pediatr (Phila)* (1980) 19, 768–9.
12. Haig GM, Brookfield EG. Increase in serum digoxin concentrations after indomethacin therapy in a full-term neonate. *Pharmacotherapy* (1992) 12, 334–6.
13. Finch MB, Johnston GD, Kelly JG, McDevitt DG. Pharmacokinetics of digoxin alone and in the presence of indomethacin therapy. *Br J Clin Pharmacol* (1984) 17, 353–5.
14. Sziegoleit W, Weiss M, Fahr A, Förster W. Are serum levels and cardiac effects of digoxin influenced by indometacin? *Pharmazie* (1986) 41, 340–2.
15. Zöller B, Engel HJ, Faust-Tinnefeldt G, Gilfrich HJ, Zimmer M. Untersuchungen zur Wechselwirkung von Isoxicam und Digoxin. *Z Rheumatol* (1984) 43, 182–4.
16. Chlud K. Zur Frage der Interaktionen in der Rheumatherapie: Untersuchungen von Isoxicam und Glibenclamid bei Diabetien mit rheumatischen Enkrankungen. *Tempo Med* (1983) 12A, 15–18.
17. Lewis GR, Jacobs SG, Vavra I. Effect of ketoprofen on serum digoxin concentrations. *Curr Ther Res* (1985) 38, 494–9.
18. Ravic M, Johnston A, Turner P. Clinical pharmacological studies of some possible interactions of lornoxicam with other drugs. *Postgrad Med J* (1990) 66 (Suppl 4), S30–S34.
19. Degner FL, Heinzel G, Narjes H, Türck D. The effect of meloxicam on the pharmacokinetics of β-acetyl-digoxin. *Br J Clin Pharmacol* (1995) 40, 486–8.
20. Baggio E, Maraffi F, Montalto C, Nava ML, Torti L, Casciarri I. A clinical assessment of the potential for pharmacological interaction between nimesulide and digoxin in patients with heart failure. *Drugs* (1993) 46 (Suppl 1), 91–4.

21. Wirth KE. Arzneimittelinteraktionen bei der Anwendung herzwirksamer Glykoside. *Med Welt* (1981) 32, 234–8.
22. Solomon HM, Reich S, Spirt N, Abrams WB. Interactions between digitoxin and other drugs *in vitro* and *in vivo*. *Ann N Y Acad Sci* (1971) 179, 362–9.
23. Rau R. Interaction study of piroxicam with digoxin. In 'Piroxicam: A New Non-steroidal Anti-inflammatory Agent.' Proc IXth Eur Cong Rheumatol, Wiesbaden, September 1979, pp 41–6. Academy Professional Information Services, NY.
24. Schwartz JI, De Smet M, Larson PJ, Verbesselt R, Ebel DL, Lins R, Lens S, Porras AG, Gertz BJ. Effect of rofecoxib on the pharmacokinetics of digoxin in healthy volunteers. *J Clin Pharmacol* (2001) 41, 107–112.
25. Doering W, Isbary J. Der Einfluß von Tiaprofensäure auf die Digoxin-konzentration im Serum. *Arzneimittelforschung* (1983) 33, 167–8.

Digitalis glycosides + Orlistat

Orlistat appears not to interact with digoxin.

Clinical evidence, mechanism, importance and management

Orlistat 120 mg three times daily for 6 days was found to have no effect on the pharmacokinetics of a single 400-microgram oral dose of **digoxin** (in soft gelatin capsules) in 12 healthy subjects.[1] This suggests that an approximate 30% reduction in dietary fat absorption induced by orlistat should not change the efficacy of **digoxin** and that no special precautions will be needed in patients who are treated with both drugs concurrently.

1. Melia AT, Zhi J, Koss-Twardy SG, Min BH, Smith BL, Freundlich NL, Arora S, Passe SM. The influence of reduced dietary fat absorption induced by orlistat on the pharmacokinetics of digoxin in healthy volunteers. *J Clin Pharmacol* (1995) 35, 840–3.

Digitalis glycosides + Penicillamine

Serum digoxin levels can be reduced by penicillamine.

Clinical evidence

While taking penicillamine 1 g daily 2 hours after taking **digoxin** orally, the serum **digoxin** levels of 10 patients measured 2, 4 and 6 hours later were reduced by 13, 20 and 39% respectively. In 10 other patients similarly treated but given **digoxin** intravenously, the serum **digoxin** levels measured 4 and 6 hours later were reduced by 23 and 64% respectively.[1] This interaction is reported by the same authors to occur in children.[2]

Mechanism

Unknown.

Importance and management

Information seems to be limited to the reports cited. Patients taking digoxin should be checked for signs of under-digitalisation if penicillamine is added. Information about digitoxin appears to be lacking.

1. Moezzi B, Fatourechi V, Khozain R, Eslami B. The effect of penicillamine on serum digoxin levels. *Jpn Heart J* (1978) 19, 366–70.
2. Moezzi B, Khozein R, Pooymehr F, Shakibi JG. Reversal of digoxin-induced changes in erythrocyte electrolyte concentrations by penicillamine in children. *Jpn Heart J* (1980) 21, 335–9.

Digitalis glycosides + Pinaverium

Plasma digoxin levels are not affected by pinaverium in patients taking either beta-acetyldigoxin or metildigoxin.

Clinical evidence, mechanism, importance and management

A single-blind study in 25 patients, taking either **beta-acetyldigoxin** or **metildigoxin** for congestive heart failure, found that pinaverium 50 mg three times daily for 12 days had no significant effect on their plasma digoxin levels.[1] No special precautions seem necessary on concurrent use.

1. Weitzel O, Seidel G, Engelbert S, Berksoy M, Eberhardt G, Bode R. Investigation of possible interaction between pinaverium bromide and digoxin. *Curr Med Res Opin* (1983) 8, 600–2.

Digitalis glycosides + Pioglitazone or Rosiglitazone

Pioglitazone and rosiglitazone do not affect the pharmacokinetics of digoxin, but they may adversely affect cardiac function in patients with cardiac failure.

Clinical evidence, mechanism, importance and management

(a) Pioglitazone

In healthy subjects pioglitazone did not alter the steady-state pharmacokinetics of **digoxin** 250 micrograms daily.[1,2]

Pioglitazone may cause fluid retention, which may cause or exacerbate heart failure.[1,3] This is not a drug-drug interaction but a disease-drug interaction.

(b) Rosiglitazone

A study in healthy subjects found that rosiglitazone 8 mg once daily for 14 days had no effect on the steady-state pharmacokinetics of **digoxin** 375 micrograms daily. Concurrent use was safe and well tolerated (aside from one patient who withdrew because of a rash).[4] However, the US makers caution rosiglitazone in those with a history of cardiac failure because it may cause fluid retention which could lead to a deterioration in cardiac function.[5] For the same reason the UK makers contraindicate concurrent use.[6] If **digoxin** or any other **digitalis glycoside** is being used to treat cardiac failure, the use of rosiglitazone would not therefore be recommended. This is not a drug-drug interaction but a disease-drug interaction.

1. Actos (Pioglitazone hydrochloride). Takeda Pharmaceutical Company Ltd. US Prescribing information, August 2004.
2. Kortboyer JM, Eckland DJA. Pioglitazone has low potential for drug interactions. *Diabetologia* (1999) 42 (Suppl 1), A228.
3. Actos (Pioglitazone hydrochloride). Takeda UK Ltd. UK Summary of product characteristics, February 2005.
4. Di Cicco RA, Miller AK, Patterson S, Freed MI. Rosiglitazone does not affect the steady-state pharmacokinetics of digoxin. *J Clin Pharmacol* (2000) 40, 1516–21.
5. Avandia (Rosiglitazone maleate). GlaxoSmithKline. US Prescribing information, March 2005.
6. Avandia (Rosiglitazone maleate). GlaxoSmithKline UK. UK Summary of product characteristics, January 2005.

Digitalis glycosides + Probenecid

Probenecid has no clinically significant effects on plasma digoxin levels.

Clinical evidence, mechanism, importance and management

A study in 2 healthy subjects taking **digoxin** 250 micrograms daily showed that two daily doses of *ColBenemid* (probenecid 500 mg with colchicine 500 micrograms) for 3 days, their plasma **digoxin** levels were slightly but not significantly raised (from 0.67 to 0.7 nanograms/ml, and from 0.6 to 0.67 nanograms/ml respectively).[1] Another study in 6 healthy subjects found that probenecid 2 g daily for 8 days had no significant effect on the pharmacokinetics of **digoxin**.[2] No special precautions would seem necessary during concurrent use.

1. Jaillon P, Weissenburger J, Cheymol G, Graves P, Marcus F. Les effets du probénécide sur la concentration plasmatique à l'équilibre de digoxine. *Therapie* (1980) 35, 655–6.
2. Hedman A, Angelin B, Arvidsson A, Dahlqvist R. No effect of probenecid on the renal and biliary clearances of digoxin in man. *Br J Clin Pharmacol* (1991) 32, 63–7.

Digitalis glycosides + Propafenone

Propafenone can increase serum digoxin levels by 30 to 90% or even more in children. A digoxin dosage reduction may be necessary.

Clinical evidence

Propafenone (increasing over 6 days to 300 mg every 8 hours) increased the mean steady-state serum levels of **digoxin** 125 to 250 micrograms daily by 83% in 5 patients. Three patients continued to take both drugs for 6 months at which point the **digoxin** levels were 63% higher. No digitalis toxicity was seen.[1] In another study, propafenone 600 mg daily in divided doses increased the steady-state serum **digoxin** levels of 10 patients by

90% (from 0.97 to 1.54 nanograms/ml), and two of them developed symptoms of toxicity (nausea, vomiting).[2] An even greater increase was seen in 3 children who showed rises in serum **digoxin** levels of 112 to 254% over 3 to 24 days when given propafenone 250 to 500 mg/m^2 daily.[3] The mean AUC of **digoxin** increased by 13.8% in 27 patients receiving propafenone 10 mg/kg daily in divided doses. However, there was great inter-individual variability, with 22 patients showing an increase in AUC, and 5 a decrease. One patient experienced **digoxin** poisoning resulting in fatal ventricular fibrillation.[4]

Propafenone 450 mg daily increased the mean steady-state serum **digoxin** levels of 12 healthy subjects by about 35% (from 0.58 to 0.78 nanograms/ml), and the cardiac effects were increased accordingly.[5] In a study in 6 subjects[6] given a single 1000-microgram intravenous dose of **digoxin**, propafenone 150 or 300 mg every 8 hours increased the AUC of **digoxin** by 28% and decreased the total clearance of **digoxin** by 21.9%. A similar study with oral **digoxin** found a 25% increase in **digoxin** AUC when healthy subjects were given propafenone.[7]

Mechanism

Not understood. One suggestion is that propafenone increases the bioavailability of the digoxin.[7] Another is that the volume of distribution and non-renal clearance of digoxin are changed by the propafenone.[6] Conversely, others reported that propafenone decreased the renal clearance of digoxin.[2,5] There is certainly some *in vitro* evidence that propafenone and its metabolite inhibit the P-glycoprotein transporter, which is concerned with digoxin secretion by the renal tubular cells.[8]

Importance and management

A very well established interaction of clinical importance. Monitor the effects of concurrent use and reduce the digoxin dosage appropriately in order to avoid toxicity. Most patients appear to be affected and dosage reductions in the range 15 to 70% were found necessary in one of the studies cited.[2] The data available suggest that the extent of the rise may possibly depend on the propafenone serum concentration rather than on its dose.[6,9]

1. Salerno DM, Granrud G, Sharkey P, Asinger R, Hodges M. A controlled trial of propafenone for treatment of frequent and repetitive ventricular premature complexes. *Am J Cardiol* (1984) 53, 77–83.
2. Calvo MV, Martin-Suarez A, Luengo CM, Avila C, Cascon M, Hurlé AD-G. Interaction between digoxin and propafenone. *Ther Drug Monit* (1989) 11, 10–15.
3. Zalzstein E, Koren G, Bryson SM, Freedom RM. Interaction between digoxin and propafenone in children. *J Pediatr* (1990) 116, 310–2.
4. Palumbo E, Svetoni N, Casini M, Spargi T, Biagi G, Martelli F, Lanzetta T. Interazione digoxina-propafenone: valori e limiti del dosaggio plasmatico dis due farmaci. *G Ital Cardiol* (1986) 16, 855–62.
5. Belz GG, Doering W, Munkes R, Matthews J. Interaction between digoxin and calcium antagonists and antiarrhythmic drugs. *Clin Pharmacol Ther* (1983) 33, 410–17.
6. Nolan PE, Marcus FI, Erstad BL, Hoyer GK, Furman C, Kirsten EB. Effects of coadministration of propafenone on the pharmacokinetics of digoxin in healthy volunteer subjects. *J Clin Pharmacol* (1989) 29, 46–52.
7. Cardaioli P, Compostella L, De Domenico R, Papalia D, Zeppellini R, Libardoni M, Pulido E, Cucchini F. Influenza del propafenone sulla farmacocinetica della digossina somministrata per via orale: studio su volontari sani. *G Ital Cardiol* (1986) 16, 237–40.
8. Woodland C, Verjee Z, Giesbrecht E, Koren G, Ito S. The digoxin-propafenone interaction: characterization of a mechanism using renal tubular cell monolayers. *J Pharmacol Exp Ther* (1997) 283, 39–45.
9. Bigot M-C, Debruyne D, Bonnefoy L, Grollier G, Moulin M, Potier J-C. Serum digoxin levels related to plasma propafenone levels during concomitant treatment. *J Clin Pharmacol* (1991) 31, 521–6.

Digitalis glycosides + Propantheline

Serum digoxin levels may be increased by at least one-third if propantheline is given with slow-dissolving forms of digoxin tablets. No clinically significant interaction is likely with digoxin given as a liquid or in soft-gelatin capsules or in the form of fast-dissolving tablets.

Clinical evidence

The serum **digoxin** levels of 9 out of 13 patients rose by 30%, from 1.02 to 1.33 nanograms/ml while taking a slow-dissolving formulation of **digoxin** tablets *(Orion)* with propantheline 15 mg three times daily for 10 days. The serum levels stayed the same in 3 patients and fell slightly in one. An associated study in 4 healthy subjects given **digoxin** in liquid form found that serum **digoxin** levels were unaffected by propantheline.[1]

Another study by the same workers showed that propantheline increased the **digoxin** serum levels of a slow-dissolving tablet formulation *(Orion)* by 40%, but had no effect on serum **digoxin** levels with a fast-dissolving tablet formulation *(Lanoxin)*.[2] In a further study, propantheline increased the AUC of **digoxin** from *Lanoxin* tablets by 24%, compared with a non-significant increase of 13% with digoxin in the form of a solution in a capsule *(Lanoxicaps)*.[3]

Mechanism

Propantheline is an anticholinergic agent, which reduces gut motility. This allows the slow-dissolving formulations of digoxin more time to pass into solution so that more is available for absorption.

Importance and management

An established interaction, but only of importance if slow-dissolving digoxin formulations are used. No interaction is likely with liquid or liquid-filled capsule forms of digoxin. With slow-dissolving forms of digoxin tablets it may be necessary to reduce the digoxin dosage. No interaction seems likely with **digitoxin** because it is better absorbed from the gut than digoxin, but this requires confirmation.

1. Manninen V, Apajalahti A, Melin J, Karesoja M. Altered absorption of digoxin in patients given propantheline and metoclopramide. *Lancet* (1973) i, 398–400.
2. Manninen V, Apajalahti A, Simonen H, Reissell P. Effect of propantheline and metoclopramide on absorption of digoxin. *Lancet* (1973) i, 1118–19.
3. Brown DD, Schmid J, Long RA, Hull JH. A steady-state evaluation of the effects of propantheline bromide and cholestyramine on the bioavailability of digoxin when administered as tablets or capsules. *J Clin Pharmacol* (1985) 25, 360–4.

Digitalis glycosides + Prostaglandins

Iloprost does not significantly change digoxin pharmacokinetics. Epoprostenol caused a small decrease in digoxin clearance in the short-term, which is of uncertain clinical importance.

Clinical evidence, mechanism, importance and management

A 6-hour intravenous infusion of **iloprost** 2 nanograms/kg per minute was given to 12 patients on **digoxin** 250 micrograms daily over a period of 20 days. The mean time to maximum serum **digoxin** was delayed by an hour, but overall the pharmacokinetics of the **digoxin** were unchanged.[1,2] No special precautions would seem to be necessary on concurrent use.

The **digoxin** clearance of 14 patients with congestive heart failure was reduced by an estimated 15% by **epoprostenol** given for 3 days, but this effect was no longer apparent by the end of 12 weeks concurrent use. The clinical relevance of this awaits evaluation but it seems unlikely to be important. However, the authors of the report suggest that the possible short-term changes in patients with high trough-serum **digoxin** levels and those prone to **digoxin** toxicity should be borne in mind when using the combination.[3]

1. Cabane J, Penin I, Bouslama K, Benchouieb A, Giral Ph, Picard O, Wattiaux MJ, Cheymol G, Souvignet G, Imbert JC. Traitement par iloprost des ischémies critiques des membres inférieurs associées à une insuffisance cardiaque. *Therapie* (1991) 46, 235–40.
2. Penin E, Cheymol G, Bouslama K, Benchouieb A, Cabane J, Souvignet G. No pharmacokinetic interaction between iloprost and digoxin. *Eur J Clin Pharmacol* (1991) 41, 505–6.
3. Carlton LD, Patterson JH, Mattson CN, Schmith VD. The effects of epoprostenol on drug disposition I. A pilot study of the pharmacokinetics of digoxin with and without epoprostenol in patients with congestive heart failure. *J Clin Pharmacol* (1996) 36, 247–56.

Digitalis glycosides + Proton pump inhibitors

A small rise in serum digoxin levels may occur with omeprazole, pantoprazole or rabeprazole, but this is not thought to be clinically significant.

Clinical evidence

(a) Lansoprazole

A study in 47 patients stabilised on **digoxin** and either lansoprazole or omeprazole found that changing the proton pump inhibitor to an equivalent dose of rabeprazole did not significantly change the mean serum **digoxin** level. However, since 12 of the patients had increases of more than 15%, the authors advised monitoring patients on digoxin if one proton pump inhibitor was replaced by another.[1]

(b) Omeprazole

One study found that omeprazole 20 mg daily for 11 days caused only minor changes in the disposition of a 1-mg oral dose of **digoxin**. On average the AUC was increased by 10%.[2] See also lansoprazole above.

(c) Pantoprazole

β-acetyldigoxin 200 micrograms twice daily was given to 18 healthy subjects, with and without pantoprazole 40 mg daily, for 5 days. The pantoprazole caused a 10% rise in the **digoxin** AUC and a 9% rise in the maximum **digoxin** serum levels, but both were considered to be clinically irrelevant. No changes in the **digoxin**-induced height reduction in the T-wave occurred.[3]

(d) Rabeprazole

A preliminary report giving few details states that rabeprazole increased the minimum **digoxin** levels by about 20%.[4] However, these changes are thought to be within the normal variations of **digoxin** levels and so are not considered clinically significant.[5] See also lansoprazole above.

Mechanism

The increase in digoxin levels with omeprazole may be the result of higher gastric pH which results in less digoxin hydrolysis and an increase in digoxin absorption.[6] Non-selective digoxin assay methods may fail to detect an interaction, whereas selective HPLC assay methods and ECG studies provide evidence that the bioavailability of digoxin may be increased by omeprazole.[6] An *in vitro* study found that omeprazole, pantoprazole and lansoprazole inhibit P-glycoprotein-mediated intestinal transport of digoxin.[7]

Importance and management

Although some studies suggest small changes in digoxin pharmacokinetics may occur these changes are usually small and unlikely to be clinically significant. No special precautions would therefore seem to be necessary if proton pump inhibitors and digoxin are given concurrently.

1. Le GH, Schaefer MG, Plowman BK, Morreale AP, Delattre M, Okino L, Felicio L. Assessment of potential digoxin-rabeprazole interaction after formulary conversion of proton-pump inhibitors. *Am J Health-Syst Pharm* (2003) 60, 1343–5.
2. Oosterhuis B, Jonkman JHG, Andersson T, Zuiderwijk PBM, Jedema JN. Minor effect of multiple dose omeprazole on the pharmacokinetics of digoxin after a single oral dose. *Br J Clin Pharmacol* (1991) 32, 569–72.
3. Hartmann M, Huber R, Bliesath H, Steinijans VW, Koch HJ, Wurst W, Kunz K. Lack of interaction between pantoprazole and digoxin at therapeutic doses in man. *Int J Clin Pharmacol Ther* (1995) 33, 481–5.
4. Humphries TJ, Nardi RV, Lazar JD, Spanyers SA. Drug-drug interaction evaluation of rabeprazole sodium: a clean/expected slate? *Gut* (1996) 39 (Suppl 3), A47.
5. Anon. Notice board. *Pharm J* (2003) 271, 541.
6. Cohen AF, Kroon R, Schoemaker HC, Hoogkamer JFW, van Vliet-Verbeek A. Effects of gastric acidity on the bioavailability of digoxin. Evidence for a new mechanism for interactions with omeprazole. *Br J Clin Pharmacol* (1991) 31, 565P.
7. Pauli-Magnus C, Rekersbrink S, Klotz U, Fromm MF. Interaction of omeprazole, lansoprazole and pantoprazole with P-glycoprotein. *Naunyn Schmiedebergs Arch Pharmacol* (2001) 364, 551–7.

Digitalis glycosides + Quinidine

In most patients the serum levels of digoxin on average doubled within five days of starting quinidine. The digoxin dosage usually needs to be halved if toxicity is to be avoided. Digitoxin levels are also increased but this occurs over a longer period of time, and to a lesser extent.

Clinical evidence

(a) Digoxin

The observation that quinidine appeared to increase serum digoxin levels prompted a retrospective study of patient records, which revealed that 25 out of 27 patients on digoxin had shown a significant rise in serum digoxin levels from 1.4 to 3.2 nanograms/ml when given quinidine. Of the patients showed a rise,16 showed typical signs of toxicity (nausea, vomiting, anorexia), which resolved in 10 when the digoxin dosage was reduced or withdrawn, and in 5 when the quinidine was withdrawn.[1]

This is one of the first reports published in 1978 (two other groups independently reported it at a similar time[2,3]) that clearly describes this interaction, although hints of its existence can be found in papers published over the previous 50 years. Since then large numbers of research reports, both retrospective and prospective, and case studies have confirmed and established the incidence and magnitude of this interaction. It occurs in over 90% of patients and, on average, there is a 100% increase in serum digoxin levels, although there are pronounced inter-individual differences, and the increase is somewhat dependent on the quinidine dose. There are numerous reports and reviews of this interaction, only a selection of which are listed here for economy of space. Two reviews published in 1982 and 1983 contain valuable bibliographies.[4,5]

(b) Digitoxin

Quinidine 750 mg daily increased the steady-state serum digitoxin levels of 8 healthy subjects by 45%, from 13.6 to 19.7 nanograms/ml, over 32 days.[6] Another study found a 31% increase in serum digitoxin levels over 10 days,[7] whereas yet another found a 115% increase.[8] A study in 5 healthy subjects found that quinidine reduced the total body clearance of digitoxin by 63%, resulting in raised serum digitoxin levels.[9]

Mechanism

Quinidine reduces the renal excretion of digoxin by 40 to 50%, and it also appears to have some effects on non-renal clearance, which includes a reduction of about 50% in digoxin excretion in the bile.[10] Quinidine displaces digoxin from tissue binding sites and significant changes in the volume of distribution occur. There is also some limited evidence that changes in the rate and extent of absorption of digoxin from the gut may have a small part to play.[11] There is some evidence that P-glycoprotein inhibition by quinidine may affect the absorption/exsorption of digoxin in the small intestine,[12] as well as reducing its renal elimination. An *in vitro* study found that quinidine inhibits P-glycoprotein-mediated transcellular transport,[13] which implies that digoxin renal tubular excretion may be inhibited by quinidine. Digoxin also appears to cause a small reduction in the renal clearance of quinidine.[14]

Quinidine appears to increase digitoxin serum levels by reducing the non-renal clearance.

Importance and management

The interaction between digoxin and quinidine is overwhelmingly well-documented, well-established and of definite clinical importance. Since serum digoxin levels are usually roughly doubled (up to fivefold increases have been seen[4]) and over 90% of patients are affected, digitalis toxicity will develop unless the dosage of digoxin is reduced (approximately halved).[1,4,15,16] A suggested rule-of-thumb is that if serum digoxin levels are no greater than 0.9 nanograms/ml the addition of quinidine is unlikely to cause cardiotoxic digoxin levels (if serum potassium levels are normal) whereas with levels of 1 nanogram/ml or more, toxic concentrations may develop.[17] Monitor the effects and readjust the dosage as necessary. Significant effects occur within a day of taking the quinidine and reach a maximum after about 3 to 6 days (quicker or slower in some patients), but digoxin levels will only stabilise when the quinidine has reached steady-state and that depends on whether a loading dose is given. The effects are to some extent dose-related but the correlation is not good: less than 400 to 500 mg of quinidine daily has minimal effects, and increasing doses up to 1200 mg has greater effects.[15,18] About 5 days are needed after withdrawing the quinidine before serum digoxin levels fall to their former levels. It has been recommended that patients with chronic renal failure should have their digoxin dosage reduced by as much as two-thirds.[19-21] An appropriate upward readjustment will be necessary if the quinidine is subsequently withdrawn.

Far less is known about the interaction between digitoxin and quinidine but similar precautions should be taken. It develops much more slowly.

1. Leahey EB, Reiffel JA, Drusin RE, Heisenbuttel RH, Lovejoy WP, Bigger JT. Interaction between quinidine and digoxin. *JAMA* (1978) 240, 533–4.
2. Ejvinsson G. Effect of quinidine on plasma concentrations of digoxin. *BMJ* (1978) i, 279–80.
3. Reid PR, Meek AG. Digoxin-quinidine interaction. *Johns Hopkins Med J* (1979) 145, 227–9.
4. Bigger JT, Leahey EB. Quinidine and digoxin. An important interaction. *Drugs* (1982) 24, 229–39.
5. Fichtl B, Doering W. The quinidine-digoxin interaction in perspective. *Clin Pharmacokinet* (1983) 8, 137–54.
6. Kuhlmann J, Dohrmann M, Marcin S. Effects of quinidine on pharmacokinetics and pharmacodynamics of digitoxin achieving steady-state conditions. *Clin Pharmacol Ther* (1986) 39, 288–94.
7. Peters U, Risler T, Grabensee B, Falkenstein U, Kroukou J. Interaktion von Chinidin und Digitoxin beim Menschen. *Dtsch Med Wochenschr* (1980) 105, 438–42.
8. Kreutz G, Keller F, Gast D and Prokein E. Digitoxin-quinidine interaction achieving steady-state conditions for both drugs. *Naunyn Schmiedebergs Arch Toxicol* (1982) 319, R82.
9. Garty M, Sood P, Rollins DE. Digitoxin elimination reduced during quinidine therapy. *Ann Intern Med* (1981) 94, 35–7.
10. Schenck-Gustafsson K, Angelin B, Hedman A, Arvidsson A, Dahlqvist R. Quinidine-induced reduction of the biliar excretion of digoxin in patients. *Circulation* (1985) 72 (Suppl), III-19.

11. Pedersen KE, Christiansen BD, Klitgaard NA, Nielsen-Kudsk F. Effect of quinidine on digoxin bioavailability. *Eur J Clin Pharmacol* (1983) 24, 41–7.
12. Su S-F, Huang J-D. Inhibition of the intestinal digoxin absorption and exsorption by quinidine. *Drug Metab Dispos* (1996) 24, 142–7.
13. Kakumoto M, Takara K, Sakaeda T, Tanigawara Y, Kita T, Okumura K. MDR1-mediated interaction of digoxin with antiarrhythmic or antianginal drugs. *Biol Pharm Bull* (2002) 25, 1604–7.
14. Rameis H. Quinidine-digoxin interaction: are the pharmacokinetics of both drugs altered? *Int J Clin Pharmacol Ther Toxicol* (1985) 23, 145–53.
15. Doering W. Quinidine-digoxin interaction: pharmacokinetics, underlying mechanism and clinical implications. *N Engl J Med* (1979) 301, 400–4.
16. Leahey EB, Reiffel JA, Heissenbuttel RH, Drusin RE, Lovejoy WP, Bigger JT. Enhanced cardiac effect of digoxin during quinidine treatment. *Arch Intern Med* (1979) 139, 519–21.
17. Friedman HS, Chen T-S. Use of control steady-state serum digoxin levels for predicting serum digoxin concentration after quinidine administration. *Am Heart J* (1982) 104, 72–6.
18. Fenster PE, Powell JR, Hager WD, Graves PE, Conrad K, Goldman S. Onset and dose dependence of digoxin-quinidine interaction. *Am J Cardiol* (1980) 45, 413.
19. Fichtl B, Doering W, Seidel H. The quinidine-digoxin interaction in patients with impaired renal function. *Int J Clin Pharmacol Ther Toxicol* (1983) 21, 229–33.
20. Fenster PE, Hager WD, Perrier D, Powell JR, Graves PE, Michael UF. Digoxin-quinidine interaction in patients with chronic renal failure. *Circulation* (1982) 66, 1277–80.
21. Woodcock BG and Rietbrock N. Digitalis-quinidine interactions. *Trends Pharmacol Sci* (1982) 3, 118–22.

Digitalis glycosides + Quinine

Some but not all patients may show a rise of more than 60% in serum digoxin levels if they are given quinine.

Clinical evidence

After taking quinine 300 mg four times daily for a day the steady-state levels of 4 subjects taking **digoxin** 250 micrograms daily rose by 63%, from 0.63 to 1.03 nanomol/l. After taking the quinine for a further 3 days the **digoxin** levels rose another 11% (to 1.1 nanomol/l). **Digoxin** renal clearance fell by 20%.[1]

Quinine sulfate 250 mg daily for 7 days increased the mean serum **digoxin** levels of 7 healthy subjects by 25%, from 0.64 to 0.8 nanograms/ml. When quinine sulfate 250 mg was given three times daily there was a further 8% rise. Considerable individual differences were seen, one subject had a 92% rise.[2] In contrast, 17 patients given quinine 750 mg daily showed only a small and statistically insignificant rise in mean serum **digoxin** levels, from 0.8 to 0.91 nanograms/ml. Serum levels were virtually unaltered in 11 patients, decreased in two and markedly increased (amount not stated) in four.[3] Another study found that **quinine** reduced the total clearance of **digoxin** by 26%.[4]

Mechanism

Not fully understood. A reduction in non-renal clearance is apparently largely responsible for the rise in serum digoxin levels with quinine.[2,4,5] This is possibly due to changes in digoxin metabolism or in its biliary excretion.[4,5]

Importance and management

An established interaction of clinical importance but only moderately documented. Monitor the effects of concurrent use and reduce the digoxin dosage where necessary. Some patients may show a substantial increase in serum digoxin levels whereas others will show only a small or moderate rise. There appear to be no case reports of digoxin toxicity arising from this interaction.

1. Aronson JK, Carver JG. Interaction of digoxin with quinine. *Lancet* (1981) i, 1418.
2. Pedersen KE, Madsen JL, Klitgaard NA, Kjaer K, Hvidt S. Effect of quinine on plasma digoxin concentration and renal digoxin clearance. *Acta Med Scand* (1985) 218, 229–32.
3. Doering W. Is there a clinically relevant interaction between quinine and digoxin in human beings? *Am J Cardiol* (1981) 48, 975–6.
4. Wandell M, Powell JR, Hager WD, Fenster PE, Graves PE, Conrad KA, Goldman S. Effect of quinine on digoxin kinetics. *Clin Pharmacol Ther* (1980) 28, 425–30.
5. Hedman A, Angelin B, Arvidsson A, Dahlqvist R, Nilsson B. Interactions in the renal and biliary elimination of digoxin: stereoselective difference between quinine and quinidine. *Clin Pharmacol Ther* (1990) 47, 20–6.

Digitalis glycosides + Quinolones

Levofloxacin, gemifloxacin, moxifloxacin and sparfloxacin do not interact pharmacokinetically with digoxin. Similarly moxifloxacin does not interact with beta-acetyldigoxin. Gatifloxacin may cause small increases in digoxin levels, which are probably not clinically significant. The effects of garenoxacin are unclear.

Clinical evidence, mechanism, importance and management

(a) Garenoxacin

In a study designed to look at the effects of garenoxacin on gut flora 16 healthy subjects were given **digoxin** 250 micrograms every 6 hours on day 1, then 250 micrograms daily to day 14, with garenoxacin 600 mg daily on days 8 to 14. Garenoxacin did not decrease (but may actually increase) the numbers of *E. lentum* in faeces (see 'Digitalis glycosides + Macrolides', p.702 for an explanation of the significance of these findings). Thus an interaction due to the effect of garenoxacin on intestinal microflora is unlikely.[1]

(b) Gatifloxacin

The vital signs of 12 healthy volunteers given gatifloxacin 400 mg daily for 7 days while taking **digoxin** 250 micrograms daily were not altered. Steady-state concentrations and the AUC of **digoxin** were increased by 12 and 19% respectively. Dosage adjustments were not considered necessary.[2]

(c) Gemifloxacin

No clinically relevant pharmacokinetic changes were seen in a study in 14 healthy elderly subjects given gemifloxacin 320 mg daily for 7 days while taking **digoxin** (*Lenoxin*) 250 micrograms daily. No clinically important changes in vital signs or ECGs were found.[3]

(d) Levofloxacin

No changes occurred in the pharmacokinetics of a single 400-microgram dose of **digoxin** (*Lanoxicaps*) when 12 healthy subjects were given levofloxacin 500 mg twice daily for 6 days.[4]

(e) Moxifloxacin

No clinically relevant changes in the steady-state pharmacokinetics of **digoxin** 250 micrograms daily in 14 healthy subjects given moxifloxacin 400 mg daily for 14 days.[5] No pharmacokinetic changes were seen in another study in 12 healthy subjects given a single 600-microgram dose of **beta-acetyldigoxin** with moxifloxacin 400 mg daily for 2 days.[6]

(f) Sparfloxacin

Sparfloxacin, 400 mg as a loading dose, followed by 200 mg daily for 9 days did not affect the pharmacokinetics of **digoxin** (*Lanoxicaps*) 300 micrograms daily in 24 healthy subjects.[7]

Mechanism, importance and management

Information about other digitalis glycosides and quinolones seems to be lacking, but bearing in mind their very extensive use, this silence in the literature would suggest that no problems normally arise. Despite *in vitro* susceptibility of *E. lentum* to a range of antibacterials including some quinolones there is currently no information to suggest such an interaction occurs between the quinolones and digoxin.[8] See 'Digitalis glycosides + Macrolides', p.702 for an explanation of the significance of *E. lentum*.

1. Nord CE, Meurling L, Russo RL, Bello A, Grasela DM, Gajjar DA. Effect of garenoxacin on Eubacteria in the normal intestinal microflora when administered concomitantly with digoxin. *J Chemother* (2003) 15, 244–7.
2. Olsen SJ, Uderman HD, Kaul S, Kollia GD, Birkhoffer MJ, Grasela DM. Pharmacokinetics of concomitantly administered gatifloxacin and digoxin. *Intersci Conf Antimicrob Agents Chemother* (1999) 39, 12.
3. Vousden M, Allen A, Lewis A, Ehren N. Lack of pharmacokinetic interaction between gemifloxacin and digoxin in healthy elderly volunteers. *Chemotherapy* (1999) 45, 485–90.
4. Chien S-C, Rogge MC, Williams RR, Natarajan J, Wong F, Chow AT. Absence of a pharmacokinetic interaction between digoxin and levofloxacin. *J Clin Pharm Ther* (2002) 27, 7–12.
5. Staß H, Frey R, Kubitza D, Möller J-G, Zühlsdorf M. Influence of orally administered moxifloxacin (MOX) on the steady state pharmacokinetics (PK) of digoxin (D) in healthy male volunteers. *J Antimicrob Chemother* (1999) 44 (Suppl A), 134–5.
6. Horstmann R, Delesen H, Dietrich H, Ochmann K, Sachse R, Staß H, Zuehlsdorf M, Kuhlmann J. No drug-drug interaction between moxifloxacin and β-acetyldigoxin. *Clin Invest Med* (1998) (Suppl), S20.
7. Johnson RD, Dorr MB, Hunt TL, Conway S, Talbot GH. Pharmacokinetic interaction of sparfloxacin and digoxin. *Clin Ther* (1999) 21, 368–79.
8. Ten Eick AP, Reed MD. Hidden dangers of coadministration of antibiotics and digoxin in children: focus on azithromycin. *Curr Ther Res* (2000) 61, 148–60.

Digitalis glycosides + Rauwolfia alkaloids

Concurrent use of digitalis glycosides and rauwolfia alkaloids is usually uneventful, but the incidence of arrhythmias appears to be increased, particularly in those with atrial fibrillation. Excessive bradycardia and syncope have also been described.

Clinical evidence

Three patients on **digoxin** and either **reserpine** or whole root ***Rauwolfia serpentina*** developed arrhythmias: atrial tachycardia with 4:1 Wenckebach irregular block; ventricular bigeminy and tachycardia; and atrial fibrillation. A large number of other patients received both drugs without problems.[1]

The incidence of premature ventricular systoles was roughly doubled in patients taking **digoxin** and **rauwolfia** compared with a similar group taking **rauwolfia** alone.[2] **Reserpine** reduced the tolerated dose of **acetyl strophanthidin** in 15 patients with congestive heart failure; 8 out of 9 with atrial fibrillation developed ECG abnormalities including complete heart block and ventricular ectopics during acute digitalisation following **reserpine** administration compared with only one of 9 without **reserpine**.[3]

A man on **digoxin** 250 and 375 micrograms on alternate days and **reserpine** 25 micrograms daily developed sinus bradycardia and carotid sinus supersensitivity. He was hospitalised because of syncope, which remitted when the **reserpine** was withdrawn.[4]

Mechanism

Not understood. A possible explanation is that because the rauwolfia alkaloids deplete the neurotransmitter from the sympathetic nerve supply to the heart, the parasympathetic vagal supply (i.e. heart slowing) has full rein. Digitalis also causes bradycardia resulting in additive bradycardia, which becomes excessive. In this situation the rate could become so slow that ectopic foci, which would normally be swamped by a faster, more normal beat, begin to fire, leading to the development of arrhythmias. Syncope could also result from the combination of bradycardia and the hypotensive effects of reserpine.

Importance and management

Some caution is advisable. One group of authors, despite having described the adverse reactions cited above,[1] conclude that time has proven the safety of the combination. However, they warn that arrhythmias must be anticipated. Particular risk of arrhythmias seems to occur in patients with atrial fibrillation, and in digitalised patients given reserpine parenterally because of the sudden release of catecholamines that takes place.[4]

1. Dick HLH, McCawley EL, Fisher WA. Reserpine-digitalis toxicity. *Arch Intern Med* (1962) 109, 503–6.
2. Schreader CJ, Etzl MM. Premature ventricular contractions due to rauwolfia therapy. *JAMA* (1956) 162, 1256.
3. Lown B, Ehrlich L, Lipschultz B, Blake J. Effect of digitalis in patients receiving reserpine. *Circulation* (1961) 24, 1185–91.
4. Bigger JT, Strauss HC. Digitalis toxicity: drug interactions promoting toxicity and the management of toxicity. *Semin Drug Treat* (1972) 2, 147–77.

Digitalis glycosides + Repaglinide

Repaglinide does not affect the pharmacokinetics of digoxin.

Clinical evidence, mechanism, importance and management

An open-label, crossover, multiple-dose trial in 14 healthy subjects found that repaglinide 2 mg three times daily before meals had no effect on the pharmacokinetics of **digoxin** 250 micrograms daily. Concurrent use was well tolerated.[1]

1. Hatorp V, Thomsen MS. Drug interaction studies with repaglinide: repaglinide on digoxin or theophylline pharmacokinetics and cimetidine on repaglinide pharmacokinetics. *J Clin Pharmacol* (2000) 40, 184–92.

Digitalis glycosides + Rifamycins

The serum levels of digitoxin can be halved by rifampicin (rifampin). There is also some evidence that digoxin serum levels may be similarly affected.

Clinical evidence

(a) Digitoxin

A comparative study in 21 patients with tuberculosis and 19 healthy subjects taking digitoxin 100 micrograms daily showed that the serum digitoxin levels of the patients on **rifampicin (rifampin)** were about half of the levels in healthy subjects not on **rifampicin** (18.4 compared with 39.1 nanograms/ml).[1] The half-life of digitoxin was reduced from 8.2 to 4.5 days by the **rifampicin**.

There are case reports confirming that **rifampicin** can markedly reduce serum digitoxin levels.[2,3]

(b) Digoxin

A woman, hospitalised for endocarditis, taking digoxin 250 to 375 micrograms daily, furosemide, aspirin, isosorbide dinitrate and potassium chloride, showed a marked fall of about 80% in her serum digoxin level when she was given **rifampicin** 600 mg daily. The serum digoxin returned to its former level over the 2 weeks following **rifampicin** withdrawal.[4] She had only moderate renal impairment (serum creatinine 2.5 mg/dl).

Another report describes 2 patients on renal dialysis whose digoxin dosage needed to be doubled while they were taking **rifampicin**, and similarly reduced when the **rifampicin** was withdrawn.[5] This confirms an earlier report.[6]

A study in 8 healthy subjects found that the AUC and maximum plasma levels of a single 1-mg oral dose of digoxin were reduced by 30 and 52% respectively by **rifampicin** 600 mg daily for 10 days.[7] A smaller 15% reduction in digoxin AUC and maximum plasma levels was seen when a single 1-mg intravenous dose of digoxin was given with the same **rifampicin** regimen.[7]

Mechanism

The interaction between digitoxin and rifampicin is almost certainly due to the increase in digitoxin metabolism caused by rifampicin, which is a potent enzyme inducing agent.[1,8] Digoxin on the other hand is largely excreted unchanged in the urine and the interaction with rifampicin appears to be mainly due to an increase in P-glycoprotein-mediated efflux by the intestinal cells.[7] Poor renal function in some patients may be an additional factor.

Importance and management

The interaction between digitoxin and rifampicin is established and clinically important. Under-digitalisation may occur unless the digitoxin dosage is increased appropriately. Good monitoring is obviously advisable.

The situation with digoxin is less clear. The documentation is very limited (most of it goes back to the 1980s) which is perhaps surprising considering how long both drugs have been available, but this would not be the first clinically relevant interaction to have been largely overlooked. It would now be prudent to monitor the concurrent use of these drugs, being alert for the need to increase the digoxin dosage. It may be that renal impairment increases the extent of this interaction. More study is needed. There does not seem to be any information regarding the other rifamycins, **rifabutin** (a weak enzyme inducer) and **rifapentine** (a moderate enzyme inducer). However, the UK makers and the UK Committee on Safety of Medicines warn that rifabutin may possibly reduce the effects of a number of drugs, including digitalis (but not digoxin).[9,10]

1. Peters U, Hausamen T-U, Grosse-Brockhoff F. Einfluβ von Tuberkulostatika auf die Pharmakokinetik des Digitoxins. *Dtsch Med Wochenschr* (1974) 99, 2381–6.
2. Boman G, Eliasson K, Odarcederlöf I. Acute cardiac failure during treatment with digitoxin - an interaction with rifampicin. *Br J Clin Pharmacol* (1980) 10, 89–90.
3. Poor DM, Self TH, Davis HL. Interaction of rifampin and digitoxin. *Arch Intern Med* (1983) 143, 599.
4. Bussey HI, Merritt GJ, Hill EG. The influence of rifampin on quinidine and digoxin. *Arch Intern Med* (1984) 144, 1021–3.
5. Gault H, Longerich L, Dawe M, Fine A. Digoxin-rifampin interaction. *Clin Pharmacol Ther* (1984) 35, 750–4.
6. Novi C, Bissoli F, Simonati V, Volpini T, Baroli A, Vignati G. Rifampin and digoxin: possible drug interaction in a dialysis patient. *JAMA* (1980) 244, 2521–2.
7. Greiner B, Eichelbaum M, Fritz P, Kreichgauer H-P, von Richter O, Zundler J, Kroemer HK. The role of intestinal P-glycoprotein in the interaction of digoxin and rifampin. J Clin Invest (1999) 104, 147–53. Correction. ibid. *(2002) 110, 571.* (2002) 110, 571.
8. Zilly W, Breimer DD, Richter E. Pharmacokinetic interactions with rifampicin. *Clin Pharmacokinet* (1977) 2, 61–70.
9. Mycobutin (Rifabutin). Pharmacia Ltd. UK Summary of product characteristics, January 2003.
10. Committee on the Safety of Medicines/Medicines Control Agency. Revised indication and drug interactions of rifabutin. *Current Problems* (1997) 23, 14.

Digitalis glycosides + Ritonavir

A woman had elevated serum digoxin levels and signs of toxicity after she was given ritonavir.

Clinical evidence

A 61-year-old HIV+ woman treated with lamivudine, indinavir, stavudine, pentamidine, warfarin and taking **digoxin** 250 micrograms daily for atrial fibrillation, presented with increasing nausea and vomiting 3 days after starting to take ritonavir 200 mg twice daily. **Digoxin** levels about 5 and 27 hours after her last dose were 7.2 nmol/l and 2.7 nmol/l respectively.[1]

A study in 12 healthy subjects found that ritonavir 300 mg twice daily for 11 days significantly increased the AUC and volume of distribution of a single 500-microgram intravenous dose of **digoxin** by 86% and 77% respectively. Non-renal and renal **digoxin** clearance was decreased by 48% and 35% respectively and its half-life increased by 156%.[2] Another study found that ritonavir 200 mg twice daily for 15 days increased the levels of a single 400-microgram oral dose of **digoxin** in 9 of 12 healthy subjects. Non-renal but not renal clearance was reduced.[3]

Mechanism

Raised digoxin levels are possibly due to inhibition of the P-glycoprotein-mediated renal transport of digoxin by ritonavir.[1] The studies in healthy subjects also suggest ritonavir-associated inhibition of P-glycoprotein.[2,3]

Importance and management

The documentation of the interaction between ritonavir and digoxin is sparse. Nevertheless it would seem prudent to closely monitor patients on digoxin when ritonavir is started or stopped.

1. Phillips EJ, Rachlis AR, Ito S. Digoxin toxicity and ritonavir: a drug interaction mediated through p-glycoprotein? *AIDS* (2003) 17, 1577–8.
2. Ding R, Tayrouz Y, Riedel K-D, Burhenne J, Weiss J, Mikus G, Haefeli WE. Substantial pharmacokinetic interaction between digoxin and ritonavir in healthy volunteers. *Clin Pharmacol Ther* (2004) 76, 73–84.
3. Penzak SR, Shen JM, Alfaro RM, Remaley AT, Natarajan V, Falloon J. Ritonavir decreases the nonrenal clearance of digoxin in healthy volunteers with known MDR1 genotypes. *Ther Drug Monit* (2004) 26, 322–30.

Digitalis glycosides + Ropinirole

Ropinirole does not significantly affect the pharmacokinetics of digoxin.

Clinical evidence, mechanism, importance and management

In a placebo-controlled study, 10 patients with Parkinson's disease were given ropinirole (initially 0.25 mg increasing to 2 mg three times daily) in addition to their standard treatment with **digoxin** 125 or 250 micrograms daily. Although ropinirole decreased the **digoxin** AUC by 10%, and the maximum plasma concentration by 25%, the **digoxin** minimum plasma concentration was not significantly altered. The authors therefore concluded that no dosage adjustment would be needed on concurrent use.[1]

1. Taylor A, Beerahee A, Citerone D, Davy M, Fitzpatrick K, Lopez-Gil A, Stocchi F. The effect of steady-state ropinirole on plasma concentrations of digoxin in patients with Parkinson's disease. *Br J Clin Pharmacol* (1999) 47, 219–22.

Digitalis glycosides + Sevelamer

The pharmacokinetics of single doses of digoxin are not affected by sevelamer.

Clinical evidence, mechanism, importance and management

In an open, randomised, crossover study a single 1-mg oral dose of **digoxin** was given with or without sevelamer 2.4 g followed by a standard breakfast. Five further doses of sevelamer were given immediately before subsequent meals over the following 2 days. During this time, the pharmacokinetic profile of **digoxin** was not altered.[1]

Sevelamer is a non-absorbed phosphate-binding polymer with bile-acid binding properties. Because the bile-acid binding resins colestyramine and colestipol may interact with **digoxin** (see 'colestyramine', (p.694) and 'colestipol', (p.694)), it was suggested that sevelamer could also interact, although this appears not to be the case. This finding requires confirmation in long-term studies.

1. Burke S, Amin N, Incerti C, Plone M, Watson N. Sevelamer hydrochloride (Renagel®), a non-absorbed phosphate-binding polymer, does not interfere with digoxin or warfarin pharmacokinetics. *J Clin Pharmacol* (2001) 41, 193–8.

Digitalis glycosides + SSRIs

Citalopram, fluvoxamine, paroxetine, and sertraline appear not to interact with digoxin, but an isolated report describes increased serum digoxin levels attributed to the use of fluoxetine.

Clinical evidence, mechanism, importance and management

A study in 11 healthy subjects showed that **citalopram** 40 mg once daily for 28 days did not have any significant effect on the pharmacokinetics of a single 1-mg dose of **digoxin** taken on day 21. No clinically significant ECG changes were observed.[1]

After taking **fluvoxamine** 100 mg daily for 15 days, the pharmacokinetics of a single 1.25-mg intravenous dose of **digoxin** were unchanged in 8 healthy subjects.[2]

A study in healthy subjects found that **paroxetine** 30 mg daily had no effect on the pharmacokinetics of **digoxin** 250 micrograms daily. The pharmacokinetics of **paroxetine** were unaffected by **digoxin**.[3]

A placebo-controlled study in 19 healthy subjects found that **sertraline**, in an initial dose of 50 mg daily titrated to 200 mg daily, had no effect on the steady-state pharmacokinetics of **digoxin**, except for a decrease in time to maximum plasma levels.[4]

In contrast, an isolated report describes a 93-year-old woman with congestive heart failure who developed increased serum **digoxin** levels on two occasions when **fluoxetine** was added.[5]

It seems unlikely that in general SSRIs will affect the steady-state serum levels of **digoxin**. No special precautions would seem to be necessary. The general importance of the case report is unknown, but it seems likely to be small.

1. Larsen F, Priskorn M, Overø KF. Lack of citalopram effect on oral digoxin pharmacokinetics. *J Clin Pharmacol* (2001) 41, 340–6.
2. Ochs HR, Greenblatt DJ, Verburg-Ochs B, Labedski L. Chronic treatment with fluvoxamine, clovoxamine and placebo: interaction with digoxin and effects on sleep and alertness. *J Clin Pharmacol* (1989) 29, 91–95.
3. Bannister SJ, Houser VP, Hulse JD, Kisicki JC, Rasmussen JGC. Evaluation of the potential for interactions of paroxetine with diazepam, cimetidine, warfarin, and digoxin. *Acta Psychiatr Scand* (1989) 80 (Suppl 350), 102–6.
4. Rapeport WG, Coates PE, Dewland PM, Forster PL. Absence of a sertraline-mediated effect on digoxin pharmacokinetics and electrocardiographic findings. *J Clin Psychiatry* (1996) 57 (Suppl 1), 16–19.
5. Leibovitz A, Bilchinsky T, Gil I, Habot B. Elevated serum digoxin level associated with coadministered fluoxetine. *Arch Intern Med* (1998) 158, 1152–3.

Digitalis glycosides + St John's wort (*Hypericum perforatum*)

Digoxin toxicity occurred in a patient on digoxin when he stopped taking St John's wort. There is good evidence that some preparations of St John's wort can reduce the blood levels of digoxin by about one-third to one-quarter.

Clinical evidence

An 80-year-old man on long-term **digoxin** and St John's wort herbal tea (2 litres daily) developed symptoms of **digoxin** toxicity (nodal bradycardia of 36 bpm and bigeminy) when he stopped taking the herbal tea.[1]

In a randomised placebo-controlled study, 93 healthy subjects were given **digoxin** alone for 7 days and then with one of ten St John's wort preparations for 14 days. Some St John's wort products including tea, juice, oil extract, and powder with low-dose hyperforin did not significantly affect the pharmacokinetics of **digoxin**. However, a high-dose hyperforin-rich extract (LI 160, Lichtwer Pharma) reduced the **digoxin** AUC, peak and trough plasma levels by 25%, 37% and 19% respectively. Comparable results were found with hypericum powder containing similar amounts of hyperforin, while hypericum powder with half the hyperforin content reduced the AUC, peak and trough plasma levels by about 18%, 21% and 13% respectively.[2]

In another study, 13 healthy subjects were given **digoxin** for 5 days until steady-state had been achieved, and then St John's wort extract (LI 160, Lichtwer Pharma) for a further 10 days. When compared with another group of 12 subjects taking digoxin and a placebo, the test group had 26.3% lower maximum plasma **digoxin** levels, 33.3% lower trough **digoxin** levels and a 25% lower AUC.[3]

Mechanism

St John's wort probably affects the activity of the P-glycoprotein drug transporter protein, which could alter the intestinal absorption of digoxin.[3,4] See also 'Drug transporter proteins', (p.8).

Importance and management

Information seems to be limited to these reports, but the interaction would appear to be established. The extent of the interaction may depend on the St John's wort preparation involved and dose used and seems to be correlated with the dose of hyperforin.[2] (See also 'Drug-herb interactions', (p.10)). Reductions in serum digoxin levels of this size are likely to diminish the control of arrhythmias or heart failure. Digoxin serum levels should therefore be well monitored if St John's wort is either started or stopped and appropriate dosage adjustments made if necessary. The recommendation of the UK Committee on Safety of Medicines is that St John's wort should not be used in patients taking digoxin.[5]

1. Anđelić S. Bigeminija – rezultat interakcije digoksina i kantariona. *Vojnosanit Pregl* (2003) 60, 361–4.
2. Mueller SC, Uehleke B, Woehling H, Petzsch M, Majcher-Peszynska J, Hehl E-M, Sievers H, Frank B, Riethling A-K, Drewelow B. Effect of St John's wort dose and preparations on the pharmacokinetics of digoxin. *Clin Pharmacol Ther* (2004) 75, 546–57.
3. Johne A, Brockmöller J, Bauer S, Maurer A, Langheinrich M, Roots I. Pharmacokinetic interaction of digoxin with an herbal extract from St John's wort (*Hypericum perforatum*). *Clin Pharmacol Ther* (1999) 66, 338–45.
4. Dürr D, Stieger B, Kullak-Ublick GA, Rentsch KM, Steinert HC, Meier PJ, Fattinger K. St John's wort induces intestinal P-glycoprotein/MDR1 and intestinal and hepatic CYP3A4. *Clin Pharmacol Ther* (2000) 68, 598–604.
5. Committee on the Safety of Medicines (UK). Message from Professor A Breckenridge (Chairman of CSM) and Fact Sheet for Health Care Professionals, 29th February 2000.

Digitalis glycosides + Statins

Atorvastatin, fluvastatin and simvastatin cause small but probably clinically unimportant increases in the serum levels of digoxin. Pravastatin and rosuvastatin appear to have no effect on digoxin pharmacokinetics.

Clinical evidence

(a) Atorvastatin

Digoxin 250 micrograms daily was given to 24 healthy subjects for 10 days, with atorvastatin 10 mg or 80 mg daily for a further 10 days. The mean steady-state **digoxin** levels were unaffected by atorvastatin 10 mg, but 80 mg caused a 20% rise in maximum **digoxin** levels and a 15% rise in the 24-hour AUC.[1]

(b) Fluvastatin

In a crossover study in 18 patients, fluvastatin 40 mg caused no significant changes in the pharmacokinetics of **digoxin** 100 to 375 micrograms daily.[2] Another similar study in patients found changes of up to 15% in maximum plasma **digoxin** levels and clearance, but these were not considered to be clinically relevant.[3]

(c) Pravastatin

Pravastatin 20 mg daily for 9 days had no significant effect on steady state levels of **digoxin** 200 micrograms daily in 18 healthy subjects.[4]

(d) Rosuvastatin

In a double-blind randomised trial 18 healthy subjects were given rosuvastatin 40 mg daily or placebo for 12 days, with a single 500-microgram dose of **digoxin** on day 8. The absorption, renal excretion, AUC and maximum serum levels of **digoxin** were unaffected by rosuvastatin.[5]

(e) Simvastatin

Plasma **digoxin** levels can be slightly raised, by about 300 picograms/ml, by simvastatin but this appears to be of little or no clinical importance.[6]

Mechanism

The small changes seen in digoxin levels are probably due to the inhibitory effects of these statins on P-glycoprotein. Pravastatin does not appear to inhibit P-glycoprotein.[7]

Importance and management

The small changes seen in the digoxin levels with statins seem unlikely to be clinically relevant in most patients. However, bear the possibility of an interaction in mind if digoxin levels are raised in patients on atorvastatin, simvastatin or fluvastatin.

1. Boyd RA, Stern RH, Stewart BH, Wu X, Reyner EL, Zegarac EA, Randinitis EJ, Whitfield L. Atorvastatin coadministration may increase digoxin concentrations by inhibition of intestinal P-glycoprotein-mediated secretion. *J Clin Pharmacol* (2000) 40, 91–8.
2. Smith HT, Jokubaitis LA, Troendle AJ, Hwang DS, Robinson WT. Pharmacokinetics of fluvastatin and specific drug interactions. *Am J Hypertens* (1993) 6 (Suppl), 375S–382S.
3. Garnett WR, Venitz J, Wilkens RC, Dimenna G. Pharmacokinetic effects of fluvastatin in patients chronically receiving digoxin. *Am J Med* (1994) 96 (Suppl 6A), 84S–86S.
4. Triscari J, Swanson BN, Willard DA, Cohen AI, Devault A, Pan HY. Steady state serum concentrations of pravastatin and digoxin when given in combination. *Br J Clin Pharmacol* (1993) 36, 263–5.
5. Martin PD, Kemp J, Dane AL, Warwick MJ, Schneck DW. No effect of rosuvastatin on the pharmacokinetics of digoxin in healthy volunteers. *J Clin Pharmacol* (2002) 42, 1352–7.
6. Garnett WR. Interactions with hydroxymethylglutaryl-coenzyme A reductase inhibitors. *Am J Health-Syst Pharm* (1995) 52, 1639–45.
7. Sakaeda T, Takara K, Kakumoto M, Ohmoto N, Nakamura T, Iwaki K, Tanigawara Y, Okumura K. Simvastatin and lovastatin, but not pravastatin, interact with MDR1. *J Pharm Pharmacol* (2002) 54, 419–23.

Digitalis glycosides + Sucralfate

Sucralfate caused only a small reduction in the absorption of digoxin in one study, but an isolated report describes a marked reduction in one patient.

Clinical evidence

Sucralfate 1 g four times daily given to 12 healthy subjects for 2 days had no effect on most of the pharmacokinetics of a single 750-microgram dose of **digoxin**. However, the AUC was reduced by 19% and the amount of **digoxin** eliminated in the urine was reduced by 12%. **Digoxin** was also absorbed faster.[1] No interaction occurred when the **digoxin** was given 2 hours before the sucralfate.[1]

One elderly patient is reported to have had subtherapeutic serum **digoxin** levels while taking sucralfate, even though the dosages were separated by 2 hours.[2]

Mechanism

Uncertain. One possibility is that the digoxin and sucralfate bind together in the gut, which reduces the digoxin absorption.

Importance and management

Information appears to be limited to the reports cited. The reduction in digoxin levels is apparently only small and therefore normally not likely to be clinically relevant, but the unexplained and isolated case suggests that clinicians should at least be aware of the possibility of an interaction.

1. Giesing DH, Lanman RC, Dimmitt DC, Runser DJ. Lack of effect of sucralfate on digoxin pharmacokinetics. *Gastroenterology* (1983) 84,1165.
2. Rey AM, Gums JG. Altered absorption of digoxin, sustained-release quinidine, and warfarin with sucralfate administration. *Ann Pharmacother* (1991) 25, 745–6.

Digitalis glycosides + Surfactants

Surfactants such as Cremophor may enhance the absorption of digoxin.

Clinical evidence, mechanism, importance and management

A double-blind, crossover, placebo-controlled study in 12 healthy subjects found that ***Cremophor RH40*** 600 mg three times daily increased the 0 to 5-hour AUC and peak plasma levels of a single 500-microgram oral dose of **digoxin** by about 22%. The absorption of **digoxin** was delayed. The pharmacodynamic effects of **digoxin** were not affected by ***Cremophor***.

It was suggested that ***Cremophor*** increases **digoxin** plasma levels by inhibiting intestinal P-glycoprotein, or that the ***Cremophor*** prolongs the dissolution of **digoxin** tablets resulting in delayed absorption from the intestines.[1]

Other surfactants inhibit P-glycoprotein mediated intestinal transport and an *in vitro* study found that the order of effectiveness for enhanced intestinal uptake of **digoxin** (starting with the most effective) was ***Labrasol***,

Imwitor 742, Acconon E, Softigen 767, Cremophor EL, Miglyol, Solutol HS 15, **Sucrose monolaurate, Polysorbate 20,** *TPGS,* **Polysorbate 80.**[2]

1. Tayrouz Y, Ding R, Burhenne J, Riedel K-D, Weiss J, Hoppe-Tichy T, Haefeli WE, Mikus G. Pharmacokinetic and pharmaceutic interaction between digoxin and Cremophor RH40. *Clin Pharmacol Ther* (2003) 73, 397–405.
2. Cornaire G, Woodley J, Hermann P, Cloarec A, Arellano C, Houin G. Impact of excipients on the absorption of P-glycoprotein substrates in vitro and in vivo. *Int J Pharm* (2004) 278, 119–31.

Digitalis glycosides + Teriparatide

Teriparatide appears not to affect the calcium-mediated pharmacodynamics of digoxin.

Clinical evidence, mechanism, importance and management

A placebo-controlled study in 15 healthy subjects given **digoxin** 500 micrograms daily, adjusted to maintain steady-state serum levels in the range 1 to 2 nanograms/ml, found that a single 20-microgram subcutaneous dose of teriparatide on day 15 or 16 did not alter the calcium-mediated effects of **digoxin** (systolic time interval), or heart rate. The transient increases in calcium observed with teriparatide were considered insufficient to increase cardiac sensitivity to **digoxin** at therapeutic dosage.[1]

1. Benson CT, Voelker JR. Teriparatide has no effect on the calcium-mediated pharmacodynamics of digoxin. *Clin Pharmacol Ther* (2003) 73, 87–94.

Digitalis glycosides + Tetracycline

Tetracycline may cause a rise in serum digoxin levels in a few patients, which is of uncertain clinical importance.

Clinical evidence

A patient on **digoxin** tablets 500 micrograms daily was given tetracycline 500 mg every 6 hours for 5 days. His urinary excretion of **digoxin** metabolites (see Mechanism) fell sharply within 2 days, and his steady-state serum **digoxin** levels rose by 43%.[1]

Another subject had a marked fall in the excretion of **digoxin** metabolites from the gut after taking tetracycline.[2]

Mechanism

Up to 10% of patients on oral digoxin excrete it in substantial amounts in the faeces and urine as inactive metabolites (digoxin reduction products or DRPs). This metabolism seems to be performed by the gut flora,[1] in particular *Eubacterium lentum*, which is anaerobic and Gram positive.[2,3] In the presence of some antibacterials, such as tetracycline, which can inhibit this organism, more digoxin becomes available for absorption, which results in a rise in serum levels. At the same time the inactive metabolites derived from the gut disappear.[2] See also 'Digitalis glycosides + Macrolides', p.702.

Importance and management

The interaction between digoxin and tetracycline is not well established and the evidence is very limited. Its general clinical importance is uncertain and it is only likely to occur with digoxin formulations with poor bioavailability. Only a small proportion of patients (about 10%) are likely to be at risk, the difficulty being that it is usually not known if a particular patient falls into this 'excreter' category or not (see Mechanism). Bear this interaction in mind in the case of an unexpected response to digoxin.

1. Lindenbaum J, Rund DG, Butler VP, Tse-Eng D, Saha JR. Inactivation of digoxin by the gut flora: reversal by antibiotic therapy. *N Engl J Med* (1981) 305, 789–94.
2. Dobkin JF, Saha JR, Butler VP, Lindenbaum J. Effects of antibiotic therapy on digoxin metabolism. *Clin Res* (1982) 30, 517A.
3. Ten Eick AP, Reed MD. Hidden dangers of coadministration of antibiotics and digoxin in children: focus on azithromycin. *Curr Ther Res* (2000) 61, 148–60.

Digitalis glycosides + Thyroid hormones and Antithyroid drugs

Thyrotoxic patients are relatively resistant to the effects of digitalis glycosides and may need reduced doses as treatment with antithyroid drugs (carbimazole, thiamazole) progresses, whereas patients with hypothyroidism may need increased doses of digitalis glycosides as treatment with thyroid hormones progresses. Carbimazole has been shown to reduce serum digoxin in healthy subjects.

Clinical evidence

(a) Carbimazole

The observation of relatively low plasma **digoxin** levels in a patient on carbimazole prompted a further study in 10 healthy subjects. In 9 out of the 10, steady-state peak serum **digoxin** levels were reduced by 23% (from 1.72 to 1.33 nanograms/ml) by a single 60-mg dose of carbimazole, but in the other subject the serum **digoxin** levels were increased. Other pharmacokinetic parameters were unaffected.

Carbimazole abolished the systolic blood pressure decrease seen in the first 3 hours with **digoxin**, and also reduced the duration of the **digoxin**-induced diastolic blood pressure fall from 12 to 6 hours. The changes in heart rates, cardiac output and stroke volumes were not statistically significant, but inter-individual differences were large.[1-3]

(b) Thiamazole

A study in 12 patients with hyperthyroidism found that normalisation of serum T3 and T4 by thiamazole treatment did not produce significant changes in the pharmacokinetics of **digoxin**.[4]

Mechanism

One explanation for the changed response to digitalis with carbimazole is that there is a direct and altered response of the heart due to the raised or lowered thyroid hormone levels. Another is that changes in glomerular filtration rate associated with hypo- or hyperthyroidism result in increased or decreased serum digoxin, respectively.[5] Why carbimazole *reduced* serum digoxin in healthy subjects (normal thyroid status) is not known.

Importance and management

As thyroid status is returned to normal by the use of drugs (antithyroid drugs or thyroid hormones), the dosage of the digitalis glycosides may need to be adjusted appropriately. Hyperthyroid patients may need to have their digitalis dosage gradually reduced as treatment proceeds (because initially they are relatively resistant to the effects of digitalis and start off needing higher doses). They are also relatively insensitive to the chronotropic effects of digitalis.[6,7] Hypothyroid patients on the other hand may need a gradually increasing dosage (because initially they are relatively sensitive to digitalis).[5,6] In either of these situations it would be prudent to monitor serum digoxin levels and glomerular filtration rate as treatment continues. The reduction of serum digoxin by carbimazole in healthy subjects does not fit with the need to decrease digoxin doses when antithyroid drugs are used in patients. Further study is needed.

1. Petereit G, Ramesh Rao B, Siepmann M, Kirch W. Influence of carbimazole on the steady state serum levels and haemodynamic effects of digoxin in healthy subjects. *Eur J Clin Pharmacol* (1995) 49, A159.
2. Rao BR, Petereit G, Ebert U, Siepmann M, Kirch W. Influence of carbimazole on the steady state serum levels and haemodynamic effects of digoxin in healthy subjects. *Therapie* (1995) 50 (Suppl), 406.
3. Rao R, Petereit G, Ebert U, Kirch W. Influence of carbimazole on serum levels and haemodynamic effects of digoxin. *Clin Drug Invest* (1997) 13, 350–4.
4. Gasińska T, Izbicka M, Dec R. Digoxin pharmacokinetics in hyperthyroid patients treated with methimazole. *J Endocrinol* (1997) 152 (Suppl), P285.
5. Croxson MS, Ibbertson HK. Serum digoxin in patients with thyroid disease. *BMJ* (1975) 3, 566–8.
6. Lawrence JR, Sumner DJ, Kalk WJ, Ratcliffe WA, Whiting B, Gray K, Lindsay M. Digoxin kinetics in patients with thyroid dysfunction. *Clin Pharmacol Ther* (1977) 22, 7–13.
7. Huffman DH, Klaassen CD, Hartman CR. Digoxin in hyperthyroidism. *Clin Pharmacol Ther* (1977) 22, 533–8.

Digitalis glycosides + Ticlopidine

Ticlopidine 250 mg twice daily for 10 days reduced the peak serum concentrations and AUC of digoxin by about 10% in 15 sub-

jects.[1] This reduction is small and unlikely to be of clinical importance.

1. Vargas R, Reitman M, Teitelbaum P, Ryan JR, McMahon FG, Jain AK, Ryan M, Regel G. Study of the effect of ticlopidine on digoxin blood levels. *Clin Pharmacol Ther* (1988) 43, 176.

Digitalis glycosides + Tiludronate

Digoxin does not appear to interact with tiludronate.

Clinical evidence, mechanism, importance and management

A study in 12 healthy subjects found that **tiludronate**, 600 mg daily for 2 days then 400 mg daily for the next 10 days, caused no significant changes in the pharmacokinetics of **digoxin** 250 micrograms daily.[1] No special precautions appear to be needed.

1. Sanofi Winthrop. Data on file, June 1996.

Digitalis glycosides + Trapidil

Trapidil does not alter serum digoxin levels.

Clinical evidence, mechanism, importance and management

Trapidil 400 mg daily for 8 days had no effect on the steady-state serum levels of **digoxin** 375 micrograms daily in 10 healthy subjects. It was noted that the positive chronotropic effect of trapidil opposed the negative chronotropic effect of **digoxin**, which should be remembered when using both drugs, but overall no adverse effects that would prevent concurrent use were noted.[1]

1. Sziegoleit W, Weiss M, Fahr A, Scharfe S. Trapidil does not affect serum levels and cardiotonic action of digoxin in healthy humans. *Jpn Circ J* (1987) 51, 1305–9.

Digitalis glycosides + Trazodone

A rise in serum digoxin levels, accompanied by toxicity in one instance, has been seen in two patients on digoxin when they were given trazodone.

Clinical evidence, mechanism, importance and management

An elderly woman stabilised on **digoxin** 125 micrograms daily (and also taking quinidine, clonidine and a triamterene/hydrochlorothiazide diuretic) complained of nausea and vomiting within a fortnight of starting to take trazodone (initially 50 mg, increasing to 300 mg daily over 11 days). Her serum **digoxin** levels had risen more than threefold, from 0.8 to 2.8 nanograms/ml. The **digoxin** was stopped and then restarted at half the original dosage, which maintained therapeutic levels.[1] The patient had poor renal function, but this did not change significantly during this incident. Another case of raised **digoxin** levels, apparently caused by trazodone, has been reported.[2]

Direct information seems to be limited to these two reports. Bear this interaction in mind in the case of an unexpected response to **digoxin**.

1. Rauch PK, Jenike MA. Digoxin toxicity possibly precipitated by trazodone. *Psychosomatics* (1984) 25, 334–5.
2. Knapp JE. Mead Johnson Pharmaceutical Newsletter, 1983.

Digitalis glycosides + Trimetazidine

Trimetazidine appears not to affect the pharmacokinetics of digoxin.

Clinical evidence, mechanism, importance and management

After taking trimetazidine 20 mg twice daily for at least 14 days the pharmacokinetics of a single 500-microgram dose of **digoxin** remained unchanged in 13 healthy subjects.[1] These results suggest that treatment with **digoxin** is unlikely to be altered in patients concurrently treated with trimetazidine, but this needs confirmation.

1. Edeki TI, Johnston A, Campbell DB, Ings RMJ, Brownsill R, Genissel P, Turner P. An examination of the possible pharmacokinetic interaction of trimetazidine with theophylline, digoxin and antipyrine. *Br J Clin Pharmacol* (1989) 26, 657P.

Digitalis glycosides + Urapidil

Urapidil does not appear to affect the pharmacokinetics of digoxin.

Clinical evidence, mechanism, importance and management

Urapidil 60 mg twice daily on days 5 to 8 had no significant effects on serum **digoxin** levels in 12 healthy subjects given 250 micrograms twice daily on day one, then 250 micrograms daily on days 2 to 8. Blood pressures and pulse rates were not significantly changed.[1] No special precautions seem necessary.

1. Solleder P, Haerlin R, Wurst W, Klingmann I, Mosberg H. Effect of urapidil on steady-state serum digoxin concentration in healthy subjects. *Eur J Clin Pharmacol* (1989) 37, 193–4.

Digitalis glycosides + Valaciclovir

Valaciclovir appears not to interact with digoxin.

Clinical evidence, mechanism, importance and management

In a randomised 4-period crossover study, 12 healthy subjects were given 1 g of oral valaciclovir alone, two 750-microgram doses of **digoxin** alone, valaciclovir 1 g after the second of two 750-microgram doses of **digoxin** given 12 hours apart, and finally valaciclovir 1 g three times daily for 8 days starting 12 hours before the first **digoxin** dose.[1]

It was found that no clinically significant changes occurred in the pharmacokinetics of either drug and no ECG changes were seen. It was concluded that no dosage adjustments of either drug are needed if given concurrently.[1] Since valaciclovir is a prodrug of **aciclovir**, it also seems unlikely that an interaction will occur between **aciclovir** and **digoxin**. Information about **digitoxin** seems to be lacking.

1. Soul-Lawton JH, Weatherley BC, Posner J, Layton G, Peck RW. Lack of interaction between valaciclovir, the L-valyl ester of aciclovir and digoxin. *Br J Clin Pharmacol* (1998) 45, 87–9.

Digitalis glycosides + Valspodar

Valspodar increases the AUC of digoxin two to threefold.

Clinical evidence, mechanism, importance and management

Twelve healthy subjects were given **digoxin** 1 mg on day 1, followed by 125 micrograms daily for the next 10 days. Starting on day 7 they were also given a single 400-mg dose of valspodar, followed by 200 mg twice daily for the following 4 days. The steady-state **digoxin** AUC was increased by 76% after the first valspodar dose, and by the end of valspodar dosing it had increased by 211%. This was apparently due to a fall in renal **digoxin** clearance of 73% and in non-renal clearance of 58%, probably because of reduced tubular secretion, and possibly reduced biliary elimination and increased intestinal absorption caused by P-glycoprotein inhibition. No symptoms of digitalis toxicity were seen and there were no changes in vital signs or ECG parameters.[1]

Information seems to be limited to this study in healthy subjects but it suggests that the **digoxin** dosage should be reduced if valspodar is given. An initial 50% reduction has been suggested.

1. Kovarik JM, Rigaudy L, Guerret M, Gerbeau C, Rost K-L. Longitudinal assessment of a P-glycoprotein-mediated drug interaction of valspodar on digoxin. *Clin Pharmacol Ther* (1999) 66, 391–400.

Digitalis glycosides + Vasodilators

Sodium nitroprusside or hydralazine can reduce serum digoxin levels but the importance of this is uncertain.

Clinical evidence, mechanism, importance and management

An experimental study in 8 patients with congestive heart failure showed that when they were given either **sodium nitroprusside** by infusion (7 to 425 micrograms/minute) or **hydralazine** by intravenous injection (5 mg every 10 to 20 minutes to a total dose of 10 to 60 mg) the total renal **digoxin** clearance was increased by about 50% by both drugs and their serum **digoxin** levels were decreased by 20% by the **nitroprusside** and 11% by the **hydralazine**.[1]

It is not known whether these changes would be sustained during chronic concurrent use, or the extent to which the **digoxin** dosage might need to be increased. More study is needed to find out if this interaction is of practical importance.

1. Cogan JJ, Humphreys MH, Carlson CJ, Benowitz NL, Rapaport E. Acute vasodilator therapy increases renal clearance of digoxin in patients with congestive heart failure. *Circulation* (1981) 64, 973–6.

Digitalis glycosides + Voriconazole

Voriconazole 200 mg twice daily for 12 days had no significant effect on the pharmacokinetics of digoxin 250 micrograms daily when given to healthy subjects for 10 days.[1] No dosage adjustments seem necessary on concurrent use.

1. Purkins L, Wood N, Kleinermans D, Nichols D. Voriconazole does not affect the steady-state pharmacokinetics of digoxin. *Br J Clin Pharmacol* (2003) 56, 45–50.

Digitalis glycosides + Ximelagatran

No significant pharmacokinetic interaction appears to occur between digoxin and ximelagatran.

Clinical evidence, mechanism, importance and management

In a double-blind, crossover study, 16 healthy subjects were given oral ximelagatran 36 mg twice daily or placebo for 8 days and a single 500-microgram oral dose of **digoxin** on day 4. Ximelagatran had no effects on the pharmacokinetics of **digoxin**. Similarly, **digoxin** had no effects on the pharmacokinetics of melagatran (the active metabolite) following oral ximelagatran administration. The anticoagulant effect of melagatran (measured as aPTT prolongation) was not altered by **digoxin**.[1]

1. Sarich TC, Schutzer K-M, Wollbratt M, Wall U, Kessler E, Eriksson UG. No pharmacokinetic or pharmacodynamic interaction between digoxin and ximelagatran, an oral direct thrombin inhibitor. *Blood* (2003) 102, 127b.

Digitalis glycosides + Zileuton

Zileuton appears not to interact with digoxin.

Clinical evidence, mechanism, importance and management

In a double-blind placebo-controlled study 12 healthy subjects were given zileuton 600 mg or a placebo every 6 hours for 13 days, with **digoxin** 250 micrograms daily from days 1 to 11. The zileuton had no effect on the steady-state **digoxin** pharmacokinetics, although the time to reach maximum plasma levels was reduced from 1.43 to 0.95 hours. Concurrent use was well tolerated.[1] This evidence suggests that no special precautions are needed if these two drugs are used together.

1. Awni WM, Hussein Z, Cavanaugh JH, Granneman GR, Dube LM. Assessment of the pharmacokinetic interaction between zileuton and digoxin in humans. *Clin Pharmacokinet* (1995) 29 (Suppl 2), 92–7.

24

Diuretics

The majority of the interactions of the diuretics appear to be pharmacodynamic in nature, that is they appear to be due to the combined effects of diuretic and the other interacting drug. Obvious examples of this would be hypotension caused by the use of a loop diuretic and a beta-blocker, or hyperkalaemia caused by an ACE inhibitor and a potassium-sparing diuretic. Some commonly accepted interactions appear to be sparsely documented, most probably as they are perceived to be a predictable effect of using two drugs with similar actions together. 'Table 24.1', (below) lists the potassium-depleting diuretics.

The interactions covered in this section are mainly those in which the diuretic is affected. There are many other interactions throughout the publication where diuretics affect the actions of other drugs.

Table 24.1 Potassium-depleting diuretics

Carbonic anhydrase inhibitors	Acetazolamide, diclofenamide (dichlorphenamide), disulfamide, ethoxzolamide, methazolamide
Loop diuretics	Azosemide, bumetanide, etacrynic acid, etozolin, furosemide, muzolimine, piretanide, torasemide
Organomercurials	Chlormerodrin, meraluride, mercaptomerin
Thiazides and related diuretics	Althiazide, ambuside, bemetizide, bendroflumethiazide, benzthiazide, benzylhydrochlorothiazide, buthiazide, chlorothiazide, chlortalidone, clopamide, clorexolone, cyclopenthiazide, cyclothiazide, epithiazide, ethiazide, fenquizone, hydrobentizide, hydrochlorothiazide, hydroflumethiazide, indapamide, mebutizide, mefruside, methylclothiazide, meticrane, metolazone, polythiazide, quinethazone, teclothiazide, trichlormethiazide, xipamide

Acetazolamide + Sodium bicarbonate

Acetazolamide is associated with development of renal calculi and it is claimed that sodium bicarbonate, even on alternate days, potentiates the risk of calculus formation.[1]

1. Rubenstein MA, Bucy JG. Acetazolamide-induced renal calculi. *J Urol (Baltimore)* (1975) 114, 610–12.

Acetazolamide + Timolol

The use of acetazolamide and timolol eye drops resulted in severe mixed acidosis in a patient with chronic obstructive pulmonary disease.

Clinical evidence, mechanism, importance and management

An elderly man with severe chronic obstructive pulmonary disease was given oral acetazolamide 750 mg daily and 0.5% timolol maleate eye drops, one drop in each eye twice daily, as premedication to reduce ocular hypertension before surgery for glaucoma. Five days later he developed progressively worsening dyspnoea and he was found to have a severe mixed acidosis.[1] This seems to have been caused by the additive effects of acetazolamide, which blocked the excretion of hydrogen ions in the kidney, and the bronchoconstrictor effects of the timolol, which was absorbed in sufficient amounts to exacerbate the airway obstruction in this patient and thereby reduced the respiration. This isolated case emphasises the potential risks of using beta-blockers in patients with obstructive pulmonary disease. The makers of acetazolamide note that it should be used with caution in those with pulmonary obstruction or emphysema because of the increased risk of acidosis.[2]

1. Boada JE, Estopa R, Izquierdo J, Dorca J, Manresa F. Severe mixed acidosis by combined therapy with acetazolamide and timolol eyedrops. *Eur J Respir Dis* (1986) 68, 226–8.
2. Diamox (Acetazolamide). Wyeth Pharmaceuticals. UK Summary of product characteristics, February 2004.

Bumetanide + Aspirin

Aspirin 640 mg four times daily reduced the 24-hour urinary output in response to bumetanide 1 mg by 18% in 8 healthy subjects.[1] The clinical significance of this interaction is unclear. See also 'Loop diuretics + NSAIDs', p.721.

1. Kaufman J, Hamburger R, Matheson J, Flamenbaum W. Bumetanide-induced diuresis and natriuresis: effect of prostaglandin synthetase inhibition. *J Clin Pharmacol* (1981) 21, 663–7.

Cyclothiazide/triamterene + Pravastatin

Reversible diabetes mellitus developed in a woman taking cyclothiazide/triamterene when she was additionally given pravastatin.

Clinical evidence, mechanism, importance and management

A 63-year-old woman who had been on cyclothiazide/triamterene and acebutolol for 4 years, developed polyuria and polydipsia within 3 weeks of starting pravastatin 20 mg daily, which gradually worsened. After another 4 months she was hospitalised for hyperglycaemia, which was treated with insulin and later glibenclamide (glyburide). The cyclothiazide/triamterene and pravastatin were stopped and gradually the diabetic symptoms began to abate. Five weeks after admission she was discharged without the need for any antidiabetic treatment with the diabetes fully resolved.[1] The detailed reasons for this reaction are not understood, but it would seem that the pravastatin increased the hyperglycaemic potential of the thiazide diuretic to the point where frank diabetes developed. This is an isolated case and there would seem to be little reason normally to avoid the concurrent use of these drugs.

1. Jonville-Bera A-P, Zakian A, Bera FJ, Carré P, Autret E. Possible pravastatin and diuretics-induced diabetes mellitus. *Ann Pharmacother* (1994) 28, 964–5.

Eplerenone + Ketoconazole or other CYP3A4 enzyme inhibitors

Ketoconazole markedly raises the AUC of eplerenone, and the maker contraindicates concurrent use. Similarly, concurrent use of other strong inhibitors of the cytochrome P450 isoenzyme CYP3A4 should be avoided. Mild to moderate inhibitors of CYP3A4 increase the AUC of eplerenone about twofold, and the dose of eplerenone should be restricted in patients on these drugs (e.g. amiodarone, diltiazem, verapamil). Grapefruit juice had a small unimportant effect.

Clinical evidence

(a) Azoles

Ketoconazole 200 mg twice daily for 7 days increased the AUC of a single 100-mg dose of eplerenone 5.4-fold in 18 healthy subjects.[1,2] **Fluconazole** 200 mg daily for 7 days increased the AUC of eplerenone 2.2-fold in 18 healthy subjects.[2] The maker predicts that **itraconazole** will have a similar effect to ketoconazole.[3]

(b) Calcium channel blockers

The steady-state AUC of eplerenone 100 mg daily was increased by about twofold by **verapamil** 240 mg daily given to 24 healthy subjects for 7 days.[2] **Diltiazem** has caused similar increases.[3]

(c) Grapefruit juice

Grapefruit juice caused only a small 25% increase in the AUC of eplerenone 100 mg.[1]

(d) Macrolides

The increase in steady-state AUC of eplerenone 100 mg daily with **erythromycin** 500 mg twice daily was 2.9-fold in 24 healthy subjects.[2] The maker predicts that **clarithromycin**,[1,3] **telithromycin**,[3] and **troleandomycin**[1] will have a greater effect. Eplerenone reduced the AUC of **erythromycin** by 14%, which was not considered clinically relevant.[2]

(e) Protease inhibitors

The increase in steady-state AUC of eplerenone 100 mg daily with **saquinavir** 1.2 g three times daily was 2.1-fold in 24 healthy subjects.[2] The maker predicts that **ritonavir** and **nelfinavir** will have a greater effect.[3] Eplerenone reduced the maximum level of **saquinavir** by 30%, and the AUC by 21%,[2] but the clinical relevance of this has not been assessed.

Mechanism

Eplerenone is metabolised by the cytochrome P450 isoenzyme CYP3A4, and therefore inhibitors of this isoenzyme raise its levels.

Importance and management

These pharmacokinetic interactions are established. Although the clinical relevance has not been assessed, it is known that the risk of hyperkalaemia with eplerenone is related to dose.[3] Consequently, in the UK the makers recommend that the dose of eplerenone should not exceed 25 mg daily in patients on mild to moderate CYP3A4 inhibitors such as **amiodarone**, diltiazem, and verapamil.[3] In the US, the maker recommends that the starting dose for hypertension should be reduced to 25 mg daily.[1] This seems as sensible precaution.

Because the increase in AUC of eplerenone with ketoconazole is so great, the makers contraindicate this combination.[1,3] They also contraindicate concurrent use of other strong inhibitors of CYP3A4, and they list itraconazole, ritonavir, nelfinavir, clarithromycin, nefazodone,[1,3] telithromycin[3] and troleandomycin.[1]

1. Inspra (Eplerenone). Pfizer Inc. US Prescribing information, May 2005.
2. Cook CS, Berry LM, Burton E. Prediction of *in vivo* drug interactions with eplerenone in man from *in vitro* metabolic inhibition data. *Xenobiotica* (2004) 34, 215–28.
3. Inspra (Eplerenone). Pfizer Ltd. UK Summary of product characteristics, October 2004.

Eplerenone + Miscellaneous

Caution is recommended when eplerenone is used with NSAIDs, alpha blockers, tricyclic antidepressants, antipsychotics, amifos-

tine and baclofen. Lithium, ciclosporin, and tacrolimus should generally not be used with eplerenone. Antacids and simvastatin had no effect on eplerenone pharmacokinetics. Eplerenone had no important effect on warfarin or contraceptive steroid pharmacokinetics, but caused a slight increase in digoxin levels.

Clinical evidence, mechanism, importance and management

(a) Antacids

The maker notes that **aluminium/magnesium**-containing antacids had no effect on the pharmacokinetics of eplerenone.[1]

(b) Ciclosporin and tacrolimus

No clinically significant pharmacokinetic interaction was noted with eplerenone was given with ciclosporin.[1,2] Nevertheless, in the UK the makers state that ciclosporin and tacrolimus may impair renal function and increase the risk of hyperkalaemia. Therefore, they recommend that concurrent use of either ciclosporin or tacrolimus with eplerenone should be avoided, or renal function and serum potassium should be closely monitored.[3] See also 'Ciclosporin + Diuretics', p.789 and 'Tacrolimus + Miscellaneous', p.823.

(c) Combined oral contraceptives

Eplerenone 100 mg daily was given to 24 healthy subjects on days 1 to 11 of taking a 28-day cycle of a combined oral contraceptive (**ethinylestradiol/norethisterone** 35 micrograms/1 mg). There was no change in the ethinylestradiol AUC, but a small 17% increase in the **norethisterone** AUC, which is unlikely to be clinically relevant.[2]

(d) Digoxin

The steady state AUC of digoxin 200 micrograms daily increased by 16% when given to healthy subjects with eplerenone 100 mg daily.[2,3] The makers warn that caution may be warranted in patients with digoxin levels near the upper end of the therapeutic range.[3]

(e) Drugs causing postural hypotension

The maker suggests that there is a risk of increased hypotensive effects and/or postural hypotension if eplerenone is used with **alpha blockers** (e.g. prazosin), **tricyclic antidepressants**, **antipsychotics**, **amifostine** and **baclofen**. They suggest increased monitoring.[3]

(f) Lithium

Serum lithium should be monitored frequently if eplerenone is given with lithium,[1,3] although, in the UK, the makers prefer avoidance of the combination.[3] This is because lithium toxicity has occurred with lithium and 'ACE inhibitors', (p.846) or 'diuretics', (p.851).

(g) NSAIDs

Because of the possibility of acute renal failure with NSAIDs, which would cause hyperkalaemia with eplerenone, the maker recommends that patients receiving NSAIDs and eplerenone be adequately hydrated and have their renal function monitored prior to starting treatment.[3]

(h) Simvastatin

Simvastatin 40 mg once daily had no effect on the pharmacokinetics of eplerenone 100 mg once daily in 18 healthy subjects. The maximum level of simvastatin was modestly decreased by 32%, and the AUC by 14%, but this was not considered clinically relevant.[2]

(i) Warfarin

Eplerenone did not alter the pharmacokinetics of warfarin to a clinically significant extent.[1,3] However, in the UK the maker still recommends caution when the warfarin dose is near the upper limit of the therapeutic range.[3]

1. Inspra (Eplerenone). Pfizer Inc. US Prescribing information, May 2005.
2. Cook CS, Berry LM, Burton E. Prediction of *in vivo* drug interactions with eplerenone in man from *in vitro* metabolic inhibition data. *Xenobiotica* (2004) 34, 215–28.
3. Inspra (Eplerenone). Pfizer Ltd. UK Summary of product characteristics, October 2004.

Eplerenone + St John's wort *(Hypericum perforatum)* or other CYP3A4 enzyme inducers

St John's wort slightly decreased the AUC of eplerenone, and the maker of eplerenone recommends avoidance. The maker also recommends the avoidance of other stronger inducers of CYP3A4 such as rifampicin because of the possible risk of decreased eplerenone efficacy.

Clinical evidence, mechanism, importance and management

St John's wort (*Hypericum perforatum*) caused a slight 30% decrease in the AUC of a single 100-mg dose of eplerenone.[1,2] Eplerenone is metabolised by the cytochrome P450 isoenzyme CYP3A4, and therefore inducers of this isoenzyme such as St John's wort would be expected to decrease its levels. In the UK, the maker predicts that a more pronounced decrease in eplerenone AUC might occur with stronger CYP3A4 inducers such as **rifampicin**.[1] Because of the possibility of decreased efficacy, they do not recommend the concurrent use of strong CYP3A4 inducers and eplerenone, and they specifically name **rifampicin**, **carbamazepine**, **phenytoin**, **phenobarbital**, and St John's wort.[1] However, it is unlikely that the decrease seen with St John's wort is clinically relevant. Further study is needed of the other potential interactions.

1. Inspra (Eplerenone). Pfizer Ltd. UK Summary of product characteristics, October 2004.
2. Inspra (Eplerenone). Pfizer Inc. US Prescribing information, May 2005.

Furosemide + Bile-acid binding resins

Colestyramine and colestipol markedly reduce the absorption and diuretic effects of furosemide. Giving the furosemide 2 to 3 hours before either of these other drugs should minimise the effects of this interaction.

Clinical evidence

Colestyramine 8 g reduced the absorption of a single 40-mg dose of furosemide in 6 healthy subjects by 95%. The 4-hour diuretic response was reduced by 77% (urinary output reduced from 1510 to 350 ml). **Colestipol** 10 g reduced the furosemide absorption by 80% and the 4-hour diuretic response by 58% (urinary output reduced from 1510 to 630 ml).[1]

Mechanism

Both colestyramine and colestipol are anionic exchange resins, which can bind furosemide within the gut, thereby by reducing its absorption and its effects.

Importance and management

An established interaction, although direct evidence seems to be limited to this study. The absorption of furosemide is relatively rapid so that giving it 2 to 3 hours before either the colestyramine or colestipol should be an effective way of overcoming this interaction. This needs confirmation. Note that it is normally recommended that other drugs are given 1 hour before or 4 to 6 hours after colestyramine and 1 hour before or 4 hours after colestipol.

1. Neuvonen PJ, Kivistö K, Hirvisalo EL. Effects of resins and activated charcoal on the absorption of digoxin, carbamazepine and frusemide. *Br J Clin Pharmacol* (1988) 25, 229–33.

Furosemide + Cloral hydrate

The intravenous injection of furosemide after treatment with cloral hydrate occasionally causes sweating, hot flushes, a variable blood pressure and tachycardia.

Clinical evidence

Six patients in a coronary care unit given an intravenous bolus of 40 to 120 mg of furosemide and who had received cloral hydrate during the previous 24 hours developed sweating, hot flushes, variable blood pressure, and tachycardia. The reaction was immediate and lasted about 15 minutes. No special treatment was given. Furosemide had caused no problems when given before the cloral hydrate was started.[1]

A retrospective study of hospital records revealed that out of 43 patients who had received both cloral hydrate and furosemide, one patient developed this reaction and 2 others may have done so.[2] The interaction has also been described in an 8-year-old boy.[3]

Mechanism

Not understood. One suggestion is that furosemide displaces trichloroacetic acid (the metabolite of cloral hydrate) from its protein binding sites, which in its turn displaces levothyroxine or alters the serum pH so that the levels of free levothyroxine rise.[1]

Importance and management

An established interaction, but information is limited to 3 reports. The incidence is uncertain but probably low. Concurrent use need not be avoided, but it would be prudent to give intravenous furosemide cautiously if cloral hydrate has been given recently. It seems possible that derivatives of cloral hydrate that break down in the body to release cloral hydrate (e.g. **dichloralphenazone**, **cloral betaine**) might interact similarly. There is no evidence that furosemide given orally or cloral hydrate given to patients already on furosemide initiates this reaction.[2]

1. Malach M, Berman N. Furosemide and chloral hydrate. Adverse drug interaction. *JAMA* (1975) 232, 638–9.
2. Pevonka MP, Yost RL, Marks RG, Howell WS, Stewart RB. Interaction of chloral hydrate and furosemide. A controlled retrospective study. *Drug Intell Clin Pharm* (1977) 11, 332–5.
3. Dean RP, Rudinsky BF, Kelleher MD. Interaction of chloral hydrate and intravenous furosemide in a child. *Clin Pharm* (1991) 10, 385–7.

Furosemide + Epoprostenol

Epoprostenol infusion did not significantly alter the pharmacokinetics of furosemide in a study modelling data from 23 patients with heart failure.[1]

1. Carlton LD, Patterson JH, Mattson CN, Schmith VD. The effects of epoprostenol on drug disposition II: a pilot study of the pharmacokinetics of furosemide with and without epoprostenol in patients with congestive heart failure. *J Clin Pharmacol* (1996) 36, 257–64.

Furosemide + Germanium

An isolated case report describes a man who became resistant to furosemide after he took germanium.

Clinical evidence, mechanism, importance and management

A 63-year-old man was hospitalised for hypertension and oedema 10 days after adding ginseng containing germanium to his usual treatment with cyclophosphamide and furosemide. He weighed almost 13 kg more than his usual weight. After treatment with intravenous furosemide he was discharged and again took ginseng with germanium. This time he gained 12 kg in weight over 14 days, despite an increase in the dose of furosemide from 80 to 240 mg twice daily. The weight gain and oedema again resolved when the ginseng and germanium was withdrawn and he was given intravenous furosemide. The authors suggest that germanium was responsible for this interaction.[1]

Note that it has been said that the use of germanium should be discouraged due to its potential to cause renal toxicity.[2]

1. Becker BN, Greene J, Evanson J, Chidsey J, Stone WJ. Ginseng-induced diuretic resistance. *JAMA* (1996) 276, 606–7.
2. Sweetman SC, editor. Martindale: The complete drug reference. 34th ed. London: Pharmaceutical Press; 2005 p. 1692.

Furosemide + Paracetamol

Paracetamol 1 g four times daily for 2 days was found to have no effect on the diuresis or natriuresis of intravenous furosemide 20 mg in 10 healthy women.[1]

1. Martin U, Prescott LF. The interaction of paracetamol with frusemide. *Br J Clin Pharmacol* (1994) 37, 464–7.

Furosemide + Phenytoin

The diuretic effects of furosemide can be reduced as much as 50% if phenytoin is also given.

Clinical evidence

The observation that dependent oedema in a group of epileptics was higher than expected, and the response to diuretic treatment seemed to be reduced, prompted further study. In 30 patients taking **phenytoin** 200 to 400 mg daily with phenobarbital 60 to 180 mg daily the maximal diuresis in response to furosemide 20 or 40 mg occurred after 3 to 4 hours instead of the usual 2 hours, and the total diuresis was reduced by 32 and 49% respectively. When intravenous furosemide 20 mg was given the total diuresis was reduced by 50%. Some of the patients were also taking carbamazepine, pheneturide, ethosuximide, diazepam or chlordiazepoxide.[1]

Another study in 5 healthy subjects given **phenytoin** 100 mg three times daily for 10 days found that the maximum serum levels of furosemide 20 mg, given orally or intravenously, were reduced by 50%.[2]

Mechanism

Not fully understood. One suggestion is that the phenytoin causes changes in the jejunal Na^+ pump activity, which reduces the absorption of the furosemide,[2] but this is not the whole story because an interaction also occurs when furosemide is given intravenously.[1] Another suggestion, based on *in vitro* evidence is that the phenytoin generates a 'liquid membrane,' which blocks the transport of the furosemide to its active site.[3]

Importance and management

Information is limited but the interaction is established. A reduced diuretic response should be expected in the presence of phenytoin. A dosage increase may be needed.

1. Ahmad S. Renal insensitivity to frusemide caused by chronic anticonvulsant therapy. *BMJ* (1974) 3, 657–9.
2. Fine A, Henderson JS, Morgan DR, Tilstone WJ. Malabsorption of frusemide caused by phenytoin. *BMJ* (1977) 2, 1061–2.
3. Srivastava RC, Bhise SB, Sood R, Rao MNA. On the reduced furosemide response in the presence of diphenylhydantoin. *Colloids and Surfaces* (1986) 19, 83–8.

Loop diuretics + Food

Some studies suggest that food modestly reduces the bioavailability and diuretic effects of furosemide. However, other studies have found that the bioavailability of furosemide and bumetanide is not affected by food.

Clinical evidence

Ten healthy subjects were given **furosemide** 40 mg with and without a standard breakfast. The food reduced the peak plasma levels of **furosemide** by 55% and the bioavailability by about 30%.[1] The results were almost identical when 5 of the subjects were given a heavy meal.[1] The diuresis over 10 hours was reduced by 21% (from 2072 to 1640 ml) and over 24 hours by 15% (from 2668 to 2270 ml) by **furosemide** taken with breakfast.[1] A comparative study in 9 and 8 healthy subjects found that the absorption of both **bumetanide** 2 mg (9 healthy subjects) and **furosemide** 40 mg (8), given as solutions, were delayed and peak plasma levels were reduced by a standard breakfast.[2] However, although food reduced the oral bioavailability of **furosemide** by about one-third, from 76% to 43%, the bioavailability of **bumetanide** was not significantly reduced (75% with food and 84% fasting). Food did not significantly alter the bioavailability of **furosemide** in two other studies.[3,4]

Mechanism

Not understood.

Importance and management

Information is limited, and contradictory. Of the four studies, only two found that the bioavailability of furosemide was reduced by food. Of the two studies that found altered bioavailability, only one assessed diuresis, and only a small change in diuretic effect was seen. The authors of this study say that furosemide should not be given with food, but this is not standard clinical practice. Food does not affect the bioavailability of bumetanide given as solution. On balance it would therefore seem that furosemide and bumetanide can be given without regard to meal times.

1. Beermann B, Midskov C. Reduced bioavailability and effect of furosemide given with food. *Eur J Clin Pharmacol* (1986) 29, 725–7.
2. McCrindle JL, Li Kam Wa TC, Barron W, Prescott LF. Effect of food on the absorption of frusemide and bumetanide in man. *Br J Clin Pharmacol* (1996) 42, 743–6.
3. Hammarlund MM, Paalzow LK, Odlind B. Pharmacokinetics of furosemide in man after intravenous and oral administration. Application of moment analysis. *Eur J Clin Pharmacol* (1984) 26, 197–207.
4. Kelly MR, Cutler RE, Forrey AW, Kimpel BM. Pharmacokinetics of orally administered furosemide. *Clin Pharmacol Ther* (1974) 15, 178–86.

Loop diuretics + H_2-blockers

Ranitidine and cimetidine may cause a moderate increase in the bioavailability of furosemide. Torasemide and cimetidine appear not to interact.

Clinical evidence, mechanism, importance and management

(a) Furosemide

In a study in 6 healthy subjects, a single 400-mg dose of **cimetidine** increased the mean AUC of furosemide by a third, although there was wide inter-patient variation. However, there were no changes in the diuretic effects of furosemide, or in the pharmacokinetics of cimetidine, and an associated study using multiple doses of **cimetidine** over 5 days found no pharmacokinetic or pharmacodynamic interaction.[1] A similar study in patients with hepatic cirrhosis also found that **cimetidine** does not interact with furosemide.[2]

Eighteen healthy subjects were given oral furosemide 40 mg one hour after intravenous **ranitidine** 50 mg or saline. The **ranitidine** increased the AUC of furosemide by 28% and the maximum serum levels by 37%.[3] The effects of furosemide could possibly be slightly increased by **ranitidine**, but the clinical importance of this is probably small. No special precautions seem necessary.

(b) Torasemide

Cimetidine 300 mg four times daily for 3 days was found to have no effect on the pharmacokinetics of a single 10-mg oral dose of torasemide in 11 healthy subjects, nor were there any changes in the volume of urine or the excretion of sodium, potassium or chloride.[4]

1. Rogers HJ, Morrison P, House FR, Bradbrook ID. Effect of cimetidine on the absorption and efficacy of orally administered furosemide. *Int J Clin Pharmacol Ther Toxicol* (1982) 20, 8–11.
2. Sanchis Closa A, Lambert C, du Souich P. Lack of effect of cimetidine on furosemide kinetics and dynamics in patients with hepatic cirrhosis. *Int J Clin Pharmacol Ther Toxicol* (1993) 31, 461–6.
3. Müller FO, De Vaal AC, Hundt KL, Luus HG. Intravenous ranitidine enhances furosemide bioavailability. *Klin Pharmakol Akt* (1993) 4, 26.
4. Kramer WG. Lack of effect of cimetidine on torasemide pharmacokinetics and pharmacodynamics in healthy subjects. 4th Int Congr Diuretics, Boca Raton, Florida Oct 11–16th 1992. Eds. Puschett JB, Greenberrg A. *Int Congr Ser 1023* (1993), 361–4.

Loop diuretics + NSAIDs

The antihypertensive and diuretic effects of loop diuretics appear to be reduced by NSAIDs, although the extent of this interaction largely depends on individual NSAIDs. See 'Table 24.2', (p.722) for a summary of the known interactions of loop, potassium-sparing and thiazide diuretics with NSAIDs. Note that diuretics increase the risk of NSAID-induced acute renal failure.

Clinical evidence

A. Bumetanide

(a) Indometacin

In two studies a single 100-mg dose of indometacin was found to reduce the bumetanide-induced output of urine, Na^+ and Cl^- (but not K^+) by about 25%.[1-3] Diuresis was reduced by 42% and weight gain was noted.[1] There are other reports confirming this interaction between bumetanide and indometacin, including a clinical study,[4] and a report of a patient who developed cardiac failure as a result of this interaction.[5]

(b) Sulindac

A study in 8 healthy subjects showed that a single 300-mg dose of sulindac did not significantly reduce the diuretic response (measured by urinary volume, sodium, potassium and chloride) to a single 1-mg dose of bumetanide.[6] However, another study in healthy subjects found that pre-treatment with sulindac 200 mg twice daily for 5 days reduced the diuretic effect of a single 1-mg dose of bumetanide (mean urine flow rate after 2 hours reduced by 21% and cumulative sodium excretion at 3 hours reduced by 22%).[7]

(c) Tolfenamic acid

A study in 8 healthy subjects found that tolfenamic acid 300 mg reduced the diuretic response (measured by urinary volume, sodium, potassium and chloride) to a single 1-mg dose of bumetanide by 34% at 2 hours.[6]

B. Furosemide

(a) Azapropazone

Ten healthy subjects had no change in their urinary excretion caused by furosemide 40 mg daily when they were also given azapropazone 600 mg twice daily. The furosemide did not antagonise the uricosuric effects of the azapropazone.[8]

(b) Diclofenac

A study in patients with heart failure and cirrhosis found that diclofenac 150 mg daily reduced the furosemide-induced excretion of sodium by 38%, but the excretion of potassium was unaltered.[9]

(c) Diflunisal

A study in 12 healthy subjects found that diflunisal 500 mg twice daily interacted with furosemide to reduce sodium excretion by 59%, but potassium excretion remained unchanged.[10]

In patients with heart failure and cirrhosis treated with furosemide, diflunisal 500 to 700 mg daily decreased the sodium excretion by 36% and the potassium excretion by 47%.[9] However, another study found no interaction.[11]

(d) Flupirtine

A study in healthy subjects found that a single 200-mg dose of flupirtine did not affect the overall furosemide diuresis, but the diuretic effect was slightly delayed.[12]

(e) Flurbiprofen

A study in 7 healthy subjects found that the increase in renal osmolal clearance of a standard water load, in response to furosemide 40 mg orally or 20 mg intravenously, fell from 105 to 19% and from 140 to 70% respectively after flurbiprofen 100 mg was given.[13]

A single-dose study in 10 healthy subjects found that flurbiprofen 100 mg reduced the urinary volume, urinary sodium and urinary potassium, in response to oral furosemide 80 mg was reduced by 10%, 9%, and 12% respectively.[14,15]

(f) Ibuprofen

An elderly man with cardiac failure taking digoxin, isosorbide dinitrate and furosemide 80 mg daily, developed symptomatic congestive heart failure with ascites when given ibuprofen 400 mg three times daily. His serum urea and creatinine levels rose and no diuresis occurred even when the furosemide dosage was doubled. Two days after withdrawing the ibuprofen, brisk diuresis took place, renal function returned to normal and his condition improved steadily.[16] Another elderly patient similarly had a poor response to furosemide (and later to metolazone as well) until ibuprofen 600 mg four times daily and at least two **aspirin** daily (for headache) were stopped.[17] This was due to hyponatraemic hypovolaemia brought on by the drug combination.

(g) Indometacin

A study in 4 healthy subjects and 6 patients with essential hypertension found that furosemide 80 mg three times daily reduced the mean blood pressure by 13 mmHg, but when indometacin 50 mg four times daily was also given the blood pressures returned to virtually pretreatment levels. Moreover the normal urinary sodium loss induced by the furosemide was significantly reduced.[18]

A study in healthy subjects and patients with congestive heart failure given furosemide found that indometacin 100 mg reduced the urinary output by 53% and also reduced the excretion of Na^+, K^+ and Cl^- by 64%, 49% and 62% respectively.[19] Another study found that indometacin reduced the urinary output in response to furosemide by 20 to 30%.[20] There are other case reports confirming the interaction between furosemide and indometacin.[21-25]

Table 24.2 Interactions of diuretics and NSAIDs

	Bumetanide	*Furosemide*	*Piretanide*	*Torasemide*	*Bemetizide*	*Bendroflume-thiazide*	*Hydrochloro-thiazide*	*Hydrochloro-thiazide + amiloride*	*Hydrochloro-thiazide + triamterene*	*Metolazone*	*Spironolactone*	*Triamterene*
Azapropazone		N/S										
Diclofenac		Excretion of Na+ ↓ 38%					N/S Weight gain	N/S				ARF
Diflunisal		Excretion of Na+ ↓ 59%					N/S					
Flupirtine		Delayed diuresis										
Flurbiprofen		Urinary volume ↓ 10%										
Ibuprofen		CCF				N/S Weight gain	↑ BP					
Indometacin	Excretion of Na+ ↓ 25%	Mean BP ↑ by 13 mmHg; Urinary output ↓ 53%; Na ↓ 64%	Excretion of Na+ ↓ 35%	Possibly as furosemide	Excretion of Na+ ↓ 47%	↑ BP by 13/9 mmHg; Weight gain	↑ BP by 6/3 mmHg	↑ BP by 13/9 mmHg		Excretion of Na+ ↓		ARF
Kebuzone							↑ SBP by 18 mmHg					
Ketoprofen		24-h Urinary output ↓ 651 ml										
Ketorolac		Diuretic effect ↓ 20%										
Lornoxicam		Diuretic effect ↓										
Meloxicam		N/S										
Mofebutazone		N/S										
Naproxen		Urinary volume ↓ 50%					↑ BP					
Phenylbutazone							↑ SBP by 18 mmHg					
Piroxicam		Diuretic effect ↓	N/S				↑ BP					
Sulindac	Na+ ↓ 22%; urine flow rate ↓ 21%	Diuretic effect ↓ 76%				Enhanced hypotensive effects	N/S	N/S		Excretion of Na+ ↓ 19%		
Tenoxicam		N/S										
Tolfenamic acid	Diuretic effect ↓ 34%											

(h) Ketoprofen

A study in 12 healthy subjects given furosemide 40 mg daily found that ketoprofen 100 mg twice daily reduced the 6-hour urine output by 67 ml, and the 24-hour output by 651 ml on the first day of treatment. However no significant differences were seen after 5 days treatment.[26]

(i) Ketorolac

Twelve healthy subjects were given oral ketorolac 30 mg four times daily, and then a single 30-mg intramuscular dose 30 minutes before a 40-mg intravenous dose of furosemide. No precise figures are given, but the maximum serum level of the furosemide, its diuretic effect and the electrolyte loss were said to be significantly reduced by the ketorolac.[27] The makers of ketorolac say that it reduces the diuretic response to furosemide by about 20%.[28] Another study in healthy elderly people found furosemide 40 mg given after they were given oral ketorolac 120 mg the day before and intramuscular ketorolac 30 mg 30 minutes before, the urinary output fell by 16% and the sodium output fell by 26% over the next 8 hours.[29]

(j) Lornoxicam

A study in 12 healthy subjects found that lornoxicam 4 mg significantly antagonised the diuretic and natriuretic effects of furosemide, but this was not quantified.[30]

(k) Meloxicam

Meloxicam 15 mg daily for 3 days had no significant effect on the pharmacokinetics of furosemide 40 mg in 12 healthy subjects. The furosemide-induced diuresis was unchanged while the cumulative urinary electrolyte excretion was somewhat lower, but this was considered to be clinically irrelevant.[31] A similar study in patients with heart failure, taking an ACE inhibitor, also found no clinically significant pharmacokinetic or pharmacodynamic interaction between furosemide and meloxicam.[32]

(l) Metamizole sodium (Dipyrone)

A study in 9 healthy subjects found that metamizole sodium 3 g daily for 3 days, reduced the clearance of intravenous furosemide 20 mg from 175 to 141 ml/minute but the diuretic effects of the furosemide were unchanged.[33]

(m) Mofebutazone

A study in 10 healthy subjects found that mofebutazone 600 mg had no effect on the diuretic effects of furosemide 40 mg. The urinary volume and excretion of sodium, potassium and chloride were unchanged.[34]

(n) Naproxen

Two elderly women with congestive heart failure did not respond to treatment with furosemide and digoxin until the naproxen they were taking was withdrawn.[16]

A single-dose study in patients with cardiac failure found that the volume of urine excreted in response to furosemide was reduced about 50% by naproxen.[20]

(o) Nimesulide

A study in 8 healthy subjects found that nimesulide 200 mg twice daily attenuated the effects of furosemide 40 mg twice daily. Subjects who had initially lost weight on furosemide regained weight, diuresis was slightly reduced and glomerular filtration rate was reduced.[35]

(p) Piroxicam

A 96-year-old woman with congestive heart failure did not adequately respond to furosemide until the dosage of piroxicam she was taking was reduced from 20 to 10 mg daily.[36]

(q) Sulindac

A study in 5 healthy subjects found that pre-treatment with two 150-mg doses of sulindac reduced the urinary volume and urinary sodium following an intravenous furosemide 80 mg by 25% and 37.5% respectively. In patients with cirrhosis and ascites, sulindac 150 mg reduced the urinary volume, urinary sodium, and urinary potassium following intravenous furosemide 80 mg by 38%, 52% and 8% respectively.[37]

(r) Tenoxicam

A study in 12 patients found that tenoxicam 20 to 40 mg daily had no significant effect on the urinary excretion of sodium or chloride due to furosemide 40 mg daily, and blood pressure, heart rate and body-weight also were not affected.[38]

C. Piretanide

(a) Indometacin

A comparative study[39] into the pharmacological mechanisms underlying the way drugs interfere with the actions of loop diuretics found that indometacin 50 mg three times daily for 2 days reduced the peak fractional excretion of sodium due to a single 6-mg dose of piretanide. The clinical importance of this change was not studied.

(b) Piroxicam

A comparative study into the pharmacological mechanisms underlying the way drugs interfere with the actions of loop diuretics found that piroxicam 20 mg twice daily for 2 days did not significantly affect the peak fractional excretion of sodium due to a single 6-mg dose of piretanide.[39]

D. Torasemide

(a) Indometacin

A study in healthy subjects suggested that indometacin did not affect the natriuretic effects of torasemide,[40] but on the basis of later work the same workers suggest that pathological factors in patients may allow an interaction similar to that with furosemide and indometacin to occur.[41]

Mechanism

Uncertain and complex. It seems almost certain that a number of different mechanisms come into play. One probable mechanism is concerned with the synthesis of renal prostaglandins which occurs when the loop diuretics cause sodium excretion. If this synthesis is blocked by drugs such as the NSAIDs, then renal blood flow and diuresis will be altered.[42]

Importance and management

NSAIDs can cause renal impairment, particularly in patients in whom prostaglandins are playing an important role in maintaining renal function. Such patients include those on diuretics. Hence the combination of diuretics and NSAIDs may increase the nephrotoxicity of NSAIDs.[25,43-45]

The antihypertensive and diuretic effects of the loop diuretics are reduced by NSAIDs. This interaction is very well documented between furosemide and indometacin and of clinical importance, whereas far less is known about the interactions with other NSAIDs. Concurrent use often need not be avoided but the effects should be checked and the furosemide dosage raised as necessary. Patients at greatest risk are likely to be the elderly with cirrhosis, cardiac failure and/or renal insufficiency. Some of the data comes from studies in healthy subjects rather than patients so that the total picture is still far from clear. Diclofenac, diflunisal, flurbiprofen, ketoprofen, ketorolac, naproxen, piroxicam and tolfenamic acid are known to interact in some individuals, but not necessarily to the same extent as indometacin. If raising the diuretic dosage is ineffective, another NSAID such as azapropazone, flupirtine, ibuprofen, metamizole sodium (dipyrone), meloxicam, sulindac or tenoxicam may not interact significantly (this is not necessarily true for patients with cirrhosis and ascites[37] or the elderly and those with coronary artery disease.[43]). Not every NSAID seems to have been investigated but be alert for this interaction with any of them. Phenylbutazone and oxyphenbutazone would be expected to interact because they cause marked sodium retention and oedema.

Much less is known about bumetanide, and even less about piretanide and torasemide, but the evidence suggests that they probably interact like furosemide with indometacin. It would therefore seem prudent to be alert for interactions with any of the NSAIDs with which furosemide interacts.

1. Aggernæs KH. Indometacinhæmning af bumetaniddiurese. *Ugeskr Laeger* (1980) 142, 691–3.
2. Brater C, Chennavasin P. Indomethacin and the response to bumetanide. *Clin Pharmacol Ther* (1980) 27, 421–5.
3. Brater DC, Fox WR, Chennavasin P. Interaction studies with bumetanide and furosemide. Effects of probenecid and of indomethacin on response to bumetanide in man. *J Clin Pharmacol* (1981) 21, 647–53.
4. Kaufman J, Hamburger R, Matheson J, Flamenbaum W. Bumetanide-induced diuresis and natriuresis: effect of prostaglandin synthetase inhibition. *J Clin Pharmacol* (1981) 21, 663–7.
5. Ahmad S. Indomethacin-bumetanide interaction: an alert. *Am J Cardiol* (1984) 54, 246–7.
6. Pentikäinen PJ, Tokola O, Vapaatalo H. Non-steroidal anti-inflammatory drugs and bumetanide response in man. Comparison of tolfenamic acid and sulindac. *Clin Pharmacol Ther* (1986) 39, 219.
7. Skinner MH, Mutterperl R, Zeitz HJ. Sulindac inhibits bumetanide-induced sodium and water excretion. *Clin Pharmacol Ther* (1987) 42, 542–6.
8. Williamson PJ, Ene MD, Roberts CJC. A study of the potential interactions between azapropazone and frusemide in man. *Br J Clin Pharmacol* (1984) 18, 619–23.
9. Jean G, Meregalli G, Vasilocò M, Silvani A, Scapaticci R, Della Ventura GF, Baiocchi C, Thiella G. Interazioni tra terapia diuretica e farmaci antiinfiammatori non steroidei. *Clin Ter* (1983) 105, 471–5.
10. Favre L, Glasson PH, Riondel A, Vallotton MB. Interaction of diuretics and non-steroidal anti-inflammatory drugs in man. *Clin Sci* (1983) 64, 407–15.
11. Tobert JA, Ostaszewski T, Reger B, Mesinger MAP, Cook TJ. Diflunisal-furosemide interaction. *Clin Pharmacol Ther* (1980) 27, 289–90.
12. Johnston A, Warrington SJ, Turner P, Riethmuller-Winzen H. Comparison of flupirtine and indomethacin on frusemide-induced diuresis. *Postgrad Med J* (1987) 63, 959–61.
13. Rawles JM. Antagonism between non-steroidal anti-inflammatory drugs and diuretics. *Scott Med J* (1982) 27, 37–40.
14. Symmons D, Kendall MJ. Non-steroidal anti-inflammatory drugs and frusemide-induced diuresis. *BMJ* (1981) 283, 988–9.
15. Symmons DPM, Kendall MJ, Rees JA, Hind ID. The effect of flurbiprofen on the responses to frusemide in healthy volunteers. *Int J Clin Pharmacol Ther Toxicol* (1983) 21, 350–4.
16. Laiwah ACY, Mactier RA. Antagonistic effect of non-steroidal anti-inflammatory drugs on frusemide-induced diuresis in cardiac failure. *BMJ* (1981) 283, 714.
17. Goodenough GK, Lutz LJ. Hyponatremic hypervolemia caused by a drug-drug interaction mistaken for syndrome of inappropriate ADH. *J Am Geriatr Soc* (1988) 36, 285–6.
18. Patak RV, Mookerjee BK, Bentzel CJ, Hysert PE, Babej M, Lee JB. Antagonism of the effects of furosemide by indomethacin in normal and hypertensive man. *Prostaglandins* (1975) 10, 649–59.
19. Sörgel F, Koob R, Gluth WP, Krüger B, Lang E. The interaction of indomethacin and furosemide in patients with congestive heart failure. *Clin Pharmacol Ther* (1985) 37, 231.
20. Faunch R. Non-steroidal anti-inflammatory drugs and frusemide-induced diuresis. *BMJ* (1981) 283, 989.
21. Allan SG, Knox J, Kerr F. Interaction between diuretics and indomethacin. *BMJ* (1981) 283, 1611.
22. Poe TE, Scott RB, Keith JF. Interaction of indomethacin with furosemide. *J Fam Pract* (1983) 16, 610–16.
23. Ritland S. Alvorlig interaksjon mellom indometacin og furosemid. *Tidsskr Nor Laegeforen* (1983) 103, 2003.
24. Nordrehaug JE. Alvorlig interaksjon mellom indometacin og furosemid. *Tidsskr Nor Laegeforen* (1983) 103, 1680–1.
25. Thomas MC. Diuretics, ACE inhibitors and NSAIDs—the triple whammy. *Med J Aust* (2000) 172, 184–5.
26. Li Kam Wa TC, Lawson M, Jackson SHD, Hitoglou-Makedou A, Turner P. Interaction of ketoprofen and frusemide in man. *Postgrad Med J* (1991) 67, 655–8.
27. Shah J, Bullingham R, Jonkman J, Curd J, Taylor R, Fratis A. PK-PD interaction of ketorolac and furosemide in healthy volunteers in a normovolemic state. *Clin Pharmacol Ther* (1994) 55, 198.
28. Toradol (Ketorolac trometamol). Roche Products Ltd. UK Summary of product characteristics, October 2002.
29. Jones RW, Notarianni LJ, Parker G. The effect of ketorolac tromethamine on the diuretic response of frusemide in healthy elderly people. *Therapie* (1995) 50 (Suppl), Abstract 98.
30. Ravic M, Johnston A, Turner P. Clinical pharmacological studies of some possible interactions of lornoxicam with other drugs. *Postgrad Med J* (1990) 66 (Suppl 4), S30–S34.
31. Müller FO, Schall R, de Vaal AC, Groenewoud G, Hundt HKL, Middle MV. Influence of meloxicam on furosemide pharmacokinetics and pharmacodynamics in healthy volunteers. *Eur J Clin Pharmacol* (1995) 48, 247–51.
32. Müller FO, Middle MV, Schall R, Terblanché J, Hundt HKL Groenewoud G. An evaluation of the interaction of meloxicam with furosemide in patients with compensated chronic cardiac failure. *Br J Clin Pharmacol* (1997) 44, 393–8.
33. Rosenkranz B, Lehr K-H, Mackert G, Seyberth HW. Metamizole-furosemide interaction study in healthy volunteers. *Eur J Clin Pharmacol* (1992) 42, 593–8.
34. Matthei U, Grabensee B, Loew D. The interaction of mofebutazone with furosemide. *Curr Med Res Opin* (1987) 10, 638–44.

35. Steinhäuslin F, Munafo A, Buclin T, Macciocchi A. Renal effects of nimesulide in furosemide-treated subjects. *Drugs* (1993) 46 (Suppl 1), 257–62.
36. Baker DE. Piroxicam-furosemide drug interaction. *Drug Intell Clin Pharm* (1988) 22, 505–6.
37. Daskalopuolos G, Kronberg I, Katkov W, Gonzalez M, Laffi G, Zipser RD. Sulindac and indomethacin suppress the diuretic action of furosemide in patients with cirrhosis and ascites: evidence that sulindac affects renal prostaglandins. *Am J Kidney Dis* (1985) 6, 217–21.
38. Hartmann D, Kleinbloesem CH, Lücker PW, Vetter G. Study on the possible interaction between tenoxicam and furosemide. *Arzneimittelforschung* (1987) 37, 1072–6.
39. Dixey JJ, Noormohamed FH, Pawa JS, Lant AF, Brewerton DA. The influence of nonsteroidal anti-inflammatory drugs and probenecid on the renal response to and kinetics of piretanide in man. *Clin Pharmacol Ther* (1988) 44, 531–9.
40. van Ganse E, Douchamps J, Deger F, Staroukine M, Verniory A, Herchuelz A. Failure of indomethacin to impair the diuretic and natriuretic effects of the loop diuretic torasemide in healthy volunteers. *Eur J Clin Pharmacol* (1986) 31 (Suppl), 43–7.
41. Herchuelz A, Derenne F, Deger F, Juvent M, van Ganse E, Staroutkine M, Verniory A, Boeynaems JM, Douchamps J. Interaction between nonsteroidal anti-inflammatory drugs and loop diuretics: modulation by sodium balance. *J Pharmacol Exp Ther* (1989) 248, 1175–81.
42. Passmore AP, Copeland CS, Johnston GD. The effects of ibuprofen and indomethacin on renal function in the presence and absence of frusemide in healthy volunteers on a restricted sodium diet. *Br J Clin Pharmacol* (1990) 29, 311–19.
43. Murray MD, Brater DC, Tierney WM, Hui SL, McDonald CJ. Ibuprofen-associated renal impairment in a large general internal medicine practice. *Am J Med Sci* (1990) 299, 222–9.
44. Blackshear JL, Davidman M, Stillman MT. Identification of risk for renal insufficiency from nonsteroidal anti-inflammatory drugs. *Arch Intern Med* (1983) 143, 1130–4.
45. Menkes CJ. Renal and hepatic effects of NSAIDs in the elderly. *Scand J Rheumatol* (1989) 83 (Suppl), 11–13.

Loop diuretics + Probenecid

Probenecid decreases the renal clearance of furosemide, but it appears not to alter its overall diuretic effect. Probenecid reduces the natriuretic effects of piretanide, but the clinical relevance of this is not known. Probenecid does not appear to significantly affect bumetanide diuresis.

Clinical evidence, mechanism, importance and management

(a) Bumetanide

Probenecid 1 g did not affect the response of 8 healthy subjects to 500 micrograms or 1 mg of intravenous bumetanide.[1] Another study reported a fall in natriuresis and in the clearance of bumetanide, but this was of minimal clinical importance.[2]

(b) Furosemide

The concurrent use of furosemide and probenecid has been closely studied to sort out renal pharmacological mechanisms of loop diuretics. One study in patients given furosemide 40 mg daily found that the addition of probenecid 500 mg twice daily for 3 days reduced their urinary excretion of sodium by about 36% (from 56.3 to 35.9 mmol daily).[3] Other studies have also found some changes in overall diuresis (a fall in some studies,[4] a rise in others,[5] and no change in others[6,7]), and a reduction of 35 to 80% in the renal clearance of furosemide.[4,6-9] One study found that probenecid 1 g increased the half-life of furosemide by 70% and decreased its oral clearance by 65%.[8] Similar results were found in another study.[10] The clinical importance of these changes is uncertain, but probably small.

(c) Piretanide

A comparative study[11] into the pharmacological mechanisms underlying the way drugs interfere with the actions of loop diuretics found that probenecid 1 g reduced the peak fractional excretion of sodium produced by a 6-mg dose of oral piretanide by 65%. Another study confirmed that probenecid reduces the natriuretic effects of piretanide.[12] The clinical importance of these changes was not studied.

1. Brater DC, Chennavasin P. Effect of probenecid on response to bumetanide in man. *J Clin Pharmacol* (1981) 21, 311–15.
2. Lant AF. Effects of bumetanide on cation and anion transport. *Postgrad Med J* (1975) 51 (Suppl 6), 35–42.
3. Hsieh Y-Y, Hsieh B-S, Lien W-P, Wu T-L. Probenecid interferes with the natriuretic action of furosemide. *J Cardiovasc Pharmacol* (1987) 10, 530–4.
4. Honari J, Blair AD, Cutler RE. Effects of probenecid on furosemide kinetics and natriuresis in man. *Clin Pharmacol Ther* (1977) 22, 395–401.
5. Brater DC. Effects of probenecid on furosemide response. *Clin Pharmacol Ther* (1978) 24, 548–54.
6. Homeida M, Roberts C, Branch RA. Influence of probenecid and spironolactone on furosemide kinetics and dynamics in man. *Clin Pharmacol Ther* (1977) 22, 402–9.
7. Smith DE, Gee WL, Brater DC, Lin ET, Benet LZ. Preliminary evaluation of furosemide-probenecid interaction in humans. *J Pharm Sci* (1980) 69, 571–5.
8. Vree TB, van den Biggelaar-Martea M, Verwey-van Wissen CPWGM. Probenecid inhibits the renal clearance of frusemide and its acyl glucuronide. *Br J Clin Pharmacol* (1995) 39, 692–5.
9. Sommers DK, Meyer EC, Moncrieff J. The influence of co-administered organic acids on the kinetics and dynamics of frusemide. *Br J Clin Pharmacol* (1991) 32, 489–93.
10. Chennavasin P, Seiwell R, Brater DC, Liang WMM. Pharmacodynamic analysis of the furosemide-probenecid interaction in man. *Kidney Int* (1979) 16, 187–95.
11. Dixey JJ, Noormohamed FH, Pawa JS, Lant AF, Brewerton DA. The influence of nonsteroidal anti-inflammatory drugs and probenecid on the renal response to and kinetics of piretanide in man. *Clin Pharmacol Ther* (1988) 44, 531–9.
12. Noormohamed FH, Lant AF. Analysis of the natriuretic action of a loop diuretic, piretanide, in man. *Br J Clin Pharmacol* (1991) 31, 463–9.

Potassium-sparing diuretics + H_2-blockers

Although minor interactions occasionally occur between diuretics and the H_2-blockers, none of these have been shown to be of clinical significance. The combinations that have been studied are; amiloride or triamterene with cimetidine, and triamterene with ranitidine. **See also 'Loop diuretics + H_2-blockers', p.721.**

Clinical evidence, mechanism, importance and management

(a) Amiloride

A study in 8 healthy subjects given amiloride 5 mg daily found that **cimetidine** 400 mg twice daily for 12 days reduced the renal clearance of amiloride by 17% and reduced the urinary excretion of amiloride from 65 to 53%. Amiloride also reduced the excretion of **cimetidine** from 43 to 32%, and the AUC was reduced by 14%.[1] No changes in the diuretic effects (urinary volume, Na^+ or K^+ excretion) occurred. It seems that each drug reduces the gastrointestinal absorption of the other drug by as yet unidentified mechanisms. The overall plasma levels of the amiloride remain unchanged, because the reduced absorption is offset by a reduction in its renal excretion. These mutual interactions do not seem to be clinically significant.

(b) Triamterene

A study in 6 healthy subjects given triamterene 100 mg daily for 4 days found that **cimetidine** 400 mg twice daily increased the triamterene AUC by 22%, reduced its metabolism (hydroxylation) by 32%, and reduced its renal clearance by 28%. There also appeared to be a reduction in the absorption of triamterene. However, the loss of sodium in the urine was not significantly changed, and the potassium-sparing effects of triamterene were not altered.[2] Because the diuretic effects of triamterene are minimally changed this interaction is unlikely to be clinically important.[2]

Ranitidine 150 mg twice daily for 4 days roughly halved the absorption (as measured by renal clearance) of triamterene 100 mg daily in 8 healthy subjects. Its metabolism was also reduced, the total effect being a 21% reduction in the AUC. As a result of the reduced plasma triamterene levels the urinary sodium loss was reduced to some extent but potassium excretion remained unchanged.[3] Overall the diuretic effects of triamterene were only mildly affected. As another study has found that a 22% reduction in the AUC of triamterene is unlikely to result in a significant change in its diuretic effects,[2] no clinically significant interaction is anticipated.

1. Somogyi AA, Hovens CM, Muirhead MR, Bochner F. Renal tubular secretion of amiloride and its inhibition by cimetidine in humans and in an animal model. *Drug Metab Dispos* (1989) 17, 190–6.
2. Muirhead MR, Somogyi AA, Rolan PE, Bochner F. Effect of cimetidine on renal and hepatic drugs elimination: studies with triamterene. *Clin Pharmacol Ther* (1986) 40, 400–7.
3. Muirhead M, Bochner F, Somogyi A. Pharmacokinetic drug interactions between triamterene and ranitidine in humans: alterations in renal and hepatic clearances and gastrointestinal absorption. *J Pharmacol Exp Ther* (1988) 244, 734–9.

Potassium-sparing diuretics + NSAIDs

The concurrent use of triamterene and indometacin may rapidly lead to acute renal failure. An isolated case of renal impairment with diclofenac has been reported in a patient taking triamterene.

Clinical evidence

(a) Spironolactone + Indometacin

A study in healthy subjects found that indometacin 150 mg daily reduced the natriuretic effect of spironolactone 300 mg daily by 54%.[1]

(b) Triamterene + Diclofenac

A patient receiving triamterene 100 mg plus trichlormethiazide 2 mg daily was given intramuscular diclofenac 75 mg before admission to hospital with breast pain. On admission serum creatinine was 91 micromol/l and after 2 days had increased to 248 micromol/l. It returned to normal over 2 weeks. Subsequent oral diclofenac produced no adverse effects. The observed deterioration in renal function was attributed to an interaction between triamterene and diclofenac.[2]

(c) Triamterene + Diflunisal

One report found that diflunisal had no effects on the pharmacokinetics of triamterene in healthy subjects, but the plasma AUC of an active metabolite, *p*-hydroxytriamterene was increased by more than fourfold.[3]

(d) Triamterene + Indometacin

A study in 4 healthy subjects found that indometacin 150 mg daily given with triamterene 200 mg daily over a 3-day period reduced the creatinine clearance in 2 subjects by 62 and 72% respectively. Renal function returned to normal after a month. Indometacin alone caused an average 10% fall in creatinine clearance, but triamterene alone caused no consistent change in renal function. No adverse reactions were seen in 18 other subjects treated in the same way with indometacin and furosemide, hydrochlorothiazide or spironolactone.[4,5] Five patients are reported to have rapidly developed acute renal failure after receiving indometacin and triamterene either concurrently or sequentially.[6-9]

Mechanism

Uncertain. One suggestion is that triamterene causes renal ischaemia for which the kidney compensates by increasing prostaglandin (PGE_2) production, thereby preserving renal blood flow. Indometacin opposes this by inhibiting prostaglandin synthesis, so that the damaging effects of triamterene on the kidney continue unchecked. Increases in pharmacologically active metabolites of triamterene due to competition for renal excretory pathways may occur but the clinical significance is uncertain.

As prostaglandins may contribute to the natriuretic effects of spironolactone, the NSAIDs may exert their effects by blocking prostaglandin synthesis. See also 'Loop diuretics + NSAIDs', p.721.

Importance and management

Information is limited to these reports, but the interaction with indometacin is established. The incidence is uncertain. Since acute renal failure can apparently develop unpredictably and very rapidly it would seem prudent to use triamterene and indometacin cautiously. The authors of the report with diclofenac suggest caution with the use of any NSAID with triamterene.[2]

1. Hofmann LM, Garcia HA. Interaction of spironolactone and indomethacin at the renal level. *Proc Soc Exp Biol Med* (1972) 141, 353–5.
2. Härkönen M, Ekblom-Kullberg S. Reversible deterioration of renal function after diclofenac in patient receiving triamterene. *BMJ* (1986) 293, 698–9.
3. Jacob SS, Franklin ME, Dickinson RG, Hooper WD. The effect of diflunisal on the elimination of triamterene in human volunteers. *Drug Metabol Drug Interact* (2000) 16, 159–71.
4. Favre L, Glasson P, Vallotton MB. Reversible acute renal failure from combined triamterene and indomethacin. A study in healthy subjects. *Ann Intern Med* (1982) 96, 317–20.
5. Favre L, Glasson PH, Riondel A, Vallotton MB. Interaction of diuretics and non-steroidal anti-inflammatory drugs in man. *Clin Sci* (1983) 64, 407–15.
6. McCarthy JT, Torres VE, Romero JC, Wochos DN, Velosa JA. Acute intrinsic renal failure induced by indomethacin: role of prostaglandin synthetase inhibition. *Mayo Clin Proc* (1982) 57, 289–96.
7. McCarthy JT. Drug-induced renal failure. *Mayo Clin Proc* (1982) 57, 463.
8. Weinberg MS, Quigg RJ, Salant DJ, Bernard DB. Anuric renal failure precipitated by indomethacin and triamterene. *Nephron* (1985) 40, 216–18.
9. Mathews A, Baillie GR. Acute renal failure and hyperkalemia associated with triamterene and indomethacin. *Vet Hum Toxicol* (1986) 28, 224–5.

Potassium-sparing diuretics + Potassium compounds

The concurrent use of spironolactone or triamterene and potassium supplements can result in severe and even life-threatening hyperkalaemia. Amiloride and eplerenone are expected to interact similarly. Potassium-containing salt substitutes can be as hazardous as potassium supplements.

Clinical evidence

In a retrospective analysis of hospitalised patients who had received spironolactone, hyperkalaemia had developed in 5.7% patients on **spironolactone** alone and 15.4% in those also taking a **potassium chloride** supplement. The incidence was 42% in those with severe azotaemia given **spironolactone** and **potassium chloride**.[1] A retrospective survey of another group of 25 patients on **spironolactone** and oral **potassium chloride** supplements found that half of them had developed hyperkalaemia.[2] Another patient developed severe hyperkalaemia and cardiotoxicity as a result of treatment with **spironolactone** and a **potassium supplement.**[3] Three patients on **furosemide** and **spironolactone** became hyperkalaemic[4,5] because they took **potassium-containing salt substitutes** (***No Salt*** in one case[4]). Two developed cardiac arrhythmias.[5] The pacemaker of a patient failed because of hyperkalaemia caused by the concurrent use of **triamterene/hydrochlorothiazide** (***Dyazide***) and **potassium chloride** (***Slow-K***).[6]

Mechanism

The effects of these potassium-sparing diuretics and potassium compounds are additive, resulting in hyperkalaemia.

Importance and management

The interaction with spironolactone is established and of clinical importance. A case has also been reported with triamterene, and **amiloride** and **eplerenone** would be expected to behave similarly. Avoid potassium compounds in patients on potassium-sparing diuretics except in cases of marked potassium depletion and where the effects can be closely monitored. Warn patients about the risks of salt substitutes containing potassium, which may increase the potassium intake by 50 to 60 mmol daily.[5] The signs and symptoms of hyperkalaemia include muscular weakness, fatigue, paraesthesia, flaccid paralysis of the extremities, bradycardia, shock and ECG abnormalities, which may develop slowly and insidiously.

1. Greenblatt DJ, Koch-Weser J. Adverse reactions to spironolactone. A report from the Boston Collaborative Drug Surveillance Program. *Clin Pharmacol Ther* (1973) 14, 136–7.
2. Simborg DN. Medication prescribing on a university medical service — the incidence of drug combinations with potential adverse interactions. *Johns Hopkins Med J* (1976) 139, 23–6.
3. Kalbian VV. Iatrogenic hyperkalemic paralysis with electrocardiographic changes. *South Med J* (1974) 67, 342–5.
4. McCaughan D. Hazards of non-prescription potassium supplements. *Lancet* (1984) i, 513–14.
5. Yap V, Patel A, Thomsen J. Hyperkalemia with cardiac arrhythmia. Induction by salt substitutes, spironolactone, and azotemia. *JAMA* (1976) 236, 2775–6.
6. O'Reilly MV, Murnaghan DP, Williams MB. Transvenous pacemaker failure induced by hyperkalemia. *JAMA* (1974) 228, 336–7.

Potassium-sparing diuretics + Total parenteral nutrition

Metabolic acidosis occurred in two patients receiving total parenteral nutrition, which was attributed to the use of triamterene or amiloride.

Clinical evidence, mechanism, importance and management

Metabolic acidosis developed in two patients receiving total parenteral nutrition associated with the concurrent use of **triamterene** or **amiloride**. The cases were complicated by a number of pathological and other factors, but it was suggested that the major reason for the acidosis was because the diuretics prevented the kidneys from responding normally to the acid load. Caution is advised during concurrent use.[1]

1. Kushner RF, Sitrin MD. Metabolic acidosis. Development in two patients receiving a potassium-sparing diuretic and total parenteral nutrition. *Arch Intern Med* (1986) 146, 343–5.

Potassium-sparing/Thiazide diuretics + Trimethoprim

Excessively low serum sodium levels have been seen in a few patients taking hydrochlorothiazide with amiloride or triamterene when given trimethoprim or co-trimoxazole.

Clinical evidence

A 75-year-old woman with multiple medical conditions taking methyldopa, levothyroxine and **co-amilozide** (**hydrochlorothiazide** with **amiloride**) developed nausea and anorexia and was found to have hyponatraemia (plasma sodium 107 mmol/l), within 4 days of starting to take trimethoprim 200 mg twice daily. The problem resolved when the diuretics and trimethoprim were stopped. When re-challenged 4 months later with trimethoprim, hyponatraemia did not occur, but it developed rapidly when **co-amilozide** was restarted.[1] The authors of this report say that they have seen several other patients who developed hyponatraemia within 4 to 12 days of starting trimethoprim or co-trimoxazole, all of whom were elderly and all but one of whom was taking a diuretic [unnamed].[1]

Another report describes hyponatraemia in two other patients after co-trimoxazole was added to treatment with **co-amilozide** or **co-triamterzide** (**hydrochlorothiazide** with **triamterene**).[2]

Mechanism

Not established. Thiazide diuretics combined with potassium-sparing diuretics are said to be particularly liable to cause hyponatraemia.[3] Trimethoprim can also cause sodium loss, and it seems likely that this can be additive with the effects of other drugs.

Importance and management

Information is very limited but it would seem prudent to be on the alert for any signs of hyponatraemia (nausea, anorexia, etc.) in any patient while taking these drugs. It should also be noted that trimethoprim has been reported to cause hyperkalaemia,[4] which in theory would be exacerbated by the presence of potassium-sparing diuretics. It may therefore be prudent to also monitor potassium levels.

1. Eastell R, Edmonds CJ. Hyponatraemia associated with trimethoprim and a diuretic. *BMJ* (1984) 289, 1658–9.
2. Hart TL, Johnston LJ, Edmonds MW, Brownscombe L. Hyponatremia secondary to thiazide-trimethoprim interaction. *Can J Hosp Pharm* (1989) 42, 243–6.
3. Hornick P. Severe hyponatraemia in elderly patients: cause for concern. *Ann R Coll Surg Engl* (1996) 78, 230–1.
4. Perazella MA. Trimethoprim-induced hyperkalaemia. Clinical data, mechanism, prevention and management. *Drug Safety* (2000) 22, 227–36.

Spironolactone + Aspirin

The antihypertensive effects of spironolactone are unaffected by aspirin in patients with hypertension, although there is evidence that the spironolactone-induced loss of sodium in the urine is reduced in healthy subjects.

Clinical evidence

(a) Effects in hypertensive patients

Five patients with low-renin essential hypertension, well-controlled for 4 months or more with spironolactone 100 to 300 mg daily, were examined in a double-blind crossover trial. Aspirin of 2.4 to 4.8 g daily given over 6-week periods had no effect on blood pressure, serum electrolytes, body-weight, blood-urea-nitrogen or plasma renin activity.[1]

(b) Effects in healthy subjects

A study in 10 healthy subjects given single 25-, 50- and 100-mg doses of spironolactone, found that a single 600-mg dose of aspirin reduced the urinary excretion of sodium.[2] In a further study in 7 of these subjects, the effectiveness of the spironolactone was reduced by 70%, and the overnight sodium excretion was reduced by one-third when they were given spironolactone 25 mg four times daily for one week followed by a single 600-mg dose of aspirin.[2]

Reductions in sodium excretion are described in other studies of this interaction.[3,4] In one of these the sodium excretion brought about by spironolactone was completely abolished when aspirin was given 90 minutes after the spironolactone, but when the drugs were given in the reverse order the inhibition of sodium excretion, which was caused by aspirin, was not completely reversed by spironolactone.[4]

Mechanism

Uncertain. There is evidence that the active secretion of canrenone (the active metabolite of spironolactone) is blocked by aspirin, but the significance of this is not entirely clear.[3]

Importance and management

An adequately but not extensively documented interaction. Despite the results of the studies in healthy subjects, the study in hypertensive patients shows that the blood pressure lowering effects of spironolactone are not affected by aspirin. Concurrent use need not be avoided, but if the diuretic response to spironolactone is less than expected, consider this interaction as a cause.

1. Hollifield JW. Failure of aspirin to antagonize the antihypertensive effect of spironolactone in low-renin hypertension. *South Med J* (1976) 69, 1034–6.
2. Tweeddale MG, Ogilvie RI. Antagonism of spironolactone-induced natriuresis by aspirin in man. *N Engl J Med* (1973) 289, 198.
3. Ramsay LE, Harrison IR, Shelton JR, Vose CW. Influence of acetylsalicylic acid on the renal handling of a spironolactone metabolite in healthy subjects. *Eur J Clin Pharmacol* (1976) 10, 43–8.
4. Elliott HC. Reduced adrenocortical steroid excretion rates in man following aspirin administration. *Metabolism* (1962) 11, 1015–18.

Spironolactone + Colestyramine

Hyperchloraemic metabolic acidosis has been seen in two patients associated with the use of colestyramine and spironolactone.

Clinical evidence, mechanism, importance and management

Two case reports describe the development of hyperchloraemic metabolic acidosis in 2 elderly patients (one with primary biliary cirrhosis the other with hepatic cirrhosis) treated with colestyramine (up to four sachets daily), who were also taking spironolactone.[1,2] One patient had mild renal impairment and upper respiratory tract infection.[1] This adverse reaction appears to be rare, but electrolyte monitoring during concurrent use has been advised.[1]

1. Eaves ER, Korman MG. Cholestyramine induced hyperchloremic metabolic acidosis. *Aust N Z J Med* (1984) 14, 670–2.
2. Clouston WM, Lloyd HM. Cholestyramine induced hyperchloremic metabolic acidosis. *Aust N Z J Med* (1985) 15, 271.

Spironolactone + Dextropropoxyphene (Propoxyphene)

A single case report describes the development of gynaecomastia and a rash in a man on spironolactone when he was given a preparation containing dextropropoxyphene.

Clinical evidence, mechanism, importance and management

A patient who had been taking spironolactone uneventfully for 4 years developed swollen and tender breasts and a rash on his chest and neck a fortnight after starting to take *Darvon Compound* (dextropropoxyphene, **aspirin**, **phenacetin** and **caffeine**). The problem disappeared when both drugs were withdrawn but the rash reappeared when the *Darvon Compound* alone was given and disappeared when it was withdrawn. No problems occurred when the spironolactone was given alone, but both the rash and the gynaecomastia recurred when the *Darvon Compound* was again added.[1] The reasons for this reaction are not understood. Gynaecomastia is a known adverse effect of spironolactone (incidence 1.2%), but the authors considered it unlikely that it should spontaneously develop after so many years of treatment. Consequently they attribute the reaction to an interaction with *Darvon Compound*, but say they cannot be sure which of the components is responsible. Concurrent use need not be avoided but prescribers should be aware of this case.

1. Licata AA, Bartter FC. Spironolactone-induced gynaecomastia related to allergic reaction to 'Darvon Compound'. *Lancet* (1976) ii, 905.

Spironolactone + Food

Food may increase the plasma levels of spironolactone, but this is probably not clinically important.

Clinical evidence, mechanism, importance and management

Food increased the plasma concentrations of canrenone (the major active metabolite of spironolactone) after a single 100-mg dose of spironolactone in healthy subjects, when compared to the fasted state.[1] However, the same research group later found that the steady-state canrenone levels did not differ when spironolactone 100 mg daily was taken at least 30 minutes before eating for 60 days compared with immediately after eating for 60 days, nor was antihypertensive efficacy altered. They suggest that the difference is due to a more specific drug assay in the second study.[2] In contrast, other authors reported that food increased the AUC of spironolactone by 71%, and of 3 of its metabolites (including canrenone) by 32% after a single dose in healthy subjects, but they did not assess whether this affected the hypotensive effect.[3] It appears from the long-term study, that food does not alter the antihypertensive efficacy of spironolactone.

1. Melander A, Danielson K, Schersten B, Thulin T, Wåhlin E. Enhancement by food of canrenone bioavailability from spironolactone. *Clin Pharmacol Ther* (1977) 22, 100–3.
2. Thulin T, Wåhlin-Boll E, Liedholm H, Lindholm L, Melander A. Influence of food intake on antihypertensive drugs: spironolactone. *Drug Nutr Interact* (1983) 2, 169–73.
3. Overdiek HW, Merkus FW. Influence of food on the bioavailability of spironolactone. *Clin Pharmacol Ther* (1986) 40, 531–6.

Thiazide diuretics + Bile-acid binding resins

The absorption of hydrochlorothiazide can be reduced by more than one-third if colestipol is given concurrently. Chlorothiazide appears to interact similarly. Colestyramine also reduces the absorption of hydrochlorothiazide by more than two-thirds. Separating the dosages of hydrochlorothiazide and colestyramine by 4 hours can reduce, but not totally overcome the effects of this interaction.

Clinical evidence

The plasma levels of **hydrochlorothiazide** were reduced by about two-thirds in 6 healthy subjects taking **colestyramine** 8 g, 2 minutes before and 6 and 12 hours after a single 75-mg oral dose of **hydrochlorothiazide**. Total urinary excretion of **hydrochlorothiazide** fell by 83%. In a parallel study with **colestipol** 10 g, the blood levels of **hydrochlorothiazide** fell by about 14% and the total urinary excretion fell by 31%.[1] A further study found that giving the **colestyramine** 4 hours after the **hydrochlorothiazide** reduced the effects of the interaction but the absorption was still reduced by one-third.[2] In another study **colestipol**, given simultaneously or one-hour later, reduced the urinary excretion of **chlorothiazide** by 58 and 54% respectively.[3]

Mechanism

Hydrochlorothiazide becomes bound to these non-absorbable anionic exchange resins within the gut, and less is available for absorption.

Importance and management

Established interactions of clinical importance. The best dosing schedule would appear to be to give hydrochlorothiazide 4 hours before colestyramine to minimise mixing in the gut. Even so a one-third reduction in thiazide absorption occurs.[2] The optimum time-interval with colestipol has not been investigated but it would be reasonable to take similar precautions. Information about other thiazides is lacking although it seems likely that they will interact similarly. Note that it is normally recommended that other drugs are given 1 hour before or 4 to 6 hours after colestyramine and 1 hour before or 4 hours after colestipol.

1. Hunninghake DB, King S, La Croix K. The effect of cholestyramine and colestipol on the absorption of hydrochlorothiazide. *Int J Clin Pharmacol Ther Toxicol* (1982) 20, 151–4.
2. Hunninghake DB, Hibbard DM. Influence of time intervals for cholestyramine dosing on the absorption of hydrochlorothiazide. *Clin Pharmacol Ther* (1986) 39, 329–34.
3. Kauffmann RE, Azarnoff DL. Effect of colestipol on gastrointestinal absorption of chlorothiazide in man. *Clin Pharmacol Ther* (1973) 14, 886.

Thiazide diuretics + Calcium/Vitamin D

Hypercalcaemia and possibly metabolic alkalosis can develop in patients given high doses of vitamin D and/or large amounts of calcium if they are additionally treated with diuretics such as the thiazides, which can reduce the urinary excretion of calcium.

Clinical evidence

(a) Calcium/vitamin D

An elderly woman on **hydrochlorothiazide** 25 mg and **triamterene** 50 mg daily for hypertension, and vitamin D_2 50 000 units with calcium 1.5 g daily for osteoporosis, became confused, disorientated and dehydrated. Her serum calcium level had risen to 13.9 mg/dl (normal range 8.2 to 10.5 mg/dl).[1]

A young woman with osteoporosis taking 3 mg of vitamin D_2 and calcium 2 g daily became hypercalcaemic when given **chlorothiazide**.[2] In a group of 12 patients treated for hypoparathyroidism with vitamin D (**dihydrotachysterol** or **ergocalciferol**), 5 patients became hypercalcaemic when treated with **bendroflumethiazide** or **methyclothiazide**.[3] A significant rise in plasma calcium levels occurred in 7 patients given vitamin D and **methyclothiazide** or **chlorothiazide**, and hypercalcaemia developed in 3 of them.[4]

(b) Calcium carbonate

A 47-year-old man was admitted to hospital complaining chiefly of dizziness and general weakness, which had begun 2 months previously. He was taking **chlorothiazide** 500 mg daily for hypertension, 'thyroid' 120 mg daily for hypothyroidism and calcium carbonate 7.5 to 10 g daily for heartburn. On examination he was found to have metabolic alkalosis with respiratory compensation, a total serum calcium concentration of 3.4 mmol/l (normal 2.15 to 2.6 mmol/l) and an abnormal ECG. He was diagnosed as having the milk-alkali syndrome. Recovery was rapid when the thiazide and calcium carbonate were withdrawn, and a sodium chloride infusion, furosemide and oral phosphates were given.[5]

An elderly woman with normal renal function on **hydrochlorothiazide** 50 mg daily and calcium 2.5 to 7.5 g daily also developed hypercalcaemia.[6]

In both cases the thiazide diuretic was thought to be implicated as the levels of calcium ingestion were in the region of the normally recommended doses.

Mechanism

The thiazide diuretics (and triamterene) can cause calcium-retention by reducing the urinary excretion. This, added to the increased intake of calcium, resulted in excessive calcium levels. Alkalosis (the milk-alkali syndrome, associated with hypercalcaemia, alkalosis, renal insufficiency) may also occur in some individuals because the thiazide limits the excretion of bicarbonate.

Importance and management

An established interaction. The incidence is unknown but the reports cited[3,4] suggest that it can be considerable if the intake of vitamin D and calcium are high. Concurrent use need not be avoided, but the serum calcium levels should be regularly monitored to ensure that they do not become excessive. There is evidence that the hypercalcaemia may be self-limiting.[3] Patients should be warned about the ingestion of very large amounts of calcium carbonate (readily available without prescription) if they are taking thiazide diuretics.

1. Drinka PJ, Nolten WE. Hazards of treating osteoporosis and hypertension concurrently with calcium, vitamin D, and distal diuretics. *J Am Geriatr Soc* (1984) 32, 405–7.
2. Parfitt AM. Chlorothiazide-induced hypercalcaemia in juvenile osteoporosis and hyperparathyroidism. *N Engl J Med* (1969) 281, 55–9.
3. Parfitt AM. Thiazide-induced hypercalcaemia in vitamin D-treated hypoparathyroidism. *Ann Intern Med* (1972) 77, 557–63.
4. Parfitt AM. Interactions of thiazide diuretics with parathyroid hormone and vitamin D. Studies in patients with hypoparathyroidism. *J Clin Invest* (1972) 51, 1879–88.
5. Gora ML, Seth SK, Bay WH, Visconti JA. Milk-alkali syndrome associated with use of chlorothiazide and calcium carbonate. *Clin Pharm* (1989) 8, 227–9.
6. Hakim R, Tolis G, Goltzman D, Meltzer S, Friedman R. Severe hypercalcemia associated with hydrochlorothiazide and calcium carbonate therapy. *Can Med Assoc J* (1979) 121, 591–4.

Thiazide and related diuretics + NSAIDs

The antihypertensive effects of the thiazides can be reduced to some extent by indometacin, but it appears to be of only moderate clinical importance and may possibly only be a transient interaction. Ibuprofen diclofenac and sulindac appear to interact to a lesser extent or not at all, and piroxicam, naproxen and phenylbutazone may interact. No adverse interaction appears to occur with diflunisal.

Clinical evidence

A. Bemetizide

(a) Indometacin

Indometacin 100 mg was found to reduce the urinary excretion of sodium and chloride caused by bemetizide by 47 and 44% respectively in healthy subjects.[1]

B. Bendroflumethiazide

(a) Ibuprofen

In a double-blind, randomised, placebo-controlled study 7 hypertensive patients, treated with bendroflumethiazide 5 to 10 mg daily were also given ibuprofen 400 mg four times daily for 2 weeks. Although some small increases in blood pressure occurred, the diastolic blood pressure of all patients remained below 90 mmHg throughout the ibuprofen phase. Overall no statistically significant weight gain was noted, although 2 patients gained more than 2 kg.[2]

(b) Indometacin

A double-blind controlled trial in 7 patients with hypertension on bendroflumethiazide 5 to 10 mg daily found that indometacin 100 mg daily for 3 weeks raised their systolic/diastolic blood pressures by 13/9 mmHg when lying and by 16/9 mmHg when standing. Body-weight increased by 1.1 kg.[3] Indometacin also attenuated the hypotensive effect of bendroflumethiazide in another study.[4]

(c) Sulindac

A brief report suggested that sulindac enhanced the hypotensive effects of bendroflumethiazide in 5 hypertensive patients.[4]

C. Hydrochlorothiazide

(a) Diclofenac

Diclofenac 25 mg three times daily was given to 8 patients with essential hypertension who were being treated with hydrochlorothiazide. Blood pressure was not significantly altered after the addition of diclofenac, but a weight gain of about 1 to 2 kg was noted, which was thought to have been caused by the sodium retaining effects of diclofenac.[5]

(b) Diflunisal

Diflunisal 375 mg twice daily caused the plasma levels of hydrochlorothiazide to rise by 25 to 30%, but this appears to be clinically unimportant.[6,7] Diflunisal also has uricosuric activity, which counteracts the uric acid retention that occurs with hydrochlorothiazide.

(c) Ibuprofen

Ibuprofen 400 mg or 600 mg three times daily for 4 weeks caused a small rise in systolic but not in diastolic pressures in two studies in patients on hydrochlorothiazide.[5,8] However, a weight gain of about 1 to 2 kg was noted in one of the studies.[5] Another study found that ibuprofen 400 mg three times daily had no effect on blood pressures controlled by triamterene with hydrochlorothiazide, although one patient had a marked fall in renal function.[9] Ibuprofen 800 mg four times daily for a week had little effect on blood pressures controlled with hydrochlorothiazide in yet another study.[10]

(d) Indometacin

A double-blind controlled trial in 7 patients with hypertension on amiloride 5 to 10 mg with hydrochlorothiazide 50 to 100 mg, found that indometacin 100 mg daily for 3 weeks raised their systolic/diastolic blood pressures by 13/9 mmHg when lying and by 16/9 mmHg when standing. Body weight increased by 1.1 kg.[3] A later study in patients on hydrochlorothiazide found a 6/3 mmHg blood pressure rise after 2 weeks of indometacin, which had gone after 4 weeks.[11] Only a 5/1 mmHg blood pressure rise was seen in another study in hypertensive patients on hydrochlorothiazide given indometacin 100 mg daily.[12] Indometacin also attenuated the hypotensive effect of hydrochlorothiazide (given with amiloride) in another study.[4]

In other studies indometacin had no effect on blood pressure in healthy subjects,[13] no effect on the sodium excretion caused by hydrochlorothiazide,[14] and did not affect the pharmacokinetics of hydrochlorothiazide.[13,14]

(e) Kebuzone

In 15 patients on hydrochlorothiazide 50 mg daily, a mean systolic blood pressure rise of 18 mmHg (from 171 to 189 mmHg) occurred when they were treated with kebuzone 750 mg daily. This rise represents about a 35% reduction in the antihypertensive effect of hydrochlorothiazide.[15]

(f) Naproxen

One study found that naproxen had no clinically relevant interaction with hydrochlorothiazide alone,[11] while another found that naproxen attenuated the antihypertensive efficacy of hydrochlorothiazide plus timolol, but how much of the attenuation is due to an interaction with the beta-blocker is unclear.[16]

(g) Phenylbutazone

In 15 patients on hydrochlorothiazide 50 mg daily, a mean systolic blood pressure rise of 18 mmHg (from 171 to 189 mmHg) occurred when they were treated with phenylbutazone 750 mg daily. This rise represents about a 35% reduction in the antihypertensive effect of hydrochlorothiazide.[15]

(h) Piroxicam

One study found that piroxicam attenuated the antihypertensive efficacy of hydrochlorothiazide plus timolol, but how much of the attenuation is due to an interaction with the beta-blocker is unclear.[16]

(i) Sulindac

Sulindac does not appear to reduce either the hypotensive or diuretic effects of hydrochlorothiazide, and may even slightly enhance the antihypertensive effects.[4,5,11,12,16,17] Another study found that sulindac did not alter the antihypertensive efficacy of hydrochlorothiazide + amiloride given with beta-blockers.[18]

D. Metolazone

(a) Indometacin

Indometacin was found to reduce the urinary sodium excretion due to metolazone by 34% in 6 healthy subjects.[19] The excretion of total potassium fell by 30%.

(b) Sulindac

Sulindac was found to reduce the urinary sodium excretion due to metolazone by 19% in 6 healthy subjects[19]. The excretion of total potassium fell by 16%.

Mechanism

Not understood. Since the prostaglandins have a role to play in renal function, drugs such as the NSAIDs, which inhibit their synthesis, might be expected to have some effect on the actions of diuretics whose effects also depend on the activity of the prostaglandins. A study in *rats* suggested that indometacin may oppose the thiazides by reducing chloride delivery to the site of thiazide action in the distal tubule.[20] The lack of effect with sulindac may be due to the absence of renal excretion of its active sulfide metabolite.[16]

Importance and management

The interaction between the thiazides and indometacin is well documented although the findings are not entirely consistent. It seems to be of only moderate clinical importance, but the effects of concurrent use should be monitored and the thiazide dosage modified if necessary. Other NSAIDs appear to interact to a lesser extent or not at all. The uricosuric effects of diflunisal may be usefully exploited to counteract the uric acid retention which occurs with hydrochlorothiazide. The effects of other NSAIDs not discussed here do not seem to have been studied.

1. Düsing R, Nicolas V, Glatte B, Glänzer K, Kipnowski J, Kramer HJ. Interaction of bemetizide and indomethacin in the kidney. *Br J Clin Pharmacol* (1983) 16, 377–84.
2. Davies JG, Rawlins DC, Busson M. Effect of ibuprofen on blood pressure control by propranolol and bendrofluazide. *J Int Med Res* (1988) 16, 173–81.
3. Watkins J, Abbott EC, Hensby CN, Webster J, Dollery CT. Attenuation of hypotensive effect of propranolol and thiazide diuretics by indomethacin. *BMJ* (1980) 281, 702–5.
4. Steiness E, Waldorff S. Different interactions of indomethacin and sulindac with thiazides in hypertension. *BMJ* (1982) 285, 1702–3.
5. Koopmans PP, Thien Th, Gribnau FWJ. The influence of ibuprofen, diclofenac and sulindac on the blood pressure lowering effect of hydrochlorothiazide. *Eur J Clin Pharmacol* (1987) 31, 553–7.
6. Tempero KF, Cirillo VJ, Steelman SL. Diflunisal: a review of the pharmacokinetic and pharmacodynamic properties, drug interactions and special tolerability studies in humans. *Br J Clin Pharmacol* (1977) 4, 31S–36S.
7. Tempero KF, Cirillo VJ, Steelman SL, Besselaar GH, Smit Sibinga CTh, De Schepper P, Tjandramaga TB, Dresse A, Gribnau FWJ. Special studies on diflunisal, a novel salicylate. *Clin Res* (1975) 23, 224A.
8. Gurwitz JH, Everitt DE, Monane M, Glynn RJ, Choodnovskiy I, Beaudet MP, Avorn J. The impact of ibuprofen on the efficacy of antihypertensive treatment with hydrochlorothiazide in elderly persons. *J Gerontol* (1996) 51A, M74–M79.
9. Gehr TWB, Sica DA, Steiger BW, Marshall C. Interaction of triamterene-hydrochlorothiazide and ibuprofen. *Clin Pharmacol Ther* (1990) 47, 200.

10. Wright JT, McKenney JM, Lehany AM, Bryan DL, Cooper LW, Lambert CM. The effect of high-dose short-term ibuprofen on antihypertensive control with hydrochlorothiazide. *Clin Pharmacol Ther* (1989) 46, 440–4.
11. Koopmans PP, Thien Th, Gribnau FWJ. Influence of non-steroidal anti-inflammatory drugs on diuretic treatment of mild to moderate essential hypertension. *BMJ* (1984) 289, 1492–4.
12. Koopmans PP, Thien Th, Thomas CMG, van den Berg RJ, Gribnau FWJ. The effects of sulindac and indomethacin on the antihypertensive and diuretic action of hydrochlorothiazide in patients with mild to moderate essential hypertension. *Br J Clin Pharmacol* (1986) 21, 417–23.
13. Koopmans PP, Kateman WGPM, Tan Y, van Ginneken CAM, Gribnau FWJ. Effects of indomethacin and sulindac on hydrochlorothiazide kinetics. *Clin Pharmacol Ther* (1985) 37, 625–8.
14. Williams RL, Davies RO, Berman RS, Holmes GI, Huber P, Gee WL, Lin ET, Benet LZ. Hydrochlorothiazide pharmacokinetics and pharmacologic effect: the influence of indomethacin. *J Clin Pharmacol* (1982) 22, 32–41.
15. Polak F. Die hemmende Wirkung von Phenylbutazon auf die durch einige Antihypertonika hervorgerufene Blutdrucksenkung bei Hypertonikern. *Z Gesamte Inn Med* (1976) 22, 375–6.
16. Wong DG, Spence JD, Lamki L, Freeman D, McDonald JWD. Effect of non-steroidal anti-inflammatory drugs on control of hypertension by beta-blockers and diuretics. *Lancet* (1986) 3, 997–1001.
17. Steiness E, Waldorff S. Different interactions of indomethacin and sulindac with thiazides in hypertension. *BMJ* (1982) 285, 1702–3.
18. Stokes GS, Brooks PM, Johnson HJ, Monaghan JC, Okoro EO, Kelly D. The effects of sulindac and diclofenac in essential hypertension controlled by treatment with a beta-blocker and/or diuretic. *Clin Exp Hypertens A* (1991) 13, 1169–78.
19. Ripley EBD, Gehr TWB, Wallace H, Wade J, Kish C, Sica DA. The effect of nonsteroidal agents (NSAIDs) on the pharmacokinetics and pharmacodynamics of metolazone. *Int J Clin Pharmacol Ther* (1994) 32, 12–18.
20. Kirchner KA, Brandon S, Mueller RA, Smith MJ, Bower JD. Mechanism of attenuated hydrochlorothiazide response during indomethacin administration. *Kidney Int* (1987) 31, 1097–1103.

Thiazide diuretics + Propantheline

Propantheline can increase the absorption of hydrochlorothiazide.

Clinical evidence, mechanism, importance and management

The absorption of hydrochlorothiazide 75 mg in 6 healthy fasting subjects was delayed and increased (AUC increased by 23% and urinary recovery increased by 36%) by propantheline 60 mg, due, it is suggested, to a slower delivery of the drug to its areas of absorption.[1] The clinical importance of this is uncertain, but it seems likely to be small.

1. Beermann B, Groschinsky-Grind M. Enhancement of the gastrointestinal absorption of hydrochlorothiazide by propantheline. *Eur J Clin Pharmacol* (1978) 13, 385–7.

25

Gastrointestinal drugs

The various gastrointestinal drug groups covered in this section are listed in 'Table 25.1'. 'Drug absorption interactions', (p.3) discusses how absorption interactions occur and contains more detailed information on some of the mechanisms of interaction covered in this section.

Table 25.1 Gastrointestinal drugs covered in this section

Group	*Drugs*
5-aminosalicylates	Balsalazide, Mesalazine, Olsalazine, Sulfasalazine
Antidiarrhoeals	Loperamide
Antimuscarinics	Pirenzepine
Bismuth compounds	Bismuth salicylate, Bismuth subnitrate, Tripotassium dicitratobismuthate
H_2-blockers	Cimetidine, Famotidine, Nizatadine, Ranitidine, Roxatidine
Mucosal protectants	Carbenoxolone, Liquorice, Sucralfate
Prokinetic drugs	Cisapride
Proton pump inhibitors	Esomeprazole, Lansoprazole, Omeprazole, Pantoprazole, Rabeprazole

Antacids + Milk

Hypercalcaemia, alkalosis and renal insufficiency (milk-alkali syndrome) developed in a man taking an antacid/liquorice preparation (*Caved-S*) and large amounts of milk.

Clinical evidence

A man presented with nausea, vomiting, constipation, polyuria and polydipsia, which was diagnosed as milk-alkali syndrome (hypercalcaemia, alkalosis, renal insufficiency) due to daily treatment with 6 tablets of ***Caved-S*** and 3.5 pints of milk for dyspepsia related to a peptic ulcer.[1] This dose of ***Caved-S*** meant he was taking 600 mg of **aluminium hydroxide**, 1200 mg of **magnesium carbonate**, 600 mg of **sodium bicarbonate** and 2280 mg of **deglycyrrhizinised liquorice** daily.

Mechanism

The hypercalcaemia occurred because the absorbed alkali decreased the excretion of calcium by the kidneys, while the intake of calcium (in the milk) remained high. The excessive amount of calcium increased the reabsorption of bicarbonate by the kidneys (through salt and water depletion) so that the alkalosis was maintained. Hypermagnesaemia may also have had a part to play.

Importance and management

The milk-alkali syndrome is well documented but very uncommon these days because there are now other and better ways of treating peptic ulcers. This case amply illustrates that while taking this or similar antiulcer preparations, well within the recommended dosage range, it is still possible to develop a serious and potentially life-threatening reaction if the intake of calcium (in milk for example) is high.

1. Gibbs CJ, Lee HA. Milk-alkali syndrome due to Caved-S. *J R Soc Med* (1992) 85, 498–9.

Bismuth compounds + Omeprazole

Omeprazole possibly causes an increase in the absorption of bismuth from tripotassium dicitratobismuthate (TDB).

Clinical evidence, mechanism, importance and management

The AUC of bismuth, after a single 240-mg dose of **tripotassium dicitratobismuthate** (**TDB**), was increased fourfold in 6 healthy subjects after taking 40 mg omeprazole daily for a week, with the last dose taken 1 hour before the bismuth compound. The maximum serum levels increased from 36.7 to 86.7 nanograms/ml, which the authors of the study point out approaches what they describe as the "toxic range" for bismuth (100 nanograms/ml and above). Reducing gastric acidity appears to maintain **TDB** in the colloidal form and increase bismuth absorption (see also 'Bismuth compounds + Ranitidine', below). The authors suggest that to avoid the possibility of systemic toxicity the dosage of the **TDB** should be halved when given with omeprazole, but this might then limit the activity of the **TDB**.[1] However, the makers say that the toxic range of bismuth is arbitrary and a small increase in absorption is not clinically significant in normal patients.[2] This would certainly seem to be the case if combined treatment is limited to the recommended 2-week regimen for resistant *Helicobacter pylori* infection. Other proton pump inhibitors would be expected to interact similarly with **TDB**.

1. Treiber G, Walker S, Klotz U. Omeprazole-induced increase in the absorption of bismuth from tripotassium dicitrato bismuthate. *Clin Pharmacol Ther* (1994) 55, 486–91.
2. Yamanouchi Pharma Ltd. Personal communication, November 1994.

Bismuth compounds + Ranitidine

Ranitidine possibly causes an increase in the absorption of bismuth from tripotassium dicitratobismuthate (TDB), but not bismuth salicylate or bismuth subnitrate.

Clinical evidence, mechanism, importance and management

The AUC of bismuth, after a single 240-mg dose of **tripotassium dicitratobismuthate** (**TDB**—*De Noltabs*), was increased fourfold in 12 healthy subjects treated with two 300-mg doses of ranitidine (one the night before and one 2 hours before the bismuth compound). The maximum serum levels were approximately doubled. The same regimen of ranitidine had no significant effect on the absorption of bismuth from **bismuth salicylate** (*Pepto-Bismol*) or **bismuth subnitrate** (*Roter tablets*).[1] The authors suggest that the reduction in gastric acidity maintains **TDB** in its colloidal form, which is more likely to be absorbed, and that this may result in increased bismuth toxicity.[1] Other H2-blockers, and other drugs that reduce gastric acidity would be expected to interact similarly (see also 'Bismuth compounds + Omeprazole', above).

However, the makers of **TDB** say that the toxic range of bismuth is arbitrary and a small increase in absorption is not clinically significant in normal patients.[2] Note that a complex of ranitidine with bismuth and citrate (**ranitidine bismuth citrate**) is available in many countries. As with all bismuth compounds, it is recommended that this is used only for limited periods (a maximum of 16 weeks in a 12-month period).[3]

1. Nwokolo CU, Prewett EJ, Sawyerr AM, Hudson M, Pounder RE. The effect of histamine H_2-receptor blockade on bismuth absorption from three ulcer-healing compounds. *Gastroenterology* (1991) 101, 889–94.
2. Yamanouchi Pharma Ltd. Personal communication, November 1994.
3. Pylorid Tablets (Ranitidine bismuth citrate). GlaxoSmithKline UK. UK Summary of product characteristics, June 2005.

Carbenoxolone + Antacids

There is some evidence that antacids may possibly reduce the bioavailability of carbenoxolone.

Clinical evidence, mechanism, importance and management

The bioavailability of carbenoxolone, in a liquid formulation, when given with **aluminium/magnesium hydroxide** antacids, was found to be approximately half that of carbenoxolone in granular and capsule formulations.[1] The extent to which antacids might reduce the ulcer-healing effects of carbenoxolone given in other formulations seems not to have been assessed, but the possibility of a reduction should be borne in mind.

1. Crema F, Parini J, Visconti M, Perucca E. Effetto degli antiacidi sulla biodisponibilità del carbenoxolone. *Farmaco (Prat)* (1987) 42, 357–64.

Carbenoxolone + Antidiabetics

Chlorpropamide appears to have an effect on the pharmacokinetics of carbenoxolone, causing a small reduction in serum levels. Tolbutamide does not appear to have any significant effect on carbenoxolone pharmacokinetics.

Clinical evidence, mechanism, importance and management

A single 500-mg dose of **tolbutamide** had no significant effect on the half-life of a single 100-mg dose of carbenoxolone in 4 healthy subjects, whereas a single 250-mg dose of **chlorpropamide** delayed the absorption of carbenoxolone and reduced its plasma levels in 6 patients taking 100 mg carbenoxolone three times daily.[1] The clinical importance of this latter interaction is uncertain.

1. Thornton PC, Papouchado M, Reed PI. Carbenoxolone interactions in man - preliminary report. *Scand J Gastroenterol* (1980) 15 (Suppl 65), 35–9.

Carbenoxolone + Antihypertensives

Carbenoxolone causes fluid retention and raises the blood pressure in some patients. This may be expected to oppose the effects of antihypertensive drugs. The potassium-depleting effects of the thiazides, related diuretics and carbenoxolone can be additive. Spironolactone or amiloride can oppose the ulcer-healing effects of carbenoxolone.

Clinical evidence, mechanism, importance and management

(a) Antihypertensives (unnamed)

Carbenoxolone can raise blood pressure. Five out of 10 patients taking 300 mg carbenoxolone daily, and 2 out of 10 patients taking 150 mg carbenoxolone daily, showed a rise in diastolic blood pressure of 20 mmHg or more.[1] Other reports[2-8] confirm that fluid retention and hypertension occur in those taking carbenoxolone, with the reported incidence of hypertension varying from as low as 4%[8] to as high as 50%,[7] and fluid retention occurring in 0%[2] to 46% of patients.[7] The reason for the blood pressure rise is that carbenoxolone has mineralocorticoid-like activity and therefore causes sodium and water retention. There appear to be few direct reports of adverse interactions between antihypertensive drugs and carbenoxolone, but patients on carbenoxolone should have regular checks on their weight and blood pressure, and carbenoxolone should be used with caution, if at all, in those with hypertension.

(b) Diuretics

Thiazide diuretics have been used to control the oedema and hypertension caused by carbenoxolone, but **spironolactone**[3] (an aldosterone-antagonist) and **amiloride**[9] are best avoided because they oppose its ulcer-healing effects. If **thiazides** or related diuretics are used it should be remembered the potassium-losing effects of the carbenoxolone and the diuretic will be additive, so that a potassium supplement may be needed to prevent hypokalaemia. For example, rhabdomyolysis and acute tubular necrosis associated with severe hypokalaemia occurred in a patient given carbenoxolone and **chlortalidone**, without a potassium supplement.[10] Other **potassium-depleting diuretics**, which might be expected to interact similarly, are listed in 'Table 24.1', (p.717). Possible alternatives to carbenoxolone are **deglycyrrhizinised liquorice** (which is an analogue of carbenoxolone, has reduced mineralocorticoid activity and therefore fewer side-effects)[7,11] the H_2-blockers, or the proton pump inhibitors.

1. Turpie AGG, Thomson TJ. Carbenoxolone sodium in the treatment of gastric ulcer with special reference to side-effects. *Gut* (1965) 6, 591.
2. Baron A, Sullivan S, eds. Carbenoxolone Sodium. London: Butterworths; 1970 p. 103–16.
3. Doll R, Langman MJS, Shawdon HH. Treatment of gastric ulcer with carbenoxolone: antagonistic effect of spironolactone. *Gut* (1968) 9, 42–5.
4. Montgomery RD, Cookson JB. Comparative trial of carbenoxolone and a deglycyrrhizinated liquorice preparation (Cavid-S). *Clin Trials J* (1972) 9, 33–5.
5. Langman MJS, Knapp DR, Wakley EJ. Treatment of chronic gastric ulcer with carbenoxolone and gefarnate: a comparative trial. *BMJ* (1973) 3, 84–6.
6. Horwich L, Galloway R. Treatment of gastric ulceration with carbenoxolone sodium: clinical and radiological evaluation. *BMJ* (1965) 2, 1274–7.
7. Fraser PM, Doll R, Langman MJS, Misiewicz JJ, Shawdon HH. Clinical trial of a new carbenoxolone analogue (BX-24), zinc sulphate, and vitamin A in the treatment of gastric ulcer. *Gut* (1972) 13, 459–63.
8. Montgomery RD. Side effects of carbenoxolone sodium: a study of ambulant therapy of gastric ulcer. *Gut* (1967) 8, 148–50.
9. Reed PI, Lewis SI, Vincent-Brown A, Holdstock DJ, Gribble RJN, Murgatroyd RE, Baron JH. The influence of amiloride on the therapeutic and metabolic effects of carbenoxolone in patients with gastric ulcer. *Scand J Gastroenterol* (1980) 15 (Suppl 65), 51–5.
10. Descamps C, Vandenbroucke JM, van Ypersele de Strihou C. Rhabdomyolysis and acute tubular necrosis associated with carbenoxolone and diuretic treatment. *BMJ* (1977) 1, 272.
11. Brogden RN, Speight TM, Avery GS. Deglycyrrhizinised liquorice: a report of its pharmacological properties and therapeutic efficacy in peptic ulcer. *Drugs* (1974) 8, 330–9.

Carbenoxolone + Phenytoin

A single 100-mg dose of phenytoin had no significant effect on the half-life of a single 100-mg dose of carbenoxolone in 4 healthy subjects.[1] This limited evidence would seem to suggest that there is no reason for avoiding concurrent use.

1. Thornton PC, Papouchado M, Reed PI. Carbenoxolone interactions in man - preliminary report. *Scand J Gastroenterol* (1980) 15 (Suppl 65), 35–9.

Cimetidine + Dimeticone

The pharmacokinetics of a 200-mg dose of cimetidine were not significantly changed by 2.25 g dimeticone in 11 healthy subjects.[1]

1. Boismare F, Flipo JL, Moore N, Chanteclair G. Etude de l'effet du diméticone sur la biodisponsibilité de la cimétidine. *Therapie* (1987) 42, 9–11.

Cimetidine + Phenobarbital

Phenobarbital modestly reduces the AUC of cimetidine, although this is probably not clinically relevant.

Clinical evidence

Phenobarbital 100 mg daily for 3 weeks reduced the AUC of a single 400-mg oral dose of cimetidine in 8 healthy subjects by 15%, and the time during which the plasma concentrations of the cimetidine exceeded 0.5 micrograms/ml (regarded as therapeutically desirable) was reduced by 11%.[1]

Phenobarbital apparently stimulates the enzymes in the gut wall so that the metabolism of the cimetidine is increased. Thus the amount of cimetidine absorbed and released into the circulation is reduced.

Direct information is very limited, but the effect of phenobarbital on cimetidine is small and unlikely to be clinically important. No special precautions seem to be necessary.

1. Somogyi A, Thielscher S, Gugler R. Influence of phenobarbital treatment on cimetidine kinetics. *Eur J Clin Pharmacol* (1981) 19, 343–7.

Cimetidine + Rifampicin (Rifampin)

Antituberculous treatment with rifampicin, isoniazid and ethambutol has been shown to increase the non-renal clearance of cimetidine by about 50%. This is probably due to enzyme induction caused by rifampicin. However, the total clearance is unchanged and so this interaction would appear to be of little clinical importance.[1]

1. Keller E, Schollmeyer P, Brandenstein U, Hoppe-Seyler G. Increased nonrenal clearance of cimetidine during antituberculous therapy. *Int J Clin Pharmacol Ther Toxicol* (1984) 22, 307–11.

Cisapride + Miscellaneous

Ketoconazole, erythromycin, and clarithromycin can cause a marked rise in serum cisapride levels, increasing the risk of serious and life-threatening ventricular arrhythmias including torsade de pointes. Nefazodone and HIV-protease inhibitors are predicted also to have this effect. Although there do not appear to be any specific reports, cisapride should not be used with other drugs that prolong the QT interval (See also 'Drugs that prolong the QT interval + Other drugs that prolong the QT interval', p.170). No clinically relevant interactions with cisapride are apparent when it is given with antacids, cimetidine, esomeprazole, fluoxetine or pantoprazole, but two isolated reports attribute cardiotoxicity to the concurrent use of cisapride, with ranitidine or diltiazem. Cisapride increases the rate of absorption of bromperidol, ciclosporin, diazepam, disopyramide, and nifedipine, but appears to have no important effect on digoxin, morphine, paracetamol (acetaminophen) or propranolol. The effects of anticoagulants may be altered by cisapride.

Clinical evidence, mechanism, importance and management

A. Interactions leading to cardiotoxicity

In many countries cisapride has been withdrawn from the market, or is only available for restricted use because of its potential to cause torsade de pointes arrhythmias, especially when cisapride serum levels are elevated.[1] This can lead to cardiac arrest and sudden death.

Both **macrolide antibacterials** (e.g. **clarithromycin**[2-6] and **erythromycin**[5-7]) and **azole antifungals** (e.g. **ketoconazole**[8,9]) are well recognised for causing this interaction with cisapride. An interaction occurs because the inhibitory effect of these drugs on the cytochrome P450 isoenzyme CYP3A4, an enzyme concerned with the metabolism of cisapride, results in raised levels of cisapride. Other drugs expected to interact similarly, because of an effect on CYP3A4, include the **HIV-protease inhibitors** and **nefazodone**.[10,11] The makers therefore contraindicate cisapride with these potent CYP3A4 inhibitors.[10] There are isolated case reports regarding ranitidine and diltiazem, but these were not considered indicative of a generalised interaction and so are discussed below under (g) Gastrointestinal drugs and under (f) Cardiovascular drugs respectively.

Many more drugs are predicted to cause torsade de pointes with cisapride due to additive effects rather than a metabolic interaction.[11] For more information on this interaction see 'Drugs that prolong the QT interval + Other drugs that prolong the QT interval', p.170.

B. General interactions

(a) Alcohol

Four studies have shown that cisapride modestly increases maximum blood alcohol levels, because it speeds up gastric emptying.[12-15] However, the effects are not as great as drinking alcohol on an empty stomach,[15] and are probably of little clinical relevance. Nevertheless, the maker of cisapride says that the sedative effects of alcohol may be enhanced.[10] There is also some evidence that alcohol may modestly increase the cisapride AUC (by 22%),[12] but the clinical relevance of this is uncertain.

(b) Analgesics

Cisapride 20 mg was found to increase the serum levels of **morphine** (20 mg ***MST Continus***, a sustained release preparation) but the effects, as measured by pupil-constriction and sedation, were unchanged.[16] Cisapride causes no significant changes in the pharmacokinetics of **paracetamol (acetaminophen)**.[17]

(c) Anticholinergics

Cisapride and drugs with anticholinergic properties have opposite effects on gastrointestinal motility. Thus one study found that cisapride 2.5 mg three times daily increased gastric emptying, which had previously been reduced by **disopyramide** 100 mg three times daily, thereby increasing the absorption and the serum levels of **disopyramide**. Its absorption rate constant was doubled and the lag time was halved. This was thought to be due to the anticholinergic side effects of disopyramide. The clinical significance of this interaction is uncertain, but you should also be aware that **disopyramide** is listed by the makers as contraindicated because of the possible risk of additive cardiotoxicity (See also 'Drugs that prolong the QT interval + Other drugs that prolong the QT interval', p.170).

(d) Anticoagulants

Twenty-two patients on **acenocoumarol** showed an increase in thrombotest values while on cisapride (10 mg three times daily for 3 weeks). These values fell when the cisapride was stopped.[18]

A study in 24 healthy subjects found that 10 mg cisapride four times daily did not significantly affect the anticoagulant effects of **phenprocoumon**.[19]

Twelve healthy subjects on **warfarin** showed a small but statistically insignificant rise in their **warfarin** requirements (from 44.5 to 49 mg) when given 10 mg cisapride daily for 25 days.[20] This contrasts with a report of a 75-year-old man with a heart valve prosthesis and well stabilised on **warfarin** whose INR rose from a range of 2.2 to 2.5 up to 10.7 within 3 weeks of stopping metoclopramide 10 mg four times daily and starting cisapride 10 mg four times daily. It seems doubtful if stopping the metoclopramide or any other factors were responsible.[21] However, it may be prudent to check the prothrombin time in the first few days after starting or stopping cisapride.[10]

(e) Anticonvulsants

Cisapride speeds up gastrointestinal motility. This would be expected to accelerate drug transit through the gut, to increase the absorption rate of some drugs and possibly reduce the extent of absorption. For this reason the makers of cisapride suggest that for drugs that need careful individual titration (e.g. some anticonvulsants) it may be useful to measure their plasma concentrations.[10] However, there seems to be no direct evidence that a clinically important interaction actually occurs with anticonvulsants. In fact, a study in a child of 3 found that 4 days after withdrawing cisapride, the total serum **phenytoin** levels and free **phenytoin** fraction were unchanged.[22]

(f) Cardiovascular drugs

Cisapride was found not to affect serum **propranolol** levels nor the blood pressure control of 9 mildly hypertensive patients receiving a sustained-release **propranolol** preparation.[23] A woman developed near syncope and a prolonged QT interval while taking cisapride and **diltiazem**. The QT interval returned to normal and the symptoms did not recur when the cisapride was stopped. This interaction was attributed to the inhibitory effect of the **diltiazem** on the activity of the cytochrome P450 isoenzyme CYP3A4, an enzyme involved in the metabolism of cisapride, resulting in a rise in the cisapride plasma levels[24] (see also A above).

A study in 20 patients with mild to moderate hypertension found that 2.5 mg of cisapride caused some increase in the effects of sustained-release **nifedipine** 20 mg. The mean reduction in blood pressure due to the **nifedipine** at 1 hour was unchanged by the presence of the cisapride, but at 3 hours the **nifedipine** effects were approximately doubled. These changes reflected an increase in the serum levels of the **nifedipine** (more than doubled at 3 hours), probably caused by increased absorption as a result of increased gastrointestinal motility.[25]

Cisapride 10 mg three times a day reduced the **digoxin** AUC and the peak serum concentrations by 12 to 13% in 6 healthy subjects given a loading dose of **digoxin** followed by 250 micrograms twice daily.[26]

After taking cisapride 10 mg three times daily for 3 days, 11 healthy subjects were additionally given **simvastatin** 20 mg twice daily for 4 more days. The AUC of cisapride was increased by 14% and the plasma concentration of the active **simvastatin** metabolite was reduced by 33%. It was concluded that this interaction may result in cisapride toxicity and a blunted effect of **simvastatin**.[27]

See also (c) Anticholinergics above.

(g) Gastrointestinal drugs

Peak serum cisapride levels are increased by 45% by **cimetidine** (possibly due to enzyme inhibition) whereas the bioavailability of **cimetidine** is reduced by 18% by cisapride.[28] Cisapride enhances the absorption rate of **ranitidine**, but reduces the AUC by 26%.[29] However, the 25% increase in the bioavailability of cisapride caused by **ranitidine**[30] was not confirmed in another study,[29] but a case report attributed an increase in the QT interval in a 39-day old infant to the concurrent use of **ranitidine**.[31] The makers of cisapride say that the changed serum levels with these H_2-blockers is unlikely to be clinically significant.[10] The concurrent use of **aluminium oxide** and **magnesium hydroxide** was found in another study not to affect the absorption of cisapride.[32] Single 20-mg doses of cisapride were given to 16 healthy subjects either alone or 1 hour after the first of three 40-mg daily doses of **pantoprazole**. No QTc changes occurred, with or without **pantoprazole**, and the only pharmacokinetic changes were a 17% fall in the maximum cisapride concentrations and an 11% increase in clearance, possibly due to gastric hypochlorhydria caused by the **pantoprazole**.[33] A study in healthy subjects found that **esomeprazole** 40 mg increased the AUC of cisapride by 32% and prolonged the elimination half-life by 31%, but the maximum serum levels remained unaltered. No increase in the QTc interval was seen.[34]

(h) Miscellaneous

A schizophrenic patient on **bromperidol** showed marked deterioration within about 5 days of additionally taking cisapride. A retrospective study showed that the serum concentrations of the **bromperidol** and its reduced metabolite had been increased by cisapride. When the cisapride was stopped his mental state recovered within a week.[35]

After taking cisapride for 2 days, 10 renal transplant patients were found to have a 24% increase in maximal serum **ciclosporin** levels, and a 50 and 38% increase in 4- and 6-hour AUCs respectively. Peak serum levels also occurred earlier.[36]

Cisapride accelerates the absorption of **diazepam** so that its sedative effects occur more quickly and may possibly be transiently increased.[37] **Fluoxetine** 20 mg daily, given with cisapride did not affect the QT interval in 12 healthy subjects.[26,31,38,39]

Cisapride 30 mg daily for 28 days was given to 15 healthy subjects to find out if it induces or inhibits liver microsomal enzymes, using **antipyrine (phenazone)** as a marker or index drug. No changes in metabolism were found.[40]

1. Ahmad SR, Wolfe SM. Cisapride and torsades de pointes. *Lancet* (1995) 345, 508.
2. van Haarst AD, van't Klooster GEA, van Gerven JMA, Schoemaker RC, van Oene JC, Burggraaf J, Coene M-C, Cohen AF. The influence of cisapride and clarithromycin on QT intervals in healthy volunteers. *Clin Pharmacol Ther* (1998) 64, 542–6.
3. Sekkarie MA. Torsades de pointes in two chronic renal failure patients treated with cisapride and clarithromycin. *Am J Kidney Dis* (1997) 30, 437–9.
4. Gray VS. Syncopal episodes associated with cisapride and concurrent drugs. *Ann Pharmacother* (1998) 32, 648–51.
5. Janssen-Cilag Ltd. Dear Doctor letter, November 1995.
6. Janssen-Cilag UK Ltd. Confidential Report from Medical Information Department and Drug Safety Unit, December 18th 1995.
7. Jenkins IR, Gibson J. Cisapride, erythromycin and arrhythmia. *Anaesth Intensive Care* (1996) 24, 728.
8. Wysowski DK, Bacsanyi J. Cisapride and fatal arrhythmia. *N Engl J Med* (1996) 335, 290–1.
9. Janssen-Cilag Ltd. Personal communication, April 1995.
10. Prepulsid (Cisapride). Janssen Pharmaceuticals. ABPI Compendium of Datasheets and Summaries of Product Characteristics 1998–9, p 569.
11. Committee on Safety of Medicines/Medicines Control Agency. Cisapride (Prepulsid): Risk of arrhythmias. *Current Problems* (1998) 24, 11.

12. Janssen Pharmaceuticals. An evaluation of possible interactions between ethanol and cisapride. Data on file (Unpublished report, N 49087), 1986.
13. Roine R, Heikkonen E, Salaspuro M. Cisapride enhances alcohol absorption and leads to high blood alcohol levels. *Gastroenterology* (1992) 102, A507.
14. Dziekan G, Contesse J, Werth B, Schwarzer G, Reinhardt WH. Cisapride increases peak plasma and saliva ethanol levels under fasting conditions. *J Intern Med* (1997) 242, 479–82.
15. Kechagias S, Jönsson K-Å, Jones AW. Impact of gastric emptying on the pharmacokinetics of ethanol as influenced by cisapride. *Br J Clin Pharmacol* (1999) 48, 728–32.
16. Rowbotham DJ, Milligan K, McHugh P. Effect of cisapride on morphine absorption after oral administration of sustained-release morphine. *Br J Anaesth* (1991) 67, 421–5.
17. Rowbotham DJ, Parnacott S, Nimmo WS. No effect of cisapride on paracetamol absorption after oral simultaneous administration. *Eur J Clin Pharmacol* (1992) 42, 235–6.
18. Janssen Pharmacetica (Jonker JJC). Effect of cisapride on anticoagulant treatment with acenocoumarol. Data on file (Clinical Research Report, R 51619-NL), August 1985.
19. Wesemeyer D, Mönig H, Gaska T, Masuch S, Seiler KU, Huss H, Bruhn HD. Der Einfluß von Cisaprid und Metoclopramid auf die Bioverfügbarkeit von Phenprocoumon. *Hamostaseologie* (1991) 11, 95–102.
20. Daneshmend TK, Mahida YR, Bhaskar NK, Hawkey CJ. Does cisapride alter the anticoagulant effect of warfarin? A pharmacodynamic assessment. British Society of Gastroenterology Spring Meeting, 12–14 April 1989.
21. Darlington MR. Hypoprothrombinemia induced by warfarin sodium and cisapride. *Am J Health-Syst Pharm* (1997) 54, 320–1.
22. Roberts GW, Kowalski SR, Calabretto JP. Lack of effect of cisapride on phenytoin free fraction. *Ann Pharmacother* (1992) 26, 1016–17.
23. Janssen Pharmaceuticals. Effect of cisapride on the plasma concentrations of a delayed formulation of propranolol and on its clinical effects on blood pressure in mildly hypertensive patients. Data on file (Study R 51619/23-NL), 1986.
24. Thomas AR, Chan L-N, Bauman JL, Olopade CO. Prolongation of the QT interval related to cisapride-diltiazem interaction. *Pharmacotherapy* (1998) 18, 381–5.
25. Satoh C, Sakai T, Kashiwagi H, Hongo K, Aizawa O, Watanabe H, Mochizuki S, Okamura T. Influence of cisapride on the pharmacokinetics and antihypertensive effect of sustained-release nifedipine. *Int Med* (1996) 35, 941–5.
26. Kirch W, Janisch HD, Santos SR, Duhrsen U, Dylewicz P, Ohnhaus EE. Effect of cisapride and metoclopramide on digoxin bioavailability. *Eur J Drug Metab Pharmacokinet* (1986) 11, 249–50.
27. Simard C, O'Hara GE, Prévost J, Guilbaud R, Massé R, Turgeon J. Study of the drug-drug interaction between simvastatin and cisapride in man. *Eur J Clin Pharmacol* (2001) 57, 229–34.
28. Kirch W, Janisch HD, Ohnhaus EE, van Peer A. Cisapride-cimetidine interaction: enhanced cisapride bioavailability and accelerated cimetidine absorption. *Ther Drug Monit* (1989) 11, 411–14.
29. Milligan KA, McHugh P, Rowbotham DJ. Effects of concomitant administration of cisapride and ranitidine on plasma concentrations in volunteers. *Br J Anaesth* (1989) 63, 628P.
30. Janssen Pharmaceuticals. Cisapride-ranitidine interaction. Data on file (Study R 51 619/74), 1986.
31. Valdes L, Champel V, Olivier C, Jonville-Bera AP, Autret E. Malaise avec allongement de l'espace QT chez un nourrisson de 39 jours traité par cisapride. *Arch Pediatr* (1997) 4, 535–7.
32. Janssen Pharmaceuticals. Unaltered oral absorption of cisapride on coadministration of antacids. Data on file (Study R 51 619/69), 1986.
33. Ferron GM, Paul JC, Fruncillo RJ, Martin PT, Yacoub L, Mayer PR. Lack of pharmacokinetic interaction between oral pantoprazole and cisapride in healthy adults. *J Clin Pharmacol* (1999) 39, 945–50.
34. Nexium (Esomeprazole). AstraZeneca. UK Summary of product characteristics, October 2004.
35. Ishida M, Iotani K, Yasui N, Inoue Y, Kaneko S. Possible interaction between cisapride and bromperidol. *Prog Neuropsychopharmacol Biol Psychiatry* (1997) 21, 235–8.
36. Finet L, Westeel PF, Hary G, Maurel M, Andrejak M, Dupas JL. Effects of cisapride on the intestinal absorption of cyclosporine in renal transplant recipients. *Gastroenterology* (1991) 100, A209.
37. Bateman DN. The action of cisapride on gastric emptying and the pharmacodynamics and pharmacokinetics of oral diazepam. *Eur J Clin Pharmacol* (1986) 30, 205–8.
38. Kuroda T, Yoshihara Y, Nakamura H, Azumi T, Inatome T, Fukuzaki H, Takanashi H, Yogo K, Akima M. Effects of cisapride on gastrointestinal motor activity and gastric emptying of disopyramide. *J Pharmacobiodyn* (1992) 15, 395–402.
39. Zhao Q, Wojcik MA, Parier J-L, Pesco-Koplowitz L. Influence of coadministration of fluoxetine on cisapride pharmacokinetics and QTc intervals in healthy volunteers. *Pharmacotherapy* (2001) 21, 149–57.
40. Davies DS, Mills FJ, Welburn PJ. Cisapride has no effect on antipyrine clearance. *Br J Clin Pharmacol* (1988) 26, 808–9.

Enteral tube feeding + Aluminium compounds

Aluminium-containing antacids and sucralfate can interact with high-protein liquid enteral feeds within the oesophagus to produce an obstructive plug.

Clinical evidence

Three patients, who were being fed with a liquid high-protein nutrient (***Fresubin liquid***) through an enteral tube, developed an obstructing protein-aluminium-complex oesophageal plug when intermittently given an aluminium/magnesium hydroxide antacid (*Alucol-Gel*).[1]

Another report also describes blockage of a nasogastric tube in a patient treated with aluminium hydroxide (*Aludrox*) and ***Nutrison***.[2] Other reports similarly describe the development of hard putty-like or creamy precipitations and encrustations that can block the oesophagus or stomach of patients treated with **sucralfate**, and ***Ensure Plus***,[3] ***Fresubin plus F***[4] or ***Osmolite***.[5] Another patient developed this precipitate when treated with ***Isocal*** and **sucralfate** with aluminium/magnesium hydroxide.[6]

Mechanism

It seems that a bezoar (a relatively insoluble complex) forms between the protein in the enteral feeds, and the aluminium from the antacids or sucralfate (sucralfate is about 18% aluminium). It thickens when the pH falls.[3]

Importance and management

An established and clinically important interaction that can result in the blockage of enteral or nasogastric tubes. The authors of one report say that high molecular protein solutions should not be mixed with antacids or followed by antacids, and if an antacid is needed, it should be given some time after the nutrients and the tube should be vigorously flushed beforehand.[1]

The authors of another report say that they feed for 18 hours daily and then give the sucralfate overnight without problems.[2]

1. Valli C, Schulthess H-K, Asper R, Escher F, Häcki WH. Interaction of nutrients with antacids: a complication during enteral tube feeding. *Lancet* (1986) i, 747–8.
2. Tomlin ME, Dixon S. Aluminium and nasogastric feeds. *Pharm J* (1996) 256, 40.
3. Rowbottom SJ, Wilson J, Samuel L, Grant IS. Total oesophageal obstruction in association with combined enteral feed and sucralfate therapy. *Anaesth Intensive Care* (1993) 21, 372–4.
4. Vohra SB, Strang TI. Sucralfate therapy - a caution. *Br J Intensive Care* (1994) 4, 114.
5. Anderson W. Esophageal medication bezoar in a patient receiving enteral feedings and sucralfate. *Am J Gastroenterol* (1989) 84, 205–6.
6. Algozzine GJ, Hill G, Scoggins WG, Marr MA. Sucralfate bezoar. *N Engl J Med* (1983) 309, 1387.

Famotidine + Probenecid

Serum famotidine levels are markedly increased by probenecid, but toxicity is not expected.

Clinical evidence, mechanism, importance and management

Probenecid 1500 mg increased the AUC of a single 20-mg dose of famotidine in 8 healthy subjects by 81%, and reduced the clearance by tubular secretion by 89%.[1] The reason appears to be that probenecid inhibits the renal secretion of famotidine, thereby reducing its loss from the body, which is consistent with the way that it affects some other drugs. The famotidine effects would be expected to be increased, but dose-related toxicity arising from this interaction seems unlikely. There would seem to be no reason for avoiding concurrent use. Other H_2-blockers may behave similarly.

1. Inotsume N, Nishimura M, Nakano M, Fujiyama S, Sato T. The inhibitory effect of probenecid on renal excretion of famotidine in young, healthy volunteers. *J Clin Pharmacol* (1990) 30, 50–56.

H_2-blockers + Antacids

The absorption of cimetidine, famotidine, nizatidine, and ranitidine may possibly be reduced to some extent by antacids, but it seems doubtful if this significantly reduces their ulcer-healing effects. Separating the dosages by 1 to 2 hours minimises any interaction. Roxatidine appears not to be affected. Cimetidine appears not to interfere with the effectiveness of *Gaviscon* (sodium alginate compound).

Clinical evidence

(a) Cimetidine

When 12 healthy subjects were given oral cimetidine 300 mg four times daily, with and without 30 ml of *Mylanta II* (**aluminium/magnesium hydroxide** mixture), the absorption of cimetidine was unaffected.[1] No interaction was found in other studies using **aluminium phosphate**[2-4] or **aluminium/magnesium hydroxide**[5] antacids.

In contrast, a number of single dose studies indicated that antacids reduce the absorption of cimetidine. The AUCs of 200- to 800-mg doses of cimetidine were reduced by an average of 19 to 34% by 10 to 45 ml doses of a variety of **aluminium/magnesium** containing antacids.[6-10] When the antacids were given 1 to 3 hours after cimetidine 'marginal' or insignificant reductions occurred in the AUCs.[7,11,12]

Gaviscon (**sodium alginate/antacid**) is an anti-reflux preparation that needs a small amount of gastric acid to be present in order for the alginic acid 'raft' to form. A study in 12 healthy subjects to find out if an

H_2-blocker would alter the effectiveness of *Liquid Gaviscon* showed that 400 mg cimetidine four times daily for 7 days caused some slight changes in gastric emptying, but the distribution of the *Gaviscon* in the fundus of the stomach was not altered.[13]

(b) Famotidine

Mylanta II (**aluminium/magnesium hydroxide** mixture) 30 ml reduced the AUC and peak serum levels of famotidine by about a third when taken simultaneously, but no significant interaction occurred when the antacid was taken 2 hours after famotidine.[14] Another study found that the peak serum levels of famotidine were reduced by about 25% by *Mylanta II* in 17 healthy subjects.[15]

In contrast, *Mylanta Double Strength* (**aluminium/magnesium hydroxide** with **simeticone**) was found to reduce the absorption of famotidine by 19%, a difference that was considered unimportant.[10] Two chewable tablets of *Mylanta II* were found to have no effect on the pharmacokinetics or pharmacodynamics of 10 or 20 mg famotidine in 18 healthy subjects.[16]

(c) Nizatidine

Mylanta Double Strength (**aluminium/magnesium hydroxide** with **simeticone**) reduced the absorption of nizatidine by 12%, which was considered clinically insignificant.[10]

(d) Ranitidine

Mylanta II (**aluminium/magnesium hydroxide** mixture) 30 ml reduced the peak ranitidine serum levels and the AUC after a single 150-mg dose by about one-third in 6 healthy subjects.[17] *Mylanta Double Strength* (**aluminium/magnesium hydroxide** with **simeticone**) reduced the absorption of ranitidine by 26%, which was not thought to be clinically significant.[10] Reductions of up to 59% were found in another study.[9] Yet another study showed that **aluminium phosphate** reduced the bioavailability of ranitidine by 30%.[4]

(e) Roxatidine

In an open-label crossover study, 24 healthy subjects were given roxatidine 150 mg with 10 ml of *Maalox* (**aluminium/magnesium hydroxide**) four times daily. The pharmacokinetics of roxatidine were unchanged, apart from a clinically insignificant lengthening of the half-life.[18]

Mechanism

Not fully understood. Changes in gastric pH caused by the antacid, and retarded gastric motility have been suggested as potential mechanisms.

Importance and management

A modest reduction in the bioavailability of cimetidine, famotidine, nizatidine and ranitidine can occur with some antacids, but none of these interactions is well established, and evidence that the ulcer-healing effects are reduced seems to be lacking. If the antacids are given 1 to 2 hours before or after the H_2-blocker (if fasting), or 1 hour after (if the blocker is taken with food), no reduction in absorption should occur.[7,14,15,19] Preliminary evidence suggests that roxatidine is unaffected, and it seems likely that this will be also be true for other H_2-blockers. The action of *Gaviscon* (sodium alginate) does not appear to be compromised by cimetidine.[13]

1. Shelly DW, Doering PL, Russell WL, Guild RT, Lopez LM, Perrin J. Effect of concomitant antacid administration on plasma cimetidine concentrations during repetitive dosing. *Drug Intell Clin Pharm* (1986) 20, 792–5.
2. Albin H, Vinçon G, Pehoucq F, Dangoumau J. Influence d'un antacide sur la biodisponibilité de la cimétidine. *Therapie* (1982) 37, 563–6.
3. Albin H, Vinçon G, Demotes-Mainard F, Begaud B, Bedjaoui A. Effect of aluminium phosphate on the bioavailability of cimetidine and prednisolone. *Eur J Clin Pharmacol* (1984) 26, 271–3.
4. Albin H, Vinçon G, Begaud B, Bistue C, Perez P. Effect of aluminum phosphate on the bioavailability of ranitidine. *Eur J Clin Pharmacol* (1987) 32, 97–99.
5. Burland WL, Darkin DW, Mills MW. Effect of antacids on absorption of cimetidine. *Lancet* (1976) ii, 965.
6. Bodemar G, Norlander B, Walan A. Diminished absorption of cimetidine caused by antacids. *Lancet* (1979) i, 444–5.
7. Steinberg WM, Lewis JH, Katz DM. Antacids inhibit absorption of cimetidine. *N Engl J Med* (1982) 307, 400–4.
8. Gugler R, Brand M, Somogyi A. Impaired cimetidine absorption due to antacids and metoclopramide. *Eur J Clin Pharmacol* (1981) 20, 225–8.
9. Desmond PV, Harman PJ, Gannoulis N, Kamm M, Mashford ML. The effect of an antacid and food on the absorption of cimetidine and ranitidine. *J Pharm Pharmacol* (1990) 42, 352–4.
10. Sullivan TJ, Reese JH, Jauregui L, Miller K, Levine L, Bachmann KA. Short report: a comparative study of the interaction between antacid and H_2-receptor antagonists. *Aliment Pharmacol Ther* (1994) 8, 123–6.
11. Russell WL, Lopez LM, Normann SA, Doering PL, Guild RT. Effect of antacids on predicted steady-state cimetidine concentrations. *Dig Dis Sci* (1984) 29, 385–9.
12. Barzaghi N, Crema F, Mescoli G, Perucca E. Effects on cimetidine bioavailability of metoclopramide and antacids given two hours apart. *Eur J Clin Pharmacol* (1989) 37, 409–10.
13. Washington N, Wilson CG, Williams DL, Robertson C. An investigation into the effect of cimetidine pre-treatment on raft formation of an anti-reflux agent. *Aliment Pharmacol Ther* (1993) 7, 553–9.
14. Barzaghi N, Gatti G, Crema F, Perucca E. Impaired bioavailability of famotidine given concurrently with a potent antacid. *J Clin Pharmacol* (1989) 29, 670–2.
15. Tupy-Visich MA, Tarzian SK, Schwartz S, Lin JH, Hessey GA, Kanovsky SM, Chremos AN. Bioavailability of oral famotidine when administered with antacid or food. *J Clin Pharmacol* (1986) 26, 555.
16. Schwartz JI, Yeh KC, Bolognese J, Laskin OL, Patterson PM, Shamblen EC, Han R, Lasseter KC. Lack of effect of chewable antacid on famotidine pharmacodynamics and pharmacokinetics. *Pharmacotherapy* (1994) 14, 375.
17. Mihaly GW, Marino AT, Webster LK, Jones DB, Louis WJ, Smallwood RA. High dose of antacid (Mylanta II) reduces the bioavailability of ranitidine. *BMJ* (1982) 285, 998–9.
18. Labs RA. Interaction of roxatidine acetate with antacids, food and other drugs. *Drugs* (1988) 35 (Suppl 3), 82–9.
19. Frislid K, Berstad A. High dose of antacid reduces bioavailability of ranitidine. *BMJ* (1983) 286, 1358.

H_2-blockers + Nicotine or Tobacco smoking

Smoking reduces the plasma levels of cimetidine and ranitidine, but does not appear to affect famotidine. Cimetidine, and to a lesser extent ranitidine, reduce the clearance of nicotine from the body.

Clinical evidence, mechanism, importance and management

(a) Nicotine

Cimetidine 600 mg twice daily for a day, prior to giving nicotine, reduced the clearance of nicotine (1 microgram/kg/minute given intravenously for 30 minutes) in 6 healthy subjects by 27 to 30%. **Ranitidine** 300 mg twice daily, for a day prior to nicotine reduced the clearance of nicotine by about 7 to 10%.[1]

The clinical significance of these finding is unclear, but those taking nicotine, either from smoking or nicotine replacement therapy may find its effects enhanced in the presence of cimetidine, ranitidine and possibly other H_2-blockers.

(b) Tobacco smoking

The healing of duodenal ulcers in patients on H_2-blockers such as **cimetidine**,[2,3] **famotidine**,[4] **nizatidine**[5] and **ranitidine**[3,4] is slower, and recurrence is more common in smokers than in non-smokers. One of the possible reasons is that smoking reduces the plasma levels of these drugs after peak levels are achieved, although peak levels occur sooner and are higher.[6] However, smoking does not appear to affect the pharmacokinetics of **famotidine** significantly.[7] It is quite possible that this is due to smoking being a risk factor for the occurrence of duodenal ulcers[2,4,5,8] rather than an interaction between smoking and H_2-blockers.

1. Bendayan R, Sullivan JT, Shaw C, Frecker RC, Sellers EM. Effect of cimetidine and ranitidine on the hepatic and renal elimination of nicotine in humans. *Eur J Clin Pharmacol* (1990) 38, 165–9.
2. Hetzel DJ, Korman MG, Hansky J, Shearman DJ, Eaves ER, Schmidt GT, Hecker R, Fitch RJ. The influence of smoking on the healing of duodenal ulcer treated with oxmetidine or cimetidine. *Aust N Z J Med* (1983) 13, 587–90.
3. Korman MG, Hansky J, Merrett AC, Schmidt GT. Ranitidine in duodenal ulcer: incidence of healing and effect of smoking. *Dig Dis Sci* (1982) 27, 712–15.
4. Reynolds JC, Schoen RE, Maislin G, Zangari GG. Risk factors for delayed healing of duodenal ulcers treated with famotidine and ranitidine. *Am J Gastroenterol* (1994) 89, 571–80.
5. Battaglia G. Risk factors of relapse in gastric ulcer: a one-year, double-blind comparative study of nizatidine versus placebo. *Ital J Gastroenterol* (1994) 26 (1 Suppl 1), 19–22.
6. Boyd EJS, Johnston DA, Wormsley KG, Jenner WN, Salanson X. The effects of cigarette smoking on plasma concentrations of gastric antisecretory drugs. *Aliment Pharmacol Ther* (1987) 1, 57–65.
7. Baak LC, Ganesh S, Jansen JBMJ, Lamers CBHW. Does smoking influence the pharmacokinetics and pharmacodynamics of the H_2-receptor antagonist famotidine. *Br J Clin Pharmacol* (1992) 33, 193–6.
8. Boyd EJS, Wilson JA, Wormsley KG. Smoking impairs therapeutic gastric inhibition. *Lancet* (1983) i, 95–7.

H_2-blockers + Sucralfate

Sucralfate normally appears not to affect the bioavailability of cimetidine, ranitidine or roxatidine, or only to reduce it moderately.

Clinical evidence, mechanism, importance and management

Most *in vitro* and human studies show that sucralfate does not affect the absorption of either **cimetidine**,[1-3] **ranitidine**,[4] or **roxatidine**,[5] but two studies found 22 to 29% reductions in **ranitidine** bioavailability due to concurrent use of sucralfate.[6,7] There is no clear reason for avoiding concurrent use.

1. Albin H, Vincon G, Lalague MC, Couzigou P, Amouretti M. Effect of sucralfate on the bioavailability of cimetidine. *Eur J Clin Pharmacol* (1986) 30, 493–4.
2. D'Angio R, Mayersohn M, Conrad KA, Bliss M. Cimetidine absorption in humans during sucralfate coadministration. *Br J Clin Pharmacol* (1986) 21, 515–20.
3. Beck CL, Dietz AJ, Carlson JD, Letendre PW. Evaluation of potential cimetidine sucralfate interaction. *Clin Pharmacol Ther* (1987) 41, 168.
4. Mullersman G, Gotz VP, Russell WL, Derendorf H. Lack of clinically significant in vitro and in vivo interactions between ranitidine and sucralfate. *J Pharm Sci* (1986) 75, 995–8.
5. Seibert-Grafe M, Pidgen A. Lack of effect of multiple dose sucralfate on the pharmacokinetics of roxatidine acetate. *Eur J Clin Pharmacol* (1991) 40, 637–8.
6. Maconochie JG, Thomas M, Michael MF, Jenner WR, Tanner RJN. Ranitidine sucralfate interaction study. *Clin Pharmacol Ther* (1987) 41, 205.
7. Kimura K, Sakai H, Yoshida Y, Kasano T, Hirose M. Effects of concomitant drugs on the blood concentration of a histamine H_2 antagonist (the 2nd report) - concomitant or time lag administration of ranitidine and sucralfate. *Nippon Shokakibyo Gakkai Zasshi* (1986) 83, 603–7.

Loperamide + Colestyramine

An isolated report, supported by an *in vitro* study, indicates that the effects of loperamide can be reduced by colestyramine.

Clinical evidence, mechanism, importance and management

A man who had undergone extensive surgery to the gut, with the creation of an ileostomy, needed treatment for excessive fluid loss. His fluid loss was observed to be "substantially less" (not precisely quantified) when given loperamide 2 mg six-hourly alone, than when loperamide was given in combination with colestyramine 2 g four-hourly.[1] The probable reason is that the colestyramine binds to the loperamide in the gut, thereby reducing its activity. An *in vitro* study using 50 ml of simulated gastric fluid showed that 64% of a 5.5-mg dose of loperamide was bound by 4 g of colestyramine.[1] Direct information is limited to this report, but what occurred is consistent with the way colestyramine interacts with other drugs. It has been suggested that the two drugs should be separated as much as possible to prevent mixing in the gut, or that the loperamide dosage should be increased.[1] It is a standard recommendation that other drugs should be avoided for 1 hour before and 4 to 6 hours after colestyramine.

1. Ti TY, Giles HG, Sellers EM. Probable interaction of loperamide and cholestyramine. *Can Med Assoc J* (1978) 119, 607–8.

Loperamide + Co-trimoxazole

Co-trimoxazole increases the plasma levels of loperamide, but no additional side-effects are seen.

Clinical evidence, mechanism, importance and management

Co-trimoxazole 960 mg twice daily was given to healthy subjects for 24 hours before and then 48 hours after taking a single 4-mg dose of loperamide (12 subjects) or loperamide oxide (a prodrug of loperamide, 10 subjects). The co-trimoxazole increased the loperamide AUC by 89% and doubled the maximum plasma levels. The loperamide oxide AUC was raised by 54% and the maximum plasma levels by 41%. It is thought that co-trimoxazole inhibits the metabolism of loperamide, possibly by reducing first pass metabolism.[1] However, despite these rises, and because loperamide has a very wide margin of safety it is thought unlikely that any dosage changes are needed.

1. Kamali F, Huang ML. Increased systemic availability of loperamide after oral administration of loperamide and loperamide oxide with cotrimoxazole. *Br J Clin Pharmacol* (1996) 41, 125–8.

Loperamide + Ritonavir

Ritonavir increases the plasma levels of loperamide, but no additional side-effects are seen.

Clinical evidence, mechanism, importance and management

In a double-blind placebo-controlled trial, 12 healthy subjects were given a single 600-mg dose of ritonavir with either loperamide 16 mg or placebo. The loperamide AUC was increased threefold and the maximum serum level by 17% by ritonavir, but no additional CNS side effects were seen. The pharmacokinetic effects were thought to be due to ritonavir inhibiting the cytochrome P450 isoenzyme CYP3A4, an enzyme involved in the metabolism of loperamide.[1] The absence of changes in pupil diameter, pain threshold and no significant difference in adverse effects suggests the combination is safe, and there is also the possibility that loperamide in reduced doses will be an effective antidiarrhoeal in the presence of ritonavir.[1]

1. Tayrouz Y, Ganssmann B, Ding R, Klingmann A, Aderjan R, Burhenne J, Haefeli WE, Mikus G. Ritonavir increases loperamide plasma concentrations without evidence for P-glycoprotein involvement. *Clin Pharmacol Ther* (2001) 70, 405–14.

Mesalazine (Mesalamine) + Ispaghula, Lactitol or Lactulose

On theoretical grounds, formulations designed to release mesalazine in response to the higher pH in the colon, should not be given with lactulose, lactitol or other preparations that lower the colonic pH. However ispaghula, which also lowers the pH in the colon, appears not to affect the bioavailability of mesalazine.

Clinical evidence, mechanism, importance and management

Asacol is a preparation of mesalazine (mesalamine) coated with an acrylic based resin (*Eudragit S*) that disintegrates above pH 7 and thereby releases the mesalazine into the terminal ileum and colon. Since the disintegration depends upon this alkaline pH, the makers of ***Asacol*** say that the concurrent use of preparations that lower the pH in the lower part of the gut should be avoided.[1] ***Salofalk*** is another preparation of mesalazine with a pH-dependent enteric coating. The question is, do any of the preparations that lower colonic pH actually interact with ***Asacol*** and ***Salofalk*** in practice?

The pH in the colon can be lowered by **lactulose** and **lactitol**, which are metabolised by gut bacteria to a number of acids (e.g. acetic, butyric, propionic, lactic).[2] In healthy subjects **lactulose** (30 to 80 g daily) has been found to cause slight falls in colonic pH;[2,3] in the right colon from about 6 to 5, and in the left colon from 7 to 6.7. **Lactitol** (40 to 180 g daily) can cause similar falls in pH.[2] **Ispaghula** can also lower colonic pH (from 6.5 to 5.8 in the right colon, and from 7.3 to 6.6 in the left colon).[4] However, a study in patients given mesalazine found that despite this colonic acidification by **ispaghula husk** (*Fybogel*), the release of mesalazine appeared not to be affected, as 24-hour faecal and urinary excretion of mesalazine metabolites were unchanged.[5]

Thus, although on theoretical grounds **ispaghula husk** would be expected to reduce the effects of mesalazine, no interaction of clinical importance seems to occur, and nobody as yet has shown that a clinically important interaction actually occurs with either **lactulose** or **lactitol**. More study is needed to find out whether these predicted but theoretical interactions are important or not.

1. Asacol (Mesalzine). Procter & Gamble Pharmaceuticals UK Ltd. UK Summary of product characteristics, April 2003.
2. Patil DH, Westaby D, Mahida YR, Palmer KR, Rees R, Clark ML, Dawson AM, Silk DBA. Comparative modes of action of lactitol and lactulose in the treatment of hepatic encephalopathy. *Gut* (1987) 28, 255–9.
3. Brown RL, Gibson JA, Sladen GE, Hicks B, Dawson AM. Effects of lactulose and other laxatives on ileal and colonic pH as measured by a radiotelemetry device. *Gut* (1974) 15, 999–1004.
4. Evans DF, Crompton J, Pye G, Hardcastle JD. The role of dietary fibre on acidification of the colon in man. *Gastroenterology* (1988) 94, A118.
5. Riley SA, Tavares IA, Bishai PM, Bennett A, Mani V. Mesalazine release from coated tablets: effect of dietary fibre. *Br J Clin Pharmacol* (1991) 32, 248–50.

Mesalazine (Mesalamine) + Proton pump inhibitors

Omeprazole does not affect the release of mesalazine from a delayed-release preparation (*Asacol*).

Clinical evidence, mechanism, importance and management

Asacol is a preparation of mesalazine (mesalamine) coated with an acrylic based resin (*Eudragit S*) that disintegrates above pH 7 and thereby releases the mesalazine into the terminal ileum and colon. The release is rapid at pH values of 7 and above, but it can also occur between pH 6 and 7. Since the proton pump inhibitors can raise the pH in the stomach to 6 and above, the potential exists for the premature release of mesalazine from *Asacol*.

However, a study in 6 healthy subjects given *Asacol* 400 mg three times daily for 3 weeks found that when they were also given omeprazole 20 mg daily during the second week, and omeprazole 40 mg daily during the third week, the steady-state pharmacokinetics of the mesalazine remained unchanged.[1] Had mesalazine been released earlier, the absorption characteristics would have changed. There would therefore appear to be no reason for avoiding the concurrent use of *Asacol* and omeprazole, and, on the basis of this study, it seems likely that other proton pump inhibitors will behave similarly. This needs confirmation.

1. Hussain FN, Ajjan RA, Moustafa M, Weir NW, Riley SA. Mesalazine release from a pH dependent formulation: effects of omeprazole and lactulose co-administration. *Br J Clin Pharmacol* (1998) 46, 173–5.

Omeprazole + Artemisinin

Artemisinin increases the metabolism of omeprazole, but the clinical significance of this is unclear.

Clinical evidence, mechanism, importance and management

A study in 9 healthy subjects found that the AUC of a single 20-mg dose of omeprazole was reduced by 35% by artemisinin 250 mg twice daily for 7 days. The pharmacokinetics of the omeprazole metabolites were unchanged, but the ratio of hydroxyomeprazole/omeprazole increased 2.2-fold in those with high levels of the cytochrome P450 isoenzyme CYP2C19 (extensive metabolisers). This suggests that artemisinin affects the pharmacokinetics of omeprazole by inducing the production of CYP2C19, an enzyme involved in its metabolism, although other isoenzymes may also be involved. Single 250-mg doses of artemisinin had no effect on the pharmacokinetics of omeprazole, which supports the proposed mechanism of enzyme induction.[1] The clinical significance of this interaction is unclear.

1. Svensson USH, Ashton M, Hai TN, Bertilsson L, Huong DX, Huong NV, Niêu NT, Sy ND, Lykkesfeldt J, Công LD. Artemisinin induces omeprazole metabolism in human beings. *Clin Pharmacol Ther* (1998) 64, 160–67.

Omeprazole + Disulfiram

An isolated case describes a catatonic reaction in a patient given omeprazole and disulfiram.

Clinical evidence, mechanism, importance and management

A patient on omeprazole 40 mg daily for 7 months was additionally given disulfiram 500 mg daily. Six days later he gradually developed confusion, which progressed into a catatonic state with muscle rigidity and trismus after 15 days. Both drugs were withdrawn and he gradually recovered. Some months later while taking disulfiram 250 mg daily, he again developed confusion, disorientation and nightmares within 72 hours of starting to take omeprazole 40 mg each morning. Again he recovered when both drugs were stopped.[1] The reason for this reaction is not understood, but the authors of the report postulate that the omeprazole may have allowed the accumulation of one of the metabolites of disulfiram, carbon disulphide, which could have been responsible for the toxic effects.[1]

This is the first and only report of a possible interaction between omeprazole and disulfiram. Other patients given both drugs are said not to have shown adverse effects.[2] The general importance of this adverse interaction is therefore uncertain, but it would now seem prudent to monitor concurrent use for any evidence of this toxicity.

1. Hajela R, Cunningham G M, Kapur B M, Peachey J E, Devenyi P. Catatonic reaction to omeprazole and disulfiram in a patient with alcohol dependence. *Can Med Assoc J* (1990) 143, 1207–8.
2. Astra Pharmaceuticals. Personal communication, 1991.

Omeprazole + SSRIs

Fluvoxamine inhibits the metabolism of omeprazole to 5-hydroxyomeprazole. Theoretically escitalopram may have the same effect. Omeprazole may increase escitalopram levels.

Clinical evidence, mechanism, importance and management

(a) Escitalopram

Although no studies appear to have been conducted, the UK maker predicts that because escitalopram and omeprazole are metabolised by the cytochrome P450 isoenzyme CYP2C19, and are mild inhibitors of CYP2C19, concurrent use may result in elevated levels of both drugs. The clinical significance of this prediction is unclear.[1]

(b) Fluvoxamine

A study in 12 healthy subjects given fluvoxamine 10 to 50 mg daily for 7 days, with a single 20-mg dose of omeprazole on day 7, found that the AUC of omeprazole was increased by 174% with fluvoxamine 10 to 20 mg and by 330% with fluvoxamine 25 to 50 mg. Fluvoxamine inhibits the metabolism of omeprazole to 5-hydroxyomeprazole by the cytochrome P450 isoenzyme CYP2C19. The clinical significance of the omeprazole/fluvoxamine interaction is not known, but the study highlights the risk of an interaction if fluvoxamine is given with drugs metabolised by CYP2C19.[2]

1. Cipralex (Escitalopram). Lundbeck Ltd. UK Summary of product characteristics, March 2004.
2. Christensen M, Tybring G, Mihara K, Yasui-Furokori N, Carrillo JA, Ramos SI, Andersson K, Dahl M-L, Bertilsson L. Low daily 10-mg and 20-mg doses of fluvoxamine inhibit the metabolism of both caffeine (cytochrome P4501A2) and omeprazole (cytochrome P4502C19). *Clin Pharmacol Ther* (2002) 71, 141–52.

Pirenzepine + Antacids

***Mylanta* reduces the bioavailability of pirenzepine by about 30%. Another antacid, *Trigastril*, modestly increases the bioavailability of pirenzepine, but these changes are probably of little clinical importance.**

Clinical evidence, mechanism, importance and management

The AUC of a single 50-mg dose of pirenzepine was reduced by about 30% in 20 healthy subjects when pirenzepine was taken with 30 ml of *Mylanta* (**aluminium/magnesium hydroxide** and **simethicone**). The **antacid** reduced the peak plasma levels of pirenzepine by about 45%.[1] Another study found that the AUC of a single 50-mg dose of pirenzepine was increased by almost 25% in 10 healthy subjects by 10 ml of an **antacid** (*Trigastril,* **aluminium/magnesium hydroxide**, **calcium carbonate**).[2] In practical terms these modest changes in bioavailability are probably too small to matter.

1. Matzek KM, MacGregor TR, Keirns JJ, Vinocur M. Effect of food and antacids on the oral absorption of pirenzepine in man. *Int J Pharmaceutics* (1986) 28, 151–5.
2. Vergin H, Herrlinger C, Gugler R. Effect of an aluminium-hydroxide containing antacid on the oral bioavailability of pirenzepine. *Arzneimittelforschung* (1989) 39, 520–3.

Pirenzepine + Cimetidine

Pirenzepine and cimetidine appear to interact together, possibly advantageously.

Clinical evidence, mechanism, importance and management

The pharmacokinetics of pirenzepine and cimetidine are not affected by the presence of the other drug, but pirenzepine increases the cimetidine-induced reduction in gastric acid secretion, which is an apparently advantageous interaction.[1]

1. Jamali F, Mahachai V, Reilly PA, Thomson ABR. Lack of pharmacokinetic interaction between cimetidine and pirenzepine. *Clin Pharmacol Ther* (1985) 38, 325–30.

Pirenzepine + Food

Food reduces the bioavailability of pirenzepine by about 30%, but this is probably of little clinical importance.

Clinical evidence, mechanism, importance and management

The AUC of a single 50-mg dose of pirenzepine was reduced by about 30% in 20 healthy subjects when pirenzepine was taken half-an-hour before food, or with food. Peak plasma levels were reduced by about 30%

and 45% respectively. The time to achieve peak levels was also reduced.[1] In practical terms this modest change in bioavailability is probably too small to matter, and in fact the makers suggest that pirenzepine should be taken half-an-hour before meals with a little fluid. The authors of this report also suggest taking it with food because compliance is better if associated with a convenient daily ritual.[1]

1. Matzek KM, MacGregor TR, Keirns JJ, Vinocur M. Effect of food and antacids on the oral absorption of pirenzepine in man. *Int J Pharmaceutics* (1986) 28, 151–5.

Proton pump inhibitors + Antacids

Pantoprazole, rabeprazole and omeprazole appear not to interact to a clinically relevant extent with *Maalox*. Antacids may cause a slight reduction in the bioavailability of lansoprazole. This is probably not clinically relevant but can be accommodated by separating their administration.

Clinical evidence, mechanism, importance and management

(a) Lansoprazole

Maalox (**aluminium/magnesium hydroxide**) 30 ml slightly reduced the AUC of a 30-mg dose of lansoprazole in a group of 12 healthy subjects by 13% (not statistically significant), and reduced the maximum plasma level by 27%. However, no changes were seen when the lansoprazole was given 1 hour after the antacid.[1] Note that in this study, the bioavailability of lansoprazole was highly variable between subjects (the AUC varied by a factor of 6), and the effect of food was greater than the effect of the antacid (see also 'Proton pump inhibitors + Food' p.739). In another study, **magaldrate** had no effect on the AUC of lansoprazole, and slightly reduced the maximum level (by 28%), but this change was not considered clinically relevant.[2] Nevertheless, the maker recommends that antacids should not be taken within an hour of lansoprazole,[3] but this seems to be an overcautious recommendation.

(b) Omeprazole

Two studies have shown that **antacids** (such as *Maalox* - **aluminium/magnesium hydroxide**) do not affect the absorption or disposition of omeprazole.[4,5] No special precautions are necessary.

(c) Pantoprazole

Pantoprazole 40 mg daily was given to 24 healthy subjects with and without 10 ml of *Maalox* (**aluminium/magnesium hydroxide**). The AUC, maximum serum levels, and the half-life of the pantoprazole were unchanged by the antacid.[6] No special precautions would seem to be necessary if pantoprazole and *Maalox* are given concurrently.

(d) Rabeprazole

In a single-dose study, 12 healthy subjects were, on separate occasions, given 20 mg of rabeprazole with, without, and 1-hour after a dose of **aluminium/magnesium hydroxide** antacid (*Maalox*).[7] The antacid had no effect on the pharmacokinetics of rabeprazole, so no special precautions would seem necessary on concurrent use.

1. Delhotal-Landes B, Cournot A, Vermerie N, Dellatolas F, Benoit M, Flouvat B. The effect of food and antacids on lansoprazole absorption and disposition. *Eur J Drug Metab Pharmacokinet* (1991), Spec No 3, 315–20.
2. Gerloff J, Barth H, Mignot A, Fuchs W, Heintze K. Does the proton pump inhibitor lansoprazole interact with antacids? *Naunyn Schmiedebergs Arch Pharmacol* (1993) 347, R31.
3. Zoton capsules (Lansoprazole). Wyeth Pharmaceuticals. UK Summary of product characteristics, September 2001.
4. Tuynman HARE, Festern HPM, Röhss K, Meuwissen SGM. Lack of effect of antacids on plasma concentrations of omeprazole given as enteric-coated granules. *Br J Clin Pharmacol* (1987) 24, 833–5.
5. Howden CW, Reid JL. The effect of antacids and metoclopramide on omeprazole absorption and disposition. *Br J Clin Pharmacol* (1988) 25, 779–80.
6. Hartmann M, Bliesath H, Huber R, Koch H, Steinijans VW, Wurst W. Lack of influence of antacids on the pharmacokinetics of the new gastric H+/K+-ATPase inhibitor pantoprazole. *Gastroenterology* (1994) 106 (Suppl), A91.
7. Yasuda S, Higashi S, Murakami M, Tomono Y, Kawaguchi M. Antacids have no influence on the pharmacokinetics of rabeprazole, a new proton pump inhibitor, in healthy volunteers. *Int J Clin Pharmacol Ther* (1999) 37, 249–53.

Proton pump inhibitors + Antibacterials

Clarithromycin almost doubles the serum levels of omeprazole and esomeprazole. A small rise in the serum levels of clarithromycin also occurs, which may be therapeutically useful. Some very limited evidence indicates that erythromycin causes a larger rise in serum omeprazole levels, without improving the gastric acid lowering effect. Roxithromycin does not appear to interact with lansoprazole or omeprazole.

Omeprazole has no effect on the plasma pharmacokinetics of oral or intravenous metronidazole.

Glossitis, stomatitis and/or black tongue developed rapidly in a small number of patients when treated with lansoprazole and antibacterials, which included amoxicillin, clarithromycin and metronidazole.

Omeprazole has no clinically important effect on the pharmacokinetics of ciprofloxacin, gemifloxacin, lomefloxacin, ofloxacin or trovafloxacin.

Clinical evidence, mechanism, importance and management

(a) Macrolides

(i) Clarithromycin. When 11 healthy subjects taking **omeprazole** 40 mg daily were also given clarithromycin 500 mg every 8 hours for 5 days, the maximum serum **omeprazole** levels rose by 30% and the 24-hour AUC rose by 89%, but the effect of **omeprazole** on gastric pH was unchanged. The maximum serum clarithromycin levels rose by 11% (from 3.8 to 4.2 micrograms/ml) and the 8-hour AUC by 15%.[1] In a similar study, approximately twofold increases in the AUC of **omeprazole** were reported.[2] Similarly, the maker notes that clarithromycin 500 mg twice daily doubled the AUC of **esomeprazole** (the *S*-isomer of **omeprazole**).[3] It is believed that clarithromycin inhibits the metabolism of **omeprazole**[1,2] and **esomeprazole**[3] by inhibiting the cytochrome P450 isoenzyme CYP3A4, an enzyme involved in their metabolism. None of the changes reported represent an adverse interaction, but they may help to explain why concurrent use is valuable in the eradication of *Helicobacter pylori* (a fact that the makers point out for **omeprazole**[4]). For mention of 6 cases of black tongue occurring with **lansoprazole** and antibacterials regimens including clarithromycin, see (c) penicillins below.

(ii) Erythromycin. A study was undertaken in a patient to confirm the *in vitro* findings that erythromycin inhibits the metabolism of **omeprazole**. After taking 500 mg of erythromycin base and 20 mg of **omeprazole** daily for 8 weeks, it was found that the AUC of **omeprazole** was increased almost fourfold, and the metabolite of **omeprazole** was undetectable. These raised **omeprazole** levels might have been expected to increase its effectiveness, but in this patient the time during which gastric pH was less than 4 decreased by 22%.[5] What is not clear is whether any of these changes are clinically important.

(iii) Roxithromycin. A study of roxithromycin 300 mg twice daily, alone, with **omeprazole** 20 mg twice daily or with **lansoprazole** 30 mg twice daily, for 6 days found no significant pharmacokinetic differences between any of the 3 regimens.[6] Therefore no precautions would seem necessary if these drugs are taken together.

(b) Metronidazole

The plasma pharmacokinetics of a single oral dose of metronidazole were unaffected by 5 days pre-treatment with **omeprazole** 20 mg twice daily in 14 healthy subjects.[7] Similar results were found in another study with oral and intravenous metronidazole, but when the gastric juice was further studied it was found that the transfer of metronidazole into the gastric juice following an intravenous dose dropped from 15.5 to 2.6% in the presence of **omeprazole**.[8] The significance of these findings is unclear, but the clinical relevance seems small. For mention of 3 cases of black tongue occurring with **lansoprazole** and antibacterials regimens including metronidazole, see (c) penicillins below.

(c) Penicillins

The reduction in gastric pH produced by **omeprazole** causes a few small changes in the pharmacokinetics of **bacampicillin** and **amoxicillin**, but their bioavailabilities are not reduced,[9-11] and the anti-*Helicobacter* effect of the **amoxicillin** is increased.

Six cases of glossitis, stomatitis and/or black tongue were reported to the Sicilian Regional Pharmacovigilance Centre in patients on **lansoprazole**, when combined with antibacterials used to treat *H. pylori* infections. All 6 patients had been given daily doses of **lansoprazole** 60 mg for a week with clarithromycin 1 g and either metronidazole 1 g (3 patients) or **amoxicillin** 2 g (3 patients), after which the antibacterials were stopped, and the **lansoprazole** continued at half the dose for periods of up to 3 weeks. The glossitis (1 patient), black tongue (3 patients) and stomatitis (2 patients) developed between days 2 and 19 of the courses of treatment.[12] Another nine cases of glossitis have been reported elsewhere with **lansoprazole** and **amoxicillin**.[13]

Just why these drugs cause these adverse effects, and whether they are due to just one drug or to an interaction is not understood. The incidence seems to be quite small, because reports of adverse reactions seem to be fairly uncommon, whereas these and related drug combinations are in increasing use for the treatment of *H. pylori* infections.

The makers say that **esomeprazole** has been shown not to have any clinically relevant effects on the pharmacokinetics of **amoxicillin**.[3] There would therefore appear to be no reason for avoiding concurrent use.

(d) Quinolones

A single-dose study found that **omeprazole** 20 or 80 mg had no significant effect on the pharmacokinetics of single doses of **ofloxacin** 400 mg, **ciprofloxacin** 500 mg or **lomefloxacin** 250 or 400 mg.[14] **Omeprazole** 40 mg caused an 18% reduction in the AUC of a single dose of **trovafloxacin** 300 mg and a 32% reduction in the maximum serum levels, but this was considered not to be of clinical significance.[15] A double-blind, randomised, crossover study in 12 healthy subjects found that the maximum serum levels and the AUC of single 320-mg doses of **gemifloxacin** were increased by 11% and 10% respectively after taking **omeprazole** 40 mg daily for 4 days. The confidence intervals indicated that the respective increases were unlikely to exceed 36% and 43%, and it was concluded that these two drugs could be given together without any need for dosage adjustments.[16]

1. Gustavson LE, Kaiser JF, Edmonds AL, Locke CS, DeBartolo ML, Schneck DW. Effect of omeprazole on concentrations of clarithromycin in plasma and gastric tissue at steady state. *Antimicrob Agents Chemother* (1995) 39, 2078–83.
2. Furuta T, Ohashi K, Kobayashi K, Iida I, Yoshida H, Shirai N, Takashima M, Kosuge K, Hanai H, Chiba K, Ishizaki T, Kaneko E. Effects of clarithromycin on the metabolism of omeprazole in relation to CYP2C19 genotype status in humans. *Clin Pharmacol Ther* (1999) 66, 265–74.
3. Nexium (Esomeprazole). AstraZeneca. UK Summary of product characteristics, October 2004.
4. Losec capsules (Omeprazole). AstraZeneca UK Ltd. UK Summary of product characteristics, March 2005.
5. Salcedo JA, Benjamin SB, Maher KA, Sukhova N. Erythromycin inhibits the metabolism of omeprazole. *Gastroenterology* (1997) 112 (4 Suppl), A277.
6. Kees F, Holstege A, Ittner KP, Zimmermann M, Lock G, Schölmerich J, Grobecker H. Pharmacokinetic interaction between proton pump inhibitors and roxithromycin in volunteers. *Aliment Pharmacol Ther* (2000) 14, 407–12.
7. David FL, Da Silva CMF, Mendes FD, Ferraz JGP, Muscara MN, Moreno H, De Nucci G, Pedrazzoli J. Acid suppression by omeprazole does not affect orally administered metronidazole bioavailability and metabolism in healthy male volunteers. *Aliment Pharmacol Ther* (1998) 12, 349–54.
8. Jessa MJ, Goddard AF, Barrett DA, Shaw PN, Spiller RC. The effect of omeprazole on the pharmacokinetics of metronidazole and hydroxymetronidazole in human plasma, saliva and gastric juice. *Br J Clin Pharmacol* (1997) 44, 245–53.
9. Paulsen O, Högland P, Walder M. No effect of omeprazole-induced hypoacidity on the bioavailability of amoxycillin and bacampicillin. *Scand J Infect Dis* (1989) 21, 219–23.
10. Cardaci G, Lambert JR, Aranda-Michel J, Underwood B. Omeprazole has no effect on the gastric mucosal bioavailability of amoxycillin. *Gut* (1995) 37 (Suppl 1), A90.
11. Goddard AF, Jessa MJ, Barrett DA, Shaw PN, Idström J-P, Wason C, Wrangstadh M, Spiller RC. Effect of omeprazole on the distribution of antibiotics in gastric juice. *Gastroenterology* (1995) 108 (Suppl), A102.
12. Greco S, Mazzaglia G, Caputi AP, Pagliaro L. Glossitis, stomatitis and black tongue with lansoprazole plus clarithromycin and other antibiotics. *Ann Pharmacother* (1997) 31, 1548.
13. Hatlebakk JG, Nesje LB, Hausken T, Bang CJ, Berstad A. Lansoprazole capsules and amoxicillin oral suspension in the treatment of peptic ulcer disease. *Scand J Gastroenterol* (1995) 30, 1053–7.
14. Stuht H, Lode H, Koeppe P, Rost KL, Schaberg T. Interaction study of lomefloxacin and ciprofloxacin with omeprazole and comparative pharmacokinetics. *Antimicrob Agents Chemother* (1995) 39, 1045–9.
15. Teng R, Dogolo LC, Willavize SA, Friedman HL, Vincent J. Effect of Maalox and omeprazole on the bioavailability of trovafloxacin. *J Antimicrob Chemother* (1997) 39 (Suppl B), 93–7.
16. Allen A, Vousden M, Lewis A. Effect of omeprazole on the pharmacokinetics of oral gemifloxacin in healthy volunteers. *Chemotherapy* (1999) 45, 496–503.

Proton pump inhibitors + Food

Food modestly reduces the bioavailability of lansoprazole, but not omeprazole.

Clinical evidence, mechanism, importance and management

A study found that food reduced **lansoprazole** bioavailability by 27%.[1] Another study found a 50% reduction in **lansoprazole** bioavailability with food.[2] The authors of both these studies therefore recommended that **lansoprazole** should not be given with food,[1,2] and the maker similarly recommends that to achieve optimal efficacy **lansoprazole** should be administered in the morning before food. A one-hour separation is probably enough to avoid the interaction.

In a study in healthy subjects, food delayed the absorption of **omeprazole**, but did not affect the total amount absorbed.[3] No special precautions are therefore needed.

1. Delhotal-Landes B, Cournot A, Vermerie N, Dellatolas F, Benoit M, Flouvat B. The effect of food and antacids on lansoprazole absorption and disposition. *Eur J Drug Metab Pharmacokinet* (1991), Spec No 3, 315–20.
2. Bergstrand R, Grind M, Nyberg G, Olofsson B. Decreased oral bioavailability of lansoprazole in healthy volunteers when given with a standardised breakfast. *Clin Drug Invest* (1995) 9, 67–71.
3. Rohss K, Andren K, Heggelund A, Lagerstrom P-O, Lundborg P. Bioavailability of omeprazole given in conjunction with food. III World Conf Clin Pharmacol Ther, Stockholm July-Aug 1986. *Acta Pharmacol Toxicol (Copenh)* (1986) 85 (Suppl 5), Abstract 207.

Sulfasalazine + Antimicrobials

The release in the colon of the active drug (5-aminosalicylic acid) from sulfasalazine is markedly reduced by the concurrent use of ampicillin or rifampicin. Metronidazole appears not to interact adversely with sulfasalazine.

Clinical evidence

(a) Ampicillin

The conversion and release of the active metabolite of sulfasalazine, 5-aminosalicylic acid, which is carried out by the bacterial microflora within the gut, was reduced by a third in 5 healthy subjects given a single 2-g dose of sulfasalazine after a 5-day course of 250 mg ampicillin four times daily.[1]

(b) Metronidazole

A study in 10 patients (7 with Crohn's disease and 5 with ulcerative colitis) on long-term sulfasalazine treatment 2 to 4 g daily found that no statistically significant changes in serum sulfapyridine levels occurred while they were additionally taking 400 mg metronidazole twice daily for 8 to 14 days.[2]

(c) Rifampicin (Rifampin)

A crossover trial in 11 patients with Crohn's disease on long term treatment with sulfasalazine found that while concurrently taking rifampicin 10 mg/kg daily and ethambutol 15 mg/kg daily their plasma levels of both 5-aminosalicylic acid and sulphapyridine fell by about 60%.[3]

Mechanism

The azo link of sulfasalazine is split by anaerobic bacteria in the colon to release sulphapyridine and 5-aminosalicylic acid, the latter being the active metabolite that acts locally in the treatment of inflammatory bowel disease. Antibacterials that decimate the gut flora can apparently reduce this conversion and this is reflected in lower plasma levels. Rifampicin also possibly increases the metabolism of the sulphapyridine.

Importance and management

Information is limited, but the interaction appears to be established. However, the extent to which these antibacterials actually reduce the effectiveness of sulfasalazine in the treatment of Crohn's disease or ulcerative colitis seems not to have been assessed, but be alert for evidence of a reduced effect if ampicillin, rifampicin or any other oral antibacterial is given. **Neomycin**, which also affects the activity of the gut microflora, has been seen to interact similarly in *animal* studies,[4] but limited evidence suggests metronidazole does not.

1. Houston JB, Day J, Walker J. Azo reduction of sulphasalazine in healthy volunteers. *Br J Clin Pharmacol* (1982) 14, 395–8.
2. Shaffer JL, Kershaw A, Houston JB. Disposition of metronidazole and its effects on sulphasalazine metabolism in patients with inflammatory bowel disease. *Br J Clin Pharmacol* (1986) 21, 431–5.
3. Shaffer JL, Houston JB. The effect of rifampicin on sulphapyridine plasma concentrations following sulphasalazine administration. *Br J Clin Pharmacol* (1985) 19, 526–8.
4. Peppercorn MA, Goldman P. The role of intestinal bacteria in the metabolism of salicylazosulfapyridine. *J Pharmacol Exp Ther* (1972) 181, 555–62.

Sulfasalazine + Cimetidine

Cimetidine does not interact with sulfasalazine.

Clinical evidence, mechanism, importance and management

In a study, 5 patients with rheumatoid arthritis were treated with sulfasalazine alone, and another 9 patients were given cimetidine 400 mg three times daily for 18 weeks as well as their usual sulfasalazine. On comparing the two groups, it was found that cimetidine did not affect the plasma or urinary levels of sulfasalazine and there were no changes in blood cell counts or haemoglobin levels. It was concluded that no clinically important interaction occurs between these two drugs.[1]

1. Pirmohamed M, Coleman MD, Galvani D, Bucknall RC, Breckenridge AM, Park BK. Lack of interaction between sulphasalazine and cimetidine in patients with rheumatoid arthritis. *Br J Rheumatol* (1993) 32, 222–6.

Sulfasalazine + Colestyramine

Animal **studies show that colestyramine can bind with sulfasalazine in the gut, thereby reducing its activity, but whether this also occurs in clinical use has not been studied.**

Clinical evidence, mechanism, importance and management

A study in *rats* found that colestyramine binds with sulfasalazine so that the azo-bond is protected against attack by the bacteria within the gut. As a result the active 5-aminosalicylic acid is not released and the faecal excretion of intact sulfasalazine increases 30-fold.[1] It seems possible that this interaction could also occur in humans, but confirmation of this is lacking. Separating the drug dosages to prevent their admixture in the gut has proved effective with other drugs that bind with colestyramine. Standard advice is to avoid other drugs for one hour before, and 4 to 6 hours after colestyramine.

1. Pieniaszek HJ, Bates TR. Cholestyramine-induced inhibition of salicylazosulfapyridine (sulfasalazine) metabolism by rat intestinal microflora. *J Pharmacol Exp Ther* (1976) 198, 240–5.

Sulfasalazine + Iron compounds

Sulfasalazine and iron appear to bind together in the gut, but whether this reduces the therapeutic response to either compound is uncertain.

Clinical evidence, mechanism, importance and management

Ferrous iron 400 mg reduced the peak serum levels of a single 50-mg/kg dose of sulfasalazine in 5 healthy subjects by 40%. The reasons are not known, but it seems likely that the sulfasalazine chelates with the **iron** in the gut and thereby interferes with its absorption.[1] The extent to which this suggested chelation affects the ability of the intestinal bacteria to split the sulfasalazine and release its locally active metabolite 5-aminosalicylic acid seems not to have been studied. Therefore the effect of this interaction on the clinical response to sulfasalazine is unclear.

1. Das KM, Eastwood MA. Effect of iron and calcium on salicylazosulphapyridine metabolism. *Scott Med J* (1973) 18, 45–50.

Sulfasalazine + Zileuton

No pharmacokinetic interaction appears to occur between sulfasalazine and zileuton.

Clinical evidence, mechanism, importance and management

In a randomised double-blind placebo controlled trial, 14 healthy subjects were given 1 g sulfasalazine 12-hourly for 8 days, with 800 mg zileuton or a placebo 12-hourly on days 3 to 8. It was found that the pharmacokinetics of the sulfasalazine and its metabolites (sulphapyridine and *N*-acetyl sulphapyridine) were not significantly changed. The study did not directly look at the pharmacokinetics of the zileuton but the parameters measured were similar to those seen in a previous study.[1] There would seem to be no reason for special precautions if both drugs are used.

1. Awni WM, Braeckman RA, Locke CS, Dubé LM, Granneman GR. The influence of multiple oral doses of zileuton on the steady-state pharmacokinetics of sulfasalazine and its metabolites, sulfapyridine and N-acetylsulfapyridine. *Clin Pharmacokinet* (1995) 29 (Suppl 2), 98–104.

26

Hormonal contraceptives and sex hormones

The oral contraceptives are of two main types: the combined oral contraceptives containing both an oestrogen and a progestogen (monophasic, biphasic, triphasic, or sequential) and the progestogen-only preparations or 'mini-pills'. Progestogen-only contraceptives are also available as parenteral preparations (implants, depot injections) and intra-uterine devices.

The oestrogen most commonly used in combined oral contraceptives is ethinylestradiol (daily dose 20 to 50 micrograms). Mestranol (a pro-drug of ethinylestradiol) is used only rarely (daily dose 50 micrograms). The progestogens used in both combined and progestogen-only oral contraceptives are commonly those derived from 19-nortestosterone and can be subdivided into first generation (e.g. etynodiol diacetate, lynestrenol, norethisterone) second generation (levonorgestrel, norgestrel) and third generation (e.g. desogestrel, gestodene, norgestimate). A patch containing ethinylestradiol and norelgestromin is also available. The progestogens used in parenteral progestogen-only contraceptives are either 19-nortestosterone derivatives (e.g. etonogestrel, norethisterone) or derived from progesterone (e.g. medroxyprogesterone acetate). Those in intra-uterine devices are 19-nortestosterone derivatives (e.g. levonorgestrel).

Combined oral preparations are most usually taken for 21 days, followed by a period of 7 days during which withdrawal bleeding occurs. Some of them include 7 inert tablets to be taken at this time so that the daily routine of taking a tablet is not broken. The combined patch is applied weekly for 3 weeks followed by a patch-free week. The oestrogenic and progestogenic components of these contraceptives act together to consistently suppress ovulation.

The progestogen-only preparations come in the form of tablets, which are taken continuously, or implants, injections or intra-uterine devices, which slowly release the progestogen over an extended period of time. They do not inhibit ovulation reliably in all cycles and probably act mainly by increasing the viscosity of the cervical mucus so that the movement of the sperm is retarded. They may also cause changes in the endometrium, which inhibit successful implantation.

Interactions

(a) Combined oral contraceptives

Almost all of the interactions of hormonal contraceptives described in this publication involve the combined oral contraceptives. Most of the clinically important interactions with the combined oral contraceptives involve increased metabolism. The major route for hepatic metabolism of ethinylestradiol is hydroxylation by the cytochrome P450 isoenzyme CYP3A4, and progestogens are also substrates for this enzyme. Thus, inducers of this enzyme can increase the clearance of the contraceptive steroids and possibly increase breakthrough bleeding and decrease contraceptive efficacy. Those that have been shown to have this effect are listed in 'Table 26.1', (below). Conversely, inhibitors of CYP3A4 may increase the incidence of adverse effects such as nausea, breast tenderness, headaches, and potentially more serious complications such as thromboembolic events, although the latter has yet to be demonstrated.

Some of the conjugated metabolites of ethinylestradiol undergo enterohepatic recirculation, and certain antibacterials are postulated to reduce this by inhibiting gut flora, thereby possibly decreasing contraceptive efficacy, although this is unproven (see 'Oral contraceptives + Antibacterials; Penicillins', p.746). Low-dose combined oral contraceptives may be more susceptible to drug interactions than standard-dose or high-dose preparations, but evidence to support this is scant. When considering any pharmacokinetic interactions, it should be noted that there is a large inter-individual variation in plasma levels of ethinylestradiol and progestogens.

(b) Progestogen-only contraceptives

There is very little direct information about interactions with the progestogen-only contraceptives (whether used orally, parenterally, or intra-uterine). It is unwise uncritically to assume that interactions known to occur with the combined oral contraceptives also occur with these. However, it seems probable that an increased risk of failure with the oral and parenteral progestogen-only contraceptives is likely with drugs that cause enzyme induction (listed in 'Table 26.1', (below)), which results in an increased clearance of the progestogen, with an accompanying loss of efficacy. The progestogen-releasing intra-uterine device is thought to have a primarily local effect, and may not be affected by enzyme-inducing drugs (see 'IUDs; Progestogen-releasing + Enzyme-inducing drugs', p.743). However, much more study is needed to clarify the situation.

(c) Emergency hormonal contraceptives

It is also not known whether interacting drugs are likely to affect the emergency (postcoital) hormonal contraceptives, although it is common practice that women taking enzyme inducing drugs (see 'Table 26.1', (below)) are given an increased dosage to accommodate the increased rate of metabolism by the liver (see 'Emergency hormonal contraceptives + Enzyme-inducing drugs', p.742).

(d) Hormone replacement therapy (HRT)

The preparations used for HRT contain oestrogens either alone or combined with progestogens. They differ from the oral contraceptives as the most commonly used estrogens in HRT are natural estrogens such as estradiol and conjugated oestrogens, and their dosages are generally lower than equivalent doses of ethinylestradiol used in combined oral contraceptives. There are only a few reports of interactions with HRT preparations, but generally they are expected to behave very much like the combined oral contraceptives.

(e) Other preparations

Cyproterone acetate combined with ethinylestradiol (co-cyprindiol) is intended for use in women with androgen-dependent skin conditions, but it also acts as an oral contraceptive and is therefore predicted to interact like conventional oestrogen-containing oral contraceptives (see 'Co-cyprindiol (Cyproterone/Ethinylestradiol) + Miscellaneous', p.742).

General references

1. Back DJ, Breckenridge AM, Crawford FE, MacIver M, Orme ML'E, Rowe PH. Interindividual variation and drug interactions with hormonal steroid contraceptives. *Drugs* (1981) 21, 46–61.
2. Shader RI, Oesterheld JR. Contraceptive effectiveness: cytochromes and induction. *J Clin Psychopharmacol* (2000) 20, 119–121.
3. Shader RI, Greenblatt DJ. More on oral contraceptives, drug interactions, herbal medicines, and hormone replacement therapy. *J Clin Psychopharmacol* (2000) 20, 397–8.
4. Elliman A. Interactions with hormonal contraception. *Br J Fam Plann* (2000) 26, 109–11.

Table 26.1 Enzyme-inducing drugs shown to reduce the efficacy and/or increase the metabolism of hormonal contraceptives

Antibacterials	Rifabutin, Rifampicin
Anticonvulsants	Barbiturates (e.g. phenobarbital, primidone), Carbamazepine, Phenytoin, Topiramate
Antifungals	Griseofulvin
Antivirals	Protease inhibitors (e.g. nelfinavir, ritonavir), Nevirapine
Other drugs	Aprepitant, Modafinil, St John's wort (*Hypericum perforatum*), Troglitazone

Co-cyprindiol (Cyproterone/Ethinylestradiol) + Miscellaneous

Co-cyprindiol (cyproterone/ethinylestradiol) is expected to interact with enzyme-inducing drugs in a similar manner to the combined oral contraceptives so that the risk of contraceptive failure is increased. Like combined oral contraceptives, there may be rare cases of contraceptive failure with broad-spectrum antibacterials. There is some evidence that co-cyprindiol also interacts with minocycline to increase facial pigmentation.

Clinical evidence, mechanism, importance and management

Co-cyprindiol is a mixture of the anti-androgenic progestogen, cyproterone acetate, 2 mg, with ethinylestradiol, 35 micrograms, which is used for the treatment of acne and moderately severe hirsutism in women who may also wish to use it as an oral contraceptive. Its contraceptive efficacy is therefore expected to be reduced by the same hepatic enzyme inducers (see 'Table 26.1', (p.741)) that interact with conventional combined oral contraceptives.[1] The precautions described in this section for the combined oral contraceptives with the various drugs listed in 'Table 26.1', (p.741) should therefore be followed.

Similarly, it is anticipated that the use of broad-spectrum antibacterials may rarely reduce the contraceptive efficacy of co-cyprindiol and the precautions under 'Oral contraceptives + Antibacterials; Tetracyclines', p.750, should be followed. Usually these precautions (additional barrier methods) are considered unnecessary after 2 weeks concurrent use. However, the maker of co-cyprindiol says that when **tetracyclines** are being taken it is advisable to use additional non-hormonal methods of contraception (except the rhythm or temperature methods) since an extremely high degree of contraceptive protection must be provided with co-cyprindiol due to the theoretical risk of cyproterone causing feminization of a male foetus. They do note that oral **tetracyclines** have not actually been shown to reduce the contraceptive efficacy of co-cyprindiol. In addition co-cyprindiol may also possibly interact with **minocycline** to accentuate facial pigmentation (see 'Tetracyclines; Minocycline + Ethinylestradiol', p.247).

The makers also point out that **combined oral contraceptives** must not be taken with co-cyprindiol.[1] To do this would be analogous to doubling the ethinylestradiol dose with consequent increased risk of adverse effects. In addition, some of the progestogens in combined oral contraceptives have weak androgenic effects, which could oppose the benefits of cyproterone.

1. Dianette (Cyproterone/ethinylestradiol), Schering Health Care Ltd. UK Summary of product characteristics, July 2004.

Emergency hormonal contraceptives + Antibacterials; Broad-spectrum

There is a theoretical possibility that the emergency (postcoital) contraceptive efficacy of norgestrel/ethinylestradiol could be affected by broad-spectrum antibacterials such as the penicillins and tetracyclines. The efficacy of levonorgestrel given for postcoital contraception is not likely to be affected by these antibacterials.

Clinical evidence, mechanism, importance and management

(a) Combined oestrogen/progestogen

The maker states that the efficacy of **norgestrel/ethinylestradiol** (***Schering PC4***) may be reduced by **ampicillin** and other antibiotics.[1] This is presumably an extrapolation from the rare cases of combined oral contraceptive failure seen with various broad-spectrum antibacterials, which have been postulated to be due to reduced enterohepatic recycling of **ethinylestradiol** (see 'Oral contraceptives + Antibacterials; Penicillins', p.746). However, it has been suggested that it is likely that sufficient hormone is absorbed initially for the emergency contraceptive to be effective[2] (it is taken as 2 doses within 12 hours of each other). The UK Family Planning Association say that there is no need to increase the dose of ***Schering PC4*** if the patient is taking antibacterials that are not enzyme inducers.[3] Note that, in any case, the use of combined oestrogen/progestogen as a postcoital contraceptive has been largely superseded by a progestogen-only preparation.

(b) Progestogen only

Levonorgestrel is metabolised to inactive substances before it is conjugated,[4] and does not therefore undergo enterohepatic recycling of the active moiety. There is no reason to expect that its efficacy as an emergency contraceptive would be affected by broad-spectrum antibacterials that alter gut flora. No special precautions are necessary.

1. Schering PC4 (Norgestrel/ethinylestradiol). Schering Health Care Ltd. UK Summary of product characteristics, July 1995.
2. Elliman A. Interactions with hormonal contraception. *Br J Fam Plann* (2000) 26, 109–11.
3. Belfield T, ed. FPA Contraceptive Handbook: a guide for family planning and other health professionals. 3rd ed. London: Family Planning Association, 1999.
4. Levonelle-2 (Levonorgestrel). Schering Health Care Ltd. UK Summary of product characteristics, October 2003.

Emergency hormonal contraceptives + Enzyme-inducing drugs

The efficacy of emergency (postcoital) hormonal contraceptives is likely to be reduced by enzyme-inducing drugs such as rifampicin and some anticonvulsants. It is usual practice to give a higher dose of the contraceptive.

Clinical evidence, mechanism, importance and management

The maker states that some enzyme-inducing drugs (see 'Table 26.1', (p.741)) might reduce the efficacy of **norgestrel/ethinylestradiol** (*Schering* PC4)[1] and **levonorgestrel** (*Levonelle-2*)[2] used as emergency contraceptives. Cases of failure of emergency contraceptives have been reported with '**St John's wort**', (p.763). Various others of these drugs have specifically been shown to decrease the levels of contraceptive steroids when used as components of combined oral contraceptives (see individual monographs). This would also be expected when they are used as postcoital contraceptives. However, it is difficult to envisage a study design that would show whether this reduced metabolism results in reduced efficacy of postcoital contraception (e.g. indicators of ovulation do not necessarily indicate likely reduced efficacy, as with combined oral contraceptives).

The UK Family Planning Association recommend that the dose of emergency hormonal contraceptive are increased by 50% if they are used in a woman on any enzyme-inducing drug known to affect oral contraceptives (see 'Table 26.1', (p.741)).[3,4] For *Schering PC4*, this involves taking 3 tablets followed 12 hours later by a further 3 tablets.[4] For **levonorgestrel-only** emergency hormonal contraception the dose should be increased to 2.25 mg (two tablets immediately followed 12 hours later by the usual dose of one tablet for *Levonelle-2*).[5] Alternatively, a copper intra-uterine device may be used. Given the potential consequences of an unwanted pregnancy, these seem sensible precautions.

1. Schering PC4 (Norgestrel/ethinylestradiol). Schering Health Care Ltd. UK Summary of product characteristics, July 1995.
2. Levonelle-2 (Levonorgestrel). Schering Health Care Ltd. UK Summary of product characteristics, October 2003.
3. Belfield T, ed. FPA Contraceptive Handbook: a guide for family planning and other health professionals. 3rd ed. London: Family Planning Association, 1999.
4. Elliman A. Interactions with hormonal contraception. *Br J Fam Plann* (2000) 26, 109–11.
5. British National Formulary. 49th ed. London: The British Medical Association and The Pharmaceutical Press; 2005. p. 407.

Gestrinone + Enzyme-inducing drugs

The makers say that rifampicin and anticonvulsants may reduce the effects of gestrinone.

Clinical evidence, mechanism, importance and management

The makers suggest that **rifampicin** and **antiepileptics** (not named, but by implication those that are enzyme-inducers, see 'Table 26.1', (p.741)) can accelerate the metabolism of gestrinone thereby reducing its effects.[1] However, there appear to be no reports that this actually occurs.[2] Good monitoring is advisable if any of these drugs is given concurrently, with dosage adjustments where it becomes clearly necessary.

1. Dimetriose (Gestrinone). Florizel Ltd. UK Summary of product characteristics, May 1997.
2. Roberts G (Roussel Labs). Personal Communication 1992.

HRT + Enzyme-inducing drugs

Enzyme-inducing drugs that increase the metabolism of contraceptive steroids might also be expected to reduce the efficacy of menopausal HRT. An isolated case describes reduced efficacy of oral conjugated oestrogens with phenytoin.

Clinical evidence, mechanism, importance and management

A report describes a 28-year-old woman taking oral **conjugated oestrogens** (*Premarin*) 1.25 mg daily after ovidectomy, who had a dramatic increase in the incidence of hot flushes when she began to take **phenytoin** 300 mg daily. Her estrone and estradiol levels were found to be very low, and they subsequently increased four to sixfold after the **phenytoin** was stopped, at which point the incidence of hot flushes decreased.[1] This seems to be the only report of this interaction.

However, it is not unreasonable to assume that enzyme-inducing drugs that increase the metabolism of contraceptive steroids (listed in 'Table 26.1', (p.741)) would also increase the metabolism of oestrogens used for HRT. Some makers state that these drugs may reduce the efficacy of HRT preparations. This would be most likely to be noticed where HRT is prescribed for menopausal vasomotor symptoms, but might be difficult to detect where the indication is osteoporosis. The interaction is not relevant to HRT applied locally for menopausal vaginitis. It has also been suggested that any interaction is less likely with transdermal HRT, which bypasses hepatic first-pass metabolism. Further study is needed to confirm the importance of this possible interaction.

1. Notelovitz M, Tjapkes J, Ware M. Interaction between estrogen and Dilantin in a menopausal woman. *N Engl J Med* (1981) 304, 788–9.

HRT + Moexipril

Moexipril is reported not to interact adversely with HRT (hormone replacement therapy).

Clinical evidence, mechanism, importance and management

A placebo-controlled study involving 95 hypertensive postmenopausal women treated with HRT found that moexipril given for 12 weeks did not affect metabolic parameters associated with cardiovascular disease and co-administration was considered safe and effective.[1] HRT had no effect on the blood pressure lowering ability of moexipril.[1]

1. Koch B, Oparil S, Stimpel M. Co-administration of an ACE-inhibitor (moexipril) and hormonal replacement therapy in postmenopausal women. *J Hum Hypertens* (1999) 13, 337–42.

IUDs; Copper + Anti-inflammatory drugs

There are a few early reports suggesting that the very occasional failure of a copper IUDs to prevent pregnancy may have been due to an interaction with a corticosteroid, aspirin or NSAID.

Clinical evidence, mechanism, importance and management

Four women have been described who, despite being fitted with copper IUDs, each had two successive pregnancies. Two were taking **corticosteroids** regularly and the other two often took **aspirin** for migraine.[1,2] Unwanted pregnancies have also been reported in 3 women with copper IUDs treated with **corticosteroids,**[3-5] and in 2 women treated with **NSAIDs** (indometacin and naproxen).[5] A later case-control study found that **aspirin** and **NSAIDs** were used more frequently in 717 women who became pregnant while using IUDs than in non-pregnant IUD users (the majority of IUDs were copper). The difference was significant only for **aspirin** (102 IUD failures, 59 controls). It is possible that this finding could have resulted from bias in recall or reporting.[2] The postulated mechanism for any interaction was that part of the efficacy of copper IUDs may be based on local inflammatory effects, and that anti-inflammatory drugs might reduce this.

The evidence for this possible interaction is very slim and inconclusive, and there appear to be no further reports of any problems. Modern copper-containing IUDs are one of the most effective methods of contraception. Also, intermittent use of anti-inflammatory drugs such as NSAIDs is widespread. One maker of copper IUDs states that the evidence does not justify general precautions.[6] No special precautions appear to be necessary.

1. Buhler M, Papiernik E. Successive pregnancies in women fitted with intrauterine devices who take anti-inflammatory drugs. *Lancet* (1983) 1, 483.
2. Papiernik R, Rozenbaum H, Amblard P, Dephot N, de Mouzon J. Intra-uterine device failure: relation with drug use. *Eur J Obstet Gynecol Reprod Biol* (1989) 32, 205–12.
3. Inkeles DM, Hansen RI. Unexpected pregnancy in a woman using an intrauterine device and receiving steroid therapy. *Ann Ophthalmol* (1982) 14, 975.
4. Zerner J, Miller AB, Festino MJ. Failure of an intrauterine device concurrent with administration of corticosteroids. *Fertil Steril* (1976) 27, 1467–8.
5. Thomas P-R, Stérilet et anti-inflammatoires: à propos de quatre observations. *Concours Med* (1977) 45, 7095–6.
6. NOVA T (copper containing intrauterine contraceptive device). Schering Health Care Limited. Technical data sheet. September 1998.

IUDs; Progestogen-releasing + Enzyme-inducing drugs

The contraceptive reliability of the progestogen-releasing IUD is not thought to be affected by the enzyme-inducing drugs (e.g. rifampicin and some anticonvulsants).

Clinical evidence, mechanism, importance and management

Some enzyme-inducing drugs increase the metabolism and reduce the efficacy of combined oral contraceptives (see 'Table 26.1', (p.741), for a list). The maker has not studied the influence of these drugs on the efficacy of the **levonorgestrel-releasing** IUD (*Mirena*),[1] and has said that they cannot be sure that the foreign body effect (i.e. the effect whereby the presence of the IUD prevents implantation) and/or locally acting hormone will provide reliable contraception when systemic hormone levels and suppression of ovaries are reduced by drug interactions.[2] However, this appears to be overly cautious. The systemic absorption of **levonorgestrel** from the IUD leads to lower blood levels than are seen with standard progestogen-only oral contraceptives.[1] In addition, women using a **levonorgestrel** IUD usually continue to ovulate.[1] Thus, the contraceptive effects of the **levonorgestrel** IUD are mainly local.[1] Also, a pilot study in 56 epileptic women using a **levonorgestrel** IUD, most of them also taking enzyme-inducing drugs, who accumulated 1075 months of use found only one apparent contraceptive failure.[3]

The UK Family Planning Association[4] consider IUDs are unlikely to be affected by enzyme-inducing drugs. They are therefore a suitable contraceptive for women on these drugs.[5] No special precautions appear to be necessary.

1. Mirena (Levonorgestrel Intrauterine System). Schering Health Care Ltd. UK Summary of product characteristics, July 2004.
2. Personal communication. Schering Health Care Limited. April 2001.
3. Bounds W, Guillebaud J. Observational series on women using the contraceptive Mirena concurrently with anti-epilepic and other enzyme-inducing drugs. *J Fam Plann Reprod Health Care* (2002) 28, 78–80.
4. Belfield T, ed. FPA Contraceptive Handbook: a guide for family planning and other health professionals. 3rd ed. London: Family Planning Association, 1999.
5. Crawford P. Interactions between antiepileptic drugs and hormonal contraception. *CNS Drugs* (2002) 16, 263–72.

Medroxyprogesterone acetate or Megestrol + Aminoglutethimide

Aminoglutethimide markedly reduces the plasma levels of medroxyprogesterone and megestrol. The dosage may need to be doubled to accommodate this interaction.

Clinical evidence

(a) Medroxyprogesterone acetate

Aminoglutethimide 250 mg two to four times daily approximately halved the plasma levels of the medroxyprogesterone acetate 500 mg three times daily in 6 postmenopausal women with breast cancer.[1] Another study in 6 postmenopausal women found that aminoglutethimide 250 mg four times daily reduced medroxyprogesterone levels by 63% after oral, but not intravenous, medroxyprogesterone therapy.[2] In another study in 6 women with advanced breast cancer, it was found that as the dosage of aminoglutethimide was gradually reduced from 250 mg twice daily and finally withdrawn, the plasma levels of medroxyprogesterone steadily climbed to threefold their initial level, although the dose remained constant at a total of 800 mg daily.[3]

(b) Megestrol

Aminoglutethimide 250 mg four times daily reduced the serum levels of megestrol 160 mg daily by 78% in 6 postmenopausal women.[2]

Mechanism

The most likely reason for this interaction is that the aminoglutethimide acts as an enzyme inducing agent, increasing the metabolism of the progestogens, thereby increasing their loss from the body.

Importance and management

Both interactions appear to be established and are possibly clinically important. A 50% reduction in the plasma levels of medroxyprogesterone and megestrol should be expected during concurrent use, and this may reduce the adrenal suppressive effect.[1] The authors of one report[3] say that to achieve adequate plasma medroxyprogesterone acetate levels in breast cancer therapy (above 100 nanograms/ml) a daily dose of 800 mg of *Provera* is probably necessary in the presence of aminoglutethimide 125 or 250 mg twice daily. This is double the usual recommended dose of this preparation.

1. Van Deijk WA, Blijham GH, Mellink WAM, Meulenberg PMM. Influence of aminoglutethimide on plasma levels of medroxyprogesterone acetate: its correlation with serum cortisol. *Cancer Treat Rep* (1985) 69, 85–90.
2. Lundgren S, Lønning PE, Aakvaag A, Kvinnsland S. Influence of aminoglutethimide on the metabolism of medroxyprogesterone acetate and megestrol acetate in postmenopausal patients with advanced breast cancer. *Cancer Chemother Pharmacol* (1990) 27, 101–5.
3. Halpenny O, Bye A, Cranny A, Feely J, Daly PA. Influence of aminoglutethimide on plasma levels of medroxyprogesterone acetate. *Med Oncol Tumor Pharmacother* (1990) 7, 241–7.

Oestrogens + Grapefruit juice

No clinically significant interaction appears to occur between grapefruit juice and a single dose of either estradiol or ethinylestradiol, although their levels are modestly increased by grapefruit juice.

Clinical evidence, mechanism, importance and management

(a) Estradiol

Grapefruit juice increased the AUC and maximum concentration of estrone, a metabolite of estradiol, but not of estradiol in women given a single 2-mg dose of estradiol.[1]

(b) Ethinylestradiol

Grapefruit juice increased the mean maximum plasma level and 0 to 8-hour AUC of ethinylestradiol by 37% and 30% in 13 healthy young women given a single 50-microgram dose of ethinylestradiol when compared with a control drink (**herb tea**). There was wide intersubject variation in the increase. The rise in the 0 to 12-hour AUC was not significant (28%). The subjects drank grapefruit juice 100 ml or control 30 minutes before the ethinylestradiol, a further 100 ml with the ethinylestradiol, and then 200 ml 3-hourly for 12 hours after taking the ethinylestradiol. It is thought that this increase in bioavailability probably occurs because grapefruit juice inhibits gut cytochrome P450 isoenzyme CYP3A4, which metabolises ethinylestradiol.[2] See also 'Grapefruit juice', (p.11).

Grapefruit juice may be taken at the same time of day as the combined oral contraceptive pill (which usually contains ethinylestradiol) but it seems unlikely that this interaction is of practical importance because the increased bioavailability is still less than the extent of known variability between individuals. However, this requires confirmation in a longer-term study. The authors suggest that diet may be a factor in the known variability of contraceptive steroid levels between individuals.[2]

1. Schubert W, Cullberg G, Edgar B, Hedner T. Inhibition of 17 beta-estradiol metabolism by grapefruit juice in ovariectomized women. *Maturitas* (1994) 20, 155–63.
2. Weber A, Jäger R, Börner A, Klinger G, Vollanth R, Matthey K, Balogh A. Can grapefruit juice influence ethinylestradiol bioavailability? *Contraception* (1996) 53, 41–7.

Oral contraceptives + Antacids

Despite *in vitro* evidence that some antacids might reduce the availability of norethisterone acetate, evidence from healthy women indicates that no interaction occurs. This also appears to be true for ethinylestradiol and levonorgestrel.

Clinical evidence, mechanism, importance and management

An *in vitro* study found that a 1% suspension of **magnesium trisilicate** in water adsorbed about 80% of **mestranol** and 50% of **norethisterone**, but minimal amounts of **ethinylestradiol**.[1,2] Similarly, another *in vitro* study reported reduced dissolution of **norethisterone acetate** from combined oral contraceptive tablets in the presence of **magnesium trisilicate, kaolin mixture,** and **aluminium hydroxide**.[3] In contrast, a single dose study in 12 healthy women given a combined oral contraceptive (**ethinylestradiol** 30 micrograms and either **norethisterone acetate** 1 mg or **levonorgestrel** 150 micrograms) with **magnesium trisilicate** 500 mg and **aluminium hydroxide** 250 mg, showed that the AUC and peak levels of all three steroids were unchanged.[4] This is in line with common experience. There do not appear to be any reports of contraceptive failure with antacids and **norethisterone acetate** or **mestranol**-containing combined oral contraceptives. No special precautions seem to be necessary.

1. Khalil SAH, Iwuagwu M. The in vitro uptake of some oral contraceptive steroids by magnesium trisilicate. *J Pharm Pharmacol* (1976) 28 (Suppl), 47P.
2. Khalil SAH, Iwuagwu M. *In vitro* uptake of oral contraceptive steroids by magnesium trisilicate. *J Pharm Sci* (1978) 67, 287–9.
3. Fadel H, Abd Elbary A, Nour El-Din E, Kassem AA. Availability of norethisterone acetate from combined oral contraceptive tablets. *Pharmazie* (1979) 34, 49–50.
4. Joshi JV, Sankolli GM, Shah RS, Joshi UM. Antacid does not reduce the bioavailability of oral contraceptive steroids in women. *Int J Clin Pharmacol Ther Toxicol* (1986) 24, 192–5.

Oral contraceptives + Anthelmintics

Early schistosomiasis and the use of praziquantel or metrifonate do not appear to alter the pharmacokinetics of combined oral contraceptives. The maker of albendazole recommends women use non-hormonal methods of contraception.

Clinical evidence, mechanism, importance and management

(a) Albendazole

The maker recommends that women taking albendazole should use non-hormonal methods of contraception during and for one month after stopping the drug. This is because albendazole is teratogenic in some *animal* species, and because there is a theoretical risk of an interaction with oral contraceptives (the maker says albendazole is a liver enzyme inducer).[1] Study is needed to confirm this.

(b) Metrifonate, Praziquantel

A study in 25 women with early active schistosomiasis (*S. haematobium* or *S. mansoni*) without signs of liver disease and 6 healthy women showed that neither the disease itself nor the concurrent use of antischistosomal drugs (a single 40-mg/kg dose of praziquantel, or metrifonate in three doses of 10 mg/kg at fortnightly intervals) had any effect on the plasma levels of steroids from a combined oral contraceptive (**ethinylestradiol/levonorgestrel** 50/500 micrograms).[2] Moreover, in another study there was no evidence that women with early active schistosomiasis without signs of liver disease were at any greater risk of hepatic impairment while using combined oral contraceptives.[3] No special precautions would therefore appear necessary in women with early active schistosomiasis taking oral contraceptives and praziquantel or metrifonate. Note that oral contraceptives are considered contraindicated in schistosomiasis with liver involvement.

1. Eskazole (Albendazole). SmithKline Beecham. UK Summary of product characteristics, August 1997.
2. El-Raghy I, Back DJ, Osman F, Orme ML'E, Fathalla M. Contraceptive steroid concentrations in women with early active schistosomiasis: lack of effect of antischistosomal drugs. *Contraception* (1986) 33, 373–7.
3. Shaaban MM, Hammad WA, Fathalla MF, Ghaneimah SA, El-Sharkawy MM, Salim TH, Liao WC, Smith SC. Effects of oral contraception on liver function tests and serum proteins in women with active schistosomiasis. *Contraception* (1982) 26, 75–82.

Oral contraceptives + Antibacterials; Cephalosporins

A few anecdotal cases of combined oral contraceptive failure have been reported with cefalexin, cefalexin with clindamycin, and

unspecified cephalosporins. The interaction (if such it is) appears to be very rare indeed.

Clinical evidence

Two pregnancies were attributed to the use of cephalosporins (unspecified) and an oral contraceptive (unspecified) in the UK Committee on Safety of Medicines adverse reactions register for the years 1968 to 1984 (61 cases were attributed to other antibacterials).[1] One case of contraceptive failure has been attributed to **cefalexin**,[2] and one to **cefalexin** used with clindamycin.[3] In a case-control study, 356 women were identified who had received oral contraceptives and antibiotics (said to be cephalosporins, penicillins, tetracyclines) over a 5-year period in 3 dermatological practices. The failure rate in these women (1.6% per year; 2 pregnancies occurred in women on a cephalosporin and 3 in women on minocycline) was indistinguishable from the failure rate seen in control patients on oral contraceptives and no antibacterials (1% per year).[4]

Mechanism

Suppression of intestinal bacteria, which results in reduced enterohepatic recirculation of ethinylestradiol and a fall in serum levels, is the suggested explanation for any interaction (see 'Oral contraceptives + Antibacterials; Penicillins', p.746).

Importance and management

The oral contraceptive/cephalosporin interactions summarised here are all that have been identified in the world's literature. These interactions are not adequately established and the whole issue remains very controversial. Bearing in mind the extremely wide use of both groups of drugs, any increased incidence of contraceptive failure above that normally seen is clearly very low indeed. On the other hand, the personal and ethical consequences of an unwanted pregnancy can be very serious. For this reason, where uncertainty remains, the UK Family Planning Association recommend that for maximal protection a second form of contraception (a barrier method) should be used routinely while taking a short course of a cephalosporin and for at least 7 days afterwards.[5] For further comment and advice see also 'Oral contraceptives + Antibacterials; Penicillins', p.746.

1. Back DJ, Grimmer SFM, Orme ML'E, Proudlove C, Mann RD, Breckenridge AM. Evaluation of Committee on Safety of Medicines yellow card reports on oral contraceptive-drug interactions with anticonvulsants and antibiotics. *Br J Clin Pharmacol* (1988) 25, 527–32.
2. DeSano EA, Hurley SC. Possible interactions of antihistamines and antibiotics with oral contraceptive effectiveness. *Fertil Steril* (1982) 37, 853–4.
3. Back DJ, Breckenridge AM, Crawford FE, MacIver M, Orme L'E, Rowe PH. Interindividual variation and drug interactions with hormonal steroids. *Drugs* (1981) 21, 46.
4. Helms SE, Bredle DL, Zajic J, Jarjoura D, Brodell RT, Krishnarao I. Oral contraceptive failure rates and oral antibiotics. *J Am Acad Dermatol* (1997) 36, 705–10.
5. Belfield T, ed. FPA Contraceptive Handbook: a guide for family planning and other health professionals. 3rd ed. London: Family Planning Association, 1999.

Oral contraceptives + Antibacterials; Macrolides

The macrolides clarithromycin, dirithromycin, roxithromycin and telithromycin appear unlikely to cause combined oral contraceptive failure. Erythromycin is also not considered to cause failure of combined oral contraceptives, but isolated anecdotal cases have been reported. An isolated case has also been reported with spiramycin.

Clinical evidence

(a) Clarithromycin

Ten women taking a combined oral contraceptive (**ethinylestradiol** with **levonorgestrel** or **desogestrel**) showed a very slight but not statistically significant rise in serum **ethinylestradiol** levels while taking clarithromycin 250 mg twice daily for 7 days. No changes in **levonorgestrel** levels occurred, but levels of the active metabolite of desogestrel were increased. Ovulation did not occur (progesterone levels remained suppressed, and follicle stimulating hormone and luteinising hormone levels were reduced). These hormonal changes suggest that clarithromycin may even increase the efficacy of combined oral contraceptives.[1]

(b) Dirithromycin

Fifteen women taking a triphasic combined oral contraceptive (**ethinylestradiol/norethisterone**) were given dirithromycin 500 mg daily for 14 days starting on day 21 of the cycle. A small but statistically significant decrease of 7.6% occurred in the mean **ethinylestradiol** AUC, but no woman ovulated (as assessed by ultrasound and ovarian hormone levels).[2]

(c) Erythromycin

Isolated cases of contraceptive failure have been attributed to erythromycin, and two pregnancies were attributed to the use of erythromycin and an oral contraceptive (unspecified) in the UK Committee on Safety of Medicines adverse reactions register for the years 1968 to 1984 (61 cases were attributed to other antibacterials).[3] Another survey of oral contraceptive failure identified 1 failure due to erythromycin (48 of 209 pill failures were attributed to antibacterials).[4] Break-through bleeding due to erythromycin has also been described in 2 cases.[5] Conversely, in 2 studies of contraceptive failures in dermatology patients, no pregnancies were identified in a total of 74 women taking erythromycin and an oral contraceptive.[6,7]

(d) Roxithromycin

While taking roxithromycin 150 mg twice daily, the anti-ovulatory effects of a triphasic combined oral contraceptive (**ethinylestradiol/levonorgestrel**) remained unchanged during one cycle in 21 healthy women. Efficacy was measured by monitoring ovulation, which was assessed by ultrasound and progesterone levels.[8]

(e) Spiramycin

One case of contraceptive failure has been attributed to concurrent treatment with spiramycin.[9]

(f) Telithromycin

Telithromycin 800 mg once daily for 10 days had no effect on the pharmacokinetics of **ethinylestradiol**, but increased the plasma levels of **levonorgestrel** in 38 healthy women on a triphasic combined oral contraceptive. None of the women ovulated, as assessed by progesterone levels.[10]

Mechanism

The macrolides such as erythromycin might possibly be expected to suppress the bacteria responsible for the entero-hepatic recycling of ethinylestradiol, but good evidence that this is clinically important is scant (see 'Hormonal contraceptives and sex hormones', (p.741)). Erythromycin (and to a lesser extent the other macrolides discussed here) also inhibit the cytochrome P450 isoenzyme CYP3A4, which is responsible for the metabolism of the contraceptive steroids. Therefore it might be expected to increase rather than reduce contraceptive efficacy. This would be expected to offset any possible reduced recycling.

Importance and management

Information on erythromycin is very limited, but the isolated reports of pregnancies with this drug, coupled with its known enzyme-inducing properties, suggest that it is unlikely to cause contraceptive failure. The UK Family Planning Association consider that it is almost certain that erythromycin does not interact with combined oral contraceptives,[11] and no special contraceptive precautions are recommended during concurrent use. Information on the other macrolides seems to be limited to the studies cited, on the basis of which no interaction appears to be likely with clarithromycin, roxithromycin and telithromycin. Dirithromycin also appears unlikely to cause oral contraceptive failure in the great majority of women. No cases of contraceptive failure with these newer macrolides appear to have been reported. If one accepts the theory that there are an, as yet, unidentifiable tiny group of women for whom enterohepatic recirculation of ethinylestradiol is important, then additional contraceptive precautions should be taken with dirithromycin, in particular, since this caused a small decrease in ethinylestradiol levels. However, if one tends to the theory that the anecdotal cases of contraceptive failure with broad-spectrum antibacterials are indistinguishable from the normal accepted failure rate, no special precautions are necessary. For discussion of the adverse hepatic interaction between oral contraceptives and the macrolide troleandomycin, see 'Oral contraceptives or HRT + Antibacterials; Troleandomycin', p.751.

1. Back DJ, Tjia J, Martin C, Millar E, Salmon P, Orme M. The interaction between clarithromycin and combined oral-contraceptive steroids. *J Pharm Med* (1991) 2, 81–7.
2. Wermeling DP, Chandler MHH, Sides GD, Collins D, Muse KN. Dirithromycin increases ethinyl estradiol clearance without allowing ovulation. *Obstet Gynecol* (1995) 86, 78–84.

3. Back DJ, Grimmer SFM, Orme ML'E, Proudlove C, Mann RD, Breckenridge AM. Evaluation of Committee on Safety of Medicines yellow card reports on oral contraceptive-drug interactions with anticonvulsants and antibiotics. *Br J Clin Pharmacol* (1988) 25, 527–32.
4. Kovacs GT, Riddoch G, Duncombe P, Welberry L, Chick P, Weisberg E, Leavesley GM, Baker HWG. Inadvertent pregnancies in oral contraceptive users. *Med J Aust* (1989) 150, 549–51.
5. Hetényi G. Possible interactions between antibiotics and oral contraceptives. *Ther Hung* (1989) 37, 86–9.
6. Hughes BR, Cunliffe WJ. Interactions between the oral contraceptive pill and antibiotics. *Br J Dermatol* (1990) 122, 717–18.
7. London BM, Lookingbill DP. Frequency of pregnancy in acne patients taking oral antibiotics and oral contraceptives. *Arch Dermatol* (1994) 130, 392–3.
8. Meyer BH, Müller FO, Wessels P, Maree J. A model to detect interactions between roxithromycin and oral contraceptives. *Clin Pharmacol Ther* (1990) 47, 671–4.
9. Pedretti E, Brunenghi GM, Morali GC. Interazione tra antibiotici e contraccettivi orali: la spiramicina. *Quad Clin Ostet Ginecol* (1991) 46, 153–4.
10. Scholtz HE, Sultan E, Wessels D, Hundt AF, Passot V, Renouz A, van Neikerk N. HMR 3647, a new ketolide antimicrobial, does not affect the reliability of low-dose, triphasic oral contraceptives. *Intersci Conf Antimicrob Agents Chemother* (1999) 39, 3.
11. Belfield T, ed. FPA Contraceptive Handbook: a guide for family planning and other health professionals. 3rd ed. London: Family Planning Association, 1999.

Oral contraceptives + Antibacterials; Metronidazole

Isolated cases of combined oral contraceptive failure have been reported with metronidazole. The interaction (if such it is) appears to be very rare indeed. In a controlled trial, metronidazole did not affect contraceptive steroid levels.

Clinical evidence, mechanism, importance and management

Metronidazole 400 mg three times daily for 6 to 8 days had no effect on the AUC of **ethinylestradiol** and **norethisterone** in 10 women taking a combined oral contraceptive. However, 2 of the 10 had a rise in plasma progesterone suggesting that ovulation may have occurred. One of a further 15 women taking metronidazole and a combined oral contraceptive also appeared to ovulate. It was noted that 1 of the 3 women who ovulated also ovulated during a cycle while not on metronidazole.[1] Another similar study in 10 women found that none ovulated while taking metronidazole and a combined oral contraceptive (**ethinylestradiol/norethisterone**).[2]

Only 3 reports of pregnancies were identified in women who took metronidazole and an oral contraceptive (unspecified) in the UK Committee on Safety of Medicines adverse reactions register for the years 1968 to 1984.[3] A survey of oral contraceptive failure identified one failure due to metronidazole (48 of a total of 209 cases were attributed to antibacterials),[4] and a follow-up study identified one further case.[5] Another survey found one failure in a woman on metronidazole, but she was also taking **doxycycline** (see 'Oral contraceptives + Antibacterials; Tetracyclines', p.750).[6] It is possible that these cases represent chance associations.

The interaction between metronidazole and combined oral contraceptives is not established, and the whole issue of any interaction with broad-spectrum antibacterials remains very controversial. Bearing in mind the extremely wide use of both metronidazole and combined oral contraceptives, any increased incidence of contraceptive failure above that seen in general usage is clearly very low indeed. However, where uncertainty remains, the UK Family Planning Authority recommend use of an additional contraceptive method when antibacterials are used (for further details see Importance and management in 'Oral contraceptives + Antibacterials; Penicillins', below).[7]

1. Joshi JV, Joshi UM, Sankholi GM, Krishna U, Mandlekar A, Chowdhury V, Hazari K, Gupta K, Sheth UK, Saxena BN. A study of interaction of low-dose combination oral contraceptive with ampicillin and metronidazole. *Contraception* (1980) 22, 643–52.
2. Viswanathan MK, Govindarajulu P. Metronidazole therapy on the efficacy of oral contraceptive steroid pills. *J Reprod Biol Comp Endocrinol* (1985) 5, 69–72.
3. Back DJ, Grimmer SFM, Orme ML'E, Proudlove C, Mann RD, Breckenridge AM. Evaluation of Committee on Safety of Medicines yellow card reports on oral contraceptive-drug interactions with anticonvulsants and antibiotics. *Br J Clin Pharmacol* (1988) 25, 527–32.
4. Kovacs GT, Riddoch G, Duncombe P, Welberry L, Chick P, Weisberg E, Leavesley GM, Baker HWG. Inadvertent pregnancies in oral contraceptive users. *Med J Aust* (1989) 150, 549–51.
5. Kakouris H, Kovacs GT. Pill failure and non-use of secondary precautions. *Br J Fam Plann* (1992) 18, 41–4.
6. Sparrow MJ. Pill method failures. *N Z Med J* (1987) 100, 102–5.
7. Belfield T, ed. FPA Contraceptive Handbook: a guide for family planning and other health professionals. 3rd ed. London: Family Planning Association, 1999.

Oral contraceptives + Antibacterials; Miscellaneous

One or two cases of combined oral contraceptive failure have been reported with chloramphenicol, clindamycin with cefalexin, dapsone, fusidic acid, isoniazid, nifurtoinol, and nitrofurantoin. These isolated cases are anecdotal and unconfirmed, and the interaction (if such it is) appears to be very rare indeed. The combination of aminosalicylic acid, isoniazid and streptomycin does not appear to affect contraceptive efficacy.

Clinical evidence, mechanism, importance and management

One woman taking a combined oral contraceptive was briefly reported to have developed breakthrough bleeding and to have become pregnant while taking **chloramphenicol**.[1,2] One or two cases of contraceptive failure have been briefly attributed to cefalexin used with **clindamycin**,[3] **dapsone**,[3] **fusidic acid**,[4] **isoniazid**,[3,5] **nifurtoinol**[6] and **nitrofurantoin**.[3,6] One case of breakthrough bleeding due to **clindamycin** and one case due to **chloramphenicol** has also been reported.[7] Conversely, no evidence of ovulation or of changes in plasma **ethinylestradiol** and **norethisterone** levels were seen in a study of 8 women taking a combined oral contraceptive and treated with **aminosalicylic acid**, **isoniazid** and **streptomycin**.[8]

The oral contraceptive/antibacterial interactions summarised here are all that have been identified in the world's literature involving the drugs cited. These interactions are not established, and given the few anecdotal cases with each drug, could just be coincidental. Any increase in the incidence of contraceptive failure above that normally anticipated is clearly very low indeed. With **isoniazid** in particular, there is evidence that the drug does not cause contraceptive failure when used in combination antitubercular therapy (without rifampicin). On the other hand, the personal and ethical consequences of an unwanted pregnancy can be very serious. For this reason, where uncertainty remains, the UK Family Planning Association recommend that for maximal protection a second form of contraception (a barrier method) should be used routinely while taking a short course of a antibiotics like these and for at least 7 days afterwards.[9] For further details see 'Oral contraceptives + Antibacterials; Penicillins', below.

Broad-spectrum antibiotics do not affect the reliability of the **progestogen-only contraceptives** (see 'Progestogen-only contraceptives + Antibacterials; Broad-spectrum', p.765).

1. Hempel E, Böhm W, Carol W, Klinger G. Medikamentöse enzyminduktion und hormonale kontrazeption. *Zentralbl Gynakol* (1973) 95, 1451–7.
2. Hempel E. Personal communication, 1975.
3. Back DJ, Breckenridge AM, Crawford FE, MacIver M, Orme ML'E, Rowe PH. Interindividual variation and drug interactions with hormonal steroid contraceptives. *Drugs* (1981) 21, 46–61.
4. Back DJ, Grimmer SFM, Orme ML'E, Proudlove C, Mann RD, Breckenridge AM. Evaluation of Committee on Safety of Medicines yellow card reports on oral contraceptive-drug interactions with anticonvulsants and antibiotics. *Br J Clin Pharmacol* (1988) 25, 527–32.
5. Kovacs GT, Riddoch G, Duncombe P, Welberry L, Chick P, Weisberg E, Leavesley GM, Baker HWG. Inadvertent pregnancies in oral contraceptive users. *Med J Aust* (1989) 150, 549–51.
6. De Groot AC, Eshuis H, Stricker BHC. Ineffectiviteit van orale anticonceptie tijdens gebruik van minocycline. *Ned Tijdschr Geneeskd* (1990) 134, 1227–9.
7. Hetényi G. Possible interactions between antibiotics and oral contraceptives. *Ther Hung* (1989) 37, 86–9.
8. Joshi JV, Joshi UM, Sankolli GM, Gupta K, Rao AP, Hazari K, Sheth UK, Saxena BN. A study of interaction of low-dose combination oral contraceptive with anti-tubercular drugs. *Contraception* (1980) 21, 617–29.
9. Belfield T, ed. FPA Contraceptive Handbook: a guide for family planning and other health professionals. 3rd ed. London: Family Planning Association, 1999.

Oral contraceptives + Antibacterials; Penicillins

Combined oral contraceptive failure has been attributed to ampicillin, amoxicillin, flucloxacillin, oxacillin, phenoxymethylpenicillin, pivampicillin and talampicillin. However, the interaction (if such it is), appears to be very rare. Controlled studies have not shown any effect of amipicillin on contraceptive steroid levels and ovarian suppression.

Clinical evidence

A case report describes 3 women taking an oral contraceptive who became pregnant when given **ampicillin**.[1] One woman had two unwanted pregnancies while taking a combined oral contraceptive (**ethinylestradi-**

ol/norethisterone). On both occasions conception occurred when she was being treated for tonsillitis.[2] Another woman on **ethinylestradiol/norethisterone** for 5 years with no history of breakthrough bleeding, lost a quantity of blood similar to a normal period loss within a day of starting to take **ampicillin** [exact dose unknown]. There was no evidence of diarrhoea or vomiting in either case.[2] One other case report attributed contraceptive failure to **oxacillin**[3] and another to an intramuscular injection of **benethamine penicillin**, **procaine penicillin** and **benzylpenicillin**.[4]

The use of a penicillin (unspecified) was implicated in 32 pregnancies in women taking an oral contraceptive (unspecified) in the UK Committee on Safety of Medicines adverse reactions register for the years 1968 to 1984 (a further 31 cases were attributed to other antibacterials).[5] In an earlier review, the penicillins in 15 cases were named as **ampicillin** alone or with fusidic acid, tetracycline or **flucloxacillin**, **amoxicillin**, **talampicillin**, **phenoxymethylpenicillin** (one also with oxytetracycline) and 'penicillin'.[6] A survey of contraceptive failure described failures due to **amoxicillin** (16 cases), **flucloxacillin**, **phenoxymethylpenicillin**, **pivampicillin** (5 cases) and **amoxicillin** with **phenoxymethylpenicillin** (1 case),[7] and a follow-up survey identified 9 further cases involving **amoxicillin** and one with 'penicillin'.[8] Another similar survey described a total of 17 cases with **amoxicillin** and 5 cases with 'penicillin',[9] and a follow-up survey identified 8 further cases with **amoxicillin** and 1 case with 'penicillin'.[10]

In contrast, 3 controlled studies have provided evidence that **ampicillin** does not alter the plasma levels of contraceptive steroids nor reduce their antiovulatory effects.[11-13] In the first study, **ampicillin** 250 mg four times daily for 16 days was given to women on **ethinylestradiol/etynodiol**. No women ovulated, as assessed by FSH, LH, and progesterone levels. Two women had breakthrough bleeding while on **ampicillin**, and one had spotting while on placebo.[11] In another study in 7 patients and 6 healthy women, **ampicillin** 500 mg three times daily for 8 days had no significant effect on the plasma levels of **ethinylestradiol** and **levonorgestrel**. However, one woman had a large fall in **ethinylestradiol** levels. Despite this, none of the women ovulated, as assessed by progesterone levels.[12] The third study in 6 women found that **ampicillin** 1 g twice daily had no effect on the plasma levels of **ethinylestradiol** and **norethisterone**, and ovulation did not occur.[13]

Mechanism

Not understood. The oestrogen component of the contraceptive undergoes enterohepatic recirculation (i.e. it is repeatedly secreted in the bile as sulfate and glucuronide conjugates, which are hydrolysed by the gut bacteria before reabsorption). One idea is that if these bacteria are suppressed by the use of an antibacterial, the steroid conjugates are not hydrolysed and are therefore only poorly reabsorbed, resulting in lower-than-normal concentrations of circulating oestrogen in some women. This may result in inadequate suppression of ovulation.[6] However, although the penicillins reduce *urinary* oestriol secretion in pregnant women,[14-18] no marked changes in *serum* ethinylestradiol levels have been found in controlled studies in women taking an oral contraceptive given ampicillin or any other broad-spectrum antibacterial (see 'tetracyclines', (p.750), 'macrolides', (p.745), 'quinolones', (below)). It may be that the enterohepatic recirculation of ethinylestradiol is not clinically important: note that women with an ileostomy have normal serum contraceptive steroid levels.[19] Alternatively, it may be that the proportion of women for whom enterohepatic recirculation is important is extremely small.[19] The progestogens do not take part in enterohepatic recirculation in their active forms.

Importance and management

The oral contraceptive/penicillins interaction is inadequately established and controversial. Almost all of the evidence is anecdotal with no controls. The total number of failures is extremely small when viewed against the number of women worldwide using combined oral contraceptives (estimated at 70 million in 1996 by WHO[20]), so most women are apparently not at risk.

On the other hand, the personal and ethical consequences of an unwanted pregnancy can be very serious. For this reason, some authorities recommend that for maximal protection a second form of contraception (a barrier method) should be used routinely while taking a short course of a penicillin,[21-23] and for at least 7 days afterwards.[21] In addition, the UK Family Planning Association (FPA) recommends that if the 7 days run beyond the end of a packet, the new packet should be started without a break, omitting any of the inactive tablets.[21] While accepting the sense of this advice, others contend that these instructions may confuse patients, and complicate pill taking, and could have the opposite effect of increasing the failure rate of oral contraceptives.[24]

The FPA also say that those on long-term antibacterials (for example for acne) need only take extra precautions for the first two weeks because, after that, the gut flora becomes resistant to the antibacterial.[21]

Broad-spectrum antibiotics do not affect the reliability of the **progestogen-only contraceptives** (see 'Progestogen-only contraceptives + Antibacterials; Broad-spectrum', p.765).

1. Dossetor J. Drug interactions with oral contraceptives. *BMJ* (1975) 4, 467–8.
2. Dossetor J. Personal communication, 1975.
3. Silber TJ. Apparent oral contraceptive failure associated with antibiotic administration. *J Adolesc Health Care* (1983) 4, 287–9.
4. Bainton R. Interaction between antibiotic therapy and contraceptive medication. *Oral Surg Oral Med Oral Pathol* (1986) 61, 453–5.
5. Back DJ, Grimmer SFM, Orme ML'E, Proudlove C, Mann RD, Breckenridge AM. Evaluation of Committee on Safety of Medicines yellow card reports on oral contraceptive-drug interactions with anticonvulsants and antibiotics. *Br J Clin Pharmacol* (1988) 25, 527–32.
6. Back DJ, Breckenridge AM, Crawford FE, MacIver M, Orme ML'E, Rowe PH. Interindividual variation and drug interactions with hormonal steroid contraceptives. *Drugs* (1981) 21, 46–61.
7. Sparrow MJ. Pill method failures. *N Z Med J* (1987) 100, 102–5.
8. Sparrow MJ. Pregnancies in reliable pill takers. *N Z Med J* (1989) 102, 575–7.
9. Kovacs GT, Riddoch G, Duncombe P, Welberry L, Chick P, Weisberg E, Leavesley GM, Baker HWG. Inadvertent pregnancies in oral contraceptive users. *Med J Aust* (1989) 150, 549–51.
10. Kakouris H, Kovacs GT. Pill failure and non-use of secondary precautions. *Br J Fam Plann* (1992) 18, 41–4.
11. Friedman CI, Huneke AL, Kim MH, Powell J. The effect of ampicillin on oral contraceptive effectiveness. *Obstet Gynecol* (1980) 55, 33–7.
12. Back DJ, Breckenridge AM, MacIver M, Orme M, Rowe PH, Staiger Ch, Thomas E, Tjia J. The effects of ampicillin on oral contraceptive steroids in women. *Br J Clin Pharmacol* (1982) 14, 43–8.
13. Joshi JV, Joshi UM, Sankholi GM, Krishna U, Mandlekar A, Chowdhury V, Hazari K, Gupta K, Sheth UK, Saxena BN. A study of interaction of low-dose combination oral contraceptive with ampicillin and metronidazole. *Contraception* (1980) 22, 643–52.
14. Willman K, Pulkkinen MO. Reduced maternal plasma and urinary estriol during ampicillin treatment. *Am J Obstet Gynecol* (1971) 109, 893–6.
15. Tikkanen MJ, Aldercreutz H, Pulkkinen MO. Effect of antibiotics on oestrogen metabolism. *BMJ* (1973) 1, 369.
16. Pulkkinen MO, Willman K. Maternal oestrogen levels during penicillin treatment. *BMJ* (1971) 4, 48.
17. Sybulski S, Maughan GB. Effect of ampicillin administration on estradiol, estriol, and cortisol levels in maternal plasma and on estriol levels in urine. *Am J Obstet Gynecol* (1976) 124, 379–81.
18. Trybuchowski H. Effect of ampicillin on the urinary output of steroidal hormones in pregnant and non-pregnant women. *Clin Chim Acta* (1973) 45, 9–18.
19. Orme M, Back DJ. Oral contraceptive steroids – pharmacological issues of interest to the prescribing physician. *Adv Contracept* (1991) 7, 325–31.
20. WHO. New program research on the safety of oral contraceptive pills. Available at: http://www.who.int/reproductive-health/hrp/progress/39/prog39.pdf (accessed 11/04/05).
21. Belfield T, ed. FPA Contraceptive Handbook: a guide for family planning and other health professionals. 3rd ed. London: Family Planning Association, 1999.
22. Hannaford PC, Webb AMC, on behalf of participants at an International workshop. Evidence-guided prescribing of combined oral contraceptives: consensus statement. *Contraception* (1996) 54, 125–9.
23. Dickinson BD, Altman RD, Nielsen NH, Sterling ML, for the Council on Scientific Affairs, American Medical Association. Drug interactions between oral contraceptives and antibiotics. *Obstet Gynecol* (2001) 98, 853–60.
24. Weaver K, Glasier A. Interaction between broad-spectrum antibiotics and the combined oral contraceptive pill. *Contraception* (1999) 59, 71–8.

Oral contraceptives + Antibacterials; Quinolones

Ciprofloxacin, moxifloxacin and ofloxacin have been shown not to affect the pharmacokinetics of the combined oral contraceptives in controlled trials. No reports of contraceptive failure appear to have been reported, and ovarian suppression is not affected.

Clinical evidence

(a) Ciprofloxacin

No ovulation occurred (as assessed by LH, FSH and estradiol levels) in 10 healthy women taking a combined oral contraceptive (**ethinylestradiol** plus **desogestrel**, **gestodene** or **levonorgestrel**) while also taking ciprofloxacin 500 mg twice daily for 7 days, starting on the first day of contraceptive intake. No breakthrough bleeding occurred.[1] Another study in 24 healthy women taking a combined oral contraceptive (**ethinylestradiol/desogestrel**) found that ciprofloxacin 500 mg twice daily for 10 days had no effect on the pharmacokinetics of **ethinylestradiol**. In addition, no subject actually ovulated, as assessed by progesterone and estradiol levels. However, 2 of the subjects were potentially ovulatory taking a placebo instead of ciprofloxacin as detected by an ultrasound of ovarian activity. A further 4 subjects taking **ciprofloxacin** and 2 on placebo had lesser indications of ovarian activity.[2]

(b) Moxifloxacin

A placebo-controlled, crossover study in 29 young healthy women taking a combined oral contraceptive (**ethinylestradiol/levonorgestrel**) found that moxifloxacin 400 mg daily on cycle days 1 to 7 had no clinically relevant effect on the pharmacokinetics of either contraceptive steroid. The hormonal parameters measured (estradiol, progesterone, LH, FSH) were also unchanged by the presence of the quinolone, indicating that ovulation continued to be suppressed.[3]

(c) Ofloxacin

Ofloxacin had no effect on ovulation suppression in 19 women taking a combined oral contraceptive (**ethinylestradiol/levonorgestrel**). In this placebo-controlled crossover study, two courses of ofloxacin 200 mg twice daily for 7 days were given on days 1 to 7 of two consecutive cycles. Ovulation was assessed by ultrasound of the ovaries, and by measuring FSH, estradiol and progesterone levels. Four of the women showed signs of ovarian activity in both the placebo and ofloxacin cycles.[4]

Mechanism

Fluoroquinolones are broad-spectrum antibacterials, and so might be expected to interrupt the enterohepatic recirculation of ethinylestradiol,[1,5] but the evidence that this is clinically important is scant (For a more detailed discussion of this mechanism see 'Oral contraceptives + Antibacterials; Penicillins', p.746).

Importance and management

The pharmacokinetic and pharmacodynamic data indicate a likely absence of interactions between combined oral contraceptives and these fluoroquinolones. In addition, reports of cases of contraceptive failure with these or any other quinolone antibiotic seem to be lacking. No special extra contraceptive precautions would therefore seem to be necessary during concurrent use. Note that the UK Family Planning Authority does not specifically apply the general recommendations for broad-spectrum antibacterials and combined oral contraceptives to quinolones.[6] However, if one accepts the theory that there are an, as yet, unidentifiable tiny group of women for whom enterohepatic recirculation of ethinylestradiol is important, then it could be argued that insufficient patients were assessed in the above studies to include anyone from this group, and that the general precautions should be applied (see 'Oral contraceptives + Antibacterials; Penicillins', p.746). However, if one tends to the theory that the anecdotal cases of contraceptive failure with broad-spectrum antibacterials are indistinguishable from the normal accepted failure rate, no special precautions are necessary with these fluoroquinolones, or indeed, any other antibacterials.

1. Maggiolo F, Puricelli G, Dottorini M, Caprioli S, Bianchi W, Suter F. The effect of ciprofloxacin on oral contraceptive steroid treatments. *Drugs Exp Clin Res* (1991) 17, 451–4.
2. Scholten PC, Droppert RM, Zwinkels MGJ, Moesker HL, Nauta JJP, Hoepelman IM. No interaction between ciprofloxacin and an oral contraceptive. *Antimicrob Agents Chemother* (1998) 42, 3266–8.
3. Staß H, Sachse R, Heinig R, Zühlsdorf M, Horstmann R. Pharmacokinetics (PK) of steroid hormones in oral contraceptives (OC) are not altered by oral moxifloxacin (MOX). *J Antimicrob Chemother* (1999) 44 (Suppl A) 138–9.
4. Csemiczky G, Alvendal C, Landgren B-M. Risk for ovulation in women taking a low-dose oral contraceptive (Microgynon) when receiving antibacterial treatment with a fluoroquinolone (ofloxacin). *Adv Contracept* (1996) 12, 101–9.
5. Back DJ, Tija J, Martin C, Millar E, Mant T, Morrison P, Orme M. The lack of interaction between temafloxacin and combined oral contraceptive steroids. *Contraception* (1991) 43, 317–23.
6. Belfield T, ed. FPA Contraceptive Handbook: a guide for family planning and other health professionals. 3rd ed. London: Family Planning Association, 1999.

Oral contraceptives + Antibacterials; Rifamycins

Combined oral contraceptives are less reliable during treatment with rifampicin. Breakthrough bleeding and spotting commonly occur, and pregnancy may not be prevented. Rifabutin also reduces the reliability of oral contraceptives, although it interacts to a lesser extent, and no contraceptive failures have yet been reported.

Clinical evidence

(a) Rifampicin

A report in 1971 noted a marked increase in the frequency of intermenstrual breakthrough bleeding (regarded as loss of reliability of the contraceptive) in women taking a combined oral contraceptive and rifampicin.[1] In a later report by the same researchers, 62 out of 88 women taking a combined oral contraceptive had menstrual cycle disorders of various kinds (spotting, bleeding, failure to menstruate) when treated with rifampicin-based antitubercular therapy, compared with only 1 of 26 treated with streptomycin-based therapy. In addition, 5 pregnancies occurred in women on rifampicin-based therapy.[2,3] Other case reports have confirmed this interaction, and there have been a total of at least 11 other pregnancies reported.[4-11] Combined oral contraceptives commonly mentioned in these reports include **ethinylestradiol** with **norgestrel** or **norethisterone**.[5,7-11]

One pharmacodynamic study found that 11 out of 21 women taking a triphasic oral contraceptive (**ethinylestradiol/levonorgestrel** 30 to 40 micrograms/50 to 125 micrograms) ovulated (assessed by increased progesterone levels) while taking rifampicin 300 mg daily.[12] In another study, 2 out of 7 women taking a combined oral contraceptive (**ethinylestradiol/norethisterone** 30 micrograms/1 mg) ovulated while taking rifampicin. In addition, rifampicin reduced the AUC of **norethisterone** by 30%.[13] Conversely, two other studies did not detect ovulation in 34 women taking a combined oral contraceptive (**ethinylestradiol/norethisterone** 35 micrograms/1 mg) taking rifampicin.[14,15] However, an increased incidence of spotting was noted in one study (36% versus 3.7% in the control cycle).[14] Furthermore, both of these studies found that rifampicin 300 mg daily for 10 days or 600 mg daily for 14 days reduced the AUC of **ethinylestradiol** by 64% and 62.5% and **norethisterone** by 60% and 49.4%. These pharmacokinetic results confirm the findings of earlier studies.[16,17] Rifampicin plasma levels[18] and efficacy[1] are reported to be unchanged by oral contraceptives.

(b) Rifabutin

In the two studies already mentioned above, rifabutin 300 mg daily for 10 or 14 days similarly reduced the plasma levels of **ethinylestradiol** and **norethisterone** in women taking a combined oral contraceptive, but to a lesser extent than **rifampicin**. The AUC for **ethinylestradiol** decreased by about 35% in both studies, and that for **norethisterone** by 20% and 14%. In one study, spotting occurred in 21.7% of women when receiving rifabutin (compared with 3.7% in the control cycle and 36% with rifampicin).[14] Ovulation did not occur with rifabutin or **rifampicin** in either study.[14,15] There appear to be no reports of contraceptive failure attributed to rifabutin.

Mechanism

Rifampicin is a potent non-specific enzyme inducer, which has been shown to increase the hydroxylation of ethinylestradiol fourfold in an *in vitro* study,[19,20] and twofold in an *in vivo* study.[21] Another study showed that the metabolism of ethinylestradiol (derived from mestranol) was similarly affected.[22] As a result, the reduced steroid levels may be insufficient to prevent the re-establishment of a normal menstrual cycle with ovulation, which would explain the breakthrough bleeding and pregnancies that have occurred. Rifabutin similarly acts as enzyme inducing agent, but it is only half as potent as rifampicin in reducing contraceptive steroid levels.[15]

Importance and management

The interaction between the combined oral contraceptives and rifampicin is well documented, well established and clinically important. Menstrual cycle disturbances in 36 to 70%,[1,2,14] and an ovulation rate of up to 52% of women taking the combination[12,13] show very clearly that women on combined oral contraceptives should use an alternative or additional form of contraception while on rifampicin, and for 4 to 8 weeks after its withdrawal.[23] The UK Family Planning Association make the same recommendation.[24]

No contraceptive failures due to rifampicin have been reported with the **progestogen-only contraceptives**, but their reliability in the presence of rifampicin is doubtful because rifampicin is known to increase the metabolism of the progestogen component of combined oral contraceptives.[13-16] The precautions suggested for the combined oral contraceptives should therefore be followed.

Direct information about the interaction between combined oral contraceptives and rifabutin seems to be limited to the pharmacodynamic studies cited, but it is supported by the well-recognised enzyme inducing properties of rifabutin, so that it would clearly be prudent for women on rifabutin to take the same precautions as with rifampicin, although the risks are lower because rifabutin is a less potent enzyme-inducing agent. No cases of contraceptive failure appear so far to have been attributed to the use of rifabutin. Nevertheless, to be on the safe side, both the makers and the UK Committee on Safety of Medicines say that patients using these contraceptives and rifabutin should be advised to use other methods of contraception.[25,26] The risk of failure with the **progestogen-only contraceptives** would also seem to be similar and the same precautions would seem to be appropriate.

1. Reimers D, Ježek A. Rifampicin und andere Antituberkulotika bei gleichzeitiger oraler Kontrazeption. *Prax Pneumol* (1971) 25, 255–62.
2. Nocke-Finck L, Breuer H, Reimers D. Wirkung von Rifampicin auf den Menstruationszyklus und die Östrogenausscheidung bei Einnahme oraler Kontrazeptiva. *Dtsch Med Wochenschr* (1973) 98, 1521–3.
3. Reimers D, Nocke-Finck L, Breuer H. Rifampicin causes a lowering in efficacy of oral contraceptives by influencing oestrogen excretion. Reports on Rifampicin: XXII International Tuberculosis Conference, Tokyo, September 1973, 87–9.
4. Kropp R. Rifampicin und Ovulationshemmer. *Prax Pneumol* (1974) 28, 270–2.
5. Bessot J-C, Vandevenne A, Petitjean R, Burghard G. Effets opposés de la rifampicine et de l'isoniazide sur le métabolisme des contraceptifs oraux? *Nouv Presse Med* (1977) 6, 1568.
6. Hirsch A. Pilules endormies. *Nouv Presse Med* (1973) 2, 2957.
7. Piguet B, Muglioni JF, Chaline G. Contraception orale et rifampicine. *Nouv Presse Med* (1975) 4, 115–16.
8. Skolnick JL, Stoler BS, Katz DB, Anderson WH. Rifampicin, oral contraceptives and pregnancy. *JAMA* (1976) 236, 1382.
9. Gupta KC, Ali MY. Failure of oral contraceptive with rifampicin. *Med J Zambia* (1980/81) 15, 23.
10. Hirsch A, Tillement JP, Chrétein J. Effects contrariants de la rifampicine sur les contraceptifs oraux: a propos de trois grossesses non désirées observées chez deux malades. *Rev Fr Mal Respir* (1975) 3, 174–82.
11. Lafaix Ch, Cadoz M, Richard A, Patouillard P. L'effect "antipilule" de la rifampicine. *Med Hyg (Geneve)* (1976) 1181, 181–2.
12. Meyer B, Müller F, Wessels P, Maree J. A model to detect interactions between roxithromycin and oral contraceptives. *Clin Pharmacol Ther* (1990) 47, 671–4.
13. Joshi JV, Joshi UM, Sankolli GM, Gupta K, Rao AP, Hazari K, Sheth UK, Saxena BN. A study of interaction of low-dose combination oral contraceptive with anti-tubercular drugs. *Contraception* (1980) 21, 617–29.
14. LeBel M, Masson E, Guilbert E, Colborn D, Paquet F, Allard S, Vallée F, Narang PK. Effects of rifabutin and rifampicin on the pharmacokinetics of ethinylestradiol and norethindrone. *J Clin Pharmacol* (1998) 38, 1042–50.
15. Barditch-Crovo P, Braun Trapnell C, Ette E, Zacur HA, Coresh J, Rocco LE, Hendrix CW, Flexner C. The effects of rifampin and rifabutin on the pharmacokinetics and pharmacodynamics of a combination oral contraceptive. *Clin Pharmacol Ther* (1999) 65, 428–38.
16. Back DJ, Breckenridge AM, Crawford F, MacIver M, Orme ML'E, Park BK, Rowe PH, Smith E. The effect of rifampicin on norethisterone pharmacokinetics. *Eur J Clin Pharmacol* (1979) 15, 193–7.
17. Back DJ, Breckenridge AM, Crawford FE, Hall JM, MacIver M, Orme ML'E, Rowe PH, Smith E, Watts MJ. The effect of rifampicin on the pharmacokinetics of ethynylestradiol in women. *Contraception* (1980) 21, 135–43.
18. Gupta KC, Joshi JV, Anklesaria PS, Shah RS, Satoskar RS. Plasma rifampicin levels during oral contraception. *J Assoc Physicians India* (1988) 36, 365–6.
19. Bolt HM, Kappus H, Bolt M. Rifampicin and oral contraception. *Lancet* (1974) i, 1280–1.
20. Bolt HM, Kappus H, Bolt M. Effect of rifampicin treatment on the metabolism of oestradiol and 17α-ethinyloestradiol by human liver microsomes. *Eur J Clin Pharmacol* (1975) 8, 301–7.
21. Bolt HM, Bolt M, Kappus H. Interaction of rifampicin treatment with pharmacokinetics and metabolism of ethinyloestradiol in man. *Acta Endocrinol (Copenh)* (1977) 85, 189–97.
22. Gelbke HP, Gethmann U, Knuppen R. Influence of rifampicin treatment on the metabolic fate of [4-^{14}C] mestranol in women. *Horm Metab Res* (1977) 9, 415–19.
23. Orme M, Back DJ. Oral contraceptive steroids – pharmacological issues of interest to the prescribing physician. *Adv Contracept* (1991) 7, 325–31.
24. Belfield T, ed. FPA Contraceptive Handbook: a guide for family planning and other health professionals. 3rd ed. London: Family Planning Association, 1999.
25. Committee on Safety of Medicines (CSM)/Medicines Control Agency (MCA). Revised indication and drug interactions of rifabutin. Current Problems 1997, 23, 14.
26. Mycobutin (Rifabutin). Pharmacia Ltd. UK Summary of product characteristics, January 2003.

Oral contraceptives + Antibacterials; Sulfonamides or Trimethoprim

Co-trimoxazole (sulfamethoxazole/trimethoprim) increases ethinylestradiol levels. However, there are about 15 anecdotal cases on record of contraceptive failure attributed to co-trimoxazole. There are also isolated cases of contraceptive failure attributed to various sulphonamides, and trimethoprim.

Clinical evidence

(a) Co-trimoxazole

Co-trimoxazole (trimethoprim/sulfamethoxazole 160/800 mg twice daily for 7 days starting on day 10 of a cycle) increased **ethinylestradiol** plasma levels by 30 to 50% in a study in 9 women taking a triphasic combined oral contraceptive (**ethinylestradiol/levonorgestrel**). **Levonorgestrel** plasma levels remained unaltered. No subjects ovulated, as assessed by progesterone and follicle stimulating hormone (FSH) levels, and FSH levels actually decreased indicating increased suppression of ovulation.[1]

In contrast, 5 cases of oral contraceptive failure attributed to the use of co-trimoxazole were identified in the UK Committee on Safety of Medicines adverse reactions register for the years 1968 to 1984 (58 cases were attributed to other antibacterials).[2,3] Contraceptive failure has been reported in another 10 patients taking co-trimoxazole,[4-8] and 3 further cases of contraceptive failure are attributed to co-trimoxazole or trimethoprim.[9]

(b) Sulphonamides

One woman on a combined oral contraceptive is briefly reported to have shown breakthrough bleeding and to have become pregnant while taking **sulfamethoxypyridazine**.[10,11] One case of a pregnancy, in a woman who had taken a sulphonamide (unspecified) and an oral contraceptive (unspecified), was identified in the UK Committee on Safety of Medicines adverse reactions register for the years 1968 to 1984 (a total of 62 cases were attributed to other antibacterials).[3] Three further cases of failure have been attributed to **sulfafurazole** (**sulfisoxazole**) and a sulphonamide (unspecified).[12]

(c) Trimethoprim

Two pregnancies were attributed to the use of trimethoprim with an oral contraceptive (unspecified) in the UK Committee on Safety of Medicines adverse reactions register for the years 1968 to 1984 (a total of 61 cases were attributed to other antibacterials).[3] Another survey of oral contraceptive failure identified one pregnancy due to trimethoprim (23 of a total of 137 cases were attributed to antibacterials),[6] while an earlier survey attributed 3 cases to either **co-trimoxazole** or trimethoprim.[9] One case with trimethoprim and one with trimethoprim plus nitrofurantoin are briefly mentioned in another report.[7]

Mechanism

A possible explanation for the rise in ethinylestradiol levels[1] is that co-trimoxazole inhibits the liver enzymes concerned with the metabolism and clearance of this estrogen from the body. Broad-spectrum antibacterials might be expected to interrupt the enterohepatic recirculation of ethinylestradiol leading to contraceptive failure, but the evidence that this is clinically important is scant (see also 'Oral contraceptives + Antibacterials; Penicillins', p.746).

Importance and management

Not established. The pharmacokinetic and pharmacodynamic evidence indicates that co-trimoxazole is not likely to reduce the effectiveness of combined oral contraceptives. Although there are a number of reports of contraceptive failure attributed to co-trimoxazole, these are anecdotal and unconfirmed. It is possible that these cases are coincidental, and fit within the normal failure rate of combined oral contraceptives. The UK Family Planning Authority considers that it is almost certain that co-trimoxazole and sulphonamides do not interact with combined oral contraceptives.[13] No special precautions appear to be necessary.

The main concern of increased levels of ethinylestradiol is whether this would increase the risk of adverse effects of the steroid. There are no data on the effect of these modest (30 to 50%) increases in steroid levels on various adverse effects. It could be argued that a 40% increase would turn a standard-strength contraceptive (35 micrograms) into a high-dose contraceptive (50 micrograms). However, early studies showed that the interindividual variation in ethinylestradiol pharmacokinetics was greater than this anyway.[2] Further study is needed on this issue.

1. Grimmer SFM, Allen WL, Back DJ, Breckenridge AM, Orme M, Tjia J. The effect of cotrimoxazole on oral contraceptive steroids in women. *Contraception* (1983) 28, 53–9.
2. Back DJ, Breckenridge AM, Crawford FE, MacIver M, Orme ML'E, Rowe PH. Interindividual variation and drug interactions with hormonal steroid contraceptives. *Drugs* (1981) 21, 46–61.
3. Back DJ, Grimmer SFM, Orme ML'E, Proudlove C, Mann RD, Breckenridge AM. Evaluation of Committee on Safety of Medicines yellow card reports on oral contraceptive-drug interactions with anticonvulsants and antibiotics. *Br J Clin Pharmacol* (1988) 25, 527–32.
4. Beeley L, Magee P, Hickey FM. *Bulletin of the West Midlands Centre for Adverse Drug Reaction Reporting* (1989) 28, 32.
5. Kovacs GT, Riddoch G, Duncombe P, Welberry L, Chick P, Weisberg E, Leavesley GM, Baker HWG. Inadvertent pregnancies in oral contraceptive users. *Med J Aust* (1989) 150, 549–51.
6. Sparrow MJ. Pregnancies in reliable pill takers. *N Z Med J* (1989) 102, 575–7.
7. De Groot AC, Eshuis H, Stricker BHC. Ineffectiviteit van orale anticonceptie tijdens gebruik van minocycline. *Ned Tijdschr Geneeskd* (1990) 134, 1227–9.
8. Kakouris H, Kovacs GT. Pill failure and non-use of secondary precautions. *Br J Fam Plann* (1992) 18, 41–4.
9. Sparrow MJ. Pill method failures. *N Z Med J* (1987) 100, 102–5.
10. Hempel E, Böhm W, Carol W, Klinger G. Medikamentöse enzyminduktion und hormonale kontrazeption. *Zentralbl Gynakol* (1973) 95, 1451–7.
11. Hempel E. Personal communication, 1975.

12. DeSano EA, Hurley SC. Possible interactions of antihistamines and antibiotics with oral contraceptive effectiveness. *Fertil Steril* (1982) 37, 853–4.

13. Belfield T, ed. FPA Contraceptive Handbook: a guide for family planning and other health professionals. 3rd ed. London: Family Planning Association, 1999.

Oral contraceptives + Antibacterials; Tetracyclines

Contraceptive failure has been attributed to doxycycline, lymecycline, oxytetracycline, minocycline, tetracycline in about 40 reported cases, 7 of which specified long-term antibacterial use, but the interaction (if such it is) appears to be very rare. Controlled trials have not shown any effect of tetracycline or doxycycline on contraceptive steroid levels.

Clinical evidence

A woman taking a combined oral contraceptive (**ethinylestradiol/levonorgestrel**) became pregnant, the evidence indicating that she had conceived during or in the week after taking **tetracycline** 500 mg six-hourly for 3 days and then 250 mg six-hourly for 2 days. There was no evidence of either nausea or vomiting, which might have been an alternative explanation for the contraceptive failure.[1] A case of breakthrough bleeding attributed to **tetracycline** was also mentioned in this report.[1] Two other case reports describe pregnancies in women taking a combined oral contraceptive and long-term **tetracycline** 500 mg daily[2] or long-term **minocycline** 100 mg daily.[3] The latter also briefly mentions 2 cases of contraceptive failure with **doxycycline.**[3]

Twelve reports of pregnancies were attributed to the use of tetracyclines (unspecified) and an oral contraceptive (unspecified) in the UK Committee on Safety of Medicines adverse reactions register for the years 1968 to 1984 (51 cases were attributed to other antibacterials).[4] In an earlier report, the tetracyclines in 6 cases were named as **tetracycline** and **oxytetracycline.**[5] A survey of oral contraceptive failure identified 7 failures due to **doxycycline**, **lymecycline** or **minocycline** (37 of a total of 163 cases were attributed to antibacterials),[6] and a follow-up survey identified 3 further cases involving short courses of **tetracycline.**[7] Similar surveys identified 5 contraceptive failures with **tetracycline,**[8-10] and 2 failures with **doxycycline.**[9] Intermenstrual bleeding was attributed to **doxycycline** or **oxytetracycline** in 3 other cases.[11]

In a dermatological practice, of 124 women taking an oral contraceptive and antibacterials (mostly tetracyclines or erythromycin), 2 became pregnant, with a calculated failure rate of 1.2%. One patient was taking long-term **minocycline** and **ethinylestradiol/norethisterone**, and one had taken a 5-day course of **oxytetracycline** while on **ethinylestradiol/levonorgestrel**. This failure rate was reported to be sixfold higher than a normal failure rate of 0.2%.[12] However, a rate of 0.2% represents perfect rather than typical use of combined oral contraceptives. In a similar analysis,[13] one of 34 women became pregnant after taking long-term **tetracycline** and **ethinylestradiol/norethisterone**. This failure rate of 1.4% was not considered to be significantly different from a normal failure rate of 0.27%. In a larger better-designed case-control study, 356 women were identified who had received oral contraceptives and antibacterials (said to be cephalosporins, penicillins, tetracyclines) over a 5-year period in 3 dermatological practices. The failure rate in these women (1.6% per year, 3 pregnancies occurred in women on long-term **minocycline** and 2 on a cephalosporin) was indistinguishable from the failure rate seen in control patients on oral contraceptives and no antibacterials (1% per year).[14]

Moreover, two controlled studies have shown that tetracyclines do not affect contraceptive steroids.[15,16] In the first, **tetracycline** 500 mg six-hourly for 10 days had no effect on the AUC of **ethinylestradiol** and **norethisterone** (measured on days 1, 5 and 10) in 7 healthy women on a combined oral contraceptive.[15] Similarly **doxycycline** 100 mg twice daily for 7 days had no effect on the serum levels of **ethinylestradiol** and **norethisterone** (measured on days 5 to 7) in 23 healthy women on a combined oral contraceptive. In addition, ovulation did not occur, as assessed by progesterone levels, but 2 women did experience breakthrough bleeding.[16]

The pharmacokinetics of **tetracycline** (4-hour AUC and peak level) were not significantly different between 7 healthy women on a combined oral contraceptive (**ethinylestradiol/norethisterone**) and 4 healthy women on no medication.[15] See 'Tetracyclines; Minocycline + Ethinylestradiol', p.247 for reports of facial pigmentation due to **minocycline** and **ethinylestradiol**.

Mechanism

Not understood. If an interaction occurs, suppression of intestinal bacteria resulting in a fall in enterohepatic recirculation of ethinylestradiol is the usual suggested explanation, but there is no evidence that this is clinically important. For a full discussion of this mechanism see 'Oral contraceptives + Antibacterials; Penicillins', p.746.

Importance and management

The oral contraceptive/tetracycline interactions summarised here are all that have been identified in the world's literature involving the drugs cited. Much of the evidence is anecdotal with insufficient controls (if any). These interactions are not adequately established and the whole issue remains controversial. Bearing in mind the extremely wide use of both drugs, any increase in the incidence of contraceptive failure above the accepted failure rate is clearly very low indeed. On the other hand, the personal and ethical consequences of an unwanted pregnancy can be very serious. For this reason, some authorities recommend that, for maximal protection, a second form of contraception (a barrier method) should be used routinely while taking a short course of tetracyclines,[17-19] and for 7 days afterwards.[17] In addition, the UK Family Planning Association (FPA) recommends that, when using a tetracycline, if the 7 days run beyond the end of a packet, the new packet should be started without a break, omitting any of the inactive tablets.[17] While accepting the sense of this advice, others contend that these instructions may confuse patients, and complicate pill taking, and could have the opposite effect of increasing the user-failure rate of oral contraceptives.[20]

In the case of long-term use of tetracyclines for acne, at least 7 cases of contraceptive failure have been reported. Nevertheless, in statistical terms the only well-designed case-controlled study in dermatological practice indicated that the incidence of contraceptive failure due to this interaction could not be distinguished from the general and recognised failure rate of oral contraceptives.[14] The UK FPA also say that those on long-term antibiotics (for example for acne) need only take extra precautions for the first 3 weeks because, after about 2 weeks, the gut flora becomes resistant to the antibiotic.[17]

Broad-spectrum antibiotics do not affect the reliability of the **progestogen-only contraceptives** (see 'Progestogen-only contraceptives + Antibacterials; Broad-spectrum', p.765).

1. Bacon JF, Shenfield GM. Pregnancy attributable to interaction between tetracycline and oral contraceptives. *BMJ* (1980) 1, 293.
2. Lequeux A. Grossesse sous contraceptif oral après prise de tétracycline. *Louvain Med* (1980) 99, 413–14.
3. de Groot AC, Eshuis H, Stricker BHC. Ineffectiviteit van orale anticonceptie tijdens gebruik van minocycline. *Ned Tijdschr Geneeskd* (1990) 134, 1227–9.
4. Back DJ, Grimmer SFM, Orme ML'E, Proudlove C, Mann RD, Breckenridge AM. Evaluation of Committee on Safety of Medicines yellow card reports on oral contraceptive-drug interactions with anticonvulsants and antibiotics. *Br J Clin Pharmacol* (1988) 25, 527–32.
5. Back DJ, Breckenridge AM, Crawford FE, MacIver M, Orme ML'E, Rowe PH. Interindividual variation and drug interactions with hormonal steroid contraceptives. *Drugs* (1981) 21, 46–61.
6. Sparrow MJ. Pill method failures. *N Z Med J* (1987) 100, 102–5.
7. Sparrow MJ. Pregnancies in reliable pill takers. *N Z Med J* (1989) 102, 575–7.
8. Kovacs GT, Riddoch G, Duncombe P, Welberry L, Chick P, Weisberg E, Leavesley GM, Baker HWG. Inadvertent pregnancies in oral contraceptive users. *Med J Aust* (1989) 150, 549–51.
9. Kakouris H, Kovacs GT. Pill failure and non-use of secondary precautions. *Br J Fam Plann* (1992) 18, 41–4.
10. DeSano EA, Hurley SC. Possible interactions of antihistamines and antibiotics with oral contraceptive effectiveness. *Fertil Steril* (1982) 37, 853–4.
11. Hetényi G. Possible interactions between antibiotics and oral contraceptives. *Ther Hung* (1989) 37, 86–9.
12. Hughes BR, Cunliffe WJ. Interactions between the oral contraceptive pill and antibiotics. *Br J Dermatol* (1990) 122, 717.
13. London BM, Lookingbill DP. Frequency of pregnancy in acne patients taking oral antibiotics and oral contraceptives. *Arch Dermatol* (1994) 130, 392–3.
14. Helms SE, Bredle DL, Zajic J, Jarjoura D, Brodell RT, Krishnarao I. Oral contraceptive failure rates and oral antibiotics. *J Am Acad Dermatol* (1997) 36, 705–10.
15. Murphy AA, Zacur HA, Charache P, Burkman RT. The effect of tetracycline on levels of oral contraceptives. *Am J Obstet Gynecol* (1991) 164, 28–33.
16. Neely JL, Abate M, Swinker M, D'Angio R. The effect of doxycycline on serum levels of ethinyl estradiol, norethindrone, and endogenous progesterone. *Obstet Gynecol* (1991) 77, 416–20.
17. Belfield T, ed. FPA Contraceptive Handbook: a guide for family planning and other health professionals. 3rd ed. London: Family Planning Association, 1999.
18. Hannaford PC, Webb AMC, on behalf of participants at an International workshop. Evidence-guided prescribing of combined oral contraceptives: consensus statement. *Contraception* (1996) 54, 125–9.
19. Dickinson BD, Altman RD, Nielsen NH, Sterling ML, for the Council on Scientific Affairs, American Medical Association. Drug interactions between oral contraceptives and antibiotics. *Obstet Gynecol* (2001) 98, 853–60.
20. Weaver K, Glasier A. Interaction between broad-spectrum antibiotics and the combined oral contraceptive pill. *Contraception* (1999) 59, 71–8.

Oral contraceptives or HRT + Antibacterials; Troleandomycin

Severe pruritus and jaundice have been observed in women taking oral contraceptives shortly after starting treatment with troleandomycin. One case has also been reported with oestrogens for hormone replacement therapy.

Clinical evidence

A report describes 10 cases of cholestatic jaundice and pruritus in women taking oral contraceptives and troleandomycin. All had been using the contraceptive for 7 to 48 months and were given the antibacterial in daily doses of 1 to 3 g. The pruritus was intense, and started within 2 to 24 days of the first dose of troleandomycin, and preceding the jaundice. In 8 of the patients the pruritus and jaundice persisted for over a month.[1] A later report and letter by the same authors describes a total of 24 cases of this reaction.[2,3]

There are numerous other reports of this adverse reaction in a total of over 40 other women.[4-12] The adverse reactions (fatigue, anorexia, severe itching, jaundice) can begin very rapidly, sometimes even within 2 days of starting the troleandomycin, and may last up to 14 weeks or more.[3,4,12] One report also describes a similar reaction in a 48-year-old woman on **oestrogens** for hormone replacement therapy.[4]

Mechanism

Uncertain. Hepatotoxicity has been associated with the use of both types of drug, but it is not common. The reaction suggests that their damaging effects on the liver may be additive or supra-additive.[10,11] Troleandomycin may cause an increase in levels of contraceptive steroids, since it is an inhibitor of hepatic enzymes.[12,13]

Importance and management

A well established, well documented and clinically important interaction. The incidence is unknown. Concurrent use should be avoided. Other macrolides may be suitable alternatives. See 'Oral contraceptives + Antibacterials; Macrolides', p.745.

1. Miguet JP, Monange C, Vuitton D, Allemand H, Hirsch JP, Carayon P, Gisselbrecht H. Ictère cholestatique survenu après administration de triacétyloléandomycine: interférence avec les contraceptifs oraux? Dix observations. *Nouv Presse Med* (1978) 7, 4304.
2. Miguet J-P, Vuitton D, Pessayre D, Allemand H, Metreau J-M, Poupon R, Capron J-P, Blanc F. Jaundice from troleandomycin and oral contraceptives. *Ann Intern Med* (1980) 92, 434.
3. Miguet J-P, Vuitton D, Allemand H, Pessayre D, Monange C, Hirsch J-P, Metreau J-M, Poupon R, Capron J-P, Blanc F. Une épidémie d'ictères due a l'association troléandomycine – contraceptifs oraux. *Gastroenterol Clin Biol* (1980) 4, 420–4.
4. Perol R, Hincky J, Desnos M. Hépatites cholestatiques lors de la prise de troléandomycine chez deux femmes prenant des estrogènes. *Nouv Presse Med* (1978) 7, 4302.
5. Goldfain D, Chauveinc L, Guillan J, Verduron J. Ictère cholestatique chez des femmes prenant simultanément de la triacétyloléandomycine et des contraceptifs oraux. *Nouv Presse Med* (1979) 8, 1099.
6. Rollux R, Plottin F, Mingat J, Bessard G. Ictère apres association estroprogestatif-troléandomycine. Trois observations. *Nouv Presse Med* (1979) 8, 1694.
7. Haber I, Hubens H. Cholestatic jaundice after triacetyloleandomycin and oral contraceptives. *Acta Gastroenterol Belg* (1980) 43, 475–82.
8. Descotes J, Evreux JC, Foyatier N, Gaumer R, Girard D, Savoye B. Trois nouvelles observations d'ictère après estroprogestatifs et troléandomycine. *Nouv Presse Med* (1979) 8, 1182–3.
9. Belgian Centre for Drug Supervison. Levertoxiciteit van troleandomycine en oestrogen. *Folia Pharmaceutica (Brussels)* (1979) 6, 64.
10. Dellas JA, Hugues FC, Roussel G, Marche J. Contraception orale et troléandomycine. Un nouveau cas d'ictère. *Therapie* (1982) 37, 443–6.
11. Girard D, Pillon M, Bel A, Petigny A, Savoye B. Hepatite au decours d'un traitment a la triacetyloleandomycine chez les jeunes femmes sous estro-progestatifs. *Lyon Mediterr Med Med Sud Est* (1980) 16, 2335–44.
12. Fevery J, Van Steenbergen W, Desmet V, Deruyttere M, De Groote J. Severe intrahepatic cholestasis due to the combined intake of oral contraceptives and triacetyloleandomycin. *Acta Clin Belg* (1983) 38, 242–5.
13. Claudel S, Euvrard P, Bory R, Chavaillon A, Paliard P. Cholestase intra-hépatique après association triacétyloléandomycine-estroprogestatif. *Nouv Presse Med* (1979) 8, 1182.

Oral contraceptives + Anticonvulsants; Barbiturates or Phenytoin

Oral contraceptives are less reliable during treatment with phenytoin and barbiturates such as phenobarbital and primidone. Intermenstrual breakthrough bleeding and spotting can take place, and pregnancies have occurred. Controlled studies have shown that phenytoin and phenobarbital can reduce contraceptive steroid levels.

Clinical evidence

An epileptic woman taking phenytoin 200 mg and **sultiame** 50 mg daily (with ferrous gluconate and folic acid) became pregnant despite the regular use of a combined oral contraceptive (**ethinylestradiol/norethisterone** 50 micrograms/3 mg).[1] Since this first report in 1972, at least 33 pregnancies have been reported in the literature in women taking a range of oral contraceptives (mostly combined) and a barbiturate (such as **phenobarbital** or **primidone**) and/or phenytoin (see 'Table 26.2', (p.752)). Note that most of these cases were with a combined oral contraceptive containing at least 50 micrograms of **ethinylestradiol**. In addition, in the UK Committee on Safety of Medicines adverse reactions register for the years 1968 to 1984, a further 25 pregnancies were identified in women who took phenytoin and an oral contraceptive, and 20 in women who took **phenobarbital** and an oral contraceptive. However, it is unclear how many of these were on monotherapy, since the authors note that some women were taking multiple anticonvulsants (combinations not stated).[2] Even so, the total number of unwanted pregnancies due to this interaction is fairly large. In this report, over half the cases of contraceptive failure with anticonvulsants related to high-dose combined oral contraceptives (50 micrograms of oestrogen). Three were in women on **progestogen-only oral contraceptives**.[2]

In one study, breakthrough bleeding (regarded as loss of reliability of the contraceptive) occurred in 30 of 51 women taking a combined oral contraceptive (**ethinylestradiol/norethisterone** or **mestranol/chlormadinone**) given **phenobarbital**.[3] In another study, 7 out of 11 patients taking **phenobarbital** and 1 of 2 taking phenytoin had breakthrough bleeding.[4] The incidence of breakthrough bleeding was 90% with preparations containing **ethinylestradiol** 30 micrograms and 29% with preparations containing 75 micrograms of ethinyloestradiol. Similarly, with preparations containing **ethinylestradiol** 50 micrograms, decreasing the dose of **norgestrel** from 500 to 125 micrograms increased breakthrough bleeding from 50 to 62%.[4]

A pharmacokinetic study in 6 women found that the AUCs of **ethinylestradiol** 50 micrograms and **levonorgestrel** 250 micrograms contained in an oral contraceptive were lowered by 49% and 42% respectively, after taking phenytoin 200 to 300 mg daily for 8 to 12 weeks.[5] In another study, **phenobarbital** 30 mg twice daily did not significantly alter the plasma levels of contraceptive steroids in 4 women on combined oral contraceptives (**ethinylestradiol** with **norethisterone** or **norgestrel**), but 2 of the women did have 54 and 60% falls in their **ethinylestradiol** levels. These 2 women had breakthrough bleeding, but ovulation suppression was maintained.[6]

Mechanism

The likeliest explanation for the unreliability and failure of oral contraceptives is that phenytoin and the barbiturates act as potent liver enzyme inducing agents, which increase the metabolism and clearance of the contraceptive steroids from the body, thereby reducing their effects, and in some instances allowing ovulation to occur.

Importance and management

The interactions between combined oral contraceptives and **phenobarbital**, phenytoin and **primidone** are clinically important and well documented. The risk of breakthrough bleeding and spotting is high (bleeding disturbances are usually regarded as an indication of reduced efficacy if cycles were previously regular[7]). However, the actual incidence of contraceptive failure when combined oral contraceptives are given with these drugs is unknown. It appears that the incidence of unintended pregnancies is quite small: in one series, a failure-rate of 3.1 per 100 woman years was calculated, compared with an expected 0.7 per 100 woman years.[8] Note that this failure-rate is still less than that seen with barrier methods such as condoms. Nevertheless, since the personal and ethical consequences of an unplanned pregnancy can be very serious, it is important to take the necessary practical steps to reduce this increased risk. Moreover, ideally, pregnancy in women with epilepsy should be planned so that therapy can be reviewed to minimise the risks of fetal malformation.[9] In this regard, it is of concern that recent surveys have shown a lack of knowledge of these interactions and their management among prescribers,[10] and the frequent use of enzyme-inducing anticonvulsants with oral contraceptives contain-

Table 26.2 Case reports of pregnancies in women on oral contraceptives taking barbiturates and/or phenytoin

Anticonvulsant	*Oestrogen*	*Progestogen*	*Number of cases*	*Refs*
Phenytoin + Sultiame	Ethinylestradiol 50 micrograms	Norethisterone 3 mg	1	1
Phenytoin + Primidone, Phenobarbital or Mephobarbital	Not stated	Not stated	7	2, 3
Primidone	Ethinylestradiol 50 or 100 micrograms	Norgestrel 0.5 mg or Megestrol 1 mg	2	4, 5
Phenytoin + Primidone or Phenobarbital	Ethinylestradiol 50 micrograms	Norgestrel 0.25 or 0.5 mg or Norethisterone 1 mg	3	4,5
Phenytoin + Primidone or Phenobarbital + Other	Ethinylestradiol 50 micrograms	Norgestrel 0.5 mg	2	4, 5
Phenytoin + Carbamazepine	Ethinylestradiol 50 micrograms	Norgestrel 0.25 mg	1	4, 5
Primidone or Phenobarbital	Ethinylestradiol	Norgestrel	3	6
Phenobarbital or Butobarbital	Ethinylestradiol or Mestranol	Norethisterone	3	7
Phenytoin	Ethinylestradiol 100 micrograms	Dimethisterone 25 mg	1	8
Phenobarbital or Mephobarbital	Ethinylestradiol 50 micrograms or Mestranol 80 micrograms	Etynodiol 1 mg or Chlormadinone 2 mg	2	8
Phenytoin + Phenobarbital	Mestranol 100 micrograms	Noretynodrel 2.5 mg	1	8
Phenobarbital	Ethinylestradiol 50 micrograms	Desogestrel 75 mg	1	9
Phenytoin + Phenobarbital	Ethinylestradiol	Levonorgestrel	1	10
Phenytoin then Carbamazepine	Ethinylestradiol	Lynestrol	1	10
Phenytoin with or without other anticonvulsants	Ethinylestradiol 30 or 50 micrograms or Mestranol 50 micrograms	Megestrol, Norethisterone, Etynodiol, Norgestrel or Levonorgestrel	25	11
Phenobarbital with or without other anticonvulsants		Progesterone only pill	20	11
Phenytoin	Ethinylestradiol 50 micrograms	Not stated	1	12
Phenytoin	Ethinylestradiol less than 50 micrograms	Not stated	2	13
Phenobarbital	Ethinylestradiol 35 micrograms ('back up' contraception also used)	Norgestimate 0.18 to 0.25 mg	1	14

1. Kenyon IE. Unplanned pregnancy in an epileptic. *BMJ* (1972) 1, 686–7.
2. Hempel E, Böhm W, Carol W, Klinger G. Medikamentöse Enzyminduktion und hormonale Kontrazeption. *Zentralbl Gynakol* (1973) 95, 1451–7.
3. Hempel E, Klinger W. Drug stimulated biotransformation of hormonal steroid contraceptives: clinical implications. *Drugs* (1976) 12, 442–8.
4. Janz D, Schmidt D. Anti-epileptic drugs and failure of oral contraceptives. *Lancet* (1974) i, 1113.
5. Janz D, Schmidt D. Antiepileptika und die Sicherheit oraler Kontrazeptiva. *Bibl Psychiatr* (1975) 151, 82–5.
6. Belaisch J, Driguez P, Janaud A. Influence de certains médicaments sur l'action des pilules contraceptives. *Nouv Presse Med* (1976) 5, 1645–6.
7. Gagnaire JC, Tchertchian J, Revol A, Rochet Y. Grossesses sous contraceptifs oraux chez les patientes recevant des barbituriques. *Nouv Presse Med* (1975) 4, 3008.
8. Coulam CB, Annegers JF. Do anticonvulsants reduce the efficacy of oral contraceptives? *Epilepsia* (1979) 20, 519–26.
9. Fanøe E. P – pillesvigt antagelig på grund af interaktion med fenemal. *Ugeskr Laeger* (1977) 139, 1485.
10. Sparrow MJ. Pill method failures. *N Z Med J* (1987) 100, 102–5.
11. Back DJ, Grimmer FM, Orme ML'E, Proudlove C, Mann RD, Breckenridge AM. Evaluation of Committee on Safety of Medicines yellow card reports on oral contraceptive-drug interactions with anticonvulsants and antibiotics. *Br J Clin Pharmacol* (1988) 25, 527–32.
12. Kovacs GT, Riddoch G, Duncombe P, Welberry L, Chick P, Weisberg E, Leavesley GM, Baker HWG. Inadvertent pregnancies in oral contraceptive users. *Med J Aust* (1989) 150, 549–51.
13. van der Graaf WT, van Loon AJ, Postmus PE, Sleijfer DT. Twee patiënten met hersenmetastasen die zwanger werden tijdens fenytoïnegebruik. *Ned Tijdschr Geneeskd* (1992) 136, 2236–8.
14. Shane-McWhorter L, Cerveny JD, MacFarlane LL, Osborn C. Enhanced metabolism of levonorgestrel during phenobarbital treatment and resultant pregnancy. *Pharmacotherapy* (1998) 18, 1360–4.

ing less that 50 micrograms of ethinylestradiol.[11] Several practical solutions have been recommended to increase the contraceptive reliability and reduce the incidence of unpleasant breakthrough bleeding:

- **Raise the dosage of ethinylestradiol** (or its equivalent) from 30 to 50 micrograms by selecting a different contraceptive preparation.[4,9,12] If breakthrough bleeding still occurs, give two doses of 30 micrograms, or 30 micrograms plus 50 micrograms,[4,9] ideally guided by measurement of progesterone levels on day 21 of the cycle to confirm ovulation suppression.[9] Reliable contraception in most patients is said to be achievable with 80 to 100 micrograms ethinylestradiol daily.[4,9,13] If these larger doses are required for good cycle control, there should be no increase in adverse effects because the enzyme-inducing effects of the anticonvulsants reduce the blood levels of the steroids. Another suggestion is 'tricycling', which is intended to reduce the number of pill-free episodes. This involves taking a monophasic combined oral contraceptive for 3 or 4 cycles without a pill-free interval, then having a shortened pill-free interval of 4 days.[12] However, note that many of the cases of unintended pregnancies were with products containing 50 micrograms of ethinylestradiol or more, and one review of contraceptive interactions suggested that women taking low-dose oestrogen contraceptives may not be at a greater risk of an interaction.[14]

- **Use an additional barrier contraceptive method** (condoms, spermicidal gel) routinely while taking any of the interacting anticonvulsants. This is most likely to be appropriate if the enzyme-inducing anticonvulsants are required only short term. After stopping the anticonvulsants, additional precautions should be used for 4 weeks to allow the liver metabolism to recover.[12]

- **Use a non-interacting form of contraceptive**. Of the non-interacting forms of contraception with high contraceptive efficacy (equivalent or better than oral contraceptives in the general population), the copper or progestogen-releasing IUDs, or the depot medroxyprogesterone injection, are suitable for use with enzyme-inducing anticonvulsants. Note that progestogen implants should **not** be used (see 'IUDs; Progestogen-releasing + Enzyme-inducing drugs', p.743, and 'Progestogen-only injections or implants + Enzyme-inducing drugs', p.765).
- Where a suitable alternative exists, **consider using a non-interacting anticonvulsant**: 'gabapentin', (p.754), 'sodium valproate', (p.755), 'tiagabine', (p.755), and 'vigabatrin', (p.756) appear not to interact with the oral contraceptives.

Almost all of the evidence cited here originates from studies on combined oral contraceptives, but the enzyme-inducing anticonvulsants can increase the metabolism of progestogens thereby reducing their efficacy, so that there is also a risk of contraceptive failure with **progestogen-only oral contraceptives**.[15] This is of particular concern since progestogen-only oral contraceptives are not as effective as combined oral contraceptives anyway. Some have suggested at least doubling the dose of the progestogen-only oral contraceptive.[9] However, others consider that this is not an option as it tends to increase the rate of irregular bleeding (a common adverse effect of these contraceptives). They consider that progestogen-only oral contraceptives are not suitable for use in women on enzyme-inducing anticonvulsants.[15]

1. Kenyon IE. Unplanned pregnancy in an epileptic. *BMJ* (1972) 1, 686–7.
2. Back DJ, Grimmer FM, Orme ML'E, Proudlove C, Mann RD, Breckenridge AM. Evaluation of Committee on Safety of Medicines yellow card reports on oral contraceptive-drug interactions with anticonvulsants and antibiotics. *Br J Clin Pharmacol* (1988) 25, 527–32.
3. Hempel E, Böhm W, Carol W, Klinger G. Medikamentöse Enzyminduktion und hormonale Kontrazeption. *Zentralbl Gynakol* (1973) 95, 1451–7.
4. Akimoto H, Kazamatsuri H, Seino M, Ward A, Eds. Advances in Epileptology: Sodium valproate and the pill. New York: Raven Press, 1982 429–32.
5. Crawford P, Chadwick DJ, Martin C, Tjia J, Back DJ, Orme M. The interaction of phenytoin and carbamazepine with combined oral contraceptive steroids. *Br J Clin Pharmacol* (1990) 30, 892–6.
6. Back DJ, Bates M, Bowden A, Breckenridge AM, Hall MJ, Jones H, MacIver M, Orme M, Perucca E, Richens A, Rowe PH, Smith E. The interaction of phenobarbital and other anticonvulsants with oral contraceptive steroid therapy. *Contraception* (1980) 22, 495–503.
7. Hempel E, Klinger W. Drug stimulated biotransformation of hormonal steroid contraceptives: clinical implications. *Drugs* (1976) 12, 442–8.
8. Coulam CB, Annegers JF. Do anticonvulsants reduce the efficacy of oral contraceptives? *Epilepsia* (1979) 20, 519–26.
9. O'Brien MD, Gilmour-White S. Epilepsy and pregnancy. *BMJ* (1993) 307, 492–5.
10. Krauss GL, Brandt J, Campbell M, Plate C, Summerfield M. Antiepileptic medication and oral contraceptive interactions: a national survey of neurologists and obstetricians. *Neurology* (1996) 46, 1534–9.
11. Shorvon SD, Tallis RC, Wallace HK. Antiepileptic drugs: coprescription of proconvulsant drugs and oral contraceptives: a national study of antiepileptic drug prescribing practice. *J Neurol Neurosurg Psychiatry* (2002) 72, 114–15.
12. Belfield T, ed. FPA Contraceptive Handbook: a guide for family planning and other health professionals. 3rd ed. London: Family Planning Association, 1999.
13. Orme M, Back DJ. Oral contraceptive steroids – pharmacological issues of interest to the prescribing physician. *Adv Contracept* (1991) 7, 325–31.
14. Szoka PR, Edgren RA. Drug interactions with oral contraceptives: compilation and analysis of an adverse experience report database. *Fertil Steril* (1988) 49 (Suppl), S31–S38.
15. McCann MF, Potter LS. Progestin-only contraception: a comprehensive review. *Contraception* (1994) 50 (Suppl 1), S1–S198.

Oral contraceptives + Anticonvulsants; Carbamazepine or Oxcarbazepine

Oral contraceptives are less reliable during treatment with carbamazepine and oxcarbazepine. Breakthrough bleeding and spotting can take place, and unintended pregnancies have occurred with carbamazepine. Controlled studies have shown that carbamazepine and oxcarbazepine can reduce contraceptive steroid levels.

Clinical evidence

(a) Carbamazepine

In an early study, 6 of 12 women taking a combined oral contraceptive (**ethinylestradiol/norethisterone**) developed spotting or breakthrough bleeding while taking carbamazepine (this is regarded as loss of reliability of the contraceptive).[1] A similar study reported breakthrough bleeding in 4 of 6 patients taking carbamazepine and a combined oral contraceptive,[2] and the same author later briefly reported 37 out of 59 patients had breakthrough bleeding on this combination.[3]

One woman on a 'low-dose' combined oral contraceptive (not specified) conceived 6 weeks after starting carbamazepine initially 200 mg daily, increased to 600 mg daily.[4] Two other cases of failure of a combined oral contraceptive containing ethinylestradiol 30 micrograms attributed to carbamazepine have been very briefly mentioned.[5,6] Six pregnancies were identified in women who took carbamazepine and an oral contraceptive (unspecified) in the UK Committee on Safety of Medicines adverse reactions register for the years 1968 to 1984. However, it is unclear how many of these 6 were receiving carbamazepine monotherapy, since the authors note that some women were taking multiple anticonvulsants.[7] Two further pregnancies have been reported in women on combined oral contraceptives and anticonvulsants including carbamazepine and **phenytoin**,[8] and one in a woman who was switched from **phenytoin** to carbamazepine.[9]

In a pharmacokinetic study, carbamazepine 300 to 600 mg daily reduced the AUC of **ethinylestradiol** by 42% and **levonorgestrel** by 40% in 4 women given a single dose of a combined oral contraceptive (**ethinylestradiol/levonorgestrel** 50/250 micrograms) before and after 8 to 12 weeks of carbamazepine therapy.[10]

(b) Oxcarbazepine

Preliminary observations revealed that 4 of 6 women receiving oxcarbazepine had breakthrough bleeding when given a combined oral contraceptive containing **ethinylestradiol** 30 micrograms. This resolved in two women when they took double the dose of **ethinylestradiol**.[3] In a pharmacokinetic study, oxcarbazepine 300 mg three times daily for 4 weeks reduced the AUCs of **ethinylestradiol** by 47% and **levonorgestrel** by 36% in 10 healthy women on a triphasic combined oral contraceptive. Three women had menstrual bleeding disturbances.[11] Similar results were reported in a later study with oxcarbazepine 1200 mg daily and a combined oral contraceptive (**ethinylestradiol/levonorgestrel** 50/250 micrograms).[12] So far, no cases of unintended pregnancy have been reported.

Mechanism

The most likely explanation for these interactions is that both carbamazepine and oxcarbazepine reduce the levels of the contraceptive steroids, presumably by inducing their metabolism. This may result in loss of contraceptive efficacy.

Importance and management

The reduction in contraceptive steroid levels caused by carbamazepine and oxcarbazepine is well established. However, the actual incidence of contraceptive failure when oral contraceptives are given with these drugs is unknown. Given the few published reports, it appears that unintended pregnancies with carbamazepine are rare (and still less frequent than that seen with barrier methods such as condoms, see also 'Oral contraceptives + Anticonvulsants; Barbiturates or Phenytoin', p.751). No pregnancies have been reported in patients taking an oral contraceptive and oxcarbazepine. Nevertheless, given the possible consequences of an unplanned and unwanted pregnancy, any reduction in the contraceptive efficacy is of concern. Several practical solutions have been recommended to increase the contraceptive reliability and reduce the unpleasant breakthrough bleeding when oral contraceptives are used with enzyme-inducing anticonvulsants such as carbamazepine and oxcarbazepine, and these are discussed in further detail under 'Oral contraceptives + Anticonvulsants; Barbiturates or Phenytoin', p.751. They include raising the dose of ethinylestradiol, using an additional barrier form of contraceptive, using an alternative non-interacting contraceptive (e.g. copper IUD, progestogen-releasing IUD), or, if appropriate, switching to a non-interacting anticonvulsant.

1. Hempel E, Klinger W. Drug stimulated biotransformation of hormonal steroid contraceptives: clinical implications. *Drugs* (1976) 12, 442–8.
2. Akimoto H, Kazamatsuri H, Seino M, Ward A, Eds. Advances in Epileptology. New York: Raven Press, 1982 429–32.
3. Sonnen AEH. Oxcarbazepine and oral contraceptives. *Acta Neurol Scand* (1990) 82 (Suppl 133) 37.
4. Rapport DJ, Calabrese JR. Interactions between carbamazepine and birth control pills. *Psychosomatics* (1989) 30, 462–4.
5. Beeley L, Magee P, Hickey FM. *Bulletin of the West Midlands Centre for Adverse Drug Reaction Reporting* (1989) 28, 21.
6. Kovacs GT, Riddoch G, Duncombe P, Welberry L, Chick P, Weisberg E, Leavesley GM, Baker HWG. Inadvertent pregnancies in oral contraceptive users. *Med J Aust* (1989) 150, 549–51.
7. Back DJ, Grimmer FM, Orme ML'E, Proudlove C, Mann RD, Breckenridge AM. Evaluation of Committee on Safety of Medicines yellow card reports on oral contraceptive-drug interactions with anticonvulsants and antibiotics. *Br J Clin Pharmacol* (1988) 25, 527–32.
8. Janz D, Schmidt D. Antiepileptika und die Sicherheit oraler Kontrazeptiva. *Bibl Psychiatr* (1975) 151, 82–5.
9. Sparrow MJ. Pill method failures. *N Z Med J* (1987) 100, 102–5.

10. Crawford P, Chadwick DJ, Martin C, Tjia J, Back DJ, Orme M. The interaction of phenytoin and carbamazepine with combined oral contraceptive steroids. *Br J Clin Pharmacol* (1990) 30, 892–6.
11. Klosterskov Jensen P, Saano V, Haring P, Svenstrup B, Menge GP. Possible interaction between oxcarbazepine and an oral contraceptive. *Epilepsia* (1992) 33, 1149–52.
12. Fattore C, Cipolla G, Gatti G, Limido GL, Sturm Y, Bernasconi C, Perucca E. Induction of ethinylestradiol and levonorgestrel metabolism by oxcarbazepine in healthy women. *Epilepsia* (1999) 40, 783–7.

Oral contraceptives + Anticonvulsants; Ethosuximide

Ethosuximide appears not to alter the efficacy of combined oral contraceptives.

Clinical evidence, mechanism, importance and management

Four pregnancies were identified in women who took ethosuximide and an oral contraceptive (unspecified) in the UK Committee on Safety of Medicines adverse reactions register for the years 1968 to 1984. However, the authors note that in only one of the cases reported was ethosuximide the sole anticonvulsant prescribed.[1] Since ethosuximide is not an inducer of hepatic enzymes, it is likely that this one case is a chance association. Another case of pregnancy in a woman who had been taking ethosuximide, phenytoin, and phenobarbital, with a combined oral contraceptive for 6 years has also been reported.[2] If indeed this case does represent an interaction, the known enzyme-inducers phenytoin and phenobarbital are more likely to be implicated than ethosuximide (see 'Oral contraceptives + Anticonvulsants; Barbiturates or Phenytoin', p.751). There do not appear to have been any pharmacokinetic/pharmacodynamic studies of the use of ethosuximide with oral contraceptives and no further case reports have been published. No special contraceptive precautions appear to be necessary on concurrent use.

1. Back DJ, Grimmer FM, Orme ML'E, Proudlove C, Mann RD, Breckenridge AM. Evaluation of Committee on Safety of Medicines yellow card reports on oral contraceptive-drug interactions with anticonvulsants and antibiotics. *Br J Clin Pharmacol* (1988) 25, 527–32.
2. Janz D, Schmidt D. Anti-epileptic drugs and failure of oral contraceptives. *Lancet* (1974) i, 1113.

Oral contraceptives + Anticonvulsants; Felbamate

Felbamate increases the clearance of gestodene from a combined oral contraceptive but it is not known if this reduces contraceptive efficacy.

Clinical evidence, mechanism, importance and management

In a randomised, double-blind placebo-controlled trial 23 healthy women were given a combined oral contraceptive (**ethinylestradiol/gestodene** 30/75 micrograms) for 3 months or more. During months 1 and 2 they were also given either felbamate in a dose of up to 2400 mg daily, or a placebo, from day 15 of month 1 to day 14 of month 2. None of the women showed any evidence of ovulation during the entire 3 months, although one had intermenstrual spotting. However, the **gestodene** AUC was reduced by 42% and the **ethinylestradiol** AUC was reduced by 13%.[1] The reasons are not understood. What this change means in terms of the reliability of the oral contraceptive is not known, but some reduction in its efficacy might be expected. More study is needed to assess the clinical relevance and to see whether other progestogens are similarly affected.

1. Saano V, Glue P, Banfield CR, Reidenberg P, Colucci RD, Meehan JW, Haring P, Radwanski E, Nomeir A, Lin C-C, Jensen PK, Affrime MB. Effects of felbamate on the pharmacokinetics of a low-dose combination oral contraceptive. *Clin Pharmacol Ther* (1995) 58, 523–31.

Oral contraceptives + Anticonvulsants; Gabapentin

In a controlled trial, gabapentin did not alter the levels of ethinylestradiol or norethisterone.

Clinical evidence, mechanism, importance and management

Gabapentin 400 mg eight-hourly for 7 days had no effect on the AUC of **ethinylestradiol** or **norethisterone** in 13 healthy women taking a combined oral contraceptive (**ethinylestradiol/norethisterone** 50 micrograms/2.5 mg). Ovulation suppression was not assessed.[1] Gabapentin does not induce hepatic enzymes responsible for the metabolism of contraceptive steroids. Thus, no special contraceptive precautions appear to be required during concurrent use.

1. Eldon MA, Underwood BA, Randinitis EJ, Sedman AJ. Gabapentin does not interact with a contraceptive regimen of norethindrone acetate and ethinyl estradiol. *Neurology* (1998) 50, 1146–8.

Oral contraceptives + Anticonvulsants; Lamotrigine

One study suggests that lamotrigine does not alter the contraceptive efficacy or plasma levels of combined oral contraceptives, although the makers say that the possibility of reduced effects can not be ruled out. Oral contraceptives may decrease the efficacy of lamotrigine.

Clinical evidence, mechanism, importance and management

(a) Contraceptive efficacy

Preliminary results of a study showed that lamotrigine 150 mg daily for 10 to 14 days had no significant effect on the mean plasma levels of **ethinylestradiol** and **levonorgestrel** in women taking a combined oral contraceptive (**ethinylestradiol/levonorgestrel** 30/150 micrograms). No ovulation occurred (assessed by progesterone levels) and no changes in menstrual pattern were observed. Furthermore, lamotrigine did not induce hepatic enzymes (assessed by 6-β-hydroxycortisol excretion).[1] However, the makers suggest that there is a possibility that contraceptive efficacy may be decreased, and advise that the use of non-hormonal contraceptives is preferable. If a hormonal contraceptive is used as the only form of contraception they advise that patients should be alert for signs of breakthrough bleeding, which may be a sign of reduced contraceptive efficacy.[2]

(b) Lamotrigine efficacy

A case report describes 7 women in whom lamotrigine plasma levels were decreased by 41 to 64% by combined oral contraceptives (**ethinylestradiol/desogestrel**, **ethinylestradiol/norethisterone**) or progestogen-only oral contraceptives (**norethisterone**). Five had increased seizure frequency or recurrence of seizures after starting an oral contraceptive and 2 had adverse effects to lamotrigine on stopping an oral contraceptive. It was suggested that oral contraceptives can increase the glucuronidation of lamotrigine, thereby increasing its clearance.[3]

The maker says that in patients already taking hormonal contraceptives lamotrigine can be started as normal. In those taking lamotrigine in addition to inducers of lamotrigine glucuronidation (phenytoin carbamazepine etc), changes in the doses of either lamotrigine or the contraceptive are unlikely to be necessary. For women not taking inducers of lamotrigine glucuronidation the lamotrigine dose may need to be increased by as much as twofold, according to clinical response.[2]

1. Holdich T, Whiteman P, Orme M, Back D, Ward S. Effect of lamotrigine on the pharmacology of the combined oral contraceptive pill. *Epilepsia* (1991) 32 (Suppl 1), 96.
2. Lamictal (Lamotrigine). GlaxoSmithKline UK. UK Summary of product characteristics, June 2005.
3. Sabers A, Buchholt JM, Uldall P, Hansen EL. Lamotrigine plasma levels reduced by oral contraceptives. *Epilepsy Res* (2001) 47, 151–4.

Oral contraceptives + Anticonvulsants; Levetiracetam

Levetiracetam appears not to alter the contraceptive efficacy and plasma levels of combined oral contraceptives.

Clinical evidence, mechanism, importance and management

The pharmacokinetics of a combined oral contraceptive (**ethinylestradiol/levonorgestrel**) were found not to be affected by levetiracetam 500 mg twice daily, nor was ovulation suppression altered (there were no changes in LH or progesterone levels). The pharmacokinetics of levetiracetam also remained unaffected.[1] These findings indicate that no special or additional precautions are needed if oral contraceptives and levetiracetam are used concurrently.

1. Giuliano RA, Hiersemenzel R, Baltes E, Johnscher G, Janik F, Weber W. Influence of a new antiepileptic drug (Levetiracetam, ucb L059) on the pharmacokinetics and pharmacodynamics of oral contraceptives. *Epilepsia* (1996) 37, 90.

Oral contraceptives + Anticonvulsants; Remacemide

Remacemide appears not to interact with combined oral contraceptives.

Clinical evidence, mechanism, importance and management

Preliminary results of a study show remacemide 200 mg twice daily for 14 days had no effect on the pharmacokinetics of **ethinylestradiol**, **desogestrel**, or **levonorgestrel** when compared with placebo in women on a combined oral contraceptive (**ethinylestradiol/levonorgestrel** 30/150 micrograms or **ethinylestradiol/desogestrel** 30/150 micrograms). Inhibition of ovulation was maintained (assessed by measurement of progesterone, follicle-stimulating hormone and luteinising hormone levels).[1] It appears that no special contraceptive precautions are needed during concurrent use.

1. Blakey GE, Lockton JA, Corfield J, Oliver SD, Back D. Absence of interaction of remacemide with oral contraceptives. *Epilepsia* (1999) 40 (Suppl 2), 95.

Oral contraceptives + Anticonvulsants; Retigabine

Retigabine did not alter the plasma levels of the components of a combined oral contraceptive.

Clinical evidence, mechanism, importance and management

Preliminary results of a study show that retigabine 150 mg three times daily had no effect on the pharmacokinetics of **ethinylestradiol** or **norgestrel** in women taking a combined oral contraceptive (**ethinylestradiol/norgestrel** 30/300 micrograms).[1] This suggests that no special contraceptive precautions are needed during concurrent use.

1. Paul J, Ferron GM, Richards L, Getsy J, Troy SM. Retigabine does not alter the pharmacokinetics of a low-dose oral contraceptive in women. *Neurology* (2001) 56 (Suppl 3), A335.

Oral contraceptives + Anticonvulsants; Rufinamide

Rufinamide caused a modest decrease in the plasma levels of the steroids in a combined oral contraceptive.

Clinical evidence, mechanism, importance and management

Preliminary results of a study show that rufinamide 800 mg twice daily for 14 days decreased the AUC of **ethinylestradiol** 35 micrograms by 22% and of **norethisterone** 1 mg by 14% in healthy women on a combined oral contraceptive. Inhibition of ovulation was not assessed.[1] These reductions in plasma levels of the contraceptive hormones are less than those shown for phenytoin and barbiturates (see 'Oral contraceptives + Anticonvulsants; Barbiturates or Phenytoin', p.751), and their clinical relevance is unknown. However, given these findings, low-dose contraceptives (**ethinylestradiol** 20 micrograms) may be considered unsuitable for use with rufinamide. Further study is needed.

1. Svendsen KD, Choi L, Chen B-L, Karolchyk MA. Single-center, open-label, multiple-dose pharmacokinetic trial investigating the effect of rufinamide administration on Ortho-Novum 1/35 in healthy women. *Epilepsia* (1998) 39 (Suppl 6), 59.

Oral contraceptives + Anticonvulsants; Valproate

Sodium valproate appears not to alter the efficacy of combined oral contraceptives. In one study, sodium valproate increased ethinylestradiol levels.

Clinical evidence, mechanism, importance and management

In a series of 32 patients taking an oral contraceptive, none of 7 on sodium valproate 600 to 1800 mg daily had breakthrough bleeding, whereas about two-thirds of those on carbamazepine or phenobarbital had breakthrough bleeding (a sign of possible reduced contraceptive efficacy). Most of these 7 patients were taking combined oral contraceptives containing 50 micrograms of **ethinylestradiol**; one was taking less than 50 micrograms, and one was on a **progestogen-only oral contraceptive**. One of the 7 patients had previously experienced breakthrough bleeding while on phenobarbital but this stopped when it was replaced with sodium valproate. Two further patients did not have breakthrough bleeding while taking sodium valproate and benzodiazepines, but breakthrough bleeding started when phenytoin was added to their therapy.[1]

In a pharmacokinetic study, sodium valproate had no effect on the AUCs of **ethinylestradiol** 50 micrograms and **levonorgestrel** 250 micrograms in women with epilepsy given a single dose of a combined oral contraceptive before, and 8 to 16 weeks after, starting sodium valproate 200 mg twice daily. A 50% *increase* in the peak plasma **ethinylestradiol** concentration was noted.[2]

Conversely, one pregnancy was identified in a woman who took sodium valproate and an oral contraceptive (unspecified) in the UK Committee on Safety of Medicines adverse reactions register for the years 1968 to 1984. However, the authors consider this one case to be a chance association.[3] Sodium valproate does not induce hepatic enzymes responsible for the metabolism of oral contraceptives. Thus sodium valproate appears not to alter the efficacy of oral contraceptives, and no special contraceptive precautions are required during concurrent use.

1. Akimoto H, Kazamatsuri H, Seino M, Ward A, Eds. Advances in Epileptology: Sodium valproate and the pill. New York: Raven Press, 1982 429–32.

2. Crawford P, Chadwick D, Cleland P, Tjia J, Cowie A, Back DJ, Orme ML'E. The lack of effect of sodium valproate on the pharmacokinetics of oral contraceptive steroids. *Contraception* (1986) 33, 23–9.

3. Back DJ, Grimmer FM, Orme L'E, Proudlove C, Mann RD, Breckenridge AM. Evaluation of Committee on Safety of Medicines yellow card reports on oral contraceptive-drug interactions with anticonvulsants and antibiotics. *Br J Clin Pharmacol* (1988) 25, 527–32.

Oral contraceptives + Anticonvulsants; Tiagabine

Tiagabine appears not to alter the contraceptive efficacy and plasma levels of combined oral contraceptives.

Clinical evidence, mechanism, importance and management

A study in 10 healthy women found that tiagabine 2 mg, four times daily from day 24 to day 7 of the next cycle, had no effect on the mean plasma levels of any of steroids in two combined oral contraceptives (**ethinylestradiol/levonorgestrel** or **ethinylestradiol/desogestrel**, both 30/150 micrograms). There was no evidence that the suppression of ovulation was altered in any way (no significant changes in the plasma concentrations of progesterone, follicle stimulating hormone and luteinising hormone were seen between the first and second cycles, and progesterone levels remained in the non-ovulatory range). Tiagabine did not induce hepatic enzymes, as assessed by 6β-hydroxycortisol excretion. Two women did develop breakthrough bleeding, but given the above findings, this was not thought to represent reduced efficacy of the contraceptive.[1] There would appear to be no reason for any special contraceptive precautions during concurrent use.

1. Mengel HB, Houston A, Back DJ. An evaluation of the interaction between tiagabine and oral contraceptives in female volunteers. *J Pharm Med* (1994) 4, 141–50.

Oral contraceptives + Anticonvulsants; Topiramate

The serum levels of ethinylestradiol are reduced by topiramate, increasing the risk of breakthrough bleeding in women taking combined oral contraceptives. It is suggested that oral contraceptives with a higher dosage of oestrogen should be used.

Clinical evidence

Eleven epileptic women stabilised on sodium valproate and taking a combined oral contraceptive (**ethinylestradiol/norethisterone** 35 micrograms/1 mg) were additionally given three escalating doses of topiramate 100, 200, 400 mg twice daily for 28-day periods. The mean AUC of the **ethinylestradiol** fell by 18%, 21% and 30%, respectively. Although no significant changes were found in the **norethisterone** AUC, the authors considered that the study was not sufficiently powered to detect small changes. No ovulation occurred, as assessed by progestogen levels, but one patient had breakthrough bleeding.[1]

Mechanism

Not understood. It is suggested that topiramate weakly induces enzymes in the liver, which increases the metabolism of the ethinylestradiol.[1]

Importance and management

An established interaction but supported by limited evidence. The modest changes in pharmacokinetics of the combined oral contraceptive seen here are lower than those seen with other enzyme-inducing anticonvulsants (e.g. see 'Oral contraceptives + Anticonvulsants; Carbamazepine or Oxcarbazepine', p.753, and 'Oral contraceptives + Anticonvulsants; Barbiturates or Phenytoin', p.751). However, it is possible that they would be sufficient to cause failure of combined oral contraceptives in rare cases, particularly at high therapeutic doses of topiramate. The makers of topiramate advise the use of a barrier contraceptive or a high-dose combined oral contraceptive (50 micrograms ethinylestradiol), and also say that patients should be told to report any changes in their bleeding patterns.[2] These seem sensible precautions. Consider also 'Oral contraceptives + Anticonvulsants; Barbiturates or Phenytoin', p.751, for other suggestions on management of interactions between enzyme-inducing anticonvulsants and oral contraceptives.

1. Rosenfeld WE, Doose DR, Walker SA, Nayak RK. Effect of topiramate on the pharmacokinetics of an oral contraceptive containing norethindrone and ethinyl estradiol in patients with epilepsy. *Epilepsia* (1997) 38, 317–23.
2. Topamax (Topiramate), Janssen-Cilag Ltd. UK Summary of product characteristics, August 2004.

Oral contraceptives + Anticonvulsants; Vigabatrin

Vigabatrin appears not to alter the pharmacokinetics of contraceptive steroids.

Clinical evidence, mechanism, importance and management

Vigabatrin 3 g daily had no statistically significant effect on the pharmacokinetics of **ethinylestradiol** and **levonorgestrel** in 13 healthy women given a single dose of a combined oral contraceptive (**ethinylestradiol/levonorgestrel** 30/150 micrograms), although 2 of the women showed a 39% and a 50% fall in the AUC of **ethinylestradiol**. Vigabatrin did not induce hepatic enzymes as assessed by antipyrine clearance and 6β-hydroxycortisol excretion.[1]

This study would seem to confirm the lack of reports of an oral contraceptive/vigabatrin interaction, but the authors of the report introduce a small note of caution because it is not clear whether the reduced **ethinylestradiol** AUCs seen in two of the women resulted from an interaction or were simply normal individual variations.[1] The UK Family Planning Association does not consider any special contraceptive precautions are necessary when vigabatrin is taken with oral contraceptives.[2]

1. Bartoli A, Gatti G, Cipolla G, Barzaghi N, Veliz G, Fattore C, Mumford J, Perucca E. A double-blind, placebo-controlled study on the effect of vigabatrin on in vivo parameters of hepatic microsomal enzyme induction and on the kinetics of steroid oral contraceptives in healthy female volunteers. *Epilepsia* (1997) 38, 702–7.
2. Belfield T, ed. FPA Contraceptive Handbook: a guide for family planning and other health professionals. 3rd ed. London: Family Planning Association, 1999.

Oral contraceptives + Antimalarials

No clinically significant interaction appears to occur between combined oral contraceptives and chloroquine or primaquine, or between oral contraceptives and mefloquine or quinine.

Clinical evidence, mechanism, importance and management

(a) Chloroquine

A pharmacokinetic study in 12 healthy women taking a combined oral contraceptive (**ethinylestradiol/norethisterone** 30 micrograms/1 mg) showed that the prophylactic use of **chloroquine phosphate**, 500 mg once a week for 4 weeks, caused a small 15% increase in the **ethinylestradiol** AUC, and no change in the **norethisterone** levels. **Chloroquine** use did not alter ovulation inhibition, as assessed by mid-luteal progesterone levels and the lack of breakthrough spotting and bleeding. In a further group of 7 women, the same combined oral contraceptive did not alter the pharmacokinetics of a single 500-mg dose of **chloroquine phosphate**.[1] Another study[2] in 6 healthy women given a single dose of a combined oral contraceptive (**ethinylestradiol/levonorgestrel** 30 micrograms/150 micrograms) confirmed that a single 300-mg dose of **chloroquine** had no significant effect on the pharmacokinetics of either the **oestrogen** or the **progestogen**. Further confirmation of the absence of an interaction comes from studies in *rhesus monkeys* infected with malaria, in which it was shown that the curative efficacy of **chloroquine** was not altered by the use of combined oral contraceptives (**ethinylestradiol/norethisterone** or **ethinylestradiol/norgestrel**).[3]

(b) Mefloquine

A study in 12 Thai women with falciparum malaria, 6 of whom were taking un-named oral contraceptives, found that their response (parasite and fever clearance) to treatment with **mefloquine** was not affected by oral contraceptives. Similarly, the pharmacokinetics of **mefloquine** were not affected by oral contraceptives in patients with malaria.[4] There would seem to be no reason for avoiding concurrent use.

(c) Primaquine

A study in 6 healthy women given a single dose of a combined oral contraceptive (**ethinylestradiol/levonorgestrel** 30 micrograms/150 micrograms) confirmed that a single 45-mg dose of **primaquine** had no significant effect on the pharmacokinetics of either the **oestrogen** or the **progestogen**.[2]

(d) Quinine

A controlled study in Thai women showed that the pharmacokinetics of single 600-mg doses of **quinine sulfate** in 7 women taking oral contraceptives were not significantly different from those in 7 other women not taking contraceptives. The contraceptives being used were combined oral contraceptives (**ethinylestradiol/levonorgestrel** or **ethinylestradiol/norgestrel**) and a progestogen-only oral contraceptive (**norethisterone**).[5] There seem to be no reports that **quinine** affects the reliability of the oral contraceptives and there would seem to be no reason for avoiding concurrent use.

1. Gupta KC, Joshi JV, Desai NK, Sankolli GM, Chowdhary VN, Joshi UM, Chitalange S, Satoskar RS. Kinetics of chloroquine and contraceptive steroids in oral contraceptive users during concurrent chloroquine prophylaxis. *Indian J Med Res* (1984) 80, 658–62.
2. Back DJ, Breckenridge AM, Grimmer SFM, Orme ML'E, Purba HS. Pharmacokinetics of oral contraceptive steroids following the administration of the antimalarial drugs primaquine and chloroquine. *Contraception* (1984) 30, 289–95.
3. Dutta GP, Puri SK, Kamboj KK, Srivastava SK, Kamboj VP. Interactions between oral contraceptives and malaria infections in rhesus monkeys. *Bull WHO* (1984) 62, 931–9.
4. Karbwang J, Looareesuwan S, Back DJ, Migasana S, Bunnag D, Breckenridge AM. Effect of oral contraceptive steroids on the clinical course of malaria infection and on the pharmacokinetics of mefloquine in Thai women. *Bull WHO* (1988) 66, 763–7.
5. Wanwimolruk S, Kaewvichit S, Tanthayaphinant O, Suwannarach C, Oranratnachai A. Lack of effect of oral contraceptive use on the pharmacokinetics of quinine. *Br J Clin Pharmacol* (1991) 31,179–81.

Oral contraceptives + Aprepitant

Aprepitant reduced the levels of ethinylestradiol in an oral contraceptive, and may therefore reduce the efficacy of oral contraceptives. Greater effects were seen in another study when dexamethasone was also given with aprepitant. Alternative or additional contraceptive methods should be used.

Clinical evidence

The makers[1,2] note that aprepitant 100 mg daily for 14 days given with a combined oral contraceptive (**ethinylestradiol/norethisterone** 35 micrograms/1 mg) decreased the AUC of **ethinylestradiol** by 43% and that of **norethisterone** by 8%. The US makers[2] give details of a study using the recommended antiemetic regimen of aprepitant 125 mg on the first day, then 80 mg daily for 2 days with **dexamethasone** 12 mg on the first day, then 8 mg daily for 3 days and ondansetron 32 mg on the first day, which was started on day 8 of a 21-day cycle of a combined oral contraceptive (**ethinylestradiol/norethisterone**). Within 2 days of starting the antiemetics (day 10) the **ethinylestradiol** AUC was 19% lower and the **norethisterone** level unchanged. However, the trough level of **ethinylestradiol** was reduced by as much as 64% and that of **norethisterone** by 60% during days 9 though to 21.

Mechanism

During the first few days of use aprepitant is an inhibitor of the cytochrome P450 isoenzyme CYP3A4, but within 2 weeks it becomes an inducer of this isoenzyme (see 'Benzodiazepines + Aprepitant', p.540). It appears that aprepitant induces the metabolism of ethinylestradiol, and reduces its levels. Dexamethasone is also an inducer of CYP3A4.

Importance and management

Although the effects of these reduced contraceptive steroids levels on ovulation were not assessed, it is likely that they could result in reduced efficacy. The maker therefore recommends that alternative or additional contraceptive methods be used during aprepitant therapy and for 2 months (UK advice)[1] or one month (US advice)[2] after the last dose of aprepitant. This seems a sensible precaution.

1. Emend (Aprepitant). Merck Sharp & Dohme Ltd. UK Summary of product characteristics, April 2005.
2. Emend (Aprepitant). Merck & Co., Inc. US prescribing information, March 2005.

Oral contraceptives or HRT + Ascorbic acid (Vitamin C)

Ascorbic acid appears not to cause any clinically important increase in serum ethinylestradiol levels but there is some evidence that ascorbic acid may modestly increase estradiol levels in women on HRT. There are a few unconfirmed anecdotal reports of contraceptive failure associated with ascorbic acid.

Clinical evidence

(a) Combined oral contraceptives

One study found that ascorbic acid 1 g raised serum **ethinylestradiol** levels by 16% at 6 hours and 48% at 24 hours post-dose in 5 women taking combined oral contraceptives.[1] However, a later well-controlled study found that ascorbic acid 1 g daily caused no significant changes in **ethinylestradiol** serum levels in 37 women taking a combined oral contraceptive (**ethinylestradiol/levonorgestrel** 30 micrograms/150 micrograms).[2]

A single case report describes a woman on a combined oral contraceptive (**ethinylestradiol/levonorgestrel**) who experienced heavy breakthrough bleeding in 3 cycles within 2 to 3 days of stopping ascorbic acid 1 g daily. This did not occur in 3 other cycles when no ascorbic acid was taken. This was postulated to be due to a fall in **ethinylestradiol** levels when the vitamin C was stopped, which could increase the risk of contraceptive failure.[3] One report attributed contraceptive failure in one case to ascorbic acid and **multivitamins**.[4] Another two studies of pregnancies in oral contraceptive users found that vitamin C had been taken in 44 of 209 cases[5] and 15 of 137 cases,[6] although other drugs/factors may possibly have been involved in some of these cases.

(b) Hormone replacement therapy

Ascorbic acid 500 mg twice daily for one month caused a non-significant 21% increase in plasma estradiol levels in 25 postmenopausal women on **transdermal estradiol** therapy. However, in the 9 women with initially low estradiol levels, ascorbic acid doubled the levels, and this reached significance.[7]

Mechanism

Both ascorbic acid and ethinylestradiol undergo sulfate conjugation. It was suggested that large doses of ascorbic acid might compete for the metabolism of ethinylestradiol, and therefore increase its levels.[1] This would be expected to increase the efficacy of the oral contraceptive. However, some have postulated that enhanced levels could be followed by rebound ovulation,[3] but there is no evidence to support this. Ascorbic acid may reverse the oxidation of oestrogens.[7]

Importance and management

Documentation about an interaction with contraceptives is limited. From the point of view of reliability, there seems to be little reason for avoiding the use of oral contraceptives and ascorbic acid. No special precautions are required.

The authors of the report on ascorbic acid and HRT say that their findings do not support the general use of ascorbic acid as an adjuvant to HRT, but that further study is needed. No special precautions are required.

1. Back DJ, Breckenridge AM, MacIver M, Orme ML'E, Purba H, Rowe PH. Interaction of ethinyloestradiol with ascorbic acid in man. *BMJ* (1981) 282, 1516.
2. Zamah NM, Hümpel M, Kuhnz W, Louton T, Rafferty J, Back DJ. Absence of an effect of high vitamin C dosage on the systemic availability of ethinyl estradiol in women using a combination oral contraceptive. *Contraception* (1993) 48, 377–91.
3. Morris JC, Beeley L, Ballantine N. Interaction of ethinyloestradiol with ascorbic acid in man. *BMJ* (1981) 283, 503.
4. DeSano EA, Hurley SC. Possible interactions of antihistamines and antibiotics with oral contraceptive effectiveness. *Fertil Steril* (1982) 37, 853–4.
5. Kovacs GT, Riddoch G, Duncombe P, Welberry L, Chick P, Weisberg E, Leavesley GM, Baker HWG. Inadvertent pregnancies in oral contraceptive users. *Med J Aust* (1989) 150, 549–51.
6. Sparrow MJ. Pregnancies in reliable pill takers. *N Z Med J* (1989) 102, 575–7.
7. Vihtamäki T, Parantainen J, Koivisto A-M, Metsä-Ketelä T, Tuimala R. Oral ascorbic acid increases plasma oestradiol during postmenopausal hormone replacement therapy. *Maturitas* (2002) 42, 129–35.

Oral contraceptives + Azoles

There are isolated reports of breakthrough bleeding and failure of combined oral contraceptives with fluconazole, itraconazole and ketoconazole. Conversely, both fluconazole and itraconazole have been shown to modestly increase serum levels of contraceptive steroids.

Clinical evidence

(a) Fluconazole

Up to 1990 the UK maker of fluconazole had received 11 reports of menstrual disorders possibly associated with single-dose fluconazole 150 mg. Eight of these were in women taking an oral contraceptive: 5 cases of break-through bleeding, 1 case of no withdrawal bleeding, and 2 cases of unintended pregnancies.[1] Three other cases of unintended pregnancy have been very briefly mentioned elsewhere.[2]

However, a single dose of fluconazole 150 mg *increased* the AUC of **ethinylestradiol** by 29% in women taking a combined oral contraceptive (**ethinylestradiol** and **norethisterone** or **levonorgestrel**).[3] Similarly, fluconazole 300 mg once weekly for 4 weeks caused a similar 24% increase in the **ethinylestradiol** AUC, and a 13% increase in the **norethisterone** AUC.[4] Moreover, the maker has data on file showing that multiple doses of fluconazole 200 mg daily raised the levels of **ethinylestradiol** by 40% and of **levonorgestrel** by 24%,[5] whereas a lower dose of fluconazole (a single 50 mg dose or 50 mg fluconazole daily for 10 days) had no significant effect on the pharmacokinetics of **ethinylestradiol** and **norgestrel**.[6] One other study in 10 women taking combined oral contraceptives found no changes in progesterone levels (suggesting no ovulation occurred) and no menstrual disorders while they were taking fluconazole 50 mg daily.[7]Furthermore, during clinical trials in which single 150-mg doses of fluconazole were used by over 700 women taking oral contraceptives, no evidence of an interaction was seen.[8]

(b) Itraconazole

A 25-year old who had been taking a combined oral contraceptive (**ethinylestradiol/levonorgestrel** 30/150 micrograms) for a year, without problems, became pregnant when she was additionally treated for 3 months with itraconazole 200 mg daily for a fungal infection. The patient was said to be compliant, had suffered no gastrointestinal upset, and was not taking any other drugs that might have accounted for the failure of the pill.[2]

The Netherlands Pharmacovigilance Foundation (LAREB) have 9 cases of menstrual changes on their records in women taking an oral contraceptive during or after taking itraconazole 100 to 400 mg daily for 1 to 4 weeks. Seven women reported delayed withdrawal bleeding (2 to 5 days). In 2 of them the menstrual flow was decreased and one transiently had a positive pregnancy test after having previously experienced an intermenstrual blood loss. The remaining two reports were of amenorrhoea during one cycle, and breakthrough bleeding. The women were taking **ethinylestradiol** plus either **desogestrel** or **levonorgestrel**.[9] A later extension of this report from LAREB, covering the period 1991 to 1997, describes 12 women taking contraceptives containing **ethinylestradiol/desogestrel**, whose withdrawal bleeding was either delayed or did not occur at all while taking itraconazole. Three other women taking **ethinylestradiol/levonorgestrel** had breakthrough bleeding, and yet another on **ethinylestradiol/cyproterone** became pregnant while taking itraconazole.[10]

However, the maker has data on file of a study showing that itraconazole 200 mg daily for 15 days had no effect on the pharmacokinetics of **ethinylestradiol**, and *increased* the bioavailability of **norethisterone** by about 40%. In this study, a single dose of **ethinylestradiol/norethisterone** was given before the first dose and with the last dose of itraconazole.[11]

(c) Ketoconazole

An early report described 7 out of 147 women taking combined oral contraceptives (**ethinylestradiol/norgestrel**) who experienced breakthrough bleeding or spotting within 2 to 5 days of starting a 5-day course of ketoconazole 400 mg daily. No pregnancies occurred.[12] One unintended pregnancy attributed to contraceptive failure due to ketoconazole has been very briefly mentioned elsewhere.[2]

Mechanism

The azole antifungals are inhibitors of the cytochrome P450 isoenzyme CYP3A4. They would therefore be expected to increase levels of contraceptive steroids, as has been shown for fluconazole and itraconazole. As such, they would not be expected to increase the incidence of breakthrough bleeding or contraceptive failure when used with combined oral contraceptives. It should be noted that the maker lists menstrual irregularities as adverse effects of ketoconazole and itraconazole, irrespective of use of combined oral contraceptives,[13,14] and menstrual disorders have also been reported with fluconazole alone.[1]

Importance and management

The picture presented by these reports is somewhat confusing and contradictory. The anecdotal reports of contraceptive failure and the cases of breakthrough bleeding would suggest that these antifungals can rarely make oral contraception less reliable in a some individuals. However, the problem with this interpretation is that the pharmacokinetic data suggest that, if anything, an *enhanced* effect of the combined oral contraceptives is likely. [Note that, of all the drugs proven to decrease the efficacy of combined oral contraceptives, all have also been shown to decrease the steroid levels]. Menstrual disorders have occurred with the azole antifungals alone, and may not be indicative of reduced contraceptive efficacy. Since there are so few reports of pregnancy, it could just be that they fall within the accepted failure rate of combined oral contraceptives, and it was just coincidental they occurred when the antifungal was being taken. Note that the makers do not advise any special precautions when taking oral contraceptives and these azole antifungals.[5,13,14] However, some consider that the data warrant consideration being given to the use of additional contraceptive measures.[10] The theoretical teratogenic risk[5,13,14] from these azole antifungals may have a bearing on this. More study is clearly needed.

The main concern of increased levels of ethinylestradiol or progestogens is whether this would increase the risk of adverse effects of the steroid. There are no data on the effect of these modest 25 to 40% increases in steroid levels on various adverse effects. It could be argued that a 40% increase would turn a standard-strength contraceptive (35 micrograms) into a high-dose contraceptive (50 micrograms). However, early studies showed that the interindividual variation in ethinylestradiol pharmacokinetics was greater than this anyway.[15] Further study is needed.

1. Pfizer Ltd. Summary of unpublished reports: female reproductive disorders possibly associated with Diflucan. Data on file (Ref DIFLU:diflu41.*1*) (1990).
2. Pillans PI, Sparrow MJ. Pregnancy associated with a combined oral contraceptive and itraconazole. *N Z Med J* (1993) 106, 436.
3. Sinofsky FE, Pasquale SA. The effect of fluconazole on circulating ethinyl estradiol levels in women taking oral contraceptives. *Am J Obstet Gynecol* (1998) 178, 300–4.
4. Hilbert J, Messig M, Kuye O, Friedman H. Evaluation of interaction between fluconazole and an oral contraceptive in healthy women. *Obstet Gynecol* (2001) 98, 218–23.
5. Diflucan (Fluconazole). Pfizer Ltd. UK Summary of product characteristics, November 2004.
6. Lazar JD, Wilner KD. Drug interactions with fluconazole. *Rev Infect Dis* (1990) 12, Suppl 3, S327–S333.
7. Devenport MH, Crook D, Wynn V, Lees LJ. Metabolic effects of low-dose fluconazole in healthy female users and non-users of oral contraceptives. *Br J Clin Pharmacol* (1989) 27, 851–9.
8. Dodd GK (Pfizer Ltd). Personal communication, 1990.
9. Meyboom RHB, van Puijenbroek EP, Vinks MHAM, Lastdrager CJ. Disturbance of withdrawal bleeding during concomitant use of itraconazole and oral contraceptives. *N Z Med J* (1997) 110, 300.
10. van Puijenbroek EP, Feenstra J, Meyboom RHB. Verstoring van de pilcyclus tijdens het gelijktijdig gebruik van itraconazol en orale anticonceptiva. *Ned Tijdschr Geneeskd* (1998) 142, 146–9.
11. Jones AR (Janssen). Personal communication, 1994.
12. Kovács I, Somos P, Hámori M. Examination of the potential interaction between ketoconazole (Nizoral) and oral contraceptives with special regard to products of low hormone content (Rigevidon, Anteovin). *Ther Hung* (1986) 34, 167–70.
13. Sporanox (Itraconazole). Janssen-Cilag Ltd. UK Summary of product characteristics, November 2002.
14. Nizoral (Ketoconazole). Janssen-Cilag Ltd. UK Summary of product characteristics, May 2001.
15. Back DJ, Breckenridge AM, Crawford FE, MacIver M, Orme ML'E, Rowe PH. Interindividual variation and drug interactions with hormonal steroids. *Drugs* (1981) 21, 46–61.

Oral contraceptives + Benzodiazepines

For discussion of the increased incidence of breakthrough bleeding seen with some benzodiazepines (chlordiazepoxide, diazepam, nitrazepam, meprobamate) when given with oral contraceptives, **see 'Benzodiazepines and related drugs + Oral contraceptives', p.550.**

Oral contraceptives + Candesartan

Candesartan cilexetil 8 mg daily had no effect on the pharmacokinetics of ethinylestradiol and levonorgestrel in a combined oral contraceptive, and no ovulation occurred during concurrent treatment.[1] No special precautions would therefore appear to be needed.

1. Jonkman JHG, van Lier JJ, van Heiningen PNM, Lins R, Sennewald R, Högemann A. Pharmacokinetic drug interaction studies with candesartan cilexetil. *J Hum Hypertens* (1997) 11 (Suppl 2), S31–S35.

Oral contraceptives + Danazol or Gestrinone

There is a theoretical risk that the effects of danazol or gestrinone and hormonal contraceptives might be altered or reduced. The makers say that women of childbearing age taking danazol or gestrinone should use an effective non-hormonal method of contraception.

Clinical evidence, mechanism, importance and management

(a) Danazol

Danazol inhibits ovulation, but it is not considered reliable enough to be used as an oral contraceptive.[1-3] Danazol should not be used in pregnancy, because it can cause virilisation of a female fetus. The makers advise the use of reliable non-hormonal contraceptive methods while taking danazol,[4,5] and by inference the avoidance of hormonal contraceptives. They say that there is a theoretical risk that danazol and exogenously administered oestrogens and/or progestogens, including oral contraceptives, might possibly compete for the same oestrogen, progestogen and androgen receptors, thereby altering the effects of both drugs.[3] This would also apply to other hormonal contraceptives such as **etonogestrel** implants and depot preparations of **medroxyprogesterone** and **norethisterone**. However, as yet there appears to be no direct evidence that any interaction actually occurs.

(b) Gestrinone

Although gestrinone, at the dose used for endometriosis, can inhibit ovulation, it is not sufficiently reliable to be used as a contraceptive. The makers strongly emphasise the importance of using a barrier method of contraception while on gestrinone because they say that not only are the effects of gestrinone possibly modified by oral contraceptives, but its use in pregnancy is totally contraindicated (high doses have been shown to be embryotoxic in some *animal* species).[6]

1. Greenblatt RB, Oettinger M, Borenstein R, Bohler CS-S. Influence of danazol (100 mg) on conception and contraception. *J Reprod Med* (1974) 13, 201–3.
2. Colle ML, Greenblatt RB. Contraceptive properties of danazol. *J Reprod Med* (1976) 17, 98–102.
3. Sterling-Winthrop, Personal communication 1990.
4. Danol (Danazol). Sanofi Synthelabo. UK Summary of product characteristics, August 2004.
5. Danocrine (Danazol). Sanofi-Synthelabo. US Prescribing information, February 2003.
6. Dimetriose (Gestrinone). Florizel Ltd. UK Summary of product characteristics, May 1997.

Oral contraceptives + Etoricoxib or Rofecoxib

Rofecoxib increases contraceptive steroid levels to a small extent, and would not therefore be expected to reduce contraceptive efficacy. Etoricoxib raises ethinylestradiol levels by 50 to 60%. Consider using a preparation with a lower ethinylestradiol dose.

Clinical evidence, mechanism, importance and management

In a placebo-controlled, crossover study in 18 healthy women taking a combined oral contraceptive (**ethinylestradiol/norethisterone** 35 micrograms/1 mg), rofecoxib 175 mg daily for 2 weeks raised the AUCs of **ethinylestradiol** and **norethisterone** by 13% and 18%, respectively. These small changes, although statistically significant, are within the accepted criteria for bioequivalence, and are unlikely to be clinically important. No abnormal menstrual bleeding was reported.[1] No special precautions are required during concurrent use.

A study in women taking a combined oral contraceptive (**ethinylestradiol/norethisterone** 35 micrograms/0.5 to 1 mg) for 21 days found that the addition of etoricoxib 120 mg with or 12 hours after the oral contraceptive increased the 24-hour steady-state levels of **ethinylestradiol** by 50 to 60% but the **norethisterone** levels were not raised to a clinically relevant extent. It is thought that etoricoxib increases **ethinylestradiol** levels because it inhibits human sulfotransferase activity. There would therefore appear to be no reason for avoiding concurrent use but the makers suggest that this increase in **ethinylestradiol** levels should be considered when choosing the oral contraceptive because of the possible increased risk of adverse events.[2] It may therefore be appropriate to use a contraceptive with a lower dose of **ethinylestradiol**.

1. Arcoxia (Etoricoxib). Merck Sharp & Dohme Ltd. UK Summary of product characteristics, May 2005.
2. Schwartz JI, Wong PH, Porras AG, Ebel DL, Hunt TR, Gertz BJ. Effect of rofecoxib on the pharmacokinetics of chronically administered oral contraceptives in healthy female volunteers. *J Clin Pharmacol* (2002) 42, 215–21.

Oral contraceptives + Ezetimibe

No significant pharmacokinetic interaction appears to occur between ezetimibe and an ethinylestradiol/norgestrel containing oral contraceptive.

Clinical evidence, mechanism, importance and management

In a randomised crossover study, 18 healthy women who had been taking a triphasic oral contraceptive (containing **ethinylestradiol/norgestrel**) were additionally given ezetimibe 10 mg daily or placebo on days 8 to 14 of two consecutive cycles. Ezetimibe did not significantly affect the pharmacokinetics of ethinylestradiol or norgestrel. No additional precautions therefore seem necessary if ezetimibe is given to women taking ethinylestradiol/norgestrel-containing contraceptives.[1]

1. Keung ACF, Kosoglou T, Statkevich P, Anderson L, Boutros T, Cutler DL, Batra V, Sellers EM. Ezetimibe does not affect the pharmacokinetics of oral contraceptives. *Clin Pharmacol Ther* (2001) 69, P55.

Oral contraceptives + Griseofulvin

The effects of the oral contraceptives may possibly be disturbed (either intermenstrual bleeding or amenorrhoea) if griseofulvin is taken concurrently. Four women on oral contraceptives have been reported who became pregnant while taking griseofulvin.

Clinical evidence

In 1984, regulatory authorities in the UK and the Netherlands noted that they had received a total of 22 reports of possible interactions between oral contraceptives and griseofulvin. These included 15 reports of transient intermenstrual bleeding and 5 of amenorrhoea occurring during the first or second cycle after starting to take griseofulvin (500 mg to 1 g daily). Four of these were re-challenged with griseofulvin (2 with intermenstrual bleeding and 2 with amenorrhoea) and all developed their original reactions. The other two women were reported to have become pregnant while taking griseofulvin and a sulphonamide ('co-trimoxazole', (p.749) in one instance and an unknown sulphonamide in the other).[1] One other case of contraceptive failure has been reported from an analysis of the UK Committee on Safety of Medicines database from 1968 to 1984,[2] but note this may already be included in the 2 already reported.[1] One other case report describes a woman taking a triphasic combined oral contraceptive who became pregnant about 2 months after she started taking griseofulvin 330 mg twice daily,[3] and another report describes a woman taking an oral contraceptive who became pregnant 6 weeks after starting to take griseofulvin 500 mg daily for 3 months and a 7-day course of 'erythromycin', (p.745).[4] Irregular menses and reduced menstrual flow have been described in another woman taking a combined oral contraceptive (**ethinylestradiol** 35 micrograms/**norethisterone** 0.5 to 1 mg) when given griseofulvin 250 to 500 mg daily. When the oral contraceptive was substituted by another with more oestrogen (**ethinylestradiol/norgestrel** 50 micrograms/500 micrograms), the menstrual cycle became normal again.[5] Break-through bleeding has also been seen in one other woman on the pill given griseofulvin.[6]

Mechanism

Not understood. Griseofulvin may possibly stimulate the activity of the liver enzymes concerned with the metabolism of the contraceptive steroids, thereby reducing their effects (see 'Hormonal contraceptives and sex hormones', (p.741)). Contraceptive failure with co-trimoxazole and other sulphonamides or erythromycin is thought unlikely (see 'Oral contraceptives + Antibacterials; Sulfonamides or Trimethoprim', p.749, and 'Oral contraceptives + Antibacterials; Macrolides', p.745).

Importance and management

Information about this interaction is very limited. The risk of contraceptive failure is uncertain but probably very small. However, it would be prudent for prescribers to warn women taking a **combined oral contraceptive** who are given griseofulvin that menstrual disturbances may possibly be signs of contraceptive unreliability, and that additional contraceptive precautions should be taken. The UK Committee on Safety of Medicines has pointed out the importance of ensuring adequate contraception during and for one month after taking griseofulvin because it can induce aneuploidy (abnormal segregation of chromosomes during cell division), which carries the potential risk of teratogenicity.[7] For maximal contraceptive protection a barrier method should be used routinely while taking griseofulvin and for a month afterwards.

The situation with **progestogen-only contraceptives** is not clear, but it has been suggested that they are not the contraceptive of choice in those taking griseofulvin, not because of reduced efficacy but because of increased menstrual irregularities.[8]

1. van Dijke CPH, Weber JCP. Interaction between oral contraceptives and griseofulvin. *BMJ* (1984) 288, 1125–6.

2. Back DJ, Grimmer SFM, Orme ML'E, Proudlove C, Mann RD, Breckenridge AM. Evaluation of Committee on Safety of Medicines yellow card reports on oral contraceptive-drug interactions with anticonvulsants and antibiotics. *Br J Clin Pharmacol* (1988) 25, 527–32.
3. Côté J. Interaction of griseofulvin and oral contraceptives. *J Am Acad Dermatol* (1990) 22, 124–5.
4. Bollen M. Use of antibiotics when taking the oral contraceptive pill. *Aust Fam Physician* (1995) 24, 928–9.
5. McDaniel PA, Caldroney RD. Oral contraceptives and griseofulvin interaction. *Drug Intell Clin Pharm* (1986) 20, 384.
6. Beeley L, Stewart P. *Bulletin of the West Midlands Centre for Adverse Drug Reaction Reporting* (1987) 25, 23.
7. Committee on Safety of Medicines/Medicines Control Agency. Griseofulvin (Fulcin, Grisovin): contraceptive precautions. *Current Problems* (1996) 22, 8.
8. McCann MF, Potter LS. Progestin-only contraception: a comprehensive review. *Contraception* (1994) 50 (Suppl 1), S1–S198.

Oral contraceptives + Immunosuppressants

No clinically relevant interactions have so far been seen between leflunomide, mycophenolate or sirolimus and combined oral contraceptives, but the makers of mycophenolate and sirolimus suggest some caution nonetheless.

Clinical evidence, mechanism, importance and management

(a) Ciclosporin

For the interactions of ciclosporin with oral contraceptives see, 'Ciclosporin + Oral contraceptives and Progestogens', p.795.

(b) Leflunomide

Leflunomide was given to healthy women taking a triphasic oral contraceptive containing 30 micrograms of **ethinylestradiol**. During the study it was found that the leflunomide had no effect on the activity of the oral contraceptive and the pharmacokinetics of the active metabolite of leflunomide (A771726) were not changed to a clinically relevant extent.[1] No special precautions would therefore appear to be needed.

(c) Mycophenolate

The makers say that no pharmacokinetic interaction was seen in a single-dose study in 15 healthy women taking mycophenolate and *Orthonovum* (**norethisterone/ethinylestradiol** 1 mg/35 micrograms).[2] A study of mycophenolate 1 g twice daily given with a combined oral contraceptive (containing **ethinylestradiol** 20 to 40 micrograms and **levonorgestrel** 50 to 150 micrograms, **desogestrel** 150 micrograms or **gestodene** 50 to 100 micrograms) over 3 consecutive menstrual cycles in 18 women not previously on immunosuppressants found no clinically relevant influence on the suppression of ovulation by the oral contraceptives.[3] However, mycophenolate was teratogenic in animal studies at doses lower than those causing maternal toxicity. The US makers say that oral contraceptives should be used with caution, and additional birth control methods considered.[4]

(d) Sirolimus

A single-dose clinical study found that the pharmacokinetics of an oral contraceptive (**ethinylestradiol/norgestrel** 30/300 micrograms) were unaffected by sirolimus. This suggests that the efficacy of the contraceptive is likely to be unchanged, but as the UK makers cautiously point out, the effects on oral contraception of using sirolimus long term are unknown.[5]

(e) Tacrolimus

The UK makers of tacrolimus say that during clinical use **ethinylestradiol** has been shown to increase tacrolimus levels, presumably because it inhibits the cytochrome P450 isoenzyme CYP3A4. *In vitro* data suggests that **gestodene** and **norethindrone** may do the same.[6] In addition, tacrolimus has the potential to interfere with the metabolism of oral contraceptives, therefore the UK makers suggest that other contraceptive measures should be used.[6]

1. Arava (Leflunomide). Sanofi-Aventis. UK Summary of product characteristics, December 2004.
2. Syntex. Data on file. A single-dose pharmacokinetic drug interaction study of oral mycophenolate mofetil and an oral contraceptive in normal subjects. (Study No. MYCS2308) 1994.
3. CellCept (Mycophenolate mofetil). Roche Products Ltd. UK Summary of product characteristics, April 2005.
4. CellCept (Mycophenolate mofetil). Roche Pharmaceuticals. US Prescribing information, October 2004.
5. Rapamune (Sirolimus). Wyeth Pharmaceuticals. UK Summary of product characteristics, September 2004.
6. Prograf (Tacrolimus). Fujisawa Ltd. UK Summary of product characteristics, June 2002.

Oral contraceptives + Leukotriene receptor antagonists

Montelukast and zafirlukast do not alter the contraceptive efficacy of oral contraceptives.

Clinical evidence, mechanism, importance and management

(a) Montelukast

The makers of montelukast say that it does not interact with an oral contraceptive (**ethinylestradiol/norethisterone** 35 micrograms/1 mg).[1,2] No special precautions are therefore needed if both drugs are used concurrently.

(b) Zafirlukast

A single-blind parallel group study in 39 healthy women taking oral contraceptives [not named] found that zafirlukast 40 mg twice daily had no effect on the serum levels of **ethinylestradiol** nor on the contraceptive efficacy.[3] This study suggests that concurrent use need not be avoided.

1. Singulair (Montelukast sodium). Merck Sharp & Dohme Ltd. UK Summary of product characteristics, November 2004.
2. Singulair (Montelukast sodium). Merck & Co., Inc. US Prescribing information, January 2005.
3. Accolate (Zafirlukast). AstraZeneca Pharmaceuticals LP. US Prescribing information, July 2004.

Oral contraceptives + Modafinil

Modafinil slightly reduced the levels of ethinylestradiol from a combined oral contraceptive.

Clinical evidence, mechanism, importance and management

Modafinil 200 mg daily for 7 days then 400 mg daily for 21 days caused an 18% decrease in the AUC and an 11% decrease in maximum plasma levels of **ethinylestradiol** in 16 healthy women on a combined oral contraceptive (**ethinylestradiol/norgestimate**). Increases in plasma FSH and LH were not significant.[1] Modafinil is an inducer of the cytochrome P450 isoenzyme CYP3A4, which is partially responsible for the metabolism of **ethinylestradiol**. These small changes are lower than those seen with other enzyme-inducing drugs known to reduce the reliability of combined oral contraceptives (e.g. see 'carbamazepine', (p.753), and 'phenytoin', (p.751)). However, it cannot be ruled out that they would be sufficient to cause failure of combined oral contraceptives in very rare cases. The UK makers of modafinil advise the use of a high-dose combined oral contraceptive (**ethinylestradiol** 50 micrograms).[2] An alternative would be the concurrent use of a barrier form of contraception.[1,3] It is also recommended that concurrent or alternative methods should be continued for up to 2 cycles after stopping modafinil.[1-3]

1. Robertson P, Hellriegel ET, Arora S, Nelson M. Effect of modafinil on the pharmacokinetics of ethinyl estradiol and triazolam in healthy volunteers. *Clin Pharmacol Ther* (2002) 71, 46–56.
2. Provigil (Modafinil). Cephalon UK Ltd. UK Summary of product characteristics, September 2004.
3. Provigil (Modafinil). Cephalon Inc. US Prescribing information, December 2004.

Oral contraceptives + Nefazodone

A woman experienced increased combined oral contraceptive adverse effects while treated with nefazodone.

Clinical evidence, mechanism, importance and management

Within a week of starting nefazodone 50 mg twice daily, a woman on a low-dose combined oral contraceptive (**ethinylestradiol** 20 micrograms/**desogestrel**) reported breast tenderness, bloating, weight gain, and increased premenstrual irritability. She had previously experienced identical symptoms while taking a combined oral contraceptive with a higher dose of oestrogen. Nefazodone was discontinued after 6 weeks, and within 24 hours the adverse effects resolved.[1] Nefazodone is a known inhibitor of the cytochrome P450 isoenzyme CYP3A4, by which **ethinylestradiol** is metabolised, and might therefore be expected to increase **ethinylestradiol** levels. However, the general importance of this case is unknown.

1. Adson DE, Kotlyar M. A probable interaction between a very low-dose oral contraceptive and the antidepressant nefazodone: a case report. *J Clin Psychopharmacol* (2001) 21, 618–19.

Oral contraceptives + NNRTIs

Nevirapine modestly reduced the plasma concentrations of ethinylestradiol and norethisterone. A barrier method of contraception should be used in addition. Efavirenz and delavirdine increased the levels of ethinylestradiol, while ethinylestradiol had no effect on efavirenz levels.

Clinical evidence, mechanism, importance and management

(a) Delavirdine

The maker of delavirdine notes that it may increase the levels of **ethinylestradiol**, but the clinical relevance of this is unknown.[1]

(b) Efavirenz

The maker notes that efavirenz *increased* the AUC of a single dose of **ethinylestradiol** by 37% while the maximum plasma levels remained unchanged. Conversely, **ethinylestradiol** had no effect on the AUC of maximum plasma levels of efavirenz. These findings suggest that efavirenz does not adversely alter the efficacy of combined oral contraceptives. Nevertheless, the maker notes that because the interaction has not been fully characterised, a reliable method of barrier contraception must be used in addition to oral contraceptives.[2,3] Note that, a barrier method would usually be considered advisable to reduce the risk of HIV transmission.

(c) Nevirapine

A study in 10 HIV+ women found that nevirapine 200 mg once daily for 2 weeks then twice daily for a further 2 weeks decreased the median AUC and elimination half life of **ethinylestradiol** by 29% and 31%, respectively, and decreased the median AUC of **norethisterone** by 19%. The women received two single doses of a combined oral contraceptive (**ethinylestradiol/norethisterone** 35 micrograms/1 mg), once 2 days before the nevirapine and once on the last day of the nevirapine therapy. Nevirapine was added to established antiretroviral therapy (commonly 3 drugs), which had been unchanged for at least 4 weeks.

It is likely that nevirapine induces the metabolism of the components of the oral contraceptive by cytochrome P450.[4] Although it is not known whether these modest reductions in levels would reduce the anti-ovulatory efficacy of the combined oral contraceptive, it would be prudent to assume they could. The makers recommend that combined oral contraceptives should not be used as the sole method of contraception in women taking nevirapine. They suggest that a barrier method (e.g. condoms) should also be used, and note that this is also advisable to reduce the risk of HIV transmission.[4-6] They also suggest that if combined oral contraceptives are used for reasons other than contraception (e.g. endometriosis), that the therapeutic effect should be monitored and the dose increased if necessary.[4,5] These precautions seem prudent.

1. Rescriptor (Delavirdine). Pharmacia & Upjohn Company. US Prescribing information, November 2003.
2. Sustiva (Efavirenz). Bristol-Myers Squibb Pharmaceuticals Ltd. UK Summary of product characteristics, March 2005.
3. Sustiva (Efavirenz). Bristol Myers Squibb Company. US Prescribing information, December 2004.
4. Mildvan D, Yarrish R, Marshak A, Hutman HW, McDonough M, Lamson M, Robinson P. Pharmacokinetic interaction between nevirapine and ethinyl estradiol/norethindrone when administered concurrently to HIV-infected women. *J Acquir Immune Defic Syndr* (2002) 29, 471–7.
5. Viramune (Nevirapine). Boehringer Ingelheim Ltd. UK Summary of product characteristics, April 2005.
6. Viramune (Nevirapine). Boehringher Ingelheim Pharmaceuticals Inc. US Prescribing information, January 2005.

Oral contraceptives + Orlistat

Orlistat does not interact with combined oral contraceptives.

Clinical evidence, mechanism, importance and management

Two groups of 10 healthy women taking a combined oral contraceptive were given **orlistat** 120 mg three times daily or a placebo on days 1 to 23 of two menstrual cycles.[1] Orlistat had no effect on ovulation (measured by luteinising hormone and progesterone levels). The contraceptives used all contained **ethinylestradiol**, but the progestogens differed: 10 with **desogestrel**, 4 **levonorgestrel**, 3 **gestodene**, 2 **cyproterone acetate**, 1 **lynestrenol**. No additional contraceptive precautions would seem necessary in women on oral contraceptives if given orlistat.

1. Hartmann D, Güzelhan C, Zuiderwijk PBM, Odink J. Lack of interaction between orlistat and oral contraceptives. *Eur J Clin Pharmacol* (1996) 50, 421–4.

Oral contraceptives + Protease inhibitors

Ethinylestradiol levels are reduced by lopinavir/ritonavir, nelfinavir and ritonavir alone, and norethisterone levels are modestly reduced by nelfinavir in patients taking combined oral contraceptives. Concurrent use of oral contraceptives with amprenavir is not recommended.
Note that whatever other methods of contraception are being used, barrier methods are also advisable to reduce the risk of HIV transmission.

Clinical evidence

(a) Amprenavir

The UK maker briefly notes that amprenavir increased the minimum plasma concentrations of **ethinylestradiol** and **norethisterone**, given as a combined oral contraceptive, by 32 and 45% respectively. Conversely the amprenavir minimum concentration and AUC were decreased by 22 and 20%, respectively.[1]

(b) Indinavir

The maker briefly notes that no clinically significant interaction was observed between indinavir and a combined oral contraceptive containing **ethinylestradiol** and **norethisterone**.[2]

(c) Lopinavir/ritonavir

A study in 12 healthy subjects found that **lopinavir/ritonavir** 400/100 mg twice daily for 14 days decreased the AUC of **ethinylestradiol** and **norethisterone**, given as a combined oral contraceptive for 21 days, by 42% and 17%, respectively.[3]

(d) Nelfinavir

The maker briefly notes that nelfinavir 750 mg three times daily for a week reduced the AUC of **ethinylestradiol** by 47% and that of **norethisterone** by 18% in women taking a combined oral contraceptive (**ethinylestradiol/norethisterone** 35/400 micrograms).[4]

(e) Ritonavir

Ritonavir 500 mg 12-hourly for 16 days decreased the AUC of **ethinylestradiol** by 41% and decreased the elimination half life from 17 to 13 hours) in a study in 23 healthy women. The women received a single dose of a combined oral contraceptive (**ethinylestradiol/ethynodiol** 50 micrograms/1 mg), 14 days before the ritonavir and on day 15 of the ritonavir therapy.[5]

Mechanism

The results for ritonavir are the opposite of those originally predicted based on *in vitro* data showing *inhibition* of ethinylestradiol metabolism (cytochrome P450 isoenzyme CYP3A mediated 2-hydroxylation).[6] It is possible that ritonavir induces rather than inhibits CYP3A after chronic use. It is also likely that ritonavir induces ethinylestradiol glucuronosyl transferase activity.[5] Nelfinavir probably interacts similarly. Amprenavir and indinavir inhibit CYP3A4.

Importance and management

Although information is limited, the pharmacokinetic interaction between the ethinylestradiol component of combined oral contraceptives and ritonavir, lopinavir/ritonavir and nelfinavir appears to be established and is likely to be clinically important. Similar decreases in plasma levels of ethinylestradiol caused by other drugs have resulted in reduced efficacy and reliability of combined oral contraceptives. Although no cases of contraceptive failure attributed to this interaction have yet been reported, to avoid this risk and that of breakthrough bleeding the makers of ritonavir recommend that the dosage of ethinylestradiol should be increased.[7] Substitute a contraceptive preparation with a higher dose of ethinylestradiol or use an alternative or additional non-hormonal form of contraception during and for one cycle after the ritonavir is stopped.[7,8] Similar advice applies to nelfinavir,[4,9] and lopinavir/ritonavir.

In contrast, amprenavir appears to increase the levels of ethinylestradiol and norethisterone, so would not be expected to decrease contraceptive efficacy. However, the levels of amprenavir are modestly reduced, and the effect of this on antiviral efficacy is unknown. The makers advise alternative methods of contraception.[1,10] There appears to be no clinically significant interaction between indinavir and combined oral contraceptives.

There is no direct information about **progestogen-only** pills but since lopinavir/ritonavir and nelfinavir cause small (less than 20%), reductions in the levels of norethisterone (given as part of a combined oral contraceptive) it is possible that these protease inhibitors could reduce the contraceptive efficacy of **progestogen-only oral contraceptives** containing norethisterone. Note that the **progestogen-only oral contraceptives** have a higher failure rate than the combined oral contraceptives anyway. It would seem prudent to use additional contraceptive measures in this situation as well. Whether this applies to other progestogens used in **progestogen-only oral contraceptives** does not appear to have been studied. However, note that whatever other methods of contraception are being used, barrier methods are also advisable to reduce the risk of HIV transmission.

1. Agenerase (Amprenavir). GlaxoSmithKline UK. UK Summary of product characteristics. December 2004.
2. Crixivan (Indinavir sulfate). Merck Sharp & Dohme Ltd. UK Summary of product characteristics, January 2005.
3. Bertz R, Hsu A, Lam W, Williams L, Renz C, Karol M, Dutta S, Carr R, Zhang Y, Wang Q, Schweitzer S, Foit C, Andre A, Bernstein B, Granneman GR, Sun E. Pharmacokinetic interaction between lopinavir/ritonavir (ABT-378r) and other non-HIV drugs (P291). *AIDS* (2000) 14 (Suppl 4), S100.
4. Viracept (Nelfinavir mesilate). Roche Products Ltd. UK Summary of product characteristics, June 2005.
5. Ouellet D, Hsu A, Qian J, Locke CS, Eason CJ, Cavanaugh JH, Leonard JM, Granneman GR. Effect of ritonavir on the pharmacokinetics of ethinyl oestradiol in healthy female volunteers. *Br J Clin Pharmacol* (1998) 46, 111–16.
6. Kumar GN, Rodrigues AD, Buko AM, Denissen JF. Cytochrome P450-mediated metabolism of the HIV-1 protease inhibitor ritonavir (ABT-538) in human liver microsomes. *J Pharmacol Exp Ther* (1996) 277, 423–31.
7. Norvir (Ritonavir). Abbott Laboratories Ltd. UK Summary of product characteristics, January 2005.
8. Norvir (Ritonavir). Abbott Laboratories. US Prescribing information, April 2005.
9. Viracept (Nelfinavir mesilate). Agouron Pharmaceuticals, Inc. US Prescribing information, September 2004.
10. Agenerase (Amprenavir). GlaxoSmithKline. US Prescribing information, May 2005.

Oral contraceptives + Proton pump inhibitors

Lansoprazole and pantoprazole appear not to interact with combined oral contraceptives.

Clinical evidence, mechanism, importance and management

(a) Lansoprazole

In a placebo-controlled crossover study 24 healthy women were given a combined oral contraceptive (**ethinylestradiol/levonorgestrel** 30/150 micrograms) for two monthly cycles, with and without lansoprazole 60 mg daily. The levels of the oral contraceptive steroids were not significantly altered by lansoprazole, nor were endogenous progesterone levels raised, suggesting that ovulation did not occur.[1] The maker has information about 3 other unpublished studies in a total of 59 women, which also found no evidence that lansoprazole interacts with oral contraceptives in any way which would affect their reliability.[2] No special precautions are necessary on concurrent use.

(b) Pantoprazole

A study over four menstrual cycles was completed by 64 pre-menopausal women. The women were confirmed to be ovulating before taking a low-dose triphasic oral contraceptive (**ethinylestradiol/levonorgestrel**), and not ovulating during contraceptive use. They continued not ovulating when pantoprazole 40 mg daily was given, so it was concluded that pantoprazole does not affect oral contraception.[3]

1. Fuchs W, Sennewald R, Klotz U. Lansoprazole does not affect the bioavailability of oral contraceptives. *Br J Clin Pharmacol* (1994) 38, 376–80.
2. Wyeth, Personal communication, February 1998.
3. Middle MV, Müller FO, Schall R, Hundt HKL, Mogilnicka EM, Beneke PC. Effect of pantoprazole on ovulation suppression by a low-dose hormonal contraceptive. *Clin Drug Invest* (1995) 9, 54–6.

Oral contraceptives + Retinoids

There seems to be no evidence that the reliability of the combined oral contraceptives is affected by acitretin, etretinate or isotretinoin, and they are the contraceptive method of choice with these teratogenic drugs. It is unclear whether the effects of the progestogen-only oral contraceptives are altered by acitretin, but, in any case, progestogen-only oral contraceptives are not generally considered reliable enough for use with these teratogenic drugs. The adverse effects of isotretinoin on lipids may be additive with those of oral contraceptives.

Clinical evidence

(a) Combined oral contraceptives

(i) Acitretin. Eight women taking a combined oral contraceptive (**ethinylestradiol/levonorgestrel**) were given acitretin 25 to 40 mg daily for at least two cycles. Suppression of ovulation was not affected by acitretin, as assessed by plasma progesterone levels.[1]

(ii) Etretinate. In another study, suppression of ovulation was not affected by **etretinate** 0.7 to 1 mg/kg in 12 women taking a combined oral contraceptive (**ethinylestradiol** plus **levonorgestrel**, **norethisterone**, **norgestrel**, or **cyproterone**).[2]

(iii) Isotretinoin. A pharmacokinetic study in 9 women taking a combined oral contraceptive showed that the plasma concentrations of **ethinylestradiol** and **levonorgestrel** were not significantly changed by the use of isotretinoin 500 micrograms/kg. Suppression of ovulation was maintained.[3]

The adverse effects of isotretinoin and combined oral contraceptives on plasma lipids may be additive. A case-control study found that women who had hypertriglyceridaemia and/or hypercholesterolaemia while taking isotretinoin were 2 to 12 times as likely to be also taking an oral contraceptive.[4]

(b) Progestogen-only oral contraceptives

One woman on a progestogen-only contraceptive (**levonorgestrel** 30 micrograms) showed a significant increase in progesterone levels after 3 cycles while taking **acitretin** 400 micrograms/kg daily. Plasma progesterone levels rose from 2.15 nanograms/ml before taking the **acitretin** to 3.87 to 13.46 nanograms/ml with **acitretin**. This rise in progesterone levels was taken as evidence that ovulation had occurred.[1]

Mechanism, importance and management

Information is limited, but it appears that these retinoids do not alter the efficacy of combined oral contraceptives. From the one available case, it is unclear whether acitretin alters the efficacy of progestogen-only oral contraceptives. However, note that **progestogen-only oral contraceptives** do not reliably suppress ovulation in all cycles, and that this is not considered their primary mechanism of action (see 'Hormonal contraceptives and sex hormones', (p.741)). The single report cannot therefore be taken as evidence that acitretin reduces the efficacy of progestogen-only contraceptives.

Also note that because the retinoids are established human teratogens, it is very important that women taking them do not become pregnant. For this reason, progestogen-only oral contraceptives are generally not considered suitable for use with retinoids.[5] Unless contraindicated, combined oral contraceptives are the method of choice.[5-7] These are started one month before the retinoids and continued for one month after stopping isotretinoin,[6,7] and for 2 years after stopping etretinate or acitretin.[5] In the USA, it is standard practice to recommend that a second form of contraception, such as a barrier method, should also be used. This is because, even though hormonal methods of contraception are highly effective, they do, on rare occasions, fail.[6] An oral contraceptive containing a non-androgenic (third generation) progestogen (e.g. desogestrel, gestodene, norgestimate) is preferred, since these have less detrimental effects on lipids,[5] and some prefer the antiandrogen cyproterone.[7]

1. Berbis Ph, Bun H, Geiger JM, Rognin C, Durand A, Serradimigni A, Hartmann D, Privat Y. Acitretin (RO10-1670) and oral contraceptives: interaction study. *Arch Dermatol Res* (1988) 280, 388–9.
2. Berbis P, Bounameaux Y, Rognin C, Hartmann D, Privat Y. Study on the influence of etretinate on biologic activity of oral contraceptives. *J Am Acad Dermatol* (1987) 17, 302–3.
3. Orme M, Back DJ, Shaw MA, Allen WL, Tjia J, Cunliffe WJ, Jones DH. Isotretinoin and contraception. *Lancet* (1984) ii, 752–3.
4. Chen Y, Xue S, Dai W, LaBraico J. Evaluation of serum triglyceride and cholesterol levels from isotretinoin therapy with concomitant oral contraceptives. *Pharmacoepidemiol Drug Safety* (1995) 4, 91–6.
5. Ceyrac DL, Serfaty D, Lefrancq H. Retinoids and contraception. *Dermatology* (1992) 184, 161–70.
6. Perlman SE, Leach EE, Dominguez L, Ruszkowski AM, Rudy SJ. "Be smart, be safe, be sure". The revised pregnancy prevention program for women on isotretinoin. *J Reprod Med* (2001), 46 (Suppl), 179–85.
7. Holmes SC, Bankowska U, Mackie RM. The prescription of isotretinoin to women: is every precaution taken? *Br J Dermatol* (1998) 138, 450–5.

Oral contraceptives + Rizatriptan

Rizatriptan appears not to interact with oral contraceptives.

Clinical evidence, mechanism, importance and management

A two-period, crossover, placebo controlled study in 20 healthy young women taking on a combined oral contraceptive (**ethinylestradiol/norethisterone** 35 micrograms/1 mg) found that the concurrent use of rizatriptan (6 days of 10 mg daily followed by 2 days of 10 mg every 4 hours for 12 hours) did not effect the pharmacokinetics of either contraceptive steroid. Blood pressure, heart rate and temperature were unaffected and adverse effects were similar to those seen with the placebo.[1] There would therefore appear to be no reason for avoiding concurrent use.

1. Shadle CR, Liu G, Goldberg MR. A double-blind, placebo-controlled evaluation of the effect of oral doses of rizatriptan 10 mg on oral contraceptive pharmacokinetics in healthy female volunteers. *J Clin Pharmacol* (2000) 40, 309–15.

Oral contraceptives + Statins

Atorvastatin and pravastatin do not seem to interact to a clinically relevant effect with combined oral contraceptives.

Clinical evidence, mechanism, importance and management

(a) Atorvastatin

A study in 12 healthy women taking a combined oral contraceptive (**ethinylestradiol/norethisterone** 35 micrograms/1 mg) found that atorvastatin 40 mg daily increased the AUC of **norethisterone** and **ethinylestradiol** by about 28% and 19% respectively, and increased their maximum plasma levels by 24% and 30% respectively.[1] These increases are only moderate and unlikely to be clinically important, but the makers say that they should be considered when selecting an appropriate oral contraceptive dosage for women given **atorvastatin**.[2,3]

(b) Pravastatin

The pharmacokinetics of a single 20-mg dose of pravastatin were found to be unaffected in 15 young women taking combined oral contraceptives (**ethinylestradiol** with **norethisterone**, **norgestrel** or **levonorgestrel**) when compared with similar women not taking contraceptives. No adverse effects attributable to concurrent use were seen.[4]

1. Yang B-B, Siedlik PH, Smithers JA, Sedman AJ, Stern RH. Atorvastatin pharmacokinetic interactions with other CYP3A4 substrates: erythromycin and ethinyl estradiol. *Pharm Res* (1996) 13 (9 Suppl), S-437.
2. Lipitor (Atorvastatin). Parke Davis. UK Summary of product characteristics, March 2005.
3. Lipitor (Atorvastatin). Pfizer Inc. US Prescribing information, July 2004.
4. Pan HY, Waclawski AP, Funke PT, Whigan D. Pharmacokinetics of pravastatin in elderly versus young men and women. *Ann Pharmacother* (1993) 27, 1029–33.

Oral contraceptives + St John's wort (*Hypericum perforatum*)

Both breakthrough bleeding and combined oral contraceptive failure have been seen in women taking St John's wort. Two cases of the failure of postcoital (emergency) hormonal contraception attributed to the use of St John's wort have also been reported.

Clinical evidence

(a) Oral contraceptive failure

The Adverse Drug Reactions Database of the Swedish Medical Products Agency has on record 2 cases of pregnancy due to failure of a combined oral contraceptive attributed to the use of products containing St John's wort (*Esbericum* and *Kira*). One woman was taking **ethinylestradiol/norethisterone** and the other **ethinylestradiol/levonorgestrel**.[1] This follows an earlier report from the Swedish MPA of 8 cases of intermenstrual bleeding in women aged 23 to 31 taking long-term oral contraceptives and St John's wort. Intermenstrual bleeding occurred within about a week of starting St John's wort in 5 of the cases, and was known to have resolved in 3 cases when the St John's wort was stopped.[2] The UK Committee on Safety of Medicines has recorded a further 7 cases of pregnancy in women taking St John's wort and oral contraceptives in the two-year period from February 2000 to February 2002.[3] Another earlier brief report describes 3 women taking a combined oral contraceptive (**ethinylestradiol/desogestrel** 30/150 micrograms) who developed breakthrough bleeding one week (2 cases) and 3 months (1 case) after starting to take St John's wort.[4]

(b) Emergency hormonal contraceptive failure

The UK Committee on Safety of Medicines has received reports of 2 women taking St John's wort who became pregnant despite taking **postcoital hormonal contraception**. One of them was also taking an oral contraceptive.[3]

Mechanism

It is believed that St John's wort can induce the cytochrome P450-mediated metabolism of the contraceptive steroids, thereby reducing their serum levels and their effects.[2,4,5] This can lead to breakthrough bleeding and, in some cases, contraceptive failure. This is consistent with the way St John's wort appears to lower the serum levels of some other drugs. Note that St John's wort is a herbal preparation, and the specific constituents responsible for enzyme induction are currently unknown. Also, the levels of individual constituents can vary between different preparations of the herb.

Importance and management

Information appears to be limited to these reports but the oral contraceptive/St John's wort interaction appears to be established. Its incidence is not known but the evidence so far suggests that breakthrough bleeding and pregnancy resulting from this interaction are uncommon. However, since it is not known who is particularly likely to be at risk, women taking oral contraceptives should either avoid St John's wort (the recommendation of the CSM/MCA in the UK[5]) or they should use an additional form of contraception.

Only two cases of postcoital (emergency) hormonal contraceptive failure attributed to an interaction with St John's wort have so far been reported. If this is, as believed, due to enzyme induction by the St John's wort (see Mechanism above), then an increase in the dosage of the postcoital hormonal contraceptive should be considered, or the copper IUD used instead. See also, 'Emergency hormonal contraceptives + Enzyme-inducing drugs', p.742.

Although the considerable worldwide popularity of St John's wort is fairly recent, it is currently the most widely used antidepressant in Germany and has been used for very many years in Germany and Austria as a herbal remedy. Yet, there seems to be no published evidence that oral contraceptive failure in those countries is more frequent than anywhere else.

This would seem to confirm that this interaction is very uncommon, or perhaps that it has failed to be identified as a possible cause.

1. Swedish Medical Products Agency. St John's wort may influence other medication. Available at http://www3.mpa.se/020206_stjohnswort.html and http://www.mpa.se/observanda/obs02/020204_fallbeskr_johannesort.shtml (accessed 15/08/02).
2. Yue Q-Y, Bergquist C, Gerdén B. Safety of St John's wort (Hypericum perforatum). *Lancet* (2000) 355, 576–7.
3. Committee on Safety of Medicines. Personal communication, February 15th, 2002.
4. Bon S, Hartmann K, Kuhn M. Johanniskraut: Ein Enzyminduktor? *Schweiz Apothekerzeitung* (1999) 16, 535–6.
5. Committee on Safety of Medicines. Message from Professor A Breckenridge (Chairman of CSM) and Fact Sheet for Health Care Professionals. Important interactions between St John's wort (*Hypericum perforatum*) preparations and prescribed medicines, 29th February 2000. Available at http://www.mca.gov.uk/mca/csm/stjohn.pdf

Oral contraceptives + Sucrose polyesters

Sucrose polyesters do not interact with oral contraceptives.

Clinical evidence, mechanism, importance and management

When 28 healthy women took 18 g of sucrose polyester (*Olestra*) daily for 28 days, the pharmacokinetics of the components of a combined oral contraceptive (**ethinylestradiol/norgestrel** 30/300 micrograms) were unchanged. Serum progesterone levels also remained unaltered, suggesting no ovulation occurred.[1] This agrees with the findings of earlier single-dose studies, which found that sucrose polyester had no effect on the bioavailability of single doses of **ethinylestradiol** or **norethisterone**.[2] No special contraceptive precautions appear to be necessary.

1. Miller KW, Williams DS, Carter SB, Jones MB, Mishell DR. The effect of olestra on systemic levels of oral contraceptives. *Clin Pharmacol Ther* (1990) 48, 34–40.
2. Roberts RJ, Leff RD. Influence of absorbable and nonabsorbable lipids and lipidlike substances on drug availability. *Clin Pharmacol Ther* (1989) 45, 299–304.

Oral contraceptives + Tobacco smoking

The risk of cardiovascular disease in women on combined oral contraceptives is greatly increased if they smoke, particularly in the older age group. Progestogen-only oral contraceptives are an alternative. There is some evidence that smoking increases the risk of breakthrough bleeding with combined oral contraceptives, although smoking appears not to alter contraceptive steroid levels.

Clinical evidence

(a) Cardiovascular effects

Early after the introduction of combined oral contraceptives it was realised that they increase the risk of cardiovascular effects such as thromboembolism, myocardial infarction, and stroke, and that the risks were markedly increased in women who also smoked.[1-5] For example, one of these studies found a relative risk of non-fatal myocardial infarction in women on the pill of 4.5 in non-smokers and 39 in heavy smokers.[4] Another study found a relative risk of subarachnoid haemorrhage in women taking oral contraceptives of 6.5 for non-smokers and 22 for smokers.[5]

(b) Contraceptive efficacy

An analysis of data from 3 large clinical trials in a total of 2956 women found that smoking was associated with an increased incidence of spotting and bleeding in users of combined oral contraceptives. The relative risk was 1.3 during the first cycle of use and increased to 1.9 by the sixth cycle.[6] Similarly, smokers were more likely to have menstrual disturbances, and combined oral contraceptive failure was 20% greater than expected in smokers in a study of women who became pregnant while on oral contraceptives.[7] This association was not noted for **progestogen-only oral contraceptive** failure.[7] Conversely, there was no increased failure rate of oral contraceptives in smokers in a large cohort study in the UK.[8]

Mechanism

(a) The cardiovascular effects reported do not appear to be attributable to any effect of smoking on the metabolism of contraceptives steroids (see below). Rather, the adverse effects of combined oral contraceptives on cardiovascular risk factors, such as plasma lipids and coagulation parameters, appear to be accentuated by smoking.

(b) Smoking increased the metabolism (2-hydroxylation) of *endogenous* estradiol in premenopausal women.[9] However, smoking does not appear to alter the levels of contraceptive steroids. In one study in 311 women on oral contraceptives, plasma levels of ethinylestradiol and norgestrel were similar in smokers and non-smokers.[10] Another study found a small increase in ethinylestradiol clearance in smokers,[11] but this is probably not clinically relevant.

Importance and management

(a) The cardiovascular interaction between smoking and combined oral contraceptives is well established. In the UK it is currently recommended that women who smoke 40 or more cigarettes a day do not receive combined oral contraceptives.[12] Similarly, those who smoke less than 40 cigarettes a day should also avoid combined oral contraceptives if they have any other risk factors for arterial disease, or if they are over 35 years of age.[12] In women who smoke for whom a combined oral contraceptive is not contraindicated, ones with the lowest doses of ethinylestradiol may be safer.[13] All smokers should be encouraged to stop.[13] In the UK, **progestogen-only oral contraceptives** are considered suitable for women who are heavy smokers,[12] although it should be remembered that they have a higher failure rate than the combined oral contraceptives.

(b) Smoking may increase the incidence of breakthrough bleeding. This may decrease the acceptability of the oral contraceptive, and lead to the use of less effective contraceptive methods.[6] However, it also raises the question of whether smoking increases the failure rate of oral contraceptives. The only evidence that this may occur is anecdotal. Further study is needed.

1. Arntzenius AC, van Gent CM, van der Voort H, Stegerhoek CI, Styblo K. Reduced high-density lipoprotein in women aged 40–41 using oral contraceptives. *Lancet* (1978) i, 1221–3.
2. Frederiksen H, Ravenholt RT. Thromboembolism, oral contraceptives and cigarettes. *Public Health Rep* (1970) 85, 197–205.
3. Collaborative Group for the study of stroke in young women. Oral contraceptives and stroke in young women: associated risk factors. *JAMA* (1975) 231, 718–22.
4. Shapiro S, Slone D, Rosenberg L, Kaufman DW, Stolley PD, Miettinen OS. Oral-contraceptive use in relation to myocardial infarction. *Lancet* (1979) i, 743–7.
5. Petitti DB, Wingerd J. Use of oral contraceptives, cigarette smoking, and risk of subarachnoid haemorrhage. *Lancet* (1978) ii, 234–6.
6. Rosenberg MJ, Waugh MS, Stevens CM. Smoking and cycle control among oral contraceptive users. *Am J Obstet Gynecol* (1996) 174, 628–32.
7. Sparrow MJ. Pregnancies in reliable pill takers. *N Z Med J* (1989) 102, 575–7.
8. Vessey MP, Villard-Mackintosh L, Jacobs HS. Anti-estrogenic effect of cigarette smoking. *N Engl J Med* (1987) 317, 769–70.
9. Michnovicz JJ, Hershcopf RJ, Naganuma H, Bradlow HL, Fishman J. Increased 2-hydroxylation of estradiol as a possible mechanism for the anti-estrogenic effect of cigarette smoking. *N Engl J Med* (1986) 315, 1305–9.
10. Crawford FE, Back DJ, Orme ML'E, Breckenridge AM. Oral contraceptive steroid plasma concentrations in smokers and non-smokers. *BMJ* (1981) 282, 1829–30.
11. Kanarkowski R, Tornatore KM, D'Ambrosio R, Gardner MJ, Jusko WJ. Pharmacokinetics of single and multiple doses of ethinyl estradiol and levonorgestrel in relation to smoking. *Clin Pharmacol Ther* (1988) 43, 23–31.
12. British National Formulary. 49th ed. London: The British Medical Association and The Pharmaceutical Press; 2005. p. 403.
13. Schiff I, Bell WR, Davis V, Kessler CM, Meyers C, Nakajima S, Sexton BJ. Oral contraceptives and smoking, current considerations: recommendations of a consensus panel. *Am J Obstet Gynecol* (1999) 180 (Part 2) S383–S384.

Oral contraceptives + Tolterodine

Tolterodine does not appear to interact with combined oral contraceptives.

Clinical evidence, mechanism, importance and management

An open-label, randomised, two-period crossover study in 24 women found that tolterodine 2 mg twice daily on days 1 to 14 for two 28-day contraceptive cycles had no effect on the pharmacokinetics of the steroids in a combined oral contraceptive (**ethinylestradiol/levonorgestrel** 30/150 micrograms). The pharmacokinetics of the tolterodine were also not relevantly changed, and the serum levels of estradiol and progesterone indicated that suppression of ovulation continued during both periods of treatment.[1] No special precautions would seem to be needed if these drugs are used concurrently.

1. Olsson B, Landgren B-M. The effect of tolterodine on the pharmacokinetics and pharmacodynamics of a combination oral contraceptive containing ethinyl estradiol and levonorgestrel. *Clin Ther* (2001) 23, 1876–88.

Oral contraceptives + Ziprasidone

Ziprasidone appears not to interact to a clinically relevant extent with oral contraceptives.

Clinical evidence, mechanism importance and management

In a double-blind, placebo-controlled, two-way crossover study, 18 women taking an oral contraceptive (**ethinylestradiol/levonorgestrel** 30/150 micrograms) for at least 3 months were also given ziprasidone 20 mg twice daily for 8 days. The only change in the pharmacokinetics of the two steroids was a 30 minute increase in the half-life of the **levonorgestrel**. No adverse effects occurred. It was concluded that combined use is safe and that ziprasidone does not affect the efficacy of this oral contraceptive[1] and is also unlikely to affect the safety of other similar contraceptives.

1. Muirhead GJ, Holt PR, Oliver S, Harness J, Anziano RJ. The effect of ziprasidone on steady-state pharmacokinetics of a combined oral contraceptive. *Eur Neuropsychopharmacol* (1996) 6 (Suppl 3), 38.

Progestogen-only contraceptives + Antibacterials; Broad-spectrum

The reliability of progestogen-only methods of hormonal contraception is not affected by broad-spectrum antibacterials such as the penicillins and tetracyclines.

Clinical evidence, mechanism, importance and management

Four of the 63 contraceptive failures attributed to antibacterials in the UK Committee on Safety of Medicines records for 1968 to 1984 occurred with a progestogen-only contraceptive (unspecified).[1] In another study, 2 of 37 cases of contraceptive failure attributed to antibacterials occurred with a progestogen-only contraceptive (unspecified).[2]

Note that the mechanism behind the rare cases of failure of *combined* oral contraceptives seen with various broad-spectrum antibacterials is postulated to be reduced enterohepatic recycling of ethinylestradiol (see 'Oral contraceptives + Antibacterials; Penicillins', p.746). Since progestogens are largely metabolised to inactive substances before they are conjugated, they do not undergo enterohepatic recycling of the active substance.

Pharmacokinetic data show that the progestogen component (**levonorgestrel, norethisterone**) of *combined* oral contraceptives is not affected by **ampicillin**,[3,4] clarithromycin,[5] **doxycycline**,[6] metronidazole,[4] moxifloxacin,[7] or **tetracycline**.[8] There is no reason to expect that the contraceptive efficacy of the various **progestogen-only methods** (tablets, implants, injections, IUDs) would be affected by broad-spectrum antibacterials that alter gut flora.

It is generally accepted that no interaction occurs,[9] and it is likely that the few cases seen with progestogen-only contraceptives are chance associations.[1] The UK Family Planning Authority do not recommend any additional contraceptive precautions with oral or any other method of progestogen-only contraception when broad-spectrum antibacterials are taken.[10] No special precautions are necessary.

1. Back DJ, Grimmer SFM, Orme ML'E, Proudlove C, Mann RD, Breckenridge AM. Evaluation of Committee on Safety of Medicines yellow card reports on oral contraceptive-drug interactions with anticonvulsants and antibiotics. *Br J Clin Pharmacol* (1988) 25, 527–32.
2. Sparrow MJ. Pill method failures. *N Z Med J* (1987) 100, 102–5.
3. Back DJ, Breckenridge AM, MacIver M, Orme M, Rowe PH, Staiger Ch, Thomas E, Tjia J. The effects of ampicillin on oral contraceptive steroids in women. *Br J Clin Pharmacol* (1982) 14, 43–8.
4. Joshi JV, Joshi UM, Sankholi GM, Krishna U, Mandlekar A, Chowdhury V, Hazari K, Gupta K, Sheth UK, Saxena BN. A study of interaction of low-dose combination oral contraceptive with ampicillin and metronidazole. *Contraception* (1980) 22, 643–52.
5. Back DJ, Tjia J, Martin C, Millar E, Salmon P, Orme M. The interaction between clarithromycin and combined oral-contraceptive steroids. *J Pharm Med* (1991) 2, 81–7.
6. Neely JL, Abate M, Swinker M, D'Angio R. The effect of doxycycline on serum levels of ethinyl estradiol, norethindrone, and endogenous progesterone. *Obstet Gynecol* (1991) 77, 416–20.
7. Staß H, Sachse R, Heinig R, Zühlsdorf M, Horstmann R. Pharmacokinetics (PK) of steroid hormones in oral contraceptives (OC) are not altered by oral moxifloxacin (MOX). *J Antimicrob Chemother* (1999) 44 (Suppl A) 138–9.
8. Murphy AA, Zacur HA, Charache P, Burkman RT. The effect of tetracycline on levels of oral contraceptives. *Am J Obstet Gynecol* (1991) 164, 28–33.
9. McCann MF, Potter LS. Progestin-only contraception: a comprehensive review. *Contraception* (1994) 50, S1–S198.
10. Belfield T, ed. FPA Contraceptive Handbook: a guide for family planning and other health professionals. 3rd ed. London: Family Planning Association, 1999.

Progestogen-only injections or implants + Enzyme-inducing drugs

Enzyme-inducing drugs appear to reduce the contraceptive reliability of the levonorgestrel implant, and pregnancies have been reported following the use of phenytoin, carbamazepine, and phenobarbital. The etonogestrel implant, and possibly the norethisterone enantate injection are expected to interact similarly. The efficacy of medroxyprogesterone depot injection does not appear to be affected by enzyme-inducing drugs.

Clinical evidence, mechanism, importance and management

(a) Implants

A woman taking **phenytoin** 300 mg daily became pregnant 9 months after the insertion of a **levonorgestrel-releasing subdermal contraceptive implant** (*Norplant*). **Levonorgestrel** levels increased by 50% after discontinuation of the **phenytoin**, and progesterone levels fell, suggesting greater suppression of ovulation.[1] In another report about women with **levonorgestrel implants**, plasma **levonorgestrel** levels were 38% lower in 6 women taking **phenytoin** alone or in combination with **carbamazepine** or valproate than in 10 subjects taking no medication. Two of the 6 women became pregnant (one on **phenytoin** and one on **phenytoin** and **carbamazepine**).[2] Similarly, one woman taking **phenobarbital** 210 mg daily became pregnant about 17 months after the insertion of a **levonorgestrel implant**.[3] Another report[4] briefly mentions that one woman on enzyme-inducing anticonvulsants became pregnant while using a **levonorgestrel implant**, and mentions that the maker had 30 other similar cases on file as of 1995. The maker of **levonorgestrel implant** (*Norplant*) advised using additional contraceptive measures during short-term use of enzyme inducers (less than 4 weeks) and for 7 days afterwards. If the enzyme inducers are used for more than 4 weeks additional precautions should be taken for 4 weeks following their withdrawal (to allow liver enzymes to recover). They stated that *Norplant* was normally inappropriate for use in long-term users of enzyme-inducing drugs.[5] [However, note that *Norplant* has now been discontinued.] Similar advice is given by the maker of **etonogestrel implant** *(Implanon)*,[6] although there are not yet any reports of drug interactions between this product and enzyme-inducing drugs. A list of enzyme-inducing drugs can be found in 'Table 26.1', (p.741)).

(b) Injectable preparations

The maker states that the clearance of **medroxyprogesterone acetate** is approximately equal to hepatic blood flow, and as such, would not be expected to be affected by drugs that alter hepatic enzyme activity. Therefore, they say that no dosage adjustment is needed.[7] Nevertheless, the UK Family Planning Association recommend that the time interval between injections should be reduced from 12 to 10 weeks in women on enzyme-inducing drugs.[8]

There are data showing that **rifamycins** can reduce the plasma levels of **norethisterone** when used as a component of combined oral contraceptives (see 'Oral contraceptives + Antibacterials; Rifamycins', p.748). The maker notes that enzyme-inducing drugs may reduce the efficacy of *Noristerat*,[9] and the UK Family Planning Association recommend that the time interval between injections should be reduced from 8 to 6 weeks in women on these drugs.[8] This seems a sensible precaution. A list of enzyme-inducing drugs can be found in 'Table 26.1', (p.741)).

1. Odlind V, Olsson S-E. Enhanced metabolism of levonorgestrel during phenytoin treatment in a woman with Norplant® implants. *Contraception* (1986) 33, 257–61.
2. Haukkamaa M. Contraception by Norplant® subdermal capsules is not reliable in epileptic patients on anticonvulsant treatment. *Contraception* (1986) 33, 559–65.
3. Shane-McWhorter L, Cerveny JD, MacFarlane LL, Osborn C. Enhanced metabolism of levonorgestrel during phenobarbital treatment and resultant pregnancy. *Pharmacotherapy* (1998) 18, 1360–4.
4. Krauss GL, Brandt J, Campbell M, Plate C, Summerfield M. Antiepileptic medication and oral contraceptive interactions: a national survey of neurologists and obstetricians. *Neurology* (1996) 46, 1534–9.
5. Norplant (Levonorgestrel) Hoechst Marion Roussel Ltd. UK Summary of product characteristics, December 1997.
6. Implanon (Etonogestrel). Organon Laboratories Ltd. UK Summary of product characteristics, December 2004.

7. Depo-Provera (Medroxyprogesterone acetate). Pharmacia Ltd. UK Summary of product characteristics, November 2004.
8. Belfield T, ed. FPA Contraceptive Handbook: a guide for family planning and other health professionals. 3rd ed. London: Family Planning Association, 1999.
9. Noristerat (Norethisterone enantate), Schering Health Care Ltd. UK Summary of product characteristics, April 2004.

Tibolone + Enzyme-inducing drugs

On theoretical grounds the makers of tibolone say that the effects of tibolone may be reduced by enzyme-inducing anticonvulsants and rifampicin.

Clinical evidence, mechanism, importance and management

The makers say that on a theoretical basis enzyme-inducing drugs such as **barbiturates, phenytoin, carbamazepine** and **rifampicin** may accelerate the metabolism of tibolone and thus decrease its efficacy.[1] However, they note that no examples of these interactions have been reported in clinical practice. Nevertheless it would be prudent to monitor concurrent use. Pharmacokinetic studies are required. A list of enzyme-inducing drugs can be found in 'Table 26.1', (p.741)).

1. Livial (Tibolone). Organon Laboratories Ltd. UK Summary of product characteristics, December 2003.

27

Immunosuppressants

The immunosuppressants dealt with in this section include the corticosteroids, ciclosporin, muromonab-CD3, mycophenolate, sirolimus and tacrolimus. When any of these drugs acts as the interacting agent the relevant monograph is categorised in the section dealing with the drug whose effects are changed. A list of the drugs that are featured here appears in 'Table 27.1', (below).

Other drugs that are also used for immunosuppression (e.g. azathioprine and methotrexate) are found in the section on antineoplastic drugs.

Table 27.1 Immunosuppressant drugs

Generic names	*Proprietary names*
Basiliximab	Simulect
Ciclosporin (Cyclosporine)	Cermox, Ciclohexal, Cicloral, Cicloralhexal, Ciclosol, Consupren, Cysporin, Deximune, Equoral, Gengraf, Immulem, Immunosporin, Imusporin, Neoral, Neoral-Sandimmun, Panimun Bioral, Restasis, Sandimmun, Sandimmun Neoral, Sandimmune, Sangcya, Sigmasporin
Corticosteroids	
Budesonide	Aero-Bud, Aerovial, Aircort, Apulein, Aquacort, Astrocast, Benacort, Benosid, Bidien, Biosonide, Budamax, Budecol, Budecort, Budefarma, Budeflam, Budenase, Budenite, Budenofalk, Budes, Budesan, Budeson, Budiair, Budicort, Budo-san, Busonid, Butacort, Butekont, Clebudan, Cortinasal, Cortivent, Cuteral, Cycortide, Dedostryl, Demotest, Desonax, Despex, Dexalocal, Easi-Cort, Eltair, Entocir, Entocord, Entocort, Esonide, Giona, Hypersol B, Inflacor, Inflammide, Inflanaze, Ixor, Kerpet, Lydenal, Miflonid, Miflonide, Miflonil, Nasocort, Nastizol Hidrospray, Neo Rinactive, Neumotex, Novopulmon, Numark, Obecirol, Obusonid, Olfex, Olfosonide, Olyspal, Pimoftal, Preferid, Proetzonide, Pulmaxan, Pulmicort, Pulmictan, Pulmo Lisoflam, Pulmotide, Resata, Respicort, Rhinocort, Rhinocort, Rhinoside, Rhinosol, Ribujet, Rino-B, Sonidal, Sonidar, Spirocort, Tafen, Udesogel, Udesospray, Vericort, Vinecort
Deflazacort	Azacortid, Calcort, Cortax, Deflan, Deflanil, Denacen, Dezacor, Dezartal, Flamirex, Flantadin, Rosilan, Zamene
Dexamethasone	Aacidexam, Adrecort, Aeroseb-Dex, afpred-DEXA, Alin, B Dexol, Baycuten, Bexine, Clenil, Cortidex, Cortidexason, Cryometasona, Dalalone, Dalamon Inyectable, Decadron, Decadronal, Decadron, Decan, Decasone, Decaspray, Decdan, Decorex, Dectancyl, Deflaren, Degabina, Dermadex, Desocort, Dexa, Dexa ANB, Dexa Loscon mono, Dexa-Allvoran, Dexabene, Dexacip, dexa-clinit, Dexacollyre, Dexacortal, Dexacort, Dexacortin, Dexacortin-K, Dexadermil, DexaEDO, Dexa-Effekton, Dexafarm, Dexaflam, Dexaflan, Dexagalen, Dexagel, Dexagrin, Dexahexal, Dexalergin, Dexalocal, Dexalone, Dexaltin, Dexamed, Dexameral, Dexameson, Dexametonal, Dexaminor, Dexamonozon, Dexanil, Dexano, Dexa-POS, Dexa-ratiopharm, Dexa-Rhinospray Mono, Dexa-sine, Dexason, Dexasone, Dexaval, Dexazen, Dexazona, Dexicar, Dexmethsone, Dexon, Dexona, Dexone, DexPak, Dexsol, Dextasona, Dexthasol, Dexton, Dibasona, Duo Decadron, Etacortilen, Fadametasona, Fortecortin, Gotabiotic D, Hexadrol, Indarzona-N, Iriniozol, Isopto Dex, Isopto Maxidex, Kaarmepakkaus, Limethason, Lipotalon, Lormine, Luxazone, Maxidex, Megacort, Mephamesone, Metax, Methaderm, Millicortenol, Minidex, Neodex, Nexadron, Oftan Dexa, Opnol, Oradexon, Polideltaxin, Ronic, Sedesterol, Soldesam, Soldesanil, Solupen N, Solurex, Solutio Cordes Dexa N, Spersadex, Sterodex, Taprodex, Taxyl, Thilodexine, Thiloxedine, Topidexa, Totocortin, Trofinan, Uni Dexametason, Visumetazone, Wymesone
Fludrocortisone	Astonin, Astonin H, Astonin-H, Cortineff, Florinef, Florinefe, Lonikan
Fluticasone	Albeoler, Allegro, Asmatil, Asmo-Lavi, Atemur, Axotide, Beconase Allergy, Brexonase, Brexovent, Brisovent, Cutivat, Cutivate, Drolasona, Eustidil, Flixoderm, Flixonase, Flixonase, Flixotaide, Flixotide, Flixotide , Flixovate, Flohale, Flomist, Flonase, Flovent, Fluinol, Flusona, Flusonal, Fluspiral, Flutaide, Flutide, Flutinase, Flutivate, Inalacor, Nasofan, Potencort, Raffonin, Rinosone, Rontilona, Seretide, Ticavent, Trialona, Ubizol, Zoflut

Continued

Table 27.1 Immunosuppressant drugs *(continued)*

Generic names	*Proprietary names*
Hydrocortisone	Acticort, Actocortina, Aftasone, A-Hydrocort, Ala-Cort, Alcortin, Alfacort, Alfacortone, Alfason, Anucort-HC, Anusol-HC, Aphilan, Apocort, Aquanil HC, Bactine, Barriere-HC, Berlison, Buccalsone, Bucort, CaldeCort, Calmicort, Calmurid, Carmol HC, Ceneo, Cetacort, Cipcorlin, Claritin Skin Itch Relief, Colifoam, Colofoam, Corlan, Cortacet, Cortaid, Cortapaisyl, Cortate, Cort-Dome, Cortef, Cortef Feminine Itch, Cortenem, Cortenema, Corticaine, Cortic, Cortidro, Cortifoam, Cortisedermyl, Cortisonal, Cortiston, Cortizone, Cortoderm, Cortop, Cortopin, Cortril, Cortropin, Covocort, Cremicort-H, Cutaderm, Cutisoft, Dermacort, Derm-Aid, Dermallerg, Dermarest Dri-Cort, Dermarest Dricort Anti-Itch, Dermaspraid Demangeaison, Dermimade Hidrocortisona, Dermirit, Dermo Posterisan, Dermocortal, Dermofenac, Dermol HC, Dermolate, Dermosa Hidrocortisona, Dhacort, Dilucort, Dioderm, DP Hydrocortisone, EarSol-HC, Ebenol, Efcortelan, Efcortesol, Efficort, Egocort, Ekzemsalbe F, Emo-Cort, Entofoam, Exe-Cort, Fadol, Fenistil, Ficortril, Filocot, Flebocortid, Foille Insetti, Fridalit, Gynecort, Hc45, Hemodren , Hemorrane, Hemril-HC, Hi-Cor, Hidalone, Hidroaltesona, Hidrocisdin, Hidrotisona, Hidyn H, Hipoge, Hycor, Hycort, Hycortin, Hyderm, Hydoftal sine neomycino, Hydracort, Hydrocort, Hydrocortistab, Hydrocortisyl, Hydrocortone, Hydrocutan, Hydrocutan mild, Hydroderm HC, Hydroderm, Hydrogalen, HydroSkin, Hydrosone, HydroVal, Hydro-Wolff, Hysone, Hytisone, Hytone, Idracemi, Isdinium, Kyypakkaus, Lacticare-HC, Lactisona, Lanacort, Laticort, Lemnis Fatty Cream HC, Lenirit, Locoid, Locoid Crelo, Locoidon, Lyo-Cortin, Massengill Medicated, Medrocil, Microsona, Mildison, Mitocortyl, Munitren H, Mylocort, Neutrogena T/Scalp, Nositrol, Novo-Hydrocort, Nutracort, Nutralona, Orabase HCA, Oralsone, Pandel, Pandermil, Penecort, Posterisan cort, Prevex HC, Procort, Proctocort, Proctocream HC 2.5%, Procutan, Recort Plus, Remederm HC, Retef, Rolak, Sanadermil, Sanatison Mono, Sarna HC, Scalpicin Capilar, Schericur, Sigmacort, Siguent Hycor, Sintotrat, Sirotamicin HC, Skincalm, Solu-Cortef, Soventol HC, Stiefcortil, Stopitch, Suniderma, Synacort, Systral Hydrocort, Tegrin-HC, Texacort, Transderma H, U-Cort, Uniderm, velopural, Vitulpas, Westcort, Wycort, Zenoxone
Methylprednisolone	Advantan, Adventan, Alergolon, A-Methapred, Asmacortone, Avancort, Cipridanol, Corticel, Cortisolona, Cryosolona, depMedalone, Depo Moderin, Depo-Medrate, Depo-Medrol, Depo-Medrone, Depo-Nisolone, Depopred, Lexxema, Lyo-drol, Medrate, Medrol, Medrone, Metilbetasone Solubile, Metilpren, Metypred, Metypresol, Metysolon, M-PredniHexal, Predmetil, Predni M, Prednilem, Radilem, Solomet, Solu-Medrol, Solu-Medrone, Solu-Moderin, Supresol, Urbason, Vanderm
Prednisolone	Adelcort, Adelone, Ak-Pred, Aprednislon, Capsoid, Cortizul, Dacortin H, Decortin H, Delta-Cortef, Deltacortril, Deltastab, Dermosolon, Dhasolone, Di-Adreson-F, Dontisolon D, duraprednisolon, Econopred, Estilsona, Farnerate, Farnezone, Fisopred, Frisolona, Gupisone, hefasolon, Hexacortone, Hydrocortancyl, Infectocortikrupp, Inflamase, Inflanefran, Inf-Oph, Key-Pred, Key-Pred-SP, Klismacort, Lenisolone, Lepicortinolo, Linola-H N, Linola-H-Fett N, Lygal Kopftinktur N, Meticortelone, Opredsone, Orapred, Panafcortelone, Pediapred, Polypred, Precortalon aquosum, Precortisyl, Prectal, Pred, Pred Fort, Pred Forte, Pred Mild, Pred Mild , Pred-Clysma, Predcor, Predenema, Predfoam, Predmix, Prednabene, Prednefrin SF, Prednersone, Prednesol, Predni, Predni H, Prednigalen, Prednihexal, Predniocil, Predni-Ophtal, Predni-POS, Prednisil, Prednisol, Prednisolut, Predone, Pred-Phosphate, Predsim, Predsol, Predsolets, Predsolone, Preflam, Prelone, Preventan, Prezolon, Rectodelt, Rectopred, Redipred, SAB-Prednase, Sintisone, Solone, Solu-Dacortin, Solu-Dacortina, Solu-Dacortine, Solu-Decortin H, Solu-Decortin-H, Solupred, Sophipren, Spiricort, Sterofrin, Ultracortene H, Ultracortenol, Ultracortenol, Walesolone, Wysolone
Prednisone	Artinizona, Bersen, Cortancyl, Corticorten, Cortiprex, Dacortin, Decortin, Deltacortene, Deltasone, Deltison, Liquid Pred, Meprosona-F, Meticorten, Nosipren, Ofisolona, Panafcort, Panasol-S, Precortil, Predeltin, Predicor, Predicorten, Predni Tablinen, Prednidib, Prednipirine, Predsone, Predval, Premagnol, Prenisonal, Procion, Pulmison, Rectodelt, Sone, Sterapred, Winpred
Daclizumab	Zenapax
Everolimus	Certican
Leflunomide	Arabloc, Arava, Filartros, Inmunoartro, Lara, Molagar
Muromonab-CD3	Cedetrin-T, Ior T3, Orthoclone, Orthoclone OKT3
Mycophenolate mofetil	CellCept, Cellmune, Mycept, Myfortic
Rituximab	Mabthera, Rituxan
Sirolimus	Rapamune
Tacrolimus	Mustopic, PanGraf, Prograf, Prograft, Protopic, Tacroz

Basiliximab + Miscellaneous

The concurrent use of basiliximab with azathioprine, muromonab-CD3 or mycophenolate is not associated with an increase in adverse effects or infections. The dose requirements of ciclosporin or tacrolimus may be altered by basiliximab. Basiliximab is reported not to interact with analgesics, anti-infective drugs, diuretics, beta-blockers or calcium channel blockers.

Clinical evidence, mechanism, importance and management

(a) Azathioprine

The total body clearance of basiliximab was reduced by 22% when azathioprine was added to regimens also including ciclosporin for microemulsion and corticosteroids. However, the use of basiliximab in triple regimens with azathioprine did not increase adverse effects or infections.[1]

(b) Ciclosporin

A study in 39 paediatric renal transplant patients taking ciclosporin found that in 24 patients, who also received basiliximab 10 or 20 mg on days 0 and 4 after transplantation, lower doses of ciclosporin resulted in significantly higher trough levels, and some evidence of early ciclosporin toxicity within the first 10 days. At days 28 to 50 ciclosporin levels declined and 20% higher doses were required to maintain adequate trough levels in the basiliximab group.[2] Another study in 54 paediatric liver transplant patients found that the addition of basiliximab to ciclosporin and corticosteroids did not significantly alter the overall ciclosporin dose requirements. However, 9 basiliximab-treated patients experienced acute rejection at 21 to 28 days after transplantation, and this was associated with low ciclosporin trough levels requiring increased ciclosporin dosage in 6 of the 9 patients.[3] It was considered that the effect on ciclosporin was due to an interleukin-2 receptor mediated alteration of the cytochrome P450 enzyme system.[2] This was considered to only play a minor role in the liver-transplant patients because of significantly lower target trough levels in these patients.[3] However, a further study found no increase in rejection episodes between days 28 to 50 in kidney-transplant patients treated with basiliximab and ciclosporin.[4]

The authors of the first study[2] recommend that the initial dose of ciclosporin should be limited to 400 mg/m^2 in children receiving renal transplants who are also treated with basiliximab. Dose reductions were not considered necessary by other authors, but close monitoring was recommended.[3,4]

(c) Muromonab-CD3

The makers of basiliximab say that patients in phase 3 studies received basiliximab with muromonab-CD3 for episodes of rejection with no increase in adverse events or infections. Human antimurine antibody responses were reported in 2 of 138 patients receiving basiliximab and 4 of 34 patients receiving basiliximab and muromonab-CD3 concurrently. Therefore, the makers say that if basiliximab has been given, muromonab-CD3 or other murine antilymphocytic antibody preparations can still subsequently be given.[1]

(d) Mycophenolate

Total body clearance of basiliximab was reduced by 51% when azathioprine was added to regimens also including ciclosporin for microemulsion and corticosteroids (see above). However, the use of basiliximab in triple regimens with mycophenolate did not increase adverse effects or infections.[1]

(e) Other drugs

The makers report that basiliximab has been used with **analgesics**, **antibacterials**, **antifungals**, **antivirals**, **diuretics, beta-blockers** and **calcium channel blockers** without any increase in adverse reactions. None of the drugs was individually named.[1]

(f) Tacrolimus

A study in 12 adult renal-transplant patients found that trough tacrolimus levels on day 3 were increased by 63% in patients also treated with basiliximab and in 50% of these patients this was associated with the development of acute tubular necrosis. By day 30, tacrolimus trough levels showed a downward trend in the basiliximab treated group, despite similar dose requirements to those on day 10. Tacrolimus dose requirements were lower in the basiliximab group compared to the control group throughout the 60-day study period.[5] Dose reductions were not considered necessary by the authors, but close monitoring was recommended.[5]

1. Simulect (Basiliximab). Novartis Pharmaceuticals UK Ltd. UK Summary of product characteristics, May 2003.
2. Strehlau J, Pape L, Offner G, Bjoern N, Ehrich JHH. Interleukin-2 receptor antibody-induced alterations of ciclosporin dose requirements in paediatric transplant patients. *Lancet* (2000) 356, 1327–8.
3. Ganschow R, Grabhorn E, Burdelski M. Basiliximab in paediatric liver-transplant recipients. *Lancet* (2001) 357, 388.
4. Vester U, Kranz B, Treichel U, Hoyer PF. Basiliximab in paediatric liver-transplant recipients. *Lancet* (2001) 357, 388–9.
5. Sifontis NM, Benedetti E, Vasquez EM. A clinically significant drug interaction between basiliximab and tacrolimus in renal transplant recipients. *Pharmacotherapy* (2001) 10, 1297.

Ciclosporin + ACE inhibitors

Acute renal failure developed in four kidney transplant patients on ciclosporin when they were given enalapril. Oliguria was seen in another patient on ciclosporin given captopril.

Clinical evidence

Two kidney transplant patients on ciclosporin developed acute renal failure 10 to 42 days after starting to take **enalapril** 5 to 10 mg twice daily. Recovery was complete when the **enalapril** was stopped in one of the patients, and when both **enalapril** and ciclosporin were stopped in the other. The latter patient had no problems when the ciclosporin was restarted. Both recovered renal function after 10 to 30 days. Neither had any previous evidence of renal artery stenosis or chronic rejection, which are conditions known to predispose to renal failure during ACE inhibitor treatment. Two other patients appeared to tolerate concurrent use well.[1] Two further kidney transplant patients developed acute renal failure when given **enalapril**. Neither had renal arterial stenosis or acute rejection.[2] The maker briefly mentions that transient oliguria was seen in a kidney transplant patient given ciclosporin and **captopril**.[3]

Mechanism

Not understood. One suggestion is that ciclosporin reduces renal blood flow and reduces perfusion through the glomerulus, which is worsened when angiotensin II is inhibited by the ACE inhibitor.[1]

Importance and management

Information is very limited indeed. The incidence of this interaction would appear to be low, nevertheless care and good monitoring are needed if captopril or enalapril and ciclosporin are used concurrently. More study is needed. Information about other ACE inhibitors is lacking but if the suggested mechanism is true, they too may possibly interact similarly. Also note that the makers of ciclosporin warn about the possible risk of hyperkalaemia with ACE inhibitors and ciclosporin as both drugs may raise potassium levels.[4] Monitor potassium levels more closely in the initial weeks of concurrent use.

1. Murray BM, Venuto RC, Kohli R, Cunningham EE. Enalapril-associated renal failure in renal transplants: possible role of cyclosporine. *Am J Kidney Dis* (1990) 16, 66–9.
2. Garcia TM, da Costa JA, Costa RS, Ferraz AS. Acute tubular renal necrosis in kidney transplant patients treated with enalapril. *Ren Fail* (1994) 16, 419–23.
3. Cockburn I. Cyclosporine A: a clinical evaluation of drug interactions. *Transplant Proc* (1986) 18 (Suppl 5), 50–5.
4. Neoral (Ciclosporin). Novartis Pharmaceuticals UK Ltd. UK Summary of product characteristics, December 2004.

Ciclosporin + Acetazolamide

There is some limited evidence that acetazolamide can cause a marked and rapid rise in ciclosporin serum levels, possibly accompanied by renal toxicity.

Clinical evidence, mechanism, importance and management

A study in 3 men found that 72 hours after they started acetazolamide [dose not stated] their trough serum ciclosporin levels rose more than six-fold, from a range of 54 to 270 nanograms/ml up to 517 to 1827 nanograms/ml.[1] Another man with a heart transplant had a fivefold increase in his serum ciclosporin levels, marked renal impairment and neurotoxicity when he was given oral acetazolamide for raised intra-ocular pressure secondary to panuveitis.[2] The increase in ciclosporin serum levels has also been seen in *animal* studies.[3]

Information seems to be limited to these reports but it seems that the concurrent use of ciclosporin and acetazolamide should be closely monitored, being alert of the need to reduce the ciclosporin dosage. The interaction can apparently develop very rapidly.

1. Tabbara KF, Al-Faisal Z, Al-Rashed W. Interaction between acetazolamide and cyclosporine. *Arch Ophthalmol* (1998) 116, 832–3.
2. Keogh A, Esmore D, Spratt P, Savdie E, McClusky P, Chang V. Acetazolamide and cyclosporine. *Transplantation* (1988) 46, 478–9.
3. El-Sayed YM, Tabbara KF, Gouda MW. Effect of acetazolamide on the pharmacokinetics of cyclosporine in rabbits. *Int J Pharmaceutics* (1995) 121, 181–6.

Ciclosporin + Aciclovir

Aciclovir does not normally seem to affect ciclosporin serum levels nor worsen renal function, but a very small number of cases of nephrotoxicity and increased serum ciclosporin levels have been seen following concurrent use.

Clinical evidence

(a) No interaction

A retrospective study of 21 kidney transplant patients on ciclosporin (serum levels in the range 100 to 250 nanograms/ml) found that oral aciclovir 800 mg four times daily for 3 months, given to 12 of them had no significant effect on their ciclosporin serum levels or on nephrotoxicity when compared with the 9 control subjects.[1]

No significant changes in renal function were seen in 11 patients on ciclosporin when they were given intravenous aciclovir 750 to 1500 mg/m^2 daily for at least 7 days to treat herpes infections.[2]

No significant changes in serum creatinine or ciclosporin levels were seen during the 14 days following kidney transplant in 17 patients given aciclovir 800 mg daily.[3] Fifty-three kidney transplant patients were given ciclosporin and aciclovir 800 to 3200 mg daily for 12 weeks. The aciclovir was withdrawn from 2 patients because of unexplained and temporary increases in serum creatinine levels. The serum ciclosporin levels were not reported.[4] Five patients (2 adults and 3 children) on ciclosporin, prednisone and azathioprine were given aciclovir 200 mg five times daily for 6 days for herpes zoster or chicken pox. Ciclosporin serum levels remained unchanged and renal function improved.[5]

(b) Toxicity

In contrast to the cases cited above, 3 of 7 bone marrow transplant patients given ciclosporin and intravenous aciclovir 500 mg/m^2 every 8 or 12 hours (depending on renal function) developed nephrotoxicity, which was fatal in one case. Histological evidence suggested ciclosporin nephrotoxicity.[6] The maker briefly notes that an increase in serum creatinine was seen in ciclosporin recipients in one report, and increased aciclovir levels accompanied by reversible acute tubular necrosis in another.[7] Yet another report describes a threefold increase in ciclosporin serum levels in a child with a heart transplant after starting intravenous aciclovir.[8]

Mechanism

Not understood, although both drugs are known to be nephrotoxic, all be it rarely in the case of aciclovir.

Importance and management

Well documented. The evidence available indicates that ciclosporin levels and renal function are usually unaltered by the concurrent use of aciclovir, but the handful of cases where problems have arisen clearly indicate that renal function should be well monitored. One group of workers recommends giving aciclovir 250 mg/m^2 given by slow infusion to well hydrated patients, with careful monitoring of serum ciclosporin levels.[2]

1. Dugandzic RM, Sketris IS, Belitsky P, Schlech WF, Givner ML. Effect of coadministration of acyclovir and cyclosporine on kidney function and cyclosporine concentrations in renal transplant patients. *DICP Ann Pharmacother* (1991) 25, 316–7.
2. Johnson PC, Kumor K, Welsh MS, Woo J, Kahan BD. Effects of coadministration of cyclosporine and acyclovir on renal function of renal allograft recipients. *Transplantation* (1987) 44, 329–31.
3. Stoffel M, Squifflet JP, Pirson Y, Lamy M, Alexandre GPJ. Effectiveness of oral acyclovir prophylaxis in renal transplant recipients. *Transplant Proc* (1987) 19, 2190–3.
4. Balfour HH, Chace BA, Stapleton JT, Simmons RL, Fryd DS. A randomized, placebo-controlled trial of oral acyclovir for the prevention of cytomegalovirus disease in recipients of renal allografts. *N Engl J Med* (1989) 320, 1381–7.
5. Hayes K, Shakuntala V, Pingle A, Dhawan IK, Masri MA. Safe use of acyclovir (Zovirax) in renal transplant patients on cyclosporine A therapy: case reports. *Transplant Proc* (1992) 24, 1926.
6. Shepp DH, Dandliker PS, Meyers JD. Treatment of varicella-zoster virus infection in severely immunocompromised patients: a randomized comparison of acyclovir and vidarabine. *N Engl J Med* (1986) 314, 208–12.
7. Cockburn I. Cyclosporine A: a clinical evaluation of drug interactions. *Transplant Proc* (1986) 18 (Suppl 5), 50–5.
8. Boardman M, Yodur Purdy C. Cyclosporine and aciclovir; report of a drug interaction. Am Soc Hosp Pharmacists Midyear Clinical Meeting, Dallas, Texas. December 1988, Abstract SP-16.

Ciclosporin + Alcohol

An isolated report describes a marked increase in serum ciclosporin levels in a patient after an episode of binge-drinking, but a subsequent study found that moderate single doses of alcohol in other patients had no such effect. Ciclosporin did not affect alcohol levels in *animals*.

Clinical evidence, mechanism, importance and management

The serum ciclosporin levels of a kidney transplant patient doubled, from 101 to 205 nanograms/ml, and remained high for about 4 days after he went on a two-day alcohol binge. A subsequent study in 8 other patients with kidney transplants found no changes in serum ciclosporin or creatinine levels when they drank 50 ml of 100% alcohol in orange juice (about equivalent to 4 oz of **whisky**).[1]

A study in *animals* found that pretreatment with oral ciclosporin had no effect on the pharmacokinetics of alcohol or acetaldehyde. This suggests that any difference in the alcohol consumption of patients on ciclosporin is unlikely to have a pharmacokinetic basis.[2]

The authors of the first study[1] say that they currently advise their renal transplant patients to avoid heavy drinking, but that an occasional drink probably does not affect ciclosporin levels.[1] See also 'Ciclosporin + Food or Drinks', p.790 for a report that red wine reduces ciclosporin levels.

1. Paul MD, Parfrey PS, Smart M, Gault H. The effect of ethanol on serum cyclosporine A levels in renal transplant patients. *Am J Kidney Dis* (1987) 10, 133–5.
2. Giles HG, Orrego H, Sandrin S, Saldivia V. The influence of cyclosporine on abstinence from alcohol in transplant patients. *Transplantation* (1990) 49, 1201–2.

Ciclosporin + Allopurinol

Isolated cases of markedly raised ciclosporin levels have been reported in patients given allopurinol.

Clinical evidence and mechanism

The ciclosporin levels of a kidney transplant patient rose by about threefold, accompanied by an increase in serum creatinine from 124 to 194 micromol/l, after allopurinol 100 mg daily was taken for 12 days.[1] Another previously stable kidney transplant patient had a two- to threefold rise in ciclosporin level when given allopurinol 200 mg daily. Her serum creatinine remained unchanged throughout.[2]

A clinical study describes a reduction in the frequency of acute kidney transplant rejections in 12 patients given ciclosporin, prednisolone and azathioprine and low dose allopurinol (25 mg on alternate days) after transplantation, compared with 15 control patients on triple therapy alone. Ciclosporin doses were adjusted to maintain levels of 100 micromol/l, and no mention was made as to whether the dose differed between the two groups.[3]

The general importance of these two reports of increased ciclosporin levels is unknown. They are probably insufficient to recommend increased monitoring of ciclosporin levels in all patients given allopurinol, but bear them in mind in the event of an unexpected response to treatment.

1. Stevens SL, Goldman MH. Cyclosporine toxicity associated with allopurinol. *South Med J* (1992) 85, 1265–6.
2. Gorrie M, Beaman M, Nicholls A, Backwell P. Allopurinol interaction with cyclosporine. *BMJ* (1994) 308, 113.
3. Chocair P, Duley J, Simmonds HA, Cameron JS, Ianhez L, Arap S, Sabbaga E. Low-dose allopurinol plus azathioprine/cyclosporin/prednisolone, a novel immunosuppressive regimen. *Lancet* (1993) 342, 83–4.

Ciclosporin + Amiodarone

Ciclosporin serum levels can be increased by amiodarone and nephrotoxicity has occurred as a result.

Clinical evidence

Eight patients with heart transplants and 3 with heart-lung transplants on ciclosporin were also given amiodarone for atrial flutter or fibrillation. Despite a 13 to 14% reduction in the ciclosporin dosage, their serum levels rose by 9%, serum creatinine levels rose by 38% (from 157 to 216 micromol/l), and blood urea nitrogen rose by 30%.[1] In another report by some of the same authors, one patient is said to have shown a 50% decrease in the clearance of ciclosporin when given amiodarone.[2] Eight other patients with heart or heart-lung transplants were effectively treated with amiodarone for atrial flutter and/or atrial fibrillation, but they had a 31% rise in serum ciclosporin levels, from 248 to 325 nanograms/ml despite a 44% reduction in the ciclosporin dosage (from 6.2 to 3.5 mg/kg daily). Serum creatinine levels rose by 39%.[3] A kidney transplant patient's serum ciclosporin levels doubled when amiodarone was given.[4] In 5 heart transplant patients amiodarone was discontinued and ciclosporin initiated, but the metabolism of ciclosporin was increased for 4 to 5 weeks (total plasma metabolites increased from 720 to 1437 nanograms/ml) and there was also an increase in the plasma concentration of amiodarone and its main metabolite, desethylamiodarone. During this period increased adverse effects, including pulmonary toxicity, were observed.[5]

Mechanism

Uncertain. A reduction[2] or an increase[5] in the metabolism of the ciclosporin by the amiodarone has been suggested. An interaction between amiodarone and phospholipids in the plasma membrane may inhibit transport processes. Blocking of the multi-drug resistance protein in the intestinal mucosa and liver by both amiodarone and ciclosporin may result in decreased excretion and increased toxicity of amiodarone as well as accumulation of ciclosporin metabolites.[5]

Importance and management

An established and clinically important interaction. Concurrent use need not be avoided but close monitoring and ciclosporin dosage reductions are needed to minimise the potential nephrotoxicity. Remember to re-adjust the dosage if the amiodarone is stopped, bearing in mind that it may take weeks before the amiodarone is totally cleared from the body.

1. Egami J, Mullins PA, Mamprin F, Chauhan A, Large SR, Wallwork J, Schofield PM. Increase in cyclosporine levels due to amiodarone therapy after heart and heart-lung transplantation. *J Am Coll Cardiol* (1993) 21, 141A.
2. Nicolau DP, Uber WE, Crumbley AJ, Strange C. Amiodarone-cyclosporine interaction in a heart transplant patient. *J Heart Lung Transplant* (1992) 11, 564–8.
3. Mamprin F, Mullins P, Graham T, Kendall S, Biocine B, Large S, Wallwork J, Schofield P. Amiodarone-cyclosporine interaction in cardiac transplantation. *Am Heart J* (1992) 123, 1725–6.
4. Chitwood KK, Abdul-Haqq AJ, Heim-Duthoy KL. Cyclosporine-amiodarone interaction. *Ann Pharmacother* (1993) 27, 569–71.
5. Preuner JG, Lehle K, Keyser A, Merk J, Rupprecht L, Goebels R. Development of severe adverse effects after discontinuing amiodarone therapy in human heart transplant recipients. *Transplant Proc* (1998) 30, 3943–4.

Ciclosporin + Amphotericin B

There is some good evidence that the risk of nephrotoxicity is increased if ciclosporin and amphotericin B are used concurrently. However, other evidence suggests that liposomal amphotericin B (*AmBisome*) does not increase nephrotoxicity or hepatotoxicity when given to infants taking ciclosporin.

Clinical evidence

(a) Evidence of toxicity

The concurrent use of ciclosporin and amphotericin B increased the incidence of nephrotoxicity in 47 patients with bone marrow transplants. Out of 10 patients who had received both drugs, 5 doubled and 3 tripled their serum creatinine levels within 5 days. In contrast only 8 out of 21 (38%) on ciclosporin alone and 3 out of 16 (19%) on methotrexate and amphotericin B doubled their serum creatinine within 14 to 30 and 5 days respectively.[1]

A study of the risk factors associated with amphotericin B identified the concurrent use of ciclosporin as posing a particularly significant risk for severe nephrotoxicity.[2] Two other studies in bone marrow transplant patients on ciclosporin found that amphotericin B contributed significantly to nephrotoxicity and renal failure.[3,4] It can apparently develop even after the amphotericin has been withdrawn.[3] Marked nephrotoxicity is described in one patient in another report.[5]

An isolated case report described severe tremors, later becoming myoclonic, attributed to the concurrent use of liposomal amphotericin B (*AmBisome*) and ciclosporin. Serum ciclosporin levels were unaltered and creatinine levels only rose slightly.[6] This alleged neurotoxicity was challenged in a letter citing 187 transplant patients on ciclosporin and *AmBisome*, none of whom developed neurotoxicity attributable to an interaction.[7]

(b) Evidence of no toxicity

A study including 8 severely ill infants undergoing bone marrow transplantation for severe immunodeficiency, found no evidence of significant nephrotoxicity or hepatotoxicity when liposomal amphotericin B (*AmBisome*) was given with ciclosporin. The average course of treatment lasted 29 days.[8]

Mechanism

Not understood. Simple additive nephrotoxicity is a likely explanation.

Importance and management

The increased nephrotoxicity associated with ciclosporin and amphotericin B appears to be established and clinically important. The authors of one report[1] say that "if amphotericin must be given, withholding ciclosporin until the serum level is less than about 150 nanograms/ml may be a means of decreasing renal toxicity without losing the immunosuppressive effect."

The reports supporting a lack of significant nephrotoxicity all used liposomal amphotericin, a formulation that is recommended when amphotericin toxicity (particularly nephrotoxicity) is considered to be a significant risk. This would seem to suggest that, in patients on ciclosporin, the less nephrotoxic forms of amphotericin are advisable.

1. Kennedy MS, Deeg HJ, Siegel M, Crowley JJ, Storb R, Thomas ED. Acute renal toxicity with combined use of amphotericin B and cyclosporine after bone marrow transplantation. *Transplantation* (1983) 35, 211–15.
2. Guglielmo BJ, Maa L, Luber AD, Lam M. Risk factors for amphotericin B- induced nephrotoxicity. *Intersci Conf Antimicrob Agents Chemother* (1997) 37, 19.
3. Tutschka PJ, Beschorner WE, Hess AD, Santos GW. Cyclosporin-A to prevent graft-versus-host-disease: a pilot study in 22 patients receiving allogeneic marrow transplants. *Blood* (1983) 61, 318–25.
4. Miller KB, Schenkein DP, Comenzo R, Erban JK, Fogaren T, Hirsch CA, Berkman E, Rabson A. Adjusted-dose continuous-infusion cyclosporin A to prevent graft-versus-host disease following allogeneic bone marrow transplantation. *Ann Hematol* (1994) 68, 15–20.
5. Conti DJ, Tolkoff-Rubin NE, Baker GP, Doran M, Cosimi AB, Delmonico F, Auchincloss H, Russell PS, Rubin RH. Successful treatment of invasive fungal infection with fluconazole in organ transplant recipients. *Transplantation* (1989) 48, 692–5.
6. Ellis ME, Spence D, Ernst P, Meunier F. Is cyclosporin neurotoxicity enhanced in the presence of liposomal amphotericin B? *J Infect* (1994) 29, 106–7.
7. Ringdén O, Andström EE, Remberger M, Svahn B-M, Tollemar J. No increase in cyclosporin neurotoxicity in transplant recipients treated with liposomal amphotericin B. *Infection* (1996) 24, 269.
8. Pasic S, Flannagan L, Cant AJ. Liposomal amphotericin (AmBisome) is safe in bone marrow transplantation for primary immunodeficiency. *Bone Marrow Transplant* (1997) 19, 1229–32.

Ciclosporin + Androgens and Anabolic steroids

Raised ciclosporin levels occurred in two patients given methyltestosterone. Hepatotoxicity has been seen in three patients given ciclosporin and norethandrolone.

Clinical evidence

(a) Methyltestosterone

A man with a kidney transplant who had been stable on ciclosporin, prednisolone and azathioprine for 23 months was given methyltestosterone 5 mg three times daily for impotence. After 4 weeks he developed anorexia and pruritus. He was found to have a raised bilirubin level and his ciclosporin level had risen from 70 to 252 nanograms/ml with an accompanying decrease in his renal function. The methyltestosterone was withdrawn and he was later restabilised on ciclosporin.[1] Another case describes abnormally high ciclosporin levels (in excess of

2000 nanograms/ml) when a patient on methyltestosterone was started on ciclosporin 15 mg/kg daily.[2]

(b) Norethandrolone

Three out of four patients with bone marrow aplasia treated with ciclosporin and prednisone developed liver toxicity. It developed in 2 of them when norethandrolone was added. No toxicity occurred when they were given either of the drugs alone.[3] Jaundice associated with toxic hepatitis that occurred in a 14-year-old girl during the post-transplant period was attributed to the concurrent use of ciclosporin and norethandrolone.[4]

Mechanism

Uncertain. In the first case, the increase in ciclosporin levels were attributed to cholestatic jaundice brought on by the methyltestosterone.[2] Both norethandrolone and ciclosporin are known to be hepatotoxic, so additive hepatotoxicity may occur.

Importance and management

Information is limited. However, it would seem prudent to avoid the use of androgens or anabolic steroids in patients on ciclosporin wherever possible. If no alternative is available it may be prudent to increase the frequency of liver function monitoring.

1. Møller BB, Ekelund B. Toxicity of cyclosporine during treatment with androgens. *N Engl J Med* (1985) 313, 1416.
2. Goffin E, Pirson Y, Geubel A, van Ypersele de Strihou C. Cyclosporine-methyltestosterone interaction. *Nephron* (1991) 59, 174–5.
3. Sahnoun Z, Frikha M, Zeghal KM, Souissi T. Toxicité hépatique de la ciclosporine et interaction médicamenteuse avec les androgènes. *Sem Hop Paris* (1993) 69, 26–8.
4. Vinot O, Cochat P, Dubourg-Derain L, Bouvier R, Vial T, Philippe N. Jaundice associated with concomitant use of norethandrolone and cyclosporine. *Transplantation* (1993) 56, 470–1.

Ciclosporin + Antibacterials; Aminoglycosides

Both *animal* and human studies indicate that nephrotoxicity may be increased by the concurrent use of ciclosporin and gentamicin. This has also been shown for tobramycin. Cases of renal impairment have been reported for amikacin and gentamicin.

Clinical evidence

A comparative study in patients given **gentamicin** 30 mg with lincomycin just before renal transplantation found that the concurrent use of ciclosporin increased the incidence of nephrotoxicity from 5 to 67%.[1] When ampicillin, ceftazidime and lincomycin were used instead of **gentamicin** the incidence of nephrotoxicity was 10%.[1] Another study describes increased nephrotoxicity associated with the concurrent use of ciclosporin and **tobramycin** in bone marrow transplant recipients.[2,3] The interaction between ciclosporin and **gentamicin** has also been well demonstrated in *animals*.[4,5] One case report describes reversible acute worsening of renal function in a renal transplant patient on ciclosporin given **gentamicin**,[6] and another case report describes impaired renal function in a heart transplant patient on ciclosporin given **amikacin**.[7]

In contrast, a retrospective analysis of the medical records of bone marrow transplant patients suggested that aminoglycosides can be safely given with a continuous infusion of ciclosporin without excessive nephrotoxicity, if the patient is carefully monitored.[8]

Mechanism

Uncertain. Since both ciclosporin and the aminoglycosides can individually be nephrotoxic, it seems that their toxicities can be additive.

Importance and management

Established and clinically important interactions. The concurrent use of ciclosporin and aminoglycosides should be avoided where possible, and only undertaken with care and very close monitoring.

1. Termeer A, Hoitsma AJ, Koene RAP. Severe nephrotoxicity caused by the combined use of gentamicin and cyclosporine in renal allograft recipients. *Transplantation* (1986) 42, 220–1.
2. Hows JM, Chipping PM, Fairhead S, Smith J, Baughan A, Gordon-Smith EC. Nephrotoxicity in bone marrow transplant recipients treated with cyclosporin A. *Br J Haematol* (1983) 54, 69–78.
3. Hows JM, Palmer S, Want S, Dearden C, Gordon-Smith EC. Serum levels of cyclosporin A and nephrotoxicity in bone marrow transplant patients. *Lancet* (1981) ii, 145–6.
4. Whiting PH, Simpson JG. The enhancement of cyclosporin A-induced nephrotoxicity by gentamicin. *Biochem Pharmacol* (1983) 32, 2025–8.
5. Ryffel B, Müller AM, Mihatsch MJ. Experimental cyclosporine nephrotoxicity: risk of concomitant chemotherapy. *Clin Nephrol* (1986) 25 (Suppl 1), S121–S125.
6. Morales JM, Andres A, Prieto C, Diaz Rolòn JA, Rodicio JL. Reversible acute renal toxicity by toxic sinergic effect between gentamicin and cyclosporine. *Clin Nephrol* (1988) 29, 272.
7. Thaler F, Gotainer B, Teodori G, Dubois C, Loirat Ph. Mediastinitis due to *Nocardia asteroides* after cardiac transplantation. *Intensive Care Med* (1992) 18, 127–8.
8. Chandrasekar PH, Cronin SM. Nephrotoxicity in bone marrow transplant recipients receiving aminoglycoside plus cyclosporine or aminoglycoside alone. *J Antimicrob Chemother* (1991) 27, 845–9.

Ciclosporin + Antibacterials; Aztreonam

Aztreonam appears not to alter ciclosporin levels.

Clinical evidence, mechanism, importance and management

A study in 20 kidney transplant patients on ciclosporin found that when aztreonam was added for the treatment of various infections the ciclosporin serum levels were not significantly changed. The ciclosporin serum levels before, during and after aztreonam treatment were 517, 534 and 592 nanograms/ml respectively.[1] On the basis of this study there would seem to be no need to take special precautions if ciclosporin and aztreonam are used concurrently.

1. Alonso Hernandez A. Effects of aztreonam on cyclosporine levels in kidney transplant patients. *Transplantology J Cell Organ Transplant* (1993) 4, 85–6.

Ciclosporin + Antibacterials; Cephalosporins

Isolated reports suggest that ceftazidime, ceftriaxone, and latamoxef may increase ciclosporin levels, whereas one report suggested ceftazidime, ceftriaxone, and cefuroxime did not, although ceftazidime caused deterioration in some measures of renal function.

Clinical evidence, mechanism, importance and management

Two kidney transplant patients had two- to fourfold rises in ciclosporin levels within 2 to 3 days of starting **ceftriaxone** 1 g twice daily. Levels fell when the antibacterial was stopped. The reason is uncertain but it was suggested that **ceftriaxone** possibly inhibits the metabolism of ciclosporin by the liver.[1] However, a report of 51 kidney transplant patients stated that **ceftriaxone** and **cefuroxime** had no effect on ciclosporin serum levels and also that they were not nephrotoxic. This report also stated that **ceftazidime** did not affect serum ciclosporin levels but it increased blood urea nitrogen and creatinine levels, indicating that it was nephrotoxic.[2] A report by the maker briefly mentions that **ceftazidime** and **latamoxef** have also been implicated in an increase in serum ciclosporin levels.[3]

Information about these cephalosporins is very limited indeed. The general relevance of these reports is uncertain, but bear them in mind in the event of unexpected response to treatment.

1. Alvarez JS, Del Castillo JAS, Ortiz MJA. Interaction between ciclosporin and ceftriaxone. *Nephron* (1991) 59, 681–2.
2. Xu F, Wu Z, Zou H. Effects on renal function and cyclosporine blood concentration by combination with three cephalosporins in renal transplant patients. *Zhongguo Kang Sheng Su Za Zhi* (1997) 22, 223–5.
3. Cockburn I. Cyclosporin A: a clinical evaluation of drug interactions. *Transplant Proc* (1986) 18 (Suppl 5), 50–5.

Ciclosporin + Antibacterials; Chloramphenicol

Four patients had a marked rise in serum ciclosporin levels when they were treated with chloramphenicol. A small study supports these findings.

Clinical evidence

A retrospective study identified 3 transplant patients on ciclosporin who had received a total of 6 courses of intravenous chloramphenicol, each lasting for at least 12 days. By day 4 of concurrent use ciclosporin levels had increased on average by 41.3%. Ciclosporin doses tended to be slightly reduced over the course of treatment, and by day 10 ciclosporin levels were about 31% below baseline.[1]

A woman with a heart-lung transplant and with a trough ciclosporin serum level of 84 nanograms/ml was started on oral chloramphenicol [dosage not stated] to treat an infection with *Xanthomonas maltophilia*. On the next day the ciclosporin levels had risen to 240 micrograms/l. The chloramphenicol was continued but the ciclosporin dosage was reduced from 300 to 225 mg daily. By day 8 the ciclosporin levels were back within the therapeutic range.[2]

Two kidney transplant patients had marked increases in serum ciclosporin levels (almost doubled in one case) when they were given chloramphenicol to treat urinary tract infections.[3]

There is another report of this interaction, but the case is greatly complicated by the presence of ciprofloxacin, vancomycin, ceftazidime and a recent course of rifampicin taken by the patient.[4]

Mechanism

Uncertain. Chloramphenicol is a recognised enzyme inhibitor and it seems possible that it may reduce the metabolism of the ciclosporin by the liver.[4]

Importance and management

Information seems to be limited to these reports so although the interaction appears to be established its incidence is obviously uncertain. It would now be prudent to monitor ciclosporin levels if systemic chloramphenicol is added, being alert for the need to reduce the ciclosporin dosage. The study[1] highlights the need to monitor levels closely throughout the whole chloramphenicol course.

It seems doubtful if there will be enough chloramphenicol absorbed from eye drops to interact with ciclosporin, but this needs confirmation.

1. Mathis AS, Shah N, Knipp GT, Friedman GS. Interaction of chloramphenicol and the calcineurin inhibitors in renal transplant recipients. *Transpl Infect Dis* (2002) 4, 169–74.
2. Steinfort CL, McConachy KA. Cyclosporin-chloramphenicol drug interaction in a heart-lung transplant recipient. *Med J Aust* (1994) 161, 455.
3. Zawadzki J, Prokurat S, Smirska E, Jelonek A. Interaction between cyclosporine A and chloramphenicol after kidney transplantation. *Pediatr Nephrol* (1991) 5, C49.
4. Bui LL, Huang DD. Possible interaction between cyclosporine and chloramphenicol. *Ann Pharmacother* (1999) 33, 252–3.

Ciclosporin + Antibacterials; Clindamycin

Two patients have had a marked reduction in serum ciclosporin levels when treated with clindamycin.

Clinical evidence, mechanism, importance and management

A lung transplant patient receiving ciclosporin in a dose to maintain levels of 100 to 150 nanograms/ml required dose increases to achieve this level when clindamycin 600 mg three times daily was given. Initially the levels were almost halved by the addition of clindamycin. Ciclosporin was reduced to the original dose when the clindamycin was stopped.[1]

In a second lung transplant patient, treatment with clindamycin 600 mg three times daily necessitated ciclosporin dose increases from 325 mg daily to 1100 mg daily over 4 weeks to maintain serum levels of about 200 nanograms/ml. The reasons for the interaction are not understood, but the authors suggest close monitoring of ciclosporin levels to prevent underdosing if clindamycin is given,[1] although this seems exceptionally cautious as these 2 cases appear to be all that have been reported.

1. Thurnheer R, Laube I, Speich R. Possible interaction between clindamycin and cyclosporin. *BMJ* (1999) 319, 163.

Ciclosporin + Antibacterials; Imipenem/cilastatin

Several transplant patients with impaired renal function have experienced adverse CNS effects (including convulsions and tremors) while taking imipenem/cilastatin and ciclosporin. Imipenem/cilastatin reduced ciclosporin levels in *animals*.

Clinical evidence, mechanism, importance and management

A woman taking ciclosporin following a kidney transplant developed a urinary-tract infection for which she was given imipenem/cilastatin 500 mg intravenously every 12 hours (dose adjusted for renal function). About 20 minutes after the second dose she became confused, disorientated, agitated, and developed motor aphasia and intense tremor. This was interpreted as being a combination of the adverse CNS effects of both drugs. The imipenem/cilastatin was not given again and the effects subsided over the next few days. However, it was noted that the ciclosporin serum levels rose over the next 4 days from about 400 to 1000 nanograms/ml.[1]

Four other transplant patients who were taking ciclosporin developed seizures when they were given imipenem/cilastatin 1 g daily, and a fifth patient developed myoclonia. These patients all had chronic renal impairment.[2] In contrast imipenem/cilastatin 2 g daily for 4 weeks, given with ciprofloxacin, was effectively and successfully used in another patient taking ciclosporin after a heart transplant. This patient was switched to imipenem/cilastatin and ciprofloxacin after developing acute renal failure on amikacin.[3] Reduced serum ciclosporin levels following the use of imipenem/cilastatin have been seen in *rats*.[4]

It should be noted that focal tremors, myoclonus and convulsions are a known adverse effects of imipenem/cilastatin and are most likely to occur in patients with reduced renal function. However, the patients cited above received imipenem/cilastatin in doses adjusted for their renal function.

The makers of imipenem/cilastatin recommend that patients who develop focal tremors, myoclonus and convulsions while receiving the antibacterial should be started on an anticonvulsant. If symptoms persist the dose should be reduced, or the drug withdrawn.[5]

1. Zazgornik J, Schein W, Heimberger K, Shaheen FAM, Stockenhuber F. Potentiation of neurotoxic side effects by coadministration of imipenem to cyclosporine therapy in a kidney transplant recipient--synergism of side effects or drug interaction? *Clin Nephrol* (1986) 26, 265–6.
2. Bösmüller C, Steurer W, Königsrainer A, Willeit J, Margreiter R. Increased risk of central nervous system toxicity inpatients treated with ciclosporin and imipenem/cilastatin. *Nephron* (1991) 58, 362–4.
3. Thaler F, Gotainer B, Teodori G, Dubois C, Loirat Ph. Mediastinitis due to *Nocardia asteroides* after cardiac transplantation. *Intensive Care Med* (1992) 18, 127–8.
4. Mraz W, Sido B, Knedel M, Hammer C. Concomitant immunosuppressive and antibiotic therapy-reduction of cyclosporine A blood levels due to treatment with imipenem/cilastatin. *Transplant Proc* (1987) 19, 4017–20.
5. Primaxin IV Injection (Imipenem monohydrate/Cilastatin sodium). Merck Sharp & Dohme Ltd. UK Summary of product characteristics, October 2003.

Ciclosporin + Antibacterials; Macrolides

Ciclosporin levels can be markedly raised by clarithromycin, erythromycin, josamycin, pristinamycin and possibly midecamycin. Rokitamycin and troleandomycin are predicted to interact similarly. Roxithromycin appears to interact minimally, while no interaction is normally seen with azithromycin, dirithromycin or spiramycin, although there are isolated reports of an interaction with azithromycin.

Clinical evidence

(a) Azithromycin

Eight healthy subjects were given ciclosporin 3.75 to 7.5 mg/kg alone and then after taking clarithromycin 250 mg every 12 hours for 7 days, erythromycin 500 mg every 8 hours, or azithromycin 500 mg initially then 250 mg daily for 4 days. Marked increases in the maximum serum levels of ciclosporin occurred when clarithromycin and erythromycin were used, but with azithromycin no changes were seen.[1] Other studies have also found no evidence of a clinically significant interaction between ciclosporin and azithromycin in a total of 62 kidney transplant patients,[2-4] but there are reports describing a marked increase in ciclosporin levels in 2 patients attributed to azithromycin.[5,6]

(b) Clarithromycin

The serum ciclosporin levels of a heart transplant patient on ciclosporin and azathioprine roughly doubled within 6 days of starting clarithromycin 500 mg twice daily. The makers of ciclosporin also have a case of increased ciclosporin serum levels after clarithromycin was started on record.[7] The trough serum ciclosporin levels of 3 kidney transplant patients doubled or tripled when they took clarithromycin 250 mg twice daily.[8] A kidney transplant patient had a doubled ciclosporin AUC when clarithromycin was given.[9] Another patient had a seven- to twelvefold rise in serum ciclosporin levels and acute renal failure within 3 weeks of starting to take clarithromycin 1 g daily.[10] Clarithromycin 250 mg twice daily approximately doubled the serum ciclosporin levels of a kidney transplant patient within 3 days[11] and increased the maximum serum levels in 8 healthy subjects by about 50% in a week.[1] A mean 30% reduction in the dosage of ciclosporin was needed in 6 transplant patients also given clarithromycin.[12] Clarithromycin 500 mg twice daily as part of a *Helicobacter pylori* eradication regimen caused a two- to threefold increase in ciclosporin levels in 27 kidney transplant patients.[13,14]

(c) Dirithromycin

Fourteen days of treatment with dirithromycin 500 mg daily did not significantly affect the pharmacokinetics of a single 15-mg/kg oral dose of ciclosporin in 8 healthy subjects.[15]

(d) Erythromycin

A study in 9 transplant patients on ciclosporin found that erythromycin increased the mean trough serum levels of the 3 patients with kidney transplants sevenfold, from 147 to 1125 nanograms/ml, and of 6 patients with heart transplants four- to fivefold, from 185 to 815 nanograms/ml. Acute nephrotoxicity occurred in all 9 patients, and 7 showed mild to severe hepatotoxicity caused by the increased ciclosporin levels.[16]

Markedly raised serum ciclosporin levels and/or toxicity have been described in a number of other studies and case reports with erythromycin given orally or intravenously to about 40 other patients.[17-31] The interaction has also been demonstrated in healthy subjects.[1,32] Oral erythromycin may possibly have a greater effect than intravenous erythromycin.[28,33] Erythromycin-related ototoxicity, possibly associated with the use of ciclosporin, has been reported in liver transplant patients.[34]

(e) Josamycin

A man with a renal transplant who was taking azathioprine, prednisone and ciclosporin 330 mg daily had a marked rise in his serum ciclosporin levels from about 90 to 600 nanograms/ml when he took josamycin 2 g daily for 5 days. He responded in the same way when later rechallenged with josamycin. Another patient also reacted in the same way.[35] Two- to fourfold rises in ciclosporin levels have been seen in 9 other patients given josamycin 2 to 3 g (50 mg/kg) daily.[36-38] Another patient had a 40% rise in ciclosporin levels when given josamycin 500 mg twice daily.[39]

(f) Midecamycin

The steady-state serum ciclosporin levels of 10 kidney transplant patients were roughly doubled when they took midecamycin 800 mg twice daily.[40] A 43-year-old kidney transplant patient on ciclosporin, azathioprine and prednisone, began further treatment on day 27 after the transplant with midecamycin diacetate 600 mg twice daily and co-trimoxazole three times daily for pneumonia. By day 33 the concentration/dose ratio of the ciclosporin had doubled, and ciclosporin levels had reached 700 nanograms/ml, accompanied by a rise in serum creatinine levels. When the midecamycin was replaced by cefuroxime, the concentrations of both ciclosporin and creatinine fell to their former levels within 3 days.[41] Ciclosporin levels in another kidney transplant patient on ciclosporin 120 mg twice daily increased from 95 to 380 nanograms/ml 3 days after starting midecamycin 800 mg twice daily.[42] Blood levels of ciclosporin in a kidney transplant patient also increased, from 97 to 203 nanograms/ml, 4 days after starting midecamycin diacetate 600 mg twice daily.[43]

(g) Pristinamycin

A kidney transplant patient had a tenfold rise in serum ciclosporin levels, from 30 to 290 nanograms/ml after taking pristinamycin 2 g daily for 8 days. Blood creatinine levels rose from 75 to 120 micromol/l. Another patient given pristinamycin 1.25 g had a rise in ciclosporin levels from 78 to 855 nanograms/ml after 6 days. Ciclosporin and creatinine levels fell to normal levels within 2 days of stopping both drugs.[44]

Pristinamycin 50 mg/kg daily raised the serum ciclosporin levels of 10 patients by 65% from 560 to 925 nanograms/ml. Ciclosporin levels fell when the pristinamycin was stopped.[45] Within 5 days of starting to take pristinamycin 4 g daily the ciclosporin levels of another patient more than doubled. His serum creatinine levels also rose. Both fell back to baseline levels within 3 days of stopping the antibacterial.[46]

(h) Roxithromycin

Eight patients with heart transplants on ciclosporin 8 mg/kg daily, prednisolone and azathioprine for at least a month, were given roxithromycin 150 mg twice daily for 11 days. A 37.5% rise in serum ciclosporin levels occurred at the time the roxithromycin was given, and a 60% rise occurred 4 hours later. Ciclosporin levels fell again when the roxithromycin was stopped. A small (10%) increase in serum creatinine levels occurred. There was no evidence of a deterioration in renal function.[47] The biological half-life of roxithromycin was found in one study to be doubled, from 17 to 34.4 hours, in patients with kidney transplants on ciclosporin.[48]

(i) Spiramycin

The ciclosporin serum levels of 6 heart transplant patients on corticosteroids, azathioprine and ciclosporin remained unchanged when given spiramycin 3 MIU twice daily for 10 days.[49] Similarly, no interaction was found between ciclosporin and spiramycin in other studies in patients with renal transplants.[50-53]

(j) Other macrolides

In vitro studies (see 'Mechanism' below) suggest that rokitamycin, and troleandomycin interact with ciclosporin in the same way as erythromycin,[54] but as yet there seems to be no direct clinical evidence of an interaction.

Mechanism

In vitro studies with human liver microsomes have found that clarithromycin, erythromycin, josamycin, rokitamycin, roxithromycin and troleandomycin (but not spiramycin) inhibit ciclosporin metabolism in the liver, which is catalysed by the cytochrome P450 isoenzyme CYP3A.[10,54] This would be expected to result in raised ciclosporin levels. Erythromycin[28] and clarithromycin[9] also possibly increase the absorption of ciclosporin from the gut by inhibiting intestinal wall metabolism. Azithromycin is believed to be metabolised by routes independent of the cytochrome system. Intravenous azithromycin was thought to have increased ciclosporin levels through P-glycoprotein inhibition and/or competition for biliary excretion in one report.[6]

Importance and management

The interaction between ciclosporin and erythromycin is well documented, well established and potentially serious. If concurrent use is thought appropriate, monitor the ciclosporin serum levels closely and reduce the dosage appropriately. A reduction of about 35% has been calculated to be necessary.[30] The dosage should be increased again when the erythromycin is stopped. The effect of intravenous erythromycin is less than oral erythromycin so if the route of administration is changed, be alert for the need to change the ciclosporin dosage.[28,33]

Information about the interactions with clarithromycin, josamycin, midecamycin, and pristinamycin is much more limited, but they appear to behave like erythromycin. The same precautions should be taken. There seems to be no direct clinical information about troleandomycin and rokitamycin but *in vitro* studies suggest that they may interact like erythromycin.[54] Be on the alert for this interaction if they are used.

Dirithromycin and spiramycin normally appear not to interact and roxithromycin appears only to interact very minimally. However, bear in mind that the roxithromycin serum levels may be increased. Although most reports suggest azithromycin does not interact, increased monitoring is recommended, because of the isolated reports of increased ciclosporin levels.[6]

1. Bottorff MB, Marien ML, Clendening C. Macrolide antibiotics and inhibition of CYP3A isozymes: differences in cyclosporin pharmacokinetics. *Clin Pharmacol Ther* (1997) 56, 224.
2. Gómez E, Sánchez JE, Aguado S, Alvarez Grande J. Interaction between azithromycin and cyclosporin? *Nephron* (1996) 73, 724.
3. Bubic-Filipi Lj, Puretic Z, Thune S, Glavas-Boras S, Pasini J, Marekovic Z. Influence of azithromycin on cyclosporin levels in patients with a kidney transplant. *Nephrol Dial Transplant* (1998) 13, A276.
4. Bachmann K, Jauregui L, Chandra R, Thakker K. Influence of a 3-day regimen of azithromycin on the disposition kinetics of cyclosporine A in stable renal transplant patients. *Pharmacol Res* (2003) 47, 549–54.
5. Ljutic D, Rumboldt Z. Possible interaction between azithromycin and cyclosporine: a case report. *Nephron* (1995) 70, 130.
6. Page RL, Ruscin JM, Fish D, LaPointe M. Possible interaction between intravenous azithromycin and oral cyclosporine. *Pharmacotherapy* (2001) 21, 1436–43.
7. Gersema LM, Porter CB, Russell EH. Suspected drug interaction between cyclosporine and clarithromycin. *J Heart Lung Transplant* (1994) 13, 343–5.
8. Ferrari SL, Goffin E, Mourad M, Wallemacq P, Squifflet J-P, Pirson Y. The interaction between clarithromycin and cyclosporine in kidney transplant recipients. *Transplantation* (1994) 58, 725–7.
9. Sketris IS, Wright MR, West ML. Possible role of intestinal P-450 enzyme system in a cyclosporine-clarithromycin interaction. *Pharmacotherapy* (1996) 16, 301–5.
10. Spicer ST, Liddle C, Chapman JR, Barclay P, Nankivell BJ, Thomas P, O'Connell PJ. The mechanism of cyclosporine toxicity induced by clarithromycin. *Br J Clin Pharmacol* (1997) 43, 194–6.
11. Treille S, Quoidbach A, Demol H, Vereerstraeten P, Abramowicz D. Kidney graft dysfunction after drug interaction between clarithromycin and cyclosporin. *Nephrol Dial Transplant* (1996) 11, 1192–3.
12. Sádaba B, López De Ocáriz A, Azanza JR, Quiroga J, Cienfuegos JA. Concurrent clarithromycin and cyclosporin A treatment. *J Antimicrob Chemother* (1998) 42, 393–5.
13. Skálová P, Marečková O, Skála I, Lácha J, Teplan V, Vítko Š, Petrásek R. Eradication of *Helicobacter pylori* with clarithromycin: danger of toxic levels of cyclosporin A. *Gut* (1998) 43 (Suppl 2), A109.
14. Skalova P, Mareckova O, Skala I, Lacha J, Teplan V, Vitko S, Petrasek R. Toxic levels of cyclosporin A after renal transplantation on clarithromycin therapy. *Nephrol Dial Transplant* (1998) 13, A256.
15. Bachmann K, Sullivan TJ, Resse JH, Miller K, Scott M, Jauregui L, Sides G. The pharmacokinetics of oral cyclosporine A are not affected by dirithromycin. *Intersci Conf Antimicrob Agents Chemother* (1994) 34, 4.
16. Jensen CWB, Flechner SM, Van Buren CT, Frazier OH, Cooley DA, Lorber MI, Kahan BD. Exacerbation of cyclosporine toxicity by concomitant administration of erythromycin. *Transplantation* (1987) 43, 263–70.

17. Kohan DE. Possible interaction between cyclosporine and erythromycin. *N Engl J Med* (1986), 314, 448.
18. Hourmant M, Le Bigot JF, Vernillet L, Sagniez G, Remi JP, Soulillou JP. Coadministration of erythromycin results in an increase of blood cyclosporine to toxic levels. *Transplant Proc* (1985) 17, 2723–7.
19. Wadhwa NK, Schroeder TJ, O'Flaherty E, Pesce AJ, Myre SA, Munda R, First MR. Interaction between erythromycin and cyclosporine in a kidney and pancreas allograft recipient. *Ther Drug Monit* (1987) 9, 123–5.
20. Murray BM, Edwards L, Morse GD, Kohli RR, Venuto RC. Clinically important interaction of cyclosporine and erythromycin. *Transplantation* (1987) 43, 602–4.
21. Griño JM, Sabate I, Castelao AM, Guardia M, Seron D, Alsina J. Erythromycin and cyclosporine. *Ann Intern Med* (1986) 105, 467–8.
22. Gonwa TA, Nghiem DD, Schulak JA, Corry RJ. Erythromycin and cyclosporine. *Transplantation* (1986) 41, 797–9.
23. Harnett JD, Parfrey PS, Paul MD, Gault MH. Erythromycin-cyclosporine interaction in renal transplant patients. *Transplantation* (1987) 43, 316–18.
24. Kessler M, Louis J, Renoult E, Vigneron B, Netter P. Interaction between cyclosporin and erythromycin in a kidney transplant patient. *Eur J Clin Pharmacol* (1986) 30, 633–4.
25. Godin JRP, Sketris IS, Belitsky P. Erythromycin-cyclosporine interaction. *Drug Intell Clin Pharm* (1986) 20, 504–5.
26. Martell R, Heinrichs D, Stiller CR, Jenner M, Keown PA, Dupre J. The effects of erythromycin in patients treated with cyclosporine. *Ann Intern Med* (1986) 104, 660–1.
27. Ptachcinski PJ, Carpenter BJ, Burckart GJ, Venkataramanan R, Rosenthal JT. Effect of erythromycin on cyclosporine levels. *N Engl J Med* (1985) 313, 1416–17.
28. Gupta SK, Bakran A, Johnson RWG, Rowland M. Erythromycin enhances the absorption of cyclosporin. *Br J Clin Pharmacol* (1988) 25, 401–2.
29. Morales JM, Andres A, Prieto C, Arenas J, Ortuño B, Praga M, Ruilope LM, Rodicio JL. Severe reversible cyclosporine-induced acute renal failure. A role for urinary PGE_2 deficiency? *Transplantation* (1988) 46, 163–5.
30. Vereerstraeten P, Thiry P, Kinnaert P, Toussaint C. Influence of erythromycin on cyclosporine pharmacokinetics. *Transplantation* (1987) 44, 155–6.
31. Ben-Ari J, Eisenstein B, Davidovits M, Shmueli D, Shapira Z, Stark H. Effect of erythromycin on blood cyclosporine concentrations in kidney transplant patients. *J Pediatr* (1988) 112, 992–3.
32. Freeman DJ, Martell R, Carruthers SG, Heinrichs D, Keown PA, Stiller CR. Cyclosporin-erythromycin interaction in normal subjects. *Br J Clin Pharmacol* (1987) 23, 776–8.
33. Zylber-Katz E. Multiple drug interactions with cyclosporine in a heart transplant patient. *Ann Pharmacother* (1995) 29, 127–31. Correction. *ibid.*; 790.
34. Moral A, Navasa M, Rimola A, García-Valdecasas JC, Grande L, Visa J, Rodés J. Erythromycin ototoxicity in liver transplant patients. *Transpl Int* (1994) 7, 62–4.
35. Kreft-Jais C, Billaud EM, Gaudry C, Bedrossian J. Effect of josamycin on plasma cyclosporine levels. *Eur J Clin Pharmacol* (1987) 32, 327–8.
36. Azanza JR, Catalán M, Alvarez MP, Sádaba B, Honorato J, Llorens R, Harreros J. Possible interaction between cyclosporine and josamycin: a description of three cases. *Clin Pharmacol Ther* (1992) 51, 572–5.
37. Torregrosa JV, Campistol JM, Franco A, Andreu J. Interaction of josamycin with cyclosporin A. *Nephron* (1993) 65, 476–7.
38. Azanza J, Catalán M, Alvarez P, Honorato J, Herreros J, Llorens R. Possible interaction between cyclosporine and josamycin. *J Heart Transplant* (1990) 9, 265–6.
39. Capone D, Gentile A, Stanziale P, Imperatore P, D'Alessandro R, D'Alto V, Basile V. Drug interaction between cyclosporine and josamycin in a kidney transplanted patient. *Fundam Clin Pharmacol* (1996) 10, 172.
40. Couet W, Istin B, Seniuta P, Morel D, Potaux L, Fourtillan JB. Effect of ponsinomycin on cyclosporin pharmacokinetics. *Eur J Clin Pharmacol* (1990) 39, 165–67.
41. Alfonso I, Alcalde G, Garcia-Sáiz M, de Cos MA, Mediavilla A. Interaction between cyclosporine a and midecamycin. *Eur J Clin Pharmacol* (1997) 52, 79–80.
42. Finielz P, Mondon J-M, Chuet C, Guiserix J. Drug interaction between midecamycin and cyclosporin. *Nephron* (1995) 70, 136.
43. Treille S, Quoidbach A, Demol H, Juvenois A, Dehout F, Abramowicz D. Kidney graft dysfunction after drug interaction between miocamycin and cyclosporin. *Transpl Int* (1999) 12, 157.
44. Gagnadoux MF, Loirat C, Pillion G, Bertheleme JP, Pouliquen M, Guest G, Broyer M. Néphrotoxicité due à l'interaction pristinamycine-cyclosporine chez le transplanté rénal. *Presse Med* (1987) 16, 1761.
45. Herbrecht R, Garcia J-J, Bergerat J-P, Oberling F. Effect of pristinamycin on cyclosporin levels in bone marrow transplant recipients. *Bone Marrow Transplant* (1989) 4, 457–8.
46. Garraffo R, Monnier B, Lapalus P, Duplay H. Pristinamycin increases cyclosporin blood levels. *Med Sci Res* (1987) 15, 461.
47. Billaud E M, Guillemain R, Fortineau N, Kitzis M-D, Dreyfus G, Amrein C, Kreft-Jaïs C, Husson J-M, Chrétien P. Interaction between roxithromycin and cyclosporin in heart transplant patients. *Clin Pharmacokinet* (1990) 19, 499–502.
48. Morávek J, Matoušovic K, Prát V, Šedivý J. Pharmacokinetics of roxithromycin in kidney grafted patients under cyclosporin A or azathioprine immunosuppression and in healthy volunteers. *Int J Clin Pharmacol Ther Toxicol* (1990) 28, 262–7.
49. Guillemain R, Billaud E, Dreyfus G, Amrein C, Kitzis M, Jebara VA and Kreft-Jais C. The effects of spiramycin on plasma cyclosporin A concentrations in heart transplant patients. *Eur J Clin Pharmacol* (1989) 36, 97–8.
50. Kessler M, Netter P, Zerrouki M, Renoult E, Trechot P, Dousset B, Jonon B, Mur JM. Spiramycin does not increase plasma cyclosporin concentrations in renal transplant patients. *Eur J Clin Pharmacol* (1988) 35, 331–2.
51. Vernillet L, Bertault-Peres P, Berland Y, Barradas J, Durand A, Olmer M. Lack of effect of spiramycin on cyclosporin pharmacokinetics. *Br J Clin Pharmacol* (1989) 27, 789–94.
52. Birmele B, Lebranchu Y, Beliveauu F, Rateau H, Furet Y, Nivet H, Bagros PH. Absence of interaction between cyclosporine and spiramycin. *Transplantation* (1989) 47, 927–8.
53. Kessler M, Netter P, Renoult E, Trechot P, Dousset B, Bannwarth B. Lack of effect of spiramycin on cyclosporin pharmacokinetics. *Br J Clin Pharmacol* (1990) 29, 370–1.
54. Marre R, de Sousa G, Orloff AM, Rahmani R. *In vitro* interaction between cyclosporin A and macrolide antibiotics. *Br J Clin Pharmacol* (1993) 35, 447–8.

Ciclosporin + Antibacterials; Metronidazole

Three reports describe an increase in ciclosporin levels in patients given metronidazole.

Clinical evidence, mechanism, importance and management

The serum ciclosporin levels of a kidney transplant patient rose from 850 to 1930 nanograms/ml when metronidazole 2.25 g daily and cimetidine 800 mg daily were started. The levels fell to about 1500 nanograms/ml when the metronidazole dosage was halved and the cimetidine stopped. Because the levels of ciclosporin were still so high, the dose of ciclosporin was reduced from 7.1 to 5.7 mg/kg daily, which resulted in a further decrease in the ciclosporin level to about 1200 to 1380 nanograms/ml. Finally the metronidazole was stopped and the ciclosporin levels fell to a range of 501 to 885 nanograms/ml.[1]

Another kidney transplant patient developed a raised serum creatinine (increased from 223 to 304 micromol/l) with virtually doubled serum ciclosporin levels metronidazole 1.5 g daily was given.[2]

Ciclosporin levels in yet another kidney transplant patient doubled (from 134 to 264 micrograms/l) accompanied by a modest elevation in serum creatinine when metronidazole 400 mg three times daily was also given. The levels fell again when metronidazole was stopped.[3]

These 3 cases appear to be the only reports of an interaction, one of which is confused by the presence of cimetidine (see also 'Ciclosporin + H_2-blockers', p.792). There is insufficient evidence to advocate monitoring every patient given the combination, but it would be prudent to at least bear this interaction in mind if using metronidazole in patients taking ciclosporin.

1. Zylber-Katz E, Rubinger D and Berlatzky Y. Cyclosporine interactions with metronidazole and cimetidine. *Drug Intell Clin Pharm* (1988) 22, 504–5.
2. Vincent F, Glotz D, Kreft-Jais C, Boudjeltia S, Duboust A, Bariety J. Insuffisance rénale aiguë chez un transplanté rénal traité par cyclosporine A et métronidazole. *Therapie* (1994) 49, 155.
3. Herzig K, Johnson DW. Marked elevation of blood cyclosporin and tacrolimus levels due to concurrent metronidazole therapy. *Nephrol Dial Transplant* (1999) 14, 521–3.

Ciclosporin + Antibacterials; Penicillins

Ampicillin does not interact adversely with ciclosporin. Increased nephrotoxicity has been seen in lung transplant patients given nafcillin prophylactically, whereas an isolated report describes a fall in ciclosporin levels in a patient treated with nafcillin. A case of raised ciclosporin levels in a patient on ticarcillin has been described.

Clinical evidence

(a) Ampicillin

Seventy-one renal transplant patients on ciclosporin had no changes in serum urea, creatinine or ciclosporin levels when ampicillin was given and later withdrawn.[1]

(b) Nafcillin

A retrospective study of 19 lung transplant patients on ciclosporin found that those given nafcillin for a week as prophylaxis against staphylococci had a greater degree of renal impairment than those not taking nafcillin. Serum creatinine levels rose steadily over 6 days until the nafcillin was stopped, whereas the patients not taking nafcillin had no changes in creatinine levels. Three of the nafcillin group temporarily needed haemodialysis. Ciclosporin doses in the nafcillin group were higher but the serum levels in both groups were not significantly different. The incidence of viral infections was also greater in the nafcillin group.[2]

A kidney transplant patient on ciclosporin and prednisone experienced a marked fall in her serum ciclosporin levels on two occasions when treated with nafcillin 2 g every 6 hours. Trough serum levels fell from 229 to 119 nanograms/ml and then to 68 nanograms/ml after 3 and 7 days of nafcillin, and rose when the nafcillin was stopped. On the second occasion ciclosporin levels fell from 272 to 42 nanograms/ml after 9 days treatment with nafcillin.[3]

(c) Ticarcillin

Rises in serum ciclosporin levels from 90 to 230 nanograms/ml, and from 120 to 300 nanograms/ml occurred in a man within 5 to 10 days of starting ticarcillin 10 g daily.[4]

Mechanism

The authors of the study[2] postulate that the nafcillin may have interfered with the ciclosporin assay, resulting in an under-estimate of the actual levels, so that the nephrotoxicity was simply due to higher ciclosporin levels.[2] The fall in ciclosporin levels in the individual patient[3] is not understood, nor is the rise in levels seen in the patient on ticarcillin.[4]

Importance and management

Information seems to be limited to the studies and cases cited. No special precautions would seem necessary with ampicillin, but an alternative to nafcillin would seem prudent for anti-staphylococcal prophylaxis. Good monitoring would seem necessary if ticarcillin is given. More study is needed.

1. Xu F, Shi XH. Interaction between ampicillin, norfloxacin and cyclosporine in renal transplant recipients. *Zhongguo Kang Sheng Su Za Zhi* (1992) 17, 290–2.
2. Jahansouz F, Kriett JM, Smith CM, Jamieson SW. Potentiation of cyclosporin nephrotoxicity by nafcillin in lung transplant recipients. *Transplantation* (1993) 55, 1045–8.
3. Veremis SA, Maddux MS, Pollak R, Mozes MF. Subtherapeutic cyclosporine concentrations during nafcillin therapy. *Transplantation* (1987) 43, 913–5.
4. Lambert C, Pointet P, Ducret F. Interaction ciclosporine-ticarcilline chez un transplanté rénal. *Presse Med* (1989) 18, 230.

Ciclosporin + Antibacterials; Quinolones

Ciclosporin serum levels are normally unchanged by the use of ciprofloxacin, but increased serum levels and nephrotoxicity may occur in a small number of patients. There is also some evidence that the immunosuppressant effects of ciclosporin are reduced by ciprofloxacin. One study, and 2 case reports describe rises in ciclosporin levels in patients given norfloxacin, but another study found no change. Similar results have been found with levofloxacin. Enoxacin, ofloxacin, pefloxacin and trovafloxacin appear not to interact significantly.

Clinical evidence

(a) Ciprofloxacin

A single-dose study in 10 healthy subjects found that after taking ciprofloxacin 500 mg twice daily for 7 days the pharmacokinetics of oral ciclosporin 5 mg/kg were unchanged.[1] Five other studies confirm the lack of a pharmacokinetic interaction in:

- 10 kidney transplant patients taking ciprofloxacin 750 mg twice daily for 13 days;[2]
- 15 kidney transplant patients on ciprofloxacin 500 mg twice daily for 7 days;[3]
- 10 bone marrow transplant patients given ciprofloxacin 500 mg twice daily for 4 days;[4]
- 4 heart transplant patients given ciprofloxacin 250 to 500 mg for 7 to 140 days;[5]
- 3 heart transplant patients given ciprofloxacin 800 to 1500 mg daily.[6]

No changes in serum ciclosporin levels or evidence of nephrotoxicity occurred.

In contrast, a handful of cases of nephrotoxicity have been reported. A heart transplant patient developed acute renal failure within 4 days of being given ciprofloxacin 750 mg every 8 hours.[7] Another patient who had undergone a kidney transplant developed reversible nephrotoxicity.[8] Decreased renal function in a heart-lung transplant patient has been described in another report.[9] This patient and another also had increased serum ciclosporin levels when given ciprofloxacin 500 mg three times daily.[9] Acute interstitial nephritis in a cardiac transplant patient has also been reported.[10-12]

A case-control study in 42 kidney transplant patients suggested that the proportion of cases experiencing at least one episode of biopsy-proved rejection within 1 to 3 months of receiving a transplant were significantly greater in those who had taken ciprofloxacin (45%) than in those who had not (19%). There was also a marked increase in the incidence of rejection associated with ciprofloxacin use (29%) compared with the controls (2%).[13]

(b) Enoxacin

Enoxacin 400 mg twice daily for 5 days had little effect on either blood or plasma levels of single doses of ciclosporin in 10 healthy subjects.[14]

(c) Levofloxacin

A single-dose study in 12 healthy subjects found that levofloxacin 500 mg had no effect on the pharmacokinetics of ciclosporin.[15] In a further study, 5 patients taking ciclosporin following a kidney transplant were given levofloxacin 500 mg twice daily for 5 days for urinary-tract infections. The maximum ciclosporin blood concentration was increased by 23% by levofloxacin. The authors concluded that this may be clinically significant, and warn about extrapolating the results from single-dose studies in healthy subjects (as above) to patients with transplants.[16]

(d) Norfloxacin

Six renal transplant patients given norfloxacin 400 mg twice daily for 3 to 23 days for urinary tract infections,[17] and 4 heart transplant patients given norfloxacin 400 mg for 7 to 140 days had no changes in serum ciclosporin levels.[5] However, two reports describe rises, one marked, in serum ciclosporin levels in a heart transplant patient and a kidney transplant patient given norfloxacin.[18] A comparative study in 5 children (mean age 8-years-old) found that while receiving norfloxacin 5 to 10 mg/kg/day their daily dose of ciclosporin was 4.5 mg/kg/day compared with another control group of 6 children not taking norfloxacin who needed 7.4 mg/kg/day.[19]

(e) Ofloxacin

Thirty-nine patients with kidney transplants taking ciclosporin and prednisolone had no evidence of nephrotoxicity nor of any other interaction when concurrently treated with ofloxacin 100 to 400 mg daily for periods of 3 to 500 days.[20]

(f) Pefloxacin

A study in kidney transplant patients taking corticosteroids, azathioprine and ciclosporin found that the pharmacokinetics of the ciclosporin were not significantly changed by pefloxacin 400 mg twice daily for 4 days.[21]

(g) Trovafloxacin

A placebo-controlled crossover study in 7 stable kidney transplant patients treated with ciclosporin (*Sandimmune*) found that the pharmacokinetics of the ciclosporin were not significantly altered by trovafloxacin 200 mg daily for 7 days.[22]

Mechanism

The interaction between ciclosporin and norfloxacin interaction probably occurs because norfloxacin inhibits the cytochrome P450 isoenzyme CYP3A4, resulting in a reduction in ciclosporin metabolism.[19] The interaction between ciclosporin and ciprofloxacin may possibly be due to some antagonism by ciprofloxacin of the ciclosporin-dependent inhibition of interleukin-2, which thereby opposes its immunosuppressant action.[13]

Importance and management

Information seems to be limited to these reports. They indicate that in children and adults the dosage of ciclosporin will probably need to be reduced in the presence of norfloxacin. Information with levofloxacin is currently limited, but a modest increase in ciclosporin levels may occur, and increased monitoring seems advisable. No pharmacokinetic interaction normally occurs between ciclosporin and ciprofloxacin but very occasionally and unpredictably an increase in serum ciclosporin levels and/or kidney toxicity occurs. There is also some evidence that the immunosuppressant effects of the ciclosporin may be reduced. Bear these interactions in mind when prescribing both drugs. There seem to be no reports of problems with enoxacin, ofloxacin, pefloxacin or trovafloxacin.

1. Tan KKC, Trull AK, Shawket S. Co-administration of ciprofloxacin and cyclosporin: lack of evidence for a pharmacokinetic interaction. *Br J Clin Pharmacol* (1989) 28, 185–7.
2. Lang J, Finaz de Villaine J, Garraffo R, Touraine J-L. Cyclosporine (cyclosporin A) pharmacokinetics in renal transplant patients receiving ciprofloxacin. *Am J Med* (1989) 87 (Suppl 5A), 82S–85S.
3. Van Buren DH, Koestner J, Adedoyin A, McCune T, MacDonell R, Johnson HK, Carroll J, Nylander W, Richie RE. Effect of ciprofloxacin on cyclosporine pharmacokinetics. *Transplantation* (1990) 50, 888–9.
4. Krüger HU, Schuler U, Proksch B, Göbel M, Ehninger G. Investigation of potential interaction of ciprofloxacin with cyclosporine in bone marrow transplant recipients. *Antimicrob Agents Chemother* (1990) 34, 1048–52.
5. Robinson JA, Venezio FR, Costanzo-Nordin MR, Pifarre R, O'Keefe PJ. Patients receiving quinolones and cyclosporine after heart transplantation. *J Heart Transplant* (1990) 9, 30–1.
6. Hooper TL, Gould FK, Swinburn CR, Featherstone G, Odom NJ, Corris PA, Freeman R, McGregor CGA. Ciprofloxacin: a preferred treatment for legionella infections in patients receiving cyclosporin A. *J Antimicrob Chemother* (1988) 22, 952–3.
7. Avent CK, Krinsky JK, Kirklin JK, Bourge RC, Figg WD. Synergistic nephrotoxicity due to ciprofloxacin and cyclosporine. *Am J Med* (1988) 85, 452–3.
8. Elston RA, Taylor J. Possible interaction of ciprofloxacin with cyclosporin A. *J Antimicrob Chemother* (1988) 21, 679–80.
9. Nasir M, Rotellar C, Hand M, Kulczycki L, Alijani MR, Winchester JF. Interaction between ciclosporin and ciprofloxacin. *Nephron* (1991) 57, 245–6.
10. Rosado LJ, Siskind MS, Copeland JG. Acute interstitial nephritis in a cardiac transplant patient receiving ciprofloxacin. *J Thorac Cardiovasc Surg* (1994) 107, 1364.
11. Bourge RC. Invited letter concerning: acute interstitial nephritis in a cardiac transplant recipients receiving ciprofloxacin. *J Thorac Cardiovasc Surg* (1994) 107, 1364–5.
12. Rosado LJ, Siskind MS, Nolan PE, Copeland JG. Invited letter concerning: acute interstitial nephritis in a cardiac transplant recipients receiving ciprofloxacin. *J Thorac Cardiovasc Surg* (1994) 107, 1365–6.

13. Wrishko RE, Levine M, Primmett DRN, Kim S, Partovi N, Lewis S, Landsberg D, Keown PA. Investigation of a possible interaction between ciprofloxacin and cyclosporine in renal transplant patients. *Transplantation* (1997) 64, 996–999.
14. Ryerson BA, Toothaker RD, Posvar EL, Sedman AJ, Koup JR. Effect of enoxacin on cyclosporine pharmacokinetics in healthy subjects. *Intersci Conf Antimicrob Agents Chemother* (1991) 31, 198.
15. Doose DR, Walker SA, Chien SC, Williams RR, Nayak RK. Levofloxacin does not alter cyclosporine disposition. *J Clin Pharmacol* (1998) 38, 90–3.
16. Federico S, Carrano R, Gentile A, Palmiero G, Basile V, Capone D. Pharmacokinetic interaction between cyclosporine and levofloxacin in kidney transplant recipients. *J Am Soc Nephrol* (2001) 12, 887A.
17. Jadoul M, Pirson Y, van Ypersele de Strihou C. Norfloxacin and cyclosporine-a safe combination. *Transplantation* (1989) 47, 747–8.
18. Thomson DJ, Menkis AH, McKenzie FN. Norfloxacin-cyclosporine interaction. *Transplantation* (1988) 46, 312–13.
19. McLellan RA, Drobitch RK, McLellan DH, Acott PD, Crocker JFS, Renton KW. Norfloxacin interferes with cyclosporine disposition in pediatric patients undergoing renal transplantation. *Clin Pharmacol Ther* (1995) 58, 322–7.
20. Vogt P, Schorn T, Frei U. Ofloxacin in the treatment of urinary tract infection in renal transplant recipients. *Infection* (1988) 16, 175–8.
21. Lang J, Finaz de Villaine J, Guemei A, Touraine JL, Faucon C. Absence of pharmacokinetic interaction between pefloxacin and cyclosporin A in patients with renal transplants. *Rev Infect Dis* (1989) 11 (Suppl 5), S1094.
22. Johnson HJ, Swan SK, Heim-Duthoy KL, Pelletier SM, Teng R, Vincent J. The effect of trovafloxacin on steady-state pharmacokinetics of cyclosporine (CSA) in stable renal transplant patients. *Pharm Res* (1997) 14 (11 Suppl), S-509.

Ciclosporin + Antibacterials; Quinupristin/Dalfopristin

In an isolated case quinupristin/dalfopristin was found to increase ciclosporin levels about threefold.

Clinical evidence, mechanism, importance and management

A kidney transplant patient maintained on ciclosporin with trough levels of between 80 and 105 nanograms/ml developed a vancomycin-resistant enterococcal infection. After a series of antibacterials had failed to clear the infection she was given intravenous quinupristin/dalfopristin 300 mg every 8 hours. After 3 days of treatment her ciclosporin trough level rose to almost 300 nanograms/ml. A ciclosporin dose reduction from 75 to 50 mg twice daily returned her levels to baseline. However, 2 days after the antibacterials were discontinued she was found to have a trough ciclosporin level of only 34 nanograms/ml. She was subsequently restabilised on her original dose of ciclosporin.[1]

This appears to be an isolated case, and its clinical significance is unknown. However, this does not appear to be a common combination, therefore, it may be prudent to monitor ciclosporin levels in any patient given quinupristin/dalfopristin until more experience has been gained.

1. Stamatakis MK, Richards JG. Interaction between quinupristin/dalfopristin and cyclosporine. *Ann Pharmacother* (1997) 31, 576–8.

Ciclosporin + Antibacterials; Rifamycins

Ciclosporin serum levels are markedly reduced by rifampicin and transplant rejection can rapidly develop. Rifamycin seems to interact similarly, but limited evidence suggests that rifabutin interacts to a lesser extent.

Clinical evidence

(a) Rifabutin

The clearance of ciclosporin in a patient with a kidney transplant doubled (from 0.3 to 0.63 L/h/kg) when isoniazid, ethambutol, pyridoxine and rifampicin 600 mg daily were given. When the antitubercular drugs were replaced by rifabutin 150 mg and clofazimine 100 mg daily the ciclosporin clearance fell to about its former levels, but after about 3 weeks rose to 0.36 L/h/kg.[1]

(b) Rifampicin (Rifampin)

A heart transplant patient on ciclosporin was started on rifampicin 600 mg daily with amphotericin B for the treatment of an *Aspergillus fumigatus* infection. Within 11 days her serum ciclosporin levels had fallen from 473 to less than 31 nanograms/ml and severe acute graft rejection occurred. The dosage of ciclosporin was increased stepwise and the levels climbed to a plateau before suddenly falling again. The dosage had to be increased to more than 30 mg/kg daily to achieve serum levels in the range 100 to 300 nanograms/ml.[2]

A considerable number of other reports about individual patients, both adult and paediatric, confirm that a very marked fall in serum ciclosporin levels occurs, often to undetectable levels, accompanied by transplantation rejection in many instances, if rifampicin is given either intravenously or orally, without raising the ciclosporin dosage.[1,3-26] Ciclosporin levels become toxic within 2 weeks of stopping the rifampicin unless the previously adjusted ciclosporin dosage is reduced.[3,5]

Three patients needed increases in the dosage of ciclosporin when given rifampicin and erythromycin, although the latter normally reduces ciclosporin requirements.[18,27,28] Another patient whose ciclosporin levels had been raised by clarithromycin had a fall in levels when rifampicin was added.[29]

(c) Rifamycin sodium

Rifamycin sodium used to irrigate a wound has been reported to reduce the serum levels of ciclosporin in a kidney transplant patient.[30]

Mechanism

Rifampicin stimulates the metabolism of the ciclosporin by the cytochrome P450 isoenzyme CYP3A[31] resulting in a marked increase in its clearance. In addition rifampicin decreases ciclosporin absorption by inducing its metabolism by the gut wall,[32] thus its effects become markedly reduced. If rifampicin is given with erythromycin or clarithromycin, the enzyme inhibitory effects of the macrolides are swamped by the more potent enzyme effects of rifampicin. Rifabutin has some enzyme inducing properties but the extent is quite small compared with rifampicin, and may be delayed.[33]

Importance and management

The interaction between ciclosporin and rifampicin is very well documented, well established and clinically important. Transplant rejection may occur unless the ciclosporin dosage is markedly increased. In one study 27% of patients on rifampicin lost grafts due to rejection, and this was directly attributed to the interaction.[21] The interaction develops within a few days (within a single day in one case[19]). Monitor the effects of concurrent use and increase the ciclosporin dosage appropriately. Three- to fivefold dosage increases (sometimes frequency-increases from two to three times daily) have proved to be effective, with daily monitoring. Remember also to reduce the dosage if the rifampicin is stopped.

The authors of one large study concluded that it is better to avoid rifampicin in patients on ciclosporin and to use other tuberculostatics instead.[21] They found that the use of three antitubercular drugs (not including rifampicin) for at least 9 months reduced mortality. Two heart transplant patients with uncomplicated tuberculosis have been successfully treated with an 18-month course of isoniazid and ethambutol.[22]

Isoniazid[11,21,22] and **ethambutol**[21,22] do not normally interact with ciclosporin. However, there is one case report describing a patient who had a gradual rise in serum ciclosporin levels when isoniazid and ethambutol were stopped,[13] and another which attributed a marked rise in ciclosporin levels to the use of isoniazid.[34] Pyrazinamide also usually appears not to interact with ciclosporin, but see 'Ciclosporin + Pyrazinamide', p.797.

Another suggested alternative is to replace the ciclosporin with azathioprine and low-dose prednisolone for immunosuppression when using rifampicin.[12]

Other rifamycins may also be an option; limited evidence suggests that rifabutin interacts minimally. However, the maker[35] and the UK Committee on Safety of Medicines[36] caution about the possibility of an interaction, and close monitoring of ciclosporin levels would still be advisable. Topical rifamycin interacted like rifampicin in one patient when it was applied to a wound.[30]

1. Vandevelde C, Chang A, Andrews D, Riggs W, Jewesson P. Rifampin and ansamycin interactions with cyclosporine after renal transplantation. *Pharmacotherapy* (1991) 11, 88–9.
2. Modry DL, Stinson EB, Oyer PE, Jamieson SW, Baldwin JC, Shumway NE. Acute rejection and massive cyclosporine requirements in heart transplant recipients treated with rifampin. *Transplantation* (1985) 39, 313–14.
3. Langhoff E, Madsen S. Rapid metabolism of cyclosporin and prednisone in kidney transplant patients on tuberculostatic treatment. *Lancet* (1983) ii, 1303.
4. Cassidy MJD, Van Zyl-Smit R, Pascoe MD, Swanepoel CR, Jacobson JE. Effect of rifampicin on cyclosporin A blood levels in a renal transplant recipient. *Nephron* (1985) 41, 207–8.
5. Coward RA, Raferty AT, Brown CB. Cyclosporin and antituberculous therapy. *Lancet* (1985) i, 1342–3.
6. Howard P, Bixler TJ, Gill B. Cyclosporine-rifampin drug interaction. *Drug Intell Clin Pharm* (1985) 19, 763–4.
7. Van Buren D, Wideman CA, Ried M, Gibbons S, Van Buren CT, Jarowenko M, Flechner SM, Frazier OH, Cooley DA, Kahan BD. The antagonistic effect of rifampin upon cyclosporine bioavailability. *Transplant Proc* (1984) 16, 1642–5.

8. Allen RDM, Hunnisett AG, Morris PJ. Cyclosporin and rifampicin in renal transplantation. *Lancet* (1985) i, 980.
9. Langhoff E, Madsen S. Rapid metabolism of cyclosporin and prednisone in kidney transplant patient receiving tuberculostatic treatment. *Lancet* (1983) ii, 1031.
10. Offermann G, Keller F, Molzahn M. Low cyclosporin A blood levels and acute graft rejection in a renal transplant recipient during rifampin treatment. *Am J Nephrol* (1985) 5, 385–7.
11. Jurewicz WA, Gunson BK, Ismail T, Angrisani L, McMaster P. Cyclosporin and antituberculous therapy. *Lancet* (1985) i, 1343.
12. Daniels NJ, Dover JS, Schachter RK. Interaction between cyclosporin and rifampicin. *Lancet* (1984) ii, 639.
13. Leimenstoll G, Schlegelberger T, Fulde R, Niedermayer W. Interaktion von Ciclosporin und Ethambutol-Isoniazid. *Dtsch Med Wochenschr* (1988) 113, 514–15.
14. Prado A, Ramirez M, Aguirre EC, Martin RS, Zucchini A. Interaccion entre ciclosporina y rifampicina en un caso de transplante renal. *Medicina (B Aires)* (1987) 47, 521–4.
15. Al-Sulaiman MH, Dhar JM, Al-Khader AA. Successful use of rifampicin in the treatment of tuberculosis in renal transplant patients immunosuppressed with cyclosporine. *Transplantation* (1990) 50, 597–8.
16. Sánchez DM, Rincón LC, Asensio JM, Serna AB. Interacción entre ciclosporina y rifampicina. *Rev Clin Esp* (1988) 183, 217.
17. Peschke B, Ernst W, Gossmann J, Kachel HG, Schoeppe W, Scheuermann EH. Antituberculous drugs in kidney transplant recipients treated with cyclosporine. *Transplantation* (1993) 56, 236–8.
18. Zylber-Katz E. Multiple drug interactions with cyclosporine in a heart transplant patient. *Ann Pharmacother* (1995) 29, 127–31. Correction. *ibid.*; 790.
19. Wandel C, Böhrer H, Böcker R. Rifampicin and cyclosporine dosing in heart transplant patients. *J Cardiothorac Vasc Anesth* (1995) 9, 621–2.
20. Capone D, Aiello C, Santoro GA, Gentile A, Stanziale P, D'Alessandro R, Imperatore P, Basile V. Drug interaction between cyclosporine and two antimicrobial agents, josamycin and rifampicin, in organ-transplanted patients. *Int J Clin Pharmacol Res* (1996) 16, 73–6.
21. Aguado JM, Herrero JA, Gavaldá J, Torre-Cisneros J, Blanes M, Rufí G, Moreno A, Gurguí A, Hayek M, Lumbreras C and the Spanish Transplantation Infection Study Group, GESITRA. Clinical presentation and outcome of tuberculosis in kidney, liver, and heart transplant recipients in Spain. *Transplantation* (1997) 63, 1276–86.
22. Muñoz P, Palomo J, Muños R, Rodríguez-Creixéms M, Pelaez T, Bouza E. Tuberculosis in heart transplant recipients. *Clin Infect Dis* (1995) 21, 398–402.
23. Freitag VL, Skifton RD, Lake KD. Effect of short-term rifampin on stable cyclosporine concentration. *Ann Pharmacother* (1999) 33, 871–2.
24. Almeida RV, Carvalho JGR, Mulinari A, Hauck P. Tuberculosis in renal transplant recipients. *J Am Soc Nephrol* (1997) 8, 709A.
25. Kim YH, Yoon YR, Kim YW, Shin JG, Cha IJ. Effects of rifampin on cyclosporine disposition in kidney recipients with tuberculosis. *Transplant Proc* (1998) 30, 3570–2.
26. Zelunka EJ. Intravenous cyclosporine-rifampin interaction in a pediatric bone marrow transplant recipient. *Pharmacotherapy* (2002) 22, 387–90.
27. Hooper TL, Gould FK, Swinburne CR, Featherstone G, Odom NJ, Corris PA, Freeman R, McGregor CGA. Ciprofloxacin: a preferred treatment for legionella infections in patients receiving cyclosporin A. *J Antimicrob Chemother* (1988) 22, 952–3.
28. Soto J, Sacristan JA, Alsar MJ. Effect of the simultaneous administration of rifampicin and erythromycin on the metabolism of cyclosporine. *Clin Transplant* (1992) 6, 312–14.
29. Plemmons RM, McAllister CK, Garces MC, Ward RL. Osteomyelitis due to *Mycobacterium haemophilum* in a cardiac transplant patient: case report and analysis of interactions among clarithromycin, rifampin and cyclosporine. *Clin Infect Dis* (1997) 24, 995–7.
30. Renoult E, Hubert J, Trechot Ph, Hestin D, Kessler M, L'Hermite J. Effect of topical rifamycin SV treatment on cyclosporin A blood levels in a renal transplant patient. *Eur J Clin Pharmacol* (1991) 40, 433–4.
31. Pichard L, Fabre JM, Domergue J, Fabre G, Saint-Aubert B, Mourad G, Maurel P. Molecular mechanism of cyclosporine A drug interactions: inducers and inhibitors of cytochrome P450 screening in primary cultures of human hepatocytes. *Transplant Proc* (1991) 23, 978–9.
32. Hebert MF, Roberts JP, Prueksaritanont T, Benet LZ. Bioavailability of cyclosporine with concomitant rifampin administration is markedly less than predicted by hepatic enzyme induction. *Clin Pharmacol Ther* (1992) 52, 453–7.
33. Perucca E, Grimaldi R, Frigo GM, Sardi A, Möning H, Ohnhaus EE. Comparative effects of rifabutin and rifampicin on hepatic microsomal enzyme activity in normal subjects. *Eur J Clin Pharmacol* (1988) 34, 595–9.
34. Diaz Couselo FA, Porato F, Turin M, Etchegoyen FP, Diez RA. Interacciones de la ciclosporina en transplantados renales. *Medicina (B Aires)* (1992) 52, 296–302.
35. Mycobutin (Rifabutin). Pharmacia Ltd. UK Summary of product characteristics, January 2003.
36. Committee on the Safety of Medicines/Medicines Control Agency. Revised indication and drug interactions of rifabutin. *Current Problems* (1997) 23, 14.

Ciclosporin + Antibacterials; Sulfonamides and/or Trimethoprim

In isolated cases, sulfadiazine given orally or sulfadimidine with trimethoprim given intravenously have caused a fall in serum ciclosporin levels. Sulfametoxydiazine possibly caused a minor fall in one case. Although co-trimoxazole increases serum creatinine levels in kidney transplant patients on ciclosporin it normally appears to be safe and effective.

Clinical evidence

(a) Co-trimoxazole

A large-scale study in 132 kidney transplant patients on ciclosporin encompassing 33 876 patient-days found that co-trimoxazole was effective and well tolerated. Ciclosporin pharmacokinetics remained unchanged. A 15% rise in serum creatinine levels occurred, which reversed when the co-trimoxazole was stopped. This rise was not interpreted as a sign of nephrotoxicity but appeared to be due to inhibition of the tubular excretion of creatinine by the co-trimoxazole.[1]

Other reports describe rises in creatinine levels (interpreted as evidence of nephrotoxicity),[2-5] interstitial nephritis,[6] granulocytopenia and thrombocytopenia[7,8] in a few patients given ciclosporin with co-trimoxazole. Apparent nephrotoxicity has also been seen with **trimethoprim** and ciclosporin.[9]

(b) Sulfadiazine or Sulfametoxydiazine

Three heart transplant patients treated for toxoplasmosis had falls in their ciclosporin levels when they were given sulfadiazine 4 to 6 g daily. Their dosage-to-level ciclosporin ratios rose by 58, 82 and 29% respectively. Two had previously been treated with sulfametoxydiazine and this had caused a minor fall in ciclosporin levels in one of these patients.[10]

Another report mentions the use of sulfadiazine in 2 transplant patients without commenting about any interaction.[11]

(c) Sulfadimidine with trimethoprim

A heart transplant patient on ciclosporin and prednisolone developed undetectable serum ciclosporin levels 7 days after starting intravenous sulfadimidine 2 g four times daily and trimethoprim 300 to 500 mg twice daily. Doubling the ciclosporin dosage had little effect and evidence of transplant rejection was seen. Within 10 days of starting to take the antibacterials orally instead of intravenously the serum ciclosporin levels returned to roughly their former levels and the rejection problems disappeared.[12]

Another report by some of the same authors describes a similar marked fall in serum ciclosporin levels in 5 heart transplant patients (one of them the same as the report already cited[12]) when given sulfadimidine and trimethoprim intravenously.[13]

However, a further report mentions the use of intravenous sulfadimidine in a transplant patient without commenting about any interaction.[11]

Mechanism

Uncertain. Co-trimoxazole and trimethoprim can raise serum creatinine levels, possibly due to inhibition of creatinine secretion by the kidney tubules.[14] The reduction in serum ciclosporin levels apparently caused by the sulfonamides is not understood.

Importance and management

The documentation is only moderate, and these interactions are not firmly established. Be aware that intravenous sulfadimidine with trimethoprim may cause a marked reduction in serum ciclosporin levels with accompanying inadequate immunosuppression. Sulfadiazine may also reduce ciclosporin levels. The evidence suggests that oral sulfadimidine with trimethoprim, sulfametoxydiazine and co-trimoxazole do not interact adversely and are normally safe and effective, although toxicity can apparently occur in a small number of patients. Until more information is available it would be prudent to keep a close check on ciclosporin levels if any sulphonamide is added to established treatment with ciclosporin.

1. Maki DG, Fox BC, Kuntz J, Sollinger HW, Belzer FO. A prospective, randomized, double-blind study of trimethoprim-sulfamethoxazole for prophylaxis of infection in renal transplantation. Side effects of trimethoprim-sulfamethoxazole interaction with cyclosporine. *J Lab Clin Med* (1992) 119, 11–24.
2. Thompson JF, Chalmers DHK, Hunnisett AGW, Wood RFM, Morris PJ. Nephrotoxicity of trimethoprim and cotrimoxazole in renal allograft recipients treated with cyclosporine. *Transplantation* (1983) 36, 204–6.
3. Ringdén O, Myrenfors P, Klintmalm G, Tydén G, Öst L. Nephrotoxicity by co-trimoxazole and cyclosporin in transplanted patients. *Lancet* (1984) i, 1016–17.
4. Klintmalm G, Säwe J, Ringdén O, von Bahr C, Magnusson A. Cyclosporine plasma levels in renal transplant patients. Association with renal toxicity and allograft rejection. *Transplantation* (1985) 39, 132–7.
5. Klintmalm G, Ringdén O, Groth CG. Clinical and laboratory signs in nephrotoxicity and rejection in cyclosporine treated renal allograft recipients. *Transplant Proc* (1983) 15 (Suppl 1), 2815–20.
6. Smith EJ, Light JA, Filo RS, Yum MN. Interstitial nephritis caused by trimethoprim-sulfamethoxazole in renal transplant recipients. *JAMA* (1980) 244, 360–1.
7. Bradley PP, Warden GD, Maxwell JG, Rothstein G. Neutropenia and thrombocytopenia in renal allograft recipients treated with trimethoprim-sulfamethoxazole. *Ann Intern Med* (1980) 93, 560–2.
8. Hulme B, Reeves DS. Leucopenia associated with trimethoprim-sulfamethoxazole after renal transplantation. *BMJ* (1971) 3, 610–2.
9. Nyberg G, Gäbel H, Althoff P, Bjoörk S, Herlitz H, Brynger H. Adverse effect of trimethoprim on kidney function in renal transplant patients. *Lancet* (1984) i, 394–5.
10. Spes CH, Angermann CE, Stempfle HU, Wenke K, Theisen K. Sulfadiazine therapy for toxoplasmosis in heart transplant recipients decreases cyclosporine concentration. *Clin Invest* (1992) 70, 752–4.
11. Wreghitt TG, Hakim M, Gray JJ, Balfour AH, Stovin PGI, Stewart S, Scott J, English TAH, Wallwork J. Toxoplasmosis in heart and lung transplant recipients. *J Clin Pathol* (1989) 42, 194–9.
12. Wallwork J, McGregor CGA, Wells FC, Cory-Pearce R, English TAH. Cyclosporin and intravenous sulphadimidine and trimethoprim therapy. *Lancet* (1983) i, 336–7.
13. Jones DK, Hakim M, Wallwork J, Higenbottam TW, White DJG. Serious interaction between cyclosporin A and sulphadimidine. *BMJ* (1986) 292, 728–9.
14. Berg KJ, Gjellestad A, Norby G, Rootwelt K, Djøseland O, Fauchald P, Mehl A, Narverud J, Talseth T. Renal effects of trimethoprim in ciclosporin- and azathioprine-treated kidney-allografted patients. *Nephron* (1989) 53, 218–22.

Ciclosporin + Anticoagulants

The ciclosporin levels of a patient fell when given warfarin. When the ciclosporin dosage was raised an increase in the warfarin dosage was needed. Another patient on warfarin also had a fall in INR when she was given ciclosporin. A further report describes a rise in serum ciclosporin levels when an unnamed anticoagulant was given. Other reports describe increased or decreased acenocoumarol effects and decreased ciclosporin levels in 2 patients.

Clinical evidence

(a) Acenocoumarol

The anticoagulant dosage of a patient on acenocoumarol needed to be reduced by about half to maintain a therapeutic INR when he was started on ciclosporin after a kidney transplant. The required dose of ciclosporin slightly decreased.[1] Conversely, a patient taking acenocoumarol 32 mg per week was started on ciclosporin for nephrotic syndrome. After 10 days his acenocoumarol dose needed to be increased to 38 mg per week to maintain a therapeutic INR, and the ciclosporin level was considered too low and so was increased from 100 to 150 mg daily. However, a further 10 days later (after the increase in acenocoumarol dose) the ciclosporin level was even lower. Eventually the patient achieved therapeutic levels in the presence of acenocoumarol with a ciclosporin dose of 200 mg daily.[2]

(b) Warfarin

A man with erythrocyte aplasia effectively treated with ciclosporin for 18 months, relapsed within a week of starting warfarin. His ciclosporin levels had fallen from a range of 300 to 350 nanograms/ml down to 170 nanograms/ml. He responded well when the ciclosporin dosage was increased from 3 to 7 mg/kg daily, but his prothrombin activity rose from 17% of control to 64% and he needed an increase in the warfarin dosage to achieve satisfactory anticoagulation. The patient was also taking phenobarbital.[3] A woman with angioimmunoblastic T-cell lymphoma on chemotherapy developed a deep vein thrombosis and was therefore treated firstly with heparin and later warfarin. When ciclosporin 300 mg daily was added, her INR decreased by about 40% and she needed a progressive warfarin dosage increase from 18.75 to 27.5 mg per week.[4] Another report briefly says that serum ciclosporin levels rose in a patient given a warfarin derivative.[5]

Mechanism

Acenocoumarol, warfarin and ciclosporin are all metabolised, at least in part, by the cytochrome P450 isoenzyme CYP3A4. It is possible that some competition occurs for metabolism, leading to increased or decreased effects of the anticoagulants and decreased ciclosporin levels.

Importance and management

Information about the interactions of the oral anticoagulants and ciclosporin seems to be limited to these reports. They simply serve to emphasise the need to monitor concurrent use because the outcome is clearly uncertain.

1. Campistol JM, Maragall D, Andreu J. Interaction between cyclosporin A and sintrom. *Nephron* (1989) 53, 291–2.
2. Borrás-Blasco J, Enriquez R, Navarro-Ruiz A, Martinez-Ramirez M, Cabezuelo JB, Gonzalez-Delgado M. Interaction between cyclosporine and acenocoumarol in a patient with nephrotic syndrome. *Clin Nephrol* (2001) 55, 338–40.
3. Snyder DS. Interaction between cyclosporine and warfarin. *Ann Intern Med* (1988) 108, 311.
4. Turri D, Lannitto E, Caracciolo C, Mariani G. Oral anticoagulants and cyclosporin A. *Haematologica* (2000) 85, 893–4.
5. Cockburn I. Cyclosporin A: a clinical evaluation of drug interactions. *Transplant Proc* (1986) 18 (Suppl 5), 50–5.

Ciclosporin + Anticonvulsants

Serum ciclosporin levels are markedly reduced by carbamazepine, phenobarbital or phenytoin. The dosage of ciclosporin may need to be increased two- to fourfold to maintain adequate immunosuppression. Oxcarbazepine may cause a small decrease in ciclosporin levels. Sodium valproate appears not to affect ciclosporin levels but two case reports suggest that it may damage renal grafts and cause hepatotoxicity in patients on ciclosporin.

Clinical evidence

(a) Carbamazepine

The ciclosporin serum levels of a kidney transplant patient fell from 346 to 64 nanograms/ml within 3 days of starting to take carbamazepine 200 mg three times daily. A week later serum levels were down to 37 nanograms/ml. They rose again when the carbamazepine was stopped but fell once more when it was restarted. The ciclosporin dosage was increased to keep the levels within the therapeutic range.[1]

The mean average steady state serum levels of ciclosporin adjusted for dose were less than 50% in a group of 3 children with kidney transplants taking carbamazepine than in 3 other matched patients not taking carbamazepine.[2] Four other individual patients have shown this interaction.[3-5] One needed her ciclosporin dosage to be doubled in order to maintain adequate serum levels while taking carbamazepine 800 mg daily.[3] When the carbamazepine was replaced by sodium valproate in 3 patients, the ciclosporin dosages could be reduced to their previous level.[3,4]

(b) Oxcarbazepine

A kidney transplant patient on ciclosporin 270 mg daily and valproate, gabapentin, prednisone, doxepin, allopurinol, levothyroxine and pravastatin was also given oxcarbazepine. Fourteen days later, with the dose of oxcarbazepine at 750 mg daily, the ciclosporin trough level fell below 100 nanograms/ml and after a further 2 days was 87 nanograms/ml. The ciclosporin dose was increased to 290 mg daily and the oxcarbazepine dose reduced to 600 mg daily. Ciclosporin levels then remained stable above 100 nanograms/ml and seizure frequency was reduced by 95%.[6]

(c) Phenobarbital

A 4-year-old child with a bone marrow transplant who was receiving phenobarbital 50 mg twice daily had serum ciclosporin levels of less than 60 nanograms/ml even after raising the ciclosporin dosage to 18 mg/kg daily. When the phenobarbital dosage was halved and later halved again the trough serum ciclosporin levels rose to 205 nanograms/ml.[7] Another report describes an increase in ciclosporin levels from 512 to 810 nanograms/ml after phenytoin and phenobarbital were replaced by sodium valproate in one patient.[8]

A threefold increase in ciclosporin clearance was seen in another child with a kidney transplant while on phenobarbital.[9] Reductions in ciclosporin levels due to phenobarbital have been described in other patients.[10-13]

(d) Phenytoin

The observation that 5 patients on ciclosporin needed dosage increases while taking phenytoin prompted a further study in 6 healthy subjects. Phenytoin 300 or 400 mg daily reduced the maximum serum ciclosporin levels and AUC 37% (from 1325 to 831 micrograms/l) and 47% respectively.[14]

Other reports describe other patients who needed two- to fourfold increases in their ciclosporin dosages when they were given phenytoin.[15-19]

Another report describes an increase in ciclosporin levels from 512 to 810 nanograms/ml after phenytoin and phenobarbital were replaced by sodium valproate.[8]

A report of severe gingival overgrowth in a kidney transplant patient was attributed to the additive adverse effects of ciclosporin and phenytoin.[20] Ciclosporin was replaced by tacrolimus, which may have fewer oral adverse effects, and almost complete reversal of gingival overgrowth was achieved within 6 months.

(e) Sodium valproate

In 4 cases an interacting anticonvulsant was successfully replaced by sodium valproate,[3,4,8] see *(a)* and *(c)* or *(d)* above. In 2 other patients, sodium valproate caused no change in ciclosporin levels.[13] However, sodium valproate may not always be without problems because interstitial nephritis was suspected in one patient with a renal graft[10] and fatal valproate-induced hepatotoxicity occurred in another.[21]

Mechanism

It is thought that phenytoin,[14,15] carbamazepine[1,2] and phenobarbital[7,11] increase the metabolism of the ciclosporin by the liver (hepatic cytochrome P450 oxygenase system) thereby increasing its loss from the body and lowering the serum levels accordingly. Oxcarbazepine produced only small reductions in ciclosporin levels, but the effect is probably due to weak induction of the cytochrome P450 isoenzyme CYP3A by oxcarbazepine.[6] Phenytoin also possibly reduces the absorption of the ciclosporin.[22]

Importance and management

None of these interactions is extensively documented but all appear to be established and of clinical importance. Serum ciclosporin levels should be well monitored if carbamazepine, phenobarbital or phenytoin are added and the ciclosporin dosage increased appropriately. Information about oxcarbazepine is very limited but small reductions in its dose, together with an increase in ciclosporin dose, may be adequate to control any interaction. However, more study is required before oxcarbazepine can be recommended as a suitable alternative.[6] The effects of the interaction may persist for a week or more after the anticonvulsant is withdrawn. Sodium valproate seems not to alter ciclosporin levels, but the case reports of nephritis and hepatotoxicity suggest some caution is warranted.

1. Lele P, Peterson P, Yang S, Jarell B, Burke JF. Cyclosporine and tegretol — another drug interaction. *Kidney Int* (1985) 27, 344.
2. Cooney GF, Mochon M, Kaiser B, Dunn SP, Goldsmith B. Effects of carbamazepine on cyclosporine metabolism in pediatric renal transplant recipients. *Pharmacotherapy* (1995) 15, 353–6.
3. Hillebrand G, Castro LA, van Scheidt W, Beukelmann D, Land W, Schmidt D. Valproate for epilepsy in renal transplant recipients receiving cyclosporine. *Transplantation* (1987) 43, 915–16.
4. Schofield OMV, Camp RDR, Levene GM. Cyclosporin A in psoriasis: interaction with carbamazepine. *Br J Dermatol* (1990) 122, 425–6.
5. Alvarez JS, Del Castillo JAC, Ortiz MJA. Effect of carbamazepine on ciclosporin blood level. *Nephron* (1991) 58, 235–6.
6. Rösche J, Fröscher W, Abendroth D, Liebel J. Possible oxcarbazepine interaction with cyclosporine serum levels: a single case study. *Clin Neuropharmacol* (2001) 24, 113–16.
7. Carstensen H, Jacobsen N, Dieperink H. Interaction between cyclosporin A and phenobarbitone. *Br J Clin Pharmacol* (1986) 21, 550–1.
8. Noguchi M, Kiuchi C, Akiyama H, Sakamaki H, Onozawa Y. Interaction between cyclosporin A and anticonvulsants. *Bone Marrow Transplant* (1992) 9, 391.
9. Burckart GJ, Venkataramanan R, Starzl T, Ptachcinski JR, Gartner JC, Rosenthal T. Cyclosporine clearance in children following organ transplantation. *J Clin Pharmacol* (1984) 24, 412.
10. Kramer G, Dillmann U, Tettenborn B. Cyclosporine-phenobarbital interaction. *Epilepsia* (1989) 30, 701.
11. Beierle FA, Bailey L. Cyclosporine metabolism impeded/blocked by co-administration of phenobarbital. *Clin Chem* (1989) 35, 1160.
12. Wideman CA. Pharmacokinetic monitoring of cyclosporine. *Transplant Proc* (1983) 15 (Suppl 1), 3168–75.
13. Matsuura T, Akiyama T, Kurita T. Interaction between phenobarbital and ciclosporin following renal transplantation: a case report. *Hinyokika Kiyo* (1990) 36, 447–50.
14. Freeman DJ, Laupacis A, Keown PA, Stiller CR, Carruthers SG. Evaluation of cyclosporin-phenytoin interaction with observations on cyclosporin metabolites. *Br J Clin Pharmacol* (1984) 18, 887–93.
15. Keown PA, Laupacis A, Carruthers G, Stawecki M, Koegler J, McKenzie FN, Wall W, Stiller CR. Interaction between phenytoin and cyclosporine following organ transplantation. *Transplantation* (1984) 38, 304–6.
16. Grigg-Damberger MM, Costanzo-Nordin R, Kelly MA, Bahamon-Dussan JE, Silver M, Zucker MJ, Celesia GG. Phenytoin may compromise efficacy of cyclosporine immunosuppression in cardiac transplant patients. *Epilepsia* (1988) 29, 693.
17. Schmidt H, Naumann R, Jaschonek K, Einsele H, Dopfer R, Ehninger G. Drug interaction between cyclosporin and phenytoin in allogeneic bone marrow transplantation. *Bone Marrow Transplant* (1989) 4, 212–13.
18. Schweitzer EJ, Canafax DM, Gillingham KJ, Najarian JS, Matas AJ. Phenytoin administration in kidney recipients on CSA immunosuppression. *J Am Soc Nephrol* (1991) 2, 816.
19. Castelao AM. Cyclosporine A – drug interactions. In Sunshine I (Ed.) Recent developments in therapeutic drug monitoring and clinical toxicology. *2nd Int Conf Therapeutic Drug Monitoring Toxicology, Barcelona, Spain* (1992) 203–9.
20. Hernandez G, Arriba L, Lucas M, de Andres A. Reduction of severe gingival overgrowth in a kidney transplant patient by replacing cyclosporin A with tacrolimus. *J Periodontol* (2000) 71, 1630–6.
21. Fischman MA, Hull D, Bartus SA, Schweizer RT. Valproate for epilepsy in renal transplant recipients receiving cyclosporine. *Transplantation* (1989) 48, 542.
22. Rowland M, Gupta SK. Cyclosporin-phenytoin interaction: re-evaluation using metabolite data. *Br J Clin Pharmacol* (1987) 24, 329–34.

Ciclosporin + Antidepressants

Four cases of raised ciclosporin levels have been seen in patients taking nefazodone and ciclosporin, one with raised creatinine levels and tremor, and one with raised liver enzymes. One case of increased ciclosporin levels has been seen with fluoxetine and one with fluvoxamine. The serotonin syndrome has been seen in a patient taking ciclosporin and sertraline. Limited evidence suggests that citalopram does not alter ciclosporin levels.

Clinical evidence, mechanism, importance and management

(a) Nefazodone

A kidney transplant patient had a 70% rise in trough serum ciclosporin levels within 3 days of starting to take nefazodone 25 mg twice daily. This was attributed to inhibition by nefazodone of the cytochrome P450 isoenzyme CYP3A4, by which ciclosporin is metabolised.[1] Another kidney transplant patient had a two- to threefold rise in ciclosporin levels associated with raised creatinine levels and marked generalised tremors after starting nefazodone 100 mg twice daily. The patient was eventually stabilised on a 50% lower dose of ciclosporin.[2] Similarly, a cardiac transplant patient on ciclosporin had a tenfold increase in ciclosporin levels shortly after the addition of nefazodone 150 mg twice daily. Levels returned to baseline over 6 days after nefazodone was stopped.[3] A patient taking nefazodone developed significantly raised AST and ALT one month after kidney transplantation. His ciclosporin level was high, at 614 nanograms/ml, and both ciclosporin and nefazodone were stopped. He had previously taken nefazodone uneventfully, and subsequently took ciclosporin uneventfully, so the raised liver enzymes were attributed to a pharmacokinetic interaction between the two drugs.[4]

Although the evidence is limited, it appears that nefazodone can cause a marked rise in ciclosporin levels, with an increase in adverse effects. Alternative antidepressants should probably be used, or concurrent therapy very well monitored.

(b) SSRIs

In 5 transplant patients the pharmacokinetics of ciclosporin were not significantly affected by **citalopram** 10 to 20 mg daily.[5]

The serum ciclosporin levels of a heart transplant patient were doubled by **fluoxetine** 20 mg daily for 10 days. They fell the ciclosporin dosage was reduced and needed to be increased again when the **fluoxetine** was stopped.[6]

A patient had increased ciclosporin and serum creatinine levels and fine tremor 2 weeks after starting **fluvoxamine** 100 mg daily, and the ciclosporin dosage was subsequently reduced by 33%.[2]

A 53-year-old man taking ciclosporin following a renal transplant developed the serotonin syndrome 5 days after starting to take **sertraline** 50 mg daily. Ciclosporin is known to increase serotonin turnover within the brain, and so the reaction was attributed to an interaction between **sertraline** and ciclosporin.[7] One report briefly mentions that a patient on ciclosporin had their antidepressant medication switched from nefazodone to **sertraline**, because **sertraline** did not affect ciclosporin levels.[3]

Information is limited, and the general importance of the cases of increased ciclosporin levels with **fluoxetine** and **fluvoxamine** is uncertain. **Citalopram**, and possibly **sertraline**, do not appear to alter ciclosporin levels. Serotonin syndrome is a rare adverse effect, usually associated with the use of more than one serotonergic drug (see 'the serotonin syndrome', (p.9)). The general importance of the case with **sertraline** and ciclosporin is unclear, but bear it in mind in the event of an unexpected response to treatment with any SSRI and ciclosporin.

1. Helms-Smith KM, Curtis SL, Hatton RC. Apparent interaction between nefazodone and cyclosporine. *Ann Intern Med* (1996) 125, 424.
2. Vella JP, Sayegh MH. Interactions between cyclosporine and newer antidepressant medications. *Am J Kidney Dis* (1998) 31, 320–3.
3. Wright DH, Lake KD, Bruhn PS, Emery RW. Nefazodone and cyclosporine drug-drug interaction. *J Heart Lung Transplant* (1999) 18, 913–15.
4. Garton T, Nefazodone and CYP450 3A4 interactions with cyclosporine and tacrolimus. *Transplantation* (2002) 74, 745.
5. Liston HL, Markowitz JS, Hunt N, DeVane CL, Boulton DW, Ashcraft E. Lack of citalopram effect on the pharmacokinetics of cyclosporine. *Psychosomatics* (2001) 42, 370–2.
6. Horton RC, Bonser RS. Interaction between cyclosporin and fluoxetine. *BMJ* (1995) 311, 422.
7. Wong EH, Chan NN, Sze KH, Or KH. Serotonin syndrome in a renal transplant patient. *J R Soc Med* (2002) 95, 304–5.

Ciclosporin + Antidiabetics

Some preliminary evidence suggests that glibenclamide (glyburide) can raise serum ciclosporin levels to a moderate extent. Glipizide caused about a twofold increase in ciclosporin levels in 2 patients, but no change was noted in a study in 11 patients.

Clinical evidence, mechanism, importance and management

A review of 6 post-transplant diabetic patients on ciclosporin found that their steady-state plasma ciclosporin levels rose by 57% when they were given **glibenclamide (glyburide)**. Hepatic and renal function were unchanged. The reason for this reaction is not known, but it is suggested that **glibenclamide** possibly inhibits the cytochrome P450 isoenzyme CYP3A4, the major isoenzyme involved in the metabolism of ciclosporin, resulting in a reduction in its clearance.[1]

The ciclosporin levels of 2 patients were more than doubled, and they needed reductions of 20 to 30% in their ciclosporin dosage when they were also given **glipizide** 10 mg daily.[2] In contrast, a study in 11 post-transplant diabetic patients found no significant alterations in ciclosporin pharmacokinetics when **glipizide** was given.[3]

This interaction is unconfirmed and of uncertain clinical significance. However, note that one of the rare adverse effects of ciclosporin is hyperglycaemia. There is insufficient evidence to recommend increased monitoring, but be aware of the potential for an interaction in the case of an unexpected response to treatment. Information about other sulphonylureas appears not to be available.

1. Islam SI, Masuda QN, Bolaji OO, Shaheen FM, Sheikh IA. Possible interaction between cyclosporine and glibenclamide in posttransplant diabetic patients. *Ther Drug Monit* (1996) 18, 624–6.
2. Chidester PD, Connito DJ. Interaction between glipizide and cyclosporine: report of two cases. *Transplant Proc* (1993) 25, 2136–7.
3. Sagedal S, Åsberg A, Hartmann A, Bergan S, Berg KJ. Glipizide treatment of post-transplant diabetes does not interfere with cyclosporine pharmacokinetics in renal allograft recipients. *Clin Transplant* (1998) 12, 553–6.

Ciclosporin + Antiretrovirals

The ciclosporin levels of one patient dramatically decreased following the addition of efavirenz, while the ciclosporin levels of another patient dramatically increased following the addition of saquinavir.

Clinical evidence

(a) Efavirenz

A patient was diagnosed as HIV+ 3 years after a kidney transplant, for which he was taking ciclosporin. He was started on efavirenz 600 mg daily, lamivudine and zidovudine, and 7 days later, after an initial rise, his ciclosporin level dropped from about 203 to 80 nanograms/ml. A nadir of 50 nanograms/ml was reached one month later.[1]

(b) Saquinavir

An HIV+ patient taking lamivudine and zidovudine, and ciclosporin for a kidney transplant, was started on saquinavir 1.2 g three times daily. Within 2 days he started to complain of fatigue, headache and gastrointestinal discomfort. On investigation his ciclosporin level was found to have risen from a range of 150 to 200 nanograms/ml up to 580 nanograms/ml, and his saquinavir AUC was increased 4.3-fold (by comparison to subjects not on ciclosporin). His ciclosporin dose was reduced from 150 mg twice daily to 75 mg twice daily, and his saquinavir dose was reduced to 600 mg three times daily, which resulted in ciclosporin levels similar to those achieved previously.[2]

Mechanism

Efavirenz induces[1] and saquinavir inhibits[2] the cytochrome P450 isoenzyme CYP3A4. Ciclosporin is extensively metabolised by CYP3A4, so any inhibition or induction of this isoenzyme is likely to increase or decrease ciclosporin levels respectively. Both ciclosporin and saquinavir are substrates for P-glycoprotein, which may explain the raised saquinavir levels.[2]

Importance and management

These appear to be the only reports of an interaction between antiretroviral drugs and ciclosporin, but what happens is in line with the known pharmacokinetic effects of these drugs. It would therefore seem prudent to monitor ciclosporin levels if efavirenz or saquinavir (and any other **protease inhibitor**) is added, withdrawn or the dose altered.

1. Tseng A, Nguyen ME, Cardella C, Humar A, Conly J. Probable interaction between efavirenz and cyclosporine. *AIDS* (2002) 16, 505–6.
2. Brinkman K, Huysmans F, Burger DM. Pharmacokinetic interaction between saquinavir and cyclosporine. *Ann Intern Med* (1998) 129, 914–15.

Ciclosporin + Azoles

The evidence suggests that all the azole antifungals can raise ciclosporin levels to a greater or lesser degree. Ketoconazole may cause rises of five- to tenfold, while itraconazole, fluconazole and voriconazole may cause rises of two- to threefold. A case report suggests that miconazole interacts similarly, while only small elevations have been reported with posaconazole. Rhabdomyolysis has been reported with the combination of ciclosporin and itraconazole, but two of these cases were complicated by the presence of statins. The antifungal activity of fluconazole may be enhanced by ciclosporin.

Clinical evidence

(a) Fluconazole

Fluconazole 200 mg daily for 14 days roughly doubled the trough serum ciclosporin levels of 8 kidney transplant patients, from 27 to 58 nanograms/ml. The AUC increased 1.8-fold but serum creatinine levels were unchanged.[1,2]

Other reports describe two- to threefold rises in serum ciclosporin levels in kidney transplant patients within 6 to 11 days of starting treatment with fluconazole 100 to 200 mg daily.[3-8] One patient developed nephrotoxicity, which resolved when the dosages of both drugs were reduced.[9]

In contrast, some patients have had little or no changes in serum ciclosporin or creatinine levels when fluconazole was given.[8,10-15] This may have been because the interaction is dose-dependent.[14,16] One study found a lack of interaction in females and African-American patients, suggesting that gender and ethnicity may also be factors.[17] Another study found that there was only a 20% increase in ciclosporin levels when intravenous ciclosporin was given with high-dose intravenous fluconazole, which was not considered clinically relevant.[18]

An *in vitro* study suggests that the activity of fluconazole against *Candida albicans* may be enhanced by ciclosporin.[19]

(b) Itraconazole

An average 56% reduction (range 33 to 84%) in the ciclosporin dosages in 4 heart-lung, 2 heart and one lung transplant patient were needed when itraconazole [dosage not stated] was given. Serum creatinine levels rose temporarily until the ciclosporin dosage had been readjusted.[20] Another report briefly mentions that the ciclosporin dosage had to be reduced by 50 to 80% when itraconazole was used.[21] Two- to threefold rises in ciclosporin levels were seen in another 2 patients given itraconazole 200 mg daily,[22,23] and in one case the raised levels persisted for more than 4 weeks after the itraconazole was stopped.[23] Intravenous itraconazole 200 mg twice daily for 2 days then 200 mg daily caused a twofold increase in the levels of intravenous ciclosporin in 2 patients.[24] Another report mentions that unspecified reductions were needed in the dose of ciclosporin after the addition of itraconazole.[25] Enhanced itraconazole absorption in the presence of a carbonated drink that increased stomach acidity was found to allow decreases in ciclosporin dose and increases in its dose interval.[26]

These reports contrast with another describing 14 bone marrow transplant patients taking ciclosporin. Those given itraconazole 100 mg twice daily had no significant changes in ciclosporin or creatinine serum levels.[27] Another patient required only a 10% reduction in ciclosporin dose when given itraconazole 400 mg daily for 40 days.[8]

Rhabdomyolysis has been reported in 3 lung transplant patients when itraconazole was used in combination with ciclosporin, but in two of these cases the concurrent use of simvastatin may have been a factor[21,28] (see also 'Statins + Azoles', p.831).

(c) Ketoconazole

Ketoconazole 200 mg daily caused a marked and rapid rise in the serum ciclosporin levels of 36 renal transplant patients. On the basis of experience with previous patients, the ciclosporin dosage was reduced by 70% when ketoconazole was started, and after a year the dosage reduction was 85% (from 420 mg to 66 mg daily). Minimal nephrotoxicity was seen.[29-31]

Other reports[8,32-46] describe essentially similar rises in serum ciclosporin levels during the use of ketoconazole. The effects of ketoconazole on ciclosporin were found to be slightly increased (from 80 to 85%) when diltiazem was also given.[47] Ketoconazole 2% cream has been found not interact with ciclosporin 1 mg/kg daily in the treatment of contact allergic dermatitis and the ciclosporin dosage does not need to be reduced.[48] Impaired glucose tolerance has been attributed to the use of ketoconazole and ciclosporin in one patient.[49]

(d) Miconazole

A single case report describes a rise of about 65% in ciclosporin serum levels within 3 days of starting intravenous miconazole 1 g every 8 hours. Ciclosporin levels rose again during subsequent treatment with miconazole.[50]

(e) Posaconazole

Posaconazole 200 mg daily was given to 4 heart transplant patients on stable doses of ciclosporin. Three of the 4 required dose reductions of between 14.3 and 26.8% to maintain ciclosporin levels.[51] Although these dosage adjustments were considered low, they do indicate that posaconazole interacts in a similar manner to the other azoles.

(f) Voriconazole

In a placebo-controlled crossover study 14 kidney transplant patients on stable doses of ciclosporin were given voriconazole 200 mg every 12 hours for 15 doses. Of the 14 patients, 7 discontinued treatment during the voriconazole phase due to adverse effects, 4 due to raised ciclosporin levels (mean 2.48-fold), one due to raised liver function, one due to asthenia, dyspnoea and oedema, and one due to an underlying condition unrelated to the voriconazole. In the remaining 7 patients voriconazole caused 1.7-fold increases in the ciclosporin AUC.[52]

Mechanism

In vitro studies show that these azole antifungals inhibit the metabolism of ciclosporin by human liver microsomal enzymes, ketoconazole being the most potent.[53,54] As a result the loss of the ciclosporin from the body is reduced and its serum levels rise. Fluconazole and ketoconazole also appear to inhibit the metabolism of ciclosporin by the gut wall.[18,42]

In the cases of rhabdomyolysis, raised ciclosporin levels may have resulted in a direct toxic effect on muscle cells.[28]

Importance and management

The interaction between ciclosporin and ketoconazole is very well established and clinically important. Ciclosporin serum levels rise rapidly and sharply, but they can be controlled by reducing the ciclosporin dosage by about 70 to 80%[8,25,29,34,46] thereby preventing kidney damage (and also saving costs). A ciclosporin dosage reduction of 68 to 89% was required over a 13-month period in one study, with no adverse changes in immunosuppressive activity, resulting in a total cost saving of about 65% because of the need to follow up more frequently and the cost of the ketoconazole.[29,30] Other studies have suggested that this interaction can be exploited to make cost savings.[43,44,46] Reviews of the pros and cons of concurrent use have been published.[31,55] Ketoconazole may possibly have a kidney-protective effect.[29,30] A study in renal transplant patients suggested that variability in absorption and in the response to metabolic inhibition by ketoconazole made the ciclosporin blood level response difficult to predict and monitor.[56] There are also other confounding factors. For example, a patient who was given ketoconazole to increase ciclosporin levels was subsequently given famotidine. The famotidine raised gastric pH, which resulted in a reduction in the ketoconazole absorption, and the ciclosporin levels consequently fell.[57]

Information about ciclosporin with fluconazole, itraconazole or miconazole is less extensive but concurrent use should be closely monitored, being alert for the need to reduce the ciclosporin dosage, in some cases by up to 50% or more, although some patients may demonstrate no significant changes at all. There is also some evidence that in the case of fluconazole, the interaction may possibly depend on its dosage,[14] gender and ethnicity,[17] and the route of ciclosporin administration.[18] Similarly, the makers of voriconazole suggest that the dose of ciclosporin should be halved when initiating voriconazole, and that ciclosporin levels should be carefully monitored during voriconazole treatment. The ciclosporin dose should be increased again as necessary if voriconazole is withdrawn.[58,59]

Additional caution is required where ciclosporin and azoles are used in patients taking statins, and either ciclosporin dose reduction[21] or replacement of ciclosporin with tacrolimus[28] has been recommended.

1. Canafax DM, Graves NM, Hilligoss DM, Carleton BC, Gardner MJ, Matas AJ. Interaction between cyclosporine and fluconazole in renal allograft recipients. *Transplantation* (1991) 51, 1014–8.
2. Canafax DM, Graves NM, Hilligoss DM, Carleton BC, Gardner MJ, Matas AJ. Increased cyclosporine levels as a result of simultaneous fluconazole and cyclosporine therapy in renal transplant recipients: a double-blind, randomized pharmacokinetic and safety study. *Transplant Proc* (1991) 23, 1041–2.
3. Torregrosa V, De la Torre M, Campistol JM, Oppenheimer F, Ricart MJ, Vilardell J, Andreu J. Interaction of fluconazole with ciclosporin A. *Nephron* (1992) 60, 125–6.
4. Sugar AM, Saunders C, Idelson BA, Bernard DB. Interaction of fluconazole and cyclosporine. *Ann Intern Med* (1989) 110, 844.
5. Barbara JAJ, Clarkson AR, LaBrooy J, McNeil JD, Woodroffe AJ. Candida albicans arthritis in a renal allograft recipient with an interaction between cyclosporin and fluconazole. *Nephrol Dial Transplant* (1993) 8, 263–6.
6. Tett S, Carey D, Lee H-S. Drug interactions with fluconazole. *Med J Aust* (1992) 156, 365.
7. Foradori A, Mezzano S, Videla C, Pefaur J, Elberg A. Modification of the pharmacokinetics of cyclosporine A and metabolites by the concomitant use of Neoral and diltiazem or ketoconazol in stable adult kidney transplants. *Transplant Proc* (1998) 30, 1685–7.
8. Koselj M, Bren A, Kandus A, Kovac D. Drug interactions between cyclosporine and rifampicin, erythromycin, and azoles in kidney recipients with opportunistic infections. *Transplant Proc* (1994) 26, 2823–4.
9. Collignon P, Hurley B, Mitchell D. Interaction of fluconazole with cyclosporin. *Lancet* (1989) i, 1262.
10. Ehninger G, Jaschonek K, Schuler U, Krüger HU. Interaction of fluconazole with cyclosporin. *Lancet* (1989) ii, 104–5.
11. Krüger HU, Schuler U, Zimmermann R, Ehninger G. Absence of significant interaction of fluconazole with cyclosporin. *J Antimicrob Chemother* (1989) 24, 781–6.
12. Conti DJ, Tolkoff-Rubin NE, Baker GP, Doran M, Cosimi AB, Delmonico F, Auchincloss H, Russell PS, Rubin RH. Successful treatment of invasive fungal infection with fluconazole in organ transplant recipients. *Transplantation* (1989) 48, 692–5.
13. Rubin RH, Debruin MF, Knirsch AK. Fluconazole therapy for patients with serious *Candida* infections who have failed standard therapies. *Intersci Conf Antimicrob Agents Chemother* (1989), 112.
14. López-Gil JA. Fluconazole-cyclosporine interaction: a dose-dependent effect? *Ann Pharmacother* (1993) 27, 427–30.
15. Lumbreras C, Cuervas-Mons V, Jara P, del Palacio A, Turrión VS, Barrios C, Moreno E, Noriega AR, Paya CV. Randomized trial of fluconazole versus nystatin for the prophylaxis of *Candida* infection following liver transplantation. *J Infect Dis* (1996) 174, 583–8.
16. Sud K, Singh B, Krishna VS, Thennarasu K, Kohli HS, Jha V, Gupta KL, Sakhuja V. Unpredictable cyclosporin-fluconazole interaction in renal transplant recipients. *Nephrol Dial Transplant* (1999) 14, 1698–1703.
17. Mathis AS, DiRenzo T, Friedman GS, Kaplan B, Adamson R. Sex and ethnicity may chiefly influence the interaction of fluconazole with calcineurin inhibitors. *Transplantation* (2001) 71, 1069–75.
18. Osowski CL, Dix SP, Lin LS, Mullins RE, Geller RB, Wingard JR. Evaluation of the drug interaction between intravenous high-dose fluconazole and cyclosporine or tacrolimus in bone marrow transplant patients. *Transplantation* (1996) 61, 1268–72.
19. Marchetti O, Moreillon P, Glauser MP, Bille J, Sanglard D. Potent synergism of the combination of fluconazole and cyclosporine in *Candida albicans*. *Antimicrob Agents Chemother* (2000) 44, 2373–81.
20. Kramer MR, Marshall SE, Denning DW, Keogh AM, Tucker RM, Galgiani JN, Lewiston NJ, Stevens DA, Theodore J. Cyclosporine and itraconazole interaction in heart and lung transplant recipients. *Ann Intern Med* (1990) 113, 327–9.
21. Malouf MA, Bicknell M, Glanville AR. Rhabdomyolysis after lung transplantation. *Aust N Z J Med* (1997) 27, 186.
22. Kwan JT C, Foxall PJD, Davidson DGC, Bending MR, Eisinger AJ. Interaction of cyclosporin and itraconazole. *Lancet* (1987) ii, 282.
23. Trenk D, Brett W, Jähnchen E, Birnbaum D. Time course of cyclosporin/itraconazole interaction. *Lancet* (1987) ii, 1335–6.
24. Leather HL, Boyette R, Wingard JR. Evaluation of the pharmacokinetic drug interaction between intravenous itraconazole and IV tacrolimus or IV cyclosporin in allogeneic bone marrow transplant patients. *Blood* (2000) 96, 390a.
25. Faggian G, Livi U, Bortolotti U, Mazzucco A, Stellin G, Chiominto B, Viviani MA, Gallucci V. Itraconazole therapy for acute invasive pulmonary aspergillosis in heart transplantation. *Transplant Proc* (1989) 21, 2506–7.
26. Wimberley SL, Haug MT, Shermock K, Maurer J, Mehta A, Schilz R, Gordon S. Enhanced cyclosporine (CSA)-itraconazole (ICZ) interaction with cola in lung transplant recipients (LTR). *Intersci Conf Antimicrob Agents Chemother* (1999) 39, 4.
27. Novakova I, Donnelly P, de Witte T, de Pauw B, Boezeman J, Veltman G. Itraconazole and cyclosporin nephrotoxicity. *Lancet* (1987) ii, 920–1.
28. Cohen E, Kramer MR, Maoz C, Ben-Dayan D, Garty M. Cyclosporin drug-interaction-induced rhabdomyolysis. A report of two cases in lung transplant recipients. *Transplantation* (2000) 70, 119–22.
29. First MR, Schroeder TJ, Weiskittel P, Myre SA, Alexander JW, Pesce AJ. Concomitant administration of cyclosporin and ketoconazole in renal transplant patients. *Lancet* (1989) ii, 1198–1201.
30. First MR, Schroeder TJ, Alexander JW, Stephens GW, Weiskittel P, Myre SA, Pesce AJ. Cyclosporine dose reduction by ketoconazole administration in renal transplant recipients. *Transplantation* (1991) 51, 365–70.
31. First MR, Schroeder TJ, Michael A, Hariharan S, Weiskittel P, Alexander JW. Cyclosporin-ketoconazole interaction. Long-term follow-up and preliminary results of a randomized trial. *Transplantation* (1993) 55, 1000–4.
32. Ferguson RM, Sutherland DER, Simmons RL, Najarian JS. Ketoconazole, cyclosporin metabolism and renal transplantation. *Lancet* (1982) ii, 882–3.
33. Morgenstern GR, Powles R, Robinson B, McElwain TJ. Cyclosporin interaction with ketoconazole and melphalan. *Lancet* (1982) ii, 1342.
34. Dieperink H, Møller J. Ketoconazole and cyclosporin. *Lancet* (1982) ii, 1217.
35. Gluckman E, Devergie A, Lokiec F, Poirier O, Baumelou A. Nephrotoxicity of cyclosporin in bone-marrow transplantation. *Lancet* (1981) ii, 144–5.
36. Shepard JH, Canafax DM, Simmons RL, Najarian JS. Cyclosporine-ketoconazole: a potentially dangerous drug-drug interaction. *Clin Pharm* (1986) 5, 468.
37. Schroeder TJ, Melvin DB, Clardy CW, Wadhwa NK, Myre SA, Reising JM, Wolf RK, Collins JA, Pesce AJ, First MR. Use of cyclosporine and ketoconazole without nephrotoxicity in two heart transplant recipients. *J Heart Transplant* (1987) 6, 84–9.
38. Girardet RE, Melo JC, Fox MS, Whalen C, Lusk R, Masri ZH, Lansing AM. Concomitant administration of cyclosporine and ketoconazole for three and a half years in one heart transplant recipient. *Transplantation* (1989) 48, 887–90.
39. Schroeder TJ, Weiskittel P, Pesce AJ, Myre SA, Alexander JW, First MR. Cyclosporine pharmacokinetics with concomitant ketoconazole therapy. *Clin Chem* (1989) 35, 1176–7.
40. Charles BG, Ravenscroft PJ, Rigby RJ. The ketoconazole-cyclosporin interaction in an elderly renal transplant patient. *Aust N Z J Med* (1989) 19, 292–3.
41. Veraldi S, Menni S. Severe gingival hyperplasia following cyclosporin and ketoconazole therapy. *Int J Dermatol* (1988) 27, 730.
42. Gomez DY, Wacher VJ, Tomlanovich SJ, Hebert MF, Benet LZ. The effects of ketoconazole on the intestinal metabolism and bioavailability of cyclosporine. *Clin Pharmacol Ther* (1995) 58, 15–9.

43. Kriett JM, Jahansouz F, Smith CM, Hayden AM, Fox KJ, Kapelanski DP, Jamieson SW. The cyclosporine-ketoconazole interaction:safety and economic impact in lung transplantation. *J Heart Lung Transplant* (1994) 13, S43.
44. Keogh A, Spratt P, McCosker C, Macdonald P, Mundy J, Kaan A. Ketoconazole to reduce the need for cyclosporine after cardiac transplantation. *N Engl J Med* (1995) 333, 628–33.
45. McLachlan AJ, Tett SE. Effect of metabolic inhibitors on cyclosporine pharmacokinetics using a population approach. *Ther Drug Monit* (1998) 20, 390–5.
46. Butman SM, Wild JC, Nolan PE, Fagan TC, Finley PR, Hicks MJ, Mackie MJ, Copeland JG. Prospective study of the safety and financial benefit of ketoconazole as adjunctive therapy to cyclosporine after heart transplantation. *J Heart Lung Transplant* (1991) 10, 351–8.
47. Hariharan S, Schroeder T, First MR. The effect of diltiazem on cyclosporin A (CYA) bioavailability in patients treated with CYA and ketoconazole. *J Am Soc Nephrol* (1992) 3, 861.
48. McLelland J, Shuster S. Topical ketoconazole does not potentiate oral cyclosporin A in allergic contact dermatitis. *Acta Derm Venereol (Stockh)* (1992) 72, 285.
49. Kiss D, Thiel G. Glucose-intolerance and prolonged renal-transplant insufficiency due to ketoconazole-cyclosporin A interaction. *Clin Nephrol* (1990) 33, 207–8.
50. Horton CM, Freeman CD, Nolan PE, Copeland JG. Cyclosporine interactions with miconazole and other azole-antimycotics: a case report and review of the literature. *J Heart Lung Transplant* (1992) 11, 1127–32.
51. Courtney RD, Statkevich P, Laughlin M, Lim J, Clement RP, Batra VK. Effect of posaconazole on the pharmacokinetics of cyclosporine. *Intersci Conf Antimicrob Agents Chemother* (2001) 41, 4.
52. Romero AJ, Le Pogamp P, Nilsson L-G, Wood N. Effect of voriconazole on the pharmacokinetics of cyclosporine in renal transplant patients. *Clin Pharmacol Ther* (2002) 71, 226–34.
53. Back DJ, Tjia JF. Comparative effects of the antimycotic drugs ketoconazole, fluconazole, itraconazole and terbinafine on the metabolism of cyclosporin by human liver microsomes. *Br J Clin Pharmacol* (1991) 32, 624–6.
54. Omar G, Whiting PH, Hawksworth GM, Humphrey MJ, Burke MD. Ketoconazole and fluconazole inhibition of the metabolism of cyclosporin A by human liver in vitro. *Ther Drug Monit* (1997) 19, 436–45.
55. Albengres E, Tillement JP. Cyclosporin and ketoconazole, drug interaction or therapeutic association? *Int J Clin Pharmacol Ther Toxicol* (1992) 30, 555–70.
56. Sorenson AL, Lovdahl M, Hewitt JM, Granger DK, Almond PS, Russlie HQ, Barber D, Matas AJ, Canafax DM. Effects of ketoconazole on cyclosporine metabolism in renal allograft recipients. *Transplant Proc* (1994) 26, 2822.
57. Karlix JL, Cheng MA, Brunson ME, Ramos EL, Howard RJ, Peterson JC, Patton PR, Pfaff WW. Decreased cyclosporine concentrations with the addition of an H_2-receptor antagonist in a patient on ketoconazole. *Transplantation* (1993) 56, 1554–5.
58. VFEND (Voriconazole). Pfizer Ltd. UK Summary of product characteristics, March 2005.
59. VFEND (Voriconazole). Pfizer Ltd. US Prescribing information, March 2005.

Ciclosporin + Benzbromarone

Benzbromarone does not interact adversely with ciclosporin.

Clinical evidence, mechanism, importance and management

Twenty-five kidney transplant patients on ciclosporin were given benzbromarone 100 mg daily to treat hyperuricaemia. The plasma uric acid levels decreased from 579 to 313 micromol/l and the 24-hour urinary uric acid secretion rose from 2082 to 3233 micromol after 4 weeks' treatment. The plasma uric acid levels normalised in 21 of the patients who had creatinine clearances of over 25 ml/minute. No significant adverse effects developed and the ciclosporin serum levels remained unchanged. The authors of the report emphasise the advantages of benzbromarone over allopurinol because of its efficacy, lack of significant adverse effects and because, unlike allopurinol, it does not interact with azathioprine, which often accompanies ciclosporin treatment.[1]

1. Zürcher RM, Bock HA, Thiel G. Excellent uricosuric efficacy of benzbromarone in cyclosporin-A-treated renal transplant patients. A prospective study. *Nephrol Dial Transplant* (1994) 9, 548–51.

Ciclosporin + Beta-blockers

There is evidence that when carvedilol is substituted for atenolol a small to moderate rise in serum ciclosporin levels occurs.

Clinical evidence, mechanism, importance and management

A study in 21 kidney transplant patients found that when **atenolol** was gradually replaced by **carvedilol** in a stepwise manner, starting with **carvedilol** 6.25 mg daily, gradually increasing to 50 mg daily, the ciclosporin dosage had to be gradually reduced. At 90 days the daily ciclosporin dosage had been reduced by 20% (from 3.7 to 3 mg/kg) to maintain levels within the therapeutic range but considerable inter-individual variations were seen.[1] The reason for this interaction is not understood. Information about other beta-blockers seems to be lacking, but be alert for this interaction if **carvedilol** is used.

1. Kaijser M, Johnsson C, Zezina L, Backman U, Dimeny E, Fellstrom B. Elevation of cyclosporin A blood levels during carvedilol treatment in renal transplant patients. *Clin Transplant* (1997) 11, 577–81.

Ciclosporin + Bifendate

Two case reports show that bifendate can cause a gradual fall in the serum levels of ciclosporin.

Clinical evidence, mechanism, importance and management

Two kidney transplant patients were successfully treated with ciclosporin and prednisolone for 30 and 36 months respectively. When they were started on bifendate 75 mg daily for the treatment of chronic hepatitis, both of them had a gradual fall in their trough serum ciclosporin levels. The ciclosporin levels of the first patient fell from 97.7 to 78 nanograms/ml at 4 weeks and to 49 nanograms/ml at 6 weeks. The other patient had a fall from 127.5 to 70.5 nanograms/ml at 8 weeks and to 45 nanograms/ml at 16 weeks. The reasons are not understood. The ciclosporin dosages remained unchanged throughout, and despite the low serum levels that occurred, no graft rejection was seen. When the bifendate was stopped, the ciclosporin levels gradually climbed again, at about the same rate as their decline, to about their former levels.[1] There would seem to be no clear reason for avoiding concurrent use but it would be prudent to monitor the outcome, being alert for the need to increase the ciclosporin dosage. Bifendate is derived from *Schisandra* and is a 'hepatonic' preparation with actions that are not understood.

1. Kim YS, Kim DH, Kim DO, Lee BK, Kim KW, Park JN, Lee JC, Choi YS, Rim H. The effect of Diphenyl-dimethyl-dicarboxylate on cyclosporine-A blood level in kidney transplants with chronic hepatitis. *Korean J Intern Med* (1997) 12, 67–9.

Ciclosporin + Bile acids or Ursodeoxycholic acid (Ursodiol)

Ursodeoxycholic acid unpredictably increases the absorption and raises the serum levels of ciclosporin in some but not all patients. Bile acids (cholic/dehydrocholic acids) appear not to interact with ciclosporin.

Clinical evidence

(a) Bile acids (Cholic/dehydrocholic acids)

Eleven healthy subjects were given a single oral dose of ciclosporin on three occasions: while fasting, with breakfast, and with breakfast plus bile acid tablets (**cholic acid** 400 mg, **dehydrocholic acid** 100 mg). The mean ciclosporin AUCs were 7283, 7453 and 9078 nanograms/ml respectively, indicating that the bile acids increased the absorption of the ciclosporin by 22%. However, a related study in 19 transplant patients found that their 12-hour trough ciclosporin serum levels were unchanged by the concurrent use of this dosage of bile acids over an 8-day period.[1]

(b) Ursodeoxycholic acid

A man who had previously had his entire ileum removed and about 1 metre of the residual jejunum anastomosed to the transverse colon, had a heart transplant. When given ursodeoxycholic acid 1 to 2 g daily it was possible to reduce his ciclosporin dosage from 1.6 to 1.2 g daily, but later when the ursodeoxycholic acid was stopped his ciclosporin serum levels became subtherapeutic and severe acute rejection developed. When ursodeoxycholic acid was restarted the ciclosporin levels rose once again, and the ciclosporin AUC was increased by over 200%.[2] The trough serum ciclosporin levels of a patient with chronic active hepatitis C increased from 150 to 500 nanograms/ml when he was treated with ursodeoxycholic acid, and it was necessary to halve his daily ciclosporin dosage to keep the ciclosporin levels at 150 nanograms/ml.[3]

In contrast, a study in 7 liver transplant patients found no statistically significant changes in mean ciclosporin levels when a single 600-mg dose of ursodeoxycholic acid was given at the same time as the ciclosporin.[4] Yet another study in 12 liver transplant patients, 6 of whom were cholestatic, found that after a single dose of ursodeoxycholic acid the ciclosporin was absorbed more rapidly in 8 patients but the mean 24-hour AUC was not significantly changed, although 7 patients had some rise. There was no consistent improvement in the ciclosporin pharmacokinetics in the cholestatic patients.[5]

Mechanism

When an interaction occurs it is thought to do so because the ursodeoxycholic acid improves micellation of the oil-containing oral ciclosporin formulation so that its absorption is increased.[2]

Importance and management

Information is limited but bile acids do not apparently interact with ciclosporin, while the interaction with ursodeoxycholic acid appears to be uncertain and unpredictable. It would therefore be prudent to monitor the effects of adding or stopping ursodeoxycholic acid in any patient on ciclosporin, being alert for the need to adjust the ciclosporin dosage. More study is needed.

1. Lindholm A, Henricsson S, Dahlqvist R. The effect of food and bile acid administration on the relative bioavailability of cyclosporin. *Br J Clin Pharmacol* (1990) 29, 541–8.
2. Gutzler F, Zimmermann R, Ring GH, Sauer P, Stiehl A. Ursodeoxycholic acid enhances the absorption of cyclosporine in a heart transplant patient with short bowel syndrome. *Transplant Proc* (1992) 24, 2620–1.
3. Sharobeem R, Bacq Y, Furet Y, Grezard O, Nivet H, Breteau M, Bagros P, Lebranchu Y. Cyclosporine A and ursodeoxycholic acid interaction. *Clin Transplant* (1993) 7, 223–6.
4. Maboundou CW, Paintaud G, Vanlemmens C, Magnette J, Bresson-Hadni S, Mantion G, Miguet JP, Bechtel PR. A single dose of ursodiol does not affect cyclosporine absorption in liver transplant patients. *Eur J Clin Pharmacol* (1996) 50, 335–7.
5. al-Quaiz MN, O'Grady JG, Tredger JM, Williams R. Variable effect of ursodeoxycholic acid on cyclosporin absorption after orthotopic liver transplantation. *Transpl Int* (1994) 7, 190–4.

Ciclosporin + Bosentan

Bosentan modestly decreases ciclosporin levels, and ciclosporin increases bosentan levels. The maker of bosentan contraindicates the combination, because of the possible increased risk of liver toxicity.

Clinical evidence, mechanism, importance and management

In a study designed to assess the effects of bosentan on ciclosporin renal toxicity, 7 healthy subjects were given bosentan 500 mg and ciclosporin 300 mg, both twice daily, for 7 days. Bosentan did maintain renal plasma flow, which is markedly decreased by ciclosporin. However, bosentan was calculated to have reduced the AUC of ciclosporin by about 50%. In addition, bosentan had no effect on the ciclosporin-induced rise in blood pressure, and headache, nausea, and vomiting were a problem with the combination. Moreover, the steady-state AUC of bosentan was raised 1.7-fold when compared with the AUC of a single dose of bosentan.[1] It should be noted that bosentan induces its own metabolism, and after 7 days plasma levels are about 50 to 65% of those seen after a single dose.[2] Therefore, the effect of ciclosporin on the bosentan AUC may be twice those described in this study (i.e. up to a fourfold increase in the AUC of bosentan). The makers of bosentan say that when bosentan is given with ciclosporin its plasma levels were markedly raised (30-fold after a single dose and three- to fourfold at steady state). They also list ciclosporin as an example of a drug, like bosentan, that inhibits the bile salt export pump, and is therefore expected to increase the risk of liver toxicity when used with bosentan. They therefore contraindicate the combination.[2] Further study is needed, as some consider the combination to have clinical potential.

1. Binet I, Wallnöfer A, Weber C, Jones R, Thiel G. Renal hemodynamics and pharmacokinetics of bosentan with and without cyclosporine A. *Kidney Int* (2000) 57, 224–31.
2. Tracleer (Bosentan monohydrate). Actelion Pharmaceuticals UK. Summary of product characteristics, September 2004.

Ciclosporin + Bupropion

An isolated case describes a large fall in ciclosporin levels in a 10-year-old given bupropion.

Clinical evidence, mechanism, importance and management

A 10-year-old boy, who had received a heart transplant 6 years previously was started on bupropion 75 mg twice daily in addition to his usual transplant medication, which included ciclosporin. After taking bupropion for 22 days, his ciclosporin level was found to be only 39 nanograms/ml. The last level taken before bupropion treatment had been 197 nanograms/ml. Despite an increase in his ciclosporin dose from 420 to 500 mg daily, the ciclosporin levels fell further, to 27 nanograms/ml. The ciclosporin dosage was then increased to 550 mg daily and the bupropion stopped.[1]

The reason for this probable interaction is unclear, although an interaction via the cytochrome P450 isoenzyme CYP3A4 is a possibility. This appears to be the only reported case of an interaction between ciclosporin and bupropion, and its general importance is unknown.

1. Lewis BR, Aoun SL, Bernstein GA, Crow SJ. Pharmacokinetic interactions between cyclosporin and bupropion or methylphenidate. *J Child Adolesc Psychopharmacol* (2001) 11, 193–8.

Ciclosporin + Busulfan and Cyclophosphamide

The development of seizures in patients taking ciclosporin after bone marrow transplants has been attributed to previous treatment with busulfan and cyclophosphamide.

Clinical evidence, mechanism, importance and management

Five of 182 patients receiving allogenic bone marrow transplants developed seizures within 22 to 61 days of starting ciclosporin and methylprednisolone. All of them had received busulfan 16 mg/kg and cyclophosphamide 120 mg/kg as preparative therapy without radiation.[1] Magnetic resonance imaging found brain abnormalities, which resolved a few days after the ciclosporin was withdrawn. The reasons are not understood, nor is the association between the use of the preparative drugs, the ciclosporin, and the development of the seizure clearly established. The authors of the report recommend that if seizures develop the ciclosporin should be stopped and anticonvulsants started.

1. Ghany AM, Tutschka PJ, McGhee RB, Avalos BR, Cunningham I, Kapoor N, Copelan EA. Cyclosporine-associated seizures in bone marrow transplant recipients given busulfan and cyclophosphamide preparative therapy. *Transplantation* (1991) 52, 310–15.

Ciclosporin + Calcium channel blockers

Diltiazem, nicardipine and verapamil markedly raise serum ciclosporin levels but also appear to possess kidney protective effects. A single case describes elevated ciclosporin levels caused by nisoldipine. Nifedipine normally appears not to interact, but rises and falls in ciclosporin levels have been seen in a few patients. Felodipine, isradipine, lacidipine and nitrendipine normally appear not to raise serum ciclosporin levels. Amlodipine has modestly increased ciclosporin levels in some studies, but not in others, and it may also have kidney-protective properties.

Clinical evidence

(a) Amlodipine

Ten hypertensive patients with kidney transplants on ciclosporin (3 of them also on azathioprine) were also given amlodipine 5 to 10 mg daily for 4 weeks. The hypertension was well controlled, the drug well tolerated, and the pharmacokinetics of the ciclosporin remained unaltered.[1] However, another study in 11 hypertensive kidney transplant patients found that amlodipine, given for 7 weeks, raised the ciclosporin levels by an average of 40%, without affecting creatinine levels.[2] A review identified two other studies that have found increases in ciclosporin levels of 23% and 43% with amlodipine, whereas four studies have found no change.[3] Amlodipine is reported to reduce ciclosporin-associated nephrotoxicity in a study in patients with psoriasis[4] and in a review of renal-transplant recipients.[3]

(b) Diltiazem

Sixty-five kidney transplant patients on ciclosporin and diltiazem needed less ciclosporin than 63 control patients not given diltiazem (7.3 compared with 9 mg/kg/day). There were considerable individual differences.[5]

Other studies clearly confirm that diltiazem can raise ciclosporin serum levels.[6-30] In some cases the serum ciclosporin levels were not only controlled by reducing the ciclosporin dosage by 30 to 60%, but it appeared that diltiazem had a kidney protective role (reduced nephrotoxicity, fewer rejection episodes and haemodialysis sessions).[10,21,31-35]

(c) Felodipine

Thirteen kidney transplant patients had no significant changes in their serum ciclosporin levels when treated with felodipine 2.5 to 10 mg daily and serum creatinine levels were also unchanged. Mean blood pressures fell from 161/100 to 152/90 mmHg.[36] Another study found no significant changes in ciclosporin levels in patients also given felodipine.[37] A single 10-mg dose of felodipine was found to have beneficial effects on blood pressure, renal haemodynamics, renal tubular sodium and water handling in ciclosporin-treated kidney transplant patients. The effects of long-term use were not studied.[38] A single-dose study in 12 healthy subjects found that the maximum serum levels of ciclosporin 5 mg/kg were slightly raised by 16% by felodipine 10 mg, while the AUC and maximum serum level of the felodipine were raised by 58% and 151% respectively, but blood pressures were unchanged.[39] The same group of workers also briefly described acute and short-term studies in groups of kidney transplant and dermatological patients, which found that felodipine 5 to 10 mg reduced blood pressure and opposed ciclosporin nephrotoxicity.[40] A study in heart transplant patients on ciclosporin found that felodipine attenuated the hypertrophic effects of ciclosporin on transplanted hearts.[41]

(d) Isradipine

Twelve kidney transplant patient had no changes in their ciclosporin levels over 4 weeks while taking up to 2.5 mg of isradipine twice daily.[42] Similar findings are noted in another study.[37] Three other studies in 31 kidney transplant patients confirmed that ciclosporin serum levels are unchanged by isradipine and blood pressures are reduced.[43-45]

(e) Lacidipine

Ten kidney transplant patients on ciclosporin, prednisone and azathioprine were started on lacidipine 4 mg daily. A very small increase in the trough serum levels (6%) and AUC (14%) of the ciclosporin occurred. The blood pressures fell from 142/93 to 125/79 mmHg, and the 14-hour urinary output rose from 1401 to 2050 ml.[46]

(f) Lercanidipine

The makers of lercanidipine contraindicate the concurrent use of ciclosporin as the plasma levels of lercanidipine were raised threefold by ciclosporin, and the ciclosporin AUC was raised by 21% by lercanidipine.[47]

(g) Nicardipine

Nicardipine 20 mg three times daily raised the serum ciclosporin levels of 9 patients by 110% (from 226 to 430 nanograms/ml, range 24 to 341%). Their serum creatinine concentrations rose from 136 to 147 micromol/l.[48]

Other studies have found increases in serum ciclosporin levels, in some cases as much as two to threefold, when nicardipine was given.[49-55]

(h) Nifedipine

Five of 9 patients who had an interaction with nicardipine (see above) had no interaction when they were given nifedipine.[48] No changes in ciclosporin levels were seen in other studies,[34,56-60] but raised[16,19] and reduced levels[61] have been reported in others. Two studies found that nifedipine appeared to protect patients against the nephrotoxicity of ciclosporin.[62,63] However, there is some evidence that the adverse effects of nifedipine (flushing, rash)[64] and gingival overgrowth may be increased.[65-68]

(i) Nisoldipine

A 46-year-old man taking azathioprine, prednisolone and ciclosporin after a kidney transplant 18 months previously was given nisoldipine 5 mg twice daily. During the following month his ciclosporin levels rose from a range of 100 to 150 micrograms/l up to 200 micrograms/l and an increase in serum creatinine levels occurred. His ciclosporin dose was gradually reduced from 325 to 250 mg daily, and his ciclosporin and creatinine levels returned to the acceptable range.[69]

(j) Nitrendipine

Nitrendipine 20 mg daily for 3 weeks had no significant effect on the serum ciclosporin levels of 16 kidney transplant patients.[70]

(k) Verapamil

Twenty-two kidney transplant patients given ciclosporin and verapamil had serum ciclosporin levels that were 50 to 70% higher than in 18 other patients not given verapamil, despite similar ciclosporin doses in both groups. Serum creatinine levels were lower in those treated with verapamil. Moreover, only 3 of the 22 had rejection episodes within 4 weeks compared with 10 out of 18 not given verapamil.[71]

Other studies have found that verapamil 120 to 320 mg daily can increase, double or even triple serum ciclosporin levels in individual patients with kidney or heart transplants.[23,37,59,61,72-76] Combined use does not apparently increase the severity or prevalence of gingival overgrowth caused by ciclosporin.[77]

Mechanism

The increased ciclosporin levels are largely due to the calcium channel blockers inhibiting ciclosporin metabolism by the liver. Diltiazem also appears to reduce ischaemia-induced renal tubular necrosis.[78] Other calcium channel blockers also seem to have a kidney-protective effect. The raised felodipine levels are possibly due to competitive inhibition by ciclosporin of intestinal and liver metabolism, or changes in P-glycoprotein activity.

Importance and management

The interactions of ciclosporin with diltiazem, nicardipine and verapamil are established and relatively well documented. Concurrent use need not be avoided, but ciclosporin levels should be well monitored and dosage reductions made as necessary. Even though ciclosporin serum levels are increased, these calcium channel blockers appear to have a kidney-protective effect. One study[79] noted that although calcium channel blockers increase ciclosporin blood levels this is of no harm to the patient, since no changes in renal function were observed. With diltiazem and verapamil the ciclosporin dosage can apparently be reduced by about 25 to 50% and possibly more with nicardipine. One case suggests that this is also true with nisoldipine. Several studies suggest that substantial cost savings can be made by combining either diltiazem[12,80,81] or verapamil[23] with ciclosporin. Take care not to substitute one diltiazem product for another after the patient has been stabilised because there is evidence that their bioequivalence differences may alter the extent of the interaction.[26,82]

The situation with nifedipine is not totally clear (no effect or decreases or increases) but it appears to have a kidney-protective effect.[60] So too does felodipine. The situation with amlodipine is also uncertain, but isradipine, lacidipine and nitrendipine appear to be non-interacting alternatives. Many of the calcium channel blockers have a kidney-protective effect.

1. Toupance O, Lavaud S, Canivet E, Bernaud C, Hotton J-M, Chanard J. Antihypertensive effect of amlodipine and lack of interference with cyclosporine metabolism in renal transplant recipients. *Hypertension* (1994) 24, 297–300.
2. Pesavento TE, Jones PA, Julian BA, Curtis JJ. Amlodipine increases cyclosporine levels in hypertensive renal transplant patients: results of a prospective study. *J Am Soc Nephrol* (1996) 7, 831–5.
3. Schrama YC, Koomans HA. Interactions of cyclosporin A and amlodipine: blood cyclosporin A levels, hypertension and kidney function. *J Hypertens* (1998) 16 (Suppl 4), S33–S38.
4. Raman GV, Campbell SK, Farrer A, Albano JDM, Cook J. Modifying effects of amlodipine on cyclosporin A-induced changes in renal function in patients with psoriasis. *J Hypertens* (1998) 16 (Suppl 4), S39–S41.
5. Kohlhaw K, Wonigeit K, Frei U, Oldhafer K, Neumann K, Pichlmayr R. Effect of calcium channel blocker diltiazem on cyclosporine A blood levels and dose requirements. *Transplant Proc* (1988) 20 (Suppl 2), 572–4.
6. Pochet JM, Pirson Y. Cyclosporin-diltiazem interaction. *Lancet* (1986) i, 979.
7. Griño JM, Sabate I, Castelao AM, Alsina J. Influence of diltiazem on cyclosporin clearance. *Lancet* (1986) i, 1387.
8. Kunzendorf U, Walz G, Neumayer H-H, Wagner K, Keller F, Offermann G. Einfluss von Diltiazem auf die Ciclosporin-Blutspiegel. *Klin Wochenschr* (1987) 65, 1101–3.
9. Sabaté I, Griñó JM, Castelao AM, Huguet J, Serón D, Blanco A. Cyclosporin-diltiazem interaction: comparison of cyclosporin levels measured with two monoclonal antibodies. *Transplant Proc* (1989) 21, 1460–1.
10. Choi KC, Kang YJ, Kim SK, Ryu SB. Effects of the calcium channel blocker diltiazem on the blood and serum levels of cyclosporin A. *Chonnam J Med Sci* (1989) 2, 131–6.
11. Campistol JM, Oppenheimer F, Vilardell J, Ricart MJ, Alcaraz A, Ponz E, Andreu J. Interaction between ciclosporin and diltiazem in renal transplant patients. *Nephron* (1991) 57, 241–2.
12. Valantine H, Keogh A, McIntosh N, Hunt S, Oyer P, Schroeder J. Cost containment-Coadministration of diltiazem with cyclosporine following cardiac transplant. *J Heart Transplant* (1990) 9, 68.
13. Bourge RC, Kirklin JK, Naftel DC, Figg WD, White-Williams C, Ketchum C. Diltiazem-cyclosporine interaction in cardiac transplant recipients: impact on cyclosporine dose and medication costs. *Am J Med* (1991) 90, 402–4.
14. Maddux MS, Veremis SA, Bauma WD, Pollak R. Significant drug interactions with cyclosporine. *Hosp Ther* (1987) 12, 56–70.
15. Brockmöller J, Neumayer H-H, Wagner K, Weber W, Heinemeyer G, Kewitz H, Roots I. Pharmacokinetic interaction between cyclosporin and diltiazem. *Eur J Clin Pharmacol* (1990) 38, 237–42.
16. Diaz C, Gillum DM. Interaction of diltiazem and nifedipine with cyclosporine in renal transplant recipients. *Kidney Int* (1989) 35, 513.
17. Wagner K, Albrecht S, Neumayer H-H. Prevention of posttransplant acute tubular necrosis by the calcium antagonist diltiazem: a prospective randomized study. *Am J Nephrol* (1987) 7, 287–91.
18. McCauley J, Ptachcinski RJ, Shapiro R. The cyclosporine-sparing effects of diltiazem in renal transplantation. *Transplant Proc* (1989) 21, 3955–7.
19. Castelao AM. Cyclosporine A - drug interactions. In Sunshine I (Ed.) Recent developments in therapeutic drug monitoring and clinical toxicology. *2nd Int Conf Therapeutic Drug Monitoring Toxicology, Barcelona, Spain* (1992) 203–9.
20. Shennib H, Auger J-L. Diltiazem improves cyclosporine dosage in cystic fibrosis lung transplant recipients. *J Heart Lung Transplant* (1994) 13, 292–6.

21. Macdonald P, Keogh A, Connell J, Harvison A, Richens D, Spratt P. Diltiazem co-administration reduces cylosporine toxicity after heart transplantation: a prospective randomised study. *Transplant Proc* (1992) 24, 2259–62.
22. Masri MA, Shakuntala V, Shanwaz M, Zaher M, Dhawan I, Yasin I, Pingle A. Pharmacokinetics of cyclosporine in renal transplant patients on diltiazem. *Transplant Proc* (1994) 26, 1921.
23. Sketris IS, Methot ME, Nicol D, Belitsky P, Knox MG. Effect of calcium-channel blockers on cyclosporine clearance and use in renal transplant patients. *Ann Pharmacother* (1994) 28, 1227–31.
24. Bleck JS, Thiesemann C, Kliem V, Christians U, Hecker H, Repp H, Frei U, Westhoff-Bleck M, Manns M, Sewing KF. Diltiazem increases blood concentrations of cyclized cyclosporine metabolites resulting in different cyclosporine metabolite patterns in stable male and female renal allograft recipients. *Br J Clin Pharmacol* (1996) 41, 551–6.
25. Morris RG, Jones TE. Diltiazem disposition and metabolism in recipients of renal transplants. *Ther Drug Monit* (1998) 20, 365–70.
26. Jones TE, Morris RG, Mathew TH. Formulation of diltiazem affects cyclosporin-sparing activity. *Eur J Clin Pharmacol* (1997) 52, 55–8.
27. Jones TE, Morris RG, Mathew TH. Diltiazem-cyclosporin pharmacokinetic interaction — dose-response relationship. *Br J Clin Pharmacol* (1997) 44, 499–504.
28. Sharma A, Bell L, Drolet D, Drouin E, Gaul M, Girardin P, Goodyer P, Schreiber R. Cyclosporine (CSA) Neoral kinetics in children treated with diltiazem. *J Am Soc Nephrol* (1996) 7, 1923.
29. Wagner C, Sperschneider H, Korn A, Christians U. Influence of diltiazem on cyclosporine metabolites in renal graft recipients treated with Sandimmun® and Neoral®. *J Am Soc Nephrol* (1997) 8, 707A.
30. Åsberg A, Christensen H, Hartmann A, Carlson E, Molden E, Berg KJ. Pharmacokinetic interactions between microemulsion formulated cyclosporine A and diltiazem in renal transplant recipients. *Eur J Clin Pharmacol* (1999) 55, 383–7.
31. Neumayer H-H, Wagner K. Diltiazem and economic use of cyclosporin. *Lancet* (1986) ii, 523.
32. Wagner K, Albrecht S, Neumayer H-H. Prevention of delayed graft function in cadaveric kidney transplantation by a calcium antagonist. Preliminary results of two prospective randomized trials. *Transplant Proc* (1986) 18, 510–15.
33. Wagner K, Albrecht S, Neumayer H-H. Prevention of delayed graft function by a calcium antagonist- a randomized trial in renal graft recipients on cyclosporine A. *Transplant Proc* (1986) 18, 1269–71.
34. Wagner K, Philipp Th, Heinemeyer G, Brockmüller F, Roots I, Neumayer HH. Interaction of cyclosporin and calcium antagonists. *Transplant Proc* (1989) 21, 1453–6.
35. Neumayer H-H, Kunzendorf U, Schreiber M. Protective effects of calcium antagonists in human renal transplantation. *Kidney Int* (1992) 41 (Suppl 36), S87–S93.
36. Cohen DJ, Teng S-N, Valeri A, Appel GB. Influence of oral felodipine on serum cyclosporine concentrations in renal transplant patients. *J Am Soc Nephrol* (1993) 4, 929.
37. Yildiz A, Sever MŞ, Türkmen A, Ecder T, Türk S, Akkaya V, Ark E. Interaction between cyclosporin A and verapamil, felodipine, and isradipine. *Nephron* (1999) 81, 117–18.
38. Pedersen EB, Sørensen SS, Eiskjær H, Skovbon H, Thomsen K. Interaction between cyclosporine and felodipine in renal transplant recipients. *Kidney Int* (1992) 41 (Suppl 36), S82–S86.
39. Madsen JK, Jensen JD, Jensen LW, Pedersen EB. Pharmacokinetic interaction between cyclosporine and the dihydropyridine calcium antagonist felodipine. *Eur J Clin Pharmacol* (1996) 50, 203–8.
40. Madsen JK, Kornerup HJ, Sørensen SS, Zachariae H, Pedersen EB. Ciclosporine nephrotoxicity can be counteracted by a calcium antagonist (felodipine) in acute and short-term studies. *J Am Soc Nephrol* (1995) 6, 1102.
41. Schwitter J, DeMarco T, Globits S, Sakuma H, Klinski C, Chatterjee K, Parmley WW, Higgins CB. Influence of felodipine on left ventricular hypertrophy and systolic function in orthoptic heart transplant recipients: possible interaction with cyclosporine medication. *J Heart Lung Transplant* (1999) 18, 1003–13.
42. Endresen L, Bergan S, Holdaas H, Pran T, Sinding-Larsen B, Berg KJ. Lack of effect of the calcium antagonist isradipine on cyclosporine pharmacokinetics in renal transplant patients. *Ther Drug Monit* (1991) 13, 490–5.
43. Martinez F, Pirson Y, Wallemacq P, van Ypersele de Strihou C. No clinically significant interaction between ciclosporin and isradipine. *Nephron* (1991) 59, 658–9.
44. Vernillet L, Bourbigot B, Codet JP, Le Saux L, Moal MC, Morin JF. Lack of effect of isradipine on cyclosporin pharmacokinetics. *Fundam Clin Pharmacol* (1992) 6, 367–74.
45. Ahmed K, Michael B, Burke JF. Effects of isradipine on renal hemodynamics in renal transplant patients treated with cyclosporine. *Clin Nephrol* (1997) 48, 307–10.
46. Ruggenenti P, Perico N, Mosconi L, Gaspari F, Benigni A, Amuchastegui CS, Bruzzi I, Remuzzi G. Calcium channel blockers protect transplant patients from cyclosporine-induced daily renal hypoperfusion. *Kidney Int* (1993) 43, 706–11.
47. Zanidip (Lercanidipine hydrochloride). Napp Pharmaceuticals Ltd. UK Summary of product characteristics, January 2004.
48. Bourbigot B, Guiserix J, Airiau J, Bressollette L, Morin JF, Cledes J. Nicardipine increases cyclosporin blood levels. *Lancet* (1986) i, 1447.
49. Cantarovich M, Hiesse C, Lockiec F, Charpentier B, Fries D. Confirmation of the interaction between cyclosporine and the calcium channel blocker nicardipine in renal transplant patients. *Clin Nephrol* (1987) 28, 190–3.
50. Kessler M, Renoult E, Jonon B, Vigneron B, Huu TC, Netter P. Interaction ciclosporine-nicardipine chez le transplanté rénal. *Therapie* (1987) 42, 273–5.
51. Deray G, Aupetit B, Martinez F, Baumelou A, Worcel A, Benhmida M, Legrand JC, Jacobs C. Cyclosporin-nicardipine interaction. *Am J Nephrol* (1989) 9, 349.
52. Kessler M, Netter P, Renoult E, Jonon B, Mur JM, Trechot P, Dousset B. Influence of nicardipine on renal function and plasma cyclosporin in renal transplant patients. *Eur J Clin Pharmacol* (1989) 36, 637–8.
53. Todd P, Garioch JJ, Rademaker M, Thomson J. Nicardipine interacts with cyclosporin. *Br J Dermatol* (1989) 121, 820.
54. Bouquet S, Chapelle G, Barrier L, Boutaud Ph, Menu P, Courtois Ph. Interactions ciclosporine-nicardipine chez un transplanté cardiaque, adaptation posologique. *J Pharm Clin* (1992) 11, 59.
55. Mabin D, Fourquet I, Richard P, Esnault S, Islam MS, Bourbigot B. Leucoencéphalopathie régressive au cours d'un surdosage en cyclosporine A. *Rev Neurol (Paris)* (1993) 149, 576–8.
56. McNally P, Mistry N, Idle J, Walls J, Feehally J. Calcium channel blockers and cyclosporine metabolism. *Transplantation* (1989) 48, 1071.
57. Rossi SJ, Hariharan S, Schroeder TJ, First MR. Cyclosporine dosing and blood levels in renal transplants receiving Procardia XL. *Clin Pharmacol Ther* (1993) 53, 238.
58. Rossi SJ, Hariharan S, Schroeder TJ, First MR. Cyclosporine dosing and blood levels in renal transplant recipients receiving Procardia XL. *J Am Soc Nephrol* (1992) 3, 877.
59. Ogborn MR, Crocker JFS, Grimm PC. Nifedipine, verapamil and cyclosporin A pharmacokinetics in children. *Pediatr Nephrol* (1989) 3, 314–16.
60. Propper DJ, Whiting PH, Power DA, Edward N, Catto GRD. The effect of nifedipine on graft function in renal allograft recipients treated with cyclosporin A. *Clin Nephrol* (1989) 32, 62–7.
61. Howard RL, Shapiro JI, Babcock S, Chan L. The effect of calcium channel blockers on the cyclosporine dose requirement in renal transplant recipients. *Ren Fail* (1990) 12, 89–92.
62. Feehally J, Walls J, Mistry N, Horsburgh T, Taylor J, Veitch PS, Bell PRF. Does nifedipine ameliorate cyclosporin A nephrotoxicity? *BMJ* (1987) 295, 310.
63. Morales JM, Andrés A, Alvarez C, Prieto C, Ortuño B, Ortuño T, Paternina ER, Hernandez Poblete G, Praga M, Ruilope LM, Rodicio JL. Calcium channel blockers and early cyclosporine nephrotoxicity after renal transplantation: a prospective randomized study. *Transplant Proc* (1990) 22, 1733–5.
64. McFadden JP, Pontin JE, Powles AV, Fry L, Idle JR. Cyclosporin decreases nifedipine metabolism. *BMJ* (1989) 299, 1224.
65. Thomason JM, Seymour RA, Rice N. The prevalence and severity of cyclosporin and nifedipine-induced gingival overgrowth. *J Clin Periodontol* (1993) 20, 37–40.
66. Jackson C, Babich S. Gingival hyperplasia: interaction between cyclosporin A and nifedipine? A case report. *N Y State Dent J* (1997) 63, 46–8.
67. Thomason JM, Ellis JS, Kelly PJ, Seymour RA. Nifedipine pharmacological variables as risk factors for gingival overgrowth in organ-transplant patients. *Clin Oral Investig* (1997) 1, 35–9.
68. Morgan JDT, Swarbrick MJ, Edwards CM, Donnelly PK. Cyclosporin, nifedipine and gingival hyperplasia: a randomized controlled study. *Transpl Int* (1994) 7 (Suppl 1), S320–S321.
69. Fourtounas C, Kopelias I, Kiriaki D, Agroyannis B. Increased cyclosporine blood levels after nisoldipine administration in a renal transplant recipient. *Transpl Int* (2002) 15, 586–8.
70. Çopur MS, Tasdemir I, Turgan Ç, Yasavul Ü, Çaglar S. Effects of nitrendipine on blood pressure and blood ciclosporin A level in patients with posttransplant hypertension. *Nephron* (1989) 52, 227–30.
71. Dawidson I, Rooth P, Fry WR, Sandor Z, Willms C, Coorpender L, Alway C, Reisch J. Prevention of acute cyclosporine-induced renal blood flow inhibition and improved immunosuppression with verapamil. *Transplantation* (1989) 48, 575–80.
72. Lindholm A, Henricsson S. Verapamil inhibits cyclosporin metabolism. *Lancet* (1987) i, 1262–3
73. Hampton EM, Stewart CF, Herrod HG, Valenski WR. Augmentation of in- vitro immunosuppressive effects of cyclosporin by verapamil. *Clin Pharmacol Ther* (1987) 41, 169.
74. Robson RA, Fraenkel M, Barratt LJ, Birkett DJ. Cyclosporin-verapamil interaction. *Br J Clin Pharmacol* (1988) 25, 402–3.
75. Angermann CE, Spes CH, Anthuber M, Kemkes BM, Theisen K. Verapamil increases cyclosporin-A blood trough levels in cardiac recipients. *J Am Coll Cardiol* (1988) 11, 206A.
76. Sabatée I, Griñó JM, Castelao AM, Ortolá J. Evaluation of cyclosporin-verapamil interaction, with observations on parent cyclosporin and metabolites. *Clin Chem* (1988) 34, 2151.
77. Cebeci I, Kantarci A, Firatli E, Çarin M, Tuncer Ö. The effect of verapamil on the prevalence and severity of cyclosporine-induced gingival overgrowth in renal allograft recipients. *J Periodontol* (1996) 67, 1201–5.
78. Oppenheimer F, Alcaraz A, Mañalich M, Ricart MJ, Vilardell J, Campistol JM, Andreu J, Talbot-Wright R, Fernandez-Cruz L. Influence of the calcium blocker diltiazem on the prevention of acute renal failure after renal transplantation. *Transplant Proc* (1992) 24, 50–1.
79. Wagner K, Henkel M, Heinemeyer G, Neumayer H-H. Interaction of calcium blockers and cyclosporine. *Transplant Proc* (1988) 20 (Suppl 2), 561–8.
80. Smith CL, Hampton EM, Pederson JA, Pennington LR, Bourne DWA. Clinical and medicoeconomic impact of the cyclosporine-diltiazem interaction in renal transplant recipients. *Pharmacotherapy* (1994) 14, 471–81.
81. Iqbal S, Holland D, Toffelmire EB. Diltiazem inhibition of cyclosporin metabolism provides cost effective therapy. *Clin Pharmacol Ther* (1995) 57, 219.
82. Cooke CE. Nontherapeutic cyclosporine levels. Sustained-release diltiazem products are not the same. *Transplantation* (1994) 57, 1687.

Ciclosporin + Chlorambucil

An isolated report describes a reduction in ciclosporin levels in a patient given chlorambucil.

Clinical evidence, mechanism, importance and management

A woman with B-chronic lymphocytic leukaemia and autoimmune haemolytic anaemia controlled with ciclosporin was started on chlorambucil 5 mg daily because of disease progression. When she reached a total dose of 200 mg of chlorambucil she suddenly relapsed, and her serum ciclosporin levels were found to have dropped to 60 nanograms/ml from a range of 200 to 400 nanograms/ml. The ciclosporin levels remained low despite a doubling of the ciclosporin dosage and withdrawal of the chlorambucil. Only after a month did the anaemia respond and the ciclosporin levels rise again.[1]

This appears to be an isolated report so the general significance of this interaction is unclear.

1. Emilia G, Messora C. Interaction between cyclosporin and chlorambucil. *Eur J Haematol* (1993) 51, 179.

Ciclosporin + Chloroquine

Three patients had rapid rises in serum ciclosporin levels, with evidence of nephrotoxicity in two of them, when they were given chloroquine. Some loss of renal function has even been seen with low doses of ciclosporin used with chloroquine for rheumatoid arthritis.

Clinical evidence

A kidney transplant patient on ciclosporin, azathioprine and prednisolone had a threefold rise in ciclosporin serum levels, from 148 to 420 nanograms/ml, accompanied by a rise in serum creatinine levels within 48 hours of starting chloroquine 900 mg daily for suspected malarial fever. On days 2 and 3 the chloroquine dosage was reduced to 300 mg daily. The ciclosporin and creatinine returned to their former levels 7 days after the chloroquine was stopped.[1]

When another kidney transplant patient on ciclosporin, azathioprine and prednisolone was given chloroquine 100 mg daily for 6 days, his ciclosporin serum levels rose from 105 to 470 nanograms/ml and his serum creatinine levels rose from 200 to 234 micromol/l, accompanied by a rise in blood pressure from 130/80 to 160/100 mmHg. These changes reversed when the chloroquine was stopped, and rose again when chloroquine was restarted.[2] The ciclosporin serum levels of another patient were doubled by chloroquine 100 mg daily.[3]

A randomised controlled study in 88 patients with recent onset rheumatoid arthritis found that the addition of ciclosporin (1.25 or 2.5 mg/kg daily) to chloroquine 100 mg daily was moderately effective, but changes in serum creatinine levels occurred. In the presence of chloroquine the creatinine was not significantly altered by placebo or ciclosporin 1.25 mg/kg, but was raised by 10 micromol/l by ciclosporin 2.5 mg/kg, indicating that some loss in renal function can occur.[4]

Mechanism

Not understood. Both chloroquine and ciclosporin can cause renal function impairment.[4]

Importance and management

Information is limited but it would now be prudent to monitor the effects of adding chloroquine in any patient on ciclosporin, being alert for any changes in renal function, even when using low doses, and additionally looking for increases in serum ciclosporin levels when using transplant doses. The authors of the study do not recommend further trials of the combination in rheumatoid arthritis.[4]

1. Nampoory MRN, Nessim J, Gupta RK, Johny KV. Drug interaction of chloroquine and ciclosporin. *Nephron* (1992) 62, 108–9.
2. Finielz P, Gendoo Z, Chuet C, Guiserix J. Interaction between cyclosporin and chloroquine. *Nephron* (1993) 65, 333.
3. Guiserix J, Aizel A. Interactions ciclosporine-chloroquine. *Presse Med* (1996) 25, 1214.
4. van den Borne BEEM, Landewé RBM, Goei The HS, Rietveld JH, Zwinderman AH, Bruyn GAW, Breedveld FC, Dijkmans BAC. Combination therapy in recent onset rheumatoid arthritis: a randomized double blind trial of the addition of low dose cyclosporine to patients treated with low dose chloroquine. *J Rheumatol* (1998) 25, 1493–8.

Ciclosporin + Clonidine

A child taking ciclosporin had a marked rise in his serum ciclosporin levels when clonidine was added.

Clinical evidence, mechanism, importance and management

A 3-year-old renal transplant patient taking ciclosporin, azathioprine and prednisone was given a combination of propranolol, hydralazine, furosemide and nifedipine postoperatively in an attempt to control his blood pressure. Minoxidil was added, but was considered unacceptable because of adverse cosmetic effects. When it was replaced with clonidine, the ciclosporin levels increased about threefold to 927 nanograms/ml, in spite of a dose reduction. Ciclosporin levels returned to the patients' normal range of 150 to 300 nanograms/ml on withdrawal of clonidine and blood pressure was controlled by the addition of an ACE inhibitor. It is possible that clonidine inhibited the metabolism of ciclosporin via the cytochrome P450 pathway.[1]

Although this appears to be the only report of the interaction there appears to be insufficient evidence to recommend increasing the monitoring of ciclosporin levels in every patient, although the possibility of an interaction should still be considered when prescribing the combination.

1. Gilbert RD, Kahn D, Cassidy M. Interaction between clonidine and cyclosporine A. *Nephron* (1995) 71, 105.

Ciclosporin + Colchicine

A number of cases of ciclosporin toxicity, multiple organ failure and serious muscle disorders (myopathy, rhabdomyolysis) have been seen when colchicine and ciclosporin were given concurrently.

Clinical evidence, mechanism, importance and management

A patient with a kidney transplant had a transient (2 to 3 day) rise in serum creatinine and serum ciclosporin levels, from 100 to 200 up to 1519 nanograms/ml the day after receiving a total of 4 mg of colchicine.[1] Another kidney transplant patient on ciclosporin, azathioprine and prednisone developed colchicine neuromyopathy (possibly rhabdomyolysis), ciclosporin nephrotoxicity and liver function abnormalities when treated with colchicine.[2] Acute myopathy (muscle weakness, myalgia) or rhabdomyolysis occurred in a further 5 patients who took ciclosporin and colchicine.[3-7] There is also a report of colchicine-induced myopathy and hepatonephropathy in a heart transplant patient who was treated with both ciclosporin and colchicine.[8]

The overall picture presented by these reports is very unclear. It is not known whether the colchicine toxicity is made worse by ciclosporin, or the ciclosporin toxicity is made worse by colchicine, or the reaction is a result of both effects. A syndrome of myopathy, gastrointestinal disturbances and mild hepatic and renal dysfunction has been described in 6 patients and was attributed to the use of colchicines with ciclosporin.[8-10] This may be due to inhibition of P-glycoprotein by ciclosporin and subsequent impairment of colchicine excretion in to the bile and urine resulting in elevated, toxic colchicine levels.[8]

If concurrent use is thought to be appropriate, it should be very carefully monitored because the outcome can be serious. Rhabdomyolysis appears to be a rare complication and the maker of ciclosporin advises a change of treatment if any signs and symptoms develop.[5] More study is needed.

1. Menta R, Rossi E, Guariglia A, David S, Cambi V. Reversible acute cyclosporin nephrotoxicity induced by colchicine administration. *Nephrol Dial Transplant* (1987) 2, 380–1.
2. Rieger EH, Halasz NA, Wahlstrom HE. Colchicine neuromyopathy after renal transplantation. *Transplantation* (1990) 49, 1196–8.
3. Lee BI, Shin SJ, Yoon SN, Choi YJ, Yang CW, Bang BK. Acute myopathy induced by colchicine in a cyclosporine-treated renal recipient. A case report and review of the literature. *J Korean Med Sci* (1997) 12, 160–1.
4. Noppen M, Velkeniers B, Dierckx R, Bruyland M, Vanhaelst L. Cyclosporine and myopathy. *Ann Intern Med* (1987) 107, 945–6.
5. Arellano F, Krupp P. Muscular disorders associated with cyclosporin. *Lancet* (1991), 337, 915.
6. Rumpf KW, Henning HV. Is myopathy in renal transplant patients induced by cyclosporin or colchicine? *Lancet* (1990) 335, 800–1.
7. Jagose JT, Bailey RR. Muscle weakness due to colchicine in a renal transplant recipient. *N Z Med J* (1997) 110, 343.
8. Gruberg L, Har-Zahav Y, Agranat O, Freimark D. Acute myopathy induced by colchicine in a cyclosporine treated heart transplant recipient: possible role of the multidrug resistance transporter. *Transplant Proc* (1999) 31, 2157–8.
9. Yussim A, Bar-Nathan N, Lustig S, Shaharabani E, Geier E, Shmuely D, Nakache R, Shapira Z. Gastrointestinal, hepatorenal, and neuromuscular toxicity caused by cyclosporine-colchicine interaction in renal transplantation. *Transplant Proc* (1994) 26, 2825–6.
10. Minetti EE, Minetti L. Multiple organ failure in a kidney transplant patient receiving both colchicine and cyclosporine. *J Nephrol* (2003) 16, 421–5.

Ciclosporin + Colestyramine

Colestyramine can interact with ciclosporin in some patients but the outcome appears to be unpredictable.

Clinical evidence, mechanism, importance and management

Four transplant patients on ciclosporin and prednisolone, given colestyramine for a week, then simultaneously with ciclosporin on the day of testing, had only a very small average increase (6%) in the AUC of ciclosporin, but one patient had a 55% increase and another a 23% decrease.[1] Another study[2] in 6 kidney transplant patients found that colestyramine 4 g daily caused no significant changes in ciclosporin pharmacokinetics. The ciclosporin was given at 8 am and 8 pm, with the colestyramine at noon.

It would seem prudent to separate administration of colestyramine and ciclosporin. It is usually advised that colestyramine is given 1 hour before or 4 to 6 hours after other drugs.

1. Keogh A, Day R, Critchley L, Duggin G, Baron D. The effect of food and cholestyramine on the absorption of cyclosporine in cardiac transplant patients. *Transplant Proc* (1988) 20, 27–30.
2. Jensen RA, Lal SM, Diaz-Arias A, James-Kracke M, Van Stone JC, Ross G. Does cholestyramine interfere with cyclosporine absorption? A prospective study in renal transplant patients. *ASAIO J* (1995) 41, M704–M706.

Ciclosporin + Corticosteroids

The concurrent use of ciclosporin and the corticosteroids is very common, but some evidence suggests that ciclosporin serum levels

are raised by corticosteroids. Ciclosporin can reduce the loss of the corticosteroids from the body and corticosteroid overdosage may occur. Convulsions have also been described during concurrent use, and the incidence of diabetes mellitus may be increased following the use of ciclosporin with methylprednisolone.

Clinical evidence

(a) Methylprednisolone

A study found that the pharmacokinetics of methylprednisolone in patients on ciclosporin and azathioprine varied widely between individual kidney transplant patients, but the mean values were similar to those found in normal subjects.[1]

The serum ciclosporin levels of 22 out of 33 patients were reported to be more than doubled by intravenous methylprednisolone. The ciclosporin dosage was reduced in 6 patients.[2,3] Other studies have found that high doses of methylprednisolone increased or more than doubled serum ciclosporin levels.[4-6] However, another study found that the clearance of ciclosporin was increased by high-dose methylprednisolone, although trough ciclosporin levels were unchanged.[7]

A report describes 4 young patients (aged 10, 12, 13 and 18-years-old) who had undergone bone marrow transplants for severe aplastic anaemia and who developed convulsions while treated with high dose methylprednisolone (5 to 20 mg/kg/day) and ciclosporin.[8] Convulsions also occurred in a 25-year-old woman given ciclosporin with high-dose methylprednisolone.[9]

A study of 314 kidney transplant patients during the period 1979 to 1987 found that the incidence of diabetes mellitus in those given ciclosporin and methylprednisolone was twice that of other patients treated with azathioprine and methylprednisolone. The diabetes developed within less than 2 months.[10]

(b) Prednisolone or Prednisone

A pharmacokinetic study in 40 patients found that the clearance of prednisolone was reduced by about 30% in those receiving ciclosporin when compared with those on azathioprine (1.9 ml/minute/kg compared with 2.6 ml/minute/kg).[11]

Another study by the same group of workers reported a 25% reduction in the clearance of prednisolone in the presence of ciclosporin in patients with kidney transplants.[12] Other studies[2,13,14] confirm that ciclosporin reduces the clearance of prednisolone by about a third, and as a result some patients develop signs of toxicity (cushingoid symptoms such as steroid-induced diabetes, osteonecrosis of the hip joints).[2] These studies have all been questioned by the authors of another study, which found that the metabolism of prednisolone was not affected by ciclosporin.[15]

A comparative study over a year, in two groups of kidney transplant patients taking ciclosporin and azathioprine, one group with and the other without prednisone, found that those taking prednisone had lower trough ciclosporin levels (about 10 to 20%) despite using the same or higher doses of ciclosporin.[16]

There is other evidence that low-dose prednisolone does not increase the immunosuppression of ciclosporin, but it can reduce ciclosporin nephrotoxicity.[17]

Mechanism

The evidence suggests that ciclosporin reduces the metabolism of the corticosteroids by the liver thereby reducing their loss from the body.[13,18]

Importance and management

None of these adverse interactions is well established, and the picture is confusing. Concurrent use is common and advantageous but be alert for any evidence of increased ciclosporin and corticosteroid effects. It is not clear whether high-dose corticosteroids cause a rise in serum ciclosporin levels or not. Ciclosporin levels measured by RIA should be interpreted with caution in patients on high-dose corticosteroids as levels of ciclosporin metabolites, which can interfere with the test, may be altered.[19] The authors of one report point out that this interaction could possibly lead to a misinterpretation of clinical data: in patients with kidney transplants a rise in serum creatinine levels is assumed to be due to rejection, unless proven otherwise. If a corticosteroid is then given, this could lead to increased ciclosporin levels, which might be interpreted as ciclosporin nephrotoxicity.[3]

1. Tornatore KM, Morse GD, Jusko WJ, Walshe JJ. Methylprednisolone disposition in renal transplant recipients receiving triple-drug immunosuppression. *Transplantation* (1989) 48, 962–5.
2. Öst L, Klintmalm G, Ringdén O. Mutual interaction between prednisolone and cyclosporine in renal transplant patients. *Transplant Proc* (1985) 17, 1252–5.
3. Klintmalm G, Säwe J. High dose methylprednisolone increases plasma cyclosporin levels in renal transplant recipients. *Lancet* (1984) i, 731.
4. Klintmalm G, Säwe J, Ringdéen O, von Bahr C, Magnusson A. Cyclosporine plasma levels in renal transplant patients. Association with renal toxicity and allograft rejection. *Transplantation* (1985) 39, 132–7.
5. Hall TG. Effect of methylprednisolone on cyclosporine blood levels. *Pharmacotherapy* (1990) 10, 248.
6. Rogerson ME, Marsden JT, Reid KE, Bewick M, Holt DW. Cyclosporine blood concentrations in the management of renal transplant recipients. *Transplantation* (1986) 41, 276–8.
7. Ptachcinski RJ, Venkataramanan R, Burckart GJ, Hakala TR, Rosenthal JT, Carpenter BJ, Taylor RJ. Cyclosporine–high-dose steroid interaction in renal transplant recipients: assessment by HPLC. *Transplant Proc* (1987) 19, 1728–9.
8. Durrant S, Chipping PM, Palmer S, Gordon-Smith EC. Cyclosporin A, methylprednisolone and convulsions. *Lancet* (1982) ii, 829–30.
9. Boogaerts MA, Zachee P, Verwilghen RL. Cyclosporin, methylprednisolone and convulsions. *Lancet* (1982) ii, 1216–17.
10. Roth D, Milgrom M, Esquenazi V, Fuller L, Burke G, Miller J. Posttransplant hyperglycaemia. Increased incidence in cyclosporine-treated renal allograft recipients. *Transplantation* (1989) 47, 278–81.
11. Langhoff E, Madsen S, Olgaard K, Ladefoged J. Clinical results and cyclosporine effect on prednisolone metabolism. *Kidney Int* (1984) 26, 642.
12. Langhoff E, Madsen S, Flachs H, Olgaard K, Ladefoged J, Hvidberg EF. Inhibition of prednisolone metabolism by cyclosporine in kidney-transplanted patients. *Transplantation* (1985) 39, 107–9.
13. Öst L. Effects of cyclosporin on prednisolone metabolism. *Lancet* (1984) i, 451.
14. Öst L. Impairment of prednisolone metabolism by cyclosporine treatment in renal graft recipients. *Transplantation* (1987) 44, 533–35.
15. Frey FJ, Schnetzer A, Horber FF, Frey BM. Evidence that cyclosporine does not affect the metabolism of prednisolone after renal transplantation. *Transplantation* (1987) 43, 494–8.
16. Hricik DE, Moritz C, Mayes JT, Schulak JA. Association of the absence of steroid therapy with increased cyclosporine blood levels in renal transplant recipients. *Transplantation* (1990) 49, 221–3.
17. Nott D, Griffin PJA, Salaman JR. Low-dose steroids do not augment cyclosporine immunosuppression but do diminish cyclosporine nephrotoxicity. *Transplant Proc* (1985) 17, 1289–90.
18. Henricsson S, Lindholm A, Aravoglou M. Cyclosporin metabolism in human liver microsomes and its inhibition by other drugs. *Pharmacol Toxicol* (1990) 66, 49–52.
19. Ptachcinski RJ, Burckart GJ, Venkataramanan R, Rosenthal JT, Carpenter BJ, Hakala TR. Effect of high-dose steroids on cyclosporine blood concentrations using RIA and HPLC analysis. *Drug Intell Clin Pharm* (1987) 21, 20A.

Ciclosporin + Danazol

Marked increases in serum ciclosporin levels have been seen in seven patients taking danazol.

Clinical evidence

A 15-year-old girl, one-year post kidney transplant, taking ciclosporin and prednisone, had a marked rise in serum ciclosporin levels over about 2 weeks (from a range of 250 to 325 up to 700 to 850 nanomol/ml) when she was given danazol 200 mg twice daily, even though the ciclosporin dosage was reduced from 350 to 250 mg daily.[1]

Similar rises in ciclosporin concentrations, from about 400 to 600 nanograms/ml, and from 150 to about 450 nanograms/ml, were seen in another patient on two occasions over about a 6-week period when given 400 mg and later 600 mg of danazol daily.[2] A 12-year-old boy needed a reduction in his ciclosporin dosage from 10 to 2 mg/kg daily when danazol 400 mg twice daily was added.[3] A marked rise in serum ciclosporin levels has been described in 2 other patients when given danazol 200 mg three[4] or four[5] times daily.

A pharmacokinetic study in one kidney transplant patient found that danazol 200 mg three times daily for 16 days reduced the ciclosporin clearance by 50%, prolonged its half-life by 66% and raised its AUC by 65%.[6]

A patient with aplastic anaemia treated with ciclosporin was subsequently treated with danazol 200 mg daily for pancytopenia and endometriosis. Within 4 days the patient had epigastric pain and elevated serum ciclosporin and creatinine levels. Danazol was stopped and the ciclosporin dose was halved. Two weeks later abrupt severe hepatic injury occurred and the patient died of hepatic failure, although this was thought to be due to danazol toxicity rather than the interaction.[7]

Mechanism

Danazol is a known inhibitor of the cytochrome P450 isoenzyme system.[3,7] Ciclosporin is predominantly metabolised by the cytochrome P450 isoenzyme CYP3A4. It therefore seems likely that danazol raises ciclosporin levels by inhibiting ciclosporin metabolism.

Importance and management

Although the information seems to be limited to these few reports the interaction is established. The ciclosporin levels of any patient who is given danazol should be carefully monitored, and dosage adjustments made as necessary.

1. Ross WB, Roberts D, Griffin PJA and Salaman JR. Cyclosporin interaction with danazol and norethisterone. *Lancet* (1986) i, 330.
2. Schröder O, Schmitz N, Kayser W, Euler HH, Löffler H. Erhöhte Ciclosporin-A-spiegel bei gleichzeitiger Therapie mit Danazol. *Dtsch Med Wochenschr* (1986) 111, 602–3.
3. Blatt J, Howrie D, Orlando S. Burckart G. Interaction between cyclosporine and danazol in a pediatric patient. *J Pediatr Hematol Oncol* (1996) 18, 95.
4. Borrás-Blasco J, Rosique-Robles JD, Peris-Marti J, Navarro-Ruiz J, Gonzalez-Delgado M, Conesa-Garcia V. Possible cyclosporin-danazol interaction in a patient with aplastic anaemia. *Am J Hematol* (1999) 62, 63–4.
5. Koneru B, Hartner C, Iwatsuki S, Starzl TE. Effect of danazol on cyclosporine pharmacokinetics. *Transplantation* (1988) 45, 1001.
6. Passfall J, Keller F. Pharmacokinetics of danazol-cyclosporin interaction. *Nephrol Dial Transplant* (1994) 9, 1055.
7. Hayashi T, Takahashi T, Minami T, Akaike J, Kasahara K, Adachi M, Hinoda Y, Takahashi S, Hirayama T, Imai K. Fatal acute hepatic failure induced by danazol in a patient with endometriosis and aplastic anemia. *J Gastroenterol* (2001) 36, 783–6.

Ciclosporin + Disopyramide

An isolated report describes the development of nephrotoxicity, which was attributed to an interaction between ciclosporin and disopyramide.

Clinical evidence, mechanism, importance and management

Ten months after receiving a kidney transplant a 40-year-old woman developed premature ventricular beats and so was started on oxprenolol in addition to her usual ciclosporin and methylprednisolone. After 2 months she had shown no improvement so she was started on disopyramide 100 mg three times daily. Over the next week her serum creatinine rose from 88 to 159 micromol/l, at which point the disopyramide was stopped. Her renal function returned to normal over the next week. As she had previously been stable on ciclosporin, and nephrotoxicity has not been reported with disopyramide, an interaction was suspected.[1]

This interaction is unconfirmed and of uncertain clinical significance. There is insufficient evidence to recommend increased monitoring, but be aware of the potential for an interaction in the case of an unexpected response to treatment.

1. Nanni G, Magalini SC, Serino F, Castagneto M. Effect of disopyramide in a cyclosporine-treated patient. *Transplantation* (1988) 45, 257.

Ciclosporin + Diuretics

Isolated cases of nephrotoxicity have been described in patients on ciclosporin when given either amiloride/hydrochlorothiazide, metolazone or mannitol. Furosemide can possibly protect the kidney against ciclosporin damage. The concurrent use of ciclosporin with thiazides, but not loop diuretics, may increase serum magnesium levels, and the concurrent use of ciclosporin with potassium-sparing diuretics may cause hyperkalaemia.

Clinical evidence, mechanism, importance and management

A 39-year-old man on ciclosporin, whose second kidney transplant functioned subnormally, and who required treatment for hypertension with atenolol and minoxidil, developed ankle oedema, which was resistant to **furosemide**, despite doses of up to 750 mg daily. When **metolazone** 2.5 mg daily was added for 2 weeks his serum creatinine levels more than doubled, from 193 to 449 micromol/l. When **metolazone** was stopped the creatinine levels fell again. Ciclosporin serum levels were unchanged and neither graft rejection nor hypovolaemia occurred.[1]

The kidney transplant of another patient on ciclosporin almost ceased to function when **mannitol** was used, and biopsy indicated severe ciclosporin nephrotoxicity. Transplant function recovered when the **mannitol** was stopped.[2] The same reaction was demonstrated in *rats*.[2]

A woman on ciclosporin had a rise in serum creatinine levels from 121 to 171 micromol/l three weeks after she started *Moduretic* (**amiloride** with [**hydro**]**chlorothiazide**). Trough serum ciclosporin levels were unchanged.[3]

Although *animal* studies suggested that **furosemide** might increase the nephrotoxicity of ciclosporin,[4] more recent human studies suggest that it may have a protective effect.[5]

Although ciclosporin and **loop diuretics** are both known to cause magnesium wasting, a review of magnesium serum levels, magnesium replacement doses and diuretic use in 50 heart transplant recipients indicated that magnesium requirements were not altered by the use of ciclosporin with **loop diuretics**. However, the concurrent use of **thiazides** with ciclosporin resulted in increases in serum magnesium and decreases in magnesium replacement.[6]

Ciclosporin alone can cause hyperkalaemia, especially if renal function is impaired. Because of this, the US makers suggest that ciclosporin should not be used with **potassium-sparing diuretics**,[7] whereas the UK makers suggest that caution is required with combined use, with close control of potassium levels.[8]

The general importance of all these adverse interactions is not clear, but good monitoring is obviously needed if diuretics are given with ciclosporin.

1. Christensen P, Leski M. Nephrotoxic drug interaction between metolazone and cyclosporin. *BMJ* (1987) 294, 578.
2. Brunner FP, Hermle M, Mihatsch MJ, Thiel G. Mannitol potentiates cyclosporine nephrotoxicity. *Clin Nephrol* (1986) 25 (Suppl 1), S130–S136.
3. Deray G, Baumelou B, Le Hoang P, Aupetit B, Girard B, Baumelou A, Legrand JC, Jacobs C. Enhancement of cyclosporin nephrotoxicity by diuretic therapy. *Clin Nephrol* (1989) 32, 47.
4. Whiting PH, Cunningham C, Thomson AW, Simpson JG. Enhancement of high dose cyclosporin A toxicity by frusemide. *Biochem Pharmacol* (1984) 33, 1075–9.
5. Driscoll DF, Pinson CW, Jenkins RL, Bistrian BR. Potential protective effects of furosemide against early cyclosporine-induced renal injury in hepatic transplant recipients. *Transplant Proc* (1989) 21, 3549–50.
6. Arthur JM, Shamin S. Interaction of cyclosporine and FK506 with diuretics in transplant patients. *Kidney Int* (2000) 58, 325–30.
7. Neoral (Ciclosporin). Novartis. US Prescribing information, March 2004.
8. Neoral (Ciclosporin). Novartis Pharmaceuticals UK Ltd. UK Summary of product characteristics, December 2004.

Ciclosporin + Fibrates

Bezafibrate significantly increased serum creatinine and tended to reduce ciclosporin levels in one study. Deterioration in renal function has also been reported in 5 patients, 4 of whom had no change in ciclosporin levels, and one of whom had increased serum ciclosporin levels. The use of fenofibrate has also been associated with reduced renal function and possibly reduced serum ciclosporin levels. Two studies found no pharmacokinetic interaction between ciclosporin and gemfibrozil while a third found gemfibrozil caused a significant reduction in ciclosporin levels.

Clinical evidence, mechanism, importance and management

(a) Bezafibrate

A kidney transplant patient had a rise in his previously stable ciclosporin serum levels from a range of 150 to 200 nanograms/ml to about 340 nanograms/ml over a 6-week period after bezafibrate 200 mg twice daily was given. The rise was accompanied by increases in blood urea nitrogen and creatinine levels. Renal biopsy found evidence of possible ciclosporin toxicity, and rejection. The patient recovered when the bezafibrate was stopped.[1]

Two other transplant patients (one kidney and the other heart) had a reversible deterioration in renal function when they were treated with bezafibrate. This was severe in one, and the other had the effect on two occasions. Neither had any changes in ciclosporin serum levels.[2,3] Two other similar cases have been reported, one of whom was subsequently treated with gemfibrozil without problems.[4]

Another study over 3 months in 40 heart transplant patients on ciclosporin found that bezafibrate was associated with a rise in serum creatinine levels, although none of the patients had to be withdrawn from the study because of this. The ciclosporin level tended to be lower (198 nanograms/ml at baseline, compared with 144 nanograms/ml after 3 months).[5]

Neither the incidence nor the reasons for these reactions are known, but because the outcome is uncertain and potentially serious, you should keep a close check on the effects of adding bezafibrate to ciclosporin in any patient. The makers of bezafibrate suggest close monitoring of renal function.[6]

(b) Fenofibrate

Fenofibrate 200 mg once daily effectively reduced the blood cholesterol levels of 10 heart transplant patients from 7.7 to 6.5 mmol/l without significantly altering serum ciclosporin levels over a 2-week period. The only possible adverse effect was an increase in creatinine levels from 145 to 157 mmol/l, suggesting some possible nephrotoxicity. No other clinically adverse effects were seen. However, the authors of this study suggested that longer follow-up studies were needed to confirm the safety of using these drugs together.[7] They followed this up with a 1-year study[8] in 43 heart transplant patients, only 14 of whom completed the study (67% withdrew for various reasons). Fourteen patients had a rise in blood creatinine levels and a decrease in renal function, which improved when the fenofibrate was stopped. There was also some evidence of a reduction in ciclosporin levels in 5 patients who developed rejection, and 14 who had to stop fenofibrate because ciclosporin levels could not be maintained without adversely affecting renal function.

The evidence from these reports emphasises the importance of monitoring the long-term concurrent use of these two drugs because there are clearly some potential hazards.

(c) Gemfibrozil

Forty kidney transplant patients taking ciclosporin had a reduction in their hypertriglyceridaemia when gemfibrozil was added, and their ciclosporin serum levels and serum creatinine remained unaltered.[9] Another study in 12 patients similarly found that gemfibrozil did not affect serum ciclosporin levels.[10]

However, in contrast to these findings, another study in 7 kidney transplant patients with hyperlipidaemia found that gemfibrozil 450 mg once or twice daily was associated with a decline in trough ciclosporin levels. Levels declined from 93 to 76 nanograms/ml after 6 weeks of treatment and after dose increases in 3 patients the level at 3 months was 88 nanograms/ml. In 8 similar patients not given gemfibrozil, and with the same ciclosporin dose throughout, trough levels changed from 99 to 98 nanograms/ml at 6 weeks and to 123 nanograms/ml at 3 months. In 2 patients there was a significant increase in serum creatinine, and biopsy revealed chronic rejection in one and ciclosporin toxicity in the other. The study was stopped at 6 months because a drug interaction was suspected. The mechanism is not known, but changes in distribution of lipoproteins during gemfibrozil treatment may cause changes in the free fraction of ciclosporin. Ciclosporin absorption may also be reduced. Close monitoring is recommended during concomitant use.[11]

1. Hirai M, Tatuso E, Sakurai M, Ichikawa M, Matsuya F, Saito Y. Elevated blood concentrations of cyclosporine and kidney failure after bezafibrate in renal graft recipient. *Ann Pharmacother* (1996) 30, 883–4.
2. Lipkin GW, Tomson CRV. Severe reversible renal failure with bezafibrate. *Lancet* (1993) 341, 371.
3. Jespersen B, Tvedegaard E. Bezafibrate induced reduction of renal function in a renal transplant recipient. *Nephrol Dial Transplant* (1995) 10, 702–3.
4. Devuyst O, Goffin E, Pirson Y, van Ypersele de Strihou C. Creatinine rise after fibrate therapy in renal graft recipients. *Lancet* (1993) 341, 840.
5. Barbir M, Hunt B, Kushwaha S, Kehely A, Prescot R, Thompson GR, Mitchell A, Yacoub M. Maxepa versus bezafibrate in hyperlipidemic cardiac transplant recipients. *Am J Cardiol* (1992) 70, 1596–1601.
6. Bezalip (Bezafibrate). Roche Products Ltd. UK Summary of product characteristics, November 2002.
7. deLorgeril M, Boissonnat P, Bizollon CA, Guidollet J, Faucon G, Guichard JP, Levy-Prades-Sauron R, Renaud S, Dureau G. Pharmacokinetics of cyclosporine in hyperlipidaemic long-term survivors of heart transplantation. Lack of interaction with the lipid-lowering agent, fenofibrate. *Eur J Clin Pharmacol* (1992) 43, 161–5.
8. Boissonnat P, Salen P, Guidollet J, Ferrara R, Dureau G, Ninet J, Renaud S, de Lorgeril M. The long-term effects of the lipid-lowering agent fenofibrate in hyperlipidemic heart transplant recipients. *Transplantation* (1994) 58, 245–7.
9. Pisanti N, Stanziale P, Imperatore P, D'Alessandro R, De Marino V, Capone D, De Marino V. Lack of effect of gemfibrozil on cyclosporine blood concentrations in kidney-transplanted patients. *Am J Nephrol* (1998) 18, 199–203.
10. Valino RN, Reiss WG, Hanes D, White M, Hoehn-Saric E, Klassen D, Bartlett S, Weir MR. Examination of the potential interaction between HMG-CoA reductase inhibitors and cyclosporine in transplant patients. *Pharmacotherapy* (1996) 16, 511.
11. Fehrman-Ekholm I, Jogestrand T, Angelin B. Decreased cyclosporine levels during gemfibrozil treatment of hyperlipidemia after kidney transplantation. *Nephron* (1996) 72, 483.

Ciclosporin + Food or Drinks

Food, milk and grapefruit juice, but not orange juice, can increase the bioavailability of ciclosporin. Lipid admixtures for parenteral nutrition appear not to affect ciclosporin pharmacokinetics. Red wine decreases ciclosporin bioavailability.

Clinical evidence

(a) Food or Milk

Patients taking ciclosporin with milk had a 39% higher AUC after food and 23% higher AUC when fasting compared with others taking ciclosporin with **orange juice**.[1] Food more than doubled the AUC of ciclosporin (bioavailability increased from 20.7 to 53%) and almost tripled its maximum serum levels, from 783 to 2062 nanograms/ml.[2] When 18 patients with kidney transplants were given ciclosporin mixed with 240 ml of chocolate milk and taken with a standard hospital **breakfast**, their peak ciclosporin levels rose by 31%, from 1120 to 1465 nanograms/ml, trough serum levels rose by 17%, from 228 to 267 nanograms/ml, and the AUC rose by 45%. Very considerable individual variations occurred.[3]

A study in 10 patients undergoing bone-marrow transplantation and given isocaloric and isonitrogenous parenteral nutrition with or without lipids found that ciclosporin pharmacokinetics are not affected by **lipid-enriched admixtures**.[4]

(b) Fruit juices

A considerable number of single and multiple dose studies in healthy subjects, transplant, and other patients with haematological diseases have shown that if oral ciclosporin is taken with 150 to 250 ml (5 to 8 ozs) of **grapefruit juice**, the trough and peak serum levels and the bioavailability of the ciclosporin may be increased. The increases reported vary very considerably. Increases in trough serum levels range from 23 to 85%,[5-12] in peak serum levels from 0 to 69%,[8-10,13-16] and in AUCs from 0 to 72%.[6-10,13,14,17,18]

In one study the AUC of the microemulsion formulation of ciclosporin was increased by 38% (range 12 to 194%) by **grapefruit juice** but the maximum levels were unchanged.[19] A further study with the microemulsion formulation found that both the peak levels and AUC were increased by **grapefruit juice**, but while increases of 39% and 60% respectively were observed in African-American patients, smaller increases of 8% and 44% were observed in Caucasian patients.[20]

A study in 6 paediatric renal transplant patients found that giving ciclosporin oral solution with **grapefruit juice** produced a significant increase (109%) in the 12-hour trough level although the AUC was not significantly changed. When ciclosporin was given as a microemulsion, **grapefruit juice** did not significantly affect the pharmacokinetics of ciclosporin.[21]

Ciclosporin levels are unaffected by **orange juice**.[6,12] **Grapefruit juice** has no effect on ciclosporin levels when the ciclosporin is given intravenously.[22]

(c) Red wine

A two-way crossover study in 12 healthy subjects given a single 8 mg/kg dose of ciclosporin with water or 350 ml (12 oz) of Californian red wine found that red wine caused a 50% increase in the oral clearance of ciclosporin. The ciclosporin AUC was reduced by 30% and the maximum blood levels were reduced by 38%, from 1258 to 779 micrograms/l. There was a high degree of variability with increases in oral clearance ranging from 1.5% to 129%, with Caucasians experiencing a greater degree of change than Asians [not-defined].[23]

Mechanism

It is suggested that grapefruit juice inhibits the activity of the cytochrome P450 isoenzyme CYP3A in the gut wall and liver. Ciclosporin is primarily metabolised by CYP3A4 and so its levels rise.

The mechanism by which red wine exerts its effect is not known. White wine does not appear to affect ciclosporin pharmacokinetics,[24] so the interaction is not believed to be an effect of alcohol (see also 'Ciclosporin + Alcohol', p.770). Antioxidants in red wine such as resveratrol may inactivate CYP3A4 and this would also be expected to increase ciclosporin levels. The solubility of ciclosporin is decreased in red wine and it is possible that substances in red wine bind ciclosporin in the gastrointestinal tract and reduce its bioavailability.[23] Another study by the same authors suggested that ciclosporin absorption is possibly impaired through P-glycoprotein activation.[25]

Importance and management

The food, milk and grapefruit juice interactions are established and clinically important. Food, milk and grapefruit juice, but not orange juice, can increase the bioavailability of ciclosporin. The situation should therefore be monitored if any changes are made to the diet of patients on ciclosporin. Patients should be warned because increased ciclosporin levels are associated with increased nephrotoxicity. Lipid admixtures in parenteral nutrition do not appear to affect ciclosporin pharmacokinetics and it is speculated that they may protect against ciclosporin-induced nephrotoxicity. Close supervision and monitoring is required. There is insufficient evidence to allow extrapolation of the results to bone-marrow transplant recipients with risk factors such as dyslipidaemia, liver or renal failure.[4]

It has been suggested that the interaction between grapefruit juice and ciclosporin could be exploited to save money. One group of authors has suggested that grapefruit juice is roughly as effective as diltiazem in raising ciclosporin serum levels, and has the advantage of being inexpensive, nutritious and lacking the systemic effects of diltiazem and ketoconazole which have been used in this way.[6] See 'Ciclosporin + Calcium channel blockers', p.784 and 'Ciclosporin + Azoles', p.781. However, it has also been pointed out that it may be risky to try to exploit this interaction in this way because the increases appear to be so variable and difficult, if not impossible, to control. This is because batches of grapefruit juice vary so much, and also considerable patient variation occurs with this interaction.[26-28] The US makers suggest that patients on ciclosporin should avoid whole grapefruit, as well as the juice.[29]

Patients may be advised to avoid alcohol after transplantation, but those who do drink should exercise caution if drinking red wine while taking ciclosporin.[23] See also 'Ciclosporin + Alcohol', p.770.

1. Keogh A, Day R, Critchley L, Duggin G, Baron D. The effect of food and cholestyramine on the absorption of cyclosporine in cardiac transplant recipients. *Transplant Proc* (1988) 20, 27–30.
2. Gupta SK, Benet LZ. Food increases the bioavailability of cyclosporin in healthy volunteers. *Clin Pharmacol Ther* (1989) 45,148.
3. Ptachcinski RJ, Venkataramanan R, Rosenthal JT, Burckart GJ, Taylor RJ, Hakala TR. The effect of food on cyclosporine absorption. *Transplantation* (1985) 40, 174–6.
4. Santos P, Lourenço R, Camilo ME, Oliveira AG, Figueira I, Pereira ME, Ferreira B, Carmo JA, Lacerda JMF. Parenteral nutrition and cyclosporine: do lipids make a difference? A prospective randomized crossover trial. *Clin Nutr* (2001) 20, 31–6.
5. Ducharme MP, Provenzano R, Dehoorne-Smith M, Edwards DJ. Trough concentrations of cyclosporine in blood following administration with grapefruit juice. *Br J Clin Pharmacol* (1993) 36, 457–9.
6. Yee GC, Stanley DL, Pessa LJ, Costa TD, Beltz SE, Ruiz J, Lowenthal DT. Effect of grapefruit juice on blood cyclosporine concentration. *Lancet* (1995) 345, 955–6.
7. Proppe DG, Hoch OD, McLean AJ, Visser KE. Influence of chronic ingestion of grapefruit juice on steady-state blood concentrations of cyclosporine A in renal transplant patients with stable graft function. *Br J Clin Pharmacol* (1995) 39, 337–8.
8. Min DI, Ku Y-M, Perry PJ, Martin MF, Lawrence G, Hunsiker LG. The effect of grapefruit juice on cyclosporine pharmacokinetics in renal allograft recipients. *Pharmacotherapy* (1996) 16, 516.
9. Herlitz H, Edgar B, Hedner T, Lidman K, Karlberg I. Grapefruit juice: a possible source of variability in blood concentration of cyclosporin A. *Nephrol Dial Transplant* (1993) 8, 375.
10. Brunner L, Munar M, Bennett W. Effect of grapefruit juice on cyclosporine pharmacokinetics in renal transplant recipients. *Pharm Res* (1997) 14 (11 Suppl), S-180–S-181.
11. Emilia G, Longo G, Bertesi M, Gandini G, Ferrara L, Valenti C. Clinical interaction between grapefruit juice and cyclosporine: is there any interest for the hematologists? *Blood* (1998) 91, 362–3.
12. Edwards DJ, Fitzsimmons ME, Schuetz EG, Yasuda K, Ducharme MP, Warbasse LH, Woster PM, Schuetz JD, Watkins P. 6',7'-dihydroxybergamottin in grapefruit juice and Seville orange juice: effects on cyclosporine disposition, enterocyte CYP3A4, and P-glycoprotein. *Clin Pharmacol Ther* (1999) 65, 237–44.
13. Ku Y-M, Min DI, Flanigan MJ. The effect of grapefruit juice on microemulsion cyclosporine (Neoral) pharmacokinetics in healthy volunteers. *Pharmacotherapy* (1998) 18, 442.
14. Proppe D, Visser K, Hoch O, Bartels R, Meier H, McLean AJ. Differential influence on cyclosporin A metabolism by chronic grapefruit juice exposure. *Eur J Clin Invest* (1996) 26 (Suppl 1), A20.
15. Ioannides-Demos LL, Christophidis N, Ryan P, Angelis P, Liolios L, McLean AJ. Dosing implications of a clinical interaction between grapefruit juice and cyclosporine and metabolite concentrations in patients with autoimmune diseases. *J Rheumatol* (1997) 24, 49–54.
16. Hollander AAMJ, van Rooij J, Lentjes EGWM, Arbouw F, van Bree JB, Schoemaker RC, van Es LA, van der Woude FJ, Cohen AF. The effect of grapefruit juice on cyclosporine and prednisone metabolism in transplant patients. *Clin Pharmacol Ther* (1995) 57, 318–24.
17. Yee GC, Adams VR, Pessa L, Braddock RJ, Ruiz J, Lowenthal DT. Comparison of one versus two doses of grapefruit juice on oral cyclosporine pharmacokinetics. *Pharmacotherapy* (1997) 17, 1112.
18. Proppe D, Visser K, Bartels R, Hoch O, Meyer H, McLean AJ. Grapefruit juice selectively modifies cyclosporin A metabolite patterns in renal transplant patients. *Clin Pharmacol Ther* (1996) 59, 138.
19. Bistrup C, Nielsen FT, Jeppesen UE, Dieperink H. Effect of grapefruit juice on Sandimmmun Neoral® absorption among stable renal allograft recipients. *Nephrol Dial Transplant* (2001) 16, 373–7.
20. Lee M, Min DI, Ku Y-M, Flanigan M. Effect of grapefruit juice on pharmacokinetics of microemulsion cyclosporine in African American subjects compared with Caucasian subjects: does ethnic difference matter? *J Clin Pharmacol* (2001) 41, 317–23.
21. Brunner LJ, Pai K-S, Munar MY, Lande MB, Olyaei AJ, Mowry JA. Effect of grapefruit juice on cyclosporin A pharmacokinetics in pediatric renal transplant patients. *Pediatr Transplant* (2000) 4, 313–21.
22. Ducharme MP, Warbasse LH, Edwards DJ. Disposition of intravenous and oral cyclosporine after administration with grapefruit juice. *Clin Pharmacol Ther* (1995) 57, 485–91.
23. Tsunoda SM, Harris RZ, Christians U, Velez RL, Freeman RB, Benet LZ, Warshaw A. Red wine decreases cyclosporine bioavailability. *Clin Pharmacol Ther* (2001) 70, 462–7.
24. Tsunoda SM, Harris RZ, Freeman RB, Warshaw A. Acute and chronic wine effects on cyclosporine disposition. *Br J Clin Pharmacol* (2000) 42.
25. Tsunoda SM, Christians U, Velez RL, Benet LZ, Harris RZ. Red wine (RW) effects on cyclosporine (CyA) metabolites. *Clin Pharmacol Ther* (2000) 67, 150.
26. Johnston A, Holt DW. Effect of grapefruit juice on blood cyclosporin concentration. *Lancet* (1995) 346, 122–3.
27. Hollander AAMJ, van der Woude FJ, Cohen AF. Effect of grapefruit juice on blood cyclosporin concentration. *Lancet* (1995) 346, 123.
28. Yee GC, Lowenthal DT. Effect of grapefruit juice on blood cyclosporin concentration. *Lancet* (1995) 346, 123–4.
29. Neoral (Ciclosporin). Novartis. US Prescribing information, March 2004.

Ciclosporin + Foscarnet

Acute but reversible renal failure occurred in two transplant patients when foscarnet was given with ciclosporin.

Clinical evidence

A man with a kidney transplant taking corticosteroids and ciclosporin developed a cytomegalovirus infection that was treated with foscarnet 85 mg/kg daily. Despite efforts to minimise the nephrotoxic effects of the foscarnet (hydration with 2.5 litres of isotonic saline daily and nifedipine 80 mg the day before and during treatment) the patient developed non-oliguric worsening of his renal function after 8 days. Nine days after stopping the foscarnet, the former renal function was restored.[1]

A liver transplant patient on steroids, azathioprine and ciclosporin was similarly treated with foscarnet 180 mg/kg daily for a hepatitis B infection. Acute renal failure occurred 5 days after the foscarnet was started, and renal function was restored 10 days after the foscarnet was stopped. The ciclosporin serum levels were therapeutic and not significantly altered at any time in either patient.[1]

Mechanism

Not understood. It seems that the nephrotoxic effects of the ciclosporin and foscarnet can be additive.

Importance and management

Direct information appears to be limited to this report, but it is consistent with the known potential toxicity of both drugs. Acute renal failure can clearly occur despite the preventative measures taken. The authors of this report[1] say that monitoring of renal function is mandatory when both drugs are given.

1. Morales JM, Muñoz MA, Fernández Zataraín G, Garcia Cantón C, García Rubiales MA, Andrés A, Aguado JM, Pinto IG. Reversible acute renal failure caused by the combined use of foscarnet and cyclosporin in organ transplanted patients. *Nephrol Dial Transplant* (1995) 10, 882–3.

Ciclosporin + Ganciclovir

Four patients given ciclosporin and ganciclovir developed an acute but reversible eye movement disorder.

Clinical evidence, mechanism, importance and management

In a USA hospital, 582 allogenic bone marrow transplants were carried out between 1988 and 1994. All the patients were given ciclosporin and about 45% also had ganciclovir at some time during the first 3 months after the transplant. Four patients (0.7%) developed an acute eye movement disorder (unilateral or bilateral sixth nerve palsies) within 4 to 34 days of starting ganciclovir. Three of the 4 patients also had bilateral ptosis. The problem cleared 24 to 48 hours after withdrawal of both drugs from 3 patients, and the withdrawal of just ciclosporin from the other patient. Objective eye movement abnormality with diplopia reoccurred in one patient when both drugs were restarted, but not when ciclosporin alone was given.[1]

The reason for this toxic reaction is not known but the authors of the report postulate a transient brain stem or neuromuscular dysfunction caused by both drugs.[1] It is an uncommon reaction and reversible, so that concurrent use need not be avoided but both drugs should be stopped if it happens. The report cited here seems to be the only report of this interaction.

1. Openshaw H, Slatkin NE, Smith E. Eye movement disorders in bone marrow transplant patients on cyclosporin and ganciclovir. *Bone Marrow Transplant* (1997) 19, 503–5.

Ciclosporin + *Geum chiloense*

A single case report describes a marked and rapid increase in the serum ciclosporin levels of a man after he drank an infusion of *Geum chiloense*.

Clinical evidence, mechanism, importance and management

A 54-year-old kidney transplant patient on ciclosporin, prednisone, azathioprine, diltiazem and nifedipine had a sudden and very marked rise in his ciclosporin levels from his usual range of 60 to 90 mg/dl up to a range of 469 to 600 mg/dl. He had been taking ciclosporin 2 to 3 mg/kg daily for 15 months since the transplant. His serum creatinine levels were found to be 115 micromol/l. It eventually turned out that about 2 weeks earlier he had started to drink an infusion of *Geum chiloense* (or *Geum quellyon),* a herbal remedy claimed to increase virility and to treat prostatism. When the herbal remedy was stopped, his serum ciclosporin levels rapidly returned to their normal values. The reasons for this apparent interaction are not known.[1]

This appears to be the only case on record but it serves, along with reports about other herbs, to emphasise that herbal remedies may not be safe just because they are 'natural'. In this instance the herbal remedy markedly increased the potential nephrotoxicity of the ciclosporin. Patients should be warned.

1. Duclos J, Goecke H. "Hierba del clavo" *(Geum chiloense)* interfiere niveles de ciclosporin: potencial riesgo para trasplantados. *Rev Med Chil* (2001) 129, 789–90.

Ciclosporin + Griseofulvin

An isolated report describes decreased ciclosporin levels in a patient given griseofulvin.

Clinical evidence, mechanism, importance and management

A 57-year-old-man, who had been stable for almost a year on ciclosporin, azathioprine and prednisolone following a kidney transplant, was started on griseofulvin 500 mg daily for onychomycosis. Two weeks later his trough ciclosporin levels had dropped from 90 to 50 nanograms/ml and remained low, despite an increase in his ciclosporin dose from 2.8 to 4.8 mg/kg. When the griseofulvin was later stopped, his ciclosporin levels rose to over 200 nanograms/ml and his dose of ciclosporin was readjusted.[1]

This appears to be the only report of an interaction with griseofulvin, and its general significance is unclear.

1. Abu-Romeh SH, Rashed A. Ciclosporin A and griseofulvin: another drug interaction. *Nephron* (1991) 58, 237.

Ciclosporin + H_2-blockers

Reports are inconsistent. Cimetidine and famotidine have been reported both to increase and not change ciclosporin levels, whereas ranitidine has only been reported to not affect ciclosporin levels. Both cimetidine and ranitidine have been reported to cause an increase in serum creatinine levels, in some but not all studies, but this may possibly not be a reliable indicator of increased nephrotoxicity. Isolated cases of thrombocytopenia and hepatotoxicity have been reported with ranitidine and ciclosporin.

Clinical evidence

(a) Cimetidine

A study in 5 liver transplant patients on ciclosporin found that three 800 mg doses of cimetidine given every 12 hours raised peak ciclosporin levels, but no changes in trough levels were seen after 4 hours. Similarly, no change in trough ciclosporin levels was seen in 2 patients who received cimetidine 400 mg four times daily for 4 weeks, and the conclusion was reached that it was safe to use cimetidine over at least a 4-week period.[1] In a retrospective study it was reported that heart transplant patients on cimetidine had a lower dosage/level quotient leading to higher serum ciclosporin levels for the same dosage.[2] Similarly, a study in 6 healthy subjects found a 30% rise in the AUC of ciclosporin 300 mg given after a 3-day course of cimetidine 400 mg daily.[3] Raised serum ciclosporin levels have also been seen in a patient when treated with cimetidine and metronidazole[4] (see 'Ciclosporin + Antibacterials; Metronidazole', p.775).

Cimetidine or **ranitidine** increased the mean serum creatinine levels in 7 kidney transplant patients on ciclosporin by 41%, from 202 to 285 micromol/l. All of the patients had a rise, whereas only 2 out of 5 other patients with heart transplants had a rise in their serum creatinine levels when given either cimetidine or **ranitidine**, nevertheless the mean rise was 37%, from 152 to 209 micromol/l. Ciclosporin levels were not altered.[5] A transient increase in creatinine serum levels at days 2 and 5 was seen in another study of 7 renal transplant patients given cimetidine 400 mg daily for 7 days. Again ciclosporin levels were not altered.[6]

Similarly, cimetidine did not alter serum ciclosporin levels in 2 studies in healthy subjects.[7,8]

(b) Famotidine

Famotidine is reported not to affect serum ciclosporin levels.[9-11] However, higher serum ciclosporin levels were found in a study of heart transplant patients given famotidine.[2] No significant changes in the pharmacokinetics of ciclosporin was seen in a single-dose study in 8 healthy subjects[8] and no changes in serum creatinine or BUN levels were seen in 7 kidney transplant patients.[11]

(c) Ranitidine

One report (see (a) above), where the effects of cimetidine and ranitidine were examined together, suggests that ranitidine raises creatinine levels in patients on ciclosporin, without affecting ciclosporin levels.[5] Similarly, several other reports say that ranitidine does not alter serum ciclosporin levels.[12-15] One also says that ranitidine does not alter creatinine levels and inulin clearance.[13]

A report describes thrombocytopenia in a man taking ciclosporin after a kidney transplant who was given ranitidine.[16] Another patient experienced hepatotoxicity while taking ciclosporin with ranitidine.[17]

Mechanism

It is not clear why these reports are inconsistent, nor how the H_2-blockers might raise serum ciclosporin levels. It has also been suggested that any rise in serum creatinine levels could simply be because these H_2-blockers compete with creatinine for secretion by the kidney tubules, and therefore rises are not an indicator of nephrotoxicity[18,19]

Importance and management

Information about the possible interactions of ciclosporin and cimetidine, famotidine or ranitidine is inconsistent, but there appear to very few reports of confirmed toxicity. Moreover the reported increases in serum creatinine levels seen with the H_2-blockers may not be a reflection of increased nephrotoxicity (see 'Mechanism'). Thus there is little to suggest that concurrent use should be avoided, but good initial monitoring is advisable.

1. Puff MR, Carey WD. The effect of cimetidine on cyclosporine A levels in liver transplant recipients: a preliminary report. *Am J Gastroenterol* (1992) 87, 287–91.
2. Reichenspurner H, Meiser BM, Muschiol F, Nollert G, Überfuhr P, Markewitz A, Wagner F, Pfeiffer M, Reichart B. The influence of gastrointestinal agents on resorption and metabolism of cyclosporine after heart transplantation: experimental and clinical results. *J Heart Lung Transplant* (1993) 12, 987–92.
3. Choi J-S, Choi I, Min DI. Effect of cimetidine on pharmacokinetics of cyclosporine in healthy volunteers. *Pharmacotherapy* (1997) 17, 1120.
4. Zylber-Katz E, Rubinger D, Berlatzky Y. Cyclosporine interactions with metronidazole and cimetidine. *Drug Intell Clin Pharm* (1988) 22, 504–5.
5. Jarowenko MV, Van Buren CT, Kramer WG, Lorber MI, Flechner SM, Kahan BD. Ranitidine, cimetidine, and the cyclosporine-treated recipient. *Transplantation* (1986) 42, 311–12.
6. Barn YM, Ramos EL, Balagtas RS, Peterson JC, Karlix JL. Cimetidine or ranitidine in prophylactic doses do not affect renal function or cyclosporine levels in renal transplant patients (RTP). *J Am Soc Nephrol* (1993) 4, 925.
7. Freeman DJ, Laupacis A, Keown P, Stiller C, Carruthers G. The effect of agents that alter drug metabolizing enzyme activity on the pharmacokinetics of cyclosporine. *Ann R Coll Physicians Surg Can* (1984) 17, 301.
8. Shaefer MS, Rossi SJ, McGuire TR, Schaaf LJ, Collier DS, Stratta RJ. Evaluation of the pharmacokinetic interaction between cimetidine or famotidine and cyclosporine in healthy men. *Ann Pharmacother* (1995) 29, 1088–91.
9. Von Schütz A, Kemkes BM. Ciclosporinspiegel unter Gabe von Famotidin. *Fortschr Med* (1990) 23, 457–8.
10. Morel D, Bannwarth B, Vinçon G, Penouil F, Elouaer-Blanc L, Aparicio M, Potaux L. Effect of famotidine on renal transplant patients treated with ciclosporine A. *Fundam Clin Pharmacol* (1993) 7, 167–70.
11. Inoue S, Sugimoto H, Nagao T, Akiyama N. Does H_2-receptor antagonist alter the renal function of cyclosporine-treated kidney grafts? *Jpn J Surg* (1990) 20, 553–8.
12. Zazgornik J, Schindler J, Gremmel F, Balcke P, Kopsa H, Derfler K, Minar E. Ranitidine does not influence the blood ciclosporin levels in renal transplant patients (RTP). *Kidney Int* (1985) 28, 401.
13. Jadoul M, Hené RJ. Ranitidine and the cyclosporine-treated recipient. *Transplantation* (1989) 48, 359.
14. Popovic J, Cameron JS. Effects of ranitidine on renal function in transplant recipients. *Nephrol Dial Transplant* (1990) 5, 980–1.
15. Tsang VT, Johnston A, Heritier F, Leaver N, Hodson ME, Yacoub M. Cyclosporin pharmacokinetics in heart-lung transplant recipients with cystic fibrosis. *Eur J Clin Pharmacol* (1994) 46, 261–5.
16. Bailey RR, Walker RJ, Swainson CP. Some new problems with cyclosporin A? *N Z Med J* (1985) 98, 915–6.

17. Hiesse C, Cantarovich M, Santelli C, Francais P, Charpentier B, Fries D, Buffet C. Ranitidine hepatotoxicity in a renal transplant patient. *Lancet* (1985) i, 1280.
18. Pachon J, Lorber MI, Bia MJ. Effects of H_2-receptor antagonists on renal function in cyclosporine-treated renal transplant patients. *Transplantation* (1989) 47, 254–9.
19. Lewis SM, McClosky WW. Potentiation of nephrotoxicity by H_2-antagonists in patients receiving cyclosporine. *Ann Pharmacother* (1997) 31, 363–5.

Ciclosporin + Melphalan

Melphalan appears to increase the nephrotoxic effects of ciclosporin.

Clinical evidence, mechanism, importance and management

A comparative study found that 13 out of 17 patients receiving bone marrow transplants and given ciclosporin 12.5 mg/kg daily with high-dose melphalan (single injection of 140 to 250 mg/m^2) developed renal failure, compared with no cases of renal failure in 7 other patients given melphalan but no ciclosporin.[1] In another study, one out of 4 patients given both drugs developed nephrotoxicity.[2] The reasons are not understood. Renal function should be monitored closely on concurrent use.

1. Morgenstern GR, Powles R, Robinson B, McElwain TJ. Cyclosporin interaction with ketoconazole and melphalan. *Lancet* (1982) ii, 1342.
2. Dale BM, Sage RE, Norman JE, Barber S, Kotasek D. Bone marrow transplantation following treatment with high-dose melphalan. *Transplant Proc* (1985) 17, 1711–13.

Ciclosporin + Metamizole sodium (Dipyrone)

The short term use of metamizole sodium appears to have no effect on the steady-state serum levels of ciclosporin.

Clinical evidence, mechanism, importance and management

A placebo-controlled, double blind crossover study in 6 kidney and 2 heart transplant patients on ciclosporin found that while they were taking metamizole sodium 500 mg three times daily for 4 days the pharmacokinetics of the ciclosporin (AUC, trough and peak serum levels, elimination half-life) were unchanged, but the time to reach maximum serum levels was slightly prolonged, from 2.1 to 3.8 hours. It is not known what the effects of longer use might be.[1,2]

1. Caraco Y, Zylber-Katz E, Levy M. The effect of dipyrone on cyclosporine A metabolism. *Eur J Clin Pharmacol* (1997) 52 (Suppl), A130.
2. Caraco Y, Zylber-Katz E, Fridlander M, Admon D, Levy M. The effect of short-term dipyrone administration on cyclosporin pharmacokinetics. *Eur J Clin Pharmacol* (1999) 55, 475–8.

Ciclosporin + Methotrexate

Previous or concurrent treatment with methotrexate may possibly increase the risk of liver and other toxicity in those given ciclosporin, but effective and valuable concurrent use has also been reported. Ciclosporin causes a moderate rise in serum methotrexate levels, but methotrexate does not appear to affect the pharmacokinetics of ciclosporin.

Clinical evidence

(a) Evidence of toxicity

A limited comparative study in patients with chronic plaque psoriasis suggested that prior treatment with methotrexate, which can cause liver damage, possibly increases the risk of ciclosporin toxicity (higher serum ciclosporin and creatinine levels, hypertension).[1] This was confirmed by another study in 4 patients with resistant psoriasis in whom ciclosporin 5 mg/kg daily given with methotrexate 2.5 mg every 12 hours for three doses at weekly intervals increased the serum levels of both drugs, and increased the adverse effects (nausea, vomiting, mouth ulcers). Rises in creatinine levels and liver enzymes (AST, ALT) also occurred.[2]

(b) Evidence of concurrent use without toxicity

In contrast to the reports cited above, a pilot study described the effective use of both drugs for the control of acute graft-versus-host disease in bone marrow transplant patients, with the ciclosporin dosage reduced by 50% to 1.5 mg/kg/day during the first 2 weeks. The methotrexate dosages were 10 to 15 mg/m^2 on days 1, 3, 6 and 11 after grafting. Hepatotoxicity appeared to be reduced.[3] Another study in three bone marrow transplant patients found that low-dose methotrexate (15 mg/m^2 on day 1, and 10 mg/m^2 on days 3, 6 and 11) given with ciclosporin did not significantly affect clinical care and no interaction of clinical significance was seen.[4]

(c) Evidence of a pharmacokinetic interaction

An open-label pharmacokinetic study in 26 patients with rheumatoid arthritis taking methotrexate and ciclosporin 1.5 mg/kg every 12 hours for 14 days, found the AUC of the methotrexate increased by 26%, whereas the serum levels of its major metabolite (7-hydroxymethotrexate), which is much less active and may be associated with toxicity, were reduced by 80%.[5] Another study in patients with rheumatoid arthritis found that the pharmacokinetics of ciclosporin after the first dose did not differ between those who had been receiving intramuscular methotrexate 10 mg each week for 6 months and those not on methotrexate.[6]

Mechanism

Not understood.

Importance and management

The reports cited here give an inconsistent picture. On the one hand there is the strong recommendation by the authors of the second study[2] that combined use should be avoided, even in patients with severe unresponsive psoriasis, whereas it seems from the other studies in patients with rheumatoid arthritis, or those undergoing bone marrow transplant[3,4] that concurrent use can be valuable, effective and apparently safe. Patients on ciclosporin should routinely be monitored for renal effects, and those on methotrexate routinely monitored for hepatotoxicity. If both drugs are used concurrently it may be worth increasing the frequency of this monitoring to aid rapid detection of any adverse effects.

1. Powles AV, Baker BS, Fry L, Valdimarsson H. Cyclosporin toxicity. *Lancet* (1990) 335, 610.
2. Korstanje MJ, van Breda Vriesman CJP, van de Staak WJBM. Cyclosporine and methotrexate: a dangerous combination. *J Am Acad Dermatol* (1990) 23, 320–1.
3. Stockschlaeder M, Storb R, Pepe M, Longton G, McDonald G, Anasetti C, Appelbaum F, Doney K, Martin P, Sullivan K, Witherspoon R. A pilot study of low-dose cyclosporin for graft-versus-host prophylaxis in marrow transplantation. *Br J Haematol* (1991) 80, 49–54.
4. Dix S, Devine SM, Geller RB, Wingard JR. Re: severe interaction between methotrexate and a macrolide antibiotic. *J Natl Cancer Inst* (1995) 87, 1641–2.
5. Fox RI, Morgan SL, Smith HT, Robbins BA, Choc MG, Baggott JE. Combined oral cyclosporin and methotrexate therapy in patients with rheumatoid arthritis elevates methotrexate levels and reduces 7-hydroxymethotrexate levels when compared with methotrexate alone. *Rheumatology (Oxford)* (2003) 42, 989–94.
6. Baraldo M, Ferraccioli G, Pea F, Gremese E, Furlanut M. Cyclosporine A pharmacokinetics in rheumatoid arthritis patients after 6 months of methotrexate therapy. *Pharm Res* (1999) 40, 483–6.

Ciclosporin + Methylphenidate

In an isolated case, the ciclosporin levels of a 10-year-old-boy were raised by 50% after he started to take methylphenidate.

Clinical evidence , mechanism, importance and management

A 10-year-old boy, who had received a heart transplant 6 years previously was started on methylphenidate 5 mg twice daily in addition to his transplant medication, which included ciclosporin. After 4 days his ciclosporin level was found to have risen from 195 to 302 nanograms/ml. His ciclosporin dosage was therefore reduced from 550 to 500 mg daily, and at the same time the methylphenidate was increased to 7.5 mg twice daily. As the next ciclosporin level was still elevated at 251 nanograms/ml, the ciclosporin dose was further reduced to 450 mg daily. The boy then remained on this dose of ciclosporin with acceptable levels, despite further dose increases in the methylphenidate to an eventual dose of 20 mg daily.[1]

The reason for this probable interaction is unclear. This appears to be the only reported case of an interaction between ciclosporin and methylphenidate, and its general importance is unknown.

1. Lewis BR, Aoun SL, Bernstein GA, Crow SJ. Pharmacokinetic interactions between cyclosporin and bupropion or methylphenidate. *J Child Adolesc Psychopharmacol* (2001) 11, 193–8.

Ciclosporin + Metoclopramide

Metoclopramide moderately increases the absorption of ciclosporin and raises its serum levels.

Clinical evidence, mechanism, importance and management

When 14 kidney transplant patients were given metoclopramide their peak serum ciclosporin levels were increased by 46%, from 388 to 567 nanograms/ml and the ciclosporin AUC was increased by 22%. The dosage of metoclopramide was 10 mg by mouth 30 minutes before, 5 mg with, and 5 mg 30 minutes after the morning dose of ciclosporin.[1] The probable reason is that the metoclopramide hastens gastric emptying and ciclosporin is largely absorbed by the small intestine. The clinical importance of this interaction is uncertain. Concurrent use should be well monitored to ensure that ciclosporin levels do not become toxic.

1. Wadhwa NK, Schroeder TJ, O'Flaherty E, Pesce AJ, Myre SA, First MR. The effect of oral metoclopramide on the absorption of cyclosporine. *Transplant Proc* (1987) 19, 1730–3.

Ciclosporin + Midazolam

On the basis of an experimental study in 9 patients it was concluded that the dosage of midazolam needs no adjustment in those on ciclosporin. Midazolam also appears to have no effect on ciclosporin.[1]

1. Li G, Treiber G, Meinshausen J, Wolf J, Werringloer J, Klotz U. Is cyclosporin A an inhibitor of drug metabolism? *Br J Clin Pharmacol* (1990) 30, 71–7.

Ciclosporin + Minoxidil

The concurrent use of ciclosporin and minoxidil can cause excessive hairiness (hypertrichosis).

Clinical evidence, mechanism, importance and management

Six male kidney transplant patients on ciclosporin (serum levels of 100 to 200 nanograms/ml) were given methyldopa, a diuretic and minoxidil 15 to 40 mg daily for intractable hypertension. After 4 weeks of treatment all of them complained of severe and unpleasant hypertrichosis. Two months after stopping the minoxidil the hypertrichosis had significantly improved.[1] Both ciclosporin and minoxidil cause hypertrichosis and it would seem that their effects may be additive. The authors of the report point out that this is not a life-threatening problem, but it limits the concurrent use of these drugs in both men and women.[1]

1. Sever MS, Sonmez YE, Kocak N. Limited use of minoxidil in renal transplant recipients because of the additive side-effects of cyclosporine on hypertrichosis. *Transplantation* (1990) 50, 536.

Ciclosporin + Modafinil

Ciclosporin serum levels were reported to be reduced by modafinil in one patient.

Clinical evidence, mechanism, importance and management

A kidney transplant patient, stabilised for 9 years on ciclosporin 200 mg daily, developed Gélineau's syndrome and was also given modafinil 200 mg daily. Within a few weeks her serum ciclosporin levels were noted to have fallen, and it was found necessary to raise her ciclosporin dosage stepwise to 300 mg daily before her serum levels were back to their former values.[1] It is thought that this interaction occurs because modafinil induces the cytochrome P450 isoenzyme CYP3A4, the major enzyme involved in the metabolism of ciclosporin. This is the first reported case of an interaction between ciclosporin and modafinil, and its general importance is unknown.

1. LeCacheux Ph, Charasse C, Mourtada R, Muh Ph, Boulahrouz R, Simon P. Gélineau's syndrome in a kidney-transplant patient. *Presse Med* (1997) 26, 466.

Ciclosporin + Morphine

An isolated report describes neuropsychosis in a patient who was given intravenous ciclosporin and morphine.

Clinical evidence, mechanism, importance and management

A patient who underwent renal transplantation was given ciclosporin 6 mg/kg daily by intravenous infusion over 2 hours and intravenous methylprednisolone postoperatively. He also received patient-controlled analgesia as bolus doses of morphine 0.5 mg to a total dose of 13 mg on the first day and 11 mg on the second day. On the third day he developed insomnia, anxiety, amnesia, aphasia and severe confusion. The morphine was discontinued and the symptoms subsided after treatment with propofol, diazepam and haloperidol. It was suggested that ciclosporin may have decreased the excitation threshold of neuronal cells, which potentiated the dysphoric effects of morphine.[1] This appears to be an isolated case and almost certainly not of general importance.

1. Lee P-C, Hung C-J, Lei H-Y, Tsai Y-C. Suspected acute post-transplant neuropsychosis due to interaction of morphine and cyclosporin after a renal transplant. *Anaesthesia* (2000) 55, 827–8.

Ciclosporin + Muromonab-CD3

Muromonab-CD3 increases serum ciclosporin levels.

Clinical evidence, mechanism, importance and management

When muromonab-CD3 5 mg daily for 10 days was given to 10 kidney transplant patients to treat acute rejection, their mean trough ciclosporin levels on day 8 were still higher than before the muromonab-CD3 was started, despite a 50% reduction in the ciclosporin dosage. When the muromonab-CD3 was withdrawn, the ciclosporin dosage needed to be increased again.[1] The reasons are not understood. It is clearly necessary to titrate the dosage of ciclosporin downwards if muromonab-CD3 is given to prevent an excessive rise in ciclosporin levels with the attendant risks of renal toxicity.

1. Vrahnos D, Sanchez J, Vasquez EM, Pollak R, Maddux MS. Cyclosporine levels during OKT3 treatment of acute renal allograft rejection. *Pharmacotherapy* (1991) 11, 278.

Ciclosporin + NSAIDs, Aspirin or Paracetamol (Acetaminophen)

Some NSAIDs (diclofenac, indometacin, ketoprofen, mefenamic acid, naproxen, piroxicam and sulindac) sometimes reduce renal function in individual patients, which is reflected in serum creatinine level rises and possibly in changes in ciclosporin levels, but concurrent use can also be uneventful. Diclofenac serum levels can be doubled. There is an isolated report of colitis in a child treated with ciclosporin and diclofenac or indometacin.

Clinical evidence

(a) Aspirin

No pharmacokinetic interaction was found when ciclosporin was given with aspirin 960 mg three times daily in healthy subjects.[1]

(b) Diclofenac

A study of 20 patients with rheumatoid arthritis given ciclosporin and diclofenac found that 7 of them had a high probability of an interaction (rises in serum creatinine levels and blood pressures), and 9 possibly had an interaction.[2] A kidney transplant patient on ciclosporin, prednisolone, digoxin, furosemide and spironolactone had a marked rise in serum creatinine levels immediately after starting to take diclofenac 25 mg three times daily. A fall in serum ciclosporin levels from 409 to 285 nanograms/ml also occurred.[3] Increased nephrotoxicity was seen in another patient taking ciclosporin for idiopathic uveitis when given diclofenac 150 mg daily.[4]

A 6-month study in 20 patients with severe rheumatoid arthritis given diclofenac 100 to 200 mg with ciclosporin 3 mg/kg daily found that the diclofenac AUC was doubled and serum creatinine levels raised from 71 to 88.4 micromol/l. The overall pattern of adverse events and laboratory abnormalities were similar to those in patients with rheumatoid arthritis treated with ciclosporin and other NSAIDs. It was suggested that it would be prudent to start with low doses of diclofenac and to monitor well.[5] A study in 24 healthy subjects found that diclofenac 50 mg every 8 hours for 8 days caused no changes in the pharmacokinetics of ciclosporin, but there was some inconclusive evidence that diclofenac serum levels were increased.[6]

A child with rheumatoid arthritis taking ciclosporin 10 mg/kg daily developed colitis when diclofenac was given. The NSAID was stopped and her symptoms resolved while still on ciclosporin.[7]

(c) Indometacin

A study in rheumatoid arthritis patients taking ciclosporin 2.5 mg/kg daily, found that creatinine clearances were reduced by 6% in those taking indometacin 50 mg four times daily, but this was not considered to be clinically important.[8] An experimental study in healthy subjects found that ciclosporin 10 mg/kg twice daily for 4 days had no effect on effective renal plasma flow (ERPF) or the glomerular filtration rate (GFR), but when indometacin 50 mg twice daily was added the ERPF fell by 32% and the GFR by 37%.[9]

A child with rheumatoid arthritis on ciclosporin 10 mg/kg daily developed colitis when **indometacin** was given. The NSAID was stopped and her symptoms resolved while still on ciclosporin.[7]

(d) Ketoprofen

A study in rheumatoid arthritis patients taking ciclosporin 2.5 mg/kg daily, found that creatinine clearances were reduced by 2.3% in those taking ketoprofen 50 mg four times daily, but this was not considered to be clinically important.[8] Another report describes increased serum creatinine levels in a patient with rheumatoid arthritis who was treated with ketoprofen.[10]

(e) Mefenamic acid

The serum ciclosporin levels of a renal transplant patient doubled, accompanied by rise in creatinine levels from 113 to 168 micromol/l within a day of starting to take mefenamic acid. Levels fell to normal within a week of stopping the mefenamic acid.[11]

(f) Naproxen

Naproxen and sulindac increased serum creatinine levels by 24% and reduced renal function (glomerular filtration rate reduced from 98 ml/minute at baseline to 67 ml/minute while on an NSAID and ciclosporin) in 11 patients with rheumatoid arthritis on ciclosporin. All patients had a clinical improvement in their rheumatoid arthritis.[12]

(g) Paracetamol (Acetaminophen)

A study in rheumatoid arthritis patients taking ciclosporin 2.5 mg/kg daily, found that creatinine clearances were reduced by 3.5% in those taking paracetamol 650 mg four times daily, but this was not considered to be clinically important.[8]

(h) Piroxicam

Piroxicam is reported to have increased the serum creatinine levels of one patient with rheumatoid arthritis by an unknown amount (but classed as a significant adverse event). This resolved when the piroxicam was withdrawn.[10]

(i) Sulindac

A study in rheumatoid arthritis patients taking ciclosporin 2.5 mg/kg daily, found that creatinine clearances were reduced by 2.6% in those taking sulindac 100 mg four times daily, but this was not considered to be clinically important.[8]

A patient with a kidney transplant had a rise in serum creatinine levels when sulindac was used. Serum ciclosporin levels fell and rose again when the sulindac was stopped.[3] Another report states that the ciclosporin levels of a woman with a kidney transplant were more than doubled within 3 days of her starting to take sulindac 150 mg twice daily.[13] Both sulindac and naproxen increased serum creatinine levels by 24% and reduced renal function (glomerular filtration rate reduced from 98 ml/minute at baseline to 67 ml/minute while on an NSAID and ciclosporin) in 11 patients on ciclosporin with rheumatoid arthritis. All patients had a clinical improvement in their rheumatoid arthritis.[12]

Another report describes increased serum creatinine levels in a patient with rheumatoid arthritis when treated with ketoprofen, but not when given sulindac.[10]

Mechanism

Uncertain. One idea is that intact kidney prostacyclin synthesis is needed to maintain the glomerular filtration rate and renal blood flow in patients given ciclosporin, which may possibly protect the kidney from the development of ciclosporin-induced nephrotoxicity. If NSAIDs that inhibit prostaglandin production in the kidney are given, the nephrotoxic effects of the ciclosporin manifest themselves, possibly independently of changes in serum ciclosporin levels.[3] A study in *rats* found that indometacin and ciclosporin together can cause rises in serum creatinine levels that are much greater than with either drug alone.[14]

The occurrence of colitis in a child receiving ciclosporin and either diclofenac or indometacin appeared to be independent of changes in ciclosporin levels and may be a result of additive effects of both drugs.[7]

Importance and management

Information about the NSAIDs listed here is sparse and limited, but the overall picture appears to be that concurrent use in rheumatoid arthritis need not be avoided but renal function should be very well monitored. The makers of ciclosporin also specifically recommend that patients with rheumatoid arthritis taking ciclosporin and an NSAID should have their hepatic function measured as well as renal function, because hepatotoxicity is a potential side effect of both drugs.[15] It has been suggested that gastrointestinal symptoms should also be carefully evaluated.[7] It is clearly difficult to generalise about what will or will not happen if any particular NSAID is given but in the case of diclofenac it has been recommended that doses at the lower end of the range should be used at the start because its serum levels can be doubled by ciclosporin.

1. Kovarik JM, Mueller EA, Gaber M, Johnston A, Jähnchen E. Pharmacokinetics of cyclosporine and steady-state aspirin during coadministration. *J Clin Pharmacol* (1993) 33, 513–21.
2. Branthwaite JP, Nicholls A. Cyclosporin and diclofenac interaction in rheumatoid arthritis. *Lancet* (1991) 337, 252.
3. Harris KP, Jenkins D, Walls J. Nonsteroidal antiinflammatory drugs and cyclosporine. A potentially serious adverse interaction. *Transplantation* (1988) 46, 598–9.
4. Deray G, Le Hoang P, Aupetit B, Achour A, Rottembourg J, Baumelou A. Enhancement of cyclosporine A nephrotoxicity by diclofenac. *Clin Nephrol* (1987) 27, 213–14.
5. Kovarik JM, Kurki P, Mueller E, Guerret M, Markert E, Alten R, Zeidler H, Genth-Stolzenburg S. Diclofenac combined with cyclosporine in treatment of refractory rheumatoid arthritis: longitudinal safety assessment and evidence of a pharmacokinetic/dynamic interaction. *J Rheumatol* (1996) 23, 2033–8.
6. Mueller EA, Kovarik JM, Koelle EU, Merdjan H, Johnston A, Hitzenberger G. Pharmacokinetics of cyclosporine and multiple-dose diclofenac during coadministration. *J Clin Pharmacol* (1993) 33, 936–43.
7. Constantopoulos A. Colitis induced by interaction of cyclosporine A and non-steroidal anti-inflammatory drugs. *Pediatr Int* (1999) 41, 184–6.
8. Tugwell P, Ludwin D, Gent M, Roberts R, Bensen W, Grace E, Baker P. Interaction between cyclosporin A and nonsteroidal antiinflammatory drugs. *J Rheumatol* (1997) 24, 1122–5.
9. Sturrock NDC, Lang CC, Struthers AD. Indomethacin and cyclosporin together produce marked renal vasoconstriction in humans. *J Hypertens* (1994) 12, 919–24.
10. Ludwin D, Bennett KJ, Grace EM, Buchanan WA, Bensen W, Bombardier C, Tugwell PX. Nephrotoxicity in patients with rheumatoid arthritis treated with cyclosporine. *Transplant Proc* (1988) 20 (Suppl 4), 367–70.
11. Agar JWMacD. Cyclosporin A and mefenamic acid in a renal transplant patient. *Aust N Z J Med* (1991) 21, 784–5.
12. Altman RD, Perez GO, Sfakianakis GN. Interaction of cyclosporine A and nonsteroidal anti-inflammatory drugs on renal function in patients with rheumatoid arthritis. *Am J Med* (1992) 93, 396–402.
13. Sesin GP, O'Keefe E, Roberto P. Sulindac-induced elevation of serum cyclosporine concentration. *Clin Pharm* (1989) 8, 445–6.
14. Whiting PH, Burke MD, Thomson AW. Drug interactions with cyclosporine. Implications from animal studies. *Transplant Proc* (1986) 18 (Suppl 5), 56–70.
15. Neoral (Ciclosporin). Novartis Pharmaceuticals UK Ltd. UK Summary of product characteristics, December 2004.

Ciclosporin + Oral contraceptives and Progestogens

Hepatotoxicity has been described in two patients given ciclosporin and oral contraceptives. Rises in serum ciclosporin levels may also occur. Some increase in ciclosporin levels has been seen with norethisterone.

Clinical evidence

(a) Contraceptives

A woman treated for uveitis with ciclosporin 5 mg/kg daily had an increase in trough serum ciclosporin levels (roughly doubled) on two occasions within 8 to 10 days of starting an oral contraceptive (**levonorgestrel/ethinylestradiol** 150/30 micrograms). She also experienced nausea, vomiting and hepatalgia, and had evidence of severe hepatotoxicity (very marked increases in AST and ALT, and rises in serum bilirubin and alkaline phosphatase).The woman had previously been on this oral contraceptive for 5 years without problems.[1]

Another report describes hepatotoxicity in a patient on ciclosporin 2 weeks after she started an oral contraceptive (**desogestrel/ethinylestradiol** 150/30 micrograms). The contraceptive was stopped, and liver enzyme levels promptly started to fall, but ciclosporin levels continued to rise, and peaked about 10 days later, at a level about threefold higher than they had been.[2]

(b) Norethisterone

A 15-year-old girl on ciclosporin who had a marked increase in serum ciclosporin levels when given 'danazol', (p.788) continued to have elevated levels, but not as high, when the danazol was replaced by norethisterone 5 mg three times daily. The levels returned to her previous normal range when the norethisterone was stopped.[3] No changes in ciclosporin levels were seen in another patient who was intermittently treated with norethisterone.[4] Two women had a mild rise in ciclosporin levels with no changes in creatinine levels when given norethisterone 10 mg daily for 10 days.[5]

Mechanism

Uncertain. It seems possible that some of these compounds inhibit the metabolism of the ciclosporin by the liver, thereby reducing its loss from the body and leading to an increase in its serum levels. The mechanism of the hepatotoxicity is not understood, but in some cases it seems that it occurs simply as a rare adverse effect of the sex hormone.

Importance and management

This interaction with oral contraceptives and norethisterone is unconfirmed and of uncertain clinical significance. There is insufficient evidence to recommend increased monitoring, but be aware of the potential for an interaction in the case of an unexpected response to treatment

1. Deray G, le Hoang P, Cacoub P, Assogba U, Grippon P, Baumelou A. Oral contraceptive interaction with cyclosporin. *Lancet* (1987) i, 158–9.
2. Leimenstoll G, Jessen P, Zabel P, Niedermayer W. Arzneimittelschaädigung der leber bei kombination von cyclosporin A und einem antikonzeptivum. *Dtsch Med Wochenschr* (1984) 109, 1989–90.
3. Ross WB, Roberts D, Griffin PJA and Salaman JR. Cyclosporin interaction with danazol and norethisterone. *Lancet* (1986) i, 330.
4. Koneru B, Hartner C, Iwatsuki S, Starzl TE. Effect of danazol on cyclosporine pharmacokinetics. *Transplantation* (1988) 45, 1001.
5. Castelao AM. Cyclosporine A — drug interactions. In Sunshine I (Ed.) Recent developments in therapeutic drug monitoring and clinical toxicology. *2nd Int Conf Therapeutic Drug Monitoring Toxicology, Barcelona, Spain* (1992) 203–9.

Ciclosporin + Orlistat

The absorption of ciclosporin is significantly reduced by orlistat. In one case, orlistat appeared to have less effect on the microemulsion formulation (*Neoral*) of ciclosporin than the standard formulation (*Sandimmun*). Nevertheless, an episode of acute graft rejection (said to be non-significant) has been reported with the microemulsion formulation.

Clinical evidence

In a heart transplant patient on ciclosporin (standard formulation), orlistat 120 mg three times daily reduced the trough blood levels of ciclosporin by 47%, to 52 nanograms/ml. The peak levels and the AUC of ciclosporin were increased by 86% and 75% respectively.[1] Another heart transplant patient taking ciclosporin (*Neoral*) had a nonsignificant acute rejection episode on routine endocardial biopsy, with trough ciclosporin levels of 38 nanograms/ml, 24 days after starting to take orlistat. Ciclosporin trough levels increased to about 90 to 110 nanograms/ml when the orlistat was stopped.[2] In a further patient taking ciclosporin (*Sandimmun*) 250 mg daily, orlistat 360 mg daily reduced the ciclosporin levels from 150 to 50 nanograms/ml. Increasing the dose of ciclosporin did not result in an increased level, so the patient was given *Neoral* instead. Adequate levels of 160 nanograms/ml were finally achieved with ciclosporin (*Neoral*) 375 mg daily.[3] Details of this patient are also briefly given elsewhere.[4] Another report describes 6 transplant recipients who developed subtherapeutic ciclosporin trough levels after also taking orlistat.[5]

Mechanism

Orlistat inhibits pancreatic lipase and prevents the absorption of dietary fat and lipophilic molecules such as ciclosporin. Absorption of ciclosporin from the oil suspension formulation (*Sandimmun*) is more dependent on the lipid absorption stage and thus may be more affected by orlistat than the microemulsion form (*Neoral*).[3]

Importance and management

Information appears to be limited to these reports, but the interaction seems to be established. It has been suggested that the effects of the interaction may be reduced by using the microemulsion formulation of ciclosporin (*Neoral*).[3] Monitoring is required if the two drugs are used together, either in the standard or microemulsion form because there is a risk of subtherapeutic levels even with the microemulsion preparation.[2] Some authors recommend avoidance of the combination.[1]

1. Nägele H, Petersen B, Bonacker U, Rödiger W. Effect of orlistat on blood cyclosporin concentration in an obese heart transplant patient. *Eur J Clin Pharmacol* (1999) 55, 667–9.
2. Schnetzler B, Kondo-Oestreicher M, Vala D, Khatchatourian G, Faidutti B. Orlistat decreases the plasma level of cyclosporine and may be responsible for the development of acute rejection episodes. *Transplantation* (2000) 70, 1540–1.
3. Le Beller C, Bezie Y, Chabatte C, Guillemain R, Amrein C, Billaud EM. Co-administration of orlistat and cyclosporine in a heart transplant recipient. *Transplantation* (2000) 70, 1541–2.
4. Chavatte C, Le Beller C, Guillemain R, Amrein C, Billaud EM. Cyclosporine/orlistat drug interaction in heart transplant recipient. *Fundam Clin Pharmacol* (2000) 14, 246.
5. Colman E, Fossler M. Reduction in blood cyclosporine concentrations by orlistat. *N Engl J Med* (2000) 342, 1141–2.

Ciclosporin + Oxybutynin

Oxybutynin appeared not to affect ciclosporin levels in two children.

Clinical evidence, mechanism, importance and management

In a retrospective analysis, one child with a kidney transplant on ciclosporin had no change in his ciclosporin level and dosage between the 2 months before and the 2 months after he started oxybutynin 2 mg twice daily. Another patient had no change in ciclosporin levels and dosage between the 3 months before and 3 months after stopping oxybutynin 5 mg twice daily.[1] This analysis was prompted by evidence suggesting oxybutynin may induce cytochrome P450 isoenzyme CYP3A4, which is involved in the metabolism of ciclosporin. Although the evidence is limited, it suggests that oxybutynin is unlikely to have an important effect on ciclosporin levels.

1. Springate JE. Oxybutynin does not affect cyclosporin blood levels. *Ther Drug Monit* (2001) 23, 155–6.

Ciclosporin + Pancreatic enzymes

Pancreatic enzyme extracts do not increase the bioavailability of ciclosporin in cystic fibrosis patients.

Clinical evidence, mechanism, importance and management

A study in heart-lung transplant patients with cystic fibrosis found that they needed almost five times the oral dose of ciclosporin of other patients, confirming other studies in these patients that had shown a very much reduced bioavailability of oral ciclosporin. This is probably a reflection of the generally poor digestion and absorption in cystic fibrosis patients. The addition of pancreatic enzymes (*Creon*) was found not to improve this poor ciclosporin bioavailability. No adverse effects were reported.[1]

1. Tsang VT, Johnston A, Heritier F, Leaver N, Hodson ME, Yacoub M. Cyclosporin pharmacokinetics in heart-lung transplant recipients with cystic fibrosis. *Eur J Clin Pharmacol* (1994) 46, 261–5.

Ciclosporin + Prazosin

Preliminary studies show that prazosin causes a small reduction in the glomerular filtration rate of kidney transplant patients taking ciclosporin.

Clinical evidence, mechanism, importance and management

A study in 8 patients with kidney transplants found that prazosin 1 mg twice daily for a week did not alter their serum ciclosporin levels, and arterial blood pressures and renal vascular resistance were reduced. However, the glomerular filtration rate (GFR) was reduced by about 10% (from 47 to 42 ml/minute).[1] Previous studies in kidney transplant patients treated with azathioprine, prednisone and prazosin found no reduction in

GFR.[2] There would seem to be no strong reasons for totally avoiding prazosin in patients on ciclosporin, but the authors of the report point out that the fall in GFR makes prazosin a less attractive antihypertensive than a calcium channel blocker.

1. Kiberd BA. Effects of prazosin therapy in renal allograft recipients receiving cyclosporine. *Transplantation* (1990) 49, 1200–1.
2. Curtis JR, Bateman FJA. Use of prazosin in management of hypertension in patients with chronic renal failure and in renal transplant recipients. *BMJ* (1975) 4, 432.

Ciclosporin + Probucol

Probucol reduces blood ciclosporin levels by about 40%.

Clinical evidence

A study in 6 heart transplant patients taking ciclosporin found that the concurrent use of probucol 500 mg every 12 hours decreased trough whole blood ciclosporin levels from 139 to 81 nanograms/ml and the 0 to 9-hour AUC by 28%. The clearance was increased by 60% and volume of distribution also increased.[1]

Another group of workers similarly found that 9 out 10 kidney transplant patients had a reduction in trough serum ciclosporin levels while being treated with probucol.[2]

Mechanism

Not understood.

Importance and management

Information appears to be limited to these studies, but the interaction appears to be well established. The ciclosporin dosage may need to be increased if probucol is added. Monitor the effects and adjust the dosage appropriately.

1. Sundararajan V, Cooper DKC, Muchmore J, Manion CV, Liguori C, Zuhdi N, Novitzky D, Chen P-N, Bourne DWA, Corder CN. Interaction of cyclosporine and probucol in heart transplant patients. *Transplant Proc* (1991) 23, 2028–32.
2. Gallego C, Sánchez P, Planells C, Sánchez S, Monte E, Romá E, Sánchez J, Pallardó LM. Interaction between probucol and cyclosporine in renal transplant patients. *Ann Pharmacother* (1994) 28, 940–2.

Ciclosporin + Propafenone

An isolated report describes a 60% increase in the ciclosporin levels of a patient who was given propafenone.

Clinical evidence

A heart transplant patient taking ciclosporin, azathioprine and prednisolone developed ventricular tachycardia 9 months after transplantation, for which he was given propafenone 600 or 750 mg daily. After the first day, his ciclosporin level had risen from about 160 to 190 nanograms/ml, and after 5 days the levels had reached around 260 nanograms/ml. Over the same time period his serum creatinine rose from 168 to 212 micromol/l. His ciclosporin dose was reduced from 240 mg daily to a final dose of 200 mg daily after which his renal function and ciclosporin levels were re-established at about the level prior to propafenone treatment.[1]

Mechanism

The authors suggest that propafenone interferes with the metabolism of ciclosporin by affecting hepatic cytochrome P450, or that propafenone may enhance the absorption of ciclosporin.

Importance and management

Information appears to be limited to this one report, the general importance of which is unknown.

1. Spes CH, Angermann CE, Horn K, Strasser T, Mudra H, Landgraf R, Theisen K. Ciclosporin-propafenone interaction. *Klin Wochenschr* (1990) 68, 872.

Ciclosporin + Proton pump inhibitors

Omeprazole normally does not appear to affect serum ciclosporin levels, but two isolated reports describe doubled serum ciclosporin levels in one patient, and more than halved serum ciclosporin levels in another. Pantoprazole does not affect serum ciclosporin levels.

Clinical evidence

(a) Omeprazole

Ten renal transplant patients had no significant changes in ciclosporin levels when given omeprazole 20 mg daily for 2 weeks.[1] Eight kidney transplant patients similarly had no significant changes in ciclosporin levels when given omeprazole 20 mg daily for 6 days.[2] No significant changes in ciclosporin levels were seen in another kidney transplant patient when omeprazole 20 mg daily was added for 8 weeks.[3]

In contrast, the serum ciclosporin levels of a liver transplant patient roughly doubled (from a range of 187 to 261 up to 510 nanograms/ml) about 2 weeks after omeprazole 40 mg daily was started. His ciclosporin levels were readjusted by reducing the dose from 130 to 80 mg twice daily. The levels then remained steady at about 171 nanograms/ml for the following 4 months.[4] In contrast, the serum ciclosporin levels of a bone marrow transplant patient fell from 254 to about 100 nanograms/ml over 14 days in the presence of omeprazole daily 40 mg. The ciclosporin levels climbed again rapidly when the omeprazole was stopped.[5]

(b) Pantoprazole

Studies in renal transplant patients have found that pantoprazole 40 mg once daily does not affect ciclosporin blood levels when given in the evening,[6] or when both drugs are given together in the morning.[7]

Mechanism

Not understood.

Importance and management

Information is limited but what is known suggests that no interaction normally occurs. Any interaction is unlikely to be of general importance, but bear the reports in mind in the case of an unexpected response to treatment. Note that, in the studies cited in which no interaction occurred, the dose of omeprazole was 20 mg daily, whereas the two cases of interaction involved 40 mg daily so some caution would be appropriate if initiating this higher dose. There would seem to be no reason for avoiding concurrent use of ciclosporin and pantoprazole.[8]

1. Blohmé I, Idström J-P, Andersson T. A study of the interaction between omeprazole and cyclosporine in renal transplant patients. *Br J Clin Pharmacol* (1993) 35, 156–60.
2. Kahn D, Manas D, Hamilton H, Pascoe MD, Pontin AR. The effect of omeprazole on cyclosporine metabolism in renal transplant recipients. *S Afr Med J* (1993) 83, 785.
3. Castellote E, Bonet J, Lauzurica R, Pastor C, Cofan F, Caralps A. Does interaction between omeprazole and cyclosporin exist? *Nephron* (1993) 65, 478.
4. Schouler L, Dumas F, Couzigou P, Janvier G, Winnock S, Saric J. Omeprazole-cyclosporin interaction. *Am J Gastroenterol* (1991) 86, 1097.
5. Arranz R, Yañez E, Franceschi JL, Fernandez-Rañada JM. More about omeprazole-cyclosporine interaction. *Am J Gastroenterol* (1993) 88, 154–5.
6. Lorf T, Ramadori G, Ringe B, Schwörer H. Pantoprazole does not affect cyclosporin A blood concentration in kidney-transplant patients. *Eur J Clin Pharmacol* (2000) 55, 733–5.
7. Lorf T, Ramadori G, Ringe B, Schwörer H. The effect of pantoprazole on tacrolimus and cyclosporin A blood concentration in transplant patients. *Eur J Clin Pharmacol* (2000) 56, 439–40.
8. Schwrer H, Lorf T, Ringe B, Ramadori G. Pantoprazole and cyclosporine or tacrolimus. *Aliment Pharmacol Ther* (2001) 15, 561–2.

Ciclosporin + Pyrazinamide

Pyrazinamide does not normally appear to interact with ciclosporin but one isolated report suggests that it may possibly have contributed to the effects of rifampicin in one patient, which resulted in lowered ciclosporin levels. Another patient developed toxic myopathy attributed to the use of pyrazinamide with ciclosporin.

Clinical evidence, mechanism, importance and management

A 12-year-old girl with a kidney transplant taking ciclosporin and prednisolone had a rejection episode while taking rifampicin and isoniazid, apparently due to the fall in serum ciclosporin levels caused by the rifampicin. The rejection settled when the rifampicin was replaced by pyrazinamide.[1] Other patients taking ciclosporin have been treated with pyrazinamide combined with ethambutol and/or streptomycin without any apparent interaction problems.[2] However, an anecdotal report suggested that when pyrazinamide was given with rifampicin with isoniazid it appeared to add to the effects of the rifampicin causing an additional reduction in serum ciclosporin levels.[3] Another report attributed the development of toxic myopathy in a kidney transplant patient to the concurrent use of pyrazinamide and ciclosporin.[4]

There would therefore seem to be no reason for avoiding pyrazinamide in patients taking ciclosporin, but be aware of these rare complications.

1. Coward RA, Raftery AT, Brown CB. Cyclosporin and antituberculous therapy. *Lancet* (1985) i, 1342–3.
2. Aguado JM, Herrero JA, Gavaldá J, Torre-Cisneros J, Blanes M, Rufí G, Moreno A, Gurguí A, Hayek M, Lumbreras C and the Spanish Transplantation Infection Study Group, GESITRA. Clinical presentation and outcome of tuberculosis in kidney, liver, and heart transplant recipients in Spain. *Transplantation* (1997) 63, 1276–86.
3. Jiménez del Cerro LA, Hernández FR. Effect of pyrazinamide on ciclosporin levels. *Nephron* (1992) 62, 113.
4. Fernández-Solà J, Campistol JM, Miró Ó, Garcés N, Soy D, Grau JM. Acute toxic myopathy due to pyrazinamide in a patient with renal transplantation and cyclosporine therapy. *Nephrol Dial Transplant* (1996) 11, 1850–2.

Ciclosporin + Quinine

An isolated case suggests that quinine reduces ciclosporin levels.

Clinical evidence, mechanism, importance and management

A man with a kidney transplant and mild cerebral falciparum malaria had a gradual decrease in his serum ciclosporin levels, from 328 to 107 nanograms/ml, over 7 days when treated with quinine 600 mg every 8 hours, and a gradual rise when the quinine was stopped.[1]

The reason for this apparently isolated report is unclear and its general importance is unknown. There is insufficient evidence to recommend increased monitoring, but be aware of the potential for an interaction in the case of an unexpected response to treatment. The effects of lower quinine doses used for cramps are unclear.

1. Tan HW, Ch'ng SL. Drug interaction between cyclosporine A and quinine in a renal transplant patient with malaria. *Singapore Med J* (1991) 32, 189–90.

Ciclosporin + Retinoids

A considerable increase in serum ciclosporin levels occurred in one patient given etretinate, but not in other studies of the combination. In two patients on isotretinoin and ciclosporin, rises in ciclosporin levels occurred, which were not attributed to the isotretinoin. Another patient on the combination had no alteration in ciclosporin levels.

Clinical evidence

(a) Etretinate

In one case, a woman with generalised pustular psoriasis had a considerable rise in her serum ciclosporin levels to 540 micrograms/l when the dosage was raised from 200 to 300 mg daily and etretinate 50 mg daily was added. It was found possible to reduce the ciclosporin dosage gradually to 150 mg daily, accompanied by a fall in the trough serum ciclosporin levels to 168 micrograms/l, without any loss in the control of the disease.[1] However, only a modest ciclosporin dosage reduction was needed in another study when etretinate was given.[2]

Other reports suggest successful uncomplicated concurrent use.

There was no improvement in a patient with erythrodermic psoriasis treated with ciclosporin 5 to 10 mg/kg daily, but ciclosporin 5 mg/kg daily with etretinate 700 micrograms/kg daily cleared the psoriasis by 90%. Reducing the dose of either drug resulted in exacerbation of symptoms.[3] Another 5 patients with plaque-type psoriasis had a relapse when the ciclosporin dosage was reduced in the presence of etretinate, but no additive therapeutic effect was seen. All of them had elevated serum creatinine levels.[4] No obvious advantages but no increase in adverse effects were found in another study that gave ciclosporin with etretinate.[5]

(b) Isotretinoin

A 27-year old man with a heart transplant on ciclosporin was given isotretinoin 40 mg daily for 2 months, then 80 mg daily up to 20 weeks. His ciclosporin trough levels remained within the recommended range, and there was no evidence of graft rejection.[6] Another man with a heart transplant on ciclosporin received isotretinoin 1 mg/kg daily for 4 months. His daily ciclosporin dose was reduced from 7 mg/kg to 6 mg/kg one month after starting isotretinoin because of a rise in ciclosporin level to 587 nanograms/ml. However, it was noted that this may have had nothing to do with the isotretinoin, since the patient required alterations in ciclosporin dose in 3 instances before isotretinoin was started. No laboratory abnormalities were noted, nor was ciclosporin toxicity seen, and the heart transplant function remained satisfactory.[7] A 13-year-old girl with aplastic anaemia on ciclosporin was given isotretinoin 40 mg daily for 20 weeks. She had a threefold increase in trough ciclosporin level at week 17, which was considered probably unrelated to isotretinoin, and was managed by reducing her ciclosporin dose. Serum lipids did not change during therapy.[8]

Mechanism

Uncertain. An *in vitro* study using human liver microsomes found that concentrations of 100 micromol of acitretin, etretinate and isotretinoin inhibited the total ciclosporin metabolism and total primary ciclosporin metabolite production to the same extent (32 to 45%).[1] These figures suggest that the retinoids may inhibit ciclosporin metabolism. However, another *in vitro* study using human liver microsomes did not show that etretinate inhibits the metabolism of ciclosporin.[9]

Importance and management

The overall picture seems to be that etretinate has only a modest effect, or no effect at all, on serum ciclosporin levels in most patients. Nevertheless, this possible interaction is worth bearing in mind because or the possibility of isolated cases of raised ciclosporin levels. There seems to be no marked therapeutic advantage in using both drugs together for psoriasis. From the cases presented, it is unclear if isotretinoin alters ciclosporin levels. In addition, it has been suggested that serum lipids should be monitored because both drugs can cause an increase.[6] **Acitretin** (the major metabolite of etretinate) probably behaves like etretinate, although this needs confirmation.

1. Shah IA, Whiting PH, Omar G, Ormerod AD, Burke MD. The effects of retinoids and terbinafine on the human hepatic microsomal metabolism of cyclosporin. *Br J Dermatol* (1993) 129, 395–8.
2. Meinardi MMHM, Bos JD. Cyclosporine maintenance therapy in psoriasis. *Transplant Proc* (1988) 20 (Suppl 4), 42–9.
3. Korstanje MJ, Bessems PJMJ, van de Staak WJBM. Combination therapy cyclosporin-etretinate effective in erythrodermic psoriasis. *Dermatologica* (1989) 179, 94.
4. Korstanje MJ, van de Staak WJBM. Combination-therapy cyclosporin-A-etretinate for psoriasis. *Clin Exp Dermatol* (1990) 15, 172–3.
5. Brechtel B, Wellenreuther U, Toppe E, Czarnetzki BM. Combination of etretinate with cyclosporine in the treatment of severe recalcitrant psoriasis. *J Am Acad Dermatol* (1994) 30, 1023–4.
6. Abel EA. Isotretinoin treatment of severe cystic acne in a heart transplant patient receiving cyclosporine: consideration of drug interactions. *J Am Acad Dermatol* (1991) 24, 511.
7. Bunker CB, Rustin MHA, Dowd PM. Isotretinoin treatment of severe acne in posttransplant patients taking cyclosporine. *J Am Acad Dermatol* (1990) 22, 693–4.
8. Hazen PE, Walker AE, Stewart JJ, Carney JF, Engstrom CW, Turgeon KL, Shurin S. Successful use of isotretinoin in a patient on cyclosporine: apparent lack of toxicity. *Int J Dermatol* (1993) 32, 466–7.
9. Webber IR, Back DJ. Effect of etretinate on cyclosporin metabolism *in vitro*. *Br J Dermatol* (1993) 128, 42–4.

Ciclosporin + Sevelamer

Sevelamer does not appear to alter ciclosporin levels.

Clinical evidence, mechanism, importance and management

The pharmacokinetics of ciclosporin were unchanged in 12 renal transplant patients taking ciclosporin, (with 6 patients also taking mycophenolate) after they took sevelamer as a single 1.6- or 1.2-mg dose then again after 4 days of treatment (same dose given three times daily).[1] Five of the patients were children (average age 15 years).[1]

No additional precautions would therefore seem to be necessary on concurrent use.

1. Pieper A-K, Buhle F, Mai I, Budde K, Neumayer HH, Haffner D, Querfeld U. Effect of sevelamer on pharmacokinetics of cyclosporin A and mycophenolate-mofetil in patients following renal transplantation. *J Am Soc Nephrol* (2002) 13, 562A.

Ciclosporin + Sodium clodronate

Clodronate appears not to alter serum ciclosporin levels.

Clinical evidence, mechanism, importance and management

Ten heart transplant patients taking ciclosporin, azathioprine and diltiazem were also given clodronate 800 mg daily for a week. No statistically significant differences were seen in their serum ciclosporin levels or AUCs while they were taking the clodronate. Three of them were also taking simvastatin, two were taking ranitidine and one was taking propafenone, furosemide and cyclophosphamide. There would seem to be no reason for avoiding concurrent use, but the authors of the report suggest that longer-term use of clodronate should be well monitored.[1] There seems to be no information about other bisphosphonates.

1. Baraldo M, Furlanut M, Puricelli C. No effect of clodronate on cyclosporin A blood levels in heart transplant patients simultaneously treated with diltiazem and azathioprine. *Ther Drug Monit* (1994) 16, 435.

Ciclosporin + Somatostatin analogues

Octreotide causes a marked fall in the serum levels of ciclosporin and inadequate immunosuppression may result. Lanreotide is predicted to interact similarly.

Clinical evidence

A diabetic man with kidney and pancreatic segment transplants was successfully immunosuppressed with azathioprine, methylprednisolone and ciclosporin. When he was also given subcutaneous **octreotide** 100 micrograms twice daily to reduce fluid collection around the pancreatic graft, his trough serum ciclosporin levels fell below the assay detection limit of 50 nanograms/ml. Serum creatinine increased dramatically, which was interpreted as a selective rejection episode of the kidney transplant. Nine other diabetics similarly treated with **octreotide** for peripancreatic fluid collection and fistulas after pancreatic transplantation also had significant falls in their serum ciclosporin levels within 24 to 48 hours, in 3 of them to undetectable levels.[1] A similar interaction was seen in another patient.[2]

The makers of **lanreotide** say that, as with other somatostatin analogues, it may reduce the absorption of ciclosporin from the gut,[3] but as yet there appear to be no reports of this interaction in practice.

Mechanism

Uncertain. A suggestion is that the octreotide reduces the intestinal absorption of the ciclosporin.[1,2]

Importance and management

The interaction between octreotide and ciclosporin is established and clinically important, although the documentation is limited. The authors of the report cited recommend that before giving octreotide the oral dosage of ciclosporin should be increased on average by 50% and the serum levels monitored daily.[1] It would be prudent to monitor the outcome of the use of lanreotide with ciclosporin.

1. Landgraf R, Landgraf-Leurs MMC, Nusser J, Hillebrand G, Illner W-D, Abendroth D, Land W. Effect of somatostatin analogue (SMS 201–995) on cyclosporine levels. *Transplantation* (1987) 44, 724–5.
2. Rosenberg L, Dafoe DC, Schwartz R, Campbell DA, Turcotte JG, Tsai S-T, Vinik A. Administration of somatostatin analog (SMS 201–995) in the treatment of a fistula occurring after pancreas transplantation. *Transplantation* (1987) 43, 764–6.
3. Somatuline LA (Lanreotide). Ipsen Ltd. UK Summary of product characteristics, August 2003.

Ciclosporin + St John's wort (*Hypericum perforatum*)

Marked reductions in serum ciclosporin levels and transplant rejection can occur with few weeks of starting St John's wort.

Clinical evidence

A marked drop in ciclosporin blood levels was identified in one kidney transplant patient as being due to the addition of St John's wort extract 300 mg three times daily. When the St John's wort was stopped the ciclosporin levels rose. The authors of this report identified another 35 kidney and 10 liver transplant patients whose ciclosporin levels had dropped by an average of 49% (range 30 to 64%) after starting St John's wort. Two of them had rejection episodes.[1,2] In addition, subtherapeutic ciclosporin levels in 7 renal transplant patients,[3-7] one liver transplant patient,[8] and 6 heart transplant patients[9-11] have been attributed to self-medication with St John's wort. Acute graft rejection episodes occurred in 7 cases,[3,5,7-9,11] and one patient subsequently developed chronic rejection, requiring a return to dialysis.[5]

These case reports are supported by a small study in which 11 renal transplant patients, with stable dose requirements for ciclosporin, were given St John's wort extract (*Jarsin 300*) 600 mg daily for 14 days. Pharmacokinetic changes were noted 3 days after the St John's wort was added. By day 10 the ciclosporin dose had to be increased from an average of 2.7 to 4.2 mg/kg daily in an attempt to keep ciclosporin levels within the therapeutic range. Two weeks after the St John's wort was stopped, only 3 patients had been successfully re-stabilised on their baseline ciclosporin dose. Additionally, the pharmacokinetics of various ciclosporin metabolites were substantially altered.[12]

Mechanism

Uncertain, but it is thought that St John's wort increases the metabolism and loss of the ciclosporin from the body,[11] perhaps by affecting the cytochrome P450 isoenzyme system.[9] It has also been suggested that St John's wort affects ciclosporin reabsorption by inducing the intestinal drug transporter, P-glycoprotein.[9,12]

Importance and management

An established and clinically important interaction. The incidence is not known, but all patients on ciclosporin should avoid St John's wort because of the potentially severity of this interaction. Transplant rejection can develop within 3 to 4 weeks. It is possible to accommodate this interaction by increasing the ciclosporin dosage[11] (possibly about doubled) but this raises the costs of an already expensive drug. Also, the varying content of natural products would make this hard to monitor. The advice of the UK Committee on Safety of Medicines is that patients on ciclosporin should avoid or stop taking St John's wort. In the latter situation the serum ciclosporin levels should be well monitored and the dosage adjusted as necessary.[13] The study described above suggests that increased monitoring will be needed for at least 2 weeks after the St John's wort is stopped.[12]

1. Breidenbach Th, Hoffmann MW, Becker Th, Schlitt H, Klempnauer J. Drug interaction of St John's wort with ciclosporin. *Lancet* (2000) 355, 1912.
2. Breidenbach T, Kliem V, Burg M, Radermacher J, Hoffmann MW, Klempnauer J. Profound drop of cyclosporin A whole blood trough levels caused by St John's wort (Hypericum perforatum). *Transplantation* (2000) 69, 2229–30.
3. Barone GW, Gurley BJ, Ketel BL, Abul-Ezz SR. Herbal supplements: a potential for drug interactions in transplant recipients. *Transplantation* (2001) 71, 239–41.
4. Mai I, Kreuger H, Budde K, Johne A, Brockmoeller J, Neumayer H-H, Roots I. Hazardous pharmacokinetic interaction of Saint John's wort (Hypericum perforatum) with the immunosuppressant cyclosporin. *Int J Clin Pharmacol Ther* (2000) 38, 500–2.
5. Barone GW, Gurley BJ, Ketel BL, Lightfoot ML, Abul-Ezz SR. Drug interaction between St John's wort and cyclosporine. *Ann Pharmacother* (2000) 34, 1013–16.
6. Moschella PA-C, Jaber BL. Interaction between cyclosporine and Hypericum perforatum (St John's wort) after organ transplantation. *Am J Kidney Dis* (2001) 38, 1105–7.
7. Turton-Weeks SM, Barone GW, Gurley BJ, Ketel BL, Lightfoot ML, Abul-Ezz SR. St John's wort: a hidden risk for transplant patients. *Prog Transplant* (2001) 11, 116–20.
8. Karliova M, Treichel U, Malagò M, Frilling A, Gerken G, Broelsch CE. Interaction of *hypericum perforatum* (St John's wort) with cyclosporin A metabolism in a patient after liver transplantation. *J Hepatol* (2000) 33, 853–5.
9. Ruschitzka F, Meier PJ, Turina M, Lüscher TF, Noll G. Acute heart transplant rejection due to Saint John's wort. *Lancet* (2000) 355, 548–9.
10. Ahmed SM, Banner NR, Dubrey SW. Low cyclosporin-A level due to Saint-John's-wort in heart-transplant patients. *J Heart Lung Transplant* (2001) 20, 795.
11. Bon S, Hartmann K, Kuhn M. Johanniskraut: ein enzyminducktor? *Schweiz Apothekerzeitung* (1999) 16, 535–6.
12. Bauer S, Störmer E, Johne A, Krüger H, Budde K, Neumayer H-H, Roots I, Mai I. Alterations in cyclosporin A pharmacokinetics and metabolism during treatment with St John's wort in renal transplant patients. *Br J Clin Pharmacol* (2003) 55, 203–11.
13. Committee on the Safety of Medicines (UK). Message from Professor A Breckenridge (Chairman of CSM) and Fact Sheet for Health Care Professionals, 29th February 2000.

Ciclosporin + Sulfasalazine

An isolated report describes elevated ciclosporin levels in a kidney transplant patient when sulfasalazine was stopped.

Clinical evidence

A patient with a kidney transplant was treated with azathioprine, ciclosporin, prednisolone and sulfasalazine 1.5 g daily. After initial adjustments the dose of ciclosporin remained at 480 mg daily for 8 months. The dose of prednisone was reduced and treatment stopped at 8 months and azathioprine was stopped at 12 months without any requirement to adjust ciclosporin dosage. Sulfasalazine was stopped 13.5 months after transplantation and the mean ciclosporin level increased from 205 nanograms/ml to 360 nanograms/ml within 5 days and to 389 nanograms/ml after 10 days. The ciclosporin dosage was reduced over the following 2 months from 9.6 mg/kg to 5.6 mg/kg to maintain blood levels at about 200 nanograms/ml.[1]

Mechanism

Not understood. The time course of the interaction, noted after 5 days probably excludes decreased absorption. It is possible that the interaction is due to induction of the cytochrome P450 enzymes.

Importance and management

Information appears to be limited to this isolated case report. There is insufficient evidence to recommend increased monitoring, but be aware of the potential for an interaction in the case of an unexpected response to treatment.

1. Du Cheyron D, Debruyne D, Lobbedez T, Richer C, Ryckelynck J-P, Hurault de Ligny B. Effect of sulfasalazine on cyclosporin blood concentration. *Eur J Clin Pharmacol* (1999) 55, 227–8.

Ciclosporin + Sulfinpyrazone

Sulfinpyrazone can reduce ciclosporin serum levels and episodes of transplant rejection have resulted.

Clinical evidence

A study in 120 heart transplant patients found that sulfinpyrazone 200 mg daily was effective in the treatment of hyperuricaemia. The mean uricaemia over a 4- to 8-month period fell by 22%, from 0.51 to 0.4 mmol/l, but unexpectedly the mean trough ciclosporin levels fell by 39%, from 183 to 121 micrograms/l, despite a 7.7% increase in the ciclosporin daily dosage. Two of the patients developed rejection: one after 4 months on sulphinpyrazone when the ciclosporin levels fell to 50 micrograms/l and the other after 7 months when the levels fell to 20 micrograms/l.[1]

Another report describes a patient who needed unusually high doses of ciclosporin while taking sulfinpyrazone,[2] while yet another report describes *increased* serum ciclosporin levels. In this latter case there is the possibility that it may have been an artefact due to interference with the assay method.[3]

Mechanism

Not understood.

Importance and management

Information appears to be limited to these reports but the interaction would seem to be established and clinically important. If sulfinpyrazone is added to established treatment with ciclosporin, be alert for the need to raise the ciclosporin dosage. The mean fall in trough ciclosporin levels seen in the major study cited was 39%.[1] This study does comment on how quickly this interaction develops but the two cases of transplant rejection occurred after 4 months and 7 months, which implies that it can possibly be slow. Long-term monitoring would therefore be a prudent precaution. The authors of this report say that sulfinpyrazone is an effective alternative to allopurinol and no additional adverse effects occur including myelotoxicity when it is used with azathioprine.

1. Caforio ALP, Gambino A, Tona F, Feltrin G, Marchini F, Pompei E, Testolin L, Angelini A, Dalla Volta S, Casarotto D. Sulfinpyrazone reduces cyclosporine levels: a new drug interaction in heart transplant recipients. *J Heart Lung Transplant* (2000) 19, 1205–8.
2. Dossetor JB, Kovithavongs T, Salkie M, Preiksaitis J. Cyclosporine-associated lymphoproliferation, despite controlled cyclosporine blood concentrations, in a renal allograft recipient. *Proc Eur Dial Transplant Assoc Eur Ren Assoc* (1985) 21, 1021–6.
3. Cockburn I. Cyclosporin A: a clinical evaluation of drug interactions. *Transplant Proc* (1986) 18 (Suppl 5), 50–5.

Ciclosporin + Ticlopidine

Two case reports describe marked falls in serum ciclosporin levels, and one study noted that trough ciclosporin levels were halved by ticlopidine. However, another study reported that ticlopidine did not affect ciclosporin bioavailability.

Clinical evidence

The serum ciclosporin levels of a patient with nephrotic syndrome were roughly halved on two occasions when he was given ticlopidine 500 mg daily.[1] Another patient with a kidney transplant had a similar fall on two occasions when ticlopidine 250 mg daily was given.[2]

Twelve heart transplant patients were given ticlopidine 250 mg twice daily. The mean whole blood trough ciclosporin levels were noted to be halved but the mean ciclosporin dosage was not altered over a 3-month period. The neutrophil, platelet and whole blood leucocyte counts and haemoglobin levels were not significantly altered, but adverse effects included epistaxis (1 patient), haematuria (1), which both necessitated a 50% dosage reduction and one neutropenia, which resolved when the ticlopidine was withdrawn.[3]

A later study by the same group in 20 heart transplant patients given ticlopidine 250 mg daily found that the bioavailability of the ciclosporin was not clearly altered by ticlopidine, although one patient was withdrawn from the study after 3 days because of a 60% fall in ciclosporin levels, attributed to poor compliance rather than an interaction. No clinically significant adverse haematological, biochemical or ECG or echocardiography changes occurred.[4]

Mechanism

Not understood.

Importance and management

Information appears to be limited to the reports cited, but the broad picture is that the concurrent use of ciclosporin and ticlopidine is normally safe and effective, but the occasional patient may unpredictably have marked reductions in serum ciclosporin levels. For this reason good monitoring is needed, particularly when ticlopidine is first added, so that any problems can be quickly identified.

1. Birmelé B, Lebranchu Y, Bagros Ph, Nivet H, Furet Y, Pengloan J. Interaction of cyclosporin and ticlopidine. *Nephrol Dial Transplant* (1991) 6, 150–1.
2. Verdejo A, de Cos MA, Zubimendi JA. Probable interaction between cyclosporin A and low dose ticlopidine. *BMJ* (2000) 320, 1037.
3. de Lorgeril M, Boissonnat P, Dureau G, Guidollet J, Renaud S. Evaluation of ticlopidine, a novel inhibitor of platelet aggregation, in heart transplant recipients. *Transplantation* (1993) 55, 1195–6.
4. Boissonnat P, de Lorgeril M, Perroux V, Salen P, Batt AM, Barthelemy JC, Brouard R, Serres E, Delaye J. A drug interaction study between ticlopidine and cyclosporin in heart transplant recipients. *Eur J Clin Pharmacol* (1997) 53, 39–45.

Ciclosporin + Trimetazidine

Trimetazidine appears not to alter the pharmacokinetics or immunosuppressive effects of ciclosporin.

Clinical evidence, mechanism, importance and management

To find out if the concurrent use of trimetazidine and ciclosporin was associated with any adverse effects, 12 kidney transplant patients on ciclosporin were given trimetazidine 40 mg twice daily for 5 days. No changes in the pharmacokinetics of the ciclosporin were seen, and there were no alterations in interleukin-2 concentrations or soluble interleukin-2 receptors.[1] An associated study by the same group of workers using two models (the lymphoproliferative response of normal human lymphocytes to phytohaemagglutinin and a delayed *mouse* hypersensitivity model) similarly found that trimetazidine did not interfere with the effects of ciclosporin.[2] It was concluded on the basis of these two studies that the concurrent use of ciclosporin and trimetazidine need not be avoided.

1. Simon N, Brunet P, Roumenov D, Dussol B, Barre J, Duche JC, Albengres E, D'Athis Ph, Crevat A, Berland Y, Tillement JP. The effects of trimetazidine-cyclosporin A coadministration on interleukin 2 and cyclosporin A blood levels in renal transplant patients. *Therapie* (1995) 50 (Suppl), 498.
2. Albengres E, Tillement JP, d'Athis P, Salducci D, Chauvet-Monges AM, Crevat A. Lack of pharmacodynamic interaction between trimetazidine and cyclosporin A in human lymphoproliferative and mouse delayed hypersensitivity response models. *Fundam Clin Pharmacol* (1996) 10, 264–8.

Ciclosporin + Vitamin E (Tocopherol)

Ciclosporin absorption is increased by vitamin E.

Clinical evidence, mechanism, importance and management

Ten healthy subjects were given a single 10-mg/kg oral dose of ciclosporin with and without a 0.1-ml/kg oral dose of vitamin E (d-alpha tocopheryl polyethylene glucose 1000 succinate). The AUC of the ciclosporin increased by 60%, and it was suggested that absorption was increased due to improved solubilisation and micelle formation within the gut, or that decreased intestinal metabolism occurred.[1] The clinical importance of this interaction awaits assessment.

1. Chang T, Benet LZ, Hebert MF. The effect of water-soluble vitamin E on cyclosporine pharmacokinetics in healthy volunteers. *Clin Pharmacol Ther* (1996) 59, 297–303.

Corticosteroids + Aminoglutethimide

The effects of dexamethasone, but not hydrocortisone, can be reduced or abolished by aminoglutethimide.

Clinical evidence

(a) Dexamethasone

Aminoglutethimide 500 to 750 mg daily reduced the half-life of dexamethasone 1 mg from 264 to 120 minutes in 6 patients.[1] In another 22 patients it was found that larger doses of dexamethasone (1.5 to 3 mg daily) compensated for the increased dexamethasone metabolism caused by aminoglutethimide and complete adrenal suppression was achieved over a prolonged period.[1] Another study found a fourfold increase in dexamethasone clearance in 10 patients on aminoglutethimide 1 g daily.[2]

A patient, dependent on dexamethasone due to brain oedema caused by a tumour, deteriorated rapidly with headache and lethargy when aminoglutethimide was also given. The problem was solved by withdrawing the aminoglutethimide and temporarily increasing the dexamethasone dosage from 6 to 16 mg daily.[3]

(b) Hydrocortisone

One study found that aminoglutethimide did not affect the response to hydrocortisone, and that hydrocortisone 40 mg was adequate replacement therapy in patients taking aminoglutethimide 1 g daily. In this study, aminoglutethimide did not affect the half-life of ^{3}H-cortisol, suggesting that it does not affect hydrocortisone metabolism.[2] Hydrocortisone 30 mg daily is normally adequate replacement in patients on aminoglutethimide, as this is the physiological dose of hydrocortisone.[4]

Mechanism

Aminoglutethimide is an enzyme inducing agent and it seems probable that it interacts by increasing the metabolism and clearance of the corticosteroids by the liver, thereby reducing their effects.[5]

Importance and management

Information is limited but the interaction between dexamethasone and aminoglutethimide is established. The reduction in the serum corticosteroid levels can be enough to reduce or even abolish the effects of corticosteroid replacement therapy[1] or to cause loss of control of a disease condition.[3] The former situation has been successfully accommodated by increasing the dosage of the dexamethasone,[1] and it would seem logical that this would also apply to disease control. Hydrocortisone is routinely used with aminoglutethimide as replacement therapy, and would seem to be a suitable alternative to dexamethasone, where clinically appropriate. Other synthetic corticosteroids are predicted to interact in the same way as dexamethasone, but this needs confirmation.

1. Santen RJ, Lipton A, Kendall J. Successful medical adrenalectomy with amino-glutethimide. Role of altered drug metabolism. *JAMA* (1974) 230, 1661–5.
2. Santen RJ, Wells SA, Runić S, Gupta C, Kendall J, Rudy EB, Samojlik E. Adrenal suppression with aminoglutethimide. I. Differential effects of aminoglutethimide on glucocorticoid metabolism as a rationale for the use of hydrocortisone. *J Clin Endocrinol Metab* (1977) 45, 469–79.
3. Halpern J, Catane R, Baerwald H. A call for caution in the use of aminoglutethimide: negative interactions with dexamethasone and beta blocker treatment. *J Med* (1984) 15, 59–63.
4. Orimeten Tablets (Aminoglutethimide). Novartis Pharmaceuticals UK Ltd. UK Summary of product characteristics, July 2000.
5. Santen RJ, Brodie AMH. Suppression of oestrogen production as treatment of breast carcinoma: pharmacological and clinical studies with aromatase inhibitors. *Clin Oncol* (1982) 1, 77–130.

Corticosteroids + Antacids

The absorption of prednisone can be reduced by large but not small doses of aluminium/magnesium hydroxide antacids. Prednisolone probably behaves similarly. Dexamethasone absorption is reduced by magnesium trisilicate.

Clinical evidence

(a) Dexamethasone

Magnesium trisilicate 5 g in 100 ml of water considerably reduced the bioavailability of a single 1-mg oral dose of dexamethasone given to 6 healthy subjects. Using the urinary excretion of 11-hydroxycorticosteroids as a measure, the reduction in bioavailability was about 75%.[1]

(b) Prednisolone or prednisone

Gastrogel (**aluminium/magnesium hydroxide** and **magnesium trisilicate**) 20 ml had no significant effect on serum levels, half-life or AUC of prednisone in 10 or 20-mg doses in 5 patients and 2 healthy subjects.[2]

Another study in 8 healthy subjects given a 20-mg dose of prednisolone found that 30 ml of **Magnesium Trisilicate Mixture BP** or *Aludrox* (**aluminium hydroxide gel**) caused small but not statistically significant changes in peak prednisolone levels and absorption. However, one subject given **magnesium trisilicate** had considerably reduced levels.[3] **Aluminium phosphate** has also been found not to affect prednisolone absorption.[4,5] In contrast, another study in healthy subjects and patients given 60 ml of *Aldrox* or *Melox* (both containing **aluminium/magnesium hydroxide**) found that the bioavailability of prednisone 10 mg was reduced by 30% on average, and even by 40% in some individuals.[6]

Mechanism

The reduction in dexamethasone absorption is attributed to adsorption onto the surface of the magnesium trisilicate.[1,7]

Importance and management

Information seems to be limited to these studies. The indication is that large doses of some antacids can reduce bioavailability, but small doses do not, although this needs confirmation. Some makers of dexamethasone suggest that the doses of antacid should be spaced as far as possible from the dexamethasone.[8,9] In other similar antacid interactions 2 to 3 hours is usually sufficient. The makers of **deflazacort** also issue a similar warning.[10] Concurrent use should be monitored to confirm that the therapeutic response is adequate. Information about the interaction of other corticosteroids and antacids is lacking.

1. Naggar VF, Khalil SA, Gouda MW. Effect of concomitant administration of magnesium trisilicate on GI absorption of dexamethasone in humans. *J Pharm Sci* (1978) 67, 1029–30.
2. Tanner AR, Caffin JA, Halliday JW, Powell LW. Concurrent administration of antacids and prednisone: effect on serum levels of prednisolone. *Br J Clin Pharmacol* (1979) 7, 397–400.
3. Lee DAH, Taylor GM, Walker JG, James VHT. The effect of concurrent administration of antacids on prednisolone absorption. *Br J Clin Pharmacol* (1979) 8, 92–4.
4. Albin H, Vinçon G, Demotes-Mainard F, Begaud B, Bedjaoui A. Effects of aluminium phosphate on bioavailability of cimetidine and prednisolone. *Eur J Clin Pharmacol* (1984) 26, 271–3.
5. Albin H, Vinçon G, Pehourcq F, Lecorre C, Fleury B, Conri C. Influence d'un anti-acide sur la biodisponibilité de la prednisolone. *Therapie* (1983) 38, 61–5.
6. Uribe M, Casian C, Rojas S, Sierra JG, Go VLW, Muñoz RM, Gil S. Decreased bioavailability of prednisone due to antacids in patients with chronic active liver disease and in healthy volunteers. *Gastroenterology* (1981) 80, 661–5.
7. Prakash A, Verma RK. *In vitro* adsorption of dexamethasone and betamethasone on antacids. *Indian J Pharm Sci* (1984) Jan-Feb, 55–6.
8. Dexamethasone. Organon Laboratories Ltd. UK Summary of product characteristics, January 2001.

9. Dexsol (Dexamethasone sodium phosphate). Rosemont Pharmaceuticals Ltd. UK Summary of product characteristics, September 2000.
10. Calcort (Deflazacort). Shire Pharmaceuticals Ltd. UK Summary of product characteristics, August 2002.

Corticosteroids + Aprepitant

In the short-term, aprepitant increased the plasma levels of dexamethasone and methylprednisolone. Dosage adjustments of these corticosteroids are recommended.

Clinical evidence

(a) Dexamethasone

In a crossover study in 20 subjects aprepitant 125 mg on day one, and 80 mg on days 2 to 5 given with a standard dexamethasone regimen (20 mg on day one, and 8 mg on days 2 to 5) increased the dexamethasone AUC by 2.2-fold on days 1 and 5. When the same dose of aprepitant was given with a reduced-dose dexamethasone regimen (12 mg on day one, and 4 mg on days 2 to 5), the dexamethasone AUC was similar to that observed with the standard dexamethasone regimen without aprepitant. All regimens in this study also included intravenous ondansetron 32 mg on day one only.[1]

(b) Methylprednisolone

In a crossover study in 10 subjects aprepitant 125 mg on day one, and 80 mg on days 2 and 3 given with a methylprednisolone regimen (125 mg intravenously on day one, and 40 mg orally on days 2 and 3) increased the methylprednisolone AUC by 1.3-fold on day one and 2.5-fold on day 3.[1]

Mechanism

Aprepitant is a moderate inhibitor of the cytochrome P450 isoenzyme CYP3A4, and probably raises levels of these corticosteroids in the short-term by inhibiting their metabolism via CYP3A4. However, if the corticosteroids were given longer term, at later time points within 2 weeks after starting aprepitant, an inductive effect on CYP3A4 may occur (see also 'Benzodiazepines + Aprepitant', p.540).

Importance and management

An established interaction of clinical importance. The maker[2,3] recommends that the usual dose of dexamethasone should be reduced by about 50% when given with aprepitant. In clinical trials a dexamethasone regimen of 12 mg on day one and 8 mg on days 2 to 4 was used, and this is the recommended regimen. The maker recommends that the usual dose of intravenous methylprednisolone be reduced by 25%, and the usual oral dose by 50%, when given with aprepitant. However, the maker also notes that during continuous treatment with methylprednisolone, levels would be expected to decrease at later time points within 2 weeks.

1. McCrea JB, Majumdar AK, Goldberg MR, Iwamoto M, Gargano C, Panebianco DL, Hesney M, Lines CR, Petty KJ, Deutsch PJ, Murphy MG, Gottesdiener KM, Goldwater DR, Blum RA. Effects of the neurokinin1 receptor antagonist aprepitant on the pharmacokinetics of dexamethasone and methylprednisolone. *Clin Pharmacol Ther* (2003) 74, 17–24.
2. Emend (Aprepitant). Merck Sharp & Dohme Ltd. UK Summary of product characteristics, April 2005.
3. Emend (Aprepitant). Merck & Co., Inc. US Prescribing information, March 2005.

Corticosteroids + Azoles; Itraconazole

There is evidence that itraconazole can increase the effects of deflazacort, dexamethasone and methylprednisolone. Prednisolone and prednisone appear to be affected to a lesser extent. Itraconazole also increased the effects of inhaled budesonide in two studies, and fluticasone in one case report. Corticosteroid toxicity may occur if the dosage is not reduced.

Clinical evidence

(a) Budesonide

In a double-blind, randomised, crossover study, 10 healthy subjects were given 1 mg of inhaled budesonide over a period of 2 minutes after taking itraconazole 200 mg daily for 5 days. The AUC of budesonide was increased 4.2-fold by the itraconazole, and the plasma cortisol levels of the patients were suppressed, indicating an increased budesonide effect.[1] Another study compared the results of the ACTH (tetracosactide) test in 25 patients taking itraconazole 400 to 600 mg daily and high-dose inhaled budesonide 800 to 1600 micrograms daily with patients treated with high-dose budesonide or itraconazole alone. Adrenal insufficiency was detected in 44% of those treated with both drugs, but in none of the patients taking itraconazole or budesonide alone.[2]

(b) Deflazacort

A patient with cystic fibrosis taking deflazacort developed Cushing's syndrome soon after starting itraconazole 200 mg twice daily, which gradually disappeared when the itraconazole was stopped.[3]

(c) Dexamethasone

A study in 8 healthy subjects found that itraconazole 200 mg daily for 4 days increased the AUC, peak plasma level and elimination half-life of a single 4.5-mg oral dose of dexamethasone by 3.7-, 1.7-, and 2.8-fold respectively. In another phase of the study itraconazole decreased systemic clearance of intravenous dexamethasone 5 mg by 68% and increased the AUC and elimination half-life 3.3- and 3.2-fold respectively. The adrenal-suppressant effects of dexamethasone were enhanced by itraconazole.[4]

(d) Fluticasone

A case report describes profound adrenal suppression with secondary Cushing's syndrome in a patient given itraconazole 200 mg twice daily and low-dose inhaled fluticasone 250 micrograms daily.[5]

(e) Methylprednisolone

A study in 14 healthy subjects found that itraconazole 400 mg for one day and then 200 mg daily for the next 3 days, increased the AUC of a single 48-mg dose of methylprednisolone more than 2.5-fold.[6] Other studies in healthy subjects have found that itraconazole decreases the clearance and increases the elimination half life and AUC of both oral and intravenous methylprednisolone. Enhanced adrenal suppression also occurred.[7,8]

A man with a lung transplant treated with methylprednisolone, ciclosporin and azathioprine was given itraconazole 200 mg twice daily to treat a suspected *Aspergillus fumigatus* infection. Three weeks later signs of corticosteroid toxicity developed, namely myopathy (confirmed by electromyography) and diabetes mellitus. Ten days after stopping the itraconazole the muscle force had improved and the daily dose of insulin had decreased from 120 to 20 units.[9]

(f) Prednisolone or prednisone

Six patients with allergic bronchopulmonary aspergillosis (3 with underlying cystic fibrosis and 3 with severe asthma) were treated with oral itraconazole 200 mg twice daily for 1 to 6 months. Four of the patients also taking systemic prednisone were able to reduce the corticosteroid dosage by 44% (from 43 to 24 mg daily) without any clinical deterioration.[10] Another study found no clinically significant pharmacokinetic interaction between itraconazole (400 mg on day one then 200 mg daily for 3 days) and a single 60-mg dose of prednisone in healthy subjects.[6]

A study in 10 healthy subjects found that itraconazole 200 mg daily for 4 days increased the AUC of a single 20-mg oral dose of prednisolone by 24%, but this was considered to be of limited clinical significance.[11]

Mechanism

Uncertain. It seems probable that the itraconazole inhibits the metabolism of these corticosteroids by the cytochrome P450 isoenzyme CYP3A4 in the liver so that they are cleared from the body less quickly and their effects are thereby increased. Prednisolone is less likely than methylprednisolone to interact with CYP3A4 inhibitors.[11]

Importance and management

These interactions appear to be established. There is currently too little data to assess the incidence, but it would now be prudent to monitor the outcome of adding itraconazole to any patient on deflazacort, dexamethasone or methylprednisolone being alert for the need to reduce the steroid dosage. Adrenal function should also be monitored in patients on inhaled budesonide or fluticasone given itraconazole. Itraconazole appears to interact with prednisone and prednisolone to a lesser extent, but this may still be clinically important in some patients. Information about other corticosteroids is lacking but good monitoring seems advisable.

1. Raaska K, Niemi M, Neuvonen M, Neuvonen PJ, Kivistö KT. Plasma concentrations of inhaled budesonide and its effects on plasma cortisol are increased by the cytochrome P4503A4 inhibitor itraconazole. *Clin Pharmacol Ther* (2002) 72, 362–9.

2. Skov M, Main KM, Sillesen IB, Müller J, Koch C, Lanng S. Iatrogenic adrenal insufficiency as a side-effect of combined treatment of itraconazole and budesonide. *Eur Respir J* (2002) 20,127–33.
3. Sauty A, Leuenberger PH, Fitting JW. Cushing's syndrome in a patient with cystic fibrosis treated with itraconazole and deflazacort for allergic bronchopulmonary aspergillosis. *Eur Respir J* (1995) 8 (Suppl 19), 441S.
4. Varis T, Kivistö KT, Backman JT, Neuvonen PJ. The cytochrome P450 3A4 inhibitor itraconazole markedly increases the plasma concentrations of dexamethasone and enhances its adrenal-suppressant effect. *Clin Pharmacol Ther* (2000) 68, 487–94.
5. Parmar JS, Howell T, Kelly J, Bilton D. Profound adrenal suppression secondary to treatment with low dose inhaled steroids and itraconazole in allergic bronchopulmonary aspergillosis in cystic fibrosis. *Thorax* (2002) 57, 749–50.
6. Lebrun-Vignes B, Corbrion Archer V, Diquet B, Levron JC, Chosidow O, Puech AJ, Warot D. Effect of itraconazole on the pharmacokinetics of prednisolone and methylprednisolone and cortisol secretion in healthy subjects. *Br J Clin Pharmacol* (2001) 51, 443–50.
7. Varis T, Kaukonen K-M, Kivistö KT, Neuvonen PJ. Plasma concentrations and effects of oral methylprednisolone are considerably increased by itraconazole. *Clin Pharmacol Ther* (1998) 64, 363–8.
8. Varis T, Kivistö KT, Backman JT, Neuvonen PJ. Itraconazole decreases the clearance and enhances the effects of intravenously administered methylprednisolone in healthy volunteers. *Pharmacol Toxicol* (1999) 85, 29–32.
9. Linthoudt H, Van Raemdonck D, Lerut T, Demedts M, Verleden G. The association of itraconazole and methylprednisolone may give rise to important steroid-related side effects. *J Heart Lung Transplant* (1996) 15, 1165.
10. Denning DW, Van Wye JE, Lewiston NJ, Stevens DA. Adjunctive therapy of allergic bronchopulmonary aspergillosis with itraconazole. *Chest* (1991) 100, 813–9.
11. Varis T, Kivistö KT, Neuvonen PJ. The effect of itraconazole on the pharmacokinetics and pharmacodynamics of oral prednisolone. *Eur J Clin Pharmacol* (2000) 56, 57–60.

Corticosteroids + Azoles; Ketoconazole

Ketoconazole reduces the metabolism and clearance of methylprednisolone. The situation with prednisone and prednisolone is uncertain. Ketoconazole modestly increases the systemic effect of inhaled budesonide, and markedly increases the AUC of oral budesonide. No clinically relevant interaction occurs with inhaled fluticasone.

Clinical evidence

(a) Budesonide

Sixteen healthy subjects were given a single 1-mg inhaled dose of budesonide after taking ketoconazole 200 mg daily for 2 days. Plasma cortisol levels and urinary cortisol excretion were used as a measure of how much budesonide was absorbed systemically, and ketoconazole was found to cause a 37% decrease in the 24-hour AUC of cortisol.[1]

Another study in 8 healthy subjects found that the AUC of a single 3-mg oral dose of budesonide was increased 6.5-fold when it was given with the last dose of ketoconazole 200 mg daily for 4 days. When budesonide was given 12 hours before the last dose of ketoconazole, the AUC was increased 3.8-fold.[2]

(b) Fluticasone

Sixteen healthy subjects were given a single 500-microgram inhaled dose of fluticasone after taking ketoconazole 200 mg daily for 2 days. Plasma cortisol levels and urinary cortisol excretion were used as a measure of how much fluticasone was absorbed systemically, and it was found that ketoconazole had no effect on fluticasone absorption.[1]

(c) Methylprednisolone

Ketoconazole 200 mg daily for 6 days increased the mean AUC of a single 20-mg intravenous dose of methylprednisolone in 6 healthy subjects by 135% and decreased the clearance by 60%. The 24-hour cortisol AUC was reduced by 44%.[3] These findings were confirmed in another study by the same group of workers.[4]

(d) Prednisolone or prednisone

Ketoconazole 200 mg daily for 6 to 7 days caused a 50% rise in the total and unbound prednisolone serum levels of 10 healthy subjects, following a dose of either oral prednisone or intravenous prednisolone.[5] In contrast, two other studies found that ketoconazole 200 mg daily for 6 days did not affect either the pharmacokinetics or the pharmacodynamics of prednisolone, as measured by the suppressive effects on serum cortisol, blood basophil and helper T-lymphocyte values of prednisolone.[6,7]

Mechanism

Ketoconazole inhibits the cytochrome P450 isoenzyme CYP3A4 in the intestinal wall and liver so that the metabolism of some oral corticosteroids is reduced.

Importance and management

The interaction between methylprednisolone and ketoconazole appears to be established and clinically important. A 50% reduction in the corticosteroid dosage is recommended in one study.[4] It has been pointed out that increased corticosteroid serum levels have an increased immunosuppressive effect, which may be undesirable in those with a fungal infection needing treatment with ketoconazole.[5] The situation with prednisone and prednisolone is as yet uncertain,[8,9] and more study is needed. The study using inhaled fluticasone or budesonide with ketoconazole indicates that no clinically important interaction occurs with fluticasone, but shows that ketoconazole increases the systemic effect of inhaled budesonide. Some makers[10,11] recommend that if the combination cannot be avoided the interval between administration of the two drugs should be as great as possible; a reduction in the dose of budesonide should also be considered. In addition, a significant interaction may occur with oral budesonide, which may be reduced by about half by separating the administration of the two drugs by 12 hours.[2]

1. Falcoz C, Lawlor C, Hefting NR, Borgstein NG, Smeets FWM, Wemer J, Jonkman JHG, House F. Effects of CYP3A4 inhibition by ketoconazole on systemic activity of inhaled fluticasone propionate and budesonide. *Eur Respir J* (1997) 10 (Suppl 25), 175S-176S.
2. Seidegård J. Reduction of the inhibitory effect of ketoconazole on budesonide pharmacokinetics by separation of their time of administration. *Clin Pharmacol Ther* (2000) 68, 13–17.
3. Glynn AM, Slaughter RL, Brass C, D'Ambrosio R, Jusko WJ. Effects of ketoconazole on methylprednisolone pharmacokinetics and cortisol secretion. *Clin Pharmacol Ther* (1986) 39, 654–9.
4. Kandrotas RJ, Slaughter RL, Brass C, Jusko WJ. Ketoconazole effects on methylprednisolone disposition and their joint suppression of endogenous cortisol. *Clin Pharmacol Ther* (1987) 42, 465–70.
5. Zürcher RM, Frey BM, Frey FJ. Impact of ketoconazole on the metabolism of prednisolone. *Clin Pharmacol Ther* (1989) 45, 366–72.
6. Yamashita SK, Ludwig EA, Middleton E, Jusko WJ. Lack of pharmacokinetic and pharmacodynamic interactions between ketoconazole and prednisolone. *Clin Pharmacol Ther* (1991) 49, 558–70.
7. Ludwig EA, Slaughter RL, Savliwala M, Brass C, Jusko WJ. Steroid-specific effects of ketoconazole disposition: unaltered prednisolone elimination. *Drug Intell Clin Pharm* (1989) 23, 858–61.
8. Jusko WJ. Ketoconazole effects on corticosteroid disposition. *Clin Pharmacol Ther* (1990) 47, 418–9.
9. Zürcher RM, Frey BM, Frey FJ. Ketoconazole effects on corticosteroid disposition. *Clin Pharmacol Ther* (1990) 47, 419–21.
10. Pulmicort (Budesonide). AstraZeneca UK Ltd. UK Summary of product characteristics, April 2005.
11. Novolizer (Budesonide). Viatris Pharmaceuticals Ltd. UK Summary of product characteristics, November 2004.

Corticosteroids + Azoles; Voriconazole

Voriconazole increased the maximum plasma levels and AUC of a single 60-mg dose of prednisolone by 11 and 34% respectively. No dosage adjustment is said to be necessary on concurrent use.[1,2]

1. VFEND (Voriconazole). Pfizer Ltd. UK Summary of product characteristics, March 2005.
2. VFEND (Voriconazole). Pfizer Ltd. US Prescribing information, March 2005.

Corticosteroids + Barbiturates

The therapeutic effects of systemic dexamethasone, methylprednisolone, prednisone and prednisolone are decreased by phenobarbital. Other barbiturates probably interact similarly, and primidone interacts like the barbiturates.

Clinical evidence

(a) Dexamethasone

A 14-year-old girl with congenital adrenal hyperplasia taking dexamethasone rapidly became over-treated (weight gain, signs of hypercortisolism) when the **primidone** 250 mg twice daily she was also taking was withdrawn over a month. Satisfactory control was only achieved when the dexamethasone dosage was reduced threefold.[1] A reduction in the effects of dexamethasone has also been described in another patient with congenital adrenal hyperplasia when treated with **primidone** for petit mal seizures.[2]

(b) Methylprednisolone

Phenobarbital increased the clearance of methylprednisolone in asthmatic children by 209%.[3]

(c) Prednisolone or prednisone

Three prednisone-dependent patients with bronchial asthma taking prednisone 10 to 40 mg daily had a marked worsening of their symptoms within a few days of starting to take **phenobarbital** 120 mg daily. There was a deterioration in their pulmonary function tests (FEV_1, degree of bronchospasm) and a rise in eosinophil counts, all of which improved when the **phenobarbital** was stopped. The prednisone clearance increased while taking the **phenobarbital**.[4] The survival of kidney transplant patients in a group of 75 children taking azathioprine and prednisone as immunosuppressants was reduced in those given **phenobarbital** 60 to 120 mg daily. Two of the 11 epileptic children were also taking phenytoin 100 mg daily.[5]

Nine patients with rheumatoid arthritis on prednisolone 8 to 15 mg daily had strong evidence of clinical deterioration (worsening joint tenderness, pain, morning stiffness, fall in grip strength) when treated with **phenobarbital** for 2 weeks (plasma concentrations 0 to 86.2 micromol/l). The prednisolone half-life fell by 25%.[6] Another study found that prednisolone elimination is increased in renal transplant patients by **phenobarbital**.[7]

In contrast, the prednisone requirements of other children were unaltered while taking a compound preparation containing **phenobarbital** 24 mg daily.[8]

Mechanism

Phenobarbital is a recognised potent liver enzyme inducer that increases the metabolism of corticosteroids, thereby reducing their effects. Pharmacokinetic studies have shown that phenobarbital reduces the half-lives of these corticosteroids and increases their clearances by 40 to 209%.[3,4,9] Primidone interacts in a similar way because it is metabolised in the body to phenobarbital.[1]

Importance and management

The interaction between the corticosteroids and phenobarbital is well documented, well established and of clinical importance. Concurrent use need not be avoided but the outcome should be monitored. Increase the corticosteroid dosage as necessary. The extent of the increase is variable. Dexamethasone,[4] hydrocortisone,[10] methylprednisolone,[3,9] prednisone[4,5] and prednisolone[3,6] are all known to be affected. Prednisone and prednisolone appear to be less affected than methylprednisolone and may be preferred.[3] Be alert for the same interaction with other corticosteroids and other barbiturates, which also are enzyme-inducing agents, although direct evidence seems to be lacking. The dexamethasone adrenal suppression test may be expected to be unreliable in those taking phenobarbital, just as it is with phenytoin, another potent enzyme-inducing agent. See 'Corticosteroids + Phenytoin', p.808.

1. Young MC, Hughes IA. Loss of therapeutic control in congenital adrenal hyperplasia due to interaction between dexamethasone and primidone. *Acta Paediatr Scand* (1991) 80, 120–4.
2. Hancock KW, Levell A. Primidone/dexamethasone interaction. *Lancet* (1978) ii, 97–8.
3. Bartoszek M, Brenner AM, Szefler SJ. Prednisolone and methylprednisolone kinetics in children receiving anticonvulsant therapy. *Clin Pharmacol Ther* (1987) 42, 424–32.
4. Brooks SM, Werk EE, Ackerman SJ, Sullivan I, Thrasher K. Adverse effects of phenobarbital on corticosteroid metabolism in patients with bronchial asthma. *N Engl J Med* (1972) 286, 1125–8.
5. Wassner SJ, Pennisi AJ, Malekzadeh MH, Fine RN. The adverse effect of anticonvulsant therapy on renal allograft survival. *J Pediatr* (1976) 88, 134–7.
6. Brooks PM, Buchanan WW, Grove M, Downie WW. Effects of enzyme induction on metabolism of prednisolone. Clinical and laboratory study. *Ann Rheum Dis* (1976) 35, 339–43.
7. Gambertoglio J, Kapusnik J, Holford N, Nishikawa R, Hau T, Birnbaum J, Amend W. Enhancement of prednisolone elimination by anticonvulsants in renal transplant recipients. *Clin Pharmacol Ther* (1982) 31, 228.
8. Falliers CJ. Corticosteroids and phenobarbital in asthma. *N Engl J Med* (1972) 287, 201.
9. Stjernholm MR, Katz FH. Effects of diphenylhydantoin, phenobarbital, and diazepam on the metabolism of methylprednisolone and its sodium succinate. *J Clin Endocrinol Metab* (1975) 41, 887–93.
10. Burstein S, Klaiber EL. Phenobarbital-induced increase in 6-β-hydroxycortisol excretion: clue to its significance in human urine. *J Clin Endocrinol Metab* (1965) 25, 293–6.

Corticosteroids + Bile-acid binding resins

Colestyramine reduces the absorption of oral hydrocortisone, but not prednisolone. Colestipol similarly affected hydrocortisone in one case.

Clinical evidence

(a) Colestyramine

Colestyramine 4 g reduced the AUC of oral **hydrocortisone** 50 mg in 10 healthy subjects by 43%. Peak levels were lower and were reached about 50 minutes later.[1] Two of the subjects were given both 4 g and 8 g of colestyramine, and their AUCs were reduced by 47 and 97%, and by 59 and 86% respectively.[1]

In contrast, 2 patients on long-term **prednisolone** had no changes in the bioavailability of an oral dose of **prednisolone** when given an 8 g dose of colestyramine.[2]

(b) Colestipol

A man with hypopituitarism taking **hydrocortisone** 20 mg each morning and 10 mg each evening became lethargic, ataxic, and developed headaches (all signs of **hydrocortisone** insufficiency) within 4 days of starting to take colestipol 15 g three times daily for hypercholesterolaemia. He responded rapidly when given intravenous **hydrocortisone** 100 mg, and was discharged with the colestipol replaced by a statin.[3]

Mechanism

It seems that hydrocortisone can become bound to colestyramine or colestipol in the gut, thereby reducing its absorption.[1,4]

Importance and management

Information is limited, but these interactions with hydrocortisone appear to be established (they are consistent with the interactions of both of these bile-acid resins with other drugs). Separate the administration of the drugs as much as possible to minimise admixture in the gut, although the authors of one report warn that this may not necessarily avoid this interaction because their data show that the colestyramine may remain in the gut for a considerable time.[1] The usual recommendation is to avoid other drugs for one hour before and 4 to 6 hours after taking colestyramine, and one hour before and 4 hours after colestipol. Monitor the effects and increase the hydrocortisone dosage if necessary. Prednisolone may be a non-interacting alternative, but the evidence is extremely limited.

1. Johansson C, Adamsson U, Stierner U, Lindsten T. Interaction of cholestyramine on the uptake of hydrocortisone in the gastrointestinal tract. *Acta Med Scand* (1978) 204, 509–12.
2. Audétat V, Paumgartner G, Bircher J. Beeinträchtigt Cholestyramin die biologische Verfügbarkeit von Prednisolon? *Schweiz Med Wochenschr* (1977) 107, 527–8.
3. Nekl KE, Aron DC. Hydrocortisone-colestipol interaction. *Ann Pharmacother* (1993) 27, 980–1.
4. Ware AJ, Combes B. Influence of sodium taurocholate, cholestyramine and Mylanta on the intestinal absorption of glucocorticoids in the rat. *Gastroenterology* (1973) 64, 1150–5.

Corticosteroids + Caffeine

The results of the dexamethasone suppression test can be falsified by the ingestion of caffeine.

Clinical evidence, mechanism, importance and management

In one study, 22 healthy subjects and 6 depressed patients were given a single 480-mg dose of caffeine or placebo at 2 pm following a single 1-mg dose of **dexamethasone** at 11 pm. Caffeine significantly increased the cortisol levels following the dexamethasone; cortisol levels taken at 4 pm were 5.3 micrograms/dl following caffeine use, compared with only 2.3 micrograms/dl with placebo.[1] Thus the equivalent of about 4 to 5 cups of coffee may effectively falsify the results of the **dexamethasone** suppression test.

1. Uhde TW, Bierer LM, Post RM. Caffeine-induced escape from dexamethasone suppression. *Arch Gen Psychiatry* (1985) 42, 737–8.

Corticosteroids + Carbamazepine

The clearance of dexamethasone, methylprednisolone and prednisolone is increased in patients taking carbamazepine. The results of the dexamethasone suppression test may be invalid in those taking carbamazepine.

Clinical evidence

A study in 8 patients on long-term treatment with carbamazepine found that the elimination half-life of **prednisolone** was shorter (1.98 hours compared to 2.73 hours), and the clearance was 42% higher than in 9 healthy subjects.[1]

A study in asthmatic children found that carbamazepine increased the clearance of **prednisolone** by 79% and increased the clearance of **methylprednisolone** by 342%.[2]

A study in 8 healthy subjects found that in the presence of carbamazepine 800 mg daily the dosage of **dexamethasone** needed to suppress cortisol secretion (as part of the **dexamethasone** adrenal suppression test) was increased two to fourfold.[3] A further study found that it took 2 to 13 days for false-positive results to occur after carbamazepine was started, and 3 to 12 days to recover when the carbamazepine was stopped.[4]

Mechanism

Carbamazepine stimulates liver enzymes, which results in the increased metabolism of the steroids.

Importance and management

Information is limited but the interaction appears to be established. Patients taking carbamazepine are likely to need increased doses of dexamethasone, methylprednisolone or prednisolone. Prednisolone is less affected than methylprednisolone and is probably preferred. The same interaction seems likely with other corticosteroids but more study is needed to confirm this. Note that hydrocortisone and prednisone are affected by another potent enzyme inducer, 'phenobarbital', (p.803).

1. Olivesi A. Modified elimination of prednisolone in epileptic patients on carbamazepine monotherapy, and in women using low-dose oral contraceptives. *Biomed Pharmacother* (1986) 40, 301–8.
2. Bartoszek M, Brenner AM, Szefler SJ. Prednisolone and methylprednisolone kinetics in children receiving anticonvulsant therapy. *Clin Pharmacol Ther* (1987) 42, 424–32.
3. Köbberling J, v zur Mühlen A. The influence of diphenylhydantoin and carbamazepine on the circadian rhythm of free urinary corticoids and on the suppressibility of the basal and the 'impulsive' activity by dexamethasone. *Acta Endocrinol (Copenh)* (1973) 72, 303–18.
4. Privitera MR, Greden JF, Gardner RW, Ritchie JC, Carroll BJ. Interference by carbamazepine with the dexamethasone suppression test. *Biol Psychiatry* (1982) 17, 611–20.

Corticosteroids + Carbimazole or Thiamazole

Prednisolone clearance is increased by the use of carbimazole or thiamazole, and therefore its dose may need increasing.

Clinical evidence

A comparative study was conducted in:

(a) 8 women taking levothyroxine with thiamazole 2.5 mg or carbimazole 5 mg daily for Graves' ophthalmology,

(b) 6 women on levothyroxine who had undergone subtotal thyroidectomy, and

(c) 6 other healthy women.

All were euthyroid. It was found that the clearance of a 540 microgram/kg dose of intravenous **prednisolone** in those in group (a) was much greater than in the other two groups (0.37, 0.24 and 0.2 l/h.kg respectively). After 6 hours the plasma **prednisolone** levels in group (a) were only about 10% of those in the healthy women and was undetectable after 8 hours, whereas total and unbound **prednisolone** levels were much higher and measurable over the 10 hour study period in groups (b) and (c).[1]

In another group of previously hyperthyroid patients, now euthyroid because of carbimazole treatment, the total **prednisolone** clearance was 0.4 l/hour.[1]

Mechanism

Not established. It seems possible that the thiamazole and carbimazole increase the metabolism of the prednisolone by the liver microsomal enzymes, thereby increasing its loss from the body.

Importance and management

Direct information seems to be limited to this study although the authors point out that there is a clinical impression that higher doses of prednisolone are needed in patients with Graves' disease. Be alert for the need to use higher doses of prednisolone in patients taking either thiamazole or carbimazole. Also note that a hypothyroid state may increase corticosteroid effects, and thus corticosteroids are cautioned in hypothyroid patients.

1. Legler UF. Impairment of prednisolone disposition in patients with Graves' disease taking methimazole. *J Clin Endocrinol Metab* (1988) 66, 221–3.

Corticosteroids + Diltiazem

Diltiazem increases the AUC of intravenous and oral methylprednisolone, but the clinical significance of this is unclear.

Clinical evidence

In a study, 5 healthy subjects were given diltiazem 180 mg daily for 4 days, then again with *intravenous* methylprednisolone 300 micrograms/kg (based on ideal body-weight) on day 5. Diltiazem increased the AUC of methylprednisolone by 50%, the half life by 37% and reduced the methylprednisolone clearance by 33%. Although the morning cortisol concentration was only 12% of that during the placebo phase, overall the suppressive effects of methylprednisolone on cortisol excretion were unchanged. The authors suggest that consideration should be given to reducing the dose of methylprednisolone in patients on diltiazem who have enhanced effects.[1] Another similar study in which patients were given diltiazem and a single 16-mg oral dose of methylprednisolone found much larger effects. The AUC of methylprednisolone was increased 2.6-fold, and the morning cortisol excretion was only 12% of that in the absence of diltiazem,[2] suggesting an enhanced effect.

Mechanism

Diltiazem is an inhibitor of the cytochrome P450 isoenzyme CYP3A4. As methylprednisolone is metabolised by CYP3A4 any inhibition of its activity would be expected to raise methylprednisolone levels.[1,2] It has been suggested that P-glycoprotein may also play a role.[1,2] Inhibition of intestinal/hepatic CYP3A4 may increase the oral bioavailability of methylprednisolone, which could contribute to the pharmacokinetic differences seen in the interaction when methylprednisolone is given orally rather than intravenously.

Importance and management

Information about the interaction between diltiazem and methylprednisolone seems limited to these two studies, but the effect of concurrent use is clear. However, the clinical significance of the raised methylprednisolone levels has not been established. Monitoring for an increase in methylprednisolone adverse effects, as suggested by one of the authors, seems a prudent measure.[1]

1. Booker BM, Magee MH, Blum RA, Lates CD, Jusko WJ. Pharmacokinetic and pharmacodynamic interactions between diltiazem and methylprednisone in healthy volunteers. *Clin Pharmacol Ther* (2002) 72, 370–82.
2. Varis T, Backman JT, Kivistö KT, Neuvonen PJ. Diltiazem and mibefradil increase the plasma concentrations and greatly enhance the adrenal-suppressant effect of oral methylprednisolone. *Clin Pharmacol Ther* (2000) 67, 215–21.

Corticosteroids + Diuretics; Potassium-depleting

Since both of these groups of drugs cause potassium loss, severe depletion may occur if they are used together.

Clinical evidence, mechanism, importance and management

There seem to be no formal clinical studies about the extent of the additive potassium depletion that can occur when potassium-depleting diuretics and corticosteroids are given together but an exaggeration of the potassium loss undoubtedly occurs (e.g. seen with **hydrocortisone** and **furosemide**[1]). One study looking at hypokalaemia with potassium-depleting diuretics found that corticosteroids were a significant risk factor for hypokalaemic events; 19.9% of patients on a potassium-depleting diuretic developed hypokalaemia, whereas 31.1% of patients on a potassium-depleting diuretic and a corticosteroid developed hypokalaemia.[2] Concurrent use should be well monitored and the potassium intake increased as appropriate to balance this loss.

The greatest potassium loss occurs with the naturally occurring corticosteroids such as **cortisone** and **hydrocortisone**. **Corticotropin (ACTH)**, which is a pituitary hormone, and **tetracosactrin** (a synthetic polypeptide) stimulate corticosteroid secretion by the adrenal cortex and can thereby indirectly cause potassium loss. **Fludrocortisone** also causes potassium loss. The synthetic corticosteroids (**glucocorticoids**) have a less marked potassium-losing effect and are therefore less likely to cause problems. These include **betamethasone**, **dexamethasone**, **prednisolone**, **prednisone** and **triamcinolone**.

The potassium-depleting diuretics (i.e. **loop diuretics** or **thiazide** and related diuretics) are listed in 'Table 24.1', (p.717). **Acetazolamide**, a weak diuretic, may also cause potassium depletion and has also been predicted to cause hypokalaemia in the presence of corticosteroids.

1. Manchon ND, Bercoff E, Lemarchand P, Chassagne P, Senant J, Bourreille J. Fréquence et gravité des interactions médicamenteuses dans une population âgée: étude prospective concernant 63 malades. *Rev Med Interne* (1989) 10, 521–5.

2. Widmer P, Maibach R, Künzi UP, Capaul R, Mueller U, Galeazzi R, Hoigné R. Diuretic-related hypokalaemia: the role of diuretics, potassium supplements, glucocorticoids and β_2-adrenoceptor agonists. *Eur J Clin Pharmacol* (1995) 49, 31–6.

Corticosteroids + Ephedrine

Ephedrine increases the clearance of dexamethasone from the body.

Clinical evidence, mechanism, importance and management

Nine asthmatic patients had a 40% increase in the clearance and a similar reduction in the half-life of **dexamethasone** when they were given ephedrine 100 mg daily for 3 weeks.[1] This would be expected to reduce the overall control of asthma, but this requires confirmation. Be alert for any evidence that the **dexamethasone** effects are reduced if both drugs are used. It is not clear whether other corticosteroids behave similarly.

1. Brooks SM, Sholiton LJ, Werk EE, Altenau P. The effects of ephedrine and theophylline on dexamethasone metabolism in bronchial asthma. *J Clin Pharmacol* (1977) 17, 308.

Corticosteroids + Glycyrrhizin (Liquorice)

Glycyrrhizin can reduce the clearance of prednisolone.

Clinical evidence, mechanism, importance and management

A study in 6 healthy subjects found that after taking 50-mg oral doses of glycyrrhizin every 8 hours for 4 doses followed by a bolus injection of **prednisolone hemisuccinate** 96 micrograms/kg, the AUC of total **prednisolone** was increased by 50% and the AUC of free **prednisolone** was increased by 55%.[1] This confirms the findings of two previous studies in which the glycyrrhizin was given by intravenous infusion.[2,3]

The probable reason for this reaction is that glycyrrhizin inhibits the metabolism of **prednisolone** by the liver so that it is cleared by the body more slowly. In one of the studies it was also found that glycyrrhizin increased the effects of **prednisolone** in some patients with rheumatoid arthritis and polyarteritis nodosa.[2]

The clinical importance of these observations is uncertain, but some increase in effects may be beneficial whereas excess effects may be toxic. Concurrent use should be well monitored.

1. Chen M-F, Shimada F, Kato H, Yano S, Kanaoka M. Effect of oral administration of glycyrrhizin on the pharmacokinetics of prednisolone. *Endocrinol Jpn* (1991) 38, 167–74.

2. Chen M-F, Shimada F, Kato H, Yano S, Kanaoka M. Effect of glycyrrhizin on the pharmacokinetics of prednisolone following low dosage of prednisolone hemisuccinate. *Endocrinol Jpn* (1990) 37, 331–41.

3. Ojima M, Itoh N, Satoh K, Fukuchi S. The effects of glycyrrhizin preparations on patients with difficult in release of steroids treatment. *Minophagen Med Rev* (1987) (Suppl 17), 120–5.

Corticosteroids + Grapefruit juice

Grapefruit juice does not affect the pharmacokinetics of prednisone or prednisolone.

Clinical evidence, mechanism, importance and management

A study in 12 kidney transplant patients taking ciclosporin and corticosteroids found that grapefruit juice, given every 3 hours for 30 hours, increased ciclosporin levels, but had no significant effect on the AUC of **prednisone** or **prednisolone**. It was concluded that grapefruit juice does not affect the metabolism of **prednisone** or **prednisolone**.[1] No special precautions are therefore needed if these corticosteroids and grapefruit juice are taken concurrently. Information about other corticosteroids is lacking.

1. Hollander AA, van Rooij J, Lentjes EGWM, Arbouw F, van Bree JB, Schoemaker RC, van Es LA, van der Woude FJ, Cohen AF. The effect of grapefruit juice on cyclosporine and prednisone metabolism in transplant patients. *Clin Pharmacol Ther* (1995) 57, 318–24.

Corticosteroids + H_2-blockers

Cimetidine does not interact with prednisolone, prednisone or dexamethasone, nor ranitidine with prednisone.

Clinical evidence, mechanism, importance and management

Prednisone is a pro-drug, which must be converted to **prednisolone** within the body to become active. A double-blind crossover study in 9 healthy subjects found that **cimetidine** 300 mg every 6 hours or **ranitidine** 150 mg twice daily for 4 days did not significantly alter the pharmacokinetics of **prednisolone** after a single 40-mg oral dose of **prednisone**.[1] Another double-blind crossover study also found that **cimetidine** 1 g daily only caused minor changes in plasma **prednisolone** levels following a 10-mg dose of enteric-coated **prednisolone**.[2] Yet another study found that 7 days of treatment with **cimetidine** 600 mg twice daily had no effect on the pharmacokinetics of a single 8-mg intravenous dose of **dexamethasone sodium phosphate**.[3]

There would therefore seem to be no reason, from the point of view of adverse interactions, for avoiding concurrent use. Information about other corticosteroids appears to be lacking, but no interaction is anticipated.

1. Sirgo MA, Rocci ML, Ferguson RK, Eshelman FN Vlasses PH. Effects of cimetidine and ranitidine on the conversion of prednisone to prednisolone. *Clin Pharmacol Ther* (1985) 37, 534–8.

2. Morrison PJ, Rogers HJ, Bradbrook ID, Parsons C. Concurrent administration of cimetidine and enteric-coated prednisolone: effect on plasma levels of prednisolone. *Br J Clin Pharmacol* (1980) 10, 87–9.

3. Peden NR, Rewhorn I, Champion MC, Mussani R, Ooi TC. Cortisol and dexamethasone elimination during treatment with cimetidine. *Br J Clin Pharmacol* (1984) 18, 101–3.

Corticosteroids + Macrolides

Troleandomycin and, to a lesser extent, clarithromycin and erythromycin can reduce the loss of methylprednisolone from the body, thereby increasing both its therapeutic and adverse effects. Prednisolone appears not to be affected by macrolides, except possibly in those also taking enzyme-inducers such as phenobarbital. Isolated case reports describe the development of acute mania and psychosis in two patients, apparently due to an interaction between prednisone and clarithromycin.

Clinical evidence

(a) Methylprednisolone

(i) Azithromycin. For mention that no interaction was reported between azithromycin and methylprednisolone, see 'Macrolides; Azithromycin + Miscellaneous', p.218.

(ii) Clarithromycin. A study in 6 asthmatic patients found that clarithromycin 500 mg twice daily for 9 days reduced the clearance of a single dose of methylprednisolone by 65% and resulted in significantly higher plasma methylprednisolone levels.[1]

(iii) Erythromycin. A study in 9 asthmatic adolescents aged 9 to 18 found that after taking erythromycin 250 mg four times daily for a week, the clearance of methylprednisolone was decreased by 46% (range 28 to 61%) and the half-life was increased by 47%, from 2.34 to 3.45 hours.[2]

(iv) Troleandomycin. A pharmacokinetic study in 4 children and 6 adult corticosteroid-dependent asthmatics found that one week of treatment with troleandomycin 14 mg/kg daily increased the half-life of methylprednisolone by 88%, from 2.46 to 4.63 hours, and reduced the total body

clearance by 64%. All 10 had cushingoid symptoms (cushingoid facies and weight gain), which resolved when the methylprednisolone dosage was reduced, without any loss in the control of the asthma.[3] Another study found that the dose of methylprednisolone could be reduced by 50% in the presence of troleandomycin, without loss of disease control.[4] Other studies have found similar effects.[5-10] However, a randomised placebo-controlled 2-year study found that although troleandomycin modestly reduced the required dose of methylprednisolone, this did not reduce corticosteroid-related adverse effects.[10] A case report describes a fatal varicella infection attributed to the potentiation of steroid effects by troleandomycin.[11]

(b) Prednisolone or prednisone

(i) Clarithromycin. A 30-year-old woman with no history of mental illness was treated for acute sinusitis with prednisone 20 mg daily for 2 days, followed by 40 mg for a further 2 days and clarithromycin 1 g daily. After 5 days she stopped taking both drugs [for unknown reasons], but a further 5 days later she was hospitalised with acute mania (disorganised thoughts and behaviour, pressured speech, increased energy, reduced need for sleep and labile effect). She spontaneously recovered after a further 5 days and had no evidence of psychiatric illness 4 months later.[12] A 50-year-old man with emphysema was given prednisone 20 mg daily to improve dyspnoea. After about 2 weeks he was also given clarithromycin 500 mg twice daily for purulent bronchitis. Shortly afterwards his family noticed psychiatric symptoms characterised by paranoia, delusions and what was described as dangerous behaviour. He recovered following treatment with low-dose olanzapine, gradual reduction of prednisone dosage and discontinuation of clarithromycin. An interaction was suspected as the patient had previously received prednisone on a number of occasions without the development of psychosis.[13]

A study in 6 asthmatic patients found that clarithromycin 500 mg twice daily for 9 days had no significant effect on prednisone pharmacokinetics.[1]

(ii) Troleandomycin. A study found that prednisolone clearance was not affected by troleandomycin in 3 patients, but was reduced by about 50% by troleandomycin in one patient who was also taking **phenobarbital**, which is an enzyme inducer.[5]

Mechanism

What is known suggests that clarithromycin, erythromycin and troleandomycin can inhibit the metabolism of methylprednisolone. The volume of distribution is also decreased.[2,3,5,14]

Importance and management

Information about the clarithromycin or erythromycin interactions with methylprednisolone is much more limited than with the interaction between troleandomycin and methylprednisolone, but they all appear to be established and of clinical importance. The effect should be taken into account during concurrent use and appropriate dosage reductions made to avoid the development of corticosteroid adverse effects. The authors of one study[3] suggest that this reduction should be empirical, based primarily on clinical symptomatology. Another group found that a 68% reduction in methylprednisolone dosage was possible within 2 weeks.[7] Troleandomycin appears to have a greater effect than erythromycin or clarithromycin.

Prednisolone seems not to interact with troleandomycin and is a non-interacting alternative, except possibly in those taking enzyme-inducers (e.g. phenobarbital).

The evidence on the interaction between prednisone and clarithromycin is limited and its general importance is uncertain, but prescribers should be aware of the reports of psychosis if both drugs are used together.

The general silence in the literature suggests that these macrolides do not normally interact with other corticosteroids but bear the possibility in mind if corticosteroid effects seem excessive. There also seems to be no information about other macrolides.

1. Fost DA, Leung DY, Martin RJ, Brown EE, Szefler SJ, Spahn JD. Inhibition of methylprednisolone elimination in the presence of clarithromycin therapy. *J Allergy Clin Immunol* (1999) 103, 1031–5.
2. LaForce CF, Szefler SJ, Miller MF, Ebling W, Brenner M. Inhibition of methylprednisolone elimination in the presence of erythromycin therapy. *J Allergy Clin Immunol* (1983) 72, 34–9.
3. Szefler SJ, Rose JQ, Ellis EF, Spector SL, Green AW, Jusko WJ. The effect of troleandomycin on methylprednisolone elimination. *J Allergy Clin Immunol* (1980) 66, 447–51.
4. Ball BD, Hill M, Brenner M, Sanks R, Szefler SJ. Critical assessment of troleandomycin in severe steroid-requiring asthmatic children. *Ann Allergy* (1988) 60, 155.
5. Szefler SJ, Ellis EF, Brenner M, Rose JQ, Spector SL, Yurchak A, Andrews F, Jusko WJ. Steroid-specific and anticonvulsant interaction aspects of triacetyloleandomycin-steroid therapy. *J Allergy Clin Immunol* (1982) 69, 455–60.
6. Itkin IH, Menzel M. The use of macrolide antibiotic substances in the treatment of asthma. *J Allergy* (1970) 45, 146–62.
7. Wald JA, Friedman BF, Farr RS. An improved protocol for the use of troleandomycin (TAO) in the treatment of steroid-requiring asthma. *J Allergy Clin Immunol* (1986) 78, 36–43.
8. Zeiger RS, Schatz M, Sperling W, Simon RA, Stevenson DD. Efficacy of troleandomycin in outpatients with severe, corticosteroid-dependent asthma. *J Allergy Clin Immunol* (1980) 66, 438–46.
9. Kamada AK, Hill MR, Brenner AM, Szefler SJ. Glucocorticoid reduction with troleandomycin in chronic, severe asthmatic children: implications for future trials and clinical application. *J Allergy Clin Immunol* (1992) 89, 285.
10. Nelson HS, Hamilos DL, Corsello PR, Levesque NV, Buchmeier AD, Bucher BL. A double-blind study of troleandomycin and methylprednisolone in asthmatic subjects who require daily corticosteroids. *Am Rev Respir Dis* (1993) 147, 398–404.
11. Lantner R, Rockoff JB, DeMasi J, Boran-Ragotzy R, Middleton E. Fatal varicella in a corticosteroid-dependent asthmatic receiving troleandomycin. *Allergy Proc* (1990) 11, 83–7.
12. Finkenbine R, Gill HS. Case of mania due to prednisone-clarithromycin interaction. *Can J Psychiatry* (1997) 42, 778.
13. Finkenbine RD, Frye MD. Case of psychosis due to prednisone-clarithromycin interaction. *Gen Hosp Psychiatry* (1998) 20, 325–6.
14. Szefler SJ, Brenner M, Jusko WJ, Spector SL, Flesher KA, Ellis EF. Dose- and time-related effect of troleandomycin on methylprednisolone elimination. *Clin Pharmacol Ther* (1982) 32, 166–171.

Corticosteroids + Mifepristone

The UK makers of mifepristone say that the efficacy of corticosteroids (included inhaled corticosteroids) are expected to be reduced in the 3 to 4 days following the use of mifepristone, because of the antiglucocorticoid activity of mifepristone.[1] Patients on corticosteroids should be monitored during this time, and consideration given to increasing the corticosteroid dose. However, the US makers contraindicate the use of mifepristone in those receiving long-term corticosteroid therapy.[2]

1. Mifegyne (Mifepristone). Exelgyn Laboratories. UK Summary of product characteristics, February 2005.
2. Mifeprex (Mifepristone). Danco Laboratories, LLC. US Prescribing information, December 2004.

Corticosteroids + NSAIDs

The concurrent use of NSAIDs and corticosteroids increases the risk of gastrointestinal bleeding and probably ulceration. Indometacin and naproxen may increase free levels of prednisolone. Rofecoxib does not affect the pharmacokinetics of either prednisone or prednisolone.

Clinical evidence, mechanism, importance and management

(a) Gastrointestinal bleeding and ulceration

A retrospective study of more than 20 000 patients who had received corticosteroids found that the incidence of upper gastrointestinal bleeding was no greater than in the control group who had not received corticosteroids (95 patients compared with 91 patients). However, the risk of bleeding was increased if the patients were also taking aspirin or other NSAIDs.[1] This is consistent with the results of another study on patients taking **prednisone** and **indometacin**,[2] and gives support to the widely held belief that the concurrent use of the NSAIDs (well-known as gastric irritants) can cause bleeding and ulceration. See also 'Aspirin or other Salicylates + Corticosteroids or Corticotropin', p.80.

(b) Pharmacokinetic interactions

A study in 11 patients with stable rheumatoid disease on regular corticosteroid therapy found that **indometacin** 75 mg or **naproxen** 250 mg twice daily for 2 weeks did not alter the total plasma levels of a single 7.5-mg dose of **prednisolone** but the amount of unbound (free) **prednisolone** increased by 30 to 60%.[3] The probable reason is that these NSAIDs displace administered and endogenous corticosteroids from their plasma protein binding sites, although the clinical relevance of this change is unclear. In a double-blind crossover study 12 healthy subjects were given **rofecoxib** 250 mg daily or placebo for 14 days with a single 30-mg dose of either intravenous **prednisolone** or oral **prednisone** on days 10 and 14. **Rofecoxib** did not affect the pharmacokinetics of the corticosteroids, even in a dose 10 times greater than that used clinically.[4]

1. Carson JL, Strom BL, Schinnar R, Sim E, Maislin G, Morse ML. Do corticosteroids really cause upper GI bleeding? *Clin Res* (1987) 35, 340A.
2. Emmanuel JH, Montgomery RD. Gastric ulcer and anti-arthritic drugs. *Postgrad Med J* (1971) 47, 227.

3. Rae SA, Williams IA, English J, Baylis EM. Alteration of plasma prednisolone levels by indomethacin and naproxen. *Br J Clin Pharmacol* (1982) 14, 459–61.
4. Schwartz JI, Mukhopadhyay S, Porras AG, Viswanathan-Aiyer K-J, Adcock S, Ebel DL, Gertz BJ. Effect of rofecoxib on prednisolone and prednisone pharmacokinetics in healthy subjects. *J Clin Pharmacol* (2003) 43, 187–92.

Corticosteroids + Omeprazole

Omeprazole had no effect on prednisone pharmacokinetics in healthy subjects, but an isolated and unexplained report describes a reduction in the effects of prednisone in a patient treated with omeprazole.

Clinical evidence, mechanism, importance and management

A placebo controlled, randomised, double-blind trial in 18 healthy subjects found that omeprazole 40 mg daily had no effect on the pharmacokinetics of a single 40-mg dose of **prednisone**.[1] This contrasts with an isolated and unexplained report of a patient suffering from pemphigus who was given **prednisone** 1 mg/kg daily, and a week later was also started on ranitidine 200 mg daily for a gastric ulcer. Four weeks later, when the skin lesions were well controlled, it was decided to replace the ranitidine with omeprazole 40 mg daily. Within 4 days the skin lesions began progressively to worsen, although the **prednisone** dosage remained unchanged. After 3 weeks it was decided to stop the omeprazole and restart the ranitidine because an adverse interaction between the **prednisone** and the omeprazole was suspected. Within about a week, the skin condition had begun to improve.[2] The suggested explanation is that the omeprazole inhibited the liver enzyme (11β-hydroxylase) that normally converts **prednisone** into its active form (prednisolone) resulting in inadequate treatment of the pemphigus.[2]

It would seem that an adverse interaction between **prednisone** and omeprazole is unlikely, but the isolated case should be borne in mind in the event of an unexpected response to treatment.

1. Cavanaugh JH, Karol M. Lack of pharmacokinetic interaction after administration of lansoprazole or omeprazole with prednisone. *J Clin Pharmacol* (1996) 36, 1064–71.
2. Joly P, Chosidow O, Laurent-Puig P, Delchier J-C, Roujeau J-C, Revuz J. Possible interaction prednisone-oméprazole dans la pemphigoïde bulleuse. *Gastroenterol Clin Biol* (1990) 14, 682–3.

Corticosteroids + Oral contraceptives or Progesterone

The serum levels of prednisone, prednisolone, cloprednol, methylprednisolone and possibly other corticosteroids are increased by oral contraceptives. In theory, both the therapeutic and toxic effects would be expected to be increased, but in practice it is uncertain whether these changes are important. Fluocortolone and oral budesonide were not affected. Progesterone appears not to affect the metabolism of prednisolone.

Clinical evidence

(a) Oral contraceptives

(i) Budesonide. The plasma levels of an oral dose of budesonide 4.5 mg daily for 7 days or in cortisol suppression in 20 women taking an oral contraceptive (**ethinylestradiol/desogestrel**) were no different when compared with 20 women not taking an oral contraceptive.[1]

(ii) Cloprednol. The clearance of cloprednol 20 mg was decreased by about one-third in 7 women on an oral contraceptive (**ethinylestradiol/norethisterone**) when compared with women not taking an oral contraceptive.[2]

(iii) Fluocortolone. A study in 7 women found that the pharmacokinetics of fluocortolone 20 mg were unaffected by an oral contraceptive (**ethinylestradiol/norethisterone**).[3]

(iv) Methylprednisolone. A study in 6 users and 6 non-users of oral contraceptives found that the clearance of methylprednisolone was decreased to about half in the oral contraceptive users. The oral contraceptive users were less sensitive to the suppressive effects of methylprednisolone on the secretion of cortisol, and had more suppression of basophils, but no changes in the T-helper cell response patterns.[4]

(v) Prednisolone or prednisone. In a placebo-controlled study, 20 healthy women took an oral contraceptive (**ethinylestradiol/desogestrel** 30/150 micrograms) for at least 4 months before being given prednisolone 20 mg daily for 7 days. The prednisolone levels were then compared with those in 20 women not taking oral contraceptives. The prednisolone AUC and steady-state levels were 2.3-fold higher in those on oral contraceptives.[1] Several other studies have found similar results, with the prednisolone AUC increasing 1.6- to sixfold,[5,6] and the clearance reducing by about 35 to 85%[5-10] in the presence of oral contraceptives containing ethinylestradiol or mestranol and various progestogens such as levonorgestrel, norgestrel and norethisterone. Similarly, a 2.3-fold increase in prednisolone AUC and a 45% decrease in clearance was seen when prednisone was given to women on an oral contraceptive.[11]

(b) Progesterone

Intravenous and oral **prednisolone** was given to 6 post-menopausal women before and after 2 months treatment with progesterone 5 mg. The pharmacokinetics of the **prednisolone** were not significantly changed.[12]

Mechanism

Not understood. The possibilities include a change in the metabolism of the corticosteroids, or in their binding to serum proteins.[11] The absence of an interaction with progesterone suggests that the oestrogenic component of the oral contraceptives is possibly responsible for any interaction.[12]

Importance and management

It is established that the pharmacokinetics of some corticosteroids are affected by oral contraceptives, but the clinical importance of any such changes is not known. The therapeutic and adverse effects would be expected to be increased but there appear to be no clinical reports of adverse reactions arising from concurrent use. In fact the authors of one study[4] concluded that women can be dosed similarly with methylprednisolone irrespective of oral contraceptive use.

However, until more is known it would be prudent to bear this interaction in mind when using any corticosteroid and oral contraceptive together. Only prednisone, prednisolone, cloprednol and methylprednisolone have been reported to interact and other corticosteroids possibly behave similarly, the exception apparently being fluocortolone and oral budesonide. Progesterone appears not to interact with prednisolone.

1. Seidegard J, Simonsson M, Edsbacker S. Effect of an oral contraceptive on the plasma levels of budesonide and prednisolone and the influence on plasma cortisol. *Clin Pharmacol Ther* (2000) 67, 373–81.
2. Legler UF. Altered cloprednol disposition in oral contraceptive users. *Clin Pharmacol Ther* (1987) 41, 237.
3. Legler UF. Lack of impairment of fluocortolone disposition in oral contraceptive users. *Eur J Clin Pharmacol* (1988) 35, 101–3.
4. Slayter KL, Ludwig EA, Lew KH, Middleton E, Ferry JJ, Jusko WJ. Oral contraceptive effects on methylprednisolone pharmacokinetics and pharmacodynamics. *Clin Pharmacol Ther* (1996) 59, 312–21.
5. Legler UF, Benet LZ. Marked alterations in prednisolone elimination for women taking oral contraceptives. *Clin Pharmacol Ther* (1982) 31, 243.
6. Olivesi A. Modified elimination of prednisolone in epileptic patients on carbamazepine monotherapy, and in women using low-dose oral contraceptives. *Biomed Pharmacother* (1986) 40, 301–8.
7. Boekenoogen SJ, Szefler SJ, Jusko WJ. Prednisolone disposition and protein binding in oral contraceptive users. *J Clin Endocrinol Metab* (1983) 56, 702–9.
8. Kozower M, Veatch L, Kaplan MM. Decreased clearance of prednisolone, a factor in the development of corticosteroid side effects. *J Clin Endocrinol Metab* (1974) 38, 407–12.
9. Legler UF, Benet LZ. Marked alterations in dose-dependent prednisolone kinetics in women taking oral contraceptives. *Clin Pharmacol Ther* (1986) 39, 425–9.
10. Meffin PJ, Wing LMH, Sallustio BC, Brooks PM. Alterations in prednisolone disposition as a result of oral contraceptive use and dose. *Br J Clin Pharmacol* (1984) 17, 655–64.
11. Frey BM, Schaad HJ, Frey FJ. Pharmacokinetic interaction of contraceptive steroids with prednisone and prednisolone. *Eur J Clin Pharmacol* (1984) 26, 505–11.
12. Tsunoda SM, Harris RZ, Mroczkowski PJ, Hebert MF, Benet LZ. Oral progesterone therapy does not affect the pharmacokinetics of prednisolone and erythromycin in post-menopausal women. *Clin Pharmacol Ther* (1995) 57, 182.

Corticosteroids + Phenytoin

The therapeutic effects of dexamethasone, methylprednisolone, prednisolone, prednisone (and probably other glucocorticoids) and fludrocortisone can be markedly reduced by phenytoin. One study suggested that dexamethasone may only modestly decrease serum phenytoin levels, but another study and two case reports suggest that an important decrease can occur. The results of the dexamethasone adrenal suppression test may prove to be unreliable in those on phenytoin.

Clinical evidence

(a) Reduced corticosteroid levels

A comparative pharmacokinetic study in 6 neurological or neurosurgical patients taking oral **dexamethasone** and phenytoin found that the average amount of **dexamethasone** that reached the general circulation was a quarter of that observed in 9 other patients taking only **dexamethasone** (mean oral bioavailability fractions of 0.21 and 0.84 respectively).[1] Another report describes patients who needed increased doses of **dexamethasone** while taking phenytoin.[2]

The **fludrocortisone** dosages of two patients required 4-fold and 10 to 20-fold increases respectively in the presence of phenytoin.[3]

Renal allograft survival is decreased in patients on **prednisone** taking phenytoin, due (it is believed) to reduced immunosuppressant effects.[4]

The results of several studies[5-9] of the effects of phenytoin on the half-lives and clearance rates of other corticosteroids are shown in 'Table 27.2', (below).

(b) Interference with the dexamethasone adrenal suppression test

A study in 7 patients found that phenytoin 300 to 400 mg daily reduced their plasma cortisol levels in response to **dexamethasone** from 22 to 19 microgram% compared with a reduction from 18 to 4 microgram% in the absence of phenytoin.[10]

Other studies confirm that plasma cortisol and urinary 17-hydroxycorticosteroid levels are suppressed far less than might be expected with small doses of **dexamethasone** (500 micrograms every 6 hours for 8 doses), but with larger doses (2 mg every 6 hours for 8 doses) suppression was normal.[11] However, one case describes a patient in whom even 16 mg of dexamethasone failed to cause cortisol depression while she was taking phenytoin, but when she was re-tested in the absence of phenytoin only 1 mg of dexamethasone was needed to elicit a response.[12]

(c) Serum phenytoin levels increased or decreased

A post-traumatic epilepsy prophylaxis study found that the serum phenytoin levels in those taking **dexamethasone** 16 to 150 mg (mean 63.6 mg) was 40% higher than those on phenytoin alone (17.3 compared with 12.5 micrograms/ml). The phenytoin was given as a loading dose of 11 mg/kg intravenously and then 13 mg/kg intramuscularly.[13]

Conversely, a retrospective study of 40 patient records indicated that **dexamethasone** reduced serum phenytoin levels. The serum phenytoin levels of 6 patients on fixed doses of phenytoin were halved by the presence of **dexamethasone**.[14] Another report describes a patient who required over 8 mg/kg of phenytoin (600 mg) to achieve therapeutic phenytoin levels in the presence of dexamethasone 16 mg. When the **dexamethasone** was increased to 28 mg daily he experienced seizures, and an increase in his phenytoin dose from 600 mg to 1 g only resulted in an increase in his levels from 13.9 to 16.4 micrograms/ml.[15] Another patient needed a large dose of phenytoin (greater than 10 mg/kg) while taking **dexamethasone**. He had an almost fourfold rise in serum phenytoin levels when **dexamethasone** was stopped.[16]

Mechanism

Phenytoin is a potent liver enzyme inducer that increases the metabolism of the corticosteroids so that they are cleared from the body more quickly, reducing both their therapeutic and adrenal suppressant effects.

Importance and management

The fall in serum corticosteroid levels is established and of clinical importance in systemic treatment, but it seems unlikely to affect the response to steroids given topically or by inhalation, intra-articular injection or enema.[17] The interaction can be accommodated in several ways:

- Increase the corticosteroid dosage proportionately to the increase in clearance (see 'Table 27.2', (below)). With prednisolone an average increase of 100% (range 58 to 260% in 5 subjects) proved effective.[17] A fourfold increase may be necessary with dexamethasone,[1] and much greater increases have been required with fludrocortisone.[3]
- Exchange the corticosteroid for another that is less affected (see 'Table 27.2', (below)). A switch from dexamethasone to equivalent doses of methylprednisolone has been reported to be effective[18] but another report found that methylprednisolone was more affected than prednisolone.[19] In another case the exchange of dexamethasone 16 mg daily for prednisone 100 mg was successful.[20]
- Exchange the phenytoin for another anticonvulsant: barbiturates (including primidone[21]) and carbamazepine, are also enzyme-inducers, but sodium valproate is a possible non-interacting alternative[2] where clinically appropriate. However, remember that corticosteroids should only be given to epileptics with care and good monitoring because of the risk that they will exacerbate the disease condition.

The effects on the dexamethasone adrenal suppression test can apparently be accommodated by using larger than usual doses of dexamethasone (2 mg every 6 hours for 8 doses)[11] or by an overnight test using 50 mg of hydrocortisone.[18]

The reports on the changes in serum phenytoin levels are inconsistent (rises and falls). The effects of concurrent use should be closely monitored.

1. Chalk JB, Ridgeway K, Brophy TRO'R, Yelland JDN, Eadie MJ. Phenytoin impairs the bioavailability of dexamethasone in neurological and neurosurgical patients. *J Neurol Neurosurg Psychiatry* (1984) 47, 1087–90.
2. McLelland J, Jack W. Phenytoin/dexamethasone interaction: a clinical problem. *Lancet* (1978) i, 1096–7.
3. Keilholz U, Guthrie GP. Case report: adverse effect of phenytoin on mineralocorticoid replacement with fludrocortisone in adrenal insufficiency. *Am J Med Sci* (1986) 291, 280–3.
4. Wassner SJ, Pennisi AJ, Malekzadeh MH, Fine RN. The adverse effect of anticonvulsant therapy on renal allograft survival. *J Pediatr* (1976) 88, 134–7.
5. Choi Y, Thrasher K, Werk EE, Sholiton LJ, Olinger C. Effect of diphenylhydantoin on cortisol kinetics in humans. *J Pharmacol Exp Ther* (1971) 176, 27–34.

Table 27.2 A comparison of the effects of phenytoin on the kinetics of different glucocorticoids (after Petereit and colleagues[1])

Corticosteroid	Daily dosage of phenytoin (mg)	Half-life without phenytoin (min)	Decreased half-life with phenytoin (%)	Increased mean clearance rate with phenytoin (%)	Refs
Hydrocortisone	300–400	60–90	–15	+25	2
Methylprednisolone	300	165	–56	+130	3
Prednisone	Prednisolone is the biologically active metabolite of prednisone so that the values for prednisone and prednisolone should be similar				4
Prednisolone	300	190–240	–45	+77	2
Dexamethasone	300	250	–51	+140	5, 6

1. Petereit LB, Meikle AW. Effectiveness of prednisolone during phenytoin therapy. *Clin Pharmacol Ther* (1977) 22, 912–6.
2. Choi Y, Thrasher K, Werk EE, Sholiton LJ, Olinger C. Effect of diphenylhydantoin on cortisol kinetics in humans. *J Pharmacol Exp Ther* (1971) 176, 27–34.
3. Stjernholm MR, Katz FH. Effects of diphenylhydantoin, phenobarbital, and diazepam on the metabolism of methylprednisolone and its sodium succinate. *J Clin Endocrinol Metab* (1975) 41, 887–93.
4. Meikle AW, Weed JA, Tyler FH. Kinetics and interconversion of prednisolone and prednisone studies with new radio-immunoassays. *J Clin Endocrinol Metab* (1975) 41, 717.
5. Brooks SM, Werk EE, Ackerman SJ, Sullivan I, Thrasher K. Adverse effects of phenobarbital on corticosteroid metabolism in patients with bronchial asthmas. *N Engl J Med* (1972) 286, 1125–8.
6. Haque N, Thrasher K, Werk EE, Knowles HC, Sholiton LJ. Studies of dexamethasone metabolism in man. Effect of diphenylhydantoin. *J Clin Endocrinol Metab* (1972) 34, 44–50.

6. Stjernholm MR, Katz FH. Effects of diphenylhydantoin, phenobarbital, and diazepam on the metabolism of methylprednisolone and its sodium succinate. *J Clin Endocrinol Metab* (1975) 41, 887–93.
7. Meikle AW, Weed JA, Tyler FH. Kinetics and interconversion of prednisolone and prednisone studies with new radio-immunoassays. *J Clin Endocrinol Metab* (1975) 41, 717.
8. Brooks SM, Werk EE, Ackerman SJ, Sullivan I, Thrasher K. Adverse effects of phenobarbital on corticosteroid metabolism in patients with bronchial asthmas. *N Engl J Med* (1972) 286, 1125–8.
9. Haque N, Thrasher K, Werk EE, Knowles HC, Sholiton LJ. Studies of dexamethasone metabolism in man. Effect of diphenylhydantoin. *J Clin Endocrinol Metab* (1972) 34, 44–50.
10. Werk EE, Choi Y, Sholiton L, Olinger C, Haque N. Interference in the effect of dexamethasone by diphenylhydantoin. *N Engl J Med* (1969) 281, 32–4.
11. Jubiz W, Meikle AW, Levinson RA, Mizutani S, West CD, Tyler FH. Effect of diphenylhydantoin on the metabolism of dexamethasone. *N Engl J Med* (1970) 283, 11–14.
12. Debrunner J, Schmid C, Schneeman M. Falsely positive dexamethasone suppression test in a patient treated with phenytoin to prevent seizures due to nocardia brain abscesses. *Swiss Med Wkly* (2002) 132, 267.
13. Lawson LA, Blouin RA, Smith RB, Rapp RP, Young AB. Phenytoin-dexamethasone interaction: a previously unreported observation. *Surg Neurol* (1981) 16, 23–4.
14. Wong DD, Longenecker RG, Liepman M, Baker S, LaVergne M. Phenytoin-dexamethasone: a possible drug-drug interaction. *JAMA* (1985) 254, 2062–3.
15. Recuenco I, Espinosa E, García B, Carcas A. Effect of dexamethasone on the decrease of serum phenytoin concentrations. *Ann Pharmacother* (1995) 29, 935.
16. Lackner TE. Interaction of dexamethasone with phenytoin. *Pharmacotherapy* (1991) 11, 344–7.
17. Petereit LB, Meikle AW. Effectiveness of prednisolone during phenytoin therapy. *Clin Pharmacol Ther* (1977) 22, 912–6.
18. Meikle AW, Stanchfield JB, West CD, Tyler FH. Hydrocortisone suppression test for Cushing syndrome: therapy with anticonvulsants. *Arch Intern Med* (1974) 134, 1068–74.
19. Bartoszek M, Brenner AM, Szefler SJ. Prednisolone and methylprednisolone kinetics in children receiving anticonvulsant therapy. *Clin Pharmacol Ther* (1987) 42, 424–32.
20. Boylan JJ, Owen DS, Chin JB. Phenytoin interference with dexamethasone. *JAMA* (1976) 235, 803–4.
21. Hancock KW, Levell MJ. Primidone/dexamethasone interaction. *Lancet* (1978) ii, 97–8.

Corticosteroids + Protease inhibitors

Several cases of Cushing's syndrome have been seen in patients using inhaled or intranasal fluticasone when ritonavir was also given. Dexamethasone may reduce levels of indinavir and saquinavir.

Clinical evidence

An HIV+ 32-year-old man who had been using intranasal **fluticasone** 200 micrograms twice daily for 3 years for allergic rhinitis, developed a cushingoid face and gained 6.5 kg in weight within 5 months of starting **ritonavir**, zidovudine and lamivudine.[1] Another HIV+ man on inhaled **beclometasone** 400 to 800 micrograms daily for asthma and intranasal **fluticasone** 800 micrograms daily for allergic rhinitis was also given **ritonavir**, **saquinavir**, stavudine and nevirapine, after which he developed mild cushingoid facial changes. Both patients had high plasma levels of **fluticasone**. The problems resolved when the **fluticasone** was withdrawn. A third HIV+ patient on inhaled **beclometasone**, intranasal **fluticasone**, **ritonavir**, zidovudine and lamivudine had increased **fluticasone** levels but no signs of Cushing's syndrome.[1]

There are reports of at least 4 other patients who have developed Cushing's syndrome within 2 to 5 months of using regimens of inhaled[2-4] or intranasal[5] **fluticasone** with **ritonavir**,[5] **ritonavir/amprenavir**,[2] **ritonavir/lopinavir**,[4] or **ritonavir/saquinavir**.[3] The interaction was confirmed in one patient by replacing the **ritonavir** with nevirapine for 3 weeks and then restarting the **ritonavir**.[5]

Mechanism

Ritonavir, and all protease inhibitors, inhibit the cytochrome P450 isoenzyme CYP3A4 to varying degrees. Fluticasone is metabolised by this isoenzyme and therefore its plasma levels rise.

Importance and management

Information is limited but the interaction between ritonavir and fluticasone appears to be an established and clinically important. The incidence is not known. Patients using these two drugs should be very well monitored for any signs of corticosteroid overdose. The problem may take months to manifest itself. Some makers of **betamethasone**[6] and **dexamethasone**[7] predict a similar interaction with ritonavir.

The makers of **dexamethasone** also state that it reduces the plasma levels of **indinavir** and saquinavir,[7] so monitor antiviral efficacy if these combinations are used.

1. Chen F, Kearney T, Robinson S, Daley-Yates PT, Waldron S, Churchill DR. Cushing's syndrome and severe adrenal suppression in patients treated with ritonavir and inhaled nasal fluticasone. *Sex Transm Infect* (1999) 75, 274.
2. Clevenbergh P, Corcostegui M, Gérard D, Hieronimus S, Mondain V, Chichmanian RM, Sadoul JL, Dellamonica P. Iatrogenic Cushing's syndrome in an HIV-infected patient treated with inhaled corticosteroids (fluticason propionate) and low dose ritonavir enhanced PI containing regimen. *J Infect* (2002) 44, 194–5.
3. Gupta SK, Dubé MP. Exogenous Cushing syndrome mimicking human immunodeficiency virus lipodystrophy. *Clin Infect Dis* (2002) 35, e69–e71.
4. Rouanet I, Peyrière H, Mauboussin JM, Vincent D. Cushing's syndrome in a patient treated by ritonavir/lopinavir and inhaled fluticasone. *HIV Med* (2003) 4, 149–50.
5. Hillebrand-Haverkort ME, Prummel MF, ten Veen JH. Ritonavir-induced Cushing's syndrome in a patient treated with nasal fluticasone. *AIDS* (1999) 13, 1803.
6. Betnesol tablets (Betamethasone sodium phosphate). Celltech Pharmaceuticals Ltd. UK Summary of product characteristics, March 2003.
7. Decadron tablets (Dexamethasone). Merck Sharpe & Dohme Ltd. UK Summary of product characteristics, October 2003.

Corticosteroids + Rifamycins

The effects of cortisone, dexamethasone, fludrocortisone, hydrocortisone, methylprednisolone, prednisone and prednisolone given systemically can be markedly reduced by rifampicin, but aldosterone appears not to be affected.

Clinical evidence

Seven patients with Addison's disease due to tuberculosis had no changes in the pharmacokinetics of infused **aldosterone** after being treated with rifampicin 600 mg daily for 6 days.[1]

A patient with Addison's disease stabilised on **cortisone** and **fludrocortisone** had typical signs of corticosteroid overdosage when the rifampicin he was taking was replaced by ethambutol.[2] Another Addisonian patient needed an increase in her dosage of **cortisone** from 37.5 to 50 mg daily, plus **fludrocortisone** 100 micrograms daily, when rifampicin 450 mg daily was started.[3] When rifampicin was added to **prednisolone** or **dexamethasone** and **fludrocortisone** it caused an Addisonian crisis in two patients.[4] A metabolic study in an Addisonian patient on **hydrocortisone** found that rifampicin shortened its half-life and reduced its AUC.[5] Rifampicin also markedly increases the clearance of **dexamethasone**.[6,7]

A child with nephrotic syndrome on **prednisolone**, accidentally given BCG vaccine, was treated with rifampicin and isoniazid to prevent possible dissemination of the vaccine. When the nephrotic condition did not respond, the **prednisolone** dosage was raised from 2 to 3 mg/kg daily without any evidence of corticosteroid overdosage. Later when the rifampicin and isoniazid were withdrawn, remission of the nephrotic condition was achieved with the original dosage of **prednisolone**.[8] A number of other reports describe a reduction in the response to **prednisone, prednisolone** or **methylprednisolone** in patients given rifampicin.[9-17] Pharmacokinetic studies in patients have shown that the AUC of **prednisolone** is reduced by about 60% by rifampicin, and the half-life is decreased by 40 to 60%.[11,15,18]

Mechanism

Rifampicin is a potent liver enzyme inducing agent which increases the metabolism of the corticosteroids by the liver,[10,19] thereby increasing their loss from the body and reducing their effects.

Importance and management

The interactions between the corticosteroids and rifampicin are established, well documented and clinically important. The need to increase the dosages of cortisone, dexamethasone, fludrocortisone, hydrocortisone, methylprednisolone, prednisolone and prednisone should be expected if rifampicin is given. It has been suggested that as an initial adjustment the dosage of prednisolone should be increased two to threefold, and reduced proportionately if the rifampicin is withdrawn.[10,11,18,20] The dosage increases needed for other corticosteroids await assessment. In the case of prednisolone the interaction develops maximally by 14 days and disappears about 14 days after withdrawal of the rifampicin.[21] There seems to be no direct information about other glucocorticoids but be alert for them to be similarly affected. It is not clear whether any of the topically applied corticosteroids will interact with rifampicin but it seems unlikely. The systemic corticosteroids are usually considered as contraindicated, or only to be used with great care, in patients with active or quiescent tuberculosis. Aldosterone does not appear to interact. There does not seem to be any information regarding the other rifamycins, **rifabutin** (a weak enzyme inducer) and **rifapentine** (a moderate enzyme inducer). However, the UK makers and the UK Committee on Safety of Medicines warn that rifabutin may possibly reduce the effects of a number of drugs, including corticosteroids.[22,23]

1. Schulte HM, Monig H, Benker G, Pagel H, Reinwein D, Ohnhaus EE. Pharmacokinetics of aldosterone in patients with Addison's disease: effect of rifampicin treatment on glucocorticoid and mineralocorticoid metabolism. *Clin Endocrinol (Oxf)* (1987) 27, 655–62.
2. Edwards OM, Courtenay-Evans RJ, Galley JM, Hunter J, Tait AD. Changes in cortisol metabolism following rifampicin therapy. *Lancet* (1974) ii, 549–51.
3. Maisey DN, Brown RC, Day JL. Rifampicin and cortisone replacement therapy. *Lancet* (1974) ii, 896–7.
4. Kyriazopoulou V, Parparousi O, Vagenakis AG. Rifampicin-induced adrenal crisis in Addisonian patients receiving corticosteroid replacement therapy. *J Clin Endocrinol Metab* (1984) 59, 1204–6.
5. Wang YH, Shi YF, Xiang HD. Effect of rifampin on the metabolism of glucocorticoids in Addison's disease. *Zhonghua Nei Ke Za Zhi* (1990) 29, 108–11,127.
6. Ediger SK, Isley WL. Rifampicin-induced adrenal insufficiency in the acquired immunodeficiency syndrome: difficulties in diagnosis and treatment. *Postgrad Med J* (1988) 64, 405–6.
7. Kawai SA. A comparative study of the accelerated metabolism of cortisol, prednisolone and dexamethasone in patients under rifampicin therapy. *Nippon Naibunpi Gakkai Zasshi* (1985) 61, 145–61.
8. Hendrickse W, McKiernan J, Pickup M, Lowe J. Rifampicin-induced non-responsiveness to corticosteroid treatment in nephrotic syndrome. *BMJ* (1979) i, 306.
9. van Marle W, Woods KL, Beeley L. Concurrent steroid and rifampicin therapy. *BMJ* (1979) i, 1020.
10. Buffington GA, Dominguez JH, Piering WF, Hebert LA, Kauffman HM, Lemann J. Interaction of rifampin and glucocorticoids. *JAMA* (1976) 236, 1958–60.
11. McAllister WAC, Thompson PJ, Al-Habet SM, Rogers HJ. Rifampicin reduces effectiveness and bioavailability of prednisolone. *BMJ* (1983) 286, 923–5.
12. Powell-Jackson PR, Gray BJ, Heaton RW, Costello JF, Williams R, English J. Adverse effect of rifampicin administration on steroid-dependent asthma. *Am Rev Respir Dis* (1983) 128, 307–10.
13. Bitaudeau Ph, Clément S, Chartier JPh, Papapietro PM, Bonnafoux A, Arnaud M, Trèves R, Desproges-Gotteron R. Interaction rifampicine-prednisolone. A propos de deux cas au cours d'une maladie de Horton. *Rev Rhum Mal Osteoartic* (1989) 56, 87–8.
14. Kawai S, Ichikawa Y. Drug interactions between glucocorticoids and other drugs. *Nippon Rinsho* (1994) 52, 773–8.
15. Carrie F, Roblot P, Bouquet S, Delon A, Roblot F, Becq-Giraudon B. Rifampin-induced nonresponsiveness of giant cell arteritis to prednisone treatment. *Arch Intern Med* (1994) 154, 1521–4.
16. Verma M, Singh T, Chhatwal J, Saini V, Pawar B. Rifampicin induced steroid unresponsiveness in nephrotic syndrome. *Indian Paediatr* (1994) 31, 1437.
17. Lin FL. Rifampin-induced deterioration in steroid-dependent asthma. *J Allergy Clin Immunol* (1996) 98, 1125.
18. Bergrem H, Refvem OK. Altered prednisolone pharmacokinetics in patients treated with rifampicin. *Acta Med Scand* (1983) 213, 339–43.
19. Sotaniemi EA, Medzihradsky F, Eliasson G. Glutaric acid as an indicator of use of enzyme-inducing drugs. *Clin Pharmacol Ther* (1974) 15, 417.
20. Löfdahl C-G, Mellstrand T, Svedmyr N, Wåhlén P. Increased metabolism of prednisolone and rifampicin after rifampicin treatment. *Am Rev Respir Dis* (1984) 129, A201.
21. Lee KH, Shin JG, Chong WS, Kim S, Lee JS, Jang IJ, Shin SG. Time course of the changes in prednisolone pharmacokinetics after co-administration or discontinuation of rifampicin. *Eur J Clin Pharmacol* (1993) 45, 287–89.
22. Mycobutin (Rifabutin). Pharmacia Ltd. UK Summary of product characteristics, January 2003.
23. Committee on the Safety of Medicines/Medicines Control Agency. Revised indication and drug interactions of rifabutin. *Current Problems* (1997) 23, 14.

Corticosteroids + Sucralfate

Sucralfate appears not to interact with prednisone.

Clinical evidence, mechanism, importance and management

Sucralfate 1 g every 6 hours had no effect on the pharmacokinetics of a single 20-mg dose of **prednisone** in 12 healthy subjects, except that the peak plasma levels were delayed by about 45 minutes when the drugs were given at the same time, but not when the sucralfate was given 2 hours after the **prednisone**.[1] No particular precautions are likely to be needed in patients given both drugs. Information about other corticosteroids is lacking.

1. Gambertoglio JG, Romac DR, Yong C-L, Birnbaum J, Lizak P, Amend WJ C. Lack of effect of sucralfate on prednisone bioavailability. *Am J Gastroenterol* (1987) 82, 42–5.

Corticosteroids + Vaccines; Live

Patients who are immunised with live vaccines while receiving immunosuppressive doses of corticosteroids may develop generalised, possibly life-threatening, infections.

Clinical evidence, mechanism, importance and management

The use of corticosteroids can reduce the number of circulating lymphocytes and suppress the normal immune response, so that concurrent immunisation with live vaccines can lead to generalised infection. It is suggested that **prednisone** in doses greater than 10 to 15 mg daily will suppress the immune response, whereas 40 to 60-mg doses on alternate days probably does not,[1] although this is debated.

A patient with lymphosarcoma and hypogammaglobulinaemia, taking **prednisone** 15 mg daily, developed a generalised vaccinial infection when she was given **smallpox vaccine**.[2] A fatal vaccinial infection developed following **smallpox vaccination** in another patient treated with **cortisone**.[3] This type of problem can be controlled with immunoglobulin to give cover against a general infection while immunity develops, and this has been successfully used in steroid-dependent patients needing **smallpox vaccination**.[4]

The principles applied to **smallpox** may be generally applicable to other live attenuated vaccines (e.g. **measles**, **mumps**, **rubella**, **poliomyelitis**, **BCG**), but no studies seem to have been done to establish what is safe.[1] It is generally accepted that patients on immunosuppressants are not given live vaccines. Problems with topical or inhaled steroids in normal dosages seem unlikely because the amounts absorbed are relatively small.[1] However, this needs confirmation. The British National Formulary states that live vaccination should be postponed for at least 3 months after stopping high-dose corticosteroids.[5]

See also 'Immunosuppressants + Vaccines', p.812.

1. Shapiro L. Questions and Answers. Live virus vaccine and corticosteroid therapy: Answered by Fauci AS, Bellanti JA, Polk IJ, Cherry JD. *JAMA* (1981) 246, 2075–6.
2. Rosenbaum EH, Cohen RA, Glatstein HR. Vaccination of a patient receiving immunosuppressive therapy for lymphosarcoma. *JAMA* (1966) 198, 737–40.
3. Olansky S, Smith JG, Hansen OCE. Fatal vaccinia associated with cortisone therapy. *JAMA* (1956) 162, 887–8.
4. Joseph MR. Vaccination of patients on steroid therapy. *Med J Aust* (1974) 2, 181.
5. British National Formulary. 49th ed. London: The British Medical Association and The Pharmaceutical Press; 2005. p. 597.

Corticosteroids + Zileuton

No clinically relevant pharmacokinetic interaction occurs between prednisone and zileuton.

Clinical evidence, mechanism, importance and management

In a randomised double-blind crossover study 16 healthy subjects were given zileuton 600 mg every 6 hours for a week, with either a 40-mg dose of **prednisone** or placebo on day 6. The pharmacokinetics of the both drugs were slightly altered but this was not considered to be clinically relevant. The **prednisone** half-life rose from 2.8 to 2.9 hours, while the zileuton AUC fell by 13% and the time to achieve maximum serum levels fell by 26%. It was concluded that concurrent use carries a minimal risk of a clinically important pharmacokinetic interaction.[1] No special precautions would appear to be needed.

1. Awni WM, Cavanaugh JH, Tzeng T-B, Witt G, Granneman GR, Dube LM. Pharmacokinetic interactions between zileuton and prednisone. *Clin Pharmacokinet* (1995) 29 (Suppl 2), 105–111.

Daclizumab + Miscellaneous

No adverse drug interactions appear to have been reported with daclizumab. Use with another antilymphocyte antibody in transplant patients on intensive immunosuppression may be a factor in fatal infection.

Clinical evidence, mechanism, importance and management

The makers of daclizumab say that because it is an immunoglobulin, no metabolic drug interactions (i.e. those mediated by inhibitory or inducing effects on cytochrome P450 enzymes) would be expected,[1,2] and none seems to have been reported. The makers say that daclizumab has been given in clinical trials with the following drugs without any adverse interactions: **aciclovir**, **azathioprine**, **antithymocyte immune globulin**, **ciclosporin**, **corticosteroids**, **ganciclovir**, **muromonab-CD3**, **mycophenolate** and **tacrolimus**.[1]

However, in one clinical trial in heart transplant patients on ciclosporin, **mycophenolate**, and corticosteroids, use of daclizumab with other antilymphocyte therapy (such as **muromonab-CD3** and **antithymocyte immunoglobulin**) appeared to be associated with a higher incidence of fatal infection: 8 of 40 patients died compared with 2 of 37 who received antilymphocyte therapy and placebo. The maker suggests that concurrent use of daclizumab with other antilymphocyte antibody therapy in patients on intensive immunosuppression may be a factor leading to fatal infection.[1,2] Caution may be warranted, and more study is needed.

1. Zenapax (Daclizumab). Roche Products Ltd. UK Summary of product characteristics, April 2004.
2. Zenapax (Daclizumab) Roche Pharmaceuticals. US Prescribing information, July 2003.

Everolimus + Ciclosporin

Ciclosporin increases the AUC of everolimus.

Clinical evidence

The possibility of a drug interaction was assessed by a crossover study in 24 healthy subjects who were given a single 2-mg dose of everolimus, alone and with single doses of a ciclosporin formulation, either *Neoral* (microemulsion) 175 mg or *Sandimmune* (corn oil suspension) 300 mg. *Neoral* increased the peak levels and AUC of everolimus by 82% and 168% respectively. *Sandimmune* did not affect the peak levels of everolimus but increased its AUC by 74%.[1]

Mechanism

Not fully understood. Both everolimus and ciclosporin are metabolised by the cytochrome P450 isoenzyme CYP3A4 and both are substrates of P-glycoprotein. Competition via one or both of these pathways in the liver or gut wall may contribute to the interaction.[1]

Importance and management

Information would seem limited to this single-dose study. However, it has been suggested if ciclosporin (either *Neoral* or *Sandimmune*) is removed from a everolimus-ciclosporin regimen, a two to threefold decrease in everolimus exposure could be expected. Monitoring is recommended.[1] Note that sirolimus (of which everolimus is a derivative) interacts similarly, see 'Sirolimus + Ciclosporin', p.817.

1. Kovarik JM, Kalbag J, Figueiredo J, Rouilly M, O'Bannon LF, Rordorf C. Differential influence of two cyclosporine formulations on everolimus pharmacokinetics: a clinically relevant pharmacokinetic interaction. *J Clin Pharmacol* (2002) 42, 95–9.

Immunosuppressants + Vaccines

The body's immune response is suppressed by immunosuppressants such as ciclosporin, mycophenolate, tacrolimus, and corticosteroids. The antibody response to vaccines may be reduced, although even partial protection may be of benefit. In general, the use of live attenuated vaccines is considered contraindicated because of the possible risk of generalised infection. See also, 'Corticosteroids + Vaccines; Live', p.811.

Clinical evidence

(a) Diptheria, tetanus, and inactivated polio vaccines

In organ transplant recipients on immunosuppressants, tetanus vaccines[1,2] and inactivated polio vaccines[1] produced protective antibody titres. The response to diphtheria vaccine was lower than in healthy controls[1] and the antibody titre had fallen below the protective level by 12 months in 38% of patients in one study,[1] and 24% in another.[2] Note that live polio vaccines are not recommended in immunosuppressed patients.

(b) Hepatitis vaccines

The antibody response to **hepatitis B vaccine** is generally poor in patients on immunosuppressants after organ transplantation,[3,4] although one research group reported a sustained antibody response in half of their patients,[5] and an overall 85% seroconversion rate was seen in one study in children (aged between 4 and 16-years-old).[6] In this latter study,[6] children on **ciclosporin** monotherapy had a higher seroconversion rate (100%) than those on **ciclosporin** and **corticosteroids** (84%) and those on **ciclosporin**, **azathioprine**, and **corticosteroids** (66%).

The antibody response to **hepatitis A vaccine** in patients on immunosuppressants after organ transplantation is variable,[7-9] and declines quicker than in healthy controls.[9] In renal transplant recipients, there is some evidence that the response is inversely related to the number of immunosuppressant drugs.[8]

(c) Influenza vaccine

A number of studies have been published on the efficacy of influenza vaccine in organ transplant recipients on immunosuppressants. Many have found a reduction in the proportion of patients developing a protective antibody titre compared with healthy control subjects,[10,11] whereas some have found no reduction.[12] A few studies have looked at the effects of individual drugs in the immunosuppressive regimen. In one comparative study in 59 kidney transplant patients, 21 patients on **ciclosporin** and **prednisone** had a significantly lower immune response to influenza vaccine (inactivated trivalent) than 38 patients on **azathioprine** and **prednisone** or 29 healthy subjects taking no drugs. All of the immune response measurements were reduced by 20 to 30% in those on **ciclosporin**.[13] In another study, 13 patients on **mycophenolate**, **ciclosporin**, and **prednisolone** had a marked reduction in antibody response to influenza vaccine when compared with 25 patients on **ciclosporin**, **azathioprine** and **prednisolone**.[14] In yet another study, patients receiving **ciclosporin** had lower antibody responses when compared with those receiving **tacrolimus**.[15] Patients on a higher dose of **prednisolone** per kg had a reduced antibody response to influenza vaccine in one study, and those on a daily dose had a reduced response compared with those on an alternate day schedule.[16]

Confirmation of the practical importance of the reduced antibody titre in some patients is described in a case report of a heart transplant patient on **ciclosporin** who did not respond to influenza vaccination while taking **ciclosporin** and **prednisone**. He had two episodes of influenza, one serologically confirmed and it was later shown that vaccination had not resulted in seroconversion.[17] Similarly, a patient on **tacrolimus** after a liver transplant developed influenza A myocarditis despite prophylactic vaccination.[18]

(d) Live vaccines

The use of live vaccines in patients on corticosteroids has caused generalised infection, see 'Corticosteroids + Vaccines; Live', p.811. Because of this risk, the use of live vaccines in patients on other immunosuppressants is not recommended, and there are few published reports. One study found that measles vaccine was effective in 7 of 18 children under 3 years old after liver transplantation, and that there were no complications directly attributable to the vaccine.[19]

(e) Pneumococcal vaccines

Good responses to pneumococcal vaccines in patients on immunosuppressant drugs after organ transplantation have been seen,[10,20] but protective antibody titres may not persist as long as in healthy subjects.[21]

Mechanism

Immunosuppression by these drugs diminishes the ability of the body to respond immunologically both to transplants and to vaccination.

Importance and management

Established and clinically important interactions. The proportion of patients developing protective antibody titres to vaccines is often reduced in patients on immunosuppressants. Nevertheless, for many vaccines, the reduced response seen is considered clinically useful, and, for example, in the case of renal transplant patients influenza vaccination is actively recommended.[22] If a vaccine is given, it may be prudent to monitor the response, so that alternative prophylactic measures can be considered where it is considered inadequate. For influenza vaccine, one suggestion is that if patients remain unprotected after a single vaccination and a booster dose, amantadine 200 mg daily should be given during an influenza epidemic. It will protect against influenza A but not B infection.[17] Note that, even where effective antibody titres are produced, these may not persist as long as in healthy subjects, and more frequent booster doses may be required.

There appears to be little published experience of the use of live vaccines in patients on non-steroidal immunosuppressants, and live vaccines should generally not be used in these patients.

The makers of **leflunomide** say that no clinical data are available on the efficacy of vaccines given to patients on leflunomide, and live vaccines are not recommended.[23,24]

1. Huzly D, Neifer S, Reinke P, Schröder K, Schönfeld C, Hofmann T, Bienzle U. Routine immunizations in adult renal transplant recipients. *Transplantation* (1997) 63, 839–45.
2. Enke BU, Bökenkamp A, Offner G, Bartmann P, Brodehl J. Response to diphtheria and tetanus booster vaccination in pediatric renal transplant recipients. *Transplantation* (1997) 64, 237–41.

3. Angelico M, Di Paolo D, Trinito MO, Petrolati A, Araco A, Zazza S, Lionetti R, Casciani CU, Tisone G. Failure of a reinforced triple course of hepatitis B vaccination in patients transplanted for HBV-related cirrhosis. *Hepatology* (2002) 35, 176–81.
4. Loinaz C, Ramón de Juanes J, Moreno Gonzalez E, López A, Lumbreras C, Gómez R, Gonzalez-Pinto I, Jiménez C, Garcia I, Fuertes A. Hepatitis B vaccination results in 140 liver transplant recipients. *Hepatogastroenterology* (1997) 44, 235–8.
5. Bienzle U, Günther M, Neuhaus R, Neuhaus P. Successful hepatitis B vaccination in patients who underwent transplantation for hepatitis B virus-related cirrhosis: preliminary results. *Liver Transpl* (2002) 8, 562–4.
6. Duca P, Del Pont JM, D'Agostino D. Successful immune response to a recombinant hepatitis B vaccine in children after liver transplantation. *J Pediatr Gastroenterol Nutr* (2001) 32, 168–70.
7. Arslan M, Wiesner RH, Poterucha JJ, Zein NN. Safety and efficacy of hepatitis A vaccination in liver transplantation recipients. *Transplantation* (2001) 72, 272–6.
8. Stark K, Günther M, Neuhaus R, Reinke P, Schröder K, Linnig S, Bienzle U. Immunogenicity and safety of hepatitis A vaccine in liver and renal transplant recipients. *J Infect Dis* (1999) 180, 2014–17.
9. Günther M, Stark K, Neuhaus R, Reinke P, Schröder K, Bienzle U. Rapid decline of antibodies after hepatitis A immunization in liver and renal transplant recipients. *Transplantation* (2001) 71, 477–90.
10. Dengler TJ, Strnad N, Buhring I, Zimmermann R, Girgsdies O, Kubler WE, Zielen S. Differential immune response to influenza and pneumococcal vaccination in immunosuppressed patients after heart transplantation. *Transplantation* (1998) 66, 1340–47.
11. Soesman NMR, Rimmelzwaan GF, Nieuwkoop NJ, Beyer WEP, Tilanus HW, Kemmeren MH, Metselaar HJ, de Man RA, Osterhaus ADME. Efficacy of influenza vaccination in adult liver transplant recipients. *J Med Virol* (2000) 61, 85–93.
12. Edvardsson VO, Flynn JT, Deforest A, Kaiser BA, Schulman SL, Bradley A, Palmer J, Polinsky MS, Baluarte HJ. Effective immunization against influenza in pediatric renal transplant recipients. *Clin Transplant* (1996) 10, 556–60.
13. Versluis DJ, Beyer WEP, Masurel N, Wenting GJ, Weimar W. Impairment of the immune response to influenza vaccination in renal transplant recipients by cyclosporine, but not azathioprine. *Transplantation* (1986) 42, 376–9.
14. Smith KGC, Isbel NM, Catton MG, Leydon JA, Becker GJ, Walker RG. Suppression of the humoral immune response by mycophenolate mofetil. *Nephrol Dial Transplant* (1998) 13, 160–4.
15. Mazzone PJ, Mossad SB, Mawhorter SD, Mehta AC, Schilz RJ, Maurer JR. The humoral immune response to influenza vaccination in lung transplant patients. *Eur Respir J* (2001) 18, 971–6.
16. Mack DR, Chartrand SA, Ruby EI, Antonson DL, Shaw BW, Heffron TG. Influenza vaccination following liver transplantation in children. *Liver Transpl Surg* (1996) 2, 431–7.
17. Beyer WEP, Diepersloot RJA, Masurel N, Simoons ML, Weimar W. Double failure of influenza vaccination in a heart transplant patient. *Transplantation* (1987) 43, 319.
18. Vilchez RA, Fung JJ, Kusne S, Influenza A myocarditis developing in an adult liver transplant recipient despite vaccination: a case report and review of the literature. *Transplantation* (2000) 70, 543–5.
19. Rand EB, McCarthy CA, Whitington PF. Measles vaccination after orthotopic liver transplantation. *J Pediatr* (1993) 123, 87–9.
20. Kazancioğlu R, Sever MŞ, Yüksel-Önel D, Eraksoy H, Yildiz A, Çelik AV, Kauacan SM, Badur S. Immunization of renal transplant recipients with pneumococcal polysaccharide vaccine. *Clin Transplant* (2000) 14, 61–5.
21. Linnemann CC, First MR, Schiffman G. Revaccination of renal transplant and hemodialysis recipients with pneumococcal vaccine. *Arch Intern Med* (1986) 146, 1554–6.
22. UK Department of Health. Adult Immunisation Update, 8 August 2003. Available at http://www.dh.gov.uk/assetRoot/04/02/99/70/04029970.pdf (accessed 11/07/05).
23. Arava (Leflunomide). Sanofi-Aventis. UK Summary of product characteristics, December 2004.
24. Arava (Leflunomide). Aventis Pharmaceuticals Inc. US Prescribing information, November 2004.

Leflunomide + Miscellaneous

The serum levels of the active metabolite of leflunomide are reduced by activated charcoal, and colestyramine. The makers advise against the concurrent use of alcohol because of the potential for hepatotoxicity. Methotrexate may also increase leflunomide hepatotoxicity, so in general the combination is not recommended, but if used increased monitoring is advised. The use of leflunomide with other DMARDs has not been studied, and is currently not advised. A case of fatal fulminant hepatic failure has been reported in a patient on leflunomide and itraconazole. The makers predict interactions between leflunomide and phenytoin or tolbutamide, and advise caution with rifampicin as it may increase leflunomide metabolite levels. No clinically relevant interaction occurs with cimetidine, corticosteroids or NSAIDs.

Clinical evidence, mechanism, importance and management

(a) Alcohol

The UK makers say that because of the potential for additive hepatotoxic effects, it is recommended that alcohol should be avoided while taking leflunomide.[1]

(b) Charcoal or Colestyramine

Studies in healthy subjects found that colestyramine 8 g three times daily reduced the serum levels of the active metabolite of leflunomide (A771726) by 48% after 24 hours and by 49 to 65% after 48 hours.[2]

Treatment with activated charcoal 50 g every 6 hours for 24 hours, either orally or by nasogastric tube, reduced A771726 levels by 37% after 24 hours and by 48% after 48 hours.[2]

These drugs are thought to bind with the A771726 in the gut, thereby interrupting the enterohepatic cycle or possibly its gastrointestinal dialysis.[1] Patients should therefore not be given either colestyramine or activated charcoal and leflunomide concurrently, unless the intention is to remove the leflunomide, for example following overdosage or when switching from leflunomide to another DMARD (see (e) and (f), below), or where there is any other good reason to clear leflunomide from the body more quickly.[1,2]

(c) Cimetidine

The makers say that no clinically significant interaction occurs between leflunomide and cimetidine.[1,2]

(d) Corticosteroids

The makers say that corticosteroids may continue to be used if leflunomide is given.[1,2]

(e) CYP2C9 substrates

The makers advise caution if leflunomide is given with **phenytoin** or **tolbutamide**.[1] The reason is that the active metabolite of leflunomide (A771726) has been shown by *in vitro* studies to be an inhibitor of the cytochrome P450 isoenzyme CYP2C9, which is concerned with the metabolism of these two drugs. If this inhibition were to occur *in vivo* it could possibly lead to a decrease in their metabolism and an increase in their toxicity. Although so far there appear to be no clinical reports of an interaction, the makers made a similar prediction with warfarin, another CYP2C9 substrate, which has been borne out in practice. See 'Anticoagulants + Leflunomide', p.289.

(f) DMARDs other than methotrexate

The makers say that the concurrent use of leflunomide and other DMARDs (they list **azathioprine, chloroquine**, **hydroxychloroquine**, intramuscular or oral **gold** and **penicillamine**) has not yet been studied but they say that combined use is currently not advisable because of the increased risk or serious adverse reactions (haemo- or hepatotoxicity). As the active metabolite of leflunomide has a long half life of 1 to 4 weeks the makers say that a washout of colestyramine or activated charcoal should be given if patients are to be started on other DMARDs.[1,2] See also (g) Methotrexate, below.

(g) Itraconazole

A 68-year-old woman who had been taking leflunomide 10 mg daily for about 4 months was started on itraconazole 300 mg daily for a fungal infection. About one month later her leflunomide dose was increased to 20 mg daily, and liver function tests were normal. The following month, she developed abdominal pain, vomiting and weakness. Despite symptomatic treatment and washout with colestyramine, fatal fulminant hepatic failure occurred. The authors of the report attribute the reaction to additive hepatotoxicity between the leflunomide and itraconazole.[3] This interaction serves to highlight the cautions about the use of other hepatotoxic agents, see (e) and (g).

(h) Methotrexate

No pharmacokinetic interaction was seen in patients while taking methotrexate (mean dose 17.2 mg per week) and leflunomide 100 mg daily for 2 days as a loading dose followed by 10 to 20 mg daily.[4] However, elevated liver enzyme levels have been seen following concurrent use.[1] By March 2001, the European Agency for the Evaluation of Medicinal Products was aware of 129 cases of serious hepatic reactions in patients on leflunomide, and 78% of these were in patients concurrently treated with hepatotoxic medications. In patients with elevated liver function tests, 58% were also being treated with methotrexate and/or NSAIDs.[5] Because of the possible risks of additive or synergistic liver toxicity or haematotoxicity, particularly when used long-term, the UK makers say that the concurrent use of methotrexate is not advisable.[1] The US makers say that if concurrent use is undertaken, chronic monitoring should be increased to monthly intervals.[2] Close liver enzyme monitoring is also recommended if switching between these drugs, and colestyramine or activated charcoal washout should be performed when switching from leflunomide to methotrexate.[1,2]

(i) NSAIDs

Leflunomide inhibits the activity of the cytochrome P450 isoenzyme CYP2C9 *in vitro* and might therefore be expected to increase the serum levels of NSAIDs that are metabolised by this isoenzyme (e.g. **diclofenac, ibuprofen**) but the makers say that no safety problems were seem in clinical trials with leflunomide and NSAIDs. No special precautions would seem to be needed if any of these or any other NSAID drugs are given concurrently.[1]

(j) Rifampicin

When a single dose of leflunomide was given to subjects after taking multiple dose rifampicin, the peak levels of the active metabolite of leflunomide (A771726) were increased by 40% but the AUC was unchanged.[1,2] The reasons are not understood. There would seem to be no reason for avoiding concurrent use, but the makers advise caution as A771721 levels may build up over time.[2] It may be prudent to increase the frequency of leflunomide monitoring if these two drugs are used together.

1. Arava (Leflunomide). Sanofi-Aventis. UK Summary of product characteristics, December 2004.
2. Arava (Leflunomide). Aventis Pharmaceuticals Inc. US Prescribing information, November 2004.
3. Legras A, Bergemer-Fouquet A-M, Jonville-Bera A-P. Fatal hepatitis with leflunomide and itraconazole. *Am J Med* (2002) 113, 352–3.
4. Weinblatt ME, Kremer JM, Coblyn JS, Maier AL, Helfgott SM, Morrell M, Byrne VM, Kaymakcian MV, Strand V. Pharmacokinetics, safety, and efficacy of combination treatment with methotrexate and leflunomide in patients with active rheumatoid arthritis. *Arthritis Rheum* (1999) 42, 1322–8.
5. EMEA. EMEA public statement on leflunomide (Arava) - severe and serious hepatic reactions. London, 12 March 2001. Available at: http://www.emea.eu.int/pdfs/human/press/pus/561101en.pdf (accessed 04/07/05).

Muromonab-CD3 + Indometacin

One report suggested that indometacin may possibly increase the incidence of encephalopathy and psychosis in patients treated with muromonab-CD3.

Clinical evidence, mechanism, importance and management

A study of patient records found that 4 out of a total of 55 kidney transplant patients (7.3%) given muromonab-CD3 and indometacin 50 mg orally or rectally every 6 to 8 hours for 48 to 72 hours developed serious encephalopathy and psychosis compared with only two out of 173 patients (1.2%) who had received muromonab-CD3 without indometacin.[1] This appears to be an isolated report, and its general significance is unknown. Indometacin has been used to reduce the adverse effects of muromonab-CD3, and in one analysis concurrent use was associated with reduced fever, headache, and gastrointestinal disturbances.[2] Muromonab-CD3 alone is associated with encephalopathy and other CNS adverse effects, and the maker warns that patients should be closely monitored for these effects.[3]

1. Chan GL, Weinstein SS, Wright CE, Bowers VD, Alveranga DY, Shires DL, Ackermann JR, LeFor WW, Kahana L. Encephalopathy associated with OKT3 administration. Possible interaction with indomethacin. *Transplantation* (1991) 52, 148–50.
2. Gaughan WJ, Francos BB, Dunn SR, Francos GC, Burke JF. A retrospective analysis of indomethacin on adverse reactions to orthoclone OKT3 in the therapy of acute renal allograft rejection. *Am J Kidney Dis* (1994) 24, 486–90.
3. Orthoclone OKT3 (muromonab-CD3). Ortho Biotech Products LP. US Prescribing information, November 2004.

Mycophenolate + Allopurinol

No clinically relevant interactions have been seen between mycophenolate mofetil and allopurinol.

Clinical evidence, mechanism, importance and management

A study in 5 kidney transplant patients with gouty arthritis, who were switched from azathioprine to mycophenolate mofetil 2 g daily (to avoid the risk of an azathioprine/allopurinol interaction), found that no adverse effects occurred when they were treated with allopurinol 100 or 200 mg daily. On average, 10 weeks after the switch had taken place, the uricaemia had dropped by 21%, mean serum creatinine levels were only slightly raised, by 12%, and white cell counts were unchanged.[1] Another study in 19 kidney transplant patients taking mycophenolate 2 g daily, ciclosporin and prednisolone also found a significant reduction in uricaemia without any adverse effects on white cell count, after 60 days treatment with allopurinol 100 mg daily.[2]

No special precautions would therefore seem necessary if allopurinol is used with mycophenolate, although the authors of both studies suggest that long-term randomised studies are needed to confirm safety.

1. Jacobs F, Mamzer-Bruneel MF, Skhiri H, Thervet E, Legendre Ch, Kreis H. Safety of the mycophenolate mofetil-allopurinol combination in kidney transplant recipients with gout. *Transplantation* (1997) 64, 1087–8.
2. Navascués RA, Gómez E, Rodriguez M, Laures AS, Baltar J, Grande JA. Safety of the allopurinol-mycophenolate mofetil combination in the treatment of hyperuricemia of kidney transplant patients. *Nephron* (2002) 91, 173–4.

Mycophenolate + Antacids

An aluminium/magnesium hydroxide antacid reduced the absorption of mycophenolate in one study, but the clinical relevance of this is uncertain.

Clinical evidence, mechanism, importance and management

When 10 ml of an **aluminium/magnesium hydroxide** antacid (*Maalox TC*) was given four times daily to 10 patients with rheumatoid arthritis, the AUC of a single 2-g dose of mycophenolate mofetil was reduced by 17% and the maximum serum concentration was reduced by 38%.[1] The clinical importance of this reduction has not been assessed, but the authors of the report suggest that since 80% of transplant patients receive antacids, in practice, this interaction is of no great significance. The US makers say that **aluminium/magnesium** antacids can be used in patients on mycophenolate, but that they should not be given simultaneously.[2] With many other (but not all) antacid interactions, a 2-hour separation is usually sufficient to avoid an interaction. It would seem prudent to check that the immunosuppressant effects of mycophenolate remain adequate in the presence of this or any other antacid.

1. Bullingham R, Shah J, Goldblum R, Schiff M. Effects of food and antacid on the pharmacokinetics of single doses of mycophenolate mofetil in rheumatoid arthritis patients. *Br J Clin Pharmacol* (1996) 41, 513–16.
2. CellCept (Mycophenolate mofetil). Roche Pharmaceuticals. US Prescribing information, October 2004.

Mycophenolate + Azathioprine

The makers have recommended that mycophenolate mofetil should not be given with azathioprine because they say that concurrent use has not been studied,[1,2] and both drugs have the potential to cause bone marrow suppression.[1]

1. CellCept (Mycophenolate mofetil). Roche Pharmaceuticals. US Prescribing information, October 2004.
2. CellCept (Mycophenolate mofetil). Roche Products Ltd. UK Summary of product characteristics, April 2005.

Mycophenolate + Ciclosporin

Ciclosporin may reduce levels of mycophenolic acid.

Clinical evidence, mechanism, importance and management

The addition of mycophenolate mofetil to ciclosporin has been found to reduce the incidence of rejection episodes in kidney transplant patients.[1] However, there are reports that trough levels of the active metabolite, mycophenolic acid, may be reduced in the presence of ciclosporin.[2] A study found that mycophenolic acid levels in transplant patients treated with mycophenolate mofetil, prednisone and ciclosporin were significantly lower than levels in patients receiving only mycophenolate mofetil and prednisone.[3]

In yet another study, 52 kidney transplant patients were treated with mycophenolate mofetil 1 g twice daily with ciclosporin and prednisone. Six months after transplantation 19 patients continued triple therapy, 19 discontinued ciclosporin and 14 discontinued prednisone. Three months later, patients in whom ciclosporin had been discontinued had higher trough mycophenolic acid levels compared to the other groups of patients. Discontinuing ciclosporin resulted in almost a doubling of mycophenolic acid trough levels.[4] Other studies note similar effects on mycophenolic acid levels in adult[5] and paediatric patients,[6] and the problems of interpreting the results of studies comparing ciclosporin or tacrolimus with mycophenolate are highlighted.[7-10] It was suggested that it could be interpreted that tacrolimus increases mycophenolic acid levels (see 'tacrolimus' (p.815)) when the correct interpretation may be that ciclosporin decreases mycophenolic acid exposure.[8]

It has also been observed that the use of the triple therapy, corticosteroids, and ciclosporin with mycophenolate mofetil rather than with azathioprine makes it possible to use a lower dose of ciclosporin.[11] The UK makers point out that as efficacy studies were conducted in patients using ciclosporin, mycophenolate and corticosteroids, the finding that ciclosporin reduces the mycophenolic acid AUC by 19 to 38% does not affect the recommended dose requirements.[12] However, other studies have noted that adjusting ciclosporin doses affects mycophenolic acid levels, and therefore the overall effect on immunosuppression needs careful monitoring.[6]

1. Sollinger HW. Mycophenolate mofetil for the prevention of acute rejection in primary care cadaveric renal allograft recipients. *Transplantation* (1995) 60, 225–32.
2. Weber SW, Keller F. Low mycophenolate predose levels with cyclosporine co-medication. *Kidney Blood Press Res* (1999) 22, 390.
3. Pou L, Brunet M, Cantarell C, Vidal E, Oppenheimer F, Monforte V, Vilardell J, Roman A, Martorell J, Capdevila L. Mycophenolic acid plasma concentrations: influence of co-medication. *Ther Drug Monit* (2001) 23, 35–8.
4. Gregoor PJ, de Sevaux RG, Hene RJ, Hesse CJ, Hilbrands LB, Vos P, van Gelder T, Hoitsma AJ, Weimar W. Effect of cyclosporine on mycophenolic acid trough levels in kidney transplant recipients. *Transplantation* (1999) 68, 1603–6.
5. Smak Gregoor PJ, Van Gelder T, Hesse CJ, van der Mast BJ, van Be NM, Weimar W. Mycophenolic acid plasma concentrations in kidney allograft recipients with or without cyclosporin: a cross-sectional study. *Nephrol Dial Transplant* (1999) 14, 706–8.
6. Filler G, Lepage N, Delisle B, Mai I. Effect of cyclosporine on mycophenolic acid area under the concentration-time curve in pediatric kidney transplant recipients. *Ther Drug Monit* (2001) 23, 514–19.
7. Hübner GI, Eismann R, Sziegoleit W. Drug interaction between mycophenolate mofetil and tacrolimus detectable within therapeutic mycophenolic acid monitoring in renal transplant patients. *Ther Drug Monit* (1999) 21, 536–9.
8. van Gelder T, Smak Gregoor PJH, Weimar W. Letter to the editor. *Ther Drug Monit* (2000) 22, 639.
9. Hübner GI, Sziegoleit W. Response to letter from van Gelder. *Ther Drug Monit* (2000) 22, 498–9.
10. Gerbase MW, Fathi M, Spiliopoulos A, Rochat T, Nicod LP. Pharmacokinetics of mycophenolic acid associated with calcineurin inhibitors: long-term monitoring in stable lung recipients with and without cystic fibrosis. *J Heart Lung Transplant* (2003) 22, 587–90.
11. Sanz Moreno C, Gomez Sanchez M, Fdez Fdez J, Botella J. Cyclosporine A (CsA) needs are reduced with substitution of azathioprine (Aza) by mycophenolate mofetil (MMF). *Nephrol Dial Transplant* (1998) 13, A260.
12. CellCept (Mycophenolate mofetil). Roche Products Ltd. UK Summary of product characteristics, April 2005.

Mycophenolate + Colestyramine

Colestyramine reduces the absorption of mycophenolate but the clinical relevance of this is uncertain.

Clinical evidence, mechanism, importance and management

Colestyramine 4 g three times daily for 4 days reduced the AUC of mycophenolic acid by 40% in a group of healthy subjects after they took a single 1.5-g oral dose of mycophenolate mofetil.[1] The UK makers advise caution,[1] while the US makers say that this combination is not recommended.[2] Separating the administration of colestyramine and mycophenolate is not likely to eliminate this interaction, as colestyramine affects the enterohepatic recirculation of mycophenolate.[2]

The clinical importance of the reduction in mycophenolic acid levels has not been assessed but, if the combination is given, it would seem prudent to confirm that the immunosuppressant effects of mycophenolate remain adequate in the presence of colestyramine.

1. CellCept (Mycophenolate mofetil). Roche Products Ltd. UK Summary of product characteristics, April 2005.
2. CellCept (Mycophenolate mofetil). Roche Pharmaceuticals. US Prescribing information, October 2004.

Mycophenolate + Iron compounds

Oral iron preparations may significantly reduce the absorption of mycophenolate.

Clinical evidence, mechanism, importance and management

A study in 7 healthy subjects found that a single dose of **ferrous sulfate** 1050 mg (210 mg of elemental iron) reduced the AUC and maximum levels of mycophenolate mofetil by more than 90%. It is possible that a chelation complex is formed between mycophenolate mofetil and iron, which reduces absorption. The authors suggest that simultaneous administration of mycophenolate mofetil and iron compounds should be avoided.[1] In other iron-chelation interactions separating administration by 2 to 3 hours has proved effective, but this needs confirmation with mycophenolate.

1. Morii M, Ueno K, Ogawa A, Kato R, Yoshimura H, Wada K, Hashimoto H, Takeda M, Tanaka K, Nakatani T, Shibakawa M. Impairment of mycophenolate mofetil absorption by iron ion. *Clin Pharmacol Ther* (2000) 68, 613–16.

Mycophenolate + Methotrexate

No clinically relevant interactions have so far been seen between mycophenolate and methotrexate.

Clinical evidence, mechanism, importance and management

A study in patients with rheumatoid arthritis found that the combination of methotrexate and mycophenolate mofetil was well-tolerated and there were no pharmacokinetic interactions.[1] There would appear to be no need for dose adjustments if both drugs are given for rheumatoid arthritis.

1. Yocum D, Kremer J, Blackburn W, Caldwell J, Furst D, Nunez M, Zuzga J, Zeig S, Gutierrez M, Merrill J, Dumont E, B Leishman. Cellcept® (mycophenolate mofetil - MMF) and methotrexate (MTX) safety and pharmacokinetic (PK) interaction study in rheumatoid arthritis patients. *Arthritis Rheum* (1999) 42 (9 Suppl), S83.

Mycophenolate + Sevelamer

Sevelamer moderately reduces mycophenolate levels.

Clinical evidence, mechanism, importance and management

The pharmacokinetics of mycophenolate were assessed in 6 renal transplant patients taking mycophenolate and ciclosporin after they also took sevelamer either as a single 1.6- or 1.2-mg dose or following 4 days of treatment (same dose given three times daily).[1] Four of the patients were children with an average age of 15 years. The AUC of mycophenolate was reduced by 25% by sevelamer.[1]

The clinical significance of this interaction is unclear, but it would seem prudent to monitor mycophenolate levels in any patient given sevelamer.

1. Pieper A-K, Buhle F, Mai I, Budde K, Neumayer HH, Haffner D, Querfeld U. Effect of sevelamer on pharmacokinetics of cyclosporin A and mycophenolate-mofetil in patients following renal transplantation. *J Am Soc Nephrol* (2002) 13, 562A.

Mycophenolate + St John's wort *(Hypericum perforatum)*

St John's wort does not appear to alter the pharmacokinetics of mycophenolate.

Clinical evidence, mechanism, importance and management

In a pharmacokinetic study, 8 stable renal transplant patients on mycophenolate and tacrolimus were given 600 mg of St John's wort extract (*Jarsin 300*) daily for 14 days. The study intended to make dose adjustments to keep the trough mycophenolic acid levels within the desired range, but dosage adjustment was not found to be necessary in any of the 8 patients.[1]

1. Mai I, Störmer E, Bauer S, Krüger H, Budde K, Roots I. Impact of St John's wort treatment on the pharmacokinetics of tacrolimus and mycophenolic acid in renal transplant patients. *Nephrol Dial Transplant* (2003) 18, 819–22.

Mycophenolate + Tacrolimus

Tacrolimus appears to increase mycophenolic acid levels, but the clinical significance of this is unclear.

Clinical evidence, mechanism, importance and management

A study in stable kidney transplant patients on long-term tacrolimus found that the addition of mycophenolate mofetil to their therapy resulted in a increase in the tacrolimus AUC, but this was not considered significant.[1] A 20% increase in tacrolimus levels is reported in a similar study in liver transplant patients.[2] The makers report that in one study in renal transplant patients receiving ciclosporin and mycophenolate mofetil, the AUC of mycophenolic acid was increased by about 30% when ciclosporin was replaced by tacrolimus.[2] Similar results are reported elsewhere,[3-5] but this may be due to a reduction in mycophenolic acid levels by ciclosporin rather than an increase in levels due to tacrolimus (see 'ciclosporin' (p.814)). It is also possible that the increased levels are a factor of increased enterohepatic recirculation of mycophenolic acid.[2]

1. Pirsch J, Bekersky I, Vincenti F, Boswell G, Woodle ES, Alak A, Kruelle M, Fass N, Facklam D, Mekki Q. Coadministration of tacrolimus and mycophenolate mofetil in stable kidney transplant patients: pharmacokinetics and tolerability. *J Clin Pharmacol* (2000) 40, 527–32.
2. CellCept (Mycophenolate mofetil). Roche Products Ltd. UK Summary of product characteristics, April 2005.
3. Hübner GI, Eismann R, Sziegoleit W. Drug interaction between mycophenolate mofetil and tacrolimus detectable within therapeutic mycophenolic acid monitoring in renal transplant patients. *Ther Drug Monit* (1999) 21, 536–9.
4. Vidal E, Cantarell C, Capdevila L, Monforte V, Roman A, Pou L. Mycophenolate mofetil pharmacokinetics in transplant patients receiving cyclosporine or tacrolimus in combination therapy. *Pharmacol Toxicol* (2000) 87, 182–4.
5. Hübner GI, Eismann R, Sziegoleit W. Drug interaction between mycophenolate mofetil and tacrolimus detectable within therapeutic mycophenolic acid monitoring in renal transplant patients. *Ther Drug Monit* (1999) 21, 536–9.

Mycophenolate + Voriconazole

Voriconazole had no effect the pharmacokinetics of a single 1-g dose of mycophenolate.[1]

1. Wood N, Abel , Fielding A, Nichols DJ, Bygrave E. Voriconazole does not affect the pharmacokinetics of mycophenolic acid. *Intersci Conf Antimicrob Agents Chemother* (2001) 41, 3.

Sirolimus + Azoles

Sirolimus levels are markedly raised by ketoconazole, and voriconazole and itraconazole appear to interact similarly. A case report suggests that fluconazole also raises sirolimus levels.

Clinical evidence

(a) Fluconazole

A patient taking sirolimus after a kidney transplant was given fluconazole 200 mg daily for oesophageal candidiasis. Because an interaction was anticipated, the sirolimus dosage was reduced from 4 to 3 mg daily. After 4 days the sirolimus level had risen from about 10 micrograms/l to 22.8 micrograms/l. The dose of sirolimus was then reduced to 2 mg daily, but by the seventh day of fluconazole treatment the sirolimus had reached 35 micrograms/l, after which they began to fall. However, the patient then had a hyperkalaemic arrest and died.[1] The sirolimus levels of another kidney transplant patient were raised almost fivefold about 3 weeks after she started to take fluconazole.[2]

(b) Itraconazole

A heart transplant patient needed only half of his normal sirolimus dose to maintain about the same trough levels when he took itraconazole 400 mg daily for a year.[2]

(c) Ketoconazole

A clinical study in 23 healthy subjects found that while taking ketoconazole 200 mg daily for 10 days, the maximum serum levels AUC following a single 5-mg dose of sirolimus were increased 4.3-fold and 10.9-fold respectively.[3]

(d) Voriconazole

Voriconazole 400 mg twice daily for 1 day, then 200 mg twice daily for 8 days markedly raised the maximum serum levels and AUC of a single 2-mg dose of sirolimus by about 5.5-fold and 10-fold respectively.[4,5] A case report describes a patient with a heart transplant who was given two doses of voriconazole 400 mg then 200 mg twice daily for 16 days. When sirolimus was started a dose of 1 mg gave a sirolimus trough level of 12.8 nanograms/ml, but after the voriconazole was stopped a dose of 3 mg only gave trough sirolimus levels of 7.4 nanograms/ml.[2] Voriconazole has been seen to markedly raise sirolimus levels in a number of other patients.[2,6]

Mechanism

Ketoconazole, itraconazole and voriconazole are potent inhibitors of the cytochrome P450 isoenzyme CYP3A4, the isoenzyme that is at least partly responsible for the metabolism of sirolimus.[7] Therefore these azoles probably causes raised sirolimus levels by inhibiting its metabolism. Fluconazole also inhibits CYP3A4, but is less potent than ketoconazole. Hence sirolimus levels rise when fluconazole is given, but the rise is not as great as that seen with ketoconazole.

Importance and management

The rises in sirolimus levels caused by voriconazole are said to be too large to be easily accommodated by reducing the dosage of the sirolimus and therefore the makers contraindicate concurrent use.[4,5]

The makers of sirolimus say that concurrent use of strong inhibitors of CYP3A4, including ketoconazole, voriconazole and itraconazole is not recommended,[7,8] but note that any patient given these drugs should have their trough sirolimus levels closely monitored both during use and after they are stopped.[7] **Clotrimazole** is predicted to interact similarly.[7,8] Fluconazole, although a weaker inhibitor of CYP3A4 than ketoconazole, voriconazole or itraconazole, has been reported to interact in two cases. Sirolimus plasma levels should be monitored during treatment with and following the withdrawal of any of these antifungals.[7]

1. Cervelli MJ. Fluconazole-sirolimus drug interaction. *Transplantation* (2002) 74, 1477–8.
2. Sádaba B, Campanero MA, Quetglas EG, Azanza JR. Clinical relevance of sirolimus drug interactions in transplant patients. *Transplant Proc* (2004) 36, 3226–8.
3. Floren LC, Christians U, Zimmerman JJ, Neefe L, Schorer R, Rushowrth D, Harper D, Renz J, Benet LZ. Sirolimus oral bioavailability increases ten-fold with concomitant ketoconazole. *Clin Pharmacol Ther* (1999) 65, 159.
4. VFEND (Voriconazole). Pfizer Ltd. UK Summary of product characteristics, March 2005.
5. VFEND (Voriconazole). Pfizer Inc. US Prescribing information, March 2005.
6. Mathis AS, Shah NK, Friedman GS. Combined use of sirolimus and voriconazole in renal transplantation: a report of two cases. *Transplant Proc* (2004) 36, 2708–9.
7. Rapamune (Sirolimus). Wyeth Pharmaceuticals. UK Summary of product characteristics, September 2004.
8. Rapamune (Sirolimus). Wyeth Laboratories. US Prescribing information, March 2005.

Sirolimus + Calcium channel blockers

Diltiazem raises sirolimus levels, and dosage adjustments may be necessary. Nicardipine and verapamil are predicted to interact similarly. Nifedipine appears not to interact with sirolimus.

Clinical evidence, mechanism, importance and management

An open, three-period, randomised, crossover study in 18 healthy subjects found that a single 120-mg oral dose of **diltiazem** affected the pharmacokinetics of a single 10-mg oral dose of sirolimus. The maximum serum levels of the sirolimus increased by 43% and its AUC increased by 60%. The pharmacokinetics of the **diltiazem** and its metabolites were unchanged. The likely reason for this interaction is that **diltiazem** inhibits the cytochrome P450 isoenzyme CYP3A4 in the intestinal wall and liver, which primarily metabolises sirolimus. **Diltiazem** may also inhibit P-glycoprotein activity, which leads to increased sirolimus absorption.[1]

This was a single-dose study, but all the evidence suggests that this interaction will also occur with multiple doses of both drugs, for which reason the makers recommend whole blood monitoring and possible sirolimus dosage reduction (based on sirolimus levels) if **diltiazem** is used concurrently.[2,3] When sirolimus oral solution 2 g daily and **verapamil** 180 mg every 12 hours were given together to 26 healthy subjects, the sirolimus maximum levels, and AUC were increased 2.3-fold, and 2.2-fold, respectively, while the maximum levels and AUC of ***(S)*-verapamil** were both increased 1.5-fold.[2,3] The maker notes that other calcium channel blockers that inhibit CYP3A4 might interact similarly, and they specifically name **nicardipine**.[2,3]

However, **nifedipine** is said not to interact,[2,3] and a study comparing 16 patients on **nifedipine** and sirolimus with 10 patients on sirolimus alone found no significant differences in sirolimus pharmacokinetics between the two groups.[4]

1. Böttinger Y, Säwe J, Brattström C, Tollemar J, Burke JT, Häss G, Zimmerman JJ. Pharmacokinetic interaction between single oral doses of diltiazem and sirolimus in healthy volunteers. *Clin Pharmacol Ther* (2001) 69, 32–40.
2. Rapamune (Sirolimus). Wyeth Laboratories. US Prescribing information, March 2005.
3. Rapamune (Sirolimus). Wyeth Pharmaceuticals. UK Summary of product characteristics, September 2004.
4. Zimmerman JJ, Kahan BD. Pharmacokinetics of sirolimus in stable renal transplant patients after multiple oral dose administration. *J Clin Pharmacol* (1997) 37, 405–15.

Sirolimus + Ciclosporin

Ciclosporin raises sirolimus serum levels, and this can be reduced by giving the drugs at least 4 hours apart. Concurrent use for longer than 3 months possibly increases renal toxicity, and should be used with caution only in those for whom the risk/benefit ratio is considered favourable. Sirolimus does not alter ciclosporin levels.

Clinical evidence

(a) Effects on ciclosporin

A double-blind randomised study found that when sirolimus was added to a ciclosporin/corticosteroid regimen in kidney transplant patients, the steady-state ciclosporin levels remained unchanged. No differences were seen in blood pressures, glomerular filtration rates, creatinine levels, triglyceride levels or liver enzymes (ALT, AST).[1] A 2-week pharmacokinetic study in 40 kidney transplant patients found that sirolimus 0.5 to 6.5 mg/m^2 given twice daily did not affect the pharmacokinetics of ciclosporin 75 to 400 mg twice daily. The patients were also taking prednisone.[2] Two related studies in kidney transplant patients confirmed the absence of an effect of sirolimus on ciclosporin pharmacokinetics.[3] Similarly, in another study, single-doses of sirolimus did not affect the pharmacokinetics of a single-doses of ciclosporin (microemulsion formulation, *Neoral*) in healthy subjects when given at the same time or 4 hours apart.[4]

(b) Effects on sirolimus

In a single-dose study in healthy subjects, ciclosporin (microemulsion formulation, *Neoral*) given 4 hours before sirolimus increased the maximum serum levels of the sirolimus 1.4-fold and the AUC 1.8-fold. When the drugs were given at the same time, the effect was even greater, with a 2.2-fold increase in maximum sirolimus level and 3.3-fold increase in AUC.[4] This study confirmed the findings of a previous multiple-dose study in kidney transplant recipients.[5] The US maker of sirolimus also presents data showing that ciclosporin (standard formulation, *Sandimmune*) given at the same time as sirolimus increased sirolimus trough levels by 67% to 86% in patients with psoriasis.[6]

Mechanism

It appears that ciclosporin inhibits the metabolism of sirolimus in the gut and liver leading to increased absorption.[4,7]

Importance and management

An established interaction. The makers recommend that sirolimus should be given 4 hours after microemulsion ciclosporin.[6,7] Despite this, it may still be necessary to reduce the sirolimus dose.[4] Moreover, the maker notes that, in patients taking sirolimus and ciclosporin for more than 3 months, higher serum creatinine levels and lower glomerular filtration rates have been seen. Until further clinical data are available, the maker does not recommend continued usage of the combination as maintenance therapy beyond 2 to 4 months,[6,7] except in patients at high risk of rejection.[6] Renal function should be closely monitored, and if serum creatinine levels increase, discontinuation of sirolimus or ciclosporin should be considered.[6] The makers say that if ciclosporin is withdrawn, the sirolimus dosage will need to be raised fourfold to take into account the absence of the interaction (twofold increase needed) and the need for increased immunosuppression (twofold increase needed). A target trough sirolimus level of 12 to 20 nanograms/ml (chromatographic assay) is recommended.[7]

1. Murgia MG, Jordan S, Kahan BD. The side effect profile of sirolimus: a phase I study in quiescent cyclosporine-prednisone-treated renal transplant patients. *Kidney Int* (1996) 49, 209–16.
2. Zimmerman JJ, Kahan BD. Pharmacokinetics of sirolimus in stable renal transplant patients after multiple oral dose administration. *J Clin Pharmacol* (1997) 37, 405–15.
3. Ferron GM, Mishina EV, Zimmerman JJ, Jusko WJ. Population pharmacokinetics of sirolimus in kidney transplant patients. *Clin Pharmacol Ther* (1997) 61, 416–28.
4. Zimmerman JJ, Harper D, Getsy J, Jusko WJ. Pharmacokinetic interactions between sirolimus and microemulsion cyclosporine when orally administered jointly and 4 hours apart in healthy volunteers. *J Clin Pharmacol* (2003) 42, 1168–76.
5. Kaplan B, Meier-Kriesche H-U, Napoli KL, Kahan BD. The effects of relative timing of sirolimus and cyclosporine microemulsion formulation coadministration on the pharmacokinetics of each agent. *Clin Pharmacol Ther* (1998) 63, 48–53.
6. Rapamune (Sirolimus). Wyeth Laboratories. US Prescribing information, March 2005.
7. Rapamune (Sirolimus). Wyeth Pharmaceuticals. UK Summary of product characteristics, September 2004.

Sirolimus + Corticosteroids

Intravenous methylprednisolone had no effect on trough sirolimus levels. Sirolimus slightly increased prednisolone levels derived from prednisone, but this is probably not clinically relevant.

Clinical evidence, mechanism, importance and management

(a) Methylprednisolone

Methylprednisolone was given as a daily intravenous bolus for 1 to 5 days (total dose of between 500 mg and 3 g) to 14 patients stabilised on sirolimus (and also taking either azathioprine or mycophenolate). Sirolimus trough concentrations were not significantly altered by the methylprednisolone.[1]

No additional precautions seem necessary on concurrent use.[1]

(b) Prednisolone or Prednisone

Only minor to moderate changes occurred in the pharmacokinetics of prednisolone in a study in kidney transplant patients on ciclosporin and prednisone 5 to 20 mg daily when sirolimus 6 to 13 mg/m^2 daily was also given, for 2 weeks.[2] The maximum serum prednisolone levels were raised by 14%, and the AUC was raised by 18%.

The clinical relevance of these findings is uncertain, but they are likely to be minor.

1. Bäckman L, Kreis H, Morales JM, Wilczek H, Taylor R, Burke JT. Sirolimus steady-state trough concentrations are not affected by bolus methylprednisolone therapy in renal allograft recipients. *Br J Clin Pharmacol* (2002) 54, 65–8.
2. Jusko WJ, Ferron GM, SM Mis, Kahan BD, Zimmerman JJ. Pharmacokinetics of prednisolone during administration of sirolimus in patients with renal transplants. *J Clin Pharmacol* (1996) 36, 1100–6.

Sirolimus + CYP3A4 enzyme inducers

Drugs that induce the cytochrome P450 isoenzyme CYP3A4 are predicted to lower sirolimus levels. Monitoring is recommended.

Clinical evidence, mechanism, importance and management

The makers point out that sirolimus is extensively metabolised by the cytochrome P450 isoenzyme CYP3A4 in the intestinal wall and by the multidrug efflux pump P-glycoprotein, so drugs that induce their activity are predicted to lower sirolimus levels.[1,2]

'Rifampicin', (p.818), and 'phenytoin', (p.818) are known potent enzyme inducers, have been seen to lower sirolimus levels, and the makers predict that **carbamazepine**, **phenobarbital**, and **St John's wort** will interact similarly.[1,2] These predictions are as yet unconfirmed, but it would certainly be prudent to monitor sirolimus levels closely if any of these drugs are used concurrently. In the case of **St John's wort**, it may be best to avoid the combination altogether. What should be remembered is that the extent of the inducing effects of these drugs is not identical, so that very marked effects like those observed with rifampicin may not occur, nevertheless the interaction may still be clinically important.

1. Rapamune (Sirolimus). Wyeth Laboratories. US Prescribing information, March 2005.
2. Rapamune (Sirolimus). Wyeth Pharmaceuticals. UK Summary of product characteristics, September 2004.

Sirolimus + CYP3A4 enzyme inhibitors

Drugs that inhibit the cytochrome P450 isoenzyme CYP3A4 are predicted to raise sirolimus levels. Monitoring is recommended.

Clinical evidence, mechanism, importance and management

The makers point out that sirolimus is extensively metabolised by cytochrome P450 isoenzyme CYP3A4 in the intestinal wall and by the multidrug efflux pump P-glycoprotein, so drugs that inhibit their activity may raise sirolimus levels.[1,2]

'Ketoconazole, voriconazole', (p.816), 'diltiazem, verapamil', (p.816) and 'erythromycin', (p.818) have been shown to raise sirolimus levels, and the makers name a number of others that also inhibit CYP3A4, which they predict will interact similarly. They list **bromocriptine**, **cimetidine**,

danazol, the **protease inhibitors** and **telithromycin**.[1,2]

These predictions are as yet unconfirmed, but it would certainly be prudent to monitor sirolimus levels closely if any of these drugs are used concurrently. What should be remembered is that the extent of the inhibitory effects of these drugs is not identical, so that very marked effects like those observed with ketoconazole may not occur, nevertheless the interaction may still be clinically important. **Grapefruit juice** inhibits CYP3A4 (potentially raising sirolimus levels), and in this case the makers recommendation is that it should be avoided.[1,2]

1. Rapamune (Sirolimus). Wyeth Laboratories. US Prescribing information, March 2005.
2. Rapamune (Sirolimus). Wyeth Pharmaceuticals. UK Summary of product characteristics, September 2004.

Sirolimus + Macrolides

Two patients had large elevations in their sirolimus levels following the addition of erythromycin. The makers predict that other macrolides will interact similarly.

Clinical evidence, mechanism, importance and management

A case report describes 2 patients on sirolimus who were also given **erythromycin** 1 g three times daily for suspected Legionella pneumonia. Despite reductions in the sirolimus dosage, both patients' sirolimus levels rose fivefold.[1]

Erythromycin is an inhibitor of the cytochrome P450 isoenzyme CYP3A4, which is the main enzyme responsible for the metabolism of sirolimus. Therefore **erythromycin** probably inhibited the metabolism of sirolimus, causing the levels to rise.

This interaction is in line with the maker's prediction. They also predict that other macrolides that inhibit the cytochrome P450 isoenzyme CYP3A4 (they name **clarithromycin** and **troleandomycin**) will interact similarly.[2,3]

1. Claesson K, Brattström C, Burke JT. Sirolimus and erythromycin interaction: two cases. *Transplant Proc* (2001) 33, 2136.
2. Rapamune (Sirolimus). Wyeth Pharmaceuticals. UK Summary of product characteristics, September 2004.
3. Rapamune (Sirolimus). Wyeth Laboratories. US Prescribing information, March 2005.

Sirolimus + Phenytoin

Two case reports describe increased sirolimus dose requirements in the presence of phenytoin. This is line with the makers prediction.

Clinical evidence, mechanism, importance and management

An 11-year-old girl with a kidney transplant taking phenytoin was started on sirolimus 30 micrograms/kg twice daily following an episode of acute rejection. The dose of sirolimus was increased tenfold over the next few weeks in an attempt to achieve the target trough level of 10 to 20 nanograms/ml, and two further episodes of acute rejection occurred. About a month after the sirolimus had been started, tacrolimus was added, and her phenytoin was stopped. Over the next few weeks her sirolimus level rose to about 40 nanograms/ml. The patient subsequently recovered.[1]

A 62-year-old woman was started on phenytoin 100 mg twice daily because she developed a seizure disorder following a liver transplant. At this time she was taking ciclosporin, but it was decided to start her on sirolimus because of neurological complications. The initial dose of 5 mg daily produced subtherapeutic sirolimus levels. She was subsequently stabilised on sirolimus 15 mg daily, with trough concentrations of less than 5 nanograms/ml. Phenytoin was stopped, and about 5 days later her trough sirolimus level was found to be around 15 to 20 nanograms/ml. After a further 5 days, the sirolimus dose was reduced to 10 mg daily. The authors of this report suggest that the initial high sirolimus dose was necessary as phenytoin, a potent inducer of the cytochrome P450 isoenzyme CYP3A4 increased the metabolism of sirolimus, which is mainly metabolised by CYP3A4. When the phenytoin was withdrawn the CYP3A4 metabolism of sirolimus returned to normal, leading to high sirolimus levels.[2]

These appear to be the only reports of this interaction, but it is in line with the maker's prediction.[3,4] It would therefore seem prudent to monitor sirolimus levels in any patient in whom phenytoin is started or withdrawn, and to adjust the dose as necessary.

1. Hodges CB, Maxwell H, Beattie TJ, Murphy AV, Jindal RM. Use of rapamycin in a transplant patient who developed ciclosporin neurotoxicity. *Pediatr Nephrol* (2001) 16, 777–8.
2. Fridell JA, Jain AKB, Patel K, Virji M, Rao KN, Fung JJ, Venkataramanan R. Phenytoin decreases the blood concentrations of sirolimus in a liver transplant recipient: a case report. *Ther Drug Monit* (2003) 25, 117–19.
3. Rapamune (Sirolimus). Wyeth Pharmaceuticals. UK Summary of product characteristics, September 2004.
4. Rapamune (Sirolimus). Wyeth Laboratories. US Prescribing information, March 2005.

Sirolimus + Rifamycins

Rifampicin (rifampin) greatly decreases sirolimus levels. Rifabutin and rifapentine are predicted to interact similarly.

Clinical evidence, mechanism, importance and management

A clinical study found that while taking multiple doses of **rifampicin** (**rifampin**), the clearance of a single 10-mg oral dose of sirolimus was increased 5.5-fold, while the AUC and the maximum serum levels were reduced by 82% and 71% respectively. The reason is that **rifampicin** is a potent inducer of cytochrome P450 isoenzyme CYP3A4, the isoenzyme by which sirolimus is metabolised.[1,2]

The makers say that concurrent use is not recommended, but if the decision is made to use both drugs they suggest that the maintenance dose of sirolimus should initially be increased eightfold, followed by trough sampling within 5 to 7 days. When the **rifampicin** is withdrawn, the sirolimus dose should be gradually reduced to the original maintenance dose.[1]

Rifabutin and **rifapentine** are predicted to also lower sirolimus levels,[1,2] but not to the same extent as **rifampicin**. However, it would still be prudent to monitor sirolimus levels closely during concurrent use.

1. Rapamune (Sirolimus). Wyeth Pharmaceuticals. UK Summary of product characteristics, September 2004.
2. Rapamune (Sirolimus). Wyeth Laboratories. US Prescribing information, March 2005.

Tacrolimus + Antacids

There is some *in vivo* and *in vitro* evidence that some antacids may possibly reduce the serum levels of tacrolimus, but the clinical importance of this awaits confirmation.

Clinical evidence, mechanism, importance and management

A very brief report states that widely variable trough plasma tacrolimus levels have been seen in patients taking **sodium bicarbonate** close to the time when the tacrolimus was given, and that the use of **sodium bicarbonate** results in lower blood concentrations of tacrolimus. No details were given.[1] The advice is that if their administration is separated by at least 2 hours, or the **sodium bicarbonate** is replaced by **sodium citrate** or **citric acid**, then stable trough serum tacrolimus levels are achieved.[1] The same 2-hour separation has also been recommended[1] for **aluminium hydroxide gel** and **magnesium oxide** because *in vitro* studies have shown that they can cause a significant reduction in tacrolimus concentrations due to pH-mediated degradation.[2]

Study is needed to confirm and assess the extent and clinical importance of these interactions, but good monitoring would be appropriate if tacrolimus is given with any antacids, being alert for the need to separate the dosages as recommended.

1. Venkataramanan R, Swaminathan A, Prasad T, Jain A, Zuckerman S, Warty V, McMichael J, Lever J, Burckart G, Starzl T. Clinical pharmacokinetics of tacrolimus. *Clin Pharmacokinet* (1995) 29, 404–30.
2. Steeves M, Abdallah HY, Venkataramanan R, Burckart GT, Ptachcinski RJ, Abu-Elmagd K, Jain AK, Fung F, Todo S, Starzl TE. In-vitro interaction of a novel immunosuppressant, FK506, and antacids. *J Pharm Pharmacol* (1991) 43, 574–7.

Tacrolimus + Antidepressants

Marked increases in tacrolimus levels and toxicity were observed in three patients when given nefazodone. Paroxetine and sertraline may not interact, but the situation is not clear.

Clinical evidence

A kidney transplant patient taking tacrolimus 5 mg daily developed delirium and renal failure 4 weeks after starting to take **nefazodone** 150 mg daily. The tacrolimus levels had been 9.4 nanograms/ml some 3 months earlier when he was on a dose of 6 mg daily, but in the presence of **nefazodone** the level was 46.4 nanograms/ml, with a tacrolimus dose of 5 mg daily. His creatinine levels had doubled. The tacrolimus level fell to 29.6 nanograms/ml within 2 days of the dose being reduced to 3 mg daily. **Nefazodone** was then replaced by **paroxetine** 20 mg daily. After 3 days the tacrolimus dose was increased to 5 mg daily and satisfactory levels of 12.4 nanograms/ml were observed.[1]

A renal transplant patient on prednisone, azathioprine and tacrolimus 5 mg daily for 2 years experienced headache, confusion and 'grey areas' in her vision within one week of starting **nefazodone** 50 mg twice daily in place of **sertraline**, for depression. Her serum creatinine had risen from 132 to 195 micromol/l and her trough tacrolimus level was greater than 30 nanograms/ml. **Nefazodone** was replaced by **sertraline**, and tacrolimus was withheld for 4 days. Signs of tacrolimus-induced neurotoxicity disappeared within 36 hours and serum creatinine and tacrolimus levels returned to pretreatment levels within 2 weeks of stopping **nefazodone**.[2]

Another patient developed raised liver enzymes and raised tacrolimus levels after taking **nefazodone** and tacrolimus for 2 weeks. When the **nefazodone** was stopped his liver enzymes normalised over the next 5 days, and his tacrolimus levels fell from 23 to 9.5 nanograms/ml over 10 days.[3]

Mechanism

Both tacrolimus and nefazodone are metabolised by the cytochrome P450 isoenzyme CYP3A4. Increased levels of tacrolimus may be due to inhibition of this isoenzyme by nefazodone. Paroxetine is a potent inhibitor of CYP2D6 with little effect on CYP3A4 and sertraline is primarily metabolised by CYP2C9 and CYP2D6 and so are unlikely to interact with tacrolimus.[1,2]

Importance and mechanism

Information appears to be limited but what is known indicates that tacrolimus levels or signs of toxicity should be well monitored if nefazodone is also given. In view of the narrow therapeutic index of tacrolimus, it may be advisable to avoid concurrent nefazodone. Paroxetine and sertraline may be suitable alternative antidepressants, but the evidence is slim, so additional monitoring may still be warranted.[1] Further study on the use of antidepressants with tacrolimus is needed.

1. Campo JV, Smith C, Perel JM. Tacrolimus toxic reaction associated with the use of nefazodone: paroxetine as an alternative agent. *Arch Gen Psychiatry* (1998) 55, 1050–1.
2. Olyaei AJ, deMattos AM, Norman DJ, Bennett WM. Interaction between tacrolimus and nefazodone in a stable renal transplant recipient. *Pharmacotherapy* (1998) 18, 1356–9.
3. Garton T, Nefazodone and CYP450 3A4 interactions with cyclosporine and tacrolimus. *Transplantation* (2002) 74, 745.

Tacrolimus + Antiretrovirals

Protease inhibitors including nelfinavir, ritonavir and saquinavir inhibit the metabolism of tacrolimus and increase its blood levels. Nucleoside reverse transcriptase inhibitors such as didanosine, stavudine and lamivudine appear not to interact with tacrolimus.

Clinical evidence, mechanism, importance and management

An HIV+ patient, with hepatitis C following a liver transplant was treated with antiviral therapy consisting of **stavudine** 30 mg twice daily, and **lamivudine** 150 mg twice daily, and **nelfinavir** 500 mg three times daily. Tacrolimus 6 mg daily was started postoperatively but high blood levels were observed and the dose was reduced over the next 3 months to a maintenance dose of 500 micrograms weekly, which achieved levels of between 7 and 25.9 nanograms/ml.[1] Another similar patient had a tacrolimus level of 10.9 nanograms/ml while taking tacrolimus 4 mg twice daily without antiretrovirals. When he was given a combination of **nelfinavir**, **stavudine** and **didanosine**, tacrolimus 500 micrograms daily produced a tacrolimus level of 23.7 nanograms/ml. When his antivirals were changed to **saquinavir**, **ritonavir**, **stavudine** and **lamivudine**, tacrolimus 1 mg twice daily resulted in tacrolimus levels in excess of 120 nanograms/ml with severe prolonged toxicity. After stabilisation of the patient, **nelfinavir**, **stavudine** and **lamivudine** were restarted. A tacrolimus dose of 500 micrograms every 3 to 5 days produced satisfactory trough tacrolimus levels of 4 to 10 nanograms/ml.[2]

A brief report describes petit mal seizures brought on by high tacrolimus levels, which were thought to be as a result of an interaction with **nelfinavir**. The patient was stabilised on once weekly tacrolimus.[3]

Mechanism

Stavudine, lamivudine and didanosine (all nucleoside reverse transcriptase inhibitors) are mainly excreted via the kidney and are unlikely to affect levels of tacrolimus. Nelfinavir, ritonavir and saquinavir (all protease inhibitors) are inhibitors of the cytochrome P450 CYP3A isoenzymes, which metabolise tacrolimus. It therefore seems likely that the protease inhibitors reduced tacrolimus metabolism resulting in the extremely high levels seen.[2]

Importance and management

An established and clinically important interaction. It is advised that when protease inhibitors are given to patients taking tacrolimus, careful monitoring and a reduction in the dose of tacrolimus is required. Nucleoside reverse transcriptase inhibitors are unlikely to contribute to the interaction.[2]

1. Schvarcz R, Rudbeck G, Söderdahl G, Ståhle L. Interaction between nelfinavir and tacrolimus after orthoptic liver transplantation in a patient coinfected with HIV and hepatitis C virus (HCV). *Transplantation* (2000) 69, 2194–5.
2. Sheikh AM, Wolf DC, Lebovics E, Goldberg R, Horowitz HW. Concomitant human immunodeficiency virus protease inhibitor therapy markedly reduces tacrolimus metabolism and increases blood levels. *Transplantation* (1999) 68, 307–9.
3. Ragni M, Dodson SF, Hunt SC, Bontempo FA, Fung JJ. Liver transplantation in a hemophilia patient with acquired immunodeficiency syndrome. *Blood* (1999) 93, 1113–14.

Tacrolimus + Azoles

When tacrolimus is given orally, its serum levels are considerably increased by oral fluconazole, and tacrolimus dose reductions may be needed. Itraconazole, ketoconazole, voriconazole, and possibly clotrimazole, also raise tacrolimus levels. There is some evidence that the levels of intravenous tacrolimus are minimally affected by fluconazole and ketoconazole.

Clinical evidence

(a) Clotrimazole

The serum levels of tacrolimus 6 mg daily rose from 3.5 to 5.6 nanograms/ml in a liver transplant patient within a day of starting clotrimazole 10 mg four times daily, and reached more than 9 nanograms/ml within 8 days. Later studies and rechallenge confirmed that the clotrimazole was responsible for the rise in tacrolimus levels. The tacrolimus AUC was nearly doubled.[1]

(b) Fluconazole

Twenty organ transplant patients (11 livers, 6 kidneys, 2 hearts and one bone marrow) taking tacrolimus were also given fluconazole 100 or 200 mg daily for various fungal infections. On day 1 the median plasma trough levels of those given fluconazole 100 mg rose 1.4-fold, and in those on 200 mg it rose 3.1-fold. The dosage of the tacrolimus was reduced to accommodate this rise, the median dosage reduction was 56% (range 0 to 88%). The highest tacrolimus level was seen within 3 days. A pharmacokinetic study in one patient found that when fluconazole 100 mg daily was stopped, the tacrolimus AUC fell by about 60%.[2]

Other studies in adult[3] and paediatric patients[4] and individual case reports[5,6] have confirmed that tacrolimus levels are increased by oral fluconazole, increasing the risk of nephrotoxicity.[4] In a retrospective study, patients given fluconazole required a 40% reduction in tacrolimus dose to achieve similar trough levels.[7]

However, one study found that if intravenous tacrolimus is given with intravenous fluconazole 400 mg, the steady-state levels of tacrolimus are only slightly increased (by about 16%), which was considered to be clinically unimportant.[8]

A bone-marrow transplant patient on tacrolimus given fluconazole for oral candidiasis experienced headache and was found to have glycosuria, increased serum creatinine and Pelger-Huet anomaly of granulocytes, which disappeared after tacrolimus was discontinued. The effects were thought to be due to tacrolimus toxicity due to an interaction with fluconazole.[9]

(c) Itraconazole

Trough blood levels of tacrolimus in a heart-lung transplant patient increased threefold from 16 to 57 nanograms/ml and serum creatinine levels also rose after she was given itraconazole 200 mg daily.[10] A renal transplant recipient on tacrolimus 6 mg daily was given itraconazole 100 mg twice daily for a urinary candida infection. Within a day, the tacrolimus trough levels increased from 12.6 to 21 nanograms/ml and the tacrolimus dose was progressively reduced to 3 mg daily. Four days after the itraconazole was discontinued tacrolimus had to be progressively increased back to its initial dose.[11] The interaction has been reported in three other renal transplant recipients.[12-14]

(d) Ketoconazole

The addition of ketoconazole 200 mg daily to tacrolimus and prednisone in a renal transplant patient resulted in an increase in tacrolimus blood levels from 11.1 to 27.9 nanograms/ml, despite a 45% decrease in the dose of tacrolimus. Eventually the dose of tacrolimus had to be reduced by 80% to keep the levels within the therapeutic range. Tacrolimus levels decreased to 5.8 nanograms/ml within a week of discontinuing ketoconazole and so the dose was raised.[15] A pharmacokinetic study in 6 healthy subjects found that ketoconazole 200 mg orally at bedtime for 12 days increased the bioavailability of single 0.1-mg/kg doses of oral tacrolimus from 14% to 30%.[16] The maker notes that the clearance of tacrolimus given intravenously was not significantly changed by ketoconazole, although it was highly variable between patients.[17]

(e) Voriconazole

A small study comparing the tacrolimus levels of two patients, one taking voriconazole 200 mg twice daily, the other placebo, found that the tacrolimus levels were nearly tenfold higher in the patient on voriconazole. This was originally designed as a larger study, but the study was stopped after the finding in these initial two subjects.[18] Another study in 14 healthy subjects found that voriconazole 400 mg twice daily on day one, then 200 mg twice daily for 6 days increased the AUC and maximum serum levels of a single 0.1-mg/kg dose of tacrolimus 3.2- and 2.3-fold respectively.[19] A liver transplant patient on tacrolimus was hospitalised with multiple complaints, and was found to have a high tacrolimus level. Tacrolimus was withheld and later restarted at 3 mg daily gradually reduced to 1.5 mg daily. When voriconazole 400 mg twice daily was started the tacrolimus dose was reduced by one-third to 0.5 mg daily, but eventually needed to be reduced to 0.15 mg daily as a result of rising tacrolimus levels.[20]

Mechanism

Fluconazole, itraconazole, ketoconazole and voriconazole inhibit the metabolism of the tacrolimus by the gut wall and/or liver (by the cytochrome P450 isoenzyme CYP3A4), and/or inhibit the activity of P-glycoprotein so that more is absorbed.[8,11,16,18] Therefore, intravenous tacrolimus is little affected.[8]

Importance and management

The interaction between tacrolimus and fluconazole is established, clinically important and can develop rapidly (within 3 days). The authors of one of the reports say that up to 200 mg of oral fluconazole daily can be used safely and effectively provided the tacrolimus dosage is reduced by half.[2] One study specifically examining dose adjustments suggests that fluconazole can be safely used if 60% of the original tacrolimus dose is given.[7] If tacrolimus is given intravenously, no clinically important interaction appears to occur.[8]

The interactions of tacrolimus with itraconazole and ketoconazole also appear to be established, and the maker states that nearly all patients will require tacrolimus dose reductions when given these drugs.[17,21] Information about clotrimazole is limited, but on the basis of the case report it would be prudent to monitor tacrolimus levels, and adjust the dose as necessary.

The makers of voriconazole advise reducing the tacrolimus dose to one-third when starting voriconazole, closely monitoring tacrolimus levels throughout, and increasing the tacrolimus dose in response to levels obtained when voriconazole is stopped.[22,23] However, greater reductions in tacrolimus dose may be needed in some patients.[18,20]

In vitro studies with human liver microsomes have shown that **miconazole**[24] also inhibits liver and small intestine microsomes that metabolise tacrolimus and it seems possible that it may interact just like fluconazole but this needs confirmation. No interaction would be expected if **miconazole** is used topically.

1. Mieles L, Venkataramanan R, Yokoyama I, Warty VJ, Starzl TE. Interaction between FK506 and clotrimazole in a liver transplant recipient. *Transplantation* (1991) 52, 1086–7.
2. Mañez R, Martin M, Raman V, Silverman D, Jain A, Warty V, Gonzalez-Pinto I, Kusne S, Starzl TE. Fluconazole therapy in transplant recipients receiving FK506. *Transplantation* (1994) 57, 1521–23.
3. Toy S, Tata P, Jain A, Patsy K, Lever J, Burckart G, Warty V, Kusne S, Abu-Elmagd K, Fung J, Starzi T, Venkataramanan R. A pharmacokinetic interaction between tacrolimus and fluconazole. *Pharm Res* (1996) 13 (9 Suppl), S435.
4. Vincent I, Furlan V, Debray D, Jacquemin E, Taburet AM. Effects of antifungal agents on the pharmacokinetics and nephrotoxicity of FK506 in paediatric liver transplant recipients. *Intersci Conf Antimicrob Agents Chemother* (1995) 35, 5.
5. Assan R, Fredj G, Larger E, Feutren G, Bismuth H. FK 506/fluconazole interaction enhances FK506 nephrotoxicity. *Diabete Metab* (1994) 20, 49–52.
6. Chamorey E, Nouveau B, Viard L, Garcia-Credoz F, Durand A, Pisano P. Interaction tacrolimus-fluconazole chez un enfant transplanté coeur-poumons. A propos d'un cas clinique. *J Pharm Clin* (1998) 17, 51–3.
7. Toda F, Tanabe K, Ito S, Shinmura H, Tokumoto T, Ishida H, Toma H. Tacrolimus trough level adjustment after administration of fluconazole to kidney recipients. *Transplant Proc* (2002) 34, 1733–5.
8. Osowski CL, Dix SP, Lin LS, Mullins RE, Geller RB, Wingard JR. Evaluation of the drug interaction between intravenous high-dose fluconazole and cyclosporine or tacrolimus in bone marrow transplant patients. *Transplantation* (1996) 61, 1268–72.
9. Gondo H, Okamura C, Osaki K, Shimoda K, Asano Y, Okamura T. Acquired Pelger-Huet anomaly in association with concomitant tacrolimus and fluconazole therapy following allogenic bone marrow transplantation. *Bone Marrow Transplant* (2000) 26, 1255–7.
10. Furlan V, Parquin F, Penaud JF, Cerrina J, Le Roy Ladurie F, Dartevelle P, Taburet AM. Interaction between tacrolimus and itraconazole in a heart-lung transplant recipient. *Transplant Proc* (1998) 30, 187–8.
11. Capone D, Gentile A, Imperatore P, Palmiero G, Basile V. Effects of itraconazole on tacrolimus blood concentrations in a renal transplant recipient. *Ann Pharmacother* (1999) 33, 1124–5.
12. Katari SR, Magnone M, Shapiro R, Jordan M, Scantlebury V, Vivas C, Gritsch A, McCauley J, Demetris AJ, Randhawa PS. Clinical features of acute reversible tacrolimus (FK506) nephrotoxicity in kidney transplant recipients. *Clin Transplant* (1997) 11, 237–42.
13. Macías MO, Salvador P, Hurtado JL, Martín I. Tacrolimus-itraconazole interaction in a kidney transplant patient. *Ann Pharmacother* (2000) 34, 536.
14. Ideura T, Muramatsu T, Higuchi M, Tachibana N, Hora K, Kiyosawa K. Tacrolimus/itraconazole interactions: a case report of ABO-incompatible living-related renal transplantation. *Nephrol Dial Transplant* (2000) 15, 1721–3.
15. Moreno M, Latorre C, Manzanares C, Morales E, Herrero JC, Dominguez-Gil B, Carreño A, Cubas A, Delgado M, Andres A, Morales JM. Clinical management of tacrolimus drug interactions in renal transplant patients. *Transplant Proc* (1999) 31, 2252–3.
16. Floren LC, Bekersky I, Benet LZ, Mekki Q, Dressler D, Lee JW, Roberts JP, Hebert MF. Tacrolimus oral bioavailability doubles with coadministration of ketoconazole. *Clin Pharmacol Ther* (1997) 62, 41–9.
17. Prograf (Tacrolimus). Fujisawa. US Prescribing information, September 2004.
18. Venkataramanan R, Zang S, Gayowski T, Singh N. Voriconazole inhibition of the metabolism of tacrolimus in a liver transplant recipient and in human liver microsomes. *Antimicrob Agents Chemother* (2002) 46, 3091–3.
19. Wood N, Tan K, Allan R, Fielding A, Nichols DJ. Effect of voriconazole on the pharmacokinetics of tacrolimus. *Intersci Conf Antimicrob Agents Chemother* (2001) 41, 2.
20. Pai MP, Allen S. Voriconazole inhibition of tacrolimus metabolism. *Clin Infect Dis* (2003) 36, 1089–91.
21. Prograf (Tacrolimus). Fujisawa Ltd. UK Summary of product characteristics, June 2002.
22. VFEND (Voriconazole). Pfizer Ltd. UK Summary of product characteristics, March 2005.
23. VFEND (Voriconazole). Pfizer Inc. US Prescribing information, March 2005.
24. Christians U, Schmidt G, Bader A, Lampen A, Schottmann R, Linck A, Sewing K-F. Identification of drugs inhibiting the *in vitro* metabolism of tacrolimus by human liver microsomes. *Br J Clin Pharmacol* (1996) 41, 187–90.

Tacrolimus + Calcium channel blockers

Nifedipine causes a moderate rise in serum tacrolimus levels and also appears to be kidney protective. Diltiazem and felodipine also appear to elevate tacrolimus levels, while nicardipine, nilvadipine and verapamil are predicted to interact similarly.

Clinical evidence

(a) Diltiazem

The trough blood levels of tacrolimus 8 mg twice daily increased from 12.9 to 55 nanograms/ml in a liver transplant patient within 3 days of him starting diltiazem (initially 5 to 10 mg/hour intravenously for one day, then 30 mg orally every 8 hours). The patient became delirious, confused and agitated. Both drugs were stopped, and over the next 3 days his mental state improved and his tacrolimus levels fell to 6.7 nanograms/ml. Tacrolimus was then restarted, gradually increasing to a dose of 5 mg twice daily, which produced levels of 9 to 10 nanograms/ml.[1]

A study in 2 liver and 2 kidney transplant patients found that diltiazem increased the AUC of tacrolimus. In the kidney transplant patients the increase appeared to be dose related; a 20-mg dose of diltiazem caused a 26 and 67% rise, while a 180-mg dose caused a 48 and 177% rise in each patient respectively. The liver transplant patients did not have any alteration in the AUC of tacrolimus until they were given higher doses of diltiazem; one patient had an 18% rise following a 120-mg dose, the other a 22% rise following a 180-mg dose.[2]

A study in 7 liver transplant patients given tacrolimus 100 micrograms/kg twice daily found that modified release diltiazem 90 mg daily did not significantly alter the absorption or metabolism of tacrolimus when compared to 7 similar patients not given diltiazem.[3] The authors of the other study[2] suggest that this lack of effect may have been because only 90 mg of diltiazem was used.

(b) Felodipine

A 13-year-old boy on tacrolimus 4 mg twice daily was given felodipine 2.5 mg daily 15 days after receiving a renal transplant. Two weeks later his tacrolimus level was reported as greater than 30 nanograms/ml (previous levels ranged from 10.6 to 20 nanograms/ml), and despite a reduction in the dose of tacrolimus to 3 mg twice daily a subsequent tacrolimus level was 53.9 nanograms/ml. He was eventually stabilised at the original tacrolimus levels on a dose of 500 micrograms twice daily. When the felodipine was stopped several months later his tacrolimus dose needed to be raised to maintain therapeutic levels.[4]

(c) Nifedipine

A 1-year retrospective study of two groups of liver transplant patients found that in the 22 patients taking nifedipine 30 or 60 mg daily there was a 55% increase in the serum tacrolimus levels after 1 month. The cumulative dosage reduction of the tacrolimus by 6 months was 25.5% in the nifedipine group and by 12 months it was 31.4% when compared with the group not taking nifedipine. The nifedipine group had improved renal function (lowered serum creatinine).[5]

Mechanism

Uncertain, but it seems likely that some calcium channel blockers inhibit the cytochrome P450 isoenzyme CYP3A4 and/or P-glycoprotein, thereby reducing the metabolism of tacrolimus leading to increased serum levels.[1,5] This is consistent with the findings of an *in vitro* study using human liver microsomes.[6]

Importance and management

In the case of nifedipine, this seems to be an established and clinically important interaction. If nifedipine is added to a tacrolimus regimen the serum levels should be well monitored and the tacrolimus dosage reduced appropriately. Although the information about diltiazem is less conclusive it would seem wise to follow the same precautions, as the effect of diltiazem on tacrolimus seems to vary greatly between the few patients studied. The makers of felodipine advise monitoring tacrolimus levels if felodipine is given.[7,8] Direct information about other calcium channel blockers appears to be lacking, but the US and UK makers of tacrolimus[9,10] predict that **nicardipine** and **verapamil** may raise tacrolimus levels by inhibiting CYP3A4 (see Mechanism), and the UK makers additionally suggest that **nilvadipine** may interact similarly.[10]

1. Hebert MF, Lam AY. Diltiazem increases tacrolimus concentrations. *Ann Pharmacother* (1999) 33, 680–2.
2. Jones TE, Morris RG. Pharmacokinetic interaction between tacrolimus and diltiazem: dose-response relationship in kidney and liver transplant recipients. *Clin Pharmacokinet* (2002) 41, 381–8.
3. Teperman L, Turgut S, Negron C, John D, Diflo T, Morgan G, Tobias H. Diltiazem is a safe drug in transplant patients on Prograf and does not affect Prograf levels. *Hepatology* (1996) 24, 180A.
4. Butani L, Berg G, Makker SP. Effect of felodipine on tacrolimus pharmacokinetics in a renal transplant recipient. *Transplantation* (2002) 73, 159.
5. Seifeldin RA, Marcos-Alvarez A, Gordon FD, Lewis WD, Jenkins RL. Nifedipine interaction with tacrolimus in liver transplant recipients. *Ann Pharmacother* (1997) 31, 571–5.
6. Iwasaki K, Matsuda H, Nagase K, Shiraga T, Tokuma Y, Uchida K. Effects of twenty-three drugs on the metabolism of FK506 by human liver microsomes. *Res Commun Chem Pathol Pharmacol* (1993) 82, 209–16.
7. Plendil (Felodipine). AstraZeneca UK Ltd. UK Summary of product characteristics, September 2003.
8. Plendil (Felodipine). AstraZeneca. US Prescribing information, November 2003.
9. Prograf (Tacrolimus). Fujisawa. US Prescribing information, September 2004.
10. Prograf (Tacrolimus). Fujisawa Ltd. UK Summary of product characteristics, June 2002.

Tacrolimus + Caspofungin

Caspofungin moderately decreases tacrolimus levels. Tacrolimus does not affect the pharmacokinetics of caspofungin.

Clinical evidence, mechanism, importance and management

The preliminary results of one study suggest that caspofungin reduces the AUC of tacrolimus by 20% in healthy subjects,[1] and reduces the trough tacrolimus levels by 26%.[2] Tacrolimus did not alter the pharmacokinetics of caspofungin.[1] The makers of caspofungin advise that tacrolimus levels should be monitored if caspofungin is given, and tacrolimus doses adjusted as appropriate.[2,3]

1. Stone J, Holland S, Wickersham P, Deutsch P, Winchell G, Hesney M, Miller R, Freeman A, Dilzer S, Lasseter K. Drug interactions between caspofungin and tacrolimus. *Intersci Conf Antimicrob Agents Chemother* (2001) 41, 1.
2. Cancidas (Caspofungin acetate). Merck Sharpe & Dohme Ltd. UK Summary of product characteristics, October 2004.
3. Cancidas (Caspofungin acetate). Merck & Co., Inc US Prescribing information, February 2005.

Tacrolimus + Ciclosporin

The makers say that tacrolimus and ciclosporin should not be used concurrently because of the increased risk of kidney damage.

Clinical evidence, mechanism, importance and management

One study found that, in patients with normal bilirubin levels, the half-life of ciclosporin was prolonged from a range of 6 to 15 hours up to 26 to 74 hours and the ciclosporin serum levels, measured by a fluorescent polarisation immunoassay, were raised by tacrolimus.[1] On the other hand another study found no changes in the pharmacokinetics of ciclosporin as measured by HPLC in patients given tacrolimus, but creatinine levels were almost doubled (suggesting kidney damage),[2] which confirmed a previous report suggesting that severe renal dysfunction may develop.[3] The suggestion is that tacrolimus inhibits ciclosporin metabolism or its absorption.[1] The makers of tacrolimus say that it should not be given with ciclosporin because of the risk of additive/synergistic nephrotoxicity, and if ciclosporin is being replaced by tacrolimus 12 to 24 hours should elapse between stopping one and starting the other.[4,5]

1. Venkataramanan R, Jain A, Cadoff E, Warty V, Iwasaki K, Nagase K, Krajack A, Imventarza O, Todo S, Fung JJ, Starzl TE. Pharmacokinetics of FK 506: preclinical and clinical studies. *Transplant Proc* (1990) 22 (Suppl 1), 52–6.
2. Jain AB, Venkataramanan R, Fung J, Burckart G, Emeigh J, Diven W, Warty V, Abu-Elmagd K, Todo S, Alessiani M, Starzl TE. Pharmacokinetics of cyclosporine and nephrotoxicity in orthoptic liver transplant patients rescued with FK 506. *Transplant Proc* (1991) 23, 2777–9.
3. McCauley J, Fung J, Jain A, Todo S, Starzl TE. The effects of FK506 on renal function after liver transplantation. *Transplant Proc* (1990) 22 (Suppl 1), 17–20.
4. Prograf (Tacrolimus). Fujisawa Ltd. UK Summary of product characteristics, June 2002.
5. Prograf (Tacrolimus). Fujisawa. US Prescribing information, September 2004.

Tacrolimus + Corticosteroids

The effects of methylprednisolone on tacrolimus are uncertain. Prednisone appears to reduce the levels of tacrolimus.

Clinical evidence, mechanism, importance and management

A review of early studies of tacrolimus stated that serum levels were said to have been increased on 10 occasions, decreased on 5 occasions, and have unaltered on 2 occasions by **methylprednisolone**.[1]

In a randomised study conducted over 3 months, 31 patients receiving tacrolimus, mycophenolate and daclizumab were compared with 34 patients receiving tacrolimus, mycophenolate and **prednisone**. Higher tacrolimus doses were required to maintain therapeutic tacrolimus concentrations in the **prednisone** group. This reached a maximum after one month, when a 30% larger tacrolimus dose was necessary.[2]

1. Venkataramanan R, Jain A, Cadoff E, Warty V, Iwasaki K, Nagase K, Krajack A, Imventarza O, Todo S, Fung JJ, Starzl TE. Pharmacokinetics of FK 506: preclinical and clinical studies. *Transplant Proc* (1990) 22 (Suppl 1), 52–6.
2. Hesselink DA, Ngyuen H, Wabbijn M, Smak Gregoor PJH, Steyerberg EW, van Riemsdijk IC, Weimar W, van Gelder T. Tacrolimus dose requirement in renal transplant recipients is significantly higher when used in combination with corticosteroids. *Br J Clin Pharmacol* (2003) 56, 327–30.

Tacrolimus + Chloramphenicol

A marked rise in serum tacrolimus levels has been reported in several patients treated with systemic chloramphenicol.

Clinical evidence, mechanism, importance and management

A retrospective study identified 3 patients on tacrolimus who had received a total of 5 courses of intravenous chloramphenicol, each lasting for at least 12 days. Tacrolimus levels were doubled by day 2, and had increased to a peak of 207% by day 6. The tacrolimus dose had been decreased by about one-third by day 12, and the tacrolimus levels were around the baseline value.[1]

An adolescent patient with a kidney transplant developed toxic tacrolimus levels on the second day of starting chloramphenicol for the treatment of a vancomycin-resistant enterococcal infection. The tacrolimus dosage had to be reduced by 83% to achieve safe serum levels, and it was found that the dose-adjusted tacrolimus AUC was 7.5-fold greater while taking the chloramphenicol.[2] Another report describes a similar interaction in a liver transplant patient on tacrolimus 4 mg twice daily. The patient was given intravenous chloramphenicol, but at the unintentionally high dose of 1850 mg every 6 hours. After about 3 days the patient complained of lethargy, fatigue, headaches and tremors so both drugs were stopped. His tacrolimus trough concentration had increased from a range of 9 to 11 nanograms/ml to more than 60 nanograms/ml. Seven days later his tacrolimus level was 8.2 nanograms/ml and his symptoms had resolved.[3]

Mechanism

Chloramphenicol (a known and potent enzyme inhibitor) is thought to raise tacrolimus levels by rapidly reducing its metabolism.[2]

Importance and management

These appear to be the only reports of this interaction, but it is consistent with the known metabolic characteristics of both drugs and therefore it is expected to be an interaction of general importance. Monitor the outcome closely if systemic chloramphenicol is given to any patient on tacrolimus, being alert for the need to reduce the tacrolimus dosage. It seems doubtful if a clinically relevant interaction will occur with topical chloramphenicol because the dosage and the systemic absorption is small, but this needs confirmation.

1. Mathis AS, Shah N, Knipp GT, Friedman GS. Interaction of chloramphenicol and the calcineurin inhibitors in renal transplant recipients. *Transpl Infect Dis* (2002) 4, 169–74.
2. Schulman SL, Shaw LM, Jabs K, Leonard MB, Brayman KL. Interaction between tacrolimus and chloramphenicol in a renal transplant recipient. *Transplantation* (1998) 65, 1397–8.
3. Taber DJ, Dupuis RE, Hollar KD, Strzalka AL, Johnson MW. Drug-drug interaction between chloramphenicol and tacrolimus in a liver transplant recipient. *Transplant Proc* (2000) 32, 660–62.

Tacrolimus + Danazol

An isolated report describes an increase in tacrolimus levels in a patient given danazol.

Clinical evidence, mechanism, importance and management

The serum levels of tacrolimus 10 mg daily rose from 0.7 to 2.7 nanograms/ml in a kidney transplant patient within 4 days of starting to take danazol 400 to 1200 mg daily. Despite a reduction in the danazol dosage to 600 mg and then 400 mg daily, her tacrolimus and creatinine serum levels remained high for a month until the danazol was withdrawn. The reason is not known, but the authors suggest that danazol possibly inhibits the metabolism (demethylation and hydroxylation) of the tacrolimus by the liver so that it is cleared from the body more slowly.[1] The general importance of this interaction is uncertain but monitor the effects of concurrent use in any patient, reducing the tacrolimus dosage as necessary.

1. Shapiro R, Venkataramanan R, Warty VS, Scantlebury VP, Rybka W, McCauley J, Fung JJ, Starzl TE. FK 506 interaction with danazol. *Lancet* (1993) 341, 1344–5.

Tacrolimus + Grapefruit juice

Grapefruit juice can markedly increase the serum levels of tacrolimus.

Clinical evidence, mechanism, importance and management

Eight liver transplant patients were given 12 oz (about 360 ml) of grapefruit juice twice daily, which they drank within 45 minutes of taking their dose of tacrolimus. After a week it was found that their 12-hour trough, and 1-hour and 4-hour tacrolimus levels were raised by 300%, 195% and 400% respectively. Two patients had headaches, one had diarrhoea and one had an increased creatinine level, that reversed, but none of the 12 developed rejection or irreversible toxicity. Two of the patients remained on the grapefruit juice and it was possible to halve their tacrolimus dosage.[1] Similarly, 6 kidney transplant patients had their dose of tacrolimus reduced by an average of 40% after taking grapefruit juice 100 ml daily for 5 days.[2]

A case report describes a kidney transplant patient on tacrolimus whose tacrolimus level rose from a range of 8 to 10 nanograms/ml up to 25.2 nanograms/ml after he ate about 100 g of **pomelo** (*Citrus grandis,* a fruit related to grapefruit).[3]

The reason for the rise in tacrolimus levels is not known, but it seems likely that it is due to inhibition of the metabolism of tacrolimus by some component of grapefruit juice and **pomelo**. In practical terms the authors of the first report suggest that this interaction means that the dosage of tacrolimus can possibly be reduced (to save money) although there is a clear need to monitor the effects closely because of the difficulties of standardising grapefruit juice.[1] However, the US makers of tacrolimus suggest that the combination should be avoided.[4]

1. Westveer MK, Farquhar ML, George P, Mayes JT. Co-administration of grapefruit juice increases tacrolimus levels in liver transplant patients. Proceedings of the 15th Annual Meeting of the American Society of Transplant Physicians 1996. Abstract P-115.
2. Michelangelo V, Piero D, Elisa C, Enrico S, Mauro B, Pietro B. Grapefruit juice and kinetics of tacrolimus. *J Am Soc Nephrol* (2001) 12, 862A.
3. Egashira K, Fukuda E, Onga T, Yogi Y, Matsuya F, Koyabu N, Ohtani H, Sawada Y. Pomelo-induced increase in the blood level of tacrolimus in a renal transplant patient. *Transplantation* (2003) 75, 1057.
4. Prograf (Tacrolimus). Fujisawa. US Prescribing information, September 2004.

Tacrolimus + Macrolides

Six patients have had marked increases in serum tacrolimus levels accompanied by evidence of renal toxicity when treated with erythromycin. The same interaction has been seen in four patients given clarithromycin, and is predicted with josamycin and troleandomycin, but not azithromycin.

Clinical evidence

(a) Azithromycin

One report briefly describes a patient taking tacrolimus following a bone marrow transplant who took a 10-day course of azithromycin [dose not stated] without any significant alteration in his serum creatinine or trough tacrolimus level.[1]

(b) Clarithromycin

A woman with a kidney transplant taking tacrolimus, prednisone and azathioprine was started on clarithromycin 500 mg twice daily for 4 days, then 250 mg daily to treat a severe *Mycoplasma pneumoniae* infection. Despite a 64% reduction in the dosage of the tacrolimus, the trough tacrolimus concentrations rose sharply, from 2.8 to 36.1 nanograms/ml by day 6 and creatinine levels increased from 309 to 442 micromol/l. The tacrolimus dosage was further reduced and then stopped, and not restarted until the clarithromycin treatment was completed.[2] In another 2 kidney transplant patients, tacrolimus levels increased by 146% and 131% respectively following 9 doses of clarithromycin 250 mg. Creatinine levels increased by 91% and 30% respectively.[3] Similarly the tacrolimus levels of a bone marrow transplant patient rose from below 1.1 to 10.1 nanograms/ml after he took clarithromycin 500 mg twice daily for about 4 days.[1]

(c) Erythromycin

A liver transplant patient on tacrolimus 6 mg twice daily for a year had a marked rise in serum tacrolimus levels from about 1.4 to 6.5 nanomol/l when intravenous ampicillin/sulbactam 3 g every 6 hours and oral erythromycin 250 mg every 6 hours were given for 4 days to treat pneumonia. Renal toxicity, demonstrated by increased blood urea and creatinine levels also occurred. The erythromycin was stopped, and the next day the tacrolimus was also stopped. Over the next week the serum levels of the tacrolimus, blood urea nitrogen and creatinine fell.[4]

A kidney transplant patient had an increase in his serum tacrolimus levels from 1.3 to 8.5 nanograms/ml 4 days after starting erythromycin 400 mg four times daily. His serum creatinine levels almost doubled.[5] A man with a kidney transplant had a sixfold rise in serum tacrolimus levels when he took erythromycin.[6] Another similar case has been described.[7] Two children aged 3 and 7-years-old also had rises in serum tacrolimus levels, which were accompanied by renal toxicity when erythromycin was added.[8]

Mechanism

The macrolides inhibit tacrolimus metabolism by the cytochrome P450 isoenzyme CYP3A. Azithromycin is less likely to interact with tacrolimus because it does not inhibit CYP3A.[9]

Importance and management

Direct information seems to be limited to these case reports. However, it would be prudent to closely monitor the effects of adding clarithromycin or erythromycin in any patient, being alert for the need to reduce the tacrolimus dosage to avoid nephrotoxicity. The makers predict that **josamycin**[10] and **troleandomycin**[11] will interact similarly and so the same precautions would also be appropriate. Most other macrolides would also be expected to interact although they do not all behave identically. Azithromycin has been predicted not to interact and the results of the case above seem to confirm this.

1. Ibrahim RB, Abella EM, Chandrasekar PH. Tacrolimus-clarithromycin interaction in a patient receiving bone marrow transplantation. *Ann Pharmacother* (2002) 36, 1971–2.
2. Wolter K, Wagner K, Philipp T, Fritschka E. Interaction between FK 506 and clarithromycin in a renal transplant patient. *Eur J Clin Pharmacol* (1994) 47, 207–8.
3. Gómez G, Álvarez ML, Errasti P, Lavilla FJ, García N, Ballester B, García I, Purroy A. Acute tacrolimus nephrotoxicity in renal transplant patients treated with clarithromycin. *Transplant Proc* (1999) 31, 2250–1.
4. Shaeffer MS, Collier D, Sorrell MF. Interaction between FK506 and erythromycin. *Ann Pharmacother* (1994) 28, 280–1.
5. Jensen C, Jordan M, Shapiro R, Scantelbury V, Hakala T, Fung J, Stasrzl T, Venkataramanan R. Interaction between tacrolimus and erythromycin. *Lancet* (1994) 344, 825.
6. Padhi ID, Long P, Basha M, Anandan JV. Interaction between tacrolimus and erythromycin. *Ther Drug Monit* (1997) 19, 120–2.
7. Moreno M, Latorre C, Manzanares C, Morales E, Herrero JC, Dominguez-Gil B, Carreño A, Cubas A, Delgado M, Andres A, Morales JM. Clinical management of tacrolimus drug interactions in renal transplant patients. *Transplant Proc* (1999) 31, 2252–3.
8. Furlan V, Perello L, Jacquemin E, Debray D, Taburet A-M. Interactions between FK506 and rifampicin or erythromycin in pediatric liver recipients. *Transplantation* (1995) 59, 1217–18.
9. Paterson DL, Singh N. Interactions between tacrolimus and antimicrobial agents. *Clin Infect Dis* (1997) 25, 1430–40.
10. Prograf (Tacrolimus). Fujisawa Ltd. UK Summary of product characteristics, June 2002.
11. Prograf (Tacrolimus). Fujisawa. US Prescribing information, September 2004.

Tacrolimus + Miscellaneous

Tacrolimus is metabolised by the cytochrome P450 isoenzyme CYP3A4, the induction and inhibition of which may affect the serum levels of tacrolimus. The makers also issue cautions about the concurrent use of tacrolimus and anticoagulants, antidiabetics, nephrotoxic or neurotoxic drugs and potassium-sparing diuretics.

Clinical evidence, mechanism, importance and management

(a) Cytochrome P450 isoenzyme CYP3A4 inducers

In vitro studies with *rat* and human liver microsomes[1,2] have found that tacrolimus is extensively metabolised by the cytochrome P450 isoenzyme CYP3A4. This means that drugs that induce CYP3A4 may potentially reduce the serum levels of tacrolimus.

Rifampicin (rifampin) and possibly **phenytoin**, known potent enzyme inducers, have been seen to lower tacrolimus levels, (see 'Tacrolimus + Rifamycins', p.824, and 'Tacrolimus + Phenytoin', p.823), and the makers suggest that **carbamazepine**, and **phenobarbital** will interact similarly.[3,4] These predictions are as yet unconfirmed, but it would certainly be prudent to monitor tacrolimus levels closely if any of these drugs are used concurrently.

(b) Cytochrome P450 isoenzyme CYP3A4 inhibitors

In vitro studies with *rat* and human liver microsomes[1,2] have found that tacrolimus is extensively metabolised by the cytochrome P450 isoenzyme CYP3A4. This means that drugs that inhibit CYP3A4 may potentially increase the serum levels of tacrolimus. Most of the known inhibitors of CYP3A4 (such as the 'azoles', (p.819), 'protease inhibitors', (p.819) and 'macrolides', (p.822)) have clearly been shown to interact with tacrolimus. The makers of tacrolimus suggest that other enzyme-inhibiting drugs may also inhibit tacrolimus metabolism, and they name **bromocriptine**, **cimetidine**, **dapsone**, **ergotamine**, **lidocaine**, **midazolam**, **quinidine** and **tamoxifen**.[3,4] These predictions are as yet unconfirmed, but it would certainly be prudent to monitor tacrolimus levels closely if any of these drugs are used concurrently.

(c) Neurotoxicity or nephrotoxicity

Other predicted interactions of tacrolimus include: additive neuro- or nephrotoxicity with **aciclovir**, **aminoglycosides**, **co-trimoxazole**, **ganciclovir**, **gyrase inhibitors** or **vancomycin** (nephrotoxicity has been seen with **amphotericin B** and tacrolimus).[3]

(d) Potassium-sparing diuretics

As tacrolimus may cause hyperkalaemia, the maker says that concurrent use of potassium-sparing diuretics should be avoided.[3]

(e) Protein-binding interactions

Because tacrolimus is extensively bound to plasma proteins, the UK makers mention the possibility of protein binding interactions with oral **anticoagulants** or **antidiabetics**,[3] (but this has largely been discredited as a mechanism, see 'Protein-binding interactions', (p.3)).

1. Shah IA, Whiting PH, Omar G, Thomson AW, Burke MD. Effects of FK 506 on human microsomal cytochrome P–450–dependent drug metabolism in vitro. *Transplant Proc* (1991) 23, 2783–5.
2. Pichard L, Fabre I, Domergue J, Joyeux H, Maurel P. Effect of FK 506 on human hepatic cytochromes P–450: interaction with CyA. *Transplant Proc* (1991) 23, 2791–3.
3. Prograf (Tacrolimus). Fujisawa Ltd. UK Summary of product characteristics, June 2002.
4. Prograf (Tacrolimus). Fujisawa. US Prescribing information, September 2004.

Tacrolimus + NSAIDs

Two liver transplant patients on tacrolimus developed acute renal failure after taking ibuprofen.

Clinical evidence, mechanism, importance and management

Two patients with liver transplants on tacrolimus developed acute but reversible renal failure, one after taking four *Motrin* (**ibuprofen**) tablets [strength not stated] and the other after three 400-mg tablets of **ibuprofen** taken over 24 hours. Both had stable renal function before taking the **ibuprofen**.[1]

NSAIDs are known to inhibit prostaglandin synthesis and as a result may decrease renal blood flow, which in certain circumstances can lead to renal failure. Renal impairment is more likely to occur in the presence of renal vasoconstrictors. Tacrolimus is known to cause renal vasoconstriction and thus the combined effects of **ibuprofen** and tacrolimus may have led to acute renal failure. Both patients also had a degree of liver impairment, which the authors suggest may have potentiated the toxicity of the tacrolimus and the **ibuprofen**.

The authors of the report say that if renal toxicity develops, the tacrolimus should be withdrawn. They used intravenous prostaglandin-E_1 effectively in one patient. They also suggest that NSAIDs should not be given to patients on tacrolimus, especially if it is being used as rescue therapy for abnormal graft function.[1] There seems as yet to be nothing documented about adverse interactions with other NSAIDs but if the suggested mechanism is true, they may possibly behave like **ibuprofen**. The UK makers of tacrolimus suggest that all NSAIDs may have additive nephrotoxic effects with tacrolimus.[2]

1. Sheiner PA, Mor E, Chodoff L, Glabman S, Emre S, Schwartz ME, Miller CM. Acute renal failure associated with the use of ibuprofen in two liver transplant recipients on FK506. *Transplantation* (1994) 57, 1132–3.
2. Prograf (Tacrolimus). Fujisawa Ltd. UK Summary of product characteristics, June 2002.

Tacrolimus + Phenytoin

An isolated report describes an increase in serum phenytoin levels attributed to the use of tacrolimus. Phenytoin decreased tacrolimus levels in one case, and has been used to reduce tacrolimus levels after an overdose.

Clinical evidence

(a) Phenytoin levels

A kidney transplant patient on phenytoin 500 and 600 mg on alternate days (and also taking azathioprine, bumetanide, digoxin, diltiazem, heparin, insulin and prednisone) had his immunosuppressant treatment changed from ciclosporin to tacrolimus 14 to 16 mg daily. About 7 weeks later he presented to hospital because of a fainting episode and his phenytoin levels were found to have risen from 18.4 to 36.2 micrograms/ml. The phenytoin was temporarily stopped until his serum levels had fallen, and he was then discharged on a reduced phenytoin dosage of 400 and 500 mg on alternate days and had no further problems.[1] The presumption is that the fainting episode was due to the raised serum phenytoin levels.

(b) Tacrolimus levels

In one renal transplant patient on phenytoin, tacrolimus 250 micrograms/kg daily was needed to give a blood level of 9 nanograms/ml. Three months later phenytoin was gradually stopped, with gradual tapering of the tacrolimus dose. The patient was eventually maintained on a tacrolimus dose of 160 micrograms/kg daily giving a blood level of 11 nanograms/ml.[2]

Another report describes the use of intravenous phenytoin infusion for treating acute tacrolimus overdose in 2 patients, with the aim of enhancing tacrolimus metabolism.[3]

Mechanism

Tacrolimus is extensively metabolised by the cytochrome P450 isoenzyme CYP3A4, and phenytoin is a known inducer of this system. Phenytoin is therefore predicted to decrease tacrolimus levels. In the first case, it was suggested that tacrolimus might have inhibited the metabolism of phenytoin, although other factors may have had some part to play in the raised phenytoin levels.[1]

Importance and management

No interaction is established, but based on the known metabolism of these drugs it would be prudent to monitor tacrolimus levels in a patient given phenytoin. Similarly, based on the single case of phenytoin toxicity, it may also be advisable to monitor phenytoin levels.

1. Thompson PA, Mosley CA. Tacrolimus-phenytoin interaction. *Ann Pharmacother* (1996) 30, 544.
2. Moreno M, Latorre C, Manzanares C, Morales E, Herrero JC, Dominguez-Gil B, Carreño A, Cubas A, Delgado M, Andres A, Morales JM. Clinical management of tacrolimus drug interactions in renal transplant patients. *Transplant Proc* (1999) 31, 2252–3.
3. Karasu Z, Gurakar A, Carlson J, Pennington S, Kerwin B, Wright H, Nour B, Sebastian A. Acute tacrolimus overdose and treatment with phenytoin in liver transplant recipients. *J Okla State Med Assoc* (2001) 94, 121–3.

Tacrolimus + Proton pump inhibitors

Lansoprazole may increase tacrolimus levels in patients with low levels of the cytochrome P450 isoenzyme CYP2C19. Omeprazole and pantoprazole are predicted to interact similarly. Rabeprazole appears not to interact with tacrolimus.

Clinical evidence

A 57-year-old woman taking tacrolimus following a kidney transplant was started on **lansoprazole** 30 mg daily 19 days after her transplant because of a peptic ulcer. After 3 days her tacrolimus level rose from a range of 16.3 to 17.6 nanograms/ml up to 26.7 nanograms/ml. The tacrolimus dose was reduced, and levels of 12 to 15.4 nanograms/ml were achieved. When **lansoprazole** was replaced by famotidine the tacrolimus levels reduced to 8 nanograms/ml. The patient was later switched from famotidine to **rabeprazole** 10 mg daily without any further alteration in tacrolimus levels.[1,2]

There is also a further report of a patient who had no significant alteration in tacrolimus levels when **rabeprazole** 10 mg daily was started and stopped.[2]

Another study in 6 transplant patients taking tacrolimus found that **pantoprazole** 40 mg once daily for 5 days did not significantly affect the trough levels of tacrolimus.[3]

Mechanism

Two of the patients reported above[1,2] had decreased activity of the cytochrome P450 isoenzyme CYP2C19, by which lansoprazole is mainly metabolised. When levels of this enzyme are low, CYP3A4 (which normally only metabolises a fraction of lansoprazole) becomes more important in the metabolism of lansoprazole, and drug interactions involving CYP3A4 become more likely. Tacrolimus is metabolised by CYP3A4, and therefore competition with lansoprazole for metabolism may have led to raised tacrolimus levels. Pantoprazole may interact similarly in poor metabolisers.[3] Rabeprazole is metabolised non-enzymatically and therefore does not seem to interact.[1,2]

Importance and management

The incidence of the interaction between tacrolimus and lansoprazole is unknown. It would seem to only occur in those with decreased CYP2C19 activity, and therefore it is not easy to predict which patients would be affected. The makers of tacrolimus say that this interaction will occur with **omeprazole**, which is metabolised in the same way as lansoprazole. It would seem prudent to monitor tacrolimus levels if either of these proton pump inhibitors is started or stopped. Although no interaction was noted in the study with pantoprazole[3] the authors do note that it may interact like lansoprazole in patients with CYP2C19 deficiency. Rabeprazole may be a suitable alternative proton pump inhibitor as limited evidence suggests that it does not interact, and nor would it be expected to do so.

1. Homma M, Itagaki F, Yuzawa K, Fukao K, Kohda Y. Effects of lansoprazole and rabeprazole on tacrolimus blood concentration: case of a renal transplant recipient with CYP2C19 gene mutation. *Transplantation* (2002) 73, 303–4.
2. Itagaki F, Homma M, Yuzawa K, Fukao K, Kohda Y. Drug interaction of tacrolimus and proton pump inhibitors in renal transplant recipients with CYP2C19 gene mutation. *Transplant Proc* (2002) 34, 2777–8.
3. Lorf T, Ramadori G, Ringe B, Schwörer H. The effect of pantoprazole on tacrolimus and cyclosporin A blood concentration in transplant recipients. *Eur J Clin Pharmacol* (2000) 56, 439–40.

Tacrolimus + Quinolones

Levofloxacin modestly raised tacrolimus levels in one study. *In vitro*, enoxacin had no effect on tacrolimus metabolism.

Clinical evidence, mechanism, importance and management

Enoxacin, the quinolone with the greatest effect on the cytochrome P450 isoenzymes, has been found in *in vitro* studies to have almost no effect on tacrolimus metabolism by the cytochrome P450 isoenzyme CYP3A4.[1] Nor, despite some changes in interleukin-2 production caused by **ciprofloxacin**, does there appear to be a clinically relevant immunological interaction, which would oppose the immunosuppressant activity of tacrolimus.[2]

However, on the basis of some quite unexpected rises in drug levels and subsequent nephrotoxicity in a handful of patients treated with another similarly metabolised immunosuppressant, ciclosporin, and quinolone antibacterials (see 'Ciclosporin + Antibacterials; Quinolones', p.776), one review suggested that good monitoring would be appropriate if tacrolimus is given with any quinolone.[3]

Later preliminary evidence, from a study in 5 kidney transplant patients,[4] which found that **levofloxacin** 500 mg twice daily for 5 days caused about a 25% increase in the 12-hour AUC and a 18% increase in the trough tacrolimus level, would seem to support this advice.

1. Iwasaki K, Matsuda H, Nagase K, Shiraga T, Tokuma Y, Uchida K. Effects of twenty-three drugs on the metabolism of FK506 by human liver microsomes. *Res Commun Chem Pathol Pharmacol* (1993) 82, 209–16.
2. Kelly PA, Burckart GJ, Anderson D, Shaprio R, Zeevi A. Ciprofloxacin does not block the antiproliferative effect of tacrolimus. *Transplantation* (1997) 63, 172–3.
3. Petersen DL, Singh N. Interactions between tacrolimus and antimicrobial agents. *Clin Infect Dis* (1997) 25, 1430–40.
4. Capone D, Carrano R, Gentile A, Palmiero G, Farella A, Andreucci VE, Basile V, Federico S. Pharmacokinetic interaction between tacrolimus and levofloxacin in kidney transplant recipients. *Nephrol Dial Transplant* (2001) 16, A207.

Tacrolimus + Rifamycins

Four liver transplant patients needed markedly increased tacrolimus dosages when rifampicin (rifampin) was added, and one renal transplant patient had markedly reduced tacrolimus levels. A pharmacokinetic study has shown rifampicin increases the

clearance and decreases the bioavailability of intravenous and oral tacrolimus. Rifabutin is unlikely to interact to the same extent, but given the magnitude of the interaction with rifampicin, caution is still warranted.

Clinical evidence

The trough serum tacrolimus concentrations of a 10-year-old boy with a liver transplant fell from 10 nanograms/ml to unmeasurable levels within 2 days of starting **rifampicin** (**rifampin**) 150 mg twice daily. His tacrolimus dosage was therefore doubled from 4 to 8 mg twice daily. When the **rifampicin** was later stopped the tacrolimus dosage had to be reduced to 3 mg twice daily to keep the serum levels within the 10 nanogram/ml range.[1]

An extremely marked reduction in serum tacrolimus levels occurred in a 10-month-old child with a liver transplant when **rifampicin** was given with tacrolimus. Tacrolimus levels fell to about a tenth of baseline levels.[2] This case has also been reported elsewhere.[3] In another case, this time in an adult, a tenfold increase was needed in the tacrolimus dosage to keep levels within the target range when **rifampicin** was started. However, despite levels with the acceptable range a biopsy showed suspected tacrolimus nephrotoxicity, which was considered to be possibly due to the cumulative tacrolimus dose, or to high levels of tacrolimus metabolites (which were not measured).[4] Another patient with a renal transplant had a decrease in tacrolimus levels from 9.2 to 1.4 nanograms/ml 2 days after starting rifampicin. **Rifampicin** was stopped and replaced by pyrazinamide, with a gradual return to the baseline tacrolimus level.[5] A study in 6 healthy subjects supports the findings of these case reports. In the study, **rifampicin** 600 mg daily significantly increased the clearance and decreased the bioavailability of both oral and intravenous tacrolimus.[6]

Mechanism

This interaction is thought to occur because rifampicin increases the metabolism of the tacrolimus by the liver and in the small bowel (by inducing the cytochrome P450 isoenzyme CYP3A4 and P-glycoprotein) so that it is cleared more rapidly.

Importance and management

What occurred in these reports is consistent with the way rifampicin interacts with many other drugs and therefore this interaction would seem to be of general clinical importance. It would be prudent to be alert for the need to raise the dosage of tacrolimus if rifampicin is added in any patient.

Direct information about **rifabutin** seems to be lacking, but any interaction with tacrolimus is likely to much less marked than with rifampicin because its enzyme inducing effects are considerably less. Nevertheless until the situation is clear it would be prudent to monitor concurrent use, being alert for the need to raise the tacrolimus dosage.

1. Furlan V, Perello L, Jacquemin E, Debray D, Taburet A-M. Interactions between FK506 and rifampicin or erythromycin in pediatric liver recipients. *Transplantation* (1995) 59, 1217–18.
2. Kiuchi T, Inomata Y, Uemoto S, Satomura K, Egawa H, Okajima H, Yamaoka Y, Tanaka K. A hepatic graft tuberculosis transmitted from a living-related donor. *Transplantation* (1997) 63, 905–7.
3. Kiuchi T, Tanaka K, Inomata Y, Uemoto S, Satomura K, Egawa H, Uyama S, Sano K, Okajima H, Yamaoka Y. Experience of tacrolimus-based immunosuppression in a living-related liver transplantation complicated with graft tuberculosis: interaction with rifampicin and side effects. *Transplant Proc* (1996) 28, 3171–2.
4. Chenhsu R-Y, Loong C-C, Chou M-H, Lin M-F, Yang W-C. Renal allograft dysfunction associated with rifampin-tacrolimus interaction. *Ann Pharmacother* (2000) 34, 27–31.
5. Moreno M, Latorre C, Manzanares C, Morales E, Herrero JC, Dominguez-Gil B, Carreño A, Cubas A, Delgado M, Andres A, Morales JM. Clinical management of tacrolimus drug interactions in renal transplant patients. *Transplant Proc* (1999) 31, 2252–3.
6. Hebert MF, Fisher RM, Marsh CL, Dressler D, Bekersky I. Effects of rifampin on tacrolimus pharmacokinetics in healthy volunteers. *J Clin Pharmacol* (1999) 39, 91–6.

Tacrolimus + Sildenafil

Sildenafil did not appear to affect the pharmacokinetics of tacrolimus. The levels of sildenafil were higher in patients on tacrolimus than in healthy subjects, but it is not clear whether this was due to tacrolimus alone. A marked blood pressure drop occurred on concurrent use.

Clinical evidence, mechanism, importance and management

In 10 men with erectile dysfunction taking tacrolimus after a kidney transplant, a single 50-mg dose of sildenafil did not affect the pharmacokinetics of tacrolimus. When the pharmacokinetics of sildenafil were compared with those quoted by the maker it was found that the maximum plasma concentration was 44% higher and the AUC was 90% larger in tacrolimus-treated patients. The AUC of the sildenafil metabolite was also raised. There are several possible reasons for these differences. The pharmacokinetics quoted by the makers are from healthy subjects, not patients, and the patients in the study were taking a multitude of other drugs, some of which could have affected sildenafil. Aside from the pharmacokinetic effects it was noted that the mean blood pressure dropped by 27/20 mmHg after sildenafil was given, which could be of significance in patients with cardiovascular disease. The authors suggest more study is needed regarding the safety of sildenafil in this type of patient and suggest that if sildenafil is used, a lower dose (25 mg) should be used.[1]

1. Christ B, Brockmeier D, Hauck EW, Friemann S. Interactions of sildenafil and tacrolimus in men with erectile dysfunction after kidney transplantation. *Urology* (2001) 58, 589–93.

Tacrolimus + Sirolimus

A single-dose study in 28 healthy subjects[1] found no pharmacokinetic interaction occurred between sirolimus and tacrolimus when they were given either at the same time, or 4 hours apart. Similarly, a multiple-dose study in 25 liver or kidney-pancreas transplant patients[2] given tacrolimus with a target trough level of 3 to 7 nanograms/ml found no nephrotoxicity and no pharmacokinetic interaction when sirolimus was also given, for 2 weeks.

1. Patat A, Zimmerman JJ, Parks V, Souan M. Lack of pharmacokinetic interaction co-administered of sirolimus and tacrolimus. *Clin Pharmacol Ther* (2003) 73, P43.
2. McAlister VC, Mahalati K, Peltekian KM, Fraser A, MacDonald AS. A clinical pharmacokinetic study of tacrolimus and sirolimus combination immunosuppression comparing simultaneous to separated administration. *Ther Drug Monit* (2002) 24, 346–50.

Tacrolimus + St John's wort *(Hypericum perforatum)*

St John's wort decreases tacrolimus levels.

Clinical evidence

In a clinical study 10 healthy subjects were given a single 100-microgram/kg dose of tacrolimus alone or after taking St John's wort 300 mg three times daily for 14 days. On average St John's wort decreased the maximum serum concentration of tacrolimus by 65% and the AUC by 32%. However, the decrease in AUC ranged from 15% to 64%, with one patient having a 31% *increase* in AUC.[1] Similar results have been found in a study in 10 renal transplant patients given St John's wort (*Jarsin300*) 600 mg daily for 2 weeks. In order to achieve target levels, the tacrolimus dose was increased in all patients from a median of 4.5 mg daily to 8 mg daily. Two weeks after stopping St John's wort, tacrolimus doses were reduced to a median of 6.5 mg daily, and to the original dose at about 4 weeks.[2]

A case report describes a 65-year-old patient taking tacrolimus following a kidney transplant. The patient started to take St John's wort (*Neuroplant*) 600 mg daily, and after one month the tacrolimus levels had dropped from a range of 6 to 10 nanograms/ml down to 1.6 nanograms/ml, with an unexpected improvement in creatinine levels. When the St John's wort was stopped, tacrolimus levels and creatinine returned to the previous range. Subsequently a lower target range of tacrolimus was set.[3]

Mechanism

St John's wort induces the cytochrome P450 isoenzyme CYP3A4 and affects the transport substance P-glycoprotein. Both CYP3A4 and P-glycoprotein are involved in the clearance of tacrolimus, so an increase in their effects would be expected to result in a decrease in tacrolimus levels.[1,3]

Importance and management

Although the evidence currently seems limited to these reports the interaction between tacrolimus and St John's wort has been predicted from the pharmacokinetics of these two drugs. Given the unpredictability of the interaction (and the variability in content of St John's wort products) it would seem prudent to avoid St John's wort in transplant patients, and possibly other types of patient taking tacrolimus. If St John's wort is withdrawn monitor tacrolimus levels and adjust the dose accordingly.

1. Hebert MF, Park JM, Chen Y-L, Akhtar S, Larson AM. Effects of St John's wort (Hypericum perforatum) on tacrolimus pharmacokinetics in healthy volunteers. *J Clin Pharmacol* (2004) 44, 89–94.
2. Mai I, Störmer E, Bauer S, Krüger H, Budde K, Roots I. Impact of St John's wort treatment on the pharmacokinetics of tacrolimus and mycophenolic acid in renal transplant patients. *Nephrol Dial Transplant* (2003) 18, 819–22.
3. Bolley R, Zülke C, Kammerl M, Fischereder M, Krämer BK. Tacrolimus-induced nephrotoxicity unmasked by induction of the CYP3A4 system with St John's wort. *Transplantation* (2002) 73, 1009.

Tacrolimus + Theophylline

An isolated report suggests that theophylline may increase serum tacrolimus levels.

Clinical evidence, mechanism, importance and management

A kidney transplant patient taking tacrolimus 7 mg daily was given theophylline 600 mg daily to treat post-transplant erythrocytosis. After 1 month the serum creatinine increased from 110 to 145 micromol/l and the tacrolimus trough blood concentration increased to 16 nanograms/ml, from a range of 5 to 15 nanograms/ml. The theophylline dosage was reduced to 300 mg daily on 4 days of each week and a month later the serum creatinine and trough tacrolimus levels were 175 micromol/l and 48.5 nanograms/ml respectively. Theophylline was discontinued and renal function and trough tacrolimus levels rapidly returned to normal. The pharmacokinetics of tacrolimus were later assessed in the same patient. Theophylline 125 mg on 4 days of the week was associated with an almost fivefold increase in the tacrolimus AUC and an increase in the peak serum tacrolimus levels from 19.3 to 37.4 nanograms/ml, without significant alterations in renal function on this occasion.[1]

Mechanism

Unclear. An *in vitro* study found that tacrolimus and theophylline exhibited a negligible effect on each others metabolism.[2] However, the authors of the case report suggest that theophylline levels in their patient could have been sufficient to inhibit the cytochrome P450 isoenzyme-mediated metabolism of tacrolimus.[1]

Importance and management

Direct information seems to be limited to this single case report. The authors conclude that low dose theophylline may be given to transplant patients with erythrocytosis provided that tacrolimus levels are closely monitored.[1] However, this interaction is unconfirmed and of uncertain clinical significance. There is insufficient evidence to recommend increased monitoring in every patient, but be aware of the potential for an interaction in the case of an unexpected response to treatment.

1. Boubenider S, Vincent I, Lambotte O, Roy S, Hiesse C, Taburet A-M, Charpentier B. Interaction between theophylline and tacrolimus in a renal transplant patient. *Nephrol Dial Transplant* (2000) 15, 1066–8.
2. Matsuda H, Iwasaki K, Shiraga T, Tozuka Z, Hata T, Guengerich FP. Interactions of FK506 (tacrolimus) with clinically important drugs. *Res Commun Mol Pathol Pharmacol* (1996) 91, 57–64.

28

Lipid-regulating drugs

This section is concerned with those drugs which are used for dyslipidaemias (i.e. disturbed levels of lipids in the blood). In the very broadest of terms (and ideally) they lower the blood levels of cholesterol and low density lipoprotein (LDL), and raise those of high density lipoprotein (HDL). Such drugs include the statins (more properly known as HMG CoA (hydroxymethylglutaryl-coenzyme A) reductase inhibitors), fibrates, bile acid binding resins (e.g. colestipol, colestyramine) and nicotinic acid (niacin) and related drugs. These are listed in 'Table 28.1', below.

Table 28.1 Lipid-regulating drugs

Group	*Drugs*
Bile-acid binding resins	Colesevelam, Colestilan, Colestipol, Colestyramine
Fibrates	Bezafibrate, Ciprofibrate, Clofibrate, Fenofibrate, Gemfibrozil
Statins	Atorvastatin, Cerivastatin, Fluvastatin, Lovastatin, Pravastatin, Simvastatin, Rosuvastatin
Miscellaneous	Acipimox, Ezetimibe, Nicotinic acid

(a) Statins

Statins are generally well-tolerated, but have two major but relatively uncommon side effects. They raise liver enzymes and can cause skeletal muscle disorders (e.g. myalgia, myopathy and rhabdomyolysis). Rhabdomyolysis is a syndrome resulting from skeletal muscle injury, which results in the release of the enzyme creatine kinase (among other things) into the circulation. Creatine kinase (CK) is also known as creatine phosphokinase (CPK). Both terms are used throughout the text, the choice being dependent on the term used in the source quoted. Rhabdomyolysis can range from asymptomatic elevations in creatine kinase to acute renal failure, and in its severest form may be life-threatening. As well as elevated creatinine kinase levels, signs and symptoms of rhabdomyolysis include muscle pain and weakness, reddish-brown urine (myoglobinuria).[1]

Just how statins cause muscle disorders is as yet unclear, although it is thought to be connected to elevated statin levels.[2] Any pharmacokinetic interactions that result in marked rises in statin levels are therefore to be regarded seriously.

One of the ways blood statin levels can become elevated is if the interacting drug inhibits the metabolism of the statin, with the result that it is cleared from the body more slowly and it begins to accumulate. Atorvastatin, lovastatin and simvastatin are all extensively metabolised by the cytochrome P450 isoenzyme CYP3A4 so that drugs that can inhibit this enzyme can cause marked rises in blood statin levels. But some of the statins are not metabolised by this enzyme so they interact differently. Fluvastatin is metabolised primarily by isoenzyme CYP2C9, rosuvastatin by CYP2C9 and CYP2C19, while the cytochrome P450 system does not appear to be involved in the metabolism of pravastatin.[3]

The statins are also P-glycoprotein substrates, and may therefore interact due to competition for this carrier, generally resulting in altered oral bioavailability.[3] Some metabolites of atorvastatin, lovastatin and simvastatin have been shown to inhibit P-glycoprotein, while fluvastatin and pravastatin seem to have little effect.[4] There appears to be no data on the effect of rosuvastatin on P-glycoprotein.[5]

The overall risk of myopathy with the statins is quite low and commonly quoted as 0.5%, although one report[6] puts the incidence of mild myopathies with the statin alone as up to 7%. The incidence seems to rise markedly if other drugs are being taken concurrently. Thus a literature review of published reports for the period 1985 to 2000 found 15 cases of rhabdomyolysis with statins alone, but 54 cases when combined with other drugs.[2]

In order to reduce the risk of myopathy the CSM advise that statins should be used with care in patients who are at increased risk of this adverse effect. Among other risk factors, they mention concomitant use with fibrates, such as 'gemfibrozil', (p.836), and with inhibitors of CYP3A4 such as 'ciclosporin', (p.834), 'macrolides', (p.838), 'azoles', (p.831), and 'protease inhibitors', (p.841). They also recommend that patients should be made aware of the risks of myopathy and rhabdomyolysis, and asked to promptly report muscle pain, tenderness or weakness, especially if accompanied by malaise, fever or dark urine.[7]

(b) Bile-acid binding resins

Bile-acid binding resins lower cholesterol by binding with bile acids in the gastrointestinal tract to form an insoluble complex that is excreted in the faeces. This predisposes them to interactions, by binding with other drugs in the same way as they do with bile acids, which prevents absorption or local action of the affected drug. These binding interactions are not covered here, but are covered under the affected drugs. A new bile-acid binding resin, colesevelam, is supposed to be devoid of clinically significant drug-binding interactions.[8]

(c) Fibrates

Fibrates are protein bound drugs that are metabolised via the cytochrome P450 isoenzyme CYP3A4. They are not generally recognised as inhibitors of this enzyme. Although protein binding contributes to their interactions, this mechanism does not usually lead to interactions of the magnitude seen with the fibrates. This leaves their mechanism of interaction largely unexplained, although recent study suggests they may act as inhibitors of glucuronidation.[9] As with the statins (see above), fibrates are also recognised as causing myopathies, and the risk of this appears to be greatly increased when they are given with statins, see 'Statins + Fibrates', p.836.

(d) Nicotinic acid

Nicotinic acid has little effect on the cytochrome P450 isoenzyme system and is therefore unlikely to result in significant pharmacokinetic interactions. It also appears to increase the risk of myopathies when given with statins, see 'Statins + Nicotinic acid (Niacin)', p.840.

This section covers interactions affecting lipid-regulating drugs. Where lipid-regulating drugs affect other drugs the interactions are covered elsewhere. The Index should be consulted for a full listing.

1. Allison RC, Bedsole DL. The other medical causes of rhabdomyolysis. *Am J Med Sci* (2003) 326, 79–88.
2. Omar MA, Wilson JP, Cox TS. Rhabdomyolysis and HMG-CoA reductase inhibitors. *Ann Pharmacother* (2001) 35, 1096–1107.
3. Williams D, Feely J. Pharmacokinetic-pharmacodynamic drug interactions with HMG-CoA reductase inhibitors. *Clin Pharmacokinet* (2002) 41, 343–70.
4. Bogman K, Peyer AK, Torok M, Kusters E, Drewe J. HMG-CoA reductase inhibitors and P-glycoprotein modulation. *Br J Pharmacol* (2001) 132, 1183–92.
5. Roach AE, Tsikouris JP, Haase KK. Rosuvastatin. A new HMG-CoA reductase inhibitor for hypercholesterolemia. *Formulary* (2002) 37, 179–85.
6. Ucar M, Mjorndal T, Dahlqvist R, HMG CoA reductase inhibitors and myotoxicity. *Drug Safety* (2000) 22, 441–57.
7. Committee on Safety of Medicines/Medicines Control Agency. HMG CoA reductase inhibitors (statins) and myopathy. *Current Problems* (2002) 28, 8–9.
8. Donovan JM, Stypinski D, Stiles MR, Olson TA, Burke SK. Drug interactions with colesevelam hydrochloride, a novel, potent lipid-lowering agent. *Cardiovasc Drugs Ther* (2000) 14, 681–90.
9. Prueksaritanont T, Zhao JJ, Ma B, Roadcap BA, Tang C, Qui Y, Liu L, Lin JH, Pearson PG, Baillie TA. Mechanistic studies on metabolic interactions between gemfibrozil and statins. *J Pharmacol Exp Ther* (2002) 301, 1042–51.

Acipimox + Colestyramine

Colestyramine does not appear to affect the pharmacokinetics of acipimox significantly.

Clinical evidence, mechanism, importance and management

A randomised crossover study in 7 healthy subjects given 150 mg of acipimox with 4 g of colestyramine, followed by two additional 4-g doses of colestyramine 8 and 16 hours later, showed that the pharmacokinetics of acipimox were slightly, but not significantly altered by the colestyramine.[1] There would seem to be no good reason for avoiding concurrent use.

1. De Paolis C, Farina R, Pianezzola E, Valzelli G, Celotti F, Pontiroli AE. Lack of pharmacokinetic interaction between cholestyramine and acipimox, a new lipid lowering agent. *Br J Clin Pharmacol* (1986) 22, 496–7.

Colestyramine + Food

Food does not interact with colestyramine.

Clinical evidence, mechanism, importance and management

A study in 10 patients with type IIA hyperlipoproteinaemia found that the efficacy of colestyramine in controlling total cholesterol and low density lipoprotein levels was unaltered whether the colestyramine was taken with or before **meals**.[1]

1. Sirtori M, Pazzucconi F, Gianfranceschi G, Sirtori CR. Efficacy of cholestyramine does not vary when taken before or during meals. *Atherosclerosis* (1991) 88, 249–52.

Ezetimibe + Ciclosporin

Ciclosporin may greatly elevate ezetimibe levels, and the combination should be used with caution.

Clinical evidence, mechanism, importance and management

In one study, 8 renal transplant patients stabilised on ciclosporin were given a single 10-mg dose of ezetimibe. When compared with other data from healthy control subjects, the AUC of ezetimibe was found to be 3.4-fold higher in the patients on ciclosporin.[1] A further patient with severe renal impairment on multiple drugs including ciclosporin also demonstrated a 12-fold increase in the AUC of ezetimibe.[1] The makers do not contraindicate the combination, but advise caution,[1] and suggest that the outcome should be carefully monitored.[2] Note that doses of ezetimibe 5 times those recommended were well-tolerated in 15 subjects when taken for 2 weeks.[1,2]

1. Ezetrol (Ezetimibe). MSD-SP Ltd. UK Summary of product characteristics, June 2005.
2. Zetia (Ezetimibe). Merck/Schering-Plough Pharmaceuticals. US Prescribing information, March 2003.

Fibrates + Bile-acid binding resins

Colestyramine does not alter the pharmacokinetics of clofibrate when given at the same time, and similarly colestipol does not alter the pharmacokinetics of clofibrate or fenofibrate. Colestipol can reduce the absorption of gemfibrozil if given at the same time, but not if separated by 2 hours.

Clinical evidence, mechanism, importance and management

(a) Clofibrate

Over a 6-day period no clinically relevant changes in the pharmacokinetics of clofibrate occurred in 24 healthy subjects, when given daily doses of 10 g of **colestipol** at the same time as 500 mg of clofibrate.[1] **Colestyramine** 4 g four times daily had no effect on the fasting plasma levels, urinary and faecal excretion, or the half-life of clofibrate in 6 patients taking 1 g of clofibrate twice daily. In this study, the morning and evening doses of **colestyramine** were taken at the same time as the clofibrate.[2] No special precautions would seem to be needed.

(b) Fenofibrate

Over a 6-day period no clinically relevant changes in the pharmacokinetics of fenofibrate occurred in 18 healthy subjects, when given daily doses of 10 g of **colestipol** at the same time as 200 mg of fenofibrate in the morning, and 5 g of **colestipol** at the same time as 100 mg of fenofibrate in the evening.[3] No special precautions would seem to be needed.

(c) Gemfibrozil

A study in 10 patients with raised serum cholesterol and triglyceride levels found that if 600 mg of gemfibrozil was given alone, 2 hours before or 2 hours after 5 g of **colestipol**, the serum gemfibrozil concentration curves were similar. However, when both drugs were given at the same time, the AUC of gemfibrozil was reduced by about a third.[4] Another study found that combined use of gemfibrozil and **colestipol** (doses not separated) enhanced the LDL-lowering effects of both drugs, but tended to mitigate the HDL-raising effects of the gemfibrozil.[5] Combined use is effective, but information is very limited about the clinical importance of the reduction in gemfibrozil bioavailability. However, the interaction can be avoided by separating the administration of the two drugs by at least 2 hours.

1. DeSante KA, DiSante AR, Albert KS, Weber DJ, Welch RD, Vecchio TJ. The effect of colestipol hydrochloride on the bioavailability and pharmacokinetics of clofibrate. *J Clin Pharmacol* (1979) 19, 721–25.
2. Sedaghat A, Ahrens EH. Lack of effect of cholestyramine on the pharmacokinetics of clofibrate in man. *Eur J Clin Invest* (1975) 5, 177–85.
3. Harvengt C, Desager JP. Lack of pharmacokinetic interaction of colestipol and fenofibrate in volunteers. *Eur J Clin Pharmacol* (1980) 17, 459–63.
4. Forland SC, Feng Y, Cutler RE. Apparent reduced absorption of gemfibrozil when given with colestipol. *J Clin Pharmacol* (1990) 30, 29–32.
5. East C, Bilheimer DW, Grundy SM. Combination drug therapy for familial combined hyperlipidemia. *Ann Intern Med* (1988) 109, 25–32.

Fibrates + Diuretics

Treatment with clofibrate in patients with nephrotic syndrome receiving furosemide (frusemide) has sometimes led to marked diuresis and severe and disabling muscular symptoms. An isolated report describes rhabdomyolysis in a patient on bezafibrate and furosemide.

Clinical evidence

(a) Bezafibrate

An isolated report attributed acute renal failure and rhabdomyolysis in a patient to treatment with 400 mg bezafibrate daily and 25 mg **furosemide** on alternate days.[1]

(b) Clofibrate

Three patients with hyperlipoproteinaemia secondary to nephrotic syndrome, receiving 80 to 500 mg **furosemide** daily, developed severe muscle pain, low lumbar backache, stiffness and general malaise with pronounced diuresis within 3 days of receiving additional treatment with 1 to 2 g of clofibrate daily. Similarly, muscle symptoms occurred within 3 days of starting clofibrate in a patient on **bendroflumethiazide** 10 mg daily. Of these four patients, three had documented raised serum transaminases or creatine phosphokinase.

Two other patients had raised levels of serum transaminases or creatine phosphokinase during treatment with clofibrate and **furosemide**.

A further study in 4 of the six patients discussed above and 4 healthy controls, free serum clofibrate was markedly higher in the patients, and this correlated with low serum albumin, and urinary clofibrate excretion was markedly delayed.[2]

Mechanism

Not understood. The marked diuresis may have been due to competition and displacement of the furosemide by the clofibrate from its plasma protein binding sites. Clofibrate occasionally causes a muscle toxicity, which could have been exacerbated by the urinary loss of Na^+ and K^+ and the increase in the half-life of clofibrate. The reason for the bezafibrate/furosemide-induced rhabdomyolysis is unknown.

Importance and management

The clinical documentation seems to be limited to these reports. It appears to be a combination of a drug-drug interaction (clofibrate/furosemide) with or without a drug-disease interaction (clofibrate/nephrotic syndrome). The authors of one report[2] suggest that serum proteins and renal function should be checked before giving clofibrate to any patient. If serum albumin is low, the total daily dosage of clofibrate should not exceed 500 mg for each 1 g per 100 ml of the albumin concentration. More study is needed.

1. Venzano C, Cordì GC, Corsi L, Dapelo M, De Micheli A, Grimaldi GP. Un caso di rabdomiolisi acuta con insufficienza renale acuta da assunzione contemporanea di furosemide e bezafibrato. *Minerva Med* (1990) 81, 909–11.
2. Bridgman JF, Rosen SM, Thorp JM. Complications during clofibrate treatment of nephrotic-syndrome hyperlipoproteinaemia. *Lancet* (1972) ii, 506–9.

Fibrates + Ezetimibe

Ezetimibe did not alter fenofibrate pharmacokinetics. Fenofibrate and gemfibrozil may modestly increase ezetimibe levels, although this is unlikely to be clinically relevant. The makers currently advise against concurrent use, because of the theoretical increased risk of gallstone formation.

Clinical evidence, mechanism, importance and management

In a randomised placebo-controlled study, 32 otherwise healthy patients with hypercholesterolaemia were given **fenofibrate** 200 mg daily, ezetimibe 10 mg daily, both drugs in combination, or placebo daily for 14 days. The combination was well-tolerated, and resulted in an increased reduction in LDL-cholesterol than that seen with either active drug alone. Ezetimibe had no effect on the pharmacokinetics of **fenofibrate,** and **fenofibrate** had no clinically relevant effect on the pharmacokinetics of ezetimibe.[1]

The makers report that **fenofibrate** and **gemfibrozil** caused 1.5- and 1.7-fold increases in ezetimibe concentrations, although these are not expected to be clinically significant.[2]

Despite these seemingly favourable results, the makers of ezetimibe do not recommend the combination until it has been further studied. This is because both fibrates and ezetimibe increase cholesterol excretion into the bile, which could promote the production of gallstones.[2]

1. Kosoglou T, Guillaume M, Sun S, Pember LJC, Reyderman L, Statkevich P, Cutler DL, Veltri EP, Affrime MB. Pharmacodynamic interaction between fenofibrate and the cholesterol absorption inhibitor ezetimibe. *Atherosclerosis* (2001) 2 (Suppl 2), 38.
2. Ezetrol (Ezetimibe). MSD-SP Ltd. UK Summary of product characteristics, June 2005.

Fibrates + Rifampicin (Rifampin)

Preliminary evidence shows that rifampicin can reduce the plasma levels of the active metabolite of clofibrate, but rifampicin apparently has no effect on gemfibrozil.

Clinical evidence, mechanism, importance and management

(a) Ciprofibrate

A 35% reduction in the steady-state plasma levels of the active metabolite of clofibrate, chlorophenoxyisobutyric acid (CIPB) was seen in 5 healthy subjects after taking 600 mg rifampicin daily for 7 days.[1] The reason appears to be that metabolism of CIPB by the liver and/or the kidneys is increased.[1] This is consistent with the well-recognised and potent enzyme inducing activity of rifampicin. On the basis of this study it would now be prudent to monitor serum lipid levels of patients if rifampicin is added, and to increase the clofibrate dosage if necessary. More study is needed to establish this interaction.

(b) Gemfibrozil

Rifampicin 600 mg daily for 6 days was found not to significantly affect the pharmacokinetics of 600 mg of gemfibrozil in 10 healthy subjects.[2] No special precautions seem necessary.

1. Houin G, Tillement J-P. Clofibrate and enzymatic induction in man. *Int J Clin Pharmacol Ther Toxicol* (1978) 16, 150–4.
2. Forland SC, Feng Y, Cutler RE. The effect of rifampin on the pharmacokinetics of gemfibrozil. *J Clin Pharmacol* (1988) 28, 930.

Fibrates; Ciprofibrate + Ibuprofen

An isolated report describes acute renal failure and rhabdomyolysis in a patient on ciprofibrate when ibuprofen was added.

Clinical evidence, mechanism, importance and management

A 29-year-old man with type M hyperlipidaemia[1] who had been receiving 100 mg of ciprofibrate daily for 6 months began to take 200 mg and then 400 mg ibuprofen daily for a painful heel. The pain became general, his urine turned 'muddy', he complained of having a 'stiff body', and he rapidly developed acute renal failure. His serum creatinine concentration was found to be 647 micromol/l and creatine kinase activity was 13,740 units/l.

The reasons for this reaction are not known, but the authors of the report postulate that the ibuprofen displaced the ciprofibrate from its binding sites, thereby turning a safe dose into a toxic one.[1] However, it should be said that this mechanism of interaction is rarely important on its own, so it seems likely that some other factors may have contributed to what happened.

This is an isolated case so that its general importance is unknown, but it is probably very small.

1. Ramachadran S, Giles PD, Hartland A. Acute renal failure due to rhabdomyolysis in presence of concurrent ciprofibrate and ibuprofen treatment. *BMJ* (1997) 314, 1593.

Fibrates; Clofibrate + Oral contraceptives

Oral contraceptives increase the loss of clofibrate from the body, but the significance of this is unclear.

Clinical evidence, mechanism, importance and management

A comparative study in men, women, and women taking combined oral contraceptives found that the clearance of clofibrate was increased by 48% in those taking combined oral contraceptives, apparently due to an increase in its metabolism (glucuronidation).[1] Another study found that combined oral contraceptives increased the excretion of clofibric acid glucuronide (the pharmacologically active form of clofibrate) by 25%.[2] None of these studies addressed the question of whether concurrent use significantly reduces clofibrate efficacy, but it would seem prudent to monitor for increases in blood lipid levels. It should be noted that combined oral contraceptives themselves can have various adverse effects on lipid levels, and these may oppose the effects of treatment.

1. Miners JO, Robson RA, Birkett DJ. Gender and oral contraceptive steroids as determinants of drug glucuronidation: effects on clofibric acid elimination. *Br J Clin Pharmacol* (1984) 18, 240–43.
2. Liu H-F, Magdalou J, Nicolas A, Lafaurie C, Siest G. Oral contraceptives stimulate the excretion of clofibric acid glucuronide in women and female rats. *Gen Pharmacol* (1991) 22, 393–7.

Fibrates; Clofibrate + Probenecid

Plasma clofibrate levels can be approximately doubled by probenecid, but the clinical significance of this is unclear.

Clinical evidence, mechanism, importance and management

A pharmacokinetic study in 4 healthy subjects taking 500 mg clofibrate 12-hourly showed that 500 mg of probenecid 6-hourly for 7 days almost doubled the steady-state clofibric acid levels, from 72 to 129 mg/l, and raised the free clofibric acid levels from 2.5 to 9.1 mg/l. The suggested reason is that the probenecid reduces the renal and metabolic clearance of the clofibrate by inhibiting its conjugation with glucuronic acid.[1] The clinical importance of this interaction is uncertain. It appears not to have been assessed.

1. Veenendaal JR, Brooks PM, Meffin PJ. Probenecid-clofibrate interaction. *Clin Pharmacol Ther* (1981) 29, 351–8.

Fibrates; Gemfibrozil + Antacids

Antacids can reduce the absorption of gemfibrozil.

Clinical evidence, mechanism, importance and management

A study in patients with kidney and liver disease showed that the concurrent use of antacids (**aluminium hydroxide, aluminium magnesium silica hydrate**) reduced the maximum plasma gemfibrozil levels by about 50 to 70%, and the AUC by about 30 to 60%. The precise values are not given in the text. The reasons for these reductions are not known, but adsorption of the gemfibrozil onto the antacids within the gut is suggested. The authors recommend that gemfibrozil is given 1 to 2 hours before antacids.[1] More study is needed to confirm these findings.

1. Knauf H, Kölle EU, Mutschler E. Gemfibrozil absorption and elimination in kidney and liver disease. *Klin Wochenschr* (1990) 68, 692–8.

Fibrates; Gemfibrozil + Psyllium

Psyllium causes a small, but almost certainly clinically unimportant, reduction in the absorption of gemfibrozil.

Clinical evidence, mechanism, importance and management

When 600 mg of gemfibrozil was taken by 10 healthy subjects with, or 2 hours after 3 g psyllium in 240 ml water, the AUC was reduced by about 10%.[1] This change in bioavailability is almost certainly too small to matter. No special precautions would seem to be necessary on concurrent use.

1. Forland SC, Cutler RE. The effect of psyllium on the pharmacokinetics of gemfibrozil. *Clin Res* (1990) 38, 94A.

Nicotinic acid (Niacin) + Aspirin

Aspirin reduces the flushing reaction that often occurs with nicotinic acid, but there is some evidence that it can also increase nicotinic acid plasma levels. The importance of this latter reaction is uncertain.

Clinical evidence, mechanism, importance and management

Nicotinic acid (70 to 100 micrograms/kg per minute as an infusion over 6 hours) was given to 6 healthy subjects. When the subjects were also given 1 g of aspirin orally 2 hours after the infusion was started, the plasma nicotinic acid levels rose markedly, due to a 30 to 54% decrease in its clearance.[1] The probable reason is that the salicylate competes with the nicotinic acid for metabolism by glycine conjugation in the liver so that the clearance of nicotinic acid is reduced, resulting in a rise in its levels. The clinical importance of this when aspirin is given to reduce the annoying nicotinic acid flushing reaction[2] is not known.

1. Ding RW, Kolbe K, Merz B, de Vries J, Weber E, Benet LZ. Pharmacokinetics of nicotinic acid-salicylic acid interaction. *Clin Pharmacol Ther* (1989) 46, 642–7.
2. Jungnickel PW, Maloley PA, Vander Tuin EL, Peddicord TE, Campbell JR. Effect of two aspirin pretreatment regimens on niacin-induced cutaneous reactions. *J Gen Intern Med* (1997) 12, 591–6.

Nicotinic acid (Niacin) + Nicotine

An isolated report describes an unpleasant flushing reaction that developed in a woman taking nicotinic acid when she started to use nicotine transdermal patches.

Clinical evidence, mechanism, importance and management

A woman was treated with 250 mg nicotinic acid twice daily for 3 years without problems, as well as nifedipine, ranitidine, colestyramine and ferrous sulfate. Following laryngectomy for cancer of the larynx, she restarted all of the drugs except the colestyramine and began to use nicotine transdermal patches 21 mg daily to try to give up smoking. On several occasions, shortly after taking the nicotinic acid, she developed unpleasant flushing episodes lasting about 30 minutes. No further episodes developed when the nicotinic acid was stopped.[1] The reasons are not understood, but flushing is a very common side-effect of nicotinic acid, and it would seem that in this case the nicotine patch may have been responsible for its emergence. This reaction is more unpleasant than serious. A comment on this report suggests that this reaction may possibly have an immunological basis.[2]

1. Rockwell KA. Potential interaction between niacin and transdermal nicotine. *Ann Pharmacother* (1993) 27, 1283–4.
2. Sudan BJL. Comment: niacin, nicotine, and flushing. *Ann Pharmacother* (1994) 28, 1113.

Statins + ACE inhibitors

In clinical trials, the safety and efficacy of statins were not altered by concurrent use of ACE inhibitors as a class. Moexipril has been reported not to interact adversely with cholesterol-lowering agents and in one study simvastatin did not alter the pharmacokinetics or ACE-inhibitory effects of ramipril. An isolated report describes severe hyperkalaemia in a diabetic when given lisinopril and lovastatin.

Clinical evidence, mechanism, importance and management

Retrospective analysis of clinical study data found no evidence that the safety of **lovastatin** was altered by the use of unspecified ACE inhibitors in 142 patients.[1] Another retrospective analysis of clinical trial data found no evidence that the safety or efficacy of **fluvastatin** was altered by the use of unspecified ACE inhibitors.[2] Likewise, the UK maker of **atorvastatin**[3] say that in clinical studies it was used concurrently with ACE inhibitors without evidence of significant adverse interactions. A study in healthy subjects found that **simvastatin** had no effect on the pharmacokinetics or ACE-inhibitory effects of **ramipril** or its metabolites.[4] Similarly, no evidence of clinically important adverse interactions was found when **moexipril** was used with **cholesterol-lowering agents** [not specifically named].[5] An isolated report describes a type I diabetic (on insulin) with hypertension and hyperlipidaemia who developed myositis and severe hyperkalaemia (serum potassium 8.4 mmol/l) when treated with **lovastatin** 20 to 40 mg daily and **lisinopril** 50 mg daily. His serum potassium returned to about 5.5 mmol/l after the **lovastatin** was stopped and the dosage of **lisinopril** lowered to 20 mg daily. About 3 months later, the patient resumed taking the **lovastatin**, but after only 2 doses he again had severe myositis and hyperkalaemia, which resolved after the **lovastatin** was discontinued. The reason seemed to be a combination of the hyperkalaemic effects of the **lisinopril**, the release of intracellular potassium into the blood stream associated with the myositis caused by the **lovastatin**, and a predisposition to hyperkalaemia due to the diabetes and mild renal impairment.[6] This is an unusual case and unlikely to be of general importance.

No special precautions would seem to be necessary if ACE inhibitors are given concurrently with statins.

1. Pool JL, Shear CL, Downton M, Schnaper H, Stinnett S, Dujovne C, Bradford RH, Chremos AN. Lovastatin and coadministered antihypertensive/cardiovascular agents. *Hypertension* (1992) 19, 242–8.
2. Peters TK, Jewitt-Harris J, Mehra M, Muratti EN. Safety and tolerability of fluvastatin with concomitant use of antihypertensive agents. An analysis of a clinical trial database. *Am J Hypertens* (1993) 6, 346S–352S.
3. Lipitor (Atorvastatin). Parke Davis. UK Summary of product characteristics, March 2005.
4. Meyer BH, Scholtz HE, Müller FO, Luus HG, de la Rey N, Seibert-Grafe M, Eckert HG, Metzger H. Lack of interaction between ramipril and simvastatin. *Eur J Clin Pharmacol* (1994) 47, 373–5.
5. Perdix (Moexipril). Schwarz Pharma Ltd. Product Monograph. Data on file, October 1995.
6. Edelman S, Witztum JL. Hyperkalemia during treatment with HMG-CoA reductase inhibitor. *N Engl J Med* (1989) 320, 1219–20.

Statins + Amiodarone

There is some evidence of a high incidence of myopathy when amiodarone is given with high doses of simvastatin. One case of myopathy and one of rhabdomyolysis have been reported in patients on the combination.

Clinical evidence, mechanism, importance and management

The makers of **simvastatin** note that in an ongoing unpublished clinical trial, myopathy (clinically significant muscle pain with a CK (creatinine kinase) at least 10 times the upper limit of normal[1]) has been reported in 6% of patients receiving **simvastatin** 80 mg daily with amiodarone.[2-4] There is some evidence from reports to the US Food and Drug Administration that concurrent use of **simvastatin** with amiodarone is associated with a higher incidence of muscle toxicity than **pravastatin**. They reported that the percentage of reports of muscle, liver, pancreas, and bone marrow toxicity associated with statins and involving concurrent amiodarone was 1% for **simvastatin** and 0.4% for **pravastatin**.[5]

A 63-year-old man developed diffuse muscle pain with generalised muscular weakness 4 weeks after starting **simvastatin** 40 mg daily, and about 2 weeks after starting amiodarone 1 g daily for 10 days, then 200 mg daily thereafter. There was a marked increase in CK, which normalised after stopping both drugs.[6] A 77-year-old man on multiple medications including amiodarone 100 mg daily and **simvastatin** 20 mg daily, developed increasing lower-extremity pain and darkening of his urine 3 weeks after his **simvastatin** dose was increased to 40 mg daily. He was diagnosed with rhabdomyolysis secondary to **simvastatin** use,[7] although a later comment suggested that amiodarone could have contributed.[8]

Amiodarone is an inhibitor of various cytochrome P450 isoenzymes. Whether it inhibits the metabolism of **simvastatin** and other extensively-metabolised statins, and thereby increases the risk of muscle toxicity, is not known. Amiodarone alone may sometimes cause myopathy.

The interaction is not established. However, one maker in the UK recommends that the dose of **simvastatin** should not exceed 20 mg daily in patients also on amiodarone unless the clinical benefit is likely to outweigh the increased risk of myopathy and rhabdomyolysis.[2] Another contraindicates the combination.[3] The US maker advises only using doses of **simvastatin** above 20 mg if the benefits outweigh the risks.[4]

Until more is known, caution is certainly warranted. **Pravastatin** appears less likely to interact.

1. Ponte CD, Wratchford P. Amiodarone's role in simvastatin-associated rhabdomyolysis. *Am J Health-Syst Pharm* (2003) 60, 1791–2.
2. Zocor (Simvastatin). Merck Sharp & Dohme Ltd. UK Summary of product characteristics, July 2004.
3. Simvador (Simvastatin). Discovery Pharmaceuticals. UK Summary of product characteristics, July 2003.
4. Zocor (Simvastatin). Merck & Co,. Inc. US Prescribing information, November 2004.
5. Alsheikh-Ali AA, Karas RH. Adverse events with concomitant amiodarone and statin therapy. *Prev Cardiol* (2005) 8, 95–7.
6. Roten L, Schoenenberger RA, Krähenbühl S, Schlienger RG. Rhabdomyolysis in association with simvastatin and amiodarone. *Ann Pharmacother* (2004) 38, 978–81.
7. Wratchford P, Ponte CD. High-dose simvastatin and rhabdomyolysis. *Am J Health-Syst Pharm* (2003) 60, 698–700.
8. de Denus S, Spinler SA. Amiodarone's role in simvastatin-associated rhabdomyolysis. *Am J Health-Syst Pharm* (2003) 60, 1791.

Statins + Antacids

An aluminium/magnesium hydroxide antacid (*Maalox*) causes a moderate reduction in the bioavailability of atorvastatin and pravastatin, but this does not appear to reduce their lipid-lowering efficacy.

Clinical evidence, mechanism, importance and management

In a multiple-dose study, 18 patients were given 10 mg of **atorvastatin** daily for 15 days followed by additional treatment with 30 ml of an **aluminium/magnesium hydroxide** antacid *(Maalox TC)* four times daily for a further 17 days. The maximum serum levels and AUC of **atorvastatin** were reduced by 34%, and the absorption rate was also reduced by the antacid. However, the LDL-cholesterol reduction remained the same.[1] The concurrent use of the same antacid *(Maalox TC)* 15 ml four times daily, given one hour before **pravastatin**, reduced the bioavailability of a single 20-mg dose of **pravastatin** by 28%. This change was less than that seen with food, which did not alter efficacy.[2]

There is therefore no need to avoid the concurrent use of **aluminium/magnesium hydroxide** antacids such as *Maalox*, nor does the dosage of **atorvastatin** or **pravastatin** need to be raised.

1. Yang B-B, Smithers JA, Abel RB, Stern RH, Sedman AJ, Olson SC. Effects of Maalox TC® on pharmacokinetics and pharmacodynamics of atorvastatin. *Pharm Res* (1996) 13 (9 Suppl), S437.
2. ER Squibb . A report on the comparative pharmacokinetics of pravastatin in the presence and absence of cimetidine or antacids in healthy male subjects. Data on file. (Protocol No 27, 201-43), 1988.

Statins + Azoles

Fluconazole modestly increases the levels of fluvastatin and rosuvastatin, but not pravastatin. Itraconazole causes a marked rise in the serum levels of atorvastatin, lovastatin, pravastatin and simvastatin, but no change in fluvastatin or rosuvastatin levels. Ketoconazole also has no significant effect on rosuvastatin levels. Rhabdomyolysis has been reported with itraconazole or ketoconazole and simvastatin, and with unnamed azoles and atorvastatin or lovastatin.

Clinical evidence

(a) Atorvastatin

Ten healthy subjects were given 200 mg of **itraconazole** daily for 5 days, and on day 4 they were additionally given a single 40-mg dose of atorvastatin. The **itraconazole** increased the AUC of atorvastatin acid and atorvastatin lactone fourfold and threefold respectively, and increased their half-lives threefold and twofold respectively. The AUC values of active and total HMG-CoA reductase inhibitors were increased 1.6- and 1.7-fold respectively.[1] In a similar study,[2] the same dose of **itraconazole** increased the AUC of atorvastatin by 150% and of atorvastatin lactone by 193%.

In a review of the FDA spontaneous reports of statin-associated rhabdomyolysis covering the period November 1997 to March 2000, an azole antifungal was potentially implicated in 2 cases involving atorvastatin.[3]

(b) Fluvastatin

A randomised double-blind trial in 12 healthy subjects found that **fluconazole** (400 mg on day 1 followed by 200 mg daily for 3 days) increased the AUC of a single 40 mg dose of fluvastatin by 84% and increased its maximum plasma level by 44%. The pharmacokinetics of the fluconazole were unaffected.[4] In a similar study using **itraconazole** 100 mg daily for 4 days, fluvastatin pharmacokinetics were largely unchanged, apart from a small increase in half life.[5]

(c) Lovastatin

Itraconazole 200 mg daily or a placebo was given to 12 healthy subjects for 4 days in a double-blind crossover study. On day 4 they were additionally given a single 40-mg oral dose of lovastatin. On average the peak plasma concentration and the 24-hour AUC of the lovastatin were increased more than 20-fold. The peak plasma concentration of the active metabolite of lovastatin, lovastatin acid, was increased 13-fold (range 10 to 23-fold) and its AUC 20-fold. The creatine kinase activity of one subject increased 10-fold, but in the other 11 subjects it remained unchanged. Brief mention is also made of severe rhabdomyolysis in one patient given lovastatin and **itraconazole**.[6] Another study also found similar pharmacokinetic changes.[5]

A 63-year-old woman who had been on 80 mg of lovastatin and 3 g of nicotinic acid daily, plus timolol and aspirin for almost 10 years without problems, developed weakness and tenderness in her arms, back and legs within two weeks of starting 100 mg **itraconazole** twice daily. A few days later her urine became brown, and positive for haem. She was diagnosed as having acute rhabdomyolysis and hepatotoxicity. The lovastatin, nicotinic acid and **itraconazole** were stopped, and she was treated with ubidecarenone. Over the next 18 days her elevated serum enzymes returned to normal, although her plasma cholesterol levels almost doubled. She was restarted on nicotinic acid 11 weeks later without problems.[7]

In a review of the FDA spontaneous reports of statin-associated rhabdomyolysis covering the period November 1997 to March 2000, an azole antifungal was potentially implicated in 6 cases involving lovastatin.[3]

(d) Pravastatin

A randomised double-blind trial in 12 healthy subjects found that **fluconazole** (400 mg on day 1 followed by 200 mg daily for 3 days) had no significant effect on the pharmacokinetics of a single 40-mg dose of pravastatin.[4]

The AUC of a single 40-mg dose of pravastatin was increased by 71% in 10 healthy subjects after taking 200 mg of **itraconazole** daily for 4 days, although this did not reach statistical significance.[8] In a similar study, the same dosage of **itraconazole** caused a modest 51% increase in the AUC of pravastatin.[2]

(e) Rosuvastatin

Fluconazole 200 mg once daily for 11 days increased the AUC and maximum plasma concentration of rosuvastatin (given on day 8) by 14% and 9% respectively in 14 healthy subjects. The proportion of circulating active HMG-CoA reductase inhibitors was not affected by **fluconazole**.[9] In similar studies by the same workers, **itraconazole**[10] and **ketoconazole**[11] also had no clinically significant effect on the levels of rosuvastatin.

(f) Simvastatin

In a two-phase crossover study, 10 healthy subjects were given 200 mg of **itraconazole** or a placebo daily for 4 days, and then on day 4 they were given a single 40-mg dose of simvastatin. The peak serum levels of total simvastatin acid (simvastatin acid + simvastatin lactone) were increased 17-fold and the AUC 19-fold. The maximum serum levels of total HMG-CoA reductase inhibitors increased about 3-fold and the AUC 5-fold.[8]

A 74-year-old who had been on 40 mg of simvastatin daily, lisinopril and aspirin for about a year without problems developed pain in his feet, and then in his arms and neck, within 3 weeks of starting **itraconazole** 200 mg daily. His urine turned brown, his muscles were tender, and abnormal serum creatine kinase and other enzyme levels were found. A diagnosis of rhabdomyolysis was made.[12] Two other similar cases have been reported in patients on simvastatin within 3 to 4 weeks of starting **ketoconazole** 200 or 400 mg daily.[13] A 70-year-old with a kidney transplant was on, among many other drugs, ciclosporin and simvastatin 40 mg daily. Despite the high dose of simvastatin, even in conjunction with ciclosporin (see also 'Statins + Ciclosporin', p.834), he had experienced no problems. Within 2 weeks of starting **itraconazole** 100 mg twice daily he developed malaise and general muscle weakness with elevated creatine kinase levels, which was diagnosed as rhabdomyolysis. His serum simvastatin levels were found to be raised, as were those of a later volunteer subject whose simvastatin serum levels rose from 0.5 to 6.5 nanogram/ml within a day of starting **itraconazole** 200 mg daily.[14] Two further similar cases have also been reported with simvastatin/ciclosporin/**itraconazole**.[15,16] In a review of the FDA spontaneous reports of statin-associated rhabdomyolysis covering the period November 1997 to March 2000, an azole antifungal was potentially implicated in 4 cases involving simvastatin.[3]

Mechanism

Fluconazole inhibits the cytochrome P450 isoenzymes CYP2C9 and CYP3A4, while itraconazole and ketoconazole are strong inhibitors of CYP3A4. Consequently their interaction profile differs amongst the various statins depending on which isoenzymes are involved in the metabolism of the statins; this has been shown in several studies.[2,4,5] From these studies it appears that the effect of itraconazole is greatest on lovastatin and simvastatin, with a marked effect on atorvastatin, a modest effect on pravastatin or rosuvastatin, and no effect on fluvastatin. Fluconazole has a marked effect on fluvastatin, but no effect on pravastatin. See 'Lipid-regulating drugs', (p.827) for further discussion on the metabolism of the statins.

Importance and management

An established interaction of clinical importance. The very marked increases in levels of lovastatin and simvastatin that can occur considerably increase the risk of severe muscle damage and use with itraconazole or ketoconazole should therefore be avoided. If a short course of an azole antifungal is considered essential, the makers suggest temporary withdrawal of the statin.[17,18] Although the increase in levels of atorvastatin are not as great, they are still marked, and the combination of azole antifungal with atorvastatin should probably also be avoided. The clinical relevance of the modest changes in fluvastatin or pravastatin levels with different azole antifungals is less clear. Note that in a review of the FDA spontaneous reports of statin-associated rhabdomyolysis for the period November 1997 to March 2000, azole antifungals were not identified as a potentially interacting drug in any of the reports for fluvastatin or pravastatin.[3] The situation with **voriconazole** is as yet unclear. The makers predict that it will interact with statins metabolised by the cytochrome P450 isoenzyme CYP3A4, resulting in elevated statin levels, and possibly rhabdomyolysis. They suggest that a dosage reduction of the statin should be considered during concurrent administration.[19,20] As yet there seem to be no reports of this interaction in practice, but the advice given seems a sensible precaution. Because of the potential seriousness of this interaction, any patient given a statin/azole combination should be told to report any unexplained muscle pain, tenderness or weakness.

1. Kantola T, Kivistö KT, Neuvonen PJ. Effect of itraconazole on the pharmacokinetics of atorvastatin. *Clin Pharmacol Ther* (1998) 64, 58–65.
2. Mazzu AL, Lasseter KC, Shamblen E, Cooper BS, Agarwal V, Lettieri J, Sundaresen P. Itraconazole alters the pharmacokinetics of atorvastatin to a greater extent than either cerivastatin or pravastatin. *Clin Pharmacol Ther* (2000) 68, 391–400.
3. Omar MA, Wilson JP. FDA adverse event reports on statin-associated rhabdomyolysis. *Ann Pharmacother* (2002) 36, 288–95.
4. Kantola T, Backman JT, Niemi M, Kivistö KT, Neuvonen PJ. Effect of fluconazole on plasma fluvastatin and pravastatin concentrations. *Eur J Clin Pharmacol* (2000) 56, 225–9.
5. Kivistö KT, Kantola T, Neuvonen PJ. Different effects of itraconazole on the pharmacokinetics of fluvastatin and lovastatin. *Br J Clin Pharmacol* (1998) 46, 49–53.
6. Neuvonen PJ, Jalava K-M. Itraconazole drastically increases plasma concentrations of lovastatin and lovastatin acid. *Clin Pharmacol Ther* (1996) 60, 54–61.
7. Lees RS, Lees AM. Rhabdomyolysis from the coadministration of lovastatin and the antifungal agent itraconazole. *N Engl J Med* (1995) 333, 664–5.
8. Neuvonen PJ, Kantola T, Kivistö KT. Simvastatin but not pravastatin is very susceptible to interaction with CYP3A4 inhibitor itraconazole. *Clin Pharmacol Ther* (1998) 332–41.
9. Cooper KJ, Martin PD, Dane AL, Warwick MJ, Schneck DW, Cantarini MV. The effect of fluconazole on the pharmacokinetics of rosuvastatin. *Eur J Clin Pharmacol* (2002) 58, 527–31.
10. Cooper KJ, Martin PD, Dane AL, Warwick MJ, Schneck DW, Cantarini MV. Effect of itraconazole on the pharmacokinetics of rosuvastatin. *Clin Pharmacol Ther* (2003) 73, 322–9.
11. Cooper KJ, Martin PD, Dane AL, Warwick MJ, Raza A, Schneck DW. Lack of effect of ketoconazole on the pharmacokinetics of rosuvastatin in healthy subjects. *Br J Clin Pharmacol* (2003) 55, 94–9.
12. Horn M. Coadministration of itraconazole with hypolipidemic agents may induce rhabdomyolysis in healthy individuals. *Arch Dermatol* (1996) 132, 1254.
13. Gilad R, Lampl Y. Rhabdomyolysis induced by simvastatin and ketoconazole treatment. *Clin Neuropharmacol* (1999) 22, 295–7.
14. Segaert MF, De Soete C, Vandewiele I, Verbanck J. Drug-interaction-induced rhabdomyolysis. *Nephrol Dial Transplant* (1996) 11, 1846–7.
15. Malouf MA, Bicknell M, Glanville AR. Rhabdomyolysis after lung transplantation. *Aust N Z J Med* (1997) 27, 186.
16. Vlahakos DV, Manginas A, Chilidou D, Zamanika C, Alivizatos PA. Itraconazole-induced rhabdomyolysis and acute renal failure in a heart transplant recipient treated with simvastatin and cyclosporine. *Transplantation* (2002) 73, 1962–4.
17. Mevacor (Lovastatin). Merck & Co., Inc. US Prescribing information, April 2005.
18. Zocor (Simvastatin). Merck Sharp & Dohme. UK Summary of product characteristics, July 2004.
19. VFEND (Voriconazole). Pfizer Ltd. UK Summary of product characteristics, March 2005.
20. VFEND (Voriconazole). Pfizer Inc. US Prescribing information, March 2005.

Statins + Beta-blockers

Propranolol does not cause any clinically relevant changes to the pharmacokinetics of fluvastatin, lovastatin or pravastatin. In clinical trials, the safety and efficacy of statins were not altered by concurrent use of beta blockers as a class.

Clinical evidence, mechanism, importance and management

The pharmacokinetics of a single 40-mg dose of **fluvastatin** was not affected by the concurrent use of 40 mg **propranolol** 12-hourly for 3 days in 24 healthy subjects.[1] Similarly, the same dose of **propranolol** caused less than an 18% reduction in the AUC of **lovastatin** (after a 20-mg dose) and its metabolites, and modestly reduced the AUC of **pravastatin** (after a 20-mg dose) and its metabolites by 16 to 23%.[2] These changes are small and unlikely to be clinically relevant.

Retrospective analysis of clinical trial data found no evidence that the safety or efficacy of **fluvastatin** was altered by the use of beta blockers (unspecified).[3] Similarly, in another analysis, there was no evidence that the safety or efficacy of **lovastatin** was altered by selective beta blockers (primarily **atenolol, metoprolol** and **labetalol**) or non-selective beta blockers (primarily **propranolol**, **nadolol** and **timolol**).[4] Likewise, the maker of **atorvastatin**[5] says that in clinical studies it was used concurrently with beta blockers without evidence of significant adverse interactions.

No special precautions would seem to be necessary if beta blockers are given concurrently with statins.

1. Smith HT, Jokubaitis LA, Troendle AJ, Hwang DS, Robinson WT. Pharmacokinetics of fluvastatin and specific drug interactions. *Am J Hypertens* (1993) 6, 375S–382S.
2. Pan HY, Triscari J, DeVault AR, Smith SA, Wang-Iverson D, Swanson BN, Willard DA. Pharmacokinetic interaction between propranolol and the HMG-CoA reductase inhibitors pravastatin and lovastatin. *Br J Clin Pharmacol* (1991) 31, 665–70.
3. Peters TK, Jewitt-Harris J, Mehra M, Muratti EN. Safety and tolerability of fluvastatin with concomitant use of antihypertensive agents. An analysis of a clinical trial database. *Am J Hypertens* (1993) 6, 346S–352S.
4. Pool JL, Shear CL, Downton M, Schnaper H, Stinnett S, Dujovne C, Bradford RH, Chremos AN. Lovastatin and coadministered antihypertensive/cardiovascular agents. *Hypertension* (1992) 19, 242–8.
5. Lipitor (Atorvastatin). Parke Davis. UK Summary of product characteristics, March 2005.

Statins + Bile-acid binding resins

Although colestyramine and colestipol reduce plasma fluvastatin and pravastatin levels, the overall total lipid-lowering effect is increased by concurrent use. Separating their administration minimises this interaction. Colestipol appears to interact with atorvastatin similarly. Colesevelam appears not to interact with lovastatin.

Clinical evidence

(a) Atorvastatin

A study in which atorvastatin and **colestipol** were given concurrently found that although the serum levels of atorvastatin were reduced by about 25%, the total reduction in the LDL-cholesterol levels was greater than when each drug was given alone.[1]

(b) Fluvastatin

Colestyramine 8 g administered at the same time as fluvastatin 20 mg decreased the AUC and the maximum plasma levels of fluvastatin in 19 healthy subjects by 89 and 96% respectively. When the fluvastatin was given 2 hours after the **colestyramine**, the AUC and the maximum plasma levels of fluvastatin were reduced by just over 50%.[2] In another study in 20 healthy subjects, the AUC and maximum plasma levels of fluvastatin were reduced by 51 and 82% respectively when fluvastatin was taken 4 hours after 8 g of **colestyramine** and a meal.[2]

Despite these marked reductions in fluvastatin bioavailability, other studies in large numbers of hypercholesterolaemic patients have shown that concurrent use has in fact additive lipid-lowering effects.[2,3] In the first of these studies, fluvastatin was administered 4 hours after **colestyramine,**[2] but the other study did not indicate whether or not doses were separated.[3]

(c) Lovastatin

An open-label crossover study in 22 healthy subjects found that the pharmacokinetics of lovastatin 20 mg given with a meal were not significantly affected when **colesevelam** 2.25 g was given at the same time.[4]

(d) Pravastatin

Thirty-three patients with primary hypercholesterolaemia were given 5, 10, or 20 mg twice daily before their morning and evening meals for 4 weeks and then for a further 4 weeks they additionally took colestyramine 24 g daily. The **colestyramine** was taken at least an hour after the pravastatin. Despite the fact that the **colestyramine** reduced the bioavailability of the pravastatin by 18 to 49%, the blood lipid level reduction caused by pravastatin was enhanced by the addition of the **colestyramine**.[5] A related study in 18 subjects found that **colestyramine** reduced the bioavailability of pravastatin by about 40% when given together, but only small and clinically insignificant pharmacokinetic changes occurred when the pravastatin was given one hour before, or 4 hours after the **colestyramine**.[6] Similarly, a multicentre study involving 311 patients found that combined use of 40 mg of pravastatin and 12 g of **colestyramine** daily was highly effective in the treatment of hypercholesterolaemia. The **colestyramine** was taken at least an hour after the pravastatin.[7]

Colestipol reduced the bioavailability of pravastatin in 18 subjects by about 50%, but no reduction in bioavailability was seen when pravastatin was given 1 hour before **colestipol** and a meal.[6]

Mechanism

It seems probable that these bile-acid binding resins bind with statins in the gut and thereby reduce the amount of statin available for absorption.

Importance and management

Established interactions but of only relatively minor importance. Despite the reduction in the bioavailability of pravastatin caused by colestyramine or colestipol, the overall lipid-lowering effect is increased by concurrent use.[5,7] The effects of the interaction can be minimised by separating their administration as described above. This can be easily achieved by taking the colestyramine or colestipol with meals, and the pravastatin at bedtime. Similarly, any interaction between fluvastatin and colestyramine can be minimised by taking fluvastatin at least 4 hours after colestyramine. There would appear to be no reason for avoiding concurrent use of atorvastatin and colestipol, nor lovastatin and colesevelam.

1. Lipitor (Atorvastatin). Parke Davis. UK Summary of product characteristics, March 2005.
2. Smith HT, Jokubaitis LA, Troendle AJ, Hwang DS, Robinson WT. Pharmacokinetics of fluvastatin and specific drug interactions. *Am J Hypertens* (1993) 6, 375S–382S.
3. Hagen E, Istad H, Ose L, Bodd E, Eriksen H-M, Selvig V, Bard JM, Fruchart JC, Borge M, Wolf M-C, Pfister P. Fluvastatin efficacy and tolerability in comparison and in combination with cholestyramine. *Eur J Clin Pharmacol* (1994) 46, 445–9.
4. Donovan JM, Kisicki JC, Stiles MR, Tracewell WG, Burke SK. Effect of colesevelam on lovastatin pharmacokinetics. *Ann Pharmacother* (2002) 36, 392–7.
5. Pan HY, DeVault AR, Swites BJ, Whigan D, Ivashkiv E, Willard DA, Brescia D. Pharmacokinetics and pharmacodynamics of pravastatin alone and with cholestyramine in hypercholesterolemia. *Clin Pharmacol Ther* (1990) 48, 201–7.
6. Pan HY, DeVault AR, Ivashkiv E, Whigan D, Brennan JJ, Willard DA. Pharmacokinetic interaction studies of pravastatin with bile-acid-binding resins. 8th International Symposium on Atherosclerosis, Rome, October 9-13, 1988. 711.
7. Pravastatin Multicenter Study Group II. Comparative efficacy and safety of pravastatin and cholestyramine alone and combined in patients with hypercholesterolemia. *Arch Intern Med* (1993) 153, 1321–9.

Statins + Calcium channel blockers

Although marked rises in statin plasma levels have been seen with lovastatin/diltiazem, simvastatin/diltiazem, simvastatin/verapamil, and isolated cases of rhabdomyolysis with atorvastatin/diltiazem and simvastatin/diltiazem, it seems that problems with combinations of statins and calcium channel blockers are rare.

Clinical evidence

(a) Atorvastatin

The makers say that **amlodipine** does not affect the pharmacokinetics of atorvastatin.[1] They also say that no clinically significant interactions were seen in clinical studies in which atorvastatin was used with antihypertensives including unspecified calcium channel blockers.[1] However, the makers do warn that drugs that are metabolised by the cytochrome P450 isoenzyme CYP3A4 (e.g. some calcium-channel blockers) do have the potential to interact.[1] This statement is supported by a case of rhabdomyolysis in a 60-year-old man, 3 weeks after **diltiazem** was added to treatment with atorvastatin 20 mg daily.[2]

(b) Fluvastatin

A retrospective study of the effects of antihypertensives on the efficacy of fluvastatin found that the concurrent use of unspecified calcium channel blockers did not significantly affect the safety or lipid lowering effects of fluvastatin, although there was a trend towards enhanced lowering of triglycerides.[3]

(c) Lovastatin

A retrospective study of the effects of lovastatin and antihypertensive medication found that when calcium channel blockers (**diltiazem**, **nifedipine** or **verapamil**) were used in combination with lovastatin there was an additional 3 to 5% lowering in the LDL-cholesterol, which was of marginal significance.[4] Pharmacokinetic studies have shown that oral **diltiazem** increases the AUC and maximum serum levels of lovastatin about fourfold.[5,6] In another study, lovastatin 20 mg and **isradipine** 5 mg was given to 12 healthy subjects either alone or together for 5 days. The lovastatin AUC was reduced by 40%, in males but not females, by the concurrent use of **isradipine**.[7]

(d) Pravastatin

A study in 10 subjects found that sustained-release **diltiazem** 120 mg twice daily had no effect on the pharmacokinetics of single-dose pravastatin.[5]

(e) Simvastatin

A single 20-mg dose of simvastatin was given to 10 healthy subjects after they had taken sustained-release **diltiazem** 120 mg twice daily, for 2 weeks. **Diltiazem** caused about a fivefold increase in the simvastatin AUC, a fourfold increase in the maximum serum levels, and a 2.5-fold increase in the half life.[8] A similar study, in which 12 subjects were given **verapamil** 80 mg three times daily found a 4.6-fold increase in the simvastatin AUC, a 2.6-fold increase in the maximum serum levels, and about a 2-fold increase in the half life.[9] An *in vitro* study using human liver microsomes also found that both **diltiazem** and **verapamil** moderately inhibited simvastatin metabolism.[10]

The clinical relevance of the **diltiazem** interaction was demonstrated in a 53-year-old man, who developed rhabdomyolysis 3 months after **diltiazem** 30 mg four times daily was added to established treatment with simvastatin 40 mg daily. Both drugs were discontinued and he recovered over the following 10 days.[11] Another similar case has also been reported.[12]

Mechanism

It is known that diltiazem, isradipine and verapamil inhibit the cytochrome P450 isoenzyme CYP3A4, and it is therefore probable that those statins which show rises in plasma levels do so because their metabolism is reduced by these calcium channel blockers. One study showed that diltiazem given orally would interact, but not when given intravenously, suggesting that it is CYP3A4 in the gut wall that is the site of the interaction.[13] See 'Lipid-regulating drugs', (p.827) for more information about the way statins are metabolised.

Importance and management

Information is limited, but what is known suggests that the concurrent use of these drugs is normally uneventful. Even with those pairs of drugs where the increases in plasma levels are quite large (lovastatin/diltiazem, simvastatin/diltiazem and simvastatin/verapamil) problems seem to be very rare. Concurrent use need not be avoided, but it has been suggested that treatment with a statin in a patient on diltiazem (and probably verapamil and isradipine) should be started with the lowest possible dose and titrated upwards, or considerably reduced[9] if for example diltiazem is started. To be absolutely on the safe side, all patients given any drug pair (statin + calcium channel blocker) should be told to be alert for any signs of possible rhabdomyolysis (i.e. otherwise unexplained muscle tenderness, pain or weakness or dark coloured urine).

1. Lipitor (Atorvastatin). Parke Davis. UK Summary of product characteristics, March 2005.
2. Lewin JJ, Nappi JM, Taylor MH. Rhabdomyolysis with concurrent atorvastatin and diltiazem. *Ann Pharmacother* (2002) 36, 1546–9.
3. Peters TK, Jewitt-Harris J, Mehra M, Muratti EN. Safety and tolerability of fluvastatin with concomitant use of antihypertensive agents. An analysis of a clinical trial database. *Am J Hypertens* (1993) 6, 346S–352S.
4. Pool JL, Shear CL, Downton M, Schnaper H, Stinnett S, Dujovne C, Bradford RH, Chremos AN. Lovastatin and coadministered antihypertensive/cardiovascular agents. *Hypertension* (1992) 19, 242–8.
5. Agbim NE, Brater DC, Hall SD. Interaction of diltiazem with lovastatin and pravastatin. *Clin Pharmacol Ther* (1996) 61, 201.
6. Jones DR, Azie NE, Masica BA, Brater DC, Hall SD. Oral but not intravenous (IV) diltiazem impairs lovastatin clearance. *Clin Pharmacol Ther* (1999) 65, 149.
7. Zhou LX, Finley DK, Hassell AE, Holtzman JL. Pharmacokinetic interaction between isradipine and lovastatin in normal, female and male volunteers. *J Pharmacol Exp Ther* (1995) 273, 121–7.
8. Mousa O, Brater DC, Sunblad KJ, Hall SD. The interaction of diltiazem with simvastatin. *Clin Pharmacol Ther* (2000) 67, 267–74.
9. Kantola T, Kivistö KT, Neuvonen PJ. Erythromycin and verapamil considerably increase serum simvastatin and simvastatin acid concentrations. *Clin Pharmacol Ther* (1998) 64, 177–82.
10. Yeo KR, Yeo WW. Inhibitory effects of verapamil and diltiazem on simvastatin metabolism in human liver microsomes. *Br J Clin Pharmacol* (2001) 51, 461–70.
11. Kanathur N, Mathai MG, Byrd RP, Fields CL, Roy TM. Simvastatin-diltiazem drug interaction resulting in rhabdomyolysis and hepatitis. *Tenn Med* (2001) 94, 339–41.
12. Peces R, Pobes A. Rhabdomyolysis associated with concurrent use of simvastatin and diltiazem. *Nephron* (2001) 89, 117–18.
13. Masica AL, Azie NE, Brater C, Hall SD, Jones DR. Intravenous diltiazem and CYP3A-mediated metabolism. *Br J Clin Pharmacol* (2000) 50, 273–6.

Statins + Ciclosporin

Ciclosporin can cause marked rises in the plasma levels of fluvastatin, lovastatin, pravastatin and simvastatin, and for some of the statins this had led to the development of serious myopathy (rhabdomyolysis) accompanied by kidney failure. Rhabdomyolysis has also been reported with atorvastatin/ciclosporin. The plasma levels of ciclosporin appear not to be affected by fluvastatin, lovastatin or pravastatin, but some moderate changes have been seen when atorvastatin or simvastatin were used.

Clinical evidence

(a) Atorvastatin

The effect of ciclosporin on atorvastatin levels does not appear to have been studied, but a case of rhabdomyolysis has been described in a woman after taking both drugs for 2 months.[1] In a review of the FDA spontaneous reports of statin-associated rhabdomyolysis covering the period November 1997 to March 2000, ciclosporin was potentially implicated in 5 cases involving atorvastatin.[2]

In a study of 10 patients on ciclosporin following a kidney transplant, 4 showed increases in their trough ciclosporin levels of between 26 and 54% when atorvastatin 10 mg was added, necessitating a dosage reduction of ciclosporin. No changes were seen in 6 other patients, and the incidence of adverse effects was no greater than in a control transplant group not given atorvastatin.[3]

(b) Fluvastatin

The AUC and maximum serum concentration of fluvastatin were found to be about 94 and 30% higher respectively in transplant patients on ciclosporin than in historical control patients not on ciclosporin.[4] Similarly, the AUC and maximum serum concentration of fluvastatin were threefold and sixfold greater in transplant patients on ciclosporin than in healthy subjects not given ciclosporin.[5] A further study in 20 renal transplant patients receiving fluvastatin 20 mg daily reported 2 patients with mild myalgia without creatine phosphokinase (CPK) rises, and a patient with elevated CPK without myalgia when ciclosporin was also given.[6]

When fluvastatin 20 mg daily was given to 16 patients on ciclosporin 21 to 103 months after renal transplantation no significant changes were seen in their ciclosporin levels, no rise was seen in CPK and no additional adverse events were reported.[7,8] Similar results were seen in another study using fluvastatin 20 mg twice daily.[9]

(c) Lovastatin

The plasma levels of lovastatin in 6 patients on ciclosporin given lovastatin 10 to 20 mg daily were about the same as those seen in healthy subjects receiving a 40 mg dose.[10] In another study in 21 renal transplant patients on ciclosporin, the maximum serum levels and AUC of lovastatin 20 mg daily were 40 and 47% higher respectively 28 days after beginning therapy than on day 1 (suggesting accumulation) and were estimated to be 20-fold higher than values reported in healthy subjects not on ciclosporin.[11] A further study found that lovastatin AUCs were five times greater in patients on ciclosporin than in patients not taking ciclosporin, irrespective of whether the patients had received transplants or were receiving other immunosuppressants.[12]

There are at least 9 documented cases of rhabdomyolysis, often resulting in acute renal failure, in patients receiving ciclosporin and lovastatin.[13-17] In each of these cases the patient was receiving lovastatin 40 to 80 mg daily. Several other studies highlight this dose-related effect. In one study, 15 patients on ciclosporin were additionally given lovastatin 20 mg daily without problem, but 4 of 5 other patients, who were receiving lovastatin 40 to 80 mg daily developed rhabdomyolysis, which was associated with renal failure in two of them.[18] A further study in 24 patients, who were either given lovastatin 10 or 20 mg daily in addition to ciclosporin. Of the 12 receiving the 20-mg dose, 7 developed either myalgia and muscle weakness or raised creatine phosphokinase levels (CPK), but only one patient from the 10-mg group did.[19]

Ciclosporin and CPK levels were not significantly changed in 6 renal transplant patients taking ciclosporin and lovastatin (10 mg for 8 weeks, then 20 mg for 12 weeks).[10] Similar results were found in another study.[20]

The incidence of myopathies with lovastatin is about 0.1 to 0.2%,[11] but in the presence of ciclosporin the incidence is said to be as high as 30%.[21]

(d) Pravastatin

Although a study in patients on ciclosporin found that the AUC of pravastatin 20 mg daily did not differ between day 1 and day 28 of therapy (suggesting no accumulation), the AUC values were estimated to be five to sevenfold higher than in patients not on ciclosporin.[11] In a review of the FDA spontaneous reports of statin-associated rhabdomyolysis covering the period November 1997 to March 2000, ciclosporin was potentially implicated in 2 cases involving pravastatin.[2] A single-dose study found that the maximum serum levels and AUC of pravastatin in a group of transplant patients on ciclosporin were sevenfold and twentyfold greater respectively than those in patients receiving pravastatin without ciclosporin.[22]

Several studies have shown no rises in creatine phosphokinase levels,[23-25] no change in ciclosporin levels[11,24] and no increase in adverse effects[11,23,26] when pravastatin in doses of 10 to 40 mg daily was given concurrently.

(e) Rosuvastatin

Rosuvastatin, which was marketed in the UK in 2003 is currently contraindicated with ciclosporin, because although ciclosporin is apparently unaffected by concurrent use, the AUC of rosuvastatin is increased sevenfold.[27]

(f) Simvastatin

A group of 20 heart transplant patients were treated with both simvastatin 10 mg daily and ciclosporin over a period of 4 months[28] and the plasma levels of simvastatin acid were at least 6 times higher in 7 patients on ciclosporin than in 7 control patients not on ciclosporin. Similarly, a study comparing 5 renal transplant patients on ciclosporin and simvastatin 20 mg daily with 5 renal transplant patients not on ciclosporin found that the AUC and maximum serum levels of simvastatin were 2.5-fold and 2-fold greater respectively in the patients on ciclosporin.[29]

There are at least 4 documented cases of rhabdomyolysis,[30-32] one fatal,[31] in patients given ciclosporin and simvastatin. In a review of the FDA spontaneous reports of statin-associated rhabdomyolysis covering the period November 1997 to March 2000, ciclosporin was potentially implicated in 31 cases involving simvastatin.[2]

In the first study cited above,[28] significant changes in ciclosporin levels and creatine kinase were seen and the combination was well tolerated. Similar results were found in another study over 8 months.[33] However, another study found that the ciclosporin levels of 12 renal transplant patients dropped from 334 to 235 micrograms/l after simvastatin 5 to 15 mg daily was added.[34] A retrospective study of 12 patients by the same authors confirmed these results.[34]

Mechanism

The marked rises in statin levels and/or toxicity (rhabdomyolysis) probably occur because both the statin and ciclosporin compete for the same metabolizing enzyme, the cytochrome P450 isoenzyme CYP3A4. The extent of the interaction seems to depend on the relative affinities of the different statins for this isoenzyme, and also on whether they can be metabolised by alternative pathways. P-glycoprotein may also have a part to play. See 'Lipid-regulating drugs', (p.827) for more information about the metabolism of the statins.

Importance and management

The interacting effect of ciclosporin on the statins is well documented, well established and clinically important. Concurrent use need not be avoided but it should be very well monitored, a precautionary recommendation being to start (or reduce) the statin to the lowest daily dose,[35,36] appropriate to the patient's condition. One of the makers suggests that the dose of simvastatin should not exceed 10 mg daily.[37] Patients should be told to report any signs of myopathy and possible rhabdomyolysis (i.e. otherwise unexplained muscle pain, tenderness or weakness or dark coloured urine). If myopathy does occur, withdrawing the statin has been shown to resolve the symptoms.

The interacting effect of the statins on ciclosporin only seems to occur with atorvastatin and simvastatin so that only with these two statins does it seem necessary to monitor ciclosporin levels more closely.

However, for other statins it would be prudent to be alert for the interactions detailed here.

1. Maltz HC, Balog DL, Cheigh JS. Rhabdomyolysis associated with concomitant use of atorvastatin and cyclosporine. *Ann Pharmacother* (1999) 33, 1176–9.
2. Omar MA, Wilson JP. FDA adverse event reports on statin-associated rhabdomyolysis. *Ann Pharmacother* (2002) 36, 288–95.
3. Renders L, Mayer-Kadner I, Koch C, Schärffe S, Burkhardt K, Veelken R, Schmieder RE, Hauser IA. Efficacy and drug interactions of the new HMG-CoA reductase inhibitors cerivastatin and atorvastatin in CsA-treated renal transplant recipients. *Nephrol Dial Transplant* (2001) 16, 141–6.
4. Goldberg R, Roth D. Evaluation of fluvastatin in the treatment of hypercholesterolemia in renal transplant recipients taking cyclosporine. *Transplantation* (1996) 62, 1559–64.
5. Park J-W, Siekmeier R, Lattke P, Merz M, Mix C, Schüler S, Jaross W. Pharmacokinetics and pharmacodynamics of fluvastatin in heart transplant recipients taking cyclosporine A. *J Cardiovasc Pharmacol Ther* (2001) 6, 351–61.
6. Goldberg RB, Roth D. A preliminary report of the safety and efficacy of fluvastatin for hypercholesterolemia in renal transplant patients receiving cyclosporine. *Am J Cardiol* (1995) 76, 107A–109A.
7. Li PKT, Mak TWL, Wang AYM, Lee YT, Leung CB, Lui SF, Lam CWK, Lai KN. The interaction of fluvastatin and cyclosporin A in renal-transplant patients. *Int J Clin Pharmacol Ther* (1995) 33, 246–8.
8. Li PKT, Mak TWL, Chan TH, Wang A, Lam CWK, Lai KN. Effect of fluvastatin on lipoprotein profiles in treating renal transplant recipients with dyslipoproteinemia. *Transplantation* (1995) 60, 652–6.
9. Holdaas H, Hartmann A, Stenstrøm J, Dahl KJ, Borge M, Pfister P. Effect of fluvastatin for safely lowering atherogenic lipids in renal transplant patients receiving cyclosporine. *Am J Cardiol* (1995) 76, 102A–106A.
10. Cheung AK, DeVault GA, Gregory MC. A prospective study on treatment of hypercholesterolemia with lovastatin in renal transplant patients receiving cyclosporine. *J Am Soc Nephrol* (1993) 3, 1884–91.
11. Olbricht C, Wanner C, Eisenhauer T, Kliem V, Doll R, Boddaert M, O'Grady P, Krekler M, Mangold B, Christians U. Accumulation of lovastatin, but not pravastatin, in the blood of cyclosporine-treated kidney graft patients after multiple doses. *Clin Pharmacol Ther* (1997) 62, 311–21.
12. Gullestad L, Nordal KP, Berg KJ, Cheng H, Schwartz MS, Simonsen S. Interaction between lovastatin and cyclosporine A after heart and kidney transplantation. *Transplant Proc* (1999) 31, 2163–5.
13. Alejandro DSJ, Petersen J. Myoglobinuric acute renal failure in a cardiac transplant patient taking lovastatin and cyclosporine. *J Am Soc Nephrol* (1994) 5, 153–160.
14. Corpier CL, Jones PH, Suki WN, Lederer ED, Quinones MA, Schmidt SW, Young JB. Rhabdomyolysis and renal injury with lovastatin use. Report of two cases in cardiac transplant recipients. *JAMA* (1988) 260, 239–41.
15. East C, Alivizatos PA, Grundy SM, Jones PH, Farmer JA. Rhabdomyolysis in patients receiving lovastatin after cardiac transplantation. *N Engl J Med* (1988) 318, 47–8.
16. Norman DJ, Illingworth DR, Munson J, Hosenpud J. Myolysis and acute renal failure in a heart-transplant recipient receiving lovastatin. *N Engl J Med* (1988) 318, 46–7.
17. Kobashigawa JA, Murphy F, Stevenson LW, Moriguchi JD, Kawata N, Chuck C, Wilmarth J, Leonard L, Drinkwater D, Laks H. Low dose of lovastatin safely lowers cholesterol after cardiac transplantation. *Circulation* (1989) 80 (Suppl II), II-641.
18. Ballantyne CM, Radovancevic B, Farmer JA, Frazier OH, Chandler L, Payton-Ross C, Cocanougher B, Jones PH, Young JB, Gotto AM. Hyperlipidemia after heart transplantation: report of a 6-year experience, with treatment recommendations. *J Am Coll Cardiol* (1992) 19, 1315–21.
19. Heroux AL, Thompson JA, Katz S, Hastillo AK, Katz M, Quigg RJ, Hess ML. Elimination of the lovastatin-cyclosporine adverse interaction in heart transplant patients. *Circulation* (1989) 80, II-641.
20. Castelao AM, Griñó JM, Andrés E, Gilvernet S, Serón D, Castiñeiras MJ, Roca M, Galcerán JM, González MT, Alsina J. HMGCoA reductase inhibitors lovastatin and simvastatin in the treatment of hypercholesterolemia after renal transplantation. *Transplant Proc* (1993) 25, 1043–6.
21. Tobert JA. Rhabdomyolysis in patients receiving lovastatin after cardiac transplantation. *N Engl J Med* (1988) 318, 48.
22. Regazzi MB, Iacona I, Campana C, Raddato V, Lesi C, Perani G, Gavazzi A, Viganò M. Altered disposition of pravastatin following concomitant drug therapy with cyclosporin A in transplant recipients. *Transplant Proc* (1993) 25, 2732–4.
23. Yoshimura N, Oka T, Okamoto M, Ohmori Y. The effects of pravastatin on hyperlipidemia in renal transplant recipients. *Transplantation* (1992) 53, 94–9.
24. Cassem JD, Hamilton MA, Albanese E, Sabad A, Kobashigawa JA. Does pravastatin affect cyclosporine pharmacokinetics in cardiac transplant recipients. *J Investig Med* (1997) 45, 139A.
25. Muhlmeister HF, Hamilton MA, Cogert GA, Cassem JD, Sabad A, Kobashigawa JA. Long-term HMG-CoA reductase inhibition appears safe and effective after cardiac transplantation. *J Investig Med* (1997) 45, 139A.
26. Kobashigawa JA, Brownfield ED, Stevenson LW, Gleeson MP, Moriguchi JD, Kawata N, Hamilton MA, Hage AS, Minkley R, Salamandra J, Ruzevich S, Drinkwater DC, Laks H. Effects of pravastatin for hypercholesterolemia in cardiac transplant recipients. *J Am Coll Cardiol* (1993) 21, 141A.
27. Crestor (Rosuvastatin calcium). AstraZeneca UK Ltd. UK Summary of product characteristics, February 2005.
28. Campana C, Iacona I, Regazzi MB, Gavazzi A, Perani G, Raddato V, Montemartini C, Viganò M. Efficacy and pharmacokinetics of simvastatin in heart transplant recipients. *Ann Pharmacother* (1995) 29, 235–9.
29. Arnadottir M, Eriksson L-O, Thysell H, Karkas JD. Plasma concentration profiles of simvastatin 3-hydroxy-3-methyl-glutaryl-coenzyme A reductase inhibitory activity in kidney transplant recipients with and without ciclosporin. *Nephron* (1993) 65, 410–13.
30. Blaison G, Weber JC, Sachs D, Korganow AS, Martin T, Kretz JG, Pasquali JL. Rhabdomyolyse causée par la simvastatine chez un transplanté cardiaque sous ciclosporine. *Rev Med Interne* (1992) 13, 61–3.
31. Weise WJ, Possidente CJ. Fatal rhabdomyolysis associated with simvastatin in a renal transplant patient. *Am J Med* (2000) 108, 351–2.
32. Meier C, Stey C, Brack T, Maggiorini M, Risti B, Krahenbuhl S. Rhabdomyolyse bei mit Simvastatin und Ciclosporin behandelten Patienten: Rolle der aktivitat des Cytochrom-P450-Enzymsystems der Leber. *Schweiz Med Wochenschr* (1995) 125, 1342–6.
33. Barbir M, Rose M, Kushwaha S, Akl S, Mitchell A, Yacoub M. Low-dose simvastatin for the treatment of hypercholesterolaemia in recipients of cardiac transplantation. *Int J Cardiol* (1991) 33, 241–6.
34. Akhlaghi F, McLachlan AJ, Keogh AM, Brown KF. Effect of simvastatin on cyclosporine unbound fraction and apparent blood clearance in heart transplant recipients. *Br J Clin Pharmacol* (1997) 44, 537–42.
35. Mevacor (Lovastatin). Merck & Co., Inc. US Prescribing information, April 2005.
36. Lipostat (Pravastatin). Bristol-Myers Squibb Pharmaceuticals Ltd. UK Summary of product characteristics, December 2004.
37. Zocor (Simvastatin). Merck Sharp & Dohme Ltd. UK Summary of product characteristics, July 2004.

Statins + Diuretics

In clinical trials, the safety and efficacy of statins were not altered by concurrent use of diuretics.

Clinical evidence, mechanism, importance and management

Retrospective analysis of clinical trial data[1] found no evidence that the safety or efficacy of **lovastatin** was altered by the use of **potassium-sparing diuretics** (hydrochlorothiazide with **triamterene** or **amiloride**), or **thiazide diuretics** (mostly **hydrochlorothiazide**). Another retrospective study of 19 patients found that the addition of **lovastatin** to diuretic treatment caused an initial 30% fall in total serum cholesterol levels for one month, followed by a rise of about 20%. In a further 13 patients, the addition of diuretic treatment to **lovastatin** caused a 20% fall in total serum cholesterol for one month and then a 20% rise back to baseline values. The diuretics used were **furosemide** (16 patients), **triamterene/hydrochlorothiazide** (7), **hydrochlorothiazide** (8), **indapamide** (1). The fall and subsequent rise in serum cholesterol levels occurred in all of the patients except just the one on **indapamide**.[2] The reason for this initial fall in cholesterol, particularly when the diuretic was added to the statin, is unknown, and the findings of this trial are difficult to interpret.

Retrospective analysis of clinical trial data found no evidence that the safety or efficacy of **fluvastatin** was altered by the use of unspecified **diuretics**.[3] Likewise, the maker of **atorvastatin**[4] says that in clinical studies it was used concurrently with unnamed **diuretics** without evidence of significant adverse interactions.

The bulk of the evidence suggests no special precautions are necessary if diuretics are given concurrently with statins.

1. Pool JL, Shear CL, Downton M, Schnaper H, Stinnett S, Dujovne C, Bradford RH, Chremos AN. Lovastatin and coadministered antihypertensive/cardiovascular agents. *Hypertension* (1992) 19, 242–8.

2. Aruna AS, Akula SK, Sarpong DF. Interaction between potassium-depleting diuretics and lovastatin in hypercholesterolemic ambulatory care patients. *J Pharm Technol* (1997) 13, 21–6.

3. Peters TK, Jewitt-Harris J, Mehra M, Muratti EN. Safety and tolerability of fluvastatin with concomitant use of antihypertensive agents. An analysis of a clinical trial database. *Am J Hypertens* (1993) 6, 346S–352S.

4. Lipitor (Atorvastatin). Parke Davis. UK Summary of product characteristics, March 2005.

Statins + Everolimus

Everolimus did not alter the pharmacokinetics or HMG-CoA reductase activity of atorvastatin or pravastatin to a clinically relevant extent in a single-dose study in healthy subjects. Everolimus pharmacokinetics were unaltered by the statins.[1]

1. Kovarik JM, Hartmann S, Hubert M, Berthier S, Schneider W, Rosenkranz B, Rordorf C. Pharmacokinetic and pharmacodynamic assessments of HMG-CoA reductase inhibitors when coadministered with everolimus. *J Clin Pharmacol* (2002) 42, 222–8.

Statins + Ezetimibe

Ezetimibe does not appear to interact adversely with atorvastatin, fluvastatin, lovastatin or simvastatin.

Clinical evidence, mechanism, importance and management

In a three-arm study, 50 patients were given **atorvastatin** or **simvastatin** 80 mg daily (17 patients), **atorvastatin** or **simvastatin** 40 mg daily with ezetimibe 10 mg daily (16 patients), or **atorvastatin** or **simvastatin** 80 mg daily with ezetimibe 10 mg daily (17 patients). No difference in adverse events was noted between each of the 3 groups and there were no significant elevations in creatine kinase. No cases of myopathy or rhabdomyolysis occurred, and the combination was well-tolerated.[1] In another study, ezetimibe 0.25 mg, 1 mg or 10 mg daily had no effect on the pharmacokinetics of **simvastatin** 10 mg daily, when both were given for 14 days. In addition, 10 and 20-mg doses of simvastatin were well-tolerated in combination with ezetimibe.[2]

In a randomised crossover study 18 healthy subjects were given either ezetimibe 10 mg daily, **lovastatin** 20 mg daily or both drugs in combination for 7 days. The combination was well tolerated, and no significant pharmacokinetic interaction was noted.[3] In a study of the same design using **fluvastatin**, similar results were found, as well as an enhanced lowering of LDL-cholesterol, which was considered to be clinically favourable.[4]

1. Gagné C, Gaudet D, Bruckert E for the Ezetimibe Study Group. Efficacy and safety of ezetimibe coadministered with atorvastatin or simvastatin in patients with homozygous familial hypercholesterolemia. *Circulation* (2002) 105, 2469–75.

2. Kosoglou T, Meyer I, Veltri EP, Statkevich P, Yang B, Zhu Y, Mellars L, Maxwell SE, Patrick JE, Cutler DL, Batra VK, Affrime MB. Pharmacodynamic interaction between the new selective cholesterol absorption inhibitor ezetimibe and simvastatin. *Br J Clin Pharmacol* (2002) 54, 309–19.

3. Reyderman L, Kosoglou T, Statkevich P, Anderson L, Boutros T, Batra V, Sieberline M. No pharmacokinetic drug interaction between ezetimibe and lovastatin. *Clin Pharmacol Ther* (2001) 69, P66.

4. Kosoglou T, Meyer I, Musiol B, Anderson L, Reyderman L, Statkevich P, Cutler DL, Veltri EP, Affrime MB. Pharmacodynamic interaction between fluvastatin and ezetimibe has favourable clinical implications. *Atherosclerosis* (2001) 2 (Suppl 2), 89.

Statins + Fibrates

The plasma levels of lovastatin and simvastatin are increased by gemfibrozil. Serious myopathy and/or rhabdomyolysis (one fatal case) have been reported. There is also an isolated case of rhabdomyolysis with atorvastatin/gemfibrozil. One report describes a rise in plasma pravastatin levels caused by gemfibrozil but no pharmacokinetic interactions occur with fluvastatin/gemfibrozil, lovastatin/bezafibrate, pravastatin/fenofibrate, or rosuvastatin/fenofibrate.

Clinical evidence

A. Bezafibrate

(a) Lovastatin

The pharmacokinetics of a single 40-mg dose of lovastatin were not altered by 3 days of bezafibrate 400 mg daily in 11 healthy subjects.[1]

B. Gemfibrozil

(a) Atorvastatin

A 43-year-old woman with multiple medical problems was taking gemfibrozil 600 mg twice daily. After a recurrent attack of pancreatitis, 10 mg atorvastatin and 2.5 mg glibenclamide (glyburide), both twice daily were added to her treatment. Later she was also given high-dose conjugated estrogens, cimetidine, fluoxetine, medroxyprogesterone, furosemide (frusemide), and trimethobenzamide suppositories. About 3 weeks after atorvastatin had been added to the gemfibrozil, she developed brown and turbid urine (suggesting urinary myoglobin), creatine kinase levels of 4633 units/l and had myalgia. She was diagnosed as having rhabdomyolysis. Her serum creatine kinase levels rapidly fell when the atorvastatin and gemfibrozil were withdrawn.[2]

(b) Fluvastatin

In a randomised crossover study 15 patients were given fluvastatin 20 mg and gemfibrozil 600 mg twice daily. The pharmacokinetics of both gemfibrozil and fluvastatin were unchanged by concurrent use and no significant adverse effects were noted.[3]

(c) Lovastatin

By 1990 the FDA had documented 12 case reports of severe myopathy or rhabdomyolysis associated with the concurrent use of lovastatin and gemfibrozil. The mean serum creatine kinase levels of the patients reached 15250 units/l. Four of those tested showed myoglobinuria and five had acute renal failure.[4] Details of cases of rhabdomyolysis associated with the concurrent use of these drugs,[5-9] three with renal failure,[6,7,9] have been described elsewhere. Other cases have been seen in patients taking lovastatin and gemfibrozil with ciclosporin.[10] In a pharmacokinetic study, 11 healthy subjects were given gemfibrozil 1200 mg daily for 3 days, with a single 40 mg dose of lovastatin on day 3. The AUC and maximum plasma level of lovastatin acid (a metabolite) were nearly threefold greater in the presence of gemfibrozil.[1]

However, in contrast, other reports[11-14] describe apparently safe and effective concurrent use under very well controlled conditions, although elevated creatine phosphokinase levels, without rhabdomyolysis, were seen in up to 8% of cases.

(d) Pravastatin

No clinically significant changes in the bioavailability of single 20-mg doses of pravastatin were seen with the concurrent use of gemfibrozil 600 mg in 18 healthy subjects.[15] A 12-week study found that pravastatin 40 mg daily and gemfibrozil 600 mg twice daily caused marked abnormalities in creatine kinase concentrations (four times the pretreatment values) in 1 of 71 patients on pravastatin alone, 1 of 73 patients on placebo, 2 of 72 patients on gemfibrozil alone, and 4 of 75 patients on combined gemfibrozil/pravastatin treatment. The differences between treatments were not statistically significant. Two patients on combination therapy had this withdrawn because of asymptomatic creatine kinase elevations. Severe myopathy or rhabdomyolysis was not seen in any patient, although 14 patients had musculoskeletal pain, but in most cases this was not considered to be related to the treatment.[16]

(e) Rosuvastatin

The makers of rosuvastatin say that concurrent use with gemfibrozil resulted in a twofold elevation in rosuvastatin levels.[17]

(f) Simvastatin

A 62-year-old man with diabetes on 20 mg simvastatin and 600 mg gemfibrozil daily (as well as acenocoumarol, glibenclamide (glyburide) and diclofenac) was hospitalised because of melaena, generalised myalgia, malaise and brown urine. Laboratory tests confirmed the diagnosis of rhabdomyolysis. He recovered when the simvastatin and gemfibrozil were stopped.[18] Another diabetic patient had been taking simvastatin and gemfibrozil 600 mg daily for two and a half years (as well as felodipine, indapamide, calcium carbonate, bumetanide, psyllium, acenocoumarol (nicoumalone) and insulin). She complained of tiredness, generalised myalgia and anuria 3 months after her dosage of simvastatin had been increased to 80 mg daily. Rhabdomyolysis with exaggerated renal insufficiency were diagnosed and confirmed. She recovered when the simvastatin and gemfibrozil were stopped.[18] A further case of rhabdomyolysis with a fatal outcome has been reported in a patient taking simvastatin 80 mg daily, 4 weeks after starting gemfibrozil.[19]

A pharmacokinetic study found that the AUC of simvastatin acid (a simvastatin active metabolite) was increased nearly twofold and the peak concentration doubled, when simvastatin was given concurrently with gemfibrozil.[20]

C. Fenofibrate

(a) Pravastatin

A single-dose study in 23 healthy subjects found that the concurrent use of pravastatin 40 mg and fenofibrate 201 mg had no effect on the pharmacokinetics of either drug, but a moderate increase in the formation of a non-toxic pravastatin metabolite was seen. This was not thought to be clinically important.[21]

(b) Rosuvastatin

A 7-day course of fenofibrate 67 mg three times daily and rosuvastatin 10 mg daily given to 14 healthy subjects resulted in only minor changes in fenofibric acid and rosuvastatin exposure, when compared to either drug given alone.[22]

D. Unspecified Fibrates

In a review[23] of the FDA spontaneous reports of statin-associated rhabdomyolysis covering the period November 1997 to March 2000, fibrates (unspecified) were potentially implicated in 10 of 73 cases of rhabdomyolysis seen with **atorvastatin**, 4 of 10 with **fluvastatin**, 5 of 40 with **lovastatin**, 6 of 71 with **pravastatin**, and 33 of 215 with **simvastatin**.

Mechanism

Not understood. Myopathy can occur with statins and fibrates alone and their effects may therefore be additive or synergistic. There is also some evidence that the fibrates may inhibit the metabolism of the statins, but *not* because they inhibit the cytochrome P450 isoenzyme CYP3A4.[1,20] More recent study has shown that gemfibrozil may inhibit the glucuronidation of some of the statin metabolites, and that gemfibrozil is an inhibitor of some of the CYP2C isoenzymes.[24]

Importance and management

The lovastatin/gemfibrozil and simvastatin/gemfibrozil interactions are established and clinically important. The FDA discourage the concurrent use of lovastatin with gemfibrozil in any patient, but suggest that it should be avoided in patients with compromised liver or renal function.[4] The UK and US makers of lovastatin and simvastatin recommends that combined use with fibrates should generally be avoided, but if the benefits are considered to outweigh the risks, a low dose of the statin should be used.[25,26]

None of the other statin/fibrate interactions are well established, (the overall incidence of myopathy with the combinations being put at 0.12%)[27] nor does there seem to be good reason for avoiding combined use where it is thought to be appropriate. However, the makers of pravastatin cautiously suggest that its use with fibrates should generally be avoided because of the risk of myopathy, except perhaps in selected patients.[28] The makers of rosuvastatin give a similar warning.[17]

As a general rule, any patient given a statin and a fibrate should be told to report any signs of myopathy and possible rhabdomyolysis (i.e. otherwise unexplained muscle pain, tenderness or weakness or dark coloured urine). If myopathy does occur, the statin should be stopped immediately.

1. Kyrklund C, Backman JT, Kivistö KT, Neuvonen M, Laitila J, Neuvonen PJ. Plasma concentrations of active lovastatin acid are markedly increased by gemfibrozil but not bezafibrate. *Clin Pharmacol Ther* (2001) 69, 340–5.
2. Duell PB, Connor WE, Illingworth DR. Rhabdomyolysis after taking atorvastatin with gemfibrozil. *Am J Cardiol* (1998) 81, 368–9.
3. Spence JD, Munoz CE, Hendricks L, Latchinian L, Khouri HE. Pharmacokinetics of the combination of fluvastatin and gemfibrozil. *Am J Cardiol* (1995) 76, 80A–83A.
4. Pierce LR, Wysowski DK, Gross TP. Myopathy and rhabdomyolysis associated with lovastatin-gemfibrozil combination therapy. *JAMA* (1990) 264, 71–75.
5. Tobert JA. Myolysis and acute renal failure in a heart-transplant recipient receiving lovastatin. *N Engl J Med* (1988) 318, 48.
6. Marais GE, Larson KK. Rhabdomyolysis and acute renal failure induced by combination lovastatin and gemfibrozil therapy. *Ann Intern Med* (1990) 112, 228–30.
7. Manoukian AA, Bhagavan NV, Hayashi T, Nestor TA, Rios C, Scottolini AG. Rhabdomyolysis secondary to lovastatin therapy. *Clin Chem* (1990) 36, 2145–7.
8. Kogan AD, Orenstein S. Lovastatin-induced acute rhabdomyolysis. *Postgrad Med J* (1990) 66, 294–6.
9. Goldman JA, Fisherman AB, Lee JE, Johnson RJ. The role of cholesterol-lowering agents in drug-induced rhabdomyolysis and polymyositis. *Arthritis Rheum* (1989) 32, 358–9.
10. East C, Alivizatos PA, Grundy SM, Jones PH, Farmer JA. Rhabdomyolysis in patients receiving lovastatin after cardiac transplantation. *N Engl J Med* (1988) 318, 47–8.
11. Illingworth DR, Bacon S. Influence of lovastatin plus gemfibrozil on plasma lipids and lipoproteins in patients with heterozygous familial hypercholesterolemia. *Circulation* (1989) 79, 590–6.
12. Glueck CJ, Oakes N, Speirs J, Tracy T, Lang J. Gemfibrozil-lovastatin therapy for primary hyperlipoproteinemias. *Am J Cardiol* (1992) 70, 1–9.
13. East C, Bilheimer DW, Grundy SM. Combination drug therapy for familial combined hyperlipidemia. *Ann Intern Med* (1988) 109, 25–32.
14. Wirebaugh SR, Shapiro ML, McIntyre TH, Whitney EJ. A retrospective review of the use of lipid-lowering agents in combination, specifically, gemfibrozil and lovastatin. *Pharmacotherapy* (1992) 12, 445–50.
15. ER Squibb. A report on the bioavailability of pravastatin in the presence and absence of gemfibrozil or probucol in healthy male subjects. Data on file (Protocol No 27, 201-18), 1988.
16. Wiklund O, Angelin B, Bergman M, Berglund L, Bondjers G, Carlsson A, Lindén T, Miettinen T, Ödman B, Olofsson S-O, Saarinen I, Sipilä R, Sjöström P, Kron B, Vanhanen H, Wright I. Pravastatin and gemfibrozil alone and in combination for the treatment of hypercholesterolemia. *Am J Med* (1993) 94, 13–20.
17. Crestor (Rosuvastatin calcium). AstraZeneca UK Ltd. UK Summary of product characteristics, February 2005.
18. Van Puijenbroek EP, Du Buf-Vereijken PWG, Spooren PFMJ, Van Doormaal JJ. Possible increased risk of rhabdomyolysis during concomitant use of simvastatin and gemfibrozil. *J Intern Med* (1996) 240, 403–4.
19. Federman DG, Hussain F, Walters JB. Fatal rhabdomyolysis caused by lipid-lowering therapy. *South Med J* (2001) 94, 1023–6.
20. Backman JT, Kyrklund C, Kivistö KT, Wang J-S, Neuvonen PJ. Plasma concentrations of active simvastatin acid are increased by gemfibrozil. *Clin Pharmacol Ther* (2001) 68, 122–9.
21. Pan W-J, Gustavson LE, Achari R, Rieser MJ, Ye X, Gutterman C, Wallin BA. Lack of a clinically significant pharmacokinetic interaction between fenofibrate and pravastatin in healthy volunteers. *J Clin Pharmacol* (2000) 40, 316–23.
22. Martin PD, Dane AL, Schneck DW, Warwick MJ. An open-label, randomized, three-way crossover trial of the effect of coadministration of rosuvastatin and fenofibrate on the pharmacokinetic properties of rosuvastatin and fenofibric acid in healthy male volunteers. *Clin Ther* (2003) 25, 459–71.
23. Omar MA, Wilson JP. FDA adverse event reports on statin-associated rhabdomyolysis. *Ann Pharmacother* (2002) 36, 288–95.
24. Prueksaritanont T, Zhao JJ, Ma B, Roadcap BA, Tang C, Qui Y, Liu L, Lin JH, Pearson PG, Baillie TA. Mechanistic studies on metabolic interactions between gemfibrozil and statins. *J Pharmacol Exp Ther* (2002) 301, 1042–51.
25. Zocor (Simvastatin). Merck Sharp & Dohme Ltd. UK Summary of product characteristics, July 2004.
26. Mevacor (Lovastatin), Merck & Co., Inc. US Prescribing information, April 2005.
27. Shek A, Ferrill J. Statin-fibrate combination therapy. *Ann Pharmacother* (2001) 35, 908–17.
28. Lipostat (Pravastatin). Bristol-Myers Squibb Pharmaceuticals Ltd. UK Summary of product characteristics, December 2004.

Statins + Fusidic acid

Two cases of rhabdomyolysis have been described in patients given atorvastatin or simvastatin with fusidic acid. Fusidic acid was also a possible contributing factor in a case described in an interaction between 'simvastatin and tacrolimus', (p.842).

Clinical evidence, mechanism, importance and management

A patient with a renal transplant and diabetes treated with various drugs was started on **atorvastatin** 10 mg daily for hyperlipidaemia. Six weeks later, because of a resistant infection, clindamycin and ciprofloxacin were discontinued and fusidic acid 1.5 g daily was started. At this time serum creatine kinase (CK) was 54 units/l. Two weeks later the patient was admitted with progressive muscle weakness and pain in both legs. His serum CK was 3550 units/l, and he also had raised myoglobin levels. Both continued to rise for 5 days after discontinuing the **atorvastatin** and fusidic acid, then gradually returned to normal over one week. Serum levels of both fusidic acid and **atorvastatin** were higher than expected, and it was considered an interaction was likely.[1] Another patient who had been taking **simvastatin** 10 mg daily for 10 months, developed rhabdomyolysis 15 days after starting fusidic acid. She recovered after stopping both drugs.[2] Fusidic acid was a possible contributing factor to another case of rhabdomyolysis seen in a patient treated with 'simvastatin and tacrolimus', (p.842). The clinical significance of this possible interaction is unclear, but it would seem wise to remind patients receiving the combination to be on the look out for the symptoms of myopathy and rhabdomyolysis.

1. Wenisch C, Krause R, Fladerer P, El Menjawi I, Pohanka E. Acute rhabdomyolysis after atorvastatin and fusidic acid therapy. *Am J Med* (2000) 109, 78.
2. Dromer C, Vedrenne C, Billey T, Pages M, Fournié B, Fournié A. Rhabdomyolyse à la simvastatine: a propos d'un cas avec revue de la littérature. *Rev Rhum Mal Osteoartic* (1992) 59, 281–3.

Statins + Grapefruit juice

Large amounts of grapefruit juice markedly increase the plasma levels of lovastatin and simvastatin, but only modestly affect the plasma levels of atorvastatin. Pravastatin seems not to interact.

Clinical evidence

(a) Atorvastatin

Twelve healthy subjects were given 200 ml double-strength grapefruit juice three times daily for 5 days. On day 3 they were given a single 40-mg dose of atorvastatin with the grapefruit juice followed by two more 200-ml doses of grapefruit juice, one after 30 minutes and the other after 90 minutes. The 72-hour AUC values of atorvastatin acid and total HMG-CoA reductase inhibitors were increased 2.5-fold and 1.5-fold respectively.[1]

(b) Lovastatin

Ten healthy subjects were given 200 ml double-strength grapefruit juice three times daily for 3 days. On day 3 they additionally took 80 mg of lovastatin with 200 ml of grapefruit juice, followed by two more 200-ml doses of grapefruit juice, one after 30 minutes and the other after 90 minutes. The mean peak serum levels of the lovastatin and its active metabolite, lovastatin acid, were increased 12-fold and 4-fold respectively, and the mean AUCs were increased 15-fold and 5-fold respectively.[2] However, another study using lovastatin 40 mg given the evening after single-strength grapefruit juice with breakfast found the AUC and maximum serum level of lovastatin were approximately doubled, and the AUC and maximum serum level of lovastatin acid were only increased 1.6-fold.[3] It has been suggested that if the grapefruit juice had been given at the same time as the lovastatin in the latter study[3] then much greater increases in the AUC and maximum serum levels would have been found.[4]

(c) Pravastatin

Grapefruit juice did not significantly affect the pharmacokinetics of a single 40-mg dose of pravastatin. In this study, 200-ml double-strength grapefruit juice was given three times daily for 2 days, and then on the third day 200 ml was given with the pravastatin and again after 30 and 90 minutes.[1]

(d) Simvastatin

Ten healthy subjects were given 200 ml double-strength grapefruit juice three times daily for 2 days. On day 3 they additionally took 60 mg of simvastatin with 200 ml of grapefruit juice, followed by two more 200-ml doses of grapefruit juice, one after 30 minutes and the other after 90 minutes. The mean peak serum levels of the simvastatin and simvastatin acid, were increased 9-fold and 7-fold respectively, and the mean AUCs were increased 16-fold and 7-fold respectively.[5] In a further study by the same research group, when simvastatin was given 24 hours after the last dose of grapefruit juice (same dosage regimen as the previous study) the effect was only 10% of that observed during concurrent use, and had disappeared within 3 to 7 days.[6] The maker notes that the effect of 240 ml standard grapefruit juice on simvastatin was minimal (13% increase in AUC of active plasma HMG-CoA reductase inhibitors).[7]

Mechanism

It seems almost certain that some components of the grapefruit juice (not yet positively identified but possibly naringenin), inhibit the activity of the cytochrome P450 isoenzyme CYP3A4 in the gut wall, thereby reducing the metabolism of the statins as they are absorbed, and allowing more to pass into the body. See 'Lipid-regulating drugs', (p.827) for more information about the metabolism of the statins.

Importance and management

Information seems to be limited to these pharmacokinetic reports (i.e. no adverse case reports) but they are consistent with the way other CYP3A4 inhibitors interact with the statins.

Large increases in the serum levels of lovastatin and simvastatin are potentially hazardous because elevated statin levels carry the risk of toxicity (muscle damage and the possible development of rhabdomyolysis). As even small quantities of grapefruit juice taken in the morning can significantly affect simvastatin levels the maker says that concurrent use should be avoided.[7]

The modest increase in atorvastatin levels when taken with high doses of grapefruit juice would seem to be clinically irrelevant, while pravastatin seems not to interact. Information about other statins appears to be lacking.

1. Lilja JJ, Kivistö KT, Neuvonen PJ. Grapefruit juice increases serum concentrations of atorvastatin and has no effect on pravastatin. *Clin Pharmacol Ther* (1999) 66, 118–27.
2. Kantola T, Kivistö KT, Neuvonen PJ. Grapefruit juice greatly increases serum concentrations of lovastatin and lovastatin acid. *Clin Pharmacol Ther* (1998) 63, 397–402.
3. Rogers JD, Zhao J, Liu L, Amin RD, Gagliano KD, Porras AG, Blum RA, Wilson MF, Stepanavage M, Vega JM. Grapefruit juice has minimal effects on plasma concentrations of lovastatin-derived 3-hydroxy-3-methylglutaryl coenzyme A reductase inhibitors. *Clin Pharmacol Ther* (1999) 66, 358–66.
4. Bailey DG, Dresser GK. Grapefruit juice-lovastatin interaction. *Clin Pharmacol Ther* (2000) 67, 690.
5. Lilja JJ, Kivistö KT, Neuvonen PJ. Grapefruit juice-simvastatin interaction: effect on serum concentrations of simvastatin, simvastatin acid, and HMG-CoA reductase inhibitors. *Clin Pharmacol Ther* (1998) 64, 477–83.
6. Lilja JJ, Kivistö KT, Neuvonen PJ. Duration of effect of grapefruit juice on the pharmacokinetics of the CYP3A4 substrate simvastatin. *Clin Pharmacol Ther* (2000) 68, 384–90.
7. Zocor (Simvastatin). Merck Sharp & Dohme Ltd. UK Summary of product characteristics, July 2004.

Statins + H_2-blockers

No clinically significant interaction appears to occur between cimetidine and atorvastatin, fluvastatin, or pravastatin, or between ranitidine and fluvastatin.

Clinical evidence, mechanism, importance and management

(a) Atorvastatin

In a crossover study, 12 healthy subjects were given 15 days of atorvastatin with and without **cimetidine** 300 mg four times daily. **Cimetidine** had no effect on the maximum serum levels or AUC of atorvastatin. **Cimetidine** had little effect on the lipid lowering ability of atorvastatin, except that the reduction in triglycerides was slightly less, but this difference was considered to be of little clinical significance.[1] There would appear to be no reason for avoiding concurrent use.

(b) Fluvastatin

The makers of fluvastatin say that its bioavailability is increased by **cimetidine** and **ranitidine**, but they say that this is of no clinical relevance.[2] No special precautions would seem to be necessary.

(c) Pravastatin

Cimetidine 300 mg four times daily for 3 days increased the bioavailability of a single 20-mg dose of pravastatin by 58%. The dose of pravastatin was given on day 3, one hour after the first dose of **cimetidine.**[3] However, the makers say that it is unlikely that the changes caused by **cimetidine** will affect the clinical efficacy of pravastatin.[3]

1. Stern RH, Gibson DM, Whitfield LR. Cimetidine does not alter atorvastatin pharmacokinetics or LDL-cholesterol reduction. *Eur J Clin Pharmacol* (1998) 53, 475–8.
2. Lescol (Fluvastatin). Novartis Pharmaceuticals UK Ltd. UK Summary of product characteristics, December 2000.
3. ER Squibb. A report on the comparative pharmacokinetics of pravastatin in the presence and absence of cimetidine or antacids in healthy male subjects. Data on file (Protocol No 27, 201-43), 1988.

Statins + Macrolides

Erythromycin causes a very marked increase in the serum levels of lovastatin and a minor increase in atorvastatin levels, but it does not interact pharmacokinetically with pravastatin. Cases of acute rhabdomyolysis have been reported with lovastatin/azithromycin, lovastatin/clarithromycin, lovastatin/erythromycin and simvastatin/roxithromycin. Macrolide antibacterials have also been potentially implicated in cases with atorvastatin and pravastatin. No significant pharmacokinetic interaction has been seen between atorvastatin/azithromycin. Atorvastatin levels are modestly raised by clarithromycin and there are some changes in lovastatin levels with roxithromycin.

Simvastatin / Clarythromycin ↑ risk myopathy (avoid concomitant use) as per BNF

Clinical evidence

(a) Azithromycin

A 51-year-old man who had been taking **lovastatin** 40 mg daily for 5 years developed muscle aches and fever one day after finishing a 5-day course of azithromycin 250 mg daily. His creatine phosphokinase concentrations were elevated and he was diagnosed as having rhabdomyolysis. This patient was also taking colestyramine, diltiazem, doxazosin, glibenclamide (glyburide), 'thyroid', allopurinol, naproxen, prednisone, loratadine and inhaled beclometasone.[1]

In a randomised study, two groups of 12 healthy subjects were given 8 days of **atorvastatin** 10 mg daily with additional azithromycin 500 mg daily or placebo for the final 3 days. When the azithromycin group were compared with the placebo group no change in **atorvastatin** pharmacokinetics were noted.[2]

(b) Clarithromycin

A 76-year-old woman who had been taking 40 mg **lovastatin** daily for 5 years developed muscle pain and weakness 2 days after completing a 10-day course of clarithromycin 500 mg twice daily. Later, when hospitalised, she was found to have elevated creatine phosphokinase concentrations and was diagnosed as having acute rhabdomyolysis. This patient was also taking famotidine, hydrochlorothiazide, triamterene, probenecid, colchicine, prednisone, aspirin, diltiazem, clonidine, insulin and inhaled salbutamol (albuterol).[1] In a similar case, a 64-year-old man with multiple pathologies, including renal impairment developed rhabdomyolysis 3 weeks after clarithromycin was added to his treatment, which included **simvastatin** 80 mg daily.[3] In a randomised study, two groups of 12 healthy subjects were given 8 days of **atorvastatin** 10 mg daily with additional clarithromycin 500 mg twice daily or placebo for the final 3 days. When the clarithromycin group were compared with the placebo group the **atorvastatin** AUC was 82% higher and the maximum serum levels 50% higher.[2]

(c) Erythromycin

Twelve healthy subjects were given a single 10-mg dose of **atorvastatin** on day 7 of an 11-day course of erythromycin 500 mg four times daily. The maximum serum **atorvastatin** levels were raised 38% by the erythromycin and the AUC was raised 33%.[4] Either **lovastatin** or **pravastatin** 40 mg daily was given to 12 healthy subjects for a week, followed by a further week with erythromycin 500 mg three times daily. The erythromycin caused the maximum serum **lovastatin** levels and the AUC to rise more than fivefold. The pharmacokinetics of the **pravastatin** remained unchanged.[5]

A man on **lovastatin** 20 mg three times daily, diltiazem, allopurinol and aspirin developed progressive weakness and diffuse myalgia after being treated with erythromycin 500 mg 6-hourly for 13 days. When admitted to hospital his creatine kinase level was high (35 200 units/l) and his urine was reddish-brown. The rhabdomyolysis was treated by stopping the lovastatin, and by giving furosemide with vigorous intravenous hydration.[6] A woman who had been on **lovastatin** for 7 years developed multiple organ toxicity (rhabdomyolysis, acute renal failure, pancreatitis, livedo reticularis and raised aminotransferase levels) when erythromycin was added.[7] Three other cases of rhabdomyolysis attributed to a **lovastatin**/erythromycin interaction have been reported,[7,8] although it should be noted that one of these patients was also taking ciclosporin.[8]

Erythromycin 500 mg four times daily for 7 days did not raise the levels of a single 80-mg dose of **rosuvastatin** in 11 healthy subjects. In fact, **rosuvastatin** levels were slightly lowered, although this was not considered to be of clinical relevance if short-term courses of erythromycin are used.[9]

(d) Roxithromycin

A 73-year-old woman, who had been stable for 6 months on a combination of gemfibrozil 600 mg twice daily, **simvastatin** 80 mg daily and diltiazem, developed muscular weakness and myalgia 7 days after starting roxithromycin. All drugs were stopped, and initially she developed myoglobinuria and had a further elevation in her creatine kinase level, but this normalised over the following 18 days. She was discharged after 6 weeks, by which time she had regained full strength.[10] In a randomised crossover study, 12 healthy subjects were given 80 mg of **lovastatin** either alone or following 5 days pre-treatment with roxithromycin 300 mg four times daily. Roxithromycin increased the maximum level and AUC of lovastatin acid by 38% and 42% and decreased the maximum level and AUC of lovastatin lactone by a similar amount.[11]

(e) Unspecified macrolides

In a review of the FDA spontaneous reports of statin-associated rhabdomyolysis covering the period November 1997 to March 2000, macrolide antibacterials (unspecified) were potentially implicated in 13 of 73 cases of rhabdomyolysis seen with **atorvastatin,** 11 of 40 with **lovastatin**, 6 of 71 with **pravastatin**, and 10 of 215 with **simvastatin**.[12]

Mechanism

It seems likely that any rises in statin levels occur because some of these macrolides inhibit their metabolism by the cytochrome P450 isoenzyme CYP3A4, leading in some instances to toxicity (myopathy and rhabdomyolysis). No interaction would be expected with pravastatin because it is not metabolised by CYP3A4. See 'Lipid-regulating drugs', (p.827) for a more detailed discussion of statin metabolism.

Importance and management

Information about the statin/macrolide interactions seems to be limited to the reports cited here. In general it appears that the macrolides raise the levels of statins metabolised by the cytochrome P450 isoenzyme CYP3A4 (i.e. atorvastatin, lovastatin and simvastatin), but not all patients are affected. It should be noted that the makers of lovastatin and simvastatin specifically recommend that these drugs are not used with erythromycin or clarithromycin, and suggest that the statin be temporarily withdrawn if these antibacterials are required.[13,14] Pravastatin is not metabolised by CYP3A4, so would not be expected to interact with macrolides via this mechanism, but potential cases have been identified. This is worth noting when considering rosuvastatin, which is also said to have a low propensity for interactions with CYP3A4.

To be on the safe side, any patient on any statin who is given a macrolide should be warned to be alert for any signs of myopathy (i.e. otherwise unexplained muscle pain, tenderness or weakness or dark coloured urine). If myopathy does occur, the statin should be stopped immediately.

1. Grunden JW, Fisher KA. Lovastatin-induced rhabdomyolysis possibly associated with clarithromycin and azithromycin. *Ann Pharmacother* (1997) 31, 859–63.
2. Amsden GW, Kuye O, Wei GCG. A study of the interaction potential of azithromycin and clarithromycin with atorvastatin in healthy volunteers. *J Clin Pharmacol* (2002) 42, 442–7.
3. Lee AJ, Maddix DS. Rhabdomyolysis secondary to a drug interaction between simvastatin and clarithromycin. *Ann Pharmacother* (2001) 35, 26–31.
4. Siedlik PH, Olson SC, Yang B-B, Stern RH. Erythromycin coadministration increases plasma atorvastatin concentrations. *J Clin Pharmacol* (1999) 39, 501–4.
5. Bottorff MB, Behrens DH, Gross A, Markel M. Differences in metabolism of lovastatin and pravastatin as assessed by CYP3A inhibition with erythromycin. *Pharmacotherapy* (1997) 17, 184.
6. Ayanian JZ, Fuchs CS, Stone RM. Lovastatin and rhabdomyolysis. *Ann Intern Med* (1988) 109, 682–3.
7. Wong PWK, Dillard TA, Kroenke K. Multiple organ toxicity from addition of erythromycin to long-term lovastatin therapy. *South Med J* (1998) 91, 202–5.
8. Corpier CL, Jones PH, Suki WN, Lederer ED, Quinones MA, Schmidt SW, Young JB. Rhabdomyolysis and renal injury with lovastatin use. Report of two cases in cardiac transplant recipients. *JAMA* (1988) 260, 239–41.
9. Cooper KJ, Martin PD, Dane AL, Warwick MJ, Raza A, Schneck DW. The effect of erythromycin on the pharmacokinetics of rosuvastatin. *Eur J Clin Pharmacol* (2003), 59, 51–6.
10. Huynh T, Cordato D, Yang F, Choy T, Johnstone K, Bagnall F, Hitchens N, Dunn R. HMG CoA reductase-inhibitor-related myopathy and the influence of drug interactions. *Intern Med J* (2002) 32, 486–90.
11. Bucher M, Mair G, Kees F. Effect of roxithromycin on the pharmacokinetics of lovastatin in volunteers. *Eur J Clin Pharmacol* (2002) 57, 787–91.
12. Omar MA, Wilson JP. FDA adverse event reports on statin-associated rhabdomyolysis. *Ann Pharmacother* (2002) 36, 288–95.
13. Mevacor (Lovastatin). Merck & Co., Inc. US Prescribing information, April 2005.
14. Zocor (Simvastatin). Merck Sharp & Dohme. UK Summary of product characteristics, July 2004.

Statins + Nefazodone

Nefazodone has been implicated in cases of muscle toxicity and rhabdomyolysis in two patients on simvastatin, two patients on lovastatin, and one patient on pravastatin.

Clinical evidence

(a) Lovastatin

In a review of the FDA spontaneous reports of statin-associated rhabdomyolysis covering the period November 1997 to March 2000, nefazodone was potentially implicated in 2 cases involving lovastatin.[1]

(b) Pravastatin

A 74-year-old man taking atenolol, aspirin and pravastatin had his treatment with citalopram replaced by nefazodone 50 mg twice daily. Because the possibility of an interaction was suspected, his plasma creatine kinase levels were monitored and were found at 36 hours to be 877 units/l (normal 0 to 190 units/l). Lactate dehydrogenase, aspartate aminotransferase and alanine aminotransferase were all slightly elevated and this was interpreted as indicating muscle toxicity. The nefazodone was withdrawn and although creatine kinase levels were falling they were still above the normal range when the pravastatin was withdrawn 14 days later. Pravastatin was subsequently re-introduced and then 75 mg venlafaxine twice daily was added without problems.[2] However, the diagnosis of muscle toxicity has been questioned, and because pravastatin levels were not measured the possibility of an interaction has also been questioned.[3]

(c) Simvastatin

A 44-year-old man who had uneventfully taken 40 mg of simvastatin daily for 19 weeks developed 'tea-coloured' urine, initially misdiagnosed as a urinary tract infection, a month after starting 100 mg of nefazodone twice daily. A month later he was also complaining of severe myalgias of the thighs and calves, and was found to have muscle weakness and tenderness. Laboratory tests confirmed a diagnosis of rhabdomyolysis and myositis. He was asymptomatic within 3 weeks of stopping both drugs, and remained problem-free 5 weeks after restarting 40 mg simvastatin daily.[4] A further case of rhabdomyolysis has been reported in a 72-year-old man on simvastatin. Symptoms developed 6 weeks after nefazodone was initiated (2 weeks after a dose increment). He recovered with rehydration after the nefazodone was stopped.[5] In a review of the FDA spontaneous reports of statin-associated rhabdomyolysis covering the period November 1997 to March 2000, nefazodone was potentially implicated in 2 cases involving simvastatin.[1]

Mechanism

Uncertain. The suggestion is that nefazodone (an inhibitor of cytochrome P450 isoenzyme CYP3A4, an enzyme involved in the metabolism of simvastatin) caused a marked increase in the serum levels of the simvastatin with accompanying toxicity.[4] The same mechanism might also account for the pravastatin/nefazodone interaction, but this is less clear-cut.[6]

See, 'Lipid-regulating drugs', (p.827) for a more detailed discussion of statin metabolism.

Importance and management

Information about statin/nefazodone interactions seems to be limited to these reports so that the risks associated with using nefazodone are uncertain, but what is known certainly suggests that concurrent use should be very well monitored. The makers of lovastatin and simvastatin advise avoiding the combination.[7,8] Note that in 2003 nefazodone was withdrawn in some countries due to cases of liver toxicity.

1. Omar MA, Wilson JP. FDA adverse event reports on statin-associated rhabdomyolysis. *Ann Pharmacother* (2002) 36, 288–95.
2. Alderman CP. Possible interaction between nefazodone and pravastatin. *Ann Pharmacother* (1999) 33, 871.
3. Bottorf MB. Comment: possible interaction between nefazodone and pravastatin. *Ann Pharmacother* (2000) 34, 538.
4. Jacobsen RH, Wang P, Glueck CJ. Myositis and rhabdomyolysis associated with concurrent use of simvastatin and nefazodone. *JAMA* (1997) 277, 296.
5. Thompson M, Samuels S. Rhabdomyolysis with simvastatin and nefazodone. *Am J Psychiatry* (2002) 159, 1067.
6. Alderman CP. Comment: possible interaction between nefazodone and pravastatin. Author's reply. *Ann Pharmacother* (2000) 34, 538 and 541.
7. Mevacor (Lovastatin), Merck & Co., Inc. US Prescribing information, April 2005.
8. Zocor (Simvastatin). Merck Sharp & Dohme. UK Summary of product characteristics, July 2004.

Statins + Nicotinic acid (Niacin)

Two cases of rhabdomyolysis and one case of myositis have been reported in patients on lovastatin and nicotinic acid (niacin).

Clinical evidence, mechanism, importance and management

Rhabdomyolysis, which developed in a patient on **lovastatin**, was attributed to the addition of nicotinic acid 2.5 g daily.[1] A similar reaction occurred in another patient taking the same combination[2] as well as in a further patient taking ciclosporin, nicotinic acid and **lovastatin**[3] (see also 'Statins + Ciclosporin', p.834). Myositis in another patient on **lovastatin** and nicotinic acid is also briefly reported.[1] These adverse reports are isolated and it is by no means certain that nicotinic acid contributed to what happened. Myopathy does occur with **lovastatin** alone,[4] with a reported incidence of 0.1%. A combined preparation of lovastatin/nicotinic acid is marketed (*Advicor,* USA), and in a 52-week study investigating efficacy and tolerability, none of the 814 patients experienced drug-induced myopathy, although 7 patients were withdrawn from the study due to elevated creatine kinase levels.[5] There do not appear to be any published reports of myopathy occurring with nicotinic acid and any other **statins**. However, in a review of the FDA spontaneous reports of statin-associated rhabdomyolysis covering the period November 1997 to March 2000, nicotinic acid was identified as a potentially interacting drug in 2 of 215 cases for **simvastatin,** 1 of 71 cases for **pravastatin,** and 1 of 40 cases for **lovastatin**. Nicotinic acid was not identified as an interacting drug in any reports for **atorvastatin** or **fluvastatin**.[6]

Nicotinic acid does not alter the bioavailability of **fluvastatin**[7] or **pravastatin**.[8]

Although these cases are isolated, to be on the safe side, if the decision is made to use nicotinic acid with a statin the outcome should be very well monitored. All patients should be warned to report promptly any unexplained muscle aches, tenderness, cramps, stiffness or weakness.

1. Reaven P, Witztum JL. Lovastatin, nicotinic acid and rhabdomyolysis. *Ann Intern Med* (1988) 109, 597–8.
2. Hill MD, Bilbao JM. Case of the month: February 1999 – 54 year old man with severe muscle weakness. *Brain Pathol* (1999) 9, 607–8.
3. Norman DJ, Illingworth DR, Munson J, Hosenpud J. Myolysis and acute renal failure in a heart-transplant recipient receiving lovastatin. *N Engl J Med* (1988) 318, 46–7.
4. Bilheimer DW. Long term clinical tolerance of lovastatin (Mevinolin) and Simvastatin (Epistatin). An overview. *Drug Invest* (1990) 2 (Suppl 2), 58–67.
5. Kashyap ML, McGovern ME, Berra K, Guyton JR, Kwiterovich PO, Harper WL, Toth PD, Favrot LK, Kerzner B, Nash SD, Bays HE, Simmons PD. Long-term safety and efficacy of a once-daily niacin/lovastatin formulation for patients with dyslipidaemia. *Am J Cardiol* (2002) 89, 672–8.
6. Omar MA, Wilson JP. FDA adverse event reports on statin-associated rhabdomyolysis. *Ann Pharmacother* (2002) 36, 288–95.
7. Smith HT, Jokubaitis LA, Troendle AJ, Hwang DS, Robinson WT. Pharmacokinetics of fluvastatin and specific drug interactions. *Am J Hypertens* (1993) 6, 375S–382S.
8. ER Squibb. A report on the effect of nicotinic acid alone and in the presence of aspirin on the bioavailability of SQ 31,000 in healthy male subjects. Data on file (Protocol No 27, 201-6), 1987.

Statins + Orlistat

No clinically relevant interaction has been seen between orlistat and either atorvastatin or pravastatin.

Clinical evidence, mechanism, importance and management

(a) Atorvastatin

In a randomised study, 32 healthy subjects were given atorvastatin 20 mg daily for 6 days, with or without orlistat 120 mg three times daily for 6 days. Orlistat had a no significant effect on the pharmacokinetics of atorvastatin.[1]

(b) Pravastatin

Orlistat 120 mg three times daily was reported to have no effect on the pharmacokinetics or lipid-lowering effects of pravastatin 40 mg daily, when both drugs were administered for 6 days in a placebo-controlled cross-over study in 24 subjects with mild hypercholesterolaemia.[2]

A review includes brief details of a comparative study in two groups of healthy subjects given pravastatin, either with orlistat or placebo. After 10 days there was no significant difference in the pravastatin AUC between the groups, but the maximum serum concentration did show a tendency to be higher in the orlistat group.[3]

1. Zhi J, Moore R, Kanitra L, Mulligan TE. Pharmacokinetic evaluation of the possible interaction between selected concomitant medications and orlistat at steady state in healthy subjects. *J Clin Pharmacol* (2002) 42, 1011–19.
2. Oo CY, Akbari B, Lee S, Nichols G, Hellmann CR. Effect of orlistat, a novel anti-obesity agent, on the pharmacokinetics and pharmacodynamics of pravastatin in patients with mild hypercholesterolaemia. *Clin Drug Invest* (1999) 17, 217–23.
3. Guerciolini R. Mode of action of orlistat. *Int J Obes* (1997) 21 (Suppl 3), S12–S23.

Statins + Phenytoin

In an isolated case, phenytoin reduced the cholesterol lowering effect of simvastatin, fluvastatin and atorvastatin.

Clinical evidence, mechanism, importance and management

A 50-year-old woman taking **simvastatin** 10 mg daily had her anticonvulsant medication changed from sodium valproate to phenytoin 325 mg daily. Over the following 3 months her total cholesterol rose from 9.4 to 15.99 mmol/l. The dose of **simvastatin** was gradually increased to 40 mg daily without significant effect on her cholesterol levels. Despite further changes (to **fluvastatin** 40 mg daily, then to **atorvastatin** 80 mg daily) her cholesterol level remained above 10 mmol/l. Finally phenytoin was discontinued and her cholesterol dropped to 6.24 mmol/l on **atorvastatin** 80 mg daily.[1] The reasons are not known, but it is possible that phenytoin induced the metabolism of the statins, so that they were cleared from the body more quickly and were therefore less effective.

This appears to be the only report of such an interaction and the clinical significance remains unclear. However, if a patient is resistant to, or becomes resistant to statin treatment consider the possibility of this interaction. More study seems warranted.

1. Murphy MJ, Dominiczak MH. Efficacy of statin therapy: possible effect of phenytoin. *Postgrad Med J* (1999) 75, 359–60.

Statins + Protease inhibitors

The levels of atorvastatin and simvastatin appear to be markedly increased by lopinavir/ritonavir, nelfinavir, ritonavir and ritonavir/saquinavir. Pravastatin seems only moderately affected. Two cases of rhabdomyolysis have been attributed to ritonavir used with simvastatin.

Clinical evidence

(a) Lopinavir/Ritonavir

Either **atorvastatin** 20 mg daily or **pravastatin** 20 mg daily were given to 24 healthy subjects for 4 days during a 14-day course of lopinavir/ritonavir 400/100 mg twice daily. The maximum serum levels and AUC of **atorvastatin** were increased by between 4.7 and 5.9-fold and the maximum serum levels and AUC of **pravastatin** were only increased by about 30%. **Atorvastatin** and **pravastatin** had no effect on the pharmacokinetics of lopinavir or ritonavir.[1]

(b) Nelfinavir

In an open label study, 32 healthy subjects were given either **atorvastatin** 10 mg daily or **simvastatin** 20 mg daily for 28 days, in combination with nelfinavir 1250 mg twice daily for the last 14 days. Nelfinavir increased the maximum serum levels and AUC of **atorvastatin** approximately twofold and the maximum serum levels and AUC of **simvastatin** approximately sixfold. No significant side effects, or any signs or rhabdomyolysis were noted throughout the study.[2]

Another study found that nelfinavir 750 mg three times daily increased the maximum serum levels and AUC of **pravastatin** 40 mg daily by 29 and 35% respectively, and increased the maximum serum levels and AUC of **atorvastatin** 40 mg daily by 32 and 209% respectively.[3] In another study, 14 healthy subjects were given nelfinavir 1250 mg twice daily for 18 days, with the addition of **pravastatin** 40 mg daily for the last 4 days. No significant change was noted in the pharmacokinetics of nelfinavir, nor of its major metabolite.[4]

(c) Ritonavir

A 51-year-old woman was admitted to hospital with a 4-day history of muscular aches and weakness. Among other drugs, she had been taking zidovudine, lamivudine, indinavir, and **simvastatin** for 2 years. Ritonavir 100 mg twice daily had been added to her usual regimen 2 weeks previously. The rhabdomyolysis was therefore attributed to a ritonavir/**simvastatin** interaction.[5] Another similar case has also been reported.[6] See also (a) above and (d) below.

(d) Saquinavir/Ritonavir

Ritonavir 300 mg twice daily and saquinavir 400 mg twice daily were given to healthy subjects twice daily for 3 days, followed by ritonavir 400 mg twice daily and saquinavir 400 mg twice daily for a further 11 days. On the last 4 days **atorvastatin**, **pravastatin**, or **simvastatin** (all 40 mg daily) were added to treatment. The mean **pravastatin** AUC was approximately halved (13 subjects), the mean **atorvastatin** AUC was increased approximately fourfold (14 subjects) and the mean **simvastatin** acid AUC was increased approximately 32-fold (14 subjects). No cases of rhabdomyolysis were noted.[4]

Mechanism

The protease inhibitors, especially ritonavir, are known to be strong inhibitors of the cytochrome P450 isoenzyme CYP3A4. The levels of statins metabolised by this isoenzyme are therefore increased. See 'Lipid-regulating drugs', (p.827) for information on the metabolism of the individual statins.

Importance and management

The statin/ protease inhibitor interactions appear to be established by the pharmacokinetic studies cited here, and supported by a few case reports. It is generally recommended that simvastatin and lovastatin be avoided in patients on HIV-protease inhibitors, and atorvastatin used in low doses (i.e.10 mg) with care. Pravastatin can be used, probably without dose adjustments, but monitoring is needed to confirm this.

1. Carr RA, Andre AK, Bertz RJ, Hsu A, Lam W, Chang M, Chen P, Williams L, Bernstein B, Sun E. Concomitant administration of ABT-378/ritonavir (ABT-378/r) results in a clinically important pharmacokinetic (PK) interaction with atorvastatin (ATO) but not pravastatin (PRA). *Intersci Conf Antimicrob Agents Chemother* (2000) 40, 334.
2. Hsyu P-H, Schultz-Smith MD, Lillibridge JH, Lewis RH, Kerr BM. Pharmacokinetic interactions between nelfinavir and 3-hydroxy-methylglutaryl coenzyme A reductase inhibitors atorvastatin and simvastatin. *Antimicrob Agents Chemother* (2001) 45, 3445–50.
3. Barry M, Belz G, Roll S, O'Grady P, Swaminathan A, Geraldes M, Mangold B. Interaction of nelfinavir with atorvastatin and pravastatin in normal healthy volunteers. *AIDS* (2000) 14 (Suppl 4), S90.
4. Fichtenbaum CJ, Gerber JG, Rosenkranz SL, Segal Y, Aberg JA, Blaschke T, Alston B, Fang F, Kosel B, Aweeka F and the NIAID AIDS Clinical Trials Group. Pharmacokinetic interactions between protease inhibitors and statins in HIV seronegative volunteers: ACTG study A5047. *AIDS* (2002) 16, 569–77.
5. Cheng CH, Miller C, Lowe C, Pearson VE. Rhabdomyolysis due to probable interaction between simvastatin and ritonavir. *Am J Health-Syst Pharm* (2002) 59, 728–30.
6. Martin CM, Hoffman V, Berggren RE. Rhabdomyolysis in a patient receiving simvastatin concurrently with highly active antiretroviral therapy. *Intersci Conf Antimicrob Agents Chemother* (2000) 40, 316.

Statins + Rifampicin (Rifampin)

Rifampicin lowers the serum levels of fluvastatin and simvastatin.

Clinical evidence, mechanism, importance and management

It was briefly mentioned in a review by the maker of **fluvastatin** that rifampicin reduced the AUC and the maximum serum levels of **fluvastatin** by 51 and 59% respectively. No further study details were given.[1] In a randomised crossover study, 5 days pre-treatment with rifampicin 600 mg daily reduced the AUCs of **simvastatin** and simvastatin acid in 10 healthy subjects by 87 and 93% respectively.[2] It might therefore be necessary to increase the dosage of **fluvastatin** and **simvastatin** if rifampicin is used concurrently, but this needs confirmation.

1. Jokubaitis LA. Updated clinical safety experience with fluvastatin. *Am J Cardiol* (1994) 73, 18D–24D.
2. Kyrklund C, Backman JT, Kivistö KT, Neuvonen M, Laitila J, Neuvonen PJ. Rifampin greatly reduces plasma simvastatin and simvastatin acid concentrations. *Clin Pharmacol Ther* (2000) 68, 592–7.

Statins + Sildenafil

A man on simvastatin developed symptoms of rhabdomyolysis after taking a single dose of sildenafil. Atorvastatin and sildenafil do not appear to interact pharmacokinetically.

Clinical evidence

A 76-year-old man who had been taking 10 mg of **simvastatin** daily for 3 years uneventfully, presented at a clinic with a 3-day history of severe and unexplained muscle aches, particularly in the lower part of his legs and feet. The problem had started within 10 hours of taking a single 50-mg dose of sildenafil. When examined he showed no muscle tenderness or swelling but his creatine phosphokinase level was slightly raised (406 units/l). There was also a mild elevation of blood urea nitrogen and an increase in creatinine and potassium levels. A tentative diagnosis of rhabdomyolysis was made, there being no other obvious identifiable cause for the myalgia. Both **simvastatin** and sildenafil were stopped, and he made a full recovery.[1] A study in 24 healthy subjects found that the pharmacokinetics of neither sildenafil (single 100-mg dose) nor **atorvastatin** (10 mg daily for 7 days) were changed by concurrent use.[2]

Mechanism, importance and management

The reasons for this possible interaction are not known. This is as yet an isolated case, and no broad generalisations can be based on such slim evidence. Patients should be warned of the risks of rhabdomyolysis when given statins. Based on the current evidence no further precautions currently seem necessary.

1. Gutierrez CA. Sildenafil-simvastatin interaction: possible cause of rhabdomyolysis? *Am Fam Physician* (2001) 63, 636–7.
2. Chung M, DiRico A, Calcagni A, Messig M, Scott R. Lack of a drug interaction between sildenafil and atorvastatin. *J Clin Pharmacol* (2000) 40, 1057.

Statins + St John's wort (*Hypericum perforatum*)

St John's wort modestly decreases the plasma level of simvastatin, but not pravastatin.

Clinical evidence, mechanism, importance and management

In a placebo-controlled crossover study, 16 healthy subjects took St John's wort 300 mg three times daily for 14 days. On day 14 half of them were given 10 mg of **simvastatin** and the other half were given 20 mg of **pravastatin**. St John's wort did not affect the plasma concentration of **pravastatin**, but it tended to reduce the **simvastatin** AUC (by 48%) and significantly reduced the AUC of its active metabolite, simvastatin hydroxy acid, by 62%.[1] The reason for this is unknown, but St John's wort may inhibit the cytochrome P450 isoenzyme CYP3A4 or have some effect on P-glycoprotein. The clinical significance of this is unclear.

1. Sugimoto K, Ohmori M, Tsuruoka S, Nishiki K, Kawaguchi A, Harada K, Arakawa M, Sakomoto K, Masada M, Miyamori I, Fujimura A. Different effects of St John's wort on the pharmacokinetics of simvastatin and pravastatin. *Clin Pharmacol Ther* (2001) 70, 518–24.

Statins + Tacrolimus

An isolated case of rhabdomyolysis occurred following the concurrent use of tacrolimus and simvastatin.

Clinical evidence, mechanism, importance and management

A 51-year-old woman, who was taking tacrolimus after a kidney transplant, was started on **simvastatin** 10 mg daily following a stroke. After 5 months, the dose was increased to 20 mg daily, and fusidic acid was started for osteomyelitis. Muscle pain developed 2 weeks later, and after a further 3 weeks she was admitted to hospital and her creatinine kinase was found to be 24,000 units/ml (reported normal range 10 to 70 units/ml) and she had renal impairment. The **simvastatin** and fusidic acid were immediately stopped and the patient recovered over the following 2 weeks. She was later treated with a combination of **fluvastatin**, tacrolimus and fusidic acid without incident, leading the authors to suspect that the rhabdomyolysis was caused by an interaction between simvastatin and tacrolimus.[1] The clinical significance of this interaction is unclear, but it would seem wise to warn patients receiving the combination to be on the look out for the symptoms of myopathy and rhabdomyolysis.

1. Kotanko P, Kiristis W, Skrabal F. Rhabdomyolysis and acute renal graft impairment in a patient treated with simvastatin, tacrolimus, and fusidic acid. *Nephron* (2002) 90, 234–5.

Statins; Atorvastatin + Delavirdine

A man developed rhabdomyolysis after taking atorvastatin and delavirdine concurrently.

Clinical evidence, mechanism, importance and management

An isolated case report describes a 63-year-old HIV+ man, who had been taking atorvastatin 20 mg daily with indinavir, lamivudine and stavudine, and who was admitted to hospital 2 months after delavirdine had been substituted for indinavir. He had a one-month history of malaise, muscle pain, vomiting, and dark urine. Laboratory tests confirmed a diagnosis of rhabdomyolysis, and he was found to have acute renal failure. All drugs were withheld, and he gradually recovered over the following month. It was suggested that delavirdine inhibited the metabolism of atorvastatin. The authors recommend great caution if this drug combination is used.[1]

1. Castro JG, Gutierrez L. Rhabdomyolysis with acute renal failure probably related to the interaction of atorvastatin and delavirdine. *Am J Med* (2002) 112, 505.

Statins; Cerivastatin + Miscellaneous

Cerivastatin has now been withdrawn by the makers because of severe muscle toxicity, but its interactions are briefly listed here for completeness.

Clinical evidence, mechanism, importance and management

A number of cases of severe rhabdomyolysis have been reported with the combination of **gemfibrozil** and cerivastatin.[1-5] This drug combination was contraindicated by the makers, who note that **gemfibrozil** 600 mg twice daily increased the AUC of cerivastatin fourfold[6] (see also 'Statins + Fibrates', p.836).

One study indicated that **ciclosporin** increased the maximum concentration and AUC of cerivastatin three to fivefold,[7,8] (therefore the maker recommended that treatment should be started at the lowest dose).[6] A case of rhabdomyolysis has been seen with this combination.[9] Cerivastatin did not affect **ciclosporin** levels.[8,10]

Tacrolimus also appears to raise cerivastatin levels.[11] A case of rhabdomyolysis has also been seen with cerivastatin and **risperidone** in combination.[12] **Erythromycin** caused a small 21% in the AUC of a single-dose of cerivastatin,[13] and a 51% increase in cerivastatin AUC on multiple dosing.[7] Similarly, **itraconazole** caused a small 38% increase in the AUC of cerivastatin.[7] Rhabdomyolysis associated with cerivastatin was reported on 215 occasions in the FDA adverse reports database for the period November 1997 to March 2000. Of these cases 22 had taken concomitant **fibrates** (unspecified), two **macrolide antibacterials**, one **ciclosporin**, and one **mibefradil**.[14]

Colestyramine causes a small reduction in the serum levels of cerivastatin, which can be avoided by separating administration.[6,7,15]

Cimetidine,[16] **digoxin**,[17] **fenofibrate**,[6] **magnesium** and **aluminium hydroxide** *(Maalox)*,[16] **nifedipine**,[18] **omeprazole**,[19] **orlistat**[20] and **warfarin**[21] do not appear to alter the pharmacokinetics of cerivastatin. Cerivastatin did not alter the pharmacokinetics of **fenofibrate**,[6] **nifedipine**,[18] or **digoxin**,[17] and did not alter the anticoagulant effect of **warfarin**.[21]

1. Pogson GW, Kindred LH, Carper BG. Rhabdomyolysis and renal failure associated with *cerivastatin-gemfibrozil* combination therapy. *Am J Cardiol* (1999) 83, 1146.
2. Bermingham PR, Whitsitt TB, Smart ML, Nowak DP, Scalley RD. Rhabdomyolysis in a patient receiving the combination of cerivastatin and gemfibrozil. *Am J Health-Syst Pharm* (2000) 57, 461–4.
3. Özdemir Ö, Boran M, Gökçe V, Uzun Y, Koçak B, Korkmaz Ş. A case with severe rhabdomyolysis and renal failure associated with cerivastatin-gemfibrozil combination therapy. *Angiology* (2000) 50, 695–7.
4. Bruno-Joyce J, Dugas JM, MacCausland OE. Cerivastatin and gemfibrozil-associated rhabdomyolysis. *Ann Pharmacother* (2001) 35, 1016–19.
5. Vascónez Espinosa F, Gómez Rodríguez N, Martín Joven A, Posada García FJ. Rabdomiólisis complicada con insuficiencia renal aguda en un paciente tratado con gemfibrozilo y cerivastatina. *Rev Clin Esp* (2001) 201, 228–9.
6. Lipobay (Cerivastatin). Bayer. UK Summary of product characteristics, June 2001.
7. Mück W. Rational assessment of the interaction profile of cerivastatin supports its low propensity for drug interactions. *Drugs* (1998) 56 (Suppl 1), 15–23.
8. Mai I, Bauer S, Fritsche J, Ochmann K, Mück W, Rohde G, Roots I, Neumayer H-H, Kuhlmann J. Single-dose pharmacokinetics of a new HMG-COA reductase inhibitor in renal transplant patients treated with cyclosporine A (CSA). *Eur J Clin Pharmacol* (1997) 52 (Suppl), A137.
9. Mora C, Rodriguez ML, Navarro JF. Cerivastatin-induced rhabdomyolysis in a renal transplant on cyclosporin. *Transplantation* (2001) 72, 551.
10. Renders L, Mayer-Kadner I, Koch C, Schärffe S, Burkhardt K, Veelken R, Schmieder RE, Hauser IA. Efficacy and drug interactions of the new HMG-CoA reductase inhibitors cerivastatin and atorvastatin in CsA-treated renal transplant recipients. *Nephrol Dial Transplant* (2001) 16, 141–6.
11. Mück W, Neal DAJ, Boix O, Voith B, Hasan R, Alexander GJM. Tacrolimus/cerivastatin interaction study in liver transplant recipients. *Br J Clin Pharmacol* (2001) 52, 213–17.
12. Giner V, Muñoz R, Redón J. Risperidone and severe cerivastatin-induced rhabdomyolysis. *J Intern Med* (2002) 251, 177–8.
13. Mück W, Ochmann K, Rhode G, Unger S, Kuhlmann J. Influence of erythromycin pre- and co-treatment on single dose pharmacokinetics of the HMG-CoA reductase inhibitor cerivastatin. *Eur J Clin Pharmacol* (1998) 53, 469–73.
14. Omar MA, Wilson JP. FDA adverse event reports on statin-associated rhabdomyolysis. *Ann Pharmacother* (2002) 36, 288–95.
15. Mück W, Ritter W, Frey R, Wetzelsberger N, Lücker PW, Kuhlmann J. Influence of cholestyramine on the pharmacokinetics of cerivastatin. *Int J Clin Pharmacol Ther* (1997) 35, 250–4.
16. Mück W, Ritter W, Dietrich H, Frey R, Kuhlmann J. Influence of the antacid Maalox and the H_2-antagonist cimetidine on the pharmacokinetics of cerivastatin. *Int J Clin Pharmacol Ther* (1997) 35, 261–4.
17. Weber P, Lettieri JT, Kaiser L, Mazzu AL. Lack of mutual pharmacokinetic interaction between cerivastatin, a new HMG-CoA reductase inhibitor, and digoxin in healthy normocholesterolemic volunteers. *Clin Ther* (1999) 21, 1563–75.
18. Sachse R, Brendel E, Mück W, Rohde G, Ochmann K, Horstmann R, Kuhlmann J. Lack of drug-drug interaction between cerivastatin and nifedipine. *Int J Clin Pharmacol Ther* (1998) 36, 409–13.
19. Sachse R, Ochmann K, Rohde G, Mück W. The effect of omeprazole pre- and cotreatment on cerivastatin absorption and metabolism in man. *Int J Clin Pharmacol Ther* (1998) 36, 517–20.

20. Mück W, Adelmann H-G, Ruf T, Unger S, Voith B. Lack of pharmacokinetic drug-drug interaction between orlistat and cerivastatin. *Clin Drug Invest* (2000) 19, 71–3.

21. Schall R, Müller FO, Hundt HKL, Ritter W, Duursema L, Groenewoud G, Middle MV. No pharmacokinetic or pharmacodynamic interaction between rivastatin and warfarin. *J Clin Pharmacol* (1995) 35, 306–13.

Statins; Lovastatin + Danazol and Doxycycline

Severe rhabdomyolysis and myoglobinuria developed in a man on lovastatin about two months after danazol was added. A short course of doxycycline may have had some part to play in what happened.

Clinical evidence, mechanism, importance and management

A 72-year-old man taking atenolol, aspirin, dipyridamole and lovastatin 20 mg twice daily was admitted to hospital after complaining of myalgia over the last 12 days, with brown urine over the last 5 days. His condition was diagnosed as severe rhabdomyolysis and myoglobinuria. About 2 months previously he had been additionally started on danazol 200 mg three times daily and prednisone, and one month previously he had received a 10-day course of doxycycline 100 mg twice daily. The aspirin and lovastatin were stopped (danazol was stopped 4 days before admission and the doxycycline was stopped 5 days before the onset of symptoms), and all the symptoms resolved. Laboratory tests were normal within 2 weeks. The reasons for this reaction are not known, but the authors postulate that danazol (and the doxycycline) were possibly hepatotoxic, and that danazol may have inhibited cytochrome P450. As a result, the metabolism of the lovastatin could have been reduced, leading to the development of lovastatin muscle toxicity. It might also be that the danazol had a direct toxic effect on the muscles.[1]

This appears to be the first and only report of this apparent interaction. Its general importance is unknown, but it would now seem prudent to monitor the concurrent use of lovastatin and either danazol or doxycycline. The authors of the report point out that other cases of severe lovastatin muscle toxicity have also been very slow to develop.

1. Dallaire M, Chamberland M, Rhabdomyolysis sévère chez un patient recevant lovastatine, danazol et doxycycline. *Can Med Assoc J* (1994) 150, 1991–4.

Statins; Lovastatin + Fibre or Pectin

Pectin and oat bran can reduce the cholesterol-lowering effects of lovastatin.

Clinical evidence, mechanism, importance and management

The serum LDL-cholesterol levels of 3 patients on 80 mg lovastatin daily showed a marked rise from 4.48 to 6.36 mmol/l when they were additionally given 15 g of pectin daily. One patient had a 59% rise in LDL-cholesterol.[1] Two other patients on lovastatin showed a rise in LDL-cholesterol from 5.03 to 6.54 mmol/l when they were additionally given 50 to 100 g of **oat bran** daily. One patient had a 41% rise in LDL cholesterol.[1] When the pectin and **oat bran** were stopped, the serum levels of the LDL-cholesterol fell. It is presumed that both pectin and **oat bran** reduced the absorption of lovastatin from the gut.[1] Evidence is still very limited but patients should be advised not to take either of these two fibres at the same time as lovastatin. Separate their ingestion as much as possible. More study is needed.

1. Richter WO, Jacob BG, Schwandt P. Interaction between fibre and lovastatin. *Lancet* (1991) 338, 706.

Statins; Pravastatin + Aspirin

Aspirin 324 mg did not significantly affect the pharmacokinetics of a single 20-mg dose of pravastatin.[1]

1. ER Squibb. A report on the effect of nicotinic acid alone and in the presence of aspirin on the bioavailability of SQ 31,000 in healthy male subjects. Data on file (Protocol No 27, 201-6), 1987.

Statins; Pravastatin + Mianserin

An isolated report describes rhabdomyolysis attributed to the long-term concurrent use of pravastatin and mianserin, triggered by a cold.

Clinical evidence, mechanism, importance and management

An isolated report describes a 72-year-old woman on pravastatin 20 mg and mianserin 10 mg daily for 2 years, who was hospitalised because of weakness in her legs that began 2 days previously, shortly after she got a cold. She could stand, but was unable to walk unaided. Laboratory data revealed evidence of increased serum enzymes, all of which suggested rhabdomyolysis. Within a week of stopping the pravastatin the leg weakness had disappeared and all of the laboratory results had returned to normal. The authors of the report attributed the toxicity to the long-term use of both drugs, ageing and the development of a cold.[1] But what part these factors and/or the presence of mianserin actually played in the development of this toxicity is not known. However, it does highlight the need to monitor for the development of muscular toxicity during the use of any of the statins, even pravastatin, which normally appears to be relatively free of adverse interactions.

1. Takei A, Chiba S. Rhabdomyolysis associated with pravastatin treatment for major depression. *Psychiatry Clin Neurosci* (1999) 53, 539.

Statins; Pravastatin + Probucol

No clinically significant changes in the bioavailability of a single 20-mg dose of pravastatin was seen in 20 healthy subjects given 500 mg probucol.[1]

1. ER Squibb. A report on the bioavailability of pravastatin in the presence and absence of gemfibrozil or probucol in healthy male subjects. Data on file (Protocol No 27, 201-18), 1988.

Statins; Simvastatin + Bosentan

Bosentan modestly reduces the AUC of simvastatin and its active metabolite, which could lead to a reduction in simvastatin efficacy.

Clinical evidence

In a three-way crossover study, 9 healthy subjects were given either bosentan 125 mg twice daily for 5.5 days, simvastatin 40 mg daily for 6 days, or both treatments together. Simvastatin had no effect on the pharmacokinetics of bosentan, but bosentan reduced the AUC of simvastatin and its β-hydroxyacid metabolite by 34 and 46% respectively.[1]

Mechanism

Bosentan is known to be a mild inducer of the cytochrome P450 isoenzyme CYP3A4, which is involved in the metabolism of simvastatin. See 'Lipid-regulating drugs', (p.827) for more information on the metabolism of all the statins.

Importance and management

A 40% reduction in the AUC of simvastatin is potentially clinically significant. If bosentan and simvastatin are used concurrently is would seem prudent to monitor the outcome to ensure simvastatin is effective.

1. Dingemanse J, Schaarschmidt D, van Giersbergen PLM. Investigation of the mutual pharmacokinetic interactions between bosentan, a dual endothelin receptor antagonist, and simvastatin. *Clin Pharmacokinet* (2003) 42, 293–301.

Statins; Simvastatin + Imatinib

Imatinib raises simvastatin serum levels, increasing the risk of toxicity.

Clinical evidence, mechanism, importance and management

In a single-dose study, 20 patients with chronic myeloid leukaemia were given simvastatin 40 mg prior to and on the last day of a 7-day course of imatinib 400 mg daily. Imatinib increased the maximum serum levels of simvastatin 2-fold and the AUC 3.5-fold. The authors conclude that caution should be taken if simvastatin and imatinib are taken concurrently.[1]

These rises increase the risk of simvastatin toxicity (myopathy/rhabdomyolysis), for which reason the simvastatin dosage should be reduced appropriately, probably by about one-half.

1. O'Brien SG, Peng B, Dutreix C, Mehring G, Milosavljev S, Capdeville R, Fischer T. A pharmacokinetic interaction of Glivec® and simvastatin, a cytochrome 3A4 substrate, in patients with chronic myeloid leukaemia. 43rd Annual Meeting of the American Society of Haematology, Orlando, Florida, USA, 2001. Abstract 593.

Statins; Simvastatin + Irbesartan

Irbesartan appears not to alter the pharmacokinetics of simvastatin.

Clinical evidence, mechanism, importance and management

A study in 12 healthy subjects found that 300 mg of irbesartan had no significant effect on the pharmacokinetics of a single 50-mg dose of simvastatin, or of its metabolite simvastatin acid, and the combination was well-tolerated.[1]

1. Marino MR, Vachharajani NN, Hadjilambris OW. Irbesartan does not affect the pharmacokinetics of simvastatin in healthy subjects. *J Clin Pharmacol* (2000) 40, 875–9.

29

Lithium

Lithium is used in the management of mania, bipolar disorder (formerly manic depression) and recurrent depressive illnesses. The dosage of lithium is adjusted to give therapeutic plasma concentrations of 0.4 to 1 mmol/l, although it should be noted that this is the range used in the UK, and other ranges have been quoted.

Lithium is given under close supervision with regular monitoring of blood concentrations, initially at least once a week, because there is a narrow margin between therapeutic concentrations and those that are toxic. Monitoring every 3 months is advised for those on stable regimens. It is usual to take serum lithium samples about 10 to 12 hours after the last oral dose.

Adverse effects that are not usually considered serious include nausea, weakness, fine tremor, mild polydipsia and polyuria. If serum concentrations rise into the 1.5 to 2 mmol/l range, toxicity usually occurs, and may present as lethargy, drowsiness, coarse hand tremor, muscular weakness, abdominal pain, nausea and vomiting or diarrhoea. Higher levels result in neurotoxicity, which manifests as confusion, nystagmus, movement disorders, and even coma or seizures. Cardiovascular symptoms may also develop and include ECG changes and circulatory problems.[1] Lithium levels of over 2 mmol/l can be extremely dangerous and therefore require urgent attention. Chronic lithium toxicity has a 9% mortality, whilst acute toxicity has a 25% mortality.[2]

In addition to the effects described above, lithium can induce diabetes insipidus and hypothyroidism in some patients, and is contraindicated in those with renal or cardiac insufficiency.

Just how lithium exerts its beneficial effects is not known, but it may compete with sodium ions in various parts of the body, and it alters the electrolyte composition of body fluids.

Most of the interactions involving lithium are discussed in this section but a few are found elsewhere in this publication. Virtually all of the reports are concerned with the carbonate, but sometimes lithium is given as the acetate, aspartate, chloride, citrate, gluconate, orotate or sulphate instead. There is no reason to believe that these lithium compounds will not interact just like lithium carbonate. The lithium compounds are listed, with their proprietary names, in 'Table 29.1', below.

1. Finley PR, Warner MD, Peabody CA. Clinical relevance of drug interactions with lithium. *Clin Pharmacokinet* (1995) 29, 172–91.
2. Vipond AJ, Bakewell S, Telford R, Nicholls AJ. Lithium toxicity. *Anaesthesia* (1996) 51, 1156–8.

Table 29.1 Lithium compounds: generic and proprietary names

Generic names	*Proprietary names*
Lithium acetate	Quilonum, Quilonorm
Lithium carbonate	Camcolit, Carbolit, Carbolith, Carbolithium, Carbolitium, Carboron, Ceglution, Contemnol, Eskalith, Hypnorex, Karlit, Lentolith, Leukominerase, Li 450, Licab, Licarb, Licarbium, Limed, Liskonum, Lit-300, Lithane, Litheum, Lithicarb, Lithobid, Lithonate, Liticarb, Litiocar, Lito, Milithin, Maniprex, Neurolepsin, Neurolithium, Phanate, Plenur, Priadel, Quilonorm, Quilonum, Teralithe
Lithium chloride	
Lithium citrate	Litarex, Li-Liquid, Priadel
Lithium gluconate	Neurolithium
Lithium glutamate	
Lithium orotate	
Lithium sulfate	Lithiofor, Lithionit

Lithium + ACE inhibitors

No important interaction between lithium compounds and ACE inhibitors occurs in most individuals, but in some the serum lithium levels can rise by about one-third. A number of cases of lithium toxicity have been reported in patients when given captopril, enalapril or lisinopril (and possibly perindopril). Risk factors seem to be poor renal function, heart failure, volume depletion, and increased age.

Clinical evidence

(a) Captopril

A patient taking lithium carbonate developed a serum lithium level of 2.35 mmol/l and toxicity (tremor, dysarthria, digestive problems) within 10 days of starting to take captopril 50 mg daily. He was restabilised on half his previous dose of lithium.[1] A retrospective study also reports a case of increased lithium levels with captopril (see under *(c) Lisinopril*, below).

(b) Enalapril

A woman taking lithium carbonate developed signs of lithium toxicity (ataxia, dysarthria, tremor, confusion) within 2 to 3 weeks of starting to take enalapril 20 mg daily. After 5 weeks her serum lithium levels had risen from 0.88 to 3.3 mmol/l, and moderate renal impairment was noted.[2] No toxicity occurred when the enalapril was later replaced by nifedipine.[2] Lithium toxicity following the use of enalapril, and associated in some cases with a decrease in renal function, has been seen in another 5 patients,[3-7] and a reduced lithium dosage was found adequate in another patient.[8] Enalapril 5 mg daily for 9 days had no effect on the mean serum lithium levels of 9 healthy young male subjects. However, one subject developed a 31% increase in lithium levels.[9]

A retrospective study also reports several cases of increased lithium levels with enalapril (see under *(c) Lisinopril*, below).

(c) Lisinopril

A retrospective study of patient records identified 20 patients who were stabilised on lithium and then started on an ACE inhibitor (13 given lisinopril, 6 enalapril and one captopril). Their serum lithium levels rose by an average of 35% (from 0.64 to 0.86 mmol/l) and there was a 26% decrease in lithium clearance. Signs and symptoms suggestive of toxicity (increased tremor, confusion, ataxia), necessitating a dosage reduction or lithium withdrawal, developed in 20% of these patients. In three patients the development of the interaction was delayed for several weeks.[10] A woman on lithium developed lithium toxicity and a trough serum level of 3 mmol/l within 3 weeks of stopping clonidine and starting lisinopril 20 mg daily.[11] Four other reports similarly describe acute lithium toxicity in four patients when they were given lisinopril.[7,12-14] One of them was also taking verapamil,[14] which has also been shown to interact with lithium, but not raise lithium levels (see 'Lithium + Calcium channel blockers' p.850).

(d) Perindopril

Toxicity took 3 months to develop in one patient[15] when given perindopril and bendroflumethiazide, which is also known to increase serum lithium levels, see 'Lithium + Diuretics; Thiazides or related', p.851.

(e) Ramipril

Ramipril has been shown to decrease renal lithium excretion in *rats*.[16]

Mechanism

Not fully understood. One suggestion is that because the ACE inhibitors reduce drinking behaviour, and both ACE inhibitors and lithium cause sodium to be lost in the urine, fluid depletion can occur. The normal compensatory reaction for this is constriction of the efferent renal arterioles to maintain the glomerular filtration rate, but this mechanism is blocked by the ACE inhibitor. Consequently the renal excretion of lithium falls and toxicity develops.

Importance and management

The lithium/ACE inhibitor interaction is established, but not of clinical importance in every patient. Generally, lithium levels can rise to some extent, but toxicity is infrequent. If any ACE inhibitor is added to established lithium treatment, monitor well for symptoms of lithium toxicity (see 'Lithium', (p.845)) and consider taking lithium levels. Be alert for the need to reduce the lithium dosage (possibly by between one-third to one-half).[11,13] The development of the interaction may be delayed, so monitoring lithium levels every week[11] or every two weeks[10] for several weeks has been advised. There are risk factors: age,[10,11] congestive heart failure,[9,11] renal insufficiency[6,11] and volume depletion[5,11] have all been implicated, and are considered as contraindications in some cases.[6,11] Only captopril, enalapril, lisinopril (and possibly perindopril) have been reported to interact, but it seems likely, given the proposed mechanism, that this interaction will occur with any other ACE inhibitor.

1. Pulik M, Lida H. Interaction lithium-inhibiteurs de l'enzyme de conversion. *Presse Med* (1988) 17, 755.
2. Douste-Blazy P, Rostin M, Livarek B, Tordjman E, Montastruc JL, Galinier F. Angiotensin converting enzyme inhibitors and lithium treatment. *Lancet* (1986) i, 1448.
3. Mahieu M, Houvenagel E, Leduc JJ, Choteau P. Lithium-inhibiteurs de l'enzyme conversion: une association á éviter? *Presse Med* (1988) 17, 281.
4. Drouet A, Bouvet O. Lithium et inhibiteurs de l'enzyme de conversion. *Encephale* (1990) 16, 51–2.
5. Navis GJ, de Jong PE, de Zeeuw D. Volume homeostasis, angiotensin converting enzyme inhibition, and lithium therapy. *Am J Med* (1989) 86, 621.
6. Simon G. Combination angiotensin converting enzyme inhibitor/lithium therapy contraindicated in renal disease. *Am J Med* (1988) 85, 893–4.
7. Correa FJ, Eiser AR. Angiotensin-converting enzyme inhibitors and lithium toxicity. *Am J Med* (1992) 93, 108–9.
8. Ahmad S. Sudden hypothyroidism and amiodarone-lithium combination: an interaction. *Cardiovasc Drugs Ther* (1995) 9, 827–8.
9. DasGupta K, Jefferson JW, Kobak KA, Greist JH. The effect of enalapril on serum lithium levels in healthy men. *J Clin Psychiatry* (1992) 53, 398–400.
10. Finley PR, O'Brien JG, Coleman RW. Lithium and angiotensin-converting enzyme inhibitors: evaluation of a potential interaction. *J Clin Psychopharmacol* (1996) 16, 68–71.
11. Baldwin CM, Safferman AZ. A case of lisinopril-induced lithium toxicity. *DICP Ann Pharmacother* (1990) 24, 946–7.
12. Griffin JH, Hahn SM. Lisinopril-induced lithium toxicity. *DICP Ann Pharmacother* (1991) 25, 101.
13. Anon. ACE inhibitors and lithium toxicity. *Biol Ther Psychiatry* (1988) 11, 43.
14. Chandragiri SS, Pasol E, Gallagher RM. Lithium, ACE inhibitors, NSAIDs, and verapamil. A possible fatal combination. *Psychosomatics* (1998) 39, 281–2.
15. Vipond AJ, Bakewell S, Telford R, Nicholls AJ. Lithium toxicity. *Anaesthesia* (1996) 51, 1156–8.
16. Barthelmebs M, Grima M, Imbs J-L. Ramipril-induced decrease in renal lithium excretion in the rat. *Br J Pharmacol* (1995) 116, 2161–5.

Lithium + Acetazolamide

There is evidence that the excretion of lithium can be increased by acetazolamide, but lithium toxicity has been seen in one patient given the combination.

Clinical evidence, mechanism, importance and management

A short-term study in 6 subjects given lithium and acetazolamide found a 27 to 31% increase in the urinary excretion of lithium.[1] A woman was successfully treated for a lithium overdose with acetazolamide, intravenous fluids, sodium bicarbonate, potassium chloride and mannitol.[2] Paradoxically lithium toxicity occurred in another patient after a months' treatment with acetazolamide. Lithium levels rose from 0.8 to 5 mmol/l, although it should be noted that the later measurement was taken 8 hours post-dose.[3] See 'Lithium', (p.845) for details of lithium monitoring.

1. Thomsen K, Schou M. Renal lithium excretion in man. *Am J Physiol* (1968) 215, 823–7.
2. Horowitz LC, Fisher GU. Acute lithium toxicity. *N Engl J Med* (1969) 281, 1369.
3. Gay C, Plas J, Granger B, Olie JP, Loo H. Intoxication au lithium. Deux interactions inédites: l'acétazolamide et l'acide niflumique. *Encephale* (1985) 11, 261–2.

Lithium + Aciclovir

An isolated case report describes lithium toxicity caused by high dose intravenous aciclovir.

Clinical evidence, mechanism, importance and management

A 42-year-old woman taking lithium carbonate 450 mg twice daily developed signs of lithium toxicity 6 days after starting treatment with intravenous aciclovir 10 mg/kg 8-hourly for a severe herpes zoster infection following chemotherapy. Her serum lithium levels had risen over fourfold to 3.4 mmol/l. The reasons are unknown but the authors of the report postulate that aciclovir may have inhibited the renal excretion of lithium.[1]

This appears to be the first and only report of this interaction, but it would now be prudent to monitor for symptoms of lithium toxicity (see 'Lithium', (p.845)) and consider taking lithium levels (every second or third day is the recommendation in this report) if high dose intravenous aciclovir is given to any patient. Oral aciclovir is predicted not to interact because of its low bioavailability, and no interaction would be expected with topical aciclovir as the plasma levels achieved by this route are minimal.

1. Sylvester RK, Leitch J, Granum C. Does acyclovir increase serum lithium levels? *Pharmacotherapy* (1996) 16, 466–8.

Lithium + Angiotensin II receptor antagonists

Lithium toxicity has been seen in individual patients given candesartan, losartan and valsartan. No interaction has yet been reported with any of the other angiotensin II receptor antagonists, but they would be expected to interact similarly.

Clinical evidence

(a) Candesartan

A 58-year-old woman on long-term lithium for depression (stable levels between 0.6 and 0.7 mmol/l), and unnamed calcium antagonists over several years for hypertension, was additionally given candesartan 16 mg daily. She was hospitalised 8 weeks later with a 10-day history of ataxia, increasing confusion, disorientation and agitation and was found to have a serum lithium level of 3.25 mmol/l. She recovered completely when all the drugs were stopped. She was later restabilised on her original lithium dosage with a change to urapidil for her hypertension.[1]

(b) Losartan

An elderly woman on lithium carbonate developed lithium toxicity (ataxia, dysarthria, and confusion) after the addition of losartan 50 mg daily. Her serum lithium levels rose from 0.63 mmol/l to 2 mmol/l over 5 weeks. When the losartan was replaced by nicardipine, her serum lithium levels were restabilised at 0.77 mmol/l within 2 weeks.[2]

(c) Valsartan

A woman with a long history of bipolar disorder was treated with lithium carbonate (serum levels consistently at 0.9 mmol/l) and a number of other drugs (L-tryptophan, lorazepam, glibenclamide, conjugated oestrogens and ciprofloxacin). Two weeks before being hospitalised for a manic relapse she was additionally started on valsartan 80 mg daily. While in hospital the ciprofloxacin was stopped, lorazepam was replaced by zopiclone, and quetiapine was added. On day 3 of her hospitalisation her serum lithium levels were 1.1 mmol/l and she became increasingly delirious, confused and ataxic over the next week. By day 11 her serum lithium levels had risen to 1.4 mmol/l. When an interaction was suspected, the valsartan was replaced by diltiazem. She later recovered and was stabilised on her original lithium carbonate dosage with levels of 0.8 mmol/l.[3]

Mechanism

Not fully understood. It could be that, as with the ACE inhibitors, angiotensin II receptor antagonists inhibit aldosterone secretion, resulting in increased sodium loss by the kidney tubules. This causes lithium retention and thus an increase in lithium levels. However, angiotensin II receptor antagonists have less effect on aldosterone then the ACE inhibitors, making a clinically significant interaction less likely. *Animal* studies show that ramipril,[4] but not losartan[5] decreases the excretion of lithium by the kidney, which would support this idea.

Importance and management

Direct information about interactions between lithium and angiotensin-II receptor antagonists seems to be limited to these three reports, although the interaction has been predicted to occur with all drugs of this class. Such sparse evidence is not enough to recommend contraindicating the concurrent use of candesartan, losartan or valsartan with lithium, but it would be prudent to monitor the outcome. The same precautions would also be appropriate with any other angiotensin-II receptor antagonist (**eprosartan**, **irbesartan**, **telmisartan**), which is the advice of the makers of these drugs, even though the risk of an interaction is probably fairly low. Ideally serum lithium levels should be monitored; one reports suggests weekly monitoring for the first month of concurrent use,[3] but any rise in serum lithium levels may be gradual so that toxicity might take as long as 3 to 7 weeks to develop fully.

Patients on lithium should be aware of the symptoms of lithium toxicity and told to immediately report them should they occur. This should be reinforced when they are given angiotensin II antagonists.

1. Zwanzger P, Marcuse A, Boerner RJ, Walther A, Rupprecht R. Lithium intoxication after administration of AT_1 blockers. *J Clin Psychiatry* (2001) 62, 208–9.
2. Blanche P, Raynaud E, Kerob D, Galezowski N. Lithium intoxication in an elderly patient after combined treatment with losartan. *Eur J Clin Pharmacol* (1997) 52, 501.
3. Leung M, Remick RA. Potential drug interaction between lithium and valsartan. *J Clin Psychopharmacol* (2000) 20, 392–3.
4. Barthelmebs M, Grima M, Imbs JL. Ramipril-induced decrease in renal excretion in the rat. *Br J Pharmacol* (1995) 116, 2161–5.
5. Barthelmebs M, Alt-Tebacher M, Madonna O, Grima M, Imbs J-L. Absence of a losartan interaction with renal lithium excretion in the rat. *Br J Pharmacol* (1995) 116, 2166–9.

Lithium + Anticonvulsants; Carbamazepine

Although combined use is beneficial in many patients, mild to severe neurotoxicity is reported to have developed in some, and possibly sinus node dysfunction in others. An isolated case of lithium toxicity has been reported, apparently caused by carbamazepine-induced renal failure.

Clinical evidence

A patient on lithium 1800 mg daily developed severe neurotoxicity (ataxia, truncal tremors, nystagmus, limb hyperreflexia, muscle fasciculation) within three days of starting to take carbamazepine 600 mg daily. Blood levels of both drugs remained within the therapeutic range. The symptoms resolved when each drug was withdrawn in turn, and re-occurred within 3 days of restarting concurrent treatment.[1] Five rapid-cycling bipolar patients developed similar neurotoxic symptoms (confusion, drowsiness, generalised weakness, lethargy, coarse tremor, hyperreflexia, cerebellar signs) when concurrently treated with lithium carbonate and carbamazepine (doses not stated). Plasma levels of both drugs remained within the accepted range.[2] Other reports describe adverse neurological effects during concurrent use, which were also not accompanied by significant changes in drug serum levels,[3-5] although in one patient raised serum levels of both drugs were seen.[6]

A nine-year study in a psychiatric hospital found that, of 5 patients on lithium who developed sinus node dysfunction, 4 were also on carbamazepine.[7] Another study in 10 patients found that carbamazepine 300 to 600 mg daily was not effective in treating the polyuria and polydipsia associated with lithium treatment, and half of the patients dropped out of the study because of ataxia, dizziness, restlessness and confusion.[8] An isolated case report describes carbamazepine-induced acute renal failure, which resulted in lithium toxicity.[9]

A systematic search through the Medline database over approximately 30 years from 1966 for reports of neurotoxic adverse effects in patients on lithium at low therapeutic concentrations found a total of 41 cases. Carbamazepine had been taken concurrently in 22% of these cases, in some instances with other potentially interacting drugs.[10]

In contrast, combined treatment in other patients is said to be well tolerated and beneficial,[11,12] but one report suggests that the dosages may need to be reduced to avoid adverse effects.[13]

Mechanism

Not understood. A paper that plotted the serum levels of lithium and carbamazepine on a two-dimensional graph failed to find evidence of synergistic toxicity.[14] Sinus node dysfunction can be caused by either lithium or carbamazepine, but this is rare. However, the effects may possibly be additive.

Importance and management

The neurotoxic interaction is established, but its incidence is not known. It may be quite small. If concurrent use is undertaken, the outcome should be closely monitored. This is particularly important because neurotoxicity can develop even though the drug serum levels remain within the accepted therapeutic range. If any neurotoxicity develops the lithium treatment should be discontinued promptly, whatever the lithium level.[10] The authors of one paper suggest that the risk factors appear to be a history of neurotoxicity with lithium, and compromised medical or neurological function.[2]

1. Chaudhry RP, Waters BGH. Lithium and carbamazepine interaction: possible neurotoxicity. *J Clin Psychiatry* (1983) 44, 30–1.

2. Shukla S, Godwin CD, Long LEB, Miller MG. Lithium-carbamazepine neurotoxicity and risk factors. *Am J Psychiatry* (1984) 141, 1604–6.
3. Andrus PF. Lithium and carbamazepine. *J Clin Psychiatry* (1984) 45, 525.
4. Marcoux AW. Carbamazepine-lithium drug interaction. *Ann Pharmacother* (1996) 30, 547.
5. Manto M-U, Jacquy J, Hildebrand J. Cerebellar ataxia in upper limbs triggered by addition of carbamazepine to lithium treatment. *Acta Neurol Belg* (1996) 96, 316–17.
6. Hassan MN, Thakar J, Weinberg AL, Grimes JD. Lithium-carbamazepine interaction: clinical and laboratory observations. *Neurology* (1987) 37 (Suppl 1), 172.
7. Steckler TL. Lithium- and carbamazepine-associated sinus node dysfunction: nine-year experience in a psychiatric hospital. *J Clin Psychopharmacol* (1994) 14, 336–9.
8. Ghose K. Effect of carbamazepine in polyuria associated with lithium therapy. *Pharmakopsychiatr Neuropsychopharmakol* (1978) 11, 241–5.
9. Mayan H, Golubev N, Dinour D, Farfel Z. Lithium intoxication due to carbamazepine-induced renal failure. *Ann Pharmacother* (2001) 35, 560–2.
10. Emilien G, Malotoeaux JM. Lithium neurotoxicity at low therapeutic doses. Hypotheses for causes and mechanism of action a following a retrospective analysis of published case reports. *Acta Neurol Belg* (1996) 96, 281–93.
11. Laird LK, Knox EP. The use of carbamazepine and lithium in controlling a case of chronic rapid cycling. *Pharmacotherapy* (1987) 7, 130–2.
12. Pies R. Combining lithium and anticonvulsants in bipolar disorder: a review. *Ann Clin Psychiatry* (2002) 14, 223–32.
13. Kramlinger KG, Post RM. The addition of lithium to carbamazepine. *Arch Gen Psychiatry* (1989) 46, 794–800.
14. McGinness J, Kishimoto A, Hollister LE. Avoiding neurotoxicity with lithium-carbamazepine combinations. *Psychopharmacol Bull* (1990) 26, 181–4.

Lithium + Anticonvulsants; Gabapentin

A single-dose study suggests that lithium does not interact with gabapentin.

Clinical evidence, mechanism, importance and management

In a double-blind study, 13 patients were given a single 600-mg dose of lithium either with or without gabapentin at steady-state. Gabapentin did not significantly alter the pharmacokinetics of the lithium, and no increase in adverse effects was noted. This study indicated that dosage adjustment appears not to be necessary if lithium is used with gabapentin, although it should be noted that this was only a single-dose investigation, and more long-term studies will be needed to confirm this lack of interaction.[1]

1. Frye MA, Kimbrell TA, Dunn RT, Piscitelli S, Grothe D, Vanderham E, Corá-Locatelli G, Post RM, Ketter TA. Gabapentin does not alter single-dose lithium pharmacokinetics. *J Clin Psychopharmacol* (1998) 18, 461–4.

Lithium + Anticonvulsants; Lamotrigine

Lamotrigine does not appear to interact with lithium to a clinically relevant extent.

Clinical evidence, mechanism, importance and management

In an open, randomised, two-period, crossover study, 20 healthy men were given 2 g of anhydrous lithium gluconate (9.8 mmol of lithium) every 12 hours for 11 doses, either with or without lamotrigine 100 mg daily. It was found that the serum lithium levels were decreased by 8.5% by lamotrigine, but these small changes were not considered to be clinically relevant.[1] No special precautions or dosage adjustments would therefore appear to be needed if these drugs are used concurrently. The lithium salt used in this study was the gluconate, but there is no reason to expect other lithium salts to behave differently.

1. Chen C, Veronese L, Yin Y. The effects of lamotrigine on the pharmacokinetics of lithium. *Br J Clin Pharmacol* (2000) 50, 193–5.

Lithium + Anticonvulsants; Phenytoin

Symptoms of lithium toxicity have been seen in some patients concurrently treated with phenytoin, although the interaction has not been clearly demonstrated. The serum lithium levels may remain the same.

Clinical evidence, mechanism, importance and management

A patient with a history of depression and convulsions was treated with increasing doses of lithium carbonate and phenytoin over a period of about 4 years. Although the serum levels of both drugs remained within the therapeutic range, he eventually began to develop symptoms of lithium toxicity (thirst, polyuria, polydipsia and tremor) that disappeared when the lithium was stopped. Later, when lithium was restarted, the symptoms returned this time abating when the phenytoin was replaced by carbamazepine. The patient then claimed that he felt normal for the first time in years.[1] Another report describes symptoms of lithium toxicity in a patient with lithium levels within the normal range. This patient was also on phenytoin.[2]

In a further case[3] a man on phenytoin became ataxic within three days of starting to take lithium. He had no other toxic symptoms and his serum lithium level was 2 mmol/l. However, as he only ever took lithium in the presence of phenytoin it is not possible to say whether the effects were as a result of an interaction, or whether toxic levels would have occurred with the lithium alone. Another similar case has also been reported.[4]

Information seems to be limited to these reports and none of them presents a clear picture of the role of phenytoin in the reactions described.[1-4] The interaction is not well established. Patients on lithium should be aware of the symptoms of lithium toxicity and told to immediately report them should they occur. This should be reinforced when they are given phenytoin. Increased serum lithium monitoring does not appear to be of value in this situation as the interaction occurred in patients with lithium levels within the normally accepted range.

1. MacCallum WAG. Interaction of lithium and phenytoin. *BMJ* (1980) 280, 610–11.
2. Spiers J, Hirsch SR. Severe lithium toxicity with "normal" serum concentrations. *BMJ* (1978) 1, 815–16.
3. Salem RB, Director K, Muniz CE. Ataxia as the primary symptom of lithium toxicity. *Drug Intell Clin Pharm* (1980) 14, 622–3.
4. Raskin DE. Lithium and phenytoin interaction. *J Clin Psychopharmacol* (1984) 4, 120.

Lithium + Anticonvulsants; Topiramate

An isolated report describes elevated serum lithium levels and evidence of toxicity in a woman five weeks after she started to take high doses of topiramate.

Clinical evidence, mechanism, importance and management

A 42-year-old woman with type II bipolar disorder was started on lithium carbonate 1500 mg and topiramate 500 mg daily, resulting in a steady-state trough serum lithium level of 0.5 mmol/l after 10 days. She was also started on citalopram 10 mg daily. The patient raised the topiramate dose to 800 mg daily in an attempt to lose weight, and 5 weeks later began to complain of severe anorexia, nausea, fatigue and impaired concentration. She had managed to lose 35 lb (almost 16 kg), weight she had gained whilst on a previous drug combination. When examined she was lethargic, with tremors, nystagmus, bradycardia and memory loss. Her trough serum lithium level had risen to 1.4 mmol/l. The symptoms disappeared over 4 days when the lithium was stopped. Two months later she was stabilised once again at 0.5 mmol/l on lithium carbonate 1200 mg and topiramate 500 mg daily.[1]

The reasons for this reaction are not known, but some of the toxicity could have been due to the adverse effects of either drug, with the weight loss possibly disturbing the sodium excretion, which could have affected the loss of lithium in the urine. This case highlights the possible risk of elevated serum lithium levels if high doses of topiramate are used. Patients on lithium should be aware of the symptoms of lithium toxicity and told to immediately report them should they occur. This should be reinforced when they are given topiramate. Consider monitoring lithium levels in patients newly started on this combination.

1. Pinninti NR, Zelinski G. Does topiramate elevate serum lithium levels? *J Clin Psychopharmacol* (2002) 22, 340.

Lithium + Anticonvulsants; Valproate

No clinically relevant adverse interaction occurs between lithium carbonate and valproate.

Clinical evidence, mechanism, importance and management

In a crossover study, 16 healthy subjects were given valproate (as valproate semisodium) or a placebo twice daily for 12 days, to which lithium carbonate 300 mg three times daily was added on days 6 to 10. The valproate serum levels and AUC rose slightly, while the serum lithium levels were unaltered. Adverse events did not change significantly. It was concluded that the concurrent use of these drugs is safe.[1] A review on the efficacy of lithium-anticonvulsant combinations in bipolar disorder lists several studies in which the combination of valproate (as valproate semisodium) and lithium has been used. On the whole the combination was considered safe, although a few patients have discontinued treatment due to intolerable adverse effects, which included gastrointestinal symptoms and tremor.[2]

1. Granneman GR, Schneck DW, Cavanaugh JH, Witt GF. Pharmacokinetic interactions and side effects resulting from concomitant administration of lithium and divalproex sodium. *J Clin Psychiatry* (1996) 57, 204–6.
2. Pies R. Combining lithium and anticonvulsants in bipolar disorder: a review. *Ann Clin Psychiatry* (2002) 14, 223–32.

Lithium + Baclofen

The hyperkinetic symptoms of two patients with Huntington's chorea taking lithium were aggravated within a few days of starting baclofen.

Clinical evidence, mechanism, importance and management

A patient with Huntington's chorea, treated with lithium and haloperidol, was additionally given baclofen, and another patient being treated with imipramine, clopenthixol, chlorpromazine and baclofen was also additionally given lithium. Within a few days both patients showed a severe aggravation of their hyperkinetic symptoms, which disappeared within 3 days of withdrawing the baclofen.[1] Other patients with Huntington's chorea showed no major changes in their mental state or movement disorders when given up to 90 mg of baclofen daily,[2,3] which suggests that an interaction with lithium may have been the cause of the hyperkinesis in these two patients. On the basis of this very limited evidence it would seem prudent to monitor the effects of concurrent use and consider stopping one of the drugs if hyperkinesis develops.

1. Andén N-E, Dalén P, Johansson B. Baclofen and lithium in Huntington's chorea. *Lancet* (1973) ii, 93.
2. Barbeau A. G.A.B.A. and Huntington's chorea. *Lancet* (1973) ii, 1499–1500.
3. Paulson GW. Lioresal in Huntington's disease. *Dis Nerv Syst* (1976) 37, 465–7.

Lithium + Benzodiazepines

Preliminary evidence suggests that alprazolam is unlikely to cause a clinically important rise in serum lithium levels. Neurotoxicity may develop if clonazepam is added to treatment with lithium carbonate and an isolated case of serious hypothermia has been reported during concurrent treatment with lithium carbonate and diazepam.

Clinical evidence, mechanism, importance and management

(a) Alprazolam

Alprazolam 2 mg daily for 4 days increased the steady-state AUC of lithium from 10.3 to 11.1 mmol/hour and reduced its urinary recovery from a 93.6 to 78.2% in 10 healthy subjects taking lithium 900 to 1500 mg daily. It is suggested that these changes are unlikely to be clinically significant, but confirmation of this is needed.[1]

(b) Clonazepam

A retrospective study of patients' records revealed 5 patients with bipolar affective disorder treated with lithium carbonate 900 to 2400 mg who had developed a neurotoxic syndrome with ataxia, dysarthria, drowsiness and confusion when their antipsychotic treatment (chlorpromazine, perphenazine, haloperidol) was replaced with clonazepam 2 to 16 mg. The syndrome was reversible. In all cases the lithium levels rose, and in two of these cases they reached toxic levels. The authors of the report suggest that the neurotoxicity was caused either by the increase in lithium levels, or by synergistic toxicity and recommend that lithium levels should be more frequently measured if clonazepam is added, and the effects of concurrent use well monitored.[2]

(c) Diazepam

A mentally retarded patient showed occasional hypothermic episodes (below 35°C) while taking lithium and diazepam, but not while on either drug alone. After taking lithium 1 g and diazepam 30 mg daily for 17 days during a test, the patient experienced a temperature fall from 35.4 to 32°C over 2 hours, and became comatose with reduced reflexes, dilated pupils, a systolic blood pressure of 40 to 60 mmHg, a pulse rate of 40 and no piloerector response.[3] The reasons for this reaction are not known. This is an isolated case so that concurrent use need not be avoided, but be alert for any evidence of hypothermia. There seems to be no evidence of this adverse interaction with any of the other benzodiazepines.

1. Evans RL, Nelson MV, Melethil S, Townsend R, Hornstra RK, Smith RB. Evaluation of the interaction of lithium and alprazolam. *J Clin Psychopharmacol* (1990) 10, 355–9.
2. Koczerginski D, Kennedy SH, Swinson RP. Clonazepam and lithium—a toxic combination in the treatment of mania? *Int Clin Psychopharmacol* (1989) 4, 195–9.
3. Naylor GJ, McHarg A. Profound hypothermia on combined lithium carbonate and diazepam treatment. *BMJ* (1977) 3, 22.

Lithium + Caffeine

The heavy consumption of caffeine-containing drinks may cause a small to moderate reduction in serum lithium levels.

Clinical evidence, mechanism, importance and management

A study in 11 psychiatric patients taking lithium 600 to 1200 mg daily who were also regular **coffee** drinkers (4 to 8 cups daily containing 70 to 120 mg caffeine per cup) showed that when the **coffee** was withdrawn, their serum lithium levels rose by an average of 24%, although the levels of 3 patients did not change.[1] These findings are consistent with another report of two patients with lithium-induced tremors that were aggravated when they stopped taking caffeine. This was attributed to a rise in serum lithium levels.[2] However, a single-dose study did not find any changes in urinary clearance of lithium in 6 subjects given caffeine 200 mg four times daily compared with a caffeine-free control period.[3]

The weight of evidence cited here suggests that although there is no need for those on lithium to avoid caffeine (**coffee**, **tea**, **cola drinks** etc.) it is not clear exactly how the caffeine affects the excretion of lithium by the kidney tubules, and in cases where a reduction in caffeine intake is desirable, it should be withdrawn cautiously. This is particularly important in those whose serum lithium levels are already high, because of the risk of toxicity. When the caffeine is withdrawn it may be necessary to reduce the dose of lithium. In addition, remember that there is a caffeine-withdrawal syndrome (headache and fatigue being the major symptoms) that might worsen some of the major psychiatric disorders (such as affective and schizophrenic disorders).[1]

1. Mester R, Toren P, Mizrachi I, Wolmer L, Karni N, Weizman A. Caffeine withdrawal increases lithium blood levels. *Biol Psychiatry* (1995) 37, 348–50.
2. Jefferson JW. Lithium tremor and caffeine intake: two cases of drinking less and shaking more. *J Clin Psychiatry* (1988) 49, 72–3.
3. Bikin D, Conrad KA, Mayersohn M. Lack of influence of caffeine and aspirin on lithium elimination. *Clin Res* (1982) 30, 249.

Lithium + Calcitonin (Salcatonin)

A study in 4 depressed women found that calcitonin (salcatonin) caused a small reduction in serum lithium levels, the clinical importance of which is not known.

Clinical evidence

Prompted by the occasional observation of decreased serum lithium levels in outpatients receiving calcitonin, a study was undertaken in 4 bipolar depressive women. The patients had been stable on lithium for 10 years and were additionally treated with salmon calcitonin (salcatonin) 100 units subcutaneously for 3 consecutive days for postmenopausal osteoporosis. It was found that their serum lithium levels fell, on average, from 0.73 to 0.59 mmol/l. The clearance of lithium in the urine was tested in 2 of the patients, and both showed increases (9.8 and 16.6%).[1]

Mechanism

Not known. Increased renal excretion and possibly some reduced intestinal absorption of the lithium is suggested by the authors of the report.[1]

Importance and management

Information seems to be limited to this study, which only lasted for 3 days. The study found only a small fall in serum lithium levels, and did not assess the effect on the control of depression. It seems likely that this interaction will not be clinically important in most patients, but as some patients may be affected, monitor the outcome of concurrent use, and consider monitoring lithium levels.

1. Passiu G, Bocchetta A, Martinelli V, Garau P, Del Zompo M, Mathieu A. Calcitonin decreases lithium plasma levels in man. Preliminary report. *Int J Clin Pharmacol Res* (1998) 18, 179–81.

Lithium + Calcium channel blockers

Concurrent use of lithium and verapamil can be uneventful, but neurotoxicity, bradycardia, choreoathetosis, and decreases in serum lithium levels have been seen in a few patients. An acute parkinsonian syndrome and marked psychosis has been seen in at least one patient on lithium and diltiazem.

Clinical evidence

(a) Diltiazem

A woman stable on lithium for several years developed marked psychosis and parkinsonism within a week of starting to take diltiazem 30 mg three times daily.[1] An acute parkinsonism syndrome developed in a 58-year-old man within four days of adding 30 mg of diltiazem three times daily to his treatment with lithium and tiotixene.[2] However, this report has been questioned as the symptoms may have been attributable to an adverse effect of the tiotixene, and, even if the lithium toxicity was genuine, it is thought to have been more likely due to the recent withdrawal of theophylline, or the patients' diuretic therapy than diltiazem.[3]

(b) Nifedipine

A patient taking lithium, who developed dysarthria and ataxia after verapamil was added to her treatment (see *(c)* below), was subsequently well controlled on lithium and nifedipine 40 mg daily.[4]

(c) Verapamil

A 42-year-old on lithium carbonate 900 mg daily developed toxicity (nausea, vomiting, muscular weakness, ataxia and tinnitus) within 9 days of starting to take verapamil 80 mg three times daily, although her bipolar depressive disorder improved. Her serum lithium levels remained unchanged at 1.1 mmol/l. The toxicity disappeared within 48 hours of stopping the verapamil, but her disorder worsened. The same pattern was repeated when verapamil was re-started and then withdrawn.[5] Another 3 cases of movement disorders following the concurrent use of lithium and verapamil have also been reported.[4,6,7] In one case the patient was restabilised by halving the dose of lithium.[6]

Conversely, a patient stable on lithium 900 to 1200 mg daily for over 8 years showed a marked fall in serum lithium levels from about 1.04 to 0.5 mmol/l when given verapamil 80 mg four times daily. He was restabilised on approximately double the dose of lithium.[8] Another patient showed an increased lithium clearance when given verapamil for three days, and a fall in serum lithium levels from 0.61 to 0.53 mmol/l.[8]

Mechanism

Not understood. However, it has been suggested that calcium channel blockers and lithium affect neurotransmitter production[1,2,7] (several pathways have been described), which results in CNS sensitivity. This produces movement disorders, which are said to mimic lithium toxicity. All the cases were remarkable in that symptoms of toxicity were present at therapeutic lithium levels, which would support this suggested mechanism.

Importance and management

The adverse reactions cited above contrast with other reports describing uneventful concurrent use.[9,10] This unpredictability emphasises the need to monitor the effects closely where it is thought appropriate to give lithium and calcium channel blockers.

1. Binder EF, Cayabyab L, Ritchie DJ, Birge SJ. Diltiazem-induced psychosis and a possible diltiazem-lithium interaction. *Arch Intern Med* (1991) 151, 373–4.
2. Valdiserri EV. A possible interaction between lithium and diltiazem: case report. *J Clin Psychiatry* (1985) 46, 540–1.
3. Flicker MR, Quigley MA, Caldwell EG. Diltiazem-lithium interaction: an opposing viewpoint. *J Clin Psychiatry* (1988) 49, 325–6.
4. Wright BA, Jarrett DB. Lithium and calcium channel blockers: possible neurotoxicity. *Biol Psychiatry* (1991) 30, 635–6.
5. Price WA, Giannini AJ. Neurotoxicity caused by lithium-verapamil synergism. *J Clin Pharmacol* (1986) 26, 717–19.
6. Price WA, Shalley JE. Lithium-verapamil toxicity in the elderly. *J Am Geriatr Soc* (1987) 35, 177–8.
7. Helmuth D, Ljaljevic Z, Ramirez L, Meltzer HY. Choreoathetosis induced by verapamil and lithium treatment. *J Clin Psychopharmacol* (1989) 9, 454–5.
8. Weinrauch LA, Belok S, D'Elia JA. Decreased serum lithium during verapamil therapy. *Am Heart J* (1984) 108, 1378–80.
9. Brotman AW, Farhadi AM, Gelenberg AJ. Verapamil treatment of acute mania. *J Clin Psychiatry* (1986) 47, 136–8.
10. Gitlin MJ, Weiss J. Verapamil as maintenance treatment in bipolar illness: a case report. *J Clin Psychopharmacol* (1984) 4, 341–3.

Lithium + Cisplatin

Isolated case reports describe either a fall or no alteration in serum lithium levels in patients given cisplatin.

Clinical evidence, mechanism, importance and management

A woman on lithium carbonate 1200 mg daily had a fall in serum lithium levels, from 1 to 0.3 mmol/l, and from 0.8 to 0.5 mmol/l, on two occasions over periods of two days when given cisplatin (100 mg/m^2 intravenously over 2 hours). To prevent cisplatin-induced renal toxicity, she was also given a fluid load over a total of 24 hours, which included one litre of sodium chloride 0.9% over 4 hours, one litre of mannitol 20% over 4 hours, and one litre of dextrose 5% in sodium chloride 0.9%. Serum lithium levels returned to normal at the end of two days. No change in the control of the psychotic symptoms was seen.[1]

A man showed a transient 64% decrease in serum lithium levels, without perceptible clinical consequences, during the first of four courses of cisplatin, bleomycin, and etoposide. The effect became less pronounced during the other courses.[2] It is not clear whether the fall in serum lithium levels in these cases was due to increased renal clearance caused by the cisplatin or sodium load, dilution from the fluid load, or a combination of all three factors.

In contrast, one patient showed clinically insignificant changes in her serum lithium levels when treated with cisplatin, but two months later her deteriorating renal function resulted in a rise in her serum lithium levels.[3]

None of these interactions was of great clinical importance, but the authors of the first report pointed out that some regimens of cisplatin involve the use of higher doses (40 mg/m^2 daily) with a sodium chloride 0.9% fluid load over 5 days, and under these circumstances it would be prudent to monitor the serum lithium levels carefully. Concurrent use should be monitored in all patients.

1. Pietruszka LJ, Biermann WA, Vlasses PH. Evaluation of cisplatin-lithium interaction. *Drug Intell Clin Pharm* (1985) 19, 31–2.
2. Beijnen JH, Bais EM, ten Bokkel Huinink WW. Lithium pharmacokinetics during cisplatin-based chemotherapy: a case report. *Cancer Chemother Pharmacol* (1994) 33, 523–6.
3. Beijnen JH, Vlasveld LT, Wanders J, ten Bokkel Huinink WW, Rodenhuis S. Effect of cisplatin-containing chemotherapy on lithium serum concentrations. *Ann Pharmacother* (1992) 26, 488–90.

Lithium + Co-trimoxazole

Two reports describe lithium toxicity, paradoxically accompanied by a fall in serum lithium levels in three patients given co-trimoxazole.

Clinical evidence, mechanism, importance and management

Two patients stabilised on lithium carbonate (serum concentration 0.75 mmol/l) showed signs of lithium toxicity (tremor, muscular weakness and fasciculation, apathy) within a few days of being given co-trimoxazole (dose not stated), yet their serum lithium levels were found to have fallen to about 0.4 mmol/l. Within 48 hours of withdrawing the co-trimoxazole, the signs of toxicity had gone and their serum lithium concentrations had returned to their former levels.[1] Another report very briefly states that ataxia, tremor and diarrhoea developed in a patient on lithium and timolol when given co-trimoxazole.[2] The reasons are not understood. The general importance of this interaction is uncertain but if concurrent use is undertaken it would clearly be prudent to monitor the clinical response because it would appear that serum level monitoring may not always be a reliable guide to toxicity.

1. Desvilles M, Sevestre P. Effet paradoxal de l'association lithium et sulfaméthoxazol-triméthoprime. *Nouv Presse Med* (1982) 11, 3267–8.
2. Edwards IR. Medicines Adverse Reactions Committee: eighteenth annual report, 1983. *N Z Med J* (1984) 97, 729–32.

Lithium + Diuretics; Loop

The concurrent use of lithium carbonate and furosemide can be safe and uneventful, but serious lithium toxicity has been described in a few individuals. Bumetanide interacts similarly.

Clinical evidence

Six healthy subjects stabilised on lithium carbonate 300 mg three times daily (mean serum levels 0.43 mmol/l) were given **furosemide** 40 mg daily for 14 days. Five experienced some minor adverse effects, probably attributable to the **furosemide**, without significant changes in serum lithium levels, but one subject experienced such a marked increase in the toxic effects of lithium that she withdrew from the study after taking both drugs for only 5 days. Her serum lithium levels were found to have risen from 0.44 to 0.71 mmol/l.[1]

There are four other case reports of individual patients who experienced serious lithium toxicity or other adverse reactions when given lithium and **furosemide**.[2-5] One of the patients was also on a salt-restricted diet,[2] which has also been implicated in episodes of lithium toxicity. In contrast, 6 patients who had been stabilised on lithium for over 6 years showed no significant changes in their serum lithium levels over a 12-week period while taking **furosemide** 20 to 80 mg daily.[6] Another study in healthy subjects also found no significant changes in lithium levels when **furosemide** 40 mg daily was given.[7] **Bumetanide** has also been responsible for the development of lithium toxicity in 2 patients[8,9] one of whom was on a salt-restricted diet.[9]

Mechanism

Not fully understood. If and when a rise in serum lithium levels occurs, it may be related to the salt depletion that can accompany the use of furosemide (see 'Lithium + Sodium compounds', below). As with the thiazides, (see 'Lithium + Diuretics; Thiazides or related', below) such an interaction would take a few days to develop. This may explain why one study in subjects given a single dose of lithium failed to demonstrate any effect on the urinary excretion of lithium after the administration of furosemide.[10]

Importance and management

Information seems to be limited to the reports cited. The incidence of this interaction is uncertain and its development unpredictable. It would therefore be imprudent to give furosemide or bumetanide to patients stabilised on lithium unless the effects can be well monitored because the occasional patient may develop serious toxicity. Patients on lithium should be aware of the symptoms of lithium toxicity and told to immediately report them should they occur. Consider monitoring lithium levels in patients newly started on this combination.

1. Jefferson JW, Kalin NH. Serum lithium levels and long-term diuretic use. *JAMA* (1979) 241, 1134–6.
2. Hurtig HI, Dyson WL. Lithium toxicity enhanced by diuresis. *N Engl J Med* (1974) 290, 748–9.
3. Oh TE. Frusemide and lithium toxicity. *Anaesth Intensive Care* (1977) 5, 60–2.
4. Grau Segura E, Pinet Ogue MC, Franco Peral M. Intoxicación por sales de litio. Presentación de un caso. *Med Clin (Barc)* (1984) 83, 294–6.
5. Thornton WE, Pray BJ. Lithium intoxication: a report of two cases. *Can Psychiatr Assoc J* (1975) 20, 281–2.
6. Saffer D, Coppen A. Frusemide: a safe diuretic during lithium therapy? *J Affect Disord* (1983) 5, 289–92.
7. Crabtree BL, Mack JE, Johnson CD, Amyx BC. Comparison of the effects of hydrochlorothiazide and furosemide on lithium disposition. *Am J Psychiatry* (1991) 148, 1060–3.
8. Kerry RJ, Ludlow JM, Owen G. Diuretics are dangerous with lithium. *BMJ* (1980) 281, 371.
9. Huang LG. Lithium intoxication with coadministration of a loop-diuretic. *J Clin Psychopharmacol* (1990) 10, 228.
10. Thomsen K, Schou M. Renal lithium excretion in man. *Am J Physiol* (1968) 215, 823–7.

Lithium + Diuretics; Potassium-sparing

There is evidence that the excretion of lithium can be increased by triamterene and serum lithium levels may rise if spironolactone is used. Amiloride is reported not to interact. See also 'Lithium + Diuretics; Loop', above, and 'Lithium + Diuretics; Thiazides or related', below.

Clinical evidence, mechanism, importance and management

Amiloride has been found to have no significant effect on serum lithium levels when used in the treatment of lithium-induced polyuria.[1,2] However, it appears in one makers summary of product characteristics[3] as a diuretic that reduces the renal clearance of lithium, thereby increasing the risk of lithium toxicity. There appears to be no evidence to confirm this alleged interaction.

One study found that **spironolactone** had no effect on the excretion of lithium,[4] whereas in another report the use of **spironolactone** 100 mg daily was accompanied by a rise in serum lithium levels from 0.63 to 0.9 mmol/l. The levels continued to rise for several days after the **spironolactone** was stopped.[5] **Triamterene**, administered to one patient taking lithium while on a salt-restricted diet, is said to have led to a strong lithium diuresis.[6]

These diuretics have been available for a very considerable time and it might have been expected that by now any serious adverse interactions with lithium would have emerged, but information is very sparse. None of the reports available gives a clear indication of the outcome of concurrent use, but some monitoring would be a prudent precaution. Patients on lithium should be aware of the symptoms of lithium toxicity and told to immediately report them should they occur.

1. Batlle DC, von Riotte AB, Gaviria M, Grupp M. Amelioration of polyuria by amiloride in patients receiving long-term lithium therapy. *N Engl J Med* (1985) 312, 408–14.
2. Kosten TR, Forrest JN. Treatment of severe lithium-induced polyuria with amiloride. *Am J Psychiatry* (1986) 143, 1563–8.
3. Midamor (Amiloride). Merck & Co Inc. US prescribing information. August November 2002.
4. Thomsen K, Schou M. Renal lithium excretion in man. *Am J Physiol* (1968) 215, 823–7.
5. Baer L, Platman SR, Kassir S, Fieve RR. Mechanisms of renal lithium handling and their relationship to mineralocorticoids: a dissociation between sodium and lithium ions. *J Psychiatr Res* (1971) 8, 91–105.
6. Williams, Katz, Shield eds. Recent Advances in the Psychobiology of the Depressive Illnesses. Washington DC: DHEW Publications, 1972 p 49–58.

Lithium + Diuretics; Thiazides or related

Thiazide and related diuretics can cause a rapid rise in serum lithium levels, leading to toxicity unless the lithium dosage is reduced appropriately. This interaction has been seen with bendroflumethiazide, chlorothiazide, chlortalidone, hydrochlorothiazide and indapamide. Other thiazides and related diuretics are expected to behave similarly.

Clinical evidence

(a) Bendroflumethiazide

A study in 22 patients, who had been treated with either bendroflumethiazide 2.5 mg or hydroflumethiazide 25 mg daily for at least 2 months, found that these diuretics caused a 24% reduction in the urinary clearance of a single 600-mg dose of lithium carbonate.[1] There is also a case report of elevated serum lithium levels,[2] and a case of lithium toxicity,[3] following the addition of bendroflumethiazide to treatment with lithium. In a further case, lithium toxicity was detected 3 months after the addition of bendroflumethiazide.[4] Lithium levels had reached 4.28 mmol/l. However, this case was complicated by the presence of perindopril, which has also been implicated in cases of raised lithium levels. See 'Lithium + ACE inhibitors', p.846.

However, in contrast to these reports, one short-term single-dose study found that bendroflumethiazide had no effect on lithium clearance.[5] However, it seems unlikely that single-dose studies will detect an interaction (see Mechanism below).

(b) Chlorothiazide

A single 300-mg dose of lithium carbonate was given to 4 healthy subjects alone and following 7 days' treatment with chlorothiazide 500 mg daily. Lithium plasma levels were increased and lithium clearance was decreased by about 26% following chlorothiazide treatment.[6]

Lithium toxicity developed in a patient on lithium after he was given chlorothiazide, triamterene and amiloride.[7] The lithium levels rose from 0.6 to 2.2 mmol/l.

A 54-year-old patient developed nephrogenic diabetes insipidus when she was treated with lithium carbonate. The addition of chlorothiazide reduced her polyuria, but resulted in an elevation in her lithium level from 1.3 to more than 2 mmol/l, with accompanying signs of toxicity. The patient was later successfully treated with chlorothiazide and a reduced dose of lithium.[8]

(c) Chlortalidone

A 58-year-old woman developed lithium toxicity within 10 days of starting chlortalidone (dose unknown).[9] Her lithium levels rose from 0.8 to 3.7 mmol/l.

(d) Hydrochlorothiazide

In a placebo-controlled study, the serum lithium levels of 13 healthy subjects on lithium 300 mg twice daily rose by 23% (from 0.3 to 0.37 mmol/l), when they were given hydrochlorothiazide 25 mg twice daily for 5 days.[10] Similar results were found in another small study.[11]

In addition to these studies at least 6 cases of lithium toxicity have been seen following the addition of hydrochlorothiazide to lithium therapy.[12-16] Hydrochlorothiazide was either given with amiloride,[12-14] spironolactone[15] or triamterene.[16] See also 'Lithium + Diuretics; Potassium-sparing', p.851.

(e) Hydroflumethiazide

A study in 22 patients who had been treated with either bendroflumethiazide 2.5 mg or hydroflumethiazide 25 mg daily for at least 2 months found that these diuretics caused a 24% reduction in the urinary clearance of a single 600-mg dose of lithium carbonate.[1]

(f) Indapamide

A 64-year-old man developed lithium toxicity one week after starting to take indapamide 5 mg daily.[17] His serum lithium level was 3.93 mmol/l.

Mechanism

Not fully understood. The interaction occurs even though the thiazides and related diuretics exert their major actions in the distal part of the kidney tubule whereas lithium is reabsorbed in the proximal part. A possible reason is that thiazide diuresis is accompanied by sodium loss which, within a few days, is compensated by retention of sodium, this time in the proximal part of the tubule. Since both sodium and lithium ions are treated similarly, the increased reabsorption of sodium would include lithium as well, hence a significant and measurable reduction in its excretion.[18]

Importance and management

Established, well-documented and potentially serious interactions. The rise in serum lithium levels and the accompanying toxicity develops most commonly within about a week to 10 days,[3,6,8-10,12,16,17] although it has been seen after 19 days[15] and 3 months.[4] Not every patient necessarily develops a clinically important interaction but it is not possible to predict which patients will be affected. Although only the diuretics named above have been implicated in this interaction it seems likely that all thiazides and related diuretics will interact similarly. None of the thiazide or related diuretics should be given to patients on lithium unless the serum lithium levels can be closely monitored and appropriate downward dosage adjustments made. The UK makers say that if a thiazide diuretic has to be prescribed for a patient on lithium, then lithium dosage should first be reduced. The patients should then be stabilised by frequent monitoring of lithium levels. Similar precautions should be exercised on diuretic withdrawal.[19] The US makers say that caution should be used.[20] Patients on lithium should be aware of the symptoms of lithium toxicity and told to immediately report them should they occur.

Concurrent use under controlled conditions has been advocated for certain psychiatric conditions and for the control of lithium-induced nephrogenic diabetes insipidus. A successful case is described above.[8] It has been suggested that a 40 to 70% reduction in the lithium dose would be needed with 500 to 1000 mg doses of chlorothiazide,[21,22] but it would seem sensible to base any dose adjustments on individual lithium levels.

1. Petersen V, Hvidt S, Thomsen K, Schou M. Effect of prolonged thiazide treatment on renal lithium clearance. *BMJ* (1974) 3, 143–5.
2. Kerry RJ, Ludlow JM, Owen G. Diuretics are dangerous with lithium. *BMJ* (1980) 281, 371.
3. Aronson JK, Reynolds DJM. ABC of monitoring drug therapy. Lithium. *BMJ* (1992) 305, 1273–6.
4. Vipond AJ, Bakewell S, Telford R, Nicholls AJ. Lithium toxicity. *Anaesthesia* (1996) 51, 1156–8.
5. Thomsen K, Schou M. Renal lithium excretion in man. *Am J Physiol* (1968) 215, 823–7.
6. Poust RI, Mallinger AG, Mallinger J, Himmelhoch JM, Neil JF, Hanin I. Effect of chlorothiazide on the pharmacokinetics of lithium in plasma and erythrocytes. *Psychopharmacol Comm* (1976) 2, 273–84.
7. Basdevant A, Beaufils M, Corvol P. Influence des diurétiques sur l'élimination rénale du lithium. *Nouv Presse Med* (1976) 5, 2085–6.
8. Levy ST, Forrest JN, Heninger GR. Lithium-induced diabetes insipidus: manic symptoms, brain and electrolyte correlates, and chlorothiazide treatment. *Am J Psychiatry* (1973) 130, 1014–18.
9. Solomon JG. Lithium toxicity precipitated by a diuretic. *Psychosomatics* (1980) 21, 425, 429.
10. Crabtree BL, Mack JE, Johnson CD, Amyx BC. Comparison of the effects of hydrochlorothiazide and furosemide on lithium disposition. *Am J Psychiatry* (1991) 148, 1060–3.
11. Jefferson JW, Kalin NH. Serum lithium levels and long-term diuretic use. *JAMA* (1979) 241, 1134–6.
12. Macfie AC. Lithium poisoning precipitated by diuretics. *BMJ* (1975) 1, 516.
13. König P, Küfferle B, Lenz G. Ein fall von Lithiumtoxikation bei therapeutischen Lithiumdosen infolge zusätzlicher Gabe eines Diuretikums. *Wien Klin Wochenschr* (1978) 90, 380–2.
14. Dorevitch A, Baruch E. Lithium toxicity induced by combined amiloride HCl-hydrochlorothiazide administration. *Am J Psychiatry* (1986) 143, 257–8.
15. Lutz EG. Lithium toxicity precipitated by diuretics. *J Med Soc New Jers* (1975) 72, 439–40.
16. Mehta BR, Robinson BHB. Lithium toxicity induced by triamterene-hydrochlorothiazide. *Postgrad Med J* (1980) 56, 783–4.
17. Hanna ME, Lobao CB, Stewart JT. Severe lithium toxicity associated with indapamide therapy. *J Clin Psychopharmacol* (1990) 10, 379–80.
18. Schwarcz G. The problem of antihypertensive treatment in lithium patients. *Compr Psychiatry* (1982) 23, 50–54.
19. Priadel (Lithium carbonate). Sanofi Synthelabo. UK Summary of product characteristics, October 2004.
20. Eskalith (Lithium carbonate). GlaxoSmithKline. US Prescribing information, September 2003.
21. Himmelhoch JM, Poust RI, Mallinger AG, Hanin I, Neil JF. Adjustment of lithium dose during lithium-chlorothiazide therapy. *Clin Pharmacol Ther* (1977) 22, 225–7.
22. Himmelhoch JM, Forrest J, Neil JF, Detre TP. Thiazide-lithium synergy in refractory mood swings. *Am J Psychiatry* (1977) 134, 149–52.

Lithium + Herbal medicines

A woman developed lithium toxicity after taking a herbal diuretic remedy.

Clinical evidence, mechanism, importance and management

A 26-year-old woman, stabilised on lithium 900 mg twice daily for 5 months with a serum level of 1.1 mmol/l and also taking hydroxyzine, lorazepam, propranolol, risperidone and sertraline, came to an emergency clinic complaining of nausea, diarrhoea, unsteady gait, tremor, nystagmus and drowsiness, (all symptoms of lithium toxicity). She had been taking a non-prescription **herbal diuretic** for the previous 2 to 3 weeks to lose weight, and she was found to have a serum lithium level of 4.5 mmol/l. This un-named herbal preparation contained **corn silk**, ***Equisetum hyemale***, **juniper**, **ovate buchu**, **parsley** and **uva ursi**, all of which are believed to have diuretic actions. The other ingredients were bromelain, paprika, potassium and vitamin B_6.[1]

The most likely explanation for what happened is that the **herbal diuretic** caused the lithium toxicity. It is impossible to know which herb or combination of herbs actually caused the toxicity, or how, but this case once again emphasises that herbal remedies are not risk-free just because they are natural. It also underscores the need for patients to avoid self-medication without first seeking informed advice and supervision if they are taking potentially hazardous drugs like lithium.

1. Pyevich D, Bogenschutz MP. Herbal diuretics and lithium toxicity. *Am J Psychiatry* (2001) 158, 1329.

Lithium + Iodides

The hypothyroid and goitrogenic effects of lithium carbonate and other iodides may be additive if given concurrently.

Clinical evidence

A man with normal thyroid function showed evidence of hypothyroidism after 3 weeks' treatment with lithium carbonate 750 to 1500 mg daily. After 2 further weeks, during which he was also treated with **potassium iodide**, the hypothyroidism became even more marked, but resolved completely within 2 weeks of the withdrawal of both drugs.[1]

A number of other reports describe the antithyroid effect of lithium when given on its own[1-8] as well as with **potassium iodide**[9,10] and possibly with **isopropamide iodide**.[11] There is also a case on record involving lithium, **isopropamide iodide** and haloperidol.[12]

Mechanism

Lithium accumulates in the thyroid gland and blocks the release of the thyroid hormones by thyroid-stimulating hormone. The mechanism is not well understood. Potassium iodide temporarily prevents the production of thyroid hormones but, as time goes on, synthesis recommences. Thus, both lithium and iodide ions can depress the production or release of the hormones and therefore have additive hypothyroid effects.

Importance and management

The incidence and clinical importance of this interaction are difficult to assess. Hypothyroidism due to lithium treatment is not infrequent (variously reported as 12 out of 33 patients,[2] two out of 56 men[6] and 20 out of 93 women[6]) but there are very few reports of hypothyroidism due to the concurrent use of these drugs. Nevertheless the outcome of concurrent use should be monitored. Only potassium iodide and isopropamide iodide have been implicated but it would seem possible with other iodides.

1. Shopsin B, Shenkman L, Blum M, Hollander CS. Iodine and lithium-induced hypothyroidism. Documentation of synergism. *Am J Med* (1973) 55, 695–9.
2. Schou M, Amidsen A, Jensen SE, Olsen T. Occurrence of goitre during lithium treatment. *BMJ* (1968) 3, 710.
3. Shopsin B, Blum M, Gershon S. Lithium-induced thyroid disturbance: case report and review. *Compr Psychiatry* (1969) 10, 215.
4. Emerson CH, Dyson WL, Utiger RD. Serum thyrotropin and thyroxine concentrations in patients receiving lithium carbonate. *J Clin Endocrinol Metab* (1973) 36, 338.
5. Candy J. Severe hypothyroidism — an early complication of lithium therapy. *BMJ* (1972) 3, 277.
6. Villeneuve A, Grantier J, Jus A, Perron D. Effect of lithium on thyroid in man. *Lancet* (1973) ii, 502.
7. Lloyde GG, Rosser RM, Crowe MJ. Effect of lithium on thyroid in man. *Lancet* (1973) ii, 619.
8. Bocchetta A, Bernardi F, Pedditizi M, Loviselli A, Velluzzi F, Martino E, Del Zompo M. Thyroid abnormalities during lithium treatment. *Acta Psychiatr Scand* (1991) 83, 193–8.
9. Luby ED, Schwartz, Rosenbaum H. Lithium-carbonate-induced myxedema. *JAMA* (1971) 218, 1298–9.
10. Spaulding SW, Burrow GN, Ramey JN, Donabedian RK. Effect of increased iodide intake on thyroid function in subjects on chronic lithium therapy. *Acta Endocrinol (Copenh)* (1977) 84, 290–6.
11. Wiener JD. Lithium carbonate-induced myxedema. *JAMA* (1972) 220, 587.
12. Luby ED, Schwartz D, Rosenbaum H. Lithium carbonate-induced myxedema. *JAMA* (1971) 218, 1298.

Lithium + Ispaghula husk or Psyllium

There is evidence that both ispaghula husk and psyllium can reduce serum lithium levels.

Clinical evidence

A 47-year-old woman recently started on lithium was found to have blood lithium levels of 0.4 mmol/l five days after an increment in her lithium dose and whilst also taking one teaspoonful of ispaghula husk twice daily. The ispaghula husk was stopped 3 days later and when the lithium levels were measured after a further four days they were found to be 0.76 mmol/l.[1]

A study in 6 subjects similarly showed that the absorption of lithium (as measured by the urinary excretion) was reduced by 14% by psyllium.[2]

Mechanism

Not understood. One idea is that the absorption of the lithium from the gut is reduced.[1,2] Another is that the ispaghula and psyllium preparations (not specifically named) might have had a high sodium content that would result in an increase in the excretion of the lithium by the kidneys.[2]

Importance and management

Information is very limited and the general importance of this interaction is uncertain, but it would now seem prudent to bear this interaction in mind in patients given ispaghula or psyllium preparations. If an interaction is suspected consider taking lithium levels and using an alternative laxative.

1. Perlman BB. Interaction between lithium salts and ispaghula husk. *Lancet* (1990) 335, 416.
2. Toutoungi M, Schulz P, Widmer J, Tissot R. Probable interaction entre le psyllium et le lithium. *Therapie* (1990) 45, 357–60.

Lithium + Levofloxacin

An isolated case of lithium toxicity has been reported in a patient taking lithium and levofloxacin.

Clinical evidence, mechanism, importance and management

A 56-year-old man taking lithium carbonate 400 mg three times daily for a bipolar disorder was admitted to hospital with bronchitis. He was started on levofloxacin 300 mg daily, and within two days was noted to have developed gait ataxia, dysarthria, coarse tremor, dizziness, vomiting, and confusion. Lithium toxicity was suspected, and because of the time course of the symptoms, an interaction with levofloxacin was considered responsible. Serum lithium levels were found to have risen from 0.89 mmol/l (measured two weeks previously) to 2.53 mmol/l, and a reduction in renal function was noted. Both drugs were stopped and the patient recovered over the following four days. His lithium level was found to be 1.12 mmol/l at that time.[1]

The mechanism of this interaction between lithium and levofloxacin is unclear, and this appears to be the only report. However, it would seem prudent to bear this interaction in mind if a patient on lithium is prescribed levofloxacin.

1. Takahashi H, Higuchi H, Shimizu T. Severe lithium toxicity induced by combined levofloxacin administration. *J Clin Psychiatry* (2000) 61, 949–50.

Lithium + Mazindol

An isolated case report describes lithium toxicity attributed to the concurrent use of mazindol.

Clinical evidence, mechanism, importance and management

A bipolar depressive woman, stabilised on lithium carbonate, showed signs of lithium toxicity within 3 days of starting to take mazindol 2 mg daily. After 3 days of concurrent treatment she became sluggish and ataxic, and after 9 days she developed twitching, limb rigidity and muscle fasciculation, and was both dehydrated and stuporose. Her serum lithium levels were found to have risen from a range of 0.4 to 1.3 mmol/l up to 3.2 mmol/l. The mazindol was stopped, and she recovered over the next 48 hours whilst being rehydrated.[1] It is not known whether this was a direct interaction between the two drugs, but the authors suggest that the anorectic effect of mazindol led to this toxicity (i.e. the reduced the intake of sodium and water caused a reduction in the renal excretion of lithium). There seem to be no other reports of interactions between lithium and other anorectic drugs confirming this possibility.

This is an isolated case and its general importance is uncertain, but bear it in mind in the case of an unexpected response to treatment. Note that mazindol is no longer recommended as an appetite suppressant.[2]

1. Hendy MS, Dove AF, Arblaster PG. Mazindol-induced lithium toxicity. *BMJ* (1980) 280, 684–5.
2. Sweetman SC, editor. Martindale: The complete drug reference. 34th ed. London: Pharmaceutical Press; 2005 p. 1589.

Lithium + Methyldopa

Lithium toxicity has been described in four patients and three healthy subjects when they were concurrently treated with methyldopa.

Clinical evidence

A manic-depressive woman, stabilised on lithium carbonate developed signs of lithium toxicity (blurred vision, hand tremors, mild diarrhoea, confusion, and slurred speech) when additionally given methyldopa 1 g daily, although her serum lithium levels remained within the range of 0.5 to 0.7 mmol/l.[1] Later the author of this report demonstrated this interaction on himself.[2] He found that within 2 days of starting to take methyldopa 1 g daily signs of lithium toxicity had clearly developed, even though his serum levels remained within the therapeutic range of 0.4 to 1 mmol/l throughout the investigation.

There are three other cases of patients who took methyldopa with lithium, and developed symptoms of lithium toxicity. In two of these cases the patients had lithium levels within the normal therapeutic range.[3-5] A small study in three healthy subjects also found that the combination of lithium and methyldopa resulted in increased confusion, sedation and dysphoria.[6]

Mechanism

Not understood.

Importance and management

Information appears to be limited to the reports cited, but the interaction would seem to be established. Avoid concurrent use whenever possible, but if this is not workable then effects should be closely monitored. Serum lithium measurements may be unreliable because toxicity can occur even though the levels remain within the normally accepted therapeutic range.

1. Byrd GJ. Methyldopa and lithium carbonate: suspected interaction. *JAMA* (1975) 233, 320.
2. Byrd GJ. Lithium carbonate and methyldopa: apparent interaction in man. *Clin Toxicol* (1977) 11, 1–4.
3. Osanloo E, Deglin JH. Interaction of lithium and methyldopa. *Ann Intern Med* (1980) 92, 433–4.
4. O'Regan JB. Adverse interaction of lithium carbonate and methyldopa. *Can Med Assoc J* (1976) 115, 385–6.
5. Yassa R. Lithium-methyldopa interaction. *Can Med Assoc J* (1986) 134, 141–2.
6. Walker N, White K, Tornatore F, Boyd JL, Cohen JL. Lithium-methyldopa interactions in normal subjects. *Drug Intell Clin Pharm* (1980) 14, 638–9.

Lithium + Metronidazole

The lithium levels of three patients rose, to toxic concentrations in two of them, after they took metronidazole.

Clinical evidence, mechanism, importance and management

A 40-year-old woman taking lithium carbonate 1800 mg daily, levothyroxine 150 micrograms daily and propranolol 60 mg daily developed signs of lithium toxicity (ataxia, rigidity, poor cognitive function, impaired co-ordination etc.) after completing a one-week course of metronidazole 500 mg twice daily. Her serum lithium levels had climbed by 46% (from 1.3 to 1.9 mmol/l).[1] Two other patients whose serum lithium levels rose by 20 and 125% respectively 5 to 12 days after finishing a one-week course of metronidazole (750 mg or 1 g daily in divided doses) are described in another report.[2] A degree of renal impairment occurred during concurrent treatment and was still present 5 and 6 months later.[2] In contrast one other patient is said to have taken both drugs together uneventfully.[1]

There seem to be no strong reasons for totally avoiding concurrent use but the outcome should be well monitored. Patients on lithium should be aware of the symptoms of lithium toxicity and told to immediately report them should they occur. This should be reinforced when they are given metronidazole. The authors of one of the reports also recommend frequent analysis of creatinine and electrolyte levels and urine osmolality in order to detect any renal problems in patients on this combination.[2]

1. Ayd JF. Metronidazole-induced lithium intoxication. *Int Drug Ther Newslett* (1982) 17, 15–16.
2. Teicher MH, Altesman RI, Cole JO, Schatzberg AF. Possible nephrotoxic interaction of lithium and metronidazole. *JAMA* (1987) 257, 3365–6.

Lithium + Mirtazapine

No clinically significant interaction appears to occur between lithium and mirtazapine.

Clinical evidence, mechanism, importance and management

In a randomised double-blind crossover study 12 healthy subjects were given lithium carbonate daily for 10 days, with a single 30-mg dose of mirtazapine or placebo on day 9. The pharmacokinetics of both mirtazapine and lithium were unaltered by concurrent use, and no pharmacodynamic changes, as studied by psychometric testing, were identified.[1]

1. Sitsen JMA, Voortman G, Timmer CJ. Pharmacokinetics of mirtazapine and lithium in healthy male subjects. *J Psychopharmacol* (2000) 14, 172–6.

Lithium + Nefazodone

No pharmacokinetic interaction occurs between lithium and nefazodone.

Clinical evidence, mechanism, importance and management

Lithium, in escalating doses from 250 mg twice daily to 500 mg twice daily, was given to 12 healthy subjects over 13 days. Lithium 500 mg twice daily was then given for a further 7 days, with the addition of nefazodone 200 mg twice daily for the last 5 days. The pharmacokinetics of both nefazodone and lithium were unaltered by concurrent use, although there were some small changes in the pharmacokinetics of the nefazodone metabolites. However, since the combination was well tolerated, no dosage adjustments were considered necessary on concurrent use.[1]

1. Laroudie C, Salazar DE, Cosson J-P, Cheuvart B, Istin B, Girault J, Ingrand I, Decourt J-P. *Eur J Clin Pharmacol* (1999) 54, 923–8.

Lithium + NSAIDs

A marked and rapid rise in serum lithium levels of 60%, with associated toxicity, may develop in patients given indometacin. A more moderate rise occurs with diclofenac and ibuprofen, but much larger rises have been seen in a few patients. Increased serum lithium levels and/or toxicity have also been seen in small numbers of patients when given celecoxib, flurbiprofen, ketoprofen, ketorolac, lornoxicam, mefenamic acid, meloxicam, naproxen, niflumic acid, phenylbutazone, piroxicam, rofecoxib or tiaprofenic acid. Sulindac is reported to increase, reduce or have no effect on serum lithium levels. It seems likely that an interaction is possible with all NSAIDs.

Clinical evidence

(a) Azapropazone

The UK summary of product characteristics for azapropazone[1] says that inhibition of renal lithium clearance by azapropazone has not been reported but the possibility of this occurring should be borne in mind, but as yet direct clinical evidence seems to be lacking.

(b) Celecoxib

A 64-year-old-woman with stable lithium levels of 0.4 to 0.6 mmol/l over the previous 12 months presented with symptoms of lithium toxicity, and a lithium level of 1.39 mmol/l. The toxicity was attributed to an interaction with celecoxib, which had been started at a dose of 200 mg twice daily about 10 weeks earlier.[2] Another similar case has been reported, in which a 58-year-old woman, with a stable serum lithium level of between 0.5 and 0.9 mmol/l, developed renal dysfunction associated with severe lithium toxicity within 5 days of starting to take celecoxib 400 mg twice daily. Her lithium level was 4 mmol/l. Of note, and a possible contributory factor, was the presence of ibuprofen, which she had taken with her lithium for several years without incident.[3]

(c) Diclofenac

Five healthy subjects stabilised on lithium sulfate showed a 26% rise in plasma lithium levels after taking diclofenac 50 mg three times daily for 7 to 10 days. Renal lithium excretion fell by 23%. The authors concluded that increases of this size were clinically significant and could lead to lithium toxicity.[4] This conclusion is supported by the case of a 57-year-old woman who was given diclofenac 75 mg daily while taking lithium carbonate 600 mg daily. The initial serum lithium level was satisfactory at 0.7 mmol/l, but 25 days later (18 days after starting the diclofenac) she developed symptoms of toxicity, with a lithium level of 1.3 mmol/l.[5]

(d) Flurbiprofen

Flurbiprofen 100 mg twice daily was given for 7 days to 11 healthy women with bipolar disorder taking lithium carbonate 600 to 1200 mg daily in a placebo-controlled study. The mean maximum plasma levels and the AUC of the lithium rose by about 18% while taking the flurbiprofen, and 4 of the women showed clinically significant serum lithium level increases, which were defined as increases of more than 25% (more than 0.2 mmol/l).[6]

(e) Ibuprofen

Three patients stabilised on lithium, with plasma levels of 0.7 to 0.9 mmol/l, were given ibuprofen 1200 or 2400 mg daily for 7 days. The serum lithium levels of one patient rose from 0.8 to 1 mmol/l and he experienced nausea and drowsiness. The two other patients (including the one on the 1200 mg ibuprofen dose) did not show this interaction.[7]

In other studies the lithium levels of patients taking ibuprofen are reported to have risen by 12 to 67%. Elevated levels occurred within 5 to 7 days,[8,9] although toxicity has been reported in one patient within 24 hours.[10] Several other reports describe cases of lithium toxicity following the use of ibuprofen.[11-13]

(f) Indometacin

The serum lithium levels of 3 subjects with stable lithium plasma levels of 0.7 to 0.9 mmol/l was increased by about 60% within 6 days of taking indometacin 150 mg daily.[7]

The serum lithium levels of healthy subjects and patients taking indometacin 50 mg three times daily were found to have risen by about 30% and 60% respectively.[14] A case report describes lithium toxicity with this combination.[15] A rise in serum lithium levels of a similar magnitude was found in another study in 10 healthy subjects taking lithium sulfate.[16]

(g) Ketoprofen

A patient stabilised on lithium carbonate showed a rise in his serum lithium levels from about 0.7 to 1.32 mmol/l over a 3-week period when treated with ketoprofen 400 mg daily.[17]

(h) Ketorolac

An 80-year-old man taking haloperidol, procyclidine, clonazepam, aspirin, digoxin and lithium (serum levels between 0.5 and 0.7 mmol/l) was additionally given indometacin 100 mg daily for arthritis, which was replaced, after 13 days, by ketorolac 30 mg daily. The next day his serum lithium level was 0.9 mmol/l and 6 days later 1.1 mmol/l. Subsequently the patient developed severe nausea and vomiting, and both drugs were stopped.[18]

A 39-year-old man was well controlled on lithium for cluster headache, but developed neurotoxicity ("shaking of the hands and legs making it difficult to go up or down steps", masking of the face and dysarthria) within 3 weeks of starting to take ketorolac 60 mg daily for low back pain. His serum lithium levels were found to have risen from about 0.6 to 0.9 mmol/l.[19]

When 5 healthy subjects were given lithium carbonate 900 mg for 7 days and ketorolac 40 mg daily for another 5 days, the 12 hour trough serum lithium levels rose from 0.5 to 0.66 mmol/l. The increase in levels ranged from 8% to 34%.[20]

(i) Lornoxicam

A study in 12 healthy subjects[21] found that lornoxicam 4 mg twice daily raised their maximum steady-state serum lithium levels by 20% (from 0.55 to 0.66 mmol/l) and the AUC by 9%. One of the subjects whose serum lornoxicam levels were unusually high showed a much greater rise in serum lithium levels and AUC of 60% and 52% respectively.

(j) Mefenamic acid

Acute lithium toxicity, accompanied by a sharp deterioration in renal function, was seen in a patient given lithium carbonate with mefenamic acid 500 mg three times daily. Withdrawal of the drugs and subsequent rechallenge confirmed this interaction.[22] Another case of toxicity was seen in a patient on lithium given mefenamic acid. Her renal function was impaired when the lithium was started, but she had been stable for about 6 months before the NSAID was added.[23] An extremely brief case report also mentions this interaction.[24]

(k) Meloxicam

A mean 21% increase in serum lithium levels from 0.54 to 0.65 mmol/l was seen in 16 healthy subjects taking lithium carbonate twice daily when they were concurrently given meloxicam 15 mg daily for 14 days. The authors concluded that there was moderate potential for an interaction.[25]

(l) Naproxen

The mean serum lithium levels of 7 patients rose by 16% (from 0.81 to 0.94 mmol/l) over a 6-day period while taking naproxen 250 mg three times daily. The range was from 0 to 42%, and 4 patients showed rises of over 20%. One patient whose levels rose from 0.95 to 1.13 mmol/l developed signs of toxicity (staggering gait and tremors).[26]

In contrast, a study in 9 healthy subjects given lithium carbonate 300 mg 12-hourly for 7 days found no evidence that naproxen 220 mg 8-hourly for a further 5 days, increased serum lithium levels.[27]

(m) Niflumic acid

An isolated report describes lithium toxicity in a woman who took niflumic acid (three capsules) and aspirin 1.5 g daily for 5 days. Her serum lithium levels rose from 0.8 to 1.6 mmol/l.[28]

(n) Oxyphenbutazone

In an apparently isolated case, a 49-year-old woman is reported to have developed nausea and vomiting associated with a rise in lithium levels following the addition of oxyphenbutazone suppositories 500 mg daily to her treatment with lithium. She responded well to a reduction in the lithium dosage.[17]

(o) Phenylbutazone

The serum lithium levels of a patient doubled from 0.7 to 1.44 mmol/l, accompanied by signs of toxicity, within 36 hours of starting treatment with phenylbutazone 750 mg daily, in the form of suppositories.[29] The renal clearance of lithium was found to have halved. The patient was also taking viloxazine, clorazepate, spironolactone, isosorbide dinitrate and dipyridamole. In contrast, a study in 6 patients with bipolar affective disorder found that 6 days' treatment with phenylbutazone 100 mg three times daily caused only a minor increase of about 0 to 15% in serum lithium levels. However some CNS-related adverse effects (drowsiness, confusion, etc.) occurred.[30]

(p) Piroxicam

A 56-year-old woman, stabilised for over 9 years on lithium with levels usually between 0.8 and 1 mmol/l, experienced lithium toxicity (unsteadiness, trembling, confusion) and was admitted to hospital on three occasions after taking piroxicam. Her serum levels on two occasions had risen to 2.7 and 1.6 mmol/l, although in the latter instance the lithium had been withdrawn the day before the levels were taken. In a subsequent study her serum lithium levels rose from 1 to 1.5 mmol/l after she took piroxicam 20 mg daily.[31]

This interaction has also been described in 3 other patients.[13,32-34]

(q) Rofecoxib

A 73-year-old man, with lithium levels of between 0.6 and 0.9 mmol/l for the past 13 years, developed symptoms of lithium toxicity (serum lithium level 1.5 mmol/l) within 9 days of starting to take rofecoxib 12.5 mg daily. Although an interaction was strongly suspected it should be noted that the patient had required his lithium dose to be successively decreased over the 13 years to maintain his lithium levels within the desired range. Captopril 6.25 mg daily had also been started during this time,[35] although it is unclear whether it had a part to play either in the lithium dose reduction or the development of an interaction.

(r) Sulindac

(i) Lithium levels reduced. A patient stabilised on lithium showed a marked fall in serum lithium levels from 0.65 to 0.39 mmol/l after 2 weeks' concurrent treatment with sulindac 100 mg twice daily. Her serum lithium levels gradually climbed over the next 6 weeks to 0.71 mmol/l and restabilised without any change in the dosage of either lithium or sulindac. She needed amitriptyline due to depression while the lithium levels were low, but bouts of depression had not been uncommon even when lithium levels were stable.[36] The serum lithium levels of another patient were approximately halved a week after his dosage of sulindac was doubled to 200 mg twice daily. He remained on both drugs, but a higher dose of lithium was needed.[36]

(ii) Lithium levels unaffected. Two small studies (in a total of 10 patients)[26,37] and a case report[38] found that serum lithium levels were unaffected by the use of sulindac.

(iii) Lithium levels increased. Two patients developed increased serum lithium levels apparently due to the use of sulindac.[39] In one case the lithium levels rose from 1 to 2 mmol/l after 19 days' treatment with sulindac 150 mg twice daily and symptoms of toxicity were seen. The levels fell to 0.8 mmol/l within 5 days of stopping the sulindac. The other patient showed a rise from 0.9 to 1.7 mmol/l within a week of adding sulindac 150 mg twice daily. The sulindac was continued and the lithium dosage was reduced from 1800 to 1500 mg daily. The serum lithium levels fell and were 1.2 mmol/l at 37 days and 1 mmol/l at 70 days. No symptoms of lithium toxicity occurred.[39]

(s) Tiaprofenic acid

A 79-year-old woman on lithium (as well as fosinopril, nifedipine, oxazepam and haloperidol) showed a rise in her trough serum lithium levels from 0.36 to 0.57 mmol/l within 3 days of starting to take tiaprofenic acid 200 mg three times daily. The serum lithium levels had risen to 0.65 mmol/l by the next day and, despite halving the lithium dosage, were found to be 0.69 mmol/l 5 days later. These rises were attributed to an interaction with the tiaprofenic acid exacerbated by the fosinopril,[40] see 'Lithium + ACE inhibitors', p.846.

(t) Valdecoxib or Parecoxib

The makers of parecoxib and valdecoxib say that valdecoxib has been shown to cause decreases in the clearance of lithium (serum clearance reduced by 25%, renal clearance reduced by 30%), resulting in a 34% increase in its serum levels. Valdecoxib pharmacokinetics were unchanged by lithium.[41,42]

Mechanism

Not understood. One suggestion is that the interacting NSAIDs inhibit the synthesis of the renal prostaglandins (PGE_2) so that the renal blood flow is reduced, thereby reducing the renal excretion of the lithium. However, this fails to explain why aspirin, which blocks renal prostaglandin synthesis by 65 to 70%, does not affect serum lithium levels.[16] It is sometimes claimed that NSAIDs cause lithium toxicity because they can reduce the excretion of lithium by the kidney tubules.

Importance and management

The documentation of these interactions is variable and limited, but what is known indicates that indometacin should be avoided unless serum lithium levels can be very well monitored and the dosage reduced appropriately. In some instances the serum lithium level rises caused by other interacting NSAIDs seem to be of little or no clinical relevance, but from some of the more detailed reports it appears that the effect of NSAIDs on lithium levels varies quite markedly from patient to patient. Although only some NSAIDs have been shown to interact it seems likely that they will all interact to a greater or lesser extent. Therefore NSAIDs should not be added to lithium unless the outcome can be well monitored (initially every few days) and serum lithium dosages reduced as necessary. The effects of sulindac appear to be unpredictable (serum levels raised, lowered or unchanged) so that good monitoring is also necessary.

Patients on lithium should be aware of the symptoms of lithium toxicity and told to immediately report them should they occur. This should be reinforced when they are given an NSAID.

1. Rheumox (Azapropazone dihydrate). Goldshield Pharmaceuticals Ltd. UK Summary of product characteristics, February 2000.
2. Gunja N, Graudins A, Dowsett R. Lithium toxicity: a potential interaction with celecoxib. *Intern Med J* (2002) 32, 494–5.
3. Slørdal L, Samstad S, Bathen J, Spigset O. A life-threatening interaction between lithium and celecoxib. *Br J Clin Pharmacol* (2003) 44, 413–14.
4. Reimann IW, Frölich JC. Effects of diclofenac on lithium kinetics. *Clin Pharmacol Ther* (1981) 30, 348–52.
5. Monji A, Maekawa T, Miura T, Nishi D, Horikawa H, Nakagawa Y, Tashiro N. Interactions between lithium and non-steroidal antiinflammatory drugs. *Clin Neuropharmacol* (2002) 25, 241–2.
6. Hughes BM, Small RE, Brink D, McKenzie ND. The effect of flurbiprofen on steady-state plasma lithium levels. *Pharmacotherapy* (1997) 17, 113–20.
7. Ragheb M, Ban TA, Buchanan D, Frolich JC. Interaction of indomethacin and ibuprofen with lithium in manic patients under a steady-state lithium level. *J Clin Psychiatry* (1980) 41, 397–8.
8. Kristoff CA, Hayes PE, Barr WH, Small RE, Townsend RJ, Ettigi PG. Effect of ibuprofen on lithium plasma and red blood cell concentrations. *Clin Pharm* (1986) 5, 51–5.
9. Ragheb M. Ibuprofen can increase serum lithium level in lithium-treated patients. *J Clin Psychiatry* (1987) 48, 161–3.
10. Bailey CE, Stewart JT, McElroy RA. Ibuprofen-induced lithium toxicity. *South Med J* (1989) 82, 1197.
11. Ayd FJ. Ibuprofen-induced lithium intoxication. *Int Drug Ther Newslett* (1985) 20, 16.
12. Khan IH. Lithium and non-steroidal anti-inflammatory drugs. *BMJ* (1991) 302, 1537–8.
13. Kelly CB, Cooper SJ. Toxic elevation of serum lithium concentration by non-steroidal anti-inflammatory drugs. *Ulster Med J* (1991) 60, 240–2.
14. Frölich JC, Leftwich R, Ragheb M, Oates JA, Reimann I, Buchanan D. Indomethacin increases plasma lithium. *BMJ* (1979) 1, 1115–16.
15. Herschberg SN, Sierles FS. Indomethacin-induced lithium toxicity. *Am Fam Physician* (1983) 28, 155–7.
16. Reimann IW, Diener U, Frölich JC. Indomethacin but not aspirin increases plasma lithium ion levels. *Arch Gen Psychiatry* (1983) 40, 283–6.
17. Singer L, Imbs JL, Danion JM, Singer P, Krieger-Finance F, Schmidt M, Schwartz J. Risque d'intoxication par le lithium en cas de traitement associé par les anti-inflammatoires non stéroïdiens. *Therapie* (1981) 36, 323–6.
18. Langlois R, Paquette D. Increased serum lithium levels due to ketorolac therapy. *Can Med Assoc J* (1994) 150, 1455–6.
19. Iyer V. Ketorolac (Toradol®) induced lithium toxicity. *Headache* (1994) 34, 442–4.
20. Cold JA, ZumBrunnen TL, Simpson MA, Augustin BG, Awad E, Jann MW. Increased lithium serum and red blood cell concentrations during ketorolac coadministration. *J Clin Psychopharmacol* (1998) 18, 33–7.
21. Ravic M, Salas-Herrera I, Johnston A, Turner P, Foley K, Rosenow D. Influence of lornoxicam a new non-steroidal anti-inflammatory drug on lithium pharmacokinetics. *Hum Psychopharmacol* (1993) 8, 289–92.
22. MacDonald J, Neale TJ. Toxic interaction of lithium carbonate and mefenamic acid. *BMJ* (1988) 297, 1339.
23. Shelley RK. Lithium toxicity and mefenamic acid: a possible interaction and the role of prostaglandin inhibition. *Br J Psychiatry* (1987) 151, 847–8.
24. Honey J. Lithium-mefenamic acid interaction: Quoted by Ayd FJ. *Int Drug Ther Newslett* (1982) 17, 16.
25. Türck D, Heinzel G, Luik G. Steady-state pharmacokinetics of lithium in healthy volunteers receiving concomitant meloxicam. *Br J Clin Pharmacol* (2000) 50, 197–204.
26. Ragheb M, Powell AL. Lithium interaction with sulindac and naproxen. *J Clin Psychopharmacol* (1986) 6, 150–4.
27. Levin GM, Grum C, Eisele G. Effect of over-the-counter dosages of naproxen sodium and acetaminophen on plasma lithium concentrations in normal volunteers. *J Clin Psychopharmacol* (1998) 18, 237–40.
28. Gay C, Plas J, Granger B, Olie JP, Loo H. Intoxication au lithium. Deux interactions inédites: l'acétazolamide et l'acide niflumique. *Encephale* (1985) 11, 261–2.
29. Singer L, Imbs JL, Schmidt M, Mack G, Sebban M, Danion JM. Baisse de la clearance rénale du lithium sous l'effet de la phénylbutazone. *Encephale* (1978) 4, 33–40.
30. Ragheb M. The interaction of lithium with phenylbutazone in bipolar affective patients. *J Clin Psychopharmacol* (1990) 10, 149–150.
31. Kerry RJ, Owen G, Michaelson S. Possible toxic interaction between lithium and piroxicam. *Lancet* (1983) i, 418–19.
32. Nadarajah J, Stein GS. Piroxicam induced lithium toxicity. *Ann Rheum Dis* (1985) 44, 502.
33. Walbridge DG, Bazire SR. An interaction between lithium carbonate and piroxicam presenting as lithium toxicity. *Br J Psychiatry* (1985) 147, 206–7.
34. Harrison TM, Wynne Davies D, Norris CM. Lithium carbonate and piroxicam. *Br J Psychiatry* (1986) 149, 124–5.
35. Lundmark J, Gunnarsson T, Bengtsson F. A possible interaction between lithium and rofecoxib. *Br J Clin Pharmacol* (2002) 53, 403–4.
36. Furnell MM, Davies J. The effect of sulindac on lithium therapy. *Drug Intell Clin Pharm* (1985) 19, 374–6.
37. Ragheb MA, Powell AL. Failure of sulindac to increase serum lithium levels. *J Clin Psychiatry* (1986) 47, 33–4.
38. Miller LG, Bowman RC, Bakht F. Sparing effect of sulindac on lithium levels. *J Fam Pract* (1989) 28, 592–3.
39. Jones MT, Stoner SC. Increased lithium concentrations reported in patients treated with sulindac. *J Clin Psychiatry* (2000) 61, 527–8.
40. Alderman CP, Lindsay KSW. Increased serum lithium concentration secondary to treatment with tiaprofenic acid and fosinopril. *Ann Pharmacother* (1996) 30, 1411–13.
41. Dynastat injection (Parecoxib sodium). Pharmacia Ltd. UK Summary of product characteristics, April 2004.
42. Bextra (Valdecoxib). Pharmacia Ltd. UK Summary of product characteristics, May 2004.

Lithium + Olanzapine

One study suggests that olanzapine does not interact with lithium. However, two case reports suggest that some patients may develop adverse reactions.

Clinical evidence, mechanism, importance and management

In an open-label study 12 healthy subjects took a single 32.4-mmol dose of lithium with olanzapine 10 mg, and after a washout period, olanzapine 10 mg daily for 8 days, with a single 32.4-mmol dose of lithium on the last day. No pharmacokinetic interactions were detected, and it was concluded that using these drugs together in recommended dosages is safe.[1] However, a 16-year old boy on lithium 1200 mg daily developed neuroleptic malignant syndrome (generalised rigidity, urinary retention, fever, tachycardia) about 2 weeks after his olanzapine dose was increased from 10 to 20 mg daily. Both drugs were stopped, and symptoms resolved over 8 days. He had previously taken olanzapine and lithium separately without problem.[2] A patient who had been diagnosed with encephalopathy and confusion while taking a combination of carbamazepine, haloperidol and lithium developed similar symptoms when he was later given lithium with olanzapine.[3]

The study suggests that normally no pharmacokinetic interaction occurs between lithium and olanzapine, but the case reports suggest that the occasional patient may develop a pharmacodynamic interaction. Concurrent use of lithium and olanzapine need not be avoided but be aware that some patients may develop adverse reactions to the combination.

1. Demolle D, Onkelinx C, Müller-Oerlinghausen B. Interaction between olanzapine and lithium in healthy male volunteers. *Therapie* (1995) 50 (Suppl), 486.
2. Berry N, Pradhan S, Sagar R, Gupta SK. Neuroleptic malignant syndrome in an adolescent receiving olanzapine-lithium combination therapy. *Pharmacotherapy* (2003) 23, 255–9.
3. Swartz CM. Olanzapine-lithium encephalopathy. *Psychosomatics* (2001) 42, 370.

Lithium + Paracetamol (Acetaminophen)

Paracetamol appears not to interact with lithium.

Clinical evidence, mechanism, importance and management

A study in 9 healthy subjects given lithium carbonate 300 mg 12-hourly to achieve steady state, followed by the addition of 650 mg of paracetamol 6-hourly for 5 days, found no evidence that paracetamol increased serum lithium levels.[1] No precautions seem necessary on concurrent use.

1. Levin GM, Grum C, Eisele G. Effect of over-the-counter dosages of naproxen sodium and acetaminophen on plasma lithium concentrations in normal volunteers. *J Clin Psychopharmacol* (1998) 18, 237–40.

Lithium + Propranolol

One study suggests that propranolol may decrease the clearance of lithium, but the significance of this is unclear. An isolated report describes marked bradycardia in a patient on lithium after he took propranolol 30 mg daily.

Clinical evidence, mechanism, importance and management

A study in an unknown number of patients found that the clearance of lithium was about 20% lower in patients taking propranolol than in patients on lithium alone.[1] However, the clinical effects of this difference were not evaluated so the significance of this finding is unclear. A 70-year-old man who had been stable on lithium for 16 years was additionally started on propranolol 30 mg daily for lithium-induced tremor. Six weeks later he was hospitalised because of vomiting, dizziness, headache and a fainting episode. His pulse rate was 35 to 40 bpm and his serum lithium level was 0.3 mmol/l. When later discharged on lithium without propranolol his pulse rate had risen to 64 to 80 bpm.

The authors attribute the bradycardia to an interaction with lithium due to the low dose of propranolol, which was considered unlikely to cause bradycardia alone. They also point out that both drugs affect the movement of calcium across cell membranes, which could account for the decreased contraction rate of the heart muscle, and thus bradycardia in this patient. They suggest careful monitoring in elderly patients with atherosclerotic cardiovascular problems.[2]

The general importance of this interaction, if it is such, is uncertain, and it seems possible with all beta-blockers because they can all cause bradycardia. However, as beta-blockers are used to treat lithium induced tremor[3] any serious problem would be expected to have come to light by now.

1. Schou M, Vestergaard P. Use of propranolol during lithium treatment: an enquiry and a suggestion. *Pharmacopsychiatry* (1987) 20, 131.
2. Becker D. Lithium and propranolol: possible synergism? *J Clin Psychiatry* (1989) 50, 473.
3. Sweetman SC, editor. Martindale: The complete drug reference. 34th ed. London: Pharmaceutical Press; 2005 p. 872.

Lithium + Quetiapine

Quetiapine slightly raises lithium levels but this is not expected to be clinically significant.

Clinical evidence, mechanism, importance and management

The steady-state serum lithium levels of 10 patients with schizophrenia, or schizoaffective or bipolar disorders were studied during and after the withdrawal of quetiapine 250 mg three times daily. The lithium 0 to 12-hour AUC and the maximum serum levels were raised by 12% and 4.5% respectively in the presence of the quetiapine, and concurrent use was well tolerated.[1] This small rise is unlikely to be clinically important. No special precautions would appear to be necessary.

1. Potkin SG, Thyrum PT, Bera R, Carreon D, Alva G, Kalali AH, Yeh C. Open-label study of the effect of combination quetiapine/lithium therapy on lithium pharmacokinetics and tolerability. *Clin Ther* (2002) 24, 1809–23.

Lithium + Salicylates

Aspirin, lysine aspirin and sodium salicylate appear not to interact with lithium.

Clinical evidence, mechanism, importance and management

In a steady-state study 10 healthy women with average plasma lithium levels of 0.63 mmol/l showed a slight rise in their renal excretion of lithium (from 22 to 23.3 ml/minute) when they were given **aspirin** 1 g four times daily for 7 days. However, no statistically significant alteration in lithium levels was found.[1]

No interaction was seen in 7 patients on lithium when given **aspirin** 975 mg four times daily for 6 days.[2] Another report states that **aspirin** 600 mg four times daily had no effect on the absorption or renal excretion of single doses of lithium carbonate given to six healthy subjects,[3] and further reports describe the absence of an interaction between lithium carbonate and **lysine aspirin**,[4] **aspirin**,[5] or **sodium salicylate**.[5]

1. Reimann IW, Diener U, Frölich JC. Indomethacin but not aspirin increases plasma lithium ion levels. *Arch Gen Psychiatry* (1983) 40, 283–6.
2. Ragheb MA. Aspirin does not significantly affect patients' serum lithium levels. *J Clin Psychiatry* (1987) 48, 425.
3. Bikin D, Conrad KA, Mayersohn M. Lack of influence of caffeine and aspirin on lithium elimination. *Clin Res* (1982) 30, 249A.
4. Singer L, Imbs JL, Danion JM, Singer P, Krieger-Finance F, Schmidt M, Schwartz J. Risque d'intoxication par le lithium en cas de traitement associé par les anti-inflammatoires non stéroïdiens. *Therapie* (1981) 36, 323–6.
5. Reimann IW, Golbs E, Fischer C, Frölich JC. Influence of intravenous acetylsalicylic acid and sodium salicylate on human renal function and lithium clearance. *Eur J Clin Pharmacol* (1985) 29, 435–41.

Lithium + Sodium compounds

The ingestion of marked amounts of sodium can prevent the establishment or maintenance of adequate serum lithium levels. Conversely, dietary salt restriction can cause serum lithium levels to rise to toxic concentrations if the lithium dosage is not reduced appropriately.

Clinical evidence

(a) Lithium response reduced by the ingestion of sodium

A 35-year-old man, initially given lithium carbonate 250 mg four times a day, achieved a serum lithium level of 0.5 mmol/l by the following morning. When the dosage frequency was progressively increased to five, and later six times a day, his serum lithium levels did not exceed 0.6 mmol/l because, unknown to his doctor, he was also taking **sodium bicarbonate**. The patient's wife said he had been taking **soda bic** for years but since he started on lithium he'd been "shovelling it in." When the **sodium bicarbonate** was stopped, relatively stable serum lithium levels of 0.8 mmol/l were achieved on the initial dosage of lithium carbonate.[1]

An investigation to find out why a number of inpatients failed either to reach or maintain adequate therapeutic serum lithium levels over a period of 2 months, revealed that a clinic nurse had been giving the patients *Efferdex*, a product containing about 50% **sodium bicarbonate**, because the patients complained of nausea. The reduction in the expected serum lithium levels was as much as 40% in some cases.[2]

Other studies confirm that the serum lithium levels can fall and the effectiveness of treatment can lessen if the intake of sodium is increased.[3-5]

(b) Lithium response increased by sodium restriction

The serum lithium levels of four patients rose more rapidly and achieved a higher peak when salt was restricted to less than 10 mmol of sodium per day than when the patients took a **dietary salt supplement**.[6]

Mechanism

The situation is complex and not fully established, but the mechanism can be broadly described in simplistic terms.

Sodium balance is controlled by the kidney; if the serum sodium is low the kidney can reabsorb more sodium to maintain the balance. The kidney excretes and reabsorbs both lithium and sodium, but it does not appear to clearly distinguish between lithium and sodium ions. Therefore, if a patient on lithium restricts sodium intake, the kidney may reabsorb both sodium and lithium, causing a rise in serum lithium levels. A corresponding decrease in lithium levels can occur when sodium intake is supplemented.[7,8]

Importance and management

Well established and clinically important interactions. The establishment and maintenance of therapeutic serum lithium levels can be jeopardised if the intake of sodium is altered. Warn patients not to take non-prescription antacids or urinary alkalinisers without first seeking informed advice. Sodium bicarbonate comes in various guises and disguises e.g. *Efferdex* (50%), *Eno's Fruit Salts* (56%), *Andrews Liver Salts* (22.6%), *Bismarex Antacid Powder* (65%), *BiSoDoL Powder* (58%). Substantial amounts also occur in some urinary alkalinising agents (e.g. *Citralka, Citravescent*).[9] There are many similar preparations available throughout the world. An antacid containing **aluminium/magnesium hydroxide** with simeticone has been found to have no effect on the bioavailability of lithium carbonate,[10] so that antacids of this type would appear to be safer alternatives.

Patients already stabilised on lithium should not begin to limit their intake of salt unless their serum lithium levels can be monitored and suitable dosage adjustments made, because their lithium levels can rise quite rapidly.

1. Arthur RK. Lithium levels and "Soda Bic". *Med J Aust* (1975) 2, 918.
2. McSwiggan C. Interaction of lithium and bicarbonate. *Med J Aust* (1978) 1, 38–9.
3. Bleiweiss H. Salt supplements with lithium. *Lancet* (1970) i, 416.
4. Demers RG, Heninger GR. Sodium intake and lithium treatment in mania. *Am J Psychiatry* (1971) 128, 100–104.
5. Baer L, Platman SR, Kassir S, Fieve RR. Mechanisms of renal lithium handling and their relationship to mineralocorticoids: a dissociation between sodium and lithium ions. *J Psychiatr Res* (1971) 8, 91–105.
6. Platman SR, Fieve RR. Lithium retention and excretion: The effect of sodium and fluid intake. *Arch Gen Psychiatry* (1969) 20, 285–9.
7. Thomsen K, Schou M. Renal lithium excretion in man. *Am J Physiol* (1968) 215, 823–7.
8. Singer I, Rotenberg D. Mechanisms of lithium action. *N Engl J Med* (1973) 289, 254–60.
9. Beard TC, Wilkinson SJ, Vial JH. Hazards of urinary alkalizing agents. *Med J Aust* (1988) 149, 723.
10. Goode DL, Newton DW, Ueda CT, Wilson JE, Wulf BG, Kafonek D. Effect of antacid on the bioavailability of lithium carbonate. *Clin Pharm* (1984) 3, 284–7.

Lithium + Spectinomycin

An isolated case report describes a patient who developed lithium toxicity when given spectinomycin.

Clinical evidence, mechanism, importance and management

A woman developed lithium toxicity (tremor, nausea, vomiting, ataxia and dysarthria) when given spectinomycin injections (dose not stated) in addition to her long-term treatment with lithium.[1] Her serum lithium levels had climbed from a range of 0.8 to 1.1 mmol/l up to 3.2 mmol/l. Spectinomycin reduces urinary output, and so it was suggested that a reduced renal clearance of lithium led to these elevated levels. Information seems to be limited to this report, but it would seem prudent to bear this interaction in mind in any patient given both drugs.

1. Conroy RW. Quoted as a personal communication by Ayd FJ. Possible adverse drug-drug interaction report. *Int Drug Ther Newslett* (1978) 13, 15.

Lithium + SSRIs

Concurrent use of lithium and SSRIs can be advantageous and largely uneventful but unexplained neurotoxicities of various kinds have occurred in a small number of patients. Increases in serum lithium levels have been seen with fluoxetine. An isolated report describes the development of symptoms similar to those of the serotonin syndrome in a patient taking lithium and paroxetine and in another patient taking lithium and fluvoxamine.

Clinical evidence

(a) Citalopram

No changes were seen in one study when lithium 30 mmol/day (as lithium sulfate 1980 mg daily) was added to citalopram 40 mg daily in 8 healthy subjects.[1] Another study, in 24 patients who had previously not responded to citalopram alone, found that the concurrent use of citalopram 40 or 60 mg and lithium carbonate 800 mg daily was effective and did not increase adverse effects.[2] Even so the makers of citalopram suggest that concurrent use should be undertaken with caution, as they are aware of reports of enhanced serotonergic effects when lithium and SSRIs are used together.[3,4]

(b) Fluoxetine

A woman with a bipolar affective disorder, successfully maintained for 20 years on lithium carbonate 1200 mg daily, developed stiffness of her arms and legs, dizziness, unsteadiness in walking and speech difficulties within a few days of starting additional treatment with fluoxetine 20 mg daily. Her serum lithium levels had risen from a range of 0.75 to 1.15 mmol/l up to 1.7 mmol/l. They fell, and the toxic symptoms disappeared, when the lithium dosage was reduced and the fluoxetine withdrawn.[5] Two other patients showed increases of about 50% in serum lithium levels and developed mania (but no lithium toxicity) about a month after starting fluoxetine 20 or 40 mg daily. The problem resolved when the lithium dosage was reduced by 40 and 30% respectively.[6] Toxicity was seen in a patient when lithium was added to fluoxetine treatment, although the serum lithium levels remained in the therapeutic range,[7] and absence seizures occurred in another patient given both drugs.[8] A woman on clonazepam developed tremor and ataxia while taking lithium carbonate 400 mg and fluoxetine 40 mg daily. The problems resolved when the lithium and fluoxetine were withdrawn.[9] Extrapyramidal effects and ataxia were seen in one patient on lithium and fluoxetine, and dystonia in another (also taking carbamazepine, captopril and trimipramine).[10] The development of the serotonin syndrome is also reported to have occurred in two patients on lithium and fluoxetine.[11,12] Heat stroke developed in a man on lithium and fluoxetine, attributed to synergistic impairment of his temperature regulatory system by the two drugs.[13]

(c) Fluvoxamine

A woman on fluvoxamine became somnolent within a day of starting additional treatment with lithium. The lithium level 20 hours after the last dose was 0.2 mmol/l. She recovered when both drugs were stopped and she was discharged on lithium alone. The excessive somnolence was considered to have been caused by increased serotonin levels caused by this drug combination.[14] A woman on long-term lithium treatment was started on fluvoxamine 50 mg daily, increased to 200 mg daily over 10 days. She gradually developed tremor, difficulties in making fine hand movements, impaired motor co-ordination and hyperreflexia. Serum lithium levels remained therapeutic throughout. The reaction was interpreted as a mild form of the serotonin syndrome.[15]

The Committee on Safety of Medicines in the UK had received 19 reports of adverse reactions when fluvoxamine was given with lithium (5 reports of convulsions and one of hyperpyrexia) by 1989.[16]

In contrast to these reports, a study in 6 patients found that lithium (dosed to achieve plasma levels of 0.3 to 0.65 mmol/l) and fluvoxamine 100 to 150 mg daily (for between 3 and 23 weeks) was safe and effective, and no adverse interaction of any kind occurred.[17] Another study in 6 depressed patients found that lithium did not affect the pharmacokinetics of fluvoxamine 100 mg daily and combined use was more effective than fluvoxamine alone.[18] It would seem therefore that concurrent use can be valuable, but there is a clear need to monitor the outcome so that any problems can be quickly identified.

(d) Paroxetine

A woman of 59 with a long-standing bipolar disorder taking lithium 400 mg and paroxetine 30 mg daily developed symptoms suggestive of the serotonin syndrome (shivering, tremor of her arms and legs, flushed face, agitation, and some impairment of mental focussing).[19] Her serum lithium and paroxetine levels were found to be 0.63 mmol/l and 690 nanograms/ml respectively (the latter being 6-fold higher than the upper levels seen in other patients). The paroxetine dosage was reduced to 10 mg daily, which reduced the serum levels to 390 nanograms/ml, whereupon she became symptom-free and her depression was relieved. It is not clear whether this reaction was due to an interaction or not. It may simply have been that the paroxetine dosage was too high, because the patient recovered when the dosage was reduced.

(e) Sertraline

In a randomised placebo controlled study, 16 healthy subjects were given lithium 600 mg twice daily for 9 days. On day eight, half of the subjects received two 100-mg doses of sertraline 8 hours apart, while the other half received placebo. Sertraline caused a statistically insignificant fall of 1.4% in steady-state lithium levels, and a statistically insignificant rise in renal lithium excretion. Seven out of the 8 taking sertraline also experienced adverse effects (mainly tremor and nausea) whereas no adverse effects were reported in the placebo group.[20] Severe priapism occurred in a patient on lithium carbonate 600 mg daily within 2 weeks of having the daily dosage of sertraline increased from 50 to 100 mg daily. It was not clear whether this was purely a reaction to the increased sertraline dosage, although it was suggested that the effect may have been due to the serotonergic effects of both drugs.[21] The makers of sertraline suggest that reports of increased tremor suggest a possible pharmacodynamic interaction, and therefore they advise caution if both drugs are used.[22]

Mechanism

Not fully understood although it seems likely that many of the symptoms could be due to the effects of both lithium and SSRIs on serotonin.

Importance and management

Concurrent use can be uneventful. A review of the safety of combined administration of lithium and SSRIs identified 503 subjects who had received the combination without any evidence of serious adverse events[23] but occasionally and unpredictably adverse reactions develop. The precise incidence is not known. If lithium is used in conjunction with an SSRI be alert for any evidence of neurotoxicity. The symptoms may include tremor, dysarthria, ataxia, confusion, and many other symptoms of the serotonin syndrome. Heat stroke has also been seen and the serum lithium levels may rise. It would clearly be prudent to monitor concurrent use carefully. For more information on the serotonin syndrome see 'Additive or synergistic interactions', (p.9).

1. Gram LF, Hansen MGJ, Sindrup SH, Brøsen K, Poulsen JH, Aaes-Jørgensen T, Overø KF. Citalopram: interaction studies with levomepromazine, imipramine, and lithium. *Ther Drug Monit* (1993) 15, 18–24.
2. Baumann P, Souche A, Montaldi S, Baettig D, Lambert S, Uehlinger C, Kasas A, Amey M, Jonzier-Perey M. A double-blind, placebo-controlled study of citalopram with and without lithium in the treatment of therapy-resistant depressive patients: a clinical, pharmacokinetic, and pharmacogenetic investigation. *J Clin Psychopharmacol* (1996) 16, 307–14.
3. Cipramil (Citalopram). Lundbeck Ltd. UK Summary of product characteristics, April 2003.
4. Celexa (Citalopram). Forest Pharmaceuticals Inc. US Prescribing information, February 2005.
5. Salama AA, Shafey M. A case of severe lithium toxicity induced by combined fluoxetine and lithium carbonate. *Am J Psychiatry* (1989) 146, 278.
6. Hadley A, Cason MP. Mania resulting from lithium-fluoxetine combination. *Am J Psychiatry* (1989) 146, 1637–8.
7. Noveske FG, Hahn KR, Flynn RJ. Possible toxicity of combined fluoxetine and lithium. *Am J Psychiatry* (1989) 146, 1515.
8. Sacristan JA, Iglesias C, Arellano F, Lequerica J. Absence seizures induced by lithium: possible interaction with fluoxetine. *Am J Psychiatry* (1991) 148, 146–7.
9. Austin LS, Arana GW, Melvin JA. Toxicity resulting from lithium augmentation of antidepressant treatment in elderly patients. *J Clin Psychiatry* (1990) 51, 344–5.
10. Coulter DM, Pillans PI. Fluoxetine and extrapyramidal side effects. *Am J Psychiatry* (1995) 152, 122–5.
11. Karle J, Bjørndal F. Serotonergt syndrom - ved kombineret behandling med litium og fluoxetin. *Ugeskr Laeger* (1995) 157, 1204–5.
12. Muly EC, McDonald W, Steffens D, Book S. Serotonin syndrome produced by a combination of fluoxetine and lithium. *Am J Psychiatry* (1993) 150, 1565.
13. Albukrek D, Moran DS, Epstein Y. A depressed workman with heatstroke. *Lancet* (1996) 347, 1016.
14. Evans M, Marwick P. Fluvoxamine and lithium: an unusual interaction. *Br J Psychiatry* (1990) 156, 286.
15. Öhman R, Spigset O. Serotonin syndrome induced by fluvoxamine-lithium interaction. *Pharmacopsychiatry* (1993) 26, 263–4.
16. Committee on the Safety of Medicines. *Current Problems* (1989) 26, 3. Correction. Ibid. 1989, 27, 3.
17. Hendrickx B, Floris M. A controlled pilot study of the combination of fluvoxamine and lithium. *Curr Ther Res* (1991) 49, 106–10.
18. Miljković BR, Pokrajac M, Timotijević I, Varagić V. The influence of lithium on fluvoxamine therapeutic efficacy and pharmacokinetics in depressed patients on combined fluvoxamine-lithium therapy. *Int Clin Psychopharmacol* (1997) 12, 207–12.
19. Sobanski T, Bagli M, Laux G, Rao ML. Serotonin syndrome after lithium add-on medication to paroxetine. *Pharmacopsychiatry* (1997) 30, 106–7.
20. Apseloff G, Wilner KD, von Deutsch DA, Henry EB, Tremaine LM, Gerber N, Lazar JD. Sertraline does not alter steady-state concentrations or renal clearance of lithium in healthy volunteers. *J Clin Pharmacol* (1992) 32, 643–6.
21. Mendelson WB, Franko T. Priapism with sertraline and lithium. *J Clin Psychopharmacol* (1994) 14, 434–5.
22. Lustral (Sertraline). Pfizer Ltd. UK Summary of product characteristics, December 2003.
23. Hawley CJ, Loughlin PJ, Quick SJ, Gale TM, Sivakumaran T, Hayes J, McPhee S, for the Hertfordshire Neuroscience Research Group. Efficacy, safety and tolerability of combined administration of lithium and selective serotonin reuptake inhibitors: a review of the current evidence. *Int Clin Psychopharmacol* (2000) 15, 197–206.

Lithium + Tetracyclines

Concurrent use is normally uneventful, but two isolated reports describe lithium toxicity, one in a woman on tetracycline, and the other in a man on doxycycline.

Clinical evidence

(a) Doxycycline

A man on long-term treatment with lithium carbonate became confused within a day of starting to take doxycycline 100 mg twice daily. By the end of a week he had developed symptoms of lithium toxicity (ataxia, dysarthria, worsened tremor, fatigue, etc.). His serum lithium levels had risen from a range of 0.8 to 1.1 mmol/l up to 1.8 mmol/l; his renal function remained normal. He recovered when the doxycycline was withdrawn.[1]

(b) Tetracycline

An isolated report describes a woman, stabilised on lithium for 3 years, with serum concentrations within the range 0.5 to 0.84 mmol/l. Within 2 days of starting to take a sustained-release form of tetracycline (*Tetrabid*) her serum lithium levels had risen to 1.7 mmol/l, and 2 days later they had further risen to 2.74 mmol/l. By then she showed clear symptoms of lithium toxicity (slight drowsiness, slurring of the speech, fine tremor and thirst).[2]

In contrast, 13 healthy subjects taking lithium carbonate 450 mg twice daily or 900 mg once daily showed a small reduction in serum lithium levels (from 0.51 to 0.47 mmol/l) when given tetracycline 500 mg twice daily for seven days.[3] The incidence of adverse reactions remained largely unchanged, except for a slight increase in CNS and gastrointestinal adverse effects.

Mechanism

Not understood. One suggested reason is that tetracycline (known to have nephrotoxic potential) may have adversely affected the renal clearance of lithium.[2]

Importance and management

These adverse interaction reports are isolated and unexplained. Two reports make the point that these drugs are used commonly for acne caused by lithium,[1,4] so any common interaction would be expected to have come to light by now. There would seem to be no reason for avoiding concurrent use of lithium and either tetracycline or doxycycline, but be aware of the potential for this rare interaction.

1. Miller SC. Doxycycline-induced lithium toxicity. *J Clin Psychopharmacol* (1997) 17, 54–5.
2. McGennis AJ. Lithium carbonate and tetracycline interaction. *BMJ* (1978) 2, 1183.
3. Fankhauser MP, Lindon JL, Connolly B, Healey WJ. Evaluation of lithium–tetracycline interaction. *Clin Pharm* (1988) 7, 314–17.
4. Jefferson JW. Lithium and tetracycline. *Br J Dermatol* (1982) 107, 370.

Lithium + Theophylline

Serum lithium levels are moderately reduced by 20 to 30% by the concurrent use of theophylline. Patients may relapse as a result.

Clinical evidence

The serum lithium levels of 10 healthy subjects on lithium carbonate 900 mg daily fell by 20 to 30%, and the urinary clearance increased by 30%, when they were given theophylline (*Theo-dur*). Steady state theophylline levels of 5.4 to 12.7 microgram/ml were achieved, and it was noted that higher theophylline levels were strongly correlated with increased lithium clearance.[1] This study has been reported in brief elsewhere.[2]

A man on theophylline was diagnosed with a bipolar disorder and started on lithium while in hospital for an exacerbation of COPD. When the dose of theophylline was raised because of a worsening in his condition, his lithium dose also had to be increased to control the emergence of manic symptoms. He received a maximum theophylline dose of 1500 mg daily, during which time he needed 2700 mg of lithium daily. When the theophylline was stopped, he only needed around 1500 mg of lithium daily to control his manic symptoms.[3] Two studies support the evidence from these cases with the finding that lithium excretion is increased by about 50% by **aminophylline** or theophylline.[4,5]

Mechanism

Uncertain. Theophylline has an effect on the renal clearance of lithium.

Importance and management

Information is very limited but the interaction appears to be established. Depressive and manic relapses may occur if the dosage of lithium is not raised appropriately when theophylline is given. Serum lithium levels should be monitored if theophylline (or aminophylline) is stopped, started, or if the dosage is altered.

1. Perry PJ, Calloway RA, Cook BL, Smith RE. Theophylline precipitated alterations of lithium clearance. *Acta Psychiatr Scand* (1984) 69, 528–37.
2. Cook BL, Smith RE, Perry PJ, Calloway RA. Theophylline-lithium interaction. *J Clin Psychiatry* (1985) 46, 278–9.
3. Sierles FS, Ossowski MG. Concurrent use of theophylline and lithium in a patient with chronic obstructive lung disease and bipolar disorder. *Am J Psychiatry* (1982) 139, 117–18.
4. Thomsen K, Schou M. Renal lithium excretion in man. *Am J Physiol* (1968) 215, 823–7.
5. Holstad SG, Perry PJ, Kathol RG, Carson RW, Krummel SJ. The effects of intravenous theophylline infusion versus intravenous sodium bicarbonate infusion on lithium clearance in normal subjects. *Psychiatry Res* (1988) 25, 203–11.

Lithium + Tricyclic and related antidepressants

A combination of tricyclic antidepressants and lithium can be successful in some patients, but a few may develop adverse effects, some of them severe. Cases of neurotoxicity, the serotonin syndrome and the neuroleptic malignant syndrome have been reported.

Clinical evidence

A study in 14 treatment-resistant depressed patients aged between 61 and 82 found that 7 showed complete improvement and 3 showed partial improvement after 3 to 21 days when given lithium and tricyclic or related antidepressants. Adverse effects of lithium occurred in 6 patients, and in 4 of these the lithium was stopped as a result. One of them was successfully restarted at a lower dose. Tremor was the most frequent adverse effect, and reversible neurotoxicity with a stroke-like syndrome was the most severe. The antidepressants used were **amitriptyline**, **doxepin**, **maprotiline** and **trazodone**.[1]

No pharmacokinetic interaction was found in 10 therapy-resistant patients with major depression who were given **amitriptyline** and lithium for 4 weeks.[2] However, seizures occurred in another patient on **amitriptyline** 300 mg daily 6 days after lithium carbonate 300 mg three times daily was added. Her lithium levels were 0.9 mmol/l. She later took **amitriptyline** 500 mg daily without adverse effect.[3]

A 65-year-old woman developed tremor, memory difficulties, disorganised thinking and auditory hallucinations when given lithium carbonate 300 mg twice daily (lithium level 0.82 mmol/l) and **nortriptyline** 50 mg daily. However, because she only ever received lithium with **nortriptyline**, the possibility that this was an effect of lithium alone cannot be excluded.[4]

A depressed man taking **clomipramine** 175 mg, levomepromazine 25 mg and flunitrazepam 2 mg daily, developed the serotonin syndrome (myoclonus, shivering, tremors, incoordination) a week after his dosage of lithium was raised from 600 to 1000 mg daily. Due to this reaction, and because his serum lithium levels were 1.6 mmol/l, the lithium was stopped. The serotonin syndrome then abated. The **clomipramine** dosage was reduced, but some mild symptoms remained until the **clomipramine** was stopped. He responded well to lithium 600 mg daily alone, without developing the serotonin syndrome.[5]

A man developed periods of confusion and disorientation 2 weeks after starting to take lithium 300 mg twice daily and **doxepin** 100 mg at bedtime, but despite the withdrawal of both drugs he developed a condition similar to the neuroleptic malignant syndrome (fever, muscle rigidity, changes in consciousness, autonomic dysfunction), which was successfully treated with dantrolene.[6] Another patient also developed neuroleptic malignant syndrome after one-week of treatment with lithium 300 mg and **amitriptyline** 25 mg, both three times daily.[7]

Mechanism

Not understood. For more information about the serotonin syndrome see 'Additive or synergistic interactions', (p.9).

Importance and management

The concurrent use of lithium and tricyclics can be valuable, but the case reports cited here clearly show the need to monitor the outcome closely so that any problems can be dealt with quickly. The incidence of these serious reactions is not known.

1. Lafferman J, Solomon K, Ruskin P. Lithium augmentation for treatment-resistant depression in the elderly. *J Geriatr Psychiatry Neurol* (1988) 1, 49–52.
2. Jaspert A, Ebert D, Loew T, Martus P. Lithium increases the response to tricyclic antidepressant medication – no evidence of influences of pharmacokinetic interactions. *Pharmacopsychiatry* (1993) 26, 165.
3. Solomon JG. Seizures during lithium-amitriptyline therapy. *Postgrad Med* (1979) 66, 145–8.
4. Austin LS, Arana GW, Melvin JA. Toxicity resulting from lithium augmentation of antidepressant treatment in elderly patients. *J Clin Psychiatry* (1990) 51, 344–5.
5. Kojima H, Terao T, Yoshimura R. Serotonin syndrome during clomipramine and lithium treatment. *Am J Psychiatry* (1993) 150, 1897.
6. Rosenberg PB, Pearlman CA. NMS-like syndrome with a lithium/doxepin combination. *J Clin Psychopharmacol* (1991) 11, 75–6.
7. Fava S, Caruana Galizia A. Neuroleptic malignant syndrome and lithium carbonate. *J Psychiatry Neurosci* (1995) 20, 305–6.

Lithium + Triptans

There are two reports of possible serotonin syndrome after the concurrent use of sumatriptan and lithium. The makers of almotriptan contraindicate the concurrent use of lithium because of a lack of safety data.

Clinical evidence, mechanism, importance and management

A comprehensive literature search published in 1998 identified only 2 patients taking **sumatriptan** and lithium concurrently who developed adverse reactions. The symptoms were suggestive of the serotonin syndrome, and were mild to moderate and self-limiting. The number of patients taking lithium and **sumatriptan** was not stated, so the incidence is unknown.[1] The conclusion was reached that **sumatriptan** can be used cautiously in patients receiving lithium.[1] The makers of **almotriptan** say that lithium is contraindicated to err on the side of caution, as patients on lithium were excluded from their clinical trials. There seem to be no reports of problems with this combination.[2] More study is needed to clarify the situation. There seems to be no information about other triptans.

1. Gardner DM, Lynd LD. Sumatriptan contraindications and the serotonin syndrome. *Ann Pharmacother* (1998) 32, 33–8.
2. Lundbeck Ltd. Personal communication, March 2001.

Lithium + Venlafaxine

No clinically significant pharmacokinetic interaction occurs between lithium and venlafaxine, although an isolated case of the serotonin syndrome has been attributed to an interaction between venlafaxine and lithium.

Clinical evidence, mechanism, importance and management

In one study 12 healthy subjects were given a single 600-mg dose of lithium carbonate on day 1 and day 8, with venlafaxine 50 mg 8-hourly from days 4 to 11. The renal clearance of venlafaxine was reduced by 50% and that of its active metabolite (*O*-desmethylvenlafaxine; ODV) was reduced by 15%. Neither of these changes was considered clinically relevant. The maximum serum levels of the lithium were increased by 10%, and the time to reach this was reduced by about 30 minutes, but these changes met the criteria for bioequivalence, and the other pharmacokinetic parameters of lithium were unchanged.[1] The general picture that emerged was that no clinically important adverse interaction normally occurs if these two drugs are used together.

However, a subsequent case report describes a 50-year-old woman who developed the serotonin syndrome 45 days after starting to take lithium and venlafaxine (10 days after the most recent dose increase of venlafaxine). Both drugs were immediately stopped and she recovered over the next 4 days. Plasma levels of venlafaxine, ODV and lithium had remained within the normal therapeutic range throughout. As she had previously experienced profound adverse effects with two SSRIs the authors concluded that the patient was unusually sensitive to serotonergic medication.[2]

There seems to be no good reason for avoiding concurrent use, but be aware that an interaction is possible and monitor the outcome carefully.

For more information about the serotonin syndrome see 'Additive or synergistic interactions', (p.9).

1. Troy SM, Parker VD, Hicks DR, Boudino FD, Chiang ST. Pharmacokinetic interaction between multiple-dose venlafaxine and single-dose lithium. *J Clin Pharmacol* (1996) 36, 175–81.
2. Mekler G, Woggon B. A case of serotonin syndrome caused by venlafaxine and lithium. *Pharmacopsychiatry* (1997) 30, 272–3.

Lithium + Ziprasidone

Ziprasidone appears not interact to a clinically relevant extent with lithium.

Clinical evidence, mechanism importance and management

An open-label, randomised, placebo-controlled study in 12 healthy subjects taking lithium carbonate 450 mg twice daily for 15 days, found that ziprasidone 20 mg twice daily on days 9 to 11, followed by 40 mg twice daily on days 12 to 15 caused only a small increase in the steady-state serum lithium levels (14% compared with 11% in the placebo group). A 5% reduction in renal clearance was seen in the ziprasidone group and a 9% reduction was seen in the placebo group. These differences were neither statistically nor clinically significant.[1] No special precautions would therefore seem to be necessary if ziprasidone is given to patients taking lithium.

1. Apseloff G, Mullet D, Wilner KD, Anziano RJ, Tensfeldt TG, Pelletier SM, Gerber N. The effects of ziprasidone on steady-state lithium levels and renal clearance of lithium. *Br J Clin Pharmacol* (2000) 49 (Suppl 1), 61S–64S.

30

MAOIs

Drugs with monoamine oxidase inhibitory activity were first developed as antidepressants because it was noticed that patients with tuberculosis given isoniazid, and more particularly iproniazid, showed some degree of mood elevation. A further development occurred when postural hypotension was seen to be one of the side-effects of treatment with iproniazid and, as a result, pheniprazine and later pargyline were introduced as antihypertensive agents.

Among the serious and unexpected problems with the first generation monoamine oxidase inhibitors (MAOIs) were the serious and potentially life-threatening interactions that occurred with the sympathomimetics found in some proprietary cough and cold remedies, and with tyramine-rich foods and drinks.

The intended target of the antidepressant MAOIs is MAO within the brain, but MAO is also found in other parts of the body. Particularly high concentrations occur in the gut and liver, where it acts as a protective detoxifying enzyme against tyramine and possibly other potentially hazardous amines that exist in foods that have undergone bacterial degradation. For this reason MAO was originally called tyramine oxidase. There are at least two forms of MAO: MAO-A metabolises (deaminates) noradrenaline (norepinephrine) and serotonin (5-HT), and MAO-B metabolises phenylethylamine. Substances like tyramine and dopamine are metabolised by both forms of MAO.

The older MAOIs (see 'Table 30.1') are non-selective or non-specific. They inhibit both isoenzymes A and B, and are mostly irreversible and long-acting, because the return of MAO activity depends upon the regeneration of new enzymes. As a result their effects (both beneficial and adverse) can last for 2 to 3 weeks after they have been withdrawn. Tranylcypromine differs in being a reversible inhibitor of MAO, so the onset and disappearance of its actions are much quicker than the other older MAOIs.

Some of the newer and more recently developed MAOIs (see 'Table 30.1') interact to a lesser extent than the first generation MAOIs. This is because they are relatively rapidly reversible and are largely selective. One group of these reversible inhibitors targets MAO-A; inhibition of this enzyme is responsible for the antidepressant effect. These selective MAO-A inhibitors (brofaromine, moclobemide, toloxatone) have been given the acronym RIMA (Reversible Inhibitors of Monoamine oxidase A). They leave MAO-B largely uninhibited so that there is still a metabolic pathway available for the breakdown of amines, such as tyramine, that can cause a rise in blood pressure. In practical terms this means that the amount of tyramine needed to cause a hypertensive crisis is about tenfold greater than with the older MAOIs.

The other MAOIs that specifically inhibit MAO-B are ineffective for the treatment of depression and are mainly used for Parkinson's disease. In low doses they inhibit MAO-B, leaving MAO-A largely uninhibited. However, selegiline loses its selectivity at doses of above 10 mg daily and will therefore be subject to the same interactions as the older MAOIs.

If you look at the SPCs issued by manufacturers, you will frequently see warnings about real and alleged interactions with MAOIs. Blackwell,[1] who has done much work on the interactions of the MAOIs, has rightly pointed out that the MAOIs are among the drugs that "...have such a long history they accumulate much myth and misinformation. Lists of side effects and interactions are lengthy but often unsupported by recent or creditable research to establish either a cause and effect relationship or to identify the underlying mechanism. Worse still, the MAOIs have developed such a sinister reputation that manufacturers often issue a reflexive admonition to avoid co-administration with new drugs."

This means that many of the warnings about potential interactions with the MAOIs may lack a sound scientific basis. Take note.

In addition to the interactions of the MAOIs described in this section, there are others dealt with elsewhere. The Index should be consulted for a full listing.

1. Blackwell B. Monoamine Oxidase Inhibitor interactions with other drugs. *J Clin Psychopharmacol* (1991) 11, 55–59.

Table 30.1 Monoamine oxidase inhibitors (MAOIs)

Generic names	*Proprietary names*
Older MAOIs	
Irreversible MAOIs	
Iproniazid	Marsilid
Isocarboxazid	Marplan
Nialamide	Niamid
Phenelzine	Nardelzine, Nardil
Reversible MAOIs	
Tranylcypromine	Jarrosom N, Jatrosom N, Parnate
Tranylcypromine with trifluoperazine	Parmodalin, Parstelin, Stelapar
Newer MAOIs	
Reversible inhibitors of MAO-A (RIMA)	
Brofaromine	
Moclobemide	Arima, Aurorix, Feraken, Manerix, Mobemide, Moclamine, Mohexal
Toloxatone	Humoryl, Umoril
Irreversible inhibitors of MAO-B	
Selegiline	Amboneural, Amindan, Antiparkin, Apomex, Atapryl, Carbex, Clondepryl, Cognitiv, Deprenyl, Deprilan, Egibren, Eldepryl, Elegelin, Elepril, Julab, Jumex, Jumexal, Jumexil, Kinline, MAOtil, Movergan, Niar, Plurimen, Regepar, Sefmex, Selecim, Seledat, Selegam, Selegos, Selemerck, Selepark, Selgene, Selgimed, Seline, Tremorex, Zelapar

MAOIs + Amantadine

An isolated report describes a rise in blood pressure in a patient on amantadine when given phenelzine.

Clinical evidence, mechanism, importance and management

A 49-year-old woman was taking amantadine 200 mg daily, haloperidol 5 mg daily and flurazepam 30 mg at night. Within 72 hours of starting to take **phenelzine** 15 mg twice daily for depression, her blood pressure rose from 140/90 to 160/110 mmHg. The **phenelzine** was withdrawn, and 24 hours later, the amantadine and haloperidol were withdrawn. The blood pressure remained elevated for a further 72 hours.[1] The reason for this hypertensive reaction is not understood. In contrast, a woman with Parkinson's disease is reported to have been given amantadine 200 mg daily and **phenelzine** 45 mg daily successfully and uneventfully.[2] The general importance of this interaction is uncertain, but bear it in mind in the case of an unusual response to treatment.

1. Jack RA, Daniel DG. Possible interaction between phenelzine and amantadine. *Arch Gen Psychiatry* (1984) 41, 726.
2. Greenberg R, Meyers BS. Treatment of major depression and Parkinson's disease with combined phenelzine and amantadine. *Am J Psychiatry* (1985) 142, 273–4.

MAOIs + Antihistamines

Most of the alleged antihistamine/MAOI interactions appear not to be based on good clinical evidence, and are probably more theoretical than real. The exception seems to be cyproheptadine, see 'MAOIs + Cyproheptadine', p.865.

Clinical evidence, mechanism, importance and management

A number of lists, charts and books about adverse interactions suggest that potentially serious interactions can occur between the MAOIs and the antihistamines. UK datasheets for various antihistamines contain a number of warnings, but, with the exception of **cyproheptadine** (see 'MAOIs + Cyproheptadine', p.865), there do not appear to be any clinical reports confirming these interactions.

The UK maker has stated that **clemastine**[1] may increase the effects of MAOIs, while **pheniramine**[2] is said to increase the sedative effects of MAOIs. The anticholinergic effects of **chlorphenamine**[3] and **diphenhydramine**[4] are said to be increased by MAOIs. **Azatadine**[5] and **mequitazine**[6] were contraindicated with MAOIs by their UK makers, while the makers of **chlorphenamine**[3] and **promethazine**[7] not only contraindicate concurrent use with MAOIs, but also extend the contraindication to the 14 days after an MAOI is stopped.

However, in correspondence with some of the makers of these antihistamines, none of them were able to quote direct clinical data in support of these statements.[8-13]

The ABPI Medicines Compendium 2002 also lists **alimemazine (trimeprazine), brompheniramine, cetirizine, fexofenadine, hydroxyzine, levocabastine, loratadine** and **mizolastine**, but no specific warning about interactions with MAOIs is given in the datasheets for any of these drugs.

Some of the drug makers contacted have written to say that the authority for their warnings is Martindale's Extra Pharmacopoeia[10] or the British National Formulary,[11] or even that it was included at the request of the Medicines Control Agency[9] or the FDA,[13] but in the absence of direct, positive and clear clinical data it is difficult to avoid the conclusion that these alleged interactions are simply part of the clinical mythology that has come to surround the MAOIs. See also Blackwell's perceptive and illuminating comment quoted in the 'introduction to this section', (p.862).

1. Tavegil (Clemastine). Novartis. ABPI Compendium of Data Sheets and Summaries of Product Characteristics 1999-2000, p.1027–8.
2. Daneral SA (Pheniramine maleate). Hoechst UK Limited. ABPI Compendium of Data Sheets and Summaries of Product Characteristics Compendium 1996–7, p. 410–11.
3. Piriton (Chlorpheniramine maleate). GlaxoSmithKline Consumer Healthcare. UK Summary of product characteristics, April 2004.
4. Nytol (Diphenydramine hydrochloride). GlaxoSmithKline Consumer Healthcare. UK Summary of product characteristics, February 2002.
5. Optimine (Azatadine maleate). Schering-Plough Ltd. UK Summary of product characteristics, July 1997.
6. Primalan (Mequitazine). Rhone-Poulenc Rorer Limited. ABPI Compendium of Data Sheets and Summaries of Product Characteristics, 1998–9, p. 1104–5.
7. Avomine (Promethazine teoclate). Manx Pharma. UK Summary of product characteristics, November 1997.
8. Intercare Products (Sandoz). Personal communication, May 1995.
9. Rhône-Poulenc Rorer, Personal communication, December 1997.
10. Glaxo Wellcome. Personal communication, December 1995.
11. Stafford Miller. Personal communication, November 1995.
12. Hoechst Roussel. Personal communication, November 1995.
13. Merck Sharp and Dohme. Personal communication, January 1996.

MAOIs + Barbiturates

Although the MAOIs can enhance and prolong the activity of barbiturates in *animals*, only a few isolated cases of adverse responses attributed to an interaction have been described in man.

Clinical evidence

One report[1] states that on three or four occasions patients taking an MAOI continued, without the prescribers knowledge, to take their usual barbiturate hypnotic and thereby ". . . unknowingly raised their dose of barbiturate by five to ten times, and as a consequence barely managed to stagger through the day". No details are given, so it is not known whether the serum barbiturate levels of these patients were measured, or whether this conclusion is only a surmise.

A patient on **tranylcypromine** was inadvertently given 250 mg of **amobarbital sodium** intravenously for sedation. Within an hour she became ataxic, and fell to the floor, repeatedly hitting her head. After complaining of nausea and dizziness the patient became semicomatose and remained in that state for a further 36 hours. To what extent the head trauma played a part is uncertain.[2]

Two other cases of coma attributed to the concurrent use of an MAOI and a barbiturate have been described.[3]

Also, a man taking **amobarbital sodium** 195 mg at night suffered severe headache, and became confused after additionally taking **phenelzine** 15 mg three times daily for 4 weeks. On admission to hospital he was comatose, and he had a temperature of 40°, blood pressure of 150/90 mmHg, tachycardia, stertorous respiration, fixed dilated pupils, exaggerated tendon reflexes and extensor plantar responses. His condition deteriorated and he died 2 hours after admission.[4] Pathology suggested a rise in intracranial pressure was responsible. The authors attribute this response to the drugs, but do not rule out a possible contribution of alcohol.[4]

Mechanism

Not known. *Animal* studies[5,6] suggest that the MAOIs have a general inhibitory action on the liver microsomal enzymes, reducing the metabolism of the barbiturates and thereby prolonging their activity. Whether this occurs in man as well is uncertain.

Importance and management

The evidence for these interactions seem to be confined to a few unconfirmed anecdotal reports. There is no well-documented evidence showing that concurrent use should be avoided, although some caution is clearly appropriate.

1. Kline NS. Psychopharmaceuticals: effects and side-effects. *Bull WHO* (1959) 21, 397.
2. Domino EF, Sullivan TS, Luby ED. Barbiturate intoxication in a patient treated with a MAO inhibitor. *Am J Psychiatry* (1962) 118, 941–3.
3. Etherington L. Personal communication, 1973.
4. MacLeod I. Fatal reaction to phenelzine. *BMJ* (1965) 1, 1554.
5. Wulfsohn NL, Politzer WM. 5-Hydroxytryptamine in anaesthesia. *Anaesthesia* (1962) 17, 64–8.
6. Buchel L, Lévy J. Mécanisme des phénomènes de synergie du sommeil expérimental. II. Étude des associations iproniazide-hypnotiques, chez le rat et la souris. *Arch Sci Physiol (Paris)* (1965) 19, 161–79.

MAOIs + Benzodiazepines

The concurrent use of MAOIs and benzodiazepines is usually safe and effective, but a very small number of adverse reactions (chorea, severe headache, massive oedema) attributed to interactions have been described.

Clinical evidence, mechanism, importance and management

A patient with depression responded well when given **phenelzine** 15 mg and **chlordiazepoxide** 10 mg three times a day, but 4 to 5 months later developed choreiform movements of moderate severity, and slight dysarthria. These symptoms subsided when both drugs were withdrawn.[1]

Two patients on **chlordiazepoxide** and either **isocarboxazid** or **phenelzine** developed severe oedema, which was attributed to the use of both drugs.[2,3] A patient on **phenelzine** 30 mg twice daily developed MAOI toxicity (excessive sweating, postural hypotension) within 10 days of increasing his daily dosage of **nitrazepam** to 15 mg. The patient was a slow acetylator, meaning metabolism of **nitrazepam** by *N*-acetyl transferase was decreased, resulting in raised levels of **nitrazepam** even before the **phenelzine** was started.[4] A patient who had been taking **phenelzine** 45 mg daily for 9 years developed a severe occipital headache after taking 500 micrograms of **clonazepam**. A similar but milder headache occurred the next night when she took the same dose. No blood pressure measurements were taken.[5] The reasons for the development of all of these reactions are unknown.

A meta-analysis of 467 patients taking moclobemide with one or more of the benzodiazepines is reported to have found that the use of benzodiazepines appeared to double the incidence of adverse effects (insomnia, restlessness, agitation, anxiety) in patients on **moclobemide**, but it is suggested that the patient groups may possibly have been different.[6] Another report found no clinically relevant interaction between **moclobemide** and benzodiazepines.[7]

The general picture portrayed by the reports in the literature is that concurrent use is usually effective and uneventful.[8-10] The adverse interaction reports cited here appear to be the exception, and it is by no means certain that all the responses were in fact due to drug interactions, however some caution is appropriate if these drugs are used together.

1. Macleod DM. Chorea induced by tranquillisers. *Lancet* (1964) i, 388–9.
2. Goonewardene A, Toghill PJ. Gross oedema occurring during treatment for depression. *BMJ* (1977) 1, 879–80.
3. Pathak SK. Gross oedema during treatment for depression. *BMJ* (1977) 1, 1220.
4. Harris AL, McIntyre N. Interaction of phenelzine and nitrazepam in a slow acetylator. *Br J Clin Pharmacol* (1981) 12, 254–5.
5. Eppel AB. Interaction between clonazepam and phenelzine. *Can J Psychiatry* (1990) 35, 647.
6. Amrein R, Güntert TW, Dingemanse J, Lorscheid T, Stabl M, Schmid-Burgk W. Interactions of moclobemide with concomitantly administered medication: evidence from pharmacological and clinical studies. *Psychopharmacology (Berl)* (1992) 106, S24–S31.
7. Zimmer R, Gieschke R, Fischbach R, Gasic S. Interaction studies with moclobemide. *Acta Psychiatr Scand* (1990) 82 (Suppl 360), 84–6.
8. Frommer EA. Treatment of childhood depression with antidepressant drugs. *BMJ* (1967) 1, 729–32.
9. Mans J, Senes M. L'isocarboxazide, le RO 5–0690 ou chlordiazépoxide, le RO-4-0403 dérivé des thioxanthènes. Étude sur leurs effets propres et leurs possibilités d'association. *J Med Bord* (1964) 141, 1909–18.
10. Suerinck A, Suerinck E. États dépressifs en milieu sanatorial et inhibiteurs de la mono-amine-oxydase. (Résultats thérapeutiques par l'association d'iproclozide et de chlordiazépoxide.) A propos de 146 observations. *J Med Lyon* (1966) 47, 573–86.

MAOIs + Buspirone

Elevated blood pressure has been reported in four patients taking buspirone and either phenelzine or tranylcypromine.

Clinical evidence, mechanism, importance and management

Four cases of significant blood pressure elevation during the use of buspirone and either **phenelzine** or **tranylcypromine** have been reported to the FDA's Spontaneous Reporting System. One patient was a 75-year-old woman and the other three patients were men aged between 30 and 42. The report does not say how much the blood pressure rose, or how quickly, and no other details are given.[1] On the basis of this rather sparse information the manufacturers of buspirone[2,3] recommend that it should not be used concomitantly with an MAOI.

1. Anon. BuSpar Update. *Psychiatry Drug Alert* (1987) 1, 43.
2. Buspar (Buspirone hydrochloride). Bristol-Myers Pharmaceuticals. UK Summary of product characteristics, July 2005.
3. Buspar (Buspirone hydrochloride). Bristol-Myers Squibb Company. US Prescribing information, November 2003.

MAOIs + Choline theophyllinate

An isolated report describes the development of tachycardia and apprehension in a patient on phenelzine after taking a cough syrup containing choline theophyllinate (oxtriphylline).

Clinical evidence, mechanism, importance and management

A woman with agoraphobia, being treated with **phenelzine** 45 mg daily, developed tachycardia, palpitations and apprehension lasting for about 4 hours after she had taken a cough syrup containing choline theophyllinate and guaifenesin. The symptoms recurred when she was again given the syrup, and yet again when given choline theophyllinate alone, but not when given guaifenesin alone.[1] The reasons are not understood.

An adverse reaction with an MAOI has also been reported with caffeine, which like choline theophyllinate is another **xanthine** (see 'MAOIs + Miscellaneous', p.868), but MAOI/**xanthine** interactions seem to be rare. It would seem prudent to check that patients given these drugs together are not experiencing any adverse effects, but there would appear to be no general need to avoid the **xanthine** bronchodilators.

1. Shader RI, Greenblatt DJ. MAOIs and drug interactions—a proposal for a clearinghouse. *J Clin Psychopharmacol* (1985) 5, A17.

MAOIs + Cloral hydrate

A case of fatal hyperpyrexia and another of serious hypertension have been linked to interactions between cloral hydrate and phenelzine, but in both cases there are other plausible explanations for the reactions seen.

Clinical evidence, mechanism, importance and management

A woman taking **phenelzine** 15 mg three times daily was found in bed deeply comatose with marked muscular rigidity, twitching down one side and a temperature of 41°C. She died without regaining consciousness. A postmortem failed to establish the cause of death, but it subsequently came to light that she had started drinking whisky again (she had been treated for alcoholism), and she had access to cloral hydrate, of which she may have taken a fatal dose.[1] Another patient, also taking **phenelzine** 15 mg three times daily and cloral hydrate for sleeping, developed an excruciating headache followed by nausea, photophobia and a substantial rise in blood pressure.[2] This latter reaction is similar to the 'cheese reaction' (interactions with 'cheese' are described on (p.876)), but at the time the authors of the report were unaware of this type of reaction so that they failed to find out if any tyramine-rich foods had been eaten on the day of the attack.[2]

There is no clear evidence that either of these adverse reactions was due to an interaction between **phenelzine** and cloral hydrate, and no other reports to suggest that an interaction between these drugs is likely.

1. Howarth E. Possible synergistic effects of the new thymoleptics in connection with poisoning. *J Ment Sci* (1961) 107, 100–103.
2. Dillon H, Leopold RL. Acute cerebro-vascular symptoms produced by an antidepressant. *Am J Psychiatry* (1965) 121, 1012–14.

MAOIs + Cocaine

An isolated report describes the delayed development of hyperpyrexia, coma, muscle tremors and rigidity after a patient on phenelzine received a cocaine spray.

Clinical evidence, mechanism, importance and management

A man on **phenelzine** 15 mg twice daily underwent vocal chord surgery. He was anaesthetised with thiopental, and later nitrous oxide and 0.5% isoflurane in oxygen. Muscle paralysis was produced with suxamethonium and gallamine. During the operation his vocal chords were sprayed with 1 ml of a 10% cocaine spray. He regained consciousness 30 minutes after the surgery and was returned to the ward, but a further 30 minutes later he was found unconscious, with generalised coarse tremors and marked muscle rigidity. His rectal temperature was 41.5°C. He was initially thought to have malignant hyperpyrexia and was treated accordingly with wet blankets, as well as with intravenous fluids and oxygen, and he largely recovered within 7 hours. However, later it seemed more likely that what occurred was probably due to an adverse interaction between the **phenelzine** and cocaine, because he had been similarly and uneventfully treated with cocaine in the absence of **phenelzine** on two previous occasions.

The reasons for the adverse reaction are not understood, but a delayed excitatory reaction due to increased 5-HT concentrations is suggested.[1] This is an isolated report and its general importance is not known.

1. Tordoff SG, Stubbing JF, Linter SPK. Delayed excitatory reaction following interaction of cocaine and monoamine oxidase inhibitor (phenelzine). *Br J Anaesth* (1991) 66, 516–8.

MAOIs + Cyproheptadine

Isolated reports describe delayed hallucinations in a patient on phenelzine and cyproheptadine, and the rapid re-emergence of depression in two other patients on brofaromine or phenelzine when given cyproheptadine.

Clinical evidence

A woman who had responded well to **brofaromine** rapidly became depressed again when given cyproheptadine. She had to be hospitalised due to suicidal ideation, but eventually she responded to treatment and received **brofaromine** and cyproheptadine for 6 months.[1] A man whose depression responded well to **phenelzine** 75 mg daily was given cyproheptadine 4 mg to treat associated sexual dysfunction and anorgasmia. Within three days of adding the cyproheptadine his depression returned, but the anorgasmia did not improve. When the cyproheptadine was stopped his depression was relieved.[2] Hallucinations developed in a woman 2 months after cyproheptadine was added to her treatment with **phenelzine**.[3] The UK makers of cyproheptadine also say that MAOIs prolong and intensify the anticholinergic effects of antihistamines,[4] but there seems to be no clinical data to support this.

Mechanism

The reversal of the effects of the brofaromine were attributed by the authors of one report[1] to the blockage of 5-HT receptors (brofaromine has both MAO-A inhibitory and 5-HT uptake inhibitory properties). Cyproheptadine has been observed to block the activity of another 5-HT uptake inhibitor (see 'SSRIs + Cyproheptadine', p.982).

Importance and management

Information seems to be limited to these reports but it would now be prudent to be alert for any adverse responses if cyproheptadine is given with any MAOI.

1. Katz RJ, Rosenthal M. Adverse interaction of cyproheptadine with serotonergic antidepressants. *J Clin Psychiatry* (1994) 55, 314–15.
2. Zubieta JK, Demitrack MA. Depression after cyproheptadine: MAO treatment. *Biol Psychiatry* (1992) 31, 1177–8.
3. Kahn DA. Possible toxic interaction between cyproheptadine and phenelzine. *Am J Psychiatry* (1987) 144, 1242–3.
4. Periactin (Cyproheptadine hydrochloride). Merck Sharp & Dohme Ltd. UK Summary of product characteristics, January 2004.

MAOIs + Dexfenfluramine or Fenfluramine

The manufacturers advise against combined use of MAOIs and fenfluramine. They also contraindicate the use of dexfenfluramine with MAOIs.

Clinical evidence, mechanism, importance and management

The recommendation of the makers is that fenfluramine should not be used in patients with a history of depression, or during treatment with antidepressants (especially the MAOIs), and there should be an interval of 3 weeks between stopping the MAOIs and starting fenfluramine.[1] Acute confusional states have been described when fenfluramine was used with **phenelzine**.[2]

The makers similarly advise against the use of dexfenfluramine with or within 2 weeks of stopping an MAOI,[3] and advise waiting 3 weeks between stopping dexfenfluramine and starting an MAOI because of the potential risk of the serotonin syndrome.[4,5]

The makers of dexfenfluramine and fenfluramine have found no clinical evidence of serious problems with either of these drugs when taken with MAOIs,[6] so that the published warnings about possible interactions would appear to be based on theoretical considerations.

Note that dexfenfluramine and fenfluramine have generally been withdrawn because their use was found to be associated with a high incidence of abnormal echocardiograms indicating abnormal functioning of heart valves.

1. Ponderax Pacaps (Fenfluramine). Servier Laboratories Ltd. ABPI Compendium of Data Sheets and Summaries of Product Characteristics 1998–9, p. 1307.
2. Brandon S. Unusual effect of fenfluramine. *BMJ* (1969) 4, 557–8.
3. Adifax (Dexfenfluramine). Servier Laboratories. ABPI Compendium of Data Sheets and Summaries of Product Characteristics 1998–9, p. 1302.
4. Dolan JA, Amchin L, Albano D. Potential hazard of serotonin syndrome associated with dexfenfluramine hydrochloride (Redux): Reply. *JAMA* (1996) 276, 1220–1.
5. Schenck CH, Mahowald MW. Potential hazard of serotonin syndrome associated with dexfenfluramine hydrochloride (Redux). *JAMA* (1996) 276, 1220.
6. Servier Laboratories Ltd. Personal communication, July 1997.

MAOIs + Dextromethorphan

Two fatal cases of hyperpyrexia and coma have occurred in patients on phenelzine who took dextromethorphan (in overdosage in one case). Three other serious but non-fatal reactions occurred in patients on dextromethorphan and isocarboxazid or phenelzine.

Clinical evidence

A woman on **phenelzine** 15 mg four times daily complained of nausea and dizziness before collapsing, 30 minutes after drinking about 55 ml of a cough mixture containing dextromethorphan. She remained hyperpyrexic (42°C), hypotensive (systolic pressure below 70 mmHg) and unconscious for 4 hours, before dying after a cardiac arrest.[1]

A 15-year-old girl taking **phenelzine** 15 mg three times daily (as well as thioridazine, procyclidine and metronidazole) took 13 capsules of *Romilar CF* (dextromethorphan hydrobromide 15 mg, phenindamine tartrate 6.25 mg, phenylephrine hydrochloride 5 mg and paracetamol (acetaminophen) 120 mg in each capsule). She became comatose, hyperpyrexic (103°F), had a blood pressure of 100/60 mmHg, a pulse of 160 bpm and later died of a cardiac arrest.[2] This case is complicated by the overdosage and multiplicity of drugs present, particularly the phenylephrine. See 'MAOIs + Phenylephrine', p.870.

A 28-year-old woman developed severe myoclonus and rigidity, and became largely unresponsive after taking **phenelzine** and *Robitussin DM* (dextromethorphan hydrobromide 15 mg + guaifenesin 100 mg).[3] Yet another patient on **phenelzine** developed muscular rigidity, uncontrollable shaking, generalised hyperreflexia and sweating when given *Robitussin DM*. Within 2 hours he had responded to 10 mg of intravenous diazepam and oral activated charcoal.[4]

A woman taking **isocarboxazid** 30 mg daily took 1 mg of diazepam and 10 ml of *Robitussin DM*. Within 20 minutes she was nauseated and dizzy, and within 45 minutes she began to have fine bilateral leg tremor and muscle spasms of the abdomen and lower back. These were followed by bilateral and persistent myoclonic jerks of legs, occasional choreoathetoid movements and marked urinary retention. These adverse effects persisted for about 19 hours, gradually becoming less severe.[5]

Mechanism

Uncertain. The authors of three of the reports[3-5] suggest that these effects may have been due to an increase in serotonin activity in the CNS. A reaction (hyperpyrexia, dilated pupils, hyperexcitability and motor restlessness) has been seen in *rabbits* treated with dextromethorphan and nialamide, phenelzine or pargyline,[6] and there is some similarity to the MAOI/pethidine interaction. See 'MAOIs + Opioids', p.869.

Importance and management

Despite the very limited information available, the severity of the reactions indicates that patients on MAOIs should avoid taking preparations containing dextromethorphan. Several different treatments have been tried, including non-specific serotonin antagonists, benzodiazepines,[3,4] chlorpromazine, dantrolene and propranolol, but results are inconsistent,[7,8] so management of any interaction mainly consists of supportive therapy.

1. Rivers N, Horner B. Possible lethal reaction between Nardil and dextromethorphan. *Can Med Assoc J* (1970) 103, 85.
2. Shamsie JC, Barriga C. The hazards of use of monoamine oxidase inhibitors in disturbed adolescents. *Can Med Assoc J* (1971) 104, 715.
3. Nierenberg DW, Semprebon M. The central nervous system serotonin syndrome. *Clin Pharmacol Ther* (1993) 53, 84–8.
4. Sauter D, Macneil P, Weinstein E, Azar A. Phenelzine sulfate-dextromethorphan interaction: a case report. *Vet Hum Toxicol* (1991) 33, 365.
5. Sovner R, Wolfe J. Interaction between dextromethorphan and monoamine oxidase inhibitor therapy with isocarboxazid. *N Engl J Med* (1988) 319, 1671.

6. Sinclair JG. Dextromethorphan-monoamine oxidase inhibitor interaction in rabbits. *J Pharm Pharmacol* (1973) 25, 803–8.
7. Sporer KA. The serotonin syndrome: implicated drugs, pathophysiology and management. *Drug Safety* (1995) 13, 94–104.
8. Corkeron MA. Serotonin syndrome—a potentially fatal complication of antidepressant therapy. *Med J Aust* (1995) 163, 481–2.

MAOIs + Dextropropoxyphene (Propoxyphene)

An isolated report describes 'leg shakes', diaphoresis and severe hypotension in a woman on phenelzine when given dextropropoxyphene. Another isolated report describes a marked increase in sedation when a woman was given phenelzine and dextropropoxyphene. An adverse reaction may possibly occur with moclobemide and dextropropoxyphene.

Clinical evidence, mechanism, importance and management

(a) Phenelzine

A woman stabilised on phenelzine 15 mg three times daily, sodium valproate, lithium and trazodone, was given (dextro)propoxyphene 100 mg and paracetamol (acetaminophen) 650 mg for back pain and headache. Some 12 hours later she was admitted to hospital for leg shakes, discomfort and weakness. She was confused and anxious, and intensely diaphoretic. The next day she became severely hypotensive (systolic BP 55 to 60 mmHg) and needed large fluid volume resuscitation in intensive care. She later recovered fully.[1] Another woman taking propranolol, an oestrogen and phenelzine became very sedated and groggy causing her to have to lie down on two occasions, both within 2 hours of taking dextropropoxyphene 100 mg and paracetamol 650 mg. She had experienced no problems with either paracetamol or dextropropoxyphene/paracetamol before starting the phenelzine.[2] The mechanisms of these interactions are not understood but some of the symptoms in the first case were not unlike those seen in the serotonin syndrome.

Apart from these two isolated reports, there seems to be no other clinical evidence of adverse interactions between irreversible MAOIs and dextropropoxyphene, nevertheless it would seem prudent to monitor the outcome well if both drugs are given.

(b) Moclobemide

There is *animal* data suggesting that the effects of dextropropoxyphene are increased by moclobemide, and there is an ambiguous reference to a patient taking both drugs who may have developed moderate agitation.[3] For these reasons it may be prudent to monitor concurrent use well.

1. Zornberg GL, Hegarty JD. Adverse interaction between propoxyphene and phenelzine. *Am J Psychiatry* (1993) 150, 1270–1.
2. Garbutt JC. Potentiation of propoxyphene by phenelzine. *Am J Psychiatry* (1987) 144, 251–2.
3. Amrein R, Güntert TW, Dingemanse J, Lorscheid T, Stabl M, Schmid-Burgk W. Interactions of moclobemide with concomitantly administered medication: evidence from pharmacological and clinical studies. *Psychopharmacology (Berl)* (1992) 106, S24–S31.

MAOIs + Disulfiram

An isolated report describes delirium in a man on lithium and disulfiram when his treatment with moclobemide was replaced by tranylcypromine.

Clinical evidence, mechanism, importance and management

A man with disulfiram implants on long-term lithium treatment was changed from **moclobemide** (dosage not stated) to 10 mg **tranylcypromine** twice daily. Within 2 days he became acutely delirious (agitated, disoriented, incoherent, visual hallucinations) and later subcomatose, with nystagmus and a downward gaze. He was successfully treated with haloperidol and promethazine, and recovered within 24 hours.[1]

The authors of this report attribute the reaction to an interaction between **tranylcypromine** and disulfiram. However, there would seem to be other possible explanations for this reaction. MAOIs have rarely been seen to interact adversely with 'lithium' (see (p.867)), and there also seems potential for an interaction between the two 'MAOIs' (see (p.867)).

This seems to be the only report of an adverse reaction between disulfiram and an MAOI so it is possible that this is just an idiosyncratic reaction, but warnings about this drug combination, based on theoretical considerations and studies in *animals*, have been made previously, and **tranylcypromine** was considered to be the MAOI that presented the greatest risk.[2] MAOIs and disulfiram are generally regarded as unsafe, but just why is not clear (apart from the general and wide-spread nervousness about giving any drug with an MAOI). It seems that this particular patient had no problems while taking **moclobemide**, which is a selective MAOI.

1. Blansjaar BA, Egberts TCG. Delirium in a patient treated with disulfiram and tranylcypromine. *Am J Psychiatry* (1995) 152, 296.
2. Ciraulo DA. Can disulfiram (Antabuse) be safely co-administered with the monoamine oxidase (MAOI) antidepressants? *J Clin Psychopharmacol* (1989) 9, 315–16.

MAOIs + Erythromycin

An isolated case report describes severe hypotension and fainting in a woman on phenelzine, which occurred shortly after she started a course of erythromycin.

Clinical evidence, mechanism, importance and management

A woman taking **phenelzine** 15 mg daily experienced three syncopal episodes four days after starting to take erythromycin 250 mg four times daily for pneumonia. When admitted to hospital her supine systolic blood pressure was only 70 mmHg. When she sat up, it was unrecordable. Although she was not dehydrated, she was given 4 litres of 0.9% sodium chloride, but without any effect on her blood pressure. Within 24 hours of stopping the **phenelzine** her blood pressure had returned to normal.[1] The reasons for this severe hypotensive reaction are not known, but it is suggested that the erythromycin may have caused rapid gastric emptying, which resulted in a very rapid absorption of the **phenelzine** (described by the author as rapid dumping into the blood stream), which resulted in the adverse effect of hypotension.[1] This seems to be the first and only report of this interaction, so that its general importance is uncertain.

1. Bernstein AE. Drug interaction. *Hosp Community Psychiatry* (1990) 41, 806–7.

MAOIs + Ginseng

Two isolated reports describe two patients on phenelzine who developed adverse effects (including headache and insomnia) after taking ginseng.

Clinical evidence, mechanism, importance and management

A 64-year-old woman treated with **phenelzine** developed headache, insomnia, and tremulousness on two occasions when ginseng was added.[1] Another depressed woman taking ginseng and bee pollen experienced a relief of her depression and became active and extremely optimistic when she was started on **phenelzine** 45 mg daily, but this was accompanied by insomnia, irritability, headaches and vague visual hallucinations. When the **phenelzine** was stopped and then re-started in the absence of the ginseng and bee pollen, her depression was not relieved.[2] It seems unlikely that the bee pollen had any part to play in these reactions and suspicion therefore falls on the ginseng. It would seem that the psychoactive effects of the ginsenosides from the ginseng and the MAOI were somehow additive. Ginseng has stimulant effects, but its adverse effects include insomnia, nervousness, hypertension and euphoria. These two cases once again illustrate that herbal medicines are not necessarily problem-free if combined with orthodox drugs.

1. Shader RI, Greenblatt DJ. Phenelzine and the dream machine—ramblings and reflections. *J Clin Psychopharmacol* (1985) 5, 65.
2. Jones BD, Runikis AM. Interaction of ginseng with phenelzine. *J Clin Psychopharmacol* (1987) 7, 201–2.

MAOIs + Linezolid

The makers contraindicate the use of linezolid with the MAOIs, including the selective MAOIs selegiline and moclobemide.

Clinical evidence, mechanism, importance and management

The UK makers contraindicate the concurrent use of linezolid and any other drug that inhibits either monoamine oxidase A or monoamine oxidase B, or within 2 weeks of taking either drug,[1] because their MAO-inhibitory activities are predicted to be additive. **Isocarboxazid**, **moclobemide**, **phenelzine** and **selegiline** are named, although if any adverse interaction were to occur it would also be likely to occur with all the MAOIs. It is not entirely clear what the outcome of any additional MAO-inhibition might be.

1. Zyvox (Linezolid). Pharmacia Ltd. UK Summary of product characteristics, November 2004.

MAOIs + Lithium

The concurrent use of phenelzine or tranylcypromine and lithium normally appears to be safe and effective. However, two cases of tardive dyskinesia have been described following the long-term use of the combination.

Clinical evidence, mechanism, importance and management

Four severely depressed patients who had failed to respond to tricyclic antidepressants or MAOIs, did so when lithium was added to their MAOI treatment. Each of them was given **phenelzine** 30 to 60 mg daily and lithium carbonate 600 to 900 mg daily. No adverse reactions were reported.[1] Eleven out of 12 patients responded better to lithium with **tranylcypromine** than to lithium with other antidepressants,[2] and a previous study had confirmed the effectiveness of concurrent treatment, apparently without toxicity.[3]

However, one report describes 2 patients with bipolar affective disorder who developed a buccolingual-masticatory syndrome after taking **tranylcypromine** 30 to 40 mg daily and lithium carbonate 900 to 1200 mg daily for 1.5 to 3 years. This reaction was attributed to dopamine receptor hypersensitivity.[4] There appear to be no other reports suggesting that the combination of MAOIs and lithium is normally unsafe.

1. Fein S, Paz V, Rao N, LaGrassa J. The combination of lithium carbonate and an MAOI in refractory depressions. *Am J Psychiatry* (1988) 145, 249–50.
2. Price LH, Charney DS, Heninger GR. Efficacy of lithium-tranylcypromine treatment in refractory depression. *Am J Psychiatry* (1985) 142, 619–23.
3. Himmelhoch JM, Detre T, Kupfer DJ, Swartzburg M, Byck R. Treatment of previously intractable depressions with tranylcypromine and lithium. *J Nerv Ment Dis* (1972) 155, 216–20.
4. Stancer HC. Tardive dyskinesia not associated with neuroleptics. *Am J Psychiatry* (1979) 136, 727.

MAOIs + MAOIs

Two patients suffered strokes (one fatal) and another experienced a hypertensive reaction when phenelzine or isocarboxazid were replaced by tranylcypromine. Moclobemide and selegiline can safely be given together or sequentially but some dietary restrictions are necessary (no tyramine-rich foods and drinks). However, because of the potential risks the makers of moclobemide contraindicate this combination. Marked orthostatic hypotension has been seen in two patients on iproniazid or tranylcypromine/trifluoperazine when given selegiline.

Clinical evidence, mechanism, importance and management

(a) Irreversible, non-selective MAOIs

A patient on **isocarboxazid** 30 mg daily was switched to **tranylcypromine** 10 mg followed by 10 mg three times daily starting the following day. Later she complained of feeling 'funny', had difficulty in talking, developed a headache, was restless, flushed, sweating, had an elevated temperature of 39.5°C, and a pulse rate of 130 bpm. She died the following day.[1] Another patient, switched from **phenelzine** 75 mg daily (by tapering the dose by 15 mg daily until discontinued) to **tranylcypromine** (starting at 10 mg daily, increasing by 10 mg daily, until a dose of 20 mg twice daily was reached) suffered a subcortical cerebral haemorrhage on the fourth day following the morning 20-mg dose of **tranylcypromine**, which resulted in total right-sided hemiplegia.[2,3] Another patient taking **phenelzine** 45 mg daily, followed by a two-day drug free period and then **tranylcypromine** 20 mg with a further 30-mg dose the next day, experienced a rise in blood pressure to 240/130 mmHg.[2]

The reasons for these reactions are not understood, but one idea is that the amfetamine-like properties of **tranylcypromine** may have had some part to play. Certainly there are cases of spontaneous rises in blood pressure and intracranial bleeding in patients given **tranylcypromine**.[4] Not all patients experience adverse reactions when switched from one MAOI to another,[5] but until more is known it would seem prudent to have a drug-free wash-out interval when doing so, and to start dosing in a conservative and step-wise manner.

(b) Reversible, selective MAOIs (RIMAs)

A study in 24 healthy subjects, designed to assess the safety and tolerability of giving **moclobemide** 100 to 400 mg and **selegiline** 5 mg twice daily, sequentially or combined, found that the adverse effects were no greater under steady-state conditions than with either drug alone, but the sensitivity to tyramine was considerably increased. The mean tyramine sensitivity factors for **moclobemide** alone, **selegiline** alone, and **moclobemide** plus **selegiline** were 2 to 3, 1.4, and 8 to 9 respectively. One subject showed a value of 18 when given both drugs.[6,7] The reason is, that when taken together, the **moclobemide** inhibits MAO-A while **selegiline** inhibits MAO-B, so that little or no MAO activity remains available to metabolise the tyramine.

In practical terms this means that patients taking **moclobemide** with **selegiline** should be given the same dietary restrictions about tyramine-rich foods and drinks (see 'tyramine-rich drinks', (p.875) and 'tyramine-rich foods', (p.876)), which relate to the non-selective MAOIs such as phenelzine and tranylcypromine, although the risks are less.[8] However, because of the potential risks the makers of **moclobemide** contraindicate this combination.[9] On the basis of work done on the *pig* (said to be similar to man in relation to the MAO isoenzymes in the brain[10]) it is suggested that if **selegiline** is replaced by **moclobemide**, the dietary restrictions can be relaxed after a wash-out period of about 2 weeks. If switching from **moclobemide** to **selegiline**, a wash-out period of 1 to 2 days is sufficient.[6]

(c) Reversible MAOIs + Irreversible MAOIs

A patient taking **iproniazid** 150 mg daily developed severe orthostatic hypotension on two occasions within an hour of taking **selegiline** 5 mg. Another patient similarly developed postural hypotension on two occasions within 2 hours of taking **selegiline** 5 mg. He had stopped taking ***Parstelin*** (**tranylcypromine** + trifluoperazine), two tablets daily, four weeks previously.[11] The reasons are not understood. This evidence suggests that **selegiline** should be given with caution to patients taking, or who have recently stopped, irreversible MAOIs.

1. Bazire SR. Sudden death associated with switching monoamine oxidase inhibitors. *Drug Intell Clin Pharm* (1986) 20, 954–6.
2. Gelenberg AJ. Switching MAOI. *Biol Ther Psychiatry* (1984) 7, 33 and 36.
3. Gelenberg AJ. Switching MAOI. The sequel. *Biol Ther Psychiatry* (1985) 8, 41.
4. Cooper AJ, Magnus RV, Rose MJ. A hypertensive syndrome with tranylcypromine medication. *Lancet* (1964) 1, 527–9.
5. True BL, Alexander B, Carter BL. Comment: switching MAO inhibitors. *Drug Intell Clin Pharm* (1986) 20, 384.
6. Dingemanse J. An update of recent moclobemide interaction data. *Int Clin Psychopharmacol* (1993) 7, 167–80.
7. Korn A, Wagner B, Moritz E, Dingemanse J. Tyramine pressor sensitivity in healthy subjects during combined treatment with moclobemide and selegiline. *Eur J Clin Pharmacol* (1996) 49, 273–8.
8. Bieck PR, Antonin KH. Tyramine potentiation during treatment with MAO inhibitors: brofaromine and moclobemide vs irreversible inhibitors. *J Neural Transm* (1989) 28 (Suppl), 21–31.
9. Manerix (Moclobemide) Roche Products Ltd. UK Summary of product characteristics, May 2004.
10. Oreland L, Jossan SS, Hartvig P, Aquilonius SM, Långström B. Turnover of monoamine oxidase B (MAO-B) in pig brain by positron emission tomography using ^{11}C-L-deprenyl. *J Neural Transm* (1990) 32 (Suppl), 55–9.
11. Pare CMB, Al Mousawi M, Sandler M, Glover V. Attempts to attenuate the 'cheese effect'. Combined drug therapy in depressive illness. *J Affect Disord* (1985) 9, 137–41.

MAOIs + Mazindol

An isolated report describes a patient on phenelzine who had a marked rise in blood pressure when given a single dose of mazindol.

Clinical evidence, mechanism, importance and management

A woman on **phenelzine** 30 mg three times a day showed a blood pressure rise from 110/60 to 200/100 mmHg within 2 hours of receiving a 10-mg test dose of mazindol. The blood pressure remained elevated for another hour, but had fallen again after another 3 hours. The patient experienced no subjective symptoms.[1] It is uncertain whether this hypertensive reaction was the result of an interaction, or simply a direct response to the mazindol alone (the dose was large compared with the manufacturers recommended dosage of 2 mg daily). The general importance is uncertain.

The manufacturers advise avoiding the combination, and that MAOIs should not be used until one month after mazindol has been stopped.[2]

1. Oliver RM. Interaction between phenelzine and mazindol: Personal communication, 1981.
2. Teronac (Mazindol). Sandoz Pharmaceuticals. ABPI Compendium of Data Sheets and Summaries of Product Characteristics 1991–2, p. 1340–1.

MAOIs + Methyldopa

The concurrent use of pargyline and methyldopa appears to be safe, although an isolated report describes the delayed development of hallucinations. The order of administration may be important. The concurrent use of antidepressant MAOIs and methyldopa may not be desirable because methyldopa can sometimes cause depression.

Clinical evidence, mechanism, importance and management

A hypertensive woman on **pargyline** 25 mg four times a day developed hallucinations about a month after starting to take methyldopa 250 mg daily, later increased to 250 mg twice daily.[1] However, a number of other reports describe no unusual reactions or toxic effects during concurrent use,[2-4] although the hypotensive response can be enhanced.[1]

The use of both drugs would therefore normally seem to be safe, but it has been suggested that the methyldopa should not be given after **pargyline** to avoid the possibility of the sudden release of the MAOI-accumulated stores of catecholamines by methyldopa.[5] There seems to be nothing documented about the use of antidepressant MAOIs with methyldopa, but the potential depressant adverse effects of methyldopa may make it an unsuitable drug for patients with depression.

1. Paykel ES. Hallucinosis on combined methyldopa and pargyline. *BMJ* (1966) 1, 803.
2. Herting RL. Monoamine oxidase inhibitors. *Lancet* (1963) i, 1324.
3. Kinross-Wright J, Charalampous KD. Concurrent administration of dopa decarboxylase and monoamine oxidase inhibitors in man. *Clin Res* (1963) 11, 177.
4. Gillespie L, Oates JA, Crout JR, Sjoerdsma A. Clinical and chemical studies with α-methyldopa in patients with hypertension. *Circulation* (1962) 25, 281–91.
5. Natajaran S. Potential danger of monoamine oxidase inhibitors and α-methyldopa. *Lancet* (1964) i, 1330.

MAOIs + Miscellaneous

No adverse interactions between the MAOIs and either anticholinergics or doxapram have been reported, although the possibility has been suggested. Bradycardia has been reported in two patients on nadolol or metoprolol and phenelzine. An isolated report suggests that the CNS stimulant effects of caffeine may possibly be increased by MAOIs.

Clinical evidence, mechanism, importance and management

Drug manufacturers often include warnings in their data sheets and package inserts about alleged interactions with the MAOIs, despite the absence of direct evidence in man that an interaction can actually take place (see Blackwell's comment at the end of the 'introduction to this section', see (p.862)). It is usually suggested that 2 weeks should elapse between stopping the MAOI and starting the other drug. This prudent precaution protects both the health of patients and the legal liability of manufacturers, but it also means that patients may sometimes be denied the use of a drug that may be perfectly safe. If you speak to the makers many will freely admit that this is the case.

(a) Anticholinergics

Although some books and lists of drug interactions state that the effects of the anticholinergic drugs (by implication those which are adverse) used in the treatment of Parkinson's disease are increased by the MAOIs, there appears to be no documented evidence of this in man, although a hyperthermic reaction has been reported in *animals*.[1] See also 'MAOIs + Antihistamines', p.863.

(b) Beta-blockers

It has been claimed[2] that MAOIs should be discontinued at least 2 weeks before starting **propranolol** therapy, but studies in *animals*[3] using **mebanazine** as a representative MAOI failed to show any undesirable property of **propranolol** following MAO inhibition. Bradycardia of 46 to 53 bpm has been described in two patients taking **nadolol** 40 mg or **metoprolol** 150 mg daily for hypertension within 8 to 11 days of starting **phenelzine** 60 mg daily. No noticeable ill effects were seen, but the authors recommend careful monitoring, particularly in the elderly, who may tolerate bradycardia poorly.[4] Until the situation is quite clear it would be prudent to monitor the concurrent use of any MAOI and beta-blocker.

(c) Caffeine

It has been claimed that a patient who normally drank 10 or 12 cups of **coffee** daily, without adverse effects, experienced extreme jitteriness during treatment with an MAOI, which subsided when the **coffee** consumption was reduced to 2 or 3 cups a day. The same reaction was also said to have occurred in other patients on MAOI who drank **tea** or some of the **'Cola' drinks**, which contain caffeine.[5] Another patient on an MAOI claimed that a single cup of **coffee** taken in the morning kept him jittery all day and up the entire night as well, a reaction that occurred on three separate occasions.[5] Apart from this report, and another[6] stating that the effects of caffeine in *rats* are enhanced by MAOIs, the literature appears to be otherwise silent about this alleged interaction. Whether this reflects its mildness and unimportance, or its rarity, is not clear.

(d) Doxapram

Based on *animal* studies, which reportedly show that the actions of doxapram are potentiated by pretreatment with MAOIs, the makers[7,8] advise that concurrent use should be undertaken with great care. It is also stated that the pressor effects of MAOIs and doxapram may be additive[8] but no clinical data in support of these statements are cited.

1. Pedersen V, Nielsen IM. Hyperthermia in rabbits caused by interaction between M.A.O.I.s, antiparkinson drugs, and neuroleptics. *Lancet* (1975) i, 409–10.
2. Frieden J. Propranolol as an antiarrhythmic agent. *Am Heart J* (1967) 74, 283–5.
3. Barrett AM, Cullum VA. Lack of inter-action between propranolol and mebanazine. *J Pharm Pharmacol* (1968) 20, 911–15.
4. Reggev A, Vollhardt BR. Bradycardia induced by an interaction between phenelzine and beta blockers. *Psychosomatics* (1989) 30, 106–8.
5. Kline NS. Psychopharmaceuticals: effects and side-effects. *Bull WHO* (1959) 21, 397–410.
6. Berkowitz BA, Spector S, Pool W. The interaction of caffeine, theophylline and theobromine with monoamine oxidase inhibitors. *Eur J Pharmacol* (1971) 16, 315–21.
7. Dopram infusion (Doxapram). Wyeth Laboratories. ABPI Compendium of Data Sheets and Summaries of Product Characteristics 1995–6, p. 1991–2.
8. Dopram (Doxapram hydrochloride). Baxter Healthcare Corporation. US Prescribing information, March 2004.

MAOIs + Monosodium glutamate

Hypertension in patients on MAOIs who have eaten certain foods (soy sauce, chicken nuggets) has been attributed in anecdotal reports to an interaction with monosodium glutamate. However a controlled study found no evidence to support this idea.

Clinical evidence

Five healthy subjects were given monosodium glutamate 400 to 1600 mg or a placebo with or without **tranylcypromine** for at least 2 weeks. Episodes of hypertension were seen in 2 subjects on **tranylcypromine** alone, but no changes in blood pressure or heart rate occurred that could be attributed to an interaction while taking monosodium glutamate as well. The largest dose of monosodium glutamate used was about twice the amount usually found in meals containing large amounts of monosodium glutamate.[1]

There are anecdotal reports of hypertensive reactions in patients on MAOIs that are attributed to interactions with the monosodium glutamate contained in **soy sauce** and **chicken nuggets**.[2,3]

Mechanism

Monosodium glutamate alone can cause a small rise in blood pressure, and MAOIs alone very occasionally cause hypertensive episodes. The reactions reported with soy sauce and chicken nuggets may possibly have been due to their high tyramine content (see 'MAOIs + Tyramine-rich foods', p.876).

Importance and management

The authors of the report cited suggest that any reaction is likely to be an idiosyncratic reaction and not due to an identifiable interaction between the MAOI and monosodium glutamate.[1] No interaction is established. It should be pointed out that the number of subjects studied was very small.

1. Balon R, Pohl R, Yeragani VK, Berchou R, Gershon S. Monosodium glutamate and tranylcypromine administration in healthy subjects. *J Clin Psychiatry* (1990) 51, 303–6.

2. Pohl R, Balon R, Berchou R. Reaction to chicken nuggets in a patient taking an MAOI. *Am J Psychiatry* (1988) 145, 651.
3. McCabe B, Tsuang MT. Dietary consideration in MAO inhibitor regimens. *J Clin Psychiatry* (1982) 43, 178–81.

MAOIs + Opioids

The concurrent use of pethidine (meperidine) and MAOIs has resulted in a serious and potentially life-threatening reaction in a few patients. Excitement, muscle rigidity, hyperpyrexia, flushing, sweating and unconsciousness occur very rapidly. Respiratory depression and hypotension are also seen. Pethidine should not be given to patients on any MAOI (selective or non-selective) or linezolid.

Limited evidence suggests that fentanyl, methadone and remifentanil do not interact with MAOIs. Morphine seems to be free from the serious interactions that occur with pethidine and MAOIs, however, hypotension (profound in one case) has been seen in two patients given morphine and an MAOI.

Clinical evidence

(a) Fentanyl

A 71-year-old woman taking ***Parstelin*** (**tranylcypromine** + trifluoperazine) was given an intravenous test dose of fentanyl 20 micrograms, and diazepam before surgery without problems. She was then given another 20-microgram intravenous dose of fentanyl during the surgery, followed by an epidural bolus infusion of fentanyl 50 micrograms 15 minutes before the end of the surgery. After surgery she was given a continuous epidural infusion of fentanyl 50 to 70 micrograms/hour for 4 days to control postoperative pain, also without problems.[1]

(b) Methadone

A patient on **methadone** maintenance therapy (30 mg daily) was successfully and uneventfully treated for depression with **tranylcypromine**, initially 10 mg gradually increased to 30 mg daily.[2]

(c) Morphine

A study in 15 patients who had been taking either **phenelzine, isocarboxazid, iproniazid** or ***Parstelin*** (**tranylcypromine** + trifluoperazine) for 3 to 8 weeks, showed no changes in blood pressure, pulse rate or state of awareness when given test doses of up to 4 mg of **morphine**.[3] Another patient on **phenelzine** is reported to have developed no problems when treated with **morphine**.[4] Other patients on MAOIs who reacted adversely to **pethidine (meperidine)**, did not do so when given **morphine**.[5,6] Two other studies reported no adverse interaction in patients on **MAOIs** given **morphine**.[7,8]

However, a patient taking **tranylcypromine** 40 mg and trifluoperazine 20 mg daily and undergoing a preoperative test with **morphine**, developed pin point pupils, became unconscious and unresponsive to stimuli, and showed a systolic blood pressure fall from 160 to 40 mmHg after receiving a total of 6 mg of **morphine** intravenously. Within 2 minutes of being given naloxone 4 mg intravenously, the patient was awake and rational with a systolic blood pressure fully restored.[9] A moderate fall in blood pressure (from 140/90 to 90/60 mmHg) was seen in another patient on a MAOI given **morphine**.[10]

(d) Pethidine

Severe, rapid and potentially fatal toxic reactions, both excitatory and depressant can occur:

A woman on **iproniazid** 50 mg twice daily stopped taking this medication, but became restless and incoherent almost immediately after being given **pethidine** 100 mg about a day and a half later for chest pain. She was comatose within 20 minutes. An hour after receiving the injection she was flushed, sweating and showed Cheyne-Stokes respiration. Her pupils were dilated and unreactive. Deep reflexes could not be initiated and plantar reflexes were extensor. Her pulse rate was 82 and blood pressure 156/110 mmHg. She was rousable within 10 minutes of receiving a 25 mg intravenous injection of prednisolone hemisuccinate.[5]

A woman who, unknown to her doctor, was taking **tranylcypromine**, was given **pethidine** 100 mg. Within minutes she became unconscious, noisy and restless, having to be held down by three people. Her breathing was stertorous and the pulse impalpable. Generalised tonic spasm developed, with ankle clonus, extensor plantar reflexes, shallow respiration and cyanosis. On admission to hospital she had a pulse rate of 160, a blood pressure of 90/60 mmHg and was sweating profusely (temperature 38.3°C). Her condition gradually improved and 4 hours after admission she was conscious but drowsy. Recovery was complete the next day.[11]

This interaction has been seen in other patients treated with **iproniazid**,[5,12-14] **pargyline**,[10,15] **phenelzine**,[6,16-20] and **mebanazine**.[21] Fatalities have occurred. It has also been seen with **selegiline**, a selective inhibitor of type B monoamine oxidase (MAO-B).[22] One report suggests that on the basis of *animal* studies the combination of **moclobemide** and **pethidine** should be avoided or used with caution.[23] A report of suspected serotonin syndrome in a 73-year-old woman, given **pethidine** in addition to her usual treatment with **moclobemide** 750 mg daily, nortriptyline 100 mg daily and lithium 750 mg daily, adds weight to this suggestion.[24]

(e) Remifentanil

A study has reported that remifentanil was used without adverse effect in the maintenance of anaesthesia in a patient taking **phenelzine**. An adverse interaction was considered unlikely with this combination.[4]

Mechanism

Not understood, despite the extensive studies undertaken.[25-27] There is some evidence that the reactions may be due to an increase in levels of 5-HT within the brain, causing the serotonin syndrome.

Importance and management

The interaction between pethidine (meperidine) and MAOIs is well-documented, serious and potentially fatal interaction, which was first observed in the mid-1950s. Its incidence is unknown, but it is probably quite low. For example, in one study 15 patients given various MAOIs and pethidine did not show the interaction,[3] and no problems were seen in another study involving 45 patients on isocarboxazid and pethidine.[8] Bear in mind that most of the older MAOI are irreversible so that an interaction is possible for many days after their withdrawal, whereas the newer selective MAOIs (e.g. moclobemide) are reversible and unlikely still to interact 48 hours after they have been stopped. Nevertheless it would be imprudent to give pethidine to any patients on an MAOI and for at least 2 weeks after it has been stopped. The makers of linezolid (a weak, reversible MAOI) contraindicate its use with pethidine because of the possibility of this reaction.[28]

The serious MAOI/pethidine interaction also casts a shadow over morphine, which probably accounts for its inclusion on a number of lists and charts of drugs said to interact with the MAOIs, despite some evidence that patients on MAOIs who had reacted adversely with pethidine did not do so when given morphine.[5,6] The hypotensive reactions cited here[9,10] are of a different character and appear to be rare. There would therefore seem to be no good reason for avoiding morphine in patients on MAOIs, but be alert for the rare adverse response. The extremely limited evidence available suggests that methadone can be given to patients on MAOIs, but a stepwise dosing would seem to be a prudent precaution. Epidural fentanyl is also suggested to be safe in patients who receive MAOIs.[1]

Sensitivity test

A sensitivity test has been suggested, but given the fact that there are many alternatives to pethidine and MAOIs readily available, and given that an interaction has been reported[29] even with the first step of the test dose (5 mg of pethidine) it would seem prudent to avoid the combination.

1. Youssef MS, Wilkinson PA. Epidural fentanyl and monoamine oxidase inhibitors. *Anaesthesia* (1988) 43, 210–12.
2. Mendelson G. Narcotics and monoamine oxidase-inhibitors. *Med J Aust* (1979) 1, 400.
3. Evans-Prosser CDG. The use of pethidine and morphine in the presence of monoamine oxidase inhibitors. *Br J Anaesth* (1968) 40, 279–82.
4. Ure DS, Gillies MA, James KS. Safe use of remifentanil in a patient treated with the monoamine oxidase inhibitor phenelzine. *Br J Anaesth* (2000) 84, 414–16.
5. Shee JC. Dangerous potentiation of pethidine by iproniazid, and its treatment. *BMJ* (1960) 2, 507–9.
6. Palmer H. Potentiation of pethidine. *BMJ* (1960) 2, 944.
7. El-Ganzouri A, Ivankovich AD, Braverman B, Land PC. Should MAOI be discontinued preoperatively? *Anesthesiology* (1983) 59, A384.
8. Ebrahim ZY, O'Hara J, Borden L, Tetzlaff J. Monoamine oxidase inhibitors and elective surgery. *Cleve Clin J Med* (1993) 60, 129–130.
9. Barry BJ. Adverse effects of MAO inhibitors with narcotics reversed with naloxone. *Anaesth Intensive Care* (1979) 7, 194.
10. Jenkins LC, Graves HB. Potential hazards of psychoactive drugs in association with anaesthesia. *Can Anaesth Soc J* (1965) 12, 121–8.
11. Denton PH, Borrelli VM, Edwards NV. Dangers of monoamine oxidase inhibitors. *BMJ* (1962) 2, 1752–3.
12. Clement AJ, Benazon D. Reactions to other drugs in patients taking monoamine-oxidase inhibitors. *Lancet* (1962) ii, 197–8.
13. Papp C, Benaim S. Toxic effects of iproniazid in a patient with angina. *BMJ* (1958) 2, 1070–2.

14. Mitchell RS. Fatal toxic encephalitis occurring during iproniazid therapy in pulmonary tuberculosis. *Ann Intern Med* (1955) 42, 417–24.
15. Vigran IM. Dangerous potentiation of meperidine hydrochloride by pargyline hydrochloride. *JAMA* (1964) 187, 953–4.
16. Taylor DC. Alarming reaction to pethidine in patients on phenelzine. *Lancet* (1962) ii, 401–2.
17. Cocks DP, Passmore-Rowe A. Dangers of monoamine oxidase inhibitors. *BMJ* (1962) 2, 1545–6.
18. Reid NCRW, Jones D. Pethidine and phenelzine. *BMJ* (1962) 1, 408.
19. Meyer D, Halfin V. Toxicity secondary to meperidine in patients on monoamine oxidase inhibitors: a case report and critical review. *J Clin Psychopharmacol* (1981) 1, 319–21.
20. Asch DA, Parker RM. Sounding board. The Libby Zion case. One step forward or two steps backward? *N Engl J Med* (1988) 318, 771–5.
21. Anon. Death from drugs combination. *Pharm J* (1965) 195, 341.
22. Zornberg GL, Bodkin JA, Cohen BM. Severe adverse interaction between pethidine and selegiline. *Lancet* (1991) 337, 246.
23. Amrein R, Güntert TW, Dingemanse J, Lorscheid T, Stabl M, Schmid-Burgk W. Interactions of moclobemide with concomitantly administered medication: evidence from pharmacological and clinical studies. *Psychopharmacology (Berl)* (1992) 106, S24–S31.
24. Gillman PK. Possible serotonin syndrome with moclobemide and pethidine. *Med J Aust* (1995) 162, 554.
25. Leander JD, Batten J, Hargis GW. Pethidine interaction with clorgyline, pargyline or 5-hydroxytryptophan: lack of enhanced pethidine lethality or hyperpyrexia in mice. *J Pharm Pharmacol* (1978) 30, 396–8.
26. Rogers KJ, Thornton JA. The interaction between monoamine oxidase inhibitors and narcotic analgesics in mice. *Br J Pharmacol* (1969) 36, 470–80.
27. Gessner PK, Soble AG. A study of the tranylcypromine-meperidine interaction: effects of *p*-chlorophenylalanine and *l*-5-hydroxytryptophan. *J Pharmacol Exp Ther* (1973) 186, 276–87.
28. Zyvox (Linezolid). Pharmacia Ltd. UK Summary of product characteristics, November 2004.
29. Churchill-Davidson HC. Anaesthesia and monoamine oxidase inhibitors. *BMJ* (1965) 1, 520.

MAOIs + Phenothiazines

The concurrent use of the MAOIs and phenothiazines is usually safe and effective. The exception appears to be levomepromazine (methotrimeprazine), which has been implicated in two fatal reactions, one with pargyline and another with tranylcypromine.

Clinical evidence, mechanism, importance and management

MAOIs and phenothiazines have been safe and effective when used together,[1-4] and a preparation containing both **tranylcypromine** and **trifluoperazine** is still marketed in some countries. **Promazine** has been used safely and effectively in the treatment of overdosage with *Parstelin* (**tranylcypromine** with **trifluoperazine**).[5] A single report[6] describes a woman on an MAOI who developed a severe occipital headache after taking 30 ml of a paediatric cough linctus. Initially this interaction was attributed to promethazine, but it is now known that the linctus in question contained **phenylpropanolamine**, which is much more likely to have been the cause.[7] See 'MAOIs + Sympathomimetics; Indirectly-acting', p.872 for the interaction with phenylpropanolamine.

However, unexplained fatalities have been reported with **levomepromazine** and **pargyline**,[8] **levomepromazine** and tranylcypromine,[9] and an unnamed MAOI/phenothiazine combination.[9]

No special precautions would normally seem to be necessary during the concurrent use of most MAOIs and phenothiazines, with the exception of **levomepromazine**, which, because it has been implicated in two fatalities, is probably best avoided.

1. Winkelman NW. Three evaluations of a monoamine oxidase inhibitor and phenothiazine combination (a methodological and clinical study). *Dis Nerv Syst* (1965) 26, 160–4.
2. Chesrow EJ, Kaplitz SE. Anxiety and depression in the geriatric and chronically ill patient. *Clin Med* (1965) 72, 1281–4.
3. Janecek J, Schiele BC, Bellville T, Anderson R. The effects of withdrawal of trifluoperazine on patients maintained on the combination of tranylcypromine and trifluoperazine. A double blind study. *Curr Ther Res* (1963) 5, 608–15.
4. Bucci L. The negative symptoms of schizophrenia and the monoamine oxidase inhibitors. *Psychopharmacology (Berl)* (1987) 91, 104–8.
5. Midwinter RE. Accidental overdose with '*Parstelin*'. *BMJ* (1962) 2, 1755–6.
6. Mitchell L. Psychotropic drugs. *BMJ* (1968) 1, 381.
7. Griffin JP, D'Arcy PF, eds. A Manual of Adverse Drug Interactions 2nd Edn Bristol: Wright; 1979 p. 174.
8. Barsa JA, Saunders JC. A comparative study of tranylcypromine and pargyline. *Psychopharmacologia* (1964) 6, 295–8.
9. McQueen EG. New Zealand Committee on Adverse Drug Reactions: fourteenth annual report 1979. *N Z Med J* (1980) 91, 226–9.

MAOIs + Phenylephrine

The concurrent use of oral phenylephrine and the older MAOIs can result in a potentially life-threatening hypertensive crisis. Phenylephrine is commonly found in proprietary cough, cold and influenza preparations. The effects of parenteral phenylephrine may be approximately doubled by MAOIs. Some interactions occur between phenylephrine and moclobemide or brofaromine, but the blood pressure response is much smaller than that seen with the older MAOIs.

Clinical evidence

(a) MAOIs

A study in four healthy subjects, given **phenelzine** 45 mg or **tranylcypromine** 30 mg daily for 7 days, found that the blood pressure rise following oral phenylephrine was grossly enhanced. In three experiments with 45 mg of phenylephrine given orally, the rise in blood pressure became potentially disastrous and had to be stopped with phentolamine. The enhancement was about 13-fold in the only experiment that was not stopped, and 6- to 35-fold in the two that were. The rise in blood pressure was accompanied by a severe headache. An approximately twofold increase was seen following parenteral administration.[1]

Another study describes a 2- to 2.5-fold increase in the effects of intravenous phenylephrine following treatment with phenelzine or tranylcypromine,[2] and an exaggerated pressor response is described in a case report.[3]

(b) Reversible inhibitors of MAO-A

No clinically important interaction occurred in healthy subjects taking **brofaromine** 75 mg twice daily when given a single 2.5-mg dose of phenylephrine (*Neo-Synephrine*) as nasal drops.[4] However, higher doses (exact amount not stated) did produce a blood pressure response,[4] with a maximum recorded diastolic blood pressure of 100 mmHg. Two studies in healthy subjects found that 100 or 200 mg of **moclobemide** three times daily for up to three weeks increased the blood pressure response to infusions of phenylephrine by up to 1.8-fold.[5,6]

Mechanism

If given by mouth phenylephrine is used in large doses because a very large proportion is destroyed by MAO in the gut and liver, and only a small amount gets into the general circulation. If MAO is inhibited, most of the oral dose escapes destruction and passes freely into circulation, hence the gross enhancement of the pressor effects. Phenylephrine has mainly direct sympathomimetic activity, but it may also have some minor indirect activity as well, which would be expected to result in the release of some of the MAOI-accumulated noradrenaline at adrenergic nerve endings. This might account for the increased response to phenylephrine given parenterally.

Importance and management

The interaction between the older (irreversible) MAOIs and oral phenylephrine is established, serious and potentially life-threatening. Phenylephrine commonly occurs in oral OTC cough, cold and influenza preparations, so patients should be strongly warned about them. Whether the effects of nasal drops and sprays are also enhanced is uncertain, but it would be prudent to avoid them until they have been shown to be safe. The response to parenteral administration is also approximately doubled, so that a dosage reduction is necessary. The few studies that are available suggest that any interaction with reversible inhibitors of MAO-A is less severe than that with MAOIs, but this needs confirmation.

Treatment

These hypertensive reactions have been controlled by intravenous phentolamine, chlorpromazine, or nifedipine. However, it is advisable to refer to current guidelines (or at least a relevant current text book) on the management of hypertensive crises for up to date advice.

In the US, the makers advise intravenous phentolamine 5 mg, given slowly to avoid excessive hypotension. Fever should be managed by means of external cooling.[7]

1. Elis J, Laurence DR, Mattie H, Prichard BNC. Modification by monoamine oxidase inhibitors of the effect of some sympathomimetics on blood pressure. *BMJ* (1967) 2, 75–8.
2. Boakes AJ, Laurence DR, Teoh PC, Barar FSK, Benedikter L, Prichard BNC. Interactions between sympathomimetic amines and antidepressant agents in man. *BMJ* (1973) 1, 311–15.
3. Jenkins LC, Graves HB. Potential hazards of psychoactive drugs in association with anaesthesia. *Can Anaesth Soc J* (1965) 12, 121–8.
4. Gleiter CH, Mühlbauer B, Gradin-Frimmer G, Antonin KH, Bieck PR. Administration of sympathomimetic drugs with the selective MAO-A inhibitor brofaromine. Effect on blood pressure. *Drug Invest* (1992) 4, 149–54.
5. Amrein R, Güntert TW, Dingemanse J, Lorscheid T, Stabl M, Schmid-Burgk W. Interactions of moclobemide with concomitantly administered medication: evidence from pharmacological and clinical studies. *Psychopharmacology (Berl)* (1992) 106, S24–S31.
6. Korn A, Eichler HG, Gasić S. Moclobemide, a new specific MAO-inhibitor does not interact with direct adrenergic agonists. The Second Amine Oxidase Workshop, Uppsala. August 1986. *Pharmacol Toxicol* (1987) 60 (Suppl I), 31.
7. Nardil (Phenelzine sulfate). Parke Davis. US Prescribing information, January 2004.

MAOIs + Rauwolfia alkaloids or Tetrabenazine

The use of drugs that have the potential to cause depression, such as the rauwolfia alkaloids or tetrabenazine, is generally contraindicated in patients needing treatment for depression. Central excitation and possibly hypertension can occur if rauwolfia alkaloids are given to patients already taking an MAOI, but is unlikely if the rauwolfia alkaloid is given first.

Clinical evidence

A chronically depressed woman treated with **nialamide** 100 mg three times daily was given **reserpine** 0.5 mg three times a day on the third day. The following day she became hypomanic and almost immediately went into frank mania.[1]

In another report,[2] a patient, who was started on tetrabenazine two days after stopping a weeks' treatment with **nialamide** 25 mg daily, collapsed 6 hours after the first dose, and demonstrated epileptiform convulsions, partial unconsciousness, rapid respiration and tachycardia.

Other reports state that the administration of **reserpine** or **tetrabenazine** after pretreatment with **iproniazid** can lead to a temporary disturbance of affect and memory, associated with autonomic excitation, delirious agitation, disorientation and illusions of experience and recognition, which lasts for up to 3 days.[3,4]

A delayed 'reserpine-reversal' was seen in three schizophrenics treated firstly with **phenelzine** for 12 weeks, then a placebo for 16 to 33 weeks, and lastly **reserpine**. Their blood pressures rose slightly and persistently, and their psychomotor activity was considerably increased, lasting in two cases throughout the 12-week period of treatment.[5]

Mechanism

Rauwolfia alkaloids such as reserpine cause adrenergic neurones to become depleted of their normal stores of noradrenaline. In this way they prevent or reduce the normal transmission of impulses at the adrenergic nerve endings of the sympathetic nervous system and thereby act as antihypertensive agents. Since the brain also possesses adrenergic neurones, failure of transmission in the CNS could account for the sedation and depression observed with these drugs. If these compounds are given to patients already taking an MAOI, large amounts of accumulated noradrenaline can be released throughout the body. In the brain, 5-HT is also released. The release of these substances results in gross central excitation and hypertension. This would account for the case reports cited and the effects seen in *animals*.[6-8] These stimulant effects are sometimes called 'reserpine-reversal' because instead of the expected sedation or depression, excitation or delayed depression is seen. It depends upon the order in which the drugs are given.

Importance and management

The administration of drugs that have the potential to cause depression is generally contraindicated in patients needing treatment for depression. However, one report suggests that if concurrent use is considered desirable, the MAOIs should be given after, and not before the other drug, so that sedation rather than excitation will occur.[9]

1. Gradwell BG. Psychotic reactions and phenelzine. *BMJ* (1960) 2, 1018.
2. Davies TS. Monoamine oxidase inhibitors and rauwolfia compounds. *BMJ* (1960) 2, 739–40.
3. Voelkel A. Klinische Wirkung von Pharmaka mit Einfluss auf den Monoaminestoffwechsel de Gehirns. *Confin Neurol* (1958) 18, 144–9.
4. Voelkel A. Clinical experiences with amine oxidase inhibitors in psychiatry. *Ann N Y Acad Sci* (1959) 80, 680–6.
5. Esser AH. Clinical observations on reserpine reversal after prolonged MAO inhibition. *Psychiatr Neurol Neurochir* (1967) 70, 59–63.
6. Shore PA, Brodie BB. LSD-like effects elicited by reserpine in rabbits pretreated with isoniazid. *Proc Soc Exp Biol Med* (1957) 94, 433–5.
7. Chessin M, Kramer ER, Scott CC. Modification of the pharmacology of reserpine and serotonin by iproniazid. *J Pharmacol Exp Ther* (1957) 119, 453–60.
8. von Euler US, Bygdeman S, Persson N-Å. Interaction of reserpine and monoamine oxidase inhibitors on adrenergic transmitter release. *Biochim Biol Sper* (1970) 9, 215–20.
9. Natarajan S. Potential danger of monoamineoxidase inhibitors and α-methyldopa. *Lancet* (1964) i, 1330.

MAOIs + Sulfafurazole

An isolated report describes a patient on phenelzine who developed weakness and ataxia after taking sulfafurazole (sulfisoxazole).

Clinical evidence, mechanism, importance and management

A woman taking **phenelzine** 15 mg three times daily complained of weakness, ataxia, vertigo, tinnitus, muscle pains and paraesthesias within 7 days of starting to take 1 g of sulfafurazole four times daily. These adverse effects continued until the 10-day sulfonamide course was completed.[1] The reasons are not understood, but as these adverse effects are a combination of the adverse effects of both drugs, it seems possible that a mutual interaction (perhaps saturation of the acetylating mechanisms in the liver) was responsible. Concurrent use need not be avoided, but prescribers should be aware of this case.

1. Boyer WF, Lake CR. Interaction of phenelzine and sulfisoxazole. *Am J Psychiatry* (1983) 140, 264–5.

MAOIs + Sympathomimetics; Directly-acting

The pressor effects of adrenaline (epinephrine), isoprenaline (isoproterenol), noradrenaline (norepinephrine) and methoxamine may be unchanged or only moderately increased in patients taking MAOIs. The increase may be somewhat greater in those who show a significant hypotensive response to the MAOI. An isolated case of tachycardia and apprehension has also been described in an asthmatic on phenelzine after taking salbutamol (albuterol). Hypomania was seen in another asthmatic after taking isoetharine. **See also 'MAOIs + Phenylephrine', p.870.**

Clinical evidence

(a) Effects in the absence of MAOI-induced hypotension

Two subjects given **phenelzine** 15 mg three times daily and another given **tranylcypromine** 10 mg three times daily for 7 days showed no significant changes in their pressor responses to either **adrenaline (epinephrine)** or **isoprenaline (isoproterenol)**.[1] In another study patients on **phenelzine** showed no significant changes in their pressor response to **noradrenaline (norepinephrine)**.[2]

Another subject on **tranylcypromine** showed a twofold increase in the pressor response in the mid-range of **noradrenaline** concentrations infused, but not in the upper or low ranges.[1]

Yet another study in 3 healthy subjects given **tranylcypromine** found that the effects of **noradrenaline** were slightly increased, while with **adrenaline** a two to four fold increase in the effects on heart rate and diastolic pressure took place, but a less marked increase in systolic pressure. **Isoprenaline** behaved very much like **adrenaline**, but there was no enhancement of systolic pressure.[3] A patient using 1% **adrenaline** eye drops twice daily showed no increase in blood pressure or heart rate when treated with **tranylcypromine** 20 mg, rising to 50 mg daily.[4] Two patients taking **nialamide** showed no augmentation of the pressor response when given **noradrenaline** or **methoxamine**.[5]

Moclobemide is reported not to interact with **noradrenaline**[6,7] or **isoprenaline**.[6] Tachycardia and apprehension has also been described in a patient on **phenelzine** who took **salbutamol (albuterol)**,[8] and hypomania has been described in a patient on **phenelzine** who took **isoetharine**.[9]

(b) Effects in the presence of MAOI-induced hypotension

In a study in 7 hypertensive patients who showed postural hypotension after being given either **pheniprazine** or **tranylcypromine**, the doses of **noradrenaline (norepinephrine)** required to produce a 25 mmHg rise in systolic pressure were reduced to 13 to 38% and the doses of **methoxamine** were reduced to 30 to 39% of those required in the absence of an MAOI.[5] However, another study found no significant change when **noradrenaline** was given to two patients treated with **pargyline**.[10]

Mechanism

These sympathomimetic amines act directly on the receptors at the nerve endings, which innervate arterial blood vessels, so that the presence of the

MAOI-induced accumulation of noradrenaline (norepinephrine) within these nerve endings would not be expected to alter the extent of direct stimulation. The enhancement seen in those patients whose blood pressure was lowered by the MAOI might possibly be due to an increased sensitivity of the receptors, which is seen if the nerves are cut, and is also seen during temporary 'pharmacological severance'. The reactions of the two patients given beta-adrenergic agonists (salbutamol, isoetharine) are not understood.

Importance and management

The evidence is limited, but the overall picture is that some slight to moderate enhancement of the effects of noradrenaline (norepinephrine) and adrenaline (epinephrine) may occur in patients who do not show MAOI-induced hypotension. However, the authors of three of the reports cited[1,3,4] are in broad agreement that problems are unlikely to occur. One group[4] says that "it seems that the use of adrenaline, whether administered in eye drops or as a component of local anaesthesia in dental and other procedures, should not be contraindicated in patients receiving MAOIs." Direct evidence about methoxamine is even more limited, but it seems to behave similarly. None of the studies demonstrated any marked changes in the effects of isoprenaline (isoproterenol).

The situation in patients who show a reduced blood pressure due to the use of an MAOI is less clear. One study found an increase in the pressor efforts of noradrenaline and methoxamine[5] in hypertensive patients on pheniprazine or tranylcypromine, whereas another[10] found no changes in the pressor effects of noradrenaline in patients on pargyline.

The cases involving salbutamol (albuterol) and isoetharine are isolated and possibly not of general importance. This needs confirmation. The interaction between phenylephrine and the MAOIs is dealt with elsewhere (see 'MAOIs + Phenylephrine', p.870).

1. Boakes AJ, Laurence DR, Teoh PC, Barar FSK, Benedikter LT, Prichard BNC. Interactions between sympathomimetic amines and antidepressant agents in man. *BMJ* (1973) 1, 311–15.
2. Elis J, Laurence DR, Mattie H, Prichard BNC. Modification by monoamine oxidase inhibitors of the effect of some sympathomimetics on blood pressure. *BMJ* (1967) 2, 75–8.
3. Cuthbert MF, Vere DW. Potentiation of the cardiovascular effects of some catecholamines by a monoamine oxidase inhibitor. *Br J Pharmacol* (1971) 43, 471P–472P.
4. Thompson DS, Sweet RA, Marzula K, Peredes JC. Lack of interaction of monoamine oxidase inhibitors and epinephrine in an older patient. *J Clin Psychopharmacol* (1997) 17, 322–3.
5. Horwitz D, Goldberg LI, Sjoerdsma A. Increased blood pressure responses to dopamine and norepinephrine produced by monoamine oxidase inhibitors in man. *J Lab Clin Med* (1960) 56, 747–53.
6. Zimmer R, Gieschke R, Fischbach R, Gasic S. Interaction studies with moclobemide. *Acta Psychiatr Scand* (1990) 82 (Suppl 360), 84–6.
7. Cusson JR, Goldenberg E, Larochelle P. Effect of a novel monoamine-oxidase inhibitor, moclobemide on the sensitivity to intravenous tyramine and norepinephrine in humans. *J Clin Pharmacol* (1991) 31, 462–7.
8. Shader RI, Greenblatt DJ. MAOIs and drug interactions—a proposal for a clearinghouse. *J Clin Psychopharmacol* (1985) 5, A17.
9. Goldman LS, Tiller JA. Hypomania related to phenelzine and isoetharine interaction in one patient. *J Clin Psychiatry* (1987) 48, 170.
10. Pettinger WA, Oates JA. Supersensitivity to tyramine during monoamine oxidase inhibition in man. *Clin Pharmacol Ther* (1968) 9, 341–4.

MAOIs + Sympathomimetics; Indirectly-acting

The concurrent use of sympathomimetic amines with indirect activity (amfetamines, ephedrine, metaraminol, phenylpropanolamine, pseudoephedrine, etc.) and the older MAOIs can result in a potentially fatal hypertensive crisis. These amines are found in many proprietary cough, cold and influenza preparations, or are used as appetite suppressants, or taken illicitly as with ecstasy (MDMA, 3,4-methylenedioxymethamfetamine). Potentially serious interactions have also been seen with brofaromine or moclobemide and indirectly-acting sympathomimetics.

Clinical evidence

(a) Non-selective MAOIs

The concurrent use of MAOIs and indirectly-acting sympathomimetics can result in a rapid and serious rise in blood pressure, accompanied by tachycardia, chest pains and severe occipital headache. Neck stiffness, flushing, sweating, nausea, vomiting, hypertonicity of the limbs, and sometimes epileptiform convulsions can occur. Fatal intracranial haemorrhage, cardiac arrhythmias and cardiac arrest may result.

A woman who, unknown to her doctors, was taking **pargyline**, was given **phenylpropanolamine** for nasal decongestion on the eve of surgery, which promptly caused a hypertensive reaction. Her blood pressure rose rapidly from 130/80 to 220/160 mmHg and she complained of occipital headache, photophobia and nausea. She also exhibited sweating and vomited. Two intravenous injections of phentolamine 5 mg partially controlled her blood pressure.[1]

A 30-year-old depressed woman who was taking **phenelzine** 15 mg three times daily and trifluoperazine 2 mg at night, acquired some **dexamfetamine sulfate** tablets from a friend and took 20 mg. Within 15 minutes she complained of severe headache, which she described as if "her head was bursting". An hour later her blood pressure was 150/100 mmHg. Later she became comatose with a blood pressure of 170/100 mmHg and died. A postmortem examination revealed a haemorrhage in the left cerebral hemisphere, disrupting the internal capsule and adjacent areas of the corpus striatum.[2] These are just two examples from many.

This interaction has been reported with **amfetamine sulfate**,[3] **d-l amfetamine**,[4] **ephedrine**,[5,6] **isometheptene mucate**,[7] **mephentermine**,[8] **metaraminol**,[9] **methylamfetamine**,[10-13] **phenylpropanolamine**,[14-18] **pseudoephedrine**,[18-21] and **methylphenidate**,[22] in patients on **tranylcypromine**,[3,5,6,10-12,15] **phenelzine**,[2,4,5,8,11-14,16-18] **isocarboxazid**,[11] **iproniazid**,[20] **mebanazine**,[14] and **pargyline**.[9] **Nialamide** is expected to behave similarly, but reports seem to be lacking. There are other reports and studies of this interaction not listed here.

Extreme hyperpyrexia, apparently without hypertension, has been described with **tranylcypromine** and **amfetamines**.[23,24]

Marked hypertension, diaphoresis, altered mental status and hypertonicity (slow forceful twisting and arching movements) occurred in one patient on **phenelzine** after taking **ecstasy** (**MDMA, 3,4-methylenedioxymethamfetamine**).[25] Increased muscle tension, decorticate-like posturing and coma occurred in another.[26] A further patient on **ecstasy** and **tranylcypromine** had a hypertensive crisis about a week after taking both drugs.[22] All three patients recovered.

(b) Selective MAOIs

No interaction was seen in subjects on **brofaromine** 75 mg twice daily for 10 days when given 75 mg of slow-release **phenylpropanolamine** (*Acutrim Late Day*), but immediate-release **phenylpropanolamine** in gelatin capsules caused a 3.3-fold increase in pressor sensitivity.[27] The pressor effects of **ephedrine** (two doses of 50 mg with a 4 hour interval) in subjects taking **moclobemide** 300 mg twice daily were increased about fourfold.[28,29]

Four patients died after taking **moclobemide** and ecstasy. The clinical evidence is limited, but in each case the forensic pathologist concluded that the cause of death was the combined use of these drugs. It was suggested that what happened is consistent with the serotonin syndrome, although the evidence is fairly slim. Two patients had taken maximum doses and two moderate overdoses of moclobemide. Post-mortem analysis also showed the presence of **amfetamines** in 3 patients and **dextromethorphan** in the fourth.[30]

Mechanism

The reaction can be attributed to overstimulation of the adrenergic receptors of the cardiovascular system.[31] During treatment with non-selective MAOIs, large amounts of noradrenaline accumulate at adrenergic nerve endings not only in the brain, but also within the sympathetic nerve endings, which innervate arterial blood vessels. Stimulation of these latter nerve endings by sympathomimetic amines with indirect actions causes the release of the accumulated noradrenaline and results in the massive stimulation of the receptors. An exaggerated blood vessel constriction occurs and the blood pressure rise is proportionately excessive. Intracranial haemorrhage can occur if the pressure is so high that a blood vessel ruptures.[2] The MAOI/ecstasy (MDMA, 3,4-methylenedioxymethamfetamine) reaction may also possibly be related to the serotonin syndrome. Ecstasy has amfetamine-like properties and acts by releasing serotonin (and possibly also dopamine) from neurones in the brain, so that increased stimulation of the serotonin receptors occurs. This possibly explains its mood-modifying effects. Monoamine oxidase inhibitors (moclobemide, phenelzine) prevent the breakdown of serotonin within neurones so that more serotonin is available for release, and in excess this can apparently result in the toxic and even fatal serotonin syndrome. The selective MAOIs, which inhibit only MAO-A (such as moclobemide), appear to behave like the irreversible non-selective MAOIs in this context.

Importance and management

(a) Non selective MAOIs

A very well-documented, serious, and potentially fatal interaction. Patients taking any of the older irreversible MAOIs, whether for depression or hypertension, should not normally take any sympathomimetic amine with indirect activity. These include the amfetamines (dexamfetamine, hydroxyamfetamine, methylamfetamine), ecstasy (MDMA, 3,4-methylenedioxymethamfetamine), ephedrine, isometheptene mucate, mephentermine, metaraminol, methylphenidate, phenylpropanolamine and pseudoephedrine. Direct evidence implicating **amfepramone (diethylpropion)**, **benzfetamine**, **chlorphentermine**, **cyclopentamine**, **mazindol**,[32] **methylephedrine**, **phendimetrazine**, **phenmetrazine** and **pholedrine** seems not to have been documented, but on the basis of their known pharmacology their concurrent administration with the MAOIs should be avoided.

Many of these sympathomimetic amines occur in OTC cough, cold and influenza preparations, and as proprietary appetite suppressants. Patients on MAOIs should be strongly warned not to take any of these drugs concurrently. A possible exception to this prohibition is that under very well controlled conditions dexamfetamine and methylphenidate may sometimes be effectively (and apparently safely) used with MAOIs for refractory depression.[33,34]

(b) Selective MAOIs

A study with brofaromine and phenylpropanolamine has demonstrated the potential for a significant interaction. Moclobemide can interact and the makers of moclobemide[35] advise avoidance of sympathomimetics such as ephedrine, pseudoephedrine and phenylpropanolamine, and it would also be prudent to avoid moclobemide with any of the other indirectly-acting sympathomimetics cited here, although the severity of the interactions with moclobemide is unlikely to be as great as that seen with the older MAOIs. However, it should be said that ephedrine and phenylephrine have been successfully and uneventfully used in the presence of moclobemide during anaesthesia to control hypotension.[36] See also 'MAOIs + Phenylephrine', p.870.

(c) Treatment

These hypertensive reactions have been controlled by intravenous phentolamine, phenoxybenzamine, intramuscular chlorpromazine, labetalol or nifedipine. However, it is advisable to refer to current guidelines (or at least a relevant current text book) on the management of hypertensive crises for up to date advice.

1. Jenkins LC, Graves HB. Potential hazards of psychoactive drugs in association with anaesthesia. *Can Anaesth Soc J* (1965) 12, 121–8.
2. Lloyd JTA, Walker DRH. Death after combined dexamphetamine and phenelzine. *BMJ* (1965) 2, 168–9.
3. Zeck P. The dangers of some antidepressant drugs. *Med J Aust* (1961) 2, 607–8.
4. Tonks CM, Livingston D. Monoamineoxidase inhibitors. *Lancet* (1963) i, 1323–4.
5. Elis J, Laurence DR, Mattie H, Prichard BNC. Modification by monoamine oxidase inhibitors of the effect of some sympathomimetics on blood pressure. *BMJ* (1967) 2, 75–8.
6. Low-Beer GA, Tidmarsh D. Collapse after "Parstelin". *BMJ* (1963) 2, 683–4.
7. Kraft KE, Dore FH. Computerized drug interaction programs: how reliable ? *JAMA* (1996) 275, 1087.
8. Stark DCC. Effects of giving vasopressors to patients on monoamine-oxidase inhibitors. *Lancet* (1962) i, 1405–6.
9. Horler AR, Wynne NA. Hypertensive crisis due to pargyline and metaraminol. *BMJ* (1965) 2, 460–1.
10. Macdonald R. Tranylcypromine. *Lancet* (1963) i, 269.
11. Mason A. Fatal reaction associated with tranylcypromine and methylamphetamine. *Lancet* (1962) i, 1073.
12. Dally PJ. Fatal reaction associated with tranylcypromine and methylamphetamine. *Lancet* (1962) i, 1235–6.
13. Nymark M, Nielsen IM. Reactions due to the combination of monoamineoxidase inhibitors with thymoleptics, pethidine, or methylamphetamine. *Lancet* (1963) ii, 524–5.
14. Tonks CM, Lloyd AT. Hazards with monoamine-oxidase inhibitors. *BMJ* (1965) 1, 589.
15. Cuthbert MF, Greenberg MP, Morley SW. Cough and cold remedies: a potential danger to patients on monoamine oxidase inhibitors. *BMJ* (1969) 1, 404–6.
16. Mason AMS, Buckle RM. "Cold" cures and monoamine-oxidase inhibitors. *BMJ* (1969) 1, 845–6.
17. Humberstone PM. Hypertension from cold remedies. *BMJ* (1969) 1, 846.
18. Harrison WM, McGrath PJ, Stewart JW, Quitkin F. MAOIs and hypertensive crises: the role of OTC drugs. *J Clin Psychiatry* (1989) 50, 64–5.
19. Wright SP. Hazards with monoamine-oxidase inhibitors: a persistent problem. *Lancet* (1978) i, 284–5.
20. Davies R. Patient medication records. *Pharm J* (1982) 228, 652.
21. Harrison W, McGrath PJ, Stewart JW, Quitkin F. MAOIs and hypertensive crisis: the role of OTC drugs. J Clin Psychiatry (1989) 50, 64–5. Correction. ibid. *(1990) 51, 212–3. [drug]* (1990) 51, 212–3. [drug]
22. Sherman M, Hauser GC, Glover BH. Toxic reactions to tranylcypromine. *Am J Psychiatry* (1964) 120, 1019–21.
23. Lewis E. Hyperpyrexia with antidepressant drugs. *BMJ* (1965) 1, 1671–2.
24. Kriskó I, Lewis E, Johnson JE. Severe hyperpyrexia due to tranylcypromine–amphetamine toxicity. *Ann Intern Med* (1969) 70, 559–64.
25. Smilkstein MJ, Smolinske SC, Rumack BH. A case of MAO inhibitor/MDMA interaction: agony after ecstasy. *Clin Toxicol* (1987) 25, 149–59.
26. Kaskey GB. Possible interaction between an MAOI and "Ecstasy". *Am J Psychiatry* (1992) 149, 411–2.
27. Gleiter CH, Mühlbauer B, Gradin-Frimmer G, Antonin KH, Bieck PR. Administration of sympathomimetic drugs with the selective MAO-A inhibitor brofaromine. Effect on blood pressure. *Drug Invest* (1992) 4, 149–54.
28. Dingemanse J. An update of recent moclobemide interaction data. *Int Clin Psychopharmacol* (1993) 7, 167–80.
29. Dingemanse J, Guentert T, Gieschke R, Stabl M. Modification of the cardiovascular effects of ephedrine by the reversible monoamine oxidase A-inhibitor moclobemide. *J Cardiovasc Pharmacol* (1996) 28, 856–61.
30. Vuori E, Henry JA, Ojanoperä I, Nieminen R, Savolainen T, Wahlsten P, Jäntti M. Death following ingestion of MDMA (ecstasy) and moclobemide. *Addiction* (2003) 98, 365–8.
31. Simpson LL. Mechanism of the adverse interaction between monoamine oxidase inhibitors and amphetamine. *J Pharmacol Exp Ther* (1978) 205, 392–9.
32. Sandoz Products Ltd. Personal communication, 1987.
33. Fawcett J, Kravitz HM, Zajecka JM, Schaff MR. CNS stimulant potentiation of monoamine oxidase inhibitors in treatment-refractory depression. *J Clin Psychopharmacol* (1991) 11, 127–32.
34. Feighner JP, Herbstein J, Damlouji N. Combined MAOI, TCA, and direct stimulant therapy of treatment-resistant depression. *J Clin Psychiatry* (1985) 46, 206–9.
35. Manerix (Moclobemide). Roche Products Ltd. UK Summary of product characteristics, May 2004.
36. Martyr JW, Orlikowski CEP. Epidural anaesthesia, ephedrine and phenylephrine in a patient taking moclobemide, a new monoamine oxidase inhibitor. *Anaesthesia* (1996) 51, 1150–2.

MAOIs + Tricyclic antidepressants

Because of the very toxic and sometimes fatal reactions (the serotonin syndrome or similar) that have very occasionally taken place in patients taking both MAOIs and tricyclic antidepressants, concurrent use is regarded as contraindicated in all but rare circumstances.

Clinical evidence

The toxic reactions have included (with variations) sweating, flushing, hyperpyrexia, restlessness, excitement, tremor, muscle twitching and rigidity, convulsions and coma. An illustrative example:

A woman who had been taking **tranylcypromine** 10 mg twice daily for about 3 weeks, stopped taking it 3 days before taking a single tablet of **imipramine**. Within a few hours she complained of an excruciating headache, and soon afterwards lost consciousness and started to convulse. The toxic reactions manifested were a temperature of 40.6°C, pulse rate of 120 bpm, severe extensor rigidity, carpal spasm, opisthotonos and cyanosis. She was treated with amobarbital and phenytoin, and her temperature was reduced with alcohol-ice-soaked towels. The treatment was effective and she recovered.[1]

Similar reactions have been recorded on a number of other occasions with normal therapeutic doses of **iproniazid**,[2] **isocarboxazid**,[2,3] **moclobemide**,[4] **pargyline**,[5] or **phenelzine**[6-13] with **imipramine**; **phenelzine** with **desipramine**[14] or **clomipramine**;[15-17] and **tranylcypromine** with **clomipramine**.[18-21]

Moclobemide is reported not to interact with **amitriptyline** or **desipramine**,[22-24] but a reaction similar to the serotonin syndrome occurred in 2 patients when **clomipramine** 50 mg daily was replaced by **moclobemide**.[25,26] A fatal serotonin syndrome is reported in a patient taking **clomipramine** and **amitriptyline**, with symptoms being manifested within 30 minutes of a 300 mg dose of **moclobemide**.[27] Four other patients developed the serotonin syndrome after taking moderate overdoses of **moclobemide** and **clomipramine**; three of them died.[28-31] A brief report notes the serotonin syndrome in a patient taking **moclobemide** and **imipramine**.[32] However, another study found that doses of up to 300 mg of **moclobemide** could be given 24 hours after the last dose of treatment with either **amitriptyline** or **clomipramine** without any major risks.[24] Another study found a 39% rise in plasma **trimipramine** levels in 15 patients and a 25% rise in plasma levels of **maprotiline** (a tetracyclic antidepressant) in 6 other patients when concurrently treated with **moclobemide**. No serious toxic reactions were reported.[33] Only a minor and clinically unimportant change in the pharmacokinetics of **amitriptyline** occurs in patients given **toloxatone**.[34]

Some other reports are confused by overdosage with one or both drugs, or by the presence of other drugs and diseases. There have been fatalities.[13,14,18,35] In some instances the drugs were not taken together, but were substituted without a washout period in between. There are far too many reports of these interactions to list all of them here, but they are extensively reviewed elsewhere.[12,36,37] Three patients with bipolar disorder developed mania when treated with **isocarboxazid** and **amitriptyline**.[38]

There are a number of other reports and reviews describing the beneficial use of MAOI/tricyclic antidepressant combinations,[36,37,39-43] and in addition, one study has reported switching 178 patients from tricyclics to MAOIs within 4 days or less. Of these patients, 63 were given the MAOI while still being tapered from the tricyclic, all without any apparent problems.[43]

Mechanism

Not understood. One idea is that both drugs cause grossly elevated monoamine levels (5-HT, noradrenaline (norepinephrine)) in the brain, which 'spill-over' into areas not concerned with mood elevation. It may be related to, or the same as the serotonin-syndrome seen with selective serotonin re-uptake inhibitors.[4,16] Some of the tricyclics (e.g. clomipramine, imipramine) are potent inhibitors of serotonin uptake. Less likely suggestions are that the MAOIs inhibit the metabolism of the tricyclic antidepressants, or that active and unusual metabolites of the tricyclic antidepressants are produced.[36]

Importance and management

An established, serious and life-threatening but apparently uncommon interaction. There is no precise information about its incidence but it is probably much lower than was originally thought. If concurrent use is to be avoided, the following guidelines[44] are recommended:

- Tricyclic antidepressants should *not* be started for 2 weeks after treatment with MAOIs has been stopped (3 weeks if starting clomipramine or imipramine).
- An MAOI should *not* be started until at least 7-14 days after a tricyclic or related antidepressant has been stopped (3 weeks in the case of clomipramine or imipramine).
- An MAOI should *not* be started for at least 2 weeks after a previous MAOI has been stopped (then started at a reduced dose).
- Moclobemide has a short duration of action so no treatment free period is required after it has been stopped before starting a tricyclic antidepressant.
- Moclobemide should *not* be started until at least a week after a tricyclic antidepressant has been stopped.

No detailed clinical work has been done to find out precisely what sets the scene when the interaction does occur, but some general empirical guidelines have been suggested so that it can, as far as possible, be avoided when concurrent treatment is thought appropriate:[11,12,36,37,45]

- Treatment with both types of drug should only be undertaken by those well aware of the problems and who can undertake adequate supervision.
- Only patients refractory to all other types of treatment should be considered.
- Tranylcypromine, phenelzine, clomipramine and imipramine appear to be high on the list of drugs which have interacted adversely. Combination of clomipramine with tranylcypromine is particularly dangerous. Amitriptyline, trimipramine and isocarboxazid are possibly safer.
- Absence of information documenting unsuitability or hazard does not necessarily imply that the two drugs may be used safely together, but may merely reflect an untried combination.[45]
- Drugs should be given orally, not parenterally.
- It seems safer to give the tricyclic antidepressants first, or together with the MAOI, than to give the MAOI first. If the patient is already taking an MAOI, it may not be safe to start the tricyclic antidepressant until recovery from MAO-inhibition is complete.
- Small doses should be given initially, increasing the levels of each drug, one at a time, over a period of 2 to 3 weeks to levels generally about half[45] those used for each one individually.

Doses of 50 and 100 mg chlorpromazine given intramuscularly have been used successfully in the treatment of this adverse interaction.[19,21] It has been suggested that dantrolene can probably be used to reduce the muscle rigidity and hyperpyrexia, and possibly methysergide, which is a 5-HT receptor antagonist.[28]

1. Brachfeld J, Wirtshafter A, Wolfe S. Imipramine-tranylcypromine incompatibility. Near-fatal toxic reaction. *JAMA* (1963) 186, 1172–3.
2. Ayd FJ. Toxic somatic and psychopathological reactions to antidepressant drugs. *J Neuropsychiatr* (1961) 2 (Suppl 1), S119–S122.
3. Kane FJ, Freeman D. Non-fatal reaction to imipramine-MAO inhibitor combination. *Am J Psychiatry* (1963), 120, 79–80.
4. Brodribb TR, Downey M, Gilbar PJ. Efficacy and adverse effects of moclobemide. *Lancet* (1994) 343, 475–6.
5. McCurdy RL, Kane FJ. Transient brain syndrome as a non-fatal reaction to combined pargyline imipramine treatment. *Am J Psychiatry* (1964), 121, 397–8.
6. Hills NF. Combining the antidepressant drugs. *BMJ* (1965) 1, 859.
7. Davies G. Side-effects of phenelzine. *BMJ* (1960) 2, 1019.
8. Howarth E. Possible synergistic effects of the new thymoleptics in connection with poisoning. *J Ment Sci* (1961) 107, 100–103.
9. Singh H. Atropine-like poisoning due to tranquillizing agents. *Am J Psychiatry* (1960) 117, 360–1.
10. Lockett MF, Milner G. Combining the antidepressant drugs. *BMJ* (1965) 1, 921.
11. Graham PM, Potter JM, Paterson JW. Combination monoamine oxidase inhibitor/tricyclic antidepressant interaction. *Lancet* (1982) ii, 440.
12. Schuckit M, Robins E, Feighner J. Tricyclic antidepressants and monoamine oxidase inhibitors. Combination therapy in the treatment of depression. *Arch Gen Psychiatry* (1971) 24, 509–14.
13. Stanley B, Pal NR. Fatal hyperpyrexia with phenelzine and imipramine. *BMJ* (1964) 2, 1011.
14. Bowen LW. Fatal hyperpyrexia with antidepressant drugs. *BMJ* (1964) 2, 1465–6.
15. Beeley L, Daly M. *Bulletin of the West Midlands Centre for Adverse Drug Reaction Reporting* (1986) 23, 16.
16. Nierenberg DW, Semprebon M. The central nervous system serotonin syndrome. *Clin Pharmacol Ther* (1993) 53, 84–8.
17. Stern TA, Schwartz JH, Shuster JL. Catastrophic illness associated with the combination of clomipramine, phenelzine, and chlorpromazine. *Ann Clin Psychiatry* (1992) 4, 81–5.
18. Beaumont G. Drug interactions with clomipramine (Anafranil). *J Int Med Res* (1973) 1, 480–4.
19. Tackley RM, Tregaskis B. Fatal disseminated intravascular coagulation following a monoamine oxidase inhibitor/tricyclic interaction. *Anaesthesia* (1987) 42, 760–3.
20. Richards GA, Fritz VU, Pincus P, Reyneke J. Unusual drug interactions between monoamine oxidase inhibitors and tricyclic antidepressants. *J Neurol Neurosurg Psychiatry* (1987) 50, 1240–1.
21. Gillman PK. Successful treatment of serotonin syndrome with chlorpromazine. *Med J Aust* (1996) 165, 345–6.
22. Zimmer R, Gieschke R, Fischbach R, Gasic S. Interaction studies with moclobemide. *Acta Psychiatr Scand* (1990) 82 (Suppl 360), 84–6.
23. Korn A, Eichler HG, Fischbach R, Gasic S. Moclobemide, a new reversible MAO inhibitor – interaction with tyramine and tricyclic antidepressants in healthy volunteers and depressive patients. *Psychopharmacology (Berl)* (1986) 88, 153–7.
24. Dingemanse J, Kneer J, Fotteler B, Groen H, Peeters PAM, Jonkman JHG. Switch in treatment from tricyclic antidepressants to moclobemide: a new generation monoamine oxidase inhibitor. *J Clin Psychopharmacol* (1995) 15, 41–8.
25. Spigset O, Mjorndal T, Lovheim O. Serotonin syndrome caused by a moclobemide-clomipramine interaction. *BMJ* (1993) 306, 248.
26. Gillman PK. Serotonin syndrome – clomipramine too soon after moclobemide? *Int Clin Psychopharmacol* (1997) 12, 339–42.
27. Kuisma MJ. Fatal serotonin syndrome with trismus. *Ann Emerg Med* (1995) 26, 108.
28. Neuvonen PJ, Pohjola-Sintonen S, Tacke U, Vuori E. Five fatal cases of serotonin syndrome after moclobemide-citalopram or moclobemide-clomipramine overdoses. *Lancet* (1993) 342, 1419.
29. Hernandez AF, Montero MN, Pla A, Villaneuva E. Fatal moclobemide overdose or death caused by serotonin syndrome? *J Forensic Sci* (1995) 40, 128–30.
30. François B, Marquet P, Desachy A, Roustan J, Lachatre G, Gastinne H. Serotonin syndrome due to an overdose of moclobemide and clomipramine: a potentially life-threatening association. *Intensive Care Med* (1997) 23, 122–4.
31. Ferrer-Dufol A, Perez-Aradros C, Murillo EC. Fatal serotonin syndrome caused by moclobemide-clomipramine overdose. *Clin Toxicol* (1998) 36, 31–2.
32. Gilbar PJ, Brodribb TR, Downey M. Serotonin syndrome due to a moclobemide-imipramine interaction: a previously unreported drug interaction? *Aust J Hosp Pharm* (1995) 25, 75.
33. König F, Wolfersdorf M, Löble M, Wößner S, Hauger B. Trimipramine and maprotiline plasma levels during combined treatment with moclobemide in therapy-resistant depression. *Pharmacopsychiatry* (1997) 30, 125–7.
34. Vandel S, Bertschy G, Perault MC, Sandoz M, Bouquet S, Chakroun R, Guibert S, Vandel B. Minor and clinically non-significant interaction between toloxatone and amitriptyline. *Eur J Clin Pharmacol* (1993) 44, 97–9.
35. Wright SP. Hazards with monoamine-oxidase inhibitors: a persistent problem. *Lancet* (1978) i, 284–5.
36. Ponto LB, Perry PJ, Liskow BI, Seaba HH. Drug therapy reviews: tricyclic antidepressant and monoamine oxidase inhibitor combination therapy. *Am J Hosp Pharm* (1977) 34, 954–61.
37. Ananth J, Luchins D. A review of combined tricyclic and MAOI therapy. *Compr Psychiatry* (1977) 18, 221–30.
38. de la Fuente JR, Berlanga C, León-Andrade C. Mania induced by tricyclic-MAOI combination therapy in bipolar treatment-resistant disorder: case reports. *J Clin Psychiatry* (1986) 47, 40–1.
39. Gander GA.The clinical value of monoamine oxidase inhibitors and tricyclic antidepressants in combination. *In 'Antidepressant Drugs' Proc 1st Int Symp Milan* (1966). Int Congr Ser No 122, p 336–43. Excerpta Medica.
40. Sargant W. Safety of combined antidepressant drugs. *BMJ* (1971) 1, 555–6.
41. White K, Pistole T, Boyd JL. Combined monoamine oxidase inhibitor-tricyclic antidepressant treatment: a pilot study. *Am J Psychiatry* (1980) 137, 1422–5.
42. Berlanga C. Ortego-Soto HA. A 3-year follow-up of a group of treatment-resistant depressed patients with a MAOI/tricyclic combination. *J Affect Disord* (1995) 34, 187–92.
43. Kahn D, Silver JM, Opler LA. The safety of switching rapidly from tricyclic antidepressants to monoamine oxidase inhibitors. *J Clin Psychopharmacol* (1989) 9, 198–202.
44. British National Formulary. 49th ed. London: The British Medical Association and The Pharmaceutical Press; 2005, pp. 197, 200, 201.
45. Sweetman SC, editor. Martindale: The complete drug reference. 34th ed. London: Pharmaceutical Press; 2005, p. 315.

MAOIs + Tryptophan

Although the concurrent use of MAOIs and tryptophan can be both safe and effective, a number of patients have developed severe behavioural and neurological signs of toxicity, and one patient died.

Clinical evidence

A man on **phenelzine** 90 mg daily developed behavioural and neurological toxicity within 2 hours of being given 6 g of tryptophan.[1] He had shivering and diaphoresis, his psychomotor retardation disappeared and he became jocular, fearful, and moderately labile. His neurological signs included bilateral Babinski signs, hyperreflexia, rapid horizontal ocular oscillations, shivering of the jaw, trunk and limbs, mild dysmetria and ataxia. The situation resolved on withdrawal of the drugs.[1]

Other reports describe patients who had severe[2] or milder[3-5] symptoms of toxicity, hypomania,[6] or delirium[7] when given **isocarboxazid**, **pargyline**, or **phenelzine** with tryptophan. Symptoms included alcohol-like intoxication, drowsiness, delirium, myoclonus, muscle twitching, hyperreflexia, jaw quivering, teeth chattering, diaphoresis and ocular oscillations.[5,8-11] One patient showed toxicity with transient hyperthermia when the dose of tryptophan was increased.[12] Fatal malignant hyperpyrexia occurred in another patient on **phenelzine**, tryptophan and lithium.[13]

In contrast however, concurrent use has been reported as both safe and effective.[14]

Table 30.2 The tyramine content of some drinks

Drink	*Tyramine content (mg/L)*	*Refs*
Beer (Canada)	6.4, 11.1, 11.2	2
Beer (UK)	1.34	5
Beer (USA)	1.8, 2.3, 4.4	1
Champagne (Canada)	0.2, 0.6	2
Chianti (Italy)		
Governo process	0.0, 1.76, 12.2, 10.36, 25.4	1–3, 5
Newer process	0.0 to 4.7	3, 5–7
Gin	0.0	7
Port	less than 0.2 (undetectable)	1
Reisling	0.6	1
Sauterne	0.4	1
Sherry (USA)	3.6	1
Sherry (Canada)	0.2	2
Sherry	2.65	7
Wine (from different regions in France)	5.02 to 13.7	4
Wine, red (Canada, France, Italy, Spain, USA)	0 to 8.64 (mean 5.18)	2, 4
Wine, red (unstated origin)	1.36	5
Wine, white (Germany, Italy, Portugal, Spain)	1.26 to 5.87 (mean 4.41)	4
Wine, white (Germany, Former Yugoslavia)	1.22	5
Vodka	0.0	7
Whiskey	0.0	7

1. Horwitz D, Lovenberg W, Engelman K, Sjoerdsma A. Monoamine oxidase inhibitors, tyramine and cheese. *JAMA* (1964) 188, 1108–10.
2. Sen NP. Analysis and significance of tyramine in foods. *J Food Sci* (1969) 34, 22–6.
3. Korn A, Eichler HG, Fischbach R, Gasic S. Moclobemide, a new reversible MAO inhibitor - interaction with tyramine and tricyclic antidepressants in healthy volunteers and depressive patients. *Psychopharmacology (Berl)* (1986) 88, 153–7.
4. Zee JA, Simard RE, L'Heureux L, Tremblay J. Biogenic amines in wines. *Am J Enol Vitic* (1983) 34, 6–9.
5. Hannah P, Glover V, Sandler M. Tyramine in wine and beer. *Lancet* (1988) i, 879.
6. Da Prada M, Zürcher G, Wüthrich I, Haefely WE. On tyramine, food, beverages and the reversible MAO inhibitor moclobemide. *J Neural Transm* (1988) (Suppl 26), 31.
7. Shulman KI, Walker SE, MacKenzine S, Knowles S. Dietary restriction, tyramine, and use of monoamine oxidase inhibitors. *J Clin Psychopharmacol* (1989) 9, 397–402.

Mechanism

Not understood. The reactions appears to be related to the serotonin syndrome, which can occur with 5-HT uptake inhibitors.

Importance and management

Information seems to be confined to the reports listed. Concurrent use can be effective in the treatment of depression,[14] but occasionally and unpredictably severe and even life-threatening toxicity occurs. The authors of the report detailed above[1] recommend that patients on MAOIs should be started on a low dose of tryptophan (0.5 g). This should be gradually increased while monitoring the mental status of the patient for changes suggesting hypomania, and neurological changes, including ocular oscillations and upper motor neurone signs. Products containing tryptophan for the treatment of depression were withdrawn in the USA, UK, and many other countries because of a possible association with the development of an eosinophilia-myalgia syndrome. However, since the syndrome appeared to have been associated with tryptophan from one manufacturer, tryptophan preparations were reintroduced in the UK in 1994 for restricted use.[15]

1. Thomas JN, Rubin EH. Case report of a toxic reaction from a combination of tryptophan and phenelzine. *Am J Psychiatry* (1984) 141, 281–3.
2. Kim SY, Mueller PD. Life-threatening interaction between phenelzine and L-tryptophan. *Vet Hum Toxicol* (1989) 31, 370.
3. Glassman AH, Platman SR. Potentiation of monoamine oxidase inhibitor by tryptophan. *J Psychiatr Res* (1969) 7, 83–8.
4. Pare CMB. Potentiation of monoamine-oxidase inhibitors by tryptophan. *Lancet* (1963) 2, 527–8.
5. Baloh RW, Dietz J, Spooner JW. Myoclonus and ocular oscillations induced by l-tryptophan. *Ann Neurol* (1982) 11, 95–7.
6. Goff DC. Two cases of hypomania following the addition of l-tryptophan to a monoamine oxidase inhibitor. *Am J Psychiatry* (1985) 142, 1487–8.
7. Alvine G, Black DW, Tsuang D. Case of delirium secondary to phenelzine/l-tryptophan combination. *J Clin Psychiatry* (1990) 51, 311.
8. Hodge JV, Oates JA, Sjoerdsma A. Reduction of the central effects of tryptophan by a decarboxylase inhibitor. *Clin Pharmacol Ther* (1964) 5, 149–55.
9. Pope HG, Jonas JM, Hudson JI, Kafka MP. Toxic reactions to the combination of monoamine oxidase inhibitors and tryptophan. *Am J Psychiatry* (1985) 142, 491–2.
10. Levy AB, Bucher P, Votolato N. Myoclonus, hyperreflexia and diaphoresis in patients on phenelzine-tryptophan combination treatment. *Can J Psychiatry* (1985) 30, 434–6.
11. Oates JA, Sjoerdsma A. Neurological effects of tryptophan in patients receiving a monoamine oxidase inhibitor. *Neurology* (1960) 10, 1076–8.
12. Price WA, Zimmer B, Kucas P. Serotonin syndrome: a case report. *J Clin Pharmacol* (1986) 26, 77–8.
13. Staufenberg EF, Tantam D. Malignant hyperpyrexia syndrome in combined treatment. *Br J Psychiatry* (1989) 154, 577–8.
14. Nelson JC. Augmentation strategies in depression 2000. *J Clin Psychiatry* (2000) 61 (Suppl 2), 13–19.
15. Sweetman SC, editor. Martindale: The complete drug reference. 34th ed. London: Pharmaceutical Press; 2005. p. 321.

MAOIs + Tyramine-rich drinks

Patients taking the older MAOIs (tranylcypromine, phenelzine, nialamide, pargyline, etc.) can suffer a serious hypertensive reaction if they drink tyramine-rich drinks (some beers, lagers or wines), but no serious interaction is likely with the newer reversible and selective MAOIs (moclobemide, etc.). The hypotensive side-effects of the MAOIs may be exaggerated in a few patients by alcohol, and they may experience dizziness and faintness after drinking relatively modest amounts.

Clinical evidence, mechanism, importance and management

(a) Hypertensive reactions

A severe and potentially life-threatening hypertensive reaction can occur in patients on MAOIs if they take alcoholic drinks containing significant amounts of tyramine. The details of this reaction, its mechanism, the names of the **older MAOIs** that interact, and the **newer reversible and selective MAOIs** that are unlikely to do so (see 'Table 30.1', (p.862)) are described in the monograph 'MAOIs + Tyramine-rich foods', p.876. A dose of 10 to 25 mg of **tyramine** is believed to be required before a serious rise in blood pressure takes place. 'Table 30.2', (above) summarises the reported tyramine-content of some drinks.[1-7] It can be used as a broad general guide when advising patients, but it cannot be an absolute guide because alcoholic drinks are the end-product of a biological fermentation process and no two batches are ever absolutely identical. For example there may be a 50-fold difference even between wines from the same grape stock.[5] There is no way of knowing for certain the **tyramine**-content of a particular drink without a detailed analysis.

(i) Ales, Beers and Lagers. Some **ales**, **beers** and **lagers** in 'social' amounts contain enough tyramine to reach the 10 to 25 mg threshold dosage, for example a litre (a little under two pints) of some samples of **Canadian ale or beer** (see 'Table 30.2', (p.875)). A man on **phenelzine** 60 mg daily developed a typical hypertensive reaction after drinking only 14 oz. (about 400 ml) of **Upper Canada lager beer on tap** (containing about 113 mg tyramine/litre).[8] **Alcohol-free beer** and **lager** may have a tyramine-content that is equal to ordinary beer and lager.[9,10] One patient on **tranylcypromine** suffered an acute cerebral haemorrhage after drinking a **de-alcoholised Irish beer**,[9] and hypertensive reactions occurred in three other patients after drinking no more than 375 ml (⅔ pint) of **alcohol-free beer or lager**[10] and a further patient developed a vascular headache after drinking 3 bottles of non-alcoholic beer.[11] A very extensive study of 79 different brands of **beer** (from Canada, England, France, Germany, Holland, Ireland, Scotland, USA) found that the tyramine content of the **bottled** and **canned beers** examined was generally too low to matter (less than 10 mg/litre), but four **beers** (all identified as being **on tap**) contained more than enough tyramine (27 to 113 mg/l) to cause a hypertensive reaction.[8] It was concluded in this report that the consumption of **canned** or **bottled beer**, including **de-alcoholised beer**, in moderation (fewer than four bottles, 1.5 litres in a four-hour period) was safe, but **ales, beers** and **lagers on tap** should be avoided.[8] However, the safety of all **de-alcoholised beers** is clearly still uncertain.

(ii) Spirits. **Gin, whisky, vodka** and **other spirits** do not contain significant amounts of tyramine because they are distilled, and the volumes drunk are relatively small.[7] There seem to be no reports of hypertensive reactions in patients taking MAOIs after drinking spirits and none would be expected.

(iii) Wines. In the context of adverse interactions with MAOIs, **Chianti** has developed a sinister reputation, because 400 ml of one early sample of **Italian Chianti wine** (see 'Table 30.2', (p.875)) contained enough **tyramine** to reach the 10 to 25 mg threshold for causing severe hypertensive reactions. However, it is claimed by the **Chianti** producers[12] and others[13] that the newer methods that have replaced the ancient 'governo alla toscana' process result in negligible amounts of **tyramine** in today's **Chianti**. This seems to be borne out by the results of analyses,[3,5-7] two of which failed to find any tyramine at all in some samples.[3,7] Some of the **other wines** listed in 'Table 30.2', (p.875) also contain **tyramine**, but patients would have to drink as much as 2 litres or more before reaching what is believed to be the threshold dosage. This suggests that small or moderate amounts (1 or 2 glasses) are unlikely to be hazardous.

(b) Hypotensive reactions

Some degree of hypotension can occur in patients on MAOIs and this may be exaggerated by the vasodilation and reduced cardiac output caused by alcohol. Patients should therefore be warned of the possibility of orthostatic hypotension and syncope if they drink.[14] They should be advised not to stand up too quickly, and to remain sitting or lying if they feel faint or begin to 'black out'.

(c) Other reactions

In addition to the hypertensive and hypotensive reactions described in (a) and (b), the possibility that the **alcohol**-induced deterioration in psychomotor skills (i.e. those associated with safe driving) might be increased by the MAOIs has also been studied. **Moclobemide** appears to have only a minor and clinically unimportant effect[15,16] and **brofaromine**[17,18] and **befloxatone**[19] do not interact with **alcohol**.

1. Horwitz D, Lovenberg W, Engelman K, Sjoerdsma A. Monoamine oxidase inhibitors, tyramine and cheese. *JAMA* (1964) 188, 1108–10.
2. Sen NP. Analysis and significance of tyramine in foods. *J Food Sci* (1969) 34, 22–6.
3. Korn A, Eichler HG, Fischbach R, Gasic S. Moclobemide, a new reversible MAO inhibitor – interaction with tyramine and tricyclic antidepressants in healthy volunteers and depressive patients. *Psychopharmacology (Berl)* (1986) 88, 153–7.
4. Zee JA, Simard RE, L'Heureux L, Tremblay J. Biogenic amines in wines. *Am J Enol Vitic* (1983) 34, 6–9.
5. Hannah P, Glover V, Sandler M. Tyramine in wine and beer. *Lancet* (1988) i, 879.
6. Da Prada M, Zürcher G, Wüthrich I, Haefely WE. On tyramine, food, beverages and the reversible MAO inhibitor moclobemide. *J Neural Transm* (1988) (Suppl 26), 31–56.
7. Shulman KI, Walker SE, MacKenzie S, Knowles S. Dietary restriction, tyramine, and use of monoamine oxidase inhibitors. *J Clin Psychopharmacol* (1989) 9, 397–402.
8. Tailor SAN, Shulman KI, Walker SE, Moss J, Gardner D. Hypertensive episode associated with phenelzine and tap beer—a reanalysis of the role of pressor amines in beer. *J Clin Psychopharmacol* (1994) 14, 5–14.
9. Murray JA, Walker JF, Doyle JS. Tyramine in alcohol-free beer. *Lancet* (1988) i, 1167–8.
10. Thakore J, Dinan TG, Kelleher M. Alcohol-free beer and the irreversible monoamine oxidase inhibitors. *Int Clin Psychopharmacol* (1992) 7, 59–60.
11. Draper R, Sandler M, Walker PL. Clinical curio: monoamine oxidase inhibitors and non-alcoholic beer. *BMJ* (1984) 289, 308.
12. Anon. Statement from the Consorzio Vino Chianti Classico, London. Undated (circa 1984).
13. Kalish G. Chianti myth. *The Wine Spectator, July 31st* (1981).
14. Anon. MAOIs — a patient's tale. *Pulse* (1981) December 5th, p 69.
15. Berlin I, Cournot A, Zimmer R, Pedarriosse A-M, Manfredi R, Molinier P, Puech AJ. Evaluation and comparison of the interaction between alcohol and moclobemide or clomipramine in healthy subjects. *Psychopharmacology (Berl)* (1990) 100, 40–5.
16. Tiller JWG. Antidepressants, alcohol and psychomotor performance. *Acta Psychiatr Scand* (1990) (Suppl 360), 13–17.
17. Gilburt SJA, Sutton JA, Hindmarch I. The pharmacodynamics of brofaromine, alone and combination with alcohol in young healthy volunteers. *Br J Clin Pharmacol* (1991) 33, 245P.
18. Kerr JS, Fairweather DB, Hindmarch I. The effects of brofaromine alone and in conjunction with alcohol on cognitive function, psychomotor performance, mood and sleep in healthy volunteers. *Hum Psychopharmacol* (1993) 8, 107–16.
19. Ramaekers JG, Muntjewerff ND, Uiterwijk MMC, van Veggel LMA, Patal A, Durrieu G, O'Hanlon JF. A study of the pharmacodynamic interaction between befloxatone and ethanol on performance and mood in healthy volunteers. *J Psychopharmacol* (1996) 10, 288–94.

MAOIs + Tyramine-rich foods

A potentially life-threatening hypertensive crisis can develop in patients on the older irreversible MAOIs (nialamide, pargyline, phenelzine, tranylcypromine, etc.) who eat tyramine-rich foods. Deaths from intracranial haemorrhage have occurred. Significant amounts of tyramine occur in some cheeses, yeast extracts (e.g. Marmite) and some types of salami. Caviar, pickled herrings, chicken and beef livers, soy sauce, avocados and other foods have been implicated in this interaction. Some of the selective MAOIs (brofaromine, moclobemide, selegiline, toloxatone) and linezolid interact to a lesser extent.

Clinical evidence

A rapid, serious, and potentially fatal rise in blood pressure can occur in patients on MAOIs who ingest tyramine-rich foods or drinks. A violent occipital headache, pounding heart, neck stiffness, flushing, sweating, nausea and vomiting may be experienced. One of the earliest recorded observations was in 1963 by a pharmacist called Rowe, who wrote to Blackwell[1] after seeing the reaction in his wife who was taking ***Parstelin*** (**tranylcypromine** with trifluoperazine).

"After **cheese on toast**; within a few minutes face flushed, felt very ill; head and heart pounded most violently, and perspiration was running down her neck. She vomited several times, and her condition looked so severe that I dashed over the road to consult her GP. He diagnosed 'palpitations' and agreed to call if the symptoms had not subsided in an hour. In fact the severity diminished and after about 3 hours she was normal, other than a severe headache — but 'not of the throbbing kind'. She described the early part of the attack 'as though her head must burst'."

Another example is that of a man on **pargyline** who, despite eating **sweitzer cheese** uneventfully on a number of previous occasions, experienced severe substernal chest pain and palpitations within 15 minutes of eating the **cheese**. His blood pressure rose to 200/114 mmHg. Two other patients experienced headache after eating **aged cheese**. Another had a severe nose-bleed and was found to have a blood pressure of 240/140 mmHg.[2]

There are too many reports of this interaction to list them here individually, but there are extensive reviews of this interaction published elsewhere.[3-5] Blackwell and his colleagues[1] discuss a series of early cases, and the reactions that led to this interaction becoming established, and another review lists 38 cases of haemorrhage and 21 deaths.[6] There have been many such reactions since. **Tranylcypromine**, **phenelzine**, **mebanazine** or **pargyline** have been implicated in this interaction with **cheese**, **yeast extracts**, **protein diet supplements**, **miso**, **pickled** and **soused herrings**, **tinned fish**, **chicken livers**, **caviar**, **soy sauce**, **avocados**, **peanuts**, **New Zealand prickly spinach**, **beef livers** and **Chianti wine**.

A phase I pharmacokinetic study in healthy subjects, given 625 mg of the weak MAOI **linezolid** twice daily, found that tyramine 100 mg raised the blood pressure by 30 mmHg but no significant rise was seen with doses of tyramine below 100 mg.[7]

Mechanism

Tyramine is formed in foods such as cheese by the bacterial degradation of milk and other proteins, firstly to tyrosine and other amino acids, and the subsequent decarboxylation of the tyrosine to tyramine. This interaction is therefore not associated with fresh foods, but with those which have been allowed to over-ripen or 'mature' in some way.[8] Tyramine is an indirectly-acting sympathomimetic amine, one of its actions being to release noradrenaline from the adrenergic neurones associated with blood vessels, which causes a rise in blood pressure by stimulating their constriction.[8]

Table 30.3 The tyramine content of some foods

Food	Tyramine content (micrograms/g)	Refs
Avocado	Higher in ripe fruit, 23, 0	1, 5, 11
Banana peel	52, 65	5, 13
Banana pulp	7, 0	5, 11, 13
Caviar (Iranian)	680	3
Cheese – see Table 30.4		
Country cured ham	not detectable	4
Farmer salami sausage	314	4
Genoa salami sausage	0 to 1237 (average 534)	4
Hard salami	0 to 392 (average 210)	4
Herring (pickled)	3030	6
Lebanon bologna	0 to 333 (average 224)	4
Liver-chicken	94 to 113	7
Liver-beef	0 to 274	8
Orange pulp	10	5
Pepperoni sausage	0 to 195 (average 39)	4
Plum, red	6	5
Sauerkraut	55	13
Soy sauce	0 to 878	12-14
Soya bean paste, fermented	206	14
Smoked landjaeger sausage	396	4
Summer sausage	184	4
Tomato	4, 0	5, 11
Thuringer cervelat	0 to 162	4
Yeast extracts		
Bovril	200 to 500	9
Bovril beef cubes	200 to 500	9
Bovril chicken cubes	50 to 200	9
Marmite (UK product)	500 to 3000	9, 11, 13
Oxo chicken cubes	130	10
Red Oxo cubes	250	10
Yoghurt	0 to 4	2, 11, 13

1. Generali JA, Hogan LC, McFarlane M, Schwab S, Hartman CR. Hypertensive crisis resulting from avocados and a MAO inhibitor. *Drug Intell Clin Pharm* (1981) 15, 904–6.
2. Horwitz D, Lovenberg W, Engelman K, Sjoerdsma A. Monoamine oxidase inhibitors, tyramine, and cheese. *JAMA* (1964) 188, 1108–10.
3. Isaac P, Mitchell B, Grahame-Smith DG. Monoamine-oxidase inhibitors and caviar. *Lancet* (1977) ii, 816.
4. Rice S, Eitenmiller RR, Koehler PE. Histamine and tyramine content of meat products. *J Milk Food Technol* (1975) 38, 256–8.
5. Udenfriend S, Lovenberg W, Sjoerdsma A. Physiologically active amines in common fruits and vegetables. *Arch Biochem* (1959) 85, 487.
6. Nuessle WF, Norman FC, Miller HE. Pickled herring and tranylcypromine reaction. *JAMA* (1965) 192, 726.
7. Heberg DL, Gordon MW, Glueck BC. Six cases of hypertensive crisis in patients on tranylcypromine after eating chicken livers. *Am J Psychiatry* (1966) 122, 933–5.
8. Boulton AA, Cookson B, Paulton R. Hypertensive crisis in a patient on MAOI antidepressants following a meal of beef liver. Can Med Assoc J (1970) 102, 1394–5.
9. Clarke A. (Bovril Ltd). Personal communication (1987).
10. Oxo Ltd. Personal communication (1987).
11. Da Prada M, Zurcher G, Wuthrich I, Haefely WE. On tyramine, food, beverages and the reversible MAO inhibitor moclobemide. *J Neural Transm* (1988) (Suppl 26), 31–56.
12. Lee S, Wing YK. MAOI and monosodium glutamate interaction. J Clin Psychiatry (1991) 52, 43.
13. Shulman KI, Walker SE, MacKenzine S, Knowles S. Dietary restriction, tyramine, and the use of monoamine oxidase inhibitors.
14. Da Prada M, Zürcher G. Tyramine content of preserved and fermented foods or condiments of Far Eastern cuisine. *Psychopharmacology (Berl)* (1992) 106, S32-S34.

Table 30.4 The tyramine content of some cheeses. This table should not be used to predict the probable tyramine content of a cheese. It is only intended to show the extent and the variation that can occur

Variety of cheese	Tyramine content (micrograms/g)	Refs
American processed	50	1
Argenti	188	3
Blue	31 to 997	2, 3, 6
Boursault	1116	2
Brick	194	3
Brie	3 to 473	1, 5, 6
Brie type (Danish)	0	2
Cambozola Blue Vein	18	6
Camembert	3 to 519	1–3, 5
Cheddar	8 to 1530	2, 5, 6
Cheshire	24 to 418	5
Cream cheese	undetectable (less than 0.2), 9	1, 6
Cottage cheese	undetectable (less than 0.2), 5	1, 5
Danish Blue	31 to 369	2, 6
d'Oka	158, 310	3
Double Gloucester	43	5
Edam	100, 214	3
Emmental	11 to 958	1, 5, 6
Feta	20, 76	5, 6
Gorgonzola	56 to 768	5, 6
Gouda	54, 95	3
Gouda type (Canadian)	20	2
Gourmandise	216	2
Gruyere	64 to 516	1, 4–6
Kashar	44 (mean of seven samples)	4
Liederkrantz	1226, 1683	3
Limburger	44 to 416	3, 5
Mozzarella	21 to 410	2, 5, 6
Munster	87 to 110	3, 5, 6
Mycella	1340	2
Parmesan	15 to 75	2, 6
Parmesan type (USA)	4, 5, 290	2
Provolone	38	2
Red Leicester	41	5
Ricotta	0	6
Romano	238	2
Roquefort	13 to 520	2, 3, 5
Stilton	466 to 2170	1, 2, 6
Swiss	50, 434	3
Tulum	208 (mean of seven samples)	4
White (Turkish)	17.5 (mean of seven samples)	4

1. Horwitz D, Lovenberg W, Engelman K, Sjoerdsma A. Monoamine oxidase inhibitors, tyramine and cheese. *JAMA* (1964) 188, 1108.
2. Sen NP. Analysis and significance of tyramine in foods. *J Food Sci* (1969) 34, 22–6.
3. Kosikowsky FV, Dahlberg AC. The tyramine content of cheese. *J Dairy Sci* (1948) 31, 293–303.
4. Kayaalp SO, Renda N, Kaymakcalan S, Özer A. Tyramine content of some cheeses. *Toxicol Appl Pharmacol* (1970) 16, 459–60.
5. Da Prada M, Z,rcher G, W,thrich I, Haefely WE. On tyramine, food, beverages and the reversible MAO inhibitor moclobemide. *J Neural Transm* (1988) (Suppl 26), 31–56.
6. Shulman KI, Walker SE, MacKenzine S, Knowles S. Dietary restriction, tyramine, and the use of monoamine oxidase inhibitors. *J Clin Psychopharmacol* (1989) 9, 397–402.

Normally any ingested tyramine is rapidly metabolised by the enzyme monoamine oxidase in the gut wall and liver before it escapes into general circulation. However, if the activity of the enzyme at these sites is inhibited (by the presence of an MAOI), any tyramine passes freely into circulation, causing not just a rise in blood pressure, but a highly exaggerated rise due to the release from the adrenergic neurones of the large amounts of noradrenaline that accumulate there during inhibition of MAO.[8] This final step in the interaction is identical to that which occurs with any other indirectly-acting sympathomimetic amine in the presence of an MAOI (see 'MAOIs + Sympathomimetics; Indirectly-acting', p.872).

Importance and management

An extremely well-documented, well-established, serious and potentially fatal hypertensive reaction can occur between the older, irreversible, non-selective MAOIs (see 'Table 30.1', (p.862)) and tyramine-rich foods. The incidence is uncertain, but estimates range from 2 to 20%[9,10] but may be lower.[9] Patients taking any of these MAOIs (**isocarboxazid**, **nialamide**, **phenelzine**, **pargyline**, **tranylcypromine**, and possibly also **iproniazid**) should not eat foods reported to contain substantial amounts of tyramine (see 'Table 30.3', (p.877) and 'Table 30.4', (p.877)). As little as 6 mg of tyramine can raise the blood pressure[11] and 10 to 25 mg would be expected to cause a serious hypertensive reaction.[11] Because tyramine levels vary so much it is impossible to guess the amount present in any food or drink. Old, over-ripe strong smelling cheeses with a salty, biting taste or those with characteristic holes due to fermentation should be avoided as they generally contain high levels of tyramine. Fresh cheeses made from pasteurised milk tend to have lower levels of tyramine.[12] The tyramine-content can even differ significantly within a single cheese between the centre with lowest levels of tyramine and the rind containing most.[12,13] There is no guarantee that patients who have uneventfully eaten these hazardous foodstuffs on many occasions may not eventually experience a full-scale hypertensive crisis, if all the many variables conspire together.[2]

A total prohibition should be imposed on the following: **cheese** and **yeast extracts** such as ***Marmite***, possibly ***Bovril*** and **pickled herrings** (see 'Table 30.3', (p.877)). Hypertensive reactions have been seen with **avocados**,[8] **beef livers**[14] and **chicken livers**,[15] **caviar**,[16] **pickled herrings**,[17] **soused herrings**,[18] **tinned fish**,[18] **peanuts**,[18] **soy sauce**,[19] **miso**,[20] **a powdered protein diet supplement** (***Ever-so-slim***),[21] **sour cream** in coffee,[18] and **New Zealand prickly spinach** (*Tetragonia tetragonoides*).[22] This is not a true spinach as found in the USA or Europe. A number of other foods should also be viewed with suspicion such as **sauerkraut**, **fermented bolognas** and **salamis**, **pepperoni**, and **summer sausage** because some of them may contain significant amounts of tyramine (see 'Table 30.3', (p.877)). Some preserved and fermented Far Eastern foods such as **soya beans**, **soya bean paste** and **soya bean condiments** also contain relatively high tyramine levels.[23] However, **yoghurt**, **fresh cream** and possibly **chocolate** are often viewed with unjustifiable suspicion. It also seems very doubtful if either **cream cheese** or **cottage cheese** represent a hazard. **Whole green bananas** contain up to 65 micrograms of tyramine per gram, but the **pulp** contains relatively small amounts. The need to plan a sensible and safe diet for those on MAOIs is clear, and over the years attempts have been made to produce simplified , practical diets for those taking MAOIs.[3,4,24]

The newer MAOIs are safer (in the context of interactions with tyramine-rich foods and drinks) than the older ones, because they are reversible and selective. Thus **brofaromine**, **moclobemide** and **toloxatone** selectively inhibit MAO-A, which leaves MAO-B still available to metabolise tyramine. This means that with **moclobemide** for example, tyramine only causes a modest rise in blood pressure if food is present.[25-28] Therefore the risk of a serious hypertensive reaction with **moclobemide**,[23,29-31] or any of the other reversible inhibitors of MAO-A, like **brofaromine**[32-34] and **toloxatone**[35,36] is very much reduced. It has been calculated that while taking **moclobemide** up to 65 mg of tyramine can be ingested before the capacity of the MAO to metabolise it becomes saturated.[37] Most patients therefore do not need to follow the special dietary restrictions required with the older irreversible MAOIs, but to be on the safe side the makers of **moclobemide** advise all patients to avoid large amounts of tyramine-rich foods, because a few individuals may be particularly sensitive to tyramine.[38] This warning would also seem appropriate for all of the other MAO-A inhibitors.

Selegiline specifically inhibits MAO-B, which leaves MAO-A still available to metabolise any tyramine. **Selegiline** 10 mg daily interacts only minimally with tyramine[39] so that the makers[40-42] say that no dietary restrictions are necessary with this dosage. However, higher doses of selegiline (30 mg daily) have been shown to increase the sensitivity to tyramine two to fourfold,[43] and a patient on only 20 mg daily is reported to have had a hypertensive reaction after eating macaroni and **cheese**.[44] A tyramine-free diet with larger **selegiline** dosages has therefore been advised.[43]

The makers of **linezolid** recommend that patients should avoid excessive amounts of **tyramine-rich food and drinks**[45,46] and should not consume more than 100 mg tyramine per meal.[46] The stringent dietary restrictions imposed on patients taking non-selective MAOIs are therefore unnecessary in those treated with linezolid, but the avoidance of very large amounts of tyramine is a prudent precaution. A severe hypertensive reaction crisis of the proportions possible with the antidepressant MAOIs seems unlikely.

Treatment

It is usual to recommend avoidance of the prohibited foods for 2 to 3 weeks after withdrawal of the MAOI to allow full recovery of the enzymes. Hypertensive reactions with MAOIs have been controlled by intravenous phentolamine, chlorpromazine, labetalol, or nifedipine. However, it is advisable to refer to current guidelines (or at least a relevant current text book) on the management of hypertensive crises for up to date advice.

1. Blackwell B, Marley E, Price J, Taylor D. Hypertensive interactions between monoamine oxidase inhibitors and foodstuffs. *Br J Psychiatry* (1967) 113, 349.
2. Hutchison JC. Toxic effects of monoamine-oxidase inhibitors. *Lancet* (1964) ii, 151.
3. Brown C, Taniguchi G, Yip K. The monoamine oxidase inhibitor-tyramine interaction. *J Clin Pharmacol* (1989) 29, 529–32.
4. Gardner DM, Shulman KI, Walker SE, Tailor SAN. The making of a user friendly MAOI diet. *J Clin Psychiatry* (1996) 57, 99–104.
5. Lippman SB, Nash K. Monoamine oxidase inhibitor update. Potential adverse food and drug interactions. *Drug Safety* (1990) 5, 195–204.
6. Sadusk JF. The physician and the Food and Drug Administration. *JAMA* (1964) 190, 907–9.
7. Antal EJ, Hendershot PE, Batts DH, Sheu W-P, Hopkins NK, Donaldson KM. Linezolid, a novel oxazolidinone antibiotic: assessment of monoamine oxidase inhibition using pressor response to oral tyramine. *J Clin Pharmacol* (2001) 41, 552–62.
8. Generali JA, Hogan LC, McFarlane M, Schwab S, Hartman CR. Hypertensive crisis resulting from avocados and a MAO inhibitor. *Drug Intell Clin Pharm* (1981) 15, 904–6.
9. Pickwell LD. Hypertensive reactions to monoamine oxidase inhibitors. *BMJ* (1964) i, 578–9.
10. Cooper AJ, Magnus RV, Rose MJ. A hypertensive syndrome with tranylcypromine medication. *Lancet* (1964) i, 527–9.
11. Horwitz D, Lovenberg W, Engelman K, Sjoerdsma A. Monoamine oxidase inhibitors, tyramine, and cheese. *JAMA* (1964) 188, 1108–10.
12. Da Prada M, Zürcher G, Wüthrich I, Haefely WE. On tyramine, food, beverages and the reversible MAO inhibitor moclobemide. *J Neural Transm* (1988) (Suppl 26), 31–56.
13. Price K, Smith SE. Cheese reaction and tyramine. *Lancet* (1971) i, 130–1.
14. Boulton AA, Cookson B, Paulton R. Hypertensive crisis in a patient on MAOI antidepressants following a meal of beef liver. *Can Med Assoc J* (1970) 102, 1394–5.
15. Hedberg DL, Gordon MW, Glueck BC. Six cases of hypertensive crisis in patients on tranylcypromine after eating chicken livers. *Am J Psychiatry* (1966) 122, 933–7.
16. Isaac P, Mitchell B, Grahame-Smith DG. Monoamine-oxidase inhibitors and caviar. *Lancet* (1977) ii, 816.
17. Nuessle WF, Norman FC, Miller HE. Pickled herring and tranylcypromine reaction. *JAMA* (1965) 192, 726–7.
18. Kelly D, Guirguis W, Frommer E, Mitchell-Heggs N, Sargant W. Treatment of phobic states with antidepressants. A retrospective study of 246 patients. *Br J Psychiatry* (1970) 116, 387–98.
19. Abrams JH, Schulman P, White WB. Successful treatment of a monoamine oxidase inhibitor-tyramine hypertensive emergency with intravenous labetalol. *N Engl J Med* (1985) 313, 52.
20. Mesmer RE. Don't mix miso with MAOIs. *JAMA* (1987) 258, 3515.
21. Zetin M, Plon L, DeAntonio M. MAOI reaction with powdered protein dietary supplement. *J Clin Psychiatry* (1987) 48, 499.
22. Comfort A. Hypertensive reaction to New Zealand prickly spinach in a woman taking phenelzine. *Lancet* (1981) ii, 472.
23. Da Prada M, Zürcher G. Tyramine content of preserved and fermented foods or condiments of Far Eastern cuisine. *Psychopharmacology (Berl)* (1992) 106, S32–S34.
24. Sullivan EA, Shulman KI. Diet and monoamine oxidase inhibitors: a re-examination. *Can J Psychiatry* (1984) 29, 707–11.
25. Korn A, Eichler HG, Fischbach R, Gasic S. Moclobemide, a new reversible MAO inhibitor – interaction with tyramine and tricyclic antidepressants in healthy volunteers and depressive patients. *Psychopharmacology (Berl)* (1986) 88, 153–7.
26. Korn A, Da Prada M, Raffesberg W, Gasic S, Eichler HG. Tyramine absorption and pressure response after MAO-inhibition with moclobemide. The Second Amine Oxidase Workshop, Uppsala, August 1986. *Pharmacol Toxicol* (1987) 60 (Suppl 1), 30.
27. Burgess CD, Mellsop GW. Interaction between moclobemide and oral tyramine in depressed patients. *Fundam Clin Pharmacol* (1989) 3, 47–52.
28. Audebert C, Blin O, Monjanel-Mouterde S, Auquier P, Pedarriosse AM, Dingemanse J, Durand A, Cano JP. Influence of food on the tyramine pressor effect during chronic moclobemide treatment of healthy volunteers. *Eur J Clin Pharmacol* (1992) 43, 507–12.
29. Berlin I, Zimmer R, Cournot A, Payan C, Pedarriosse AM, Puech AJ. Determination and comparison of the pressor effect of tyramine during long-term moclobemide and tranylcypromine treatment in healthy volunteers. *Clin Pharmacol Ther* (1989) 46, 344–51.
30. Simpson GM, Gratz SS. Comparison of the pressor effect of tyramine after treatment with phenelzine and moclobemide in healthy male volunteers. *Clin Pharmacol Ther* (1992) 52, 286–91.
31. Warrington SJ, Turner P, Mant TGK, Morrison P, Haywood G, Glover V, Goodwin BL, Sandler M, St John-Smith P, McClelland GR. Clinical pharmacology of moclobemide, a new reversible monoamine oxidase inhibitor. *J Psychopharmacol* (1991) 5, 82–91.
32. Bieck PR, Firkusny L, Schick C, Antonin K-H, Nilsson E, Schulz R, Schwenk M, Wollmann H. Monoamine oxidase inhibition by phenelzine and brofaromine in healthy volunteers. *Clin Pharmacol Ther* (1989) 45, 260–9.
33. Bieck PR, Antonin KH. Tyramine potentiation during treatment with MAO inhibitors: brofaromine and moclobemide vs irreversible inhibitors. *J Neural Transm* (1989) (Suppl 28), 21–31.
34. Bieck PR, Antonin K-H, Schmidt E. Clinical pharmacology of reversible monoamine oxidase-A inhibitors. *Clin Neuropharmacol* (1993) 16 (Suppl 2), S34–S41.

35. Tipton KF, Dostert P, Strolin Benedetti M, eds. Monoamine Oxidase and Disease: Prospects for therapy with reversible inhibitors. London: Academic Press; 1984 p. 429–41.
36. Provost J-C, Funck-Brentano C, Rovei V, D'Estanque J, Ego D, Jaillon P. Pharmacokinetic and pharmacodynamic interaction between toloxatone, a new reversible monoamine oxidase-A inhibitor, and oral tyramine in healthy subjects. *Clin Pharmacol Ther* (1992) 52, 384–93.
37. Karet FE, Dickerson JEC, Brown J, Brown MJ. Bovril and moclobemide: a novel therapeutic strategy for central autonomic failure. *Lancet* (1994) 344, 1263–5.
38. Manerix (Moclobemide). Roche Products Ltd. UK Summary of product characteristics, May 2004.
39. Elsworth JD, Glover V, Reynolds GP, Sandler M, Lees AJ, Phuapradit P, Shaw KM, Stern GM, Kumar P. Deprenyl administration in man: a selective monoamine oxidase B inhibitor without the 'cheese effect'. *Psychopharmacology (Berl)* (1978) 57, 33–8.
40. Eldepryl (Selegiline hydrochloride). Orion Pharma (UK) Ltd. UK Summary of product characteristics, October 2003.
41. Zelapar (Selegiline hydrochloride). Zeneus Pharma Ltd. UK Summary of product characteristics, February 2003.
42. Eldepryl (Selegiline hydrochloride). Somerset Pharmaceuticals Inc. US Prescribing information, July 1998.
43. Prasad A, Glover V, Goodwin BL, Sandler M, Signy M, Smith SE. Enhanced pressor sensitivity to oral tyramine challenge following high dose selegiline treatment. *Psychopharmacology (Berl)* (1988) 95, 540–3.
44. McGrath PJ, Stewart JW, Quitkin FM. A possible l-deprenyl induced hypertensive reaction. *J Clin Psychopharmacol* (1989) 9, 310–11.
45. Zyvox (Linezolid). Pharmacia Ltd. UK Summary of product characteristics, November 2004.
46. Zyvox (Linezolid). Pharmacia & Upjohn. US Prescribing information, September 2004.

Moclobemide + Cimetidine

Cimetidine increases the plasma levels of moclobemide. Moclobemide dosage reductions are recommended.

Clinical evidence, mechanism, importance and management

After taking cimetidine 200 mg five times daily for two weeks the maximum plasma levels of a single 100-mg dose of moclobemide in 8 healthy subjects was increased by 39% and the clearance was reduced by 52%.[1] The probable reason is that the cimetidine (a well-recognised enzyme inhibitor) reduces the first-pass metabolism of the moclobemide.

It has been recommended that if moclobemide is added to treatment with cimetidine it should be started at the lowest therapeutic dose, and titrated as required. If cimetidine is added to treatment with moclobemide, the dosage of the latter should initially be reduced by 50% and later adjusted as necessary.[2]

There appears to be nothing to suggest that an adverse interaction occurs with any other MAOI and cimetidine.

1. Schoerlin M-P, Mayersohn M, Hoevels B, Eggers H, Dellenbach M, Pfefen J-P. Cimetidine alters the disposition kinetics of the monoamine oxidase-A inhibitor moclobemide. *Clin Pharmacol Ther* (1991) 49, 32–8.
2. Amrein R, Güntert TW, Dingemanse J, Lorscheid T, Stabl M, Schmid-Burgk W. Interactions of moclobemide with concomitantly administered medication: evidence from pharmacological and clinical studies. *Psychopharmacology (Berl)* (1992) 106, S24–S31.

Moclobemide + Miscellaneous

No serious adverse interactions were seen in patients and subjects given moclobemide with the drugs named below, and no special precautions would seem to be necessary if they are used with moclobemide.

Clinical evidence, mechanism, importance and management

There was no evidence of any adverse interaction when moclobemide 150 to 675 mg daily was given for 3 to 52 weeks to 50 patients on **lithium**.[1]

A study in 24 healthy subjects found that moclobemide 150 mg three times daily for 7 days had no effect on the absorption or disposition of **ibuprofen**, and the amount of **ibuprofen**-induced blood loss was unaffected.[2]

Studies in healthy subjects found that moclobemide 200 mg three times daily for 2 weeks increased the hypotensive effect of **metoprolol** (systolic 10 to 15 mmHg lower, diastolic 5 to 10 mmHg lower), but no comparable effects were seen when moclobemide was given with **hydrochlorothiazide** or **nifedipine**. No orthostatic hypotension occurred with any of the drug combinations.[1]

A study in 14 patients with decompensated heart failure found that moclobemide 100 mg three times daily for 8 days caused a non-significant 14% fall (from 0.99 to 0.85 nanograms/ml) in their serum **beta-acetyldigoxin** levels. No adverse effects attributable to an interaction were seen.[1]

A study in 7 women taking combined **oral contraceptives** found no evidence of any significant alterations in estradiol, progesterone, follicle stimulating hormone or luteinising hormone levels while taking moclobemide 200 mg three times daily for one cycle. No serious adverse reactions occurred. It was considered that the efficacy of the **oral contraceptives** is likely to be maintained during concurrent use.[1]

No serious adverse effects were seen in 110 patients given moclobemide 150 to 400 mg daily with **acepromazine**, **aceprometazine**, **alimemazine** (**trimeprazine**), **bromperidol**, **chlorpromazine**, **chlorprothixene**, **clothiapine**, **clozapine**, **cyamemazine**, **flupenthixol**, **fluphenazine**, **fluspirilene**, **haloperidol**, **levomepromazine** (**methotrimeprazine**), **penfluridol**, **pipamperone**, **prothipendyl**, **sulpiride**, **thioridazine** or **zuclopenthixol** (**clopenthixol**). There was however some evidence that hypotension, tachycardia, sleepiness, tremor and constipation were more common.[1]

No serious adverse effects were reported in extensive clinical trials of moclobemide when used in patients taking **antiparkinsonian drugs**, **antibacterials**, **anticonvulsants**, **hormones** and others, but none was specifically named.[1]

1. Amrein R, Güntert TW, Dingemanse J, Lorscheid T, Stabl M, Schmid-Burgk W. Interactions of moclobemide with concomitantly administered medication: evidence from pharmacological and clinical studies. *Psychopharmacology (Berl)* (1992) 106, S24–S31.
2. Güntert TW, Schmitt M, Dingemanse J, Jonkman JHG. Influence of moclobemide on ibuprofen-induced faecal blood loss. *Psychopharmacology (Berl)* (1992) 106, S40–S42.

31

Neuromuscular blockers and anaesthetics

This section is concerned with the interactions where the effects of neuromuscular blocking drugs and anaesthetics, both general and local, are affected by the presence of other drugs. Where the neuromuscular blocking drugs or anaesthetics are responsible for an interaction they are dealt with under the heading of the drug affected. Barbiturates used as anaesthetics (e.g. thiopental) are largely covered here, whereas those used predominantly for their antiepileptic or sedative properties (e.g. phenobarbital or secobarbital) are dealt with in the appropriate sections. See the Index for a full listing.

The modes of action of the two types of neuromuscular blocker are discussed in the monograph 'Neuromuscular blockers + Neuromuscular blockers', p.913. The different types of blocker are listed in 'Table 31.1'.

The general and local anaesthetics mentioned in this section are listed in 'Table 31.2', (p.881). Some of them are also used as antiarrhythmic agents and these are dealt with in 'Antiarrhythmics', (p.156).

Table 31.1 Neuromuscular blockers

Generic names	*Proprietary names*
Competitive (Non-depolarising) blockers – Aminosteroid type	
Pancuronium bromide	Bromurex, Curon-B, Pancuron, Pancurox, Panlem, Pavulon
Pipecuronium bromide	Arduan, Arpilon
Rapacuronium	
Rocuronium	Esmeron, Zemuron
Vecuronium bromide	Curlem, Norcuron
Competitive (Non-depolarising) blockers – Benzylisoquinolinium type	
Alcuronium chloride	Alloferin, Alloferine
Atracurium besilate	Atracur, Faulcurium, Ifacur, Mycurium, Relatrac, Sitrac, Trablok, Tracrium
Cisatracurium besilate	Nimbex, Nimbium
Doxacurium chloride	Nuromax
Gallamine triethiodide	Flaxedil, Miowas G
Metocurine	
Mivacurium	Mivacron, Novacrium
Tubocurarine chloride (*d*-Tubocurarine chloride)	Curarine, Tubarine
Depolarising blockers	
Suxamethonium bromide/chloride (Succinylcholine)	Anectine, Celocurin, Celocurine, Curacit, Ethicholine, Lysthenon, Midarine, Mioflex, Myoplegine, Myotenlis, Pantolax, Quelicin, Scoline, Succicuran, Succinolin, Succinyl, Sukolin, Uxicolin

Table 31.2 Anaesthetics

Generic names	*Proprietary names*
General anaesthetics	
Inhalation	
Cyclopropane	
Diethyl ether (Ether)	
Desflurane	Sulorane, Suprane
Enflurane	Alyrane, Efrane, Enfluthane, Enfran, Ethrane
Halothane	Fluothane
Isoflurane	AErrane, Forane, Forene, Forthane, Isoflurane, Isothane, Sofloran
Methoxyflurane	Brevimytal, Brevital, Brietal
Nitrous oxide	Entonox (N_2O/O_2)
Sevoflurane	Sevorane, Ultane
Trichloroethylene	
Parenteral	
Alphaxalone/Alphadolone	
Etomidate	Amidate, Hypnomidate, Radenarcon
Ketamine	Brevinaze, Calypsol, Ketalar, Ketalin, Ketanest, Ketolar, Velonarcon
Methohexital	
Propofol	Ansiven, Cryotol, Diprivan, Diprofol, Disoprivan, Fresofol, Ivofol, Klimofol, Pofol, Pronest, Propocam, Recofol
Sodium oxybate	Alcover, Gamma-OH, Somsanit, Xyrem
Thiopental (Thiopentone)	Farmotal, Intraval, Nesdonal, Pentothal, Sodipental, Tiobarbital, Trapanal
Local anaesthetics	
Articaine	Alfacaina, Alphacaine, Articaina C/E, Astracaine, Cartidont, Citocartin, Meganest, Predesic, Primacaine, Rudocaine, Septanest, Septocaine, Ubistesin, Ultracain, Ultracain Dental, Ultracain D-S, Ultracain D-Suprarenin, Ultracain hyperbar
Bupivacaine	Bicain, Bucain, Bupiforan, Bupyl, Buvacaina, Carbostesin, Dolanaest, Duracain, Kamacaine, Macaine, Marcain, Marcaina, Marcaine, Neocaina, Sensorcaine, Svedocain Sin Vasoconstr
Chloroprocaine	Ivracain, Nesacain, Nesacaine
Etidocaine	
Levobupivacaine	
Lidocaine (Lignocaine)	Basicaina, Curadent, Dentipatch, Dilocaine, Docaine, Duo-Trach Kit, Dynexan, Ecocain, ELA-Max, Esracain, Gelicain, Laryng-O-Jet, Licain, Lident Adrenalina, Lident Andrenor, Lidesthesin, Lidocation, Lidocaton, Lidodan, Lidoject, Lidonostrum, Lidosen, Lidrian, Lignospan, Lignostab-A, Lincaina, Linisol, Llorentecaina Noradrenal, Luan, Mesocaine, Neo-Lidocaton, Neo-Sinedol, Neo-Xylestesin, Nervocaine, Nurocain, Octocaine, Odontalg, Ortodermina, Peterkaien, Pisacaina, Rapidocaine, Remicaine, Rowo-629, Sagittaproct, Sedagul, Xilo-Mynol, Xilonibsa, Xylanaest, Xylesine, Xylestesin, Xylocain, Xylocaina, Xylocaine, Xylocitin, Xyloneural, Xylonor, Xylotox
Mepivacaine	Carbocain, Carbocaina, Carbocaine, Carbocaine with Neo-Cobefrin, Isocaine, Isogaine, Meaverin, Meaverin hyperbar, Mecain, Mepicain, Mepicaton, Mepident, Mepiforan, Mepihexal, Mepinaest, Mepivastesin, Mepi-Mynol, Mepyl, Optocain, Pericaina, Polocaine, Scandicain, Scandicaine, Scandinibsa, Scandinor, Scandonest, Tevacaine
Prilocaine	Citanest, Citanest Dental, Citanest Octapresin, Citocaina, Eutecaina, Xylonest
Procaine	Anestesia Loc Braun C/A, Aqucilina, Atralcilina, Cibramicina, Cilicaine Syringe, Crysticillin, Farmaproina, Geroaslan H3, Gerovital H3, Hewedolor Procain, Jenacillin O, Lenident, Lophakomp-Procain N, Novanaest, Novocain, Novocillin, Procaneural, Procillin, Sodilin, Wycillin
Propoxycaine	
Ropivacaine	Narop, Naropeine, Naropin, Naropina
Surface anaesthetics	
Cocaine	

Anaesthetics, general + Alcohol

Those who regularly drink alcohol may need more thiopental or propofol than those who do not. It is also probably unsafe to drink for several hours following anaesthesia because of the combined central nervous depressant effects.

Clinical evidence, mechanism, importance and management

A study in 532 healthy patients, aged from 20 to over 80 years, found that those who normally drank alcohol (more than 40 g weekly, roughly 400 ml of wine) needed more **thiopental** to achieve anaesthesia than non-drinkers. After adjusting for differences in age and weight distribution, men who were heavy drinkers (more than 40 g alcohol daily) needed 33% more **thiopental** for induction than non-drinkers, and women drinkers needed 44% more.[1] Chronic alcohol intake is known to increase barbiturate metabolism by cytochrome P450 enzymes.[2]

Another study found that 26 chronic alcoholics (drinkers of about 40 g of alcohol daily, with no evidence of liver impairment) needed about one-third more **propofol** to induce anaesthesia than another 20 patients who only drank socially, however, there was great interindividual variation in the alcoholic group.[3]

When 12 healthy subjects were given 0.7 g/kg alcohol 4 hours after receiving 5 mg/kg of 2.5% **thiopental**, body sway and lightheadedness were accentuated.[4] This suggests that an interaction may occur if an ambulatory patient drinks alcohol within 4 hours of receiving an induction dose of **thiopental**. Patients should be cautioned not to drink alcohol following anaesthesia and surgery. The UK makers of propofol advise avoiding alcohol for 8 hours before and after the use of any anaesthetic.[5]

The maker notes that the metabolism of **sevoflurane** may be increased by known inducers of the cytochrome P450 isoenzyme CYP2E1 including alcohol and isoniazid. See 'Anaesthetics, general + Isoniazid', p.886. This may increase the risk of kidney damage because of an increase in plasma fluoride, although no cases appear to have been reported.

1. Dundee JW, Milligan KR. Induction dose of thiopentone: the effect of alcohol intake. *Br J Clin Pharmacol* (1989) 27, 693P–694P.
2. Weathermon R, Crabb DW. Alcohol and medication interactions. *Alcohol Res Health* (1999) 23, 40–54.
3. Fassoulaki A, Farinotti R, Servin F, Desmonts JM. Chronic alcoholism increases the induction dose of propofol in humans. *Anesth Analg* (1993) 77, 553–6.
4. Lichtor JL, Zacny JP, Coalson DW, Flemming DC, Uitvlugt A, Apfelbaum JL, Lane BS, Thisted RA. The interaction between alcohol and the residual effects of thiopental anesthesia. *Anesthesiology* (1993) 79, 28–35.
5. Diprivan (Propofol). AstraZeneca UK Ltd. UK Summary of product characteristics, February 2004.

Anaesthetics, general + Anaesthetics, general

The required dose of propofol will be lower if it is given with nitrous oxide or halogenated anaesthetics and synergy has been reported between propofol and etomidate. The dose requirement of inhalational anaesthetics and barbiturate anaesthetics is reduced by nitrous oxide. The effect of ketamine may be prolonged by barbiturate anaesthetics. An isolated report described myoclonic seizures in a man anaesthetised with *Alfathesin* (alfaxalone/alfadolone) when additionally given enflurane.

Clinical evidence, mechanism, importance and management

In general, the combined effects of general anaesthetics are at least additive. Concurrent administration of either **halothane** or **isoflurane** increased serum concentrations of **propofol** by about 20% during maintenance of general anaesthesia in 20 healthy patients.[1] The US maker of **propofol** notes that **inhalational anaesthetics** such as these would be expected to increase the effects of **propofol**. The maker also states that the dosage of **propofol** required may be reduced if given with supplemental **nitrous oxide**.[2]

Nitrous oxide usually reduces the MAC of **inhalational anaesthetics** in a simple additive manner; an inspired concentration of 60 to 70% nitrous oxide is commonly used with volatile anaesthetics.[3] Similarly, concurrent administration of **nitrous oxide** reduces the dose of intravenous **barbiturate anaesthetics** required for anaesthesia.[4]

Synergy has been reported between **propofol** and **etomidate**–patients given induction doses of either **etomidate** or **propofol** alone required about a 15% higher dose than those given half etomidate and half propofol in sequence.[5]

For reports of enhanced sedation when midazolam is given with **propofol, thiopental** or other anaesthetics, see 'Anaesthetics, general + Benzodiazepines', p.884.

The makers of **ketamine** note that **barbiturates** may prolong the effect of **ketamine** and delay recovery.[6,7]

Myoclonic activity occurred in a healthy 23-year-old man after anaesthesia was induced with 2.5 ml of ***Alfathesin*** (**alfaxalone/alfadolone**) given intravenously over 2 minutes, and then maintained with 2% **enflurane** in oxygen. The myoclonic activity subsided after stopping the **enflurane**, and anaesthesia was maintained with **nitrous oxide/oxygen**. The myoclonus recurred when the **enflurane** was restarted, but it resolved when the **enflurane** was replaced with **halothane**.[8] Since both *Alfathesin* and **enflurane** can cause CNS excitation, it seemed possible that these effects might be additive, and it was suggested that concurrent use should be avoided, particularly in patients with known convulsive disorders.[8] *Alfathesin* has, however, been withdrawn from general use.

1. Grundmann U, Ziehmer M, Kreienmeyer J, Larsen R, Altmayer P. Propofol and volatile anaesthetics. *Br J Anaesth* (1994) 72 (Suppl 1) 88.
2. Diprivan (Propofol). AstraZeneca. US Prescribing information, July 2004.
3. Dale O. Drug interactions in anaesthesia: focus on desflurane and sevoflurane. *Baillieres Clin Anaesthesiol* (1995) 9, 105–17.
4. Aitkenhead AR, ed. Textbook of anaesthesia. 4th ed. Edinburgh: Churchill Livingstone; 2001 P. 172–4
5. Drummond GB, Cairns DT. Do propofol and etomidate interact kinetically during induction of anaesthesia? *Br J Anaesth* (1994) 73, 272P.
6. Ketalar (Ketamine). Pfizer Ltd. UK Summary of product characteristics, August 2003.
7. Ketalar (Ketamine). Monarch Pharmaceuticals. US Prescribing information, April 2004.
8. Hudson R, Ethans CT. Alfathesin and enflurane: synergistic central nervous system excitation? *Can Anaesth Soc J* (1981) 28, 55–6.

Anaesthetics, general + Anaesthetics, local

An isolated report describes convulsions associated with the use of propofol with topical cocaine. Cocaine abuse may also increase the risk of cardiovascular complications during inhalational anaesthesia. The dosage of propofol may need to be reduced after administration of bupivacaine or lidocaine (e.g. during regional anaesthetic techniques). Similarly, epidural lidocaine reduces sevoflurane requirements, and is likely to have the same effect on other inhalational anaesthetics.

Clinical evidence, mechanism, importance and management

(a) Cocaine

A patient with no history of epilepsy, undergoing septorhinoplasty for cosmetic reasons, was premedicated with papaveretum and hyoscine, and intubated after **propofol** and suxamethonium (succinylcholine) were given. Anaesthesia was maintained with **nitrous oxide/oxygen** and 2% **isoflurane**. During anaesthesia a paste containing 10% **cocaine** was applied to the nasal mucosa. During recovery the patient experienced a dystonic reaction, which developed into a generalised convulsion. The authors of the report suggest that a possible interaction between the **propofol** and **cocaine** might have been responsible, although they also suggest that the convulsions may have been an adverse effect of the propofol.[1]

Reviews of the anaesthetic implications of illicit drug use have stated that anaesthetists should be aware of the medical complications of cocaine abuse such as myocardial ischaemia, hypertension and tachycardia due to sympathetic nervous system stimulation.[2,3] It was suggested that concurrent use of **cocaine** and **inhalational anaesthetics**, such as **halothane**, that are known to significantly sensitise the myocardium to circulating catecholamines, should be avoided, and that other halogenated agents should be used with caution.[2,3] Theoretically, **isoflurane** would be a better choice of inhalational agent since it has less cardiovascular effects.[2] **Ketamine** should also be avoided because of its sympathomimetic effects. **Nitrous oxide**, **thiopental** and fentanyl were considered to be useful agents in general anaesthesia for patients who regularly abuse **cocaine**.[2,3]

(b) Lidocaine or Bupivacaine

A double-blind, randomised study of 17 patients requiring ventilatory support demonstrated that hourly laryngotracheal instillation of 5 ml of 1% lidocaine significantly reduced the dose of **propofol** required to maintain adequate sedation (overall reduction of 50%) when compared with pre-study values.[4]

In a placebo-controlled, double-blind study of 90 patients undergoing minor gynaecological surgery, intramuscular administration of 4% lidocaine (1 to 3 mg/kg) 10 minutes before induction of anaesthesia or 0.5% bupivacaine (500 to 1000 micrograms/kg) 30 minutes before induction of anaesthesia, significantly enhanced the hypnotic effect of intravenous **propofol** in a dose-dependent manner. Only the lowest doses of lidocaine and bupivacaine tested (500 and 250 micrograms/kg, respectively) lacked a significant effect on the hypnotic dose of **propofol**. The highest doses of lidocaine and bupivacaine (3 and 1 mg/kg, respectively) reduced the hypnotic requirements for **propofol** by 34.4% and 39.6%, respectively. The dose of **propofol** should therefore be modified after intramuscular administration of lidocaine or bupivacaine.[5] The UK maker of propofol also notes that required doses may be lower when general anaesthesia is used in association with regional anaesthetic techniques.[6]

A randomised, double-blind, placebo-controlled study involving 44 patients demonstrated that lidocaine epidural anaesthesia (15 ml of 2% plain lidocaine) reduced the MAC of **sevoflurane** required for general anaesthesia by approximately 50% (from 1.18 to 0.52%). This implies that a markedly lesser amount of **inhalational anaesthetic** provides adequate anaesthesia during combined epidural-general anaesthesia than for general anaesthesia alone.[7]

(c) Sympathomimetics in local anaesthetics

Note that sympathomimetics such as adrenaline (epinephrine) used with local anaesthetics may interact with inhalational anaesthetics such as halothane to increase the risk of arrhythmias, although lidocaine may reduce this risk, see 'Anaesthetics, general + Sympathomimetics', p.891.

1. Hendley BJ. Convulsions after cocaine and propofol. *Anaesthesia* (1990) 45, 788–9.
2. Voigt L. Anesthetic management of the cocaine abuse patient. *J Am Assoc Nurse Anesth* (1995) 63, 438–43.
3. Culver JL, Walker JR. Anesthetic implications of illicit drug use. *J Perianesth Nurs* (1999) 14, 82–90.
4. Mallick A, Smith SN, Bodenham AR. Local anaesthesia to the airway reduces sedation requirements in patients undergoing artificial ventilation. *Br J Anaesth* (1996) 77, 731–4.
5. Ben-Shlomo I, Tverskoy M, Fleyshman G, Cherniavsky G. Hypnotic effect of i.v. propofol is enhanced by i.m. administration of either lignocaine or bupivacaine. *Br J Anaesth* (1997) 78, 375–7.
6. Diprivan (Propofol). AstraZeneca UK Ltd. UK Summary of product characteristics, February 2004.
7. Hodgson PS, Liu SS, Gras TW. Does epidural anesthesia have general anesthetic effects? *Anesthesiology* (1999) 91, 1687–92.

Anaesthetics, general + Anticholinesterases

Inhalation anaesthetics may impair the efficacy of anticholinesterases in reversing neuromuscular blockade. Physostigmine pretreatment increased propofol requirements by 20% in one study.

Clinical evidence, mechanism, importance and management

(a) Inhalational anaesthetics

Inhalational anaesthetics can impair **neostigmine** reversal of neuromuscular blockade. In one study, the reversal of blockade by pancuronium with **neostigmine** was prolonged when using **enflurane** compared with fentanyl or **halothane**.[1] Another study demonstrated that the reversal of **vecuronium** block with **neostigmine** 40 micrograms/kg was more dependent on the concentration of **sevoflurane** than the degree of block present. At the lowest concentration of **sevoflurane** (0.2 MAC), adequate reversal was obtained in all patients within 15 minutes, but with increasing concentrations (up to 1.2 MAC) satisfactory restoration of neuromuscular function was not achieved within 15 minutes, probably because of a greater contribution of **sevoflurane** to the degree of block.[2] Note that inhalation anaesthetics potentiate neuromuscular blockers, see 'Anaesthetics, general + Neuromuscular blockers', p.888.

(b) Intravenous anaesthetics

A study of 40 patients found that **physostigmine** pre-treatment (2 mg intravenously 5 minutes before induction) increased **propofol** requirements by 20%.[3]

1. Delisle S, Bevan DR. Impaired neostigmine antagonism of pancuronium during enflurane anaesthesia in man. *Br J Anaesth* (1982) 54, 441–5.
2. Morita T, Kurosaki D, Tsukagoshi H, Shimada H, Sato H, Goto F. Factors affecting neostigmine reversal of vecuronium block during sevoflurane anaesthesia. *Anaesthesia* (1997) 52, 538–43.
3. Fassoulaki A, Sarantopoulos C, Derveniotis C. Physostigmine increases the dose of propofol required to induce anaesthesia. *Can J Anaesth* (1997) 44, 1148–51.

Anaesthetics, general + Antiemetics

Metoclopramide pre-treatment reduces the dosage requirements of propofol and thiopental. Droperidol acts similarly with thiopental. Ondansetron does not appear to interact with thiopental.

Clinical evidence

(a) Metoclopramide or Droperidol

In a randomised, placebo-controlled, double-blind study of 60 surgical patients, half of whom were given metoclopramide 150 micrograms/kg 5 minutes before induction, it was found that the induction dose of **propofol** was reduced by 24% in the group given metoclopramide.[1] Similar results were seen in another study of 21 patients pre-treated with metoclopramide.[2] The **propofol** requirements were reduced by 24.5% with metoclopramide 10 mg and by 41.2% with 15 mg. In a randomised, double-blind, placebo-controlled study in 96 women patients, both metoclopramide and droperidol reduced the amount of **thiopental** needed to induce anaesthesia by about 45%.[3]

(b) Ondansetron

Ondansetron 100 or 200 micrograms/kg administered intravenously 5 minutes before **thiopental** induction did not influence the hypnotic requirements of the **thiopental**, in a double-blind, placebo-controlled, randomised study of 168 female patients.[4]

Mechanism

The exact mechanism by which metoclopramide reduces propofol or thiopental dose requirements is unclear, but it appears to involve the blockade of dopamine (D_2) receptors.

Importance and management

Although the evidence is limited these interactions with metoclopramide/thiopental, metoclopramide/propofol and droperidol/thiopental would appear to be established. Droperidol has not been studied with propofol, but, on the basis of other interactions it would be expected to behave like metoclopramide. When patients are pretreated with either metoclopramide or droperidol, be alert for the need to use less propofol and thiopental to induce anaesthesia. Ondansetron appears not to interact.

1. Page VJ, Chhipa JH. Metoclopramide reduces the induction dose of propofol. *Acta Anaesthesiol Scand* (1997) 41, 256–9.
2. Santiveri X, Castillo J, Buil JA, Escolano F, Castaño J. Efectos de la metoclopramida sobre las dosis hipnóticas de propofol. *Rev Esp Anestesiol Reanim* (1996) 43, 297–8.
3. Mehta D, Bradley EL, Kissin I. Metoclopramide decreases thiopental hypnotic requirements. *Anesth Analg* (1993) 77, 784–7.
4. Kostopanagiotou G, Pouriezis T, Theodoraki K, Kottis G, Andreadou I, Smyrniotis V, Papadimitriou L. Influence of ondansetron on thiopental hypnotic requirements. *J Clin Pharmacol* (1998) 38, 825–9.

Anaesthetics, general + Antihypertensives

Concurrent use of general anaesthetics and antihypertensives generally need not be avoided but it should be recognised that the normal homoeostatic responses of the cardiovascular system will be impaired (see also 'Anaesthetics, general + Beta-blockers', p.885, and 'Anaesthetics, general + Calcium channel blockers', p.885). Marked hypotension has been seen in patients on ACE inhibitors during anaesthetic induction. Profound hypotension may occur in patients on alfuzosin during general anaesthesia.

Clinical evidence, mechanism, importance and management

The antihypertensive drugs differ in the way they act, but they all interfere with the normal homoeostatic mechanisms that control blood pressure and, as a result, the reaction of the cardiovascular system during anaesthesia to fluid and blood losses, body positioning, etc. is impaired to some extent. For example, enhanced hypotension was seen in a study of the calcium channel blocker **nimodipine** during general anaesthesia (see 'Anaesthetics, general + Calcium channel blockers', p.885), and marked hypotension has also been seen with ACE inhibitors in this setting (see below). This instability of the cardiovascular system needs to be recognised and allowed for, but it is widely accepted that antihypertensive treatment should normally be continued.[1-3] In some cases there is a real risk in stopping, for example a hypertensive rebound can occur if **clonidine** or the **beta-blockers** are suddenly withdrawn. See also 'Anaesthetics, general + Beta-blockers', p.885.

(a) ACE inhibitors

Severe and unexpected hypotension has been seen during anaesthetic induction in patients on **captopril**.[4] Marked hypotension (systolic BP 75 mmHg) occurred in a 42-year-old man on **enalapril** when anaesthetised with **propofol**, which did not respond to surgical stimulation. He responded slowly to the infusion of one litre of Hartmann's solution.[5] In a randomised clinical study, the incidence of hypotension during anaesthetic induction was higher in patients who had taken **captopril** or **enalapril** on the day of surgery than in those who had stopped these drugs 12 or 24 hours prior to surgery.[6] Another experimental study found that a single dose of **captopril** at induction of anaesthesia caused a small reduction in cerebral blood flow when compared with control patients or patients given metoprolol.[7] Although information is limited, there would seem to be the need to take particular care with patients on ACE inhibitors, but there is insufficient evidence to generally recommend discontinuing ACE inhibitors before surgery. One recommendation is that intravenous fluids should be given to all patients on ACE inhibitors who are anaesthetised.[5] Others consider that hypotension occurring at anaesthetic induction in those on ACE inhibitors can readily be treated with low doses of methoxamine.[3]

(b) Alpha blockers

The UK makers of **alfuzosin** note that administration of general anaesthetics to patients receiving **alfuzosin** could cause profound hypotension, and they recommend that **alfuzosin** be withdrawn 24 hours before surgery.[8]

1. Craig DB, Bose D. Drug interactions in anaesthesia: chronic antihypertensive therapy. *Can Anaesth Soc J* (1984) 31, 580–8.
2. Foëx P, Cutfield GR, Francis CM. Interactions of cardiovascular drugs with inhalational anaesthetics. *Anasth Intensivmed* (1982) 150, 109–28.
3. Anon. Drugs in the peri-operative period: 4 – Cardiovascular drugs. *Drug Ther Bull* (1999) 37, 89–92.
4. McConachie I, Healy TEJ. ACE inhibitors and anaesthesia. *Postgrad Med J* (1989) 65, 273–4.
5. Littler C, McConachie I, Healy TEJ. Interaction between enalapril and propofol. *Anaesth Intensive Care* (1989) 17, 514–15.
6. Coriat P, Richer C, Douraki T, Gomez C, Hendricks K, Giudicelli J-F, Viars P. Influence of chronic angiotensin-converting enzyme inhibition on anesthetic induction. *Anesthesiology* (1994) 81, 299–307.
7. Jensen K, Bunemann L, Riisager S, Thomsen LJ. Cerebral blood flow during anaesthesia: influence of pretreatment with metoprolol or captopril. *Br J Anaesth* (1989) 62, 321–3.
8. Xatral XL (Alfuzosin). Sanofi-Aventis. UK Summary of product characteristics, April 2004.

Anaesthetics, general + Antipsychotics

An isolated report describes a grand mal seizure in a man on chlorpromazine and flupenthixol when he was anaesthetised with enflurane.

Clinical evidence, mechanism, importance and management

An isolated report[1] describes an unexpected grand mal seizure in a schizophrenic patient without a history of epilepsy when given **enflurane** anaesthesia. He was taking **chlorpromazine** 50 mg three times daily (irregularly) and **flupenthixol** 40 mg intramuscularly every 2 weeks. The suggested reason is that the **enflurane** had a synergistic effect with the two antipsychotics, all of which are known to lower the seizure threshold. The general importance of this interaction is not known.

Droperidol reduces the dose requirements of thiopental, see 'Anaesthetics, general + Antiemetics', p.883.

1. Vohra SB. Convulsions after enflurane in a schizophrenic patient receiving neuroleptics. *Can J Anaesth* (1994) 41, 420–2.

Anaesthetics, general + Aspirin or Probenecid

The induction of anaesthesia with midazolam is more rapid in patients who have been pretreated with aspirin or probenecid. The anaesthetic dosage of thiopental is reduced, and its effects prolonged by pretreatment with aspirin or probenecid.

Clinical evidence

(a) Midazolam

A study in patients about to undergo surgery found that pretreatment with aspirin 1 g (given as intravenous **lysine acetylsalicylate**) 1 minute before induction, or oral probenecid 1 g given one hour before induction, shortened the induction time with intravenous midazolam 300 micrograms/kg given over 20 seconds. Only 60% were 'asleep' within 3 minutes of midazolam alone, but 80 to 81% were 'asleep' within 3 minutes of midazolam given after the aspirin or probenecid pretreatment.[1]

(b) Thiopental

The same study[1] cited above found that similar pretreatment with aspirin reduced the dosage of 2.5% thiopental by 34% from 5.3 to 3.5 mg/kg. Initially thiopental 2 mg/kg was given followed by increments of 25 mg until the eyelash reflex was abolished.[1] The same study[1] also found that oral probenecid 1 g given one hour before anaesthesia reduced the thiopental dosage by 23% from 5.3 to 4.1 mg/kg.

A further double-blind study in 86 women found that probenecid given 3 hours before surgery prolonged the duration of anaesthesia with thiopental 7 mg/kg. In patients premedicated with pethidine 1 mg/kg, atropine 7.5 micrograms/kg and either 500 mg or 1 g of probenecid, the duration of anaesthesia was prolonged by 65% and 46% respectively. Without the pethidine, 500 mg of probenecid caused a 26% prolongation. In patients without pethidine and given only 4 mg/kg of thiopental, but no surgical stimulus during anaesthesia, probenecid increased the duration of anaesthesia by 109%.[2]

Mechanism

Not understood. It has been suggested that the aspirin and the probenecid increase the amount of free (and active) midazolam and thiopental in the plasma since they compete for the binding sites on the plasma albumins.[1,3]

Importance and management

Information is limited but what is known shows that the effects of both midazolam and thiopental are increased by aspirin and probenecid. Be alert for the need to reduce the dosages. However, note also that regular aspirin use may increase the risk of bleeding during surgery, and in some situations this may justify avoidance of aspirin in the week before surgery.[4]

1. Dundee JW, Halliday NJ, McMurray TJ. Aspirin and probenecid pretreatment influences the potency of thiopentone and the onset of action of midazolam. *Eur J Anaesthesiol* (1986) 3, 247–51.
2. Kaukinen S, Eerola M, Ylitalo P. Prolongation of thiopentone anaesthesia by probenecid. *Br J Anaesth* (1980) 52, 603–7.
3. Halliday NJ, Dundee JW, Collier PS, Howard PJ. Effects of aspirin pretreatment on the *in vitro* serum binding of midazolam. *Br J Clin Pharmacol* (1985) 19, 581P–582P.
4. Anon. Drugs in the peri-operative period: 4 – Cardiovascular drugs. *Drug Ther Bull* (1999) 37, 89–92.

Anaesthetics, general + Benzodiazepines

Midazolam markedly potentiates the anaesthetic action of halothane. Similarly, the effects of propofol or thiopental and midazolam given concurrently are greater than would be expected by simple addition, although the extent varies between the endpoints measured (analgesic, motor, hypnotic).

Clinical evidence

(a) Halothane

Midazolam markedly potentiated the anaesthetic action of halothane in a study in 50 women undergoing surgery. A mean **midazolam** dose of 278 micrograms/kg reduced the halothane MAC by 51.3%.[1]

(b) Propofol

Two studies found that if propofol and **midazolam** were given together, the hypnotic and anaesthetic effects were greater than would be expected by the simple additive effects of both drugs.[2,3] In one of these studies, the ED_{50} for hypnosis was 44% less than that expected of the individual agents and the addition of **midazolam** 130 micrograms/kg caused a 52% reduction in the ED_{50} of propofol required for anaesthesia.[2] A pharmacokinetic study showed a very modest 20% increase in the levels of free **midazolam** in the plasma when it was given with propofol, but it was considered too small to explain the considerable synergism.[4] In a further double-blind, placebo-controlled study in 24 patients, premedication with intravenous **midazolam** 50 micrograms/kg given 20 minutes before induction of anaesthesia, reduced the propofol dose requirements for multiple anaesthetic end-points including hypnotic, motor, EEG and analgesia. However, the potentiating effect and the mechanism of the interaction appeared to vary with the anaesthetic end-point and the dose of propofol. Notably, the interaction was most marked for analgesia.[5] Another double-blind, placebo-controlled study in 60 children aged 1 to 3 years demonstrated that **midazolam** 500 micrograms/kg given by mouth approximately 30 minutes before the induction of anaesthesia delayed early recovery from anaesthesia induced with propofol and maintained with **sevoflurane** and **nitrous oxide/oxygen**. However, the time to hospital discharge was not prolonged.[6]

(c) Thiopental

Thiopental has been shown to act synergistically with **midazolam** at induction of anaesthesia in two studies.[7,8] In one of these studies, **midazolam** reduced the dose of thiopental required to produce anaesthesia by 50%.[8] In a further double-blind, placebo-controlled study in 23 patients, premedication with intravenous **midazolam** 50 micrograms/kg, given 20 minutes before the induction of anaesthesia, reduced the thiopental dose requirements for multiple anaesthetic end-points including hypnotic, motor, EEG and analgesia. Potentiation was greatest for the motor end-point (about 40%) and smallest for analgesia (18%).[9]

Mechanism

Propofol, barbiturates and halothane appear to interact with benzodiazepines through their effects on the gamma-aminobutyric acid (GABA) receptor.

Importance and management

The interactions between propofol or thiopental and midazolam are well established. This synergy has been utilised for the induction of anaesthesia.[10]

1. Inagaki Y, Sumikawa K, Yoshiya I. Anesthetic interaction between midazolam and halothane in humans. *Anesth Analg* (1993) 76, 613–17.
2. Short TG, Chui PT. Propofol and midazolam act synergistically in combination. *Br J Anaesth* (1991) 67, 539–45.
3. McClune S, McKay AC, Wright PMC, Patterson CC, Clarke RSJ. Synergistic interactions between midazolam and propofol. *Br J Anaesth* (1992) 69, 240–5.
4. Teh J, Short TG, Wong J, Tan P. Pharmacokinetic interactions between midazolam and propofol: an infusion study. *Br J Anaesth* (1994) 72, 62–5.
5. Wilder-Smith OHG, Ravussin PA, Decosterd LA, Despland PA, Bissonnette B. Midazolam premedication reduces propofol dose requirements for multiple anesthetic endpoints. *Can J Anesth* (2001) 48, 439–45.
6. Viitanen H, Annila P, Viitanen M, Yli-Hankala A. Midazolam premedication delays recovery from propofol-induced sevoflurane anesthesia in children 1-3 yr. *Can J Anesth* (1999) 46, 766–71.
7. Tverskoy M, Fleyshman G, Bradley EL, Kissin I. Midazolam–thiopental anesthetic interaction in patients. *Anesth Analg* (1988) 67, 342–5.
8. Short TG, Galletly DC, Plummer JL. Hypnotic and anaesthetic action of thiopentone and midazolam alone and in combination. *Br J Anaesth* (1991) 66, 13–19.
9. Wilder-Smith OHG, Ravussin PA, Decosterd LA, Despland PA, Bissonnette B. Midazolam premedication and thiopental induction of anaesthesia: interactions at multiple end-points. *Br J Anaesth* (1999) 83, 590–5.
10. Orser BA, Miller DR. Propofol-benzodiazepine interactions: insights from a "bench to bedside" approach. *Can J Anesth* (2001) 48, 431–4.

Anaesthetics, general + Beta-blockers

Anaesthesia in the presence of beta-blockers normally appears to be safer than withdrawal of the beta-blocker before anaesthesia, provided certain inhalational anaesthetics are avoided (methoxyflurane, cyclopropane, ether, trichloroethylene) and atropine is used to prevent bradycardia. See also 'Anaesthetics, general + Antihypertensives', p.883 and 'Anaesthetics, general + Timolol', p.892.

Clinical evidence and mechanism

It used to be thought that beta-blockers should be withdrawn from patients before surgery because of the risk that their cardiac depressant effects would be additive with those of inhalational anaesthetics, reducing cardiac output and lowering blood pressure, but it seems to depend on the anaesthetic used.[1] Lowenstein has drawn up a ranking order of compatibility (from the least to the most compatible) as follows: **methoxyflurane**, **ether**, **cyclopropane**, **trichloroethylene**, **enflurane**, **halothane**, **isoflurane**.[1]

(a) Cyclopropane, Ether, Methoxyflurane, Trichloroethylene

A risk of cardiac depression certainly seems to exist with cyclopropane and ether because their depressant effects on the heart are normally counteracted by the release of catecholamines, which would be blocked by the presence of a beta-blocker. There is also some evidence (clinical and/or *animal*) that unacceptable cardiac depression may occur with methoxyflurane and trichloroethylene when a beta-blocker is present (reviewed by Foëx et al.[2,3]). For these four inhalational anaesthetics it has been stated that an absolute indication for their use should exist before giving them in combination with a beta-blocker.[1]

(b) Enflurane, Halothane, Isoflurane

Although a marked reduction in cardiac performance has been described in a study in *dogs* given **propranolol** and enflurane (reviewed by Foëx et al.[2,3]) these drugs have been widely used without apparent difficulties.[1] Normally beta-blockers and halothane or isoflurane appear to be safe (reviewed by Foëx et al.[2,3]). On the positive side there appear to be considerable benefits to be gained from the continued use of beta-blockers during anaesthesia. Their sudden withdrawal from patients treated for angina or hypertension can result in the development of acute and life-threatening cardiovascular complications whether the patient is undergoing surgery or not. In the peri-operative period patients benefit from beta-blockade because it can minimise the effects of sympathetic overactivity of the cardiovascular system during anaesthesia and surgery (for example during endotracheal intubation, laryngoscopy, bronchoscopy and various surgical manoeuvres), which can cause cardiac arrhythmias and hypertension.

Importance and management

The consensus of opinion is that beta-blockers should not be withdrawn before anaesthesia and surgery[4] because of the advantages of maintaining blockade, and because the risks accompanying withdrawal are considerable. But, if inhalational anaesthetics are used, it is important to select the safest anaesthetics (isoflurane, halothane), and avoid those that appear to be most risky (methoxyflurane, ether, cyclopropane, trichloroethylene), as well as ensuring that the patient is protected against bradycardia by atropine. See also 'Anaesthetics, general + Antihypertensives', p.883 and 'Anaesthetics, general + Timolol', p.892.

1. Smith NT, Miller RD, Corbascio AN, eds. Beta-adrenergic blockers in Drug Interactions in Anesthesia. Philadelphia: Lea and Febiger; 1981 P. 83–101.
2. Foëx P, Cutfield GR, Francis CM. Interactions of cardiovascular drugs with inhalational anaesthetics. *Anasth Intensivmed* (1982) 150, 109–28.
3. Foëx P, Francis CM, Cutfield GR. The interactions between β-blockers and anaesthetics. Experimental observations. *Acta Anaesthesiol Scand* (1982) (Suppl 76), 38–46.
4. Anon. Drugs in the peri-operative period: 4 – Cardiovascular drugs. *Drug Ther Bull* (1999) 37, 89–92.

Anaesthetics, general + Calcium channel blockers

Impaired myocardial conduction has been seen in two patients on diltiazem after they were anaesthetised with enflurane, and prolonged anaesthesia has been seen with verapamil and etomidate, but it has been suggested that the concurrent use of anaesthetics and calcium channel blockers is normally without problems.

Clinical evidence, mechanism, importance and management

The author of a review about calcium channel blockers and anaesthetics concludes that concurrent use in patients with reasonable ventricular function is normally beneficial, except where there are other complicating factors. Thus he warns about possible decreases in ventricular function in patients undergoing open chest surgery given *intravenous* **verapamil** or **diltiazem**.[1] A report describes a patient on **diltiazem** and atenolol who had impaired AV and sinus node function before anaesthesia, which worsened following the use of **enflurane**.[2] Another patient also on **diltiazem** demonstrated severe sinus bradycardia, which progressed to asystole when **enflurane** was used.[2] The authors of this latter report suggest that **enflurane** and **diltiazem** can have additive depressant effects on myocardial conduction. Two cases of prolonged anaesthesia and Cheynes-Stokes respiration have been reported in patients who were undergoing cardioversion. Both received **verapamil** and were induced with **etomidate**.[3] Enhanced hypotension was seen in a study in which patients were given intravenous **nimodipine** during general anaesthesia including either **halothane** or **isoflurane**.[4] Some caution is clearly appropriate, especially with intravenous calcium channel blockers given during surgery, but general experience suggests that long-term treatment with calcium channel blockers need not be avoided in most patients undergoing anaesthesia.

1. Merin RG. Calcium channel blocking drugs and anesthetics: is the drug interaction beneficial or detrimental? *Anesthesiology* (1987) 66, 111–13.
2. Hantler CB, Wilton N, Learned DM, Hill AEG, Knight PR. Impaired myocardial conduction in patients receiving diltiazem therapy during enflurane anesthesia. *Anesthesiology* (1987) 67, 94–6.
3. Moore CA, Hamilton SF, Underhill AL, Fagraeus L. Potentiation of etomidate anesthesia by verapamil: a report of two cases. *Hosp Pharm* (1989) 24, 24–5.
4. Müller H, Kafurke H, Marck P, Zierski J, Hempelmann G. Interactions between nimodipine and general anaesthesia – clinical investigations in 124 patients during neurosurgical operations. *Acta Neurochir (Wien)* (1988) 45 (Suppl), 29–35.

Anaesthetics, general + Dexmedetomidine

Dexmedetomidine can reduce the dose requirements of thiopental, isoflurane and other similar anaesthetics.

Clinical evidence, mechanism, importance and management

Dexmedetomidine reduced the **thiopental** dose requirement for EEG burst suppression by 30% in 7 patients when compared with 7 control patients given placebo. In this study, dexmedetomidine was administered for 35 minutes before anaesthesia and during anaesthesia at a dose of 100 nanograms/kg/minute for the first 10 minutes, 30 nanograms/kg/minute for the following 15 minutes, and 6 nanograms/kg/minute thereafter. There was no pharmacodynamic synergism, and pharmacokinetic analysis showed that dexmedetomidine significantly reduced the **thiopental** distribution, probably due to reduced cardiac output and decreased regional blood flow.[1]

In another study, dexmedetomidine reduced the ED_{50} dose requirement of **isoflurane** for anaesthesia (motor response) in 9 healthy subjects. Dexmedetomidine plasma levels of 0.35 and 0.75 nanograms/mL reduced the requirements for **isoflurane** by about 30% and 50%, respectively. Subjects who had received dexmedetomidine took longer to wake up.[2] Dexmedetomidine has sedative, analgesic and anxiolytic effects[3] and therefore, like other sedatives, may reduce the dose requirements of anaesthetics. However, it may also affect the distribution of **thiopental** and possibly other **intravenous anaesthetics**.

1. Bührer M, Mappes A, Lauber R, Stanski DR, Maitre PO. Dexmedetomidine decreases thiopental dose requirement and alters distribution pharmacokinetics. *Anesthesiology* (1994) 80, 1216–27.
2. Khan ZP, Munday IT, Jones RM, Thornton C, Mant TG, Amin D. Effects of dexmedetomidine on isoflurane requirements in healthy volunteers. 1: Pharmacodynamic and pharmacokinetic interactions. *Br J Anaesth* (1999) 83, 372–80.
3. Bhana N, Goa KL, McClellan KJ. Dexmedetomidine. *Drugs* (2000) 59, 263–8.

Anaesthetics, general + Herbal medicines

Animal **data suggest valerian may prolong the effect of thiopental. Based on pharmacology, it has been predicted that kava kava and St John's wort may also prolong of the effects of anaesthetic agents. The American Society of Anesthesiologists recommends that all herbal medicines be stopped two weeks prior to elective surgery.**

Clinical evidence and mechanism

An ethanol extract of **valerian** *(Valeriana officinalis)* was shown to modestly prolong **thiopental** anaesthesia in *mice*, possibly via its effects on the GABA-benzodiazepine receptor.[1]

There is one case report of **kava kava** potentiating benzodiazepines (see 'Benzodiazepines + Kava', p.547), and it has been suggested that it could potentiate other CNS depressants including **barbiturates**[2,3] (e.g. **thiopental**), and may prolong or potentiate the effects of **anaesthetics**.[4-6] Kava may act via GABA receptors, and kavalactones (one group of active constituents) also have skeletal muscle relaxant and local anaesthetic properties.[2,3] Toxic doses can produce muscle weakness and paralysis.[2,3]

It has been suggested that **St John's wort** *(Hypericum perforatum)* may prolong anaesthesia,[4-7] but there are no reports of this. This appears to have been based on the possibility that **St John's wort** acts as an MAOI,[5,7,8] and the limited evidence that MAOIs may cause hepatic enzyme inhibition and potentiate the effects of barbiturates (see 'MAOIs + Barbiturates', p.863). However, there is now increasing evidence that **St John's wort** induces hepatic enzymes, and might therefore increase the metabolism of **barbiturates**, which suggests it could increase requirements for **thiopental** anaesthesia. The possible MAOI activity of **St John's wort** has led to the recommendation that the same considerations apply as for other MAOIs and general anaesthetics,[7,8] see 'Anaesthetics, general + MAOIs', p.887. However, St John's wort may not have any MAOI activity.[9]

Importance and management

Not established. The evidence presented suggests that some caution may be warranted in patients using valerian, kava kava, or St John's wort given general anaesthetics. Many other herbs have the potential to cause problems in the care of patients undergoing surgery (other than via drug interactions with anaesthetic agents) and these have been reviewed.[5-7] Because of the limited information, the American Society of Anesthesiologists have recommended discontinuation of all herbal medicines 2 weeks before an elective anaesthetic[4,6] and if there is any doubt about the safety of a product, this may be a prudent precaution.[5]

1. Hiller K-O, Zetler G. Neuropharmacological studies on ethanol extracts of *Valeriana officinalis* L.; behavioural and anticonvulsant properties. *Phytother Res* (1996) 10,145–51.
2. Anon. Piper methysticum (kava kava). *Altern Med Rev* (1998) 3, 458–60.
3. Pepping J. Kava: *Piper methysticum*. *Am J Health-Syst Pharm* (1999) 56, 957–8 and 960.
4. Larkin, M. Surgery patients at risk for herb–anaesthesia interactions. *Lancet* (1999) 354, 1362.
5. Cheng B, Hung CT, Chiu W. Herbal medicine and anaesthesia. *Hong Kong Med J* (2002) 8, 123–30.
6. Leak JA. Perioperative considerations in the management of the patient taking herbal medicines. *Curr Opin Anaesthesiol* (2000) 13, 321–5.
7. Lyons TR. Herbal medicines and possible anesthesia interactions. *AANA J* (2002) 70, 47–51.
8. Klepser TB, Klepser ME. Unsafe and potentially safe herbal therapies. *Am J Health-Syst Pharm* (1999) 56, 125–38.
9. Miller LG. Herbal medicinals. Selected clinical considerations focusing on known or potential drug-herb interactions. *Arch Intern Med* (1998) 158, 2200–11.

Anaesthetics, general + Isoniazid

Isoniazid may increase the metabolism of enflurane, isoflurane or sevoflurane and thereby increase plasma-fluoride concentrations. However, this does not seem to have resulted in clinically important renal impairment.

Clinical evidence, mechanism, importance and management

A 46-year-old woman underwent anaesthesia for renal transplantation 6 days after commencement of isoniazid 300 mg daily. Anaesthesia was induced with intravenous thiopental and maintained for 4 hours with 60% nitrous oxide, fentanyl and **isoflurane**. Serum fluoride ion concentrations increased from 4.3 micromol preoperatively to approximately 30 micromol between 2 and 8 hours after commencing isoflurane administration, however, no impairment of renal function occurred. A second patient who was given 5 times the first patient's exposure to **isoflurane** and who had received isoniazid for 13 years showed no increase in serum fluoride concentrations over preoperative values, but did show an increase in trifluoroacetic acid levels.[1]

When **enflurane** was administered to 20 patients who had been receiving isoniazid 300 mg daily for one week up to one year, 9 showed an increase in peak fluoride ion levels. These 9 patients had a fourfold higher fluoride level than 36 control subjects not taking isoniazid and the 11 other subjects on isoniazid. By 48 hours after anaesthesia, there was no difference in fluoride levels. Despite the increase in fluoride levels, there was no change in renal function.[2]

The manufacturers of sevoflurane have reported that the metabolism of **sevoflurane** may be increased by inducers of the cytochrome P450 isoenzyme CYP2E1 including isoniazid.[3,4]

Isoniazid may increase the metabolism of **enflurane, isoflurane** or **sevoflurane** in some patients (probably related to isoniazid acetylator phenotype[2]) and so increase the release of fluoride ions that may cause nephrotoxicity; however, there do not appear to be any reports of a significant clinical effect on renal function.

1. Gauntlett IS, Koblin DD, Fahey MR, Konopka K, Gruenke LD, Waskell L, Eger EI. Metabolism of isoflurane in patients receiving isoniazid. *Anesth Analg* (1989) 69, 245–9.
2. Mazze RI, Woodruff RE, Heerdt ME. Isoniazid-induced enflurane defluorination in humans. *Anesthesiology* (1982) 57, 5–8.
3. Sevoflurane. Abbott Laboratories Ltd. UK Summary of product characteristics, November 2003.
4. Ultane (Sevoflurane). Abbott Laboratories. US Prescribing information, August 2003.

Anaesthetics, general + Levothyroxine

Marked hypertension and tachycardia occurred in two patients taking levothyroxine when given ketamine.

Clinical evidence, mechanism, importance and management

Two patients on thyroid replacement treatment with levothyroxine developed severe hypertension (240/140 and 210/130 mmHg respectively) and tachycardia (190 and 150 bpm) when given **ketamine**. Both were effectively treated with 1 mg of intravenous propranolol.[1] It was not clear whether this was an interaction or simply a particularly exaggerated response to **ketamine**, but care is clearly needed if **ketamine** is given to patients in this category.

1. Kaplan JA, Cooperman LH. Alarming reactions to ketamine in patients taking thyroid medication — treatment with propranolol. *Anesthesiology* (1971) 35, 229–30.

Anaesthetics, general + MAOIs

It is generally recommended that MAOIs should be withdrawn 2 weeks before anaesthesia, although there is some evidence that this may be unnecessary in most patients. However, individual cases of both hypo- and hypertension have been seen and MAOIs can interact dangerously with other drugs sometimes used during surgery (particularly pethidine (meperidine) and ephedrine).

Clinical evidence and mechanism

The absence of problems during emergency general anaesthesia in 2 patients on MAOIs prompted further study in 6 others on long-term treatment with unnamed MAOIs. All 6 were premedicated with 10 to 15 mg of diazepam 2 hours before surgery, induced with **thiopental**, given suxamethonium (succinylcholine) before intubation, and maintained with **nitrous oxide/oxygen** with either **halothane** or **isoflurane**. Pancuronium was used for muscle relaxation, and morphine was given postoperatively. One patient experienced hypotension that responded to repeated 100-microgram intravenous doses of phenylephrine without hypertensive reactions. No other untoward events occurred either during or after the anaesthesia.[1]

No adverse reactions occurred in 27 other patients on MAOIs (**tranylcypromine**, **phenelzine**, **isocarboxazid**, **pargyline**) when anaesthetised.[2] No problems were seen in *dogs* on **tranylcypromine** anaesthetised with **enflurane** and fentanyl and then give the vasopressors noradrenaline (norepinephrine) and ephedrine.[3] Two single case reports describe the safe and uneventful use of **propofol** in a patient on **phenelzine**[4] and another on **tranylcypromine**.[5] The latter was also given alfentanil. No problems were seen in one patient on **tranylcypromine** when given **ketamine**[6] and in another on **selegiline** when given fentanyl, **isoflurane** and midazolam.[7] No problems were seen in another patient on **phenelzine** when anaesthetised firstly with **sevoflurane** in oxygen, followed by **isoflurane**, oxygen, air and an infusion of **remifentanil**.[8] Unexplained hypertension has been described in a patient taking **tranylcypromine** when **etomidate** and **atracurium** were used.[9] **Moclobemide** was stopped on the morning of surgery in a patient who was anaesthetised with **propofol** and later **isoflurane** in **nitrous oxide** and oxygen. **Atracurium,** morphine and droperidol were also used. No adverse reactions occurred.[10] Ketorolac, **propofol** and midazolam were used uneventfully in one patient on **phenelzine**.[11]

There are a few anecdotal reports of MAOIs potentiating the effects of amobarbital, butobarbital and secobarbital–see 'MAOIs + Barbiturates', p.863.

Importance and management

The BNF[12] states that 'in view of their hazardous interactions MAOIs should normally be stopped 2 weeks before surgery.' However, there seems to be little documentary evidence that the withdrawal of MAOI before anaesthesia is normally necessary. Scrutiny of reports[13] alleging an adverse reaction usually shows that what happened could be attributed to an interaction between other drugs used during the surgery (e.g. either 'directly-acting sympathomimetics', (p.871) or 'indirectly-acting sympathomimetics', (p.872), or 'pethidine', (p.869)) rather than with the anaesthetics. The authors of the reports cited here offer the opinion that 'general and regional anaesthesia may be provided safely without discontinuation of MAOI therapy, provided proper monitoring, adequate preparation, and prompt treatment of anticipated reactions are utilised'.[1,2] This implies that the possible interactions between the MAOI and other drugs are fully recognised, but be alert for the rare unpredictable response.

1. El-Ganzouri A, Ivankovich AD, Braverman B, Land PC. Should MAOI be discontinued preoperatively? *Anesthesiology* (1983) 59, A384.
2. El-Ganzouri AR, Ivankovich AD, Braverman B, McCarthy R. Monoamine oxidase inhibitors: should they be discontinued preoperatively? *Anesth Analg* (1985) 64, 592–6.
3. Braverman B, Ivankovich AD, McCarthy R. The effects of fentanyl and vasopressors on anesthetized dogs receiving MAO inhibitors. *Anesth Analg* (1984) 63, 192.
4. Hodgson CA. Propofol and mono-amine oxidase inhibitors. *Anaesthesia* (1992) 47, 356.
5. Powell H. Use of alfentanil in a patient receiving monoamine oxidase inhibitor therapy. *Br J Anaesth* (1990) 64, 528–9.
6. Doyle DJ. Ketamine induction and monoamine oxidase inhibitors. *J Clin Anesth* (1990) 2, 324–5.
7. Noorily SH, Hantler CB, Sako EY. Monoamine oxidase inhibitors and cardiac anesthesia revisited. *South Med J* (1997) 90, 836–8.
8. Ure DS, Gillies MA, James KS. Safe use of remifentanil in a patient treated with the monoamine oxidase inhibitor phenelzine. *Br J Anaesth* (2000) 84, 414–16.
9. Sides CA. Hypertension during anaesthesia with monoamine oxidase inhibitors. *Anaesthesia* (1987) 42, 633–5.
10. McFarlane HJ. Anaesthesia and the new generation monoamine oxidase inhibitors. *Anaesthesia* (1994) 49, 597–9.
11. Fischer SP, Mantin R, Brock-Utne JG. Ketorolac and propofol anesthesia in a patient taking chronic monoamine oxidase inhibitors. *J Clin Anesth* (1996) 8, 245–7.
12. British National Formulary. 49th ed. London: The British Medical Association and The Pharmaceutical Press; 2005. p. 619.
13. Stack CG, Rogers P, Linter SPK. Monoamine oxidase inhibitors and anaesthesia: a review. *Br J Anaesth* (1988) 60, 222–7.

Anaesthetics, general + Methylphenidate

A single report described difficulty in sedating a child taking methylphenidate, and a possible delayed interaction between ketamine and methylphenidate, which resulted in nausea, vomiting and dehydration. Administration of methylphenidate after ketamine anaesthesia increased the incidence of vomiting, excessive talking, and limb movements in one study. Methylphenidate should probably be withheld before surgery using inhalational anaesthetics, because of the potential risk of hypertension and/or arrhythmias.

Clinical evidence, mechanism, importance and management

A 6-year-old boy weighing 22 kg, who was receiving methylphenidate 5 mg twice daily for attention deficit disorder, was found to be difficult to sedate for an echocardiogram. Sedation was attempted with oral cloral hydrate 75 mg/kg without success. One week later he received midazolam 20 mg orally, but was only mildly sedated 20 minutes later and would not lie still. Despite an additional oral dose of midazolam 10 mg mixed with oral **ketamine** 60 mg the child was still alert and uncooperative 20 minutes later. He was finally given intravenous glycopyrronium (glycopyrrolate) 100 micrograms followed by intravenous midazolam 5 mg given over 5 minutes and was successfully sedated. He recovered from sedation uneventfully, but developed nausea, vomiting and lethargy after discharge from hospital, which responded to rehydration treatment.[1] In a double-blind study, methylphenidate was given as a single 20-mg intravenous dose to try and speed recovery at the end of **ketamine** anaesthesia for short urological procedures. However, methylphenidate did not improve recovery, and increased the incidence of vomiting, excessive talking, and limb movements.[2]

In the first case, the stimulant effect of the methylphenidate was thought to have antagonised the sedative effect of the midazolam and **ketamine**. The methylphenidate may also have delayed the absorption of the oral drugs. In addition, methylphenidate may inhibit liver microsomal enzymes and could therefore possibly delay elimination of both **ketamine** and midazolam so that hazardous plasma concentrations could develop.[1]

These appear to be the only reports, so any effect is not established. Be aware that methylphenidate may possibly antagonise the effect of sedative drugs, and may also be associated with an increased incidence of vomiting. Note that methylphenidate is an indirect-acting sympathomimetic, and as such might be expected to increase the risk of hypertension and arrhythmias if used with **inhalational anaesthetics** (see 'Anaesthetics, general + Sympathomimetics', p.891). Because of this, the maker of one brand of methylphenidate recommends that, if surgery with halogenated anaesthetics is planned, methylphenidate treatment should not be given on the day of surgery.[3] Taken together, these reports suggest this advice may be a prudent precaution for any form of sedation and/or general anaesthesia.

1. Ririe DG, Ririe KL, Sethna NF, Fox L. Unexpected interaction of methylphenidate (Ritalin®) with anaesthetic agents. *Paediatr Anaesth* (1997) 7, 69–72.
2. Attalah MM, Saied MMA, Yahya R, Ibrahiem EI. Ketamine anesthesia for short transurethral urologic procedures. *Middle East J Anesthesiol* (1993) 12, 123–33.
3. Concerta XL (Methylphenidate). Janssen-Cilag Ltd. UK Summary of product characteristics, March 2004.

Anaesthetics, general + Neuromuscular blockers

The inhalational anaesthetics increase neuromuscular blockade to differing extents, but nitrous oxide appears not to interact significantly. Ketamine has been reported to potentiate atracurium. Propofol does not appear to interact with vecuronium. Bradycardia has been seen in patients given vecuronium with etomidate and thiopental. Propofol can cause serious bradycardia if given with suxamethonium (succinylcholine) without adequate anticholinergic premedication, and asystole has been seen with fentanyl, propofol and suxamethonium given sequentially.

Clinical evidence, mechanism, importance and management

A. Neuromuscular blockade

(a) Inhalational anaesthetics

Neuromuscular blockade is increased by inhalational anaesthetics, the greater the dosage of the anaesthetic the greater the increase in blockade. In broad terms **desflurane, ether, enflurane, isoflurane, methoxyflurane** and **sevoflurane** have a greater effect than **halothane**, which is more potent than **cyclopropane**, whereas **nitrous oxide** appears not to interact significantly with competitive blockers.[1-7] The mechanism is not fully understood but seems to be multifactorial. It has been suggested that: the anaesthetic may have an effect via the CNS (including depression of spinal motor neurones); an effect on the neuromuscular junction (including a decrease in the release of acetylcholine and in the sensitivity of the motor end-plate to acetylcholine); and it may affect the muscle tissue itself.[6,8]

The dosage of the neuromuscular blocker may need to be adjusted according to the anaesthetic in use. For example, the dosage of **atracurium** can be reduced by 25 to 30% if, instead of balanced anaesthesia (with **thiopental**, fentanyl and **nitrous oxide/oxygen**),[9] **enflurane** is used, and by up to 50% if **isoflurane** or **desflurane** are used.[4,10,11] In one study, **enflurane** and **isoflurane** reduced the **vecuronium** infusion rate requirements by as much as 70%, when compared with fentanyl anaesthesia.[12] Another study demonstrated that although **halothane** and **isoflurane** could both increase the neuromuscular potency of **vecuronium**, only **isoflurane** prolonged the recovery from neuromuscular blockade.[13]

The duration of exposure to the anaesthetic and the duration of effect of the various neuromuscular blockers also appear to affect the degree of potentiation that occurs.[8,14] In a study in which the muscle relaxant was administered shortly (about 5 minutes) after the start of inhalational anaesthesia, **enflurane** prolonged the action of **atracurium, pipecuronium** and **pancuronium**, but did not significantly affect **vecuronium**. However, **halothane** did not significantly prolong the clinical duration of any of the neuromuscular blockers.[14] It was suggested that more prolonged exposure to the anaesthetic, allowing equilibration of the anaesthetic to the tissues, might result in more significant potentiation of the neuromuscular blocking agents. In addition, the duration of effect of the **vecuronium** may have been too short for interaction with a volatile anaesthetic that had not had time to equilibrate with the tissues.[14] The duration of exposure to **sevoflurane** also influences the dose-response of **vecuronium,** but it has been suggested that sevoflurane-induced potentiation of neuromuscular blockers might be more rapid than with other inhalational anaesthetics.[8] In one study when the volatile anaesthetics were administered approximately 10 minutes before the neuromuscular blocker, **sevoflurane** was reported to increase and prolong the blockade of **rocuronium** more than **isoflurane** or **propofol**.[15] However, another study using steady-state conditions after a 40-minute equilibration period of the inhalation anaesthetic, found no significant difference between **desflurane, isoflurane** and **sevoflurane** in relation to potency, infusion requirements or recovery characteristics of **rocuronium**; the potency of rocuronium was increased by 25 to 40% under inhalational anaesthesia compared with **propofol**.[16] Another study demonstrated considerable prolongation of neuromuscular blockade with **rapacuronium** in the presence of **sevoflurane**; the recovery times were approximately doubled compared with published literature using thiopental/opioid-nitrous oxide anaesthesia. This led to the study being prematurely terminated as spontaneous recovery of neuromuscular function was required after short surgical procedures.[17] Marked potentiation of neuromuscular block following the combination of **sevoflurane** and a small dose of **cisatracurium** 25 micrograms/kg) has been reported in a myasthenic patient.[18]

Although it is generally assumed that **nitrous oxide** does not affect the potency of neuromuscular blockers, one study found that the administration of **nitrous oxide** increased **suxamethonium (succinylcholine)** neuromuscular blockade.[19]

(b) Intravenous anaesthetics

Ketamine prolonged the duration of neuromuscular blockade induced by **atracurium**,[20] but at clinically relevant doses **ketamine** did not influence **suxamethonium** (**succinylcholine**)-induced neuromuscular blockade.[21] However, the UK makers of **suxamethonium** still warn of a possible interaction because they say that **ketamine** may reduce normal plasma cholinesterase activity.[22]

In *animals,* **ketamine** and **thiopental** potentiated the neuromuscular blocking effects of **rocuronium**, whereas **propofol** had no effect.[23]

The original formulation of **propofol** in *Cremophor* was found to increase the blockade due to **vecuronium**,[24] but the more recent formulation in soybean oil and egg phosphatide has been found in an extensive study not to interact with **vecuronium**.[25]

B. Bradycardia, asystole or arrhythmias

Serious sinus bradycardia (heart rates of 30 to 40 bpm) developed rapidly in two young women when they were anaesthetised with a slow intravenous injection of **propofol** 2.5 mg/kg, followed by **suxamethonium (succinylcholine)** 1.5 mg/kg. This was controlled with 600 micrograms of intravenous atropine. Four other patients premedicated with 600 micrograms of intramuscular atropine given 45 minutes before induction of anaesthesia showed no bradycardia.[26] It would appear that **propofol** lacks central vagolytic activity and can exaggerate the muscarinic effects of **suxamethonium**.[26] Another report describes asystole in a woman when given an anaesthetic induction sequence of fentanyl, **propofol** and **suxamethonium**.[27] Bradycardia and asystole has also been seen following the sequential administration of **propofol** and fentanyl in 2 patients.[28,29] All of these three drugs (fentanyl, **propofol, suxamethonium**) alone have been associated with bradycardia and their effects can apparently be additive.

Bradycardia and asystole occurred in another patient given **propofol**, fentanyl and **atracurium**.[30] The authors of one report suggest that atropine or glycopyrrolate pretreatment should attenuate or prevent such reactions.[27]

Bradycardia occurring during anaesthetic induction with **vecuronium** and **etomidate**, or to a lesser extent **thiopental**, has also been reported, particularly in patients also receiving fentanyl,[31] see also 'Neuromuscular blockers + Opioids', p.914.

C. Muscle effects

In children receiving suxamethonium, those who had anaesthesia induced and maintained with **halothane** had much higher levels of serum myoglobulin than those undergoing intravenous induction with **thiopental** followed by **halothane**. This suggests that prior use of halothane may have potentiated suxamethonium-induced muscle damage.[32]

1. Schuh FT. Differential increase in potency of neuromuscular blocking agents by enflurane and halothane. *Int J Clin Pharmacol Ther Toxicol* (1983) 21, 383–6.
2. Fogdall RP, Miller RD. Neuromuscular effects of enflurane, alone and combined with *d*-tubocurarine, pancuronium, and succinylcholine, in man. *Anesthesiology* (1975) 42, 173–8.
3. Miller RD, Way WL, Dolan WM, Stevens WC, Eger EI. Comparative neuromuscular effects of pancuronium, gallamine, and succinylcholine during Forane and halothane anesthesia in man. *Anesthesiology* (1971) 35, 509–14.
4. Lee C, Kwan WF, Chen B, Tsai SK, Gyermek L, Cheng M, Cantley E. Desflurane (I-653) potentiates atracurium in humans. *Anesthesiology* (1990) 73, A875.
5. Izawa H, Takeda J, Fukushima K. The interaction between sevoflurane and vecuronium and its reversibility by neostigmine in man. *Anesthesiology* (1992) 77, A960.
6. Østergaard D, Engbaek J, Viby-Mogensen J. Adverse reactions and interactions of the neuromuscular blocking drugs. *Med Toxicol Adverse Drug Exp* (1989) 4, 351–68.
7. Vanlinthout LEH, Booij LHDJ, van Egmond J, Robertson EN. Effect of isoflurane and sevoflurane on the magnitude and time course of neuromuscular block produced by vecuronium, pancuronium and atracurium. *Br J Anaesth* (1996) 76, 389–95.
8. Suzuki T, Iwasaki K, Fukano N, Hariya S, Saeki S, Ogawa S. Duration of exposure to sevoflurane affects dose–response relationship of vecuronium. *Br J Anaesth* (2000) 85, 732–4.
9. Ramsey FM, White PA, Stullken EH, Allen LL, Roy RC. Enflurane potentiation of neuromuscular blockade by atracurium. *Anesthesiology* (1982) 57, A255.
10. Sokoll MD, Gergis SD, Mehta M, Ali NM, Lineberry C. Safety and efficacy of atracurium (BW33A) in surgical patients receiving balanced or isoflurane anesthesia. *Anesthesiology* (1983) 58, 450–5.

11. Smiley RM, Ornstein E, Mathews D, Matteo RS. A comparison of the effects of desflurane and isoflurane on the action of atracurium in man. *Anesthesiology* (1990) 73, A882.
12. Cannon JE, Fahey MR, Castagnoli KP, Furuta T, Canfell PC, Sharma M, Miller RD. Continuous infusion of vecuronium: the effect of anesthetic agents. *Anesthesiology* (1987) 67, 503–6.
13. Pittet J-F, Melis A, Rouge J-C, Morel DR, Gemperle G, Tassonyi E. Effect of volatile anesthetics on vecuronium-induced neuromuscular blockade in children. *Anesth Analg* (1990) 70, 248–52.
14. Swen J, Rashkovsky OM, Ket JM, Koot HWJ, Hermans J, Agoston S. Interaction between nondepolarizing neuromuscular blocking agents and inhalational anesthetics. *Anesth Analg* (1989) 69, 752–5.
15. Lowry DW, Mirakhur RK, McCarthy GJ, Carroll MT, McCourt KC. Neuromuscular effects of rocuronium during sevoflurane, isoflurane, and intravenous anesthesia. *Anesth Analg* (1998) 87, 936–40.
16. Bock M, Klippel K, Nitsche B, Bach A, Martin E, Motsch J. Rocuronium potency and recovery characteristics during steady-state desflurane, sevoflurane, isoflurane or propofol anaesthesia. *Br J Anaesth* (2000) 84, 43–7.
17. Cara DM, Armory P, Mahajan RP. Prolonged duration of neuromuscular block with rapacuronium in the presence of sevoflurane. *Anesth Analg* (2000) 91, 1392–3.
18. Baraka AS, Taha SK, Kawkabani NI. Neuromuscular interaction of sevoflurane - cisatracurium in a myasthenic patient. *Can J Anesth* (2000) 47, 562–5.
19. Szalados JE, Donati F, Bevan DR. Nitrous oxide potentiates succinylcholine neuromuscular blockade in humans. *Anesth Analg* (1991) 72, 18–21.
20. Toft P, Helbo-Hansen S. Interaction of ketamine with atracurium. *Br J Anaesth* (1989) 62, 319–20.
21. Helbo-Hansen HS, Toft P, Kirkegaard Neilsen H. Ketamine does not affect suxamethonium-induced neuromuscular blockade in man. *Eur J Anaesthesiol* (1989) 6, 419–23.
22. Anectine (Suxamethonium). GlaxoSmithKline. UK Summary of product characteristics, April 2003.
23. Muir AW, Anderson KA, Pow E. Interaction between rocuronium bromide and some drugs used during anaesthesia. *Eur J Anaesthesiol* (1994) 11 (Suppl 9), 93–8.
24. Robertson EN, Fragen RJ, Booij LHDJ, van Egmond J, Crul JF. Some effects of diisopropyl phenol (ICI 35 868) on the pharmacodynamics of atracurium and vecuronium in anaesthetized man. *Br J Anaesth* (1983) 55, 723–7.
25. McCarthy GJ, Mirakhur RK, Pandit SK. Lack of interaction between propofol and vecuronium. *Anesth Analg* (1992) 75, 536–8.
26. Baraka A. Severe bradycardia following propofol-suxamethonium sequence. *Br J Anaesth* (1988) 61, 482–3.
27. Egan TD, Brock-Utne JG. Asystole after anesthesia induction with a fentanyl, propofol, and succinylcholine sequence. *Anesth Analg* (1991) 73, 818–20.
28. Guise PA. Asystole following propofol and fentanyl in an anxious patient. *Anaesth Intensive Care* (1991) 19, 116–18.
29. Dorrington KL. Asystole with convulsion following a subanaesthetic dose of propofol plus fentanyl. *Anaesthesia* (1989) 44, 658–9.
30. Ricós P, Trillo L, Crespo MT, Guilera N, Puig MM. Bradicardia y asistolia asociadas a la administración simultánea de propofol y fentanilo en la inducción anestésica. *Rev Esp Anestesiol Reanim* (1994) 41, 194–5.
31. Inoue K, El-Banayosy A, Stolarski L, Reichelt W. Vecuronium induced bradycardia following induction of anaesthesia with etomidate or thiopentone, with or without fentanyl. *Br J Anaesth* (1988) 60, 10–17.
32. Laurence AS, Henderson P. Serum myoglobin after suxamethonium administration to children: effect of pretreatment before i.v. and inhalation induction. *Br J Anaesth* (1986) 58, 126P.

Anaesthetics, general + Opioids

The respiratory depressant effects of ketamine and morphine may be additive. The dose requirements of propofol may be lower after opioid administration. Opisthotonos or grand mal seizures have rarely been associated with the use of propofol with alfentanil and/or fentanyl. The effects of inhalational anaesthetics may be enhanced by opioid analgesics.

Clinical evidence, mechanism, importance and management

(a) Inhalational anaesthetics

Opioid analgesics have been reported to reduce the MAC values of inhalational anaesthetics, e.g. **fentanyl** has been shown to lower the MAC value of **desflurane,** probably in a dose-dependent manner (reviewed by Dale[1]). However, 100 microgram/kg doses of **morphine** given during anaesthesia did not extend the awakening concentration of **sevoflurane**.[2]

(b) Ketamine

Ketamine is a respiratory depressant like **morphine**, but less potent, and its effects can be additive with morphine.[3]

(c) Propofol

A 71-year-old man undergoing a minor orthopaedic operation was given a 500-microgram intravenous injection of **alfentanil** followed by a slow injection of propofol 2.5 mg/kg. Approximately 15 seconds after the propofol, the patient developed strong bilateral fits and grimaces for 10 seconds. Anaesthesia was maintained with nitrous oxide/oxygen and halothane and there were no other intra- or postoperative complications. The patient had no history of convulsions.[4] Propofol has also been associated with opisthotonos (a spasm where the head and heels bend backwards and the body arches forwards) in two patients given **fentanyl** with or without **alfentanil**.[5] These are rare cases, and any association with the opioid remains unknown.

Alfentanil has been found to reduce the amount of propofol needed for loss of eyelash reflex and loss of consciousness, as well as increasing the blood pressure fall produced by propofol.[6] Propofol inhibits both **alfentanil** and **sufentanil** metabolism causing an increase in plasma concentrations of these opioids, while **alfentanil** also increases propofol concentrations (reviewed by Vuyk[7]). Pretreatment with **fentanyl** may also decrease the propofol requirements for induction of anaesthesia,[7] and increase blood concentrations of propofol;[8] however, another study was unable to confirm an effect on blood propofol concentrations.[9] **Remifentanil** has been reported to reduce the dose of propofol needed for anaesthesia and also to reduce the recovery time.[10]

The maker notes that the required induction dose of propofol may be reduced in patients who have received opioids, and that these agents may increase the anaesthetic and sedative effects of propofol, and also cause greater reductions in blood pressure and cardiac output. They also state that the rate of propofol administration for maintenance of anaesthesia may be reduced in the presence of supplemental analgesics such as opioids.[11]

1. Dale O. Drug interactions in anaesthesia: focus on desflurane and sevoflurane. *Baillieres Clin Anaesthesiol* (1995) 9, 105–17.
2. Katoh T, Suguro Y, Kimura T, Ikeda K. Morphine does not affect the awakening concentration of sevoflurane. *Can J Anaesth* (1993) 40, 825–8.
3. Bourke DL, Malit LA, Smith TC. Respiratory interactions of ketamine and morphine. *Anesthesiology* (1987) 66, 153–6.
4. Wittenstein U, Lyle DJR. Fits after alfentanil and propofol. *Anaesthesia* (1989) 44, 532–3.
5. Laycock GJA. Opisthotonos and propofol: a possible association. *Anaesthesia* (1988) 43, 257.
6. Vuyk J, Griever GER, Engbers FHM, Burm AGL, Bovill JG, Vletter AA. The interaction between propofol and alfentanil during induction of anesthesia. *Anesthesiology* (1994) 81, A400.
7. Vuyk J. Pharmacokinetic and pharmacodynamic interactions between opioids and propofol. *J Clin Anesth* (1997) 9, 23S–26S.
8. Cockshott ID, Briggs LP, Douglas EJ, White M. Pharmacokinetics of propofol in female patients. Studies using single bolus injections. *Br J Anaesth* (1987) 59, 1103–10.
9. Dixon J, Roberts FL, Tackley RM, Lewis GTR, Connell H, Prys-Roberts C. *Br J Anaesth* (1990) 64, 142–7.
10. O'Hare R, Reid J, Breslin D, Hayes A, Mirakhur RK. Propofol–remifentanil interaction: influence on recovery. *Br J Anaesth* (1999) 83, 180P.
11. Diprivan (Propofol). AstraZeneca. US Prescribing information, July 2004.

Anaesthetics, general + Parecoxib or Valdecoxib

Limited evidence suggests parecoxib does not affect the pharmacokinetics or clinical effects of propofol. Valdecoxib and parecoxib do not appear to interact with nitrous oxide and isoflurane.

Clinical evidence, mechanism, importance and management

A randomised, placebo-controlled, double-blind, crossover study in 12 healthy subjects found that pretreatment with 40 mg of parecoxib given intravenously one hour before a 2 mg/kg intravenous bolus of **propofol** did not significantly affect the pharmacokinetics of the **propofol**. Moreover, parecoxib did not alter the clinical effects of **propofol** (e.g. the time to loss of consciousness or the speed of awakening).[1] These limited data suggest that no special precautions should be required during concomitant use.

The UK makers of parecoxib and valdecoxib say that no formal interaction studies have been done with inhalational anaesthetics, but in surgical studies, where either drug had been given preoperatively, there was no evidence of pharmacodynamic interactions in patients who had been given **nitrous oxide** and **isoflurane**.[2,3]

1. Ibrahim A, Park S, Feldman J, Karim A, Kharasch ED. Effects of parecoxib, a parenteral COX-2-specific inhibitor, on the pharmacokinetics and pharmacodynamics of propofol. *Anesthesiology* (2002) 96, 88–95.
2. Dynastat injection (Parecoxib sodium). Pharmacia Ltd. UK Summary of product characteristics, April 2004.
3. Bextra (Valdecoxib). Pharmacia Ltd. UK Summary of product characteristics, May 2004.

Anaesthetics, general + Phenylephrine, topical

Phenylephrine eye drops caused marked cyanosis and bradycardia in a baby, and hypertension in a woman, undergoing general anaesthesia.

Clinical evidence, mechanism, importance and management

A 3-week-old baby anaesthetised with **halothane** and **nitrous oxide/oxygen** became cyanosed shortly after the instillation of two drops of 10%

phenylephrine solution in one eye. The heart rate decreased from 160 to 60 bpm, S-T segment and T wave changes were seen, and blood pressure measurements were unobtainable. The baby recovered uneventfully when anaesthesia was stopped and oxygen administered. It was suggested that the phenylephrine caused severe peripheral vasoconstriction, cardiac failure and reflex bradycardia.[1] A 54-year-old woman anaesthetised with **isoflurane** developed hypertension (a rise from 125/70 to 200/90 mmHg) shortly after having two drops of 10% phenylephrine in one eye, which responded to nasal glyceryl trinitrate (nitroglycerin) and increasing concentrations of isoflurane.[1] The authors of this report consider that general anaesthesia may have contributed to the systemic absorption of the phenylephrine. They suggest that phenylephrine should be administered 30 to 60 minutes prior to anaesthesia, and not during anaesthesia. However, if it is necessary, use the lowest concentrations of phenylephrine (2.5%). They also point out that the following are effective mydriatics: single drop combinations of 0.5% cyclopentolate and 2.5% phenylephrine or 0.5% tropicamide and 2.5% phenylephrine.

Phenylephrine is a sympathomimetic, and as such may carry some risk of potentiating arrhythmias if used with inhalational anaesthetics such as halothane –see 'Anaesthetics, general + Sympathomimetics', p.891. However, it is considered that it is much less likely than adrenaline (epinephrine) to have this effect, since it has primarily alpha-agonist activity.[2]

1. Van der Spek AFL, Hantler CB. Phenylephrine eyedrops and anesthesia. *Anesthesiology* (1986) 64, 812–14.
2. Smith NT, Miller RD, Corbascio AN, eds. Sympathomimetic drugs, in Drug Interactions in Anesthesia. Philadelphia: Lea and Febiger; 1981 P. 55–82.

Anaesthetics, general + Phenytoin, Phenobarbital or Rifampicin (Rifampin)

Phenytoin toxicity occurred in a child following halothane anaesthesia. A near fatal hepatic reaction occurred in a woman given rifampicin (rifampin) after halothane anaesthesia, and hepatitis occurred in a patient given phenobarbital following halothane anaesthesia. See also 'Anaesthetics, general + Isoniazid', p.886 and 'Anaesthetics, general; Methoxyflurane + Antibacterials or Barbiturates', p.893.

Clinical evidence

A 10-year-old girl on long-term treatment with phenytoin 300 mg daily was found to have phenytoin plasma levels of 25 micrograms/ml before surgery. Three days after anaesthesia with **halothane** her plasma phenytoin levels had risen to 41 micrograms/ml and she had marked signs of phenytoin toxicity.[1]

A woman on promethazine and phenobarbital 60 mg three times daily died from **halothane** associated hepatitis within six days of having **halothane** for the first time.[2] A nearly fatal shock-producing hepatic reaction occurred in a woman four days after having **halothane** anaesthesia immediately followed by a course of rifampicin 600 mg daily and isoniazid 300 mg daily.[3]

Mechanism

It seems possible that the general toxic effects of halothane on the liver can slow the normal rate of phenytoin metabolism. One suggested explanation for the increased adverse effects on the liver is that, just as in *animals*, pretreatment with phenobarbital and phenytoin increases the rate of drug metabolism and the hepatotoxicity of halogenated hydrocarbons including chloroform and carbon tetrachloride.[4] As well as increased metabolism, the halothane-rifampicin interaction might also involve additive hepatotoxicity.

Importance and management

No firm conclusions can be drawn from these isolated cases, but they serve to emphasise the potential hepatotoxicity of these anaesthetics with other drugs. It has been suggested that patients on enzyme inducing drugs such as phenobarbital and phenytoin may constitute a high-risk group for liver damage after halogenated anaesthetics.[5] See also 'Anaesthetics, general + Isoniazid', p.886 and 'Anaesthetics, general; Methoxyflurane + Antibacterials or Barbiturates', p.893.

1. Karlin JM, Kutt H. Acute diphenylhydantoin intoxication following halothane anesthesia. *J Pediatr* (1970) 76, 941–4.
2. Patial RK, Sarin R, Patial SB. Halothane associated hepatitis and phenobarbitone. *J Assoc Physicians India* (1989) 37, 480.
3. Most JA, Markle GB. A nearly fatal hepatotoxic reaction to rifampin after halothane anesthesia. *Am J Surg* (1974) 127, 593–5.
4. Garner RC, McLean AEM. Increased susceptibility to carbon tetrachloride poisoning in the rat after pretreatment with oral phenobarbitone. *Biochem Pharmacol* (1969) 18, 645–50.
5. Sweetman SC, editor. Martindale: The complete drug reference. 34th ed. London: Pharmaceutical Press; 2005 p. 1300.

Anaesthetics, general + Sparteine sulfate

Patients induced with thiamylal sodium showed a marked increase in cardiac arrhythmias when they were given intravenous sparteine sulfate, but those given thiopental or etomidate did not.

Clinical evidence, mechanism, importance and management

A group of 109 women undergoing dilatation and curettage were premedicated with atropine and fentanyl, induced with either 2% **thiamylal sodium** (5 mg/kg), 0.2% **etomidate** (0.3 mg/kg) or 2.5% **thiopental** (4 mg/kg), and given mask anaesthesia with **nitrous oxide/oxygen**. During the surgical procedure they were given a slow intravenous injection of sparteine sulfate 100 mg. Fourteen out of 45 patients given **thiamylal sodium** developed cardiac arrhythmias, 10 had bigeminy and 4 had frequent ventricular premature contractions, whereas only two patients given the other induction agents (**etomidate** or **thiopental**) showed any cardiac arrhythmias. It is not understood why sparteine should interact with **thiamylal sodium** in this way. Although the arrhythmias were effectively treated with lidocaine, the authors of this report suggest that the concurrent use of these drugs should be avoided.[1]

1. Cheng C-R, Chen S-Y, Wu K-H, Wei T-T. Thiamylal sodium with sparteine sulfate inducing dysrhythmia in anesthetized patients. *Ma Zui Xue Za Zhi* (1989) 27, 297–8.

Anaesthetics, general + SSRIs

One patient had a seizure following the concurrent use of methohexital and paroxetine.

Clinical evidence, mechanism, importance and management

A generalised tonic-clonic seizure occurred in a 42-year-old woman immediately after being anaesthetised with 120 mg of intravenous **methohexital** for the last in a series of six electroconvulsive therapies. She had been receiving **paroxetine** 40 mg daily throughout the series.[1] The authors suggest that paroxetine should be administered with caution in patients receiving ECT or methohexital anaesthesia.[1] Note that this appears to be an isolated report.

1. Folkerts H. Spontaneous seizure after concurrent use of methohexital anesthesia for electroconvulsive therapy and paroxetine: a case report. *J Nerv Ment Dis* (1995) 183, 115–16.

Anaesthetics, general + Sulfonamides

The anaesthetic effects of thiopental are increased but shortened by pretreatment with sulfafurazole. Phenobarbital appears not to affect the pharmacokinetics of sulfafurazole or sulfisomidine.

Clinical evidence

A study in 48 patients showed that the prior intravenous administration of **sulfafurazole** 40 mg/kg reduced the required anaesthetic dosage of **thiopental** by 36%, but the duration of action was shortened.[1] This interaction has also been observed in *animal* experiments.[2] A study in children showed that **phenobarbital** did not affect the pharmacokinetics of **sulfafurazole** or **sulfisomidine**.[3]

Mechanism

It has been suggested that sulfafurazole successfully competes with thiopental for plasma protein binding sites,[4] the result being that more free and active barbiturate molecules remain in circulation to exert their anaesthetic effects and smaller doses are therefore required.

Importance and management

The evidence for the sulfafurazole/thiopental interaction is limited, but it appears to be strong. Less thiopental than usual may be required to achieve adequate anaesthesia, but since the awakening time is shortened repeated doses may be needed. Barbiturates appear not to interact pharmacokinetically with the sulfonamides.

1. Csögör SI, Kerek SF. Enhancement of thiopentone anaesthesia by sulphafurazole. *Br J Anaesth* (1970) 42, 988–90.
2. Csögör SI, Pálffy B, Feszt G, Papp J. Influence du sulfathiazol sur l'effet narcotique du thiopental et de l'hexobarbital. *Rev Roum Physiol* (1971) 8, 81–5.
3. Krauer B. Vergleichende Untersuchung der Eliminationskinetik zweier Sulfonamide bei Kindern mit und ohne Phenobarbitalmedikation. *Schweiz Med Wochenschr* (1971) 101, 668–71.
4. Csögör SI, Papp J. Competition between sulphonamides and thiopental for the binding sites of plasma proteins. *Arzneimittelforschung* (1970) 20, 1925–7.

Anaesthetics, general + Sympathomimetics

Patients anaesthetised with inhalational anaesthetics (particularly cyclopropane and halothane, and to a lesser extent desflurane, enflurane, ether, isoflurane, methoxyflurane, sevoflurane) can develop cardiac arrhythmias if given adrenaline (epinephrine) or noradrenaline (norepinephrine) unless the dosages are very low. Children appear to be less susceptible. Two patients developed arrhythmias when terbutaline was used with halothane. The possibility of other sympathomimetic agents interacting with inhalation anaesthetics should be borne in mind. See also 'Anaesthetics, general + Phenylephrine, topical', p.889.

Clinical evidence, mechanism, importance and management

(a) Adrenaline (Epinephrine) or Noradrenaline (Norepinephrine)

As early as 1895, Oliver and Schäfer observed that an adrenal extract could cause ventricular fibrillation in a *dog* anaesthetised with chloroform,[1] and it is now very well recognised that similar cardiac arrhythmias can be caused by adrenaline and noradrenaline in humans when anaesthetised with **inhalational anaesthetics**. The mechanism appears to be a sensitisation of the myocardium to β-adrenergic stimulation, caused by the **inhalational anaesthetic** agent. The likelihood of arrhythmias is increased by hypoxia and marked hypercapnia. It has been reported that the highest incidence of complications has been in patients anaesthetised with **cyclopropane**, but that the incidence is also high with **trichloroethylene** and **halothane**.[2] A suggested[3] listing of inhalational anaesthetics in order of decreasing sensitivity is as follows:

cyclopropane, **halothane**, **enflurane/methoxyflurane**, **isoflurane**, **ether**. **Sevoflurane** appeared to behave like **isoflurane** in one clinical study,[4] and **desflurane** was also similar to **isoflurane** in another.[5]

The following recommendation has been made if adrenaline is used to reduce surgical bleeding in patients anaesthetised with **halothane/nitrous oxide/oxygen**: the dosage should not exceed 10 ml of 1:100,000 in any given 10 minute period, nor 30 ml per hour (i.e. about a 100 microgram bolus or 1.5 micrograms/kg/10 minutes for a 70 kg person), and adequate alveolar ventilation must be assured.[6] This dosage guide should also be safe for use with other inhalational anaesthetics since **halothane** is more arrhythmogenic than the others,[3] with the exception of **cyclopropane**, which is no longer widely used. However, some have suggested that concurrent **halothane** and adrenaline may have been a contributing factor in 3 deaths in patients undergoing tooth implant surgery.[7] Others consider that if adrenaline is used for haemostasis during surgery, **isoflurane** or **sevoflurane** carry less risk of cardiac arrhythmias than **halothane**.[8] Solutions containing 0.5% **lidocaine** with adrenaline 1:200,000 also appear to be safe because lidocaine may help to control the potential dysrhythmic effects. For example, a study in 19 adult patients anaesthetised with **halothane** showed that the dose of adrenaline needed to cause three premature ventricular contractions in half the group was 2.11 micrograms/kg in saline, but 3.69 micrograms/kg in 0.5% **lidocaine**. Note that both these values were less than that in 16 patients anaesthetised with **isoflurane** (6.72 micrograms/kg), demonstrating **isoflurane** was still safer.[9] It should be borne in mind that the arrhythmogenic effects of adrenaline are increased if sympathetic activity is increased, and in hyperthyroidism and hypercapnia.[3]

Children appear to be much less susceptible than adults. A retrospective study of 28 children showed no evidence of arrhythmia during **halothane** anaesthesia with adrenaline doses of up to 8.8 micrograms/kg, and a subsequent study on 83 children (three months to 17 years) found that 10 micrograms/kg doses of adrenaline were safe.[10]

(b) Terbutaline

Two patients developed ventricular arrhythmias while anaesthetised with **halothane** and nitrous oxide/oxygen when given terbutaline 250 to 350 micrograms subcutaneously for wheezing. Both developed unifocal premature ventricular contractions followed by bigeminy, which responded to lidocaine.[11] Halothane was replaced by **enflurane** in one case, which allowed the surgery to be completed without further incident.[11]

(c) Other sympathomimetics

Other drugs that stimulate the sympathetic nervous system might also cause hypertension and ventricular arrhythmias during anaesthesia with inhalational anaesthetics. Examples include 'theophylline', (below), 'methylphenidate', (p.887), and cocaine (see 'Anaesthetics, general + Anaesthetics, local', p.882).

An isolated case of fatal cardiac arrest has been attributed to **halothane** anaesthesia in a woman taking **fenfluramine**.[12] Note that **fenfluramine** was generally withdrawn in 1997 because its use was found to be associated with a high incidence of abnormal echocardiograms indicating abnormal functioning of heart valves.

1. Oliver G, Schäfer EA. The physiological effects of extracts of the suprarenal capsules. J Physiol (1895) 18, 230–76.
2. Gibb D. Drug interactions in anaesthesia. *Clin Anaesthesiol* (1984) 2, 485–512.
3. Smith NT, Miller RD, Corbascio AN, eds. Sympathomimetic drugs, in Drug Interactions in Anesthesia. Philadelphia: Lea and Febiger; 1981 P. 66–82.
4. Navarro R, Weiskopf RB, Moore MA, Lockhart S, Eger EI, Koblin D, Lu G, Wilson C. Humans anesthetized with sevoflurane or isoflurane have similar arrhythmic response to epinephrine. *Anesthesiology* (1994) 80, 545–9.
5. Moore MA, Weiskopf RB, Eger EI, Wilson C, Lu G. Arrhythmogenic doses of epinephrine are similar during desflurane or isoflurane anesthesia in humans. *Anesthesiology* (1993) 79, 943–7.
6. Katz RL, Matteo RS, Papper EM. The injection of epinephrine during general anesthesia with halogenated hydrocarbons and cyclopropane in man. 2. Halothane. *Anesthesiology* (1962) 23, 597–600.
7. Buzik SC. Fatal interaction? Halothane, epinephrine and tooth implant surgery. *Can Pharm J* (1990) 123, 68–9 and 81.
8. Ransom ES, Mueller RA. Safety considerations in the use of drug combinations during general anaesthesia. *Drug Safety* (1997) 16, 88–103.
9. Johnston RR, Eger EI, Wilson C. A comparative interaction of epinephrine with enflurane, isoflurane, and halothane in man. *Anesth Analg* (1976) 55, 709–12.
10. Karl HW, Swedlow DB, Lee KW, Downes JJ. Epinephrine–halothane interactions in children. *Anesthesiology* (1983) 58, 142–5.
11. Thiagarajah S, Grynsztejn M, Lear E, Azar I. Ventricular arrhythmias after terbutaline administration to patients anesthetized with halothane. *Anesth Analg* (1986) 65, 417–8.
12. Bennett JA, Eltringham RJ. Possible dangers of anaesthesia in patients receiving fenfluramine. *Anaesthesia* (1977) 32, 8–13.

Anaesthetics, general and/or Neuromuscular blockers + Theophylline

Cardiac arrhythmias can develop during the concurrent use of halothane and aminophylline but this is possibly less likely with isoflurane. One report attributes seizures to an interaction between ketamine and aminophylline. Supraventricular tachycardia occurred in a patient on aminophylline when given pancuronium. Isolated cases suggest the effects of pancuronium, but not vecuronium, can be opposed by aminophylline.

Clinical evidence, mechanism, importance and management

(a) Development of arrhythmias

A number of reports describe arrhythmias apparently due to an interaction between **halothane** and theophylline or aminophylline. One describes intraoperative arrhythmias in three out of 45 adult asthmatics who had received preoperative theophylline/aminophylline then **halothane** anaesthesia.[1] Nine other patients developed heart rates exceeding 140 bpm when given aminophylline and **halothane**, whereas no tachycardia occurred in 22 other patients given only **halothane**.[1] There are other reports of individual adult and child patients who developed ventricular tachycardias attributed to this interaction.[2-5] One child had a cardiac arrest.[5] The same interaction has been reported in *animals*.[6,7] One suggested reason for the interaction with halothane is that theophylline causes the release of endogenous catecholamines (adrenaline (epinephrine), noradrenaline (norepinephrine)), which are known to sensitise the myocardium (see also 'Anaesthetics, general + Sympathomimetics', above). Another report describes supraventricular tachycardia in a patient on aminophylline who was anaesthetised with **thiopental** and fentanyl, and then given **pancuronium**. Three minutes later his heart rate rose to 180 bpm and an ECG revealed that it was supraventricular in origin.[8] The authors of this report attributed this reaction to an interaction between the **pancuronium** and the aminophylline, because previous surgery with these drugs in the absence of aminophylline had been without incident.[8]

The authors of one of the reports advise the avoidance of concurrent use i.e. to wait approximately 13 hours after the last dose of aminophylline before using **halothane**[2] but another[9] says that: "... my own experience with the liberal use of these drugs has convinced me of the efficacy and wide margin of safety associated with their use in combination." A possibly safer anaesthetic may be **isoflurane**, which in studies with *dogs* has been shown not to cause cardiac arrhythmias in the presence of aminophylline.[10]

(b) Development of seizures

Over a period of 9 years, tachycardia and extensor-type seizures were observed in four patients on theophylline or aminophylline, who were initially anaesthetised with **ketamine**, and later with **halothane** or **enflurane**.[11] Based on subsequent study in *mice*, the authors attributed the seizures to an interaction between **ketamine** and theophylline or aminophylline and they suggest that the combination should perhaps be avoided in some, or antiseizure premedication be used in patients at risk. However, this appears to be an isolated report. Note that, in *mice*, **ketamine** had no effect on aminophylline-induced seizures.[12]

(c) Altered neuromuscular blockade

Marked resistance to the effects of **pancuronium** was seen in one patient on an aminophylline infusion, but no resistance was seen when **vecuronium** was given instead.[13] Two other patients are reported to have shown a similar resistance but they had also had hydrocortisone, which could have had a similar effect[14,15] (see also 'Neuromuscular blockers + Corticosteroids', p.906). These appear to be the only reports of such an interaction.

A study in *rabbits* showed that, at therapeutic concentrations of theophylline, the effects of **tubocurarine** were increased,[16] but there do not appear to have been any studies done in humans.

1. Barton MD. Anesthetic problems with aspirin-intolerant patients. *Anesth Analg* (1975) 54, 376–80.
2. Roizen MF, Stevens WC. Multiform ventricular tachycardia due to the interaction of aminophylline and halothane. *Anesth Analg* (1978) 57, 738–41.
3. Naito Y, Arai T, Miyake C. Severe arrhythmias due to the combined use of halothane and aminophylline in an asthmatic patient. *Jpn J Anesthesiol* (1986) 35, 1126–9.
4. Bedger RC, Chang J-L, Larson CE, Bleyaert AL. Increased myocardial irritability with halothane and aminophylline. *Anesth Prog* (1980) 27, 34–6.
5. Richards W, Thompson J, Lewis G, Levy DS, Church JA. Cardiac arrest associated with halothane anesthesia in a patient receiving theophylline. *Ann Allergy* (1988) 61, 83–4
6. Takaori M, Loehning RW. Ventricular arrhythmias induced by aminophylline during halothane anaesthesia in dogs. *Can Anaesth Soc J* (1967) 14, 79–86.
7. Stirt JA, Berger JM, Roe SD, Ricker SM, Sullivan SF. Halothane-induced cardiac arrhythmias following administration of aminophylline in experimental animals. *Anesth Analg* (1981) 60, 517–20.
8. Belani KG, Anderson WW, Buckley JJ. Adverse drug interaction involving pancuronium and aminophylline. *Anesth Analg* (1982) 61, 473–4.
9. Zimmerman BL. Arrhythmogenicity of theophylline and halothane used in combination. *Anesth Analg* (1979) 58, 259–60.
10. Stirt JA, Berger JM, Sullivan SF. Lack of arrhythmogenicity of isoflurane following administration of aminophylline in dogs. *Anesth Analg* (1983) 62, 568–71.
11. Hirshman CA, Krieger W, Littlejohn G, Lee R, Julien R. Ketamine-aminophylline-induced decrease in seizure threshold. *Anesthesiology* (1982) 56, 464–7.
12. Czuczwar SJ, Janusz W, Wamil A, Kleinrok Z. Inhibition of aminophylline-induced convulsions in mice by antiepileptic drugs and other agents. *Eur J Pharmacol* (1987) 144, 309–15.
13. Daller JA, Erstad B, Rosado L, Otto C, Putnam CW. Aminophylline antagonizes the neuromuscular blockade of pancuronium but not vecuronium. *Crit Care Med* (1991) 19, 983–5.
14. Doll DC, Rosenberg H. Antagonism of neuromuscular blockage by theophylline. *Anesth Analg* (1979) 58, 139–40.
15. Azar I, Kumar D, Betcher AM. Resistance to pancuronium in an asthmatic patient treated with aminophylline and steroids. *Can Anaesth Soc J* (1982) 29, 280–2.
16. Fuke N, Martyn J, Kim C, Basta S. Concentration-dependent interaction of theophylline with *d*-tubocurarine. *J Appl Physiol* (1987) 62, 1970–4.

Anaesthetics, general + Timolol

Marked bradycardia and hypotension occurred in a man using timolol eye drops when he was anaesthetised.

Clinical evidence, mechanism, importance and management

A 75-year-old man being treated with timolol eye drops for glaucoma developed bradycardia and severe hypotension when anaesthetised (agent not named), and responded poorly to intravenous atropine, dextrose-saline infusion and elevation of his feet.[1] It would seem that there was sufficient systemic absorption of the timolol for its effects to be additive with the anaesthetic and cause marked depression of cardiac activity. The authors of this report suggest that if patients are to be anaesthetised, low concentrations of timolol should be used (possibly withhold the drops pre-operatively), and that "... induction agents should be used judiciously and beta-blocking antagonists kept readily available." It is easy to overlook the fact that systemic absorption from eye drops can be remarkably high. See also 'Anaesthetics, general + Beta-blockers', p.885.

1. Mostafa SM, Taylor M. Ocular timolol and induction agents during anaesthesia. *BMJ* (1985) 290, 1788.

Anaesthetics, general + Trichloroethane

Two patients with chronic cardiac toxicity after repeated exposure to trichloroethane had a deterioration in cardiac function following halothane anaesthesia.

Clinical evidence, mechanism, importance and management

Two patients who had been repeatedly exposed to trichloroethane (one during solvent abuse including *Tipp-Ex* typewriter correcting fluid thinner and the other due to industrial exposure including *Genklene* for degreasing steel) showed evidence of chronic cardiac toxicity. In both cases there was circumstantial evidence of cardiac deterioration after routine anaesthesia with **halothane**. Some **solvents** have a close chemical similarity to **inhalational anaesthetic** drugs, particularly the halogenated hydrocarbons, and these related compounds might have a toxic interaction.[1]

1. McLeod AA, Marjot R, Monaghan MJ, Hugh-Jones P, Jackson G. Chronic cardiac toxicity after inhalation of 1,1,1-trichloroethane. *BMJ* (1987) 294, 727–9.

Anaesthetics, general and/or Neuromuscular blockers + Tricyclic and related antidepressants

Tricyclic antidepressants may increase the risk of arrhythmias and hypotension during anaesthesia. Tachyarrhythmias have been seen in patients on imipramine who were given halothane and pancuronium. Some very limited evidence suggests that amitriptyline may increase the likelihood of enflurane-induced seizure activity. A man taking maprotiline and lithium developed a tonic-clonic seizure when given propofol. Tricyclics cause an increase in the duration of barbiturate anaesthesia and lower doses of barbiturates should be used.

Clinical evidence, mechanism, importance and management

(a) Development of arrhythmias

Two patients who were taking **nortriptyline** or **nortriptyline** with fluphenazine developed prolonged cardiac arrhythmias during general anaesthesia with **halothane**.[1] Two further patients taking **imipramine** developed marked tachyarrhythmias when anaesthetised with **halothane** and given **pancuronium**.[2] This adverse interaction was subsequently clearly demonstrated in *dogs*.[2] The authors concluded on the basis of their studies that:

- **pancuronium** should be given with caution to patients taking any **tricyclic antidepressant** if **halothane** is used;
- **gallamine** probably should be avoided but **tubocurarine** may be an acceptable alternative to **pancuronium**;
- **pancuronium** is probably safe in the presence of a tricyclic if **enflurane** is used.

However, this last conclusion does not agree with that reached by the authors of another report[3], who found an increased risk of seizures.

Some manufacturers[4] have recommended stopping tricyclics several days before elective surgery where possible. However, the BNF advises that tricyclic antidepressants need not be stopped, but there may be an increased risk of arrhythmias and hypotension (and dangerous interaction with vasopressor drugs–see 'Tricyclic antidepressants + Sympathomimetics; Directly-acting', p.1001). Therefore, the anaesthetist should be informed if they are not stopped.[5]

(b) Development of seizures

(i) Enflurane + Tricyclics. Two patients taking **amitriptyline** developed clonic movements of the leg, arm and hand during surgery while anaesthetised with enflurane and **nitrous oxide**. The movements stopped when the

enflurane was replaced by **halothane**.[3] A possible reason is that **amitriptyline** can lower the seizure threshold at which enflurane-induced seizure activity occurs. It is suggested that it may be advisable to avoid enflurane in patients needing tricyclic antidepressants, particularly in those who have a history of seizures, or when hyperventilation or high concentrations of enflurane are likely to be used.[3]

(ii) Propofol + Maprotiline. A man with a bipolar mood disorder on maprotiline 200 mg four times daily and lithium carbonate 300 mg daily, underwent anaesthesia during which he received fentanyl, **tubocurarine** and propofol 200 mg. Shortly after the injection of the propofol the patient complained of a burning sensation in his face. He then became rigid, his back and neck extended and his eyes turned upwards. After 15 seconds, rhythmic twitching developed in his eyes, arms and hands. This apparent seizure lasted about 1 minute until suxamethonium (succinylcholine) was given and his trachea was intubated. The patient regained consciousness after several minutes and the surgery was cancelled.[6] It is not known whether the reaction was due to an interaction between propofol and the antidepressants, or due to just one of the drugs because both propofol[7,8] and maprotiline[9] have been associated with seizures. However, the authors of this report suggest that it would now be prudent to avoid using propofol in patients taking drugs that significantly lower the convulsive threshold. More study of this possible interaction is needed.

(c) Increased duration of anaesthesia

In a review of electroconvulsive therapy and anaesthetic considerations, it was noted that tricyclics interact with **barbiturates** resulting in an increased sleep time and duration of anaesthesia, and therefore lower doses of barbiturate anaesthetics such as **thiopental** should be employed.[10]

1. Plowman PE, Thomas WJW. Tricyclic antidepressants and cardiac dysrhythmias during dental anaesthesia. *Anaesthesia* (1974) 29, 576–8.
2. Edwards RP, Miller RD, Roizen MF, Ham J, Way WL, Lake CR, Roderick L. Cardiac responses to imipramine and pancuronium during anesthesia with halothane or enflurane. *Anesthesiology* (1979) 50, 421–5.
3. Sprague DH, Wolf S. Enflurane seizures in patients taking amitriptyline. *Anesth Analg* (1982) 61, 67–8.
4. Amitriptylline oral solution. Rosemont Pharmaceuticals Ltd. UK Summary of product characteristics, May 2004.
5. British National Formulary. 49th ed. London: The British Medical Association and The Pharmaceutical Press; 2005. p. 619.
6. Orser B, Oxorn D. Propofol, seizure and antidepressants. *Can J Anaesth* (1994) 41, 262.
7. Bevan JC. Propofol-related convulsions. *Can J Anaesth* (1993) 40, 805–9.
8. Committee on Safety of Medicines. Propofol – convulsions, anaphylaxis and delayed recovery from anaesthesia. *Current Problems* (1989) 26.
9. Jabbari B, Bryan GE, Marsh EE, Gunderson CH. Incidence of seizures with tricyclic and tetracyclic antidepressants. *Arch Neurol* (1985) 42, 480–1.
10. Gaines GY, Rees DI. Electroconvulsive therapy and anesthetic considerations. *Anesth Analg* (1986) 65, 1345–56.

Anaesthetics, general; Methoxyflurane + Antibacterials or Barbiturates

The nephrotoxic effects of methoxyflurane appear to be increased by the use of tetracyclines, and possibly some aminoglycoside antibacterials and barbiturates.

Clinical evidence, mechanism, importance and management

Methoxyflurane has been withdrawn in many countries because it causes kidney damage. This damage can be exacerbated by the concurrent use of other nephrotoxic drugs or possibly by the chronic use of hepatic enzyme-inducing drugs. Five out of 7 patients anaesthetised with methoxyflurane who had been given **tetracycline** before or after surgery showed rises in blood urea nitrogen, and three died. Post-mortem examination showed pathological changes (oxalosis) in the kidneys.[1] Another study identified renal tubular necrosis associated with calcium oxalate crystals in six patients who had been anaesthetised with methoxyflurane and given **tetracycline** (four patients) and **penicillin** with **streptomycin** (two patients).[2] Other reports support the finding of increased nephrotoxicity with **tetracycline**.[3-5] Another study suggested that **penicillin**, **streptomycin** and **chloramphenicol** appear not to increase the renal toxicity of methoxyflurane,[1] but **gentamicin** and **kanamycin** possibly do so.[6] There is also some evidence that **barbiturates** can exacerbate the renal toxicity because they enhance the metabolism of the methoxyflurane and increase the production of nephrotoxic metabolites.[7,8]

The risk of kidney damage with methoxyflurane would therefore appear to be increased by some of these drugs and the concurrent use of **tetracycline** or **nephrotoxic antibiotics** should be avoided. Similarly, methoxyflurane should only be used with great caution, if at all, following the chronic use of hepatic enzyme-inducing drugs.

1. Kuzucu EY. Methoxyflurane, tetracycline, and renal failure. *JAMA* (1970) 211, 1162–4.
2. Dryden GE. Incidence of tubular degeneration with microlithiasis following methoxyflurane compared with other anesthetic agents. *Anesth Analg* (1974) 53, 383–5.
3. Albers DD, Leverett CL, Sandin JH. Renal failure following prostatovesiculectomy related to methoxyflurane anesthesia and tetracycline—complicated by Candida infection. *J Urol (Baltimore)* (1971) 106, 348–50.
4. Proctor EA, Barton FL. Polyuric acute renal failure after methoxyflurane and tetracycline. *BMJ* (1971) 4, 661–2.
5. Stoelting RK, Gibbs PS. Effect of tetracycline therapy on renal function after methoxyflurane anesthesia. *Anesth Analg* (1973) 52, 431–5.
6. Cousins MJ, Mazze RI. Tetracycline, methoxyflurane anaesthesia, and renal dysfunction. *Lancet* (1972) i, 751–2.
7. Churchill D, Yacoub JM, Siu KP, Symes A, Gault MH. Toxic nephropathy after low-dose methoxyflurane anesthesia: drug interaction with secobarbital? *Can Med Assoc J* (1976) 114, 326–33.
8. Cousins MJ, Mazze RI. Methoxyflurane nephrotoxicity: a study of dose response in man. *JAMA* (1973) 225, 1611–16.

Anaesthetics, local + Acetazolamide

Limited evidence suggests an increase in the half-life of procaine in patients given acetazolamide.

Clinical evidence, mechanism, importance and management

The mean **procaine** half-life in 6 healthy subjects was increased by 66% (from 1.46 to 2.43 minutes) 2 hours after being given acetazolamide 250 mg orally. This appears to be because the hydrolysis of the **procaine** is inhibited by the acetazolamide.[1] As the evidence of this interaction is limited to one report, its general significance is unclear.

1. Calvo R, Carlos R, Erill S. Effects of disease and acetazolamide on procaine hydrolysis by red blood cell enzymes. *Clin Pharmacol Ther* (1980) 27, 179–83.

Anaesthetics, local + Alcohol and Antirheumatics

Limited evidence suggests that the failure rate of spinal anaesthesia with bupivacaine may be markedly increased in patients who are receiving antirheumatic drugs and/or who drink alcohol.

Clinical evidence, mechanism, importance and management

The observation that regional anaesthetic failures seemed to be particularly high among patients undergoing orthopaedic surgery who were suffering from rheumatic joint diseases, prompted further study of a possible interaction involving antirheumatic drugs and alcohol. It was found that the failure rate of low-dose spinal anaesthesia with an average volume of 2 ml of 0.5% **bupivacaine** increased from 5% in the control group (no alcohol or long-term treatment) to 32% to 42% in those who had been taking antirheumatic drugs (**indometacin** or unspecified) for at least six months or who drank at least 80 g of ethanol daily, or both. The percentage of those patients who had a reduced response (i.e. an extended latency period and/or a reduced duration of action) also increased from 3% to 39 to 42%.[1] The reasons are not understood. This appears to be the only report of such an effect.

For the effect of alcohol on the surface anaesthetic cocaine, see 'Alcohol + Cocaine', p.48.

1. Sprotte G, Weis KH. Drug interaction with local anaesthetics. *Br J Anaesth* (1982) 54, 242P–243P.

Anaesthetics, local + Anaesthetics, local

Mixtures of local anaesthetics are sometimes used to exploit the most useful characteristics of each drug. This normally seems to be safe although it is sometimes claimed that it increases the risk of toxicity. There is a case report of a man who developed toxicity when bupivacaine and mepivacaine were mixed together. Spinal bupivacaine followed by epidural ropivacaine may also interact to produce profound motor blockade. However, the effectiveness of bupivacaine in epidural anaesthesia may be reduced if it is preceded by chloroprocaine.

Clinical evidence and mechanism

(a) Evidence of no interaction

A study designed to assess the possibility of adverse interactions retrospectively studied the records of 10,538 patients over the period 1952 to 1970 who had been given **tetracaine** combined with **chloroprocaine, lidocaine**, **mepivacaine, prilocaine** or **propoxycaine** for caudal, epidural, or peripheral nerve block. The incidence of systemic toxic reactions was found to be no greater than when used singly and the conclusion was reached that combined use was advantageous and safe.[1] An *animal* study using combinations of **bupivacaine, lidocaine** and **chloroprocaine** also found no evidence that the toxicity was greater than if the anaesthetics were used singly.[2] **Lidocaine** does not affect the pharmacokinetics of **bupivacaine** in man.[3]

(b) Evidence of reduced analgesia

A study set up to examine the clinical impression that **bupivacaine** given epidurally did not relieve labour pain effectively if preceded by **chloroprocaine** confirmed that this was so. Using an initial 10-ml dose of 2% **chloroprocaine** followed by an 8-ml dose of 0.5% **bupivacaine**, the pain relief was less and the block took longer to occur, had a shorter duration of action and had to be augmented more frequently than if only **bupivacaine** was used.[4] This interaction could not be corrected by adjusting the pH of the local anaesthetics.[5]

(c) Evidence of enhanced effect/toxic interaction

There is a single case report of a patient given 0.75% **bupivacaine** and 2% **mepivacaine** who demonstrated lethargy, dysarthria and mild muscle tremor, which the authors of the report correlated with a marked increase in the percentage of unbound (active) **mepivacaine**. They attributed this to its displacement by the **bupivacaine** from protein binding sites.[6] **Bupivacaine** has also been shown *in vitro* to displace **lidocaine** from α_1-acid glycoprotein.[7] Two cases of prolonged, profound motor blockade with patient-controlled epidural analgesia using 0.1% **ropivacaine**, following spinal **bupivacaine** for caesarean section have been reported. Including these two patients, a total of 11 out of 23 patients given regional anaesthesia with **bupivacaine** had clinical evidence of motor weakness at 8 hours after starting **ropivacaine**.[8]

Importance and management

Well examined interactions. The overall picture is that combined use does not normally result in increased toxicity, although there may be some exceptions. For example, until more is known, caution should be exercised when administering epidural **ropivacaine** postoperatively to patients who have had bupivacaine spinal anaesthesia, as unexpected motor block may occur.[8] Reduced effectiveness might be seen if bupivacaine is preceded by chloroprocaine.

1. Moore DC, Bridenbaugh LD, Bridenbaugh PO, Thompson GE, Tucker GT. Does compounding of local anesthetic agents increase their toxicity in humans? *Anesth Analg* (1972) 51, 579–85.
2. de Jong RH, Bonin JD. Mixtures of local anesthetics are no more toxic than the parent drugs. *Anesthesiology* (1981) 54, 177–81.
3. Freysz M, Beal JL, D'Athis P, Mounie J, Wilkening M, Escousse A. Pharmacokinetics of bupivacaine after axillary brachial plexus block. *Int J Clin Pharmacol Ther Toxicol* (1987) 25, 392–5.
4. Hodgkinson R, Husain FJ, Bluhm C. Reduced effectiveness of bupivacaine 0.5% to relieve labor pain after prior injection of chloroprocaine 2%. *Anesthesiology* (1982) 57, A201.
5. Chen B-J, Kwan W-F. pH is not a determinant of 2-chloroprocaine-bupivacaine interaction: a clinical study. *Reg Anesth* (1990) 15 (Suppl 1), 25.
6. Hartrick CT, Raj PP, Dirkes WE, Denson DD. Compounding of bupivacaine and mepivacaine for regional anesthesia. A safe practice? *Reg Anesth* (1984) 9, 94–7.
7. Goolkasian DL, Slaughter RL, Edwards DJ, Lalka D. Displacement of lidocaine from serum α_1-acid glycoprotein binding sites by basic drugs. *Eur J Clin Pharmacol* (1983) 25, 413–17.
8. Buggy DJ, Allsager CM, Coley S. Profound motor blockade with epidural ropivacaine following spinal bupivacaine. *Anaesthesia* (1999) 54, 895–8.

Anaesthetics, local + Antihypertensives

Severe hypotension and bradycardia have been seen in patients on captopril or verapamil during epidural anaesthesia with bupivacaine, but not with verapamil and epidural lidocaine. Acute hypotension also occurred in a man on prazosin during epidural anaesthesia with bupivacaine. See also 'Anaesthetics, local + Beta-blockers', p.895.

Clinical evidence

(a) ACE inhibitors

An 86-year-old man who had been receiving **captopril** 25 mg twice daily and bendrofluazide 25 mg daily [sic] for hypertension, underwent a transurethral resection of prostate under spinal anaesthesia using 3 to 3.5 ml of 'heavy' **bupivacaine** 0.5%. At the end of surgery, he was returned to the supine position and suddenly developed a severe sinus bradycardia (35 bpm), his arterial blood pressure fell to 65/35 mmHg and he became unrousable. Treatment with head-down tilt, oxygen and 1.2 mg of atropine produced rapid improvement in cardiovascular and cerebral function. A further hypotensive episode (without bradycardia) occurred approximately one hour later, which responded rapidly to 4 mg of methoxamine.[1]

(b) Alpha blockers

A man on **prazosin** (5 mg three times daily for hypertension) developed marked hypotension (BP 60/40 mmHg) within 3 to 5 minutes of receiving 100 mg of **bupivacaine** through an L3–4 lumbar epidural catheter.[2] He was unresponsive to intravenous phenylephrine (five 100-microgram boluses) but his blood pressure rose within 3 to 5 minutes of starting an infusion of adrenaline (epinephrine) 0.05 micrograms/kg/minute.

(c) Beta-blockers

See 'Anaesthetics, local + Beta-blockers', p.895.

(d) Anaesthetics, local + Verapamil

Four patients on long-term verapamil treatment developed severe hypotension (systolic pressures as low as 60 mmHg) and bradycardia (48 bpm) 30 to 60 minutes after epidural block with **bupivacaine** 0.5% with adrenaline (epinephrine). This was totally resistant to atropine and ephedrine, and responded only to calcium gluconate or chloride. No such interaction was seen in a similar group of patients when epidural **lidocaine** was used.[3]

Animal experiments have shown that the presence of verapamil increases the toxicity of **lidocaine**, and greatly increases the toxicity of **bupivacaine**, and that pretreatment with calcium chloride blocked this effect.[4]

Mechanism

Spinal anaesthesia can produce bradycardia and a fall in cardiac output resulting in arterial hypotension, which may be magnified by the action of the antihypertensive agent, and by hypovolaemia. Other factors probably contributed to the development of this interaction in these particular patients.

Importance and management

Direct information seems to be limited to the reports cited. Their general relevance is uncertain, but they serve to emphasise the importance of recognising that all antihypertensive drugs interfere in some way with the normal homoeostatic mechanisms that control blood pressure, so that the normal physiological response to hypotension during epidural anaesthesia may be impaired. In this context lidocaine would appear to be preferable to bupivacaine. Intravenous calcium effectively controls the hypotension and bradycardia produced by verapamil toxicity by reversing its calcium channel blocking effects.[5] Particular care would seem to be important with any patient given epidural anaesthesia while taking these antihypertensives. See also 'Anaesthetics, general + Antihypertensives', p.883.

1. Williams NE. Profound bradycardia and hypotension following spinal anaesthesia in a patient receiving an ACE inhibitor: an important 'drug' interaction? *Eur J Anaesthesiol* (1999) 16, 796–8.
2. Lydiatt CA, Fee MP, Hill GE. Severe hypotension during epidural anesthesia in a prazosin-treated patient. *Anesth Analg* (1993) 76, 1152–3.
3. Collier C. Verapamil and epidural bupivacaine. *Anaesth Intensive Care* (1984) 13, 101–8.
4. Tallman RD, Rosenblatt RM, Weaver JM, Wang Y. Verapamil increases the toxicity of local anesthetics. *J Clin Pharmacol* (1988) 28, 317–21.
5. Coaldrake LA. Verapamil overdose. *Anaesth Intensive Care* (1984) 12, 174–5.

Anaesthetics, local + Azoles or Macrolides

Itraconazole may reduce the clearance of bupivacaine, and itraconazole, ketoconazole or clarithromycin may affect ropivacaine metabolism, but the clinical importance of these interactions appears to be limited.

Clinical evidence, mechanism, importance and management

(a) Bupivacaine

Pretreatment with **itraconazole** 200 mg once daily by mouth for 4 days reduced the clearance of bupivacaine 0.3 mg/kg given intravenously over 60 minutes by 20 to 25% in a double-blind, placebo-controlled, crossover study in 7 healthy subjects. The increase in plasma concentrations of bupivacaine should be taken into account when **itraconazole** is used concurrently, although the interaction is probably of limited clinical significance.[1]

(b) Ropivacaine

Pretreatment with **itraconazole** 200 mg daily or **clarithromycin** 250 mg twice daily for 4 days did not significantly affect the pharmacokinetics of ropivacaine 600 microgram/kg given intravenously to 8 healthy subjects, however, there was considerable interindividual variation. A small but insignificant increase of 20% in the AUC of ropivacaine occurred, and the peak plasma concentrations of the metabolite 2′,6′-pipecoloxylidide were significantly decreased by clarithromycin and itraconazole by 44% and 74% respectively. Both itraconazole and clarithromycin inhibit the formation of this metabolite by the cytochrome P450 isoenzyme CYP3A4.[2] Similar results were found with **ketoconazole** and ropivacaine.[3] Potent inhibitors of CYP3A4 appear to cause only a minor decrease in clearance of ropivacaine, which is unlikely to be of clinical relevance.[3]

1. Palkama VJ, Neuvonen PJ, Olkkola KT. Effect of itraconazole on the pharmacokinetics of bupivacaine enantiomers in healthy volunteers. *Br J Anaesth* (1999) 83, 659–61.
2. Jokinen MK, Ahonen J, Neuvonen PJ, Olkkola KT. Effect of clarithromycin and itraconazole on the pharmacokinetics of ropivacaine. *Pharmacol Toxicol* (2001) 88, 187–91.
3. Arlander E, Ekström G, Alm C, Carrillo JA, Bielenstein M, Böttiger Y, Bertilsson L, Gustafsson LL. Metabolism of ropivacaine in humans is mediated by CYP1A2 and to a minor extent by CYP3A4: An interaction study with fluvoxamine and ketoconazole as in vivo inhibitors. *Clin Pharmacol Ther* (1998) 64, 484–91.

Anaesthetics, local + Benzodiazepines

Diazepam may increase the maximum plasma concentrations of bupivacaine, but its rate of elimination may also be increased. Midazolam has been reported to cause a modest decrease in lidocaine but not mepivacaine levels. Spinal anaesthesia with tetracaine may increase the sedative effects of midazolam. A case of possible lidocaine toxicity has been described in a woman on sertraline given flurazepam before intraoperative lidocaine.

Clinical evidence, mechanism, importance and management

(a) Effect of benzodiazepines on local anaesthetics

Twenty-one children aged 2 to 10 years were given single 1-ml/kg caudal injections of a mixture of 0.5% **lidocaine** and 0.125% **bupivacaine** for regional anaesthesia. Pretreatment with **diazepam** 10 mg rectally half-an-hour before the surgery had no significant effect on the plasma concentrations of **lidocaine**, but the AUC and maximum plasma **bupivacaine** concentrations were increased by 70 to 75%.[1] In another study, prior administration of intravenous **diazepam** in adult patients slightly, but not significantly, increased the mean maximum plasma concentrations of epidural **bupivacaine** or **etidocaine**. However, the elimination half-lives of both anaesthetics were significantly decreased by about a half.[2]

A study in 20 children aged 2 to 7 years receiving caudal block with 1 ml/kg of a solution containing 0.5% **lidocaine** and 0.125% **bupivacaine**, found that **midazolam** 400 micrograms/kg given rectally half-an-hour before surgery caused a slight but not significant reduction in the AUC and serum levels of **bupivacaine**, whereas the **lidocaine** AUC was reduced by 24%.[3] In contrast, **midazolam** 400 micrograms/kg given rectally as a premedication was found to have no significant effect on plasma **mepivacaine** levels.[4]

There has been a single report of possible **lidocaine** toxicity following tumescent liposuction in a patient given perioperative sedation with **flurazepam** 30 mg orally. Ten hours after the completion of the procedure, in which a total of 58 mg/kg of lidocaine was used, the patient had nausea and vomiting, unsteady gate, mild confusion, and speech impairment. Her lidocaine level was 6.3 mg/L (levels greater than 6 mg/L were considered to be associated with an increased risk of toxicity). The patient was also on long-term treatment with sertraline. The authors suggested that sertraline and **flurazepam** may have had an additive effect on reducing the rate of **lidocaine** metabolism via inhibition of cytochrome P450 isoenzyme CYP3A4.[5]

The clinical importance of these interactions is uncertain, but anaesthetists should be aware that increased **bupivacaine** plasma concentrations have been observed with **diazepam**, and reduced **lidocaine** concentrations with **midazolam**. More study is needed.

(b) Effect of local anaesthetics on benzodiazepines

Twenty patients undergoing surgery were given repeated 1-mg intravenous doses of **midazolam** as induction anaesthesia every 30 seconds until they failed to respond to three repeated commands to squeeze the anaesthetist's hand. This was considered as the induction end-point 'titrated' dose. It was found that the 10 who had been given prior spinal anaesthesia with **tetracaine** 12 mg needed only half the dose of **midazolam** (7.6 mg) than the 10 other patients who had not received a spinal injection (14.7 mg). The reasons are not known. The authors of this report simply advise care in this situation.[6]

1. Giaufre E, Bruguerolle B, Morisson-Lacombe G, Rousset-Rouviere B. The influence of diazepam on the plasma concentrations of bupivacaine and lignocaine after caudal injection of a mixture of the local anaesthetics in children. *Br J Clin Pharmacol* (1988) 26, 116–18.
2. Giasi RM, D'Agostino E, Covino BG. Interaction of diazepam and epidurally administered local anesthetic agents. *Reg Anesth* (1980) 5, 8–11.
3. Giaufre E, Bruguerolle B, Morisson-Lacombe G, Rousset-Rouviere B. The influence of midazolam on the plasma concentrations of bupivacaine and lidocaine after caudal injection of a mixture of the local anesthetics in children. *Acta Anaesthesiol Scand* (1990) 34, 44–6.
4. Giaufre E, Bruguerolle B, Morisson-Lacombe G, Rousset-Rouviere B. Influence of midazolam on the plasma concentrations of mepivacaine after lumbar epidural injection in children. *Eur J Clin Pharmacol* (1990) 38, 91–2.
5. Klein JA, Kassarjdian N. Lidocaine toxicity with tumescent liposuction: a case report of probable drug interactions. *Dermatol Surg* (1997) 23, 1169–74.
6. Ben-David B, Vaida S, Gaitini L. The influence of high spinal anesthesia on sensitivity to midazolam sedation. *Anesth Analg* (1995) 81, 525–8.

Anaesthetics, local + Beta-blockers

Propranolol reduces the clearance of bupivacaine and so theoretically the toxicity of bupivacaine may be increased. There has been a single report of enhanced bupivacaine cardiotoxicity in a patient also receiving metoprolol and digoxin. Propranolol and some other beta-blockers increase plasma-lidocaine concentrations, see 'Lidocaine + Beta-blockers', p.174. The coronary vasoconstriction caused by cocaine is increased by propranolol. Beta-blockers may interact with adrenaline (epinephrine)-containing local anaesthetics, see also 'Beta-blockers + Sympathomimetics; Directly-acting', p.643.

Clinical evidence, mechanism, importance and management

(a) Bupivacaine + Propranolol

The clearance of bupivacaine was reduced by about 35% in 6 healthy subjects given bupivacaine 30 to 50 mg intravenously over 10 to 15 minutes after taking 40 mg propranolol six-hourly for a day. The reason is thought to be that the propranolol inhibits the activity of the liver microsomal enzymes, thereby reducing the metabolism of the bupivacaine. Changes in blood flow to the liver are unlikely to affect bupivacaine metabolism substantially because it is relatively poorly extracted from the blood. The clinical importance of this interaction is uncertain, but it is suggested that an increase in local anaesthetic toxicity might occur and caution should be exercised if multiple doses of bupivacaine are given.[1] Propranolol and some other beta-blockers are known to reduce the metabolism of lidocaine—see 'Lidocaine + Beta-blockers', p.174.

(b) Bupivacaine + Metoprolol

There is a case report of possible enhanced bupivacaine cardiotoxicity in a patient who was receiving enalapril 5 mg daily, metoprolol 25 mg twice daily and digoxin 250 micrograms four times a day (serum digoxin level 1.1 nanograms/ml). Cardiac arrest occurred 15 minutes after injection of 0.5% bupivacaine with adrenaline (epinephrine) for intercostal nerve block (total dose 100 mg). The cardiodepressant effects of metoprolol, digoxin and bupivacaine may have combined to produce toxicity at a dose of bupivacaine not usually considered toxic. The authors caution that patients on digoxin/calcium channel blocker and/or beta-blockers should be considered at higher risk for bupivacaine cardiotoxicity.[2]

(c) Cocaine + Propranolol

A study in 30 patients being evaluated for chest pain found that 2 mg/kg of a 10% intranasal solution of cocaine reduced coronary sinus flow by about 14% and coronary artery diameter by 6 to 9%. The coronary vascular resistance increased by 22%. The addition of propranolol

400 microgram/minute by intracoronary infusion, (to a total of 2 mg) reduced coronary sinus flow by a further 15% and increased the coronary vascular resistance by 17%. The probable reason is that the cocaine stimulates the alpha-receptors (vasoconstrictor) of the coronary blood vessels. When the beta-receptors are blocked by propranolol, the resultant unopposed alpha-adrenergic stimulation may lead to enhanced coronary vasoconstriction (see also 'Beta-blockers + Sympathomimetics; Directly-acting', p.643). The clinical importance of these findings is uncertain but the authors of the report suggest that beta-blockers should be avoided in patients with myocardial ischaemia or infarction associated with the use of cocaine.[3]

(d) Lidocaine and Adrenaline (Epinephrine) + Beta-blockers

In a double-blind, randomised, crossover study in 10 healthy subjects, the upper lateral incisor teeth were anaesthetised using lidocaine with or without adrenaline (epinephrine). The mean duration of pulpal and soft-tissue anaesthesia using 1 ml of 2% lidocaine containing 1:100,000 adrenaline was increased by 58% (17 minutes) and 19% (16.5 minutes), respectively, in subjects pretreated with **nadolol** 80 mg orally compared with placebo. Pretreatment with the beta-blocker did not affect the duration of anaesthesia when lidocaine without adrenaline was used.[4] It is likely that the combined effects of adrenaline and **nadolol** caused increased local vasoconstriction, which resulted in the lidocaine persisting for longer. When a small amount of local anaesthetic with adrenaline is injected for dental procedures, this study shows that an increased duration of analgesia may result. However, note that, with larger doses of adrenaline, serious hypertension and bradycardia have resulted from the interaction between non-selective beta blockers and adrenaline (see 'Beta-blockers + Sympathomimetics; Directly-acting', p.643). The authors conclude that, for dental procedures, the minimum amount of local anaesthetic containing the lowest concentration of adrenaline should be used. Alternatively, if excessive bleeding is unlikely, a local anaesthetic without adrenaline is preferred.[4]

1. Bowdle TA, Freund PR, Slattery JT. Propranolol reduces bupivacaine clearance. *Anesthesiology* (1987) 66, 36–8.
2. Roitman K, Sprung J, Wallace M, Matjasko J. Enhancement of bupivacaine cardiotoxicity with cardiac glycosides and β-adrenergic blockers: a case report. *Anesth Analg* (1993) 76, 658–61.
3. Lange RA, Cigarroa RG, Flores ED, McBride W, Kim AS, Wells PJ, Bedotto JB, Danziger RS, Hillis LD. Potentiation of cocaine-induced coronary vasoconstriction by beta-adrenergic blockade. *Ann Intern Med* (1990) 112, 897–903.
4. Zhang C, Banting DW, Gelb AW, Hamilton JT. Effect of β-adrenoreceptor blockade with nadolol on the duration of local anesthesia. *J Am Dent Assoc* (1999) 130, 1773–80.

Anaesthetics, local + Fluvoxamine

Fluvoxamine inhibits the clearance of ropivacaine; therefore, prolonged administration of ropivacaine should be avoided in patients treated with fluvoxamine.

Clinical evidence, mechanism, importance and management

Fluvoxamine decreased the mean total plasma clearance of **ropivacaine** by 68% from 354 to 112 ml/minute, and almost doubled the **ropivacaine** half life in a randomised, crossover study in 12 healthy subjects. Fluvoxamine was given at a dose of 25 mg twice daily for 2 days, and a single 40 mg intravenous dose of **ropivacaine** was given over 20 minutes one hour after the morning dose of fluvoxamine on the second day.[1]

Fluvoxamine is a potent inhibitor of the cytochrome P450 isoenzyme CYP1A2 and so reduces the metabolism of **ropivacaine** to its major metabolite 3-hydroxyropivacaine.

The UK maker recommends that prolonged administration of **ropivacaine** should be avoided in patients concurrently treated with potent CYP1A2 inhibitors such as fluvoxamine.[2]

1. Arlander E, Ekström G, Alm C, Carrillo JA, Bielenstein M, Böttiger Y, Bertilsson L, Gustafsson LL. Metabolism of ropivacaine in humans is mediated by CYP1A2 and to a minor extent by CYP3A4: An interaction study with fluvoxamine and ketoconazole as in vivo inhibitors. *Clin Pharmacol Ther* (1998) 64, 484–91.
2. Naropin (Ropivacaine). AstraZeneca UK Ltd. UK Summary of product characteristics, March 2004.

Anaesthetics, local + H_2-blockers

Some studies suggest that both cimetidine and ranitidine can raise plasma bupivacaine levels, whereas other evidence suggests that no significant interaction occurs. Neither H_2-blocker appears to significantly affect lidocaine when used as an anaesthetic, but see also 'Lidocaine + H_2-blockers', p.176.

Clinical evidence

(a) Cimetidine + Bupivacaine

Pretreatment with cimetidine 300 mg intramuscularly 1 to 4 hours before epidural anaesthesia with 0.5% bupivacaine (for caesarean section) had no effect on the pharmacokinetics of bupivacaine in 16 women or their foetuses when compared with 20 control women, although the maternal unbound bupivacaine plasma levels rose by 22%.[1] These findings were confirmed in two similar studies[2,3] in which women were pretreated with cimetidine before caesarean section, and a further study[4] in 7 healthy subjects (6 women and one man) given two oral doses of cimetidine 400 mg before intramuscular bupivacaine. However, four healthy male subjects who were given cimetidine 400 mg at 10 pm the previous evening and 8 am on the study day, followed by a 50-mg infusion of bupivacaine at 11 am, showed a 40% increase in the bupivacaine AUC compared with placebo.[5]

(b) Cimetidine + Lidocaine

No changes in the pharmacokinetics of 400 mg of lidocaine 2% (administered with adrenaline (epinephrine) 1:200,000) were seen in five women given epidural anaesthesia for caesarean section after a single 400-mg oral dose of cimetidine given about 2 hours preoperatively.[6] Another very similar study in 9 women found no statistically significant rises in whole blood lidocaine levels (although they tended to be higher) in the presence of cimetidine 300 mg, given intramuscularly, at least an hour preoperatively.[7]

(c) Ranitidine + Bupivacaine

Pretreatment with oral ranitidine 150 mg 1.5 to 2 hours before bupivacaine for extradural anaesthesia for caesarean section, increased the maximum plasma levels of bupivacaine in 10 patients by about 36%, compared with 10 patients given no pretreatment.[3] Another study found that two oral doses of ranitidine 150 mg caused a 25% increase in the mean AUC of bupivacaine, but this was not statistically significant.[5] No increased bupivacaine toxicity was described in any of these reports. However, two other studies in 36 and 28 women, respectively, (undergoing caesarean section) found no measurable effect on the bupivacaine disposition when given ranitidine 150 mg the night before and on the morning of anaesthesia[2] or **ranitidine** 50 mg intramuscularly 2 hours before anaesthesia.[8]

(d) Ranitidine + Lidocaine

No changes in the pharmacokinetics of 400 mg of lidocaine 2%, (administered with adrenaline (epinephrine) 1:200,000) were seen in 7 women given epidural anaesthesia for caesarean section after a single 150-mg oral dose of ranitidine given about 2 hours preoperatively.[6] A similar study in 8 women also found no statistically significant rises in whole blood lidocaine levels in the presence of ranitidine 150 mg given orally at least 2 hours preoperatively.[7]

Mechanism

Not understood. A reduction in the metabolism of the bupivacaine by the liver caused by the cimetidine is one suggested explanation. Protein binding displacement is another.

Importance and management

A confusing situation. No clinically important interaction has been established, but be alert for any evidence of increased bupivacaine toxicity resulting from raised total plasma levels and rises in unbound bupivacaine levels during concurrent use. Cimetidine (but not ranitidine) has been shown to raise plasma lidocaine levels when lidocaine is used as an antiarrhythmic agent (see 'Lidocaine + H_2-blockers', p.176), but this was not demonstrated in the studies cited above.

1. Kuhnert BR, Zuspan KJ, Kuhnert PM, Syracuse CD, Brashear WT, Brown DE. Lack of influence of cimetidine on bupivacaine levels during parturition. *Anesth Analg* (1987) 66, 986–90.
2. O'Sullivan GM, Smith M, Morgan B, Brighouse D, Reynolds F. H_2 antagonists and bupivacaine clearance. *Anaesthesia* (1988) 43, 93–5.
3. Flynn RJ, Moore J, Collier PS, McClean E. Does pretreatment with cimetidine and ranitidine affect the disposition of bupivacaine? *Br J Anaesth* (1989) 62, 87–91.
4. Pihlajamäki KK, Lindberg RLP, Jantunen ME. Lack of effect of cimetidine on the pharmacokinetics of bupivacaine in healthy subjects. *Br J Clin Pharmacol* (1988) 26, 403–6.
5. Noble DW, Smith KJ, Dundas CR. Effects of H-2 antagonists on the elimination of bupivacaine. *Br J Anaesth* (1987) 59, 735–7.

6. Flynn RJ, Moore J, Collier PS, Howard PJ. Single dose oral H_2-antagonists do not affect plasma lidocaine levels in the parturient. *Acta Anaesthesiol Scand* (1989) 33, 593–6.
7. Dailey PA, Hughes SC, Rosen MA, Healey K, Cheek DBC, Shnider SM. Effect of cimetidine and ranitidine on lidocaine concentrations during epidural anesthesia for cesarean section. *Anesthesiology* (1988) 69, 1013–17.
8. Brashear WT, Zuspan KJ, Lazebnik N, Kuhnert BR, Mann LI. Effect of ranitidine on bupivacaine disposition. *Anesth Analg* (1991) 72, 369–76.

Anaesthetics, local + Quinolones

It is likely that enoxacin will inhibit the metabolism of ropivacaine; therefore, prolonged administration of ropivacaine should be avoided in patients treated with enoxacin.

Clinical evidence, mechanism, importance and management

Ropivacaine is extensively metabolised in the liver via the cytochrome P450 isoenzyme CYP1A2 to form the major metabolite 3-hydroxyropivacaine. On the basis of data with 'fluvoxamine', (p.896), the UK manufacturer of **ropivacaine** has recommended that prolonged administration of ropivacaine should be avoided in patients concurrently treated with strong CYP1A2 inhibitors such as **enoxacin**.[1]

1. Naropin (Ropivacaine). AstraZeneca UK Ltd. UK Summary of product characteristics, March 2004.

Anaesthetics, local + Rifampicin (Rifampin) and/or Tobacco smoking

Rifampicin increases the metabolism of ropivacaine, but this probably has little clinical relevance to its use as a local anaesthetic. Smoking appears to have only a minor effect on ropivacaine pharmacokinetics. Tobacco smoking may enhance cocaine-associated myocardial ischaemia.

Clinical evidence, mechanism, importance and management

(a) Cocaine

In a study involving 42 smokers (36 with proven coronary artery disease) the mean product of the heart rate and systolic arterial pressure increased by 11% after intranasal cocaine 2 mg/kg, by 12% after one cigarette and by 45% after both cocaine use and one cigarette. Compared with baseline measurements, the diameters of non-diseased coronary arterial segments decreased on average by 7% after cocaine use, 7% after smoking and 6% after cocaine and smoking; however, the diameters of diseased segments decreased by 9%, 5% and 19%, respectively.[1] Cigarette smoking increases myocardial oxygen demand and induces coronary-artery vasoconstriction through an alpha-adrenergic mechanism similar to cocaine and therefore tobacco smoking may enhance cocaine-associated myocardial ischaemia.[1,2]

(b) Ropivacaine

A study in 10 healthy nonsmokers and 8 healthy smokers given ropivacaine 600 micrograms/kg by intravenous infusion over 30 minutes showed that smoking increased the urinary excretion of the metabolite 3-hydroxyropivacaine and decreased the urinary excretion of 2′,6′-pipecoloxylidide by 62%, but did not significantly affect the ropivacaine AUC. However, pretreatment with rifampicin 600 mg daily by mouth for 5 days increased the clearance (by 93% and 46%) and decreased the AUC by 52% and 38% and half-life of ropivacaine in both nonsmokers and smokers, respectively.[3] Ropivacaine undergoes oxidative hepatic metabolism mainly by the cytochrome P450 isoenzymes CYP1A2 and CYP3A4. Cigarette smoking may increase CYP1A2-mediated metabolism of ropivacaine, and the elimination of ropivacaine may be considerably accelerated by rifampicin, which is a potent cytochrome P450 enzyme inducer. However, in clinical use the local anaesthetic is administered near the nerves to be desensitised and induction of isoenzymes is not likely to affect the local anaesthetic before it enters the systemic blood circulation.[3] This interaction is therefore of little clinical relevance.

Rifampicin may also increase the metabolism of lidocaine to a minor extent, see 'Lidocaine + Rifampicin (Rifampin)', p.178, and smoking may reduce the *oral* bioavailability of 'lidocaine', (p.178).

1. Moliterno DJ, Willard JE, Lange RA, Negus BH, Boehrer JD, Glamann DB, Landau C, Rossen JD, Winniford MD, Hillis LD. Coronary-artery vasoconstriction induced by cocaine, cigarette smoking, or both. *N Engl J Med* (1994) 330, 454–9.
2. Hollander JE. The management of cocaine-associated myocardial ischemia. *N Engl J Med* (1995) 333, 1267–72.
3. Jokinen MJ, Olkkola KT, Ahonen J, Neuvonen PJ. Effect of rifampin and tobacco smoking on the pharmacokinetics of ropivacaine. *Clin Pharmacol Ther* (2001) 70, 344–50.

Botulinum toxin + Miscellaneous

Theoretically, the neuromuscular blocking effects of botulinum toxin can be increased by other drugs with neuromuscular blocking effects such as the aminoglycosides and muscle relaxants, but no such interactions have been reported.

Clinical evidence, mechanism, importance and management

A case report describes a 5-month-old baby boy who was admitted to hospital because of lethargy, poor feeding, constipation and muscle weakness (later identified as being due to a ***Clostridium botulinum*** **infection**). An hour after starting intravenous treatment with ampicillin and **gentamicin** 7.5 mg/kg daily in divided doses every 8 hours for presumed sepsis, he stopped breathing and died. The reason appeared to be the additive neuromuscular blocking effects of the systemic botulinum toxin produced by the *Clostridium botulinum* infection and the **gentamicin**.[1] *Animal* studies confirm that **gentamicin** and **tobramycin** potentiate the neuromuscular blocking effects of systemically administered botulinum toxin (used to mimic botulism),[1] and there is every reason to believe that any of the other drugs known to cause neuromuscular blockade (**aminoglycosides**, conventional **neuromuscular blockers**, etc.) will behave similarly. However, note that clinically, botulinum A toxin is injected for local effect in specific muscles, and is not used systemically; therefore, the situation is not analogous to that described in the case of the child with systemic botulism.

Up until 2002, the UK makers of botulinum A toxin stated in their prescribing information that the **aminoglycosides** and **spectinomycin** were contraindicated. They also advised caution with **polymyxins, tetracyclines** and **lincomycin**, and a reduced starting dose with **muscle relaxants** with a long-lasting effect, or the use of an intermediate action drug such as vecuronium or atracurium.[2] Later prescribing information notes that no interactions of clinical significance have been reported, and the cautions have been reduced to a general statement of the theoretical possibility of potentiation.[3] Similarly the UK makers of botulinum B caution use with aminoglycosides or other drugs that affect neuromuscular transmission.[4]

1. Santos JI, Swensen P, Glasgow LA. Potentiation of *Clostridium botulinum* toxin by aminoglycoside antibiotics: clinical and laboratory observations. *Pediatrics* (1981) 68, 50–4.
2. Botox (Botulinum A toxin). Allergan Ltd. UK Summary of product characteristics, December 2002.
3. Botox (Botulinum A toxin). Allergan Ltd. UK Summary of product characteristics, April 2005.
4. Neurobloc (Botulinum B toxin). Elan Pharma Ltd. UK Summary of product characteristics, July 2003.

Bupivacaine + Calcium channel blockers

On theoretical grounds the potentially serious cardiac depressant effects of intravenous bupivacaine may be enhanced in patients taking calcium channel blockers.

Clinical evidence, mechanism, importance and management

A number of factors (e.g. hypoxia, hyperkalaemia, acidosis, pregnancy and age)[1] can enhance the myocardial depression of intravenous bupivacaine, and studies in *dogs* have now confirmed the suspicion that calcium channel blockers such as **nifedipine**[1] and **verapamil**[2] can do the same. Elderly patients with impaired cardiovascular function on calcium channel blockers would therefore appear to be at considerable risk if bupivacaine is accidentally given intravenously during regional anaesthesia, but so far there appear to be no clinical reports of this adverse interaction.

1. Howie MB, Mortimer W, Candler EM, McSweeney TD, Frolicher DA. Does nifedipine enhance the cardiovascular depressive effects of bupivacaine? *Reg Anesth* (1989) 14, 19–25.
2. Liu P, Feldman HS, Covino BM, Giasi R, Covion, BG. Acute cardiovascular toxicity of intravenous amide local anesthetics in anesthetized ventilated dogs. *Anesth Analg* (1982) 61, 317–22.

Cocaine + Adrenaline (Epinephrine)

Arrhythmias occurred in 3 patients given a concentrated nasal paste containing cocaine and adrenaline (epinephrine).

Clinical evidence, mechanism, importance and management

Two children and one adult patient undergoing general anaesthesia developed arrhythmias shortly after nasal application of a paste containing cocaine 25% and adrenaline (epinephrine) 0.18%. All 3 patients received doses of cocaine that exceeded the maximum dose (1.5 mg/kg) currently recommended in the BNF[1] for healthy adults.

Cocaine has sympathomimetic actions (tachycardia, peripheral vasoconstriction, and hypertension). Combined use with sympathomimetics such as adrenaline increases these effects, and the risk of life-threatening arrhythmias. This risk may be further increased if halothane anaesthesia is used (two of the above cases received halothane[2]). See also 'Anaesthetics, general + Anaesthetics, local', p.882 and 'Anaesthetics, general + Sympathomimetics', p.891.

The use of adrenaline with topical cocaine is controversial. Some consider that the addition of adrenaline is of doubtful value and that the combination should not be used, especially in the form of a concentrated paste.[2] However, others consider the combination to be safe and useful.[3] Whether or not adrenaline is combined with cocaine, the BNF considers that topical cocaine should be used only by those skilled in the precautions needed to minimise absorption and the consequent risk of arrhythmias.[1]

Note also that the use of local anaesthetics containing adrenaline should be avoided in patients who abuse cocaine, unless it is certain that they have not used cocaine for at least 24 hours.[4]

1. British National Formulary. 49th ed. London: The British Medical Association and The Pharmaceutical Press; 2005. p. 637.
2. Nicholson KEA, Rogers JEG. Cocaine and adrenaline paste: a fatal combination? *BMJ* (1995) 311, 250–1.
3. De R, Uppal HS, Shehab ZP, Hilger AW, Wilson PS, Courteney-Harris R. Current practices of cocaine administration by UK otorhinolaryngologists. *J Laryngol Otol* (2003) 117, 109–12.
4. Goulet J-P, Pérusse R, Turcotte J-Y. Contraindications to vasoconstrictors in dentistry: part III. *Oral Surg Oral Med Oral Pathol* (1992) 74, 692–7.

Neuromuscular blockers + Aminoglycosides

The aminoglycoside antibacterials possess neuromuscular blocking activity. Appropriate measures should be taken to accommodate the increased neuromuscular blockade and the prolonged and potentially fatal respiratory depression that can occur if these antibacterials are used with conventional neuromuscular blocking drugs of any kind.

Clinical evidence

Two examples from many:

A 38-year-old patient anaesthetised with **cyclopropane** experienced severe respiratory depression after intraperitoneal administration of **neomycin** solution 500 mg. She had also received **suxamethonium (succinylcholine)** and **tubocurarine**. This antibacterial-induced neuromuscular blockade was resistant to treatment with edrophonium.[1]

A 71-year-old woman received a standard bowel preparation consisting of oral erythromycin and **neomycin** (a total of 3 grams). Surgery was postponed for one day and she received a second similar bowel preparation pre-operatively. Anaesthesia was induced with sufentanil and etomidate and maintained with isoflurane and sufentanil. **Rocuronium** (total dose of 60 mg over 2 hours) was used to facilitate tracheal intubation and maintain muscle relaxation. Despite clinical appearance of reversal of neuromuscular blockade after the intravenous administration of neostigmine 3.5 mg and glycopyrrolate 400 micrograms, the patient complained of dyspnoea and required reintubation twice. The effects of additional doses of neostigmine were inconsistent and administration of edrophonium 50 mg or calcium chloride 500 mg intravenously caused no improvement.[2]

Many other reports confirm that some degree of respiratory depression or paralysis can occur if aminoglycosides are given to anaesthetised patients. When a conventional blocker is also used, the blockade is deepened and recovery prolonged. If the antibacterial is given towards the end of surgery the result can be that a patient who is recovering normally from neuromuscular blockade suddenly develops serious apnoea which can lead on to prolonged and in some cases fatal respiratory depression. Pittinger[3] lists more than a 100 cases in the literature over the period 1956 to 1970 involving:

- **tubocurarine** with **neomycin** or **streptomycin**,
- **gallamine** with **neomycin**, **kanamycin** or **streptomycin**,
- **suxamethonium** with **neomycin**, **kanamycin** or **streptomycin**.

The routes of antibacterial administration were oral, intraperitoneal, oesophageal, intraluminal, retroperitoneal, intramuscular, intrapleural, cystic, beneath skin flaps, extradural and intravenous. Later reports involve:

- **pancuronium**; with **amikacin**,[4] **gentamicin**,[5] **neomycin**,[6] or **streptomycin**,[7,8]
- **pipecuronium** with **netilmicin**,[9]
- **suxamethonium** with **dibekacin**,[10]
- **tubocurarine**; with **amikacin**,[11] **dibekacin**,[10,12] **framycetin** (eye irrigation),[13] **ribostamycin**,[10,12] or **tobramycin**,[14]
- **vecuronium**; with **amikacin/polymyxin**,[15] **gentamicin**,[16,17] **gentamicin/clindamycin**,[18] or **tobramycin**.[17,19]

Aminoglycosides and neuromuscular blockers that have been reported not to interact are as follows:

- **tobramycin** with **alcuronium**,[20] **atracurium**[17] or **suxamethonium**,[10]
- **gentamicin** with **atracurium**,[17]
- **ribostamycin** with **suxamethonium**.[10]

Mechanism

The aminoglycosides appear to reduce or prevent the release of acetylcholine at neuromuscular junctions (related to an impairment of calcium influx) and they may also lower the sensitivity of the post-synaptic membrane, thereby reducing transmission. These effects would be additive with those of conventional neuromuscular blockers, which act at the post-synaptic membrane.

Importance and management

Extremely well documented, very long established, clinically important and potentially serious interactions. Ten out of the 111 cases cited by Pittinger[3] were fatal, related directly or indirectly to aminoglycoside-induced respiratory depression. Concurrent use need not be avoided, but be alert for increased and prolonged neuromuscular blockade with every aminoglycoside and neuromuscular blocker although the potencies of the aminoglycosides differ to some extent. In *animal* studies at concentrations representing the maximum therapeutic levels, the neuromuscular blocking potency of various aminoglycosides was rated (from highest to lowest) neomycin, streptomycin, gentamicin, kanamycin.[21] The postoperative recovery period should also be closely monitored because of the risk of recurarisation if the aminoglycoside is given during surgery. High-risk patients appear to be those with renal disease and hypocalcaemia who may have elevated serum antibacterial levels, and those with pre-existing muscular weakness. Treatment of the increased blockade with anticholinesterases and calcium has met with variable success because the response seems to be inconsistent.

1. LaPorte J, Mignault G, L'Allier R, Perron P. Un cas d'apnée à la néomycine. *Union Med Can* (1959) 88, 149–52.
2. Hasfurther DL, Bailey PL. Failure of neuromuscular blockade reversal after rocuronium in a patient who received oral neomycin. *Can J Anaesth* (1996) 43, 617–20.
3. Pittinger CB, Eryasa Y, Adamson R. Antibiotic-induced paralysis. *Anesth Analg* (1970) 49, 487–501.
4. Monsegur JC, Vidal MM, Beltrán J, Felipe MAN. Parálisis neuromuscular prolongada tras administración simultánea de amikacina y pancuronio. *Rev Esp Anestesiol Reanim* (1984) 31, 30–3.
5. Regan AG, Perumbetti PPV. Pancuronium and gentamicin interaction in patients with renal failure. *Anesth Analg* (1980) 59, 393.
6. Giala M, Sareyiannis C, Cortsaris N, Paradelis A, Lappas DG. Possible interaction of pancuronium and tubocurarine with oral neomycin. *Anaesthesia* (1982) 37, 776.
7. Giala MM, Paradelis AG. Two cases of prolonged respiratory depression due to interaction of pancuronium with colistin and streptomycin. *J Antimicrob Chemother* (1979) 5, 234–5.
8. Torresi S, Pasotti EM. Su un caso di curarizzazione prolungata da interazione tra pancuronio e streptomicina. *Minerva Anestesiol* (1984) 50, 143–5.
9. Stanley JC, Mirakhur RK, Clarke RSJ. Study of pipecuronium-antibiotic interaction. *Anesthesiology* (1990) 73, A898.
10. Arai T, Hashimoto Y, Shima T, Matsukawa S, Iwatsuki K. Neuromuscular blocking properties of tobramycin, dibekacin and ribostamycin in man. *Jpn J Antibiot* (1977) 30, 281–4.
11. Singh YN, Marshall IG, Harvey AL. Some effects of the aminoglycoside antibiotic amikacin on neuromuscular and autonomic transmission. *Br J Anaesth* (1978) 50, 109–17.
12. Hashimoto Y, Shima T, Matsukawa S, Iwatsuki K. Neuromuscular blocking properties of some antibiotics in man. *Tohoku J Exp Med* (1975) 117, 339–400.
13. Clark R. Prolonged curarization due to intraocular soframycin. *Anaesth Intensive Care* (1975) 3, 79–80.

14. Waterman PM, Smith RB. Tobramycin-curare interaction. *Anesth Analg* (1977) 56, 587–8.
15. Kronenfeld MA, Thomas SJ, Turndorf H. Recurrence of neuromuscular blockade after reversal of vecuronium in a patient receiving polymyxin/amikacin sternal irrigation. *Anesthesiology* (1986) 65, 93–4.
16. Harwood TN, Moorthy SS. Prolonged vecuronium-induced neuromuscular blockade in children. *Anesth Analg* (1989) 68, 534–6.
17. Dupuis JY, Martin R, Tétrault J-P. Atracurium and vecuronium interaction with gentamicin and tobramycin. *Can J Anaesth* (1989) 36, 407–11.
18. Jedeikin R, Dolgunski E, Kaplan R, Hoffman S. Prolongation of neuromuscular blocking effect of vecuronium by antibiotics. *Anaesthesia* (1987) 42, 858–60.
19. Vanacker BF, Van de Walle J. The neuromuscular blocking action of vecuronium in normal patients and in patients with no renal function and interaction vecuronium-tobramycin in renal transplant patients. *Acta Anaesthesiol Belg* (1986) 37, 95–9.
20. Boliston TA, Ashman R. Tobramycin and neuromuscular blockade. *Anaesthesia* (1978) 33, 552.
21. Caputy AJ, Kim YI, Sanders DB. The neuromuscular blocking effects of therapeutic concentrations of various antibiotics on normal rat skeletal muscle: a quantitative comparison. *J Pharmacol Exp Ther* (1981) 217: 369–78.

Neuromuscular blockers + Anaesthetics, local

The neuromuscular blockade due to suxamethonium (succinylcholine) can be increased and prolonged by lidocaine, procaine and possibly procainamide. Lidocaine, procaine and procainamide all have some neuromuscular blocking activity and may theoretically also enhance the block produced by competitive neuromuscular blockers. Increased toxicity occurred when mivacurium and prilocaine were given together for regional anaesthesia.

Clinical evidence

A patient anaesthetised with fluroxene and nitrous oxide demonstrated 100% blockade with **suxamethonium** (**succinylcholine**) and **tubocurarine**. About 50 minutes later when twitch height had fully returned and tidal volume was 400 ml, she was given lidocaine 50 mg intravenously for premature ventricular contractions. She immediately stopped breathing and the twitch disappeared. About 45 minutes later the tidal volume was 450 ml. Later it was found that the patient had a dibucaine number (a measure of cholinesterase activity) of 23%.[1]

A study in 10 patients has confirmed that lidocaine and procaine prolong the apnoea following the use of **suxamethonium** 700 micrograms/kg. A dose-relationship was established. The duration of apnoea was approximately doubled by 5 mg/kg of lidocaine or 2.2 mg/kg of procaine intravenously, and tripled by 16.6 mg/kg and 11.2 mg/kg, respectively, although the effects of procaine at higher doses were more marked.[2]

Procainamide has been reported to increase the effects of **suxamethonium** in *animals*,[3] increase muscle weakness in a myasthenic patient[4] and reduce plasma cholinesterase activity in healthy subjects.[5] An *animal* study demonstrated potentiation of the neuromuscular blocking effect of **tubocurarine** by lidocaine alone and combined with antibiotics having neuromuscular blocking activity (**neomycin** or **polymyxin B**).[6]

In a study of 10 healthy subjects, prolonged muscle weakness and symptoms of local anaesthetic toxicity were experienced after deflation of the tourniquet when 40 ml of **prilocaine** 0.5% and **mivacurium** 600 micrograms were used together for intravenous regional anaesthesia of the forearm. Administration of **prilocaine** or **mivacurium** alone did not produce these effects. The slow recovery suggested that **mivacurium** was not broken down in the ischaemic limb,[7] but inhibition of plasma cholinesterase by **prilocaine** would not fully explain the prolonged weakness once the cuff was deflated.[8]

Mechanism

Uncertain. Some local anaesthetics (ester-type[9]) such as procaine appear to inhibit plasma cholinesterase,[10] which might prolong the activity of suxamethonium. There may additionally be competition between suxamethonium and procaine for hydrolysis by plasma cholinesterase, which metabolises them both.[2,5] These effects are particularly important in patients with abnormal plasma cholinesterase.[11] Therapeutic procainamide plasma concentrations of 5 to 10 micrograms/ml have been found to inhibit cholinesterase activity by 19 to 32%.[5]

All local anaesthetics have some neuromuscular blocking activity and may enhance the block produced by competitive neuromuscular blockers if given in sufficient doses.[11,12] Procainamide also has acetylcholine receptor channel blocking activity.[12]

Importance and management

Information is limited but the suxamethonium/lidocaine and suxamethonium/procaine interactions appear to be established and of clinical importance. Be alert for signs of increased blockade and/or recurarisation with apnoea during the recovery period from suxamethonium blockade if either drug is used.

Despite the potential for an interaction between suxamethonium and procainamide, no marked interaction has yet been reported. Nevertheless be aware that some increase in the neuromuscular blocking effects is possible.

Lidocaine, procaine and procainamide all have some neuromuscular blocking activity and may also enhance the block produced by competitive neuromuscular blockers if given in sufficient doses. However, again, there seems to be an absence of reports of this, probably because the amount of local anaesthetic absorbed into the circulation following a local block is usually modest.[12]

Animal studies indicate that low and otherwise safe doses of lidocaine given with other drugs having neuromuscular blocking activity (e.g. polymyxin B, aminoglycosides) may possibly be additive with conventional neuromuscular blockers and cause problems.[6]

1. Smith NT, Miller RD, Corbascio AN, eds. Neuromuscular blocking drugs, in Drug Interactions in Anesthesia. Philadelphia: Lea and Febiger; 1981 p. 249.
2. Usubiaga JE, Wikinski JA, Morales RL, Usubiaga LEJ. Interaction of intravenously administered procaine, lidocaine and succinylcholine in anesthetized subjects. *Anesth Analg* (1967) 46, 39–45.
3. Cuthbert MF. The effect of quinidine and procainamide on the neuromuscular blocking action of suxamethonium. *Br J Anaesth* (1966) 38, 775–9.
4. Drachman DA, Skom JH. Procainamide—a hazard in myasthenia gravis. *Arch Neurol* (1965) 13, 316–20.
5. Kambam JR, Naukam RJ, Sastry BVR. The effect of procainamide on plasma cholinesterase activity. *Can J Anaesth* (1987) 34, 579–81.
6. Brueckner J, Thomas KC, Bikhazi GB, Foldes FF. Neuromuscular drug interactions of clinical importance. *Anesth Analg* (1980) 59, 533–4.
7. Torrance JM, Lewer BMF, Galletly DC. Low-dose mivacurium supplementation of prilocaine i.v. regional anaesthesia. *Br J Anaesth* (1997) 78, 222–3.
8. Torrance JM, Lewer BMF, Galletly DC. Interactions between mivacurium and prilocaine. *Br J Anaesth* (1997) 79, 262.
9. Sweetman SC, editor. Martindale: The complete drug reference. 34th ed. London: Pharmaceutical Press: 2005. p. 1408.
10. Reina RA, Cannavà N. Interazione di alcuni anestetici locali con la succinilcolina. *Acta Anaesthesiol Ital* (1972) 23, 1–10
11. Østergaard D, Engbaek J, Viby-Mogensen J. Adverse reactions and interactions of the neuromuscular blocking drugs. *Med Toxicol Adverse Drug Exp* (1989) 4, 351–68.
12. Feldman S, Karalliedde L. Drug interactions with neuromuscular blockers. *Drug Safety* (1996) 15, 261–73.

Neuromuscular blockers + Anticholinesterases

Anticholinesterases oppose the actions of competitive neuromuscular blockers (e.g. tubocurarine) and can therefore be used as an antidote to restore muscular activity following their use. Conversely, anticholinesterases increase and prolong the actions of the depolarising neuromuscular blockers (e.g. suxamethonium (succinylcholine)). Anticholinesterases used to treat Alzheimer's disease may interact with neuromuscular blockers. See also 'Neuromuscular blockers + Ecothiopate iodide', p.907 and 'Neuromuscular blockers + Insecticides', p.909.

Clinical evidence, mechanism, importance and management

There are two main types of neuromuscular blockers: competitive (non-depolarising) and depolarising, see 'Neuromuscular blockers + Neuromuscular blockers', p.913:

(a) Competitive (non-depolarising) neuromuscular blockers

Competitive (non-depolarising) neuromuscular blockers (e.g. **tubocurarine** and others listed in 'Table 31.1', (p.880)) compete with acetylcholine for receptors on the motor endplate. Anticholinesterases (e.g. **ambenonium**, **edrophonium**, **neostigmine**, **physostigmine**, **pyridostigmine**, etc.) can be used as an antidote to this kind of neuromuscular blockade, because they inhibit the enzymes that destroy acetylcholine so that the concentration of acetylcholine at the neuromuscular junction builds up. In this way the competition between the molecules of the blocker and the acetylcholine for occupancy of the receptors swings in favour of the acetylcholine so that transmission is restored. These drugs are used routinely following surgery to reactivate paralysed muscles. Note that inhalational anaesthetics can impair this effect of anticholinesterases on neuromuscular blockers (see 'Anaesthetics, general + Anticholinesterases', p.883).

(b) Depolarising neuromuscular blockers

The depolarising blockers (**suxamethonium** (**succinylcholine**) and others listed in 'Table 31.1', see (p.880)) act like acetylcholine to depolarise the motor endplate, but unlike acetylcholine, they are not immediately removed by cholinesterase. The anticholinesterase drugs increase the concentration of acetylcholine at the neuromuscular junction, which enhances and prolongs this type of blockade, and therefore anticholinesterases cannot be used as an antidote for this kind of blocker. Care should be taken if an anticholinesterase has been administered to antagonise a competitive neuromuscular block prior to administration of **suxamethonium**, as the duration of the **suxamethonium** block may be prolonged.[1] See also 'Neuromuscular blockers + Ecothiopate iodide', p.907.

(c) Tacrine and other anticholinesterases used in Alzheimer's

Tacrine, like other anticholinesterases, has been used *intravenously* in anaesthetic practice to reverse the effects of competitive (non-depolarising) blockers such as **tubocurarine**[2] and to prolong the effects of depolarising blockers such as **suxamethonium**.[2-6] For example, one study found that only one-third of the normal dosage of **suxamethonium** was needed in the presence of 15 mg of intravenous tacrine.[7] However, tacrine is now more commonly used *orally* for its central effects in the treatment of Alzheimer's disease. You should therefore be alert for changes in the effects of both types of neuromuscular blocking drugs in patients in whom tacrine is being used for the treatment of Alzheimer's. Other cholinesterase inhibitors used for Alzheimer's disease (including galantamine, rivastigmine and possibly donepezil) will behave like tacrine. For a report of prolonged neuromuscular block in a patient on long-term **donepezil** therapy who received **suxamethonium (succinylcholine), pancuronium** and **neostigmine** see 'Anticholinesterases + Other Anticholinesterases, Cholinergics or Anticholinergics', p.251.

(d) Organophosphorus compounds

The organophosphorus pesticides are potent anticholinesterases used in agriculture and horticulture to control insects on crops and in veterinary practice to control various ectoparasites. They are applied as sprays and dips. Anyone who is exposed to these toxic pesticides may therefore show changes in their responses to neuromuscular blockers (see 'Neuromuscular blockers + Insecticides', p.909). Widely used organophosphorus pesticides include **azamethiphos, bromophos, chlorpyrifos, clofenvinfos, coumafos, cythioate, dichlorvos, dimethoate, dimpylate, dioxation, ethion, famphur, fenitrothion, fenthion, heptenophos, iodofenphos, malathion, naled, parathion, phosmet, phoxim, pirimiphos-methyl, propetamphos, pyraclofos, temefos.**[8] A number of the **nerve gases** (such as **sarin, soman, tabun** and **VX**) are also potent anticholinesterases.

1. Fleming NW, Macres S, Antognini JF, Vengco J. Neuromuscular blocking action of suxamethonium after antagonism of vecuronium by edrophonium, pyridostigmine or neostigmine. *Br J Anaesth* (1996) 77, 492–5.
2. Hunter AR. Tetrahydroaminacrine in anaesthesia. *Br J Anaesth* (1965) 37, 505–13.
3. Oberoi GS, Yaubihi N. The use of tacrine (THA) and succinylcholine compared with alcuronium during laparoscopy. *P N G Med J* (1990) 33, 25–8.
4. Davies-Lepie SR. Tacrine may prolong the effect of succinylcholine. *Anesthesiology* (1994) 81, 524.
5. Norman J, Morgan M. The effect of tacrine on the neuromuscular block produced by suxamethonium in man. *Br J Anaesth* (1975) 47, 1027.
6. Lindsay PA, Lumley J. Suxamethonium apnoea masked by tetrahydroaminacrine. *Anaesthesia* (1978) 33, 620–2.
7. El-Kammah BM, El-Gafi SH, El-Sherbiny AM, Kader MMA. Biochemical and clinical study for the role of tacrine as succinylcholine extender. *J Egypt Med Assoc* (1975) 58, 559–67.
8. Sweetman SC, editor. Martindale: The complete drug reference. 34th ed. London: Pharmaceutical Press; 2005. p. 1499.

Neuromuscular blockers + Anticonvulsants

The effects of many competitive neuromuscular blockers are reduced and shortened if carbamazepine or phenytoin are given for longer than one week, but they appear to be increased if phenytoin is given acutely (e.g. during surgery). Carbamazepine and phenytoin appear not to interact with mivacurium.

Clinical evidence

(a) Carbamazepine given long term: neuromuscular blocking effects reduced

The recovery from neuromuscular blockade with **pancuronium** in 18 patients undergoing craniotomy for tumours, seizure foci or cerebrovascular surgery was on average 65% shorter in those taking carbamazepine.[1] Another 9 patients undergoing surgery and neuromuscular blockade with **doxacurium** and on carbamazepine for at least a week took 66 minutes to reach 50% recovery compared with 161 minutes in the control group.[2] Similar findings were obtained in another study.[3] Further studies found that carbamazepine significantly shortened the recovery time from **vecuronium** blockade in adults[4] and in children.[5] Several reports and studies have demonstrated a shorter duration of action of **rocuronium** following long-term carbamazepine,[6-9] although preliminary investigations found no effect.[10,11] Reduced duration of action has also been reported with **rapacuronium** in a patient on carbamazepine.[12] The effects of **pipecuronium** are also reduced by carbamazepine.[13,14] In one study it was found that the onset time for **pipecuronium** blockade was lengthened (although this was not statistically significant) in patients with therapeutic plasma concentrations of anticonvulsant (carbamazepine or phenytoin), but not in those with subtherapeutic levels. However, a shorter duration of action was seen regardless of anticonvulsant levels.[14] One study found that the recovery time from intravenous **atracurium** 500 micrograms/kg was significantly shorter in 14 patients on long-term carbamazepine therapy when compared with 21 nonepileptic patients; the recovery index (time between 25% and 75% recovery of baseline electromyogram values) was 5.93 and 8.02 minutes, respectively.[15] However, other studies have reported no effect, see (d) below.

(b) Phenytoin given long-term: neuromuscular blocking effects reduced

In the preliminary report of a study the reduction in the time to recover from 25 to 75% of the response to ulnar nerve stimulation in patients who had received phenytoin for longer than one week was: **metocurine** 58%, **pancuronium** 40%, **tubocurarine** 24%, **atracurium** 8% (the last two were not statistically significant).[16] The **metocurine** results are published in full elsewhere.[17] In another study approximately 80% more **pancuronium** was needed by 9 patients on long-term phenytoin than in 18 others not receiving phenytoin (58 and 32 micrograms/kg/hour, respectively).[18] Resistance to **pancuronium** and a shortening of the recovery period due to long-term phenytoin[3,19] or unspecified anticonvulsants[20] has also been described in other reports. **Doxacurium,**[2,3] **pipecuronium,**[13,14] **rapacuronium** (case report),[12] **rocuronium**[21,22] and **vecuronium**[5,23-25] are affected like pancuronium. In one study it was found that the onset time for **pipecuronium** blockade was lengthened (although this was not statistically significant) for patients with therapeutic plasma concentrations of anticonvulsants (phenytoin or carbamazepine), but not in those with subtherapeutic levels. However, a shorter duration of action occurred regardless of the anticonvulsant level.[14]

A reduced recovery time from **atracurium**-induced neuromuscular blockade was found in one study in patients on long-term anticonvulsants including phenytoin[15] but other studies have reported no effect, see (d) below.

(c) Phenytoin given short term: neuromuscular blocking effects increased

A retrospective review of 8 patients on long-term phenytoin treatment (greater than 2 weeks) and 3 others given phenytoin within 8 hours of surgery showed that the average doses of **vecuronium** used from induction to extubation were 155 micrograms/kg/hour (long term) and 61.5 micrograms/kg/hour (acute).[26] Others have reported similar results.[24] Another study found that the sensitivity of patients to **vecuronium** was increased by phenytoin given intravenously during surgery,[27] and this has also been seen in *animal* studies with **tubocurarine**.[28] Similarly, a study of 20 patients undergoing craniotomy showed that phenytoin (10 mg/kg given over approximately 30 minutes) administered during the operation augmented the neuromuscular block produced by **rocuronium**.[29]

(d) Anticonvulsants given long term: neuromuscular blocking effects unaffected

Long-term (greater than 4 weeks) **carbamazepine** appears not to affect **mivacurium**-induced neuromuscular blockade.[30] Similarly, a study in 32 patients who had been taking **carbamazepine** alone or with **phenytoin** or **valproic acid** for greater than 2 weeks found no resistance to **mivacurium**,[31] although in an earlier preliminary study by the same research group of 13 patients on **unspecified anticonvulsants** a trend towards a shorter recovery from **mivacurium** was seen (not statistically significant).[32] **Carbamazepine** has also been reported to have no effect on **atracurium**[4,33] and two studies suggest that **atracurium** is normally minimally affected by **phenytoin**.[23,34] However, one study[15] found that the recovery time from **atracurium** blockade was significantly reduced in patients on long-term anticonvulsant therapy, see (a) and (b) above.

(e) Anticonvulsants given long term: neuromuscular blocking effects increased

Eight patients who had been on **phenytoin** and/or **carbamazepine** for at least one month took longer to recover from **suxamethonium** (**succinylcholine**) blockade compared with 9 control patients; the time for return to baseline twitch height was 14.3 and 10 minutes, respectively. The slight prolongation of **suxamethonium** action was considered to have few clinical implications.[35]

Mechanism

Not fully understood, but it appears to be multifactorial. Suggestions to account for the reduced response with chronic anticonvulsants include: induction of liver enzyme activity (phenytoin and carbamazepine are both potent inducers of cytochrome P450 isoenzymes), which would increase the metabolism and clearance of the neuromuscular blocker; anticonvulsant-induced changes at the neuromuscular junction, including reduced acetylcholine release and increased number of acetylcholine receptors on the muscle membrane (up-regulation), with decreased sensitivity; and changes in plasma protein binding.[5,35,36] It has been shown that carbamazepine doubles the clearance of vecuronium[5,37,38] and phenytoin therapy possibly increases the plasma clearance of pancuronium[19] and rocuronium.[21]

Importance and management

Established and clinically important interactions. More is known about phenytoin and carbamazepine than other anticonvulsants.

Anticipate the need to use more (possibly up to twice as much) doxacurium, metocurine, pancuronium, pipecuronium, rocuronium and vecuronium in patients given these anticonvulsants for more than a week,[24] and expect an accelerated recovery. The effects on tubocurarine and atracurium appear only to be small or moderate, whereas mivacurium appears not to interact.

Anticipate the need to use a smaller neuromuscular blocker dosage, or prepare for a longer recovery time if phenytoin is given acutely.

1. Roth S, Ebrahim ZY. Resistance to pancuronium in patients receiving carbamazepine. *Anesthesiology* (1987) 66, 691–3.
2. Ornstein E, Matteo RS, Weinstein JA, Halevy JD, Young WL, Abou-Donia MM. Accelerated recovery from doxacurium-induced neuromuscular blockade in patients receiving chronic anticonvulsant therapy. *J Clin Anesth* (1991) 3, 108–11.
3. Desai P, Hewitt PB, Jones RM. Influence of anticonvulsant therapy on doxacurium and pancuronium-induced paralysis. *Anesthesiology* (1989) 71, A784.
4. Ebrahim Z, Bulkley R, Roth S. Carbamazepine therapy and neuromuscular blockade with atracurium and vecuronium. *Anesth Analg* (1988) 67, S55.
5. Soriano SG, Sullivan LJ, Venkatakrishnan K, Greenblatt DJ, Martyn JAJ. Pharmacokinetics and pharmacodynamics of vecuronium in children receiving phenytoin or carbamazepine for chronic anticonvulsant therapy. *Br J Anaesth* (2001) 86, 223–9.
6. Baraka A, Idriss N. Resistance to rocuronium in an epileptic patient on long-term carbamazepine therapy. *Middle East J Anesthesiol* (1996) 13, 561–4.
7. Loan PB, Connolly FM, Mirakhur RK, Kumar N, Farling P. Neuromuscular effects of rocuronium in patients receiving beta-adrenoreceptor blocking, calcium entry blocking and anticonvulsant drugs. *Br J Anaesth* (1997) 78, 90–1.
8. Spacek A, Neiger FX, Krenn CG, Hoerauf K, Kress HG. Rocuronium-induced neuromuscular block is affected by chronic carbamazepine therapy. *Anesthesiology* (1999) 90, 109–12.
9. Soriano SG, Kaus SJ, Sullivan LJ, Martyn JAJ. Onset and duration of action of rocuronium in children receiving chronic anticonvulsant therapy. *Paediatr Anaesth* (2000) 10, 133–6.
10. Spacek A, Neiger FX, Katz RL, Watkins WD, Spiss CK. Chronic carbamazepine therapy does not affect neuromuscular blockade by rocuronium. *Anesth Analg* (1995) 80 (Suppl 2), S463.
11. Spacek A, Neiger FX, Krenn C-G, Spiss CK, Kress HG. Does chronic carbamazepine therapy influence neuromuscular blockade by rocuronium? *Anesthesiology* (1997) 87, A833.
12. Tobias JD, Johnson JO. Rapacuronium administration to patients receiving phenytoin or carbamazepine. *J Neurosurg Anesthesiol* (2001) 13, 240–2.
13. Jellish WS, Modica PA, Tempelhoff R. Accelerated recovery from pipecuronium in patients treated with chronic anticonvulsant therapy. *J Clin Anesth* (1993) 5, 105–8.
14. Hans P, Ledoux D, Bonhomme V, Brichant JF. Effect of plasma anticonvulsant level on pipecuronium-induced neuromuscular blockade: preliminary results. *J Neurosurg Anesthesiol* (1995) 7, 254–8.
15. Tempelhoff R, Modica PA, Jellish WS, Spitznagel EL. Resistance to atracurium-induced neuromuscular blockade in patients with intractable seizure disorders treated with anticonvulsants. *Anesth Analg* (1990) 71, 665–9.
16. Ornstein E, Matteo RS, Silverberg PA, Schwartz AE, Young WL, Diaz J. Chronic phenytoin therapy and nondepolarizing muscular blockade. *Anesthesiology* (1985) 63, A331.
17. Ornstein E, Matteo RS, Young WL, Diaz J. Resistance to metocurine-induced neuromuscular blockade in patients receiving phenytoin. *Anesthesiology* (1985) 63, 294–8.
18. Chen J, Kim YD, Dubois M, Kammerer W, Macnamara TE. The increased requirement of pancuronium in neurosurgical patients receiving Dilantin chronically. *Anesthesiology* (1983) 59, A288.
19. Liberman BA, Norman P, Hardy BG. Pancuronium-phenytoin interaction: a case of decreased duration of neuromuscular blockade. *Int J Clin Pharmacol Ther Toxicol* (1988) 26, 371–4.
20. Messick JM, Maass L, Faust RJ, Cucchiara RF. Duration of pancuronium neuromuscular blockade in patients taking anticonvulsant medication. *Anesth Analg* (1982) 61, 203–4.
21. Szenohradszky J, Caldwell JE, Sharma ML, Gruenke LD, Miller RD. Interaction of rocuronium (ORG 9426) and phenytoin in a patient undergoing cadaver renal transplantation: a possible pharmacokinetic mechanism? *Anesthesiology* (1994) 80, 1167–70.
22. Hernández-Palazón J, Tortosa JA, Martínez-Lage JF, Pérez-Ayala M. Rocuronium-induced neuromuscular blockade is affected by chronic phenytoin therapy. *J Neurosurg Anesthesiol* (2001) 13, 79–82.
23. Ornstein E, Matteo RS, Schwartz AE, Silverberg PA, Young WL, Diaz J. The effect of phenytoin on the magnitude and duration of neuromuscular block following atracurium or vecuronium. *Anesthesiology* (1987) 67, 191–6.
24. Platt PR, Thackray NM. Phenytoin-induced resistance to vecuronium. *Anaesth Intensive Care* (1993) 21, 185–91.
25. Caldwell JE, McCarthy GJ, Wright PMC, Szenohradszky J, Sharma ML, Gruenke LD, Miller RD. Influence of chronic phenytoin administration on the pharmacokinetics and pharmacodynamics of vecuronium. *Br J Anaesth* (1999) 83, 183P–184P.
26. Baumgardner JE, Bagshaw R. Acute versus chronic phenytoin therapy and neuromuscular blockade. *Anaesthesia* (1990) 45, 493–4.
27. Gray HSJ, Slater RM, Pollard BJ. The effect of acutely administered phenytoin on vecuronium-induced neuromuscular blockade. *Anaesthesia* (1989) 44, 379–81.
28. Gandhi IC, Jindal MN, Patel VK. Mechanism of neuromuscular blockade with some antiepileptic drugs. *Arzneimittelforschung* (1976) 26, 258–61.
29. Spacek A, Nickl S, Neiger FX, Nigrovic V, Ullrich O-W, Weindlmayr-Goettel M, Schwall B, Taeger K, Kress HG. Augmentation of the rocuronium-induced neuromuscular block by the acutely administered phenytoin. *Anesthesiology* (1999) 90, 1551–5.
30. Spacek A, Neiger FX, Spiss CK, Kress HG. Chronic carbamazepine therapy does not influence mivacurium-induced neuromuscular block. *Br J Anaesth* (1996) 77, 500–2.
31. Jellish WS, Thalji Z, Brundidge PK, Tempelhoff R. Recovery from mivacurium-induced neuromuscular blockade is not affected by anticonvulsant therapy. *J Neurosurg Anesthesiol* (1996) 8, 4–8.
32. Thalji Z, Jellish WS, Murdoch J, Tempelhoff R. The effect of chronic anticonvulsant therapy on recovery from mivacurium induced paralysis. *Anesthesiology* (1993) 79 (Suppl 3A), A965.
33. Spacek A, Neiger FX, Spiss CK, Kress HG. Atracurium-induced neuromuscular block is not affected by chronic anticonvulsant therapy with carbamazepine. *Acta Anaesthesiol Scand* (1997) 41, 1308–11.
34. deBros F, Okutani R, Lai A, Lawrence KW, Basta S. Phenytoin does not interfere with atracurium pharmacokinetics and pharmacodynamics. *Anesthesiology* (1987) 67, A607.
35. Melton AT, Antognini JF, Gronert GA. Prolonged duration of succinylcholine in patients receiving anticonvulsants: evidence for mild up-regulation of acetylcholine receptors? *Can J Anaesth* (1993) 40, 939–42.
36. Kim CS, Arnold FJ, Itani MS, Martyn JAJ. Decreased sensitivity to metocurine during long-term phenytoin therapy may be attributable to protein binding and acetylcholine receptor changes. *Anesthesiology* (1992) 77, 500–6.
37. Alloul K, Varin F, Whalley D, Chutway F. Carbamazepine induced changes on vecuronium pharmacokinetics in anesthetized patients. *Clin Pharmacol Ther* (1994) 55, 143.
38. Alloul K, Varin F, Chutway F, Ebrahim Z, Whalley D. Carbamazepine effect on vecuronium pharmacokinetic-pharmacodynamic modeling in anesthetized patients. *Anesthesiology* (1994) 81, A414.

Neuromuscular blockers + Antineoplastics

The effects of suxamethonium (succinylcholine) can be increased and prolonged in patients treated with cyclophosphamide because their plasma cholinesterase levels are depressed. Respiratory insufficiency and prolonged apnoea have been reported. *Animal* data suggests that thiotepa may also enhance the effects of suxamethonium. An isolated report describes a marked increase in the neuromuscular blocking effects of pancuronium in a myasthenic patient when given thiotepa, but normally it appears not to interact with competitive neuromuscular blocking agents.

Clinical evidence

(a) Cyclophosphamide

Respiratory insufficiency and prolonged apnoea occurred in a patient on two occasions while receiving cyclophosphamide and undergoing anaesthesia during which **suxamethonium** (**succinylcholine**) and **tubocurarine** were used. Plasma cholinesterase levels were found to be low. Anaesthesia without the **suxamethonium** was uneventful. Seven out of 8 patients subsequently examined also showed depressed plasma cholinesterase levels while taking cyclophosphamide.[1]

Respiratory depression and low plasma cholinesterase levels have been described in other reports in patients receiving cyclophosphamide.[2-4] Similarly, in the discussion of an *in vitro* study, the authors report preliminary results from a study in patients, showing a 35 to 70% reduction in cholinesterase activity for several days.[2]

(b) Thiotepa

A myasthenic patient rapidly developed very prolonged respiratory depression when given thiotepa intraperitoneally after receiving **pancuronium**.[5] Thiotepa has also been shown to increase the duration of **suxamethonium** (**succinylcholine**) neuromuscular blockade in *dogs*.[6] However, an *in vitro* study showed that thiotepa was a poor inhibitor of plasma cholinesterase.[2]

Mechanism

Cyclophosphamide inhibits the activity of plasma cholinesterase,[4] and as a result the metabolism of the suxamethonium is reduced and its actions are enhanced and prolonged. Other alkylating agents also reported to reduce plasma cholinesterase activity include **mustine** (**chlormethine**).

Importance and management

The interaction between suxamethonium and cyclophosphamide is well documented and established. It is of clinical importance, but whether all patients are affected to the same extent is uncertain. The depression of the plasma cholinesterase levels may last several days, possibly weeks, so that ideally plasma cholinesterase levels should be checked before using suxamethonium. In patients taking cyclophosphamide it should certainly be used with caution, and the dosage should be reduced.[2] Some have suggested that concurrent use should be avoided.[1] *Animal* data suggest thiotepa may enhance the effects of suxamethonium. The general silence in the literature would seem to indicate that no special precautions are normally necessary, however, patients with malignant tumours often have a reduced plasma cholinesterase activity, so care should be taken in these patients.[7]

1. Walker IR, Zapf PW, Mackay IR. Cyclophosphamide, cholinesterase and anaesthesia. *Aust N Z J Med* (1972) 3, 247–51.
2. Zsigmond EK, Robins G. The effect of a series of anti-cancer drugs on plasma cholinesterase activity. *Can Anaesth Soc J* (1972) 19, 75–82.
3. Mone JG, Mathie WE. Qualitative and quantitative defects of pseudocholinesterase activity. *Anaesthesia* (1967) 22, 55–68.
4. Wolff H. Die Hemmung der Serumcholinesterase durch Cyclophosphamid (Endoxan®). *Klin Wochenschr* (1965) 43, 819–21.
5. Bennett EJ, Schmidt GB, Patel KP, Grundy EM. Muscle relaxants, myasthenia, and mustards? *Anesthesiology* (1977) 46, 220–1
6. Cremonesi E, Rodrigues I de J. Interação de agentes curarizantes com antineoplásico. *Rev Bras Anestesiol* (1982) 32, 313–15.
7. Viby Mogensen J. Cholinesterase and succinylcholine. *Dan Med Bull* (1983) 30, 129–50.

Neuromuscular blockers + Antipsychotics

An isolated report describes prolonged apnoea in a patient given promazine while recovering from neuromuscular blockade with suxamethonium (succinylcholine). Recovery from the neuromuscular blocking effects of suxamethonium is prolonged by fentanyl/droperidol.

Clinical evidence

(a) Suxamethonium (succinylcholine) + Promazine

A woman, recovering from surgery during which she had received suxamethonium, was given promazine 25 mg intravenously for sedation. Within 3 minutes she had become cyanotic and apnoeic, and required assisted respiration for 4 hours.[1]

(b) Suxamethonium (succinylcholine) + Fentanyl/droperidol

The observation that patients who had received *Innovar* (fentanyl/droperidol) before anaesthesia appeared to have prolonged suxamethonium effects, seen as apnoea, prompted further study of this possible interaction.[2] An average delay in recovery from neuromuscular blockade of 36% to 80% was seen in two studies.[2,3] Another study[4] showed that the droperidol component of *Innovar* was probably responsible for this interaction.

Mechanism

Not understood. It has been suggested that promazine[1] and droperidol[4] depress plasma cholinesterase levels, which would reduce the metabolism of the suxamethonium and thereby prolong recovery. It has also been suggested that droperidol might act as a membrane stabiliser at neuromuscular junctions.[4]

Importance and management

Some caution would seem appropriate if promazine is given to any patient who has had suxamethonium. There seems to be no information about other phenothiazines and other neuromuscular blockers.

Delayed recovery should be anticipated in patients on suxamethonium if droperidol is used. This is an established interaction.

1. Regan AG, Aldrete JA. Prolonged apnea after administration of promazine hydrochloride following succinylcholine infusion. *Anesth Analg* (1967) 46, 315–18.
2. Wehner RJ. A case study: the prolongation of Anectine® effect by Innovar®. *J Am Assoc Nurse Anesth* (1979) 47, 576–9.
3. Moore GB, Ciresi S, Kallar S. The effect of Innovar® versus droperidol or fentanyl on the duration of action of succinylcholine. *J Am Assoc Nurse Anesth* (1986) 54, 130–6.
4. Lewis RA. A consideration of prolonged succinylcholine paralysis with Innovar®: is the cause droperidol or fentanyl? *J Am Assoc Nurse Anesth* (1982) 50, 55–9.

Neuromuscular blockers + Aprotinin

Apnoea developed in a number of patients after being given aprotinin while recovering from neuromuscular blockade with suxamethonium (succinylcholine) with or without tubocurarine.

Clinical evidence

Three patients undergoing surgery who had received **suxamethonium (succinylcholine)**, alone or with **tubocurarine**, were given aprotinin intravenously in doses of 2500 to 12 000 KIU (kallikrein inactivator units) at the end of, or shortly after, the operation when spontaneous breathing had resumed. In each case respiration rapidly became inadequate and apnoea lasting periods of 7, 30 and 90 minutes occurred.[1] Seven other cases have been reported elsewhere.[2]

Mechanism

Not fully understood. Aprotinin is only a very weak inhibitor of serum cholinesterase (100,000 KIU caused a maximal 16% inhibition in man)[3] and on its own would have little effect on the metabolism of suxamethonium. But it might tip the balance in those whose cholinesterase was already very depressed.

Importance and management

The incidence of this interaction is uncertain but probably low. Only a few cases have been reported. It seems probable that it only affects those whose plasma cholinesterase levels are already very low for other reasons. No difficulties should arise in those whose plasma cholinesterase levels are normal.

1. Chasapakis G, Dimas C. Possible interaction between muscle relaxants and the kallikrein-trypsin inactivator "Trasylol". *Br J Anaesth* (1966) 38, 838–9.
2. Marcello B, Porati U. Trasylol e blocco neuromuscolare. *Minerva Anestesiol* (1967) 33, 814–15.
3. Doenicke A, Gesing H, Krumey I, Schmidinger St. Influence of aprotinin (Trasylol) on the action of suxamethonium. *Br J Anaesth* (1970) 42, 948–60.

Neuromuscular blockers + Benzodiazepines

A few studies report that diazepam and other benzodiazepines increase the effects of neuromuscular blockers, but many others found that they do not. If an interaction occurs, the response is likely to be little different from the individual variations in response of patients to neuromuscular blockers.

Clinical evidence

(a) Increased blockade

A comparative study of 10 patients given **gallamine** and 4 others given **gallamine** and **diazepam** 150 to 200 micrograms/kg) intravenously showed that the **diazepam** prolonged the duration of activity of the blocker by a factor of three, and doubled the depression of the twitch response.[1] Persistent muscle weakness and respiratory depression was seen in 2 other patients on **tubocurarine** after premedication with **diazepam.**[2] A small reduction (approximately 10%) in neuromuscular blocker requirement has been described with **diazepam** and **tubocurarine**[3] or **suxamethonium (succinylcholine)**, but see also (b) below.[4]

Another study found that recovery to 25% and 75% of the twitch height after **vecuronium** was prolonged approximately 25% by 15 mg of intravenous **midazolam**, compared with control patients.[5] The same study found about a 20% prolongation of recovery from the effects of **atracurium** by **midazolam**. However, the increased recovery time due to **midazolam** was not statistically significant when compared with control patients, but was significantly longer when compared with patients receiving 20 mg of intravenous **diazepam**.[5] See also (b) below.

(b) Reduced blockade or no effect

The duration of paralysis due to **suxamethonium** was reduced in one study by 20% when **diazepam** (150 micrograms/kg) was used and the recovery time was shortened.[1] **Diazepam** also slightly reduced the time to 25% and 75% recovery of twitch height in patients given **vecuronium** by about 15% (not statistically significant).[5] In *animals*, **diazepam** increased the mean dose of **rocuronium** required by 13%, but this was not statistically significant.[6]

In other studies **diazepam** was found to have no significant effect on the blockade due to **alcuronium**,[7] **atracurium**,[5] **gallamine**,[8] **pancuronium**,[7] **suxamethonium**[7,9] or **tubocurarine**.[7-10] **Lorazepam** and **lormetazepam** have been reported to have little or no effects on **atracurium** or **vecuronium**,[5] and **midazolam** to have no effect on **suxamethonium** or **pancuronium**.[11]

Mechanism

Not understood. One suggestion is that where some alteration in response is seen it may be a reflection of a central depressant action rather than a direct effect on the myoneural junction.[8] Another study suggests instead a direct action on the muscle.[12]

Importance and management

There is no obvious explanation for these discordant observations. What is known shows that the benzodiazepines may sometimes unpredictably alter the depth and prolong the recovery period from neuromuscular blockade, but the extent may not be very great and may possibly be little different from the individual variations in the response of patients to neuromuscular blockers.

1. Feldman SA, Crawley BE. Interaction of diazepam with the muscle-relaxant drugs. *BMJ* (1970) 2, 336–8.
2. Feldman SA, Crawley BE. Diazepam and muscle relaxants. *BMJ* (1970) 1, 691.
3. Stovner J, Endresen R. Intravenous anaesthesia with diazepam. *Acta Anaesthesiol Scand* (1966) 24 (Suppl), 223–7.
4. Jörgensen H. Premedicinering med diazepam, Valium®. Jämförelse med placebo i en dubbel-blind-undersökning. *Nord Med* (1964) 72, 1395–9.
5. Driessen JJ, Crul JF, Vree TB, van Egmond J, Booij LHDJ. Benzodiazepines and neuromuscular blocking drugs in patients. *Acta Anaesthesiol Scand* (1986) 30, 642–6.
6. Muir AW, Anderson KA, Pow E. Interaction between rocuronium bromide and some drugs used during anaesthesia. *Eur J Anaesthesiol* (1994) 11 (Suppl 9), 93–8.
7. Bradshaw EG, Maddison S. Effect of diazepam at the neuromuscular junction. A clinical study. *Br J Anaesth* (1979) 51, 955–60.
8. Dretchen K, Ghoneim MM, Long JP. The interaction of diazepam with myoneural blocking agents. *Anesthesiology* (1971) 34, 463–8.
9. Stovner J, Endresen R. Diazepam in intravenous anaesthesia. *Lancet* (1965) ii, 1298–9.
10. Hunter AR. Diazepam (Valium) as a muscle relaxant during general anaesthesia: a pilot study. *Br J Anaesth* (1967) 39, 633–7.
11. Tassonyi E. Effects of midazolam (Ro 21-3981) on neuromuscular block. *Pharmatherapeutica* (1984) 3, 678–81.
12. Ludin HP, Dubach K. Action of diazepam on muscular contraction in man. *Z Neurol* (1971) 199, 30–8.

Neuromuscular blockers + Beta-agonist bronchodilators

Bambuterol can prolong the recovery time from neuromuscular blockade with suxamethonium (succinylcholine) or mivacurium. A case report describes modestly enhanced blockade with pancuronium or vecuronium following intravenous salbutamol administration.

Clinical evidence

(a) Bambuterol

A double-blind study in 25 patients found that the recovery time from neuromuscular blockade with **suxamethonium** (**succinylcholine**) was prolonged by about 30% in those who had received 10 mg of bambuterol 10 to 16 hours before surgery, and by about 50% in those who had received 20 mg of bambuterol.[1]

This confirms two previous studies,[2,3] one of which found that 30 mg of bambuterol given about 10 hours before surgery approximately doubled the duration of **suxamethonium** blockade.[2] Furthermore, in 7 patients who were heterozygous for abnormal plasma cholinesterase, 20 mg of bambuterol taken 2 hours before surgery prolonged **suxamethonium** blockade 2 to 3 times, and in 4 patients a phase II block occurred.[4]

Similar results have been found in a study involving 27 patients given **mivacurium**. A marked decrease in plasma cholinesterase activity, leading to reduced clearance and prolonged elimination half-life of **mivacurium,** occurred following 20 mg of bambuterol administered orally 2 hours before induction of anaesthesia. The duration of action of **mivacurium** was prolonged three- to fourfold compared with placebo.[5]

(b) Salbutamol

A case report describes a 28-year-old man undergoing elective surgery who was given 3 intravenous doses of salbutamol 125 micrograms over 3.5 hours for treatment and prophylaxis of bronchospasm. Muscle relaxation was maintained with **pancuronium** and then **vecuronium**. The neuromuscular blockade (measured by the force of contraction of the adductor pollicis in response to ulnar nerve stimulation) increased following salbutamol injection, from 45 to 66% during **pancuronium** blockade and from 66 to 86% following **vecuronium**. In addition, recovery of neuromuscular function after neostigmine appeared to be slower than expected.[6]

Mechanism

Bambuterol is an inactive prodrug which is slowly converted enzymatically in the body to its active form, terbutaline. The carbamate groups that are split off can selectively inhibit the plasma cholinesterase that is necessary for the metabolism of suxamethonium and mivacurium. As a result, the metabolism of these neuromuscular blockers is reduced and their effects are thereby prolonged. The effect appears to be related to the dose of the bambuterol and the time lag after administration; maximal depression of plasma cholinesterase activity appears to occur approximately 2 to 6 hours following oral administration, but is still markedly depressed after 10 hours.[2]

The effect of intravenous salbutamol was probably a direct effect at the neuromuscular junction.[6]

Importance and management

The interaction with bambuterol is an established interaction, which anaesthetists should be aware of. It may be more important where other factors reduce plasma cholinesterase activity or affect the extent of blockade in other ways (e.g. subjects heterozygous for abnormal plasma cholinesterase). This interaction only applies to beta-agonists that are metabolised to carbamic acid (bambuterol appears to be the only one available).

The interaction between intravenous salbutamol and pancuronium or vecuronium appears to be limited to this single report and is probably of only minor clinical importance.

1. Staun P, Lennmarken C, Eriksson LI, Wirén J-E. The influence of 10 mg and 20 mg of bambuterol on the duration of succinylcholine-induced neuromuscular blockade. *Acta Anaesthesiol Scand* (1990) 34, 498–500.
2. Fisher DM, Caldwell JE, Sharma M, Wirén J-E. The influence of bambuterol (carbamylated terbutaline) on the duration of action of succinylcholine-induced paralysis in humans. *Anesthesiology* (1988) 69, 757–9.
3. Bang U, Viby-Mogensen J, Wirén JE, Skovgaard LT. The effect of bambuterol (carbamylated terbutaline) on plasma cholinesterase activity and suxamethonium-induced neuromuscular blockade in genotypically normal patients. *Acta Anaesthesiol Scand* (1990) 34, 596–9.
4. Bang U, Viby-Mogensen J, Wirén JE. The effect of bambuterol on plasma cholinesterase activity and suxamethonium-induced neuromuscular blockade in subjects heterozygous for abnormal plasma cholinesterase. *Acta Anaesthesiol Scand* (1990) 34, 600–4.
5. Østergaard D, Rasmussen SN, Viby-Mogensen J, Pedersen NA, Boysen R. The influence of drug-induced low plasma cholinesterase activity on the pharmacokinetics and pharmacodynamics of mivacurium. *Anesthesiology* (2000) 92, 1581–7.
6. Salib Y, Donati F. Potentiation of pancuronium and vecuronium neuromuscular blockade by intravenous salbutamol. *Can J Anaesth* (1993) 40, 50–3.

Neuromuscular blockers + Beta-blockers

Increases or decreases (often only modest) in the extent of neuromuscular blockade have been seen in patients treated with beta-blockers. The bradycardia and hypotension sometimes caused by anaesthetics and beta-blockers (see also 'Anaesthetics, general + Beta-blockers', p.885) is not counteracted by atracurium.

Clinical evidence

(a) Reduced neuromuscular blockade

The effects of **suxamethonium** (**succinylcholine**) were slightly, but not significantly, reduced in 8 patients given a dose of **propranolol** of 1 mg/15 kg body weight intravenously 15 minutes pre-operatively. In another 8 patients, **propranolol**, given intravenously 20 to 40 minutes after the onset of action of **tubocurarine**, was also observed to shorten the recovery from **tubocurarine**.[1] Another study described a shortened recovery period from **tubocurarine** due to **oxprenolol** or **propranolol**, but **pindolol** only slightly affected a few subjects.[2]

(b) Increased neuromuscular blockade

Two patients with thyrotoxicosis showed prolonged neuromuscular blockade with **tubocurarine** after they had received **propranolol** 120 mg daily for 14 days prior to surgery.[3] In 8 patients, intravenous **esmolol** 300 to 500 microgram/kg/minute reduced the increase in heart rate during intubation, and slightly but significantly prolonged the recovery from blockade with **suxamethonium** by approximately 3 minutes when compared with 8 patients given placebo.[4]

(c) Bradycardia and hypotension

Eight out of 42 patients on unnamed beta-blockers given **atracurium** developed bradycardia (less than 50 bpm) and hypotension (systolic pressure less than 80 mmHg). Most of them had been premedicated with diazepam, induced with methohexital, and maintained with droperidol, fentanyl and nitrous oxide/oxygen. A further 24 showed bradycardia, associated with hypotension on 9 occasions. All responded promptly to 300 to 600 micrograms of intravenous atropine.[5]

Another patient using 0.5% **timolol eye drops** for glaucoma similarly developed bradycardia and hypotension when **atracurium** was used.[6] Bradycardia and hypotension have been seen in 2 other patients, one given **alcuronium** while using **timolol eye drops** for glaucoma, and the other given **atracurium** while using **atenolol** for hypertension.[7]

For reports of bradycardia associated with **vecuronium** and opioids in patients also receiving beta-blockers, see 'Neuromuscular blockers + Opioids', p.914.

(d) No interaction

A study of 16 patients who had been taking various beta-blockers (**propranolol** 5, **atenolol** 5, **metoprolol** 2, **bisoprolol** 2, **oxprenolol** 1, **celiprolol** 1) for longer than one month found no difference in onset and duration of action of **rocuronium** when compared with a control group.[8] Similarly, intra-operative **esmolol** did not affect the onset and recovery time from **suxamethonium** (**succinylcholine**) blockade in patients with normal plasma cholinesterase (pseudocholinesterase) activity,[9] but see also (b) above.

Mechanism

The changes in the degree of blockade are not understood but it appears to occur at the neuromuscular junction. It has been seen in *animal* studies.[10,11] The bradycardia and hypotension (c) were probably due to the combined depressant effects on the heart of the anaesthetics and the beta-blocker not being offset by atracurium, which has little or no effect on the vagus nerve at doses within the recommended range. Note that neuromuscular blockers with vagolytic activity can cause tachycardia and hypotension.

Importance and management

Information is fairly sparse, but these interactions appear normally to be of relatively minor importance. Be aware that changes in neuromuscular blockade (increases or decreases) can occur if beta-blockers are used, but they seem to be unpredictable, and then often only modest in extent. The possible combined cardiac depressant effects of beta-blockade and anaesthesia are well known (see 'Anaesthetics, general + Beta-blockers', p.885). These effects may not be prevented when a neuromuscular blocker is used that has little or no effect on the vagus (such as atracurium or vecuronium). See also 'Beta-blockers + Anticholinesterases', p.626.

1. Varma YS, Sharma PL, Singh HW. Effect of propranolol hydrochloride on the neuromuscular blocking action of d-tubocurarine and succinylcholine in man. *Indian J Med Res* (1972) 60, 266–72.
2. Varma YS, Sharma PL, Singh HW. Comparative effect of propranolol, oxprenolol and pindolol on neuromuscular blocking action of d-tubocurarine in man. *Indian J Med Res* (1973) 61, 1382–6.
3. Rozen MS, Whan FM. Prolonged curarization associated with propranolol. *Med J Aust* (1972) 1, 467–8.
4. Murthy VS, Patel KD, Elangovan RG, Hwang T-F, Solochek SM, Steck JD, Laddu AR. Cardiovascular and neuromuscular effects of esmolol during induction of anesthesia. *J Clin Pharmacol* (1986) 26, 351–7.
5. Rowlands DE. Drug interaction? *Anaesthesia* (1984) 39, 1252.
6. Glynne GL. Drug interaction? *Anaesthesia* (1984) 39, 293.
7. Yate B, Mostafa SM. Drug interaction? *Anaesthesia* (1984) 39, 728–9.
8. Loan PB, Connolly FM, Mirakhur RK, Kumar N, Farling P. Neuromuscular effects of rocuronium in patients receiving beta-adrenoreceptor blocking, calcium entry blocking and anticonvulsant drugs. *Br J Anaesth* (1997) 78, 90–1.
9. McCammon RL, Hilgenberg JC, Sandage BW, Stoelting RK. The effect of esmolol on the onset and duration of succinylcholine-induced neuromuscular blockade. *Anesthesiology* (1985) 63, A317.
10. Usubiaga JE. Neuromuscular effects of beta-adrenergic blockers and their interaction with skeletal muscle relaxants. *Anesthesiology* (1968) 29, 484–92.
11. Harrah MD, Way WL, Katzung BG. The interaction of d-tubocurarine with antiarrhythmic drugs. *Anesthesiology* (1970) 33, 406–10.

Neuromuscular blockers + Bretylium

In theory there is the possibility of increased and prolonged neuromuscular blockade if bretylium is given with neuromuscular blockers.

Clinical evidence, mechanism, importance and management

Although case reports seem to be lacking, there is some evidence from *animal* studies that the effects of **tubocurarine** can be increased and prolonged by bretylium.[1] There is a theoretical possibility that if the bretylium were to be given during surgery to control arrhythmias, its effects (which are delayed) might be additive with the residual effects of the neuromuscular blocker during the recovery period, resulting in apnoea. This needs confirmation.

1. Welch GW, Waud BE. Effect of bretylium on neuromuscular transmission. *Anesth Analg* (1982) 61, 442–4.

Neuromuscular blockers + Calcium channel blockers

Limited evidence indicates that intra-operative intravenous diltiazem, nicardipine, nifedipine and verapamil can increase the neuromuscular blocking effects of vecuronium and other competitive neuromuscular blockers. However, intravenous nimodipine did not alter vecuronium effects in one study. An isolated case report describes potentiation of tubocurarine/pancuronium by oral verapamil. However, long-term oral nifedipine did not alter vecuronium or atracurium effects, and long-term therapy with various calcium channel blockers did not interact with rocuronium. Calcium channel blockers do not increase the plasma potassium rise due to suxamethonium (succinylcholine).

Clinical evidence

(a) Competitive (non-depolarising) neuromuscular blockers + intravenous calcium channel blockers

A study in 24 surgical patients[1] anaesthetised with nitrous oxide and isoflurane found that **diltiazem** 5 or 10 micrograms/kg/minute decreased the **vecuronium** requirements by up to 50%. Another study in 24 surgical patients showed that **diltiazem** 5 mg bolus followed by a 4-microgram/kg/minute infusion decreased the **vecuronium** requirements by 45% when compared with a control group (no **diltiazem**) or those receiving **diltiazem** at half the infusion dose.[2] Reductions in the requirements for **vecuronium** were also noted in other surgical patients receiving intravenous **diltiazem** or **nicardipine**.[3] A study in patients given **vecuronium** 100 micrograms/kg for tracheal intubation found that **nicardipine** 10 micrograms/kg shortened the onset of blockade to the same extent as other patients given a higher dose of **vecuronium** 150 micrograms/kg alone. Recovery times were unaffected by the **nicardipine**.[4] Yet another study showed that **nicardipine** reduced the requirements for **vecuronium** in a dose-dependent manner; nicardipine 1, 2 and 3 micrograms/kg/minute reduced the vecuronium dose requirement to 79%, 60% and 53% of control, respectively.[5] A study involving 44 patients anaesthetised with isoflurane in nitrous oxide/oxygen found that 1 mg of intravenous **nifedipine** prolonged the neuromuscular blockade due to **atracurium** from 29 to 40 minutes, and increased the neuromuscular blockade of **atracurium** or **vecuronium** from 75 to 90%.[6] In contrast, a study involving 20 patients demonstrated that an intravenous infusion of **nimodipine** had no significant effect on the time course of action of **vecuronium**.[7]

A 66-year-old woman with renal impairment, receiving 5 mg of intravenous **verapamil** three times a day for supraventricular tachycardia, underwent abdominal surgery during which she was initially anaesthetised with thiopental and then maintained on nitrous oxide/oxygen with fentanyl. **Vecuronium** was used as the muscle relaxant. The effects of the **vecuronium** were increased and prolonged, and at the end of surgery reversal of the blockade using neostigmine was difficult and extended.[8] Intravenous **verapamil** alone caused respiratory failure in a patient with poor neuromuscular transmission (Duchenne's dystrophy).[9] Note that *in vitro* and *animal* studies have confirmed an increase in the neuromuscular blocking effects of **tubocurarine, pancuronium, vecuronium, atracurium** and **suxamethonium** (**succinylcholine**) by **diltiazem**, **verapamil** and **nifedipine**.[9-11]

(b) Competitive (non-depolarising) neuromuscular blockers + oral calcium channel blockers

A report describes increased neuromuscular blockade in a patient on long-term **verapamil** 40 mg three times daily who was given **pancuronium** 2 mg and **tubocurarine** 5 mg, which was difficult to reverse with neostigmine, but which responded well to edrophonium.[12] However, the authors of this report say that many patients on long-term **verapamil** do not show a clinically significant increased sensitivity to muscle relaxants.[12] This case also contrasts with another study in which 30 predominantly elderly patients on chronic **nifedipine** treatment (mean daily dose 33 mg) showed no changes in the time of onset to maximum block nor the duration of clinical relaxation in response to **atracurium** or **vecuronium** compared with 30 control patients.[13] Similarly, a study of 17 patients taking calcium channel blockers (**nifedipine** 12, **diltiazem** 2, **nicardipine** 2, **amlodipine** 1) found no changes in the neuromuscular blocking effects of **rocuronium**.[14]

(c) Suxamethonium + oral calcium channel blockers

A comparative study in 21 patients taking calcium channel blockers long term (**diltiazem, nifedipine, verapamil**) and 15 other patients not taking calcium channel blockers found that, although suxamethonium (succinylcholine) caused a modest average peak rise of 0.5 mmol/l in plasma potassium levels, there were no differences between the two groups.[15] See also (a) above.

Mechanism

Not fully understood. One explanation for the increased blockade is as follows. Nerve impulses arriving at nerve endings release calcium ions, which in turn causes the release of acetylcholine. Calcium channel blockers can reduce the concentration of calcium ions within the nerve so that less acetylcholine is released. This would be additive with the effects of a neuromuscular blocker.[11,12]

Importance and management

Direct information so far seems to be limited. Be alert for increased neuromuscular blockade in any patient given intravenous nicardipine, nifedipine, verapamil or any other calcium channel blocker during surgery. However, this may not apply to nimodipine. From the limited evidence available it appears that increased blockade is not likely in patients on long-term oral calcium channel blockers, although one case has been reported with verapamil.

It would seem from the study[15] quoted above that patients on chronic calcium channel blocker treatment are at no greater risk of hyperkalaemia with suxamethonium than other patients.

1. Sumikawa K, Kawabata K, Aono Y, Kamibayashi T, Yoshiya I. Reduction in vecuronium infusion dose requirements by diltiazem in humans. *Anesthesiology* (1992) 77, A939.
2. Takasaki Y, Naruoka Y, Shimizu C, Ochi G, Nagaro T, Arai T. Diltiazem potentiates the neuromuscular blockade by vecuronium in humans. *Jpn J Anesthesiol* (1995) 44, 503–7.
3. Takiguchi M, Takaya T. Potentiation of neuromuscular blockade by calcium channel blockers. *Tokai J Exp Clin Med* (1994) 19, 131–7.
4. Yamada T, Takino Y. Can nicardipine potentiate vecuronium induced neuromuscular blockade? *Jpn J Anesthesiol* (1992) 41, 746–50.
5. Kawabata K, Sumikawa K, Kamibayashi T, Kita T, Takada K, Mashimo T, Yoshiya I. Decrease in vecuronium infusion dose requirements by nicardipine in humans. *Anesth Analg* (1994) 79, 1159–64.
6. Jelen-Esselborn S, Blobner M. Wirkungsverstärkung von nichtdepolarisierenden Muskelrelaxanzien durch Nifedipin i.v. in Inhalationsanaesthesie. *Anaesthesist* (1990) 39, 173–8.
7. Aysel'I, HepağuŞlar H, Balcioğlu T, Uyar M. The effects of nimodipine on vecuronium-induced neuromuscular blockade. *Eur J Anaesthesiol* (2000) 17, 383–9.
8. van Poorten JF, Dhasmana KM, Kuypers RSM, Erdmann W. Verapamil and reversal of vecuronium neuromuscular blockade. *Anesth Analg* (1984) 63, 155–7.
9. Durant NN, Nguyen N, Katz RL. Potentiation of neuromuscular blockade by verapamil. *Anesthesiology* (1984) 60, 298–303.
10. Bikhazi GB, Leung I, Foldes FF. Interaction of neuromuscular blocking agents with calcium channel blockers. *Anesthesiology* (1982) 57, A268.
11. Wali FA. Interactions of nifedipine and diltiazem with muscle relaxants and reversal of neuromuscular blockade with edrophonium and neostigmine. *J Pharmacol* (1986) 17, 244–53.
12. Jones RM, Cashman JN, Casson WR, Broadbent MP. Verapamil potentiation of neuromuscular blockade: failure of reversal with neostigmine but prompt reversal with edrophonium. *Anesth Analg* (1985) 64, 1021–5.
13. Bell PF, Mirakhur RK, Elliott P. Onset and duration of clinical relaxation of atracurium and vecuronium in patients on chronic nifedipine therapy. *Eur J Anaesthesiol* (1989) 6, 343–6.
14. Loan PB, Connolly FM, Mirakhur RK, Kumar N, Farling P. Neuromuscular effects of rocuronium in patients receiving beta-adrenoreceptor blocking, calcium entry blocking and anticonvulsant drugs. *Br J Anaesth* (1997) 78, 90–1.
15. Rooke GA, Freund PR, Tomlin J. Calcium channel blockers do not enhance increases in plasma potassium after succinylcholine in humans. *J Clin Anesth* (1994) 6, 114–18.

Neuromuscular blockers + Chloroquine or Quinine

A report describes respiratory insufficiency during the recovery period following surgery, attributed to the use of chloroquine diorotate. An isolated report describes recurarisation and dyspnoea in a patient given intravenous quinine after recovering from neuromuscular blockade with suxamethonium (succinylcholine) and pancuronium.

Clinical evidence, mechanism, importance and management

(a) Chloroquine

Studies were carried out on the possible neuromuscular blocking actions of chloroquine diorotate in *animals,* because it was noticed that when it was used in the peritoneal cavity to prevent adhesions following abdominal surgery in man, it caused respiratory insufficiency during the recovery period. These studies found that it had a non-depolarising blocking action at the neuromuscular junction, which was opposed by neostigmine.[1] It would seem therefore that during the recovery period the effects of the chloroquine can be additive with the residual effects of the conventional neuromuscular blocker used during the surgery.

Although this appears to be the only report of this interaction, it is consistent with the way chloroquine can unmask or aggravate myasthenia gravis, or oppose the effects of drugs used in its treatment. Be alert for this reaction if chloroquine is used.

(b) Quinine

A 47-year-old man with acute pancreatitis, taking quinine 600 mg three times daily, was given penicillin and gentamicin intravenously before undergoing surgery during which **pancuronium** and **suxamethonium** (**succinylcholine**) were used uneventfully. After the surgery the neuromuscular blockade was reversed with neostigmine and atropine, and the patient awoke and was breathing well. A 6-hour intravenous infusion of quinine 500 mg was started 90 minutes postoperatively. Within 10 minutes (after receiving about 15 mg quinine) he became dyspnoeic, his breathing became totally ineffective and he needed re-intubation. Muscle flaccidity persisted for 3 hours.[2] The reason for this reaction is not fully understood. A possible explanation is that it may have been the additive neuromuscular blocking effects of the gentamicin (well recognised as having neuromuscular blocking activity—see 'Neuromuscular blockers + Aminoglycosides', p.898) and the quinine (an optical isomer of quinidine—see 'Neuromuscular blockers + Quinidine', p.915) and the residual effects of the **pancuronium** and **suxamethonium**.

There seem to be no other reports of problems in patients on neuromuscular blockers when given quinine, but this isolated case serves to emphasise the importance of being alert for any signs of recurarisation in patients concurrently treated with one or more drugs possessing some neuromuscular blocking activity.

1. Jui-Yen T. Clinical and experimental studies on mechanism of neuromuscular blockade by chloroquine diorotate. *Jpn J Anesthesiol* (1971) 20, 491–503.
2. Sher MH, Mathews PA. Recurarization with quinine administration after reversal from anaesthesia. *Anaesth Intensive Care* (1983) 11, 241–3.

Neuromuscular blockers + Clonidine

There is limited evidence that clonidine modestly increases the duration of action of vecuronium.

Clinical evidence, mechanism, importance and management

In a study of 16 surgical patients, 8 received oral clonidine 4 to 5.5 micrograms/kg 90 minutes before their operation. Anaesthesia was induced by thiamylal and maintained by nitrous oxide/isoflurane/oxygen supplemented by fentanyl. Following administration of **vecuronium** the duration of neuromuscular blockade was increased by 26.4% in the clonidine group.[1]

The reasons are not understood. The clinical importance of this interaction would appear to be small.

1. Nakahara T, Akazawa T, Kinoshita Y, Nozaki J. The effect of clonidine on the duration of vecuronium-induced neuromuscular blockade in humans. *Jpn J Anesthesiol* (1995) 44, 1458–63.

Neuromuscular blockers + Corticosteroids

Two reports describe antagonism of the neuromuscular blocking effects of pancuronium by high-dose prednisone or prednisolone and hydrocortisone. A third report in a patient with adrenocortical insufficiency describes reversal of pancuronium block with hydrocortisone. Some evidence suggests the dosage of vecuronium may need to be almost doubled in those receiving intramuscular betamethasone. However, prolonged coadministration of high-dose corticosteroids and neuromuscular blockers may increase the risk of myopathy, resulting in prolonged paralysis following the discontinuation of the neuromuscular blocker.

Clinical evidence

(a) Neuromuscular blocking effects

A man undergoing surgery who was on **prednisone** 250 mg daily by mouth, had good muscular relaxation in response to intravenous **pancuronium** 8 mg (100 micrograms/kg) early in the operation, but an hour later began to show signs of inadequate relaxation and continued to do so for the next 75 minutes despite being given four additional 2-mg doses of **pancuronium**.[1] Another patient on large doses of **hydrocortisone**, **prednisolone** and aminophylline proved to be resistant to the effects of **pancuronium**.[2] A hypophysectomised man on **cortisone** developed profound paralysis when given **pancuronium**, which was rapidly reversed with 100 mg of **hydrocortisone sodium succinate**.[3]

Inadequate neuromuscular blockade (presenting as unexpected movements) occurred in 2 patients during neurosurgery who had received **vecuronium**. They had both been given a preoperative course of **betamethasone** 4 mg four times daily to reduce raised intracranial pressure.[4] This prompted a retrospective search of the records of 50 other patients, which revealed that those given intramuscular **betamethasone** preoperatively had needed almost double the dose of **vecuronium** (134 compared with 76 micrograms/kg/hour).[4]

These reports contrast with another,[5] in which 25 patients who had no adrenocortical dysfunction or histories of corticosteroid therapy were given **pancuronium**, **metocurine**, **tubocurarine** or **vecuronium**. They showed no changes in their neuromuscular blockade when given a single intravenous dose of **dexamethasone** 400 micrograms/kg or **hydrocortisone** 10 mg/kg.

(b) Increased risk of myopathy

A report describes 3 patients in status asthmaticus who developed acute reversible myopathy after treatment with high-dose intravenous **methylprednisolone** 320 to 750 mg daily and steroidal neuromuscular blockers (**vecuronium** or **pancuronium**), used concurrently for at least 8 days.[6] A review of the literature from 1977 to 1995 found over 75 cases of prolonged weakness associated with combined use of neuromuscular blockers and **corticosteroids**.[7] This condition has been referred to as 'blocking agent–corticosteroid myopathy' (BACM). Prior to 1994, virtually all cases involved either **pancuronium** or **vecuronium**, leading some authors to suggest that **atracurium** might be safer as it does not have the steroidal structure of these neuromuscular blockers.[6] However, there have since been reports of prolonged paralysis associated with extended treatment with high-dose **corticosteroids** and **atracurium**.[8,9]

Mechanism

Not understood.

For the partial reversal of neuromuscular blockade, one idea, based on *animal* studies, is that adrenocortical insufficiency causes a defect in neuromuscular transmission, which is reversed by the corticosteroids.[3] Another idea is the effects seen are connected in some way with the steroid nucleus of the pancuronium and vecuronium and are mediated presynaptically.[4,10]

The increased myopathy may be due to an additive effect as both neuromuscular blockers and corticosteroids can cause myopathy. Results of an *in vitro* study suggested that the combination of vecuronium and methylprednisolone might augment pharmacologic denervation, which may lead to myopathy and contribute to the prolonged weakness observed in some critically ill patients.[11]

Importance and management

The evidence for antagonism of neuromuscular blocking effects seems to be limited to the reports cited, and involve only pancuronium and vecuronium. Careful monitoring is clearly needed if either is used in patients who have been treated with corticosteroids, being alert for the need to increase the dosage of the neuromuscular blocker. Note that *animal* studies suggest that atracurium may also possibly be affected by betamethasone to the same extent as vecuronium.[10] However, also be aware that prolonged coadministration of competitive neuromuscular blockers and corticosteroids, particularly in patients in intensive care, may result in a marked prolongation of muscle weakness (several months' rehabilitation have been needed in some cases[6]). The complex state of the critically ill patient means that the effects of neuromuscular blockers may be unpredictable.

1. Laflin MJ. Interaction of pancuronium and corticosteroids. *Anesthesiology* (1977) 47, 471–2.
2. Azar I, Kumar D, Betcher AM. Resistance to pancuronium in an asthmatic patient treated with aminophylline and steroids. *Can Anaesth Soc J* (1982) 29, 280–2.
3. Meyers EF. Partial recovery from pancuronium neuromuscular blockade following hydrocortisone administration. *Anesthesiology* (1977) 46, 148–50.
4. Parr SM, Galletly DC, Robinson BJ. Betamethasone-induced resistance to vecuronium: a potential problem in neurosurgery? *Anaesth Intensive Care* (1991) 19, 103–5.
5. Schwartz AE, Matteo RS, Ornstein E, Silverberg PA. Acute steroid therapy does not alter nondepolarizing muscle relaxant effects in humans. *Anesthesiology* (1986) 65, 326–7.
6. Griffin D, Fairman N, Coursin D, Rawsthorne L, Grossman JE. Acute myopathy during treatment of status asthmaticus with corticosteroids and steroidal muscle relaxants. *Chest* (1992) 102, 510–14.
7. Fischer JR, Baer RK. Acute myopathy associated with combined use of corticosteroids and neuromuscular blocking agents. *Ann Pharmacother* (1996) 30, 1437–45.
8. Branney SW, Haenel JB, Moore FA, Tarbox BB, Schreiber RH, Moore EE. Prolonged paralysis with atracurium infusion: a case report. *Crit Care Med* (1994) 22, 1699–1701.
9. Meyer KC, Prielipp RC, Grossman JE, Coursin DB. Prolonged weakness after infusion of atracurium in two intensive care unit patients. *Anesth Analg* (1994) 78, 772–4.
10. Robinson BJ, Lee E, Rees D, Purdie GL, Galletly DC. Betamethasone-induced resistance to neuromuscular blockade: a comparison of atracurium and vecuronium in vitro. *Anesth Analg* (1992) 74, 762–5.
11. Kindler CH, Verotta D, Gray AT, Gropper MA, Yost CS. Additive inhibition of nicotinic acetylcholine receptors by corticosteroids and the neuromuscular blocking drug vecuronium. *Anesthesiology* (2000) 92, 821–32.

Neuromuscular blockers + Danazol or Tamoxifen

Two isolated case reports describe prolonged atracurium effects attributed to tamoxifen and danazol.

Clinical evidence, mechanism, importance and management

A case report describes a 67-year-old mastectomy patient on methyldopa, hydrochlorothiazide, triamterene and long-term tamoxifen 10 mg twice daily who showed prolonged neuromuscular blockade to a single 500-microgram/kg dose of **atracurium**, which the authors suggest might be due to an interaction between **atracurium** and tamoxifen.[1] The authors also point out an earlier report[2] of prolonged **atracurium** blockade where the patient was taking danazol. These interactions appear not to be of general importance.

1. Naguib M, Gyasi HK. Antiestrogenic drugs and atracurium – a possible interaction? *Can Anaesth Soc J* (1986) 33, 682–3.
2. Bizzarri-Schmid MD, Desai SP. Prolonged neuromuscular blockade with atracurium. *Can Anaesth Soc J* (1986) 33, 209–12.

Neuromuscular blockers + Dantrolene

One patient showed increased vecuronium effects when given dantrolene, whereas two others showed no changes.

Clinical evidence, mechanism, importance and management

A 60-year-old woman, given a total of 350 mg of dantrolene orally during the 28 hours before surgery to prevent malignant hyperthermia, showed increased neuromuscular blockade and a slow recovery rate when **vecuronium** was used subsequently.[1] This report contrasts with another describing two patients on long-term dantrolene 20 to 50 mg daily who showed no changes in **vecuronium**-induced neuromuscular blockade during or after surgery.[2] Dantrolene is a muscle relaxant that acts directly on the muscle by lowering intracellular calcium concentrations in skeletal muscle; it reduces the release of calcium from the sarcoplasmic reticulum. It may also possibly inhibit calcium-dependent pre-synaptic neurotransmitter release.[3] Be alert for any increased effects if both drugs are used.

1. Driessen JJ, Wuis EW, Gielen MJM. Prolonged vecuronium neuromuscular blockade in a patient receiving orally administered dantrolene. *Anesthesiology* (1985) 62, 523–4.
2. Nakayama M, Iwasaki H, Fujita S, Narimatsu E, Namiki A. Neuromuscular effects of vecuronium in patients receiving long-term administration of dantrolene. *Jpn J Anesthesiol* (1993) 42, 1508–10.
3. Dantrium (Dantrolene). Procter & Gamble Pharmaceuticals UK Ltd. UK Summary of product characteristics, October 2002

Neuromuscular blockers + Dexmedetomidine

Dexmedetomidine caused a minor increase in plasma rocuronium concentrations.

Clinical evidence, mechanism, importance and management

A study in 10 healthy subjects under general anaesthesia with alfentanil, propofol and nitrous oxide/oxygen, demonstrated that an intravenous infusion of dexmedetomidine (950 to 990 nanograms/kg) increased plasma **rocuronium** concentrations by 7.6%, which was not clinically significant, and decreased the twitch tension from 51% to 44% after 45 minutes. Dexmedetomidine also decreased finger blood flow and increased systemic blood pressure. It was suggested these pharmacokinetic changes occurred due to peripheral vasoconstriction.[1]

1. Talke PO, Caldwell JE, Richardson CA, Kirkegaard-Nielsen H, Stafford M. The effects of dexmedetomidine on neuromuscular blockade in human volunteers. *Anesth Analg* (1999) 88, 633–9.

Neuromuscular blockers + Dexpanthenol

An isolated report of an increase in the neuromuscular blocking effects of suxamethonium (succinylcholine) was attributed to the concurrent use of dexpanthenol in one patient, but a further study of pantothenic acid failed to confirm this interaction.

Clinical evidence, mechanism, importance and management

A study in 6 patients under general anaesthesia showed that their response to **suxamethonium** (**succinylcholine**) was unaffected by the infusion of 500 mg of **pantothenic acid**.[1] This study was conducted in response to an earlier case report, which reported respiratory depression requiring re-intubation following the use of intramuscular **dexpanthenol** shortly after stopping a **suxamethonium** infusion.[1]

Apart from the single unconfirmed report there seems to be little other reason for avoiding concurrent use or for taking particular precautions. However the US maker of **dexpanthenol** recommends that it should not be administered within one hour of **suxamethonium**.[2]

1. Smith RM, Gottshall SC, Young JA. Succinylcholine-pantothenyl alcohol: a reappraisal. *Anesth Analg* (1969) 48, 205–208.
2. Dexpanthenol. In: AHFS Drug Information, 2004. American Society of Health-System Pharmacists, Inc. p. 3496–3498.

Neuromuscular blockers + Disopyramide

An isolated case report suggests that disopyramide may oppose the effects of neostigmine used to reverse neuromuscular blockade with vecuronium.

Clinical evidence, mechanism, importance and management

A case report[1] suggests that the normal antagonism by neostigmine of **vecuronium** neuromuscular blockade may be opposed by therapeutic serum levels of disopyramide (5 micrograms/ml). Disopyramide has also been shown to decrease the antagonism by **neostigmine** of the neuromuscular blockade of tubocurarine on the *rat* phrenic nerve-diaphragm preparation.[2] The general clinical importance of these observations are not known.

1. Baurain M, Barvais L, d'Hollander A, Hennart D. Impairment of the antagonism of vecuronium-induced paralysis and intra-operative disopyramide administration. *Anaesthesia* (1989) 44, 34–6.
2. Healy TEJ, O'Shea M, Massey J. Disopyramide and neuromuscular transmission. *Br J Anaesth* (1981) 53, 495–8.

Neuromuscular blockers + Ecothiopate iodide

The neuromuscular blocking effects of suxamethonium (succinylcholine) are markedly increased and prolonged in patients under treatment with ecothiopate iodide. The dosage of suxamethonium should be reduced appropriately.

Clinical evidence

In 1965 Murray McGavi[1] showed that ecothiopate iodide eye drops could markedly lower pseudocholinesterase levels. He warned that ". . . within a few days of commencing therapy, levels are reached at which protracted apnoea could occur, should these patients require general anaesthesia in which muscle relaxation is obtained with **succinylcholine**". Cases of apnoea due to this interaction were reported the following year,[2,3] and other cases have been subsequently reported.[4,5] In one case a woman given **suxamethonium** (**succinylcholine**) 200 mg showed apnoea for 5½ hours.[2] Other studies have confirmed that ecothiopate given orally[6] or as eye drops[7] markedly reduced the levels of plasma cholinesterase, and can prolong recovery after **suxamethonium**.[6] On discontinuing ecothiopate, it takes several weeks to 2 months for enzyme activity to return to normal.[7]

Mechanism

Suxamethonium is metabolised in the body by plasma cholinesterase. Ecothiopate iodide depresses the levels of this enzyme so that the metabolism of the suxamethonium is reduced and its effects are thereby enhanced and prolonged.[3,6] One study in 71 patients found that two drops of 0.06% ecothiopate iodide three times weekly in each eye caused a twofold reduction in plasma cholinesterase (pseudocholinesterase) activity in about one-third of the patients, and a fourfold reduction in 1 in 7 patients.[8]

Importance and management

An established, adequately documented and clinically important interaction. The dosage of suxamethonium should be reduced appropriately because of the reduced plasma cholinesterase levels caused by ecothiopate. The study cited above[8] suggests that prolonged apnoea is likely in about 1 in 7 patients. One report describes the successful use of approximately one-fifth of the normal dosage of suxamethonium in a patient receiving 0.125% ecothiopate iodide solution, one drop twice a day in both eyes, and with a plasma cholinesterase activity 62% below normal. Recovery from the neuromuscular blockade was rapid and uneventful.[9] Another report describes the successful and uneventful use of atracurium instead.[5] **Mivacurium** is also metabolised by plasma cholinesterase, and would be expected to interact with ecothiopate similarly to suxamethonium.[10] See also 'Neuromuscular blockers + Anticholinesterases', p.899.

1. McGavi DDM. Depressed levels of serum-pseudocholinesterase with ecothiophate-iodide eyedrops. *Lancet* (1965) ii, 272–3.
2. Gesztes T. Prolonged apnoea after suxamethonium injection associated with eye drops containing an anticholinesterase agent. *Br J Anaesth* (1966) 38, 408–409.
3. Pantuck EJ. Ecothiopate iodide eye drops and prolonged response to suxamethonium. *Br J Anaesth* (1966) 38, 406–407.
4. Mone JG, Mathie WE. Qualitative and quantitative defects of pseudocholinesterase activity. *Anaesthesia* (1967) 22, 55–68.
5. Messer GJ, Stoudemire A, Knos G, Johnson GC. Electroconvulsive therapy and the chronic use of pseudocholinesterase-inhibitor (echothiophate iodide) eye drops for glaucoma. A case report. *Gen Hosp Psychiatry* (1992) 14, 56–60.
6. Cavallaro RJ, Krumperman LW, Kugler F. Effect of echothiophate therapy on the metabolism of succinylcholine in man. *Anesth Analg* (1968) 47, 570–4.
7. de Roetth A, Dettbarn W-D, Rosenberg P, Wilensky JG, Wong A. Effect of phospholine iodide on blood cholinesterase levels of normal and glaucoma subjects. *Am J Ophthalmol* (1965) 59, 586–92.
8. Eilderton TE, Farmati O, Zsigmond EK. Reduction in plasma cholinesterase levels after prolonged administration of echothiophate iodide eyedrops. *Can Anaesth Soc J* (1968) 15, 291–6.
9. Donati F, Bevan DR. Controlled succinylcholine infusion in a patient receiving echothiophate eye drops. *Can Anaesth Soc J* (1981) 28, 488–90.
10. Feldman S, Karalliedde L. Drug interactions with neuromuscular blockers. *Drug Safety* (1996) 15, 261–73.

Neuromuscular blockers + Furosemide

The effects of the neuromuscular blockers may possibly be changed by furosemide.

Clinical evidence

(a) Increased neuromuscular blockade

Three patients receiving kidney transplants[1] showed increased neuromuscular blockade with **tubocurarine** (seen as a pronounced decrease in twitch tension) when given furosemide 40 or 80 mg and mannitol 12.5 g intravenously. One of them showed the same reaction when later given only 40 mg of furosemide but no mannitol. The residual blockade was easily antagonised with pyridostigmine 14 mg or neostigmine 3 mg with atropine 1.2 mg.

(b) Decreased neuromuscular blockade

Ten neurosurgical patients given furosemide 1 mg/kg 10 minutes before induction of anaesthesia, took 14.7 minutes to recover from 95 to 50% blockade with **pancuronium** (as measured by a twitch response) compared with 21.8 minutes in 10 similar patients who had not received furosemide.[2]

Mechanism

Uncertain. *Animal* studies indicate that what happens probably depends on the dosage of furosemide: 0.1 to 10 micrograms/kg increased the blocking effects of tubocurarine and suxamethonium (succinylcholine) whereas 1 to 4 mg/kg opposed the blockade.[3] One suggestion is that low doses of furosemide may inhibit protein kinase causing a reduction in neuromuscular transmission, whereas higher doses cause inhibition of phosphodiesterase resulting in increased cyclic AMP activity and causing antagonism of neuromuscular blockade. It has also been suggested that large doses of loop diuretics may affect the renal excretion of neuromuscular blockers that are cleared by this route, resulting in more rapid recovery from the blockade.[3]

Importance and management

The documentation is very limited. Be on the alert for changes in the response to any blocker if furosemide is used.

1. Miller RD, Sohn YJ, Matteo RS. Enhancement of *d*-tubocurarine neuromuscular blockade by diuretics in man. *Anesthesiology* (1976) 45, 442–5.
2. Azar I, Cottrell J, Gupta B, Turndorf H. Furosemide facilitates recovery of evoked twitch response after pancuronium. *Anesth Analg* (1980) 59, 55–7.
3. Scappaticci KA, Ham JA, Sohn YJ, Miller RD, Dretchen KL. Effects of furosemide on the neuromuscular junction. *Anesthesiology* (1982) 57, 381–8.

Neuromuscular blockers + H_2-blockers

One report says that recovery from the neuromuscular blocking effects of suxamethonium (succinylcholine) is prolonged by cimetidine, but this may possibly have been due to the presence of metoclopramide. Four other reports say that no interaction occurs between suxamethonium and either cimetidine, famotidine or ranitidine. Cimetidine, but not ranitidine, has been reported to increase the effects of vecuronium, and neither affects atracurium. Cimetidine does not affect rocuronium.

Clinical evidence

(a) Evidence of increased neuromuscular blockade

A study in 10 patients given **cimetidine** 300 mg orally at bedtime and another 300 mg 2 hours before anaesthesia, showed that while the onset of action of **suxamethonium (succinylcholine)** 1.5 mg/kg intravenously was unchanged when compared with 10 control patients, the time to recover 50% of the twitch height was prolonged 2 to 2.5 times (from 8.6 to 20.3 minutes). One patient took 57 minutes to recover. His plasma cholinesterase levels were found to be normal.[1] It was later reported that some patients were also taking **metoclopramide**, which is known to interact in this way.[2] See also 'Neuromuscular blockers + Metoclopramide', p.911.

Another study[3] in 24 patients found that **cimetidine** 400 mg significantly prolonged the recovery (T1–25 period) from **vecuronium**, but few patients showed any response to **cimetidine** 200 mg or **ranitidine** 100 mg. This slight prolongation of action of **vecuronium** due to **cimetidine** was confirmed in another placebo-controlled study (mean time to return of T1 was 30 versus 22.5 minutes).[4] A study using a *rat* phrenic nerve diaphragm preparation found that **cimetidine** increased the neuromuscular blocking effects of **tubocurarine** and **pancuronium**, but there seem to be no reports confirming this in man.[5]

(b) Evidence of unchanged neuromuscular blockade

A study in 10 patients given **cimetidine** 400 mg orally at bedtime and 400 mg 90 minutes before anaesthesia found no evidence of an effect on the neuromuscular blockade caused by **suxamethonium**, nor on its duration or recovery period when compared with 10 control patients.[6] Another controlled study in patients given **cimetidine** 300 mg or **ranitidine** 150 mg the night before and 1 to 2 hours before surgery found no evidence that the duration of action of **suxamethonium** or the activity of plasma cholinesterase were altered.[2] A study in 15 patients undergoing caesarean section also found no evidence that either **cimetidine** or **ranitidine** affected the neuromuscular blocking effects of **suxamethonium.**[7] A study in 70 patients[8] found no changes in the neuromuscular blocking effects of **suxamethonium** in those given **cimetidine** 400 mg, **ranitidine** 80 mg or **famotidine** 20 mg.

Cimetidine and **ranitidine** appear not to affect **atracurium**, nor does **cimetidine** affect **rocuronium**,[9] or **ranitidine** affect **vecuronium**.[4] Another study found that premedication with **ranitidine** did not affect **vecuronium** blockade in postpartum patients, but that the neuromuscular blockade was prolonged in these patients compared with nonpregnant controls.[10]

Mechanism

Not understood. Studies with human plasma failed to find any evidence that cimetidine in normal serum concentrations inhibits the metabolism of suxamethonium,[2,11] however, metoclopramide does. *In vitro* studies with very high cimetidine concentrations found inhibition of plasma cholinesterase (pseudocholinesterase) activity.[12] The cimetidine/vecuronium interaction is not understood, but it has been suggested that cimetidine may reduce the hepatic metabolism of vecuronium.[4]

Importance and management

Information seems to be limited to the reports cited. The most likely explanation for the discord between the cimetidine/suxamethonium results is that in the one study reporting increased suxamethonium effects[1] some of the patients were also given metoclopramide, which can inhibit plasma cholinesterase and prolong the effects of suxamethonium[2,8] (see also 'Neuromuscular blockers + Metoclopramide', p.911). In four other studies, cimetidine and other H_2-blockers did not alter suxamethonium effects. Therefore, it seems unlikely that an interaction exists. There is some evidence that cimetidine may slightly prolong the effects of vecuronium, but ranitidine appears not to interact. Atracurium and rocuronium appear not to be affected. Overall these possible interactions seem to be of little clinical significance.

1. Kambam JR, Dymond R, Krestow M. Effect of cimetidine on duration of action of succinylcholine. *Anesth Analg* (1987) 66, 191–2.
2. Woodworth GE, Sears DH, Grove TM, Ruff RH, Kosek PS, Katz RL. The effect of cimetidine and ranitidine on the duration of action of succinylcholine. *Anesth Analg* (1989) 68, 295–7.
3. Tryba M, Wruck G. Interaktionen von H_2-Antagonisten und nichtdepolarisierenden Muskelrelaxantien. *Anaesthesist* (1989) 38, 251–4.
4. McCarthy G, Mirakhur RK, Elliott P, Wright J. Effect of H_2-receptor antagonist pretreatment on vecuronium- and atracurium-induced neuromuscular block. *Br J Anaesth* (1991) 66, 713–15.
5. Galatulas I, Bossa R, Benvenuti C. Cimetidine increases the neuromuscular blocking activity of aminoglycoside antibiotics: antagonism by calcium. *Chem Indices Mec Proc Symp* (1981) 321–5.
6. Stirt JA, Sperry RJ, DiFazio CA. Cimetidine and succinylcholine: potential interaction and effect on neuromuscular blockade in man. *Anesthesiology* (1988) 69, 607–8.
7. Bogod DG, Oh TE. The effect of H_2 antagonists on duration of action of suxamethonium in the parturient. *Anaesthesia* (1989) 44, 591–3.
8. Turner DR, Kao YJ, Bivona C. Neuromuscular block by suxamethonium following treatment with histamine type 2 antagonists or metoclopramide. *Br J Anaesth* (1989) 63, 348–50.
9. Latorre F, de Almeida MCS, Stanek A, Weiler N, Kleemann PP. Beeinflussung der Pharmakodynamik von Rocuronium durch Cimetidin. *Anaesthesist* (1996) 45, 900–2.
10. Hawkins JL, Adenwala J, Camp C, Joyce TH. The effect of H_2-receptor antagonist premedication on the duration of vecuronium-induced neuromuscular blockade in postpartum patients. *Anesthesiology* (1989) 71, 175–7.
11. Cook DR, Stiller RL, Chakravorti S, Mannenhira T. Cimetidine does not inhibit plasma cholinesterase activity. *Anesth Analg* (1988) 67, 375–6.
12. Hansen WE, Bertl S. The inhibition of acetylcholinesterase and pseudocholinesterase by cimetidine. *Arzneimittelforschung* (1983) 33, 161–3.

Neuromuscular blockers + Immunosuppressants

There is limited evidence that the neuromuscular blocking effects of atracurium, pancuronium and vecuronium may be increased in some patients treated with ciclosporin. There is also some evidence of reduced neuromuscular blockade with azathioprine and antilymphocyte immunoglobulins, and other evidence that there is no clinically relevant interaction with azathioprine.

Clinical evidence

(a) Azathioprine or Antilymphocyte immunoglobulins

A retrospective study found that patients on azathioprine or antilymphocyte immunoglobulins following organ transplantation needed an increased dosage of unspecified **muscle relaxants** to achieve satisfactory muscle relaxation.[1] A control group of 74 patients on no immunosuppression needed 0 to 15 mg doses of **non-depolarising muscle relaxants**; 13 patients on azathioprine needed 12.5 to 25 mg; 11 patients on antilymphocyte immunoglobulins (antilymphocyte globulin) needed 10 to 20 mg and two patients on azathioprine and guanethidine needed 55 and 90 mg.[1] However, a controlled study of 28 patients undergoing renal transplantation, who were receiving **atracurium, pancuronium** or **vecuronium** at a constant infusion rate, found that injection of azathioprine 3 mg/kg given over 3 minutes caused a rapid, but only small and transient decrease of neuromuscular blockade. Ten minutes after the end of the injection of azathioprine, residual interaction was only detectable in those patients who had received **pancuronium**.[2]

(b) Ciclosporin

A retrospective study found 4 of 36 patients receiving **atracurium** and 4 of 29 patients receiving **vecuronium** experienced prolonged neuromuscular blockade after anaesthesia for kidney transplantation. Respiratory failure occurred more often in patients who received intravenous ciclosporin during surgery.[3] Extended recovery times after **atracurium** and **vecuronium** are described in another report in renal transplant patients who had been receiving oral ciclosporin.[4] Similarly, prolonged duration of action of **vecuronium** was noted in 7 kidney transplant recipients compared with patients with normal renal function, and ciclosporin was considered to be a factor in this.[5] Two case reports describe prolonged neuromuscular blockade attributed to intravenous ciclosporin.

In the first report,[6] a woman with a 2-year renal transplant underwent surgery during which **pancuronium** 5.5 mg was used as the neuromuscular blocker. She was also infused with ciclosporin before and after surgery. The surgery lasted four hours and no additional doses of pancuronium were given. Residual paralysis was inadequately reversed with neostigmine and atropine, and so edrophonium was given prior to extubation. However, she had to be re-intubated 20 minutes later because of increased respiratory distress.

In the second report,[7] a 15-year-old girl on intravenous ciclosporin with serum levels of 138 micrograms/litre was anaesthetised using fentanyl, thiopental and **vecuronium** 100 micrograms/kg. Anaesthesia was maintained with nitrous oxide, oxygen and isoflurane. Attempts were later made to reverse the blockade with edrophonium, atropine and neostigmine but full neuromuscular function was not restored until 3 hours and 20 minutes after the **vecuronium** was given. Another report describes prolongation of the effects of **vecuronium** in a renal-transplant recipient on oral ciclosporin, azathioprine, and prednisolone.[8]

Mechanism

The reasons for the reduction in neuromuscular blockade with azathioprine and antilymphocyte immunoglobulins are not understood. It has been suggested that azathioprine may inhibit phosphodiesterase at the motor nerve terminal resulting in increased release of acetylcholine.[9]

The ciclosporin interaction may be partly due to the vehicle used in intravenous preparations. One idea is that *Cremophor*, a surface-active agent used as a solvent for the ciclosporin, may increase the effective concentration of pancuronium at the neuromuscular junction.[6] Both compounds have been observed in *animal* studies to increase vecuronium blockade[10] and *Cremophor* has also been seen to decrease the onset time of pancuronium blockade in patients given *Cremophor*-containing anaesthetics.[11] However this is not the entire answer because the interaction has also been seen with oral ciclosporin, which does not contain *Cremophor*.[8]

Importance and management

Direct information seems to be limited to the reports cited, and the interactions are not established. Although retrospective data suggest that azathioprine and antilymphocyte immunoglobulins can cause a reduction in the effects of neuromuscular blockers, and in some cases the dosage may need to be increased two- to fourfold,[1] the only prospective study found that the interaction with azathioprine was not clinically significant.[2] The general importance of the ciclosporin interaction is also uncertain, but be alert for an increase in the effects of atracurium, pancuronium or vecuronium in any patient receiving ciclosporin. Not all patients appear to develop this interaction.[3] More study is needed.

1. Vetten KB. Immunosuppressive therapy and anaesthesia. *S Afr Med J* (1973) 47, 767–70.
2. Gramstad L. Atracurium, vecuronium and pancuronium in end-stage renal failure. Dose-response properties and interactions with azathioprine. *Br J Anaesth* (1987) 59, 995–1003.
3. Sidi A, Kaplan RF, Davis RF. Prolonged neuromuscular blockade and ventilatory failure after renal transplantation and cyclosporine. *Can J Anaesth* (1990) 37, 543–8.
4. Lepage JY, Malinowsky JM, de Dieuleveult C, Cozian A, Pinaud M, Souron R. Interaction cyclosporine atracurium et vecuronium. *Ann Fr Anesth Reanim* (1989) 8 (Suppl), R135.
5. Takita K, Goda Y, Kawahigashi H, Okuyama A, Kubota M, Kemmotsu O. Pharmacodynamics of vecuronium in the kidney transplant recipient and the patient with normal renal function. *Jpn J Anesthesiol* (1993) 42, 190–4.
6. Crosby E, Robblee JA. Cyclosporine-pancuronium interaction in a patient with a renal allograft. *Can J Anaesth* (1988) 35, 300–2.
7. Wood GG. Cyclosporine-vecuronium interaction. *Can J Anaesth* (1989) 36, 358.
8. Ganjoo P, Tewari P. Oral cyclosporine-vecuronium interaction. *Can J Anaesth* (1994) 41, 1017.
9. Viby-Mogensen J. Interaction of other drugs with muscle relaxants. *Semin Anesth* (1985) 4, 52–64.
10. Gramstad L, Gjerløw JA, Hysing ES, Rugstad HE. Interaction of cyclosporin and its solvent, cremophor, with atracurium and vecuronium: studies in the cat. *Br J Anaesth* (1986) 58, 1149–55.
11. Gramstad L, Lilleaasen P, Minsaas B. Onset time for alcuronium and pancuronium after cremophor-containing anaesthetics. *Acta Anaesthesiol Scand* (1981) 25, 484–6.

Neuromuscular blockers + Insecticides

Exposure to organophosphorus insecticides such as malathion and dimpylate (diazinon) can markedly prolong the neuromuscular blocking effects of suxamethonium (succinylcholine).

Clinical evidence

A man admitted to hospital for an appendectomy became apnoeic during the early part of the operation when given **suxamethonium** (**succinylcholine**) 100 mg to facilitate tracheal intubation, and remained so throughout the 40 minutes of surgery. Restoration of neuromuscular activity occurred about 180 minutes after administration of the **suxamethonium**. Later studies showed that he had an extremely low plasma cholinesterase activity (3 to 10%) although he had a normal phenotype. It subsequently turned out that he had been working with **malathion** for 11 weeks without any protection.[1]

Another report describes a man whose recovery from neuromuscular blockade with **suxamethonium** was very prolonged. He had attempted suicide approximately 2 weeks earlier with **dimpylate** (**diazinon**), a household insecticide. His pseudocholinesterase was found to be 2.5 units/l (normal values 7 to 19) and his dibucaine number (a measurement of cholinesterase activity) was too low to be measured.[2]

Mechanism

Malathion and dimpylate are organophosphorus insecticides, which inhibit the activity of plasma cholinesterase, thereby reducing the metabolism of the suxamethonium and prolonging its effects.

Importance and management

An established and well understood interaction. Particular care should be exercised if suxamethonium is used in individuals known to have been exposed to **organophosphorus pesticides** such as malathion and dimpylate (diazinon). Pesticides of this type are widely used in agricultural, horticultural and veterinary practice in **sprays** and **sheep dips** (see 'Neuromuscular blockers + Anticholinesterases', p.899). These anticholinesterases are expected to interact with other depolarising neuromuscular blockers in just the same way, but to oppose the actions of competitive (non-depolarising) neuromuscular blockers.

1. Guillermo FP, Pretel CMM, Royo FT, Macias MJP, Ossorio RA, Gomez JAA, Vidal CJ. Prolonged suxamethonium-induced neuromuscular blockade associated with organophosphate poisoning. *Br J Anaesth* (1988) 61, 233–6.
2. Ware MR, Frost ML, Berger JJ, Stewart RB, DeVane CL. Electroconvulsive therapy complicated by insecticide ingestion. *J Clin Psychopharmacol* (1990) 10, 72–3.

Neuromuscular blockers + Lansoprazole

There is some evidence that lansoprazole increases the duration of action of vecuronium.

Clinical evidence, mechanism, importance and management

In a study of 50 adult surgical patients, half of whom received lansoprazole 30 mg on the night before their operation, it was found that there was no significant difference between the time of onset of neuromuscular blockade by **vecuronium** in the two groups but lansoprazole increased the duration by about 34%.[1] This needs confirmation but be alert for this interaction in any patient treated with lansoprazole.

1. Ahmed SM, Panja C, Khan RM, Bano S. Lansoprazole potentiates vecuronium paralysis. *J Indian Med Assoc* (1997) 95, 422–3.

Neuromuscular blockers + Lithium

The concurrent use of neuromuscular blockers and lithium is normally safe and uneventful, but four patients on lithium have been described who experienced prolonged blockade and respiratory difficulties after receiving standard doses of pancuronium or suxamethonium (succinylcholine) or both.

Clinical evidence

A manic depressive woman on lithium carbonate with a serum lithium concentration of 1.2 mmol/l, underwent surgery and was given thiopental, 310 mg of **suxamethonium (succinylcholine)** over a period of 2 hours and 500 micrograms of **pancuronium**. Prolonged neuromuscular blockade with apnoea occurred.[1]

Three other patients on lithium are described elsewhere who experienced enhanced neuromuscular blockade when given **pancuronium** alone[2] or with **suxamethonium**,[3] or **suxamethonium** alone.[4] The authors of one of these reports[3] say that "...We have seen potentiation of the neuromuscular blockade produced by **succinylcholine** in several patients taking lithium carbonate. . . " but give no further details. In contrast, a retrospective analysis of data from 17 patients on lithium carbonate, who received **suxamethonium** during a total of 78 ECT treatments, failed to reveal any instances of unusually prolonged recovery.[5] A lithium/**pancuronium**[1] and lithium/**suxamethonium**[6,7] interaction has been demonstrated in *dogs,* and a lithium/**tubocurarine** interaction in *cats*,[8] but no clear interaction has been demonstrated with any other neuromuscular blocker.[7,9] A case of lithium toxicity has been described in a woman on lithium and **suxamethonium**, but it is doubtful if it arose because of an interaction.[10]

Mechanism

Uncertain. One suggestion is that, when the interaction occurs, it may be due to changes in the electrolyte balance caused by the lithium, which results in changes in the release of acetylcholine at the neuromuscular junction.[8,11]

Importance and management

Information is limited. There are only four definite reports of this interaction in man and good evidence that no adverse interaction normally occurs. Concurrent use need not be avoided but it would be prudent to be on the alert for this interaction in any patient on lithium who is given any neuromuscular blocker.

1. Hill GE, Wong KC, Hodges MR. Potentiation of succinylcholine neuromuscular blockade by lithium carbonate. *Anesthesiology* (1976) 44, 439–42.
2. Borden H, Clarke MT, Katz H. The use of pancuronium bromide in patients receiving lithium carbonate. *Can Anaesth Soc J* (1974) 21, 79–82.
3. Rosner TM, Rosenberg M. Anesthetic problems in patients taking lithium. *J Oral Surg* (1981) 39, 282–5.
4. Rabolini V, Gatti G. Potenziamento del blocco neuro-muscolare di tipo depolarizzante da sali di litio (relazione su un caso). *Anest Rianim* (1988) 29, 157–9.
5. Martin BA, Kramer PM. Clinical significance of the interaction between lithium and a neuromuscular blocker. *Am J Psychiatry* (1982) 139, 1326–8.
6. Reimherr FW, Hodges MR, Hill GE, Wong KC. Prolongation of muscle relaxant effects by lithium carbonate. *Am J Psychiatry* (1977) 134, 205–6.
7. Hill GE, Wong KC, Hodges MR. Lithium carbonate and neuromuscular blocking agents. *Anesthesiology* (1977) 46, 122–6.
8. Basuray BN, Harris CA. Potentiation of d-tubocurarine (d-Tc) neuromuscular blockade in cats by lithium chloride. *Eur J Pharmacol* (1977) 45, 79–82.
9. Waud BE, Farrell L, Waud DR. Lithium and neuromuscular transmission. *Anesth Analg* (1982) 61, 399–402.
10. Jephcott G, Kerry RJ. Lithium: an anaesthetic risk. *Br J Anaesth* (1974) 46, 389–90.
11. Dehpour AR, Samadian T, Roushanzamir F. Interaction of aminoglycoside antibiotics and lithium at the neuromuscular junctions. *Drugs Exp Clin Res* (1992) 18, 383–7.

Neuromuscular blockers + Magnesium compounds

The effects of mivacurium, rocuronium, tubocurarine, vecuronium, and probably other competitive neuromuscular blockers can be increased and prolonged by magnesium sulfate given parenterally. There is some evidence that magnesium may interact similarly with suxamethonium (succinylcholine), but also evidence from well-controlled trials that it does not.

Clinical evidence

(a) Depolarising neuromuscular blockers

An early study in 59 women undergoing caesarean section showed that those given magnesium sulfate for eclampsia and pre-eclampsia needed less **suxamethonium (succinylcholine)** than control patients (4.73 compared with 7.39 mg/kg/hour).[1] A 71-year-old woman given magnesium sulfate and lidocaine for ventricular tachycardia underwent emergency cardioversion and showed delayed onset and prolonged neuromuscular blockade when given **suxamethonium**.[2] Increased blockade by magnesium has been demonstrated with **suxamethonium** in *animals*.[3,4]

However, a randomised study involving 20 patients found that pretreatment with a single bolus dose of 60-mg/kg magnesium sulfate did not significantly affect the onset or prolong the block produced by **suxamethonium**.[5] Similar results were found in a non-randomised study[6] and in a double-blind randomised study.[7] In randomised studies, administration of magnesium sulfate has also been reported to reduce **suxamethonium**-associated fasciculations[7] and reduce the increase in serum potassium concentrations produced by **suxamethonium**.[5]

(b) Competitive (non-depolarising) neuromuscular blockers

A pregnant 40-year-old with severe pre-eclampsia and receiving magnesium sulfate by infusion, underwent emergency caesarean section during which she was initially anaesthetised with thiopental, maintained with nitrous oxide/oxygen and enflurane, and given firstly **suxamethonium** and later **vecuronium** as muscle relaxants. At the end of surgery she rapidly recovered from the anaesthesia but the neuromuscular blockade was very prolonged (an eight-fold increase in duration).[8] In a series of randomised studies involving 125 patients, pretreatment with intravenous magnesium sulfate 40 mg/kg reduced the dose requirement of **vecuronium** by 25%, approximately halved the time to the onset of action, and prolonged the duration of action from 25.2 to 43.3 minutes.[9] Another study found that pretreatment with 40 mg/kg of magnesium sulfate, but not 20 mg/kg, decreased the onset and prolonged the recovery time from **vecuronium** blockade.[10] Evidence of enhanced **vecuronium** neuromuscular blockade by magnesium sulfate is described in one other study,[6] and case report.[11] Another study in 20 patients showed that recurarisation (sufficient to compromise respiration) occurred when magnesium sulfate 60 mg/kg was administered in the postoperative period, shortly after recovery from neuromuscular block with **vecuronium**.[12] Neostigmine-induced recovery from **vecuronium** block was attenuated by about 30% in patients pretreated with magnesium sulfate in a randomised study. The authors demonstrated this was due to slower spontaneous recovery and not decreased response to neostigmine.[13]

A fourfold increase in the duration of neuromuscular blockade of **rocuronium** 0.9 mg/kg was reported in a pregnant woman receiving magnesium sulfate.[14] A further randomised placebo-controlled study confirmed that pretreatment with magnesium sulfate 60 mg/kg increased the duration of neuromuscular block produced by **rocuronium** (time to initial recovery increased from 25.1 to 42.1 minutes), but the onset time was not affected.[15]

The infusion rate of **mivacurium** required to obtain relaxation in women undergoing a caesarean section was about threefold lower in 12 women who had received magnesium sulfate for pre-eclampsia than in 12 women who had not.[16]

Prolonged neuromuscular block with **rapacuronium** has also been reported in a patient undergoing emergency caesarean section who received magnesium sulfate and clindamycin, although the clindamycin was thought to be mainly responsible (see also 'Neuromuscular blockers + Miscellaneous anti-infectives', p.912).[17]

Prolonged neuromuscular blockade has been described in two women with pre-eclampsia given magnesium sulfate and either **tubocurarine** alone or with **suxamethonium**.[3] Increased blockade by magnesium has been demonstrated with **tubocurarine** in *animals*.[3,4]

Mechanism

Not fully understood. Magnesium sulfate has direct neuromuscular blocking activity by inhibiting the normal release of acetylcholine from nerve endings, reducing the sensitivity of the postsynaptic membrane and depressing the excitability of the muscle membranes. These effects are seen when serum magnesium levels rise above the normal range (hypermagnesaemia) and are possibly simply additive (or possibly more than additive) with the effects of competitive neuromuscular blockers.

Importance and management

The interaction between competitive (non-depolarising) neuromuscular blockers and parenteral magnesium is established. Magnesium may decrease the time to onset (vecuronium but not rocuronium), prolong the duration of action and reduce the dose requirement of competitive neuromuscular blockers. Be alert for an increase in the effects of any competitive neuromuscular blocker if intravenous magnesium sulfate has been used, and anticipate the need to reduce the dose. Some have suggested that the decreased time to onset with vecuronium may be of use clinically to improve the intubating conditions for rapid sequence induction if suxamethonium is not suitable.[9] Intravenous calcium gluconate was used to assist recovery in one case of prolonged block.[3] Also be aware that recurarisation may occur when intravenous magnesium compounds are used in the postoperative period.[12] Hypermagnesaemia can occur in patients receiving magnesium in antacids, enemas or parenteral nutrition, especially if there is impaired renal function, but an interaction would not normally be expected as oral magnesium compounds generally result in lower systemic levels than intravenous magnesium due to poor absorption.[18]

The interaction between magnesium and suxamethonium is not established. Although some *animal* and clinical evidence suggests potentiation of suxamethonium can occur, well-controlled studies have not confirmed this. Therefore some authors consider that magnesium sulfate does not significantly affect the clinical response to suxamethonium.[6,19]

1. Morris R, Giesecke AH. Potentiation of muscle relaxants by magnesium sulfate therapy in toxemia of pregnancy. *South Med J* (1968) 61, 25–8.
2. Ip-Yam C, Allsop E. Abnormal response to suxamethonium in a patient receiving magnesium therapy. *Anaesthesia* (1994) 49, 355–6.
3. Ghoneim MM, Long JP. The interaction between magnesium and other neuromuscular blocking agents. *Anesthesiology* (1970) 32, 23–7.
4. Giesecke AH, Morris RE, Dalton MD, Stephen CR. Of magnesium, muscle relaxants, toxemic parturients, and cats. *Anesth Analg* (1968) 47, 689–95.
5. James MFM, Cork RC, Dennett JE. Succinylcholine pretreatment with magnesium sulfate. *Anesth Analg* (1986) 65, 373–6.
6. Baraka A, Yazigi A. Neuromuscular interaction of magnesium with succinylcholine-vecuronium sequence in the eclamptic parturient. *Anesthesiology* (1987) 67, 806–8.
7. Stacey MRW, Barclay K, Asai T, Vaughan RS. Effects of magnesium sulphate on suxamethonium-induced complications during rapid-sequence induction of anaesthesia. *Anaesthesia* (1995) 50, 933–6.
8. Sinatra RS, Philip BK, Naulty JS, Ostheimer GW. Prolonged neuromuscular blockade with vecuronium in a patient treated with magnesium sulfate. *Anesth Analg* (1985) 64, 1220–2.
9. Fuchs-Buder T, Wilder-Smith OHG, Borgeat A, Tassonyi E. Interaction of magnesium sulphate with vecuronium-induced neuromuscular block. *Br J Anaesth* (1995) 74, 405–9.
10. Okuda T, Umeda T, Takemura M, Shiokawa Y, Koga Y. Pretreatment with magnesium sulphate enhances vecuronium-induced neuromuscular block. *Jpn J Anesthesiol* (1998) 47, 704–8.
11. Hino H, Kaneko I, Miyazawa A, Aoki T, Ishizuka B, Kosugi K, Amemiya A. Prolonged neuromuscular blockade with vecuronium in patient with triple pregnancy treated with magnesium sulfate. *Jpn J Anesthesiol* (1997) 46, 266–70.
12. Fuchs-Buder T, Tassonyi E. Magnesium sulphate enhances residual neuromuscular block induced by vecuronium. *Br J Anaesth* (1996) 76, 565–6.
13. Fuchs-Buder T, Ziegenfuß T, Lysakowski K, Tassonyi E. Antagonism of vecuronium-induced neuromuscular block in patients pretreated with magnesium sulphate: dose-effect relationship of neostigmine. *Br J Anaesth* (1999) 82, 61–5.
14. Gaiser RR, Seem EH. Use of rocuronium in a pregnant patient with an open eye injury, receiving magnesium medication, for preterm labour. *Br J Anaesth* (1996) 77, 669–71.
15. Kussman B, Shorten G, Uppington J, Comunale ME. Administration of magnesium sulphate before rocuronium: effects on speed of onset and duration of neuromuscular block. *Br J Anaesth* (1997) 79, 122–4.
16. Ahn EK, Bai SJ, Cho BJ, Shin Y-S. The infusion rate of mivacurium and its spontaneous neuromuscular recovery in magnesium-treated parturients. *Anesth Analg* (1998) 86, 523–6.
17. Sloan PA, Rasul M. Prolongation of rapacuronium neuromuscular blockade by clindamycin and magnesium. *Anesth Analg* (2002) 94, 123–4.
18. Cammu G. Interactions of neuromuscular blocking drugs. *Acta Anaesthesiol Belg* (2001) 52, 357–63.
19. Guay J, Grenier Y, Varin F. Clinical pharmacokinetics of neuromuscular relaxants in pregnancy. *Clin Pharmacokinet* (1998) 34, 483–96.

Neuromuscular blockers + MAOIs

Three patients showed an enhancement of the effects of suxamethonium (succinylcholine) during concurrent treatment with phenelzine.

Clinical evidence, mechanism, importance and management

Two patients, one taking **phenelzine** and the other who had ceased to do so six days previously, developed apnoea following ECT during which **suxamethonium** (**succinylcholine**) was used. Both responded to injections of nikethamide and positive pressure ventilation with oxygen.[1] A later study observed the same response in another patient taking **phenelzine**.[2] This would appear to be explained by the finding that **phenelzine** caused a reduction in the levels of plasma cholinesterase (pseudocholinesterase) in 4 out of 10 patients studied. Since the metabolism of **suxamethonium** depends on this enzyme, reduced levels of the enzyme would result in a reduced rate of **suxamethonium** metabolism and in a prolongation of its effects. None of 12 other patients taking **tranylcypromine, isocarboxazid** or **mebanazine** showed reduced plasma cholinesterase levels.[2]

It would clearly be prudent to be on the alert for this interaction in patients on **phenelzine**. **Phenelzine** may be anticipated to react similarly with **mivacurium** as it is also metabolised by plasma cholinesterase.[3] On the basis of limited evidence this interaction seems less likely to occur with the other MAOIs cited.

1. Bleaden FA, Czekanska G. New drugs for depression. *BMJ* (1960) 1, 200.
2. Bodley PO, Halwax K, Potts L. Low serum pseudocholinesterase levels complicating treatment with phenelzine. *BMJ* (1969) 3, 510–12.
3. Feldman S, Karalliedde L. Drug interactions with neuromuscular blockers. *Drug Safety* (1996) 15, 261–73.

Neuromuscular blockers + Metoclopramide

The neuromuscular blocking effects of suxamethonium (succinylcholine) and mivacurium can be slightly increased and prolonged in patients taking metoclopramide, although this may be clinically relevant only in short procedures.

Clinical evidence

Metoclopramide 10 mg given intravenously 1 to 2 hours before induction of anaesthesia prolonged the time to 25% recovery after **suxamethonium** (**succinylcholine**) by 1.83 minutes (23%) in 19 patients when compared with 21 control patients.[1,2] A larger 20-mg dose of metoclopramide prolonged the time to recovery by 56% in a further 10 patients.[1] In another study by the same research group, the recovery from neuromuscular blockade (time from 95% to 25% suppression of the activity of the adductor pollicis muscle) due to **suxamethonium** was prolonged by 67% in 11 patients who were given metoclopramide 10 mg intravenously during surgery one minute before the **suxamethonium**.[3]

A randomised, placebo-controlled, double-blind study in 30 patients demonstrated that 150 micrograms/kg of intravenous metoclopramide given prior to anaesthetic induction about 10 minutes before **mivacurium** 150 micrograms/kg prolonged the duration of action of **mivacurium** by approximately 30%.[4]

Mechanism

Metoclopramide is postulated to reduce the activity of plasma cholinesterase, which is responsible for the metabolism of suxamethonium and mivacurium. One *in vitro* study found that a metoclopramide concentration of 800 nanograms/ml inhibited plasma cholinesterase activity by 50%. However, a 10-mg dose of metoclopramide in adult patients weighing 50 to 70 kg produces peak plasma concentrations five times less than this (140 nanograms/ml).[5] In an *in vivo* study, metoclopramide had only minimal inhibitory effects on plasma cholinesterase, and there was no difference in plasma cholinesterase levels in patients who had received metoclopramide and those who had not.[4]

Importance and management

The metoclopramide/suxamethonium interaction is an established but not extensively documented interaction of only moderate or minor clinical importance. However anaesthetists should be aware that some enhancement of blockade can occur. The mivacurium/suxamethonium interaction has only more recently been demonstrated, and again is likely to be of modest importance. However, the authors note that an increase in duration of neuromuscular block of only a few minutes could be clinically relevant in short procedures.[4] The authors of the suxamethonium reports also point out that plasma cholinesterase activity is reduced in pregnancy and so suxamethonium sensitivity is more likely in obstetric patients. Ester-type local anaesthetics also depend on plasma cholinesterase activity for metabolism[1,5] and their effects would therefore be expected to be additive with the effects of metoclopramide, see 'Neuromuscular blockers + Anaesthetics, local', p.899.

1. Kao YJ, Tellez J, Turner DR. Dose-dependent effect of metoclopramide on cholinesterases and suxamethonium metabolism. *Br J Anaesth* (1990) 65, 220–4.
2. Turner DR, Kao YJ, Bivona C. Neuromuscular block by suxamethonium following treatment with histamine type 2 antagonists or metoclopramide. *Br J Anaesth* (1989) 63, 348–50.
3. Kao YJ, Turner DR. Prolongation of succinylcholine block by metoclopramide. *Anesthesiology* (1989) 70, 905–8.
4. Skinner HJ, Girling KJ, Whitehurst A, Nathanson MH. Influence of metoclopramide on plasma cholinesterase and duration of action of mivacurium. *Br J Anaesth* (1999) 82, 542–5.
5. Kambam JR, Parris WCV, Franks JJ, Sastry BVR, Naukam R, Smith BE. The inhibitory effect of metoclopramide on plasma cholinesterase activity. *Can J Anaesth* (1988) 35, 476–8.

Neuromuscular blockers + Miscellaneous anti-infectives

Colistin, colistimethate sodium, polymyxin B, clindamycin, lincomycin, some penicillins (apalcillin, azlocillin, mezlocillin, piperacillin) and vancomycin possess some neuromuscular blocking activity. Increased and prolonged neuromuscular blockade is possible if these antibacterials are used with anaesthetics and conventional neuromuscular blocking drugs. In theory amphotericin B might also interact, but the tetracyclines probably do not. No interaction is seen with cefuroxime, chloramphenicol or metronidazole. See also 'Neuromuscular blockers + Aminoglycosides', p.898.

Clinical evidence

(a) Amphotericin B

Amphotericin B can induce hypokalaemia resulting in muscle weakness,[1] which might be expected to enhance the effects of neuromuscular blockers, but there appear to be no reports in the literature confirming that this actually takes place.

(b) Cephalosporins

No change in neuromuscular blockade was seen in patients given intravenous **cefuroxime** shortly before **pipecuronium**[2] or **rocuronium**[3] in a controlled study. Similarly, intravenous **cefoxitin** given before, during and after surgery was not associated with a clinically important prolongation of **vecuronium** blockade,[4] see (f) below.

(c) Chloramphenicol

No interaction was seen in myasthenic patients given chloramphenicol.[5]

(d) Clindamycin, Lincomycin

Enhanced blockade has been demonstrated in patients given **pancuronium** and lincomycin, which was reversed by neostigmine.[6] Respiratory paralysis was seen 10 minutes after lincomycin 600 mg was given intramuscularly in a man recovering from blockade with **tubocurarine**[7] and this interaction was confirmed in another report.[8] Other case reports[9-11] and clinical studies[12] describe minor to marked increases in neuromuscular blockade in patients on **pancuronium**,[10] **pipecuronium**,[12] **rapacuronium**[11] or **suxamethonium (succinylcholine)**[9] when treated with **clindamycin**. One patient developed very prolonged blockade after being unintentionally given clindamycin 2400 mg instead of 600 mg shortly after recovery from **suxamethonium** and **tubocurarine**.[13] Prolongation of the neuromuscular blocking effects of **vecuronium** has also been reported in a patient who received both clindamycin and gentamicin.[14]

(e) Metronidazole

An increase in the neuromuscular blocking effects of **vecuronium** with metronidazole has been reported in *cats*,[15] but a later study in patients failed to find any evidence of an interaction,[16] and another study with **rocuronium** also found no evidence of an interaction with metronidazole.[3] Similarly, no interaction was seen with **rocuronium** and metronidazole/**cefuroxime**.[3] Another study found no significant interaction between **pipecuronium** and metronidazole.[2]

(f) Penicillins

A study in patients showed that the neuromuscular blocking effects of **vecuronium** were prolonged by a number of penicillins: **apalcillin** 26%, **azlocillin** 55%, **mezlocillin** 38%, and **piperacillin** 46%.[17] Reinstitution of neuromuscular blockade and respiratory failure occurred in a patient given **piperacillin** 3 g by intravenous infusion postoperatively following reversal of **vecuronium** blockade.[18] However, a randomised, double-blind study involving 30 patients showed that **piperacillin** or **cefoxitin**, administered by intravenous infusion, pre- and intraoperatively, were not associated with clinically important prolongation of neuromuscular block induced by **vecuronium**. Of 27 patients who could be evaluated, 22 showed a modest overall decrease in recovery time and 5 patients (2 patients after receiving **piperacillin** and 3 patients after **cefoxitin**) exhibited a slight prolongation in recovery time, but these patients all responded readily to administration of neostigmine or other anticholinesterase and subsequent recurarisation did not occur.[4]

No interaction was seen in myasthenic patients given **ampicillin**.[19]

(g) Polymyxins

In a literature review of antibiotic-neuromuscular blocker interactions 17 cases over the period 1956 to 1970 period were identified in which **colistin (polymyxin E)** or **colistimethate sodium**, with or without conventional neuromuscular blockers, were responsible for the development of increased blockade and respiratory muscle paralysis. Some of the patients had renal disease.[20] A later report describes prolonged respiratory depression in a patient on **pancuronium** and **colistin**.[21] Calcium gluconate was found to reverse the blockade.[21] A placebo-controlled study found that one million units of **colistin** also considerably prolonged the recovery time from **pipecuronium** blockade.[12] Six cases of enhanced neuromuscular blockade involving **polymyxin B** have also been reported.[20] An increase in the blockade due to **pancuronium** by **polymyxin B** and bacitracin wound irrigation is described in another report; pyridostigmine, neostigmine and edrophonium were ineffective antagonists of this block and only partial improvement occurred after calcium chloride was administered.[22] Prolonged and fatal apnoea occurred in another patient on **suxamethonium** when his peritoneal cavity was instilled with a solution containing 100 mg of **polymyxin B** and 100,000 units of bacitracin.[23]

(h) Tetracyclines

Four cases of enhanced neuromuscular blockade with **rolitetracycline** or **oxytetracycline** in myasthenic patients have been reported[20] but there seem to be no reports of interactions in normal patients given neuromuscular blocking drugs.

(i) Vancomycin

A man recovering from neuromuscular blockade with **suxamethonium** (with some evidence of residual Phase II block) developed almost total muscle paralysis and apnoea when given an intravenous infusion of vancomycin. He recovered spontaneously when the vancomycin was stopped, but it took several hours.[24] The neuromuscular blockade due to **vecuronium** was increased in a patient when given an infusion of vancomycin (1 g in 250 ml saline over 35 minutes).[25] Transient apnoea and apparent cardiac arrest have also been described in a patient following an intravenous injection of 1-g vancomycin given over 2 minutes.[26] However, in both of these cases[25,26] the vancomycin was given more rapidly than the current recommendations. It is now known that rapid infusion of vancomycin can provoke histamine release, which can result in apnoea, hypotension, anaphylaxis and muscular spasm, effects similar to those seen in these two patients.

Mechanism

Not fully understood but several sites of action at the neuromuscular junction (pre and/or post, effects on ion-channels or receptors) have been suggested.

The neuromuscular blocking properties of the polymyxins (polymyxin B, colistin, colistimethate sodium) involve a number of mechanisms, which may explain the difficulty in reversing the blockade.[27]

Importance and management

The interactions involving polymyxin B, colistin, colistimethate sodium, lincomycin, and clindamycin are established and clinically important. The incidence is uncertain. Concurrent use need not be avoided, but be alert for increased and prolonged neuromuscular blockade. The recovery period should be well monitored because of the risk of recurarisation. Check the outcome of using amphotericin. No interaction would be expected with the tetracyclines, cefuroxime, metronidazole or metronidazole/cefuroxime, and probably with ampicillin and chloramphenicol, but some caution would seem appropriate with apalcillin, azlocillin, mezlocillin and piperacillin. The situation with vancomycin is less clear. The evidence does suggest a link between vancomycin and increased neuromuscular blockade following the use of suxamethonium, and possibly vecuronium. However, vancomycin is given routinely as antibiotic prophylaxis before surgical procedures. The sparsity of reports therefore suggests that in practice vancomycin rarely causes a clinically significant interaction with neuromuscular blockers.

1. Drutz DJ, Fan JH, Tai TY, Cheng JT, Hsieh WC. Hypokalemic rhabdomyolysis and myoglobinuria following amphotericin B therapy. *JAMA* (1970) 211, 824–6.
2. Stanley JC, Mirakhur RK, Clarke RSJ. Study of pipecuronium-antibiotic interaction. *Anesthesiology* (1990) 73, A898.
3. Cooper R, Maddineni VR, Mirakhur RK. Clinical study of interaction between rocuronium and some commonly used antimicrobial agents. *Eur J Anaesthesiol* (1993) 10, 331–5.
4. Condon RE, Munshi CA, Arfman RC. Interaction of vecuronium with piperacillin or cefoxitin evaluated in a prospective, randomized, double-blind clinical trial. *Am Surg* (1995) 61, 403–6.
5. Gibbels E. Weitere Beobachtungen zur Nebenwirkung intravenöser Reverin-Gaben bei Myasthenia gravis pseudoparalytica. *Dtsch Med Wochenschr* (1967) 92, 1153–4.
6. Booij LHDJ, Miller RD, Crul JF. Neostigmine and 4-aminopyridine antagonism of lincomycin-pancuronium neuromuscular blockade in man. *Anesth Analg* (1978) 57, 316–21.
7. Samuelson RJ, Giesecke AH, Kallus FT, Stanley VF. Lincomycin-curare interaction. *Anesth Analg* (1975) 54, 103–5.
8. Hashimoto Y, Iwatsuki N, Shima T, Iwatsuki K. Neuromuscular blocking properties of lincomycin and Kanendomycin® in man. *Jpn J Anesthesiol* (1971) 20, 407–11.
9. Avery D, Finn R. Succinylcholine-prolonged apnea associated with clindamycin and abnormal liver function tests. *Dis Nerv Syst* (1977) 38, 473–5.
10. Fogdall RP, Miller RD. Prolongation of a pancuronium-induced neuromuscular blockade by clindamycin. *Anesthesiology* (1974) 41, 407–8.
11. Sloan PA, Rasul M. Prolongation of rapacuronium neuromuscular blockade by clindamycin and magnesium. *Anesth Analg* (2002) 94, 123–4.
12. de Gouw NE, Crul JF, Vandermeersch E, Mulier JP, van Egmond J, Van Aken H. Interaction of antibiotics on pipecuronium-induced neuromuscular blockade. *J Clin Anesth* (1993) 5, 212–5.
13. Al Ahdal O, Bevan DR. Clindamycin-induced neuromuscular blockade. *Can J Anaesth* (1995) 42, 614–7.
14. Jedeikin R, Dolgunski E, Kaplan R, Hoffman S. Prolongation of neuromuscular blocking effect of vecuronium by antibiotics. *Anaesthesia* (1987) 42, 858–60.
15. McIndewar IC, Marshall RJ. Interactions between the neuromuscular blocking drug ORG NC 45 and some anaesthetic, analgesic and antimicrobial agents. *Br J Anaesth* (1981) 53, 785–92.
16. d'Hollander A, Agoston S, Capouet V, Barvais L, Bomblet JP, Esselen M. Failure of metronidazole to alter a vecuronium neuromuscular blockade in humans. *Anesthesiology* (1985) 63, 99–102.
17. Tryba M. Wirkungsverstärkung nicht-depolarisierender Muskelrelaxantien durch Acylaminopenicilline. Untersuchungen am Beispiel von Vecuronium. *Anaesthesist* (1985) 34, 651–55.
18. Mackie K, Pavlin EG. Recurrent paralysis following piperacillin administration. *Anesthesiology* (1990) 72, 561–3.
19. Wullen F, Kast G, Bruck A. Über Nebenwirkungen bei Tetracyclin-Verabreichung an Myastheniker. *Dtsch Med Wochenschr* (1967) 92, 667–9.
20. Pittinger CB, Eryasa Y, Adamson R. Antibiotic-induced paralysis. *Anesth Analg* (1970) 49, 487–501.
21. Giala MM, Paradelis AG. Two cases of prolonged respiratory depression due to interaction of pancuronium with colistin and streptomycin. *J Antimicrob Chemother* (1979) 5, 234–5.
22. Fogdall RP, Miller RD. Prolongation of a pancuronium-induced neuromuscular blockade by polymyxin B. *Anesthesiology* (1974) 40, 84–7.
23. Small GA. Respiratory paralysis after a large dose of intraperitoneal polymyxin B and bacitracin. *Anesth Analg* (1964) 43, 137–9.
24. Albrecht RF, Lanier WL. Potentiation of succinylcholine-induced phase II block by vancomycin. *Anesth Analg* (1993) 77, 1300–1302.
25. Huang KC, Heise A, Shrader AK, Tsueda K. Vancomycin enhances the neuromuscular blockade of vecuronium. *Anesth Analg* (1990) 71, 194–6.
26. Glicklich D, Figura I. Vancomycin and cardiac arrest. *Ann Intern Med* (1984) 101, 880–1.
27. Østergaard D, Engbaek J, Viby-Mogensen J. Adverse reactions and interactions of the neuromuscular blocking drugs. *Med Toxicol Adverse Drug Exp* (1989) 4, 351–68.

Neuromuscular blockers + Neuromuscular blockers

Combinations of competitive neuromuscular blockers may have additive or synergistic effects, however, the sequence of administration may also affect the interaction. Prior administration of a small dose of a competitive neuromuscular blocker (e.g. vecuronium) generally reduces the effects of a depolarising blocker (e.g. suxamethonium), but if the depolarising blocker is given during recovery from a competitive neuromuscular blocker, antagonism, enhancement or a combination of the two may occur. The effects of a competitive blocker may be increased if it is given after a depolarising blocker.

Clinical evidence, mechanism, importance and management

Neuromuscular blockers are of two types: competitive (non-depolarising) and depolarising:

The **competitive** or **non-depolarising** blockers (**atracurium** and others listed in 'Table 31.1', (p.880)) compete with acetylcholine for the receptors on the endplate of the neuromuscular junction. Thus the receptors fail to be stimulated and muscular paralysis results. Competitive neuromuscular blockers may be divided by chemical structure into the **aminosteroid** group (e.g. **pancuronium**) and the **benzylisoquinolinium** group (e.g. **atracurium**), see also 'Table 31.1', (p.880).

The **depolarising** blockers (**suxamethonium** (**succinylcholine**) and **decamethonium**) also occupy the receptors on the endplate but they act like acetylcholine to cause depolarisation. However, unlike acetylcholine, they are not immediately removed by cholinesterase so that the depolarisation persists and the muscle remains paralysed.

(a) Competitive neuromuscular blockers + Competitive neuromuscular blockers

Combinations of **competitive** (non-depolarising) **neuromuscular blockers** may have additive or synergistic effects. Structural differences between the interacting neuromuscular blockers may have an effect; it has been suggested that structurally similar neuromuscular blockers tend to produce an additive response, whereas structurally different blockers may be synergistic.[1,2] For example, additive effects have been found between the structurally similar combinations of:

- **atracurium** and **cisatracurium**[3] or **mivacurium**,[4]
- **pancuronium** and **vecuronium**,[5]
- **tubocurarine** and **metocurine**.[1]

Potentiation of neuromuscular blockade or synergy has been reported between the structurally different combinations of:

- **cisatracurium** and **rocuronium**,[3,6] or **vecuronium**,[3]
- **metocurine** and **pancuronium**,[1]
- **mivacurium** and **pancuronium**[2] or **rocuronium**,[7]
- **tubocurarine** and **pancuronium**[1] or **vecuronium**.[8]

However, contrary to the prediction, synergism has been reported with the structurally similar combinations of:

- **cisatracurium** and **mivacurium**,[3]
- **tubocurarine** and **atracurium**.[8]

In addition to affecting response, the initial blocker may modify the duration of action of the supplemental blocker.[9,10] The blocking action of **pancuronium** was shortened when it was given during **vecuronium**-induced partial neuromuscular blockade.[10] Conversely, the duration of action of **mivacurium**[2,11] or **vecuronium**[10] was lengthened if they were given after **pancuronium**-induced neuromuscular block. Therefore, care should be taken if a small dose of a short-acting blocker is given near the end of an operation in which a longer-acting blocker has already been given.

(b) Competitive then depolarising neuromuscular blockers

The combination of a **competitive** and a **depolarising neuromuscular blocker** has an intrinsic antagonistic effect. This interaction has been used clinically to reduce muscle fasciculations caused by **suxamethonium**. A small dose of **competitive neuromuscular blocker** given shortly before the **suxamethonium** generally reduces effects and the duration of action of the suxamethonium.[12] However, following **pancuronium** pretreatment, the duration of **suxamethonium** blockade appears to be prolonged,[12] and this is probably due to the inhibition of cholinesterase by pancuronium.[13] Antagonism of **decamethonium** has also been demonstrated when administered after a small dose of **vecuronium**.[14]

If **suxamethonium** is given during the recovery from a paralysing dose of a **competitive neuromuscular blocker**, the resultant neuromuscular block is influenced by the depth of residual block and the dose of suxamethonium used.[15,16] In a study involving 38 patients recovering from **atracurium** 400 micrograms/kg, lower intravenous doses of **suxamethonium** 0.25 to 1 mg/kg mainly antagonised the partial block, whereas higher doses 1.5 to 3 mg/kg usually enhanced the blockade.[15] However, the degree of recovery from the underlying block also influences the effects of **suxamethonium**: early on when the residual block is still considerable, suxamethonium may appear to have no effect or produce a partial antagonism of the block, but later, a biphasic response may be seen (antagonism of the competitive block initially before superimposing a depolarising block); a combination of antagonism and enhancement may also occur in different muscle groups.[16] Partial antagonism of **vecuronium** block has been seen in 5 patients given **decamethonium** during the recovery from vecuronium block.[17] The neuromuscular blockade will also be affected by the competitive neuromuscular blocker used and whether or not an anticholinesterase has been given.[15,16] See also, 'Neuromuscular blockers + Anticholinesterases', p.899.

Suxamethonium and **decamethonium** would be expected to antagonise **competitive neuromuscular blockers** due to their opposite mechanisms of action (suxamethonium and decamethonium exert a receptor agonist-type activity whereas competitive blockers exhibit receptor antagonism). However, the depolarising blockers may also reverse a competitive block by enhancing the effect of acetylcholine postsynaptically.[17,18]

(c) Depolarising then competitive neuromuscular blockers

In general, when a **competitive blocker** is given following **suxamethonium,** the onset time may be reduced and the potency or duration of the block may be increased, although not always significantly. In a study involving 350 patients, prior administration of **suxamethonium** 1 mg/kg significantly accelerated the onset of neuromuscular blockade with **atracurium, pancuronium, pipecuronium** and **vecuronium**, when these were given after full recovery from the suxamethonium block. However, the duration of blockade was only significantly prolonged with **vecuronium.**[19] One study found potentiation of **vecuronium** when it was given up to 30 minutes after full recovery from a single intravenous dose of **suxamethonium** 1 mg/kg.[20] Another study found the effects of **vecuronium** or **pancuronium** were potentiated for at least 2 hours after full recovery from an intubating dose of suxamethonium.[21] Another study showed that the effect of prior administration of **suxamethonium** on **atracurium** neuromuscular block appears to depend on the level of recovery from suxamethonium. As with previous studies, the onset of atracurium blockade was shortened when given after full recovery from the suxamethonium. However, this effect was less apparent when the atracurium was given before full suxamethonium recovery.[22] Pretreatment with **suxamethonium** reduced the time to onset of **cisatracurium** block, but did not potentiate it or prolong recovery.[23] A study in *animals* suggested **rocuronium** is not affected by **suxamethonium**.[24]

Prior administration of **decamethonium** 100 micrograms/kg caused a sevenfold increase in sensitivity to **vecuronium** (reducing the ED_{50} from 24 to 3.5 micrograms/kg).[17]

It has been suggested that depolarising neuromuscular blockers such as decamethonium and suxamethonium may have a presynaptic action resulting in reduced acetylcholine output.[17] Although not always clinically significant, be aware that a reduction in the dose of competitive blocker may be necessary following administration of a depolarising neuromuscular blocker.

1. Lebowitz PW, Ramsey FM, Savarese JJ, Ali HH. Potentiation of neuromuscular blockade in man produced by combinations of pancuronium and metocurine or pancuronium and *d*-tubocurarine. *Anesth Analg* (1980) 59, 604–9.
2. Kim KS, Shim JC, Kim DW. Interactions between mivacurium and pancuronium. *Br J Anaesth* (1997) 79, 19–23.
3. Kim KS, Chun YS, Chon SU, Suh JK. Neuromuscular interaction between cisatracurium and mivacurium, atracurium, vecuronium or rocuronium administered in combination. *Anaesthesia* (1998) 53, 872–8.
4. Naguib M, Abdulatif M, Al-Ghamdi A, Selim M, Seraj M, El-Sanbary M, Magboul MA. Interactions between mivacurium and atracurium. *Br J Anaesth* (1994) 73, 484–9.
5. Ferres CJ, Mirakhur RK, Pandit SK, Clarke RSJ, Gibson FM. Dose-response studies with pancuronium, vecuronium and their combination. *Br J Clin Pharmacol* (1984) 18, 947–50.
6. Naguib M, Samarkandi AH, Ammar A, Elfaqih SR, Al-Zahrani S, Turkistani A. Comparative clinical pharmacology of rocuronium, cisatracurium, and their combination. *Anesthesiology* (1998) 89, 1116–24.
7. Naguib M. Neuromuscular effects of rocuronium bromide and mivacurium chloride administered alone and in combination. *Anesthesiology* (1994) 81, 388–95.
8. Middleton CM, Pollard BJ, Healy TEJ, Kay B. Use of atracurium or vecuronium to prolong the action of tubocurarine. *Br J Anaesth* (1989) 62, 659–63.
9. Okamoto T, Nakai T, Aoki T, Satoh T. Interaction between vecuronium and pancuronium. *Jpn J Anesthesiol* (1993) 42, 534–9.
10. Rashkovsky OM, Agoston S, Ket JM. Interaction between pancuronium bromide and vecuronium bromide. *Br J Anaesth* (1985) 57, 1063–6.
11. Erkola O, Rautoma P, Meretoja OA. Mivacurium when preceded by pancuronium becomes a long-acting muscle relaxant. *Anesthesiology* (1996) 84, 562–5.
12. Ferguson A, Bevan DR. Mixed neuromuscular block. The effect of precurarization. *Anaesthesia* (1981) 36, 661–6.
13. Stovner J, Oftedal N, Holmboe J. The inhibition of cholinesterases by pancuronium. *Br J Anaesth* (1975) 47, 949–54.
14. Campkin NTA, Hood JR, Feldman SA. Resistance to decamethonium neuromuscular block after prior administration of vecuronium. *Anesth Analg* (1993) 77, 78–80.
15. Scott RPF, Norman J. Effect of suxamethonium given during recovery from atracurium. *Br J Anaesth* (1988) 61, 292–6.
16. Black AMS. Effect of suxamethonium given during recovery from atracurium. *Br J Anaesth* (1989) 62, 348–9.
17. Feldman S, Fauvel N. Potentiation and antagonism of vecuronium by decamethonium. *Anesth Analg* (1993) 76, 631–4.
18. Braga MFM, Rowan EG, Harvey AL, Bowman WC. Interactions between suxamethonium and non-depolarizing neuromuscular blocking drugs. *Br J Anaesth* (1994) 72, 198–204.
19. Swen J, Koot HWJ, Bencini A, Ket JM, Hermans J, Agoston S. The interaction between suxamethonium and the succeeding non-depolarizing neuromuscular blocking agent. *Eur J Anaesthesiol* (1990) 7, 203–9.
20. d'Hollander AA, Agoston S, De Ville A, Cuvelier F. Clinical and pharmacological actions of a bolus injection of suxamethonium: two phenomena of distinct duration. *Br J Anaesth* (1983) 55, 131–4.
21. Ono K, Manabe N, Ohta Y, Morita K, Kosaka F. Influence of suxamethonium on the action of subsequently administered vecuronium or pancuronium. *Br J Anaesth* (1989) 62, 324–6.
22. Roed J, Larsen PB, Olsen JS, Engbæk J. The effect of succinylcholine on atracurium-induced neuromuscular block. *Acta Anaesthesiol Scand* (1997) 41, 1331–4.
23. Pavlin EG, Forrest AP, Howard M, Quessy S, McClung C. Prior administration of succinylcholine does not affect the duration of Nimbex (51W89) neuromuscular blockade. *Anesth Analg* (1995) 80, S374.
24. Muir AW, Anderson KA, Pow E. Interaction between rocuronium bromide and some drugs used during anaesthesia. *Eur J Anaesthesiol* (1994) 11 (Suppl 9), 93–8.

Neuromuscular blockers + Ondansetron

Ondansetron does not affect neuromuscular blockade with atracurium.

Clinical evidence, mechanism, importance and management

A double-blind placebo-controlled study of 30 patients undergoing elective surgery found that intravenous ondansetron 8 or 16 mg given over 5 minutes had no effect on subsequent neuromuscular blockade with **atracurium**.[1] No special precautions would therefore seem necessary. The authors suggest that no interaction is likely with other non-depolarising neuromuscular blockers, but this needs confirmation.

1. Lien CA, Gadalla F, Kudlak TT, Embree PB, Sharp GJ, Savarese JJ. The effect of ondansetron on atracurium-induced neuromuscular blockade. *J Clin Anesth* (1993) 5, 399–403.

Neuromuscular blockers + Opioids

A woman experienced hypertension and tachycardia when she was given pancuronium after induction of anaesthesia with morphine and nitrous oxide/oxygen. Bradycardia has been reported with vecuronium and alfentanil, fentanyl, or sufentanil, sometimes in patients receiving beta-blockers and/or calcium channel blockers.

Clinical evidence, mechanism, importance and management

(a) Pancuronium

A woman about to receive a coronary by-pass graft was premedicated with **morphine** 10 mg and hyoscine 400 micrograms, intramuscularly, one hour before the induction of anaesthesia. **Morphine** 1 mg/kg was then slowly infused while the patient was ventilated with 50% nitrous oxide/oxygen. With the onset of neuromuscular relaxation with pancuronium 150 micrograms/kg, her blood pressure rose sharply from 120/60 to 200/110 mmHg and her pulse rate increased from 54 to 96 bpm, persisting for several minutes but restabilising when 1% halothane was added.[1] The suggested reason is that pancuronium can antagonise the vagal tone (heart slowing) induced by the **morphine**, thus allowing the blood pressure and heart rate to rise. The authors of the report point out the undesirability of this in those with coronary heart disease.

(b) Vecuronium

Two patients, one aged 72 and the other aged 84, undergoing elective carotid endarterectomy developed extreme bradycardia following induction with **alfentanil** and vecuronium; both were premedicated with **morphine**. The first was taking **propranolol** 20 mg 8-hourly and as the drugs were injected his heart rate fell from 50 to 35 bpm, and his blood pressure fell from 160/70 to 75/35 mmHg. He responded to atropine, ephedrine and phenylephrine. The other patient was taking nifedipine and quinidine. His heart rate fell from 89 to 43 bpm, and his blood pressure dropped from 210/80 to 120/45 mmHg. Both heart rate and blood pressures recovered following skin incision.[2]

Bradycardia in the presence of vecuronium has been seen during anaesthetic induction with other drugs including **fentanyl**,[3,4] and **sufentanil** (in 3 patients on beta-blockers with or without diltiazem).[5] The lack of vagolytic effects associated with vecuronium may mean that opioid-induced bradycardia is unopposed.[4,5] The beta-blockers and diltiazem may also have played a part in the bradycardia seen in some of these patients[5] (see also 'Neuromuscular blockers + Beta-blockers', p.903). Be alert for this effect if vecuronium is given with any of these agents. Atropine 500 micrograms given intravenously at the time of induction may prevent the bradycardia.[4]

For reports of bradycardia occurring with **atracurium** or **suxamethonium** used with propofol and **fentanyl**, see 'Anaesthetics, general + Neuromuscular blockers', p.888.

1. Grossman E, Jacobi AM. Hemodynamic interaction between pancuronium and morphine. *Anesthesiology* (1974) 40, 299–301.
2. Lema G, Sacco C, Urzúa J. Bradycardia following induction with alfentanil and vecuronium. *J Cardiothorac Vasc Anesth* (1992) 6, 774–5.
3. Mirakhur RK, Ferres CJ, Clarke RSJ, Bali IM, Dundee JW. Clinical evaluation of Org NC 45. *Br J Anaesth* (1983) 55, 119–24.
4. Inoue K, El-Banayosy A, Stolarski L, Reichelt W. Vecuronium induced bradycardia following induction of anaesthesia with etomidate or thiopentone, with or without fentanyl. *Br J Anaesth* (1988) 60, 10–17.
5. Starr NJ, Sethna DH, Estafanous FG. Bradycardia and asystole following the rapid administration of sufentanil with vecuronium. *Anesthesiology* (1986) 64, 521–3.

Neuromuscular blockers + Quinidine

The effects of both depolarising (e.g. suxamethonium (succinylcholine)) and competitive (e.g. tubocurarine) neuromuscular blockers can be increased by quinidine. Recurarisation and apnoea have been seen in patients when quinidine was given during the recovery period from neuromuscular blockade.

Clinical evidence

A patient given **metocurine** during surgery regained her motor functions and was able to talk coherently during the recovery period. However, within 15 minutes of additionally being given quinidine sulphate 200 mg by injection she developed muscular weakness and respiratory depression. She needed intubation and assisted respiration for a period of two and a half hours. Edrophonium and neostigmine were used to aid recovery.[1]

This interaction has also been described in case reports involving **tubocurarine**[2] and **suxamethonium (succinylcholine)**,[3,4] and has been confirmed in *animal* studies.[5-7]

Mechanism

Not fully understood, but it has been shown that quinidine can inhibit the enzyme (choline acetyltransferase), which is concerned with the synthesis of acetylcholine at nerve endings.[8] Neuromuscular transmission would be expected to be reduced if the synthesis of acetylcholine is reduced. Quinidine also inhibits the activity of plasma cholinesterase, which is concerned with the metabolism of suxamethonium.[4]

Importance and management

The interaction between quinidine and neuromuscular blockers is an established interaction of clinical importance, but the documentation is limited. The incidence is uncertain, but it was seen in one report cited[3] to a greater or lesser extent in five of the six patients studied. It has only been reported clinically with metocurine, tubocurarine and suxamethonium, but it occurs in *animals* with **gallamine**, and it seems possible that it could occur clinically with any depolarising or non-depolarising neuromuscular blocker. Be alert for increased neuromuscular blocking effects during and after surgery.

1. Schmidt JL, Vick NA, Sadove MS. The effect of quinidine on the action of muscle relaxants. *JAMA* (1963) 183, 669–71.
2. Way WL, Katzung BG, Larson CP. Recurarization with quinidine. *JAMA* (1967) 200, 163–4.
3. Grogono AW. Anaesthesia for atrial defibrillation: effect of quinidine on muscular relaxation. *Lancet* (1963) ii, 1039–40.
4. Kambam JR, Franks JJ, Naukam R, Sastry BVR. Effect of quinidine on plasma cholinesterase activity and succinylcholine neuromuscular blockade. *Anesthesiology* (1987) 67, 858–60.
5. Miller RD, Way WL, Katzung BG. The neuromuscular effects of quinidine. *Proc Soc Exp Biol Med* (1968) 129, 215–18.
6. Miller RD, Way WL, Katzung BG. The potentiation of neuromuscular blocking agents by quinidine. *Anesthesiology* (1967) 28, 1036–41.
7. Cuthbert MF. The effect of quinidine and procainamide on the neuromuscular blocking action of suxamethonium. *Br J Anaesth* (1966) 38, 775–9.
8. Kambam JR, Day P, Jansen VE, Sastry BVR. Quinidine inhibits choline acetyltransferase activity. *Anesthesiology* (1989) 71, A819.

Neuromuscular blockers + Testosterone

An isolated report describes marked resistance to the effects of suxamethonium (succinylcholine) and vecuronium, apparently due to the long-term use of testosterone.

Clinical evidence, mechanism, importance and management

A woman transsexual who had been receiving testosterone enantate 200 mg intramuscularly twice monthly for 10 years was resistant to 100 mg of intravenous **suxamethonium (succinylcholine)**, and needed 100 micrograms/kg of intravenous **vecuronium** for effective tracheal intubation before surgery. During the surgery it was found necessary to use a total of 22 mg of **vecuronium** over a 50-minute period to achieve acceptable relaxation of the abdominal muscles for hysterectomy and salpingo-oophorectomy to be carried out. The reasons are not understood.[1]

1. Reddy P, Guzman A, Robalino J, Shevde K. Resistance to muscle relaxants in a patient receiving prolonged testosterone therapy. *Anesthesiology* (1989) 70, 871–3.

Neuromuscular blockers + Tobacco smoking

There is some evidence that smokers may need more vecuronium and less atracurium, but rocuronium appears to be unaffected by smoking.

Clinical evidence, mechanism, importance and management

Variable results have been reported on the effect of smoking on neuromuscular blocking agents. The amount of **atracurium** required was about 25% lower in smokers compared with non-smokers.[1] However, in another study, smokers required more **vecuronium** than non-smokers did (96.8 compared with 72.11 micrograms/kg/hour, respectively; a 34% increase).[2] In yet another study, the onset and recovery times from the neuromuscular blocking effects of **rocuronium** 600 micrograms/kg were reported to be not significantly affected by smoking more than 10 cigarettes daily.[3]

Tobacco smoke contains many different compounds and has enzyme-inducing properties, which may affect the dose requirements of neuromuscular blockers. In addition, the time interval in refraining from smoking will affect plasma nicotine concentrations; small doses of nicotine may stimulate the neuromuscular junction, but larger doses may block transmission.[2] More studies are needed.

1. Kroeker KA, Beattie WS, Yang H. Neuromuscular blockade in the setting of chronic nicotine exposure. *Anesthesiology* (1994) 81, A1120.
2. Teiriä H, Rautoma P, Yli-Hankala A. Effect of smoking on dose requirements for vecuronium. *Br J Anaesth* (1996) 76, 154–5.
3. Latorre F, de Almeida MCS, Stanek A, Kleemann PP. Die Wechselwirkung von Rocuronium und Rauchen. Der Einfluß des Rauchens auf die neuromuskuläre Übertragung nach Rocuronium. *Anaesthesist* (1997) 46, 493–5.

Neuromuscular blockers + Trimetaphan

Trimetaphan can increase the effects of suxamethonium (succinylcholine), which may result in prolonged apnoea. This may possibly occur with other neuromuscular blocking drugs (seen also with alcuronium).

Clinical evidence

A man undergoing neurosurgery was given **tubocurarine** and **suxamethonium (succinylcholine)**. Neuromuscular blockade was prolonged postoperatively, lasting about 2.5 hours, and was attributed to the concurrent use of trimetaphan 4500 mg over a 90-minute period. Later when he underwent further surgery using essentially the same anaesthetic techniques and drugs, but with a very much smaller dose of trimetaphan (35 mg over a 10-minute period), the recovery was normal.[1]

Nine out of 10 patients receiving ECT treatment and given **suxamethonium** showed an almost 90% prolongation in apnoea (from 142 to 265 seconds) when trimetaphan 10 to 20 mg was used instead of 1.2 mg of atropine.[2] Prolonged apnoea has been seen in another patient given **suxamethonium** and trimetaphan.[3] On the basis of an *in vitro* study it was calculated that a typical dose of trimetaphan would double the duration of paralysis due to **suxamethonium**.[4] Prolonged neuromuscular blockade was also seen in a man given **alcuronium** and trimetaphan.[5]

Mechanism

Not fully understood. Trimetaphan can inhibit plasma cholinesterase to some extent,[2,5] which would reduce the metabolism of the suxamethonium and thereby prolong its activity. Studies in *rats*[6,7] and case reports[8] also indicate that trimetaphan has direct neuromuscular blocking activity. Its effects are at least additive with the neuromuscular blocking effects of the aminoglycosides.[7]

Importance and management

Information is limited but the interaction appears to be established. If trimetaphan and suxamethonium are used concurrently, be alert for enhanced and prolonged neuromuscular blockade. This has also been seen with alcuronium, and trimetaphan may interact with other competitive neuromuscular blockers.[5] Respiratory arrest has been seen when large doses of trimetaphan were given in the absence of a neuromuscular blocker, so that caution is certainly needed.[8] *Animal* studies suggested that the blockade might not be reversed by neostigmine or calcium chloride,[7] but neostigmine and calcium gluconate were successfully used to reverse the effects of alcuronium and trimetaphan in one case.[5]

1. Wilson SL, Miller RN, Wright C, Hasse D. Prolonged neuromuscular blockade associated with trimethaphan: a case report. *Anesth Analg* (1976) 55, 353–6.
2. Tewfik GI. Trimetaphan. Its effect on the pseudo-cholinesterase level of man. *Anaesthesia* (1957) 12, 326–9.
3. Poulton TJ, James FM, Lockridge O. Prolonged apnea following trimethaphan and succinylcholine. *Anesthesiology* (1979) 50, 54–6.
4. Sklar GS, Lanks KW. Effects of trimethaphan and sodium nitroprusside on hydrolysis of succinylcholine *in vitro*. *Anesthesiology* (1977) 47, 31–3.
5. Nakamura K, Koide M, Imanaga T, Ogasawara H, Takahashi M, Yoshikawa M. Prolonged neuromuscular blockade following trimetaphan infusion. *Anaesthesia* (1980) 35, 1202–7.
6. Pearcy WC, Wittenstein ES. The interactions of trimetaphan (Arfonad), suxamethonium and cholinesterase inhibitor in the rat. *Br J Anaesth* (1960) 32, 156–9.
7. Paradelis AG, Crassaris LG, Karachalios DN, Triantaphyllidis CJ. Aminoglycoside antibiotics: interaction with trimethaphan at the neuromuscular junctions. *Drugs Exp Clin Res* (1987) 13, 233–6.
8. Dale RC, Schroeder ET. Respiratory paralysis during treatment of hypertension with trimethaphan camsylate. *Arch Intern Med* (1976) 136, 816–18.

Neuromuscular blockers + Ulinastatin

Ulinastatin delays the onset and hastens the recovery from vecuronium neuromuscular block.

Clinical evidence, mechanism, importance and management

A randomised, placebo-controlled study involving 60 patients found that a 5000 unit/kg intravenous bolus dose of the protease inhibitor ulinastatin given before induction of anaesthesia and 2 minutes before intravenous **vecuronium** 100 micrograms/kg, delayed the onset of neuromuscular blockade compared with placebo (250 compared with 214 seconds). The recovery from neuromuscular block (measured as return of post-tetanic count) was significantly shorter after ulinastatin than placebo (11 compared with 17.7 minutes). The effects of ulinastatin were thought to be due to an increase in the release of acetylcholine at the neuromuscular junction and enhanced **vecuronium** elimination due to increases in liver blood flow and urine volume.[1]

1. Saitoh Y, Fujii Y, Oshima T. The ulinastatin-induced effect on neuromuscular block caused by vecuronium. *Anesth Analg* (1999) 89, 1565–9.

32

Respiratory drugs

This section includes the diverse drugs that are principally used in the management of asthma and chronic obstructive pulmonary disease (COPD), with the exception of corticosteroids, which are covered elsewhere.

(a) Antimuscarinic bronchodilators

The parasympathetic nervous system is involved in the regulation of bronchomotor tone and antimuscarinic drugs have bronchodilator properties. Ipratropium bromide and other antimuscarinic bronchodilators used in COPD are listed in 'Table 32.1', (below). A wide range of drugs have antimuscarinic (anticholinergic) adverse effects. Enhanced antimuscarinic effects occur when drugs with these properties are given concurrently, see 'Anticholinergics + Anticholinergics', p.501. However, these interactions do not usually occur with drugs such as ipratropium given by inhalation.

(b) Beta-2 agonist bronchodilators

Salbutamol and terbutaline are examples of short-acting beta-agonists that selectively stimulate the beta-2 receptors in the bronchi causing bronchodilation. They are used in the treatment of asthma and the management of COPD. Long-acting beta-2 agonists such as salmeterol are used in patients with asthma who also require anti-inflammatory therapy. 'Table 32.1', (below) lists the beta-2 agonists along with their proprietary names. The beta-2 agonists represent a significant improvement on isoprenaline (isoproterenol), which also stimulates beta-1 receptors in the heart, and on ephedrine, which also stimulates alpha receptors as well. The beta-2 agonists can cause hypokalaemia, which can be increased by the concurrent use of 'potassium-depleting drugs', (p.920).

(c) Leukotriene receptor antagonists

Montelukast and zafirlukast block the effects of cysteinyl leukotrienes. They are used in the treatment of asthma either alone or with inhaled corticosteroids. They should not be used to relieve an acute asthma attack. Both drugs are metabolised in the liver by the cytochrome P450 isoenzymes. There is therefore a possibility that interactions could occur with other drugs that undergo metabolism by these isoenzymes but there is little clinical evidence of such interactions.

(d) Xanthines

The main xanthines used in medicine are theophylline and aminophylline, the latter generally being preferred when greater water solubility is needed (e.g. in the formulation of injections). Xanthines are given in the treatment of asthma because they relax the bronchial smooth muscle. In an attempt to improve upon theophylline, various different derivatives have been made, such as diprophylline and enprofylline. 'Table 32.1', (below) lists these xanthines along with their proprietary names.

Caffeine is also a xanthine and it is principally used as a central nervous system stimulant, increasing wakefulness, and mental and physical activity. It is most commonly taken in the form of tea, coffee, cola drinks ('*Coke*') and cocoa. 'Table 32.2', (p.918) lists the usual caffeine content of these drinks. Caffeine is also included in hundreds of non-prescription analgesic preparations with aspirin, codeine and/or paracetamol, but whether it enhances the analgesic effect is debatable. Caffeine is also used to assess the activity of hepatic enzyme systems (particularly the cytochrome P450 isoenzyme CYP1A2) and can usefully demonstrate altered liver function, notably from drugs, as well as disease states.

Interactions. Theophylline is metabolised by the cytochrome P450 isoenzymes in the liver, principally CYP1A2, to demethylated and hydroxylated products. Many drugs interact with theophylline by inhibition or potentiation of its metabolism. Theophylline has a narrow therapeutic range, and small increases in serum levels can result in toxicity. Moreover, symptoms of serious toxicity such as convulsions and arrhythmias can occur before minor symptoms suggestive of toxicity. Within the context of interactions, aminophylline behaves like theophylline, because it is a complex of theophylline with ethylenediamine. Caffeine also undergoes extensive hepatic metabolism, principally by CYP1A2, and interacts with many drugs, but it has a wider therapeutic range. However, other xanthines may act differently (e.g. diprophylline does not undergo hepatic metabolism), so it should not be assumed that they all share common interactions. Note though, that all xanthines can potentiate hypokalaemia caused by other drugs, and that the toxic effects of different xanthines are additive.

Table 32.1 *Respiratory drugs*

Generic names	*Proprietary names*
Aminophylline	Alergo Filinal, Aminocont, Aminoima, Aminoliv, Aminomal, Amnivent, Anti-Asmatico, Asmafin, Asmapen, Asmeton, Asmodrin, Asmoquinol, Asthma-Hilfe, Cardiomin, Cardirenal, Diaphyllin, Diphenamill, Dispneitrat, Drafilyn-Z, Emergent-Ez, Escophylline, Eufilina, Euphyllin, Fadafilina, Fileen, Filotempo, Genasma, Larjanfilina, Limptar, Lotussin Expectorant, Minoton, Mundiphyllin, Myocardon, Natrophylline Compound, Neophyllin, Paliatil, Peterphyllin, Pharophyllin, Phyllocontin, Phyllotemp, Repasma, Syntophyllin, Tefamin, Teofylamin, Truphylline, Unifilin
Bambuterol	Bambec, Bambudil, Montair Plus, Oxeol
Diprophylline (Diphylline)	Alergical Expect, Astho-Med, Austrophyllin, Bronsal, Cort-Inal, Dilor, Dyflex-G, Dy-G, Dylix, Fluidin Mucolitico, Katasma, Lufyllin, Neufil, Noradran, Novofilin, Panfil G, Philinal, Philinet, Silbephylline
Doxofylline	Ansimar
Enprofylline	
Fenoterol	Alveofen, Atrovent, Berodual, Berodualin, Berotec, Bromifen, Bronchodual, Ditec, Dosberotec, Duotec, Duovent, Feno, Fenovent, Fenozan, Fymnal, Inhalex, Iprafen, Parsistene, Partusisten, Sabax Nebrafen
Formoterol	Asmatec, Assieme, Atimos, Broncoral, Delnil, Duova, Eolus, Fluir, Foracort, Foradil, Foradile, Foraseq, Foratec, Fordilen, Neblik, Neumoterol, Oxez, Oxeze, Oxis, Rilast, Simbicort, Sinestic, Symbicord, Symbicort, Xanol

Continued

Table 32.1 *Respiratory drugs (continued)*

Generic names	*Proprietary names*
Ipratropium	Aerovent, Alvent, Apo-Ipravent, Apoven, Apovent, Atem, Atrodual, Atronase, Atrovent, Berodual, Berodualin, Berovent, Breva, Bronchodual, Combivent, Di-Promal, Dospir, Duolin, DuoNeb, Duovent, Fenovent, Inhalex, Ipra, Iprabon, Iprafen, Ipranase, Ipraneo, Ipratrin, Ipravent, Ipvent, Itrop, Neorinol, Novo-Ipramide, ratio-Ipra Sal UDV, Respontin, Rhinovent, Rinatec, Rinovagos, Sabax Nebrafen
Isoetharine	
Isoprenaline (Isoproterenol)	Aldo Asma, Aleudrina, Ciapar, Frenal Compositum, Imuprel, Isobutil, Isolin, Isuprel, Medihaler-Iso, Prelus, Proterenal, Saventrine, Zantril
Montelukast	Kipres, Lukair, Lukasm, Montair, Montegen, Singulair
Orciprenaline	Adco-Linctopent, Alotec, Alupent, Benylin Chesty, Bisolvon Linctus DA, Broncodual Compuesto, Bronkese Compound, Cloval Compuesto, Flemeze, Orcinol, Pulbronc, Silomat DA, Solvanol, Tusabron, Vapoflu
Pirbuterol	Exirel, Maxair
Reproterol	Aarane, Allergospasmin, Bronchospasmin
Rimiterol	
Ritodrine	Materlac, Miodrina, Miolene, Pre-Par, Ritopar, Yutopar
Salbutamol (Albuterol)	Ac-Butamol, Accuneb, Aerocort, Aerodine, Aeroflux, Aero-Jet, Aerolin, Aero-Ped, Aero-Plus, Aero-Sal, Aerosoma, Aerotamol, Aerotide, Aerotrat, Airomir, Airsalbu, Albutamol, Aldobronquial, Almasal, Ambrodil-S, Amcof, Amocasin, Apo-Salvent, Apsomol, Ascoril Expectorant, Asmaliv, Asmasal, Asmatol, Asmavent, Asmol, Assal, Asthacrom, Asthalin, Asthavent, Asthmalitan, Asthmolin, Asthmotrat, Atrodual, Axalin, Azmasol, Beatolin, Beclasma, Belomet, Berovent, Biorenyn, Biovent, Breva, Bronchilet, Broncho Fertiginhalat, Broncho Inhalat, Bronchospray, Broncoterol, Broncovaleas, Budesal, Butahale, Butalin, Butamol, Buto Asma, Butosol, Butotal, Butovent, Buventol, Clenil Compositum, Cobamol, Combivent, Cybutol, Deletus A, Dilamol, Di-Promal, Dospir, Duolin, DuoNeb, Duopack, Ecosal, Ecovent, Epaq, Etinoline, Exafil, Fatigan Bronquial, Fesema, Gerivent, Herolan Aerosol, Huma-Salmol, Intal Plus, Kentamol, Kofarest, Loftan, Medihaler, Medolin, Microterol, Mucolinc, Normobron, Okaril, Oladin, Padiamol, Pentamol, Plenaer, Propavente, Proventil, Pulmoflux, Pulmo-Rest, Pulvinal Salbutamol, ratio-Ipra Sal UDV, Redol Comp, Respax, Respiret, Respiroma, Respolin, Royalin, Salamol, Salapin, Salbetol, Salbu, Salbubreathe, Salbuhexal, Salbulair, Salbulind, Salbumol, Salbunova, Salbupp, Salburin, Salbusian, Salbutac, Salbutalan, Salbutalin, Salbutam, Salbutamax, Salbutol, Salbutol Beclo, Salbuvent, Salda, Salmaplon, Salmax, Salmol, Salmundin, Salsol, Salvuron, Sinasmal, Steri-Neb Salamol, Sultanol, Teoden, Theo-Asthalin, Tussiliv, Venderol, Ventadur, Ventamol, Venterol, Ventexxair, Venteze, Ventide, Ventilan, Ventilastin, Ventmax, Ventodisk, Ventolin, Ventoline, Ventomol, Ventorlin, Violin, Volmac, Volmax, VoSpire, Zarent, Zenmolin, Zibil
Salmeterol	Abrilar, Advair, Aeromax, Aliflus, Anasma, Arial, Atmadisc, Beglan, Betamican, Brexotide, Brisair, Brisomax, Dilamax, Inaladuo, Inaspir, Kolpovent, Maizar, Plusvent, Salmetedur, Salmeter, Seretaide, Seretide, Serevent, Serobid, Seroflo, Ultrabeta, Veraspir, Viani, Xemos
Terbutaline	Aerodur, Ascoril +, Asmaline, Asmotone Plus, Asthamsian, Ataline, Benylin Bronchospect, Brethine, Bricalin, Bricanyl, Bricanyl comp, Bricanyl Composto, Bricarex, Broncholine, Bronchonyl, Bronchoped, Bronchosolvin, Bro-Zedex, Bucanil, Bucaril, Butaline, Butylin, Cencanyl, Cof QX, Cofbron, Contimit, Dhatalin, Dracanyl, Grilinctus-BM, Lanterbine, Monovent, Mucaryl-AX, Mucosol, Okaril Plus, Proasma-T, Sulterline, Taziken, Tedipulmo, Terbasmin, Terbosil, Terbron, Terbul, Terbulin, Terbuno, Terbuta, Tergil, Terpect, Terphylate, Terphylin, Theobric, Tolbin, Toscof, Tuspel Plus, Vida-Butaline
Theophylline	Aberten, Accurbron, Actophlem, Aerobin, Aerodyne, Aerolate, Afonilum, Afonilum novo, afpred-THEO, Airbronal, Alcophyllex, Alcophyllin, Alergin, Almarion, Almasal, Ambredin, Aminoefedrison NF, Aminofilin, Aminomal, Apo-Theo, Asianbron, Asmabiol, Asmalix, Asmapax, Asmasolon, Asthma, Asthmino, Bermacia, Bronchil, Broncho-Euphyllin, Bronchoparat, Bronchoretard, Broncofol, Brondil, Bronkasma, Bronquisedan, Bronquitos, Cadiphylate, Codrinan, Contiphyllin, CP-Theo, Crisasma, Cronasma, Dericip, Deriphyllin, Derm'attive, Dexa Aminofilin, Dexa Teosona, Diatussin, Diffumal, Dilatrane, Do-Do ChestEze, Drilyna, Duraphyllin, Egifilin, Elixifilin, Elixine, Elixomin, Elixophyllin, Endotussin, Eufilina, Euphyllin, Euphyllina, Euphylline, Euphylong, Fatigan Bronquial, Franol, Frivent, Glyceryl-T, Glyphyllin, Gulamyl, Histafilin, Hydrophed, Inastmol, Lepobron, Marax, Mediphyllin Chrono, Metexol, Mila-Asma, Microphyllin, Nefoben, Nirason N, Novaphylline, Novofilin, Novo-Theophyl, Nuelin, Oxantil, Phylobid, Phyloday, Pneumogeine, Polyphed, Prelus, Primatene, Pulmeno, Pulmophyllin, Pulmo-Timelets, Quadrinal, Qualiton, Quibron, ratio-Theo-Bronc, Respicur, Retafyllin, Sedacris, Slo-Bid, Slo-Phyllin, Slo-Theo, Sodip-phylline, Solosin, Solphyllex, Solphyllin, Spophyllin, Talofilina, Tedralan, Tedrigen, Tefamin, Temaco, Teodosis, Teolixir, Teolong, Teonibsa, Teophyl, Teosona, Teoston, Teotard, Teovent, Tergil-T, Teromol, Theo, Theo-Asthalin, Theobid, Theobric, Theochron, Theoday, Theodrine, Theo-Dur, Theodur, Theofol, Theolair, Theolin, Theolong, Theomax DF, Theoped, Theophar, Theophen, Theophtard, Theophyllard, Theoplus, Theospirex, Theostat, Theotard, Theotrim, Tromphyllin, T-Phyl, Unicontin, Uni-Dur, Unifyl, Unilair, Uniphyl, Uniphyllin, UniXan, Uromil, Vent Retard, Xanthium, Zepholin
Tulobuterol	Atenos, Brelomax, Bremax, Hokunalin, Respacal
Zafirlukast	Accolate, Accoleit, Aeronix, Olmoran, Resma, Vanticon, Zafarismal, Zafirst, Zuvair

Table 32.2 Caffeine-containing herbs and caffeine-containing drinks

Source	*Caffeine-content*	*Caffeine-content of drink*
Cocoa[1]		up to 30 mg/100 ml
Coffee beans[2]	1–2%	up to 100 mg/100 ml, decaffeinated about 3 mg/100 ml
Guarana[3*]	2.5–7.0%	
Kola (Cola)[2]	1.5–2.5%	up to 20 mg/100 ml in '*Cola*' drinks
Maté[2]	0.2–2.0%	
Tea[2]	1–5%	up to 60 mg/100 ml

* Note that guarana contains guaranine (which is known to be identical to caffeine) as well as small quantities of other xanthines.

1. Information taken from research conducted by the US Department of Nutritional Services. Available at http://www.holymtn.com/tea/caffeine_content.htm (Accessed 09/08/05).
2. Sweetman SC, editor. Martindale: The complete drug reference. 34th ed. London: Pharmaceutical Press; 2005 p. 1765.
3. Houghton P. Herbal products 7. Guarana. *Pharm J* (1995) 254, 435–6.

Antiasthma drugs + Beta-blockers

Non-cardioselective beta-blockers (e.g. propranolol, timolol, see 'Table 20.2', (p.623)) should not be used in asthmatic subjects because they may cause serious bronchoconstriction, even if given as eye drops. Non-cardioselective beta-blockers oppose the bronchodilator effects of beta-agonist bronchodilators, and higher doses may be required to reverse bronchospasm. Even cardioselective blockers (e.g. atenolol, see 'Table 20.1', (p.623)) can sometimes cause acute bronchospasm in asthmatics. However, cardioselective beta-blockers do not generally inhibit the bronchodilator effect of beta-agonist bronchodilators (e.g. isoprenaline, salbutamol).

Clinical evidence

(a) Cardioselective beta-blockers

A review of 29 studies (including 19 single-dose studies) on the use of cardioselective beta-blockers in patients with reversible airway disease indicated that in patients with mild to moderate disease, the short-term use of cardioselective beta-blockers does not cause significant adverse respiratory effects. Information on the effects in patients with more severe or less reversible disease or on the frequency or severity of acute exacerbations was not available.[1] Another review indicated that when low doses of cardioselective beta-blockers are prescribed in patients with mild, intermittent or persistent asthma, or moderate persistent asthma and heart failure or myocardial infarction the benefits of treatment outweigh risks. However, it was considered that further study is required to establish long-term safety, and also that beta-blockers should be avoided in severe persistent asthma.[2]

The cardioselective beta-blockers would not be expected to affect the beta-receptors in the bronchi, but bronchospasm can sometimes occur following their use by asthmatics and others with obstructive airways diseases, particularly if high doses are used. Deterioration of asthma was reported in a patient taking oral **betaxolol** with **theophylline** and **pranlukast**, although **betaxolol** is considered to be highly cardioselective and less likely to cause pulmonary adverse effects than other cardioselective beta-blockers.[3]

No adverse interaction normally occurs between beta-agonist sympathomimetic bronchodilators and cardioselective beta-blockers. This has been demonstrated in studies with **celiprolol**[4] or **metoprolol**[5,6] with **isoprenaline** (**isoproterenol**) infusion or inhalation; **celiprolol** with **terbutaline** infusion or inhalation;[7] and **atenolol** or **celiprolol** with **salbutamol** (**albuterol**) inhalation.[4,8,9] In contrast, another study found that the increase in forced expiratory volume (FEV) with **terbutaline** inhalation and infusion was reduced by about 300 ml by **atenolol** and **metoprolol**, and the authors considered that this would be clinically relevant in severe asthma.[10]

(b) Non-selective beta-blockers

Non-selective beta-blockers (e.g. **propranolol**) are contraindicated in asthmatic subjects because they can cause bronchospasm, reduce lung ventilation and may possibly precipitate a severe asthmatic attack in some subjects. An example of the danger is illustrated by an asthmatic patient who developed fatal status asthmaticus after taking just one dose of **propranolol**.[11] Another case report describes a patient with bronchial asthma on **salbutamol** who collapsed and died after taking three 20-mg **propranolol** tablets which had been supplied in error instead of 20-mg prednisone tablets.[12] The makers of **propranolol** note that from 1965 to 1996, the UK Committee on Safety of Medicines had received 51 reports of bronchospasm due to **propranolol**, 13 of them fatal, and 5 of them in patients who had a history of asthma, bronchospasm or wheeze.[13] They also highlight the dangers in their patient information leaflets.[13,14]

The non-cardioselective beta-blockers **oxprenolol**[8] and **propranolol**[4-8] oppose the effects of bronchodilators such as **isoprenaline**,[4-6] **salbutamol** (**albuterol**),[4,8] and **terbutaline**.[7] Even eye drops containing the non-selective beta-blockers **timolol**[15,16] and **metipranolol**[17] have been reported to precipitate acute bronchospasm. In patients with heart failure treated with **carvedilol**, 3 of 12 with concurrent asthma had wheezing requiring **carvedilol** withdrawal. In contrast, only 1 of 31 patients with COPD had wheezing.[18]

Mechanism

Non-selective beta-blockers, intended for their actions on the heart, also block the beta-2 receptors in the bronchi so that the normal bronchodilation, which is under the control of the sympathetic nervous system, is reduced or abolished. As a result the bronchoconstriction of asthma can be made worse. Cardioselective beta-blockers on the other hand, preferentially block beta-1 receptors in the heart, with less effect on the beta-2 receptors, so that beta-2 stimulating bronchodilators such as isoprenaline, salbutamol and terbutaline continue to have bronchodilator effects.

Importance and management

A well established drug-disease interaction. In 1996, the UK Committee on Safety of Medicines (CSM)[19] re-issued the following advice: "Beta-blockers, including those considered to be cardioselective, should not be given to patients with a history of asthma/bronchospasm." Non-cardioselective beta-blockers (listed in 'Table 20.2', (p.623)) should certainly be avoided in asthmatics and those with chronic obstructive pulmonary disease, whether given systemically or in eye-drops, because serious and life-threatening bronchospasm may occur. The cardioselective beta-blockers (listed in 'Table 20.1', (p.623)) are generally safer but not entirely free from risk in some patients, particularly in high dosage. In contrast to the 1996 recommendations of the CSM on cardioselective beta-blockers, one recent review[1,20] recommends that "cardioselective beta-blockers should not be withheld from patients with mild to moderate reversible airway disease". However, some concern has been expressed that this conclusion was based on results from short-term studies and state that the question of safety in asthmatics over the long term has not been answered.[21] Further, there are no studies to suggest the safety of cardioselective beta blockers in patients with exacerbations of asthma,[22] and even a highly cardioselective drug such as betaxolol may cause bronchospasm.[3] In 1999, the American College of Cardiology and American Heart Association stated that the benefits of using beta-blockers in acute myocardial infarction strongly outweigh the risk of adverse events in patients with COPD or asthma. A cardioselective beta-blocker should be used, and the patients pulmonary function monitored.[23]

Celiprolol (a cardioselective blocker) appears to be exceptional in causing mild bronchodilatation in asthmatics and not bronchoconstriction, but some caution is still necessary as this requires confirmation.[9]

The bronchoconstrictive effects of the beta-blockers can be opposed by beta-2 agonist bronchodilators such a salbutamol, but as the makers point out, large doses may be needed and they suggest that ipratropium and intravenous aminophylline may also be needed.[13]

1. Salpeter S, Ormiston T, Salpeter EE. Cardioselective β-blockers in patients with reversible airway disease: a meta-analysis. *Ann Intern Med* (2002) 137, 715–25.
2. Self T, Soberman JE, Bubla JM, Chafin CC. Cardioselective beta-blockers in patients with asthma and concomitant heart failure or history of myocardial infarction: when do benefits outweigh risks? *J Asthma* (2003) 40, 839–45.
3. Miki A, Tanaka Y, Ohtani H, Sawada Y. Betaxolol-induced deterioration of asthma and a pharmacodynamic analysis based on β-receptor occupancy. *Int J Clin Pharmacol Ther* (2003) 41, 358–64.
4. Doshan HD, Rosenthal RR, Brown R, Slutsky A, Applin WJ, Caruso FS. Celiprolol, atenolol and propranolol: a comparison of pulmonary effects in asthmatic patients. *J Cardiovasc Pharmacol* (1986) 8 (Suppl 4), S105–S108.
5. Thiringer G, Svedmyr N. Interaction of orally administered metoprolol, practolol and propranolol with isoprenaline in asthmatics. *Eur J Clin Pharmacol* (1976) 10, 163–70.
6. Johnsson G, Svedmyr N, Thiringer G. Effects of intravenous propranolol and metoprolol and their interaction with isoprenaline on pulmonary function, heart rate and blood pressure in asthmatics. *Eur J Clin Pharmacol* (1975) 8, 175–80.
7. Matthys H, Doshan HD, Rühle K-H, Applin WJ, Braig H, Pohl M. Bronchosparing properties of celiprolol, a new β_1, α_2 blocker, in propranolol-sensitive asthmatic patients. *J Cardiovasc Pharmacol* (1986) 8 (Suppl 4), S40–S42.
8. Fogari R, Zoppi A, Tettamanti F, Poletti L, Rizzardi G, Fiocchi G. Comparative effects of celiprolol, propranolol, oxprenolol, and atenolol on respiratory function in hypertensive patients with chronic obstructive lung disease. *Cardiovasc Drugs Ther* (1990) 4, 1145–50.
9. Pujet JC, Dubreuil C, Fleury B, Provendier O, Abella ML. Effects of celiprolol, a cardioselective beta-blocker, on respiratory function in asthmatic patients. *Eur Respir J* (1992) 5, 196–200.
10. Löfdahl C-G, Svedmyr N. Cardioselectivity of atenolol and metoprolol. A study in asthmatic patients. *Eur J Respir Dis* (1981) 62, 396–404.
11. Anon. Beta-blocker caused death of asthmatic. *Pharm J* (1991) 247, 185.
12. Spitz DJ. An unusual death in an asthmatic patient. *Am J Forensic Med Pathol* (2003) 24, 271–2.
13. Fallowfield JM, Marlow HF. Propranolol is contraindicated in asthma. *BMJ* (1996) 313, 1486.
14. Inderal (Propranolol hydrochloride). AstraZeneca. UK Patient information leaflet, 2002.
15. Charan NB, Lakshminarayan S. Pulmonary effects of topical timolol. *Arch Intern Med* (1980) 140, 843–4.
16. Jones FL, Ekberg NL. Exacerbation of obstructive airway disease by timolol. *JAMA* (1980) 244, 2730.
17. Vinti H, Chichmanian RM, Fournier JP, Pesce A, Taillan B, Fuzibet JG, Cassuto JP, Dujardin P. Accidents systémiques des bêta-bloquants en collyres. A propos de six observations. *Rev Med Interne* (1989) 10, 41–4.
18. Kotlyar E, Keogh AM, Macdonald PS, Arnold RH, McCaffrey DJ, Glanville AR. Tolerability of carvedilol in patients with heart failure and concomitant chronic obstructive pulmonary disease or asthma. *J Heart Lung Transplant* (2002), 21, 1290–5.

19. Committee on Safety of Medicines/Medicines Control Agency. Reminder: Beta-blockers contraindicated in asthma. *Current Problems* (1996) 22, 2.
20. Salpeter SR, Ormiston TM. Use of β-blockers in patients with reactive airway disease. *Ann Intern Med* (2003) 139, 304.
21. Shulan DJ, Katlan M, Lavsky-Shulan M. Use of β-blockers in patients with reactive airway disease. *Ann Intern Med* (2003) 139, 304.
22. Epstein PE. Fresh air and β-blockade. *Ann Intern Med* (2002) 137, 766–7.
23. Ryan TJ, Antman EM, Brooks NH, Califf RM, Hillis LD, Hiratzka LF, Rapaport E, Riegel B, Russell RO, Smith EE 3rd, Weaver WD, Gibbons RJ, Alpert JS, Eagle KA, Gardner TJ, Garson A Jr, Gregoratos G, Ryan TJ, Smith SC Jr. 1999 update: ACC/AHA guidelines for the management of patients with acute myocardial infarction. A report of the American College of Cardiology/American Heart Association Task Force on Practice Guidelines (Committee on Management of Acute Myocardial Infarction). *J Am Coll Cardiol* (1999) 34, 890–911.

Antiasthma drugs + Betel nuts

The chewing of betel nuts may worsen the symptoms of asthma.

Clinical evidence

A study of a possible interaction with betel nuts was prompted by the observation of 2 Bangladeshi patients with severe asthma that appeared to have been considerably worsened by chewing betel nuts. One out of 4 other asthmatic patients who regularly chewed betel nuts developed severe bronchoconstriction (a 30% fall in the FEV_1) on two occasions when given betel nuts to chew, and all 4 patients said that prolonged betel nut chewing induced coughing and wheezing. A double-blind study found that the inhalation of **arecoline** (the major constituent of the nut) caused bronchoconstriction in 6 of 7 asthmatics, and 1 of 6 healthy control subjects.[1]

Mechanism

Betel nut 'quids' consist of areca nut (*Areca catechu*) wrapped in betel vine leaf (*Piper betle*) and smeared with a paste of burnt (slaked) lime. It is chewed for the euphoric effects of the major constituent, arecoline, a cholinergic alkaloid, which appears to be absorbed through the mucous membrane of the mouth. Arecoline has identical properties to pilocarpine and normally has only mild systemic cholinergic properties; however asthmatic subjects seem to be particularly sensitive to the bronchoconstrictor effects of this alkaloid and possibly other substances contained in the nut.

Importance and management

Direct evidence appears to be limited to the report cited, but the interaction seems to be established. It would not normally appear to be a serious interaction, but asthmatics should be encouraged to avoid betel nuts. This is a drug-disease interaction rather than a drug-drug interaction.

1. Taylor RFH, Al-Jarad N, John LME, Conroy DM, Barnes NC. Betel-nut chewing and asthma. *Lancet* (1992) 339, 1134–6.

Antiasthma drugs + NSAIDs

Aspirin and many other NSAIDs can cause bronchoconstriction in some asthmatic patients. Aspirin, nimesulide and piroxicam appear not to alter theophylline pharmacokinetics.

Clinical evidence, mechanism, importance and management

(a) NSAIDs in asthma

About 10% of asthmatics are hypersensitive to **aspirin**, and in some individuals life-threatening bronchoconstriction can occur. This is not a drug-drug interaction but an adverse response of asthmatic patients to **aspirin**, whether taking an anti-asthmatic drug or not. The reasons are not fully understood. Those known to be sensitive to **aspirin** may also possibly react to other NSAIDs, in particular the **acetylated salicylates**, the **indole** and **indene acetic acids**, and the **propionic acid derivatives** (see 'Table 5.1', (p.73)). The **fenamates**, **oxicams**, **pyrazolones** and **pyrazolidinediones** are better tolerated.[1] The nonacetylated salicylates (**sodium salicylate**, **salicylamide**, **choline magnesium trisalicylate**) are normally well tolerated. Aspirin-sensitive individuals are also less likely to react to **nimesulide**.[1]

In 60 patients with proven **aspirin**-sensitivity, **celecoxib** 100 mg on day one and 200 mg on day two caused no decline in forced expiratory volume. **Celecoxib** is a selective inhibitor of cyclo-oxygenase-2 and this supports the suggestion that inhibition of cyclo-oxygenase-1 may be critical factor in the precipitation of respiratory reactions in **aspirin**-exacerbated respiratory disease.[2] This suggests that **celecoxib** may be an alternative in patients who are known to be aspirin sensitive. Nevertheless, the maker of **celecoxib** contraindicates its use in patients who are sensitive to aspirin or NSAIDs.[3]

(b) NSAIDs with theophylline

Piroxicam 20 mg daily for 7 days had no effect on the pharmacokinetics of theophylline (given as a single 6-mg/kg intravenous dose of aminophylline) in 6 healthy subjects.[4] **Enteric-coated aspirin** 650 mg daily for 4 weeks had no effect on the steady-state serum levels of theophylline in 8 elderly patients (aged 60 to 81) with chronic obstructive pulmonary disease.[5] **Nimesulide** 100 mg twice daily for 7 days did not affect lung function in 10 patients with chronic obstructive airways disease taking slow-release theophylline 200 mg twice daily, although there was a slight, clinically insignificant fall in theophylline levels, possibly due to enzyme induction. The pharmacokinetics of the nimesulide were unchanged.[6]

Apart from checking that the patient is not sensitive to **aspirin** or any other NSAID (see above), there would seem to be no reason for avoiding **aspirin** or **piroxicam** in patients taking theophylline.

1. Bianco S, Robuschi M, Petrigni G, Scuri M, Pieroni MG, Refini RM, Vaghi A, Sestini PS. Efficacy and tolerability of nimesulide in asthmatic patients intolerant to aspirin. *Drugs* (1993) 46 (Suppl 1), 115–120.
2. Woessner KM, Simon RA, Stevenson DD. The safety of celecoxib in patients with aspirin-sensitive aspirin. *Arthritis Rheum* (2002) 46, 2201–6.
3. Celebrex (Celecoxib). Pharmacia Ltd. UK Summary of product characteristics, March 2003.
4. Maponga C, Barlow JC, Schentag JJ. Lack of effect of piroxicam on theophylline clearance in healthy volunteers. *DICP Ann Pharmacother* (1990) 24, 123–6.
5. Daigneault EA, Hamdy RC, Ferslew KE, Rice PJ, Singh J, Harvill LM, Kalbfleisch JH. Investigation of the influence of acetylsalicylic acid on the steady state of long-term therapy with theophylline in elderly male patients with normal renal function. *J Clin Pharmacol* (1994) 34, 86–90.
6. Auteri A, Blardi P, Bruni F, Domini L, Pasqui AL, Saletti M, Verzuri MS, Scaricabarozzi I, Vargui G, Di Perri T. Pharmacokinetics and pharmacodynamics of slow-release theophylline during treatment with nimesulide. *Int J Clin Pharmacol Res* (1991) 11, 211–7.

Beta-agonist bronchodilators + Potassium-depleting drugs

Beta-agonists (e.g. fenoterol, terbutaline, salbutamol (albuterol), see 'Table 32.1', (p.917)) can cause hypokalaemia. This can be increased by other potassium-depleting drugs such as the corticosteroids, diuretics (bendroflumethiazide, furosemide, see 'Table 24.1', (p.717)) and 'theophylline', (p.930). The risk of serious cardiac arrhythmias in asthmatic patients may be increased.

Clinical evidence

(a) Corticosteroids

(i) Hypokalaemia. The hypokalaemic effects of beta agonists may be increased by corticosteroids. Twenty-four healthy subjects had a fall in serum potassium levels when given either **salbutamol** (**albuterol**) 5 mg or **fenoterol** 5 mg by nebuliser over 30 minutes. These falls were increased after taking **prednisone** 30 mg daily for a week. The greatest fall (from 3.75 to 2.78 mmol/l) was found 90 minutes after **fenoterol** and **prednisone** were taken. The ECG effects observed included ectopic beats and transient T wave inversion, but no significant interaction was noted for ECG disturbances in these healthy subjects.[1]

(ii) Anti-inflammatory/bronchodilator effects. A marked rise in asthma deaths was noted in New Zealand in the 1980s. A case-control study found that the risk of death was increased in oral corticosteroid-dependent asthmatics (severe asthma) who were also taking inhaled **fenoterol**.[2] This, and other data, suggested the possibility that combined use of short-acting beta-2 agonists and corticosteroids might be deleterious in some situations, prompting numerous studies, which were reviewed in 2000.[3] The overall findings were that, although inhaled corticosteroids do not prevent the pro-inflammatory effects of short-acting beta-2 agonists, the combination is beneficial in the treatment of asthma at usual therapeutic doses of both drugs. The authors caution that this might not apply with excessive use of short-acting beta-2 agonists.[3]

The addition of a long-acting beta-2 agonist (e.g. **salmeterol**) to therapy in patients with chronic asthma inadequately controlled by inhaled corticosteroids and 'as required' short-acting beta-2 agonists is beneficial.[3,4]

(b) Diuretics

The serum potassium level of 15 healthy subjects was measured after inhaling **terbutaline** 5 mg with either a placebo, **furosemide** 40 mg daily, or **furosemide** 40 mg with **triamterene** 50 mg daily for 4 days. With **terbutaline** alone the potassium levels fell from 3.88 to 3.35 mmol/l; after taking **furosemide** as well they fell to 3.13 mmol/l; and after **furosemide** and **triamterene** they fell to 3.29 mmol/l. These falls were reflected in some ECG (T wave) changes.[5]

After seven days' treatment with **bendroflumethiazide** 5 mg daily for a week the serum potassium levels of 10 healthy subjects had fallen from 3.78 to 3.07 mmol/l. After taking 100 micrograms to 2 mg of inhaled **salbutamol** (**albuterol**) as well, the levels fell to 2.72 mmol/l. ECG changes consistent with hypokalaemia and hypomagnesaemia were seen.[6]

Other diuretics that can cause potassium loss include **bumetanide**, **furosemide**, **etacrynic acid**, the **thiazides**, and many other related diuretics, see 'Table 24.1', (p.717).

(c) Theophylline

The concurrent use of **salbutamol** (**albuterol**) or **terbutaline** and theophylline can cause an additional fall in serum potassium levels, and other beta-2 agonists will interact similarly. See 'Theophylline + Beta-agonist bronchodilators', p.930.

Mechanism

Additive potassium-depleting effects.

Importance and management

Established interactions. The UK Committee on Safety of Medicines[7] advises that, since potentially serious hypokalaemia may result from beta-2 agonist therapy, particular caution is required in severe asthma, as this effect may be potentiated by theophylline and its derivatives, corticosteroids, diuretics, and by hypoxia. Plasma potassium concentrations should therefore be monitored in severe asthma. Hypokalaemia may result in cardiac arrhythmias in patients with ischaemic heart disease and may also affect the response of patients to drugs such as the digitalis glycosides and antiarrhythmics. The combined use of beta-2 agonists and corticosteroids in asthma is usually beneficial.

1. Taylor DR, Wilkins GT, Herbison GP, Flannery EM. Interaction between corticosteroid and β-agonist drugs. Biochemical and cardiovascular effects in normal subjects. *Chest* (1992) 102, 519–24.
2. Crane J, Pearce N, Flatt A, Burgess C, Jackson R, Kwong T, Ball M, Beasley R. Prescribed fenoterol and death from asthma in New Zealand, 1981–1983: case-control study. *Lancet* (1989) i, 917–22.
3. Taylor DR, Hancox RJ. Interactions between corticosteroids and β agonists. *Thorax* (2000) 55, 595–602.
4. Shrewsbury S, Pyke S, Britton M. Meta-analysis of increased dose of inhaled steroid or addition of salmeterol in symptomatic asthma (MIASMA). *BMJ* (2000) 320, 1368–73.
5. Newnham DM, McDevitt DG, Lipworth BJ. The effects of frusemide and triamterene on the hypokalaemic and electrocardiographic responses to inhaled terbutaline. *Br J Clin Pharmacol* (1991) 32, 630–2.
6. Lipworth BJ, McDevitt DG, Struthers AD. Prior treatment with diuretic augments the hypokalemic and electrocardiographic effects of inhaled albuterol. *Am J Med* (1989) 86, 653–7.
7. Committee on Safety of Medicines. β_2 agonists, xanthines and hypokalaemia. *Current Problems* (1990) 28.

Caffeine + Allopurinol

Allopurinol may invalidate the results of studies using caffeine as a probe drug for determining acetylator status or activity of the cytochrome P450 isoenzyme CYP1A2.

Clinical evidence, mechanism, importance and management

In 21 healthy subjects, allopurinol 300 mg daily for 8 days altered the levels of urinary caffeine metabolites after a single 200-mg dose of caffeine. In particular, the metabolic ratio used to determine whether people are fast or slow acetylators was substantially changed. Thus, allopurinol may invalidate the results of phenotyping with the urinary caffeine test. In addition, the caffeine metabolite ratio used to express the activity of the cytochrome P450 isoenzyme CYP1A2 was not stable when allopurinol was used.[1] This interaction is of relevance to research rather than clinical practice.

1. Fuchs P, Haefeli WE, Ledermann HR, Wenk M. Xanthine oxidase inhibition by allopurinol affects the reliability of urinary caffeine metabolic ratios as markers for *N*-acetyltransferase 2 and CYP1A2 activities. *Eur J Clin Pharmacol* (1999) 54, 869–76.

Caffeine + Anticonvulsants

Phenytoin can increase the loss of caffeine from the body, and possibly invalidates the caffeine breath test. Whether carbamazepine increases caffeine metabolism is unclear. Valproate appears not to have any effect.

Clinical evidence

The clearance of caffeine was about twofold higher, and its half-life was about 50% shorter, in patients with epilepsy taking **phenytoin** than in healthy subjects on no medications. In the same study, there were no significant differences in caffeine pharmacokinetics between healthy subjects and patients receiving **carbamazepine** or **sodium valproate**.[1] Conversely, **carbamazepine** was considered to have induced the metabolism of caffeine in 5 children with epilepsy, as assessed by the caffeine breath test.[2] In another study, there was a reduction in the AUC of **carbamazepine** when it was given with caffeine in healthy subjects, but caffeine had no effect on the pharmacokinetics of **sodium valproate**.[3]

Mechanism

Phenytoin acts as an enzyme inducer, thereby increasing the metabolism and loss of caffeine from the body. Carbamazepine has the same effect.

Importance and management

Phenytoin may possibly invalidate the caffeine breath test, but normally no special precautions are needed if both drugs are taken. The interaction between carbamazepine and caffeine requires further study.

1. Wietholtz H, Zysset T, Kreiten K, Kohl D, Büchsel R, Matern S. Effect of phenytoin, carbamazepine, and valproic acid on caffeine metabolism. *Eur J Clin Pharmacol* (1989) 36, 401–6.
2. Parker AC, Pritchard P, Preston T, Choonara I. Induction of CYP1A2 activity by carbamazepine in children using the caffeine breath test. *Br J Clin Pharmacol* (1998) 45, 176–8.
3. Vaz J, Kulkarni C, David J, Joseph T. Influence of caffeine on pharmacokinetic profile of sodium valproate and carbamazepine in normal healthy volunteers. *Indian J Exp Biol* (1998) 36, 112–14.

Caffeine + Antifungals

Fluconazole and terbinafine cause a modest rise in serum caffeine levels. Ketoconazole appears to have less effect.

Clinical evidence, mechanism, importance and management

A study in 6 young subjects (average age 24) given **fluconazole** 400 mg daily and 5 elderly subjects (average age 69) given **fluconazole** 200 mg daily for 10 days found that fluconazole reduced the clearance of the caffeine from the plasma by an average of 25% (32% in the young and 17% in the old).[1] In a single-dose study in 8 healthy subjects, **terbinafine** 500 mg and **ketoconazole** 400 mg decreased caffeine clearance by 21% and 10% respectively, and increased the half-life by 31% and 16%, respectively.[2]

It seems unlikely that these moderately increased serum caffeine levels will have a clinically important effect, but this needs confirmation.

1. Nix DE, Zelenitsky SA, Symonds WT, Spivey JM, Norman A. The effect of fluconazole on the pharmacokinetics of caffeine in young and elderly subjects. *Clin Pharmacol Ther* (1992) 51, 183.
2. Wahlländer A, Paumgartner G. Effect of ketoconazole and terbinafine on the pharmacokinetics of caffeine in healthy volunteers. *Eur J Clin Pharmacol* (1989) 37, 279–83.

Caffeine + Cimetidine

The clearance of caffeine is decreased by cimetidine but this seems unlikely to be clinically significant.

Clinical evidence, mechanism, importance and management

Cimetidine 1 g daily for 6 days increased the half-life of a single 300-mg dose of caffeine in 5 subjects by about 70% and reduced caffeine clearance.[1] In another study, cimetidine 1.2 g daily for 4 days increased the caffeine half-life by 45% in 6 smokers and by 96% in 6 non-smokers. The caffeine clearance was reduced by 31% in the smokers and by 42% in the non-smokers.[2] A further study found that the caffeine half-life was increased by 59% and the clearance decreased by 40% by cimetidine.[3] Conversely, in a further study in children, cimetidine was not found to affect caffeine metabolism as assessed by the caffeine breath test.[4]

The changes seen in some studies probably occurred because cimetidine, a well-known non-specific enzyme inhibitor reduced metabolism of the caffeine by the liver, resulting in its accumulation in the body.

Any increased caffeine effects are normally unlikely to be of much importance in most people, but they might have a small part to play in exaggerating the undesirable effects of caffeine from drinks (e.g. tea, coffee, cola drinks) and analgesics, which are sometimes formulated with caffeine.

1. Broughton LJ, Rogers HJ. Decreased systemic clearance of caffeine due to cimetidine. *Br J Clin Pharmacol* (1981) 12, 155–9.
2. May DC, Jarboe CH, VanBakel AB, Williams WM. Effects of cimetidine on caffeine disposition in smokers and nonsmokers. *Clin Pharmacol Ther* (1982) 31, 656–61.
3. Beach CA, Gerber N, Ross J, Bianchine JR. Inhibition of elimination of caffeine by cimetidine in man. *Clin Res* (1982) 30, 248A.
4. Parker AC, Pritchard P, Preston T, Dalzell AM, Choonara I. Lack of inhibitory effect of cimetidine on caffeine metabolism in children using the caffeine breath test. *Br J Clin Pharmacol* (1997) 43, 467–70.

Caffeine + Class I antiarrhythmics

Caffeine clearance is reduced by 30 to 60% by mexiletine, resulting in raised serum caffeine levels. Whether this might result in caffeine toxicity is uncertain. Lidocaine, flecainide and tocainide appear not to affect caffeine clearance. Caffeine did not alter mexiletine levels.

Clinical evidence

(a) Mexiletine

The clearance of caffeine was reduced by 48% in a study in 7 patients with cardiac arrhythmias taking long-term mexiletine 600 mg daily.[1] In 5 healthy subjects given a single 200-mg dose of mexiletine the clearance of a single 366-mg dose of caffeine was reduced by 57%, from 126 to 54 ml/minute, and the elimination half-life rose from 246 to 419 minutes.[1] The clearance of mexiletine was not affected by caffeine. A preliminary report of this study also noted that fasting caffeine levels were almost six-fold higher during the mexiletine treatment period (1.99 compared with 0.35 micrograms/ml).[2]

Another study in 14 healthy subjects, caffeine 100 mg four times daily for 2 days before and 2 days after mexiletine did not cause any significant changes in the plasma levels of a single 200-mg dose of mexiletine.[3] Although not specifically monitored, caffeine levels tended to be increased by the mexiletine.

(b) Other antiarrhythmics

Single doses of **lidocaine** 200 mg, **flecainide** 100 mg and **tocainide** 500 mg had no effect on caffeine clearance in 7 healthy subjects given a single 366-mg dose of caffeine.[2]

Mechanism

It is likely that, as with theophylline (see 'Theophylline + Mexiletine or Tocainide', p.944), mexiletine inhibits the hepatic metabolism of caffeine.

Importance and management

The interaction between caffeine and mexiletine appears to be established, but its clinical importance is uncertain. Some of the adverse effects of mexiletine might be partially due to caffeine-retention (from drinking tea, coffee, cola drinks, etc.).[1] In excess, caffeine can cause jitteriness, tremor and insomnia. It has also been suggested that the caffeine test for liver function might be impaired by mexiletine.[1] Be alert for these possible effects.

1. Joeres R, Klinker H, Heusler H, Epping J, Richter E. Influence of mexiletine on caffeine elimination. *Pharmacol Ther* (1987) 33, 163–9.
2. Joeres R, Richter E. Mexiletine and caffeine elimination. *N Engl J Med* (1987) 317, 117.
3. Labbé L, Abolfathi Z, Robitaille NM, St-Maurice F, Gilbert M, Turegon J. Stereoselective disposition of the antiarrhythmic agent mexiletine during the concomitant administration of caffeine. *Ther Drug Monit* (1999) 21, 191–9.

Caffeine + Disulfiram

Disulfiram reduces the loss of caffeine from the body, which might complicate the withdrawal from alcohol.

Clinical evidence, mechanism, importance and management

A study in healthy subjects and recovering alcoholics found that disulfiram 250 or 500 mg daily reduced the clearance of caffeine by about 30%, but a few of the alcoholics had a more than 50% reduction.[1] As a result the levels of caffeine in the body increased. Raised levels of caffeine can cause irritability, insomnia and anxiety, similar to the symptoms of alcohol withdrawal. As coffee consumption is often particularly high among recovering alcoholics, there is the risk that they may turn to alcohol to calm themselves down. To avoid this possible complication it might be wise for recovering alcoholics not to drink too much tea or coffee. Decaffeinated coffee and tea are widely available.

1. Beach CA, Mays DC, Guiler RC, Jacober CH, Gerber N. Inhibition of elimination of caffeine by disulfiram in normal subjects and recovering alcoholics. *Clin Pharmacol Ther* (1986) 39, 265–70.

Caffeine + Fluvoxamine

The clearance of caffeine is considerably reduced by fluvoxamine. An increase in the stimulant and adverse effects of caffeine would be expected.

Clinical evidence

In a randomised crossover study, fluvoxamine 50 mg daily for 4 days and then 100 mg daily for a further 8 days was given to 8 healthy subjects, with a single 200-mg oral dose of caffeine before and on day 8 of fluvoxamine use. Fluvoxamine reduced the total clearance of caffeine by about 80% (from 107 to 21 ml/minute) and increased its half-life from 5 to 31 hours. Specifically, the clearance of caffeine by *N*3-, *N*1- and *N*7-demethylation was decreased.[1] Another study in 30 patients found a positive correlation between plasma fluvoxamine and plasma caffeine levels, suggesting that the interaction is dose related.[2] A further study found that low non-therapeutic doses of fluvoxamine 10 or 20 mg daily were sufficient to markedly inhibit caffeine metabolism.[3]

Mechanism

Fluvoxamine is a potent inhibitor of the cytochrome P450 isoenzyme CYP1A2, which is the principal enzyme concerned with the metabolism of caffeine. As a result the caffeine is cleared from the body much more slowly and accumulates.[1-3]

Importance and management

The interaction would seem to be established, even though few studies exist. There are no reports of caffeine toxicity arising from this interaction, but an increase in the stimulant and adverse effects of caffeine (headache, jitteriness, restlessness, insomnia) is possible if patients continue to drink normal amounts of caffeine-containing drinks (tea, coffee, cola-drinks, etc.) or take caffeine-containing medications. They should be warned to reduce their caffeine intake if problems develop. It has been suggested that some of the adverse effects of fluvoxamine (i.e. nervousness, restlessness and insomnia) could in fact be caused by caffeine toxicity. However, a preliminary study suggested that caffeine intake had a limited effect on the frequency of adverse effects of fluvoxamine.[4]

1. Jeppesen U, Loft S, Poulsen HE, Brøsen K. A fluvoxamine-caffeine interaction study. *Pharmacogenetics* (1996) 6, 213–222.
2. Yoshimura R, Ueda N, Nakamura J, Eto S, Matsushita. Interaction between fluvoxamine and cotinine or caffeine. *Neuropsychobiology* (2002) 45, 32–5.
3. Christensen M, Tybring G, Mihara K, Yasui-Furokori N, Carrillo JA, Ramos SI, Andersson K, Dahl M-L, Bertilsson L. Low daily 10-mg and 20-mg doses of fluvoxamine inhibit the metabolism of both caffeine (cytochrome P4501A2) and omeprazole (cytochrome P4502C19). *Clin Pharmacol Ther* (2002) 71, 141–52.
4. Spigset O. Are adverse drug reactions attributed to fluvoxamine caused by concomitant intake of caffeine? *Eur J Clin Pharmacol* (1998) 54, 665–6.

Caffeine + Grapefruit juice

Grapefruit juice does not interact to a clinically relevant extent with caffeine.

Clinical evidence, mechanism, importance and management

Grapefruit juice, at a dose of 1.2 litres, decreased the clearance of caffeine from coffee by 23% and prolonged its half-life by 31% in 12 healthy subjects, but these changes were not considered clinically relevant.[1] A crossover study in 6 healthy subjects given caffeine 3.3 mg/kg found that multiple doses of grapefruit juice (equivalent to 6 glasses) caused a non-significant increase in the AUC of caffeine. No changes in ambulatory systolic or diastolic blood pressure or heart rate were seen.[2]

1. Fuhr U, Klittich K, Staib AH. Inhibitory effect of grapefruit juice and the active component, naringenin on CYP1A2 dependent metabolism of caffeine in man. *Br J Clin Pharmacol* (1993) 35, 431–6. [Title corrected by erratum]
2. Maish WA, Hampton EM, Whitsett TL, Shepard JD, Lovallo WR. Influence of grapefruit juice on caffeine pharmacokinetics and pharmacodynamics. *Pharmacotherapy* (1996) 16, 1046–52.

Caffeine + HRT or Oral contraceptives

The half-life of caffeine is prolonged to some extent in women taking combined oral contraceptives or HRT.

Clinical evidence

(a) Contraceptives

The clearance of a single 162-mg dose of caffeine was reduced, the half-life prolonged (7.9 compared with 5.4 hours), and the plasma levels raised in 9 women taking low-dose combined oral contraceptives for at least 3 months, when compared with 9 other women not taking an oral contraceptive.[1] This finding was confirmed in 3 other studies,[2-4] which found that caffeine elimination was prolonged from 4 to 6 hours before the use of combined oral contraceptives to about 9 hours by the end of the first cycle, and to about 11 hours by the end of the third cycle.[3,4] A further study found that there was little difference between the effects of two oral contraceptives (**ethinylestradiol** 30 micrograms with **gestodene** 75 micrograms or **levonorgestrel** 125 micrograms). Both increased the half-life of caffeine by a little over 50%, but the maximum serum levels were unchanged.[5]

(b) HRT

In one study, 12 healthy postmenopausal women were given a single 200-mg dose of caffeine after taking **estradiol** (*Estrace*) for 8 weeks, titrated to give **estradiol** plasma concentrations of 50 to 150 picograms/ml. The metabolism of caffeine was reduced by 29% overall. If the data for 2 subjects who were found to have taken extra caffeine during the study period are excluded, the caffeine metabolism showed an even greater average reduction, of 38%.[6]

Mechanism

Uncertain. Estrogens can inhibit the cytochrome P450 isoenzyme CYP1A2, by which caffeine is metabolised, which may explain its accumulation in the body.

Importance and management

An established interaction that is probably of limited clinical importance. Women taking oral contraceptives containing estrogens or HRT who take caffeine-containing analgesics or drink caffeine-containing drinks (tea, coffee, cola drinks, etc.) may find the effects of caffeine increased and prolonged. In excess caffeine can cause jitteriness and insomnia.

1. Abernethy DR, Todd EL. Impairment of caffeine clearance by chronic use of low-dose oestrogen-containing oral contraceptives. *Eur J Clin Pharmacol* (1985) 28, 425–8.
2. Patwardhan RV, Desmond PV, Johnson RF, Schenker S. Impaired elimination of caffeine by oral contraceptive steroids. *J Lab Clin Med* (1980) 95, 603–8.
3. Meyer FP, Canzler E, Giers H, Walther H. Langzeituntersuchung zum Einfluß von Non-Ovlon auf die Pharmakokinetik von Coffein im intraindividuellen Vergleich. *Zentralbl Gynakol* (1988) 110, 1449–54.
4. Rietveld EC, Broekman MMM, Houben JJG, Eskes TKAB, van Rossum JM. Rapid onset of an increase in caffeine residence time in young women due to oral contraceptive steroids. *Eur J Clin Pharmacol* (1984) 26, 371–3.
5. Balogh A, Klinger G, Henschel L, Börner A, Vollanth R, Kuhnz W. Influence of ethinylestradiol-containing combination oral contraceptives with gestodene or levonorgestrel on caffeine elimination. *Eur J Clin Pharmacol* (1995) 48, 161–6.
6. Pollock BG, Wylie M, Stack JA, Sorisio DA, Thompson DS, Kirshner MA, Folan MM, Condifer KA. Inhibition of caffeine metabolism by estrogen replacement therapy in postmenopausal women. *J Clin Pharmacol* (1999) 39, 936–40.

Caffeine + Idrocilamide

Oral idrocilamide reduces the clearance of caffeine, which can lead to caffeine toxicity.

Clinical evidence, mechanism, importance and management

The possibility that caffeine ingestion might have had some part to play in the development of psychiatric disorders seen in patients on idrocilamide, prompted a pharmacokinetic study in 4 healthy subjects. While taking oral idrocilamide 400 mg three times a day the half-life of caffeine (150 to 200 mg of caffeine from one cup of coffee) was prolonged from about 7 to 59 hours. The overall clearance of caffeine was decreased by about 90%.[1,2]

Idrocilamide can inhibit the cytochrome P450 isoenzyme CYP1A2 by which caffeine is metabolised, leading to its accumulation.

Evidence is limited but the interaction appears to be established. Patients on oral idrocilamide should probably avoid caffeine, including caffeine-containing drinks (tea, coffee, cola drinks, etc.), or only take very small amounts, otherwise caffeine toxicity may develop. Decaffeinated teas and coffee are widely available. Some medicines may contain caffeine, so these should also be used with care.

1. Brazier JL, Descotes J, Lery N, Ollagnier M, Evreux J-C. Inhibition by idrocilamide of the disposition of caffeine. *Eur J Clin Pharmacol* (1980) 17, 37–43.
2. Evreux JC, Bayere JJ, Descotes J, Lery N, Ollagnier M, Brazier JL. Les accidents neuro-psychiques de l'idrocilamide: conséquence d'une inhibition due métabolisme de la caféine? *Lyon Med* (1979) 241, 89–91.

Caffeine + Psoralens

Oral methoxsalen and 5-methoxypsoralen markedly reduce caffeine clearance but the clinical significance of this is uncertain. Topical methoxsalen did not interact.

Clinical evidence

A single 1.2-mg/kg oral dose of **methoxsalen** (8-methoxypsoralen) given to 5 subjects with psoriasis 1 hour before a single 200-mg oral dose of caffeine reduced the caffeine clearance by 69%. The elimination half-life of caffeine over the period from 2 to 16 hours after taking the **methoxsalen** increased tenfold (from 5.6 to 57 hours).[1] In a similar study, 8 patients with psoriasis were given caffeine 200 mg with or without **5-methoxypsoralen** 1.2 mg/kg. The AUC of caffeine increased by about threefold and there was a threefold decrease in clearance.[2]

A study in patients on PUVA therapy (**methoxsalen** either as oral therapy in 4 patients or topical therapy as a bath in 7 patients, plus UVA) found that the clearance or a single 150-mg dose of caffeine was markedly reduced in the patients given oral **methoxsalen** but not altered in those given topical **methoxsalen**.[3]

Mechanism

Both methoxsalen and 5-methoxypsoralen inhibit the hepatic metabolism of caffeine by the cytochrome P450 isoenzyme CYP1A2, thereby markedly reducing caffeine loss from the body.[2,3]

Importance and management

The practical consequences of this interaction are as yet uncertain, but it seems possible that the toxic effects of caffeine will be increased. In excess, caffeine (including that from tea, coffee and cola-drinks) can cause jitteriness, headache and insomnia. The interaction is less likely with topical methoxsalen.

1. Mays DC, Camisa C, Cheney P, Pacula CM, Nawoot S, Gerber N. Methoxsalen is a potent inhibitor of the metabolism of caffeine in humans. *Clin Pharmacol Ther* (1987) 42, 621–6.

2. Bendriss EK, Bechtel Y, Bendriss A, Humbert P, Paintaud G, Megnette J, Agache P, Bechtel PR. Inhibition of caffeine metabolism by 5-methoxypsoralen in patients with psoriasis. *Br J Clin Pharmacol* (1996) 41, 421–4.
3. Tantcheva-Poór I, Servera-Llaneras M, Scharffetter-Kochanek K, Fuhr U. Liver cytochrome P450 CYP1A2 is markedly inhibited by systemic but not by bath PUVA in dermatological patients. *Br J Dermatol* (2001) 144, 1127–32.

Caffeine + Quinolones

Enoxacin markedly increases caffeine levels. The effects of caffeine derived from drinks such as tea, coffee or cola, would be expected to be increased. Pipemidic acid interacts to a lesser extent, and ciprofloxacin, norfloxacin and pefloxacin interact less still. Fleroxacin, lomefloxacin, ofloxacin, rufloxacin, and trovafloxacin appear not to interact.

Clinical evidence

The effects of various quinolones on the pharmacokinetics of caffeine[1-13] are summarised in 'Table 32.3', (p.925). In one study ciprofloxacin and fleroxacin increased caffeine levels more in women than men, but this difference in effect was not significant when the results were normalised to 70 kg body-weight.[13]

Mechanism

It would seem that the metabolism (*N*-demethylation) of caffeine is markedly reduced by some quinolones (notably pipemidic acid and enoxacin) resulting in greater levels and possibly greater effects. Other quinolones have either a much smaller effect or no effect at all. The quinolones appear to competitively inhibit the cytochrome P450 isoenzyme CYP1A2[14] by which caffeine is metabolised.

Importance and management

Established interactions. Based on the results of two studies, on a scale of 100 to 0, the relative potencies of these quinolones as inhibitors of caffeine elimination have been determined as follows: enoxacin 100, pipemidic acid 29, ciprofloxacin 11, norfloxacin 9 and ofloxacin 0.[15] From further studies, clinafloxacin appears to be similar to enoxacin, pefloxacin to norfloxacin (to which it is metabolised), and fleroxacin, lomefloxacin, rufloxacin, and trovafloxacin appear to behave like ofloxacin. Patients taking enoxacin, and possibly clinafloxacin, might be expected to experience an increase in the effects of caffeine (such as headache, jitteriness, restlessness, insomnia) if, for example, they continue to drink normal amounts of caffeine-containing drinks (tea, coffee, cola drinks, etc.). They should be warned to cut out or reduce their intake of caffeine if this occurs. The authors of one report[1] suggest that patients with hepatic disorders, cardiac arrhythmias or latent epilepsy should avoid caffeine if they take enoxacin for a week or more. The effects of pipemidic acid are less, and those of ciprofloxacin, norfloxacin and pefloxacin are probably of little or no clinical importance. Fleroxacin, lomefloxacin, ofloxacin, rufloxacin, and trovafloxacin do not interact.

1. Staib AH, Stille W, Dietlein G, Shah PM, Harder S, Mieke S, Beer C. Interaction between quinolones and caffeine. *Drugs* (1987) 34 (Suppl 1), 170–4.
2. Carbó M, Segura J, De la Torre R, Badenas JM, Camí J. Effect of quinolones on caffeine disposition. *Clin Pharmacol Ther* (1989) 45, 234–40.
3. Harder S, Staib AH, Beer C, Papenburg A, Stille W, Shah PM. 4-Quinolones inhibit biotransformation of caffeine. *Eur J Clin Pharmacol* (1988) 35, 651–6.
4. Stille W, Harder S, Mieke S, Beer C, Shah PM, Frech K, Staib AH. Decrease of caffeine elimination in man during co-administration of 4-quinolones. *J Antimicrob Chemother* (1987) 20, 729–34.
5. Healy DP, Schoenle JR, Stotka J, Polk RE. Lack of interaction between lomefloxacin and caffeine in normal volunteers. *Antimicrob Agents Chemother* (1991) 35, 660–4.
6. Peloquin CA, Nix DE, Sedman AJ, Wilton JH, Toothaker RD, Harrison NJ, Schentag JJ. Pharmacokinetics and clinical effects of caffeine alone and in combination with oral enoxacin. *Rev Infect Dis* (1989) II (Suppl 5), S1095.
7. Healy DP, Polk RE, Kanawati L, Rock DT, Mooney ML. Interaction between oral ciprofloxacin and caffeine in normal volunteers. *Antimicrob Agents Chemother* (1989) 33, 474–8.
8. Nicolau DP, Nightingale CH, Tessier PR, Fu Q, Xuan D-w, Esguerra EM, Quintiliani R. The effect of fleroxacin and ciprofloxacin on the pharmacokinetics of multiple dose caffeine. *Drugs* (1995) 49 (Suppl 2), 357–9.
9. LeBel M, Teng R, Dogolo LC, Willavize S, Friedman HL, Vincent J. The influence of steady-state trovafloxacin on the steady-state pharmacokinetics of caffeine in healthy subjects. *Pharm Res* (1996) 13 (Suppl 9), S434.
10. Randinitis EJ, Koup JR, Rausch G, Vassos AB. Effect of (CLX) administration on the single-dose pharmacokinetics of theophylline and caffeine. *Intersci Conf Antimicrob Agents Chemother* (1998) 38, 6.
11. Cesana M, Broccali G, Imbimbo BP, Crema A. Effect of single doses of rufloxacin on the disposition of theophylline and caffeine after single administration. *Int J Clin Pharmacol Ther Toxicol* (1991) 29, 133–8.
12. Kinzig-Schippers M, Fuhr U, Zaigler M, Dammeyer J, Rüsing G, Labedzki A, Bulitta J, Sörgel F. Interaction of pefloxacin and enoxacin with the human cytochrome P450 enzyme CYP1A2. *Clin Pharmacol Ther* (1999) 65, 262–74.
13. Kim M-Y, Nightingale CH, Nicolau DP. Influence of sex on the pharmacokinetic interaction of fleroxacin and ciprofloxacin with caffeine. *Clin Pharmacokinet* (2003), 42, 985–96.
14. Fuhr U, Wolff T, Harder S, Schymanski P, Staib AH. Quinolone inhibition of cytochrome P450-dependent caffeine metabolism in human liver microsomes. *Drug Metab Dispos* (1990) 18, 1005–10.
15. Barnett G, Segura J, de la Torre R, Carbó M. Pharmacokinetic determination of relative potency of quinolone inhibition of caffeine disposition. *Eur J Clin Pharmacol* (1990) 39, 63–9.

Caffeine + Venlafaxine

Venlafaxine does not affect the pharmacokinetics of caffeine.

Clinical evidence, mechanism, importance and management

Venlafaxine 37.5 mg twice daily for 3 days then 75 mg twice daily for 4 days did not affect the AUC or clearance of caffeine 200 mg daily (equivalent to about 3 cups of coffee) in 15 healthy subjects. A slight but significant decrease in the half-life from 6.1 to 5.5 hours was noted.[1] On the basis of this study, no special precautions are needed if both drugs are taken together.

1. Amchin J, Zarycranski W, Taylor KP, Albano D, Klockowski PM. Effect of venlafaxine on CYP1A2-dependent pharmacokinetics and metabolism of caffeine. *J Clin Pharmacol* (1999) 39, 252–9.

Caffeine + Verapamil

A small and relatively unimportant decrease in the clearance of caffeine may occur in patients given verapamil.

Clinical evidence, mechanism, importance and management

Verapamil 80 mg three times daily for 2 days decreased the total clearance of a single 200-mg dose of caffeine by 25%, and increased its half-life by 25% (from 4.6 to 5.8 hours) in 6 healthy subjects.[1] These changes are small, and unlikely to be of much importance in most patients.

1. Nawoot S, Wong D, Mays DC, Gerber N. Inhibition of caffeine elimination by verapamil. *Clin Pharmacol Ther* (1988) 43, 148.

Doxofylline + Miscellaneous

There is some limited evidence that erythromycin may increase the effects of doxofylline, but the clinical importance of this is uncertain. Digoxin initially raises, then lowers serum doxofylline levels, but the bronchodilator effects do not appear to be significantly affected. Allopurinol and lithium carbonate appear to have no significant effects on doxofylline.

Clinical evidence, mechanism, importance and management

Healthy subjects were given doxofylline 400 mg three times daily either alone or with **allopurinol** 100 mg once daily, **erythromycin** 400 mg three times daily or **lithium carbonate** 300 mg three times daily. None of the pharmacokinetic parameters measured, including the maximum serum levels, were significantly altered by any of these drugs apart from the AUC of doxofylline, which was raised by about 40% by **allopurinol**, 70% by **erythromycin**, and 35% by **lithium carbonate**. Only the **erythromycin** result was significant.[1]

The clinical significance of these changes is uncertain, and their mechanism is not understood. Until the situation is much clearer it would be prudent to check the outcome of adding **erythromycin** to established treatment with doxofylline, being alert for evidence of increased effects.

In a comparative study in 9 patients on doxofylline 800 mg daily, **digoxin** 500 micrograms daily was given to 5 patients. It was found that the **digoxin** increased the serum levels of doxofylline by 50% on the first day of treatment, 3 hours after administration, and reduced doxofylline levels by about 30% at steady-state (day 30). Nevertheless, the bronchodilating effects of the doxofylline were little different between the two groups. It was concluded that concurrent use is normally safe and effective, but the initial

Table 32.3 Effect of quinolones on caffeine pharmacokinetics in healthy subjects

Quinolone[a]	*Daily caffeine intake*[b]	*Change in AUC*	*Change in clearance*	*Refs*
Ciprofloxacin				
100 mg twice daily	220 to 230 mg	+17%		1
250 mg twice daily	220 to 230 mg	+57%	–33%	1, 2, 3
500 mg twice daily	230 mg	+58%		1
500 mg twice daily	100 mg three times daily	+127%	–49%	4
750 mg (3 x 12-hourly doses)	100 mg	+59%	–45%	5
Clinafloxacin				
400 mg twice daily	200 mg		–84%	6
Enoxacin				
100 mg twice daily	230 mg	+138%		1
200 mg twice daily	230 mg	+176%		1
400 mg twice daily	220 to 230 mg	+346%	–78%	1, 2, 3
400 mg twice daily	200 mg daily	+370%	–79%	7
400 mg twice daily	183 mg daily		–83%	8
Fleroxacin				
400 mg daily	100 mg three times daily	+18%	No change	4
Lomefloxacin				
400 mg daily	200 mg daily	No change	No change	9
Norfloxacin				
200 mg twice daily	230 mg	+16%		1
800 mg twice daily	350 mg	+52%	–35%	10
Ofloxacin				
200 mg twice daily	220 to 230 mg	No change	No change	1, 2, 3
Pefloxacin				
400 mg twice daily	183 mg daily		–47%	8
Pipemidic acid				
400 mg twice daily	230 mg	+179%		1
800 mg twice daily	350 mg	+119%	–63%	10
Rufloxacin				
400 mg (single dose)	200 mg	–18%	No change	11
Trovafloxacin				
200 mg daily	183 mg daily	+17%		12

[a] Unless otherwise stated quinolones were given for 3 to 5 days.
[b] Unless otherwise stated caffeine was given as a single dose.

1. Harder S, Staib AH, Beer C, Papenburg A, Stille W, Shah PM. 4-Quinolones inhibit biotransformation of caffeine. *Eur J Clin Pharmacol* (1988) 35, 651–6.
2. Staib AH, Stille W, Dietlein G, Shah PM, Harder S, Mieke S, Beer C. Interaction between quinolones and caffeine. *Drugs* (1987) 34 (Suppl 1), 170–4.
3. Stille W, Harder S, Mieke S, Beer C, Shah PM, Frech K, Staib AH. Decrease of caffeine elimination in man during co-administration of 4-quinolones. *J Antimicrob Chemother* (1987) 20, 729–34.
4. Nicolau DP, Nightingale CH, Tessier PR, Fu Q, Xuan D-W, Esguerra EM, Quintiliani R. The effect of fleroxacin and ciprofloxacin on the pharmacokinetics of multiple dose caffeine. *Drugs* (1995) 49 (Suppl 2), 357–9.
5. Healy DP, Polk RE, Kanawati L, Rock DT, Mooney ML. Interaction between oral ciprofloxacin and caffeine in normal volunteers. *Antimicrob Agents Chemother* (1989) 33, 474–8.
6. Randinitis EJ, Koup JR, Rausch G, Vassos AB. Effect of (CLX) administration on the single-dose pharmacokinetics of theophylline and caffeine. *Intersci Conf Antimicrob Agents Chemother* (1998) 38, 6.
7. Peloquin CA, Nix DE, Sedman AJ, Wilton JH, Toothaker RD, Harrison NJ, Schentag JJ. Pharmacokinetics and clinical effects of caffeine alone and in combination with oral enoxacin. *Rev Infect Dis* (1989) II (Suppl 5), S1095.
8. Kinzig-Schippers M, Fuhr U, Zaigler M, Dammeyer J, Rüsing G, Labedzki A, Bulitta J, Sörgel F. Interaction of pefloxacin and enoxacin with the human cytochrome P450 enzyme CYP1A2. *Clin Pharmacol Ther* (1999) 65, 262–74.
9. Healy DP, Schoenle JR, Stotka J, Polk RE. Lack of interaction between lomefloxacin and caffeine in normal volunteers. *Antimicrob Agents Chemother* (1991) 35, 660–4.
10. Carbó M, Segura J, De la Torre R, Badenas JM, Camí J. Effect of quinolones on caffeine disposition. *Clin Pharmacol Ther* (1989) 45, 234-40.
11. Cesana M, Broccali G, Imbimbo BP, Crema A. Effect of single doses of rufloxacin on the disposition of theophylline and caffeine after single administration. *Int J Clin Pharmacol Ther Toxicol* (1991) 29, 133–8.
12. LeBel M, Teng R, Dogolo LC, Willavize S, Friedman HL, Vincent J. The influence of steady-state trovafloxacin on the steady-state pharmacokinetics of caffeine in healthy subjects. *Pharm Res* (1996) 13 (Suppl 9), S434.

doxofylline dose should be chosen to avoid too high a serum level on the first day, and pulmonary function should be well monitored.[2]

1. Harning R, Sekora D, O'Connell K, Wilson J. A crossover study of the effect of erythromycin, lithium carbonate, and allopurinol on doxofylline pharmacokinetics. *Clin Pharmacol Ther* (1994) 55, 158.
2. Provvedi D, Rubegni M, Biffignandi P. Pharmacokinetic interaction between doxofylline and digitalis in elderly patients with chronic obstructive bronchitis. *Acta Ther* (1990) 16, 239–46.

Ipratropium bromide + Salbutamol (Albuterol)

Acute angle-closure glaucoma developed rapidly in eight patients given nebulised ipratropium and salbutamol. Increased intra-ocular pressure has been reported in others. No interaction has been seen when the drugs are given by inhaler.

Clinical evidence

Five patients with an acute exacerbation of chronic obstructive airways disease, given nebulised ipratropium and salbutamol, developed acute angle-closure glaucoma, four of them within 1 to 36 hours of starting treatment. Two of the patients had a history of angle-closure glaucoma prior to admission.[1] Three other similar cases of acute angle-closure glaucoma due to concurrent use are reported elsewhere.[2,3] An increase in intra-ocular pressure has also been reported in other patients given both drugs by nebuliser.[4]

Mechanism

This reaction appears to occur because the anticholinergic action of the ipratropium causes semi-dilatation of the pupil, partially blocking the flow of aqueous humour from the posterior to the anterior chamber, thereby bowing the iris anteriorly and obstructing the drainage angle. The salbutamol increases the production of aqueous humour and makes things worse. Additional factors are that higher levels of both drugs are achieved by using a nebuliser, and that some drug may escape round the edge of the mask and have a direct action on the eye.[1]

Importance and management

An established but uncommon interaction, which appears to occur mainly in patients already predisposed to angle-closure glaucoma. The authors of the first report[1] advise care in the placing of the mask to avoid the escape of droplets (the use of goggles and continuing the application of any glaucoma treatment is also effective[4]) and, if possible, the avoidance of their concurrent use by nebuliser in patients predisposed to angle-closure glaucoma. They point out that no cases of glaucoma have been reported with either drug given by inhaler.[1]

1. Shah P, Dhurjon L, Metcalfe T, Gibson JM. Acute angle closure glaucoma associated with nebulised ipratropium bromide and salbutamol. *BMJ* (1992) 304, 40–1.
2. Packe GE, Cayton RM, Mashoudi N. Nebulised ipratropium bromide and salbutamol causing closed-angle glaucoma. *Lancet* (1984) ii, 691.
3. Reuser T, Flanagan DW, Borland C, Bannerjee DK. Acute angle closure glaucoma occurring after nebulized bronchodilator treatment with ipratropium bromide and salbutamol. *J R Soc Med* (1992) 85, 499–500.
4. Kalra L, Bone M. The effect of nebulized bronchodilator therapy on intraocular pressures in patients with glaucoma. *Chest* (1988) 93, 739–41.

Montelukast + Miscellaneous

There is an isolated report of severe oedema in a patient on oral prednisone and montelukast, but studies suggest that concurrent use of prednisolone or prednisone are useful and well-tolerated. Montelukast in normal doses does not interact to a clinically relevant extent with loratadine, phenobarbital, salbutamol (albuterol) or terfenadine, and no important interaction seems likely with phenytoin or rifampicin (rifampin).

Clinical evidence, mechanism, importance and management

(a) Corticosteroids

A double-blind, placebo-controlled, parallel study in healthy subjects (55 on montelukast and 36 on a placebo) found that the plasma profiles of oral **prednisone** 20 mg and of intravenous **prednisolone** 250 mg were unaffected by montelukast 200 mg daily for 6 weeks.[1] Other studies in patients using inhaled and/or oral corticosteroids have found that concurrent use is useful and well tolerated.[2-4]

However, an isolated report describes a case of marked peripheral oedema possibly linked to **prednisone** and montelukast. A 23-year-old patient with severe allergic and exercise-induced asthma and rhinoconjunctivitis treated with salmeterol and fluticasone by inhalation and oral cetirizine was given **prednisone** 40 mg daily for one week then 20 mg daily for a further week. When **prednisone** was stopped, severe asthma reoccurred and he was given **prednisone** 60 mg daily for one week then 40 mg daily for a further week and montelukast 10 mg daily. After 10 days of treatment he developed severe peripheral oedema, gaining 13 kg in weight. Renal and cardiovascular function were normal. **Prednisone** was stopped and the asthma was controlled by continued montelukast therapy and the excess weight was lost as the oedema resolved. The patient had good tolerance of both **prednisone** and montelukast alone. Corticosteroid-induced renal tubular sodium and fluid retention may have occurred when montelukast was also given.[5]

This isolated report is of uncertain general relevance. Usually, no special precautions appear to be needed if these drugs are used concurrently, and the makers say that montelukast can be used as add-on therapy in patients using inhaled corticosteroids.[6]

(b) Miscellaneous drugs

A study in patients with moderately severe asthma found no adverse interactions when **salbutamol** (**albuterol**) was given with montelukast 100 mg or 250 mg, with or without inhaled corticosteroids.[7] The makers say that montelukast can be used as an add-on for the treatment of patients taking **beta-agonist drugs**.[6] No adverse interactions were seen in large numbers of patients given montelukast 10 or 20 mg and **loratadine** 10 mg, and the combination was found to be beneficial in the treatment of allergic rhinitis and conjunctivitis.[8]

(c) Phenobarbital, Phenytoin, Rifampicin (Rifampin)

Montelukast 10 mg was given to 14 healthy subjects before and after they took phenobarbital 100 mg daily for 14 days. It was found that the geometric mean AUC and maximum serum levels of the montelukast were reduced by 38% and 20% respectively, but it was concluded that no montelukast dosage adjustment is needed.[9] The reason for these reductions is almost certainly because phenobarbital induces the cytochrome P450 isoenzyme CYP3A4 so that the montelukast metabolism is increased. The makers therefore caution the use of montelukast and inducers of CYP3A4 such as phenytoin, phenobarbital and rifampicin, especially in children.[6] However, there is so far no clinical evidence that the montelukast dosage needs adjustment in the presence of any of these drugs.

(d) Terfenadine

Healthy subjects were given terfenadine 60 mg 12-hourly for 14 days, with montelukast 10 mg daily from day 8 to day 14. It was found that the terfenadine pharmacokinetics and the QTc interval were unaltered by concurrent use.[10] No special precautions are needed if both drugs are given concurrently.

1. Noonan T, Shingo S, Kundu S, Reiss TF. A double-blind, placebo-controlled, parallel-group study in healthy male volunteers to investigate the safety and tolerability of 6 weeks of administration of MK-0476, and in subgroups, the effect of 6 weeks of administration of MK-0476 on the single dose pharmacokinetics of po and iv theophylline and corticosteroids. Merck Sharp & Dohme. Data on file.
2. Dahlén S-E, Malmström K, Nizankowska E, Dahlén B, Kuna P, Kowalski M, Lumry WR, Picado C, Stevenson DD, Bousquet J, Pauwels R, Holgate ST, Shahane A, Zhang J, Reiss TF, Szczeklik A. Improvement of aspirin-intolerant asthma by montelukast, a leukotriene antagonist. *Am J Respir Crit Care Med* (2002) 165, 9–14.
3. Knorr B, Matz J, Bernstein JA, Nguyen H, Seidenberg BC, Reiss TF, Becker A, for the Pediatric Montelukast Study Group. Montelukast for chronic asthma in 6- to 14-year-old children. A randomized, double-blind trial. *JAMA* (1998) 279, 1181–6.
4. Phipatanakul W, Greene C, Downes SJ, Cronin B, Eller TJ, Schneider LC, Irani A-M. Montelukast improves asthma control in asthmatic children maintained on inhaled corticosteroids. *Ann Allergy Asthma Immunol* (2003) 91, 49–54.
5. Geller M. Marked peripheral edema associated with montelukast and prednisone. *Ann Intern Med* (2000) 132, 924.
6. Singulair (Montelukast sodium). Merck Sharp & Dohme Ltd. UK Summary of product characteristics, November 2004.
7. Botto A, Kundu S, Reiss T. A double-blind, placebo-controlled, 3-period, crossover study to investigate the bronchodilating ability of oral doses of MK-0476 and to investigate the interaction with inhaled albuterol in moderately severe asthmatic patients. Merck Sharp & Dohme. Data on file (Protocol 066) 1996.
8. Malstrom K, Meltzer E, Prenner B, Lu S, Weinstein S, Wolfe J, Wei LX, Reiss TF. Effects of montelukast (a leukotriene receptor antagonist), loratadine, montelukast + loratadine and placebo in seasonal allergic rhinitis and conjunctivitis. *J Allergy Clin Immunol* (1998) 101, S97.
9. Holland S, Shahane A, Rogers JD, Porras A, Grasing K, Lasseter K, Pinto M, Freeman A, Gertz B, Amin R. Metabolism of montelukast (M) is increased by multiple doses of phenobarbital (P). *Clin Pharmacol Ther* (1998) 63, 231.
10. Holland S, Gertz B, DeSmet M, Michiels N, Larson P, Freeman A, Keymeulen B. Montelukast (MON) has no effect on terfenadine (T) pharmacokinetics (PK) or QTc. *Clin Pharmacol Ther* (1998) 63, 232.

Terbutaline + Magnesium sulfate

Terbutaline and parenteral magnesium sulfate appear not to interact adversely.

Clinical evidence, mechanism, importance and management

Eight healthy adults were given two subcutaneous doses of terbutaline 250 micrograms 30 minutes apart, with and without intravenous magnesium sulfate 4 g in 250 ml of saline over the same 30-minute period.[1] Most of the effects of the terbutaline were found to be moderately increased by magnesium sulfate at 60 minutes (RR interval further decreased by 90 milliseconds; QTc interval further increased by 10 milliseconds; diastolic pressure further decreased by 8 mmHg; increase in systolic pressure reduced by about 5 mmHg; serum calcium further decreased by 0.13 mg/dl; serum glucose further increased by 9 mg/dl) but these changes were all considered to be small. The conclusion was reached that there appear to be no good reasons for avoiding their concurrent use, for example in the emergency treatment of asthma and other conditions.

1. Skorodin MS, Freebeck PC, Yetter B, Nelson JE, Van de Graaff WB, Walsh JM. Magnesium sulfate potentiates several cardiovascular and metabolic actions of terbutaline. *Chest* (1994) 105, 701–5.

Theophylline + Aciclovir

Preliminary evidence suggests that aciclovir can increase the serum levels of theophylline.

Clinical evidence

Prompted by a case of increased theophylline adverse effects in a patient given aciclovir, a study was carried out in 5 healthy subjects who were given single 320-mg doses of theophylline (as 400 mg of aminophylline) before and with the sixth dose of aciclovir 800 mg five times daily for 2 days. The AUC of the theophylline was increased by 45% and the total body clearance was reduced by 30%, when aciclovir was added.[1]

Mechanism

Uncertain, but the evidence suggests that aciclovir inhibits the oxidative metabolism of theophylline, resulting in accumulation.[1]

Importance and management

Evidence appears to be limited to this report, but the interaction seems to be established. Be alert for an increase in adverse effects of theophylline (nausea, headache, tremor) if aciclovir is added to established treatment, and consider monitoring levels. More study is needed.

1. Maeda Y, Konishi T, Omoda K, Takeda Y, Fukuhara S, Fukuzawa M, Ohune T, Tsuya T, Tsukiai S. Inhibition of theophylline metabolism by aciclovir. *Biol Pharm Bull* (1996) 19, 1591–5.

Theophylline + Allopurinol

Evidence from clinical studies and a single case report indicate that the effects of theophylline may be increased by allopurinol.

Clinical evidence

The peak plasma levels of theophylline 450 mg daily rose by 38% in a patient who took allopurinol for 3 days.[1] Allopurinol 300 mg twice daily for 14 days increased the half-life of a single 5-mg/kg oral dose of theophylline by 25%, and increased the AUC by 27% in 12 healthy subjects.[2] Similar increases were seen when a second dose of theophylline was given 28 days after starting the allopurinol.[2]

However, in 2 other studies allopurinol 300 mg daily for 7 days did not have any effect on the pharmacokinetics of theophylline following a single 5-mg/kg intravenous dose of aminophylline.[3,4] Similarly, steady-state theophylline concentrations were not affected by allopurinol 100 mg three times daily in 4 subjects. However, there was an alteration in the proportion of different urinary theophylline metabolites: methyluric acid decreased and methylxanthine increased.[4]

Mechanism

Uncertain. Allopurinol, a xanthine oxidase inhibitor, can block the conversion of methylxanthine to methyluric acid, but this had no effect on theophylline plasma levels in two studies. One suggestion is that allopurinol inhibits oxidative metabolism of theophylline by the liver.[1]

Importance and management

Evidence appears to be limited to a single case report and the studies in healthy subjects. The interaction only appears to be of moderate importance. Nevertheless, it would seem prudent to check for any signs of theophylline overdosage (headache, nausea, tremor) during concurrent use, particularly in situations where the metabolism of the theophylline may already be reduced (other drugs or diseases), or where high doses of allopurinol are used. For mention that allopurinol may invalidate the results of phenotyping tests using caffeine, see 'Caffeine + Allopurinol', p.921.

1. Barry M, Feeley J. Allopurinol influences aminophenazone elimination. *Clin Pharmacokinet* (1990) 19, 167–9.
2. Manfredi RL, Vesell ES. Inhibition of theophylline metabolism by long-term allopurinol administration. *Clin Pharmacol Ther* (1981) 29, 224–9.
3. Vozeh S, Powell JR, Cupit GC, Riegelman S, Sheiner LB. Influence of allopurinol on theophylline disposition in adults. *Clin Pharmacol Ther* (1980) 27, 194–7.
4. Grygiel JJ, Wing LMH, Farkas J, Birkett DJ. Effects of allopurinol on theophylline metabolism and clearance. *Clin Pharmacol Ther* (1979) 26, 660–7.

Theophylline + Alosetron

Alosetron does not alter theophylline pharmacokinetics.

Clinical evidence, mechanism, importance and management

Alosetron 1 mg twice daily or a placebo was given to 10 healthy women for 16 days, with oral theophylline 200 mg twice daily from day 8 to day 16. No clinically relevant changes in the pharmacokinetics of the theophylline were seen, and concurrent use was well tolerated. The effect of theophylline on alosetron pharmacokinetics was not measured but the authors of the report say that no metabolic interaction seems likely.[1] No special precautions would therefore appear to be needed if these drugs are used together.

1. Koch KM, Ricci BM, Hedayetullah NS, Jewel D, Kersey KE. Effect of alosetron on theophylline pharmacokinetics. *Br J Clin Pharmacol* (2001) 52, 596–600.

Theophylline + Aminoglutethimide

Theophylline clearance is increased by aminoglutethimide, which may result in a moderate reduction in its serum levels and therapeutic effects.

Clinical evidence, mechanism, importance and management

Aminoglutethimide 250 mg four times a day increased the clearance of sustained release theophylline 200 mg twice daily by 18 to 43% in 3 patients.[1] Theophylline clearance was assessed before starting aminoglutethimide as well as during weeks 2 to 12 of combined therapy.

It seems probable that aminoglutethimide, a known enzyme-inducing agent, increases the metabolism of theophylline by the liver, thereby increasing its loss from the body. The clinical importance is uncertain, but it seems likely that the effects of theophylline would be reduced to some extent. Monitor the effects and if necessary take theophylline levels. Increase the theophylline dosage accordingly.

1. Lønning PE, Kvinnsland S, Bakke OM. Effect of aminoglutethimide on antipyrine, theophylline and digitoxin disposition in breast cancer. *Clin Pharmacol Ther* (1984) 36, 796–802.

Theophylline + Amiodarone

An isolated case report describes raised theophylline levels and toxicity in an elderly man when amiodarone was given.

Clinical evidence, mechanism, importance and management

An 86-year-old man on furosemide, digoxin, domperidone and sustained-release theophylline developed signs of theophylline toxicity when amiodarone 600 mg daily was given. After 9 days his serum theophylline levels had doubled, from 93 to 194 micromol/l. The toxicity disappeared when the theophylline was stopped.[1] The reason for this adverse reaction is not understood but a reduction in the metabolism of the theophylline by the liver is suggested.[1] There was no evidence of liver dysfunction. This is an isolated case and its general importance is uncertain. More study is needed.

1. Soto J, Sacristán JA, Arellano F, Hazas J. Possible theophylline-amiodarone interaction. *DICP Ann Pharmacother* (1990) 24, 1115.

Theophylline + Ampicillin/Sulbactam or Amoxicillin

Neither ampicillin with or without sulbactam nor amoxicillin alters the pharmacokinetics of theophylline.

Clinical evidence, mechanism, importance and management

A retrospective study in asthmatic children aged 3 months to 6 years found that the mean half-life of theophylline did not differ between those treated with ampicillin and those not.[1] The pharmacokinetics of theophylline 8.5 mg/kg daily were not altered in 12 adult patients with chronic obstructive pulmonary disease when they were given ampicillin 1 g plus sulbactam 500 mg 12-hourly for 7 days.[2]

A study in 9 healthy adult subjects showed that amoxicillin 750 mg daily for 9 days did not affect the pharmacokinetics of theophylline 540 mg twice daily.[3,4]

No special precautions would seem to be necessary during concurrent use of these antibacterials and theophylline. However, note that acute infections *per se* can alter theophylline pharmacokinetics.

1. Kadlec GJ, Ha LT, Jarboe CH, Richards D, Karibo JM. Effect of ampicillin on theophylline half-life in infants and young children. *South Med J* (1978) 71, 1584.
2. Cazzola M, Santangelo G, Guidetti E, Mattina R, Caputi M, Girbino G. Influence of sulbactam plus ampicillin on theophylline clearance. *Int J Clin Pharmacol Res* (1991) 11, 11–15.
3. Jonkman JHG, van der Boon WJV, Schoenmaker R, Holtkamp A, Hempenius J. Lack of effect of amoxicillin on theophylline pharmacokinetics. *Br J Clin Pharmacol* (1985) 19, 99–101.
4. Jonkman JHG, van der Boon WJV, Schoenmaker R, Holtkamp AH, Hempenius J. Clinical pharmacokinetics of amoxycillin and theophylline during cotreatment with both medicaments. *Chemotherapy* (1985) 31, 329–35.

Theophylline + Antacids

The extent of absorption of theophylline from the gut does not appear to be significantly affected by aluminium or magnesium hydroxide antacids.

Clinical evidence, mechanism, importance and management

In a study in 12 healthy subjects, there was no difference in the steady-state maximum serum concentrations or AUC of theophylline given as *Nuelin-Depot* or *Theodur* when an antacid (*Novalucid*, containing **aluminium/magnesium hydroxide** and **magnesium carbonate**) was given. However, the antacid caused a faster absorption of theophylline from *Nuelin-Depot*, which resulted in greater fluctuations in the serum levels. It was considered that the adverse effects of theophylline might be increased in those patients with serum levels at the top of the range.[1] Similar results have been found in single-dose studies when aminophylline[2] and *Theodur*[3] were given with **aluminium/magnesium hydroxide** antacids, and in multiple dose studies in patients when *Armophylline*,[4] *Aminophyllin*[5] or *Theodur*[5] were given with **aluminium/magnesium hydroxide** antacids. Care should be taken extrapolating this information to other sustained release preparations of theophylline, but generally speaking no special precautions seem to be necessary if antacids are given with theophylline.

1. Myhre KI, Walstad RA. The influence of antacid on the absorption of two different sustained-release formulations of theophylline. *Br J Clin Pharmacol* (1983) 15, 683–7.
2. Arnold LA, Spurbeck GH, Shelver WH, Henderson WM. Effect of an antacid on gastrointestinal absorption of theophylline. *Am J Hosp Pharm* (1979) 36, 1059–62.
3. Darzentas LJ, Stewart RB, Curry SH, Yost RL. Effect of antacid on bioavailability of a sustained-release theophylline preparation. *Drug Intell Clin Pharm* (1983) 17, 555–7.
4. Muir JF, Peiffer G, Richard MO, Benhamou D, Adrejak M, Hary L, Moore N. Lack of effect of magnesium-aluminium hydroxide on the absorption of theophylline given as a pH-dependent sustained release preparation. *Eur J Clin Pharmacol* (1993) 44, 85–8.
5. Reed RC, Schwartz HJ. Lack of influence of an intensive antacid regimen on theophylline bioavailability. *J Pharmacokinet Biopharm* (1984) 12, 315–331.

Theophylline + Anthelmintics; Benzimidazoles

Theophylline serum levels can be markedly increased by tiabendazole and toxicity may develop. Neither albendazole nor mebendazole appear to interact with theophylline.

Clinical evidence

(a) Albendazole

A study in 6 healthy subjects found that the pharmacokinetics of a single dose of theophylline were unaffected by a single 400-mg dose of albendazole.[1]

(b) Mebendazole

A study in 6 healthy subjects found that the pharmacokinetics of a single dose of intravenous aminophylline were unaffected by mebendazole 100 mg twice daily for 3 days.[1] The absence of a significant interaction was reported in another similar study using the same mebendazole dosage.[2]

(c) Tiabendazole

An elderly man on prednisone, furosemide, terbutaline and orciprenaline was switched from oral aminophylline to an intravenous infusion, giving a stable serum level of 21 micrograms/ml after 48 hours. When he was also given tiabendazole 4 g daily for 5 days for persistence of a *Strongyloides stercoralis* infestation he developed theophylline toxicity (severe nausea) and his serum levels were found to be 46 micrograms/ml. Three months previously, he had been treated with tiabendazole 3 g daily for 3 days without any symptoms of toxicity (no theophylline levels were measured).[3] The theophylline levels of another patient rose from 15 to 22 micrograms/ml when he was given tiabendazole 1.8 g twice daily for 3 days, despite a dosage reduction of one-third, made in anticipation of the interaction. Theophylline levels were still elevated 2 days after the tiabendazole was stopped, and the theophylline dose was further reduced. Levels returned to normal after 5 days, and the theophylline dose was eventually increased again.[4]

A retrospective study of patients given theophylline and tiabendazole found that 9 out of 40 (23%) had developed elevated serum theophylline levels and of those, 5 experienced significant toxicity, with 3 requiring hospitalisation. The other 31 patients did not have theophylline levels taken.[5] A further report describes a patient on intravenous aminophylline who had an increase in theophylline levels from 18 to 26 micrograms/ml within 2 days of starting tiabendazole 1.5 g twice daily.[2] The authors of this report then studied 6 healthy subjects who received a single dose of aminophylline before and while taking tiabendazole 1.5 g twice daily for 3 days. Three of the subjects had to discontinue the study because of severe nausea, vomiting or dizziness. In the remaining three, tiabendazole markedly affected the pharmacokinetics of aminophylline; the half-life increased from 6.7 to 18.6 hours, the clearance fell by 66% and the elimination rate constant decreased by 65%.[2]

Mechanism

Uncertain. It is suggested that tiabendazole inhibits the metabolism of theophylline by the liver thereby prolonging its stay in the body and raising its serum levels. The nausea and vomiting may have been due to the adverse effects of both the theophylline and the tiabendazole.

Importance and management

The interaction between theophylline and tiabendazole is established and of clinical importance. Monitor theophylline levels and reduce the theophylline dosage accordingly. A 50% theophylline dosage reduction has been suggested,[4] or, where practical, stopping theophylline for 2 to 3 days while giving the tiabendazole.[5] Where albendazole or mebendazole are suitable alternative anthelmintics, these may be preferred since no special precautions would seem to be needed if either of these is given to patients taking theophylline or aminophylline.

1. Adebayo GI, Mabadeje AFB. Theophylline disposition — effects of cimetidine, mebendazole and albendazole. *Aliment Pharmacol Ther* (1988) 2, 341–6.
2. Schneider D, Gannon R, Sweeney K, Shore E. Theophylline and antiparasitic drug interactions. A case report and a study of the influence of thiabendazole and mebendazole on theophylline pharmacokinetics in adults. *Chest* (1990) 97, 84–7.
3. Sugar AM, Kearns PJ, Haulk AA, Rushing JL. Possible thiabendazole-induced theophylline toxicity. *Am Rev Respir Dis* (1980) 122, 501–3.

4. Lew G, Murray WE, Lane JR, Haeger E. Theophylline—thiabendazole drug interaction. *Clin Pharm* (1989) 8, 225–7.
5. German T, Berger R. Interaction of theophylline and thiabendazole in patients with chronic obstructive lung disease. *Am Rev Respir Dis* (1992) 145, A807.

Theophylline + Antihistamines or other anti-allergic drugs

Azelastine, ketotifen, mequitazine, mizolastine, pemirolast potassium, repirinast, and terfenadine appear not to alter the pharmacokinetics of theophylline.

Clinical evidence, mechanism, importance and management

Azelastine 2 mg twice daily had no significant effect on the clearance of theophylline 300 mg twice daily in 10 subjects with bronchial asthma. One patient had a 20.8% increase and another a 25.3% decrease.[1]

Two studies, one in healthy adults[2] and one in asthmatic children,[3] showed that **ketotifen** did not affect the pharmacokinetics of a single oral dose of theophylline[2] or aminophylline.[3] It was suggested that concurrent use might actually decrease the CNS adverse effects of each drug.[2]

The pharmacokinetics of theophylline at steady state were not significantly affected when **mequitazine** 6 mg daily was given to 7 asthmatic patients for 3 weeks.[4]

Mizolastine 10 mg daily had virtually no effect on the steady-state pharmacokinetics of theophylline in 17 healthy subjects, although a 13% increase in mean trough level and an 8% increase in the AUC was seen. These changes were not considered clinically relevant.[5]

Pemirolast potassium 10 mg daily for 4 days was found to have no significant effect on the steady-state serum levels or clearance of theophylline in 7 healthy subjects.[6]

Repirinast 300 mg daily had no effect on the pharmacokinetics of theophylline in 10 asthmatics given a single dose of aminophylline.[7] Another study in 7 asthmatics found that **repirinast** [dosage not clearly stated] for 3 weeks had no effect on the pharmacokinetics of theophylline 400 to 800 mg in two divided doses.[8]

The pharmacokinetics of a single 250-mg dose of theophylline were unchanged by **terfenadine** 120 mg twice daily for 16 days in 10 healthy subjects.[9] Similarly, **terfenadine** 60 mg twice daily did not affect the steady-state pharmacokinetics of theophylline 4 mg/kg daily.[10]

No special precautions seem to be necessary if any of these drugs is given with theophylline.

1. Asamoto H, Kokura M, Kawakami A, Sasaki Y, Fujii H, Sawano T, Iso S, Ooishi T, Horiuchi Y, Ohara N, Kitamura Y, Morishita H. Effect of azelastine on theophylline clearance in asthma patients. *Arerugi* (1988) 37, 1033–7.
2. Matejcek M, Irwin P, Neff G, Abt K, Wehrli W. Determination of the central effects of the asthma prophylactic ketotifen, the bronchodilator theophylline, and both in combination: an application of quantitative electroencephalography to the study of drug interactions. *Int J Clin Pharmacol Ther Toxicol* (1985) 23, 258–66.
3. Garty M, Scolnik D, Danziger Y, Volovitz B, Ilfeld DN, Varsano I. Non-interaction of ketotifen and theophylline in children with asthma - an acute study. *Eur J Clin Pharmacol* (1987) 32, 187–9.
4. Hasegawa T, Takagi K, Kuzuya T, Nadai M, Apichartpichean R, Muraoka I. Effect of mequitazine on the pharmacokinetics of theophylline in asthmatic patients. *Eur J Clin Pharmacol* (1990) 38, 255–8.
5. Pinquier JL, Salva P, Deschamps C, Ascalone V, Costa J. Effect of mizolastine, a new non sedative H1 antagonist on the pharmacokinetics of theophylline. *Therapie* (1995) 50 (Suppl), 148.
6. Hasegawa T, Takagi K, Nadai M, Ogura Y, Nabeshima T. Kinetic interaction between theophylline and a newly developed anti-allergic drug, pemirolast potassium. *Eur J Clin Pharmacol* (1994) 46, 55–8.
7. Nagata M, Tabe K, Houya I, Kiuchi H, Sakamoto Y, Yamamoto K, Dohi Y. The influence of repirinast, an anti-allergic drug, on theophylline pharmacokinetics in patients with bronchial asthma. *Nihon Kyobu Shikkan Gakkai Zasshi* (1991) 29, 413–9.
8. Takagi K, Kuzuya T, Horiuchi T, Nadai M, Apichartpichean R, Ogura Y, Hasegawa T. Lack of effect of repirinast on the pharmacokinetics of theophylline in asthmatic patients. *Eur J Clin Pharmacol* (1989) 37, 301–3.
9. Brion N, Naline E, Beaumont D, Pays M, Advenier C. Lack of effect of terfenadine on theophylline pharmacokinetics and metabolism in normal subjects. *Br J Clin Pharmacol* (1989) 27, 391–5.
10. Luskin SS, Fitzsimmons WE, MacLeod CM, Luskin AT. Pharmacokinetic evaluation of the terfenadine-theophylline interaction. *J Allergy Clin Immunol* (1989) 83, 406–11.

Theophylline + Azoles

Theophylline levels are normally unaffected or only minimally affected by either fluconazole or ketoconazole. An isolated report describes a rise in serum theophylline levels due to fluconazole, and another describes falls in theophylline levels in three patients on ketoconazole.

Clinical evidence

(a) Fluconazole

A crossover study in 5 healthy subjects found that fluconazole 100 mg given every 12 hours for 3 days, with the final dose on day 4, caused only a non-significant 16% decrease in the clearance of a single 300-mg oral dose of aminophylline.[1] Another study in 10 healthy subjects found that fluconazole 100 mg daily for a week had no significant effect on the serum levels of theophylline 150 mg twice daily.[2] The clearance of a single 6-mg/kg oral dose of theophylline was reduced by 13.4% in 9 subjects who took fluconazole 400 mg daily for 10 days.[3] However, an isolated and brief report says that one of 2 patients given theophylline and fluconazole showed a rise [amount not specified] in serum theophylline levels.[4]

(b) Ketoconazole

No significant changes in the pharmacokinetics of a single 3-mg/kg intravenous dose of theophylline (given as aminophylline) were seen in 12 healthy subjects who took a single 400-mg dose of ketoconazole, or in 4 subjects who took ketoconazole 400 mg daily for 5 days.[5] Similar results were found in another study in 10 healthy subjects who took **ketoconazole** 200 mg daily for 7 days.[6] Ketoconazole 400 mg daily for 6 days increased the half-life of a single 250-mg oral dose of theophylline by 21.7% in 6 healthy subjects, but had no effect on its clearance.[7] However, a case report describes a man whose serum theophylline levels fell sharply from about 16.5 to 9 mg/l (normal range 10 to 20 mg/l) over the 2 hours immediately after taking 200 mg of ketoconazole. A less striking fall was seen in 2 other patients.[8]

Mechanism

These antifungals appear to have minimal effects on the cytochrome P450 isoenzyme CYP1A, which is concerned with the oxidative metabolism of theophylline.[1,7] It is not clear why a few individuals show some changes in theophylline levels.

Importance and management

Information seems to be limited to these reports. Neither fluconazole nor ketoconazole normally appears to interact to a relevant extent in most patients. However, it seems that very occasionally some changes occur so bear this interaction in mind in the case of unexpected theophylline levels, adverse effects or uncontrolled symptoms. Other azole antifungals such as itraconazole and voriconazole, which are substrates for and inhibitors of CYP2C19, CYP2C9, and/or CYP3A4, are also unlikely to interact with theophylline.

1. Konishi H, Morita K, Yamaji A. Effect of fluconazole on theophylline disposition in humans. *Eur J Clin Pharmacol* (1994) 46, 309–12.
2. Feil RA, Rindone JP, Morrill GB, Habib MP. Effect of low-dose fluconazole on theophylline serum concentrations in healthy volunteers. *J Pharm Technol* (1995) 11, 267–9.
3. Foisy MM, Nix D, Middleton E, Kotas T, Symonds WT. The effects of single dose fluconazole (SD FLU) versus multiple dose fluconazole (MD FLU) on the pharmacokinetics (PK) of theophylline (THL) in young healthy volunteers. *Intersci Conf Antimicrob Agents Chemother* (1995) 39, 7.
4. Tett S, Carey D, Lee H-S. Drug interactions with fluconazole. *Med J Aust* (1992) 156, 365.
5. Brown MW, Maldonado AL, Meredith CG, Speeg KV. Effect of ketoconazole on hepatic oxidative drug metabolism. *Clin Pharmacol Ther* (1985) 37, 290–7.
6. Heusner JJ, Dukes GE, Rollins DE, Tolman KG, Galinsky RE. Effect of chronically administered ketoconazole on the elimination of theophylline in man. *Drug Intell Clin Pharm* (1987) 21, 514–17.
7. Naline E, Sanceaume M, Pays M, Advenier C. Application of theophylline metabolite assays to the exploration of liver microsome oxidative function in man. *Fundam Clin Pharmacol* (1988) 2, 341–51.
8. Murphy E, Hannon D, Callaghan B. Ketoconazole—theophylline interaction. *Ir Med J* (1987) 80, 123–4.

Theophylline + Barbiturates

Theophylline serum levels can be reduced by phenobarbital or pentobarbital. A single report describes a similar interaction with secobarbital and it would be expected to occur with other barbiturates.

Clinical evidence

(a) Pentobarbital

A single case report describes a man on intravenous aminophylline who had a 95% rise in the clearance of theophylline when treated with high-dose intravenous pentobarbital.[1] In healthy subjects pentobarbital 100 mg daily for 10 days increased the clearance of oral theophylline by a mean of 40% and reduced the AUC by 26%, although there were marked intersubject differences.[2]

(b) Phenobarbital

After taking phenobarbital (2 mg/kg daily to a maximum of 60 mg) for 19 days the mean steady-state serum theophylline levels in 7 asthmatic children aged 6 to 12 years were reduced by 30%, and the clearance was increased by 35% (range 12 to 71%).[3] In contrast, two earlier studies (one by the same group of authors) found no significant change in the pharmacokinetics of theophylline, in asthmatic children given phenobarbital 2 mg/kg daily, or 16 or 32 mg three times daily.[4,5]

The mean theophylline clearance, from a single intravenous dose of aminophylline was increased by 34% in healthy adult subjects given phenobarbital.[6] In another study the clearance of theophylline was increased by 17% by phenobarbital for 2 weeks, although this was not significant.[7] The effects of phenobarbital can be additive with the effects of phenytoin and smoking; one patient required 4 g of theophylline daily to maintain therapeutic serum levels and to control her asthma.[8]

One retrospective study found that premature infants needed a higher dose of intravenous aminophylline for neonatal apnoea when they were given phenobarbital,[9] but a later prospective study failed to confirm this.[10] A study in one set of newborn twins given intravenous aminophylline found that the serum theophylline levels of the twin given phenobarbital were about half those of the twin not given phenobarbital.[11]

(c) Secobarbital

The clearance of theophylline increased by 337% over a 4-week period in a child treated with periodic doses of secobarbital and regular doses of **phenobarbital**.[12]

Mechanism

Barbiturates are potent liver enzyme inducing agents, which possibly increase the metabolism of theophylline by the liver, thereby hastening its removal from the body. This has been shown in *animal* studies, although *N*-demethylation (the main metabolic route for theophylline) was not affected.[13]

Importance and management

A moderately well documented, established and clinically important interaction. Patients treated with phenobarbital or pentobarbital may need above-average doses of theophylline to achieve and maintain adequate serum levels. Concurrent use should be monitored and appropriate dosage increases made. All of the barbiturates can cause enzyme induction and may, to a greater or lesser extent, be expected to behave similarly. This is illustrated by the single report involving secobarbital. However, direct information about other barbiturates seems to be lacking.

1. Gibson GA, Blouin RA, Bauer LA, Rapp RP, Tibbs PA. Influence of high-dose pentobarbital on theophylline pharmacokinetics: A case report. *Ther Drug Monit* (1985) 7, 181–4.
2. Dahlqvist R, Steiner E, Koike Y, von Bahr C, Lind M, Billing B. Induction of theophylline metabolism by pentobarbital. *Ther Drug Monit* (1989) 11, 408–10.
3. Saccar CL, Danish M, Ragni MC, Rocci ML, Greene J, Yaffe SJ, Mansmann HC. The effect of phenobarbital on theophylline disposition in children with asthma. *J Allergy Clin Immunol* (1985) 75, 716–9.
4. Goldstein EO, Eney RD, Mellits ED, Solomon H, Johnson G. Effect of phenobarbital on theophylline metabolism in asthmatic children. *Ann Allergy* (1977) 39, 69.
5. Greene J, Danish M, Ragni M, Lecks H, Yaffe S. The effect of phenobarbital upon theophylline elimination kinetics in asthmatic children. *Ann Allergy* (1977) 39, 69.
6. Landay RA, Gonzalez MA, Taylor JC. Effect of phenobarbital on theophylline disposition. *J Allergy Clin Immunol* (1978) 62, 27–9.
7. Piafsky KM, Sitar DS, Ogilvie RI. Effect of phenobarbital on the disposition of intravenous theophylline. *Clin Pharmacol Ther* (1977) 22, 336–9.
8. Nicholson JP, Basile SA, Cury JD. Massive theophylline dosing in a heavy smoker receiving both phenytoin and phenobarbital. *Ann Pharmacother* (1992) 26, 334–6.
9. Yazdani M, Kissling GE, Tran TH, Gottschalk SK, Schuth CR. Phenobarbital increases the theophylline requirement of premature infants being treated for apnea. *Am J Dis Child* (1987) 141, 97–9.
10. Kandrotas RJ, Cranfield TL, Gal P, Ransom J, Weaver RL. Effect of phenobarbital administration on theophylline clearance in premature neonates. *Ther Drug Monit* (1990) 12, 139–43.
11. Delgado E, Carrasco JM, García B, Pérez E, García Lacalle C, Bermejo T, De Juana P. Interacción teofilina-fenobarbital en un neonato. *Farm Clin* (1996) 13, 142–5.
12. Paladino JA, Blumer NA, Maddox RR. Effect of secobarbital on theophylline clearance. *Ther Drug Monit* (1983) 5, 135–9.
13. Williams JF, Szentivanyi A. Implications of hepatic drug-metabolizing activity in the therapy of bronchial asthma. *J Allergy Clin Immunol* (1975) 55, 125.

Theophylline + BCG vaccine

There is evidence that BCG vaccine can increase the half-life of theophylline, but the clinical importance of this is uncertain.

Clinical evidence, mechanism, importance and management

Two weeks after 12 healthy subjects received vaccination against tuberculosis with 0.1 ml of BCG vaccine, the clearance of single 128-mg doses of theophylline (as choline theophyllinate) was reduced by 21% and the theophylline half-life was prolonged by 14% (range: 10% reduction to 47% increase).[1] It therefore seems possible that the occasional patient may develop some signs of theophylline toxicity if their serum levels are already towards the top end of the therapeutic range but most patients are unlikely to be affected.

1. Gray JD, Renton KW, Hung OR. Depression of theophylline elimination following BCG vaccination. *Br J Clin Pharmacol* (1983) 16, 735–7.

Theophylline + Beta-agonist bronchodilators

The concurrent use of xanthines such as theophylline and beta-agonist bronchodilators is a useful option in the management of asthma and chronic obstructive pulmonary disease, but potentiation of some adverse reactions can occur, the most serious being hypokalaemia and tachycardia, particularly with high-dose theophylline. Some patients may show a significant fall in serum theophylline levels if given oral or intravenous salbutamol (albuterol) or intravenous isoprenaline (isoproterenol).

Clinical evidence

(a) Formoterol

In a single-dose study, 8 healthy subjects were given oral doses of theophylline 375 mg and formoterol 144 micrograms. Combined use caused no significant pharmacokinetic interaction, but a significantly greater drop in the potassium level was seen, when compared with either drug given alone.[1]

(b) Isoprenaline (Isoproterenol)

The infusion of isoprenaline increased the clearance of theophylline (given as intravenous aminophylline) by a mean of 19% in 6 children with status asthmaticus and respiratory failure. Two of them had increases in clearance of greater than 30%.[2] Another study in 12 patients with status asthmaticus found that an isoprenaline infusion (mean maximum rate 0.77 micrograms/kg per minute) caused a mean fall in serum theophylline levels of almost 6 micrograms/ml.[3] The levels rose again when isoprenaline was stopped.[3] A critically ill patient on intravenous aminophylline, phenytoin and nebulised terbutaline showed a marked increase in theophylline clearance of 354% when an isoprenaline infusion and intravenous methylprednisolone were added to the regimen.[4]

(c) Orciprenaline (Metaproterenol)

Orciprenaline 20 mg given every 8 hours by mouth, or 1.95 mg given every 6 hours by inhalation for 3 days had no effect on the pharmacokinetics of theophylline (given as a single intravenous dose of aminophylline) in 6 healthy subjects.[5] This confirms a previous finding in asthmatic children, in whom it was shown that oral orciprenaline did not alter steady-state serum theophylline levels.[6]

(d) Salbutamol (Albuterol)

(i) Effects on heart rate or potassium levels. Pretreatment with oral theophylline for 9 days significantly increased the hypokalaemia and tachycardia caused by an infusion of salbutamol (4 micrograms/kg loading dose then 8 micrograms/kg for an hour) in healthy subjects.[7] A potentially dangerous additive increase in heart rate of about 35 to 40% was seen in one study in 9 patients with COPD given infusions of aminophylline and salbutamol.[8] Similarly, heart rate was significantly higher in 15 asthmatic children given single doses of oral theophylline and salbutamol (109 bpm) when compared with a control group given oral theophylline alone (91 bpm).[9] However, another study found that neither the occurrence nor the severity of arrhythmias seemed to be changed when oral theophylline was added to inhaled salbutamol therapy in 18 patients with COPD and heart disease.[10] Respiratory arrest possibly related to hypokalaemia occurred in a 10-year-old girl given theophylline and salbutamol.[11]

(ii) Effects on theophylline levels. Reduced theophylline levels (clearance increased by a mean of 14%, and in 3 cases by greater than 30%) were seen when salbutamol was given orally to 10 healthy volunteers, but no changes in clearance were seen when salbutamol was given by inhalation.[12] Another study reported a 25% reduction in serum theophylline levels in 10

patients who took oral salbutamol 16 mg.[13] A child of 19 months given intravenous theophylline needed a threefold increase in theophylline dosage when an infusion of salbutamol was added because of an increase in the theophylline clearance.[14] Peak flow readings were decreased in 15 children (aged 5 to 13 years) given single doses of oral salbutamol and theophylline, but theophylline levels were not significantly decreased.[9] These reports contrast with another study in 8 healthy subjects, which found no change in the steady-state pharmacokinetics of oral theophylline given with oral salbutamol.[15]

(e) Terbutaline

In 7 healthy subjects pretreatment with oral theophylline for at least 4 days significantly increased the fall in serum potassium levels and rises in blood glucose, pulse rates and systolic blood pressures caused by an infusion of terbutaline.[16] A study in children given slow-release formulations of both theophylline and terbutaline found no increases in reported adverse effects and simple additive effects on the control of their asthma.[17]

Oral terbutaline decreased serum theophylline levels by about 10% in 6 asthmatics, but the control of asthma was improved.[18] Another study in asthmatic children, found that terbutaline elixir 75 micrograms/kg three times daily reduced steady-state serum levels of theophylline by 22%, but the symptoms of cough and wheeze improved.[19] Yet another study found no changes in the pharmacokinetics of aminophylline in asthmatic children given terbutaline.[20]

(f) Unspecified beta$_2$-agonists

In 1990, the UK Committee on Safety of Medicines noted that of 26 reports they had on record of hypokalaemia with **xanthines** or beta-2 agonists [both unnamed], 9 occurred in patients receiving both groups of drugs. In 5 of these 9 cases, the hypokalaemia had no clinical consequence. However, in 2 cases it resulted in cardiorespiratory arrest, in one case confusion, and in one case intestinal pseudo-obstruction.[21]

Mechanism

Beta$_2$-agonists can cause hypokalaemia, particularly when they are given parenterally or by nebuliser. Xanthines such as theophylline can also cause hypokalaemia, and this is a common feature of theophylline toxicity. The potassium lowering effects of both these groups of drugs are additive. Why some beta-agonists lower serum theophylline levels is not known.

Importance and management

Concurrent use is beneficial, but the reports outlined above illustrate some of the disadvantages and adverse effects that have been identified. In particular, it has been suggested that the use of intravenous beta-agonists in acutely ill patients on theophylline may be hazardous because of the risk of profound hypokalaemia and cardiac arrhythmias.[7,16] Monitoring of serum potassium in these situations was suggested.[16] Moreover, the CSM in the UK particularly recommend monitoring potassium levels in those with severe asthma as the hypokalaemic effects of beta$_2$-agonists can be potentiated by theophylline and its derivatives, corticosteroids, diuretics and hypoxia.[21]

1. van den Berg BTJ, Derks MGM, Koolen MGJ, Braat MCP, Butter JJ, van Boxtel CJ. Pharmacokinetic/pharmacodynamic modelling of the eosinopenic and hypokalemic effects of formoterol and theophylline combination in healthy men. *Pulm Pharmacol Ther* (1999) 12, 185–92.
2. Hemstreet MP, Miles MV, Rutland RO. Effect of intravenous isoproterenol on theophylline kinetics. *J Allergy Clin Immunol* (1982) 69, 360–4.
3. O'Rourke PP, Crone RK. Effect of isoproterenol on measured theophylline levels. *Crit Care Med* (1984) 12, 373–5.
4. Griffith JA, Kozloski GD. Isoproterenol-theophylline interaction: possible potentiation by other drugs. *Clin Pharm* (1990) 9, 54–7.
5. Conrad KA, Woodworth JR. Orciprenaline does not alter theophylline elimination. *Br J Clin Pharmacol* (1981) 12, 756–7.
6. Rachelefsky GS, Katz RM, Mickey MR, Siegel SC. Metaproterenol and theophylline in asthmatic children. *Ann Allergy* (1980) 45, 207–12.
7. Whyte KF, Reid C, Addis GJ, Whitesmith R, Reid JL. Salbutamol induced hypokalaemia: the effect of theophylline alone and in combination with adrenaline. *Br J Clin Pharmacol* (1988) 25, 571–8.
8. Georgopoulos D, Wong D, Anthonisen NR. Interactive effects of systemically administered salbutamol and aminophylline in patients with chronic obstructive pulmonary disease. *Am Rev Respir Dis* (1988) 138, 1499–1503.
9. Dawson KP, Fergusson DM. Effects of oral theophylline and oral salbutamol in the treatment of asthma. *Arch Dis Child* (1982) 57, 674–6.
10. Poukkula A, Korhonen UR, Huikuri H, Linnaluoto M. Theophylline and salbutamol in combination in patients with obstructive pulmonary disease and concurrent heart disease: effect on cardiac arrhythmias. *J Intern Med* (1989) 226, 229–34.
11. Epelbaum S, Benhamou PH, Pautard JC, Devoldere C, Kremp O, Piussan C. Arrêt respiratoire chez une enfant asthmatique traitée par bêta-2-mimétiques et théophylline. Rôle possible de l'hypokaliémie dans les décès subits des asthmatiques. *Ann Pediatr (Paris)* (1989) 36, 473–5.
12. Amitai Y, Glustein J, Godfrey S. Enhancement of theophylline clearance by oral albuterol. *Chest* (1992) 102, 786–9.
13. Terra Filho M, Santos SRCJ, Cukier A, Verrastro C, Carvalho-Pinto RM, Fiss E, Vargas FS.Efeitos dos agonistas beta-2-adrenérgicos por via oral, sobre os níveis séricos de teofilina. *Rev Hosp Clin Fac Med Sao Paulo* (1991) 46, 170–2.
14. Amirav I, Amitai Y, Avital A, Godfrey S. Enhancement of theophylline clearance by intravenous albuterol. *Chest* (1988) 94, 444–5.
15. McCann JP, McElnay JC, Nicholls DP, Scott MG, Stanford CF. Oral salbutamol does not affect theophylline kinetics. *Br J Pharmacol* (1986) 89 (Proc Suppl), 715P.
16. Smith SR, Kendall MJ. Potentiation of the adverse effects of intravenous terbutaline by oral theophylline. *Br J Clin Pharmacol* (1986) 21, 451–3.
17. Chow OKW, Fung KP. Slow-release terbutaline and theophylline for the long-term therapy of children with asthma: A latin square and factorial study of drug effects and interactions. *Pediatrics* (1989) 84, 119–25.
18. Garty MS, Keslin LS, Ilfeld DN, Mazar A, Spitzer S, Rosenfeld JB. Increased theophylline clearance by terbutaline in asthmatic adults. *Clin Pharmacol Ther* (1988) 43, 150.
19. Danziger Y, Garty M, Volwitz B, Ilfeld D, Versano I, Rosenfeld JB. Reduction of serum theophylline levels by terbutaline in children with asthma. *Clin Pharmacol Ther* (1985) 37, 469–71.
20. Wang Y, Yin A, Yu Z. Effects of bricanyl on the pharmacokinetics of aminophylline in asthmatic patients [In Chinese]. *Zhongguo Yiyuan Yaoxue Zazhi* (1992) 12, 389–90.
21. Committee on Safety of Medicines. β$_2$-Agonists, xanthines and hypokalaemia. *Current Problems* (1990) 28.

Theophylline + Beta-blockers

Propranolol reduces the clearance of theophylline. More importantly, non-cardioselective beta-blockers such as nadolol and propranolol, listed in 'Table 20.2', (p.623), should not be given to asthmatic patients because they can cause bronchospasm. The concurrent use of theophylline and cardioselective beta-blockers such as atenolol, bisoprolol or metoprolol, listed in 'Table 20.1', (p.623), is not totally contraindicated, but some caution is still appropriate. Neither atenolol or bisoprolol affected the pharmacokinetics of theophylline. See also 'Antiasthma drugs + Beta-blockers', p.919.

Clinical evidence

(a) Pharmacokinetics

A study in 8 healthy subjects (6 of whom smoked 10 to 30 cigarettes daily) found that the clearance of a single dose of theophylline (as intravenous aminophylline) was reduced by 37% by **propranolol** 40 mg six-hourly. **Metoprolol** 50 mg six-hourly, did not alter the clearance in the group as a whole, but the smokers showed an 11% reduction in clearance.[1] Another study found that the steady-state plasma clearance of theophylline in 7 healthy subjects was reduced by 30% by **propranolol** 40 mg every 8 hours, and by 52% by **propranolol** 240 mg every 8 hours.[2] However, a further study found no significant pharmacokinetic interaction between theophylline and **propranolol**.[3] Three other studies found that the cardioselective beta-blockers **atenolol** 50 to 150 mg,[4,5] and **bisoprolol** 10 mg,[6] and the non-selective beta-blocker **nadolol** 80 mg[4] did not affect the pharmacokinetics of theophylline.

(b) Pharmacodynamics

Beta-blockers, particularly those that are not cardioselective, can cause bronchoconstriction, which opposes the bronchodilatory effects of theophylline. See 'betaxolol with theophylline and pranlukast', (p.919) for mention of a patient who had deterioration of asthma with this combination.

In a study in 8 healthy subjects, both **propranolol** 40 mg every 6 hours and **metoprolol** 50 mg every 6 hours prevented the mild inotropic effect seen with theophylline alone.[7]

Propranolol infusion reduced hypokalaemia and tachycardia that occurred after a theophylline overdose.[8,9] **Esmolol** has been used similarly.[10]

Mechanism

Propranolol possibly affects the clearance of theophylline by inhibiting its metabolism (demethylation and hydroxylation).[2,11]

Importance and management

The risk of severe, possibly even fatal bronchospasm when beta-blockers are used in asthmatics would seem to be far more important than any pharmacokinetic interaction with theophylline. See the warning in 'Antiasthma drugs + Beta-blockers', p.919. Therefore the non-cardioselective beta-blockers, such as propranolol, are contraindicated in patients with asthma or chronic obstructive pulmonary disease (COPD). Bronchospasm can occur with beta-blockers, given by any route of administration, even topically as eye drops. Cardioselective beta-blockers have less effect on the airways, but can still cause bronchoconstriction.

1. Conrad KA, Nyman DW. Effects of metoprolol and propranolol on theophylline elimination. *Clin Pharmacol Ther* (1980) 28, 463–7.
2. Miners JO, Wing LMH, Lillywhite KJ, Robson RA. Selectivity and dose-dependency of the inhibitory effect of propranolol on theophylline metabolism in man. *Br J Clin Pharmacol* (1985) 20, 219–23.
3. Minton NA, Turner J, Henry JA. Pharmacodynamic and pharmacokinetic interactions between theophylline and propranolol during dynamic exercise. *Br J Clin Pharmacol* (1995) 40, 521P.
4. Corsi CM, Nafziger AN, Pieper JA, Bertino JS. Lack of effect of atenolol and nadolol on the metabolism of theophylline. *Br J Clin Pharmacol* (1990) 29, 265–8.
5. Cerasa LA, Bertino JS, Ludwig EA, Savliwala M, Middleton E, Slaughter RL. Lack of effect of atenolol on the pharmacokinetics of theophylline. *Br J Clin Pharmacol* (1988) 26, 800–802.
6. Warrington SJ, Johnston A, Lewis Y, Murphy M. Bisoprolol: Studies of potential interactions with theophylline and warfarin in healthy volunteers. *J Cardiovasc Pharmacol* (1990) 16 (Suppl 5), S164–S168.
7. Conrad KA, Prosnitz EH. Cardiovascular effects of theophylline. Partial attenuation by beta-blockade. *Eur J Clin Pharmacol* (1981) 21, 109–114.
8. Kearney TE, Manoguerra AS, Curtis GP, Ziegler MG. Theophylline toxicity and the beta-adrenergic system. *Ann Intern Med* (1985) 102, 766–9.
9. Amin DN, Henry JA. Propranolol administration in theophylline overdose. *Lancet* (1985) i, 520–1.
10. Seneff M, Scott J, Freidman B, Smith M. Acute theophylline toxicity and the use of esmolol to reverse cardiovascular instability. *Ann Emerg Med* (1990) 19, 671–3.
11. Greenblatt DJ, Franke K, Huffman DH. Impairment of antipyrine clearance in humans by propranolol. *Circulation* (1978) 57, 1161–4.

Theophylline + Caffeine

Consumption of caffeine-containing beverages can raise serum theophylline levels, but the clinical relevance of this is unclear.

Clinical evidence, mechanism, importance and management

Caffeine can decrease the clearance of theophylline by 18 to 29%, prolong its half-life by up to 44% and increase its average serum levels by as much as 23%.[1-3] In addition, caffeine plasma levels were increased about two-fold when theophylline was given.[2] In these studies, caffeine was given in the form of tablets[1,2] or as 2 to 7 cups of instant coffee.[3] In one study, 2 of the subjects who did not normally drink coffee experienced headaches and nausea.[2]

The probable mechanism of the interaction is that the 2 drugs compete for the same metabolic pathway resulting in a reduction in metabolism and accumulation. In addition, when caffeine levels are high, a small percentage of it is converted to theophylline. There would, however, seem to be no good reason for those on theophylline to avoid caffeine (in **coffee**, **tea**, **cola drinks**, medications, etc.), but if otherwise unexplained adverse effects occur it might be worth checking if caffeine is responsible. In addition, caffeine intake could have an impact on the interaction of theophylline with other drugs.

1. Loi CM, Jue SG, Bush ED, Crowley JJ, Vestal RE. Effect of caffeine dose on theophylline metabolism. *Clin Res* (1987) 35, 377A.
2. Jonkman JHG, Sollie FAE, Sauter R, Steinijans VW. The influence of caffeine on the steady-state pharmacokinetics of theophylline. *Clin Pharmacol Ther* (1991) 49, 248–55.
3. Sato J, Nakata H, Owada E, Kikuta T, Umetsu M, Ito K. Influence of usual intake of dietary caffeine on single-dose kinetics of theophylline in healthy human subjects. *Eur J Clin Pharmacol* (1993) 44, 295–8.

Theophylline + Calcium channel blockers

Giving calcium channel blockers to patients on theophylline normally has no adverse effect on the control of asthma, despite the small or modest alteration that occur in serum theophylline levels with diltiazem, felodipine, nifedipine and verapamil. However, there are isolated case reports of unexplained theophylline toxicity in two patients given nifedipine and two patients given verapamil. Isradipine appears not to interact.

Clinical evidence

(a) Diltiazem

Diltiazem 90 mg twice daily for 10 days reduced the clearance of theophylline (given as a single 6-mg/kg dose of aminophylline) by 21%, and increased its half-life from 6.1 to 7.5 hours in 9 healthy subjects.[1] A 12% fall in the clearance of a single 5-mg/kg oral dose of theophylline was found when healthy subjects were given diltiazem 90 mg three times daily.[2] In 8 patients with asthma or chronic obstructive pulmonary disease (COPD), diltiazem 60 mg three times daily for 5 days reduced the clearance of steady-state theophylline (given as a continuous infusion of aminophylline 12 mg/kg/day) by 22% and increased its half-life from 5.7 to 7.5 hours.[3]

Conversely, other studies found no significant changes in peak steady-state theophylline levels in 18 patients with asthma given diltiazem 240 to 480 mg daily for 7 days,[4] or in 7 healthy subjects given diltiazem 120 mg twice daily for 7 days.[5] Similarly, there was no significant change in the half-life or clearance of theophylline (given as a single 250-mg intravenous dose of aminophylline) in healthy subjects given diltiazem 120 mg three times daily for 6 days.[6]

(b) Felodipine

Felodipine 5 mg eight-hourly for 4 days reduced the plasma AUC of theophylline (given as theophylline aminopropanol; *Oxyphylline*) in 10 healthy subjects by 18.3%, but had no effect on metabolic or renal clearance.[7]

(c) Isradipine

A three-way crossover study in 11 healthy subjects found that isradipine 2.5 or 5 mg every 12 hours for 6 days had no significant effect on the pharmacokinetics of a single 5-mg/kg dose of aminophylline oral solution.[8]

(d) Nifedipine

In one study, slow-release nifedipine 20 mg twice daily reduced the mean steady-state theophylline levels of 8 asthmatics by 30%, from 9.7 to 6.8 micrograms/ml. Levels fell by 50, 56 and 64% in three of the patients, but no changes in the control of the asthma (as measured by peak flow determinations and symptom scores) were seen.[9] However, many other studies have found no changes, or only small to modest changes, in the pharmacokinetics of theophylline (given as oral theophylline or as intravenous lysine theophylline[10] or aminophylline[11]) in healthy subjects[5,10-12] or asthmatic patients[4,13,14] when given nifedipine. The control of the asthma was unchanged by nifedipine.[13,14] Yet another study found that the combined use of slow-release theophylline and nifedipine improved pulmonary function and blood pressure control.[15]

In contrast, there are 2 case reports of patients who developed theophylline toxicity (theophylline levels raised to 30 and 41 micrograms/ml), apparently due to the addition of nifedipine.[16,17] In one case, the toxicity recurred on rechallenge, and resolved when the theophylline dosage was reduced by 60%.[17] During a Swan Ganz catheter study of patient response to nifedipine for pulmonary hypertension, 2 patients developed serious nifedipine adverse effects, which responded to intravenous aminophylline.[18]

(e) Verapamil

In one study, verapamil 80 mg every 6 hours for 2 days had no effect on the pharmacokinetics of theophylline (200 mg aminophylline every 6 hours) given to 5 asthmatics, and no effect on their spirometry (FVC, FEV_1, FEF_{25-75}).[19] Similarly, another study found verapamil 80 mg every 8 hours had no effect on the steady-state levels of sustained-release theophylline 3 mg/kg per day in healthy subjects.[20] In contrast, numerous other studies in healthy subjects (given intravenous or oral aminophylline or theophylline) have found modest reductions in theophylline clearance of between 8% and 23% with verapamil 40 to 120 mg every 6 to 8 hours.[2,6,12,21-23] One study showed that the extent of reduction in clearance depended on the verapamil dosage.[23] An isolated report describes a woman on digoxin and sustained release theophylline who developed signs of toxicity (tachycardia, nausea, vomiting) after starting to take verapamil 80 mg, increased to 120 mg every 8 hours. Her theophylline serum levels doubled over a 6-day period. Theophylline was later successfully reintroduced at one-third of the original dosage.[24] Another isolated report describes a patient who needed 50% less theophylline while taking verapamil 120 mg daily.[25]

Mechanism

It is believed that diltiazem and verapamil can, to a limited extent, decrease the metabolism of theophylline by the liver, possibly by inhibiting the cytochrome P450 isoenzyme CYP1A2.[26] Similarly, nifedipine may alter hepatic theophylline metabolism,[12] or it may increase the volume of distribution of theophylline.[10,11] Felodipine possibly reduces theophylline absorption.[7]

Importance and management

Adequately documented. The results are not entirely consistent but the overall picture is that the concurrent use of theophylline and these calcium channel blockers is normally safe. Despite the small or modest decreases in the clearance or absorption of theophylline seen with diltiazem, felodipine and verapamil, and the quite large reductions in serum levels seen in one study with nifedipine, no adverse changes in the control of the asthma were seen in any of the studies. However, very occasionally and unpredictably theophylline levels have risen enough to cause toxicity in patients given nifedipine (2 case reports) or verapamil (2 case reports), so that it would be prudent to be aware of this possibility of an interaction when prescribing these drugs.

1. Nafziger AN, May JJ, Bertino JS. Inhibition of theophylline elimination by diltiazem therapy. *J Clin Pharmacol* (1987) 27, 862–5.
2. Sirmans SM, Pieper JA, Lalonde RL, Smith DG, Self TH. Effect of calcium channel blockers on theophylline disposition. *Clin Pharmacol Ther* (1988) 44, 29–34.
3. Soto J, Sacristan JA, Alsar MJ. Diltiazem treatment impairs theophylline elimination in patients with bronchospastic airway disease. *Ther Drug Monit* (1994) 16, 49–52.
4. Christopher MA, Harman E, Hendeles L. Clinical relevance of the interaction of theophylline with diltiazem or nifedipine. *Chest* (1989) 95, 309–13.
5. Smith SR, Haffner CA, Kendall MJ. The influence of nifedipine and diltiazem on serum theophylline concentration-time profiles. *J Clin Pharm Ther* (1989) 14, 403–8.
6. Abernethy DR, Egan JM, Dickinson TH, Carrum G. Substrate-selective inhibition by verapamil and diltiazem: differential disposition of antipyrine and theophylline in humans. *J Pharmacol Exp Ther* (1988) 244, 994–9.
7. Bratel T, Billing B, Dahlqvist R. Felodipine reduces the absorption of theophylline in man. *Eur J Clin Pharmacol* (1989) 36, 481–5.
8. Perreault MM, Kazierad DJ, Wilton JH, Izzo JL. The effect of isradipine on theophylline pharmacokinetics in healthy volunteers. *Pharmacotherapy* (1993) 13, 149–53.
9. Smith SR, Wiggins J, Stableforth DE, Skinner C, Kendall MJ. Effect of nifedipine on serum theophylline concentrations and asthma control. *Thorax* (1987) 42, 794–6.
10. Jackson SHD, Shah K, Debbas NMG, Johnston A, Peverel-Cooper CA, Turner P. The interaction between i.v. theophylline and chronic oral dosing with slow release nifedipine in volunteers. *Br J Clin Pharmacol* (1986) 21, 389–92.
11. Adebayo GI, Mabadeje AFB. Effect of nifedipine on antipyrine and theophylline disposition. *Biopharm Drug Dispos* (1990) 11, 157–64.
12. Robson RA, Miners JO, Birkett DJ. Selective inhibitory effects of nifedipine and verapamil on oxidative metabolism: effects on theophylline. *Br J Clin Pharmacol* (1988) 25, 397–400.
13. Garty M, Cohen E, Mazar A, Ilfeld DN, Spitzer S, Rosenfeld JB. Effect of nifedipine and theophylline in asthma. *Clin Pharmacol Ther* (1986) 40, 195–8.
14. Yilmaz E, Canberk A, Eroğlu L. Nifedipine alters serum theophylline levels in asthmatic patients with hypertension. *Fundam Clin Pharmacol* (1991) 5, 341–5.
15. Spedini C, Lombardi C. Long-term treatment with oral nifedipine plus theophylline in the management of chronic bronchial asthma. *Eur J Clin Pharmacol* (1986) 31, 105–6.
16. Parrillo SJ, Venditto M. Elevated theophylline blood levels from institution of nifedipine therapy. *Ann Emerg Med* (1984) 13, 216–17.
17. Harrod CS. Theophylline toxicity and nifedipine. *Ann Intern Med* (1987) 106, 480.
18. Kalra L, Bone MF, Ariaraj SJP. Nifedipine-aminophylline interaction. *J Clin Pharmacol* (1988) 28, 1056–7.
19. Gotz VP, Russell WL. Effect of verapamil on theophylline disposition. *Chest* (1987) 92, 75S.
20. Rindone JP, Zuniga R, Sock JA. The influence of verapamil on theophylline serum concentrations. *Drug Metabol Drug Interact* (1989) 7, 143–7.
21. Nielsen-Kudsk JE, Buhl JS, Johannessen AC. Verapamil-induced inhibition of theophylline elimination in healthy humans. *Pharmacol Toxicol* (1990) 66, 101–3.
22. Gin AS, Stringer KA, Welage LS, Wilton JH, Matthews GE. The effect of verapamil on the pharmacokinetic disposition of theophylline in cigarette smokers. *J Clin Pharmacol* (1989) 29, 728–32.
23. Stringer KA, Mallet J, Clarke M, Lindenfeld JA. The effect of three different oral doses of verapamil on the disposition of theophylline. *Eur J Clin Pharmacol* (1992) 43, 35–8.
24. Burnakis TG, Seldon M, Czaplicki AD. Increased serum theophylline concentrations secondary to oral verapamil. *Clin Pharm* (1983) 2, 458–61.
25. Bangura L, Malesker MA, Dewan NA. Theophylline and verapamil: Clinically significant drug interaction. *J Pharm Technol* (1997) 13, 241–3.
26. Fuhr U, Woodcock BG, Siewert M. Verapamil and drug metabolism by the cytochrome P450 isoform CYP1A2. *Eur J Clin Pharmacol* (1992) 42, 463–4.

Theophylline + Carbamazepine

Two case reports describe a marked fall in serum theophylline levels when carbamazepine was given. Another single case report and a pharmacokinetic study describe a fall in serum carbamazepine levels when theophylline was given.

Clinical evidence

(a) Theophylline serum levels reduced

An 11-year-old girl with asthma was stable for 2 months with theophylline, until the phenobarbital she was taking was replaced by carbamazepine. The asthma worsened, her theophylline serum levels became subtherapeutic and the half-life of the theophylline was reduced from 5.25 to 2.75 hours. Asthmatic control was restored, and the half-life returned to pre-treatment levels 3 weeks after the carbamazepine was replaced by ethotoin.[1] The clearance of theophylline in an adult patient was doubled by carbamazepine 600 mg daily.[2]

(b) Carbamazepine serum levels reduced

The trough carbamazepine levels of a 10-year-old girl were roughly halved when she was given theophylline for 2 days, and she experienced a grand mal seizure. Her serum theophylline levels were also unusually high at 142 micromol/l (equivalent to 26 micrograms/ml) for the 5 mg/kg dosage she was taking, so it may be that the convulsions were as much due to this as to the fall in carbamazepine levels.[3]

A single-dose pharmacokinetic study in healthy subjects found that the AUC and maximum serum levels of carbamazepine were reduced by 31% and 45% respectively by oral aminophylline.[4]

Mechanism

Not established, but it seems probable that each drug increases the liver metabolism and clearance of the other drug, resulting in a reduction in their effects.[1,3] It is also possible that aminophylline interferes with the absorption of carbamazepine.[4]

Importance and management

Information seems to be limited to the reports cited so that the general importance is uncertain. Concurrent use need not be avoided, but it would be prudent to check that the serum concentrations of each drug (and their effects) do not become subtherapeutic.

1. Rosenberry KR, Defusco CJ, Mansmann HC, McGeady SJ. Reduced theophylline half-life induced by carbamazepine therapy. *J Pediatr* (1983) 102, 472–4.
2. Reed RC, Schwartz HJ. Phenytoin-theophylline-quinidine interaction. *N Engl J Med* (1983) 308, 724–5.
3. Mitchell EA, Dower JC, Green RJ. Interaction between carbamazepine and theophylline. *N Z Med J* (1986) 99, 69–70.
4. Kulkarni C, Vaz J, David J, Joseph T. Aminophylline alters pharmacokinetics of carbamazepine but not that of sodium valproate — a single dose pharmacokinetic study in human volunteers. *Indian J Physiol Pharmacol* (1995) 39, 122–6.

Theophylline + Cephalosporins

Ceftibuten and cefalexin appear not to interact with theophylline. Cefaclor has been implicated in two cases of theophylline toxicity in children, but studies in adult subjects found no pharmacokinetic interaction.

Clinical evidence, mechanism, importance and management

Ceftibuten 200 mg twice daily for 7 days was found to have no significant effect on the pharmacokinetics of a single intravenous dose of theophylline given to 12 healthy subjects.[1] A study in 9 healthy adults given a single 5-mg/kg intravenous dose of aminophylline found that **cefalexin** 500 mg, then 250 mg every 6 hours for 48 hours, had no significant effect on the kinetics of theophylline.[2]

A case report,[3] and a brief summary in the introduction of a study,[4] have suggested that **cefaclor** might have been responsible for the development of theophylline toxicity in 2 children. However, a single-dose study[4,5] and a steady-state study[6] in healthy adults found that **cefaclor** 750 mg daily for 8 and 9 days respectively had no effect on the pharmacokinetics of oral or intravenous theophylline. Although the pharmacokinetics of theophylline differ in adults and children a significant interaction with **cefaclor** seems unlikely.

No special precautions seem to be necessary with any of these antibacterials. Note that acute infections *per se* can alter theophylline pharmacokinetics.

1. Bachmann K, Schwartz J, Jauregui L, Martin M, Nunlee M. Failure of ceftibuten to alter single dose theophylline clearance. *J Clin Pharmacol* (1990) 30, 444–8.
2. Pfeifer HJ, Greenblatt DJ, Friedman P. Effects of three antibiotics on theophylline kinetics. *Clin Pharmacol Ther* (1979) 26, 36–40.
3. Hammond D, Abate MA. Theophylline toxicity, acute illness, and cefaclor administration. *DICP Ann Pharmacother* (1989) 23, 339–40.
4. Jauregui L, Bachmann K, Forney R, Bischoff M, Schwartz J. The impact of cefaclor on the pharmacokinetics of theophylline. *Recent Adv Chemother Proc Int Congr Chemother 14th Antimicrob Section 1* (1985) 694–5.
5. Bachmann K, Schwartz J, Forney RB, Jauregui L. Impact of cefaclor on the pharmacokinetics of theophylline. *Ther Drug Monit* (1986) 8, 151–4.
6. Jonkman JHG, van der Boon WJV, Schoenmaker R, Holtkamp A, Hempenius J. Clinical pharmacokinetics of theophylline during co-treatment with cefaclor. *Int J Clin Pharmacol Ther Toxicol* (1986) 24, 88–92.

Theophylline + Clopidogrel or Ticlopidine

Ticlopidine reduces the loss of theophylline from the body and is expected to raise its serum levels. Clopidogrel, an analogue of ticlopidine, appears not to interact.

Clinical evidence, mechanism, importance and management

(a) Clopidogrel

Clopidogrel 75 mg daily for 10 days did not alter the steady-state pharmacokinetics of theophylline given to 12 healthy subjects.[1] No problems are therefore anticipated with the concurrent use of these two drugs.

(b) Ticlopidine

Ticlopidine 250 mg twice daily for 10 days reduced the clearance of a single 5-mg/kg oral dose of theophylline in 10 healthy subjects by 37% and increased the half-life by 44%, from 514 to 731 minutes.[2] The reason is not known but it seems possible that ticlopidine inhibits the metabolism of theophylline by the liver. Information is limited, but it would now seem prudent to monitor the effects of concurrent use. It may be necessary to reduce the dosage of theophylline, particularly when serum levels are already at the top end of the range.

1. Caplain H, Thebault J-J, Neccari J. Clopidogrel does not affect the pharmacokinetics of theophylline. *Semin Thromb Hemost* (1999) 24, 65–8.
2. Colli A, Buccino G, Cocciolo M, Parravicini R, Elli GM, Scaltrini G. Ticlopidine-theophylline interaction. *Clin Pharmacol Ther* (1987) 41, 358–62.

Theophylline + Corticosteroids

Theophylline and corticosteroids have established roles in the management of asthma and their concurrent use is not uncommon. There are isolated reports of increases in serum theophylline levels (sometimes associated with toxicity) when oral or parenteral corticosteroids are given, but other reports show no changes. The general clinical importance of these findings is uncertain. Both theophylline and corticosteroids can cause hypokalaemia, which may be additive.

Clinical evidence

(a) Increased serum theophylline levels

Three patients in status asthmaticus with relatively stable serum concentrations of theophylline were given a 500-mg intravenous bolus of **hydrocortisone** followed 6 hours later by 200 mg given every 2 hours for 3 doses. In each case the serum theophylline levels rose from about 20 to between 30 and 50 micrograms/ml. At least 2 of the patients complained of nausea and headache.[1] Another study in 10 children (aged 2 to 6) with status asthmaticus showed that intramuscular **methylprednisolone** tended to increase the half-life of theophylline (given as oral aminophylline or theophylline).[2] A further study also reported that when intravenous aminophylline was given to 16 children taking corticosteroids (route and type not specified) the theophylline half-life was prolonged, from 5 to 6.2 hours, and the clearance was reduced by about one-third when compared with 10 children not taking corticosteroids.[3]

(b) Reduced serum theophylline levels

An 88% increase in the clearance of a single dose of intravenous aminophylline was seen in one of 3 healthy subjects when pretreated with oral **methylprednisolone**.[4] There was no significant change in clearance in the other 2 subjects.

(c) Theophylline levels unchanged

Seven healthy subjects given sustained relase theophylline had no significant change in steady-state theophylline clearance when they were given single doses of intravenous **methylprednisolone** 1.6 mg/kg and **hydrocortisone** 33 mg/kg in a crossover study, although there was a trend towards increased clearance.[5] Another study in 6 healthy subjects showed that a single 20-mg oral dose of **prednisone** had no significant effect on the pharmacokinetics of a single 200-mg oral dose of aminophylline.[6] The pharmacokinetics of a single 5.6-mg/kg intravenous dose of aminophylline was unchanged in 9 patients with chronic airflow obstruction when they were given **prednisolone** 20 mg daily for 3 weeks.[7] Intravenous bolus doses of 500 mg or 1 g of **hydrocortisone** did not affect theophylline levels in patients taking choline theophyllinate 400 mg every 12 hours for 8 days.[8] The elimination half-life of theophylline (given as intravenous aminophylline) was no different in premature infants who had been exposed to **betamethasone** *in utero* than in those who had not, although the exposed neonates had a wider range of theophylline metabolites indicating greater hepatic metabolism.[9,10]

In one study it was briefly mentioned that theophylline did not appear to affect **dexamethasone** metabolism.[11]

Mechanism

Not understood.

Importance and management

The concurrent use of theophylline and corticosteroids is common and therapeutically valuable, whereas the few reported interactions of theophylline with oral or parenteral corticosteroids are poorly documented and their clinical importance is difficult to assess because both increases, small decreases and no changes in the serum levels of theophylline have been seen. It is also questionable whether the results of studies in healthy subjects can validly be extrapolated to patients with status asthmaticus. There do not appear to be any data on the effect of *inhaled* corticosteroids on the clearance of theophylline. Both theophylline and corticosteroids can cause hypokalaemia, and the possibility that this may be potentiated by concurrent use should be considered.

1. Buchanan N, Hurwitz S, Butler P. Asthma—a possible interaction between hydrocortisone and theophylline. *S Afr Med J* (1979) 56, 1147–8.
2. De La Morena E, Borges MT, Garcia Rebollar C, Escorihuela R. Efecto de la metil-prednisolona sobre los niveles séricos de teofilina. *Rev Clin Esp* (1982) 167, 297–300.
3. Elvey SM, Saccar CL, Rocci ML, Mansmann HC, Martynec DM, Kester MB. The effect of corticosteroids on theophylline metabolism in asthmatic children. *Ann Allergy* (1986) 56, 520.
4. Squire EN, Nelson HS. Corticosteroids and theophylline clearance. *N Engl Reg Allergy Proc* (1987) 8, 113–15.
5. Leavengood DC, Bunker-Soler AL, Nelson HS. The effect of corticosteroids on theophylline metabolism. *Ann Allergy* (1983) 50, 249–51.
6. Anderson JL, Ayres JW, Hall CA. Potential pharmacokinetic interaction between theophylline and prednisone. *Clin Pharm* (1984) 3, 187–9.
7. Fergusson RJ, Scott CM, Rafferty P, Gaddie J. Effect of prednisolone on theophylline pharmacokinetics in patients with chronic airflow obstruction. *Thorax* (1987) 42, 195–8.
8. Tatsis G, Orphanidou D, Douratsos D, Mellissinos C, Pantelakis D, Pipini E, Jordanoglou J. The effect of steroids on theophylline absorption. *J Int Med Res* (1991) 19, 326–9.
9. Jager-Roman E, Doyle PE, Thomas D, Baird-Lambert J, Cvejic M, Buchanan N. Increased theophylline metabolism in premature infants after prenatal betamethasone administration. *Dev Pharmacol Ther* (1982) 5, 127–35.
10. Baird-Lambert J, Doyle PE, Thomas D, Jager-Roman E, Cvejic M, Buchanan N. Theophylline metabolism in preterm neonates during the first weeks of life. *Dev Pharmacol Ther* (1984) 7, 239–44.
11. Brooks SM, Sholiton LJ, Werk EE, Altenau P. The effects of ephedrine and theophylline on dexamethasone metabolism in bronchial asthma. *J Clin Pharmacol* (1977) 17, 308.

Theophylline + Co-trimoxazole

Co-trimoxazole does not alter the pharmacokinetics of theophylline.

Clinical evidence, mechanism, importance and management

Co-trimoxazole 960 mg twice daily for 8 days had no effect on the pharmacokinetics of theophylline after a single 341-mg intravenous dose of aminophylline in 6 healthy subjects.[1] Another study found that co-trimoxazole 960 mg twice daily for 5 days had no effect on the pharmacokinetics of a single 267-mg oral dose of theophylline in 8 healthy subjects.[2] No special precautions would seem necessary if these drugs are given concurrently. However, note that acute infections *per se* can alter theophylline pharmacokinetics.

1. Jonkman JHG, Van Der Boon WJV, Schoenmaker R, Holtkamp AH, Hempenius J. Lack of influence of co-trimoxazole on theophylline pharmacokinetics. *J Pharm Sci* (1985) 74, 1103–4.
2. Lo KF, Nation RL, Sansom LN. Lack of effect of co-trimoxazole on the pharmacokinetics of orally administered theophylline. *Biopharm Drug Dispos* (1989) 10, 573–80.

Theophylline + Dextropropoxyphene (Propoxyphene)

Dextropropoxyphene does not significantly alter steady-state theophylline levels.

Clinical evidence, mechanism, importance and management

Pre-treatment with dextropropoxyphene 65 mg every 8 hours for 5 days did not significantly change the total plasma clearance of theophylline 125 mg every 8 hours at steady state in 6 healthy subjects.[1] There was a small reduction in the formation of the hydroxylated metabolite of theophylline. There would seem to be no need to avoid concurrent use or to take particular precautions.

1. Robson RA, Miners JO, Whitehead AG, Birkett DJ. Specificity of the inhibitory effect of dextropropoxyphene on oxidative drug metabolism in man: effects on theophylline and tolbutamide disposition. *Br J Clin Pharmacol* (1987) 23, 772–5.

Theophylline + Disulfiram

Theophylline clearance is decreased by disulfiram.

Clinical evidence

After taking disulfiram 250 mg daily for a week, the clearance of a 5-mg/kg intravenous dose of theophylline was decreased by a mean of about 21% (range 14.6 to 29.6%) in 20 recovering alcoholics. Those taking disulfiram 500 mg daily showed a mean decrease of 32.5% (range 21.6 to 49.6%).[1] Smoking appeared to have no important effects on the extent of this interaction.

Mechanism

Disulfiram inhibits the liver enzymes concerned with the both the hydroxylation and demethylation of theophylline, thereby reducing its clearance from the body.

Importance and management

Information appears to be limited to this study but it would seem to be an established and clinically important interaction. Monitor the serum levels of theophylline and its effects if disulfiram is added, anticipating the need to reduce the theophylline dosage, bearing in mind that the extent of this interaction appears to depend upon the dosage of disulfiram used.

1. Loi C-M, Day JD, Jue SG, Bush ED, Costello P, Dewey LV, Vestal RE. Dose-dependent inhibition of theophylline metabolism by disulfiram in recovering alcoholics. *Clin Pharmacol Ther* (1989) 45, 476–86.

Theophylline + Donepezil

An open-label crossover study in 12 healthy subjects found that donepezil 5 mg daily for 10 days had no significant effects on the pharmacokinetics of theophylline. Dose modification or additional monitoring is not required during concurrent use.[1]

1. Tiseo PJ, Foley K, Friedhoff LT. Concurrent administration of donepezil HCl and theophylline; assessment of pharmacokinetic changes following multiple-dose administration in healthy volunteers. *Br J Clin Pharmacol* (1998) 46 (Suppl 1), 35–9.

Theophylline + Doxapram

Doxapram pharmacokinetics are unchanged by theophylline in premature infants, but agitation and increased muscle activity may occur in adults.

Clinical evidence, mechanism, importance and management

Intravenous theophylline does not affect the pharmacokinetics of doxapram given to treat apnoea in premature infants. No adjustment of the dosage of doxapram is needed in the presence of theophylline.[1] However, the makers of doxapram say that there may be an interaction between doxapram and aminophylline or theophylline, which is manifested by agitation and increased skeletal muscle activity. Care should be taken if these drugs are used together.[2]

1. Jamali F, Coutts RT, Malek F, Finer NN, Peliowski A. Lack of a pharmacokinetic interaction between doxapram and theophylline in apnea of prematurity. *Dev Pharmacol Ther* (1991) 16, 78–82.
2. Dopram (Doxapram hydrochloride). Baxter Healthcare Corporation. US Prescribing information, March 2004.

Theophylline + Enoximone

Aminophylline possibly reduces the beneficial cardiovascular effects of enoximone.

Clinical evidence, mechanism, importance and management

An experimental study into the mechanism of action of enoximone in 14 patients with ischaemic or idiopathic dilative cardiomyopathy found that pretreatment with aminophylline 7 mg/kg intravenously over 15 minutes reduced the beneficial haemodynamic effects of enoximone 1 mg/kg intravenously over 15 minutes.[1] The reason appears to be that each drug competes for inhibition of cAMP specific phosphodiesterases in cardiac and vascular smooth muscle. The clinical importance of this awaits evaluation.

1. Morgagni GL, Bugiardini R, Borghi A, Pozzati A, Ottani F, Puddu P. Aminophylline counteracts the hemodynamic effects of enoximone. *Clin Pharmacol Ther* (1990) 47, 140.

Theophylline + Ephedrine

Some data suggest that an increased frequency of adverse effects occurs when ephedrine is used with theophylline.

Clinical evidence, mechanism, importance and management

A double-blind randomised study in 23 children aged 4 to 14 found that when ephedrine was combined with theophylline (in a ratio of 25 mg ephedrine to 130 mg theophylline), the number of adverse reactions increased significantly when compared with each drug taken separately. Moreover, the combination was no more effective than theophylline alone. The combination was associated with insomnia (14 patients), nervousness (13) and gastrointestinal complaints (18), including vomiting (12). The serum theophylline levels were unchanged by ephedrine.[1] A previous study by the same authors in 12 asthmatic children given ephedrine and aminophylline produced similar results.[2] In contrast, a later study suggested that ephedrine 25 mg every 8 hours given with aminophylline did produce improvements in spirometry and no adverse effects were seen. However, it was calculated that the theophylline dosage used was about half that used in the previous study.[3]

In the treatment of asthma, ephedrine has been largely superseded by more selective sympathomimetics, which have fewer adverse effects. Ephedrine is still an ingredient of a number of cough and cold remedies, when it may be combined with theophylline (e.g. *Franol*).

1. Weinberger M, Bronsky E, Bensch GW, Bock GN, Yecies JJ. Interaction of ephedrine and theophylline. *Clin Pharmacol Ther* (1975) 17, 585–92.
2. Weinberger MM, Bronsky EA. Evaluation of oral bronchodilator therapy in asthmatic children. *J Pediatr* (1974) 84, 421–7.
3. Tinkelman DG, Avner SE. Ephedrine therapy in asthmatic children. Clinical tolerance and absence of side effects. *JAMA* (1977) 237, 553–7.

Theophylline + Food

The effect of food on theophylline bioavailability is unclear. In general it appears that fat or fibre in food has no effect, while high-protein and high-carbohydrate diets decrease and increase the theophylline half-life respectively. Significant changes in theophylline bioavailability have been seen with both enteral feeds and total parenteral nutrition.

Clinical evidence

(a) Theophylline and food

The bioavailability of theophylline from sustained release preparations has been shown to be reduced,[1] increased,[1,2] or unaffected[3-5] when given immediately after **breakfast**. Dose dumping, leading to signs of theophylline toxicity, was seen in 3 children with asthma who were given a dose of *Uniphyllin* immediately after **breakfast**.[5] The **fat** content[6,7] or **fibre** content[8] of meals does not seem to significantly affect theophylline absorption. **High-protein** meals appear to decrease theophylline half-life,[9,10] whereas **high-carbohydrate** meals seem to increase it.[10] There was no difference in theophylline metabolism in one study when patients were changed from a **high-carbohydrate/low-protein** diet to a **high-protein/low-carbohydrate** diet.[11] One study found that changing from a **high-protein** to a **high-carbohydrate** meal had an effect on the metabolism of theophylline similar to that of cimetidine, and that the effects of the meal change and cimetidine were additive.[12] The effects of **spicy food** have been studied, but the clinical significance of the changes are uncertain.[13]

(b) Theophylline and enteral feeds

A patient with chronic obstructive pulmonary disease had a 53% reduction in his serum theophylline levels accompanied by bronchospasm when he was fed continuously through a nasogastric tube with ***Osmolite***. The interaction occurred with both theophylline tablets (*Theo-Dur*) and liquid theophylline, but not when the theophylline was given intravenously as aminophylline. It was also found that the interaction could be avoided by interrupting feeding 1 hour either side of the oral liquid theophylline dose.[14] Conversely, hourly administration of 100 ml of ***Osmolite*** did not affect the extent of theophylline absorption from a slow-release preparation (*Slo-bid Gyrocaps*) in healthy subjects, although the rate of absorption was slowed.[15] Similarly, hourly administration of 100 ml of ***Ensure*** for 10 hours did not affect the rate or extent of absorption of theophylline from *Theo-24* tablets in healthy subjects.[16]

(c) Theophylline and parenteral nutrition

An isolated report describes an elderly woman treated with aminophylline by intravenous infusion who showed a marked fall in her serum theophylline levels (from 16.3 to 6.3 mg/l) when the amino acid concentration of her parenteral nutrition regimen was increased from 4.25 to 7%.[17] A study in 7 patients with malnutrition (marasmus-kwashiorkor) found only a small, probably clinically irrelevant increase in the elimination of a single intravenous dose of theophylline when they were fed intravenously.[18]

Mechanism

Not fully understood. As with any sustained-release formulation, the presence of food in the gut may alter the rate or extent of drug absorption by altering gastrointestinal transit time. It has been suggested that high-protein diets stimulate liver enzymes thereby increasing the metabolism of the theophylline and hastening its loss from the body. High carbohydrate diets have the opposite effect. The cytochrome P450 isoenzyme CYP1A2 (the principal enzyme involved in the metabolism of theophylline) is known to be induced by chemicals contained in cruciferous vegetables[19] or formed by the action of high temperatures or smoke on meat.[20] This suggestion is supported by a study in which charcoal-grilled (broiled) beef decreased theophylline half-life by an average of 22%.[21] Further, high doses of daidzein, the principal isoflavone in soybeans, may inhibit CYP1A2 resulting in an increase in theophylline levels and half-life of about 33% and 41% respectively.[22]

Importance and management

The theophylline-food interactions have been thoroughly studied but there seems to be no consistent pattern in the way the absorption of different theophylline preparations is affected. Be alert for any evidence of an inadequate response that can be related to food intake. Avoid switching between different preparations, and monitor the effects if this is necessary. Consult the product literature for any specific information on food and encourage patients to take their theophylline consistently in relation to meals where this is considered necessary. Advise patients not make major changes in their diet without consultation. Monitor the effects of both enteral and parenteral nutrition, since theophylline dosage adjustments may be required.

1. Karim A, Burns T, Wearley L, Streicher J, Palmer M. Food-induced changes in theophylline absorption from controlled-release formulations. Part I. Substantial increased and decreased absorption with Uniphyl tablets and Theo-Dur Sprinkle. *Clin Pharmacol Ther* (1985) 38, 77–83.
2. Vaughan L, Milavetz G, Hill M, Weinberger M, Hendeles L. Food-induced dose-dumping of Theo-24, a 'once-daily' slow-release theophylline product. *Drug Intell Clin Pharm* (1984) 18, 510.
3. Johansson Ö, Lindberg T, Melander A, Wåhlin-Boll E. Different effects of different nutrients on theophylline absorption in man. *Drug Nutr Interact* (1985) 3, 205–11.
4. Sips AP, Edelbroek PM, Kulstad S, de Wolff FA, Dijkman JH. Food does not effect bioavailability of theophylline from Theolin Retard. *Eur J Clin Pharmacol* (1984) 26, 405–7.
5. Steffensen G, Pedersen S. Food induced changes in theophylline absorption from a once-a-day theophylline product. *Br J Clin Pharmacol* (1986) 22, 571–7.
6. Thebault JJ, Aiache JM, Mazoyer F, Cardot JM. The influence of food on the bioavailability of a slow release theophylline preparation. *Clin Pharmacokinet* (1987) 13, 267–72.
7. Lefebvre RA, Belpaire FM, Bogaert MG. Influence of food on steady state serum concentrations of theophylline from two controlled-release preparations. *Int J Clin Pharmacol Ther Toxicol* (1988) 26, 375–9.
8. Fassihi AR, Dowse R, Robertson SSD. Effect of dietary cellulose on the absorption and bioavailability of theophylline. *Int J Pharmaceutics* (1989) 50, 79–82.
9. Kappas A, Anderson KE, Conney AH, Alvares AP. Influence of dietary protein and carbohydrate on antipyrine and theophylline metabolism in man. *Clin Pharmacol Ther* (1976) 20, 643–53.
10. Feldman CH, Hutchinson VE, Pippenger CE, Blumenfeld TA, Feldman BR, Davis WJ. Effect of dietary protein and carbohydrate on theophylline metabolism in children. *Pediatrics* (1980) 66, 956–62.
11. Thompson PJ, Skypala I, Dawson S, McAllister WAC, Turner Warwick M. The effect of diet upon serum concentrations of theophylline. *Br J Clin Pharmacol* (1983) 16, 267–70.
12. Anderson KE, McCleery RB, Vesell ES, Vickers FF, Kappas A. Diet and cimetidine induce comparable changes in theophylline metabolism in normal subjects. *Hepatology* (1991) 13, 941–6.
13. Bouraoui A, Toumi A, Bouchahcha S, Boukef K, Brazier JL. Influence de l'alimentation épicée et piquante sur l'absorption de la théophylline. *Therapie* (1986) 41, 467–71.
14. Gal P, Layson R. Interference with oral theophylline absorption by continuous nasogastric feedings. *Ther Drug Monit* (1986) 8, 421–3.
15. Bhargava VO, Schaaf LJ, Berlinger WG, Jungnickel PW. Effect of an enteral nutrient formula on sustained-release theophylline absorption. *Ther Drug Monit* (1989) 11, 515–19.
16. Plezia PM, Thornley SM, Kramer TH, Armstrong EP. The influence of enteral feedings on sustained-release theophylline absorption. *Pharmacotherapy* (1990) 10, 356–61.
17. Ziegenbein RC. Theophylline clearance increase from increased amino acid in a CPN regimen. *Drug Intell Clin Pharm* (1987) 21, 220–1.
18. Cuddy PG, Bealer JF, Lyman EL, Pemberton LB. Theophylline disposition following parenteral feeding of malnourished patients. *Ann Pharmacother* (1993) 27, 846–51.
19. Pantuck EJ, Pantuck CB, Garland WA, Min BH, Wattenberg LW, Anderson KE, Kappas A, Conney AH. Stimulatory effect of Brussels sprouts and cabbage on human drug metabolism. *Clin Pharmacol Ther* (1979) 25, 88–95.
20. Kleman MI, Overvik E, Poellinger L, Gustafsson JA. Induction of cytochrome P4501A isoenzymes by heterocyclic amines and other food-derived compounds. *Princess Takamatsu Symp* (1995) 23, 163–71.
21. Kappas A, Alvares AP, Anderson KE, Pantuck EJ, Pantuck CB, Chang R, Conney AH. Effect of charcoal-broiled beef on antipyrine and theophylline metabolism. *Clin Pharmacol Ther* (1979) 23, 445–50.
22. Peng W-X, Li H-D, Zhou H-H. Effect of daidzein on CYP1A2 activity and pharmacokinetics of theophylline in healthy volunteers. *Eur J Clin Pharmacol* (2002) 59, 237–41.

Theophylline + Furosemide

Furosemide is reported to increase, decrease or to have no effect on serum theophylline levels. Both theophylline and diuretics can cause hypokalaemia, which may be additive.

Clinical evidence

In 8 asthmatics the mean peak serum level of a 300-mg dose of sustained release theophylline was reduced by 41%, from 12.14 to 7.16 micrograms/ml by a single 25-mg oral dose of furosemide.[1] Conversely, 10 patients with asthma, chronic bronchitis or emphysema, receiving a continuous maintenance infusion of aminophylline, had a 21% rise in their serum theophylline levels, from 13.7 to 16.6 micrograms/ml, 4 hours after being given a 40-mg intravenous dose of furosemide over 2 minutes.[2] A study in 12 healthy subjects failed to find any change in steady-state plasma theophylline levels when two 20-mg doses of oral furosemide were given 4 hours apart.[3]

Four premature neonates, two given oral and two given intravenous theophylline and furosemide had a fall in steady-state serum theophylline levels from 8 micrograms/ml down to 2 to 3 micrograms/ml when the furosemide was given within 30 minutes of the theophylline.[4]

A randomised placebo-controlled study in 24 infants receiving ECMO (extracorporeal membrane oxygenation) found that theophylline 2 mg/kg enhanced the response to diuresis with furosemide 1 mg/kg. If the response were maintained over a 24-hour period an extra 110 ml of fluid would have been lost.[5]

Mechanism

Not understood, although in theory furosemide may cause increased renal excretion of theophylline, which could explain the reduced levels.

Importance and management

Information is limited and the outcome of concurrent use is inconsistent and uncertain. If both drugs are used be aware for the potential for changes in serum theophylline levels. Consider measuring levels, and make appropriate dosage adjustments as necessary. Both theophylline and diuretics can cause hypokalaemia, and the possibility that this may additive on concurrent use should be considered. More study is needed to assess the clinical significance of the effects of theophylline and furosemide on diuresis.

1. Carpentiere G, Marino S, Castello F. Furosemide and theophylline. *Ann Intern Med* (1985) 103, 957.
2. Conlon PF, Grambau GR, Johnson CE, Weg JG. Effect of intravenous furosemide on serum theophylline concentration. *Am J Hosp Pharm* (1981) 38, 1345–7.
3. Jänicke U-A, Gundert-Remy U. Failure to detect a clinically significant interaction between theophylline and furosemide. *Naunyn Schmiedebergs Arch Pharmacol* (1986) 332 (Suppl), R100.
4. Toback JW, Gilman ME. Theophylline-furosemide inactivation? *Pediatrics* (1983) 71, 140–1.
5. Lochan SR, Adeniyi-Jones S, Assadi FK, Frey BM, Marcus S, Baumgart S. Coadministration of theophylline enhances diuretic response to furosemide in infants during extracorporeal membrane oxygenation: a randomized controlled pilot study. *J Pediatr* (1998) 133, 86–9.

Theophylline + Grapefruit juice

Grapefruit juice does not significantly alter theophylline pharmacokinetics.

Clinical evidence, mechanism, importance and management

In one study, 12 healthy subjects were given a single 200-mg oral dose of theophylline solution (*Euphyllin*) diluted in either 100 ml of grapefruit juice or water, followed by 900 ml more juice or water over the next 16 hours. The pharmacokinetics of the theophylline were found to be unchanged by the grapefruit juice.[1]

The authors of this study had previously shown that grapefruit juice had a small effect on the pharmacokinetics of 'caffeine', (p.923), and that one of the constituents of grapefruit juice (naringenin) inhibited the cytochrome P450 isoenzyme CYP1A2 *in vitro* (the principal enzyme in theophylline metabolism). However, most clinically relevant interactions between drugs and grapefruit juice are considered to be mediated via inhibition of intestinal CYP3A4.

There would seem to be no reason why patients on theophylline should avoid grapefruit juice.

1. Fuhr U, Maier A, Keller A, Steinijans VW, Sauter R, Staib AH. Lacking effect of grapefruit juice on theophylline pharmacokinetics. *Int J Clin Pharmacol Ther* (1995) 33, 311–14.

Theophylline + Griseofulvin

Griseofulvin appears not to alter the pharmacokinetics of theophylline to a clinically relevant extent.

Clinical evidence, mechanism, importance and management

A study was initiated because it was suspected that griseofulvin might possibly interact with theophylline. In 12 healthy subjects griseofulvin 500 mg daily for 8 days reduced the half-life of theophylline from 6.6 to 5.7 hours, and increased the clearance of two of its metabolites, after a single oral dose of aminophylline (*Teofylamin*). However, these changes are far too small to usually have any clinical relevance.[1] There would appear to be no reason for avoiding concurrent use.

1. Rasmussen BB, Jeppesen U, Gaist D, Brøsen K. Griseofulvin and fluvoxamine interactions with the metabolism of theophylline. *Ther Drug Monit* (1997) 19, 56–62.

Theophylline + H_2-blockers

Cimetidine raises theophylline serum levels and toxicity may develop. However, the extent of the interaction is unlikely to be clinically relevant in most patients with low-dose (e.g. non-prescription) cimetidine. Famotidine, nizatidine, ranitidine and roxatidine appear not to interact.

Clinical evidence

(a) Cimetidine

A number of case reports describe significantly increased theophylline levels, including many that were toxic, in patients (adults and children) given oral or intravenous aminophylline or theophylline and cimetidine.[1-6] A few cases describe serious effects such as seizures.[3,4]

In a large number of pharmacokinetic studies healthy subjects were given oral or intravenous aminophylline or theophylline[7-15] and patients were given oral or intravenous theophylline[16-20] with oral cimetidine 800 to 1200 mg daily in divided doses for 4 to 10 days. It was clearly shown that cimetidine prolonged the theophylline half-life by about 30 to 65% and reduced theophylline clearance by about 20 to 40%. Steady-state serum theophylline levels were raised about one-third.[16,17,20] The effect of cimetidine was maximal in 3 days in the one study assessing this.[16] The extent of the interaction did not differ between cimetidine 1200 mg and 2400 mg daily in one study,[10] although 2 further studies found that cimetidine 800 mg daily had less effect than cimetidine 1200 mg daily.[12,21] A study investigating low-dose cimetidine (200 mg twice daily; non-prescription dosage) found only a 12% decrease in theophylline clearance.[22]

Two studies found that the effect of cimetidine did not differ between young and elderly subjects,[12,23] whereas another found it was more pronounced in the elderly.[21] The effects of cimetidine did not differ between smokers and non-smokers in one study,[24] but were more pronounced in smokers in another.[25] In further study the effects of cimetidine were not affected by gender.[21] Three studies found that the inhibitory effects of cimetidine and ciprofloxacin were additive.[23,26,27]

Three studies found that intravenous cimetidine also inhibited the clearance of theophylline (given as intravenous aminophylline or sustained release theophylline).[28-30] In one of these, oral and intravenous cimetidine reduced theophylline clearance to the same extent, but when clearance was corrected for the lower bioavailability of the oral cimetidine, oral cimetidine resulted in a greater inhibition than intravenous cimetidine.[28] Another study found that the effects of a continuous infusion of cimetidine 50 mg/hour were similar to those of an intermittent infusion of 300 mg every 6 hours.[29]

In contrast, a further study[31] in healthy subjects found no clinically important interaction between intravenous aminophylline and an intravenous cimetidine infusion, but the aminophylline was given only 12 hours after starting the cimetidine, which may be insufficient for cimetidine to have had an effect. Similarly, a more recent study in 18 critically ill patients given a continuous intravenous infusion of cimetidine 50 mg/hour and low-dose aminophylline 10.8 mg/hour for just 48 hours found no clinically important interaction.[32]

(b) Famotidine

Famotidine 40 mg twice daily for 5 days had no effect on the pharmacokinetics of theophylline (given as intravenous aminophylline) in 10 healthy subjects.[14] In another study, 16 patients with bronchial asthma or chronic obstructive pulmonary disease (COPD) found that famotidine 20 mg twice daily for 3 days or more did not affect the clearance of theophylline.[33] Two further studies also found no interaction between intravenous theophylline and famotidine 20 or 40 mg twice daily for 4 or 9 days in COPD patients.[19,34] In a post-marketing surveillance study it was noted that 4 asthmatics on theophylline had been treated with famotidine 40 mg daily for 4 to 8 weeks without any problems.[35] In contrast, in a patient with COPD and liver impairment, serum levels and AUC after an intravenous dose of theophylline were raised by 78% and the clearance was halved by famotidine 40 mg daily for 8 days.[36] A later study by the same authors in 7 patients with COPD similarly treated, but with normal liver function, found that the AUC of theophylline was increased by 56% and the clearance was reduced by 35% by famotidine.[37]

(c) Nizatidine

A study in 17 patients with chronic obstructive pulmonary disease found that nizatidine 150 mg twice daily for a month had no effect on the steady-state pharmacokinetics of theophylline.[20] However, there were 6 reports of apparent interactions in the FDA Spontaneous Adverse Drug Reaction Database up to the end of August 1989. Four patients on theophylline developed elevated serum theophylline levels, with symptoms of toxicity in at least one case, when given nizatidine. The problems resolved when either both drugs, or just nizatidine were stopped.[38]

(d) Ranitidine

Many studies in healthy subjects (given intravenous aminophylline or theophylline by mouth)[10,11,15,39-41] and patients (given sustained-release theophylline)[17,20,42-45] have failed to find that ranitidine affects the pharmacokinetics of theophylline, even in daily doses far in excess of those used clinically (up to 4200 mg of ranitidine daily).[39] However, there are 7 reports describing a total of 10 patients, who developed theophylline toxicity when given ranitidine with sustained-release theophylline[46-51] or intravenous aminophylline.[52] The validity of a number of these reports has been questioned,[53-56] with the authors subsequently modifying some.[57,58]

(e) Roxatidine

Roxatidine 150 mg daily did not affect the clearance of theophylline.[59] Similarly, roxatidine 150 mg twice daily did not significantly change the pharmacokinetics of a single 250-mg intravenous dose of aminophylline in 9 healthy subjects.[60]

Mechanism

Cimetidine is an enzyme inhibitor that reduces the metabolism (predominantly *N*-demethylation)[61] of theophylline by the liver, thereby prolonging its stay in the body and raising its serum levels. Famotidine, nizatidine and ranitidine do not have enzyme-inhibiting effects so that it is not clear why they sometimes appear to behave like cimetidine.

Importance and management

The interaction between theophylline and cimetidine is very well documented (not all the references being listed here), very well established and clinically important. Theophylline serum levels normally rise by about one-third, but much greater increases have been seen in individual patients. Monitor theophylline levels, noting that one study found the peak effect was reached in 3 days. Initial theophylline dose reductions of 30 to 50% have been suggested to avoid toxicity.[4] Alternatively, use one of the other H_2-blockers (see also below). The effect of low-dose (e.g. non-prescription) cimetidine is unlikely to be clinically relevant unless theophylline levels are at the higher end of the therapeutic range. The situation with famotidine, nizatidine and ranitidine is not totally clear. They would not be expected to interact because they are not enzyme inhibitors like cimetidine, but very occasionally and unpredictably they appear to do so, nevertheless current opinion is that normally no special precautions are needed.[54] Roxatidine appears not to interact.

1. Weinberger MM, Smith G, Milavetz G, Hendeles L. Decreased theophylline clearance due to cimetidine. *N Engl J Med* (1981) 304, 672.
2. Campbell MA, Plachetka JR, Jackson JE, Moon JF, Finley PR. Cimetidine decreases theophylline clearance. *Ann Intern Med* (1981) 95, 68–9.
3. Lofgren RP, Gilbertson RA. Cimetidine and theophylline. *Ann Intern Med* (1982) 96, 378.
4. Bauman JH, Kimelblatt BJ, Carracio TR, Silverman HM, Simon GI, Beck GJ. Cimetidine-theophylline interaction. Report of four patients. *Ann Allergy* (1982) 48, 100–102.
5. Fenje PC, Isles AF, Baltodano A, MacLeod SM, Soldin S. Interaction of cimetidine and theophylline in two infants. *Can Med Assoc J* (1982) 126, 1178.
6. Uzzan D, Uzzan B, Bernard N, Caubarrere I. Interaction médicamenteuse de la cimétidine et de la théophylline. *Nouv Presse Med* (1982) 11, 1950.
7. Jackson JE, Powell JR, Wandell M, Bentley J, Dorr R. Cimetidine decreases theophylline clearance. *Am Rev Respir Dis* (1981) 123, 615–17.
8. Roberts RK, Grice J, Wood L, Petroff V, McGuffie C. Cimetidine impairs the elimination of theophylline and antipyrine. *Gastroenterology* (1981) 81, 19–21.
9. Reitberg DP, Bernhard H, Schentag JJ. Alteration of theophylline clearance and half-life by cimetidine in normal volunteers. *Ann Intern Med* (1981) 95, 582–5.
10. Powell JR, Rogers JF, Wargin WA, Cross RE, Eshelman FN. Inhibition of theophylline clearance by cimetidine but not ranitidine. *Arch Intern Med* (1984) 144, 484–6.
11. Ferrari M, Angelini GP, Barozzi E, Olivieri M, Penna S, Accardi R. A comparative study of ranitidine and cimetidine effects on theophylline metabolism. *G Ital Mal Torace* (1984) 38, 31–4.
12. Cohen IA, Johnson CE, Berardi RR, Hyneck ML, Achem SR. Cimetidine-theophylline interaction: effects of age and cimetidine dose. *Ther Drug Monit* (1985) 7, 426–34.
13. Mulkey PM, Murphy JE, Shleifer NH. Steady-state theophylline pharmacokinetics during and after short-term cimetidine administration. *Clin Pharm* (1983) 2, 439–41.
14. Lin JH, Chremos AN, Chiou R, Yeh KC, Williams R. Comparative effect of famotidine and cimetidine on the pharmacokinetics of theophylline in normal volunteers. *Br J Clin Pharmacol* (1987) 24, 669–72.
15. Adebayo GI. Effects of equimolar doses of cimetidine and ranitidine on theophylline elimination. *Biopharm Drug Dispos* (1989) 10, 77–85.
16. Vestal RE, Thummel KE, Musser B, Mercer GD. Cimetidine inhibits theophylline clearance in patients with chronic obstructive pulmonary disease: A study using stable isotope methodology during multiple oral dose administration. *Br J Clin Pharmacol* (1983) 15, 411–18.
17. Boehning W. Effect of cimetidine and ranitidine on plasma theophylline in patients with chronic obstructive airways disease treated with theophylline and corticosteroids. *Eur J Clin Pharmacol* (1990) 38, 43–5.
18. Roberts RK, Grice J, McGuffie C. Cimetidine-theophylline interaction in patients with chronic obstructive airways disease. *Med J Aust* (1984) 140, 279–80.
19. Bachmann K, Sullivan TJ, Reese JH, Jauregui L, Miller K, Scott M, Yeh KC, Stepanavage M, King JD, Schwartz J. Controlled study of the putative interaction between famotidine and theophylline in patients with chronic obstructive pulmonary disease. *J Clin Pharmacol* (1995) 35, 529–35.
20. Bachmann K, Sullivan TJ, Mauro LS, Martin M, Jauregui L, Levine L. Comparative investigation of the influence of nizatidine, ranitidine, and cimetidine on the steady-state pharmacokinetics of theophylline in COPD patients. *J Clin Pharmacol* (1992) 32, 476–82.
21. Seaman JJ, Randolph WC, Peace KE, Frank WO, Dickson B, Putterman K, Young MD. Effects of two cimetidine dosage regimens on serum theophylline levels. *Postgrad Med Custom Comm* (1985) 78, 47–53.
22. Nix DE, Di Cicco RA, Miller AK, Boyle DA, Boike SC, Zariffa N, Jorkasky DK, Schentag JJ. The effect of low-dose cimetidine (200 mg twice daily) on the pharmacokinetics of theophylline. *J Clin Pharmacol* (1999) 39, 855–65.
23. Loi C-M, Parker BM, Cusack BJ, Vestal RE. Aging and drug interactions.III. Individual and combined effects of cimetidine and ciprofloxacin on theophylline metabolism in healthy male and female nonsmokers. *J Pharmacol Exp Ther* (1997) 280, 627–37.
24. Cusack BJ, Dawson GW, Mercer GD, Vestal RE. Cigarette smoking and theophylline metabolism: effects of cimetidine. *Clin Pharmacol Ther* (1985) 37, 330–6.
25. Grygiel JJ, Miners JO, Drew R, Birkett DJ. Differential effects of cimetidine on theophylline metabolic pathways. *Eur J Clin Pharmacol* (1984) 26, 335–40.
26. Davis RL, Quenzer RW, Kelly HW, Powell JR. Effect of the addition of ciprofloxacin on theophylline pharmacokinetics in subjects inhibited by cimetidine. *Ann Pharmacother* (1992) 26, 11–13.
27. Loi C-M, Parker BM, Cusack BJ, Vestal RE. Individual and combined effects of cimetidine and ciprofloxacin on theophylline metabolism in male nonsmokers. *Br J Clin Pharmacol* (1993) 36, 195–200.
28. Cremer KF, Secor J, Speeg KV. Effect of route of administration on the cimetidine-theophylline drug interaction. *J Clin Pharmacol* (1989) 29, 451–6.
29. Gutfeld MB, Welage LS, Walawander CA, Wilton JH, Harrison NJ. The influence of intravenous cimetidine dosing regimens on the disposition of theophylline. *J Clin Pharmacol* (1989) 29, 665–9.
30. Krstenansky PM, Javaheri S, Thomas JP, Thomas RL. Effect of continuous cimetidine infusion on steady-state theophylline concentration. *Clin Pharm* (1989) 8, 206–9.
31. Gaska JA, Tietze KJ, Rocci ML, Vlasses PH. Theophylline pharmacokinetics: effect of continuous versus intermittent cimetidine IV infusion. *J Clin Pharmacol* (1991) 31, 668–72.
32. Mojtahedzadeh M, Sadray S, Hadjibabaie M, Fasihi M, Rezaee S. Determination of theophylline clearance after cimetidine infusion in critically ill patients. *J Infus Nurs* (2003) 26, 234–8.
33. Asamoto H, Kokura M, Kawakami A, Sawano T, Sasaki Y, Kohara N, Kitamura Y, Oishi T, Morishita H. Effect of famotidine on theophylline clearance in asthma and COPD patients. *Arerugi* (1987) 36, 1012–17.
34. Verdiani P, DiCarlo S, Baronti A. Famotidine effects on theophylline pharmacokinetics in subjects affected by COPD. Comparison with cimetidine and placebo. *Chest* (1988) 94, 807–10.
35. Chichmanian RM, Mignot G, Spreux A, Jean-Girard C, Hofliger P. Tolérance de la famotidine. Étude due réseau médecins sentinelles en pharmacovigilance. *Therapie* (1992) 47, 239–43.
36. Dal Negro R, Turco P, Pomari C, Trevisan F. Famotidina e teofillina: interferenza farmacocinetica cimetidino-simile? *G Ital Mal Torace* (1988) 42, 185–6.
37. Dal Negro R, Pomari C, Turco P. Famotidine and theophylline pharmacokinetics. An unexpected cimetidine-like interaction in patients with chronic obstructive pulmonary disease. *Clin Pharmacokinet* (1993) 24, 255–8.
38. Shinn AF. Unrecognized drug interactions with famotidine and nizatidine. *Arch Intern Med* (1991) 151, 810–14.
39. Kelly HW, Powell JR, Donohue JF. Ranitidine at very large doses does not inhibit theophylline elimination. *Clin Pharmacol Ther* (1986) 39, 577–81.
40. McEwen J, McMurdo MET, Moreland TA. The effects of once-daily dosing with ranitidine and cimetidine on theophylline pharmacokinetics. *Eur J Drug Metab Pharmacokinet* (1988) 13, 201–5.
41. Kehoe WA, Sands CD, Feng Long L, Hui Lan H, Harralson AF. The effect of ranitidine on theophylline metabolism in healthy ethnic Koreans. *Pharmacotherapy* (1994) 14, 373.
42. Seggev JS, Barzilay M, Schey G. No evidence for interaction between ranitidine and theophylline. *Arch Intern Med* (1987) 147, 179–80.
43. Zarogoulidis K, Economidis D, Paparoglou A, Pneumaticos I, Sevastou P, Tsopouridis A, Papaioanou A. Effect of ranitidine on theophylline plasma levels in patients with COPD. *Eur Respir J* (1988) 1 (Suppl 2), 195S.
44. Pérez-Blanco FJ, Huertas González JM, Morata Garcia de la Puerta IJ, Saucedo Sánchez R. Interacción de ranitidina con teofilina. *Rev Clin Esp* (1995) 195, 359–60.
45. Cukier A, Vargas FS, Santos SRCJ, Donzella H, Terra-Filho M, Teixeira LR, Light RW. Theophylline-ranitidine interaction in elderly COPD patients. *Braz J Med Biol Res* (1995) 28, 875–9.
46. Fernandes E, Melewicz FM. Ranitidine and theophylline. *Ann Intern Med* (1984) 100, 459.
47. Gardner ME, Sikorski GW. Ranitidine and theophylline. *Ann Intern Med* (1985) 102, 559.
48. Roy AK, Cuda MP, Levine RA. Induction of theophylline toxicity and inhibition of clearance rates by ranitidine. *Am J Med* (1988) 85, 525–7.
49. Dietemann-Molard A, Popin E, Oswald-Mammosser M, Colas des Francs V, Pauli G. Intoxication à la théophylline par interaction avec la ranitidine à dose élevée. *Presse Med* (1988) 17, 280.
50. Skinner MH, Lenert L, Blaschke TF. Theophylline toxicity subsequent to ranitidine administration: a possible drug-drug interaction. *Am J Med* (1989) 86, 129–32.
51. Hegman GW, Gilbert RP. Ranitidine-theophylline interaction — fact or fiction? *DICP Ann Pharmacother* (1991) 25, 21–5.
52. Murialdo G, Piovano PL, Costelli P, Fonzi S, Barberis A, Ghia M. Seizures during concomitant treatment with theophylline and ranitidine: a case report. *Ann Ital Med Int* (1990) 5, 413–17.
53. Muir JG, Powell JR, Baumann JH. Induction of theophylline toxicity and inhibition of clearance rates by ranitidine. *Am J Med* (1989) 86, 513–14.
54. Kelly HW. Comment: ranitidine does not inhibit theophylline metabolism. *Ann Pharmacother* (1991) 25, 1139.
55. Williams DM, Figg WD, Pleasants RA. Comment: ranitidine does not inhibit theophylline metabolism. *Ann Pharmacother* (1991) 25, 1140.
56. Dobbs JH, Smith RN. Ranitidine and theophylline. *Ann Intern Med* (1984) 100, 769.
57. Roy AK. Induction of theophylline toxicity and inhibition of clearance rates by ranitidine. *Am J Med* (1989) 86, 513.
58. Hegman GW. Comment: ranitidine does not inhibit theophylline metabolism. *Ann Pharmacother* (1991) 25, 1140–41.
59. Labs RA. Interaction of roxatidine acetate with antacids, food and other drugs. *Drugs* (1988) 35 (Suppl 3), 82–9.
60. Yoshimura N, Takeuchi H, Ogata H, Ishioka T, Aoi R. Effects of roxatidine acetate hydrochloride and cimetidine on the pharmacokinetics of theophylline in healthy subjects. *Int J Clin Pharmacol Ther Toxicol* (1989) 27, 308–12.
61. Naline E, Sanceaume M, Pays M, Advenier C. Application of theophylline metabolite assays to the exploration of liver microsome oxidative function in man. *Fundam Clin Pharmacol* (1988) 2, 341–51.

Theophylline + Idrocilamide

Idrocilamide given orally can increase serum theophylline levels.

Clinical evidence, mechanism, importance and management

Idrocilamide 600 mg daily for 3 days then 1200 mg for 4 days by mouth increased the half-life of a single dose of theophylline 2.5-fold, from 8.5 to 21.6 hours in 6 healthy subjects and reduced the clearance by 67%.[1] This is due to a reduction in the liver metabolism caused by the idrocilamide (see also 'Caffeine + Idrocilamide', p.923). Information is very limited but it indicates that concurrent use should be closely monitored.

Anticipate the need to reduce the theophylline dosage with oral idrocilamide.

1. Lacroix C, Nouveau J, Hubscher Ph, Tardif D, Ray M, Goulle JP. Influence de l'idrocilamide sur le metabolisme de la theophylline. *Rev Pneumol Clin* (1986) 42, 164–6.

Theophylline + Imipenem

Seizures developed in three patients on aminophylline or theophylline when given imipenem.

Clinical evidence, mechanism, importance and management

Two patients on intravenous aminophylline developed seizures within 11 to 56 hours of starting treatment with imipenem 500 mg given every 6 to 8 hours intravenously. Seizures developed in a third patient on theophylline after 6 days. In all 3, seizures occurred 2 to 3 hours after a dose of imipenem.[1] The reasons are not known. Theophylline serum levels appeared to be unchanged.[1] In an analysis of data from 1754 patients who had received imipenem in dose-ranging studies, 3% had seizures, and imipenem was judged to be associated with a third of these cases. However, the concurrent use of theophylline or aminophylline was not found to be a significant risk factor for the development of seizures with imipenem.[2] The general importance of these observations is uncertain but be aware of the cases mentioned.

1. Semel JD, Allen N. Seizures in patients simultaneously receiving theophylline and imipenem or ciprofloxacin or metronidazole. *South Med J* (1991) 84, 465–8.
2. Calandra G, Lydick E, Carrigan J, Weiss L, Guess H. Factors predisposing to seizures in seriously ill infected patients receiving antibiotics: experience with imipenem/cilastatin. *Am J Med* (1988) 84, 911–18.

Theophylline + Influenza vaccines

Normally none of the influenza vaccines (whole-virion, split-virion and surface antigen) interact with theophylline, but there are 3 reports describing rises in serum theophylline levels in a few patients attributed to the use of an influenza vaccine, accompanied by toxicity in some instances.

Clinical evidence

(a) Evidence of no interaction

Mean steady-state serum theophylline levels were not altered by a trivalent split-virion influenza vaccine (*Fluzone*) in 12 patients with asthma, although 1 patient had an increase in levels (see (b), below). Levels were measured before vaccination and 1, 3, 7 and 14 days after vaccination.[1] Similarly, no evidence of a rise in theophylline levels was found in a number of other studies in healthy subjects, both adults and children, on maintenance theophylline or aminophylline therapy, given various trivalent split-virion vaccines including *Fluzone*,[2] *Fluogen*,[3-5] *Influvac*,[6] *Mutagrip*[7] and various unnamed trivalent split-virion vaccines.[8-11] In addition, no change in the pharmacokinetics of theophylline (given as oral aminophylline) was found after use of a whole-virion vaccine[12] in healthy adults. No evidence of serious theophylline toxicity was seen in 119 elderly people on maintenance theophylline given an unspecified influenza vaccine.[13]

(b) Evidence of an interaction

Three patients who had been taking oral choline theophyllinate (oxtriphylline) 200 mg (equivalent to 128 mg of theophylline) every 6 hours for at least 7 days had a rise in their serum theophylline levels of 219, 89 and 85% respectively, within 12 to 24 hours of receiving 0.5 ml trivalent split-virion influenza vaccine (*Fluogen*, Parke Davis). In some cases effects persisted for up to 72 hours, and two patients showed signs of theophylline toxicity. A subsequent study in 4 healthy subjects found that the same dose of vaccine more than doubled the half-life of theophylline, from 3.3 to 7.3 hours and halved its clearance.[14]

A girl had a rise in theophylline levels from 20 to 34 micrograms/ml (with no sign of toxicity) within 5 hours of being given a trivalent split-virion vaccine.[15] In a study where 11 of 12 patients had no increase in theophylline levels after vaccination with *Fluzone*, one woman showed a rise in levels (from 10 to 24.5 micrograms/ml) accompanied by headaches and palpitations.[1]

The clearance of theophylline (given as choline theophyllinate) was reduced by 25% one day after influenza vaccination (trivalent influenza vaccine, *Fluogen*, Parke Davis) in 8 healthy subjects, but this was of borderline significance. Theophylline metabolism had returned to pre-vaccination levels after 7 days.[16]

Mechanism

Uncertain. If an interaction occurs, it has been suggested it is probably due to inhibition of the liver enzymes concerned with the metabolism of theophylline, possibly secondary to interferon production, resulting in theophylline accumulation in the body.[14,16] One suggestion is that vaccine contaminants, which are potent interferon-inducing agents, may be responsible (rather than the vaccine itself), so that an interaction would seem to be less likely with modern highly-purified subunit vaccines.[17] In one study where an interaction occurred, an increase in serum interferon levels was detected,[16] whereas, in two of the studies showing no interaction, no interferon production was detected.[5,12] Influenza infection *per se* can result in decreased theophylline clearance and theophylline toxicity.[18]

Importance and management

A very thoroughly investigated interaction, the weight of evidence being that no adverse interaction normally occurs with any type of influenza vaccine in children, adults or the elderly. Even so, bearing in mind the occasional and unexplained reports of an interaction[1,14,15] it would seem prudent to monitor the effects of concurrent use (for nausea headaches, palpitations), although problems are very unlikely to arise now that purer vaccines are available (see 'Mechanism').

1. Fischer RG, Booth BH, Mitchell DQ, Kibbe AH. Influence of trivalent influenza vaccine on serum theophylline levels. *Can Med Assoc J* (1982) 126, 1312–13.
2. Goldstein RS, Cheung OT, Seguin R, Lobley G, Johnson AC. Decreased elimination of theophylline after influenza vaccination. *Can Med Assoc J* (1982) 126, 470.
3. San Joaquin VH, Reyes S, Marks MI. Influenza vaccination in asthmatic children on maintenance theophylline therapy. *Clin Pediatr (Phila)* (1982) 21, 724–6.
4. Bukowskyj M, Munt PW, Wigle R, Nakatsu K. Theophylline clearance. Lack of effect of influenza vaccination and ascorbic acid. *Am Rev Respir Dis* (1984) 129, 672–5.
5. Grabowski N, May JJ, Pratt DS, Richtsmeier WJ, Bertino JS, Sorge KF. The effect of split virus influenza vaccination on theophylline pharmacokinetics. *Am Rev Respir Dis* (1985) 131, 934–8.
6. Winstanley PA, Tjia J, Back DJ, Hobson D, Breckenridge AM. Lack of effect of highly purified subunit influenza vaccination on theophylline metabolism. *Br J Clin Pharmacol* (1985) 20, 47–53.
7. Jonkman JHG, Wymenga ASC, de Zeeuw RA, van der Boon WVJ, Beugelink JK, Oosterhuis B, Jedema JN. No effect of influenza vaccination on the theophylline pharmacokinetics as studied by ultraviolet spectrophotometry, HPLC, and EMIT assay methods. *Ther Drug Monit* (1988) 10, 345–8.
8. Stults BM, Hashisaki PA. Influenza vaccination and theophylline pharmacokinetics in patients with chronic obstructive lung disease. *West J Med* (1983) 139, 651–4.
9. Gomolin IH, Chapron DJ, Luhan PA. Lack of effect of influenza vaccine on theophylline levels and warfarin anticoagulation in the elderly. *J Am Geriatr Soc* (1985) 33, 269–72.
10. Feldman CH, Rabinowitz A, Levison M, Klein R, Feldman BR, Davis WJ. Effects of influenza vaccine on theophylline metabolism in children with asthma. *Am Rev Respir Dis* (1985) 131 (4 Suppl), A9.
11. Bryett KA, Levy J, Pariente R, Gobert P, Falquet JCV. Influenza vaccine and theophylline metabolism. Is there an interaction? *Acta Ther* (1989) 15, 49–58.
12. Hannan SE, May JJ, Pratt DS, Richtsmeier WJ, Bertino JS. The effect of whole virus influenza vaccination on theophylline pharmacokinetics. *Am Rev Respir Dis* (1988) 137, 903–6.
13. Patriarca PA, Kendal AP, Stricof RL, Weber JA, Meissner MK, Dateno B. Influenza vaccination and warfarin or theophylline toxicity in nursing-home residents. *N Engl J Med* (1983) 308, 1601–2.
14. Renton KW, Gray JD, Hall RI. Decreased elimination of theophylline after influenza vaccination. *Can Med Assoc J* (1980) 123, 288–90.
15. Walker S, Schreiber L, Middelkamp JN. Serum theophylline levels after influenza vaccination. *Can Med Assoc J* (1981) 125, 243–4.
16. Meredith CG, Christian CD, Johnson RF, Troxell R, Davis GL, Schenker S. Effects of influenza virus vaccine on hepatic drug metabolism. *Clin Pharmacol Ther* (1985) 37, 396–401.
17. Winstanley PA, Back DJ, Breckenridge AM. Inhibition of theophylline metabolism by interferon. *Lancet* (1987) ii, 1340.
18. Kraemer MJ, Furukawa CT, Koup JR, Shapiro GG, Pierson WE, Bierman CW. Altered theophylline clearance during an influenza B outbreak. *Pediatrics* (1982) 69, 476–80.

Theophylline + Interferon alfa

Theophylline clearance is reduced by interferon alfa. One study found that it was halved.

Clinical evidence

A study in 5 patients with stable chronic active hepatitis B and 4 healthy subjects showed that 20 hours after being given a single 9- or 18-million-unit intramuscular injection of interferon (recombinant human interferon alfa A; Hoffman La Roche), the clearance of theophylline (given as intravenous aminophylline) was approximately halved (range 33 to 81%) in 8 of them. The mean theophylline elimination half-life was increased from 6.3 to 10.7 hours (1.5 to sixfold increases). One healthy subject showed no change. In the healthy subjects, 4 weeks after the study, the theophylline clearances were noted to have returned to their former values.[1]

Another study, in 11 healthy subjects given interferon alfa (*Roferon-A*; Hoffman La Roche) 3 million units daily for 3 days, found that the terminal half-life and AUC of the theophylline (given as aminophylline) were only increased by 10 to 15%, with a similar decrease in clearance.[2] Interferon alfa (*Intron-A*; Schering) 3 million units given 3 times a week for 2 weeks decreased the clearance of a single 150-mg oral dose of theophylline by 33% in 7 patients with cancer.[3]

Mechanism

Interferon alfa inhibits the liver enzymes[4] concerned with the metabolism of some drugs, including theophylline, so that it is cleared from the body more slowly and accumulates.

Importance and management

Direct information appears to be limited to these reports, only one of which found clear evidence of a clinically important interaction. So far there appear to be no reports of toxicity but it would seem prudent to monitor concurrent use closely (nausea, headaches, palpitations), taking theophylline levels if necessary. Patients with enhanced metabolism (e.g. smokers) are predicted to be most at risk.[1]

1. Williams SJ, Baird-Lambert JA, Farrell GC. Inhibition of theophylline metabolism by interferon. *Lancet* (1987) ii, 939–41.
2. Jonkman JHG, Nicholson KG, Farrow PR, Eckert M, Grasmeijer G, Oosterhuis B, De Noorde OE, Guentert TW. Effects of α-interferon on theophylline pharmacokinetics and metabolism. *Br J Clin Pharmacol* (1989) 27, 795–802.
3. Israel BC, Blouin RA, McIntyre W, Shedlofsky SI. Effects of interferon-α monotherapy on hepatic drug metabolism in cancer patients. *Br J Clin Pharmacol* (1993) 36, 229–35.
4. Williams SJ, Farrell GC. Inhibition of antipyrine metabolism by interferon. *Br J Clin Pharmacol* (1986) 22, 610–12.

Theophylline + Ipriflavone

An isolated report describes increased theophylline levels in a patient given ipriflavone.

Clinical evidence, mechanism, importance and management

The theophylline serum levels of a patient with chronic obstructive pulmonary disease, taking sustained-release theophylline 300 mg twice daily, rose from 9.5 to 17.3 micrograms/ml in the presence of ipriflavone 600 mg daily for about 4 weeks. No symptoms of toxicity occurred. The serum theophylline levels returned to roughly the initial level when the ipriflavone was stopped, and rose again when it was restarted.[1] *In vitro* studies with human liver microsomes suggest that ipriflavone can inhibit the cytochrome P450 isoenzyme CYP1A2 and the demethylation of theophylline,[2,3] which would reduce the loss of theophylline from the body.

Although so far only one case of this interaction has been reported, the *in vitro* studies suggest that it would be prudent to monitor the theophylline levels of any patient given ipriflavone, making any dosage reductions as necessary.

1. Takahashi J, Kawakatsu K, Wakayama T, Sawaoka H. Elevation of serum theophylline levels by ipriflavone in a patient with chronic obstructive pulmonary disease. *Eur J Clin Pharmacol* (1992) 43, 207–8.
2. Monostory K, Vereczkey L. The effect of ipriflavone and its main metabolites on theophylline biotransformation. *Eur J Drug Metab Pharmacokinet* (1996) 21, 61–6.
3. Monostory K, Vereczkey L, Lévai F, Szatmári I. Ipriflavone as an inhibitor of human cytochrome P450 enzymes. *Br J Pharmacol* (1998) 123, 605–10.

Theophylline + Isoniazid ± other antimycobacterials

Two short-term studies found that theophylline serum levels were slightly increased and clearance decreased by isoniazid. An isolated report describes theophylline toxicity in a patient one month after starting to take theophylline with isoniazid. However, another short-term study found that isoniazid slightly increased rather than decreased theophylline clearance. Isoniazid and rifampicin-containing therapy increased theophylline clearance during the initial few days of tuberculosis treatment in one study, but there is some evidence that it decreases it within 4 weeks in another. See also 'Theophylline + Rifamycins', p.952.

Clinical evidence

(a) Isoniazid alone

Theophylline toxicity has been described in one patient receiving concurrent treatment with isoniazid 5 mg/kg daily and theophylline, and this subsequently recurred on re-challenge.[1]

In 7 healthy subjects, high-dose isoniazid (10 mg/kg daily) for 10 days increased the 0 to 6-hour AUC of theophylline by only 8% (from 274 to 296 micromol/h/l). The theophylline was given as an intravenous infusion of aminophylline and the plasma levels after 6 hours were 22% higher (58 micromol/l compared with 48.5 micromol/l). Five subjects also showed an increase in isoniazid half-life and AUC, but these were not statistically significant.[2] Another study found that 400 mg isoniazid daily for 2 weeks reduced the mean clearance of theophylline (given as intravenous aminophylline) in 13 healthy subjects by 21%.[3]

However, another study in 4 healthy subjects given 300 mg isoniazid daily for 6 days, found that the clearance of theophylline given orally was increased by 16%, but no consistent changes were seen in any of the other pharmacokinetic parameters measured.[4]

(b) Isoniazid with other antimycobacterials

A study[5] in patients taking a combination of isoniazid, rifampicin, ethambutol and pyrazinamide for pulmonary tuberculosis and intravenous aminophylline 7.35 mg/kg daily for 7 days found the clearance of theophylline progressively increased, and was 53% faster on day 7. In contrast, in an earlier study by the same authors, after 4 weeks of the same antimycobacterials (isoniazid, rifampicin, ethambutol with or without pyrazinamide) the theophylline clearance in patients on long-term theophylline was about 35% slower than in a control group of similar patients not taking antimycobacterials.[6] A single report describes unexpectedly *high* serum theophylline levels 4 days after theophylline 300 mg twice daily was started in an alcoholic patient with hepatic impairment who had begun rifampicin and isoniazid 2 weeks previously.[7]

Mechanism

Unknown. It has been suggested that isoniazid inhibits the metabolism of theophylline by the liver, thereby reducing its loss from the body and increasing its plasma levels. However, see 'Importance and management', below.

With combined therapy, it was suggested that the effects of 'rifampicin', (p.952) might be more apparent during the initial 7 days, but that by week 4 the effect of isoniazid might predominate because of its reduced inactivation by rifampicin combined with a reduction in effect of rifampicin by auto-induction of its metabolism.[6]

Importance and management

The reason for the inconsistent results with isoniazid alone is not understood, nor is this interaction well established. It has been suggested that it may take 3 to 4 weeks for any significant increase in theophylline levels to occur.[1] However, if enzyme inhibition was the cause, the effects would be expected more rapidly than this. All of the studies cited covered a period of only 6 to 14 days, whereas the case report describes the effects over a period up to 55 days.[1] It has also been suggested that the dose of isoniazid may be important, with clearance of theophylline being unaffected by 'usual doses' of isoniazid, but reduced by larger doses.[8]

Isoniazid is usually given as part of combination chemotherapy in the treatment of tuberculosis and the effects of other drugs such as 'rifampicin', (p.952) may also need to be considered. With combined therapy, there is some evidence that in the short-term theophylline levels will decrease, but may increase during long-term therapy, but this requires confirmation.The outcome of concurrent isoniazid and theophylline use is uncertain and may be affected by other co-administered antitubercular therapy, but it would clearly be prudent to be alert for any evidence of changes in theophylline levels and toxicity if isoniazid is given.

1. Torrent J, Izquierdo I, Cabezas R, Jané F. Theophylline-isoniazid interaction. *DICP Ann Pharmacother* (1989) 23, 143–5.
2. Höglund P, Nilsson L-G, Paulsen O. Interaction between isoniazid and theophylline. *Eur J Respir Dis* (1987) 70, 110–16.
3. Samigun, Mulyono, Santoso B. Lowering of theophylline clearance by isoniazid in slow and rapid acetylators. *Br J Clin Pharmacol* (1990) 29, 570–3.
4. Thompson JR, Burckart GJ, Self TH, Brown RE, Straughn AB. Isoniazid-induced alterations in theophylline pharmacokinetics. *Curr Ther Res* (1982) 32, 921–5.
5. Ahn HC, Lee YC. The clearance of theophylline is increased during the initial period of tuberculosis treatment. *Int J Tuberc Lung Dis* (2003) 7, 587–91.
6. Ahn HC, Yang JH, Lee HB, Rhee YK, Lee YC. Effect of combined therapy of oral anti-tubercular agents on theophylline pharmacokinetics. *Int J Tuberc Lung Dis* (2000) 4, 784–7.

7. Dal Negro R, Turco P, Trevisan F, De Conti F. Rifampicin-isoniazid and delayed elimination of theophylline: a case report. *Int J Clin Pharmacol Res* (1988) 8, 275–7.
8. Thompson JR, Self TH. Theophylline and isoniazid. *Br J Clin Pharmacol* (1990) 30, 909.

Theophylline + Leukotriene receptor antagonists

Montelukast does not appear to alter theophylline levels. A single case report describes a rapid rise in theophylline levels after the addition of zafirlukast. Zafirlukast levels are modestly reduced by theophylline, but this does not appear to be clinically important.

Clinical evidence

(a) Montelukast

The pharmacokinetics of a single intravenous dose of theophylline were not significantly changed in a group of 16 healthy subjects after they took montelukast 10 mg daily for 10 days, but when they were given doses of montelukast 200 and 600 mg daily, the AUC of theophylline was reduced by 43 and 66% respectively. These doses are 20 and 60-fold higher than the usual 10 mg daily dose.[1]

(b) Zafirlukast

When zafirlukast was given with theophylline, the mean serum levels of zafirlukast were reduced by 30%, but the serum theophylline levels remained unchanged.[2] In contrast, an isolated report describes a 15-year-old asthmatic taking sustained release theophylline 300 mg twice daily (as well as inhaled fluticasone, salbutamol (albuterol) and salmeterol, and oral prednisolone) who became nauseous shortly after zafirlukast (dose not stated) was added to her treatment. An increase in her theophylline level from 11 to 24 mg/l was noted. The theophylline was stopped, and later attempts to reintroduce theophylline at lower doses resulted in the same dramatic increases in serum theophylline levels.[3]

Mechanism

Not understood.

Importance and management

Information about interactions between theophylline and montelukast seems to be limited. The studies indicate that when using normal clinical doses of montelukast no special precautions or dosage alterations are needed. Similarly, no adverse interaction would normally seem to occur with zafirlukast and theophylline; the isolated case is of doubtful general significance.

1. Malmstrom K, Schwartz J, Reiss TF, Sullivan TJ, Reese JH, Jauregui L, Miller K, Scott M, Shingo S, Peszek I, Larson P, Ebel D, Hunt TL, Huhn RD, Bachmann K. Effect of montelukast on single-dose theophylline pharmacokinetics. *Am J Ther* (1998) 5, 189–95.
2. Accolate (Zafirlukast). AstraZeneca UK Ltd. UK Summary of product characteristics, December 2004.
3. Katial RK, Stelzle RC, Bonner MW, Marino M, Cantilena LR, Smith LJ. A drug interaction between zafirlukast and theophylline. *Arch Intern Med* (1998) 158, 1713–5.

Theophylline + Loperamide

Loperamide delays the absorption of theophylline from a sustained-release preparation.

Clinical evidence, mechanism, importance and management

A study of the effects of altering the transit time of drugs through the small intestine found that when 12 healthy subjects were given high-dose loperamide (8 mg six-hourly for a total of 8 doses), the rate, but not extent, of absorption of a single 600-mg dose of sustained-release theophylline (*Theo-24*) was decreased. The maximum serum theophylline levels were reduced from 4.6 to 3.2 micrograms/ml, and this peak level occurred at 20 hours instead of 11 hours. One suggested reason is that loperamide inhibits the movement of the gut, thereby decreasing the dissolution rate of the *Theo-24* pellets.[1] More study is needed to establish the clinical significance of the interaction in patients on long-term theophylline therapy.

1. Bryson JC, Dukes GE, Kirby MG, Heizer WD, Powell JR. Effect of altering small bowel transit time on sustained release theophylline absorption. *J Clin Pharmacol* (1989) 29, 733–8.

Theophylline + Macrolides

Troleandomycin can increase serum theophylline levels, causing toxicity if the dosage is not reduced. Azithromycin, clarithromycin, dirithromycin, josamycin, midecamycin, rokitamycin, spiramycin, and telithromycin normally only cause modest changes in theophylline levels or do not interact at all. There are unexplained and isolated case reports of theophylline toxicity with josamycin and with clarithromycin. Roxithromycin usually has no relevant interaction but a significant increase in theophylline levels was seen in one study. See also 'Theophylline + Macrolides; Erythromycin', p.942.

Clinical evidence

(a) Azithromycin

In an analysis of the safety data from clinical trials of azithromycin, there was no evidence that the plasma levels of theophylline were affected in patients treated with both drugs.[1] Similarly, no adverse effects were reported in another clinical study of patients on azithromycin and theophylline.[2] Azithromycin 250 mg twice daily did not affect the clearance or serum levels of theophylline in patients with asthma.[3] However, a 68-year-old man had a marked but transient fall in his serum theophylline level when azithromycin was withdrawn, and this was confirmed on rechallenge.[4] The same authors conducted a study in 4 healthy subjects given azithromycin 500 mg on day 1 then 250 mg daily for 4 days and sustained-release theophylline 200 mg twice daily. Theophylline levels were slightly elevated during azithromycin therapy, and a transient drop occurred 5 days after azithromycin withdrawal.[5]

(b) Clarithromycin

Clarithromycin 250 mg twice daily for 7 days had no effect on the steady-state serum theophylline levels of 10 elderly patients with COPD.[6] Similarly, two other studies found that clarithromycin had little or no effect on theophylline pharmacokinetics.[3,7] Another study in healthy subjects given clarithromycin 500 mg twice daily for 4 days found a 17% rise in the AUC and an 18% rise in the maximum plasma levels of theophylline, but this was considered clinically unimportant.[8] A similar number of patients required an adjustment in theophylline dosage when treated with clarithromycin in two clinical trials in patients with an acute bacterial exacerbation of chronic bronchitis.[9,10] However, there are isolated reports of possible theophylline toxicity, including a case of rhabdomyolysis with renal failure requiring haemodialysis.[11,12] For a report of theophylline toxicity in a patient taking clarithromycin and levofloxacin, see 'Theophylline + Quinolones', p.951.

(c) Dirithromycin

In one study, 13 healthy subjects showed a fall in steady-state theophylline trough serum level of 18%, and a fall in peak serum level of 26% while taking dirithromycin 500 mg daily for 10 days, although this was not considered clinically relevant.[13] No significant changes in theophylline pharmacokinetics were seen in 14 patients with COPD when given dirithromycin 500 mg daily for 10 days.[14] This is supported by a similar single-dose study in 12 healthy subjects.[15]

(d) Josamycin

No clinically significant changes in serum theophylline levels were seen in 5 studies in patients (both adults and children)[16-18] or healthy subjects[19] given josamycin, but a modest rise was described in one study in children.[20] Another study reported a 23% reduction in the levels of theophylline (given as intravenous aminophylline) in 5 patients with particularly severe respiratory impairment, but no significant effect in 5 other patients with less severe disease.[21] However, an isolated report describes theophylline toxicity in a 80-year-old man who was given josamycin.[22]

(e) Midecamycin/Midecamycin diacetate

In one study, 18 asthmatic children showed a slight decrease in serum theophylline levels when they were given midecamycin 40 mg/kg daily for 10 days for a bronchopulmonary infection, but no changes were seen in 5 healthy adult subjects.[23]

Similarly, no significant changes in serum theophylline levels were seen in 20 patients on slow-release theophylline (*Theo-dur*) 300 mg twice daily, or intravenous theophylline 4 mg/kg three times daily, when they were given midecamycin diacetate (miocamycin; ponsinomycin) 1200 mg daily for 10 days.[24] A number of other studies confirm the absence of a clinically important interaction between oral or intravenous theophylline or intravenous aminophylline and midecamycin diacetate in children and adults.[25-28]

(f) Rokitamycin

Two studies in 12 adults with COPD and 11 elderly patients on theophylline found no significant changes in serum theophylline levels when they were given rokitamycin 600 to 800 mg daily for a week.[29,30]

(g) Roxithromycin

One study in 12 healthy subjects and another in 16 patients with chronic obstructive pulmonary disease found only minor increases in steady-state theophylline levels when they were given roxithromycin 150 mg twice daily, which were not considered clinically relevant.[31,32] Another study in 5 healthy subjects similarly showed that roxithromycin 300 mg twice daily did not affect the pharmacokinetics of theophylline.[33] However, another study reported a significant increase in serum theophylline levels in 14 patients with asthma who were given roxithromycin 150 mg twice daily, but since the amount was not stated it is difficult to assess the clinical relevance of this finding.[3]

(h) Spiramycin

A study in 15 asthmatic patients on theophylline showed that spiramycin 1 g twice daily for at least 5 days had no significant effect on their steady-state serum theophylline levels.[34]

(i) Telithromycin

A study in 24 healthy subjects given theophylline found that telithromycin 800 mg daily for 4 days did not increase exposure to theophylline to a clinically significant extent.[35]

(j) Troleandomycin

A series of 8 patients with severe chronic asthma found that troleandomycin 250 mg four times daily caused an average reduction in the clearance of theophylline (given as intravenous aminophylline) of 50%. One of them had a theophylline-induced seizure after 10 days, with a serum theophylline level of 43 micrograms/ml (normal range 10 to 20 micrograms/ml). The theophylline half-life in this patient had increased from 4.6 to 11.3 hours.[36] Other studies in healthy subjects[23,37] and patients[18] given oral theophylline have also found reductions in theophylline clearance and marked rises in serum theophylline levels and half-life due to troleandomycin, even at low doses.[38]

Mechanism

It is believed that troleandomycin forms inactive cytochrome P450-metabolite complexes within the liver, the effect of which is to reduce the metabolism (*N*-demethylation and 8-hydroxylation)[37] of theophylline, thereby reducing its loss from the body. Josamycin, midecamycin, clarithromycin, and roxithromycin are thought to rarely form complexes, and azithromycin, dirithromycin, rokitamycin and spiramycin are not thought to inactivate cytochrome P450.[39]

Importance and management

The interaction between theophylline and troleandomycin is established and well documented. If troleandomycin is added, monitor the levels of theophylline closely and adjust the dose as necessary. Reductions of 25 to 50% may be needed.[38,40] The situation with roxithromycin is uncertain since only 1 of 4 studies suggested an interaction, but it would be prudent to be alert for the need to reduce the theophylline dosage. Alternative macrolides that usually interact only moderately, or not at all are azithromycin, clarithromycin, dirithromycin, josamycin, midecamycin, rokitamycin and spiramycin. Telithromycin may also be a suitable alternative. However, even with these macrolides it would still be prudent to monitor the outcome because a few patients, especially those with theophylline levels at the high end of the range, may need some small theophylline dosage adjustments. In the case of azithromycin, care should be taken in adjusting the dose based on theophylline levels taken after about 5 days of concurrent use, as they may only be a reflection of a transient drop. In addition, acute infection *per se* may alter theophylline pharmacokinetics.

1. Hopkins S. Clinical toleration and safety of azithromycin. *Am J Med* (1991) 91 (Suppl 3A), 40S–45S.
2. Davies BI, Maesen FPV, Gubbelman R. Azithromycin (CP-62,993) in acute exacerbations of chronic bronchitis: an open, clinical, microbiological and pharmacokinetic study. *J Antimicrob Chemother* (1989) 23, 743–51.
3. Rhee YK, Lee HB, Lee YC. Effects of erythromycin and new macrolides on the serum theophylline level and clearance. *Allergy* (1998) 53 (Suppl 43), 142.
4. Pollak PT, Slayter KL. Reduced serum theophylline concentrations after discontinuation of azithromycin: evidence for an usual interaction. *Pharmacotherapy* (1997) 17, 827–9.
5. Pollack PT, MacNeil DM. Azithromycin-theophylline inhibition-induction interaction. *Clin Pharmacol Ther* (1999) 65, 144.
6. Gaffuri-Riva V, Crippa F, Guffanti EE. Theophylline interaction with new quinolones and macrolides in COPD patients. *Am Rev Respir Dis* (1991) 143, A498.
7. Gillum JG, Israel DS, Scott RB, Climo MW, Polk RE. Effect of combination therapy with ciprofloxacin and clarithromycin on theophylline pharmacokinetics in healthy volunteers. *Antimicrob Agents Chemother* (1996) 40, 1715–16.
8. Ruff F, Chu S-Y, Sonders RC, Sennello LT. Effect of multiple doses of clarithromycin (C) on the pharmacokinetics (Pks) of theophylline (T). *Intersci Conf Antimicrob Agents Chemother* (1990) 30, 213.
9. Bachand RT. Comparative study of clarithromycin and ampicillin in the treatment of patients with acute bacterial exacerbations of chronic bronchitis. *J Antimicrob Chemother* (1991) 27 (Suppl A), 91–100.
10. Aldons PM. A comparison of clarithromycin with ampicillin in the treatment of outpatients with acute bacterial exacerbation of chronic bronchitis. *J Antimicrob Chemother* (1991) 27 (Suppl A), 101–8.
11. Abbott Labs. Personal communication, February 1995.
12. Shimada N, Omuro H, Saka S, Ebihara I, Koide H. A case of acute renal failure with rhabdomyolysis caused by the interaction of theophylline and clarithromycin. *Nippon Jinzo Gakkai Shi* (1999) 41, 460–3.
13. Bachmann K, Nunlee M, Martin M, Sullivan T, Jauregui L, DeSante K, Sides GD. Changes in the steady-state pharmacokinetics of theophylline during treatment with dirithromycin. *J Clin Pharmacol* (1990) 30, 1001–5.
14. Bachmann K, Jauregui L, Sides G, Sullivan TJ. Steady-state pharmacokinetics of theophylline in COPD patients treated with dirithromycin. *J Clin Pharmacol* (1993) 33, 861–5.
15. McConnell SA, Nafziger AN, Amsden GW. Lack of effect of dirithromycin on theophylline pharmacokinetics in healthy volunteers. *J Antimicrob Chemother* (1999) 43, 733–6.
16. Ruff F, Prosper M, Puget JC. Théophylline et antibiotiques. Absence d'interaction avec la josamycine. *Therapie* (1984) 39, 1–6.
17. Jiménez Baos R, Casado de Frías E, Cadórniga R, Moreno M. Estudio de posibles interacciones entre josamicina y teofilina en niños. *Rev Farmacol Clin Exp* (1985) 2, 345–8.
18. Brazier JL, Kofman J, Faucon G, Perrin-Fayolle M, Lepape A, Lanoue R. Retard d'élimination de la théophylline dû á la troléandomycine. Absence d'effet de la josamycine. *Therapie* (1980) 35, 545–9.
19. Selles JP, Panis G, Jaber H, Bres J, Armando P. Influence of josamycine on theophylline kinetics. *Proceedings of the 13th International Congress on Chemotherapy, Vienna* (1983) Aug 28–Sept 2, 15–20.
20. Vallarino G, Merlini M, Vallarino R. Josamicina e teofillinici nella patologia respiratoria pediatrica. *G Ital Chemioter* (1982) 29 (Suppl 1), 129–33.
21. Bartolucci L, Gradoli C, Vincenzi V, Iapadre M, Valori C. Macrolide antibiotics and serum theophylline levels in relation to the severity of the respiratory impairment: a comparison between the effects of erythromycin and josamycin. *Chemioterapia* (1984) 3, 286–90.
22. Barbare JC, Martin F, Biour M. Surdosage en théophylline at anomalies des tests hépatiques associés à la prise de josamycine. *Therapie* (1990) 45, 357–58.
23. Lavarenne J, Paire M, Talon O. Influence d'un nouveau macrolide, la midécamycine, sur les taux sanguins de théophylline. *Therapie* (1981) 36, 451–6.
24. Rimoldi R, Bandera M, Fioretti M, Giorcelli R. Miocamycin and theophylline blood levels. *Chemioterapia* (1986) 5, 213–16.
25. Principi N, Onorato J, Giuliani MG, Vigano A. Effect of miocamycin on theophylline kinetics in children. *Eur J Clin Pharmacol* (1987) 31, 701–4.
26. Couet W, Ingrand I, Reigner B, Girault J, Bizouard J, Fourtillan JB. Lack of effect of ponsinomycin on the plasma pharmacokinetics of theophylline. *Eur J Clin Pharmacol* (1989) 37, 101–4.
27. Dal Negro R, Turco P, Pomari C, de Conti F. Miocamycin doesn't affect theophylline serum levels in COPD patients. *Int J Clin Pharmacol Ther Toxicol* (1988) 26, 27–9.
28. Principi N, Onorato J, Giuliani M, Viganó A. Effect of miocamycin on theophylline kinetics in asthmatic children. *Chemioterapia* (1987) 6 (Suppl 2), 339–40.
29. Ishioka T. Effect of a new macrolide antibiotic, 3'-O-propionyl-leucomycin A5 (Rokitamycin), on serum concentrations of theophylline and digoxin in the elderly. *Acta Ther* (1987) 13, 17–23.
30. Cazzola M, Matera MG, Paternò E, Scaglione F, Santangelo G, Rossi F. Impact of rokitamycin, a new 16-membered macrolide, on serum theophylline. *J Chemother* (1991) 3, 240–4.
31. Saint-Salvi B, Tremblay D, Surjus A, Lefebvre MA. A study of the interaction of roxithromycin with theophylline and carbamazepine. *J Antimicrob Chemother* (1987) 20 (Suppl B), 121–9.
32. Bandera M, Fioretti M, Rimoldi R, Lazzarini A, Anelli M. Roxithromycin and controlled release theophylline, an interaction study. *Chemioterapia* (1988) 7, 313–16.
33. Hashiguchi K, Niki Y, Soejima R. Roxithromycin does not raise serum theophylline levels. *Chest* (1992) 102, 653–4.
34. Debruyne D, Jehan A, Bigot M-C, Lechevalier B, Prevost J-N, Moulin M. Spiramycin has no effect on serum theophylline in asthmatic patients. *Eur J Clin Pharmacol* (1986) 30, 505–7.
35. Bhargava V, Leroy B, Shi J, Montay G. Effect of telithromycin on the pharmacokinetics of theophylline in healthy volunteers. *Intersci Conf Antimicrob Agents Chemother* (2002) 42, 28.
36. Weinberger M, Hudgel D, Spector S, Chidsey C. Inhibition of theophylline clearance by troleandomycin. *J Allergy Clin Immunol* (1977) 59, 228–31.
37. Naline E, Sanceaume M, Pays M, Advenier C. Application of theophylline metabolite assays to the exploration of liver microsome oxidative function in man. *Fundam Clin Pharmacol* (1988) 2, 341–51.
38. Kamada AK, Hill MR, Brenner AM, Szefler SJ. Effect of low-dose troleandomycin on theophylline clearance: implications for therapeutic drug monitoring. *Pharmacotherapy* (1992) 12, 98–102.
39. Periti P, Mazzei T, Mini E, Novelli A. Pharmacokinetic drug interactions of macrolides. Clin Pharmacokinet (1992) 23, 106–31. Correction. *ibid.* (1993) 24, 70.
40. Eitches RW, Rachelefsky GS, Katz RM, Mendoza GR, Siegel SC. Methylprednisolone and troleandomycin in treatment of steroid-dependent asthmatic children. *Am J Dis Child* (1985) 139, 264–8.

Theophylline + Macrolides; Erythromycin

Theophylline serum levels can be increased by erythromycin. Toxicity may develop in those patients whose serum levels are at the higher end of the therapeutic range unless the dosage is reduced. The onset may be delayed for several days, and not all pa-

tients demonstrate this interaction. Erythromycin levels may possibly fall to subtherapeutic concentrations. For the effect of other macrolides, see 'Theophylline + Macrolides', p.941.

Clinical evidence

(a) Theophylline serum levels increased

The peak serum theophylline levels of 12 patients with COPD given aminophylline 4 mg/kg orally every 6 hours were raised by 28% by erythromycin stearate 500 mg every 6 hours, given for 2 days. The clearance was reduced by 22%. Only one patient developed clinical signs of toxicity, although the authors suggest this may because the patients had low theophylline levels (11 micrograms/ml) to start with and they may not have been studied for long enough to detect the full effect of the erythromycin.[1] Several single-dose studies in healthy or asthmatic adults given aminophylline or theophylline have demonstrated this interaction[2-6] and multiple-dose studies with aminophylline have also shown altered theophylline pharmacokinetics.[7,8] A multiple-dose study in asthmatic children showed a 40% rise in the levels of theophylline (given as intravenous aminophylline).[9] There was often wide inter-subject variability, and not all patients demonstrated the interaction.[1,4,6-9] In addition to the studies, there are several case reports where erythromycin was thought to have caused previously therapeutic theophylline concentrations to rise to toxic levels. In 3 cases the level rose twofold, with accompanying symptoms of toxicity,[10-12] and in one case the patient developed a fatal cardiac arrhythmia.[13]

Conversely, several studies in both healthy adults,[14-17] and adults with COPD[5,18] did not demonstrate any clinically significant interaction, although two of these studies did find reduced clearance of theophylline in some subjects.[14,18]

(b) Erythromycin serum levels reduced

The peak serum levels of erythromycin 500 mg 8-hourly were almost halved and the 0 to 8-hour AUC was reduced by 38% when 6 healthy subjects were given a single 250-mg intravenous dose of theophylline.[6] Another pharmacokinetic study found that serum erythromycin levels fell by more than 30% when intravenous theophylline was given with oral erythromycin.[8] Earlier studies using intravenous erythromycin found no significant pharmacokinetic changes. The renal clearance was increased, but this did not affect the overall clearance.[17,19]

Mechanism

(a) Not fully understood. It seems most likely that erythromycin inhibits the metabolism of theophylline by the liver resulting in a reduction in its clearance from the body and a rise in its serum levels.

(b) It seems most likely that theophylline can affect the absorption of oral erythromycin.[17]

Importance and management

(a) The effects of erythromycin on theophylline are established (but still debated) and well documented. Not all the reports are referenced here. It does not seem to matter which erythromycin salt is used. Monitor theophylline levels and anticipate the need to reduce the theophylline dosage to avoid toxicity. Not all patients will show this interaction but remember it may take several days (most commonly 2 to 7 days) to manifest itself. Limited evidence suggests that levels may return to normal 2 to 7 days after stopping erythromycin.[10-12] There are many factors, such as smoking,[3,18] which affect theophylline kinetics, and which may play a role in altering the significance of the interaction in different patients. Those particularly at risk are patients with already high serum theophylline levels and/or taking high dosages (20 mg/kg body-weight or more). Where concurrent treatment cannot be avoided, a 25% reduction in theophylline dose has been recommended for patients with levels in the 15 to 20 micrograms/ml range,[1,2,20] but little dosage adjustment is probably needed for those at the lower end of the range, (below 15 micrograms/ml) unless toxic symptoms appear.[1,4] In practice erythromycin can probably be safely started with theophylline, with levels monitored after 48 hours and appropriate dosage adjustments then made.

(b) The fall in erythromycin levels caused by theophylline is not well documented, but what is known suggests that it may be clinically important. Be alert for any evidence of an inadequate response to the erythromycin and increase the dosage or change the antibacterials if necessary. Intravenous erythromycin appears not to be affected.

1. Reisz G, Pingleton SK, Melethil S, Ryan PB. The effect of erythromycin on theophylline pharmacokinetics in chronic bronchitis. *Am Rev Respir Dis* (1983) 127, 581–4.
2. Prince RA, Wing DS, Weinberger MM, Hendeles LS, Riegleman S. Effect of erythromycin on theophylline kinetics. *J Allergy Clin Immunol* (1981) 68, 427–31.
3. May DC, Jarboe CH, Ellenberg DT, Roe EJ, Karibo J. The effects of erythromycin on theophylline elimination in normal males. *J Clin Pharmacol* (1982) 22, 125–30.
4. Zarowitz BJM, Szefler SJ, Lasezkay GM. Effect of erythromycin base on theophylline kinetics. *Clin Pharmacol Ther* (1981) 29, 601–5.
5. Richer C, Mathieu M, Bah H, Thuillez C, Duroux P, Giudicelli J-F. Theophylline kinetics and ventilatory flow in bronchial asthma and chronic airflow obstruction: Influence of erythromycin. *Clin Pharmacol Ther* (1982) 31, 579–86.
6. Iliopoulou A, Aldhous ME, Johnston A, Turner P. Pharmacokinetic interaction between theophylline and erythromycin. *Br J Clin Pharmacol* (1982) 14, 495–9.
7. Branigan TA, Robbins RA, Cady WJ, Nickols JG, Ueda CT. The effects of erythromycin on the absorption and disposition kinetics of theophylline. *Eur J Clin Pharmacol* (1981) 21, 115–20.
8. Paulsen O, Höglund P, Nilsson L-G, Bengtsson H-I. The interaction of erythromycin with theophylline. *Eur J Clin Pharmacol* (1987) 32, 493–8.
9. LaForce CF, Miller MF, Chai H. Effect of erythromycin on theophylline clearance in asthmatic children. *J Pediatr* (1981) 99, 153–6.
10. Cummins LH, Kozak PP, Gillman SA. Erythromycin's effect on theophylline blood level. *Pediatrics* (1977) 59, 144–5.
11. Cummins LH, Kozak PP, Gillman SA. Theophylline determinations. *Ann Allergy* (1976) 37, 450–51.
12. Green JA, Clementi WA. Decrease in theophylline clearance after the administration of erythromycin to a patient with obstructive lung disease. *Drug Intell Clin Pharm* (1983) 17, 370–2.
13. Andrews PA. Interactions with ciprofloxacin and erythromycin leading to aminophylline toxicity. *Nephrol Dial Transplant* (1998) 13, 1006–8.
14. Pfeifer HJ, Greenblatt DJ, Friedman P. Effects of three antibiotics on theophylline kinetics. *Clin Pharmacol Ther* (1979) 26, 36–40.
15. Kelly SJ, Pingleton SK, Ryan PB, Melethil S. The lack of influence of erythromycin on plasma theophylline levels. *Chest* (1980) 78, 523.
16. Maddux MS, Leeds NH, Organek HW, Hasegawa GR, Bauman JL. The effect of erythromycin on theophylline pharmacokinetics at steady state. *Chest* (1982) 81, 563–5.
17. Pasic J, Jackson SHD, Johnston A, Peverel-Cooper CA, Turner P, Downey K, Chaput de Saintonge DM. The interaction between chronic oral slow-release theophylline and single-dose intravenous erythromycin. *Xenobiotica* (1987) 17, 493–7.
18. Stults BM, Felice-Johnson J, Higbee MD, Hardigan K. Effect of erythromycin stearate on serum theophylline concentration in patients with chronic obstructive lung disease. *South Med J* (1983) 76, 714–18.
19. Hildebrandt R, Möller H, Gundert-Remy U. Influence of theophylline on the renal clearance of erythromycin. *Int J Clin Pharmacol Ther Toxicol* (1987) 25, 601–4.
20. Aronson JK, Hardman M, Reynolds DJM. ABC of monitoring drug therapy. Theophylline. *BMJ* (1992) 305, 1355–8.

Theophylline + Methotrexate

Methotrexate causes a modest reduction in the theophylline clearance. Theophylline may reduce methotrexate-induced neurotoxicity, but there is the possibility that it may also reduce methotrexate efficacy.

Clinical evidence

(a) Effects on theophylline

The apparent clearance of theophylline (given as oral aminophylline, choline theophyllinate or theophylline) was reduced by 19% in 8 patients with severe steroid-dependent asthma after 6 weeks' treatment with intramuscular methotrexate 15 mg weekly. Three patients complained of nausea and the theophylline dosage was reduced in one of them.[1]

(b) Effects on methotrexate

Four of 6 patients aged 3 to 16 years with acute lymphoblastic leukaemia with high-dose methotrexate-induced neurotoxicity had complete resolution of their symptoms when they were given a 2.5-mg/kg aminophylline infusion over 1 hour. The other 2 had some improvement. One patient also had symptom-relief with rapid-release theophylline.[2] Similar results were reported for another child who developed neurotoxicity after high-dose methotrexate. In this case, aminophylline was reported not to alter methotrexate levels.[3]

Mechanism

It is not known why theophylline clearance is altered. Methotrexate neurotoxicity may be linked with increased levels of adenosine. Theophylline is a competitive antagonist for adenosine receptors at serum concentrations within the therapeutic range used in asthma therapy.[2]

Importance and management

The clinical importance of reduced theophylline clearance is uncertain. Although aminophylline may reduce methotrexate-induced neurotoxicity, it should be borne in mind that *animal* studies suggest that the efficacy of methotrexate in rheumatoid arthritis and psoriasis may be reduced by theophylline and caffeine.[4] Although there is some evidence that theophylline does not alter the cytotoxic effects of methotrexate, this requires confirmation.[2]

1. Glynn-Barnhart AM, Erzurum SC, Leff JA, Martin RJ, Cochran JE, Cott GR, Szefler SJ. Effect of low-dose methotrexate on the disposition of glucocorticoids and theophylline. *J Allergy Clin Immunol* (1991) 88, 180–6.
2. Bernini JC, Fort DW, Griener JC, Kane BJ, Chappell WB, Kamen BA. Aminophylline for methotrexate-induced neurotoxicity. *Lancet* (1995) 345, 544–7.
3. Peyriere H, Poiree M, Cociglio M, Margueritte G, Hansel S, Hillaire-Buys D. Reversal of neurologic disturbances related to high-dose methotrexate by aminophylline. *Med Pediatr Oncol* (2001) 36, 662–4.
4. Montesinos MC, Yap JS, Desai A, Posadas I, McCrary CT, Cronstein BN. Reversal of anti-inflammatory effects of methotrexate by the nonselective adenosine receptor antagonists theophylline and caffeine: evidence that the anti-inflammatory effects of methotrexate are mediated via multiple adenosine receptors in rat adjuvant arthritis. *Arthritis Rheum* (2000) 43, 656–63.

Theophylline + Methoxsalen

Oral methoxsalen markedly increases theophylline levels.

Clinical evidence, mechanism, importance and management

In a single dose study, when 3 healthy subjects were given a 1.2-mg/kg oral dose of methoxsalen, with theophylline 600 mg one hour later, the AUC of theophylline was raised 1.7-fold, 2.1-fold and 2.7-fold, in the 3 subjects, respectively.[1] Methoxsalen probably inhibits the metabolism of theophylline by the cytochrome P450 isoenzyme CYP1A2. Although information is limited, the findings support what is known about caffeine and 'psoralens', (p.923). Theophylline dose reductions are likely to be required during concurrent use.

1. Apseloff G, Shepard DR, Chambers MA, Nawoot S, Mays DC, Gerber N. Inhibition and induction of theophylline metabolism by 8-methoxypsoralen. In vitro study in rats and humans. *Drug Metab Dispos* (1990) 18, 298–303.

Theophylline + Metoclopramide

Metoclopramide appears not to interact with slow-release theophylline.

Clinical evidence, mechanism, importance and management

A single 10-mg dose of metoclopramide taken 20 minutes before 600 mg of slow-release theophylline (*Theo-Dur*), caused a small 14.5% reduction in the bioavailability of the theophylline in 8 healthy subjects. This was not statistically significant. However, adverse effects (nausea, headache, tremors, CNS stimulation) were seen more often in those taking metoclopramide than in those taking placebo, possibly because metoclopramide caused an earlier rise in theophylline levels, and because the effects of the two drugs may be additive.[1] A later study found that metoclopramide 15 mg every 6 hours had no effect on the rate or extent of absorption of 600 mg of sustained-release theophylline (*Theo-24*) in 12 healthy subjects.[2] A similar lack of interaction was found in another study using *Theo-Dur*.[3] There would seem to be no reason for avoiding concurrent use.

1. Steeves RA, Robinson JD, McKenzie MW, Justus PG. Effects of metoclopramide on the pharmacokinetics of a slow-release theophylline product. *Clin Pharm* (1982) 1, 356–60.
2. Bryson JC, Dukes GE, Kirby MG, Heizer WD, Powell JR. Effect of altering small bowel transit time on sustained release theophylline absorption. *J Clin Pharmacol* (1989) 29, 733–8.
3. Sommers DK, Meyer EC, Van Wyk M, Moncrieff J, Snyman JR, Grimbeek RJ. The influence of codeine, propantheline and metoclopramide on small bowel transit and theophylline absorption from a sustained-release formulation. *Br J Clin Pharmacol* (1992) 33, 305–8.

Theophylline + Metronidazole

No interaction of clinical importance normally takes place if metronidazole is given to patients taking theophylline, but an isolated report describes seizures in one patient also taking ciprofloxacin.

Clinical evidence, mechanism, importance and management

There were no significant changes in the pharmacokinetics of theophylline after a single intravenous dose of aminophylline in 5 women taking metronidazole 250 mg three times a day for trichomoniasis.[1] Another study in 10 healthy subjects confirmed this finding.[2] However, an acutely ill elderly woman on theophylline had a generalised seizure while being treated with metronidazole and ciprofloxacin, despite her theophylline level being within the therapeutic range (10 to 20 micrograms/ml).[3] Both ciprofloxacin and, more rarely, metronidazole are associated with seizures.[3] Although the evidence is limited, no special precautions would seem to be necessary during concurrent use.

1. Reitberg DP, Klarnet JP, Carlson JK, Schentag JJ. Effect of metronidazole on theophylline pharmacokinetics. *Clin Pharm* (1983) 2, 441–4.
2. Adebayo GI, Mabadeje AFB. Lack of inhibitory effect of metronidazole on theophylline disposition in healthy subjects. *Br J Clin Pharmacol* (1987) 24, 110–13.
3. Semel JD, Allen N. Seizures in patients simultaneously receiving theophylline and imipenem or ciprofloxacin or metronidazole. *South Med J* (1991) 84, 465–8.

Theophylline + Mexiletine or Tocainide

Serum theophylline levels are increased by mexiletine and toxicity may occur. Tocainide has only a small and probably clinically unimportant effect on theophylline.

Clinical evidence

(a) Mexiletine

A man developed theophylline toxicity within a few days of starting to take mexiletine 200 mg three times daily. His serum theophylline level rose from 15.3 to 25 micrograms/ml, but fell to 14.2 micrograms/ml, and the symptoms of toxicity resolved, when the theophylline dosage was reduced by two-thirds.[1]

Other case reports describe 1.5 to threefold increases in theophylline serum levels (accompanied by clear signs of toxicity in some instances) in a total of 9 patients who were given mexiletine.[2-6] Theophylline dose reductions of 50% were required in 3 cases,[2,6] although 2 of the patients that did not require dose reductions had initial theophylline levels below the therapeutic range.[3] The arrhythmia of one patient was aggravated even at therapeutic serum theophylline levels, and mexiletine was discontinued.[4]

In 15 healthy subjects, mexiletine 200 mg three times a day for 5 days reduced the clearance of a single 5-mg/kg intravenous dose of theophylline by 46% in the women and 40% in the men. The theophylline half-life was prolonged by 96% (from 7.4 to 14.5 hours) in the women and 71% (from 8.7 to 14.9 hours) in the men.[7] Two further studies in healthy subjects given theophylline with mexiletine for 5 days found a reduction in steady-state theophylline clearance of 44 and 43%, and an increase in the AUC of 58 and 65%, respectively.[8,9]

(b) Tocainide

After taking tocainide 400 mg every 8 hours for 5 days, the pharmacokinetics of a single 5-mg/kg intravenous dose of theophylline was measured in 8 healthy subjects. The clearance was decreased by about 10% and the half-life slightly prolonged (from 9.7 to 10.4 hours), but these changes were not thought to be large enough to warrant altering theophylline doses.[10]

Mechanism

Mexiletine inhibits the metabolism (demethylation) of theophylline by the liver, thereby reducing its loss from the body and increasing its effects.[7,9,11] It is possible that the interaction is due to competitive inhibition of the cytochrome P450 isoenzyme CYP1A2.[12] Studies in *rats* have shown that tocainide has a substantially smaller effect on CYP1A1 than mexiletine.[13]

Importance and management

The interaction between theophylline and mexiletine is established and of clinical importance. Monitor concurrent use and reduce the theophylline dosage as necessary to prevent the development of theophylline toxicity. It has been suggested that 50% dose reductions may be necessary.[7] It seems doubtful if the interaction between theophylline and tocainide is clinically important but this needs confirmation.

1. Katz A, Buskila D, Sukenik S. Oral mexiletine-theophylline interaction. *Int J Cardiol* (1987) 17, 227–8.
2. Stanley R, Comer T, Taylor JL, Saliba D. Mexiletine-theophylline interaction. *Am J Med* (1989) 86, 733–4.
3. Ueno K, Miyai K, Seki T, Kawaguchi Y. Interaction between theophylline and mexiletine. *DICP Ann Pharmacother* (1990) 24, 471–2.

4. Kessler KM, Interian A, Cox M, Topaz O, De Marchena EJ, Myerburg RJ. Proarrhythmia related to a kinetic and dynamic interaction of mexiletine and theophylline. *Am Heart J* (1989) 117, 964–6.
5. Kendall JD, Chrymko MM, Cooper BE. Theophylline-mexiletine interaction: a case report. *Pharmacotherapy* (1992) 12, 416–18.
6. Inafuku M, Suzuki T, Ohtsu F, Hariya Y, Nagasawa K, Yoshioka Y, Nakahara Y, Hayakawa H. The effect of mexiletine on theophylline pharmacokinetics in patients with bronchial asthma. *J Cardiol* (1992) 22, 227–33.
7. Loi C-M, Wei X, Vestal RE. Inhibition of theophylline metabolism by mexiletine in young male and female nonsmokers. *Clin Pharmacol Ther* (1991) 49, 571–80.
8. Stoysich AM, Mohiuddin SM, Destache CJ, Nipper HC, Hilleman DE. Influence of mexiletine on the pharmacokinetics of theophylline in healthy volunteers. *J Clin Pharmacol* (1991) 31, 354–7.
9. Hurwitz A, Vacek JL, Botteron GW, Sztern MI, Hughes EM, Jayaraj A. Mexiletine effects on theophylline disposition. *Clin Pharmacol Ther* (1991) 50, 299–307.
10. Loi C-M, Wei X, Parker BM, Korrapati MR, Vestal RE. The effect of tocainide on theophylline metabolism. *Br J Clin Pharmacol* (1993) 35, 437–40.
11. Ueno K, Miyai K, Kato M, Kawaguchi Y, Suzuki T. Mechanism of interaction between theophylline and mexiletine. *DICP Ann Pharmacother* (1991) 25, 727–30.
12. Nakajima M, Kobayashi K, Shimada N, Tokudome S, Yamamoto T, Kuroiwa Y. Involvement of CYP1A2 in mexiletine metabolism. *Br J Clin Pharmacol* (1998) 46, 55–62.
13. Wei X, Loi C-M, Jarvi EJ, Vestal RE. Relative potency of mexiletine, lidocaine, and tocainide as inhibitors of rat liver CYP1A1 activity. *Drug Metab Dispos* (1995) 23, 1335–8.

Theophylline + Moracizine

Moracizine modestly increases the theophylline clearance. In contrast, more recent *animal* data suggest that moracizine inhibits theophylline metabolism.

Clinical evidence

Single oral doses of aminophylline and a sustained-release theophylline preparation (*TheoDur*) were given to 12 healthy subjects. After additionally taking moracizine 250 mg three times daily for 2 weeks, the AUC of theophylline was reduced by 32 and 36%, theophylline was clearance increased by 44 and 66%, and the elimination half-life decreased by 33 and 20% respectively.[1]

Mechanism

Uncertain. Moracizine is an enzyme-inducer and appears to increase the metabolism of theophylline.[1] In contrast, more recent *in vitro* and *animal* data show moracizine to be an inhibitor of the cytochrome P450 isoenzyme CYP1A2, which is the main isoenzyme involved in the metabolism of theophylline.[2]

Importance and management

Information seems to be limited to this study. The clinical importance of this interaction has not been assessed, but monitor the effects of concurrent use and be alert for the need to adjust the theophylline dose. More study is needed.

1. Pieniaszek HJ, Davidson AF, Benedek IH. Effect of moricizine on the pharmacokinetics of single-dose theophylline in healthy subjects. *Ther Drug Monit* (1993) 15, 199–203.
2. Konishi H, Morita K, Minouchi T, Yamaji A. Moricizine, an antiarrhythmic agent, as a potent inhibitor of hepatic microsomal CYP1A. *Pharmacology* (2002) 66, 190–8.

Theophylline + Nefazodone

Nefazodone appears not to interact adversely with theophylline.

Clinical evidence, mechanism, importance and management

Nefazodone 200 mg twice daily for 7 days had no effect on the pharmacokinetics or pharmacodynamics of theophylline 600 to 1200 mg daily in patients with chronic obstructive airways disease, nor was there any effect on their FEV_1 values.[1] No special precautions would seem necessary if both drugs are used.

1. Dockens RC, Rapoport D, Roberts D, Greene DS, Barbhaiya RH. Lack of an effect of nefazodone on the pharmacokinetics and pharmacodynamics of theophylline during concurrent administration in patients with chronic obstructive airways disease. *Br J Clin Pharmacol* (1995) 40, 598–601.

Theophylline + Non-prescription theophylline products

Patients on theophylline should not take other medications containing theophylline (some of which are non-prescription products) unless the total dosage of theophylline can be adjusted appropriately.

Clinical evidence, mechanism, importance and management

A patient on theophylline developed elevated serum theophylline levels of 35.7 micrograms/ml while taking *Quinamm* for leg cramps (old formulation containing quinine 260 mg and aminophylline 195 mg). This case report highlights the need to avoid the inadvertent intake of additional doses of theophylline if toxicity is to be avoided. The newer formulation of *Quinamm* does not contain theophylline.[1] Note that non-prescription preparations containing theophylline are available in many countries. For example, some cough and cold preparations in the UK contain theophylline (e.g. *Do-Do Chesteze, Franol*). Patients should be warned.

1. Shane R. Potential toxicity of theophylline in combination with *Quinamm*. *Am J Hosp Pharm* (1982) 39, 40.

Theophylline + Olanzapine

There appears to be no significant pharmacokinetic interaction between theophylline and olanzapine.

Clinical evidence, mechanism, importance and management

A study in 18 healthy subjects given olanzapine 5 mg on day one, 7.5 mg on day 2 and then 10 mg daily for 7 days showed no significant changes in the pharmacokinetics of theophylline (given as a single 350-mg intravenous dose of aminophylline). The pharmacokinetics of olanzapine also appeared to be unchanged when used together. No special precautions would appear to be necessary on concurrent use. The authors also conclude[1] that olanzapine would not be expected to affect the pharmacokinetics of other drugs that are (like theophylline) substrates for the cytochrome P450 isoenzyme CYP1A2.

1. Macias WL, Bergstrom RF, Cerimele BJ, Kassahun K, Tatum DE, Callaghan JT. Lack of effect of olanzapine on the pharmacokinetics of a single aminophylline dose in healthy men. *Pharmacotherapy* (1998) 18, 1237–48.

Theophylline + Oral contraceptives

Theophylline clearance is reduced to some extent in women taking a combined oral contraceptive, but no toxicity has been reported.

Clinical evidence

The total plasma clearance of a single 4-mg/kg oral dose of aminophylline was about 30% lower in 8 women on a combined oral contraceptive (**ethinylestradiol/norgestrel**, *Ovral*) than in 8 other women not on oral contraceptives (35.1 compared with 53.1 ml/h/kg).[1] The theophylline half-life was also prolonged by about 30%, from 7.34 to 9.79 hours. Similar results were found in other studies in subjects given intravenous or oral aminophylline and combined oral contraceptives (**ethinylestradiol/norgestrel**, *Ovral* and **mestranol/etynodiol diacetate**, *Ovulen* or unnamed products).[2,3] In contrast, no significant differences were seen in the pharmacokinetics of theophylline (given as intravenous aminophylline) in 10 adolescent women (15 to 18 years) on low-dose combined or sequential oral contraceptives (**ethinylestradiol/norethisterone**), when compared with age matched controls.[4] However, the clearance of oral theophylline was found to be reduced by 33% after 3 to 4 months' use of a **triphasic** combined oral contraceptive in the same women.[5] In a retrospective analysis of factors affecting theophylline clearance, the use of oral contraceptives was associated with a reduced theophylline clearance in women who smoked.[6]

Mechanism

Uncertain, but it seems possible that the oestrogenic component may inhibit the metabolism of the theophylline by the liver microsomal enzymes, thereby reducing its clearance.

Importance and management

An established interaction, but there seem to be no reports of theophylline toxicity resulting from concurrent use. Women on combined oral contraceptives may need less theophylline than those not taking oral contraceptives. There is a small risk that patients with serum theophylline levels at the top end of the range may show some toxicity when oral contraceptives are added. It has been proposed that the effects may be more apparent with long-term, high-dose contraceptive use.[1,4]

1. Tornatore KM, Kanarkowski R, McCarthy TL, Gardner MJ, Yurchak AM, Jusko WJ. Effect of chronic oral contraceptive steroids on theophylline disposition. *Eur J Clin Pharmacol* (1982) 23, 129–34.
2. Roberts RK, Grice J, McGuffie C, Heilbronn L. Oral contraceptive steroids impair the elimination of theophylline. *J Lab Clin Med* (1983) 101, 821–5.
3. Gardner MJ, Tornatore KM, Jusko WJ, Kanarkowski R. Effects of tobacco smoking and oral contraceptive use on theophylline disposition. *Br J Clin Pharmacol* (1983) 16, 271–80.
4. Koren G, Chin TF, Correia J, Tesoro A, MacLeod S. Theophylline pharmacokinetics in adolescent females following coadministration of oral contraceptives. *Clin Invest Med* (1985) 8, 222–6.
5. Long DR, Roberts EA, Brill-Edwards M, Quaggin S, Correia J, Koren G, MacLeod SM. The effect of the oral contraceptive Ortho 7/7/7® on theophylline (T) clearance in non-smoking women aged 18–22. *Clin Invest Med* (1987) 10 (4 Suppl B), B59.
6. Jusko WJ, Gardner MJ, Mangione A, Schentag JJ, Koup JR, Vance JW. Factors affecting theophylline clearances: age, tobacco, marijuana, cirrhosis, congestive heart failure, obesity, oral contraceptives, benzodiazepines, barbiturates, and ethanol. *J Pharm Sci* (1979) 68, 1358–66.

Theophylline + Ozagrel

Ozagrel appears not to alter theophylline pharmacokinetics.

Clinical evidence, mechanism, importance and management

Ozagrel 200 mg twice daily was given to 4 patients with asthma taking sustained-release theophylline. After 24 weeks the ozagrel was stopped, and the pharmacokinetics of theophylline did not significantly change. Similarly, in another 8 patients with bronchial asthma, there were no significant differences in the pharmacokinetics of theophylline (given as a single infusion of aminophylline) before and after 7 days treatment with ozagrel 200 mg twice daily.[1] No special precautions would seem to be needed during concurrent use.

1. Kawakatsu K, Kino T, Yasuba H, Kawaguchi H, Tsubata R, Satake N, Oshima S. Effect of ozagrel (OKY-046), a thromboxane synthetase inhibitor, on theophylline pharmacokinetics in asthmatic patients. *Int J Clin Pharmacol Ther Toxicol* (1990) 28, 158–63.

Theophylline + Pentoxifylline

Pentoxifylline can raise serum theophylline serum levels.

Clinical evidence, mechanism, importance and management

The mean trough steady-state theophylline serum levels of 9 healthy subjects given sustained-release theophylline *(TheoDur)* 200 or 300 mg twice daily for 7 days were 30% higher while they were taking pentoxifylline 400 mg three times daily. However, the change in levels ranged from a 12.8% decrease to a 94.8% increase. The subjects complained of insomnia, nausea, diarrhoea and tachycardia more frequently while taking both drugs, but this did not reach statistical significance.[1] The mechanism of this interaction is not understood, although pentoxifylline is also a xanthine derivative. Patients should be well monitored for theophylline adverse effects (headache, nausea, palpitations) while taking both drugs. More study is needed to clarify this highly variable interaction.

1. Ellison MJ, Horner RD, Willis SE, Cummings DM. Influence of pentoxifylline on steady-state theophylline serum concentrations from sustained-release formulations. *Pharmacotherapy* (1990) 10, 383–6.

Theophylline + Phenylpropanolamine

There is evidence that phenylpropanolamine can reduce the clearance of theophylline.

Clinical evidence, mechanism, importance and management

A single 150-mg oral dose of phenylpropanolamine decreased the clearance of theophylline (given as a single 4-mg/kg intravenous dose of aminophylline 1 hour after the phenylpropanolamine) by 50% in 8 healthy subjects.[1] Such a large reduction would be expected to cause a marked rise in serum theophylline levels, but so far no studies of this potentially clinically important interaction seem to have been carried out in patients. Be alert for evidence of toxicity if both drugs are used. More study is needed. See also 'Sympathomimetics + Caffeine', p.968.

1. Wilson HA, Chin R, Adair NE, Zaloga GP. Phenylpropanolamine significantly reduces the clearance of theophylline. *Am Rev Respir Dis* (1991) 143, A629.

Theophylline + Phenytoin

The serum levels of theophylline can be markedly reduced by phenytoin. Dosage increases may be needed to maintain therapeutic concentrations. Some limited evidence suggests that theophylline may also reduce phenytoin levels.

Clinical evidence

(a) Reduced phenytoin serum levels

A preliminary report noted that the seizure frequency of an epileptic woman on phenytoin 100 mg four times daily increased when she was given intravenous and later oral theophylline. Her serum phenytoin levels had more than halved, from 15.7 micrograms/ml to around 5 to 8 micrograms/ml. An increase in the phenytoin dosage to 200 mg three times daily raised her serum phenytoin levels to only 7 to 11 micrograms/ml until the drugs were given 1 to 2 hours apart. The patient then developed phenytoin toxicity with a serum level of 33 micrograms/ml. A subsequent single-dose study in 4 healthy subjects confirmed higher serum levels of both drugs were achieved when the theophylline and phenytoin were given 2 hours apart rather than simultaneously.[1]

A later preliminary study in 14 subjects by some of the same authors, showed that, after 2 weeks of concurrent use, the mean serum phenytoin levels of 5 of the subjects rose by 40% and a mean levels of the whole group rose by about 27% when the theophylline was stopped. Urinary concentrations of a phenytoin metabolite were raised.[2]

(b) Reduced theophylline serum levels

The observation that a patient on phenytoin had lower than expected theophylline levels prompted a study in 10 healthy subjects. After taking phenytoin for 10 days the clearance of theophylline (after a single intravenous dose of aminophylline) was increased by 73%, and both the AUC and the half-life were reduced by about 50%.[3] Another study in 6 healthy subjects showed that after taking phenytoin 300 mg daily for 3 weeks the mean clearance of theophylline (after a single intravenous dose of aminophylline) was increased by 45% (range 31 to 65%).[4] Similar results were found in a further study.[5] Other reports on individual asthmatic patients have shown that phenytoin can cause about a 1.3 to 3.5-fold increase in the clearance of theophylline.[6-8] Another study[9] and a case report[10] show that the reduction in theophylline levels caused by phenytoin can be additive with the effects of smoking. Consider also 'Theophylline + Tobacco or Cannabis smoking', p.956.

Mechanism

Uncertain. It has been suggested that theophylline either impairs phenytoin absorption or induces phenytoin metabolism, but neither suggestion seem likely.

It seems probable that phenytoin, a known enzyme-inducing agent, increases the metabolism of theophylline by hepatic cytochrome P450 isoenzyme CYP1A2, thereby hastening its clearance from the body.

Importance and management

The effect of phenytoin on theophylline is established and of clinical importance. Patients given both drugs should be monitored to confirm that theophylline therapy remains effective. Ideally the serum levels should be measured to confirm that they remain within the therapeutic range. Dosage increases of theophylline of up to 50% or more may be required.[11] The effect of theophylline on phenytoin is not established and the documentation is limited. It may be prudent to monitor phenytoin levels as well. Separating the doses appears to minimise any interaction.

1. Wada JA, Perry JK, eds. Advances in Epileptology: Phenytoin-theophylline interaction; a case report. New York: Raven Press; 1980 p. 505.
2. Taylor JW, Hendeles L, Weinberger M, Lyon LW, Wyatt R, Riegelman S. The interaction of phenytoin and theophylline. *Drug Intell Clin Pharm* (1980) 14, 638.
3. Marquis J-F, Carruthers SG, Spense JD, Brownstone YS, Toogood JH. Phenytoin-theophylline interaction. *N Engl J Med* (1982) 307, 1189–90.
4. Miller M, Cosgriff J, Kwong T, Morken DA. Influence of phenytoin on theophylline clearance. *Clin Pharmacol Ther* (1984) 35, 666–9.
5. Adebayo GI. Interaction between phenytoin and theophylline in healthy volunteers. *Clin Exp Pharmacol Physiol* (1988) 15, 883–7.
6. Sklar SJ, Wagner JC. Enhanced theophylline clearance secondary to phenytoin therapy. *Drug Intell Clin Pharm* (1985) 19, 34–6.
7. Reed RC, Schwartz HJ. Phenytoin-theophylline-quinidine interaction. *N Engl J Med* (1983) 308, 724–5.
8. Landsberg K, Shalansky S. Interaction between phenytoin and theophylline. *Can J Hosp Pharm* (1988) 41, 31–2.
9. Crowley JJ, Cusack BJ, Jue SG, Koup JR, Vestal RE. Cigarette smoking and theophylline metabolism: effects of phenytoin. *Clin Pharmacol Ther* (1987) 42, 334–40.
10. Nicholson JP, Basile SA, Cury JD. Massive theophylline dosing in a heavy smoker receiving both phenytoin and phenobarbital. *Ann Pharmacother* (1992) 26, 334–6.
11. Slugg PH, Pippenger CE. Theophylline and its interactions. *Cleve Clin Q* (1985) 52, 417–24.

Theophylline + Pirenzepine

Pirenzepine does not appear to alter theophylline pharmacokinetics.

Clinical evidence, mechanism, importance and management

Pirenzepine 50 mg twice daily for 5 days had no effect on the pharmacokinetics of theophylline (given as aminophylline 6.5 mg/kg, intravenously) in 5 healthy subjects.[1] This would suggest that no special precautions are needed on concurrent use.

1. Sertl K, Rameis H, Meryn S. Pirenzepin does not alter the pharmacokinetics of theophylline. *Int J Clin Pharmacol Ther Toxicol* (1987) 25, 15–17.

Theophylline + Pneumococcal vaccine

Pneumococcal vaccination appears not to affect theophylline pharmacokinetics.

Clinical evidence, mechanism, importance and management

The pharmacokinetics of oral theophylline 250 mg three times daily for 10 days were unaltered in 6 healthy subjects the day after they received 0.5 ml of a pneumococcal vaccine, and a week later.[1] These findings need confirmation in patients, but what is known suggests that no special precautions are needed during concurrent use.

1. Cupit GC, Self TH, Bekemeyer WB. The effect of pneumococcal vaccine on the disposition of theophylline. *Eur J Clin Pharmacol* (1988) 34, 505–7.

Theophylline or Diprophylline + Probenecid

Serum levels of theophylline are unaffected by probenecid, but serum diprophylline levels can be raised.

Clinical evidence

(a) Diprophylline

A study in 12 healthy subjects showed that the half-life of a single 20-mg/kg oral dose of diprophylline was doubled (from 2.6 to 4.9 hours) and the clearance approximately halved by probenecid 1 g, resulting in raised serum diprophylline levels.[1]

(b) Theophylline

A study in 7 healthy subjects found that probenecid 1 g given 30 minutes before a 5.6-mg/kg oral dose of aminophylline had no significant effect on the pharmacokinetics of theophylline.[2]

Mechanism

Diprophylline is largely excreted unchanged by the kidneys, and probenecid inhibits its renal tubular secretion.[3] Theophylline is largely cleared from the body by hepatic metabolism, and would therefore not be expected to be affected by probenecid.

Importance and management

Based on the findings of this single-dose study, it would seem to be prudent to monitor serum diprophylline levels if probenecid is started or stopped. No special precautions are needed if theophylline and probenecid are given concurrently.

1. May DC, Jarboe CH. Effect of probenecid on dyphylline elimination. *Clin Pharmacol Ther* (1983) 33, 822–5.
2. Chen TWD, Patton TF. Effect of probenecid on the pharmacokinetics of aminophylline. *Drug Intell Clin Pharm* (1983) 17, 465–6.
3. Nadai M, Apichartpichean R, Hasegawa T, Nabeshima T. Pharmacokinetics and the effect of probenecid on the renal excretion mechanism of diprophylline. *J Pharm Sci* (1992) 81, 1024–7.

Theophylline + Propafenone

Two isolated reports describe raised serum theophylline levels, with symptoms of toxicity, in two patients when given propafenone.

Clinical evidence

In a 71-year-old man propafenone 150 mg daily raised the levels of sustained-release theophylline 300 mg twice daily from a range of 10.2 to 12.8 micrograms/ml to 19 micrograms/ml with signs of theophylline toxicity. The day after propafenone was withdrawn the level fell to 10.8 micrograms/ml. When the propafenone was later restarted the theophylline levels rose to 17.7 micrograms/ml within one week, but fell when the theophylline dosage was reduced to 200 mg twice daily.[1]

In another report, a 63-year-old man showed a marked reduction in the clearance of sustained-release theophylline and a rise in theophylline levels from 10.8 mg/l to a maximum of 20.3 mg/l over 7 days when he took propafenone 150 mg every 8 hours, increasing to 300 mg every 8 hours.[2] Theophylline was discontinued.

Mechanism

Uncertain. It has been suggested that propafenone may reduce the metabolism of theophylline by the liver, thereby reducing its loss from the body.

Importance and management

Information is limited to these two reports, but it would seem prudent to monitor the effect of adding propafenone to established treatment with theophylline in any patient. Be alert for increased serum levels and signs of toxicity. Controlled studies are needed to further investigate this potential interaction.

1. Lee BL, Dohrmann ML. Theophylline toxicity after propafenone treatment: evidence for drug interaction. *Clin Pharmacol Ther* (1992) 51, 353–5.
2. Spinler SA, Gammaitoni A, Charland SL, Hurwitz J. Propafenone-theophylline interaction. *Pharmacotherapy* (1993) 13, 68–71.

Theophylline + Protease inhibitors

Ritonavir can reduce the serum levels of theophylline. Indinavir appears not to interact.

Clinical evidence, mechanism, importance and management

(a) Indinavir

A study in 12 healthy subjects given a single 250-mg oral dose of theophylline before and after 5 days' treatment with indinavir 800 mg three times a day found an 18% increase in AUC for theophylline, which was not considered clinically significant.[1] Further research is needed to confirm the safety in clinical practice, but it would seem unlikely that special precautions are necessary during concurrent use.

(b) Ritonavir

In a placebo-controlled study, 27 subjects on theophylline 3 mg/kg every 8 hours were given ritonavir 300 mg increased to 500 mg twice daily for 10 days. Ritonavir reduced the maximum and minimum steady-state theophylline levels by 32% and 57%, respectively. The interaction achieved its maximal effects 6 days after starting ritonavir.[2] Information is very limited but the interaction appears to be established. Be alert for the need to increase the theophylline dosage if ritonavir and theophylline are used concurrently.

1. Mistry GC, Laurent A, Sterrett AT, Deutsch PJ. Effect of indinavir on the single-dose pharmacokinetics of theophylline in healthy subjects. *J Clin Pharmacol* (1999) 39, 636–42.
2. Hsu A, Granneman GR, Witt G, Cavanaugh JH, Leonard J. Assessment of multiple doses of ritonavir on the pharmacokinetics of theophylline. *11th Int Conf AIDS, Vancouver* (1996) 1, 89.

Theophylline + Proton pump inhibitors

Omeprazole and lansoprazole may cause a small increase in theophylline clearance, which is unlikely to be clinically relevant. Pantoprazole and rabeprazole do not appear to interact with theophylline.

Clinical evidence

(a) Lansoprazole

Lansoprazole 60 mg daily for 9 days caused only a very slight reduction in the steady state theophylline serum levels of 14 healthy subjects.[1] Other studies have also shown little or no change in theophylline pharmacokinetics on concurrent use.[2-5]

(b) Omeprazole

The changes in the half-life and clearance of theophylline caused by omeprazole were found to be small and clinically unimportant in two studies.[6,7] No changes in the steady-state pharmacokinetics of theophylline were found in other studies.[5,8,9] However, one study found that omeprazole produced an 11% increase in the clearance of theophylline in poor metabolisers of omeprazole (i.e. those with low levels of the cytochrome P450 isoenzyme CYP2C19),[10] which seems unlikely to be clinically significant.

(c) Pantoprazole

A crossover study in 8 healthy subjects showed that intravenous pantoprazole 30 mg daily had no clinically important effect on the pharmacokinetics of theophylline given by infusion. No clinically relevant changes in blood pressure, heart rate, ECG and routine clinical laboratory parameters were seen.[11] Other studies have also found no significant change in theophylline pharmacokinetics on concurrent use with pantoprazole.[4,5]

(d) Rabeprazole

A single 250-mg oral dose of theophylline was given to 25 patients before and after taking rabeprazole 20 mg or a placebo daily for 7 days. No significant changes in the pharmacokinetics of theophylline were seen.[12,13]

Mechanism, importance and management

Lansoprazole possibly induces cytochrome P450 isoenzyme CYP1A2 to a small extent, but this is unlikely to be significant unless an individual is particularly sensitive to this effect.[1] Other proton pump inhibitors are likely to interact, and so no special precautions would seem necessary on concurrent use.

1. Granneman GR, Karol MD, Locke CS, Cavanaugh JH. Pharmacokinetic interaction between lansoprazole and theophylline. *Ther Drug Monit* (1995) 17, 460–4.
2. Kokufu T, Ihara N, Sugioka N, Koyama H, Ohta T, Mori S, Nakajima K. Effects of lansoprazole on pharmacokinetics and metabolism of theophylline. *Eur J Clin Pharmacol* (1995) 48, 391–5.
3. Ko J-W, Jang I-J, Shin S-G, Flockhart DA. Effect of lansoprazole on theophylline clearance in extensive and poor metabolizers of cytochrome P450 2C19. *Clin Pharmacol Ther* (1998) 63, 217.
4. Pan WJ, Goldwater DR, Zhang Y, Pilmer BL, Hunt RH. Lack of a pharmacokinetic interaction between lansoprazole or pantoprazole and theophylline. *Aliment Pharmacol Ther* (2000) 14, 345–52.
5. Dilger K, Zheng Z, Klotz U. Lack of drug interaction between omeprazole, lansoprazole, pantoprazole and theophylline. *Br J Clin Pharmacol* (1999) 48, 438–44.
6. Oosterhuis B, Jonkman JHG, Andersson T, Zuiderwijk PBM. No influence of single intravenous doses of omeprazole on theophylline elimination kinetics. *J Clin Pharmacol* (1992) 32, 470–5.
7. Sommers De K, van Wyk M, Snyman JR, Moncrieff J. The effects of omeprazole-induced hypochlorhydria on absorption of theophylline from a sustained-release formulation. *Eur J Clin Pharmacol* (1992) 43, 141–3.
8. Taburet AM, Geneve J, Bocquentin M, Simoneau G, Caulin C, Singlas E. Theophylline steady state pharmacokinetics is not altered by omeprazole. *Eur J Clin Pharmacol* (1992) 42, 343–5.
9. Pilotto A, Franceschi M, Lagni M, Fabrello R, Fortunato A, Meggiato T, Soffiati G, Oliani G, Di Mario F. The effect of omeprazole on serum concentrations of theophylline, pepsinogens A and C, and gastrin in elderly duodenal ulcer patients. *Am J Ther* (1995) 2, 43–6.
10. Cavuto NJ, Sukhova N, Hewett J, Balian JD, Woosley RL, Flockhart MD. Effect of omeprazole on theophylline clearance in poor metabolizers of omeprazole. *Clin Pharmacol Ther* (1995) 57, 215.
11. Schulz H-U, Hartmann M, Steinijans VW, Huber R, Lührmann B, Bliessath H, Wurst W. Lack of influence of pantoprazole on the disposition kinetics of theophylline in man. *Int J Clin Pharmacol Ther Toxicol* (1991) 29, 369–75.
12. Humphries TJ, Nardi RV, Spera AC, Lazar JD, Laurent AL, Spanyers SA. Coadministration of rabeprazole sodium (E3810) does not effect the pharmacokinetics of anhydrous theophylline or warfarin. *Gastroenterology* (1996) 110 (Suppl), A138.
13. Humphries TJ, Nardi RV, Lazar JD, Spanyers SA. Drug-drug interaction evaluation of rabeprazole sodium: a clean/expected slate? *Gut* (1996) 39 (Suppl 3), A47.

Theophylline + Pyrantel

A single case report describes increased serum theophylline levels in a child when given pyrantel.

Clinical evidence

An 8-year-old boy with status asthmaticus was treated firstly with intravenous aminophylline and then switched to sustained-release oral theophylline on day 3, at which point his serum theophylline level was 15 micrograms/ml. On day 4, at the same time as his second theophylline dose, he was given a single 160-mg dose of pyrantel (for an *Ascaris lumbricoides* infection). About 2.5 hours later his serum theophylline level was 24 micrograms/ml, and a further 1.5 hours later it had risen to 30 micrograms/ml. No further theophylline was given and no symptoms of theophylline toxicity occurred. The patient was discharged later in the day without theophylline.[1]

Mechanism

Not understood. One suggestion is that the pyrantel inhibited the liver enzymes concerned with the metabolism of the theophylline, thereby reducing its loss from the body. However, this is unlikely as the interaction occurred so rapidly. Another suggestion was that pyrantel may have increased drug release from the sustained-release theophylline preparation.

Importance and management

Information is limited to this single case report. No general conclusions can be based on such slim evidence, but concurrent use should be well monitored because, in this case, the serum theophylline concentration increase was very rapid. More study is needed.

1. Hecht L, Murray WE, Rubenstein S. Theophylline-pyrantel pamoate interaction. *DICP Ann Pharmacother* (1989) 23, 258.

Theophylline + Pyridoxal

No adverse interaction occurs if pyridoxal (a vitamin B_6 substance) and theophylline are taken concurrently. Some reduction in theophylline-induced hand tremor may occur.

Clinical evidence, mechanism, importance and management

In a crossover study, 15 young healthy adults were given theophylline (*Theo-Dur*) for 4 weeks, with the dose adjusted to give plasma levels of 10 mg/l, combined with daily doses of either a placebo or a vitamin B_6 supplement containing pyridoxal hydrochloride 15 mg. A variety of psychomotor and electrophysiological tests and self-report questionnaires failed to distinguish between the effects of the placebo or the vitamin B_6 supplement, except that the hand tremor induced by the theophylline tended to be reduced.[1] There would seem to be no reason for avoiding concurrent use and it may even have some advantage.

1. Bartel PR, Ubbink JB, Delport R, Lotz BP, Becker PJ. Vitamin B-6 supplementation and theophylline-related effects in humans. *Am J Clin Nutr* (1994) 60, 93–9.

Table 32.4 Effect of quinolones on theophylline pharmacokinetics in order of magnitude of the potential interaction

Quinolone (daily dose)	*Increase in theophylline level*	*Increase in AUC*	*Decrease in clearance*	*Refs*
Enoxacin 600 to 1200 mg	72 to 243%	84 to 248%	42 to 74%	1–8
Pipemidic acid 800 to 1500 mg	71%	76 to 79%	49%	3, 9
Clinafloxacin 400 to 800 mg			46 to 69%	10
Grepafloxacin 200 to 600 mg	28 to 82%	93 to 113%	33 to 54%	11, 12
Ciprofloxacin 600 to 1500 mg	17 to 50%	22 to 52%	18 to 31%	2, 3, 13–18
Pazufloxacin 500 mg	up to 27%	up to 33%	25%	19
Pefloxacin 400 to 800 mg	17 to 20%	19 to 53%	29%	2, 3
Norfloxacin 600 to 800 mg	up to 22%	up to 17%	up to 15%	7, 16, 20–23
Prulifloxacin 600 mg		16%	15%	24
Ofloxacin 400 to 600 mg	up to 10%	up to 10%	up to 12%	2, 3, 7, 22, 25–27
Trovafloxacin 200 to 300 mg		up to 8%		28, 29
Fleroxacin 400 mg	No significant change	up to 8%	up to 6%	30–33
Flumequine 1200 mg	No significant change	No significant change	No significant change	34
Gatifloxacin 400 mg	No significant change	No significant change		35
Gemifloxacin 400 to 600 mg	No significant change	No significant change		36
Levofloxacin 300 to 1000 mg	No significant change	No significant change	No significant change	11, 37, 38
Lomefloxacin 400 to 800 mg	No significant change	No significant change	No significant change	9, 15, 39–42
Moxifloxacin 200 to 400 mg	No significant change	No significant change	No significant change	43
Nalidixic acid 400 to 600 mg		No significant change	No significant change	2, 16
Rufloxacin 200 to 400 mg	No significant change	No significant change	No significant change	44, 45
Sparfloxacin 200 to 400 mg	No significant change	No significant change	No significant change	46–49

1. Wijnands WJA, Vree TB, van Herwaarden CLA. Enoxacin decreases the clearance of theophylline in man. *Br J Clin Pharmacol* (1985) 20, 583–8.
2. Wijnands WJA, Vree TB, van Herwaarden CLA. The influence of quinolone derivatives on theophylline clearance. *Br J Clin Pharmacol* (1986) 22, 677–83.
3. Niki Y, Soejima R, Kawane H, Sumi M, Umeki S. New synthetic quinolone antibacterial agents and serum concentration of theophylline. *Chest* (1987) 92, 663–9.
4. Beckmann J, Elsäßer W, Gundert-Remy U, Hertrampf R. Enoxacin – a potent inhibitor of theophylline metabolism. *Eur J Clin Pharmacol* (1987) 33, 227–30.
5. Takagi K, Hasegawa T, Yamaki K, Suzuki R, Watanabe T, Satake T. Interaction between theophylline and enoxacin. *Int J Clin Pharmacol Ther Toxicol* (1988) 26, 288–92.
6. Rogge MC, Solomon WR, Sedman AJ, Welling PG, Koup JR, Wagner JG. The theophylline-enoxacin interaction: II. Changes in the disposition of theophylline and its metabolites during intermittent administration of enoxacin. *Clin Pharmacol Ther* (1989) 46, 420–8.
7. Sano M, Kawakatsu K, Ohkita C, Yamamoto I, Takeyama M, Yamashina H, Goto M. Effects of enoxacin, ofloxacin and norfloxacin on theophylline disposition in humans. *Eur J Clin Pharmacol* (1988) 35, 161–5.
8. Sörgel F, Mahr G, Granneman GR, Stephan U, Nickel P, Muth P. Effects of 2 quinolone antibacterials, temafloxacin and enoxacin, on theophylline pharmacokinetics. *Clin Pharmacokinet* (1992) 22 (Suppl 1), 65–74.
9. Staib AH, Harder S, Fuhr U, Wack C. Interaction of quinolones with the theophylline metabolism in man: investigations with lomefloxacin and pipemidic acid. *Int J Clin Pharmacol Ther Toxicol* (1989) 27, 289–93.
10. Randinitis EJ, Alvey CW, Koup JR, Rausch G, Abel R, Bron NJ, Hounslow NJ, Vassos AB, Sedman AJ. Drug interactions with clinafloxacin. *Antimicrob Agents Chemother* (2001) 45, 2543–52.
11. Niki Y, Hashiguchi K, Okimoto N, Soejima R. Quinolone antimicrobial agents and theophylline. *Chest* (1992) 101, 881.
12. Efthymiopoulos C, Bramer SL, Maroli A, Blum B. Theophylline and warfarin interaction studies with grepafloxacin. *Clin Pharmacokinet* (1997) 33 (Suppl 1), 39–46.
13. Nix DE, DeVito JM, Whitbread MA, Schentag JJ. Effect of multiple dose oral ciprofloxacin on the pharmacokinetics of theophylline and indocyanine green. *J Antimicrob Chemother* (1987) 19, 263–9.

Continued

Table 32.4 Effect of quinolones on theophylline pharmacokinetics in order of magnitude of the potential interaction *(continued)*

14. Schwartz J, Jauregui L, Lettieri J, Bachmann K. Impact of ciprofloxacin on theophylline clearance and steady-state concentrations in serum. *Antimicrob Agents Chemother* (1988) 32, 75–7.
15. Robson RA, Begg EJ, Atkinson HC, Saunders DA, Frampton CM. Comparative effects of ciprofloxacin and lomefloxacin on the oxidative metabolism of theophylline. *Br J Clin Pharmacol* (1990) 29, 491–3.
16. Prince RA, Casabar E, Adair CG, Wexler DB, Lettieri J, Kasik JE. Effect of quinolone antimicrobials on theophylline pharmacokinetics. *J Clin Pharmacol* (1989) 29, 650–4.
17. Batty KT, Davis TME, Ilett KF, Dusci LJ, Langton SR. The effect of ciprofloxacin on theophylline pharmacokinetics in healthy subjects. *Br J Clin Pharmacol* (1995) 39, 305–11.
18. Gillum JG, Israel DS, Scott RB, Climo MW, Polk RE. Effect of combination therapy with ciprofloxacin and clarithromycin on theophylline pharmacokinetics in healthy volunteers. *Antimicrob Agents Chemother* (1996) 40, 1715–16.
19. Niki Y, Watanabe S, Yoshida K, Miyashita N, Nakajima M, Matsushima T. Effect of pazufloxacin mesilate on the serum concentration of theophylline. *J Infect Chemother* (2002) 8, 33–6.
20. Bowles SK, Popovski Z, Rybak MJ, Beckman HB, Edwards DJ. Effect of norfloxacin on theophylline pharmacokinetics at steady state. *Antimicrob Agents Chemother* (1988) 32, 510–12.
21. Sano M, Yamamoto I, Ueda J, Yoshikawa E, Yamashina H, Goto M. Comparative pharmacokinetics of theophylline following two fluoroquinolones co-administration. *Eur J Clin Pharmacol* (1987) 32, 431–2.
22. Ho G, Tierney MG, Dales RE. Evaluation of the effect of norfloxacin on the pharmacokinetics of theophylline. *Clin Pharmacol Ther* (1988) 44, 35–8.
23. Davis RL, Kelly HW, Quenzer RW, Standefer J, Steinberg B, Gallegos J. Effect of norfloxacin on theophylline metabolism. *Antimicrob Agents Chemother* (1989) 33, 212–4.
24. Fattore C, Cipolla G, Gatti G, Bartoli A, Orticelli G, Picollo R, Millerioux L, Ciotolli GB, Perucca E. Pharmacokinetic interactions between theophylline and prulifloxacin in healthy volunteers. *Clin Drug Invest* (1998) 16, 387–92.
25. Gregoire SL, Grasela TH, Freer JP, Tack KJ, Schentag JJ. Inhibition of theophylline clearance by coadministered ofloxacin without alteration of theophylline effects. *Antimicrob Agents Chemother* (1987) 31, 375–8.
26. Al-Turk WA, Shaheen OM, Othman S, Khalaf RM, Awidi AS. Effect of ofloxacin on the pharmacokinetics of a single intravenous theophylline dose. *Ther Drug Monit* (1988) 10, 160–3.
27. Fourtillan JB, Granier J, Saint-Salvi B, Salmon J, Surjus A, Tremblay D, Vincent du Laurier M, Beck S. Pharmacokinetics of ofloxacin and theophylline alone and in combination. *Infection* (1986) 14 (Suppl 1), S67–S69.
28. Dickens GR, Wermeling D, Vincent J. Phase I pilot study of the effects of trovafloxacin (CP-99,219) on the pharmacokinetics of theophylline in healthy men. *J Clin Pharmacol* (1997) 37, 248–52.
29. Vincent J, Teng R, Dogolo LC, Willavize SA, Friedman HL. Effect of trovafloxacin, a new fluoroquinolone antibiotic, on the steady-state pharmacokinetics of theophylline in healthy volunteers. *J Antimicrob Chemother* (1997) 39 (Suppl B), 81–6.
30. Niki Y, Tasaka Y, Kishimoto T, Nakajima M, Tsukiyama K, Nakagawa Y, Umeki S, Hino J, Okimoto N, Yagi S, Kawane H, Soejima R. Effect of fleroxacin on serum concentration of theophylline. *Chemotherapy* (1990) 38, 364–71.
31. Seelmann R, Mahr G, Gottschalk B, Stephan U, Sörgel F. Influence of fleroxacin on the pharmacokinetics of theophylline. *Rev Infect Dis* (1989) 11 (Suppl 5), S1100.
32. Soejima R, Niki Y, Sumi M. Effect of fleroxacin on serum concentrations of theophylline. *Rev Infect Dis* (1989) 11 (Suppl 5), S1099.
33. Parent M, St-Laurent M, LeBel M. Safety of fleroxacin coadministered with theophylline to young and elderly volunteers. *Antimicrob Agents Chemother* (1990) 34, 1249–53.
34. Lacarelle B, Blin O, Auderbert C, Auquier P, Karsenty H, Horriere F, Durand A. The quinolone, flumequine, has no effect on theophylline pharmacokinetics. *Eur J Clin Pharmacol* (1994) 46, 477–8.
35. Stahlberg HJ, Göhler K, Guillaume M, Mignot A. Effects of gatifloxacin (GTX) on the pharmacokinetics of theophylline in healthy young volunteers. *J Antimicrob Chemother* (1999) 44 (Suppl A), 136.
36. Davy M, Allen A, Bird N, Rost KL, Fuder H. Lack of effect of gemifloxacin on the steady-state pharmacokinetics of theophylline in healthy volunteers. *Chemotherapy* (1999) 45, 478–84.
37. Okimoto N, Niki Y, Soejima R. Effect of levofloxacin on serum concentration of theophylline. *Chemotherapy* (1992) 40, 68–74.
38. Gisclon LG, Curtin CR, Fowler CL, Williams RR, Hafkin B, Natarajan J. Absence of a pharmacokinetic interaction between intravenous theophylline and orally administered levofloxacin. *J Clin Pharmacol* (1997) 37, 744–50.
39. Nix DE, Norman A, Schentag JJ. Effect of lomefloxacin on theophylline pharmacokinetics. *Antimicrob Agents Chemother* (1989) 33, 1006–8.
40. Wijnands GJA, Cornel JH, Martea M, Vree TB. The effect of multiple-dose oral lomefloxacin on theophylline metabolism in man. *Chest* (1990) 98, 1440–4.
41. LeBel M, Vallé F, St-Laurent M. Influence of lomefloxacin on the pharmacokinetics of theophylline. *Antimicrob Agents Chemother* (1990) 34, 1254–6.
42. Kuzuya T, Takagi K, Apichartpichean R, Muraoka I, Nadai M, Hasegawa T. Kinetic interaction between theophylline and a newly developed quinolone, NY-198. *J Pharmacobiodyn* (1989) 12, 405–9.
43. Stass H, Kubitza D. Lack of pharmacokinetic interaction between moxifloxacin, a novel 8-methoxyfluoroquinolone, and theophylline. *Clin Pharmacokinet* (2001) 40 (Suppl 1) 63–70.
44. Cesana M, Broccali G, Imbimbo BP, Crema A. Effect of single doses of rufloxacin on the disposition of theophylline and caffeine after single administration. *Int J Clin Pharmacol Ther Toxicol* (1991) 29, 133–8.
45. Kinzig-Schippers M, Fuhr U, Cesana M, Müller C, Staib AH, Rietbrock S. Sörgel F. Absence of effect of rufloxacin on theophylline pharmacokinetics in steady state. *Antimicrob Agents Chemother* (1998) 42, 2359–64.
46. Takagi K, Yamaki K, Nadai M, Kuzuya T, Hasegawa T. Effect of a new quinolone, sparfloxacin, on the pharmacokinetics of theophylline in asthmatic patients. *Antimicrob Agents Chemother* (1991) 35, 1137–41.
47. Okimoto N, Niki Y, Sumi M, Nakagawa Y, Soejima R. Effect of sparfloxacin on plasma concentration of theophylline. *Chemotherapy* (Tokyo) (1991) 39 (Suppl 4), 158–60.
48. Mahr G, Seelmann R, Gottschalk B, Stephan U, Sörgel F. No effect of sparfloxacin (SPFX) on the metabolism of theophylline (THE) in man. *Intersci Conf Antimicrob Agents Chemother* (1990) 30, 296.
49. Yamaki K, Miyatake H, Taki F, Suzuki R, Takagi K, Satake T. Studies on sparfloxacin (SPFX) against respiratory tract infections and its effect on theophylline pharmacokinetics. *Chemotherapy* (1991) 39 (Suppl 4), 280–5.

Theophylline + Quinolones

Theophylline serum levels can be markedly increased in most patients by enoxacin. Pipemidic acid and clinafloxacin probably interact similarly. Theophylline levels can also be markedly increased in some patients by ciprofloxacin, and possibly pefloxacin. Norfloxacin, ofloxacin, pazufloxacin, or prulifloxacin normally cause a much smaller rise in theophylline levels. However, serious toxicity has been seen in few patients given norfloxacin. Fleroxacin, flumequine, gatifloxacin, gemifloxacin, levofloxacin, lomefloxacin, moxifloxacin, nalidixic acid, rufloxacin, sparfloxacin and trovafloxacin appear not to interact.

Clinical evidence

A. Pharmacokinetic studies

For comparison, the affects of the quinolones on the pharmacokinetics of theophylline in clinical studies in healthy subjects or patients are listed in 'Table 32.4', (p.949).

B. Case reports

(a) Ciprofloxacin

There are numerous cases that describe the interaction between ciprofloxacin and theophylline or aminophylline, which commonly report large increases in serum theophylline levels (32 to 478% or 1.3 to 5.6-fold increases), often associated with toxicity.[1-11] From 1987 to 1988, the UK Committee on Safety of Medicines had received 8 reports of clinically important toxic interactions between these two drugs, with one fatal case.[1] By 1991, the US Food and Drugs Administration had 39 reports of the interaction, with three deaths.[9]

An elderly woman on theophylline developed toxic serum levels and died shortly after starting to take ciprofloxacin.[7] Seizures, associated with toxic levels of theophylline, were described in a number of the case reports.[5,9-11] Seizures have also occurred when ciprofloxacin was used with theophylline or aminophylline, even when theophylline levels were within the therapeutic range (10 to 20 micrograms/ml).[9,12,13] Ciprofloxacin and toxic levels of theophylline are both known to cause seizures independently. It was suggested that, in the case of seizures, there may be a pharmacodynamic interaction between theophylline and fluoroquinolones as well as a pharmacokinetic interaction.[9] In each case seizures began within 1 to 7 days of starting the combination and were reported as being either partial or grand mal. The addition of clarithromycin does not appear to increase the effects of ciprofloxacin on theophylline.[14]

(b) Clinafloxacin

The apparently stable serum theophylline levels of a 78-year-old man with steroid dependent chronic obstructive pulmonary disease were approximately doubled after he received intravenous clinafloxacin 200 mg every 12 hours for 5 days. Two theophylline doses were withheld, and then the dosage was reduced from 300 mg every 8 hours to 200 mg every 8 hours. Within another 5 days his serum theophylline levels had returned to his previous steady-state level.[15]

(c) Enoxacin

Some patients in early studies of enoxacin experienced adverse effects (serious nausea and vomiting, tachycardia, seizures)[16,17] and this was found to be associated with unexpectedly high plasma theophylline levels.[16,18]

(d) Levofloxacin

Levofloxacin has not significantly altered the pharmacokinetics of theophylline, see 'Table 32.4', (p.949). However, a 59-year-old man developed theophylline toxicity 7 and 5 days after starting clarithromycin and levofloxacin respectively. His theophylline clearance decreased by about 40% when compared to the value before starting these drugs. The theophylline dosage was reduced. After stopping the levofloxacin, the theophylline level fell, and the theophylline clearance returned to the initial value, even though clarithromycin was continued.[19]

(e) Norfloxacin

No clinically significant changes in theophylline levels occurred in a patient given norfloxacin who subsequently showed marked changes when given ciprofloxacin.[3] This report and the studies in 'Table 32.4', (p.949) contrast with the US Food and Drug Administration records of 3 patients (up to 1989)[20] and 9 patients (up to 1991)[9] who experienced marked increases in theophylline levels ranging from 64 to 171% (mean 103%). Three developed seizures and one died.[9]

(f) Pefloxacin

An isolated report describes convulsions in a patient attributed to the use of theophylline with pefloxacin.[21]

Mechanism

The interacting quinolones appear to inhibit the metabolism (*N*-demethylation) of theophylline to different extents (some hardly at all), so that it is cleared from the body more slowly and its serum levels rise. The quinolones are known to inhibit the cytochrome P450 isoenzyme CYP1A2 by which theophylline is metabolised. Although neither levofloxacin and clarithromycin alone usually interact, the case report suggests that together they may.[19] There is some evidence that combined use of theophyllines and quinolones may amplify the epileptogenic activity of the quinolones.[9,22]

Importance and management

The interactions of enoxacin and ciprofloxacin with theophylline are well documented, well established and of clinical importance. The effect of enoxacin is marked and occurs in most patients, whereas the incidence with ciprofloxacin is uncertain and problems do not develop in all patients. Nevertheless, be alert for this interaction in any patient if ciprofloxacin is started. The risk seems greatest in the elderly[23] and those with theophylline levels already towards the top end of the therapeutic range. Toxicity may develop rapidly (within 2 to 3 days) unless the dosage of theophylline is reduced.

With enoxacin, it has been suggested that the dose of theophylline should be reduced by 50%,[18,24-26] although reductions of 75% may possibly be necessary for those with high theophylline clearances.[26] Alterations in the theophylline dose should be based on careful monitoring of theophylline levels. New steady-state serum theophylline levels are achieved within about 2 to 3 days of starting and stopping enoxacin.[26,27]

With ciprofloxacin, some recommend an initial reduction in theophylline dose, in the order of 30 to 50%.[9,28,29] However, since a proportion of patients will not require a dose reduction, others suggest that the dose should be modified based on the theophylline level on day 2 of ciprofloxacin therapy.[11,24,30-32]

Direct information about clinafloxacin and pipemidic acid is more limited, but they also appear to cause a considerable rise in serum theophylline levels, similar to enoxacin.

Keep a check on the effects if norfloxacin, ofloxacin, pazufloxacin, or pefloxacin are used because theophylline serum levels may possibly rise to a small extent (10 to 22%), but these antibacterials normally appear to be much safer. However, be aware that norfloxacin has caused a much larger rise on occasions.[9,20] Fleroxacin, flumequine, gatifloxacin, gemifloxacin, levofloxacin, lomefloxacin, moxifloxacin, nalidixic acid, rufloxacin, sparfloxacin and trovafloxacin appear not to interact significantly, and no special precautions seem necessary with these drugs. However, note that acute infection can alter theophylline pharmacokinetics. Further, a report of theophylline toxicity in a patient has been attributed to inhibition of its metabolism by the combination of levofloxacin and clarithromycin.[19] The makers of some quinolones include a warning in their product literature about the risk of combining theophylline with quinolones because of their potential additive effects on reducing the seizure threshold. Convulsions have been reported with theophylline and ciprofloxacin, norfloxacin or pefloxacin. With some of these cases it is difficult to know whether what happened was due to increased theophylline levels, to patient pre-disposition, to potential additive effects on the seizure threshold, or to all three factors combined. However, the literature suggests that seizures attributed to concurrent use are relatively rare, so that the general warning about the risks with all quinolones may possibly be an overstatement.

1. Bem JL, Mann RD. Danger of interaction between ciprofloxacin and theophylline. *BMJ* (1988) 296, 1131.
2. Thomson AH, Thomson GD, Hepburn M, Whiting B. A clinically significant interaction between ciprofloxacin and theophylline. *Eur J Clin Pharmacol* (1987) 33, 435–6.
3. Richardson JP. Theophylline toxicity associated with the administration of ciprofloxacin in a nursing home patient. *J Am Geriatr Soc* (1990) 38, 236–8.
4. Duraski RM. Ciprofloxacin-induced theophylline toxicity. *South Med J* (1988) 81,1206.
5. Holden R. Probable fatal interaction between ciprofloxacin and theophylline. *BMJ* (1988) 297, 1339.
6. Rybak MJ, Bowles SK, Chandraseker PH, Edwards DJ. Increased theophylline concentrations secondary to ciprofloxacin. *Drug Intell Clin Pharm* (1987) 21, 879–81.

7. Paidipaty B, Erickson S. Ciprofloxacin-theophylline drug interaction. *Crit Care Med* (1990) 18, 685–6.
8. Spivey JM, Laughlin PH, Goss TF, Nix DE. Theophylline toxicity secondary to ciprofloxacin administration. *Ann Emerg Med* (1991) 20, 1131–4.
9. Grasela TH, Dreis MW. An evaluation of the quinolone-theophylline interaction using the Food and Drug Administration spontaneous reporting system. *Arch Intern Med* (1992) 152, 617–621.
10. Schlienger RG, Wyser C, Ritz R, Haefeli WE. Der klinisch-pharmakologische fall (4). Epileptischer Anfall als unerwünschte Arzneimittelwirkung bei Theophyllinintoxikation. *Schweiz Rundsch Med Prax* (1996) 85, 1407–12.
11. Andrews PA. Interactions with ciprofloxacin and erythromycin leading to aminophylline toxicity. *Nephrol Dial Transplant* (1998) 13, 1006–8.
12. Semel JD, Allen N. Seizures in patients simultaneously receiving theophylline and imipenem or ciprofloxacin or metronidazole. *South Med J* (1991) 84, 465–8.
13. Bader MB. Role of ciprofloxacin in fatal seizures. *Chest* (1992) 101, 883–4.
14. Gillum JG, Israel DS, Scott RB, Climo MW, Polk RE. Effect of combination therapy with ciprofloxacin and clarithromycin on theophylline pharmacokinetics in healthy volunteers. *Antimicrob Agents Chemother* (1996) 40, 1715–16.
15. Matuschka PR, Vissing RS. Clinafloxacin-theophylline drug interaction. *Ann Pharmacother* (1995) 29, 378–80.
16. Wijnands WJA, van Herwaarden CLA, Vree TB. Enoxacin raises plasma theophylline concentrations. *Lancet* (1984) ii, 108–9.
17. Davies BI, Maesen FPV, Teengs JP. Serum and sputum concentrations of enoxacin after single oral dosing in a clinical and bacteriological study. *J Antimicrob Chemother* (1984) 14 (Suppl C), 83–9.
18. Wijnands WJA, Vree TB, van Herwaarden CLA. Enoxacin decreases the clearance of theophylline in man. *Br J Clin Pharmacol* (1985) 20, 583–8.
19. Nakamura H, Ohtsuka T, Enomoto H, Hasegawa A, Kawana H, Kuriyama T, Ohmori S, Kitada M. Effect of levofloxacin on theophylline clearance during theophylline and clarithromycin combination therapy. *Ann Pharmacother* (2001) 35, 691–3.
20. Green L, Clark J. Fluoroquinolones and theophylline toxicity: norfloxacin. *JAMA* (1989) 262, 2383.
21. Conri C, Lartigue MC, Abs L, Mestre MC, Vincent MP, Haramburu F, Constans J. Convulsions chez une malade traitée par péfloxacine et théophylline. *Therapie* (1990) 45, 358.
22. Segev S, Rehavi M, Rubinstein E. Quinolones, theophylline, and diclofenac interactions with the γ-aminobutyric acid receptor. *Antimicrob Agents Chemother* (1988) 32, 1624–6.
23. Raoof S, Wollschlager C, Khan FA. Ciprofloxacin increases serum levels of theophylline. *Am J Med* (1987) 82 (Suppl 4A), 115–18.
24. Wijnands WJA, Vree TB, van Herwaarden CLA. The influence of quinolone derivatives on theophylline clearance. *Br J Clin Pharmacol* (1986) 22, 677–83.
25. Takagi K, Hasegawa T, Yamaki K, Suzuki R, Watanabe T, Satake T. Interaction between theophylline and enoxacin. *Int J Clin Pharmacol Ther Toxicol* (1988) 26, 288–92.
26. Koup JR, Toothaker RD, Posvar E, Sedman AJ, Colburn WA. Theophylline dosage adjustment during enoxacin coadministration. *Antimicrob Agents Chemother* (1990) 34, 803–7.
27. Rogge MC, Solomon WR, Sedman AJ, Welling PG, Koup JR, Wagner JG. The theophylline-enoxacin interaction: II. Changes in the disposition of theophylline and its metabolites during intermittent administration of enoxacin. *Clin Pharmacol Ther* (1989) 46, 420–8.
28. Robson RA, Begg EJ, Atkinson HC, Saunders DA, Frampton CM. Comparative effects of ciprofloxacin and lomefloxacin on the oxidative metabolism of theophylline. *Br J Clin Pharmacol* (1990) 29, 491–3.
29. Prince RA, Casabar E, Adair CG, Wexler DB, Lettieri J, Kasik JE. Effect of quinolone antimicrobials on theophylline pharmacokinetics. *J Clin Pharmacol* (1989) 29, 650–4.
30. Nix DE, DeVito JM, Whitbread MA, Schentag JJ. Effect of multiple dose oral ciprofloxacin on the pharmacokinetics of theophylline and indocyanine green. *J Antimicrob Chemother* (1987) 19, 263–9.
31. Schwartz J, Jauregui L, Lettieri J, Bachmann K. Impact of ciprofloxacin on theophylline clearance and steady-state concentrations in serum. *Antimicrob Agents Chemother* (1988) 32, 75–7.
32. Batty KT, Davis TME, Ilett KF, Dusci LJ, Langton SR. The effect of ciprofloxacin on theophylline pharmacokinetics in healthy subjects. *Br J Clin Pharmacol* (1995) 39, 305–11.

Theophylline + Repaglinide

Repaglinide 2 mg three times a day for 4 days did not significantly affect the steady-state pharmacokinetics of theophylline in 14 healthy subjects, although the peak plasma concentration was slightly reduced.[1] No special precautions would appear to be necessary during concurrent use.

1. Hartop V, Thomsen MS. Drug interaction studies with repaglinide: repaglinide on digoxin or theophylline pharmacokinetics and cimetidine on repaglinide pharmacokinetics. *J Clin Pharmacol* (2000) 40, 184–92.

Theophylline + Ribavirin

Ribavirin does not alter theophylline levels.

Clinical evidence, mechanism, importance and management

Oral ribavirin 200 mg every 6 hours had no effect on the plasma theophylline levels of 13 healthy subjects given immediate or sustained-release aminophylline. Similarly, ribavirin 10 mg/kg daily did not affect the plasma theophylline levels in 6 children with influenza and asthma.[1] No special precautions seem necessary on concurrent use.

1. Fraschini F, Scaglione F, Maierna G, Cogo R, Furcolo F, Gattei R, Borghi C, Palazzini E. Ribavirin influence on theophylline plasma levels in adult and children. *Int J Clin Pharmacol Ther Toxicol* (1988) 26, 30–2.

Theophylline + Rifamycins

Rifampicin (rifampin) lowers the serum levels of theophylline. Rifabutin appears to have little effect. For the effect of rifampicin in combination with isoniazid, see 'Theophylline + Isoniazid ± other antimycobacterials', p.940.

Clinical evidence

(a) Rifabutin

After taking rifabutin 300 mg daily for 12 days the AUC of a single 5-mg/kg dose of theophylline was reduced by 6% in 11 healthy subjects, which was not significant. The half-life and clearance of theophylline were not affected.[1]

(b) Rifampicin (Rifampin)

After taking rifampicin 600 mg daily for a week the AUC of theophylline (given as sustained-release aminophylline 450 mg) was reduced by 18% in 7 healthy subjects. A parallel study in another 8 healthy subjects given the same dosage of rifampicin showed that the metabolic clearance of theophylline (given as intravenous aminophylline 5 mg/kg) was increased by 45%.[2]

Similarly, other studies in healthy subjects given oral or intravenous theophylline or intravenous aminophylline and rifampicin 300 to 600 mg daily for 6 to 14 days found 25 to 82% rises in theophylline clearance, and 19 to 31% decreases in half-life.[1,3-8] A 61% fall in the 5-hour postdose serum levels of theophylline (given as choline theophyllinate) occurred in a 15-month-old boy when he was given a 4-day course of rifampicin 20 mg/kg daily as meningitis prophylaxis.[9]

For reports of changes (increases and decreases) in serum levels of theophylline with concurrent rifampicin and isoniazid, see 'Theophylline + Isoniazid ± other antimycobacterials', p.940.

Mechanism

Rifampicin is a potent liver enzyme inducing agent, which increases the metabolism of the theophylline, thereby speeding up its clearance from the body resulting in reduced serum levels.[4] High theophylline levels in the isolated case may have been due to liver impairment brought about by the combined use of rifampicin and isoniazid, or alcoholism.[9] Rifabutin is a much less potent liver enzyme-inducing agent than rifampicin and consequently has less of an effect on theophylline metabolism.

Importance and management

The interaction between theophylline and rifampicin is established. The levels and therapeutic effects of theophylline are likely to be reduced during concurrent treatment, and this effect can usually be detected within 36 hours.[9] The wide range of increases in clearance that have been reported (25 to 82%) and the large inter-subject variation make it difficult to predict the increase in theophylline dosage required, but in some instances a twofold increase may be needed.[4] Monitor theophylline levels if rifampicin is started or stopped. The effects of other concurrent drugs such as isoniazid on theophylline levels should also be borne in mind (see 'Theophylline + Isoniazid ± other antimycobacterials', p.940) as they may also influence the levels of theophylline. Monitoring is advised.

The effects of rifabutin are considerably less than rifampicin, with the one available study showing no significant interaction. On the basis of this, no special precautions appear to be necessary, but it may be prudent to monitor the efficacy of theophylline on concurrent use.

1. Gillum JG, Sesler JM, Bruzzese VL, Israel DS, Polk RE. Induction of theophylline clearance by rifampin and rifabutin in healthy male volunteers. *Antimicrob Agents Chemother* (1996) 40, 1866–9.
2. Powell-Jackson PR, Jamieson AP, Gray BJ, Moxham J, Williams R. Effect of rifampicin administration on theophylline pharmacokinetics in humans. *Am Rev Respir Dis* (1985) 131, 939–40.
3. Straughn AB, Henderson RP, Lieberman PL, Self TH. Effect of rifampin on theophylline disposition. *Ther Drug Monit* (1984) 6, 153–6.
4. Robson RA, Miners JO, Wing LMH, Birkett DJ. Theophylline-rifampicin interaction: non-selective induction of theophylline metabolic pathways. *Br J Clin Pharmacol* (1984) 18, 445–8.
5. Löfdahl CG, Mellstrand T, Svedmyr N. Increased metabolism of theophylline by rifampicin. *Respiration* (1984) 46 (Suppl 1), 104.
6. Hauser AR, Lee C, Teague RB, Mullins C. The effect of rifampin on theophylline disposition. *Clin Pharmacol Ther* (1983) 33, 254.
7. Boyce EG, Dukes GE, Rollins DE, Sudds TW. The effect of rifampin on theophylline kinetics. *J Clin Pharmacol* (1986) 26, 696–9.

8. Rao S, Singh SK, Narang RK, Rajagopalan PT. Effect of rifampicin on theophylline pharmacokinetics in human beings. *J Assoc Physicians India* (1994) 42, 881–2.
9. Brocks DR, Lee KC, Weppler CP, Tam YK. Theophylline-rifampin interaction in a pediatric patient. *Clin Pharm* (1986) 5, 602–4.

Theophylline + Ropinirole

Theophylline and ropinirole do not interact pharmacokinetically.

Clinical evidence, mechanism, importance and management

In one study, 12 patients with parkinsonism were given ropinirole, increased from 0.5 mg to 2 mg three times daily over 28 days, then continued for a further 19 days. The pharmacokinetics of theophylline, given as a single intravenous dose of aminophylline, were assessed before the ropinirole was started and on day 27. The pharmacokinetics of ropinirole were then assessed before, during, and after, the use of oral controlled-release theophylline twice daily for 13 days (dose titrated to achieve plasma levels in the range 8 to 15 micrograms/ml). In both cases it was found that the pharmacokinetics of neither drug was altered, and concurrent use was well tolerated.[1] There would therefore appear to be no reason to take special precautions if both drugs are used concurrently, and no need to adjust the dosage of either drug. An interaction had originally been suspected because both drugs are metabolised by the cytochrome P450 isoenzyme CYP1A2.

1. Thalamas C, Taylor A, Brefel-Courbon C, Eagle S, Fitzpatrick K, Rascol O. Lack of pharmacokinetic interaction between ropinirole and theophylline in patients with Parkinson's disease. *Eur J Clin Pharmacol* (1999) 55, 299–303.

Theophylline + SSRIs

Theophylline serum levels can be markedly and rapidly increased by fluvoxamine. Toxicity will develop if the theophylline dosage is not suitably reduced. Some preliminary clinical evidence suggests that fluoxetine and citalopram may not interact, and *in vitro* evidence suggests that paroxetine and sertraline are also unlikely to interact.

Clinical evidence

(a) Citalopram

In a study in 13 healthy subjects citalopram 40 mg daily for 21 days (to achieve steady-state) did not affect the pharmacokinetics of a single 300-mg oral dose of theophylline.[1]

(b) Fluoxetine

The pharmacokinetics of theophylline were unchanged in 8 healthy subjects when they were given a 6-mg/kg infusion of aminophylline over 30 minutes, 8 hours after a single 40-mg dose of fluoxetine.[2]

(c) Fluvoxamine

The effect of fluvoxamine on theophylline pharmacokinetics has been characterised in two studies in healthy subjects. In the first study the AUC of theophylline (given as a single 442-mg oral dose of aminophylline) was increased almost threefold, the clearance was reduced by 62% and the half-life was prolonged from 7.4 to 32.1 hours by fluvoxamine 50 mg daily for 3 days then 100 mg daily for 13 days.[3] In the second study, the clearance of theophylline (given as a single 300-mg oral dose of aminophylline) was reduced by about 70% and the half-life was increased from 6.6 to 22 hours by fluvoxamine 50 to 100 mg daily for 7 days.[4]

A number of case reports have described fluvoxamine-induced theophylline toxicity. Agitation and tachycardia (120 bpm) developed in an 83-year-old man about a week after he started to take fluvoxamine 100 mg daily. His serum theophylline levels were found to have risen from under 15 mg/l to 40 mg/l.[5] A 70-year-old man similarly developed theophylline toxicity, with theophylline levels of 177 micromol/l, when fluvoxamine was added. Subsequently the theophylline concentrations were found to parallel a number of changes in the fluvoxamine dosage.[6] The clearance of theophylline in an 84-year-old man was approximately halved while he was taking fluvoxamine.[7] An 11-year-old boy complained of headaches, tiredness and vomiting within a week of starting to take fluvoxamine. His serum theophylline levels were found to have doubled, from 14.2 to 27.4 mg/l.[8] A 78-year-old woman became nauseous within 2 days of starting to take fluvoxamine 50 mg daily, and by day 6, when the fluvoxamine was stopped, her serum theophylline levels were found to have increased about threefold.[9] She experienced a seizure, became comatose, and had supraventricular tachycardia (200 bpm) requiring intravenous digoxin and verapamil. She recovered uneventfully.

Mechanism

In vitro studies with human liver microsomes have shown that fluvoxamine inhibits the cytochrome P450 isoenzyme CYP1A2, the principal enzyme responsible for the metabolism of theophylline,[10,11] which results in raised theophylline levels and toxicity. The other SSRIs, citalopram, fluoxetine, **paroxetine** and **sertraline** only weakly inhibited this enzyme *in vitro*, and consequently would not be expected to interact.[10,11]

Importance and management

The interaction between fluvoxamine and theophylline is established and clinically important. The UK Committee on Safety of Medicines advise that concurrent use should usually be avoided, but that if this is not possible, reduce the theophylline dosage to a half when fluvoxamine is added.[12] Monitor well. There is good *in vitro* evidence to suggest that fluvoxamine is the only SSRI likely to interact (because it is the only one that affects CYP1A2). This would seem to be borne out by the general silence in the literature about problems with any of the other SSRIs.

1. Møller SE, Larsen F, Pitsiu M, Rolan PE. Effect of citalopram on plasma levels of oral theophylline. *Clin Ther* (2000) 22, 1494–1501.
2. Mauro VF, Mauro LS, Klions HA. Effect of single dose fluoxetine on aminophylline pharmacokinetics. *Pharmacotherapy* (1994) 14, 367.
3. Donaldson KM, Wright DM, Mathlener IS, Harry JD. The effect of fluvoxamine at steady state on the pharmacokinetics of theophylline after a single dose in healthy male volunteers. *Br J Clin Pharmacol* (1994) 37, 492P.
4. Rasmussen BB, Jeppesen U, Gaist D, Brøsen K. Griseofulvin and fluvoxamine interactions with the metabolism of theophylline. *Ther Drug Monit* (1997) 19, 56–62.
5. Diot P, Jonville AP, Gerard F, Bonnelle M, Autret E, Breteau M, Lemarie E, Lavandier M. Possible interaction entre théophylline et fluvoxamine. *Therapie* (1991) 46, 170–71.
6. Thomson AH, McGovern EM, Bennie P, Caldwell G, Smith M. Interaction between fluvoxamine and theophylline. Pharm J (1992) 249, 137. Correction. *ibid.* (1992) 249, 214.
7. Puranik A, Fitzpatrick R, Ananthanarayanan TS. Monitor serum theophylline. *Care Elder* (1993) 5, 237.
8. Sperber AD. Toxic interaction between fluvoxamine and sustained released theophylline in an 11-year-old boy. *Drug Safety* (1991) 6, 460–2.
9. van den Brekel AM, Harrington L. Toxic effects of theophylline caused by fluvoxamine. *Can Med Assoc J* (1994) 151, 1289–90.
10. Brøsen K, Skjelbo E, Rasmussen BB, Poulsen HE, Loft S. Fluvoxamine is a potent inhibitor of cytochrome P4501A2. *Biochem Pharmacol* (1993) 45, 1211–14.
11. Rasmussen BB, Mäenpää J, Pelkonen O, Loft S, Poulsen HE, Lykkesfeldt J, Brøsen K. Selective serotonin reuptake inhibitors and theophylline metabolism in human liver microsomes: potent inhibition by fluvoxamine. *Br J Clin Pharmacol* (1995) 39, 151–9.
12. Committee on Safety of Medicines/Medicines Control Agency. Fluvoxamine increases plasma theophylline levels. *Current Problems* (1994) 20, 12.

Theophylline + St John's wort *(Hypericum perforatum)*

A patient needed a marked increase in the dosage of theophylline while taking St John's wort, but no pharmacokinetic interaction was found in a 2-week study in healthy subjects.

Clinical evidence

A woman, who had previously been stabilised for several months on theophylline 300 mg twice daily, was found to need a markedly increased theophylline dosage of 800 mg twice daily to achieve serum levels of 9.2 micrograms/ml. It turned out that 2 months previously she had additionally started to take 300 mg of a St John's wort supplement (0.3% hypericin) each day. When she stopped taking the St John's wort, her serum theophylline levels doubled within a week to 19.6 micrograms/ml and her theophylline dosage was consequently reduced. This patient was also taking a whole spectrum of other drugs (amitriptyline, furosemide, ibuprofen, inhaled triamcinolone, morphine, potassium, prednisone, salbutamol (albuterol), valproic acid, zolpidem and zafirlukast) and was also a smoker. No changes in the use of these drugs or altered compliance were identified that might have offered an alternative explanation for the changed theophylline requirements.[1]

However, a study in 12 healthy subjects found that a preparation of St John's wort 300 mg (about 0.8 mg hypericin per caplet; 0.27%) three times daily for 15 days had no significant effects on the plasma level of a single 400-mg oral dose of theophylline.[2]

Mechanism

Uncertain. *In vitro* data suggest one component of St John's wort (hypericin) can act as an inducer of the cytochrome P450 isoenzyme CYP1A2.[1] It has also been suggested that treatment with St John's wort for 15 days was unlikely to induce the isoenzymes sufficiently to cause changes in plasma theophylline.[2] The patient in the case report had been taking St John's wort for 2 months, although at a lower dose, therefore differences in duration of treatment may account for the discrepancy. This is supported by studies in which 4-week[3] but not 2-week treatment[4] with St John's wort modestly increased the paraxanthine/caffeine ratio, used as a measure of CYP1A2 activity.

Importance and management

Direct information about this apparent interaction between theophylline and St John's wort appears to be limited. No pharmacokinetic interaction was noted in healthy subjects, but the case report describes a marked decrease in theophylline levels. Mechanistic studies suggest a modest interaction at most. Furthermore most clinically significant interactions with St John's wort are mediated by the cytochrome P450 isoenzyme CYP3A4. However, it would be prudent to monitor the effects and serum levels of theophylline if St John's wort is started or stopped, and patients should be warned of the possible effects of concurrent use. In 2000, the UK Committee on Safety of Medicines recommended that patients on theophylline should not take St John's wort. In those patients already taking the combination, the St John's wort should be stopped and the theophylline dosage monitored and adjusted if necessary.[5,6] More study is needed.

1. Nebel A, Schneider BJ, Baker RK, Kroll DJ. Potential metabolic interaction between St John's wort and theophylline. *Ann Pharmacother* (1999) 33, 502.
2. Morimoto T, Kotegawa T, Tsutsumi K, Ohtani Y, Imai H, Nakano S. Effect of St John's wort on the pharmacokinetics of theophylline in healthy volunteers. *J Clin Pharmacol* (2004) 44, 95–101.
3. Gurley BJ, Gardner SF, Hubbard MA, Williams DK, Gentry WB, Cui Y, Ang CYW. Cytochrome P450 phenotypic ratios for predicting herb-drug interactions in humans. *Clin Pharmacol Ther* (2002) 72, 276–287.
4. Wang Z, Gorski JC, Hamman MA, Huang S-M, Lesko LJ, Hall SD. The effects of St John's wort (*Hypericum perforatum*) on human cytochrome P450 activity. *Clin Pharmacol Ther* (2001) 70, 317–326.
5. Committee on Safety of Medicines (UK). Message from Professor A Breckenridge (Chairman of CSM) and Fact Sheet for Health Care Professionals, 29th February 2000.
6. Committee on Safety of Medicines/Medicines Control Agency. Reminder: St John's wort *(Hypericum perforatum)* interactions. *Current Problems* (2000) 26, 6–7.

Theophylline + Succimer

A single case report describes a 36% reduction in the serum theophylline levels of a man treated with succimer.

Clinical evidence, mechanism, importance and management

A 65-year old man with chronic obstructive airways disease and chronic lead intoxication was given a 19-day course of lead chelation with succimer. His theophylline concentration was found to be reduced from about 11 to 7 micrograms/ml on day 6 and remained at this level until about 9 days after the course of succimer was completed, when it returned to pretreatment levels. His clinical status did not alter despite these changes; possibly because he was also taking prednisone.[1] The reason for these alterations is not understood.

The general importance of this interaction is not known, but it would now be prudent to monitor the situation closely if succimer is added to established treatment with theophylline.

1. Harchelroad R. Pharmacokinetic interaction between dimercaptosuccinic acid (DMSA) and theophylline (THEO). *Vet Hum Toxicol* (1994) 36, 376.

Theophylline + Sucralfate

Two studies found that sucralfate caused only minor changes in theophylline pharmacokinetics, but another suggests that the absorption of sustained-release theophylline is significantly reduced by sucralfate.

Clinical evidence, mechanism, importance and management

No clinically important changes occurred in the absorption of a single 5-mg/kg dose of an oral non-sustained release theophylline preparation (*Slo-Phyllin*) in 8 healthy subjects given at the same time as sucralfate 1 g four times daily. A slight 5% decrease in the AUC was detected.[1] Another study found that sucralfate 1 g four times daily reduced the AUC of a single dose of a sustained-release theophylline preparation (*Theodur*) by 9% (timing of the theophylline dose in relation to the sucralfate dose not noted).[2] In contrast, another group of workers found that when sucralfate 1 g was given 30 minutes before a 350 mg dose of sustained-release theophylline (*PEG capsules*), the theophylline AUC was reduced by 40%.[3] The reasons are not understood.

Many patients are given sustained-release theophylline preparations, but neither of these studies clearly shows what is likely to happen in clinical practice, so be alert for any evidence of a reduced response to theophylline. Usually, separating the administration of sucralfate from other drugs by 2 hours is considered sufficient to avoid interactions that occur by reduced absorption.[4] However, the study showing decreased theophylline absorption did not examine the effect of separating the doses. Further study is needed.

1. Cantral KA, Schaaf LJ, Jungnickel PW, Monsour HP. Effect of sucralfate on theophylline absorption in healthy volunteers. *Clin Pharm* (1988) 7, 58–61.
2. Kisor DF, Livengood B, Vieira-Fattahi S, Sterchele JA. Effect of sucralfate administration on the absorption of sustained released theophylline. *Pharmacotherapy* (1990) 10, 253.
3. Fleischmann R, Bozler G, Boekstegers P. Bioverfügbarkeit von Theophylline unter Ulkustherapeutika. *Verh Dtsch Ges Inn Med* (1984) 90, 1876–9.
4. Antepsin (Sucralfate). Chugai Pharma UK Ltd. UK Summary of product characteristics, January 2004.

Theophylline + Sulfinpyrazone

Sulfinpyrazone can cause a small reduction in serum theophylline levels.

Clinical evidence, mechanism, importance and management

The total clearance of theophylline 125 mg every 8 hours for 4 days was increased by 22% (range 8.5 to 42%) in 6 healthy subjects given sulfinpyrazone 200 mg every 6 hours.[1] This appeared to be the sum of an increase in the metabolism of the theophylline by the liver and a decrease in its renal clearance.

Information seems to be limited to this study. The fall in serum theophylline levels is unlikely to be clinically relevant in most patients, but it may possibly affect a few. Be aware of this interaction if both drugs are used.

1. Birkett DJ, Miners JO, Attwood J. Evidence for a dual action of sulphinpyrazone on drug metabolism in man: theophylline-sulphinpyrazone interaction. *Br J Clin Pharmacol* (1983) 15, 567–9.

Theophylline + Tacrine

The serum levels of theophylline are increased by tacrine.

Clinical evidence, mechanism, importance and management

Healthy subjects were given theophylline 158 mg alone or while taking tacrine 20 mg every 6 hours. The clearance of the theophylline was reduced by 50%, probably because the tacrine inhibits its metabolism by the cytochrome P450 isoenzyme CYP1A2 in the liver.[1] Be alert for the need to reduce the theophylline dosage to avoid toxicity if tacrine is added. More study of this interaction is needed in patients given multiple doses of both drugs.

1. deVries TM, Siedlik P, Smithers JA, Brown RR, Reece PA, Posvar EL, Sedman AJ, Koup JR, Forgue ST. Effect of multiple-dose tacrine administration on single-dose pharmacokinetics of digoxin, diazepam, and theophylline. *Pharm Res* (1993) 10 (10 Suppl), S-333.

Theophylline + Tamsulosin

No clinically relevant pharmacokinetic interaction occurs between theophylline and tamsulosin.

Clinical evidence, mechanism, importance and management

In a double-blind study 10 healthy subjects were given tamsulosin 400 micrograms 30 minutes after breakfast for 2 days then 800-microgram doses on the following 5 days with a single 5-mg/kg dose of intravenous theophylline one hour after the last dose of tamsulosin. The pharmacokinetics of theophylline and tamsulosin were not affected by concurrent use. Theophylline is mainly metabolised by the cytochrome isoenzyme CYP1A2, while tamsulosin is metabolised by CYP3A4 and CYP2D6 and therefore a pharmacokinetic interaction would not be expected.[1] The safety of combined use was considered acceptable and dose adjustments were not considered necessary during concurrent use.[1]

1. Miyazawa Y, Starkey LP, Forrest A, Schentag JJ, Kamimura H, Swarz H, Ito Y. Effects of the concomitant administration of tamsulosin (0.8 mg/day) on the pharmacokinetics and safety profile of theophylline (5 mg/kg): a placebo-controlled evaluation. *J Int Med Res* (2002) 30, 34–43.

Theophylline + Tegaserod

Tegaserod appears not to alter the pharmacokinetics of theophylline.

Clinical evidence, mechanism, importance and management

In 18 healthy subjects, the pharmacokinetics of a single 600-mg dose of controlled-release theophylline were unchanged when given with three doses of tegaserod 6 mg (the first was given about 24 hours before the theophylline, the second simultaneously, and the third 12 hours later). It was suggested that no dose adjustment is required when drugs metabolised via the cytochrome P450 isoenzyme CYP1A2 such as theophylline are given with tegaserod.[1]

1. Zhou H, Khalilieh S, Svendsen K, Pommier F, Osborne S, Appel-Dingemanse S, Lasseter K, McLeod JF. Tegaserod coadministration does not alter the pharmacokinetics of theophylline in healthy subjects. *J Clin Pharmacol* (2001) 41, 987–93.

Theophylline + Teicoplanin

Clinical studies in 20 patients with chronic obstructive pulmonary disease found that teicoplanin 200 mg twice daily and aminophylline 240 mg twice daily (both given as intravenous infusions) had no significant effect on the steady-state pharmacokinetics of either drug.[1] No special precautions would seem necessary during concurrent use.

1. Angrisani M, Cazzola M, Loffreda A, Losasso C, Lucarelli C, Rossi F. Clinical pharmacokinetics of teicoplanin and aminophylline during cotreatment with both medicaments. *Int J Clin Pharmacol Res* (1992) 12, 165–71.

Theophylline + Terbinafine

Preliminary evidence indicates that terbinafine can increase the serum levels of theophylline to some extent, but the clinical importance of this is uncertain.

Clinical evidence, mechanism, importance and management

In an open-label, randomised crossover study 12 healthy subjects were given a single 5-mg/kg oral dose of theophylline (as aminophylline) before and after taking terbinafine 250 mg daily for 3 days. The AUC and half-life of theophylline were increased by 16% and 23% respectively, and the theophylline clearance was reduced by 14%. It was suggested[1] that this is due to the inhibitory effect of terbinafine on the activity of the cytochrome P450 isoenzyme CYP1A2, which is the main isoenzyme involved in the metabolism of theophylline. The changes seen were only relatively small, but the study periods only lasted 3 days, so that the effects of longer concurrent use are uncertain but a clinically significant interaction seems unlikely. More study is needed.

1. Trépanier EF, Nafziger AN, Amsden GW. Effect of terbinafine on theophylline pharmacokinetics in healthy volunteers. *Antimicrob Agents Chemother* (1998) 42, 695–7.

Theophylline + Tetracyclines

Serum theophylline levels increased in two patients who were also given minocycline or tetracycline. Some controlled studies have shown both increases and decreases in theophylline clearance with doxycycline and tetracycline, with no significant changes overall.

Clinical evidence

(a) Doxycycline

A study in 10 asthmatic subjects given doxycycline 100 mg twice daily on day 1 and then 100 mg daily for 4 days found that the mean serum theophylline level was not significantly altered. However, there was large inter-individual variation, with 4 subjects showing rises of more than 20% (range 24 to 31%) and 2 having decreases of 22 and 33%.[1] Fluctuations of this size are not unusual with theophylline. Another study in 8 healthy subjects given doxycycline 100 mg daily for 7 days with theophylline 350 mg twice daily failed to find any significant changes in theophylline pharmacokinetics.[2]

(b) Minocycline

The serum theophylline levels of a 70-year-old woman with normal liver function increased from 9.8 to 15.5 micrograms/ml after she was given minocycline 100 mg twice daily by infusion for 6 days. The serum concentration was 10.9 micrograms/ml 14 days after the minocycline was stopped.[3]

(c) Tetracycline

After taking tetracycline hydrochloride 250 mg four times daily for 8 days a patient with chronic obstructive pulmonary disease (COPD) showed evidence of theophylline toxicity. After 10 days of tetracycline her serum theophylline levels had risen from about 13 mg/l to 30.8 mg/l. Both drugs were stopped, and after 24 hours her theophylline level was 12.4 mg/l. A later rechallenge in this patient confirmed that the tetracycline was responsible for the raised theophylline levels.[4]

In an earlier study in 8 healthy subjects tetracycline 250 mg four times daily for 7 days did not affect the mean pharmacokinetics of theophylline (given as a single intravenous dose of aminophylline), although there was large inter-individual variation. Four subjects had a decrease in clearance of over 15%, (32% in one subject), and conversely, one subject had a 21% increase in clearance.[5] Other studies in subjects and patients given tetracycline for shorter periods have also not found important interactions. A study in 9 healthy adults given single 5-mg/kg intravenous doses of aminophylline found that tetracycline 250 mg six-hourly for 48 hours had no significant effect on theophylline pharmacokinetics.[6] Five non-smoking patients with COPD or asthma had an average rise in serum theophylline levels of 14% after 5 days' treatment with tetracycline 250 mg four times a day, and an 11% decrease in clearance. However, when a sixth patient was included (a smoker) the results were no longer statistically significant.[7]

Mechanism

Not understood. Inhibition of theophylline metabolism and clearance by the tetracyclines has been suggested.[4]

Importance and management

Information seems to be limited. There are two isolated cases of increased theophylline levels with minocycline and tetracycline, but controlled studies have not shown any significant changes in overall theophylline pharmacokinetics. It has been suggested that a clinically important interaction may possibly only occur in a few patients.[1,4] Further study is needed. There seems to be no evidence of adverse interactions with any of the other tetracyclines. However, note that acute infections *per se* can alter theophylline pharmacokinetics.

1. Seggev JS, Shefi M, Schey G, Farfel Z. Serum theophylline concentrations are not affected by coadministration of doxycycline. *Ann Allergy* (1986) 56, 156–7.
2. Jonkman JHG, van der Boon WJV, Schoenmaker R, Holtkamp A, Hempenius J. No influence of doxycycline on theophylline pharmacokinetics. *Ther Drug Monit* (1985) 7, 92–4.
3. Kawai M, Honda A, Yoshida H, Goto M, Shimokata T. Possible theophylline-minocycline interaction. *Ann Pharmacother* (1992) 26, 1300–1.
4. McCormack JP, Reid SE, Lawson LM. Theophylline toxicity induced by tetracycline. *Clin Pharm* (1990) 9, 546–9.
5. Mathis JW, Prince RA, Weinberger MM, McElnay JC. Effect of tetracycline hydrochloride on theophylline kinetics. *Clin Pharm* (1982) 1, 446–8.
6. Pfeifer HJ, Greenblatt DJ, Friedman P. Effects of three antibiotics on theophylline kinetics. *Clin Pharmacol Ther* (1979) 26, 36–40.
7. Gotz VP, Ryerson GG. Evaluation of tetracycline on theophylline disposition in patients with chronic obstructive airways disease. *Drug Intell Clin Pharm* (1986) 20, 694–7.

Theophylline + Thyroid or Antithyroid compounds

Thyroid dysfunction may modestly affect theophylline requirements. There are two isolated cases of theophylline toxicity during treatment for correction of thyroid dysfunction.

Clinical evidence

The theophylline elimination rate constant after a single intravenous dose of aminophylline was found to be greater in hyperthyroid patients (0.155 h^{-1}) than in euthyroid (0.107 h^{-1}) or hypothyroid patients (0.060 h^{-1}); some other pharmacokinetic parameters were also changed.[1] The authors concluded that thyroid dysfunction may modestly alter theophylline requirements. It is therefore also likely that drug-induced changes in the thyroid status may alter the amount of theophylline needed to maintain therapeutic levels.

(a) Antithyroid compounds

The serum theophylline level of an asthmatic patient was found to have doubled, from 15.2 to 30.9 micrograms/ml, accompanied by toxicity, 3 months after treatment for hyperthyroidism with **radioactive iodine** (^{131}I). At this point the patient was hypothyroid, and after treatment with levothyroxine was started, his serum theophylline returned to about the level prior to radioactive iodine treatment (13.9 micrograms/ml).[2] Five hyperthyroid patients showed a 20% reduction in theophylline clearance and a rise in theophylline half-life, from 4.6 to 5.9 hours, when they were treated with **carbimazole** 45 mg and propranolol 60 mg daily. In this study, a single intravenous dose of aminophylline was given before the treatment of thyrotoxicosis and after the euthyroid state had been achieved.[3]

(b) Thyroid hormones

One week after starting to take theophylline 1 g daily, a patient who was hypothyroid (serum thyroxine 1.4 micrograms/100 ml, normal range 4 to 11 micrograms/100 ml) developed severe theophylline toxicity, with serum levels of 34.7 micrograms/ml, manifested by ventricular fibrillation (from which he was successfully resuscitated) and repeated seizures over 24 hours. After 2 months treatment with **thyroid hormones**, which increased his serum thyroxine levels to 4.3 micrograms/100 ml, his serum theophylline level was 13.2 micrograms/ml, 10 days after reinstitution of the same theophylline dosage.[4]

Mechanism

Thyroid status may affect the rate at which theophylline is metabolised. In hyperthyroidism it is increased, whereas in hypothyroidism it is decreased.

Importance and management

It is established that changes in thyroid status may affect how the body handles theophylline. Monitor the effects and anticipate the possible need to begin to reduce the theophylline dosage if treatment for hyperthyroidism is started (e.g. with radioactive iodine, carbimazole, **thiamazole**, **propylthiouracil**, etc.). Similarly anticipate the possible need to increase the theophylline dosage if treatment is started for hypothyroidism (e.g. with levothyroxine). Stabilisation of the thyroid status may take weeks or even months to achieve so that if monitoring of the theophylline dosage is considered necessary, it will need to extend over the whole of this period.

1. Pokrajac M, Simić D, Varagić VM. Pharmacokinetics of theophylline in hyperthyroid and hypothyroid patients with chronic obstructive pulmonary disease. *Eur J Clin Pharmacol* (1987) 33, 483–6.
2. Johnson CE, Cohen IA. Theophylline toxicity after iodine 131 treatment for hyperthyroidism. *Clin Pharm* (1988) 7, 620–2.
3. Vozeh S, Otten M, Staub J-J, Follath F. Influence of thyroid function on theophylline kinetics. *Clin Pharmacol Ther* (1984) 36, 634–40.
4. Aderka D, Shavit G, Garfinkel D, Santo M, Gitter S, Pinkhas J. Life-threatening theophylline intoxication in a hypothyroidic patient. *Respiration* (1983) 44, 77–80.

Theophylline + Tobacco or Cannabis smoking

Tobacco or cannabis smokers, and non-smokers heavily exposed to tobacco smoke, may need more theophylline than non-smokers to achieve the same therapeutic benefits, because the theophylline is cleared from the body more quickly. This may also occur in those who chew tobacco or take snuff but not if they chew nicotine gum.

Clinical evidence

A study found that the mean half-life of theophylline (given as a single oral dose of aminophylline) was 4.3 hours in a group of tobacco smokers (20 to 40 cigarettes a day) compared with 7 hours in a group of non-smokers, and that theophylline clearance was higher (mean 126%) and more variable in the smokers.[1] Almost identical results were found in an earlier study,[2] and a number of later studies in subjects given oral or intravenous theophylline or aminophylline confirm these findings.[3-7] The ability of smoking to increase theophylline clearance occurs irrespective of age,[4] gender,[3,6] and in the presence of congestive heart failure or liver dysfunction.[7]

A similar high clearance of theophylline (given as intravenous aminophylline) has been seen in a patient who chewed tobacco (1.11 compared with the more usual 0.59 ml/kg/minute).[8] The half-life of theophylline (given as intravenous aminophylline) in passive smokers (non-smokers regularly exposed to tobacco smoke in the air they breathe, for 4 hours a day in this study) is reported to be shorter than in non-smokers (6.93 hours compared with 8.69 hours).[9] The clearance of theophylline (given as intravenous aminophylline) was also found to be greater (1.36 compared to 0.09 ml/kg/minute), and steady-state serum theophylline levels lower, in asthmatic children exposed to passive tobacco smoke than in similar children not so exposed.[10]

One study found that tobacco or cannabis smoking similarly caused higher total clearances of theophylline (given as oral aminophylline) than in non-smokers (about 74 compared with 52 ml/kg/hour), and that clearance was even higher (93 ml/kg/hour) in those who smoked both.[5] A later analysis by the same authors, of factors affecting theophylline clearance, found that smoking 2 or more joints of cannabis weekly was associated with a higher total clearance of theophylline than non-use (82.9 versus 56.1 ml/kg/hour).[11]

In one study, 3 of 4 patients who stopped smoking for 3 months (confirmed by serum thiocyanate levels) had a longer theophylline half-life, but only 2 had a slight decrease in theophylline clearance.[1] In another study, ex-smokers who had quit heavy smoking 2 years previously had values for theophylline clearance and half-life that were intermediate between non-smokers and current heavy smokers.[3] Conversely, in another study, 7 hospitalised smokers who abstained from smoking for 7 days had a 35.8% increase in theophylline half-life and a 37.6% decrease in clearance (although clearance after abstinence was still higher than values usually found in non-smokers).[12]

Mechanism

Tobacco and cannabis smoke contain polycyclic hydrocarbons, which act as liver enzyme inducing agents, and this results in a more rapid clearance of theophylline from the body. Both the *N*-demethylation and 8-hydroxylation of theophylline is induced.[13]

Importance and management

Established interaction of clinical importance. Heavy smokers (20 to 40 cigarettes daily) may need much greater theophylline dosage than non-smokers,[1] and increased doses are likely for those who chew tobacco or take snuff,[8] but not for those who chew nicotine gum.[12,14] In patients who stop smoking, a reduction in the theophylline dosage of up to 25 to 33% may be needed after a week,[12] but full normalisation of hepatic function appears to take many months.[1,3] Less is known about the effects of smoking cannabis, but be alert for the need to increase the theophylline dosage in regular users.

Investigators of the possible interactions of theophylline with other drugs should take smoking habits into account when selecting their subjects.[6,9,10]

1. Hunt SN, Jusko WJ, Yurchak AM. Effect of smoking on theophylline disposition. *Clin Pharmacol Ther* (1976) 19, 546–51.
2. Jenne J, Nagasawa H, McHugh R, MacDonald F, Wyse E. Decreased theophylline half-life in cigarette smokers. *Life Sci* (1975) 17, 195–8.
3. Powell JR, Thiercelin J-F, Vozeh S, Sansom L, Riegelman S. The influence of cigarette smoking and sex on theophylline disposition. *Am Rev Respir Dis* (1977) 116, 17–23.
4. Cusack B, Kelly JG, Lavan J, Noel J, O'Malley K. Theophylline kinetics in relation to age: the importance of smoking. *Br J Clin Pharmacol* (1980) 10, 109–14.
5. Jusko WJ, Schentag JJ, Clark JH, Gardner M, Yurchak AM. Enhanced biotransformation of theophylline in marihuana and tobacco smokers. *Clin Pharmacol Ther* (1978) 24, 406–10.

6. Jennings TS, Nafziger AN, Davidson L, Bertino JS. Gender differences in hepatic induction and inhibition of theophylline pharmacokinetics and metabolism. *J Lab Clin Med* (1993) 122, 208–16.
7. Harralson AF, Kehoe WA, Chen J-D. The effect of smoking on theophylline disposition in patients with hepatic disease and congestive heart failure. *J Clin Pharmacol* (1996) 36, 862.
8. Rockwood R, Henann N. Smokeless tobacco and theophylline clearance. *Drug Intell Clin Pharm* (1986) 20, 624–5.
9. Matsunga SK, Plezia PM, Karol MD, Katz MD, Camilli AE, Benowitz NL. Effects of passive smoking on theophylline clearance. *Clin Pharmacol Ther* (1989) 46, 399–407.
10. Mayo PR. Effect of passive smoking on theophylline clearance in children. *Ther Drug Monit* (2001) 23, 503–5.
11. Jusko WJ, Gardner MJ, Mangione A, Schentag JJ, Koup JR, Vance JW. Factors affecting theophylline clearances: age, tobacco, marijuana, cirrhosis, congestive heart failure, obesity, oral contraceptives, benzodiazepines, barbiturates, and ethanol. *J Pharm Sci* (1979) 68, 1358–66.
12. Lee BL, Benowitz NL, Jacob P. Cigarette abstinence, nicotine gum, and theophylline disposition. *Ann Intern Med* (1987) 106, 553–5.
13. Grygiel J, Birkett DJ. Cigarette smoking and theophylline clearance and metabolism. *Clin Pharmacol Ther* (1981) 30, 491–6.
14. Benowitz NL, Lee BL, Jacob P. Nicotine gum and theophylline metabolism. *Biomed Pharmacother* (1989) 43, 1–3.

Theophylline + Trimetazidine

Trimetazidine appears not to alter theophylline pharmacokinetics.

Clinical evidence, mechanism, importance and management

After taking trimetazidine 20 mg twice daily for at least 14 days the pharmacokinetics of a single 375-mg dose of theophylline remained unchanged in 13 healthy subjects.[1] These results suggest that treatment with theophylline is unlikely to be altered in patients concurrently treated with trimetazidine, but this needs confirmation in multiple-dose studies.

1. Edeki TI, Johnston A, Campbell DB, Ings RMJ, Brownsill R, Genissel P, Turner P. An examination of the possible pharmacokinetic interaction of trimetazidine with theophylline, digoxin and antipyrine. *Br J Clin Pharmacol* (1989) 26, 657P.

Theophylline + Vidarabine

A single case report describes a woman who showed a rise in serum theophylline levels when treated with aminophylline oral liquid and vidarabine.

Clinical evidence, mechanism, importance and management

A woman treated with ampicillin, gentamicin, clindamycin, digoxin and aminophylline oral liquid for congestive heart failure, chronic pulmonary disease and suspected sepsis developed elevated serum theophylline levels (an increase from 14 mg/l to 24 mg/l) four days after starting to take vidarabine 400 mg daily for herpes zoster.[1] The suggested reason is that the vidarabine inhibited the metabolism of the theophylline. Whether this is an interaction is uncertain, but it would now seem prudent to bear this interaction in mind if vidarabine is given with aminophylline or theophylline.

1. Gannon R, Sullman S, Levy RM, Grober J. Possible interaction between vidarabine and theophylline. *Ann Intern Med* (1984) 101, 148–9.

Theophylline + Viloxazine

Viloxazine increases serum theophylline levels, and toxicity may occur.

Clinical evidence

A study in 8 healthy subjects given a single 200-mg dose of theophylline confirmed that pretreatment with viloxazine 100 mg three times daily for 3 days increased the 24-hour AUC of theophylline by 47%, and increased its maximum serum concentration and reduced its clearance.[1] An elderly woman hospitalised for respiratory failure and treated with a variety of drugs including theophylline, developed acute theophylline toxicity (a grand mal seizure) 2 days after starting to take viloxazine 200 mg daily. Her serum theophylline levels had increased threefold, from about 10 to 28 mg/l, but the levels were reduced when the viloxazine was withdrawn.[2] Nausea and vomiting, associated with raised serum theophylline levels, occurred in another patient treated with viloxazine. Theophylline was stopped, and then reintroduced at one quarter of the original dose. The theophylline level then became subtherapeutic when the viloxazine was stopped.[3] A further case report in an elderly man describes a marked rise in serum theophylline levels to toxic concentrations (55.3 micrograms/ml) when viloxazine, 100 mg increased to 300 mg daily, was started.[4]

Mechanism

It is suggested that the viloxazine competitively antagonises the metabolism of the theophylline by the liver, thereby reducing its loss from the body and resulting in an increase in its serum levels.

Importance and management

Information seems to be limited to these reports but it would appear to be a clinically important interaction. Theophylline serum levels should be well monitored if viloxazine is added, anticipating the need to reduce the dosage.

1. Perault MC, Griesemann E, Bouquet S, Lavoisy J, Vandel B. A study of the interaction of viloxazine with theophylline. *Ther Drug Monit* (1989) 11, 520–2.
2. Laaban JP, Dupeyron JP, Lafay M, Sofeir M, Rochemaure J, Fabiani P. Theophylline intoxication following viloxazine induced decrease in clearance. *Eur J Clin Pharmacol* (1986) 30, 351–3.
3. Thomson AH, Addis GJ, McGovern EM, McDonald NJ. Theophylline toxicity following coadministration of viloxazine. *Ther Drug Monit* (1988) 10, 359–60.
4. Vial T, Bertholon P, Lafond P, Pionchon C, Grangeon C, Bruel M, Antoine JC, Ollagnier M, Evreux JC. Surdosage en théophylline secondaire à un traitement par viloxazine. *Rev Med Interne* (1994) 15, 696–8.

Theophylline + Zileuton

Zileuton raises theophylline levels and increases the incidence of adverse effects.

Clinical evidence

In a double-blind crossover study, 13 healthy subjects were given 200 mg of theophylline (*Slo-Phyllin*) four times daily for 5 days and either zileuton 800 mg twice daily or a placebo. The zileuton caused a 73% rise in the mean steady-state peak serum levels of the theophylline (from 12 to 21 mg/l), a 92% increase in the AUC, and halved the apparent plasma clearance. During the use of zileuton the incidence of adverse effects increased (headache, gastrointestinal effects), which was attributed to theophylline toxicity, and this caused 3 of the original 16 subjects to withdraw from the study.[1]

Mechanism

Not fully established but it seems highly likely that the zileuton inhibits the metabolism of the theophylline by the cytochrome P450 enzymes (probably the isoenzymes CYP1A2 and CYP3A) so that its serum levels rise.

Importance and management

Information is limited but the interaction appears to be established and of clinical importance. Concurrent use need not be avoided but monitor theophylline levels and reduce the dosage of theophylline as necessary. The report[1] quoted above suggests that the typical asthma patient will initially need the theophylline dosage to be halved. This is based on the results of a trial of over 1000 patients given zileuton 600 mg four times daily without apparent problems when this course of action was followed.[1]

1. Granneman GR, Braeckman RA, Locke CS, Cavanaugh JH, Dubé LM, Awni WM. Effect of zileuton on theophylline pharmacokinetics. *Clin Pharmacokinet* (1995) 29 (Suppl 2), 77–83.

Zafirlukast + Miscellaneous

Zafirlukast plasma levels are decreased by erythromycin and terfenadine and increased by aspirin, but none of these changes appears to be clinically important. No interaction has been found with azithromycin or clarithromycin.

Clinical evidence, mechanism, importance and management

(a) Aspirin

Zafirlukast 40 mg daily given with aspirin 650 mg four times daily is reported to have resulted in a mean increase in plasma zafirlukast levels of 45%. No further details are available.[1,2] The clinical importance of this interaction awaits assessment but the makers do not suggest any alteration in the zafirlukast dosage.[3]

(b) Macrolides

A study in 11 asthmatic patients found that **erythromycin** 500 mg three times daily for 5 days reduced the mean plasma levels of zafirlukast 40 mg by about 40%.[1,2] This reduction in levels would be expected to reduce its antiasthmatic effects. If these drugs are given concurrently, be alert for a reduced response. However, note that the makers do not suggest any alteration in the zafirlukast dosage.[3]

A study in 12 healthy subjects found that zafirlukast 20 mg twice daily for 12 days did not significantly affect the pharmacokinetics of single 500-mg doses of **azithromycin** and **clarithromycin**, even though zafirlukast is an inhibitor of the cytochrome P450 isoenzyme CYP3A4 by which these macrolides are metabolised.[4] See also section (c) below.

(c) Miscellaneous drugs

The makers[2] say that although zafirlukast is known to inhibit the cytochrome P450 isoenzyme CYP2C9, there have been no formal interaction studies with other drugs that are metabolised by this isoenzyme. Zafirlukast is also an inhibitor of the cytochrome P450 isoenzyme CYP3A4 *in vitro*. Whether these predictions lead to clinically significant drug interactions awaits formal evaluation from clinical studies, but if zafirlukast is added to treatment with drugs that are metabolised by these isoenzymes it would be prudent to monitor for an increase in their effects. However, in one study zafirlukast had no effect on the CYP3A4 substrates azithromycin and clarithromycin, see (b) Macrolides, above, nor terfenadine, see (d) below.

(d) Terfenadine

A study in 16 healthy men given zafirlukast 320 mg daily found that terfenadine 60 mg twice daily reduced the mean maximum serum levels of the zafirlukast by 66% and reduced its AUC by 54%. Terfenadine serum levels remained unchanged and no ECG alterations occurred.[1] The reduction in zafirlukast serum levels would be expected to reduce its antiasthmatic effects, but this needs assessment in asthmatic patients. If both drugs are given be alert for a reduced response, but there is no need to avoid concurrent use. More study is needed.

1. Accolate (Zafirlukast). AstraZeneca Pharmaceuticals LP. US Prescribing information, July 2004.
2. Accolate (Zafirlukast). AstraZeneca UK Ltd. UK Summary of product characteristics, December 2004.
3. Zeneca Pharmaceuticals, Personal communication, July 1997.
4. Garey KW, Peloquin CA, Godo PG, Nafziger AN, Amsden GW. Lack of effect of zafirlukast on the pharmacokinetics of azithromycin, clarithromycin and 14-hydroxyclarithromycin in healthy volunteers. *Antimicrob Agents Chemother* (1999) 43, 1152–5.

33

Sympathomimetics

Noradrenaline (norepinephrine) is the principal neurotransmitter involved in the final link between nerve endings of the sympathetic nervous system and the adrenergic receptors of the organs or tissues innervated. The effects of stimulating this system can be reproduced or mimicked by exogenous noradrenaline and by a number of other drugs that also stimulate these receptors. The drugs that behave in this way are described as 'sympathomimetics' and act either directly, like noradrenaline, on the adrenergic receptors, or indirectly by releasing stored noradrenaline from the nerve endings. Some drugs do both. This is very simply illustrated in 'Figure 33.1'.

The adrenergic receptors of the sympathetic system are not identical but can be subdivided into two main types, namely alpha and beta receptors, which can then be further subdivided. The sympathomimetics are categorised in 'Table 33.1', p.960), and a brief summary of the principal effects of stimulation of these receptors is listed below:

- alpha-1 (vasoconstriction, increased blood pressure and sometimes reflex bradycardia; contraction of smooth muscle; mydriasis in the eye)
- alpha-2 (role in feedback inhibition of neurotransmitter release; inhibition of insulin release)
- beta-1 (increased rate and force of contraction or the heart)
- beta-2 (vasodilatation and bronchodilatation; uterine relaxation and decreased gastrointestinal motility; release of insulin)

A third distinct group of receptors, which occur primarily within the CNS and may be affected by some sympathomimetics, are known as dopamine receptors.

It is therefore possible to broadly categorise the sympathomimetics into groups according to their activity. The value of this categorisation is that individual sympathomimetic drugs can be selected for their stimulant actions on particular organs or tissues.

This section is generally concerned with the interactions of sympathomimetics that have predominately cardiovascular actions (mainly through stimulation of alpha-1 and/or beta-1 receptors), those used as decongestants (through stimulation of alpha receptors with or without beta activity) and also sympathomimetics with central stimulant actions. Interactions involving beta-agonists, such as salbutamol, which selectively stimulate the beta-2 receptors in bronchi causing bronchodilation, are mainly covered in 'Respiratory drugs', (p.917). Interactions involving dopaminergics, such as levodopa, are dealt with in 'Antiparkinsonian and related drugs', (p.499).

Although many of the sympathomimetics are covered in this section it is important to appreciate that they have a very wide range of actions and uses. One should not, therefore, extrapolate the interactions seen with one drug to any other without fully taking into account their differences.

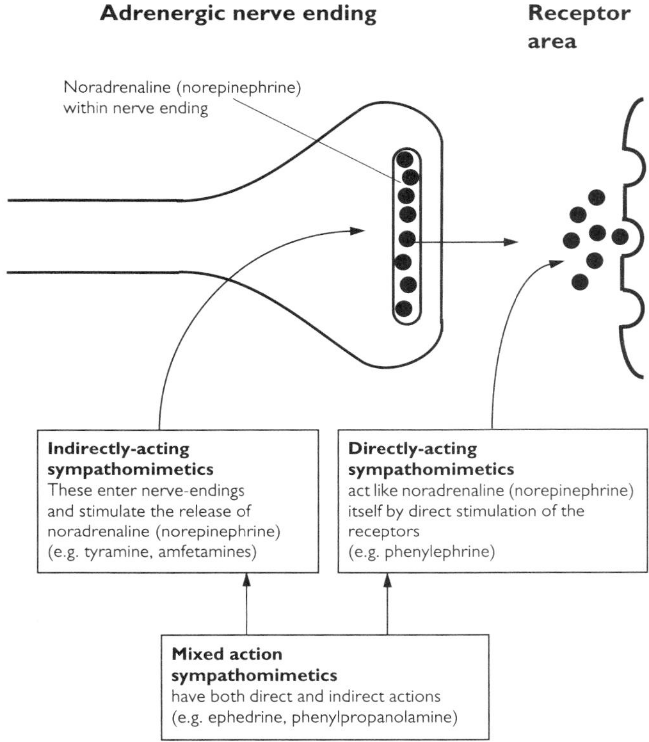

Fig. 33.1 A very simple illustration of the modes of action of indirectly-acting, directly-acting and mixed action sympathomimetics at adrenergic neurones.

Table 33.1 A categorisation of some sympathomimetic drugs

Drug	*Receptors stimulated*
Direct stimulators of alpha and beta receptors	
Adrenaline (Epinephrine)	Beta more marked than alpha
Mainly direct stimulators of alpha receptors	
Phenylephrine	Predominantly alpha
Methoxamine	Predominantly alpha
Metaraminol	Predominantly alpha
Noradrenaline (Norepinephrine)	Predominantly alpha
Mainly direct stimulators of beta-1 receptors	
Dopamine	Predominantly beta-1, some alpha
Dobutamine	Predominantly beta-1, some beta-2 and alpha
Direct stimulators of beta-1 and beta-2 receptors (beta-agonist bronchodilators)	
Bambuterol	Predominantly beta-2
Fenoterol	Predominantly beta-2
Formoterol	Predominantly beta-2
Isoetharine	Predominantly beta-2
Isoprenaline (Isoproterenol)	Beta-1 and beta-2
Orciprenaline	Predominantly beta-2
Pirbuterol	Predominantly beta-2
Reproterol	Predominantly beta-2
Rimiterol	Predominantly beta-2
Ritodrine	Predominantly beta-2
Salbutamol (Albuterol)	Predominantly beta-2
Salmeterol	Predominantly beta-2
Terbutaline	Predominantly beta-2
Tulobuterol	Predominantly beta-2
Direct and indirect stimulators of alpha and beta receptors	
Ephedrine	Alpha and beta
Etefedrine	Alpha and beta
Phenylpropanolamine	Alpha and beta
Pseudoephedrine	Alpha and beta
Mainly indirect stimulators of alpha and beta receptors	
Amfetamine (Amphetamine)	Alpha and beta – also central stimulant
Mephentermine	Alpha and beta – also central stimulant
Methylphenidate	Alpha and beta – also central stimulant
Tyramine	Alpha and beta

Amfetamines + Cocaine

An ischaemic stroke occurred in a patient following combined amfetamine and cocaine abuse. Cocaine inhibits the demethylenation of ecstasy (MDMA, 3,4-methylenedioxymethamfetamine) *in vitro* but the clinical significance of this is unknown.

Clinical evidence, mechanism, importance and management

A 16-year-old boy developed unsteadiness and double vision 5 minutes after intranasal inhalation of a small amount of amfetamine 'cut' with cocaine. Cranial MRI (magnetic resonance imaging) revealed a mesencephalic lesion that was seen to have decreased 12 days later, and he became symptom-free after 3 weeks. The ischaemic lesion was thought to be due to vasospasm caused by synergistic stimulation of the sympathetic nervous system: amfetamine causes the release of adrenaline (epinephrine) and noradrenaline (norepinephrine), while cocaine prevents their reuptake.[1]

An *in vitro* study showed that cocaine (a potent inhibitor of the cytochrome P450 isoenzyme CYP2D6) inhibited the CYP2D6-mediated demethylenation of **ecstasy (MDMA, 3,4-methylenedioxymethamfetamine)**. Therefore, theoretically, the use of cocaine would be expected to increase plasma and CNS concentrations of **ecstasy**[2] but it is not known if this is significant in practice.

1. Strupp M, Hamann GF, Brandt T. Combined amphetamine and cocaine abuse caused mesencephalic ischemia in a 16-year-old boy – due to vasospasm? *Eur Neurol* (2000) 43, 181–2.
2. Ramamoorthy Y, Yu A, Suh N, Haining RL, Tyndale RF, Sellers EM. Reduced (±)-3,4-methylenedioxymethamphetamine ("Ecstasy") metabolism with cytochrome P450 2D6 inhibitors and pharmacogenetic variants *in vitro*. *Biochem Pharmacol* (2002) 63, 2111–19.

Amfetamines or related drugs + Lithium

The effects of the amfetamines can be opposed by lithium.

Clinical evidence, mechanism, importance and management

Two depressed patients stopped abusing **metamfetamine** with cannabis, and **phenmetrazine** with 'other diet pills' because, while taking lithium carbonate, they were unable to get 'high'. Another patient complained that she felt no effects from amfetamines taken for weight reduction, including no decrease in appetite, until lithium carbonate was withdrawn.[1] A controlled study in 9 depressed patients confirmed that lithium attenuates the effects of **amfetamine**.[2] The reasons for these reactions are not known, but one suggestion is that amfetamines and lithium have mutually opposing pharmacological actions on noradrenaline (norepinephrine) release and uptake at adrenergic neurones.[1] Information is very limited, but be alert for evidence of reduced amfetamine effects in the presence of lithium.

1. Flemenbaum A. Does lithium block the effects of amphetamine? A report of three cases. *Am J Psychiatry* (1974) 131, 820–1.
2. Van Kammen DP, Murphy D. Attenuation of the euphoriant and activating effects of *d*- and *l*-amphetamine by lithium carbonate treatment. *Psychopharmacologia* (1975) 44, 215–24.

Amfetamines or related drugs + Phenothiazines

The appetite suppressant and other effects of amfetamines, chlorphentermine and phenmetrazine are opposed by chlorpromazine. The antipsychotic effects of chlorpromazine can be opposed by dexamfetamine.

Clinical evidence

In a placebo-controlled study 10 obese schizophrenic patients treated with drugs including **chlorpromazine**, **thioridazine**, imipramine and chlordiazepoxide did not respond to treatment with **dexamfetamine** for obesity. The expected sleep disturbance was also not seen.[1] In a double-blind, placebo-controlled study involving 76 patients, **chlorpromazine** was found to diminish the weight-reducing effect of **phenmetrazine**,[2] and in another study the effects of both **phenmetrazine** and **chlorphentermine** on the control of obesity were found to be reduced by **chlorpromazine**.[3] Similarly, antagonism of the effects of **amfetamines** by **chlorpromazine** has been described in other reports.[4,5]

A study involving 462 patients taking **chlorpromazine** 200 to 600 mg daily indicated that the addition of **dexamfetamine** 10 to 60 mg daily had a detrimental effect on the control of their schizophrenic symptoms.[6]

Mechanism

Not understood. It is known that chlorpromazine can inhibit adrenergic and dopaminergic activity, which could explain some part of the antagonism of the amfetamines, the euphoriant effects of which are said to be mediated by central dopamine receptors.

Importance and management

Established interactions. These reports suggest that it is not beneficial to attempt to treat patients on chlorpromazine with amfetamines, such as dexamfetamine, or other central stimulants such as phenmetrazine. In one study, thioridazine also appeared to interact. However, it is not clear whether this interaction takes place with phenothiazines other than chlorpromazine, but it seems possible, especially if the suggested mechanism is correct.

This interaction was deliberately exploited, with success, in the treatment of 22 children poisoned with various amfetamines or related compounds (amfetamine, dexamfetamine, **metamfetamine**, phenmetrazine).[4]

There seem to be no reports about interactions between other drugs related to dexamfetamine (such as benzfetamine, fenproporex, phendimetrazine, phentermine) and chlorpromazine, but it would be prudent to be alert for a similar interaction.

1. Modell W, Hussar AE. Failure of dextroamphetamine sulfate to influence eating and sleeping patterns in obese schizophrenic patients: clinical and pharmacological significance. *JAMA* (1965) 193, 275–8.
2. Reid AA. Pharmacological antagonism between chlorpromazine and phenmetrazine in mental hospital patients. *Med J Aust* (1964) 10, 187–8.
3. Sletten IW, Ognjanov V, Menendez S, Sundland D, El-Toumi A. Weight reduction with chlorphentermine and phenmetrazine in obese psychiatric patients during chlorpromazine therapy. *Curr Ther Res* (1967) 9, 570–5.
4. Espelin DE, Done AK. Amphetamine poisoning: effectiveness of chlorpromazine. *N Engl J Med* (1968) 278, 1361–65.
5. Jönsson L-E. Pharmacological blockade of amphetamine effects in amphetamine dependent subjects. *Eur J Clin Pharmacol* (1972) 4, 206–11.
6. Casey JF, Hollister LE, Klett CJ, Lasky JJ, Caffey EM. Combined drug therapy of chronic schizophrenics. Controlled evaluation of placebo, dextro-amphetamine, imipramine, isocarboxazid and trifluoperazine added to maintenance doses of chlorpromazine. *Am J Psychiatry* (1961) 117, 997–1003.

Amfetamines + Phenylpropanolamine

The effects of levamfetamine were attenuated in a hyperactive child by a nasal decongestant containing chlorphenamine and phenylpropanolamine.

Clinical evidence, mechanism, importance and management

Maintenance therapy with **levamfetamine succinate** 42 mg daily in a 12-year-old hyperactive boy was found to be ineffective on two occasions when he took ***Contac*** cold capsules and ***Allerest*** tablets for colds. Both of these proprietary nasal decongestants contain phenylpropanolamine and chlorphenamine.[1] The reason for this interaction is not understood. There is too little information to make any statement about the general importance of this reaction.

1. Huestis RD, Arnold LE. Possible antagonism of amphetamine by decongestant-antihistamine compounds. *J Pediatr* (1974) 85, 579.

Amfetamines or related drugs + Protease inhibitors

A man taking ritonavir suffered a fatal serotonergic reaction after taking ecstasy (MDMA, 3,4-methylenedioxymethamfetamine). A similar fatal reaction occurred with metamfetamine and ritonavir.

Clinical evidence

(a) Ecstasy (MDMA, 3,4-methylenedioxymethamfetamine)

An HIV+ man taking lamivudine and zidovudine was additionally started on **ritonavir** 600 mg twice daily. About a fortnight later he went to a club and took **ecstasy**, in a dose estimated to be about 180 mg. He soon became unwell, and when seen by a nurse in the club was hypertonic, tachypnoeic (45 breaths/minute), tachycardic (more than 140 bpm), cyanosed and diaphoretic. He had a tonic-clonic seizure, his pulse rose to 200 bpm, he then vomited, had a cardiorespiratory arrest and died. A post mortem showed blood-alcohol concentrations of 24 mg% and an **ecstasy** level of 4.56 micrograms/ml, which was almost 10 times greater than might have been expected from the dose he had taken. The authors say that death was consistent with a severe serotonergic reaction.[1] Another report verifies that high ecstasy levels (4.05 micrograms/ml) result in these life-threatening symptoms.[2]

A patient with AIDS, treated with **ritonavir** and **saquinavir**, experienced agitation that lasted for over a day, following a small dose of **ecstasy**. He then experienced a nearly fatal reaction to a small dose of **sodium oxybate (GHB, gamma-hydroxybutyrate, γ-hydroxybutyrate)**, becoming unresponsive within 20 minutes of ingestion of the drug and exhibiting a brief episode of repetitive clonic contractions.[3]

(b) Metamfetamine

A 49-year-old HIV+ man taking protease inhibitors was found dead after injecting himself twice with metamfetamine as well as sniffing **amyl nitrate**. He had been taking an antiretroviral regimen of **ritonavir** 400 mg twice daily, soft gel **saquinavir** 400 mg twice daily and stavudine 40 mg twice daily for 4 months. Toxicology detected metamfetamine 500 nanograms/ml in the blood (considered to be in the fatal range, especially when used with other unnamed drugs). Cannabinoids and traces of diazepam and nordiazepam were also found in this patient.[4]

Mechanism

Ritonavir inhibits the cytochrome P450 isoenzyme CYP2D6, which is responsible for the demethylenation of ecstasy, so concurrent use leads to a sharp rise in ecstasy plasma levels. Poor liver function (due to alcoholism) may have been a contributory factor in one patient,[1] and further CYP inhibition by nitric oxide (the metabolite of amyl nitrate) may have contributed to another case.[4] An additional factor is that ecstasy may show non-linear pharmacokinetics.[5] Metamfetamine is also metabolised by CYP2D6 and its levels would therefore similarly be raised by ritonavir.

Importance and management

Although there are few reported cases, what happens is consistent with the known toxic effects and pharmacology of the drugs concerned. In addition, protease inhibitors may theoretically inhibit the metabolism of ecstasy via other isoenzymes (CYP3A4, CYP2B6), which could therefore also lead to increased levels.

It has been suggested that patients who are prescribed protease inhibitor drugs are made aware of the potential risks of using any form of recreational drugs metabolised by CYP2D6.[4] In particular, some authors recommend that patients taking ritonavir should avoid using ecstasy, metamfetamine and other amfetamines.[6] Open discussions of illicit drug use would enable carers to warn patients that the use of these drugs may be even more dangerous while taking protease inhibitors. Appropriate precautions, apart from avoidance, include a reduction of the usual dose of ecstasy to about 25%, taking breaks from dancing, checking that a medical team are on site, maintaining adequate hydration by avoiding alcohol, and replenishing fluids regularly.[6]

1. Henry JA, Hill IR. Fatal interaction between ritonavir and MDMA. *Lancet* (1998) 352, 1751–2.
2. Roberts L, Wright H. Survival following intentional massive overdose of 'Ecstasy'. *J Accid Emerg Med* (1993) 11, 53–4.
3. Harrington RD, Woodward JA, Hooton TM, Horn JR. Life-threatening interactions between HIV-1 protease inhibitors and the illicit drugs MDMA and SYMBOL 103 "Symbol" 12-hydroxybutyrate. *Arch Intern Med* (1999) 159, 2221–4.
4. Hales G, Roth N, Smith D. Possible fatal interaction between protease inhibitors and methamphetamine. *Antivir Ther* (2000) 5,19.
5. de la Torre, R, Ortuño J, Mas M, Farré M, Segura J. Fatal MDMA intoxication. *Lancet* (1999) 353, 593.
6. Antoniou T, Tseng AL. Interactions between recreational drugs and antiretroviral agents. *Ann Pharmacother* (2002) 36, 1598–1613.

Amfetamines + Urinary acidifiers or alkalinisers

The loss of amfetamines in the urine is increased by urinary acidifiers (ammonium chloride) and reduced by urinary alkalinisers (sodium bicarbonate).

Clinical evidence

A study in 6 healthy subjects given **dexamfetamine** 10 to 15 mg showed that when the urine was made alkaline (about pH 8) by giving **sodium bicarbonate**, only 3% of the original dose of amfetamine was excreted over a 16-hour period, compared with 55% when the urine was made acidic (about pH 5) by taking **ammonium chloride**.[1]

Similar results have been reported elsewhere.[2] Psychoses resulting from amfetamine retention in patients with **alkaline urine** has been described.[3]

Mechanism

Amfetamines are bases, which are excreted by the kidneys. If the urine is alkaline most of the drug exists in the unionised form, which is readily reabsorbed by the kidney tubules so that little is lost. In acid urine, little of the drug is in the unionised form so that little can be reabsorbed and much of it is lost. For more detail see 'changes in urinary pH', (p.7).

Importance and management

A well established and well understood interaction but reports of problems in practice seem rare. The interaction has been exploited to clear amfetamines from the body more rapidly in cases of overdosage by acidifying the urine with ammonium chloride. Conversely it can represent an undesirable interaction if therapeutic doses of amfetamines are excreted too rapidly. Care is needed to ensure that amfetamine toxicity does not develop if the urine is made alkaline with sodium bicarbonate or **acetazolamide**.

1. Beckett AH, Rowland M, Turner P. Influence of urinary pH on excretion of amphetamine. *Lancet* (1965) i, 303.
2. Rowland M, Beckett AH. The amphetamines: clinical and pharmacokinetic implications of recent studies of an assay procedure and urinary excretion in man. *Arzneimittelforschung* (1966) 16, 1369–73.
3. Änggård E, Jönsson L-E, Hogmark A-L, Gunne L-M. Amphetamine metabolism in amphetamine psychosis. *Clin Pharmacol Ther* (1973) 14, 870–80.

Atomoxetine + Miscellaneous

The maker contraindicates the concurrent use of atomoxetine and MAOIs on theoretical grounds. Atomoxetine did not alter desipramine pharmacokinetics and would therefore not be expected to affect other substrates of the cytochrome P450 isoenzyme CYP2D6. Atomoxetine did not alter midazolam pharmacokinetics and would therefore not be expected to affect other CYP3A4 substrates. Antacids and omeprazole do not alter atomoxetine bioavailability.

Clinical evidence, mechanism, importance and management

(a) Antacids or Omeprazole

The maker notes that neither **aluminium/magnesium hydroxide** nor omeprazole affected atomoxetine bioavailability.[1,2] No special precautions appear to be necessary on concurrent use.

(b) Desipramine and other substrates of the cytochrome P450 isoenzyme CYP2D6

Atomoxetine 40 or 60 mg twice daily for 13 days was given to 21 subjects who were extensive metabolisers of CYP2D6, with a single 50-mg dose of desipramine on day 4. Atomoxetine had no effect on desipramine pharmacokinetics.[3]

Desipramine is extensively metabolised by CYP2D6, and can be used as a probe drug for assessment of the effect of drugs on this isoenzyme in extensive metabolisers (see 'Genetic factors', (p.4)). It was concluded that atomoxetine, even at the maximum recommended dose, does not cause clinically relevant inhibition of CYP2D6 *in vivo*, and so will not affect the pharmacokinetics of other CYP2D6 substrates.[3] For a list of CYP2D6 substrates, see 'Table 1.3', (p.6).

(c) MAOIs

The maker contraindicates the concurrent use of atomoxetine with MAOIs, or within 2 weeks of stopping an MAOI,[1,2] because other drugs that affect brain monoamine levels have caused serious reactions when taken with MAOIs.[2]

(d) Midazolam and other substrates of the cytochrome P450 isoenzyme CYP3A4

Atomoxetine 60 mg twice daily for 12 days, with a single 5-mg oral dose of midazolam on days 6 and 12, was given to 6 subjects who were poor metabolisers of CYP2D6. Atomoxetine increased the maximum level and AUC of midazolam by about 16%, which was not statistically or clinically significant.[3]

Midazolam is extensively metabolised by CYP3A4, and can be used as a probe drug for assessment of the effect of drugs on this isoenzyme. Poor metabolisers of CYP2D6 were chosen for this study, because they have much higher levels of atomoxetine than extensive metabolisers of CYP2D6. It was concluded that atomoxetine, even at the maximum recommended dose, does not cause clinically relevant inhibition of CYP3A4 *in vivo*, and so will not affect the pharmacokinetics of other CYP3A4 substrates.[3] For a list of CYP3A4 substrates, see 'Table 1.4', (p.6).

1. Strattera (Atomoxetine hydrochloride). Eli Lilly and Company Ltd. UK Summary of product characteristics, January 2005.
2. Strattera (Atomoxetine hydrochloride). Eli Lilly and Company. US Prescribing information, April 2005.
3. Sauer J-M, Long AJ, Ring B, Gillespie JS, Sanburn NP, DeSante KA, Petullo D, VandenBranden MR, Jensen CB, Wrighton SA, Smith BP, Read HA, Witcher JW. Atomoxetine hydrochloride: clinical drug-drug interaction prediction and outcome. *J Pharmacol Exp Ther* (2004) 308, 410–18.

Atomoxetine + Other sympathomimetics or Pressor drugs

Atomoxetine potentiated the increase in heart rate and blood pressure seen with intravenous salbutamol. No increase in cardiovascular effects was seen when atomoxetine was given with methylphenidate. Atomoxetine is predicted to have additive effects with pressor agents and other sympathomimetics.

Clinical evidence, mechanism, importance and management

Atomoxetine is a sympathomimetic that acts as a noradrenaline reuptake inhibitor. As such, it causes a modest increase in pulse and/or blood pressure in many patients.[1,2] It can also cause hypotension.[1,2]

(a) Methylphenidate

The maker briefly notes that concurrent use of methylphenidate and atomoxetine did not increase cardiovascular effects beyond that seen with methylphenidate alone.[2]

(b) Pressor drugs

The maker recommends caution if atomoxetine is given concurrently with pressor drugs, because of the possible additive effects on blood pressure.[1,2]

(c) Salbutamol (albuterol)

The maker notes that atomoxetine 60 mg twice daily for 5 days potentiated the increase in heart rate and blood pressure seen with an infusion of salbutamol 600 micrograms over 2 hours.[2] Because of this, they recommend caution when atomoxetine is used in patients on intravenous or oral salbutamol or other $beta_2$-agonists[1,2] (for a list, see 'Table 32.1', (p.917)). The UK maker also extends this precaution to high-dose nebulised salbutamol.[1]

(d) Other sympathomimetics

The maker recommends caution when atomoxetine is given concurrently with other drugs that affect noradrenaline, because of the potential for additive or synergistic pharmacological effects. Examples they name are antidepressants such as **imipramine**, **venlafaxine** and **mirtazapine**, and the decongestants **pseudoephedrine** or **phenylephrine.**[1] Until more is known, this would seem a sensible precaution.

1. Strattera (Atomoxetine hydrochloride). Eli Lilly and Company Ltd. UK Summary of product characteristics, January 2005.
2. Strattera (Atomoxetine hydrochloride). Eli Lilly and Company. US Prescribing information, April 2005.

Atomoxetine + Paroxetine and other CYP2D6 enzyme inhibitors

Paroxetine markedly increases atomoxetine levels in extensive metabolisers of the cytochrome P450 isoenzyme CYP2D6. There is a possibility that this may increase adverse effects, and a slower titration of atomoxetine dose is suggested for patients on paroxetine and other CYP2D6 inhibitors.

Clinical evidence

Paroxetine 20 mg daily for 17 days, with atomoxetine 20 mg twice daily on days 12 to 17, was given to 22 healthy subjects who were extensive metabolisers of the cytochrome P450 isoenzyme CYP2D6. Paroxetine increased the AUC of atomoxetine 6.5-fold, increased the maximum plasma level by 3.5-fold, and increased the elimination half-life by 2.5-fold compared with atomoxetine alone. No changes in paroxetine pharmacokinetics were seen.[1] The pharmacokinetics of atomoxetine with paroxetine in these subjects was similar to that previously seen with atomoxetine alone in poor metaboliser subjects.[1,2]

Mechanism

Atomoxetine is extensively metabolised by CYP2D6,[3] an isoenzyme that shows polymorphism, with up to 10% of the population lacking an active form (poor metabolisers). Paroxetine inhibits CYP2D6, and thereby increases atomoxetine levels in those with an extensive metaboliser phenotype. It would not be expected to have any effect in poor metabolisers.

Importance and management

An established pharmacokinetic interaction. Paroxetine effectively changes patients from an extensive metaboliser phenotype to a poor metaboliser phenotype, so markedly raising atomoxetine levels. Although the clinical relevance has not been directly assessed, the maker notes that some adverse effects of atomoxetine were up to twice as frequent in poor metaboliser patients in clinical trials.[2] Because of this, they suggest that patients already on CYP2D6 inhibitors should undergo a slower titration of atomoxetine dose than usual,[4] with the dose only increased if symptoms fail to improve and if the initial dose is well tolerated.[2] This seems a sensible precaution. They specifically mention paroxetine, **fluoxetine**,[2,4] and **quinidine**.[2] For a list of inhibitors of CYP2D6, see 'Table 1.3', (p.6). It would also seem prudent to be alert to the possibility of an increase in adverse effects if CYP2D6 inhibitors are added to established atomoxetine treatment.

1. Belle DJ, Ernest CS, Sauer J-M, Smith BP, Thomasson HR, Witcher JW. Effect of potent CYP2D6 inhibition by paroxetine on atomoxetine pharmacokinetics. *J Clin Pharmacol* (2002) 42, 1219–27.
2. Strattera (Atomoxetine hydrochloride). Eli Lilly and Company. US prescribing information, April 2005.
3. Sauer J-M, Ponsler GD, Mattiuz EL, Long AJ, Witcher JW, Thomasson HR, Desante KA. Disposition and metabolic fate of atomoxetine hydrochloride: the role of CYP2D6 in human disposition and metabolism. *Drug Metab Dispos* (2003) 31, 98–107.
4. Strattera (Atomoxetine hydrochloride). Eli Lilly and Company Ltd. UK Summary of product characteristics, January 2005.

Dobutamine and/or Dopamine + Cimetidine

An exaggerated hypertensive response to dobutamine occurred in a patient taking cimetidine while undergoing anaesthetic induction. Another case report describes supraventricular tachycardia in a patient on dobutamine and dopamine when given cimetidine.

Clinical evidence, mechanism, importance and management

A patient developed unexpectedly marked hypertension of 210/100 mmHg in response to a 5 microgram/kg/minute dobutamine infusion following induction of anaesthesia (with midazolam, fentanyl, vecuronium and oxygen) for coronary artery bypass grafting. The infusion was stopped and over the next 15 minutes the blood pressure fell to 90/50 mmHg. A new infusion had the same hypertensive effect, and his blood pressure was subsequently controlled at 120/80 mmHg with dobutamine 1 microgram/kg/minute.[1]The authors of the report suggest that this exaggerated response to dobutamine may have been due to cimetidine

1 g daily, which the patient was also taking. They postulate that the cimetidine may possibly have inhibited the metabolism and clearance of the dobutamine by the liver, thereby increasing its effects.[1]

A post-operative patient on dopamine and dobutamine infusions developed a supraventricular tachycardia 30 seconds after an intravenous injection of cimetidine. Similar episodes of tachycardia occurred on rechallenge with both drugs, but not when each drug was given separately.[2]

These are isolated cases and the general importance is not known.

1. Baraka A, Nauphal M, Arab W. Cimetidine–dobutamine interaction? *Anaesthesia* (1992) 47, 965–6.
2. Grozel JM, Mignotte H, Descotes J. Une nouvelle interaction médicamenteuse: dopamine-cimétidine? *Nouv Presse Med* (1980) 9, 3548.

Dobutamine + Dipyridamole

The addition of dipyridamole to dobutamine for echocardiography can cause potentially hazardous hypotension.

Clinical evidence, mechanism, importance and management

Ten patients with a low probability of coronary artery disease underwent dobutamine echocardiography. Five were given dobutamine alone, while the other 5 had a low intravenous dose of dipyridamole added to the maximal dose of dobutamine to see whether the sensitivity of the test could be improved. Four of the patients given both drugs experienced severe hypotension while no hypotension was seen in the control group. The conclusion was reached that this combination of drugs can be hazardous and should not be used in patients suspected of coronary heart disease.[1]

1. Shaheen J, Rosenmann D, Tzivoni D. Severe hypotension induced by combination of dobutamine and dipyridamole. *Isr J Med Sci* (1996) 32, 1105–7.

Dobutamine + Theophylline

A man taking theophylline developed marked tachycardia when treated with dobutamine.

Clinical evidence, mechanism, importance and management

An asthmatic patient taking sustained-release theophylline 150 mg twice daily, digoxin and spironolactone was anaesthetised for an aortic valve replacement with fentanyl, midazolam and pipecuronium. Following induction, intubation, and ventilation with 100% oxygen, his systolic blood pressure fell from 120 to 80 mmHg, and his heart rate slowed from 70 to 50 bpm. Dobutamine was given at 5 micrograms/kg per minute, and after 2 to 3 minutes his heart rate rose to 150 bpm and his systolic pressure rose to 190 mmHg. The authors of the report[1] attribute the tachycardia to a dobutamine/theophylline interaction, possibly resulting from a synergistic increase in cyclic AMP levels in cardiac muscle and/or theophylline-induced potentiation of catecholamine action. They advise the careful titration of dobutamine in any asthmatic taking theophylline, particularly if a slow-release preparation is being used. More study of this apparent interaction is needed.

1. Baraka A, Darwish R, Rizkallah P. Excessive dobutamine-induced tachycardia in the asthmatic cardiac patient: possible potentiation by theophylline therapy. *J Cardiothorac Vasc Anesth* (1993) 7, 641–2.

Dopamine + Ergometrine (Ergonovine)

An isolated report attributes the development of gangrene and subsequently fatal septicaemia to the infusion of dopamine following the use of ergometrine.

Clinical evidence, mechanism, importance and management

One patient developed gangrene of the hands and feet after being given an infusion of dopamine following the use of ergometrine.[1] This would seem to have resulted from the additive peripheral vasoconstrictor effects of both drugs, which reduced the circulation to such an extent that gangrene and then fatal septicaemia developed. It would seem prudent to avoid concurrent use or monitor the outcome extremely closely.

1. Buchanan N, Cane RD, Miller M. Symmetrical gangrene of the extremities associated with the use of dopamine subsequent to ergometrine administration. *Intensive Care Med* (1977) 3, 55–6.

Dopamine + Phenytoin

There is some limited evidence that patients needing dopamine to support their blood pressure can become severely hypotensive if they are also given phenytoin.

Clinical evidence, mechanism, importance and management

Five critically ill patients treated with a number of different drugs, were given dopamine to maintain an adequate blood pressure. When seizures developed they were additionally given intravenous phenytoin at an infusion rate of 5 to 25 mg/minute. Their previously stable blood pressures then fell rapidly, and two patients died from cardiac arrest. A similar reaction was demonstrated in *dogs* made hypovolaemic and hypotensive by bleeding.[1] However, another study in *dogs* was unable to find evidence of this serious adverse interaction,[2] and no evidence of marked hypotension occurred in a patient with cardiogenic shock on dopamine and dobutamine when a phenytoin infusion was added.[3]

The documentation of this adverse interaction is limited to this single report but phenytoin is known to cause hypotension if it is given rapidly, particularly in gravely ill patients. Blood pressure is doubtless being monitored in patients receiving dopamine, and should be measured when phenytoin is given intravenously. However, more frequent monitoring may be necessary, as this interaction develops rapidly.

1. Bivins BA, Rapp RP, Griffen WO, Blouin R, Bustrack J. Dopamine-phenytoin interaction. A cause of hypotension in the critically ill. *Arch Surg* (1978) 113, 245–9.
2. Smith RD, Lomas TE. Modification of cardiovascular responses to intravenous phenytoin by dopamine in dogs: evidence against an adverse interaction. *Toxicol Appl Pharmacol* (1978) 45, 665–73.
3. Torres E, Garcia B, Sosa P, Alba D. No interaction between dopamine and phenytoin. *Ann Pharmacother* (1995) 29, 1300–1.

Dopamine + Selegiline

A case report describes a hypertensive reaction attributed to the concurrent use of dopamine and selegiline.

Clinical evidence, mechanism, importance and management

A 75-year-old man who was receiving selegiline 5 mg twice daily for Parkinson's disease, was started on intravenous dopamine 3.5 micrograms/kg per minute due to a decline in blood pressure and urine output following a serious road traffic accident. Twenty minutes after the infusion was started his blood pressure had hardly changed, but 30 minutes later it had risen from 108/33 to 228/50 mmHg. The dopamine infusion was discontinued and the blood pressure decreased to 121/40 mmHg over the next 30 minutes. The dopamine infusion was reinstituted twice more at lower doses (1.03 and 0.9 micrograms/kg per minute), but each time similar reactions occurred. The exaggerated vasopressor response was thought to be due to inhibition of dopamine metabolism by selegiline.[1]

The authors of the report[1] and the makers of selegiline recommend that dopamine should be used cautiously,[2] if at all,[3] in patients who are chronically receiving selegiline or who have received selegiline in the 2 weeks prior to dopamine therapy. In addition, the makers of dopamine warn that in patients who have received **MAOIs** within the previous 2 to 3 weeks, the initial dose of dopamine should be no greater than 10% of the usual dose.[4]

1. Rose LM, Ohlinger MJ, Mauro VF. A hypertensive reaction induced by concurrent use of selegiline and dopamine. *Ann Pharmacother* (2000) 34, 1020– 4.
2. Eldepryl (Selegiline). Orion Pharma (UK) Ltd. UK Summary of product characteristics, October 2003.
3. Zelapar (Selegiline hydrochloride). Zeneus Pharma Ltd. UK Summary of product characteristics, February 2003.
4. Dopamine Sterile Concentrate. Mayne Pharma plc. UK Summary of product characteristics, April 2003.

Dopamine + Tolazoline

Acute and eventually fatal hypotension occurred in a patient given dopamine and tolazoline.

Clinical evidence

A patient on ventilatory support following surgery was given dopamine on the third postoperative day. Pulmonary arterial pressure had been steadily rising since the surgery, so on day 4 he was given a slow bolus injection of tolazoline 2 mg/kg. Systemic arterial pressure immediately fell to 50/30 mmHg so the dopamine infusion was increased, but the arterial pressure then fell even further to 38/15 mmHg. The dopamine was stopped and ephedrine, methoxamine and fresh frozen plasma were given. Two hours later his blood pressure was 70/40 mmHg. Two further attempts were made to infuse dopamine, but the arterial pressure fell to 40/15 mmHg on the first occasion, and to 38/20 mmHg on the second. The patient died following a cardiac arrest.[1]

Mechanism

Not fully understood. Dopamine has both alpha (vasoconstrictor) and beta (vasodilator) activity. With the alpha effects on the systemic circulation competitively blocked by the tolazoline, its vasodilatory actions would predominate, resulting in paradoxical hypotension.

Importance and management

Information is limited but this interaction would appear to be established. The authors of this report warn that infusion of dopamine should not be considered for several hours after giving even a small single dose of tolazoline. They point out that impaired renal function often accompanies severe respiratory failure, which may significantly prolong the half-life of tolazoline and its effects.

1. Carlon GC. Fatal association of tolazoline and dopamine. *Chest* (1979) 76, 336.

Ecstasy (MDMA, 3,4-methylenedioxymethamfetamine) + SSRIs

The psychological effects of ecstasy (MDMA, 3,4-methylenedioxymethamfetamine) may be reduced by the prior use of citalopram. It seems likely that other SSRIs will also reduce or block some of the effects of ecstasy, but increased serotonin effects may, in theory, also be possible. An isolated report describes a neurotoxic reaction in a man on citalopram when he took unknown amounts of ecstasy. Fluoxetine and paroxetine may decrease the metabolism of ecstasy.

Clinical evidence

(a) Ecstasy effects reduced

A double-blind placebo-controlled psychometric study in 16 healthy subjects found that ecstasy 1.5 mg/kg produced an emotional state with heightened mood, increased self-confidence and extroversion, moderate derealisation and an intensification of sensory perception. Most of these effects were found to be markedly reduced by pretreatment with **citalopram** 40 mg by intravenous infusion, although the duration of the effects was prolonged by up to 2 hours.[1] However, an account of 4 ecstasy users who had taken **fluoxetine** 20 mg prior to ecstasy 100 to 250 mg, reported that they still experienced the subjective effects of euphoria, but one commented that the overall acute experience was "slightly calmer". Some of the adverse effects such as jaw clenching and insomnia were also attenuated and recovery was more rapid.[2]

(b) Neurotoxic reaction

When a man on **citalopram** 60 mg daily additionally took unknown amounts of ecstasy he became aggressive, agitated, severely grandiose, restless and performed compulsive movements in a peculiar and joyless dancelike manner. He lacked normal movement control and said he could see little bugs. He was treated with haloperidol and chlordiazepoxide, and improved within 2 days of replacing the **citalopram** with promazine.[3] This appears to be the first and only report of this reaction, but there have been isolated reports of neurotoxicity with other sympathomimetics and SSRIs, see 'SSRIs + Sympathomimetics', p.987.

(c) Pharmacokinetic interactions

An *in vitro* study demonstrated that **fluoxetine** and **paroxetine** inhibited the demethylenation of ecstasy. As this may be the major metabolic pathway of ecstasy, both drugs may theoretically be predicted to increase the concentration of ecstasy *in vivo*.[4]

Mechanism

Complex. It has been suggested that the psychological and neurotoxic effects of ecstasy may be caused by serotonin release in the brain.[2,5] This could potentially be blocked by serotonin reuptake inhibitors (such as citalopram) resulting in reduced ecstasy effects. However, ecstasy is also thought to inhibit serotonin reuptake,[5] so use with the SSRIs could increase serotonin effects, which could result in neurotoxicity.[6] Furthermore, the SSRIs (to varying degrees) inhibit the cytochrome P450 isoenzyme CYP2D6, by which ecstasy is metabolised, so concurrent use could result in increased ecstasy levels.

Importance and management

The ecstasy/citalopram study was primarily undertaken to find out how ecstasy works, but on the basis of these results and *animal* studies it seems likely that patients already taking citalopram may not be able to get as 'high' on usual doses of ecstasy, and some adverse effects may also be reduced. Furthermore, if the proposed mechanism of interaction is correct, the same is also likely to be true if they are taking any other SSRI (such as fluoxetine, **fluvoxamine**, paroxetine, **sertraline**). However, be aware of possible pharmacokinetic interactions with some SSRIs that are potent CYP2D6 inhibitors (e.g. fluoxetine, paroxetine), which may increase ecstasy levels. There is also a risk of increased serotonergic activity and there have been a few reports of interactions involving other sympathomimetics and SSRIs or related drugs, see 'Phentermine + Fluoxetine', p.967.

The neurotoxic reaction cited seems to be an isolated case but it illustrates some of the risks attached to using 'recreational' drugs by patients already taking other medications, particularly antidepressant and psychotropic drugs that affect the same receptors in the CNS.

1. Liechti ME, Baumann C, Gamma A, Vollenweider FX. Acute psychological effects of 3,4-methylenedioxymethamphetamine (MDMA, "Ecstasy") are attenuated by the serotonin uptake inhibitor citalopram. *Neuropsychopharmacology* (2000) 22, 513–21.
2. McCann UD, Ricaurte GA. Reinforcing subjective effects of (±) 3,4-methylenedioxymethamphetamine ("Ecstasy") may be separable from its neurotoxic actions: clinical evidence. *J Clin Psychopharmacol* (1993) 13, 214–17.
3. Lauerma H, Wuorela M, Halme M. Interaction of serotonin reuptake inhibitor and 3,4-methylenedioxymethamphetamine? *Biol Psychiatry* (1998) 43, 929.
4. Ramamoorthy Y, Yu A, Suh N, Haining RL, Tyndale RF, Sellers EM. Reduced (±)-3,4-methylenedioxymethamphetamine ("Ecstasy") metabolism with cytochrome P450 2D6 inhibitors and pharmacogenetic variants *in vitro*. *Biochem Pharmacol* (2002) 63, 2111–19.
5. Lyles J, Cadet JL. Methylenedioxymethamphetamine (MDMA, Ecstasy) neurotoxicity: cellular and molecular mechanisms. *Brain Res Brain Res Rev* (2003) 42, 155–68.
6. Oesterheld JR, Armstrong SC, Cozza KL. Ecstasy: pharmacodynamic and pharmacokinetic interactions. *Psychosomatics* (2004) 45, 84–7.

Ephedrines + Miscellaneous

Alkalinisation of the urine by sodium bicarbonate or other urinary alkalinisers causes retention of ephedrine and pseudoephedrine in the body, leading to the possible development of toxicity (tremors, anxiety, insomnia, tachycardia). Acidification of the urine with ammonium chloride has the opposite effect. Kaolin does not appear to interact significantly with pseudoephedrine but aluminium hydroxide may possibly cause a more rapid onset of action.

Clinical evidence

(a) Ephedrine

When the urine was made acidic (about pH 5) with **ammonium chloride**, the excretion of ephedrine in the urine of three healthy subjects was two to fourfold higher than when the urine was made alkaline (about pH 8) with **sodium bicarbonate**.[1]

(b) Pseudoephedrine

A patient with renal tubular acidosis and persistently alkaline urine developed unexpected toxicity when given therapeutic doses of pseudoephedrine. Therefore 8 adult and child subjects were studied to establish the possible effects of changing the urinary pH on pseudoephedrine elimination. When the urinary pH was adjusted using **ammonium chloride** or **sodium bicarbonate**, within the approximate range of 5.7 to 7.8, the half-life of a single dose of pseudoephedrine (about 5 mg/kg) was found to increase from 1.9 hours at the lowest pH to 21 hours at the highest pH.[2]

This confirms an earlier study in which it was found that at a urinary pH of 8, the half-life of pseudoephedrine was 16, 9.2 and 15 hours, respectively in 3 subjects. At a urinary pH of about 5, the half-life was 4.8, 3 and 6.4 hours, respectively.[3] **Sodium bicarbonate** was given to raise urinary pH and **ammonium chloride** to lower urinary pH.

Another study in 6 healthy subjects found that **sodium bicarbonate** 5 g initially increased the excretion rates of a single 60-mg dose of pseudoephedrine, but as the urinary pH increased the excretion of pseudoephedrine was reduced.[4] The same study also found that 30 ml of **aluminium hydroxide gel** did not affect the total amount of pseudoephedrine absorbed over 24 hours, but the rate of absorption was significantly increased during the first 3 hours.[4]

In a study of 6 healthy subjects 30 ml of a 30% suspension of **kaolin** was found to cause a small decrease of about 10% in the absorption of a single 60-mg dose of pseudoephedrine. The rate of absorption was also decreased.[4]

Mechanism

The ephedrines are basic drugs, which are mainly excreted unchanged in the urine. In acid urine, most of the drug is ionised in the tubular filtrate and unable to diffuse passively back into the circulation, and is therefore lost in the urine. In alkaline urine, it mostly exists in the lipid-soluble form which is retained. As a result it is lost much more slowly and accumulates.

The increased rate of absorption of pseudoephedrine in the gut seen with sodium bicarbonate and aluminium hydroxide is probably also due to pH rises which favour the formation of the lipid-soluble absorbable form of pseudoephedrine. The reduced absorption with kaolin is probably due to adsorption of the pseudoephedrine onto the surface of the kaolin.

Importance and management

The ephedrines/urinary alkaliniser interaction is established but reports of adverse reactions in patients appear to be rare. Monitor the outcome of alkalinising the urine for any evidence of toxicity due to drug retention (tremor, anxiety, insomnia, tachycardia, etc.), reducing the dosage if necessary. **Acetazolamide** makes the urine alkaline and would be expected to interact with the ephedrines in the same way as sodium bicarbonate. Acidification of the urine with ammonium chloride increases the loss of the ephedrines in the urine and could be exploited in cases of drug overdosage. Aluminium hydroxide may possibly cause a more rapid onset of pseudoephedrine activity (but this needs confirmation) whereas the effects of kaolin on absorption are small and unlikely to be clinically important.

1. Wilkinson GR, Beckett AH. Absorption, metabolism and excretion of the ephedrines in man. I. The influence of urinary pH and urine volume output. *J Pharmacol Exp Ther* (1968) 162, 139–47.
2. Brater DC, Kaojarern S, Benet LZ, Lin ET, Lockwood T, Morris RC, McSherry EJ, Melmon KL. Renal excretion of pseudoephedrine. *Clin Pharmacol Ther* (1980) 28, 690–4.
3. Kuntzman RG, Tsai I, Brand L, Mark LC. The influence of urinary pH on the plasma half-life of pseudoephedrine in man and dog and a sensitive assay for its determination in human plasma. *Clin Pharmacol Ther* (1971) 12, 62–7.
4. Lucarotti RL, Colaizzi JL, Barry H, Poust RI. Enhanced pseudoephedrine absorption by concurrent administration of aluminium hydroxide gel in humans. *J Pharm Sci* (1972) 61, 903–5.

Inotropes + Calcium compounds

Calcium chloride infusions reduce the cardiotonic effects of adrenaline (epinephrine) and dobutamine but not those of amrinone.

Clinical evidence, mechanism, importance and management

In a double-blind, randomised, cross-over study in 12 patients following coronary artery bypass grafting, calcium chloride 10 mg/kg bolus followed by 2 mg/kg per hour infusion was found to attenuate the effects of **adrenaline** (**epinephrine**) 10 and 30 nanograms/kg per minute for 8 minutes each. **Adrenaline** alone produced a significant increase in the cardiac index, but following the calcium infusion **adrenaline** had no significant effect and the maximal **adrenaline**-induced increase in cardiac index was reduced by 70%. **Adrenaline** 30 nanograms/kg per minute alone increased mean arterial blood pressure from 87 to 95 mmHg; calcium chloride also raised blood pressure from 85 to 93 mmHg, but after calcium, **adrenaline** had no further significant effect on blood pressure.[1]

Some of these workers also studied the mode of action of **dobutamine** in 22 patients recovering from coronary artery bypass surgery. It was found that an infusion of calcium chloride (1 mg/kg per minute initially, then 0.25 mg/kg per minute) reduced the increase in cardiac output produced by an infusion of **dobutamine** 2.5 to 5 micrograms/kg per minute by 30%. The cardiotonic actions of **amrinone** (a phosphodiesterase inhibitor) in a group of 24 similar patients were unaffected by the calcium infusion.[2]

Just how the calcium alters the effects of **adrenaline** and **dobutamine** is not known, but since they are both beta-receptor agonists it is reasonable to postulate that calcium interferes with the signal transduction through the beta-adrenergic receptor complex. The clinical importance of these findings is uncertain.

1. Zaloga GP, Strickland RA, Butterworth JF, Mark LJ, Mills SA, Lake CR. Calcium attenuates epinephrine's ß-adrenergic effects in postoperative heart surgery patients. *Circulation* (1990) 81, 196–200.
2. Butterworth JF, Zaloga GP, Prielipp RC, Tucker WY, Royster RL. Calcium inhibits the cardiac stimulating properties of dobutamine but not of amrinone. *Chest* (1992) 101, 174–80.

Methylphenidate + Carbamazepine

Carbamazepine may reduce methylphenidate levels.

Clinical evidence, mechanism, importance and management

A 7-year-old boy with attention deficit disorder taking carbamazepine 1 g daily for grand mal epilepsy was referred because of unmanageable behaviour. He failed to respond to methylphenidate in doses of up to 30 mg every 4 hours, and his blood levels of both methylphenidate and its metabolites were undetectable. The authors attributed this to the carbamazepine.[1] Similarly, symptoms of attention deficit hyperactivity disorder worsened in a 13-year-old girl taking methylphenidate after she also took carbamazepine. Methylphenidate serum concentrations decreased markedly and the dose of methylphenidate had to be increased from 20 to 60 mg three times daily to regain the benefit she had before the addition of carbamazepine.[2] However, another report describes 4 out of 7 children taking methylphenidate and carbamazepine in whom the combination was successful. Blood levels of methylphenidate were apparently not measured.[3] Despite these conflicting results, and the sparsity of the information, it would seem wise to monitor the response to methylphenidate treatment carefully in patients taking carbamazepine.

1. Behar D, Schaller J, Spreat S. Extreme reduction of methylphenidate levels by carbamazepine. *J Am Acad Child Adolesc Psychiatry* (1998) 37, 1128–9.
2. Schaller JL, Behar D. Carbamazepine and methylphenidate in ADHD. *J Am Acad Child Adolesc Psychiatry* (1999) 38, 112–13.
3. Gross-Tsur V. Carbamazepine and methylphenidate. *J Am Acad Child Adolesc Psychiatry* (1999) 38, 637.

Methylphenidate + Clonidine

Much publicised fears about the serious consequences of using methylphenidate with clonidine appear to be unfounded. There is limited evidence that concurrent use can be both safe and effective.

Clinical evidence, mechanism, importance and management

There have been fears about serious adverse events when methylphenidate is taken with clonidine,[1] due to reports of 3 deaths in children taking both drugs. One child died from ventricular fibrillation due to cardiac abnormalities, one from cardiac arrest attributed to an overdose of fluoxetine, and the third death was unexplained. Studies of these 3 cases and one other failed to establish any link between the use of methylphenidate with clonidine and these deaths, the final broad conclusion being that the event was largely a media-inspired scare story built on inconclusive evidence.[2,3] A small scale pilot study in 24 patients suggested that the combination is both safe and effective for the treatment of attention deficit hyperactivity disorder,[4] and the makers of one formulation of methylphenidate[1] said that they were not aware of any reports describing adverse events when *Concerta XL* (methylphenidate) was used with clonidine.

1. Janssen-Cilag. Personal communication, April 2002.
2. Popper CW. Editorial commentary. Combining methylphenidate and clonidine: pharmacologic questions and news reports about sudden death. *J Child Adolesc Psychopharmacol* (1995) 5, 157–66.
3. Fenichel RR. Special communication. Combining methylphenidate and clonidine: the role of post-marketing surveillance. *J Child Adolesc Psychopharmacol* (1995) 5, 155–6.
4. Connor DF, Barkley RA, Davis HT. A pilot study of methylphenidate, clonidine, or the combination in ADHD comorbid with aggressive oppositional defiant or conduct disorder. *Clin Pediatr (Phila)* (2000) 39, 15–25.

Modafinil + Dexamfetamine

No pharmacokinetic interaction appears to occur between modafinil and dexamfetamine.

Clinical evidence, mechanism, importance and management

In a steady-state study, 23 healthy subjects were given modafinil 200 mg daily for 7 days, followed by 400 mg daily for 3 weeks. During the last week, 10 of the subjects were also given dexamfetamine 20 mg daily, 7 hours after their modafinil dose. Dexamfetamine caused no significant change in the pharmacokinetics of modafinil and the combination was well tolerated. In addition, the pharmacokinetics of dexamfetamine did not appear to be affected by modafinil when compared with values reported in the literature.[1] Similar results were found in a single dose study.[2] No additional precautions appear to be necessary on concurrent use.

1. Hellriegel ET, Arora S, Nelson M, Robertson P. Steady-state pharmacokinetics and tolerability of modafinil administered alone or in combination with dextroamphetamine in healthy volunteers. *J Clin Pharmacol* (2002) 42, 448–58.
2. Wong YN, Wang L, Hartman L, Simcoe D, Chen Y, Laughton W, Eldon R, Markland C, Grebow P. Comparison of the single-dose pharmacokinetics and tolerability of modafinil and dextroamphetamine administered alone or in combination in healthy male volunteers. *J Clin Pharmacol* (1998) 38, 971–8.

Modafinil + Methylphenidate

No pharmacokinetic interaction appears to occur between modafinil and methylphenidate.

Clinical evidence, mechanism, importance and management

Single doses of modafinil 200 mg and methylphenidate 40 mg were given together without any clinically relevant changes in the pharmacokinetic profile of either drug.[1] In a steady-state study, 30 healthy subjects were given modafinil 200 mg daily for 7 days, followed by 400 mg daily for 3 weeks. During the last week, 16 of the subjects were also given methylphenidate 20 mg daily, 8 hours after their modafinil dose. Methylphenidate caused no significant change in the pharmacokinetics of modafinil. In addition, the pharmacokinetics of methylphenidate did not appear to be affected by modafinil when compared with values reported in the literature.[2] No special precautions would appear to be necessary on concurrent use.

1. Wong YN, King SP, Laughton WB, McCormick GC, Grebow PE. Single-dose pharmacokinetics of modafinil and methylphenidate given alone or in combination in healthy male volunteers. *J Clin Pharmacol* (1998) 38, 276–82.
2. Hellriegel ET, Arora S, Nelson M, Robertson P. Steady-state pharmacokinetics and tolerability of modafinil given alone or in combination with methylphenidate in healthy volunteers. *J Clin Pharmacol* (2001) 41, 895–904.

Phenmetrazine + Amobarbital

The CNS adverse effects and the weight-reducing effects of phenmetrazine are reduced by amobarbital.

Clinical evidence, mechanism, importance and management

A comparative study in 50 overweight adults of the effects of phenmetrazine 25 mg three times daily with or without amobarbital 30 mg three times daily found that although the adverse CNS effects, particularly insomnia, headache and nervousness, were decreased by the presence of the barbiturate, the weight-reducing effects were also decreased (by 65%).[1]

1. Hadler AJ. Phenmetrazine vs. phenmetrazine with amobarbital for weight reduction: a double-blind study. *Curr Ther Res* (1969) 11, 750–4.

Phentermine + Fluoxetine

An isolated report describes phentermine toxicity in a woman several days after she stopped taking fluoxetine.

Clinical evidence, mechanism, importance and management

A 22-year-old woman who had successfully and uneventfully taken fluoxetine 20 mg daily for 3 months, stopped the fluoxetine and then 8 days later took a single 30-mg tablet of phentermine. Within a few hours she experienced racing thoughts, stomach cramps, palpitations (pulse 84 bpm), tremors, dry eyes and diffuse hyperreflexia. The problems had all resolved the following day after she took lorazepam 1.5 mg. The authors of this report suggested that the residual inhibitory effects of the fluoxetine on liver cytochrome P450 enzymes led to decreased phentermine metabolism, resulting in increased phentermine levels and sympathetic hyperstimulation. It is known that fluoxetine and its active metabolite are only cleared from the body slowly and can persist for weeks. The authors also alternatively wondered whether some of the symptoms might have fitted the serotonin syndrome.[1]

Although this is an isolated case and its general importance is unknown, the authors of the report draw attention to the possible risks of taking SSRIs and sympathomimetic drugs used for controlling diet.

A neurotoxic reaction has also been reported with ecstasy and citalopram, see 'Ecstasy (MDMA, 3,4-methylenedioxymethamfetamine) + SSRIs', p.965.

1. Bostwick JM, Brown TM. A toxic reaction from combining fluoxetine and phentermine. *J Clin Psychopharmacol* (1996) 16, 189–90.

Phenylephrine + Atropine

The hypertensive and other serious adverse effects of phenylephrine absorbed from eye drops can be markedly increased by atropine.

Clinical evidence

A brief report describes 7 cases of pseudo-phaeochromocytoma with severe rises in blood pressure and tachycardia in young adults and children undergoing eye operations when treated with phenylephrine 10% eye drops and atropine. Only two of them had any pre-existing cardiovascular illness (moderate hypertension). All were under general anaesthesia with propofol, phenoperidine and vecuronium, and premedicated with intramuscular atropine, and some were later given more intravenous atropine because of the bradycardia when the oculomotor muscles were stretched. The total atropine doses were less than 10 micrograms/kg in adults and 20 micrograms/kg in the children. At least 0.4 ml of phenylephrine 10% was used. In three cases left ventricular failure and pulmonary oedema occurred, which needed monitoring in intensive care.[1]

In a study of this interaction, 6 healthy subjects were given a phenylephrine infusion before and after being given three intravenous doses of atropine (20, 10, and 10 micrograms/kg) at 90, 120 and 150 minutes. It was found that phenylephrine 420 nanograms/kg per minute raised the diastolic and systolic blood pressures by 4 mmHg before using atropine, and 17 mmHg after atropine was given. For safety reasons the increases in blood pressure were limited to 30 mmHg above the base line.[2]

Mechanism

Phenylephrine causes vasoconstriction, which can raise the blood pressure. Normally this would be limited by a baroreflex mediated by the vagus nerve, but if this cholinergic mechanism is blocked by atropine, the rise in blood pressure is largely uncontrolled. Severe hypertension may occur, and other adverse cardiac events such as acute cardiac failure may follow.

Importance and management

A surprisingly large amount of phenylephrine can be absorbed from eye drops, and the potential adverse effects of this (severe hypertension, cardiac arrhythmias, myocardial infarction) are now well documented.[3-5] The reports cited here are good evidence that these risks are increased by the presence of atropine, and the interaction is clearly potentially serious. The authors of one of the reports[1] suggest that the risks can be reduced by reducing the concentrations of phenylephrine used, swabbing to minimise the amount that drains into the nasolachrymal duct to the nasal mucosa where rapid absorption occurs, and reducing the drop size by using a thin-walled cannula.[6] Other suggestions for reducing systemic absorption are punctal plugging, nasolachrymal duct compression, and lid closure after instillation of the eye drop.[6]

1. Daelman F, Andréjak M, Rajaonarivony D, Bryselbout E, Jezraoui P, Ossart M. Phenylephrine eyedrops, systemic atropine and cardiovascular adverse events. *Therapie* (1994) 49, 467.
2. Levine MAH, Leenen FHH. Role of vagal activity in the cardiovascular responses to phenylephrine in man. *Br J Clin Pharmacol* (1992) 33, 333–6.
3. Fraunfelder FT, Scafidi AF. Possible adverse effects from topical ocular 10% phenylephrine. *Am J Ophthalmol* (1978) 85, 447–53.
4. Van der Spek AFL, Hantler CB. Phenylephrine eyedrops and anesthesia. *Anesthesiology* (1986) 64, 812–14.
5. Lai Y-K. Adverse effect of intraoperative phenylephrine 10%: case report. *Br J Ophthalmol* (1989) 73, 468–9.
6. Craig EW, Griffiths PG. Effect on mydriasis of modifying the volume of phenylephrine drops. *Br J Ophthalmol* (1991) 75, 222–3.

Phenylpropanolamine + Indinavir

A report describes a hypertensive crisis in a patient receiving indinavir when phenylpropanolamine was additionally given.

Clinical evidence, mechanism, importance and management

A 28-year-old woman was prescribed HIV-prophylaxis following a needle stick injury. She was initially treated with zidovudine, indinavir and lamivudine, but after one week stavudine was substituted for zidovudine as she was experiencing nausea and vomiting. Six hours after taking *Tavist-D* (clemastine with phenylpropanolamine) for a sinus complaint she had a feeling of chest tightness associated with difficulty in breathing, and shortly afterwards she experienced left-sided upper extremity weakness, followed by a severe right-sided temporal headache. Her blood pressure was 220/120 mmHg, but returned to normal within 4 hours, and the neurological deficit resolved over the next 8 hours. However, 12 hours later, the same neurological deficit recurred, although no increase in blood pressure was noted. The neurological deficit was thought to be due to reversible cerebral vasoconstriction, secondary to sympathomimetic toxicity. She was treated with nimodipine 60 mg every 4 hours and aspirin 325 mg daily, and her symptoms did not recur.[1]

The patient had been taking phenylpropanolamine intermittently for several years without any adverse reaction and it was thought that the recent addition of the anti-HIV regimen potentiated the effect of the phenylpropanolamine.[1] It seems likely that the indinavir was responsible for the interaction as it is a potent enzyme inhibitor. This is an isolated report and its general significance is not known, but it would be prudent to be alert for this interaction in patients given both drugs.

1. Khurana V, de la Fuente M, Bradley TP. Hypertensive crisis secondary to phenylpropanolamine interacting with triple-drug therapy for HIV prophylaxis. *Am J Med* (1999) 106, 118–19.

Phenylpropanolamine + Indometacin

An isolated report describes a patient on phenylpropanolamine who developed serious hypertension after taking a single dose of indometacin, but a controlled study in other subjects failed to find any evidence of an adverse interaction.

Clinical evidence

A woman who had been taking phenylpropanolamine 85 mg daily for several months as an appetite suppressant, developed a severe bifrontal headache within 15 minutes of taking indometacin 25 mg. Thirty minutes later her systolic blood pressure was 210 mmHg and the diastolic blood pressure was unrecordable. A later study in this patient confirmed that neither drug on its own caused this response, but when taken together the blood pressure rose to a maximum of 200/150 mmHg within half an hour of taking the indometacin, and was associated with bradycardia. The blood pressure was rapidly reduced by phentolamine.[1]

In contrast, a controlled study in 14 healthy young women found no evidence that sustained-release indometacin 75 mg twice daily given with sustained-release phenylpropanolamine 75 mg daily caused a rise in blood pressure.[2]

Mechanism

Not understood.

Importance and management

Direct information seems to be limited to these reports. They suggest that an adverse hypertensive response is very unlikely in most individuals given these drugs, but it should be borne in mind that phenylpropanolamine, even on its own, can sometimes cause severe hypertension.[3-5]

1. Lee KY, Beilin LJ, Vandongen R. Severe hypertension after ingestion of an appetite suppressant (phenylpropanolamine) with indomethacin. *Lancet* (1979) i, 1110–11.
2. McKenney JM, Wright JT, Katz GM, Goodman RP. The effect of phenylpropanolamine on 24-hour blood pressure in normotensive subjects administered indomethacin. *DICP Ann Pharmacother* (1991) 25, 234–9.
3. Livingston PH. Transient hypertension and phenylpropanolamine. *JAMA* (1966) 196, 1159.
4. Duvernoy WFC. Positive phentolamine test in hypertension induced by a nasal decongestant. *N Engl J Med* (1969) 280, 877.
5. Shapiro SR. Hypertension due to anorectic agent. *N Engl J Med* (1969) 280, 1363.

Ritodrine + Miscellaneous

Supraventricular tachycardia developed in a woman on ritodrine when she was given glycopyrronium (glycopyrrolate). Tachycardia has also been reported with ritodrine and atropine in two patients. The abuse of cocaine does not appear to increase the incidence of adverse effects in patients given ritodrine.

Clinical evidence, mechanism, importance and management

Premature labour in a 39-year-old woman who was 28 weeks pregnant was arrested with an intravenous infusion of ritodrine hydrochloride. Two weeks later while she was on the maximum dose of ritodrine (300 micrograms/minute) her uterine contractions began again and she was scheduled for emergency caesarean section. The ritodrine was discontinued 40 minutes before the operation. It was noted in the operating room that she had copious oral secretions so she was given 100% oxygen by mask and **glycopyrronium** (**glycopyrrolate**) 200 micrograms intravenously. Shortly afterwards she developed supraventricular tachycardia (a rise from 80 up to 180 bpm), which was converted to sinus tachycardia of 130 bpm with propranolol 500 micrograms intravenously in divided doses.[1]

The reason for this reaction is not understood. Ritodrine alone has been responsible for tachyarrhythmias and one possible explanation for this interaction is that the effects of these two drugs were additive. For further comment on the interaction between a sympathomimetic and antimuscarinic agent, see 'Phenylephrine + Atropine', p.967. Two other cases of tachyarrhythmias have been described in patients premedicated with **atropine** who were given ritodrine as a single intravenous bolus.[2] Information is very limited and the interaction is not well established but some caution is clearly appropriate if both drugs are used. The authors of the first report advise avoidance.

A study in 51 pregnant patients given ritodrine for premature labour found no evidence of an increase in adverse effects in 17 of the patients who had been abusing **cocaine**.[3]

1. Simpson JI, Giffin JP. A glycopyrrolate-ritodrine drug-drug interaction. *Can J Anaesth* (1988) 35, 187–9.
2. Sheybany S, Murphy JF, Evans D, Newcombe RG, Pearson JF. Ritodrine in the management of fetal distress. *Br J Obstet Gynaecol* (1982) 89, 723–6.
3. Darby MJ, Mazdisnian F. Does recent cocaine use increase the risk of side effects with β-adrenergic tocolysis? *Am J Obstet Gynecol* (1991) 164, 377.

Sympathomimetics + Caffeine

Phenylpropanolamine can raise blood pressure and in some cases this may be further increased by caffeine. Combined use resulted in hypertensive crises in a few individuals. Ephedrine may interact similarly. Phenylpropanolamine can markedly raise plasma caffeine levels, and isolated reports describe the development of acute psychosis with caffeine and phenylpropanolamine or ephedrine.

Clinical evidence

(a) Ephedrine

Several patients have experienced severe adverse effects (subarachnoid haemorrhage, cardiac arrest, hypertension, tachycardia and neurosis) after taking ephedrine or **ephedra** alkaloids with caffeine.[1,2] However, it is not possible to definitively say that these effects were the result of an interaction because none of the patients took either drug separately. Nevertheless, given the way phenylpropanolamine interacts (see below) an interaction seems likely.

Two episodes of acute psychosis occurred in a 32-year-old man following the consumption of ***'vigueur fit'*** tablets (containing **ephedra** alkaloids and caffeine), ***'Red Bull'*** (containing caffeine) and **alcohol**. He had no previous record of aberrant behaviour despite regularly taking 6 to 9 tablets of ***'vigueur fit'*** daily (about twice the recommended dose). However, on this occasion, over a 10-hour period, he consumed 3 or 4 bottles of ***'Red Bull'*** (containing about 95 mg of caffeine per 250-mg bottle) and enough **alcohol** to reach a blood-alcohol level of about 335 mg%. No more episodes occurred after he stopped taking the alkaloid tablets. **Ephedra** alkaloids (ephedrine and **pseudoephedrine**) may cause psychosis and it appears that their effects may be exaggerated by interaction with caffeine and **alcohol**.[3]

(b) Phenylpropanolamine

The mean blood pressure of 16 healthy subjects rose by 11/12 mmHg after they took caffeine 400 mg, by 12/13 mmHg after they took phenylpropanolamine 75 mg, and by 12/11 mmHg when both drugs were taken. Phenylpropanolamine 150 mg caused a greater rise of 36/18 mmHg. One of the subjects had a hypertensive crisis after phenylpropanolamine 150 mg and again 2 hours after caffeine 400 mg. This needed antihypertensive treatment.[4] The same group of workers describe a similar study in which the AUC of caffeine 400 mg increased more than threefold, and the mean peak caffeine concentration increased almost fourfold (from 2.1 to 8 micrograms/ml) after phenylpropanolamine 75 mg was given.[5] Additive increases in blood pressure are described in another report.[6]

Mania with psychotic delusions occurred in a healthy woman (who normally drank 7 to 8 cups of **coffee** daily) within 3 days of starting to take a phenylpropanolamine-containing decongestant. She recovered within a week of stopping both the **coffee** and the phenylpropanolamine.[7]

Mechanism

Uncertain. Simple additive hypertensive effects would seem to be part of the explanation. The effects of caffeine may compound the effects of the sympathomimetics on the cardiovascular and central nervous systems by blocking adenosine receptors (causing vasoconstriction) and also augmenting the release of catecholamines.[1,3]

Importance and management

Fairly well established interactions. These studies illustrate the potential hazards of these drugs, even in normal healthy individuals. However, it has to be said that there seem to be no other reports of adverse interactions, which is perhaps surprising bearing in mind that coffee/caffeine is very widely used and ephedrine and phenylpropanolamine have also been widely available over the counter. One possible explanation for this could be that these interactions may go unrecognised or be attributed to one drug only e.g. phenylpropanolamine, whereas caffeine has also been taken either as part of the preparation[1,8] or in beverages (often not reported).

Nevertheless, serious adverse events have been reported with caffeine and phenylpropanolamine or dietary supplements containing ephedra alkaloids (sometimes called ma huang) and therefore these preparations may pose a serious health risk to some users.[1] The risk may be affected by individual susceptibility, the additive stimulant effects of caffeine, the variability in the contents of alkaloids in non-prescription dietary supplements, or pre-existing medical conditions.[1]

The authors of one report[4] advised that likely users of phenylpropanolamine (those with allergies or the overweight) and those particularly vulnerable (elderly or hypertensive patients) should be warned about taking more than the recommended dose of phenylpropanolamine, and also about taking caffeine at the same time, because of the possible risk of intracranial haemorrhage.

1. Haller CA, Benowitz NL. Adverse cardiovascular and central nervous system events associated with dietary supplements containing ephedra alkaloids. *N Engl J Med* (2000) 343, 1833–8.
2. Astrup A, Breum L, Toubro S, Hein P, Quaade F. The effect and safety of an ephedrine/caffeine compound compared to ephedrine, caffeine and placebo in obese subjects on an energy restricted diet. A double blind trial. *Int J Obes Relat Metab Disord* (1992) 16, 269–77.
3. Tormey WP, Bruzzi A. Acute psychosis due to the interaction of legal compounds – ephedra alkaloids in 'Vigueur Fit' tablets, caffeine in 'Red Bull' and alcohol. *Med Sci Law* (2001) 41, 331–6.
4. Lake CR, Zaloga G, Bray J, Rosenberg D, Chernow B. Transient hypertension after two phenylpropanolamine diet aids and the effects of caffeine: a placebo-controlled follow-up study. *Am J Med* (1989) 86, 427–32.
5. Lake CR, Rosenberg DB, Gallant S, Zaloga G, Chernow B. Phenylpropanolamine increases plasma caffeine levels. *Clin Pharmacol Ther* (1990) 47, 675–85.
6. Brown NJ, Ryder D, Branch RA. A pharmacodynamic interaction between caffeine and phenylpropanolamine. *Clin Pharmacol Ther* (1991) 50, 363–71.
7. Lake CR. Manic psychosis after coffee and phenylpropanolamine. *Biol Psychiatry* (1991) 30, 401–4.
8. Lake CR, Gallant S, Masson E, Miller P. Adverse drug effects attributed to phenylpropanolamine: a review of 142 case reports. *Am J Med* (1990) 89, 195– 208.

Sympathomimetics + Clonidine

Experimental studies in patients show that pretreatment with clonidine can increase the blood pressure responses to ephedrine and phenylephrine, but not those of noradrenaline (norepinephrine). In the context of adverse reactions these increases appear to be of little clinical importance.

Clinical evidence, mechanism, importance and management

A study in 77 patients (38 premedicated with clonidine 5 micrograms/kg and famotidine 20 mg, and a control group of 39 given only famotidine, 90 minutes before induction of general anaesthesia) found that the rise in blood pressure caused by intravenous **phenylephrine** 2 micrograms/kg was augmented by clonidine. However, the overall response to **noradrenaline (norepinephrine)** 0.5 micrograms/kg was not significantly affected, although 2 to 4 minutes after administration the mean arterial blood pressure was raised in the clonidine group. The reasons are not understood. There were no significant differences between the groups in terms of the incidence of hypertension, arrhythmias or bradycardia.[1] A similar and related study by the same group of workers, using enflurane and nitrous oxide/oxygen for anaesthesia, found that the mean maximum blood pressure increases in the group premedicated with clonidine and given **phenylephrine** 2 micrograms/kg intravenously were 26% and 32% respectively, for awake and anaesthetised subjects, and 13% and 18% respectively, in the group not given clonidine.[2] The authors of the first report[1] suggested that the increase in pressor response was unlikely to be clinically significant. Similar additional effects on blood pressure were found in patients given intravenous **ephedrine** 100 micrograms/kg after pretreatment with clonidine.[3]

1. Tanaka M, Nishikawa T. Effects of clonidine premedication on the pressor response to α-adrenergic agonists. *Br J Anaesth* (1995) 75, 593–7.
2. Inomata S, Nishikawa T, Kihara S, Akiyoshi Y. Enhancement of pressor response to intravenous phenylephrine following oral clonidine medication in awake and anaesthetized patients. *Can J Anaesth* (1995) 42, 119–25.
3. Nishikawa T, Kimura T, Taguchi N, Dohi S. Oral clonidine preanesthetic medication augments the pressor responses to intravenous ephedrine in awake or anesthetized patients. *Anesthesiology* (1991) 74, 705–10.

Sympathomimetics; Directly-acting + Guanethidine

The pressor effects of noradrenaline (norepinephrine), phenylephrine, metaraminol and similar direct-acting sympathomimetics can be increased in the presence of guanethidine. The mydriatic effects are similarly enhanced and prolonged.

Clinical evidence

(a) Pressor responses

A study in 6 normotensive subjects, given guanethidine 200 mg on the first day of study and 100 mg daily for the next 2 days, showed that their mean arterial blood pressure when given an infusion of **noradrenaline (norepinephrine)** in a range of doses was increased by 6% to 18% (a 6 to 20 mmHg increase). Moreover cardiac arrhythmias appeared at lower doses of **noradrenaline** and with greater frequency than in the absence of guanethidine, and were more serious in nature.[1]

In another report, a patient on guanethidine 20 mg daily was given intramuscular **metaraminol** 10 mg, which rapidly caused a blood pressure rise to 220/130 mmHg accompanied by severe headache and extreme angina.[2] An increase in blood pressure from 165/90 to 170/110 mmHg was also seen in a patient on guanethidine who, prior to surgery, was treated with **phenylephrine eye drops**.[3]

(b) Mydriatic responses

The mydriasis due to **phenylephrine** administered as a 10% **eye drop** solution was observed to be prolonged for up to 10 hours in a patient receiving guanethidine for hypertension.[4] This enhanced mydriatic response has been described in another study using guanethidine eye drops with **adrenaline (epinephrine)**, **phenylephrine** or **methoxamine** eye drops.[5]

Mechanism

If sympathetic nerves are cut surgically, the receptors that they normally stimulate become hypersensitive. By preventing the release of noradrenaline from adrenergic neurones, guanethidine and other adrenergic neurone blockers cause a temporary 'drug-induced sympathectomy', which is also accompanied by hypersensitivity of the receptors. Hence the increased response to the stimulation of the receptors by directly acting sympathomimetics.

Importance and management

An established, well-documented and potentially serious interaction. Since the pressor effects can be grossly exaggerated, dosages of directly-acting sympathomimetics (alpha-agonists) should be reduced appropriately. In addition it should be remembered that the incidence and severity of heart arrhythmias is increased.[1] Considerable care is required. Direct evidence seems to be limited to noradrenaline (norepinephrine), phenylephrine and metaraminol, but **dopamine** and **methoxamine** possess direct sympathomimetic activity and may be expected to interact similarly. No interaction would be expected with the **beta-agonist drugs** used for the treatment of asthma (such as **terbutaline**, **salbutamol**). If as a result of this interaction the blood pressure becomes grossly elevated, it can be controlled by giving an alpha-adrenergic blocker such as phentolamine.[6] Phenylephrine is contained in a number of non-prescription cough and cold preparations, which may contain 12 mg in a dose. Given as a single-dose, this dose is only likely to cause a moderate blood pressure rise compared with the marked rise seen in subjects on **debrisoquine** given single 0.75-mg/kg doses of phenylephrine (roughly 50 mg in a 70-kg individual).[6] However, this requires confirmation, particularly since the non-prescription products may be taken up to 4 times daily for up to 7 days.

An exaggerated pressor response is clearly much more potentially serious than enhanced and prolonged mydriasis, but the latter is also possible and undesirable. The same precautions apply about using smaller amounts of the sympathomimetic drugs. Note that many indirect-acting sympathomimetics can antagonise the blood pressure lowering effect of guanethidine, see 'Guanethidine + Amfetamines and related drugs', p.669.

1. Mulheims GH, Entrup RW, Paiewonsky D, Mierzwiak DS. Increased sensitivity of the heart to catecholamine-induced arrhythmias following guanethidine. *Clin Pharmacol Ther* (1965) 6, 757–62.
2. Stevens FRT. A danger of sympathomimetic drugs. *Med J Aust* (1966) 2, 576.
3. Kim JM, Stevenson CE, Mathewson HS. Hypertensive reactions to phenylephrine eyedrops in patients with sympathetic denervation. *Am J Ophthalmol* (1978) 85, 862–8.
4. Cooper B. Neo-synephrine (10%) eye drops. *Med J Aust* (1968) 55, 420.
5. Sneddon JM, Turner P. The interactions of local guanethidine and sympathomimetic amines in the human eye. *Arch Ophthalmol* (1969) 81,622–7.
6. Allum W, Aminu J, Bloomfield TH, Davies C, Scales AH, Vere DW. Interaction between debrisoquine and phenylephrine in man. *Br J Clin Pharmacol* (1974) 1, 51–7.

Sympathomimetics + Lithium

The pressor effects of noradrenaline (norepinephrine) and phenylephrine are slightly reduced by lithium carbonate. The pressor effects of tyramine are not affected by lithium.

Clinical evidence, mechanism, importance and management

A study in 8 patients with manic depression found that after taking lithium carbonate for 7 to 10 days (serum level range 0.72 to 1.62 mmol/l) the dosage of **noradrenaline (norepinephrine)** had to be increased by 1.8 micrograms in 7 patients to maintain a blood pressure increase of 25 mmHg. The pressor effect of the **noradrenaline** was reduced 22% by the lithium.[1] Another study in 17 depressed patients with serum lithium levels in the range 0.8 to 1.2 mmol/l found that 12% more **noradrenaline** and 31% more **phenylephrine** was needed to raise the blood pressure by 30 mmHg,[2] The reasons are not known. In both of these studies the pressor effects of **tyramine** were found to be unaffected by the presence of the lithium.[1,2]

These decreases in the pressor response to **noradrenaline** and to **phenylephrine** in the presence of lithium carbonate are both relatively small and it seems unlikely that they will present any problems in practice.

For reduced amfetamine effects in the presence of lithium, see 'Amfetamines or related drugs + Lithium', p.961.

1. Fann WE, Davis JM, Janowsky DS, Cavanaugh JH, Kaufmann JS, Griffith JD, Oates JA. Effects of lithium on adrenergic function in man. *Clin Pharmacol Ther* (1972) 13, 71–7.
2. Ghose K. Assessment of peripheral adrenergic activity and its interactions with drugs in man. *Eur J Clin Pharmacol* (1980) 17, 233–8.

Sympathomimetics + Rauwolfia alkaloids

The pressor and other effects of directly acting sympathomimetics such as adrenaline (epinephrine) are slightly increased in the presence of the rauwolfia alkaloids. The effects of indirectly acting sympathomimetics or those with mixed activity, such as the amfetamines may be reduced or abolished by the rauwolfia alkaloids.

Clinical evidence

Eleven patients taking **reserpine** were found to have an increase in blood pressures of 30/12 mmHg when they were pretreated with **phenylephrine** 10% eye drops, whereas no significant increase in blood pressure occurred in 176 patients who received **phenylephrine** eye drops but were not on **reserpine**.[1] After 7 healthy subjects took **reserpine** 0.25 to 1 mg daily for 2 weeks the pressor responses to **noradrenaline (norepinephrine)** was increased by 20 to 40% but their responses to **tyramine** (an indirectly-acting amine) were reduced by about 75%.[2] A man taking **reserpine** who became hypotensive while undergoing surgery failed to respond to an intravenous injection of **ephedrine**, but did so after 30 minutes treatment with **noradrenaline**, presumably because the stores of **noradrenaline** at adrenergic neurones had become replenished.[3] The mydriatic effects of **ephedrine** have also been shown to be antagonised by pretreatment with **reserpine**.[4] However, in contrast, one report claimed that ephedrine 25 mg given orally or intramuscularly, once or twice a day, proved to be an effective treatment for reserpine-induced hypotension and bradycardia in schizophrenic patients.[5]

Experiments with *dogs* have demonstrated that **adrenaline (epinephrine)**, **noradrenaline** and **phenylephrine** (all sympathomimetics with direct actions) remain effective vasopressors after treatment with **reserpine**, and their actions are enhanced to some extent, whereas the vasopressor actions of **ephedrine**, **amfetamine**, **metamfetamine**, **tyramine** and **mephentermine** (all sympathomimetics with indirect actions) are reduced or abolished by **reserpine**.[6-8]

Mechanism

The rauwolfia alkaloids cause adrenergic neurones to lose their stores of noradrenaline (**norepinephrine**), so that they can no longer stimulate adrenergic receptors and transmission ceases. Indirectly-acting sympathomimetics, which work by stimulating the release of stored noradrenaline, may therefore be expected to become ineffective. In contrast, the effects of directly-acting sympathomimetics should remain unchanged or possibly even enhanced because of the supersensitivity of the receptors, which occurs when they are deprived of stimulation by noradrenaline for any length of time. Drugs with mixed direct and indirect actions, such as ephedrine, should fall somewhere between the two, although the reports cited seem to indicate that ephedrine has predominantly indirect activity.[3,4]

Importance and management

These are established interactions, but the paucity of clinical information suggests that in practice they do not present many problems. If a pressor drug is required, a directly acting drug such as noradrenaline (**norepinephrine**) or phenylephrine may be expected to be effective. **Metaraminol** has also been successfully used as a pressor drug in reserpine-treated patients.[9] The receptors may show some supersensitivity so that a dosage reduction may be required.

1. Kim JM, Stevenson CE, Mathewson HS. Hypertensive reactions to phenylephrine eyedrops in patients with sympathetic denervation. *Am J Ophthalmol* (1978) 85, 862–8.
2. Abboud FM, Eckstein JW. Effects of small oral doses of reserpine on vascular responses to tyramine and norepinephrine in man. *Circulation* (1964) 29, 219–23.
3. Ziegler CH, Lovette JB. Operative complications after therapy with reserpine and reserpine compounds. *JAMA* (1961) 176, 916–19.
4. Sneddon JM, Turner P. Ephedrine mydriasis in hypertension and the response to treatment. *Clin Pharmacol Ther* (1969) 10, 64–71.
5. Noce RH, Williams DB, Rapaport W. Reserpine (Serpasil) in the management of the mentally ill. *JAMA* (1955) 158, 11–15.
6. Stone CA, Ross CA, Wenger HC, Ludden CT, Blessing JA, Totaro JA, Porter CC. Effect of α-methyl-3,4-dihydroxyphenylalanine (methyldopa), reserpine and related agents on some vascular responses in the dog. *J Pharmacol Exp Ther* (1962) 136, 80–8.
7. Eger EI, Hamilton WK. The effect of reserpine on the action of various vasopressors. *Anesthesiology* (1959) 20, 641–5.
8. Moore JI, Moran NC. Cardiac contractile force responses to ephedrine and other sympathomimetic amines in dogs after pretreatment with reserpine. *J Pharmacol Exp Ther* (1962) 136, 89–96.
9. Smessaert AA, Hicks RG. Problems caused by rauwolfia drugs during anesthesia and surgery. *N Y State J Med* (1961) 61, 2399–2403.

Tyramine-rich foods + Cimetidine

A woman taking cimetidine experienced a severe headache and hypertension when she drank *Bovril* and ate some cheese.

Clinical evidence, mechanism, importance and management

A 77-year-old woman with hiatus hernia, who had been taking cimetidine 400 mg four times daily for three years, experienced a severe frontal headache and hypertension, which appeared to be related to the ingestion of a cup of ***Bovril*** and some **English cheddar cheese**, both of which can contain substantial amounts of tyramine.[1] Although the authors point out the similarity between this reaction and that seen in patients on MAOIs who eat tyramine-rich foods (see 'MAOIs + Tyramine-rich foods', p.876), there is no satisfactory explanation for what occurred. This is an isolated report and there is no reason why patients in general on cimetidine should avoid tyramine-rich foods.

1. Griffin MJJ, Morris JS. MAOI-like reaction associated with cimetidine. *Drug Intell Clin Pharm* (1987) 21, 219.

34

Tricyclics, SSRIs and related antidepressants

The development of the tricyclic antidepressants arose out of work carried out on phenothiazine compounds related to chlorpromazine. The earlier molecules possessed two benzene rings joined by a third ring of carbon atoms, with sometimes a nitrogen, and had antidepressant activity (hence their name). Some of the later antidepressants have one, two or even four rings. 'Table 34.1', (below) lists the common tricyclic antidepressants, the selective serotonin re-uptake inhibitors (SSRIs) and a number of other compounds that are also used for depression.

Antidepressant activity of tricyclic antidepressants

The tricyclic antidepressants inhibit the activity of the 'uptake' mechanism by which some chemical transmitters (serotonin (5-HT) or noradrenaline (norepinephrine)) re-enter nerve endings in the CNS. In this way they raise the concentrations of the chemical transmitter in the receptor area. If depression represents some inadequacy in transmission between the nerves in the brain, increasing the amount of transmitter may go some way towards reversing this by improving transmission.

Other properties of tricyclic antidepressants

The tricyclics also have antimuscarinic (sometimes referred to as anticholinergic or atropine-like) activity and can cause dry mouth, blurred vision, constipation, urinary retention and an increase in ocular tension. Postural hypotension and cardiotoxic effects may also occur, but they are less frequent. Among the CNS adverse effects are sedation, the precipitation of seizures in certain individuals, and extrapyramidal reactions.

Selective serotonin re-uptake inhibitor antidepressants (SSRIs)

These antidepressants act on neurones in a similar way to the tricyclics but they selectively inhibit the re-uptake of serotonin (5-hydroxytryptamine or 5-HT). They have fewer antimuscarinic effects and are also less sedative and cardiotoxic.

Other antidepressant drugs

These include the tetracyclic antidepressants, mianserin and maprotiline, which have actions similar to those of the tricyclic antidepressants. However, while the tetracyclics are more sedating, their antimuscarinic effects are less marked. Maprotiline inhibits the re-uptake of noradrenaline (norepinephrine) and has weak affinity for central adrenergic (α_1) receptors. Mianserin does not prevent peripheral re-uptake of noradrenaline; it blocks presynaptic adrenergic (α_2) receptors and increases the turnover of brain noradrenaline. It is also an antagonist of serotonin receptors in some parts of the brain.

Mirtazapine is a piperazinoazepine and an analogue of mianserin. It is a pre-synaptic adrenergic α_2-antagonist that increases central noradrenergic and serotonergic transmission. It is a potent inhibitor at histamine (H_1) receptors and this accounts for its sedative properties. It has little antimuscarinic activity.

Nefazodone is a phenylpiperazine structurally related to trazodone. Both block the re-uptake of serotonin at pre-synaptic neurones and both block α_1-adrenoceptors, but have no apparent effect on dopamine. Unlike trazodone, nefazodone blocks the re-uptake of noradrenaline. Compared to the tricyclics, neither drug has very significant antimuscarinic effects, but trazodone also has marked sedative properties.

Reboxetine is a potent inhibitor of noradrenaline re-uptake. It has a weak effect on serotonin re-uptake and no significant affinity for muscarinic receptors.

Venlafaxine, a phenylethylamine derivative, is a serotonin and noradrenaline re-uptake inhibitor (SNRI); it weakly inhibits dopamine re-uptake. Compared with the tricyclics, it lacks significant sedative and antimuscarinic effects.

Table 34.1 Cyclic and other antidepressants

Generic names	*Proprietary names*
Tricyclic compounds	
Amitriptyline	Adepril, ADT, Amineurin, Amitrip, Amytril, Anapsique, Deprelio, Elatrol, Elatrolet, Elavil, Endep, Laroxyl, Maxivalet, Noriline, Novoprotect, Polytanol, Protanol, Redomex, Saroten, Sarotena, Sarotex, Stelminal, Syneudon, Teperin, Trepiline, Tripsol, Tripsyline, Tripta, Triptizol, Triptyl, Triptyline, Tryptal, Tryptanol, Tryptizol, Tryptomer, Uxen
Amoxapine	Asendin, Asendis, Defanyl, Demolox
Butriptyline	
Clomipramine	Anafranil, Atenual, Ausentron, Clofranil, Clopress, Equinorm, Hydiphen, Maronil, Placil, Zoiral
Desipramine	Deprexan, Distonal, Nebril, Norpramin, Nortimil, Pertofran, Petylyl
Dibenzepin	Noveril
Dimetacrine	
Dosulepin	Dopress, Dothapax, Dothep, Espin, Idom, Prepadine, Prothiaden, Protiaden, Protiadene, Thaden
Doxepin	Anten, Aponal, Deptran, Doneurin, Doxal, Doxe, Doxederm, Doxepia, espadox, Gilex, Mareen, Quitaxon, Sinequan, Sinquan, Sinquane, Spectra, Xepin, Zonalon

Continued

Table 34.1 Cyclic and other antidepressants *(continued)*

Generic names	*Proprietary names*
Imipramine	Antidep, Celamine, Depramina, Depsonil, Elepsin, Ethipramine, Imipra, Melipramin, Melipramine, Mipralin, Praminan, Primonil, Pryleugan, Sermonil, Talpramin, Tofranil, Tofranil-PM, Topramine
Lofepramine	Deftan, Deprimil, Emdalen, Feprapax, Gamanil, Gamonil, Tymelyt
Melitracen	Dixeran
Nortriptyline	Allegron, Ateben, Aventyl, Norfenazin, Noritren, Norline, Norpress, Norterol, Nortrilen, Nortylin, Nortyline, Ortrip, Pamelor, Paxtibi, Sensaval, Sensival
Protriptyline	Vivactil
Trimipramine	Apo-Trimip, Eldoral, Herphonal, Rhotrimine, Sapilent, Stangyl, Surmontil, Trimidura, Trimine, Trimineurin, Tripress, Tydamine
Tetracyclic compounds	
Maprotiline	Aprotilin, Deprilept, Ludiomil, Maludil, Maprolu, Maprotibene, Melodil
Mianserin	Athimil, Athymil, Bonserin, Depnon, Hopacem, Lantanon, Lerivon, Lumin, Mealin, Miabene, Mianeurin, Miaxan, Ornate , Prevalina, Prisma, Servin, Tolimed, Tolmin, Tolvin, Tolvon
Bicyclic compounds	
Viloxazine	Vivalan
SSRIs (Selective serotonin re-uptake inhibitors)	
Citalopram	Actipram, Akarin, Alutan, Apertia, Celapram, Celexa, Cilex, Cilift, Cimal, Ciprager, Cipram, Cipramil, Cipramil, Cipramil, Ciprapine, Citadep, Citadur, Citadura, Citaham, Citalec, Citalhexal, Citalon, Citarcana, Citavie, Citopam, Citor, Citrol, Claropram, Denyl, Desital, Elopram, Emocal, Finap, Genprol, Humorap, Lontax, Pram, Prisdal, Prisma, Recital, Semax, Sepram, Serital, Seropram, Setronil, Talam, Talohexal, Talomil, Temperax, Zebrak, Zentius
Escitalopram	Cipralex, Entact, Lexapro, Lexapro, Recita, S-Citadep, Seroplex, Sipralexa
Femoxetine	
Fluoxetine	Actan, Actisac, Adofen, Afeksin, Affectine, Affex, Alental, Animex-On, Anisimol, Anzac, Apo-Fluoxetine, Astrin, Atd, Auroken, Auscap, Axtin, Azur, Biozac, Captaton, Clexiclor, Clinium, Cloriflox, CP-Fluoxet, Daforin, Dagrilan, Deprax, Deprenon, Depress, Deprex, Deprexen, Deprexin, Deproxin, Deprozan, Depzac, Diesan, Digassim, Dinalexin, Dominium, Eburnate, Equilibrane, Eufor, Exostrept, Fefluzin, Felicium, Flocet, Flonital, Florexal, Flotina, Floxet, Fluctin, Fluctine, Fludac, Flumed, Flumirex, Fluneurin, Fluocim, Fluogal, Fluohexal, Fluopiram, Fluox, Fluoxac, Fluoxal, fluox-basan, Fluoxebell, FluoxeLich, Fluoxemerck, Fluoxe-Q, Fluoxeren, Fluoxgamma, Fluoxibene, Fluoxifar, Fluoxin, Fluoxine, Fluoxistad, Fluoxityrol, Fluox-Puren, Fluoxstad, Flusac, Flusol, Flustad, Flutin, Flutine, Fluval, Fluxadir, Fluxantin, Flux, Fluxene, Fluxet, Fluxetil, Fluxetin, Fluxil, FluxoMed, Fluxonil, Fluzac, Fokeston, Folizol, Fondur, Fontex, Fonzac, Foxetin, Framex, FXT, Gerozac, Ibixetin, Ladose, Lapsus, Lecimar, Lorien, Lovan, Loxetine, Luramon, Magrilan, Milezin, Mitilase, Mutan, Nervosal, Neupax, Nodepe, Nopres, Nortec, Norzac, NuFluo, Nuzac, Nuzak, Orthon, Oxetine, Oxsac, Platin, Plazeron, Plinzene, Portal, Positivum, Pragmaten, Prizma, Prodep, Prohexal, Prozac, Prozamel, Prozatan, Prozen, Prozit, Psipax, Psiquial, Ranflocs, Reneuron, Salipax, Sanzur, Sarafem, Sartuzin, Saurat, Selectus, Seromex, Seronil, Seroscand, Siquial, Sostac, Stephadilat-S, Stressless, Tremafarm, Tuneluz, Unprozy, Verotina, Xeredien, Zactin, Zaxetina, Zinovat
Fluvoxamine	Dumirox, Dumyrox, Faverin, Favoxil, Felixsan, Fevarin, Flox-ex, Floxyfral, Fluvohexal, Fluvoxadura, Fluvoxin, Fluvoxin, Luvox, Maveral, Movox, Myroxine
Paroxetine	Allenopar, Aparo, Aropax, Aroxat, Bectam, Casbol, Cebrilin, Daparox, Denerval, Deroxat, Divarius, Ennos, Euplix, Eutimil, Frosinor, Glaxopar, Meloxat, Motivan, Optipar, Oxepar, Oxet, Oxetine, Paluxetil, Pamoxet, Parexat, Pari, Parocetan, Paroglax, ParoLich, Paroser, Parotin, Parox, Paroxat, Paroxedura, Paroxiflex, Paxetil, Paxil, Paxtine, Paxxet, Pexeva, Pondera, Posivyl, Psicoasten, Rexetin, Seretran, Sereupin, Serodur, Seroxat, Tagonis, Traviata, Xet, Xetin
Sertraline	Altruline, Anilar, Aremis, Asentra, Atenix, Besitran, Bicromil, Deprax, Eleval, Emergen, Gladem, Implicane, Inosert, Insertec, Irradial, Lowfin, Lustral, Novativ, Sedoran, Sercerin, Serdep, Serivo, Serlain, Serlife, Serlift, Serta, Stimuloton, Tatig, Tolrest, Tresleen, Xydep, Zoloft
Other compounds	
Iprindole	
Mirtazapine	Avanza, Ciblex, Comenter, Divaril, Miro, Mirtaril, Mirtaz, Mirtazon, Norset, Promyrtil, Remergil, Remergon, Remeron, Rexer, Tazamel, Vastat, Zispin, Zuleptan
Nefazodone	Deprefax
Reboxetine	Davedax, Edronax, Irenor, Narebox, Norebox, Prolift, Solvex
Trazodone	Azona, Deprax, Depsan, Desirel, Desyrel, Donaren, Molipaxin, Taxagon, Thombran, Trazodil, Trazolan, Trazone, Tritico AC, Triticum, Trittico
Venlafaxine	Depurol, Dobupal, Efectin, Efexor, Efexor XR, Effexor, Elafax, Faxine, Flavix, Norpilen, Sentidol, Trevilor, Vandral, Venla, Venlax, Venlor, Viepax

Bupropion + Guanfacine

A grand mal seizure in a child, which was attributed to an interaction between bupropion and guanfacine, was later identified as being more probably due to a bupropion overdose.

Clinical evidence, mechanism, importance and management

A girl of 10 being treated for attention deficit hyperactivity disorder was prescribed increasing doses of bupropion up to 100 mg three times daily, to which guanfacine, initially 500 micrograms twice daily then 500 micrograms three times daily, was added. Ten days later she had a grand mal seizure attributed by the author of the report to an interaction between the two drugs.[1,2] This was challenged in subsequent correspondence.[3] However, two years later the author of the original report wrote to say that he had now discovered that the girl had in fact taken 500 mg of bupropion and 5 mg of guanfacine before the seizure took place so that what happened was much more likely to have been due to an overdose of the bupropion than to an interaction with guanfacine.[4] Bupropion is associated with seizures at high doses. There is insufficient evidence to suggest that the concurrent use of these two drugs should be avoided.

1. Tilton P. Bupropion and guanfacine. *J Am Acad Child Adolesc Psychiatry* (1998) 37, 682–3.
2. Tilton P. Seizure associated with bupropion and guanfacine. *J Am Acad Child Adolesc Psychiatry* (1999) 38, 3.
3. Namerow LB. Seizure associated with bupropion and guanfacine. *J Am Acad Child Adolesc Psychiatry* (1999) 38, 2.
4. Tilton P. Seizure after guanfacine plus bupropion: correction. *J Am Acad Child Adolesc Psychiatry* (2000) 39, 1341.

Bupropion + Miscellaneous

Bupropion is contraindicated with MAOIs, although some evidence suggests that serious problems are unlikely. Carbamazepine or valproate may cause marked changes in the plasma levels of bupropion and its metabolites. There is a report of hypomania in a patient taking bupropion and lamotrigine. There are isolated reports of psychosis, mania and seizures associated with the use of bupropion and fluoxetine. An isolated report describes acute liver failure with concurrent bupropion and carbimazole. The makers also issue warnings about the concurrent use of bupropion with drugs that can lower the convulsive threshold, amantadine, levodopa, ritonavir, drugs metabolised by the cytochrome P450 isoenzymes CYP2D6 and CYP2B6, the possible use of nicotine and following tobacco withdrawal. Cimetidine does not interact.

Clinical evidence, mechanism, importance and management

(a) Anticonvulsants

(i) Carbamazepine, Phenobarbital, Phenytoin. The makers warn about the outcome of using enzyme-inducing anticonvulsants such as carbamazepine, phenytoin and phenobarbital, which are expected to increase the metabolism of bupropion.[1,2] One study found that carbamazepine at steady state decreased the maximum plasma levels and AUC of bupropion and two of its metabolites (threohydrobupropion and erythrohydrobupropion) by about 81 to 96%. These two metabolites have only 10 to 50% of the potency of the parent compound. However, the AUC of another metabolite, hydroxybupropion (which has the same potency as the parent compound) was increased by 50% and its maximum serum levels by 71%.[3] Two patients with bipolar illness have been described who were initially given bupropion 450 mg daily, later increased up to 600 mg daily. They had undetectable bupropion plasma levels while taking carbamazepine but their plasma levels of hydroxybupropion were markedly increased.[4] What the sum of all these changes is likely to mean is uncertain, but good monitoring for any evidence of reduced efficacy and/or increased toxicity (due to the raised hydroxybupropion) is clearly needed. The same good monitoring would also be appropriate with phenytoin and phenobarbital but clinical studies appear to be lacking and the outcome equally uncertain.

(ii) Sodium valproate, Lamotrigine. A study found that the AUC of hydroxybupropion, an active metabolite of bupropion, almost doubled when bupropion was given with valproate at steady-state, but the pharmacokinetics of the parent compound and the two other less active metabolites were unaffected.[3] An increase in valproate levels of almost 30% was seen in another report in one patient.[4] The reasons for these changes are not known, nor is it clear what the clinical outcome of concurrent use is likely to be, but good monitoring for evidence of changed efficacy and possibly increased adverse effects would seem appropriate.

A 23-year-old patient with a DSM-IV diagnosis of major depression showed partial improvement with cognitive therapy and bupropion 300 mg daily for 6 months. There was no further improvement with an increased dose of bupropion to 400 mg daily for 3 months. Her mood improved when she was also given lamotrigine 25 mg at night and there was further improvement in mood, decreased anxiety and increased energy when lamotrigine was increased to 50 mg daily for 3 weeks. However, when the dose was increased to 75 mg daily she reported decreased sleep, increased energy, mood lability and increased spending, which was diagnosed as hypomania. The symptoms resolved over about 2 weeks when the lamotrigine dose was reduced to 50 mg at bedtime. Antidepressants in high doses or in combination can induce hypomania and in this case the effect was attributed to the potentiating antidepressant properties of lamotrigine.[5]

(b) Antiparkinsonian drugs

The makers say that the concurrent use of bupropion and **levodopa** or **amantadine** should be undertaken with caution because limited clinical data suggests a higher incidence of undesirable effects (nausea, vomiting, excitement, restlessness, postural tremor) in patients given bupropion with either drug. Good monitoring is therefore appropriate and patients should be given small initial bupropion doses, which are increased gradually.[1,2]

(c) Antiretroviral drugs

In vitro data indicate that the antiretroviral drugs **efavirenz**, **nelfinavir** and **ritonavir** are capable of inhibiting the cytochrome P450 isoenzyme CYP2B6, which is the isoenzyme primarily involved in bupropion metabolism.[6] The potential therefore exists for a serious drug interaction with an increase in bupropion concentrations and the risk of seizures. A retrospective study identified 10 HIV+ patients who had taken bupropion 150 mg once or twice daily together with **nelfinavir, ritonavir** or **efavirenz** for 3 weeks to 2 years (median 8 months) without having seizures. However, the number of patients was small and the 2 patients who received **ritonavir** were only given 100 mg twice daily.[7]

The UK makers of **ritonavir** contraindicate the concurrent use of bupropion[8] on theoretical grounds. They predict that the metabolism mediated by the cytochrome P450 isoenzyme CYP2D6 might possibly be inhibited, leading to increased levels and toxicity. But the makers of bupropion do not mention the possibility of an interaction with **ritonavir** in their product literature[1,2] and there seem to be no reports of an adverse interaction. Further study is needed.

(d) Carbimazole

A 41-year-old man treated for hyperthyroidism with carbimazole 15 mg daily and propranolol 10 mg daily for 5 years received a 10-day course of bupropion 150 mg daily to aid smoking cessation. Ten weeks after completing the course of bupropion he was admitted to hospital with severe jaundice, nausea, dyspepsia, lethargy, and epigastric pain of 5 days' duration. The only other medication he had taken was paracetamol (acetaminophen) 500 mg to 1 g daily for up to 2 days about 2 weeks before admission. Both carbimazole and propranolol were discontinued. He developed acute liver failure and rapid deterioration of renal function complicated by sepsis and coagulopathy. Liver biopsy showed evidence of non-specific drug-induced acute liver injury. The patient died 19 days after the onset of symptoms. Both bupropion and carbimazole may cause liver damage. In this case the hepatotoxicity was attributed to bupropion or a combined toxic effect of bupropion and carbimazole. The potential for serious hepatotoxicity should be borne in mind if bupropion is given with other hepatotoxic drugs.[9]

(e) Cimetidine

A randomised, open-label, two period crossover study in 24 healthy subjects found no evidence of any clinically relevant interaction between a single 300-mg dose of bupropion (sustained release preparation) and cimetidine 800 mg.[10] No special precautions would seem to be necessary on concurrent use.

(f) Cytochrome P450 isoenzyme CYP2D6 inducers, inhibitors and substrates

A pharmacokinetic study in healthy subjects known to be extensive metabolisers of CYP2D6 found that bupropion doubled the maximum plasma levels of **desipramine** and increased its AUC fivefold.[1] Another study in a 64-year-old woman on **imipramine** 150 to 200 mg daily found that when bupropion 225 mg daily was added, there was a fourfold rise in the plasma levels of **imipramine** and **desipramine** but no problems were reported. A comparison of the estimated clearances were: **imipramine** alone 1.7 ml/minute; **desipramine** alone 1.7 ml/minute; **imipramine** with bupropion 0.73 ml/minute; and **desipramine** with bupropion 0.31 ml/minute.[11] *In vitro* studies[1] have shown that both bupropion and its metabolite are inhibitors of CYP2D6 so the explanation would seem to be that bupropion inhibited CYP2D6, the isoenzyme involved with the metabolism of these tricyclics, so that they were cleared from the body more slowly.

Formal interaction studies with other drugs metabolised by CYP2D6 have not been carried out by the makers but they predict that a number of drugs may be similarly affected, which might in theory result in a rise in their plasma levels. In addition to **desipramine** they list **imipramine**, **nortriptyline**, SSRIs (**fluoxetine**, **paroxetine**, **sertraline**), antipsychotics (**haloperidol**, **risperidone**, **thioridazine**), beta-blockers (**metoprolol**) and type Ic antiarrhythmics (**flecainide**, **propafenone**). The recommendation is that if any of these drugs is added to treatment with bupropion, doses at the lower end of the range should be used. If bupropion is added to existing treatment, decreased dosages should be considered.[1,2] However, there appear to be no reports of problems with the concurrent use of any of these drugs.

The makers also advise caution if bupropion is used with drugs such as **orphenadrine**, **cyclophosphamide** and **ifosfamide**. The reason is that bupropion is metabolised to its major metabolite hydroxybupropion by CYP2B6 and these drugs affect this isoenzyme.[1]

It should be emphasised that all of the predictions, recommendations and precautions quoted here are largely based on *in vitro* studies, not on clinical studies, and thus far there appear to be no reports of problems arising from the concurrent use of these drugs with bupropion.

(g) Drugs and circumstances that can lower the convulsive threshold

There is a small dose-related risk of seizures with bupropion. At a dose of 300 mg the risk is 0.1%, which increases to 0.4% at a dose of 450 mg, and increases tenfold between doses of 450 and 600 mg.[2] The makers caution the use of other drugs that lower the convulsive threshold, the concern being that these drugs might further lower the convulsive threshold. The US[2] and UK[1] makers list **antipsychotics**, **antidepressants**, **systemic steroids** and **theophylline**. The UK makers additionally list **antimalarials**, **tramadol**, **quinolones** and **sedating antihistamines**. Caution is also urged with regard to conditions that may lower the convulsive threshold, including the use of anorectic agents or stimulants, and diabetes treated with hypoglycaemics or insulin.[1,2]

(h) Fluoxetine

The day after stopping fluoxetine 60 mg daily, a 41-year-old man was started on 75 mg and later 100 mg of bupropion three times daily. After 10 days he became edgy and anxious and after 12 days he developed myoclonus. After 14 days he became severely agitated and psychotic, with delirium and hallucinations. His behaviour returned to normal 6 days after the bupropion was stopped.[12] It was suggested that the residual fluoxetine may have inhibited the metabolism of the bupropion, leading to toxic levels.[12] Another patient maintained on lithium carbonate for bipolar disorder developed anxiety, panic and eventually mania a little over a week after stopping fluoxetine and starting bupropion.[13] Yet another patient developed a grand mal seizure after being given fluoxetine and bupropion 300 mg daily.[14]

Information is very limited but these reports suggest that if concurrent or sequential use is thought appropriate, the outcome should be well monitored. More study is needed.

(i) MAOIs

In an uncontrolled trial, 10 patients were treated for major affective disorder (8 unipolar, 2 bipolar) with bupropion in daily doses of 225 to 450 mg and various MAOIs (**isocarboxazid** (1 patient), **phenelzine** (5), **tranylcypromine** (2), **selegiline** (2)). Four were transferred from the MAOI to bupropion without any washout period, and the other 6 were given both drugs concurrently. No untoward cardiovascular events occurred, except for one patient on bupropion and **selegiline**, who experienced orthostatic hypotension. Notable weight loss occurred in two others when transferred from the MAOI to bupropion.[15]

Despite this clear (though very limited) clinical evidence of apparent safety, the makers of bupropion are apparently wary of a possible interaction with MAOIs because of the toxicity seen in studies in *rats* when **phenelzine** and bupropion were given concurrently.[2] Thus at the moment they contraindicate bupropion with MAOIs and recommend that at least 14 days should elapse between stopping irreversible MAOIs and starting bupropion.[1,2] This precaution would therefore apply particularly to the older MAOIs (**phenelzine**, **tranylcypromine**, **isocarboxazid** etc). For reversible MAOIs, the makers advise that a 24-hour period is sufficient.[1]

(j) Nicotine

Nicotine transdermal patches are reported not to affect the pharmacokinetics of bupropion or its metabolites.[1] The makers of bupropion say that limited data suggest that giving up smoking is more easily achieved if bupropion is taken while using a nicotine transdermal system, but they recommend weekly monitoring to check for any evidence of a blood pressure increase.[1] The same warning would also seem to be applicable to the use of nicotine in any other form (oral or nasal).

(k) Pseudoephedrine

A 21-year-old man presented in a hospital emergency department with severe chest pain, radiating pain into both arms and between the shoulder blades, diaphoresis and shortness of breath. Initially this was diagnosed as acute myocardial infarction, but a later angiogram showed normal coronary arteries and it was concluded that these symptoms were due to acute myocardial ischaemia apparently brought on by the combined use of pseudoephedrine (9 tablets of 30 mg) over the previous 3 days, bupropion for smoking cessation and **nicotine** (he smoked 25 cigarettes daily). The authors of the report postulate that all these drugs acted on the alpha receptors of the coronary arteries to cause vasospasm and acute ischaemia. He had been taking both drugs and erythromycin for 3 days, and had taken pseudoephedrine on numerous previous occasions without problems. He recovered fully.[16]

This is an isolated case from which no general conclusions can be drawn, but some warning might be appropriate for patients who might already be at risk of coronary ischaemia.

(l) Tobacco withdrawal

Patients who give up smoking may find that the dosages of some of their medications are more than they actually need. The reason is that tobacco smoke contains compounds that induce the metabolism and loss from the body of certain drugs. Thus when smoking stops, the inducer is removed, the metabolism slows down and less of the drug is needed. The components of tobacco smoke are not potent enzyme inducers so that tobacco withdrawal does not usually have a marked effect, but the makers of bupropion draw attention to the following drugs that may possibly be affected by tobacco withdrawal: clomipramine, clozapine, flecainide, fluvoxamine, imipramine, olanzapine, pentazocine, theophylline and tacrine.[1] Check on patients' responses to these drugs after tobacco withdrawal and make any necessary downward dosage adjustments.

1. Zyban (Bupropion). GlaxoSmithKline. UK Summary of product characteristics, July 2005.
2. Zyban SR (Bupropion). GlaxoSmithKline. US Prescribing Information, January 2005.
3. Ketter TA, Jenkins JB, Schroeder DH, Pazzaglia PJ, Marangell LB, George MS, Callahan AM, Hinton ML, Chao J, Post RM. Carbamazepine but not valproate induced bupropion metabolism. *J Clin Psychopharmacol* (1995) 15, 327–33.
4. Popli AP, Tanquary J, Lamparella V, Masand PS. Bupropion and anticonvulsant drug interactions. *Ann Clin Psychiatry* (1995) 7, 99–101.
5. Margolese HC, Beauclair L, Szkrumelak N, Chouinard G. Hypomania induced by adjunctive lamotrigine. *Am J Psychiatry* (2003) 160, 183–4.
6. Hesse LM, von Moltke LL, Shader RI, Greenblatt DJ. Ritonavir, efavirenz, and nelfinavir inhibit CYP2B6 activity in vitro: potential drug interactions with bupropion. *Drug Metab Dispos* (2001) 29, 100–102.
7. Park-Wyllie LY, Antoniou T. Concurrent use of bupropion with CYP2B6 inhibitors, nelfinavir, ritonavir and efavirenz: a case series. *AIDS* (2003) 17, 638–40.
8. Norvir (Ritonavir). Abbott Laboratories Ltd. UK Summary of product characteristics, January 2005.
9. Ai-Leng K, Lai-San T, Kang-Hoe L, Gek-Kee L. Acute liver failure with concurrent bupropion and carbimazole therapy. *Ann Pharmacother* (2003) 37, 220–3.
10. Corrigan B, Hsyu PH, Kustra R, Duncan B, Dunn J, Griffin R. A randomized, crossover study to evaluate the pharmacokinetic effect of cimetidine on *Wellbutrin* (bupropion HCl) sustained release in healthy subjects. *Pharm Res* (1997) 14 (11 Suppl), S-560.
11. Shad MU, Preskorn SH. A possible bupropion and imipramine interaction. *J Clin Psychopharmacol* (1997) 17, 118–19.
12. van Putten T, Shaffer I. Delirium associated with bupropion. *J Clin Psychopharmacol* (1990) 10, 234.
13. Zubieta JK, Demitrack MA. Possible bupropion precipitation of mania and a mixed affective state. *J Clin Psychopharmacol* (1991) 11, 327–8.
14. Ciraulo DA, Shader RI. Fluoxetine drug-drug interactions.II. *J Clin Psychopharmacol* (1990) 10, 213–17.
15. Abuzzahab Sr, FS. Combination therapy: monoamino oxidase inhibitors and bupropion HCl. *Neuropsychopharmacology* (1994) 10, (3S Pt 2), 74S.
16. Pederson KJ, Kuntz DH, Garbe GJ. Acute myocardial ischemia associated with ingestion of bupropion and pseudoephedrine in a 21-year-old man. *Can J Cardiol* (2001) 17, 599–601.

Duloxetine + Miscellaneous

The maker of duloxetine contraindicates concurrent use of duloxetine and MAOIs because of the theoretical risk of serotonin syndrome. Similarly they recommend caution with other serotonergic drugs including St John's wort, venlafaxine, triptans, tramadol, pethidine, and tryptophan.
Concurrent use of ciprofloxacin and enoxacin (cytochrome P450 CYP1A2 inhibitors) should be avoided because of the likelihood of markedly increased duloxetine levels. Quinidine (a CYP2D6 inhibitor) may increase duloxetine levels. Concurrent use of thioridazine (CYP2D6 substrate) is not recommended and caution is suggested for propafenone and flecainide, because duloxetine is likely to increase their levels. Duloxetine did not alter theophylline levels, and antacids and famotidine did not affect duloxetine pharmacokinetics.

Clinical evidence

(a) Antacids and H_2-blockers

Aluminium/magnesium-containing antacids and famotidine had no effect on the rate or extent of absorption of a single 40-mg dose of duloxetine.[1-3] No special precautions appear to be necessary on concurrent use.

(b) Cytochrome P450 isoenzyme CYP1A2 inhibitors

Fluvoxamine, a potent inhibitor of the cytochrome P450 isoenzyme CYP1A2, markedly increased levels of duloxetine, and concurrent use should be avoided, see 'Duloxetine + SSRIs', p.976. Other CYP1A2 inhibitors are predicted to interact similarly, and should also be avoided. The maker specifically names **ciprofloxacin** and **enoxacin**.[1,2] For a list of CYP1A2 inhibitors, see 'Table 1.2', (p.4).

(c) Cytochrome P450 isoenzyme CYP2D6 inhibitors

The cytochrome P450 isoenzyme CYP2D6 inhibitor paroxetine, increased levels of duloxetine, see 'Duloxetine + SSRIs', p.976, and other CYP2D6 inhibitors are predicted to interact similarly. The maker specifically names **quinidine**.[3] For a list of CYP2D6 inhibitors, see 'Table 1.3', (p.6).

(d) Cytochrome P450 isoenzyme CYP2D6 substrates

Duloxetine is a moderate inhibitor of the cytochrome P450 isoenzyme CYP2D6, as shown by its effect on 'tolterodine', (p.1038) and 'desipramine', (p.996). The maker advises caution if duloxetine is given with drugs that are predominantly metabolised by CYP2D6 and have a narrow therapeutic index.[1-3] The US maker specifically contraindicates **thioridazine** because of the risk of arrhythmias with elevated levels of this drug.[3] They also caution the concurrent use of **propafenone** or **flecainide**.[3] For a list of CYP2D6 substrates, see 'Table 1.3', (p.6).

(e) MAOIs

The makers contraindicate the use of duloxetine with non-selective irreversible MAOIs, and for 14 days after discontinuing an MAOI. This is because of the possible risk of serotonin syndrome.[1-3] Although the risk would be lower with selective, reversible MAOIs such as **moclobemide**, the maker still says concurrent use is not recommended.[1,2]

(f) Other serotonergic drugs

Because the concurrent use of more than one serotonergic drug has rarely resulted in 'the serotonin syndrome', (p.9), the maker advises caution if duloxetine is used with 'SSRIs', (below), 'tricyclic antidepressants', (p.996), **St John's wort**, **venlafaxine**, or **triptans**, **tramadol**, **pethidine**, and **tryptophan**.[1,2]

(g) Theophylline and other cytochrome P450 isoenzyme CYP1A2 substrates

The maker notes that the pharmacokinetics of theophylline were not significantly affected by duloxetine 60 mg twice daily in healthy male subjects.[1-3] This is despite duloxetine being an inhibitor of CYP1A2 *in vitro*.[3] No special precautions would appear to be needed. The US maker notes that duloxetine is unlikely to have an important effect on the metabolism of other CYP1A2 substrates,[3] although the UK maker says that an effect cannot be excluded in women.[1,2] For a list of CYP1A2 substrates, see 'Table 1.2', (p.4).

1. Cymbalta (Duloxetine hydrochloride). Eli Lilly and Company Ltd. UK Summary of product characteristics, December 2004.
2. Yentreve (Duloxetine hydrochloride). Eli Lilly and Company Ltd. UK Summary of product characteristics, August 2004.
3. Cymbalta (Duloxetine hydrochloride). Eli Lilly and Company. US Prescribing information, January 2005.

Duloxetine + SSRIs

Combined use of duloxetine with other serotonergic drugs such as the SSRIs should be undertaken with caution because of the possible increased risk of the serotonin syndrome. Fluvoxamine should not be used with duloxetine, because it markedly increases its levels. Low-dose paroxetine caused a modest increase in duloxetine AUC, and fluoxetine is predicted to interact similarly.

Clinical evidence

(a) Fluvoxamine

Fluvoxamine 100 mg once daily increased the AUC of duloxetine five- to sixfold, and decreased clearance by about 77% in 14 healthy subjects.[1-3]

(b) Paroxetine

The concurrent use of paroxetine 20 mg once daily and duloxetine 40 mg once daily increased the AUC of duloxetine at steady state by about 60% in healthy subjects.[4]

Mechanism

Fluvoxamine is a potent inhibitor of the cytochrome P450 isoenzyme CYP1A2, by which duloxetine is metabolised.[3] Other SSRIs have minimal effects on this isoenzyme. Paroxetine is a potent inhibitor of CYP2D6, which also has a role in duloxetine metabolism.[3] Other SSRIs such as fluoxetine also inhibit this isoenzyme.

Importance and management

The pharmacokinetic interactions are established. Although the clinical relevance of the increases in duloxetine levels have not been assessed, the maker considers that the rise with fluvoxamine is so marked that the combination should be avoided.[1-3] The rise in duloxetine levels with paroxetine 20 mg daily is probably not clinically relevant, but the maker notes that greater increases would be expected with higher doses.[3] Fluoxetine would be expected to interact similarly.[3] Caution is warranted.

Although no cases of 'the serotonin syndrome', (p.9) have been reported for duloxetine combined with other serotonergic drugs such as SSRIs, the maker notes that combined use should be undertaken with caution.[1,2]

1. Cymbalta (Duloxetine hydrochloride). Eli Lilly and Company Ltd. UK Summary of product characteristics, December 2004.
2. Yentreve (Duloxetine hydrochloride). Eli Lilly and Company Ltd. UK Summary of product characteristics, August 2004.
3. Cymbalta (Duloxetine hydrochloride). Eli Lilly and Company. US Prescribing information, January 2005.
4. Skinner MH, Kuan H-Y, Pan A, Sathirakul K, Knadler MP, Gonzales CR, Yeo KP, Reddy S, Lim M, Ayan-Oshodi M, Wise SD. Duloxetine is both an inhibitor and a substrate of cytochrome P4502D6 in healthy volunteers. *Clin Pharmacol Ther* (2003) 73, 170–7.

Maprotiline + Oral contraceptives or Tobacco smoking

Neither tobacco smoking nor the oral contraceptives affect maprotiline.

Clinical evidence, mechanism, importance and management

A study in women showed that, over a 28-day period, the use of oral contraceptives did not significantly affect the steady-state blood levels of maprotiline 75 mg given at night, nor was its therapeutic effectiveness changed.[1] Smoking also has no effect on maprotiline efficacy and blood levels.[1,2]

1. Luscombe DK. Interaction studies: the influence of age, cigarette smoking and the oral contraceptive on blood concentrations of maprotiline. In 'Depressive Illness — Far Horizons?' McIntyre JNM (ed), Cambridge Med Publ, Northampton 1982, p 61–2.
2. Holman RM. Maprotiline and cigarette smoking: an interaction study: clinical findings. In 'Depressive Illness — Far Horizons?' McIntyre JNM (ed), Cambridge Med Publ, Northampton 1982, p 66–7.

Maprotiline + Propranolol

Maprotiline toxicity, attributed to the concurrent use of propranolol, has been described in three patients.

Clinical evidence

A patient experienced maprotiline toxicity (dizziness, hypotension, dry mouth, blurred vision, etc.) after taking propranolol 120 mg daily for two weeks. His trough maprotiline levels had risen by 40%. The levels fell and the adverse effects disappeared when the propranolol was withdrawn.[1] Another patient on propranolol 120 mg daily began to experience visual hallucinations and psychomotor agitation within a few days of starting to take maprotiline 200 mg daily.[2] Another man on haloperidol, benzatropine, triamterene, hydrochlorothiazide and propranolol became disorientated, agitated and uncooperative, with visual hallucinations and incoherent speech, within a week of starting to take maprotiline 150 mg daily. These symptoms disappeared when all the drugs were withdrawn. Reintroduction of the antihypertensive drugs with haloperidol and desipramine proved effective and uneventful.[3]

Mechanism

Not understood. A suggested reason is that the propranolol reduces the blood flow to the liver so that the metabolism of the maprotiline is reduced, leading to its accumulation in the body.

Importance and management

Information seems to be limited to the cases cited. The general importance of this interaction is uncertain, but if concurrent use is thought appropriate the outcome should be well monitored. The authors of one of the reports[2] say that simultaneous use is inadvisable.

1. Tollefson G, Lesar T. Effect of propranolol on maprotiline clearance. *Am J Psychiatry* (1984) 141, 148–9.
2. Saiz-Ruiz J, Moral L. Delirium induced by association of propranolol and maprotiline. *J Clin Psychopharmacol* (1988) 8, 77–8.
3. Malek-Ahmadi P, Tran T. Propranolol and maprotiline toxic interaction. *Neurobehav Toxicol Teratol* (1985) 7, 203.

Maprotiline or Mianserin + Sympathomimetics

No adverse interaction would usually be expected in patients on maprotiline or mianserin who are treated with sympathomimetic amines.

Clinical evidence, mechanism, importance and management

The pressor (increased blood pressure) responses to **tyramine** and **noradrenaline** (**norepinephrine**) in depressed patients remained virtually unchanged after 14 days of treatment with mianserin 60 mg daily.[1-4] In 5 healthy subjects on maprotiline the pressor response to **tyramine** was reduced threefold while the **noradrenaline** response remained unchanged.[5]

The practical importance of these observations is that, unlike the tricyclic antidepressants, no special precautions normally seem necessary if patients on maprotiline or mianserin are given **noradrenaline** or other directly-acting sympathomimetics. Similarly, none of the dietary precautions against eating **tyramine**-rich foods or drinks, or the administration of indirectly-acting sympathomimetics such as **phenylpropanolamine** in cough and cold remedies, need to be imposed.

1. Ghose K, Coppen A, Turner P. Autonomic actions and interactions of mianserin hydrochloride (Org GB94) and amitriptyline in patients with depressive illness. *Psychopharmacology (Berl)* (1976) 49, 201–4.
2. Coppen A, Ghose K, Swade C, Wood K. Effect of mianserin hydrochloride on peripheral uptake mechanisms for noradrenaline and 5-hydroxytryptamine in man. *Br J Clin Pharmacol* (1978) 5, 13S–17S.
3. Ghose K. Studies on the interaction between mianserin and noradrenaline in patients suffering from depressive illness. *Br J Clin Pharmacol* (1977) 4, 712–14.
4. Coppen AJ, Ghose K. Clinical and pharmacological effects of treatment with a new antidepressant. *Arzneimittelforschung* (1976) 26, 1166–7.
5. Briant RH, George CF. The assessment of potential drug interactions with a new tricyclic antidepressant drug. *Br J Clin Pharmacol* (1974) 1, 113–18.

Mianserin + Anticonvulsants

Plasma levels of mianserin can be markedly reduced by the concurrent use of phenytoin, phenobarbital or carbamazepine.

Clinical evidence

A comparative study[1,2] in 6 epileptics and 6 healthy subjects showed that **phenytoin** with either **phenobarbital** or **carbamazepine** markedly reduced the plasma levels of a single dose of mianserin. The mean half-life of mianserin was reduced by 75% (from 16.9 to 4.8 hours) and the AUC was reduced by 86%. Another study in 4 patients found that **carbamazepine** reduced serum mianserin concentrations by 70%.[3]

Mechanism

It seems probable that these anticonvulsants increase the metabolism of mianserin by the liver, thereby increasing its loss from the body.

Importance and management

Information appears to be limited to these studies, but the interaction appears to be established and of clinical importance. Monitor concurrent use and increase the dosage of mianserin as necessary.

1. Nawishy S, Hathway N, Turner P. Interactions of anticonvulsant drugs with mianserin and nomifensine. *Lancet* (1981) ii, 871–2.
2. Richens A, Nawishy S, Trimble M. Antidepressant drugs, convulsions and epilepsy. *Br J Clin Pharmacol* (1983) 15, 295S–298S.
3. Leinonen E, Lillsunde P, Laukkanen V, Ylitalo P. Effects of carbamazepine on serum antidepressant concentrations in psychiatric patients. *J Clin Psychopharmacol* (1991) 11, 313–18.

Mirtazapine + Miscellaneous

The sedative effects of mirtazapine may be increased by alcohol and the benzodiazepines. Cimetidine increases the bioavailability of mirtazapine. Concurrent administration of mirtazapine with amitriptyline may have a small effect on plasma concentrations of either drug. Pharmacokinetic interactions may occur between mirtazapine and inhibitors or inducers of the cytochrome P450 isoenzyme CYP3A4. The makers say that two weeks should elapse between taking an MAOI and mirtazapine. Mirtazapine can cause slight increases in INR in warfarin-treated patients.

Clinical evidence, mechanism, importance and management

(a) Alcohol

Mirtazapine does not affect the absorption of alcohol but it adds to its CNS depressant actions,[1] which underlies the maker's advice to avoid concurrent use.[2]

(b) Amitriptyline

In a single-blind three-way crossover study involving 24 healthy subjects, mirtazapine 15 to 30 mg daily, amitriptyline 25 to 75 mg daily or both drugs were given for periods of 9 days and in addition, 8 subjects received placebo. Amitriptyline increased the maximum plasma levels of mirtazapine, in male subjects only, by 36%. Mirtazapine increased the maximum plasma levels of amitriptyline in male subjects by 23% but in female subjects the maximum plasma levels were decreased by 23%. Other pharmacokinetic parameters and tolerability were not affected by concurrent administration.[3]

(c) Anticonvulsants

In a placebo-controlled study healthy subjects were given **carbamazepine** (at steady state) with mirtazapine for 7 days. It was found that **carbamazepine** (an inducer of cytochrome P450 isoenzyme CYP3A4) decreased the AUC and maximum plasma levels of mirtazapine, by 63 and 44% and increased the peak levels of demethylmirtazapine. Another related study showed that mirtazapine did not affect the pharmacokinetics of **carbamazepine** (a CYP3A4 substrate).[4]

A study in 9 healthy subjects given **phenytoin** 200 mg daily for 17 days and, from day 9, mirtazapine 15 mg daily for 2 days then 30 mg daily for 5 days, found that mirtazapine had no effect on the steady-state pharmacokinetics of **phenytoin**.[5] In a second associated study, 8 healthy subjects were given mirtazapine 15 mg daily for 2 days then 30 mg daily for

15 days with **phenytoin** 200 mg daily on days 8 to 17, it was found that the AUC and maximum plasma levels of mirtazapine were decreased by 47% and 33%, respectively, by **phenytoin**, an inducer of CYP3A4.[5]

The makers advise that if **carbamazepine** or other drugs that induce drug metabolism are given with mirtazapine, the mirtazapine dose may have to be increased. Further, if treatment with an inducer is stopped, mirtazapine dosage may have to be reduced.[2]

(d) Benzodiazepines

The impairment of psychomotor performance and learning caused by **diazepam** is increased by mirtazapine and therefore the makers warn that the sedative effects of benzodiazepines in general may be potentiated,[2] although the pharmacokinetics of neither mirtazapine nor **diazepam** are affected by concurrent use.[6]

(e) Cimetidine

In a double-blind cross-over study in 12 healthy subjects, placebo or cimetidine 800 mg twice daily were given for 14 days. Mirtazapine 30 mg was given at night on days 6 to 12. Concurrent administration of cimetidine with mirtazapine increased the AUC and peak plasma levels of mirtazapine by 54% and 22% respectively. Trough and average mirtazapine plasma levels, at steady state, were increased by 61% and 54%, respectively, during concurrent cimetidine administration. Mirtazapine did not affect the pharmacokinetics of cimetidine.[7] The makers advise that mirtazapine dosage may need to be reduced during concurrent treatment and increased when cimetidine treatment is stopped.[2]

(f) Cytochrome P450 isoenzyme CYP3A4 inhibitors

Ketoconazole is reported to increase peak plasma levels and AUC of mirtazapine by about 30% and 45% respectively.[2] The makers advise caution when strong inhibitors of the cytochrome isoenzyme CYP3A4 such as **azole antifungals**, **HIV-protease inhibitors**, **erythromycin**, or **nefazodone** are administered with mirtazapine.[2]

(g) MAOIs

No adverse mirtazapine/MAOI interactions have been reported[8] but to be on the safe side the makers say that the concurrent use of mirtazapine and the MAOIs should be avoided both during and within two weeks of stopping treatment.[2] This is a general warning that most of the makers of antidepressants issue.

(h) Rifampicin (Rifampin)

The makers advise that if drugs such as rifampicin that induce drug metabolism are given with mirtazapine, the mirtazapine dose may have to be increased. Further, if treatment with an inducer is stopped, mirtazapine dosage may have to be reduced.[2]

(i) Risperidone

A pilot study in 6 psychiatric patients treated with risperidone 1 to 3 mg twice a day for 1 to 4 weeks followed by 2 to 4 weeks of combined treatment with mirtazapine 15 to 30 mg at night, found that mirtazapine did not affect the plasma concentrations of risperidone or its 9-hydroxy metabolite. Data from another patient suggest that the addition of risperidone to mirtazapine treatment does not result in clinically relevant changes in plasma levels of mirtazapine. No clinically relevant differences in adverse effects were observed in the combined treatment phase compared with the single drug treatment phase, but the number of patients was limited and further study is needed.[9]

(j) Warfarin

Mirtazapine may cause small but clinically insignificant increases in INR in patients treated with warfarin.[2]

1. Sitsen JMA, Zivkov M. Mirtazapine — clinical profile. *CNS Drugs* (1995) 4 (Suppl 1), 39–48.
2. Zispin (Mirtazapine). Organon Laboratories Ltd. UK Summary of product characteristics, June 2003.
3. Sennef C, Timmer CJ, Sitsen JMA. Mirtazapine in combination with amitriptyline: a drug-drug interaction study in healthy subjects. *Hum Psychopharmacol* (2003) 18, 91–101.
4. Sitsen JMA, Maris FA, Timmer CJ. Drug-drug interaction studies with mirtazapine and carbamazepine in healthy male subjects. *Eur J Drug Metab Pharmacokinet* (2001) 26, 109–21.
5. Spaans E, van den Heuvel MW, Schnabel PG, Peeters PAM, Chin-Kon-Sung UG, Colbers EPH, Sitsen JMA. Concomitant use of mirtazapine and phenytoin: a drug-drug interaction study in healthy male subjects. *Eur J Clin Pharmacol* (2002) 58, 423–9.
6. Mattila M, Mattila MJ, Vrijmoed-de Vries M, Kuitunen T. Actions and interactions of psychotropic drugs on human performance and mood: single doses of ORG 3770, amitriptyline and diazepam. *Pharmacol Toxicol* (1989) 65, 81–8.
7. Sitsen JMA, Maris FA, Timmer CJ. Concomitant use of mirtazapine and cimetidine: a drug-drug interaction study in healthy male subjects. *Eur J Clin Pharmacol* (2000) 56, 389–94.
8. Akzo Nobel, Organon Laboratories Ltd. Personal communication, January 1999.
9. Loonen AJM, Doorschot CH, Oostelbos MCJM, Sitsen JMA. Lack of drug interactions between mirtazapine and risperidone in psychiatric patients: a pilot study. *Eur Neuropsychopharmacol* (1999) 10, 51–7.

Mirtazapine + SSRIs

SSRIs may increase plasma levels of mirtazapine and there are two reports of the serotonin syndrome and one of hypomania associated with combined use.

Clinical evidence

(a) Fluoxetine

There is an isolated report[1] of the serotonin syndrome in a 75-year-old woman when fluoxetine 20 mg daily was discontinued and mirtazapine 30 mg daily started soon afterwards [exact interval not stated]. Symptoms including dizziness, headache, nausea, dry mouth, anxiety, agitation, suicidal ideas and difficulty in walking occurred within hours of the first dose of mirtazapine. Symptoms worsened until mirtazapine was discontinued on day 5, after which an improvement was noticed. Fluoxetine was restarted on day 7.

(b) Fluvoxamine

A 26-year-old woman with a 12-year history of anorexia nervosa, treated with fluvoxamine 200 mg daily, developed symptoms consistent with the serotonin syndrome (tremors, restlessness, twitching, flushing, diaphoresis, nausea) about 4 days after starting mirtazapine 30 mg daily.[2] A 17-year-old boy treated with mirtazapine 30 mg daily experienced increased anxiety when fluvoxamine 100 mg daily was also given. Mirtazapine serum levels were increased threefold. In a second patient treated with mirtazapine 15 mg daily, the addition of fluvoxamine 50 mg daily resulted in a fourfold increase in serum mirtazapine concentrations, accompanied by mood improvements.[3]

(c) Paroxetine

A study in 21 healthy subjects given mirtazapine 30 mg, paroxetine 40 mg or a combination of both, daily for 9 days, found that paroxetine inhibited the metabolism of mirtazapine (AUCs of mirtazapine increased by about 17%). Mirtazapine did not alter the pharmacokinetics of paroxetine. The results of psychometric assessments suggested that concurrent use of mirtazapine and paroxetine did not alter cognitive function, or cause major changes in mood or sleep, compared with the administration of either drug alone.[4]

(d) Sertraline

A woman on sertraline 250 mg daily was additionally started on mirtazapine 15 mg daily because of inadequately controlled depression. Within 4 days she showed hypomanic symptoms and she stopped taking the mirtazapine. The hypomania resolved within 3 days but her depression then recurred.[5]

Mechanism

The cytochrome P450 isoenzyme CYP2D6 is inhibited by fluoxetine and paroxetine and CYP1A2 is inhibited by fluvoxamine. Both of these isoenzymes are involved in the metabolism of mirtazapine, which may explain the raised mirtazapine levels reported. Both SSRIs and mirtazapine affect serotonin transmission, which may lead to increased serotonin levels[1,2] and therefore cause the symptoms described as the serotonin syndrome. For more about the serotonin syndrome see 'Additive or synergistic interactions', (p.9).

Importance and management

These isolated reports would seem to suggest that combined use of mirtazapine and the SSRIs can lead to the serotonin syndrome. However, whether these are cases of the serotonin syndrome has been disputed.[6] Low body-weight, decrease in total body fat and a decrease in the volume of distribution of a fat-soluble drug such as fluvoxamine may also have contributed in one case.[2] This and other reports of anxiety and hypomania highlight the need for some caution during concurrent use. More study is required.

1. Benazzi F. Serotonin syndrome with mirtazapine-fluoxetine combination. *Int J Geriatr Psychiatry* (1998) 13, 495–6.
2. Demers JC, Malone M. Serotonin syndrome induced by fluvoxamine and mirtazapine. *Ann Pharmacother* (2001) 35, 1217–20.
3. Anttila SAK, Rasanen I, Leinonen EVJ. Fluvoxamine augmentation increases serum mirtazapine concentrations three- to fourfold. *Ann Pharmacother* (2001) 35, 1221–3.
4. Ruwe FJL, Smulders RA, Kleijn HJ, Hartmans HLA, Sitsen JMA. Mirtazapine and paroxetine: a drug-drug interaction study in healthy subjects. *Hum Psychopharmacol* (2001) 16, 449–59.
5. Soutullo CA, McElroy SL, Keck PE. Hypomania associated with mirtazapine augmentation of sertraline. *J Clin Psychiatry* (1998) 59, 320.
6. Isbister GK, Dawson AH, Whyte IM. Comment: serotonin syndrome induced by fluvoxamine and mirtazapine. *Ann Pharmacother* (2001) 35, 1674–5.

Nefazodone + Antidepressants

An isolated report describes a woman who developed marked and acute hypotension and weakness when her treatment with desipramine, fluoxetine and venlafaxine was replaced by nefazodone. Isolated cases describe the serotonin syndrome in other patients. An elderly patient on nefazodone developed symptoms diagnosed as the serotonin syndrome when St John's wort was taken concurrently.

Clinical evidence, mechanism, importance and management

(a) Amitriptyline

A woman who had been taking amitriptyline 10 mg at night and thioridazine developed the serotonin syndrome after taking half a tablet of nefazodone [dosage unspecified].[1]

(b) Fluoxetine

A woman with a one-year history of DSM-IV major depressive disorder and panic disorder was treated with daily doses of **desipramine** 75 mg, fluoxetine 20 mg, **venlafaxine** 37.5 mg, **clonazepam** 3 mg and **valproate** 400 mg with no adverse effects except a dry mouth and sexual difficulties.[2] The first three drugs were stopped and replaced by nefazodone 100 mg twice daily started about 12 hours later. Within an hour of the first dose she felt very weak and her blood pressure was found to have fallen to only 90/60 mmHg (normally 120/90 mmHg). On waking the next day she had severe weakness, unsteady gait, a pale, cool and sweaty skin, and paraesthesia. During the day she took two further 100-mg doses of nefazodone and her condition persisted and worsened with continuing hypotension. The nefazodone was discontinued and by the following day the weakness had improved; disappearing over the next few days. Within a week nefazodone 200 mg daily was reintroduced without problems.

The US makers of nefazodone note that nefazodone does not alter the pharmacokinetics of fluoxetine, but fluoxetine increases the AUC of the metabolites of nefazodone by up to 6-fold.[3] When nefazodone was given to patients who had been taking fluoxetine for 7 days adverse effects (including headache and nausea) were increased. The makers advise allowing a washout of at least one week (more may be needed depending on dose and individual patient characteristics) to minimise these effects.[3] They also note that **desipramine** increases nefazodone metabolite levels (by up to 50%), but no dosage adjustments are required on concurrent use.[3] It therefore seems likely that fluoxetine was the interacting drug, but it is impossible to rule out a contribution from the other drugs.

(c) MAOIs

The makers state that nefazodone should not be used with or within 2 weeks of discontinuing treatment with an MAOI. Conversely at least one week should be allowed after stopping nefazodone before starting an MAOI.[2,3] There appears to be no direct clinical or other evidence that an adverse interaction occurs.

(d) Paroxetine

A woman was withdrawn from nefazodone after 6 months, tapering over the last fortnight to 75 mg 12-hourly. Within a day she started paroxetine 20 mg daily and valproic acid, and was admitted the next day with muscle rigidity, uncoordinated muscle tremors, flailing arms and twitching legs, diaphoresis and agitation. This was identified as the serotonin syndrome. Rechallenge with paroxetine 7 days later was uneventful.[4]

(e) St John's wort

An elderly patient on nefazodone 100 mg twice daily, developed symptoms similar to the serotonin syndrome within 3 days of starting additional treatment with St John's wort 300 mg three times daily. The symptoms included nausea, vomiting, and restlessness. She was asked to stop both medications, but continued the St John's wort and her symptoms gradually improved over a 1-week period.[5]

(f) Trazodone

A woman receiving irbesartan for hypertension was also treated for depression with nefazodone at an initial dosage of 200 mg daily, followed by 400 mg daily for about 5 weeks. Four days after the dose was increased to 500 mg daily, and trazodone 25 to 50 mg daily also added as a hypnotic, she was admitted to hospital with a blood pressure of 240/120 mmHg. She was confused, had difficulty concentrating and had numbness on the right side of her lips, nose and right-hand fingers, flushed pruritic skin, nausea and loose stools. On examination she was restless, hyperreflexic and diaphoretic. Nefazodone and trazodone were discontinued. She recovered after treatment with labetalol, clonidine, amlodipine and increased irbesartan dosage. Although trazodone is used with other serotonergic agents, it is important to be aware that this may lead to the potentially fatal serotonin syndrome.[6] For more on the serotonin syndrome see 'Additive or synergistic interactions', (p.9).

1. Chan BSH, Graudins A, Whyte IM, Dawson AH, Braitberg G, Duggin GG. Serotonin syndrome resulting from drug interactions. *Med J Aust* (1998) 169, 523–5.
2. Benazzi F. Dangerous interaction with nefazodone added to fluoxetine, desipramine, venlafaxine, valproate and clonazepam combination therapy. *J Psychopharmacol* (1997) 11, 190–1.
3. Nefazodone hydrochloride. Watson Laboratories Inc. US Prescribing information, June 2004.
4. John L, Perreault MM, Tao T, Blew PG. Serotonin syndrome associated with nefazodone and paroxetine. *Ann Emerg Med* (1997) 29, 287–9.
5. Lantz MS, Buchalter E, Giambanco V. St. John's wort and antidepressant drug interactions in the elderly. *J Geriatr Psychiatry Neurol* (1999) 12, 7–10.
6. Margolese HC, Chouinard G. Serotonin syndrome from addition of low-dose trazodone to nefazodone. *Am J Psychiatry* (2000) 157, 1022.

Nefazodone + Miscellaneous

Nefazodone appears not to interact adversely with alcohol, cimetidine, phenytoin, propranolol or warfarin. The maker warns about a possible interaction with haloperidol but this appears to be largely theoretical.

Clinical evidence, mechanism, importance and management

(a) Alcohol

Nefazodone 400 mg was found not to increase the sedative-hypnotic effects of alcohol,[1] but even so the makers of nefazodone say that it would be prudent to avoid concurrent use,[2,3] because alcohol use is not advised in depressed patients.[3]

(b) Cimetidine

No changes in the steady-state pharmacokinetics of either cimetidine or nefazodone were seen in a week long study in 18 healthy subjects given cimetidine 300 mg four times daily and nefazodone 200 mg 12-hourly. No special precautions would seem to be necessary if both drugs are used concurrently.[4]

(c) Haloperidol

After taking nefazodone 200 mg twice daily for about 7 days to achieve steady-state pharmacokinetics, the AUC of haloperidol 5 mg in 12 healthy subjects was found to be increased by 36% but the maximum plasma levels of haloperidol were unaltered. The pharmacokinetics of the nefazodone were unaltered.[5] The makers advise caution when using these two drugs together,[2] and suggest that dosage adjustments may be necessary,[3] but it seems fairly unlikely that the change is enough to be of clinical relevance.

(d) Phenytoin

Nefazodone 200 mg twice daily for 7 days had no effect on the pharmacokinetics of a single 300-mg dose of phenytoin in healthy subjects, and no changes in vital signs, ECGs or other physical measurements were seen. There was no evidence that a clinically significant interaction was likely.[6]

(e) Propranolol

A study in 18 healthy subjects found that 200 mg of nefazodone 12-hourly reduced the AUC of propranolol 40 mg 12-hourly by 14% and decreased the maximum plasma levels by 29%, but no clinically significant changes in the response to propranolol or relevant adverse responses were seen. The pharmacokinetics of the nefazodone were largely unchanged.[7] No special precautions would therefore seem to be necessary if both drugs are used.

(f) Warfarin

In one study, 17 healthy subjects stabilised on enough warfarin to achieve a prothrombin ratio of 1.2 to 1.5 for 14 days were then additionally given nefazodone 200 mg or placebo 12-hourly for a further 7 days. No clinically significant changes occurred in the plasma warfarin levels or in their prothrombin ratios.[8] No special precautions would seem necessary if both drugs are used.

1. Frewer LJ, Lader M. The effects of nefazodone, imipramine and placebo, alone and combined with alcohol, in normal subjects. *Int Clin Psychopharmacol* (1993) 8, 13–20.
2. Dutonin (Nefazodone) Bristol-Myers Squibb Pharmaceuticals Ltd. UK Summary of product characteristics, June 2002.
3. Nefazodone hydrochloride. Watson Laboratories Inc. US Prescribing information, June 2004.
4. Barbhaiya RH, Shukla UA, Greene DS. Lack of interaction between nefazodone and cimetidine: a steady state pharmacokinetic study in humans. *Br J Clin Pharmacol* (1995) 40, 161–5.
5. Barbhaiya RH, Shukla UA, Greene DS, Breuel H-P, Midha KK. Investigation of pharmacokinetic and pharmacodynamic interactions after coadministration of nefazodone and haloperidol. *J Clin Psychopharmacol* (1996) 16, 26–34.
6. Marino MR, Langenbacher KM, Hammett JL, Nichola P, Uderman HD. The effect of nefazodone on the single-dose pharmacokinetics of phenytoin in healthy male subjects. *J Clin Psychopharmacol* (1997) 17, 27–33.
7. Salazar DE, Marathe PH, Fulmor IE, Lee JS, Raymond RH, Uderman HD. Pharmacokinetic and pharmacodynamic evaluation during coadministration of nefazodone and propranolol in healthy men. *J Clin Pharmacol* (1995) 35, 1109–18.
8. Salazar DE, Dockens RC, Milbrath RL, Raymond RH, Fulmor IE, Chaikin PC, Uderman HD. Pharmacokinetic and pharmacodynamic evaluation of warfarin and nefazodone coadministration in healthy subjects. *J Clin Pharmacol* (1995) 35, 730–8.

Reboxetine + Miscellaneous

Few clinically relevant interactions have yet been identified with reboxetine. Ketoconazole may inhibit the metabolism of reboxetine and the makers advise avoidance of concurrent use with azole antifungals, macrolide antibacterials and fluvoxamine. Reboxetine does not interact with alcohol although the makers advise caution, and no interaction has been seen with the MAOIs. Even so, the makers currently advise avoidance.

Clinical evidence, mechanism, importance and management

Reboxetine appears to be relatively free from adverse drug interactions. Studies with human liver microsomes using concentrations of reboxetine eight times greater than maximum plasma levels found that it has no inhibitory effects on the cytochrome P450 isoenzymes (CYP1A2, CYP2C9, CYP2D6, CYP2E1, CYP3A4) which are responsible for the metabolism of the majority of other drugs.[1]

(a) Alcohol

A study in 10 healthy subjects found that reboxetine does not affect cognitive or psychomotor function, and there is no interaction with alcohol,[2] nevertheless the makers say that patients should be cautioned if operating machinery or driving.[3]

(b) Cytochrome P450 isoenzyme CYP2D6 mediated interactions

Reboxetine has been shown *in vitro* to inhibit CYP2D6 at concentrations exceeding those achieved in clinical use.[3] However, a study[4] in healthy subjects found that reboxetine 8 mg daily did not interact with **dextromethorphan** suggesting that there are unlikely to be clinically significant interactions with CYP2D6 substrates. CYP2D6 is not involved in reboxetine metabolism.[3]

(c) Cytochrome P450 isoenzyme CYP3A4 mediated interactions

Reboxetine has been shown *in vitro* to inhibit CYP2D6 at concentrations exceeding those achieved in clinical use. This isoenzyme is also the primary enzyme involved in reboxetine metabolism.[3] This *in vitro* data is supported by a study in 11 healthy subjects that found that **ketoconazole** 200 mg daily for 5 days decreased the clearance of single doses of reboxetine 4 mg, taken on the second day. The adverse effect profile of reboxetine was not altered, but it was concluded that caution should be used and a reduction in reboxetine dosage considered if it is given with **ketoconazole**.[5] The makers recommend that potent inhibitors of CYP3A4, including **azole antifungals**, **fluvoxamine**, **macrolides** (**erythromycin**) and **nefazodone**, should not be given with reboxetine.[3] However, note that **fluvoxamine** is more usually considered a potent inhibitor of CYP1A2 and is generally considered a weak inhibitor of CYP3A4.

(d) Lorazepam

A mild to moderate drowsiness and an orthostatic increase in heart rate has been seen in healthy subjects when reboxetine and lorazepam were given concurrently, but no pharmacokinetic interaction occurred.[3]

(e) Miscellaneous drugs

The makers point out the possibility of hypokalaemia if reboxetine is used with **potassium-depleting diuretics**. Experience with reboxetine suggests it reduces potassium by 0.8 mmol/l, starting after 14 weeks of use. The makers also suggest that concurrent use of reboxetine and **ergot derivatives** might result in increased blood pressure although no clinical data are quoted.[3]

(f) Other antidepressants

A study in 30 healthy subjects given reboxetine 4 mg twice daily and **fluoxetine** 20 mg daily found no significant changes in the pharmacokinetics of either drug.[6] No data seem to be available about the concurrent use of reboxetine with **MAOIs** and at the moment the makers currently advise the avoidance of **fluvoxamine** (see above) and **MAOIs** to be on the safe side.[3]

1. Dostert P, Benedetti MS, Poggesi I. Review of the pharmacokinetics and metabolism of reboxetine, a selective noradrenaline reuptake inhibitor. *Eur Neuropsychopharmacol* (1997) 7 (Suppl 1), S23–S35.
2. Kerr JS, Powell J, Hindmarch I. The effects of reboxetine and amitriptyline, with and without alcohol on cognitive function and psychomotor performance. *Br J Clin Pharmacol* (1996) 42, 239–41.
3. Edronax (Reboxetine). Pharmacia Ltd. UK Summary of product characteristics, September 2004.
4. Avenoso A, Facciolà G, Scordo MG, Spina E. No effect of the new antidepressant reboxetine on CYP2D6 activity in healthy volunteers. *Ther Drug Monit* (1999) 21, 577–9.
5. Herman BD, Fleishaker JC, Brown MT. Ketoconazole inhibits the clearance of the enantiomers of the antidepressant reboxetine in humans. *Clin Pharmacol Ther* (1999) 66, 374–9.
6. Fleishaker JC, Herman BD, Pearson LK, Ionita A, Mucci M. Evaluation of the potential pharmacokinetic/pharmacodynamic interaction between fluoxetine and reboxetine in healthy volunteers. *Clin Drug Invest* (1999) 18, 141–50.

SSRIs + Benzatropine

Seven patients developed delirium when given fluoxetine, paroxetine or sertraline with benzatropine, in the presence of perphenazine or haloperidol. Other patients remained symptom free.

Clinical evidence, mechanism, importance and management

Five patients became confused and developed delirium when given an antipsychotic, an SSRI (4 on **fluoxetine** and one on **paroxetine**) and benzatropine. No peripheral anticholinergic toxicity was seen. The delirium developed within 2 days in two cases, but took several weeks to appear in another. The authors of the report attributed this to an interaction between the SSRIs and benzatropine, speculating that the SSRIs may have inhibited the metabolism of the benzatropine thereby increasing its toxicity. Alternatively they suggest a possible additive central anticholinergic effect. They also very briefly mention two other patients who became delirious when given an unnamed antipsychotic and either **sertraline** or **paroxetine** with benzatropine.[1] It is noteworthy that 4 of the first group of patients were given perphenazine and one haloperidol,[1] both of which have been involved in additive anticholinergic interactions (see 'Antipsychotics + Anticholinergics', p.529). Also note that adverse interactions have been reported with the use of 'antipsychotics and SSRIs', (p.533). Another case of delirium associated with the use of **paroxetine** and benzatropine has been described.[2]

In contrast, another report describes 12 patients on **fluoxetine** and perphenazine who also received benzatropine 1 mg daily without showing signs of delirium.[3,4] The general clinical importance of this interaction is therefore very uncertain indeed, but it would now seem prudent to be alert for evidence of confusion and possible delirium in patients given SSRIs with benzatropine, particularly if they are also taking other psychotropics that may have anticholinergic actions. The authors of the first report say that they have not seen delirium with combinations of SSRIs (not named) and other anticholinergic drugs such as biperiden and diphenhydramine.[1]

1. Roth A, Akyol S, Nelson JC. Delirium associated with the combination of a neuroleptic, an SSRI, and benztropine. *J Clin Psychiatry* (1994) 55, 492–5.

2. Armstrong SC, Schweitzer SM. Delirium associated with paroxetine and benztropine combination. *Am J Psychiatry* (1997) 154, 581–2.
3. Rothschild AJ, Samson JA, Bessette MP, Carter-Campbell JT. Efficacy of the combination of fluoxetine and perphenazine in the treatment of psychotic depression. *J Clin Psychiatry* (1993) 54, 338–42.
4. Rothschild AJ. Delirium: an SSRI-benztropine adverse effect? *J Clin Psychiatry* (1995) 56, 537.

SSRIs + Benzodiazepines or related drugs

On the whole, no clinically significant interaction appears to occur between the SSRIs and the benzodiazepines or related drugs such as cloral hydrate or zaleplon. However, there is some evidence to suggest that the metabolism of some benzodiazepines (such as alprazolam, bromazepam, diazepam) may be reduced by some SSRIs (such as fluoxetine, fluvoxamine and paroxetine). There is some evidence to support the suggestion that sedation is likely to be increased by the concurrent use of SSRIs and benzodiazepines. Rare cases of hallucinations have been seen with zolpidem and some SSRIs.

Clinical evidence

(a) Citalopram

The UK makers of citalopram say that no pharmacodynamic interactions have been noted in clinical studies in which citalopram was given with benzodiazepines,[1] although the US makers point out that caution should be used with citalopram and any CNS active drug.[2] A general study in psychiatric patients found that when data on benzodiazepines was pooled, they caused a modest 23% increase in serum citalopram levels, which is almost certainly too small to be clinically relevant. **Alprazolam** was the only benzodiazepine to cause an elevation of citalopram levels (by 13%) when analysed alone.[3] A study in 17 healthy subjects found no pharmacokinetic interaction between **triazolam** and citalopram, and it was suggested that **triazolam** and other substrates of the cytochrome P450 isoenzyme CYP3A4 are unlikely to have pharmacokinetic interactions with citalopram.[4]

(b) Fluoxetine

The concurrent use of fluoxetine 60 mg daily has been found to reduce the clearance of **alprazolam** 1 mg four times daily by about 21% and to increase its plasma levels by about 30%. These changes were accompanied by increased psychomotor impairment.[5] This appears to be due to reduced **alprazolam** metabolism.[6]

Fluoxetine 30 mg, given daily for 1 or 8 days, had no effect on the pharmacokinetics of **diazepam** 10 mg.[7] A later study by the same group, using 60 mg of fluoxetine suggested that the **diazepam** half-life and AUC were increased, possibly because the fluoxetine decreased the metabolism of **diazepam**. However, they concluded that this was not of any clinical significance.[8] Another study found that fluoxetine 60 mg alone did not affect psychomotor performance but fluoxetine 60 mg plus **diazepam** 5 mg significantly impaired the divided attention tracking test and vigilance test more than with **diazepam** 5 mg alone.[9] Other studies found that the pharmacokinetics of **clonazepam**,[10] **estazolam**,[11] **midazolam**,[12,13] **triazolam**,[14] and **zolpidem**[15,16] were not significantly affected by fluoxetine.

In contrast, isolated cases of visual hallucinations lasting up to 7 hours have been reported in patients on **zolpidem** who were taking fluoxetine.[17] Marked drowsiness occurred for a whole day in a patient taking fluoxetine 20 mg daily after being given **cloral hydrate** 500 mg the night before. She later tolerated **cloral hydrate** 1 g in the absence of fluoxetine without adverse effects.[18]

(c) Fluvoxamine

In 60 healthy subjects fluvoxamine 50 mg daily for 3 days then 100 mg daily for 7 days, doubled the plasma levels of alprazolam 1 mg four times daily given on days 7 to 10. The alprazolam clearance was more than halved. Psychomotor performance and memory were found to be significantly worsened, even after only one day of the combination.[19] A study in 23 Japanese patients found that fluvoxamine increased plasma levels of **alprazolam** by 58%. There was wide interpatient variability, possibly associated with differences in the cytochrome P450 isoenzyme CYP2C19 levels in these patients (see 'Genetic factors', (p.4)), although it is unclear exactly what impact this isoenzyme has on the interaction.[20]

Fluvoxamine 50 mg twice daily increased the plasma levels of a single 12-mg dose of **bromazepam** in 12 healthy subjects by 36% and increased the AUC almost 2.5-fold. Some increased impairment in cognitive function was seen.[21]

Fluvoxamine has been found not to interact adversely with **cloral hydrate**.[22] Fluvoxamine (50 mg on day one, 100 mg on day 2, then 150 mg daily thereafter) for 16 days decreased the clearance of a single 10-mg dose of **diazepam** given on day 4 in 8 healthy subjects by about 65%. The half-life was increased from 51 to 118 hours, and the AUC was increased threefold.[23]

Fluvoxamine 50 mg twice daily caused a very small, non-significant, increase in the serum levels and AUC of a single 4-mg dose of **lorazepam** in 12 healthy subjects.[21]

A study in 10 healthy subjects[13] found that fluvoxamine 50 mg twice daily for 8 days then 100 mg twice daily for 6 days had minimal effects on the pharmacokinetics of a single 10-mg dose of **midazolam** given on day 12.

In a placebo-controlled study in 12 healthy subjects it was found that fluvoxamine 25 mg twice daily for 14 days had no effect on the pharmacokinetics of a single 20-mg dose of **quazepam**. However, formation of the metabolite 2-oxoquazepam was decreased, and there was a minor decrease in the sedative effects of **quazepam** at 4 hours, although these changes were considered to be of little clinical significance.[24]

(d) Paroxetine

No important changes in the pharmacokinetics of paroxetine were seen when 12 healthy subjects given paroxetine 30 mg daily were also given **diazepam** 5 mg three times a day. Adverse events were not increased by the combination.[25] In another study it was found that paroxetine did not increase the impairment of a number of psychomotor tests caused by **oxazepam**.[26] *In vitro* studies using human liver microsomal enzymes have shown that paroxetine inhibits the metabolism of **alprazolam** mediated by the cytochrome P450 subfamily CYP3A,[27,28] so that some increased **alprazolam** effects are possible if both drugs are used concurrently. An isolated report describes worsening anxiety, agitation, mild abdominal cramps and diaphoresis in a woman on paroxetine, shortly after taking **clonazepam** (dosage stated as one tablet). This toxic response was suggested as being the serotonin syndrome, although in fact many of the usual signs were absent and moreover, **clonazepam** has actually been used to treat the myoclonus that occurs in the serotonin syndrome. She was effectively treated with **lorazepam**.[29]

In a double-blind study in healthy subjects it was found that paroxetine 20 mg for 9 days had no effect on the pharmacokinetics of **zaleplon** 20 mg, and psychomotor performance was unaffected by concurrent use.[30]

An isolated report describes a healthy 16-year-old girl with depression who took paroxetine 20 mg daily for 3 days, and then on the evening of the third night a single 10-mg dose of **zolpidem**. Within 1 hour she began to hallucinate, then became disorientated and was unable to recognise members of her family. She recovered spontaneously within 4 hours.[31]

(e) Sertraline

No clinically relevant effects were found in interaction studies in which sertraline was given with a single intravenous dose of **diazepam**.[32,33] One *in vitro* study in human liver microsomes suggested that sertraline inhibits the metabolism of **alprazolam**,[6] whereas another suggested no interaction occurred.[34] *In vivo* studies largely demonstrate a lack of interaction. For example, a pharmacokinetic study in 10 healthy subjects found that sertraline 50 to 150 mg daily had no effect on the pharmacokinetics of **alprazolam**, although some small decreases in a driving simulation score were seen at the 100- and 150-mg doses of sertraline.[35] Similarly, sertraline 50 mg daily had no effect on the pharmacokinetics of **alprazolam** 1 mg daily in 12 healthy subjects, after 2 weeks of concurrent use.[34]

A study in 13 subjects given daily doses of **clonazepam** 1 mg with sertraline 100 mg for 10 days found no evidence that the addition of sertraline to clonazepam made the subjects more sedated or less able to carry out simple psychometric tests.[36]

Sertraline appears to have no clinically significant effects on the pharmacokinetics of **zolpidem**,[37] but isolated cases of visual hallucinations lasting up to 7 hours have been reported in patients on **zolpidem** who were taking sertraline.[17]

Mechanism

The evidence suggests that fluvoxamine inhibits the metabolism of those benzodiazepines that undergo oxidation (e.g. alprazolam,[28] bromazepam, diazepam) thereby increasing and prolonging their effects, but not those that are metabolised by glucuronidation (e.g. lorazepam). Zaleplon is metabolised by aldehyde oxidase and therefore does not interact.

Importance and management

Evidence is limited, but what is known suggests that the dosages of alprazolam, bromazepam, diazepam and other similarly metabolised benzodiazepines (e.g. nitrazepam) should be reduced, probably by half, in the presence of fluvoxamine to avoid adverse effects (drowsiness, reduced psychomotor performance and memory). Fluvoxamine is unlikely to affect lorazepam and other benzodiazepines metabolised by glucuronidation (e.g. lormetazepam, oxazepam, temazepam) or midazolam. It seems unlikely that sertraline will affect any of the benzodiazepines and it may therefore be a useful alternative to fluvoxamine. Nevertheless, the makers of sertraline say that it should not be given with benzodiazepines or other tranquillisers in patients who drive or operate machinery.[38]

The hallucinations seen with the SSRIs and zolpidem appear rare, and reactions of this kind have been seen with zolpidem alone. The concurrent use of these drugs need not be avoided, but bear this possible interaction in mind if hallucinations occur.

1. Cipramil (Citalopram). Lundbeck Ltd. UK Summary of product characteristics, April 2003.
2. Celexa (Citalopram). Forest Pharmaceuticals Inc. US Prescribing information, February 2005.
3. Leinonen E, Lepola U, Koponen H, Kinnunen I. The effect of age and concomitant treatment with other psychoactive drugs on serum concentrations of citalopram measured with a non-enantioselective method. *Ther Drug Monit* (1996) 18, 111–17.
4. Nolting A, Abramowitz W. Lack of interaction between citalopram and the CYP3A4 substrate triazolam. *Pharmacotherapy* (2000) 20, 750–5.
5. Lasher TA, Fleishaker JC, Steenwyk RC, Antal EJ. Pharmacokinetic pharmacodynamic evaluation of the combined administration of alprazolam and fluoxetine. *Psychopharmacology (Berl)* (1991) 104, 323–7.
6. von Moltke LL, Greenblatt DJ, Cotreau-Bibbo MM, Harmatz JS, Shader RI. Inhibitors of alprazolam metabolism *in vitro*: effect of serotonin-reuptake-inhibitor antidepressants, ketoconazole and quinidine. *Br J Clin Pharmacol* (1994) 38, 23–31.
7. Lemberger L, Bergstrom RF, Wolen RL, Farid NA, Enas GG, Aronoff GR. Fluoxetine: clinical pharmacology and physiologic disposition. *J Clin Psychiatry* (1985) 46, 3 (Sec 2), 14–19.
8. Lemberger L, Rowe H, Bosomworth JC, Tenbarge JB, Bergstrom RF. The effect of fluoxetine on the pharmacokinetics and psychomotor responses of diazepam. *Clin Pharmacol Ther* (1988) 43, 412–19.
9. Moskowitz H, Burns M. The effects on performance of two antidepressants, alone and in combination with diazepam. *Prog Neuropsychopharmacol Biol Psychiatry* (1988) 12, 783–92.
10. Greenblatt DJ, Preskorn SH, Cotreau MM, Horst WD, Harmatz JS. Fluoxetine impairs clearance of alprazolam but not of clonazepam. *Clin Pharmacol Ther* (1992) 52, 479–86.
11. Cavanaugh J, Schneck D, Eason C, Hansen M, Gustavson L. Lack of effect of fluoxetine on the pharmacokinetics (PK) and pharmacodynamics (PD) of estazolam. *Clin Pharmacol Ther* (1994) 55, 141.
12. Lam YWF, Alfaro CL, Ereshefsky L, Miller M. Effect of antidepressants and ketoconazole on oral midazolam pharmacokinetics. *Clin Pharmacol Ther* (1998) 63, 229.
13. Lam YWF, Alfaro CL, Ereshefsky L, Miller M. Pharmacokinetics and pharmacodynamic interactions of oral midazolam with ketoconazole, fluoxetine, fluvoxamine, and nefazodone. *J Clin Pharmacol* (2003) 43, 1274–82.
14. Wright CE, Lasher-Sisson TA, Steenwyk RC, Swanson CN. A pharmacokinetic evaluation of the combined administration of triazolam and fluoxetine. *Pharmacotherapy* (1992) 12, 103–6.
15. Piergies AA, Sweet J, Johnson M, Roth-Schechter BF, Allard S. The effect of co-administration of zolpidem with fluoxetine: pharmacokinetics and pharmacodynamics. *Int J Clin Pharmacol Ther* (1996) 34, 178–83.
16. Allard S, Sainati S, Roth-Schechter B, Macintyre J. Minimal interaction between fluoxetine and multiple-dose zolpidem in healthy women. *Drug Metab Dispos* (1998) 26, 617–22.
17. Elko CJ, Burgess JL, Robertson WO. Zolpidem-associated hallucinations and serotonin reuptake inhibition: a possible interaction. *Clin Toxicol* (1998) 36, 195–203.
18. Devarajan S. Interaction of fluoxetine and chloral hydrate. *Can J Psychiatry* (1992) 37, 590–1.
19. Fleishaker JC, Hulst LK. A pharmacokinetic and pharmacodynamic evaluation of the combined administration of alprazolam and fluvoxamine. *Eur J Clin Pharmacol* (1994) 46, 35–9.
20. Suzuki Y, Shioiri T, Muratake T, Kawashima Y, Sato S, Hagiwara M, Inoue Y, Shimoda K, Someya T. Effects of concomitant fluvoxamine on the metabolism of alprazolam in Japanese psychiatric patients: interaction with CYP2C19 mutated alleles. *Eur J Clin Pharmacol* (2003) 58, 829–33.
21. Van Harten J, Holland RL, Wesnes K. Influence of multiple-dose administration of fluvoxamine on the pharmacokinetics of the benzodiazepines bromazepam and lorazepam: a randomised, cross-over study. *Eur Neuropsychopharmacol* (1992) 2, 381.
22. Benfield P, Ward A. Fluvoxamine, a review of its pharmacodynamic and pharmacokinetic properties and therapeutic efficacy in depressive illness. *Drugs* (1986) 32, 313–34.
23. Perucca E, Gatti G, Cipolla G, Spina E, Barel S, Soback S, Gips M, Bialer M. Inhibition of diazepam metabolism by fluvoxamine: a pharmacokinetic study in normal volunteers. *Clin Pharmacol Ther* (1994) 56, 471–6.
24. Kanda H, Yasui-Furukori N, Fukasawa T, Aoshima T, Suzuki A, Otani K. Interaction study between fluvoxamine and quazepam. *J Clin Pharmacol* (2003) 43, 1392–7.
25. Bannister SJ, Houser VP, Hulse JD, Kisicki JC, Rasmussen JGC. Evaluation of the potential for interactions of paroxetine with diazepam, cimetidine, warfarin, and digoxin. *Acta Psychiatr Scand* (1989) 80 (Suppl 350), 102–6.
26. Cooper SM, Jackson D, Loudon JM, McClelland GR, Raptopoulos P. The psychomotor effects of paroxetine alone and in combination with haloperidol, amylobarbitone, oxazepam, or alcohol. *Acta Psychiatr Scand* (1989) 80 (Suppl 350), 53–55.
27. Greenblatt DJ, von Moltke LL, Harmatz JS, Ciraulo DA, Shader RI. Alprazolam pharmacokinetics, metabolism, and plasma levels: clinical implications. *J Clin Psychiatry* (1993) 54 (Suppl), 4–11.
28. von Moltke LL, Greenblatt DJ, Court MH, Duan SX, Harmatz JS, Shader RI. Inhibition of alprazolam and desipramine hydroxylation *in vitro* by paroxetine and fluvoxamine: comparison with other selective serotonin reuptake inhibitor antidepressants. *J Clin Psychopharmacol* (1995) 15, 125–31.
29. Rella JG, Hoffman RS. Possible serotonin syndrome from paroxetine and clonazepam. *Clin Toxicol* (1998) 36, 257–8.
30. Darwish M. Overview of drug interaction studies with zaleplon. Poster presented at 13th Annual Meeting of Associated Professional Sleep Studies (APSS), Orlando, Florida, June 23rd, 1999.
31. Katz SE. Possible paroxetine-zolpidem interaction. *Am J Psychiatry* (1995) 152, 1689.
32. Warrington SJ. Clinical implications of the pharmacology of sertraline. *Int Clin Psychopharmacol* (1991) 6 (Suppl 2), 11–21.
33. Gardner MJ, Baris BA, Wilner KD, Preskorn SH. Effect of sertraline on the pharmacokinetics and protein binding of diazepam in healthy volunteers. *Clin Pharmacokinet* (1997) 32 (Suppl 1), 43–9.
34. Preskorn SH, Greenblatt DJ, Harvey AT. Lack of effect of sertraline on the pharmacokinetics of alprazolam. *J Clin Psychopharmacol* (2000) 20, 585–6.
35. Hassan PC, Sproule BA, Herrmann N, Reed K, Naranjo CA. Dose-response evaluation of sertraline-alprazolam interaction in humans. *Clin Pharmacol Ther* (1998) 63, 185.
36. Kroboth PD, Bonate PL, Smith RB, Suarez E. Clonazepam (Klonopin®) and sertraline (Zoloft®): absence of drug interaction in a multiple dose study. *Clin Pharmacol Ther* (1997), 61, 178.
37. Allard S, Sainati S, Roth-Schechter BF. Coadministration of short-term zolpidem with sertraline in healthy women. *J Clin Pharmacol* (1999) 39, 184–91.
38. Lustral (Sertraline). Pfizer Ltd. UK Summary of product characteristics, December 2003.

SSRIs + Cyproheptadine

Three reports say that cyproheptadine can oppose the antidepressant effects of fluoxetine, and another describes the same effect with paroxetine.

Clinical evidence

(a) Fluoxetine

Three depressed men complained of anorgasmia when treated with fluoxetine. When this was treated with cyproheptadine their depressive symptoms returned, decreasing again when cyproheptadine was stopped.[1] Two women also complained of anorgasmia within 1 to 3 months of starting treatment with fluoxetine 40 to 60 mg daily for bulimia nervosa. When cyproheptadine was added to treat this sexual dysfunction, the urge to binge on food returned in both of them and one experienced increased depression. These symptoms resolved 4 to 7 days after stopping cyproheptadine treatment.[2] A woman successfully treated with fluoxetine 40 mg daily showed a re-emergence of her depressive symptoms on two occasions within 36 hours of starting to take cyproheptadine.[3] In a further case, a woman who responded well to fluoxetine 20 mg daily for depression had a recurrence of her depression after she began to take cyproheptadine for migraine. Increasing the dose of fluoxetine to 40 mg daily controlled the depressive symptoms while cyproheptadine was continued for migraine.[4] In contrast, no exacerbation of depression was seen in a study in which both cyproheptadine and fluoxetine were used in 2 patients.[5]

(b) Paroxetine

The depression of a woman, which had responded well to paroxetine 20 mg daily, re-emerged and worsened, and was accompanied by confusion and psychotic symptoms, within 2 days of starting to take cyproheptadine 2 mg twice daily for the treatment of anorgasmia.[6] Psychotic symptoms resolved 2 days after stopping cyproheptadine.

Mechanism

Although the mechanism is not fully understood, it has been suggested that because cyproheptadine is a serotonin antagonist it blocks or opposes the serotoninergic effects of these SSRIs.[1-3,6]

Importance and management

Direct information about this interaction appears to be limited to these studies although cyproheptadine has also been found to oppose the antidepressant effects of MAOIs (see 'MAOIs + Cyproheptadine', p.865). One of the studies suggests that not every patient is affected.[5] If concurrent use is thought appropriate, the outcome should be very well monitored for evidence of a reduced antidepressant response.

1. Feder R. Reversal of antidepressant activity of fluoxetine by cyproheptadine in three patients. *J Clin Psychiatry* (1991) 52, 163–4.
2. Goldbloom DS, Kennedy SH. Adverse interaction of fluoxetine and cyproheptadine in two patients with bulimia nervosa. *J Clin Psychiatry* (1991) 52, 261–2.
3. Katz RJ, Rosenthal M. Adverse interaction of cyproheptadine with serotonergic antidepressants. *J Clin Psychiatry* (1994) 55, 314–15.

4. Boon F. Cyproheptadine and SSRIs. *J Am Acad Child Adolesc Psychiatry* (1999) 38, 112.
5. McCormick S, Olin J, Brotman AW. Reversal of fluoxetine-induced anorgasmia by cyproheptadine in two patients. *J Clin Psychiatry* (1990) 51, 383–4.
6. Christensen RC. Adverse interaction of paroxetine and cyproheptadine. *J Clin Psychiatry* (1995) 56, 433–4.

SSRIs + Dextromethorphan

Three reports describe the development of a serotonin-like syndrome in two patients on paroxetine and one on fluoxetine after taking dextromethorphan.

Clinical evidence

(a) Fluoxetine

A woman who had been on fluoxetine 20 mg daily for 17 days took two teaspoonfuls of a cough syrup containing dextromethorphan, and two more the next morning with the next dose of fluoxetine. Within 2 hours vivid hallucinations developed (bright colours, distortions of shapes and sizes), which lasted 6 to 8 hours. The patient said they were similar to her past experience with LSD 12 years earlier.[1] The reasons for this reaction are uncertain. This seems to be the first and only report of this interaction. No mention was made of adverse effects in the report of an extensive metabolic study[2] in which depressed patients on fluoxetine were given a single 30-mg dose of dextromethorphan, nevertheless concurrent use should be well monitored. In this latter study the dextromethorphan was being used as an indicator or marker of changes in enzyme activity, and it was confirmed that fluoxetine inhibits the activity of cytochrome P450 isoenzyme CYP2D6, an enzyme involved in the *O*-demethylation of dextromethorphan.[2]

(b) Paroxetine

A man with multiple medical problems was admitted to hospital as an emergency, mainly because of vomiting blood. He was taking diazepam, diltiazem, glyceryl trinitrate, paroxetine, piroxicam, ranitidine and ticlopidine. Four days previously he had begun to take ***Nyquil***, a non-prescription remedy for colds, containing dextromethorphan, pseudoephedrine, paracetamol (acetaminophen) and doxylamine. After two days he developed shortness of breath, nausea, headache and confusion, and on admission he was also diaphoretic, tremulous, tachycardic and hypertensive. Later he became rigid. The eventual diagnosis was that he was suffering from the serotonin syndrome, attributed to an interaction between paroxetine and dextromethorphan in the presence of vascular disease. He was treated successfully with lorazepam 16 mg intravenously over 1 hour. The bleeding was thought to be from a small prepyloric ulcer.[3]

The authors of this report very briefly describe another patient on paroxetine who developed symptoms consistent with the serotonin syndrome within a few hours of taking a non-prescription cough remedy containing dextromethorphan and guaifenesin. She needed intensive care treatment.[4]

Mechanism

Not understood. The symptoms that developed were attributed by the authors of the report to the serotonin syndrome, caused by the additive effects of the SSRIs and dextromethorphan on serotonin transmission. It has also been suggested that paroxetine inhibited the cytochrome P450 isoenzyme CYP2D6, by which dextromethorphan is metabolised, resulting in increased dextromethorphan levels.[4,5] Fluoxetine also inhibits CYP2D6.

Importance and management

These seem to be, so far, the only reports of the serious serotonin syndrome being attributed to an interaction between an SSRI and dextromethorphan. The general importance of this apparent interaction is therefore very uncertain. The SSRIs are now very widely prescribed and dextromethorphan is a not uncommon ingredient of non-prescription medicines. More study is therefore needed to establish this apparent interaction, but in the meantime it would seem prudent for patients on paroxetine to be cautious using dextromethorphan-containing products because the serotonin syndrome, if it occurs, can be serious. It is not clear whether other SSRIs would interact with dextromethorphan similarly, but it has been predicted that **sertraline** and **fluvoxamine** are less likely to do so.[5] This prediction has been challenged.[4] The outcome will largely depend on the mechanism of this interaction as **sertraline** and **fluvoxamine** do not usually have clinically significant effects on CYP2D6.

1. Achamallah NS. Visual hallucinations after combining fluoxetine and dextromethorphan. *Am J Psychiatry* (1992) 149, 1406.
2. Otton SV, Wu D, Joffe RT, Cheung SW, Sellers EM. Inhibition by fluoxetine of cytochrome P450 2D6 activity. *Clin Pharmacol Ther* (1993) 53, 401–9.
3. Skop BP, Finkelstein JA, Mareth TR, Magoon MR, Brown TM. The serotonin syndrome associated with paroxetine, an over-the-counter cold remedy, and vascular disease. *Am J Emerg Med* (1994) 12, 642–4.
4. Skop BP, Brown TM, Mareth TR. The serotonin syndrome associated with paroxetine. *Am J Emerg Med* (1995) 13, 606–7.
5. Harvey AT, Burke M. Comment on: The serotonin syndrome associated with paroxetine, an over-the-counter-cold remedy, and vascular disease. *Am J Emerg Med* (1995) 13, 605–6.

SSRIs + H_2-blockers

Citalopram, escitalopram, femoxetine, paroxetine and sertraline levels are moderately increased by cimetidine but the only effect appears to be a slight increase in adverse effects with sertraline.

Clinical evidence

(a) Citalopram

Twelve healthy subjects were given citalopram 40 mg daily for 21 days and then for the next 8 days they were additionally given **cimetidine** 400 mg twice daily. The **cimetidine** caused a 29% decrease in the oral clearance of the citalopram, a 39% rise in its maximum serum levels and a 43% increase in its AUC. Some changes in the renal clearance of the citalopram metabolites were also seen.[1]

(b) Escitalopram

Cimetidine 400 mg daily for 8 days raised the AUC and maximum serum levels of escitalopram by 43 and 39% respectively.[2]

(c) Femoxetine

Cimetidine 1 g daily for 7 days raised the steady-state plasma trough levels of femoxetine 600 mg daily in 6 healthy subjects by 140% (from 10 to 24 nanograms/ml). The AUC was increased but not significantly, and no increase in adverse effects was seen.[3]

(d) Paroxetine

Cimetidine 200 mg four times daily for 8 days did not affect the mean pharmacokinetic values or bioavailability of single 30-mg doses of paroxetine in 10 healthy subjects. However, 2 subjects showed AUC increases of 55% and 81% while on **cimetidine** and 4 others also showed some increases.[4] Another study in 11 healthy subjects found that **cimetidine** 300 mg three times a day increased the AUC of paroxetine 30 mg daily by 50% after 1 week of concurrent use.[5]

(e) Sertraline

In a randomised, two-way crossover study, 12 healthy subjects were given single 100-mg oral doses of sertraline after taking either **cimetidine** 800 mg or a placebo at bedtime for seven days. The **cimetidine** increased the sertraline AUC by 50%, it increased the maximum serum sertraline levels by 24%, and increased the half-life by 26%. There was a small increase in sertraline adverse effects (not specified) while taking the **cimetidine**.[6] The makers note that cimetidine can cause a substantial decrease in sertraline clearance.[7]

Mechanism

The apparent reason for all these changes is that cimetidine inhibits the activity of cytochrome P450 so that the metabolism of the SSRIs is reduced, and as a result their serum concentrations rise.

Importance and management

The authors of the citalopram study say that while cimetidine certainly causes an increase in the serum levels of citalopram, the extent is only moderate and because the drug is well tolerated and there are very considerable pharmacokinetic variations between individual subjects, they consider that there is no need to reduce the citalopram dosage.[1] This advice is most likely applicable to escitalopram, the *S*-isomer of citalopram.

The authors of the femoxetine study recommend that the initial femoxetine dosage should be reduced from 600 to 400 mg daily.[3]

Information on the concurrent use of cimetidine and paroxetine or sertraline seems to be limited and the makers of sertraline[7,8] note that the clinical significance of the changes in clearance are not known. However, it would be prudent to monitor the outcome for excessive adverse effects (dry mouth, nausea, diarrhoea, dyspepsia, tremor, ejaculatory delay, sweating) if cimetidine is used with either of these SSRIs. Reduce the sertraline or paroxetine dosage if necessary.

If the suggested mechanism of interaction is true, one of the other H_2-blockers that lack enzyme inhibitory activity, such as **ranitidine** or **famotidine**, might be a non-interacting alternative for cimetidine. This needs confirmation.

1. Priskorn M, Larsen F, Segonzac A, Moulin M. Pharmacokinetic interaction study of citalopram and cimetidine in healthy subjects. *Eur J Clin Pharmacol* (1997) 52, 241–2.
2. Lexapro (Escitalopram). Forest Pharmaceuticals Inc. US Prescribing information, August 2004.
3. Schmidt J, Sørensen AS, Gjerris A, Rafaelsen OJ, Mengel H. Femoxetine and cimetidine: interaction in healthy volunteers. *Eur J Clin Pharmacol* (1986) 31, 299–302.
4. Greb WH, Buscher G, Dierdorf H-D, Köster FE, Wolf D, Mellows G. The effect of liver enzyme inhibition by cimetidine and enzyme induction by phenobarbitone on the pharmacokinetics of paroxetine. *Acta Psychiatr Scand* (1989) 80 (Suppl 350), 95–8.
5. Bannister SJ, Houser VP, Hulse JD, Kisicki JC, Rasmussen JGC. Evaluation of the potential for interactions of paroxetine with diazepam, cimetidine, warfarin, and digoxin. *Acta Psychiatr Scand* (1989) 80 (Suppl 350), 102–6.
6. Invicta Pharmaceuticals. Phase 1 study to assess the potential of cimetidine to alter the disposition of sertraline in normal, healthy male volunteers. Data on file (Study 050-019), 1991.
7. Lustral (Sertraline). Pfizer Ltd. UK Summary of product characteristics, December 2003.
8. Zoloft (Sertraline). Pfizer Inc. US Prescribing information, February 2005.

SSRIs + Lysergide (LSD)

Three patients with a history of lysergide (lysergic acid diethylamide, LSD) abuse experienced the new onset or worsening of the LSD flashback syndrome when given fluoxetine, paroxetine or sertraline. Grand mal convulsions occurred in one patient on LSD when given fluoxetine. In contrast, one study found that SSRIs reduced or eliminated the subjective responses to LSD.

Clinical evidence

A girl of 18 with depression, panic and anxiety disorders, and with a long history of illicit drug abuse experienced a 15-hour LSD flashback within 2 days of starting to take **sertraline** 50 mg daily. Another flashback lasting a day occurred when the **sertraline** was replaced by **paroxetine**. No further flashbacks occurred when the SSRIs were stopped. A youth of 17 with depression, also with a long history of illicit drug abuse (including LSD), began to experience LSD flashbacks 2 weeks after starting to take **paroxetine**. His father, a chronic drug abuser, had been treated with both **fluoxetine** and **paroxetine** for depression and had also reported new onset of a flashback syndrome.[1] An isolated report describes grand mal convulsions in a patient while taking **fluoxetine**, tentatively attributed to the concurrent abuse of LSD.[2] In contrast, a retrospective study found that 28 of 32 subjects (88%) who self-administered LSD and who had taken an SSRI (**fluoxetine**, **paroxetine** or **sertraline**) or trazodone for more than 3 weeks had a subjective decrease or virtual elimination of their responses to LSD. However, another subject who had taken **fluoxetine** for only one week had an increased response to LSD.[3]

Mechanism

Not understood. Lysergide increases serotonin in the brain, and one suggestion is that when the serotonin re-uptake is blocked in the brain, there is an increased stimulation of 5-HT_1 and 5-HT_2 receptors.[1] Changes in brain catecholamine systems may also be involved.[3]

Importance and management

Information is very limited and conflicting. The authors of the first report suggest that patients who are given SSRIs should be warned about the possibility of flashback or hallucinations if they have a known history of LSD abuse. It might be better to use other antidepressants that do not act through a 5-HT mechanism.

1. Markel H, Lee A, Holmes RD, Domino EF. Clinical and laboratory observations. LSD flashback syndrome exacerbated by selective serotonin reuptake inhibitor antidepressants in adolescents. *J Pediatr* (1994) 125, 817–9.
2. Picker W, Lerman A, Hajal F. Potential interaction of LSD and fluoxetine. *Am J Psychiatry* (1992) 149, 843–4.
3. Bonson KR, Buckholtz JW, Murphy DL. Chronic administration of serotonergic antidepressants attenuates the subjective effects of LSD in humans. *Neuropsychopharmacology* (1996) 14, 425–36.

SSRIs + Macrolides

An isolated case report describes apparent acute fluoxetine toxicity in a man brought about by the addition of clarithromycin. Another isolated report describes the development of what is thought to be the serotonin syndrome in a 12-year-old boy on sertraline and erythromycin.

Clinical evidence

(a) Fluoxetine

A 53-year-old-man on long-term fluoxetine 80 mg and nitrazepam 10 mg at bedtime for depression and insomnia, was additionally started on **clarithromycin** 250 mg twice daily for a respiratory infection. Within a day he started to become increasingly confused and after 3 days was admitted to hospital with a diagnosis of psychosis and delirium. When no organic cause for the delirium could be found, all his medications were stopped, and **erythromycin** was started. His mental state returned to normal after 36 hours. Once the antibacterial course had finished, the fluoxetine and nitrazepam were restarted and no further problems occurred.[1]

(b) Sertraline

A 12-year-old boy with severe obsessive-compulsive disorder and simple phobia, responded to sertraline 12.5 mg daily, titrated over 12 weeks to 37.5 mg daily. He began to feel mildly nervous within 4 days of additionally starting **erythromycin** 400 mg daily for an infection. Over the next 10 days his nervousness grew, culminating in panic, restlessness, irritability, agitation, paraesthesias, tremulousness, decreased concentration and confusion. The symptoms abated within 72 hours of stopping both drugs.[2]

Mechanism

The authors attribute what was seen to fluoxetine toxicity in the first case, and to the serotonin syndrome in the second case. They postulated that erythromycin (a known and potent inhibitor of cytochrome P450 isoenzyme CYP3A4) and the related macrolide clarithromycin, reduced the metabolism of the SSRIs, thereby raising their serum levels and precipitating the observed toxicity.[1,2]

Importance and management

These are isolated reports and their general importance is unknown. Nor is it unequivocally established that the second case was the serotonin syndrome and not an idiosyncratic reaction. Nevertheless, these cases suggest that it would now be prudent to monitor well if erythromycin (or possibly one of the related macrolides such as clarithromycin) is added to fluoxetine or sertraline.

1. Pollak PT, Sketris IS, MacKenzie SL, Hewlett TJ. Delirium probably induced by clarithromycin in a patient receiving fluoxetine. *Ann Pharmacother* (1995) 29, 486–8.
2. Lee DO, Lee CD. Serotonin syndrome in a child associated with erythromycin and sertraline. *Pharmacotherapy* (1999) 19, 894–6.

SSRIs + MAOIs

A number of case reports describe the serotonin syndrome in patients given a variety of SSRIs with MAOIs: some have been fatal. Concurrent use is contraindicated. Some studies suggest that moclobemide may not interact with the SSRIs, but there have been case reports of the serotonin syndrome and concurrent use is contraindicated.

Clinical evidence, mechanism, importance and management

(a) MAOIs (non-selective)

(i) Escitalopram. The makers of escitalopram contraindicate the concurrent use of MAOIs because of the risk of the serotonin syndrome.[1,2]

(ii) Fluoxetine. A very high incidence (25 to 50%) of adverse effects occurred in 12 patients taking fluoxetine 10 to 100 mg daily with either **phenelzine** 30 to 60 mg daily or **tranylcypromine** 10 to 140 mg daily, and in 6 other patients started on either of these MAOIs 10 days or more after stopping the fluoxetine. There were mental changes such as hypomania, racing thoughts, agitation, restlessness and confusion. The physical symptoms included myoclonus, hypertension, tremor, teeth chattering and diarrhoea.[3]

A detailed review of cases reported to the makers described 8 acute cases, 7 of them fatal, in patients given fluoxetine with either **tranylcypromine** or **phenelzine**.[4] Uncontrollable shivering, teeth chattering, double vision, nausea, confusion, and anxiety developed in a woman given **tranylcypromine** after stopping fluoxetine. The problem resolved within a day of stopping the **tranylcypromine**, and did not recur when fluoxetine was tried again 6 weeks later.[5]

A number of other reports describe similar reactions in patients given fluoxetine and **tranylcypromine**,[5-10] some occurring up to 6 weeks after the SSRI was stopped,[8] and several resulting in fatalities.[5,9]

(iii) Fluvoxamine. The Committee on Safety of Medicines in the UK has warned of possible adverse reactions if fluvoxamine is given with antidepressants such as the MAOIs.[11] This seems to be a reasonable extrapolation from the serious serotonin syndrome reaction seen with fluoxetine and the MAOIs.

(iv) Sertraline. A man on **tranylcypromine** and clonazepam was additionally given sertraline 25 to 50 mg daily. Within 4 days he began to experience chills, increasing confusion, sedation, exhaustion, unsteadiness and incoordination. Other symptoms included impotence, urinary hesitancy and constipation. These problems rapidly resolved when the sertraline was stopped and the **tranylcypromine** dosage reduced from 30 to 20 mg daily.[12]

A woman with a major depressive disorder taking lithium, thioridazine, doxepin and **phenelzine** was additionally started on sertraline 100 mg daily for worsening depression. Within 3 hours she became semi-comatose, with a temperature of 41°C, a heart rate of 154 bpm and symptoms of rigidity and shivering. She was treated with diazepam, midazolam, ice-packs and dantrolene.[13] Two other similar cases, involving sertraline with **isocarboxazid**[14] and **phenelzine**[15] have been reported. The latter case was fatal.[15]

(b) Befloxatone

A double-blind study in 41 healthy subjects found that when they were given **fluoxetine** 40 mg daily for 7 days, then 20 mg for 9 days, immediately followed by befloxatone (2.5, 5, 10 or 20 mg daily) for 5 days, no unusual adverse reactions occurred and no changes in body temperature, haemodynamics or ECGs were seen.[16] However, note that although studies have not found an interaction between moclobemide and **fluoxetine** cases of the serotonin syndrome have been reported.

(c) Moclobemide

(i) Citalopram. Three patients developed the serotonin syndrome (tremor, convulsions, hyperthermia, unconsciousness) and died 3 to 16 hours after taking overdoses of moclobemide and citalopram.[17] It is not clear whether the same would happen if this drug combination were to be taken in normal therapeutic doses, but additional indirect evidence suggests it may not be safe.

(ii) Escitalopram. The makers of escitalopram contraindicate the concurrent use of MAOIs because of the risk of the serotonin syndrome.[1,2]

(iii) Fluoxetine. A placebo-controlled trial in 18 healthy subjects found that the concurrent use of fluoxetine 20 mg and moclobemide 100 to 600 mg daily for 9 days gave no evidence of an adverse interaction.[18] Other studies, in healthy subjects and patients similarly found no evidence of the serotonin syndrome.[19,20]

A post-marketing analysis found that at least 30 patients switched from fluoxetine to moclobemide within a week had experienced no ill-effects.[18,21]

However, three patients have developed the serotonin syndrome[22-24] and one developed agitation and confusion[25] following the use of moclobemide and fluoxetine. A study suggests that the combination may cause a high rate of adverse effects (insomnia, dizziness, nausea and headache).[22]

(iv) Fluvoxamine. When 13 of 22 healthy subjects on fluvoxamine 100 mg daily for 9 days were additionally given increasing doses (50 to 400 mg daily) of moclobemide for 4 days from day 7, no serious adverse reactions occurred. Any adverse events were mild to moderate (some increase in headaches, fatigue, dizziness, all of which may occur with both drugs alone) and there was no evidence of the serious serotonin syndrome.[18,26] An open study in 6 depressed patients given moclobemide 225 to 800 mg daily and fluvoxamine 50 to 200 mg daily found a marked improvement. Insomnia was the commonest adverse effect (treated with trazodone) but none of the patients showed any evidence of the serotonin syndrome.[27] Similar results were found in other studies.[20,28]

(v) Paroxetine. An open 6-week study in 19 patients with major depression on paroxetine (or fluoxetine) 20 mg daily to which was added up to 600 mg of moclobemide daily, indicated that it was possibly effective.[29] An extension of this study with 50 patients is reported elsewhere.[22] A range of adverse effects occurred in some patients, the clearest one being insomnia, and the serotonin syndrome was seen in one patient.[22,29] The serotonin syndrome was not seen in another study, where low initial doses and gradual up-titration of both paroxetine and moclobemide was used.[20]

(vi) Sertraline. In one study, 31 severely ill patients were given moclobemide 35 to 800 mg daily with sertraline 25 to 100 mg daily, initially using lower-than-usual starting doses of both drugs and then gradually titrating them slowly upwards. The other SSRIs used were fluoxetine, fluvoxamine and paroxetine. There was no evidence of the serotonin syndrome.[20] An open study in 5 depressed patients given moclobemide 150 to 600 mg daily and sertraline 25 to 200 mg daily found improvements ranging from minimal to complete remission. Insomnia was the commonest adverse effect (treated with trazodone) but none of the patients showed any evidence of the serotonin syndrome.[27]

(d) Selegiline

See 'Selegiline + Antidepressants', p.514 for the interactions between SSRIs and selegiline.

Mechanism

MAO-B is involved in the metabolism of serotonin, so combined use with SSRIs may lead to excessive serotonin levels, which result in the serotonin syndrome. However, as moclobemide (an MAO-A) inhibitor) also interacts, this seems unlikely to be the full story. For more information about the serotonin syndrome see 'Additive or synergistic interactions', (p.9).

Importance and management

Direct information about the interaction between MAOIs and SSRIs is limited, and given that the combination is contraindicated, further reports seem unlikely. However, it is clear that severe, sometimes fatal interactions occur, so these reports should certainly be taken seriously. The makers say that the concurrent use of citalopram, escitalopram, fluvoxamine, paroxetine or sertraline and MAOIs is contraindicated and that these SSRIs should not be given within 14 days of discontinuing an irreversible MAOI nor should any type of MAOI be added until paroxetine or sertraline has been stopped for 14 days,[30-33] or citalopram, escitalopram or fluvoxamine have been stopped for 7 days,[1,34,35] (14 days in the US).[2,36]

The makers of fluoxetine recommend that (a) at least five weeks should elapse between stopping the fluoxetine and starting the MAOI because the effects of fluoxetine are very persistent, and (b) two weeks between stopping an MAOI and starting fluoxetine. A longer interval is suggested if long-term or high-dose fluoxetine has been used.[37,38]

It used to be thought that moclobemide, a selective reversible inhibitor of MAO-A, could be given to patients on fluoxetine, but the need to manage concurrent use with considerable care was emphasised.[22,39] However, the three (possibly four) cases of serotonin syndrome cited[22-25] suggest that this combination is not necessarily safe, and it should be noted that the makers contraindicate the use of fluoxetine in combination with moclobemide. They state that fluoxetine may be started the day after moclobemide is stopped.[37] However, the makers of citalopram, fluvoxamine, paroxetine and sertraline suggest an interval of 1 day if starting the SSRI after moclobemide, but 14 days if starting moclobemide after the SSRI.[1,30,31,34,35]

1. Cipralex (Escitalopram). Lundbeck Ltd. UK Summary of product characteristics, March 2004.
2. Lexapro (Escitalopram). Forest Pharmaceuticals Inc. US Prescribing information, August 2004.
3. Feighner JP, Boyer WF, Tyler DL, Neborsky RJ. Adverse consequences of fluoxetine-MAOI combination therapy. *J Clin Psychiatry* (1990) 51, 222–5.
4. Beasley CM, Masica DN, Heiligenstein JH, Wheadon DE, Zerbe RL. Possible monoamine oxidase inhibitor — serotonin uptake inhibitor interaction: fluoxetine clinical data and preclinical findings. *J Clin Psychopharmacol* (1993) 13, 312–20.

5. Sternbach H. Danger of MAOI therapy after fluoxetine withdrawal. *Lancet* (1988) ii, 850–1.
6. Ooi, TK. The serotonin syndrome. *Anaesthesia* (1991) 46, 507–8.
7. Spiller HA, Morse S, Muir C. Fluoxetine ingestion: A one year retrospective study. *Vet Hum Toxicol* (1990) 32, 153–5.
8. Coplan JD, Gorman JM. Detectable levels of fluoxetine metabolites after discontinuation: an unexpected serotonin syndrome. *Am J Psychiatry* (1993) 150, 837.
9. Kline SS, Mauro LS, Scala-Barnett DM, Zick D. Serotonin syndrome versus neuroleptic malignant syndrome as a cause of death. *Clin Pharm* (1989) 8, 510–14.
10. Miller F, Friedman R, Tanenbaum J, Griffin A. Disseminated intravascular coagulation and acute myoglobinuric renal failure: a consequence of the serotonergic syndrome. *J Clin Psychopharmacol* (1991) 11, 277–9.
11. Committee on Safety of Medicines. Current Problems, May 1989, 26, 3. Correction. Ibid., December 1989, 27, 3.
12. Bhatara VS, Bandettini FC. Possible interaction between sertraline and tranylcypromine. *Clin Pharm* (1993) 12, 222–5.
13. Graber MA, Hoehns TB, Perry PJ. Sertraline-phenelzine drug interaction: a serotonin syndrome reaction. *Ann Pharmacother* (1994) 28, 732–5.
14. Brannan SK, Talley BJ, Bowden CL. Sertraline and isocarboxazid cause a serotonin syndrome. *J Clin Psychopharmacol* (1994) 14, 144–5.
15. Keltner N. Serotonin syndrome: a case of fatal SSRI/MAOI interaction. *Perspect Psychiatr Care* (1994) 30, 26–31.
16. Pinquier JL, Caplain H, Durrieu G, Zieleniuk I, Rosenzweig P. Safety and pharmacodynamic study of befloxatone after fluoxetine withdrawal. *Clin Pharmacol Ther* (1998) 63, 187.
17. Neuvonen PJ, Pohjola-Sintonen S, Tacke U, Vuori E. Five fatal cases of serotonin syndrome after moclobemide-citalopram or moclobemide-clomipramine overdoses. *Lancet* (1993) 342, 1419.
18. Dingemanse J. An update of recent moclobemide interaction data. *Int Clin Psychopharmacol* (1993) 7, 167–80.
19. Dingemanse J, Wallnöfer A, Gieschke R, Guentert T, Amrein R. Pharmacokinetic and pharmacodynamic interactions between fluoxetine and moclobemide in the investigation of development of the "serotonin syndrome". *Clin Pharmacol Ther* (1998) 63, 403–13.
20. Bakish D, Hooper CL, West DL, Miller C, Blanchard A, Bashir F. Moclobemide and specific serotonin re-uptake inhibitor combination treatment of resistant anxiety and depressive disorders. *Hum Psychopharmacol* (1995) 10, 105–9.
21. Dingemanse J, Guentert TW, Moritz E, Eckernas S-A. Pharmacodynamic and pharmacokinetic interactions between fluoxetine and moclobemide. *Clin Pharmacol Ther* (1993) 53, 178.
22. Hawley CJ, Quick SJ, Ratnam S, Pattinson HA, McPhee S. Safety and tolerability of combined treatment with moclobemide and SSRIs: a systematic study of 50 patients. *Int Clin Psychopharmacol* (1996) 11, 187–91.
23. Benazzi F. Serotonin syndrome with moclobemide-fluoxetine combination. *Pharmacopsychiatry* (1996) 29, 162.
24. Liebenberg R, Berk M, Winkler G. Serotonergic syndrome after concomitant use of moclobemide and fluoxetine. *Hum Psychopharmacol* (1996) 11, 146–7.
25. Chan BSH, Graudins A, Whyte IM, Dawson AH, Braitberg G, Duggin GG. Serotonin syndrome resulting from drug interactions. *Med J Aust* (1998) 169, 523–5.
26. Wallnöfer A, Guentert TW, Eckernäs SA, Dingemanse J. Moclobemide and fluvoxamine coadministration: a prospective study in healthy volunteers to investigate the potential development of the 'serotonin syndrome'. *Hum Psychopharmacol* (1995) 10, 25–31.
27. Joffe RT, Bakish D. Combined SSRI-moclobemide treatment of psychiatric illness. *J Clin Psychiatry* (1994) 55, 24–5.
28. Ebert D, Albert R, May A, Stosiek I, Kaschka W. Combined SSRI-RIMA treatment in refractory depression. Safety data and efficacy. *Psychopharmacology (Berl)* (1995) 119, 342–4.
29. Hawley CJ, Ratnam S, Pattinson HA, Quick SJ, Echlin D. Safety and tolerability of combined treatment with moclobemide and SSRIs: a preliminary study of 19 patients. *J Psychopharmacol* (1996) 10, 241–5.
30. Seroxat (Paroxetine). GlaxoSmithKline. UK Summary of product characteristics, April 2005.
31. Lustral (Sertraline). Pfizer Ltd. UK Summary of product characteristics, December 2003.
32. Zoloft (Sertraline). Pfizer Inc. US Product information, February 2005.
33. Paxil (Paroxetine). GlaxoSmithKline. US Prescribing information, January 2005.
34. Cipramil (Citalopram). Lundbeck Ltd. UK Summary of product characteristics, April 2003.
35. Faverin (Fluvoxamine). Solvay Healthcare Ltd. UK Summary of product characteristics, November 2004.
36. Celexa (Citalopram). Forest Pharmaceuticals Inc. US Prescribing information, February 2005.
37. Prozac (Fluoxetine). Eli Lilly and Company Ltd. UK Summary of product characteristics, September 2004.
38. Prozac (Fluoxetine). Eli Lilly and Company. US Prescribing information, January 2005.
39. Mitchell PB. Drug interactions of clinical significance with selective serotonin reuptake inhibitors. *Drug Safety* (1997) 17, 390–406.

SSRIs + Metoclopramide

There is a report of the serotonin syndrome in one patient on sertraline when metoclopramide was added. Extrapyramidal symptoms have occurred in patients given fluoxetine, fluvoxamine or sertraline with metoclopramide.

Clinical evidence, mechanism, importance and management

Two patients developed extrapyramidal symptoms while taking **fluoxetine** and metoclopramide.[1,2]

A 14-year-old boy receiving **fluvoxamine** 50 mg daily for anorexia nervosa was, after day 7, given metoclopramide 10 mg three times daily. On the third day of concurrent use he developed acute movement disorders including acute dystonia, jaw rigidity, horizontal nystagmus, uncontrolled tongue movements and dysarthria. A pharmacokinetic interaction was considered unlikely. Both drugs can cause extrapyramidal reactions; metoclopramide by blocking dopamine D_2 receptors in the basal ganglia, and **fluvoxamine** by inhibition of dopamine neurotransmission.[3]

In another report a woman with gastro-oesophageal reflux, controlled with metoclopramide 15 mg four times daily, developed symptoms consistent with a mandibular dystonia (periauricular pain, jaw tightness, the sensation of her teeth clenching and grinding) 2 days after starting **sertraline** 50 mg daily. A 50-mg dose of diphenhydramine resolved the problem within 30 minutes, but the same symptoms recurred the next day, 8 hours after taking **sertraline**. The symptoms were relieved by 2 mg of oral benzatropine.

A possible explanation for this extrapyramidal reaction is that the serotonin inhibition by the **sertraline** increased the dopamine antagonism of the metoclopramide, producing enough dopaminergic inhibition to cause the dystonia.[4]

Another patient taking **sertraline** 100 mg daily for depression over an 18-month period developed agitation, dysarthria, diaphoresis, and a movement disorder within 2 hours of a single 10-mg intravenous dose of metoclopramide. The symptoms, diagnosed as the serotonin syndrome with serious extrapyramidal movement disorder, resolved within 6 hours of treatment with diazepam.[5]

Information seems to be limited to these reports, but they highlight the fact that care should be taken if two drugs with the potential to cause the same adverse effects are used together. Some monitoring would be advisable if an SSRI/metoclopramide drug combination is used.

1. Coulter DM, Pillans PI. Fluoxetine and extrapyramidal side effects. *Am J Psychiatry* (1995) 152, 122–5.
2. Fallon BA, Liebowitz MR. Fluoxetine and extrapyramidal symptoms in CNS lupus. *J Clin Psychopharmacol* (1991) 11, 147–8.
3. Palop V, Jimenez MJ, Catalán C, Martínez-Mir I. Acute dystonia associated with fluvoxamine-metoclopramide. *Ann Pharmacother* (1999) 33, 382.
4. Christensen RC, Byerly MJ. Mandibular dystonia associated with the combination of sertraline and metoclopramide. *J Clin Psychiatry* (1996) 57, 596.
5. Fisher AA, Davis MW. Serotonin syndrome caused by selective serotonin reuptake-inhibitors–metoclopramide interaction. *Ann Pharmacother* (2002) 36, 67–71.

SSRIs + SSRIs

An isolated report describes an adverse reaction (hypertension, tachycardia, fever, auditory hallucinations and confusion) in a man when he started sertraline within a day of stopping fluoxetine. A small study found that the concurrent use of citalopram and fluvoxamine was beneficial.

Clinical evidence, mechanism, importance and management

(a) Citalopram + Fluvoxamine

A study in 7 depressed patients who had not responded to 3 weeks' treatment with citalopram 40 mg daily found that the addition of **fluvoxamine** 50 to 100 mg daily for another 3 weeks improved the control of the depression. Plasma *S*-and *R*-citalopram levels rose two- to threefold. None of the patients developed the serotonin syndrome, and no changes in vital signs or ECGs were seen.[1] More study of combined use is needed.

(b) Fluoxetine + Sertraline

One of 16 healthy subjects who began to take sertraline 50 mg daily on the day after stopping a 2-week trial of fluoxetine 20 mg daily, rapidly developed hypertension, tachycardia, fever, auditory hallucinations and confusion. Most of these symptoms disappeared 48 hours after stopping the sertraline, but the confusion took a week to subside.[2] The other 15 subjects showed no clinically significant adverse effects. This subject was later found to have a history of psychosis so that the picture is a little confused, but the rapid abatement of the symptoms when the sertraline was stopped suggests that they were due either to the sertraline alone, or to an interaction with the residual fluoxetine.

It is therefore not clear whether a washout period is needed between these two drugs, but a decision on this will depend on the severity of the depression in the particular patient being treated. The makers of sertraline imply caution when they say that the duration of a washout period when switching from one SSRI to another has not yet been established.[3,4]

1. Bondolfi G, Chautems C, Rochat B, Bertschy G, Baumann P. Non-response to citalopram in depressive patients: pharmacokinetic and clinical consequences of a fluvoxamine augmentation. *Psychopharmacology (Berl)* (1996) 128, 421–5.
2. Rosenblatt JE, Rosenblatt NC. How long a hiatus between discontinuing fluoxetine and beginning sertraline? *Curr Affect Illn* (1992) 11, 2.
3. Lustral (Sertraline). Pfizer Ltd. UK Summary of product characteristics, December 2003.
4. Zoloft (Sertraline). Pfizer Inc. US Prescribing information, February 2005.

SSRIs + St John's wort (*Hypericum perforatum*)

Four patients on sertraline developed symptoms diagnosed as the serotonin syndrome after also taking St John's wort. Another patient on St John's wort developed severe sedation after taking a single dose of paroxetine.

Clinical evidence

(a) Paroxetine

In one report, a woman stopped taking paroxetine 40 mg daily after 8 months, and 10 days later started to take 600 mg of St John's wort powder daily. No problems occurred until the next night when she took a single 20-mg dose of paroxetine because she thought it might help her sleep. The following day at noon she was found still to be in bed, rousable but incoherent, groggy and slow moving and almost unable to get out of bed. Two hours later she still complained of nausea, weakness and fatigue, but her vital signs and mental status were normal. Within 24 hours all symptoms had resolved.[1]

(b) Sertraline

Four elderly patients on sertraline developed symptoms characteristic of the serotonin syndrome within 2 to 4 days of starting additional treatment with St John's wort 300 mg, either two or three times daily. The symptoms included dizziness, nausea, vomiting, headache, anxiety, confusion, restlessness and irritability. Two of them were treated with oral cyproheptadine 4 mg either two or three times daily, and the symptoms of all of them resolved within a week. They later resumed treatment with sertraline without problems.[2]

Mechanism

Not understood. A very brief and undetailed report, which says that the serotonin syndrome has been seen with St John's wort alone,[3] raises the possibility that additive serotonergic effects are the explanation for what occurred in the patients described here.

Importance and management

Information appears to be limited to these reports but these interactions between paroxetine or sertraline and St John's wort would seem to be established. The incidence is not known but it is probably small, nevertheless because of the potential severity of the reaction it would seem prudent to avoid concurrent use. The advice of the Committee on Safety of Medicines in the UK is that St John's wort should be stopped if patients are taking any SSRI because of the risk of increased serotonergic effects and an increased incidence of adverse reactions.[4]

1. Gordon JB. SSRIs and St. John's wort: possible toxicity? *Am Fam Physician* (1998) 57, 950–3.
2. Lantz MS, Buchalter E, Giambanco V. St. John's wort and antidepressant drug interactions in the elderly. *J Geriatr Psychiatry Neurol* (1999) 12, 7–10.
3. Demott K. St. John's wort tied to serotonin syndrome. *Clin Psychiatry News* (1998) 26, 28.
4. Committee on Safety of Medicines (UK). Message from Professor A Breckenridge (Chairman of CSM) and Fact Sheet for Health Care Professionals, 29th February 2000.

SSRIs + Sympathomimetics

Isolated reports describe delirium in one patient and a seizure in another during concurrent treatment with methylphenidate and sertraline, as well as schizophrenia and symptoms of amfetamine toxicity in two others on amfetamine and fluoxetine. There is an isolated report of the serotonin syndrome associated with concurrent citalopram and dexamfetamine.

Clinical evidence, mechanism, importance and management

(a) Amfetamine

A man who had taken a small, unspecified, but previously tolerated dose of amfetamine developed signs of amfetamine overdosage (restlessness, agitation, hyperventilation, etc.) while taking **fluoxetine** 60 mg daily. Another man on **fluoxetine** 20 mg daily developed symptoms of schizophrenia after taking two unspecified doses of amfetamine.[1] The postulated reason for this effect is that **fluoxetine** inhibits the cytochrome P450 isoenzyme CYP2D6, which is involved in the metabolism of amfetamine, thereby increasing amfetamine levels.[2] The general importance of these apparent interactions is uncertain.

(b) Dexamfetamine

A patient who had the serotonin syndrome with concurrent 'venlafaxine', (p.1007) and dexamfetamine experienced a second episode when **citalopram** rather than venlafaxine was added to his dexamfetamine therapy for adult attention deficit hyperactivity disorder.[3]

(c) Methylphenidate

A 61-year-old man with major depression was prescribed **sertraline** 50 mg daily without response. Three months later the dose was increased to 100 mg daily and methylphenidate 2.5 mg daily was started. His symptoms improved and the dose of methylphenidate was increased to 2.5 mg twice daily and then 5 mg twice daily. After several days at the higher dose, the patient experienced visual hallucinations and confusion. The methylphenidate was discontinued and a day later the psychosis resolved. He was maintained on **sertraline** 100 mg daily and his mood and motivation remained good.[4]

An isolated report describes a tonic-clonic seizure in a 13-year-old boy after approximately two weeks' of treatment with **sertraline** 25 to 50 mg daily and methylphenidate 80 mg daily. He had been receiving methylphenidate without significant adverse effects for about 10 months before the seizure and following discontinuation of the **sertraline** experienced no further seizures.[5]

In contrast, beneficial augmentation of effects has been reported with methylphenidate and SSRIs (**fluoxetine**, **paroxetine**, **sertraline**) without significant adverse effects.[6,7]

(d) Phenylpropanolamine

A 16-year-old girl with an eating disorder, taking **fluoxetine** 20 mg once daily, developed vague medical complaints of dizziness, 'hyper' feelings, diarrhoea, palpitations and a reported weight loss of 14 lbs within two weeks. The author of the report suggested that these effects might have been the result of an interaction with phenylpropanolamine (1 to 2 capsules of ***Dexatrim*** once daily), which the patient was surreptitiously taking, associated with a restricted food and fluid intake.[8]

1. Barrett J, Meehan O, Fahy T. SSRI and sympathomimetic interaction. *Br J Psychiatry* (1996) 168, 253.
2. Glue P. SSRI and sympathomimetic interaction. *Br J Psychiatry* (1996) 168, 653.
3. Prior FH, Isbister GK, Dawson AH, Whyte IM. Serotonin toxicity with therapeutic doses of dexamphetamine and venlafaxine. *Med J Aust* (2002) 176, 240–1.
4. McGlohn SE, Bostwick JM. Sertraline with methylphenidate in an ICU patient. *Psychosomatics* (1995) 36, 584–5.
5. Feeney DJ, Klykylo WM. Medication-induced seizures. *J Am Acad Child Adolesc Psychiatry* (1997) 36, 1018–19.
6. Gammon GD, Brown TE. Fluoxetine and methylphenidate in combination for treatment of attention deficit disorder and comorbid depressive disorder. *J Child Adolesc Psychopharmacol* (1993) 3, 1–10.
7. Stoll AL, Pillay SS, Diamond L, Workum SB, Cole JO. Methylphenidate augmentation of serotonin selective reuptake inhibitors: a case series. *J Clin Psychiatry* (1996) 57, 72–6.
8. Walters AM. Sympathomimetic-fluoxetine interaction. *J Am Acad Child Adolesc Psychiatry* (1992) 31, 565–6.

SSRIs + Tryptophan

Central and peripheral toxicity developed in five patients on fluoxetine when given tryptophan. On theoretical grounds an adverse reaction seems possible between fluvoxamine (and probably other SSRIs) and tryptophan.

Clinical evidence

(a) Fluoxetine

Concurrent use of tryptophan with fluoxetine 20 mg daily is said to be tolerated.[1] A more recent placebo-controlled double-blind study involving 30 patients with depression found that concurrent tryptophan 2 g daily during the initial phase of treatment with fluoxetine 20 mg daily was beneficial and well-tolerated,[2] but problems have been seen when higher doses of both drugs have been given together. Five patients on fluoxetine 50 to 100 mg daily for at least three months developed a number of reactions including central toxicity (agitation, restlessness, aggressive behaviour, worsening of obsessive-compulsive disorders) and peripheral toxicity (abdominal cramps, nausea, diarrhoea) within a few days of starting tryptophan 1 to 4 g daily. These symptoms disappeared when the tryptophan was stopped. Some of the patients had taken tryptophan in the absence of fluoxetine without problems.[3]

(b) Fluvoxamine

A warning by the CSM in the UK about the risks of giving fluvoxamine with tryptophan appears to be an extrapolation from the serious reaction (the serotonin syndrome) which has been seen with fluoxetine[4] (see (a) above).

Mechanism and importance and management

The reason for this reaction is not understood, but the authors point out that the symptoms resemble the serotonin syndrome seen in *animals* when serotonin levels are increased, and warn against the concurrent use of tryptophan with fluoxetine or other serotonin re-uptake inhibitors.[3] This caution is echoed by most of the makers of the SSRIs.

Products containing tryptophan for the treatment of depression were withdrawn in the USA, UK, and many other countries because of a possible association with the development of an eosinophilia-myalgia syndrome. However, since the syndrome appeared to have been associated with tryptophan from one manufacturer, tryptophan preparations were reintroduced in the UK in 1994 for restricted use.[5]

1. Ciraulo DA, Shader RI. Fluoxetine drug-drug interactions II. *J Clin Psychopharmacol* (1990) 10, 213–17.
2. Levitan RD, Shen J-H, Jindal R, Driver HS, Kennedy SH, Shapiro CM. Preliminary randomized double-blind placebo-controlled trial of tryptophan combined with fluoxetine to treat major depressive disorder: antidepressant and hypnotic effects. *J Psychiatry Neurosci* (2000) 25, 337–46.
3. Steiner W, Fontaine R. Toxic reaction following the combined administration of fluoxetine and L-tryptophan: five case reports. *Biol Psychiatry* (1986) 21, 1067–71.
4. Committee on Safety of Medicines. Current Problems, May 1989, 26, 3. Correction. Ibid., December 1989, 27, 3.
5. Sweetman SC, editor. Martindale: The complete drug reference. 34th ed. London: Pharmaceutical Press; 2005. p. 321.

SSRIs; Citalopram + Miscellaneous

The UK makers of citalopram say that no pharmacodynamic interactions have been noted in clinical studies in which citalopram was given with analgesics, antihistamines, antihypertensives or other cardiovascular drugs, but none of the individual drugs are named.[1]

1. Cipramil (Citalopram). Lundbeck Ltd. UK Summary of product characteristics, April 2003.

SSRIs; Fluoxetine + Cannabis

An isolated report describes mania in a patient on fluoxetine after she smoked cannabis.

Clinical evidence, mechanism, importance and management

A 21-year-old woman with a 9-year history of bulimia and depression was treated with fluoxetine 20 mg daily. A month later, about two days after smoking two 'joints' of cannabis (**marijuana**), she experienced a persistent sense of well-being, increased energy, hypersexuality and pressured speech. These symptoms progressed into grandiose delusions, for which she was hospitalised. Her mania and excitement were controlled with lorazepam and perphenazine, and she largely recovered after about 8 days. The reasons for this reaction are not understood but the authors of the report point out that one of the active components of cannabis, **dronabinol** (**Δ^9-tetrahydrocannabinol**), is, like fluoxetine, a potent inhibitor of serotonin uptake. Thus a synergistic effect on central serotonergic neurones might have occurred.[1] This seems to be the first and only report of an apparent adverse interaction between cannabis and fluoxetine, but it emphasises the risks of concurrent use.

1. Stoll AL, Cole JO, Lukas SE. A case of mania as a result of fluoxetine-marijuana interaction. *J Clin Psychiatry* (1991) 52, 280–1.

SSRIs; Fluoxetine + Itraconazole

Anorexia developed in a patient on fluoxetine when itraconazole was started, and it disappeared when the itraconazole was stopped.

Clinical evidence, mechanism, importance and management

A man taking fluoxetine 20 mg daily, diazepam and several anti-asthmatic drugs (salbutamol (albuterol), salmeterol, budesonide, theophylline) was started on itraconazole 200 mg daily for allergic bronchopulmonary aspergillosis. Within 1 to 2 days he developed anorexia without nausea. He stopped the itraconazole after a week, and the anorexia resolved 1 to 2 days later. The author of the report suggested that itraconazole, a potent enzyme inhibitor, increased the levels of the fluoxetine metabolite, norfluoxetine, which resulted in the anorexia.[1] Anorexia is a recognised adverse effect of fluoxetine. However, drug levels were not taken, so this suggestion has not been confirmed.

This report and the conclusions reached are uncertain, but they draw attention to the possibility of a fluoxetine/itraconazole interaction. Monitor well if both drugs are used. More study is needed.

1. Black PN. Probable interaction between fluoxetine and itraconazole. *Ann Pharmacother* (1995) 29, 1048–9.

SSRIs; Fluoxetine + Miscellaneous

Fluoxetine normally appears not to interact with chlorothiazide. Spontaneous movements have been seen with patients on fluoxetine anaesthetised with propofol. There is *in vitro* evidence that the effects of flecainide and mexiletine may possibly be increased by fluoxetine, and also evidence that the effects of fluoxetine are increased by aminoglutethimide.

Clinical evidence, mechanism, importance and management

(a) Aminoglutethimide

A patient with severe obsessive-compulsive disorder, resistant to clomipramine combined with SSRIs, improved when given fluoxetine 40 mg daily and aminoglutethimide 250 mg four times daily. Over a four-and-a-half year period, whenever attempts were made to reduce the dosage of either drug, the patient started to relapse.[1] Thus at least one patient has taken both drugs together without problems, and the evidence suggests that the aminoglutethimide has a potentiating effect on the fluoxetine. However, more study is needed to confirm the efficacy and safety of this drug combination in other patients.

(b) Chlorothiazide

Fluoxetine is reported not to affect the pharmacokinetics of chlorothiazide.[2] No special precautions would seem necessary on concurrent use.

(c) Flecainide or Mexiletine

Studies in patients and *in vitro* investigations using human liver microsomes have shown that fluoxetine and its metabolite, norfluoxetine have a strong inhibitory effect on the activity of cytochrome P450 isoenzyme CYP2D6 in the liver.[3,4] The practical consequences of this are that the effects of other drugs whose liver metabolism depends on this particular isoenzyme are likely to be increased and prolonged.

Flecainide and mexiletine are predominantly or partly metabolised by CYP2D6 but there appear to be no clinical cases of interactions between these drugs and fluoxetine. However, fluoxetine does interact with propafenone, which is also metabolised by CYP2D6 so it would seem prudent to be alert for increased and prolonged effects if fluoxetine is added. See 'Propafenone + SSRIs', p.186.

(d) Propofol

Two women in their mid-twenties, who had been on fluoxetine 20 mg daily for 4 to 6 months, had pronounced involuntary upper limb movements lasting 20 to 30 seconds immediately after anaesthetic induction with 180 mg of propofol (2 to 2.5 mg/kg). The movements ceased spontaneously and the rest of the anaesthesia and surgery were uneventful. Neither had any history of epilepsy or movement disorders. It is not clear whether this was a propofol/fluoxetine interaction or just a rare (but previously reported) reaction to propofol.[5]

1. Chouinard G, Bélanger M-C, Beauclair L, Sultan S, Murphy BEP. Potentiation of fluoxetine by aminoglutethimide, an adrenal steroid suppressant, in obsessive-compulsive disorder resistant to SSRIs: a case report. *Prog Neuropsychopharmacol Biol Psychiatry* (1996) 20, 1067–79.
2. Lemberger L, Bergstrom RF, Wolen RL, Farid NA, Enas GG, Aronoff GR. Fluoxetine: clinical pharmacology and physiologic disposition. *J Clin Psychiatry* (1985) 46, 14–19.
3. Otton SV, Wu D, Joffe RT, Cheung SW, Sellers EM. Inhibition by fluoxetine of cytochrome P450 2D6 activity. *Clin Pharmacol Ther* (1993) 53, 401–9.
4. Brøsen K, Skjelbo E. Fluoxetine and norfluoxetine are potent inhibitors of P450IID6 — the source of the sparteine/debrisoquine oxidation polymorphism. *Br J Clin Pharmacol* (1991) 32, 136–7.
5. Armstrong TSH, Martin PD. Propofol, fluoxetine and spontaneous movement. *Anaesthesia* (1997) 52, 809–10.

SSRIs; Fluvoxamine + Miscellaneous

Preliminary evidence suggests that smokers may possibly need a moderate increase in the dose of fluvoxamine. Grapefruit juice appears to raise fluvoxamine levels, but the clinical significance of this is unclear.

Clinical evidence, mechanism, importance and management

(a) Grapefruit juice

A randomised, placebo-controlled, cross-over study in 10 healthy subjects found that 250 ml of grapefruit juice three times daily for 6 days increased the AUC of a single 75-mg dose of fluvoxamine by 60% and increased the maximum plasma levels by 33%, probably by inhibition of fluvoxamine metabolism. The clinical significance of this interaction is uncertain because a wide range of fluvoxamine plasma levels have been found at therapeutic doses. More study is needed.[1]

(b) Tobacco smoking

A comparative study in 12 smokers and 12 non-smokers given single 50-mg oral doses of fluvoxamine found that smoking reduced the fluvoxamine AUC and the maximum serum concentrations by about 30%.[2] What this means in practice is uncertain, but there may possibly be the need to raise the dosage of fluvoxamine to accommodate this interaction. More study is needed to assess the clinical importance of this interaction.

1. Hori H, Yoshimura R, Ueda N, Eto S, Shinkai K, Sakata S, Ohmori O, Terao T, Nakamura J. Grapefruit juice-fluvoxamine interaction. Is it risky or not? *J Clin Psychopharmacol* (2003) 23, 422–4.
2. Spigset O, Carleborg L, Hedenmalm K, Dahlqvist R. Effect of cigarette smoking on fluvoxamine pharmacokinetics in humans. *Clin Pharmacol Ther* (1995) 58, 399–403.

SSRIs; Paroxetine + Aprepitant

The US maker of aprepitant notes that the concurrent use of paroxetine 20 mg daily and aprepitant 85 or 170 mg daily reduced the AUC of both drugs by about 25%, and the maximum serum levels by about 20%.[1] These changes are unlikely to be clinically important.

1. Emend (Aprepitant). Merck & Co., Inc. US Prescribing information, March 2005.

SSRIs; Paroxetine + Miscellaneous

Paroxetine appears not to interact to a clinically important extent with aluminium hydroxide, amobarbital or food, but phenobarbital may reduce the AUC of paroxetine. The antidepressant effects of paroxetine may be reversed by interferon.

Clinical evidence, mechanism, importance and management

(a) Aluminium hydroxide

Aludrox (aluminium hydroxide) 15 ml twice daily increased the absorption of a single 30-mg dose of paroxetine in healthy subjects by about 12%, and increased the maximum plasma concentration by 14%.[1] This is unlikely to be clinically important. No particular precautions would seem to be necessary on concurrent use.

(b) Barbiturates

Phenobarbital 100 mg once daily given to 10 healthy subjects for 14 days caused reductions of 10 to 86% in the AUC of paroxetine in 6 subjects, but the mean values were unaltered. One subject showed a 56% *increase* in AUC.[2] The sedative effects and impairment of psychomotor performance caused by **amobarbital** 100 mg were not increased by paroxetine 30 mg.[3] An isolated report describes a spontaneous tonic-clonic seizure in a woman on paroxetine immediately after she was given **methohexital** but before electrical stimulation in the course of an ECT series. Previous ECTs under **methohexital** anaesthesia had been uneventful.[4] The general importance of this reaction is uncertain but some caution would seem appropriate. Two cases of hepatitis in young women were considered to be caused by the concurrent use of ***Atrium*** (a barbiturate complex) and paroxetine, which are both hepatotoxic.[5]

(c) Food or drink

A study in healthy subjects found that the absorption of paroxetine was not markedly changed by food. A 40% reduction in absorption was seen when paroxetine was taken with one litre of **milk**,[1] but few people are likely to drink such a large amount regularly, and so this interaction is unlikely to be clinically significant.

(d) Interferon

A 31-year-old woman, whose mood and other depressive symptoms improved during treatment with paroxetine 50 mg daily and trazodone 50 mg at night, was later found to have essential thrombocytopenia. After unsuccessful treatment with dipyridamole, she was given **interferon alfa**, stabilised at 3 million units 3 times weekly. After 3 months her depressive symptoms returned, and worsened over a period of 6 months, despite increased doses of trazodone and cognitive therapy. **Interferon alfa** was discontinued and replaced by hydroxycarbamide, and then anagrelide. After a good response to a course of ECT, her depressive symptoms were controlled by paroxetine 50 mg daily and trazodone 150 mg at night.[6]

Interferon is associated with a risk of depression, but in this case it appeared to reverse the antidepressant response to paroxetine. It was suggested that this may have been due to the capacity of interferon to impair serotonin synthesis, by inducing enzymes that degrade the serotonin precursor tryptophan.

1. Greb WH, Brett MA, Buscher G, Dierdorf H-D, von Schrader HW, Wolf D, Mellows G, Zussman BD. Absorption of paroxetine under various dietary conditions and following antacid intake. *Acta Psychiatr Scand* (1989) 80 (Suppl 350), 99–101.
2. Greb WH, Buscher G, Dierdorf H-D, Köster FE, Wolf D, Mellows G. The effect of liver enzyme inhibition by cimetidine and enzyme induction by phenobarbitone on the pharmacokinetics of paroxetine. *Acta Psychiatr Scand* (1989) 80 (Suppl 350), 95–8.
3. Cooper SM, Jackson D, Loudon JM, McClelland GR, Raptopoulos P. The psychomotor effects of paroxetine alone and in combination with haloperidol, amylobarbitone, oxazepam, or alcohol. *Acta Psychiatr Scand* (1989) 80 (Suppl 350), 53–55.
4. Folkerts H. Spontaneous seizure after concurrent use of methohexital anesthesia for electroconvulsive therapy and paroxetine: a case report. *J Nerv Ment Dis* (1995) 183, 115–16.
5. Cadranel J-F, Di Martino V, Cazier A, Pras V, Bachmeyer C, Olympio P, Gonzenbach A, Mofredj A, Coutarel P, Devergie B, Biour M. *Atrium* and paroxetine-related severe hepatitis. *J Clin Gastroenterol* (1999) 28, 52–5.
6. McAllister-Williams RH, Young AH, Menkes DB. Antidepressant response reversed by interferon. *Br J Psychiatry* (2000) 176, 93.

Trazodone + Fluoxetine

Trazodone and fluoxetine have been used concurrently with advantage, but some patients develop increased adverse effects.

Clinical evidence, mechanism, importance and management

A patient on trazodone showed a 31% increase in the antidepressant/dose ratio when given fluoxetine 40 mg daily. She became sedated and developed an unstable gait.[1] Another study in patients found that fluoxetine increases plasma trazodone levels.[2]

A man with traumatic brain injury showed new-onset dysarthria and speech blocking when fluoxetine was added to trazodone. His speech returned to normal when the fluoxetine was stopped.[3] Five out of 16 patients taking fluoxetine stopped taking trazodone 25 to 75 mg, which was given for insomnia, because of excessive sedation the next day.[4] Three out of 8 patients had improvement in sleep and depression when given both drugs but the other 5 were either unaffected or had intolerable adverse effects (headaches, dizziness, daytime sedation, fatigue).[5] However, another report described advantageous concurrent use in 6 patients without an increase in adverse effects.[6]

These cases and studies suggest that the concurrent use of trazodone and fluoxetine can be useful and uneventful but it would seem prudent to monitor the outcome for any evidence of increased adverse effects (excessive sedation). There seems to be no information regarding other SSRIs.

1. Aranow RB, Hudson JI, Pope HG, Grady TA, Laage TA, Bell IR, Cole JO. Elevated antidepressant plasma levels after addition of fluoxetine. *Am J Psychiatry* (1989) 146, 911–13.
2. Maes M, Westenberg H, Vandoolaeghe E, Demedts P, Wauters A, Neels H, Meltzer HY. Effects of trazodone and fluoxetine in the treatment of major depression: therapeutic pharmacokinetic and pharmacodynamic interactions through formation of meta-chlorophenylpiperazine. *J Clin Psychopharmacol* (1997) 17, 358–64.
3. Patterson DE, Braverman SE, Belandres PV. Speech dysfunction due to trazodone-fluoxetine combination in traumatic brain injury. *Brain Inj* (1997) 11, 287–91.
4. Metz A, Shader RI. Adverse interactions encountered when using trazodone to treat insomnia associated with fluoxetine. *Int Clin Psychopharmacol* (1990) 5, 191–4.
5. Nierenberg AA, Cole JO, Glass L. Possible trazodone potentiation of fluoxetine: a case series. *J Clin Psychiatry* (1992) 53, 83–5.
6. Swerdlow NR, Andia AM. Trazodone-fluoxetine combination for treatment of obsessive-compulsive disorder. *Am J Psychiatry* (1989) 146, 1637.

Trazodone + Haloperidol

Low dose haloperidol is reported not to interact to a clinically relevant extent with trazodone.

Clinical evidence, mechanism, importance and management

Nine depressed patients who had been taking trazodone 150 to 300 mg at bedtime for 2 to 19 weeks were additionally given haloperidol 4 mg daily for a week. Plasma trazodone concentrations were not significantly changed but levels of its metabolite (*m*-chlorophenylpiperazine) were slightly raised (from 78 to 92 nanograms/ml). This study[1] was done to investigate the way trazodone is metabolised, but it also demonstrated that no clinically relevant pharmacokinetic interaction occurs between these two drugs at these dosages.

1. Mihara K, Otani K, Ishida M, Yasui N, Suzuki A, Ohkubo T, Osanai T, Kaneko S, Sugawara K. Increases in plasma concentration of m-chlorophenylpiperazine, but not trazodone, with low-dose haloperidol. *Ther Drug Monit* (1997) 19, 43–5.

Trazodone + Lysergide (LSD)

A retrospective study found that 28 of 32 subjects (88%) who self-administered LSD and who had taken an SSRI or trazodone for more than 3 weeks had a subjective decrease or virtual elimination of their responses to LSD.[1]

1. Bonson KR, Buckholtz JW, Murphy DL. Chronic administration of serotonergic antidepressants attenuates the subjective effects of LSD in humans. *Neuropsychopharmacology* (1996) 14, 425–36.

Trazodone + Sympathomimetics

A single report describes toxicity in a woman on trazodone when she took pseudoephedrine.

Clinical evidence, mechanism, importance and management

A study in healthy subjects given trazodone 50 mg three times a day found that the pressor response to **tyramine** remained unchanged, whereas the response to **noradrenaline** (**norepinephrine**) was reduced.[1] However, an isolated report describes a woman who had been taking trazodone 250 mg daily for two years who took two doses of an OTC medicine containing **pseudoephedrine**. Within 6 hours she experienced dread, anxiety, panic, confusion, depersonalisation and the sensation that parts of her body were separating. None of these symptoms had been experienced in the past when she was taking either preparation alone.[2] The reasons for this reaction are not understood.

It appears that reactions between sympathomimetics and trazodone are rare, but the case report indicates that the occasional patient may possibly experience unpleasant adverse effects.

1. Larochelle P, Hamet P, Enjalbert M. Responses to tyramine and norepinephrine after imipramine and trazodone. *Clin Pharmacol Ther* (1979) 26, 24–30.
2. Weddige RL. Possible trazodone-pseudoephedrine toxicity: a case report. *Neurobehav Toxicol Teratol* (1985) 7, 204.

Trazodone + Tryptophan

Concurrent use can effectively control aggression and agitation in patients with mental disorders, but a single case report describes the development of anorexia, psychosis and hypomania in one patient.

Clinical evidence, mechanism, importance and management

Trazodone with tryptophan has been used to treat aggressive behaviour in patients with dementia, mental retardation and other mental disorders.[1] There is also a report of the combination being used successfully to treat agitation in a patient with cognitive defects associated with a stroke,[2] although the rationale for the use of the combination in this patient has been criticised.[3] A single report describes the effective use of trazodone 100 mg and tryptophan 500 mg, both three times weekly with clonazepam in a mildly mentally retarded patient with schizophrenia and congenital defects. However, the patient stopped eating and lost 4.5 kg in three weeks and developed signs of psychosis or hypomania and soon afterwards she became drowsy and withdrawn. When the drugs were withdrawn the aggressive behaviour restarted, but she responded again to lower doses of trazodone and tryptophan although the signs of psychosis re-emerged.[4]

1. Wilcock GK, Stevens J, Perkins A. Trazodone/tryptophan for aggressive behaviour. *Lancet* (1987) i, 929–30.
2. Hottin P. Pharmacothérapie pour contrôler l'agitation chez les patients ayant des déficits cognitifs. *Can J Psychiatry* (1990) 35, 270–2.
3. Signer SF. Controlling agitation in patients with cognitive impairment. *Can J Psychiatry* (1991) 36, 312–13.
4. Patterson BD, Srisopark MM. Severe anorexia and possible psychosis or hypomania after trazodone-tryptophan treatment of aggression. *Lancet* (1989) i, 1017.

Tricyclic antidepressants + ACE inhibitors

Preliminary evidence from two patients suggests that enalapril may increase the effects of clomipramine, resulting in toxicity.

Clinical evidence

Two patients taking **enalapril** (one on 20 mg daily and the other taking 20 mg five times weekly) were given **clomipramine** for depression. The **clomipramine** dosage of one of them was increased from 25 to 50 mg, and 10 days later he became euphoric and exalted. The problem resolved when the **clomipramine** dosage was reduced to 25 mg again. The other patient had been stable on **enalapril** for over a year when **clomipramine** and disulfiram 400 mg daily were added. Within two weeks he developed confusion, irritability and insomnia. These adverse effects diminished when the **clomipramine** dosage was reduced to 50 mg daily.[1]

Mechanism

The ratio of clomipramine to its metabolite (desmethylclomipramine) is normally less than 1, but both of these patients demonstrated a ratio of more than 1. This suggests that the normal metabolism (demethylation) of the clomipramine was inhibited, thus allowing the clomipramine to accumulate and its toxic effects to manifest themselves. In the second patient the disulfiram may also have had a minor additional enzyme inhibitory effect.[1]

Importance and management

Information is limited to these two cases and the interaction is not firmly established. More study is needed. There seems to be nothing documented about adverse effects from the concurrent use of the other ACE inhibitors and tricyclic antidepressants, although postural hypotension is a possibility.

1. Toutoungi M. Potential effect of enalapril on clomipramine metabolism. *Hum Psychopharmacol* (1992) 7, 347–9.

Tricyclic antidepressants + Azoles; Fluconazole

Markedly increased serum amitriptyline levels developed in four patients and increased serum nortriptyline levels in another patient when they were concurrently treated with fluconazole. There is a report of prolonged QT interval and torsades de pointes associated with concurrent amitriptyline and fluconazole.

Clinical evidence

(a) Amitriptyline

A man with AIDS given fluconazole 200 mg daily and amitriptyline 25 mg then 50 mg three times a day developed mental changes and visual hallucinations within 3 days. His serum amitriptyline levels were found to be 724 nanograms/ml (therapeutic levels 150 to 250 nanograms/ml). The confusion resolved within 4 days of stopping the amitriptyline when the levels had fallen to 270 nanograms/ml. Another man with AIDS given amitriptyline 50 mg daily showed a smaller rise in amitriptyline levels (from 185 to 349 nanograms/ml) over a 33-day period when given fluconazole (loading dose of 200 mg, followed by 100 mg daily). Yet another patient with end-stage renal disease and on peritoneal dialysis and taking amitriptyline 100 mg daily showed grossly elevated serum amitriptyline levels (1464 nanograms/ml) and delirium 6 days after starting fluconazole (1 g orally initially, then 200 to 400 mg daily).[1]

A 12-year-old boy with prostatic rhabdomyosarcoma taking amitriptyline (initially 25 mg at bedtime, increased gradually to 75 mg twice daily) for neuropathic pain experienced episodes of syncope when fluconazole 200 mg daily was administered for periodic mucositis secondary to chemotherapy. Previous treatment with fluconazole without amitriptyline had not caused any problems. Syncope in this patient was considered to be due to elevated amitriptyline serum levels. No further episodes occurred when amitriptyline was discontinued.[2]

There is also a report of prolonged QT interval and torsades de pointes in a 57- year-old woman caused by the concurrent use of fluconazole and amitriptyline; other medications included sertraline, lisinopril and an iron supplement. Symptoms began 2 weeks after initiation of amitriptyline and were consistent with tricyclic toxicity, and resolved after discontinuation of the amitriptyline and reduction of the fluconazole dose to 200 mg daily. The presence of hypokalaemia and sertraline (which can increase serum tricyclic levels) may have additionally contributed to this patient's arrhythmia.[3]

(b) Nortriptyline

An elderly woman on nortriptyline 75 mg daily and other drugs (ciclosporin, morphine, metoclopramide, bumetanide as well as an unnamed antibacterial) was additionally started on fluconazole (loading dose of 200 mg, followed by 100 mg daily). After 13 days' concurrent use her trough serum nortriptyline levels had risen by 70% (from 149 to 252 nanograms/ml).[4]

Mechanism

Not understood, but it has been suggested that the fluconazole inhibits the cytochrome P450 isoenzymes CYP2C9, CYP2C19, CYP3A4 and possibly CYP2D6, which are concerned with the metabolism of these tricyclics, and as a result their serum levels rise.[1,2]

Importance and management

Information about the tricyclic/fluconazole interactions seems to be limited to these reports, which, bearing in mind the widespread use of these drugs, would suggest that these interactions are uncommon. Nevertheless it would now seem prudent to be on the alert for this interaction with any tricyclic antidepressant and fluconazole. More study is needed.

1. Newberry DL, Bass SN, Mbanefo CO. A fluconazole/amitriptyline drug interaction in three male adults. *Clin Infect Dis* (1997) 24, 270–1.
2. Robinson RF, Nahata MC, Olshefski RS. Syncope associated with concurrent amitriptyline and fluconazole therapy. *Ann Pharmacother* (2000) 34, 1406–9.
3. Dorsey ST, Biblo LA. Prolonged QT interval and torsades de pointes caused by the combination of fluconazole and amitriptyline. *Am J Emerg Med* (2000) 18, 227–9.
4. Gannon RH, Anderson ML. Fluconazole-nortriptyline drug interaction. *Ann Pharmacother* (1992) 26, 1456–7.

Tricyclic antidepressants + Azoles; Ketoconazole

Ketoconazole appears not to interact with desipramine, and only interacts to a small and clinically irrelevant extent with imipramine.

Clinical evidence, mechanism, importance and management

Two groups of 6 healthy subjects were given a single 100-mg dose of either **imipramine** or **desipramine** alone, and then again on day 10 of a 14 day course of ketoconazole 200 mg once daily. It was found that the ketoconazole caused the oral clearance of the **imipramine** to fall by 17%, its half-life to rise by 15% and the AUC of **desipramine**, derived from the **imipramine**, to fall by 9%. No significant changes in the pharmacokinetics of the **desipramine** were seen.[1]

These findings show that ketoconazole inhibits the demethylation of **imipramine** without affecting the 2-hydroxylation of **imipramine** and **desipramine**, and confirms that cytochrome P450 isoenzyme CYP3A4 has a role in the metabolism of these tricyclic antidepressants.[1] However, in practical terms it would seem that any changes are small and unlikely to be of any clinical significance. No special precautions would appear necessary if ketoconazole is used with either of these two drugs. Information about other tricyclics seems to be lacking.

1. Spina E, Avenoso A, Campo GM, Scordo MG, Caputi AP, Perucca E. Effect of ketoconazole on the pharmacokinetics of imipramine and desipramine in healthy subjects. *Br J Clin Pharmacol* (1997) 43, 315–8.

Tricyclic antidepressants + Baclofen

An isolated report describes a patient with multiple sclerosis on baclofen who was unable to stand within a few days of starting to take nortriptyline, and later imipramine.

Clinical evidence, mechanism, importance and management

A man with multiple sclerosis, who was taking baclofen 10 mg four times a day to relieve spasticity, complained of leg weakness and was unable to stand within 6 days of starting to take **nortriptyline** 50 mg at bedtime. His muscle tone returned 48 hours after stopping the **nortriptyline**. Two weeks later he was given **imipramine** 75 mg daily and once again his muscle tone was lost.[1] The reason is not understood. There seems to be nothing documented about any other tricyclic antidepressant and baclofen. Prescribers should be aware of this report if considering the use of both drugs, but its general importance is not known. It is probably small.

1. Silverglat MJ. Baclofen and tricyclic antidepressants: possible interaction. *JAMA* (1981) 246, 1659.

Tricyclic antidepressants + Barbiturates

The plasma levels of amitriptyline, imipramine and nortriptyline can be reduced by the concurrent use of barbiturates. A reduced therapeutic response would be expected. The tricyclics also lower the convulsive threshold and may be inappropriate for patients with convulsive disorders.

Clinical evidence

A comparative study in 5 pairs of twins given **nortriptyline** found that the twins concurrently treated with unnamed barbiturates developed considerably lower steady-state plasma **nortriptyline** levels.[1]

Similar observations have been made in patients and healthy subjects taking **nortriptyline** with **amobarbital**[2,3] or **pentobarbital**,[4] and **protriptyline** with **amobarbital sodium**.[5] Another showed a reduction in blood **imipramine** levels of about 50% (and loss of antidepressant control) within 2 weeks of starting to take about 400 mg of **butalbital** daily.[6]

Mechanism

The barbiturates are potent liver enzyme inducing agents (possibly of cytochrome P450 isoenzyme CYP1A2), and may therefore increase the metabolism and clearance of the tricyclic antidepressants from the body.

Importance and management

The tricyclic antidepressant/barbiturate interaction is established. By no means every drug pair has been studied but since the barbiturates as a whole are potent liver enzyme inducers one should be alert for this interaction with any of them. Some reduction in the effects of the tricyclic would be expected, but the general clinical importance is uncertain.

Tricyclics lower the convulsive threshold. Toxic overdosage with the tricyclics can cause convulsions and other effects, including respiratory depression. Although barbiturates have anticonvulsant effects concurrent use may increase respiratory depression.

1. Alexanderson B, Price Evans DA, Sjöqvist F. Steady-state plasma levels of nortriptyline in twins: influence of genetic factors and drug therapy. *BMJ* (1969) 4, 764–8.
2. Burrows GD, Davies B. Antidepressants and barbiturates. *BMJ* (1971) 4, 113.
3. Silverman G, Braithwaite R. Interaction of benzodiazepines and tricyclic antidepressants. *BMJ* (1972) 4, 111.
4. Steiner E, Koike Y, Lind M, von Bahr C. Increased nortriptyline metabolism after treatment with pentobarbital in man. *Acta Pharmacol Toxicol (Copenh)* (1986) 59 (Suppl 4), 91.
5. Moody JP, Whyte SF, MacDonald AJ and Naylor GJ. Pharmacokinetic aspects of protriptyline plasma levels. *Eur J Clin Pharmacol* (1977) 11, 51–6.
6. Garey KW, Amsden GW, Johns CA. Possible interaction between imipramine and butalbital. *Pharmacotherapy* (1997) 17, 1041–2.

Tricyclic antidepressants + Benzodiazepines or related drugs

Concurrent use is not uncommon and normally appears to be uneventful. A combined preparation of amitriptyline and chlordiazepoxide (*Limbitrol*) is available but its advantages have been questioned. However, three patients became drowsy, forgetful and appeared uncoordinated and drunk while taking amitriptyline and chlordiazepoxide, and four others showed toxic effects while taking *Limbitrol*. Diazepam may increase the risks of carrying out complex tasks (e.g. driving) if added to amitriptyline as may other combinations of benzodiazepines and tricyclics.

Clinical evidence

(a) Amitriptyline + Chlordiazepoxide

Clinical trials on large numbers of patients have shown that the incidence of adverse reactions while taking amitriptyline and chlordiazepoxide was no greater than might have been expected with either of the drugs used alone,[1,2] but a few adverse reports have been documented. A depressed patient on amitriptyline 150 mg and chlordiazepoxide 40 mg daily became confused, forgetful and uncoordinated. He acted as though he was drunk.[3] Two other patients taking amitriptyline and chlordiazepoxide experienced drowsiness, memory impairment, slurring of the speech and an inability to concentrate. Both were unable to work and one described himself as feeling drunk.[4] Four patients on ***Limbitrol*** are reported to have experienced some manifestations of toxicity (delusions, confusion, agitation, disorientation, dry mouth, blurred vision).[5] Some of these effects seem to arise from increased CNS depression (possibly additive) and/or an increase in the anticholinergic adverse effects of the tricyclic.

(b) Other tricyclics and benzodiazepines

Studies on the effects of **chlordiazepoxide**, **diazepam**, **nitrazepam** and **oxazepam** on the steady-state plasma levels of **nortriptyline** and **amitriptyline**;[6,7] of **diazepam** and **chlordiazepoxide** on **nortriptyline**;[8] and of **alprazolam** on **clomipramine**[9] or **nortriptyline**[10] all failed to find any interactions. **Alprazolam** seems to raise **imipramine** levels by about 20 to 30%,[11] but an *in vitro* study with human liver microsomes found that **alprazolam** does not affect the metabolism (hydroxylation) of **desipramine**.[10] Another study demonstrated an increase in **amitriptyline** levels when **diazepam** was given,[12] and two others found that the addition of **diazepam** to **amitriptyline** 50 to 75 mg further reduced attention and the performance of a number of psychomotor tests.[13,14] A single 75-mg dose of **imipramine** had no effect on the pharmacokinetics of **zaleplon** 20 mg, and psychomotor tests showed only short term additive effects lasting 1 to 2 hours.[15] A single-dose study using **zolpidem** 20 mg and **imipramine** 75 mg found no effect on the pharmacokinetics of either drug. However, **imipramine** increased the sedative effects of **zolpidem**, and anterograde amnesia was seen.[16] Visual hallucinations have been seen in one patient given **zolpidem** and **desipramine**.[17] An isolated report describes a patient taking **desipramine** 300 mg daily whose serum **desipramine** levels were halved when he was given **clonazepam** 3 mg daily and rose again when it was withdrawn.[18] In a study in 10 healthy subjects, when **zopiclone** and **trimipramine** were given concurrently for a week, the bioavailability of **zopiclone** was reduced by almost 14% and the bioavailability of the **trimipramine** by almost 27%, but neither of these changes were statistically significant.[19] **Triazolam** is effective in treating insomnia in depressed patients on **imipramine**, and does not reduce the effects of the antidepressant.[20,21] **Lorazepam** may be useful for anxiety or insomnia in elderly depressed patients without impairing the response to treatment with **nortriptyline**.[22]

Mechanism

Uncertain. Additive CNS depression and increased anticholinergic effects are a possibility with some combinations..

Importance and management

There seems to be no reason for avoiding the concurrent use of benzodiazepines and tricyclics although the advantages and disadvantages remain the subject of debate. Other tricyclic antidepressant/benzodiazepine combinations would not be expected to behave differently from those described here. Some patients will possibly experience increased drowsiness and inattention with the more sedative antidepressants such as amitriptyline, particularly during the first few days, and this may be exaggerated by benzodiazepines such as diazepam. Driving risks may therefore be increased.

1. Haider I. A comparative trial of Ro4–6270 and amitriptyline in depressive illness. *Br J Psychiatry* (1967) 113, 993–8.
2. General Practitioner Clinical Trials. Chlordiazepoxide with amitriptyline in neurotic depression. *Practitioner* (1969) 202, 437–40.
3. Kane FJ, Taylor TW. A toxic reaction to combined Elavil-Librium therapy. *Am J Psychiatry* (1963) 119, 1179–80.
4. Abdou FA. Elavil-Librium combination. *Am J Psychiatry* (1964) 120, 1204.
5. Beresford TP, Feinsilver DL, Hall RCW. Adverse reactions to a benzodiazepine-tricyclic antidepressant compound. *J Clin Psychopharmacol* (1981) 1, 392–4.
6. Silverman G, Braithwaite RA. Benzodiazepines and tricyclic antidepressant plasma levels. *BMJ* (1973) 3, 18–20.
7. Otani K, Nordin C, Bertilsson L. No interaction of diazepam on amitriptyline disposition in depressed patients. *Ther Drug Monit* (1987) 9, 120–2.
8. Gram LF, Overo KF and Kirk L. Influence of neuroleptics and benzodiazepines on metabolism of tricyclic antidepressants in man. *Am J Psychiatry* (1974) 131, 863.
9. Carson SW, Wright CE, Millikin SP, Lyon J, Chambers JH. Pharmacokinetic evaluation of the combined administration of alprazolam and clomipramine. *Clin Pharmacol Ther* (1992) 51, 154.
10. Bertilsson L, Åberg-Wistedt A, Lidén A, Otani K, Spina E. Alprazolam does not inhibit the metabolism of nortriptyline in depressed patients or inhibit the metabolism of desipramine in human liver microsomes. *Ther Drug Monit* (1988) 10, 231–3.
11. Grasela TH, Antal EJ, Ereshefsky L, Wells BG, Evans RL, Smith RB. An evaluation of population pharmacokinetics in therapeutic trials. Part II. Detection of a drug-drug interaction. *Clin Pharmacol Ther* (1987) 42, 433–41.
12. Dugal R, Caille G, Albert J-M, Cooper SF. Apparent pharmacokinetic interaction of diazepam and amitriptyline in psychiatric patients: a pilot study. *Curr Ther Res* (1975) 18, 679–87.
13. Patat A, Klein MJ, Hucher M, Granier J. Acute effects of amitriptyline on human performance and interactions with diazepam. *Eur J Clin Pharmacol* (1988) 35, 585–92.
14. Moskowitz H, Burns M. The effects on performance of two antidepressants, alone and in combination with diazepam. *Prog Neuropsychopharmacol Biol Psychiatry* (1988) 12, 783–92.
15. Darwish M. Overview of drug interaction studies with zaleplon. Poster presented at 13th Annual Meeting of Associated Professional Sleep Studies (APSS), Orlando, Florida, June 23rd, 1999.
16. Sauvanet JP, Langer SZ, Morselli PL, eds. Imidazopyridines in Sleep Disorders. New York: Raven Press; 1988 p. 165–73.
17. Elko CJ, Burgess JL, Robertson WO. Zolpidem-associated hallucinations and serotonin reuptake inhibition: a possible interaction. *Clin Toxicol* (1998) 36, 195–203.
18. Deicken RF. Clonazepam-induced reduction in serum desipramine concentration. *J Clin Psychopharmacol* (1988) 8, 71–3.
19. Caille G, Du Souich P, Spenard J, Lacasse Y, Vezina M. Pharmacokinetic and clinical parameters of zopiclone and trimipramine when administered simultaneously to volunteers. *Biopharm Drug Dispos* (1984) 5, 117–25.
20. Cohn JB. Triazolam treatment of insomnia in depressed patients taking tricyclics. *J Clin Psychiatry* (1983) 44, 401–6.
21. Dominguez RA, Jacobson AF, Goldstein BJ, Steinbook RM. Comparison of triazolam and placebo in the treatment of insomnia in depressed patients. *Curr Ther Res* (1984) 36, 856–65.
22. Buysse DJ, Reynolds CF, Houck PR, Perel JM, Frank E, Begley AE, Mazumdar S, Kupfer DJ. Does lorazepam impair the antidepressant response to nortriptyline and psychotherapy? *J Clin Psychiatry* (1997) 58, 426–432.

Tricyclic antidepressants + Butyrophenones

Serum desipramine levels can be considerably increased in a few patients by the concurrent use of haloperidol. This may have caused a grand mal seizure in one case but toxic reactions appear to be uncommon. Desipramine and bromperidol appear not to interact.

Clinical evidence

(a) Bromperidol

When 13 schizophrenics on bromperidol 12 to 24 mg daily for 1 to 20 weeks were additionally given **desipramine** 50 mg daily for a week, bromperidol plasma levels remained unchanged and no adverse clinical events were seen.[1]

(b) Haloperidol

(i) Desipramine. A comparative study in patients on similar doses of desipramine (2.5 to 2.55 mg/kg) showed that the two patients concurrently treated with haloperidol had steady-state plasma desipramine levels that were more than double those of 15 others not taking haloperidol (255 compared with 110 nanograms/ml).[2]
A case report describes a patient who had a grand mal seizure when concurrently treated with desipramine and haloperidol. Her serum desipramine levels were unusually high at 610 nanograms/ml.[3]

(ii) Imipramine. The urinary excretion of a test dose of ^{14}C-imipramine given to two schizophrenic patients was reduced by about 35 to 40% when they took haloperidol 12 to 20 mg daily.[4] The plasma metabolite levels of ^{14}C-nortriptyline of another schizophrenic fell while taking haloperidol 16 mg daily, whereas plasma levels of unchanged nortriptyline rose.[5]

Mechanism

Haloperidol reduces the metabolism of the tricyclic antidepressants, thereby reducing their loss from the body, which results in a rise in their plasma levels.

Importance and management

The tricyclic antidepressant/haloperidol interaction is established though its documentation is sparse. Concurrent use is common whereas adverse reactions are not, but be aware that serum desipramine levels may be elevated. This may have been the cause of the grand mal seizure in the case cited.[3] Imipramine appears to interact similarly. Monitor the outcome if haloperidol is added to established treatment with tricyclic antidepressants.

Desipramine appears not to interact adversely with bromperidol. See also 'Drugs that prolong the QT interval + Other drugs that prolong the QT interval', p.170, for information on a possible pharmacodynamic interaction.

1. Suzuki A, Otani K, Ishida M, Yasui N, Kondo T, Mihara K, Kaneko S, Inoue Y. No interaction between desipramine and bromperidol. *Prog Neuropsychopharmacol Biol Psychiatry* (1996) 20, 1265–71.
2. Nelson JC, Jatlow PI. Neuroleptic effect on desipramine steady-state plasma concentrations. *Am J Psychiatry* (1980) 137, 1232–4.
3. Mahr GC, Berchou R, Balon R. A grand mal seizure associated with desipramine and haloperidol. *Can J Psychiatry* (1987) 32, 463–4.
4. Gram LF, Overø KF. Drug interaction: inhibitory effect of neuroleptics on metabolism of tricyclic antidepressants in man. *BMJ* (1972) 1, 463–5.
5. Gram LF, Overø KF, Kirk L. Influence of neuroleptics and benzodiazepines on metabolism of tricyclic antidepressants in man. *Am J Psychiatry* (1974) 131, 863–6.

Tricyclic antidepressants + Calcium channel blockers

Diltiazem and verapamil can increase plasma imipramine levels, possibly accompanied by undesirable ECG changes. Two isolated reports describe increased nortriptyline and trimipramine levels in two patients given diltiazem.

Clinical evidence

(a) Imipramine

Twelve healthy subjects were given a 7-day course of **verapamil** 120 mg 8-hourly and 13 healthy subjects were given a 7-day course of **diltiazem** 90 mg 8-hourly. The AUCs of a single 100-mg dose of imipramine given on day 4 were increased by 15% by **verapamil**, and 30% by **diltiazem**. One hour after taking imipramine (2 hours after taking the calcium channel blockers), the average PR interval on the ECG was greater than 200 milliseconds, which represented first-degree heart block. Two subjects developed second-degree heart block after concurrent imipramine and **verapamil**.[1]

(b) Nortriptyline

A diabetic patient on glipizide and aspirin was started on nortriptyline, and, at the same time, his treatment with **nifedipine** was replaced by **diltiazem** 180 mg daily initially, raised to 240 mg daily after a week. Several changes in the nortriptyline dosage were made over a 4-week period because its plasma levels became unexpectedly high (the ratio of plasma nortriptyline to its dosage were approximately doubled).[2]

(c) Trimipramine

A depressed woman on **trimipramine** 125 mg daily developed high plasma levels of 546 micrograms/l while taking **diltiazem** 60 mg three times daily. Two weeks later they reached 708 micrograms/l, despite a reduction in the **trimipramine** dosage to 75 mg daily. She showed no toxicity and her ECG was normal.[3]

Mechanism

It has been suggested that diltiazem and verapamil increase the bioavailability of imipramine by decreasing its clearance. The ECG changes appear to result from the increased imipramine levels and the additive effects of both drugs on the atrioventricular conduction time. Diltiazem may similarly affect nortriptyline and trimipramine.

Importance and management

Information appears to be limited to these reports so that the general clinical importance of each of these interactions is uncertain. However it would now seem prudent to be alert for evidence of increases in the levels of tricyclic antidepressants if calcium channel blockers are added. The evidence of heart block with imipramine/diltiazem is of particular concern. More study is needed to evaluate these and other potential interactions between these two groups of drugs.

1. Hermann DJ, Krol TF, Dukes GE, Hussey EK, Danis M, Han Y-H, Powell JR, Hak LJ. Comparison of verapamil, diltiazem, and labetalol on the bioavailability and metabolism of imipramine. *J Clin Pharmacol* (1992) 32, 176–83.
2. Krähenbühl S, Smith-Gamble V, Hoppel CL. Pharmacokinetic interaction between diltiazem and nortriptyline. *Eur J Clin Pharmacol* (1996) 49, 417–19.
3. Cotter PA, Raven PW, Hudson M. Asymptomatic tricyclic toxicity associated with diltiazem. *Ir J Psychol Med* (1996) 13, 168–9.

Tricyclic antidepressants + Cannabis

Tachycardia has been described in patients taking tricyclic antidepressants when they smoked cannabis.

Clinical evidence, mechanism, importance and management

A 21-year-old woman student on **nortriptyline** 30 mg daily experienced marked tachycardia (an increase from 90 to 160 bpm) after smoking a cannabis cigarette. It was controlled with propranolol.[1] A man of 26 complained of restlessness, dizziness and tachycardia (120 bpm) after smoking cannabis while taking **imipramine** 50 mg daily.[2] Four adolescents aged 15 to 18 treated for attention-deficit hyperactivity disorder with tricyclic antidepressants showed transient cognitive changes, delirium and tachycardia after smoking cannabis.[3]

Increased heart rates are well-documented adverse effects of both the tricyclic antidepressants and cannabis, and what occurred was probably due to the additive beta-adrenergic and anticholinergic effects of the tricyclics, with the beta-adrenergic effect of the cannabis. Direct information is limited but it has been suggested that concurrent use should be avoided.[1] An increased heart rate would be expected with other anticholinergics and cannabis.

1. Hillard JR, Vieweg WVR. Marked sinus tachycardia resulting from the synergistic effects of marijuana and nortriptyline. *Am J Psychiatry* (1983) 140, 626–7.
2. Kizer KW. Possible interaction of TCA and marijuana. *Ann Emerg Med* (1980) 9, 444.
3. Wilens TE, Biederman J, Spencer TJ. Case study: adverse effects of smoking marijuana while receiving tricyclic antidepressants. *J Am Acad Child Adolesc Psychiatry* (1997) 36, 45–8.

Tricyclic antidepressants + Carbamazepine

The serum levels of amitriptyline, desipramine, doxepin, imipramine and nortriptyline, but possibly not clomipramine, can be reduced (halved or more) by the concurrent use of carbamazepine but there is evidence that this is not necessarily clinically important. An isolated report describes carbamazepine toxicity in a patient shortly after she started to take desipramine.

Clinical evidence

(a) Carbamazepine levels increased

A woman on long-term treatment with carbamazepine developed toxicity (nausea, vomiting, blurred vision with visual hallucinations, slurred speech, ataxia) within 6 days of starting to take **desipramine** daily (3 days at 150 mg daily). Her carbamazepine blood levels were found to have doubled from 7.7 to 15 micrograms/ml.[1]

(b) Tricyclic levels increased

In contrast to (a), a study confirming the value of carbamazepine and **clomipramine** in the treatment of post-herpetic neuralgia found that carbamazepine appeared to raise both **clomipramine** plasma levels and those of its major metabolite (desmethylclomipramine).[2]

(c) Tricyclic levels reduced

A study found that the addition of carbamazepine reduced the serum levels of **nortriptyline** to 42% and of **amitriptyline** plus **nortriptyline** to 40% in 8 psychiatric patients. In 17 other patients on **doxepin** the addition of carbamazepine reduced serum **doxepin** levels to 46% and of **doxepin** plus **nordoxepin** to 45%.[3] A retrospective study of very large numbers of patients confirmed that carbamazepine approximately halves the serum levels of **amitriptyline** and **nortriptyline**.[4] An elderly woman needed her **nortriptyline** dosage to be increased from 75 to 150 mg daily to achieve effective antidepressant serum levels when carbamazepine 500 to 600 mg daily was added.[5]

In a study in 36 children (aged 5 to 16) with attention-deficit disorder on **imipramine**, or **imipramine** and carbamazepine for 1 to 6 months, the imipramine dosage was significantly higher in the combined treatment group, even though the plasma levels were significantly lower. Twelve children matched on imipramine dosage per kg had total plasma antidepressant levels that were approximately half those found in other children not taking carbamazepine.[6,7] A study[8] in 6 healthy subjects found that carbamazepine 200 mg twice daily for a month increased the apparent oral clearance of a single 100-mg dose of **desipramine** (given on day 24) by 31% and shortened its half-life from 22.1 to 17.8 hours. A patient given **desipramine** and carbamazepine is reported to have had exceptionally low serum **desipramine** levels and cardiac complaints, which may have been due to the presence of increased levels of the hydroxy metabolite of **desipramine**.[9]

A study in 13 patients with endogenous depression (DSM-III-R) on **imipramine**, which confirmed that carbamazepine reduced the total serum levels of **imipramine** and desipramine, found that levels of the pharmacologically active free drugs remained unchanged.[10,11] Moreover 10 of the patients demonstrated a positive therapeutic response (greater than a 50% decrease in the Hamilton Depression Rating Scale) and a reduction in adverse drug reactions.[10]

Mechanism

It seems likely that the carbamazepine (a recognised enzyme-inducing agent) increases the metabolism and loss of these tricyclics from the body, thereby reducing their serum levels. The reason for the increased serum carbamazepine and clomipramine levels is not understood.

Importance and management

The reduction in the serum levels of amitriptyline, desipramine, doxepin, imipramine and nortriptyline caused by the interaction with carbamazepine appears to be established but the clinical importance is very much less certain. Evidence from one study,[10] that achieved a beneficial response in patients on tricyclics and carbamazepine suggests that it is possibly not necessary to increase the tricyclic dosage to accommodate this interaction. Certainly if carbamazepine is added to treatment with any of these tricyclics, check the therapeutic response first before you raise the tricyclic dosage. Remember too that the tricyclics can lower the convulsive threshold and should therefore be used with caution in patients with epilepsy.

1. Lesser I. Carbamazepine and desipramine: a toxic reaction. *J Clin Psychiatry* (1984) 45, 360.
2. Gerson GR, Jones RB, Luscombe DK. Studies on the concomitant use of carbamazepine and clomipramine for the relief of post-herpetic neuralgia. *Postgrad Med J* (1977) 53 (Suppl 4), 104–9.
3. Leinonen E, Lillsunde P, Laukkanen V, Ylitalo P. Effects of carbamazepine on serum antidepressant concentrations in psychiatric patients. *J Clin Psychopharmacol* (1991) 11, 313–18.
4. Jerling M, Bertilsson L, Sjöqvist F. The use of therapeutic drug monitoring data to document kinetic drug interactions: an example with amitriptyline and nortriptyline. *Ther Drug Monit* (1994) 16, 1–12.
5. Brøsen K, Kragh-Sørensen P. Concomitant intake of nortriptyline and carbamazepine. *Ther Drug Monit* (1993) 15, 258–60.
6. Brown CS, Wells BG, Self TH, Jabbour JT. Influence of carbamazepine on plasma imipramine concentration in children with attention-deficit hyperactivity disorder. *Pharmacotherapy* (1988) 8, 135.
7. Brown CS, Wells BG, Cold JA, Froemming JH, Self TH, Jabbour JT. Possible influence of carbamazepine on plasma imipramine concentrations in children with attention deficit hyperactivity disorder. *J Clin Psychopharmacol* (1990) 10, 359–62.
8. Spina E, Avenoso A, Campo GM, Caputi AP, Perucca E. The effect of carbamazepine on the 2-hydroxylation of desipramine. *Psychopharmacology (Berl)* (1995) 117, 413–16.
9. Baldessarini RJ, Teicher MH, Cassidy JW, Stein MH. Anticonvulsant cotreatment may increase toxic metabolites of antidepressants and other psychotropic drugs. *J Clin Psychopharmacol* (1988) 8, 381–2.
10. Szymura-Oleksiak J, Wyska E, Wasieczko A. Effects of carbamazepine coadministration on free and total serum concentrations of imipramine and its metabolites. *Eur J Clin Pharmacol* (1997) 52 (Suppl) A141.
11. Szymura-Oleksiak J, Wyska E, Wasieczko A. Pharmacokinetic interaction between imipramine and carbamazepine in patients with major depression. *Psychopharmacology (Berl)* (2001) 154, 38–42.

Tricyclic antidepressants + Colestyramine

Colestyramine causes a moderate fall in the plasma levels of imipramine. *In vitro* evidence suggests that amitriptyline, desipramine and nortriptyline probably interact like imipramine. One patient controlled on doxepin who had an unusual gut pathology became depressed again when colestyramine was added.

Clinical evidence

Six depressed patients were treated with **imipramine** 75 to 150 mg, usually twice daily. When colestyramine 4 g three times daily was added for 5 days, their plasma **imipramine** levels fell by an average of 23% (range 11 to 30%) and their plasma desipramine levels fell, although this was less consistent and said not to be statistically significant. The effect of these reduced levels on the control of the depression was not assessed.[1]

A man whose depression was controlled with **doxepin** relapsed within a week of starting to take colestyramine 6 g twice daily. Within 3 weeks of increasing the dosage separation of the two drugs from 4 to 6 hours his combined serum antidepressant levels (i.e. **doxepin** plus *n*-desmethyldoxepin) had risen from 39 to 81 nanograms/ml and his depression had improved. Reducing the colestyramine dosage to a single 6-g dose daily, separated from the **doxepin** by 15 hours, resulted in a further rise in his serum antidepressant levels to 117 nanograms/ml accompanied by relief of his depression.[2]

Mechanism

It seems almost certain that these tricyclics become bound to the colestyramine (an anion-exchange resin) within the gut, thereby reducing their absorption. An *in vitro* study[3] with simulated gastric fluid (1.2 mol/l HCl) found an approximately 79 to 90% binding with colestyramine at pH 1 with amitriptyline, desipramine, doxepin, imipramine and nortriptyline, a 36 to 48% binding at pH 4, and a 62 to 76% binding at pH 6.5. In an earlier study,[4] binding of these tricyclics at pH 1 had ranged from 76 to 100%.

Importance and management

The imipramine/colestyramine interaction is established but of uncertain clinical importance because the fall in the plasma imipramine levels quoted above was only moderate (23%) and the effects were not measured. The single case involving doxepin[2] was unusual because the patient had an abnormal gastrointestinal tract (hemigastrectomy with pyloroplasty and chronic diarrhoea). Nevertheless it would now be prudent to be alert for any evidence of a reduced antidepressant response if colestyramine is given concurrently. A simple way of minimising the admixture of the drugs in the gut is to separate their administration. It is usually suggested that these drugs should be given 1 hour before or 4 to 6 hours after colestyramine. There seems to be no direct clinical information about other tricyclics but the *in vitro* studies cited in Mechanism, which involved **amitriptyline**, **desipramine** and **nortriptyline**, suggest that they also probably interact like imipramine. This needs confirmation.

1. Spina E, Avenoso A, Campo GM, Caputi AP, Perucca E. Decreased plasma concentrations of imipramine and desipramine following cholestyramine intake in depressed patients. *Ther Drug Monit* (1994) 16, 432–4.
2. Geeze DS, Wise MG, Stigelman WH. Doxepin-cholestyramine interaction. *Psychosomatics* (1988) 29, 233–6.
3. Bailey DN. Effect of pH changes and ethanol on the binding of tricyclic antidepressants to cholestyramine in simulated gastric fluid. *Ther Drug Monit* (1992) 14, 343–6.
4. Bailey DN, Coffee JJ, Anderson B, Manoguerra AS. Interactions of tricyclic antidepressants with cholestyramine in vitro. *Ther Drug Monit* (1992) 14, 339–42.

Tricyclic and related antidepressants + Co-trimoxazole

Four patients on tricyclic antidepressants and one on viloxazine relapsed when given co-trimoxazole.

Clinical evidence, mechanism, importance and management

Four patients taking tricyclic antidepressants (**imipramine**, **clomipramine**, **dibenzepin**) and one taking **viloxazine** relapsed into depression when they were concurrently treated with co-trimoxazole (trimethoprim with sulfamethoxazole) for 2 to 9 days.[1] The reasons are not known. This seems to be the first and only report of a possible interaction between these drugs so that its general importance is very uncertain.

1. Brion S, Orssaud E, Chevalier JF, Plas J, Waroquaux O. Interaction entre le cotrimoxazole et les antidépresseurs. *Encephale* (1987) 13, 123–6.

Tricyclic antidepressants + Dexamfetamine or Methylphenidate

Methylphenidate can cause a very marked increase in the plasma levels of imipramine resulting in clinical improvement. No significant pharmacokinetic interaction has been reported between desipramine and methylphenidate. Methylphenidate may accelerate the response to tricyclic antidepressants but adverse effects were reported. Two adolescents experienced severe mood deterioration, and hypertensive episodes occurred in 3 other patients while taking methylphenidate and tricyclics. An isolated report describes a blood dyscrasia in a child given methylphenidate and imipramine.

Clinical evidence

A study in 'several patients' demonstrated a dramatic increase in the plasma levels of **desipramine** and **imipramine** during concurrent treatment with **imipramine** and methylphenidate. In one patient on **imipramine** 150 mg daily it was observed that methylphenidate 20 mg daily increased the plasma levels of **imipramine** from 100 to 700 micrograms/l and of **desipramine** from 200 to 850 micrograms/l over a period of 16 days.[1]

Similar effects have been described in other reports.[2-5] It seems that elevation of drug levels takes several days to occur, and several days to wear off.[3] A 9-year-old and a 15-year-old exhibited severe behavioural problems until the **imipramine** and methylphenidate they were taking were stopped.[6] In contrast, a retrospective review in 142 children and adolescents taking either **desipramine** alone, or **desipramine** with dexamfetamine or methylphenidate, indicated the absence of a clinically significant interaction between **desipramine** and either stimulant. Pharmacokinetic parameters were similar in each group.[7] In one patient on **desipramine** 250 mg daily, concurrent methylphenidate 40 mg daily resulted in a small decrease in serum **desipramine** levels, but a marked improvement in mood.[8]

A study of the combined use of tricyclic antidepressants (**desipramine**, **imipramine**, **nortriptyline**, **doxepin**) with methylphenidate 5 to 15 mg twice daily was undertaken in 20 of 41 patients with depression who responded to a test dose of methylphenidate. Combined use accelerated the antidepressant response to tricyclics with 6 of 20 patients responding after 1 week and 10 of 16 after 2 weeks. Adverse effects included insomnia, dizziness, hypotension and dry mouth. Methylphenidate was discontinued after less than 2 weeks concurrent use in 3 patients because of increased anxiety, irritability and hypomania.[9] There is also a report of more frequent adverse effects in 10 paediatric patients treated with concurrent methylphenidate and **desipramine** than with methylphenidate alone.[10] Three patients on tricyclic antidepressants and with labile blood pressure experienced hypertensive episodes when methylphenidate was also given. They responded to withdrawal of methylphenidate and two patients had further hypertensive episodes when rechallenged with methylphenidate.[11] An isolated report describes leucopenia, anaemia, eosinophilia and thrombocytosis in a child of 10 when given **imipramine** and methylphenidate.[12]

Mechanism

In vitro experiments with human liver slices indicate that methylphenidate inhibits the metabolism of imipramine, resulting in raised blood levels.[3] The accelerated response to tricyclic antidepressants may also be partly due to increased serum levels in the presence of methylphenidate, although the adverse effects observed were not entirely consistent with elevated levels of tricyclics.[9] There are also reports suggesting that methylphenidate does not significantly affect desipramine levels.[8,10] The blood dyscrasia may have been due to the rare additive effects of both drugs.[12]

Importance and management

Information is limited. Some therapeutic improvement including accelerated response is seen in some patients. This is may be partially because of the very marked rise in the blood levels of the antidepressant due to methylphenidate, but may also be due to an effect on mood attributable to methylphenidate alone. Concurrent use may cause adverse effects sufficiently severe to necessitate withdrawal of methylphenidate, but it is not certain whether they can be attributed to increases in serum levels of tricyclic antidepressants alone. There is evidence that the pharmacokinetics of desipramine are not significantly affected by either methylphenidate or dexamfetamine. Information about other tricyclic antidepressants is lacking. It has been suggested that concurrent use in children and adolescents may be undesirable, due to case reports of adverse behavioural effects.[6]

1. Sellers EM. Ed. Clinical Pharmacology of Psychoactive Drugs.Toronto: Alcoholism and Drug Addiction Research Foundation; 1975 p 183–202.
2. Cooper TB, Simpson GM. Concomitant imipramine and methylphenidate administration: a case report. *Am J Psychiatry* (1973) 130, 721.
3. Wharton RN, Perel JM, Dayton PG, Malitz S. A potential clinical use for methylphenidate with tricyclic antidepressants. *Am J Psychiatry* (1971) 127, 1619–25.
4. Zeidenberg P, Perel JM, Kanzler M, Wharton RN, Malitz S. Clinical and metabolic studies with imipramine in man. *Am J Psychiatry* (1971) 127, 1321–6.
5. Cooper TB, Simpson GM. Concomitant imipramine and methylphenidate administration: a case report. *Am J Psychiatry* (1973) 130, 721.
6. Grob CS, Coyle JT. Suspected adverse methylphenidate-imipramine interactions in children. *J Dev Behav Pediatr* (1986) 7, 265–7.
7. Cohen LG, Prince J, Biederman J, Wilens T, Faraone SV, Whitt S, Mick E, Spencer T, Meyer MC, Polisner D, Flood JG. Absence of effect of stimulants on the pharmacokinetics of desipramine in children. *Pharmacotherapy* (1999) 19, 746–52.
8. Drimmer EJ, Gitlin MJ, Gwirtsman HE. Desipramine and methylphenidate combination treatment for depression: case report. *Am J Psychiatry* (1983) 140, 241–2.
9. Gwirtsman HE, Szuba MP, Toren L, Feist M. The antidepressant response to tricyclics in major depressives is accelerated with adjunctive use of methylphenidate. *Psychopharmacol Bull* (1994) 30, 157–64.
10. Pataki CS, Carlson GA, Kelly KL, Rapport MD, Biancaniello TM. Side effects of methylphenidate and desipramine alone and in combination in children. *J Am Acad Child Adolesc Psychiatry* (1993) 32, 1065–72.
11. Flemenbaum A. Hypertensive episodes after adding methylphenidate (Ritalin) to tricyclic antidepressants. *Psychosomatics* (1972) 13, 265–8.
12. Burke MS, Josephson A, Lightsey A. Combined methylphenidate and imipramine complication. *J Am Acad Child Adolesc Psychiatry* (1995) 34, 403–4.

Tricyclic antidepressants + Dextropropoxyphene (Propoxyphene)

An elderly patient on doxepin experienced increased lethargy and daytime sedation when additionally given dextropropoxyphene.

There is some evidence that dextropropoxyphene may cause moderate rises in the serum concentrations of amitriptyline and nortriptyline, possibly accompanied by increased adverse effects.

Clinical evidence

An elderly man on **doxepin** 150 mg daily developed lethargy and daytime sedation when he started to take dextropropoxyphene 65 mg every 6 hours. His plasma **doxepin** levels rose by almost 150% (from 20 to 48.5 nanograms/ml) and desmethyldoxepin levels were similarly increased (from 8.8 to 20.7 nanograms/ml).[1]

The **amitriptyline** concentration/dose ratio in 12 patients given **amitriptyline** and dextropropoxyphene was raised from 2.57 to 3.04 nanomoles/mg per day when compared with other patients on **amitriptyline** alone. Similarly, the plasma concentration of the **amitriptyline** metabolite **nortriptyline** was raised from 210 to 275 nanomoles in 14 patients treated with **amitriptyline** and dextropropoxyphene.[2] In patients treated with **nortriptyline** and dextropropoxyphene, the **nortriptyline** plasma levels were raised by 16% when compared to those in individuals not taking dextropropoxyphene.[2]

Fifteen patients with rheumatoid arthritis given 25-mg doses of **amitriptyline** and dextropropoxyphene (up to 65 mg three times daily) experienced some drowsiness and mental slowness. They complained of being clumsier and had more pain, but these effects were said to be mild.[3]

Mechanism

The available evidence suggests that dextropropoxyphene inhibits liver metabolism of other drugs such as phenazone (antipyrine)[1] by inhibiting the activity of the cytochrome P450 isoenzyme CYP2D6, and as a result the serum levels of the tricyclic antidepressants rise.

Importance and management

The general clinical significance of these interactions is uncertain but be alert for any evidence of increased CNS depression and increased tricyclic antidepressant adverse effects if dextropropoxyphene is added. In this context it is worth noting that one report found that the incidence of hip fractures in the elderly was found to be increased by a factor of 1.6 in those taking dextropropoxyphene, and further increased to 2.6 when antidepressants, benzodiazepines or antipsychotics were added,[4] suggesting that combined use makes patients drowsier and clumsier and therefore more accident-prone. Information about other tricyclics appears to be lacking.

1. Abernethy DR, Greenblatt DJ, Steel K. Propoxyphene inhibition of doxepin and antipyrine metabolism. *Clin Pharmacol Ther* (1982) 31, 199.
2. Jerling M, Bertilsson L, Sjöqvist F. The use of therapeutic drug monitoring data to document kinetic drug interactions: an example with amitriptyline and nortriptyline. *Ther Drug Monit* (1994) 16, 1–12.
3. Saarialho-Kere U, Julkunen H, Mattila MJ, Seppälä T. Psychomotor performance of patients with rheumatoid arthritis: cross-over comparison of dextropropoxyphene, dextropropoxyphene plus amitriptyline, indomethacin and placebo. *Pharmacol Toxicol* (1988) 63, 286–92.
4. Shorr RI, Griffin MR, Daugherty JR, Ray WA. Opioid analgesics and the risk of hip fracture in the elderly: codeine and propoxyphene. *J Gerontol* (1992) 47, M111–M115.

Tricyclic antidepressants + Disulfiram

Disulfiram reduces the clearance of imipramine and desipramine from the body. The concurrent use of amitriptyline and disulfiram is reported to cause a therapeutically useful increase in the effects of disulfiram but organic brain syndrome has been seen in two patients.

Clinical evidence, mechanism, importance and management

It has been noted that **amitriptyline** increases the effects of both **disulfiram** and citrated calcium carbimide without any increase in adverse effects.[1] However, there is also some evidence that an adverse interaction can occur. A study in two men showed that while taking disulfiram 500 mg daily, the AUC of **imipramine** 12.5 mg given intravenously after an overnight fast increased by 32.5 and 26.7% respectively, and of **desipramine** 12.5 mg given intravenously in one subject by 32.3%.[2] Peak plasma levels were also increased. The suggested reason is that the disulfiram inhibits the metabolism of the antidepressants by the liver. There is also a report of a man taking disulfiram who, when given **amitriptyline**, complained of dizziness, visual and auditory hallucinations, and who became disorientated to person, place and time. A similar reaction was seen in another patient.[3] Concurrent use should therefore be well monitored for any evidence of toxicity. More study is needed to establish the importance and extent of this interaction.

1. MacCallum WAG. Drug interactions in alcoholism treatment. *Lancet* (1969) i, 313.
2. Ciraulo DA, Barnhill J, Boxenbaum H. Pharmacokinetic interaction of disulfiram and antidepressants. *Am J Psychiatry* (1985) 142, 1373–4.
3. Maany I, Hayashida M, Pfeffer SL, Kron RE. Possible toxic interaction between disulfiram and amitriptyline. *Arch Gen Psychiatry* (1982) 39, 743–4.

Tricyclic antidepressants + Duloxetine

Duloxetine markedly increased the AUC of desipramine, and the maker recommends caution with this and other tricyclics metabolised by the cytochrome P450 isoenzyme CYP2D6. They also say that combined use of duloxetine with other serotonergic drugs such as the tricyclics should be undertaken with caution because of the theoretical increased risk of serotonin syndrome.

Clinical evidence

Duloxetine 60 mg twice daily increased the AUC of a 50-mg single dose of **desipramine** by 2.9-fold in subjects who were extensive metabolisers of the cytochrome P450 isoenzyme CYP2D6.[1]

Mechanism

Desipramine is extensively metabolised by the cytochrome P450 isoenzyme CYP2D6, and can be used as a probe drug for assessment of the effect of drugs on this isoenzyme in extensive metabolisers (see 'Genetic factors', (p.4)).

Importance and management

The pharmacokinetic interaction with desipramine is established. Although the clinical relevance of the increased levels has not been assessed, the maker recommends caution if duloxetine is given to patients on desipramine and other tricyclic antidepressants that are metabolised by CYP2D6 including **nortriptyline**, **amitriptyline** and **imipramine**.[2]

Although no cases of 'the serotonin syndrome', (p.9) have been reported for duloxetine combined with other serotonergic drugs, the maker notes that combined use with tricyclics like **clomipramine** or **amitriptyline** should be undertaken with caution.[3,4]

1. Skinner MH, Kuan H-Y, Pan A, Sathirakul K, Knadler MP, Gonzales CR, Yeo KP, Reddy S, Lim M, Ayan-Oshodi M, Wise SD. Duloxetine is both an inhibitor and a substrate of cytochrome P4502D6 in healthy volunteers. *Clin Pharmacol Ther* (2003) 73, 170–7.
2. Cymbalta (Duloxetine hydrochloride). Eli Lilly and Company. US Prescribing information, January 2005.
3. Cymbalta (Duloxetine hydrochloride). Eli Lilly and Company Ltd. UK Summary of product characteristics, December 2004.
4. Yentreve (Duloxetine hydrochloride). Eli Lilly and Company Ltd. UK Summary of product characteristics, August 2004.

Tricyclic antidepressants + Food

Some preliminary evidence suggests that very high fibre diets can reduce the serum levels of doxepin and desipramine, and thereby oppose their action. The bioavailability of amitriptyline may be affected by food.

Clinical evidence, mechanism, importance and management

Three patients showed no response to **doxepin** or **desipramine** and had reduced serum tricyclic antidepressant levels while taking very high **fibre diets** (**wheat bran**, **wheat germ**, **oat bran**, **rolled oats**, **sunflower seeds**, **coconut shreds**, **raisins**, **bran muffins**). When the diet was changed or stopped, the serum tricyclic antidepressant levels rose and the depression was relieved.[1] The reasons are not known. This interaction may possibly provide an explanation for otherwise unaccountable relapses or inadequate responses to tricyclic antidepressant treatment. Another study found that **breakfast** had no effect on the bioavailability of **imipramine**, on its peak concentrations or the time to peak concentrations in 12 healthy subjects following a 50-mg oral dose.[2] A study in 9 healthy subjects given a single 25-mg dose of **amitriptyline** in the fasting state and with a standardised **breakfast** found that there were no consistent significant changes in the bioavailability of **amitriptyline** or its main metabolite **nortriptyl-**

ine. Similar results were found in a parallel study in which the same subjects were given a single 25-mg dose of **nortriptyline**. However, there were large interindividual changes in the AUC of **amitriptyline** after food, ranging from an increase of 94% to a decrease of about 40%. The largest food-related **amitriptyline** AUC *increases* occurred among the subjects with the lowest fasting AUC values and the only major food-related *decrease* occurred in the subject with the largest fasting AUC. It was concluded that for an individual patient, the timing of **amitriptyline** administration in relation to food intake should be standardised to avoid large variations in drug levels.[3]

1. Stewart DE. High-fiber diet and serum tricyclic antidepressant levels. *J Clin Psychopharmacol* (1992) 12, 438–40.
2. Abernethy DR, Divoll M, Greenblatt DJ, Shader RI. Imipramine pharmacokinetics and absolute bioavailability: effect of food. *Clin Res* (1983) 31, 626A.
3. Liedholm H, Lidén A. Food intake and the presystemic metabolism of single doses of amitriptyline and nortriptyline. *Fundam Clin Pharmacol* (1998) 12, 636–42.

Tricyclic antidepressants + H_2-blockers

The concurrent use of cimetidine can raise the plasma levels of amitriptyline, desipramine, doxepin, imipramine and nortriptyline. Toxicity may develop if the dosage of the tricyclic antidepressant is not reduced appropriately. Other tricyclic antidepressants are expected to interact similarly. Ranitidine does not interact.

Clinical evidence

(a) Amitriptyline

After a group of healthy subjects took **cimetidine** 1.2 g daily for two days, the peak plasma levels and the AUC of a single 25-mg dose of amitriptyline were raised by 37% and 80% respectively.[1]

Another study by the same authors found that **ranitidine** does not interact with amitriptyline.[2]

(b) Desipramine

After taking **cimetidine** 1 g daily for 4 days, the plasma desipramine levels of 8 patients taking 100 to 250 mg daily were raised by 51%, and its hydroxylated metabolite (2-hydroxydesipramine) was raised by 46%.[3] Another study showed that this interaction only occurs in those individuals who are 'rapid' hydroxylators.[4]

(c) Doxepin

A study in 10 healthy subjects given a single 100-mg oral dose of doxepin 12 hours after starting to take **cimetidine** 300 mg every 6 hours showed that the peak plasma level and AUC of doxepin were raised by 28% and 31% respectively.[5]

In another study **cimetidine** 1.2 g daily was found to double the steady-state plasma levels of doxepin 50 mg daily, whereas **ranitidine** 300 mg daily had no effect.[6] A patient being treated with doxepin complained that the normally mild adverse effects (urinary hesitancy, dry mouth and decreased visual acuity) became incapacitating when additionally treated with **cimetidine**. His serum doxepin levels were found to be elevated.[7]

(d) Imipramine

After taking **cimetidine** 1.2 g daily for 3 days, the peak plasma levels and the AUC of imipramine in 12 healthy subjects following a single 100-mg dose were raised by 65% and 172% respectively. After taking **ranitidine** 300 mg daily for 3 days the pharmacokinetics of imipramine were unaltered.[8] These findings with **cimetidine** confirm those of previous studies.[9,10]

There are case reports of patients taking imipramine who developed severe anticholinergic adverse effects (dry mouth, urine retention, blurred vision) associated with very marked rises in serum imipramine levels when concurrently treated with **cimetidine**.[11,12]

(e) Nortriptyline

After taking **cimetidine** 1.2 g daily for 2 days, the peak plasma nortriptyline levels of 6 healthy subjects were not significantly raised, but the AUC was increased by 20%.[9]

A case report describes a patient whose serum nortriptyline levels were raised about one-third while taking **cimetidine**.[13] Another patient complained of abdominal pain and distention (but no other anticholinergic adverse effects) when treated with nortriptyline and **cimetidine**.[14]

Mechanism

Cimetidine is a potent liver enzyme inhibitor, which reduces the metabolism of the tricyclic antidepressants, and may also reduce the hepatic clearance of these drugs. This results in a rise in their serum levels. Ranitidine does not interact because it is not an enzyme inhibitor.

Importance and management

The interactions with cimetidine are well established, well documented and of clinical importance. The incidence is uncertain but a study with desipramine[4] showed that only 'rapid' hydroxylators demonstrate this interaction so that not all patients will be affected. Those taking amitriptyline, desipramine, doxepin, imipramine or nortriptyline who are given cimetidine should be monitored for evidence of increased toxicity (an excessive increase in mouth dryness, urine retention, blurred vision, constipation, tachycardia, postural hypotension). Other tricyclic antidepressants would be expected to be similarly affected. Ideally the antidepressant plasma levels should be monitored. Reduce the dosage of the antidepressant by 33 to 50% where necessary or replace the cimetidine with ranitidine, which, because it is not an enzyme inhibitor, does not interact with amitriptyline, doxepin or imipramine and would not be expected to interact with other tricyclic antidepressants. Other H_2-blockers which do not cause enzyme inhibition include **famotidine** and **nizatidine** and would therefore not be expected to interact with the tricyclic antidepressants.

1. Curry SH, DeVane CL, Wolfe MM. Cimetidine interaction with amitriptyline. *Eur J Clin Pharmacol* (1985) 29, 429–33.
2. Curry SH, DeVane CL, Wolfe MM. Lack of interaction of ranitidine with amitriptyline. *Eur J Clin Pharmacol* (1987) 32, 317–20.
3. Amsterdam JD, Brunswick DJ, Potter L, Kaplan MJ. Cimetidine-induced alterations in desipramine plasma concentrations. *Psychopharmacology (Berl)* (1984) 83, 373–5.
4. Steiner E, Spina E. Differences in the inhibitory effect of cimetidine on desipramine metabolism between rapid and slow debrisoquin hydroxylators. *Clin Pharmacol Ther* (1987) 42, 278–82.
5. Abernethy DR, Todd EL. Doxepin-cimetidine interaction: increased doxepin bioavailability during cimetidine treatment. *J Clin Psychopharmacol* (1986) 6, 8–12.
6. Sutherland DL, Remillard AJ, Haight KR, Brown MA, Old L. The influence of cimetidine versus ranitidine on doxepin pharmacokinetics. *Eur J Clin Pharmacol* (1987) 32, 159–64.
7. Brown MA, Haight KR, McKay G. Cimetidine-doxepin interaction. *J Clin Psychopharmacol* (1985) 5, 245–7.
8. Wells BG, Pieper JA, Self TH, Stewart CF, Waldon SL, Bobo L, Warner C. The effect of ranitidine and cimetidine on imipramine disposition. *Eur J Clin Pharmacol* (1986) 31, 285–90.
9. Henauer SA, Hollister LE. Cimetidine interaction with imipramine and nortriptyline. *Clin Pharmacol Ther* (1984) 35, 183–7.
10. Abernethy DR, Greenblatt DJ, Shader RI. Imipramine-cimetidine interaction: impairment of clearance and enhanced absolute bioavailability. *J Pharmacol Exp Ther* (1984) 229, 702–705.
11. Shapiro PA. Cimetidine-imipramine interaction: case report and comments. *Am J Psychiatry* (1984) 141, 152.
12. Miller DD, Macklin M. Cimetidine-imipramine interaction: a case report. *Am J Psychiatry* (1983) 140, 351–2.
13. Miller DD, Macklin M. Cimetidine-imipramine interaction: case report and comments. Reply. *Am J Psychiatry* (1984) 141, 153.
14. Lerro FA. Abdominal distention syndrome in a patient receiving cimetidine-nortriptyline therapy. *J Med Soc New Jers* (1983) 80, 631–2.

Tricyclic antidepressants + Isoprenaline

Although amitriptyline alone and imipramine with isoprenaline (isoproterenol) have been used safely and with advantage in the treatment of asthma, an isolated fatality has been reported arising from concurrent over-use of amitriptyline and isoprenaline.

Clinical evidence, mechanism, importance and management

Amitriptyline alone[1,2] and **imipramine** with isoprenaline[3] have been shown to be beneficial in the treatment of asthma, and in a study of possible adverse interactions between **imipramine** and isoprenaline, no abnormalities of heart rhythm were seen, although one out of the 4 healthy subjects studied showed potentiation of isoprenaline-induced tachycardia.[4] However, a woman taking *Tedral* (theophylline, ephedrine and phenobarbital), twice daily, died as a result of aspiration of vomit in response to cardiac arrhythmias induced by the use of **amitriptyline** and isoprenaline.[5] It was estimated that she had taken more than 40 doses of isoprenaline 125 micrograms, daily for several days prior to her death. **Amitriptyline**, isoprenaline, ephedrine and the fluorocarbon inhaler propellant appear to have had additive cardiotoxic effects. This fatal interaction would seem to be due to the over-use of these drugs. However, the case serves to emphasise the risk attached to the over-use of isoprenaline inhalers if cardiotoxic drugs such as the tricyclic antidepressants are being used concurrently.

1. Ananth J. Antiasthmatic effect of amitriptyline. *Can Med Assoc J* (1974) 110, 1131–3.

2. Meares RA, Mills JE, Horvath TB, Atkinson JM, Pun L-Q, Rand MJ. Amitriptyline and asthma. *Med J Aust* (1971) 2, 25–8.
3. Mattila MJ, Muittari A. Modification by imipramine of the bronchodilator response to isoprenaline in asthmatic patients. *Ann Med Intern Fenn* (1968) 57, 185–7.
4. Boakes AJ, Laurence DR, Teoh PC, Barar FSK, Benedikter LT, Prichard BNC. Interactions between sympathomimetic amines and antidepressant agents in man. *BMJ* (1973) 1, 311–15.
5. Kadar D. Amitriptyline and isoproterenol: fatal drug combination. *Can Med Assoc J* (1975) 112, 556–7.

Tricyclic antidepressants + Macrolides

Troleandomycin increases the plasma levels of imipramine, and an isolated report suggests that josamycin may possibly increase amitriptyline serum levels. Erythromycin may interact with clomipramine, but was not found to interact with other tricyclic antidepressants.

Clinical evidence, mechanism, importance and management

(a) Erythromycin

Six days' treatment with erythromycin 250 mg four times daily was found not to affect the plasma levels of 8 patients taking tricyclic antidepressants (**desipramine**, **imipramine**, **doxepin**, **nortriptyline**).[1] Behavioural changes have been reported in a 15-year-old patient when erythromycin was added to a regimen of **clomipramine** and risperidone,[2] resulting in symptoms compatible with the serotonin syndrome, although mental confusion and autonomic instability were absent.[3] It seems likely that erythromycin increased **clomipramine** levels by inhibiting its metabolism by the cytochrome P450 isoenzyme CYP3A4.[4] **Clomipramine** levels may also have been raised by competition with risperidone for metabolism by CYP2D6. However, caution is recommended with concurrent use of erythromycin (and other macrolides) with psychotropic drugs that are metabolised by cytochrome P450 isoenzymes.[2,3]

(b) Josamycin

A patient taking **amitriptyline** showed a marked increase in total **amitriptyline/nortriptyline** serum levels after being treated with josamycin but no toxicity was reported. It was suggested that josamycin had inhibited amitriptyline metabolism.[5] This is only an isolated case but be alert for any evidence of increased tricyclic effects if josamycin is given.

(c) Troleandomycin

A study in 9 healthy Chinese men found that when they were given troleandomycin 250 mg daily for 2 days before a single 100-mg oral dose of **imipramine**, the AUC of the **imipramine** was increased by 59% and its oral clearance was reduced by 30%. It is thought that troleandomycin inhibits the *N*-demethylation of imipramine by inhibiting the cytochrome P450 isoenzyme subfamily CYP3A.[6] The clinical importance of this interaction is uncertain, but good monitoring is advisable.

1. Amsterdam JD, Maislin G. Effect of erythromycin on tricyclic antidepressant metabolism. *J Clin Psychopharmacol* (1991) 11, 203–6.
2. Fisman S, Reniers D, Diaz P. Erythromycin interaction with risperidone or clomipramine in an adolescent. *J Child Adolesc Psychopharmacol* (1996) 6, 133–8.
3. Fisman S, Diaz P. Erythromycin and clomipramine: Noncompetitive inhibition of demethylation. Reply. *J Child Adolesc Psychopharmacol* (1996) 6, 213.
4. Oesterheld JR. Erythromycin and clomipramine: Noncompetitive inhibition of demethylation. *J Child Adolesc Psychopharmacol* (1996) 6, 211–12.
5. Sánchez Romero A, Calzado Solaz C. Posible interacción entre josamicina y amitriptilina. *Med Clin (Barc)* (1992) 98, 279.
6. Wang J-S, Wang W, Xie H-G, Huang S-L, Zhou H-H. Effect of troleandomycin on the pharmacokinetics of imipramine in Chinese: the role of CYP3A. *Br J Clin Pharmacol* (1997) 44, 195–8.

Tricyclic antidepressants + Oestrogens or Oral contraceptives

There is evidence that oestrogens can sometimes reduce the effects of imipramine, yet at the same time paradoxically cause imipramine toxicity. The general clinical importance of this interaction has yet to be evaluated.

Clinical evidence

A study in women taking **imipramine** 150 mg daily for primary depression found that those given **ethinylestradiol** 25 or 50 micrograms for one week showed greater improvement than those given **imipramine** alone. However, after 2 weeks, those given **ethinylestradiol** 50 micrograms daily for 2 weeks showed less improvement than other women given only 25 micrograms or a placebo.[1] In an earlier associated study the 5 patients on **imipramine** 150 mg and **ethinylestradiol** 50 micrograms developed signs of **imipramine** toxicity (severe lethargy (4 patients), hypotension (4), coarse tremor (2), mild depersonalisation (2)) that was dealt with by halving the **imipramine** dose.[1] Another study found that oral contraceptives increased the absolute bioavailability of **imipramine** by 60%.[2]

Long-standing **imipramine** toxicity was relieved in a woman taking **imipramine** 100 mg daily when her dosage of conjugated oestrogen was reduced to a quarter.[3] In contrast, several studies that showed that serum **clomipramine** levels were raised or remained unaffected by the concurrent use of oestrogen-containing contraceptives failed to confirm that tricyclic antidepressant toxicity occurs more often in those on the pill than those who are not.[4-7] Akathisia in 3 patients has been attributed to an interaction between conjugated oestrogens and **amitriptyline** or **clomipramine**.[8]

Mechanism

Among the possible reasons for these effects are that the oestrogens increase the bioavailability of imipramine,[2] or inhibit its metabolism.[9]

Importance and management

These interactions are inadequately established. There is no obvious reason for avoiding concurrent use, but it would seem reasonable to be alert for any evidence of toxicity and/or lack of response to tricyclic antidepressant treatment. One study suggested that the imipramine dosage should be reduced by about one-third.[2] More study is needed.

1. Prange AJ, Wilson IC, Alltop LB. Estrogen may well affect response to antidepressant. *JAMA* (1972) 219, 143–4.
2. Abernethy DR, Greenblatt DJ, Shader RI. Imipramine disposition in users of oral contraceptive steroids. *Clin Pharmacol Ther* (1984) 35, 792–7.
3. Khurana RC. Estrogen-imipramine interaction. *JAMA* (1972) 222, 702–3.
4. Beaumont G. Drug interactions with clomipramine (Anafranil). *J Int Med Res* (1973) 1, 480–84.
5. Gringras M, Beaumont G, Grieve A. Clomipramine and oral contraceptives: an interaction study — clinical findings. *J Int Med Res* (1980) 8 (Suppl 3), 76–80.
6. Luscombe DK, Jones RB. Effects of concomitantly administered drugs on plasma levels of clomipramine and desmethylclomipramine in depressive patients receiving clomipramine therapy. *Postgrad Med J* (1977) 53 (Suppl 4), 77.
7. John VA, Luscombe DK, Kemp H. Effects of age, cigarette smoking and the oral contraceptive on the pharmacokinetics of clomipramine and its desmethyl metabolite during chronic dosing. *J Int Med Res* (1980) 8 (Suppl 3), 88–95.
8. Krishnan KRR, France RD, Ellinwood EH Jr. Tricyclic-induced akathisia in patients taking conjugated estrogens. *Am J Psychiatry* (1984) 141, 696–7.
9. Somani SM, Khurana RC. Mechanism of estrogen-imipramine interaction. *JAMA* (1973) 223, 560.

Tricyclic antidepressants + Quinidine

Quinidine can reduce the loss of desipramine, imipramine, nortriptyline and trimipramine from the body, thereby increasing their serum levels.

Clinical evidence

Quinidine 50 mg given 1 hour before a single 50-mg dose of **nortriptyline** increased its AUC in 5 healthy subjects fourfold, and the half-life threefold (from 14.2 to 44.7 hours).[1] The clearance fell from 5.4 to 1.9 ml/minute.

Another study in healthy subjects found that quinidine 200 mg daily reduced the clearance of single 100-mg doses of **imipramine** by 30% and of **desipramine** 100 mg by 85%.[2] A further study in 2 healthy subjects similarly found that quinidine 50 mg almost doubled the half-life of a single 75-mg dose of **trimipramine**, which was reflected in some waking EEG changes.[3]

Mechanism

Quinidine reduces the metabolism (hydroxylation) of these tricyclic antidepressants, by inhibiting the cytochrome P450 isoenzyme CYP2D6, and thereby reduces their loss from the body.[4,5]

Importance and management

The clinical importance of these interactions awaits assessment, but be alert for evidence of increased tricyclic antidepressant effects and possibly the toxicity if quinidine is added. One report suggested steady-state increases of 30% with imipramine and more than 500% with desipramine in extensive metabolisers.[2] More study is needed. There seems to be no information about other tricyclics. See also 'Drugs that prolong the QT interval + Other drugs that prolong the QT interval', p.170 for a possible pharmacodynamic interaction between these drugs.

1. Ayesh R, Dawling S, Widdop B, Idle JR, Smith RL. Influence of quinidine on the pharmacokinetics of nortriptyline and desipramine. *Br J Clin Pharmacol* (1988) 25, 140P–141P.
2. Brøsen K, Gram LF. Quinidine inhibits the 2-hydroxylation of imipramine and desipramine, but not the demethylation of imipramine. *Eur J Clin Pharmacol* (1989) 37, 155–60.
3. Eap CB, Laurian S, Souche A, Koeb L, Reymond P, Buclin T, Baumann P. Influence of quinidine on the pharmacokinetics of trimipramine and on its effect on the waking EEG of healthy volunteers. A pilot study on two subjects. *Neuropsychobiology* (1992) 25, 214–20.
4. Pfandl B, Mörike K, Winne D, Schareck W, Breyer-Pfaff U. Stereoselective inhibition of nortriptyline hydroxylation in man by quinidine. *Xenobiotica* (1992) 22, 721–30.
5. Von Moltke LL, Greenblatt DJ, Cotreau-Bibbo MM, Duan SX, Harmatz JS, Shader RI. Inhibition of desipramine hydroxylation *in vitro* by serotonin-reuptake-inhibitor antidepressants, and by quinidine and ketoconazole: a model system to predict drug interactions *in vivo*. *J Pharmacol Exp Ther* (1994) 268, 1278–83.

Tricyclic antidepressants + Rifampicin (Rifampin)

Three patients showed a marked reduction in serum nortriptyline or amitriptyline levels when given rifampicin.

Clinical evidence

A man with tuberculosis needed 175-mg doses of **nortriptyline** to achieve therapeutic serum concentrations while taking isoniazid 300 mg, rifampicin (rifampin) 600 mg, pyrazinamide 1.5 g and pyridoxine 25 mg daily. Three weeks after stopping the antitubercular drugs, the patient suddenly became drowsy and his **nortriptyline** serum levels were found to have risen from 193 to 562 nanomol/l and later to 671 nanomol/l. It was then found possible to maintain his **nortriptyline** serum levels in the range 150 to 500 nanomol/l with only 75 mg of **nortriptyline** daily.[1] A woman on **amitriptyline** and fluoxetine showed a marked fall in plasma **amitriptyline** levels when she was treated with rifampicin 600 mg, isoniazid 200 mg and ethambutol 1.2 g daily. When these antitubercular drugs were stopped, her **amitriptyline** plasma levels rose once again.[2] In a further case in a 43-year-old woman on **nortriptyline** 50 mg daily, serum concentrations were not detectable when rifampicin 600 mg daily was given concurrently. Increasing the dose of **nortriptyline** to 75 mg daily failed to produce detectable serum levels. Two weeks after discontinuation of rifampicin, **nortriptyline** concentrations increased significantly.[3]

Mechanism

It seems highly probable that rifampicin (a well recognised and potent enzyme inducer) increased the metabolism of nortriptyline and amitriptyline by the liver and hastened their loss from the body.

Importance and management

Information about the tricyclic antidepressant/rifampicin interaction seems to be limited to just these three reports, which is a little surprising since both have been widely used for a considerable time. This suggests that generally this interaction may have limited clinical importance. However, bear this interaction in mind if patients on rifampicin seem unresponsive to treatment with tricyclics. Increase the tricyclic dosage if necessary, and remember to readjust the dose if rifampicin is stopped.

1. Bebchuk JM, Stewart DE. Drug interaction between rifampin and nortriptyline: a case report. *Int J Psychiatry Med* (1991) 21, 183–7.
2. Bertschy G, Vandel S, Perault MC. Un cas d'interaction métabolique: amitriptyline, fluoxétine, antituberculeux. *Therapie* (1994) 49, 509–12.
3. Self T, Corley CR, Nabhan S, Abell T. Case report: interaction of rifampin and nortriptyline. *Am J Med Sci* (1996) 311, 80–1.

Tricyclic and related antidepressants + SSRIs

The levels of the tricyclic antidepressants can be raised by the SSRIs, but the extent varies greatly, from 20% to tenfold. Tricyclic toxicity has been seen in a number of cases. Tricyclics may increase the levels of citalopram and possibly fluvoxamine, but the significance of this is unclear. There are several case reports of the serotonin syndrome following concurrent and even sequential use of the SSRIs and tricyclics.

Clinical evidence

(a) Citalopram

In one study[1] citalopram caused an increase of about 50% in the AUC of **desipramine**, and a reduction in the levels of the subsequently formed metabolite of **desipramine** (the primary metabolite of imipramine) after a single 100-mg oral dose of **imipramine**. In contrast, 5 patients on **amitriptyline**, **clomipramine** or **maprotiline** showed no changes in their plasma tricyclic antidepressant levels when citalopram 20 to 60 mg daily was added.[2] In another general study, in which 18 patients were given citalopram and tricyclic antidepressants, serum levels of citalopram were doubled in those receiving the tricyclic **clomipramine**; pooled results for all the tricyclics showed a 44% rise in serum citalopram levels.[3] An increase of this size is of doubtful clinical importance with citalopram.

A case report describes elevated **desipramine** levels in a patient on paroxetine that resolved when the patient was switched to citalopram.[4]

(b) Escitalopram

Escitalopram 20 mg daily for 21 days increased the maximum serum levels and AUC of a single 50-mg dose of **desipramine** by 40 and 100% respectively.[5]

(c) Fluoxetine

Four patients on daily doses of **desipramine** 300 mg, **imipramine** 150 mg or **nortriptyline** 100 mg showed two to fourfold increases in plasma tricyclic antidepressant levels within 1 to 2 weeks of starting fluoxetine 10 to 60 mg daily. Two of them developed anticholinergic adverse effects (constipation, urinary hesitancy).[6]

A number of other reports and studies clearly confirm that marked increases occur in the levels of **amitriptyline**,[7-11] **clomipramine**,[8,12] **desipramine**,[13-22] **imipramine**[8,17-19,23,24] and **nortriptyline**,[15,16,25-27] accompanied by toxicity, if fluoxetine is added without reducing the dosage of the tricyclic antidepressant. Delirium and seizures have also been described,[18,28] and a death has been attributed to chronic **amitriptyline** toxicity caused by fluoxetine.[29] The pharmacokinetics of fluoxetine appear not to be affected by **amitriptyline**.[11]

A migraine-like stroke developed in a woman 48 hours after her long-standing therapy with fluoxetine 100 mg daily was changed to **clomipramine** 200 mg daily only 24 hours later.[30]

(d) Fluvoxamine

The **amitriptyline** plasma levels of 8 patients rose (range 15 to 233%) when given fluvoxamine 100 to 300 mg daily. Even larger rises in serum **clomipramine** levels occurred (up to eightfold) in four others given fluvoxamine 100 to 300 mg daily. The tricyclic dosages remained the same or were slightly lower. No toxicity was seen.[31-33]

A number of other reports and studies confirm that increases occur in the levels of **amitriptyline**,[34-37] **clomipramine**,[34-39] **desipramine**,[40-43] **imipramine**,[34,35,40-44] **maprotiline**[34] and **trimipramine**[45] in the presence of fluvoxamine. This interaction seems severe with **clomipramine** (a 10-fold rise in one case)[39] and mild with **desipramine**.[42,43] One study also suggested that fluvoxamine levels may be raised.[34]

(e) Paroxetine

A study in 17 healthy subjects who were extensive metabolisers and on **desipramine** 50 mg daily found that when additionally given paroxetine 20 mg daily for 10 days the maximum plasma levels of the **desipramine** rose by 358%, the trough plasma levels by 511% and the AUC by 421%. An approximately tenfold increase in the maximum serum levels and the AUC of the paroxetine also occurred.[46] Paroxetine has also been shown to increase the levels of **clomipramine**,[47] **desipramine**,[4] **imipramine**[48,49] and **trimipramine**.[50] This resulted in a variety of adverse effects including dizziness,[47] confusion,[4] sedation[50] and memory impairment.[50]

A 21-year-old man developed the serotonin syndrome when he took one tablet of paroxetine only one day after stopping **desipramine**, which he had taken for 5 days. He recovered after treatment with cyproheptadine.[51] A woman on paroxetine 30 mg daily developed the serotonin syndrome (tachycardia, delirium, bizarre movements, myoclonus) within 2 hours of taking a single 50-mg dose of **imipramine**. She recovered when treated with intravenous fluids, sedation and cyproheptadine.[52]

(f) Sertraline

Sertraline 50 mg daily increased the maximum plasma levels of **desipramine** 50 mg daily by 31% at steady-state in 9 healthy subjects and increased the AUC by 23%.[22] A later related study in 17 healthy subjects by the same group of workers found that, using the same drug dosages, sertraline increased the **desipramine** maximum plasma levels by 44%, the minimum levels by 19% and the AUC by 37%. The maximum plasma levels and AUC of the sertraline were increased about twofold.[46] Other studies have found that sertraline increases **desipramine**,[53-56] **imipramine**[53] and **nortriptyline**[57] levels, but it has been suggested that sertraline has no effect on **imipramine** levels.[58,59]

A woman who had been taking sertraline 50 mg daily (as well as morphine sulfate and periciazine) developed the serotonin syndrome within 3 days of starting to take **amitriptyline** 75 mg daily. She recovered when all of the psychotropic drugs were withdrawn.[60]

Mechanism

Fluoxetine, paroxetine, and to a lesser extent sertraline and citalopram, inhibit the cytochrome P450 isoenzyme CYP2D6, which is involved in the metabolism of the tricyclic antidepressants. Hence these SSRIs cause tricyclic levels to rise. Fluvoxamine causes a similar effect, possibly by inhibiting the latter stages of metabolism through CYP1A2 and CYP3A4.

The serotonin syndrome possibly develops because both the tricyclics and SSRIs affect serotonin transmission, which may result in increased serotonin levels. For more about the serotonin syndrome see 'Additive or synergistic interactions', (p.9).

Importance and management

The interactions of the SSRIs and tricyclic antidepressants are established and of clinical significance. The SSRIs increase tricyclic levels, with fluvoxamine, fluoxetine and paroxetine apparently having the greatest effects. The increased tricyclic levels can be beneficial.[34,37,61] However, it has been suggested that patients given fluoxetine should have their tricyclic dose reduced to a quarter.[17] Similar recommendations have been made with fluvoxamine (reduction in tricyclic dose to a third)[40] and sertraline.[62] It would also seem prudent to consider a dosage reduction of the tricyclic if paroxetine is added. Some suggest that a small initial dose of the SSRI should also be used.[62]

Patients on any combination of tricyclic and SSRI should be monitored for adverse effects (e.g. dry mouth, sedation, confusion) with tricyclic levels monitored where possible. Remember that the active metabolite of fluoxetine has a half-life of 7 to 15 days, and so any interaction may persist for some time after the fluoxetine is withdrawn,[63-65] and may occur on sequential use.

The serotonin syndrome seems to occur rarely but patients and prescribers should be aware of the symptoms so that prompt action can be taken if problems occur. For more about the serotonin syndrome see 'Additive or synergistic interactions', (p.9).

1. Gram LF, Hansen MG, Sindrup SH, Brøsen K, Poulsen JH, Aaes-Jørgensen T, Overø KF. Citalopram: interaction studies with levomepromazine, imipramine and lithium. *Ther Drug Monit* (1993) 15, 18–24.
2. Baettig D, Bondolfi G, Montaldi S, Amey M, Baumann P. Tricyclic antidepressant plasma levels after augmentation with citalopram: a case study. *Eur J Clin Pharmacol* (1993) 44, 403–5.
3. Leinonen E, Lepola U, Koponen H, Kinnunen I. The effect of age and concomitant treatment with other psychoactive drugs on serum concentrations of citalopram measured with a non-enantioselective method. *Ther Drug Monit* (1996) 18, 111–17.
4. Ashton AK. Lack of desipramine toxicity with citalopram. *J Clin Psychiatry* (2000) 61, 144.
5. Lexapro (Escitalopram). Forest Pharmaceuticals Inc. US Prescribing information, August 2004.
6. Aranow RB, Hudson JI, Pope HG, Grady TA, Laage TA, Bell IR, Cole JO. Elevated antidepressant plasma levels after addition of fluoxetine. *Am J Psychiatry* (1989) 146, 911–13.
7. March JS, Moon RL, Johnston H. Fluoxetine-TCA interaction. *J Am Acad Child Adolesc Psychiatry* (1990) 29, 985–6.
8. Vandel S, Bertschy G, Bonin B, Nezelof S, François TH, Vandel B, Sechter D, Bizouard P. Tricyclic antidepressant plasma levels after fluoxetine addition. *Neuropsychobiology* (1992) 25, 202–7.
9. El-Yazigi A, Chaleby K, Gad A, Raines DA. Steady-state pharmacokinetics of fluoxetine and amitriptyline in patients treated with a combination of these drugs. *Pharm Res* (1993) 10 (10 Suppl), S-309.
10. Bertschy G, Vandel S, Perault MC. Un cas d'interaction métabolique: amitriptyline, fluoxétine, antituberculeux. *Therapie* (1994) 49, 509–12.
11. El-Yazigi A, Chaleby K, Gad A, Raines DA. Steady-state kinetics of fluoxetine and amitriptyline in patients treated with a combination of these drugs as compared with those treated with amitriptyline alone. *J Clin Pharmacol* (1995) 35, 17–21.
12. Balant-Gorgia AE, Ries C, Balant LP. Metabolic interaction between fluoxetine and clomipramine: A case report. *Pharmacopsychiatry* (1996) 29, 38–41.
13. Bell IR, Cole JO. Fluoxetine induces elevation of desipramine level and exacerbation of geriatric nonpsychotic depression. *J Clin Psychopharmacol* (1988) 8, 447–8.
14. Goodnick PJ. Influence of fluoxetine on plasma levels of desipramine. *Am J Psychiatry* (1989) 146, 552.
15. Vaughan DA. Interaction of fluoxetine with tricyclic antidepressants. *Am J Psychiatry* (1988) 145, 1478.
16. von Ammon Cavanaugh S. Drug-drug interactions of fluoxetine with tricyclics. *Psychosomatics* (1990) 31, 273–6.
17. Westermeyer J. Fluoxetine-induced tricyclic toxicity: extent and duration. *J Clin Pharmacol* (1991) 31, 388–92.
18. Preskorn SH, Beber JH, Faul JC, Hirschfeld RMA. Serious adverse effects of combining fluoxetine and tricyclic antidepressants. *Am J Psychiatry* (1990) 147, 532.
19. Bergstrom RF, Peyton AL, Lemberger L. Quantification and mechanism of the fluoxetine and tricyclic antidepressant interaction. *Clin Pharmacol Ther* (1992) 51, 239–48.
20. Nelson JC, Mazure CM, Bowers MB, Jatlow PI. A preliminary, open study of the combination of fluoxetine and desipramine for rapid treatment of major depression. *Arch Gen Psychiatry* (1991) 48, 303–7.
21. Wilens TE, Biederman J, Baldessarini RJ, McDermott SP, Puopolo PR, Flood JG. Fluoxetine inhibits desipramine metabolism. *Arch Gen Psychiatry* (1992) 49, 752.
22. Preskorn SH, Alderman J, Chung M, Harrison W, Messig M, Harris S. Pharmacokinetics of desipramine coadministered with sertraline or fluoxetine. *J Clin Psychopharmacol* (1994) 14, 90–8.
23. Faynor SM, Espina V. Fluoxetine inhibition of imipramine metabolism. *Clin Chem* (1989) 35, 1180.
24. Hahn SM, Griffin JH. Comment: fluoxetine adverse effects and drug interactions. *DICP Ann Pharmacother* (1991) 25, 1273–4.
25. Kahn DG. Increased plasma nortriptyline concentration in a patient cotreated with fluoxetine. *J Clin Psychiatry* (1990) 51, 36.
26. Schraml F, Benedetti G, Hoyle K, Clayton A. Fluoxetine and nortriptyline combination therapy. *Am J Psychiatry* (1989) 146, 1636–7.
27. Downs JM, Downs AD, Rosenthal TL, Deal N, Akiskal HS. Increased plasma tricyclic antidepressant concentrations in two patients concurrently treated with fluoxetine. *J Clin Psychiatry* (1989) 50, 226–7.
28. Sternbach H. Fluoxetine-clomipramine interaction. *J Clin Psychiatry* (1995) 56, 171–2.
29. Preskorn SH, Baker B. Fatality associated with combined fluoxetine-amitriptyline therapy. *JAMA* (1997) 277, 1682.
30. Molaie M. Serotonin syndrome presenting with migraine like stroke. *Headache* (1997) 37, 519–21.
31. Vandel S, Bertschy G, Allers G. Fluvoxamine tricyclic antidepressant interaction. *Therapie* (1990) 45, 21.
32. Bertschy G, Vandel S, Vandel B, Allers G, Vomat R. Fluvoxamine-tricyclic antidepressant interaction. An accidental finding. *Eur J Clin Pharmacol* (1991) 40, 119–120.
33. Bertschy G, Vandel S, Nezelof S, Bizouard P, Bechtel P. L'interaction fluvoxamine-antidépresseurs tricycliques. *Therapie* (1993) 48, 63–4.
34. Härtter S, Wetzel H, Hammes E, Hiemke C. Inhibition of antidepressant demethylation and hydroxylation by fluvoxamine in depressed patients. *Psychopharmacology (Berl)* (1993) 110, 302–8.
35. Szegedi A, Wetzel H, Leal M, Härtter S, Hiemke C. Combination treatment with clomipramine and fluvoxamine: drug monitoring, safety, and tolerability data. *J Clin Psychiatry* (1996) 57, 257–64.
36. Vandel S, Bertschy G, Baumann P, Bouquet S, Bonin B, Francois T, Sechter D, Bizouard P. Fluvoxamine and fluoxetine: Interaction studies with amitriptyline, clomipramine and neuroleptics in phenotyped patients. *Pharmacol Res* (1995) 31, 347–53.
37. Vandel P, Bonin B, Bertschy G, Baumann P, Bouquet S, Vandel S, Sechter D, Bizouard P. Observations of the interaction between tricyclic antidepressants and fluvoxamine in poor metabolisers of dextromethorphan and mephenytoin. *Therapie* (1997) 52, 74–6.
38. Conus P, Bondolfi G, Eap CB, Macciardi F, Baumann P. Pharmacokinetic fluvoxamine-clomipramine interaction with favorable therapeutic consequences in therapy-resistant depressive patient. *Pharmacopsychiatry* (1996) 29, 108–110.
39. Roberge C, Lecordier-Maret F, Beljean-Leymarie M, Heriault F, Starace J. Major drug interaction between fluvoxamine and clomipramine: about a case report. *J Pharm Clin* (1998) 17, 117–19.
40. Spina E, Campo GM, Avenoso A, Pollicino MA, Caputi AP. Interaction between fluvoxamine and imipramine/desipramine in four patients. *Ther Drug Monit* (1992) 14, 194–6.
41. Maskall DD, Lam RW. Increased plasma concentration of imipramine following augmentation with fluvoxamine. *Am J Psychiatry* (1993) 150, 1566.
42. Spina E, Pollicino AM, Avenso A, Campo GM, Caputi AP. Fluvoxamine-induced alterations in plasma concentrations of imipramine and desipramine in depressed patients. *Int J Clin Pharmacol Res* (1993) 13, 167–71.
43. Spina E, Pollicino AM, Avenoso A, Campo GM, Perucca E, Caputi AP. Effect of fluvoxamine on the pharmacokinetics of imipramine and desipramine in healthy subjects. *Ther Drug Monit* (1993) 15, 243–6.
44. Xu ZH, Huang S-L, Zhou H-H. Inhibition of imipramine *N*-demethylation by fluvoxamine in Chinese young men. *Acta Pharmacol Sin* (1996) 17, 399–402.
45. Seifritz E, Holsboer-Trachsler E, Hemmeter U, Eap CB, Baumann P. Increased trimipramine plasma levels during fluvoxamine comedication. *Eur Neuropsychopharmacol* (1994) 4, 15–20.
46. Alderman J, Preskorn SH, Greenblatt DJ, Harrison W, Penenberg D, Allison J, Chung M. Desipramine pharmacokinetics when coadministered with paroxetine or sertraline in extensive metabolizers. *J Clin Psychopharmacol* (1997) 17, 284–91.
47. Skjelbo EF, Brøsen K. Interaktion imellem paroxetin og clomipramin som mulig årsag til indlæggelse på medicinsk afdeling. *Ugeskr Laeger* (1998) 160, 5665–6.
48. Albers LJ, Reist C, Helmeste D, Vu R, Tang SW. Paroxetine shifts imipramine metabolism. *Psychiatry Res* (1996) 59, 189–96.
49. Yoon YR, Shim JC, Shin JG, Shon JH, Kim YH, Cha IJ. Drug interaction between paroxetine and imipramine. Kor Soc Pharmacol Meeting, Seoul, S Korea, October 1997, p168.
50. Leinonen E, Koponen HJ, Lepola U. Paroxetine increases serum trimipramine concentration. A report of two cases. *Hum Psychopharmacol* (1995) 10, 345–7.
51. Chan BSH, Graudins A, Whyte IM, Dawson AH, Braitberg G, Duggin GG. Serotonin syndrome resulting from drug interactions. *Med J Aust* (1998) 169, 523–5.
52. Weiner AL, Tilden FF, McKay CA. Serotonin syndrome: case report and review of the literature. *Conn Med* (1997) 61, 717–21.
53. Kurtz DL, Bergstrom RF, Goldberg MJ, Cerimele BJ. The effect of sertraline on the pharmacokinetics of desipramine and imipramine. *Clin Pharmacol Ther* (1997) 62, 145–56.
54. Zussman BD, Davie CC, Fowles SE, Kumar R, Lang U, Wargenau M, Sourgens H. Sertraline, like other SSRIs, is a significant inhibitor of desipramine metabolism in vivo. *Br J Clin Pharmacol* (1995) 39, 550P–551P.
55. Lydiard RB, Anton RF, Cunningham T. Interactions between sertraline and tricyclic antidepressants. *Am J Psychiatry* (1993) 150, 1125–6.
56. Barros J, Asnis G. An interaction of sertraline and desipramine. *Am J Psychiatry* (1993) 150, 1751.
57. Solai LK, Mulsant BH, Pollock BG, Sweet RA, Rosen J, Yu K, Reynolds CF. Effect of sertraline on plasma nortriptyline levels in depressed elderly. *J Clin Psychiatry* (1997) 58, 440–3.
58. Erikson SM, Carson SW, Grimsley S, Carter JG, Kumar A, Jann MW. Effect of sertraline on steady-state serum concentrations of imipramine and its metabolites. *Pharmacotherapy* (1994) 14, 368.
59. Jann MW, Carson SW, Grimsley SR, Erikson S, Kumar A, Carter JG. Effects of sertraline upon imipramine pharmacodynamics. *Clin Pharmacol Ther* (1995) 57, 207.
60. Alderman CP, Lee PC. Comment: serotonin syndrome associated with combined sertraline-amitriptyline treatment. *Ann Pharmacother* (1996) 30, 1499–1500.

61. Wetzel H, Härtter A, Szegedi A, Hammes E, Leal M, Hiemke C. Fluvoxamine co-medication to tricyclic antidepressants: metabolic interactions, clinical efficiency and side-effects. *Pharmacopsychiatry* (1993) 26, 211.
62. Eiber R, Escande M. Associations et interactions: les antidépresseurs tricycliques et les inhibiteurs spécifiques de la recapture de la sérotonine. *Encephale* (1999) 25, 584–9.
63. Downs JM, Dahmer SK. Fluoxetine and elevated plasma levels of tricyclic antidepressants. *Am J Psychiatry* (1990) 147, 1251.
64. Skowron DM, Gutierrez MA, Epstein S. Precaution with titrating nortriptyline after the use of fluoxetine. *DICP Ann Pharmacother* (1990) 24, 1008.
65. Müller N, Brockmöller J, Roots I. Extremely long plasma half-life of amitriptyline in a woman with the cytochrome P450IID6 29/29-kilobase wild-type allele — a slowly reversible interaction with fluoxetine. *Ther Drug Monit* (1991) 13, 533–6.

Tricyclic antidepressants + St John's wort (*Hypericum perforatum*)

The plasma levels of amitriptyline can be reduced by St John's wort and nortriptyline seems to be similarly affected, but the clinical importance of this interaction is unknown.

Clinical evidence

Twelve depressed patients were given 75 mg of **amitriptyline** twice daily and 900 mg of St John's wort extract (*Lichtwer Pharma, Berlin*) daily for at least 14 days. The 0 to 12 hour AUC of the **amitriptyline** was reduced by 21.7% and the AUC of **nortriptyline** by 40.6%.[1]

Mechanism

Not known, but there is evidence that St John's wort is an enzyme inducer, which can increase liver metabolism, thereby reducing the plasma levels of both amitriptyline and its metabolite (nortriptyline).

Importance and management

The interaction appears to be established, but its clinical importance is uncertain. Both the tricyclics and St John's wort are antidepressants, but whether the final sum of this interaction is more or less antidepressant activity is not known. It was not assessed in this study.[1] Other tricyclics probably interact similarly because they too can be affected by enzyme inducing agents (and nortriptyline clearly is). Monitor antidepressant efficacy if St John's wort is given with any tricyclic. More study is needed.

1. Roots I, Johne A, Schmider J, Brockmöller J, Maurer A, Störmer E, Donath F. Interaction of a herbal extract from St. John's wort with amitriptyline and its metabolites. *Clin Pharmacol Ther* (2000) 67, 159.

Tricyclic antidepressants + Sympathomimetics; Directly-acting

Patients on tricyclic antidepressants show a grossly exaggerated response (hypertension, cardiac arrhythmias, etc.) to parenteral noradrenaline (norepinephrine), adrenaline (epinephrine) and to a lesser extent to phenylephrine. Local anaesthetics containing these vasoconstrictors do not seem to be associated with the same problems. Felypressin may be a safe alternative. Doxepin appears not to interact to the same extent as most tricyclic antidepressants.

Clinical evidence

The effects of intravenous infusions of **noradrenaline** (**norepinephrine**) were increased approximately ninefold, and of **adrenaline** (**epinephrine**) approximately threefold, in 6 healthy subjects who had been taking **protriptyline** 60 mg daily for 4 days.[1,2]

The pressor effects of intravenous infusions of **noradrenaline** were increased four to eightfold, of **adrenaline** two to fourfold, and of **phenylephrine** two to threefold in 4 healthy subjects who had been taking **imipramine** 75 mg daily for 5 days. There were no noticeable or consistent changes in their response to **isoprenaline** (**isoproterenol**).[3]

Five patients taking **nortriptyline**, **desipramine** or other unnamed tricyclic antidepressants experienced adverse reactions, some of them severe (throbbing headache, chest pain) following the injection of ***Xylestesin*** (lidocaine with 1:25,000 **noradrenaline**) during dental treatment.[4] Several episodes of marked increases in blood pressure, dilated pupils, intense malaise, violent but transitory tremor and palpitations have been reported in patients taking unnamed tricyclic antidepressants when they were given local anaesthetics containing **adrenaline** or **noradrenaline** for dental treatment.[5]

There are other reports describing this interaction of **noradrenaline** with **imipramine**,[6,7] **desipramine**,[7,8] **nortriptyline**,[9] **protriptyline**[8] and **amitriptyline**;[7,8] of **adrenaline** with **amitriptyline**,[10] and of **corbadrine** with **desipramine** (in *dogs*).[11]

Mechanism

The tricyclics and some related antidepressants block or inhibit the uptake of noradrenaline (norepinephrine) into adrenergic neurones. Thus the most important means by which noradrenaline is removed from the adrenoceptor area is inactivated and the concentration of noradrenaline outside the neurone can rise. If more noradrenaline (or one of the other directly acting alpha or alpha/beta agonists) is infused into the body, the adrenoceptors of the cardiovascular system concerned with raising blood pressure become grossly stimulated by this superabundance of amines, and the normal response is therefore exaggerated.

Importance and management

A well documented, well established and potentially serious interaction. The parenteral administration of noradrenaline (norepinephrine), adrenaline (epinephrine), phenylephrine or any other sympathomimetic amines with predominantly direct activity should be avoided in patients treated with tricyclic antidepressants. If these sympathomimetics must be used, the rate and amount injected must be very much reduced to accommodate the exaggerated responses that will occur. However, the situation where adrenaline or noradrenaline are used with a local anaesthetic for surface or infiltration anaesthesia, or nerve block is less clear. The cases cited are all from the 1960s or 1970s, and the preparations concerned contained concentrations of adrenaline or noradrenaline several times greater than those used currently. However, it should be noted that preparations such as *Xylocaine* with adrenaline still carry a caution in their UK product information about their use with tricyclic antidepressants.[12] Anecdotal evidence suggests that local anaesthetics containing sympathomimetics are, in practice, commonly used in patients receiving tricyclic antidepressants,[13] so the sparsity of reports, especially recent ones, would add weight to the argument that the interaction is only rarely significant. However, it would still seem advisable to be aware of the potential for interaction. Aspiration has been recommended to avoid inadvertent intravenous administration. **Felypressin** has been shown to be a safe alternative.[14-16] If an adverse interaction occurs it can be controlled by the use of an alpha-receptor blocking agent such as phentolamine.

Doxepin in doses of less than 150 to 200 mg daily blocks neuronal uptake much less than other tricyclic antidepressants and so is unlikely to show this interaction to the same degree, but in larger doses it will interact like other tricyclics.[17,18] The pressor response to noradrenaline is also not significantly increased in the presence of **iprindole**.[19] It does not seem to have been established whether the response to oral doses or nasal drops containing phenylephrine is enhanced by the presence of a tricyclic, but there seem to be no reports of problems.

1. Svedmyr N. The influence of a tricyclic antidepressive agent (protriptyline) on some of the circulatory effects of noradrenaline and adrenaline in man. *Life Sci* (1968) 7, 77–84.
2. Svedmyr N. Potentieringsrisker vid tillförsel av katekolaminer till patienter som behandlas med tricykliska antidepressiva medel. *Lakartidningen* (1968) 65 (Suppl 1), 72–6.
3. Boakes AJ, Laurence DR, Teoh PC, Barar FSK, Benedikter LT, Prichard BNC. Interactions between sympathomimetic amines and antidepressant agents in man. *BMJ* (1973) 1, 311–15.
4. Boakes AJ, Laurence DR, Lovel KW, O'Neil R, Verrill PJ. Adverse reactions to local anaesthetic/vasoconstrictor preparations. A study of the cardiovascular responses to Xylestesin and Hostacain-with-Noradrenaline. *Br Dent J* (1972) 133, 137–40.
5. Dam WH. Personal communication cited by Kristoffersen MB. Antidepressivas potensering af katekolaminvirkning. *Ugeskr Laeger* (1969) 131, 1013–14.
6. Gershon S, Holmberg G, Mattsson E, Mattsson N, Marshall A. Imipramine hydrochloride. Its effects on clinical, autonomic and psychological functions. *Arch Gen Psychiatry* (1962) 6, 96–101.
7. Fischbach R, Harrer G, Harrer H. Verstärkung der noradrenalin-wirkung durch psychopharmaka beim menschen. *Arzneimittelforschung* (1966) 16, 263–5.
8. Mitchell JR, Cavanaugh JH, Arias L, Oates JA. Guanethidine and related agents. III. Antagonism by drugs which inhibit the norepinephrine pump in man. *J Clin Invest* (1970) 49, 1596–1604.
9. Persson G, Siwers B. The risk of potentiating effect of local anaesthesia with adrenalin in patients treated with tricyclic antidepressants. *Swed Dent J* (1975) 68, 9–18.
10. Siemkowicz E. Hjertestop efter amitriptylin og adrenalin. *Ugeskr Laeger* (1975) 137, 1403–4.
11. Dreyer AC, Offermeier J. The influence of desipramine on the blood pressure elevation and heart rate stimulation of levonordefrin and felypressin alone and in the presence of local anaesthetics. *J Dent Assoc S Afr* (1986) 41, 615–18.

12. Xylocaine 2% with adrenaline 1:200,000 (Lidocaine with adrenaline). AstraZeneca UK Ltd. UK Summary of product characteristics, December 2004.
13. Brown RS, Lewis VA. More on the contraindications to vasoconstrictors in dentistry. *Oral Surg Oral Med Oral Pathol* (1993) 76, 2–3.
14. Aellig WH, Laurence DR, O'Neil R, Verrill PJ. Cardiac effects of adrenaline and felypressin as vasoconstrictors in local anaesthesia for oral surgery under diazepam sedation. *Br J Anaesth* (1970) 42, 174–6.
15. Goldman V, Astrom A, Evers H. The effect of a tricyclic antidepressant on the cardiovascular effects of local anaesthetic solutions containing different vasoconstrictors. *Anaesthesia* (1971) 26, 91.
16. Perovic J, Terzic M, Todorovic L. Safety of local anaesthesia induced by prilocaine with felypressin in patients on tricyclic antidepressants. *Bull Group Int Rech Sci Stomatol Odontol* (1979) 22, 57–62.
17. Fann WE, Cavanaugh JH, Kaufmann JS, Griffith JD, Davis JM, Janowsky DS, Oates JA. Doxepin: effects on transport of biogenic amines in man. *Psychopharmacologia* (1971) 22, 111–25.
18. Oates JA, Fann WE, Cavanaugh JH. Effect of doxepin on the norepinephrine pump. *Psychosomatics* (1969) 10, 12–13.
19. Fann WE, Davis JM, Janowsky DS, Kaufmann JS, Griffith JD, Oates JA. Effect of iprindole on amine uptake in man. *Arch Gen Psychiatry* (1972) 26, 158–62.

Tricyclic antidepressants + Sympathomimetics; Indirectly-acting

The effects of indirectly acting sympathomimetics (amfetamines, phenylpropanolamine, pseudoephedrine, tyramine, etc.) would be expected to be reduced by the tricyclic antidepressants, but so far only one case, involving ephedrine and amitriptyline, seems to have been reported.

Clinical evidence, mechanism, importance and management

Indirectly-acting sympathomimetic amines like **tyramine** exert their effects by causing the release of **noradrenaline** (**norepinephrine**) from adrenergic neurones rather than by a direct stimulant action on the receptors. In the presence of a tricyclic antidepressant, the uptake of these amines into adrenergic neurones is partially or totally prevented and the **noradrenaline**-releasing effects are therefore blocked. The reduction in the pressor response to **tyramine** due to this interaction has been used in monitoring the efficacy of treatment with the tricyclic antidepressants,[1] but **tyramine** itself is only used as a research tool, or as a model drug to test the behaviour of indirectly acting sympathomimetics. The activity of other similar sympathomimetics that are used therapeutically might therefore be expected to be blocked by the tricyclics in just the same way, but only an isolated case seems to have been reported.[2]

An elderly woman on **amitriptyline** 75 mg daily developed hypotension (70 mmHg systolic) during subarachnoid anaesthesia. Her blood pressure rose only minimally when given intravenous boluses of **ephedrine** (a mixed action sympathomimetic) totalling 90 mg but she responded normally when given **adrenaline** (**epinephrine**) a directly-acting sympathomimetic.[2]

This single case appears to be the only report of this type of interaction occurring in a clinical situation. Bearing in mind how long and how widely both groups of drugs have been in use, the absence of any other reports would suggest that any interaction between them is rarely of practical importance, even so some drug makers include this largely theoretical interaction on their data sheets.

1. Mulgirigama LD, Pare CMB, Turner P, Wadsworth J, Witts DJ. Tyramine pressor responses and plasma levels during tricyclic antidepressant therapy. *Postgrad Med J* (1977) 53 (Suppl 4), 30–4.
2. Serle DG. Amitriptyline and ephedrine in subarachnoid anesthesia. *Anaesth Intensive Care* (1985) 13, 214.

Tricyclic antidepressants + Thioxanthenes

Flupentixol did not inhibit the metabolism of imipramine in two patients but high levels of imipramine and desipramine were found in another patient.

Clinical evidence, mechanism, importance and management

A study using ^{14}C-**imipramine** showed that, unlike the situation between the 'tricyclic antidepressants and phenothiazines', (p.570) **flupentixol** 3 to 6 mg daily did not inhibit the metabolism of **imipramine** in 2 patients.[1] However, there is an isolated report of very high plasma levels of **imipramine** and its metabolite **desipramine** in a patient with schizophrenia given concurrent **flupentixol decanoate** 40 mg intramuscularly once every 2 weeks and **imipramine** 150 mg daily, which may be due to competitive inhibition of the hepatic microsomal enzymes.[2]

1. Gram LF, Overø KF. Drug interaction: inhibitory effect of neuroleptics on metabolism of tricyclic antidepressants in man. *BMJ* (1972) 1, 463–5.
2. Cook PE, Dermer SW, Cardamone J. Imipramine-flupenthixol decanoate interaction. *Can J Psychiatry* (1986) 31, 235–7.

Tricyclic antidepressants + Thyroid preparations

The antidepressant response to imipramine, amitriptyline and possibly other tricyclics can be accelerated by the use of thyroid preparations. Isolated cases of paroxysmal atrial tachycardia, thyrotoxicosis and hypothyroidism due to concurrent therapy have been described.

Clinical evidence, mechanism, importance and management

The addition of **liothyronine** 25 micrograms daily was found to increase the speed and efficacy of **imipramine** in relieving depression.[1] Similar results have been described in other studies with **desipramine**[2] or **amitriptyline**[3] but the reasons are not understood. One possible explanation is that the patients had overt or subclinical hypothyroidism, which after correction with **liothyronine** allowed them to overcome an impaired response to tricyclic antidepressants.[4] However, adverse reactions have also been seen. A patient being treated for both hypothyroidism and depression with thyroid 60 mg and **imipramine** 150 mg daily complained of dizziness and nausea. She was found to have developed paroxysmal atrial tachycardia.[5] A 10-year-old girl with congenital hypothyroidism, well controlled on desiccated thyroid 150 mg daily, developed severe thyrotoxicosis after taking **imipramine** 25 mg daily for 5 months for enuresis. The problem disappeared when the **imipramine** was withdrawn.[6] In another patient the effect of **levothyroxine** was lost and hypothyroidism developed when given **dosulepin**.[7] Normally an advantageous interaction,[8] in which **liothyronine** appears to have a significantly greater antidepressant potentiating effect than **levothyroxine**.[9] These apparent interactions remain unexplained. There would seem to be no good reason, generally speaking, for avoiding concurrent use unless problems arise.

1. Wilson IC, Prange AJ, McClane TK, Rabon AM, Lipton MA. Thyroid-hormone enhancement of imipramine in nonretarded depressions. *N Engl J Med* (1970) 282, 1063–7.
2. Extein I. Case reports of l-triiodothyronine potentiation. *Am J Psychiatry* (1982) 139, 966–7.
3. Wheatley D. Potentiation of amitriptyline by thyroid hormone. *Arch Gen Psychiatry* (1972) 26, 229–33.
4. Berlin I, Corruble E. Thyroid hormones and antidepressant response. *Am J Psychiatry* (2002) 159, 1441.
5. Prange AJ. Paroxysmal auricular tachycardia apparently resulting from combined thyroid-imipramine treatment. *Am J Psychiatry* (1963) 119, 994–5.
6. Colantonio LA, Orson JM. Triiodothyronine thyrotoxicosis. Induction by desiccated thyroid and imipramine. *Am J Dis Child* (1974) 128, 396–7.
7. Beeley L, Beadle F, Lawrence R. *Bulletin of the West Midlands Centre for Adverse Drug Reaction Reporting* (1984) 19, 11.
8. Altshuler LL, Bauer M, Frye MA, Gitlin MJ, Mintz J, Szuba MP, Leight KL, Whybrow PC. Does thyroid supplementation accelerate tricyclic antidepressant response? A review and meta-analysis of the literature. *Am J Psychiatry* (2001) 158, 1617–22.
9. Joffe RT, Singer W. A comparison of triiodothyronine and thyroxine in the potentiation of tricyclic antidepressants. *Psychiatry Res* (1990) 32, 241–51.

Tricyclic antidepressants + Tobacco smoking

Smoking reduces the plasma levels of amitriptyline, clomipramine, desipramine, imipramine and nortriptyline, but the concentration of the free and unbound antidepressant rises, which appears to offset the effects of this interaction.

Clinical evidence

Two studies failed to find any difference between the steady-state **nortriptyline** plasma levels of smokers and non-smokers,[1,2] but others have found that smoking lowers the plasma levels of **amitriptyline**, **clomipramine**,[3] **desipramine**, **imipramine**[4] and **nortriptyline**.[5] For example a 25% reduction in plasma **nortriptyline** levels was found in one study,[5] and a 45% reduction in total **imipramine** plus **desipramine** levels in another.[4]

Mechanism

The probable reason is that some of the components of tobacco smoke are enzyme inducing agents, which increase the metabolism of these antidepressants by the liver.

Importance and management

These interactions are established but it might wrongly be concluded from the figures quoted that smokers need larger doses to control their depression. Preliminary data show that the plasma concentrations of free (and pharmacologically active) nortriptyline are greater in smokers than non-smokers (10.2% compared with 7.4%), which probably offsets the fall in total plasma levels.[5] Thus the lower plasma levels in smokers may be as therapeutically effective as the higher levels in non-smokers, so that there is probably no need to raise the dosage to accommodate this interaction.

1. Norman TR, Burrows GD, Maguire KP, Rubinstein G, Scoggins BA, Davies B. Cigarette smoking and plasma nortriptyline levels. *Clin Pharmacol Ther* (1977) 21, 453–6.
2. Alexanderson B, Price Evans DA, Sjöqvist F. Steady-state plasma levels of nortriptyline in twins: influence of genetic factors and drug therapy. *BMJ* (1969) 4, 764–8.
3. John VA, Luscombe DK, Kemp H. Effects of age, cigarette smoking and the oral contraceptive on the pharmacokinetics of clomipramine and its desmethyl metabolite during chronic dosing. *J Int Med Res* (1980) 8 (Suppl 3), 88–95.
4. Perel JM, Hurwic MJ, Kanzler MB. Pharmacodynamics of imipramine in depressed patients. *Psychopharmacol Bull* (1975) 11, 16–18.
5. Perry PJ, Browne JL, Prince RA, Alexander B, Tsuang MT. Effects of smoking on nortriptyline plasma concentrations in depressed patients. *Ther Drug Monit* (1986) 8, 279–84.

Tricyclic antidepressants + Urinary acidifiers or alkalinisers

The blood levels of desipramine, nortriptyline and other tricyclic antidepressants are not significantly affected by agents that alter urinary pH.

Clinical evidence, mechanism, importance and management

Because the tricyclics are bases it might be expected that changes in the urinary pH would have an effect on their excretion, but in fact the excretion of unchanged drug is small (less than 5% with **nortriptyline** and **desipramine**) compared with the amounts metabolised by the liver.[1] Only in the case of hepatic dysfunction is simple urinary clearance likely to take on a more important role.

1. Sjöqvist F, Berglund F, Borgå O, Hammer W, Andersson S, Thorstrand C. The pH-dependent excretion of monomethylated tricyclic antidepressants. *Clin Pharmacol Ther* (1969) 10, 826–33.

Tricyclic antidepressants + Valproate

Amitriptyline and nortriptyline plasma levels can be increased by sodium valproate and valpromide. Valproate pharmacokinetics may be moderately affected by amitriptyline. An isolated report attributes a paradoxical rise in serum desipramine levels to the withdrawal of sodium valproate.

Clinical evidence

(a) Sodium or Semisodium valproate

In one study, 15 healthy subjects were given a single 50-mg dose of **amitriptyline** 2 hours after taking the ninth dose of semisodium valproate 500 mg 12-hourly. The maximum plasma levels and AUC of **amitriptyline** were raised by 19% and 30% respectively. The corresponding values for the **nortriptyline** metabolite were 28% and 55% respectively.[1] A study in 6 patients with depression found that **amitriptyline** 100 mg daily for 3 weeks produced a 43% increase in the volume of distribution and a 16% increase in the plasma half-life of a single 400-mg intravenous dose of sodium valproate. The AUC and total body clearance of valproate were not significantly changed.[2]

One patient developed delirium within 3 days, and another developed grossly elevated **nortriptyline** plasma levels (393 nanograms/ml, about threefold higher than the normal range) and evidence of toxicity (tremulousness of hands and fingers) about one week after starting valproate 750 to 1000 mg daily. The toxicity rapidly disappeared when both drugs were stopped. Another patient also developed elevated **nortriptyline** plasma levels, attributed to the addition of valproate.[3] A patient on **clomipramine** 150 mg daily suffered feelings of numbness and sleep disturbances attributed to elevated serum levels of **clomipramine** and **desmethylclomipramine,** caused by the administration of valproate 1 to 1.4 g daily. Halving the dose of **clomipramine** restored serum concentrations to therapeutic levels.[4]

(b) Valproic acid

A woman on thiothixene developed elevated and potentially toxic serum **desipramine** levels (a rise from 259 to 324 mg/l) at the end of a 3-month period during which valproic acid was gradually withdrawn and replaced by clorazepate. The authors of the report attributed this reaction to the valproic acid withdrawal.[5]

(c) Valpromide

The addition of valpromide 600 mg daily for 10 days caused a 65% rise in the plasma levels of **nortriptyline** (from 61 to 100.5 nanograms/ml) and a 50% rise in the levels of **amitriptyline** (from 70.5 to 105.5 nanograms/ml) in 10 patients.[6,7]

Mechanism

Uncertain. Inhibition of the metabolism of these tricyclics by the valproate has been suggested.[3,4]

Importance and management

Information seems to be limited to these reports. It would now seem prudent to monitor the plasma levels of amitriptyline or nortriptyline if valproate is added, and to reduce the dosage of the amitriptyline if necessary. The clinical relevance of these increases is uncertain; the rises seem to be only moderate in most patients, but the gross rises seen in one patient emphasise the need to monitor concurrent use well. Information about other tricyclic antidepressants seems to be lacking.

1. Wong SL, Cavanaugh J, Shi H, Awni WM, Granneman GR. Effects of divalproex sodium on amitriptyline and nortriptyline pharmacokinetics. *Clin Pharmacol Ther* (1996) 60, 48–53.
2. Pisani F, Primerano G, D'Agostino AA, Spina E, Fazio A. Valproic acid-amitriptyline interaction in man. *Ther Drug Monit* (1986) 8, 382–3.
3. Fu C, Katzman M, Goldbloom DS. Valproate/nortriptyline interaction. *J Clin Psychopharmacol* (1994) 14, 205–6.
4. Fehr C, Gründer G, Hiemke C, Dahmen N. Increase in serum clomipramine concentrations caused by valproate. *J Clin Psychopharmacol* (2000) 20, 493–4.
5. Joseph AB, Wroblewski BA. Potentially toxic serum concentrations of desipramine after discontinuation of valproic acid. *Brain Inj* (1993) 7, 463–5.
6. Bertschy G, Vandel S, Jounet JM, Allers G. Interaction valpromide-amitriptyline. Augmentation de la biodisponibilité de l'amitriptyline et de la nortriptyline par le valpromide. *Encephale* (1990) 16, 43–5.
7. Vandel S, Bertschy G, Jounet JM, Allers G. Valpromide increases the plasma concentrations of amitriptyline and its metabolite nortriptyline in depressive patients. *Ther Drug Monit* (1988) 10, 386–9.

Tricyclic antidepressants + Venlafaxine

Venlafaxine can cause a marked increase in the anticholinergic adverse effects of clomipramine, desipramine and nortriptyline. There are isolated reports of seizures in a patient taking venlafaxine and trimipramine and the serotonin syndrome in another patient on venlafaxine, amitriptyline and pethidine.

Clinical evidence

A 74-year-old man on venlafaxine 150 mg daily and thioridazine had his treatment changed to daily doses of venlafaxine 75 mg, **desipramine** 50 mg, haloperidol 500 micrograms and alprazolam 250 micrograms. Within 5 days he exhibited severe anticholinergic effects (acute confusion, delirium, stupor, urinary retention and paralytic ileus). He had previously had few problems with venlafaxine combined with haloperidol and alprazolam.[1] A 75-year-old man on haloperidol, alprazolam and venlafaxine developed urinary retention and became delirious when **desipramine** was added.[2] A woman on **nortriptyline** 20 mg and fluoxetine 20 mg daily with only mild anticholinergic effects developed much more severe effects (dry mouth, worsened constipation, blurred vision) over 4 weeks following the replacement of the fluoxetine by venlafaxine 75 mg daily.[3] A 73-year-old man on fluoxetine 20 mg and **nortriptyline** 20 mg daily developed constipation, blurred vision and a dry mouth within a week of starting venlafaxine. A 61-year-old man on **clomipramine** 150 mg daily similarly developed anticholinergic effects (dry mouth, constipation, urinary retention) within a week of starting to take venlafaxine. These adverse effects disappeared when the venlafaxine was stopped.[2]

A 69-year-old man with bipolar disorder, who had been taking venlafaxine up to 337.5 mg daily, thioridazine 25 mg at night, and sodium valproate 1.2 g daily for several months with no adverse motor symptoms, experienced extrapyramidal effects 3 to 4 days after the venlafaxine had been gradually replaced by **nortriptyline** 50 mg daily. Symptoms persisted despite withdrawal of thioridazine, but improved on reduction of the **nortriptyline** dosage to 20 mg daily.[4] The cause of the reaction was not known, but it was suggested that there may have been an interaction between venlafaxine and **nortriptyline** possibly modulated by thioridazine or sodium valproate.

A 25-year-old woman on venlafaxine 150 mg daily and **trimipramine** 50 mg daily for depression developed seizures within 11 days of the **trimipramine** dose being increased to 100 mg daily. Both drugs were stopped and the patient had no further seizures.[5]

There is also a report of the serotonin syndrome occurring in a 21-year-old patient when **amitriptyline** 10 mg at night was added to the range of medications she was receiving, which included venlafaxine 37.5 mg daily, pethidine (meperidine) 400 mg daily and fluconazole 200 mg daily.[6]

Mechanism

Not fully established but it is suggested that a possible major mechanism is that venlafaxine can inhibit the metabolism of these tricyclics by the cytochrome P450 isoenzyme CYP2D6, leading to an increase in their serum levels and a marked increase in their anticholinergic adverse effects.[2] Some of the patients were elderly, which may have increased their sensitivity to these adverse effects.

Both venlafaxine and trimipramine can cause seizures, although usually after overdose. Either a pharmacokinetic interaction involving inhibition of drug metabolism by the isoenzyme CYP2D6, or a pharmacodynamic interaction may have resulted in seizures.[5]

The serotonin syndrome has been reported in patients on venlafaxine, amitriptyline and pethidine alone or with other serotonergic drugs. All three can increase serotonergic activity by inhibition of serotonin re-uptake at presynaptic neurones. In addition this case is complicated by the fact that the metabolism of amitriptyline can be inhibited by fluconazole.[6] See also 'Tricyclic antidepressants + Azoles; Fluconazole', p.991.

Importance and management

Information appears to be limited to these reports, three of which are by the same author. The incidence is not known but if venlafaxine and any tricyclic antidepressant are given concurrently, be alert for any evidence of increased anticholinergic adverse effects. Although there appears to be only one report, the possibility of an increased risk of seizures with concurrent use should be borne in mind. It may be necessary to withdraw one or other of the two drugs. The report of the serotonin syndrome highlights the need for caution when one or more serotonergic drugs are given.

1. Benazzi F. Anticholinergic toxic syndrome with venlafaxine-desipramine combination. *Pharmacopsychiatry* (1998) 31, 36–7.
2. Benazzi F. Venlafaxine drug-drug interactions in clinical practice. *J Psychiatry Neurosci* (1998) 23, 181–2.
3. Benazzi F. Venlafaxine-fluoxetine-nortriptyline interaction. *J Psychiatry Neurosci* (1997) 22, 278–9.
4. Conforti D, Borgherini G, Fiorellini Bernardis LA, Magni G. Extrapyramidal symptoms associated with the adjunct of nortriptyline to a venlafaxine-valproic acid combination. *Int Clin Psychopharmacol* (1999) 14, 197–8.
5. Schlienger RG, Klink MH, Eggenberger C, Drewe J. Seizures associated with therapeutic doses of venlafaxine and trimipramine. *Ann Pharmacother* (2000) 34, 1402–5.
6. Dougherty JA, Young H, Shafi T. Serotonin syndrome induced by amitriptyline, meperidine, and venlafaxine. *Ann Pharmacother* (2002) 36, 1647–8.

Tricyclic antidepressants; Amitriptyline + Ethchlorvynol

Transient delirium has been attributed to the concurrent use of amitriptyline and ethchlorvynol,[1] but no details were given and there appear to be no other reports confirming this alleged interaction.

1. Hussar DA. Tabular compilation of drug interactions. *Am J Pharm* (1969) 141, 109–156.

Tricyclic antidepressants; Amitriptyline + Fenfluramine

Some say that concurrent use is safe and effective while others say that fenfluramine can cause depression and should therefore not be used when tricyclics are given for depression.

Clinical evidence, mechanism, importance and management

Exacerbation of depression has been seen in some patients given fenfluramine[1] and several cases of withdrawal depression have been observed in patients on amitriptyline and fenfluramine, following episodes of severe depression.[2] The manufacturers say that fenfluramine should not be used in patients with a history of depression or while being treated with antidepressants.[3] On the other hand it has also been claimed that fenfluramine can be used safely and effectively with tricyclic antidepressants.[4,5] One report describes a rise in the plasma levels of amitriptyline when fenfluramine 60 mg daily was given to patients on amitriptyline 150 mg daily.[6]

However, you should note that fenfluramine was widely withdrawn in 1997 because its use was found to be associated with a high incidence of abnormal echocardiograms indicating abnormal functioning of heart valves.

1. Gaind R. Fenfluramine (Ponderax) in the treatment of obese psychiatric out-patients. *Br J Psychiatry* (1969) 115, 963–4.
2. Harding T. Fenfluramine dependence. *BMJ* (1971) 3, 305.
3. ABPI Data Sheet Compendium, 1998–99 p 1307. Datapharm publications, London.
4. Pinder RM, Brogden RN, Sawyer PR, Speight TM, Avery GS. Fenfluramine: a review of its pharmacological properties and therapeutic efficacy in obesity. *Drugs* (1975) 10, 241–323.
5. Mason EC. Servier Laboratories Ltd. Personal Communication, February 1976.
6. Gunne L-M, Antonijevic S, Jonsson J. Effect of fenfluramine on steady state plasma levels of amitriptyline. *Postgrad Med J* (1975) 51 (Suppl 1), 117.

Tricyclic antidepressants; Amitriptyline + Furazolidone

A report describes the development of toxic psychosis, hyperactivity, sweating and hot and cold flushes in a woman on amitriptyline when given furazolidone with diphenoxylate and atropine.

Clinical evidence, mechanism, importance and management

A depressed woman taking daily doses of conjugated oestrogen substances 1.25 mg and amitriptyline 75 mg, was additionally given furazolidone 300 mg daily and diphenoxylate with atropine sulphate. Two days later she began to experience blurred vision, profuse perspiration followed by alternate chills and hot flushes, restlessness, motor activity, persecutory delusions, auditory hallucinations and visual illusions. The symptoms cleared within a day of stopping the furazolidone.[1] The reasons are not understood but the authors point out that furazolidone has MAO-inhibitory properties and that the symptoms were similar to those seen when the tricyclic antidepressants and MAOIs interact. However the MAO-inhibitory activity of furazolidone normally develops over several days. Whether the concurrent use of atropine and amitriptyline (both of which have anticholinergic activity) had some part to play in the reaction is uncertain. No firm conclusions can be drawn from this slim evidence, but prescribers should be aware of this case when considering the concurrent use of tricyclic antidepressants and furazolidone.

1. Aderhold RM and Muniz CE. Acute psychosis with amitriptyline and furazolidone. *JAMA* (1970) 213, 2080.

Tricyclic antidepressants; Amitriptyline + Sucralfate

Sucralfate causes a marked reduction in the absorption of amitriptyline.

Clinical evidence, mechanism, importance and management

When a single 75-mg dose of amitriptyline was taken by 6 healthy subjects with a single 1-g dose of sucralfate, the AUC of the amitriptyline was reduced by 50% (from 680 to 320 nanograms hours/ml).[1] Concurrent use should be monitored to confirm that the therapeutic effects of the antidepressant are not lost. An increase in the dosage may be needed. There seems to be nothing documented about other tricyclics.

1. Ryan R, Carlson J, Farris F. Effect of sucralfate on the absorption and disposition of amitriptyline in humans. *Fedn Proc* (1986) 45, 205.

Tricyclic antidepressants; Clomipramine + Ademetionine

A severe reaction, diagnosed as the serotonin syndrome, developed in a woman on ademetionine shortly after her clomipramine dosage was raised.

Clinical evidence, mechanism, importance and management

An elderly woman with a major affective disorder was treated with intramuscular ademetionine 100 mg daily and clomipramine 25 mg daily for 10 days. About 2 to 3 days after the clomipramine dosage was raised to 75 mg daily, she became progressively agitated, anxious and confused. On admission to hospital she was stuporous, with a pulse rate of 130 bpm, a respiratory rate of 30 breaths per minute, and she had diarrhoea, myoclonus, generalised tremors, rigidity, hyperreflexia, shivering, profound diaphoresis and dehydration. Her temperature rose from 40.5 to 43°C. She had no infection, and the diagnosis was of serotonin syndrome (see 'Additive or synergistic interactions', (p.9) for more information about the serotonin syndrome). The drugs were withdrawn and she was given dantrolene 50 mg intravenously every 6 hours for 48 hours. She made a complete recovery.[1] The reason for this severe adverse reaction is not understood.

1. Iruela LM, Minguez L, Merino J, Monedero G. Toxic interaction of *S*-adenosylmethionine and clomipramine. *Am J Psychiatry* (1993) 150, 522.

Tricyclic antidepressants; Clomipramine + Modafinil

Clomipramine serum levels were reported to be increased by modafinil in one patient. However, a study found no pharmacokinetic interaction.

Clinical evidence, mechanism, importance and management

In a placebo-controlled crossover study, 18 patients were given a single 50-mg dose of clomipramine on day 1 and modafinil 200 mg daily on days 1 to 3. No pharmacokinetic changes were found to have occurred with either of the two drugs.[1] However, a single case report describes a patient on clomipramine 75 mg daily who showed a rise in serum clomipramine and desmethylclomipramine levels when modafinil 200 mg was added.[2] It was suggested that she had low levels of the cytochrome P450 isoenzyme CYP2D6 (a 'poor metaboliser') so that the additional inhibition of CYP2C19 by modafinil resulted in elevated serum levels.

Information about other tricyclic antidepressants is lacking, but the makers of modafinil point out that other poor metabolisers (about 7 to 10% of the Caucasian population) may possibly also show increased serum tricyclic antidepressant levels in the presence of modafinil.[3] Therefore monitoring concurrent use would seem to be a prudent precaution.

1. Wong YN, Gorman S, Simcoe D, McCormick GC, Grebow P. A double-blind placebo-controlled crossover study to investigate the kinetics and acute tolerability of modafinil and clomipramine alone and in combination in healthy male volunteers. Association of Professional Sleep Societies meeting, San Francisco, June 1997, Abstract 117.
2. Grözinger M, Härtter S, Hiemke C, Griese E-U, Röschke J. Interaction of modafinil and clomipramine as comedication in a narcoleptic patient. *Clin Neuropharmacol* (1998) 21, 127–9.
3. Provigil (Modafinil). Cephalon Inc. US Prescribing information, December 2004.

Tricyclic antidepressants; Desipramine + Methadone

Methadone can double the serum levels of desipramine.

Clinical evidence

The mean serum levels of desipramine 2.5 mg/kg daily were approximately doubled in 5 men after they took methadone 500 micrograms/kg daily for 2 weeks. Previous observations in patients given both drugs had shown that desipramine levels were higher than expected and desipramine side-effects developed at relatively low doses.[1]

Further evidence of an increase in plasma desipramine levels due to **methadone** is described in another study.[2]

Mechanism

Not understood. It is suggested that the methadone may possibly inhibit the hydroxylation of the desipramine, thereby reducing its loss from the body.[2]

Importance and management

Information seems to be limited to these two studies but the interaction would seem to be established. Monitor the effects of concurrent use and anticipate the need to reduce the desipramine dosage. There seems to be nothing reported about the effects of methadone on other tricyclic antidepressants.

1. Maany I, Dhopesh V, Arndt IO, Burke W, Woody G, O'Brien CP. Increase in desipramine serum levels associated with methadone treatment. *Am J Psychiatry* (1989) 146, 1611–13.
2. Kosten TR, Gawin FH, Morgan C, Nelson JC, Jatlow P. Desipramine and its 2-hydroxy metabolite in patients taking or not taking methadone. *Am J Psychiatry* (1990) 147, 1379–80.

Tricyclic antidepressants; Desipramine + Propafenone

An isolated report describes markedly raised serum desipramine levels in a patient who also took propafenone.

Clinical evidence, mechanism, importance and management

A man with major depression responded well to desipramine 175 mg daily with serum desipramine levels in the range 500 to 1000 nanomol/l. When he was treated for paroxysmal atrial fibrillation with digoxin 250 micrograms daily and propafenone 150 mg twice daily and 300 mg at night he developed markedly elevated serum desipramine levels (2092 nanomol/l) and toxicity (dry mouth, sedation, shakiness) while taking desipramine 150 mg daily. The adverse effects resolved when the desipramine was stopped for 5 days, but when it was restarted at 75 mg daily his serum desipramine levels were still raised (1130 nanomol/l).

The raised desipramine levels are thought to result from decreased metabolism and clearance, caused by propafenone.[1] The general importance of this case is uncertain, but be alert for signs of desipramine toxicity in any patient given propafenone concurrently. Adjust the desipramine dosage appropriately.

1. Katz MR. Raised serum levels of desipramine with the antiarrhythmic propafenone. *J Clin Psychiatry* (1991) 52, 432–3.

Tricyclic antidepressants; Doxepin + Tamoxifen

An isolated report describes a reduction in doxepin serum levels attributed to the concurrent use of tamoxifen.

Clinical evidence, mechanism, importance and management

A 79-year-old woman with a long history of bipolar (manic-depressive) disorder, stabilised on lithium carbonate and doxepin 200 mg at bedtime and also taking propranolol, was additionally started on tamoxifen 20 mg daily after a mastectomy for breast cancer. It was noted that her total blood levels of doxepin and its major metabolite were reduced about 25% over the next 11 months. The control of her depression remained unchanged. The reasons for this apparent interaction are not known.[1] The makers of tamoxifen have another undetailed and isolated report of a possible interaction.[2]

This appears to be the first and only clear report of an interaction between a tricyclic antidepressant and tamoxifen so that its general importance is not known.

1. Jefferson JW. Tamoxifen-associated reduction in tricyclic antidepressant levels in blood. *J Clin Psychopharmacol* (1995) 15, 223–4.
2. Zeneca, Personal communication. November 1995.

Tricyclic antidepressants; Imipramine + Beta-blockers

Propranolol increased the plasma imipramine levels in two children. Labetalol has been found to increase plasma imipramine levels in adults. The clinical importance of these interactions is uncertain.

Clinical evidence

(a) Labetalol

After taking 200 mg of labetalol 12-hourly for four days, the AUC of a single 100-mg dose of imipramine in 13 healthy subjects was increased by 53% compared with a placebo.[1] The maximum plasma level increased by 28%.

(b) Propranolol

A 9-year-old boy was given propranolol for the control of anger and aggression, and imipramine for stress and depression. When his imipramine dosage was raised from 60 to 80 mg daily and his propranolol from 360 to 400 mg daily, his imipramine/desipramine levels rose sharply from a total of 139 to 469 nanograms/ml. Reducing the imipramine to 60 mg and raising the propranolol to 440 mg daily only reduced the total imipramine/desipramine levels to 426 nanograms/ml. Another imipramine reduction to 40 mg and an increase in propranolol to 480 mg daily resulted in a final total imipramine/desipramine level of 207 nanograms/ml. No significant adverse effects or heart block occurred.[2]

A 9-year-old girl taking imipramine 75 mg daily with a total imipramine/desipramine level of 260 nanograms/ml, showed a marked rise to 408 nanograms/ml within three days of starting propranolol 10 mg three times daily. Two days after stopping the imipramine, her desipramine level (imipramine not measured) had fallen from 382 to 222 nanograms/ml.[2]

Mechanism

Uncertain. The suggestion is that these drugs compete for metabolism (hydroxylation) by the same cytochrome P450 isoenzymes (CYP2D6 and CYP2C8) in the liver, with imipramine being the 'loser', resulting in its accumulation in the body.[2]

Importance and management

Information seems to be limited to these two studies. The clinical importance of this interaction is uncertain, but it would now be prudent to monitor the outcome if propranolol or labetalol is added to treatment with imipramine. Ideally the plasma imipramine levels should be measured. There seems to be no information as yet about other beta-blockers or tricyclic antidepressants.

1. Hermann DJ, Krol TF, Dukes GE, Hussey EK, Danis M, Han Y-H, Powell JR, Hak LJ. Comparison of verapamil, diltiazem, and labetalol on the bioavailability and metabolism of imipramine. *J Clin Pharmacol* (1992) 32, 176–83.
2. Gillette DW, Tannery LP. Beta blocker inhibits tricyclic metabolism. *J Am Acad Child Adolesc Psychiatry* (1994) 33, 223–4.

Tricyclic antidepressants; Imipramine + Vinpocetine

Vinpocetine is reported not to affect plasma imipramine levels.

Clinical evidence, mechanism, importance and management

The steady-state plasma levels of **imipramine** 25 mg three times daily of 18 healthy subjects were unaffected by **vinpocetine** 10 mg three times daily, taken concurrently for 10 days.[1] No special precautions would seem to be necessary. There seems to be nothing documented about any of the other tricyclic antidepressants.

1. Hitzenberger G, Schmid R, Braun W, Grandt R. Vinpocetine therapy does not change imipramine pharmacokinetics in man. *Int J Clin Pharmacol Ther Toxicol* (1990) 28, 99–104.

Venlafaxine + Benzodiazepines

No important interaction normally appears to occur between venlafaxine and alprazolam or diazepam.

Clinical evidence, mechanism, importance and management

A double blind study in 18 healthy subjects taking venlafaxine 50 mg 8-hourly found that **diazepam** 10 mg did not impair the pharmacokinetics of venlafaxine or its major active metabolite (*O*-desmethylvenlafaxine), nor were the pharmacokinetics of the active metabolite of **diazepam** (**desmethyldiazepam**) affected. **Diazepam** affected the performance of a battery of pharmacodynamic tests, but the addition of venlafaxine had no further effects.[1]

A study in 16 healthy subjects found that venlafaxine 75 mg twice daily reduced the AUC of a single 2-mg oral dose of **alprazolam** by 29% and reduced its half-life by 21%, but the performance of some psychometric tests were only minimally changed.[2] These two studies suggest that no special precautions are necessary during the concurrent use of venlafaxine and these benzodiazepines.

1. Troy SM, Lucki I, Peirgies AA, Parker VD, Klockowski PM, Chiang ST. Pharmacokinetic and pharmacodynamic evaluation of the potential drug interaction between venlafaxine and diazepam. *J Clin Pharmacol* (1995) 35, 410–19.
2. Amchin J, Zarycranski W, Taylor KP, Albano D, Klockowski PM. Effect of venlafaxine on the pharmacokinetics of alprazolam. *Psychopharmacol Bull* (1998) 34, 211–19.

Venlafaxine + Cimetidine

Cimetidine does not appear to affect the pharmacokinetics of venlafaxine to a clinically significant extent.

Clinical evidence, mechanism, importance and management

Cimetidine 800 mg once daily for 5 days was found to reduce the oral clearance of venlafaxine 50 mg 8-hourly by 40%, and to increase the AUC by 62% in 18 healthy subjects. It had no effect on the formation or elimination of venlafaxine's major active metabolite (*O*-desmethylvenlafaxine; ODV). A composite of plasma concentrations for venlafaxine and ODV was found to be increased by only 13%. Thus the overall pharmacological activity of the two was only slightly increased by cimetidine[1] and no special precautions would seem to be necessary. However, the makers of venlafaxine suggest that the elderly and those with hepatic dysfunction may possibly show a more pronounced effect.[2,3]

1. Troy SM, Rudolph R, Mayersohn M, Chiang ST. The influence of cimetidine on the disposition kinetics of the antidepressant venlafaxine. *J Clin Pharmacol* (1998) 38, 467–74.
2. Efexor (Venlafaxine hydrochloride). Wyeth Pharmaceuticals. UK Summary of product characteristics, December 2004.
3. Effexor XR (Venlafaxine). Wyeth Pharmaceuticals Inc. US Prescribing information, January 2005.

Venlafaxine + Co-amoxiclav

An isolated case of the serotonin syndrome has been attributed to the concurrent use of venlafaxine and co-amoxiclav.

Clinical evidence, mechanism, importance and management

A 56-year-old man taking venlafaxine 37.5 mg twice daily for 10 months was given a course of co-amoxiclav (**amoxicillin** with **clavulanate**) 375 mg three times daily to treat gingivitis and a dental abscess. Within 3 hours of a dose of co-amoxiclav he developed tingling in the tip of his tongue, intense paraesthesia in the fingers, severe abdominal cramps, profuse diarrhoea, cold sweats, and uncontrollable shivering and tremor. He was also agitated and frightened, but not confused. The symptoms lasted for 6 hours and were initially assumed to be due to gastroenteritis. However, 2 months later while still on venlafaxine, he developed identical symptoms after a single dose of co-amoxiclav, which were then diagnosed as the serotonin syndrome. The patient had taken co-amoxiclav without problem when not taking venlafaxine and after the second episode continued venlafaxine without further episodes of the serotonin syndrome. Venlafaxine is metabolised mainly by the cytochrome P450 isoenzyme CYP2D6, but co-amoxiclav is not a substrate for this isoenzyme and its ability to inhibit CYP2D6 is not known. It is probable that many patients have received both venlafaxine and co-amoxiclav without adverse effects, so the general importance of this isolated report is unknown, but it seems likely to be small.[1]

1. Connor H. Serotonin syndrome after single doses of co-amoxiclav during treatment with venlafaxine. *J R Soc Med* (2003) 96, 233–4.

Venlafaxine + Dexamfetamine

An isolated case of the serotonin syndrome have been attributed to the concurrent use of dexamfetamine and venlafaxine.

Clinical evidence, mechanism, importance and management

A 32-year-old patient taking dexamfetamine 5 mg three times daily for adult attention deficit hyperactivity disorder presented with marked agitation, anxiety, shivering and tremor 2 weeks after also taking venlafaxine 75 mg to 150 mg daily. Other symptoms included generalised hypertonia, hyperreflexia, frequent myoclonic jerking, tonic spasm of the orbicularis oris muscle, and sinus tachycardia. His symptoms resolved completely when both drugs were withdrawn and cyproheptadine to a total dose of 32 mg over 3 hours was given. Dexamfetamine was restarted after 3 days. It was suggested that the combination of serotonin re-uptake blockade and either presynaptic release of serotonin or monoamine oxidase inhibition by dexamfetamine can cause increased serotonin in the CNS. Caution is advised when dexamfetamine is given with venlafaxine.[1]

1. Prior FH, Isbister GK, Dawson AH, Whyte IM. Serotonin toxicity with therapeutic doses of dexamphetamine and venlafaxine. *Med J Aust* (2002) 176, 240–1.

Venlafaxine + MAOIs

Serious and potentially life-threatening reactions (the serotonin syndrome) can develop if venlafaxine and non-selective, irreversible MAOIs (isocarboxazid, phenelzine, tranylcypromine) are given concurrently or even sequentially if insufficient time is left in between. The situation with the reversible, selective MAOI moclobemide, in therapeutic doses, is uncertain.

Clinical evidence

A. Irreversible non-selective MAOIs

(a) Isocarboxazid

A man with recurrent depression on isocarboxazid 30 mg daily was additionally given venlafaxine 75 mg. After the second dose he developed agitation, hypomania, diaphoresis, shivering and dilated pupils. These symptoms subsided when the venlafaxine was stopped. He subsequently developed myoclonic jerks and diaphoresis when given both drugs.[1]

(b) Phenelzine

A woman who had stopped taking phenelzine 45 mg daily 7 days previously, developed sweating, lightheadedness and dizziness within 45 minutes of taking a single 37.5-mg dose of venlafaxine. In the emergency department she was found to be lethargic, agitated and extremely diaphoretic. The agitation was treated with lorazepam. A week later, after she had recovered she was again started on the same regimen of venlafaxine without problems.[2] A man similarly developed the serotonin syndrome when he started venlafaxine the day after he stopped taking phenelzine.[3] A woman developed the serotonin syndrome within less than an hour of taking phenelzine and venlafaxine together,[4] and 4 other patients have been described who similarly developed the reaction when phenelzine was replaced by venlafaxine.[5]

Twelve days after an overdose of phenelzine (53 tablets of 15 mg) as well as benztropine, haloperidol and lorazepam, a 31-year-old man was started on venlafaxine 75 mg every 12 hours in addition to existing treatment with olanzapine and diazepam. About an hour after the first dose, he developed leg shakiness and stiffness, diaphoresis, blurred vision, difficulty breathing, chills, nausea and palpitations. Venlafaxine and olanzapine were discontinued and the man recovered within 24 hours, after treatment with intravenous fluids, propranolol and paracetamol.[6]

(c) Tranylcypromine

A woman who had been taking tranylcypromine for 3 weeks developed a serious case of the serotonin syndrome within 4 hours of inadvertently taking a single tablet of venlafaxine. She recovered within 24 hours when treated with ice packs, a cooling blanket, diazepam and dantrolene.[7] The serotonin syndrome developed in a man on tranylcypromine within 2 hours of taking half a venlafaxine tablet.[8]

B. Selective MAOIs

(a) Moclobemide

A 32-year-old man taking moclobemide 20 mg twice daily and diazepam developed the serotonin syndrome 40 minutes after taking a single 37.5-mg dose of venlafaxine.[9] Another man very rapidly developed the serotonin syndrome after taking considerable overdoses of moclobemide (3 g) and venlafaxine (2.625 g).[10]

(b) Selegiline

See 'Selegiline + Antidepressants', p.514 for the interactions between venlafaxine and selegiline.

Mechanism

The serotonin syndrome is thought to occur because venlafaxine can both inhibit serotonin re-uptake (its antidepressant activity is related to this activity) and because its metabolism is inhibited by MAOIs. The result is an increase in the concentrations of serotonin apparently causing overstimulation of the 5-HT_{1A} receptors in the brain and spinal cord.[11] For more about the serotonin syndrome see 'Additive or synergistic interactions', (p.9).

Importance and management

An established, serious and potentially life-threatening interaction. The makers of venlafaxine say that adverse reactions, some serious, have been seen in patients who had recently stopped taking an MAOI and started venlafaxine, or who had stopped venlafaxine and then started an MAOI. Some have been fatal.[11-13] They recommend that venlafaxine should not be used in combination with an MAOI or within 14 days of stopping treatment with the MAOI.[12,13] Based on the half-life of venlafaxine they say that at least 7 days should elapse between stopping venlafaxine and starting an MAOI. The makers do not distinguish in this recommendation between the irreversible older MAOIs and the newer, reversible, selective MAOIs such as moclobemide. In theory the latter are probably less likely to interact, however for the time being it would be prudent to take the same precautions recommended for the non-selective MAOIs. In one of the studies it was suggested that a wash-out period of several weeks is required between stopping MAOIs such as phenelzine and initiating a second serotonergic agent such as venlafaxine.[6]

1. Klysner R, Larsen JK, Sørensen P, Hyllested M, Pedersen BD. Toxic interaction of venlafaxine and isocarboxazide. *Lancet* (1995) 346, 1298–9.
2. Phillips SD, Ringo P. Phenelzine and venlafaxine interaction. *Am J Psychiatry* (1995) 152, 1400–1401.
3. Heisler MA, Guidry JR, Arnecke B. Serotonin syndrome induced by administration of venlafaxine and phenelzine. *Ann Pharmacother* (1996) 30, 84.
4. Weiner LA, Smythe M, Cisek J. Serotonin syndrome secondary to phenelzine-venlafaxine interaction. *Pharmacotherapy* (1998) 18, 399–403.
5. Diamond S, Pepper BJ, Diamond ML, Freitag FG, Urban GJ, Erdemoglu AK. Serotonin syndrome induced by transitioning from phenelzine to venlafaxine: four patient reports. *Neurology* (1998) 51, 274–6.
6. Mason PJ, Morris VA, Balcezak TJ. Serotonin syndrome. Presentation of 2 cases and review of the literature. *Medicine* (2000) 79, 201–9.
7. Hodgman M, Martin T, Dean B, Krenzelok E. Severe serotonin syndrome secondary to venlafaxine and maintenance tranylcypromine therapy. *J Toxicol Clin Toxicol* (1995) 33, 554.
8. Brubacher JR, Hoffman RS, Lurin MJ. Serotonin syndrome from venlafaxine-tranylcypromine interaction. *Vet Hum Toxicol* (1996) 38, 358–61.
9. Chan BSH, Graudins A, Whyte IM, Dawson AH, Braitberg G, Duggin GG. Serotonin syndrome resulting from drug interactions. *Med J Aust* (1998) 169, 523–5.
10. Roxanas MG, Machado JFD. Serotonin syndrome in combined moclobemide and venlafaxine ingestion. *Med J Aust* (1998) 168, 523–4.
11. Wyeth Laboratories. Personal communication, March 1995.
12. Efexor (Venlafaxine hydrochloride). Wyeth Pharmaceuticals. UK Summary of product characteristics, December 2004.
13. Effexor XR (Venlafaxine). Wyeth Pharmaceuticals Inc. US Prescribing information, January 2005.

Venlafaxine + Metoclopramide

An isolated case of the serotonin syndrome has been attributed to the concurrent use of metoclopramide and venlafaxine.

Clinical evidence, mechanism, importance and management

A 32-year-old woman with depression who had been taking venlafaxine 225 mg daily in divided doses for 3 years was admitted to hospital after a fall. She developed a movement disorder and a period of unresponsiveness after being given a 10-mg intravenous dose of metoclopramide. After a second dose of metoclopramide the symptoms recurred and were associated with confusion, agitation, fever, diaphoresis, tachypnoea, tachycardia, and hypertension. The symptoms were consistent with the serotonin syndrome, with a serious extrapyramidal movement disorder. The venlafaxine was withheld and she was given diazepam. The symptoms resolved over the next two days, after which she continued to take venlafaxine.[1] Information seems to be limited to this report, and the general significance of this interaction is unclear.

1. Fisher AA, Davis MW. Serotonin syndrome caused by selective serotonin reuptake-inhibitors–metoclopramide interaction. *Ann Pharmacother* (2002) 36, 67–71.

Venlafaxine + Miscellaneous

No important interactions normally appear to occur with venlafaxine and ACE inhibitors, beta-blockers, diuretics, hypoglycaemic agents or oral contraceptives. Some caution is thought appropriate with triptans.

Clinical evidence, mechanism, importance and management

(a) Antidiabetics

During clinical trials, 18 diabetic patients took venlafaxine and hypoglycaemic agents (not specifically named). There was a slightly higher incidence of adverse effects (nausea, somnolence, dry mouth, confusion, insomnia, impotence, decreased libido) but the makers say there was no reason to suggest that an interaction occurred.[1] Information is clearly still very limited but there is nothing to suggest that special precautions are necessary during concurrent use.

(b) Antihypertensives

During the phase II and III clinical trials of venlafaxine, 267 patients were also taking antihypertensive medications (**beta-blockers**, **diuretics**, **ACE-inhibitors**, etc.). Specific drugs were not named in the report.[1] There was nothing to suggest that adverse interactions of any kind occurred, but no pharmacokinetic studies were undertaken.[1]

(c) Contraceptives, oral

The makers of venlafaxine say that no systematic studies have been carried out on a possible interaction with oral contraceptives, but during the phase II and phase III clinical trials several women were taking oral contraceptives, and the inference to be drawn is that no problems arose.[2] In effect nobody yet really knows whether they interact, but they appear not to do so.

(d) Triptans

The makers caution the use of drugs that affect serotonergic transmission, such as the triptans.[3,4] This is because of the possible risks of the serotonin syndrome. For more about the serotonin syndrome see 'Additive or synergistic interactions', (p.9).

(e) Other drugs

Other *in vivo* and *in vitro* studies with venlafaxine have shown that it either does not, or only weakly inhibits the activity of the cytochrome P450 isoenzymes CYP2C9, CYP2D6, CYP1A2 and CYP3A3/4. This means that it is likely to be free, or largely free from clinically relevant drug-drug interactions due to changes (induction or inhibition) in drug metabolism.[5] However, some studies suggest that the metabolism of venlafaxine may be inhibited by drugs such as **diphenhydramine**, which are inhibitors of CYP2D6, especially in patients who are extensive metabolisers (i.e. have normal levels) of this isoenzyme.[6-8]

1. Wyeth Laboratories. Data on file (Study S).
2. Wyeth Laboratories. Personal communication, March 1995.
3. Efexor (Venlafaxine hydrochloride). Wyeth Pharmaceuticals. UK Summary of product characteristics, December 2004.
4. Effexor XL (Venlafaxine). Wyeth Pharmaceuticals Inc. US Prescribing information, January 2005.
5. Ereshefsky L. Drug-drug interactions involving antidepressants: focus on venlafaxine. *J Clin Psychopharmacol* (1996) 16 (Suppl 2), 37S–50S.
6. Lessard E, Yessine MA, Hamelin BA, Gauvin C, Labbe L, O'Hara G, LeBlanc J, Turgeon J. Diphenhydramine alters the disposition of venlafaxine through inhibition of CYP2D6 activity in humans. *J Clin Psychopharmacol* (2001) 21, 175–84.
7. Eap CB, Bertel-Laubscher R, Zullino D, Amey M, Baumann P. Marked increase of venlafaxine enantiomer concentrations as a consequence of metabolic interactions: A case report. *Pharmacopsychiatry* (2000) 33, 112–15.
8. Fogelman S, Schmider J, Greenblatt DJ, Shader RI. Inhibition of venlafaxine metabolism in vitro by index inhibitors and by SSRI antidepressants. *Clin Pharmacol Ther* (1997) 61, 181.

Venlafaxine + Propafenone

An isolated report describes psychosis in a patient during concurrent treatment with venlafaxine and propafenone.

Clinical evidence, mechanism, importance and management

A 67-year-old woman with bipolar disorder treated with venlafaxine 300 mg daily experienced symptoms of paranoia, visual hallucinations and marked confusion, about 2 weeks after starting propafenone 600 mg daily for intermittent atrial fibrillation. Serum levels of venlafaxine had increased from 85 nanograms/ml to 520 nanograms/ml (upper level of normal range 150 nanograms/ml) and levels of the metabolite O-desmethylvenlafaxine had increased but were still within normal ranges. Venlafaxine was stopped for a few days then restarted at the lower dose of 75 mg daily and her mental condition (diagnosed as organic psychosis) improved. However, as she also had orthostatic hypotension her propafenone dosage was subsequently reduced to 300 mg daily, which necessitated dosage adjustments of venlafaxine because of a marked drop in serum level. When propafenone was again increased to 600 mg daily the venlafaxine had to be reduced to 50 mg daily.[1] The reasons for the interaction are not known. Information is limited to this single case report, but bear this interaction in mind in the case of an unexpected response to treatment.

1. Pfeffer F, Grube M. An organic psychosis due to a venlafaxine-propafenone interaction. *Int J Psychiatry Med* (2001) 31, 427–32.

Venlafaxine + SSRIs

Anticholinergic side-effects can develop in patients on fluoxetine when venlafaxine is added. The serotonin syndrome developed in one patient when fluoxetine was stopped and venlafaxine started, and in another when paroxetine was stopped and venlafaxine started.

Clinical evidence

(a) Anticholinergic adverse effects

A woman on **fluoxetine** 20 mg and clonazepam 1 mg daily developed blurred vision, dry mouth, constipation, dizziness, insomnia and a hand tremor within a week of additionally starting venlafaxine 37.5 mg daily. These symptoms worsened by the second week and persisted until the venlafaxine was stopped.[1,2]

Four patients aged 21, 24, 51 and 70 on **fluoxetine** developed anticholinergic adverse effects (constipation, blurred vision, urinary retention and dry mouth) within a week of adding venlafaxine, which persisted until the venlafaxine was stopped.[3] A 61-year-old man on **fluoxetine** 20 mg daily had extreme difficulty in urinating within 2 days of additionally starting to take venlafaxine 37.5 mg daily. The effect became intolerable after 10 days but no other obvious anticholinergic adverse effects (blurred vision, constipation, dry mouth, tachycardia) were seen. This patient had some prostate enlargement and had previously had some moderate urinary problems when treated with **fluoxetine** and nortriptyline.[2,4]

(b) Serotonin syndrome

A 39-year-old woman with depression and panic attacks was treated with cimetidine, trazodone, clonazepam and **fluoxetine**. Within 24 hours of abruptly stopping the latter two drugs and starting lorazepam and venlafaxine, she developed the serotonin syndrome (diaphoresis, tremors, slurred speech, myoclonus, restlessness and diarrhoea).[5]

A 21-year-old woman whose long-term treatment with **paroxetine** was stopped a week before starting venlafaxine (37.5 mg daily for 5 days then 75 mg daily for 2 days) developed vomiting, dizziness, incoordination, falling, anxiety and electric shock sensations in her arms and legs within 3 days of starting venlafaxine. She stopped venlafaxine after 7 days of treatment, but symptoms persisted for 5 days until treated with cyproheptadine.[6]

Mechanism

One possible explanation is that fluoxetine inhibits the cytochrome P450 isoenzyme CYP2D6, which is concerned with the metabolism of venlafaxine, leading to an increase in its serum levels and in its usually minimal anticholinergic adverse effects.[1-4] An alternative explanation is that these adverse effects are due to an adrenergic mechanism.[4] For more about the serotonin syndrome see 'Additive or synergistic interactions', (p.9).

Importance and management

Information about the adverse anticholinergic syndrome due to a fluoxetine/venlafaxine interaction seems to be limited to these reports, all by the same author. The incidence is not known, but if venlafaxine and fluoxetine are given concurrently, be alert for any evidence of increased anticholinergic adverse effects. It may be necessary to withdraw one or other of the two drugs. You should also be aware that the development of the serotonin syndrome has been attributed to the sequential use of fluoxetine and venlafaxine in one patient, and paroxetine and venlafaxine in another. The makers of venlafaxine caution its use with other drugs that affect serotonergic transmission, such as the SSRIs[7,8] because of the potential risks of the serotonin syndrome.

1. Benazzi F. Severe anticholinergic side effects with venlafaxine-fluoxetine combination. *Can J Psychiatry* (1997) 42, 980–1.
2. Benazzi F. Venlafaxine-fluoxetine interaction. *J Clin Psychopharmacol* (1999) 19, 96–8.
3. Benazzi F. Venlafaxine drug-drug interactions in clinical practice. *J Psychiatry Neurosci* (1998) 23, 181–2.
4. Benazzi F. Urinary retention with venlafaxine-fluoxetine combination. *Hum Psychopharmacol* (1998) 13, 139–40.
5. Bhatara VS, Magnus RD, Paul KL, Preskorn SH. Serotonin syndrome induced by venlafaxine and fluoxetine: a case study in polypharmacy and potential pharmacodynamic and pharmacokinetic mechanisms. *Ann Pharmacother* (1998) 32, 432–6.
6. Chan BSH, Graudins A, Whyte IM, Dawson AH, Braitberg G, Duggin GG. Serotonin syndrome resulting from drug interactions. *Med J Aust* (1998) 169, 523–5.
7. Effexor XL (Venlafaxine). Wyeth Pharmaceuticals Inc. US Prescribing information, January 2005.
8. Efexor (Venlafaxine hydrochloride). Wyeth Pharmaceuticals. UK Summary of product characteristics, December 2004.

35

Miscellaneous drugs

Acamprosate + Miscellaneous

Acamprosate does not interact with alcohol, barbiturates, diazepam, disulfiram, imipramine, meprobamate, or oxazepam.

Clinical evidence, mechanism, importance and management

A 15-day study in 591 patients, to assess the effects of the concurrent use of acamprosate with other drugs commonly used in the management of alcohol withdrawal, found no evidence of additional adverse effects with **meprobamate**, **oxazepam**, or the barbiturate complex **tetrabamate** (that includes **phenobarbital**).[1] Other studies found that acamprosate caused no clinically relevant changes in **imipramine** pharmacokinetics; **disulfiram** did not alter acamprosate pharmacokinetics; and the pharmacokinetics of both **alcohol** and acamprosate and **diazepam** and acamprosate were unchanged by concurrent use.[2]

No special precautions would therefore appear to be needed with any of these drugs.

1. Aubin HJ, Lehert P, Beaupère B, Parot P, Barrucand D. Tolerability of the combination of acamprosate with drugs used to prevent alcohol withdrawal syndrome. *Alcoholism* (1995) 31, 25–38.
2. Saivin S, Hulot T, Chabac S, Potgieter A, Durbin P, Houin G. Clinical pharmacokinetics of acamprosate. *Clin Pharmacokinet* (1998) 35, 331–45.

Allopurinol + Aluminium hydroxide

Three haemodialysis patients showed a marked reduction in the effects of allopurinol while concurrently taking aluminium hydroxide. Separating the doses by 3 hours reduced the effects of this interaction.

Clinical evidence

Three patients on chronic haemodialysis, taking 5.7 g of aluminium hydroxide daily and allopurinol 300 mg daily for high phosphate and uric acid levels, failed to show any fall in their hyperuricaemia until the aluminium hydroxide was given 3 hours before the allopurinol, whereupon their uric acid levels fell by 40 to 65%. When one patient again took both preparations together, her uric acid levels began to rise.[1]

Mechanism

Not understood, but aluminium/allopurinol binding resulting in impaired absorption seems likely.

Importance and management

Information seems to be limited to this report. Renal patients on large doses of aluminium should be advised to separate the administration of these two drugs by 3 hours or more to avoid admixture in the gut. The effects of lower doses of aluminium and the effects in patients with normal renal function do not appear to have been studied. Monitor the outcome.

1. Weissman I, Krivoy N. Interaction of aluminum hydroxide and allopurinol in patients on chronic hemodialysis. *Ann Intern Med* (1987) 107, 787.

Allopurinol + Iron compounds

No adverse interaction occurs if iron and allopurinol are given concurrently.

Clinical evidence, mechanism, importance and management

Some early *animal* studies, where allopurinol was given in very large doses, suggested that allopurinol might have an inhibitory effect on the release of **iron** from hepatic stores. It was feared that this might result in hepatic iron overload. This led the makers of allopurinol in some countries to issue a warning about their concurrent use.[1] However, it appears that no special precautions are needed.[1-3]

1. Ascione FJ. Allopurinol and iron. *JAMA* (1975) 232, 1010.
2. Emmerson BT. Effects of allopurinol on iron metabolism in man. *Ann Rheum Dis* (1966) 25, 700–703.
3. Davis PS, Deller DJ. Effect of a xanthine-oxidase inhibitor (allopurinol) on radioiron absorption in man. *Lancet* (1966) ii, 470–2.

Allopurinol + Probenecid

The theoretical possibility of an adverse interaction between allopurinol and probenecid, which could lead to uric acid precipitation in the kidneys, appears not to occur in practice. Probenecid markedly increases the serum levels of allopurinol riboside, which may be advantageous in some circumstances.

Clinical evidence, mechanism, importance and management

(a) Allopurinol

Probenecid appears to increase the renal excretion of the active metabolite of allopurinol, oxipurinol,[1] while allopurinol is thought to inhibit the metabolism of probenecid.[2] Allopurinol can increase the half life and raise the serum plateau levels of probenecid by about 50 and 20% respectively.[2] It has been suggested that this might lead to an increase in the excretion of uric acid, which could result in the precipitation of uric acid in the kidneys. However, the clinical importance of these mutual interactions seems to be minimal. No problems were reported in two studies in patients given 100 to 600 mg of allopurinol and 500 to 2500 mg of probenecid daily for between 8 and 16 weeks.[3]

(b) Allopurinol riboside

A study in 3 healthy subjects found that probenecid halved the clearance, increased the peak plasma levels and AUC, and extended the half life of allopurinol riboside.[4] In some circumstances such an interaction may be advantageous as there is some evidence that the cure rate of American trypanosomiasis (Chagas' disease) and cutaneous leishmaniasis is better when the two drugs are used together.[4,5]

1. Elion GB, Yü T-F, Gutman AB, Hitchings GH. Renal clearance of oxipurinol, the chief metabolite of allopurinol. *Am J Med* (1968) 45, 69–77.
2. Horwitz D, Thorgeirsson SS, Mitchell JR. The influence of allopurinol and size of dose on the metabolism of phenylbutazone in patients with gout. *Eur J Clin Pharmacol* (1977) 12, 133–6.
3. Yü T-F, Gutman AB. Effect of allopurinol (4-hydroxypyrazolo(3,4-d)pyrimidine) on serum and urinary uric acid in primary and secondary gout. *Am J Med* (1964) 37, 885–98.
4. Were JBO, Shapiro TA. Effects of probenecid on the pharmacokinetics of allopurinol riboside. *Antimicrob Agents Chemother* (1993) 37, 1193–6.
5. Saenz RE, Paz HM, Johnson CM, Marr JJ, Nelson DJ, Pattishall KH, Rogers MD. Treatment of American cutaneous leishmaniasis with orally administered allopurinol riboside. *J Infect Dis* (1989) 160, 153–8.

Allopurinol + Tamoxifen

A single case report describes allopurinol hepatotoxicity in a man given tamoxifen.

Clinical evidence, mechanism, importance and management

An elderly man who had been on 300 mg of allopurinol daily for 12 years developed fever and marked increases in his serum levels of lactic dehydrogenase and alkaline phosphatase within a day of starting to take 10 mg of tamoxifen twice daily.[1] He rapidly recovered when the allopurinol was stopped. The reasons for the reaction are not understood, but the authors suggested that the increased hepatotoxic effect may have resulted from tamoxifen inhibiting allopurinol metabolism, thereby increasing the serum levels of allopurinol and its metabolite. The general importance of this isolated report is not known.

1. Shah KA, Levin J, Rosen N, Greenwald E, Zumoff B. Allopurinol hepatotoxicity potentiated by tamoxifen. *N Y State J Med* (1982) 82, 1745–6.

Allopurinol + Thiazide diuretics

Severe allergic reactions to allopurinol have been seen in a few patients also given thiazide diuretics in the presence of renal impairment.

Clinical evidence, mechanism, importance and management

Most patients tolerate allopurinol very well, but life-threatening hypersensitivity reactions (e.g. rash, vasculitis, hepatitis, eosinophilia, progressive renal impairment, etc.) develop very occasionally with doses of 200 to 400 mg of allopurinol daily.[1] A report of six such hypersensitivity reactions found that all of the reported cases were associated with pre-existing renal impairment, and in half of these, the patients were taking thiazide diuretics.[1] Another report describes two patients who developed a hypersensitivity vasculitis while taking allopurinol and **hydrochlorothiazide**.[2] The excretion of oxipurinol (the major metabolite of allopurinol) is impaired in renal failure, but studies indicate that in healthy subjects with normal renal function, thiazide diuretics, such as hydrochlorothiazide, do not appear to affect the plasma levels of oxipurinol or its excretion.[3,4] However, other studies have shown that the effects of allopurinol on pyrimidine metabolism are enhanced by the use of thiazides (i.e. they potentially increase hyperuricaemia, which may lead to renal damage).[5] Some caution is therefore appropriate if both drugs are used, particularly if renal function is abnormal, but more study is needed to confirm this possible interaction.

1. Hande KR, Noone RM, Stone WJ. Severe allopurinol toxicity. Description and guidelines for prevention in patients with renal insufficiency. *Am J Med* (1984) 76, 47–56.
2. Young JL, Boswell RB, Nies AS. Severe allopurinol hypersensitivity. Association with thiazides and prior renal compromise. *Arch Intern Med* (1974) 134, 553–8.
3. Hande KR. Evaluation of a thiazide-allopurinol drug interaction. *Am J Med Sci* (1986) 292, 213–16.
4. Löffler W, Landthaler R, de Vries JX, Walter-Sack I, Ittensohn A, Voss A, Zöllner N. Interaction of allopurinol and hydrochlorothiazide during prolonged oral administration of both drugs in normal subjects. I. Uric acid kinetics. *Clin Invest* (1994) 72, 1071–5.
5. Wood MH, O'Sullivan WJ, Wilson M, Tiller DJ. Potentiation of an effect of allopurinol on pyrimidine metabolism by chlorothiazide in man. *Clin Exp Pharmacol Physiol* (1974) 1, 53–8.

Alprostadil + Miscellaneous

Intracavernosal alprostadil and other drugs used for erectile dysfunction should not be given concurrently.

Clinical evidence, mechanism, importance and management

There appear to be no published reports of adverse interactions between intracavernous alprostadil (prostaglandin E_1) and other drugs, but the makers say that smooth muscle relaxants such as **papaverine** and other drugs used to induce erections such as **alpha blocking drugs** (e.g. intracavernosal **phentolamine**, **thymoxamine**) should not be used concurrently because of the risks of priapism (painful prolonged abnormal erection).[1]

1. Viridal Duo (Alprostadil). Schwarz Pharma Ltd. UK Summary of product characteristics, January 2005.

Aluminium hydroxide + Citrates or Vitamin C (Ascorbic acid)

Patients with renal failure, given aluminium and oral citrate, can develop a potentially fatal encephalopathy due to a very marked rise in blood aluminium levels. There is evidence that vitamin C may interact similarly. Some also suggest that those with normal renal function should not take aluminium antacids within 2 to 3 hours of foods and drinks that contain citrates. It is worth noting that formulations of a wide-range of drugs (including many non-prescription preparations) contain citrates as the effervescing or dispersing agent.

Clinical evidence

(a) Citrates

Following the death of 4 renal patients due to hyperaluminaemia, possibly exacerbated by the concurrent use of aluminium hydroxide and citrate (**Shohl's**) solution,[1,2] a study was conducted in 34 renal patients and 5 healthy subjects to assess the possibility of an interaction.[2] It was found that in the patients, increased serum aluminium levels were correlated with increased citrate intake. In the healthy subjects, aluminium levels were 11 micrograms/l at baseline, rising to 44 micrograms/l on the administration of aluminium hydroxide, and rising to 98 micrograms/l when citrate was given concurrently. It was also found that aluminium clearance had dramatically increased in the presence of citrate.[2] Patients with renal failure are unlikely to be able to increase renal aluminium clearance, and so the effect of citrate in patients may be even more dramatic. Another report claims to have noticed this interaction in another 8 renal patients, all of whom died.[3]

A tenfold rise in serum aluminium levels that occurred in a haemodialysis patient given **effervescent co-codamol**, was attributed to the presence of sodium citrate in the formulation, which is used to produce the effervescence.[4]

(b) Vitamin C (Ascorbic acid)

A study in 13 healthy subjects given aluminium hydroxide 900 mg three times daily found that vitamin C 2 g daily increased the urinary excretion of aluminium threefold.[5] Ascorbic acid significantly increases the concentration of aluminium in the liver, brain, and bones of *rats* given aluminium hydroxide.[6]

Mechanism

Studies in healthy subjects clearly demonstrate that citrate markedly increases the absorption of aluminium from the gut.[2,7,8] The absorption is increased threefold if taken with lemon juice,[9] eight to tenfold if taken with orange juice,[10,11] and five to fiftyfold if taken with citrate,[2,7,8,10] but the reason is not understood. It could be that a highly soluble aluminium citrate complex is formed.[3,7]

Importance and management

(a) Patients with renal impairment

The aluminium/citrate interaction in patients with renal failure is established and clinically important. It is potentially fatal. Concurrent use should be strictly avoided. The authors of one report emphasise the risks associated with any of the commonly used citrates (sodium, calcium or potassium citrates, citric acid, Shohl's solution (citric acid/sodium citrate), etc).[7] Remember too that some effervescent and dispersible tablets (including many proprietary non-prescription analgesics, indigestion and hangover remedies such as *Alka-Seltzer*) contain citric acid or citrates,[4,12] and they may also occur in soft drinks.[12] Haemodialysis patients should be strongly warned about these. The aluminium/vitamin C interaction is not yet well established, but the information available so far suggests that this combination should also be avoided. It is not clear whether orange juice is also unsafe but the available evidence suggests that concurrent administration is probably best avoided.

(b) Patients with normal renal function

The importance of the aluminium/citrate interaction in subjects with normal renal function is by no means clear, because it is still not known whether increased aluminium absorption results in aluminium accumulation over the long term, in those with normal renal function.[11] However, some authors have recommended that food or drinks containing citric acid (citrus fruits and fruit juices) should not be taken at the same time as aluminium-containing medicines, but that their ingestion should be separated by 2 to 3 hours.[11]

1. Bakir AA, Hryhorczuk DO, Berman E, Dunea G. Acute fatal hyperaluminemic encephalopathy in undialyzed and recently dialyzed uremic patients. *Trans Am Soc Artif Intern Organs* (1986) 32, 171–6.
2. Bakir AA, Hryhorczuk DO, Ahmed S, Hessl SM, Levy PS, Spengler R, Dunea G. Hyperaluminemia in renal failure: the influence of age and citrate intake. *Clin Nephrol* (1989) 31, 40–4.
3. Kirschbaum HB, Schoolwerth AC. Acute aluminum toxicity associated with oral citrate and aluminum-containing antacids. *Am J Med Sci* (1989) 297, 9–11.
4. Main J, Ward MK. Potentiation of aluminium absorption by effervescent analgesic tablets in a haemodialysis patient. *BMJ* (1992) 304, 1686.
5. Domingo JL, Gomez M, Llobet JM, Richart C. Effect of ascorbic acid on gastrointestinal aluminium absorption. *Lancet* (1991) 338, 1467.
6. Domingo JL, Gomez M, Llobet JM, Corbella J. Influence of some dietary constituents on aluminum absorption and retention in rats. *Kidney Int* (1991) 39, 598–601.
7. Coburn JW, Mischel MG, Goodman WG, Salusky IB. Calcium citrate markedly enhances aluminum absorption from aluminium hydroxide. *Am J Kidney Dis* (1991) 17, 708–11.
8. Walker JA, Sherman RA, Cody RP. The effect of oral bases on enteral aluminum absorption. *Arch Intern Med* (1990) 150, 2037–9.
9. Slanina P, Frech W, Ekström L-G, Lööf L, Slorach S, Cedergren A. Dietary citric acid enhances absorption of aluminum in antacids. *Clin Chem* (1986) 32, 539–41.
10. Weberg R, Berstad A. Gastrointestinal absorption of aluminium from single doses of aluminium containing antacids in man. *Eur J Clin Invest* (1986) 16, 428–32.
11. Fairweather-Tait S, Hickson K, McGaw B, Reid M. Orange juice enhances aluminium absorption from antacid preparation. *Eur J Clin Nutr* (1994) 48, 71–3.
12. Dorhout Mees EJ, Başçi A. Citric acid in calcium effervescent tablets may favour aluminium intoxication. *Nephron* (1991) 59, 322.

Aprepitant + CYP2C9 enzyme substrates

Aprepitant slightly reduced plasma levels of 'warfarin', (p.265) and 'tolbutamide' (p.421), because it is an inducer of the cytochrome P450 isoenzyme CYP2C9. The makers therefore recommend caution when aprepitant is given with other drugs that are known to be metabolised by CYP2C9, because of the possibility of lower plasma levels of these drugs.[1,2] They specifically mention phenytoin.[1,2] Other CYP2C9 substrates are listed in 'Table 1.3', (p.6). However, note that the UK maker strongly advises avoiding the concurrent use of phenytoin, since this is expected to markedly reduce aprepitant levels.[1]

1. Emend (Aprepitant). Merck Sharp & Dohme Ltd. UK Summary of product characteristics, April 2005.
2. Emend (Aprepitant). Merck & Co., Inc. US Prescribing information, March 2005.

Aprepitant + CYP3A4 enzyme substrates

Aprepitant can increase the levels of CYP3A4 substrates in the short-term, then reduce them within 2 weeks. Caution is advised. Note that the makers of aprepitant specifically contraindicate its concurrent use with pimozide, terfenadine, astemizole or cisapride.

Clinical evidence, mechanism, importance and management

In the first few days of use, aprepitant markedly increased levels of midazolam, a probe drug substrate for the cytochrome P450 isoenzyme CYP3A4. Then, within 2 weeks a reduction in levels was seen, see 'Benzodiazepines + Aprepitant', p.540. Aprepitant is therefore both an inhibitor and an inducer of CYP3A4.

Because of this, aprepitant is expected to increase drug levels of other CYP3A4 substrates during treatment by up to about threefold, and the maker recommends caution.[1,2] They specifically recommend caution with **ergot derivatives**. Moreover, because of the risk of life-threatening torsade de points arrhythmias with increased levels of **pimozide**, **terfenadine**, **astemizole** or **cisapride**, they specifically contraindicate the concurrent use of aprepitant with these CYP3A4 substrates. For a list of CYP3A4 substrates, see 'Table 1.4', (p.6). See also 'antineoplastics', (p.451), 'corticosteroids', (p.802), 'contraceptives', (p.757), and 'calcium channel blockers', (p.651).

Within 2 weeks of aprepitant therapy, a reduced level of CYP3A4 substrates might occur, and caution is also advised during this time.

1. Emend (Aprepitant). Merck Sharp & Dohme Ltd. UK Summary of product characteristics, April 2005.
2. Emend (Aprepitant). Merck & Co., Inc. US Prescribing information, March 2005.

Aprepitant + Ketoconazole and other CYP3A4 enzyme inhibitors

Ketoconazole markedly increases aprepitant levels. The maker recommends caution when aprepitant is used with ketoconazole or other strong inhibitors of CYP3A4.

Clinical evidence, mechanism, importance and management

The makers note that when a single 125-mg dose of aprepitant was given on day 5 of a 10-day regimen of ketoconazole 400 mg daily, the AUC of aprepitant was increased by about fivefold, and the half-life by about threefold.[1,2]

Ketoconazole is an inhibitor of the cytochrome P450 isoenzyme CYP3A4, by which aprepitant is metabolised.

Although the effects of these increases has not been assessed, such marked increases in levels could increase adverse effects. The makers recommend caution when aprepitant is given with ketoconazole and other drugs that are strong inhibitors of CYP3A4. They specifically name **ritonavir**, **clarithromycin**,[1,2] **telithromycin**,[1] **itraconazole**, **nefazodone**, **troleandomycin**, and **nelfinavir**.[2] For the effect of diltiazem (a moderate CYP3A4 inhibitor), see 'Calcium channel blockers + Aprepitant', p.651. Other inhibitors of CYP3A4 are listed in 'Table 1.4', (p.6).

1. Emend (Aprepitant). Merck Sharp & Dohme Ltd. UK Summary of product characteristics, April 2005.
2. Emend (Aprepitant). Merck & Co., Inc. US Prescribing information, March 2005.

Aprepitant + Rifampicin (Rifampin) and CYP3A4 enzyme inducers

Rifampicin markedly reduced the AUC of aprepitant, and reduced efficacy would be expected. In the UK, the maker recommends that concurrent use of aprepitant and other strong inducers of CYP3A4 should be avoided.

Clinical evidence, mechanism, importance and management

The makers note that when a single 375-mg dose of aprepitant was given on day 9 of a 14-day regimen of rifampicin 600 mg daily, the AUC of aprepitant was decreased about 11-fold (91%), and the half-life about threefold (68%).[1,2]

Rifampicin is an inducer of the cytochrome P450 isoenzyme CYP3A4, by which aprepitant is metabolised.

Although not assessed, this marked reduction in aprepitant levels could result in reduced efficacy. In the UK, the maker recommends that concurrent use of aprepitant and strong inducers of CYP3A4 such as rifampicin be avoided.[1] They also name **phenytoin** (but see also 'Aprepitant + CYP2C9 enzyme substrates', above), **carbamazepine**, and **phenobarbital**, and also recommend that concurrent use of **St John's wort** is avoided.[1] Other inducers of CYP3A4 are listed in 'Table 1.4', (p.6).

1. Emend (Aprepitant). Merck Sharp & Dohme Ltd. UK Summary of product characteristics, April 2005.
2. Emend (Aprepitant). Merck & Co., Inc. US Prescribing information, March 2005.

Baclofen + Ibuprofen

A man developed baclofen toxicity when given ibuprofen.

Clinical evidence, mechanism, importance and management

An isolated report describes a man taking baclofen 20 mg three times a day, who developed baclofen toxicity (confusion, disorientation, bradycardia, blurred vision, hypotension and hypothermia) after taking 8 doses of ibuprofen 600 mg three times daily. It appeared that the toxicity was caused by ibuprofen-induced acute renal insufficiency leading to baclofen accumulation.[1] Renal insufficiency is a relatively rare side-effect of ibuprofen. The general importance of this interaction is likely to be very small. There appears to be no information about baclofen and other NSAIDs, and little reason for avoiding concurrent use.

1. Dahlin PA, George J. Baclofen toxicity associated with declining renal clearance after ibuprofen. *Drug Intell Clin Pharm* (1984) 18, 805–8.

Baclofen + Tizanidine

No clinically significant pharmacokinetic interaction appears to occur between baclofen and tizanidine.

Clinical evidence, mechanism, importance and management

In a randomised three-period study, 15 healthy subjects were given baclofen 10 mg three times daily and tizanidine 4 mg three times daily, together and alone, for 7 consecutive doses. None of the pharmacokinetic parameters of either drug were changed by more than 30%, a figure calculated to indicate the presence of an interaction.[1] No changes in the dosages of either drug are therefore likely to be needed if they are taken concurrently.

1. Shellenberger MK, Groves L, Shah J, Novak GD. A controlled pharmacokinetic evaluation of tizanidine and baclofen at steady state. *Drug Metab Dispos* (1999) 27, 201–204.

Benzbromarone + Aspirin

Aspirin antagonises the uricosuric effects of benzbromarone.

Clinical evidence, mechanism, importance and management

A single dose of benzbromarone 160 mg increased the percent ratio of urate to creatinine clearance by 371% at its peak in 6 subjects with gout. However, when the same dose of benzbromarone was given with a single 600-mg dose of aspirin, the peak ratio of urate to creatinine clearance with benzbromarone 160 mg was reduced by about 75%.[1] In another study aspirin, in divided doses of 650 mg, up to a total of 5.2 g daily, was given to 29 healthy subjects on benzbromarone 40 to 80 mg daily. The urate lowering effects of benzbromarone were most affected by aspirin 2.7 g; alone, benzbromarone reduced the urate levels by 60%, but in the presence of aspirin 2.7 g the levels were only reduced by 48%.[2] Aspirin and other **salicylates** antagonise the effects of uricosuric drugs such as benzbromarone, and should generally be avoided in those with hyperuricaemia or gout (see also 'Aspirin or other Salicylates + Probenecid', p.82).

1. Sinclair DS, Fox IH. The pharmacology of hypouricemic effect of benzbromarone. *J Rheumatol* (1975) 2, 437–45.
2. Sorensen LB, Levinson DJ. Clinical evaluation of benzbromarone. *Arthritis Rheum* (1976) 19, 183–90.

Benzbromarone + Chlorothiazide

Benzbromarone lowers uric acid levels in those on chlorothiazide, without affecting diuretic activity.[1,2]

1. Heel RC, Brogden RN, Speight TM, Avery GS. Section 4.5 Effect on diuretic-induced hyperuricaemia. In: Benzbromarone: a review of its pharmacological properties and therapeutic use in gout and hyperuricaemia. *Drugs* (1977) 14, 349–66.
2. Gross A, Giraud V. Über die Wirkung von Benzbromaron auf Urikämie und Urikosurie. *Med Welt* (1972) 23, 133–6.

Benzbromarone + Pyrazinamide

Pyrazinamide commonly causes hyperuricaemia and may therefore antagonise the uricosuric effect of benzbromarone. Benzbromarone may have modest efficacy in reducing hyperuricaemia caused by pyrazinamide.

Clinical evidence, mechanism, importance and management

A single dose of pyrazinamide completely abolished the uricosuric effect of a single 160-mg dose of benzbromarone in 5 subjects with hyperuricaemia and gout.[1] Other authors also briefly mention the same finding.[2] However in another study, when benzbromarone 50 mg daily for 8 to 10 days was given to 10 patients taking 35 mg/kg pyrazinamide daily for tuberculosis, uric acid levels were reduced by an average of 24.3%, and returned to normal levels in four of them.[3] It is unclear from these studies whether or not pyrazinamide abolishes the uricosuric effects of benzbromarone. However, pyrazinamide commonly causes hyperuricaemia, and would be expected to antagonise the effects of uricosuric drugs such as benzbromarone, it should be avoided in patients with hyperuricaemia and gout (see also 'Pyrazinamide + Antigout drugs', p.227). Benzbromarone may have modest efficacy in reducing hyperuricaemia caused by pyrazinamide, but further study is necessary.

1. Sinclair DS, Fox IH. The pharmacology of hypouricemic effect of benzbromarone. *J Rheumatol* (1975) 2, 437–45.
2. Sorensen LB, Levinson DJ. Clinical evaluation of benzbromarone. *Arthritis Rheum* (1976) 19, 183–90.
3. Kropp R. Zur urikosurischen Wirkung von Benzbromaronum an Modell der pyrizinamidbedingten Hyperurikämie. *Med Klin* (1970) 65, 1448–50.

Betahistine + Terfenadine

A single report describes the re-emergence of labyrinthine symptoms in a patient taking betahistine when given terfenadine.

Clinical evidence, mechanism, importance and management

An isolated and very brief report describes a patient whose labyrinthine symptoms [vertigo, dizziness, nausea and vomiting], controlled by betahistine, returned during concurrent use of terfenadine and other unspecified drugs.[1] This interaction had been predicted on theoretical grounds because betahistine, being an analogue of histamine, would be expected to interact like this with any antihistamine.[2] The use of antihistamines should be carefully considered in patients taking betahistine.

1. Beeley L, Cunningham H, Brennan A. *Bulletin of the West Midlands Centre for Adverse Drug Reaction Reporting* (1993) 36, 28.
2. Serc (Betahistine). Solvay Healthcare Ltd. UK Summary of product characteristics, April 2003.

Bisphosphonates + Aspirin or NSAIDs

The concurrent use of alendronate and NSAIDs may possibly increase the risk of gastric mucosal damage, but this is not yet established. NSAIDs may exacerbate the renal dysfunction sometimes seen with clodronate. Indometacin raises tiludronate bioavailability. Aspirin and diclofenac do not appear to interact with tiludronate.

Clinical evidence, mechanism, importance and management

(a) Alendronate

A short-term study in 26 healthy subjects found that gastric ulcers developed in 8% of those given alendronate alone, in 12% of those given **naproxen** alone, and 38% of those given both drugs.[1] In a case-control study,[2] the risk of having an acid-related upper gastrointestinal disorder with alendronate was increased with concurrent use of NSAIDs (relative risk 1.7). However, analysis of data from a very large long-term placebo-controlled trial found no evidence that the risk of upper gastrointestinal adverse effects with concurrent use of NSAIDs and alendronate was any greater than with NSAIDs and placebo.[3] Note that this finding has been questioned,[4] and some of the issues responded to.[5]

Alendronate is commonly known to be associated with oesophageal adverse effects, and there are strict dosing instructions to minimise this risk.[6] It may also cause local irritation of the stomach, although its potential to cause gastric ulcers is not considered established.[3,6]

The status of this interaction is currently controversial. Some consider that alendronate should not be used in patients receiving NSAIDs,[4] while others urge caution in their use together.[1,2] However, some consider that there is no evidence that alendronate adds to the known gastrointestinal toxicity of NSAIDs,[5] and the maker issues no caution about concurrent use of NSAIDs.[6] Until further evidence is available, it would seem sensible to monitor the concurrent use of alendronate and NSAIDs carefully.

(b) Clodronate

The maker notes that patients receiving NSAIDs in addition to clodronate have developed renal dysfunction, although a synergistic action has not been established.[7] Clodronate alone may cause renal impairment, and the makers suggest that renal function should be assessed before giving clodronate.[7] This would seem particularly important in those on NSAIDs.

(c) Risedronate

The maker notes that despite aspirin and NSAIDs being used by 33% and 45% of patients, respectively, in phase III osteoporosis studies of risedronate no clinically relevant interactions were noted.[8]

(d) Tiludronate

Single-dose studies in 12 healthy subjects found that **diclofenac** 25 mg and aspirin 600 mg had no significant effect on the pharmacokinetics of tiludronate. On the other hand, **indometacin** 50 mg increased the maximum serum concentration and the AUC of tiludronate about twofold when these drugs were taken together, but not when separated by 2 hours. For this reason the makers advise that **indometacin** and tiludronate should be given 2 hours apart.[9]

1. Graham DY, Malaty HM. Alendronate and naproxen are synergistic for development of gastric ulcers. *Arch Intern Med* (2001) 161, 107–110.
2. Ettinger B, Pressman A, Schein J. Clinic visits and hospital admissions for care of acid-related upper gastrointestinal disorders in women using alendronate for osteoporosis. *Am J Manag Care* (1998) 4, 1377–82.
3. Bauer DC, Black D, Ensrud K, Thompson D, Hochberg M, Nevitt M, Musliner T, Freedholm D, for the Fracture Intervention Trial Research Group. Upper gastrointestinal tract safety profile of alendronate. *Arch Intern Med* (2000) 160, 517–25.
4. Rothschild BM. Alendronate and nonsteroidal anti-inflammatory drug interaction safety is not established. *Arch Intern Med* (2000) 160, 1702.
5. Bauer DC, for the Fracture Intervention Trial Research Group. Alendronate and nonsteroidal anti-inflammatory drug interaction safety is not established: a reply. *Arch Intern Med* (2000) 160, 2686.
6. Fosamax (Alendronate sodium). Merck Sharp & Dohme Ltd. UK Summary of product characteristics, April 2004.
7. Bonefos capsules (Sodium clodronate). Boehringer Ingelheim Ltd. UK Summary of product characteristics, July 2002.
8. Actonel (Risedronate sodium). Procter & Gamble Pharmaceuticals UK Limited. UK Summary of product characteristics, January 2005.
9. Sanofi Winthrop. Data on file, June 1996.

Bisphosphonates + Polyvalent cations

The oral absorption of bisphosphonates is reduced by *Maalox* and by other antacids, calcium-rich foods, calcium supplements, iron preparations, magnesium-containing laxatives or milk. Administration should be separated to avoid a reduction in absorption.

Clinical evidence

(a) Clodronate

In a randomised study in 31 healthy subjects the AUC of clodronate was reduced to 10% of the optimum level when it was taken with breakfast. Delaying administration until 2 hours after breakfast only slightly improved the AUC (34% of optimum). The best AUC was achieved when clodronate was given 2 hours before breakfast, although the AUC one hour before was similar (91% of optimum).[1]

(b) Tiludronate

The maximum serum levels and AUC of tiludronate in 12 healthy subjects were halved when *Maalox* (**aluminium/magnesium hydroxide**) was taken one hour before tiludronate, but the bioavailability was only slightly affected when *Maalox* was taken 2 hours after the tiludronate.[2]

Mechanism

The bisphosphonates can form complexes with a number of polyvalent metallic ions (e.g. Al^{3+}, Ca^{2+}, Fe, Mg^{2+}), which can impair their absorption.

Importance and management

Established and important interactions, although the documentation is limited. Bisphosphonates should be prevented from coming into contact with a range of preparations such as **antacids** (containing **aluminium, bismuth**, **calcium**, **magnesium**), **laxatives** (containing magnesium), **iron preparations** and **calcium** or other **mineral supplements**. **Food**, **milk** and **dairy products** in particular, contain calcium, and may also impair absorption.

Recommendations on the timing of administration of bisphosphonates in relation to food and other drugs varies. The makers of **alendronate**[3] suggest that, in order to avoid absorption interactions, patients should wait at least 30 minutes after taking alendronate before taking any other drug or food, and that alendronate should be taken with plain water only. The makers of tiludronate[4] recommend that it is taken with water on an empty stomach (at least two hours before or after meals). In addition, they recommend administration of **tiludronate** and antacids or calcium salts should be separated by 2 hours. The makers of clodronate[5] suggest leaving 1 hour between the administration of food and clodronate. The makers of **risedronate**[6] recommend it is taken with water at least 30 minutes before the first food or drink of the day. Alternatively, they say it should be given at least 2 hours from any food or drink at any other time of the day, at least 30 minutes before going to bed. Similarly, the makers of **etidronate**[7] recommend it is given on an empty stomach at least 2 hours from any food or medicines containing polyvalent cations (as listed above).

1. Laitinen K, Patronen A, Harju P, Löyttyniemi E, Pylkkänen L, Kleimola T, Perttunen K. Timing of food intake has a marked effect on the bioavailability of clodronate. *Bone* (2000) 27, 293–6.
2. Sanofi Winthrop. Data on file, June 1996.
3. Fosamax (Alendronate sodium). Merck Sharp & Dohme Ltd. UK Summary of product characteristics, April 2004.
4. Skelid (Disodium tiluronate). Sanofi Synthelabo. UK Summary of product characteristics, December 2001.
5. Bonefos capsules (Sodium clodronate). Boehringer Ingelheim Ltd. UK Summary of product characteristics, July 2002.
6. Actonel (Risedronate sodium). Procter & Gamble Pharmaceuticals UK Limited. UK Summary of product characteristics, January 2005.
7. Didronel (Etidronate disodium). Procter & Gamble Pharmaceuticals UK Ltd. UK Summary of product characteristics, October 2002.

Bisphosphonates; Clodronate + Aminoglycosides

Severe hypocalcaemia occurred in two patients treated with sodium clodronate when they were given netilmicin or amikacin.

Clinical evidence

A 62-year-old woman with multiple myeloma was given sodium clodronate 2400 mg daily for osteolysis and bone pain. After 7 days she developed grand mal seizures, and her serum calcium was found to be 1.72 mmol/l (normal range 2.25 to 2.6 mmol/l). Despite daily calcium infusions her calcium remained low. The authors state that symptomatic hypocalcaemia with clodronate is rare, and attributed the dramatic response in this patient to an interaction with a course of **netilmicin** given 5 days earlier for septicaemia.[1]

A 69-year-old man with prostate cancer had been on sodium clodronate 2400 mg daily for bone pain for 13 months, and serum calcium levels had always remained within normal limits. After being admitted with febrile neutropenia following a course of chemotherapy, the clodronate was withdrawn and he was given intravenous **amikacin** and ceftazidime. After 7 days he became unconscious, and developed spontaneous twitching movements in his arms and legs. His calcium was found to be 1.39 mmol/l and he was diagnosed with hypocalcaemic tetany. He was given calcium infusions, and his serum calcium returned to normal over the next 12 hours.[2]

Mechanism

Not fully understood, but one suggestion is that any fall in blood calcium levels brought about by the use of clodronate is normally balanced to some extent by the excretion of parathyroid hormone, which raises blood calcium levels. However, the aminoglycoside antibacterials can damage the kidneys, not only causing the loss of calcium, but of magnesium as well. Any hypomagnesaemia inhibits the activity of the parathyroid gland, so that the normal homoeostatic response to hypocalcaemia is reduced or even abolished.[1,2] Clodronate itself can sometimes be nephrotoxic.

Importance and management

Direct information seems to be limited to these two reports. Biochemical hypocalcaemia is believed to occur in about 10% of patients on bisphosphonates,[3] but symptomatic hypocalcaemia is said to be rare.[2] It seems therefore that the addition of the aminoglycoside in these two cases precipitated severe clinical hypocalcaemia. The authors of both reports therefore advise care if bisphosphonates are given with aminoglycosides, and recommend close monitoring of calcium and magnesium levels. They also point out that the renal loss of calcium and magnesium can continue for weeks after aminoglycosides are stopped, and that bisphosphonates can also persist in bone for weeks.[1,2] This means that the interaction is potentially possible whether the drugs are given concurrently or sequentially.

1. Pedersen-Bjergaard U, Myhre J. Severe hypoglycaemia (sic) after treatment with diphosphonate and aminoglycoside. *BMJ* (1991) 302, 295.
2. Mayordomo JI, Rivera F. Severe hypocalcaemia after treatment with oral clodronate and aminoglycoside. *Ann Oncol* (1993) 4, 432–5.
3. Jodrell DI, Iveson TJ, Smith IE. Symptomatic hypocalcaemia after treatment with high-dose aminohydroxypropylidene diphosphonate. *Lancet* (1987) i, 622.

Cannabis + Disulfiram

An isolated case report describes a hypomanic-like reaction in a man on disulfiram when he used cannabis.

Clinical evidence, mechanism, importance and management

A man with a 10-year history of drug abuse (alcohol, amfetamines, cocaine, cannabis) being treated with disulfiram 250 mg daily, experienced a hypomanic-like reaction (euphoria, hyperactivity, insomnia, irritability) on two occasions, associated with the concurrent use of cannabis. The patient said that he felt as though he had been taking amfetamine.[1] The reason for this reaction is not understood. Other patients given both of these drugs did not experience this reaction.[2]

1. Lacoursiere RB, Swatek R. Adverse interaction between disulfiram and marijuana: a case report. *Am J Psychiatry* (1983) 140, 243–4.
2. Rosenberg CM, Gerrein JR, Schnell C. Cannabis in the treatment of alcoholism. *J Stud Alcohol* (1978) 39, 1955–8.

Charcoal + Miscellaneous

Charcoal adsorbs some drugs and in large doses (8 to 50 g) it can markedly reduce their absorption by the gut, but smaller doses (1 to 2 g) of charcoal possibly interact minimally, or not at all.

Clinical evidence

In vitro studies have found that **carbutamide**, **chlorpropamide**, **tolazamide**, **tolbutamide**, **glibenclamide** and **glipizide** are all extensively adsorbed onto activated charcoal.[1] An antiemetic complementary remedy containing activated charcoal completely negated the effect of **mitobronitol** 125 mg used to treat primary thrombocythaemia in one patient.[2] A number of other studies[3-14] have shown a variety of drugs to be affected by charcoal. See 'Table 35.1', (below). In contrast, charcoal 1 g has been reported not to affect the pharmacokinetics of **ciprofloxacin** 500 mg, although repeated or higher doses may have more of an effect.[15,16]

Table 35.1 Drug interactions with activated charcoal

Activated charcoal administration	*Effects*	*Refs*
Aspirin		
+ charcoal 50 g	Absorption of a 1 g dose decreased 70% by charcoal	1
+ charcoal 50 g 1 h later	Absorption of a 1 g dose decreased 10% by charcoal	1
+ charcoal 10 g	Absorption of a 975 mg dose decreased 70% by charcoal	2
Carbamazepine		
+ charcoal 50 g	Absorption of a 400 mg dose decreased 92% by charcoal	3
+ charcoal 118 g in 5 divided doses after 10 to 48 h	Half-life reduced from 32 to 17.6 h	4
Chlorpropamide		
+ charcoal 50 g	Absorption of a 250 mg dose reduced 90% by charcoal	5
Dapsone		
+ charcoal 118 g in 5 divided doses after 10 to 48 h	Half-life reduced from 32 to 17.6 h	4
Digoxin		
+ charcoal 50 g	Absorption of a 500 microgram dose decreased 98% by charcoal	1
+ charcoal 50 g 1 h later	Absorption of a 500 microgram dose decreased 40% by charcoal	1
+ charcoal 8 g	Absorption of a 500 microgram dose decreased 98% by charcoal	3
Furosemide (Frusemide)		
+ charcoal 8 g	Absorption of a 40 mg dose reduced 99% by charcoal	3
Glipizide		
+ charcoal 8 g	Absorption of a 10 mg dose reduced 81% by charcoal	6
Nizatidine		
+ charcoal 2 g 1 h later	Absorption of a 150 mg dose reduced 30% by charcoal	7
Paracetamol (Acetaminophen)		
+ charcoal 10 g	Absorption of a 2 g dose decreased 63% by charcoal	8
+ charcoal 10 g 1 h later	Absorption of a 2 g dose decreased 23% by charcoal	8
Paroxetine		
+ charcoal 20 g 20 and 40 min later	Paroxetine became undetectable in the plasma	9
Phenobarbital (Phenobarbitone)		
+ charcoal 118 g in 5 divided doses after 10 to 48 h	Half-life reduced from 110 to 19.8 h	4

Continued

Table 35.1 Drug interactions with activated charcoal *(continued)*

Activated charcoal administration	*Effects*	*Refs*
Phenylbutazone		
+ charcoal 118 g in 5 divided doses after 10 to 48 h	Half-life reduced from 51.5 to 36.7 h	4
Phenytoin (Diphenylhydantoin)		
+ charcoal 50 g	Absorption of a 500 mg dose decreased 98% by charcoal	1
+ charcoal 50 g 1 h later	Absorption of a 500 mg dose decreased 80% by charcoal	1
Rifampicin (Rifampin)		
+ charcoal 15 g	Urinary recovery reduced to 1.2%	10
+ charcoal 7.5 g	Urinary recovery reduced to 4.2%	10
Sodium valproate		
+ charcoal 50 g	Absorption of a 300 mg dose decreased 65% by charcoal	11
Theophylline		
+ charcoal 140 g in divided doses over 12 h	Half-life reduced from 6.4 to 3.3 h AUC nearly halved	12
Tolbutamide		
+ charcoal 50 g	Absorption of a 500 mg dose decreased 90% by charcoal	11

1. Neuvonen PJ, Elfving SM, Elonen E. Reduction of absorption of digoxin, phenytoin and aspirin by activated charcoal in man. *Eur J Clin Pharmacol* (1978) 13, 213–18.
2. Juhl RP. Comparison of kaolin-pectin and activated charcoal for inhibition of aspirin absorption. *Am J Hosp Pharm* (1979) 36, 1097–8.
3. Neuvonen P J, Kivistö K, Hirvisalo E L. Effects of resins and activated charcoal on the adsorption of digoxin, carbamazepine and frusemide. *Br J Clin Pharmacol* (1988) 25, 229–3.
4. Neuvonen PJ, Elonen E, Mattila MJ. Orally given charcoal increases the rate of elimination of phenobarbital, carbamazepine, phenylbutazone, and dapsone in man. *Clin Pharmacol Ther* (1980) 27, 275–6.
5. Neuvonen P J, Kärkkäinen S. Effects of charcoal, sodium bicarbonate and ammonium chloride on chlorpropamide kinetics. *Clin Pharmacol Ther* (1983) 33, 386–93.
6. Kivistö KT, Neuvonen PJ. The effect of cholestyramine and activated charcoal on glipizide absorption. *Br J Clin Pharmacol* (1990) 30, 733–6.
7. Knadler MP, Bergstrom RF, Callaghan JT, Obermeyer BD, Rubin A. Absorption studies of the H2-blocker nizatidine. *Clin Pharmacol Ther* (1987) 42, 514–20.
8. Dordoni B, Willson RA, Thompson RPH, Williams R. Reduction of absorption of paracetamol by activated charcoal and cholestyramine: a possible therapeutic measure. *BMJ* (1973) 3, 86–7.
9. Greb WH, Buscher G, Dierdorf H-D, von Schrader HW, Wolf D. Ability of charcoal to prevent absorption of paroxetine. *Acta Psychiatr Scand* (1989) 80 (Suppl 350), 156–7.
10. Orisakwe OE, Dioka CE, Okpogba AN, Orish CN, Ofoefule SI. Effect of activated charcoal on rifampicin absorption in man. *Tokai J Exp Clin Med* (1996) 21, 51–4.
11. Neuvonen PJ, Kannisto H, Hirvisalo EL. Effect of activated charcoal on absorption of tolbutamide and valproate in man. *Eur J Clin Pharmacol* (1983) 24, 243–6.
12. Berlinger WG, Spector R, Goldberg MJ, Johnson GF, Quee CK, Berg MJ. Enhancement of theophylline clearance by oral activated charcoal. *Clin Pharmacol Ther* (1983) 33, 351–4.

Mechanism

Activated charcoal can adsorb gases, toxins and drugs onto its surface so that less is available for absorption through the gut wall. Separating the dosages reduces admixture in the gut.

Importance and management

Very well established interactions. Most of the reports are about the treatment of drug poisoning and overdoses, where relatively large amounts of charcoal (50 g or more) are given to adsorb as much of the drug as possible. In this situation, it is generally recommended that other drugs required concurrently are given parenterally. In addition, activated charcoal should not be used concurrently with specific oral antidotes such as methionine, although in the US oral acetylcysteine and charcoal are used concurrently with no apparent reduction in effects.

There seems to be little reported about the effects of small doses of charcoal (1 to 2 g daily) given to absorb intestinal gas or for the treatment of diarrhoea and dysentery, except that ciprofloxacin[15] is apparently not affected by 1 g charcoal, while **nizatidine** absorption is reduced by about 30%.[9] More study is needed to define the situation more clearly and to find out the extent to which separating the dosages to prevent admixture in the gut reduces the effects of this interaction. A one hour separation was partially effective with **paracetamol**.[8]

1. Kannisto H, Neuvonen PJ. Adsorption of sulphonylureas onto activated charcoal *in vitro*. *J Pharm Sci* (1984) 73, 253–6.
2. Windrum P, Hull DR, Morris TCM. Herb-drug interactions. *Lancet* (2000) 355, 1019–20.
3. Neuvonen PJ, Elfving SM, Elonen E. Reduction of absorption of digoxin, phenytoin and aspirin by activated charcoal in man. *Eur J Clin Pharmacol* (1978) 13, 213–18.
4. Kivistö KT, Neuvonen PJ. The effect of cholestyramine and activated charcoal on glipizide absorption. *Br J Clin Pharmacol* (1990) 30, 733–6.
5. Neuvonen PJ, Kärkkäinen S. Effects of charcoal, sodium bicarbonate, and ammonium chloride on chlorpropamide kinetics. *Clin Pharmacol Ther* (1983) 33, 386–93.
6. Neuvonen PJ, Kivistö K, Hirvisalo E L. Effects of resins and activated charcoal on the absorption of digoxin, carbamazepine and frusemide. *Br J Clin Pharmacol* (1988) 25, 229–33
7. Neuvonen PJ, Kannisto H, Hirvisalo EL. Effect of activated charcoal on absorption of tolbutamide and valproate in man. *Eur J Clin Pharmacol* (1983) 24, 243–6.
8. Dordoni B, Willson RA, Thompson RPH, Williams R. Reduction of absorption of paracetamol by activated charcoal and cholestyramine: a possible therapeutic measure. *BMJ* (1973) 3, 86–7.
9. Knadler MP, Bergstrom RF, Callaghan JT, Obermeyer BD, Rubin A. Absorption studies of the H_2-blocker nizatidine. *Clin Pharmacol Ther* (1987) 42, 514–20.
10. Juhl RP. Comparison of kaolin-pectin and activated charcoal for inhibition of aspirin absorption. *Am J Hosp Pharm* (1979) 36, 1097–8.
11. Neuvonen PJ, Elonen E, Mattila MJ. Orally given charcoal increases the rate of elimination of phenobarbital, carbamazepine, phenylbutazone, and dapsone in man. *Clin Pharmacol Ther* (1980) 27, 275–6.
12. Berlinger WG, Spector R, Goldberg MJ, Johnson GF, Quee CK, Berg MJ. Enhancement of theophylline clearance by oral activated charcoal. *Clin Pharmacol Ther* (1983) 33, 351–4.
13. Greb WH, Buscher G, Dierdorf H-D, von Schrader HW, Wolf D. Ability of charcoal to prevent absorption of paroxetine. *Acta Psychiatr Scand* (1989) 80 (Suppl 350), 156–7.
14. Orisakwe OE, Dioka CE, Okpogba AN, Orish CN, Ofoefule SI. Effect of activated charcoal on rifampicin absorption in man. *Tokai J Exp Clin Med* (1996) 21, 51–4.
15. Torre D. Influence of charcoal on ciprofloxacin activity. *Rev Infect Dis* (1988) 10, 1231.
16. Torre D, Sampietro C, Rossi S, Bianchi W, Maggiolo F. Ciprofloxacin and activated charcoal: pharmacokinetic data. *Rev Infect Dis* (1989) 11 (Suppl 5), S1015–S1016.

Chlorzoxazone + Disulfiram

Disulfiram markedly increases the plasma levels of chlorzoxazone.

Clinical evidence, mechanism, importance and management

A study in 6 healthy subjects to identify the activity of cytochrome P4502E1 found that a single 500-mg dose of disulfiram markedly inhibited the metabolism of a single 750-mg dose of chlorzoxazone (clearance reduced by 85%, half-life increased from 0.92 to 5.1 hours, and a two-fold increase in peak plasma levels).[1]

No increased side-effects were seen while using these single doses, but an increase in toxicity would be expected (sedation, headache, nausea) with multiple doses. Be alert for the need to reduce the chlorzoxazone dosage if disulfiram is given concurrently.

1. Kharasch ED, Thummel KE, Mhyre J, Lillibridge JH. Single-dose disulfiram inhibition of chlorzoxazone metabolism: a clinical probe for P450 2E1. *Clin Pharmacol Ther* (1993) 53, 643–50.

Chlorzoxazone + Isoniazid

The side-effects of chlorzoxazone may be increased in some patients (particularly slow-acetylators of isoniazid) if they also receive isoniazid.

Clinical evidence, mechanism, importance and management

Five out of 10 healthy slow acetylators of isoniazid experienced an increase in the side effects of a 750-mg dose of chlorzoxazone (sedation, headache, nausea) after taking isoniazid 300 mg daily for 7 days. These symptoms disappeared within 2 days of withdrawing the isoniazid.[1] This appears to be because isoniazid inhibits the activity of cytochrome P450 isoenzyme CYP2E1, the enzyme that mediates the metabolism of chlorzoxazone, and the clearance of chlorzoxazone is consequently reduced (in this case by 58%). Following withdrawal of isoniazid, the metabolism of chlorzoxazone is increased.[1]

In practical terms this means that it may be necessary to reduce the chlorzoxazone dosage in some patients if they also receive isoniazid. However, only half of this group of slow acetylators developed adverse effects, and fast acetylators would not be expected to demonstrate this interaction. There is no quick and easy way to find out a patient's acetylator status. In the absence of this information you will need to monitor concurrent use carefully.

1. Zand R, Nelson SD, Slattery JT, Thummel KE, Kalhorn TF, Adams SP, Wright JM. Inhibition and induction of cytochrome P4502E1-catalyzed oxidation by isoniazid in humans. *Clin Pharmacol Ther* (1993) 54, 142–9.

CNS depressants + CNS depressants

The concurrent use of two or more drugs that depress the CNS may be expected to result in increased CNS depression. This may have undesirable and even life-threatening consequences.

Clinical evidence, mechanism, importance and management

Many drugs have the propensity to cause depression of the central nervous system, resulting in drowsiness, sedation, respiratory depression and at the extreme, death. If more than one CNS depressant is taken, their effects may be additive. It is not uncommon for patients, particularly the elderly, to be taking half-a-dozen drugs or more (and possibly alcohol as well). Such patients are therefore at risk of cumulative CNS depression ranging from mild drowsiness through to a befuddled stupor, which can make the performance of the simplest everyday task more difficult or even impossible. The importance of this will depend on the context: it may considerably increase the risk of accident in the kitchen, at work, in a busy street, driving a car, or handling other potentially dangerous machinery where alertness is at a premium. It has been estimated that as many as 600 traffic accident fatalities each year in the UK can be attributed to the sedative effects of psychoactive drugs.[1] In a Spanish study of fatal road traffic accidents, blood samples were analysed from 9.7% of drivers killed in road accidents over a 10 year period. Of these drivers, medicines were detected in 4.7% (269 cases), and of these benzodiazepines were the most common (73%). Other drugs present in 6% to 12% of cases included antidepressants, analgesics, anti-epileptics, barbiturates and antihistamines. Of the benzodiazepine cases, almost three quarters had another substance detected, mainly illicit drugs (cocaine, opiates, or cannabis) or alcohol. Only 7.7% had benzodiazepines and another medicinal drug alone.[2] **Alcohol** almost certainly makes things worse.

An example of the lethal effects of combining an **antihistamine**, a **benzodiazepine** and **alcohol** is briefly mentioned in the monograph 'Alcohol + Antihistamines', p.39. A less spectacular but socially distressing example is that of a woman accused of shop-lifting while in a confused state arising from the combined sedative effects of *Actifed*, a *Beechams Powder* and *Dolobid* (containing **triprolidine**, **salicylamide** and **diflunisal** respectively).[3]

Few if any well-controlled studies have investigated the cumulative or additive detrimental effects of CNS depressants (except with **alcohol**), but the following is a list of some of the groups of drugs that to a greater or lesser extent possess CNS depressant activity and which may be expected to interact in this way: **alcohol**, **opioid analgesics**, **anticonvulsants**, **antidepressants**, **antihistamines**, **antiemetics**, **antipsychotics**, **anxiolytics** and **hypnotics**. Some of the interactions of **alcohol** with these drugs are dealt with in individual monographs.

1. Anon. Sedative effects of drugs linked to accidents. *Pharm J* (1994) 253, 564.
2. Carmen del Río M, Gómez J, Sancho M, Alvarez FJ. Alcohol, illicit drugs and medicinal drugs in fatally injured drivers in Spain between 1991 and 2000. *Forensic Sci Int* (2002) 127, 63–70.
3. Herxheimer A, Haffner BD. Prosecution for alleged shoplifting: successful pharmacological defence. *Lancet* (1982) i, 634.

Colchicine + Macrolides

Two isolated case reports describe acute life-threatening colchicine toxicity caused by the addition of erythromycin or clarithromycin.

Clinical evidence, mechanism, importance and management

A woman with familial Mediterranean fever and amyloidosis, who was taking colchicine 1 mg daily, developed acute and life-threatening colchicine toxicity 16 days after starting to take **erythromycin** 2 g daily. This patient had both cholestasis and renal impairment, factors that would be expected to reduce colchicine clearance and therefore predispose her to colchicine toxicity.[1] However, the reaction was attributed, at least in part, to the **erythromycin**. It was suggested that **erythromycin** may have inhibited the hepatic metabolism of colchicine, or produced a more generalised hepatotoxicity as colchicine levels rose from between 9 to 12.6 nanograms/ml to 22 nanograms/ml after the addition of **erythromycin**.[1]

In a second case, a 67-year-old man on CAPD taking colchicine 500 micrograms twice daily was admitted with symptoms of colchicine toxicity (including pancytopenia) 4 days after starting a course of **clarithromycin** 500 mg twice daily for an upper respiratory tract infection. All drugs were stopped and supportive treatment given, but he later died from multi-organ failure.[2]

Information on this interaction is limited, but it appears that macrolide antibacterials can provoke acute colchicine toxicity, at the very least in pre-disposed individuals. If any patient is given colchicine and a macrolide, be aware of the potential for toxicity, especially in patients with pre-existing renal impairment.

1. Caraco Y, Putterman C, Rahamimov R, Ben-Chetrit E. Acute colchicine intoxication - possible role of erythromycin administration. *J Rheumatol* (1992) 19, 494–6.
2. Dogukan A, Oymak FS, Taskapan H, Güven M, Tokgoz B, Utas C. Acute fatal colchicine intoxication in a patient on continuous ambulatory peritoneal dialysis (CAPD). Possible role of clarithromycin administration. *Clin Nephrol* (2001) 55, 181–2.

Contrast media; Iopanoic acid + Colestyramine

A single report describes poor radiographic visualisation of the gall bladder in a man due to an interaction between iopanoic acid and colestyramine within the gut.

Clinical evidence, mechanism, importance and management

The cholecystogram of a man on colestyramine with post-gastrectomy syndrome who was given oral iopanoic acid as an x-ray contrast medium, suggested that he had an abnormal and apparently collapsed gall bladder. A week after stopping the colestyramine a repeat cholecystogram gave excellent visualisation of a gall bladder of normal appearance.[1] The same effects have been observed experimentally in *dogs*.[1] The reason seems to be that the colestyramine binds with the iopanoic acid in the gut so that little is absorbed and little is available for secretion in the bile, hence the poor visualisation of the gall bladder.

On the basis of reports about other drugs that similarly bind to colestyramine, it seems probable that this interaction could be avoided if the administration of the iopanoic acid and the colestyramine were to be separated as much as possible. Whether other oral acidic x-ray contrast media bind in a similar way to colestyramine is uncertain, but this possibility should be considered.

1. Nelson JA. Effect of cholestyramine on telepaque oral cholecystography. *Am J Roentgenol Radium Ther Nucl Med* (1974) 122, 333–4.

Contrast media; Metrizamide + Phenothiazines

Two isolated case reports describe epileptiform reactions in two patients when metrizamide was used in the presence of chlorpromazine or dixyrazine.

Clinical evidence, mechanism, importance and management

A patient on long-term treatment with **chlorpromazine** 75 mg daily had a grand mal seizure three-and-a-half hours after being given metrizamide (16 ml of 170 mg iodine per ml by the lumbar route). He had another seizure 5 hours later.[1] One out of 34 other patients demonstrated epileptogenic activity on an EEG when given metrizamide for lumbar myelography. The patient was taking **dixyrazine** 10 mg three times daily.[2] A clinical study of 26 patients given **levomepromazine** for the relief of lumbago-sciatic pain found no evidence of an increased risk of epilepsy after receiving metrizamide.[3] It is reported that the US makers say that chlorpromazine should be stopped prior to giving metrizamide because of a risk of convulsions.[4] Note that metrizamide should not be given into the CNS as it is now recognised that neurotoxicity can occur following the use of hypertonic contrast media by this route.[4]

1. Hindmarsh T, Grepe A and Widen L. Metrizamide-phenothiazine interaction. Report of a case with seizures following myelography. *Acta Radiol Diagnosis* (1975) 16, 129–34.
2. Hindmarsh T. Lumbar myelography with meglumine iocarmate and metrizamide. *Acta Radiol Diagnosis* (1975) 16, 209–22.
3. Standnes B, Oftedal S-I, Weber H. Effect of levomepromazine on EEG and on clinical side effects after lumbar myelography with metrizamide. *Acta Radiol Diagnosis* (1982) 23, 111–14.
4. Sweetman SC, editor. Martindale: The complete drug reference. 34th ed. London: Pharmaceutical Press; 2005 pp. 679, 1060.

Cyclobenzaprine + Fluoxetine and Droperidol

A patient on cyclobenzaprine and fluoxetine developed torsade de pointes arrhythmia and ventricular fibrillation when droperidol was added.

Clinical evidence, mechanism, importance and management

A 59-year-old woman on long-term treatment with fluoxetine and cyclobenzaprine, who had a prolonged baseline QTc interval of 497 milliseconds, was additionally given droperidol before surgery on her Achilles tendon. During the surgery she developed torsade de pointes arrhythmia, which progressed to ventricular fibrillation. On the first postoperative day after the cyclobenzaprine had been withdrawn, her QTc interval had decreased towards normal (440 milliseconds).[1]

A likely explanation is that her cyclobenzaprine serum levels were already raised by fluoxetine (a known inhibitor of cytochrome P450 isoenzyme CYP2D6, an enzyme involved in the metabolism of cyclobenzaprine) and as a result her QTc interval was already prolonged. Cyclobenzaprine is structurally like the tricyclic antidepressants and shares their adverse effects, including their dysrhythmic potentialities, so that the addition of the droperidol, also known to prolong the QT interval, simply further extended the QTc interval and precipitated the torsade de pointes. This case not only illustrates the existence of an interaction between cyclobenzaprine and fluoxetine, but also the life-threatening risks of adding other drugs that can further prolong the QT interval.

1. Michalets EL, Smith LK, Van Tassel ED. Torsade de pointes resulting from the addition of droperidol to an existing cytochrome P450 drug interaction. *Ann Pharmacother* (1998) 32, 761–5.

Dantrolene + Metoclopramide

Metoclopramide increases the bioavailability of dantrolene.

Clinical evidence, mechanism, importance and management

A study in 7 paraplegics and 6 quadriplegics with spinal cord injury found that a single 10-mg intravenous dose of metoclopramide increased the bioavailability of a single 100-mg oral dose of dantrolene by 57%. The reasons are not known, although it was suggested that absorption may have been affected. The clinical relevance of this interaction is uncertain but the authors of the study suggest that patients should be well monitored if metoclopramide is added or withdrawn from patients who are being treated with dantrolene.[1]

1. Gilman TM, Segal JL, Brunnemann SR. Metoclopramide increases the bioavailability of dantrolene in spinal cord injury. *J Clin Pharmacol* (1996) 36, 64–71.

Desferrioxamine (Deferoxamine) + Prochlorperazine

Prochlorperazine caused unconsciousness in two patients being treated with desferrioxamine.

Clinical evidence, mechanism, importance and management

Administration of prochlorperazine to 2 patients receiving desferrioxamine resulted in unconsciousness for 48 to 72 hours. It was suggested that the drug combination resulted in increased removal of iron from the central nervous system, thereby impairing noradrenergic and serotonergic systems.[1] It has also been suggested that desferrioxamine-induced damage of the retina may be more likely in the presence of phenothiazines.[2] It would seem wise to avoid the concurrent use of desferrioxamine and prochlorperazine, but there seems to be no direct evidence of adverse interactions with any of the other phenothiazines.

1. Blake DR, Winyard P, Lunec J, Williams A, Good PA, Crewes SJ, Gutteridge JMC, Rowley D, Halliwell B, Cornish A, Hider RC. Cerebral and ocular toxicity induced by desferrioxamine. *Q J Med* (1985) 56, 345–55.
2. Pall H, Blake DR, Good PA, Wynyard P, Williams AC. Copper chelation and the neuro-ophthalmic toxicity of desferrioxamine. *Lancet* (1986) ii, 1279.

Desferrioxamine (Deferoxamine) + Vitamin C (Ascorbic acid)

High-dose vitamin C may cause cardiac disorders in some patients treated with desferrioxamine.

Clinical evidence, mechanism, importance and management

Vitamin C is given with desferrioxamine to patients with iron overload because it mobilises iron stores and thus promotes the excretion of iron. One study in 11 patients with thalassaemia noted that a striking deterioration in left ventricular function occurred when the patients were given 500 mg of vitamin C with intramuscular desferrioxamine. In most patients left ventricular function returned to normal when the vitamin C was stopped.[1] For this reason it has been suggested that vitamin C should be used with desferrioxamine with caution,[2] only where there is a demonstrated need,[3] and in the lowest possible dose.[1] The makers of desferrioxamine recommend that a maximum daily dose of 200 mg of vitamin C should be used, and that vitamin C should not be given within the first month of desferrioxamine treatment.[4]

1. Henry W. Echocardiographic evaluation of the heart in thalassemia major. *Ann Intern Med* (1979) 91, 892–4.
2. Cohen A, Cohen IJ, Schwartz E. Scurvy and altered iron stores in thalassemia major. *N Engl J Med* (1981) 304, 158–60.
3. Nienhuis AW. Vitamin C and iron. *N Engl J Med* (1981) 304, 170–1.
4. Desferal Vials (Desferrioxamine mesilate). Novartis Pharmaceuticals UK Ltd. UK Summary of product characteristics, February 2004.

Dexfenfluramine or Fenfluramine + Other anorectics

Fenfluramine and dexfenfluramine have generally been withdrawn worldwide because of the occurrence of serious and sometimes fatal valvular heart disease (aortic, mitral, tricuspid or mixed valve disease). Pulmonary hypertension has also sometimes been seen. These serious adverse effects occurred when these drugs were taken alone, and when combined with phentermine as *Fen-phen* and *Dexfen-phen*, but not with phentermine alone.[1-5]

There is also an isolated case of cardiomyopathy attributed to the use of fenfluramine with mazindol.[6] Prior to withdrawal of the drug from the market, the makers of fenfluramine recommended that concurrent use with other centrally acting anorectics should be avoided.[7]

1. Committee on Safety of Medicines/Medicines Control Agency. Fenfluramine and dexfenfluramine withdrawn. *Current Problems* (1997) 23, 12.
2. Food and Drugs Administration. FDA announces withdrawal fenfluramine and dexfenfluramine (Fen-Phen). September 15th, 1997.
3. Connolly HM, Crary JL, McGoon MD, Hensrud DD, Edwards BS, Edwards WD, Schaff HV. Valvular heart disease associated with fenfluramine-phentermine. *N Engl J Med* (1997) 337, 581–8.
4. Mark EJ, Patals ED, Chang HT, Evans RJ, Kessler SC. Fatal pulmonary hypertension associated with short-term use of fenfluramine and phentermine. *N Engl J Med* (1997) 337, 602–6.
5. Graham DJ, Green L. Further cases of valvular heart disease associated with fenfluramine-phentermine. *N Engl J Med* (1997) 337, 635.
6. Gillis D, Wengrower D, Witztum E, Leitersdorf E. Fenfluramine and mazindol: acute reversible cardiomyopathy associated with their use. *Int J Psychiatry Med* (1985) 15, 197–200.
7. Ponderax Pacaps (Fenfluramine). Servier Laboratories Limited. ABPI Compendium of Datasheets and Summaries of Product Characteristics 1997–8, 1307.

Dextromethorphan + Amiodarone

Amiodarone can increase the serum levels of dextromethorphan.

Clinical evidence

A study in 8 patients with cardiac arrhythmias found that amiodarone (1 g daily for 10 days followed by 200 to 400 mg daily for a mean duration of 76 days) changed their excretion of dextromethorphan 40 mg and its metabolite. The amount of unchanged dextromethorphan in the urine rose by nearly 150%, whereas the amount of its metabolite (dextrorphan) fell by about 25%.[1]

Mechanism

In vitro studies using liver microsomes have shown that amiodarone inhibits the metabolism (*O*-demethylation) of dextromethorphan by decreasing the activity of the cytochrome P450 isoenzyme CYP2D6 within the liver.[1] Thus the dextromethorphan is cleared from the body more slowly.

Importance and management

Information seems to be limited to this study. The clinical implications are (a) that amiodarone may interfere with the results of phenotyping if dextromethorphan is used to determine CYP2D6 activity, and (b) that dextromethorphan toxicity (excitation, confusion) may possibly develop in patients taking amiodarone. Be alert for any signs of toxicity if both are used. As yet, too little is known about this interaction to say by how much the dextromethorphan dosage should be reduced. Remember that dextromethorphan occurs in a considerable number of proprietary cough preparations.

1. Funck-Brentano C, Jacqz-Aigrain E, Leenhardt A, Roux A, Poirier J-M, Jaillon P. Influence of amiodarone on genetically determined drug metabolism in humans. *Clin Pharmacol Ther* (1991) 50, 259–66.

Dextromethorphan + Quinidine

Quinidine markedly increases the plasma levels of dextromethorphan.

Clinical evidence

A study found that 3 out of 6 patients given dextromethorphan 60 mg twice daily had steady-state plasma levels of less than 5 nanograms/ml 12 hours after the dose. The plasma dextromethorphan levels averaged only 12 nanograms/ml in the group as a whole. However, after being given quinidine 75 mg twice daily for a week, with only half the dose of dextromethorphan, their serum levels averaged 38 nanograms/ml.[1] Some of the patients experienced dextromethorphan toxicity (nervousness, tremors, restlessness, dizziness, shortness of breath, confusion etc).[1]

Mechanism

Quinidine inhibits the cytochrome P450 isoenzyme CYP2D6, which is involved with the metabolism of the dextromethorphan by the liver.[1] As a result, the dextromethorphan accumulates, its serum levels rise and its toxic effects manifest themselves.

Importance and management

An established and clinically important interaction, but with limited documentation. If the combination is thought necessary, a low dose of dextromethorphan is advisable. Concurrent use should be well monitored for evidence of toxicity (see above).

1. Zhang Y, Britto MR, Valderhaug KL, Wedlund PJ, Smith RA. Dextromethorphan: enhancing its systemic availability by way of low-dose quinidine-mediated inhibition of cytochrome P4502D6. *Clin Pharmacol Ther* (1992) 51, 647–55.

Dolasetron + Miscellaneous

Dolasetron appears to be free from clinically significant pharmacokinetic interactions, but it is predicted to interact pharmacodynamically with drugs that prolong the QT interval.

Clinical evidence, mechanism, importance and management

(a) Cimetidine

A study in 18 healthy subjects given dolasetron 200 mg daily found that cimetidine 300 mg four times daily for 7 days increased the AUC and maximum plasma level of the active metabolite of dolasetron, hydrodolasetron, by 24 and 15% respectively, probably due to the inhibitory effect of cimetidine on the cytochrome P450-mediated metabolism of dolasetron. As 400-mg oral doses of dolasetron have been shown to be well tolerated (the usual oral dose is up to 200 mg) these changes were not considered to be clinically significant.[1] Therefore no special precautions appear necessary if cimetidine and dolasetron are used concurrently.

(b) Drugs that affect the QT interval

Prolongation of the QTc interval, which appears to be dose related, has been seen following the use of dolasetron.[2,3] As a consequence, and because of the lack of further information, the UK makers contraindicate[2] and the US makers advise caution[3] the concurrent use of dolasetron and **class I or class III antiarrhythmics**. Both makers also advise caution with all drugs that may prolong the QT interval. These include **diuretics**,[3] which may prolong the QT interval by inducing hypokalaemia. For further information on drug interactions involving the QT interval see 'Drugs that prolong the QT interval + Other drugs that prolong the QT interval', p.170.

(c) Food

In a single-dose study, 23 healthy subjects were given 200 mg of dolasetron orally either alone, or following a **high-fat breakfast** (containing fat 55 g, protein 33 g and carbohydrate 58 g). Although there was a slight delay in absorption, both were considered to be bioequivalent. Therefore dolasetron may be given without regard to meals.[4]

(d) Rifampicin

A study in 17 healthy subjects given dolasetron 200 mg daily found that rifampicin (rifampin) 600 mg daily for 7 days decreased the AUC and maximum plasma level of the active metabolite of dolasetron, hydrodolasetron, by 28 and 17% respectively, probably due to induction of hydrodolasetron metabolism by rifampicin.[1] These changes were not considered to be clinically significant and therefore no special precautions appear necessary if rifampicin and dolasetron are used concurrently.

(e) Verapamil

In one case a 61-year-old woman taking verapamil developed complete heart block following the administration of dolasetron, although this was not proven to be as a result of an interaction.[3] In other patients taking verapamil, no effect was seen on the clearance of hydrodolasetron (the active metabolite of dolasetron).[3]

(f) Miscellaneous drugs

Because the active metabolite of dolasetron is eliminated by multiple routes, and because no clinically significant interaction occurs with the known enzyme inhibitor cimetidine, or the known enzyme inducer rifampicin (see (a) and (d) above respectively), the makers say that the potential for clinically significant pharmacokinetic interactions is low.[2,3] In patients taking **ACE inhibitors**, **diltiazem**, **furosemide**, **glibenclamide** (**glyburide**), **nifedipine** or **propranolol**, no effect was shown on the clearance of hydrodolasetron (the active metabolite of dolasetron) and therefore no problems would be expected on concurrent use.[3] **Atenolol** reduced the clearance of hydrodolasetron by 27%, but this was not considered to be clinically significant.[3]

1. Dimmitt DC, Cramer MB, Keung A, Arumugham T, Weir SJ. Pharmacokinetics of dolasetron with coadministration of cimetidine or rifampin in healthy subjects. *Cancer Chemother Pharmacol* (1999) 43, 126–32.
2. Anzemet (Dolasetron mesilate). Amdipharm. UK Summary of product characteristics, December 2003.
3. Anzemet (Dolasetron mesylate). Aventis Pharmaceuticals Inc. US Prescribing information, March 2003.
4. Lippert C, Keung A, Arumugham T, Eller M, Hahne W, Weir S. The effect of food on the bioavailability of dolasetron mesylate tablets. *Biopharm Drug Dispos* (1998) 19, 17–19.

Dutasteride + Miscellaneous

Preliminary evidence suggests that diltiazem and verapamil, inhibitors of cytochrome P450 isoenzyme CYP3A4, cause moderate increases in dutasteride levels. Dosage adjustments may therefore be needed with potent inhibitors of CYP3A4 such as indinavir, itraconazole, ketoconazole, nefazodone and ritonavir. No clinically significant interaction appears to occur between dutasteride and: ACE inhibitors, beta-blockers, alpha-blockers, amlodipine, calcium channel blockers, corticosteroids, digoxin, diuretics, lipid regulating drugs, NSAIDs, phosphodiesterase inhibitors, quinolone antibacterials, salicylates, tamsulosin, terazosin, or warfarin. There is no interaction when dutasteride is given one hour before colestyramine. Antacids, H_2-blockers, and proton pump inhibitors are predicted not to interact.

Clinical evidence, mechanism, importance and management

(a) Alpha blockers

A study in 24 subjects given dutasteride 500 micrograms daily for 14 days found that when given with either **tamsulosin** 400 micrograms or **terazosin** (titrated to 10 mg) once daily for 14 days, the pharmacokinetics of the drugs remained unchanged.[1] Furthermore, a clinical study in 327 men demonstrated that the combination of **tamsulosin** and dutasteride was well-tolerated over a period of 6 months.[1,2] No additional precautions seem necessary on concurrent use. Consider also 'Finasteride + Alpha blockers', p.1021.

(b) Colestyramine

The absorption of dutasteride 5 mg was not affected when it was given one hour before a single 12-g dose of colestyramine.[1,2] No precautions seem necessary if this dosing interval is observed.[1]

(c) Cytochrome P450 isoenzyme CYP3A4 inhibitors and substrates

When dutasteride was given with **amlodipine** (4 subjects), **diltiazem** (5 subjects) or **verapamil** (6 subjects) during dose-ranging studies, **amlodipine** did not significantly affect the clearance of dutasteride but **diltiazem** and **verapamil** were associated with a decrease of 44 and 37% respectively. This was thought to be due to the inhibitory effect of **diltiazem** and **verapamil** on P-glycoprotein and the cytochrome P450 isoenzyme CYP3A4.[1] Dutasteride has a wide safety margin, so these changes were not thought to be clinically significant. However, the makers warn that potent CYP3A4 inhibitors (they name **indinavir**, **itraconazole**, **ketoconazole**, **nefazodone** and **ritonavir**) may cause a clinically significant increase in dutasteride levels, and so they suggest reducing the dosing frequency if increased dutasteride side effects occur.[2]

(d) Digoxin

A 35-day placebo controlled study in healthy subjects taking digoxin found that its pharmacokinetics were unchanged by a loading dose of dutasteride 25 mg [sic] on day 15, followed by dutasteride 500 micrograms daily on days 16 to 35.[1] No special precautions would appear to be necessary on concurrent use.

(e) Warfarin

Dutasteride, given in combination with warfarin for 35 days had no effect on the pharmacokinetics of *(S)*- or *(R)*-warfarin, and the prothrombin time was unaffected by the presence of dutasteride.[1] No special precautions would appear to be necessary on concurrent use.

(f) Miscellaneous drugs

During clinical trials with dutasteride, no clinically relevant adverse interactions were attributed to the concurrent use of **ACE inhibitors** (390 patients), **beta-blockers** (386 patients), **calcium channel blockers** (394 patients – but see also (c) above), **corticosteroids** (395 patients), **diuretics** (264 patients), **lipid lowering drugs** (493 patients), **NSAIDs** (599 patients), **phosphodiesterase inhibitors** (230 patients), **quinolone antibacterials** (301 patients), or **salicylates** (821 patients).[1] Individual drugs were not named. The UK makers also predict that because dutasteride is formulated in solution in a gelatin capsule, pH changes are unlikely to affect its dissolution significantly, an it will therefore not interact with **antacids**, **H_2-blockers** or **proton pump inhibitors**.[1]

1. GlaxoSmithKline. Personal Communication, August 2003.
2. Avodart (Dutasteride). GlaxoSmithKline UK. UK Summary of product characteristics, May 2005.

Enteric coated, delayed release preparations + Antacids

It is thought that enteric-coated, delayed-release preparations may possibly dissolve prematurely if they are taken at the same time as antacids, but positive confirmatory evidence of this seems to be lacking.

Clinical evidence, mechanism, importance and management

A number of drugs may damage the stomach wall (the NSAIDs for example) and for this reason some of them are given an enteric coating to resist gastric acid to prevent their release until they reach the more alkaline conditions within the small intestine. Other drugs are formulated as delayed release preparations to ensure that the drug is released at the optimum site for absorption. There is a British National Formulary 'Cautionary and Advisory label' (No.5) that advises patients not to take them at the same time of day as indigestion remedies.[1] The belief is that a rise in pH caused by the antacid might result in the premature dissolution of the preparation.

What is not clear is whether any rise in pH caused by antacids actually causes premature dissolution of these preparations. Confirmatory clinical and experimental evidence of this seems to be lacking. Moreover, antacids usually do not cause a marked change in the gastric pH. On the other hand the proton pump inhibitors cause marked and long lasting changes in pH, which would be much more likely to affect the enteric-coating, but there are no BNF warnings about using these drugs concurrently.

1. British National Formulary. 49th ed. London: The British Medical Association and The Pharmaceutical Press; 2005. p. 819.

Ethylene dibromide + Disulfiram

The very high incidence of malignant tumours in *rats* exposed to both ethylene dibromide and disulfiram is the basis of the recommendation that concurrent exposure to these compounds should be avoided.

Clinical evidence, mechanism, importance and management

Research conducted to establish occupational safety of exposure to ethylene dibromide showed that the incidence of malignant tumours in *rats* exposed to 20 ppm ethylene dibromide (7 hours daily, 5 days weekly), while receiving a diet containing 0.05% disulfiram by weight, is very high indeed.[1,2] The reasons are not understood. In addition to the precautions needed to protect workers from the toxic effects of ethylene dibromide, it has been strongly recommended that disulfiram should not be given to those who may be exposed to this compound.[2] This information is also summarised in another report.[3]

1. Plotnick HB. Carcinogenesis in rats of combined ethylene dibromide and disulfiram. *JAMA* (1978) 239, 1609.

2. Anon. Ethylene dibromide and disulfiram toxic interaction. NIOSH Current Intelligence Bulletin. *US Department of Health, Education and Welfare Publication* (1978) No 78-145.

3. Stein HP, Bahlman LJ, Leidel NA, Parker JC, Thomas AW, Millar JD. Ethylene dibromide and disulfiram toxic interaction. *Am Ind Hyg Assoc J* (1978) 39, A35–A37.

Evening primrose oil + Phenothiazines

Although seizures have occurred in a few schizophrenics on phenothiazines and evening primrose oil, no adverse effects were seen in others, and there appears to be no firm evidence that evening primrose oil should be avoided by epileptic patients.

Clinical evidence

Twenty-three patients were enrolled in a placebo-controlled trial of evening primrose oil in schizophrenia. During the treatment phase, patients were given 8 capsules of *Efamol* in addition to their normal medication. Seizures developed in 3 patients, one during treatment with placebo. The other two patients were on evening primrose oil, one was receiving **fluphenazine decanoate** 50 mg once every 2 weeks and the other **fluphenazine decanoate** 25 mg once every 2 weeks with **thioridazine**, which was later changed to **chlorpromazine**.[1] In another study, 3 long-stay hospitalised schizophrenics were treated with evening primrose oil. Their schizophrenia became much worse and all 3 patients showed EEG evidence of temporal lobe epilepsy.[2]

In contrast, no seizures or epileptiform events were reported in a cross-over study of 48 patients (most of them schizophrenics) on **phenothiazines** when they were additionally treated with evening primrose oil for 4 months.[3] Concurrent use was also apparently uneventful in another study in schizophrenic patients.[4]

Mechanism

Not understood. One suggestion is that evening primrose oil possibly increases the well-recognised epileptogenic effects of the phenothiazines, rather than having an epileptogenic action of its own.[1] Another idea is that it might unmask temporal lobe epilepsy.[1,2]

Importance and management

The phenothiazine/evening primrose oil interaction is not well established, nor is its incidence known, but clearly some caution is appropriate during concurrent use in schizophrenic patients, because seizures may develop in a few individuals. There seems to be no way of identifying the patients at particular risk. The extent to which the underlying disease condition might affect what happens is also unclear.

No **anticonvulsant**/evening primrose oil interaction has been established and the reports cited above[1,2] appear to be the sole basis for the suggestion that evening primrose oil should be avoided by epileptics. No seizures appear to have been reported in patients on evening primrose oil not taking phenothiazines. The makers of *Epogam*, an evening primrose oil preparation, claim that it is known to have improved the control of epilepsy in patients previously uncontrolled with conventional anti-epileptic drugs, and other patients are said to have had no problems during concurrent treatment.[5] Even so, until the situation is formally examined it would seem prudent to monitor concurrent use.

1. Holman CP, Bell AFJ. A trial of evening primrose oil in the treatment of chronic schizophrenia. *J Orthomol Psychiatry* (1983) 12, 302–4.

2. Vaddadi KS. The use of gamma-linolenic acid and linoleic acid to differentiate between temporal lobe epilepsy and schizophrenia. *Prostaglandins Med* (1981) 6, 375–9.

3. Vaddadi KS, Courtney P, Gilleard CJ, Manku MS, Horrobin DF. A double-blind trial of essential fatty acid supplementation in patients with tardive dyskinesia. *Psychiatry Res* (1989) 27, 313–23.

4. Vaddadi KS, Horrobin DF. Weight loss produced by evening primrose oil administration in normal and schizophrenic individuals. *IRCS Med Sci* (1979) 7, 52.

5. Scotia Pharmaceuticals Ltd. Personal Communication, January 1991.

Finasteride + Alpha blockers

No clinically important interaction has been found to occur with finasteride and doxazosin. In one study terazosin did not interact with finasteride, but in another there was a suggestion of modestly increased finasteride levels.

Clinical evidence, mechanism, importance and management

In a parallel study, 48 healthy subjects were divided into three groups. One group took **terazosin** 10 mg daily for 18 days, another took finasteride 5 mg daily for 18 days, and the third group took both drugs. The pharmacokinetics and pharmacodynamics of both drugs remained unchanged, and the serum levels of testosterone and dihydrotestosterone were also unaltered by concurrent use.[1] However, another study, comparing groups of healthy subjects on finasteride and alpha blockers found that after 5 days of combined therapy the finasteride/**terazosin** group had an 11% lower maximum plasma level of finasteride and a 12% higher AUC, compared with the group taking finasteride alone (both differences were not statistically significant). Conversely, after 10 days of combined therapy, the maximum finasteride level was 16% higher and the AUC 31% higher, which was statistically significant. The levels of the finasteride/**doxazosin** group were not significantly different. The clinical significance of the possible modest increased finasteride levels with **terazosin** is not clear,[2] but is likely to be small.

1. Samara E, Hosmane B, Locke C, Eason C, Cavanaugh J, Granneman GR. Assessment of the pharmacokinetic-pharmacodynamic interaction between terazosin and finasteride. *J Clin Pharmacol* (1996) 36, 1169–78.

2. Vashi V, Chung M, Hilbert J, Lawrence V, Phillips K. Pharmacokinetic interaction between finasteride and terazosin, but not finasteride and doxazosin. *J Clin Pharmacol* (1998) 38, 1072–6.

Folic acid + Adsorbents

***In vitro* studies show that folic acid is markedly adsorbed by magnesium trisilicate and edible clay.[1] This would be expected to reduce its absorption from the gut, but the clinical importance of this awaits assessment.**

1. Iwuagwu MA, Jideonwo A. Preliminary investigations into the in-vitro interaction of folic acid with magnesium trisilicate and edible clay. *Int J Pharmaceutics* (1990) 65, 63–7.

Folic acid + Sulfasalazine

Sulfasalazine can reduce the absorption of folic acid.

Clinical evidence, mechanism, importance and management

The absorption of folic acid was reduced by about a third (from 65% to 44.5%) in patients with ulcerative and granulomatous colitis when compared with healthy subjects, and even further reduced (down to 32%) while taking sulfasalazine.[1] The clinical importance of this is uncertain, but it should be borne in mind when both drugs are given together.

1. Franklin JL, Rosenberg IH. Impaired folic acid absorption in inflammatory bowel disease: effects of salicylazosulfapyridine (Azulfidine). *Gastroenterology* (1973) 64, 517–25.

Glucagon + Beta-blockers

The hyperglycaemic effects of glucagon may be reduced by propranolol.

Clinical evidence, mechanism, importance and management

The hyperglycaemic activity of glucagon was reduced in the presence of **propranolol** in 5 healthy subjects.[1] Blood sugar levels increased by about 45% in the presence of glucagon, but when propranolol was also given the increase was only about 15%. The reason is uncertain, but one suggestion is that the **propranolol** inhibits the effects of the catecholamines that are released by glucagon. The clinical importance of this interaction is uncertain.

1. Messerli FH, Kuchel O, Tolis G, Hamet P, Frayasse J, Genest J. Effects of β-adrenergic blockage on plasma cyclic AMP and blood sugar responses to glucagon and isoproterenol in man. *Int J Clin Pharmacol Biopharm* (1976) 14, 189–94.

5-HT$_3$ receptor antagonists + Aprepitant

Aprepitant had no clinically relevant effect on the pharmacokinetics of granisetron, ondansetron or palonosetron.

Clinical evidence, mechanism, importance and management

In a study in healthy subjects aprepitant 375 mg on day one, then 250 mg on days 2 to 5 caused a minor 15% increase in the AUC of intravenous **ondansetron** 32 mg given on day one.[1] In another study, aprepitant 125 mg on day one, then 80 mg on days 2 and 3 had no effect on the pharmacokinetics of oral **granisetron** 2 mg given on day one.[1] Similarly, aprepitant 125 mg on day one, then 80 mg on days 2 and 3 had no effect on the pharmacokinetics of a single 250-microgram intravenous dose of **palonosetron** given on day one to healthy subjects.[2]

No dosage adjustment is required when aprepitant is given with **ondansetron**, **granisetron** or **palonosetron**.

1. Blum RA, Majumdar A, McCrea J, Busillo J, Orlowski LH, Panebianco D, Hesney M, Petty KJ, Goldberg MR, Murphy MG, Gottesdiener KM, Hustad CM, Lates C, Kraft WK, Van Buren S, Waldman SA, Greenberg HE. Effects of aprepitant on the pharmacokinetics of ondansetron and granisetron in healthy subjects. *Clin Ther* (2003) 25, 1407–19.
2. Shah AK, Hunt TL, Gallagher SC, Cullen MT. Pharmacokinetics of palonosetron in combination with aprepitant in healthy volunteers. *Curr Med Res Opin* (2005) 21, 595–601.

Iron compounds + Antacids

The absorption of iron and the expected haematological response can be reduced by the concurrent use of antacids. Separate their administration as much as possible.

Clinical evidence

(a) Aluminium and magnesium hydroxides, sodium bicarbonate and calcium carbonate

A study in healthy subjects who were mildly iron-deficient (due to blood donation or menstruation) found that one teaspoonful of *Mylanta II* (**aluminium/magnesium hydroxide** + simeticone) had little effect on the absorption of 10 or 20 mg **ferrous sulfate** at 2 hours. However, **sodium bicarbonate** 1 g almost halved the absorption of **ferrous sulfate**, and **calcium carbonate** 500 mg reduced it by two-thirds. Iron absorption from a **multivitamin** and **mineral** preparation was little affected by whether or not the tablet contained **calcium carbonate**.[1] Another study found that an antacid containing **aluminium/magnesium hydroxides** and **magnesium carbonate** reduced the absorption of **ferrous sulfate** and **ferrous fumarate** (both containing 100 mg of ferrous iron) in healthy iron-replete subjects by 37% and 31% respectively.[2] Poor absorption of iron during treatment with **sodium bicarbonate** and **aluminium hydroxide** has been described elsewhere.[3,4] One study did not find that the absorption of **ferrous sulfate** (iron 10 mg/kg) was affected by doses of **magnesium hydroxide** (5 mg for every 1 mg of iron) when given 30 minutes apart.[5] However, it has been suggested that iron absorption was not measured for a sufficient period to fully rule out a reduction in absorption.[6]

(b) Magnesium trisilicate

When oral iron failed to cause an expected rise in haemoglobin levels in patients taking non-absorbable alkalis such as magnesium trisilicate, a study was undertaken in 9 patients. Each patient was given 5 mg of isotopically labelled **ferrous sulfate** after a 35-g dose of magnesium trisilicate. The magnesium reduced the absorption of iron from an average of 30 to 12%, the reduction being small in some patients, but one individual showed a fall from 67 to 5%.[7]

Mechanism

Uncertain. One suggestion is that magnesium sulphate changes ferrous sulphate into less easily absorbed salts, or increases its polymerisation.[7] Carbonates possibly cause the formation of poorly soluble iron complexes.[3] Aluminium hydroxide is believed to precipitate iron as the hydroxide and ferric ions can become intercalated into the aluminium hydroxide crystal lattice,[8] leaving less available for absorption.

Importance and management

Information is limited and difficult to assess because of the many variables (e.g. different dosages ranging from very small to those mimicking overdose, and a mix of subjects and patients). However, a reasonable 'blanket precaution' to achieve maximal absorption would be to separate the administration of iron preparations and antacids as much as possible to avoid admixture in the gut. This may not prove to be necessary with some preparations.

1. O'Neil-Cutting MA, Crosby WH. The effect of antacids on the absorption of simultaneously ingested iron. *JAMA* (1986) 255, 1468–70.
2. Ekenved G, Halvorsen L, Sölvell L. Influence of a liquid antacid on the absorption of different iron salts. *Scand J Haematol* (1976) 28 (Suppl), 65–77.
3. Benjamin BI, Cortell S, Conrad ME. Bicarbonate-induced iron complexes and iron absorption: one effect of pancreatic secretions. *Gastroenterology* (1967) 35, 389–96.
4. Rastogi SP, Padilla F, Boyd CM. Effect of aluminum hydroxide on iron absorption. *J Arkansas Med Soc* (1976) 73, 133–4.
5. Snyder BK, Clark RF. Effect of magnesium hydroxide administration on iron absorption after a supratherapeutic dose of ferrous sulfate in human volunteers: a randomized controlled trial. *Ann Emerg Med* (1999) 33, 400–405.
6. Wallace KL, Curry SC, LoVecchio F, Raschke RA. Effect of magnesium hydroxide on iron absorption after ferrous sulfate. *Ann Emerg Med* (1999) 34, 685–6.
7. Hall GJL, Davis AE. Inhibition of iron absorption by magnesium trisilicate. *Med J Aust* (1969) 2, 95–6.
8. Coste JF, De Bari VA, Keil LB, Needle MA. *In-vitro* interactions of oral hematinics and antacid suspensions. *Curr Ther Res* (1977) 22, 205–15.

Iron compounds or Vitamin B$_{12}$ + Chloramphenicol

In addition to the serious and potentially fatal bone marrow depression that can occur with chloramphenicol, it may also cause a milder, reversible bone marrow depression, which can oppose the treatment of anaemias with iron or vitamin B$_{12}$.

Clinical evidence

Ten out of 22 patients on **iron dextran** for iron-deficiency anaemia and also given chloramphenicol, failed to show the expected haematological response to the iron.[1] Four patients on vitamin B$_{12}$ for pernicious anaemia were all similarly refractory to treatment until the chloramphenicol was withdrawn.[1]

Mechanism

Chloramphenicol can cause two forms of bone marrow depression. One is serious and irreversible, and can result in fatal aplastic anaemia, whereas the other is probably unrelated, milder and reversible, and appears to occur at chloramphenicol serum levels of 25 micrograms/ml or more. The reason is, that chloramphenicol can inhibit protein synthesis, the first sign of which is a fall in the reticulocyte count, which reflects inadequate red cell maturation. This response to chloramphenicol has been seen in *animals*,[2] healthy individuals,[3] a series of patients with liver disease,[4] and in anaemic patients[1] being treated with iron dextran or vitamin B$_{12}$.

Importance and management

An established interaction of clinical importance. The authors of one study recommend that chloramphenicol dosages of 25 to 30 mg/kg are usually adequate for treating infections without running the risk of elevating serum levels to 25 micrograms/ml or more, which is when this type of marrow depression can occur.[5] Monitor the effects of using iron or B$_{12}$ concurrently. A preferable alternative would be to use a different antibacterial. Note that chloramphenicol should not be used in patients with pre-existing bone-marrow depression or blood dyscrasias.

1. Saidi P, Wallerstein RO, Aggeler PM. Effect of chloramphenicol on erythropoiesis. *J Lab Clin Med* (1961) 57, 247–56.
2. Rigdon RH, Crass G, Martin N. Anemia produced by chloramphenicol (Chloromycetin) in the duck. *AMA Arch Pathol* (1954) 58, 85–93.
3. Jiji RM, Gangarosa EJ, de la Macorra F. Chloramphenicol and its sulfamoyl analogue. Report of reversible erythropoietic toxicity in healthy volunteers. *Arch Intern Med* (1963) 111, 116–28.
4. McCurdy PR. Chloramphenicol bone marrow toxicity. *JAMA* (1961) 176, 588–93.
5. Scott JL, Finegold SM, Belkin GA, Lawrence JS. A controlled double-blind study of the hematologic toxicity of chloramphenicol. *N Engl J Med* (1965) 272, 1137–42.

Iron compounds + Coffee or Tea

Coffee may possibly contribute towards the development of iron-deficiency anaemia in pregnant women, and reduce the levels of iron in breast milk. As a result their babies may also be iron-deficient. Tea may also possibly be associated with microcytic anaemia in children.

Clinical evidence

(a) Coffee

A controlled study among pregnant women in Costa Rica found that coffee consumption was associated with reductions in the haemoglobin levels and haematocrits of the mothers during pregnancy, and of their babies shortly after birth, despite the fact that the women were taking 200 mg **ferric sulphate** and 500 micrograms of folate daily. The babies also had a slightly lower birth weight (3189 g vs 3310 g). Almost a quarter of the mothers were considered as having iron-deficiency anaemia (haemoglobin levels of less than 11 g/dl) compared with none among the control group of non-coffee drinkers. Levels of iron in breast milk were reduced by about one third. The coffee drinkers drank more than 450 ml of coffee daily, equivalent to more than 10 g ground coffee.[1]

(b) Tea

A much higher incidence of microcytic anaemia has been described in tea-drinking infants in Israel. The 'tea-drinkers' consumed a median of 250 ml tea each day, and the incidence of anaemia was 64%, which was about twice that of the non-tea drinking control group (31%).[2] A case report describes impaired response to iron, given to correct an iron-deficiency anaemia, in the presence of 2 litres of black tea taken daily. The patient recovered when the black tea was stopped.[3] Another report describes no change in the absorption of **iron supplements** in daily doses of 2 to 15.8 mg/kg in 10 iron-deficient tea-drinking children, although the children were only given 150 ml of tea.[4]

Mechanism

Tannins are thought to form insoluble complexes with iron and thus reduce its absorption.[2,4]

Importance and management

The general importance of these findings is uncertain, but be aware that coffee or tea consumption may contribute to iron-deficiency anaemia. Note that tea and coffee are not generally considered to be suitable drinks for babies and children, because of their effects on iron absorption. More study is needed.

1. Muñoz LM, Lönnerdal B, Keen CL, Dewey KG. Coffee consumption as a factor in iron deficiency anemia among pregnant women and their infants in Costa Rica. *Am J Clin Nutr* (1988) 48, 645–51.
2. Merhav H, Amitai Y, Palti H, Godfrey S. Tea drinking and microcytic anemia in infants. *Am J Clin Nutr* (1985) 41, 1210–13.
3. Mahlknecht U, Weidmann E, Seipelt G. Black tea delays recovery from iron-deficiency anaemia. *Haematologica* (2001) 86, 559.
4. Koren G, Boichis H, Keren G. Effects of tea on the absorption of pharmacological doses of an oral iron preparation. *Isr J Med Sci* (1982) 18, 547.

Iron compounds + Colestyramine

Colestyramine binds with ferrous sulphate in the gut and reduces its absorption, but the clinical importance of this is uncertain.

Clinical evidence, mechanism, importance and management

Studies have shown that colestyramine binds with iron, and in *rats* this was found to halve the absorption of a single 100-microgram dose of **ferrous sulphate**.[1] Nobody seems to have checked on the general clinical importance of this in patients. Until more is known it would seem prudent to separate the dosages of the iron and colestyramine to avoid mixing in the gut, thereby minimising the effects of this possible interaction. The standard recommendation is to avoid other drugs one hour before or 4 to 6 hours after colestyramine.

1. Thomas FB, McCullough F, Greenberger NJ. Inhibition of the intestinal absorption of inorganic and hemoglobin iron by cholestyramine. *J Lab Clin Med* (1971) 78, 70–80.

Iron compounds + H_2-blockers

Apart from a brief and unconfirmed report alleging that cimetidine reduced the response to ferrous sulphate in three patients, there appears to be no other evidence that H_2-blockers reduce the absorption of iron to a clinically relevant extent. Iron causes only a small and clinically irrelevant reduction in the serum levels of cimetidine and famotidine.

Clinical evidence, mechanism, importance and management

(a) Effect on iron

A brief report describes 3 patients taking **cimetidine** 1 g and **ferrous sulfate** 600 mg daily whose ulcers healed after 2 months, but their anaemia and altered iron metabolism persisted. When the **cimetidine** was reduced to 400 mg daily, but with the same dose of iron, the blood picture resolved satisfactorily within a month.[1] The author of the report attributed this response to the **cimetidine**-induced rise in gastric pH, which reduced the absorption of the iron. However, this suggested mechanism was subsequently disputed, as medicinal iron is already in the most absorbable form, Fe^{2+}, and so does not need an acidic environment to aid absorption.[2] A study in patients with iron deficiency, or iron deficiency anaemia, found that the concurrent use of **famotidine**, **nizatidine**, or **ranitidine**, did not affect their response to 2400 mg of **iron succinyl-protein complex** (equivalent to 60 mg of iron twice daily).[3] No special precautions would seem necessary on concurrent use.

(b) Effect on H_2-blockers

In a series of 3 studies, healthy subjects were given a 300-mg tablet of **cimetidine** with either a 300-mg tablet of **ferrous sulfate** or 300 mg of **ferrous sulfate** in solution. The reductions in the AUC and the maximum serum levels of the **cimetidine** were small (less than 16%). In the third experiment they were given **famotidine** 40 mg with a 300-mg tablet of **ferrous sulfate**. Again, the AUC and maximum serum level reductions were also very small (10% or less). These small reductions are almost certainly due to the formation of a weak complex between the iron and these H_2-blockers.[4] An *in vitro* study with **ranitidine** found that, while it also binds with iron, it forms a very weak complex, and is less likely to bind than **cimetidine** or **famotidine**.[4] It was concluded that no clinically relevant interaction occurs between **ferrous sulfate** and any of these H_2-blockers.[4]

1. Esposito R. Cimetidine and iron-deficiency anaemia. *Lancet* (1977) ii, 1132.
2. Rosner F. Cimetidine and iron absorption. *Lancet* (1978) i, 95.
3. Bianchi FM, Cavassini GB, Leo P. Iron protein succinylate in the treatment of iron deficiency: Potential interaction with H_2-receptor antagonists. *Int J Clin Pharmacol Ther Toxicol* (1993) 31, 209–17.
4. Partlow ES, Campbell NRC, Chan SC, Pap KM, Granberg K, Hasinoff BB. Ferrous sulfate does not reduce serum levels of famotidine or cimetidine after concurrent ingestion. *Clin Pharmacol Ther* (1996) 59, 389–93.

Iron compounds + Neomycin

Neomycin may alter the absorption of iron.

Clinical evidence, mechanism, importance and management

A study in 6 patients found that neomycin markedly reduced the absorption of iron ($iron^{59}$ as **ferrous citrate**) in 4 patients, but increased the absorption in the other 2 patients who initially had low serum iron levels. None of the patients were anaemic at any time.[1] The importance of this is uncertain, but monitor the outcome of concurrent use.

1. Jacobson ED, Chodos RB, Faloon WW. An experimental malabsorption syndrome induced by neomycin. *Am J Med* (1960) 28, 524–33.

Iron compounds + Vitamin E

Vitamin E impaired the response to iron in a group of anaemic children.

Clinical evidence, mechanism, importance and management

A group of 26 anaemic children aged 7 to 40 months were given **iron dextran** 5 mg/kg daily for 3 days. Vitamin E 200 units daily was also given to 9 of the children, starting 24 hours before the **iron dextran** and continued for a total of 4 days. It was noted that after 6 days, those on vitamin E had a reticulocyte response of only 4.4% compared with 14.4% in the patients not given vitamin E. The vitamin E group also had reduced haemoglobin levels and a lower haematocrit. The reasons are not understood. Check for any evidence of a reduced haematological response in anaemic patients given iron and vitamin E. The authors of the report point out that this dosage of vitamin E was well above the recommended daily dietary intake.[1]

1. Melhorn DK, Gross S. Relationships between iron-dextran and vitamin E in iron deficiency anemia in children. *J Lab Clin Med* (1969) 74, 789–802.

Methoxsalen + Phenytoin

The serum levels of methoxsalen can be markedly reduced by the concurrent use of phenytoin. This resulted in failure of treatment for psoriasis in one patient.

Clinical evidence, mechanism, importance and management

A patient with epilepsy failed to respond to treatment for psoriasis with PUVA (12 treatments of methoxsalen 30 mg given orally and ultraviolet A irradiation) while taking phenytoin 250 mg daily. Methoxsalen serum levels were normal in the absence of phenytoin, but abnormally low while taking phenytoin,[1] due, it is suggested, to the enzyme inducing effects of the phenytoin. This interaction could lead to serious erythema and blistering if the phenytoin dose is reduced during therapy, as methoxsalen levels rise and therefore photosensitivity caused by the methoxsalen may be increased. Concurrent use should be avoided or very closely monitored.

1. Staberg B, Hueg B. Interaction between 8-methoxypsoralen and phenytoin. Consequence for PUVA therapy. *Acta Derm Venereol* (1985) 65, 553–5.

Metyrapone + Cyproheptadine

Cyproheptadine may interfere with the metyrapone test.

Clinical evidence, mechanism, importance and management

Pretreatment with cyproheptadine 4 mg six-hourly, 2 days before and throughout a standard metyrapone test (750 mg four-hourly for 6 doses), reduced the metyrapone-induced urinary 17-hydroxycorticosteroid response in 9 healthy subjects by 32%, and also reduced the serum 11-deoxycortisol response.[1] Consequently the results of metyrapone tests for Cushing's syndrome will be unreliable in patients taking cyproheptadine and therefore it should be withdrawn prior to the test.

1. Plonk J, Feldman JM, Keagle D. Modification of adrenal function by the anti-serotonin agent cyproheptadine. *J Clin Endocrinol Metab* (1976) 42, 291–5.

Metyrapone + Phenytoin

The results of the metyrapone test are unreliable in patients taking phenytoin.

Clinical evidence, mechanism, importance and management

A study in 5 healthy subjects and 3 patients taking phenytoin 300 mg showed that their serum metyrapone levels 4 hours after taking a regular 750-mg dose were very low when compared with a control group (6.5 compared with 48.2 micrograms/100 ml). The response to metyrapone (i.e. the fall in circulation glucocorticoids) is related to serum levels and was therefore proportionately lower.[1] Other reports confirm that the urinary steroid response is subnormal in patients taking phenytoin.[2,3] The reason is, that phenytoin is a potent liver enzyme inducer that increases the metabolism of the metyrapone, thereby reducing the size of the effect.[1,4] Because of this, the results of the metyrapone test for Cushing's syndrome are invalid. Doubling the dose of metyrapone from 750 mg four-hourly to two-hourly has been shown to give results similar to those in subjects not taking phenytoin.[1] However, the maker recommends that phenytoin and **barbiturates** are withdrawn prior to the test.[5]

1. Meikle AW, Jubiz W, Matsukura S, West CD, Tyler FH. Effect of diphenylhydantoin on the metabolism of metyrapone and release of ACTH in man. *J Clin Endocrinol Metab* (1969) 29, 1553–8.
2. Krieger DT. Effect of diphenylhydantoin on pituitary-adrenal interrelations. *J Clin Endocrinol Metab* (1962) 22, 490–3.
3. Werk EE, Thrasher K, Choi Y, Sholiton LJ. Failure of metyrapone to inhibit 11-hydroxylation of 11-deoxycortisol during drug therapy. *J Clin Endocrinol Metab* (1967) 27, 1358–60.
4. Jubiz W, Levinson RA, Meikle AW, West CD, Tyler FH. Absorption and conjugation of metyrapone during diphenylhydantoin therapy: mechanism of the abnormal response to oral metyrapone. *Endocrinology* (1970) 86, 328–31.
5. Metopirone (Metyrapone). Alliance Pharmaceuticals. UK Summary of product characteristics, February 2005.

Mifepristone + Aspirin or NSAIDs

The makers of mifepristone say that the antiprostaglandin effects of NSAIDs including aspirin could theoretically decrease the efficacy of mifepristone. They recommend using non-NSAID analgesics.[1]

1. Mifegyne (Mifepristone). Exelgyn Laboratories. UK Summary of product characteristics, February 2005.

Modafinil + Miscellaneous

The makers advise vigilance if anticonvulsants, particularly phenytoin, are used with modafinil. No pharmacokinetic interaction appears to occur with triazolam. There is speculation, based on *in vitro* studies, about some possible interactions with other drugs. For other interactions of modafinil see also 'dexamfetamine', (p.967), and 'methylphenidate', (p.967).

Clinical evidence, mechanism, importance and management

Due to the enzyme inducing potential of modafinil, the makers say that care should be observed with co-administration of **phenytoin**.[1] There is *in vitro* evidence to indicate that modafinil may possibly inhibit the metabolism of **phenytoin** by the cytochrome P450 isoenzymes CYP2C9 and CYP2C19, there is some reason for monitoring concurrent use for evidence of increased **phenytoin** effects and toxicity.[2] In the case of concurrent use with the potent enzyme inducer **phenobarbital** *animal* studies suggest that it is the serum levels of modafinil that may be reduced rather than those of **phenobarbital**.[3]

There is no clinical evidence of a **warfarin**/modafinil interaction, but because **warfarin** can be metabolised by the cytochrome P450 isoenzyme CYP2C9 (which is inhibited by modafinil) the US product information suggests that concurrent use should be monitored.[2] Similarly there is no clinical evidence of interactions with potent inhibitors of CYP3A4 (e.g. **itraconazole**, **ketoconazole**), which might increase the effects of modafinil, or with potent enzyme inducers (**carbamazepine**, **phenobarbital**, **rifampicin (rifampin)**), which might reduce the effects of modafinil, but the US product information includes them under the heading of drug interactions.[2] Such interactions seem unlikely because CYP3A4 is not the only cytochrome P450 isoenzyme that is involved in the metabolism of modafinil. Nor does it seem likely that the serum levels of **theophylline** will be reduced to a clinically relevant extent by the modest enzyme inducing effects of modafinil. The makers report that single-dose studies in normal subjects given 400 mg of modafinil with 125 micrograms of **triazolam** found that the maximum plasma concentration of triazolam was reduced by 42% and its elimination half-life was reduced by about 1 hour and they consider dosage adjustments may be necessary.[2]

All of these 'interactions' are only tentative predictions based on *in vitro* evidence and confirmation in practice is awaited.

1. Provigil (Modafinil). Cephalon UK Ltd. UK Summary of product characteristics, September 2004.
2. Provigil (Modafinil), Cephalon. US prescribing information, December 2004.
3. Moachon G, Kanmacher I, Clenet M, Matinier D. Pharmacokinetic profile of modafinil. *Drugs Today* (1996) 32 (Suppl 1), 23–33.

Nicotine + Vasopressin

A case report described marked hypotension and bradycardia in a young woman during surgery, attributed to the combined effects of vasopressin and the nicotine from a transdermal patch.

Clinical evidence

A 22-year-old woman in good health was anaesthetised for surgery with nitrous oxide/oxygen and isoflurane. Twenty minutes after induction she was given an injection of 0.2 units of vasopressin into the cervix. Within seconds she developed severe hypotension and bradycardia, and over the next 30 minutes blood pressures as low as 70/35 mmHg and heart rates as low as 38 bpm were recorded. She was treated with atropine and adrenaline (epinephrine), and eventually made a full recovery. This patient was wearing a transdermal nicotine patch.[1]

Mechanism

The circulatory collapse was attributed by the authors to the combined effects of the injected vasopressin and the nicotine from the transdermal patch. Both of these drugs can increase afterload and cause coronary artery vasoconstriction.[1]

Importance and management

This is an isolated report and any interaction is therefore not well established. Nevertheless the recommendation of the authors seems sensible, namely that nicotine patches should be removed the night before or 24 hours before surgery, and that patients should be asked to avoid smoking before surgery to make sure that nicotine levels are minimal. More study is needed.

1. Groudine SB, Morley JN. Recent problems with paracervical vasopressin: a possible synergistic reaction with nicotine. *Med Hypotheses* (1996) 47, 19–21.

Ondansetron + Food or Antacids

Food slightly increases the bioavailability of ondansetron, but an antacid was found to have no effect.

Clinical evidence, mechanism, importance and management

When 12 healthy subjects were given an 8 mg ondansetron tablet 5 minutes after a **meal**, its bioavailability was slightly increased (AUC + 17%) but the coadministration of a **aluminium/magnesium hydroxide** antacid (*Maalox*) had no effect.[1]

1. Bozigian HP, Pritchard JF, Gooding AE, Pakes GE. Ondansetron absorption in adults: effect of dosage form, food, and antacids. *J Pharm Sci* (1994) 83, 1011–13.

Oxybutynin + CYP3A4 enzyme inhibitors

Itraconazole can increase the serum levels of oxybutynin, but adverse effects are not increased. This interaction is considered to be of only minor clinical relevance.

Clinical evidence, mechanism, importance and management

A single 5-mg dose of oxybutynin was given to 10 healthy subjects after they had taken **itraconazole** 200 mg or a placebo daily for 4 days. The peak serum levels and the AUC of the oxybutynin were approximately doubled, while the pharmacokinetics of the active metabolite of oxybutynin were unchanged. The sum of the oxybutynin and its metabolite concentrations were on average about 13% higher than with the placebo. No increase in adverse effects was seen. This interaction is almost certainly due to **itraconazole** inhibiting the metabolism of oxybutynin by the cytochrome P450 isoenzyme CYP3A4, in the intestinal wall and liver. The authors of this report consider that this interaction is only of minor importance and, because **itraconazole** is a known and potent enzyme inhibitor, they also predict that other CYP3A4 inhibitors that are less potent (they cite **erythromycin**, **diltiazem**, **verapamil**) are unlikely to interact with oxybutynin significantly.[1]

1. Lukkari E, Juhakoski A, Aranko K, Neuvonen PJ. Itraconazole moderately increases serum concentrations of oxybutynin but does not affect those of the active metabolite. *Eur J Clin Pharmacol* (1997) 52, 403–6.

Oxygen; hyperbaric + Miscellaneous

It has been suggested, but not confirmed, that because increased levels of carbon dioxide in the tissues can increase the 'sensitivity' to oxygen-induced convulsions, carbonic anhydrase-inhibitors such as acetazolamide are contraindicated in those given hyperbaric oxygen, because they cause carbon dioxide to persist in the tissues. Nor should hyperbaric oxygen be given during opioid or barbiturate withdrawal because the convulsive threshold of such patients is already low.[1]

1. Gunby P. HBO can interact with preexisting patient conditions. *JAMA* (1981) 246, 1177–8.

Papaverine + Diazepam

Two men given normal test doses of papaverine for the investigation of impotence had prolonged erections attributed to the concurrent use of diazepam.

Clinical evidence, mechanism, importance and management

Undesirably prolonged erections (duration of 5 and 6 hours) occurred in 2 patients who had been given 5 or 10 mg of diazepam intravenously for anxiety before a 60-mg intracavernosal injection of papaverine.[1] Papaverine acts by relaxing the arterioles that supply the corpora so that the pressure rises. The increased pressure in the corpora compresses the trabecular venules so that the pressure continues to maintain the erection. Diazepam also relaxes smooth muscle and it would seem that this can be additive with the effects of papaverine. The authors of the report say that caution should be exercised in the choice of papaverine dosage in patients on anxiolytics (i.e. use less) although these two cases involving diazepam seem to be the only ones recorded.[1]

1. Vale JA, Kirby RS, Lees W. Papaverine, benzodiazepines, and prolonged erections. *Lancet* (1991) 337, 1552.

Penicillamine + Antacids

The absorption of penicillamine from the gut can be reduced by 30 to 40% if antacids containing aluminium/magnesium hydroxide are taken concurrently.

Clinical evidence

Maalox-plus (**aluminium/magnesium hydroxide**, **simeticone**) 30 ml reduced the absorption of a single 500-mg dose of penicillamine in 6 healthy subjects by a third.[1] Another study found that 30 ml of *Aludrox* (**aluminium/magnesium hydroxide**) reduced the absorption of penicillamine by about 40%.[2]

Mechanism

The most likely explanation is that the penicillamine forms less soluble chelates with magnesium and aluminium ions in the gut, which reduces its absorption.[2] Another idea is that the penicillamine is possibly less stable at the higher pH values caused by the antacid.[1]

Importance and management

An established interaction of clinical importance. If maximal absorption is needed the administration of the two drugs should be separated to avoid mixing in the gut. Two hours or so has been found enough for most other drugs which interact similarly. There seems to be nothing documented about other antacids.

1. Osman MA, Patel RB, Schuna A, Sundstrom WR, Welling PG. Reduction in oral penicillamine absorption by food, antacid and ferrous sulphate. *Clin Pharmacol Ther* (1983) 33, 465–70.
2. Ifan A, Welling PG. Pharmacokinetics of oral 500-mg penicillamine: effect of antacids on absorption. *Biopharm Drug Dispos* (1986) 7, 401–5.

Penicillamine + Food

Food can reduce the absorption of penicillamine by as much as a half.

Clinical evidence

The presence of food reduced the plasma levels of penicillamine 500 mg by about 50% (from 3.05 to 1.52 micrograms/ml) in healthy subjects. The total amount absorbed was similarly reduced.[1,2] These figures are in good agreement with previous findings.[3]

Mechanism

Uncertain. One suggestion is that food delays stomach emptying so that the penicillamine is exposed to more prolonged degradation in the stomach.[2] Another idea is that the protein in food reduces penicillamine absorption.

Importance and management

An established interaction. If maximal effects are required the penicillamine should not be taken with food.

1. Schuna A, Osman MA, Patel RB, Welling PG, Sundstrom WR. Influence of food on the bioavailability of penicillamine. *J Rheumatol* (1983) 10, 95–7.
2. Osman MA, Patel RB, Schuna A, Sundstrom WR, Welling PG. Reduction in oral penicillamine absorption by food, antacid and ferrous sulphate. *Clin Pharmacol Ther* (1983) 33, 465–70.
3. Bergstrom RF, Kay DR, Harkcom TM, Wagner JG. Penicillamine kinetics in normal subjects. *Clin Pharmacol Ther* (1981) 30, 404–13.

Penicillamine + Iron compounds

The absorption of penicillamine can be reduced as much as two-thirds by oral iron compounds.

Clinical evidence

Ferrous iron (as *Fersamal*) 90 mg reduced the absorption of penicillamine 250 mg in 5 healthy subjects by about two-thirds (using the cupruretic effects of penicillamine as a measure).[1]

A two-thirds reduction in absorption has been described in 6 other subjects given penicillamine 500 mg and **ferrous sulfate** 300 mg.[2] Other studies confirm this interaction.[3,4] There is also evidence that the withdrawal of iron from patients stabilised on penicillamine can lead to the development of toxicity (nephropathy) unless the penicillamine dosage is reduced.[5]

Mechanism

It is believed that the iron and penicillamine form a chemical complex or chelate within the gut, which is less easily absorbed.

Importance and management

An established and clinically important interaction. For maximal absorption give the iron at least 2 hours after the penicillamine. This should reduce their admixture in the gut.[1] Do not withdraw iron suddenly from patients stabilised on penicillamine because the marked increase in absorption that follows may precipitate penicillamine toxicity. The toxic effects of penicillamine seem to be dependent on the size of the dose and possibly also related to the rate at which the dosage is increased.[5] Only ferrous sulfate and fumarate have been studied but other iron compounds would be expected to interact similarly.

1. Lyle WH. Penicillamine and iron. *Lancet* (1976) ii, 420.
2. Osman MA, Patel RB, Schuna A, Sundstrom WR, Welling PG. Reduction in oral penicillamine absorption by food, antacid, and ferrous sulphate. *Clin Pharmacol Ther* (1983) 33, 465–70.
3. Lyle WH, Pearcey DF, Hui M. Inhibition of penicillamine-induced cupruresis by oral iron. *Proc R Soc Med* (1977) 70 (Suppl 3), 48–9.
4. Hall ND, Blake DR, Alexander GJM, Vaisey C, Bacon PA. Serum SH reactivity: a simple assessment of D-penicillamine absorption? *Rheumatol Int* (1981) 1, 39–41.
5. Harkness JAL, Blake DR. Penicillamine nephropathy and iron. *Lancet* (1982) ii, 1368–9.

Penicillamine + Miscellaneous

Penicillamine plasma levels are increased by chloroquine and to a lesser extent by indometacin. An increase in penicillamine toxicity is possible. An isolated report describes penicillamine-induced breast enlargement in a woman given a combined oral contraceptive.

Clinical evidence, mechanism, importance and management

Studies in which **chloroquine** was given to patients on penicillamine found that it was more effective, less effective, or indistinguishable from penicillamine alone. However in some instances penicillamine toxicity was reported to be increased.[1] A pharmacokinetic study in patients with rheumatoid arthritis on penicillamine 250 mg daily found that a single 250-mg dose of **chloroquine phosphate** increased the AUC by 34%, and raised the peak plasma levels by about 55%.[1] It seems possible therefore that any increased toxicity is simply a reflection of increased plasma penicillamine levels. Be alert for evidence of toxicity if both drugs are used.

Indometacin has been found to increase the AUC of penicillamine by 26% and the peak plasma levels by about 22%.[1]

A woman with Wilson's disease began to develop dark facial hair about 10 months after starting to take penicillamine 1.25 to 1.5 g daily. After 20 months her testosterone levels were found to be slightly raised, and she was started on a **combined oral contraceptive**, but within a month her breasts began to enlarge and become more tender, and after a further 6 months the penicillamine was replaced by trientine hydrochloride.[2] The reasons are not understood, but the authors of the report suggest that the penicillamine was the prime cause of the macromastia, but it possibly needed the presence of a 'second trigger' (i.e. the **oral contraceptive**) to set things in motion.[2]

There are 12 other cases of macromastia and gynaecomastia on record associated with the use of penicillamine, in some of which the second trigger may possibly have been a **corticosteroid** or **cimetidine**.[2] Macromastia appears to be an unusual adverse effect of penicillamine and there would seem to be no general reason for patients taking penicillamine to avoid **oral contraceptives**.

1. Seideman P, Lindström B. Pharmacokinetic interactions of penicillamine in rheumatoid arthritis. *J Rheumatol* (1989) 16, 473–4.
2. Rose BI, LeMaire WJ, Jeffers LJ. Macromastia in a woman treated with penicillamine and oral contraceptives. *J Reprod Med* (1990) 35, 43–5.

PUVA therapy + Herbal medicines or Foods

Two case reports describe photosensitivity, one in a patient taking rue (*Ruta graveolens*) and another in a patient who ate large amounts of celery soup.

Clinical evidence, mechanism, importance and management

A 35-year-old woman taking methoxsalen and undergoing PUVA for psoriasis unexpectedly developed increased photosensitivity. Over the previous weekend and on the morning of therapy she had been drinking a concoction of **rue (*Ruta graveolens*)**.[1] This plant naturally contains 5-methoxypsoralen so it would appear that a pharmacodynamic interaction occurred, which resulted in the photosensitivity.

The authors note that other herbal products contain photosensitising substances (e.g. those containing members of the **Umbelliferae** family; such as **celery**, or ***Chlorella*** species), and so suggest that patients undergoing PUVA should be warned about the potential interactions.[1] This warning appears justified by the case of a woman taking methoxsalen and undergoing PUVA, who developed photosensitivity after eating a large quantity of soup containing **celery**, parsnip and parsley.[2]

1. Puig L. Pharmacodynamic interaction with phototoxic plants during PUVA therapy. *Br J Dermatol* (1997) 136, 973–4.
2. Boffa MJ, Gilmour E, Ead RD. Celery soup causing severe phototoxicity during PUVA therapy. *Br J Dermatol* (1996) 135, 330–45.

Raloxifene + Miscellaneous

The absorption of raloxifene is reduced by colestyramine, and their concurrent use is not recommended. No clinically relevant interactions occur with aluminium/magnesium hydroxide, ampicillin, oral antibacterials, antihistamines, aspirin, benzodiazepines, calcium carbonate, digoxin, H_2-blockers, ibuprofen or paracetamol (acetaminophen).

Clinical evidence, mechanism, importance and management

(a) Antacids

The makers of raloxifene report that in studies, an antacid containing **aluminium/magnesium hydroxide** given 1 hour before and 2 hours after raloxifene had no effect on its absorption. Also, no interaction was seen with **calcium carbonate**.[1] There would therefore appear to be no reason for avoiding concurrent use.

(b) Colestyramine

The makers report that the concurrent use of colestyramine twice daily reduced the absorption of raloxifene by about 40% due to an interruption in enterohepatic cycling.[1] It is recommended that these two drugs should not be used concurrently.[1,2]

(c) Miscellaneous drugs

Ampicillin is reported to reduce the maximum serum levels of raloxifene, but the extent of the absorption and the elimination rate are unaffected.[1] Raloxifene is reported not to affect the steady-state AUC of **digoxin** over an 11-day period, while the maximum serum levels of **digoxin** were increased by only 5%. No clinically relevant changes in the plasma levels of raloxifene were seen in trials in which other drugs were also used. These drugs included **oral antibacterials** (not named), **antihistamines** (not named), **aspirin**, **benzodiazepines** (not named), **H_2-blockers** (not named), NSAIDs (**ibuprofen**, **naproxen**), and **paracetamol** (**acetaminophen**).[1] There would therefore appear to be no reason for avoiding the concurrent use of any of these drugs with raloxifene.

1. Eli Lilly and Company Limited. Personal communication, September 1998.
2. Evista (Raloxifene). Eli Lilly and Company Ltd. UK Summary of product characteristics, July 2003.

Retinoids + Food

Fatty foods increase the absorption of acitretin and etretinate. Food increases the absorption of isotretinoin. It is recommended that acitretin, etretinate and isotretinoin are taken with food.

Clinical evidence, mechanism, importance and management

The absorption of **acitretin** was increased by 90% and the peak plasma concentrations were increased by 70% when **acitretin** 50 mg was taken by 18 healthy subjects with a **standard breakfast**. The **breakfast** consisted of two poached eggs, two slices of toast, two pats of margarine and 8 oz (about 240 ml) of skimmed milk.[1] Other studies have found that **high fat meals**, and **milk** cause about a two to fivefold increase in the absorption of **etretinate** when compared with **high carbohydrate meals** or when fasting.[2,3] Similarly, the UK maker of **isotretinoin** notes that **food** (not specified) doubles the bioavailability of **isotretinoin**.[4] It is thought that because these retinoids are lipid soluble they become absorbed into the lymphatic system by becoming incorporated into the bile-acid micelles of the **fats** in the food. In this way losses due to first-pass liver metabolism and gut wall metabolism are minimised, and bioavailability increased. The makers of **acitretin** recommend taking it with **meals** or with **milk**,[5] and the makers of **isotretinoin** recommend taking it with food.[4] Similar recommendations were made with **etretinate**.[6]

1. McNamara PJ, Jewell RC, Jensen BK, Brindley CJ. Food increases the bioavailability of acitretin. *J Clin Pharmacol* (1988) 28, 1051–5.
2. DiGiovanna JJ, Cross EG, McClean SW, Ruddel ME, Gantt G, Peck GL. Etretinate: effect of milk intake on absorption. *J Invest Dermatol* (1984) 82, 636–40.
3. Colburn WA, Gibson DM, Rodriguez LC, Buggé CJL, Blumenthal HP. Effect of meals on the kinetics of etretinate. *J Clin Pharmacol* (1985) 25, 583–9.
4. Isotretinoin. Beacon Pharmaceuticals. UK Summary of product characteristics, June 2005.
5. Neotigason (Acitretin). Roche Products Ltd. UK Summary of product characteristics, August 2004.
6. Tigason (Etretinate). Roche Products Ltd. ABPI Datasheet Compendium, 1993–1994, p.1347–9.

Retinoids + Tetracyclines

The development of 'pseudotumour cerebri' (benign intracranial hypertension) has been associated with the concurrent use of isotretinoin and tetracyclines.

Clinical evidence, mechanism, importance and management

The concurrent use of **isotretinoin** and a **tetracycline** has resulted in the development of 'pseudotumour cerebri' (i.e. a clinical picture of cranial hypertension with headache, dizziness and visual disturbances). By 1983, the FDA had received reports of 10 patients with 'pseudotumour cerebri' and/or papilloedema associated with the use of **isotretinoin**. Four had retinal haemorrhages, and 5 of the 10 were also being treated with a **tetracycline**.[1] The makers also have similar reports on file of 3 patients given **isotretinoin** and either **minocycline** or **tetracycline**.[2] The same reaction has been seen in 2 patients given **etretinate** with **minocycline** or prednisolone.[3] It seems that the tetracyclines and retinoids have an additive effect in increasing intracranial pressure. The makers of **isotretinoin** contraindicate its use with tetracyclines.[4]

1. Anon. Adverse effects with isotretinoin. *FDA Drug Bull* (1983) 13, 21–3.
2. Shalita AR, Cunningham WJ, Leyden JJ, Pochi PE, Strauss JS. Isotretinoin treatment of acne and related disorders: an update. *J Am Acad Dermatol* (1983) 9, 629–38.
3. Viraben R, Mathieu C, Fonton B. Benign intracranial hypertension during etretinate therapy for mycosis fungoides. *J Am Acad Dermatol* (1985) 13, 515–17.
4. Isotretinoin. Beacon Pharmaceuticals. UK Summary of product characteristics, June 2005.

Retinoids + Vitamin A (Retinol)

A condition similar to vitamin A (retinol) overdosage may occur if isotretinoin and vitamin A are given concurrently.

Clinical evidence, mechanism, importance and management

Combined treatment with isotretinoin and **vitamin A** may result in a condition similar to overdosage with **vitamin A**. Concurrent use should therefore be avoided or very closely monitored because changes in bone structure can occur, including premature fusion of the epiphyseal discs in children.[1] The makers of **isotretinoin** say that high doses of **vitamin A** should be avoided.[2]

1. Milstone LM, McGuire J, Ablow RC. Premature epiphyseal closure in a child receiving oral 13-*cis*-retinoic acid. *J Am Acad Dermatol* (1982) 7, 663–6.
2. Isotretinoin. Beacon Pharmaceuticals. UK Summary of product characteristics, June 2005.

Sevelamer + Miscellaneous

Sevelamer has been shown not to alter the pharmacokinetics of enalapril, metoprolol or warfarin and seems unlikely to alter the absorption of other drugs, but monitoring is advisable until more clinical experience has been gained.

Clinical evidence, mechanism, importance and management

Concurrent administration of single doses of sevelamer hydrochloride 2.418 g (equivalent to 6 capsules) and **enalapril** 20 mg did not alter the AUC of **enalapril** or its active metabolite, enalaprilat, in 28 healthy subjects.[1] Similarly, concurrent administration of single doses of sevelamer 2.418 g and **metoprolol** 100 mg did not alter the AUC of **metoprolol** in 31 healthy subjects.[1] The makers also report that other studies in healthy subjects have shown that the pharmacokinetics of a single oral dose of **warfarin** 30 mg were not statistically changed by the presence of 2.418 g sevelamer hydrochloride (equivalent to 6 capsules). Five more 2.418 g doses of the sevelamer were given over 2 days to check whether it had any effect on the enterohepatic circulation. No effect was seen.[2,3] Thus it appears that sevelamer does not bind to these drugs within the gut to reduce their absorption. The makers similarly report that in *dogs* the peak serum drug levels and AUCs of single doses of **calcitriol**, **estrone**, **levothyroxine**, **propranolol**, **tetracycline**, **valproic acid**, **verapamil** and **warfarin** were not altered by sevelamer.[2] While the results of *animal* studies should never be extrapolated uncritically to the human situation, since in this instance no significant chemical or physiochemical binding apparently occurred between sevelamer and any of these drugs in the gut (and already demonstrated in the case of **warfarin**), this suggests that interactions with these drugs in the human gut are also unlikely.

So far the general picture is that interactions within the gut are not expected, but until more clinical experience is gained the makers suggest in the US product information[4] that "... when administering any other oral drug for which alterations in blood levels could have a clinically significant effect on safety or efficacy, the drug should be administered at least 1 hour before or 3 hours after *Renagel Capsules* (sevelamer)." If there is any evidence of reduced efficacy when other drugs are used concurrently, following this advice would seem sensible and practical.

1. Burke SK, Amin NS, Incerti C, Plone MA, Lee JW. Sevelamer hydrochloride (Renagel®), a phosphate-binding polymer, does not alter the pharmacokinetics of two commonly used antihypertensives in healthy volunteers. *J Clin Pharmacol* (2001) 41, 199–205.
2. Renagel (Sevelamer). Genzyme. UK Summary of product characteristics, January 2000.
3. Genzyme BV. Personal communication, May 2000.
4. Renagel Capsules (Sevelamer hydrochloride). Genzyme. US Prescribing information, October 2004.

Sibutramine + Azoles

Ketoconazole modestly increases steady-state levels of sibutramine and its active metabolites. The makers recommend caution when sibutramine is used with itraconazole or ketoconazole.

Clinical evidence, mechanism, importance and management

Twelve obese patients were given sibutramine 20 mg daily for 7 days, then together with 200 mg **ketoconazole** twice daily for a further 7 days. **Ketoconazole** caused moderate increases in the serum levels of sibutramine and its two metabolites (AUC and maximum serum level increases of 58 and 36% for metabolites M1, and 20 and 19% for M2, probably through inhibition of cytochrome P450 isoenzyme CYP3A4). Small increases in heart rates were seen (+2.5 bpm at 4 hours and +1.4 bpm at 8 hours), while ECG parameters were unchanged.[1] Sibutramine alone can cause an increase in heart rate, and a rate increase of 10 bpm is an indication to withdraw the drug. Therefore, the makers in the UK[2] suggest caution should be exercised when sibutramine is used with **ketoconazole**. They also suggest that due to its ability to inhibit CYP3A4 **itraconazole** should also be used with caution.

1. Hinson JL, Leone MB, Kisiki MJ, Moult JT, Trammel A and Faulkner RD. Steady-state interaction study of sibutramine (Meridia) and ketoconazole in uncomplicated obese subjects. *Pharm Res* (1996) 13 (9 Suppl), S116.
2. Reductil (Sibutramine). Abbott Laboratories Ltd. UK Summary of product characteristics, February 2004.

Sibutramine + Macrolides

Although no interaction appears to occur between sibutramine and erythromycin, the makers still caution the use of sibutramine with clarithromycin, erythromycin and troleandomycin.

Clinical evidence, mechanism, importance and management

Twelve obese patients were given sibutramine 20 mg daily for 7 days, then together with **erythromycin** 500 mg three times daily for a further 7 days. It was found that apart from some slight and unimportant changes in the pharmacokinetics of the metabolites of sibutramine (probably caused by some inhibition of the cytochrome P450 isoenzyme CYP3A4), the pharmacokinetics of sibutramine were not significantly altered by **erythromycin**. No blood pressure changes were seen and only very small and clinically irrelevant increases in the QTc interval and heart rate occurred.[1] The extent of any interaction appears to be too small to matter,[1] and there would seem to be no reason for avoiding the concurrent use of these two drugs. Despite this the UK makers still say that caution should be exercised, probably because sibutramine is principally metabolised by CYP3A4.[2] They also extrapolate their caution to the CYP3A4 inhibitors **clarithromycin** and **troleandomycin**.

1. Hinson JL, Leone MB, Leese PT, Moult JT, Carter FJ, Faulkner RD. Steady-state interaction study of sibutramine (Meridia) and erythromycin in uncomplicated obese subjects. *Pharm Res* (1996) 13 (9 Suppl), S116.
2. Reductil (Sibutramine). Abbott Laboratories Ltd. UK Summary of product characteristics, February 2004.

Sibutramine + Miscellaneous

On theoretical grounds the makers contraindicate the concurrent use of sibutramine with MAOIs, and they say that it should not be given with serotonergic drugs because of the risk of the serious serotonin syndrome. A case of hypomania has been reported with citalopram and sibutramine. The makers say that the use of sibutramine with other centrally acting appetite suppressants is contraindicated and they caution about drugs that raise blood pressure or heart rate. No clinically relevant interactions have been seen between sibutramine and cimetidine, and no interaction occurs with oral contraceptives. For other interactions of sibutramine see also 'azoles', and 'macrolides', (above).

Clinical evidence, mechanism, importance and management

(a) Cimetidine

When cimetidine 400 mg twice daily and sibutramine 15 mg once daily were given concurrently to 12 healthy subjects, there were some very small changes in the combined sibutramine metabolites. Their maximum serum levels and AUCs were increased by 3.4 and 7.3% respectively.[1] These changes are too small to be of clinical significance, and there is no reason for avoiding the concurrent use of these two drugs.

(b) Centrally acting appetite suppressants, and drugs that raise blood pressure or heart rate

The makers say that the concurrent use of sibutramine and other centrally acting appetite suppressants is contraindicated. No work has been done to see what happens if sibutramine is given with **decongestants, cough, cold** and **allergy medications**, but the makers say that caution should be used if used concurrently because of the risk of raised blood pressure or heart rate. The makers in the UK and US both list **ephedrine** and **pseudoephedrine**,[1,2] while in the UK **xylometazoline**[2] is included, and in the US **phenylpropanolamine**.[1]

(c) Inducers of the cytochrome P450 isoenzyme CYP3A4

The makers in the UK point out that **carbamazepine**, **dexamethasone**, **phenobarbital**, **phenytoin** and **rifampicin** are all inducers of CYP3A4, an isoenzyme involved in the metabolism of sibutramine.[2] These drugs might therefore possibly increase the metabolism of sibutramine resulting in a fall in its serum levels. However, this has not been studied experimentally and, at the present time, the existence, the extent and the possible clinical relevance of any such interaction is unknown.

(d) Inhibitors of cytochrome P450 isoenzyme CYP3A4

The UK makers advise that caution is needed with concurrent use of **ciclosporin**, since it is an inhibitor of CYP3A4, the principal isoenzyme involved in the metabolism of sibutramine.[2] However, other CYP3A4 inhibitors do not seem to interact to a clinically relevant extent with sibutramine, or only interact modestly (see 'Sibutramine + Azoles', and 'Sibutramine + Macrolides', above), so it seems unlikely that **ciclosporin** will behave very differently.

(e) MAOIs

There are no reports of adverse reactions between sibutramine and the MAOIs. However, sibutramine inhibits serotonin reuptake, and because the serious serotonin syndrome can occur when MAOIs and SSRIs are used together, the makers warn that concurrent use of sibutramine and MAOIs is contraindicated. They say that 14 days should elapse between stopping either drug and starting the other.[1,2]

(f) Oral contraceptives

A crossover study in 12 subjects found that sibutramine 15 mg daily over 8 weeks had no clinically significant effect on the ovulation inhibitory effects of an oral contraceptive, and it was concluded that there is no need to use alternative contraceptive methods while taking sibutramine.[1]

(g) Serotonergic drugs

Because sibutramine inhibits serotonin uptake, and because the serious serotonin syndrome has been seen when serotonergic drugs were taken with SSRIs, the makers say that sibutramine should not be taken with any serotonergic drugs.[1,2] They name **dextromethorphan**, **dihydroergotamine**, **fentanyl**, **pentazocine**, **pethidine** (**meperidine**), **SSRIs**, **sumatriptan**, and **tryptophan**. The US makers also include **lithium** in their list,[1] and see also (e) above. The extent of the risk with these serotonergic drugs is not known, but because of the potential severity of the reaction this warning would seem to be a prudent precaution. A report describes a possible case of this interaction in a clinical setting. A 43-year-old woman taking **citalopram** 40 mg daily was additionally given sibutramine 10 mg daily. Within a few hours of taking the first dose of sibutramine she developed racing thoughts, hyperactivity, psychomotor agitation, shivering and diaphoresis, which continued for the 3 days that she continued to take sibutramine.[3]

1. Meridia (Sibutramine). Abbot Laboratories. Product Information, July 2001.
2. Reductil (Sibutramine). Abbott Laboratories Ltd. UK Summary of product characteristics, February 2004.
3. Benazzi F. Organic hypomania secondary to sibutramine-citalopram interaction. *J Clin Psychiatry* (2002) 63, 165.

Sildenafil + Cardiovascular drugs

The makers contraindicate the concurrent use of sildenafil and organic nitrates (glyceryl trinitrate, isosorbide dinitrate, isosorbide mononitrate etc) because potentially serious hypotension can occur and myocardial infarction may possibly be precipitated. Postural hypotension may also occur with higher doses of sildenafil given at the same time as doxazosin. There is no evidence of important interactions with other non-nitrate antihypertensive vasodilator drugs.

Clinical evidence

(a) Organic nitrates

Two double-blind placebo-controlled studies in groups of 15 or 16 men with angina found that the blood pressure falls seen when taking nitrates and a single 50-mg dose of sildenafil were approximately doubled. Those given sildenafil and **isosorbide dinitrate** 20 mg twice daily showed a mean blood pressure fall of 44/26 mmHg compared with 22/13 mmHg with placebo. Those who used 500 micrograms of sublingual **glyceryl trinitrate** 1 hour before the sildenafil showed a mean blood pressure fall of 36/21 mmHg compared with 26/11 mmHg with **glyceryl trinitrate** and placebo. Individual blood pressure falls as great as 84/52 mmHg were seen.[1]

A postmarketing report from the FDA for the period late March to July 1998 briefly lists 69 US fatalities after taking sildenafil. These were mostly in middle-aged and elderly men (average age 64), 12 of whom had also taken **glyceryl trinitrate** (**nitroglycerin**) or a **nitrate** medication, but it is not clear what part (if any) the **nitrates** played in the deaths.[2]

In a limited and preliminary study it was reported that no blood pressure alteration was seen when a small dose of **glyceryl trinitrate** (amount not specified) was administered in the form of a dermal patch while subjects were taking 50 mg of sildenafil. In addition, the beneficial effects of the **glyceryl trinitrate** on the radial artery pressure waveform were approximately doubled, and persisted for up to 8 hours.[3]

Sildenafil has been investigated as an adjunct to **inhaled nitric oxide** in the management of pulmonary hypertension.[4,5] Although use was beneficial in one case, a study in 15 infants found significant hypotension, which along with a decrease in oxygenation, was considered sufficiently detrimental for the study to be stopped early.[5] [Nitric oxide is not to be confused with the anaesthetic **nitrous oxide**, which it not a nitric oxide donor and therefore poses no risk,[6] see Mechanism below.]

The ACC/AHA Expert consensus document provides a useful list of many of the organic nitrates available.[6]

(b) Other antihypertensives

Retrospective analysis of pooled data from various clinical trials suggests that patients on non-nitrate antihypertensives (**ACE inhibitors**, **alpha-blockers**, **beta-blockers**, **calcium channel blockers**, **diuretics**) showed no significant difference in side effect profile, blood pressure, or heart rate when also taking sildenafil or placebo.[7] The makers say that this is also true for **adrenergic neurone blockers** and **angiotensin II antagonists.** They also quote a study where 100 mg of sildenafil was given to hypertensive patients on the calcium channel blocker **amlodipine.** The mean additional fall in blood pressure (8/7 mmHg) was of the same magnitude as that seen when sildenafil was given alone to healthy subjects.[8] However, in another study with the alpha-blocker **doxazosin**, when sildenafil (at doses greater than 25 mg) was given simultaneously with **doxazosin** 4 mg, there were infrequent reports of symptomatic postural hypotension within 1 to 4 hours of dosing. This did not occur with sildenafil 25 mg.[9]

The makers report that **ACE inhibitors**, **calcium channel blockers** and **thiazide** and **related diuretics** do not affect the pharmacokinetics of sildenafil, whereas the AUC of the active metabolite of sildenafil is increased by 62% by **loop** and **potassium-sparing diuretics** and by 102% by **non-selective beta-blockers**.[9]

Mechanism

Sexual stimulation causes the endothelium of the penis to release nitric oxide (NO), which in turn activates guanylate cyclase to increase the production of cyclic guanosine monophosphate (cGMP). This relaxes the blood vessel musculature of the corpus cavernosum thus allowing it to fill with blood and causing an erection. The erection ends when the guanosine monophosphate is removed by an enzyme (type 5 cGMP phosphodiesterase, or PDE5). Sildenafil inhibits this enzyme thereby increasing and prolonging the effects of the guanosine monophosphate. Because this vasodilation is usually fairly localised (sildenafil is highly selective for PDE5) it normally only causes mild to moderate falls in blood pressure (on average about 10 mmHg) with mild headache or flushing. However, if other nitrates (e.g. glyceryl trinitrate) are taken concurrently, high levels of nitric oxide enter the circulation, and this markedly increases systemic vasodilation and hence the hypotensive effect.

Importance and management

The sildenafil/nitrate interaction is established, clinically important, potentially serious and even possibly fatal. Sildenafil and organic nitrates of any form should not be used concurrently[8] (within 24 hours of each other[6]) because of the risk of precipitating serious hypotension, or even myocardial infarction.[10] Consequently, sildenafil should not be used in patients using nitrates in any form. In contrast to the situation with nitric oxide donor drugs, there appears to be no reason for patients taking non-nitrate vasodilator antihypertensives (those cited in (c) above) to avoid sildenafil.[7,11] However, caution may be required with some alpha blockers. The US prescribing information states that, based on infrequent reports of symptomatic hypotension seen with concurrent use of doxazosin, doses of sildenafil above 25 mg should not be taken within 4 hours of an alpha-blocker.[9]

It is not yet known whether **nicorandil** interacts with sildenafil to a clinically relevant extent or not, but because part of its vasodilatory actions are (like conventional nitrates) mediated by the release of nitric oxide, to be on the safe side, the makers say that the use of **nicorandil** with sildenafil is contraindicated.[12,13]

1. Webb DJ, Muirhead G, Wulff M, Sutton A, Levi R, Dinsmore WW. Sildenafil citrate potentiates the hypotensive effects of nitric oxide donor drugs in male patients with stable angina. *J Am Coll Cardiol* (2000) 36, 25–31.
2. FDA (US Food and Drug Administration) postmarketing information sildenafil citrate (Viagra): Postmarketing safety of sildenafil citrate (Viagra). Reports of death in Viagra users received from marketing (late March) through July 1998. August 27th 1998.
3. O'Rourke M, Jiang X-J. Sildenafil/nitrate interaction. *Circulation* (2000) 101, e90.
4. Bigatello LM, Hess D, Dennehy KC, Medoff BD, Hurford WE. Sildenafil can increase the response to inhaled nitric oxide. *Anesthesiology* (2000) 92, 1827–9.
5. Stocker C, Penny DJ, Brizard CP, Cochrane AD, Soto R, Shekerdemian LS. Intravenous sildenafil and inhaled nitric oxide: a randomised trial in infants after cardiac surgery. *Intensive Care Med* (2003) 29, 1996–2003.
6. ACC/AHA Expert consensus document. Use of sildenafil (Viagra) in patients with cardiovascular disease. *J Am Coll Cardiol* (1999) 33, 273–82.
7. Zusman RM, Prisant LM, Brown MJ. Effect of sildenafil citrate on blood pressure and heart rate in men with erectile dysfunction taking concomitant antihypertensive medication. *J Hypertens* (2000) 18, 1865–9.
8. Viagra (Sildenafil citrate). Pfizer Ltd. UK Summary of product characteristics, April 2005.
9. Viagra (Sildenafil citrate). Pfizer. US Prescribing information, April 2005.
10. Viagra (Sildenafil). Pfizer Inc. Dear Doctor letter, May 1998.
11. Kloner RA, Siegel RL. Sildenafil and nonnitrate antihypertensive medications. *JAMA* (2000) 283, 201–2.
12. Aventis Pharma, Personnal communication, February 2000.
13. Ikorel (Nicorandil). Rhone-Poulenc Rorer Ltd. UK Summary of product characteristics, June 2004.

Sildenafil + Dihydrocodeine

Two men using sildenafil had prolonged erections following orgasm while also taking dihydrocodeine.

Clinical evidence, mechanism, importance and management

Two men, successfully treated with 100-mg doses of sildenafil for erectile dysfunction, experienced prolonged erections after orgasm while also taking 30 to 60 mg of dihydrocodeine 6-hourly for soft tissue injuries. One of them had two erections lasting 4 and 5 hours, and this did not occur on subsequent occasions when the dihydrocodeine was stopped. The other had 2 to 3 hour erections on three occasions during the first week of dihydrocodeine use, but no problems over the next two weeks while continuing to take the dihydrocodeine.[1] The reasons are not understood.

According to the makers of sildenafil, priapism (painful prolonged abnormal erection) associated with its use is rare, and there appear to be no other reports about a sildenafil/dihydrocodeine interaction. Excessively prolonged erections can have serious consequences and may need urgent treatment. Therefore, the authors suggest it would now be prudent to warn patients about this possible (though remote) problem if **opiates** are being used, and advise them to contact the prescriber if priapism occurs.[1]

1. Goldmeier D, Lamba H. Prolonged erections produced by dihydrocodeine and sildenafil. *BMJ* (2002) 324, 1555.

Sildenafil + Ecstasy (MDMA, 3,4-methylenedioxymethamfetamine)

The abuse of sildenafil and ecstasy has been reported to result in serious headache and priapism requiring emergency treatment.

Clinical evidence, mechanism, importance and management

A journalist's account, based purely on anecdotal reports, claims that the illicit use of sildenafil with ecstasy causes "hammerheading" because of the pounding headache and the prolonged and painful penile erections that require emergency medical treatment.[1] The report does not say how much of each of these drugs is taken to produce these adverse effects. The outcome can clearly be unpleasant, painful and, the priapism, potentially serious.

1. Breslau K, Peraino K, Fantz A. The 'sextasy' craze. Newsweek, June 3, 2002, 30.

Sildenafil + Grapefruit juice

Grapefruit juice modestly increases the absorption of sildenafil.

Clinical evidence, mechanism, importance and management

Grapefruit juice 250 ml was given to 24 healthy subjects one hour before and with a 50-mg dose of sildenafil. The AUC of sildenafil was increased by 23% by grapefruit juice, but the maximum plasma level was not significantly changed. Inter-individual variation in sildenafil pharmacokinetics was also increased by grapefruit juice. The authors suggest that although the slight rise in AUC is unlikely to be clinically significant, the combination is best avoided due to the increased variability in sildenafil pharmacokinetics.[1]

1. Jetter A, Kinzig-Schippers M, Walchner-Bonjean M, Hering U, Bulitta J, Schreiner P, Sörgel F, Fuhr U. Effects of grapefruit juice on the pharmacokinetics of sildenafil. *Clin Pharmacol Ther* (2002) 71, 21–9.

Sildenafil + Miscellaneous

Erythromycin, an inhibitor of the cytochrome P450 isoenzyme CYP3A4, markedly increases the serum levels of sildenafil; other potent CYP3A4 inhibitors such as itraconazole and ketoconazole are predicted to behave similarly. A low starting dose of sildenafil is recommended in the presence of all these drugs. Cimetidine modestly increases sildenafil levels. It is not entirely clear whether an increased sildenafil dosage is needed if enzyme inducers such as rifampicin are used. No clinically relevant interactions occur with alcohol, aluminium/magnesium hydroxide, azithromycin, barbiturates, phenytoin, SSRIs, tolbutamide, tricyclic antidepressants or warfarin. For other interactions of sildenafil, see also 'cardiovascular drugs', (p.1029), 'dihydrocodeine', (p.1029), 'grapefruit juice', (above), and 'protease inhibitors', (below).

Clinical evidence, mechanism, importance and management

A. Interacting drugs

(a) Cytochrome P450 inhibitors

Erythromycin (a specific inhibitor of cytochrome P450 isoenzyme CYP3A4) 500 mg twice daily for 5 days was found to increase the AUC of single 100-mg doses of sildenafil almost threefold because it reduces the metabolism and loss of sildenafil from the body.[1] Other more potent CYP3A4 inhibitors such as **itraconazole** and **ketoconazole** are predicted to have even greater effects. Because of the expected increased efficacy and incidence of side-effects due to these interactions, the makers recommend that a low starting dose of 25 mg sildenafil should be used if any of these drugs is being used concurrently.[2,3] For information on the CYP3A4 inhibitor, **ritonavir**, see 'Sildenafil + Protease inhibitors', below.

Cimetidine 800 mg was found to increase sildenafil concentrations (following a 50-mg dose) by 56%, probably because **cimetidine** is a non-specific cytochrome P450 inhibitor.[3] No recommendation is made about **cimetidine** in the US prescribing information,[3] but the UK SPC[2] includes it in the general warning with **erythromycin** and **ketoconazole** (i.e. use a low starting dose of 25 mg), although it seems doubtful if the extent of the increased effects due to **cimetidine** is likely to matter very much.

(b) Cytochrome P450 inducers

In the US prescribing information it is predicted that cytochrome P450 isoenzyme CYP3A4 inducers such as **rifampicin** (**rifampin**) will reduce the serum levels of sildenafil, so that it may therefore be necessary to use a larger dose in patients on **rifampicin**.[3] However, in the UK SPC the makers say that although no specific interaction studies have been carried out, population pharmacokinetic analysis suggests that no interaction occurs with inducers of cytochrome P450 metabolism (and they specifically cite **rifampicin** and **barbiturates**).[2] They also say that no interaction was seen with **phenytoin**.[2]

B. Non-interacting drugs

In vivo studies have shown no significant interactions with **warfarin** 40 mg or **tolbutamide** 250 mg, probably because sildenafil is only a weak inhibitor of cytochrome P450 isoenzyme CYP2C9. Clinical trial data similarly indicate that **SSRIs** and **tricyclic antidepressants** (inhibitors of CYP2D6) do not have any effect on the pharmacokinetics of sildenafil. The bioavailability of sildenafil is not affected by single doses of an **aluminium/magnesium hydroxide** antacid, and sildenafil has been found not to increase the hypotensive effects of **alcohol** (80 mg%) in healthy subjects.[2,3] **Azithromycin** 500 mg once daily for 3 days had no effect on the pharmacokinetics of a single 100-mg dose of sildenafil in healthy subjects.[1]

In vitro studies have shown that sildenafil is only a weak inhibitor of the cytochrome P450 isoenzymes CYP1A2, CYP2C9, CYP2C19, CYP2D6, CYP2E1 and CYP3A4, and it is predicted therefore that sildenafil is unlikely to alter the metabolism of drugs metabolised by these isoenzymes.[2,3]

1. Muirhead GJ, Faulkner S, Harness JA, Taubel J. The effects of steady-state erythromycin and azithromycin on the pharmacokinetics of sildenafil citrate in healthy volunteers. *Br J Clin Pharmacol* (2002) 53, 37S–43S.
2. Viagra (Sildenafil citrate). Pfizer Ltd. UK Summary of product characteristics, April 2005.
3. Viagra (Sildenafil citrate). Pfizer. US Prescribing information, September 2002.

Sildenafil + Protease inhibitors

Indinavir, saquinavir and ritonavir cause marked rises in serum sildenafil levels. A fatal heart attack occurred in a man on ritonavir and saquinavir after taking sildenafil. Concurrent use of HIV-protease inhibitors need not be avoided (except, probably, in the case of ritonavir), but the sildenafil dosage should be reduced.

Clinical evidence

(a) Indinavir

A study in 6 HIV+ patients found that 25 mg of sildenafil did not significantly alter the plasma levels of indinavir. However, the sildenafil AUC was about 4.4-fold higher than the AUC in historical control patients taking sildenafil (data normalised to a 25 mg dose) without indinavir.[1]

(b) Ritonavir

In a randomised, placebo-controlled, double-blind, crossover study, 28 healthy subjects were given sildenafil 100 mg before and after taking ritonavir for 7 days (300, 400 and 500 mg twice daily on days 1, 2 and 3 to 7 respectively). It was found that the sildenafil AUC was increased 11-fold and the maximum serum levels 3.9-fold, but the incidence and severity of sildenafil side-effects and the steady-state levels of ritonavir remained unchanged.[2] However, the clinical significance of this interaction is highlighted by a case report of a 47-year-old man, with no cardiovascular risk factors apart from smoking, who had a fatal heart attack after taking sildenafil 25 mg while he was also on ritonavir and saquinavir. One hour after the ninth dose, he had onset of severe chest pain, and he died soon after.[3]

(c) Saquinavir

In a randomised, placebo-controlled, double-blind crossover study, 28 healthy subjects were given sildenafil 100 mg before and after taking saquinavir 1.2 g three times daily for 7 days. It was found that the sildenafil AUC was increased 3.1-fold and the maximum serum levels 2.4-fold, but the incidence and severity of sildenafil side-effects and the steady-state levels of saquinavir remained unchanged.[2] Also see (b) above.

Mechanism

HIV-protease inhibitors inhibit the activity of the cytochrome P450 isoenzyme CYP3A4, an enzyme responsible for the metabolism of sildenafil. This results in an increase in serum levels of sildenafil.[2] Of the HIV-protease inhibitors currently available, ritonavir is the most potent CYP3A4 inhibitor, followed by indinavir, nelfinavir, amprenavir, and then saquinavir.

Importance and management

Information appears to be limited to the studies and case cited, but the interactions would seem to be established and of clinical importance. Because of the very marked rises in sildenafil levels, concurrent use of ritonavir and sildenafil is not advised.[4] If the decision is taken to use sildenafil in a patient on ritonavir, the dose of sildenafil should not exceed a single 25-mg dose in a 48-hour period,[2,4,5] but note that the fatality described above[3] occurred despite the use of this dose. For other CYP3A4 inhibitors such as saquinavir, the recommendation is that a low starting dose (25 mg) should be considered.[2,4,5] The authors of the indinavir study suggest that a 12.5 mg starting dose may be more appropriate in those on indinavir, and that the maximum dosage frequency be reduced to once or twice weekly.[1] Direct evidence for other HIV-protease inhibitors is lacking but they would be expected to interact similarly (see Mechanism above) and it would seem consistent to follow the broad principle of starting with a low sildenafil dosage. Consider also 'Sildenafil + Miscellaneous', p.1030, which discusses the interactions of sildenafil with other CYP3A4 inhibitors.

1. Merry C, Barry MG, Ryan M, Tjia JF, Hennessy M, Eagling V, Mulcahy F, Back DJ. Interaction of sildenafil and indinavir when co-administered to HIV positive patients. AIDS (Hagerstown) 1999, 13, F101–F107.
2. Muirhead GJ, Wulff MB, Fielding A, Kleinermans D, Buss N. Pharmacokinetic interactions between sildenafil and saquinavir/ritonavir. *Br J Clin Pharmacol* (2000) 50, 99–107.
3. Hall MCS, Ahmad S. Interaction between sildenafil and HIV-1 combination therapy. *Lancet* (1999) 353, 2071–2.
4. Viagra (Sildenafil citrate). Pfizer Ltd. UK Summary of product characteristics, April 2005.
5. Viagra (Sildenafil citrate). Pfizer. US Prescribing information, September 2002.

Sodium polystyrene sulphonate + Antacids

The concurrent use of antacids with sodium polystyrene sulphonate can result in metabolic alkalosis.

Clinical evidence, mechanism, importance and management

A man with hyperkalaemia developed metabolic alkalosis when given 30 g of sodium polystyrene sulphonate with 30 ml of **magnesium hydroxide** mixture three times daily.[1] Alkalosis has also been described in a study on a number of patients given this cation exchange resin with *Maalox* (**magnesium/aluminium hydroxide**) and **calcium carbonate**.[2] The suggested reason is that the breakdown of the **magnesium hydroxide** usually requires equal amounts of bicarbonate and hydrogen ions, and so does not cause any acid-base disturbance. However, when sodium polystyrene sulphonate is given, it binds the **magnesium**, while the hydroxide is neutralised by the hydrogen ions. This results in a relative excess of bicarbonate ions, which are absorbed, leading to metabolic alkalosis. This interaction appears to be established. Concurrent use should be undertaken with caution and serum electrolytes should be closely monitored. Administration of the resin rectally as an enema can avoid the problem.

1. Fernandez PC, Kovnat PJ. Metabolic acidosis reversed by the combination of magnesium and a cation-exchange resin. *N Engl J Med* (1972) 286, 23–4.
2. Schroeder ET. Alkalosis resulting from combined administration of a 'nonsystemic' antacid and a cation-exchange resin. *Gastroenterology* (1969) 56, 868–74.

Sodium polystyrene sulphonate + Sorbitol

Potentially fatal colonic necrosis may occur if sodium polystyrene sulphonate is given as an enema with sorbitol.

Clinical evidence

Five patients with uraemia developed severe colonic necrosis after being given enemas containing sodium polystyrene sulphonate and sorbitol for the treatment of hyperkalaemia. Four of the 5 died as a result. Associated studies in uraemic *rats* found that all of them died over a 2-day period after being given enemas of sodium polystyrene sulphonate with sorbitol. Extensive haemorrhage and transmural necrosis developed. No deaths occurred after enemas without sorbitol were given.[1]

Mechanism

Not understood.

Importance and management

Information is very limited and the interaction is not firmly established, nevertheless its seriousness indicates that sodium polystyrene sulphonate should not be given as an enema in aqueous vehicles containing sorbitol. More study is needed.

1. Lillemoe KD, Romolo JL, Hamilton SR, Pennington LR, Burdick JF, Williams GM. Intestinal necrosis due to sodium polystyrene (Kayexalate) in sorbitol enemas: clinical and experimental support for the hypothesis. *Surgery* (1987) 101, 267–72.

Solifenacin + Ketoconazole or other CYP3A4 enzyme inhibitors

Ketoconazole markedly increases solifenacin levels, and the solifenacin dose should be limited if ketoconazole or other potent inhibitors of the cytochrome P450 isoenzyme CYP3A4 are used.

Clinical evidence, mechanism, importance and management

The makers note that ketoconazole 200 mg daily increased the AUC of solifenacin twofold, while ketoconazole 400 mg daily increased the AUC by threefold.[1] Solifenacin is principally metabolised by the cytochrome P450 isoenzyme CYP3A4, which ketoconazole inhibits.

Although the clinical relevance of this interaction has not been assessed, the makers recommend that the daily dose of solifenacin succinate is limited to 5 mg if it is given with ketoconazole or other potent inhibitors of CYP3A4.[1,2] In addition, in patients with have severe renal impairment or moderate hepatic impairment, the combined use of solifenacin and potent CYP3A4 inhibitors is contraindicated.[1] The UK maker specifically names **itraconazole**, **nelfinavir** and **ritonavir**.[1] For a list of CYP3A4 inhibitors, see 'Table 1.4', (p.6).

1. Vesicare (Solifenacin succinate). Yamanouchi Pharma Ltd. UK Summary of product characteristics, August 2004.
2. Vesicare (Solifenacin succinate). GlaxoSmithKline. US Prescribing information, November 2004.

Solifenacin + Miscellaneous

The maker notes that solifenacin had no significant effect on the pharmacokinetics of digoxin, the pharmacokinetics of an oral contraceptive (ethinylestradiol/levonorgestrel) or the pharma-

cokinetics or effect of warfarin.[1,2] Food did not affect solifenacin pharmacokinetics.[3]

1. Vesicare (Solifenacin succinate). Yamanouchi Pharma Ltd, UK Summary of product characteristics, August 2004.
2. Vesicare (Solifenacin succinate). GlaxoSmithKline. US Prescribing information, November 2004.
3. Uchida T, Krauwinkel WJ, Mulder H, Smulders RA. Food does not affect the pharmacokinetics of solifenacin, a new muscarinic receptor antagonist: results of a randomized crossover trial. *Br J Clin Pharmacol* (2004) 58, 4–7.

Strontium ranelate + Miscellaneous

Food, dairy products and calcium supplements markedly reduce the absorption of strontium ranelate, and administration should be separated by at least 2 hours. Aluminium and magnesium antacids only slightly reduce strontium ranelate absorption. Strontium ranelate is predicted to reduce the absorption of the quinolones and the tetracyclines, and strontium should be stopped while these antibacterials are required. Vitamin D does not affect strontium ranelate bioavailability.

Clinical evidence, mechanism, importance and management

(a) Antacids

The maker notes that **aluminium/magnesium hydroxide** slightly reduced the absorption of strontium ranelate (AUC decreased by 20 to 25%) when given at the same time or 2 hours before the strontium. However, when the antacid was given 2 hours after strontium, absorption was barely affected.[1] Therefore, the makers recommend that antacids should be taken 2 hours after strontium ranelate. However, because it is also recommended that strontium ranelate is taken at bedtime, they say that if this is impractical, concurrent intake is acceptable.[1] Note that **calcium**-containing antacids would have a greater effect, see (b) below, and concurrent intake would not be recommended.

(b) Food, dairy products, and calcium supplements

The makers note that food, milk, dairy products, and calcium supplements reduce the bioavailability of strontium ranelate by about 60 to 70% when compared with administration 3 hours after a meal.[1] This is because divalent cations such as calcium form complexes with strontium ranelate so preventing its absorption. Therefore, strontium ranelate should not be taken within 2 hours of eating. The maker recommends that it should be taken at bedtime, at least 2 hours after eating.[1]

(c) Quinolones and tetracyclines

The maker predicts that strontium will complex with quinolones and tetracyclines, so preventing their absorption. Because of this, they recommend that when treatment with quinolones or tetracyclines is required, strontium ranelate therapy should be temporarily suspended.[1]

(d) Vitamin D

The maker notes that vitamin D supplements had no effect on strontium ranelate bioavailability.[1]

1. Protelos (Strontium ranelate). Servier Laboratories Ltd. UK Summary of product characteristics, September 2004.

Sucrose polyesters + Orlistat

A single case report suggests that concurrent use of orlistat and sucrose polyesters (*Olestra* – used in some foods as a fat substitute) can result in additive gastrointestinal adverse effects (soft, fatty/oily stools, increased flatus and abdominal pain). In the case in question, symptoms resolved when the patient stopped eating *Olestra*-containing food while continuing to take orlistat.[1]

1. Heck AM, Calis KA, McDuffie JR, Carobene SE, Yanovski JA. Additive gastrointestinal effects with concomitant use of olestra and orlistat. *Ann Pharmacother* (2002) 36, 1003–5.

Sulfinpyrazone + NSAIDs

The uricosuric effects of sulfinpyrazone are not opposed by the concurrent use of flufenamic acid, meclofenamic acid or mefenamic acid.[1,2] Consider also 'Aspirin or other Salicylates + Sulfinpyrazone', p.82).

1. Latham BA, Radcliff F, Robinson RG. The effect of mefenamic acid and flufenamic acid on plasma uric acid levels. *Ann Phys Med* (1966) 8, 242–3.
2. Robinson RG, Radcliff FJ. The effect of meclofenamic acid on plasma uric acid levels. *Med J Aust* (1972) 1, 1079–80.

Sulfinpyrazone + Probenecid

Probenecid reduces the urinary excretion of sulfinpyrazone, but the overall uric acid clearance remains unaltered.

Clinical evidence, mechanism, importance and management

A study in 8 patients with gout showed that while probenecid was able to inhibit the renal tubular excretion of sulfinpyrazone, reducing it by about 75%, the maximal uric acid clearance was about the same as when either drug was given alone.[1] There would therefore seem to be no advantage in using these drugs together. Whether the toxic effects of sulfinpyrazone are increased seems not to have been studied.

1. Perel JM, Dayton PG, Snell MM, Yü TF, Gutman AB. Studies of interactions among drugs in man at the renal level: probenecid and sulphinpyrazone. *Clin Pharmacol Ther* (1969) 10, 834–40.

Tadalafil + Miscellaneous

Potentially significant hypotension may occur in some subjects given nitrates and tadalafil. The combination of nitrates and tadalafil is contraindicated. The hypotensive effects of doxazosin are increased to some degree by tadalafil. Tadalafil levels are reduced by rifampicin, and probably also by other potent CYP3A4 inducers, and this may reduce efficacy. Tadalafil levels are raised by ketoconazole, and probably by other CYP3A4 inhibitors, but this is almost certainly not clinically important. No clinically relevant interactions occur with alcohol, amlodipine, antacids, aspirin, bendrofluazide, enalapril, lovastatin metoprolol, midazolam, nizatidine, tamsulosin, theophylline or warfarin.

Clinical evidence, mechanism, importance and management

(a) Alcohol

Studies in subjects with blood alcohol levels of 80 mg% found that the effects of alcohol on cognitive function were unchanged by 10 mg of tadalafil, and the effect of alcohol on blood pressure was unchanged by 20 mg of tadalafil. The serum levels of tadalafil were found to be unaltered 3 hours after taking the alcohol.[1] For all these reasons, concurrent use need not be avoided.

(b) Antacids

An open-label, randomised, crossover study in 12 healthy subjects found that 20 ml of *Maalox* (**aluminium/magnesium hydroxide**) reduced the mean maximum serum level of a single 10-mg dose of tadalafil by 30%. Although peak tadalafil levels were delayed by 2.5 hours, the total amount of tadalafil absorbed was unchanged. None of the changes caused were considered to be clinically relevant, and there would appear to be no reason for avoiding concurrent use.[2]

(c) Antihypertensive drugs

A placebo-controlled, randomised, two-period crossover study in 18 healthy subjects found that a single 20-mg dose of tadalafil increased the blood pressure reducing effects of doxazosin following 7 days treatment with **doxazosin** 8 mg daily. The mean maximum systolic/diastolic falls for the combination compared with the tadalafil placebo were 3.6/2.8 mmHg when lying and 9.6/5.3 mmHg when standing. Some of the subjects felt dizzy, but none of them fainted.[1] The makers suggest that concurrent use is not advisable.[1]

Studies by the makers found that 10 to 20 mg doses of tadalafil did not change the effects of a range of antihypertensive drugs, representing several drug classes. These were **amlodipine** (calcium channel blocker), **enalapril** (ACE inhibitor), **metoprolol** (beta-blocker), **bendroflumethiazide** (thiazide diuretic) and unnamed **angiotensin II inhibitors**.[1,2] A small and clinically irrelevant effect was seen with 10 or 20 mg of tadalafil and **tamsulosin**.[1,2] The makers say that tadalafil 20 mg with antihypertensive drugs in general may induce a small fall in blood pressure, but this is unlikely to be clinically relevant. They also say that the adverse effects seen in phase III clinical trials were the same, whether tadalafil was taken with or without antihypertensive drugs.[1] There would therefore appear to be no reason for avoiding the concurrent use of any of these drugs nor (the implication is) with other drugs that fall into these drug classes. However, it should be noted that some calcium channel blockers (e.g. **nifedipine**, **verapamil**) are known to have effects on the cytochrome P450 isoenzyme CYP3A4, an enzyme involved in the metabolism of tadalafil, and so may have the potential to interact, although see (f) below.

(d) Aspirin

A randomised, double-blind, parallel group study on a total of 28 subjects found that 10-mg doses of tadalafil did not increase the bleeding time after taking aspirin 300 mg daily for 5 days.[2] There would seem to be no reason for taking special precautions if both drugs are used.

(e) Cytochrome P450 CYP3A4 inducers

A study[2] in 12 healthy subjects found that **rifampicin** 600 mg daily given for 13 days decreased the AUC of a single 10-mg dose of tadalafil by 88%. The reason is that **rifampicin** induces the activity of the cytochrome P450 isoenzyme CYP3A4, an enzyme concerned with the metabolism of tadalafil, and as a result it is cleared from the body more quickly and its serum levels fall. It is unlikely therefore that 10-mg doses of tadalafil would be as effective as usual. Other CYP3A4 inducers such as **carbamazepine**, **phenobarbital** and **phenytoin** are predicted by the makers to do the same, but the extent of the reduction in AUC is uncertain.[1,2] The makers of tadalafil do not give any recommendations about how this interaction should be handled, but one simple answer would be increase the tadalafil dosage if it seemed to be ineffective.

(f) Cytochrome P450 CYP3A4 inhibitors

An open label, randomised study[2] in 12 healthy subjects found that 7 days' treatment with **ketoconazole** 200 mg daily increased the AUC of a single 10-mg dose of tadalafil by 107%. This is thought to be because **ketoconazole** inhibits the activity of CYP3A4, an enzyme concerned with the metabolism of tadalafil, and as a result it is cleared from the body more slowly. The makers predict that other CYP3A4 inhibitors will probably do the same, the examples they list being **clarithromycin**, **erythromycin**, **grapefruit juice**, **itraconazole**, **ritonavir**, and **saquinavir**.[1,2] However, rises in serum levels of the order of 100% are unlikely to be of clinical relevance because other studies have shown that very large doses of tadalafil (multiple daily doses of 100 mg in patients, single 500-mg doses in healthy subjects) only produced adverse events similar those seen with 10 to 20-mg doses.[1] The makers[1] say that very common adverse reactions are headache and dyspepsia, while common reactions include dizziness, flushing, nasal decongestion, back pain and myalgia. These events were described as being 'transient and generally mild or moderate'. There would therefore appear to be no reason for avoiding any of these drugs unless adverse reactions become unacceptable.

(g) Cytochrome P450 CYP3A4 substrates

An open label study in 12 healthy subjects found that while taking tadalafil 10 mg daily for 14 consecutive days, the pharmacokinetics of single 15-mg doses of **midazolam** were unchanged. A similar study in 6 healthy subjects also found 20 mg tadalafil daily for 14 days did not affect the pharmacokinetics of 40 mg doses of **lovastatin**. Since both **midazolam** and **lovastatin** are metabolised by CYP3A4, it is concluded from these two studies that the absence of any interaction shows that tadalafil does not inhibit or induce the activity of this cytochrome.[2] No special precautions are therefore needed if either of these drugs is given with tadalafil.

(h) Nitrates

In a two-part double-blind randomised, placebo-controlled trial, 51 patients with chronic stable angina were given 5 mg or 10 mg of tadalafil or a placebo, followed 2 hours later by a single 400-microgram dose of sublingual **glyceryl trinitrate**. Another 45 similar patients were given 30 or 60 mg oral **isosorbide mononitrate** in place of glyceryl trinitrate one hour after the tadalafil. It was found that the presence of the tadalafil had minimal effects on the decrease in blood pressure caused by these nitrates.[3] Another similar study in 49 patients compared the effects of tadalafil 10 mg in combination with sublingual **glyceryl trinitrate** (400 micrograms[2]). Again, it was found that the presence of the tadalafil had minimal effects on the mean maximum decreases in blood pressure but it was noted that 23 patients given tadalafil had a standing systolic blood pressure of 85 mmHg or less following the administration of the nitrate.[4] It is for this reason that the makers of tadalafil contraindicate the use of **organic nitrates**.[2] That is to say, the contraindication covers the use of these drugs in all patients although only some are likely to be affected. The explanation for the way sildenafil interacts with nitrates (see 'Mechanism' in the monograph entitled 'Sildenafil + Cardiovascular drugs', p.1029) is equally true for tadalafil.

(i) Nizatidine

An open-label, randomised, three-period crossover study in 12 healthy subjects found that nizatidine 300 mg reduced the mean maximum serum levels of tadalafil by 14% following a single 10-mg dose, but other pharmacokinetic parameters including the extent of absorption were largely unchanged. None of the changes caused were considered to be clinically relevant and there would appear to be no reason for avoiding concurrent use.[2]

It would not be unreasonable to conclude from these results that any alterations in the absorption of tadalafil are not caused by changes in gastric pH,[2] and a further tentative conclusion might be that other drugs that change the gastric pH are also unlikely to interact by this mechanism.

(j) Theophylline

A double-blind, placebo-controlled, randomised, crossover study in 17 healthy subjects given enough oral theophylline (a non-selective phosphodiesterase inhibitor) to achieve steady-state levels of about 12 mg/L found that when also given tadalafil 10 mg daily for 7 days the pharmacokinetics of both drugs remained unchanged. There was a small increase of 3.5 bpm in the heart rate, which was considered to be clinically irrelevant in the healthy subjects,[2] but the makers advise that this should be considered when both drugs are used concurrently.[1]

(k) Warfarin

A double blind, placebo-controlled, randomised, crossover study in which a single-dose of warfarin was given on day 7 of 12 consecutive days treatment with either tadalafil 10 mg or placebo found that tadalafil did not affect the AUCs of either (*S*)-warfarin and (*R*)-warfarin, and prothrombin times were unchanged. There would therefore appear to be no reason for taking special precautions if both drugs are used.[1,2]

(l) Miscellaneous interactions

Some of the studies briefly described above show that tadalafil is affected by cytochrome CYP3A4 inducers and inhibitors, but it has also been shown that tadalafil acts neither as an enzyme inducer nor as an inhibitor of the cytochrome P450 isoenzymes CYP1A2, CYP2D6, CYP2E1 or CYP2C9.[2] This means that it will almost certainly not interact by causing enzyme induction or inhibition of any drugs that are primarily metabolised by these isoenzymes.

1. Cialis (Tadalafil). Eli Lilly and Company Ltd. UK Summary of product characteristics, October 2004.
2. Eli Lilly and Company. Personal communication, March 2003.
3. Kloner RA, Emmick J, Bedding A et al. Pharmacodynamic interactions between tadalafil and nitrates. *Int J Impot Res* (2002) 14 (Suppl 3) S29.
4. Kloner RA, Mitchell MI, Bedding A, Emmick J. Pharmacodynamic interactions between tadalafil and nitrates compared with sildenafil. *J Urol (Baltimore)* (2002) 167 (Suppl) 176–7.

Tedisamil + Beta-blockers

Atenolol does not have additive effects on the bradycardia and QT-prolonging effects of tedisamil in healthy subjects.

Clinical evidence, mechanism, importance and management

There was no evidence of excessive bradycardia or QT interval prolongation in 10 healthy subjects given twice daily doses of tedisamil 100 mg and **atenolol** 50 mg of tedisamil alone or in combination with **atenolol** increased the QT interval by 12%, whereas **atenolol** given alone had no effect. The fall in heart rate was not significantly different for either of the drugs given alone or when given together.[1] It seems likely that apart from sotalol, which is known to prolong the QT interval, most other beta-blockers will behave like **atenolol**. However, the authors of this report were at pains to point out that this study was in healthy subjects and that studies are now needed in patients with myocardial ischaemia to confirm the safety of this drug combination.

1. Démolis J-L, Martel C, Funck-Brentano C, Sachse A, Weimann H-J, Jaillon P. Effects of tedisamil, atenolol and their combination on heart and rate-dependent QT interval in healthy volunteers. *Br J Clin Pharmacol* (1997) 44, 403–9.

Thymoxamine + Miscellaneous

The makers say that intracavernosal injections of thymoxamine should not be given in combination with other drugs used for erectile dysfunction, and should be avoided by patients taking alpha- or beta-blockers. Care should also be taken in those receiving other antihypertensives such as ACE inhibitors or calcium channel blockers.

Clinical evidence, mechanism, importance and management

Thymoxamine is an alpha-1, and to a lesser extent, an alpha-2 blocker which, if injected into the corpus cavernosum, can be used to treat erectile dysfunction. It causes relaxation of the smooth muscle fibres of the corpus cavernosum, thereby increasing the flow of blood and dilatation which results in erection of the penis. These vasodilatory effects are intended to be localised, but since some of the drug can escape into the circulation causing more general systemic effects. Therefore the makers of intracavernosal thymoxamine say that the concurrent use of other alpha-blockers (they list **alfuzosin**, **doxazosin**, **prazosin**, **terazosin** and **urapidil**) and **beta-blockers** should be avoided because of the risks of additive and possibly severe orthostatic hypotension. They also suggest that if thymoxamine is to be used by patients unavoidably taking other antihypertensives (they cite **ACE inhibitors** and **calcium channel blockers**), precautions should be taken in case of potentiation of the antihypertensive effect.[1] This means, presumably, ensuring that marked hypotension (manifested as dizziness, fainting) is not a problem. The makers of intracavernosal thymoxamine also say that it should not be used in combination with other drugs used for erectile dysfunction.[1] These other drugs would include **alprostadil**, **papaverine**, **phentolamine** and the **phosphodiesterase inhibitors** such as **sildenafil**.

1. Érecnos (Moxisylyte hydrochloride). Fournier Pharmaceuticals. UK Summary of product characteristics, June 1997.

Thyroid hormones + Antacids

A few reports describe reduced levothyroxine effects in patients given antacids.

Clinical evidence, mechanism, importance and management

A man with hypothyroidism controlled by 150 micrograms of **levothyroxine** daily developed high serum TSH levels (a rise from 1.1 up to 36 mIU/L) while taking an **aluminium/magnesium hydroxide** antacid (*Silain-Gel*), and on two subsequent occasions when rechallenged. The reasons are not understood. Although he remained asymptomatic throughout,[1] the rise in the levels of TSH indicated that the dosage of the **levothyroxine** had become insufficient in the presence of the antacid. Two similar cases have also been reported, where the presence of an **aluminium/magnesium** antacid or **magnesium oxide** reduced the response to **levothyroxine**. One patient required four times her normal dose of **levothyroxine**.[2]

The general importance of this interaction is not known, but be alert for the need to increase the **levothyroxine** dosage in any patient given antacids. More study is needed.

1. Sperber AD, Liel Y. Evidence for interference with the intestinal absorption of levothyroxine sodium by aluminum hydroxide. *Arch Intern Med* (1991) 152, 183–4.
2. Mersebach H, Rasmussen ÅK, Kirkegaard L, Feldt-Rasmussen U. Intestinal adsorption of levothyroxine by antacids and laxatives: case stories and *in vitro* experiments. *Pharmacol Toxicol* (1999) 84, 107–9.

Thyroid hormones + Anticonvulsants

An isolated report describes a patient, previously well maintained on levothyroxine (thyroxine), who developed clinical hypothyroidism when phenytoin was given. Both carbamazepine and phenytoin can reduce endogenous serum thyroid hormone levels, but clinical hypothyroidism caused by an interaction seems to be rare.

Clinical evidence

A patient with hypothyroidism, successfully treated with 150 micrograms of **levothyroxine** daily for 4 years, developed hypothyroidism when given 300 mg of **phenytoin** daily. Doubling the **levothyroxine** dosage proved to be effective. Later this interaction was confirmed when stopping and restarting the **phenytoin** produced the same effect.[1]

A number of other reports describe very significant reductions in endogenous markers of thyroid function in subjects and patients when treated with **phenytoin**[2-5] or **carbamazepine**,[4-6] but not **sodium valproate**.[5] However, there seems to be only two cases in which reversible hypothyroidism was seen, one with **carbamazepine** and **phenytoin**, and the other with **carbamazepine** alone.[7] There is also a report of an arrhythmia in a patient with hypothyroidism and rheumatic heart disease given **phenytoin**; this was attributed to the displacement of protein bound **levothyroxine** by **phenytoin** leading to an increase in free **levothyroxine** in the plasma.[8] This report was later criticised by others, who suggested that the arrhythmia, if indeed there was one, was caused directly by the cardiac actions of **phenytoin**.[9,10]

Mechanism

Both phenytoin and carbamazepine can increase the metabolism of endogenous thyroid hormones, thereby reducing their plasma levels. Phenytoin can also displace levothyroxine and triiodothyronine from thyroxine binding globulin.[11]

Importance and management

Despite very clear evidence that both carbamazepine and phenytoin can cause a marked reduction in endogenous serum thyroid hormone levels, the development of clinical hypothyroidism seems to be very rare, and there seems to be only one case on record of an interaction between levothyroxine and phenytoin. There seems to be little reason for avoiding concurrent use, but the outcome should be monitored. Increase the levothyroxine dosage if necessary. See also 'Thyroid hormones + Barbiturates', below.

1. Blackshear JL, Schultz AL, Napier JS, Stuart DD. Thyroxine replacement requirements in hypothyroid patients receiving phenytoin. *Ann Intern Med* (1983) 99, 341–2.
2. Hansen JM, Skovsted L, Lauridsen UB, Kirkegaard C, Siersbæk-Nielsen K. The effect of diphenylhydantoin on thyroid function. *J Clin Endocrinol Metab* (1974) 39, 785–9.
3. Oppenheimer JH, Fisher LV, Nelson KM, Jailer JW. Depression of the serum protein-bound iodine level by diphenylhydantoin. *J Clin Endocrinol Metab* (1961) 21, 252–62.
4. Rootwelt K, Ganes T, Johannessen SI. Effect of carbamazepine, phenytoin and phenobarbitone on serum levels of thyroid hormones and thyrotropin in humans. *Scand J Clin Lab Invest* (1978) 38, 731–6.
5. Larkin JG, Macphee GJA, Beastall GH, Brodie MJ. Thyroid hormone concentrations in epileptic patients. *Eur J Clin Pharmacol* (1989) 36, 213–16.
6. Connell JMC, Rapeport WG, Gordon S, Brodie MJ. Changes in circulating thyroid hormones during short-term hepatic enzyme induction with carbamazepine. *Eur J Clin Pharmacol* (1984) 26, 453–6.
7. Aanderud S, Strandjord RE. Hypothyroidism induced by anti-epileptic therapy. *Acta Neurol Scand* (1980) 61, 330–2.
8. Fulop M, Widrow DR, Colmers RA, Epstein EJ. Possible diphenylhydantoin-induced arrhythmia in hypothyroidism. *JAMA* (1966) 196, 454–6.
9. Farzan S. Diphenylhydantoin and arrhythmia. *JAMA* (1966) 197, 133.
10. Gaspar HL. Diphenylhydantoin and arrhythmia. *JAMA* (1966) 197, 133.
11. Franklyn JA, Sheppard MC, Ramsden DB. Measurement of free thyroid hormones in patients on long-term phenytoin therapy. *Eur J Clin Pharmacol* (1984) 26, 633–4.

Thyroid hormones + Barbiturates

An isolated report describes a reduction in the response to levothyroxine when a woman was additionally treated with a barbiturate. See also 'Thyroid hormones + Anticonvulsants', above.

Clinical evidence, mechanism, importance and management

An elderly woman on 300 micrograms of **levothyroxine** daily for hypothyroidism complained of severe breathlessness within a week of reducing her nightly dose of *Tuinal* (**secobarbital** 100 mg + **amobarbital** 100 mg) from two capsules to one capsule. She was subsequently found to be thyrotoxic. She became symptom-free again when the dosage of the **levothyroxine** was halved.[1] The reason is not known, but **phenobarbital** has been shown to reduce the serum levels of endogenous thyroid hormones in some studies,[2] and it seems possible that in this case these other two barbiturates acted in the same way, probably by enzyme induction. The general importance of this interaction is almost certainly small, but be alert for any evidence of changes in thyroid status if barbiturates are added or withdrawn from patients being treated with **levothyroxine**. See also 'Thyroid hormones + Anticonvulsants', p.1034.

1. Hoffbrand BI. Barbiturate/thyroid-hormone interaction. *Lancet* (1979) ii, 903–4.
2. Ohnhaus EE, Studer H. A link between liver microsomal enzyme activity and thyroid hormone metabolism in man. *Br J Clin Pharmacol* (1983) 15, 71–6.

Thyroid hormones + Calcium carbonate

The efficacy of levothyroxine can be reduced by the concurrent use of calcium carbonate. Separating the dosages avoids this interaction.

Clinical evidence

Twenty patients with hypothyroidism were treated with **levothyroxine** alone, to which 1200 mg of calcium carbonate daily was then added for 3 months. While taking the calcium carbonate their mean free thyroxine levels fell from 16.7 to 15.4 picomol/L and rose again to 18 picomol/L when it was stopped. The mean total thyroxine levels over the same period were about 118, 111 and 120 nanomol/L respectively and the mean TSH levels were 1.6, 2.7 and 1.4 mIU/L respectively.[1]

A woman with thyroid cancer given **levothyroxine** 125 micrograms daily, to suppress serum TSH levels, showed a reduced response (fatigue, weight gain) when she took *Tums* containing calcium carbonate for the prevention of osteoporosis. She often took the two together. Over a 5-month period her serum TSH levels rose from 0.08 mIU/L to 13.3 mIU/L. Within 3 weeks of stopping the calcium carbonate, her serum TSH levels had fallen to 0.68 mIU/L.[2] Other reports have described 4 patients who had elevations in their TSH levels while taking calcium carbonate concurrently with **levothyroxine**. All levels returned to normal when administration was separated by about 4 hours.[2-4]

Mechanism

In vitro studies indicate that levothyroxine is adsorbed onto calcium carbonate when the pH is low (as in the stomach), which would reduce the amount available for absorption.[1]

Importance and management

An established interaction, which seems to be of limited clinical significance. The study quoted[1] shows that the mean reduction in the absorption of levothyroxine is quite small, but the case histories[2,3] show that some individuals can experience a reduction in the absorption that is clinically important. Since it is impossible to predict which patients are likely to be affected significantly, the cautious approach would be to advise all patients to separate the dosages of the two preparations by at least 4 hours to avoid admixture in the gut. This interaction would be expected to occur with calcium carbonate in any form but it is not known whether other thyroid hormone preparations interact in the same way as levothyroxine.

1. Singh N, Singh PN, Hershmann JM. Effect of calcium carbonate on the absorption of levothyroxine. *JAMA* (2000) 283, 2822–25.
2. Schneyer CR. Calcium carbonate and reduction of levothyroxine efficacy. *JAMA* (1998) 279, 750.
3. Butner LE, Fulco PP, Feldman G. Calcium carbonate-induced hypothyroidism. *Ann Intern Med* (2000) 132, 595.
4. Csako G, McGriff NJ, Rotman-Pikielny P, Sarlis NJ, Pucino F. Exaggerated levothyroxine malabsorption due to calcium carbonate supplementation in gastrointestinal disorders. *Ann Pharmacother* (2001) 35, 1578–83.

Thyroid hormones + Colestyramine

The absorption of thyroid extract, levothyroxine (thyroxine), and tri-iodothyronine from the gut is reduced by the concurrent use of colestyramine. Separate the dosages by 4 to 6 hours to minimise the interaction.

Clinical evidence

When a patient with hypothyroidism, taking **levothyroxine**, showed a fall in his basal metabolic rate when given colestyramine, a further study was made on two similar patients taking 60 mg of **thyroid extract** or 100 micrograms **levothyroxine sodium** daily, and on five normal subjects. Colestyramine 4 g four times daily reduced their absorption of **levothyroxine**[131], the amount recovered in the faeces being roughly doubled. One of the patients showed a worsening of her hypothyroidism. Giving the **levothyroxine** 4 to 5 hours after the colestyramine reduced but did not completely prevent the interaction.[1]

Another report describes a patient on **levothyroxine** whose thyroid-stimulating hormone (TSH) levels rose when given colestyramine, and fell again when it was stopped, indicating an impairment of **levothyroxine** absorption.[2]

Mechanism

Colestyramine binds to levothyroxine in the gut, thereby reducing its absorption. Since levothyroxine probably also undergoes enterohepatic recirculation, continued contact with the colestyramine is possible.

Importance and management

An established interaction (although the documentation is very limited) and of clinical importance. *In vitro* tests show that tri-iodothyronine interacts similarly.[1] The interaction can be minimised by separating the dosages by 4 to 6 hours (but see 'Mechanism'). Even so, the outcome should be monitored so that any necessary thyroid hormone dosage adjustments can be made.

1. Northcutt RC, Stiel JN, Hollifield JW, Stant EG. The influence of cholestyramine on thyroxine absorption. *JAMA* (1969) 208, 1857–61.
2. Harmon SM, Seifert CF. Levothyroxine-cholestyramine interaction reemphasized. *Ann Intern Med* (1991) 115, 658–9.

Thyroid hormones + Ferrous sulphate

Ferrous sulphate causes a reduction in the effects of levothyroxine in patients treated for hypothyroidism.

Clinical evidence

Fourteen patients with primary hypothyroidism showed an increase in TSH levels from 1.6 to 5.4 mIU/L when given 300 mg of **ferrous sulfate** daily for 12 weeks along with their usual **levothyroxine** dose. The symptoms of hypothyroidism in 9 patients worsened.[1] In another report a woman with hypothyroidism, on **levothyroxine**, showed a very marked rise in TSH levels when given **ferrous sulfate**. Her **levothyroxine** dosage needed to be raised from 175 to 200 micrograms daily.[2]

Mechanism

The addition of iron to levothyroxine *in vitro* was found to produce a poorly soluble purple iron-levothyroxine complex suggesting that this might also occur in the gut.[1]

Importance and management

Information is limited to these reports but it appears to be a clinically important interaction. Monitor the effects of concurrent use and separate the doses by 2 hours or more on the assumption that reduced absorption accounts for this interaction. Monitor well. The same precautions would seem appropriate with any other iron preparation.

1. Campbell NRC, Hasinoff BB, Stalts H, Rao B, Wong NCW. Ferrous sulfate reduces thyroxine efficacy in patients with hypothyroidism. *Ann Intern Med* (1992) 117, 1010–3.
2. Schlienger JL. Accroissement des besoins en thyroxine par le sulfate de fer. *Presse Med* (1994) 23, 492.

Thyroid hormones + H_2-blockers

Cimetidine, but not ranitidine, causes a small reduction in the absorption of levothyroxine.

Clinical evidence, mechanism, importance and management

When 10 women with simple goitre were given 400 mg of **cimetidine** 90 minutes before a single capsule of **levothyroxine**, the absorption of **levothyroxine** was reduced over the first 4 hours by about 21%. The reasons are not understood. A single 300-mg dose of **ranitidine** was found not to affect the **levothyroxine** absorption in a matched group of 10 women.[1]

The clinical importance of this interaction with **cimetidine** awaits assessment, but it is probably not great. Nevertheless it would be prudent to monitor the outcome if both drugs are used, being alert for the need to increase the **levothyroxine** dosage.

1. Jonderko G, Jonderko K, Marcisz CZ, Kotulska A. Effect of cimetidine and ranitidine on absorption of [^{125}I] levothyroxine administered orally. *Acta Pharmacol Sin* (1992) 13, 391–4.

Thyroid hormones + Lovastatin

An isolated report describes raised serum thyroid hormone levels and evidence of thyrotoxicosis in a man on levothyroxine (thyroxine) additionally given lovastatin. In contrast another isolated case report describes hypothyroidism in a woman on levothyroxine when given lovastatin.

Clinical evidence, mechanism, importance and management

A 54-year-old diabetic man taking 150 micrograms of **levothyroxine** (thyroxine) daily for Hashimoto's thyroiditis, and a number of other drugs (gemfibrozil, clofibrate, propranolol, diltiazem, quinidine, aspirin, dipyridamole, insulin) was started on 20 mg of lovastatin daily. Weakness and muscle aches (with a normal creatinine phosphokinase) developed within 2 to 3 days and over a 27-day period he lost 10% of his body weight. His serum **levothyroxine** levels rose from 11.3 to 27.2 micrograms/dl. The author of the report postulated that the lovastatin may have displaced the thyroid hormones from their binding sites, thereby increasing their effects and causing this acute thyrotoxic state. It was suggested that the patient did not have any cardiac symptoms because of his pre-existing drug regimen.[1] In contrast, a woman with goitrous hypothyroidism due to Hashimoto's thyroiditis, which was being treated with 125 micrograms of **levothyroxine sodium** daily, developed evidence of hypothyroidism (elevated TSH) on two occasions when additionally treated with 20 or 60 mg of lovastatin daily. No clinical signs of hypothyroidism developed, apart from some increased fatigue, and possibly an increased sensitivity to insulin. The author suggests lovastatin may have influenced the absorption or clearance of **levothyroxine**.[2]

When the second report was published, the makers of lovastatin reported that at that time (August 1989) more than 1 million patients had taken lovastatin, and hypothyroidism had only been reported in 3 patients.[3] It seems that any interaction is a very rare event and consequently unlikely to happen in most patients. No special precautions would therefore seem to be necessary.

1. Lustgarten BP. Catabolic response to lovastatin therapy. *Ann Intern Med* (1988) 109, 171–2.
2. Demke DM. Drug interaction between thyroxine and lovastatin. *N Engl J Med* (1989) 321, 1341–2.
3. Gormley GJ, Tobert JA. Drug interaction between thyroxine and lovastatin. *N Engl J Med* (1989) 321, 1342.

Thyroid hormones + Protease inhibitors

A man needed to have his levothyroxine dosage doubled when given ritonavir/saquinavir, whereas a woman possibly had a similar reaction when given indinavir then nelfinavir. Another woman needed a markedly reduced dose of levothyroxine when given indinavir.

Clinical evidence, mechanism, importance and management

An HIV+ man, stabilised on **levothyroxine** for autoimmune thyroiditis, developed an enlarged thyroid gland and marked lethargy about a month after his HIV treatment was changed to include stavudine, lamivudine, **saquinavir** and **ritonavir**. It became necessary to double his maintenance dose of levothyroxine to re-stabilise him. When the **ritonavir** and **saquinavir** were withdrawn and replaced by **indinavir**, the patient was able to go back to the original dose of **levothyroxine**. It is thought that this interaction occurred because **ritonavir** *increases* the activity of the glucuronosyl transferases, which are concerned with the metabolism (conjugation) of levothyroxine.[1] Although this case suggested that **indinavir** did not interact with **levothyroxine**, a further case suggests the opposite. A 36-year-old HIV+ woman taking **levothyroxine** 750 micrograms daily (following partial thyroid gland destruction for Grave's disease) was started on stavudine, lamivudine and **indinavir**. After about 7 weeks she presented with symptoms of hyperthyroidism (including nervousness, palpitations and weight loss). Serum TSH was low and thyroxine was high. After stepped dose decreases she was finally restabilised on **levothyroxine** 120 micrograms daily, with normal thyroid indices. The authors postulated that **indinavir** *reduces* the activity of glucuronosyl transferases (in contrast to **ritonavir**).[2] Conversely, in another woman a 4-week course of antiretroviral prophylaxis, including 2 weeks of **indinavir** then 2 weeks of **nelfinavir**, tended to reduce the efficacy of thyroid hormone replacement with **levothyroxine** 125 micrograms daily. She was fatigued and had elevated TSH and hypercholesterolaemia, which resolved after the antiretroviral therapy was stopped.[3]

Direct information of the interactions of protease inhibitors and thyroid hormones seems limited. Whether or not an interaction occurs seems to depend on the individual protease inhibitor, how it affects glucuronidation, and how much remaining thyroid function a patient has.[3] Until more is known about this interaction it would seem prudent to monitor thyroid function more closely if a protease inhibitor is given to a patient with pre-existing thyroid dysfunction.

1. Tseng A, Fletcher D. Interaction between ritonavir and levothyroxine. *AIDS* (1998) 12, 2235–6.
2. Lanzafame M, Trevenzoli M, Faggian F, Marcati P, Gatti F, Carolo G, Concia E. Interaction between levothyroxine and indinavir in a patient with HIV infection. *Infection* (2002) 30, 54–5.
3. Nerad JL, Kessler HA. Hypercholesterolemia in a health care worker receiving thyroxine after postexposure prophylaxis for human immunodeficiency virus infection. *Clin Infect Dis* (2001) 32, 1635–6.

Thyroid hormones + Rifampicin (Rifampin)

Two case reports suggest that rifampicin might possibly reduce the effects of thyroid hormones.

Clinical evidence, mechanism, importance and management

A woman with Turner's syndrome, who had undergone a total thyroidectomy and who was being treated with 100 micrograms of **levothyroxine** (thyroxine) daily, showed a marked fall in serum **levothyroxine** levels and free **levothyroxine** index with a dramatic rise in TSH levels when given rifampicin. However, no symptoms of clinical hypothyroidism developed, and the drop in serum **levothyroxine** occurred prior to starting rifampicin, which may reflect the clinical picture of an acute infection.[1] Another case describes a fall in TSH levels when rifampicin was discontinued.[2] A possible reason for the changes is that rifampicin, being a potent enzyme inducing agent, can markedly increase the metabolism of many drugs and thereby reduce their effects. Rifampicin has been found to reduce endogenous serum thyroxine levels in healthy subjects[3] and possibly in patients.[2] There seem to be no reports of adverse effects in other patients given both drugs and the evidence for this interaction is by no means conclusive. Although rifampicin can affect thyroid hormones, it appears that healthy individuals can compensate for this. Since hypothyroid patients may not be able to compensate in the same way, bear this interaction in mind if rifampicin is given to a patient on **levothyroxine**.

1. Isley WL. Effect of rifampin therapy on thyroid function tests in a hypothyroid patient on replacement L-thyroxine. *Ann Intern Med* (1987) 107, 517–18.
2. Nolan SR, Self TH, Norwood JM. Interaction between rifampin and levothyroxine. *South Med J* (1999) 92, 529–31.
3. Ohnhaus EE, Studer H. A link between liver microsomal enzyme activity and thyroid hormone metabolism in man. *Br J Clin Pharmacol* (1983) 15, 71–6.

Thyroid hormones + Sertraline

The effects of levothyroxine can be opposed in some patients by the concurrent use of sertraline.

Clinical evidence, mechanism, importance and management

Nine patients with hypothyroidism were noted to have elevated TSH levels (indicating a decrease in the efficacy of their treatment with **levothyroxine** when they also received sertraline. Two other patients with thyroid cancer, whose TSH levels had been deliberately depressed, developed TSH levels in the normal range while taking sertraline. None of the patients showed any signs of hypothyroidism at the time, and all of them had been taking the same dose of **levothyroxine** for at least 6 months. TSH levels up to almost 17 mIU/L (normal range 0.3 to 5 mIU/L) were seen in some patients. The **levothyroxine** dosages were increased by 11 to 50%, until the TSH levels were back to normal. The authors of this report say that they know of 3 patients whose TSH levels were unaltered by sertraline.[1]

The makers of **sertraline** say that their early-alert safety database to the end of July 1997 had identified 14 cases of hypothyroidism where a possible relation to **sertraline** could not be excluded. Seven of the patients were taking **levothyroxine**.[2]

The mechanism of this interaction (if such it is) is not known, but these cases draw attention to the need to monitor the effects of adding **sertraline** in patients taking **thyroid hormones**, the dosage of which may need to be increased. More study is needed.

1. McCowen KC, Spark R. Elevated serum thyrotropin in thyroxine-treated patients with hypothyroidism given sertraline. *N Engl J Med* (1997) 337, 1010–11.
2. Clary CM, Harrison WM. Elevated serum thyrotropin in thyroxine-treated patients with hypothyroidism given sertraline. *N Engl J Med* (1997) 337, 1011.

Thyroid hormones + Sodium polystyrene sulphonate

A woman with hypothyroidism controlled with levothyroxine relapsed when concurrently treated with sodium polystyrene sulphonate.

Clinical evidence

A woman taking 150 micrograms of **levothyroxine** daily for hypothyroidism, following total thyroidectomy, later developed renal failure and required dialysis. She was also taking digoxin, clofibrate, calcium carbonate, ferrous sulphate, nicotinic acid, folic acid, and magnesium sulphate. Because of persistent hyperkalaemia she took **sodium polystyrene sulphonate** 15 g daily. After 6 months, she developed lethargy, hoarse voice, facial fullness and weight gain (all symptoms of hypothyroidism). These symptoms resolved within 6 weeks of raising the **levothyroxine** dosage to 200 micrograms daily and separating its administration from the **sodium polystyrene sulphonate** by 10 hours (previously taken at the same time).[1]

Mechanism

Sodium polystyrene sulphonate is a cation-exchange resin that is used to bind potassium ions in exchange for sodium. An *in vitro* study found that when levothyroxine 200 micrograms was dispersed in 100 ml water with 15 g sodium polystyrene sulphonate, the concentration of the levothyroxine at pH 2 fell by 93% and at pH 7 by 98%.[1] This drop in concentration would almost certainly occur in the gut as well, thereby markedly reducing the amount of levothyroxine available for absorption.

Importance and management

Information seems to be limited to this study, but the interaction would appear to be of general importance. Separate the dosages of levothyroxine and sodium polystyrene sulphonate as much as possible (10 hours seems to be effective) and monitor the thyroid function to confirm that this is effective.

1. McLean M, Kirkwood I, Epstein M, Jones B, Hall C. Cation-exchange resin and inhibition of intestinal absorption of thyroxine. *Lancet* (1993) 341, 1286.

Thyroid hormones + Sucralfate

An isolated report describes a marked reduction in the effects of levothyroxine in a patient taking sucralfate.

Clinical evidence, mechanism, importance and management

A woman with hypothyroidism did not respond to **levothyroxine** despite taking 4.8 micrograms/kg daily while on sucralfate. Her response remained inadequate (TSH levels high, thyroxine levels low) even when the **levothyroxine** was taken 2.5 hours after the sucralfate, but when levothyroxine was taken 4.5 hours before the sucralfate, the thyroxine and TSH levels gradually became normal. A later *in vitro* study demonstrated that sucralfate binds strongly to **levothyroxine**, and it is presumed that this can also occur in the gut, thereby reducing its absorption.[1] Although this seems to be the first and only report of this interaction, it would now seem prudent not to take sucralfate until a few hours after the **levothyroxine**. Patients should be advised accordingly and the response well monitored.

1. Havrankova J, Lahaie R. Levothyroxine binding by sucralfate. *Ann Intern Med* (1992) 117, 445–6.

Tizanidine + Miscellaneous

Tizanidine may increase the effects of antihypertensive drugs (there is one case report with lisinopril) and may also increase the effects of sedative drugs and alcohol. Oral contraceptives can reduce the serum levels of tizanidine. No interaction occurs with paracetamol (acetaminophen).

Clinical evidence, mechanism, importance and management

Tizanidine can cause a reduction in blood pressure (seen in 7 to 12% of patients)[1] for which reason the makers suggest that it may possibly increase the effects of **antihypertensive drugs**, including **diuretics**. There is one case report of such an interaction in a 10-year-old child taking **lisinopril**, who developed severe hypotension within a week of starting tizanidine. In this case it was suggested that the combined effects of ACE inhibition and alpha-agonist effects prevented the usual sympathetic response to hypotension (that is, it was not thought to be due to simple additive hypotensive effects).[2] The makers also say that the concurrent use of **beta-blockers** and **digoxin** may potentiate hypotension and bradycardia,[3] but there do not appear to be any reports of problems with concurrent use.

One of the most common side-effects of tizanidine is somnolence or drowsiness (occurring in up to 50% of patients[1]) for which reason the makers warn about the possibility of increased sedation with other **sedative drugs**, and **alcohol**.[3] There is pharmacokinetic evidence that the clearance of tizanidine is reduced by about 50% in women taking **oral contraceptives**, but the clinical relevance of this is uncertain. No clinically important tizanidine/**oral contraceptive** interactions have been reported in clinical trials.[3] A trial in 20 healthy subjects found that no clinically significant interaction occurred between 325 mg of **paracetamol** (**acetaminophen**) and 4 mg of tizanidine.[1]

1. Wagstaff AJ, Bryson HM. Tizanidine. A review of its pharmacology, clinical efficacy and tolerability in the management of spasticity associated with cerebral and spinal disorders. *Drugs* (1997) 53, 435–52.
2. Johnson TR, Tobias JD. Hypotension following the initiation of tizanidine in a patient treated with an angiotensin converting enzyme inhibitor for chronic hypertension. *J Child Neurol* (2000) 15, 818–19.
3. Zanaflex (Tizanidine hydrochloride). Elan Pharma Ltd. UK Summary of product characteristics, February 2003.

Tolrestat + Aspirin

The pharmacokinetics of both drugs are changed by concurrent use, but the extent is small and unlikely to be clinically relevant.

Clinical evidence, mechanism, importance and management

Eighteen healthy subjects were given tolrestat 400 mg daily or 975 mg aspirin 8-hourly on study days 1 to 5, then both drugs together for days 6 to 10, and finally one or other of the drugs for days 11 to 15. The AUCs of the aspirin and tolrestat were raised 16% and 18% respectively, and the maximum serum levels raised 9% and lowered 2% respectively. These changes were due to reductions in the renal clearances of both drugs.[1] The clinical importance of these alterations has not been evaluated in diabetics, but all of them are quite small and unlikely to be clinically relevant. This needs confirmation.

1. Garg V, Parker V, Turner MB, Burghart P, Fruncillo R, Battle M, Chiang S. Pharmacokinetic interaction between aspirin and tolrestat in normal volunteers. *Pharm Res* (1995) 12 (9 Suppl), S-392

Tolterodine + CYP3A4 enzyme inhibitors

Ketoconazole can increase tolterodine levels in those who are deficient in cytochrome P450 isoenzyme CYP2D6 (poor metabolisers). The makers currently say that potent CYP3A4 inhibitors such as clarithromycin, erythromycin, itraconazole and ketoconazole, and HIV-protease inhibitors should be used with caution or avoided because of a risk of increased tolterodine effects.

Clinical evidence, mechanism, importance and management

A study[1] in 8 healthy subjects who were deficient in cytochrome P450 isoenzyme CYP2D6 (poor metabolisers) found that after taking 200 mg of **ketoconazole** daily for 4 days the clearance of a single 2-mg dose of tolterodine was reduced by 61% and its AUC was increased 2.5-fold. A subsequent multiple-dose study in 6 of the original subjects given tolterodine 1 mg twice daily (half the usual dose) found similar increased levels. In this study, ketoconazole 200 mg once daily caused a 2.1-fold increase in tolterodine AUC, and a 2.2-fold increase in the AUC of the active moiety (unbound tolterodine plus metabolite).[1]

Although tolterodine is normally metabolised to its active metabolite by CYP2D6, in those with low levels of this isoenzyme (about 5 to 10% of the population), metabolism by CYP3A4, becomes more important. It should be noted that tolterodine levels are already higher in poor CYP2D6 metabolisers than extensive metabolisers[2] but are likely to rise even further when a potent CYP3A4 inhibitor such as **ketoconazole** blocks this other route of metabolism. The UK makers consider that this increase in levels represents a risk of overdose in poor CYP2D6 metabolisers. Consequently, they do not recommend the use of potent CYP3A4 inhibitors with tolterodine in any patient (note that metaboliser status is rarely known). They name **clarithromycin**, **erythromycin**, **ketoconazole**, and **itraconazole**, and **HIV-protease** inhibitors.[3] However, the US makers[2] recommend only that the dose of tolterodine be reduced to 1 mg twice daily in patients currently taking drugs that are potent inhibitors of CYP3A4, and this seems the more sensible advice. It may be prudent to assess experience of adverse effects in these patients, and to reduce the dose further or withdraw the drug if it is not tolerated.

1. Brynne N, Forslund C, Hallén B, Gustafsson LL, Bertilsson L. Ketoconazole inhibits the metabolism of tolterodine in subjects with deficient CYP2D6 activity. *Br J Clin Pharmacol* (1999) 48, 564–72.
2. Detrol (Tolterodine). Pharmacia & Upjohn Company. US prescribing information, July 2003.
3. Detrusitol (Tolterodine). Pharmacia Ltd. UK Summary of product characteristics, October 2004.

Tolterodine + Duloxetine

Duloxetine increased the maximum levels of tolterodine by 64%, but this was not considered to be clinically significant.

Clinical evidence, mechanism, importance and management

In a crossover placebo-controlled study, 14 healthy subjects received duloxetine 40 mg twice daily and tolterodine 2 mg twice daily for 5 days. Duloxetine increased the steady-state AUC of tolterodine by 71% and its maximum level by 64%. However, duloxetine had no effect on the pharmacokinetics of 5-hydroxymethyl-tolterodine the active metabolite of tolterodine.[1]

Duloxetine is an inhibitor of the cytochrome P450 isoenzyme CYP2D6, by which tolterodine is metabolised.

The increases in tolterodine levels were not considered to be clinically relevant, and no routine dosage adjustment of tolterodine dosage was considered necessary when given with duloxetine.[1] Consider also 'Tolterodine + Fluoxetine', p.1038.

1. Hua TC, Pan A, Chan C, Poo YK, Skinner MH, Knadler MP, Gonzales CR, Wise SD. Effect of duloxetine on tolterodine pharmacokinetics in healthy volunteers. *Br J Clin Pharmacol* (2004) 57, 652–6.

Tolterodine + Fluoxetine

Although fluoxetine can markedly inhibit the metabolism of tolterodine in some patients this is unlikely to cause a clinically important increase in the effects of tolterodine.

Clinical evidence, mechanism, importance and management

Thirteen psychiatric patients with symptoms of urinary incontinence were treated with tolterodine 2 mg twice daily for 5 doses, followed by fluoxetine 20 mg daily for 3 weeks, and then for a further 3 days with tolterodine and fluoxetine concurrently. Nine of the 13 completed the trial, the other 4 withdrew because of fluoxetine-related side effects. Fluoxetine is an inhibitor of the cytochrome P450 isoenzyme CYP2D6, the main enzyme involved in the metabolism of tolterodine. However, levels of this enzyme can vary between individuals and in the 7 patients with high CYP2D6 levels ('extensive metabolisers') there was a 4.8-fold increase in the AUC of tolterodine and a minor reduction in its active and equipotent metabolite. In contrast the AUC of tolterodine increased by about 25% in 2 patients with low levels of CYP2D6 ('poor metabolisers'). These changes in AUC represent an increase of about 25% in active moiety (unbound tolterodine plus metabolite) for both poor and extensive metabolisers, a figure within normal variation.[1]

In practical terms this means that the anticholinergic (antimuscarinic) effects of the tolterodine are only moderately increased, and it seems unlikely that any tolterodine dosage changes are likely to be needed. Consider also 'Anticholinergics + Anticholinergics', p.501.

1. Brynne N, Svanström C, Åberg-Wistedt A, Hallén B, Bertilsson L. Fluoxetine inhibits the metabolism of tolterodine—pharmacokinetic implications and proposed clinical relevance. *Br J Clin Pharmacol* (1999) 48, 553–63.

Trientine + Miscellaneous

Trientine can possibly chelate with iron thereby reducing its absorption. On theoretical grounds a similar chelation interaction may occur with calcium and magnesium antacids.

Clinical evidence, mechanism, importance and management

(a) Iron preparations

Trientine is a copper chelating agent used for Wilson's disease. One of the side-effects of trientine is that it can cause iron deficiency, probably because it chelates with iron in the gut and thereby reduces its absorption. It is usual to make good this iron deficiency where necessary by giving an iron supplement. The makers suggest that the iron supplement should be given at a different time of the day from trientine to minimise their admixture in the gut.[1] A separation of at least 2 hours is effective with other drugs that interact with iron due to binding or chelation in the gut, and it seems likely that this will also be effective with this drug combination.

(b) Magnesium and calcium antacids

The makers say that there is no evidence that calcium or magnesium antacids alter the efficacy of trientine, but on theoretical grounds they might possibly form a chelate with the trientine in the gut.[1] It is therefore suggested that their administration should be separated.

1. Trientine dihydrochloride. Product summary, August 2000.

Ursodeoxycholic acid (Ursodiol) + Colestilan

The absorption of ursodeoxycholic acid can be more than halved by colestilan if taken together.

Clinical evidence, mechanism, importance and management

Following a test meal with an overnight fast, 5 healthy subjects were given 200 mg of ursodeoxycholic acid alone or with 1.5 g colestilan granules. It was found that the ursodeoxycholic acid serum levels at 30 minutes were reduced by the colestilan by more than 50% in 4 out of the 5 subjects, and the mean level was decreased from 9.2 to 3.4 micromol/l. The mechanism of this interaction would appear to be that the colestilan, being an ion exchange resin, binds with the ursodeoxycholic acid in the intestine and thereby reduces its absorption. The authors of this report recommend that in order to reduce the effects of this interaction, these two drugs should be given at least 2 hours apart so that admixture in the gut is minimised.[1]

1. Takikawa H, Ogasawara T, Sato A, Ohashi M, Hasegawa Y, Hojo M. Effect of colestimide on intestinal absorption of ursodeoxycholic acid in men. *Int J Clin Pharmacol Ther* (2001) 39, 558–60.

Vardenafil + Miscellaneous

Vardenafil is contraindicated with nitrates, and concomitant use with alpha blockers is also not recommended, because of the potential for additive hypotensive effects. Indinavir, itraconazole, ketoconazole and ritonavir cause large elevations in vardenafil levels, and concomitant use requires dosage restrictions and is contraindicated in men aged over 75 years. Erythromycin increases vardenafil levels to a lesser extent, but dosage restrictions may still be needed. Similarly, grapefruit juice is predicted to increase vardenafil levels, and avoidance is recommended. Nifedipine causes moderate additive blood pressure decreases and heart rate increases with vardenafil, suggesting this may occur with other antihypertensives. The US makers suggest the avoidance of some antiarrhythmics because of fears of possible QT interval prolongation. No clinically significant interaction has been seen between vardenafil and alcohol, ACE inhibitors, antacids, aspirin, beta-blockers, cimetidine, digoxin, diuretics, food, glibenclamide (glyburide) metformin, ranitidine, sulphonylureas or warfarin.

Clinical evidence, mechanism, importance and management

(a) Alcohol

Alcohol (mean blood level of 73 mg/dl) did not affect the pharmacokinetics of vardenafil 20 mg. The effects of alcohol on heart rate and blood pressure were also not affected by vardenafil. There would therefore seem to be no need to avoid the combination.[1]

(b) Antacids

In a two-way crossover study a single 20-mg dose of vardenafil was given to 12 healthy subjects with 10 ml of an **aluminium/magnesium hydroxide** antacid (*Maalox 70*). The bioavailability of vardenafil was not significantly altered by the antacid, therefore no additional precautions are needed if used together.[2]

(c) Antiarrhythmics (class Ia and III)

Vardenafil 10 mg and 80 mg caused very small (4 and 6 millisecond) increases in the corrected QT interval in healthy subjects.[3] Because of this, the US prescribing information (but not the UK maker) recommends that vardenafil is not used in those taking class Ia antiarrhythmics (e.g. quinidine, procainamide) or class III (e.g. amiodarone, sotalol) antiarrhythmics, which are also known to prolong the QT interval.[3] Note that prolongation of the QT interval is associated with an increased risk of the potentially fatal torsade de pointes arrhythmia (see also 'Drugs that prolong the QT interval + Other drugs that prolong the QT interval', p.170).

(d) Antidiabetics

The makers say that the pharmacokinetics of **glibenclamide** (**glyburide**) were not affected by a single dose of vardenafil 20 mg,[1] and that vardenafil had no effect on glibenclamide pharmacodynamics (glucose and insulin levels).[3] Also, although no specific pharmacokinetic study has been conducted, the makers say that population pharmacokinetic analysis suggests that **sulphonylureas** (not named) and **metformin** have no effect on vardenafil pharmacokinetics. No additional precautions therefore seem necessary on concurrent use.[1]

(e) Antihypertensives

Significant hypotension (standing systolic blood pressure 85 mmHg or less) developed in 2 out of 9, and 6 out of 8 healthy subjects given vardenafil 10 or 20 mg respectively and **terazosin** 10 mg simultaneously. Similarly, when administration was separated by 6 hours, seven of 28 subjects had significant hypotension.[3] In another study significant hypotension occurred in one of 24 subjects when given vardenafil 20 mg and **tamsulosin** 400 micrograms separated by 6 hours and in 2 of 16 subjects when given the drugs simultaneously.[3] The UK makers say that vardenafil should only be given to patients stabilised on alpha blockers. The dose should not exceed 5 mg and should not be given within 6 hours of the alpha blocker (with the exception of tamsulosin).[1]

In a randomised, double blind, crossover study, 22 patients with hypertension, stabilised on slow release **nifedipine** 30 or 60 mg daily were given a single 20-mg dose of vardenafil, or placebo. Vardenafil slightly decreased the maximum plasma levels and relative bioavailability of **nifedipine**, as well as causing a further decrease in supine blood pressure of about 6/5 mmHg. Heart rate was increased by 4 bpm.[4] Vardenafil alone may decrease blood pressure, and the US product information cautions that vardenafil may add to the blood pressure lowering effects of **antihypertensive drugs**.[3]

The makers say that, although not specifically studied, population pharmacokinetic analysis suggests that **ACE inhibitors**, **beta-blockers**, and **diuretics** had no effect on vardenafil pharmacokinetics.[1]

(f) Aspirin

The makers say that, population pharmacokinetic analysis suggests that aspirin had no effect on vardenafil pharmacokinetics. In addition, vardenafil 10 mg did not potentiate the bleeding time caused by aspirin 162 mg. No additional precautions therefore seem necessary on concurrent use.[1]

(g) Azoles

Ketoconazole, a potent inhibitor of the cytochrome P450 isoenzyme CYP3A4, in a dose of 200 mg daily, increased the AUC of a 5-mg dose of vardenafil tenfold, and increased the maximum plasma levels fourfold. Although not specifically studied, **itraconazole**, also a CYP3A4 inhibitor, is expected to cause similar rises in vardenafil levels. The UK makers therefore advise avoiding these combinations in all patients, but in patients over 75 years, the use of **ketoconazole** or **oral itraconazole** with vardenafil is specifically contraindicated.[1] In contrast, the US prescribing information recommends dose restrictions as follows: the dose of vardenafil should not exceed 5 mg in 24 hours when used with **ketoconazole** 200 mg daily, and a 2.5-mg dose should not be exceeded when used with **ketoconazole** 400 mg daily. The same advice is given for **itraconazole**.[3]

(h) Digoxin

In a placebo-controlled study, 19 healthy subjects were given digoxin 375 micrograms daily for 28 days, with vardenafil 20 mg once daily on alternate days from day 16 to day 28. The pharmacokinetics of digoxin were not significantly changed by vardenafil, and there was no alteration in vital signs, ECG readings and laboratory parameters (not stated). The incidence of mild to moderate headache rose slightly from 7 out of 19 with the placebo to 13 out of 19 with digoxin.[5] There would therefore appear to be no reason to monitor digoxin levels while taking vardenafil concurrently.

(i) Erythromycin

Erythromycin 500 mg three times daily increased the AUC of a 5-mg dose of vardenafil fourfold, and increased the maximum plasma levels threefold.[1] The UK makers say that vardenafil dosage adjustment 'might be necessary' when used with erythromycin, and the US prescribing information specifically recommends that the dose of vardenafil should not exceed 5 mg in 24 hours.[3]

(j) Food

In a single-dose study, healthy subjects were given a single 20-mg dose of vardenafil on four occasions; after an overnight fast, on an empty stomach, following a **high-fat breakfast** (fat 58 g), or following a **moderate-fat evening meal** (fat 23 g). No pharmacokinetic changes were noted in the fasting or moderate-fat periods. Although the **high-fat breakfast** caused a slight decrease and a slight delay in the absorption of vardenafil this was not considered to be sufficient to warrant changing the dosing time or making dosage adjustments. Therefore vardenafil may be given without regard to meals.[6]

(k) Grapefruit juice

Because grapefruit juice is a moderate inhibitor of CYP3A4 gut wall metabolism, concurrent use with vardenafil (which is metabolised by CYP3A4) may lead to elevations in vardenafil serum levels. The makers therefore say the combination should be avoided.[1]

(l) H_2-blockers

In a three-way crossover study, a single 20-mg dose of vardenafil was given to 10 healthy subjects following a 3-day course of **cimetidine** 400 mg twice daily, **ranitidine** 150 mg twice daily or with no pre-treatment. **Cimetidine** slightly increased the relative bioavailability of vardenafil (by about 12%, not considered clinically relevant), while **ranitidine** had no effect. It was concluded that any alterations in the absorption of vardenafil are not caused by changes in gastric pH.[7] No special precautions appear to be necessary during concurrent use.

(m) Nitrates

A single 400-microgram dose of sublingual **glyceryl trinitrate** (nitroglycerin) given to 18 healthy subjects 1 to 24 hours after a single 10-mg dose of vardenafil was found to be no different to placebo in causing changes in heart rate and blood pressure.[1,8] However, a 20-mg single dose of vardenafil did potentiate (degree not stated) the blood pressure lowering effects and increases in heart rate seen with sublingual **nitrates** (400 micrograms) when this was taken 1 and 4 hours after the vardenafil. These effects were not seen when the **nitrate** was taken 24 hours after the vardenafil dose.[3] The makers therefore say that the combination of vardenafil and nitrates (taken either regularly and/or intermittently) is contraindicated because of the potential hypotensive effects.[1,3] Consider also 'Sildenafil + Cardiovascular drugs', p.1029, and 'Tadalafil + Miscellaneous', p.1032.

(n) Protease inhibitors

When a single-dose of vardenafil 10 mg was given with **indinavir** 800 mg three times daily, the AUC of vardenafil was increased sixteenfold, and the maximum plasma level was increased sevenfold.[1,3] Moreover, **ritonavir** 600 mg twice daily produced a 49-fold increase in the AUC of vardenafil, and prolonged the half-life to 26 hours.[3] The UK maker therefore advises avoiding the combination in all patients, but in patients over 75 years, the use of **indinavir** or **ritonavir** with vardenafil is specifically contraindicated.[1] In contrast, the US prescribing information recommends dose restrictions as follows: the dose of vardenafil should not exceed 2.5 mg in 24 hours when used with **indinavir**, and should not exceed 2.5 mg in 72 hours when used with **ritonavir**.[3]

(o) Warfarin

No pharmacokinetic interaction was observed between vardenafil and warfarin.[1] No additional precautions therefore seem necessary on concurrent use.

1. Levitra (Vardenafil hydrochloride trihydrate). Bayer plc. UK Summary of product characteristics, March 2005.
2. Rohde G, Wensing G, Sachse R. The pharmacokinetics of vardenafil, a new selective PDE5 inhibitor, are not affected by the antacid, Maalox 70. *Pharmacotherapy* (2001) 21, 1254.
3. Levitra (Vardenafil). Bayer pharmaceuticals Corporation. US prescribing information, August 2003.
4. Rohde G, Jordaan PJ. Influence of vardenafil on blood pressure and pharmacokinetics in hypertensive patients on nifedipine therapy. 31th Annual Meeting of the American College of Clinical Pharmacology, San Francisco, California, 2002.
5. Rohde G, Bauer R-J, Unger S, Ahr G, Wensing G. Vardenafil, a new selective PDE5 inhibitor, produces no interaction with digoxin. *Pharmacotherapy* (2001) 21, 1254.
6. Rajagopalan P, Mazzu A, Xia C, Dawkins R, Sundaresan P. Effect of high-fat breakfast and moderate-fat evening meal on the pharmacokinetics of vardenafil, an oral phosphodiesterase-5 inhibitor for the treatment of erectile dysfunction. *J Clin Pharmacol* (2003) 43, 1–8.
7. Rohde G, Wensing G, Unger S, Sachse R. The pharmacokinetics of vardenafil, a new selective PDE5 inhibitor, is minimally affected by coadministration with cimetidine or ranitidine. *Pharmacotherapy* (2001) 21, 1254.
8. Mazzu AL, Nicholls AJ, Zinny M. Vardenafil, a new selective PDE-5 inhibitor, interacts minimally with nitroglycerin in healthy middle-aged male subjects. *Int J Impot Res* (2001) 13 (Suppl 5) S64.

Vesnarinone + Miscellaneous

Erythromycin increases the bioavailability of vesnarinone whereas famotidine decreases the rate but not the extent of its absorption from the gut. The clinical relevance of these interactions is uncertain.

Clinical evidence, mechanism, importance and management

A study in 12 healthy subjects found that 500 mg **erythromycin** three times daily for a week increased the AUC of a single 60-mg dose of vesnarinone by 65% and the maximum serum levels by 11%. Systemic clearance was reduced by 36%. It was concluded from this and other *in vitro* studies that the cytochrome P450 isoenzymes CYP3A4 and CYP2E1 are involved in the metabolism of vesnarinone.[1,2] Whether this interaction with **erythromycin**, (or potentially with other inhibitors of CYP3A4) is likely to be clinically important is not yet known, but it would seem prudent to be alert for any evidence of vesnarinone toxicity if used concurrently.

A single-blind, randomised two-way crossover study was carried out in 12 healthy subjects to study the effects of changes in gastric pH on the absorption of vesnarinone. Using a pH monitor to ensure that the pH had risen from less than 2 to greater than 6, in the presence of the **famotidine** it was found that the maximum serum vesnarinone levels fell by 25% (from 3.33 to 2.5 micrograms/ml), the AUC fell by less than 2%, while the time to maximum serum levels rose from about 6 to 24 h.[3] Thus these changes in gastric pH prolong the rate but not the extent of the absorption of vesnarinone. What this is likely to mean in practical terms awaits clinical assessment. Other drugs which raise gastric pH (e.g. other **H_2-blockers**, **proton pump inhibitors**) would be expected to act like famotidine.

1. Wandel C, Lang CC, Cowart DS, Girard AF, Bramer S, Flockhart DA, Wood AJ. Effect of CYP3A inhibition on vesnarinone metabolism in humans. *Clin Pharmacol Ther* (1998) 63, 506–11.
2. Wandel C, Lang CC, Cowart D, Girard A, Bramer S, Wood AJJ. CYP3A inhibition increases plasma levels of vesnarinone in humans. *Clin Pharmacol Ther* (1997) 61, 204.
3. Cowart D, Koneru B, Bramer S, Noorisa M, Kisicki J. Effect of gastric pH on the absorption and oral pharmacokinetics of the inotropic agent vesnarinone. *Clin Pharmacol Ther* (1997) 61, 157.

Vinpocetine + Antacids

Magnesium/aluminium hydroxide gel (1 sachet four times daily) had no significant effects on the serum levels of vinpocetine (20 mg three times daily) in 18 healthy subjects.[1] No special precautions seem necessary if they are taken together.

1. Lohmann A, Grobara P, Dingler E. Investigation of the possible influence of the absorption of vinpocetine with concomitant application of magnesium-aluminium-hydroxide gel. *Arzneimittelforschung* (1991) 41, 1164–7.

Vitamin A (Retinol) + Neomycin

Neomycin can markedly reduce the absorption of vitamin A (retinol) from the gut.

Clinical evidence, mechanism, importance and management

Neomycin 2 g markedly reduced the absorption of a test dose of vitamin A in 5 healthy subjects. It is suggested that this was due to a direct chemical interference between the neomycin and bile in the gut, which disrupted the absorption of fats and fat-soluble vitamins.[1] The extent to which chronic treatment with neomycin (or other aminoglycosides) would impair the treatment of vitamin A deficiency has not been determined.

1. Barrowman JA, D'Mello A, Herxheimer A. A single dose of neomycin impairs absorption of vitamin A (Retinol) in man. *Eur J Clin Pharmacol* (1973) 5, 199–201.

Vitamin B_{12} + Miscellaneous

Although neomycin, aminosalicylic acid and the H_2-blockers can reduce the absorption of vitamin B_{12} from the gut, no interaction is likely because B_{12} is usually given by injection.

Clinical evidence, mechanism, importance and management

Neomycin causes a generalised malabsorption syndrome, which has been shown[1] to reduce the absorption of vitamin B_{12}. **Colchicine** has also been shown to decrease B_{12} absorption.[1] **Aminosalicylic acid** reduces vitamin B_{12} absorption for reasons that are not understood, but which are possibly related to a mild generalised malabsorption syndrome.[2] Review of the literature[3] suggests that H_2-blockers (such as **cimetidine** and **ranitidine**) can also reduce vitamin B_{12} absorption, primarily because they reduce gastric acid production. The acid is needed to aid the release of B_{12} from dietary protein sources. There is therefore a possibility that on long-term use patients could become vitamin B_{12} deficient.

Within the context of adverse drug interactions, none of these drugs is normally likely to interact adversely because, for anaemia, vitamin B_{12} is usually given parenterally for convenience and to avoid well-established problems with absorption.

1. Faloon WW, Chodos RB. Vitamin B_{12} absorption studies using colchicine, neomycin and continuous 57Co B_{12} administration. *Gastroenterology* (1969) 56, 1251.
2. Palva IP, Rytkönen U, Alatulkkila M, Palva HLA. Drug-induced malabsorption of vitamin B_{12}. V. Intestinal pH and absorption of vitamin B_{12} during treatment with para-aminosalicylic acid. *Scand J Haematol* (1972) 9, 5–7.
3. Force RW, Nahata MC. Effect of histamine H_2-receptor antagonists on vitamin B_{12} absorption. *Ann Pharmacother* (1992) 26, 1283–6.

Vitamin C (Ascorbic acid) + Salicylates

Aspirin reduces the absorption of ascorbic acid by about a third. Serum salicylate levels do not appear to be affected by ascorbic acid.

Clinical evidence, mechanism, importance and management

A study in healthy subjects found that the absorption of a single 500-mg dose of ascorbic acid was about a third lower in those given 900 mg **aspirin** concurrently, and the urinary excretion was about 50% lower.[1] The clinical importance of this is uncertain. It has been suggested that the normal physiological requirement of 30 to 60 mg of ascorbic acid daily may need to be increased to 100 to 200 mg daily in the presence of **aspirin**.[1] More study is needed. Another study in 9 healthy subjects found that ascorbic acid 1 g three times daily did not significantly affect serum salicylate levels given as **choline salicylate**.[2]

1. Basu TK. Vitamin C-aspirin interactions. *Int J Vitam Nutr Res* (1982) 23 (Suppl), 83–90.
2. Hansten PD, Hayton WL. Effect of antacid and ascorbic acid on serum salicylate concentration. *J Clin Pharmacol* (1980) 24, 326–31.

Vitamin D substances; Alfacalcidol + Danazol

An isolated report describes hypercalcaemia in a woman on alfacalcidol when additionally treated with danazol.

Clinical evidence, mechanism, importance and management

A woman with idiopathic hypoparathyroidism, treated with alfacalcidol, developed hypercalcaemia when she was additionally given danazol 400 mg daily for endometriosis. She needed a reduction in the dosage of alfacalcidol from 4 to 0.75 micrograms daily. When the danazol was stopped 6 months later, the alfacalcidol dosage was raised to 4 micrograms daily and she remained normocalcaemic.[1] The reasons are not understood. The general importance of this apparent interaction is limited as it appears to be an isolated case.

1. Hepburn NC, Abdul-Aziz LAS, Whiteoak R. Danazol-induced hypercalcaemia in alphacalcidol-treated hypoparathyroidism. *Postgrad Med J* (1989) 65, 849–50.

Vitamin D substances + Phenytoin

The long-term use of phenytoin and other anticonvulsants can disturb vitamin D and calcium metabolism and may result in osteomalacia. There are a few reports of patients taking vitamin D supplements who responded poorly to vitamin replacement while taking phenytoin or barbiturates. Serum phenytoin levels are not altered by vitamin D.

Clinical evidence

(a) Effect of phenytoin on vitamin D

A 16-year-old with grand mal epilepsy and idiopathic hypoparathyroidism failed to respond adequately to daily doses of **alfacalcidol** 10 micrograms and 6 to 12 g of calcium, apparently due to the concurrent use of phenytoin 200 mg and primidone 500 mg daily. However, treatment with **dihydrotachysterol** 0.6 to 2.4 mg daily produced normal calcium levels.[1]

Other reports describe patients whose response to usual doses of vitamin D was poor, because of concurrent anticonvulsant treatment with phenytoin and phenobarbital or primidone.[2-4] Other reports clearly show low serum calcium levels,[5,6] low serum vitamin D levels,[7] osteomalacia,[6] and bone structure alterations[5,7] while taking phenytoin alone.

(b) Effect of vitamin D on phenytoin

A controlled trial in 151 epileptic patients on phenytoin and calcium showed that the addition of 2000 units of vitamin D_2 daily over a 3-month period had no significant effect on serum phenytoin levels.[8]

Mechanism

The enzyme-inducing effects of phenytoin and other anticonvulsants increase the metabolism of the vitamin D, thereby reducing its effects and disturbing calcium metabolism.[3] In addition, phenytoin may possibly reduce the absorption of calcium from the gut.[1]

Importance and management

The disturbance of calcium metabolism by phenytoin and other anticonvulsants is very well established, but there are only a few reports describing a poor response to vitamin D. The effects of concurrent treatment should be well monitored. Those who need vitamin D supplements may possibly need greater than usual doses.

1. Rubinger D, Korn-Lubetzki I, Feldman S, Popovtzer MM. Delayed response to 1 α-hydroxycholecalciferol therapy in a case of hypoparathyroidism during anticonvulsant therapy. *Isr J Med Sci* (1980) 16, 772–4.
2. Asherov J, Weinberger A, Pinkhas J. Lack of response to vitamin D therapy in a patient with hypoparathyroidism under anticonvulsant drugs. *Helv Paediatr Acta* (1977) 32, 369–73.
3. Chan JCM, Oldham SB, Holick MF, DeLuca HF. 1-α-Hydroxyvitamin D_3 in chronic renal failure. A potent analogue of the kidney hormone, 1,25-dihydroxycholecalciferol. *JAMA* (1975) 234, 47–52.
4. Maclaren N, Lifshitz F. Vitamin D-dependency rickets in institutionalized, mentally retarded children on long term anticonvulsant therapy. II. The response to 25-hydroxycholecalciferol and to vitamin D_2. *Pediatr Res* (1973) 7, 914–22.
5. Mosekilde L, Melsen F. Anticonvulsant osteomalacia determined by quantitative analyses of bone changes. Population study and possible risk factors. *Acta Med Scand* (1976) 199, 349–55.
6. Hunter J, Maxwell JD, Stewart DA, Parson V, Williams R. Altered calcium metabolism in epileptic children on anticonvulsants. *BMJ* (1971) 4, 202–4.
7. Hahn TJ, Avioli LV. Anticonvulsant osteomalacia. *Arch Intern Med* (1975) 135, 997–1000.
8. Christiansen C, Rødbro P. Effect of vitamin D_2 on serum phenytoin. A controlled therapeutical trial. *Acta Neurol Scand* (1974) 50, 661–4.

Vitamin K + Antibacterials

Seven patients in intensive care failed to respond to intravenous vitamin K for hypoprothrombinaemia while receiving gentamicin and clindamycin.

Clinical evidence, mechanism, importance and management

Some patients, particularly those in intensive care who are not eating, can quite rapidly develop acute vitamin K deficiency, which leads to prolonged prothrombin times and possibly bleeding.[1,2] This can normally be controlled by giving vitamin K parenterally. However, one report describes 7 such patients, all with normal liver function, who unexpectedly failed to respond to intravenous **phytomenadione**. Examination of their records showed that all were receiving **gentamicin** and **clindamycin**.[2] Just why, or if, these two antibacterials oppose the effects of vitamin K is not understood. More study is needed.

1. Ham JM. Hypoprothrombinaemia in patients undergoing prolonged intensive care. *Med J Aust* (1971) 2, 716–18.
2. Rodriguez-Erdmann F, Hoff JV, Carmody G. Interaction of antibiotics with vitamin K. *JAMA* (1981) 246, 937.

Vitamins + Orlistat

It is recommended that multivitamin preparations should be taken at least 2 hours after orlistat or at bedtime.

Clinical evidence, mechanism, importance and management

There is good evidence that patients taking orlistat long-term have **vitamin A, D, E, K** and **beta-carotene** levels in the normal range.[1] However, because orlistat may potentially impair the absorption of these fat-soluble vitamins (it blocks the ingestion of about one third of dietary fats) the makers recommend that any **multivitamin preparations** should be taken at least 2 hours after orlistat or at bedtime[1] to ensure maximum vitamin absorption. A study in healthy subjects found that about two-thirds of a supplemental dose of **beta-carotene** were absorbed in the presence of orlistat.[2]

1. Xenical (Orlistat). Roche Products Ltd. UK Summary of product characteristics, June 2005.
2. Zhi J, Melia AT, Koss-Twardy SG, Arora S, Patel IH. The effect of orlistat, an inhibitor of dietary fat absorption, on the pharmacokinetics of β-carotene in healthy volunteers. *J Clin Pharmacol* (1996) 36, 152–9.

Zinc sulphate + Calcium salts

Calcium salts reduce the absorption of zinc.

Clinical evidence, mechanism, importance and management

Elemental calcium in doses of 600 mg (either as **calcium carbonate** or **calcium citrate**) was given to 9 healthy women with single 20-mg oral doses of zinc sulphate.[1] The AUC of zinc was reduced by 72% by **calcium carbonate** and by 80% by **calcium citrate**. The reason is not understood, nor is the clinical importance of this interaction known, but it would seem prudent to separate the administration of zinc from the administration of any calcium salts. Two to three hours separation is often sufficient to achieve maximal absorption with interactions like this. More study of this interaction is needed to confirm the extent and to determine if separation of the doses is an adequate precaution.

1. Argiratos V, Samman S. The effect of calcium carbonate and calcium citrate on the absorption of zinc in healthy female subjects. *Eur J Clin Nutr* (1994) 48, 198–204.

Index

All of the pairs of drugs included in the text of this book are listed in this index. They may also be listed under the group names if two or more members of the group interact or if only general information is available. **You should always look up the names of both individual drugs and their groups to ensure that you have access to all the information in this book.** You can possibly get a lead on the way unlisted drugs behave if you look up those which are related or the appropriate drug group, but bear in mind that none of them are identical and any conclusions reached should only be tentative.

Whereas both recommended International Non-proprietary Names (rINNs) and United States Approved Names (USANs) have been used in the text, entries in the index are to be found under the rINN with cross-references provided for USANs, British Approved Names, and some other widely used synonyms. Brand names have been avoided but tables of international proprietary names/generic names are included in the introductory sections of most chapters. You can find these tables by looking up the group names of the drugs in question (e.g. Anticoagulants, Anticonvulsants, etc.) or by looking on the first few pages of each chapter.

C

G

H

I

O

P

Q

R

S

X